at a glance

D1353691

STEDMAN'S WORDFINDER

A unique dictionary-within-a-dictionary that serves as a master cross-reference index of multiword terms. For additional information see page xiv, in the front of the dictionary.

Use it:

- To find where multiword terms are defined
- As a handy spelling checker for modifiers

To find multiword terms in boldface, look under the organizing term shown in regular type.

To find	Look under (in A–Z section)
accelerator	factor; fibers; globulin; nerve
accessory	adrenal; gland; ligaments; molecules; nerve; organs of the eye; spleen; symptom
adrenergic	blockade; bronchodilators; fibers; receptors
frontal	area; artery; bone; cortex; crest; lobe of cerebrum; nerve; plane; pole of cerebrum; sinus; suture
muscle	hemoglobin; plate; serum; spasm; tone
open	biopsy; comedo; dislocation; drainage; flap; fracture; hospital; pneumothorax; reduction of fractures; tuberculosis; wound
organic	acid; chemistry; compound; contracture; delusions; disease; evolution; murmur; vertigo
physical	activity; agent; allergy; diagnosis; fitness; map; medicine; sign; therapy

MEDICAL PREFIXES, SUFFIXES, AND COMBINING FORMS

Listing of the 400 most common medical word parts begins on page xxv, in the front of the dictionary. These are prefixes, suffixes, and combining forms that make up 90 to 95 percent of medical vocabulary.

Throughout the A–Z section symbol △.

△ **a-** not, without, -less
△ **ab-** from, away from, off
△ **abs-** from, away from, off
△ **-ad** toward, in the direction of; -ward
△ **ad-** increase, adherence, motion toward; very
△ **alge-** pain
△ **algesi-** pain
△ **algio-** pain

Index to multiword entries immediately before A–Z

26 color anatomy plates from A.D.A.M.® with index Insert A

How to use Stedman's Concise

STEDMAN'S
CONCISE
MEDICAL & ALLIED HEALTH
DICTIONARY

ILLUSTRATED
THIRD EDITION

EDITOR

John H. Dirckx, M.D.

Director, University of Dayton Health Center
Dayton, Ohio

SANS
TACHE

Williams & Wilkins
A WAVERLY COMPANY

BALTIMORE • PHILADELPHIA • LONDON • PARIS • BANGKOK
BUENOS AIRES • HONG KONG • MUNICH • SYDNEY • TOKYO • WROCLAW

Editor: John H. Dirckx, M.D.
Senior Acquisitions Editor: Elizabeth Randolph
Project Manager: Marjory Spraycar
Managing Editor: Vincent Ercolano
Art Director: Jonathan Dimes
Copy Editor: Harriet Felscher
Design: Dan Pfisterer
Production Coordinator: Marette Magargle-Smith
Printing Coordinator: Brian Smith
On-Line Editors: Barbara Ferretti, Ruth Kendall
Proofreaders: Audrey Knox, Jolanta Obrebska, Margaret Swanson,
          Natalie Tyler, Barbara Werner

Illustrations: Neil O. Hardy
          Additional artwork by Michael Schenk, Mary Anna Barratt-Dimes,
          Caitlin Duckwall, and Rob Duckwall.

          Graphic assistance by In-Tandem Design and Hope Jester.

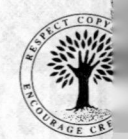
Printed in the United States of America

First Edition,

Library of Congress Cataloging-in-Publication Data

ISBN 0-683-23125-1

Stedman's concise medical dictionary : illustrated. — 3rd ed. /
    editor, John H. Dirckx.
        p.   cm.
    ISBN 0-683-23125-1
    1. Medicine—Dictionaries.   I. Dirckx, John H., 1938–   .
II. Stedman, Thomas Lathrop, 1853–1938.   III. Title: Concise medical
dictionary
    [DNLM]:   1. Dictionaries, Medical.   W 13 S8125 1997]
R121.S8   1997
610'.3—dc20
DNLM/DLC
for Library of Congress   96-31924
                                                       CIP

*The publishers have made every effort to trace the copyright holders for borrowed material. If they have inadvertently ov
looked any, they will be pleased to make the necessary arrangements at the first opportunity.*

To purchase additional copies of this book, please call **(410) 528–4223** or fax us at **(410) 528–8550.**

For information regarding translation rights, please address our International Rights Department by fax at **(410) 528–85**

Distribution Rights
The publisher has produced this special edition for sale outside of the United States of America. Sale of this edition with
the United States of America is prohibited by the publisher.

96 97 98 99
2 3 4 5 6 7 8 9

CONTENTS

A MESSAGE FROM THE PUBLISHER

Featuring 40,000 entries and more than 350 illustrations, *Stedman's Concise Medical Dictionary, Illustrated, Third Edition,* gives health professionals access to the core language of medicine and allied health. A compact counterpart to *Stedman's Medical Dictionary, Stedman's Concise* meets the quick-reference needs of students and practitioners throughout the health professions, with particular emphasis on athletic training, audiology, clinical laboratory sciences, dental assisting, dental hygiene, exercise science, health information management, medical assisting (including medical terminology), nutrition, occupational therapy, pharmacy and pharmacy technology, physical therapy, radiography and radiologic technology, respiratory therapy, and speech-language pathology.

Health Professions Consultants

To strengthen the health professions emphasis of *Stedman's Concise,* we nearly doubled the number of consultants in this edition, from 9 to 17, representing 15 fields. Well regarded as both scholars and practitioners, these consultants evaluated the preceding edition of the *Concise,* checking for the presence of key terms in their professions and refining definitions. In addition, the consultants generated approximately 600 new terms and definitions. About 1,000 new entries have also been added to this new edition of the *Concise* from *Stedman's Medical Dictionary* (26th ed.).

More Color—More Illustrations

This new edition offers more than 350 photographs, radiographs, and illustrations, most in full color. Our 17 consultants played an important part in selecting the images to be included. The art program features images from two award-winning sources, medical illustrator Neil Hardy and A.D.A.M.®, the medical education software company. The A.D.A.M.® art is showcased in a quick-reference, 32-page anatomical atlas section. This edition of the *Concise* also includes a full-color insert containing about 90 illustrations depicting various medical technologies and imaging techniques.

Users of the dictionary can easily track down any image using the Illustrations Index (with page references) in the front section of the book. In the A-Z section, a symbol alongside an entry—a white letter "i" in a solid blue square (🛈)—indicates that it is illustrated, either at the entry or in the inserts or appendices.

Updated Appendices

...ounding out the book is a set of more than two dozen appendices. This section includes lists, ...les, tables, and more than 30 illustrations that provide immediate access to information that stu-...ts and practitioners alike can put to use in the classroom, laboratory, or clinic. See Contents: ...Appendices.

Find it Faster

...ed users' word searches, green "precision" thumb tabs have been printed on every page of ...k (with the exception of a few opening pages). In the A-Z section, each thumb tab consists ...st two letters of the last entry on the page. Elsewhere, thumb tabs identify appendices, ...r inserts, and components of the book's opening section such as **Stedman's** ...der. Located just before the A-Z section **Stedman's WordFinder** serves as an index to ...ord terms in the dictionary as well as a quick spelling reference.

Acknowledgments

...s & Wilkins are grateful, first and foremost, to John H. Dirckx—physician and ety-...the skill, experience, and learning he has brought to his service as principal editor ...ion of *Stedman's Concise Medical Dictionary.*

We thank our consultants in the medical specialties for writing and revising the thousands of entries in this and other Stedman's dictionaries, providing a base from which to work. We are grateful as well to our consultants in the health professions for reviewing the content of *Stedman's Concise*. We especially appreciate all they have done to enable this dictionary to meet the needs of audiences from a wide variety of health professions.

The quality and consistency of the art program would not have been possible without the outstanding efforts of Jonathan Dimes at Williams & Wilkins. Our medical assisting and medical terminology consultant, Marjorie Canfield Willis, provided valuable input in the selection of art. And thanks to the diligence of Managing Editor Vincent Ercolano, the input from our many consultants was seamlessly incorporated into this edition of *Stedman's Concise*.

Your Medical Word Resource Publisher

We strive to provide students, practitioners, and educators with the most up-to-date and accurate medical-language references available. We welcome your suggestions for improvements, changes, corrections, and additions—whatever will make this Stedman's product more useful to you.

Elizabeth Randolph
Senior Acquisitions Editor
WILLIAMS & WILKINS
Baltimore, Maryland

EDITOR'S PREFACE

This third edition of *Stedman's Concise Medical Dictionary* provides access to a carefully selected core language of medicine in a format that will be of particular value to students and practitioners in the health professions. The 17-member board of consultants in the health professions contributed about 600 new entries and also revised more than 100 existing ones pertaining to their fields. They also performed a truly editorial role by advising on the range of terms to be defined, the optimum scope and content of entries, and the relevance of each feature of the dictionary to their respective fields.

There is a saying that selection means rejection. For each entry added to this new edition of the *Concise,* existing material had to be abridged or deleted. This process has entailed some hard choices. For instance, entries for individual drug entities have been largely deleted, on the assumption that students and practitioners in pharmacy and pharmacy technology are accustomed to using more comprehensive sources of drug information than a medical dictionary. Please note that conciseness implies not merely brevity but also simplicity and directness. Each definition has been pared down to its essence; readers can get at the information they need unimpeded by elaborate examples and little-used alternate definitions.

Unlike editors of general dictionaries, lexicographers in scientific and technical fields are still expected to perform a prescriptive function, upholding standards of correctness and consistency. Here the problem is that the nomenclature of nearly every biomedical field is unstable. A term can have one meaning in formal usage and quite another in the jargon of practitioners. Furthermore, both meanings may vary widely from the term's etymologic or historical sense. For instance, the naming of diseases is utterly chaotic, the product of a largely spontaneous evolution over the past 25 centuries. Taking an authoritative stand on medical language's myriad points of terminology and usage demands circumspection, command of a wide range of references, and conversance with changes in standards and conventions. In the face of this requirement, this new edition of *Stedman's Concise* is well served by its consultants, who bring strong backgrounds in scholarship and practice in their respective fields.

This edition of *Stedman's Concise* incorporates several innovations. Main entries for gross anatomical structures are now given under their English names. This change, which follows the usage in the 26th edition of *Stedman's Medical Dictionary,* is precisely the reverse of the practice that prevailed almost universally as recently as a half-decade ago. Also in emulation of *Stedman's Medical Dictionary,* entries for most hereditary diseases and conditions now include M.I.M. numbers (six-digit codes as given in V. A. McKusick et al., *Mendelian Inheritance in Man,* 10th ed., Williams & Wilkins, 1992), and entries for dyes and stains now include five-digit identifying numbers according to the international Colour Index (C.I.). The number of illustrations has more than doubled, with thematic inserts—one an anatomical atlas and the other devoted to medical technologies and imaging techniques—included for the first time.

The editors, designers, and other publishing professionals at Williams & Wilkins worked in concert with the consultants and with me to make the third edition of *Stedman's Concise Medical Dictionary* a complete, accurate, keenly focused resource—one, readers will find, that makes every word and every symbol count.

John H. Dirckx, M.D.
Dayton, Ohio

CONSULTANTS IN THE HEALTH PROFESSIONS

Dorothea Cavallucci, BS, CDA, EFDA, RDH　　*Dental Assisting*

Program Director of Dental Assisting, Assistant Professor of Dental Assisting and Dental Hygiene, Harcum College, Bryn Mawr, PA

Wendy C. Hildenbrand, OTR　　*Occupational Therapy*

Teaching Associate, University of Kansas Medical Center, Kansas City, KS

Nicholas M. Hipskind, PhD, CCC-A　　*Audiology*

Associate Professor, Hearing Clinic Director, Department of Speech and Hearing Sciences, Indiana University, Bloomington, IN

Wanda H. Howell, PhD, RD, CNSD　　*Nutrition*

Assistant Professor, Department of Nutritional Sciences, University of Arizona, Tucson, AZ

Scott Irwin, PT, CCS　　*Physical Therapy*

Assistant Professor of Physical Therapy, North Georgia College, Dahlonega, GA, Instructor in Physical Therapy, Emory University Programs in Physical Therapy, Atlanta, GA

Catherine Kurimchak, MS, RT(R) (ARRT)　　*Radiography and Radiologic*
Radiologic Technology Program Faculty,　　*Technology*
Community College of Philadelphia, Philadelphia, PA

Malissa Martin, EdD, ATC　　*Athletic Training*

Assistant Professor, Department of Physical Education, Director, Athletic Training Program, University of South Carolina, Columbia, SC 29208

William D. McArdle, PhD　　*Exercise Science*

Professor, Department of Family, Nutrition, and Exercise Sciences, Queens College of the City University of New York, Flushing, NY

Shirlyn B. McKenzie, PhD, CLS(NCA),　　*Clinical Laboratory Sciences*
MT(ASCP)SH

Professor and Chair, Department of Clinical Laboratory Sciences, University of Texas Health Science Center at San Antonio, San Antonio, TX

Robert J. Michocki, PharmD, BCPS　　*Pharmacy and Pharmacy Technology*

Professor, Department of Pharmacy Practice and Science, University of Maryland, School of Pharmacy, Baltimore, MD

Trina L. Schulz, MS, OTR *Occupational Therapy*

Clinical Director of Occupational Therapy, University of Kansas Medical Center, Kansas City, KS

Robin Sylvis, RDH, MS *Dental Hygiene*

Associate Professor of Dental Hygiene, Clinic Director, Dental Hygiene Program, Harcum College, Bryn Mawr, PA

Susan M. Turley, MA, RN, ART, CMT *Health Information Management*

Health information management and medical transcription, Professor, Health Information Management, Stephens College, Columbia, MO

Jack Wanger, MBA, RRT, RPFT *Respiratory Therapy*

Manager and Technical Director, Pulmonary Physiology Unit, National Jewish Center for Immunology and Respiratory Medicine, Denver, CO

Marjorie Canfield Willis, CMA-AC *Medical Terminology and Medical Assisting*

Professor of Allied Health, Director, Medical Assisting Program, Director, Medical Transcription Program, School of Allied Health Professions, Orange Coast College, Costa Mesa, CA

Amy B. Wohlert, PhD, CCC-SLP *Speech-Language Pathology*

Assistant Professor, Department of Audiology and Speech Sciences, Purdue University, West Lafayette, IN

Lynda D. Woodruff, PhD, PT *Physical Therapy*

Professor of Physical Therapy, Division of Graduate Studies, North Georgia College, Dahlonega, GA

Robert M. Goldwyn, MD *Plastic and Reconstructive Surgery*
Clinical Professor of Surgery, Harvard Medical School, Head, Division of Plastic Surgery, Beth Israel Hospital, Boston, MA

Nicholas M. Greene, MD *Anesthesiology*
Professor Emeritus of Anesthesiology, Yale University School of Medicine, New Haven, CT

Steven I. Gutman, MD, MBA *Laboratory Medicine*
Medical Officer, Division of Clinical Laboratory Devices, Office of Device Evaluation, Food and Drug Administration, Rockville, MD

Duane E. Haines, PhD *Neuroanatomy*
Professor of Anatomy and Chairman, Department of Anatomy, University of Mississippi Medical Center, Jackson, MS

Donald Heyneman, PhD *Parasitology*
Professor of Parasitology Emeritus, Associate Dean for Health and Medical Sciences Emeritus, School of Public Health, University of California, Berkeley/University of California, San Francisco, Joint Medical Program

Steven E. Hyler, MD *Psychiatry*
Associate Professor of Clinical Psychiatry, Columbia University, New York State Psychiatric Institute, New York, NY

Iain Kalfas, MD, FACS *Neurosurgery*
Head, Section of Spinal Surgery, Department of Neurosurgery, Cleveland Clinic Foundation, Cleveland, OH

John M. Last, MD, FRACP, FRCPC *Medical Statistics and Epidemiology*
Professor Emeritus, Department of Epidemiology and Community Medicine, University of Ottawa, Ottawa, Ontario, Canada

Stanley S. Lefkowitz, PhD *Immunology/Virology*
Professor, Department of Microbiology and Immunology, Texas Tech University Health Sciences Center, Lubbock, TX

Alan T. Marty, MD, FACS, FCCP, FACC, FCCM *Thoracic Surgery*
Consultant, Indiana University Medical School, Evansville, IN

Joseph P. Matarazzo, PhD *Psychology*
Professor of Medical Psychology, Chairman, Department of Medical Psychology, Oregon Health Sciences University, Portland, OR

David N. Menton, PhD *Histology*
Associate Professor of Anatomy, Washington University School of Medicine, St. Louis, MO

Edmond A. Murphy, MD *Genetics*
Professor Emeritus, The Johns Hopkins University School of Medicine, Baltimore, MD

Martin L. Nusynowitz, MD *Nuclear Medicine*
Professor, Radiology, Internal Medicine, and Pathology, University of Texas Medical Branch at Galveston, Galveston, TX

Thomas Poirier, MD, PhD *Bacteriology*
Division of Infectious Disease, College of Medicine, University of Florida, Gainesville, FL, Florida Infection Physicians, Gainesville, FL

Richard Prayson, MD *Neuropathology*
Department of Anatomic Pathology, The Cleveland Clinic Foundation, Cleveland, OH

Arthur Raines, PhD *Pharmacology and Toxicology*
Professor of Pharmacology and Neurology, Department of Pharmacology, Georgetown University Medical Center, Washington, DC

Alvin L. Rogers, PhD *Mycology*
Professor Emeritus, Medical Mycology, Michigan State University, East Lansing, MI

Clarence T. Sasaki, MD *Otorhinolaryngology*
Charles W. Ohse Professor of Surgery and Chief, Section of Otolaryngology, Yale University School of Medicine, New Haven, CT

George S. Schuster, DDS, MS, PhD *Dentistry*
Ione and Arthur Merritt Professor and Acting Chairman, Department of Oral Biology, Medical College of Georgia School of Dentistry, Augusta, GA

Sheldon M. Schuster, PhD *Biotechnology*
Professor, Biochemistry and Molecular Biology, Program Director, Biotechnology Program, University of Florida, Gainesville, FL

Donald P. Speer, BS, MD *Orthopaedics*
Professor of Surgery and Anatomy, Associate Head for Academic Affairs, Department of Surgery, University of Arizona College of Medicine, Tucson, AZ

David H. Spodick MD, DSc *Cardiology*
Professor of Medicine, University of Massachusetts Medical School, Lecturer in Medicine, Tufts University School of Medicine, Lecturer in Medicine, Boston University School of Medicine, Director of Clinical Cardiology and Director of Cardiovascular Fellowship Training, St. Vincent Hospital, Worcester, MA

Martha E. Sucheston, PhD *Embryology*
Associate Professor, Cell Biology, Neurobiology, and Anatomy, Powelson Professor

of Medicine, Director, MEDPATH, Ohio State University College of Medicine, Columbus, OH

Michael L. Steer, MD   *General Surgery*
Professor of Surgery, Harvard Medical School, Chief of General Surgery and Associate Surgeon-In-Chief, Beth Israel Hospital, Boston, MA

H. Stanley Thompson, MD   *Ophthalmology*
Professor of Ophthalmology, University of Iowa College of Medicine, Iowa City, IA

Asa J. Wilbourn, MD   *Neurology*
Director, EMG Laboratory, The Cleveland Clinic Foundation, Associate Clinical Professor of Neurology, Case Western Reserve University School of Medicine, Cleveland, OH

Colin Wood, MD   *Dermatology*
Professor Emeritus of Pathology, University of Maryland School of Medicine, Baltimore, MD

Organization of the Vocabulary

Is using **Stedman's Concise** *like using a general English dictionary?* For single-word entries, yes. As in any other dictionary, single-word entries are organized alphabetically. Alphabetization is letter by letter as spelled (not word by word), without regard to variables such as punctuation, spaces, and numbers. For example:

> amylogenic
>
> amylo-1,6-glucosidase
>
> amyloid
>
> OR
>
> diphasic
>
> 2,5-diphenyloxazole
>
> diphosgene

How is using **Stedman's Concise** *different from using a general dictionary?* Medical concepts often consist of more than one word, and finding such terms—for example, *myocardial infarction*—is different in *Stedman's Concise*. In general, *Stedman's Concise* groups multiple-word terms under the primary noun as the **main entry**. Consider these examples:

To find	Look under
myocardial infarction	infarction
hemorrhagic fever	
paratyphoid fever	fever
Q fever	
carcinoid tumor	
giant cell tumor of bone	tumor
Wilms' tumor	

Where will I find multiple-word chemical and drug terms? Location of multiple-word chemical and drug terms generally is determined by the first word of a term. For example:

To find	Look under
Agent Orange	Agent Orange
(a specific compound)	

If the term includes a general noun that can be considered a kind or type, look for it under the noun. For example:

To find	Look under
adrenergic blocking agent	agent
(a type of agent)	

Where will I find definitions of medical abbreviations and symbols? **Stedman's Concise** contains 400 medical abbreviations, acronyms, and symbols. You will find them listed:

- as entries in the dictionary
- within definitions of full words
- separately in appendices (Common Abbreviations Used in Medical Orders, Common Medical Abbreviations, and Symbols; see Contents: The Appendices for page numbers)

How to Use Stedman's WordFinder

What if I'm not sure where to find a multiple-word term and its definition? Turn to **Stedman's WordFinder,** which immediately precedes the A-Z section of the dictionary. For example, if you need to find the term *subacute migratory panniculitis,* check for the first word *subacute* in **Stedman's WordFinder**. The **WordFinder** shows all the *Stedman Concise* terms beginning with *subacute* (the word is listed in bold) and where to find the definitions (look for the noun in non-boldface type *panniculitis*). It's like having an index to the whole dictionary at your fingertips. In another example—if you were seeking a term related to the spine, you would find the word *spinal* in the **WordFinder,** and at that *spinal* entry you would find an alphabetical listing of all the words associated with *spinal* as multiple-word terms in *Stedman's Concise,* beginning with *analgesia* and ending with *veins.*

Using the **WordFinder** saves time two ways: first, because you can look in one place for all the headings related to the spine instead of trying to guess what those headings might be; and, second, because you can use the first word of a multiple-word term to find the head word where it will be defined. **Stedman's WordFinder** is a word-search index that you find only in *Stedman's.*

What if I just need to check the spelling of a term? **Stedman's WordFinder** also acts as a quick spelling reference for terms containing more than one word.

Synonyms and Cross-References

What is the significance of synonyms? Synonyms, which are words that have identical meanings, are abundant in the English language: cat and feline, car and automobile, etc. Synonyms are likewise common in medical English. To conserve space, the editors of the *Concise* have placed the definition of terms that are synonyms at just one of those terms—the preferred term. When you look up a term and find a synonym cross-reference printed in blue, you'll know that you need only look up the term in blue to find the definition. For example:

> **abscess**
> collar-button a. SYN: shirt-stud a.
>
> **shirt-stud a.** two a.'s connected by a narrow channel, usually formed by rupture through an overlying fascia; SYN: collar-button a.
>
> **acariasis** any disease caused by mites, usually a skin infestation; also mange; scabies; SYN: acaridiasis; acarinosis
>
> **acaridiasis** SYN: acariasis
>
> **acarinosis** SYN: acariasis

How are the three kinds of cross-references different from each other? *Synonyms* are terms whose meanings are the same, such as *shirt-stud abscess* and *collar-button abscess.* The abbreviation SYN at the beginning of an entry says that the term that follows (set in blue type) not only means the same, but that you can turn to that term (the one in blue) for the definition. SYN at the end of a definition indicates that the term or terms that follow (set in regular type) may be used to mean the same as the bold entry. A *see* reference points to a word that is related in meaning. For example, the entry for *semilunar cartilage* has a *see* reference to *meniscus,* which has a general meaning of *crescent,* used for several structures, including cartilage. The *see also* reference is a for-your-information reference, linking a general term to a specific term in the same category. For example, *blood group* includes a *see also* reference to the term *blood type.*

Does the dictionary show me how to pronounce words? Yes. Pronunciations appear in parentheses after main-entry words.

The following pronunciation key provides examples of vowel and consonant sounds encountered in the phonetic system. No attempt has been made to accommodate the slurred sounds common in speech or regional variations in speech sounds. Note that a vowel with a breve (˘) is used for the indefinite vowel sound of the schwa (ə). Native pronunciation of foreign words is approximated as closely as possible.

Pronunciation Key

Vowels

ā	day, mate, care, dairy, aorta, ape, ate, face, way, sail, air, aero, behave, gauge, heir, beige, eight, their, they, suede
a	mat, hat, plaid, act, para, damage, banana
ă	abortion, media, banana, about, alone, aorta, para, hepatitis, cephalo, damage, mountain, equal
ah	father, hurrah, wasp, wander, yacht
ar	far, artery, guard, cart, heart
aw	fall, cause, taught, tall, talk, calm, raw, thaw, lawyer, saw, auto
ē	be, bee, meet, deer, bleed, equal, key, fetal, even, perineo, prosthesis, team, ear, beat, bacteria, anterior, pity, busy, -logy, meridian, machine
ĕ	taken, system, synthesis, genesis
er	term, err, merry, operation, father, earn, learn, firm, thirst, myrtle
ī	pie, pine, fire, high, side, ice, bite, height, buy, hyper, deny, pylon
i	pit, mirror, tip, fit, differ, habit, easily, perineo, -ism, archi-, sieve, build, pyramid, physical, women, walking
ĭ	pencil
ō	no, note, fore, for, so, toe, open, bone, phone, perineo, thorus, road, boat, owe, snow, soul, four, sew
o	not, rotten, box, bother, cot, on, oncology, ought, fought, broad
ŏ	occult, lemon, collect, love, son, ton, flood, does, rough
ow	cow, brow, power, plow, now, out, bough, hour, loud, thou
oy	boy, troy, toy, void, mastoid, oil, coin, buoy, Freud
ū	food, ooze, pool, to, too, tool, prove, move, canoe, rule, lupus, June, fruit, acoustic, dew, new, grew
u	wood, foot, wool, took, wolf, would, pull, put
ŭ	but, sun, bud, cup, up, humdrum, fudge, lupus, occult, adjust, us, couple, traction, adjust, uterus
yū	dispute, pure, unit, union, curable, future, uterus, youth, beauty, cue, feud, fuse, few, view

Consonants

b	bad, table, tab		f	fit, differ, if, rough, phone
ch	child, teacher, much		g	got, bigger, leg
n	no, sunset, on		h	hit, behave
ng	single, ring		j	jade, adjust, germ, edge
d	dog, ladder, led		k	cat, action, kept, wake, book, chronic
dh	this, rhythm, smooth			

ks	exquisite, excellent, tax	t	ten, button, cat
kw	exquisite, acquire, quit	th	thin, ether, with
l	law, alone, all	v	very, liver, gave
m	me, simple, him	w	we, away
p	pan, upper, top	y	yes, lawyer
r	rot, hurry, near	z	zero, maze, those, braces, says, browse
s	so, passing, miss, cent, dancing		
sh	should, tension, plantation	zh	azure, measure

In some words the initial sound is not that of the initial letter(s), or the initial letter(s) is not sounded or has a different sound, as in the following examples:

aerobe (ar´ob)

eimeria (ime´re-a)

gnathic (nath´ik)

knuckle (nuk-l)

oedipism (ed´i-pizm)

phthalein (thal´e-in)

pneumonia (nu-mo´ne-a)

psychology (si-kol´o-je)

ptosis (to´sis)

xanthoma (zan-tho´ma)

MEDICAL ETYMOLOGY

Most of the main entries in the dictionary include information about the origins of a word from Greek, Latin, or another language—information that is known as the *etymology* of a word.

Etymologies appear in square brackets at the end of main-entry definitions and are presented in a special format. For example, the following information accompanies the entry *eccrine*:

[G. ek-krino, to single out, separate, expel, secrete]

The letter *G* indicates that the word is of Greek origin; an *L* indicates Latin origin.

Etymologies are your shortcuts to learning more words with less effort. They will help you retain the meaning of the word the first time you look it up and will help you distinguish between words that are similar in spelling but different in meaning.

Will etymology help me to learn medical terminology? Yes. Ninety to ninety-five percent of our medical and technical scientific vocabulary comes from Greek and Latin sources. Most of the words from this vocabulary can be separated into prefixes, suffixes, and combining forms—the building blocks of medical language. On average, learning one of these "building block" words will help you learn about 50 different medical words. And just 500 Greek and 500 Latin word components account for the vast bulk of all the medical words you are likely to encounter in any single health field.

Where do I find these building blocks? They are the individual main entries that are marked with a △ symbol in the A-Z section of the dictionary; they are also listed in Medical Prefixes, Suffixes, and Combining Forms, in the front of the dictionary.

Please explain some of the most common abbreviations, acronyms, and symbols in the dictionary. There are five that are used throughout the dictionary.

The abbreviation SYN at the beginning of an entry not only shows that the term that follows means the same, but tells you to turn to this term for the definition. At the end of a definition, SYN means that the term or terms that follow can be used interchangably, although the boldface term with the definition may be preferred by many users.

The acronym NA, in brackets, follows the pronunciation of certain Latin words or terms. [NA] indicates that a term derives from the Nomina Anatomica, a universally accepted system of anatomical terminology written in Latin.

The acronym MIM stands for *Mendelian Inheritance in Man*. It sometimes appears after terms, followed by six digits and in some cases by an asterisk as well. The MIM is a standard reference source for traits in humans that have been shown to be mendelian or are thought on reasonable grounds to be so. The six digits constitute a catalog number; the asterisk indicates that a trait has been firmly established by molecular biology or by extensive clinical studies.

The △ symbol appears in the margin to the left of some terms. It indicates that an entry is a "building block" term, i.e., a prefix, suffix, or combining form.

The symbol ⋮ in the margin to the left of some terms indicates that an entry is illustrated, either on the same page or in an insert or in the appendices.

ILLUSTRATIONS INDEX

The Illustrations Index provides a quick way to find any image in this book. The page number accompanying each term listed below tells you where an illustration of that term is found. A page number preceded by the letter A indicates that the image can be found in the first color insert, the 32-page anatomical atlas. A page number preceded by the letter B indicates that the image can be found in the second color insert, a 16-page section dedicated to diagnostic medicine and imaging techniques. When you look up a word in the A-Z section, you can tell if it is illustrated—either at the word itself or in the inserts or appendices—if it is accompanied by this symbol: ■.

INTRODUCTION

ARTWORK CREDITS

All artwork in the A-Z section and diagnostic imaging insert was created by Neil O. Hardy, Westport, CT, except the following:

pure tone **audiogram.** Courtesy of Nick Hipskind, PhD, Indiana University, and adapted by Mary Anna Barratt-Dimes, Parkton, MD.

human **calorimeter,** bomb **calorimeter, hand** deformities and fractures, muscles of **mastication, rigidity.** Michael Schenk, Jackson, MS.

rating of perceived **exertion.** Mary Anna Barratt-Dimes.

lesions, rhythm. From Willis, ME: *Medical terminology: The language of health care.* Baltimore: Williams & Wilkins, 1996.

lung volume compartments. Adapted by Mary Anna Barratt-Dimes. From Forster, RE, DuBois, AB, Briscoe, WA, & Fisher, AB: *The lung: Physiologic basis of pulmonary function tests* (3rd ed.). Chicago: Year Book Medical Publishers, 1986.

developmental **milestones.** Michael Schenk, adapted from Klein, MD, Ossman, NH, & Tracey, B: *Normal development copybook.* Tucson, AZ: Therapy Skill Builders, 1991.

nutrition absorption, **obesity.** Neil O. Hardy, adapted from Whitney, Cataldo, Debrayne, & Rolfes: *Nutrition for health and health care.* St. Paul, MN: West, 1995.

nutrition support **route.** Mary Anna Barratt-Dimes, adapted from *Journal of Parenteral and Enteral Nutrition,* 17(4 suppl): 1SA–52SA, July-August 1993.

osteoarthritis. Rob Duckwall, Baltimore.

pinch. Michael Schenk, adapted from Erhardt, R: *Developmental hand dysfunction* (2nd ed.). San Antonio, TX: Therapy Skill Builders, 1994.

eating-right **pyramid.** Source: US Department of Agriculture.

tympanogram. Adapted by Mary Anna Barratt-Dimes from Martin, FN: *Introduction to audiology,* (5th ed.). Englewood Cliffs, NJ: Prentice Hall, 1994.

All artwork in the anatomy insert, Imagery © 1996 A.D.A.M. Software, Inc. Atlanta. All Rights Reserved.

All artwork in the appendix, Radiographic Anatomy and Positioning, from Eisenberg, RL, Dennis, CA, & May, CR, *Radiographic Positioning* (2nd ed.). Boston: Little, Brown, 1995.

PHOTOGRAPHY CREDITS

All photographs in the A-Z section and diagnostic imaging insert from *Roche Lexikon Medizin* (3rd ed.), Munich, Germany: Urban & Schwarzenberg, 1993, except the following:

AIDS (Kaposi's sarcoma, hairy leukoplakia), infectious **diseases** (pediculosis capitis, pediculosis pubis, HSV-2), toxic epidermal **necrolysis,** Kaposi's **sarcoma.** From Sanders, CV, & Nesbitt, Jr., LT: *The skin and infection: A color atlas and text.* Baltimore: Williams & Wilkins, 1995.

basophil, eosinophil, mitochondrion, monocyte, neutrophil. From Gartner, LP, & Hiatt, JL: *Color atlas of histology* (2nd ed.). Baltimore: Williams & Wilkins, 1994.

brain. From Haines, DL: *Neuroanatomy: An atlas of structures, sections, and systems.* Baltimore: Williams & Wilkins, 1995.

bronchoscopy. Photo provided by Temple University Hospital, Philadelphia.

basal cell **carcinoma,** squamous cell **carcinoma.** Courtesy of the Skin Cancer Foundation, New York.

carina, vocal **fold, trachea, bronchus.** From Feinsilver, SH, & Fein, A. *A textbook on bronchoscopy.* Baltimore: Williams & Wilkins, 1995.

cholelithiasis, gastritis, magnetic resonance **imaging,** colon **polypectomy, sonogram,** esophageal **varices.** Courtesy of Mission Hospital Regional Medical Center, Mission Viejo, CA.

cholesteatoma, otitis externa, **otitis** media, tympanic **membrane, tympanoschlerosis.** Courtesy of Michael Hawke, MD, Toronto.

Philadelphia **chromosome** translocation, **abnormalities of erythrocytes** (microcytosis, macrocytosis, poikilocytosis, anisocytosis, sickle cell anemia, hemolytic anemia, aplastic anemia, microcytic anemia), **thalassemia.** From McKenzie, S, Clare, N, Burns, C, Larson, L, & Metz, J: *Textbook of hematology* (2nd ed.). Baltimore: Williams & Wilkins, 1996.

colonoscope. Courtesy of Olympus America, Inc., Melville, NY.

retinal **detachment,** normal **retina.** Courtesy of Scheie Eye Institute, Philadelphia.

Alzheimer's **disease, neoplasia** (squamous cell carcinoma, nodular melanoma, Bowen disease, liposarcoma, lymphoma, neuroblastoma, teratoma, Wilms tumor). From Damjanov, I: *Histopathology: A color atlas and textbook.* Baltimore: Williams & Wilkins, 1996.

echocardiology, Doppler **ultrasonography.** Courtesy of Acuson Corporation, Mountain View, CA.

echocardiogram, barium **enema.** Courtesy of Orange Coast College, Costa Mesa, CA.

electroencephalography. Courtesy of Burdick Corporation, Milton, WI.

exostosis, cephalometric **film, myositis** ossificans. From Yochum, TR, & Rowe, LJ: *Essentials of skeletal radiology* (2nd. ed.). Baltimore: Williams & Wilkins, 1996.

film (occlusal, bitewing, periapical). Courtesy of Dorothea Cavallucci, CDA, EFDA, RDH, Harcum College, Bryn Mawr, PA.

gonococci. From McClatchey, KD.: *Clinical laboratory medicine.* Baltimore: Williams & Wilkins, 1994.

pyogenic **granuloma,** seborrheic **keratoses.** From Rassner, G: *Atlas of dermatology.* Munich, Germany: Urban & Schwarzenberg, 1983.

magnetic resonance **imaging,** lung **scan,** MRI **scan,** computed **tomography,** positron emission **tomography** (PET). Photos and images provided by General Electric Medical Systems, Milwaukee, WI.

primary **lesions** (macule, patch, papule, plaque, nodule, tumor, wheal, vesicle, bulla, pustule); secondary **lesions** (erosion, ulcer, fissure, scale, crust, keloid); vascular **lesions** (cherry angioma, ecchymosis, telangiectasia). From the American Academy of Dermatology, Schamburg, IL.

lung. From Eroschenko, VP: *di Fiore's atlas of histology with functional correlations* (8th ed.). Baltimore: Williams & Wilkins, 1996.

malignant **melanoma.** Courtesy of the American Cancer Society, Inc., Atlanta, GA.

microglia. From Parent, A: *Human neuroanatomy* (9th ed.). Baltimore: Williams & Wilkins, 1995.

muscle fiber. From Ross, MH, Romrell, LJ, & Kaye, G: *Histology: A text and atlas* (3rd ed.). Baltimore: Williams & Wilkins, 1994.

small bowel **obstruction,** CT **scan,** upper gastrointestinal **series.** From Brant, WE, & Helms, CA: *Fundamentals of diagnostic radiology.* Baltimore: Williams & Wilkins, 1994.

ophthalmoscope, ophthalmoscopy, otoscope, otoscopy. Courtesy of Welch Allyn, Inc., Skaneateles Falls, NY.

petechia, syphilis. Courtesy of Laurence J. & Richard D. Underwood, Mission Viejo, CA.

lobar **pneumonia.** From Boyd, SH: *Boyd's introduction to the study of disease* (11th ed.). Philadelphia: Lea & Febiger, 1992.

sonography. Courtesy of Advanced Technology Laboratory, Bothell, WA.

open circuit **spirometry, urography.** From McArdle, WD, Katch, FI, & Katch, VL: *Essentials of exercise physiology*. Baltimore: Williams & Wilkins, 1994.

bone **scan.** Courtesy of Hoag Memorial Presbyterian Hospital, Newport Beach, CA.

PET **scan.** Courtesy of Newport Diagnostic Center, Newport Beach, CA.

ventilation-profusion **scan.** Courtesy of Felix Wang, MD, Orange, CA.

computed **tomography.** Courtesy of Philips Medical Systems, Shelton, CT.

MEDICAL PREFIXES, SUFFIXES, AND COMBINING FORMS

a- not, without, less

ab- from, away from, off

abs- from, away from, off

ad- increase, adherence, motion toward; very

-ad toward, in the direction of; -ward

alge- pain

algesi- pain

algio- pain

algo- pain

ambi- around, on (both) sides, on all sides, both

amyl- starch, polysaccharide nature or origin

amylo- starch, polysaccharide nature or origin

an- not, without, -less

ana- up, toward, apart

ante- before

anti- 1 against, opposing; 2 curative; 3 an antibody

apo- separated from, derived from

arteri- artery

arterio- artery

arthr- a joint, an articulation

arthro- a joint, an articulation

-ase an enzyme

-ate a salt or ester of an "*-ic*" acid

aut- self, same

auto- self, same

bacteri- bacteria

bacterio- bacteria

bi- twice, double

bio- life

blasto- budding by cells or tissue

bronch- bronchus

bronchi- bronchus

broncho- bronchus

carcin- cancer

carcino- cancer

cardi- 1 the heart; 2 esophageal opening of stomach

cardio- 1 the heart; 2 esophageal opening of stomach

cata- down

cephal- the head

cephalo- the head

chem- chemistry

chemo- chemistry

chlor- 1 green; 2 chlorine

chloro- 1 green; 2 chlorine

chol- bile

chondrio- 1 cartilage; 2 granular; 3 gritty

chondro- 1 cartilage; 2 granular; 3 gritty

chrom- color

chromat- color

chromo- color

-cidal killing, destroying

-cide killing, destroying

cis- on this side, on the near side

co- with, together, in association, very, complete

col- with, together, in association, very, complete

com- with, together, in association, very, complete

con- with, together, in association, very, complete

cor- with, together, in association, very, complete

crani- cranium

cranio- cranium

cry- cold

cryo- cold

cycl- 1 a circle, a cycle; 2 the ciliary body

cyst- the bladder; the cystic duct; a cyst

cysti- the bladder; the cystic duct; a cyst

cysto- the bladder; the cystic duct; a cyst

cyt- cell

-cyte cell

cyto- cell

dactyl- the fingers, the toes

dactylo- the fingers, the toes

de- away from, cessation

derm- skin

derma- skin

dermat- skin

dermato- skin

dermo- skin

dextr- right, toward or on the right side

dextro- right, toward or on the right side

di- separation, taking apart, reversal, not, un-

dif- separation, taking apart, reversal, not, un-

dir- separation, taking apart, reversal, not, un-

dis- separation, taking apart, reversal, not, un-

duodeno- the duodenum

-dynia pain

dynamo- force, energy

dys- bad, difficult

ect- outer, on the outside

ecto- outer, on the outside

encephal- the brain

encephalo- the brain

end- within, inner

endo- within, inner

enter- the intestines

entero- the intestines

epi- upon, following, subsequent to

ergo- work

erythr- red, redness

erythro- red, redness

esthesio- sensation, perception

eu- good, well

ex- out of, from, away from

exo- exterior, external, outward

extra- without, outside of

ferri- the presence in a compound of a ferric ion

ferro- metallic iron, the divalent ion Fe^{2+}

fibr- fiber

fibro- fiber

-form in the form or shape of
galact- milk
galacto- milk
-gen 1 producing, coming to be; **2** precursor of
gen- 1 producing, coming to be; **2** precursor of
gloss- the tongue
glosso- the tongue
gluco- glucose
glyco- sugars
gnath- the jaw
gnatho- the jaw
-gram a recording
granul- granular, granule
granulo- granular, granule
-graph a recording instrument
gyn- woman
gyne- woman
gyneco- woman
gyno- woman
hem- blood
hema- blood
hemat- blood
hemato- blood
hemi- one-half
hemo- blood
hepat- the liver
hepatico- the liver
hepato- the liver
hidr- sweat
hidro- sweat
hist- tissue
histio- tissue
histo- tissue
hydr- water; hydrogen
hydro- water; hydrogen
hyper- excessive, above normal
hypo- beneath; diminution, deficiency; the lowest
hyster- 1 uterus; hysteria; **2** late, following
hystero- 1 uterus; hysteria; **2** late, following
-ia a condition
-iasis a condition, a state
-ic pertaining to

-ics organized knowledge, practice, treatment
ileo- the ileum
infra- below
inter- between, among
intra- within
irid- the iris
irido- the iris
ischi- the ischium
ischio- the ischium
-ism 1 condition, disease; **2** a practice, doctrine
-ismus spasm; contraction
iso- 1 equal, like; **2** "isomer of"; **3** sameness
-ite the nature of, resembling
-ites -y, -like
-itides plural of -itis
-itis inflammation
karyo- nucleus
kerat- the cornea
kerato- the cornea
kin- movement
kine- movement
kinesi- motion
kinesio- motion
kineso- motion
kino- movement
lact- milk
lacti- milk
lacto- milk
laryng- the larynx
laryngo- the larynx
latero- lateral, to one side, a side
-lepsis a seizure
-lepsy seizure
lepto- light, slender, thin, frail
leuk- white
leuko- white
linguo- the tongue
lip- fat, lipid
lipo- fat, lipid
lith- a stone, calculus, calcification
litho- a stone, calculus, calcification
-log speech, words
log- speech, words
-login 1 study of; **2** collecting

logo- speech, words
-logy 1 study of; **2** collecting
lymph- lymph
lympho- lymph
lys- lysis, dissolution
lyso- lysis, dissolution
macr- large; long
macro- large; long
mast- breast
masto- breast
meg- 1 large, oversize; **2** one million
mega- 1 large, oversize; **2** one million
megal- large
megalo- large
-megaly large
melan- black
melano- black
mening- meninges
meningo- meninges
mes- 1 middle, mean, intermediacy; **2** mesentery
meso- 1 middle, mean, intermediacy; **2** mesentery
meta- 1 after, behind; **2** joint action, sharing
micr- 1 smallness; **2** one-millionth; **3** microscopic
micro- 1 smallness; **2** one-millionth; **3** microscopic
mon- single
mono- single
morph- form, shape, structure
morpho- form, shape, structure
myx- mucus
myxo- mucus
necr- death, necrosis
necro- death, necrosis
nephr- the kidney
nephro- the kidney
neur- a nerve, the nervous system
neuri- a nerve, the nervous system
neuro- a nerve, the nervous system
oculo- eye, ocular

odont- tooth
odonto- tooth
odyn- pain
odyno- pain
-oid resemblance to
olig- few, little
oligo- few, little
-oma tumor, neoplasm
-omata plural of -oma
oncho- onco-
onco- tumor, bulk, volume
-one a ketone (—CO—) group
onych- fingernail, toenail
onycho- fingernail, toenail
oo- egg, ovary
oophor- ovary
oophoro- ovary
ophthalm- the eye
ophthalmo- the eye
orchi- testis
orchido- testis
orchio- testis
-oses plural of -osis
-osis process, condition, state
ossi- bone
osseo- bony
ost- bone
oste- bone
osteo- bone
ovari- ovary
ovario- ovary
ovi- egg
ovo- egg
oxa- the presence or addition of oxygen atom(s)
oxo- addition of oxygen
oxy- sharp; acid; acute; shrill; quick; oxygen
pachy- thick
pan- all, entire
pant- all, entire
panto- all, entire
para- 1 abnormal; 2 involvement of two like parts
path- disease
patho- disease
-pathy disease
ped- 1 child; 2 foot
pedi- 1 child; 2 foot
pedo- 1 child; 2 foot

-penia deficiency
per- through, thoroughly, intensely
peri- around, about
-pexy fixation, usually surgical
phaco- 1 lens-shaped; 2 relation to a lens
-phage eating, devouring
-phagia eating, devouring
phago- eating, devouring
-phagy eating, devouring
pharmaco- drugs, medicine
pharyng- the pharynx
pharyngo- the pharynx
phleb- vein
phlebo- vein
phon- sound, speech
phono- sound, speech
phor- carrying, bearing; a carrier, a bearer; phoria
phoro- carrying, bearing; a carrier, a bearer; phoria
phos- light
phot- light
photo- light
phren- 1 diaphragm; 2 the mind; 3 phrenic
phreni- 1 diaphragm; 2 the mind; 3 phrenic
-phrenia of mind
phrenico- 1 diaphragm; 2 the mind; 3 phrenic
phreno- 1 diaphragm; 2 the mind; 3 phrenic
physi- 1 physical; 2 natural; 3 the science of physics
physio- 1 physical; 2 natural; 3 the science of physics
physo- 1 tendency to swell or inflate; 2 air, gas
phyt- plants
phyto- plants
-plasia formation
plasma- plasma
plasmat- plasma
plasmato- plasma
plasmo- plasma
-plegia paralysis
pleur- rib, side, pleura
pleura- rib, side, pleura

pleuro- rib, side, pleura
pluri- several, more
-pnea breath, respiration
pneo- breath, respiration
pneum- 1 air, gas; 2 the lungs; 3 breathing
pneuma- 1 air, gas; 2 the lungs; 3 breathing
pneumat- 1 air, gas; 2 the lungs; 3 breathing
pneumato- 1 air, gas; 2 the lungs; 3 breathing
pod- foot, foot-shaped
-pod foot, foot-shaped
podo- foot, foot-shaped
-poiesis production
poly- 1 multiplicity; 2 "polymer of"
post- after, behind, posterior
pre- anterior, before
pro- 1 before, forward; 2 precursor of
proct- the anus, the rectum
procto- the anus, the rectum
psych- the mind
psyche- the mind
psycho- the mind
pyel- (renal) pelvis
pyelo- (renal) pelvis
pyo- suppuration, an accumulation of pus, pus
pyreto- fever
pyro- fire, heat, fever
rachi- the spine
rachio- the spine
radio- 1 radiation, chiefly x-ray; 2 radius
re- again, backward
rect- the rectum
recto- the rectum
retro- backward, behind
rhin- the nose
rhino- the nose
-rrhagia discharge
-rrhaphy surgical suturing
-rrhea a flowing, a flux
salping- a tube
salpingo- a tube
sarco- muscular substance, fleshlike

schisto- split, cleft
schiz- split, cleft, division
schizo- split, cleft, division
scler- hardness (induration), sclerosis, the sclera
sclero- hardness (induration), sclerosis, the sclera
-scope an instrument for viewing
-scopy the use of an instrument for viewing
semi- one-half; partly
sial- saliva, the salivary glands
sialo- saliva, the salivary glands
sigmoid- sigmoid, the sigmoid colon
sigmoido- sigmoid, the sigmoid colon
sito- food, grain
somat- the body, bodily
somato- the body, bodily
somatico- the body, bodily
spasmo- spasm
spermato- semen, spermatozoa
spermo- semen, spermatozoa
sperma- semen, spermatozoa
splanchn- the viscera
splanchni- the viscera
splanchno- the viscera
splen- the spleen
spleno- the spleen
staphyl- a grape, a bunch of grapes; staphylococci

staphylo- a grape, a bunch of grapes; staphylococci
-stat an agent to prevent changing or moving
steno- narrowness, constriction
stheno- strength, force, power
stom- mouth
stoma- mouth
stomat- mouth
stomato- mouth
sub- beneath, less than normal, inferior
super- in excess, above, superior, in the upper part
sy- together
syl- together
sym- together
syn- together
sys- together
thel- the nipples
thelo- the nipples
therm- heat
thermo- heat
thorac- the chest, the thorax
thoracico- the chest, the thorax
thoraco- the chest, the thorax
thromb- blood clot
thrombo- blood clot
thyr- the thyroid gland
thyro- the thyroid gland
toco- childbirth
-tome 1 a cutting instrument; 2 a segment, section
-tomy a cutting operation
tono- tone, tension, pressure
top- place, topical

topo- place, topical
tox- a toxin, a poison
toxi- a toxin, a poison
toxico- a toxin, a poison
toxo- a toxin, a poison
trache- the trachea
tracheo- the trachea
trans- across, through, beyond
trich- the hair, a hairlike structure
trichi- the hair, a hairlike structure
-trichia the hair, a hairlike structure
tricho- the hair, a hairlike structure
-trophic food, nutrition
tropho- food, nutrition
-trophy food, nutrition
-tropic turning toward, affinity
uri- uric acid
uric- uric acid
urico- uric acid
vas- a duct, a blood vessel
vasculo- a blood vessel
vaso- a duct, a blood vessel
vesic- a vesica, a vesicle
vesico- a vesica, a vesicle
xanth- yellow, yellowish
xantho- yellow, yellowish
zo- an animal, animal life
zoo- an animal, animal life
zym- fermentation, enzymes
zymo- fermentation, enzymes

A

α: fetoprotein; thalassemia

α-: fetoproteins; streptococci

A: bands; cells; chain; fibers; A-aO₂: difference

Abbott's: method

abdominal: angina; cavity; fissure; guarding; hernia; hysterectomy; hysterotomy; ostium of uterine tube; pad; pregnancy; pressure; regions; respiration; section

abdominothoracic: arch

abducent: nerve

abductor digiti minimi: muscle of foot; muscle of hand

abductor hallucis: muscle

Abell-Kendall: method

aberrant: goiter

abnormal: occlusion

ABO hemolytic: disease of the newborn

aborted: systole

abortive: transduction

ABR: audiometry

abraded: wound

abscopal: effect

absence: seizure

absolute: humidity; hyperopia; leukocytosis; scale; temperature; unit; zero

absorbable gelatin: film

absorbancy: index

absorbed: dose

absorption: chromatography; coefficient; lines; spectrum

abstract: thinking

acanthomeatal: line

accelerator: factor; fibers; globulin; nerve

accessory: adrenal; gland; ligaments; molecules; nerve; organs of the eye; spleen; symptom

accessory cephalic: vein

accessory hemiazygos: vein

accessory obturator: artery

accessory pancreatic: duct

accessory phrenic: nerves

accessory vertebral: vein

accidental: hypothermia

accommodation: reflex

accommodative: asthenopia

accommodative convergence-accommodation: ratio

accordion: graft

accoucheur's: hand

accretionary: growth

acetabular: fossa

acetone: body

acetyl-activating: enzyme

achievement: age; quotient; test

Achilles: reflex; tendon

acholuric: jaundice

achondroplastic: dwarfism

achrestic: anemia

achromatic: lens; objective; vision

acid: cell; fuchsin; indigestion; phosphatase; stain; tide

acid-ash: diet

acid-base: balance

acidic: dyes

acidified serum: test

acidophil: adenoma

acid perfusion: test

acinar: cell

acinic cell: adenocarcinoma

acinotubular: gland

acinous: cell; gland

acne: keloid

Acosta's: disease

acoustic: aphasia; meatus; nerve; neurilemoma; neuroma; radiation

acoustic reflex: threshold

acoustic trauma: deafness

acquired: character; drives; hyperlipoproteinemia; immunity; nevus; toxoplasmosis in adults

acquired epileptic: aphasia

acquired immunodeficiency: syndrome

Acrel's: ganglion

acrocentric: chromosome

acromial: angle; process

acromioclavicular: joint

acromiothoracic: artery

acrosomal: cap; granule; vesicle

ACTH-producing: adenoma

actin: filament

actinic: dermatitis; granuloma; keratosis

action: current; potential

activated clotting: time

activated partial thromboplastin: time

active: anaphylaxis; congestion; hyperemia; immunity; methyl; principle; repressor; site; splint; transport

active chronic: hepatitis

activities of daily living: scale

activity: adaptation; analysis; coefficient; group; synthesis

activity pattern: analysis

actual: cautery

acupuncture: anesthesia

acute: abdomen; alcoholism; inflammation; malaria; rhinitis; trypanosomiasis; tuberculosis

acute adrenocortical: insufficiency

acute African sleeping: sickness

acute anterior: poliomyelitis

acute ascending: paralysis

acute bulbar: poliomyelitis

acute care: hospital

acute compression: triad

acute contagious: conjunctivitis

acute disseminated: encephalomyelitis

acute epidemic: leukoencephalitis

acute fulminating: meningococcemia

acute hemorrhagic: conjunctivitis; pancreatitis

acute idiopathic: polyneuritis

acute intermittent: porphyria

acute isolated: myocarditis

acute necrotizing: encephalitis

acute necrotizing hemorrhagic: encephalomyelitis

acute necrotizing ulcerative: gingivitis

acute promyelocytic: leukemia

acute pulmonary: alveolitis

acute respiratory: failure

acute situational: reaction

acute yellow: atrophy of the liver

acyclic: compound

acyl carrier: protein

Adams-Stokes: disease; syndrome

adansonian: classification

adaptive: hypertrophy

adaptive behavior: scales

addisonian: crisis

Addison's: anemia; disease

additive: effect

adductor: canal

adductor brevis: muscle

adductor hallucis: muscle

adductor longus: muscle

adductor magnus: muscle

adductor pollicis: muscle

adenoid: facies; tissue

adenoid cystic: carcinoma

adenoid squamous cell: carcinoma

adenomatoid: tumor

adenomatoid odontogenic: tumor

adenomatous: goiter; polyp

adequate: stimulus

adhesion: molecules

adhesive: bandage; capsulitis; otitis; pericarditis; peritonitis; pleurisy; vaginitis

adhesive absorbent: dressing

Adie: syndrome

Adie's: pupil

adipokinetic: hormone

adipose: cell; degeneration; fossae; infiltration; tissue

adiposogenital: dystrophy

adjustment: disorders

admitting: physician

adnexal: adenoma

adolescent: medicine

adoptive: immunotherapy

adrenal: crisis; gland; hypertension; rest

adrenal androgen-stimulating: hormone

adrenergic: blockade; bronchodilators; fibers; receptors

β-adrenergic: receptors

α-adrenergic: receptors

β-adrenergic blocking: agent

α-adrenergic blocking: agent

adrenergic blocking: agent

adrenergic neuronal blocking: agent

adrenocortical: insufficiency

adrenocorticotropic: hormone

adrenocorticotropic releasing: factor

adrenogenital: syndrome

adrenomedullary: hormones

adrenomimetic: amine

Adson's: test

adsorption: theory of narcosis

adult: rickets

adult lactase: deficiency

adult-onset: diabetes

adult pseudohypertrophic muscular: dystrophy

adult respiratory distress: syndrome

adult T-cell: leukemia; lymphoma

advanced multiple-beam equalization: radiography

advancement: flap

adventitial: cell; neuritis

adventitious: cyst

adventitious lung: sounds

adverse: reaction

adverse drug: event; reaction

adynamic: ileus

A-E: amputation

aerobic: respiration

aerosol: generator

affective: disorders; psychosis

afferent: fibers; lymphatic; nerve; vessel

afferent glomerular: arteriole

AFORMED: phenomenon

African: trypanosomiasis

African sleeping: sickness

after-: pains

afunctional: occlusion

agitated: depression

agranular endoplasmic: reticulum

Ahumada-Del Castillo: syndrome

air: bronchogram; cells; conduction; embolism; pollution; sickness; splint; vesicles

air-bone: gap

air-conditioner: lung

air contrast: enema

airplane: splint

airway: anatomy; obstruction; resistance

A-K: amputation

akamushi: disease

Akerlund: deformity

akinetic: mutism

alar: spine

alarm: reaction

alaryngeal: speech

albino: rats

albumin-globulin: ratio

Alcock's: canal

alcohol amnestic: syndrome

alcoholic: cirrhosis

Alder's: anomaly

aldosterone: antagonist

Aleppo: boil

aleukemic: leukemia

Alexander's: deafness

algid: stage

alignment: curve

alimentary: canal; glycosuria; hyperinsulinism; lipemia; pentosuria; system; tract

alkali: metal; reserve

alkaline: earths; phosphatase; tide

alkaline-ash: diet

alkaline earth: elements
allantoic: fluid; sac; stalk; vesicle
allantoid: membrane
allantoidoangiopagous: twins
allelic: gene
allergenic: extract
allergic: conjunctivitis; eczema; extract; purpura; reaction; rhinitis
allergic contact: dermatitis
alligator: forceps
all or none: law
allogeneic: graft
allograft: rejection
allosteric: site
Almeida's: disease
alpha: angle; cells; fibers; granule; particle; rhythm; wave
ALT:AST: ratio
alternate cover: test
alternating: current; pulse; tremor
alternative: medicine
altitude: sickness
alveolar: abscess; air; cell; duct; gas; gingiva; gland; macrophage; point; process; sac; ventilation
alveolar air: equation
alveolar-arterial oxygen: difference
alveolar-arterial oxygen tension: difference
alveolar-capillary: membrane
alveolar cell: carcinoma
alveolar dead: space
alveolar soft part: sarcoma
alveolocapillary: block
alveolodental: ligament; membrane
Alzheimer's: dementia; disease
amalgam: tattoo
amaurotic: pupil
amber: codon
ambiguous external: genitalia
Ambu: bag

ambulatory: care; surgery
ambulatory patient: group
amebic: abscess; colitis; dysentery; granuloma
ameboid: cell; movement
ameloblastic: fibroma; fibrosarcoma; layer; odontoma; sarcoma
ameloblastic adenomatoid: tumor
amenorrhea-galactorrhea: syndrome
American: leishmaniasis
American College of Sports: Medicine
American Health Information Management: Association
American Law Institute: rule
Ames: test
Ammon's: horn
amnestic: aphasia; syndrome
amniotic: bands; cavity; fluid; fold; sac
amphibolic: fistula
amphoric: rale; resonance
amphotropic: virus
amplitude of: accommodation
ampullar: pregnancy
ampullary: crest
amputation: neuroma
amygdaloid: body
amylase-creatinine clearance: ratio
amyloid: degeneration; kidney; nephrosis; tumor
amyotrophic lateral: sclerosis
anabolic: steroid
anaclitic: depression
anacrotic: pulse
anaerobic: respiration; threshold
anagen: effluvium
anal: atresia; canal; columns; ducts; fissure; fistula; pecten; phase; pit; plate; reflex; sinuses; verge
analeptic: enema
analytical: psychology
anamnestic: reaction
anaphylactic: antibody; shock
anaphylactoid: purpura; shock
anaplastic: cell

anastomotic: branch; ulcer
anatomical: pathology; position; sphincter; wart
anatomical dead: space
anchor: splint
anconeus: muscle
Anderson: splint
androgen binding: protein
androgenic: alopecia; steroid
android: pelvis
anechoic: chamber
anemic: anoxia; halo; hypoxia; infarct; murmur
anesthesia: record
anesthetic: depth; gas; index; leprosy
aneurysmal: bruit; varix
aneurysmal bone: cyst
anginose: scarlatina
angiogenesis: factor
angiography: catheter
angioimmunoblastic: lymphadenopathy with dysproteinemia
angioneurotic: edema
angioplasty: balloon
angiotensin-converting: enzyme
angiotensin-converting enzyme: inhibitors
angle of: convergence
angle-closure: glaucoma
Angle's: classification of malocclusion
Ångström: unit
angular: artery; cheilitis; curvature; gyrus; spine; stomatitis; vein
anicteric virus: hepatitis
animal: model; pole
anion: gap
anion-exchange: resin
Anitschkow: cell; myocyte
ankle: bone; joint; reflex
ankylosing: spondylitis
annealing: lamp
annular: cataract; ligament; scotoma
annuloaortic: ectasia
anococcygeal: nerves
anocutaneous: line

anogenital: raphe
anomalous: complex; corre-
    spondence
anomic: aphasia
anosognosic: epilepsy
anovular: menstruation
anoxic: anoxia
Anrep: phenomenon
anserine: bursa
antagonistic: muscles
antalgic: gait
antegonial: notch
antegrade: urography
anterior: border of tibia;
    chamber of eye; column;
    commissure; embryotoxon;
    funiculus; horn; lobe of
    hypophysis; pyramid;
    rhinoscopy; scleritis;
    staphyloma
anterior auricular: muscle;
    nerves
anterior cardinal: veins
anterior cerebral: vein
anterior ciliary: artery
anterior condyloid: foramen
anterior cruciate: ligament
anterior elastic: lamina of
    cornea
anterior focal: point
anterior intercostal: veins
anterior interosseous: nerve
anterior labial: veins
anterior lacrimal: crest
anterior limiting: layer of
    cornea; ring
anterior lingual: gland
anterior nasal: spine
anterior ocular: segment
anterior pituitary: gonado-
    tropin
anterior pituitary-like: hor-
    mone
anterior spinocerebellar:
    tract
anterior tibial compart-
    ment: syndrome
anterior vertebral: vein
anterograde: amnesia; block
anteroposterior: projection
anthropoid: pelvis

antianxiety: agent
anti-basement membrane:
    antibody; glomerulonephritis
antibiotic: enterocolitis
antibody: excess
antidiuretic: hormone
antigen: excess; unit
antigen-antibody: reaction
antigenic: determinant; drift;
    shift
antigen-sensitive: cell
antihemophilic: factor A;
    globulin A; globulin B
antihuman: globulin
antilymphocyte: serum
antinuclear: antibody; factor
antiphospholipid antibody:
    syndrome
antipsychotic: agent
antiseptic: dressing
antiserum: anaphylaxis
antisocial: personality
antisocial personality: disorder
antitoxin: unit
antitragicus: muscle
antitrypsin: deficiency
α-1 antitrypsin deficiency:
    panniculitis
antiviral: protein
anxiety: disorders; hysteria;
    neurosis; reaction
aortic: arch; atresia; body;
    bulb; dissection; hiatus;
    insufficiency; murmur; nip-
    ple; notch; orifice; sinus;
    stenosis; valve; vestibule
aortoiliac: bypass
aortoiliac occlusive: disease
aortorenal: bypass
AP: projection
apatite: calculus
apex: beat; pneumonia
Apgar: score
aphakic: eye
aphthous: stomatitis
apical: cap; foramen of tooth;
    gland; granuloma; pulse; space
apical periodontal: cyst
aplanatic: lens
aplastic: anemia; lymph
apneic: pause

apneustic: breathing
apochromatic: objective
apocrine: adenoma; carcino-
    ma; chromhidrosis; gland;
    metaplasia
aponeurotic: fibroma
apothecaries': weight
appendiceal: abscess
appendicular: artery; mus-
    cle; skeleton; vein
applanation: tonometer
apple jelly: nodules
apposition: suture
appositional: growth
approximation: suture
aptitude: test
APUD: cells
aquagenic: pruritus
aqueous: chambers; humor;
    phase
arachnoid: cyst; granula-
    tions; membrane; villi
Aran-Duchenne: disease
arcuate: arteries of kidney;
    artery; fibers; nuclei; veins
    of kidney; zone
areolar: glands; tissue
areolar venous: plexus
argentaffin: cells
arginine: vasopressin
Argyll Robertson: pupil
aristotelian: method
arithmetic: mean
Arneth: count; index
Arnold-Chiari: malformation
aromatic: compound; series
aromatic ammonia: spirit
arrector pili: muscles
Arrhenius-Madsen: theory
arterial: blood; canal; capil-
    lary; circle of cerebrum;
    cone; duct; forceps; line;
    nephrosclerosis; sclerosis;
    spider; tension
arteriolar: nephrosclerosis;
    network
arteriosclerotic: aneurysm
arteriovenous: anastomosis;
    aneurysm; fistula; shunt
arteriovenous carbon diox-
    ide: difference

arteriovenous oxygen: difference
arthritic general: pseudoparalysis
arthrodial: joint
articular: capsule; cartilage; corpuscles; disc; lamella; muscle; nerve; rheumatism
articularis cubiti: muscle
articularis genu: muscle
articular vascular: network of elbow
articulatory: apraxia
artificial: ankylosis; heart; insemination; kidney; larynx; pacemaker; pneumothorax; radioactivity; respiration; selection; ventilation
aryepiglottic: fold; muscle
arytenoid: cartilage
asbestos: bodies
ascending: artery; branch of the inferior mesenteric artery; colon; degeneration
ascending lumbar: vein
ascending pharyngeal: artery
Aschoff: bodies
aseptic: necrosis; surgery
asexual: dwarfism; generation; reproduction
aspiration: biopsy; pneumonia
assimilation: pelvis
assist-control: ventilation
assisted: respiration; ventilation
assistive listening: device
association: areas; cortex; fibers; test
associative: aphasia
assortative: mating
asteroid: body; hyalosis
astigmatic: lens
atactic: abasia
ataxic: aphasia; dysarthria; gait
atheromatous: degeneration
athlete's: foot; heart
athletic: training

atomic: number; weight
atomic absorption: spectrophotometry
atomic mass: number; unit
atonic: bladder
atopic: allergy; cataract; dermatitis; keratoconjunctivitis
atraumatic: suture
atrial: arteries; auricle; complex; dissociation; extrasystole; fibrillation; flutter
atrial capture: beat
atrial chaotic: tachycardia
atrial fusion: beat
atrial septal: defect
atrioventricular: block; bundle; canal; dissociation; extrasystole; node; septum; valves
atrioventricular canal: cushions
atrioventricular junctional: bigeminy; rhythm
atrioventricular nodal: extrasystole
atrophic: arthritis; excavation; gastritis; rhinitis; vaginitis
attached: gingiva
attack: rate
attending: physician; staff
attention deficit: disorder
attention deficit hyperactivity: disorder
attenuated: virus
attraction: sphere
atypical: lipoma; measles; mycobacteria; pneumonia
atypical verrucous: endocarditis
auditory: agnosia; aphasia; area; capsule; cortex; defensiveness; field; hairs; nerve; ossicles; pits; reflex; tube; vertigo; vesicle
auditory brainstem response: audiometry
auditory receptor: cells
Auer: bodies; rods
augmentation: mammaplasty
augmentative and alternative: communication

aural: rehabilitation
auricle: hematoma
auricular: cartilage; point; tubercle
auriculotemporal: nerve
auropalpebral: reflex
auscultatory: alternans; gap; percussion
Austin Flint: murmur; phenomenon
Australian X: disease
authoritarian: personality
authority: figure
autochthonous: ideas
autocrine: hypothesis
autodermic: graft
autoerythrocyte: sensitization
autoerythrocyte sensitization: syndrome
autogeneic: graft
autogenous: vaccine
autoimmune: disease
autoimmune hemolytic: anemia
autologous: graft
autolytic: enzyme
automated differential leukocyte: counter
automatic: beat; speech
autonomic: ganglia; imbalance; plexuses
autonomic nervous: system
autonomic neurogenic: bladder
autoplastic: graft
autopolymer: resin
auto-positive end-expiratory: pressure
autosomal: gene
A-V: block; interval
avascular: necrosis
aversion: therapy
avian leukosis-sarcoma: complex; virus
Avogadro's: constant; number
avoidant: personality
avoirdupois: weight
avulsed: wound
avulsion: fracture

WORDFINDER

axial: angle; current; filament; hyperopia; loading; muscle; plate; point; skeleton
axial pattern: flap
axillary: artery; cavity; lymph nodes; nerve; vein
axis: deviation; shift
axis-traction: forceps
axon: hillock; terminals
axoplasmic: transport
Ayerza's: disease; syndrome
azure lunules of: nails
azygos: lobe of lung; vein

B

β: thalassemia
β_1F: globulin
β_1C: globulin
β_1E: globulin
β-: fetoproteins
B: cells; chain; fibers; lymphocyte
B19: virus
Babbington: nebulizer
Babinski's: sign
baby: tooth
bacillary: angiomatosis; dysentery; layer
back: pressure
backboard: splint
background: radiation
backward heart: failure
bacterial: capsule; endarteritis; endocarditis; plaque; vaginosis; virus
bacterial food: poisoning
bacteriocinogenic: plasmids
bacteriogenic: agglutination
bag of: waters
Baker's: cyst
balanced: anesthesia; diet; occlusion; polymorphism; translocation
balancing side: condyle
Balkan: frame; splint
ball: valve
ball-and-socket: joint
balloon-tip: catheter
ballotable: patella
Bamberger-Marie: disease
Bamberger's: sign

bamboo: hair; spine
band: cell
Bandl's: ring
band-shaped: keratopathy
Bang's: bacillus
Bankart's: lesion
Bannister's: disease
Bárány's caloric: test
bare lymphocyte: syndrome
barium: enema
Barlow's: disease
barometric: pressure
Barr chromatin: body
barrel: chest
Barrett's: esophagus
barrier: contraceptive
Bartholin's: cyst; gland
Barth's: hernia
Barton's: bandage; fracture
basal: anesthesia; body; cell; ganglia; granule; lamina of; ciliary body lamina of neural tube; layer; layer of choroid; rod; vein of Rosenthal
basal cell: carcinoma; epithelioma; nevus
basal cell nevus: syndrome
basal joint: reflex
basal tentorial: branch of internal carotid artery
base: deficit; excess; line; pair; units
baseball: finger
basement: membrane
basibregmatic: axis
basic: dyes; fuchsin; stain
basic fuchsin-methylene blue: stain
basic personality: type
basicranial: axis; flexure
basifacial: axis
basilar: artery; lamina; membrane; meningitis; vertebra
basilic: vein
basivertebral: vein
basket: cell
basophil: adenoma
basophilic: leukemia; leukocyte; leukopenia
basosquamous: carcinoma
Bassini's: operation

bath: itch; pruritus
bathing trunk: nevus
battle: fatigue; neurosis
battledore: placenta
Battle's: sign
Baudelocque's: operation
Bauer's: syndrome
Bayle's: disease
bayonet: forceps; hair
BCR/ABL: gene
β-δ: thalassemia
B-E: amputation
beaded: hair
beaked: pelvis
beaker: cell
bearing-down: pain
Bechterew-Mendel: reflex
Bechterew's: disease
Beckwith-Wiedemann: syndrome
bed: rest; sore
Bednar's: aphthae
Beer's: law
Beevor's: sign
behavior: disorder; modification; therapy
behavioral: epidemic; genetics; immunogen; pathogen; psychology
Behring's: law
Bell's: law; muscle; palsy
bell-shaped: curve
Bence Jones: proteinuria; reaction
Bender gestalt: test
bending: fracture
Benedict's: test
benign: hypertension; lymphocytoma cutis; tetanus; tumor
benign inoculation: lymphoreticulosis; reticulosis
benign myalgic: encephalomyelitis
benign paroxysmal postural: vertigo
benign positional: vertigo
benign prostatic: hyperplasia
Bennett's: fracture
bentiromide: test

bentonite flocculation: test
benzene: ring
Berger's: disease
berloque: dermatitis
Bernard-Cannon: homeostasis
Bernhardt's: disease
Bernoulli's: law
Bernstein: test
berry: aneurysm
Besnier-Boeck-Schaumann: disease; syndrome
beta: cells; fibers; granule; particle; ray; rhythm; wave
Bethesda: system; unit
Betke-Kleihauer: test
Betz: cells
Beuren: syndrome
biauricular: axis
biaxial: joint
bi-bi: reaction
BICAP: cautery
biceps: reflex
biceps brachii: muscle
biceps femoris: muscle
Bichat's: fissure; membrane
bicipital: rib
biconcave: lens
bicondylar: joint
biconvex: lens
bicornate: uterus
bicuspid: tooth; valve
bidirectional ventricular: tachycardia
bidiscoidal: placenta
Biernacki's: sign
Bier's: method
bifid: tongue
bifocal: lens
big: ACTH
bigeminal: pulse; rhythm
bilateral: coordination; hermaphroditism
bile: acids; duct; pigments; salts
bilevel positive airway: pressure
bilharzial: dysentery
biliary: atresia; canaliculus; cirrhosis; duct; ductules
bilirubin: encephalopathy

bilocular: joint
bimalleolar: fracture
bimanual: version
binary: digit; fission
binaural: diplacusis
Binet: scale; test
binocular: microscope; vision
Binswanger's: disease; encephalopathy
biochemical: profile
biologic: evolution; indicator
biological: sampling; vector
biomechanical: frame of reference
biomedical: model
biopsychosocial: model
Biot's: breathing; respiration
biparietal: diameter
bipolar: cautery; cell; disorder; lead; neuron
bird-breeder's: lung
bird shot: retinochoroiditis
birth: amputation; canal; control; palsy; rate; trauma; weight
bisferious: pulse
bismuth: line
bite: analysis
bitewing: film; radiograph
biuret: reaction; test
bivalent: chromosome
B-K: amputation
black: cataract; death; eye; lung; tongue
blackwater: fever
Blainville: ears
Blair-Brown: graft
Blalock-Taussig: operation; shunt
bland: diet
blanket: suture
blast: cell; injury
blastodermic: vesicle
bleeding: time
blind: fistula; spot
blind loop: syndrome
blistering distal: dactylitis
block: anesthesia
blocking: activity; agent; antibody
Blocq's: disease

blood: albumin; blister; capillary; count; cyst; disk; doping; dyscrasia; gases; group; plasma; poisoning; pressure; relationship; sugar; type; vessel
blood-air: barrier
blood-aqueous: barrier
blood-brain: barrier
blood-cerebrospinal fluid: barrier
blood gas: analysis
blood group: antigen
blood group-specific: substances A and B
bloodless: operation
blood plasma: fractions
blood pool: imaging
blood urea: nitrogen
Blount's: disease
blow-out: fracture
blue: baby; cataract; line; nevus; pus; spot
blueberry muffin: baby
blue dome: cyst
blue-green: bacteria
blue rubber-bleb: nevi
Blumberg's: sign
blunted: affect
blunt-ended: DNA
Bochdalek's: hernia
Bodansky: unit
body: cavity; image; scheme
body mass: index
body surface: area
Boerhaave's: syndrome
Bohr: effect; effect
bomb: calorimeter
Bombay: blood type
bone: block; canaliculus; conduction; forceps; marrow; matrix; scan; spur; tissue
bone marrow: transplantation
bony: ankylosis; labyrinth; palate
bony semicircular: canals
booster: dose

borderline personality: disorder
Borg: scale
Bornholm: disease
Bornholm disease: virus
Botallo's: duct
botryoid: sarcoma
botulinus: toxin
Bourdon: gauge
boutonneuse: fever
boutonnière: deformity
bovine: babesiosis
bovine serum: albumin
bow-: leg
Bowditch's: law
bowel: bypass; sounds
Bowen's: disease
bowler's: thumb
Bowman's: membrane
boxer's: fracture
Boyden: meal
Boyle's: law
Bozeman-Fritsch: catheter
Bozeman's: position
brachial: artery; plexus; veins
brachialis: muscle
brachiocephalic: arteritis; trunk; veins
brachioradialis: muscle
Bracht: maneuver
brachypellic: pelvis
Bradford: frame
brain: concussion; stem; sugar; swelling; wave
Brain's: reflex
brainstem evoked response: audiometry
braking: radiation
brancher glycogen storage: disease
branchial: clefts
branchiomotor: nuclei
Brandt-Andrews: maneuver
brass founder's: fever
brawny: edema
Braxton Hicks: sign
break-even: point
breast: bone; pump
breath-holding: test
breathing: bag; reserve

breech: presentation
Bremsstrahlung: radiation
Brenner: tumor
Breslow's: thickness
Breus: mole
Bricker: operation
bridle: suture
Brill's: disease
Brill-Zinsser: disease
Briquet's: disease
British thermal: unit
brittle: bones; diabetes
broad: ligament of the uterus; spectrum
Broadbent's: sign
broad spectrum: antibiotic
Broca's: aphasia; area; center
bromphenol: test
Brompton: cocktail
bronchial: adenoma; arteriography; asthma; glands; hygiene; pneumonia; veins
bronchic: cells
bronchiolar: carcinoma
bronchiolo-alveolar: carcinoma
bronchoalveolar: lavage
bronchocentric: granulomatosis
bronchoesophageal: muscle
bronchogenic: carcinoma; cyst
bronchopleural: fistula
bronchopulmonary: dysplasia; lymph nodes; segment; sequestration
Brønsted: acid; base; theory
bronze: diabetes
bronzed: disease
brow: presentation
brown: induration of the lung
brownian: movement
Brudzinski's: sign
Brunn's: membrane
brush: biopsy; border; catheter
Bryant's: triangle
bubble gum: dermatitis
bubble-through: humidifier
bubonic: plague
buccal: artery; glands; nerve
buccinator: muscle
buck: tooth

bucket-handle: tear
Buck's: extension
Bucky: diaphragm
Buerger's: disease
buffalo: neck
buffer: value
buffy: coat
bulbar: myelitis; palsy; paralysis
bulbocavernosus: muscle
bulbourethral: gland
bulbous: bougie
bull: neck
bulldog: forceps
bullet: forceps
bullous: emphysema; impetigo of newborn; keratopathy; pemphigoid
bullous congenital ichthyosiform: erythroderma
bundle-branch: block
Bunsen's solubility: coefficient
bunyavirus: encephalitis
buried: flap; suture
Burkitt's: lymphoma
bursal: synovitis
Busse-Buschke: disease
butterfly: pattern
button: suture
buttress: plate

C

C: fibers
cable: graft
Cabot's ring: bodies
Cagot: ear
Cain: complex
caisson: disease
cake: kidney
calcaneal: petechiae; spur
calcareous: degeneration; infiltration
calcarine: sulcus
calcifying and keratinizing odontogenic: cyst
calcifying odontogenic: cyst
calcium: pump
calcium channel: blocker
calcium channel-blocking: agent

Caldwell-Luc: operation
Caldwell-Moloy: classification
calf: bone
California: virus
Call-Exner: bodies
caloric: nystagmus; test
Calori's: bursa
Calot's: triangle
camp: fever
cAMP receptor: protein
camptomelic: dwarfism
cancellous: bone; tissue
cancer: family
cancer antigen 125: test
canine: tooth
canker: sores
cannonball: pulse
Cannon's: point
cantering: rhythm
canthomeatal: plane
cantilever: bridge
capeline: bandage
capillary: arteriole; attraction; bed; drainage; filling; fracture; fragility; hemangioma; lake; loops; vein
capitate: bone
capsular: antigen; cataract; ligament; space
capsule: forceps
capsulolenticular: cataract
car: sickness
carbamino: compound
carbohydrate: loading
carbon dioxide: cycle
carbon dioxide combining: power
carbon monoxide: hemoglobin; poisoning
carcinoembryonic: antigen
carcinoid: syndrome; tumor
cardiac: arrest; arrhythmia; asthma; catheter; cirrhosis; cycle; decompression; dysrhythmia; edema; ganglia; gating; gland; histiocyte; index; insufficiency; jelly; murmur; muscle; neurosis; notch; orifice; part of;

stomach; plexus; reserve; souffle; sphincter; tamponade
cardiac valvular: incompetence
cardinal: ligament; points; symptom; veins
cardioesophageal: junction
cardiogenic: shock
cardiophrenic: angle
cardioplegic: arrest
cardiopulmonary: bypass; murmur; resuscitation
cardiothoracic: ratio
cardiovascular: system
Carey Coombs: murmur
Carhart: notch
carinate: abdomen
Carlen's: tube
caroticotympanic: nerve
carotid: body; bruit; canal; ganglion; sheath; sinus; triangle
carotid-cavernous: fistula
carotid sinus: reflex; syncope; syndrome
carp: mouth
carpal: bones; joints; tunnel
carpal tunnel: syndrome
carpometacarpal: joints
carpopedal: contraction; spasm
carrier: screening
carrying: angle
cartilage: bone; capsule; lacuna; matrix; space
cartilaginous: joint
cascade: stomach
case fatality: rate
caseous: degeneration; necrosis; osteitis
Castle's intrinsic: factor
castration: cells; complex
catabolite (gene) activator: protein
catarrhal: gastritis; inflammation
catastrophic: reaction
catatonic: rigidity; schizophrenia
categorical: trait
caterpillar: flap
catheter: embolus
cation-exchange: resin

cat-scratch: disease; fever
caudal: anesthesia; flexure
caudal transverse: fissure
caudate: lobe; nucleus; process
cauliflower: ear
cavernous: angioma; body; hemangioma; nerves of clitoris; nerves of penis; rale; sinus; veins of penis
cavernous sinus: branch of internal carotid artery
cavopulmonary: anastomosis
cavosurface: angle
C-banding: stain
cecocentral: scotoma
celiac: artery; disease; ganglia; lymph nodes; trunk
celiac (nervous): plexus
celiac plexus: reflex
cell: body; bridges; culture; cycle; fusion; inclusions; line; membrane; wall
cell adhesion: molecule
cell-mediated: immunity; reaction
cellular: biology; immunodeficiency with abnormal immunoglobulin synthesis; infiltration; pathology
CELO: virus
Celsius: scale
cement: line
cementodentinal: junction
cementoenamel: junction
center of: gravity
centimeter-gram-second: system; unit
central: amputation; apnea; artery of retina; canal; deafness; ganglioneuroma; gyri; necrosis; osteitis; paralysis; scotoma; spindle; sulcus; vein of retina; veins of liver; vein of suprarenal gland; vision
central auditory nervous: system
central cord: syndrome
central nervous: system

WORDFINDER

central ossifying: fibroma
central palmar: space
central retinal: fovea
central venous: catheter; pressure
centric: fusion; occlusion
centrifugal: nerve
centrilobular: emphysema
centripetal: nerve
centroacinar: cell
centromedian nucleus
cephalic: flexure; pole; presentation; tetanus; vein; version
cephalocaudal: axis
ceratocricoid: muscle
cerebellar: cortex; fissures; gait; hemisphere; peduncle; tonsil
cerebral: aqueduct; cortex; death; decompression; dominance; dysplasia; edema; gigantism; hemisphere; hemorrhage; hernia; localization; palsy; peduncle; vesicle
cerebral amyloid: angiopathy
cerebrospinal: axis; fluid; meningitis; pressure
cerebrospinal fluid: rhinorrhea
cerebrovascular: accident
certified: milk
certified pasteurized: milk
ceruminous: glands
cervical: canal; flexure; glands; line; loop; nerves; plexus; pregnancy; rib
cervical intraepithelial: neoplasia
cervical rib: syndrome
cervicothoracic: ganglion
cesarean: hysterectomy; section
Cestan-Chenais: syndrome
Chaddock: reflex; sign
Chagas-Cruz: disease
chain: reaction; reflex
challenge: diet
Chandler: syndrome

character: disorder; neurosis
characteristic: radiation
characterizing: group
Charcot-Leyden: crystals
Charcot-Marie-Tooth: disease
Charcot's: disease; joint; syndrome; triad
Charles: law
cheese worker's: lung
chemical: antidote; attraction; dermatitis; diabetes; energy; peritonitis; potential; repair
chemiluminescence: immunoassay
cherry: angioma
cherry-red: spot
cherry-red spot myoclonus: syndrome
chest: leads; tube; wall
Cheyne-Stokes: respiration
chicken: breast
chicken fat: clot
chickenpox: virus
chief: agglutinin; cell; complaint
child: abuse
childbed: fever
childhood: apraxia
childhood absence: epilepsy
Chinese restaurant: syndrome
chip: graft; syringe
chi-square: test
chloride: shift
chlorine: acne
chocolate: cyst
choked: disk
cholangiolitic: cirrhosis; hepatitis
choledochal: cyst
choleraic: diarrhea
cholestatic: jaundice
cholesterinized: antigen
cholesterol: embolism
cholinergic: blockade; fibers; receptors; urticaria
cholinesterase: inhibitor
chondral: fracture
chondrification: center
chondrodystrophic: dwarfism
chondroectodermal: dysplasia
chondroid: tissue

chondromyxoid: fibroma
Chopart's: amputation; joint
choreic: abasia; movement
choriocapillary: layer
chorionic: epithelioma; gonadotropin; villi
chorionic gonadotropic: hormone
chorionic growth: hormone-prolactin
chorionic villus: biopsy
choroid: glomus; plexus; tela of fourth ventricle; tela of third ventricle
Christmas: disease; factor
chromaffin: body; cell; tissue; tumor
chromatic: aberration; vision
chromatin: body
chromophil: adenoma
chromophobe: adenoma; cells
chromosomal: deletion; region; syndrome; trait
chromosomal instability: syndromes
chromosome: aberration; band; satellite; walking
chronic: alcoholism; bronchitis; inflammation; malaria; shock; trypanosomiasis; ulcer
chronic adrenocortical: insufficiency
chronic atrophic: thyroiditis
chronic desquamative: gingivitis
chronic erythremic: myelosis
chronic fibrosing: pancreatitis
chronic granulomatous: disease
chronic interstitial: salpingitis
chronic mountain: sickness
chronic obstructive pulmonary: disease
chronic progressive external: ophthalmoplegia
chronic relapsing: pancreatitis

chronologic: age
Chvostek's: sign
chyle: vessel
chylous: ascites
cicatricial: alopecia; pemphigoid
cigarette: drain
ciliary: body; disk; ganglion; glands; movement; muscle; process; ring; veins; zone; zonule
ciliated: epithelium
ciliospinal: center; reflex
cineplastic: amputation
cingulate: gyrus; sulcus
circle absorption: anesthesia
circuit: training
circuit resistance: training
circuit weight: training
circular: amputation; dichroism; folds; sinus
circulatory: system
circumanal: glands
circumferential: fibrocartilage; lamella
circumflex scapular: artery
circumscribed: myxedema
circumventricular: organs
cirsoid: aneurysm
cisternal: puncture
citric acid: cycle
citrovorum: factor
clamp: forceps
clang: association
Clapton's: line
Clark's: level
clasp-knife: rigidity; spasticity
class I: antigens
class II: antigens
class III: antigens
classic: migraine
claw: foot; hand
clear: cell; layer of epidermis
clearing: factors
cleavage: cavity; division; lines; product; site; spindle
cleft: hand; lip; palate; spine; tongue
clenched fist: sign
client-centered: therapy

clinical: anatomy; diagnosis; fitness; genetics; lethal; medicine; nurse specialist; pathology; psychology; thermometer
clinoid: process
clip: forceps
cloacal: membrane
clonal selection: theory
clonic: convulsion; spasm; state
cloning: vector
Cloquet's: hernia
closed: anesthesia; comedo; dislocation; drainage; fracture; hospital; reduction of fractures; surgery
closed chain: compound
closed chest: massage
closed circuit: method; spirometry
closed-circuit helium: dilution
closed head: injury
close pack: position
closing: snap; volume
closure: principle
clotting: factor
cloudy: swelling
club: foot; hair; hand
clubbed: digits; fingers
cluster: headache
CO_2: analyzer
coagulation: necrosis; time
coaptation: splint; suture
coated: tongue
Cobb: syndrome
cobbler's: suture
coccygeal: body; ganglion; nerve; plexus; sinus
coccygeus: muscle
cochlear: canal; canaliculus; duct; implant; joint; nerve
cochleopalpebral: reflex
coding: sequence
Codman's: triangle
codominant: inheritance; trait
Coe: virus
Cogan-Reese: syndrome
cognitive: dissonance; therapy
cognitive laterality: quotient
cogwheel: respiration; rigidity
cold: abscess; agglutination;

agglutinin; nodule; sore; stage; therapy; ulcer; urticaria
cold cure: resin
coliform: bacilli
collagen: diseases; fiber
collagenous: colitis
collar: bone
collar-button: abscess
collateral: artery; circulation; hyperemia; inheritance; sulcus; vessel
collective: unconscious
Colles': fracture
colloid: acne; bath; carcinoma; degeneration; goiter
colloidal: gel; solution
colony-forming: unit
colony-stimulating: factors
color: agnosia; blindness; chart; hearing; scotoma; taste
Colorado tick: fever
Colorado tick fever: virus
colored: vision
colostomy: bag
column: chromatography
columnar: epithelium
coma: aberration; scale
combined: glaucoma; immunodeficiency; pregnancy; version
Comby's: sign
comfort: zone
comitant: strabismus
comma: bacillus
commando: procedure
comminuted: fracture
commissural: fibers
common: antigen; migraine; pathway of coagulation
common basal: vein
common bile: duct
common facial: vein
common flexor: sheath
common hepatic: duct
communicable: disease
communicating: artery; branch; hydrocephalus
communication: disorder
communicative: disorder

community: psychiatry; psychology

Comolli's: sign

compact: bone; substance

comparative: anatomy; pathology

compartment: syndrome

compensated: acidosis; alkalosis

compensation: neurosis

compensatory: circulation; hypertrophy; movement; pause; polycythemia

competitive: inhibition

competitive binding: assay

complement: fixation; unit

complemental: air

complementary: air; DNA; hypertrophy

complement binding: assay

complement chemotactic: factor

complement-fixation: test

complement-fixing: antibody

complete: antibody; antigen; blood count; carcinogen; denture; fistula; hernia; transduction

complete A-V: block

complex: odontoma

complex learning: processes

complex partial: seizure

complex precipitated: epilepsy

composite: flap; graft

compound: aneurysm; dislocation; fracture; gland; heterozygote; joint; microscope; odontoma

compound hyperopic: astigmatism

compound myopic: astigmatism

compressible: volume

compression: cyanosis; fracture; neuropathy; paralysis; syndrome; therapy

compulsive: idea; neurosis; personality

computed: tomography

computer-based patient: record

computerized axial: tomography

concave: lens

concavoconcave: lens

concavoconvex: lens

concealed: hemorrhage

concentric: contraction; hypertrophy; lamella

concept: formation

concomitant: symptom

concordance: rate

concordant: alternans; alternation

concrete: thinking

concurrent: disinfection

conditioned: reflex; response; stimulus

conduct: disorder

conducting: system of heart

conduction: analgesia; anesthesia; aphasia

conductive: deafness; hearing loss; heat

condylar: canal; fossa; joint; process

condyloid: canal; process

cone: cell; granule

confocal: microscope

congenital: afibrinogenemia; amputation; anemia; glaucoma; hypothyroidism; megacolon; nevus; nystagmus; paramyotonia; stridor; syphilis; toxoplasmosis; valve

congenital diaphragmatic: hernia

congenital ectodermal: defect; dysplasia

congenital erythropoietic: porphyria

congenital Heinz body hemolytic: anemia

congenital hemolytic: anemia

congenital hypoplastic: anemia

congenital ichthyosiform: erythroderma

congenital pyloric: stenosis

congenital virilizing adrenal: hyperplasia

congestive: splenomegaly

congestive heart: failure

congophilic: angiopathy

conical: cornea; papillae

conjoined: anastomosis; twins

conjugate: deviation of the eyes; foramen; nystagmus; point

conjugate acid-base: pair

conjugated: antigen; hapten; protein

conjugated double: bonds

conjugative: plasmid

conjunctival: reflex; ring; sac; varix; veins

connecting: cartilage

connective: tissue; tumor

Conn's: syndrome

consecutive: amputation

consistency: principle

constitutional: reaction; symptom

constriction: ring

constrictive: bronchiolitis; pericarditis

consulting: staff

consumption: coagulopathy

contact: allergy; cheilitis; dermatitis; inhibition; lens; splint

contact-type: dermatitis

contagious: disease

content: analysis

contig: map

continuous: capillary; murmur; suture

continuous ambulatory peritoneal: dialysis

continuous bar: retainer

continuous positive airway: pressure

continuous positive pressure: breathing; ventilation

contraceptive: device; sponge

contracted: kidney; pelvis

contractual: psychiatry

contralateral: hemiplegia

contrast: bath; medium; stain

contrecoup: injury; injury of brain

control: experiment; group; syringe
controlled: respiration; substance; ventilation
controlled mechanical: ventilation
convective: heat
conventional: signs; thoracoplasty
convergence: excess; insufficiency
convergent: evolution; strabismus
conversion: disorder; hysteria; reaction
conversion hysteria: neurosis
conversive: heat
convex: lens
convexoconcave: lens
convexoconvex: lens
convoluted: part of kidney lobule; tubule
Cooley's: anemia
Coombs': serum; test
coracoacromial: ligament
coracobrachialis: muscle
coracoclavicular: ligament
coracoid: process
cord: blood
cordate: pelvis
cordiform: uterus
core: temperature
Cori: cycle
Cori's: disease
corneal: astigmatism; corpuscles; graft; layer; pannus; reflex; space; staphyloma
corneocyte: envelope
corniculate: cartilage
cornual: pregnancy
coronal: plane; suture
coronary: angiography; artery; bypass; cataract; failure; groove; insufficiency; occlusion; sinus; thrombosis
coronary care: unit
coronoid: process
corpuscular: radiation

corpus luteum: hormone
Corrigan's: sign
corrugator supercilii: muscle
cortical: arteries; audiometry; blindness; bone; cataract; deafness; hormones; lobules of kidney; substance
corticosteroid-binding: globulin
corticotropin-like intermediate-lobe: peptide
corticotropin releasing: factor; hormone
Corti's: arch; canal; membrane; organ; tunnel
Corvisart's: facies
cosmetic: surgery
costal: angle; arch; cartilage
costoaxillary: vein
costocervical: artery; trunk
costoclavicular: ligament
costophrenic: angle
costotransverse: ligament
Cotte's: operation
cotton-fiber: embolism
cotton-wool: patches
cotyloid: cavity; joint
cough: reflex
countercurrent: mechanism
counting: chamber
coup: injury of brain
coupled: pulse; rhythm
coupling: factors
Courvoisier's: gallbladder
Couvelaire: uterus
covert: sensitization
cover-uncover: test
Cowper's: gland
Coxsackie: encephalitis; virus
crack: cocaine
cracked: heel
cradle: cap
Crampton: test
cranial: arteritis; bones; cavity; flexure; nerves; root of accessory nerve; sutures; vertebra
craniofacial dysjunction: fracture
craniometric: points
cravat: bandage

C-reactive: protein
creatine kinase: isoenzymes
creatinine: clearance
cremaster: muscle
cremasteric: artery; reflex
crepitant: rale
crescendo: angina; murmur
crescent cell: anemia
CREST: syndrome
Creutzfeldt-Jakob: disease
crib: death
cribriform: plate of ethmoid bone
cricoid: cartilage
cricothyroid: muscle
cri-du-chat: syndrome
Crigler-Najjar: disease; syndrome
criminal: abortion; psychology
critical: organ; temperature
critical care: unit
critical micelle: concentration
crocodile tears: syndrome
Crohn's: disease
Crooke's hyaline: change
cross: flap; infection; reaction; section; tolerance
crossed: diplopia; embolism; eyes; reflex
crossed extension: reflex
crossed renal: ectopia
cross-over: study
cross-reacting: agglutinin; antibody
cross-sectional: study
cross-table lateral: projection
croup-associated: virus
croupous: membrane
crown-heel: length
crown-rump: length
cruciate: anastomosis; ligaments; ligaments of knee; muscle
crural: hernia; sheath
crural interosseous: nerve
crush: syndrome

Cruveilhier-Baumgarten: murmur; sign
Cruveilhier's: disease
Cruz: trypanosomiasis
crypt: abscesses
cryptogenic: septicemia
cubic: centimeter
cubital: joint; nerve
cuboid: bone
cuboidal: epithelium
Cullen's: sign
cultural: shock
culture: medium
cumulative: action; effect
cumulative trauma: disorders
cuneate: fasciculus; funiculus; nucleus
cuneiform: bone; cartilage
cup biopsy: forceps
cup:disc: ratio
cupping: glass
cupular: cecum of the cochlear duct
cupuliform: cataract
curative: dose
Curling's: ulcer
currant jelly: clot
curvature: aberration; hyperopia; myopia
Cushing's: basophilism; disease; syndrome; medicamentosa
cusp: height
cutaneous: ancylostomiasis; horn; larva migrans; leishmaniasis; muscle; nerve; tuberculosis; vasculitis
cutis: plate
cyanotic: induration
cyclic: compound
cyclist's: palsy
cyclothymic: disorder; personality
cylindrical: lens
cylindromatous: carcinoma
cynic: spasm
cystic: acne; artery; disease of the breast; duct; fibrosis; fibrosis of the pan-

creas; goiter; lymph node; veins
cystine: calculus
cystoduodenal: ligament
cystoid: maculopathy
cystoscopic: urography
cytogenic: reproduction
cytologic: smear
cytomegalic inclusion: disease
cytomegalovirus: disease
cytopathogenic: virus
cytophilic: antibody
cytoplasmic: bridges; inheritance
cytoplasmic inclusion: bodies
cytoreductive: therapy
cytotoxic: reaction
cytotropic: antibody
Czerny-Lembert: suture
Czerny's: suture

D

Dalrymple's: sign
Dalton's: law
Dandy: operation
Dandy-Walker: syndrome
Dane: particles
dark: adaptation
dark-adapted: eye
dark-field: microscope
Darling's: disease
Darwinian: evolution
darwinian: reflex; tubercle
date: boil
datum: plane
daughter: cell; cyst; star
Daviel's: operation
dawn: phenomenon
day: blindness
dead: pulp; space
dead-end: host
deamidizing: enzymes
deaminating: enzymes
death: instinct; rate
debranching: enzymes
debulking: operation
decay: constant; theory
decerebrate: rigidity
decidual: cell
deciduous: dentition; membrane; tooth
declamping: phenomenon; shock

decompression: sickness
decorticate: rigidity
decubitus: film; projection; ulcer
deep: artery of clitoris; artery of penis; fascia; fascia of thigh; reflex; vein of penis; veins of clitoris
deep cerebral: veins
deep cervical: vein
deep dorsal: vein of clitoris; vein of penis
deep facial: vein
deep femoral: vein
deep inguinal: ring
deep lingual: artery; vein
deep temporal: nerves
deep transverse perineal: muscle
defective: bacteriophage; virus
defense: mechanism
defensive: medicine
deferent: duct
deficiency: disease; symptom
definitive: host
degenerative joint: disease
degloving: injury
Dejerine-Sottas: disease
delayed: allergy; dentition; flap; graft; reaction
Delbet's: sign
delphian: node
delta: agent; antigen; bilirubin; cell; granule; hepatitis; rhythm; wave
deltoid: ligament; muscle
demand: pacemaker
demand oxygen delivery: device
dematiaceous: fungi
demigauntlet: bandage
demyelinating: disease
dendriform: keratitis
dendritic: cells; process; spines
dendritic corneal: ulcer
dengue: fever; virus
dengue hemorrhagic: fever
Denis Browne: splint
Dennie's: line

dental: abscess; anatomy; ankylosis; arch; assistant; bulb; calculus; crypt; follicle; forceps; formula; geriatrics; granuloma; hygienist; implants; ledge; papilla; plaque; pulp; ridge; sac; surgeon; syringe

dentate: gyrus; nucleus of cerebellum; suture

dentigerous: cyst

dentin: bridge; dysplasia

dentinal: canals; sheath; tubules

dentinal lamina: cyst

dentinoenamel: junction

denture: base; border; foundation; stability

Denver Developmental Screening: Test

deoxy: sugar

dependent: drainage; edema; personality

depolarizing: block

depressed skull: fracture

depressor: fibers

depressor anguli oris: muscle

depressor labii inferioris: muscle

depressor septi: muscle

depressor supercilii: muscle

depth: perception

de Quervain's: disease; tenosynovitis

dermal: graft; papillae; sinus

dermoid: cyst; tumor

Desault's: bandage

Descemet's: membrane

descending: colon; degeneration

descending genicular: artery

desmoid: tumor

desmoplastic: fibroma; trichoepithelioma

detached: retina

detector: coil

developmental: age; anatomy; anomaly; apraxia of speech; disability; dyspraxia of speech; grooves; lines; milestones; psychology

Devic's: disease

devil's: grip

diabetic: acidosis; amyotrophy; coma; dermopathy; diet; glomerulosclerosis; neuropathy; retinopathy

diachronic: study

diagnosis related: group

diagnostic: specificity; ultrasound

diagonal: conjugate

dialysis: dementia

dialysis encephalopathy: syndrome

Diana: complex

diaper: dermatitis; rash

diaphragmatic: flutter; hernia; ligament of the mesonephros; pleurisy

diarthrodial: joint

diastolic: murmur; pressure; thrill

diatomaceous: earth

dicarboxylic acid: cycle

Dick: test

Dickens: shunt

dicrotic: notch; pulse

dietary: amenorrhea; fiber

Dietl's: crisis

differential: diagnosis

differential ureteral catheterization: test

diffuse: abscess; injuries

diffuse cutaneous: leishmaniasis; mastocytosis

diffuse idiopathic skeletal: hyperostosis

diffuse obstructive: emphysema

diffuse waxy: spleen

diffusible: stimulant

diffusing: capacity

diffusion: anoxia; coefficient; hypoxia; respiration

digastric: fossa; muscle; triangle

digestive: system; tract

digital: crease; radiography; reflex

digital subtraction: angiography

dihydric: alcohol

dilated: pore

dilator: muscle

dilator pupillae: muscle

dilute Russell's viper venom: test

dinitrophenylhydrazine: test

dinner: pad

dioptric: aberration

diphtheria toxoid, tetanus toxoid, and pertussis: vaccine

diphtheritic: membrane

diploic: vein

dipolar: ions

direct: calorimetry; current; flap; fracture; laryngoscopy; ophthalmoscope; transfusion; vision

direct nuclear: division

direct reacting: bilirubin

disciform: degeneration; keratitis

disclosing: agent; solution

discoid: lupus erythematosus

discontinuation: test

discordant: alternans; alternation

discriminant: stimulus

disease: determinants

disk: syndrome

dislocation: fracture

disorganized: schizophrenia

dispersion: medium

displaced: fracture

dissecting: aneurysm; cellulitis

dissection: tubercle

disseminated: lupus erythematosus; tuberculosis

disseminated intravascular: coagulation

dissociated: anesthesia; nystagmus

dissociation: movement; sensibility

dissociative: anesthesia; reaction

distal: end; ileitis; occlusion

distant: flap

distortion: aberration
disulfide: bond
divergence: insufficiency
divergent: strabismus
diving: goiter; reflex
dizygotic: twins
djenkol: poisoning
DMFS caries: index
dmfs caries: index
DNA: helix; polymorphism; virus
DNA-RNA: hybrid
dolichoectatic: artery
dolichopellic: pelvis
doll's eye: sign
dominance of: traits
dominant: character; eye; gene; hemisphere; idea; inheritance; trait
Donath-Landsteiner: antibody; phenomenon
Donders': law
Doppler: echocardiography; effect; shift; ultrasonography
Doppler color: flow
dorsal: artery of clitoris; artery of penis; flexure; nerve of clitoris; nerve of penis; nucleus of vagus nerve; root
dorsal digital: artery; nerves of foot; nerves of hand
dorsalis pedis: artery
dorsal nasal: artery
dorsal radiocarpal: ligament
dorsal scapular: artery; nerve; vein
Dorset's culture egg: medium
dorsolateral: fasciculus
dose equivalent: limits
double: bond; helix; pneumonia; product; refraction; stain; vision
double blind: experiment
double-channel: catheter
double compartment: hydrocephalus
double contrast: enema
double flap: amputation

double-masked: experiment
doubly: heterozygous
doubly armed: suture
douche: bath
Douglas: bag
dowager's: hump
Down: syndrome
Downey: cell
drainage: tube
drawer: sign; test
dreamy: state
drepanocytic: anemia
dressing: forceps
Dressler: beat
Drinker: respirator
drop: attack; foot; hand
droplet: infection
drug: abuse; eruption; psychosis; rash; resistance; tetanus
drum: membrane
dry: abscess; cough; gangrene; joint; pleurisy; rale; synovitis; vomiting
Dubois': abscesses; disease
Dubowitz: score
Duchenne: dystrophy
Duchenne-Aran: disease
Duchenne-Erb: paralysis
Ducrey's: bacillus
ductless: glands
Dugas': test
Duhring's: disease
dumping: syndrome
duodenal: ampulla; cap; glands
duodenojejunal: flexure
duplex: kidney; ultrasonography; uterus
Dupuy-Dutemps: operation
Dupuytren's: amputation; contracture
dural: sheath
dural venous: sinuses
duration: tetany
Durham: rule
dust: cell
duty: cycle
dynamic: equilibrium; ileus; movement; psychiatry; psychology; refraction; splint

dysharmonious: correspondence
dyskinesia: syndrome
dysplastic: nevus
dysplastic nevus: syndrome
dysthymic: disorder
dystonic: reaction
dystrophic: calcification

E

ear: bones
ear lobe: crease
eating: epilepsy
eating-right: pyramid
Eaton: agent
EB: virus
Ebola: virus
Ebstein's: anomaly; disease; sign
eccentric: contraction; hypertrophy; occlusion
ecchymotic: mask
eccrine: gland; poroma
echinococcus: cyst
ECHO: virus
Eck: fistula
eclipse: period
ecotropic: virus
ectatic: emphysema
ectopic: beat; pregnancy; schistosomiasis; tachycardia; testis
Eder-Pustow: bougie
Edison: effect
effective: conjugate; dose; temperature
effective osmotic: pressure
effective renal blood: flow
effective renal plasma: flow
efferent: ductules of testis; nerve; vessel
efferent glomerular: arteriole
effervescent: salts
egg: albumin; membrane
eggshell: calcification
ego: ideal; identity
ego-dystonic: homosexuality
Egyptian: ophthalmia
Ehrlich's inner: body
eighth cranial: nerve

Einthoven's: law; triangle
Eisenmenger's: complex
ejaculatory: duct
ejection: murmur; period
elastic: bandage; cartilage; fibers; lamella; laminae of arteries; layers of arteries; membrane; tissue
elastoid: degeneration
elastotic: degeneration
elbow: bone; joint
elbowed: bougie
elder: abuse
elective: abortion; mutism
Electra: complex
electrical: alternans; alternation of heart; axis; diastole; failure; systole
electroconvulsive: therapy
electrode catheter: ablation
electrodermal: audiometry
electroencephalographic: dysrhythmia
electrohydraulic shock wave: lithotripsy
electromagnetic: radiation; spectrum
electromechanical: dissociation
electromotive: force
electron: microscope; radiography
electronic cell: counter
electron spin: resonance
electrophrenic: respiration
electroshock: therapy
electrostatic: bond
elementary: granule; particle
elephantoid: fever
elevator: muscle of scapula; muscle of soft palate; muscle of upper eyelid
elimination: diet
Elliot's: operation
ellipsoidal: joint
elliptical: amputation
elongation: factor
Embden-Meyerhof: pathway
emboliform: nucleus

embryo: transfer
embryonal: area; carcinoma; leukemia; rhabdomyosarcomas; tumor
embryonic: membrane; shield
embryopathic: cataract
emergency: theory
EMG: biofeedback
emissary: vein
emotional: deprivation; disorder
empiric: risk
empirical: formula
enamel: cap; crypt; germ; layer; membrane; organ
enarthrodial: joint
encephalomyocarditis: virus
encounter: group
encysted: calculus
end: artery; bud; bulb; organ; stage
end-diastolic: volume
endemic: disease; hematuria; neuritis; stability; typhus
endobronchial: tube
endochondral: bone; ossification
endocrine: glands; system
endogenic: toxicosis
endogenous: depression; hyperglyceridemia; infection; pyrogens
endolymphatic: duct; sac
endometrial stromal: sarcoma
endometrioid: carcinoma; tumor
endomyocardial: fibrosis
endoplasmic: reticulum
endorectal pull-through: procedure
endoscopic: biopsy
endoscopic retrograde: cholangiopancreatography
endothelial: dystrophy of cornea; leukocyte; myeloma
endothoracic: fascia
endotracheal: anesthesia; intubation; tube
end-systolic: volume
energy balance: equation
ensiform: process

enteric: fever; tuberculosis; viruses
enteric coated: tablet
entericoid: fever
enteric orphan: viruses
enteroendocrine: cells
enterogastric: reflex
enterogenous: cyanosis; cysts
enterohemorrhagic: *Escherichia coli*
enterohepatic: circulation
enteroinvasive: *Escherichia coli*
enteropathogenic: *Escherichia coli*
enterotoxigenic: *Escherichia coli*
entrapment: neuropathy
environmental: psychology
enzootic: stability
enzygotic: twins
enzyme: immunoassay
enzyme-linked immunosorbent: assay
enzyme-multiplied: immunoassay technique
eosin-methylene blue: agar
eosinophil: adenoma
eosinophil chemotactic: factor of anaphylaxis
eosinophilia-myalgia: syndrome
eosinophilic: granuloma; leukemia; leukocyte; leukocytosis; leukopenia; pneumonia
eosinophilic pustular: folliculitis
ependymal: cell
epicanthal: fold
epicranial: aponeurosis
epicranius: muscle
epicritic: sensibility
epidemic: disease; hemoglobinuria; keratoconjunctivitis; myalgia; myositis; neuromyasthenia; parotiditis; pleurodynia; polyarthritis; roseola; typhus
epidemic gastroenteritis: virus

WORDFINDER

epidemic hemorrhagic: fever
epidemic keratoconjunctivitis: virus
epidemic parotitis: virus
epidemic pleurodynia: virus
epidemiological: genetics
epidermal: cyst; ridges
epidermoid: carcinoma; cyst
epidural: anesthesia; block; cavity; hematoma
epigastric: fossa; hernia; region
epiglottic: cartilage
epileptogenic: zone
epiotic: center
epiphyseal: fracture
epiphysial: arrest; cartilage; line; plate
epiploic: foramen
episcleral: artery; space; veins
epithelial: dystrophy; lamina; pearl; plug
epithelioid: cell
epitympanic: recess
Epstein-Barr: virus
equatorial: plane; plate; staphyloma
equilibrium: dialysis
equine infectious: anemia
Erb: palsy; paralysis
Erb-Westphal: sign
erectile: tissue
erector: muscles of hairs; muscle of spine
erector spinae: muscles
ergogenic: aid
erogenous: zone
E-rosette: test
eruptive: xanthoma
erythema: dose
erythremic: myelosis
erythrocyte: indices
erythrocyte sedimentation: rate
erythrocytic: series
erythrogenic: toxin
erythropoietic: porphyria; protoporphyria

escape: beat; rhythm
esophageal: achalasia; hiatus; lead; reflux; speech; varices; veins
esophagogastric: junction
essential: amino acids; dysmenorrhea; hypertension; oils; pruritus; telangiectasia; thrombocytopenia; tremor
Esser: graft
Estlander: operation
estrous: cycle
ethereal: oil
ethmoid: bone
ethmoid air: cells
ethmoidal: crest; foramen; infundibulum; labyrinth; veins
eunuchoid: gigantism
euplastic: lymph
eustachian: tube
eutectic: alloy
evoked: response
evolutionary: fitness
Ewart's: sign
Ewing's: tumor
exchange: transfusion
excision: biopsy
excitable: area
excitation: wave
excitatory postsynaptic: potential
excited: state
exciting: eye
excitor: nerve
excitoreflex: nerve
excretory: duct; ducts of lacrimal gland; gland
exercise: physiology; prescription
exercise-induced: anemia; asthma; bronchospasm
exercise radionuclide: angiocardiography
exercise stress: test
exfoliative: cytology; dermatitis; gastritis
exocrine: gland
exoerythrocytic: stage
exogenous: depression; fibers; hyperglyceridemia; pyrogens

exophthalmic: goiter; ophthalmoplegia
experimental: error; group; medicine; psychology
experimenter: effects
expiratory: stridor
expiratory reserve: volume
expired: gas
exposure: dose; keratitis
expressed skull: fracture
expression: vector
expressive: aphasia
expulsive: pains
extended radical: mastectomy
extensor: muscle of fingers; muscle of little finger; retinaculum
extensor carpi radialis brevis: muscle
extensor carpi radialis longus: muscle
extensor carpi ulnaris: muscle
extensor digiti minimi: muscle
extensor digitorum: muscle
extensor digitorum brevis: muscle
extensor digitorum longus: muscle
extensor hallucis brevis: muscle
extensor hallucis longus: muscle
extensor indicis: muscle
external: base of skull; capsule; conjugate; ear; fistula; fixation; genitalia; nose; ophthalmopathy; ophthalmoplegia; os of uterus; phase; respiration; traction
external carotid: nerves
external cephalic: version
external nasal: veins
external oblique: muscle
external obturator: muscle
external occipital: crest
external pudendal: arteries; veins
external urethral: orifice

extinction: coefficient

extracapsular: ankylosis; ligaments

extracellular: enzyme; fluid; toxin

extrachromosomal: element; inheritance

extracorporeal: circulation

extracorporeal-membrane: oxygenation

extracorporeal shock wave: lithotripsy

extracting: forceps

extraction: coefficient; ratio

extradural: hemorrhage

extramammary Paget: disease

extraocular: muscles

extraperitoneal: fascia

extrapyramidal: disease; dyskinesias

extrapyramidal motor: system

extrasaccular: hernia

extrasensory: perception

extrathoracic airway: obstruction

extravascular: fluid

extrinsic: factor; sphincter

extrinsic allergic: alveolitis

extrinsic coagulation: pathway

extrinsic incubation: period

exudation: cyst

exudative: inflammation; retinitis

eye: cup; speculum; tooth

eye-closure pupil: reaction

eyelash: sign

F

F: factor; plasmid

F-: actin

Fab: fragment

face: presentation

facial: artery; axis; bones; canal; hemiplegia; nerve; palsy; paralysis; spasm; tic; vein

facilitated: communication

factorial: experiments

facultative: anaerobe; hyperopia; parasite

Faden: suture

fagot: cell

Fahrenheit: scale

falciform: ligament; ligament of liver; process

falciparum: malaria

fallopian: tube

Fallot's: triad

false: anemia; aneurysm; ankylosis; blepharoptosis; cast; conjugate; diverticulum; hematuria; hermaphroditism; image; joint; membrane; neuroma; pelvis; pregnancy; ribs; suture; waters

false-negative: reaction

false-positive: reaction

false vocal: cord

familial: aggregation; dysautonomia; goiter; hypercholesterolemia; hypercholesterolemia with hyperlipemia; hyperchylomicronemia; hypertriglyceridemia; jaundice; screening

familial amyloid: neuropathy

familial fat-induced: hyperlipemia

familial hypertrophic: cardiomyopathy

familial nonhemolytic: jaundice

familial paroxysmal: polyserositis

familial periodic: paralysis

familial pseudoinflammatory macular: degeneration

family: medicine; practice; therapy

far: point

Farabeuf's: triangle

far-and-near: suture

farmer's: lung

fascia: graft

fascial: sheath of eyeball

fascicular: degeneration; graft

fast: smear

fastigial: nucleus

fat: cell; embolism; necrosis; pad; tide

fatality: rate

fat-free body: mass

fat-soluble: vitamins

fat-storing: cell

fatty: acid; cirrhosis; degeneration; heart; hernia; infiltration; kidney; liver; metamorphosis; oil

fatty acid oxidation: cycle

faucial: tonsil

faulty: union

Fc: fragment

febrile: convulsion

fecal: abscess; fistula; vomiting

Fechner-Weber: law

feedback: inhibition; mechanism

feeding: tube

feline infectious: anemia

female: catheter; pseudohermaphroditism

female pattern: alopecia

femininity: complex

femoral: artery; canal; hernia; nerve; sheath; triangle; vein

fenestrated: capillary; membrane

fern: test

Ferrein's: pyramid

fertile: period

festinating: gait

fetal: death; dystocia; hydrops; medicine; membrane; placenta; souffle; wastage

fetal alcohol: syndrome

fever: blister

fiberoptic endoscopic: examination of swallowing

fibrillary: astrocyte; contractions

fibrin: calculus

fibrin/fibrinogen degradation: products

fibrinoid: degeneration

fibrinolytic: purpura

fibrinous: bronchitis; inflammation; pericarditis; pleurisy; polyp

fibroid: adenoma; cataract
fibrolamellar liver cell: carcinoma
fibrositic: headache
fibrous: ankylosis; capsule; capsule of kidney; capsule of liver; degeneration; dysplasia of bone; goiter; joint; tissue; tubercle; union
fibrous articular: capsule
fibrous cortical: defect
fibular: artery; veins
Ficoll-Hypaque: technique
field: block
fifth: disease
figure-ground: perception
figure-of-8: bandage
Filatov: flap
Filatov-Dukes': disease
Filatov-Gillies: flap
filial: generation
filiform: bougie; papillae
filling: defect
filtering: operation
filtration: angle; coefficient; fraction
fine needle: biopsy
finger: agnosia
finger-nose: test
finger-thumb: reflex
finger-to-finger: test
first: molar
first degree: prolapse
first heart: sound
Fishberg concentration: test
fission: product
fissured: fracture; tongue
five-year survival: rate
fixation: nystagmus
fixator: muscle
fixed: idea; macrophage; pupil; virus
fixed drug: eruption
fixed partial: denture
fixed-rate: pacemaker
flaccid: dysarthria
flagellar: antigen
flail: chest; joint
flank: position

flap: amputation; operation
flapless: amputation
flapping: tremor
flash: blindness; method
flat: bone; chest; condyloma; electroencephalogram; flap; pelvis; plate; wart
Fleischner: lines
Fletcher: factor
Flexner's: bacillus
flexor: reflex; retinaculum of lower limb
flexor carpi radialis: muscle
flexor carpi ulnaris: muscle
flexor digiti minimi brevis: muscle of foot; muscle of hand
flexor digitorum brevis: muscle
flexor digitorum longus: muscle
flexor digitorum profundus: muscle
flexor digitorum superficialis: muscle
flexor hallucis brevis: muscle
flexor hallucis longus: muscle
flexor pollicis brevis: muscle
flexor pollicis longus: muscle
flight of: ideas
flight or fight: response
Flint's: murmur
flip: angle
floating: cartilage; kidney; patella; ribs; spleen
floor: plate
flotation: constant; method
flow: cytometry
fluorescence: microscopy
fluorescence in situ: hybridization
fluorescent: screen; stain
fluorescent antibody: technique
fluorescent treponemal antibody-absorption: test
fluxionary: hyperemia
foam: cells
foamy: viruses
focal: amyloidosis; depth; distance; epilepsy; glomeru-

lonephritis; infection; injury; necrosis; point; reaction
focal-film: distance
focal segmental: glomerulosclerosis
Fogarty: catheter
folded-lung: syndrome
Foley: catheter
foliate: papillae
folic acid: antagonists
Folin's: test
folk: medicine
follicle-stimulating: hormone; hormone-releasing hormone
follicle-stimulating hormone-releasing: factor
follicular: cell; cyst; cystitis; goiter; lymphoma; stigma
following: bougie
food: ball; poisoning
foot: process
footling: presentation
foot-pound-second: system; unit
forced: beat; feeding
forced expiratory: flow; time; volume
forced vital: capacity
forceps: delivery
Fordyce's: spots
foreign: body
foreign body: granuloma
Forel's: decussation
forensic: dentistry; medicine; psychiatry; psychology
forequarter: amputation
form: constancy
formalin: pigment
fornicate: gyrus
Fort Bragg: fever
fortification: spectrum
forward heart: failure
Foster: frame
Fothergill's: disease; neuralgia; operation
founder: principle
fountain: decussation; syringe
Fourier: analysis

WORDFINDER

fourth: disease; ventricle
fourth heart: sound
Fowler's: position
fragile: site
fragile X: chromosome; syndrome
fragility: test
frank breech: presentation
Frank-Starling: curve
fraternal: twins
Frazier-Spiller: operation
Fredet-Ramstedt: operation
Fredrickson's: classification
free: association; energy; flap; gingiva; graft; macrophage; radical
free induction: decay
free nerve: endings
freeway: space
Freiberg's: disease
Frejka pillow: splint
French: scale
French-American-British: classification system
freudian: psychoanalysis
friction: rub; sound
Friedman: curve
Friedreich's: ataxia; sign
frontal: area; artery; bone; cortex; crest; lobe of cerebrum; nerve; plane; pole of cerebrum; sinus; suture
frontal lobe: epilepsy
frontoanterior: position
frontoposterior: position
frontotransverse: position
Frost: suture
frosted: liver
frozen: pelvis; section
fruit: sugar
fuller's: earth
full-thickness: graft
functional: activity; anatomy; blindness; congestion; deafness; disease; disorder; dysmenorrhea; murmur; neurosurgery; occlusion; splint; test
functional residual: air; capacity
fundamental: frequency

fungiform: papillae
fungus: ball
funicular: graft; process
funnel: breast; chest
funnel-shaped: pelvis
fused: kidney
fusiform: aneurysm; gyrus
fusion: beat
fusospirochetal: gingivitis
Futcher's: line

G

γ-: fetoproteins
G: cells
G_{M2}: gangliosidosis
G_{M1}: gangliosidosis
G-: actin
gag: reflex
galactophorous: ducts
galactose: cataract
gallop: rhythm
galvanic skin: response
Gambian: trypanosomiasis
gamekeeper's: thumb
gamma: angle; camera; fibers
gangliated: nerve
ganglion: cell; cyst
ganglionic: blockade; branches of maxillary nerve; branch of internal carotid artery
ganglionic blocking: agent
gangrenous: stomatitis
Ganser's: syndrome
gap: junction; phenomenon
Gardner-Diamond: syndrome
gas: abscess; bacillus; chromatography; gangrene; peritonitis
gas-liquid: chromatography
gastric: analysis; arteries; bypass; digestion; feeding; fistula; glands; indigestion; stapling; tetany; vertigo
gastric inhibitory: peptide; polypeptide
gastrocnemius: muscle
gastrocolic: reflex
gastroduodenal: artery
gastroenteritis: virus type A; virus type B
gastroepiploic: arteries
gastroesophageal: hernia

gastroesophageal reflux: disease
gastroileac: reflex
gastrointestinal: tract
gastro-omental: arteries
gate-control: theory
gated radionuclide: angiocardiography
gating: mechanism
Gaucher: cells
Gaucher's: disease
gauntlet: bandage
gaussian: distribution
Gavard's: muscle
gay bowel: syndrome
G-banding: stain
gelatinous: substance
gel diffusion precipitin: tests
genal: glands
gender: identity; role
gene: expression; therapy
gene dosage: compensation
general: anatomy; anesthesia; anesthetic; immunity; stimulant
general adaptation: reaction; syndrome
general duty: nurse
generalized: anaphylaxis; lentiginosis
generalized anxiety: disorder
generalized Shwartzman: phenomenon
generalized tonic-clonic: epilepsy; seizure
genetic: amplification; association; code; determinant; female; fitness; lethal; load; psychology
genial: tubercle
genicular: arteries
geniculate: body; ganglion; neuralgia
genioglossus: muscle
geniohyoid: muscle
genital: cord; corpuscles; furrow; herpes; organs; phase; ridge; system; tract; wart

genitofemoral: nerve
genitourinary: system
genucubital: position
genupectoral: position
geographic: keratitis; tongue
geometric: isomerism; mean
germ: cell; disk; layer; line;
  membrane
German: measles
German measles: virus
germinal: area; cell; disk;
  epithelium; localization;
  pole
gestalt: phenomenon; psy-
  chology; therapy
gestational: age; diabetes;
  edema; proteinuria
Ghon's: focus; tubercle
Ghon's primary: lesion
ghost: cell; corpuscle
giant: cell; condyloma;
  urticaria
giant axonal: neuropathy
giant cell: arteritis; carcinoma; fibroma; granuloma;
  myeloma; tumor of bone;
  tumor of tendon sheath
Gibson: murmur
Giemsa: stain
Gierke's: disease
Gilles de la Tourette's: syndrome
gingival: abscess; margin;
  massage; sulcus
ginglymoid: joint
girdle: anesthesia; sensation
glandular: epithelium
Glanzmann's: disease;
  thrombasthenia
glaserian: fissure
glass ionomer: cement
glassy: membrane
glaucomatous: cataract; cup;
  excavation; halo
Glenn's: operation
glenohumeral: joint; ligaments
glenoid: fossa; labrum
glia: cells
gliding: joint
global: aphasia

glomerular: capsule; nephritis
glomerular filtration: rate
glomerulosa: cell
glomus: tumor
glomus jugulare: tumor
glossopharyngeal: breathing;
  nerve
glottal: attack
glove: anesthesia
glover's: suture
glucose oxidase: method
glucose-6-phosphate dehydrogenase: deficiency
glucose transport: maximum
glucosidase: inhibitors
β-D-glucuronidase: deficiency
gluteal: fold; furrow
gluten: enteropathy
gluten-free: diet
gluteus maximus: muscle
gluteus medius: muscle
gluteus minimus: muscle
glycogen: granule; loading
glycosylated: hemoglobin
glycotropic: factor
goblet: cell
Goldblatt: hypertension;
  kidney
Goldflam: disease
Goldstein's toe: sign
Golgi: apparatus
Golgi-Mazzoni: corpuscle
Golgi's: stain
Golgi tendon: organ
Golgi type I: neuron
Golgi type II: neuron
gonadal: cords; dysgenesis;
  ridge
gonadotropic: hormone
gonadotropin-releasing: factor; hormone
gonococcal: arthritis; conjunctivitis
gonorrheal: ophthalmia
Goodell's: sign
Goodenough draw-a-man:
  test
Gouley's: catheter
gouty: arthritis; tophus
Gowers': syndrome
graafian: follicle

gracile: fasciculus; nucleus
gracilis: muscle
graded exercise: test
grade I: astrocytoma
grade II: astrocytoma
grade III: astrocytoma
grade IV: astrocytoma
graduated: tenotomy
Graefe's: operation; sign
graft versus host: disease;
  reaction
Graham's: law
Graham Steell's: murmur
gram: calorie; equivalent
gram-: ion
Gram's: stain
grand: mal
granddaughter: cyst
granny: knot
granular: conjunctivitis; cortex; leukocyte; ophthalmia;
  pits
granular cell: tumor
granular endoplasmic:
  reticulum
granulation: tissue
granule: cells
granulocyte colony-stimu-
  lating: factor
granulocyte-macrophage
  colony-stimulating: factor
granulocytic: leukemia; sarcoma; series
granulomatous: colitis;
  encephalomyelitis; enteritis; inflammation
granulosa: cell
granulosa cell: tumor
grasp: reflex
grasping: reflex
gravel: voice
Graves': disease
gravid: uterus
gravitational: insecurity;
  ulcer
gray: cataract; columns;
  degeneration; fibers; hepatization; induration; matter;
  substance; syndrome
gray-scale: ultrasonography
great: foramen

great adductor: muscle
great auricular: nerve
great cardiac: vein
great cerebral: vein of Galen
greater: curvature of stomach; omentum; pelvis; trochanter; wing of sphenoid bone
greater alar: cartilage
greater multangular: bone
greater palatine: canal; foramen; nerve
greater posterior rectus: muscle of head
greater splanchnic: nerve
greater vestibular: gland
Greenfield: filter
greenstick: fracture
grenz: ray
Gritti-Stokes: amputation
gross: anatomy
ground: bundles; lamella; state; substance
ground-glass: pattern
group: agglutination; agglutinin; antigens; practice
group A streptococcal necrotizing: fasciitis
group model: health maintenance organization
growing: pains
growth: hormone; hormone-inhibiting hormone; hormone-releasing hormone; rate
growth hormone-producing: adenoma
growth hormone-releasing: factor
growth-onset: diabetes
gum: line; resection
Gunn's: sign
gunstock: deformity
gurgling: rale
gustatory: cells; hyperhidrosis; rhinorrhea
Guthrie: test
gutta-percha: points
gutter: dystrophy of cornea; fracture; wound
gynecoid: pelvis

H

H: agglutinin; antigen; band
HA1: virus
HA2: virus
haarscheibe: tumor
habit: spasm
habitual: abortion; pitch
HACEK: group
***Haemophilus influenzae* type B:** vaccine
Hageman: factor
hair: ball; cells; follicle; papilla; root; whorls
hairline: fracture
hairy: cells; leukoplakia; mole; tongue
hairy cell: leukemia
Haldane: effect
half-: life; time
half and half: nail
half-value: layer
Haller's: circle
Hallervorden-Spatz: syndrome
halo: effect; nevus; sign
Halsted's: operation; suture
hamate: bone
Hamburger's: law
Hamman's: disease; murmur; syndrome
hammer: toe
hamstring: muscles; tendon
hand-foot-and-mouth: disease
Hand-Schüller-Christian: disease
hangman's: fracture
Hansen's: bacillus; disease
Harada's: syndrome
hard: chancre; corn; palate; pulse; tubercle; ulcer
Hardy-Rand-Ritter: test
Hardy-Weinberg: law
harlequin: fetus
harmonic: mean; suture
harmonious: correspondence
Harrison's: groove
Hartmann's: operation; pouch
Hartnup: disease; syndrome
Hashimoto's: disease; struma; thyroiditis
Hasson: cannula

Haverhill: fever
haversian: canals; lamella; spaces; system
hay: fever
head: cap; fold
head-dropping: test
health: record
health-related physical: fitness
heart: beat; failure; massage; rate; sac
heart-lung: machine
heat: capacity; cramps; exhaustion; lamp; rash; stroke; urticaria
heavy: chain
heavy chain: disease
hebephrenic: schizophrenia
Heberden's: nodes
heel: bone; spur; tendon
Hegglin's: anomaly
height of: contour
Heimlich: maneuver
Heinz-Ehrlich: body
HeLa: cells
helicopod: gait
helium: therapy
Hellin's: law
Helmholtz: energy
helper: cell; virus
hemadsorption: virus type 1; virus type 2
hematogenous: jaundice; metastasis
hematopoietic: gland; system
hematopoietic growth: factor
hematoxylin and eosin: stain
hemiazygos: vein
hemic: murmur
hemiplegic: gait
Hemoccult: test
hemochorial: placenta
hemoendothelial: placenta
hemoglobinuric: nephrosis
hemolysin: unit
β-hemolytic: streptococci
hemolytic: anemia; disease of newborn; jaundice; splenomegaly

WORDFINDER

hemolytic uremic: syndrome
hemorrhagic: ascites; colitis; cyst; cystitis; disease of the newborn; endovasculitis; fever; fever with renal syndrome; infarct; measles; plague; shock
hemorrhoidal: zone
hemostatic: forceps
Henderson-Hasselbalch: equation
Henle's: loop; sheath
Henoch-Schönlein: purpura
Henry's: law
Hensen's: cell; node
heparin: lock
hepatic: adenoma; coma; duct; encephalopathy; flexure; lobule; porphyria; veins
hepatic portal: vein
hepatitis A: virus
hepatitis B: virus
hepatitis B core: antigen
hepatitis B e: antigen
hepatitis B immune: globulin
hepatitis B surface: antigen
hepatitis C: virus
hepatitis D: virus
hepatitis delta: virus
hepatitis E: virus
hepatocellular: carcinoma; jaundice
hepatogenous: jaundice
hepatojugular: reflux
hepatolenticular: degeneration
hepatopancreatic: ampulla
hepatorenal: syndrome
herd: immunity; instinct
hereditary: chorea; clubbing; spherocytosis
hereditary cerebellar: ataxia
hereditary spinal: ataxia
Hering-Breuer: reflex
hernial: sac
herniated: disk
herpes: virus
herpes simplex: encephalitis; virus

herpes zoster: virus
herpetic: keratitis; keratoconjunctivitis; whitlow
herpetiform: aphthae
Herxheimer's: reaction
Hesselbach's: hernia; triangle
heterochromic: uveitis
heterocytotropic: antibody
heterogeneous: radiation; system
heterogenetic: antigen; parasite
heterogenic enterobacterial: antigen
heterologous: graft; stimulus; tumor; twins
heterometric: autoregulation
heterotypic: cortex
heterotypical: chromosome
heteroxenous: parasite
hexokinase: method
hexone: bases
Heyer-Pudenz: valve
Hey's: amputation
hiatal: hernia
high: enema
high endothelial postcapillary: venules
high energy: phosphates
high energy phosphate: bond
highest intercostal: vein
high-fiber: diet
high-frequency: ventilation
high molecular weight: kininogen
Highmore's: body
high-performance liquid: chromatography
high-resolution computed: tomography
high steppage: gait
Hill: operation
Hill's: equation; sign
Hill-Sachs: lesion
Hilton's: law
Hilton's white: line
hilus: cells
hindfoot: valgus; varus
hinge: joint; region
hinged: flap
hip: bone; joint
hippocampal: sulcus

hippocratic: face; facies; fingers; nails
hippocratic succussion: sound
Hirschsprung's: disease
His': line
His bundle: electrogram
Histalog: test
histamine: test
histaminic: headache
histocompatibility: complex; testing
histoid: leprosy
histologic: accommodation
histotoxic: anoxia
HLA: complex; typing
HMG-CoA reductase: inhibitors
hobnail: cells; liver
Hodgkin's: disease
Hodgson's: disease
Hoffa's: operation
Hoffmann's: reflex; sign
Hofmeister's: operation
Hogben: number
holandric: gene
holistic: medicine
Hollenhorst: plaques
hollow: bone
hollow-cathode: lamp
Holmes-Adie: pupil; syndrome
Holmes-Rahe: questionnaire
holocrine: gland
Holter: monitor
Holthouse's: hernia
Holzknecht: unit
Homans': sign
homeometric: autoregulation
homocytotropic: antibody
homogeneous: radiation; system
homologous: chromosomes; graft; stimulus; tumor
homonymous: images
homoplastic: graft
homosexual: panic
honeycomb: lung; pattern
Hong Kong: influenza
Hooke's: law
hookworm: disease

WORDFINDER

horizontal: fissure of cerebellum; heart; overlap; plane; tear; transmission

horizontal maxillary: fracture

Horner's: pupil; syndrome; teeth

Horner-Trantas: dots

horny: layer

horseradish: peroxidases

horseshoe: fistula; kidney

Hortega: cells

hospital: formulary; record

hot: flash; flush; nodule; spot

hot-wire flow-measuring: device

hourglass: contraction; murmur; stomach

house: staff

housemaid's: knee

Howell-Jolly: bodies

Howship's: lacunae

human: calorimeter; genetics; herpesvirus 1; herpesvirus 2; herpesvirus 3; herpesvirus 4; herpesvirus 5; herpesvirus 6; insulin

human antihemophilic: factor

human chorionic: gonadotropin; somatomammotropin

human chorionic somatomammotropic: hormone

human diploid cell: vaccine

human gamma: globulin

human granulocytic: ehrlichiosis

human immunodeficiency: virus

human lymphocyte: antigens

human menopausal: gonadotropin

human monocytic: ehrlichiosis

human papilloma: virus

human placental: lactogen

human plasma protein: fraction

human T-cell lymphoma/ leukemia: virus

humeral: joint

humoral: immunity

hunger: contractions; pain

Hunner's: ulcer

Hunter's: canal

hunting: response

Huntington's: chorea; disease

Hunt's: neuralgia; syndrome

Hurler's: syndrome

Hürthle cell: adenoma; carcinoma; tumor

Hutchinson-Gilford: disease

Hutchinson's: facies; mask; pupil; teeth; triad

Hutchinson's crescentic: notch

H-Y: antigen

hyaline: bodies; cartilage; degeneration; membrane; tubercle

hyaloid: artery; body; fossa

hydatid: cyst; disease; fremitus; thrill

hydatidiform: mole

hydrodynamic: nebulizer

hydrogen: bond; donor; ion; pump; transport

hydropic: degeneration

17-hydroxycorticosteroid: test

hyoglossal: membrane; muscle

hyoglossus: muscle

hyoid: arch; bone

hyperbaric: chamber; oxygen

hyperbaric oxygen: therapy

hyperchromic: anemia

hyperendemic: disease

hypereosinophilic: syndrome

hyperextension-hyperflexion: injury

hyperfunctional: occlusion

hypergonadotropic: eunuchoidism

hyperimmunoglobulin E: syndrome

hyperkalemic periodic: paralysis

hyperkinetic: dysarthria; syndrome

hyperlucent: lung

hypermature: cataract

hypernatremic: encephalopathy

hyperopic: astigmatism

hyperosmolar (hyperglycemic) nonketotic: coma

hyperplastic: gingivitis; polyp; pulpitis

hyperreactive malarious: splenomegaly

hypersensitivity: pneumonitis

hypertensive: arteriopathy; arteriosclerosis; retinopathy

hypertrophic: arthritis; cardiomyopathy; rhinitis

hypertrophic pulmonary: osteoarthropathy

hypertrophic pyloric: stenosis

hyperventilation: tetany

hypnagogic: hallucination

hypnogenic: spot

hypnopompic: hallucination

hypochondriac: region

hypochondriacal: melancholia

hypochromic: anemia

hypodermic: syringe; tablet

hypogastric: nerve

hypoglossal: canal; nerve; nucleus

hypoglycemic: coma

hypokalemic periodic: paralysis

hypokinetic: dysarthria

hypopharyngeal: diverticulum

hypophysial: cachexia; fossa; syndrome

hypoplastic: anemia

hypostatic: congestion; ectasia; pneumonia

hypothalamic: infundibulum

hypothalamohypophysial portal: system

hypothenar: eminence

hypothetical mean: organism

hypovolemic: shock

hypoxic: hypoxia; nephrosis
hysterical: blindness; joint; psychosis

I

I: band; cell
iatrogenic: transmission
ICAO standard: atmosphere
Iceland: disease
ichthyosiform: erythroderma
icterohemorrhagic: fever
ICU: psychosis
identical: twins
identity: crisis; disorder
ideokinetic: apraxia
idiomuscular: contraction
idiopathic: aldosteronism; hypercalcemia of infants; neuralgia
idiopathic hypertrophic subaortic: stenosis
idiopathic pulmonary: fibrosis
idiopathic thrombocytopenic: purpura
idioventricular: rhythm
ileal: arteries; veins
ileocecal: orifice; valve
ileocolic: artery; valve; vein
iliac: bone; colon; crest; muscle
iliacus: muscle
iliococcygeal: muscle
iliococcygeus: muscle
iliocostal: muscle
iliocostalis: muscle
iliocostalis cervicis: muscle
iliocostalis lumborum: muscle
iliofemoral: ligament; triangle
iliohypogastric: nerve
ilioinguinal: nerve
iliolumbar: artery; vein
iliopectineal: line
iliopsoas: muscle
iliotibial: tract
iliotrochanteric: ligament
image: amplifier
immature: cataract
immediate: allergy; auscultation; denture; flap; percussion; reaction; transfusion

immersion: foot; objective
immovable: joint
immune: adherence; adsorption; complex; reaction; response; serum; surveillance; system
immune complex: disease
immune electron: microscopy
immune response: genes
immune thrombocytopenic: purpura
immunochemical: assay
immunofluorescent: stain
immunologic: tolerance
immunological: mechanism; paralysis; surveillance
immunologic pregnancy: test
immunoperoxidase: technique
immunoproliferative: disorders
immunoradiometric: assay
impacted: fetus; fracture; tooth
imperfect: fungus; stage
imperforate: anus
impingement: syndrome
implant: denture
implanted: suture
impressive: aphasia
impulse control: disorder
impulsive: obsession
impure: flutter
inactivated poliovirus: vaccine
inactive: repressor
inadequate: personality; stimulus
inborn: errors of metabolism
incarcerated: hernia
incident: point
incidental: parasite
incisal guide: angle
incised: wound
incision: biopsy
incisional: hernia
incisive: bone; canal; foramen; papilla
incisive canal: cyst
incisor: tooth
inclusion: bodies; cell; conjunctivitis
inclusion body: disease
incompetent cervical: os

incomplete: abortion; antibody; antigen; fistula
incomplete foot: presentation
incubation: period
incubative: stage
independent living: model
independent practice association: health maintenance organization
index: case; finger
index extensor: muscle
indifferent: gonad; tissue
indirect: calorimetry; fracture; laryngoscopy; ophthalmoscope; transfusion; vision
indirect hemagglutination: test
indirect nuclear: division
indirect reacting: bilirubin
individual: psychology
individualized education: program
individuation: field
indolent: bubo
induced: abortion; enzyme; erythrocythemia; hypotension
induction: period
industrial: disease; hygiene
indwelling: catheter
inert: gases
inertia: time
infantile: acropustulosis; autism; eczema; hypothyroidism; osteomalacia; scurvy; sexuality
infantile neuroaxonal: dystrophy
infantile purulent: conjunctivitis
infantile spinal muscular: atrophy
infant mortality: rate
infected: abortion
infection: immunity
infection-exhaustion: psychosis
infectious: disease; endocarditis; mononucleosis

WORDFINDER

infectious bovine: kerato-conjunctivitis
infectious eczematoid: dermatitis
infectious hepatitis: virus
infectious papilloma: virus
infective: embolism
inferior: ganglion of glossopharyngeal nerve; vena cava
inferior alveolar: artery; nerve
inferior basal: vein
inferior cerebellar: peduncle
inferior cerebral: veins
inferior constrictor: muscle of pharynx
inferior dental: arch
inferior epigastric: vein
inferior extensor: retinaculum
inferior gemellus: muscle
inferiority: complex
inferior labial: vein
inferior longitudinal: fasciculus
inferior macular: arteriole
inferior medullary: velum
inferior nasal: concha
inferior oblique: muscle
inferior olivary: nucleus
inferior pelvic: aperture
inferior rectal: nerves
inferior rectus: muscle
inferior temporal: line; sulcus
inferior thalamic: peduncle
inferior thalamostriate: veins
infiltration: anesthesia
infinite: distance
inflammatory: carcinoma; lymph; pseudotumor; rheumatism
inflammatory papillary: hyperplasia
influenza: viruses
influenzal: pneumonia
information: theory
infraclavicular: fossa
infranodal: extrasystole

infraorbital: artery; canal; foramen; nerve
infrared: microscope
infraspinatus: bursa; muscle
infratemporal: crest; fossa
infratrochlear: nerve
infundibular: stalk; stem
infusion-aspiration: drainage
ingrown: hairs; nail
inguinal: canal; hernia; ligament; region; triangle; trigone
inhalation: analgesia; anesthesia; anesthetic
inherited: character
inhibitory: fibers; nerve; obsession
inhibitory postsynaptic: potential
initiating: agent
initiation: codon; factor
inlay: graft
innate: immunity
innocent: murmur
innominate: artery; bone; veins
inorganic: acid; chemistry; compound; orthophosphate
insensible: perspiration
insertion: sequences
insertional: mutagenesis
inspiratory: capacity; stridor
inspiratory reserve: volume
inspired: gas
insufflation: anesthesia
insular: gyri
insulin: resistance; shock
insulin-antagonizing: factor
insulin-dependent: diabetes mellitus
insulin-like: activity
insulin-like growth: factors
intelligence: quotient
intensive care: unit
intention: spasm; tremor
interalveolar: septum
interarch: distance
interatrial: septum
intercalated: disk; ducts
intercapillary: glomerulosclerosis
intercapitular: veins

intercarotid: body
intercarpal: joints; ligaments
intercavernous: sinuses
intercellular: bridges; canaliculus
intercostal: membranes; nerves; space
intercostobrachial: nerves
interdental: canals; papilla; septum; splint
interfacial: canals
interglobular: dentin
interim: denture
interlaminar: jelly
interlobar: duct; veins of kidney
interlobular: arteries; duct; emphysema; pleurisy; veins of kidney; veins of liver
intermaxillary: bone; suture
intermediary: nerve
intermediate: heart; host; nerve; trait
intermediate basilic: vein
intermediate cephalic: vein
intermediate cuneiform: bone
intermediate vastus: muscle
intermediolateral: nucleus
intermediomedial: nucleus
intermenstrual: pain
intermetacarpal: joints
intermetatarsal: joints
intermittent: claudication; compression; cramp; tetanus
intermittent acute: porphyria
intermittent explosive: disorder
intermittent mandatory: ventilation
intermittent positive pressure: breathing; ventilation
intermuscular: septum
internal: base of skull; capsule; ear; energy; fistula; fixation; hemorrhage; medicine; ophthalmopathy; ophthalmoplegia; phase; respiration; traction

internal adhesive: pericarditis
internal auditory: veins
internal carotid: nerve
internal cephalic: version
internal cerebral: veins
internal iliac: artery; vein
internal intercostal: muscle
internal oblique: muscle
internal obturator: muscle
internal occipital: crest
internal pudendal: artery; vein
internal urethral: orifice
internasal: suture
International: System of Units
international: unit
International System of: Units
internodal: segment
internuncial: neuron
interobserver: error
interocclusal: distance
interosseous: cartilage
interparietal: suture
interpeduncular: fossa; nucleus
interpelviabdominal: amputation
interphalangeal: joints of hand
interpleural: space
interpolated: extrasystole
interproximal: space
interradicular: space
interrupted: suture
interspinal: muscles; plane
interspinales: muscles
interstitial: cells; cystitis; disease; emphysema; fluid; gastritis; growth; hernia; keratitis; lamella; nephritis; neuritis; pregnancy; tissue
interstitial cell-stimulating: hormone
interstitial plasma cell: pneumonia
intertarsal: joints
intertransversarii: muscles
intertransverse: muscles

intertrochanteric: crest; line
intertubercular: sheath
interureteric: fold
intervenous: tubercle
interventricular: foramen; septum
intervertebral: disc; vein
intervillous: lacuna; spaces
intestinal: anastomosis; angina; arteries; atresia; digestion; emphysema; fistula; follicles; glands; villi
intra-aortic: balloon
intra-aortic balloon: pump
intra-atrial: conduction
intracapsular: ligaments
intracardiac: catheter
intracellular: canaliculus; fluid; toxin
intracranial: cavity; hemorrhage; pressure
intracutaneous: reaction
intradermal: injection; nevus
intrafusal: fibers
intraligamentary: pregnancy
intralobular: duct
intramural: hematoma; pregnancy
intranasal: anesthesia
intraobserver: error
intraocular: pressure
intraoral: anesthesia
intraparietal: sulcus
intraparotid: plexus of facial nerve
intrapartum: hemorrhage
intrathoracic airway: obstruction
intrauterine: amputation; devices; fracture
intrauterine contraceptive: devices
intravascular: ligature
intravenous: anesthesia; anesthetic; bolus; cholangiography; drip; urography
intravenous regional: anesthesia
intraventricular: block; conduction
intravital: stain

intrinsic: dysmenorrhea; factor; PEEP; reflex; sphincter
intrinsic coagulation: pathway
intuitive: stage
inulin: clearance
invert: sugar
involuntary: muscles
involutional: depression; melancholia
iodide: acne
iodinated ^{131}I human serum: albumin
iodinated ^{125}I serum: albumin
iodine: stain
ion exchange: chromatography
ion-exchange: resin
ionic: strength
ionization: chamber
ionizing: radiation
iridocorneal: angle
iridocorneal endothelial: syndrome
IRI/G: ratio
iris: pits
iris-nevus: syndrome
iron: lung
iron deficiency: anemia
iron-storage: disease
irreducible: hernia
irregular: astigmatism; bone; dentin
irreversible: pulpitis
irritable: colon
irritant contact: dermatitis
irritation: fibroma
Irvine-Gass: syndrome
ischemic: contracture of the left ventricle; hypoxia; necrosis
ischial: bone; bursa; spine
ischiatic: hernia
ischiocavernous: muscle
Ishihara: test
island: flap
islet: cell
isoelectric: line; period; point
isogeneic: graft
isolated: proteinuria

isolated explosive: disorder
isologous: graft
isometric: contraction; exercise; period of cardiac cycle
isoperistaltic: anastomosis
isophane: insulin
isoplastic: graft
isosbestic: point
isotonic: contraction
^{131}**I uptake:** test

J

J: chain; point
jacksonian: epilepsy; seizure
Jackson's: membrane
Janeway: lesion
Japanese B: encephalitis
Japanese B encephalitis: virus
jargon: aphasia
Jarisch-Herxheimer: reaction
Jarvik artificial: heart
jaw: bone; reflex
jaw-winking: syndrome
jejunal: arteries
jejunal and ileal: veins
jejunoileal: bypass; shunt
Jensen's: disease
jerky: nystagmus
jersey: finger
jet: nebulizer
Jewett and Strong: staging
Jocasta: complex
jock: itch
Jod-Basedow: phenomenon
Joffroy's: sign
joint: capsule; effusion; extension
Joint Commission on Accreditation of Healthcare: Organizations
Jones': fracture
Joubert's: syndrome
Joule's: equivalent
jugal: bone; point
jugular: foramen; fossa; gland; glomus; nerve; pulse
jugulodigastric: lymph node
jugulo-omohyoid: lymph node
jump: flap

jumping: disease
junction: nevus
junctional: epithelium; rhythm
jungian: psychoanalysis
junk: DNA
juvenile: arthritis; cataract; cell; pelvis; periodontitis
juvenile myoclonic: epilepsy
juvenile-onset: diabetes
juvenile spinal muscular: atrophy
juxta-esophageal pulmonary: lymph nodes
juxtaglomerular: cells; granules

K

K: cells
Kanner's: syndrome
kaolin clotting: time
Kaposi's: sarcoma
kappa: angle
Karnofsky: scale
Kartagener's: syndrome; triad
Kasai: operation
Kawasaki's: syndrome
Kayser-Fleischer: ring
Kearns-Sayre: syndrome
Kehr's: sign
Kelly's: operation
Kelvin: scale
Kemp: echo
keratic: precipitates
keratin: pearl
keratinous: cyst
keratogenous: membrane
keratohyalin: granules
keratoid: exanthema
Kerley B: lines
Kernig's: sign
ketogenic: diet
ketone: body
key-in-lock: maneuver
Kiel: classification
Kienböck's: unit
Kiernan's: space
Kiesselbach's: area
killer: cells
kilogram: calorie
kilovolt: peak
Kimmelstiel-Wilson: disease; syndrome

kinematic: chain; viscosity
kinesthetic: sense
kinetic: energy
Kleihauer-Betke: technique
Klinefelter's: syndrome
Klumpke: palsy
knee: complex; joint; presentation; reflex
knee-chest: position
knee-elbow: position
knee-jerk: reflex
knuckle: pads
Koch's: bacillus
Koch's old: tuberculin
Koch's original: tuberculin
Koch-Weeks: bacillus
Kock: pouch
Kohlrausch's: muscle
Kondoleon: operation
Korean hemorrhagic: fever
Korean hemorrhagic fever: virus
Korotkoff: sounds; sounds
Korotkoff's: test
Korsakoff's: psychosis; syndrome
Kraske's: operation
Krause's end: bulbs
Krebs: cycle
Krebs-Henseleit: cycle
Krukenberg's: amputation; spindle; tumor
Kupffer: cells
Kussmaul: respiration
Kussmaul's: coma; disease; sign
Kveim: antigen; test
kyphotic: pelvis

L

L: doses
L$_r$: dose
labial: hernia; splint
labor: pains
laboratory: diagnosis
labyrinthine: artery; nystagmus; veins; vertigo
Lachman: test
lacrimal: apparatus; artery; bone; canaliculus; caruncle; fold; fossa; gland;

lake; nerve; papilla; punctum; sac; vein

β-lactamase: inhibitors

lactate: threshold

lactation: amenorrhea

lacteal: vessel

lactiferous: ducts; sinus

lactogenic: hormone

lacunar: amnesia; ligament

ladder: splint

Laënnec's: cirrhosis

Lafora: body

Laki-Lorand: factor

Lamaze: method

lambdoid: suture

Lambrinudi: operation

lamellar: bone; cataract

lamellated: corpuscles

lamina: propria

laminar: flow

laminated: clot; epithelium

Lancefield: classification

Landau-Kleffner: syndrome

Landry: syndrome

Landry's: paralysis

Langenbeck's: triangle

lanugo: hair

laparoscopic: cholecystotomy; knot

laparotomy: pad

large: calorie; intestine

large cell: carcinoma; lymphoma

Laron type: dwarfism

Larrey's: amputation

Larson-Johansson: disease

laryngeal: papillomatosis; prominence; stenosis; syncope

Lassa: fever; virus

late: rickets; systole

latency: period; phase

latent: allergy; carrier; content; diabetes; gout; hyperopia; image; learning; nystagmus; period; reflex; schizophrenia; stage

lateral: aberration; cartilage of nose; column; cord of brachial plexus; folds; funiculus; hermaphro-

ditism; meniscus; pinch; plate; ventricle

lateral cerebral: sulcus

lateral cuneiform: bone

lateral geniculate: body

lateral humeral: epicondylitis

lateral longitudinal: stria

lateral occipital: artery

lateral rectus: muscle; muscle of the head

lateral recumbent: position

lateral sacral: crests; veins

lateral thalamic: peduncle

lateral vastus: muscle

lateral venous: lacunae

latissimus dorsi: muscle

LCAT: deficiency

LE: cell

lead: encephalitis; encephalopathy; poisoning

Lear: complex

learned: drive

learning: disability

leather-bottle: stomach

LE cell: test

lecithin/sphingomyelin: ratio

Lefort I: fracture

left: heart; lobe of liver; ventricle

left colic: flexure

left gastric: artery; vein

left heart: bypass

left hepatic: duct

left-to-right: shunt

left umbilical: vein

left ventricular: failure

left-ventricular assist: device

left ventricular ejection: time

legal: blindness; medicine

Legg-Calvé-Perthes: disease

Legg-Perthes: disease

Legg's: disease

Legionnaire's: disease

Leiner's: disease

Leishman-Donovan: body

Lembert: suture

Lennox: syndrome

Lennox-Gastaut: syndrome

lens: capsule; pits; stars; vesicle

lenticular: astigmatism; loop; nucleus; process of incus

lentiform: nucleus

leonine: facies

LEOPARD: syndrome

lepromatous: leprosy

lepromin: test

leptospiral: jaundice

Leriche's: syndrome

Leri's: sign

lesser: curvature of stomach; omentum; pelvis; trochanter; wing of sphenoid bone

lesser alar: cartilages

lesser palatine: foramina; nerves

Lesser's: triangle

lesser splanchnic: nerve

lesser vestibular: glands

lethal: dose; factor; gene; mutation

lethal midline: granuloma

leukemic: retinopathy

leukemoid: reaction

leukocyte adhesion: deficiency

leukocyte esterase: test

leukocytoclastic: vasculitis

leukopenic: index; leukemia

levator: muscle of thyroid gland

levator anguli oris: muscle

levator ani: muscle

levator labii superioris: muscle

levator labii superioris alaeque nasi: muscle

levator palpebrae superioris: muscle

levator prostatae: muscle

levator scapulae: muscle

levator veli palatini: muscle

Levin: tube

Lev's: syndrome

Lewis: acid; base

Lhermitte's: sign

Libman-Sacks: endocarditis; syndrome

licensed practical: nurse

lichenoid: dermatosis; keratosis

lienal: artery

lienteric: diarrhea
life: instinct; stress; table
life-span: development
light: adaptation; chain; reflex; treatment
light-adapted: eye
light chain-related: amyloidosis
Likert: scale
limb: bud; lead
limb-girdle muscular: dystrophy
limbic: system
limit: testing
line: spectrum
linear: accelerator; atrophy; fracture
lingual: artery; follicles; frenulum; goiter; gyrus; nerve; papilla; tonsil; vein
linkage: disequilibrium; marker
linking: number
lip: reflex
lipedematous: alopecia
lipid: granulomatosis; pneumonia
lipoid: granuloma; nephrosis; theory of narcosis
lipomatous: infiltration
lipotropic: hormone
lipotropic pituitary: hormone
liquefactive: necrosis
liquid-liquid: chromatography
Lisch: nodule
Lisfranc's: amputation
Lister's: method
Listing's: law
lithotomy: position
little: ACTH
Little League: elbow; shoulder
Littré's: hernia
Litzmann: obliquity
live: vaccine
liveborn: infant
livedoid: dermatitis
liver: acinus; spot
lobar: pneumonia

lobular: glomerulonephritis
local: anaphylaxis; anesthesia; asphyxia; death; flap; immunity; reaction; stimulant
localized: mucinosis; scleroderma
localized nodular: tenosynovitis
localizing: symptom
locked: knee
locked-in: syndrome
long: bone; gyrus of insula; muscle of head; muscle of neck
long-acting thyroid: stimulator
long adductor: muscle
long extensor: muscle of toes
long flexor: muscle of great toe; muscle of thumb; muscle of toes
longissimus capitis: muscle
longissimus cervicis: muscle
longissimus thoracis: muscle
longitudinal: aberration; dissociation; fracture; lie; ligament; relaxation; section; tear
longitudinal pontine: fasciculi
long levatores costarum: muscles
long radial extensor: muscle of wrist
long-term: memory
long thoracic: nerve
longus capitis: muscle
longus colli: muscle
loop: diuretic; excision
loop electrocautery excision: procedure
loose: associations
Lou Gehrig's: disease
lower: airway; extremity; limb
lower esophageal: sphincter
lower motor: neuron
lower nodal: rhythm
lowest splanchnic: nerve
low purine: diet
low salt: diet
Lr: dose
Ludwig's: angina; ganglion
Luer: syringe
luetic: mask

lumbar: artery; flexure; hernia; nerves; plexus; puncture; rheumatism; rib; triangle; veins
lumbar iliocostal: muscle
lumbar splanchnic: nerves
lumbocostal: ligament
lumbocostoabdominal: triangle
lumbrical: muscles of foot; muscles of hand
luminous: intensity
lunate: bone
lupoid: hepatitis; sycosis
lupus: anticoagulant; nephritis
lupus band: test
lupus erythematosus: cell
lupus erythematosus cell: test
luteal: cell; phase
luteinizing: hormone; hormone-releasing hormone
luteinizing hormone/follicle-stimulating hormone-releasing: factor
luteinizing hormone-releasing: factor
Lutembacher's: syndrome
luteoplacental: shift
luteotropic: hormone
Lutz-Splendore-Almeida: disease
Lyme: arthritis; disease
lymph: capillary; corpuscle; follicle; gland; node; nodule; vessels
lymphatic: duct; leukemia; node; plexus; sinus; system; tissue
lymph node permeability: factor
lymphoblastic: leukemia; lymphoma
lymphocytic: adenohypophysitis; choriomeningitis; hypophysitis; leukemia; series
lymphocytic choriomeningitis: virus
lymphogenous: metastasis

Lyon: hypothesis
lysogenic: bacterium
lysosomal: disease

M

M: band; line
MacConkey: agar
Macewen's: sign; triangle
Mach: effect
machinery: murmur
macrobiotic: diet
macrocytic: anemia
macrophage colony-stimu-
lating: factor
macroscopic: anatomy
macular: amyloidosis; arteries; dystrophy; leprosy
Madelung's: deformity
Mad Hatter: syndrome
Madura: boil
magnetic resonance:
imaging
magnification: radiography
mainstream: aerosol
major: agglutinin
major histocompatibility:
complex
major salivary: glands
major sublingual: duct
malabsorption: syndrome
malar: bone
malariae: malaria
malarial: crescent
male pattern: alopecia
Malgaigne's: luxation
malignant: anemia; bubo;
dyskeratosis; granuloma;
hepatoma; histiocytosis;
hypertension; hyperther-
mia; jaundice; lymphoma;
melanoma; melanoma in
situ; nephrosclerosis;
tumor
malignant ciliary: epithelioma
malignant fibrous: histiocytoma
malignant tertian: malaria
mallet: finger
Mallory: bodies
Mallory-Weiss: lesion; syndrome; tear

malpighian: bodies; capsule;
pyramid; stigmas; stratum
mamillary: body; ducts; line
mamillothalamic: fasciculus
mammary: ducts; fold; gland;
line; ridge
mammary duct: ectasia
managed: care
Manchester: operation
mandibular: arch; cartilage;
fossa; joint; lymph node;
nerve; process
mandibuloacral: dysplasia
manic: episode
manic-depressive: psychosis
manifest: content; hyperopia
manifesting: heterozygote
Manson's: disease
mantle: radiotherapy
Mantoux: test
manual: ventilation
Marburg: disease; virus
Marburg virus: disease
Marcacci's: muscle
march: fracture; hemoglobinuria
Marchiafava-Bignami: disease
Marcus Gunn: phenomenon;
syndrome
Marcus Gunn's: sign
Marfan's: syndrome
marginal tentorial: branch of
internal carotid artery
marker: trait
masculine: pelvis; uterus
masked: virus
masklike: face
masochistic: personality
mass: hysteria; peristalsis
masseter: muscle
masseteric: artery; nerve
mast: cell; leukocyte
mast cell: leukemia
Master: test
master: gland
master patient: index
Master's two-step exercise:
test
masticatory: force; system
mastoid: antrum; bone;
canaliculus; foramen; process

mastoid air: cells
matched: groups
maternal: dystocia; placenta
matrix: band; calculus
mattress: suture
maturation: arrest; index
mature: bacteriophage;
cataract
maturity-onset: diabetes
Mauriac's: syndrome
Mauriceau's: maneuver
Mauthner's: sheath
maxillary: artery; gland;
nerve; process; sinus; vein
maximal: dose
maximum: velocity
maximum breathing:
capacity
maximum expiratory:
pressure
maximum inspiratory:
pressure
maximum permissible: dose
maximum voluntary: ventilation
Mayer's: reflex
Mayo-Robson's: position
Mayo's: operation
May-White: syndrome
McArdle's: disease
McArdle-Schmid-Pearson:
disease
McBurney's: point; sign
McCune-Albright: syn-
drome
McMurray: test
McRoberts: maneuver
McVay's: operation
M:E: ratio
meadow: dermatitis
mean: calorie
mean corpuscular: hemoglobin; volume
mean corpuscular hemoglo-
bin: concentration
measles: virus
mechanical: antidote; dys-
menorrhea; ileus; jaundice;
vector; ventilation
Meckel: scan
Meckel's: diverticulum

WORDFINDER

meconium: aspiration; ileus; peritonitis
medial: cord of brachial plexus; epicondylitis; ligament; meniscus
medial collateral: ligament
medial cuneiform: bone
medial forebrain: bundle
medial geniculate: body
medial longitudinal: fasciculus; stria
medial occipital: artery
medial rectus: muscle
medial vastus: muscle
median: artery; groove of tongue; nerve; plane; rhinoscopy; section
median antebrachial: vein
median cubital: vein
median rhomboid: glossitis
median sacral: crest; vein
mediastinal: emphysema; fibrosis; space; veins
mediate: auscultation; percussion
medical: assistant; diathermy; genetics; psychology; record
mediotarsal: amputation
Mediterranean exanthematous: fever
medullary: arteries of brain; carcinoma; cavity; cone; membrane; plate; pyramid; ray; space; striae of fourth ventricle; stria of thalamus; substance
medullary sponge: kidney
Medusa: head
megacystic: syndrome
megakaryocytic: leukemia
megaloblastic: anemia
meibomian: cyst; glands
Meissner's: corpuscle
melanocyte-stimulating: hormone
melanotic: carcinoma
melanotic neuroectodermal: tumor of infancy
melanotropin release-inhibiting: hormone

melanotropin-releasing: factor; hormone
Meleney's: ulcer
melting: point
membrane: bone; potential
membrane-coating: granule
membrane expansion: theory
membranoproliferative: glomerulonephritis
membranous: cataract; dysmenorrhea; glomerulonephritis; labyrinth; laryngitis; ossification
Mendel-Bechterew: reflex
mendelian: inheritance
Mendelsohn: maneuver
Ménétrier's: disease
Ménière's: disease
meningeal: veins
meningitic: streak
meningococcal: meningitis
meniscus: lens
menstrual: cycle; period
mental: age; artery; disease; disorder; foramen; health; hygiene; illness; image; nerve; point; retardation; scotoma; spine; symphysis
mentalis: muscle
mentoanterior: position
mentoposterior: position
mentotransverse: position
Mercier's: bar
mercury: poisoning
meridional: aberration
merocrine: gland
mesangial: nephritis
mesangial proliferative: glomerulonephritis
mesencephalic: flexure; tegmentum
mesial: angle; occlusion
mesocaval: shunt
mesoglial: cells
mesomelic: dwarfism
mesometanephric: carcinoma
mesonephric: duct; fold; ridge
messenger: RNA
metabisulfite: test
metabolic: acidosis; alkalosis; coma; craniopathy;

encephalopathy; equivalent; mucinosis
metacarpal: bone
metacarpophalangeal: joints
metacentric: chromosome
metachromatic: bodies; leukodystrophy; stain
metaherpetic: keratitis
metameric nervous: system
metanephric: duct
metaphysial: dysostosis; dysplasia
metaplastic: anemia; carcinoma; ossification; polyp
metastatic: abscess; calcification
metatarsal: artery; bone
metatarsophalangeal: joints
meter: angle
metered-dose: inhaler
metopic: suture
metric: system
Mexican hat: cell
Meynert's: decussation
Michaelis: constant
Michaelis-Menten: hypothesis
microangiopathic hemolytic: anemia
micro-Astrup: method
microcytic: anemia
microglandular: adenosis
micromelic: dwarfism
micromyeloblastic: leukemia
microscopic: anatomy
middle: ear
middle cardiac: vein
middle cerebellar: peduncle
middle colic: artery
middle constrictor: muscle of pharynx
middle genicular: artery
middle meningeal: veins
middle nasal: concha
middle rectal: lymph node
middle temporal: vein
midlife: crisis
midline: myelotomy
midsagittal: plane
migraine: headache

migrating: abscess
Mikulicz': aphthae
Miles': operation
miliary: abscess; embolism; fever; pattern
milieu: therapy
milk: crust; ducts; fever; line; sugar; tooth
milk-alkali: syndrome
Miller-Abbott: tube
MIM: number
Minamata: disease
mineral: water
miner's: lung
minimal: dose
minimal brain: dysfunction
minimal infecting: dose
minimal lethal: dose
minimal reacting: dose
minimum data: set
Minnesota Multiphasic Personality: Inventory
Minnesota multiphasic personality inventory: test
minor: agglutinin; hysteria
minor salivary: glands
minor sublingual: ducts
minute: volume
mirror: speech
mirror-image: cell
missed: abortion; labor
missense: mutation
Mitchell's: disease
mite: typhus
mitochondrial: chromosome
mitotic: figure; rate; spindle
mitral: insufficiency; murmur; orifice; stenosis; valve
mitral valve: prolapse
mixed: aphasia; astigmatism; gland; leukemia; nerve; paralysis; tumor
mixed agglutination: reaction; test
mixed connective-tissue: disease
mixed expired: gas
mixed lymphocyte: culture
mixed lymphocyte culture: test

M'Naghten: rule
Mobitz: block
modal: frequency; pitch
modified radical: mastectomy
Mohs': chemosurgery
moist: gangrene; rale
Mokola: virus
molar: tooth
molar absorption: coefficient
molecular: biology; disease; layer of cerebellum; movement; rotation; weight
molecular weight: ratio
Moloney: test
molybdenum target: tube
Mondini: dysplasia
Mondor's: disease
Monge's: disease
mongolian: spot
moniliform: hair
monoamine oxidase: inhibitor
monoamniotic: twins
monochromatic: aberration
monoclonal: antibody; immunoglobulin
monocular: diplopia
monocytic: leukemia
monocytoid: cell
monohydric: alcohol
mononuclear phagocyte: system
monopolar: cautery
monozygotic: twins
mood-congruent: hallucination
mood-incongruent: hallucination
moon: face
morbid: obesity
morbidity: rate
morcellation: operation
Morgagni's: cataract; disease; syndrome
morning: sickness
Moro's: reflex
morphogenetic: movement
mortality: rate
mortise: joint
Morton's: neuralgia; syndrome; toe

Morvan's: disease
mosaic: inheritance; pattern; wart
Moss: tube
mother: cell; cyst; yaw
motion: sickness
motor: aphasia; area; ataxia; cortex; decussation; endplate; fibers; image; nerve; neuron; paralysis; plate; point; unit; urgency
motor neuron: disease
motor speech: center
mottled: enamel
mountain: sickness
mouse-tooth: forceps
mouth-to-mouth: respiration; resuscitation
movable: joint; spleen
movement: system
mucinous: carcinoma
mucociliary: transport
mucocutaneous: junction; leishmaniasis
mucocutaneous lymph node: syndrome
mucoid: degeneration
mucomembranous: enteritis
mucoserous: cells
mucous: cell; colitis; cyst; gland; glands of auditory tube; plug
mucous connective: tissue
mud: fever
Mueller electronic: tonometer
Mueller-Hinton: medium
multangular: bone
multiaxial: joint
multifactorial: inheritance
multifidus: muscle
multifocal: lens
multiformat: camera
multilamellar: body
multilocular: cyst
multinodular: goiter
multiple: fission; fracture; myeloma; myositis; neuritis; personality; pregnancy; sclerosis; stain; vision
multiple ego: states

multiple endocrine deficiency: syndrome
multiple epiphysial: dysplasia
multiple intestinal: polyposis
multiple mucosal neuroma: syndrome
multiple puncture tuberculin: test
multiplicative: division
multipolar: cell; neuron
multivalent: vaccine
mumps: virus
mumps skin test: antigen
mural: endocarditis; thrombosis; thrombus
murine: typhus
Murphy: drip
Murphy's: sign
Murray Valley: encephalitis
muscle: fiber, hemoglobin; plate; serum; spasm; tone
muscular: asthenopia; atrophy; coat; dystrophy; endurance; power; relaxant; sense; strength; system; tissue; triangle
musculocutaneous: nerve
musculophrenic: artery; veins
musculospiral: paralysis
musculotubal: canal
mushroom: poisoning
Musset's: sign
Mustard: operation
mutant: gene
mutation: rate
mutilating: keratoderma
mutual: resistance
myasthenic: facies; syndrome
mycoplasmal: pneumonia
mycotic: aneurysm
myelin: sheath
myeloblastic: leukemia
myelocytic: leukemia
myelodysplastic: syndrome
myeloid: metaplasia; sarcoma; series; tissue

myelophthisic: anemia
myeloproliferative: syndromes
myenteric: plexus
mylohyoid: muscle; nerve
myo-: inositol
myocardial: infarction; insufficiency
myocardial depressant: factor
myoclonic astatic: epilepsy
myoclonus: epilepsy
myofacial pain-dysfunction: syndrome
myofunctional: therapy
myoid: cells
myoneural: blockade; junction
myopic: astigmatism; crescent
myosin: filament
myotatic: contraction; irritability; reflex
myxoid: cyst
myxomembranous: colitis
myxopapillary: ependymoma

N

nabothian: cyst; follicle
Naegeli: syndrome
Naffziger: operation
Nägele: obliquity
nail: bed; fold; pits
naked: virus
narcotic: blockade; reversal
narrow-angle: glaucoma
nasal: bone; capsule; cavity; crest; emission; escape; meatus; muscle; pits; point; reflex; septum; spine of frontal bone; spines
nasalis: muscle
nasal septal: cartilage
nasociliary: nerve
nasofrontal: vein
nasogastric: tube
nasolabial: lymph node
nasolacrimal: canal; duct
nasopalatine: nerve
nasopharyngeal: leishmaniasis
nasotracheal: tube
Nasse's: law
natural: antibody; dyes; immunity; pitch; selection
natural killer: cells

navicular: abdomen; bone; fossa of urethra
near: point
necrogenic: wart
necrotic: cirrhosis; inflammation; pulp
necrotizing: arteriolitis; enterocolitis
necrotizing ulcerative: gingivitis
needle: bath; biopsy; forceps
negative: accommodation; convergence; electrode; scotoma; stain
negative base: excess
negative end-expiratory: pressure
negative pressure: ventilation
Negri: bodies
Nelson: syndrome
neonatal: anemia; diagnosis; hepatitis; herpes; hyperbilirubinemia; medicine; tetany
neonatal mortality: rate
nephritic: syndrome
nephrogenic: diabetes insipidus
nephronic: loop
nephrostomy: tube
nephrotic: syndrome
nerve: avulsion; block; conduction; decompression; plexus
nerve block: anesthesia
nervous: bladder; indigestion; lobe of hypophysis; system
network model: health maintenance organization
Neufeld: reaction
Neufeld capsular: swelling
neural: arch; crest; folds; groove; plate; spine
neural crest: syndrome
neuralgic: amyotrophy
neurenteric: cysts
neurilemma: cells
neuritic: plaque

neurodevelopmental: treatment
neurogenic: bladder
neurolemma: cells
neuroleptic: agent
neuroleptic malignant: syndrome
neuromuscular: spindle; system
neuroparalytic: keratitis; keratopathy
neuropathic: arthropathy; bladder; joint
neuropsychologic: disorder
neurotendinous: spindle
neurotrophic: keratitis
neutral: mutation; occlusion; stain
neutralization: plate; test
neutralizing: antibody
neutrophilic: leukocyte
nevus: cell
New Hampshire: rule
Newtonian: constant of gravitation
New World: leishmaniasis
New York Heart Association: classification
Niemann-Pick: cell
night: blindness; vision
Nikolsky's: sign
ninhydrin: reaction
nipple: line; shield
Nissl: bodies; granules; substance
nitro: dyes
nitrogen: balance; cycle; equivalent; narcosis
nitroprusside: test
NK: cells
noble: gases
nocturnal: enuresis; myoclonus
nodal: point
nodding: spasm
nodose: rheumatism
nodular: amyloidosis; leprosy; lymphoma
noise: pollution
nominal: aphasia

nonbacterial verrucous: endocarditis
noncommunicating: hydrocephalus
noncompetitive: inhibition
nonconjugative: plasmid
noncovalent: bond
nondepolarizing: block
nonessential: amino acids
nonfenestrated: forceps
non-Hodgkin's: lymphoma
nonimmune: serum
non-insulin-dependent: diabetes mellitus
nonisolated: proteinuria
nonlamellar: bone
nonmedullated: fibers
nonobstructive: jaundice
nonoral: communication
nonosteogenic: fibroma
nonpenetrant: trait
nonpenetrating: wound
nonpitting: edema
nonpropositional: speech
nonprotein: nitrogen
non-rapid eye: movement
nonrebreathing: anesthesia
nonsense: triplet
nonsexual: generation
nonspecific: protein
nonsteroidal anti-inflammatory: drugs
nonthrombocytopenic: purpura
nontoxic: goiter
nontropical: sprue
nonverbal: communication
nonvital: pulp
normal: antibody; antitoxin; concentration; distribution; occlusion; opsonin; range; serum; solution; values
normal human: plasma
normal human serum: albumin
normal pressure: hydrocephalus
normochromic: anemia
normocytic: anemia
normokalemic periodic: paralysis
North American: blastomycosis

Northern blot: analysis
Norwalk: virus
notifiable: disease
nuchal: ligament; plane
nuclear: cataract; envelope; family; jaundice; medicine; membrane; ophthalmoplegia; RNA; spindle; stain
nuclear:cytoplasmic: ratio
nuclear inclusion: bodies
nuclear magnetic: resonance
nuclear medicine: technologist
null: cells; hypothesis
nummular: eczema; sputum
nursemaid's: elbow
nutrient: arteries of humerus; artery; artery of femur; artery of fibula; canal; foramen; vessel
nutritive: equilibrium
Nysten's: law

O

O: agglutinin; antigen
oat: cell
oat cell: carcinoma
object: relationship
objective: sensation; symptom
obligate: aerobe; anaerobe; parasite
oblique: amputation; diameter; fracture; lie; section; vein of left atrium
obliterative: bronchitis
obsessive-compulsive: disorder; neurosis
obstetric: conjugate
obstetrical: binder; forceps; hand; palsy; paralysis
obstructive: apnea; dysmenorrhea; hydrocephalus; jaundice; murmur; thrombus; uropathy
obstructive ventilatory: defect
obturating: embolism
obturator: artery; canal; crest; foramen; hernia; nerve; vein
obturator externus: muscle

obturator internus: muscle
occipital: artery; bone; lobe of cerebrum; pole of cerebrum; sinus; vein
occipital cerebral: veins
occipital lobe: epilepsy
occipitoanterior: position
occipitofrontal: diameter; muscle
occipitofrontalis: muscle
occipitomental: diameter; projection
occipitoposterior: position
occipitotransverse: position
occlusal: analysis; equilibration; film; force; imbalance; position
occlusive: dressing; ileus; meningitis
occult: blood; fracture; PEEP
occult cleft: palate
occupational: behavior; disease; role; science; therapy
ochre: codon
ocular: albinism; humor; hypertelorism; tension; vertigo
oculomotor: nerve; nucleus
oculopharyngeal: dystrophy
odontoblastic: layer
odontogenic: cyst; keratocyst
odontoid: process of epistropheus
oedipal: phase
Oedipus: complex
official: formula
Ogino-Knaus: rule
Ogura: operation
OKT: cells
Old World: leishmaniasis
olfactory: bulb; epithelium; foramen; glands; membrane; nerves; sulcus
olfactory receptor: cells
oligoclonal: band
Ollier: graft
Ollier-Thiersch: graft
omega-oxidation: theory
omental: bursa; graft
omnifocal: lens
omohyoid: muscle

omphalomesenteric: duct
oncocytic hepatocellular: tumor
oncofetal: antigens; marker
oncogenic: virus
oncotic: pressure
one-carbon: fragment
on-off: phenomenon
Onuf's: nucleus
opal: codon
opalescent: dentin
open: biopsy; comedo; dislocation; drainage; flap; fracture; hospital; pneumothorax; reduction of fractures; tuberculosis; wound
open-angle: glaucoma
open chain: compound
open chest: massage
open circuit: method; spirometry
open-circuit nitrogen: washout
open drop: anesthesia
open head: injury
open heart: surgery
opening: snap
operating: microscope
operator: gene
ophthalmic: artery; nerve; solutions; vesicle
opiate: receptors
opioid: antagonists
Oppenheim's: disease; syndrome
opponens digiti minimi: muscle
opponens pollicis: muscle
oppositional: disorder
opsonic: index
optic: axis; canal; capsule; chiasm; cup; decussation; disk; foramen; nerve; neuritis; papilla; radiation; tract
optical: aberration; activity; density; image; isomerism; keratoplasty; rotation
optimal: pitch
optimum: dose
optokinetic: nystagmus
oral: apraxia; biology; cavity;

contraceptive; defensiveness; hygiene; pathology; phase; surgery; vestibule
oral motor: apraxia
oral poliovirus: vaccine
orbicular: zone
orbicularis oculi: muscle
orbicularis oris: muscle
orbital: cavity; gyri; muscle; plane; process
orbitalis: muscle
orbitomeatal: line; plane
organ: culture
organic: acid; chemistry; compound; contracture; delusions; disease; evolution; murmur; vertigo
organic brain: syndrome
organic mental: disorder
organoid: tumor
organ-specific: antigen
orienting: reflex; response
orotracheal: tube
Oroya: fever
orphan: disease; drugs; products; viruses
orthograde: degeneration
orthopaedic: surgery
orthostatic: hypotension
oscillating: vision
oscillatory: potential
Osgood-Schlatter: disease
Osler: node
Osler's: disease; sign
Osler-Vaquez: disease
osmotic: diuretics; fragility; pressure
osseous: lacuna; tissue
osseous hydatid: cyst
osseous spiral: lamina
ossific: center
osteoclast activating: factor
osteogenetic: fibers; layer
osteogenic: sarcoma
osteoid: osteoma
osteomalacic: pelvis
osteopathic: medicine; physician
osteoprogenitor: cell
Ostwald's solubility: coefficient

otic: capsule; ganglion; vesicle
otitic: meningitis
otoacoustic: emissions
Otto's: disease
Ouchterlony: technique
outlet forceps: delivery
oval: amputation; window
ovarian: artery; cycle; cyst; fossa; pregnancy
overanxious: disorder
overlay: denture
overload: principle
overt: homosexuality
overuse: syndrome
ovular: membrane
ox: heart
oxalate: calculus
oxazin: dyes
oxidative: phosphorylation
oxygen: capacity; concentrator; consumption; content; debt; deficit; toxicity
oxygen affinity: hypoxia
oxyhemoglobin dissociation: curve
oxyntic: cell
oxyphil: cells
oxyphilic: leukocyte

P

P: wave
PA: projection
pacchionian: bodies
pacemaker: lead
pacing: catheter
pacinian: corpuscles
pagetoid: cells
Paget's: disease
painful: heel
pain-pleasure: principle
palatal: reflex
palatine: bone; process; raphe; spines; tonsil; uvula; vein
palatoglossal: arch
palatoglossus: muscle
palatopharyngeal: arch; muscle
palatopharyngeus: muscle
palliative: treatment
palmar: arch; pinch

palmar interosseous: muscle
palmar radiocarpal: ligament
palmar ulnocarpal: ligament
palmate: folds
palpatory: percussion
palpebral: arteries; fissure; veins
pampiniform: plexus
pancake: kidney
Pancoast: syndrome
pancreatic: calculus; cystoduodenostomy; digestion; duct; veins
pancreaticoduodenal: veins
panic: attack; disorder
panlobular: emphysema
pannicular: hernia
panoramic: radiograph
panoramic x-ray: film
pansystolic: murmur
pantaloon: hernia
PAP: technique
Pap: smear
Pap: test
Papanicolaou: stain
paper: chromatography
paper mill worker's: disease
papillary: adenocarcinoma; adenoma of large intestine; carcinoma; ducts; hidradenoma; muscle; stasis; tumor
papillary cystic: adenoma
Pappenheimer: bodies
papular: mucinosis; tuberculid; urticaria
papulonecrotic: tuberculid
para-aortic: bodies
parabasal: body
paracentral: fissure
parachute: reflex
parachute mitral: valve
paracoccidioidal: granuloma
paradoxical: contraction; pulse; reflex; respiration; sleep
paradoxical diaphragm: phenomenon
parafollicular: cells
parahippocampal: gyrus
parainfluenza: viruses
parallax: test

paralytic: dementia; ileus
paramesonephric: duct
paranasal: sinuses
paraneoplastic: encephalomyelopathy; syndrome
paranoid: personality; schizophrenia
paraperitoneal: hernia
parasinoidal: sinuses
parasitic: cyst; melanoderma
parasympathetic: ganglia; nerve
parasympathetic nervous: system
parataxic: distortion
parathyroid: gland; hormone; tetany
paratyphoid: fever
paraumbilical: veins
paraurethral: ducts
paraventricular: nucleus
paravertebral: ganglia
parenchymatous: degeneration; goiter; hemorrhage; neuritis
parent: cyst
parental: generation
parenteric: fever
parietal: bone; cell; fistula; foramen; hernia; lobe of; cerebrum lymph nodes; thrombus; wall
parieto-occipital: sulcus
Parinaud's: syndrome
Parinaud's oculoglandular: syndrome
parkinsonian: dysarthria
Parkinson's: disease; facies
parotid: duct; gland; notch; papilla; veins
paroxysmal: tachycardia
paroxysmal cold: hemoglobinuria
paroxysmal nocturnal: dyspnea; hemoglobinuria
parrot: fever
parrot's beak: tear
partial: agglutinin; antigen; denture; pressure; seizure; volume

partial rebreathing: mask
partial-thickness: flap; graft
partial thromboplastin: time
partition: chromatography
parturient: canal
Pascal's: law
Passavant's: cushion
Passavoy: factor
passive: anaphylaxis; atelectasis; clot; congestion; hemagglutination; hyperemia; immunity; movement
passive-aggressive: personality
patch: test
patella-femoral: syndrome
patellar: ligament; reflex
patellofemoral: joint; syndrome
patent: medicine
pathogenic: occlusion
pathognomonic: symptom
pathologic: calcification; fracture; myopia
pathological: anatomy
pathologic retraction: ring
patient controlled: analgesia
Patrick's: test
patterned: alopecia
pattern sensitive: epilepsy
Payne: operation
Payr's: sign
peak: flowmeter
peak expiratory: flow
pectinate: line; muscles; zone
pectineal: ligament; muscle
pectineus: muscle
pectoral: girdle; region; veins
pedicle: flap
pedigree: analysis
peer-review: organization
pegged: tooth
Pel-Ebstein: disease; fever
Pellegrini's: disease
pellucid: zone
pelvic: axis; cavity; cellulitis; diaphragm; fascia; ganglia;

girdle; peritonitis; plane of greatest dimensions; plane of least dimensions; pole; version
pelvic inflammatory: disease
pelvivertebral: angle
pendular: nystagmus
penetrating: wound
penile: raphe
Penrose: drain
pentose phosphate: pathway
pep: pills
peptic: cell; digestion; ulcer
peptide: bond
perceptual: processing
percutaneous transhepatic: cholangiography
percutaneous transluminal: angioplasty
perfect: fungus; stage
perforated: ulcer
perforating: abscess; arteries; fibers; veins; wound
periapical: curettage; film; granuloma; radiograph
periapical cemental: dysplasia
periappendiceal: abscess
periarterial: plexus; sympathectomy
periarticular: abscess
pericardiacophrenic: artery; veins
pericardial: cavity; decompression; effusion; fremitus; murmur; veins
perichondral: bone
pericytic: venules
peridental: membrane
peri-infarction: block
perilymphatic: duct; space
perinatal: medicine
perineal: artery; hernia; nerves; raphe; section
perineural: anesthesia
periodic: disease; neutropenia; paralysis
periodontal: ligament; membrane
periosteal: bud; elevator; graft
periosteoplastic: amputation
peripheral: scotoma; vision

peripheral nervous: system
peripheral ossifying: fibroma
peritoneal: cavity; dialysis
peritoneovenous: shunt
peritonsillar: abscess
peritubular contractile: cells
permanent: cartilage; dentition; tooth
permeability: coefficient; constant
pernicious: anemia; vomiting
peroneal: artery; retinaculum; veins
peroneal muscular: atrophy
peroneus tertius: muscle
persistent: cloaca; truncus arteriosus
persistent anterior hyperplastic primary: vitreous
persistent chronic: hepatitis
persistent posterior hyperplastic primary: vitreous
personal: equation; space
personality: disorder; formation; profile
Peruvian: wart
pervasive developmental: disorder
petechial: hemorrhage
Peters': ovum
petit: mal
Petit's lumbar: triangle
petro-occipital: fissure
petrotympanic: fissure
petrous: part of internal carotid artery; part of temporal bone
Peyer's: patches
Peyronie's: disease
Pfeiffer's: bacillus
phacogenic: glaucoma
phacomorphic: glaucoma
phagedenic: ulcer
phagocytic: index; pneumonocyte
phakic: eye
phallic: phase
phantom: corpuscle; limb; tumor

WORDFINDER

phantom limb: pain
pharmaceutical: care
pharmacopeial: gel
pharyngeal: bursa; flap; opening of auditory tube; reflex; tonsil; veins
pharyngoconjunctival: fever
pharyngoesophageal: diverticulum
phase: image; microscope
phase I: block
phase II: block
Phemister: graft
phenol: coefficient
phenotypic: value
phenylhydrazine: hemolysis
Philadelphia: chromosome
phlegmonous: abscess
phlorizin: glycosuria
phlyctenular: keratitis
phosphate: diabetes
phosphotungstic acid: hematoxylin
photic: driving
photochromic: lens
photodynamic: sensitization
photogenic: epilepsy
photo-patch: test
photopic: adaptation; eye; vision
photoradiation: therapy
photoreceptor: cells
phrenic: ganglia; nerve
phrenicocolic: ligament
phrenicopleural: fascia
physical: activity; agent; allergy; diagnosis; fitness; map; medicine; sign; therapy
physician office: laboratory
physiologic: antidote; congestion; hypertrophy; icterus; jaundice; leukocytosis; occlusion; scotoma; unit
physiological: drives; saline; sphincter
physiologic dead: space
physiologic rest: position
physiologic retraction: ring
Pick: cell

Pick's: atrophy
pickwickian: syndrome
picrocarmine: stain
piebald: eyelash; skin
Pierre Robin: syndrome
piezogenic pedal: papule
pigeon: breast
pigmentary: retinopathy
pigmented villonodular: synovitis
pigtail: catheter
pilar: cyst; tumor of scalp
pileous: gland
pillow: splint
pill-rolling: tremor
pilomotor: reflex
pilonidal: sinus
Pinard's: maneuver
pincer: nail
pinch: graft
pineal: body; gland; stalk
pinhole: pupil
pink: disease
Pins': syndrome
piriform: muscle
piriformis: muscle
piriform neuron: layer
Pirogoff's: amputation
pisiform: bone
pitch: wart
pitted: keratolysis
pitting: edema
Pittsburgh: pneumonia
Pittsburgh pneumonia: agent
pituitary: cachexia; diverticulum; dwarfism; gigantism; gland; myxedema; stalk
pituitary gonadotropic: hormone
pituitary growth: hormone
pivot: joint
placental: barrier; circulation; dystocia; membrane; presentation
placental growth: hormone
plain: film
Planck's: constant
plane: joint; suture
planoconcave: lens
planoconvex: lens
plantar: arch; fibromatosis;

muscle; reflex; space; wart
plantar calcaneonavicular: ligament
plantar interosseous: muscle
plantaris: muscle
plasma: cell; fibronectin; membrane; proteins
plasma accelerator: globulin
plasma cell: leukemia; mastitis; myeloma
plasmacrit: test
plasma renin: activity
plasma thromboplastin: antecedent
plasminogen: activator
plaster: bandage
plastic: pleurisy; surgery
plateau: pressure; pulse
platelet: factor 3; factor 4
platelet-activating: factor
platelet-aggregating: factor
platelet neutralization: procedure
platelet tissue: factor
platelike: atelectasis
platypellic: pelvis
platypelloid: pelvis
platysma: muscle
play: therapy
pleasure: principle
pleiotropic: gene
pleomorphic: lipoma
pleural: cavity; effusion; fluid; fremitus; space
pleuritic: rub
pleuroesophageal: muscle
pleuropneumonia-like: organisms
plexiform: neurofibroma; neuroma
Plummer-Vinson: syndrome
pneumatic: bone; otoscopy; tonometer
Pneumocystis carinii: pneumonia
pneumogastric: nerve
pneumonic: plague
pocket: dosimeter
pocketed: calculus
podalic: version

podiatric: medicine
point: angle; epidemic; mutation
Poiseuille's: law; space
poker: spine
polar: body; cataract; star
polarized: light
poliomyelitis: virus
poliovirus: vaccines
Politzer: bag
polyacrylamide gel: electrophoresis
polyaxial: joint
polychromatic: cell
polychromatophil: cell
polyclonal: gammopathy
polycystic: disease of kidneys; kidney; liver; ovary
polycystic ovary: syndrome
polymerase chain: reaction
polymorphonuclear: leukocyte
polymorphous light: eruption
polyneuritic: psychosis
polyphenic: gene
polyvalent: allergy; serum; vaccine
pomade: acne
Pomeroy's: operation
Pompe's: disease
pontine: flexure; nuclei
pontomedullary: groove
poorly differentiated lymphocytic: lymphoma
popliteal: artery; fossa; groove; muscle; vein
popliteus: muscle
population: genetics
portacaval: shunt
portal: canals; circulation; fissure; hypertension; lobule of liver; system; triad; vein
portal hypophysial: circulation
portal-systemic: encephalopathy
port-wine: mark; stain
position: effect; sense
positional: nystagmus

positive: accommodation; convergence; scotoma; stain
positive end-expiratory: pressure
positive-negative pressure: breathing
positive pressure: ventilation
positron emission: tomography
postadrenalectomy: syndrome
postcapillary: venules
postcentral: area; gyrus; sulcus
postcommissurotomy: syndrome
postconcussion: syndrome
postcostal: anastomosis
posterior: arch of atlas; asynclitism; chamber of eye; column; column of spinal cord; cord of brachial plexus; embryotoxon; funiculus; horn; lobe of hypophysis; rhinoscopy; scleritis; segment of eyeball; staphyloma; vein of left ventricle
posterior auricular: nerve
posterior cerebral: commissure
posterior cruciate: ligament
posterior elastic: lamina of cornea
posterior focal: point
posterior intercostal: veins
posterior interosseous: nerve
posterior labial: commissure; veins
posterior lacrimal: crest
posterior limiting: layer of cornea
posterior nasal: spine
posterior sagittal: diameter
posterior septal: artery of nose
posterior spinocerebellar: tract
posterolateral: sulcus
postextrasystolic: pause
postextrasystolic T: wave
postgastrectomy: syndrome
posthepatitic: cirrhosis
posthypnotic: suggestion
postmature: infant
postmortem: delivery; livedo; lividity; rigidity; wart

postnasal: drip
postnecrotic: cirrhosis
postpartum: hemorrhage; psychosis
postpericardiotomy: pericarditis; syndrome
postsynaptic: membrane
post-term: infant
posttraumatic: delirium; dementia; epilepsy; syndrome
posttraumatic stress: disorder
postural: alignment; contraction; drainage; position; syncope; vertigo
posture: sense
postvaccinal: encephalomyelitis
potassium sparing: diuretics
potential: energy
Potter-Bucky: diaphragm
Potts': operation
Pott's: disease; fracture
Poupart's: ligament; line
Powassan: encephalitis
P-R: interval
Prague: maneuver; pelvis
preautomatic: pause
precentral: area; gyrus; sulcus
precipitate: labor
precipitin: test
precocious: puberty
precollagenous: fibers
preconceptual: stage
precordial: leads
precostal: anastomosis
precursory: cartilage
predictive: value
preexcitation: syndrome
preferred provider: organization
prefrontal: area
prelogical: thinking
premature: birth; delivery; ejaculation; labor; systole
premaxillary: bone
premenstrual: syndrome; tension
premolar: tooth

WORDFINDER

prenatal: diagnosis
prepatellar: bursa
prepatent: period
preputial: calculus; glands
prepyloric: vein
presacral: neurectomy; sympathectomy
presenile: dementia
pressor: amine; base; fibers; nerve
pressure: alopecia; dressing; epiphysis; paralysis; point; reversal; sense; sore; stasis; tapping; ventilator
pressure support: ventilation
pressure-volume: index
presumed ocular: histoplasmosis
presynaptic: membrane
presystolic: gallop; murmur; thrill
preterm: infant
pretibial: fever; myxedema
preventive: dentistry; medicine
prevertebral: ganglia
Price-Jones: curve
prickle: cell
prickle cell: layer
prickly: heat
primary: adhesion; alcohol; aldosteronism; amenorrhea; amine; amyloidosis; anesthetic; atelectasis; care; complex; dementia; dentin; dentition; deviation; digestion; disease; dysmenorrhea; fissure of cerebellum; gain; hemochromatosis; hemorrhage; lysosomes; nondisjunction; oocyte; process; spermatocyte; syphilis; tooth; tuberculosis; union
primary adrenocortical: insufficiency
primary atypical: pneumonia
primary brain: vesicle
primary care: physician

primary herpetic: stomatitis
primary immune: response
primary lateral: sclerosis
primary ovarian: follicle
primary pulmonary: lobule
primary senile: dementia
primary sex: characters
primitive: groove; gut; knot; node; streak
primordial ovarian: follicle
princeps pollicis: artery
principal: diagnosis; point
principal optic: axis
Prinzmetal's: angina
prion: protein
prism: diopter
private: hospital
private duty: nurse
privileged: site
proacrosomal: granules
probe: syringe
problem-oriented: record
procerus: muscle
procursive: epilepsy
prodromal: stage
productive: cough
profunda brachii: artery
profunda femoris: artery
progestational: hormone
progressive: cataract; staining
progressive bulbar: paralysis
progressive hypertrophic: polyneuropathy
progressive multifocal: leukoencephalopathy
progressive muscular: atrophy
progressive-resistance: exercise
projectile: vomiting
projection: fibers
prolactin-inhibiting: factor; hormone
prolactin-producing: adenoma
prolactin-releasing: factor; hormone
proliferative: inflammation; retinopathy
prominent: heel
promontory: flush
promoting: agent
pronator quadratus: muscle

pronator teres: muscle
proparathyroid: hormone
properdin: factor A; factor B; factor D; factor E; system
prophylactic: treatment
propositional: speech
proprietary: medicine
proprioceptive: mechanism; sensibility
proprioceptive neuromuscular: facilitation
proserum prothrombin conversion: accelerator
prospective payment: system
prostate: gland
prostate-specific: antigen
prostatic: calculus; ducts; ductules; fluid; massage; sinus; utricle
prostatic intraepithelial: neoplasia
prosthetic: group
protection: test
protective laryngeal: reflex
protein: metabolism
protein-losing: enteropathy
prothrombin: accelerator; fragment 1.2; test; time
protodiastolic: gallop
proton: pump
protopathic: sensibility
protoplasmic: astrocyte
protruded: disk
protrusive: occlusion
protuberant: abdomen
proud: flesh
pruritic urticarial: papules and plaques of pregnancy
psammoma: bodies
psammomatous: meningioma
pseudobulbar: palsy; paralysis
pseudomembranous: bronchitis; colitis; enteritis; enterocolitis; gastritis; inflammation
pseudostratified: epithelium
psi: phenomenon

psoas: abscess
psoriatic: arthritis
psychiatric: rehabilitation
psychic: trauma
psychoanalytic: psychiatry; therapy
psychogenic: deafness; pain; vomiting
psychogenic pain: disorder
psychomotor: epilepsy; seizure
psychosexual: development; dysfunction
psychosomatic: disorder; medicine
pterygoid: canal; nerve; process
pterygopalatine: canal; ganglion
pubic: angle; arch; bone; crest; region; symphysis
public: health
pubococcygeal: muscle
pubococcygeus: muscle
puboprostatic: muscle
puborectal: muscle
puborectalis: muscle
pubovaginal: muscle
pubovaginalis: muscle
pubovesical: muscle
pubovesicalis: muscle
Puchtler-Sweat: stain for basement membranes; stain for hemoglobin and hemosiderin
pudendal: canal; cleft; nerve
puerperal: eclampsia; fever; septicemia; tetanus
Puestow: procedure
pulmonary: acinus; adeno-matosis; alveolus; artery; circulation; edema; embolism; emphysema; hamartoma; hypertension; insufficiency; ligament; murmur; plexus; stenosis; toilet; trunk; valve; veins; ventilation
pulmonary alveolar: microlithiasis; proteinosis

pulmonary capillary wedge: pressure
pulmonary dysmaturity: syndrome
pulmonary function: techni-cian; technologist; test
pulp: amputation; canal; cavi-ty; chamber; horn; test
pulse: deficit; generator; oximeter; pressure; rate; wave
pulse-field gel: electrophoresis
pulse height: analyzer
pulseless: disease
pulsion: diverticulum
pump: lung
punch: biopsy; grafts
punchdrunk: syndrome
punctate: hemorrhage; hyalosis
puncture: wound
pupillary: distance; membrane; reflex; zone
pupillary-skin: reflex
pupillotonic: pseudostrabismus
pure: absence; culture; tone
pure tone: audiogram
purse-string: instrument; suture
purulent: inflammation; oph-thalmia; pleurisy; synovitis
Putnam-Dana: syndrome
Putti-Platt: operation
pyelovenous: backflow
pyemic: abscess; embolism
pyloric: antrum; canal; cap; constriction; glands; orifice; sphincter; stenosis; vein
pyogenic: granuloma
pyramid: sign
pyramidal: bone; cataract; cells; decussation; fracture; lobe of; thyroid gland mus-cle; muscle of auricle; radia-tion; tract
pyramidal auricular: muscle
pyramidalis: muscle

Q

Q: fever; wave
Q-: angle
Q-banding: stain
QRS: complex

Q-T: interval
quadrangular: lobule
quadrate: lobe
quadratus femoris: muscle
quadratus lumborum: muscle
quadratus plantae: muscle
quadriceps: muscle of thigh; reflex
quadriceps femoris: muscle
quadrigeminal: rhythm
quadripedal extensor: reflex
qualitative: analysis
quality: control
quantitative: analysis
quantum: theory; yield
quartan: malaria
Queckenstedt-Stookey: test
quellung: phenomenon; reac-tion; test
Quick's: method; test
quiet: lung
Quincke's: pulse; sign
quotidian: malaria

R

R: wave
rabies: virus
raccoon: eyes
racemose: aneurysm; gland
rachitic: pelvis; rosary
racket: amputation
radial: artery; keratotomy; nerve; veins
radial collateral: artery
radial flexor: muscle of wrist
radial growth: phase
radialis indicis: artery
radial recurrent: artery
radiant: intensity
radiate: crown; ligament of head of rib
radiation: biology; dermato-sis; sickness; therapy
radical: hysterectomy; mas-tectomy
radicular: fila
radioactive: constant; iso-tope
radioallergosorbent: test
radiocarpal: joint

WORDFINDER

radiographic: artifact; contrast; density
radioimmunosorbent: test
radiologic: distortion; technologist
radiological: anatomy; enteroclysis
radionuclide: angiocardiography
Ramsay Hunt's: syndrome
Ramstedt: operation
random: mating; sampling
random pattern: flap
range of: accommodation
Ranvier's: node
Raoult's: law
raphe: nuclei
rapid: canities
rapid eye: movements
Rapoport: test
Rapoport-Leubering: shunt
rare: earths
rat-bite: fever
rate: constants
Rathke's: pouch
rational: formula; therapy
Raynaud's: disease; phenomenon; syndrome
R-banding: stain
reaction: formation; time
reactive: depression; hyperemia
reactive airways: disease
reaginic: antibody
reality: principle; testing
rearfoot: pronation; supination
rebound: phenomenon; tenderness
rebreathing: anesthesia; technique; volume
recapitulation: theory
receptive: aphasia
receptor: protein
recessive: character; inheritance; trait
reciprocal: forces; transfusion; translocation
Recklinghausen's: disease of bone; tumor
recognition: factors

recombinant: DNA; vector
recommended daily: allowance
reconstructive: mammaplasty; surgery
recrudescent: typhus
rectal: ampulla; anesthesia; columns
rectococcygeal: muscle
rectococcygeus: muscle
rectourethral: muscle
rectourethralis: muscle
rectouterine: muscle; pouch
rectovaginal: septum
rectovesical: muscle; pouch; septum
rectovesicalis: muscle
rectus: muscle of abdomen; muscle of thigh
rectus abdominis: muscle
rectus capitis anterior: muscle
rectus capitis lateralis: muscle
rectus capitis posterior major: muscle
rectus capitis posterior minor: muscle
rectus femoris: muscle
recurrence: risk
recurrent aphthous: ulcers
recurrent herpetic: stomatitis
recurrent ulcerative: stomatitis
recurrent ulnar: artery
red: corpuscle; hepatization; induration; muscle; neuralgia; nucleus; pulp; reflex
red blood: cell
reduced: hematin; hemoglobin
reducible: hernia
reduction: deformity; mammaplasty
re-entrant: mechanism
reference: range; values
referred: pain; sensation
reflectance: spectrophotometry
reflected inguinal: ligament
reflection: coefficient
reflex: arc; cough; epilepsy; inhibition; symptom
reflex neurogenic: bladder
reflex sympathetic: dystrophy

reflux: esophagitis; otitis media
refractive: index; keratoplasty; keratotomy
refractory: anemia; period; state
refrigeration: anesthesia
regenerative: polyp
regional: anatomy; anesthesia; enteritis; hypothermia
regional granulomatous: lymphadenitis
registered: nurse
regression: analysis
regressive: staining
regular: astigmatism
regulator: gene
regulatory: disorder; sequence
regurgitant: murmur
regurgitation: jaundice
Reid's base: line
Reissner's: membrane
Reiter's: disease; syndrome
relapsing: fever; polychondritis
relapsing febrile nodular nonsuppurative: panniculitis
relative: accommodation; humidity; leukocytosis; polycythemia; scotoma; specificity
relative molecular: mass
relaxant: reversal
relaxation: suture; time
releasing: factors; hormone
Remak's: sign
removable: bridge
removable partial: denture
renal: amyloidosis; artery; calculus; columns; corpuscle; cortex; fascia; ganglia; glycosuria; hematuria; hypertension; hypoplasia; medulla; osteodystrophy; papilla; pelvis; pyramid; rickets; sinus; tubules; veins
renal tubular: acidosis

WORDFINDER

renin-angiotensin-aldo-sterone: system
renovascular: hypertension
reparative: dentin
repetition: time
replacement: therapy
replicative: form
reportable: disease
repressible: enzyme
repressor: gene
reproductive: cycle; system
reserve: air; force
reservoir: bag; host
reservoir oxygen-conserving: device
residual: abscess; air; capacity; schizophrenia; urine; volume
resin: cement
resistance: plasmids; thermometer
resistance-transfer: factor
resolving: power
resonant: frequency
resorption: lacunae
respiration: rate
respiratory: acidosis; alkalosis; bronchioles; capacity; care; center; compliance; enzyme; frequency; pause; pigments; quotient; scleroma; system; therapist; therapy; tract
respiratory care: practitioner
respiratory enteric orphan: virus
respiratory exchange: ratio
respiratory minute: volume
restiform: body
resting: tremor
resting tidal: volume
restorative: dentistry
restriction: endonuclease; enzyme; site
restriction fragment length: polymorphism
restriction-site: polymorphism
restrictive ventilatory: defect

retained: menstruation
retarded: dentition
rete: ridges
retention: cyst; jaundice; suture; vomiting
reticular: degeneration; dystrophy of cornea; fibers; formation; membrane; substance; tissue
reticular activating: system
reticulated: bone
reticulocyte production: index
reticuloendothelial: system
reticulospinal: tract
retinal: adaptation; detachment
retroauricular: lymph nodes
retrobulbar: anesthesia; neuritis
retrocollic: spasm
retrocuspid: papilla
retrograde: amnesia; beat; block; embolism; hernia; menstruation; urography
retrohyoid: bursa
retromandibular: vein
retromolar: pad
retroperitoneal: fibrosis; space
retropubic: space
retrospective: falsification
retrusive: occlusion
Rett's: syndrome
return: extrasystole
reverse: osmosis; transcriptase
reversed: coarctation; peristalsis
reverse Eck: fistula
reverse passive: hemagglutination
reversibility: principle
reversible: calcinosis
Reye's: syndrome
Rhese: projection
rheumatic: arteritis; endocarditis; fever; pneumonia
rheumatic heart: disease
rheumatoid: arthritis; factors; nodules; spondylitis
Rh-immune: globulin
rhinal: sulcus
Rh null: syndrome
Rhodesian: trypanosomiasis

rhombencephalic: isthmus; tegmentum
rhomboid: fossa; ligament
rhomboidal: sinus
rhonchal: fremitus
rhythm: method
ribosomal: RNA
Richter's: hernia
Rideal-Walker: coefficient
rider's: bone
Riedel's: lobe; thyroiditis
Rieder: cells
Rieder cell: leukemia
Riegel's: pulse
right: heart; lobe of liver; ventricle
right colic: flexure
right gastric: artery; vein
right heart: bypass
right hepatic: duct
right-left: discrimination
right lymphatic: duct
right-to-left: shunt
right ventricular: failure
ring: abscess; chromosome; finger; scotoma; syringe
Rinne's: test
Riolan's: anastomosis
risorius: muscle
RNA: virus
RNA tumor: viruses
robertsonian: translocation
Robinson: index
Rocky Mountain spotted: fever
rod: cell; granule
rodent: ulcer
roentgen: ray
Roger's: disease; murmur
Rokitansky's: disease; pelvis
rolandic: epilepsy
Rolando's: area
roller: bandage
Romberg's: sign
roof: plate
root: amputation; canal of tooth; resection; sheath
root caries: index
rooting: reflex
rose: spots
Rose's: position

Rossolimo's: reflex; sign
Ross River: virus
rotary: joint
rotating: anode
rotation: flap
rotational: nystagmus
rotator: cuff of shoulder; muscles
rotatores: muscles
rotatory: nystagmus
rote: learning
rouleaux: formation
round: atelectasis; heart; ligament of femur; ligament of liver; ligament of uterus; window
Rous-associated: virus
Rous sarcoma: virus
Roux-en-Y: anastomosis
rubber-bulb: syringe
rubber dam clamp: forceps
rubella: virus
rubella HI: test
rubeola: virus
rubrospinal: decussation
runaway: pacemaker
ruptured: disk
Russell: bodies
Russell's: sign; syndrome
rusty: sputum
Ruysch's: membrane; muscle

S

S: wave
saber: shin; tibia
Sabouraud's dextrose: agar
saccular: aneurysm; gland; nerve
sacral: canal; crest; flexure; flexure of rectum; foramen; nerves; plexus
sacral splanchnic: nerves
sacroanterior: position
sacroposterior: position
sacrotransverse: position
sacrouterine: fold
saddle: head; joint; nose
saddle block: anesthesia
Saemisch's: section
Saenger's: sign

safety: lens
sagittal: axis; plane; suture
sago: spleen
Saint's: triad
saline: agglutinin; solution
salivary: digestion; fistula
salivary gland: disease
salpingopharyngeal: muscle
salpingopharyngeus: muscle
salt: wasting
saltatory: conduction; evolution; spasm
salt-losing: nephritis
same-day: surgery
Santorini's: duct
saphenous: nerve; opening
sarcoidal: granuloma
sarcoplasmic: reticulum
sartorius: muscle
satellite: abscess
saturated: color; fatty acid; solution
saturation: index
Saundby's: test
Savary: bougies
scalenus medius: muscle
scalp: hair
scanning: speech
scanning electron: microscope
scanning equalization: radiography
Scanzoni's: maneuver
scaphoid: abdomen; bone; scapula
scapulocostal: syndrome
scapulohumeral: rhythm
scapulothoracic: joint
scar: carcinoma
scarlet: fever
Scarpa's: fascia; fluid; membrane; triangle
scarring: alopecia
Scheuermann's: disease
Schick: test
Schilder's: disease
Schiller's: test
Schilling: test
Schilling's: blood count
schistosomal: dermatitis
schizo-affective: psychosis
schizoid: personality

schizotypical: personality
Schlemm's: canal
Schmidt-Lanterman: incisures
school: phobia
Schultz-Charlton: reaction
Schwalbe's: ring
Schwann: cells
Schwartze: sign
sciatic: foramen; hernia; nerve
scimitar: sign
scintillating: scotoma
scintillation: camera; counter
scirrhous: carcinoma
scleral: staphyloma; sulcus; veins
sclerosing: adenosis; hemangioma; keratitis; osteitis
sclerotic: bodies; dentin
sclerotic cemental: mass
scoliotic: pelvis
scombroid: poisoning
scotopic: adaptation; eye; vision
Scott: operation
scout: film
scratch: test
screen: memory
screening: test
scrotal: hernia; raphe; septum
scrub: nurse; typhus
sea gull: murmur
seasonal affective: disorder
sebaceous: adenoma; cyst; epithelioma; follicles; glands
seborrheic: blepharitis; dermatitis; dermatosis; keratosis
second: molar; tooth
secondary: adhesion; alcohol; aldosteronism; amenorrhea; amine; amyloidosis; anesthetic; atelectasis; axis; cataract; degeneration; dementia; dentin; dentition; deviation; digestion; disease; drives; dysmenorrhea; encephalitis;

follicle; gain; glaucoma; gout; hemochromatosis; hemorrhage; lysosomes; mucinosis; nondisjunction; oocyte; process; saturation; spermatocyte; syphilis; tuberculosis; union

secondary abdominal: pregnancy

secondary adrenocortical: insufficiency

secondary immune: response

secondary sex: characters

secondary tympanic: membrane

second degree: prolapse

second degree A-V: block

second heart: sound

second-look: operation

secretory: carcinoma; nerve; otitis media

sector: scan

sedimentation: coefficient; constant; rate

segmental: anesthesia; arteries of kidney; fracture; neuritis

segmentation: cavity

segmented: cell

segregation: analysis; ratio

Seldinger: technique

selection: coefficient

selective: inhibition; stain

selective serotonin reuptake: inhibitor

self: concept

self-registering: thermometer

self-retaining: catheter

Sellick's: maneuver

semicircular: ducts

semi-closed: anesthesia

semihorizontal: heart

semilunar: bone; cartilage; fibrocartilage; hiatus; line; valve

semilunar conjunctival: fold

semimembranosus: muscle

seminal: colliculus; duct; fluid; gland; granule; lake; vesicle

seminiferous: epithelium; tubule

seminiferous tubule: dysgenesis

semi-open: anesthesia

semipolar: bond

semispinalis capitis: muscle

semispinalis cervicis: muscle

semispinalis thoracis: muscle

semitendinosus: muscle

semivertical: heart

Sengstaken-Blakemore: tube

senile: amyloidosis; arteriosclerosis; cataract; dementia; hemangioma; lentigo; melanoderma; plaque; psychosis; retinoschisis; tremor; vaginitis

sense: organs

sensible: perspiration

sensitized: antigen; cell

sensorimotor: area

sensorineural: deafness

sensory: aphasia; cortex; deprivation; epilepsy; ganglion; image; integration; nerve; neuronopathy; paralysis; processing; registration; urgency

sensory speech: center

sentinel: gland; pile; tag

separation: anxiety

septate: uterus

septic: abortion; fever; infarct; phlebitis; shock

septicemic: abscess

septo-optic: dysplasia

serial: dilution; extraction; radiography; section

serofibrinous: pleurisy

seromucous: gland

serous: cell; cyst; gland; inflammation; ligament; membrane; meningitis; otitis; pleurisy; synovitis

serrate: suture

serratus anterior: muscle

Sertoli-cell-only: syndrome

serum: accelerator; agglutinin; albumin; disease; nephritis; reaction; shock; sickness

serum accelerator: globulin

serum hepatitis: virus

serum prothrombin conversion: accelerator

sesamoid: bone

setting sun: sign

Sever's: disease

sex: cell; chromatin; chromosomes; determination; hormones; linkage; ratio; reversal; role

sex-influenced: inheritance

sex-limited: inheritance

sex-linked: character; inheritance

sexual: abuse; dimorphism; generation; infantilism; intercourse; reproduction; selection

sexually transmitted: disease

Sézary: cell

shadow: test

shagreen: skin

shallow: breathing

shave: biopsy

Sheehan's: syndrome

shell: nail; shock

Shenton's: line

Shiga-Kruse: bacillus

shin: bone

shirt-stud: abscess

shock: lung; therapy; treatment

short: bone; gyri of insula

short adductor: muscle

short bowel: syndrome

short extensor: muscle of great toe; muscle of toes

short flexor: muscle of great toe; muscle of little finger; muscle of little toe; muscle of thumb; muscle of toes

short gastric: arteries; veins

short gut: syndrome

short radial extensor: muscle of wrist

short-term: memory

short-term exposure: limit

shot-silk: retina

shoulder: complex; girdle; joint; presentation

shoulder-girdle: syndrome

WORDFINDER

Shwartzman: phenomenon
Shy-Drager: syndrome
Siamese: twins
sibilant: rale
sibling: rivalry
sicca: complex
sick: headache; role
sick building: syndrome
sickle: cell
sickle cell: anemia; crisis; disease; hemoglobin; retinopathy
sickle cell C: disease
sickle cell-thalassemia: disease
side: chain
sideroblastic: anemia
siderotic: cataract
sidestream: aerosol
sigmoid: arteries; colon; sinus; veins
signal: node
signal-to-noise: ratio
signet ring: cells
silent: area; aspiration
silent myocardial: infarction
silhouette: sign of Felson
silo-filler's: lung
silver-fork: deformity; fracture
silver protein: stain
simian: virus
Simmonds': disease
simple: absence; dislocation; epithelium; fission; fracture; glaucoma; goiter; joint; mastectomy; microscope; protein
simple squamous: epithelium
Sims': position
sincipital: presentation
Sindbis: fever; virus
sine: wave
singer's: nodules
single: bond
single photon emission computed: tomography
sinoatrial: block
sinuatrial: node
sinus: arrest; arrhythmia; pause; rhythm

SISI: test
Sister Joseph's: nodule
in situ: hybridization
situational: psychosis
sitz: bath
sixth: disease
sixth-year: molar
Sjögren's: syndrome
skeletal: extension; muscle; traction
skim: milk
skin: dose; ridges; tag; test; traction
skinfold: measurements
skodaic: resonance
slant: culture
sleep: apnea; paralysis
sleeping: sickness
slew: rate
sliding: flap; hernia
slipped: hernia
slipping: rib
slipping rib: cartilage
slit: lamp
slow: virus
slow channel-blocking: agent
slow-reacting: substance
slow virus: disease
small: calorie; intestine
small cardiac: vein
small cell: carcinoma
smaller posterior rectus: muscle of head
small increment sensitivity: index
smallpox: virus
smear: culture
Smith-Indian: operation
Smith's: fracture
smoldering: leukemia
smooth: diet; muscle
smudge: cells
snapping hip: syndrome
sniff: test
snout: reflex
snow: blindness
Soave: operation
social: psychiatry
socialized: medicine
sodium: pump
sodium-potassium: pump

soft: chancre; corn; diet; palate; tubercle; ulcer; wart
solar: cheilitis; elastosis; urticaria
soleus: muscle
solitary: tract
solitary bone: cyst
solitary lymphatic: follicles
solubility: test
soluble: RNA
somatic: antigen; cells; crossing-over; death; delusion; mutation; nerve; pain; reproduction; swallow
somatic motor: nuclei
somatic mutation: theory of cancer
somatic sensory: cortex
somatization: disorder
somatotropic: hormone
somatotropin release-inhibiting: factor; hormone
somatotropin-releasing: factor; hormone
Somogyi: effect; phenomenon; unit
Sonne: bacillus
sonorous: rale
sore: throat
source-to-image-receptor: distance
South African tick-bite: fever
South American: blastomycosis; trypanosomiasis
Southern blot: analysis
spallation: product
Spanish: influenza
sparing: action
spasmodic: dysmenorrhea; dysphonia
spastic: abasia; dysarthria; dysphonia; gait; hemiplegia; ileus
spatial: relation
speaker's: nodules
special: anatomy; sense
species-specific: antigen
specific: action; activity; extinction; gravity; immu-

nity; opsonin; parasite; reaction

specific absorption: coefficient

specific dynamic: action

specificity of training: principle

speculum: forceps

speech: bulb; centers; frequencies; mechanism; pathology; perception

Spens': syndrome

spermacytic: seminoma

spermatic: cord; duct

sphenoid: bone; crest

sphenoidal: angle of parietal bone; conchae; sinus; spine

sphenopalatine: artery; foramen

sphenoparietal: sinus

spherical: aberration; lens

spherocytic: anemia

spheroid: joint

sphincter: muscle; muscle of pupil

sphincter of Oddi: dysfunction

sphygmic: interval

spica: bandage

spider: angioma; nevus; telangiectasia

Spigelius': lobe

spike: potential

spike and wave: complex

spin: density; echo

spinal: analgesia; anesthesia; block; canal; column; cord; curvature; decompression; fusion; ganglion; headache; instability; muscle of neck; nerves; paralysis; reflex; stenosis; tap; veins

spinal cord: concussion

spinalis capitis: muscle

spinalis cervicis: muscle

spinalis thoracis: muscle

spindle: cell

spindle cell: carcinoma; lipoma

spinocerebellar: ataxia

spinothalamic: tract

spinous: layer; process

spiral: bandage; canal of modiolus; fold of cystic duct; fracture; ganglion of cochlea; joint; ligament of cochlea; organ; vein of modiolus

spirit: lamp

Spitz: nevus

splanchnesthetic: sensibility

splanchnic: anesthesia; ganglion; wall

splenic: artery; flexure; pulp; sinus; vein

splenic lymph: follicles

splenius: muscle of head; muscle of neck

splenius capitis: muscle

splenius cervicis: muscle

splenorenal: ligament; shunt

splinter: hemorrhages

split: hand; pelvis

split-thickness: flap; graft

splitting of heart: sounds

spondylolisthetic: pelvis

sponge: bath

spongiform: encephalopathy

spongy: bone; substance

spontaneous: abortion; amputation; gangrene of newborn; generation; mutation; pneumothorax; speech; version

spontaneous intermittent mandatory: ventilation

spoon: nail

sports: anemia; medicine

spot: test for infectious mononucleosis

spotted: fever

spouse: abuse

sprain: fracture

spring: conjunctivitis

spurious: ankylosis

squamoparietal: suture

squamous: cell; epithelium; metaplasia; metaplasia of amnion; suture

squamous cell: carcinoma

squamous odontogenic: tumor

squinting: patella

stab: cell; culture; drain

stable: isotope

staccato: speech

staff: cell

staff model: health maintenance organization

staghorn: calculus

stagnant: anoxia

staircase: phenomenon

standard: atmosphere; bicarbonate; deviation; pressure; solution; temperature; volume

standard error of: difference

Stanford-Binet intelligence: scale

stapedius: muscle

stapes: mobilization

Starling's: curve; hypothesis; law

startle: epilepsy; reflex

starvation: diabetes

stasis: dermatitis; eczema

state-dependent: learning

statokinetic: reflex

steady: state

Stearns alcoholic: amentia

Steinberg thumb: sign

stellate: abscess; block; cell; fracture; hair; reticulum; veins; venules

Stellwag's: sign

stem: cell

stem cell: leukemia

stenosal: murmur

Stensen's: duct

steppage: gait

stercoraceous: vomiting

stercoral: abscess; ulcer

stereochemical: formula

stereoscopic: microscope; vision

stereotactic: instrument; surgery

stereotaxic: surgery

sterile: cyst

sternal: angle; line; muscle; plane; puncture

sternalis: muscle

sternoclavicular: angle; joint

WORDFINDER

sternocleidomastoid: muscle; vein

sternohyoid: muscle

sternomastoid: muscle

sternothyroid: muscle

steroid: acne; hormones; ulcer

Stevens-Johnson: syndrome

Stewart-Holmes: sign

Stewart-Treves: syndrome

sticky-ended: DNA

stiff: neck

stiff-man: syndrome

still: layer

stillborn: infant

Still's: disease; murmur

stimulus: control

stimulus sensitive: myoclonus

stitch: abscess

St. Louis encephalitis: virus

stock: culture; vaccine

Stockholm: syndrome

stocking: anesthesia

stoichiometric: number

Stokes: amputation

Stokes-Adams: syndrome

stoma: button

stomach: ache; pump; tube

stomal: ulcer

stomatognathic: system

stone: heart

Stookey-Scarff: operation

storage: disease

straight: gyrus; sinus

straight seminiferous: tubule

strain: fracture

strangulated: hernia

strap: cell

stratified: epithelium

straw: itch

straw-bed: itch

strawberry: hemangioma; mark; nevus; tongue

stray: light

streak: culture

streaming: movement

street: drug; virus

streptococcus erythrogenic: toxin

stress: fracture; reaction; test; ulcer

stress urinary: incontinence

stretch: receptors; reflex

striate: body; veins

striated: border; duct; muscle

string: sign

stroboscopic: microscope

stroke: volume

stroke work: index

structural: formula; gene; isomerism

Stryker: frame

Stuart: factor

stump: cancer

styloglossus: muscle

stylohyoid: muscle

styloid: process; process of radius; process of temporal bone; process of ulna

stylomastoid: artery; foramen; vein

stylopharyngeal: muscle

stylopharyngeus: muscle

subacromial: bursa

subacute: inflammation

subacute bacterial: endocarditis

subacute combined: degeneration of the spinal cord

subacute granulomatous: thyroiditis

subacute migratory: panniculitis

subacute necrotizing: myelitis

subacute sclerosing: panencephalitis

subacute spongiform: encephalopathy

subaortic: stenosis

subarachnoid: space

subarcuate: fossa

subcallosal: gyrus

subcapsular: cataract

subchorial: lake; space

subclavian: artery; muscle; nerve; steal; vein

subclavius: muscle

subclinical: diabetes

subcostal: artery; muscle; nerve; plane

subcutaneous: emphysema; flap; mastectomy; operation; tenotomy; tissue; veins of abdomen

subdeltoid: bursa

subdural: hematoma; hemorrhage; space

subendocardial: layer

subendothelial: layer

subgingival: curettage

subjective: sensation; symptom

subleukemic: leukemia

sublingual: artery; cyst; fossa; gland; nerve; vein

submammary: mastitis

submandibular: duct; fossa; ganglion; gland; triangle

submental: artery; vein

submucosal: plexus

submucous cleft: palate

suboccipital: nerve

suboccipitobregmatic: diameter

subperiosteal: amputation

subpubic: angle

subscapular: artery; muscle

subscapularis: muscle

subsegmental: atelectasis

subsidiary atrial: pacemaker

substance: abuse; dependence

substance abuse: disorders

substernal: goiter

substitution: product; therapy; transfusion

subtalar: joint

subtendinous: bursa of gastrocnemius muscle; bursa of the tibialis anterior muscle

subtendinous iliac: bursa

subthalamic: nucleus

subungual: hematoma; melanoma

subunit: vaccine

subvocal: speech

succussion: sound

sucking: wound

suction: catheter; drainage

sudden: death

sudden infant death: syndrome

Sudeck's: atrophy

sudomotor: fibers

suffocative: goiter

summation: gallop

summer: diarrhea

sump: drain; syndrome

sun: stroke

sun protection: factor

superciliary: arch

superconducting: magnet

superficial: fascia; fascia of perineum; reflex; vein

superficial brachial: artery

superficial dorsal: veins of penis

superficial epigastric: vein

superficial flexor: muscle of fingers

superficial inguinal: ring

superficial transverse perineal: muscle

superior: ganglion of glossopharyngeal nerve; ganglion of vagus nerve; vein of vermis; vena cava

superior alveolar: nerves

superior auricular: muscle

superior basal: vein

superior cerebellar: artery; peduncle

superior cerebral: veins

superior constrictor: muscle of pharynx

superior dental: arch

superior epigastric: veins

superior extensor: retinaculum

superior frontal: gyrus

superior gemellus: muscle

superiority: complex

superior labial: vein

superior limbic: keratoconjunctivitis

superior longitudinal: fasciculus

superior macular: arteriole

superior medullary: velum

superior nasal: concha

superior oblique: muscle

superior orbital: fissure

superior pelvic: aperture

superior rectus: muscle

superior temporal: line; sulcus

superior thalamostriate: vein

superior vena cava: syndrome

supersaturated: solution

supinator: muscle

supplemental: air

suppression: amblyopia

suppressor: mutation

suppurative: arthritis; gingivitis; hyalitis; inflammation; nephritis

supracervical: hysterectomy

supraclavicular: triangle

supraclinoid: aneurysm

supracondylar: process

supraglottic: swallow

supramarginal: gyrus

supramastoid: crest

suprameatal: triangle

supranormal: excitability

supranuclear: paralysis

supraoptic: commissures; nucleus of hypothalamus

supraorbital: artery; foramen; margin; nerve; vein

supraorbitomeatal: plane

suprapatellar: bursa

suprapubic: cystotomy

suprarenal: cortex; gland; medulla

suprascapular: artery; nerve; vein

supraspinatus: muscle

supraspinous: muscle

supratrochlear: artery; nerve; veins

supravaginal: portion of cervix

supravalvar: stenosis

supraventricular: crest

supravital: stain

supreme nasal: concha

sural: artery; nerve; region

surface: anatomy; biopsy; coil; epithelium; tension

surface thalamic: veins

surgeon's: knot

surgical: abdomen; anatomy; anesthesia; diathermy;

emphysema; microscope; pathology; prosthesis; splint

surrogate: mother

suspended: animation

suspensory: bandage; ligament of axilla; ligament of eyeball; ligament of lens; ligament of ovary; ligaments of breast; muscle of duodenum

sustained-action: tablet

sustained-release: tablet

sutural: bones; ligament

Svedberg: unit

swallowing: reflex

swamp: fever

Swan-Ganz: catheter

sweat: glands; pore

sweat gland: carcinoma

Swift's: disease

swimmer's: ear; itch

swimming pool: conjunctivitis

switching: site

Swyer-James: syndrome

Sydenham's: chorea

Syme's: amputation

symmetrical: gangrene

sympathetic: amine; ganglia; nerve; ophthalmia; trunk; uveitis

sympathetic nervous: system

sympathomimetic: amine

symptom: complex

symptomatic: porphyria; pruritus; reaction

synaptic: cleft; conduction; vesicles

synaptinemal: complex

synarthrodial: joint

synchondrodial: joint

synchronic: study

synchronized intermittent mandatory: ventilation

syncytial: knot

syndesmodial: joint

synergistic: muscles

synovial: bursa; crypt; cyst; fluid; hernia; joint; liga-

ment; membrane; sheath;
sheaths of digits of foot;
sheaths of digits of hand
synthesis: period
synthetic: dyes
syphilitic: aneurysm; leukoderma; roseola
systematized: delusion
systemic: anaphylaxis; circulation; lupus erythematosus
systemic vascular: resistance
systolic: murmur; pressure;
thrill

T

T: antigens; cell; lymphocyte; tubule; wave
T-: binder
tabetic: arthropathy; neurosyphilis
tachycardia: window
tachycardia-bradycardia:
syndrome
tactile: agnosia; anesthesia;
corpuscle; defensiveness;
fremitus; image; meniscus;
papilla
tail: bud; fold
Takayasu's: arteritis; disease; syndrome
talc: operation
talocalcaneal: joint
talocalcaneonavicular: joint
talocrural: joint
Tamm-Horsfall: mucoprotein
Tanner: stage
Tanner growth: chart
tapir: mouth
TAR: syndrome
tardive: cyanosis
target: cell; gland; organ;
response
target heart rate: range
tarry: cyst
tarsal: bones; cyst; glands;
joints; sinus
tarsometatarsal: joints; ligaments
tart: cell
taste: bud; cells; hairs
Taussig-Bing: syndrome

tautomeric: fibers
Tay-Sachs: disease
T-cell: receptor
T cytotoxic: cells
teaching: hospital
Teale's: amputation
tear: gas; sac; stone
teardrop: cell
tectonic: keratoplasty
tectorial: membrane of
cochlear duct
TED: hose
tegmental: decussations;
nuclei; syndrome
telangiectatic: angioma; fibroma; wart
telangiectatic osteogenic: sarcoma
telencephalic: flexure
telogen: effluvium
temperate: bacteriophage
temporal: arteritis; bone; fossa;
lobe; muscle; plane; pole of
cerebrum; process
temporalis: muscle
temporal lobe: epilepsy
temporary: cartilage; denture;
parasite; tooth
temporomandibular: joint;
nerve
temporomandibular joint:
dysfunction
**temporomandibular joint
pain-dysfunction:** syndrome
temporoparietal: muscle
temporoparietalis: muscle
tenaculum: forceps
tendinous: arch; arch of pelvic
fascia; cords; synovitis
tendon: cells; recession; reflex
tennis: elbow; thumb
tension: curve; headache;
suture
tensor: muscle of soft palate;
muscle of tympanic mem-
brane
tensor fasciae latae: muscle
tensor tympani: muscle
tensor veli palati: muscle
tentorial: sinus
teratoid: tumor

teres major: muscle
teres minor: muscle
terminal: artery; bar; boutons; bronchiole; disinfection; filum; hair; infection;
line; nerves; nuclei; sinus;
stria
termino-terminal: anastomosis
territorial: matrix
tertiary: alcohol; amine;
dentin
tessellated: fundus
test: meal; profile; solution;
tube
testicular: artery; cord
testicular feminization: syndrome
testis: ectopia
test-tube: baby
tetanus: toxin
text: blindness
thalamic: peduncle
thalamostriate: veins
Thayer-Martin: agar
T helper: cells
thematic apperception:
test
thenar: eminence
therapeutic: abortion; crisis;
drug; index; range; ratio
thermal: anesthesia; capacity
thermionic: emission
thermoluminescent:
dosimeter
theta: rhythm; wave
thiazin: dyes
thigh: bone
thin: section
thin-layer: chromatography
third: disease; molar; ventricle; ventriculostomy
third degree: prolapse
third heart: sound
third peroneal: muscle
Thomas: splint
Thoma's: ampulla
Thompson's: test
thoracic: cage; cavity; duct;
nucleus; wall
thoracic cardiac: nerves

thoracic longissimus: muscle
thoracic outlet: syndrome
thoracic spinal: nerves
thoracoacromial: artery; vein
thoracodorsal: artery; nerve
thoracoepigastric: vein
thoracolumbar: fascia
thready: pulse
three-glass: test
threshold: stimulus; substance; trait
threshold limit: value
thrombocytic: series
thrombocytopenia-absent radius: syndrome
thrombocytopenic: purpura
thrombopenic: purpura
thrombotic thrombocytopenic: purpura
through: drainage
thumb: forceps
thymic: alymphoplasia; corpuscle; veins
thymus: gland
thyroarytenoid: muscle
thyrocardiac: disease
thyrocervical: trunk
thyroepiglottic: muscle
thyrohyoid: muscle
thyroid: bruit; cartilage; gland; storm
thyroid-stimulating: hormone; immunoglobulins
thyrotoxic: crisis
thyrotropin-releasing: hormone
thyrotropin-releasing hormone stimulation: test
tibial: nerve
tibial collateral: ligament
tick: fever; paralysis; typhus
tick-borne: encephalitis (Eastern subtype)
tick-borne encephalitis: virus
tidal: air; drainage; volume
tight: junction
tilt: test
tine: test

Tinel's: sign
tip: pinch
tissue: culture; lymph; respiration; tension
tissue plasminogen: activator
tissue-specific: antigen
tissue thromboplastin inhibition: time
T-lymphocyte antigen: receptor
TMJ: syndrome
TNM: staging
tobacco: heart
Todd's: paralysis
tolbutamide: test
tolerance: dose
Tolosa-Hunt: syndrome
tongue thrust: therapy
tonic: contraction; convulsion; epilepsy; pupil; spasm
tonic neck: reflex
tonoclonic: spasm
tonsillar: crypt; fossa
tooth: bud; germ; pulp; socket
tophaceous: gout
topical: anesthesia
topographic: anatomy
topographical: orientation
TORCH: syndrome
torsion: fracture; spasm
torsional: deformity
torus: fracture
total: aphasia; communication; hyperopia; transfusion
total body: hypothermia
total end-diastolic: diameter
total end-systolic: diameter
total iron binding: capacity
total joint: arthroplasty
total lung: capacity
total parenteral: nutrition
Tourette: syndrome
Touton giant: cell
Tovell: tube
toxic: cirrhosis; goiter; hemoglobinuria; megacolon; nephrosis; neuritis; shock; tetanus; unit
toxic epidermal: necrolysis
toxic shock: syndrome
toxin: unit

Toynbee: maneuver
trabecular: bone; reticulum
trace: elements
tracheal: cartilages; tube; veins
trachealis: muscle
trachelobregmatic: diameter
tracheoesophageal: puncture
tracheotomy: tube
trachoma: bodies
trachomatous: conjunctivitis; keratitis
traction: diverticulum; epiphysis
tragicus: muscle
training: group
training-sensitive: zone
transactional: analysis
trans-airway: pressure
transcellular: fluids
transcutaneous blood gas: monitor
transducer: cell
transesophageal: echocardiography
transfer: factor; RNA
transference: neurosis
transferrin: saturation
transfixion: suture
transforming: factor
transfusion: nephritis
transhiatal: esophagectomy
transient: hypogammaglobulinemia of infancy
transient acantholytic: dermatosis
transient global: amnesia
transient ischemic: attack
transition: mutation
transitional: denture; epithelium; gyrus; zone
transitional cell: carcinoma
transjugular intrahepatic portosystemic: shunt
transparent: dentin; septum
transport: maximum; medium
transposable: element
transsynaptic: degeneration
transthoracic: esophagectomy

transtracheal oxygen: therapy

transurethral: resection

transversalis: fascia

transverse: amputation; artery of neck; colon; diameter; foramen; fracture; hermaphroditism; lie; ligament of elbow; ligament of knee; muscle of abdomen; muscle of chin; muscle of nape; muscle of tongue; plane; presentation; process; relaxation; section; sinus; vein of face; veins of neck

transverse carpal: ligament

transverse cervical: artery; nerve; veins

transverse facial: artery; vein

transverse horizontal: axis

transverse pericardial: sinus

transverse perineal: ligament

transverse rectal: folds

transverse rhombencephalic: flexure

transverse scapular: artery

transverse tarsal: joint

transverse temporal: gyri

transversion: mutation

transversospinal: muscle

transversospinalis: muscle

transversus abdominis: muscle

transversus menti: muscle

transversus nuchae: muscle

transversus thoracis: muscle

trapezium: bone

trapezius: muscle

trapezoid: bone; ligament; line

Traube-Hering: curves; waves

traumatic: amenorrhea; amnesia; amputation; anesthesia; asphyxia; discopathy; encephalopathy; neuri-

tis; neuroma; neurosis; tetanus

traumatogenic: occlusion

traveler's: diarrhea

trench: fever; mouth

Trendelenburg's: sign; test

trial: denture; frame; lenses

triangular: bandage; bone; muscle

tricarboxylic acid: cycle

triceps: muscle of arm; muscle of calf; reflex

triceps brachii: muscle

triceps surae: muscle; reflex

trichomonal: vaginitis

trichrome: stain

tricuspid: atresia; insufficiency; murmur; orifice; stenosis; valve

trifacial: neuralgia

trifocal: lens

trigeminal: cave; ganglion; nerve; neuralgia; pulse; rhizotomy; rhythm

trigger: area; point; zone

triggered: activity

trihydric: alcohol

Tripier's: amputation

triple: bond; response; vision

tripod: fracture

triquetral: bone

trisomy 21: syndrome

triton: tumor

trochlear: nerve; spine

trochoid: joint

trophic: ulcer

trophoblastic: lacuna

trophoneurotic: leprosy

tropical: abscess; acne; anemia; bubo; diarrhea; diseases; eosinophilia; lichen; medicine; sore; sprue; typhus; ulcer

tropical splenomegaly: syndrome

Trousseau's: sign

true: ankylosis; diverticulum; ribs

true vocal: cord

tsutsugamushi: disease

tubal: ligation; pregnancy

tubed: flap

tubercle: bacillus

tuberculin: test

tuberculoid: leprosy

tuberculous: abscess; enteritis; meningitis; spondylitis; wart

tuboabdominal: pregnancy

tubo-ovarian: pregnancy

tuboreticular: structure

tubular: carcinoma; cyst; forceps; gland; vision

tubuloacinar: gland

tubulointerstitial: nephritis

tufted: cell

tumor: antigens; marker; stage; virus

tumor angiogenic: factor

tumor-specific transplantation: antigens

tumor suppressor: gene

tuning: fork

tunnel: vision

turbulent: flow

turf: toe

turnaround: time

Turner's: syndrome; tooth

turnover: number

tussive: fremitus

twelfth-year: molar

twilight: state

twin-twin: transfusion

twisted: hairs

two-carbon: fragment

two-dimensional: echocardiography

two-glass: test

two-step exercise: test

two-way: catheter

tympanic: bone; canaliculus; cavity; ganglion; membrane; nerve; opening of auditory tube; plexus; ring; sinus; veins

tympanitic: resonance

tympanomastoid: fissure

tympanostomy: tube

Tyndall: phenomenon

type: culture

type 1: glycogenosis

type 2: glycogenosis

type 3: glycogenosis
type 4: glycogenosis
type 5: glycogenosis
type 6: glycogenosis
type A: behavior; personality
type B: behavior
type I: diabetes
type I familial: hyperlipoproteinemia
type II: diabetes
type II familial: hyperlipoproteinemia
type III familial: hyperlipoproteinemia
type IV familial: hyperlipoproteinemia
type V familial: hyperlipoproteinemia
typhoid: bacillus; fever

U

U: wave
ulcerating: granuloma of
pudenda
ulcerative: colitis; stomatitis
ulceromembranous: gingivitis
ulnar: artery; nerve; veins
ulnar extensor: muscle of
wrist
ulnar flexor: muscle of wrist
ulnar nerve compression:
syndrome
ultrashortwave: diathermy
ultrasonic: nebulizer
ultrasound: cardiography
ultrastructural: anatomy
ultraviolet: keratoconjunctivitis; microscope
umber: codon
umbilical: artery; cord; hernia; ring; vein; vesicle
unbalanced: translocation
unciform: bone; fasciculus
uncinate: fasciculus; gyrus
uncompensated: alkalosis
unconditioned: reflex;
response; stimulus
undescended: testis
undetermined: nitrogen
undifferentiated type:
fevers

undulant: fever
undulating: membrane; pulse
uniaxial: joint
unicameral bone: cyst
unicellular: gland
unicorn: uterus
unilateral: anesthesia; hermaphroditism
unilateral hyperlucent: lung
unilateral lobar: emphysema
unilocular: cyst; joint
uninhibited neurogenic:
bladder
uninterrupted: suture
unipolar: leads; neuron
unit: membrane; record
univalent: antibody
universal: donor
unmyelinated: fibers
unsaturated: fatty acid
unstable: angina
unsystematized: delusion
upper: airway; extremity; limb
upper gastrointestinal: series
upper nodal: rhythm
ur-: defenses
urea: clearance; cycle; frost;
nitrogen
uremic: coma
ureteric: orifice
ureteropelvic: junction
ureterorenal: reflux
urethral: artery; caruncle;
crest; glands; groove; hematuria; papilla; valves
urethrovaginal: fistula
urge: incontinence
urinary: bladder; calculus;
nitrogen; sand; stuttering;
system; tract
urinary tract: infection
urogenital: canal; diaphragm;
ridge; system
USP: unit
usual interstitial: pneumonia
of Liebow
uterine: artery; calculus; cavity; contraction; glands;
ostium of uterine tubes; segments; sinus; souffle; tube;
veins

uteroplacental: sinuses
uterovesical: ligament;
pouch
utricular: nerve
utriculoampullar: nerve
uveoparotid: fever
uvular: muscle

V

V: wave
vaccine: lymph
VACTERL: syndrome
vagabond's: disease
vagal: trunk
vaginal: artery; atresia;
celiotomy; gland; hysterectomy; hysterotomy; nerves;
orifice; portion of cervix
vagrant's: disease
vagus: nerve; pulse
Valentine's: position
valgus: laxity
vallate: papilla
Valsalva: maneuver
valvular: endocarditis; insufficiency; regurgitation
van Buchem's: syndrome
vanishing: lung
vanishing lung: syndrome
variant: angina pectoris
varicella: encephalitis
varicella-zoster: virus
varicose: aneurysm; ulcer;
veins
variegate: porphyria
variola: virus
varus: laxity
vascular: cataract; circle of
optic nerve; dementia;
lacuna; lamina of choroid;
leiomyoma; nerve; polyp;
ring; spider; system; tunic
of eye; zone
vascularized: graft
vasoactive: amine
vasoactive intestinal:
polypeptide
vasodepressor: syncope
vasoformative: cell
vasomotor: imbalance;
nerve; paralysis; rhinitis
vastus intermedius: muscle

WORDFINDER

vastus lateralis: muscle
vastus medialis: muscle
VDRL: test
vector: cardiography
vegetal: pole
vegetative: bacteriophage; endocarditis
velopharyngeal: insufficiency
venereal: bubo; disease; ulcer; wart
veno-occlusive: disease of the liver
venous: admixture; angle; blood; capillary; hum; hyperemia; insufficiency; pulse; sinuses; star
ventilation-perfusion: scan
ventilation/perfusion: ratio
ventilatory: threshold
ventral: horn; plate; root
ventral thalamic: peduncle
ventricular: arteries; band of larynx; complex; conduction; escape; extrasystole; fibrillation; flutter; fold; preload; rhythm
ventricular assist: device
ventricular fusion: beat
ventricular septal: defect
Venturi: mask
verbal: apraxia; dyspraxia
vermicular: movement; pulse
vermiform: appendix
vermilion: border
vernal: conjunctivitis
Vernet's: syndrome
verrucous: hemangioma; nevus; xanthoma
vertebral: arch; artery; canal; column; foramen; formula; nerve; ribs; vein
vertebrated: catheter
vertebroarterial: foramen
vertebrocostal: trigone
vertex: presentation
vertical: heart; muscle of tongue; nystagmus; overlap; strabismus; transmission

vertical banded: gastroplasty
vertical growth: phase
vesical: calculus; diverticulum; hematuria; triangle; veins
vesicle: hernia
vesicoureteral: reflux; valve
vesicouterine: fistula
vesicular: murmur; resonance; respiration; transport
vesicular ovarian: follicle
vesiculotympanitic: resonance
vestibular: canal; crest; fold; ganglion; membrane; nerve; neuronitis; nystagmus; organ; veins
vestibulocochlear: nerve; nuclei
vestibulospinal: reflex; tract
vestigial: organ
veterinary: medicine
vibrating: line
vicarious: hypertrophy; menstruation
vicious: circle; union
villous: adenoma; carcinoma; tenosynovitis
Vincent's: angina; disease
viral: dysentery; envelope; hemagglutination; hepatitis; hepatitis type A; hepatitis type B; hepatitis type D; tropism
"viral" spongiform: encephalopathy
Virchow's: node
virulent: bacteriophage
virus: keratoconjunctivitis
virus-transformed: cell
visceral: anesthesia; cleft; layer; layer of serous pericardium; leishmaniasis; lymph nodes; pain; sense; swallow
visible: spectrum
visual: agnosia; angle; aphasia; area; axis; closure; cortex; field; memory; orientation; pigments; purple; violet
visual evoked: potential
visual receptor: cells
vital: capacity; index; pulp; signs; stain; statistics

vitality: test
vitamin B$_{12}$: neuropathy
vitamin D: milk
vitamin D-resistant: rickets
vitelline: membrane; pole
vitellointestinal: cyst
vitreous: body; detachment; hernia; humor; lamella; membrane
vivax: malaria
in vivo: fertilization
vocal: fold; fremitus; ligament; muscle; nodules; process of arytenoid cartilage; resonance
vocalis: muscle
voiding: cystogram
volatile: oil
volitional: tremor
Volkmann's: contracture
volume: index; ventilator
volumetric: analysis; solution
voluntary: muscle
vomerine: cartilage
vomiting: reflex
von Gierke's: disease
von Graefe's: sign
von Willebrand's: disease
vortex: veins
vorticose: veins
vulnerable: phase
vulsella: forceps

W

walk-through: angina
wallerian: degeneration
waltzed: flap
wandering: abscess; cell; goiter; kidney; pacemaker
war: neurosis
water: itch
water-hammer: pulse
Waterhouse-Friderichsen: syndrome
Waters': projection
watershed: infarction
water-trap: stomach
Watson-Crick: helix
waxy: degeneration; kidney; spleen
wear-and-tear: pigment

webbed: fingers; neck
Weber-Fechner: law
Weber's: paradox; syndrome
Wechsler intelligence: scales
wedge: bone; pressure; resection
wedge-and-groove: joint; suture
Wegener's: granulomatosis
Weil-Felix: reaction; test
Weill-Marchesani: syndrome
Weil's: disease
Weitbrecht's: foramen
well-differentiated lymphocytic: lymphoma
Wenckebach: block; period
Wernicke-Korsakoff: encephalopathy; syndrome
Wernicke's: area; center; disease; encephalopathy; reaction; sign; syndrome
Wertheim's: operation
Westergren: method
Western blot: analysis; test
western equine: encephalomyelitis
Westgard: rules
Westphal's: sign
Westphal-Strümpell: disease
wet: gangrene; lung; nurse
Wharton's: duct; jelly
wheal-and-erythema: reaction
wheal-and-flare: reaction
whiplash: injury
Whipple's: operation
white: corpuscle; fiber; gangrene; graft; infarct; line; line of anal canal; matter; muscle; piedra; pulp; substance

white blood: cell
Whitehead's: operation
whole: blood
whole-body: counter
whooping: cough
wild: type
Wilms': tumor
Wilson: block
Wilson's: disease
windchill: index
winged: catheter; scapula
wink: reflex
Wirsung's: canal
wiry: pulse
wisdom: tooth
Wissler's: syndrome
witch's: milk
withdrawal: symptoms; syndrome
Wolfe: graft
wolffian: body; cyst; duct; rest
Wolff-Parkinson-White: syndrome
Wolff's: law
Wood's: lamp; light
work of: breathing
workload: unit
wormian: bones
wound: clip
woven: bone
Wright's: stain
wrist: joint; sign
writing: hand
wry: neck
Wyburn-Mason: syndrome

X

X: chromosome
x-: ray
xanthene: dyes
xenotropic: virus
xiphoid: cartilage; process
X-linked: gene; hypogamma-globulinemia
XO: syndrome

x-ray: microscope
XXY: syndrome
XYY: syndrome

Y

Y: cartilage
yellow: atrophy of the liver; cartilage; fever; fibers; hepatization
Y-linked: gene
yolk: membrane; sac; stalk
Young-Helmholtz: theory of color vision
Y-shaped: ligament

Z

Z: band; filament; line
Z-: DNA
Zenker's: degeneration; diverticulum
zero end-expiratory: pressure
zeta sedimentation: ratio
Zinn's: membrane
Zollinger-Ellison: syndrome
zonal: necrosis
zonular: cataract; spaces
zoo blot: analysis
zoonotic: potential
zoonotic cutaneous: leishmaniasis
zwitter: hypothesis
zygomatic: arch; bone; nerve; process of maxilla
zygomaticofacial: foramen
zygomatico-orbital: artery; foramen
zygomaticotemporal: foramen
zygomaticus major: muscle
zygomaxillary: point
zymogenic: cell

WORDFINDER

α (al′fa). SEE alpha.

A 1. adenine; alanine. **2.** As a subscript, refers to alveolar *gas*. **3.** Symbol (usually capitalized italic) for absorbance. **4.** Symbol for adenosine or adenylic acid in polynucleotides; alanine in polypeptides; first substrate in a multisubstrate enzyme-catalyzed reaction.

Å angstrom.

°A Degree absolute; replaced by K (kelvin).

A⁻ anion.

A. absorbance.

a 1. Ante; area; asymmetric; auris. **2.** Symbol for atto-. **3.** As a subscript, refers to systemic arterial blood.

a specific absorption *coefficient*. Abbreviation for absorptivity.

a-, an-. Not, without, -less; equivalent to L. *in-* and E. *un-*. [G. not, un-; usually *an-* before a vowel]

AA, aa amino acid; aminoacyl.

AAC augmentative and alternative *communication*.

AAMT American Association for Medical Transcription.

AASH adrenal androgen-stimulating *hormone*.

Ab antibody.

ab-, abs-. 1. From, away from, off. **2.** Prefix applied to electrical units in the CGS-electromagnetic system to distinguish them from units in the CGS-electrostatic system (prefix stat-) and those in the metric system or SI system (no prefix). [L. *ab*, from; usually *abs-* before c, q, and t; often *a-*before m, p, or v]

ab·am·pere (ab-am′pēr). Electromagnetic unit of current equal to 10 absolute amperes; a current that exerts a force of 2π dynes on a unit magnetic pole at the center of a circle of wire 1 cm in radius.

abap·i·cal (ă-bap′i-kăl). Opposite the apex.

abar·og·no·sis (ā-bar′og-nō′sis). Loss of ability to appreciate the weight of objects held in the hand, or to differentiate objects of different weights. When the primary senses are intact, a. is caused by a lesion of the contralateral parietal lobe. [G. *a-* priv. + *baros*, weight, + *gnōsis*, knowledge]

aba·sia (ă-bā′zē-ă). Inability to walk. SEE gait. [G. *a-* priv. + *basis*, step]

  atactic a., ataxic a., difficulty in walking due to ataxia of the legs.

  choreic a., a. related to choreiform movements of the legs.

  spastic a., a. due to a spastic contraction of the muscles when an attempt is made to walk.

  a. trep·i·dans, a. due to trembling of the lower limbs.

aba·si·a-asta·si·a. SEE astasia-abasia.

aba·sic (ă-bā′sik). **1.** Affected by, or associated with, abasia; also abatic (ă-bat′ik). **2.** Refers to loss of pyrimidine sites in DNA.

ab·ax·i·al, ab·ax·ile (ab-ak′sē-ăl, -ak′sīl). **1.** Lying outside the axis of any body or part. **2.** Situated at the opposite extremity of the axis of a part.

ab·do·men (ab-dō′men, ab′dō-men) [NA]. The part of the trunk that lies between the thorax and the pelvis. The a. is considered by some anatomists to include the pelvis (abdominopelvic cavity). It includes the greater part of the abdominal cavity (cavum abdominis [NA]), and is divided by arbitrary planes into nine regions. SEE ALSO abdominal *regions*, under region. SYN venter (1). [L. *abdomen*, etym. uncertain]

  acute a., any serious acute intra-abdominal condition (such as appendicitis) attended by pain, tenderness, and muscular rigidity, and for which emergency surgery must be considered. SYN surgical a.

  carinate a., a sloping of the sides with prominence of the central line of the a.

  navicular a., SYN scaphoid a.

  protuberant a., unusual or prominent convexity of the a., due to excessive subcutaneous fat, poor muscle tone, or an increase in intra-abdominal content.

  scaphoid a., a condition in which the anterior abdominal wall is sunken and presents a concave rather than a convex contour. SYN navicular a.

  surgical a., SYN acute a.

ab·dom·i·nal (ab-dom′i-năl). Relating to the abdomen.

abdomino-, abdomin-. The abdomen, abdominal. [L. *abdomen, abdominis*]

ab·dom·i·no·cen·te·sis (ab-dom′i-nō-sen-tē′sis). Paracentesis of the abdomen. [abdomino- + G. *kentēsis*, puncture]

ab·dom·i·no·cy·e·sis (ab-dom′i-nō-sī-ē′sis). **1.** SYN abdominal *pregnancy*. **2.** SYN secondary abdominal *pregnancy*. [abdomino- + G. *kyēsis*, pregnancy]

ab·dom·i·no·cys·tic (ab-dom-i-nō-sis′tik). SYN abdominovesical. [abdomino- + G. *kystis*, bladder]

ab·dom·i·no·gen·i·tal (ab-dom′i-nō-gen′i-tăl). Relating to the abdomen and the genital organs.

ab·dom·i·no·hys·ter·ec·to·my (ab-dom′i-nō-his-ter-ek′tō-mē). SYN abdominal *hysterectomy*.

ab·dom·i·no·hys·ter·ot·o·my (ab-dom′i-nō-his-ter-ot′ō-mē). SYN abdominal *hysterotomy*.

ab·dom·i·no·pel·vic (ab-dom′i-nō-pel′vik). Relating to the abdomen and pelvis, especially the combined abdominal and pelvic cavities.

ab·dom·i·no·per·i·ne·al (ab-dom′i-nō-pār-i-nē′ăl). Relating to both abdomen and perineum.

ab·dom·i·no·plas·ty (ab-dom′i-nō-plas-tē). An operation performed on the abdominal wall for esthetic purposes. [abdomino- + G. *plastos*, formed]

ab·dom·i·nos·co·py (ab-dom-i-nos′kŏ-pē). SYN peritoneoscopy. [abdomino- + G. *skopeō*, to examine]

ab·dom·i·no·scro·tal (ab-dom′i-nō-skrō′tăl). Relating to the abdomen and the scrotum.

ab·dom·i·no·tho·rac·ic (ab-dom′i-nō-thō-ras′ik). Relating to both abdomen and thorax.

ab·dom·i·no·vag·i·nal (ab-dom′i-nō-vag′i-năl). Relating to both abdomen and vagina.

ab·dom·i·no·ves·i·cal (ab-dom′i-nō-ves′i-kăl).

ab

Relating to the abdomen and urinary bladder, or to the abdomen and gallbladder. SYN abdomino-cystic.

ab•duce (ab-dūs′). SYN abduct.

ab•du•cens (ab-dū′senz). SYN abducent (1). [L.]
  a. oc′uli, SYN lateral rectus *muscle.*

ab•du•cent (ab-dū′sent). **1.** Abducting; drawing away, especially away from the median plane. SYN abducens. **2.** SYN abducent *nerve.* [L. *abducens*]

ab•duct (ab-dŭkt′). To move away from the median plane. SYN abduce.

ab•duc•tion (ab-dŭk′shŭn). **1.** Movement of a body part away from the median plane (of the body, in the case of limbs; of the hand or foot, in the case of digits). **2.** Monocular rotation (duction) of the eye toward the temple. **3.** A position resulting from such movement. Cf. adduction. [L. *abductio*]

ab•duc•tor (ab-dŭk′ter, -tōr). A muscle that draws a part away from the median plane; or, in the case of the digits, away from the normal axis of the middle finger or the second toe.

Abell-Kendall meth•od. See under method.

ab•er•rant (ab-er′ant). **1.** Wandering off; said of certain ducts, vessels, or nerves deviating from the normal course or pattern. **2.** Differing from the normal; in botany or zoology, said of certain atypical individuals in a species. **3.** SYN ectopic (1). [L. *aberrans*]

ab•er•ra•tion (ab-er-ā′shŭn). **1.** Deviating from the normal course or pattern. **2.** Deviant development or growth. SEE ALSO chromosome. [L. *aberratio*]

  chromatic a., the difference in focus or magnification of an image arising because of a difference in the refraction of different wavelengths composing white light. SYN chromatism (2).

  chromosome a., any deviation from the normal number or morphology of chromosomes; also the phenotypic consequences thereof.

  coma a., the distortion of image formation created when a bundle of light rays enters an optical system not parallel to the optic axis. [G. *komē,* hair, foliage]

  curvature a., lack of spatial correspondence causing the image of a straight extended object to appear curved.

  dioptric a., SYN spherical a.

  distortion a., the faulty formation of an image arising because the magnification of the peripheral part of an object is different from that of the central part when viewed through a lens.

  lateral a., in spherical a., the distance between paraxial focus of central rays on the optic axis.

  longitudinal a., in spherical a., the distance separating the focus of paraxial and peripheral rays on the optic axis.

  meridional a., an a. produced in the plane of a single meridian of a lens.

  monochromatic a., a defect in an optical image arising because of the nature of lenses; the main types are spherical, coma, curvature, and distortion a., and astigmatism of oblique pencils.

  optical a., failure of rays from a point source to form a perfect image after traversing an optical system.

  spherical a., a monochromatic a. occurring in refraction at a spherical surface in which the paraxial and peripheral rays focus along the axis at different points. SYN dioptric a.

abe•ta•lip•o•pro•tein•e•mia (ā-bā′tă-lip′ō-prō′tēn-ē′mē-ă) [MIM*200100]. A disorder characterized by an absence from plasma of low density lipoproteins that migrate electrophoretically as beta globules, presence of acanthocytes in blood, retinal pigmentary degeneration, malabsorption, engorgement of upper intestinal absorptive cells with dietary triglycerides, and neuromuscular abnormalities; autosomal recessive inheritance. [G. *a-,* priv., + β, + lipoprotein + *-emia,* blood]

ABG (air-bone gap) Arterial blood gas. SEE blood *gases,* under *gas.*

abi•ot•ic (ā-b-ī-ot′ik). **1.** Incompatible with life. **2.** Without life.

ab•i•ot•ro•phy (ab-ē-ot′rō-fē). An age-dependent manifestation of a genetically determined trait that has been latent from the time of conception. [G. *a-* priv. + *bios,* life, + *trophē,* nourishment]

abl. An oncogene found in the Abelson strain of mouse leukemia virus and involved in the Philadelphia chromosome translocation in chronic granulocytic leukemia.

ab•late (ab-lāt′). To remove, or to destroy the function of. [L. *au- fero,* pp. *ab-latus,* to take away]

ab•la•tion (ab-lā′shun). Removal of a body part or the destruction of its function, as by a surgical procedure, morbid process, or noxious substance. [L. see ablate]

  electrode catheter a., a method of ablating the site of origin of arrhythmias whereby high energy electric shocks are delivered by intravascular catheters.

ab•ner•val (ab-ner′văl). Away from a nerve; denoting specifically a current of electricity passing through a muscular fiber in a direction away from the point of entrance of the nerve fiber. SYN abneural (1).

ab•neu•ral (ab-nūr′ăl). **1.** SYN abnerval. **2.** Away from the neural axis. [L. *ab,* away from, + G. *neuron,* nerve]

ab•nor•mal•i•ty (ab-nōr-mal′i-tē). **1.** The state or quality of being abnormal. **2.** An anomaly, deformity, malformation, impairment, or dysfunction.

ab•o•rad, ab•o•ral (ab-ō′rad, -răl). In a direction away from the mouth; opposite of orad. [L. *ab,* from, + *os (or-),* mouth]

abort (ă-bōrt′). **1.** To give birth to an embryo or fetus before it is viable. **2.** To arrest a disease in its earliest stages. **3.** To arrest in growth or development; to cause to remain rudimentary. **4.** To remove products of conception prior to viability. [L. *aborior,* to fail at onset]

abor•ti•fa•cient (ă-bōr-ti-fā′shent). **1.** Producing abortion. SYN abortive (3). **2.** An agent that produces abortion. [L. *abortus,* abortion, + *facio,* to make]

abor•tion (ă-bōr′shŭn). **1.** Expulsion from the uterus of an embryo or fetus prior to the stage of viability at about 20 weeks of gestation (fetus weighs less than 500 g). Premature infants are those born after the stage of viability but prior to 37 weeks. A. may be either spontaneous (occurring from natural causes) or induced (artificial or therapeutic). **2.** The product of such nonviable birth. **3.** The arrest of any action or process before its normal completion.

criminal a., termination of pregnancy without legal justification.

elective a., an a. without medical justification but done in a legal way, as in the United States.

habitual a., a condition in which a woman has had three or more consecutive, spontaneous a.'s.

incomplete a., a. in which part of the products of conception have been passed but part (usually the placenta) remains in the uterus.

induced a., a. brought on deliberately by drugs or mechanical means.

infected a., a septic complication of an a.

missed a., a. in which the fetus dies but is retained *in utero* for two months or longer.

septic a., an infected a. complicated by fever, endometritis, and parametritis.

spontaneous a., a. that has not been artificially induced.

therapeutic a., a. induced because of the mother's physical or mental health, or to prevent birth of a deformed child or a child resulting from rape.

abor·tion·ist (ă-bōr′shŭn-ist). One who interrupts a pregnancy.

abor·tive (ă-bōr′tiv). **1.** Not reaching completion; said of a disease subsiding before it has completed its course. **2.** SYN rudimentary. **3.** SYN abortifacient (1). [L. *abortivus*]

abor·tus (ă-bōr′tŭs). Any product (or all products) of an abortion. [L.]

ABP androgen binding *protein.*

ABR auditory brainstem response.

abra·chia (ă-brā′kē-ă). Congenital absence of arms. SEE amelia. [G. *a-* priv. + *brachiōn*, arm]

abra·chi·o·ce·pha·lia (-se-fā′lē-ă). SEE abrachiocephaly.

abra·chi·o·ceph·a·ly, abra·chi·o·ce·pha·lia (ă-brā′kē-ō-sef′ă-lē, -se-fā′lē-ă). Congenital absence of arms and head. [G. *a-* priv. + *brachiōn*, arm, + *kephalē*, head]

abrade (ă-brād′). **1.** To wear away by mechanical action. **2.** To scrape away the surface layer from a part. [L. *ab-rado*, pp. *-rasus*, to scrape off]

abra·sion (ă-brā′zhŭn). **1.** An excoriation, or circumscribed removal of the superficial layers of skin or mucous membrane. SYN abraded wound. **2.** A scraping away of a portion of the surface. **3.** DENTISTRY the pathological grinding or wearing away of tooth substance by incorrect tooth-brushing methods, foreign objects, bruxism, or similar causes. SYN grinding. Cf. attrition. [SEE abrade]

abra·sive (a-brā′siv). **1.** Causing abrasion. **2.** Any material used to produce abrasions. **3.** A substance used in dentistry for abrading, grinding, or polishing.

abra·sive·ness (ă-brā′siv-nes). **1.** That property of a substance which causes surface wear by friction. **2.** The quality of being able to scratch or wear away another material.

ab·re·ac·tion (ab-rē-ak′shŭn). In freudian psychoanalysis, an emotional release or catharsis associated with the recollection of previously repressed unpleasant experiences.

ab·rup·tio pla·cen·tae (ab-rŭp′shē-ō pla-sen′tē). Premature detachment of a normally situated placenta.

🛈 **ab·scess** (ab′ses). **1.** A circumscribed collection of purulent exudate appearing in an acute or chronic localized infection, caused by tissue destruction and frequently associated with swelling and other signs of inflammation. **2.** A cavity formed by liquefaction necrosis within solid tissue. [L. *abscessus,* a going away]

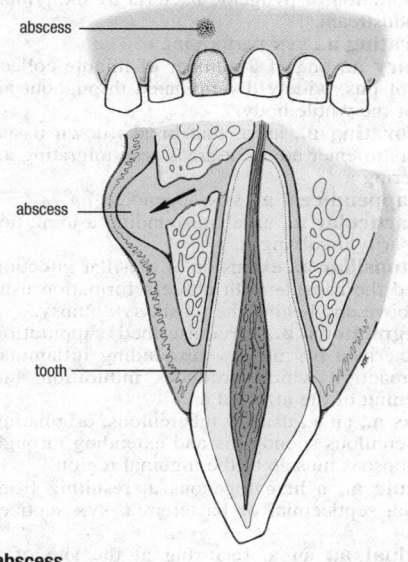

abscess

alveolar a., an a. situated within the alveolar process of the jaws, most often caused by extension of infection from an adjacent nonvital tooth. SYN dental a., dentoalveolar a.

amebic a., an area of liquefaction necrosis of the liver or other organ containing amebae, often following amebic dysentery. SYN tropical a.

appendiceal a., an intraperitoneal a., usually in the right iliac fossa, resulting from extension of infection in acute appendicitis, especially with perforation of the appendix. SYN periappendiceal a.

cold a., (1) an a. without heat or other usual signs of inflammation; (2) SYN tuberculous a.

collar-button a., an a. consisting of two cavities connected by a narrow channel, usually formed by rupture of an a. through an overlying fascia. SYN shirt-stud a.

crypt a.'s, a.'s in crypts of Lieberkühn, a characteristic feature of ulcerative colitis.

dental a., dentoalveolar a., SYN alveolar a.

diffuse a., a collection of pus not circumscribed by a well-defined capsule.

dry a., the remains of an a. after the pus is absorbed.

Dubois' a.'s, small cysts of the thymus containing polymorphonuclear leukocytes but lined by squamous epithelium; reported in congenital syphilis but also found in the absence of syphilis. SYN Dubois' disease.

fecal a., SYN stercoral a.

gas a., an a. containing gas caused by *Enterobacter aerogenes*, *Escherichia coli*, or other gas-forming microorganisms.

gingival a., an a. confined to the gingival soft tissue.

metastatic a., a secondary a. formed, at a distance from the primary focus, as a result of the transportation of pyogenic bacteria by the lymph or bloodstream.

migrating a., SYN perforating a.

miliary a., one of a number of minute collections of pus, widely disseminated throughout an area or the whole body.

perforating a., an a. that breaks down tissue barriers to enter adjacent areas. SYN migrating a., wandering a.

periappendiceal a., SYN appendiceal a.

periarticular a., an a. surrounding a joint, not necessarily involving it.

peritonsillar a., extension of tonsillar infection beyond the capsule with abscess formation usually above and behind the tonsil. SYN quinsy.

phlegmonous a., circumscribed suppuration characterized by intense surrounding inflammatory reaction which produces induration and thickening of the affected area.

psoas a., an a., usually tuberculous, originating in tuberculous spondylitis and extending through the iliopsoas muscle to the inguinal region.

pyemic a., a hematogenous a. resulting from pyemia, septicemia, or bacteremia. SYN septicemic a.

residual a., an a. recurring at the site of a former a. resulting from persistence of microbes and pus.

ring a., an acute purulent inflammation of the corneal periphery in which a necrotic area is surrounded by an annular girdle of leukocytic infiltration.

satellite a., an a. closely associated with a primary a.

septicemic a., SYN pyemic a.

shirt-stud a., SYN collar-button a.

stellate a., a star-shaped necrotic area surrounded by histiocytes, seen within swollen inguinal lymph nodes in lymphogranuloma venereum.

stercoral a., a collection of pus and feces. SYN fecal a.

stitch a., an a. around a suture.

tropical a., SYN amebic a.

tuberculous a., an a. caused by the tubercle bacillus. SYN cold a. (2).

wandering a., SYN perforating a.

ab•scis•sion (ab-si′shŭn). Cutting away. [L. *abscindo*, pp. -*scissus*, to cut away from]

ab•sco•pal (ab-skō′păl, -skop′ăl). Denoting the effect that irradiation of a tissue has on remote nonirradiated tissue. [ab- + G. *skopos*, target, + -al]

ab•sence (ab′sens). Paroxysmal attacks of impaired consciousness, occasionally accompanied by spasm or twitching of cephalic muscles, which usually can be brought on by hyperventilation. [L. *absentia*]

pure a., SYN simple a.

simple a., a brief clouding of consciousness accompanied by the abrupt onset of 3/sec spikes and waves on EEG. SYN pure a.

Ab•sid•ia (ab-sid′ē-ă). A genus of fungi commonly found in nature. Thermophilic species survive in compost piles at temperatures exceeding 45°C and may cause zygomycosis in humans.

ab•sorb (ab-sōrb′). **1.** To take in by absorption. **2.** To reduce the intensity of transmitted light. [L. *ab-sorbeo*, pp. -*sorptus*, to suck in]

ab•sor•bance (*A*, *A*) (ab-sōr′bans). SPECTROPHOTOMETRY, 2 minus the log of the percentage transmittance of light. SYN absorbancy, absorbency, extinction (2), optical density.

ab•sor•ban•cy (ab-sōr′ban-sē). SYN absorbance.

ab•sorb•en•cy (ab-sōr′ben-sē). SYN absorbance.

ab•sor•bent (ab-sōr′bent). **1.** Having the power to absorb, soak up, or take into itself a gas, liquid, light rays, or heat. SYN absorptive. **2.** Any substance possessing such power. **3.** Material (usually caustic) for removal of carbon dioxide from circuits in which rebreathing occurs; *e.g.,* anesthesia equipment.

ab•sorp•tion (ab-sōrp′shŭn). **1.** The taking in, incorporation, or reception of gases, liquids, light, or heat. Cf. adsorption. **2.** RADIOLOGY the uptake of energy from radiation by the tissue or medium through which it passes. **3.** MEDICAL PHYSICS the number of disintegrations per second of a radionuclide. Radioactivity. Unit (SI): becquerel. [L. *absorptio*, fr. *absorbeo*, to swallow]

ab•sorp•tive (ab-sōrp′tiv). SYN absorbent (1).

ab•sorp•tiv•i•ty (*a*) (ab-sōrp-tiv′i-tē). **1.** SYN specific absorption *coefficient*. **2.** SYN molar absorption *coefficient*.

ab•sti•nence (ab′sti-nens). Refraining from the use of certain articles of diet, alcoholic beverages, illegal drugs, or from sexual intercourse. [L. *abs-tineo,* to hold back, fr. *teneo,* to hold]

ab•strac•tion (ab-strak′shŭn). **1.** Distillation or separation of the volatile constituents of a substance. **2.** Exclusive mental concentration. **3.** The making of an abstract from the crude drug. **4.** Malocclusion in which the teeth or associated structures are lower than their normal occlusal plane. **5.** The process of selecting a certain aspect of a concept from the whole. [L. *abs-traho,* pp. -*tractus,* to draw away]

ab•ter•mi•nal (ab-ter′mi-năl). In a direction away from the end and toward the center; denoting the course of an electrical current in a muscle. [L. *ab,* from, + *terminus,* end]

γ-Abu γ-aminobutyric acid.

abu•lia (ă-bū′lē-ă). **1.** Loss or impairment of the ability to perform voluntary actions or to make decisions. **2.** Reduction in speech, movement, thought, and emotional reaction; a common result of bilateral frontal lobe disease. [G. *a-* priv. + *boulē,* will]

abu•lic (ă-bū′lik). Relating to, or suffering from, abulia.

abuse (ă-byūs′). **1.** Misuse, wrong use, especially excessive use, of anything. **2.** Injurious, harmful, or offensive treatment, as in child a. or sexual a.

child a., the psychological, emotional, and sexual a. of a child, typically by a parent, stepparent, or parent surrogate. SEE domestic violence.

drug a., habitual use of drugs not needed for therapeutic purposes, such as solely to alter one's mood, affect, or state of consciousness, or to affect a body function unnecessarily (as in laxative a.); non-medical use of drugs.

elder a., the physical or emotional a., including financial exploitation, of an elderly person, by one or more of the individual's children, nursing home caregivers, or others.

sexual a., SEE domestic violence.

spouse a., spousal a., SEE domestic violence.

substance a., maladaptive pattern of drug or alcohol use that may lead to social, occupational, psychological, or physical problems.

abut•ment (ă-bŭt′ment). DENTISTRY a natural tooth or implanted tooth substitute, used for the support or anchorage of a fixed or removable prosthesis.

AC alternating *current.*

Ac actinium; acetyl.

AC/A Accommodative covergence-accommodation *ratio.*

acal•cu•lia (ā′kal-kyū′lē-a). A form of aphasia characterized by the inability to perform simple mathematical problems; found with lesions of the cerebral hemispheres, and often an early sign of dementia. [G. *a-* priv. + L. *calculo,* to reckon]

acan•tha (ă-kan′thă). **1.** A spine or spinous process. **2.** The spinous process of a vertebra. [G. *akantha,* a thorn]

acan•thes•the•sia (ă-kan-thes-thē′zē-ă). Paresthesia in which there is the sensation of a pinprick. [G. *akantha,* thorn, + *aisthēsis,* sensation]

acan•thi•on (ă-kan′thē-on). The tip of the anterior nasal spine. [G. *akantha,* thorn]

△**acantho-.** A spinous process; spiny, thorny. [G. *akantha,* a thorn, the backbone, the spine, fr. *akē,* a point, + *anthos,* a flower]

acan•tho•cyte (ă-kan′thō-sīt). An erythrocyte characterized by spiny cytoplasmic projections. SYN acanthrocyte. [acantho- + G. *kytos,* cell]

acan•tho•cy•to•sis (ă-kan′thō-sī-tō′sis). A rare condition in which the majority of erythrocytes are acanthocytes; a regular feature of abetalipoproteinemia. SYN acanthrocytosis.

acan•thoid (ă-kan′thoyd). Spine-shaped.

ac•an•thol•y•sis (ak-an-thol′i-sis). Separation of individual epidermal keratinocytes from their neighbors, as in conditions such as pemphigus vulgaris and Darier's disease. [acantho- + G. *lysis,* loosening]

ac•an•tho•ma (ak-an-thō′mă). A tumor formed by proliferation of epithelial squamous cells. SEE ALSO keratoacanthoma. [acantho- + G. *-oma,* tumor]

acan•thor•rhex•is (ă-kan-thō-rek′sĭs). Rupture of the intercellular bridges of the prickle cell layer of the epidermis, as in contact-type dermatitis. SEE spongiosis. [acantho + G. *rhexis,* rupture]

ac•an•tho•sis (ak-an-thō′sis). An increase in the thickness of the stratum spinosum of the epidermis. [acantho- + G. *-osis,* condition]

  a. ni′gricans, an eruption of velvet warty benign growths and hyperpigmentation occurring in the skin of the axillae, neck, anogenital area, and groins; in adults, may be associated with internal malignancy, endocrine disorders, or obesity; a benign (juvenile) type occurs in children. [L. fr. *niger,* black]

ac•an•thot•ic (ak-an-thot′ik). Pertaining to or characteristic of acanthosis.

acan•thro•cyte (a-kan′thrō-sīt). SYN acanthocyte.

acan•thro•cy•to•sis (ă-kan′thrō-sī-tō′sis). SYN acanthocytosis.

acap•nia (ă-kap′nē-ă). Absence of carbon dioxide in the blood; sometimes used erroneously for hypocapnia. [G. *a-* priv. + *kapnos,* smoke]

acar•dia (ā-kar′dē-ă). Congenital absence of the heart; a condition sometimes occurring in monozygotic twins or in the smaller of conjoined twins when its partner monopolizes the placental blood supply. [G. *a-* priv. + *kardia,* heart]

ac•a•ri•a•sis (ak-ar-ī′ă-sis). Any disease caused by mites, usually a skin infestation. SEE mange. SYN acaridiasis, acarinosis.

acar•i•cide (ă-kar′i-sīd). An agent that kills acarines; commonly used to denote chemicals that kill ticks. [Mod. L. *acarus,* a mite, fr. G. *akari* + L. *caedo,* to cut, kill]

ac•a•rid (ak′ă-rid). A general term for a member of the family Acaridae or for a mite. [G. *akari,* mite]

Acar•i•dae (ă-kar′i-dē). A family of the order Acarina, a large group of exceptionally small mites, usually 0.5 mm or less, abundant in dried fruits and meats, grain, meal, and flour; frequently a cause of severe dermatitis among persons hypersensitized by frequent handling of infested products.

ac•ar•i•di•a•sis (ak′ar-i-dī′ă-sis). SYN acariasis.

Ac•a•ri•na (ak-ă-rī′nă). An order of Arachnida that includes the mites and ticks. [G. *akari,* a mite]

ac•a•rine (ak′ă-rīn). A member of the order Acarina.

ac•ar•i•no•sis (ak′ă-ri-nō′sis, ă-kar′i-). SYN acariasis.

ac•a•ro•der•ma•ti•tis (ak′ă-rō-der-mă-tī′tis). A skin inflammation or eruption produced by a mite. [G. *akari,* mite, + *derma* (*dermat-*), skin]

ac•a•ro•pho•bia (ak′ă-rō-fō′bē-ă). Morbid fear of small parasites, small particles, or itching. [G. *akari,* mite, + *phobos,* fear]

Ac•a•rus (ak′ă-rŭs). A genus of mites of the family Acaridae. [G. *akari,* mite]

acar•y•ote (ă-kar′ē-ōt). SYN akaryocyte.

ac•cel•er•ant (ak-sel′er-ant). SYN accelerator.

ac•cel•er•a•tor (ak-sel′er-ā-ter). **1.** Anything that increases rapidity of action or function. **2.** PHYSIOLOGY a nerve, muscle, or substance that quickens movement or response. **3.** A catalytic agent used to hasten a chemical reaction. **4.** NUCLEAR PHYSICS a device that accelerates charged particles (*e.g.,* protons) to high speed in order to produce nuclear reactions in a target, often for the production of radionuclides or for radiation therapy. SYN accelerant. [L. *accelerans,* pres. p. of *ac-celero,* to hasten, fr. *celer,* swift]

  linear a., a device imparting high velocity and energy to atomic and subatomic particles; an important device for radiation therapy.

proserum prothrombin conversion a. (PPCA), SYN *factor* VIII.
prothrombin a., SYN *factor* V.
serum a., SYN *factor* VII.
serum prothrombin conversion a. (SPCA), SYN *factor* VII.

ac·cen·tu·a·tor (ak-sent'yū-ā-ter). A substance, such as aniline, the presence of which allows a combination between a tissue or histologic element and a stain that might otherwise be impossible. [L. *accentus,* accent, fr. *cano,* to sing]

ac·cep·tor (ak-sep'ter). A compound that will take up a chemical group (*e.g.,* an amine group, a methyl group, a carbamoyl group) from another compound (the donor). [L. *ac-cipio,* pp. *-ceptus,* to accept]

ac·cess (ak'ses). A way or means of approach or admittance. DENTISTRY **1.** The space required for visualization and for manipulation of instruments to remove decay and prepare a tooth for restoration. **2.** The opening in the crown of a tooth required to allow adequate admittance to the pulp space to clean, shape, and seal the root canal(s). [L. *accessus*]

ac·ces·so·ry (ak-ses'ō-rē). ANATOMY denoting certain muscles, nerves, glands, etc., that are auxiliary or supernumerary to some similar, generally more important thing. [L. *accessorius,* fr. *accedo,* pp. *-cessus,* to move toward]

ac·ci·dent (ak'si-dent). An unanticipated but often predictable event leading to injury, *e.g.,* in traffic, industry, or a domestic setting, or such an event developing in the course of a disease. [L. *ac-cido,* to happen]
  cerebrovascular a. (CVA), an imprecise term for cerebral stroke.

acclimation. SYN acclimatization.

acclimatization (ă-klī-mă-ti-zā'shŭn). Physiological adaptation to a variation in environmental factors such as temperature, climate, or altitude. SYN acclimation.

ac·com·mo·da·tion (ă-kom'ŏ-dā'shŭn). **1.** The act or state of adjustment or adaptation; especially change in the shape of the ocular lens for various focal distances. **2.** SENSORIMOTOR THEORY the alteration of schemata or cognitive expectations to conform with experience. [L. *ac-commodo,* pp. *-atus,* to adapt, fr. *modus,* a measure]
  amplitude of a., the difference in refractivity of the eye at rest and when fully accommodated.
  histologic a., change in shape of cells to meet altered physical conditions, as the flattening of cuboidal cells in cysts as a result of pressure.
  negative a., the decrease of a. that occurs when shifting from near vision to distance vision.
  positive a., increased refractivity of the eye that occurs when shifting from the distance to a near object.
  range of a., the distance between an object viewed with minimal refractivity of the eye and one viewed with maximal accommodation.
  relative a., quantity of a. required for single binocular vision for any specified distance, or for any particular degree of convergence.

ac·com·mo·da·tive (ă-kom'ŏ-dā-tiv). Relating to accommodation.

ac·cre·tio cor·dis (ă-krē'shē-ō kōr'dis). Adhe-

sion of the pericardium to adjacent extracardiac structures.

ac·cre·tion (ă-krē'shŭn). **1.** Increase by addition to the periphery of material of the same nature as that already present; *e.g.,* the manner of growth of crystals. **2.** DENTISTRY foreign material (usually plaque or calculus) collecting on the surface of a tooth or in a cavity. **3.** A growing together. [L. *accretio,* fr. *ad,* to, + *crescere,* to grow]

ac·cur·a·cy (ak'kyŭ-ră-sē). The degree to which a measurement represents the true value of the attribute that is being measured. In the laboratory a. of a test is determined when possible by comparing results from the test in question with results generated from an established reference method.

acel·lu·lar (ā-sel'yū-lăr). **1.** Devoid of cells. **2.** A term applied to unicellular organisms that do not become multicellular and are complete within a single cell unit. [G. *a-* priv. + L. *cellula,* a small chamber]

acen·tric (ā-sen'trik). Lacking a center. CYTOGENETICS denoting a chromosome fragment without a centromere. [G. *a-* priv. + *kentron,* center]

ace·pha·lia, aceph·a·lism (ă-se-fā'lē-ă, ă-sef'ă-lizm). SYN acephaly.

aceph·a·lo·car·dia (ă-sef'ă-lō-kar'dē-ă). Absence of head and heart in a parasitic twin. [G. *a-* priv. + *kephalē,* head, + *kardia,* heart]

aceph·a·lo·chei·ria, aceph·a·lo·chi·ria (ă-sef'ă-lō-kī'rē-ă). Congenital absence of head and hands. [G. *a-* priv. + *kephalē,* head, + *cheir,* hand]

aceph·a·lo·gas·ter·ia (ă-sef'ă-lō-gas-tēr'ē-ă). Congenital absence of head, thorax, and abdomen in a parasitic twin with pelvis and legs only.

aceph·a·lo·po·dia (ă-sef'ă-lō-pō'dē-ă). Congenital absence of head and feet. [G. *a-* priv. + *kephalē,* head, + *pous,* foot]

aceph·a·lo·sto·mia (ă-sef'ă-lō-stō'mē-ă). Congenital absence of the greater part of the head with, however, the presence of a mouthlike opening. [G. *a-* priv. + *kephalē,* head, + *stoma,* mouth]

aceph·a·lo·tho·ra·cia (ă-sef'ă-lō-thōr-ā'sē-ă). Congenital absence of head and thorax. [G. *a-* priv. + *kephalē,* head, + *thorax,* chest]

aceph·a·lous (ă-sef'ă-lŭs). Headless.

aceph·a·lus (ă-sef'ă-lŭs). A headless fetus. [G. *a-* priv. + *kephalē,* head]

aceph·a·ly (ă-sef'ă-lē). Congenital absence of the head. SYN acephalia, acephalism. [G. *a-* priv. + *kephalē,* head]

△**acet-, aceto-.** Combining forms denoting the two-carbon fragment of acetic acid.

ac·e·tab·u·la (as-ĕ-tab'yū-lă). Plural of acetabulum.

ac·e·tab·u·lar (as-ĕ-tab'yū-lăr). Relating to the acetabulum.

ac·e·tab·u·lec·to·my (as'ĕ-tab-yū-lek'tō-mē). Excision of the acetabulum. [acetabulum + G. *ektomē,* excision]

ac·e·tab·u·lo·plas·ty (as-ĕ-tab'yū-lō-plas-tē). Any operation aimed at restoring the acetabulum to as near a normal state as possible. [acetabulum + G. *plastos,* formed]

ac·e·tab·u·lum, pl. **ac·e·tab·u·la** (as-ĕ-tab'yū-lŭm, -lă) [NA]. A cup-shaped depression on the external surface of the hip bone, with which the head of the femur articulates. SYN cotyloid cavity. [L. a shallow vinegar vessel or cup]

ac•e•tal (as′e-tal). Product of the addition of 2 moles of alcohol to one of an aldehyde. SEE ALSO hemiacetal, hemiketal, ketal.

ac•e•tate (as′e-tāt). CH_3COO^-; a salt or ester of acetic acid.
  a. thiokinase, SYN *acetyl-CoA* ligase.

ac•e•tate-CoA ligase. SYN *acetyl-CoA* ligase.

ac•e•tate thi•o•ki•nase. See under acetate.

△**aceto-.** SEE acet-.

ac•e•to•ac•e•tate (as′e-tō-as′e-tāt). A salt or ion of acetoacetic acid. A ketone body formed in ketogenesis.

ac•e•to•a•ce•tic ac•id (as′e-tō-a-sē′tik). CH_3COCH_2COOH; one of the ketone bodies, formed in excess and appearing in the urine in starvation or diabetic acidosis. SYN diacetic acid.

ac•e•to•a•ce•tyl-CoA (as′e-tō-a-sē′til). Intermediate in the oxidation of fatty acids and in the formation of ketone bodies; also formed from two molecules of acetyl-CoA; major role is condensation with acetyl-CoA to form the important β-hydroxy-β-methylglutaryl-CoA.
  a.-CoA thiolase, SYN *acetyl-CoA* acetyltransferase.

ac•e•tone (as′e-tōn). CH_3COCH_3; a colorless, volatile, inflammable liquid; small amounts are found in normal urine, but larger quantities occur in urine and blood of diabetic persons, sometimes imparting an ethereal odor to the urine and breath. Used as a solvent in some pharmaceutical and commercial preparations.

ac•e•ton•e•mia (as′ĕ-tō-nē′mē-ă). The presence of acetone or acetone bodies in relatively large amounts in the blood. [acetone + G. *haima,* blood]

ac•e•to•nu•ria (as′e-tō-nūr′ē-ă). Excretion in the urine of large amounts of acetone. [acetone + G. *ouron,* urine]

acetowhitening. Whitening of skin or mucous membrane after application of dilute acetic acid, an indication of hyperplasia, dysplasia, or neoplasia; used particularly to identify genital warts on the skin and the uterine cervix.

ace•tyl (Ac) (as′e-til). CH_3CO-; the radical; an acetic acid molecule from which the hydroxyl group has been removed.

acet•y•lase (a-set′il-ās). Any enzyme catalyzing acetylation or deacetylation, as in the formation of *N*-acetylglutamate from glutamate plus acetyl-CoA, or the reverse; a.'s are usually called acetyl-transferases.

acet•y•la•tion (a-set-i-lā′shŭn). Formation of an acetyl derivative.

ace•tyl•cho•line (ACH, Ach) (as-e-til-kō′lēn). (2-acetoxyethyl)trimethylammonium ion; the neurotransmitter substance at cholinergic synapses, which causes cardiac inhibition, vasodilation, gastrointestinal peristalsis, and other parasympathetic effects.

ace•tyl-CoA. Condensation product of coenzyme A and acetic acid, symbolized as $CoA-COCH_3$; intermediate in transfer of two-carbon fragment, notably in its entrance into the tricarboxylic acid cycle and in fatty acid synthesis.

a.-CoA acetyltransferase, an acetyltransferase forming acetoacetyl-CoA from two molecules of a.-CoA, releasing one CoA. A key step in ketogenesis and sterol synthesis. SYN acetoacetyl-CoA thiolase, a.-CoA thiolase.

a.-CoA ligase, a ligase that catalyzes the reaction of acetate and CoA and ATP to form AMP, pyrophosphate, and a.-CoA. A key step in the activation of acetate. SYN acetate thiokinase, acetate-CoA ligase, acetyl-activating enzyme, a.-CoA synthetase.

a.-CoA synthetase, SYN a.-CoA ligase.

a.-CoA thiolase, SYN a.-CoA acetyltransferase.

ace•tyl•trans•fer•ase (as′e-til-trans′fer-ās). Any enzyme transferring acetyl groups from one compound to another. SEE ALSO *choline* acetyltransferase. SYN transacetylase.

AcG, ac-g accelerator *globulin.*

ACH, Ach acetylcholine.

Ach SEE ACH.

acha•la•sia (ak-ă-lā′-zē-ă). Failure to relax; referring especially to visceral openings such as the pylorus, cardia, or any other sphincter muscles. [G. *a-* priv. + *chalasis,* a slackening]
  esophageal a., an obstruction to the passage of food that develops in the terminal esophagus, caused by an autonomic nervous system abnormality. SYN cardiospasm.

ache (āk). A dull, poorly localized pain, usually one of less than severe intensity.
  stomach a., pain in the abdomen, usually arising in the stomach or intestine.

achei•rop•o•dy, achi•rop•o•dy (ă-kī-rop′ō-dē, ă-kī-rop′ō-dē) [MIM*200500]. Congenital absence of the hands and feet; autosomal recessive inheritance. [G. *a-* priv. + *cheir,* hand, + *podos,* foot]

achei•rous, achi•rous (ă-kī′rŭs). Characterized by or relating to acheiria (1).

achil•lo•bur•si•tis (ă-kil′ō-ber-sī′tis). Inflammation of a bursa in proximity to the tendo calcaneus. SYN retrocalcaneobursitis.

achil•lo•dyn•ia (ă-kil-ō-din′ē-ă). Pain due to inflammation of the bursa between the calcaneus and the tendo calcaneus (achillobursitis). [Achilles (tendon) + G. *odynē,* pain]

ach•il•lor•rha•phy (ă-kil-ōr′ă-fē). Suture of the tendo calcaneus. [Achilles (tendon) + G. *rhaphē,* a sewing]

achil•lo•ten•ot•o•my (ă-kil′ō-ten-ot′ō-mē). SYN achillotomy. [Achilles (tendon) + G. *tenōn,* tendon, + *tomē,* a cutting]

ach•il•lot•o•my (ă-kil-ot′ō-mē). Division of the tendo calcaneus. SYN achillotenotomy. [Achilles (tendon) + G. *tomē,* incision]

achlor•hy•dria (ā-klōr-hī′drē-ă). Absence of hydrochloric acid from the gastric juice. [G. *a-* priv. + chlorhydric (acid)]

achlor•o•phyl•lous (ā-klōr-ŏf′ĭ-lŭs). Without chlorophyll, as in fungi.

acho•lia (ă-kō′lē-ă). Suppressed or absent secretion of bile. [G. *a-* priv. + *cholē,* bile]

achol•ic (ă-kol′ik). Without bile, as in a. (pale) stools.

achol•u•ria (ā-kō-lū′rē-ă). Absence of bile pigments from the urine in certain cases of jaundice. [G. *a-* priv. + *cholē,* bile, + *ouron,* urine]

achol•u•ric (ā-kō-lū'rik). Without bile in the urine.

achon•dro•gen•e•sis (ă-kon-drō-jen'ĕ-sis) [MIM*200600 *200720]. Dwarfism accompanied by various bone aplasias of all four limbs, a normal or enlarged skull, and a short trunk with delayed ossification of the lower spine. [G. *a*-priv. + *chondros*, cartilage, + *genesis*, origin]

achon•dro•pla•sia (ă-kon-drō-plā'zē-ă) [MIM* 100800]. A type of chondrodystrophy characterized by an abnormality in conversion of cartilage into bone, predominantly affecting long bones, in which epiphysial growth is retarded and ceases early, resulting in dwarfism apparent at birth, with short extremities but normal trunk. [G. *a*-priv. + *chondros*, cartilage, + *plasis*, a molding]

achon•dro•plas•tic (ă-kon-drō-plas'tik). Relating to or characterized by achondroplasia.

achro•ma•cyte (ă-krō'mă-sīt). SYN achromocyte.

ach•ro•mat•ic (ak-rō-mat'ik). **1.** Colorless. **2.** Not staining readily. **3.** Refracting light without chromatic aberration. [G. *a*- priv. + *chrōma*, color]

achro•ma•tism (ă-krō'mă-tizm). **1.** The quality of being achromatic. **2.** The annulment of chromatic aberration by combining glasses of different refractive indexes and different dispersion.

achro•mat•o•cyte (ā-krō-mat'ō-sīt). SYN achromocyte.

achro•mat•o•phil (ă-krō-mat'ō-fil). **1.** Not being colored by histologic or bacteriologic stains. SYN achromophilic, achromophilous. **2.** A cell or tissue that cannot be stained in the usual way. SYN achromophil. [G. *a*- priv. + *chrōma*, color, + *philos*, fond]

achro•ma•top•sia, achro•ma•top•sy (ă-krō-mă-top'sē-ă, ă-krō'mă-top-sē) [MIM*216900]. A severe congenital deficiency in color perception, often associated with nystagmus and reduced visual acuity. SYN achromatic vision, monochromatism (2). [G. *a*- priv. + *chrōma*, color, + *opsis*, vision]

achro•ma•tous (ă-krō'mă-tŭs). Colorless.

achro•ma•tu•ria (ă-krō-mă-tū'rē-ă). The passage of colorless or very pale urine. [G. *a*- priv. + *chrōma*, color, + *ouron*, urine]

achro•mia (ă-krō'mē-ă). **1.** Depigmentation; absence or loss of natural pigmentation of the skin and iris. SEE ALSO depigmentation. **2.** Lack of capacity to accept stains in cells or tissue. [G. *a*-priv. + *chrōma*, color]

achro•mic (ā-krō'mik). Colorless.

achro•mo•cyte (ă-krō'mō-sīt). A hypochromic, crescent-shaped erythrocyte, probably resulting from artifactual rupture of a red cell. SYN achromacyte, achromatocyte, ghost corpuscle, phantom corpuscle. [G. *a*- priv. + *chrōma*, color, + *kytos*, hollow (cell)]

achro•mo•phil (ă-krō'mō-fil). SYN achromatophil.

achro•mo•phil•ic, achro•moph•i•lous (ā-krō-mō-fil'ik, ā-krō-mof'i-lŭs). SYN achromatophil (1).

achy•lia (ă-kī'lē-ă). **1.** Absence of gastric juice or other digestive secretions. **2.** Absence of chyle. [G. *a*- priv. + *chylos*, juice]

achy•lous (ă-kī'lŭs). **1.** Lacking in gastric juice or

other digestive secretions. **2.** Having no chyle. [G. *achylos*, without juice]

ac•id (as'id). **1.** A compound yielding a hydrogen ion in a polar solvent (*e.g.*, in water); a.'s form salts by replacing all or part of the ionizable hydrogen with an electropositive element or radical. **2.** In popular language, any chemical compound that has a sour taste (given by the hydrogen ion). **3.** Sour; sharp to the taste. **4.** Relating to a.; giving an a. reaction. For individual acids, see specific names. [L. *acidus*, sour]

bile a.'s, steroid a.'s found in bile; *e.g.*, taurocholic and glycocholic a.'s, used therapeutically when biliary secretion is inadequate and for biliary colic. Their physiological roles include fat emulsification.

Brønsted a., an a. that is a proton donor.

fatty a., SEE fatty acid.

inorganic a., an a. made up of molecules not containing organic radicals; *e.g.*, HCl, H_2SO_4, H_3PO_4.

Lewis a., an a. that is an electron pair acceptor.

organic a., an a. made up of molecules containing organic radicals; *e.g.*, acetic a., citric a., which contain the ionizable —COOH group.

ac•i•de•mia (as-i-dē'mē-ă). An increase in the H-ion concentration of the blood or a fall below normal in pH, despite shifts in bicarbonate concentration. Individual types of a. are listed by specific name, *e.g.*, isovaleric acidemia, aminoacidemia, etc. [acid + G. *haima*, blood]

lactic a. (lak'tik-as-i-dē'mē-ă), The presence of dextrorotatory lactic acid in the circulating blood. [lactic acid + G. *haima*, blood]

ac•id-fast (as'id-fast). Denoting bacteria that are not decolorized by acid-alcohol after having been stained with dyes such as basic fuchsin; *e.g.*, the mycobacteria and a few nocardiae.

acid•i•fy (a-sid'i-fī). **1.** To render acid. **2.** To become acid.

acid•i•ty (a-sid'i-tē). **1.** The state of being acid. **2.** The acid content of a fluid.

ac•i•do•phil, ac•i•do•phile (ă-sid'ō-fil, ă-sid'ō-fīl). **1.** SYN acidophilic. **2.** One of the acid-staining cells of the anterior pituitary. **3.** A microorganism that grows well in a highly acid medium. [acid + G. *philos*, fond]

ac•i•do•phil•ic (as'i-dō-fil'ik, ă-sid'ō-fil-ik). Having an affinity for acid dyes; denoting a cell or tissue element that stains with an acid dye, such as eosin. SYN acidophil (1), acidophile, oxychromatic.

ac•i•do•sis (as-i-dō'sis). Actual or relative decrease of alkali in body fluids; depending on the degree of compensation for the a., the pH of body fluids may be normal or decreased; an accumulation of acid metabolites often is present. [acid + G. -*ōsis*, condition]

compensated a., an a. in which the pH of body fluids is normal; compensation is achieved by respiratory or renal mechanisms.

diabetic a., decreased pH and bicarbonate concentration in the body fluids caused by accumulation of ketone bodies in diabetes mellitus.

metabolic a., decreased pH and bicarbonate concentration in the body fluids caused either by the accumulation of acids or by abnormal losses of fixed base from the body, as in diarrhea or renal disease.

renal tubular a., a clinical syndrome characterized by decreased ability to acidify urine, and by low plasma bicarbonate and high plasma chloride concentrations, often with hypokalemia.

respiratory a., a. caused by retention of carbon dioxide; due to inadequate pulmonary ventilation or hypoventilation, with decrease in blood pH unless compensated by renal retention of bicarbonate.

acid sulfate. SYN bisulfate.

ac·id·u·lous (a-sid′yū-lŭs). Acid or sour.

ac·i·du·ria (as-i-dū′rē-ă). **1.** Excretion of an acid urine. **2.** Excretion of an abnormal amount of any specified acid. Individual types of a. are prefixed by the specific acid; *e.g.,* aminoaciduria, ketoaciduria. [acid + G. *ouron,* urine]

ac·i·du·ric (as-i-dū′rik). Pertaining to bacteria that tolerate an acid environment. [acid + L. *duro,* to endure]

ac·i·nar (as′i-nar). Pertaining to the acinus. SYN acinic.

ac·i·ni (as′i-nī). Plural of acinus.

acin·ic (a-sin′ik). SYN acinar.

acin·i·form (a-sin′i-fŏrm). SYN acinous. [L. *acinus,* grape, + *forma,* shape]

ac·i·ni·tis (as-in-ī′tis). Inflammation of an acinus.

ac·i·nose (as′i-nōs). SYN acinous.

ac·i·nous (as′i-nŭs). Resembling an acinus or grape-shaped structure. SYN aciniform, acinose.

ac·i·nus, gen. and pl. **ac·i·ni** (as′i-nŭs, -nī) [NA]. One of the minute grape-shaped secretory portions of an acinous gland. [L. berry, grape]

liver a., the smallest functional unit of the liver, comprising all of the liver parenchyma supplied by a terminal branch of the portal vein and hepatic artery.

pulmonary a., that part of the airway consisting of a respiratory bronchiole and all of its branches. SYN primary pulmonary lobule.

ac·la·sis (ak′lă-sis). A state of continuity between normal and abnormal tissue. [G. *a-* priv. + *klasis,* a breaking away, a fragment]

ac·mes·the·sia (ak-mes-thē′zē-ă). **1.** Sensitivity to pinprick. **2.** A cutaneous sensation of a sharp point. [G. *acmē,* point, + *aisthēsis,* sensation]

ac·ne (ak′nē). An inflammatory follicular, papular, and pustular eruption involving the pilosebaceous apparatus. [probably a corruption (or copyist's error) of G. *akmē,* point of efflorescence]

chlorine a., SYN chloracne.

colloid a., SYN colloid *milium.*

a. congloba′ta, severe cystic a., characterized by cystic lesions, abscesses, communicating sinuses, and thickened, nodular scars; usually sparing the face.

a. cosmet′ica, low-grade, non-inflammatory acne lesions from repeated application of comedogenic agents in cosmetics.

cystic a., severe a. in which the predominant lesions are follicular cysts which rupture and scar.

a. erythemato′sa, SYN rosacea.

a. fulminans (ak′nē ful′mi-nanz), severe scarring a. in teenaged males, which may be associated with fever, polyarthralgia, crusted ulcerative lesions, weight loss, and anemia. [*fulmen, fulminis,* thunder, lightning]

a. indura′ta, deeply seated a., with large papules and pustules, large scars, and hypertrophic scars.

iodide a., a follicular eruption on the face, trunk, and extremities, due to injection or ingestion of iodide in a hypersensitive individual. SEE ALSO iododerma.

a. kerato′sa, an eruption of papules consisting of horny plugs projecting from the hair follicles, accompanied by inflammation.

a. medicamento′sa, a. caused or exacerbated by drugs.

a. papulo′sa, a. vulgaris in which papular lesions predominate.

pomade a., a. commonly found on the forehead and temples of black males after repeated application of hair creams.

a. puncta′ta, a. with black comedones.

a. pustulo′sa, a. vulgaris in which pustular lesions predominate.

a. rosa′cea, SYN rosacea.

steroid a., folliculitis similar to a. vulgaris, but resulting from topical or oral administration of steroids; comedones are rare.

tropical a., a severe type of a. of the entire trunk, shoulders, upper arms, buttocks, and thighs; occurs in hot, humid climates.

a. variolifor′mis, a pyogenic infection involving follicles occurring chiefly on the forehead and temples, followed by scar formation.

a. vulga′ris, an eruption, predominantly of the face, upper back, and chest, composed of comedones, cysts, papules, and pustules on an inflammatory base; the condition occurs in a majority of cases during puberty and adolescence, due to androgenic stimulation of sebum secretion, with plugging of follicles by keratinization, associated with proliferation of *Propionibacterium acnes.*

ac·ne·form (ak′nē-fŏrm). Resembling acne. SYN acneiform.

ac·ne·i·form (ak-nē′i-fŏrm). SYN acneform.

*cis-*ac·o·nit·ic ac·id (ak-ō-nit′ik). Dehydration product of citric acid; an intermediate in the tricarboxylic acid cycle.

aco·rea (ă-kō′rē-ă). Congenital absence of the pupil of the eye. [G. *a-* priv. + *korē,* pupil]

-acousis. 1. Suffix referring to hearing and the ability to hear. **2.** SYN hearing. SEE audio-, audition.

acous·tic (ă-kūs′tik). Pertaining to hearing and the perception of sound. [Gr. *akoustikos*]

acous·tics (ă-kūs′tiks). The science concerned with sounds and their perception. [G. *akoustikos,* relating to hearing]

ACP acyl carrier *protein.*

ac·quired (ă-kwīrd′). Denoting a disease, condition, or abnormality, that is not inherited. [L. *acquiro* (*adq-*), to obtain, fr. *quaero,* to seek]

ac·qui·si·tion (ak-wi-zish′ŭn). PSYCHOLOGY the empirical demonstration of an increase in the strength of the conditioned response in successive trials of pairing the conditioned and unconditioned stimuli.

ACR American College of Radiology.

ac·ral (ak′răl). Relating to or affecting the peripheral parts, *e.g.*, limbs, fingers, ears, etc. [G. *akron,* extremity]

Acra·nia (ă-krā′nē-ă). A group of the phylum Chordata whose members possess a notochord, gill slits, and nerve cord but no vertebrae, ribs, or skull; *e.g., Amphioxus,* tunicates, and acorn worms. [G. *a-* priv. + *kranion,* skull]

acra·nia (ă-krā′nē-ă). Complete or partial absence of a skull; associated with anencephaly. [G. *a-* priv. + *kranion,* skull]

acra·ni·al (ă-krā′nē-ăl). Having no cranium; relating to acrania or an acranius.

Ac·re·mo·ni·um (ak-rĕ-mō′nē-ŭm). A genus of fungi (family Moniliaceae, order Moniliales) that causes keratomycosis and eumycotic mycetoma; produces the antibiotic cephalosporin.

ac·ri·dine orange (ak′ri-dēn aw′renj) [C.I. 46005]. 10-azaanthracene; a basic fluorescent dye useful as a metachromatic stain for nucleic acids; also used in screening cervical smears for abnormal and malignant cells.

△**acro-.** Combining form meaning: **1.** Extremity, tip, end, peak, topmost. **2.** Extreme. [G. *akron,* highest point, extremity; *akros,* topmost, outermost, inmost, extreme, tip]

ac·ro·ag·no·sis (ak′rō-ag-nō′sis). Loss or impairment of the sensory recognition of a limb. Absence of acrognosis.

ac·ro·an·es·the·sia (ak′rō-an-es-thē′zē-ă). Anesthesia of one or more of the extremities. [acro- + G. *an-* priv. + *aisthēsis* sensation]

ac·ro·a·tax·ia (ak′rō-ă-tak′sē-ă). Ataxia affecting the distal portion of the extremities, *i.e.,* hands and fingers, feet, and toes. Cf. proximoataxia. [acro- + ataxia]

ac·ro·blast (ak′rō-blast). Component of the developing spermatid composed of numerous Golgi elements; it contains the proacrosomal granules. [acro- + G. *blastos,* germ]

ac·ro·brach·y·ceph·a·ly (ak′rō-brak-i-sef′ă-lē). Type of craniosynostosis with premature closure of the coronal suture. [acro- + G. *brachys,* short, + *kephalē,* head]

ac·ro·cen·tric (ak-rō-sen′trik). Having the centromere close to one end; said of a normal chromosome. [acro- + G. *kentron,* center]

ac·ro·ce·pha·lia (ak-rō-se-fā′lē-ă). SYN oxycephaly.

ac·ro·ce·phal·ic (ak-rō-se-fal′ik). SYN oxycephalic.

ac·ro·ceph·a·lo·syn·dac·ty·ly (ak′rō-sef′ă-lō-sin-dak′ti-lē). A group of congenital syndromes characterized by peaking at the head and fusion or webbing of digits. [acrocephaly + G. *syn,* together, + *daktylos,* finger]

ac·ro·ceph·a·lous (ak-rō-sef′ă-lŭs). SYN oxycephalic.

ac·ro·ceph·a·ly (ak′rō-sef′ă-lē). SYN oxycephaly. [acro- + G. *kephalē,* head]

ac·ro·chor·don (ak-rō-kōr′don). SYN skin *tag.* [acro- + G. *chordē,* cord]

ac·ro·cy·a·no·sis (ak′rō-sī-ă-nō′sis). A circulatory disorder in which the hands, and less commonly the feet, are persistently cold and blue; some forms are related to Raynaud's phenomenon. [acro- + G. *kyanos,* blue, + *-osis,* condition]

ac·ro·cy·a·not·ic (ak′rō-sī-ă-not′ik). Characterized by acrocyanosis.

ac·ro·der·ma·ti·tis (ak′rō-der-mă-tī′tis). Inflammation of the skin of the extremities. [acro- + G. *derma,* skin, + *-itis,* inflammation]

   a. chron′ica atroph′icans, a late skin manifestation of Lyme disease, appearing first on the feet, hands, elbows or knees, and composed of indurated, erythematous plaques that become atrophic.

   a. contin′ua, SYN *pustulosis* palmaris et plantaris.

   a. per′stans, SYN *pustulosis* palmaris et plantaris.

ac·ro·der·ma·to·sis (ak′rō-der-mă-tō′sis). Any cutaneous affection involving the more distal portions of the extremities. [acro- + G. *derma,* skin, + *-osis,* condition]

ac·ro·dyn·ia (ak-rō-din′ē-ă). **1.** Pain in peripheral or acral parts of the body. **2.** A syndrome caused almost exclusively by mercury poisoning: in children, characterized by erythema of the extremities, chest, and nose, polyneuritis, and gastrointestinal symptoms; in adults, by anorexia, photophobia, sweating, and tachycardia. SYN dermatopolyneuritis, erythredema, pink disease, Swift's disease. [acro- + G. *odynē,* pain]

ac·ro·es·the·sia (ak′rō-es-thē′zē-ă). **1.** An extreme degree of hyperesthesia. **2.** Hyperesthesia of one or more of the extremities. [acro- + G. *aisthēsis,* sensation]

ac·rog·no·sis (ak-rog-nō′sis). Cenesthesia, or normal sensory perception, of the extremities. [acro- + G. *gnōsis,* knowledge]

ac·ro·ker·a·to·sis (ak′rō-ker-ă-tō′sis). Nodular overgrowth of the horny layer of the skin on the fingers and toes, and occasionally on the ear and nose. [acro- + G. *keras,* horn, + *-osis,* condition]

ac·ro·me·gal·ic (ak′rō-mĕ-gal′ik). Pertaining to or characterized by acromegaly.

ac·ro·meg·a·ly (ak-rō-meg′ă-lē). A disorder marked by progressive enlargement of the head, face, hands, and feet, due to excessive secretion of somatotropin; organomegaly and metabolic disorders occur; diabetes mellitus may develop. [acro- + G. *megas,* large]

ac·ro·mel·al·gia (ak-rō-mel-al′jē-ă). SEE erythromelalgia. [acro- + G. *melos,* limb, + *algos,* pain]

ac·ro·mel·ic (ak-rō-mel′ik). Affecting the terminal part of a limb. [acro- + G. *melos,* limb]

ac·ro·mes·o·me·lia (ak′rō-mē-sō-mē′lē-ă) [MIM*201250]. A form of dwarfism in which shortening is striking in the most distal segment of the limbs; autosomal recessive inheritance. [acro- + G. *melos,* limb, + *ia,* condition]

ac·ro·met·a·gen·e·sis (ak′rō-met-ă-jen′ĕ-sis). Abnormal growth of the extremities resulting in deformity. [acro- + G. *meta,* beyond, + *genesis,* origin]

acro·mi·al (ă-krō′mē-ăl). Relating to the acromion.

acro·mi·o·cla·vic·u·lar (ă-krō′mē-ō-kla-vik′yū-lăr). Relating to the acromion and the clavicle; denoting the articulation and ligaments between the clavicle and the acromion of the scapula. SYN scapuloclavicular (1).

acro·mi·o·cor·a·coid (ă-krō-mē-ō-kōr′ă-koyd). SYN coracoacromial.

acro·mi·o·hu·mer·al (ă-krō′mē-ō-hyū′mer-ăl). Relating to the acromion and the humerus.

acro·mi·on (ă-krō′mē-on) [NA]. The lateral end of the spine of the scapula, which projects as a broad flattened process overhanging the glenoid fossa; it articulates with the clavicle and gives attachment to part of the deltoid and trapezius muscles. SYN acromial process. [G. *akrōmion*, fr. *akron*, tip, + *ōmos*, shoulder]

acro·mi·o·scap·u·lar (ă-krō′mē-ō-skap′yū-lăr). Relating to both the acromion and body of the scapula.

acro·mi·o·tho·rac·ic (ă-krō′mē-ō-thō-ras′ik). SYN thoracoacromial.

ac·ro·my·o·to·nia (ak′rō-mī-ō-tō′nē-ă). Myotonia affecting the extremities only, resulting in spastic deformity of the hand or foot. SYN acromyotonus. [acro- + G. *mys*, muscle, + *tonos*, tension]

ac·ro·my·ot·o·nus (ak-rō-mī-ot′ō-nŭs). SYN acromyotonia.

ac·ro·par·es·the·sia (ak′rō-par-es-thēs′ē-a). **1.** Paresthesia of one or more of the extremities. **2.** Nocturnal paresthesia involving the hands, most often of middle-aged women; formerly attributed to a lesion in the thoracic outlet, but now known to be a classic symptom of carpal tunnel syndrome. [acro- + paresthesia]

ac·ro·pho·bia (ak-rō-fō′bē-ă). Morbid fear of heights. [acro- + G. *phobos*, fear]

ac·ro·pus·tu·lo·sis (ak′rō-pŭs-tyū-lō′sis). Pustular eruptions of the hands and feet, often a form of psoriasis. [acro- + pustulosis]

    infantile a., a recurrent papulopustular and crusting pruritic eruption, usually in black children.

ac·ro·scle·ro·der·ma (ak′rō-sklēr-ō-der′mă). SYN acrosclerosis. [acro- + G. *sklēros*, hard, + *derma*, skin]

ac·ro·scle·ro·sis (ak′rō-sklĕ-rō′sis). Stiffness and tightness of the skin of the fingers, with atrophy of the soft tissue and osteoporosis of the distal phalanges of the hands and feet; a limited form of progressive systemic sclerosis occurring with Raynaud's phenomenon. SEE CREST *syndrome*. SYN acroscleroderma, sclerodactyly′, sclerodactylia.

ac·ro·sin (ak′rō-sin). A serine proteinase in spermatozoa similar in specificity to trypsin.

ac·ro·some (ak′rō-sōm). A cap-like organelle that surrounds the anterior two-thirds of the nucleus of a sperm cell. Within this cap are enzymes that are thought to facilitate entry of the sperm into the ovum. [acro- + G. *soma*, body]

acrot·ic (ă-krot′ik). Marked by weakness or absence of the pulse; pulseless. [G. *a-* priv. + *krotos*, a striking]

ac·ro·tism (ak′rō-tizm). Absence or imperceptibility of the pulse. [G. *a-* priv. + *krotos*, a striking]

ACSM American College of Sports *Medicine*.

ACT activated clotting *time*.

ACTH adrenocorticotropic *hormone*.

    big ACTH, a form of ACTH, produced by certain tumors, not immunochemically distinguishable from little ACTH but not exerting any of the biological effects characteristic of ACTH.

    little ACTH, the conventional ACTH molecule when contrasted with big ACTH.

ac·tin (ak′tin). One of the protein components into which actomyosin can be split; it can exist in a fibrous form (F-actin) or a globular form (G-actin).

    F-a., the association of G-a. subunits into a fibrous (F) protein.

    G-a., the globular (G) subunits of the a. molecule, having a molecular weight of 57,000 and containing one molecule of ATP.

ac·tin·ic (ak-tin′ik). Relating to the chemically active rays of the electromagnetic spectrum particularly to sunlight. [G. *aktis* (*aktin-*), a ray]

ac·tin·ides (ak′tin-īdz). Those elements with atomic numbers 89 to 103, corresponding to the lanthanides in the Periodic Table. [*actinium*, first element of the series]

ac·tin·i·um (Ac) (ak-tin′ē-ŭm). An element, atomic no. 89, atomic wt. 227.05; it possesses no stable isotopes and exists in nature only as a disintegration product of uranium and thorium. [G. *aktis*, a ray]

△**actino-.** Combining form meaning a ray, as of light; applied to any form of radiation or to any structure with radiating parts. SEE ALSO radio-. [G. *aktis*, *aktinos*, a ray of light, a beam.]

Ac·ti·no·ba·cil·lus (ak′tin-ō-bă-sil′lŭs). A genus of nonmotile, nonsporeforming, aerobic, facultatively anaerobic bacteria (family Brucellaceae) containing Gram-negative rods interspersed with coccal elements. The metabolism of these bacteria is fermentative. They are pathogenic to animals. The type species is *A. lignieresii*. [actino- + L. *bacillus*, a little rod]

    A. actinomycetemcom′itans, a species of doubtful taxonomic position; frequently associated with human periodontal disease as well as subacute and chronic endocarditis; occurs with actinomycetes in actinomycotic lesions.

ac·ti·no·der·ma·ti·tis (ak′ti-nō-der-mă-tī′tis). SYN photodermatitis.

Ac·ti·no·mad·u·ra (ak′ti-nō-mad′yū-ră). A genus of aerobic, Gram-positive, non-acid-fast fungi whose filaments fragment into spores. *A. pelletieri* is an agent of mycetoma. [actino- + *Madura*, India]

Ac·ti·no·my·ces (ak′ti-nō-mī′sēz). A genus of slow-growing, nonmotile, nonsporeforming, anaerobic to facultatively anaerobic bacteria (family Actinomycetaceae) containing Gram-positive, irregularly staining filaments. These organisms can cause chronic suppurative infection in humans. The type species is *A. bovis*. [actino- + G. *mykēs*, fungus]

    A. bo′vis, a species of bacteria causing actinomycosis in cattle; infection in humans is not established; it is the type species of its genus.

    A. israe′lii, a species of bacteria causing human actinomycosis and, occasionally, infections in cattle.

Ac·ti·no·my·ce·ta·ce·ae (ak′ti-nō-mī′sē-tā′sē-ē). A family of nonsporeforming, nonmotile, facultatively anaerobic bacteria (order Actinomycetales) containing Gram-positive, non-acid-fast, predominantly diphtheroid cells which tend to form branched filaments. This family contains the genera *Actinomyces* (type genus), *Arachnia*, *Bacterionema*, *Bifidobacterium*, and *Rothia*.

Ac•ti•no•my•ce•ta•les (ak'ti-nō-mī'sē-tā'lēz). An order of bacteria consisting of moldlike, rod-shaped, clubbed or filamentous forms with tendency to branching; it includes the families Mycobacteriaceae, Actinomycetaceae, Streptomycetaceae, and Nocardiaceae.

ac•ti•no•my•cetes (ak'ti-nō-mī-sē'tēz). A term used to refer to members of the genus *Actinomyces;* sometimes improperly used to refer to any member of the family Actinomycetaceae or order Actinomycetales.

ac•ti•no•my•co•ma (ak'ti-nō-mī-kō'mă). A swelling caused by an actinomycete. SEE mycetoma. [actino- + G. *mykēs,* fungus, + *-oma,* tumor]

ac•ti•no•my•co•sis (ak'ti-nō-mī-kō'sis). A disease primarily of cattle and humans caused by *Actinomyces bovis* in cattle and by *A. israelii* and *Arachnia propionica* in humans. These actinomycetes are part of the normal bacterial flora of the mouth and pharynx, but they may produce chronic destructive abscesses or granulomas which eventually discharge a viscid pus containing minute yellowish granules (sulfur granules). In humans, the disease commonly affects the cervicofacial area, abdomen, or thorax. [actino- + G. *mykēs,* fungus, + *-osis,* condition]

ac•ti•no•my•cot•ic (ak'ti-nō-mī-kot'ik). Relating to actinomycosis.

ac•ti•no•ther•a•py (ak'ti-nō-thār'ă-pē). DERMATOLOGY ultraviolet light therapy.

ac•tion (ak'shŭn). **1.** The performance of any function, the manner of such performance, or its result. **2.** The exertion of any force or power, physical, chemical, or mental. [L. *actio,* from *ago,* pp. *actus,* to do]

  cumulative a., SYN cumulative *effect.*

  sparing a., the manner in which a nonessential nutritive component, by its presence in the diet, lowers the dietary requirement for an essential component.

  specific a., the a. of a drug or a method of treatment which has a direct and especially curative effect upon a disease.

  specific dynamic a. (SDA), increase of heat production caused by the ingestion of food, especially of protein.

ac•ti•va•tion (ak-ti-vā'shŭn). **1.** The act of rendering active. **2.** An increase in the energy content of an atom or molecule, through the raising of temperature, absorption of light photons, or other means. **3.** Techniques of stimulating the brain by light, sound, electricity, or chemical agents, in order to elicit abnormal activity in the electroencephalogram. **4.** Stimulation of peripheral nerve fibers to the point that action potentials are initiated. **5.** Stimulation of cell division in an ovum by fertilization or by artificial means. **6.** The act of making radioactive.

ac•ti•va•tor (ak'ti-vā-tōr). **1.** A substance that renders another substance, or catalyst, active, or that accelerates a process or reaction. **2.** The fragment, produced by chemical cleavage of a proac-

tivator, that induces the enzymic activity of another substance. **3.** An apparatus for making substances radioactive. **4.** A removable type of myofunctional orthodontic appliance that acts as a passive transmitter of force, produced by the function of the activated muscles, to the teeth and alveolar process that are in contact with it.

  plasminogen a., a proteinase converting plasminogen to plasmin by cleavage of a single (usually Arg-Val) bond in the former. SYN urokinase.

  tissue plasminogen a., thrombolytic serine protease catalyzing the enzymatic conversion of plasminogen to plasmin; a genetically engineered protein used as a thrombolytic agent in patients with thrombotic occlusion of a coronary or cerebral artery.

ac•tiv•i•ty (ak-tiv'i-tē). **1.** ELECTROENCEPHALOGRAPHY the presence of neurogenic electrical energy. **2.** PHYSICAL CHEMISTRY an ideal concentration for which the law of mass action will apply perfectly; the ratio of the a. to the true concentration is the a. coefficient (γ), which becomes 1.00 at infinite dilution. **3.** For enzymes, the amount of substrate consumed (or product formed) in a given time under given conditions; turnover number.

  blocking a., repression or elimination of electrical activity in the brain by the arrival of a sensory stimulus.

  functional a., (1) an activity that improves performance or prevents dysfunction; **(2)** an activity that allows one to meet the demands of the environment and daily life.

  insulin-like a. (ILA), a measure of substances, usually in plasma, that exert biologic effects similar to those of insulin in various bioassays; sometimes used as a measure of plasma insulin concentrations; always gives higher values than immunochemical techniques for the measurement of insulin.

  optical a., the ability of a compound in solution to rotate the plane of polarized light.

  physical a., any body movement produced by muscles that results in energy expenditure. SEE exercise.

  plasma renin a. (PRA), estimation of renin in plasma by measuring the rate of formation of angiotensin I or II.

  specific a., (1) radioactivity per unit mass of the stated element or compound; **(2)** for an enzyme, the amount of substrate consumed (or product formed) in a given time under given conditions per milligram of protein; **(3)** a. per unit mass of the stated radionuclide.

  triggered a., one or a series of spontaneously generated heart beats originating from an action potential that produces an after-depolarization which reaches activation threshold.

activity grading. changing incrementally the process, tools, materials, or environment of a given activity in order to increase or decrease performance demands gradually, and in order ultimately to ensure best performance.

ac•to•my•o•sin (ak'-tō-mī'ō-sin). A protein complex composed of actin and myosin; the essential contractile substance of muscle fiber.

acu•i•ty (ă-kyū'i-tē). Sharpness, clearness, distinctness. **2.** Severity. [thr. Fr., fr. L. *acuo,* pp. *acutus,* sharpen]

acu•le•ate (ă-kyū′lē-āt). Pointed; covered with sharp spines. [L. *aculeatus,* pointed, fr. *acus,* needle]

acu•mi•nate (ă-kyū′mi-nāt). Pointed; tapering to a point. [L. *acumino,* pp. *-atus,* to sharpen]

a•cu•pres•sure (ak′yū-pree′shoor). Application of pressure in sites used for acupuncture with therapeutic intent.

ac•u•punc•ture (ak-yū-punk′chūr). Puncture with long, fine needles: **1.** An ancient Asian system of healing. **2.** More recently, acupuncture anesthesia or analgesia. [L. *acus,* needle, + puncture]

acute (ă-kyūt′). **1.** Referring to a health effect, brief, not chronic; sometimes loosely used to mean severe. **2.** Referring to exposure, brief, intense, short-term; sometimes specifically referring to brief exposure of high intensity. [L. *acutus,* sharp]

acy•a•not•ic (ă-sī-ă-not′ik). Characterized by absence of cyanosis.

ac•yl (as′il). An organic radical derived from an organic acid by the removal of the carboxylic hydroxyl group.

ac•yl•am•i•dase (as-il-am′i-dās). SYN amidase.

ac•yl-CoA. $RCH_2COSCoA$ or $RCH_2CO\sim SCoA$; condensation product of a carboxylic acid and coenzyme A; metabolic intermediate of importance, notably in the oxidation and synthesis of fat.

ac•yl•trans•fer•as•es (as-il-trans′fer-ā-sez) [EC class 2.3]. Enzymes catalyzing the transfer of an acyl group from an acyl-CoA to various acceptors. SYN transacylases.

acys•tia (ā-sis′tē-ă). Congenital absence of the urinary bladder. [G. *a-* priv. + *kystis,* bladder]

△**ad-.** To, toward; increase; adherence; near; very. Prefix denoting increase, adherence, to, toward; increase; adherence; near; very. [L. *ad,* to, toward;]

△**-ad.** In anatomical nomenclature, -ward; toward or in the direction of the part indicated by the main portion of the word. [L. *ad,* to]

ADA American Dental Association; Americans with Disabilities Act.

adac•ty•lous (ā-dak′tĭ-lŭs). Without fingers or toes.

adac•ty•ly (ā-dak′ti-lē). Congenital absence of digits (fingers or toes). [G. *a-* priv. + *daktylos,* digit]

Adam's ap•ple. SYN laryngeal *prominence.*

ad•am•site (DM) (ad′ăm-sīt). A vomiting agent that has been used in military training and in riot control. [Roger *Adams,* Am. chemist]

ad•ap•ta•tion (ad-ap-tā′shŭn). **1.** Preferential survival of members of a species because of a phenotype that gives them an enhanced capacity to withstand the environment. **2.** An advantageous change in function or constitution of an organ or tissue to meet new conditions. **3.** Adjustment of the sensitivity of the retina to light intensity. **4.** A property of certain sensory receptors that modifies the response to repeated or continued stimuli at constant intensity. **5.** The fitting, condensing, or contouring of a restorative material, foil, or shell to a tooth or cast so as to be in close contact. **6.** The dynamic process wherein the thoughts, feelings, behavior, and biophysiologic mechanisms of the individual continually change to adjust to a constantly changing environment. **7.** A homeostatic response. [L. *ad-apto,* pp. *-atus,* to adjust]

  activity a., the process that changes an aspect of an activity to make successful performance possible and thus to accomplish a particular therapeutic goal.

  dark a., the visual adjustment occurring under reduced illumination in which the retinal sensitivity to light is increased. SEE ALSO dark-adapted *eye.* SYN scotopic a.

  light a., the visual adjustment occurring under increased illumination in which the retinal sensitivity to light is reduced. SEE ALSO light-adapted *eye.* SYN photopic a.

  photopic a., SYN light a.

  retinal a., adjustment to degree of illumination.

  scotopic a., SYN dark a.

adapt•er, adap•tor (a-dap′ter, -tōr). **1.** A connecting part, joining two pieces of apparatus. **2.** A converter of electric current to a desired form.

ad•ap•tom•e•ter (ad-ap-tom′ĕ-ter). A device for determining the course of retinal dark adaptation and for measuring the minimum light threshold.

add. L. *adde,* add; L. *addantur,* let them be added; *addendus,* to be added; *addendo,* by adding.

ad•dict (ad′ikt). A person who is habituated to a substance or practice, especially one considered harmful or illegal.

ad•dic•tion (ă-dik′shŭn). Habitual psychological and physiological dependence on a substance or practice that is beyond voluntary control. [L. *ad-dico,* pp. *-dictus,* consent, fr. *ad-* + *dico,* to say]

ad•di•tive (ad′i-tiv). **1.** A substance not naturally a part of a material (*e.g.,* food) but deliberately added to fulfill some specific purpose (*e.g.,* preservation). **2.** Tending to add or be added; denoting addition. **3.** In metrical studies (*e.g.,* genetics, epidemiology, physiology, statistics), having the property that the total combined effect of two or more factors equals the sum of their individual effects in isolation. Cf. synergism.

ad•duct (a-dŭkt′). To draw toward the median plane. [L. *ad-duco,* pp. *-ductus,* to bring toward]

ad•duc•tion (ă-dŭk′shŭn). **1.** Movement of a body part toward the median plane (of the body, in the case of limbs; of the hand or foot, in the case of digits). **2.** Monocular rotation (duction) of the eye toward the nose. **3.** A position resulting from such movement. Cf. abduction.

ad•duc•tor (ă-dŭk′ter, tōr). A muscle that draws a part toward the median plane; or, in the case of the digits, toward the normal axis of the middle finger or the second toe.

Ade adenine.

△**aden-.** SEE adeno-.

aden•dric (ā-den′drik). SYN adendritic.

aden•drit•ic (ā-den-drit′ik). Without dendrites. SYN adendric. [G., *a-* priv. + *dendron,* tree]

ad•e•nec•to•my (ad-ĕ-nek′tō-mē). Excision of a gland. [aden- + G. *ektomē,* excision]

ad•e•nec•to•pia (ad′ĕ-nek-tō′pē-ă). Presence of a

gland other than in its normal anatomical position. [aden- + G. *ek,* out of, + *topos,* place]

aden•i•form (ă-den′i-fōrm). SYN adenoid (1).

ad•e•nine (A, Ade) (ad′ĕ-nēn). One of the two major purines (the other being guanine) found in both RNA and DNA, and also in various free nucleotides.

  a. deoxyribonucleotide, SYN deoxyadenylic acid.

  a. nucleotide, SYN adenylic acid.

ad•e•ni•tis (ad-ĕ-nī′tis). Inflammation of a lymph node or of a gland. [aden- + G. *-itis,* inflammation]

ad•e•ni•za•tion (ad-ĕ-nī-zā′shŭn). Conversion into a glandlike structure.

⌂**adeno-, aden-.** Combining forms denoting gland, glandular; corresponds to L. *glandul-, glandi-.* [G. *adēn, adenos* a gland]

ad•e•no•ac•an•tho•ma (ad′ĕ-nō-ak-an-thō′mă). A malignant neoplasm consisting chiefly of glandular epithelium (adenocarcinoma), usually well differentiated, with foci of metaplasia to squamous (or epidermoid) neoplastic cells. SYN adenoid squamous cell carcinoma.

ad•e•no•blast (ad′ĕ-nō-blast). A proliferating embryonic cell with the potential to form glandular parenchyma. [adeno- + G. *blastos,* germ]

ad•e•no•car•ci•no•ma (ad′ĕ-nō-kar-si-nō′mă). A malignant neoplasm of epithelial cells in glandular or glandlike pattern.

  acinic cell a., an a. arising from secreting cells of a racemose gland, particularly the salivary glands.

  papillary a., an a. containing finger-like processes of vascular connective tissue covered by neoplastic epithelium, projecting into cysts or the cavity of glands or follicles.

ad•e•no•cel•lu•li•tis (ad′ĕ-nō-sel-yū-lī′tis). Inflammation of a gland, usually a lymph node, and of the adjacent connective tissue.

ad•e•no•chon•dro•ma (ad′ĕ-nō-kon-drō′mă). SYN pulmonary *hamartoma.* [adeno- + G. *chondros,* cartilage, + *-oma,* tumor]

ad•e•no•cys•to•ma (ad′ĕ-nō-sis-tō′mă). Adenoma in which the neoplastic glandular epithelium forms cysts.

ad•e•no•cyte (ad′ĕ-nō-sīt). A secretory cell of a gland. [adeno- + G. *kytos,* a hollow (cell)]

ad•e•no•fi•bro•ma (ad′ĕ-nō-fī-brō′mă). A benign neoplasm composed of glandular and fibrous tissues, with a relatively large proportion of glands.

ad•e•no•fi•bro•my•o•ma (ad′ĕ-nō-fī′brō-mī-ō′mă). SYN adenomatoid *tumor.*

ad•e•no•fi•bro•sis (ad′ĕ-nō-fī-brō′sis). SYN sclerosing *adenosis.*

ad•e•nog•en•ous (ad-ĕ-noj′en-ŭs). Having an origin from glandular tissue.

ad•e•no•hy•po•phy•si•al (ad′ĕ-nō-hī-pō-fiz′ē-ăl). Relating to the adenohypophysis.

ad•e•no•hy•poph•y•sis (ad′ĕ-nō-hī-pof′i-sis) [NA]. The anterior pituitary gland. It consists of the distal part, intermediate part, and infundibular part. SEE ALSO hypophysis. SYN lobus anterior hypophyseos [NA], anterior lobe of hypophysis ✕.

ad•e•no•hy•poph•y•si•tis (ad′ĕ-nō-hī-pof-ĭ-sī′tis). Inflammatory reaction or sepsis affecting the anterior pituitary gland, often related to pregnancy.

  lymphocytic a., a diffuse lymphocytic infiltration of the adenohypophysis, often related to pregnancy; probably a disturbance in the immune system.

ad•e•noid (ad′ĕ-noyd). **1.** Glandlike; of glandular appearance. SYN adeniform, lymphoid (2). **2.** SEE adenoids. [adeno- + G. *eidos,* appearance]

ad•e•noid•ec•to•my (ad′ĕ-noy-dek′tō-mē). An operation for the removal of adenoid growths in the nasopharynx. [adenoid + G. *ektomē,* excision]

ad•e•noid•i•tis (ad′ĕ-noy-dī′tis). Inflammation of nasopharyngeal lymphoid tissue.

ad•e•noids (ad′ĕ-noydz). **1.** A normal collection of unencapsulated lymphoid tissue in the nasopharynx. Also called pharyngeal tonsils. **2.** Common terminology for the large (normal) pharyngeal tonsils of children. [G. *adēn,* gland, + *-eidos,* resemblance]

ad•e•no•li•po•ma (ad′ĕ-nō-li-pō′mă). A benign neoplasm composed of glandular and adipose tissues. [G. *adēn,* gland, + *lipos,* fat, + *-oma,* tumor]

ad•e•no•lip•o•ma•to•sis (ad′ĕ-nō-lip′ō-mă-tō′sis). A condition characterized by development of multiple adenolipomas.

ad•e•no•ma (ad-ĕ-nō′mă). An ordinarily benign neoplasm of epithelial tissue in which the tumor cells form glands or glandlike structures in the stroma; usually well circumscribed, tending to compress rather than infiltrate or invade adjacent tissue. [adeno- + G. *-oma,* tumor]

  acidophil a., a tumor of the adenohypophysis in which cell cytoplasm stains with acid dyes; often growth-hormone producing. SYN eosinophil a.

  ACTH-producing a., a pituitary tumor composed of corticotrophs that produce ACTH, often a basophilic adenoma; may give rise to Cushing's disease or Nelson's syndrome.

  adnexal a., an a. arising in, or forming structures resembling, skin appendages.

  apocrine a., SYN papillary *hidradenoma.*

  basophil a., a tumor of the adenohypophysis in which the cell cytoplasm stains with basic dyes, often ACTH-producing.

  bronchial a., a benign or malignant polypoid epithelial tumor of bronchial mucosa, arising deep to the surface epithelium, possibly from mucous glands or their ducts.

  chromophil a., any a. composed of cells that stain readily.

  chromophobe a., chromophobic a., a tumor of the adenohypophysis whose cells do not stain with either acid or basic dyes.

  eosinophil a., SYN acidophil a.

  fibroid a., a. fibro′sum, SYN fibroadenoma.

  growth hormone-producing a., an a. that produces the clinical picture of gigantism or acromegaly, although a third of the cells have no granules or are a mixture of acidophils and chromophobes; some tumors may secrete both growth hormone and prolactin; often an acidophil or eosinophil adenoma.

  hepatic a., a benign tumor of the liver, usually occurring in women in association with lengthy oral contraceptive use.

Hürthle cell a., an uncommon type of thyroid tumor characterized by abundant eosinophilic cytoplasm containing numerous mitochondria. Often malignant with widespread metastases; rarely takes up radioiodine.

papillary cystic a., an a. in which the lumens of the acini are frequently distended by fluid, and the neoplastic epithelial elements tend to form irregular, fingerlike projections.

papillary a. of large intestine, SYN villous a.

prolactin-producing a., a pituitary adenoma composed of prolactin-producing cells; it gives rise to symptoms of nonpuerperal amenorrhea and galactorrhea (Forbes-Albright syndrome) in women and to impotence in men. SYN prolactinoma.

sebaceous a., a benign neoplasm of sebaceous tissue, with a predominance of mature secretory sebaceous cells.

villous a., a solitary sessile, often large, tumor of colonic mucosa composed of mucinous epithelium covering delicate vascular projections; malignant change occurs frequently. SYN papillary a. of large intestine.

ad•e•no•ma•toid (ad-ĕ-nō′mă-toyd). Resembling an adenoma.

ad•e•no•ma•to•sis (ad′ĕ-nō-mă-tō′sis). A condition characterized by multiple glandular overgrowths.

pulmonary a., a neoplastic disease in which the alveoli and distal bronchi are filled with mucus and mucus-secreting columnar epithelial cells; characterized by abundant, extremely tenacious sputum, chills, fever, cough, dyspnea, and pleuritic pain.

ad•e•nom•a•tous (ad-ĕ-nō′mă-tŭs). Relating to an adenoma, and to some types of glandular hyperplasia.

ad•e•no•mere (ad′ĕ-nō-mēr). Structural unit in the parenchyma of a developing gland which becomes the functional portion of the organ. [adeno- + G. *meros,* part]

ad•e•no•my•o•ma (ad′ĕ-nō-mī-ō′mă). A benign neoplasm of muscle (usually smooth muscle) with glandular elements; occurs most frequently in uterus and uterine ligaments. [G. *adēn,* gland, + *mys,* muscle, + *-oma,* tumor]

ad•e•no•my•o•sis (ad′ĕ-nō-mī-ō′sis). The ectopic occurrence or diffuse implantation of adenomatous tissue in muscle (usually smooth muscle). [G. *adēn,* gland, + *mys,* muscle, + *-osis* condition]

ad•e•nop•a•thy (ad-ĕ-nop′ă-thē). Swelling or morbid enlargement of the lymph nodes. [adeno- + G. *pathos,* suffering]

ad•e•no•sal•pin•gi•tis (ad′ĕ-nō-sal-pin-jī′tis). SYN *salpingitis* isthmica nodosa.

ad•e•no•sar•co•ma (ad′ĕ-nō-sar-kō′mă). A malignant neoplasm arising simultaneously or consecutively in mesodermal tissue and glandular epithelium of the same part.

aden•o•sine (Ado) (ă-den′ō-sēn). A condensation product of adenine and D-ribose; a nucleoside found among the hydrolysis products of all nucleic acids and of the various adenine nucleotides.

a. diphosphate, SEE adenosine 5′-diphosphate.

a. monophosphate (AMP), adenosine-5′-monophosphate. SEE adenylic acid.

a. phosphate, specifically, adenosine 3′- or 5′-phosphate. SEE adenylic acid.

a. 5′-phosphosulfate (APS), An intermediate in the formation of PAPS (active sulfate).

a. triphosphate, SYN adenosine 5′-triphosphate.

aden•o•sine 3′,5′-cy•clic monophos•phate (cAMP). An activator of phosphorylase kinase and an effector of other enzymes, formed in muscle from ATP by adenylate cyclase and broken down to 5′-AMP by a phosphodiesterase; sometimes referred to as the "second messenger." A related compound (2′,3′) is also known. SYN cyclic AMP.

aden•o•sine 5′-di•phos•phate (ADP). A condensation product of adenosine with pyrophosphoric acid, formed from ATP by the hydrolysis of the terminal phosphate group of the latter compound.

ad•e•no•sine tri•phos•pha•tase (ATPase) (a-den′ō-sēn-trī-fos′fă-tās). An enzyme in muscle (myosin) and elsewhere that catalyzes the release of the terminal phosphate group of adenosine 5′-triphosphate.

aden•o•sine 5′-tri•phos•phate (ATP). adenosine (5) pyrophosphate; adenosine with triphosphoric acid esterfied at its 5′ position; immediate precursors of adenine nucleotides in RNA. The primary energy currency of a cell. SYN adenosine triphosphate.

ad•e•no•sis (ad-ĕ-nō′sis). A rarely used term for a more or less generalized glandular disease.

microglandular a., a. of the breast in which irregular clusters of small tubules are present in adipose or fibrous tissues, resembling tubular carcinoma but lacking stromal fibroblastic proliferation.

sclerosing a., a nodular, benign breast lesion occurring most frequently in relatively young women and consisting of hyperplastic distorted lobules of acinar tissue with increased collagenous stroma; the changes may be difficult to distinguish microscopically from carcinoma. Also, a benign nodular microscopic lesion of the prostate consisting of acinar tissue with increased stroma; the basal cell layer shows characteristic smooth muscle metaplasia. SYN adenofibrosis.

ad•e•not•o•my (ad-ĕ-not′ō-mē). Incision of a gland. [adeno- + G. *tomē,* a cutting]

ad•e•no•ton•sil•lec•to•my (ad′ĕ-nō-ton-si-lek′tō-mē). Operative removal of tonsils and adenoids.

Ad•e•no•vi•ri•dae (ad′ĕ-nō-vir′i-dē). A family of double-stranded DNA viruses, commonly known as adenoviruses, that develop in the nuclei of infected cells in mammals and birds.

ad•e•no•vi•rus (ad′ĕ-nō-vī′rŭs). Adenoidal-pharyngeal-conjunctival or A-P-C virus; any virus of the family Adenoviridae. More than 40 types are known to infect man causing upper respiratory symptoms, acute respiratory disease, conjunctivitis, gastroenteritis, hemorrhagic cystitis, and serous infections in neonates. SYN adenoidal-pharyngeal-conjunctival virus. [G. *adēn,* gland, + virus]

ad•e•nyl (ad′e-nil). The radical or ion of adenine.

aden·y·late (a-den′i-lāt). Salt or ester of adenylic acid.

a. cyclase, an enzyme acting on ATP to form 3′,5′-cyclic AMP plus pyrophosphate. A crucial step in the regulation and formation of second messengers. SYN 3′,5′-cyclic AMP synthetase.

a. kinase, adenylic acid kinase; a phosphotransferase that catalyzes the reversible phosphorylation of a molecule of ADP by MgADP, yielding MgATP and AMP.

ad·e·nyl·ic ac·id (ad-e-nil′ik). A condensation product of adenosine and phosphoric acid; a nucleotide found among the hydrolysis products of all nucleic acids. SEE ALSO AMP. SYN adenine nucleotide.

a·deps, gen. **adi·pis**, **adi·pes** (ad′eps, ad′i-pis, -pēz). **1.** Denoting fat or adipose tissue. **2.** The rendered fat of swine, lard, used in the preparation of ointments. SYN lard. SEE ALSO a. lanae. [L. lard, fat]

a. lanae, the greasy substance obtained from the wool of the sheep *Ovis aries* (family Bovidae). Used as an emollient base for creams and ointments. [L. fat of wool]

ader·mia (ă-der′mē-ă). Congenital defect or absence of skin. [G. *a*- priv. + *derma*, skin]

ader·mo·gen·e·sis (ă-der-mō-jen′ĕ-sis). Failure or imperfection in the regeneration of the skin, especially the imperfect repair of a cutaneous defect. [G. *a*- priv. + *derma*, skin, + *genesis*, origin]

ad·her·ence (ad-hēr′ens). **1.** The act or quality of sticking to something. SEE ALSO adhesion. **2.** The extent to which a patient continues treatment under limited supervision. Cf. compliance (2), maintenance. [L. *adhaereo*, to stick to]

immune a., the binding of antigen-antibody complexes or cells coated with antibodies or complement to cells bearing the appropriate complement or Fc receptors.

ad·he·sion (ad-hē′zhŭn). **1.** The process of adhering or uniting of two surfaces or parts, especially the union of the opposing surfaces of a wound. SYN conglutination (1). **2.** In the plural, inflammatory bands that connect opposing serous surfaces. **3.** Physical attraction of unlike molecules for one another. **4.** Molecular attraction existing between the surfaces of bodies in contact. [L. *adhaesio*,, fr. *adhaereo*, to stick to]

primary a., SYN *healing* by first intention.

secondary a., SYN *healing* by second intention.

ad·he·si·ot·o·my (ad-hē-sē-ot′ō-mē). Surgical section or lysis of adhesions.

ad·he·sive (ad-hē′siv). **1.** Relating to, or having the characteristics of, an adhesion. **2.** Any material that adheres to a surface or causes adherence between surfaces.

ad·i·ad·o·cho·ki·ne·sis (ă-dī′ă-dō-kō-kin-ē′sis). Inability to perform rapid alternating movements, a sign of cerebellar dysfunction. Cf. diadochokinesia. [G. *a*- priv. + *diadochos*, successive, + *kinēsis*, movement]

adi·a·pho·re·sis (ā′dī-ă-fō-rē′sis). SYN anhidrosis. [G. *a*- priv. + *diaphorēsis*, perspiration]

adi·a·pho·ria (ă-dī-ă-fō′rē-ă). Failure to respond to stimulation after a series of previously applied stimuli. [G. *a*- priv. + *dia*, through, + *phoros*, bearing]

⌂**adip-, adipo-.** Fat, fatty. Corresponds to G. lip-, lipo-. SEE ALSO lipo-. [L. *adeps, adipis*, soft animal fat, lard, grease]

adi·pes (-pēz).

adi·pis (ad′i-pis).

⌂**adipo-.** SEE adip-.

ad·i·po·cel·lu·lar (ad′i-pō-sel′yū-lăr). Relating to both fatty and cellular tissues, or to connective tissue with many fat cells.

ad·i·po·cer·a·tous (ad-i-pō-ser′ă-tŭs). Relating to adipocere. SYN lipoceratous.

ad·i·po·cere (ad′i-pō-sēr). A fatty substance of waxy consistency into which dead animal tissues (as those of a corpse) are sometimes converted when kept from the air under certain favoring conditions of temperature. SYN lipocere. [adipo- + L. *cera*, wax]

ad·i·po·cyte (ad′i-pō-sīt). SYN fat *cell*.

ad·i·po·gen·e·sis (ad′i-pō-jen′ĕ-sis). SYN lipogenesis.

ad·i·po·gen·ic, ad·i·pog·e·nous (ad′i-pō-jen′ik, ad-i-poj′ĕ-nŭs). SYN lipogenic.

ad·i·poid (ad′i-poyd). SYN lipoid. [adipo- + G. *eidos*, resemblance]

ad·i·po·ki·net·ic (ad′i-pō-ki-net′ik). Denoting a substance or factor that causes mobilization of stored lipid. [adipo- + G. *kinēsis*, movement]

ad·i·po·ki·nin (ad-i-pō-kī′nin). An anterior pituitary hormone that causes mobilization of fat from adipose tissue. SYN adipokinetic hormone.

ad·i·pose (ad′i-pōs). Denoting fat.

ad·i·po·sis (ad-i-pō′sis). Excessive local or general accumulation of fat in the body. SYN lipomatosis, liposis (1), steatosis (1). [adipo- + G. *-osis*, condition]

a. cardi′aca, SYN fatty *heart* (2).

ad·i·pos·i·ty (ad-i-pos′i-tē). **1.** SYN obesity. **2.** Excessive accumulation of lipids in a site or organ.

ad·i·po·su·ria (ad′i-pō-sū′rē-ă). SYN lipuria. [adipo- + G. *ouron*, urine]

ad·i·tus, pl. **ad·i·tus** (ad′i-tŭs) [NA]. SYN aperture, inlet. [L. access, fr. *ad-eo*, pp. *-itus*, go to]

ad·ju·vant (ad′jū-vănt). **1.** A substance added to a drug product formulation which affects the action of the active ingredient in a predictable way. **2.** IMMUNOLOGY a vehicle used to enhance antigenicity; *e.g.,* a suspension of minerals (alum, aluminum hydroxide or phosphate) on which antigen is adsorbed; or water-in-oil emulsion in which antigen solution is emulsified in mineral oil (Freund's incomplete a.), sometimes with the inclusion of killed mycobacteria (Freund's complete a.) to further enhance antigenicity. [L. *adjuvo*, pres. p. *-juvans*, to give aid to]

ADL. activities of daily living. SEE activities of daily living *scale*.

ad lib. L. *ad libitum*, freely, as desired.

admixture (ad-miks-chur). A product of mixing.

venous a., the mingling in the pulmonary circulation of arterial blood and desaturated blood resulting from ventilation-perfusion mismatching (reduced ventilation with full perfusion).

ad·ner·val (ad-ner′văl). SYN adneural.

ad·neu·ral (ad-nūr′ăl). **1.** Lying near a nerve. **2.** In the direction of a nerve; said of an electric current passing through muscular tissue toward the point of entrance of the nerve. SYN adnerval.

ad•nexa, sing. **ad•nex•um** (ad-nek′să, -sŭm). Parts accessory to the main organ or structure. SEE ALSO appendage. SYN annexa. [L. connected parts]

ad•nex•al (ad-nek′săl). Relating to the adnexa. SYN annexal.

ad•nex•um (ad-nek′sŭm). Singular of adnexa.

Ado adenosine.

ad•o•les•cence (ad-ō-les′ens). The period of life beginning with puberty and ending with physical maturity. [L. *adolescentia*]

ad•o•les•cent (ad-ō-les′ent). **1.** Pertaining to adolescence. **2.** An individual in that stage of development.

ADP adenosine 5′-diphosphate.

ADR adverse drug *reaction.*

△**adren-.** SEE adreno-.

ad•re•nal (ă-drē′năl). **1.** Near or upon the kidney; denoting the suprarenal (adrenal) gland. **2.** A suprarenal gland or separate tissue or product thereof. [L. *ad*, to, + *ren*, kidney]

 accessory a., an island of cortical tissue separate from the adrenal gland, usually found in the retroperitoneal tissues, kidney, or genital organs. SYN adrenal rest.

ad•re•nal•ec•to•my (ă-drē-năl-ek′tō-mē). Removal of one or both adrenal glands. [adrenal + G. *ektomē*, excision]

ad•ren•a•line. SYN epinephrine.

adre•nal•i•tis (ă-drē-năl-ī′tis). Inflammation of the adrenal gland.

adre•na•lop•a•thy (ă-drē-nă-lop′ă-thē). Any pathologic condition of the adrenal glands. SYN adrenopathy. [adrenal + G. *pathos*, suffering]

ad•re•ner•gic (ad-rĕ-ner′jik). **1.** Relating to nerve cells or fibers of the autonomic nervous system that employ norepinephrine as their neurotransmitter. Cf. cholinergic. **2.** Relating to drugs that mimic the actions of the sympathetic nervous system. SEE α-adrenergic *receptors,* under *receptor,* β-adrenergic *receptors,* under *receptor.* [adren- + G. *ergon,* work]

adren•ic (ă-drē′nik). Relating to the suprarenal gland.

△**adreno-, adrenal-, adren-.** Relating to the adrenal gland. [L. *ad,* to, near, + *renes,* the kidneys, + -o- + -*alis,* pertaining to]

adre•no•cep•tive (ă-dren-ō-sep′tiv). Referring to chemical sites in effectors with which the adrenergic mediator unites. Cf. cholinoceptive.

adre•no•cor•ti•cal (ă-drē-nō-kōr′ti-kăl). Pertaining to suprarenal cortex.

adre•no•cor•ti•co•mi•met•ic (ă-drē′nō-kōr′ti-kō-mi-met′ik). Mimicking or producing effects similar to adrenocortical function. [adrenal + cortex + G. *mimētikos,* imitating]

adre•no•gen•ic, adre•nog•e•nous (ă-drē-nō-jen′ik, a-drĕ-noj′ē-nŭs). Of adrenal origin. [adreno- + G. -*gen,* producing]

adre•no•lyt•ic (ă-dren-ō-lit′ik). Denoting antagonism to or inhibition or blockade of the action of epinephrine, norepinephrine, and related sympathomimetics. SEE ALSO adrenergic blocking *agent.* [adreno- + G. *lysis,* loosening, dissolution]

adre•no•meg•a•ly (ă-drē-nō-meg′ă-lē). Enlarge-

ment of the adrenal glands. [adreno- + G. *megas,* big]

adre•no•mi•met•ic (ă-drē′nō-mi-met′ik). Having an action similar to that of the compounds epinephrine and norepinephrine; a term proposed to replace the less specific term, sympathomimetic. Cf. adrenergic, cholinomimetic. [adreno- + G. *mimētikos,* imitative]

adre•no•my•e•lo•neu•rop•a•thy (ad-rē′nō-mī′e-lō-nū-rop′ă-thē). A disorder of adult males, consisting of long-standing adrenal insufficiency, hypogonadism, progressive myelopathy, peripheral neuropathy, and sphincter disturbances; considered a variant of adrenoleukodystrophy. [adreno- + G. *myelos,* medulla, + *neuron,* nerve, + *pathos,* suffering]

adre•nop•a•thy (ă-drē-nop′ă-thē). SYN adrenalopathy.

adre•no•re•cep•tors (ă-drē′nō-rē-sep′terz). SYN adrenergic *receptors,* under *receptor.*

adre•no•tro•pin (ă-drē-nō-trō′pin). SYN adrenocorticotropic *hormone.*

ad sat. L. *ad saturatum,* to saturation.

ad•sorb (ad-sōrb′). To take up by adsorption. [L. *ad,* to, + *sorbeo,* to suck in]

ad•sorb•ent (ad-sōr′bent). **1.** A solid substance with the property of attaching other substances to its surface without covalent bonding. **2.** An antigen or antibody used in immune adsorption.

ad•sorp•tion (ad-sōrp′shŭn). The property of a solid substance to attract and hold to its surface a gas, liquid, or a substance in solution or in suspension. Cf. absorption. [L. *ad,* to, + *sorbeo,* to suck up]

 immune a., (1) removal of antibody from antiserum by use of specific antigen. **(2)** removal of antigen by specific antiserum.

adst. feb. (L.) adstante febre, when fever is present.

ad•ter•mi•nal (ad-ter′mi-năl). In a direction toward the nerve endings, muscular insertions, or the extremity of any structure.

adult (ă-dŭlt′). **1.** Fully grown and physically mature. **2.** A fully grown and mature individual. [L. *adultus,* grown up fr. *adolesco,* to grow up]

adul•ter•ant (ă-dŭl′ter-ănt). An impurity; an additive that is considered to have an undesirable effect or to dilute the active material so as to reduce its therapeutic or monetary value.

adul•ter•a•tion (ă-dŭl-ter-ā′shŭn). The alteration of any substance by the deliberate addition of a component not ordinarily part of that substance; usually used to imply that the substance is debased as a result.

ad us. ext. (L.) ad usum externum, for external use.

advance directive. A legal document with written instructions signed by the patient (or the patient's next of kin if the patient cannot sign) as to what type of care measures and services are or are not to be provided to prolong life in the event of a life-threatening illness. SYN durable power of attorney.

ad•vanced life sup•port. Definitive emergency medical care that includes defibrillation, airway management, and use of drugs and medications. Cf. basic life support.

ad·vance·ment (ad-vans'ment). Surgical procedure in which a ligamentous or partially tendinous insertion or a skin flap is partially severed or released from its attachment and sutured to a more distal point.

ad·ven·ti·tia (ad-ven-tish'ă). The outermost connective tissue covering of any organ, vessel, or other structure not covered by a serosa. SYN membrana adventitia (1). [L. *adventicius,* coming from abroad, foreign, fr. *ad,* to + *venio,* to come]

ad·ven·ti·tial (ad-ven-tish'ăl). Relating to the outer coat or adventitia of a blood vessel or other structure. SYN adventitious (3).

ad·ven·ti·tious (ad-ven-tish'ŭs). **1.** Arising from an external source or occurring in an unusual place or manner. SEE ALSO extrinsic. **2.** Occurring accidentally or spontaneously, as opposed to natural causes or hereditary. **3.** SYN adventitial.

△**ae-.** For words so beginning and not found here, see under e-.

Aedes (ā-ē'dēz). A widespread genus of small mosquitoes frequently found in tropical and subtropical regions; various species are vectors for yellow fever, dengue, and other human diseases. [G. *aēdēs,* unpleasant, unfriendly]

△**aer-, aero-.** The air, a gas; aerial, gassy. [G. *aēr* (L. *aer*), air]

aer·ate (ār'āte). **1.** To supply (blood) with oxygen. **2.** To expose to the circulation of air for purification. **3.** To supply or charge (liquid) with a gas, especially carbon dioxide.

△**aero-.** SEE aer-.

aer·obe (ār'ōb). **1.** An organism that can live and grow in the presence of oxygen. **2.** An organism that can use oxygen as a final electron acceptor in a respiratory chain. [aero- + G. *bios,* life]

obligate a., an organism which cannot live or grow in the absence of oxygen.

aer·o·bic (ār-ō'bik). **1.** Living in air. **2.** Relating to an aerobe. SYN aerophilic, aerophilous.

aer·o·bi·o·sis (ār-ō-bī-ō'sis). Existence in an atmosphere containing oxygen. [aero- + G. *biōsis,* mode of living]

aer·o·bi·ot·ic (ār-ō-bī-ot'ik). Relating to aerobiosis.

aer·o·cele (ār'ō-sēl). Distention of a small natural cavity with gas. [aero- + G. *kēlē,* tumor]

aer·o·col·pos (ār-ō-kol'pos). Distention of the vagina with gas. [aero- + G. *kolpos,* lap, hollow]

aer·o·don·tal·gia (ār'ō-don-tal'jē-ă). Dental pain caused by either increased or reduced atmospheric pressure. [aero- + G. *odous,* tooth, + *algos,* pain]

aer·o·dy·nam·ics (ār'ō-dī-nam'iks). The study of air and other gases in motion, the forces that set them in motion, and the results of such motion. [aero- + G. *dynamis,* force]

aer·o·pha·gia, aer·oph·a·gy (ār-ō-fā'jē-ă, -of'ă-jē). An abnormal swallowing of air as seen in crib-biting and wind-sucking. [aero- + G. *phagō,* to eat]

aer·o·phil, aer·o·phile (ār'ō-fil, -fīl). **1.** Air-loving. **2.** An aerobic organism (aerobe), especially an obligate aerobe. [aero- + G. *philos,* fond]

aer·o·phil·ic, aer·oph·i·lous (ār-ō-fil'ik, ār-of'i-lŭs). SYN aerobic.

aer·o·pho·bia (ār-ō-fō'bē-ă). Morbid dread of fresh air or of air in motion. [aero- + G. *phobos,* fear]

aer·o·pi·e·so·ther·a·py (ār'ō-pī-ē'sō-thār'ă-pē). Treatment of disease by compressed (or rarified) air. [aero- + G. *piesis,* pressure, + *therapeia,* medical treatment]

aer·o·si·nus·i·tis (ār-ō-sī-nŭ-sī'tis). Inflammation of the paranasal sinuses caused by pressure difference within the sinus relative to ambient pressure, secondary to obstruction of the sinus orifice, sometimes due to high altitude flying or by descent from high altitude. SYN barosinusitis.

aer·o·sol (ār'ō-sol). **1.** Liquid or particulate matter dispersed in air in the form of a fine mist for therapeutic, insecticidal, or other purposes. **2.** A product that is packaged under pressure and contains therapeutically or chemically active ingredients intended for topical application, inhalation, or introduction into body orifices. [aero- + solution]

mainstream a., a system for administering an aerosol that directs the mainstream of inspired airflow through the aerosol generator.

sidestream a., a system for administering an aerosol that adds the aerosol through a side connection into the mainstream of inspired airflow.

aer·o·ti·tis me·dia (ār-ō-tī'tis mē'dē-ă). An acute or chronic inflammation of the middle ear caused by a reduction in pressure in the tympanic cavity relative to ambient pressure, secondary to auditory tube obstruction; often occurs on descent from high altitude. SYN barotitis media. [aero- + G. *ous,* ear, + *-itis,* inflammation]

aes·cu·la·pi·an (es-kyū-lā'pē-an). Relating to Aesculapius, the art of medicine, or a medical practitioner. [L. *Aesculapius,* G. *Asklēpios,* the god of medicine]

AFB Acid-fast bacillus. SEE acid-fast.

afe·brile (ā-feb'ril). SYN apyretic.

afe·tal (ă-fē'tăl). Without relation to a fetus or intrauterine life.

af·fect (af'fekt). The emotional feeling, tone, and mood attached to a thought, including its external manifestations. [L. *affectus,* state of mind, fr. *afficio,* to have influence on]

blunted a., a disturbance in mood seen in schizophrenic patients manifested by shallowness and a severe reduction in the expression of feeling.

af·fec·tion (ă-fek'shŭn). **1.** A moderate feeling of tenderness, caring, or love. **2.** An abnormal condition of body or mind. [L. *affectio,* fr. *af-ficio,* to affect, influence]

af·fec·tive (af-fek'tiv). Pertaining to mood, emotion, feeling, sensibility, or a mental state.

af·fer·ent (af'er-ent). Inflowing; conducting toward a center, denoting certain arteries, veins, lymphatics, and nerves. Opposite of efferent. SYN centripetal (1). [L. *afferens,* fr. *af-fero,* to bring to]

af·fin·i·ty (ă-fin'i-tē). **1.** CHEMISTRY The force that impels certain atoms to unite with certain others. **2.** Selective staining of a tissue by a dye. **3.** The strength of binding between a Fab site of an antibody and an antigenic determinant. [L. *affinis,* neighboring, fr. *ad,* to, + *finis,* end, boundary]

afi·bril·lar (ā-fī′bri-lăr). Denoting a biological structure that does not contain fibrils.

afi·brin·o·gen·e·mia (ā-fī′brin-ō-jĕ-nē′mē-ă). The absence of fibrinogen in the plasma. SEE ALSO hypofibrinogenemia.

  congenital a. [MIM*202400], a rare disorder of blood coagulation in which little or no fibrinogen can be found in plasma.

Afipia felis. A Gram-negative bacterium that causes one form of cat-scratch *disease.*

AFP Abbreviation for α-*fetoproteins.* SEE fetoproteins.

af·ter·birth (af′ter-berth). The placenta and membranes that are extruded from the uterus after birth. SYN secundines.

af·ter·im·age (af′ter-im′ij). Persistence of a visual response after cessation of the stimulus.

af·ter·im·pres·sion (af′ter-im-presh′ŭn). SYN aftersensation.

af·ter·load (af′ter-lōd). **1.** The arrangement of a muscle so that, in shortening, it lifts a weight from an adjustable support or otherwise does work against a constant opposing force to which it is not exposed at rest. **2.** The load or force thus encountered in shortening.

af·ter·pains (af′ter-pānz). Painful cramplike contractions of the uterus occurring after childbirth.

af·ter·per·cep·tion (af′ter-per-sep′shŭn). Subjective persistence of a stimulus after its cessation. Cf. palinopsia.

af·ter·po·ten·tial (af′ter-pō-ten′shăl). The small change in electrical potential in a stimulated nerve that follows the main, or spike, potential; it consists of an initial negative deflection followed by a positive deflection in the oscillograph record.

af·ter·sen·sa·tion (af′ter-sen-sā′shŭn). Subjective persistence of sensation after cessation of stimulus. SYN afterimpression.

af·ter·sound (af′ter-sownd). Subjective persistence of an auditory stimulus after cessation of the stimulus.

af·ter·taste (af′ter-tāst). Subjective persistence of a gustatory stimulus after contact with the stimulating substance has ceased.

Ag 1. silver (argentum). **2.** antigen.

ag·a·lac·tia (ă-gal-ak′shē-ă). Absence of milk in the breasts after childbirth. SYN agalactosis. [G. *a-* priv. + *gala* (*galakt-*), milk]

aga·lac·tor·rhea (ā-ga-lak-tō-rē′ă). Absence of the secretion or flow of breast milk. [G. *a-* priv. + *gala,* milk, + *rhoia,* a flow]

ag·a·lac·to·sis (ă-gal-ak-tō′sis). SYN agalactia.

ag·a·lac·tous (ă-gal-ak′tŭs). Relating to agalactia, or to the diminution or absence of breast milk.

agam·ic (ā-gam′ik). Denoting nonsexual reproduction, as by fission, budding, etc. SYN agamous.

agam·ma·glob·u·lin·e·mia (ā-gam′ă-glob′yū-li-nē′mē-ă). Absence of, or extremely low levels of, the gamma fraction of serum globulin; sometimes used loosely to denote absence of immunoglobulins in general. SEE ALSO hypogammaglobulinemia.

ag·a·mous (ag′ă-mŭs). SYN agamic. [G. *agamos,* unmarried]

agan·gli·on·ic (ā-gang-glē-on′ik). Without ganglia.

agan·gli·o·no·sis (ā-gang′glē-ō-nō′sis). The state of being without ganglia; *e.g.,* absence of ganglion cells from the myenteric plexus as a characteristic of congenital megacolon. [G. ā- priv. + ganglion + *-osis,* condition]

agar (ah′gar, ā′gar). A polysaccharide derived from seaweed; used as a solidifying agent in culture media. [Bengalese]

  eosin-methylene blue a., a. composed of peptone, lactose, and sucrose and containing eosin and methylene blue, used to distinguish between lactose-fermenting and non-lactose-fermenting Gram-negative bacteria.

  MacConkey a., medium containing peptone, lactose, bile salts, neutral red, and crystal violet, used to identify Gram-negative bacilli and characterize them according to their status as lactose fermenters. Fermenters appear as red colonies while nonfermenters are colorless.

  Sabouraud's dextrose a., a dextrose peptone medium that supports the growth of most pathogenic fungi.

  Thayer-Martin a., a Mueller-Hinton a. with 5% heat-hemolyzed sheep blood and antibiotics, used for transport and primary isolation of *Neisseria gonorrhoeae* and *Neisseria meningitidis.*

agas·tric (ă-gas′trik). Without stomach or digestive tract. [G. *a-* priv. + *gastēr,* belly]

age (āj). **1.** The period that has elapsed since birth. **2.** One of the periods into which human life is divided, distinguished by physical evolution, equilibrium, and involution; *e.g.,* the seven a.'s of man are: infancy, childhood, adolescence, maturity, middle life, senescence, and senility. **3.** To grow old; to gradually develop changes in structure that are not due to preventable disease or trauma and that are associated with decreased functional capacity and an increased probability of death. **4.** To cause artificially the appearance characteristic of one who has lived long or of a thing that has existed for a long time. **5.** DENTISTRY to heat an alloy for amalgam so as to make it set more slowly, increase strength, reduce flow, and have a stable shelf life. Aging occurs by relieving internal strains. [F. *âge,* L. *aetas*]

  achievement a., the relationship between the chronologic age and the age of achievement, as established by standard achievement tests.

  chronologic a. (CA), a. expressed in years and months; used as a measurement against which to evaluate a child's mental a. in computing the Stanford-Binet intelligence quotient.

  developmental a., (1) age estimated by anatomic development since implantation; **(2) (DA),** age of an individual estimated from the degree of anatomic, physiologic, mental, and emotional maturation.

  gestational a., the a. of a fetus expressed in elapsed time since conception; usually measured from the first day of the last normal menstrual period.

  mental a. (MA), a measure, expressed in years and months, of a child's intelligence relative to age norms as determined by testing with the Stanford-Binet intelligence scale.

ag

agen•e•sis (ă-jen′ĕ-sis). Absence, failure of formation, or imperfect development of any part. [G. *a-* priv. + *genesis,* production]

agen•i•tal•ism (ă-jen′i-tal-izm). Congenital absence of genitalia.

agen•o•so•mia (ă-gen-ō-sō′mē-ă). Markedly defective formation or absence of the genitalia in a fetus; usually accompanied by protrusion of the abdominal viscera through an incomplete abdominal wall. [G. *a-* priv. + *genos,* sex, + *soma,* body]

agent (ā′jent). **1.** An active force or substance capable of producing an effect. For agents not listed here, see the specific name. **2.** Referring to disease, a factor such as a microorganism, chemical substance, or form of radiation whose presence or absence (as in deficiency diseases) is essential for the occurrence of a disease. [L. *ago,* pres. p. *agens* (*agent-*), to perform]

adrenergic blocking a., a compound that selectively blocks or inhibits responses to sympathetic adrenergic nerve activity (sympatholytic a.) and to epinephrine, norepinephrine, and other adrenergic amines (adrenolytic a.); two distinct classes exist, alpha- and beta-adrenergic receptor blocking a.'s.

α-adrenergic blocking a., an agent that competitively blocks α-adrenergic receptors; used in the treatment of hypertension.

β-adrenergic blocking a., a class of drugs that compete with β-adrenergic agonists for available receptor sites; some compete for both β_1 and β_2 receptors (*e.g.,* propranolol) while others are primarily either β_1 (*e.g.,* metoprolol) or β_2 blockers; used in the treatment of a variety of cardiovascular diseases where β-adrenergic blockade is desirable. SYN beta-blocker.

adrenergic neuronal blocking a., a drug that prevents the release of norepinephrine from sympathetic nerve terminals.

antianxiety a., a functional category of drugs useful in the treatment of anxiety and able to reduce anxiety at doses which do not cause excessive sedation (*e.g.,* diazepam). SYN anxiolytic (1).

antipsychotic a., a functional category of neuroleptic drugs that are helpful in the treatment of psychosis and have a capacity to ameliorate thought disorders (*e.g.,* chlorpromazine, haloperidol). SYN antipsychotic (1).

blocking a., a class of drugs that inhibit (block) a biologic activity or process; frequently called "blockers."

calcium channel-blocking a., a class of drugs that have the ability to inhibit movement of calcium ions across the cell membrane; of value in the treatment of cardiovascular disorders. SYN slow channel-blocking a.

delta a., SYN hepatitis D *virus.*

disclosing a., selective dye in solution, tablet, or lozenge form used to visualize and identify bacterial plaque on the surfaces of the teeth.

Eaton a., SYN *Mycoplasma pneumoniae.*

ganglionic blocking a., an a. that impairs the passage of impulses in autonomic ganglia.

initiating a., SEE initiation.

neuroleptic a., SYN neuroleptic (1).

physical a., a form of acoustical, aqueous, electrical, mechanical, thermal, or light energy applied to living tissues in a systematic manner to alter physiological processes, in conjunction with or for therapeutic purposes. SEE modality.

Pittsburgh pneumonia a., SYN *Legionella micdadei.*

promoting a., SEE promotion.

slow channel-blocking a., SYN calcium channel-blocking a.

ageu•sia (ă-gū′sē-ă). Loss of the sense of taste. [G. *a-* priv. + *geusis,* taste]

ag•glu•ti•nant (ă-glū′ti-nant). A substance that holds parts together or causes agglutination. [L. *ad,* to + *gluten,* glue]

ag•glu•ti•na•tion (ă-glū-ti-nā′shŭn). **1.** The process by which suspended bacteria, cells, or other particles are caused to adhere and form clumps; similar to precipitation, but the particles are larger and are in suspension rather than being in solution. For specific a. reactions in the various blood groups, see Blood Groups appendix. **2.** Adhesion of the surfaces of a wound. [L. *ad,* to, + *gluten,* glue]

bacteriogenic a., the clumping of erythrocytes as a result of effects of bacteria or their products.

cold a., a. of red blood cells by their own serum (see autoagglutination), or by any other serum when the blood is cooled below body temperature; seen occasionally in the blood of normal persons or as a pathologic finding in mycoplasmal pneumonia, infectious mononucleosis, certain protozoan infections, or lymphoproliferative neoplasms. SEE autoagglutination.

group a., a. by antibodies specific for minor (group) antigens common to several microorganisms, each of which possesses its own major specific antigen.

ag•glu•ti•na•tive (ă-glū′ti-nă-tiv). Causing, or able to cause, agglutination.

ag•glu•ti•nin (ă-glū′ti-nin). **1.** An antibody that causes clumping or agglutination of the bacteria or other cells which either stimulated the formation of the a., or contain immunologically similar, reactive antigen. **2.** A substance, other than a specific agglutinating antibody, that causes organic particles to agglutinate.

chief a., SYN major a.

cold a., an antibody which reacts more efficiently at temperatures below 37°C.

cross-reacting a., SYN group a.

group a., an immune a. specific for a group antigen. SYN cross-reacting a.

H a., (1) an a. that is formed as the result of stimulation by, and which reacts with, the thermolabile antigen(s) in the flagella of motile strains of microorganisms; (2) see ABO blood group, Blood Groups appendix.

major a., immune a. present in greatest quantity in an antiserum and evoked by the most dominant of a mosaic of antigens. SYN chief a.

minor a., immune a. present in an antiserum in lesser concentration than the major a. SYN partial a.

O a., (1) an a. that is formed as the result of stimulation by, and that reacts with, the relatively thermostable antigen(s) in the cell bodies of microorganisms; **(2)** see ABO blood group, Blood Groups appendix.

  partial a., SYN minor a.

  saline a., an antibody which causes agglutination of erythrocytes when they are suspended either in saline or in a protein medium. SYN complete antibody.

  serum a., an antibody which coats erythrocytes; the cells do not agglutinate when suspended in saline, but do agglutinate when suspended in serum or other protein media such as albumin. SYN incomplete antibody (2).

ag·glu·tin·o·gen (ă-glū-tin′ō-jen). An antigenic substance that stimulates the formation of specific agglutinin, which, under certain conditions, causes agglutination of cells that contain the antigen or particles coated with the antigen. SYN agglutogen. [agglutinin + G. *-gen,* production]

ag·glu·tin·o·gen·ic (ă-glū′tin-ō-jen′ik). Capable of causing the production of an agglutinin. SYN agglutogenic.

ag·glu·tin·o·phil·ic (ă-glū′tin-ō-fil′ik). Readily undergoing agglutination. [agglutination + G. *phileō,* to love]

ag·glu·to·gen (ă-glū′tō-jen). SYN agglutinogen.

ag·glu·to·gen·ic (ă-glū-tō-jen′ik). SYN agglutinogenic.

ag·gre·gate (ag′rĕ-gāt). **1.** To unite or come together in a mass or cluster. **2.** The total of individual units making up a mass or cluster. [L. *aggrego,* pp. *-atus,* to add to, fr. *grex* (greg-), a flock]

ag·gre·ga·tion (ag-rĕ-gā′shŭn). A crowded mass of independent but similar units; a cluster.

  familial a., occurrence of a trait in more members of a family than can be readily accounted for by chance; presumptive but not cogent evidence of the operation of genetic factors.

ag·gres·sion (ă-gresh′ŭn). A domineering, forceful, or assaultive verbal or physical action toward another person as the motor component of anger, hostility, or rage. [L. *aggressio,* fr. *aggredior,* to accost, attack]

ag·gres·sive (ă-gres′iv). **1.** Denoting aggression. **2.** Denoting a competitive forcefulness or invasiveness, as of a behavioral pattern, a pathogenic organism, or a disease process.

ag·ing (ā′jing). **1.** The process of growing old, especially by failure of replacement of cells in sufficient number to maintain full functional capacity; particularly affects cells (*e.g.,* neurons) incapable of mitotic division. **2.** The gradual deterioration of a mature organism resulting from time-dependent, irreversible changes in structure. **3.** In the cardiovascular system, the progressive replacement of functional cell types by fibrous connective tissue. **4.** A demographic term, meaning an increase over time in the proportion of older persons in the population.

agit. ante us. (L.) agita ante usum, shake before using.

agit. bene. (L.) agita bene, shake well.

aglos·so·sto·mia (ă-glos-ō-stō′mē-ă). Congenital absence of the tongue, with a malformed (usually closed) mouth. [G. *a-* priv. + *glōssa,* tongue, + *stoma,* mouth]

ag·lu·ti·tion (ā-glū-tish′ŭn). SYN dysphagia.

agly·cos·u·ria (ā-glī-kō-sū′rē-ă). Absence of carbohydrate in the urine.

agly·cos·u·ric (ă-glī-kō-sū′rik). Relating to aglycosuria.

ag·na·thia (ag-nā′thē-ă). Congenital absence of the lower jaw, usually accompanied by approximation of the ears. SEE ALSO otocephaly, synotia. [G. *a-* priv. + *gnathos,* jaw]

ag·na·thous (ag′nā-thŭs). Relating to agnathia.

ag·no·gen·ic (ag-nō-jen′ik). SYN idiopathic. [G. *a-* priv. + *gnosis,* knowledge, + *genesis,* origin]

ag·no·sia (ag-nō′zē-ă). Impairment of ability to recognize, or comprehend the meaning of, various sensory stimuli, not attributable to disorders of the primary receptors or general intellect; a.'s are receptive defects caused by lesions in various portions of the cerebrum. [G. ignorance; from *a-* priv. + *gnōsis,* knowledge]

  auditory a., inability to recognize sounds, words, or music; caused by a lesion of the auditory cortex of the temporal lobe.

  color a., inability to name or identify colors; caused by lesions of the dominant occipital and temporal lobes.

  finger a., inability to name or recognize individual fingers, of one's own or of other persons; most often caused by lesion of or near the angular gyrus of the dominant hemisphere.

  tactile a., inability to recognize objects by touch, in the presence of intact cutaneous and proprioceptive hand sensation; caused by a lesion in the contralateral parietal lobe. SYN astereognosis.

  visual a., inability to recognize objects by sight; usually caused by bilateral parieto-occipital lesions.

△**-agogue, -agog.** Leading, promoting, stimulating; a promoter or stimulant of. [G. *agōgos,* leading forth, fr. *agō,* to lead.]

agom·pho·sis, agom·phi·a·sis (ag-om-fō′sis, fī′ă-sis). SYN anodontia. [G. *a-* priv. + *gomphos,* peg, bolt]

ago·nad·al (ă-gon′ă-dăl). Denoting the absence of gonads.

ag·o·nist (ag′on-ist). **1.** Denoting a muscle in a state of contraction, with reference to its opposing muscle, or antagonist. **2.** A drug capable of combining with receptors to initiate drug actions; it possesses affinity and intrinsic activity. [G. *agōn,* a contest]

ag·o·ra·pho·bia (ag′ōr-ă-fō′bē-ă). A mental disorder characterized by an irrational fear of leaving the familiar setting of home, or venturing into the open; often associated with panic attacks. [G. *agora,* marketplace, + *phobos,* fear]

agor·a·pho·bic (ă-gōr-ă-fō′bik). Relating to or characteristic of agoraphobia.

△**-agra.** Sudden onslaught of acute pain. [G. *agra,* a hunting, a catching, a trap]

agram·ma·tism (ā-gram′ă-tizm). A form of aphasia characterized by an inability to construct a grammatical sentence, and the use of unintelligible or incorrect words; caused by a lesion in the dominant temporal lobe. SYN jargon aphasia.

agran·u·lo·cyte (ă-gran′yū-lō-sīt). A nongranular leukocyte. [G. *a-* priv. + L. *granulum,* granule, + G. *kytos,* cell]

agran·u·lo·cy·to·sis (ă-gran′yū-lō-sī-tō′sis). An acute condition characterized by pronounced leukopenia; infected ulcers are likely to develop in the throat, intestinal tract, and other mucous membranes, as well as in the skin.

agran·u·lo·plas·tic (ă-gran′yū-lō-plas′tik). Capable of forming nongranular cells, and incapable of forming granular cells. [G. *a-* priv. + L. *granulum,* granule, + G. *plastikos,* formative]

agraph·ia (ă-graf′ē-ă). Inability to write properly in the absence of abnormalities of the limb; often accompanies aphasia and alexia; caused by lesions in various portions of the cerebrum. SYN anorthography, logagraphia. [G. *a-* priv. + *graphō,* to write]

agraph·ic (ă-graf′ik). Relating to or marked by agraphia.

agre·tope (ag-rē′tōp). That part of a processed antigen that binds to the major histocompatibility complex molecule. [*antigen* + *restriction* + *-tope*]

agy·ria (ă-jī′rē-ă). Congenital lack or underdevelopment of the convolutional pattern of the cerebral cortex. SYN lissencephalia. [G. *a-* priv. + *gyros,* circle]

AHF antihemophilic *factor* A.

AHIMA American Health Information Management *Association.*

AID artificial insemination donor.

ergogenic aid, application of a nutritional, physical, mechanical, psychologic, or pharmacologic procedure or aid to improve physical work capacity or athletic performance.

⊞**AIDS** (ādz). A syndrome of the immune system characterized by opportunistic diseases, including candidiasis, *Pneumocystis carinii* pneumonia, oral hairy leukoplakia, herpes zoster, Kaposi's sarcoma, toxoplasmosis, isosporiasis, cryptococcosis, non-Hodgkin's lymphoma, and tuberculosis. The syndrome is caused by the human immunodeficiency virus (HIV-1, HIV-2), which is transmitted in body fluids (notably blood and semen) through sexual contact, sharing of contaminated needles (by IV drug abusers), accidental needle sticks, contact with contaminated blood, or transfusion of contaminated blood or blood products. Hallmark of the immunodeficiency is depletion of $T4^+$ helper/inducer lymphocytes, primarily the result of selective tropism of the virus for the lymphocytes. SYN acquired immunodeficiency syndrome.

AIH artificial insemination (homologous).

ai·lu·ro·pho·bia (ī′lū-rō-fō′bē-ă, ā′lu-). Morbid fear of or aversion to cats. [G. *ailouros,* cat, + *phobos,* fear]

AIR 5-aminoimidazole ribose 5′-phosphate; 5-aminoimidazole ribotide.

air (ār). **1.** A mixture of odorless gases found in the atmosphere in the following approximate percentages: oxygen, 20.95; nitrogen, 78.08; argon 0.93; carbon dioxide, 0.03; other gases, 0.01. **2.** SYN ventilate. [G. *aēr;* L. *aer*]

alveolar a., SYN alveolar *gas.*

complemental a., SYN inspiratory reserve *volume.*

complementary a., SYN inspiratory *capacity.*

functional residual a., SYN functional residual *capacity.*

a. hunger, extremely deep ventilation such as occurs in patients with acidosis attempting to increase ventilation of alveoli and exhale more carbon dioxide. SEE ALSO Kussmaul *respiration.*

reserve a., SYN expiratory reserve *volume.*

residual a., SYN residual *volume.*

supplemental a., SYN expiratory reserve *volume.*

tidal a., SYN tidal *volume.*

Airbrasive (ār-brā′sive). Air-powered teeth-polishing device using air and water pressure to deliver a stream of specially processed sodium bicarbonate slurry mixture through a handpiece nozzle.

air·trap·ping (ār-trap′ing). Slow or incomplete emptying of air from all or part of a lung on expiration; implies obstruction of regional airways or emphysema.

air·way (ār′wā). **1.** Any part of the respiratory tract through which air passes during breathing. **2.** In anesthesia or resuscitation, a device for correcting obstruction to breathing, especially an oropharyngeal and nasopharyngeal a., endotracheal a., or tracheotomy tube.

lower a., the portion of the respiratory tract that extends from the subglottis to and including the terminal bronchioles.

a. management, assistance given to a patient in maintaining a patent airway, with or without intubation.

upper a., the portion of the respiratory tract that extends from the nares or mouth to and including the larynx.

akar·y·o·cyte (ā-kar′ē-ō-sīt). A cell without a nucleus, such as the erythrocyte. SYN acaryote, akaryote. [G. *a-* priv. + *karyon,* kernel, + *kytos,* a hollow (cell)]

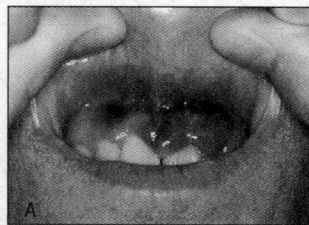
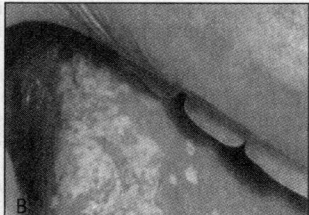
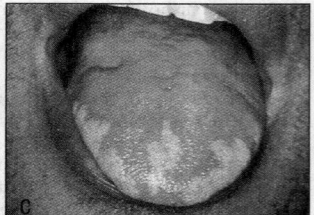

AIDS: oral lesions associated with AIDS: (A) Kaposi's sarcoma, (B) candida albicans, (C) hairy leukoplakia

akar•y•ote (ā-kar′ē-ōt). SYN akaryocyte. [G. *a*-priv. + *karyon,* kernel]

a•ka•thi•sia (ak-ă-thiz′ē-ă). A syndrome characterized by an inability to remain in a sitting posture, with motor restlessness and a feeling of muscular quivering; may appear as a side effect of antipsychotic and neuroleptic medication. [G. *a*- priv. + *kathisis,* a sitting]

aker•a•to•sis (ă-ker-ă-tō′sis). Deficiency or absence of the horny layer of the epidermis.

aki•ne•sia (ā-ki-nē′sē-ă, ā-kī-). Absence or loss of the power of voluntary movement, due to an extrapyramidal disorder. SYN akinesis. [G. *a*-priv. + *kinēsis,* movement]

aki•ne•sic (ā-ki-nē′sik, ā-kī-). SYN akinetic.

aki•ne•sis (ā-ki-nē′sis, ā-kī-). SYN akinesia.

akin•es•the•sia (ā-kin′es-thē′zē-ă). Inability to perceive movement or position. [G. *a*- priv. + *kinēsis,* motion, + *aisthēsis,* sensation]

aki•net•ic (ā-ki-net′ik, -kī-net′ik). Relating to or suffering from akinesia. SYN akinesic.

Al aluminum.

ALA δ-aminolevulinic acid. Cf. Ala.

Ala alanine or its mono- or diradical.

ala, gen. and pl. **alae** (ā′lă, ā′lē). [NA] SYN wing. [L. wing]

ala•lia (ă-la′lē-ă). Mutism; inability to speak. SEE aphonia. [G. *a*- priv. + *lalia,* talking]

al•a•nine (A, Ala) (al′ă-nēn). 2-aminopropionic acid; α-aminopropionic acid; one of the amino acids widely occurring in proteins.

al•a•nine ami•no•trans•fer•ase (ALT) (al′ă-nēn ă-mē′nō-trans′fer-āz). An enzyme transferring amino groups from L-alanine to 2-ketoglutarate, or the reverse (from L-glutamate to pyruvate); serum concerntration is increased in viral hepatitis and myocardial infarction. SYN glutamic-pyruvic transaminase, serum glutamic-pyruvic transaminase.

al•a•nyl (al′ă-nil). The acyl radical of alanine.

alar (ā′lăr). **1.** Relating to a wing; winged. **2.** SYN axillary. **3.** Relating to the wings (alae) of such structures as the nose, sphenoid, sacrum, etc.

ALARA. Acronym for a philosophy of use of radiation based on using dosages *as low as rea-*sonably *a*hchievable to attain the desired diagnostic, therapeutic, or other goal.

al•ba (al′bă). SYN white *matter.* [fem. of L. *albus,* white]

al•bi•cans, pl. **al•bi•can•tia** (al′bi-kanz, -kan′tē-ă). **1.** SYN white. **2.** SYN *corpus* albicans. [L.]

al•bi•du•ria (al-bi-dū′rē-ă). The passing of pale or white urine of low specific gravity, as in chyluria. SYN albinuria. [L. *albidus,* whitish, + G. *ouron,* urine]

al•bi•nism (al′bi-nizm). A group of inherited (usually autosomal recessive) disorders with deficiency or absence of pigment in the skin, hair, and eyes, or eyes only, due to an abnormality in production of melanin. SEE ocular a., piebaldism. [albino + ism]

　ocular a. [MIM*300650 &], absence of pigment chiefly in the iris, choroid, and retinal pigment epithelium with deafness; X-linked inheritance.

al•bi•no (al-bī′nō). An individual with albinism.

[Pg., little white one, fr. *albo,* white, fr. L. *albus* + *-ino,* dim. suffix]

al•bi•not•ic (al-bi-not′ik). Pertaining to albinism.

al•bi•nu•ria (al-bi-nū′rē-ă). SYN albiduria.

al•bu•gin•ea (al-byū-jin′ē-ă). A white fibrous tissue layer, such as the tunica albuginea. SEE *tunica* albuginea. [L. *albugineus,* fr. *albugo,* white spot]

al•bu•men (al-byū′men). SYN ovalbumin. [see albumin]

al•bu•min (al-byū′min). A type of simple protein, varieties of which are widely distributed throughout the tissues and fluids of plants and animals; a.'s are soluble in pure water, precipitable from solution by strong acids, and coagulable by heat in acid or neutral solution. [L. *albumen* (*-min-*), the white of egg]

　blood a., SYN serum a.

　bovine serum a. (BSA), a source of a. commonly used in *in vitro* biological studies.

　egg a., SYN ovalbumin.

　iodinated [131]**I human serum a.,** a sterile, buffered, isotonic solution prepared to contain not less than 10 mg of radioiodinated normal human serum a. per ml, and adjusted to provide not more than 1 mCi of radioactivity per ml; used as a diagnostic aid in the measurement of blood volume and cardiac output.

　iodinated [125]**I serum a.,** a sterile, buffered, isotonic solution prepared to contain not less than 10 mg of radioiodinated normal human serum albumin per ml, and adjusted to provide not more than 1 mCi of radioactivity per ml; used as a diagnostic aid in determining blood volume and cardiac output.

　normal human serum a., a sterile preparation of serum a. obtained by fractionating blood plasma proteins from healthy persons; used as a transfusion material and to treat edema due to hypoproteinemia.

　serum a., the principal protein in plasma, present in blood plasma and in serous fluids. Participates in fatty acid transport and helps regulate the osmotic pressure of blood. SYN blood a., seralbumin.

al•bu•mi•noid (al-byū′min-oyd). **1.** Resembling albumin. **2.** Any protein. **3.** A simple type of protein, insoluble in neutral solvents, present in horny and cartilaginous tissues and in the lens of the eye; *e.g.,* keratin, elastin, collagen. SYN scleroprotein.

al•bu•min•ous (al-byū′min-ŭs). Relating to, containing, or consisting of albumin.

al•bu•min•ur•ia (al-byū-mi-nū′rē-ă). Presence of protein in urine, chiefly albumin but also globulin; usually indicative of disease, but sometimes resulting from a temporary or transient dysfunction. SYN proteinuria (2). [albumin + G. *ouron,* urine]

al•bu•min•ur•ic (al-byū-mi-nū′rik). Relating to or characterized by albuminuria.

al•cap•ton (al-kap′tŏn). SYN homogentisic acid.

al•cap•ton•u•ria, al•kap•ton•u•ria (al-kap-tō-nū′rē-ă). Excretion of homogentisic acid (alkapton) in the urine due to congenital lack of the enzyme homogentisate 1,2-dioxygenase; urine turns dark if allowed to stand; may recur and subside at irregular intervals; arthritis and ochronosis are late complications. [alkapton + G. *ouron,* urine]

al·co·hol (al′kō-hol). **1.** One of a series of organic chemical compounds in which a hydrogen (H) attached to carbon is replaced by a hydroxyl (OH); a.'s react with acids to form esters and with alkali metals to form alcoholates. For individual a.'s not listed here, see specific name. **2.** CH_3CH_2OH; made from carbohydrates by fermentation and synthetically from ethylene or acetylene. It has been used in beverages and as a solvent, vehicle, and preservative; medicinally, it is used externally as a rubefacient, coolant, and disinfectant, and internally as an analgesic, stomachic, sedative, and antipyretic. SYN ethanol, ethyl alcohol. **3.** The azeotropic mixture of CH_3CH_2OH and water (92.3% by weight of ethanol). [Ar. *al,* the, + *kohl,* fine antimonial powder, the term being applied first to a fine powder, then to anything impalpable (spirit)]

dihydric a., a. containing two OH groups in its molecule; *e.g.,* ethylene glycol.

monohydric a., an a. containing one OH group.

primary a., an a. characterized by the univalent radical, —CH_2OH.

secondary a., an a. characterized by the bivalent atom group, —CH(OH)—.

tertiary a., methanol bearing three substitutes on its carbon atom.

trihydric a., an a. containing three OH groups; *e.g.,* glycerol.

al·co·hol de·hy·dro·gen·ase (al′ko-hol dē-hī-droj′en-āz). An oxidoreductase that reversibly converts an alcohol to an aldehyde (or ketone) with NAD⁺ as the H acceptor. For example, ethanol + NAD⁺ ↔ acetaldehyde + NADH. Plays an important role in alcoholism.

al·co·hol·ic (al-kō-hol′ik). **1.** Relating to, containing, or produced by alcohol. **2.** One who suffers from alcoholism. **3.** One who abuses or is dependent upon alcohol.

al·co·hol·ism (al′kō-hol-izm). Chronic alcohol abuse, dependence, or addiction; chronic excessive drinking of alcoholic beverages resulting in impairment of health and/or social or occupational functioning, and increasing adaptation to the effects of alcohol requiring increasing doses to achieve and sustain a desired effect.

acute a., a temporary deterioration in mental function, accompanied by muscular incoordination and paresis, induced by the rapid ingestion of alcoholic beverages. SYN intoxication (2).

chronic a., a pathologic condition, affecting chiefly the nervous and gastroenteric systems, associated with impairment in social and occupational functioning, caused by the habitual use of alcoholic beverages in toxic amounts.

al·co·hol·y·sis (al-kō-hol′i-sis). Splitting of a chemical bond with the addition of the elements of alcohol at the point of splitting. [alcohol + G. *lysis,* dissolution]

ALD assistive listening *device.*

al·de·hyde (al′dĕ-hīd). A compound containing the radical —CH=O, reducible to an alcohol (—CH_2OH), oxidizable to a carboxylic acid (—COOH); *e.g.,* acetaldehyde.

al·do·pen·tose (al-dō-pen′tōs). A monosaccharide with five carbon atoms, of which one is a (potential) aldehyde group; *e.g.,* ribose.

al·dose (al′dōs). A monosaccharide potentially containing the characteristic group of the aldehydes, —CHO; a polyhydroxyaldehyde.

al·dos·ter·one (al-dos′ter-ōn). A hormone produced by the adrenal cortex; its major action is to facilitate potassium exchange for sodium in the distal renal tubule, causing sodium reabsorption and potassium and hydrogen loss; the principal mineralocorticoid.

al·do·ste·ron·ism (al-dos′ter-on-izm). A disorder caused by excessive secretion of aldosterone. SYN hyperaldosteronism.

idiopathic a., SYN primary a.

primary a., an adrenocortical disorder caused by excessive secretion of aldosterone and characterized by headaches, nocturia, polyuria, fatigue, hypertension, potassium depletion, hypokalemic alkalosis, hypervolemia, and decreased plasma renin activity; may be associated with small benign adrenocortical adenomas. SYN Conn's syndrome, idiopathic a.

secondary a., a. resulting not from a defect intrinsic to the adrenal cortex but from a stimulation of hormonal secretion caused by extra-adrenal disorders; associated with increased plasma renin activity and occurs in heart failure, nephrotic syndrome, cirrhosis, and hypoproteinemia.

alec·i·thal (ă-les′i-thal). Without yolk; denoting ova with little or no deutoplasm. [G. *a-* priv. + *lekithos,* yolk]

aleu·ke·mia (ă-lū-kē′mē-ă). **1.** Literally, a lack of leukocytes in the blood. The term is generally used to indicate varieties of leukemic disease in which the white blood cell count in circulating blood is normal or even less than normal (*i.e.,* no leukocytosis), but a few young leukocytes are observed; sometimes used more restrictedly for unusual instances of leukemia with no leukocytosis and no young forms in the blood. **2.** Leukemic changes in bone marrow associated with a subnormal number of leukocytes in the blood. SEE ALSO subleukemic *leukemia.* [G. *a-* priv. + *leukos,* white, + *haima,* blood]

aleu·ke·mic (ā-lū-kē′mik). Pertaining to aleukemia.

aleu·ke·moid (ā-lū-kē′moyd). Resembling aleukemia symptomatically.

aleu·kia (ā-lū′kē-ă). Absence or extremely decreased number of leukocytes in the circulating blood; sometimes also termed aleukemic myelosis. [G. *a-* priv. + *leukos,* white]

aleu·ko·cyt·ic (ā-lū-kō-sit′ik). Manifesting absence or extremely reduced numbers of leukocytes in blood or lesions.

aleu·ko·cy·to·sis (ā-lū-kō-sī-tō′sis). Absence or great reduction of white blood cells in the circulating blood, or the lack of leukocytes in an anatomical lesion. [G. *a-* priv. + *leukos,* white, + *kytos,* a hollow (cell)]

alex·ia (ă-lek′sē-ă). An inability to comprehend the meaning of written or printed words and sentences, caused by a cerebral lesion. Also called **optical a., sensory a.,** or **visual a.,** in distinction to **motor a.** (anarthria), in which there is loss of the power to read aloud although the significance of what is written or printed is understood. SYN text blindness, word blindness, visual aphasia (1). [G. *a*- priv. + *lexis,* a word or phrase]

alex·ic (ă-lek'sik). Pertaining to alexia.

alex·i·thy·mia (ă-lek-si-thī'mē-ă). Difficulty in recognizing and describing one's emotions, defining them in terms of somatic sensations or behavioral reactions. [G. *a*- priv. + *lexis,* word, + -*thymia,* feelings, passion]

al·gae (al'jē). A division of eukaryotic, photosynthetic, nonflowering organisms that includes many seaweeds. [pl. of L. *alga,* seaweed]

al·gal (al'găl). Resembling or pertaining to algae.

△**alge-, algesi-, algio-, algo-.** Pain; corresponds to L. dolor-. [G. *algos,* a pain]

△**algesi-.** SEE alge-.

al·ge·sia (al-jē'zē-ă). ~~SYN algesthesia.~~ [G. *algēsis,* a sense of pain]

al·ge·sic (al-jēz-ik). **1.** Painful; related to or causing pain. **2.** Relating to hypersensitivity to pain. SYN algetic.

al·ge·sim·e·ter (al-jē-sim'ĕ-ter). SYN algesiometer.

al·ge·si·o·gen·ic (al-jē'zē-ō-jen'ik). Pain-producing. SYN algogenic. [G. *algēsis,* sense of pain, + -*gen,* production]

al·ge·si·om·e·ter (al-jē-zē-om'ĕ-ter). An instrument for measuring the degree of sensitivity to a painful stimulus. SYN algesimeter, algometer, odynometer. [G. *algēsis,* sense of pain, + *metron,* measure]

al·ges·the·sia (al-jes-thē'zē-ă). **1.** The appreciation of pain. **2.** Hypersensitivity to pain. SYN algesia, algesthesis. [G. *algos,* pain, + *aisthēsis,* sensation]

al·ges·the·sis (al-jes-thē'sis). SYN algesthesia.

al·get·ic (al-jet'ik). SYN algesic.

△**-algia.** Pain, painful condition. [G. *algos,* a pain]

△**algio-.** SEE alge-.

△**algo-.** SEE alge-.

al·go·gen·ic (al-gō-jen'ik). SYN algesiogenic.

al·go·lag·nia (al-gō-lag'nē-ă). Form of sexual perversion in which the infliction or the experiencing of pain increases the pleasure of the sexual act or causes sexual pleasure independent of the act; includes both sadism (active a.) and masochism (passive a.). SYN algophilia (2). [algo- + G. *lagneia,* lust]

al·gom·e·ter (al-gom'ĕ-ter). SYN algesiometer. [algo- + G. *metron,* measure]

al·go·phil·ia (al-gō-fil'ē-ă). **1.** Pleasure experienced in the thought of pain in others or in oneself. **2.** SYN algolagnia. [algo- + G. *phileō,* to love]

al·go·pho·bia (al-gō-fō'bē-ă). Abnormal fear of or sensitiveness to pain. [algo- + G. *phobos,* fear]

al·go·rithm (al'gō-rithm). A process consisting of steps, each depending on the outcome of the previous one. In clinical medicine, a step-by-step protocol for management of a health care problem; in computed tomography, the formulas used for calculation of the final image from the x-ray transmission data. [Mediev. L. *algorismus,* after

Muhammad ibn-Musa *al-Khwarizmi,* Arabian mathematician, + G. *arithmos,* number]

al·go·vas·cu·lar (al-gō-vas'kyū-lăr). Relating to changes in the lumen of the blood vessels occurring under the influence of pain. [G. *algos,* pain]

alien·a·tion (ā-lē-en-ā'shŭn). A condition characterized by lack of meaningful relationships with others, sometimes resulting in depersonalization and estrangement from others. [L. *alieno,* pp. -*atus,* to make strange]

ali·e·nia (ā-li-ē'nē-ă). Congenital absence of the spleen. [G. *a*- priv. + L. *lien,* spleen]

al·i·form (al'i-fōrm). Wing-shaped. [L. *ala,* + *forma,* shape]

alignment (ă-līn'ment). **1.** The longitudinal position of a bone or limb. **2.** DENTISTRY The arrangement of the teeth in relation to the supporting structures and the adjacent and opposing dentitions.

postural alignment, ~~maintenance of biomechanical integrity among body parts.~~

al·i·men·ta·ry (al-i-men'ter-ē). Relating to food or nutrition. [L. *alimentarius,* fr. *alimentum,* nourishment]

al·i·men·ta·tion (al-i-men-tā'shŭn). Providing nourishment. SEE ALSO feeding.

al·i·na·sal (al'i-nā'săl). Relating to the wings of the nose (alae nasi), or flaring portions of the nostrils. [L. *ala,* + *nasus,* nose]

al·i·phat·ic (al-i-fat'ik). Denoting the acyclic carbon compounds, most of which belong to the fatty acid series. [G. *aleiphar* (*aleiphat-*), fat, oil]
  a. acids, The acids of nonaromatic hydrocarbons (*e.g.,* acetic, propionic, butyric acids); the so-called fatty acids of the formula R–COOH, where R is a nonaromatic (aliphatic) hydrocarbon.

al·i·quant (al'ĭ-kwant). In chemistry and immunology, pertaining to a portion that results from dividing the whole in a manner that some is left after the a.'s (equal in volume or weight) have been apportioned.

al·i·quot (al'i-kwot). In chemistry and immunology, pertaining to a portion of the whole; loosely, any one of two or more samples of something, of the same volume or weight. [L. a few, several]

al·i·sphe·noid (al-i-sfē'noyd). Relating to the greater wing of the sphenoid bone. [L. *ala,* + *sphēn,* wedge]

aliz·a·rin (ă-liz'ă-rin) [C.I. 58000]. 1,2-Dihydroxyanthraquinone; a red dye that occurs in the root of madder as orange needles, slightly soluble in water; used by the ancients as a dye. Now made synthetically from anthracene and used in the manufacture of dyes, *e.g.,* a. blue, a. orange, "Turkey red." As an indicator, it is yellow below pH 5.5 and red above pH 6.8; other modified a.'s have other colors and change color at other pH values.

al·ka·le·mia (al-kă-lē'mē-ă). A decrease in H-ion concentration of the blood or a rise in pH, irrespective of alterations in the level of bicarbonate ion. [alkali + G. *haima,* blood]

al·ka·les·cent (al-ka-les'ent). **1.** Slightly alkaline. **2.** Becoming alkaline.

al·ka·li, pl. **al·ka·lis, al·ka·lies** (al'kă-lī, -līz). **1.** A strongly basic substance yielding hydroxide ions (OH⁻) in solution; *e.g.,* sodium hydroxide, potassium hydroxide. **2.** SYN base (3). **3.** SYN alkali *metal.* [Ar., *al,* the, + *qalīy,* soda ash]

al·ka·line (al′kă-līn). Relating to or having the reaction of an alkali.

al·ka·lin·i·ty (al-kă-lin′i-tē). The state of being alkaline.

al·ka·li·nu·ria (al′kă-li-nū′rē-ă). The passage of alkaline urine. SYN alkaluria. [alkaline + G. *ouron,* urine]

al·ka·loid (al′kă-loyd). Originally, any one of hundreds of plant products distinguished by alkaline (basic) reactions, but now restricted to heterocyclic nitrogen-containing and often complex structures possessing pharmacological activity; their trivial names usually end in -ine (*e.g.,* morphine, atropine, colchicine). A.'s are synthesized by plants and are found in the leaf, bark, seed, or other parts, usually constituting the active principle of the crude drug; they are a loosely defined group, but may be classified according to the chemical structure of their main nucleus. For medicinal purposes, due to improved water solubility, the salts of a.'s are usually used. SEE ALSO individual a. or a. class.

al·ka·lo·sis (al-kă-lō′sis). A disorder characterized by H-ion loss or base excess in body fluids (metabolic a.), or caused by CO_2 loss due to hyperventilation (respiratory a.).

  compensated a., a. in which there is a change in bicarbonate but the pH of body fluids approaches normal; respiratory a. may be compensated by increased production of metabolic acids or increased renal excretion of bicarbonate; metabolic a. is rarely compensated by hypoventilation.

  metabolic a., an a. associated with an increased arterial bicarbonate concentration, resulting from an excessive intake of alkaline materials or an excessive loss of acid in the urine or through persistent vomiting; the base excess and standard bicarbonate are both elevated. SEE ALSO compensated a.

  respiratory a., a. resulting from abnormal loss of CO_2 produced by hyperventilation, either active or passive, with concomitant reduction in arterial bicarbonate concentration. SEE ALSO compensated a.

  uncompensated a., a. in which the pH of body fluids is elevated because of lack of the compensatory mechanisms of compensated a.

al·ka·lot·ic (al-kă-lot′ik). Relating to alkalosis.

al·ka·lu·ria (al-kă-lū′rē-ă). SYN alkalinuria.

al·kane (al′kān). The general term for a saturated acyclic hydrocarbon; *e.g.,* propane, butane.

al·kap·ton (al-kap′tŏn). SYN homogentisic acid. [alkali + G. *kaptō,* to suck up greedily]

al·kene (al′kēn). An acyclic hydrocarbon containing one or more double bonds; *e.g.,* ethene, propene. SYN olefin.

al·ke·nyl (al′ken-il). The radical of an alkene.

al·kide (al′kīd). SYN alkyl (2).

al·kyl (al′kil). **1.** A hydrocarbon radical of the general formula C_nH_{2n+1}. **2.** A compound, such as tetraethyl lead, in which a metal is combined with alkyl radicals. SYN alkide.

al·kyl·a·tion (al′ki-lā′shŭn). Substitution of an alkyl radical for a hydrogen atom; *e.g.,* introduction of a side chain into an aromatic compound.

ALL acute lymphocytic *leukemia.*

al·la·ches·the·sia (al′ă-kes-thē′zē-ă). A condition in which a tactile sensation is referred to a point other than that to which the stimulus is applied. [G. *allachē,* elsewhere, + *aisthēsis,* sensation]

allanto-, allant-. Allantois; allantoid; sausage. [G. *allas, allantos,* sausage]

al·lan·to·cho·ri·on (ă-lan-tō-kōr′ē-on). Extraembryonic membrane formed by the fusion of the allantois and chorion.

al·lan·to·ic (ă-lan-tō′ik). Relating to the allantois.

al·lan·toid (ă-lan′toyd). **1.** Sausage-shaped. **2.** Relating to, or resembling, the allantois. [allanto- + G. *eidos,* appearance]

al·lan·to·in·u·ria (ă-lan′tō-in-yū′rē-ă). The urinary excretion of allantoin; normal in most mammals, abnormal in humans. [allantoin + G. *ouron,* urine]

al·lan·to·is (ă-lan′tō-is). A fetal membrane developing from the hindgut (or yolk sac, in humans). In humans it is vestigial; externally, in mammals, it contributes to the formation of the umbilical cord and placenta. SYN allantoid membrane. [allanto- + G. *eidos,* appearance]

al·lele (ă-lēl′). Any one of two or more different genes that may occupy the same locus on a specific chromosome. As autosomal chromosomes are paired, each autosomal gene is represented twice in normal somatic cells. If the same a. occupies both units of the locus, the individual or cell is homozygous for this a. If the a.'s are different, the individual or cell is heterozygous for both a.'s. SEE ALSO DNA markers. SYN allelomorph. [G. *allēlōn,* reciprocally]

al·le·lic (ă-lē′lik). Relating to an allele.

al·le·lo·morph (ă-lē′lō-mōrf). SYN allele. [G. *allēlōn,* reciprocally, + *morphē,* shape]

al·le·lo·tax·is, al·le·lo·taxy (ă-lēl-ō-taks′is, -taks′ē). Development of an organ from a number of embryonal structures or tissues. [G. *allēlōn,* reciprocally, + *taxis,* an arranging]

al·ler·gen (al′er-jen). Term for an incitant of altered reactivity (allergy), an antigenic substance. [allergy + G. *-gen,* producing]

al·ler·gen·ic (al-er-jen′ik). SYN antigenic.

al·ler·gic (ă-ler′jik). Relating to any response stimulated by an allergen.

al·ler·gic sa·lute (ă-ler′jik sal-oot′). A characteristic wiping or rubbing of the nose with a transverse or upward movement of the hand, as seen in children with allergic rhinitis.

al·ler·gist (al′er-jist). One who specializes in the treatment of allergies.

al·ler·gy (al′er-jē). **1.** Hypersensitivity caused by exposure to a particular antigen (allergen) resulting in a marked increase in reactivity to that antigen upon subsequent exposure sometimes resulting in harmful consequences. SEE ALSO allergic *reaction,* anaphylaxis, immune. **2.** That branch of medicine concerned with the study, diagnosis, and treatment of allergic manifestations. **3.** An acquired hypersensitivity to certain drugs and biologic materials. [G. *allos,* other, + *ergon,* work]

atopic a., SEE atopy.

contact a., SYN allergic contact *dermatitis.*

delayed a., a type IV allergic reaction; so called because in a sensitized subject the reaction becomes evident hours after contact with the allergen (antigen), reaches its peak after 36 to 48 hours, then recedes slowly. Associated with cell-mediated responses. SEE ALSO delayed *reaction.* Cf. immediate a.

immediate a., a type I allergic reaction; so called because in a sensitized subject the reaction becomes evident usually within minutes after contact with the allergen (antigen), reaches its peak within an hour or so, then rapidly recedes. SEE ALSO immediate *reaction,* anaphylaxis. Cf. delayed a.

latent a., a. that causes no signs or symptoms but can be revealed by means of certain immunologic tests with specific allergens.

physical a., excessive response to factors in the environment such as heat or cold.

polyvalent a., allergic response manifested simultaneously for several or numerous specific allergens.

al·lied health pro·fes·sion·al. An individual trained to perform services in the care of patients; includes a variety of therapy technicians (*e.g.,* pulmonary), radiology technicians, physical therapists, etc.

all or none. SEE Bowditch's *law.*

allo-. 1. Other; differing from the normal or usual. 2. Chemical prefix formerly used with amino acids whenever their side chain contained an asymmetric carbon; for example, the alloisoleucines and allothreonines. [G. *allos,* other]

al·lo·an·ti·body (al-ō-an′ti-bod-ē). An antibody specific for an alloantigen. Isoantibody is sometimes used in this sense.

al·lo·an·ti·gen (al-ō-an′ti-jen). An antigen that occurs in some, but not in other members of the same species. Isoantigen is sometimes used in this sense.

al·lo·chei·ria (al-ō-kī′rē-ă). SEE allochiria.

al·lo·chi·ria, al·lo·chei·ria (al′-ō-kī′rē-ă, al-ō-kī′rē-ă). A form of allachesthesia in which the sensation of a stimulus in one limb is referred to the contralateral limb. SYN Bamberger's sign (2). [allo- + G. *cheir,* hand]

al·lo·cor·tex (al′ō-kōr′teks). O. Vogt's term denoting several regions of the cerebral cortex, in particular the olfactory cortex and the hippocampus, characterized by fewer cell layers than the isocortex; SEE ALSO cerebral *cortex.* SYN heterotypic cortex. [allo- + L. *cortex,* bark (cortex)]

al·lo·dip·loid (al-ō-dip′loyd). SEE alloploid.

al·lo·dyn·ia (al-ō-din′ē-ă). Condition in which ordinarily nonpainful stimuli evoke pain. [allo- + G. *odynē,* pain]

al·lo·e·rot·ic (al′ō-ĕ-rot′ik). Pertaining to or characterized by alloerotism. SYN heteroerotic.

al·lo·er·o·tism (al-ō-ār′ō-tizm). Sexual attraction toward another person. Cf. autoerotism. SYN heteroerotism. [allo- + G. *erōs,* love]

al·lo·graft (al′ō-graft). A graft transplanted between genetically nonidentical individuals of the same species. SYN allogeneic graft, homologous graft, homoplastic graft.

al·lo·ker·a·to·plas·ty (al-ō-ker′ă-tō-plas-tē). Replacement of opaque corneal tissue with a transparent prosthesis, usually plastic.

al·lo·la·lia (al-ō-lā′lē-ă). Any speech defect, especially one caused by a cerebral disorder. [allo- + G. *lalia,* talking]

al·lom·er·ism (ă-lom′er-izm). The state of differing in chemical composition but having the same crystalline form. [allo- + G. *meros,* part]

al·lo·mor·phism (al-ō-mōr′fizm). 1. Change of shape in cells due to mechanical causes, such as flattening from pressure, or to progressive metaplasia, such as the change of bile duct cells into liver cells. 2. The state of being similar in chemical composition but differing in form (especially crystalline). [allo- + G. *morphē,* form]

al·lo·path·ic (al-ō-path′ik). Relating to allopathy.

al·lop·a·thy (al-op′ă-thē). A therapeutic system in which a disease is treated by producing a second condition that is incompatible with or antagonistic to the first. Cf. homeopathy. SYN heteropathy (2). [allo- + G. *pathos,* suffering]

al·lo·plast (al′ō-plast). 1. A graft of an inert metal or plastic material. 2. A relatively inert foreign body used for implantation into tissues. [allo- + G. *plastos,* formed]

al·lo·plas·ty (al′ō-plas-tē). Repair of defects by allotransplantation.

al·lo·ploid (al′ō-ployd). Relating to a hybrid individual or cell with two or more sets of chromosomes derived from two different ancestral species. [allo- + -ploid]

al·lo·ploi·dy (al-ō-ploy′dē). The condition of being alloploid.

al·lo·pol·y·ploid (al-ō-pol′i-ployd). An alloploid having three or more haploid sets of chromosomes. [allo- + polyploid]

al·lo·pol·y·ploi·dy (al-ō-pol′i-ploy-dē). The condition of being allopolyploid.

al·lo·psy·chic (al-ō-sī′kik). Denoting the mental processes in their relation to the outer world. [allo- + G. *psychē,* mind]

al·lo·rhyth·mia (al-ō-rith′mē-ă). An irregularity in the cardiac rhythm that repeats itself any number of times. [allo- + G. *rhythmos,* rhythm]

al·lo·rhyth·mic (al-ō-rith′mik). Relating to or characterized by allorhythmia.

al·lo·some (al′ō-sōm). One of the chromosomes differing in appearance or behavior from the autosomes and sometimes unequally distributed among the germ cells. SYN heterochromosome, heterotypical chromosome. [allo- + G. *sōma,* body]

al·lo·ste·ric (al-ō-stār′ik). Pertaining to or characterized by allosterism.

al·lo·ster·ism, al·lo·ste·ry (ă-los′ter-izm, -los′ter-ē). The influencing of an enzyme activity, or the binding of a ligand to a protein, by a change in the conformation of the protein, brought about by the binding of a substrate or other effector at a site (allosteric site) other than the active site of the protein. Cf. hysteresis.

al·lo·tope (al′ō-tōp). The antigenic determinant of an allotype. [allo- + -tope]

al

al·lo·trans·plan·ta·tion (al'ō-tranz-plan-ta' shŭn). Transplantation of an allograft.

al·lo·trope (al'ō-trōp). An element in one of the allotropic forms that it may assume. [allo- + G. *tropos,* a turning]

al·lo·tro·pic (al-ō-trop'ik). 1. Relating to allotropism. 2. Denoting a type of personality characterized by a preoccupation with the reactions of others.

al·lot·ro·pism, al·lot·ro·py (ă-lot'rō-pizm, -lot' rō-pē). The existence of certain elements, in several forms differing in physical properties; *e.g.,* carbon black, graphite, and diamond are all pure carbon. [allo- + G. *tropos,* a turning]

al·lo·type (al'ō-tīp). Any one of the genetically determined antigenic differences within a given class of immunoglobulin that occur among members of the same species. SEE ALSO antibody. [allo- + G. *typos,* model]

al·lo·typ·ic (al-ō-tip'ik). Pertaining to an allotype.

al·low·ance (a'lau-antz). 1. Permission. 2. A portion allotted.

  recommended daily a. (RDA), the amount of daily nutrient intake judged to be adequate for the maintenance of good nutrition in an average adult.

al·lox·u·re·mia (al-oks-yū-rē'mē-ă, al-ok-sū-rē' mē-ă). The presence of purine bases in the blood. [alloxan + G. *haima,* blood]

al·lox·u·ria (al-oks-yū'rē-ă, al-ok-sū'rē-ă). The presence of purine bodies in the urine. [alloxan + G. *ouron,* urine]

al·loy (al'oy). A substance composed of a mixture of two or more metals.

  eutectic a., an a., generally brittle and subject to tarnish and corrosion, with a fusion temperature lower than that of any of its components; used in dentistry mainly in solders.

alo·gia (ă-lō'jē-ă). 1. SYN aphasia. 2. Inability to speak due to mental deficiency or an episode of dementia. [G. *a-* priv. + *logos,* speech]

al·o·pe·cia (al-ō-pē'shē-ă). Loss of hair. SYN baldness. [G. *alōpekia,* a disease like fox mange, fr. *alōpēx,* a fox]

  a. adnata, underdevelopment of the lashes. SEE ALSO a. congenitalis. SYN madarosis.

  androgenic a., gradual decrease of scalp hair density in adults as a result of familial increased susceptibility of hair follicles to androgen secretion following puberty. SEE female pattern a., male pattern a. SYN a. hereditaria, patterned a.

  a. area′ta [MIM*104000], a condition of undetermined etiology characterized by circumscribed, nonscarring, usually asymmetrical areas of baldness on the scalp, eyebrows, and bearded portion of the face. SYN a. circumscripta.

  a. cap′itis tota′lis, SYN a. totalis.

  cicatricial a., SYN scarring a. [L. *cicatrix, cicatricis,* scar + suffix *-al,* characterized by]

  a. circumscrip′ta, SYN a. areata.

  a. congenita′lis [MIM*104130], absence of all hair at birth, associated with psychomotor epilepsy.

  female pattern a., diffuse partial hair loss in the centroparietal area of the scalp, with preserva-

tion of the frontal and temporal hair lines; the most frequent type of androgenic a. in women.

  a. heredita′ria [MIM*109200], SYN androgenic a.

  lipedematous a., a. with itching, soreness, or tenderness of the scalp in black women; the scalp is thickened and soft, subcutaneous fat is increased, and the hair is sparse and short.

  male pattern a., the most common form of androgenic a., seen in men as receding frontal and bilateral triangular temple hair lines, and a balding patch on the vertex, which may progress to complete a.

  a. margina′lis, hair loss at the hair line, a condition most commonly seen in blacks; commonly transient and caused by chronic traction, although long-continued traction may cause permanent a.

  a. medicamento′sa, diffuse hair loss, most notably of the scalp, caused by administration of various types of drugs.

  patterned a., SYN androgenic a.

  a. pityro′des, a loss of hair, of the body as well as of the scalp, accompanied by an abundant branlike desquamation.

  pressure a., loss of hair over a circumscribed area usually on the posterior scalp, resulting from the continuous pressure on the occiput in a lengthy operative procedure, or unconsciousness following a drug overdose.

  scarring a., a. in which hair follicles are irreversibly destroyed by scarring processes including trauma, burns, lupus erythematosus, lichen planopilaris, scleroderma, folliculitis decalvans, or of uncertain cause (pseudopelade). SYN cicatricial a.

  a. symptomat′ica, a. occurring in the course of various constitutional or local diseases, or following prolonged febrile illness.

  a. tota′lis, total loss of hair of the scalp either within a very short period of time or from progression of localized a., especially a. areata. Cf. a. universalis. SYN a. capitis totalis.

  a. universa′lis, total loss of hair from all parts of the body. Cf. a. totalis.

al·o·pe·cic (al-ō-pē'sik). Relating to alopecia.

alpha (α) (al'fă) 1. First letter of the Greek alphabet; used as a classifier in the nomenclature of many sciences. 2. Symbol for Bunsen's solubility *coefficient.* 3. CHEMISTRY denotes the first in a series, a position immediately adjacent to a carboxyl group, the first of a series of closely related compounds, an aromatic substituent on an aliphatic chain, or the direction of a chemical bond away from the viewer. 4. Abbreviation for alpha *particle.* 5. CHEMISTRY symbol for angle of optical *rotation;* degree of dissociation. For terms with the prefix α, see the specific term.

Al·pha·vi·rus (al'fă-vī-rŭs). One of the genera of the family Togaviridae that was formerly classified as part of the "group A" arboviruses and includes the viruses that cause eastern equine, western equine, and Venezuelan encephalitis.

ALS amyotrophic lateral *sclerosis*; antilymphocyte *serum.*

ALT alanine aminotransferase.

al·ter·nans (awl-ter'nanz). Alternating; used as a noun in the sense of *pulsus* alternans. [L.]

auscultatory a., alternation in the intensity of heart sounds or murmurs in the presence of a regular cardiac rhythm.

concordant a., simultaneous occurrence of right ventricular and pulmonary artery a. with left ventricular and peripheral pulsus a.

discordant a., presence of right ventricular and pulmonary artery a. with peripheral pulsus a., but with the strong beat of the right ventricle coinciding with the weak beat of the left and vice versa.

electrical a., electrical alternation of the heart.

al·ter·na·tion (awl-ter-nā′shŭn). The occurrence of two things or phases in succession and recurrently; used interchangeably with alternans.

concordant a., a. in either the mechanical or electrical activity of the heart, occurring in both systemic and pulmonary circulations.

discordant a., a. in cardiac activities of either the systemic or the pulmonary circulation, but not of both, or in both but oppositely directed in each.

electrical a. of heart, a disorder in which the ventricular or atrial complexes or both are regular in time but of alternating pattern; detected by electrocardiography.

alu·mi·no·sis (ă-lū-min-ō′sis). A pneumoconiosis caused by inhalation of aluminum particles.

alu·mi·num (Al) (ă-lū′min-ŭm). A white silvery metal of very light weight; atomic no. 13, atomic wt. 26.981539. Many salts and compounds are used in medicine and dentistry. [L. *alumen,* alum]

al·vei (al′vē-ī). Plural of alveus.

al·ve·o·al·gia (al′vē-ō-al′jē-ă). A postoperative complication of tooth extraction in which the blood clot in the socket disintegrates, resulting in focal osteomyelitis and severe pain. SYN alveolalgia. [alveolus + G. *algos,* pain]

al·ve·o·lal·gia (al′vē-ō-lal′jē-ă). SYN alveoalgia.

al·ve·o·lar (al-vē′ō-lăr). Relating to an alveolus.

al·ve·o·lec·to·my (al′vē-ō-lek′tō-mē). Surgical excision of a portion of the dentoalveolar process at the time of tooth removal to facilitate a dental prosthesis. [alveolus + G. *ektomē,* excision]

al·ve·o·li (al-vē′ō-lī). Plural of alveolus.

al·ve·o·lin·gual (al′vē-o-ling′gwăl). SYN alveolo-lingual.

al·ve·o·li·tis (al′vē-ō-lī′tis). 1. Inflammation of alveoli. 2. Inflammation of a tooth socket.

acute pulmonary a., acute inflammation involving formation of exudate in pulmonary alveoli and impaired gas exchange; may result in necrosis with hemorrhage into the lungs; occurs in Goodpasture's syndrome, in association with a glomerulonephritis.

extrinsic allergic a., pneumoconiosis resulting from hypersensitivity to organic dust, usually specified according to occupational exposure; in the acute form, respiratory symptoms and fever start several hours after exposure to the dust; in the chronic form, there is eventual diffuse pulmonary fibrosis after exposure over several years.

◬**alveolo-.** An alveolus, the alveolar process; alveolar. [L. *alveolus,* a concave vessel, a bowl, a basin, fr. *alveus,* a trough, + *-olus,* small, little; akin to *alvus,* the belly, the womb]

al·ve·o·lo·cla·sia (al-vē′ō-lō-klā′zē-ă). Destruc-tion of the alveolus. [alveolo- + G. *klasis,* breaking]

al·ve·o·lo·den·tal (al-vē′ō-lō-den′tăl). Relating to the alveoli and the teeth.

al·ve·o·lo·la·bi·al (al-vē′ō-lō-lā′bē-ăl). Relating to the labial or vestibular (outer) surface of the alveolar processes of the upper or lower jaw.

al·ve·o·lo·lin·gual (al-vē′ō-lō-ling′gwăl). Relating to the lingual (inner) surface of the alveolar process of the lower jaw. SYN alveolingual.

al·ve·o·lo·pal·a·tal (al-vē′ō-lō-pal′ă-tăl). Relating to the palatal surface of the alveolar process of the upper jaw.

al·ve·o·lo·plas·ty (al-vē′ō-lō-plas-tē). Surgical preparation of the alveolar ridges for the reception of dentures; shaping and smoothing of socket margins after extraction of teeth with subsequent suturing to insure optimal healing. SYN alveo-plasty. [alveolo- + G. *plassō,* to form]

al·ve·o·lot·o·my (al-vē-ō-lot′ō-mē). Surgical opening into a dental alveolus to allow drainage of pus from a periapical or other intraosseous abscess. [alveolo- + G. *tomē,* incision]

al·ve·o·lus, gen. and pl. **al·ve·o·li** (al-vē′ō-lŭs, -ō-lī) [NA]. A small cell, cavity, or socket. **1.** SYN pulmonary a. **2.** One of the terminal secretory portions of an alveolar or racemose gland. **3.** One of the honeycomb pits in the wall of the stomach. **4.** SYN tooth *socket.* [L. dim. of *alveus,* trough, hollow sac, cavity]

pulmonary a., one of the thin-walled saclike terminal dilations of the respiratory bronchioles, alveolar ducts, and alveolar sacs across which gas exchange occurs between alveolar air and the pulmonary capillaries. SYN alveoli pulmonis [NA], alveolus (1) [NA], air cells (1), air vesicles, bronchic cells.

alveoli pulmo′nis [NA], SYN pulmonary a.

al·ve·o·plas·ty (al′vē-ō-plas-tē). SYN alveolo-plasty.

al·ve·us, pl. **al·vei** (al′vē-ŭs, -vē-ī). A channel or trough. [L. tray, trough, cavity, fr. *alvus,* belly]

alym·pho·cy·to·sis (ă-lim′fō-sī-tō′sis). Absence or great reduction of lymphocytes.

alym·pho·pla·sia (ă-lim-fō-plā′zē-ă). Aplasia or hypoplasia of lymphoid tissue.

thymic a., hypoplasia with absence of Hassall's corpuscles and deficiency of lymphocytes in the thymus and usually in lymph nodes, spleen, and gastrointestinal tract; there is peripheral lymphopenia and often hypogammaglobulinemia and absence of plasma cells; presents in early infancy with respiratory infections and leads to death within a few months.

Am americium.

am ammeter.

AMA. American Medical Association.

am·a·crine (am′ă-krin). **1.** A cell or structure lacking a long, fibrous process. **2.** Denoting such a cell or structure. [G. *a-* priv. + *makros,* long, + *is (in-),* fiber]

amal·gam (ă-mal′gam). An alloy of an element or a metal with mercury. In dentistry, primarily of two types: silver-tin alloy, containing small amounts of copper, zinc and perhaps other metals, and a second type containing more copper (12 to 30% by weight); they are used for restoring teeth and making dies. [G. *malagma,* a soft mass]

Am·a·ni·ta (am-ă-nī'tă). A genus of fungi, many members of which are highly poisonous. [G. *amanitai,* fungi]

  A. musca'ria, a toxic species of mushroom with yellow to red pileus and white gills; it contains muscarine, which produces psychosis-like states and other symptoms.

  A. phalloi'des, a species containing poisonous principles, including phalloidin and amanitin, that cause gastroenteritis, hepatic necrosis, and renal necrosis.

amas·tia (ă-mas'tē-ă). Absence of the breasts. SYN amazia. [G. *a-* priv. + *mastos,* breast]

amas·ti·gote (ă-mas'ti-gōt). SYN Leishman-Donovan *body.* [G. *a-* priv. + *mastix,* whip]

am·au·ro·sis (am-aw-rō'sis). Blindness, especially that occurring without apparent change in the eye itself, as from a brain lesion. [G. *amauros,* dark, obscure, + *-osis,* condition]

  a. fu'gax, transient blindness that may result from carotid artery insufficiency, retinal artery embolus, or centrifugal force (visual blackout in flight).

am·au·rot·ic (am-aw-rot'ik). Relating to or suffering from amaurosis.

ama·zia (ă-mā'zē-ă). SYN amastia.

am·ba·geu·sia (am-bă-gū'sē-ă). Loss of taste from both sides of the tongue. [L. *ambo,* both, + G. *a-* priv. + *geusis,* taste]

AMBER (am'ber) advanced multiple-beam equalization *radiography.*

△**ambi-.** Around; on all (both) sides; both, double; corresponds to G. amphi-. [L., around, about, akin to *ambo,* both]

am·bi·dex·ter·i·ty (am-bi-deks-ter'i-tē). The ability to use both hands with equal ease.

am·bi·dex·trous (am-bi-deks'trŭs). Having equal facility in the use of both hands.

am·bi·ent (am'bē-ent). Surrounding, encompassing; pertaining to the environment in which an organism or apparatus functions. [L. *ambiens,* going around]

am·bi·lat·er·al (am-bi-lat'er-ăl). Relating to both sides. [ambi- + L. *latus,* side]

am·bi·le·vous (am-bi-lē'vŭs). Awkwardness in the use of both hands. [ambi- + L. *laevus,* left]

am·bi·sex·u·al (am-bi-seks'yū-ăl). **1.** Denoting sexual characteristics found in both sexes, *e.g.,* breasts, pubic hair. **2.** Slang term for bisexual.

am·biv·a·lence (am-biv'ă-lens). The coexistence of antithetical attitudes or emotions toward a given person or thing, or idea, as in the simultaneous feeling and expression of love and hate toward the same person. [ambi- + L. *valentia,* strength]

am·biv·a·lent (am-biv'ă-lent). Relating to or characterized by ambivalence.

△**ambly-.** Dullness, dimness; blunt, dull, dim, dimmed. [G. *amblys,* blunt, dulled; faint, dim]

am·bly·a·phia (am-blī-ā'fē-ă). Diminution in tactile sensibility. [ambly- + G. *haphē,* touch]

am·bly·geus·tia (am-bli-gūs'tē-ă). A diminution in the sense of taste. [ambly- + G. *geusis,* taste]

Am·bly·om·ma (am-blē-om'ă). A genus of hard ticks characterized by eyes, festoons, and deeply

imbedded ventral plates near the festoons in males. [ambly- + G. *omma,* eye, vision]

am·bly·o·pia (am-blē-ō'pē-ă). Poor vision in one eye, without detectable cause, that cannot be corrected with a lens; almost synonymous with suppression a. [G. *amblyōpia,* dimness of vision, fr. *amblys* dull, + *ōps,* eye]

  suppression a., suppression of the central vision in one eye when the images from the two eyes are so different that they cannot be fused into one. This may be due to: 1) faulty image formation (sensory a.); 2) a large difference in refraction between the two eyes (anisometropic a.); or 3) the two eyes pointing in different directions (strabismic a.). Most suppression a. can be reversed if appropriately treated before age 6.

am·bly·o·pic (am-blē-ō'pik). Relating to, or suffering from, amblyopia.

am·bly·o·scope (am'blē-ō-skōp). A reflecting stereoscope used to evaluate or stimulate binocular vision. [amblyopia + G. *skopeō,* to view]

am·bo·cep·tor (am'bō-sep-tŏr). Complement-fixing antibody; now used chiefly to denote the anti-sheep erythrocyte antibody used in the hemolytic system of complement-fixation tests. [ambo- + L. *capio,* to take]

ambulation (am-byū-lā'shŭn). The activity of moving or walking about. [L. *ambulo,* to walk]

am·bu·la·to·ry, am·bu·lant (am'byū-lă-tōr-ē, am'byū-lant). Walking about or able to walk about; denoting a patient who is not confined to bed or hospital as a result of disease or surgery. [L. *ambulans,* walking]

ame·ba, pl. **ame·bae, ame·bas** (ă-mē'bă, -bē, -băz). Common name for *Amoeba* and similar naked, lobose, sarcodine protozoa.

am·e·bi·a·sis (ă-mē-bī'ă-sis). Infection with *Entamoeba histolytica* or other pathogenic amebas. [ameba + G. *-iasis,* condition]

ame·bic (ă-mē'bik). Relating to, resembling, or caused by amebas.

ame·bi·ci·dal (ă-mē-bi-sī'dăl). Destructive to amebas.

ame·bi·cide (ă-mē'bi-sīd). Any agent that causes the destruction of amebas. [ameba + L. *caedo,* to kill]

ame·bi·form (ă-mē'bi-fōrm). Of the shape or appearance of an ameba. [ameba + L. *forma,* shape]

ame·bo·cyte (ă-mē'bō-sīt). **1.** A wandering cell found in invertebrates. **2.** An *in vitro* tissue culture leukocyte. [ameba, + *kytos,* cell]

ame·boid (ă-mē'boyd). **1.** Resembling an ameba in appearance or characteristics. **2.** Of irregular outline with peripheral projections; denoting the outline of a form of colony in plate culture. [ameba + G. *eidos,* appearance]

am·e·bo·ma (ă-mē-bō'mă). A nodular, tumor-like focus of proliferative inflammation sometimes developing in chronic amebiasis, especially in the wall of the colon. SYN amebic granuloma. [ameba + G. *-oma,* tumor]

am·e·bu·ria (am-ē-byū'rē-ă). The presence of amebas in the urine. [ameba + G. *ouron,* urine]

ame·lia (ă-mē'lē-ă) [MIM104400]. Congenital absence of a limb or limbs. [G. *a-* priv. + *melos,* a limb]

am•e•lo•blast (ă-mel′ō-blast, am-ĕ-lō′blast). One of the columnar epithelial cells of the inner layer of the enamel organ of a developing tooth, concerned with the formation of enamel. [Early E. *amel*, enamel, + G. *blastos*, germ]

am•e•lo•blas•to•ma (am′ĕ-lō-blas-tō′mă). A benign odontogenic epithelial neoplasm; it behaves as a slowly growing expansile radiolucent tumor, occurs most commonly in the posterior regions of the mandible, and has a marked tendency to recur if inadequately excised. [ameloblast + G. *-oma*, tumor]

am•e•lo•den•tin•al (am′ĕ-lō-den′ti-năl). SYN dentinoenamel.

am•e•lo•gen•e•sis (am′ĕ-lō-jen′ĕ-sis). The deposition and maturation of enamel. SYN enamelogenesis.

amen•or•rhea (ă-men-ō-rē′ă). Absence or abnormal cessation of the menses. [G. *a-* priv. + *mēn*, month, + *rhoia*, flow]

dietary a., loss of menstrual function due to severe weight loss or gain.

lactation a., physiological suppression of menses while nursing.

primary a., a. in which the menses have never occurred.

secondary a., a. in which the menses appeared at puberty but subsequently ceased.

traumatic a., absence of menses because of endometrial scarring or cervical stenosis resulting from injury or disease.

amen•or•rhe•al, amen•or•rhe•ic (ă-men-ō-rē′ăl, -rē′ik). Relating to, accompanied by, or due to amenorrhea.

amen•tia (ă-men′shē-ă). **1.** SYN mental *retardation*. **2.** SYN dementia. [L. madness, fr. *ab*, from, + *mens*, mind]

Stearns alcoholic a., a temporary alcoholic mental disorder resembling delirium tremens but lasting for a longer time and showing a greater degree of amnesia and other mental defects.

amen•ti•al (ă-men′shē-al). Pertaining to amentia.

American Association for Medical Transcription (AAMT). Professional association for medical transcriptionists. SEE medical transcriptionist.

Amer•i•can Law In•sti•tute rule. See under rule.

American Manual Alphabet. Specific hand and finger positions used to represent each of the letters of the alphabet, used in conjunction with American Sign Language and other sign languages. SEE ALSO augmentative and alternative *communication*, fingerspelling, sign language.

Americans with Disabilities Act. Federal legislation (Public Law 101-336, enacted in 1990) guaranteeing persons with disabilities equal access to employment, education, public accommodations, transportation, telecommunications, and government services at all levels.

am•er•i•ci•um (Am) (am′ĕ-ris′ē-ŭm). An element obtained by the bombardment of uranium with neutrons or β decay of plutoniums 241, 242, and 243; atomic no. 95; atomic weight 243.06. ^{241}Am (half-life of 432.2 years) has been used in the diagnosis of bone disorders. ^{243}Am has a half-life of 7370 years. [the Americas]

ame•tria (ă-mē′trē-ă). Congenital absence of the uterus. [G. *a-* priv. + *mētra*, uterus]

am•e•tro•pia (am-ĕ-trō′pē-ă). Any refractive error that prevents objects from being focused on the retina. [G. *ametros*, disproportionate, fr. *a-* priv. + *metron*, measure, + *ōps*, eye]

am•e•tro•pic (am-ĕ-trō′pik). Relating to, or suffering from, ametropia.

△**-amic.** Chemical suffix denoting the replacement of one COOH group of a dicarboxylic acid by a carboxamide group (—$CONH_2$); applied only to trivial names (*e.g.,* succinamic acid).

ami•cro•bic (ā-mī-krō′bik). Not microbic; not related to or caused by microorganisms.

am•i•dase (am′i-dās). An enzyme that catalyzes the hydrolysis of monocarboxylic amides to free acid plus NH_3; ω-a. acts on amides such as α-ketoglutaramic acid and α-ketosuccinamic acid. SYN acylamidase.

am•i•das•es. SYN amidohydrolases.

am•ide (am′īd, am′id). A substance formally derived from ammonia through the substitution of one or more of the hydrogen atoms by acyl groups, R—CO—NH_2, or from a carboxylic acid by replacement of a carboxylic OH by NH_2. Replacement of one hydrogen atom constitutes a **primary a.**; that of two hydrogen atoms, a **secondary a.**; and that of three atoms, a **tertiary a.**.

am•i•dine (am′i-din). The monovalent radical —C(NH)-NH_2.

△**amido-.** Prefix denoting the amide radical, R-CO-NH- or R-SO_2-NH-, etc. [am(monia) + -id(e) + -o-]

ami•do•hy•dro•las•es (am′i-dō-hī′drō-lā-sez) [EC class 3.5.1 and 3.5.2]. Enzymes hydrolyzing C-N bonds of amides and cyclic amides; *e.g.,* asparaginase, barbiturase, urease, amidase. SYN amidases, deamidases, deamidizing enzymes.

amim•ia (ā-mim′ē-a). **1.** Inability to express ideas by nonverbal communication, such as gestures or signs. **2.** Asymbolia; the inability to comprehend the meaning of gestures, signs, symbols, or pantomime. [G. *a-* priv. + *minos*, a mimic]

am•i•nate (am′i-nāt). To combine with ammonia.

amine (ă-mēn′, am′in). A substance formally derived from ammonia by the replacement of one or more of the hydrogen atoms by hydrocarbon or other radicals. The substitution of one hydrogen atom constitutes a **primary a.**, *e.g.,* NH_2CH_3; that of two atoms, a **secondary a.**, *e.g.,* $NH(CH_3)_2$; that of three atoms, a **tertiary a.**, *e.g.,* $N(CH_3)_3$; and that of four atoms, a **quaternary ammonium ion**, *e.g.,* $^+N(CH_3)_4$, a positively charged ion isolated only in association with a negative ion. The a.'s form salts with acids.

adrenomimetic a., SYN sympathomimetic a.

a. oxidase (flavin-containing), an oxidoreductase containing flavin and oxidizing amines with the aid of O_2 and water to aldehydes or ketones with the release of NH_3 and H_2O_2. Acted upon by antidepressants.

pressor a., SYN pressor *base*.

primary a.,

secondary a.,

sympathetic a., SYN sympathomimetic a.

sympathomimetic a., an agent that evokes responses similar to those produced by adrenergic nerve activity (*e.g.,* epinephrine, ephedrine, iso-proterenol). SYN adrenomimetic a., sympathetic a.

tertiary a.,

vasoactive a., a substance, such as histamine or serotonin, that contains amino groups and is pharmacologically characterized by its action on the blood vessels (altering vascular caliber or permeability).

amine ox•i•dase (fla•vin•con•tain•ing). See under amine.

△**amino-.** Prefix denoting a compound containing the radical, —NH₂. [am(monia) + in(e) + -o-]

ami•no ac•id (AA, aa) (ă-mē'nō). An organic acid in which one of the hydrogen atoms on a carbon atom has been replaced by NH₂. Usually refers to an aminocarboxylic acid. However, taurine is also an a. a. SEE ALSO α-amino acid.

 a. a. dehydrogenases, enzymes catalyzing the oxidative deamination of amino acids to the corresponding oxo (keto) acids. Cf. a. a. oxidases.

 essential a. a.'s, α-amino acids nutritionally required by an organism and which must be supplied in its diet (*i.e.,* cannot be synthesized by the organism) either as free a. a. or in proteins.

 nonessential a. a.'s, those a. a.'s that may be synthesized by an organism and are thus not required as such in its diet.

 a. a. oxidases, flavoenzymes oxidizing, with O₂ and H₂0, either L- or D-amino acids specifically, to the corresponding 2-keto acids, NH₃ and H₂O₂. Cf. a. a. dehydrogenases.

α**-ami•no ac•id.** Typically, an amino acid of the general formula R-CHNH₂-COOH (*i.e.,* the NH₂ in the α position); the L forms of these are the hydrolysis products of proteins.

ami•no•ac•i•de•mia (ă-mē'nō-as-i-dē'mē-ă, am'i-nō-). The presence of excessive amounts of specific amino acids in the blood. [amino acid + G. *haima,* blood]

ami•no•ac•i•du•ria (am'i-nō-as-i-dū'rē-ă). Excretion of amino acids in the urine, especially in excessive amounts. [amino acid + G. *ouron,* urine]

ami•no•ac•yl (AA, aa) (ă-mē'nō-as'il). The radical formed from an amino acid by removal of OH from a COOH group.

ami•no•ac•yl•ase (ă-mē'nō-as'i-lās). An enzyme catalyzing hydrolysis of a wide variety of *N*-acyl amino acids to the corresponding amino acid and an acid anion.

p-**ami•no•ben•zo•ic acid (PABA)** (ă-mē'nō-ben-zō'ik). A factor in the vitamin B complex, a part of all folic acids and required for its formation; neutralizes the bacteriostatic effects of the sulfonamides since it furnishes an essential growth factor for bacteria, with the use of which sulfonamides interfere; used as an ultraviolet screen in lotions and creams.

γ-**ami•no•bu•tyr•ic ac•id** (γ-**Abu**) (ă-mē'nō-byū-tēr'ik). 4-aminobutyric acid; a constituent of the central nervous system; quantitatively the principal inhibitory neurotransmitter. Used in the treatment of a number of disorders (*e.g.,* epilepsy).

5-ami•no•im•id•az•ole ri•bose 5′-phos•phate (AIR) (ă-mē'nō-im-id-az'ōl). 5-amino-1-β-D-ribofuranosylimidazole 5′-phosphate; an interme-diate in the biosynthesis of purines. SYN 5-amino-imidazole ribotide.

5-a•mi•no•i•mid•a•zole ri•bo•tide (AIR). SYN 5-aminoimidazole ribose 5′-phosphate.

δ-**ami•no•lev•u•lin•ic ac•id (ALA)** (ă-mē'nō-lev-yū-lin'ik). An acid formed by δ-aminolevulinate synthase from glycine and succinyl-coenzyme A; a precursor of porphobilinogen, hence an important intermediate in the biosynthesis of hematin. ALA levels are elevated in cases of lead poisoning.

am•i•nol•y•sis (am-i-nol'i-sis). Replacement of a halogen in an alkyl or aryl molecule by an amine radical, with elimination of hydrogen halide.

ami•no•pep•ti•das•es (ă-mē'nō-pep'ti-dās-ez) [EC sub-group 3.4.11]. Enzymes catalyzing the breakdown of a peptide, removing the amino acid at the amino end of the chain (*i.e.,* an exopeptidase); found in intestinal secretions.

am•i•noph•er•as•es (am-i-nof'er-ās-ez). SYN aminotransferases.

α-**ami•no•suc•cin•ic ac•id** (ă-mē'nō-sŭk-sin'ik). SYN aspartic acid.

ami•no•trans•fer•as•es (ă-mē'nō-trans'fer-ās-ez) [EC sub-group 2.6.1]. Enzymes transferring amino groups between an amino acid to (usually) a 2-keto acid. SYN aminopherases, transaminases.

am•i•nu•ria (am-i-nū'rē-ă). Excretion of amines in the urine. [amine + G. *ouron,* urine]

ami•to•sis (am-i-tō'sis). Direct division of the nucleus and cell, without the complicated changes in the nucleus that occur in the ordinary process of cell reproduction. SYN direct nuclear division. [G. *a-* priv. + mitosis]

ami•tot•ic (am-i-tot'ik). Relating to or marked by amitosis.

am•me•ter (am) (am'mē-ter). An instrument for measuring strength of electric current in amperes.

am•mo•ne•mia, am•mo•ni•e•mia (am-ō-nē'mē-ă). The presence of ammonia or some of its compounds in the blood, thought to be formed from the decomposition of urea; it usually results in subnormal temperature, weak pulse, gastroenteric symptoms, and coma. [ammonia + G. *haima,* blood]

am•mo•nia-ly•as•es (ă-mō'nē-ă-lī'ās-ēz). Enzymes removing ammonia or an amino compound nonhydrolytically by rupture of a C—N bond leaving a double bond.

△**ammonio-.** Combining form indicating an ammonium group.

am•mo•ni•um (ă-mō'nē-ŭm). The ion, NH₄⁺, formed by combination of NH₃ and H⁺; behaves as a univalent metal in forming ammonium compounds.

am•mo•ni•u•ria (ă-mō-nē-yū'rē-ă). Excretion of urine that contains an excessive amount of ammonia. [ammonia + G. *ouron,* urine]

am•mo•nol•y•sis (ă-mō-nol'i-sis). The breaking of a chemical bond with the addition of the elements of ammonia (NH₂ and H) at the point of breakage. [ammonia + G. *lysis,* dissolution]

am•ne•sia (am-nē'zē-ă). A disturbance in the memory of information stored in long-term memory, in contrast to short-term memory, manifested by total or partial inability to recall past experiences. [G. *amnēsia,* forgetfulness] anterograde a., a. in reference to events occurring after the trauma or disease that caused the condition.

lacunar a., localized a., a. in reference to isolated events.

retrograde a., a. in reference to events that occurred before the trauma or disease (*e.g.*, cerebral concussion) that caused the condition.

transient global a., a memory disorder seen in middle aged and elderly persons characterized by an episode of a. and bewilderment which persists for several hours; during the episode the patient has a memory defect for present and recent past events, but is fully alert, oriented, capable of high-level intellectual activity, and has a normal neurological examination.

traumatic a., the loss or disturbance of memory following an insult or injury to the brain of the type that accompanies a head injury, or excessive use of alcohol, or following the cessation of alcohol ingestion or other psychoactive drugs; or loss or disturbance of memory of the type seen in hysteria and other forms of dissociative disorders.

am•ne•si•ac (am-nē'sē-ak). One suffering from amnesia.

am•ne•sic (am-nē'sik). Relating to or characterized by amnesia. SYN amnestic (1).

am•nes•tic (am-nes'tik). 1. SYN amnesic. 2. An agent causing amnesia. 3. A disorder in which the essential feature is an impairment of the memory function.

△amnio-. The amnion. [G. *amnion*]

☐ am•ni•o•cen•te•sis (am'nē-ō-sen-tē'sis). Transabdominal aspiration of fluid from the amniotic sac for diagnostic purposes. [amnio- + G. *kentēsis*, puncture]

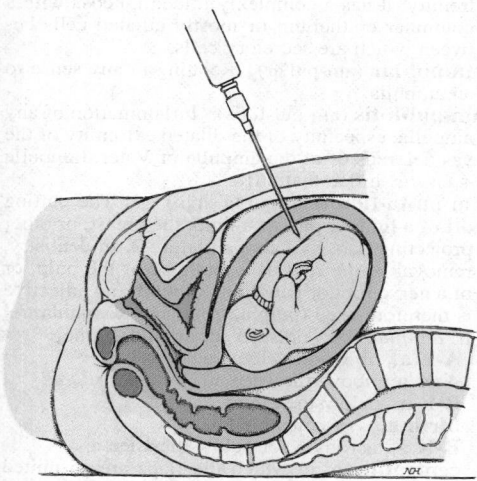

amniocentesis: performed at 15 weeks

am•ni•o•cho•ri•al, am•ni•o•cho•ri•on•ic (am' nē-ō-kōr'ē-ăl, -kōr-ē-on'ik). Relating to both amnion and chorion.

am•ni•o•gen•e•sis (am'nē-ō-jen'ě-sis). Formation of the amnion. [amnio- + G. *genesis*, production]

am•ni•o•ma (am-nē-ō'mă). Broad flat tumor of the skin resulting from antenatal adhesion of the amnion. [amnio- + G. *-oma*, tumor]

am•ni•on (am'nē-on). Innermost of the extraembryonic membranes enveloping the embryo *in utero* and containing the amniotic fluid; it consists of an internal embryonic layer with its ectodermal component, and an external somatic mesodermal component; in the later stages of pregnancy the amnion expands to come in contact with and partially fuse to the inner wall of the chorionic vesicle; derived from the trophoblast cells. SYN amniotic sac. [G. the membrane around the fetus, fr. *amnios*, lamb]

a. nodo′sum, nodules in the a. that consist of typical stratified squamous epithelium. SYN squamous metaplasia of amnion.

am•ni•on•ic (am-nē-on'ik). Relating to the amnion. SYN amniotic.

am•ni•o•ni•tis (am'nē-ō-nī'tis). Inflammation resulting from infection of the amniotic sac, which, in turn, usually results from premature rupture of the membranes (a condition often associated with neonatal infection). [amnion + G. *-itis*, inflammation]

am•ni•or•rhea (am-nē-ō-rē'ă). Escape of amniotic fluid. [amnio- + G. *rhoia*, flow]

am•ni•or•rhex•is (am-nē-ō-rek'sis). Rupture of the amniotic membrane. [amnio- + G. *rhēxis*, rupture]

am•ni•o•scope (am'nē-ō-skōp). An endoscope for studying amniotic fluid through the intact amniotic sac.

am•ni•os•co•py (am-nē-os'kō-pē). Examination of the amniotic fluid in the lowest part of the amniotic sac by means of an endoscope introduced through the cervical canal. [amnio- + G. *skopeō*, to view]

am•ni•ot•ic (am-nē-ot'ik). SYN amnionic.

am•ni•o•tome (am'nē-ō-tōm). An instrument for puncturing the fetal membranes. [amnio- + G. *tomē*, cutting]

am•ni•ot•o•my (am-nē-ot'ō-mē). Artificial rupture of the fetal membranes as a means of inducing or expediting labor.

A-mode. In diagnostic ultrasound, a one-dimensional presentation of a reflected sound wave in which echo amplitude (A) is displayed along the vertical axis and time of rebound (depth) along the horizontal axis; the echo information is presented from interfaces along a single line in the direction of the sound beam.

Amoe•ba (ă-mē'bă). A genus of naked, lobose, pseudopod-forming protozoa of the class Sarcodina (or Rhizopoda), that are abundant soil-dwellers, especially in rich organic debris, and are also commonly found as parasites. The typical amebic parasites of man are now placed in the genera *Entamoeba*, *Endolimax*, and *Iodamoeba*. [Mod. L. fr. G. *amoibē* change]

amorph (ā'mōrf). An allele that has no phenotypically recognizable product and therefore its existence can be inferred on molecular evidence only. [G. *a-* neg. + *morphē*, form, shape]

amor•phia, amor•phism (ă-mōr'fē-ă, -fizm).

Condition of being amorphous (1). [G. *a*- priv. + *morphē*, form]

amor·phous (ă-mōr'fŭs). **1.** Without definite shape or visible differentiation in structure. **2.** Not crystallized.

AMP *adenosine* monophosphate; specifically, the 5'-monophosphate unless modified by a numerical prefix. SEE adenylic acid.

Ampère, André-Marie, French physicist, 1775–1836. SEE ampere.

am·pere (A) (am-pēr'). The practical unit of electrical current; the absolute, practical a. originally was defined as having the value of 1/10 of the electromagnetic unit (see abampere and coulomb). Present definitions are: **1.** The practical unit of electrical current; the absolute, practical a. originally was defined as having the value of 1/10 of the electromagnetic unit (see abampere and coulomb). **2.** Legal definition: the current that, flowing for 1 second, will deposit 1.118 mg of silver from silver nitrate solution. **3.** Scientific (SI) definition: the current that, if maintained in two straight parallel conductors of infinite length and of negligible circular cross-sections and placed 1 m apart in a vacuum, produces between them a force of 2×10^{-7} N/m of length. [A. *Ampère*]

△**amph-.** SEE amphi-, ampho-.

△**amphi-.** On both sides, surrounding, double; corresponds to L. *ambi*-. [G. *amphi*, *amphi*-, on both sides, about, around]

am·phi·ar·thro·di·al (am'fi-ar-thrō'dē-ăl). Relating to a symphysis (1) (amphiarthrosis).

am·phi·as·ter (am-fi-as'ter). The double-star figure formed by the two astrospheres and their connecting spindle fibers during mitosis. [amphi- + G. *aster*, star]

am·phi·cen·tric (am-fi-sen'trik). Centering at both ends, said of a rete mirabile that begins by the vessel breaking up into a number of branches and ends by the branches joining again to form the same vessel. [amphi- + G. *kentron*, center]

△**ampho-.** On both sides, surrounding, double. [G. *amphō*, both]

am·pho·cyte (am'fō-sīt). SYN amphophil (2).

am·pho·phil, am·pho·phile (am'fō-fil, -fīl). **1.** Having an affinity for both acid and basic dyes. SYN amphophilic, amphophilous. **2.** A cell that stains readily with either acid or basic dyes. SYN amphocyte. [ampho- + G. *philos*, fond]

am·pho·phil·ic, am·phoph·i·lous (am-fō-fil'ik, am-fof'i-lŭs). SYN amphophil (1).

am·phor·ic (am-fōr'ik). Denoting a hollow sound heard on percussion and auscultation of the thorax over a pulmonary cavity or pneumothorax. [G. *amphora*, a jar]

am·pho·ter·ic (am-fō-tār'ik). Having two opposite characteristics, especially having the capacity of reacting as either an acid or a base. [G. *amphoteroi* (pl.), both, fr. *amphō*, both]

amphoterism (am-fo-ter-izm). The property of being amphoteric.

am·pli·fi·ca·tion (am'pli-fi-kā'shŭn). The process of making larger, as in increasing an auditory or visual stimulus to enhance its perception. [L. *amplificatio*, an enlarging]

genetic a., a process for producing an increase in pertinent genetic material, particularly for increasing the proportion of plasmid DNA to that of bacterial DNA. Includes the production of extrachromosomal copies of the genes for RNA.

am·pli·fi·er. **1.** A device that increases the magnification of a microscope. **2.** An electronic apparatus that increases the strength of input signals.

image amplifier, a device for converting a low light level fluoroscopic image to one that can be seen by the eye in a lighted environment; usually consists of an electronic light amplifier chained to a television tube.

am·pul·la, gen. and pl. **am·pul·lae** (am-pul'lă, -ē) [NA]. A saccular dilation of a canal or duct. [L. a two-handled bottle]

a. of ductus deferens, the dilation of the ductus deferens where it approaches its contralateral partner just before it is joined by the duct of the seminal vesicle.

duodenal a., the dilated portion of the superior part of the duodenum; SYN a. duodeni [NA]. SEE ALSO duodenal *cap*.

a. duode'ni [NA], SYN duodenal a.

hepatopancreatic a., the dilation within the major duodenal papilla that normally receives both the common bile duct and the main pancreatic duct.

rectal a., a dilated portion of the rectum just above the anal canal.

a. of the semicircular ducts, a nearly spherical enlargement of one end of each of the three semicircular ducts, anterior, posterior, and lateral, where they connect with the utricle. Each contains a neuroepithelial crista ampullaris.

Thoma's a., a dilation of the arterial capillary beyond the sheathed artery of the spleen.

a. of uterine tube, the wide portion of the uterine (fallopian) tube near the fimbriated extremity; it has a complexly folded mucosa with a columnar epithelium of mostly ciliated cells between which are secretory cells.

am·pul·lar (am-pul'ăr). Relating in any sense to an ampulla.

am·pul·li·tis (am-pul-lī'tis). Inflammation of any ampulla, especially of the dilated extremity of the vas deferens or of the ampulla of Vater. [ampulla + G. *itis*, inflammation]

am·pu·ta·tion (am-pyū-tā'shŭn). **1.** The cutting off of a limb or part of a limb, the breast, or other projecting part. SYN congenital a. **2.** In dentistry, removal of the root of a tooth, or of the pulp, or of a nerve root or ganglion; a modifying adjective is therefore used (pulp a.; root a.). [L. *amputatio*, fr. *am-puto*, pp. *-atus*, to cut around, prune]

A-E a., *a*bove-the-*e*lbow a.

A-K a., *a*bove-the-*k*nee a.

B-E a., *b*elow-the-*e*lbow a.

birth a., SYN congenital a.

B-K a., acronym for *b*elow-the-*k*nee a.

central a., a. in which the flaps are so united that the cicatrix runs across the end of the stump.

Chopart's a., a. through the midtarsal joint; *i.e.,* between the tarsal navicular and the calcaneocuboid joints. SYN mediotarsal a.

cineplastic a., a method of a. of an extremity whereby the muscles and tendons are so arranged in the stump that they are able to execute independent movements and to communicate motion to a specially constructed prosthetic apparatus. SYN cineplastics, kineplastics.

circular a., a. performed by a circular incision through the skin, the muscles being similarly divided higher up, and the bone higher still.

congenital a., a. produced *in utero;* attributed to the pressure of constricting bands (amniotic). SYN amputation (1), birth a., intrauterine a., spontaneous a. (1).

consecutive a., a revision or secondary amputation of a limb.

a. in continuity, a. through a segment of a limb, not at a joint.

double flap a., a. in which a flap is cut from the soft parts on either side of the limb.

Dupuytren's a., a. of the arm at the shoulder joint.

elliptical a., circular a. in which the sweep of the knife is not exactly vertical to the axis of the limb, the outline of the cut surface being therefore elliptical.

flap a., an a. in which flaps of the muscular and cutaneous tissues are made to cover the end of the bone. SYN flap operation (1).

flapless a., an a. without any tissue to cover the stump

forequarter a., amputation of the arm with removal of the scapula and a portion of the clavicle.

Gritti-Stokes a., supracondylar a. of the femur, the patella being preserved and applied to the end of the bone, its articular cartilage being removed so as to obtain union.

Hey's a., a. of the foot in front of the tarsometatarsal joint.

interpelviabdominal a., SYN hemipelvectomy.

intrauterine a., SYN congenital a.

Krukenberg's a., a cineplastic a. at the carpus with the distal end of the forearm used to create a fork-like stump; especially valuable in the blind because the stump has proprioception.

Larrey's a., a. at the shoulder joint.

Lisfranc's a., a. of the foot at the tarsometatarsal joint, the sole being preserved to make the flap.

mediotarsal a., SYN Chopart's a.

oblique a., a. in which the line of section through an extremity is at other than a right angle; this yields an oval appearance to the cut surface (hence sometimes, though rarely, referred to as an oval a.).

oval a., (1) a. in which the flaps are obtained by oval incisions through the skin and muscle; **(2)** rarely used term for oblique a.

periosteoplastic a., SYN subperiosteal a.

Pirogoff's a., a. of the foot; the lower articular surfaces of the tibia and fibula are sawed through and the ends covered with a portion of the os calcis which has also been sawed through from above posteriorly downward and forward.

pulp a., SYN pulpotomy.

racket a., a circular or slightly oval a., in which a long incision is made in the axis of the limb.

root a., surgical removal of one or more roots of a multirooted tooth, the remaining root

canal(s) usually being treated endodontically. SYN radectomy, radiectomy, radisectomy.

spontaneous a., (1) SYN congenital a. **(2)** a. as the result of a pathologic process rather than external trauma.

Stokes a., a modification of the Gritti-Stokes a. in that the line of section of the femur is slightly higher.

subperiosteal a., a. in which the periosteum is stripped back from the bone and replaced afterward, forming a periosteal flap over the cut end. SYN periosteoplastic a.

Syme's a., a. of the foot at the ankle joint, the malleoli being sawed off, and a flap being made with the soft parts of the heel.

Teale's a., (1) a. of the forearm in its lower half, or of the thigh, with a long posterior rectangular flap and a short anterior one; **(2)** a. of the leg, with a long anterior rectangular flap and a short posterior one.

transverse a., a. in which the line of section through the extremity is at right angles to the long axis.

traumatic a., a. resulting from accidental or nonsurgical injury; may be complete or incomplete.

Tripier's a., a modification of Chopart's a., in that a part of the calcaneus is also removed.

am•pu•tee (am′pyū-tē). A person with an amputated limb or part of limb.

amu atomic mass *unit*.

amu•sia (ă-myū′zē-ă). A form of aphasia characterized by an inability to produce or recognize music. [G. *a-* priv. + *mousa*, music]

amy•e•lia (ă-mī-ē′lē-ă). Congenital absence of the spinal cord, found in association with anencephaly. [G. *a-* priv. + *myelos*, marrow]

amy•el•ic (ă-mī-ē′lik). SYN amyelous.

amy•e•li•nat•ed (ă-mī′ĕ-li-nā′ted). SYN unmyelinated.

amy•e•li•na•tion (ă-mī′ĕ-li-nā′shŭn). Failure of formation of myelin sheath of a nerve.

amy•e•lin•ic (ă-mī′ĕ-lin′ik). SYN unmyelinated.

amy•e•lo•ic, amy•e•lon•ic (ă-mī-ĕ-lō′ik, ă-mī-ĕ-lon′ik). **1.** SYN amyelous. **2.** In hematology, sometimes used to indicate the absence of bone marrow or the lack of functional participation of bone marrow in hemopoiesis. [G. *a-* priv. + *myelos*, marrow]

amy•e•lous (ă-mī′ĕ-lŭs). Without spinal cord. SYN amyelic, amyeloic (1), amyelonic.

amyg•da•la, gen. and pl. **amyg•da•lae** (ă-mig′dă-lă, -lē). Denoting the cerebellar tonsil, as well as the lymphatic tonsils (pharyngeal, palatine, lingual, laryngeal, and tubal). [L. fr. G. *amygdalē*, almond; in Mediev. & Mod. L., a tonsil]

amyg•da•loid (ă-mig′dă-loyd). Resembling an almond or a tonsil. [amygdala + G. *eidos*, appearance]

am•yl (ā′mil). The radical formed from a pentane, C_5H_{12}, by removal of one H. Several isomeric forms exist. SYN pentyl (1).

△**amyl-. 1.** SEE amylo-. **2.** Pentyl- SEE amyl.

am•y•la•ceous (am′i-lā′shŭs). Starchy.

am•y•lase (am′il-ās). One of a group of amylolytic enzymes that cleave starch, glycogen, and related 1,4-α-glucans.

am·y·la·su·ria (am-i-lā-sū′rē-ă). The excretion of amylase (sometimes termed diastase) in the urine, especially increased amounts in acute pancreatitis. SYN diastasuria.

am·y·lin (am′i-lin). The cellulose of starch; the insoluble envelope of starch grains.

△**amylo-.** Starch, of polysaccharide nature or origin. [G. *amylon,* unmilled; starch, fr. *a-* + *mylē,* a mill]

am·y·lo·gen·e·sis (am-i-lō-jen′ĕ-sis). Biosynthesis of starch. [amylo- + G. *genesis,* production]

am·y·lo·gen·ic (am-i-lō-jen′ik). Relating to amylogenesis.

am·y·loid (am′i-loyd). **1.** Any of a group of chemically diverse proteins that appears microscopically homogeneous, but is composed of linear nonbranching aggregated fibrils arranged in sheets when seen under the electron microscope; it stains dark brown with iodine, produces a characteristic green color in polarized light after staining with Congo red, is metachromatic with either methyl violet (pink-red) or crystal violet (purple-red), and fluoresces yellow after thioflavine T staining; a. occurs characteristically as pathologic extracellular deposits (amyloidosis), especially in association with reticuloendothelial tissue; the chemical nature of the proteinaceous fibrils is dependent upon the underlying disease process. **2.** Resembling or containing starch. [amylo- + G. *eidos,* resemblance]

am·y·loi·do·sis (am′i-loy-dō′sis). **1.** A disease characterized by extracellular accumulation of amyloid in various organs and tissues of the body; may be primary or secondary. **2.** The process of deposition of amyloid protein. [amyloid + G. *-osis,* condition]

   a. of aging, characterized by deposition of Congo-red staining material, derived from a variety of proteins, especially in nervous tissue, myocardium and pancreas. Associated with Alzheimer's syndrome; intractable congestive heart failure may result.

   focal a., SYN nodular a.

   light chain-related a., a form of primary a. in which the fibrillar amyloid deposits are derived from the light chains of immunoglobulin; seen in B-lymphocyte and plasma-cells dyscrasias.

   macular a., a localized form of a. cutis characterized by pruritic symmetrical brown reticulated macules, especially on the upper back; microscopically, amyloid is deposited as small subepidermal globules.

   nodular a., a localized form of a. in which amyloid occurs as masses or nodules beneath the skin or mucous membranes, *e.g.,* in the larynx. SYN amyloid tumor, focal a.

   primary a., a. not associated with other recognized disease. Tends to involve arterial walls and mesenchymal tissues in the tongue, lungs, intestinal tract, skin, skeletal muscle, and myocardium; the amyloid frequently does not manifest the usual affinity for Congo red, and sometimes provokes a foreign-body type of inflammatory reaction.

   renal a., renal deposits of amyloid, especially in glomerular capillary walls, which may cause

albuminuria and the nephrotic syndrome. SYN amyloid nephrosis (1).

   secondary a., a. occurring in association with another chronic inflammatory disease; organs chiefly involved are the liver, spleen, and kidneys, and the adrenal glands less frequently.

   senile a., a common form of a. in very old people, usually mild and limited to the heart. SEE ALSO a. of aging.

am·y·lol·y·sis (am-i-lol′i-sis). Hydrolysis of starch into soluble products. [amylo- + G. *lysis,* dissolution]

am·y·lo·lyt·ic (am-i-lō-lit′ik). Relating to amylolysis.

am·y·lo·pec·tin (am-i-lō-pek′tin). A branched-chain polyglucose (glucan) in starch containing both 1,4 and 1,6 linkages. Cf. amylose.

am·y·lor·rhea (am′i-lō-rē′ă). Passage of undigested starch in the stools, implying a deficiency of amylase activity in the intestine. [amylo- + G. *rhoia,* flow]

am·y·lose (am′i-lōs). An unbranched polyglucose (glucan) in starch, similar to cellulose, containing α(1→4) linkages. Cf. amylopectin.

am·y·lo·su·ria (am′i-lō-sū′rē-ă). Excretion of starch in the urine. SYN amyluria.

am·y·lu·ria (am-i-lū′rē-ă). SYN amylosuria.

amy·o·es·the·sia, amy·o·es·the·sis (ă-mī′ō-es-thē′zē-ă, -thē′sis). Absence of muscle sensation. [G. *a-* priv. + *mys,* muscle, + *aisthēsis,* perception]

amy·o·sta·sia (ă-mī-ō-stā′zē-ă). Difficulty in standing, due to muscular tremor or incoordination. [G. *a-* priv. + *mys,* muscle, + *stasis,* standing]

amy·o·stat·ic (ă-mī-ō-stat′ik). Showing muscular tremors.

amy·os·the·nia (ă-mī′os-thē′nē-ă). Muscular weakness. [G. *a-* priv. + *mys,* muscle, + *sthenos,* strength]

amy·os·then·ic (ă-mī-os-then′ik). Relating to or causing muscular weakness.

amy·o·taxy, amy·o·tax·ia (ă-mī′ō-tak-sē, ă-mī-ō-tak′sē-ă). Muscular ataxia. [G. *a-* priv. + *mys,* muscle, + *taxis,* order]

amy·o·to·nia (ă-mī-ō-tō′nē-ă). Generalized absence of muscle tone, usually associated with flabby musculature and an increased range of passive movement at joints. [G. *a-* priv. + *mys,* muscle, + *tonos,* tone]

   a. congen′ita, (1) atonic pseudoparalysis of congenital origin (neither familial nor hereditary), observed especially in infants and characterized by absence of muscular tone only in muscles innervated by the spinal nerves. SYN myatonia congenita, Oppenheim's disease, Oppenheim's syndrome. **(2)** an indefinite term for a number of congenital neuromuscular disorders that cause generalized myotonia in young children and have a benign course.

amy·o·tro·phic (ă-mī-ō-trō′fik). Relating to muscular atrophy.

amy·ot·ro·phy (ă-mī-ot′rō-fē). Muscular wasting or atrophy. [G. *a-* priv. + *mys,* muscle, + *trophē,* nourishment]

   diabetic a., a type of diabetic neuropathy that primarily affects elderly patients with diabetes mellitus; clinically characterized by unilateral or bilateral anterior thigh pain, weakness, and atrophy; one type of diabetic polyradiculopathy. Sometimes referred to, erroneously, as diabetic femoral neuropathy.

neuralgic a., a neurological disorder, of unknown cause, characterized by the sudden onset of severe pain, usually about the shoulder and often beginning at night, soon followed by weakness and wasting of various forequarter muscles, particularly shoulder girdle muscles; both sporadic and familial in occurrence with the former much more common; often preceded by some antecedent event, such as an upper respiratory infection, hospitalization, vaccination, or nonspecific trauma; usually attributed to a brachial plexus lesion, because the nerve fibers involved are most often derived from the upper trunk, but actually multiple proximal mononeuropathies. SYN shoulder-girdle syndrome.

amyx·or·rhea (ă-mik-sō-rē′ă). Absence of the normal secretion of mucus. [G. *a-* priv. + *myxa,* mucus, + *rhoia,* flow]

△**an-.** SEE a-.

△**ana-.** Prefix: up, toward, apart; not to be confused with *an-* (a form of the prefix *a-,* without, used before a vowel). [G. *ana,* up]

an·a·bi·o·sis (an′ă-bī-ō′sis). Resuscitation after apparent death. [G. a reviving, fr. *ana,* again, + *biōsis,* life]

an·a·bol·ic (an-ă-bol′ik). Relating to or promoting anabolism.

anab·o·lism (ă-nab′ō-lizm). 1. The building up in the body of complex chemical compounds from simpler compounds (*e.g.,* proteins from amino acids), usually with the use of energy. Cf. catabolism, metabolism. 2. The sum of synthetic metabolic reactions. [G. *anabolē,* a raising up]

anab·o·lite (ă-nab′ō-līt). Any substance formed as a result of anabolic processes.

an·a·cid·i·ty (an-ă-sid′i-tē). Absence of acidity; used especially to denote absence of hydrochloric acid in the gastric juice.

anac·la·sis (ă-nak′lă-sis). 1. Reflection of light or sound. 2. Refraction of the ocular media. [G. a bending back, reflection]

an·a·clit·ic (an-ă-klit′ik). Leaning or depending upon; in psychoanalysis, relating to the dependence of the infant on the mother or mother substitute. SEE anaclitic *depression.* [G. *ana,* toward, + *klinō,* to lean]

an·a·crot·ic (an-ă-krot′ik). Referring to the upstroke or ascending limb of the arterial pulse tracing; an abbreviated form for anadicrotic, twice beating on the upstroke. SYN anadicrotic.

anac·ro·tism (ă-nak′rō-tizm). Peculiarity of the pulse wave. SEE anacrotic *pulse.* SYN anadicrotism. [G. *ana,* up, + *krotos,* a beat]

an·a·cu·sis (an′ă-kū′sis). Absence of the ability to perceive sound. SYN anakusis. [G. *an-* priv. + *akousis,* hearing]

an·a·di·crot·ic (an-ă-dī-krot′ik). SYN anacrotic.

an·a·di·cro·tism (an-ă-dik′rō-tizm). SYN anacrotism. [G. *ana,* up, + *di-krotos,* double beating]

an·ad·re·nal·ism (an-ă-drē′năl-izm). Complete lack of adrenal function.

an·aer·obe (an′ār-ōb, an-ār′ōb). A microorganism that can live and grow in the absence of oxygen. [G. *an-* priv. + *aēr,* air, + *bios,* life]

facultative a., an a. that grows in the presence of air or under conditions of reduced oxygen tension.

obligate a., an a. that will grow only in the absence of free oxygen.

an·aer·o·bic (an-ār-ō′bik). Relating to an anaerobe; living without oxygen.

an·aer·o·bi·o·sis (an-ār-ō-bī-ō′sis). Existence in an oxygen-free atmosphere. [G. *an-* priv. + *aēr,* air, + *biōsis,* way of living]

an·aer·o·gen·ic (an-ār-ō-jen′ik). Not producing gas. [G. *an-* priv. + *aēr,* air, + *-gen,* producing]

an·a·gen (an′ă-jen). Growth phase of the hair cycle, lasting about 3 to 6 years in human scalp hair. [G. *ana,* up, + *-gen,* producing]

an·a·ku·sis (an-ă-kū′sis). SYN anacusis.

anal (ā′năl). Relating to the anus.

an·al·bu·mi·ne·mia (an′al-bū-mi-nē′mē-ă). Absence of albumin from the serum. [G. *an-* priv. + albumin + G. *haima,* blood]

an·a·lep·tic (an-ă-lep′tik). 1. Strengthening, stimulating, or invigorating. 2. A restorative remedy. 3. A central nervous system stimulant, particularly used to denote agents that reverse depressed central nervous system function. [G. *analēptikos,* restorative]

an·al·ge·sia (an-ăl-jē′zē-ă). A neurologic or pharmacologic state in which painful stimuli are so moderated that, though still perceived, they are no longer painful. Cf. anesthesia. [G. insensibility, fr. *an-* priv. + *algēsis,* sensation of pain]

a. al′gera, SYN a. dolorosa.

conduction a., SYN regional *anesthesia.*

a. doloro′sa, spontaneous pain in a body area that lacks sensation. SYN a. algera.

inhalation a., a. produced by inhalation of a central nervous system depressant gas (especially nitrous oxide) or vapor.

patient-controlled a. (PCA), a method for control of pain based upon a pump for the constant intravenous or, less frequently, epidural infusion of a dilute narcotic solution that includes a mechanism for the self-administration at predetermined intervals of a predetermined amount of the narcotic solution should the infusion fail to relieve pain.

spinal a., SEE spinal *anesthesia.*

an·al·ge·sic (an-ăl-jē′zik). 1. A compound capable of producing analgesia, *i.e.,* one that relieves pain by altering perception of nociceptive stimuli without producing anesthesia or loss of consciousness. 2. Characterized by reduced response to painful stimuli. SYN antalgic.

anal·i·ty (ā-nal′i-tē). Referring to the psychic organization derived from, and characteristic of, the freudian anal period of psychosexual development.

an·al·ler·gic (an-ă-ler′jik). Not allergic.

an·a·log (an′ă-log). 1. One of two organs or parts in different species of animals or plants which differ in structure or development but are similar in function. 2. A compound that resembles another in structure but is not necessarily an isomer; a.'s are often used to block enzymatic reactions by combining with enzymes. SYN analogue. [G. *analogos,* proportionate]

anal·o·gous (ă-nal′ō-gŭs). Possessing a functional resemblance, but having a different origin or structure.

an·a·logue (an′ă-log). SYN analog.

an·al·pha·lip·o·pro·tein·e·mia (an-al′fă-lip′ō-prō′tēn-ē′mē-ă) [MIM*205400]. Familial high density lipoprotein deficiency; a heritable disorder of lipid metabolism characterized by almost complete absence from plasma of high density lipoproteins, and by storage of cholesterol esters in foam cells, tonsillar enlargement, an orange or yellow-gray color of the pharyngeal and rectal mucosa, hepatosplenomegaly, lymph node enlargement, corneal opacity, and peripheral neuropathy; autosomal recessive inheritance. [G. *an-,* priv., + *alpha,* α, + lipoprotein + *-emia,* blood]

anal·y·sand (ă-nal′i-sand). In psychoanalysis, the person being analyzed. [analysis + L. *-andus,* gerundive ending]

anal·y·sis, pl. **anal·y·ses** (ă-nal′i-sis, -sēz). **1.** The breaking up of a chemical compound or mixture into simpler elements; a process by which the composition of a substance is determined. **2.** The examination and study of a whole in terms of the parts composing it. **3.** SEE psychoanalysis. [G. a breaking up, fr. *ana,* up, + *lysis,* a loosening]

activity a., the process of examining an activity or movement pattern in order to distinguish its component parts.

activity pattern a., any method of determining the type, amount, and organization of activity that occupies the lives of individuals on a recurring basis.

bite a., SYN occlusal a.

blood gas a., the direct electrode measurement of the partial pressure of oxygen and carbon dioxide in the blood.

content a., any of a variety of techniques for classification and study of the verbal products of normal or of psychologically disabled individuals.

Fourier a., a mathematical approximation of a function as the sum of periodic functions (sine waves) of different frequencies; used in reconstruction of images in computed tomography and magnetic resonance imaging and in analysis of any kind of signal for its frequency content.

gastric a., measurement of pH and acid output of stomach contents; basal acid output can be determined by collecting the overnight gastric secretion or by a 1-hr collection; maximal acid output is determined following injection of histamine; output is measured by titration with a strong base.

Northern blot a., a procedure similar to the Southern blot a., used mostly to separate and identify RNA fragments; typically via transferring RNA fragments from an agarose gel to a nitrocellulose filter followed by detection with a suitable probe. [Coined to distinguish it from eponymic Southern blot a.]

occlusal a., a study of the relations of the occlusal surfaces of opposing teeth and their effect upon related structures. SYN bite a.

pedigree a., the formal study of the pattern of a trait in a pedigree to determine such properties as its mode of inheritance, age of onset, and variability in phenotype.

qualitative a., determination of the nature, as opposed to the quantity, of each of the elements composing a substance.

quantitative a., determination of the amount, as well as the nature, of each of the elements composing a substance.

regression a., the statistical method of finding the "best" mathematical model to describe one variable as a function of another.

segregation a., in genetics, the enumeration of progeny according to distinct and mutually exclusive phenotypes; used as a test of a putative pattern of inheritance, *e.g.,* mendelian, dominant autosomal, epistatic, age-dependent.

Southern blot a., a procedure to separate and identify DNA sequences; DNA fragments are separated by electrophoresis on an agarose gel, transferred (blotted) onto a nitrocellulose or nylon membrane, and hybridized with complementary (labeled) nucleic acid probes.

transactional a., a psychotherapy system, used in both individual and group treatment, involving a systematic understanding of the qualities of interpersonal interactions in the treatment sessions; includes four components: 1) structural analysis of intrapsychic phenomena; 2) transactional a. proper, determination of the currently dominant ego state (parent, child, or adult) of each participant; 3) game analysis, identification of the games played in their interactions and of the gratifications provided; 4) script analysis, uncovering of the causes of the patient's emotional problems.

a. of variance (ANOVA), a statistical technique that isolates and assesses the contribution of categorical independent variables to variation in the mean of a continuous dependent variable.

volumetric a., quantitative a. by the addition of graduated amounts of a standard test solution to a solution of a known amount of the substance analyzed, until the reaction is just at an end; depends upon the stoichiometric nature of the reaction between the test solution and the unknown.

Western blot a., a procedure in which proteins separated by electrophoresis in polyacrylamide gels are transferred (blotted) onto nitrocellulose or nylon membranes and identified by specific complexing with antibodies that are either pre- or post-tagged with a labeled secondary protein. SEE ALSO immunoblot. SYN Western blot, Western blotting. [Coined to distinguish it from eponymic Southern blot a.]

zoo blot a., a procedure using Southern blot a. to test the ability of a nucleic acid probe from one species to hybridize with the DNA fragment of another species.

an·a·lyst (an′ă-list). **1.** One who makes analytical determinations. **2.** Psychoanalyst.

an·a·lyte (an′ă-līt). A material or substance whose presence or concentration in a specimen is determined by analysis.

an·a·lyt·ic, an·a·lyt·i·cal (an-ă-lit′-ik, -i-kăl). **1.** Relating to analysis. **2.** Relating to psychoanalysis.

an·a·lyz·er, an·a·lyz·or (an′ă-līz-er, -ŏr). **1.**

Any instrument that performs an analysis. **2.** The prism in a polariscope by means of which the polarized light is examined. **3.** The neural basis of the conditioned reflex; includes all of the sensory side of the reflex arc and its central connections. **4.** A device that electronically determines the frequency and amplitude of a particular channel of an electroencephalogram.

CO₂ a., SYN capnometer.

pulse height a., electronic circuitry that determines the energy of scintillations recorded by a detector, allowing use of a discriminator to select for photons of a specific type.

an•am•ne•sis (an-am-nē′sis). **1.** The act of remembering. **2.** The medical or developmental history of a patient. [G. *anamnēsis*, recollection]

an•am•nes•tic (an-am-nes′tik). **1.** Assisting the memory. SYN mnemonic. **2.** Relating to the medical history of a patient.

an•a•phase (an′ă-fāz). The stage of mitosis or meiosis in which the chromosomes move from the equatorial plate toward the poles of the cell. In mitosis a full set of daughter chromosomes (46 in humans) moves toward each pole. In the first division of meiosis one member of each homologous pair (23 in humans), consisting of two chromatids united at the centromere, moves toward each pole. In the second division of meiosis the centromere divides, and the two chromatids separate with one moving to each pole. [G. *ana*, up, + *phasis*, appearance]

an•a•phia (an-ā′fē-ă, an-af′ē-ă). Absence of the sense of touch. [G. *an-* priv. + *haphē*, touch]

an•aph•ro•di•si•ac (an′af-rō-diz′ē-ak). **1.** Repressing or destroying sexual desire. **2.** An agent that lessens or abolishes sexual desire. [G. *an-* priv. + *aphrodisia*, sexual pleasure]

an•a•phy•lac•tic (an′ă-fī-lak′tik). Relating to anaphylaxis; manifesting extremely great sensitivity to foreign protein or other material.

an•a•phy•lac•to•gen (an′ă-fī-lak′tō-jen). A substance (antigen) capable of rendering an individual susceptible to anaphylaxis; a substance (antigen) that will cause an anaphylactic reaction in such a sensitized individual.

an•a•phy•lac•to•gen•e•sis (an′ă-fī-lak-tō-jen′ē-sis). The production of anaphylaxis.

an•a•phy•lac•to•gen•ic (an′ă-fī-lak-tō-jen′ik). Producing anaphylaxis; pertaining to substances (antigens) that result in an individual becoming susceptible to anaphylaxis.

an•a•phy•lac•toid (an′ă-fī-lak′toyd). Resembling anaphylaxis. [anaphylaxis + G. *eidos*, resemblance]

an•a•phyl•a•tox•in (an′ă-fil-ă-tok′sin). **1.** A substance postulated to be the immediate cause of anaphylactic shock and that is assumed to result from the *in vivo* combination of specific antibody and the specific sensitizing material. **2.** The small fragment (C3a) split from the third component (C3) of complement, which produces a local wheal following intracutaneous injection. SYN anaphylotoxin. [anaphylaxis + toxin]

an•a•phy•lax•is (an′ă-fī-lak′sis). The immediate, transient kind of immunologic (allergic) reaction characterized by contraction of smooth muscle and dilation of capillaries due to release of phar-

macologically active substances (histamine, bradykinin, serotonin, and slow-reacting substance), classically initiated by the combination of antigen (allergen) with mast cell-fixed, cytophilic antibody (chiefly IgE); the reaction can be initiated, also, by relatively large quantities of serum aggregates (antigen-antibody complexes, and others) that seemingly activate complement leading to production of anaphylatoxin, a reaction sometimes termed "aggregate a." [G. *ana*, away from, back from, + *phylaxis*, protection]

active a., reaction following inoculation of antigen in a subject previously sensitized to the specific antigen, in contrast to passive a.

antiserum a., SYN passive a.

generalized a., the immediate response, involving smooth muscles and capillaries throughout the body, that follows injection of antigen (allergen). SEE ALSO anaphylactic *shock*. SYN systemic a.

local a., the immediate, transient kind of response that follows the injection of antigen (allergen) into the skin of a sensitized individual and is limited to the area surrounding the site of inoculation. SEE ALSO skin *test*.

passive a., a reaction resulting from inoculation of antigen in an animal previously inoculated intravenously with specific antiserum from another animal, a latent period being required between the two inoculations. SYN antiserum a.

systemic a., SYN generalized a.

an•a•phyl•o•tox•in (an′ă-fil-ō-tok′sin). SYN anaphylatoxin.

an•a•pla•sia (an-ă-plā′sē-ă). Loss of structural differentiation, especially as seen in most, but not all, malignant neoplasms. SYN dedifferentiation (2). [G. *ana*, again, + *plasis*, a molding]

an•a•plas•tic (an-ă-plas′tik). **1.** Relating to anaplasty. **2.** Characterized by or pertaining to anaplasia. **3.** Growing without form or structure.

an•a•poph•y•sis (an-ă-pof′i-sis). An accessory spinal process of a vertebra, found especially in the thoracic or lumbar vertebrae. [G. *ana*, back, + *apophysis*, offshoot]

anap•tic (ă-nap′tik). Relating to anaphia.

an•a•rith•mia (an-ă-rith′mē-ă). Aphasia characterized by an inability to count or use numbers. [G. *an-* priv. + *arithmos*, number]

an•ar•thria (an-ar′thrē-a). Loss of the power of articulate speech. SEE ALSO aphasia, alexia, dysarthria. [G. fr. *an-anthos*, without joints; (of sound) inarticulate]

an•a•sar•ca (an-ă-sar′kă). A generalized infiltration of edema fluid into subcutaneous connective tissue. [G. *ana*, through, + *sarx* (*sark-*), flesh]

an•a•sar•cous (an-ă-sar′kŭs). Characterized by anasarca.

an•as•tig•mats. **1.** Lenses in which astigmatism is corrected. **2.** Lenses in which both astigmatism and field curvature are corrected.

anas•to•mose (ă-nas′tō-mōs). **1.** To open one structure into another directly or by connecting channels, said of blood vessels, lymphatics, and hollow viscera; also incorrectly applied to nerves. **2.** To unite by means of an anastomosis, or connection between formerly separate structures.

anas•to•mo•sis, pl. **anas•to•mo•ses** (ă-nas′tō-mō′sis, -sez). **1.** A natural communication, direct or indirect, between two blood vessels or other tubular structures. Also incorrectly applied to nerves. SEE communication. **2.** An operative union of two hollow or tubular structures. **3.** An opening created by surgery, trauma, or disease between two or more normally separate spaces or organs. [G. *anastomōsis,* from *anastomoō,* to furnish with a mouth]

arteriovenous a., vessels through which blood is shunted from arterioles to venules without passing through the capillaries.

cavopulmonary a., a means of palliating cyanotic heart disease by anastomosing the right pulmonary artery to the superior vena cava.

conjoined a., the joining together of two small blood vessels by side-to-side elliptical a. to create a single larger stoma for subsequent end-to-end a.

cruciate a., crucial a., a four-way a. between branches of the first perforating branch of the deep femoral, inferior gluteal and medial and lateral circumflex femoral arteries, located posterior to the upper part of the femur.

intestinal a., SYN enteroenterostomy.

isoperistaltic a., an a. allowing flow of contents in the same and normal direction.

postcostal a., longitudinal a. of intersegmental arteries giving rise to the vertebral artery.

precostal a. (prē-kos-tal), longitudinal a. of intersegmental arteries in the embryo that gives rise to the thyrocervical and costocervical trunks.

Riolan's a., the specific portion of the marginal artery of the colon connecting the middle and left colic arteries.

Roux-en-Y a., a. of the distal end of the divided jejunum to the stomach, bile duct, or another structure, with implantation of the proximal end into the side of the jejunum at a suitable distance below the first a., the bowel then forming a Y-shaped pattern.

termino-terminal a., an operation by which the central end of an artery is connected with the peripheral end of the corresponding vein, and the peripheral end of the artery with the central end of the vein.

anas•to•mot•ic (a-nas-tō-mot′ik). Pertaining to an anastomosis.

an•a•tom•i•cal (an′ă-tom′i-kăl). **1.** Relating to anatomy. **2.** SYN structural. **3.** Denoting a strictly morphological feature distinct from its physiological or surgical considerations, *e.g.,* anatomical neck of humerus, anatomical dead space, anatomical lobulation of the liver.

anat•o•mist (ă-nat′ŏ-mist). A specialist in the science of anatomy.

anat•o•my (ă-nat′ŏ-mē). **1.** The morphologic structure of an organism. **2.** The science of the morphology or structure of organisms. **3.** SYN dissection. **4.** A work describing the form and structure of an organism and its various parts. [G. *anatomē,* dissection, from *ana,* apart, + *tomē,* a cutting]

airway a., the tracheobronchial structure, similar to an inverted tree, containing three types of airways: cartilaginous airways (trachea, main stem bronchi, and approximately five generations of small bronchi); membranous bronchioles (ap-

proximately eight generations of non-cartilaginous airways); and respiratory bronchioles (approximately five generations of gas-exchange or alveolar ducts).

clinical a., the practical application of anatomical knowledge to diagnosis and treatment.

comparative a., the comparative study of animal structure with regard to homologous organs or parts.

dental a., that branch of gross a. concerned with the morphology of teeth, their location, position, and relationships.

developmental a., a. of the structural changes of an individual from fertilization to adulthood; includes embryology, fetology, and postnatal development.

functional a., a. studied in its relation to function.

general a., the study of gross and microscopic structures as well as of the composition of the body, its tissues and fluids.

gross a., general a., so far as it can be studied without the use of the microscope; commonly used to denote the study of a. by dissection of a cadaver. SYN macroscopic a.

macroscopic a., SYN gross a.

microscopic a., the branch of a. in which the structure of cells, tissues, and organs is studied with the light microscope. SEE ALSO histology.

pathological a., SYN anatomical *pathology.*

radiological a., the study of bodily structure using radiographs and other imaging methods.

regional a., an approach to anatomical study based on regions, parts, or divisions of the body (*e.g.,* the foot or the inguinal region), emphasizing the relationships of various systemic structures (*e.g.,* muscles, nerves, and arteries) within that area; distinguished from systemic anatomy. SYN topographic a.

special a., the a. of certain definite organs or groups of organs involved in the performance of special functions; descriptive a. dealing with the separate systems.

surface a., the study of the configuration of the surface of the body, especially in its relation to deeper parts.

surgical a., applied a. in reference to surgical diagnosis and treatment.

topographic a., SYN regional a.

ultrastructural a., the ultramicroscopic study of structures too small to be seen with a light microscope.

an•a•tri•crot•ic (an′ă-trī-krot′ik). Characterized by anatricrotism; denoting a sphygmographic tracing with three waves on the ascending limb.

an•a•tric•ro•tism (an′ă-trik′rō-tizm). A condition of the pulse manifested by a triple beat on the ascending limb of the sphygmographic tracing. [G. *ana,* up, + *tri-,* thrice, + *krotos,* beating]

an•chor•age (ang′kōr-ij). **1.** Operative fixation of loose or prolapsed abdominal or pelvic organs. **2.** The part to which anything is fastened. In dentistry, a tooth or an implanted tooth substitute with which a fixed or removable partial denture, crown, or restoration is retained. **3.** The nature and degree of resistance to displacement offered by an anatomical unit when used for the purpose of effecting tooth movement. [L. *ancora,* fr. G. *ankyra,* anchor]

an•cil•lary (an'si-lār-ē). Auxiliary, accessory, or secondary. [L. *ancillaris,* relating to a maid-servant]

ancillary services. diagnostic or therapeutic a. s.'s provided by a physician for inpatients or outpatients as an adjunct to basic medical or surgical services.

an•cip•i•tal, an•cip•i•tate, an•cip•i•tous (an-sip'i-tăl, -i-tāt, -i-tŭs). Two-headed; two-edged. [L. *anceps,* two-headed]

an•co•nad (ang'kō-nad). Toward the elbow. [G. *ankōn,* elbow, + L. *ad,* to]

an•co•nal, an•co•ne•al (ang'kŏ-năl, ang-kō'nē-ăl). 1. Relating to the elbow (ancon). 2. Relating to the anconeus muscle.

◇**ancylo-.** SEE ankylo-.

An•cy•los•to•ma (an-si-los'tō-mă, an-ki-). A genus of Nematoda, the Old World hookworm, the members of which are parasitic in the duodenum. They attach themselves to the mucous membrane, suck blood, and may cause anemia. The eggs are passed with the feces, and the larvae develop in moist soil to become infectious third-stage (filariform) larvae that enter the human body through the skin and possibly in drinking water; they migrate by the bloodstream to lung alveoli, are carried to bronchi and trachea, swallowed, and passed to the intestine, where they mature. SEE ALSO ancylostomiasis, *Necator.* [G. *ankylos,* curved, hooked, + *stoma,* mouth]

A. brazilien'se, a species characterized by one pair of ventral buccal teeth, normally an intestinal parasite of dogs and cats but also found in humans as a cause of human cutaneous larva migrans.

A. cani'num, a species possessing three pairs of ventral teeth in the oral cavity; common in dogs, but also occurring in human skin as a cause of cutaneous larva migrans.

A. duodena'le, the Old World hookworm of humans, a species widespread in temperate areas, in contrast to the more tropical distribution of the New World hookworm, *Necator americanus.* It is the only hookworm found in the U.S.

an•cy•lo•sto•mi•a•sis (an'si-lō-stō-mī'ă-sis, an'ki-). Hookworm disease caused by *Ancylostoma duodenale* and characterized by eosinophilia, anemia, emaciation, dyspepsia, and, in children with severe chronic infections, swelling of the abdomen with mental and physical maldevelopment.

cutaneous a., cutaneous larva migrans caused by larvae of hookworms. SYN swimmer's itch (1), water itch (1).

an•cy•roid (an'si-royd). Shaped like the fluke of an anchor; denoting the cornua of the lateral ventricles of the brain and the coracoid process of the scapula. [G. *ankyra,* anchor, + *eidos,* resemblance]

◇**andro-.** Masculine. [G. *anēr, andros,* a male human being]

an•dro•blas•to•ma (an'drō-blas-tō'mă). 1. A testicular tumor microscopically resembling fetal testis, with varying proportions of tubular and stromal elements; the tubules contain Sertoli cells, which may cause feminization. 2. SYN arrhenoblastoma. [G. *anēr (andro-),* man, + *blastos,* germ, + *-oma,* tumor]

an•dro•gen (an'drō-jen). Generic term for an agent, usually a hormone (*e.g.,* androsterone, testosterone), that stimulates activity of the accessory male sex organs, promotes development of male sex characteristics, or prevents changes in the latter that follow castration; natural a.'s are steroids, derivatives of androstane.

an•drog•y•nous (an-droj'i-nŭs). Pertaining to androgyny.

an•drog•y•ny (an-droj'i-nē). 1. SYN female *pseudohermaphroditism.* 2. Having both masculine and feminine characteristics, as in attitudes and behaviors that contain features of stereotyped, culturally sanctioned sexual roles of both male and female. [andro- + G. *gynē,* woman]

an•dro•mor•phous (an-drō-mōr'fŭs). Having a male form or habitus. [andro- + G. *morphē,* form]

an•dro•pho•bia (an-drō-fō'bē-ă). Morbid fear of men, or of the male sex, resulting in avoidance of situations where men are present. [andro- + G. *phobos,* fear]

an•dro•stane (an'drō-stān). The parent hydrocarbon of the androgenic steroids.

an•dro•stane•di•ol (an-drō-stān'dī-ol). 5α-Androstane-3β,17β-diol; a steroid metabolite, of which 5β isomers are also known.

an•dro•stane•di•one (an-drō-stān'dī-ōn). 5α-Androstane-3,17-dione; a steroid metabolite, of which the 5β isomer is also known.

an•dro•stene (an'drō-stēn). Androstane with an unsaturated (*i.e.,* —CH=CH—) bond in the molecule.

an•dro•stene•di•ol (an-drō-stēn'dī-ol). 5-Androsten-3β,17β-diol; a steroid metabolite differing from androstanediol by possessing a double bond between C-5 and C-6.

an•dro•stene•di•one (an-drō-stēn'dī-ōn). 4-Androstene-3,17-dione; an androgenic steroid of weaker biological potency than testosterone; secreted by the testis, ovary, and adrenal cortex.

an•dros•ter•one (an-dros'ter-ōn). *cis*-Androsterone; 3α-hydroxy-5α-androstan-17-one; (3α-hydroxyetioallocholan-17-one; 3-epihydroxyetioallocholan-17-one); a steroid metabolite, found in male urine, having weak androgenic potency. Formed in testes from progesterone.

an•e•cho•ic (an-ĕ-kō'ik). The property of appearing echo-free or without echoes on a sonographic image; a clear cyst appears anechoic. [G. *an-* priv. + echo + ic]

ane•mia (ă-nē'mē-ă). Any condition in which the number of red blood cells per cu mm, the amount of hemoglobin in 100 ml of blood, and the volume of packed red blood cells per 100 ml of blood are less than normal; clinically, generally pertaining to the concentration of oxygen-transporting material in a designated volume of blood, in contrast to total quantities as in oligocythemia, oligochromemia, and oligemia. A. is frequently manifested by pallor of the skin and mucous membranes, shortness of breath, palpitations of the heart, soft systolic murmurs, lethargy, and fatigability. [G. *anaimia,* fr. *an-* priv. + *haima,* blood]

achrestic a., a form of chronic progressive macrocytic a. that can be fatal in which the changes in bone marrow and circulating blood closely resemble those of pernicious a., but in which there is only transient or no response to therapy with vitamin B$_{12}$; glossitis, gastrointestinal disturbances, central nervous system disease, and pyrexia are not observed, and there is only little bleeding or hemolysis. [G. *a-* priv. + *chrēsis,* a using]

Addison's a., SYN pernicious a.

aplastic a., a. characterized by a greatly decreased formation of erythrocytes and hemoglobin, usually associated with pronounced granulocytopenia and thrombocytopenia, as a result of hypoplastic or aplastic bone marrow.

autoimmune hemolytic a., (1) a. caused by severe hemolysis in cold hemagglutinin disease; **(2)** (warm antibody type) acquired hemolytic a. due to serum autoantibodies that react with the patient's red blood cells, antigenic specificity being chiefly in the Rh complex; it may be idiopathic or secondary to neoplastic, autoimmune, or other disease.

congenital a., SYN *erythroblastosis* fetalis.

congenital Heinz body hemolytic a., a group of congenital hemolytic a.'s caused by inheritance of an unstable hemoglobin variant. An amino acid substitution in one of the hemoglobin chains prevents the hemoglobin from folding into its normal conformation, alters the alpha-helix structure or subunit interaction sites, or affects the binding of heme to globin. The hemoglobin denatures into Heinz bodies, which attach to the cell membrane and cause membrane injury and premature destruction of the cell.

congenital hemolytic a., accelerated destruction of red blood cells due to an inherited defect, such as in the membrane in hereditary spherocytosis.

congenital hypoplastic a. [MIM*205900], congenital nonregenerative, familial hypoplastic, or pure red cell a.; erythrogenesis imperfecta; Diamond-Blackfan syndrome; a. resulting from congenital hypoplasia of the bone marrow, which is grossly deficient in erythroid precursors while other elements are normal; a. is progressive and severe, but leukocyte and platelet counts are normal or slightly reduced; survival of transfused erythrocytes is normal.

Cooley's a., SYN *thalassemia* major.

crescent cell a., SYN sickle cell a.

drepanocytic a., SYN sickle cell a.

equine infectious a., a worldwide infectious disease of horses and other equids, caused by equine infectious a. virus and a member of the family Retroviridae, marked by general debility, remittent fever, staggering gait, progressive a., and loss of flesh; it is transmitted by bloodsucking insects and by contact, oral infection, or the use of unsterilized syringes and needles. SYN swamp fever (1).

exercise-induced a., reduction in hemoglobin concentration to levels approaching clinical a., believed due to intense exercise training; generally occurs in the early phase of training and parallels the disproportionately large expansion

in plasma volume in relation to total hemoglobin with training. SEE ALSO anemia. SYN sports a.

false a., SYN pseudoanemia.

feline infectious a. (FIA), an acute or chronic a. of domestic cats caused by the rickettsia *Haemobartonella felis.*

hemolytic a., any a. resulting from an increased rate of erythrocyte destruction.

hyperchromic a., hyperchromatic a., a. characterized by a decrease in the ratio of the weight of hemoglobin to the volume of the erythrocyte, *i.e.,* the mean corpuscular hemoglobin concentration is less than normal.

hypochromic a., a. characterized by a decrease in the ratio of the weight of hemoglobin to the volume of the erythrocyte, *i.e.,* the mean corpuscular hemoglobin concentration is less than normal.

hypoplastic a., progressive nonregenerative a. resulting from greatly depressed, inadequately functioning bone marrow; as the process persists, aplastic a. may occur.

iron deficiency a., hypochromic microcytic a. characterized by low serum iron, increased serum iron-binding capacity, decreased serum ferritin, and decreased marrow iron stores.

macrocytic a., any a. in which the average size of circulating erythrocytes is greater than normal, *i.e.,* the mean corpuscular volume is 94 cu μm or more (normal range, 82 to 92 cu μm), including such syndromes as pernicious a., sprue, celiac disease, macrocytic a. of pregnancy, a. of diphyllobothriasis, and others.

malignant a., SYN pernicious a.

megaloblastic a., any a. in which there is a predominant number of megaloblastic erythroblasts, and relatively few normoblasts, among the hyperplastic erythroid cells in the bone marrow (as in pernicious a.).

metaplastic a., pernicious a. in which the various formed elements in the blood are changed, *e.g.,* multisegmented, unusually large neutrophils (macropolycytes), immature myeloid cells, bizarre platelets.

microangiopathic hemolytic a., hemolysis due to narrowing or obstruction of small blood vessels usually due to inflammation, causing fragmentation and distortion in the shape of red blood cells.

microcytic a., any a. in which the average size of circulating erythrocytes is smaller than normal, *i.e.,* the mean corpuscular volume is 80 cu μm or less (normal range, 82 to 92 cu μm).

myelophthisic a., myelopathic a., SYN leukoerythroblastosis.

neonatal a., SYN *erythroblastosis* fetalis.

normochromic a., any a. in which the concentration of hemoglobin in the erythrocytes is within the normal range, *i.e.,* the mean corpuscular hemoglobin concentration is from 32 to 36%.

normocytic a., any a. in which the erythrocytes are normal in size, *i.e.,* the mean corpuscular volume ranges from 82 to 92 cu μm.

pernicious a. [MIM*361000], a chronic progressive a. of older adults due to failure of absorption of Vitamin B$_{12}$, usually resulting from a defect of the stomach accompanied by mucosal atrophy and associated with lack of secretion of "intrinsic" factor; characterized by numbness and tingling, weakness, and a sore smooth tongue, as well as dyspnea after slight exertion, faintness, pallor of the skin and mucous membranes, anorexia, diarrhea, loss of weight, and fever; laboratory studies usually reveal greatly decreased red blood cell counts, low levels of hemoglobin, numerous characteristically oval shaped macrocytic erythrocytes, and hypo- or achlorhydria, in association with a predominant number of megaloblasts and relatively few normoblasts in the bone marrow; the leukocyte count in peripheral blood may be less than normal, with relative lymphocytosis and hypersegmented neutrophils; a low level of vitamin B_{12} is found in peripheral red blood cells; administration of vitamin B_{12} results in a characteristic reticulocyte response, relief from symptoms, and an increase in erythrocytes, provided that pernicious a. is not complicated by another disease. SYN Addison's a., malignant a.

refractory a., progressive a. unresponsive to therapy other than transfusion.

sickle cell a. [MIM*141900], an autosomal dominant a. [MIM141900] characterized by crescent- or sickle-shaped erythrocytes and by accelerated hemolysis, due to substitution of a single amino acid (valine for glutamic acid) in the sixth position of the beta chain of hemoglobin; affected homozygotes have 85-95% Hb S and severe anemia, while heterozygotes (said to have sickle cell trait) have 40-45% Hb S, the rest being normal Hb A; low oxygen tension causes polymerization of the abnormal beta chains, thus distorting the shape of the red blood cells to the sickle form. Homozygotes develop "crises" episodes of severe pain due to microvascular occlusions, bone infarcts, leg ulcers, and atrophy of the spleen associated with increased susceptibility to bacterial infections, especially streptococcal pneumonia. Occurs almost exclusively in blacks. SYN crescent cell a., drepanocytic a., sickle cell disease.

sideroblastic a., sideroachrestic a., refractory a. characterized by the presence of sideroblasts in the bone marrow.

spherocytic a., SYN hereditary *spherocytosis.*

sports a., SYN exercise-induced a.

tropical a., various syndromes frequently observed in persons in tropical climates, usually resulting from nutritional deficiencies or hookworm or other parasitic diseases.

ane•mic (ă-nē′mik). Pertaining to or manifesting the various features of anemia.

an•e•mo•pho•bia (an′ē-mō-fō′bē-ă). Morbid fear of wind. [G. *anemos,* wind, + *phobos,* fear]

an•en•ce•phal•ic (an-en-se-fal′ik). Relating to anencephaly.

an•en•ceph•a•ly (an′en-sef′ă-lē). Congenital defective development of the brain, with absence of the bones of the cranial vault and absent or rudimentary cerebral and cerebellar hemispheres, brainstem, and basal ganglia. [G. *an-* priv. + *enkephalos,* brain]

aneph•ric (ă-nef′rik). Lacking kidneys. [*a-* priv. + G. *nephros,* kidney]

an•er•ga•sia (an-er-gā′zē-ă). Absence of psychic

activity as the result of organic brain disease. [G. *an-* priv. + *ergasia,* work]

an•er•gas•tic (an-er-gas′tik). Pertaining to or characterized by anergasia.

an•er•gic (an-er′jik). Relating to, or marked by, anergy.

an•er•gy (an′er-jē). **1.** Absence of ability to generate a sensitivity reaction in a subject to substances expected to be antigenic (immunogenic, allergenic) in that individual. **2.** Lack of energy. [G. *an-* priv. + *energeia,* energy, from *ergon,* work]

an•e•ryth•ro•pla•sia (an′ĕ-rith-rō-plā′zē-ă). A condition in which there is no formation of red blood cells. [G. *an-* priv. + erythro(cyte) + G. *plasis,* a molding]

an•e•ryth•ro•plas•tic (an′ĕ-rith-rō-plas′tik). Pertaining to or characterized by anerythroplasia.

an•es•the•ki•ne•sia (an-es′thē-ki-nē′zē-ă). Combined sensory and motor paralysis. [G. *an-* priv. + *aisthēsis,* sensation, + *kinēsis,* movement]

an•es•the•sia (an′es-thē′zē-ă). **1.** Loss of sensation resulting from pharmacologic depression of nerve function or from neurological dysfunction. **2.** Broad term for anesthesiology as a clinical specialty. [G. *anaisthēsia,* fr. *an-* priv. + *aisthēsis,* sensation]

acupuncture a., percutaneous insertion of, and stimulation by, needles placed in critical areas of the body to produce loss of sensation in another area.

balanced a., a technique of general a. based on the concept that administration of a mixture of small amounts of several neuronal depressants summates the advantages, but not the disadvantages of, the individual components of the mixture.

basal a., parenteral administration of one or more sedatives to produce a state of depressed consciousness short of a general a.

block a., SYN conduction a.

caudal a., regional a. by injection of local anesthetic solution into the epidural space via the sacral hiatus.

circle absorption a., inhalation a. in which a circuit with carbon dioxide absorbent is used for complete (closed) or partial (semiclosed) rebreathing of exhaled gases.

closed a., inhalation a. in which there is total rebreathing of all exhaled gases, except carbon dioxide which is absorbed; gas flow into the anesthetic circuit consists only of oxygen, in amounts equal to the patient's metabolic consumption, plus small amounts of other gases (*e.g.,* nitrous oxide) which undergo continued uptake by and distribution in the patient.

conduction a., regional a. in which local anesthetic solution is injected about nerves to inhibit nerve transmission; includes spinal, epidural, nerve block, and field block a., but not local or topical a. SYN block a.

dissociated a., loss of some types of sensation with persistence of others; most often used in context of nerve blocks, wherein a loss of sensation for pain and temperature occurs without loss of tactile sense.

dissociative a., a form of general a., but not

necessarily complete unconsciousness, characterized by catalepsy, catatonia, and amnesia, especially that produced by phenylcyclohexylamine compounds, including ketamine.

a. doloro′sa, severe spontaneous pain occurring in an anesthetic area.

endotracheal a., inhalation a. technique in which anesthetic and respiratory gases pass through a tube placed in the trachea via the mouth or nose.

epidural a., regional a. produced by injection of local anesthetic solution into the peridural space.

general a., loss of ability to perceive pain associated with loss of consciousness produced by intravenous or inhalation anesthetic agents.

girdle a., a. distributed as a band encircling the trunk.

glove a., loss of sensation in the distal upper extremity, *i.e.,* the hand and fingers.

infiltration a., a. produced by injection of local anesthetic solution directly into an area that is painful or about to be operated upon.

inhalation a., general a. resulting from breathing of anesthetic gases or vapors.

insufflation a., maintenance of inhalation a. by delivery of anesthetic gases or vapors directly to the airway of a spontaneously breathing patient.

intranasal a., (1) insufflation a. in which an inhalation anesthetic is added to inhaled air passing through the nose or nasopharynx; **(2)** a. of nasal passages by infiltration and topical application of local anesthetic solution to nasal mucosa.

intraoral a., (1) insufflation a. in which an inhalation anesthetic is added to inhaled air passing through the mouth; **(2)** regional a. of the mouth and associated structures when local anesthetic solutions are used by topical application to oral mucosa, by local infiltration, or as nerve blocks.

intravenous a., general a. produced by injection of central nervous system depressants into the venous circulation.

intravenous regional a., regional a. by intravenous injection of local anesthetic solution distal to an occlusive tourniquet in an extremity previously exsanguinated by pressure or gravity. SYN Bier's method (1).

local a., a general term referring to topical, infiltration, field block, or nerve block a. but usually not to spinal or epidural a.

nerve block a., conduction a. in which local anesthetic solution is injected about nerves, nerve trunks, or nerve plexuses.

nonrebreathing a., a technique for inhalation a. in which valves exhaust all exhaled air from the circuit.

open drop a., inhalation a. by vaporization of a liquid anesthetic placed drop by drop on a gauze mask covering the mouth and nose.

patient-controlled a. (PCA), a method for control of pain based upon a pump for the constant intravenous or, less frequently, epidural infusion of a dilute narcotic solution that includes a mechanism for the self-administration at predetermined intervals of a predetermined amount

of the narcotic solution should the infusion fail to relieve pain.

perineural a., a. produced by injection of an anesthetic agent around a nerve.

rebreathing a., a technique for inhalation a. in which a portion or all of the gases that are exhaled are subsequently inhaled after carbon dioxide has been absorbed.

rectal a., general a. produced by instillation into the rectum of a solution containing a central nervous system depressant.

refrigeration a., SYN cryoanesthesia.

regional a., use of local anesthetic solution(s) to produce circumscribed areas of loss of sensation; a generic term including conduction, nerve block, spinal, epidural, field block, infiltration, and topical a. SYN conduction analgesia.

retrobulbar a., injection of a local anesthetic behind the eye to produce sensory denervation of the eye.

saddle block a., a form of spinal a. limited in area to the buttocks, perineum, and inner surfaces of the thighs.

segmental a., loss of sensation limited to an area supplied by one or more spinal nerve roots.

semi-closed a., inhalation a. using a circuit in which a portion of the exhaled air is exhausted from the circuit and a portion is rebreathed following absorption of carbon dioxide.

semi-open a., inhalation a. in which a portion of inhaled gases is derived from an anesthesia circuit while the remainder consists of room air.

spinal a., (1) loss of sensation produced by injection of local anesthetic solution(s) into the spinal subarachnoid space; **(2)** loss of sensation produced by disease of the spinal cord.

splanchnic a., loss of sensation in areas of the visceral peritoneum innervated by the splanchnic nerves. SYN visceral a.

stocking a., loss of sensation in the distal lower extremity, *i.e.,* the foot and toes.

surgical a., (1) any a. administered for the performance of an operative procedure, as differentiated from obstetrical, diagnostic, and therapeutic a.; **(2)** loss of sensation with muscle relaxation adequate for an operative procedure.

tactile a., loss or impairment of the sense of touch.

thermal a., thermic a., loss of temperature appreciation.

topical a., superficial loss of sensation in conjunctiva, mucous membranes or skin, produced by direct application of local anesthetic solutions, ointments, or jellies.

traumatic a., loss of sensation resulting from nerve injury.

unilateral a., SYN hemianesthesia.

visceral a., SYN splanchnic a.

an•es•the•si•ol•o•gist (an′es-thē-zē-ol′ō-jist). **1.** A physician specializing solely in anesthesiology and related areas. **2.** An individual with a doctorate degree who is board-certified and legally qualified to administer anesthetics and related techniques. Cf. anesthetist.

an•es•the•si•ol•o•gy (an′es-thē-zē-ol′ō-jē). The medical specialty concerned with the pharmacological, physiological, and clinical basis of anesthesia and related fields, including resuscitation, intensive respiratory care, and the management of acute and chronic pain. [anesthesia + G. *logos*, treatise]

an•es•thet•ic (an-es-thet′ik). **1.** A compound that reversibly depresses neuronal function, producing loss of ability to perceive pain and/or other sensations. **2.** Collective designation for anesthetizing agents administered to an individual at a particular time. **3.** Characterized by loss of sensation or capable of producing loss of sensation. **4.** Associated with or due to the state of anesthesia.

    general a., a compound that produces loss of sensation associated with loss of consciousness.

    inhalation a., a gas or a liquid with sufficient vapor pressure to produce general anesthesia when breathed.

    intravenous a., a compound that produces anesthesia when injected intravenously.

    primary a., the compound that contributes most to loss of sensation when a mixture of anesthetics is administered.

    secondary a., a compound that contributes to, but is not primarily responsible for, loss of sensation when two or more anesthetics are simultaneously administered.

anes•the•tist (ă-nes′thĕ-tist). One who administers an anesthetic, whether an anesthesiologist, a physician who is not an anesthesiologist, a nurse a., or an anesthesia assistant.

anes•the•ti•za•tion (ă-nes′thĕ-ti-zā′shun). The act of producing loss of sensation.

anes•the•tize (ă-nes′thĕ-tīz). To produce loss of sensation.

an•e•to•der•ma (an-ĕ-tō-der′mă). Atrophoderma in which the skin becomes baglike and wrinkled. [G. *anetos*, relaxed, + *derma*, skin]

an•eu•ploid (an′yū-ployd). Having an abnormal number of chromosomes not an exact multiple of the haploid number, as contrasted with abnormal numbers of complete haploid sets of chromosomes, such as diploid, triploid, etc. [G. *an-* priv. + euploid]

an•eu•ploi•dy (an′yū-ploy-dē). State of being aneuploid.

an•eu•rysm (an′yū-rizm). Circumscribed dilation of an artery or a cardiac chamber, usually due to an acquired or congenital weakness of the wall of the artery or chamber. [G. *aneurysma (-mat-)*, a dilation, fr. *eurys*, wide]

    arteriosclerotic a., the most common type of a., occurring in the abdominal aorta and other large arteries, primarily in the elderly.

    arteriovenous a., **(1)** a dilated arteriovenous shunt. **(2)** communication between an artery and a vein, sometimes congenital.

    berry a., a small saccular a. of a cerebral artery that resembles a berry. Such a.'s frequently rupture causing subarachnoid hemorrhage.

    cirsoid a., dilation of a group of blood vessels owing to congenital malformation with arteriovenous shunting. SYN racemose a.

    compound a., an a. in which some of the coats of the artery are ruptured, others intact.

    dissecting a., splitting or dissection of an arterial wall by blood entering through an intimal tear

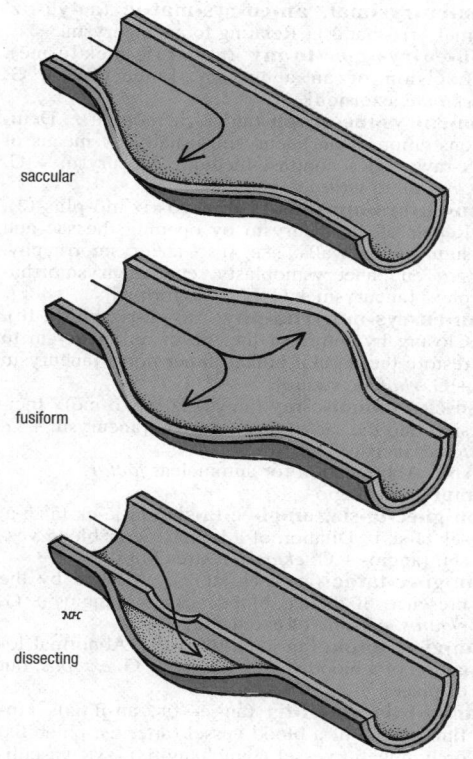

saccular

fusiform

dissecting

aneurysm

or by interstitial hemorrhage; more common in the aorta.

    false a., **(1)** pulsating, encapsulated hematoma in communication with the lumen of a ruptured vessel; **(2)** ventricular pseudoaneurysm, a cardiac rupture contained and loculated by pericardium, which forms its external wall. **(3)** an a. whose walls consist of adventitia and periarterial fibrous tissue and hematoma.

    fusiform a., an elongated spindle-shaped dilation of an artery.

    mycotic a., an a. caused by the growth of fungi within the vascular wall, usually following impaction of a septic embolus; also used to refer to the growth of bacteria within the vascular wall of an a.; may result from impaction of septic embolus or from primary infection of the vessel wall.

    racemose a., SYN cirsoid a.

    saccular a., sacculated a., a saclike bulging on one side of an artery.

    supraclinoid a., an intracranial a. located immediately above the anterior clinoid process of the sphenoid bone.

    syphilitic a., an a., usually involving the thoracic aorta, resulting from tertiary syphilitic aortitis.

    varicose a., a blood-containing sac, communicating with both an artery and a vein.

an·eu·rys·mal, an·eu·rys·mat·ic (an-yū-riz′ măl, -riz-mat′ik). Relating to an aneurysm.

an·eu·rys·mec·to·my (an-yū-riz-mek′tō-mē). Excision of an aneurysm. [aneurysm + G. *ektomē*, excision]

an·eu·rys·mo·graph (an′yū-riz′mōg′răf). Demonstration of an aneurysm, usually by means of x-rays and a contrast medium. [aneurysm + G. *graphō*, to write]

an·eu·rys·mo·plas·ty (an-yū-riz′mō-plas-tē). Repair of an aneurysm by opening the sac and suturing its walls. SEE ALSO aneurysmorrhaphy. SYN endoaneurysmoplasty, endoaneurysmorrhaphy. [aneurysm + G. *plastos*, formed]

an·eu·rys·mor·rha·phy (an′yū-riz-mōr′ă-fē). Closure by suture of the sac of an aneurysm to restore the normal lumen dimensions. [aneurysm + G. *rhaphē*, suture]

an·eu·rys·mot·o·my (an′yū-riz-mot′ō-mē). Incision into the sac of an aneurysm. [aneurysm + G. *tomē*, incision]

ANF Abbreviation for antinuclear *factor*.

△**angi-.** SEE angio-.

an·gi·ec·ta·sia, an·gi·ec·ta·sis (an-jē-ek-tā′zē-ă, -ek′tă-sis). Dilation of a lymphatic or blood vessel. [angio- + G. *ektasis*, a stretching]

an·gi·ec·tat·ic (an-jē-ek-tat′ik). Marked by the presence of dilated blood vessels. [angio- + G. *ektatos*, capable of extension]

an·gi·ec·to·pia (an-jē-ek-tō′pē-ă). Abnormal location of a blood vessel. [angio- + G. *ektopos*, out of place]

an·gi·i·tis, an·gi·tis (an-jē-ī′tis, an-jī′tis). Inflammation of a blood vessel (arteritis, phlebitis) or lymphatic vessel (lymphangitis). SYN vasculitis. [angio- + G. *-itis*, inflammation]

an·gi·na (an′ji-nă, an-jī′nă). **1.** A severe, often constricting pain; usually refers to a. pectoris. **2.** Old term for a sore throat from any cause. [L. quinsy]

abdominal a., a. abdom′inis, intermittent abdominal pain, frequently occurring at a fixed time after eating, caused by inadequacy of the mesenteric circulation from arteriosclerosis or other arterial disease. SYN intestinal a.

crescendo a., a. pectoris that occurs with increasing frequency, intensity, or duration.

a. cru′ris, intermittent claudication of the leg.

intestinal a., SYN abdominal a.

a. inver′sa, SYN Prinzmetal's a.

Ludwig's a., a cellulitis, usually of odontogenic origin, bilaterally involving the submaxillary, sublingual, and submental spaces, resulting in painful swelling of the floor of the mouth, elevation of the tongue, dysphasia, dysphonia, and (at times) compromise of the airway. [W.F. Ludwig]

a. pec′toris, severe constricting pain in the chest, often radiating from the precordium to a shoulder (usually left) and down the arm, due to ischemia of the heart muscle usually caused by coronary disease. SYN stenocardia.

Prinzmetal's a., a form of a. pectoris, characterized by pain that is not precipitated by cardiac work, is of longer duration, is usually more severe, and is associated with unusual electrocardiographic manifestations including elevated ST segments in leads that are ordinarily depressed in typical a., and usually without reciprocal ST changes; occurring at night in bed in EKG leads in which sT segment depression occurs in typical a. SYN a. inversa, variant a. pectoris.

unstable a., (1) a. pectoris characterized by pain in the chest of coronary origin occurring in response to progressively less exercise or fewer other stimuli than ordinarily required to produce a.; often leading to myocardial infarction, if untreated, and caused by coronary artery spasm rather than increased myocardial oxygen and demand. **(2)** a. that has not achieved a constant or reproducible pattern in 30 or 60 days.

variant a. pectoris, SYN Prinzmetal's a.

Vincent's a., an ulcerative infection of the oral soft tissues including the tonsils and pharynx caused by fusiform and spirochetal organisms; it is usually associated with necrotizing ulcerative gingivitis and may progress to noma. Death from suffocation or sepsis may occur.

walk-through a., a circumstance in which despite continuing activity, such as walking, the pain of a. pectoris diminishes or disappears.

an·gi·nal (an′ji-năl, an-jī′). Relating to angina in any sense.

an·gi·ni·form (an-jin′i-fōrm). Resembling angina.

an·gi·noid (an′jin-oid). Rarely used term for resembling an angina, especially angina pectoris.

an·gi·nose, an·gi·nous (an′ji-nōs, -ji-nŭs). Rarely used term for relating to any angina.

△**angio-, angi-.** Blood or lymph vessels; a covering, an enclosure; corresponds to L. vas-,vaso-, vasculo-. [G. *angeion*, a vessel or cavity of the body, fr. *angos*, a vessel, vat, bucket, + *-eion*, small, little]

an·gi·o·blast (an′jē-ō-blast). **1.** A cell taking part in blood vessel formation. SYN vasoformative cell. **2.** Primordial mesenchymal tissue from which embryonic blood cells and vascular endothelium are differentiated. [angio- + G. *blastos*, germ]

an·gi·o·blas·to·ma (an′jē-ō-blas-tō′mă). SYN hemangioblastoma.

an·gi·o·car·di·og·ra·phy (an′jē-ō-kar-dē-og′ră-fē). X-ray imaging of the heart and great vessels made visible by injection of a radiopaque solution. SEE coronary *angiography*. [angio- + G. *kardia*, heart, + *graphō*, to write]

exercise radionuclide a., radionuclide a. while performing exercise, such as on a treadmill or bicycle.

gated radionuclide a., radionuclide a. using cardiac gating to combine images from several cardiac cycles to improve the quality of the images of separate phases (*e.g.,* systole and diastole).

radionuclide a., the display, by means of a stationary scintillation camera device, of the passage of a bolus of a rapidly injected radiopharmaceutical.

an·gi·o·car·di·o·ki·net·ic, an·gi·o·car·di·o·ci·net·ic (an′jē-ō-kar′dē-ō-ki-net′ik, -dē-ō-si-net′ik). Causing dilation or contraction in the heart and blood vessels. [angio- + G. *kardia*, heart, + *kinēsis*, movement]

an·gi·o·car·di·op·a·thy (an′jē-ō-kar-dē-op′ă-thē). Disease affecting both heart and blood vessels. [angio- + G. *kardia,* heart, + *pathos,* disease]

an·gi·o·dys·pla·sia (an′jē-ō-dis-plā′zē-ă). Degenerative or congenital structural abnormality of the normally distributed vasculature.

an·gi·o·dys·tro·phy, an·gi·o·dys·tro·phia (an′jē-ō-dis′trō-fē, -dis-trō′fē-ă). Defective formation or growth associated with marked vascular changes. [angio- + G. *dys-,* bad, + *trophē,* nourishment]

an·gi·o·e·de·ma (an′jē-ō-ě-dē′mă). Recurrent large circumscribed areas of subcutaneous edema of sudden onset, usually disappearing within 24 hours; seen mainly in young women, frequently as an allergic reaction to foods or drugs. SYN angioneurotic edema, Bannister's disease, giant urticaria.

an·gi·o·en·do·the·li·o·ma·to·sis (an′jē-ō-en-dō-thē′lē-ō-mă-tō′-sis). Proliferation of endothelial cells within blood vessels.

an·gi·o·fi·bro·ma (an′jē-ō-fī-brō′mă). SYN telangiectatic *fibroma.*

an·gi·o·fi·bro·sis (an′jē-ō-fī-brō′sis). Fibrosis of the walls of blood vessels.

an·gi·o·gen·ic (an′jē-ō-jen′ik). **1.** Relating to angiogenesis. **2.** Of vascular origin.

an·gi·o·gli·o·ma (an′jē-ō-glī-ō′mă). A mixed glioma and angioma.

an·gi·o·gram (an′jē-ō-gram). Radiograph obtained by angiography. [angio- + G. *gramma,* a writing]

an·gi·o·graph·ic (an-jē-ō-graf′ik). Relating to or utilizing angiography.

an·gi·og·ra·phy (an-jē-og′ră-fē). Radiography of vessels after the injection of a radiopaque contrast material; usually requires percutaneous insertion of a radiopaque catheter and positioning under fluoroscopic control. SEE ALSO arteriography, venography. [angio- + G. *graphō,* to write]

coronary a., imaging of the circulation of the myocardium by injection of contrast medium, usually by selective catheterization of each coronary artery, formerly by injection at the root of the aorta.

digital subtraction a. (DSA), computer-assisted roentgenographic a. permitting visualization of vascular structures without superimposed bone and soft tissue density; images made before and after contrast injection allow subtraction (separation and removal) of opacities not enhanced by the contrast medium. Other image-processing can be performed. Contrast material may be injected intravenously or in lower-than-usual amount intra-arterially.

an·gi·oid (an′jē-oyd). Resembling blood vessels; an arborizing pattern. [angio- + G. *eidos,* resemblance]

a. streaks, breaks in Bruch's membrane visible in the peripapillary fundus oculi, and sometimes mistaken for choroidal vessels.

an·gi·o·ker·a·to·ma (an′jē-ō-ker-ă-tō′mă). A superficial capillary telangiectasis, over which there is a wartlike hyperkeratosis and acanthosis. SYN telangiectatic wart. [angio- + G. *keras,* horn, + *-ōma,* tumor]

an·gi·o·ker·a·to·sis (an′jē-ō-ker-ă-tō′sis). The occurrence of multiple angiokeratomas.

an·gi·o·ki·ne·sis (an′jē-ō-ki-nē′sis). SYN vasomotion. [angio- + G. *kinēsis,* movement]

an·gi·o·ki·net·ic (an′jē-ō-ki-net′ik). SYN vasomotor. [angio- + G. *kinētikos,* pertaining to movement]

an·gi·o·lith (an′jē-ō-lith). An arteriolith or a phlebolith. [angio- + G. *lithos,* stone]

an·gi·o·lith·ic (an′jē-ō-lith′ik). Relating to an angiolith.

an·gi·ol·o·gy (an-jē-ol′ō-jē). The science concerned with the blood vessels and lymphatics in all their relations. [angio- + G. *logos,* treatise, discourse]

an·gi·o·lu·poid (an′jē-ō-lū′poyd). A sarcoid-like eruption of the skin in which the granulomatous telangiectatic papules are distributed over the nose and cheeks. [angio- + L. *lupus,* wolf, + G. *eidos,* resemblance]

an·gi·ol·y·sis (an-jē-ol′i-sis). Obliteration of a blood vessel, such as occurs in the newborn infant after tying of the umbilical cord. [angio- + G. *lysis,* destruction]

an·gi·o·ma (an-jē-ō′mă). A swelling or tumor due to proliferation, with or without dilation, of the blood vessels (hemangioma) or lymphatics (lymphangioma). [angio- + G. *-ōma,* tumor]

cavernous a., vascular malformation composed of sinusoidal vessels without a large feeding artery.

cherry a., SYN senile *hemangioma.*

a. serpigino′sum, the presence of rings of red dots on the skin, especially in female children, which tend to widen peripherally, due to dilatation of superficial capillaries. SYN essential telangiectasia (2).

spider a., a telangiectatic arteriole in the skin with radiating capillary branches simulating the legs of a spider; characteristic, but not pathognomonic, of parenchymatous liver disease; also seen in pregnancy, often disappearing after delivery, and at times in normal persons. SYN arterial spider, spider nevus, spider telangiectasia, spider (2), vascular spider.

telangiectatic a., a. composed of dilated vessels.

an·gi·o·ma·toid (an-jē-ō′mă-toyd). Resembling a tumor of vascular origin.

an·gi·o·ma·to·sis (an′jē-ō-mă-tō′sis). A condition characterized by multiple angiomas.

bacillary a., an infection of immunocompromised patients by a newly recognized Rickettsial species *Rochalimaea henselae,* characterized by fever and granulomatous cutaneous nodules, and peliosis hepatis in some cases. Skin biopsy shows vascular proliferation and infiltration of vessel walls by neutrophils and clumps of organisms seen with Warthin-Starry silver staining.

an·gi·o·ma·tous (an-jē-ō′mă-tŭs). Relating to or resembling an angioma.

an·gi·o·neu·rec·to·my (an′jē-ō-nū-rek′tō-mē). **1.** Excision of the vessels and nerves of a part. [angio- + G. *neuron,* nerve, + *ektomē,* excision] **2.** Excision of a segment of the spermatic cord to produce sterility. [G. *neuron,* cord] [angio- + G. *neuron,* nerve, + *ektomē,* excision]

an·gi·op·a·thy (an-jē-op′ă-thē). Any disease of

the blood vessels or lymphatics. [angio- + G. *pathos*, suffering]

cerebral amyloid a., a pathological condition of small cerebral vessels characterized by deposits of amyloid in the vessel walls, which may lead to infarcts or hemorrhage; may also occur in Alzheimer's disease. SEE ALSO congophilic a.

congophilic a., a condition of blood vessels characterized by deposits in the vessel walls of a substance, usually amyloid, that takes a Congo red stain. SEE ALSO cerebral amyloid a.

an·gi·o·phac·o·ma·to·sis, an·gi·o·phak·o·ma·to·sis (an′jē-ō-fak′ō-mă-tō′sis). The angiomatous phacomatoses: von Hippel-Landau's disease and the Sturge-Weber syndrome.

an·gi·o·plas·ty (an′jē-ō-plas-tē). Reconstitution or recanalization of a blood vessel; may involve balloon dilation, mechanical stripping of intima, forceful injection of fibrinolytics, or placement of a stent. [angio- + G. *plastos*, formed, shaped]

percutaneous transluminal a. (PTA), an operation for enlarging a narrowed vascular lumen by inflating and withdrawing through the stenotic region a balloon on the tip of an angiographic catheter; may include positioning of an intravascular stent.

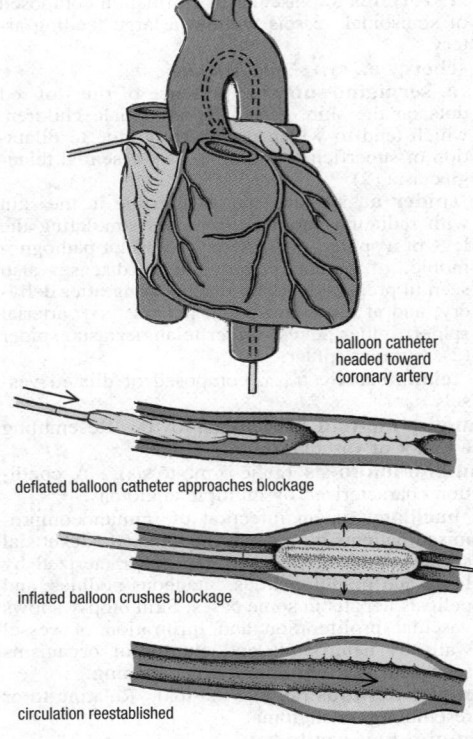

balloon catheter headed toward coronary artery

deflated balloon catheter approaches blockage

inflated balloon crushes blockage

circulation reestablished

percutaneous transluminal angioplasty

an·gi·o·poi·e·sis (an′jē-ō-poy-ē′sis). Formation of blood or lymphatic vessels. SYN vasifaction, vasoformation. [angio- + G. *poiesis*, making]

an·gi·o·poi·et·ic (an′jē-ō-poy-et′ik). Relating to angiopoiesis. SYN vasifactive, vasoformative.

an·gi·or·rha·phy (an-jē-ōr′ă-fē). Suture repair of any vessel, especially of a blood vessel. [angio- + G. *rhaphē*, a seam]

an·gi·o·sar·co·ma (an′jē-ō-sar-kō′mă). A rare malignant neoplasm occurring most often in the breast and skin, and believed to originate from the endothelial cells of blood vessels; microscopically composed of closely packed round or spindle-shaped cells, some of which line small spaces resembling vascular clefts.

an·gi·os·co·py (an-jē-os′kō-pē). **1.** Visualization with a microscope of the passage of substances (*e.g.,* contrast media, radiopaque agents) through capillaries after intravenous injection. **2.** Visualization of the interior of blood vessels, especially the pulmonary arteries, using a fiberoptic catheter inserted through a peripheral artery. [angio- + G. *skopeō*, to view]

an·gi·o·sco·to·ma (an′jē-ō-skō-tō′mă). Ribbon-shaped defect of the visual fields caused by the retinal vessels overlying photoreceptors. [angio- + G. *skotōma*, dizziness, vertigo]

an·gi·o·sco·tom·e·try (an′jē-ō-skō-tom′ĕ-trē). The measurement or projection of the angioscotoma pattern.

an·gi·o·spasm (an′jē-ō-spazm). SYN vasospasm.

an·gi·o·spas·tic (an′jē-ō-spas′tik). SYN vasospastic.

an·gi·o·ste·no·sis (an′jē-ō-stĕ-nō′sis). Narrowing of one or more blood vessels. [angio- + G. *stenōsis*, a narrowing]

an·gi·o·ten·sin (an-jē-ō-ten′sin). A family of peptides with vasoconstrictive activity, produced by action of renin on angiotensinogen.

a. III amide, a synthetic substance closely related to naturally occurring angiotensin II; it is a potent vasopressor useful in certain types of shock and circulatory collapse.

an·gi·o·ten·sin·o·gen·ase (an′jē-ō-ten-sin′ō-jen-ās). SYN renin.

an·gi·ot·o·my (an-jē-ot′ō-mē). Sectioning of a blood vessel, or the creation of an opening into a vessel prior to its repair. [angio- + G. *tomē*, cutting]

an·gi·o·to·nia (an′jē-ō-tō′nē-ă). SYN vasotonia.

an·gi·o·tro·phic (an′jē-ō-trof′ik). Rarely used term for vasotrophic. [angio- + G. *trophē*, nourishment]

Angle, Edward Hartley, U.S. orthodontist, 1855–1930. SEE A.'s *classification* of malocclusion.

carrying A., the angle between the humerus and ulna when the arm is in anatomical position.

Q-A., the A. formed by the line of traction of the quadriceps tendon on the patella and the line of traction of the patellar tendon on the tibial tubercle.

an·gle (θ) (ang′gl). The meeting point of two lines or planes; the figure formed by the junction of two lines or planes; the space bounded on two sides by lines or planes that meet. For a.'s not listed below, see the descriptive term; *e.g.,* axio-incisal, distobuccal, labiogingival, linguogingival (2), mesiogingival, proximobuccal, etc. SYN angulus [NA]. [L. *angulus*]

acromial a., the prominent angle at the junction

of the posterior and lateral borders of the acromion. SYN angulus acromialis [NA].

alpha a., (1) the a. between the visual and optic axes as they cross at the nodal point of the eye; **(2)** the a. between the visual line and the major axis of the corneal ellipse.

axial a., an a. formed by two surfaces of a body, the line of union of which is parallel with its axis; the axial a.'s of a tooth are the distobuccal, distolabial, distolingual, mesiobuccal, mesiolabial, and mesiolingual.

cardiophrenic a., the a. between the heart and the diaphragm at either lateral end of the cardiac projection on imaging (usually the chest x-ray film). The right cardiophrenic a. is normally indistinguishable from the cardiohepatic a. radiographically.

cavosurface a., the a. formed by the junction of a cavity wall and the surface of the tooth.

costal a., the rather abrupt change in curvature of the body of a rib posteriorly, such that the neck and head of the rib are directed upward. SYN angulus costae [NA].

costophrenic a., costophrenic sulcus as seen on chest radiograph.

a. of eccentricity, in strabismus, the a. between the line of fixation and the line of normal foveal fixation.

filtration a., SYN iridocorneal a.

flip a., in a magnetic resonance imaging sequence, the rotation of the average axis of the protons induced by radiofrequency signals; low angles are used in rapid-imaging sequences and to show a signal from flowing blood.

gamma a., the a. formed between a line joining the fixation point to the center of the eye and the optic axis.

incisal guide a., the a. formed with the horizontal plane by drawing a line in the sagittal plane between incisal edges of the maxillary and mandibular central incisors when the teeth are in centric occlusion.

iridocorneal a., the acute angle between the iris and the cornea at the periphery of the anterior chamber of the eye. SYN angulus iridocornealis [NA], a. of iris, filtration a.

a. of iris, SYN iridocorneal a.

a. of jaw, SYN a. of mandible.

kappa a., the a. between the pupillary axis and the visual axis; it is positive when the pupillary axis is nasal to the visual axis, and negative when the pupillary axis is temporal to the visual axis.

a. of mandible, the angle formed by the lower margin of the body and the posterior margin of the ramus of the mandible. SYN angulus mandibulae [NA], a. of jaw.

mesial a., the a. formed by the meeting of the mesial with the labial (or buccal) or lingual surface of a tooth.

meter a., the amount of convergence required to view binocularly an object 1 meter distant and exerting 1 diopter of accommodation.

pelvivertebral a., the a. made by the pelvis as defined by the plane of the superior pelvic aperture with the general axis of the trunk or vertebral column.

point a., the junction of three surfaces of the crown of a tooth, or of the walls of a cavity.

pubic a., SYN subpubic a.

sphenoidal a. of parietal bone, the anterior inferior angle of the parietal bone.

sternal a., the angle between the manubrium and the body of the sternum at the manubriosternal junction. Marks the level of the second costal cartilage (rib) for counting ribs or intercostal spaces. Denotes level of aortic arch, bifurcation of trachea, and T4/T5 intervertebral disc. SYN angulus sterni [NA].

sternoclavicular a., the a. formed by the junction of the clavicle with the sternum.

subpubic a., the a. formed between the inferior rami of the pubic bones. In the female, the angle approximates that a. between the widely extended thumb and index finger (90°); in the male, it approximates the a. between the widely abducted index and middle fingers (60°). SEE ALSO pubic *arch*. SYN angulus subpubicus [NA], pubic a.

a. of torsion, the amount of rotation of a long bone along its axis or between two axes, measured in degrees.

venous a., (1) the junction of the internal jugular and subclavian veins, toward which converge the external and the anterior jugular and the vertebral veins, the thoracic duct in the left a. and the right lymphatic duct in the right a.; **(2)** in neuroradiology, the a. of union of the superior thalamostriate vein (vena terminalis) with the internal cerebral vein, usually closely behind the interventricular foramen of Monro.

visual a., the a. formed at the retina by the meeting of lines drawn from the periphery of the object seen.

Ångström, Anders J., Swedish physicist, 1814–1874. SEE angstrom.

ang•strom (Å) (ang′strŏm). A unit of wavelength, 10^{-10} m, roughly the diameter of an atom; equivalent to 0.1 nm. [A.J. Ångström]

an•gu•la•tion (ang′gū-lā′shŭn). Formation of an angle; an abnormal angle or bend in an organ.

an•gu•lus, gen. and pl. **an•gu•li** (ang′gyū-lŭs, -lī) [NA]. SYN angle. [L.]

a. acromia′lis [NA], SYN acromial *angle.*

a. cos′tae [NA], SYN costal *angle.*

a. iridocornea′lis [NA], SYN iridocorneal *angle.*

a. mandib′ulae [NA], SYN *angle* of mandible.

a. ster′ni [NA], SYN sternal *angle.*

a. subpu′bicus [NA], SYN subpubic *angle.*

an•he•do•nia (an-hē-dō′nē-ă). Absence of pleasure from the performance of acts that would ordinarily be pleasurable. [G. *an-* priv. + *hedonē,* pleasure]

an•hi•dro•sis (an-hĭ-drō′sis). Inability to tolerate heat; absence of sweat glands. SYN adiaphoresis. [G. *an-* priv. + *hidrōs,* sweat]

an•hi•drot•ic (an-hĭ-drot′ik). **1.** Relating to, or characterized by, anhidrosis. **2.** Denoting a reduction or absence of sweat glands, characteristic of congenital ectodermal defect and anhidrotic ectodermal dysplasia.

an•hy•drase (an-hī′drās). An enzyme that catalyzes the removal of water from a compound;

most such enzymes are now known as hydrases, hydro-lyases, or dehydratases.

an·hy·dra·tion (an-hī-drā'shŭn). SYN dehydration (1).

an·hy·dride (an-hī'drĭd). An oxide that can combine with water to form an acid or that is derived from an acid by the abstraction of water.

△**anhydro-**. Chemical prefix denoting the removal of water. Cf. pyro- (2). [G. *an-* priv., + *hydōr,* water]

an·hy·drous (an-hī'drŭs). Containing no water, especially water of crystallization.

an·i·lide (an'i-lid). An *N*-acyl aniline; *e.g.,* acetanilide.

ani·linc·tion, ani·linc·tus (ā-ni-lingk'shŭn, -lingk'tŭs). SYN anilingus.

an·i·line (an'i-lin, -lēn). C₆H₅(NH₂); an oily, colorless or brownish liquid, of aromatic odor and acrid taste, that is the parent substance of many synthetic dyes. Aniline is highly toxic and may cause industrial poisoning. [Ar. *an-nil,* indigo]

ani·lin·gus (ā-ni-ling'gŭs). Sexual stimulation by licking or kissing the anus. SYN anilinction, anilinctus. [L. *anus,* + *lingo,* to lick]

an·il·ism (an'i-lizm). Chronic aniline poisoning characterized by gastric and cardiac weakness, vertigo, muscular depression, intermittent pulse, and cyanosis.

an·i·ma (an'i-mă). **1.** The soul or spirit. SEE animus (4). **2.** In jungian psychology, the inner self, in contrast to persona; a female archetype in a man. Cf. animus (5). [L. breath, soul]

an·i·mal (an'i-măl). **1.** A living, sentient organism that has membranous cell walls, requires oxygen and organic foods, and is capable of voluntary movement, as distinguished from a plant or mineral. **2.** One of the lower a. organisms as distinguished from humans. [L.]

an·i·ma·tion (an-i-mā'shŭn). **1.** The state of being alive. **2.** Liveliness; high spirits. [L. *animo,* pp. *-atus,* to make alive; *anima,* breath, soul]

suspended a., a temporary state resembling death, with cessation of respiration; may also refer to certain forms of hibernation in animals or to endospore formation by some bacteria.

an·i·mus (an'i-mŭs). **1.** An animating or energizing spirit. **2.** Intention to do something; disposition. **3.** In psychiatry, a spirit of active hostility or grudge. **4.** The ideal image toward which a person strives. **5.** In jungian psychology, a male archetype in a woman. Cf. anima (2). [L. *animus,* breath, rational soul in man, will]

an·i·on (A⁻) (an'ī-on). An ion that carries a negative charge, going therefore to the positively charged anode; in salts, acid radicals are a.'s.

a. exchange, the process by which an anion in a mobile (liquid) phase exchanges with another anion previously bound to a solid, positively charged phase, the latter being an anion exchanger. Anion exchange may also be used chromatographically, to separate anions, and medicinally, to remove an anion (*e.g.,* Cl⁻) from gastric contents or bile acids in the intestine.

an·i·rid·ia (an-i-rid'ē-ă) [MIM*106200]. Absence of the iris. Cf. irideremia. [G. *an-* priv. + irid- + -ia]

an·is·ei·ko·nia (an'ĭ-sī-kō'nē-ă). An ocular condition in which the image of an object in one eye differs in size or shape from the image of the same object in the fellow eye. [G. *anisos,* unequal, + *eikōn,* an image]

△**aniso-**. Unequal, dissimilar, unlike. [G. *anisos,* unequal, fr. *an-,* not, + *isos,* equal]

an·i·so·ac·com·mo·da·tion (an-ī'sō-ă-kom-ō-dā'shŭn). Variation between the two eyes in accommodation capacity. [aniso- + L. *accommodo,* to adapt]

an·i·so·chro·mat·ic (an-ī'sō-krō-mat'ik). Not uniformly of one color.

an·i·so·co·ria (an-ī-sō-kō'rē-ă). A condition in which the two pupils are not of equal size. [aniso- + G. *korē,* pupil]

▌**an·i·so·cy·to·sis** (an-ī'sō-sī-tō'sis). Considerable variation in the size of cells that are normally uniform, especially with reference to red blood cells. [aniso- + G. *kytos,* cell, + *-osis,* condition]

an·i·so·dac·ty·lous (an-ī'sō-dak'ti-lŭs). Relating to anisodactyly.

an·i·so·dac·ty·ly (an-ī'sō-dak'ti-lē). Unequal length in corresponding fingers. [aniso- + G. *daktylon,* finger]

an·i·sog·a·my (an'-i-sog'ă-mē). Fusion of two gametes unequal in size or form; fertilization as distinguished from isogamy or conjugation. [aniso- + G. *gamos,* marriage]

an·i·sog·na·thous (an-i-sog'nă-thŭs). Having jaws of unequal size, the upper being wider than the lower. [aniso- + G. *gnathos,* jaw]

an·i·so·kar·y·o·sis (an-ī'sō-kar-ē-ō'sis). Variation in size of nuclei, greater than the normal range for a tissue. [aniso- + G. *karyon,* nut (nucleus), + *-osis,* condition]

an·i·so·mas·tia (an-i-sō-mas'tē-ă). Breasts of unequal size. [aniso- + G. *mastos,* breast]

an·i·so·me·lia (an-i-sō-mē'lē-ă). A condition of inequality between two paired limbs. [aniso- + G. *melos,* limb]

an·i·so·me·tro·pia (an-ī'sō-me-trō'pē-ă). A difference in the refractive power of the two eyes. [aniso- + G. *metron,* measure, + *ōps,* sight]

an·i·so·me·tro·pic (an-ī'sō-me-trop'ik). **1.** Relating to anisometropia. **2.** Having eyes of unequal refractive power.

an·i·so·pi·e·sis (an-ī-sō-pī-ē'sis). Unequal arterial blood pressure on the two sides of the body. [aniso- + G. *piesis,* pressure]

an·i·so·sphyg·mia (an-ī-sō-sfig'mē-ă). Difference in volume, force, or time of the pulse in the corresponding arteries on two sides of the body, *e.g.,* the two radials, or femorals. [aniso- + G. *sphygmos,* pulse]

an·i·sos·then·ic (an-ī-sos-then'ik). Of unequal strength; denoting two muscles or groups of muscles that are either paired or are antagonists. [aniso- + G. *sthenos,* strength]

an·i·so·ton·ic (an-ī-sō-ton'ik). Not having equal tension; having unequal osmotic pressure. [aniso- + G. *tonus,* tension]

an·kle (ang'kl). **1.** SYN ankle joint. **2.** The region of the a. joint. **3.** SYN talus.

△**ankylo-**. Bent, crooked, stiff, fused, fixed, closed SEE ALSO ancylo-. [G. *ankylos,* bent, crooked; *ankylōsis,* stiffening of the joints, fr. *ankos,* a bend, a hollow]

an·ky·lo·glos·sia (ang'ki-lō-glos'ē-ă) [MIM 106280]. Partial or complete fusion of the tongue to the floor of the mouth; abnormal shortness of the frenulum linguae. SYN tongue-tie. [ankylo- + G. *glōssa,* tongue]

an·ky·lo·poi·et·ic (ang'ki-lō-poy-et'ik). Forming ankylosis.

an·ky·losed (ang'ki-lōst). Stiffened; bound by adhesions; denoting a joint in a state of ankylosis.

an·ky·lo·sis (ang'ki-lō'sis). Stiffening or fixation of a joint as the result of a disease process, with fibrous or bony union across the joint. [G. *anky-lōsis,* stiffening of a joint]

  artificial a., SYN arthrodesis.

  bony a., SYN synostosis.

  dental a., rigid fixation of a tooth to the surrounding alveolus as a result of ossification of the ligament; prevents eruption and orthodontic movement.

  extracapsular a., stiffness of a joint due to induration or heterotopic ossification of the surrounding tissues. SYN spurious a.

  false a., SYN fibrous a.

  fibrous a., stiffening of a joint due to the presence of fibrous bands between and about the bones forming the joint. SYN false a., pseudankylosis.

  spurious a., SYN extracapsular a.

  true a., SYN synostosis.

an·ky·lot·ic (ang-ki-lot'ik). Characterized by or pertaining to an ankylosis.

an·la·ge, pl. **an·la·gen** (ahn'lah-ge, -gen). **1.** SYN primordium. **2.** In psychoanalysis, genetic predisposition to a given trait or personality characteristic. [Ger. plan, outline]

an·nec·tent (a-nek'tent). Connected with; joined. [L. *an-necto,* pres. p. *-nectere,* pp. *-nexus,* to join to]

an·nexa (a-nek'să). SYN adnexa.

an·nex·al (a-neks-ăl). SYN adnexal.

an·nu·lar (an'yū-lăr). Ring-shaped. [L. *anulus,* ring]

an·nu·lo·plasty (an'yū-lō-plas-tē). Reconstruction of the ring (or annulus) of an incompetent cardiac valve. [L. *anulus,* ring, + G. *plastos,* formed]

an·nu·lor·rha·phy (an-yū-lōr'ă-fē). Closure of a hernial ring by suture. [L. *anulus,* ring, + G. *rhaphē,* seam]

an·nu·lus (an'yū-lŭs) [NA]. SYN ring. SEE ALSO ring.

  a. abdomina'lis, SYN deep inguinal ring.

  a. conjuncti'vae [NA], SYN conjunctival ring.

  a. inguina'lis profun'dus [NA], SYN deep inguinal ring.

  a. inguina'lis superficia'lis [NA], SYN superficial inguinal ring.

  a. tympan'icus [NA], SYN tympanic ring.

  a. umbilica'lis [NA], SYN umbilical ring.

ano·coc·cyg·e·al (a-nō-kok-sij'ē-ăl). Relating to both anus and coccyx.

an·ode (an'ōd). **1.** The positive pole of a galvanic battery or the electrode connected with it; an electrode toward which negatively charged ions (anions) migrate; a positively charged electrode. **2.** The portion, usually made of tungsten, of an x-ray tube from which x-rays are released by bombardment by cathode rays (electrons). [G. *anodos,* a way up, fr. *ana,* up, + *hodos,* a way]

  rotating a., in diagnostic radiography, modern x-ray tubes that have a mushroom-shaped anode that rotates rapidly to avoid local heat buildup from electron impact during x-ray generation.

an·o·derm (ā'nō-derm). Lining of the anal canal immediately inferior to the dentate line and extending for about 1.5 cm to the anal verge; it is devoid of hair and sebaceous and sweat glands; it is especially vulnerable to abrasion (as from rough toilet paper), chemical irritants (soaps), and is well-provided with tactile and nociceptive (pain, itch) endings innervated by the inferior rectal (pudendal) nerve.

an·o·don·tia (an-ō-don'shē-ă). Congenital absence of the teeth; developmental, not due to extraction or impaction. SYN agomphosis, agomphiasis. [G. *an-* priv. + *odous,* tooth]

ano·gen·i·tal (ā'nō-jen'ĭ-tăl). Relating in any way to both the anal and the genital regions.

anom·a·lad (ă-nom'ă-lad). A malformation together with its subsequently derived structural changes. [SEE anomaly]

anom·a·ly (ă-nom'ă-lē). Deviation from the average or norm; anything that is structurally unusual or irregular or contrary to a general rule. Congenital defects are an example of the definition of anomaly. [G. *anōmalia,* irregularity]

  Alder's a., coarse azurophilic granulation of leukocytes, especially granulocytes, which may be associated with gargoylism and Morquio's disease.

  developmental a., an a. established during intrauterine life; a congenital a.

  Ebstein's a., congenital downward displacement of the tricuspid valve into the right ventricle. SYN Ebstein's disease.

  Hegglin's a., a disorder in which neutrophils and eosinophils contain basophilic structures known as Döhle or Amato bodies and in which there is faulty maturation of platelets, with thrombocytopenia.

an·o·mer (an'ō-mer). One of two sugar molecules that are epimeric at the hemiacetal or hemiketal carbon atom. SEE ALSO sugars. Cf. epimer.

ano·mia (ă-nō'mē-ă). SYN nominal *aphasia.* [G. *a-* priv. + *ōnoma,* name]

an·o·nych·ia, an·o·ny·cho·sis (an-ō-nik'ē-ă, an-ō-nī-kō'sis). Absence of the nails. [G. *an-* priv. + *onyx* (*onych-*), nail]

anon·y·ma (ă-non'i-mă). Without name; a term formerly applied to the large vessels in the thorax (now called the brachiocephalic trunk and vein) and the hip bone. SYN innominate. [G. *an-* priv. + *onyma,* name]

Anoph·e·les (ă-nof'ĕ-lēz). A genus of mosquitoes. The sporogenous cycle of the malarial parasite is passed in the body cavity of female mosquitoes of certain species of this genus. [G. *anōphelēs,* useless, harmful, fr. *an-* priv. + *ōpheleō,* to be of use]

anoph·e·line (ă-nof'ĕ-līn). Referring to the *Anopheles* mosquito.

an·oph·thal·mia (an-of-thal'mē-ă). Congenital absence of all tissues of the eyes. [G. *an-* priv. + *ophthalmos,* eye]

ano•plas•ty (ā'nō-plas-tē). Plastic surgery of the anus. [L. *anus* + G. *plastos,* formed]

an•or•chia (an-ōr'kē-ă). SYN anorchism.

an•or•chism (an-ōr'kizm). Absence of the testes; may be congenital or acquired. SYN anorchia. [G. *an-* priv. + *orchis,* testicle]

ano•rec•tal (ā'nō-rek'tăl). Relating to both anus and rectum.

an•o•rec•tic, an•o•ret•ic (an-ō-rek'tic, -ret'ik). **1.** Relating to, characteristic of, or suffering from anorexia, especially anorexia nervosa. **2.** An agent that causes anorexia. SYN anorexic.

an•o•rex•ia (an-ō-rek'sē-ă). Diminished appetite; aversion to food. [G. fr. *an-* priv. + *orexis,* appetite]

    a. nervo'sa, a personality disorder manifested by extreme fear of becoming obese and an aversion to eating, usually occurring in young women and often resulting in life-threatening weight loss, accompanied by a disturbance in body image, hyperactivity, and amenorrhea.

an•o•rex•i•ant (an-ō-rek'sē-ănt). A drug ("diet pills"), process, or event that leads to anorexia.

an•o•rex•ic (an-ō-rek'sik). SYN anorectic.

an•or•gas•my, an•or•gas•mia (an-ōr-gaz'mē, -gaz'mē-ă). Failure to experience an orgasm; may be biogenic (secondary to a physical disorder or medication), psychogenic (secondary to psychological or situational factors), or a combination of the two. [G. *an-* priv. + orgasm + -ia]

an•or•thog•ra•phy (an-ōr-thog'ră-fē). SYN agraphia. [G. *an-* priv. + *orthos,* straight, + *graphō,* to write]

ano•scope (ā'nō-skōp). A short speculum for examining the anal canal and lower rectum.

ano•sig•moid•os•co•py (ā'nō-sig-moy-dos'-kŏ-pē). Endoscopy of the anus, rectum and sigmoid colon.

an•os•mia (an-oz'mē-ă). Loss of the sense of smell. It may be due to lesion of the olfactory nerve, obstruction of the nasal fossae, or functional, without any apparent causative lesion. [G. *an-* priv. + *osmē,* sense of smell]

an•os•mic (an-oz'mik). Relating to anosmia.

ano•sog•no•sia (ă-nō'sog-nō'sē-ă). Ignorance of the presence of disease, specifically of paralysis. Most often seen in patients with non-dominant parietal lobe lesions, who deny their hemiparesis. [G. *a-* priv. + *nosos,* disease, + *gnōsis,* knowledge]

ano•sog•no•sic (ă-nō-sog-nō'sik). Relating to anosognosia.

ano•spi•nal (ā'nō-spī'năl). Relating to the anus and the spinal cord.

an•os•to•sis (an-os-tō'sis). Failure of ossification. [G. *an-* priv. + *osteon,* bone]

an•o•tia (an-ō'shē-ă). Congenital absence of one △ or both auricles of the ears. [G. *an-* priv. + *ous,* ear]

ANOVA *analysis* of variance.

ano•ves•i•cal (ā'nō-ves'i-kăl). Relating in any way to both anus and urinary bladder.

an•ov•u•lar (an-ov'yū-lăr). Absence of discharge of an ovum from the ovary during an ovarian cycle.

an•ov•u•la•tion (an-ov-yū-lā'shŭn). Suspension or cessation of ovulation.

an•ox•e•mia (an-ok-sē'mē-ă). Absence of oxygen in arterial blood; formerly often used to include moderate decrease in oxygen now properly distinguished as hypoxemia. [G. *an-* priv. + oxygen + G. *haima,* blood]

an•ox•ia (an-ok'sē-ă). Absence or almost complete absence of oxygen from inspired gases, arterial blood, or tissues; to be differentiated from hypoxia. [G. *an-* priv. + oxygen]

    anemic a., anemic hypoxia in which oxygen is almost completely lacking.

    anoxic a., hypoxic hypoxia in which oxygen is almost completely lacking.

    diffusion a., diffusion hypoxia severe enough to result in the absence of oxygen in alveolar gas.

    histotoxic a., poisoning of the respiratory enzyme systems of the tissues, as in the inhibition of cytochrome oxidase by cyanides; owing to the inability of tissue cells to utilize oxygen, its tension in arterial and capillary blood is usually greater than normal.

    stagnant a., stagnant hypoxia severe enough to result in the absence of oxygen in tissues.

an•ox•ic (an-ok'sik). Denoting or characteristic of anoxia.

an•sa, gen. and pl. **an•sae** (an'să, -sē) [NA]. Any anatomical structure in the form of a loop or an arc. SEE ALSO loop. [L. loop, handle]

    a. cervica'lis [NA], a loop in the cervical plexus consisting of fibers from the first three cervical nerves. Fibers from a loop between the C-1 and C-2 spinal nerves accompany the hypoglossal nerve for a short distance, leaving it as the superior root of the a. cervicalis. Fibers from a loop between the C-2 and C-3 spinal nerves form the inferior root of the a. cervicalis. Most commonly, the roots merge, forming the a. cervicalis, which gives rise to branches innervating infrahyoid muscles. SYN cervical loop.

    ansae nervo'rum spina'lium, SYN loops of spinal nerves, under loop.

    a. peduncula'ris [NA], a complex fiber bundle curving around the medial edge of the internal capsule and connecting the anterior part of the temporal lobe (temporal cortex), amygdala, and olfactory cortex with the mediodorsal nucleus of the thalamus; it enters the thalamus as a component of the inferior thalamic peduncle which also contains a major part of the fibers connecting the mediodorsal nucleus to the orbitofrontal cortex.

    a. subcla'via [NA], a nerve cord connecting the middle cervical and stellate sympathetic ganglia, forming a loop around the subclavian artery.

an•sate (an'sāt). SYN ansiform.

an•si•form (an'si-fōrm). In the shape of a loop or arc. SYN ansate. [L. *ansa,* handle, + *forma,* shape]

△ **ant-.** SEE anti-.

ant•ac•id (ant-as'id). **1.** Neutralizing an acid. **2.** Any agent that reduces or neutralizes acidity, as of the gastric juice or any other secretion. SYN antiacid.

an•tag•o•nism (an-tag'on-izm). **1.** Denoting mutual opposition in action between structures, agents, diseases, or physiologic processes. Cf. synergism. **2.** The situation in which the combined effect of two or more factors is smaller than the solitary effect of any one of the factors.

SYN mutual resistance. [G. *antagōnisma,* from *anti,* against, + *agōnizomai,* to fight, fr. *agōn,* a contest]

an•tag•o•nist (an-tag′ŏ-nist). Something opposing or resisting the action of another; certain structures, agents, diseases, or physiologic processes that tend to neutralize or impede the action or effect of others. Cf. synergist.

    aldosterone a., an agent that opposes the action of the adrenal hormone aldosterone on renal tubular mineralocorticoid retention; these agents, *e.g.,* spironolactone, are useful in treating the hypertension of primary hyperaldosteronism, or the sodium retention of secondary hyperaldosteronism.

    folic acid a.'s, modified pterins, such as aminopterin and amethopterin, that interfere with the action of folic acid and thus produce the symptoms of folic acid deficiency; have been used in cancer chemotherapy.

    opioid a.'s, agents such as naloxone and naltrexone which have high affinity for opiate receptors but do not activate these receptors. These drugs block the effects of exogenously administered opioids such as morphine, heroin, meperidine, and methadone, or of endogenously released endorphins and enkephalins.

ant•al•gic (ant-al′jik). SYN analgesic (2).

△**ante-.** Before, in front of (in time or place or order). SEE ALSO pre-, pro- (1). [L. *ante,* before, in front of]

an•te•brach•i•al (an′te-brā′kē-ăl). Relating to the forearm.

an•te•bra•chi•um (an-te-brā′kē-ŭm) [NA]. SYN forearm. [ante- + L. *brachium,* arm]

an•te•ced•ent (an-te-sē′dent). A precursor. [L. *antecedo,* to go before]

    plasma thromboplastin a. (PTA), SYN *factor* XI.

an•te ci•bum (an′tē sī′bŭm). Before a meal. The plural is ante cibos, before meals. [L.]

an•te•cu•bi•tal (an-te-kyū′bi-tăl). In front of the elbow. [ante- + L. *cubitum,* elbow]

an•te•flex•ion (an-te-flek′shŭn). A bending forward; a sharp forward curve or angulation; denoting especially the normal forward bend in the uterus at the junction of corpus and cervix uteri.

an•te•grade (an′tĕ-grād). In the direction of normal movement, as in blood flow or peristalsis. [ante- + L. *gradior,* to walk]

an•te•mor•tem (an′te-mōr-tem). Before death. Cf. postmortem. [ante- + L. *mors (mort-),* death]

an•te•na•tal (an-te-nā′tăl). SYN prenatal. [ante- + L. *natus,* birth]

an•te•par•tum (an′te-par-tŭm). Before labor or childbirth. Cf. intrapartum, postpartum. [ante- + L. *pario,* pp. *partus,* to bring forth]

an•te•py•ret•ic (an′te-pī-ret′ik). Before the occurrence of fever; before the period of reaction following shock. [ante- + G. *pyretos,* fever]

an•te•ri•or (an-tēr′ē-ōr). **1** [NA]. HUMAN ANATOMY Denoting the front surface of the body; often used to indicate the position of one structure relative to another, *i.e.,* situated nearer the front part of the body. SYN ventral (2). **2.** Near the head or rostral end of certain embryos. **3.** Before, in relation to time or space. [L.]

△**antero-.** Anterior. [L. *anterior,* more before, earlier, fr. *ante,* before, + -r- -*ior,* more]

an•ter•o•grade (an′ter-ō-grād). **1.** Moving forward. Cf. antegrade. **2.** Extending forward from a particular point in time; used in reference to amnesia. [L. *gradior,* pp. *gressus,* to step, go]

an•ter•o•in•fe•ri•or (an′ter-ō-in-fēr′ē-ōr). In front and below.

an•ter•o•lat•er•al (an′ter-ō-lat′er-ăl). In front and away from the middle line.

an•ter•o•me•di•al (an′ter-ō-mē′dē-ăl). In front and toward the middle line.

an•ter•o•me•di•an (an′ter-ō-mē′dē-an). In front and in the central line.

an•ter•o•pos•te•ri•or (an′ter-ō-pos-tēr-ē-er). **1.** Relating to both front and rear. **2.** In x-ray imaging, describing the direction of the beam through the patient from anterior to posterior.

an•ter•o•su•pe•ri•or (an′ter-ō-sū-pē′rē-er). In front and above.

an•te•sys•to•le (an-te-sis′tō-lē). Premature activation of the ventricle, responsible for the pre-excitation syndrome of the Wolff-Parkinson-White or Lown-Ganong-Levine types.

anteversion (an-tē-ver′zhŭn). Forward displacement or turning forward of a body segment without bending. [L. *ante,* before, forward, + *verto, versus,* to turn]

an•te•vert•ed (an-te-vert′ed). Tilted forward; in a position of anteversion.

ant•he•lix (ant′hē-liks, an′thē-liks) [NA]. SYN antihelix. [anti- + G. *helix,* coil]

an•thel•min•thic (ant-hel-min′thik). SYN anthelmintic (1).

an•thel•min•tic (ant-hel-min′tik, an-thel-). **1.** An agent that destroys or expels intestinal worms. SYN anthelminthic, helminthagogue. **2.** Having the power to destroy or expel intestinal worms. [anti- + G. *helmins,* worm]

an•thrac•ic (an-thras′ik). Relating to anthrax.

an•thra•coid (an′thră-koyd). Resembling a carbuncle or cutaneous anthrax. [G. *anthrax,* carbuncle, + *eidos,* resemblance]

an•thra•co•sil•i•co•sis (an′thră-kō-sil′i-kō′sis). Pneumoconiosis from accumulation of carbon and silica in the lungs from inhaled coal dust; the silica content produces fibrous nodules. [anthraco- + silicosis]

an•thra•co•sis (an-thră-kō′sis). Pneumoconiosis from accumulation of carbon from inhaled smoke or coal dust in the lungs. SYN melanedema, miner's lung (1). [anthraco- + G. -*osis,* condition]

an•thrax (an′thraks). A disease in humans caused by infection with *Bacillus anthracis;* marked by hemorrhage and serous effusions in various organs and body cavities and by symptoms of extreme prostration. SYN carbuncle (2). [G. *anthrax (anthrak-),* charcoal, coal, a carbuncle]

△**anthropo-.** Human. [G. *anthrōpos,* a human being (of either sex)]

an•thro•po•cen•tric (an′thrō-pō-sen′trik). With a human bias, under the assumption that humankind is the central fact of the universe. [anthropo- + G. *kentron,* center]

an•thro•poid (an′thrō-poyd). **1.** Resembling man in structure and form. **2.** One of the monkeys resembling man; an ape. [G. *anthrōpo-eidēs,* man-like]

an·thro·pol·o·gy (an-thrō-pol'ō-jē). The branch of science concerned with origin and development of humans in all their physical, social, and cultural relationships. [anthropo- + G. *logos,* treatise]

an·thro·po·met·ric (an-thrō-pō-met'rik). Relating to anthropometry.

an·thro·pom·e·try (an-thrō-pom'ĕ-trē). The branch of anthropology concerned with comparative measurements of the human body. [anthropo- + G. *metron,* measure]

an·thro·po·mor·phism (an'thrō-pō-mōr'fizm). Ascription of human shape or qualities to nonhuman creatures or inanimate objects. [anthropo- + G. *morphē,* form]

an·thro·po·phil·ic (an'thrō-pō-fil'ik). Human-seeking or human-preferring, especially with reference to: 1) bloodsucking arthropods, denoting the preference of a parasite for the human host as a source of blood or tissues over an animal host; and 2) dermatophytic fungi which grow preferentially on humans rather than other animals. [anthropo- + G. *phileō,* to love]

an·thro·po·zo·o·no·sis (an'thrō-pō-zō'ō-nō'sis). A zoonosis maintained in nature by animals and transmissible to man; *e.g.,* rabies, brucellosis. [anthropo- + G. *zōon,* animal, + *nosos,* disease]

△**anti-.** **1.** Against, opposing, or, in relation to symptoms and diseases, curative. **2.** Prefix denoting an antibody (immunoglobulin) specific for the thing indicated; *e.g.,* antitoxin (antibody specific for a toxin). [G. *anti,* against, opposite, instead of]

an·ti·ac·id (an-tē-as'id). SYN antacid.

an·ti·ad·ren·er·gic (an'tē-ad-rĕ-ner'jik). Antagonistic to the action of sympathetic or other adrenergic nerve fibers. SEE ALSO sympatholytic.

an·ti·ag·glu·ti·nin (an'tē-ă-glū'ti-nin). A specific antibody that inhibits or destroys the action of an agglutinin.

an·ti·an·a·phy·lax·is (an'tē-an'ă-fī-lak'sis). SYN desensitization (1).

an·ti·a·ne·mic (an'tē-ă-nē'mik). Pertaining to factors or substances that prevent or correct anemic conditions.

an·ti·an·ti·body (an'tē-an'tē-bod-ē). Antibody specific for another antibody.

an·ti·an·ti·tox·in (an'tē-an-tē-tok'sin). An antiantibody that inhibits or counteracts the effects of an antitoxin.

an·ti·bac·te·ri·al (an'tē-bak-tēr'ē-ăl). Destructive to or preventing the growth of bacteria.

an·ti·bi·o·sis (an'tē-bī-ō'sis). **1.** An association of two organisms which is detrimental to one of them, in contrast to probiosis. **2.** Production of an antibiotic by bacteria or other organisms inhibitory to other living things, especially among soil microbes. [anti- + G. *biōsis,* life]

an·ti·bi·ot·ic (an'tē-bī-ot'ik). **1.** Relating to antibiosis. **2.** Prejudicial to life. **3.** A soluble substance derived from a mold or bacterium that inhibits the growth of other microorganisms. **4.** Relating to such an action.

    broad spectrum a., an a. having a wide range of activity against both Gram-positive and Gram-negative organisms.

an·ti·body (Ab) (an'tē-bod-i). An immunoglobulin molecule with a specific amino acid sequence evoked in man or other animals by an antigen, and characterized by reacting specifically with the antigen in some demonstrable way, antibody and antigen each being defined in terms of the other. It is believed that antibodies may also exist naturally, without being present as a result of the stimulus provided by the introduction of an antigen: 1) in the broad sense any body or substance, soluble or cellular, which is evoked by the stimulus provided by the introduction of antigen and which reacts specifically with antigen in some demonstrable way; 2) one of the classes of globulins (immunoglobulins) present in the blood serum or body fluids of an animal as a result of antigenic stimulus or occurring "naturally." Different genetically inherited determinants, Gm (found on IgG H chains), Am (found on IgA H chains), and Km (found on K-type L chains and formerly called InV), control the antigenicity of the antibody molecule; subclasses are denoted either alphabetically or numerically (*e.g.,* G3mb1 or G3m5). The various classes differ widely in their ability to react in different kinds of serologic tests. SEE ALSO immunoglobulin.

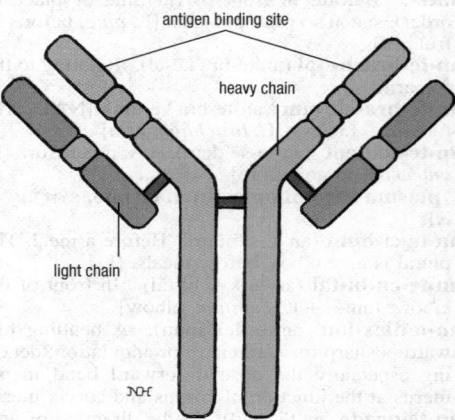

antibody

    anaphylactic a., SYN cytotropic a.

    anti-basement membrane a., autoantibodies to renal glomerular basement membrane antigens.

    antinuclear a., an a. showing an affinity for cell nuclei, demonstrated by exposing a cell substrate to the serum to be tested, followed by exposure to an antihuman-globulin serum; found in the serum of a high proportion of patients with systemic lupus erythematosus, rheumatoid arthritis, and certain collagen diseases, in some of their healthy relatives, and in about 1% of normal individuals.

    blocking a., (1) a. which, in certain concentrations, does not cause precipitation after combining with specific antigen, and which, in this combined state, "blocks" activity of additional a. added to increase the concentration to a level at which precipitation would ordinarily occur; **(2)** the IgG class of immunoglobulin which combines specifically with an atopic allergen but does not elicit a type I allergic reaction, the combined IgG a. "blocking" available IgE class (reaginic) a. activity.

complement-fixing a., a. that combines with and sensitizes antigen leading to the activation of complement, which may result in cell lysis.

complete a., SYN saline *agglutinin.*

cross-reacting a., (1) a. specific for group antigens, *i.e.,* those with identical functional groups; **(2)** a. for antigens that have functional groups of closely similar, but not identical, chemical structure.

cytophilic a., SYN cytotropic a.

cytotropic a., a. that has an affinity for certain kinds of cells, in addition to and unrelated to its specific affinity for the antigen that induced it, because of the properties of the Fc portion of the heavy chain. SEE ALSO heterocytotropic a., homocytotropic a. SYN anaphylactic a., cytophilic a.

Donath-Landsteiner a., an IgG a. associated with paroxysmal cold hemoglobinuria. The antibody is biphasic, reacting with erythrocytes at temperatures below 15° C, which fixes complement to the cell membrane. Upon warming to body temperature, the a. detaches, but the terminal complement components are activated on the cell membrane, causing hemolysis. SEE ALSO hemoglobinuria.

heterocytotropic a., a cytotropic a. (chiefly of the IgG class) similar in activity to homocytotropic a., but having an affinity for cells of a different species rather than for cells of the same or a closely related species.

homocytotropic a., a. of the IgE class that has an affinity for tissues (notably mast cells) of the same or a closely related species and that, upon combining with specific antigen, triggers the release of pharmacological mediators of anaphylaxis from the cells to which it is attached. SYN reaginic a.

incomplete a., (1) SYN univalent a. **(2)** SYN serum *agglutinin.*

monoclonal a., an a. produced by a clone or genetically homogeneous population of hybrid cells *i.e.,* hybridoma; hybrid cells are cloned to establish cell lines producing a specific a. that is chemically and immunologically homogeneous; a mainstay of immunological research and medical diagnosis. SEE ALSO cluster of differentiation.

natural a., SYN normal a.

neutralizing a., a form of a. that reacts with an infectious agent (usually a virus) and destroys or inhibits its infectivity and virulence.

normal a., a. demonstrable in the serum or plasma of various persons or animals not known to have been stimulated by specific antigen, either artificially or as the result of naturally occurring contact. SYN natural a.

reaginic a., SYN homocytotropic a.

univalent a., an "incomplete" form of a. that may coat antigen, but which according to the "lattice theory" does not have a second receptor for attachment to another molecule of antigen; in

the case of Rh+ erythrocytes, such an anti-Rh antibody may coat the cells but not cause them to agglutinate in saline; however, agglutination does occur when such coated cells are suspended in serum or other protein media, such as albumin, therefore called serum agglutinin. SYN incomplete a. (1).

an·ti·cho·lin·er·gic (an'tē-kol-i-ner'jik). Antagonistic to the action of parasympathetic or other cholinergic nerve fibers (*e.g.,* atropine).

an·ti·cho·lin·es·ter·ase (an'tē-kō-lin-es'ter-ās). One of the drugs that inhibit or inactivate acetylcholinesterase, either reversibly (*e.g.,* physostigmine) or irreversibly (*e.g.,* tetraethyl pyrophosphate).

an·ti·cli·nal (an-tē-klī'năl). Inclined in opposite directions, as two sides of a pyramid. [anti- + G. *klinō,* to incline]

an·ti·co·ag·u·lant (an'tē-kō-ag'yū-lant). **1.** Preventing coagulation. **2.** An agent having such action (*e.g.,* warfarin).

lupus a., antiphospholipid antibody causing elevation in partial thromboplastin time; associated with venous and arterial thrombosis.

an·ti·co·don (an-tē-kō'don). The trinucleotide sequence complementary to a codon found in one loop of a tRNA molecule; *e.g.,* if a codon is A-G-C, its anticodon is U (or T)-C-G. The complementarity principle arises from Watson-Crick base-pairing, in which A is complementary to U (or T) and G is complementary to C. Sometimes called "nodoc".

an·ti·com·ple·ment (an-tē-kom'plĕ-ment). A substance that combines with a complement and neutralizes its action by preventing its union with an antibody.

an·ti·con·vul·sant (an'tē-kon-vŭl'sant). **1.** Preventing or arresting seizures. **2.** An agent having such action.

an·ti·de·pres·sant (an'tē-dē-pres'ănt). **1.** Counteracting depression. **2.** An agent used in treating depression.

an·ti·di·u·re·sis (an'tē-dī-yū-rē'sis). Reduction of urinary volume.

an·ti·di·u·ret·ic (an'tē-dī-yū-ret'ik). A drug or hormone that reduces urine production by the kidneys.

an·ti·dot·al (an-tē-dō'tăl). Relating to or acting as an antidote.

an·ti·dote (an'tē-dōt). An agent that neutralizes a poison or counteracts its effects. [G. *antidotos,* fr. *anti,* against, + *dotos,* what is given, fr. *didōmi,* to give]

chemical a., a substance that unites with a poison to form an innocuous chemical compound.

mechanical a., a substance that prevents the absorption of a poison.

physiologic a., an agent that produces systemic effects contrary to those of a given poison.

an·ti·drom·ic (an-tē-drom'ik). Moving in the direction opposite to normal; said of impulses in nerves and in the conduction system of the heart.

an·ti·e·met·ic (an'tē-ĕ-met'ik). **1.** Preventing or arresting vomiting. **2.** A remedy that tends to control nausea and vomiting. [anti- + G. *emetikos,* emetic]

an·ti·en·zyme (an-tē-en'zīm). An agent or principle that retards, inhibits, or destroys the activity of an enzyme; may be an inhibitory enzyme or an antibody to an enzyme.

an•ti•es•tro•gen (an'tē-es'trō-jen). Any substance capable of preventing full expression of the biological effects of estrogenic hormones on responsive tissues.

an•ti•fe•brile (an-tē-fē'brīl, -feb'ril). SYN antipyretic (1). [anti- + L. *febris,* fever]

an•ti•fi•bri•nol•y•sin (an'tē-fī-bri-nol'i-sin). SYN antiplasmin.

an•ti•fi•bri•no•lyt•ic (an'tē-fī-brin-ō-lit'ik). Denoting a substance that decreases the breakdown of fibrin; *e.g.,* aminocaproic acid.

an•ti•gen (Ag) (an'ti-jen). Any substance that, as a result of coming in contact with appropriate cells, induces a state of sensitivity and/or immune responsiveness after a latent period (days to weeks) and which reacts in a demonstrable way with antibodies and/or immune cells of the sensitized subject *in vivo* or *in vitro.* Modern usage tends to retain the broad meaning of a., employing the terms "antigenic determinant" or "determinant group" for the particular chemical group of a molecule that confers antigenic specificity. SEE ALSO hapten. SYN immunogen. [anti(body) + G. -*gen,* producing]

blood group a., generic term for any inherited antigen found on the surface of erythrocytes that determines a blood grouping reaction with specific antiserum; a.'s of the ABO and Lewis blood groups may be found also in saliva and other body fluids. See also Blood Groups appendix.

capsular a., that found only in the capsules of certain microorganisms; *e.g.,* the specific polysaccharides of various types of pneumococci.

carcinoembryonic a. (CEA), a glycoprotein constituent of the glycocalyx of embryonic endodermal epithelium, generally absent from adult cells with the exception of some carcinomas. It may also be detected in the serum of patients with colon cancer.

cholesterinized a., cardiolipin to which cholesterol has been added.

class I a.'s, cell-membrane–bound glycoproteins that are coded by genes of the major histocompatibility complex.

class II a.'s, a cell-membrane glycoprotein encoded by genes of the major histocompatibility complex. These antigens are distributed on a.-presenting cells such as macrophages, B cells, and dendritic cells.

class III a.'s, non–cell-membrane molecules that are encoded by the S region of the major histocompatibility complex. These a.'s are not involved in determining histocompatibility and include the complement proteins.

common a., cross-reacting a. (epitope), a common a. that occurs in two or more different molecules or organisms. SYN heterogenic enterobacterial a.

complete a., any a. capable of stimulating the formation of antibody with which it reacts *in vivo* or *in vitro,* as distinguished from incomplete a. (hapten).

conjugated a., SYN conjugated *hapten.*

delta a., SYN hepatitis D *virus.*

flagellar a., the heat-labile a.'s associated with bacterial flagella, in contrast to somatic a. SEE ALSO H a.

group a.'s, a.'s that are shared by related genera of microorganisms.

H a., (1) the a. in the flagella of motile bacteria; SEE ALSO O a. (1). **(2)** the chemical precursor of a.'s of the ABO blood group locus.

hepatitis B core a. (HB$_c$Ab, HB$_c$Ag), the a. found in the core of the Dane particle (which is the complete virus) and also in hepatocyte nuclei in hepatitis B infections.

hepatitis B e a. (HBe, HB$_e$Ag), an a., or group of a.'s, associated with hepatitis B infection and distinct from the surface a. (HB$_s$Ag) and the core a. (HB$_c$Ag). Its presence indicates that the virus is replicating and the individual is potentially infectious.

hepatitis B surface a. (HB$_s$Ag), a. of the small (20 nm) spherical and filamentous forms of hepatitis B a., and a surface a. of the larger (42 nm) Dane particle (complete infectious hepatitis B virus). SEE ALSO hepatitis B e a.

heterogenetic a., an a. which is possessed by a variety of phylogenetically unrelated species; *e.g.,* the various organ- or tissue-specific a.'s, the alpha- and beta-crystalline protein of the lens of the eye, and Forssman a.

heterogenic enterobacterial a., SYN common a.

human lymphocyte a.'s (HLA) [MIM* 142560], system designation for the gene products of at least four linked loci (A, B, C, and D) and a number of subloci on the sixth human chromosome which have a strong influence on human allotransplantation, transfusions, and certain disease associations.

H-Y a., an a. factor, dependent on the Y chromosome, responsible for the differentiation of the human embryo into the male phenotype by inducing the initially bipotential embryonic gonad to develop into a testis; in the absence of this a., the indifferent gonad develops into an ovary.

incomplete a., SYN hapten.

Kveim a., a saline suspension of human sarcoid tissue prepared from the spleen of an individual with active sarcoidosis; used in the Kveim test.

mumps skin test a., a suspension of killed mumps virus used to determine susceptibility to mumps or to confirm previous exposure.

O a., (1) somatic a. of enteric gram-negative bacteria. External part of cell wall lipopolysaccharide; SEE ALSO H a. (1). **(2)** see ABO blood group, Blood Groups appendix.

oncofetal a.'s, tumor-associated a.'s present in fetal tissue but not in normal adult tissue, including α-fetoprotein and carcinoembryonic a.

organ-specific a., a heterogenetic antigen with organ specificity; *e.g.,* in addition to species-specific a., kidney of one species contains a. that is identical to that in kidney of other species. SYN tissue-specific a.

partial a., SYN hapten.

prostate-specific a. (PSA), a single chain 31 kilodalton glycoprotein with 240 amino acid residues and 4 carbohydrate side chains that is a kallikrein protease; found in normal seminal fluid and produced by the prostatic epithelial cells. Elevated levels of PSA in blood serum are associated with prostatic enlargement and prostatic adenocarcinoma, and this allows early detection of cancer in many cases. In about 70% of cases, the rise is due to a cancerous condition. Thus, some studies have suggested that PSA testing may supplement an older test for prostatic acid phosphate (PAP), previously a fairly reliable gauge of metastatic prostate cancer. However, because no large-scale clinical studies have been completed, the medical and economic value of PSA testing remains uncertain.

sensitized a., the complex formed when a. combines with specific antibody; so called because the a., by the mediation of antibody, is rendered sensitive to the action of complement.

somatic a., an a. located in the cell wall of a bacterium in contrast to one in the flagella (flagellar a.) or in a capsule (capsular a.).

species-specific a., antigenic components in tissues and fluids by means of which various species may be immunologically distinguished; *e.g.,* serum albumin of horses is immunologically different from that of man, dogs, sheep.

T a.'s, tumor antigens associated wtih replication and transformation by certain DNA tumor viruses, including adenoviruses and papovaviruses. SEE ALSO β-hemolytic *streptococci,* under *streptococcus,* tumor a.'s.

tissue-specific a., SYN organ-specific a.

tumor a.'s, (1) a.'s that may be frequently associated with tumors or may be specifically found on tumor cells of the same origin (tumor specific); **(2)** tumor antigens may also be associated with replication and transformation by certain DNA tumor viruses, including adenoviruses and papovaviruses. SYN neoantigens. SEE ALSO T a.'s.

tumor-specific transplantation a.'s (TSTA), surface a.'s of DNA tumor virus-transformed cells, which elicit an immune rejection of the virus-free cells when transplanted into an animal that has been immunized against the specific cell-transforming virus.

an•ti•ge•ne•mia (an′ti-jĕ-nē′mē-ă). Persistence of antigen in circulating blood; *e.g.,* HB$_s$-antigenemia (presence of hepatitis B virus surface antigen in serum). [antigen + G. *haima,* blood]

an•ti•gen•ic (an-ti-jen′ik). Having the properties of an antigen (allergen). SYN allergenic, immunogenic.

an•ti•ge•nic•i•ty (an′ti-jĕ-nis′i-tē). The state or property of being antigenic. SYN immunogenicity.

an•ti-HB$_c$. Antibody to the hepatitis B core antigen (HB$_c$Ag).

an•ti-HB$_s$. Antibody to the hepatitis B surface *antigen* (HB$_s$Ag).

an•ti•he•lix (an-tē-hē′liks). An elevated ridge of cartilage anterior and roughly parallel to the posterior portion of the helix of the auricle. SYN anthelix [NA].

an•ti•hem•ag•glu•ti•nin (an′tē-hē-mă-glū′ti-nin, an′tē-hem-ă-). A substance (including antibody) that inhibits or prevents hemagglutination.

an•ti•he•mo•ly•sin (an′tē-hē-mol′i-sin, an′tē-

hem-ol′-). A substance (including antibody) that inhibits or prevents the effects of hemolysin.

an•ti•he•mo•lyt•ic (an′tē-hē-mō-lit′ik, an′tē-hem-ō-). Preventing hemolysis.

an•ti•hem•or•rhag•ic (an′tē-hem-ō-rāj′ik). Arresting hemorrhage. SYN hemostatic (2).

an•ti•his•ta•mines (an-tē-his′tă-mēnz). Drugs having an action antagonistic to that of histamine; used in the treatment of allergy symptoms.

an•ti•his•ta•min•ic (an′tē-his-tă-min′ik). **1.** Tending to neutralize or antagonize the action of histamine or to inhibit its production in the body. **2.** An agent having such an effect, used to relieve the symptoms of allergy.

an•ti•hor•mones (an-tē-hōr′mōnz). Substances demonstrable in serum that inhibit or prevent the usual effects of certain hormones, *e.g.,* specific antibodies.

an•ti•hy•per•ten•sive (an′tē-hī-per-ten′siv). Indicating a drug or mode of treatment that reduces the blood pressure of hypertensive individuals.

an•ti•in•flam•ma•to•ry (an′tē-in-flam′ă-tō-rē). Reducing inflammation by acting on body mechanisms, without directly antagonizing the causative agent; denoting agents such as glucocorticoids and aspirin.

an•ti•lith•ic (an-tē-lith′ik). **1.** Preventing the formation of calculi or promoting their dissolution. **2.** An agent so acting. [anti- + G. *lithos,* stone]

an•ti•ly•sin (an-tē-lī′sin). An antibody that inhibits or prevents the effects of lysin.

an•ti•mere (an′ti-mēr). **1.** A segment of an animal body formed by planes cutting the axis of the body at right angles. **2.** One of the symmetrical parts of a bilateral organism. **3.** The right or left half of the body. [anti- + G. *meros,* a part]

an•ti•me•tab•o•lite (an′tē-me-tab′ō-līt). A substance that competes with, replaces, or antagonizes a particular metabolite; *e.g.,* ethionine is an a. of methionine.

an•ti•mi•cro•bi•al (an′tē-mī-krō′bē-ăl). Tending to destroy microbes, to prevent their multiplication or growth, or to prevent their pathogenic action.

an•ti•mon•gol•oid (an-tē-mon′gō-loyd). The condition in which the lateral portion of the palpebral fissure is lower than the medial portion.

an•ti•mo•ny (Sb) (an′ti-mō-nē). A metallic element, atomic no. 51, atomic wt. 121.757, valences 0, −3, +3, +5; used in alloys; toxic and irritating to the skin and mucous membranes. [G. *anti + monos,* not found alone]

an•ti•mu•ta•gen (an-tē-myū′tă-jen). A factor that reduces or interferes with the mutagenic actions of effects of a substance.

an•ti•my•cot•ic (an′-tē-mī-kot′ik). Antagonistic to fungi. [anti- + G. *mykēs,* fungus]

an•ti•ne•o•plas•tic (an′tē-nē-ō-plas′tik). Preventing the development, maturation, or spread of neoplastic cells.

an•tin•i•on (an-tin′ē-on). The space between the eyebrows; the point on the skull opposite the inion. SEE ALSO glabella. [anti- + G. *inion,* nape of the neck]

an•ti•on•co•gene (an-tē-on′kō-jēn). A tumor-suppressing gene involved in controlling cellular growth; inactivation of this type of gene leads to deregulated cellular proliferation, as in cancer. SYN tumor suppressor gene (2).

an·ti·par·a·sit·ic (an'tē-par-ă-sit'ik). Destructive to parasites.

an·ti·pe·dic·u·lot·ic (an'tē-pe-dik-yū-lot'ik). Effective in the treatment of pediculosis, especially denoting such an agent.

an·ti·per·i·stal·sis (an'tē-per-i-stal'sis). SYN reversed *peristalsis*.

an·ti·per·i·stal·tic (an'tē-per-i-stal'tik). 1. Relating to antiperistalsis. 2. Impeding or arresting peristalsis.

an·ti·per·spi·rant (an-tē-per'spi-rant). 1. Having an inhibitory action upon the secretion of sweat. 2. An agent having such an action (*e.g.*, aluminum chloride).

an·ti·phlo·gis·tic (an'tē-flō-jis'tik). 1. Older term denoting preventing or relieving inflammation. 2. An agent that reduces inflammation. [anti- + G. *phogistos*, burnt up]

an·ti·plas·min (an-tē-plaz'min). A substance that inhibits or prevents the effects of plasmin; found in plasma and some tissues, especially the spleen and liver. SYN antifibrinolysin.

a₂ antiplasmin (al-fa-tu-an-te-plaz-min). A major protease inhibitor of plasmin and plasminogen, key components of the fibrinolytic system. Also inhibits other serine proteases, including the coagulation contact factors, factor Xa, and thrombin.

an·ti·port (an'tē-pōrt). The coupled transport of two different molecules or ions through a membrane in opposite directions by a common carrier mechanism (antiporter). Cf. symport, uniport. [anti- + L. *porto*, to carry]

an·ti·pro·throm·bin (an'tē-prō-throm'bin). An anticoagulant that inhibits or prevents the conversion of prothrombin into thrombin; examples are heparin, which is present in various tissues (especially in liver), and dicoumarin, which is isolated from partially decomposed sweet clover.

an·ti·pru·rit·ic (an'tē-prū-rit'ik). 1. Preventing or relieving itching. 2. An agent that relieves itching.

an·ti·psy·chot·ic (an'tē-sī-kot'ik). 1. SYN antipsychotic *agent*. 2. Denoting the actions of such an agent.

an·ti·py·ret·ic (an'tē-pī-ret'ik). 1. Reducing fever. SYN antifebrile, antithermic, febrifugal. 2. An agent that reduces fever (*e.g.*, acetaminophen, aspirin). SYN febrifuge. [anti- + G. *pyretos*, fever]

an·ti·scor·bu·tic (an'tē-skōr-byū'tik). 1. Preventive or curative of scurvy (scorbutus). 2. A treatment for scurvy (*e.g.*, vitamin C).

an·ti·se·cre·to·ry (an'tē-sē-krē'tō-rī). Inhibitory to secretion, said of certain drugs that reduce or suppress gastric secretion (*e.g.*, ranitidine, omeprazole).

an·ti·sep·sis (an-tē-sep'sis). Prevention of infection by inhibiting the growth of infectious agents. SEE ALSO disinfection. [anti- + G. *sēpsis*, putrefaction]

an·ti·sep·tic (an-tē-sep'tik). 1. Relating to antisepsis. 2. An agent or substance capable of effecting antisepsis.

an·ti·se·rum (an-tē-sē'rŭm). Serum that contains demonstrable antibody or antibodies specific for

one or more antigens; may be prepared from the blood of animals inoculated with an antigenic material or from the blood of animals and persons that have been stimulated by natural contact with an antigen (as by an attack of disease). SYN immune serum.

an·ti·so·cial (an-tē-sō'shŭl). Opposed to the rights of individuals or to the legal norms of society. Cf. asocial.

an·ti·spas·mod·ic (an'tē-spaz-mod'ik). 1. Preventing or alleviating muscle spasms (cramps). 2. An agent that quiets spasm.

an·ti·strep·to·coc·cic (an'tē-strep-tō-kok'sik). Destructive to streptococci or antagonistic to their toxins.

antithermic (an-ti-ther-mik). SYN antipyretic (1). [*anti-* + G. *therme, heat, warmth,* + *-ic*]

an·ti·tox·ic (an-tē-tok'sik). Neutralizing the action of a poison; specifically, relating to an antitoxin. SEE ALSO antidotal.

an·ti·tox·in (an-tē-tok'sin). Antibody formed in response to antigenic poisonous substances of biologic origin, such as bacterial exotoxins, phytotoxins, and zootoxins; in general usage, serum from humans or animals (usually horses) immunized by injections of the specific toxoid. A. neutralizes the pharmacologic effects of its specific toxin. [anti- + G. *toxikon*, poison]

  normal a., serum that is capable of neutralizing an equivalent quantity of a normal toxin solution.

an·ti·tra·gus (an-tē-trā'gŭs) [NA]. A projection of the cartilage of the auricle, in front of the tail of the helix, just above the lobule, and posterior to the tragus from which it is separated by the intertragic notch. [G. *anti-tragos*, the eminence of the external ear, fr. *anti*, opposite, + *tragos*, a goat, the tragus]

an·ti·trep·o·ne·mal (an'tē-trep-ō-nē'mǎl). SYN treponemicidal.

an·ti·tro·pic (an-tē-trō'pik). Similar, bilaterally symmetrical, but in an opposite location (as in a mirror image), *e.g.*, the right thumb in relation to the left thumb.

an·ti·tryp·sic (an-tē-trip'sik). SYN antitryptic.

an·ti·tryp·sin (an-tē-trip'sin). A substance that blocks the action of trypsin.

an·ti·tryp·tic (an-tē-trip'tik). Possessing properties of antitrypsin. SYN antitrypsic.

an·ti·tus·sive (an-tē-tŭs'iv). 1. Relieving cough. 2. A cough remedy (*e.g.*, codeine). [anti- + L. *tussis*, cough]

an·ti·ven·in (an-tē-ven'in). An antitoxin specific for an animal or insect venom. [anti- + L. *venenum*, poison]

an·ti·vi·ral (an-tē-vī'rǎl). Opposing a virus; interfering with its replication; weakening or abolishing its action.

an·ti·vi·ta·min (an-tē-vī'tǎ-min). A substance that prevents a vitamin from exerting its typical biological effects. Most a.'s have chemical structures like those of vitamins and appear to function as competitive antagonists.

an·tra (-trǎ).

an·tra (an'trǎ). Plural of antrum.

an·tral (an'trǎl). Relating to an antrum.

an·trec·to·my (an-trek'tō-mē). 1. Removal of the walls of an antrum. 2. Removal of the antrum (distal half) of the stomach. [antrum + G. *ektomē*, excision]

an•tri (-trī).

⌂**antro-.** An antrum. [L. *antrum,* from G. *antron,* a cave]

an•tro•du•o•de•nec•to•my (an'trō-dū-ō-dĕ-nek'tō-mē). Surgical removal of the antrum of the stomach and the ulcer-bearing part of the duodenum.

an•tro•na•sal (an-trō-nā'săl). Relating to a maxillary sinus and the corresponding nasal cavity.

an•tro•scope (an'trō-skōp). An instrument to aid in the visual examination of any cavity, particularly the antrum of Highmore (maxillary sinus). [antro- + G. *skopeō,* to view]

an•tros•co•py (an-tros'cō-pē). Examination of any cavity, especially the antrum of Highmore, by means of an antroscope.

an•tros•to•my (an-tros'tō-mē). Formation of a permanent opening into any antrum. [antro- + G. *stoma,* mouth]

an•trot•o•my (an-trot'ō-mē). Incision through the wall of any antrum. [antro- + G. *tomē,* incision]

an•tro•tym•pan•ic (an'trō-tim-pan'ik). Relating to the mastoid antrum and the tympanic cavity.

an•trum, gen. **an•tri,** pl. **an•tra** (an'trŭm, -trī, -tră). [NA] Any nearly closed cavity, particularly one with bony walls. **2.** SYN pyloric a. [L. fr. G. *antron,* a cave]

   mastoid a., a cavity in the petrous portion of the temporal bone, communicating posteriorly with the mastoid cells and anteriorly with the epitympanic recess of the middle ear via the aperture of the mastoid a.

   pyloric a., the initial portion of the pyloric part of the stomach, which may temporarily become partially or completely shut off from the remainder of the stomach during digestion by peristaltic contraction of the prepyloric "sphincter"; it is sometimes demarcated from the second part of the pyloric part of the stomach (pyloric canal) by a slight groove. SYN antrum (2).

ANUG acute necrotizing ulcerative *gingivitis.*

an•u•lus, pl. **an•u•li** (an'yū-lŭs, -lī) [NA]. ⋆official alternate term for ring. [L.]

an•u•ria (an-yū'rē-ă). Absence of urine formation.

an•u•ric (an-yūr'ik). Relating to anuria.

anus, gen. **ani,** pl. **ani** (ā'nŭs, -nī, -nī) [NA]. The lower opening of the digestive tract, lying in the cleft between the buttocks, through which fecal matter is extruded. [L.]

   imperforate a., (1) SYN anal *atresia.* **(2)** SYN ectopic (1).

an•vil. SYN incus.

anx•i•e•ty (ang-zī'ĕ-tē). **1.** Apprehension of danger and dread accompanied by restlessness, tension, tachycardia, and dyspnea unattached to a clearly identifiable stimulus. **2.** EXPERIMENTAL PSYCHOLOGY a drive or motivational state learned from and thereafter associated with previously neutral cues. [L. *anxietas,* anxiety, fr. *anxius,* distressed, fr. *ango,* to press tight, to torment]

   separation a., a child's apprehension or fear associated with removal from or loss of a parent or significant other.

anx•i•o•lyt•ic (ang'zē-ō-lit'ik). **1.** SYN antianxiety *agent.* **2.** Denoting the actions of such an agent. [anxiety + G. *lysis,* a dissolution or loosening]

aor•ta, gen. and pl. **aor•tae** (ā-ōr'tă, ā-ōr'tē) [NA]. A large artery which is the main trunk of the systemic arterial system, arising from the left ventricle and ending at the lumbar vertebra by dividing to form the right and left common iliac arteries. The a. is formed from: ascending a.; aortic arch; and descending a., which is divided into the thoracic a. and the abdominal a. [Mod. L. fr. G. *aortē,* from *aeirō,* to lift up]

aor•tal (ā-ōr'tăl). SYN aortic.

aor•tal•gia (ā-ōr-tal'jē-ă). Pain assumed to be due to aneurysm or other pathologic conditions of the aorta. [aorta + G. *algos,* pain]

aor•tic (ā-ōr'tik). Relating to the aorta or the a. orifice of the left ventricle of the heart. SYN aortal.

aor•ti•tis (ā-ōr-tī'tis). Inflammation of the aorta.

aor•to•cor•o•nary (ā-ōr'tō-kōr'ō-nār-ē). Relating to the aorta and the coronary arteries.

aor•to•gram (ā-ōr'tō-gram). The image or set of images resulting from aortography.

aor•tog•ra•phy (ā-ōr-tog'ră-fē). **1.** Radiographic imaging of the aorta and its branches by injection of contrast medium. **2.** Imaging of the aorta by ultrasound or magnetic resonance. [aorta + G. *graphō,* to write]

aor•top•a•thy (ā-ōr-top'ă-thē). Disease affecting the aorta. [aorta + G. *pathos,* suffering]

aor•to•plas•ty (ā-ōr'tō-plas'tē). A procedure for surgical repair of the aorta.

aor•tor•rha•phy (ā-ōr-tōr'ă-fē). Suture of the aorta. [aorta + G. *rhaphē,* seam]

aor•to•scle•ro•sis (ā-ōr'tō-skler-ō'sis). Arteriosclerosis of the aorta.

aor•tot•o•my (ā-ōr-tot'ō-mē). Incision of the aorta. [aorta + G. *tomē,* a cutting]

apall•es•the•sia (ă-pal-es-thē'zē-ă). SYN pallanesthesia. [G. *a-* priv. + *pallo,* to tremble, quiver, + *aisthēsis,* feeling]

apar•a•lyt•ic (ā-par'ă-lit'ik). Without paralysis; not causing paralysis.

ap•a•thet•ic (ap-ă-thet'ik). Exhibiting apathy; indifferent.

ap•a•thism (ap'ă-thizm). A sluggishness of reaction. Cf. erethism.

ap•a•thy (ap'ă-thē). Indifference; absence of interest in the environment. Often one of the earliest signs of cerebral disease. [G. *apatheia,* fr. *a-* priv. + *pathos,* suffering]

apel•lous (ă-pel'ŭs). **1.** Without skin. **2.** Without foreskin; circumcised. [G. *a-* not + L. *pellis,* skin]

ape•ri•od•ic (ā-pēr-ē-od'ik). Not occurring periodically.

aper•i•stal•sis (ā'per-i-stal'sis). Absence of peristalsis.

aper•to•gnath•ia (ă-per-tō-nath'ē-ă). An open bite deformity, a type of malocclusion characterized by premature posterior occlusion and absence of anterior occlusion. [L. *apertus,* open, + G. *gnathos,* jaw]

ap•er•tu•ra, pl. **ap•er•tu•rae** (ap-er-tū'ră, -rē) [NA]. SYN aperture. [L. fr. *aperio,* pp. *apertus,* to open]

a. pel′vis infe′rior [NA], SYN inferior pelvic *aperture*.

a. pel′vis supe′rior [NA], SYN superior pelvic *aperture*.

ap·er·ture (ap′er-chūr). **1.** An inlet or entrance to a cavity or channel; in anatomy, an open gap or hole. **2.** The diameter of the objective of a microscope. SYN aditus [NA], apertura [NA], opening. [L. *apertura*, an opening]

inferior pelvic a., the lower opening of the true pelvis, bounded anteriorly by the pubic arch, laterally by the rami of the ischium and the sacrotuberous ligament on either side, and posteriorly by these ligaments and the tip of the coccyx. SYN apertura pelvis inferior [NA].

superior pelvic a., the upper opening of the true pelvis, bounded anteriorly by the pubic symphysis and the pubic crest on either side, laterally by the iliopectineal lines, and posteriorly by the promontory of the sacrum. SYN apertura pelvis superior [NA].

apex, gen. **ap·i·cis,** pl. **ap·i·ces** (ā′peks, ap′i-sis, ap′i-sēs) [NA]. The extremity of a conical or pyramidal structure, such as the heart or the lung. [L. summit or tip]

apex·car·di·og·ra·phy (ā′peks-kar′dē-og-ră-fē). Noninvasive graphic recording of cardiac pulsations from the region of the apex, usually of the left ventricle, and resembling the ventricular pressure curve.

apex·i·fi·ca·tion (ā-pek′si-fi-kā′shŭn). Induced tooth root development or closure of the root apex by hard tissue deposition.

APG ambulatory patient *group*.

apha·gia (ă-fā′jē-ă). Inability to eat. [G. *a-* priv. + *phagō*, to eat]

apha·kia (ă-fā′kē-ă). Absence of the lens of the eye. [G. *a-* priv. + *phakos*, lentil, anything shaped like a lentil]

apha·lan·gia (ă-fă-lan′jē-ă). Congenital absence of a digit, or more specifically, absence of one or more of the long bones (phalanges) of a finger or toe. [G. *a-* priv. + phalanx]

apha·sia (ă-fā′zē-ă). Impaired or absent comprehension or production of, or communication by, speech, writing, or signs, due to an acquired lesion of the dominant cerebral hemisphere. SYN alogia (1), dysphasia, dysphrasia, logagnosia, logamnesia, logasthenia. [G. speechlessness, fr. *a-* priv. + *phasis,* speech]

acoustic a., SYN auditory a.

acquired epileptic a., SYN Landau-Kleffner *syndrome*.

amnestic a., amnesic a., SYN nominal a.

anomic a., SYN nominal a.

associative a., SYN conduction a.

ataxic a., SYN motor a.

auditory a., an impairment in comprehension of the auditory forms of language and communication, including the ability to write from dictation in the presence of normal hearing. Spontaneous speech, reading, and writing are not affected. SYN acoustic a.

Broca's a., SYN motor a.

conduction a., a form of a. in which the patient understands spoken and written words, is aware of his deficit, and can speak and write, but skips

or repeats words, or substitutes one word for another (paraphasia); word repetition is severely impaired. The responsible lesion is in the associate tracts connecting the various language centers. SYN associative a.

expressive a., SYN motor a.

global a., in which all aspects of speech and communication are severely impaired. At best, patients can understand or speak only a few words or phrases; they cannot read or write. SYN mixed a., total a.

impressive a., SYN sensory a.

jargon a., SYN agrammatism.

mixed a., SYN global a.

motor a., a type of a. in which there is a deficit in speech production or language output, often accompanied by a deficit in communicating by writing, signs, etc. The patient is aware of the impairment. SYN ataxic a., Broca's a., expressive a.

nominal a., an a. in which the principal deficit is difficulty in naming persons and objects seen, heard, or felt; due to lesions in various portions of the language area. SYN amnestic a., amnesic a., anomia, anomic a.

receptive a., SYN sensory a.

sensory a., a. in which there is impairment in the comprehension of spoken and written words, associated with effortless, articulated, but paraphrastic, speech and writing; malformed words, substitute words, and neologisms are characteristic. When severe, and speech is incomprehensible, it is called jargon a. The patient often appears unaware of the deficit. SYN impressive a., receptive a.

total a., SYN global a.

visual a., (1) SYN alexia. **(2)** improperly used as a synonym for anomia.

apha·si·ac, apha·sic (ă-fā′zē-ak, ă-fā′sik). Relating to or suffering from aphasia. SYN dysphasic.

apha·si·ol·o·gist (ă-fā′zē-ol′ŏ-gist). A specialist who deals with speech disorders caused by dysfunction of the language areas of the brain.

apha·si·ol·o·gy (ă-fā′zē-ol′ŏ-gē). The science of speech disorders caused by dysfunction of the cerebral language areas.

aphe·mia (ă-fē′mē-ă). Obsolete term for a form of motor aphasia in which the ability to express ideas in spoken words is lost. [a- priv. + G. *phēmē,* voice]

apher·e·sis (ă-fer-ē′sis). Extraction of certain fluid or cellular elements from withdrawn blood, which is then reinfused into the donor or patient; performed therapeutically to remove harmful elements from the blood, and also to obtain immune globulins. [G. *aphairesis,* withdrawal]

apho·nia (ă-fō′nē-ă). Loss of the voice as a result of disease or injury to the larynx. [G. *a-* priv. + *phōnē,* voice]

aphon·ic (ă-fon′ik). Relating to aphonia.

aphra·sia (ă-frā′zē-ă). Inability to speak, from any cause. [G. *a-* priv. + *phrasis,* speaking]

aph·ro·di·si·ac (af-rō-diz′ē-ak). **1.** Increasing sexual desire. **2.** Anything that arouses or increases sexual desire.

aph·tha, pl. **aph·thae** (af′thă, af′thē). **1.** In the singular, a small ulcer on a mucous membrane. **2.**

In the plural, stomatitis characterized episodes of painful oral ulcers of unknown etiology that are covered by gray exudate, are surrounded by an erythematous halo, and heal spontaneously in one to two weeks. SYN aphthae minor, aphthous stomatitis, canker sores, recurrent aphthous ulcers, recurrent ulcerative stomatitis, ulcerative stomatitis. [G. ulceration]

Bednar's aphthae, traumatic ulcers located bilaterally on either side of the midpalatal raphe in infants.

herpetiform aphthae, a variant of oral aphthae, of unknown etiology, characterized by up to several dozen ulcers, 2-3 mm in diameter, organized in a clustered herpetiform distribution.

aphthae ma′jor, a severe form of aphthae characterized by unusually numerous, large, deep, and frequent ulcers; healing may take as long as six weeks and results in scarring. SYN Mikulicz' aphthae, periadenitis mucosa necrotica recurrens.

Mikulicz' aphthae, SYN aphthae major.

aphthae mi′nor, SYN aphtha (2).

aph•thoid (af′thoyd). Resembling aphthae.

aph•tho•sis (af-thō′sis). Any condition characterized by the presence of aphthae.

aph•thous (af′thŭs). Characterized by or relating to aphthae or aphthosis.

ap•i•cal (ap′i-kăl). **1.** Relating to the apex or tip of a pyramidal or pointed structure. **2.** Situated nearer to the apex of a structure in relation to a specific reference point; opposite of basal.

ap•i•cec•to•my (ap-i-sek′tō-mē). **1.** Opening and exenteration of air cells in the apex of the petrous part of the temporal bone. **2.** In dental surgery, an obsolete synonym for apicoectomy. [L. apex, summit or tip, + G. ektomē, excision]

ap•i•ces (ap′i-sēs). Plural of apex.

ap•i•ci•tis (ap-i-sī′tis). Inflammation of the apex of a structure or organ.

⟡apico-. An apex; apical [L. apex, apicis, a summit or a tip + -o-]

ap•i•co•ec•to•my (ap′i-kō-ek′tō-mē). Surgical removal of a dental root apex. SYN root resection. [apico- + G. ektomē, excision]

ap•i•col•y•sis (ap-i-kol′i-sis). Surgical collapse of the upper portion of the lung by the operative detachment of the parietal pleura allowing a medial displacement of the pulmonary apex. [apico- + G. lysis, destruction]

ap•i•cot•o•my (ap-i-kot′ō-mē). Incision into an apical structure. [apico- + G. tomē, a cutting]

ap•la•nat•ic (ap-la-nat′ik). Pertaining to aplanatism, or to an aplanatic lens.

apla•sia (ă-plā′zē-ă). **1.** Defective development or congenital absence of an organ or tissue. **2.** HEMATOLOGY incomplete, retarded, or defective development, or cessation of the usual regenerative process. [G. a- priv. + plasis, a molding]

aplas•tic (ā-plas′tik, ă-). Pertaining to aplasia, or conditions characterized by defective regeneration, as in a. anemia.

ap•nea (ap′nē-ă). Absence of breathing. [G. apnoia, want of breath]

  central a., a. as the result of medullary depression which inhibits respiratory movement.

  obstructive a., peripheral a., a. either as the result of obstruction of the air passages or inadequate respiratory muscle activity.

  sleep a., central and/or peripheral a. during sleep, associated with frequent awakening and often with daytime sleepiness.

ap•ne•ic (ap′nē-ik). Related to or suffering from apnea.

ap•neu•mia (ap-nū′mē-ă). Congenital absence of the lungs. [G. a- priv. + pneumōn, lung]

ap•neu•sis (ap-nū′sis). An abnormal respiratory pattern consisting of a pause at full inspiration; cramp caused by a lesion at the mid or caudal pontine level of the brainstem. [G. a- priv. + pneusis, a breathing, fr. pneō, to breathe]

⟡apo-. Combining form meaning, usually, separated from or derived from. [G. apo, away from, off; apo- becomes ap-, especially before a vowel or h]

ap•o•crine (ap′ō-krin). Denoting a mechanism of glandular secretion in which the apical portion of secretory cells is shed and incorporated into the secretion. SEE ALSO apocrine gland. [G. apo-krinō, to separate]

a•po•dal (ă-pō′dal). Relating to apodia. [G. a- priv. + pous, foot]

apo•dia (ă-pō′dē-ă). Congenital absence of feet. [G. a- priv. + pous, foot]

ap•o•en•zyme (ap′ō-en-zīm). The protein portion of an enzyme as contrasted with the nonprotein portion, or coenzyme, or prosthetic portion (if present).

ap•o•fer•ri•tin (ap-ō-fer′i-tin). A protein in the intestinal wall that combines with a ferric hydroxide-phosphate compound to form ferritin, the first stage in the absorption of iron.

ap•o•lip•o•pro•tein (ap′ō-lip-ō-prō′tēn). The protein component of lipoprotein complexes that is a normal constituent of plasma chylomicrons, HDL, LDL, and VLDL in man.

ap•o•neu•rec•to•my (ap′ō-nū-rek′tō-mē). Excision of an aponeurosis. [aponeurosis + G. ektomē, excision]

ap•o•neu•ror•rha•phy (ap′ō-nū-rōr′ă-fē). SYN fasciorrhaphy. [aponeurosis + G. rhaphē, suture]

ap•o•neu•ro•ses (-sēz).

ap•o•neu•ro•sis, pl. **ap•o•neu•ro•ses** (ap′ō-nū-rō′sis, -sēz) [NA]. A fibrous sheet or flat, expanded tendon, giving attachment to muscular fibers and serving as the means of origin or insertion of a flat muscle; it sometimes also performs the office of a fascia for other muscles. [G. the end of the muscle where it becomes tendon, fr. apo, from, + neuron, sinew]

  epicranial a., the aponeurosis or intermediate tendon connecting the frontalis and occipitalis muscles to form the epicranius. SYN galea (2).

ap•o•neu•ro•si•tis (ap′ō-nū-rō-sī′tis). Inflammation of an aponeurosis.

ap•o•neu•rot•ic (ap′ō-nū-rot′ik). Relating to an aponeurosis.

ap•o•neu•rot•o•my (ap′ō-nū-rot′ō-mē). Incision of an aponeurosis.

apoph•y•sis, pl. **apoph•y•ses** (ă-pof′i-sis, -sēz). An outgrowth or projection, especially one from a bone. A bony process or outgrowth that lacks an independent center of ossification. [G. an offshoot]

apoph·y·si·tis (ă-pof-i-sī′tis). Inflammation of any apophysis.

ap·o·plec·tic (ap-ŏ-plek′tik). Relating to, suffering from, or predisposed to apoplexy.

ap·o·pro·tein (ap-ō-prō′tēn). A polypeptide chain (protein) not yet complexed with the prosthetic group that is necessary to form the active holoprotein.

ap·o·re·pres·sor (ap′ō-rē-pres′er). SYN inactive *repressor*.

ap·o·stax·is (ap-ō-staks′is). Slight hemorrhage, or bleeding by drops. [G. a trickling down]

apos·thia (ă-pos′thē-ă). Congenital absence of the prepuce. [G. a- priv. + *posthē*, foreskin]

ap·pa·ra·tus (ap-ă-rā′tŭs). 1. A collection of instruments adapted for a special purpose. 2. An instrument made up of several parts. 3 [NA]. A group or system of glands, ducts, blood vessels, muscles, or other anatomical structures involved in the performance of some function. SEE ALSO system. [L. equipment. fr. *ap-paro*, pp. *-atus*, to prepare]

   Golgi a., a membranous system of cisternae and vesicles located between the nucleus and the secretory pole or surface of a cell; concerned with the investment and intracellular transport of membrane-bounded secretory proteins.

   lacrimal a., consisting of the lacrimal gland, the lacrimal lake, the lacrimal canaliculi, the lacrimal sac, and the nasolacrimal duct.

ap·pend·age (ă-pen′dij). Any part, subordinate in function or size, attached to a main structure. SEE ALSO adnexa. SYN appendix (1). [L. *appendix*]

   a.'s of skin, the hairs, nails, and sweat, sebaceous, and mammary glands.

ap·pen·dec·to·my (ap-pen-dek′tō-mē). Surgical removal of the vermiform appendix. SYN appendicectomy. [appendix + G. *ektomē*, excision]

ap·pen·di·cal (ă-pen′di-kăl). SYN appendiceal.

ap·pen·dic·e·al (ă-pen-dis′ē-ăl). Relating to an appendix. SYN appendical.

ap·pen·di·cec·to·my (ap-pen-di-sek′tō-mē). SYN appendectomy.

ap·pen·di·ci·tis (ă-pen-di-sī′tis). Inflammation of the vermiform appendix. [appendix + G. *-itis*, inflammation]

△**appendico-.** An appendix, usually the vermiform appendix. [L. *appendix, appendicis* an appendage, fr. *appendo*, to hang something onto something, fr. *ad-, ap-*, to, onto, + *pendo*, to hang, + *-o-*]

ap·pen·di·co·lith (ă-pen′dĭ-kō-lith). A calcified concretion in the appendix visible on an abdominal radiograph. [appendico- + G. *lithos*, stone]

ap·pen·di·co·li·thi·a·sis (ă-pen′di-kō-li-thī′ă-sis). The presence of concretions in the vermiform appendix. [appendico- + G. *lithos*, stone]

ap·pen·di·col·y·sis (ă-pen-di-kol′i-sis). An operation for freeing the appendix from adhesions. [appendico- + G. *lysis*, a loosening]

ap·pen·di·cos·to·my (ă-pen-di-kos′tō-mē). An operation for opening into the intestine through the tip of the vermiform appendix, previously attached to the anterior abdominal wall. [appendico- + G. *stoma*, mouth]

ap·pen·dic·u·lar (ap′en-dik′yū-lăr). 1. Relating to an appendix or appendage. 2. Relating to the limbs, as opposed to axial, which refers to the trunk and head.

ap·pen·dix, gen. **ap·pen·di·cis**, pl. **ap·pen·di·ces** (ă-pen′diks, -di-sis, -di-sēs). 1 [NA]. SYN appendage. 2. Specifically, the vermiform appendix. [L. appendage, fr. *ap-pendo*, to hang something on]

   a. epiplo′ica, pl. **appen′dices epiplo′icae** [NA], one of a number of little processes or sacs of peritoneum filled with adipose tissue and projecting from the serous coat of the large intestine, except the rectum; they are most evident on the transverse and sigmoid colon, being most numerous along the free tenia.

   vermiform a., a wormlike intestinal diverticulum extending from the blind end of the cecum; it varies in length and ends in a blind extremity. SYN a. vermiformis [NA].

   a. vermifor′mis [NA], SYN vermiform a.

ap·per·cep·tion (ap-er-sep′shŭn). 1. The final stage of attentive perception in which something is clearly apprehended and thus is relatively prominent in awareness; the full apprehension of any psychic content. 2. The process of referring the perception of ideas to one's own personality. [L. *ad*, to, + *per- cipio*, pp. *-ceptus*, to take wholly, perceive]

ap·per·cep·tive (ap-er-sep′tiv). Relating to, involved in, or capable of apperception.

ap·pe·tite (ap′ĕ-tīt). A desire or motive derived from a biologic or psychological need for food, water, sex, or affection; a desire or longing to satisfy any conscious physical or mental need. [L. *ad-peto*, pp. *-petitus*, to seek after, desire]

ap·pla·na·tion (ap′lan-ā′shŭn). TONOMETRY the flattening of the cornea by pressure. Intraocular pressure is directly proportional to external pressure, and inversely proportional to the area flattened. SEE ALSO applanation *tonometer*. [L. *ad*, toward, + *planum*, plane]

ap·pla·nom·e·try (ap-lan-om′ĕ-trē). Use of an applanation tonometer.

ap·pli·ance (ă-plī′ans). A device used to provide function to a part, or for therapeutic purposes. [fr, O. Fr. *aplier*, to apply, fr. L. *applico*, to fold together]

ap·pli·ca·tor (ap′li-kā-tōr). A slender rod of wood, flexible metal, or synthetic material, at one end of which is attached a pledget of cotton or other substance for making local applications to any accessible surface. [L. *ap-plico*, to attach to]

ap·po·si·tion (ap-ō-zish′ŭn). 1. The placing in contact of two substances. 2. The condition of being placed or fitted together. 3. The relationship of fracture fragments to one another. 4. The process of thickening of the cell wall. [L. *ap-pono*, pp. *-positus*, to place at or to]

ap·prox·i·mate (ă-prok′si-māt). To bring close together. DENTISTRY 1. Proximate, denoting the contact surfaces, either mesial or distal, of two adjacent teeth. 2. Close together; denoting the teeth in the human jaw, as distinguished from the separated teeth in certain of the lower animals. [L. *ad*, to, + *proximus*, nearest]

ap·prox·i·ma·tion (ă-prok-si-mā′shŭn). In surgery, bringing tissue edges into desired apposition for suturing.

aprac•tic (ă-prak′tik). SYN apraxic.

aprax•ia (ă-prak′sē-ă). **1.** A disorder of voluntary movement, consisting of impairment in the performance of skilled or purposeful movements, notwithstanding the preservation of comprehension, muscular power, sensibility, and coordination in general; due to acquired cerebral disease. **2.** A psychomotor defect in which the proper use of an object can not be carried out although the object can be named and its uses described. [G. *a-* priv. + *prattō,* to do]

    articulatory a., SYN verbal a.

    childhood a., SYN developmental a. of speech.

    developmental a. of speech (DAS), severe articulatory disturbance in childhood characterized by multiple and inconsistent errors in production of voluntary sequences of phonemes, but not due to weakness or spasticity of speech musculature (*i.e.,* not dysarthria). SYN childhood a., developmental dyspraxia of speech.

    ideokinetic a., ideomotor a., a form of a. in which simple acts are incapable of being performed, presumably because the connections between the cortical centers that control volition and the motor cortex are interrupted.

    oral a., reduced ability, due to cortical sensorimotor damage, to perform voluntary movements of the oral musculature, especially sequenced movements. Often occurs with apraxia of speech. SEE ALSO apraxia. SYN oral motor a.

    oral motor a., SYN oral a.

    a. of speech, SYN verbal a.

    verbal a., speech disorder due to cortical sensorimotor damage that impairs the ability to program speech musculature for volitional production of sequenced phonemes. Often accompanies motor a. SEE apraxia, oral a., developmental a. of speech. SYN a. of speech, articulatory a., dyspraxia of speech, verbal dyspraxia.

aprax•ic (ă-prak′sik). Marked by or pertaining to apraxia. SYN apractic.

aproc•tia (ă-prok′shē-ă). Congenital absence or imperforation of the anus. [G. *a-* priv. + *prōktos,* anus]

apronectomy. Surgical excision of a redundant and dependent panniculus adiposus of the abdominal wall, which is commonly called an apron.

ap•ro•so•pia (ap-rō-sō′pē-ă). Congenital absence of the greater part or all of the face, usually associated with other malformations. [G. *a-* priv. + *prosōpon,* face]

APS (antiphospholipid antibody syndrome) adenosine 5′-phosphosulfate.

aPS antiphospholipid antibody *syndrome.*

aPTT activated partial thromboplastin *time.*

APUD. Proposed designation for a group of cells in different organs secreting polypeptide hormones. Cells in this group have certain biochemical characteristics in common, the first letters of which form the name: they contain amines, such as catecholamine and 5-hydroxytryptamine, take up precursors of these amines *in vivo,* and contain amino-acid decarboxylase. [*a*mine *p*recursor *u*ptake, *d*ecarboxylase]

apy•ret•ic (ā-pī-ret′ik). Without fever, denoting

apyrexia; having a normal body temperature. SYN afebrile.

apy•rex•ia (ā-pī-rek′sē-ă). Absence of fever. [G. *a-* priv. + *pyrexis,* fever]

aq. Abbreviation for L. *aqua,* water.

aq. dest. Abbreviation for L. *aqua destillata,* distilled water.

aq•ua•pho•bia (ak-wă-fō′bē-ă). Morbid fear of water. [L. *aqua,* water, + G. *phobos,* fear]

aq•ue•duct (ak′we-dŭkt). A conduit or canal. SYN aqueductus [NA]. [L. *aquaeductus*]

    cerebral a., an ependyma-lined canal in the mesencephalon about 20 mm long, connecting the third to the fourth ventricle.

aq•ue•duc•tus, pl. **aq•ue•duc•tus** (ak-we-dŭk′tŭs) [NA]. SYN aqueduct. [L. fr. *aqua,* water, + *ductus,* a leading, fr. *duco,* pp. *ductus,* to lead]

    a. coch′leae, SYN perilymphatic *duct.*

aque•ous (ak′wē-ŭs, ā′kwē-ŭs). Watery; of, like, or containing water.

Ar argon.

△**arab-.** Gum arabic; similar gummy substances. [G. *Araps, Arabos,* an Arab]

arachnase (ă-rak′nāz). A positive control plasma for the monitoring of clotting-endpoint coagulation tests used in the detection of circulating lupus anticoagulants: it is a normal plasma that contains a venom extract from the brown recluse spider, *Loxosceles reclusa,* which mimics the presence of a lupus anticoagulant (LA) in a variety of clotting-endpoint tests.

arach•ne•pho•bia (ă-rak-nē-fō′bē-ă). Morbid fear of spiders. SYN arachnophobia. [G. *arachne,* spider, + *phobos,* fear]

Arach•ni•da (ă-rak′ni-dă). A class of arthropods in the subphylum Chelicerata, consisting of spiders, scorpions, harvestmen, mites, ticks, and allies. [G. *arachnē,* spider]

arach•no•dac•ty•ly (ă-rak-nō-dak′ti-lē). A condition in which the hands and fingers, and often the feet and toes, are abnormally long and slender; a characteristic of Marfan's syndrome and kindred hereditary disorders of connective tissue. [G. *arachnē,* spider, + *daktylos,* finger]

arach•noid (ă-rak′noyd). A delicate fibrous membrane forming the middle of the three coverings of the central nervous system. Its external surface is closely applied (but not attached) to the internal surface of the dura mater, with only a potential space (subdural space) intervening. Thus, in a spinal puncture, dura mater and a. are penetrated simultaneously as if a single layer. SEE ALSO leptomeninges. SYN arachnoidea, arachnoides [NA], arachnoid membrane. [G. *arachnē,* spider, cobweb, + *eidos,* resemblance]

ar•ach•noi•dea, ar•ach•noi•des (ă-rak-noyd′ē-ă, -dēz) [NA]. SYN arachnoid. [Mod. L. *arachnoideus* fr. G. *arachnē,* spider, + *eidos,* resemblance]

arach•noid•i•tis (ă-rak-noy-dī′tis). Inflammation of the arachnoid membrane often with involvement of the subjacent subarachnoid space. SEE ALSO leptomeningitis. [arachnoidea + *-itis,* inflammation]

arach•no•pho•bia (ă-rak-nō-fō′bē-ă). SYN arachnephobia.

ar•bor, pl. **ar•bo•res** (ar′bōr, ar-bō′rēz). In anatomy, a treelike structure with branchings. [L. tree]

ar·bo·res·cent (ar-bō-res'ent). SYN dendriform.

ar·bo·ri·za·tion (ar'bōr-i-zā'shŭn). **1.** The terminal branching of nerve fibers or blood vessels in a branching treelike pattern. **2.** The branched pattern formed by a dried smear of cervical mucus, indicating the effect of estrogen unopposed by progesterone.

ar·bo·rize (ar'bōr-īz). To spread in a treelike branching pattern.

ar·bo·vi·rus (ar'bō-vī'rŭs). A large, heterogeneous group of RNA viruses. There are over 500 species, which have been recovered from arthropods, bats, and rodents. These taxonomically diverse viruses are unified by an epidemiological concept, *i.e.,* transmission between vertebrate hosts by blood-feeding arthropod vectors, such as mosquitoes, ticks, sandflies, and midges. In most instances diseases produced by these viruses are mild and difficult to distinguish from illnesses caused by viruses of other taxonomic groups. Infections may be separated into several clinical syndromes: undifferentiated type fevers (systemic febrile disease), hepatitis, hemorrhagic fevers, and encephalitides. [*ar,* arthropod, + *bo,* borne, + virus]

arc (ark). **1.** A curved line or segment of a circle. **2.** Continuous luminous passage of an electric current in a gas or vacuum between two or more separated carbon or other electrodes. [L. *arcus,* a bow]

reflex a., the route followed by nerve impulses in the production of a reflex act, from the peripheral receptor organ through the afferent nerve to the central nervous system synapse and then through the efferent nerve to the effector organ.

Ar·can·o·bac·te·ri·um (ar-kā'nō-bac-tēr'ē-ŭm). A genus of nonmotile, facultatively anaerobic bacteria containing Gram-positive slender irregular rods, sometimes showing clubbed ends. These organisms are obligate parasites of the pharynx in farm animals and humans, occasionally causing lesions on the pharynx or skin. The type species is *A. haemolyticum.*

arch. Any structure resembling a bent bow or an arch; an arc. In anatomy, any vaulted or archlike structure. SEE arcus. SYN arcus [NA]. [thru O. Fr. fr. L. *arcus,* bow]

abdominothoracic a., a bell-shaped line defined by the lower end of the sternum and the costal a.'s on each side, constituting a boundary line between the anterolateral portions of the thoracic and abdominal walls.

aortic a., **(1)** the curved portion between the ascending and descending parts of the aorta; it begins as a continuation of the ascending aorta posterior to the sternal angle, runs posteriorly and slightly to the left as it passes over the root of the left lung, and becomes the descending aorta as it reaches and begins to course along the vertebral column; it gives rise to the brachiocephalic trunk, the left common carotid and left subclavian arteries; **(2)** any member of the several pairs of arterial channels encircling the embryonic pharynx in the mesenchyme of the brachial a.'s; there are potentially six pairs, but in mammals the fifth

pair is poorly developed or absent. The first and second pairs are functional only in very young embryos; the third pair is involved in the formation of the carotids; the fourth a. on the left is incorporated in the a. of the aorta; the sixth pair forms the proximal part of the pulmonary arteries.

Corti's a., the a. formed by the junction of the heads of Corti's inner and outer pillar cells.

costal a., that portion of the inferior aperture of the thorax formed by the articulated cartilages of the seventh to tenth (false) ribs.

dental a., the curved composite structure of the natural dentition and the residual ridge, or the remains thereof after the loss of some or all of the natural teeth.

a. of foot, SYN *arcus* pedis.

hyoid a., the second visceral, or branchial, a; the second postoral a. in the branchial a. series.

inferior dental a., the teeth supported by the alveolar part of the mandible, whether the 10 deciduous teeth or the 16 permanent teeth.

mandibular a., the first postoral a. in the branchial a. series. SYN mandibular process.

neural a., SYN vertebral a.

palatoglossal a., one of a pair of ridges or folds of mucous membrane passing from the soft palate to the side of the tongue; it encloses the palatoglossus muscle and forms the anterior margin of the tonsillar fossa. Also demarcates the oral cavity from the isthmus of fauces.

palatopharyngeal a., one of a pair of ridges or folds of mucous membrane which pass downward from the posterior margin of the soft palate to the lateral wall of the pharynx. It encloses the palatopharyngeus muscle and forms the posterior margin of the tonsillar fossa. It also demarcates the isthmus of the fauces from the oropharynx.

palmar a., SYN *arcus* palmaris.

plantar a., **(1)** the arterial arch formed by the lateral plantar artery running across the bases of the metatarsal bones and anastomosing with the dorsalis pedis artery; **(2)** either of two bony a.'s of the foot, longitudinal a. or transverse a.

posterior a. of atlas, the posterior arch of the atlas that connects the lateral masses of the atlas posteriorly, forming the posterior wall of the vertebral canal at this level.

pubic a., the arch formed by the symphysis, bodies and inferior rami of the pubic bones. SEE ALSO subpubic *angle.*

superciliary a., a fullness extending laterally from the glabella on either side, above the orbital margin of the frontal bone.

superior dental a., the teeth supported by the alveolar process of the two maxillae, whether the 10 deciduous teeth or the 16 permanent teeth.

tendinous a., **(1)** a white, fibrous band attached to bone and/or muscle, arching over and thus protecting neurovascular elements passing beneath it from injurious compression; **(2)** a linear thickening of the deep fascia of a muscle which provides attachment for ligaments and/or muscle fibers.

tendinous a. of pelvic fascia, a linear thickening of the superior fascia of the pelvic diaphragm extending posteriorly from the body of the pubis alongside the bladder (and vagina in the female) and giving attachment to the supporting ligaments of the pelvic viscera.

a. of thoracic duct, SEE thoracic *duct.*

vertebral a., the posterior projection from the body of a vertebra that encloses the vertebral foramen; it consists of paired pedicles and laminae; the spinous, transverse, and articular processes arise from the arch. In aggregate, the venous a.'s—and the ligamenta flava that unite them—form the posterior wall of the vertebral (spinal) canal. SYN neural a.

zygomatic a., the arch formed by the temporal process of the zygomatic bone that joins the zygomatic process of the temporal bone. SYN zygoma (2).

arch-, arche-, archi-, archo-. Combining forms meaning primitive, or ancestral; also first, or chief. primitive, ancestral; first, chief, extreme. [G. *archē,* origin, beginning, + -o-]

arche-. SEE arch-.

ar•che•o•ki•net•ic (ar-kē-ō-ki-net′ik). Denoting a low and primitive type of motor nerve mechanism, such as is found in the peripheral and the ganglionic nervous systems. Cf. neokinetic, paleokinetic. [G. *archaios,* ancient, + *kinētikos,* relating to movement]

ar•che•type (ar′kē-tīp). **1.** A primitive structural plan from which various modifications have evolved. **2.** JUNGIAN PSYCHOLOGY structural manifestation of the collective unconscious. SYN imago (2). [G. *archetypos,* pattern, model, fr. *archē,* beginning, + *typtō,* to stamp out]

archi-. SEE arch-.

arch•wire (arch′wīr). A device consisting of a wire conforming to the alveolar or dental arch, used as an anchorage in correcting irregularities in the position of the teeth.

ar•ci•form (ar′si-fōrm). SYN arcuate.

arc•ta•tion (ark-tā′shŭn). A narrowing, contraction, stricture, or coarctation. [L. *arto* (improp. *arcto*), pp. *-atus,* to tighten]

ar•cu•ate (ar′kyū-āt). Denoting a form that is arched or has the shape of a bow. SYN arciform. [L. *arcuatus,* bowed]

ar•cu•a•tion (ar-kyū-ā′shŭn). A bending or curvature.

ar•cus (ar′kŭs) [NA]. SYN arch. [L. a bow]

arcus cornea′lis, an opaque, grayish ring at the periphery of the cornea just within the sclerocorneal junction, of frequent occurrence in the aged; it results from a deposit of fatty granules in, or hyaline degeneration of, the lamellae and cells of the cornea. SYN anterior embryotoxon, gerontoxon.

arcus palmaris, (1) arcus palmaris profundus (deep); the arterial arch located deep to the long flexor tendons in the hand, formed by the radial artery and the deep palmar branch of the ulnar artery; **(2)** arcus palmaris superficialis: the arterial arch in the hand located superficial to the long flexor tendons, formed principally by the ulnar artery and usually completed by a communication with the superficial palmar branch of the radial artery. SYN palmar arch.

arcus pedis, (1) longitudinalis: consisting of a medial longitudinal arch, including the calcaneus,

talus, navicular, three cuneiform bones, and the three medial metatarsals, and a lateral longitudinal arch formed by calcaneus, cuboid and two lateral metatarsals; **(2)** transversalis: formed by the proximal parts of the metatarsal bones, the three cuneiform bones, and the cuboid. SYN arch of foot.

ARDS adult respiratory distress *syndrome.*

ar•ea (a), pl. **ar•e•ae** (ār′ē-ă, -ē). **1** [NA]. Any circumscribed surface or space. **2.** All of the part supplied by a given artery or nerve. **3.** A part of an organ having a special function, as the motor a. of the brain. SEE ALSO regio, region, space, spatium, zone. [L. a courtyard]

association areas, SYN association *cortex.*

auditory a., SYN auditory *cortex.*

body surface a., the a. of the external surface of the body, expressed in square meters (m^2); used to estimate metabolic, electrolyte, and nutritional requirements and lung size and function.

Broca's a., SYN Broca's *center.*

a. of cardiac dullness, a triangular a. determined by percussion of the front of the chest; it corresponds to the part of the heart that is not covered by lung tissue.

embryonal a., embryonic a., the a. of the blastoderm on either side of, and immediately cephalic to, the primitive streak where the component cell layers have become thickened.

excitable a., SYN motor *cortex.*

frontal a., SYN frontal *cortex.*

germinal a., a. germinati′va, the place in the blastoderm where the embryo begins to be formed.

Kiesselbach's a., an a. on the anterior portion of the nasal septum rich in capillaries (Kiesselbach's plexus) and often the seat of epistaxis.

motor a., SYN motor *cortex.*

postcentral a., the cortex of the postcentral gyrus.

precentral a., the cortex of the precentral gyrus.

prefrontal a., SEE frontal *cortex.*

Rolando's a., SYN motor *cortex.*

sensorimotor a., the precentral and postcentral gyri of the cerebral cortex.

silent a., any a. of the cerebrum or cerebellum in which lesions cause no definite sensory or motor symptoms.

trigger a., SYN trigger *point.*

visual a., SYN visual *cortex.*

Wernicke's a., SYN Wernicke's *center.*

are•flex•ia (ā-rē-flek′sē-ă). Absence of reflexes.

Are•na•vi•ri•dae (ă-rē-nă-vir′i-dē). A family of RNA viruses, many of which are parasites of rodents, that includes lymphocytic choriomeningitis virus, Lassa virus, and the Tacaribe virus complex. [L. *arena (harena),* sand]

Are•na•vi•rus (ă-rē′nă-vī′rŭs). A genus in the family Arenaviridae that is associated with lymphocytic choriomeningitis and a number of hemorrhagic fevers.

are•o•la, pl. **are•o•lae** (ă-rē′ō-lă, -lē). **1** [NA]. Any small area. **2.** One of the spaces or interstices in areolar tissue. **3.** SYN a. of nipple. **4.** A pigmented, depigmented, or erythematous zone surrounding a papule, pustule, wheal, or cutaneous neoplasm. SYN halo (3). [L. dim. of *area*]

  a. mam′mae [NA], SYN a. of nipple.

  a. of nipple, a circular pigmented area surrounding the nipple or papilla mammae; its surface is dotted with little projections due to the presence of areolar glands beneath. SYN a. mammae [NA], a. papillaris, areola (3).

  a. papilla′ris, SYN a. of nipple.

  a. umbilici, a pigmented ring around the umbilicus in the pregnant woman.

are·o·lar (ă-rē′ō-lăr). Relating to an areola.

ARF acute respiratory *failure.*

ar·ga·sid (ar-gas′id). Common name for members of the family Argasidae.

Argas·i·dae (ar-gas′i-dē). Family of ticks, the soft ticks, so called because of their wrinkled appearance that fills out when the tick is engorged with blood. Argasid ticks, chiefly species of *Ornithodoros,* harbor and transmit spirochetes of the genus *Borrelia* that cause relapsing fever in birds and mammals.

ar·gen·taf·fin, ar·gen·taf·fine (ar-jen′tă-fin, -fēn). Pertaining to cells or tissue elements that reduce silver ions in solution, thereby becoming stained brown or black. [L. *argentum,* silver, + *affinitas,* affinity]

ar·gen·taf·fi·no·ma (ar′jen-tă-fi-nō′mă, -taf-i-nō′ mă). SYN carcinoid *tumor.*

ar·gen·to·phil, ar·gen·to·phile (ar-jen′tō-fil, -fīl). SYN argyrophil.

ar·gi·nase (ar′ji-nās). An enzyme of the liver that catalyzes the hydrolysis of L-arginine to L-ornithine and urea; a key enzyme of the urea cycle.

ar·gi·nine (ar′ji-nēn). 2-amino-5-guanidinopentanoic acid; one of the amino acids occurring among the hydrolysis products of proteins, particularly abundant in the basic proteins such as histones and protamines. A dibasic amino acid.

ar·gi·ni·no·suc·cin·ic ac·id (ar′ji-ni-nō-sŭk-sin′ ik). Formed as an intermediate in the conversion of L-citrulline to L-arginine in the urea cycle.

ar·gi·ni·no·suc·cin·ic·ac·i·du·ria (ar-ji-nin′ō-sŭk-sin′ik-as-i-dū′rē-ă) [MIM*207900]. An autosomal recessive disorder characterized by excessive urinary excretion of argininosuccinic acid, epilepsy, ataxia, mental retardation, liver disease, and friable, tufted hair; presumed to be the consequence of a deficiency of an enzyme responsible for splitting argininosuccinic acid to arginine and fumaric acid.

ar·gon (Ar) (ar′gon). A gaseous element, atomic no. 18, atomic wt. 39.948, present in the dry atmosphere in the proportion of about 0.94%; one of the noble gases. [G. ntr. of *argos,* lazy, inactive, fr. *a-* priv. + *ergon,* work]

ar·gyr·ia (ar-jir′ē-ă, -jī′rē-ă). A slate-gray or bluish discoloration of the skin and deep tissues, due to the deposit of silver, occurring after medicinal administration of a soluble silver salt. SYN argyrism. [G. *argyros,* silver]

ar·gyr·ic (ar-jir′ik). Relating to argyria.

ar·gy·rism (ar′ji-rizm). SYN argyria.

ar·gyr·o·phil, ar·gyr·o·phile (ar-jī′rō-fil, -fīl). Pertaining to tissue elements that are capable of impregnation with silver ions and being made visible after an external reducing agent is used.

SYN argentophil, argentophile. [G. *argyros,* silver, + *philos,* fond]

arhin·ia (ă-rin′ē-ă). Congenital absence of the nose. SYN arrhinia.

ari·bo·fla·vin·o·sis (ă-rī′bō-flā-vi-nō′sis). A commonly used term for hyporiboflavinosis.

A·ri·zo·na (ar′i-zō′nă). A genus of motile, peritrichous, nonsporeforming, aerobic to facultatively anaerobic bacteria (family Enterobacteriaceae) containing Gram-negative rods. These organisms have been isolated from a wide variety of animals, including humans; they may cause gastroenteritis in humans and frequently are involved in localized lesions in humans and lower animals. There is a single species, *A. hinshawii.*

arm. 1. The segment of the upper limb between the shoulder and the elbow; commonly used to mean the whole upper limb. SYN brachium (1) [NA], brachio- (1). **2.** An anatomical extension resembling an arm. **3.** A specifically shaped and positioned extension of a removable partial denture framework. [L. *armus,* forequarter of an animal; G. *harmos,* a shoulder joint]

ar·ma·men·tar·i·um (ar′mă-men-tār′ē-ŭm). All the therapeutic means available to the health practitioner for professional practice. [L. an arsenal, fr. *armamenta,* implements, tackle, fr. *arma,* armor, arms]

ar·o·mat·ic (ar-ō-mat′ik). **1.** Having an agreeable, somewhat pungent, spicy odor. **2.** One of a group of vegetable drugs having a fragrant odor and slightly stimulant properties. **3.** SEE cyclic *compound.* [G. *arōmatikos,* fr. *arōma,* spice, sweet herb]

ar·rec·tor, pl. **ar·rec·to·res** (ă-rek′tōr, ă-rek-tō′ rēz). SYN erector. [L. that which raises, fr. *arrigo,* pp. *-rectus,* to raise up]

ar·rest (ă-rest′). **1.** To stop, check, or restrain. **2.** A stoppage; interference with, or checking of, the regular course of a disease, a symptom, or the performance of a function. **3.** Inhibition of a developmental process, usually at the ultimate stage of development; premature a. may lead to a congenital abnormality. [O. Fr. *arester,* fr. LL. *adresto,* to stop behind]

  cardiac a. (CA), complete cessation of cardiac activity either electric, mechanical, or both; may be purposely induced for therapeutic reasons.

  cardioplegic a., stoppage of electrical and mechanical cardiac activity, used by surgeons when operating upon the heart.

  epiphysial a., early and premature fusion between epiphysis and diaphysis.

  maturation a., cessation of complete differentiation of cells at an immature stage; in spermatogenic maturation a., the seminiferous tubules contain spermatocytes, but no spermatozoa develop.

  sinus a., cessation of sinus activity; the ventricles may continue to beat under ectopic atrial, A-V junctional, or idioventricular control.

ar·rhe·no·blas·to·ma (ă-rē′nō-blas-tō′mă). A rare ovarian tumor that produces masculinization and often contains tubules and luteinized cells. SYN androblastoma (2), gynandroblastoma (1). [G. *arrhēn,* male, + *blastos,* germ, + *-ōma,* tumor]

ar·rhin·ia (ă-rin′ē-ă). SYN arhinia. [G. *a*- priv. + *rhis* (*rhin*-), nose]

ar·rhyth·mia (ă-rith′mē-ă). Loss of rhythm; denoting especially an irregularity of the heartbeat. See also entries under rhythm. Cf. dysrhythmia. [G. *a*- priv. + *rhythmos*, rhythm]

   cardiac a., SEE cardiac *dysrhythmia*.

   sinus a., a cyclic variation in heart rate, usually normal and linked to respiratory movements.

ar·rhyth·mic (ă-ridh′mik, ā-). Marked by loss of rhythm; pertaining to arrhythmia.

ar·rhyth·mo·gen·ic (ă-ridh-mō-jen′ik). Capable of inducing cardiac arrhythmias. [G. *a*- priv. + *rhythmos*, rhythm, + -*gen*, production]

ar·se·nic (As) (ar′sĕ-nik). A metallic element, atomic no. 33, atomic wt. 74.92159; forms a number of poisonous compounds, some of which are used in medicine. [L. *arsenicum*, G. *arsenikon*, fr. Pers. *zarnik*]

ar·se·nic (ar-sen′ik). Denoting the element arsenic or one of its compounds, especially arsenic acid.

ar·sen·i·cal (ar-sen′i-kăl). **1.** A drug or agent, the effect of which depends on its arsenic content. **2.** Denoting or containing arsenic.

ART acoustic reflex *threshold*.

ar·te·fact (ar′tĕ-fakt). SYN artifact.

◇arteri-. SEE arterio-.

ar·te·ria, gen. and pl. **ar·te·ri·ae** (ar-tēr′ē-ă, ar-tēr′ĭ-e) [NA]. SYN artery. SEE ALSO branch. [L. from G. *artēria*, the windpipe, later an artery as distinct from a vein]

   a. angula′ris [NA], SYN angular *artery*.

   a. appendicula′ris [NA], SYN appendicular *artery*.

   a. arcua′ta [NA], SYN arcuate *artery*.

   arte′riae arcua′tae renis [NA], SYN arcuate *arteries* of kidney, under *artery*.

   a. ascen′dens, [NA] SYN ascending *artery*.

   arteriae atria′les, SYN atrial *arteries*, under *artery*.

   a. axilla′ris [NA], SYN axillary *artery*.

   a. basila′ris [NA], SYN basilar *artery*.

   a. brachia′lis [NA], SYN brachial *artery*.

   a. bucca′lis [NA], SYN buccal *artery*.

   a. bul′bi pe′nis [NA], SYN *artery* of bulb of penis.

   a. bul′bi vestib′uli [NA], SYN *artery* of bulb of vestibule.

   a. cana′lis pterygoid′ei [NA], SYN *artery* of pterygoid canal.

   a. celi′aca, SYN celiac *trunk*.

   a. centra′lis ret′inae [NA], SYN central *artery* of retina.

   a. cremaster′ica [NA], SYN cremasteric *artery*.

   a. cys′tica [NA], SYN cystic *artery*.

   a. dorsa′lis clitor′idis [NA], SYN dorsal *artery* of clitoris.

   a. duc′tus deferen′tis [NA], SYN *artery* of ductus deferens.

   a. episclera′lis [NA], SYN episcleral *artery*.

   a. facia′lis [NA], SYN facial *artery*.

   a. femora′lis [NA], SYN femoral *artery*.

   a. gastroduodena′lis [NA], ⋆official alternate term for gastroduodenal *artery*.

   a. hyaloi′dea [NA], SYN hyaloid *artery*.

   arte′riae ilea′les [NA], SYN ileal *arteries*, under *artery*.

   a. ileocol′ica [NA], SYN ileocolic *artery*.

   a. iliolumba′lis [NA], SYN iliolumbar *artery*.

   a. infraorbita′lis [NA], SYN infraorbital *artery*.

   arteriae interlobula′res [NA], SYN interlobular *arteries*, under *artery*.

   arteriae jejuna′les [NA], SYN jejunal *arteries*, under *artery*.

   a. lacrima′lis [NA], SYN lacrimal *artery*.

   a. liena′lis, ⋆official alternate term for splenic *artery*.

   a. ligamen′ti tere′tis u′teri [NA], SYN *artery* of round ligament of uterus.

   a. lingua′lis [NA], SYN lingual *artery*.

   a. luso′ria, an aberrant right subclavian artery arising from the descending aorta; it passes posterior to the esophagus, often producing dysphagia.

   a. masseter′ica [NA], SYN masseteric *artery*.

   a. maxilla′ris [NA], SYN maxillary *artery*.

   a. media′na, SYN median *artery*.

   a. menta′lis [NA], SYN mental *artery*.

   a. musculophren′ica [NA], SYN musculophrenic *artery*.

   a. nutri′cia [NA], SYN nutrient *artery*.

   a. obturato′ria [NA], SYN obturator *artery*.

   a. obturato′ria accesso′ria [NA], SYN accessory obturator *artery*.

   a. occipita′lis [NA], SYN occipital *artery*.

   a. ophthal′mica [NA], SYN ophthalmic *artery*.

   a. ova′rica [NA], SYN ovarian *artery*.

   arte′riae palpebra′les [NA], SYN palpebral *arteries*, under *artery*.

   arte′riae perforan′tes [NA], SYN perforating *arteries*, under *artery*.

   a. pericardiacophren′ica [NA], SYN pericardiacophrenic *artery*.

   a. perinea′lis [NA], SYN perineal *artery*.

   a. perone′a [NA], SYN peroneal *artery*.

   a. pharyn′gea ascen′dens [NA], SYN ascending pharyngeal *artery*.

   a. poplit′ea [NA], SYN popliteal *artery*.

   a. profun′da clitor′idis [NA], SYN deep *artery* of clitoris.

   a. profun′da pe′nis [NA], SYN deep *artery* of penis.

   a. pulmona′lis, SYN pulmonary *trunk*.

   a. radia′lis [NA], SYN radial *artery*.

   a. rena′lis [NA], SYN renal *artery*.

   arte′riae sigmoi′deae [NA], SYN sigmoid *arteries*, under *artery*.

   a. sphe′nopalati′na [NA], SYN sphenopalatine *artery*.

   a. stylomastoi′dea [NA], SYN stylomastoid *artery*.

   a. subcla′via [NA], SYN subclavian *artery*.

   a. subcosta′lis [NA], SYN subcostal *artery*.

   a. sublingua′lis [NA], SYN sublingual *artery*.

   a. submenta′lis [NA], SYN submental *artery*.

   a. subscapula′ris [NA], SYN subscapular *artery*.

   a. supraorbita′lis [NA], SYN supraorbital *artery*.

   a. suprascapula′ris [NA], SYN suprascapular *artery*.

a. supratrochlea′ris [NA], SYN supratrochlear *artery*.

a. sura′lis [NA], SYN sural *artery*.

a. testicula′ris [NA], SYN testicular *artery*.

a. thoracoacromia′lis [NA], SYN thoracoacromial *artery*.

a. thoracodorsa′lis [NA], SYN thoracodorsal *artery*.

a. transver′sa col′li [NA], ⭑official alternate term for transverse cervical *artery*.

a. transver′sa facie′i [NA], SYN transverse facial *artery*.

a. ulna′ris [NA], SYN ulnar *artery*.

a. umbilica′lis [NA], SYN umbilical *artery*.

a. urethra′lis [NA], SYN urethral *artery*.

a. uteri′na [NA], SYN uterine *artery*.

a. vagina′lis [NA], SYN vaginal *artery*.

arte′riae ventricula′res [NA], SYN ventricular *arteries*, under *artery*.

a. vertebra′lis [NA], SYN vertebral *artery*.

a. zygomat′ico-orbita′lis [NA], SYN zygomatico-orbital *artery*.

ar•te•ri•al (ar-tē′rē-ăl). Relating to one or more arteries or to the entire system of arteries.

ar•te•ri•ec•to•my (ar-tēr-ē-ek′tō-mē). Excision of part of an artery. [L. *arteria*, artery, + G. *ektomē*, excision]

△**arterio-, arteri-.** Artery. [L. *arteria*, fr. G. *artēria*, a windpipe, an artery]

ar•te•ri•o•cap•il•lary (ar-tēr′ē-ō-cap′i-lār-ē). Relating to both arteries and capillaries.

ar•te•ri•o•gram (ar-tēr′ē-ō-gram). Radiographic demonstration of an artery after injection of contrast medium. [arterio- + G. *gramma*, something written]

ar•te•ri•o•graph•ic (ar-tēr′ē-ō-graf′ik). Relating to or utilizing arteriography.

🔳**ar•te•ri•og•ra•phy** (ar-tēr-ē-og′ră-fē). Visualization of an artery or arteries by x-ray imaging after injection of a radiopaque contrast medium. [arterio- + G. *graphō*, to write]

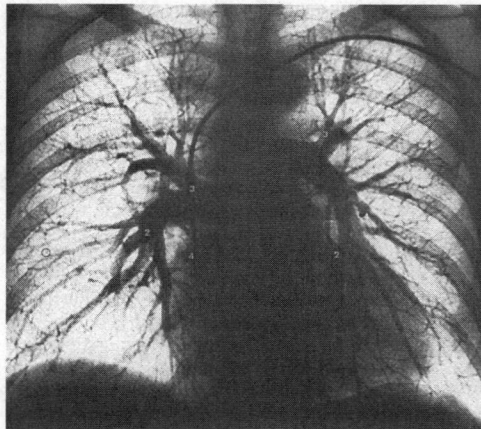

arteriography: normal finding for the pulmonary arteries

bronchial a., radiography of bronchial arteries by selective injection of the intercostal arteries from which they arise.

ar•te•ri•o•la, pl. **ar•te•ri•o•lae** (ar-tēr-ē-ō′lă, -ō′lē) [NA]. SYN arteriole. [Mod. L. dim. of *arteria*, artery]

a. macula′ris infe′rior [NA], SYN inferior macular *arteriole*.

a. macula′ris supe′rior [NA], SYN superior macular *arteriole*.

ar•te•ri•o•lar (ar-ter-ē-ō′lăr). Of or pertaining to an arteriole or the arterioles collectively.

🔳**ar•te•ri•ole** (ar-tēr′ē-ōl). A minute artery with a tunica media comprising only one or two layers of smooth muscle cells; a terminal artery continuous with the capillary network. SYN arteriola [NA].

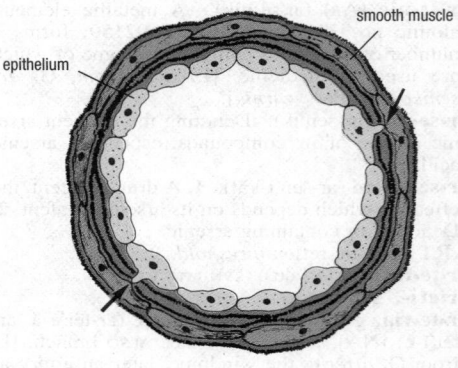

arteriole: arrows show points of contact between epithelium and smooth muscle

afferent glomerular a., a branch of an interlobular artery of the kidney that conveys blood to the glomerulus. SYN vas afferens [NA].

capillary a., a minute artery that terminates in a capillary.

efferent glomerular a., the vessel that carries blood from the glomerular capillary network to the capillary bed of the proximal convoluted tubule. SYN vas efferens (2) [NA], efferent vessel.

inferior macular a., *origin*, central artery of retina; *distribution*, inferior part of macula. SYN arteriola macularis inferior [NA].

superior macular a., *origin*, central artery of retina; *distribution*, upper part of macula. SYN arteriola macularis superior [NA].

ar•te•ri•o•lith (ar-tēr′ē-ō-lith). A calcareous deposit in an arterial wall or thrombus. [L. *arteria*, artery, + G. *lithos*, a stone]

ar•ter•i•o•li•tis (ar-tēr′ē-ō-lī′tis). Inflammation of the wall of the arterioles. [L. *arteriola*, arteriole, + G. *-itis*, inflammation]

necrotizing a., necrosis in the media of arterioles, characteristic of malignant hypertension. SYN arteriolonecrosis.

△**arteriolo-.** The arterioles. [Modern L. *arteriola*, arteriole]

ar•te•ri•o•lo•ne•cro•sis (ar-tēr-ē-ō′lō-nĕ-krō′sis). SYN necrotizing *arteriolitis*. [L. *arteriola*, arteriole, + G. *nekrōsis*, a killing]

ar•te•ri•o•lo•neph•ro•scle•ro•sis (ar-tēr-ē-ō′lō-nef′rō-skler-ō-sis). SYN arteriolar *nephrosclerosis*.

ar·te·ri·o·lo·scle·ro·sis (ar-tēr-ē-ō′lō-skler-ō′sis). Arteriosclerosis affecting mainly the arterioles, seen especially in chronic hypertension.

ar·te·ri·o·mo·tor (ar-tēr′ē-ō-mō′ter). Causing changes in the caliber of an artery; vasomotor with special reference to the arteries.

ar·te·ri·o·neph·ro·scle·ro·sis (ar-tēr′ē-ō-nef′rō-skler-ō′sis). SYN arterial *nephrosclerosis.*

ar·te·ri·op·a·thy (ar-tēr-ē-op′ă-thē). Any disease of the arteries. [arterio- + G. *pathos,* suffering]

  hypertensive a., arterial degeneration resulting from hypertension.

ar·te·ri·o·plas·ty (ar-tēr′ē-ō-plas-tē). Any operation for the reconstruction of the wall of an artery. [arterio- + G. *plastos,* formed]

ar·te·ri·o·pres·sor (ar-tēr′ē-ō-pres′ser). Causing increased arterial blood pressure.

ar·te·ri·or·rha·phy (ar-tēr-ē-ōr′ă-fē). Suture of an artery. [arterio- + G. *rhaphē,* seam]

ar·te·ri·or·rhex·is (ar-tēr′ē-ō-rek′sis). Rupture of an artery. [arterio- + G. *rhēxis,* rupture]

ar·te·ri·o·scle·ro·sis (ar-tēr′ē-ō-skler-ō′sis). Hardening of the arteries; types generally recognized are: atherosclerosis, Mönckeberg's a., and arteriolosclerosis. SYN arterial sclerosis. [arterio- + G. *sklērōsis,* hardness]

  hypertensive a., progressive increase in muscle and elastic tissue of arterial walls, resulting from hypertension; in longstanding hypertension, elastic tissue forms numerous concentric layers in the intima and there is replacement of muscle by collagen fibers and hyaline thickening of the intima of arterioles; such changes can develop with increasing age in the absence of hypertension and may then be referred to as senile a.

  a. oblit′erans, a. producing narrowing and occlusion of the arterial lumen.

  senile a., a. similar to hypertensive a., but as a result of advanced age rather than hypertension.

ar·te·ri·o·scle·rot·ic (ar-tēr′ē-ō-skler-ot′ik). Relating to or affected by arteriosclerosis.

ar·te·ri·o·spasm (ar-tēr′ē-ō-spazm). Spasm of an artery or arteries.

ar·te·ri·o·ste·no·sis (ar-tēr′ē-ō-stĕ-nō′sis). Narrowing of the caliber of an artery, either temporary, through vasoconstriction, or permanent, through arteriosclerosis. [arterio- + G. *stenosis,* a narrowing]

ar·te·ri·ot·o·my (ar-tēr-ē-ot′ō-mē). Any surgical incision into the lumen of an artery, *e.g.,* to remove an embolus. [arterio- + G. *tomē,* incision]

ar·te·ri·o·ve·nous (A-V) (ar-tēr′ē-ō-vē′nŭs). Relating to both an artery and a vein or to both arteries and veins in general; both arterial and venous, as an "arteriovenous (A-V) anastomosis."

ar·te·ri·tis (ar-ter-ī′tis). Inflammation involving an artery or arteries. [L. *arteria,* artery, + G. *-itis,* inflammation]

  brachiocephalic a., giant-cell a. seen in older adults; characterized by inflammatory lesions in medium sized arteries, most commonly in the head, neck and/or shoulder girdle area. Erythrocyte sedimentation rate is elevated. Visual loss can occur.

  cranial a., SYN temporal a.

  giant cell a., SYN temporal a.

  a. oblit′erans, obliterating a., SYN *endarteritis* obliterans.

  rheumatic a., a. due to rheumatic fever; Aschoff bodies are frequently found in the adventitia of small arteries, especially in the myocardium, and may lead to fibrosis and constriction of the lumens.

  Takayasu's a., a progressive obliterative arteritis of unknown origin involving fibrosis and luminal narrowing that affects the aorta and its branches; more common in females. SYN pulseless disease, Takayasu's disease, Takayasu's syndrome.

  temporal a., a subacute, granulomatous a. involving the external carotid arteries, especially the temporal artery; occurs in elderly persons and may be manifested by constitutional symptoms, particularly severe headache, and sometimes sudden unilateral blindness. Shares many of the symptoms of polymyalgia rheumatica. SYN cranial a., giant cell a.

ar·tery (ar′ter-ē). A relatively thick-walled, muscular, pulsating blood vessel conveying blood in a direction away from the heart. With the exception of the pulmonary and umbilical arteries, the arteries convey red or aerated blood. At the major arteries, the arterial branches are listed separately following the designation *branches.* SYN arteria [NA]. [L. *arteria,* fr. G. *artēria*]

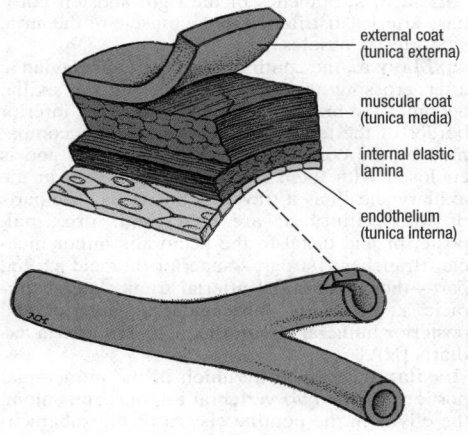

external coat (tunica externa)

muscular coat (tunica media)

internal elastic lamina

endothelium (tunica interna)

artery: showing layers of wall

  accessory obturator a., term applied to the anastomosis of the pubic branch of the inferior epigastric a. with the pubic branch of the obturator a. when it contributes a significant supply through the obturator canal. SYN arteria obturatoria accessoria [NA].

  acromiothoracic a., SYN thoracoacromial a.

  angular a., the terminal branch of the facial artery; *distribution,* muscles and skin of side of nose; *anastomoses,* lateral nasal, and dorsal artery of nose and palpebrals from the ophthalmic a., thereby providing an external-internal carotid arterial anastomosis; SYN arteria angularis [NA].

  a. of angular gyrus, the last branch of the

terminal part of the middle cerebral artery distributed to parts of the temporal parietal and occipital lobes.

anterior ciliary a., one of several arteries derived from muscular branches of the ophthalmic which perforate the anterior part of the sclera and anastomose with posterior ciliary arteries.

appendicular a., the branch of the ileocolic artery that descends posterior to the terminal ileum in the mesoappendix to supply the vermiform appendix. SYN arteria appendicularis [NA].

arcuate a., *origin,* dorsalis pedis; *branches,* passes laterally dorsal to the bases of the metatarsals, giving rise to the 2nd, 3rd, and 4th dorsal metatarsal a.'s at the level of the medial cuneiform bone. SYN arteria arcuata [NA].

arcuate a.'s of kidney, curved a.'s at the corticomedullary border, arising from interlobar a.'s and giving rise to interlobular a.'s. SYN arteriae arcuatae renis [NA].

ascending a., the branch of the inferior branch of the ileocolic artery that passes superiorly up the ascending colon to communicate with a branch of the right colic artery and supplying the ascending colon. SYN arteria ascendens.

ascending pharyngeal a., *origin,* external carotid; *distribution,* wall of pharynx and soft palate, posterior cranial fossa. SYN arteria pharyngea ascendens [NA].

atrial a.'s, branches of the right and left coronary arteries distributed to the muscle of the atria. SYN arteriae atriales.

axillary a., the continuation of the subclavian a. after crossing the first rib to enter the axilla; becomes the brachial a. upon passing the inferior border of the teres major muscle. It is accompanied by the cords of the brachial plexus, and is enclosed with them and the axillary vein in the axillary sheath as it traverses the axilla. The parts of the axillary a. are described: proximal, posterior and distal to the pectoralis minor muscle. Branches: 1st part—superior thoracic a.; 2nd part—thoracoacromial arterial trunk, lateral thoracic a.; 3rd part—subscapular a., anterior and posterior humeral circumflex a.'s. SYN arteria axillaris [NA].

basilar a., formed by union of the intracranial portions of the two vertebral arteries; runs along the clivus in the pontine cistern of the subarachnoid space from the lower to the upper border of the pons, where it bifurcates into the two posterior cerebral arteries; *branches,* anterior, inferior, cerebellar, labyrinthine, pontine, mesencephalic, and superior cerebellar. SYN arteria basilaris [NA].

brachial a., *origin,* is a continuation of the axillary beginning at the inferior border of the teres major muscle; *branches,* deep brachial, superior ulnar collateral, inferior ulnar collateral, muscular, and nutrient; terminates in the cubital fossa by bifurcating into radial and ulnar a.'s. SYN arteria brachialis [NA].

buccal a., buccinator a., *origin,* maxillary; *distribution,* buccinator muscle, skin, and mucous membrane of cheek; *anastomoses,* buccal branch of facial. SYN arteria buccalis [NA].

a. of bulb of penis, a branch of the internal

pudendal artery which supplies the bulb of the penis including the bulbar urethra. SYN arteria bulbi penis [NA].

a. of bulb of vestibule, the branch of the internal pudendal artery in the female that supplies the bulb of the vestibule. SYN arteria bulbi vestibuli [NA].

celiac a., SYN celiac *trunk.*

central a. of retina, a branch of the ophthalmic artery which penetrates the optic nerve 1 cm behind the eye to enter the eye at the optic papilla in the retina; it divides into superior and inferior temporal and nasal branches. SYN arteria centralis retinae [NA].

circumflex scapular a., *origin,* subscapular; *distribution,* muscles of shoulder and scapular region; *anastomoses,* branches of suprascapular and transverse cervical.

collateral a., **(1)** one that runs parallel with a nerve or other structure; **(2)** one through which a collateral circulation is established.

communicating a., an a. that connects two larger a.'s.

cortical a.'s, branches of the anterior, middle, and posterior cerebral a.'s that supply the cerebral cortex.

▣**coronary a.,** **(1)** right coronary artery: *origin,* right aortic sinus; *distribution,* it passes around the right side of the heart in the coronary sulcus, giving branches to the right atrium and ventricle, including the atrioventricular branches and the posterior interventricular branch. **(2)** left coronary artery: *origin,* left aortic sinus; *distribution,* divides into two major branches, anterior interventricular which descends in anterior interventricular sulcus, and circumflex branch which passes to the diaphragmatic surface of left ventricle; it gives atrial, ventricular, and atrioventricular branches.

costocervical a., SYN costocervical *trunk.*

cremasteric a., *origin,* inferior epigastric; *distribution,* coverings of spermatic cord; *anastomoses,* external pudendal, spermatic, and perineal a. SYN arteria cremasterica [NA].

cystic a., *origin,* right branch of hepatic; *distribution,* gall bladder and visceral surface of the liver. SYN arteria cystica [NA].

deep a. of clitoris, the deep terminal branch of the internal pudendal artery in the female; it supplies the crus of the clitoris. SYN arteria profunda clitoridis [NA].

deep a. of penis, *origin,* terminal branch (with dorsal a. of penis) of the internal pudendal artery; *distribution,* corpus cavernosum of the penis via capillary beds and via helicine arteries and arteriovenous anastomoses to produce erection. SYN arteria profunda penis [NA].

deep lingual a., termination of lingual artery, *distribution,* muscles and mucous membrane of under surface of tongue.

descending genicular a., *origin,* femoral, in adductor canal; *distribution,* penetrates vasoadductor fascia to supply knee joint and adjacent parts; *anastomoses,* medial superior genicular, medial inferior genicular, lateral superior genicular, lateral inferior genicular and anterior tibial recurrent a.'s, *i.e.,* articular network of knee.

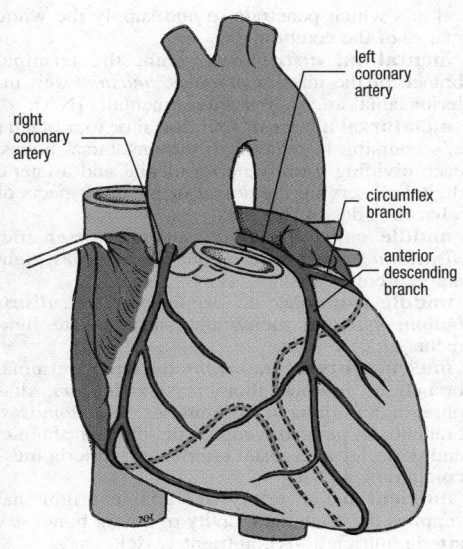

right coronary artery

left coronary artery

circumflex branch

anterior descending branch

coronary arteries

dolichoectatic a., a distorted, dilated, and elongated artery commonly compressing a neural structure.

dorsal a. of clitoris, one of the two terminal branches of the internal pudendal artery in the female, the other being the deep a. of the clitoris. SYN arteria dorsalis clitoridis [NA].

dorsal a. of penis, the dorsal terminal branch of the internal pudendal artery in the male.

dorsal digital a., one of the collateral digital branches of the dorsal metatarsal arteries in the foot, and/or of the dorsal metacarpal arteries in the hand.

dorsal nasal a., origin, ophthalmic; external artery of the nose; distribution, skin of side of root of nose; anastomoses, angular a.

dorsal scapular a., origin, subclavian or as the deep branch of the transverse cervical; distribution, passes deep to the rhomboid muscles, supplying them and other muscles and skin along the vertebral border of the scapula; anastomoses, suprascapular and scapular circumflex.

dorsalis pedis a., continuation of anterior tibial artery after crossing ankle; branches, lateral tarsal, arcuate, dorsal metatarsal; anastomoses, with the lateral plantar to form the plantar arch.

a. of ductus deferens, origin, anterior division of internal iliac, or sometimes superior vesical; distribution, ductus deferens, seminal vesicles, testicle, ureter; anastomoses, testicular, cremasteric a.'s. SYN arteria ductus deferentis [NA].

end a., an a. with insufficient anastomoses to maintain viability of the tissue supplied if occlusion of the a. occurs. SYN terminal a.

episcleral a., one of many small branches of the anterior ciliary a.'s that arise as they perforate the sclera near the corneoscleral junction, and course on the sclera. SYN arteria episcleralis [NA].

external pudendal a.'s, origin, femoral; distribution, skin over pubis, skin over penis and skin of scrotum or labium majus via anterior scrotal (labial) arteries; anastomoses, dorsal artery of penis or clitoris, posterior scrotal or labial arteries.

facial a., origin, external carotid; branches, ascending palatine, tonsillar and glandular branches, submental, inferior labial, superior labial, masseteric, buccal, lateral nasal branches, and angular. SYN arteria facialis [NA].

femoral a., origin, continuation of external iliac, beginning at inguinal ligament; branches, external pudendal, superficial epigastric, superficial circumflex iliac, profunda femoris, descending genicular, terminating as the popliteal a. as it passes through the adductor hiatus to enter the popliteal space. SYN arteria femoralis [NA].

fibular a., SYN peroneal a.

frontal a., SYN supratrochlear a.

gastric a.'s, a.'s supplying the stomach along the lesser curvature.

gastroduodenal a., origin, hepatic; terminal branches, right gastroepiploic, superior pancreaticoduodenal. SYN arteria gastroduodenalis✶ [NA].

gastroepiploic a.'s, a.'s which supply the stomach and greater omentum as they course along the greater curvature of the stomach. SYN gastro-omental a.'s.

gastro-omental a.'s, SYN gastroepiploic a.'s.

genicular a.'s, a.'s contributing to the articular network of the knee.

hyaloid a., the terminal branch of the primitive ophthalmic artery, which forms in the embryo an extensive ramification in the primary vitreous and a vascular tunic around the lens; by $8\frac{1}{2}$ months, these vessels have atrophied almost completely, but a few persistent remnants are evident entoptically as muscae volitantes. SYN arteria hyaloidea [NA].

ileal a.'s, origin, superior mesenteric; distribution, ileum; anastomoses, other branches of superior mesenteric. SYN arteriae ileales [NA].

ileocolic a., origin, superior mesenteric, often by a common trunk with the right colic; distribution, terminal part of ileum, cecum, vermiform appendix, and ascending colon; anastomoses, right colic and ileal. SYN arteria ileocolica [NA].

iliolumbar a., origin, internal iliac; distribution, pelvic muscles and bones; anastomoses, deep circumflex iliac, lumbar. SYN arteria iliolumbalis [NA].

inferior alveolar a., origin, 1st part of maxillary artery; distribution, through mandibular foramen/canal to lower teeth and chin; branches, a. to mylohyoid, mental a., dental a.'s.

infraorbital a., origin, third part of maxillary; distribution, upper canine and incisor teeth, inferior rectus and inferior oblique muscles, lower eyelid, lacrimal sac, maxillary sinus, and upper lip; anastomoses, branches of ophthalmic, facial, superior labial, transverse facial, and buccal. SYN arteria infraorbitalis [NA].

innominate a., obsolete term for brachiocephalic trunk.

interlobular a.'s, a.'s that pass between lobules of an organ. SYN arteriae interlobulares [NA].

ar

internal iliac a., *origin*, common iliac; *branches*, iliolumbar, lateral sacral, obturator, superior gluteal, inferior gluteal, umbilical, superior vesical, inferior vesical, middle rectal, and internal pudendal.

internal pudendal a., *origin*, internal iliac; *branches*, inferior rectal, perineal, posterior scrotal (or labial), urethral, artery of bulb of penis (or of vestibule), deep artery of penis (or clitoris), dorsal artery of penis (or clitoris).

intestinal a.'s, SEE ileal a.'s, jejunal a.'s.

jejunal a.'s, *origin*, superior mesenteric; *distribution*, jejunum; *anastomoses*, by a series of arches with each other and with ileal arteries. SYN arteriae jejunales [NA].

labyrinthine a., internal acoustic meatal branch, a branch of the basilar artery that enters the labyrinth through the internal acoustic meatus.

lacrimal a., *origin*, ophthalmic; *distribution*, lacrimal gland, lateral and superior rectus muscles, superior eyelid, forehead, and temporal fossa. SYN arteria lacrimalis [NA].

lateral occipital a., one of the terminal branches of the posterior cerebral artery; it supplies, by several named branches, the lateral portions of the temporal lobe.

left gastric a., *origin*, celiac; *distribution*, cardia of stomach at lesser curvature, abdominal part of the esophagus, and, frequently, a portion of the left lobe of the liver via an aberrant left hepatic branch; *anastomoses*, esophageal, right gastric.

lienal a., SYN splenic a.

lingual a., *origin*, external carotid; *distribution*, runs along under surface of tongue, terminates as deep lingual a.; *branches*, suprahyoid and dorsal lingual branches and sublingual artery. SYN arteria lingualis [NA].

lumbar a., *origin*, abdominal aorta; one of four or five pairs; *distribution*, lumbar vertebrae, muscles of back, abdominal wall; *anastomoses*, intercostal, subcostal, superior and inferior epigastric, deep circumflex iliac, and iliolumbar.

macular a.'s, SEE inferior macular *arteriole*, superior macular *arteriole*.

masseteric a., *origin*, maxillary; *distribution*, deep surface of masseter muscle; *anastomoses*, branches of transverse facial and masseteric branches of facial. SYN arteria masseterica [NA].

maxillary a., *origin*, external carotid; *branches*, deep auricular, anterior tympanic, middle meningeal, inferior alveolar, masseteric, deep temporal, buccal, posterior superior alveolar, infraorbital, descending palatine, artery of pterygoid canal, sphenopalatine. SYN arteria maxillaris [NA].

medial occipital a., one of the terminal branches of the posterior cerebral artery; it is distributed, by several named branches, to the posterior corpus callosum and the medial and superolateral portions of the occipital lobe including the visual cortex.

median a., *origin*, anterior interosseous; *distribution*, accompanies median nerve to palm; *anastomoses*, branches of superficial palmar arch. SYN arteria mediana.

medullary a.'s of brain, branches of the cortical a.'s which penetrate to and supply the white matter of the cerebrum.

mental a., *distribution*, chin; the terminal branch of the inferior alveolar; *anastomoses*, inferior labial artery. SYN arteria mentalis [NA].

metatarsal a., one of four dorsal or four plantar a.'s coursing in relation to the metatarsal bones, each dividing distally into a medial and a lateral digital a., serving the dorsal or plantar aspects of adjacent sides of two toes.

middle colic a., *origin*, superior mesenteric; *distribution*, transverse colon; *anastomoses*, right and left colic.

middle genicular a., *origin*, popliteal; *distribution*, synovial membrane and cruciate ligaments of knee joint.

musculophrenic a., *origin*, the lateral terminal branch of internal thoracic; *distribution*, diaphragm and intercostal muscles; *anastomoses*, branches of pericardiacophrenic, inferior phrenic, and posterior intercostal arteries. SYN arteria musculophrenica [NA].

nutrient a., an artery of variable origin that supplies the medullary cavity of a long bone. SYN arteria nutricia [NA], nutrient vessel.

nutrient a. of femur, one of two a.'s, superior and inferior, arising from the first and third perforating a.'s respectively (sometimes second and fourth).

nutrient a. of fibula, *origin*, peroneal (fibular); *distribution*, fibula.

nutrient a.'s of humerus, *origin*, deep brachial; *distribution*, the medullary cavity of the humerus.

obturator a., *anastomoses*, iliolumbar, inferior epigastric, medial circumflex femoral; *origin*, anterior division of the internal iliac; *distribution*, ilium, pubis, obturator and adductor muscles; *branches*, pubic, acetabular, anterior, and posterior. SYN arteria obturatoria [NA].

occipital a., *origin*, external carotid; *branches*, sternocleidomastoid, meningeal, auricular, occipital, mastoid, and descending. SYN arteria occipitalis [NA].

ophthalmic a., *origin*, internal carotid; *branches*, ciliary, central artery of retina, anterior meningeal, lacrimal, conjunctival, episcleral, supraorbital, ethmoidal, palpebral, dorsal nasal, and supratrochlear. SYN arteria ophthalmica [NA].

ovarian a., *origin*, aorta; *distribution*, ureter, ovary, ovarian ligament and uterine tube; *anastomoses*, uterine. SYN arteria ovarica [NA].

palpebral a.'s, branches of the ophthalmic supplying the upper and lower eyelids, consisting of two sets, lateral and medial. SYN arteriae palpebrales [NA].

a. of the pancreatic tail, *origin*, splenic artery near the left gastroepiploic; *distribution*, the tail of the pancreas; *anastomoses*, with other pancreatic arteries.

a.'s of penis, SEE dorsal a. of penis, deep a. of penis.

perforating a.'s, *origin*, a. profunda femoris; *distribution*, as three or four vessels that pass through the aponeurosis of the adductor magnus to the posterior and anterior compartments of the thigh. SYN arteriae perforantes [NA].

pericardiacophrenic a., *origin,* internal thoracic; *distribution,* pericardium, diaphragm, and pleura; *anastomoses,* musculophrenic, inferior phrenic, mediastinal and pericardial branches of the internal thoracic. SYN arteria pericardiacophrenica [NA].

perineal a., *origin,* internal pudendal; *distribution,* superficial structures of the perineum; *anastomoses,* external pudendal arteries. SYN arteria perinealis [NA].

peroneal a., *origin,* posterior tibial; *distribution,* soleus, tibialis posterior, flexor longus hallucis, peroneal muscles, inferior tibiofibular articulation, and ankle joint; *anastomoses,* anterior lateral malleolar, lateral tarsal, lateral plantar, dorsalis pedis. SYN arteria peronea [NA], fibular a.

popliteal a., continuation of femoral a. in the popliteal space, bifurcating (at the lower border of the popliteus muscle as it passes deep to the arcus tendineus of the soleus muscle) into the anterior and posterior tibial a.'s; *branches,* lateral and medial superior genicular, middle genicular, lateral and medial inferior genicular, and sural arteries. SYN arteria poplitea [NA].

posterior septal a. of nose, a branch of the sphenopalatine artery that supplies the nasal septum and accompanies the nasopalatine nerve.

princeps pol′licis a., *origin,* radial (deep palmar (arterial) arch); *distribution,* palmar surface and sides of thumb; *anastomoses,* a.'s on dorsum of thumb.

profunda brachii a., *origin,* brachial; *distribution,* humerus and muscles and integument of arm; *anastomoses,* posterior circumflex humeral, radial recurrent, recurrent interosseous, ulnar collateral, *i.e.,* articular vascular *network* of elbow.

profunda fem′oris a., *origin,* femoral; *branches,* lateral circumflex femoral, medial circumflex femoral, terminating in three or four perforating a.'s.

a. of pterygoid canal, *origin:* usually arises from the third part of the maxillary artery, but frequently from the greater palatine artery, within the pterygopalatine fossa. Passes posteriorly to run through the pterygoid canal with the corresponding nerve, supplying the contents and wall of the canal, the mucous membrane of the upper pharynx, the auditory tube and the tympanic cavity. SYN arteria canalis pterygoidei [NA].

pulmonary a., SYN pulmonary *trunk.*

radial a., *origin,* brachial; *branches,* radial recurrent, dorsal metacarpal, dorsal digital, princeps pollicis, radial index, palmar metacarpal, and muscular, carpal, and perforating. SYN arteria radialis [NA].

radial collateral a., the anterior terminal branch of the profunda brachii, anastomosing with the radial recurrent, forming part of the articular network of the elbow.

radial recurrent a., *origin,* radial; *distribution,* ascends around lateral side of elbow joint; *anastomoses,* radial collateral, interosseous recurrent.

radialis indicis a., *origin,* radial; *distribution,* radial side of index finger.

recurrent ulnar a., *origin,* ulnar artery; *distribution,* two branches, anterior and posterior, pass medially in front of and behind the elbow joint;

anastomoses, superior and inferior ulnar collateral, *i.e.,* with articular vascular *network* of elbow.

renal a., *origin,* aorta; *branches,* segmental, ureteral, and inferior suprarenal; *distribution,* kidney. SYN arteria renalis [NA].

right gastric a., *origin,* hepatic; *distribution,* pyloric portion of stomach on the lesser curvature; *anastomoses,* left gastric.

a. of round ligament of uterus, *origin,* inferior epigastric; *distribution,* round ligament of uterus. SYN arteria ligamenti teretis uteri [NA].

a. to sciatic nerve, *origin,* inferior gluteal; *distribution,* sciatic nerve; *anastomoses,* branches of profunda femoris.

segmental a.'s of kidney, the branches of the renal artery that supply the anatomical segments of kidney. Usually five in number, they are end a.'s and give off interlobar, arcuate, and interlobular a.'s in sequence. The latter send afferent arterioles to the glomeruli as well as branches to the kidney capsule. The segmental a.'s of the kidney are identified as: (1) anterior inferior (arteriae segmenti anterioris inferioris renis [NA]); (2) anterior superior (arteriae segmenti anterioris superioris renis [NA]); (3) inferior (arteriae segmenti inferioris renis [NA]); (4) posterior (arteriae segmenti posterioris renis [NA]); and (5) superior (arteriae segmenti superioris renis [NA]).

short gastric a.'s, four or five small arteries given off from the splenic, passing via the gastrosplenic ligament to the fundus of the stomach along the greater curvature, and anastomosing with the other arteries in that region.

sigmoid a.'s, *origin,* inferior mesenteric; *distribution,* descending colon and sigmoid flexure; *anastomoses,* left colic, superior rectal. SYN arteriae sigmoideae [NA].

sphenopalatine a., *origin,* third part of maxillary; *distribution,* posterior portion of lateral nasal wall and septum; *anastomoses,* branches of descending palatine, superior labial, and infraorbital. SYN arteria sphenopalatina [NA].

splenic a., *origin,* celiac trunk; *branches,* pancreatic, left gastroepiploic, short gastric, and (proper) splenic. SYN arteria lienalis★, lienal a.

stylomastoid a., *origin,* posterior auricular; *distribution,* external acoustic meatus, mastoid cells, semicircular canals, stapedius muscle, and vestibule; *anastomoses,* tympanic branches of internal carotid and ascending pharyngeal, and labyrinthine a.'s. SYN arteria stylomastoidea [NA].

subclavian a., *origin,* right from brachiocephalic, left from arch of aorta; *branches,* vertebral, thyrocervical trunk, internal thoracic; costocervical trunk, descending scapular; it continues as the axillary a. after crossing the first rib. SYN arteria subclavia [NA].

subcostal a., *origin,* thoracic aorta; *distribution,* inferior to twelfth rib in a manner similar to posterior intercostal arteries. SYN arteria subcostalis [NA].

sublingual a., *origin,* lingual; *distribution,* extrinsic muscles of tongue, sublingual gland, mucosa of region; *anastomoses,* the artery of opposite side and submental. SYN arteria sublingualis [NA].

submental a., *origin*, facial; *distribution*, mylohyoid muscle, submandibular and sublingual glands, and structures of lower lip; *anastomoses*, inferior labial, mental branch of inferior dental and sublingual. SYN arteria submentalis [NA].

subscapular a., *origin*, axillary; *branches*, circumflex scapular, thoracodorsal; *distribution*, muscles of shoulder and scapular region; *anastomoses*, branches of transverse cervical, suprascapular, lateral thoracic, and intercostals. SYN arteria subscapularis [NA].

superficial brachial a., an occasional variation in which the brachial artery lies superficial to the median nerve in the arm.

superior cerebellar a., *origin*, basilar; *distribution*, upper surface of cerebellum, colliculi, and most of the cerebellar nuclei; *anastomoses*, posterior inferior cerebellar.

supraorbital a., *origin*, ophthalmic; *distribution*, frontalis muscle and scalp; *anastomoses*, branches of the superficial temporal and supratrochlear. SYN arteria supraorbitalis [NA].

suprascapular a., *origin*, thyrocervical trunk; *distribution*, clavicle, scapula, muscles of shoulder, and shoulder joint; *anastomoses*, transverse cervical circumflex scapular. SYN arteria suprascapularis [NA], transverse scapular a.

supratrochlear a., *origin*, ophthalmic; *distribution*, anterior portion of scalp; *anastomoses*, branches of supraorbital. SYN arteria supratrochlearis [NA], frontal a.

sural a., one of four or five arteries arising (sometimes by a common trunk) from the popliteal; *distribution*, muscles and integument of the calf; *anastomoses*, posterior tibial, medial, and lateral inferior genicular. SYN arteria suralis [NA].

terminal a., SYN end a.

testicular a., *origin*, aorta; *branches*, ureteral, cremasteric, epididymal; *distribution*, testicle and parts designated by names of branches; *anastomoses*, branches of renal, inferior epigastric, deferential. SYN arteria testicularis [NA].

thoracoacromial a., *origin*, axillary; *distribution*, muscles and skin of shoulder and upper chest; *anastomoses*, branches of superior thoracic, internal thoracic, lateral thoracic, posterior and anterior circumflex humeral, and suprascapular. SYN arteria thoracoacromialis [NA], acromiothoracic a.

thoracodorsal a., *origin*, subscapular; *distribution*, muscles of upper part of back; *anastomoses*, branches of lateral thoracic. SYN arteria thoracodorsalis [NA].

transverse cervical a., *origin*, thyrocervical trunk; *branches*, superficial (superficial cervical) and deep (descending scapular). SYN arteria transversa colli ✭ [NA], transverse a. of neck.

transverse facial a., *origin*, superficial temporal; *distribution*, parotid gland, parotid duct, masseter muscle, and overlying skin; *anastomoses*, infraorbital and buccal branches of maxillary, and buccal and masseteric branches of facial. SYN arteria transversa faciei [NA].

transverse a. of neck, SYN transverse cervical a.

transverse scapular a., SYN suprascapular a.

ulnar a., *origin*, brachial; *branches*, ulnar recurrent, common interosseous, dorsal and palmar carpal, deep palmar, and superficial palmar arch with its digital branches. SYN arteria ulnaris [NA].

umbilical a., before birth the a. is a continuation of the internal iliac; after birth it is obliterated between the bladder and umbilicus, forming the medial umbilical ligament, the remaining portion, between the internal iliac artery and bladder, being reduced in size and giving off the superior vesical arteries. SYN arteria umbilicalis [NA].

urethral a., *origin*, perineal artery; *distribution*, membranous urethra. SYN arteria urethralis [NA].

uterine a., *origin*, internal iliac; *distribution*, uterus, upper part of vagina, round ligament, and medial part of uterine (fallopian) tube; *anastomoses*, ovarian, vaginal, inferior epigastric. Supplies maternal circulation to placenta during pregnancy. SYN arteria uterina [NA].

vaginal a., *origin*, internal iliac; *distribution*, vagina, base of bladder, rectum; *anastomoses*, uterine, internal pudendal. SYN arteria vaginalis [NA].

ventricular a.'s, branches of the right and left coronary arteries distributed to the muscle of the ventricles. SYN arteriae ventriculares [NA].

vertebral a., the first branch of the subclavian artery; for descriptive purposes, divided into four parts: 1) prevertebral part, the portion before it enters the foramen of the transverse process of the sixth cervical vertebra; 2) transversarial part, the portion in the transverse foramina of the first six cervical vertebrae; 3) suboccipital (atlantic) part, the portion running along the posterior arch of the atlas; and 4) intracranial part, the portion within the cranial cavity to its union with the artery from the other side to form the basilar artery. SYN arteria vertebralis [NA].

zygomatico-orbital a., *origin*, superficial temporal, sometimes middle temporal; *distribution*, orbicularis oculi muscle and portions of the orbit; *anastomoses*, lacrimal and palpebral branches of ophthalmic. SYN arteria zygomatico-orbitalis [NA].

△**arthr-.** SEE arthro-.

ar•thral•gia (ar-thral′jē-ă). Pain in a joint, especially one not inflammatory in character. SYN arthrodynia. [G. *arthron*, joint, + *algos*, pain]

ar•thral•gic (ar-thral′jik). Relating to or affected with arthralgia. SYN arthrodynic.

ar•threc•to•my (ar-threk′tō-mē). Excision of a joint. [G. *arthron*, joint, + *ektomē*, excision]

ar•thrit•ic (ar-thrit′ik). Relating to arthritis.

ar•thri•tis, pl. **ar•thrit•i•des** (ar-thrī′tis, ar-thrit′i-dēz). Inflammation of a joint or a state characterized by inflammation of joints. SYN articular rheumatism. [G. fr. *arthron*, joint, + -*itis*, inflammation]

atrophic a., obsolete term for a. without new bone formation, now usually called rheumatoid a.

a. defor′mans, SYN rheumatoid a.

gonococcal a., joint space infection in humans caused by disseminated *Neisseria gonorrhoeae;* characteristically monarticular, but may be polyarticular.

gouty a., inflammation of the joints in gout.

hypertrophic a., SYN osteoarthritis.

juvenile a., juvenile rheumatoid a., chronic

a. beginning in childhood, most cases of which are pauciarticular, *i.e.*, affecting few joints. Several patterns of illness have been identified: in one subset, primarily affecting girls, iritis is common and antinuclear antibody is usually present; another subset, primarily affecting boys, frequently includes spinal a. resembling ankylosing spondylitis; some cases are true rheumatoid a. beginning in childhood and characterized by the presence of rheumatoid factor and destructive deforming joint changes, often undergoing remission at puberty. SEE ALSO Still's *disease*.

Lyme a., the arthritic manifestation of Lyme disease.

psoriatic a., the concurrence of psoriasis and polyarthritis, resembling rheumatoid a. but thought to be a specific disease entity, seronegative for rheumatoid factor and often involving the digits.

rheumatoid a., a systemic disease, occurring more often in women, which affects connective tissue; a. is the dominant clinical manifestation, involving many joints, especially those of the hands and feet, accompanied by thickening of articular soft tissue, with extension of synovial tissue over articular cartilages, which become eroded; the course is variable but often is chronic and progressive, leading to deformities and disability. SYN a. deformans, nodose rheumatism (1).

suppurative a., acute inflammation of synovial membranes, with purulent effusion into a joint, due to bacterial infection. SYN purulent synovitis, pyarthrosis.

♻**arthro-, arthr-.** A joint, an articulation; corresponds to L. articul-. [G. *arthron*, a joint, fr. *araiskō*, to join, to fit together]

ar·thro·cele (ar'thrō-sēl). 1. Hernia of the synovial membrane through the capsule of a joint. 2. Any swelling of a joint. [arthro- + G. *kēlē*, hernia, tumor]

ar·thro·cen·te·sis (ar'thrō-sen-tē'sis). Aspiration of fluid from a joint through a needle. [arthro- + G. *kentēsis*, puncture]

ar·thro·chon·dri·tis (ar'thrō-kon-drī'tis). Inflammation of an articular cartilage. [arthro- + G. *chondros*, cartilage, + -*itis*, inflammation]

ar·thro·cla·sia (ar-thrō-klā'zē-ă). Forcible breaking up of adhesions in ankylosis. [arthro- + G. *klasis*, a breaking]

Arth·ro·der·ma (ar'thrō-der'mă). A genus of ascomycetous fungi composed of the anamorph genera *Microsporium* and *Trichoderma* species.

ar·throd·e·sis (ar-throd'ĕ-sis, ar-thrō-dē'sis). The stiffening of a joint by operative means. SYN artificial ankylosis, syndesis. [arthro- + G. *desis*, a binding together]

ar·thro·dia (ar-thrō'dē-ă). SYN plane *joint*. [G. *arthrōdia*, a gliding joint, fr. *arthron*, joint, + *eidos*, form]

ar·thro·di·al (ar-thrō'dē-ăl). Relating to arthrodia.

ar·thro·dyn·ia (ar-thrō-din'ē-ă). SYN arthralgia. [arthro- + G. *odynē*, pain]

ar·thro·dyn·ic (ar-thrō-din'ik). SYN arthralgic.

ar·thro·dys·pla·sia (ar'thrō-dis-plā'zē-ă). Hereditary congenital defect of joint development. [arthro- + G. *dys*, bad, + *plasis*, a molding]

ar·thro·en·dos·co·py (ar'thrō-en-dos'kŏ-pē). SYN arthroscopy.

ar·thro·gram (ar'thrō-gram). Roentgenogram of a joint; usually implies the introduction of a contrast agent into the joint capsule. [arthro- + G. *gramma*, a writing]

ar·throg·ra·phy (ar-throg'ră-fē). Radiography of a joint after injecting one or more contrast media into the joint. [arthro- + G. *graphō*, to describe]

ar·thro·gry·po·sis (ar'thrō-gri-pō'sis). Congenital defect of the limbs characterized by contractures of joints. [arthro- + G. *gryphōsis*, a crooking]

a. mul'tiplex congen'ita, limitation of range of joint motion and contractures present at birth, usually involving multiple joints; a syndrome probably of diverse etiology that may result from changes in spinal cord, muscle, or connective tissue.

arthrokinematics (ar-thrō-kin-ĕ-mat'iks). The study of movements between adjoining articular (joint) surfaces. [arthro- + G. *kinēma, kinēmatos*, movement, + -*ics*]

ar·throl·y·sis (ar-throl'i-sis). Restoration of mobility in stiff and ankylosed joints. [arthro- + G. *lysis*, a loosening]

ar·throm·e·ter (ar-throm'ĕ-ter). SYN goniometer (3).

ar·throm·e·try (ar-throm'ĕ-trē). Measurement of the range of movement in a joint. [arthro- + G. *metron*, measure]

ar·thro-oph·thal·mop·a·thy (ar'thrō-of'thal-mop'ă-thē) [MIM*108300]. Disease affecting joints and eyes. [arthro- + ophthalmo- + G. *pathos*, suffering]

ar·throp·a·thy (ar-throp'ă-thē). Any disease affecting a joint. [arthro- + G. *pathos*, suffering]

neuropathic a., SYN neuropathic *joint*.

tabetic a., a neuropathic a. that occurs with tabes dorsalis. SEE ALSO neuropathic *joint*. SYN Charcot's joint.

ar·thro·plas·ty (ar'thrō-plas-tē). 1. Creation of an artificial joint to correct ankylosis. 2. An operation to restore as far as possible the integrity and functional power of a joint. [arthro- + G. *plastos*, formed]

total joint a., a. in which both joint surfaces are replaced with artificial materials, usually metal and high-density plastic.

ar·thro·pneu·mo·ra·di·og·raph·y (ar'thrō-nū'mō-rā-dē-og'ra-fē). Radiographic examination of a joint after it has been injected with air. [arthro- + pneumo- + radiography]

ar·thro·pod (ar'thrō-pod). A member of the phylum Arthropoda. [arthro- + G. *pous*, foot]

Ar·throp·o·da (ar-throp'ŏ-dă). A phylum of the Metazoa that includes the classes Crustacea (crabs, shrimps, crayfish, lobsters), Insecta, Arachnida (spiders, scorpions, mites, ticks), Chilopoda (centipedes), Diplopoda (millipedes), Merostomata (horseshoe crabs), and various other extinct or lesser known groups. A. forms the largest assemblage of living organisms, 75% insects, of which over a million species are known. [arthro- + G. *pous*, foot]

ar·thro·po·di·a·sis (ar'thrō-pō-dī'ă-sis). Direct effects of arthropods upon vertebrates, including acariasis, allergy, dermatosis, entomophobia, and actions of contact toxins.

ar•thro•py•o•sis (ar′thrō-pī-ō′sis). Suppuration in a joint. [arthro- + G. *pyōsis,* suppuration]

ar•thro•scle•ro•sis (ar′thrō-skler-ō′sis). Stiffness of the joints, especially in the aged. [arthro- + G. *sklērōsis,* hardening]

ar•thro•scope (ar′thrō-skōp). An endoscope for examining the interior of a joint.

ar•thros•co•py (ar-thros′kŏ-pē). Endoscopic examination of the interior of a joint. SYN arthroendoscopy. [arthro- + G. *skopeō,* to view]

▯**ar•thro•sis** (ar-thrō′sis). **1.** SYN joint. [G. *arthrōsis,* a jointing] **2.** A degenerative disorder of a joint. [arthro- + G. *-osis,* condition]

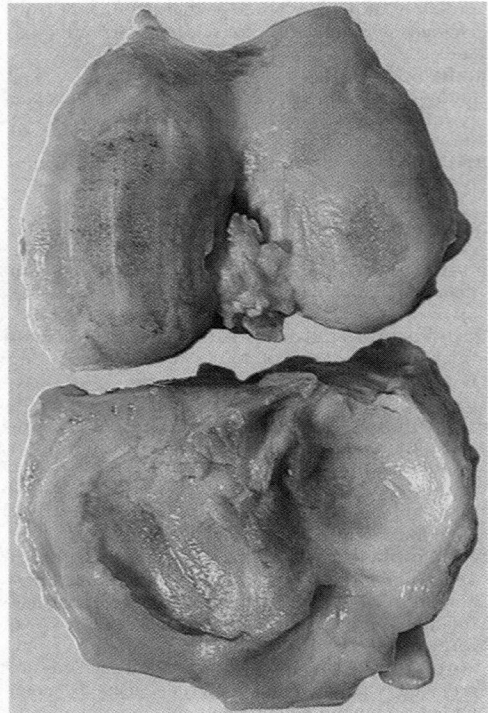

arthrosis: the cartilage of the knee is nearly destroyed

ar•thros•to•my (ar-thros′tō-mē). Establishment of a temporary opening into a joint cavity. [arthro- + G. *stoma,* mouth]

ar•thro•sy•no•vi•tis (ar′thrō-sin-ō-vī′tis). Inflammation of the synovial membrane of a joint.

ar•throt•o•my (ar-throt′ō-mē). Cutting into a joint. [arthro- + G. *tome,* a cutting]

ar•throx•e•sis (ar-throk′sĕ-sis). Removal of diseased tissue from a joint by means of the sharp spoon or other scraping instrument. [arthro- + G. *xesis,* a scraping]

ar•tic•u•lar (ar-tik′yū-lăr). Relating to a joint.

ar•tic•u•late (ar-tik′yū-lit). **1.** SYN articulated. **2.** Capable of distinct and connected speech. (ar-tik′yū-lāt). **3.** To join or connect together loosely

to allow motion between the parts. **4.** To speak distinctly and connectedly. [L. *articulo,* pp. *-atus,* to articulate]

ar•tic•u•lat•ed (ar-tik′yū-lā-ted). Jointed. SYN articulate (1).

ar•tic•u•la•tio, pl. **ar•tic•u•la•ti•o•nes** (ar-tik-yū-lā′shē-ō, -lā-shē-ō′nēz) [NA]. SYN joint. [L. a forming of vines]

ar•tic•u•la•tion (ar-tik-yū-lā′shŭn). **1.** SYN joint. **2.** A joining or connecting together loosely so as to allow motion between the parts. **3.** Distinct connected speech or enunciation. **4.** In dentistry, the contact relationship of the occlusal surfaces of the teeth during jaw movement. [see articulatio]

ar•tic•u•la•tor (ar-tik′yū-lā-tŏr). A mechanical device which represents the temporomandibular joints and jaw members to which maxillary and mandibular casts may be attached.

articulators. Organs of the speech mechanism that form the configurations required for production of meaningful speech sounds, *i.e.,* the teeth, lips, mandible, tongue, velum, and pharynx. SEE ALSO speech *mechanism.*

ar•ti•fact (ar′ti-fakt). **1.** Anything, especially in a histologic specimen or a graphic record, that is caused by the technique used or is not a natural occurrence, but is merely incidental. **2.** A skin lesion produced or perpetuated by self-inflicted action, as in dermatitis artefacta. SYN artefact. [L. *ars,* art, + *facio,* pp. *factus,* to make]

  radiographic a., blemish on a radiograph caused by heat, light, damaged screens, dust, or improper handling of the x-ray film.

ar•ti•fac•ti•tious (ar′ti-fak-tish′ŭs). SYN artifactual.

ar•ti•fac•tu•al (ar-ti-fak′chyū-ăl). Produced or caused by an artifact. SYN artifactitious.

ar•yl (ar′il). An organic radical derived from an aromatic compound by removing a hydrogen atom.

ar•yl•sul•fa•tase (ar-il-sŭl′fă-tās). An enzyme that cleaves phenol sulfates, including cerebroside sulfates (*i.e.,* a phenol sulfate + H_2O → a phenol + sulfate anion). Some a.'s are inhibited by sulfate (type II) and some are not (type I). SYN sulfatase (2).

ar•y•te•noid (ar-i-tē′noyd). Denoting a cartilage (arytenoid cartilage) and muscles (oblique and transverse arytenoid muscles) of the larynx.

ar•y•te•noi•dec•to•my (ar′ĭ-tē-noy-dek′tō-mē). Excision of an arytenoid cartilage, usually in bilateral vocal fold paralysis, to improve breathing. [arytenoid + G. *ektomē,* excision]

ar•yt•e•noi•di•tis (ă-rit′ĕ-noy-dī′tis). Inflammation of an arytenoid cartilage or its mucosal cover.

ar•y•te•noi•do•pexy (ar′ĭ-tĕ-noy′dō-pek′sē). Fixation by surgery of cartilages or muscles of arytenoids. [arytenoid + G. *pēxis,* fixation]

A.S. *auris sinistra* [L.], left ear.

As arsenic.

as•bes•tos (as-bes′tŏs). Product obtained from fibrous hydrated silicates divided into amphiboles and serpentines; it is insoluble and is used to provide tensile strength and moldability, thermal insulation, and resistance to fire, heat, and corrosion; inhalation of a. particles can cause asbestosis and cancer of the lung and pleura. [G. unquenchable; so called in the erroneous belief that when heated, it could not be quenched]

as•bes•to•sis (as-bes-tō'sis). Pneumoconiosis due to inhalation of asbestos fibers suspended in the ambient air; sometimes complicated by pleural mesothelioma or bronchogenic carcinoma; ferruginous bodies are the histologic hallmark of exposure to asbestos.

as•ca•ri•a•sis (as-kă-rī'ă-sis). Disease caused by infection with *Ascaris* or related ascarid nematodes. [G. *askaris,* an intestinal worm, + *-iasis,* condition]

as•car•i•cide (as-kar'i-sīd). **1.** Causing the death of ascarid nematodes. **2.** An agent having such properties. [ascarid + L. *caedo,* to kill]

As•ca•ris (as'kă-ris). A genus of large, heavy-bodied roundworms parasitic in the small intestine; abundant in humans and many other vertebrates. [G. *askaris,* an intestinal worm]

📷 ***A. lumbricoi'des,*** a large roundworm of humans, one of the commonest human parasites; various symptoms such as restlessness, fever, and diarrhea are attributed to its presence, but usually it causes no definite symptoms.

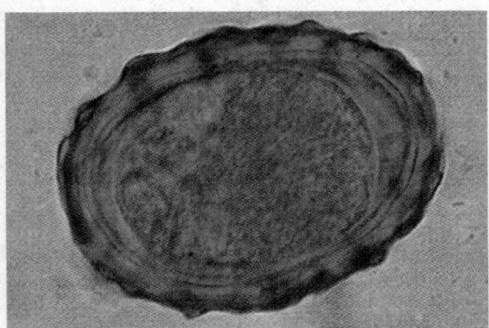

Ascaris lumbricoides (egg)

as•ci•tes (ă-sī'tēz). Accumulation of serous fluid in the peritoneal cavity. SYN hydroperitoneum, hydroperitonia. [L. fr. G. *askos,* a bag, + *-ites*]

   chylous a., a. chylo'sus, presence in the peritoneal cavity of a milky fluid containing suspended fat, ordinarily caused by an obstruction or injury of the thoracic duct or cisterna. SYN chyloperitoneum.

   hemorrhagic a., bloody or blood-stained serous fluid, frequently resulting from metastatic carcinoma, in the peritoneal cavity.

ascit•ic (ă-sit'ik). Relating to ascites.

As•co•my•ce•tes (as'kō-mī-sē'tēz). A class of fungi characterized by the presence of asci and ascospores. Such fungi have generally two distinct reproductive phases, the sexual or perfect stage and the asexual or imperfect stage. *Ajellomyces capsulatum* and *Ajellomyces dermatitidis* are pathogenic members of this class. [G. *askos,* a bag, + *mykēs,* mushroom]

as•cor•bate (as-kōr'bāt). A salt or ester of ascorbic acid.

   a. oxidase, a copper-containing enzyme that catalyzes the oxidation of L-ascorbic acid with O_2 to L-dehydroascorbic acid. Some forms of a. use $NADP^+$ as well. Used as an antitumor enzyme.

ascor•bic ac•id (as-kōr'bik). 2,3-didehydro-L-*threo*-hexono-1,4-lactone; used in preventing scurvy, as a strong reducing agent, and as an antioxidant in foodstuffs. SYN vitamin C. [G. *a*-priv. + Mod.L. *scorbutus,* scurvy, fr. Germanic]

△**-ase.** A termination denoting an enzyme, suffixed to the name of the substance (substrate) upon which the enzyme acts; *e.g.,* phosphatase, lipase, proteinase. May also indicate the reaction catalyzed *e.g.,* decarboxylase, oxidase. [Fr. *(diast)-ase,* an amylase that converts starch to maltose, fr. G. *diastasis,* separation, fr. *dia-,* through, apart, + *stasis,* a standing]

as•e•ma•sia, ase•mia (as-ĕ-mā'zē-ă, ă-sē'mē-ă). SYN asymbolia. [G. *a*- priv. + *sēmasia,* the giving of a signal, fr. *sēma,* sign]

asep•sis (ă-sep'sis, ā-). A condition in which living pathogenic organisms are absent; a state of sterility (2). [G. *a*- priv. + *sēpsis,* putrefaction]

asep•tic (ă-sep'tik, ā-). Marked by or relating to asepsis.

asex•u•al (ā-seks'yū-ăl). **1.** Referring to reproduction without nuclear fusion in an organism. **2.** Having no sexual desire or interest. [G. *a*- priv. + sexual]

ASL (sign language) sign language.

aso•cial (ā-sō'shŭl). Not social; withdrawn from society; indifferent to social rules or customs; *e.g.,* a recluse, a regressed schizophrenic person, a schizoid personality. Cf. antisocial.

Asp aspartic acid or its radical forms.

as•par•tate (as-par'tāt). A salt or ester of aspartic acid.

   a. aminotransferase (AST), an enzyme catalyzing the reversible transfer of an amine group from L-glutamic acid to oxaloacetic acid, forming α-ketoglutaric acid and L-aspartic acid; a diagnostic aid in viral hepatitis and in myocardial infarction. SYN glutamic-oxaloacetic transaminase, serum glutamic-oxaloacetic transaminase.

as•par•tic ac•id (Asp) (as-par'tik). The L-isomer is one of the amino acids occurring in proteins. SYN α-aminosuccinic acid.

β-as•par•tyl(ace•tyl•glu•cos•a•mine) (as-par'til-as'e-til-glū'kō-să-mēn). A compound of *N*-acetylglucosamine and asparagine, linked via the amide nitrogen of the latter and carbon-1 of the former. An important structural linkage in many glycoproteins.

as•pect (as'pekt). **1.** Appearance; looks. **2.** A side or surface of an object or structure, as viewed from a specified direction. [L. *aspectus,* fr. *a-spicio,* pp. *-spectus,* to look at]

as•per•gil•lo•ma (as'per-ji-lō'mă). **1.** An infectious granuloma caused by *Aspergillus.* **2.** A variety of bronchopulmonary aspergillosis; a ball-like mass of *Aspergillis fumigatus* colonizing an existing cavity in the lung. [aspergillus + *-oma,* tumor]

as•per•gil•lo•sis (as'per-ji-lō'sis). The presence of *Aspergillus* in the tissues or on a mucous surface of humans and animals, and the symptoms produced thereby.

As•per•gil•lus (as-per-jil′ŭs). A genus of fungi that contains many species, a number of them with black, brown, or green spores. A few species are pathogenic for man. [Med. L. a sprinkler, fr. L. *aspergo,* to sprinkle]

as•phyx•ia (as-fik′sē-ă). Impairment of ventilatory exchange of oxygen and carbon dioxide; combined hypercapnia and hypoxia or anoxia. [G. *a-* priv. + *sphyzō,* to throb]

a. liv′ida, a form of a. neonatorum in which the skin is cyanotic, but the heart is strong and the reflexes are preserved.

local a., stagnation of the circulation, sometimes resulting in local gangrene, especially of the fingers; one of the symptoms usually associated with Raynaud's disease.

a. neonato′rum, a. occurring in the newborn.

traumatic a., cyanotic a. due to trauma; the extravasation of blood into the skin and conjunctivae, produced by a sudden mechanical increase in venous pressure, analogous to the Rumpel-Leede test; it is common in those who have been hanged, and is seen occasionally in crush injuries. SYN pressure stasis.

as•phyx•i•al (as-fik′sē-ăl). Relating to asphyxia.

as•phyx•i•ate (as-fik′sē-āt). To induce asphyxia.

as•phyx•i•a•tion (as-fik-sē-ā′shŭn). The production of, or the state of, asphyxia.

as•pi•rate. 1 (as′pi-rāt). To remove by aspiration. **2** (as′pi-rit). The substance removed by aspiration. [L. *a-spiro,* pp. *-atus,* to breathe on, give the H sound]

as•pi•ra•tion (as-pi-rā′shŭn). **1.** Removal, by suction, of a gas or fluid from a body cavity, from unusual accumulations, or from a container. **2.** The inspiratory sucking into the airways of fluid or foreign body, as of vomitus. **3.** A surgical technique for cataract, requiring a small corneal incision, severance of the lens capsule, fragmentation of the lens material, and removal with a needle. [L. *aspiratio,* fr. *aspiro,* to breathe on]

meconium a., intrauterine a. by the fetus of amniotic fluid contaminated by meconium resulting from fetal hypoxic distress.

silent a., movement of a liquid or solid bolus into the trachea below the vocal cords, without clinical signs such as coughing, choking, color change, or change in respirations.

as•pi•ra•tor (as′pi-rā-ter, -tōr). An apparatus for removing fluid by aspiration from any of the body cavities; it consists usually of a hollow needle or trocar and cannula, connected by tubing with a container vacuumized by a syringe or reversed air (suction) pump.

asple•nia (ă-splē′nē-ă). Congenital absence of the spleen.

asplen•ic (ă-splen′ik). Having no spleen.

as•sas•sin bug (ă-sas′in). An insect of the family Reduviidae that inflicts irritating, painful bites in animals and man; related to the cone-nosed bugs (triatomines), a vector of American trypanosomiasis. [Fr., fr. It. *assassino,* fr. Ar. *hashshāshin,* those addicted to hashish]

as•say (as′sā, ă-sā′). **1.** Test of purity; trial. **2.** To ‑‑‑‑ to subject to analysis. **3.** The quantita- ‑‑‑‑ evaluation of a substance for ‑‑‑‑ results of such an

evaluation. [M.E., fr. O.Fr. *essaier,* fr. L.L. *exagium,* a weighing]

competitive binding a., an a. in which a binder competes for labeled versus unlabeled ligand; following separation of free and bound ligand, the ligand is quantitated by relating bound and unbound ratios to known standards. SEE ALSO enzyme-linked immunosorbent a., immunoassay, enzyme-multiplied *immunoassay* technique, radioimmunoassay.

complement binding a., a test for the detection of immune complexes.

enzyme-linked immunosorbent a. (ELISA), a sensitive method for serodiagnosis of specific infectious diseases; an *in vitro* competitive binding a. in which an enzyme and its substrate rather than a radioactive substance serve as the indicator system; in positive tests, the two yield a colored or other easily recognizable substance; the enzyme is linked to known immunoglobulin (or antigen) and in positive tests remains as part of the antigen-antibody complex available to react with its substrate when added.

immunochemical a., SYN immunoassay.

immunoradiometric a., a procedure in which an unknown antigen binds to an excess of antibody that has a radioactive label. The unbound antibody is removed in a subsequent step. The amount of antigen present is directly proportional to the amount of measured radioactivity.

as•sim•i•la•tion (ă-sim-i-lā′shŭn). **1.** Incorporation of digested materials from food into the tissues. **2.** Amalgamation and modification of newly perceived information and experiences into the existing cognitive structure. [L. *as-similo,* pp. *-atus,* to make alike]

as•sis•tant. Provider of support services to a health professional.

dental a., a person trained to provide support to a dentist with general tasks ranging from clerical work and assistance at chairside to laboratory and radiographic work.

medical a., a person who assists a physician by performing administrative and routine technical tasks.

as•so•ci•a•tion (ă-sō-sē-ā′shŭn). **1.** A connection of persons, things, or ideas by some common factor. **2.** A functional connection of two ideas, events, or psychological phenomena established through learning or experience. SEE ALSO conditioning. **3.** Statistical dependence between two or more events, characteristics, or other variables. [L. *as-socio,* pp. *-sociatus,* to join to; *ad* + *socius,* companion]

American Health Information Management A. (AHIMA), professional a. for members of the health information management profession. SEE health information management.

clang a., psychic a.'s resulting from sounds; often encountered in the manic phase of manic-depressive psychosis.

free a., an investigative psychoanalytic technique in which the patient verbalizes, without reservation or censor, the passing contents of his or her mind; the conflicts verbalized are the basis of the psychoanalyst's interpretations.

genetic a., the occurrence together in a population, more often than can be readily explained by chance, of two or more traits of which at least one is known to be genetic.

loose a.'s, a manifestation of a thought disorder whereby the patient's responses do not relate to the interviewer's questions or one paragraph, sentence, or phrase is not logically connected to those that occur before or after.

as·sort·ment (ă-sōrt′ment). In genetics, the relationship between nonallelic genetic traits that are transmitted from parent to child more or less independently in accordance with the degree of linkage between the respective loci.

AST *aspartate* aminotransferase.

asta·sia (ă-stā′zē-ă). Inability, through muscular incoordination, to stand. [G. unsteadiness, from *a*-priv. + *stasis,* standing]

asta·sia-aba·sia (ă-stā′zē-ă-ă-bā′zē-ă). Inability to stand or walk in a normal manner; the gait is bizarre and often the patient sways and nearly falls, but recovers at the last moment; a symptom of hysteria-conversion reaction. SYN Blocq's disease.

astat·ic (ā-stat′ik). Pertaining to astasia.

as·ta·tine (At) (as′tă-tēn). An artificial radioactive element of the halogen series; atomic no. 85, atomic wt. 211. [G. *astatos,* unstable]

aste·a·to·sis (ă-stē-ă-tō′sis). Diminished or arrested secretion of the sebaceous glands. [G. *a*-priv. + *stear* (*steat*-), fat]

as·ter (as′ter). SYN astrosphere. [Mod. L. fr. G. *astēr,* a star]

aster·e·og·no·sis (ă-stēr-og-nō′sis). SYN tactile *agnosia.* [G. *a*- priv. + *stereos,* solid + *gnōsis,* knowledge]

as·te·ri·on (ăs-tē′rē-on). A craniometric point at the junction of the lambdoid, occipitomastoid, and parietomastoid sutures. [G. *asterios,* starry]

aster·ix·is (as-ter-ik′sis). Involuntary jerking movements, especially in the hands, due to arrhythmic lapses of sustained posture; seen primarily with metabolic and toxic encephalopathies, especially hepatic encephalopathy. SYN flapping tremor. [G. *a*- priv. + *stērixis,* fixed position]

aster·nal (ā-ster′năl). **1.** Not related to or connected with the sternum, *e.g.,* a. rib. **2.** Without a sternum. [G. *a*- priv. + *sternon,* chest]

aster·nia (ă-ster′nē-ă). Congenital absence of the sternum.

as·the·nia (as-thē′nē-ă). Weakness or debility. [G. *astheneia,* weakness, fr. *a*- priv. + *sthenos,* strength]

as·then·ic (as-then′ik). **1.** Relating to asthenia. **2.** Denoting a thin, delicate body habitus.

as·the·no·pia (as-thē-nō′pē-ă). Subjective symptoms of ocular fatigue, discomfort, lacrimation, and headaches arising from use of the eyes. SYN eyestrain. [G. *astheneia,* weakness, + *ōps,* eye]

accommodative a., a. due to errors of refraction and excessive contraction of the ciliary muscle.

muscular a., a. due to imbalance of the extrinsic ocular muscles.

as·the·nop·ic (as-thĕ-nop′ik). Relating to or suffering from asthenopia.

as·the·no·sper·mia (as-thē-nō-sper′mē-ă). Loss

or reduction of motility of the spermatozoa, frequently associated with infertility. [G. *astheneia,* weakness, + *sperma,* seed, semen]

asth·ma (az′mă). Originally, a term used to mean "difficult breathing"; now used to denote bronchial a. SYN reactive airways disease. [G.]

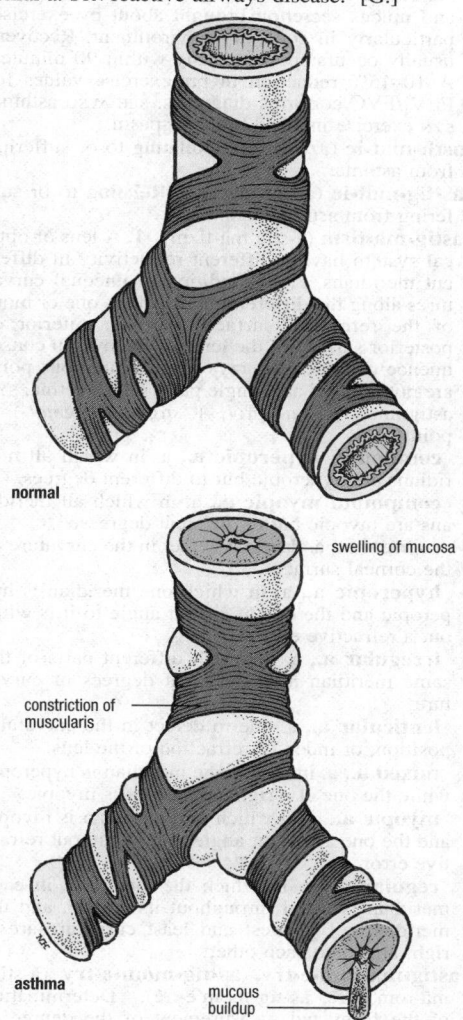

normal

swelling of mucosa

constriction of muscularis

asthma

mucous buildup

asthma: showing changes in bronchiole during asthma attack

bronchial a., a condition of the lungs in which there is widespread narrowing of airways, varying over short periods of time either spontaneously or as a result of treatment, due in varying degrees to contraction (spasm) of smooth muscle, edema of the mucosa, chronic or recurrent local inflammation of the submucosa with eventual fibrosis, and excessive mucus in the lumen of the bronchi and bronchioles; these changes are caused by the local release of spasmogens and vasoactive substances (*e.g.,* histamine, or certain leukotrienes or prostaglandins) in the course of an allergic process.

cardiac a., an asthmatic attack due to the pulmonary congestion and edema of left ventricular failure.

exercise-induced a., bronchial spasm, edema, and mucus secretion brought about by exercise, particularly in cool, dry environment. Recovery usually occurs spontaneously within 90 minutes. A 10–15% reduction in pre-exercise values for FEV_1/FVC confirms diagnosis. SEE ALSO asthma. SYN exercise-induced bronchospasm.

asth•mat•ic (az-mat′ik). Relating to or suffering from asthma.

as•tig•mat•ic (as′tig-mat′ik). Relating to or suffering from astigmatism.

astig•ma•tism (ă-stig′mă-tizm). **1.** A lens or optical system having different refractivity in different meridians. **2.** A condition of unequal curvatures along the different meridians in one or more of the refractive surfaces (cornea, anterior or posterior surface of the lens) of the eye, in consequence of which the rays from a luminous point are not focused at a single point on the retina. SYN astigmia. [G. *a*- priv. + *stigma* (*stigmat*-), a point]

compound hyperopic a., a. in which all meridians are hyperopic but to different degrees.

compound myopic a., a. in which all meridians are myopic but to different degrees.

corneal a., a. due to a defect in the curvature of the corneal surface.

hyperopic a., a. in which one meridian is hyperopic and the one at a right angle to it is without a refractive error.

irregular a., a. in which different parts of the same meridian have different degrees of curvature.

lenticular a., a. due to defect in the curvature, position, or index of refraction of the lens.

mixed a., a. in which one meridian is hyperopic while the one at a right angle to it is myopic.

myopic a., a. in which one meridian is myopic and the one at a right angle to it is without refractive error.

regular a., a. in which the curvature in each meridian is equal throughout its course, and the meridians of greatest and least curvature are at right angles to each other.

astig•ma•tom•e•try, as•tig•mom•e•try (ă-stig-mă-tom′ĕ-trē, as-tig-mom′ĕ-trē). Determination of the form and measurement of the degree of astigmatism.

astig•mia (ă-stig′mē-ă). SYN astigmatism.

asto•mia (ă-stō′mē-ă). Congenital absence of a mouth. [G. *a*- priv. + *stoma*, mouth]

as•trag•a•lar (as-trag′ă-lar). Relating to the astragalus or talus.

as•trag•a•lec•to•my (as-trag-ă-lek′tō-mē). Removal of the astragalus, or talus. [astragalus, + G. *ektomē*, excision]

as•tral (as′trăl). Relating to an astrosphere.

as•tric•tion (as-trik′shŭn). **1.** Astringent action. **2.** Compression to arrest hemorrhage.

as•trin•gent (as-trin′jent). **1.** Causing contraction of the tissues, arrest of secretion, or control of

bleeding. **2.** An agent having these effects. [L. *astringens*]

as•tro•blast (as′trō-blast). A primitive cell developing into an astrocyte. [G. *astron*, star, + *blastos*, germ]

as•tro•blas•to•ma (as′trō-blas-tō′mă). A relatively poorly differentiated glioma composed of young, immature, neoplastic cells of the astrocytic series, frequently arranged radially with short fibrils terminating on small blood vessels. [astro- + G. *blastos*, germ, + *-oma*, tumor]

as•tro•cyte (as′trō-sīt). One of the large neuroglia cells of nervous tissue. SEE ALSO neuroglia. SYN astroglia, macroglia. [G. *astron*, star, + *kytos*, hollow (cell)]

fibrillary a., fibrous a., a stellate astrocytic cell with long processes found mainly in the white matter of the brain and spinal cord and characterized by having bundles of glial filaments in its cytoplasm; origin of most astrocytomas.

protoplasmic a., one form of a., found mainly in gray matter, having few fibrils and numerous branching processes.

as•tro•cy•to•ma (as′trō-sī-tō′mă). A glioma derived from astrocytes; in persons less than 20 years of age, a.'s usually arise in a cerebellar hemisphere; in adults, a.'s usually occur in the cerebrum, sometimes growing rapidly and invading extensively. [G. *astron*, star, + *kytos*, cell, + *-oma*, tumor]

grade I a., solid or cystic a. of high differentiation or low grade.

grade II a., a. of low to intermediate grade.

grade III a., a. of intermediate grade. SEE ALSO glioblastoma multiforme.

grade IV a., SYN glioblastoma multiforme.

as•trog•lia (as-trog′lē-ă). SYN astrocyte. [G. *astron*, star, + neuroglia]

as•tro•sphere (as′trō-sfēr). A set of radiating microtubules extending outward from the cytocentrum and centrosphere of a dividing cell. SYN aster, attraction sphere. [G. *astron*, star, + *sphaira*, ball]

asym•bo•lia (ā-sim-bō′lē-ă). A form of aphasia in which the significance of signs and symbols is not appreciated. SYN asemasia, asemia. [G. *a*- priv. + *symbolon*, an outward sign]

asym•met•ric (a) (ā-sim-et′rik). Not symmetrical; denoting a lack of symmetry between two or more like parts.

asym•me•try (ā-sim′e-trē). **1.** Lack of symmetry; disproportion between two normally alike parts. **2.** Significant difference in amplitude or frequency of EEG activity recorded simultaneously from the two sides of the brain under identical conditions.

asymp•tom•at•ic (ā′simp-tō-mat′ik). Without symptoms, or producing no symptoms.

asymp•tot•ic (ā′simp-tot′ik). Pertaining to a limiting value, for example of a dependent variable, when the independent variable approaches zero or infinity.

asyn•cli•tism (ă-sin′kli-tizm). Absence of synclitism or parallelism between the axis of the presenting part of the child and the pelvic planes in childbirth. SYN obliquity. [G. *a*- priv. + *syn-klinō*, to incline together]

posterior a., SYN Litzmann *obliquity*.

asyn•de•sis (ă-sin'dĕ-sis). **1.** Rarely used term for a mental defect in which separate ideas or thoughts cannot be joined into a coherent concept. **2.** A breaking up of the connecting links in language, said to be characteristic of the language disturbance of schizophrenics. [G. *a-* priv. + *syn,* together, + *desis,* binding]

asyn•ech•ia (ā-si-nek'ē-ă). Discontinuity of structure. [G. *a-* priv. + *synecheia,* continuity]

asyn•er•gic (ā'sin-er'jik). Characterized by asynergia.

asyn•er•gy (ă-sin'er-jē). Lack of coordination among various muscle groups during the performance of complex movements, resulting in loss of skill and speed. When severe, results in decomposition of movement, wherein complex motor acts are performed in a series of isolated movements; caused by cerebellar disorders.

asys•tem•at•ic (ā'sis-tĕ-mat'ik). Not systematic; not relating to one system or set of organs.

asys•to•le (ă-sis'tō-lē). Absence of contractions of the heart. [G. *a-* priv, + *systolē,* a contracting]

asys•tol•ic (ă-sis-tol'ik). **1.** Relating to asystole. **2.** Not systolic.

AT The adenine-thymine hydrogen-bonded base pair observed in double-stranded polynucleotides.

At astatine.

at•a•vism (at'ă-vizm). The appearance in an individual of characteristics presumed to have been present in some remote ancestor; reversion to an earlier biological type. [L. *atavus,* a remote ancestor]

at•a•vis•tic (at-ă-vis'tik). Relating to atavism.

atax•ia (ă-tak'sē-ă). An inability to coordinate muscle activity, causing jerkiness, incoordination, and inefficiency of voluntary movement. Most often due to disorders of the cerebellum or the posterior columns of the spinal cord; may involve limbs, head, or trunk. SYN incoordination. [G. *a-*prov. + *taxis,* order]

　Friedreich's a., SYN hereditary spinal a.

　hereditary cerebellar a., **(1)** a disease of later childhood and early adult life, marked by ataxic gait, hesitating and explosive speech, nystagmus, and sometimes optic neuritis. **(2)** collective term for a number of hereditary disorders in which cerebellar signs are the most prominent finding.

　hereditary spinal a. [MIM*229300], sclerosis of the posterior and lateral columns of the spinal cord, occurring in children and marked by a. in the lower extremities, extending to the upper, followed by paralysis and contractures. SEE ALSO spinocerebellar a. SYN Friedreich's a.

　motor a., a. developing upon attempting to perform coordinated muscular movements.

　spinocerebellar a., the most common hereditary a., with onset in middle to late childhood, manifested as limb a., nystagmus, kyphoscoliosis, and pes cavus; the major pathological changes are found in the posterior columns of the spinal cord.

　a. telangiectasia, ataxia-telangiectasia, a slowly progressive multisystem disorder with a. appearing with the onset of walking; telangiectases of the conjunctiva and skin; athetosis and nystagmus; and recurrent infections of the respiratory system caused by immunoglobulin deficiencies. Approximately 70% of the patients have an IgA deficiency concomitant with decreased T helper cell function.

atax•i•a•pha•sia (ă-tak'sē-ă-fā'zē-ă). Inability to form connected sentences, although single words may be used intelligibly. [G. *a-* priv. + *taxis,* order, + *phasis,* an affirmation, speech]

atax•ia-tel•an•gi•ec•ta•sia. SEE *ataxia* telangiectasia.

atax•ic (ă-tak'sik). Relating to, marked by, or suffering from ataxia.

atax•i•o•phe•mia (ă-tak-sē-ō-fē'mē-ă). Incoordination of the muscles concerned in speech production. [G. *a-* priv. + *taxis,* order, + *phēmē,* voice, speech]

△**-ate.** Termination used as a replacement for "-ic acid" when the acid is neutralized (*e.g.,* sodium acetate) or esterified (*e.g.,* ethyl acetate).

at•el•ec•ta•sis (at-ĕ-lek'tă-sis). Absence of gas from a part or the whole of the lungs, due to failure of expansion or resorption of gas from the alveoli. [G. *atelēs,* incomplete, + *ektasis,* extension]

　passive a., the pulmonary collapse that occurs due to a space-occupying intrathoracic process such as pneumothorax or hydrothorax.

　platelike a., SYN subsegmental a.

　primary a., nonexpansion of the lungs after birth, found in all stillborn infants and in liveborn infants who die before respiration is established.

　round a., SYN folded-lung *syndrome*.

　secondary a., pulmonary collapse at any age, but particularly of infants, due to hyaline membrane disease or elastic recoil of the lungs while dying from other causes.

　subsegmental a., collapse of the portion of the lung distal to an obstructed subsegmental bronchus, manifested as a linear opacity on a chest radiograph. SEE Fleischner *lines,* under *line.* SYN platelike a.

at•e•lec•tat•ic (at-ĕ-lek-tat'ik). Relating to atelectasis.

ate•lia (ă-tē'lē-ă). SYN ateliosis.

atel•i•o•sis (ă-tē'lē-ō'sis). Incomplete development of the body or any of its parts, as in infantilism and dwarfism. SYN atelia. [G. *atelēs,* incomplete, + *-osis,* condition]

atel•i•ot•ic (ă-tē-lē-ot'ik). Marked by ateliosis.

athe•lia (ă-thē-lē-ă). Congenital absence of the nipples. [G. *a-* priv. + *thēlē,* nipple]

△**athero-.** Gruel-like, soft, pasty materials; atheroma, atheromatous. [G. *athērē,* gruel, porridge]

ath•er•o•em•bo•lism (ath'er-ō-em'bō-lizm). Cholesterol embolism, with or without calcific matter, originating from an atheroma of the aorta or other diseased artery.

ath•er•o•gen•e•sis (ath'er-ō-jen'ĕ-sis). Formation of atheroma, important in the pathogenesis of arteriosclerosis.

ath•er•o•gen•ic (ath-er-ō-jen'ik). Having the capacity to initiate, increase, or accelerate the process of atherogenesis.

ath•er•o•ma (ath-er-ō'mă). The lipid deposits in the intima of arteries, producing a yellow swelling on the endothelial surface; a characteristic of atherosclerosis. [G. *athērē,* gruel, + *-ōma,* tumor]

ath·er·om·a·tous (ath-er-ō′mă-tŭs). Relating to or affected by atheroma.

ath·er·o·scle·ro·sis (ath′er-ō-skler-ō′sis). Arteriosclerosis characterized by irregularly distributed lipid deposits in the intima of large and medium-sized arteries; such deposits provoke fibrosis and calcification. Atherosclerosis is set in motion when cells lining the arteries are damaged as a result of high blood pressure, smoking, toxic substances in the environment, and other agents. Plaques develop when high density lipoproteins accumulate at the site of arterial damage and platelets act to form a fibrous cap over this fatty core. Deposits impede or eventually shut off blood flow. See free radicals, low-fat diets.

ath·er·o·scle·rot·ic (ath′er-ō-skler-ot′ik). Relating to or characterized by atherosclerosis.

ath·e·toid (ath′ĕ-toyd). Resembling athetosis.

ath·e·to·sic, ath·e·tot·ic (ath-ĕ-tō′sik, -tot′ik). Pertaining to, or marked by, athetosis.

ath·e·to·sis (ath-ĕ-tō′sis). Slow, writhing, involuntary movements of flexion, extension, pronation, and supination of the fingers and hands, and sometimes of the toes and feet. Usually caused by an extrapyramidal lesion. [G. *athetos,* without position or place]

athletic trainer. an individual skilled in the prevention, evaluation, treatment, and rehabilitation of athletic injuries.

athy·mia (ă-thī′mē-ă). **1.** Absence of affect or emotivity; morbid impassivity. **2.** Congenital absence of the thymus gland, often with associated immunodeficiency. SYN athymism. [G. *a*-priv. + *thymos,* mind, also thymus]

athy·mism (ă-thī′mizm). SYN athymia (2).

athy·roid·ism (ă-thī′royd-izm). Congenital absence of the thyroid gland or suppression or absence of its hormonal secretion. SEE hypothyroidism.

athy·rot·ic (ă-thī-rot′ik). Relating to athyroidism.

ATL adult T-cell *leukemia* or adult T-cell *lymphoma.*

at·lan·tad (at-lan′tad). In a direction toward the atlas.

at·lan·tal (at-lan′tăl). Relating to the atlas.

△**atlanto-, atlo-.** The atlas (the bone that supports the head). [G. *Atlas, Atlantos,* Atlas, the mythical Titan who supported the heavens on his shoulders]

at·lan·to·ax·i·al (at-lan′tō-ak′sē-ăl). Pertaining to the atlas and the axis; denoting the joint between the first two cervical vertebrae. SYN atloaxoid.

at·las (at′las) [NA]. First cervical vertebra, articulating with the occipital bone and rotating around the dens of the axis. [G. *Atlas,* in Greek mythology a Titan who supported the heavens on his shoulders]

△**atlo-.** SEE atlanto-.

at·lo·ax·oid (at-lō-ak′soyd). SYN atlantoaxial.

atm standard *atmosphere.*

△**atmo-.** Prefix denoting steam or vapor; or derived by action of steam or vapor. [G. *atmos,* steam, vapor]

at·mos·phere (at′mŏs-fēr). **1.** Any gas surrounding a given body; a gaseous medium. **2.** A unit of air pressure. SEE ALSO standard a. [atmo- + G. *sphaira,* sphere]

  ICAO standard a., the standard a. adopted by the International Civil Aviation Organization, used for calibrating altimeters and for expressing hypobaric chamber pressures in terms of equivalent altitude.

  standard a. (atm), (**1**) the pressure of the a. at mean sea level, equivalent to 1,013,250 dynes/cm^2 or 101,325 Pa (N/m^2 in the SI system); (**2**) a standardized expression of the relation of barometric pressure, temperature, and other atmospheric variables as a function of altitude above sea level.

at·om (at′ŏm). The once ultimate particle of an element, believed to be as indivisible as its name indicates. Discovery of radioactivity demonstrated the existence of subatomic particles, notably protons, neutrons, and electrons, the first two comprising most of the mass of the atomic nucleus. We now know that subatomic particles are further divisible ino hadrons, leptons, and quarks. [G. *atomos,* indivisible, uncut]

atom·ic (ă-tom′ik). Relating to an atom.

at·om·iz·er (at′ŏm-ī-zer). A device used to reduce liquid medication to fine particles in the form of a spray or aerosol; useful in delivering medication to the nose and throat. SEE ALSO nebulizer, vaporizer. [G. *atomos,* indivisible particle]

aton·ic (ă-ton′ik). Relaxed; without normal tone or tension.

at·o·ny (at′ŏ-nē). Relaxation, flaccidity, or lack of tone or tension. [G. *atonia,* languor]

at·o·pen (at′ŏ-pen). The excitant causing any form of atopy.

atop·ic (ă-top′ik). Relating to or marked by atopy. [G. *atopos,* out of place; strange]

atop·og·no·sia, atop·og·no·sis (ă-top-og-nō′zē-ă, -og-nō′sis). Sensory inattention; inability to locate a sensation properly. Usually caused by a contralateral parietal lobe lesion. [G. *a*- priv. + *topos,* place, + *gnōsis,* knowledge]

at·o·py (at′ō-pē). A genetically determined state of hypersensitivity to environmental allergens. Type I allergic reaction is associated with the IgE antibody and a group of diseases, principally asthma, hay fever, and atopic dermatitis. [G. *atopia,* strangeness, fr. *a*- priv. + *topos,* a place]

atox·ic (ā-tok′sik). Not toxic.

ATP adenosine 5′-triphosphate.

ATPase adenosine triphosphatase.

ATPS Symbol indicating that a gas volume has been expressed as if it were *s*saturated with water vapor at the *a*mbient *t*emperature and barometric *p*ressure; the condition of an expired gas equilibrated in a *s*pirometer.

atre·sia (ă-trē′zē-ă). Absence of a normal opening or normally patent lumen. [G. *a*- priv. + *trēsis,* a hole]

  anal a., a. a′ni, congenital absence of an anal opening due to the presence of a membranous septum (persistence of the cloacal membrane) or a complete absence of the anal canal. SYN imperforate anus (1), proctatresia.

  aortic a., congenital absence of the normal valvular orifice into the aorta.

  biliary a., a. of the major bile ducts, causing

cholestasis and jaundice, which does not become apparent until several days after birth; periportal fibrosis develops and leads to cirrhosis, with proliferation of small bile ducts unless these are also atretic; giant cell transformation of hepatic cells also occurs. Cf. neonatal *hepatitis*.

intestinal a., an obliteration of the lumen of the small intestine, with the ileum involved in 50% of cases and the jejunum and duodenum next in frequency; most frequent cause of intestinal obstruction in the newborn; etiology may be related to a failure of recanalization during early development or to some impairment of blood supply during intrauterine life.

tricuspid a., congenital lack of the tricuspid orifice.

vaginal a., congenital or acquired imperforation or occlusion of the vagina, or adhesion of the walls of the vagina. SYN colpatresia.

atret•ic (ă-tret′ik). Relating to atresia. SYN imperforate.

△**atreto-.** Lack of an opening. [G. *atrētos,* imperforate fr. *a-,* not + *trētos,* perforated, fr. *tetrainō, titrēmi,* to bore through, to pierce.]

atria (ā′trē-ă). Plural of atrium.

atri•al (ā′trē-ăl). Relating to an atrium.

atrich•ia (ă-trik′ē-ă). Absence of hair, congenital or acquired. SYN atrichosis. [G. *a-* priv. + *thrix* (*trich-*), hair]

atri•cho•sis (at-ri-kō′sis). SYN atrichia.

at•ri•chous (at′ri-kŭs). Without hair.

△**atrio-.** The atrium; atrial. [L. *atrium,* an entrance hall]

atri•o•meg•a•ly (ā′trē-ō-meg′ă-lē). Enlargement of the atrium. [atrio- + G. *megas,* great]

atri•o•sep•to•plas•ty (ā′trē-ō-sep′tō-plas-tē). Surgical repair of an atrial septal defect. [atrio- + L. *septum,* partition, + G. *plastos,* formed]

atri•o•sep•tos•to•my (ā′trē-ō-sep-tos′tō-mē). Establishment of a communication between the two atria of the heart. [atrio- + L. *septum,* partition, + G. *stoma,* mouth]

atri•o•ven•tric•u•lar (A-V) (ā′trē-ō-ven-trik′yū-lar). Relating to both the atria and the ventricles of the heart, especially to the ordinary, orthograde transmission of conduction or blood flow.

atri•um, pl. **atria** (ā′trē-ŭm, ā′trē-ă). **1** [NA]. A chamber or cavity to which are connected several chambers or passageways. **2.** SYN a. of heart. **3.** That part of the tympanic cavity that lies immediately deep to the eardrum. **4.** In the lung, a subdivision of the alveolar duct from which alveolar sacs open. [L. entrance hall]

a. cor′dis [NA], SYN a. of heart.

a. of heart, the upper chamber of each half of the heart. SYN a. cordis [NA], atrium (2).

atro•phia (ă-trō′fē-ă). SYN atrophy. [G. fr. *a-* priv. + *trophē,* nourishment]

atroph•ic (ă-trof′ik). Denoting atrophy.

at•ro•phied (at′rō-fēd). Characterized by atrophy.

at•ro•pho•der•ma (at′rō-fō-der′mă). Atrophy of the skin that may occur either in discrete localized areas or in widespread areas. SEE ALSO anetoderma.

at•ro•pho•der•ma•to•sis (at′rō-fō-der-mă-tō′sis).

Any cutaneous disorder in which a prominent symptom is skin atrophy.

at•ro•phy (at′rō-fē). A wasting of tissues, organs, or the entire body, as from death and reabsorption of cells, diminished cellular proliferation, decreased cellular volume, pressure, ischemia, malnutrition, lessened function, or hormonal changes. SYN atrophia. [G. *atrophia,* fr. *a-* priv. + *trophē,* nourishment]

acute yellow a. of the liver, a lesion in which there is extensive and rapid death of parenchymal cells of the liver, sometimes with fatty degeneration; may result from fulminant viral infection or chemical poisoning; associated with jaundice. SYN Rokitansky's disease.

infantile spinal muscular a. [MIM*253300], transmitted as autosomal recessive on chromosome 5q. Progressive dysfunction of the anterior horn cells in the spinal cord and brainstem cranial nerves with profound weakness and bulbar dysfunction occurring in the first two years of life. Three groups, based on age of clinical onset, are recognized.

juvenile spinal muscular a. [MIM*253600], slowly progressive proximal muscular weakness and wasting, beginning in childhood, caused by degeneration of motor neurons in the anterior horns of the spinal cord; onset usually between 2 and 17 years of age; usually autosomal recessive inheritance.

linear a., SYN *striae* cutis distensae, under *stria.*

muscular a., wasting of muscular tissue.

peroneal muscular a. [MIM*118200 to 118220], a group of familial peripheral neuromuscular disorders, sharing the common feature of marked wasting of the distal parts of the extremities, particularly the peroneal muscle groups, resulting in "stork legs." SYN Charcot-Marie-Tooth disease.

Pick's a., circumscribed a. of the cerebral cortex.

progressive muscular a., SYN amyotrophic lateral *sclerosis.*

Sudeck's a., a. of bones, commonly of the carpal or tarsal bones, following a slight injury such as a sprain. SEE ALSO causalgia, reflex sympathetic *dystrophy.*

yellow a. of the liver, SEE acute yellow a. of the liver.

at•tack (ă-tak′). The occurrence of some disorder or episode, ordinarily with dramatic and sudden onset, such as an a. of shingles or heart a.

drop a., an episode of sudden falling that occurs during standing or walking, without warning and without loss of consciousness, vertigo, or postictal behavior. The patients are usually elderly and have normal electroencephalograms; of unknown cause.

glottal a., excessive glottal closure prior to phonation resulting in loud and sudden voice onset. SYN coup de glotte.

panic a., sudden onset of intense apprehension, fear, terror, or impending doom accompanied by increased autonomic nervous system activity and by various constitutional disturbances, depersonalization, and derealization.

transient ischemic a. (TIA), a sudden focal

loss of neurological function with complete recovery usually within 24 hours; caused by a brief period of inadequate perfusion in a portion of the territory of the carotid or vertebral basilar arteries.

at·ten·u·a·tion (ă-ten-yū-ā'shŭn). **1.** The act of attenuating. **2.** Diminution of virulence in a strain of an organism, obtained through selection of variants which occur naturally or through experimental means. **3.** Loss of energy of a beam of radiant energy due to absorption, scattering, beam divergence, and other causes as the beam propagates through a medium. **4.** Regulation of termination of transcription; involved in control of gene expression in specific tissues.

at·ti·cot·o·my (at-i-kot'ō-mē). Operative opening into the tympanic attic. [attic + G. *tomē*, incision]

at·ti·tude (at'i-tūd). **1.** Position of the body and limbs. **2.** Manner of acting. **3.** PSYCHOLOGY a predisposition to behave or react in a certain way toward persons, objects, institutions, or issues. [Mediev. L. *aptitudo*, fr. L. *aptus*, fit]

atto- (a). Prefix used in the SI and metric systems to signify one quintillionth (10^{-18}). [Danish *atten*, eighteen]

at·trac·tion (ă-trak'shŭn). A property or force by which anything tends to cause something else to approach it. [L. *at-traho*, pp. *-tractus*, to draw toward]

    capillary a., the force that causes fluids to rise up very fine tubes or pass through the pores of a loose material.

    chemical a., the force impelling atoms of different elements or molecules to unite to form new substances or compounds.

at·tri·tion (ă-trish'ŭn). **1.** Wearing away by friction or rubbing. **2.** In dentistry, physiological loss of tooth structure caused by the abrasive character of food or from bruxism. Cf. abrasion. [L. *attero*, pp. *-tritus*, to rub against, rub away]

at wt atomic *weight.*

atyp·i·cal (ā-tip'i-kal). Not typical; not corresponding to the normal form or type. [G. *a-* priv. + *typikos*, conformed to a type]

Au gold (aurum).

au·dile (aw'dil). **1.** Relating to audition. **2.** Denoting the type of mental imagery in which one recalls most readily that which has been heard rather than seen or read. Cf. motile. **3.** SYN auditive.

audio-. The sense of hearing. [L. *audio*, to hear]

au·di·o·an·al·ge·sia (aw'dē-ō-an-ăl-jē'zē-ă). Use of music or sound delivered through earphones to mask pain during dental or surgical procedures.

au·di·o·gen·ic (awd'ē-ō-jen'ik). **1.** Caused by sound, especially a loud noise. **2.** Sound-producing. [audio- + G. *genesis*, production]

au·di·o·gram (aw'dē-ō-gram). The graphic record drawn from the results of hearing tests with the audiometer; charts the threshold of hearing at various frequencies against sound intensity in decibels. [audio- + G. *gramma*, a drawing]

pure tone a., an a. in which the threshold for pure tone stimuli is charted in decibels of hearing level down the vertical axis, the horizontal axis

being the frequency that is usually measured in octave steps from 125 Hz to 8 kHz.

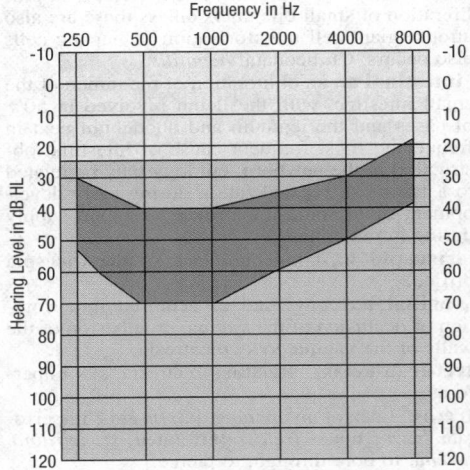

pure tone audiogram: yellow area indicates limits of normal hearing; dark green area illustrates the frequency and intensity of the English phonemes; the grid is 20 dB / octave

au·di·ol·o·gist (aw-dē-ol'ōjist). A specialist in evaluation and rehabilitation of those whose communication disorders center in whole or in part in the hearing function.

au·di·ol·o·gy (aw-dē-ol'ō-jē). The study of hearing disorders through the identification and measurement of hearing function loss as well as the rehabilitation of persons with hearing impairments.

au·di·om·e·ter (aw-dē-om'ĕ-ter). An electrical instrument for measuring the threshold of hearing for pure tones of frequencies generally varying from 128 to 8000 Hz (recorded in decibels). [audio- + G. *metron*, measure]

au·di·o·met·ric (aw'dē-ō-met'rik). Related to measurement of hearing levels.

au·di·om·e·try (aw-dē-om'ĕ-trē). Use of the audiometer.

    auditory brainstem response a. (ABR), ABR a., an electrophysiologic measure of auditory function utilizing responses produced by the auditory nerve and the brainstem to repetitive acoustic stimuli. SYN brainstem evoked response a., BSER a.

    brainstem evoked response a., BSER a., SYN auditory brainstem response a.

    cortical a., measurement of the potentials that arise in the auditory system above the level of the brainstem.

    electrodermal a., a form of electrophysiologic a. used to determine hearing thresholds by measuring changes in skin resistance as a conditioned response to noise stimuli.

au·di·o·vi·su·al (aw'dē-ō-vizh'yū-ăl). Pertaining to a communication or teaching technique that combines both audible and visible symbols.

au·di·tion (aw-dish'ŭn). SYN hearing. [L. *auditio*, a hearing, fr. *audio*, to hear]

au·di·tive (aw'di-tiv). One who recalls most readily that which has been heard. SYN audile (3).

au·di·to·ry (aw'di-tōr-ē). Pertaining to the sense of hearing or to the organs of hearing. [L. *audio*, pp. *auditus*, to hear]

au·ra, pl. **au·rae** (aw'ră, -rē). **1.** Subjective symptoms occurring at the onset of a partial epileptic seizure; often characteristic for the brain region involved in the seizure, *e.g.*, visual aura, occipital lobe auditory aura, temporal lobe. **2.** Subjective symptoms at the onset of a migraine headache. [L. breeze, odor, gleam of light]

au·ral (aw'răl). **1.** Relating to the ear (auris). **2.** Relating to an aura.

⌂**auri-**. Combining form denoting the ear. SEE ALSO ot-, oto-. [L. *auris*, an ear.]

au·ri·cle (aw'ri-kl). **1** [NA]. The projecting shell-like structure on the side of the head, constituting, with the external acoustic meatus, the external ear. SYN auricula (1), pinna (1). **2.** SYN a. of atrium.

  atrial a., SYN a. of atrium.

  a. of atrium, a small conical ("ear-shaped") pouch projecting from the upper anterior portion of each atrium of the heart, increasing slightly the atrial volume. SYN atrial a., auricle (2), auricula (2).

au·ric·u·la, pl. **au·ric·u·lae** (aw-rik'yū-lă, -lē). **1** [NA]. SYN auricle (1). **2.** SYN *auricle* of atrium. [L. the external ear, dim. of *auris*, ear]

au·ric·u·lar (aw-rik'yū-lăr). Relating to the ear, or to an auricle in any sense.

au·ric·u·la·re, pl. **au·ric·u·lar·ia** (aw-rik-yū-lā'rē, -rē-ă). A craniometric point at the center of the opening of the external acoustic meatus; or, in certain cases, the middle of the upper edge of this opening. SYN auricular point. [L. *auricularis*, pertaining to the ear]

au·ric·u·lar·ia (-rē-ă).

au·ric·u·lo·tem·po·ral (aw-rik'yū-lō-tem'pō-răl). Relating to the auricle or pinna of the ear and the temporal region.

au·ris, pl. **au·res** (aw'ris, aw'rēz) [NA]. SYN ear. [L.]

au·rum (aw'rŭm). SYN gold. [L.]

aus·cul·tate, aus·cult (aws'kŭl-tāt, aws-kŭlt'). To perform auscultation.

▪**aus·cul·ta·tion** (aws-kŭl-tā'shŭn). Listening to the sounds made by various body structures and functions as a diagnostic method, usually with a stethoscope. [L. *ausculto*, pp. *-atus*, to listen to]

  immediate a., direct a., a. by application of the ear to the surface of the body.

  mediate a., a. performed with the use of a stethoscope.

aus·cul·ta·to·ry (aws-kŭl'tă-tō-rē). Relating to auscultation.

⌂**aut-**. SEE auto-.

au·tism (aw'tizm). A tendency to morbid self-absorption at the expense of regulation by outward reality. [G. *autos*, self]

  infantile a., a severe emotional disturbance of childhood characterized by qualitative impairment in reciprocal social interaction and in communication, language, and social development. SYN Kanner's syndrome.

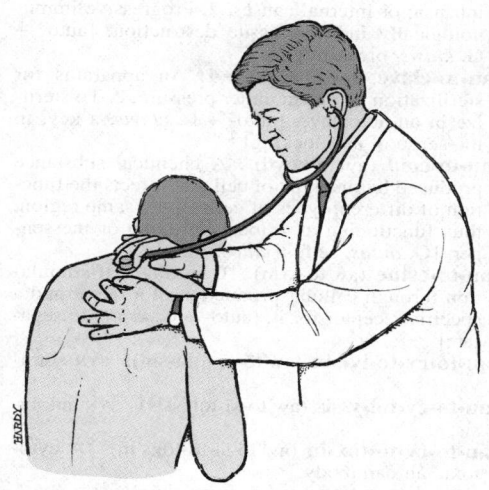

auscultation: mediate

au·tis·tic (aw-tis'tik). Pertaining to or characterized by autism.

⌂**auto-, aut-**. Prefixes meaning self, same. [G. *autos*, self]

au·to·ag·glu·ti·na·tion (aw'to-ă-glū-ti-nā'shŭn). **1.** Nonspecific agglutination or clumping together of cells (*e.g.*, bacteria, erythrocytes) due to physical-chemical factors. **2.** The agglutination of red blood cells by specific autoantibody present in one's own serum.

au·to·ag·glu·ti·nin (aw'tō-ă-glū'ti-nin). An agglutinating autoantibody.

au·to·al·ler·gic (aw'tō-ă-ler'jik). Pertaining to autoallergy.

au·to·al·ler·gy (aw-tō-al'er-jē). An altered reactivity in which antibodies (autoantibodies) are produced against an individual's own tissues, causing a destructive rather than a protective effect. SYN autoimmunity.

au·to·an·ti·body (aw-tō-an'ti-bod-ē). Antibody occurring in response to antigenic constituents of the host's tissue, and which reacts with the inciting tissue component.

au·to·an·ti·gen (aw-to-an'ti-jen). A "self" antigen; any tissue constituent that evokes an immune response by the host.

au·to·ca·tal·y·sis (aw'tō-kă-tal'i-sis). A reaction in which one or more of the products formed acts to catalyze the reaction; beginning slowly, the rate of such a reaction rapidly increases. Cf. chain *reaction*.

au·to·cat·a·lyt·ic (aw'tō-kat-ă-lit'ik). Relating to autocatalysis.

au·toch·thon·ous (aw-tok'thon-ŭs). **1.** Native to the place inhabited; aboriginal. **2.** Originating in the place where found; said of a disease originating in the part of the body where found, or of a disease acquired in the place where the patient is. [auto- + G. *chthon*, land, ground, country]

au·toc·la·sis, au·to·cla·sia (aw-tok'lă-sis, aw-tō-klā'zē-ă). **1.** A breaking up or rupturing from intrinsic or internal causes. **2.** Progressive immunologically induced tissue destruction. [auto- + G. *klasis,* breaking]

au•to•clave (aw′tō-klāv). **1.** An apparatus for sterilization by steam under pressure. **2.** To sterilize in an autoclave. [auto- + L. *clavis,* a key, in the sense of self-locking]

au•to•coid (aw′tō-koyd). A chemical substance produced by one type of cell that affects the function of different types of cells in the same region, thus functioning as a local hormone or messenger. [G. *autos,* self, + *eidos,* form]

au•to•crine (aw′tō-krin). Denoting self-stimulation through cellular production of a factor and a specific receptor for it. [auto- + G. *krinō,* to separate]

au•to•cy•tol•y•sin (aw′tō-sī-tol′i-sin). SYN autolysin.

au•to•cy•tol•y•sis (aw′tō-sī-tol′i-sis). SYN autolysis.

au•to•cy•to•tox•in (aw′tō-sī-tō-toks′in). A cytotoxic autoantibody.

au•to•di•ges•tion (aw′tō-dī-jes′chŭn). SYN autolysis.

au•to•ech•o•la•lia (aw′tō-ek-ō-lā′lē-ă). A morbid repetition of another person's or one's own words. [auto- + echolalia]

au•to•e•rot•ic (aw′tō-ĕ-rot′ik). Pertaining to autoerotism.

au•to•er•o•tism (aw-tō-ār′ō-tizm). **1.** Sexual arousal or gratification using one's own body, as in masturbation. **2.** Sexual self-love. SEE ALSO narcissism (1). Cf. alloerotism. [auto- + G. *erōtikos,* relating to love]

au•tog•a•my (aw-tog′ă-mē). A form of self-fertilization in which fission of the cell nucleus occurs without division of the cell, the two pronuclei so formed reuniting to form the synkaryon; in other cases, the cell body also divides, but the two daughter cells immediately conjugate. [auto- + G. *gamos,* marriage]

au•to•graft (aw′tō-graft). A tissue or an organ transferred by grafting into a new position in the body of the same individual. SYN autogeneic graft, autologous graft, autoplastic graft, autotransplant. [auto- + A.S. *graef*]

au•to•hem•ag•glu•ti•na•tion (aw′tō-hē′mă-glūti-nā′shŭn). Autoagglutination of erythrocytes.

au•to•he•mo•ly•sin (aw′tō-hē-mol′i-sin). An autoantibody that causes lysis of erythrocytes in the same individual in whose body the lysin is formed.

au•to•he•mol•y•sis (aw′tō-hē-mol′i-sis). Hemolysis occurring in certain diseases as a result of an autohemolysin.

au•to•im•mune (aw-tō-i-myūn′). Arising from and directed against the individual's own tissues, as in autoimmune disease.

au•to•im•mu•ni•ty (aw′tō-i-myū′ni-tē). IMMUNOLOGY the condition in which one's own tissues are subject to deleterious effects of the immune system, as in autoallergy and in autoimmune disease; immune response against the body's own tissues. SYN autoallergy.

au•to•im•mu•ni•za•tion (aw′tō-im′yū-ni-zā′shŭn). Induction of autoimmunity.

au•to•im•mu•no•cy•to•pe•nia (aw-tō-im′yū-nō-sī-tō-pē′nē-ă). Anemia, thrombocytopenia, and leukopenia resulting from cytotoxic autoimmune reactions.

au•to•in•fec•tion (aw′tō-in-fek′shŭn). **1.** Reinfection by microbes or parasitic organisms on or within the body that have already passed through an infective cycle, such as a succession of boils, or a new infective cycle with production of a new generation of larvae and adults. **2.** Self-infection by direct contagion as with parasite eggs passed in the infectious state transmitted by fingernails (anal-oral route). SYN autoreinfection.

au•to•in•fu•sion (aw′tō-in-fyū′zhŭn). Forcing the blood from the extremities or other areas such as the spleen, as by the application of a bandage or pressure device, to raise the blood pressure and fill the vessels in the vital centers; resorted to after excessive loss of blood or other body fluids. Cf. autotransfusion.

au•to•in•oc•u•la•tion (aw′tō-in-ok-yū-lā′shŭn). A secondary infection originating from a focus of infection already present in the body.

au•to•in•tox•i•cant (aw′tō-in-toks′i-kant). An endogenous toxic agent that causes autointoxication.

au•to•in•tox•i•ca•tion (aw′tō-in-toks-i-kā′shŭn). A disorder resulting from absorption of the waste products of metabolism, decomposed matter from the intestine, or the products of dead and infected tissue as in gangrene. SYN endogenic toxicosis.

au•to•i•sol•y•sin (aw′tō-ī-sol′i-sin). An antibody that in the presence of complement causes lysis of cells in the individual in whose body the lysin is formed, as well as in others of the same species.

au•to•ker•a•to•plas•ty (aw-tō-ker′ă-tō-plas-tē). Grafting of corneal tissue from one eye of a patient to the fellow eye. [auto- + G. *keras,* horn, + *plastos,* formed]

au•to•ki•ne•sia, au•to•ki•ne•sis (aw-tō-ki-ne′sē-ă, aw-tō-ki-nē′sis). Voluntary movement. [auto- + G. *kinēsis,* movement]

au•to•ki•net•ic (aw-tō-kĭ-net′ik). Relating to autokinesis.

au•tol•o•gous (aw-tol′ŏ-gŭs). **1.** Occurring naturally and normally in a certain type of tissue or in a specific structure of the body. **2.** Sometimes used to denote a neoplasm derived from cells that occur normally at that site, *e.g.,* a squamous cell carcinoma in the upper esophagus. **3.** TRANSPLANTATION referring to a graft in which the donor and recipient areas are in the same individual. [auto- + G. *logos,* relation]

au•tol•y•sate (aw-tol′i-sāt). The mixture of substances resulting from autolysis.

au•tol•y•sin (aw-tol′i-sin). An antibody that causes lysis of the cells and tissues in the body of the individual in whom the lysin is formed. SYN autocytolysin.

au•tol•y•sis (aw-tol′i-sis). **1.** Enzymatic digestion of cells (especially dead or degenerate) by enzymes present within them (autogenous). **2.** Destruction of cells as a result of a lysin formed in those cells or others in the same organism. SYN autocytolysis, autodigestion, isophagy. [auto- + G. *lysis,* dissolution]

au•to•lyt•ic (aw-tō-lit′ik). Pertaining to or causing autolysis.

au•tom•a•tism (aw-tom′ă-tizm). **1.** The state of being independent of the will or of central innervation; applicable, for example, to the heart's action. **2.** An epileptic attack consisting of stereotyped psychic, sensory, or motor phenomena carried out in a state of impaired consciousness and of which the individual usually has no knowledge. **3.** A condition in which an individual is consciously or unconsciously, but involuntarily, compelled to the performance of certain motor or verbal acts, often purposeless and sometimes foolish or harmful. SYN telergy. [G. *automatos*, self-moving, + -in]

au•to•nom•ic (aw-tō-nom′ik). Relating to the autonomic nervous system.

au•to•nom•o•tro•pic (aw′tō-nom-ō-trop′ik). Acting on the autonomic nervous system. [autonomic + G. *trepo*, to turn]

au•to•ox•i•da•tion (aw′tō-oks-i-dā′shŭn). The direct combination of a substance with molecular oxygen at ordinary temperatures. SYN autoxidation.

auto-PEEP auto-positive end-expiratory *pressure.*

au•to•pha•gia (aw-tō-fā′jē-ă). **1.** Biting one's own flesh; *e.g.,* as a symptom of Lesch-Nyhan syndrome. **2.** Maintenance of the nutrition of the whole body by metabolic consumption of some of the body tissues. **3.** SYN autophagy. [auto- + G. *phagō*, to eat]

au•to•pha•gic (aw-tō-fā′jik). Relating to or characterized by autophagia.

au•toph•a•gy (aw-tof′ă-jē). Segregation and disposal of damaged organelles within a cell. SYN autophagia (3). [auto- + G. *phagō*, to eat]

au•to•plas•tic (aw′tō-plas-tik). Relating to autoplasty.

au•to•plas•ty (aw′tō-plas-tē). Repair of defects by autotransplantation.

au•top•sy (aw′top-sē). An examination of the organs of a dead body to determine the cause of death or to study the pathologic changes present. SYN necropsy. [G. *autopsia*, seeing with one's own eyes]

au•to•ra•di•o•graph (aw-tō-rā′dē-ō-graf). Image of the distribution and concentration of radioactivity in a tissue or other substance made by placing a photographic emulsion on the surface of, or in close proximity to, the substance.

au•to•ra•di•og•ra•phy (aw′tō-rā-dē-og′ră-fē). The process of producing an autoradiograph. SYN radioautography.

au•to•reg•u•la•tion (aw′tō-reg-yū-lā′shŭn). **1.** The tendency of the blood flow to an organ or part to remain at or return to the same level despite changes in the pressure in the artery which conveys blood to it. **2.** In general, any biologic system equipped with inhibitory feedback systems such that a given change tends to be largely or completely counteracted; *e.g.,* baroreceptor reflexes form a basis for autoregulation of the systemic arterial blood pressure.

heterometric a., intrinsic regulation of the strength of cardiac contraction as a function of diastolic fiber length (volume), independent of afterload, autonomic nerves, and other extrinsic influences. Heterometric a. is also known as the length-tension relationship, the relationship of end diastolic volume to end diastolic pressure, Starling's law of the heart, and the Frank-Starling mechanism.

homeometric a., intrinsic regulation of strength of cardiac contraction in response to influences that do not depend on change in fiber length, *i.e.,* the Frank-Starling mechanism, (*e.g.,* the Anrep effect in which strength increases in response to increased afterload, and the Bowditch staircase effect (treppe) in which strength increases in response to increased heart rate) and do not depend on extrinsic regulation (*e.g.,* in which strength increases in response to sympathetic nerve stimulation or norepinephrine).

au•to•re•in•fec•tion (aw′tō-rē-in-fek′shŭn). SYN autoinfection.

au•to•re•pro•duc•tion (aw′tō-rē-prō-duk′shŭn). The ability of a gene or virus, or nucleoprotein molecule generally, to bring about the synthesis of another molecule like itself from smaller molecules within the cell.

au•to•se•rum (aw-tō-sē′rŭm). Serum obtained from the patient's own blood and used in autoserotherapy.

au•to•site (aw′tō-sīt). That member of abnormal, unequal conjoined twins that is able to live independently and nourish the other member (parasite) of the pair. [auto- + G. *sitos*, food]

au•to•so•mal (aw-tō-sō′măl). Pertaining to an autosome.

au•to•some (aw′tō-sōm). Any chromosome other than a sex chromosome; a.'s normally occur in pairs in somatic cells and singly in gametes. [auto- + G. *sōma*, body]

au•to•sug•ges•tion (aw′tō-sŭg-jes′chŭn). **1.** Constant dwelling upon an idea or concept, thereby inducing some change in the mental or bodily functions. **2.** Reproduction in the brain of impressions previously received which become then the starting point of new acts or ideas.

au•to•top•ag•no•sia (aw′tō-top′ag-nō′zē-ă). Inability to recognize or to orient any part of one's own body; caused by a parietal lobe lesion. Cf. somatotopagnosis. [auto- + G. *topos*, place, + G. *a-* priv. + gnōsis]

au•to•tox•ic (aw-tō-toks′ik). Relating to autointoxication.

au•to•trans•fu•sion (aw′tō-tranz-fyū′zhŭn). Withdrawal and reinjection/transfusion of the patient's own blood. Cf. autoinfusion.

au•to•trans•plant (aw-tō-tranz′plant). SYN autograft.

au•to•trans•plan•ta•tion (aw′tō-tranz-plan-tā′shŭn). The performance of an autograft.

au•to•troph (aw′tō-trōf). A microorganism that uses only inorganic materials as its source of nutrients; carbon dioxide serves as the sole carbon source. [auto- + G. *trophē*, nourishment]

au•to•tro•phic (aw-tō-trof′ik). **1.** Self-nourishing. The ability of an organism to produce food from inorganic compounds. **2.** Pertaining to an autotroph.

au•tox•i•da•tion (aw-tok-si-dā′shŭn). SYN autoxidation.

⌂**auxano-, auxo-, aux-.** Increase, *e.g.,* in size, intensity, speed. [G. *auxanō,* to increase]

aux·an·o·gram (awk-san′ō-gram). A plate culture of bacteria in which variable conditions are provided in order to determine the effect of these conditions on the growth of the bacteria. [auxano- + G. *gramma,* something written]

aux·an·o·graph·ic (awk′san-ō-graf′ik). Pertaining to auxanogram or auxanography.

aux·a·nog·ra·phy (awk-să-nog′ră-fē). The study, using auxanograms, of the effects of different conditions on the growth of bacteria.

aux·e·sis (awk-sē′sis). Increase in size, especially as in hypertrophy. [G. increase]

aux·il·ia·ry (og-zil′yă-rē). **1.** Functioning in an augmenting capacity; supplementary. **2.** Functioning as a subordinate; secondary.

aux·i·lyt·ic (awk′si-lit′ik). Increasing the destructive power of a lysin, or favoring lysis. [G. *auxō,* to increase, + *lysis,* dissolution]

⌂**auxo-.** SEE auxano-.

aux·o·chrome (awk′sō-krōm). The chemical group within a dye molecule by which the dye is bound to reactive end groups in tissues. [auxo- + G. *chrōma,* color]

aux·o·ton·ic (awk-sō-ton′ik). Denoting the condition in which a contracting muscle shortens against an increasing load. Cf. isometric (2), isotonic (3).

aux·o·troph (awk′sō-trōf). A mutant microorganism that requires some nutrient that is not required by the organism (prototroph) from which the mutant was derived. [auxo- + G. *trophē,* nourishment]

aux·o·tro·phic (awk-sō-trof′ik, -trō′fik). Pertaining to an auxotroph.

A–V arteriovenous; atrioventricular.

avas·cu·lar (ă-vas′kyū-ler, ā-). Without blood or lymphatic vessels; may be a normal state as in certain forms of cartilage, or the result of disease.

avas·cu·lar·i·za·tion (ă-vas′kyū-lar-ī-zā′shŭn, ā-). **1.** Expulsion of blood from a part, as by means of an Esmarch tourniquet or arterial compression. **2.** Loss of vascularity, as by scarring.

aVF, aVL, aVR Augmented electrocardiographic leads from the foot (left), left arm, and right arm, respectively.

avi·an (ā′vē-ăn). Pertaining to birds. [L. *avis,* bird]

avidity. A measure of the binding strength of a multivalent antibody to a multivalent antigen. SEE ALSO affinity.

avir·u·lent (ā-vir′yū-lent). Not virulent.

avi·ta·min·o·sis (ā-vī′tă-min-ō′sis). Properly, hypovitaminosis.

av·oir·du·pois (av′er-du-poyz′). A system of weights in which 16 ounces make a pound, equivalent of 453.59237 g. See Weights and Measures appendix. [Fr. to have weight, corrupted fr. O. Fr. *avoir,* property, + *de,* of, + *pois,* weight]

AVP antiviral *protein;* arginine *vasopressin.*

avul·sion (ă-vŭl′shŭn). A tearing away or forcible separation. Cf. evulsion. [L. *a-vello,* pp. *-vulsus,* to tear away]

  nerve a., the tearing away of a peripheral nerve

at its point of origin from its parent nerve due to traction.

AW atomic *weight.*

ax axis.

axen·ic (ā-zen′ik). Sterile, denoting especially a pure culture; *e.g.,* a protozoan culture free from bacteria. Also used to denote "germ-free" animals born and raised in a sterile environment. [G. *a-* priv. + *xenos,* foreign]

ax·es (ak′sēz). Plural of axis.

ax·i·al (ak′sē-ăl). **1.** Relating to an axis. SYN axile. **2.** Relating to or situated in the central part of the body, in the head and trunk as distinguished from the limbs, *e.g.,* axial skeleton. **3.** DENTISTRY relating to or parallel with the long axis of a tooth. **4.** RADIOLOGY an axial image is one obtained by rotating around the axis of the body, producing a transverse planar image, *i.e.,* a section transverse to the axis.

ax·if·u·gal (ak-sif′yū-găl). Extending away from an axis or axon. SYN axofugal. [L. *axis + fugio,* to flee from]

ax·ile (ak′sīl). SYN axial (1).

ax·il·la, gen. and pl. **ax·il·lae** (ak′sil′ă, ak-sil′ē). The space below the shoulder joint, bounded by the pectoralis major anteriorly, the latissimus dorsi posteriorly, the serratus anterior medially, and the humerus laterally; it has a superior opening between the clavicle, scapula, and first rib (cervicoaxillary canal), and an inferior opening covered by the axillary fascia; it contains the axillary artery and vein, the infraclavicular part of the brachial plexus, axillary lymph nodes and vessels, and areolar tissue. SYN axillary cavity. [L.]

ax·il·lary (ak′sil-ār-ē). Relating to the axilla. SYN alar (2).

⌂**axio-.** An axis. SEE ALSO axo-. [L. *axis*]

ax·i·o·plasm (ak′sē-ō-plazm). SYN axoplasm.

ax·i·o·ver·sion (ak′sē-ō-ver′zhŭn). Abnormal inclination of the long axis of a tooth.

ax·ip·e·tal (ak-sip′ĕ-tăl). SYN centripetal (2). [L. *axis + peto,* to seek]

ax·is (ax), pl. **ax·es** (ak′sis, ak′sēz). **1.** A straight line passing through a spherical body between its two poles, and about which the body may revolve. **2.** The central line of the body or any of its parts. **3.** The vertebral column. **4.** The central nervous system. **5** [NA]. The second cervical vertebra. SYN epistropheus, vertebra dentata. **6.** An artery that divides, immediately upon its origin, into a number of branches, *e.g.,* celiac axis. SEE trunk. [L. axle, axis]

  basibregmatic a., a line extending from the basion to the bregma.

  basicranial a., a line drawn from the basion to the midpoint of the sphenoethmoidal suture.

  basifacial a., a line drawn from the subnasal point to the midpoint of the sphenoethmoidal suture. SYN facial a.

  biauricular a., a straight line joining the two auricles.

  cephalocaudal a., Long axis of the body; the imaginary straight line in the median plane which runs from the apex of the skull through the center of the perineum and continuing between the lower limbs.

cerebrospinal a., the central nervous system; the brain and spinal cord.

electrical a., the net direction of the electromotive forces developed in the heart during its activation, usually represented in the frontal plane.

facial a., SYN basifacial a.

optic a., the a. of the eye connecting the anterior and posterior poles; it usually diverges from the visual a. by five degrees or more.

pelvic a., a hypothetical curved line joining the center point of each of the four planes of the pelvis, marking the center of the pelvic cavity at every level. SYN plane of pelvic canal.

principal optic a., a line passing through the center of the lens of a refracting system at right angles to its surface.

sagittal a., DENTISTRY the line in the frontal plane around which the working side condyle rotates during mandibular movement.

secondary a., any ray passing through the optical center of a lens.

transverse horizontal a., an imaginary line around which the mandible may rotate through the horizontal plane.

visual a., the straight line extending from the object seen, through the center of the pupil, to the macula lutea of the retina.

△**axo-.** Axis; axion. [G. *axōn*, axis]

ax•o•ax•on•ic (ak′sō-ak-son′ik). Relating to synaptic contact between the axon of one nerve cell and that of another. SEE synapse.

ax•o•den•drit•ic (ak′sō-den-drit′ik). Pertaining to the synaptic relationship of an axon with a dendrite of another neuron. SEE synapse.

ax•of•u•gal (ak-sof′yū-găl). SYN axifugal. [axo- + L. *fugio*, to flee]

ax•o•lem•ma (ak′sō-lem′ă). The plasma membrane of the axon. SYN Mauthner's sheath. [axo- + G. *lemma*, husk]

ax•ol•y•sis (ak-sol′i-sis). Destruction or dissolution of a nerve axon. [axo- + G. *lysis*, dissolution]

ax•on (ak′son). The single process of a nerve cell that under normal conditions conducts nervous impulses away from the cell body and its remaining processes (dendrites). A.'s 0.5 μm thick or over are generally enveloped by a segmented myelin sheath provided by oligodendroglia cells (in brain and spinal cord) or Schwann cells (in peripheral nerves). Nerve cells synaptically transmit impulses to other nerve cells or to effector cells (muscle cells, gland cells) exclusively by way of the synaptic terminals of their a. [G. *axōn*, axis]

ax•o•nal (ak′sō-năl). Pertaining to an axon.

ax•o•neme (ak′sō-nēm). **1.** The central thread running in the axis of the chromosome. **2.** SYN axial *filament*. **3.** The distinctive array of microtubules in the core of eukaryotic cilia and flagella comprising a central pair surrounded by a sheaf of nine doublet microtubules. [axo- + G. *nēma*, a thread]

ax•on•og•ra•phy (ak-sŏ-nog′ră-fē). The recording of electrical changes in axons.

ax•on•ot•me•sis (ak′son-ot-mē′sis). Interruption of the axons of a nerve followed by complete degeneration of the peripheral segment, without severance of the supporting structure of the nerve; such a lesion may result from pinching, crushing, or prolonged pressure. SEE ALSO neurapraxia, neurotmesis. [axon + G. *tmēsis*, a cutting]

ax•op•e•tal (ak-sop′ĕ-tăl). Extending in a direction toward an axon. [axo- + L. *peto*, to seek]

ax•o•plasm (ak′sō-plazm). Neuroplasm of the axon. SYN axioplasm.

ax•o•so•mat•ic (ak-sō-sō-mat′ik). Relating to the synaptic relationship of an axon with a nerve cell body. SEE synapse. [axo- + G. *sōma*, body]

aze•o•trope (ā-zē′ō-trōp). A mixture of two or more liquids that boils without change in proportion of the liquids, either in the liquid or the vapor phase. [G. *a-* priv. + *zeō*, to boil, + *tropos*, a turning]

aze•o•tro•pic (ā-zē-ō-trop′ik). Denoting or characteristic of an azeotrope.

az•i•do•thy•mi•dine (AZT) (az′i-dō-thī′mi-dēn). SEE AZT.

△**azo-.** Prefix denoting the presence in a molecule of the group ≡C–N=N–C≡. Cf. diazo-. [Fr. *azote*, nitrogen]

az•ole (az′ōl). SYN pyrrole.

a•zo•o•sper•mia (ā-zō-ō-sper′mē-ă). Absence of living spermatozoa in the semen; failure of spermatogenesis. [G. *a-* priv. + *zōon*, animal, + *sperma*, seed]

az•o•pro•tein (az-ō-prō′tēn). Any of the modified proteins produced by treatment with diazonium derivatives of various aromatic amines; used to elicit antibody formation and demonstrate antibody specificity.

az•o•te•mia (az-ō-tē′mē-ă). SYN uremia. [azo- (azote) + G. *haima*, blood]

az•o•tem•ic (az-ō-tēm′ik). Relating to azotemia.

azo•tu•ria (az-ō-tūr′ē-ă). An increased elimination of urea in the urine. [azo- (azote) + G. *ouron*, urine]

AZT Azidothymidine; a thymidine analogue that is an inhibitor of replication of HIV virus *in vitro* and is used in the management of AIDS.

az•ure (azh′yūr). A term for a group of basic blue methylthionine or phenothiazine dyes; used as biological stains, especially in blood and nuclear stains.

az•u•res•in (azh′yū-res′in). A complex of azure A and carbacrylic resin; used as an indicator for the detection of gastric achlorhydria without intubation.

az•u•ro•phil, az•u•ro•phile (azh′yū-rō-fil, -fīl). Staining readily with an azure dye, denoting especially the hyperchromatin and reddish purple granules of certain blood cells. [azure + G. *philos*, fond]

azy•go•gram (az′i-gō-gram). Radiographic demonstration of the azygos venous system after injection of contrast medium. [azygos + G. *gramma*, a writing]

azy•gog•ra•phy (az′i-gog′ră-fē). Radiography of the azygos venous system after injection of contrast medium.

az•y•gos (az′ī-gos). **1.** An unpaired (azygous) anatomical structure. **2.** SYN azygos *vein*. [G. *a-* priv. + *zygon*, a yoke]

az•y•gous (az′ī-gŭs, ă-zī′gŭs). Unpaired; single. [G. *azygos*]

B

β (bā'ta). beta. SEE beta.

β⁺. positron.

B 1. boron; aspartic acid; bromouridine; second substrate in a multisubstrate enzyme-catalyzed reaction. **2.** As a subscript, refers to barometric pressure.

b. 1. As a subscript, refers to blood. **2.** Abbreviation for bis [L.], twice.

Ba barium.

Ba·be·sia (bă-bē'zē-ă). The economically most important genus of the family Babesiidae; characterized by multiplication in host red blood cells to form pairs and tetrads; it causes babesiosis (piroplasmosis) in most types of domestic animals, and two species cause disease in splenectomized or normal people; vectors are ixodid or argasid ticks. [V. *Babès*]

B. micro'ti, a malaria-like protozoan naturally parasitizing certain rodents; a number of human cases have been reported from Nantucket and Martha's Vineyard islands and nearby coastal New England. The local tick vector is *Ixodes dammini,* whose numbers and infection levels have greatly increased in recent years with the increase in the deer population, which serves as an abundant blood source for *I. dammini.* SEE ALSO *Borrelia burgdorferi.*

ba·be·si·o·sis (bă-bē'zē-ō'sis). A disease caused by infection with a species of *Babesia,* the infection being transmitted by ticks. In animals, the disease is characterized by fever, malaise, listlessness, severe anemia, and hemoglobulinuria; the death rate frequently is higher in adult than in young animals.

bovine b., an infectious disease of cattle caused by *Babesia* species and transmitted by ticks. SYN tick fever (3).

ba·by (bā'bē). An infant; a newborn child.

blue b., a child born cyanotic because of a congenital cardiac or pulmonary defect causing incomplete oxygenation of the blood.

blueberry muffin b., jaundice and purpura, especially of the face in the newborn, which may result from intrauterine viral infection.

test-tube b., popular term for a b. born after uterine implantation of a maternal ovum fertilized *in vitro.*

bac·cate (bak'āt). Berry-like. [L. *bacca,* berry]

bac·ci·form (bak'sĭ-fōrm). Berry-shaped. [L. *bacca,* berry]

Ba·cil·la·ce·ae (bă-si-lā'sē-ē). A family of aerobic or facultatively anaerobic, sporeforming, ordinarily motile bacteria (order Eubacteriales) containing Gram-positive rods. Some species are pathogenic. Ordinarily two genera, *Bacillus* and *Clostridium,* are included. The type genus is *Bacillus.*

ba·cil·lar, bac·il·la·ry (bas'i-lar, bas'i-lā-rē). Shaped like a rod; consisting of rods or rodlike elements.

bac·il·le·mia (bas-i-lē'mē-ă). The presence of rod-shaped bacteria in the circulating blood. [bacillus + G. *haima,* blood]

ba·cil·li (bă-sil'ī). Plural of bacillus.

ba·cil·li·form (ba-sil'i-fōrm). Rod-shaped. [L. *bacillus,* a rod, + *forma,* form]

ba·cil·lin (ba-sil'in). An antibiotic substance produced by *Bacillus subtilis.*

bac·il·lo·sis (bas-i-lō'sis). A general infection with bacilli.

bac·il·lu·ria (bas-i-lū'rē-ă). The presence of bacilli in the urine. [bacillus + G. *ouron,* urine]

Ba·cil·lus (ba-sil'ŭs). A genus of aerobic or facultatively anaerobic, sporeforming, ordinarily motile bacteria containing Gram-positive rods. Motile cells are peritrichous. A few species are animal pathogens; some species produce antibodies. The type species is *B. subtilis.* [L. dim. of *baculus,* rod, staff]

B. ce'reus, a species that causes an emetic type and a diarrheal type of food poisoning in humans, and can cause infections in humans and other mammals.

B. sphae'ricus, a species that is an insect pathogen and that has been associated with human and other mammalian infections, especially in compromised hosts.

ba·cil·lus, pl. **ba·cil·li** (ba-sil'ŭs, -ī). **1.** A vernacular term used to refer to any member of the genus *Bacillus.* **2.** Term formerly used to refer to any rod-shaped bacterium. [L. dim. of *baculus,* a rod, staff]

Bang's b., SYN *Brucella abortus.*

coliform bacilli (kō'li-fōrm, kol'i-fōrm), common name for *Escherichia coli* that is used as an indicator of fecal contamination of water, measured in terms of coliform count. Occasionally used to refer to all lactose-fermenting enteric bacteria.

comma b., SYN *Vibrio cholerae.*

Ducrey's b., SYN *Haemophilus ducreyi.*

Flexner's b., SYN *Shigella flexneri.*

gas b., SYN *Clostridium perfringens.*

Hansen's b., SYN *Mycobacterium leprae.*

Koch's b., (1) SYN *Mycobacterium tuberculosis.* **(2)** SYN *Vibrio cholerae.*

Koch-Weeks b., SYN *Haemophilus aegypticus.*

Pfeiffer's b., SYN *Haemophilus influenzae.*

Shiga-Kruse b., SYN *Shigella dysenteriae.*

Sonne b., SYN *Shigella sonnei.*

tubercle b., (1) SYN *Mycobacterium tuberculosis.* **(2)** SYN *Mycobacterium bovis.* **(3)** SYN *Mycobacterium avium.*

typhoid b., SYN *Salmonella typhi.*

back·ache (bak'āk). Nonspecific term used to describe back pain; generally refers to pain below the cervical level.

back·bone (bak'bōn). SYN vertebral *column.*

back·cross (bak'kros). Mating of an individual heterozygous at one or more loci to an individual homozygous at the same loci.

back-extrapolation. A process to determine the onset of exhalation during the forced expiratory vital capacity maneuver; excessive back extrapolation volume (usually expressed as a percentage of the forced vital capacity) is an indication of hesitation or false starting.

back·flow. The reversal of the normal flow of a current. SEE ALSO regurgitation.

pyelovenous b., retrograde movement of fluid (urine or injected contrast materials) from renal pelvis into renal venous system. This occurs under conditions of distal obstruction or injection of solutions into renal collecting system.

back·pro·jec·tion (bak′prō-jek′shŭn). In computed tomography or other imaging techniques requiring reconstruction from multiple projections, an algorithm for calculating the contribution of each voxel of the structure to the measured ray data, in order to generate an image; the oldest and simplest method of image reconstruction.

bac·te·re·mia (bak-tēr-ē′mē-ă). The presence of viable bacteria in the circulating blood; may be transient following trauma such as dental or other iatrogenic manipulation or may be persistent or recurrent as a result of infection. SYN bacteriemia. [bacteria + G. *haima,* blood]

⌂**bacteri-.** SEE bacterio-.

bac·te·ria (bak-tēr′ē-ă). Plural of bacterium.

blue-green b., SEE Cyanobacteria.

bac·te·ri·al (bak-tēr′ē-ăl). Relating to bacteria.

bac·te·ri·cid·al (bak-tēr′i-sī′dăl). Causing the death of bacteria. Cf. bacteriostatic. SYN bacteriocidal.

bac·te·ri·cide (bak-tēr′i-sīd). An agent that destroys bacteria. SYN bacteriocide. [bacteria + L. *caedo,* to kill]

bac·ter·id (bak′ter-id). **1.** A recurrent or persistent eruption of discrete sterile pustules of the palms and soles, thought to be an allergic response to bacterial infection at a remote site. **2.** A dissemination of a previously localized bacterial skin infection. [bacteria + -*id* (1)]

bac·te·ri·e·mia (bak-tēr-ē-ē′mē-ă). SYN bacteremia.

⌂**bacterio-, bacteri-.** Bacteria. [see bacterium]

bac·te·ri·o·cid·al (bak-tēr′ē-ō-sī′dăl). SYN bactericidal.

bac·ter·i·o·cide (bak-tēr′ē-ō-sīd). SYN bactericide.

bac·te·ri·o·cid·in (bak-tēr′ē-ō-sī′din). Antibody having bactericidal activity.

bac·te·ri·o·cin·o·gens (bak-tēr′ē-ō-sin′ō-jenz). SYN bacteriocinogenic *plasmids,* under *plasmid.*

bac·te·ri·o·cins (bak-tēr′ē-ō-sinz). Proteins produced by certain bacteria that exert a lethal effect on closely related bacteria; in general, b.'s have a narrower range of activity than antibiotics do and are more potent.

bac·te·ri·o·gen·ic (bak-tēr′ē-ō-jen′ik). Caused by bacteria.

bac·te·ri·o·log·ic, bac·te·ri·o·log·i·cal (bak′tēr-ē-ō-loj′ik, -i-kăl). Relating to bacteria or to bacteriology.

bac·te·ri·ol·o·gist (bak′ter-ē-ol′ŏ-jist). One who primarily studies or works with bacteria.

bac·te·ri·ol·o·gy (bak-tēr-ē-ol′ŏ-jē). The branch of science concerned with the study of bacteria. [bacterio- + G. *logos,* study]

bac·te·ri·o·ly·sin (bak-tēr-ē-ol′i-sin). Specific antibody that combines with bacterial cells (*i.e.,* antigen) and, in the presence of complement, causes lysis or dissolution of the cells.

bac·te·ri·ol·y·sis (bak-tēr-ē-ol′i-sis). The dissolution of bacteria, *e.g.,* by means of hypotonic solutions or by specific antibody and complement. [bacterio- + G. *lysis,* dissolution]

bac·te·ri·o·lyt·ic (bak-tēr-ē-ō-lit′ik). Pertaining to lytic destruction of bacteria; manifesting the ability to cause dissolution of bacterial cells.

bac·te·ri·o·pexy (bak-tēr′ē-ō-pek-sē). Immobilization of bacteria by phagocytic cells. [bacterio- + G. *pēxis,* fixation]

bac·te·ri·o·phage (bak-tēr′ē-ō-fāj). A virus with specific affinity for bacteria. B.'s have been found in essentially all groups of bacteria; like other viruses they contain either RNA or DNA (but never both) and vary in structure from simple to complex; their relationships to host bacteria are specific and may be genetically intimate. B.'s are named after the bacterial species, group, or strain for which they are specific, *e.g.,* corynebacteriophage, coliphage. SEE ALSO coliphage. SYN phage. [bacterio- + G. *phagō,* to eat]

defective b., a temperate b. mutant whose genome does not contain all of the normal components and cannot become a fully infectious virus, yet can replicate indefinitely in the bacterial genome as defective probacteriophage; many defective b.'s are mediators of transduction.

mature b., the complete, infective form of b.

temperate b., b. whose genome incorporates with, and replicates with, that of the host bacterium; dissociation (and resultant development of vegetative b.) occurs at a slow rate resulting occasionally in lysis of a bacterium and release of mature b., thus rendering the bacterial culture capable of inducing general lysis if transferred to a culture of a susceptible bacterial strain.

vegetative b., the form of b. in which the b. nucleic acid (lacking its coat) multiplies freely within the host bacterium, independently of bacterial multiplication.

virulent b., a b. that regularly causes lysis of the bacteria that it infects.

bac·te·ri·op·so·nin (bak-tēr-ē-op′sō-nin). An opsonin acting upon bacteria.

bac·te·ri·o·sis (bak-tēr-ē-ō′sis). A localized or generalized bacterial infection.

bac·te·ri·o·stat·ic (bak-tēr′ē-ō-stat′ik). Inhibiting or retarding the growth of bacteria.

bac·te·ri·um, pl. **bac·te·ria** (bak-tēr′ē-ŭm, -ă). A unicellular prokaryotic microorganism that usually multiplies by cell division and has a cell wall that provides a constancy of form; may be aerobic or anaerobic, motile or nonmotile, and free-living, saprophytic, parasitic, or pathogenic. SEE ALSO Cyanobacteria. [Mod. L. fr. G. *baktērion,* dim. of *baktron,* a staff]

lysogenic b., (1) a b. in the symbiotic condition in which its genome includes the genome (probacteriophage) of a temperate bacteriophage; in occasional instances the probacteriophage dissociates from the bacterial genome, develops into vegetative bacteriophage, and then matures, causing lysis of the respective host b. and release into the culture medium of infective temperate bacteriophage; (2) formerly, a pseudolysogenic bacterial strain, *i.e.,* a "carrier" strain of bacteriophage of low infectivity.

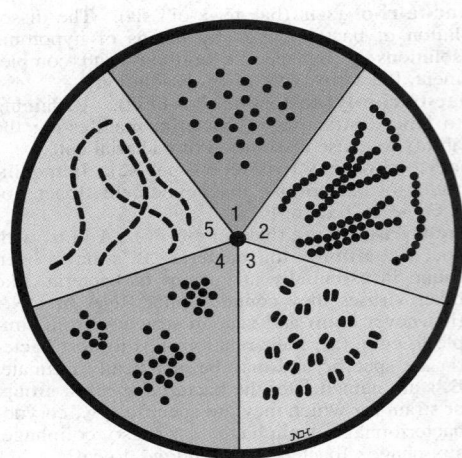

bacteria: (1) cocci, (2) streptococci, (3) diplococci, (4) staphylococci, (5) bacilli

bac•te•ri•u•ria (bak-tēr-ē-ū′rē-ă). The presence of bacteria in the urine.

Bac•te•roi•des (bak-ter-oy′dēz). A genus of obligate anaerobic, non–spore-forming bacteria containing Gram-negative rods. They are part of the normal flora of the oral, respiratory, intestinal, and urogenital cavities of humans and animals; some species are pathogenic. The type species is *B. fragilis.* [G. *bacterion* + *eidos,* form]

B. capillo′sus, a species isolated from human cysts and wounds, the mouth, and feces.

B. di′siens, a species isolated from abdominal and urogenital infections, and from the mouth.

B. frag′ilis, a species that is one of the predominant organisms in the lower intestinal tract of man and other animals; also found in specimens from appendicitis, peritonitis, rectal abscesses, pilonidal cysts, surgical wounds, and lesions of the urogenital tract; it is the type species of the genus *B.*

B. melaninogenicus, SYN *Prevotella melaninogenica.*

B. o′ris, a species isolated from the gingival crevice, systemic infections, face, neck, and chest abscesses, wound drainages, and blood and various bodily fluids.

B. thetaiotamicron, a species implicated in intra-abdominal infections.

BAER Brainstem auditory evoked response. SEE evoked *response.*

bag. A pouch, sac, or receptacle. [A.S. *baelg*]

Ambu b., proprietary name for a self-reinflating b. with nonrebreathing valves to provide positive pressure ventilation during resuscitation with oxygen or air.

breathing b., a collapsible reservoir from which gases are inhaled and into which gases may be exhaled during general anesthesia or artificial ventilation. SYN reservoir b.

colostomy b., a bag worn over an artificial anus to collect feces.

Douglas b., a large b. in which expired gas is collected for several minutes to determine oxygen consumption in humans under conditions of actual work. [C.G. Douglas]

Politzer b., a pear-shaped rubber b. used for forcing air through the auditory tube by the Politzer method.

reservoir b., SYN breathing b.

b. of waters, colloquialism for the amniotic sac and contained amniotic fluid.

bag•as•so•sis (bag-ă-sō′sis). Extrinsic allergic alveolitis following exposure to sugar cane fiber (bagasse); variously attributed to inhalation of spores of soil fungi and, particularly, thermophilic actinomycetes.

BAL bronchoalveolar *lavage.*

△**balan-.** SEE balano-.

bal•ance (bal′ans). 1. An apparatus for weighing; *e.g.,* scales. 2. The normal state of action and reaction between two or more parts or organs of the body. 3. Quantities, concentrations, and proportionate amounts of bodily constituents. 4. The difference between intake and utilization, storage, or excretion of a substance by the body. SEE ALSO equilibrium. [L. *bi-,* twice, + *lanx,* dish, scale]

acid-base b., the normal b. between acid and base in the blood plasma, expressed in the hydrogen ion concentration or pH, resulting from the relative amounts of acidic and basic materials ingested and produced by body metabolism, compared to the relative amounts of acidic and basic materials excreted from the body and consumed by body metabolism; the normal state of acid-base b. is not one of neutrality, with equal concentrations of hydrogen and hydroxyl ions, but a more alkaline state with a certain excess of hydroxyl ions.

nitrogen b., the difference between the total nitrogen intake by an organism and its total nitrogen loss. A normal, healthy adult has a zero nitrogen b.; the b. may become negative (more excreted than taken in).

ba•lan•ic (ba-lan′ik). Relating to the glans penis or glans clitoridis. [G. *balanos,* acorn, glans]

bal•a•ni•tis (bal-ă-nī′tis). Inflammation of the glans penis or clitoris. [G. *balanos,* acorn, glans, + *-itis,* inflammation]

△**balano-, balan-.** Glans penis. [G. *balanos,* acorn, glans]

bal•a•no•plas•ty (bal′an-ō-plas-tē). Surgical reconstruction of the glans penis. [balano- + G. *plastos,* formed]

bal•a•no•pos•thi•tis (bal′an-ō-pos-thī′tis). Inflammation of the glans penis and overlying prepuce. [balano- + G. *posthē,* prepuce, + *-itis,* inflammation]

bal•an•ti•di•a•sis (bal′an-ti-dī′ă-sis). A disease caused by the presence of *Balantidium coli* in the large intestine; characterized by diarrhea, dysentery, and occasionally ulceration.

Ba•lan•ti•di•um (bal-an-tid′ē-ŭm). A genus of ciliates (family Balantidiidae) found in the digestive tract of vertebrates and invertebrates. [G. *balantidion,* dim of *ballantion,* a bag]

B. co′li, a very large parasitic ciliate species, usually 50 to 80 μm in length, reaching up to 200 μm in pigs, found in the cecum or large intestine, swimming actively in the lumen; usually harmless in man but may invade and ulcerate the intestinal wall, producing a colitis resembling amebic dysentery.

bald•ness (bawld'nes). SYN alopecia.

ball. **1.** A round mass. SEE bezoar. **2.** In veterinary medicine, a large pill or bolus.

  food b., SYN phytobezoar.

  fungus b., a compact mass of fungal mycelium and cellular debris, 1 to 5 cm in diameter, residing within a lung cavity; usually produced by *Aspergillus fumigatus*. SEE ALSO aspergilloma (2).

  hair b., SYN trichobezoar.

bal•lis•mus (bal-iz'mŭs). A type of involuntary movement affecting the proximal limb musculature, manifested as jerking, flinging movements of the extremity; caused by a lesion of or near the contralateral subthalamic nucleus. Usually only one side of the body is involved, resulting in hemiballismus. [G. *ballismos*, a jumping about]

bal•loon (bă-lūn). **1.** An inflatable spherical or ovoid device used to retain tubes or catheters in, or provide support to, various body structures. **2.** A distensible device used to stretch or occlude a stenotic viscus or blood vessel. **3.** To distend a body cavity with a gas or fluid to facilitate its examination, dilate a structure, or occlude its lumen. [Fr. *ballon*, fr. It. *ballone*, fr. *balla*, ball, fr. Germanic]

  angioplasty b., a b. near the tip of an angiographic catheter, designed to distend narrowed vessels. SEE balloon-tip *catheter.*

  intra-aortic b., an externally and intermittently inflatable balloon placed into the descending aorta and which, on activation during diastole, augments blood pressure and organ perfusion by its pulsatile thrust; then, on deflation, decreases the cardiac work with each systole—the so-called counterpulsation principle—by reducing cardiac afterload.

bal•loon•sep•tos•to•my (bă-lūn'sep-tos'tō-mē). Creation of an artificial interatrial septal defect by cardiac catheterization during which an inflated balloon is pulled across the interatrial septum through the foramen ovale; used in cases of transposition of the great vessels and tricuspid atresia.

bal•lotte•ment (bal-ot-maw'). Maneuver used in physical examination to estimate the size, shape, or consistency of an organ not near the surface, particularly when there is ascites, by a rhythmic, thrusting motion of the hand or fingers similar to that involved in bouncing a ball. [Fr. *balloter*, to toss up]

balm (bawlm). **1.** An ointment, especially a fragrant one. **2.** A soothing application. [L. *balsamum*, fr. G. *balsamon*, the balsam tree]

band. **1.** Any appliance or part of an apparatus that encircles or binds a part of the body. SEE ALSO zone. **2.** Any ribbon-shaped or cordlike anatomical structure that encircles or binds another structure or that connects two or more parts. SEE fascia, line, linea, stria, tenia. **3.** A narrow strip containing one or more macromolecules (on occasions, small molecules) detected in electrophoresis or certain types of chromatography.

  A b.'s, the dark-staining anisotropic cross striations in the myofibrils of muscle fibers, comprising regions of overlapping thick (myosin) and thin (actin) filaments.

  amniotic b.'s, strands of amniotic tissue adherent to the embryo or fetus; they may cause constriction of embryonic limbs. SEE ALSO congenital *amputation.* SYN constriction ring (2).

  chromosome b., a region of darker or contrasting staining across the width of a chromosome; the pattern of b.'s is characteristic for most chromosomes. SEE banding.

  H b., the paler area in the center of the A b. of a striated muscle fiber, comprising the central portion of thick (myosin) filaments that are not overlapped by thin (actin) filaments.

  I b., a light b. on each side of the Z line of striated muscle fibers, comprising a region of the sarcomere where thin (actin) filaments are not overlapped by thick (myosin) filaments.

  M b., SYN M *line.*

  matrix b., a metal or plastic b. secured around the crown of a tooth to confine restorative material to be adapted into a prepared cavity.

  oligoclonal b., small discrete b.'s in the gamma globulin region of the spinal fluid electrophoresis, indicating local central nervous system production of IgG; b.'s are frequently seen in patients with multiple sclerosis but can also be found in other diseases of the central nervous system including syphilis, sarcoidosis, and chronic infection or inflammation.

  ventricular b. of larynx, SYN vestibular *fold.*

  Z b., SYN Z *line.*

ban•dage (ban'dij). **1.** A piece of cloth or other material, of varying shape and size, applied to a body part to make compression, absorb drainage, prevent motion, retain surgical dressings. **2.** To cover a body part by application of a b.

  adhesive b., a dressing of plain absorbent gauze affixed to plastic or fabric coated with a pressure-sensitive adhesive.

  Barton's b., a figure-of-8 b. supporting the mandible below and anteriorly; used in mandibular fracture.

  capeline b., a b. covering the head or an amputation stump like a cap. [L. *capella*, a cap]

  cravat b., a b. made by bringing the point of a triangular b. to the middle of the base and then folding lengthwise to the desired width.

  demigauntlet b., a gauntlet b. that covers only the hand, leaving the fingers exposed.

  Desault's b., a b. for fracture of the clavicle; the elbow is bound to the side, with a pad placed in the axilla.

  elastic b., a b. containing stretchable material; used to make local pressure.

  figure-of-8 b., a b. applied alternately to two parts, usually two segments of a limb above and below the joint, in such a way that the turns describe the figure 8; used primarily for the treatment of fractures of the clavicle.

  gauntlet b., a figure-of-8 b. covering the hand and fingers.

  plaster b., a roller b. impregnated with plaster of Paris and applied moist; used to make a rigid dressing for a fracture or diseased joint.

  roller b., a strip of material, of variable width,

rolled into a compact cylinder to facilitate its application.

spica b., successive strips of material applied to the body and the first part of a limb, or to the hand and a finger, which overlap slightly in a V to resemble an ear of grain. [L. *spica,* ear of grain]

spiral b., an oblique b. encircling a limb, the successive turns overlapping those preceding.

suspensory b., a bag of expansile fabric for supporting the scrotum and its contents.

triangular b., a piece of cloth cut in the shape of a right-angled triangle, used as a sling.

band•ing. The process of differential staining of chromosomes to reveal characteristic patterns of bands that permit identification of individual chromosomes and recognition of missing segments; each of the 22 pairs of human chromosomes and the X and Y chromosomes has an identifying b. pattern.

bar. 1. A unit of pressure equal to 1 megadyne (10^6 dyne) per cm^2 in the CGS system, 0.9869233 atmosphere, or 10^5 Pa (N/m^2) in the SI system. **2.** A metal segment of greater length than width that serves to connect two or more parts of a removable partial denture. **3.** A segment of tissue or bone that unites two or more similar structures.

Mercier's b., SYN interureteric *fold.*

terminal b., dark spots or b. (depending on the plane of section) in the lateral boundary between the apical ends of columnar epithelial cells.

bar•ag•no•sis (bar-ag-nō'sis). Loss of ability to appreciate the weight of objects held in the hand, or to differentiate objects of different weights. When the primary senses are intact, caused by a lesion of the contralateral parietal lobe. [G. *baros,* weight + *a-* priv., + *gnōsis,* a knowing]

bar•bi•tu•rism (bar'bi-chyūr-izm). Chronic poisoning by any of the derivatives of barbituric acid; symptoms include cutaneous eruption, chills, fever, and headache.

bar•bo•tage (bar-bō-tahzh'). A method of spinal anesthesia in which a portion of the anesthetic solution is injected into the cerebrospinal fluid, which is then aspirated back into the syringe and reinjected. [Fr. *barboter,* to dabble]

bar•es•the•sia (bar-es-thē'zē-ă). SYN pressure *sense.* [G. *baros,* weight, + *aisthēsis,* sensation]

bar•es•the•si•om•e•ter (bar'es-thē'zē-om'ĕ-ter). An instrument for measuring the pressure sense. [G. *baros,* weight, + *aisthēsis,* sensation, + *metron,* measure]

bar•i•at•ric (bar-ē-at'rik). Relating to bariatrics.

bar•i•at•rics (bar-ē-at'riks). That branch of medicine concerned with the management of obesity. [G. *baros,* weight, + *iatreia,* medical treatment]

bar•i•um (Ba) (ba'rē-ŭm, bā'rē-ŭm). A metallic, alkaline, divalent earth element; atomic no. 56, atomic wt. 137.327. Salts are often used in diagnosis. [G. *barys,* heavy]

b. swallow, oral administration of b. sulfate suspension for radiographic investigation of the hypopharynx and esophagus.

⚠**baro-.** Weight, pressure. [G. *baros,* weight]

bar•o•cep•tor (bar'ō-sep-ter, -tōr). SYN baroreceptor.

bar•og•no•sis (bar'og-nō'sis). Ability to appreciate the weight of objects, or to differentiate objects of different weights. [G. *baros,* weight, + *gnōsis,* knowledge]

bar•o•phil•ic (bar'ō-fil'ik). Thriving under high environmental pressure; applied to microorganisms. [G. *baros,* weight, + *phileō,* to love]

bar•o•re•cep•tor (bar'ō-rē-sep'ter, -tōr). **1.** In general, any sensor of pressure changes. **2.** Sensory nerve ending in the wall of the auricles of the heart, vena cava, aortic arch, and carotid sinus, sensitive to stretching of the wall resulting from increased pressure from within, and functioning as the receptor of central reflex mechanisms that tend to reduce that pressure. SYN baroceptor, pressoreceptor. [G. *baros,* weight, + receptor]

bar•o•re•flex (bar-ō-rē'fleks). A reflex triggered by stimulation of a baroreceptor.

bar•o•si•nus•i•tis (bar'ō-sī-nus-ī'tis). SYN aerosinusitis. [G. *baros,* weight, pressure, + sinusitis]

bar•o•stat (bar'ō-stat). A pressure-regulating device or structure. [G., *baros,* weight, pressure, + *statos,* made to stand]

bar•o•tax•is (bar-ō-tak'sis). Reaction of living tissue to changes in pressure. [G. *baros,* weight, + *taxis,* order]

bar•o•ti•tis me•dia (bar-ō-tī'tis mē'dē-ă). SYN aerotitis media.

bar•o•trau•ma (băr'ō-traw'mă). **1.** Injury to the middle ear or paranasal sinuses, resulting from imbalance between ambient pressure and that within the affected cavity. **2.** Lung injury that occurs when a patient is on a ventilator and is subjected to excessive airway pressure (pulmonary barotrauma). [G. *baros,* weight, + trauma]

bar•ri•er (bar'ē-er). **1.** An obstacle or impediment. **2.** PSYCHIATRY a conflictual agent that blocks behavior which could help resolve a personal struggle. [M.E., fr. O.Fr. *barriere,* fr. L.L. *barraria*]

blood-air b., the material intervening between alveolar air and the blood; it consists of a nonstructural film or surfactant, alveolar epithelium, basement lamina, and endothelium.

blood-aqueous b., a selectively permeable b. between the capillary bed in the ciliary body and the aqueous humor.

blood-brain b. (BBB), a selective mechanism opposing the passage of most ions and large-molecular weight compounds from the blood to brain tissue.

blood-cerebrospinal fluid b., blood-CSF b., a b. located at the tight junctions which surround and connect the cuboidal epithelial cells on the surface of the choroid plexus; capillaries and connective tissue stroma of the choroid do not represent a b. to protein tracers or dyes.

placental b., SYN placental *membrane.*

bar•tho•lin•i•tis (bar-tō-lin-ī'tis). Inflammation of a vulvovaginal (Bartholin's) gland.

Bar•ton•el•la (bar-tō-nel'ă). A genus of bacteria closely resembling *Rickettsia* in staining properties, morphology, and mode of transmission between hosts. Organisms usually reside extracellularly in arthropod hosts and intracellularly in mammalian hosts. The type of species is *Rochalimaea quintana.* [A. L. *Barton*]

B. bacillifor′mis, a species found in the blood, lymph nodes, spleen, and liver in Oroya fever and in blood and eruptive elements in verruga peruana.

B. henselae, a recently recognized species, formerly classified as a riskettsialike organism in the genus *Rochalimaea;* causes bacillary angiomatosis, particularly in immunocompromised persons, and a form of cat-scratch disease.

bar•ton•el•lo•sis (bar-tō-nel-ō′sis). A disease, endemic in certain valleys of the Andes in Peru, Chile, Ecuador, Bolivia, and Colombia, caused by *Bartonella bacilliformis,* which is transmitted by the bite of the nocturnally biting sandfly, *Phlebotomus verrucarum;* occurs in three forms: 1) Oroya fever; 2) verruga peruana; 3) a combination or sequence of these.

△**baryto-.** Prefix indicating the presence of barium in a mineral.

ba•sad (bā′sad). In a direction toward the base of any object or structure.

ba•sal (bā′săl). **1.** Situated nearer the base of a pyramid-shaped organ in relation to a specific reference point; opposite of apical. **2.** In dentistry, denoting the floor of a cavity in the grinding surface of a tooth. **3.** Denoting a standard or reference state of a function, as a basis for comparison.

base (bās). **1.** The lower part or bottom; the part of a pyramidal or cone-shaped structure opposite the apex; the foundation. SYN basis [NA]. **2.** In pharmacy, the chief ingredient of a mixture. **3.** In chemistry, an electropositive element (cation) that unites with an anion to form a salt; a compound ionizing to yield hydroxyl ion. SYN alkali (2). SEE ALSO Brønsted b., Lewis b. **4.** Nitrogen-containing organic compounds (*e.g.,* purines, pyrimidines, amines, alkaloids, ptomaines) that act as Brønsted b.'s. **5.** Cations, or substances forming cations. [L. and G. *basis*]

Brønsted b., any molecule or ion that combines with a proton; *e.g.,* OH^-, CN^-, NH_3; this definition replaces the older and more limited concepts of base (3).

denture b., (**1**) that part of a denture which rests on the oral mucosa and to which teeth are attached; (**2**) that part of a complete or partial denture which rests upon the basal seat and to which teeth are attached. SYN saddle (2).

external b. of skull, external aspect of the b. of skull

b. of heart, that part of the heart that lies opposite the apex, formed mainly by the left atrium but to a small extent by the posterior part of the right atrium; it is directed backward and to the right and is separated from the vertebral column by the esophagus and aorta. SYN basis cordis [NA].

hexone b.'s, histone b.'s, the α-amino acids arginine, histidine, and lysine, which are basic by virtue of the presence in the side chains of a guanidine, imidazole, and amine group, respectively.

internal b. of skull, the interior aspect of the skull b. on which the brain rests; the floor of the cranial cavity. SEE ALSO b. of skull.

Lewis b., a b. that is an electron-pair donor.

b. of lung, the lower concave part of the lung that rests upon the convexity of the diaphragm. SYN basis pulmonis [NA].

pressor b., (**1**) one of several products of intestinal putrefaction believed to cause functional hypertension when absorbed; (**2**) any alkaline substance that raises blood pressure. SYN pressor amine.

b. of skull, the sloping floor of the cranial cavity. It comprises both the external b. of skull (external view) and the internal b. of skull (internal view). SYN basis cranii.

b. of stapes, the flat portion of the stapes that fits in the oval window. SYN basis stapedis [NA], footplate (1), foot-plate.

base•plate (bās′plāt). A temporary form representing the base of a denture; used for making maxillomandibular (jaw) relation records and for the arrangement of teeth.

△**basi-, baso-, basio-.** Base; basis. [G. and L. *basis*]

ba•sic (bā′sik). Relating to a base.

ba•sic•i•ty (bā-sis′i-tē). **1.** The valence or combining power of an acid, or the number of replaceable atoms of hydrogen in its molecule. **2.** The characteristic(s) of being a chemical base.

ba•sic life sup•port. Emergency cardiopulmonary resuscitation, control of bleeding, treatment of shock, acidosis, and poisoning, stabilization of injuries and wounds, and basic first aid.

Ba•sid•i•ob•o•lus (ba-sid′ē-ob-ō-lŭs). A genus of fungi. *B. haptosporus* has been isolated from cases of zygomycosis (entomophthoramycosis basidiobolae). [Mod. L. *basidium,* dim. of G. *basis,* base, + L. *bolus,* fr. G. *bolos,* lump or clod]

Ba•sid•i•o•my•co•ta (bă-sid′ē-ō-mī-kō-tă). A phylum of fungi characterized by a spore-bearing organ, the basidium, that is usually a clavate cell that bears basidiospores after karyogamy and meiosis.

ba•sid•i•um, pl. **ba•sid•ia** (ba-sid′ē-ŭm, -ă). A cell or spore-bearing organ, usually club-shaped, that is characteristic of the Basidiomycota. It bears basidiospores externally after karyogamy and meiosis. It is composed of a swollen terminal cell situated on a slender stalk, and gives rise to slender filaments (sterigmata), usually four in number, from the ends of which the basidiospores are developed. [L., fr G. *basis,* base]

ba•si•fa•cial (bā′si-fā′shăl). Relating to the lower portion of the face.

bas•i•lar, bas•i•la•ris (bas′i-lăr, bas-i-lā′ris). Relating to the base of a pyramidal or broad structure.

ba•si•lat•er•al (bā′si-lat′er-ăl). Relating to the base and one or more sides of any part.

ba•si•lem•ma (bā-si-lem′ă). SYN basement *membrane.* [basi- + G. *lemma,* rind]

△**basio-.** SEE basi-.

ba•si•on (bā′sē-on) [NA]. The middle point on the anterior margin of the foramen magnum, opposite the opisthion. [G. *basis,* a base]

ba•sip•e•tal (bā-sip′ĕ-tăl). **1.** In a direction toward the base. **2.** Pertaining to asexual conidial production in fungi, in which successive budding of the basal conidium forms in unbranched chain with the youngest at the base. [basi- + L. *peto,* to seek]

bas·i·pho·bia (bās-i-fō′bē-ă). Morbid fear of walking. [G. *basis,* a stepping, + *phobos,* fear]

ba·sis (bā′sis) [NA]. SYN base (1). [L. and G.]
  b. cor′dis [NA], SYN *base of heart.*
  b. cra′nii, SYN *base of skull.*
  b. pulmo′nis [NA], SYN *base of lung.*
  b. stape′dis [NA], SYN *base of stapes.*

ba·si·sphe·noid (bā′si-sfē′noyd). Relating to the base or body of the sphenoid bone.

⌂**baso-.** SEE basi-.

ba·so·e·ryth·ro·cyte (bā′sō-e-rith′rō-sīt). A red blood cell that manifests changes of basophilic degeneration, such as basophilic stippling, punctate basophilia, or basophilic granules.

ba·so·e·ryth·ro·cy·to·sis (bā′sō-ĕ-rith′rō-sī-tō′sis). An increase of red blood cells with basophilic degenerative changes, frequently observed in hypochromic anemia.

ba·so·lat·er·al (bā-sō-lat′er-ăl). Basal and lateral; specifically used to refer to one of the two major cytological divisions of the amygdaloid complex.

🔲**ba·so·phil, ba·so·phile** (bā′sō-fil, -fīl). 1. A cell with granules that stain specifically with basic dyes. 2. SYN basophilic. 3. A phagocytic leukocyte of the blood characterized by basophilic granules containing heparin and histamine; except for its segmented nucleus, it is morphologically and physiologically similar to the mast cell though they originate from different stem cells in the bone marrow. [baso- + G. *phileo,* to love]

ba·so·phil·ia (bā-sō-fil′ē-ă). 1. A condition in which there are more than the usual number of basophilic leukocytes in the circulating blood (basophilic leukocytosis) or an increase in the proportion of parenchymatous basophilic cells in an organ (in the bone marrow, basophilic hyperplasia). 2. A condition in which basophilic erythrocytes are found in circulating blood, as in certain instances of leukemia, advanced anemia, malaria, and plumbism. SYN basophilism.

ba·so·phil·ic (bā′sō-fil′ik). Denoting tissue components having an affinity for basic dyes. SYN basophil (2), basophile.

ba·so·phil·ism (bā-sof′i-lizm). SYN basophilia.
  Cushing's b., SYN Cushing's *syndrome.*

bath. 1. Immersion of the body or any of its parts in water or any other yielding or fluid medium, or application of such medium in any form to the body or any of its parts. 2. Apparatus used in giving a b. of any form. 3. Fluid used for maintenance of metabolic activities or growth of living organisms, *e.g.,* cells derived from body tissue. [A.S. *baeth*]
  colloid b., a b. prepared by adding soothing agents such as sodium bicarbonate or oatmeal to the b. water to relieve skin irritation and pruritus.
  contrast b., a b. in which a part is immersed in hot water for a period of a few minutes and then in cold, the hot and cold periods alternated regularly at intervals, usually half-hours; used to increase the blood flow to the part.
  douche b., the local application of water in the form of a large jet or stream.

needle b., a b. in which water is projected forcibly against the body in many very fine jets.

sitz b., immersion of only the perineum and buttocks, with the legs being outside the tub. [Ger. *sitzen,* to sit]

sponge b., a b. in which the body is washed with a wet sponge or cloth.

bath·mo·tro·pic (bath-mō-trō′pik). Influencing nervous and muscular irritability in response to stimuli. [G. *bathmos,* threshold, + *trope,* a turning]

⌂**batho-.** Depth. SEE ALSO bathy-. [G. *bathos,* depth]

bath·o·pho·bia (bath-ō-fō′bē-ă). Morbid fear of deep places or of looking into them. [G. *bathos,* depth, + *phobos,* fear]

⌂**bathy-.** Depth. SEE ALSO batho-. [G. *bathys,* deep]

bath·y·an·es·the·sia (bath′ē-an-es-thē′zē-ă). Loss of deep sensibility, *i.e.,* from muscles, ligaments, tendons, bones, and joints. [G. *bathys,* deep, + *an-* priv. + *aisthesis,* sensation]

bath·y·es·the·sia (bath′ē-es-thē′zē-ă). General term for all sensation from the tissues beneath the skin, *i.e.,* muscles, ligaments, tendons, bones and joints. SEE ALSO myesthesia. [G. *bathys,* deep, + *aisthesis,* sensation]

bath·y·hy·per·es·the·sia (bath-ē-hī′per-es-thē′zē-ă). Exaggerated sensitiveness of deep structures, *e.g.,* muscular tissue. [G. *bathys,* deep, + *hyper,* above, + *aisthesis,* sensation]

bath·y·hyp·es·the·sia (bath-ē-hip′es-thē′zē-ă). Impairment of sensation in the structures beneath the skin, *e.g.,* muscle tissue. [G. *bathys,* deep, + *hypo,* under, + *aisthesis,* sensation]

bat·tery (bat′er-ē). A group or series of tests administered for analytic or diagnostic purposes. [M.E. *batri,* beaten metal, fr. O.Fr. *batre,* to beat]

BBB blood-brain *barrier.*

BBOT 2,5-bis(5-*t*-butylbenzoxazol-2-yl)thiophene, a liquid scintillator.

BE barium *enema.*

bead·ed (bēd′ed). 1. Marked by numerous small rounded projections, often arranged in a row like a string of beads. 2. Applied to a series of noncontinuous bacterial colonies along the line of inoculation in a stab culture. 3. Denoting stained bacteria in which more deeply stained granules occur at regular intervals in the organism.

beam (bēm). 1. Any bar whose curvature changes under load. DENTISTRY frequently used instead of "bar." 2. A collimated emission of light or other radiation, such as an x-ray b. [O.H.G. *Boum*]

bear·ing down. Expulsive effort of a parturient woman in the second stage of labor.

beat (bēt). 1. To strike; to throb or pulsate. 2. A stroke, impulse, or pulsation, as of the heart or pulse. 3. Activity of a cardiac chamber produced by catching a stimulus generated elsewhere in the heart. [A.S. *beatan*]
  apex b., the visible and/or palpable pulsation made by the apex of the left ventricle as it strikes the chest wall in systole; normally in the fifth intercostal space, about 10 cm to the left of the median line.
  atrial capture b., the cardiac cycle resulting when, after a period of A-V dissociation, the atria regain control of the ventricles; atrial depolariza-

tion due to retrograde transmission from a ventricular ectopic beat or an electronically paced ventricular impulse.

atrial fusion b., a b. that occurs when the atria are activated in part by the sinus impulse and in part by an ectopic or retrograde impulse from A-V junction or ventricle.

automatic b., in contrast to forced b., an ectopic b. that arises *de novo* and is not precipitated by the preceding b.; thus escaped and parasystolic b.'s are automatic.

Dressler b., fusion b. interrupting a ventricular tachycardia and producing a normally narrow QRS complex as a result of the fusion of two impulses, one impulse from the ventricular tachycardia and the other from a supraventricular focus; Dressler b.'s strongly support the diagnosis of ventricular tachycardia by interruption of it.

ectopic b., a cardiac b. originating elsewhere than at the sinoatrial node.

escape b., escaped b., an automatic b., usually arising from the A-V junction or ventricle, occurring after the next expected normal b. has defaulted; it is therefore always a late b., terminating a longer cycle than the normal.

forced b., (1) an extrasystole supposedly precipitated in some way by the preceding normal b. to which it is coupled; **(2)** an extrasystole caused by artificial stimulation of the heart.

fusion b., a b. triggered by more than a single electrical impulse, when the wave fronts coincide to act together on a single final pathway of activity; in the electrocardiogram, the atrial or ventricular complex when either atria or ventricles are activated jointly by two simultaneous or nearly simultaneous invading impulses.

heart b., a complete cardiac cycle, including spread of the electrical impulse and the consequent mechanical contraction.

retrograde b., a b. occurring as an electrical activation of a portion of a heart chamber cephalad to the chamber of origin, *e.g.,* an atrial b. triggered by an impulse originating in the ventricle.

ventricular fusion b., a fusion b. that occurs when the ventricles are activated partly by the descending sinus or A-V junctional impulse and partly by an ectopic ventricular impulse.

Becquerel, Antoine H., French physicist and Nobel laureate, 1852–1908. SEE becquerel.

bec•que•rel (bek-ă-rel′). The SI unit of measurement of radioactivity, equal to 1 disintegration per second; 1 Bq = 0.027 × 10^{-9} Ci. SEE ALSO absorption. [A.H. *Becquerel*]

bed (bĕd). **1.** In anatomy, a base or structure that supports another structure. **2.** A piece of furniture used for rest, recuperation, or treatment.

capillary b., the capillaries considered collectively and their volume capacity for blood.

nail b., the area of the corium on which the nail rests; it is extremely sensitive and presents numerous longitudinal ridges on its surface. SYN matrix unguis [NA], keratogenous membrane.

bed•bug. SYN *Cimex lectularius.*

bed•sore (bed′sōr). SYN decubitus *ulcer.*

bed-wet•ting. SYN nocturnal *enuresis.*

be•hav•ior (be-hāv′yer). **1.** Any response emitted

by or elicited from an organism. **2.** Any mental or motor act or activity. **3.** Specifically, parts of a total response pattern. [M.E., fr. O. Fr. *avoir,* to have]

occupational b., organization and b. based on skills, knowledge, and attitudes that make functioning in life roles possible.

type A b., a b. pattern characterized by aggressiveness, ambitiousness, restlessness, and a strong sense of time urgency; associated with increased risk for coronary heart disease.

type B b., a b. pattern characterized by the absence or obverse of type A b. characteristics.

be•hav•ior•al (bē-hāv′yer-ăl). Pertaining to behavior.

be•hav•ior•al sci•enc•es. A collective term for those disciplines or branches of science, such as psychology, sociology, and anthropology, that derive their theories and methods from the study of the behavior of living organisms.

be•hav•ior•ism (bē-hāv′yer-izm). A branch of psychology that formulates, through systematic observation and experimentation, the laws and principles which underlie the behavior of man and animals; its major contributions have been made in the areas of conditioning and learning. SYN behavioral psychology.

bel. Unit expressing the relative intensity of a sound. The intensity in bels is the logarithm (to the base 10) of the ratio of the power of the sound to that of a reference sound. Ordinarily, the reference sound is assumed to be one with a power of 10^{-16} watts per sq cm, approximately the threshold of a normal human ear at 1000 Hz. [A.G. *Bell*, Scottish-U.S. scientist, 1847–1922]

belch•ing. SYN eructation. [A.S. *baelcian*]

belle in•dif•fér•ence. SEE la belle indifférence.

bel•ly (bel′ē). **1.** The abdomen. **2.** The wide swelling part of a muscle. SYN venter (2). **3.** Popularly, the stomach or womb. [O.E. *belig, bag*]

bel•o•ne•pho•bia (bel′ō-nē-fō′bē-ă). Morbid fear of needles, pins, and other sharp-pointed objects. [G. *belonē,* needle, + *phobos,* fear]

bends (bendz). Colloquialism for Caisson sickness; decompression *sickness.* [fr. convulsive posture of those so afflicted]

be•nign (bē-nīn′). Denoting the mild character of an illness or the nonmalignant character of a neoplasm. [thru O. Fr., fr. L. *benignus,* kind]

ben•tir•o•mide (ben-tir′ō-mīd). 4-[[(2-Benzoylamino)-3-(4-hydroxyphenyl)-1- oxopropyl]-amino]benzoic acid; a peptide used in a screening test for exocrine pancreatic insufficiency and to monitor the adequacy of supplemental pancreatic therapy.

△**benz-.** Combining form denoting benzene.

ben•zo•yl (ben′zō-il). The benzoic acid radical, C_6H_5CO—, forming benzoyl compounds.

ben•zyl•i•dene (ben-zil′i-dēn). The hydrocarbon radical, C_6H_5CH=.

ben•zyl•ox•y•car•bon•yl (Z) (ben′zil-ok-sē-kar′bon-il). Amino-protecting radical used (as the chloride) in peptide synthesis, yielding $PhCH_2OCO$—NHR.

be•reave•ment (bĕ-rēv-ment). An acute state of intense psychological sadness and suffering experienced after the tragic loss of a loved one or some priceless possession. [M.E., *bireven*, to deprive, + -ment]

ber·i·beri, beri beri (ber′ē-ber′ē). A nutritional deficiency syndrome occurring in endemic form in eastern and southern Asia, sporadically in other parts of the world, and sometimes in alcoholics, resulting mainly from a dietary deficiency of thiamine; characterized by painful polyneuritis, and edema resulting from a high-output form of heart failure. SYN endemic neuritis. [Singhalese, extreme weakness]

beri beri. SEE beriberi.

berke·li·um (Bk) (berk′lē-um). An artificial transuranium radioactive element; atomic no. 97, atomic wt. 247.07. [*Berkeley*, Calif., city where first prepared]

Ber·lin blue (ber-lin′ bloo) [C.I. 77510]. Ferric ferrocyanide; a dye used to color injection masses for blood vessels and lymphatics, and in staining of siderocytes. SYN Prussian blue.

be·ryl·li·o·sis (be-ril-ē-ō′sis). Beryllium poisoning characterized by granulomatous fibrosis of the lungs from chronic inhalation of beryllium.

be·ryl·li·um (be-ril′ē-ŭm). A white metal element belonging to the alkaline earths; atomic no. 4., atomic wt. 9.012182. [G. *beryllos*, beryl]

bes·ti·al·i·ty (bes-tē-al′i-tē). Sexual relations between a human and an animal. SYN zooerastia. [L. *bestia*, beast]

beta (β) (bā′ta). **1.** Second letter of the Greek alphabet. **2.** CHEMISTRY denotes the second in a series, the second carbon from a functional (*e.g.*, carboxylic) group, or the direction of a chemical bond toward the viewer. For terms with the prefix β, see the specific term.

be·ta-block·er (bā′tă-blok′er). SYN β-adrenergic blocking *agent*.

be·ta·cism (bā′tă-sizm). A defect in speech in which the sound of *b* is given to other consonants. [G. *bēta*, the second letter of the alphabet]

be·ta·ine (bē′tă-ēn). **1.** An oxidation product of choline and a transmethylating intermediate in metabolism. **2.** A class of compounds related to b.(1) (*i.e.*, $R_3 N^=-CHR'-COO^-$).

be·ta·tron (bā′tă-tron). A circular electron accelerator that is a source of either high energy electrons or x-rays.

Betke-Kleihauer test. See under test.

be·zoar (bē′zōr). A concretion formed in the alimentary canal of animals, and occasionally humans; formerly considered to be a useful medicine with magical properties and apparently still used for this purpose in some places; according to the substance forming the ball, may be termed trichobezoar (hairball), trichophytobezoar (hair and vegetable fiber mixed), or phytobezoar (foodball). [Pers. *padzahr*, antidote]

Bi bismuth.

△**bi-.** **1.** Prefix meaning twice or double, referring to double structures, dual actions, etc. **2.** In chemistry, used to denote a partially neutralized acid (an acid salt); *e.g.*, bisulfate. Cf. bis-, di-. [L.]

bi·ar·tic·u·lar (bī′ar-tik′yū-lăr). SYN diarthric.

bi·as (bī′-as). **1.** Systematic discrepancy between a laboratory measurement and the true value; may be constant or proportionate and may ad-

versely affect test results. **2.** Deviation of results or inferences from the truth, or processes leading to such deviation; any trend in the collection, analysis, interpretation, publication, or review of data that can lead to conclusions that are systematically different from the truth. [Fr. *biais*, obliquity, perh. fr. L. *bifax*, two-faced]

bi·cam·er·al (bī-kam′er-ăl). Having two chambers; denoting especially an abscess divided by a more or less complete septum. [bi- + L. *camera*, chamber]

bi·cap·su·lar (bī-kap′sū-lăr). Having a double capsule.

bi·car·bon·ate (bī-kar′bon-āt). HCO_3^-; the ion remaining after the first dissociation of carbonic acid; a central buffering agent in blood.

  standard b., the plasma b. concentration of a sample of whole blood that has been equilibrated at 37°C with a carbon dioxide pressure of 40 mm Hg and an oxygen pressure greater than 100 mm Hg; abnormally high or low values indicate metabolic alkalosis or acidosis, respectively.

bi·car·di·o·gram (bī-kar′dē-ō-gram). The composite curve of an electrocardiogram representing the combined effects of the right and left ventricles.

bi·cel·lu·lar (bī-sel′yū-lăr). Having two cells or subdivisions.

bi·ceps (bī′seps). A muscle with two origins or heads. Commonly used to refer to the biceps brachii muscle. [bi- + L. *caput*, head]

bi·cip·i·tal (bī-sip′i-tăl). **1.** Two-headed. **2.** Relating to a biceps muscle. [bi- + L. *caput*, head]

bi·clo·nal (bī-klō′năl). Pertaining to or characterized by biclonality.

bi·clon·al·i·ty (bī-klōn-al′i-tē). A condition in which some cells have markers of one cell line and other cells have markers of another cell line, as in biclonal leukemias.

bi·con·cave (bī-kon′kāv). Concave on two sides; denoting especially a form of lens. SYN concavo-concave.

bi·con·vex (bī-kon′veks). Convex on two sides; denoting especially a form of lens. SYN convexo-convex.

bi·cor·nous, bi·cor·nu·ate, bi·cor·nate (bī-kōr′nŭs, -nū-āt, -nāt). Two-horned; having two processes or projections. [bi- + L. *cornu*, horn]

△**bicro-.** SYN pico- (2).

bi·cron (bī′kron). SYN picometer.

bi·cus·pid (bī-kŭs′pid). **1.** Having two points, prongs, or cusps. **2.** Teeth having two cusps. Humans have eight: two in front of each group of molars. SEE bicuspid *tooth*. [bi- + L. *cuspis*, point]

bi·dac·ty·ly (bī-dak′ti-lē). Abnormality in which the medial digits are lacking, with only the first and fifth represented. SEE ALSO ectrodactyly. [bi- + G. *daktylos*, finger]

BIDS [MIM*234050] Acronym for *b*rittle hair, *i*mpaired intelligence, *d*ecreased fertility, and *s*hort stature; usually manifested as an inherited deficiency of a high-sulfur protein.

bi·fid (bī′fid). Split or cleft; separated into two parts. [L. *bifidus*, cleft in two parts]

bi·fo·cal (bī-fō′kăl). Having two foci.

bi·fo·rate (bī-fō′rāt). Having two openings. [bi- + L. *foro*, pp. -atus, to bore, pierce]

bi·fur·cate, bi·fur·cat·ed (bī-fer′kāt, -kā-ted). Forked; two-pronged; having two branches. [bi- + L. *furca,* fork]

bi·fur·ca·tion (bī-fer-kā′shŭn). A forking; a division into two branches.

bi·gem·i·ny (bī-jem′i-nē). Pairing; especially, the occurrence of heartbeats in pairs. [bi- + L. *geminus,* twin]

  atrioventricular junctional b., paired beats, each pair consisting of an A-V nodal extrasystole coupled to a beat of the dominant, usually sinus, rhythm.

bi·lat·er·al (bī-lat′er-ăl). Relating to, or having, two sides. [bi- + L. *latus,* side]

bile (bīl). The yellowish brown or green fluid secreted by the liver and discharged into the duodenum, where it aids in the emulsification of fats, increases peristalsis, and retards putrefaction; contains sodium glycocholate and sodium taurocholate, cholesterol, biliverdin and bilirubin, mucus, fat, lecithin, cells, and cellular debris. [L. *bilis*]

△**bili-.** Bile. [L. *bilis,* bile]

bil·i·ary (bil′ē-ār-ē). Relating to bile or the biliary tract. SYN bilious (1).

bil·i·gen·e·sis (bil-i-jen′ĕ-sis). Bile production. [bili- + G. *genesis,* production]

bil·i·gen·ic (bil-i-jen′ik). Bile-producing.

bil·ious (bil′yŭs). **1.** SYN biliary. **2.** Relating to or characteristic of biliousness. **3.** Formerly, denoting a temperament characterized by a quick, irritable temper. SYN choleric.

bil·i·ra·chia (bil-i-rā′kē-ă). Occurrence of bile pigments in the spinal fluid. [bili- + G. *rhachis,* spine]

bil·i·ru·bin (bil-i-rū′bin). A yellow bile pigment found as sodium bilirubinate (soluble), or as an insoluble calcium salt in gallstones, formed from hemoglobin during normal and abnormal destruction of erythrocytes by the reticuloendothelial system. Excess b. is associated with jaundice. [bili- + L. *ruber,* red]

  delta b., the fraction of b. covalently bound to albumin.

  direct reacting b., the fraction of serum b. which has been conjugated with glucuronic acid in the liver cell to form b. diglucuronide; so called because it reacts directly with the Ehrlich diazo reagent; increased levels are found in hepatobiliary diseases, especially of the obstructive variety.

  indirect reacting b., the fraction of serum b. which has not been conjugated with glucuronic acid in the liver cell; so called because it reacts with the Ehrlich diazo reagent only when alcohol is added; increased levels are found in hepatic disease and hemolytic conditions.

bil·i·ru·bi·ne·mia (bil′i-rū-bin-ē′mē-ă). The presence of bilirubin in the blood, where it is normally present in relatively small amounts; the term is usually used in relation to increased concentrations observed in various pathologic conditions where there is excessive destruction of erythrocytes or interference with the mechanism of excretion in the bile. Determination of the quantity of bilirubin in the blood serum reveals two fractions, namely direct reacting (conjugated)

and indirect reacting (nonconjugated) bilirubin; determination of conjugated and total bilirubin in serum is an important and frequently used clinical laboratory test. [bilirubin + G. *haima,* blood]

bil·i·ru·bin·oids (bil-i-rū′bin-oydz). Generic term denoting intermediates in the conversion of bilirubin to stercobilin by reductive enzymes in intestinal bacteria; most are found in normal urine and feces.

bil·i·ru·bi·nu·ria (bil′i-rū-bi-nū′rē-ă). The presence of bilirubin in the urine. [bilirubin + G. *ouron,* urine]

bil·i·u·ria (bil-ē-yū′rē-ă). The presence of various bile salts, or bile, in the urine. SYN choleuria, choluria. [bili- + G. *ouron,* urine]

bi·lo·bate, bi·lobed (bī-lō′bāt, bī′lōbd). Having two lobes.

bi·lob·u·lar (bī-lob′yū-lăr). Having two lobules.

bi·loc·u·lar, bi·loc·u·late (bī-lok′yū-lăr, -yū-lāt). Having two compartments or spaces. [bi- + L. *loculus,* dim. of *locus,* a place]

bi·man·u·al (bī-man′yū-ăl). Relating to, or performed by, both hands. [bi- + L. *manus,* hand]

bi·mas·toid (bī-mas′toyd). Relating to both mastoid processes.

bi·max·il·lary (bī-mak′si-lār-e). Relating to both the right and left maxillae; sometimes used when describing something affecting both halves of the upper jaw.

bi·na·ry (bī′nār-ē). **1.** Comprising two components, elements, molecules, etc. **2.** Denoting a choice of two mutually exclusive outcomes for one event (*e.g.,* male or female; heads or tails; affected or unaffected). [L. *binarius,* consisting of two, fr. *bini,* two at a time]

bin·au·ral (bin-aw′răl). Relating to both ears. SYN binotic. [L. *bini,* a pair, + *auris,* ear]

bind·er (bīnd′er). **1.** A broad bandage, especially one encircling the abdomen. **2.** Anything that binds.

  obstetrical b., a supporting garment covering the abdomen from the ribs to the trochanters, tightly pinned at the back, affording support after childbirth or, rarely, during childbirth.

  T-b., two strips of cloth at right angles; used for retaining a dressing, as on the perineum.

bin·oc·u·lar (bin-ok′yū-lăr). Adapted to the use of both eyes; said of an optical instrument. [L. *bini,* paired, + *oculus,* eye]

bi·no·mi·al (bī-nō′mē-ăl). A set of two terms or names; in the probabilistic or statistical sense it corresponds to a Bernoulli trial. [bi- + G. *nomos,* name]

bin·ot·ic (bin-ot′ik). SYN binaural. [L. *bini,* a pair, + G. *ous (ōt-),* ear]

bi·nu·cle·ar, bi·nu·cle·ate (bī-nū′klē-ăr, -klē-āt). Having two nuclei.

bi·nu·cle·o·late (bī-nū′klē-ō-lāt). Having two nucleoli.

△**bio-.** Combining form denoting life. [G. *bios,* life]

bi·o·a·cous·tics (bī′ō-ă-kūs′tiks). The science dealing with the effects of sound or vibration on living organisms.

bi·o·as·say (bī-ō-as′ā). Determination of the potency or concentration of a compound by its effect upon animals, isolated tissues, or microorganisms, as contrasted with analysis of its chemical or physical properties.

bi·o·a·vail·a·bil·i·ty (bī'ō-ă-vāl'ă-bil'i-tē). The physiological availability of a given amount of a drug, as distinct from its chemical potency; proportion of the administered dose which is absorbed into the bloodstream.

bi·o·chem·i·cal (bī-ō-kem'i-kăl). Relating to biochemistry.

bi·o·chem·is·try (bī-ō-kem'is-trē). The chemistry of living organisms and of the chemical, molecular, and physical changes occurring therein.

bi·o·cid·al (bī-ō-sī'dăl). Destructive of life; particularly pertaining to microorganisms. [bio- + L. *caedo,* to kill]

bi·o·cy·ber·net·ics (bī'ō-sī-ber-net'iks). The science of communication and control within a living organism, particularly on a molecular basis.

bi·o·de·grad·a·ble (bī'ō-dē-grād'ă-bl). Denoting a substance that can be chemically degraded or decomposed by natural effectors (*e.g.,* weather, soil bacteria, plants, animals).

bi·o·de·gra·da·tion. SYN biotransformation.

bi·o·feed·back (bī-ō-fēd'bak). A training technique that enables an individual to gain some element of voluntary control over autonomic body functions; based on the learning principle that a desired response is learned when received information such as a recorded increase in skin temperature (feedback) indicates that a specific thought complex or action has produced the desired physiological response.

EMG b., a form of b. that uses an electromyographic measure of muscle tension as the physical symptom to be deconditioned, such as tension in the frontalis muscle in the head which can cause headaches.

bi·o·gen·e·sis (bī-ō-jen'ĕ-sis). **1.** The principle that life originates from preexisting life only and never from nonliving material. SEE recapitulation *theory.* **2.** SYN biosynthesis. [bio- + G. *genesis,* origin]

bi·o·ge·net·ic (bī'ō-jĕ-net'ik). Relating to biogenesis.

bi·o·in·stru·ment (bī'ō-in'strŭ-ment). A sensor or device attached to or embedded in the body to record and transmit physiologic data to a receiving station.

bi·o·ki·net·ics (bī'ō-ki-net'iks). The study of the growth changes and movements that developing organisms undergo. [bio- + G. *kinēsis,* motion]

bi·o·log·ic, bi·o·log·i·cal (bī'ō-loj'ik, -loj'i-kăl). Relating to biology.

bi·ol·o·gist (bī-ol'ō-jist). A specialist or expert in biology.

bi·ol·o·gy (bī-ol'ō-jē). The science concerned with the phenomena of life and living organisms. [bio- + G. *logos,* study]

cellular b., SYN cytology.

molecular b., study of phenomena in terms of molecular interactions; it differs from biochemistry in that it emphasizes chemical interactions involved in the replication of DNA, its "transcription" into RNA, and its "translation" into or expression in protein.

oral b., that aspect of b. devoted to the study of biological phenomena associated with the oral

cavity in health and disease (*e.g.,* dental caries, mastication, periodontal disease).

radiation b., science that studies the biological effects of ionizing radiation.

bi·o·mass (bī'ō-mas). The total weight of all living things in a given area, biotic community, species population, or habitat; a measure of total biotic productivity.

bi·ome (bī'ōm). The total complex of biotic communities occupying and characterizing a particular geographic area or zone. [bio- + -ome]

bi·o·me·chan·ics (bī-ō-me-kan'iks). The science concerned with the action of forces, internal or external, on the living body.

bi·o·med·i·cal (bī-ō-med'i-kăl). **1.** Pertaining to aspects of the biologic sciences that relate to or underlie medicine. **2.** Biological and medical, *i.e.,* encompassing both the science(s) and the art of medicine.

bi·o·mem·brane (bī-ō-mem'brān). A structure bounding a cell or cell organelle; it contains lipids, proteins, glycolipids, steroids, etc. SYN membrana [NA], membrane (2).

bi·o·me·tri·cian (bī-ō-me-trish'ăn). One who specializes in the science of biometry.

bi·om·e·try (bī-om'ĕ-trē). The application of statistical methods to the study of numerical data based on biological observations and phenomena. [bio- + G. *metron,* measure]

bi·o·mi·cro·scope (bī-ō-mī'krō-skōp). SYN slit-lamp.

bi·o·mi·cros·co·py (bī'ō-mī-kros'kŏ-pē). **1.** Microscopic examination of living tissue in the body. **2.** Examination of the cornea, aqueous humor, lens, vitreous humor, and retina by use of a slitlamp combined with a binocular microscope.

bi·o·ne·cro·sis (bī-ō-ne-krō'sis). SYN necrobiosis.

bi·on·ic (bī-on'ik). Relating to or developed from bionics.

bi·on·ics (bī-on'iks). **1.** The science of biologic functions and mechanisms as applied to electronic technology. **2.** The science of applying the knowledge gained by studying the characteristics of living organisms to the formulation of nonorganic devices and techniques. [bio- + electronics]

bi·o·phar·ma·ceu·tics (bī'ō-far-mă-sū'tiks). The study of the physical and chemical properties of a drug, and its dosage form, as related to the onset, duration, and intensity of drug action.

bi·o·phys·ics (bī-ō-phyz'iks). **1.** The study of biological processes and materials by means of the theories and tools of physics. **2.** The study of physical processes (*e.g.,* electricity, luminescence) occurring in organisms.

■ **bi·op·sy** (bī'op-sē). **1.** Process of removing tissue from living patients for diagnostic examination. **2.** A specimen obtained by b. [bio- + G. *opsis,* vision]

aspiration b., SYN needle b.

brush b., b. obtained by passing a bristled catheter into a tubular or hollow organ to remove cells from suspected areas of disease.

chorionic villus b., transcervical or transabdominal sampling of the chorionic villi for genetic analysis.

endoscopic b., b. obtained by instruments

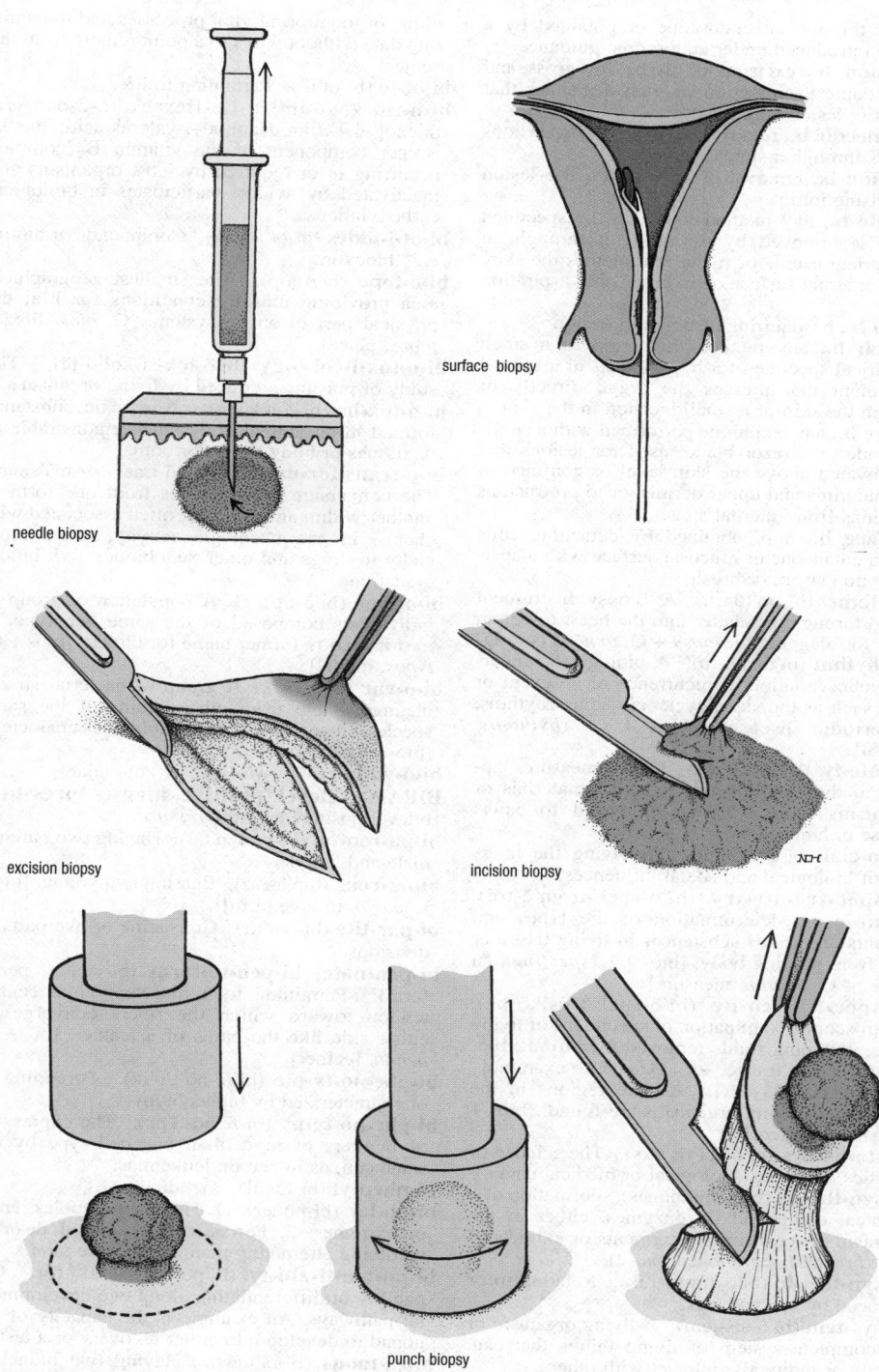

surface biopsy

needle biopsy

excision biopsy

incision biopsy

punch biopsy

biopsy

passed through an endoscope or obtained by a needle introduced under endoscopic guidance.

excision b., excision of tissue for gross and microscopic examination in such a manner that the entire lesion is removed.

fine needle b., removal of tissue or suspensions of cells through a small needle.

incision b., removal of only a part of a lesion by incising into it.

needle b., any method in which the specimen for b. is removed by aspirating it through an appropriate needle or trocar that pierces the skin, or the external surface of an organ. SYN aspiration b.

open b., b. requiring a surgical incision.

punch b., any method that removes a small cylindrical specimen for b. by means of a special instrument that pierces the organ directly or through the skin or a small incision in the skin.

shave b., a b. technique performed with a surgical blade or a razor blade; used for lesions that are elevated above the skin level or confined to the epidermis and upper dermis, or to protrusions of lesions from internal sites.

surface b., a b. obtained by detaching cells from a cutaneous or mucosal surface with a spatula, cotton swab, or brush.

bi·op·tome (bī-op′tōm). A biopsy instrument passed through a catheter into the heart to obtain tissue for diagnosis. [*biop*sy + G. *tomē,* a cutting]

bi·o·rhythm (bī′ō-rith-m). A biologically inherent cyclic variation or recurrence of an event or state, such as the sleep cycle, circadian rhythms, or periodic diseases. [bio- + G. *rhythmos,* rhythm]

bi·o·safe·ty (b-ī′ō-saf′tē). Safety measures applied to the handling of biological materials or organisms with a known potential to cause disease in humans.

bi·o·so·cial (bī-ō-sō′shŭl). Involving the interplay of biological and social influences.

bi·o·spec·trom·e·try (bī′ō-spek-trom′ĕ-trē). Spectroscopic determination of the types and amounts of various substances in living tissue or fluid from a living body. [bio- + L. *spectrum,* an image, + G. *metron,* measure]

bi·o·spec·tros·co·py (bī′ō-spek-tros′kō-pē). Spectroscopic examination of specimens of living tissue, including fluids removed therefrom. [bio- + L. *spectrum,* image, + G. *skopeō,* to examine]

bi·o·sphere (bī′ō-sfēr). All the regions in the world where living organisms are found. [bio- + G. *sphaira,* sphere]

bi·o·sta·tis·tics (bī′ō-stă-tis′tiks). The science of statistics applied to biological or medical data.

bi·o·syn·the·sis (bī-ō-sin′thĕ-sis). Formation of a chemical compound by enzymes, either in the organism (*in vivo*) or by fragments or extracts of cells (*in vitro*). SYN biogenesis (2).

bi·o·syn·thet·ic (bī′ō-sin-thet′ik). Relating to or produced by biosynthesis.

bi·o·sys·tem (bī′ō-sis-tem). A living organism or any complete system of living things that can, directly or indirectly, interact with others.

bi·o·ta (bī-ō′tă). The collective flora and fauna of a region. [Mod. L., fr. G. *bios,* life]

bi·o·te·lem·e·try (bī-ō-tel-em′ĕ-trē). The technique of monitoring vital processes and transmitting data without wires to a point remote from the subject.

bi·ot·ic (bī-ot′ik). Pertaining to life.

bi·o·tin (bī′ō-tin). *cis*-Hexahydro-2-oxo-1*H*-thieno[3,4-*d*]imidazoline-4-valeric acid; the D-isomer component of the vitamin B_2 complex occurring in or required by most organisms and inactivated by avidin; participates in biological carboxylations.

bi·ot·i·nides (bī-ot′i-nīdz). Compounds of biotin; *e.g.,* biocytin.

bi·o·tope (bī′ō-tōp). The smallest geographical area providing uniform conditions for life; the physical part of an ecosystem. [G. *bios,* life, + *topos,* place]

bi·o·tox·i·col·o·gy (bī′ō-tok-si-kol′ō-jē). The study of poisons produced by living organisms.

bi·o·tox·in (bī-ō-tok′sin). Any toxic substance formed in an animal body, and demonstrable in its tissues or body fluids, or both.

bi·o·trans·for·ma·tion (bī′ō-trans-fōr-mā′shŭn). The conversion of molecules from one form to another within an organism, often associated with change in pharmacologic activity; refers especially to drugs and other xenobiotics. SYN biodegradation.

bi·o·type (bī′ō-tīp). **1.** A population or group of individuals composed of the same genotype. **2.** BACTERIOLOGY former name for biovar. [bio- + G. *typos,* model]

bi·o·var (bī′ō-var). A group of bacterial strains distinguishable from other strains of the same species on the basis of physiological characters. [bio- + *variant*]

bi·o·vu·lar (bī′ov-yū-lar). SYN diovular.

BiPAP (bilevel positive airway pressure) bilevel positive airway *pressure*.

bi·pa·ren·tal (bī-pa-ren′tăl). Having two parents, male and female.

bip·a·rous (bip′ă-rŭs). Bearing two young. [bi- + L. *pario,* to give birth]

bi·par·tite (bī-par′tīt). Consisting of two parts or divisions.

bi·pen·nate, bi·pen·ni·form (bī-pen′āt, pen′i-fōrm). Pertaining to a muscle with a central tendon toward which the fibers converge on either side like the barbs of a feather. [bi- + L. *penna,* feather]

bi·phe·no·ty·pic (bī′fē-nō-tip′ik). Pertaining to or characterized by biphenotypy.

bi·phe·no·ty·py (bī-fē′nō-tī′pē). The expression of markers of more than one cell type by the same cell, as in certain leukemias.

bi·phen·yl (bī-fen′il). SYN diphenyl.

bi·po·lar (bī-pō′ler). **1.** Having two poles, ends, or extremes. **2.** Pertaining to a mood disorder involving alternating mania and depression.

bi·po·ten·ti·al·i·ty (bī′pō-ten-shē-al′i-tē). Capability of differentiating along two developmental pathways. An example is the capacity of the gonad to develop into either an ovary or a testis.

bi·ra·mous (bī-rā′mŭs). Having two branches. [bi- + L. *ramus,* branch]

bi·re·frin·gence (bī-rē-frin′jens). SYN double refraction.

bi·re·frin·gent (bī-rē-frin′-jent). Refracting twice; splitting a ray of light in two.

birth (berth). **1.** Passage of the offspring from the uterus to the outside world; the act of being born. **2.** Specifically, complete expulsion or extraction of a fetus from its mother.

premature b., b. of an infant after viability has been achieved with gestation of at least 20 weeks or birth weight of at least 500 g, but before 37 weeks.

birth·mark (berth′mark). A persistent visible lesion, usually on the skin, identified at or near birth; commonly due to nevus or hemangioma. SEE nevus (1).

△**bis-.** **1.** Prefix signifying two or twice. **2.** CHEMISTRY used to denote the presence of two identical but separated complex groups in one molecule. Cf. bi-, di-. [L.]

2,5-bis(5-*t*-bu·tyl·ben·zox·a·zol-2-yl)thi·o·phene (BBOT). A scintillator used in radioactivity measurements by scintillation counting.

bis in die (bis in dī′ē). Twice a day. [L.]

bi·sex·u·al (bī-seks′yū-ăl). **1.** Having gonads of both sexes. SEE ALSO hermaphroditism. **2.** Denoting an individual who engages in both heterosexual and homosexual relations.

bis·fer·i·ous (bis-fēr′ē-ŭs). Striking twice; said of the pulse. [L. *bis*, twice, + *ferio*, to strike]

bis·il·i·ac (bis-il′ē-ak). Relating to any two corresponding iliac parts or structures, as the iliac bones or iliac fossae.

bis·muth (Bi) (biz′mŭth). A trivalent metallic element; atomic no. 83, atomic wt. 20.98037. Several of its salts are used in medicine. [Ger. *Wismut, weisse Masse*, white mass]

bis·mu·tho·sis (bis-mŭ-thō′sis). Chronic bismuth poisoning.

bis·muth·yl (biz′mŭ-thil). The group, BiO^+, that behaves chemically as the ion of a univalent metal; its salts are subsalts of bismuth.

bis·tou·ry (bis′tū-rē). A long, narrow-bladed knife, with a straight or curved edge and sharp or blunt point (probe-point); used for opening or slitting cavities or hollow structures. [Fr. *bistouri*, fr. It. dialect *bistori*, perh. fr. *Pistoia*, Italy]

bi·sul·fate (bī-sŭl′fāt). A salt containing HSO_4^-. SYN acid sulfate.

bi·sul·fide (bī-sŭl′fīd). A compound of the anion HS^-; an acid sulfide.

bi·sul·fite (bī-sŭl′fīt). A salt or ion of HSO_3^-.

bite (bīt). **1.** To incise or seize with the teeth. **2.** The act of incision or seizure with the teeth. **3.** A morsel of food held between the teeth. **4.** Term used to denote the amount of pressure developed in closing the jaws. **5.** Undesirable jargon for terms such as interocclusal record, maxillomandibular registration, denture space, and interarch distance. **6.** A wound or puncture of the skin made by animal or insect. SEE bites. [A.S. *bītan*]

bite·plate, bite·plane (bīt′plāt, bīt′plān). A removable appliance that incorporates a plane of acrylic designed to occlude with the opposing teeth.

bites (bīts). Penetration of the skin (puncture or laceration) causing reactions that result from 1) mechanical injury; 2) injection of toxic material such as snake or scorpion venom; 3) injection of antigenic substance, especially by insect or arthropod bites, capable of inducing and eliciting allergic sensitization; 4) introduction of otherwise saprophytic flora such as *Staphylococcus pyogenes* in the instance of human bites; 5) invasion of the tissue as in myiasis; 6) transmission of disease such as typhus and rabies. [see bite]

bite·wing (bīt′wing). SEE bitewing *radiograph*.

bi·tro·chan·ter·ic (bī-trō-kan-ter′ik). Relating to two trochanters, either to the two trochanters of one femur or to both greater trochanters.

bi·u·ret (bī-ū-ret′). $NH(CONH_2)_2$; obtained by eliminating one NH_3 between two urea molecules. Used in protein determinations. SYN carbamoylurea.

bi·va·lence, bi·va·len·cy (bī-vā′lens, bī-vā′len-sē). A combining power (valence) of 2. SYN divalence, divalency.

bi·va·lent (bī-vā′lent, biv′ă-lent). **1.** Having a combining power (valence) of 2. SYN divalent. **2.** CYTOLOGY a structure consisting of two paired homologous chromosomes, each split into two sister chromatids, as seen during the pachytene stage of prophase in meiosis.

bi·ven·tral (bī-ven′tral). SYN digastric (1).

Bk berkelium.

black·head (blak′hed). **1.** SYN open *comedo*. **2.** SYN histomoniasis.

black·out (blak′owt). **1.** Temporary loss of consciousness due to decreased blood flow to the brain. **2.** Momentary loss of consciousness as in an absence. **3.** Temporary loss of vision, without alteration of consciousness, due to positive (> normal) g (gravity) forces; caused by temporary decreased blood flow in the central retinal artery, and seen mostly in aviators. **4.** A transient episode that occurs during a state of intense intoxication (alcoholic b.) for which the person has no recall, although not unconscious (as observed by others).

blad·der (blad′er). A distensible musculomembranous organ serving as a receptacle for fluid, as the gallbladder. SEE detrusor. SYN vesica (1). [A.S. *blaedre*]

atonic b., a large, dilated, and nonemptying urinary b.; usually due to disturbance of innervation or to chronic obstruction.

autonomic neurogenic b., malfunctioning urinary b., secondary to low spinal cord lesions.

nervous b., a b. condition in which there is a need to urinate frequently but with failure to empty the b. completely.

neurogenic b., SYN neuropathic b.

neuropathic b., any defective functioning of bladder due to impaired innervation, *e.g.*, cord b., neuropathic b. SYN neurogenic b.

reflex neurogenic b., an abnormal condition of urinary b. function whereby the b. is cut off from upper motor neuron control, but where the lower motor neuron arc is still intact.

uninhibited neurogenic b., a condition, either congenital or acquired, of abnormal urinary b. function whereby normal inhibitory control of detrusor function by the central nervous system is impaired or underdeveloped, resulting in precipitant or uncontrolled micturition and/or anuresis.

urinary b., a musculomembranous elastic bag

serving as a storage place for the urine. SYN vesica urinaria [NA].

blank. A solution consisting of all of the analytical components except the compound to be measured; this is used to establish a baseline of measurement intensity against which the compound of interest is compared. [M.E. white, fr. O.Fr. *blanc*, fr. Germanic]

⌂**-blast.** An immature precursor cell of the type indicated by the preceding word. [G. *blastos*, germ]

blas·te·ma (blas-tē'mă). **1.** The primordial cellular mass (precursor) from which an organ or part is formed. **2.** A cluster of cells competent to initiate the regeneration of a damaged or ablated structure. [G. a sprout]

blas·tem·ic (blas-tem'ik). Relating to the blastema.

⌂**blasto-.** Pertaining to the process of budding by cells or tissue. [G. *blastos*, germ]

blas·to·cele (blas'tō-sēl). The cavity in the blastula of a developing embryo. SYN cleavage cavity, segmentation cavity. [blasto- + G. *koilos*, hollow]

blas·to·cel·ic (blas-tō-sē'lik). Relating to the blastocele.

Blas·to·co·nid·i·um (blas'tō-cŏ-nid'ē-ŭm). A holoblastic conidium that is produced singly or in chains, and detached at maturity leaving a bud scar, as in the budding of a yeast cell. [blasto- + conidium]

blas·to·cyst (blas'tō-sist). The modified blastula stage of mammalian embryos, consisting of the inner cell mass and a thin trophoblast layer enclosing the blastocele. SYN blastodermic vesicle. [blasto- + G. *kystis*, bladder]

blas·to·cyte (blas'tō-sīt). An undifferentiated blastomere of the morula or blastula stage of an embryo. [blasto- + G. *kytos*, cell]

blas·to·cy·to·ma (blas'tō-sī-tō'mă). SYN blastoma.

blas·to·derm, blas·to·der·ma (blas'tō-derm, -tō-der'ma). The thin, disk-shaped cell mass of a young embryo and its extraembryonic extensions over the surface of the yolk; when fully formed, all three primary germ layers (ectoderm, endoderm, and mesoderm) are present. SYN germ membrane, germinal membrane. [blasto- + G. *derma*, skin]

blas·to·der·mal, blas·to·der·mic (blas-tō-der' măl, -der'mik). Relating to the blastoderm.

blas·to·disk (blas'tō-disk). **1.** The disk of active cytoplasm at the animal pole of a telolecithal egg. **2.** The blastoderm, especially in very young stages when its extent is small.

blas·to·gen·e·sis (blas-tō-jen'ĕ-sis). **1.** Reproduction of unicellular organisms by budding. **2.** Development of an embryo during cleavage and germ layer formation. **3.** Transformation of small lymphocytes of human peripheral blood in tissue culture into large, morphologically primitive blast-like cells capable of undergoing mitosis. [blasto- + G. *genesis*, origin]

blas·to·ge·net·ic, blas·to·gen·ic (blas'tō-je-net' ik, -tō-jen'ik). Relating to blastogenesis.

blas·to·ma (blas-tō'mă). A neoplasm composed chiefly or entirely of immature undifferentiated

cells (*i.e.*, blast forms), with little or virtually no stroma. SYN blastocytoma. [blasto- + G. *-oma*, tumor]

blas·to·mere (blas'tō-mēr). One of the cells into which the egg divides after its fertilization. [blasto- + G. *meros*, part]

Blas·to·my·ces der·ma·tit·i·dis (blas-tō-mī'sēz der-mă-tit'i-dis). A dimorphic soil fungus that causes blastomycosis. It grows in mammalian tissues as budding cells and in culture as a white to buff-colored filamentous fungus bearing spherical or ovoid conidia. [blasto- + G. *mykēs*, fungus]

blas·to·my·co·sis (blas-tō-mī-kō'sis). A chronic granulomatous and suppurative disease caused by *Blastomyces dermatitidis;* originates as a respiratory infection and disseminates, usually with pulmonary, osseous, and/or cutaneous involvement predominating. Formerly called North American b., the disease now has been found in African states as well as in Canada and the U.S.

North American b., SEE blastomycosis.

South American b., SYN paracoccidioidomycosis.

blas·to·pore (blas'tō-pōr). The opening into the archenteron formed by invagination of the blastula to form a gastrula. [blasto- + G. *poros*, opening]

blas·tu·la (blas'tyū-lă). An early stage of an embryo formed by the rearrangement of the blastomeres of the morula to form a hollow sphere. [G. *blastos*, germ]

blas·tu·lar (blas'tyū-lar). Pertaining to the blastula.

blas·tu·la·tion (blas-tyū-lā'shŭn). Formation of the blastula or blastocyst from the morula.

bleb (blĕb). A large flaccid vesicle.

bleed (blēd). To lose blood as a result of rupture or severance of blood vessels.

blem·ish (blĕ'mish). **1.** A small circumscribed alteration of the skin considered to be unesthetic but insignificant. **2.** To alter the skin, rendering an unesthetic appearance.

⌂**blenno-, blenn-.** Mucus. [G. *blenna, blennos*]

blen·no·gen·ic (blen-ō-jen'ik). SYN muciparous. [blenno- + G. *-gen*, to produce]

blen·nog·e·nous (ble-noj'ĕ-nŭs). SYN muciparous.

blen·noid (blen'oyd). SYN muciform. [blenno- + G. *eidos*, resemblance]

⌂**blephar-.** SEE blepharo-.

bleph·ar·ad·e·ni·tis (blef'ar-ad-ĕ-nī'tis). Inflammation of the meibomian glands or the marginal glands of Moll or Zeis. SYN blepharoadenitis. [blephar- + G. *adēn*, gland, + *-itis*, inflammation]

bleph·a·rec·to·my (blef'a-rek'tō-mē). Excision of all or part of an eyelid. [blepharo- + G. *ektomē*, excision]

bleph·ar·e·de·ma (blef'ar-ĕ-dē'mă). Edema of the eyelids, causing swelling and often a baggy appearance.

bleph·a·ri·tis (blef'ă-rī'tis). Inflammation of the eyelids. [blepharo- + G. *-itis*, inflammation]

seborrheic b., a common type of chronic inflammation of the margins of the eyelids with erythema and white scales; often with an associated seborrheic dermatitis of scalp and face.

⌂blepharo-, blephar-. Eyelid. [G. *blepharon*, an eyelid]

bleph•a•ro•ad•e•ni•tis (blef′ă-rō-ad-ĕ-nī′tis). SYN blepharadenitis.

bleph•a•ro•ad•e•no•ma (blef′ă-rō-ad-ĕ-nō′mă). A tumor or adenoma of a gland of the eyelid. [blepharo- + G. *adēn*, gland, + *-oma*, tumor]

bleph•a•ro•chal•a•sis (blef′ă-rō-kal′ă-sis). Redundancy of the skin of the upper eyelids so that a fold of skin hangs down, often concealing the tarsal margin when the eye is open. [blepharo- + G. *chalasis*, a slackening]

bleph•a•ro•col•o•bo•ma (blef′ă-rō-kol-ō-bō′mă). A defect of the eyelid; may be congenital or acquired. [blepharo- + coloboma]

bleph•a•ro•con•junc•ti•vi•tis (blef′ă-rō-kon-jŭnk-ti-vī′tis). Inflammation of the palpebral conjunctiva.

bleph•a•ro•ker•a•to•con•junc•ti•vi•tis (blef′ă-rō-ker′ă-tō-kon-jŭnk′ti-vī′tis). An inflammation involving the eyelids, cornea, and conjunctiva.

bleph•a•ro•phi•mo•sis (blef′ă-rō-fi-mō′sis). Decrease in the size of the palpebral aperture without fusion of lid margins. SYN blepharostenosis. [blepharo- + G. *phimōsis*, an obstruction]

bleph•a•ro•plas•tic (blef′ă-rō-plas′tik). Relating to blepharoplasty.

bleph•a•ro•plas•ty (blef′ă-ro-plast-tē). Any operation for the correction of a defect in the eyelids. [blepharo- + G. *plassō*, to form]

bleph•a•ro•ple•gia (blef′ă-rō-plē′jē-ă). Paralysis of an eyelid. [blepharo- + G. *plēgē*, stroke]

bleph•a•rop•to•sis, bleph•ar•op•to•sia (blef′ă-rop′tō-sis, -rop-tō′sē-ă). Drooping of the upper eyelid. SYN ptosis (2). [blepharo- + G. *ptōsis*, a falling]

b. adipo′sa, b. causing skin to hang over the free border of the eyelid.

false b., SYN pseudoptosis.

bleph•a•ro•spasm, bleph•a•ro•spas•mus (blef′ă-rō-spazm, -spaz′mŭs). Involuntary spasmodic contraction of the orbicularis oculi muscle.

bleph•a•ro•stat (blef′ă-rō-stat). SYN eye *speculum*. [blepharo- + G. *statos*, fixed]

bleph•a•ro•ste•no•sis (blef′ă-rō-ste-nō′sis). SYN blepharophimosis. [blepharo- + G. *stenōsis*, a narrowing]

bleph•a•ro•syn•ech•ia (blef′ă-rō-sin-ek′ē-ă). Adhesion of the eyelids to each other or to the eyeball. [blepharo- + G. *synecheia*, continuity, fr. *syn-echō*, to hold together]

bleph•a•rot•o•my (blef-ă-rot′ō-mē). A cutting operation on an eyelid. [blepharo- + G. *tomē*, incision]

blind (blīnd). Unable to see; without useful sight. SEE blindness.

blind•ness (blīnd′nes). **1.** Loss of the sense of sight; absolute b. denotes total absence of perception. SEE ALSO amblyopia, amaurosis. **2.** Loss of visual appreciation of objects although visual acuity is normal. **3.** Absence of the appreciation of sensation, *e.g.*, taste b. SYN typhlosis.

color b., misleading term for anomalous or deficient color vision; complete color b. is the absence of one of the primary cone pigments of the retina. SEE protanopia, deuteranopia, tritanopia.

cortical b., loss of sight due to an organic lesion in the visual cortex.

day b., SYN hemeralopia.

flash b., a temporary loss of vision produced when retinal light-sensitive pigments are bleached by light more intense than that to which the retina is physiologically adapted at that moment.

functional b., apparent loss of vision related to suggestibility.

hysterical b., loss of vision or blurring of vision following a highly traumatic event.

legal b., generally, visual acuity of less than 6/60 or 20/200 using Snellen test types, or visual field restriction to 20° or less in the better eye; the criteria used to define legal b. vary.

night b., SYN nyctalopia.

snow b., severe photophobia secondary to ultraviolet keratoconjunctivitis.

text b., word b., SYN alexia.

blis•ter (blis′ter). **1.** A fluid-filled thin-walled structure under the epidermis. **2.** To form a b. with heat or some other vesiculating agent.

blood b., a b. containing blood; resulting from a pinch or crushing injury.

fever b., colloquialism for herpes simplex of the lips.

blis•ter•ing. SYN vesiculation (1).

bloat, bloat•ing (blōt, blōt′ing). Abdominal distention from swallowed air or intestinal gas.

block. 1. To obstruct; to arrest passage through. **2.** A condition in which the passage of an electrical impulse is arrested, wholly or in part, temporarily or permanently. **3.** SYN atrioventricular b. [Fr. *bloquer*]

alveolo-capillary b., the presence of material that impairs the diffusion of gases between the air in the alveolar spaces and the blood in alveolar capillaries; b. can be caused by edema, cellular infiltration, fibrosis, or tumor, and results in undersaturation of peripheral arterial blood with oxygen.

alveolocapillary b., the presence of material that impairs the diffusion of gases between the air in the alveolar spaces and the blood in alveolar capillaries; b. can be caused by edema, cellular infiltration, fibrosis, or tumor, and results in undersaturation of peripheral arterial blood with oxygen.

anterograde b., conduction b. of an impulse traveling in its ordinary direction, for example, from the sinoatrial node toward the ventricular myocardium.

atrioventricular b., partial or complete b. of electric impulses originating in the atrium or sinus node preventing them from reaching the atrioventricular node and ventricles. In first degree A-V block, there is prolongation of A-V conduction time (P-R interval); in second degree A-V b., some but not all atrial impulses fail to reach the ventricles, thus some ventricular beats are dropped; in complete A-V b., complete atrioventricular dissociation (2) occurs; no impulses can reach the ventricles despite even a slow ventricular rate (under 45 per minute); atria and ventricles beat independently. SYN block (3).

bone b., a surgical procedure in which the bone

bl

adjacent to the joint is modified to limit the motion of the joint mechanically.

bundle-branch b., intraventricular b. due to interruption of conduction in one of the two main branches of the bundle of His and manifested in the electrocardiogram by marked prolongation of the QRS complex.

complete A-V b., SEE atrioventricular b.

depolarizing b., skeletal muscle paralysis associated with loss of polarity of the motor endplate, as occurs following administration of succinylcholine.

epidural b., an obstruction in the epidural space; used inaccurately to refer to epidural anesthesia.

field b., regional anesthesia produced by infiltration of local anesthetic solution into tissues surrounding an operative field.

intraventricular b., I-V b., delayed conduction within the ventricular conducting system or myocardium, including bundle-branch, peri-infarction b.'s, the fascicular b.'s, excitation, and the W-P-W (pre-excitation) syndrome.

Mobitz b., second degree atrioventricular b. in which there is a ratio of two or more atrial deflections (P waves) to ventricular responses.

nerve b., interruption of conduction of impulses in peripheral nerves or nerve trunks by injection of anesthetic.

nondepolarizing b., skeletal muscle paralysis unaccompanied by changes in polarity of the motor endplate, as occurs following administration of tubocurarine.

peri-infarction b., an electrocardiographic abnormality associated with an old myocardial infarct and caused by delayed activation of the myocardium in the region of the infarct; characterized by an initial vector directed away from the infarcted region with the terminal vector directed toward it.

phase I b., inhibition of nerve impulse transmission across the myoneural junction associated with depolarization of the motor endplate, as in the muscle paralysis produced by succinylcholine.

phase II b., inhibition of nerve impulse transmission across the myoneural junction unaccompanied by depolarization of the motor endplate, as in the muscle paralysis produced by tubocurarine.

retrograde b., impaired conduction backward from the ventricles or A-V node into the atria.

second degree A-V b., SEE atrioventricular b.

sinoatrial b., S-A b., sinus b., blockade of the impulse leaving the sinus node before it can activate atrial muscle.

spinal b., an obstruction to the flow of cerebrospinal fluid in the spinal subarachnoid space; used inaccurately to refer to spinal anesthesia.

stellate b., injection of local anesthetic solution in the vicinity of the stellate ganglion.

Wenckebach b., a form of b. in any cardiac tissue (most often the atrioventricular junction) in which there is progressive lengthening of conduction until a beat is dropped.

Wilson b., the commonest form of right bundle-branch b., characterized in lead I by a tall slender R wave followed by a wider S wave of lower voltage.

block•ade (blok′ād). **1.** Intravenous injection of colloidal dyes or other substances whereby the reaction of the reticuloendothelial cells to other influences (*e.g.,* by phagocytosis) is temporarily prevented. **2.** Arrest of peripheral nerve conduction or transmission at autonomic synaptic junctions, autonomic receptor sites, or myoneural junctions by a drug.

adrenergic b., selective inhibition by a drug of the responses of effector cells to adrenergic sympathetic nerve impulses (sympatholytic) and to epinephrine and related amines (adrenolytic).

cholinergic b., (1) inhibition by a drug of nerve impulse transmission at autonomic ganglionic synapses (ganglionic b.), at postganglionic parasympathetic effector cells (*e.g.,* by atropine), and at myoneural junctions (myoneural b.); **(2)** the inhibition of a cholinergic agent.

ganglionic b., inhibition of nerve impulse transmission at autonomic ganglionic synapses by drugs such as nicotine or hexamethonium.

myoneural b., inhibition of nerve impulse transmission at myoneural junctions by a drug such as curare.

narcotic b., the use of drugs to inhibit the effects of narcotic substances, as with naloxone.

block•er (blok′er). **1.** An instrument used to obstruct a passage. **2.** SEE blocking *agent.*

calcium channel b., a class of drugs with the capacity to prevent calcium ions from passing through biologic membranes. These agents are used to treat hypertension, angina pectoris, and cardiac arrhythmias; examples include nifedipine, diltiazem, and verapamil.

blood (blŭd). The fluid and its suspended formed elements that are circulated through the heart, arteries, capillaries, and veins; b. is the means by which 1) oxygen and nutritive materials are transported to the tissues, and 2) carbon dioxide and various metabolic products are removed for excretion. The b. consists of a pale yellow or grayyellow fluid, plasma, in which are suspended red b. cells (erythrocytes), white b. cells (leukocytes), and platelets. SEE ALSO arterial b., venous b. [A.S. blōd]

arterial b., b. that is oxygenated in the lungs, found in the left chambers of the heart and in the arteries, and relatively bright red.

cord b., b. present in the umbilical vessels at the time of delivery.

occult b., b. in the feces in amounts too small to be seen but detectable by chemical tests.

venous b., b. which has passed through the capillaries of various tissues, except the lungs, and is found in the veins, the right chambers of the heart, and the pulmonary arteries; it is usually dark red as a result of a lower content of oxygen.

whole b., b. drawn from a selected donor under rigid aseptic precautions; contains citrate ion or heparin as an anticoagulant; used as a b. replenisher.

blood bank. A place, usually a separate part or division of a hospital laboratory or a separtate free-standing facility, in which blood is collected from donors, typed, separated into several components, stored, and/or prepared for transfusion to recipients.

blood boosting. SYN blood *doping.*

blood count. Calculation of the number of red (RBC) or white (WBC) blood cells in a cubic millimeter of blood, by means of counting the cells in an accurate volume of diluted blood, stained film of blood, or by flow cytometry.

blood group. A system of genetically determined antigens or agglutinogens located on the surface of the erythrocyte. Because of the antigen differences existing between individuals, b. g.'s are significant in blood transfusions, maternal-fetal incompatibilities (erythroblastosis fetalis), tissue and organ transplantation, disputed paternity cases, and in genetic and anthropologic studies; certain b. g.'s have been supposed to be related to susceptibility or resistance to certain diseases. Often used as synonymous with blood type. See Blood Groups appendix for individual groups.

blood group·ing. The classification of blood samples by means of laboratory tests of their agglutination reactions with respect to one or more blood groups.

blood·let·ting (blŭd′let-ing). Removing blood, usually from a vein; used in congestive heart failure and polycythemia.

blood·shot (blŭd′shot). Denoting locally congested smaller blood vessels of a part (*e.g.,* the conjunctiva) which are dilated and visible.

blood·stream (blŭd′strēm). The flowing blood as it is encountered in the circulatory system as distinguished from blood that has been removed from the circulatory system or sequestered in a part.

blood type. The specific reaction pattern of erythrocytes of an individual to the antisera of one blood group; *e.g.,* the ABO blood group consists of four major b. t.'s: O, A, B, and AB. This classification depends on the presence or absence of two major antigens: A or B. Type O occurs when neither is present and type AB when both are present. See Blood Groups appendix.

Bombay b. t., b. t. of individuals who possess the genes for A and B antigens but are unable to express the genes because they lack the gene for H antigen, a required precursor of A and B. Individuals with this blood type frequently have anti-H in their blood.

blood ves·sel. A tube (artery, capillary, vein, or sinus) conveying blood.

blot. SEE Northern blot *analysis,* Southern blot *analysis,* Western blot *analysis,* zoo blot *analysis.*

blow-bottles. A device used to maintain optimal lung expansion in the postsurgical patient; it consists of two containers connected by a tube; one container is initially filled with water; with a series of slow, forced exhalations (each preceded by a deep inspiration), the patient forces the water from the first chamber into the second.

blunt-end. Refers to double-stranded DNA in which there are no unpaired bases at the end.

blush (blŭsh). **1.** A sudden and brief redness of the face and neck due to emotion. **2.** In angiography, used metaphorically to describe neovascularity or, in some cases, extravasation. [M.E., fr. O.E. *blyscan,*]

BMI body mass *index.*

B-mode. A two-dimensional diagnostic ultrasound presentation of echo-producing interfaces in a single plane; the intensity of the echo is represented by modulation of the brightness (B) of the spot, and the position of the echo is determined from the position of the transducer and the transit time of the acoustical pulse.

body (bod′ē). **1.** The head, neck, trunk, and extremities. The human body, consisting of head (caput), neck (collum), trunk (truncus), and limbs (membra). **2.** The material part of a human, as distinguished from the mind and spirit. **3.** The principal mass of any structure. **4.** A thing; a substance. SEE ALSO corpus, soma. SYN corpus (1) [NA]. [A.S. *bodig*]

acetone b., SYN ketone b.

amygdaloid b., a rounded mass of gray matter in the temporal lobe internal to the cortex of the uncus and immediately anterior to the inferior horn of the lateral ventricle; its major afferents are olfactory and its efferent connections are with the hypothalamus and mediodorsal nucleus of the thalamus and it is also reciprocally associated with the cortex of the temporal lobe; it is subdivided into two major nuclear groups; basolateral and corticormedial.

aortic b., one of several aggregations of chromaffin cells lying close to the aorta and containing chemoreceptors that respond primarily to decreases in blood oxygen tension. SYN corpora para-aortica, glomus aorticum.

asbestos b.'s, ferruginous b.'s with asbestos fibers as a core; a histologic hallmark of exposure to asbestos.

Aschoff b.'s, a form of granulomatous inflammation observed in acute rheumatic carditis.

asteroid b., (1) an eosinophilic inclusion resembling a star with delicate radiating lines, occurring in a vacuolated area of cytoplasm of a multinucleated giant cell; (2) a structure that is characteristic of sporotrichosis when found in the skin or secondary lesions of this mycosis; in tissue, it surrounds the 3- to 5-μm in diameter ovoid yeast of *Sporothrix schenkii.*

Auer b.'s, rod-shaped structures of uncertain nature in the cytoplasm of immature myeloid cells, especially myeloblasts, in acute myelocytic leukemia. SYN Auer rods.

Barr chromatin b., SYN sex *chromatin.*

basal b., an elongated centriolar structure situated at the base of each cilium at the apical margin of a cell. SYN basal granule.

Cabot's ring b.'s, ring-shaped or figure-of-eight structures that stain red with Wright's stain, found in red blood cells in severe anemias, possibly a remnant of the nuclear membrane.

Call-Exner b.'s, small fluid-filled spaces between granulosal cells in ovarian follicles and in ovarian tumors of granulosal origin; they may form a rosette-like structure.

carotid b., a small epithelioid structure located just above the bifurcation of the common carotid artery on each side. It serves as a chemoreceptor organ responsive to oxygen lack, carbon dioxide excess, and increased hydrogen ion concentration. SYN intercarotid b.

cavernous b., SEE *corpus* cavernosum clitoridis, *corpus* cavernosum penis.

cell b., the part of the cell containing the nucleus.

chromaffin b., SYN paraganglion.

chromatin b., the genetic apparatus of bacteria. SEE nucleus (2).

ciliary b., a thickened portion of the vascular tunic of the eye between the choroid and the iris; it consists of three parts or zones: orbiculus ciliaris, corona ciliaris, and ciliary muscle. SYN corpus ciliare [NA].

coccygeal b., an arteriovenous (arteriolovenular) anastomosis supplied by the middle sacral artery and located on the pelvic surface of the coccyx. It was formerly called a gland (of Luschka) or a glomus and included with the paraganglia.

cytoplasmic inclusion b.'s, SEE inclusion b.'s.

Ehrlich's inner b., a round oxyphil b. found in the red blood cell in hemolysis due to a specific blood poison. SYN Heinz-Ehrlich b.

foreign b., anything in the tissues or cavities of the b. that has been introduced there from without, and that is not rapidly absorbable.

geniculate b., SEE lateral geniculate b., medial geniculate b.

Heinz-Ehrlich b., SYN Ehrlich's inner b.

Highmore's b., SYN *mediastinum* testis.

Howell-Jolly b.'s, spherical or ovoid eccentrically located granules, approximately 1 μm in diameter, occasionally observed in the stroma of circulating erythrocytes after splenectomy or in megaloblastic or severe hemolytic anemia.

hyaline b.'s, homogeneous eosinophilic inclusions in the cytoplasm of epithelial cells; in renal tubules, hyaline b.'s represent droplets of protein reabsorbed from the lumen. SEE ALSO Mallory b.'s, drusen.

hyaloid b., SYN vitreous b.

b. of hyoid bone, the body of the hyoid bone, from which the greater and lesser horns extend.

inclusion b.'s, distinctive structures frequently formed in the nucleus or cytoplasm (occasionally in both locations) in cells infected with certain filtrable viruses, observed especially in nerve, epithelial, or endothelial cells.

intercarotid b., SYN carotid b.

ketone b., one of a group of ketones that includes acetoacetic acid, β-hydroxybutyric acid, and acetone; high levels are found in tissues and body fluids in ketosis. SYN acetone b.

Lafora b. [MIM*254780], an intraneural intracytoplasmic inclusion b. composed of acid mucopolysaccharides, seen in familial myoclonus epilepsy.

lateral geniculate b., the lateral one of a pair of small oval masses that protrude slightly from the posteroinferior aspects of the thalamus; its main (dorsal) subdivision serves as a processing station in the major pathway from the retina to the cerebral cortex, receiving fibers from the optic tract and giving rise to the geniculocalcarine radiation to the visual cortex in the occipital lobe. SYN corpus geniculatum laterale [NA].

Leishman-Donovan b., the intracytoplasmic, nonflagellated leishmanial form of certain intracellular parasites, such as species of *Leishmania* or the intracellular form of *Trypanosoma cruzi*. SYN amastigote.

Mallory b.'s, large, poorly defined accumulations of eosinophilic material in the cytoplasm of damaged hepatic cells in certain forms of cirrhosis and marked fatty change especially due to alcoholism.

malpighian b.'s, SYN splenic lymph *follicles*, under *follicle*.

mamillary b., a small, round, paired cell group that protrudes into the interpeduncular fossa from the inferior aspect of the hypothalamus. It receives hippocampal fibers through the fornix and projects fibers to the anterior thalamic nuclei and into the brainstem tegmentum. SYN corpus mamillare [NA].

medial geniculate b., the medial one of a pair of prominent cell groups in the posteroinferior parts of the thalamus; it functions as the last of a series of processing stations along the auditory conduction pathway to the cerebral cortex, receiving the brachium of the inferior colliculus and giving rise to the auditory radiation to the auditory cortex in the superior temporal gyrus. SYN corpus geniculatum mediale [NA].

metachromatic b.'s, concentrated deposits consisting primarily of polymetaphosphate and occurring in many bacteria as well as in algae, fungi, and protozoa; m. b.'s differ in staining properties from the surrounding protoplasm. SEE metachromasia.

multilamellar b., SYN cytosome (2).

Negri b.'s, eosinophilic, sharply outlined, pathognomonic inclusion b.'s (2 to 10 μm in diameter) found in the cytoplasm of certain nerve cells containing the virus of rabies, especially in Ammon's horn of the hippocampus.

Nissl b.'s, SYN Nissl *substance*.

nuclear inclusion b.'s, SEE inclusion b.'s.

pacchionian b.'s, SYN arachnoid *granulations*, under *granulation*.

Pappenheimer b.'s, phagosomes, containing ferruginous granules, found in red blood cells in diseases such as sideroblastic anemia, hemolytic anemia, and sickle cell disease.

parabasal b., part of the giant mitochondrion of certain parasitic flagellates. The parabasal b. plus the basal b. were previously thought to comprise a kinetoplast, but kinetoplast is now restricted to part of the DNA giant mitochondrion.

para-aortic b.'s, small masses of chromaffin tissue found near the sympathetic ganglia along the aorta; they are more prominent during fetal life. The chromaffin cells secrete noradrenalin; chemoreceptive endings monitor levels of blood gases.

pineal b., a small, unpaired, flattened body, shaped somewhat like a pine cone, attached at its anterior pole to the region of the posterior and habenular commissures, and lying in the depression between the two superior colliculi below the splenium of the corpus callosum; it is a glandular structure, composed of follicles containing epithelioid cells and lime concretions called brain sand; despite its attachment to the brain, it appears to receive nerve fibers exclusively from the peripheral autonomic nervous system. It produces melatonin. SYN corpus pineale [NA], conarium, pineal gland.

polar b., one of two small cells formed by the first and second meiotic division of oocytes; the first is usually released just prior to ovulation, the second not until discharge of the ovum from the ovary.

psammoma b.'s, (1) mineralized b.'s occurring in the meninges, choroid plexus, and in certain meningiomas; composed usually of a central capillary surrounded by concentric whorls of meningocytes in various stages of hyaline change and mineralization; can also occur in benign and malignant epithelial tumors (often papillary) or with chronic inflammation; (2) SYN *corpora* arenacea, under *corpus*. (3) SYN calcospherite.

restiform b., a lateral (larger) subdivision of the inferior cerebellar peduncle composed of a variety of fibers including, but not limited to, olivo-, reticulo-, cuneo-, trigemino-, and dorsal spinocerebellar.

Russell b.'s, small, discrete, variably sized, spherical, intracytoplasmic, acidophilic, hyaline b.'s that stain deeply with fuchsin; they occur frequently in plasma cells in chronic inflammation.

sclerotic b.'s, vegetative rounded muriform cells of dematiaceous fungi, characteristic of the causal agents of chromoblastomycosis.

b. of stomach, the part of the stomach that lies between the fundus above and the pyloric antrum below; its boundaries are poorly defined.

striate b., the caudate and lentiform (lenticular) nuclei; the striate appearance on section is caused by slender fascicles of myelinated fibers. SYN corpus striatum [NA].

trachoma b.'s, distinctive, complex, intracytoplasmic forms found in the conjunctival epithelial cells of persons in the acute phase of trachoma.

vitreous b., a transparent jelly-like substance filling the interior of the eyeball behind the lens of the eye; it is composed of a delicate network (vitreous stroma) enclosing in its meshes a watery fluid (vitreous humor). SYN corpus vitreum [NA], hyaloid b., vitreous (2), vitreum.

wolffian b., SYN mesonephros.

boil (boyl). SYN furuncle. [A.S. *byl*, a swelling]

Aleppo b., the lesion occurring in cutaneous leishmaniasis. SEE cutaneous *leishmaniasis*.

date b., Delhi b., Jericho b., the lesion occurring in cutaneous leishmaniasis.

Madura b., SYN mycetoma (1).

bo·lus (bō′lŭs). **1.** A single, relatively large quantity of a substance, usually one intended for therapeutic use, such as a b. dose of a drug. **2.** A masticated morsel of food or another substance ready to be swallowed, such as a b. of barium for x-ray studies. **3.** In high-energy radiation therapy, a quantity of tissue-equivalent material placed next to the irradiated region to increase the dose of secondary radiation to the superficial tissues. [L. fr. G. *bōlos*, lump, clod]

intravenous b., a relatively large volume of fluid or dose of a drug or test substance given intravenously and rapidly to hasten or magnify a response; in radiology, rapid injection of a large dose of contrast medium to increase opacification of blood vessels.

bond. In chemistry, the force holding two neighboring atoms in place and resisting their separation; a b. is electrovalent if it consists of the attraction between oppositely charged groups, or covalent if it results from the sharing of one, two, or three pairs of electrons by the bonded atoms.

conjugated double b.'s, two or more double b.'s separated by each single b.

disulfide b., a single bond between two sulfurs; specifically, the —S—S— link binding two peptide chains (or different parts of one peptide chain).

double b., a covalent b. resulting from the sharing of two pairs of electrons; *e.g.,* $H_2C=CH_2$ (ethylene).

electrostatic b., b. between atoms or groups carrying opposite charges (or, in some cases, partial charges).

high energy phosphate b., SEE high energy *phosphates,* under *phosphate.*

hydrogen b., a b. arising from the sharing of a hydrogen atom, covalently bound to an electronegative element (*e.g.,* N or O), with another electronegative element (*e.g.,* N, O, or a halogen).

noncovalent b., b. in which electrons are not shared between atoms; *e.g.,* electrostatic b., hydrogen b.

peptide b., the common link (—CO—NH—) between amino acids in proteins, formed by elimination of H_2O between the —COOH of one amino acid and the H_2N— of another.

semipolar b., a b. in which the two electrons shared by a pair of atoms belonged originally to only one of the atoms; often represented by a small arrow pointing toward the electron receiver; *e.g.,* nitric acid, $O(OH)N{\rightarrow}O$; phosphoric acid, $(OH)_3P{\rightarrow}O$.

single b., a covalent b. resulting from the sharing of one pair of electrons; *e.g.,* $H_3C—CH_3$ (ethane).

triple b., a covalent b. resulting from the sharing of three pairs of electrons; *e.g.,* $HC{\equiv}CH$ (acetylene).

bone (bōn). **1.** A hard connective tissue consisting of cells embedded in a matrix of mineralized ground substance and collagen fibers. The fibers are impregnated with a form of calcium phosphate similar to hydroxyapatite as well as with substantial quantities of carbonate, citrate sodium, and magnesium; by weight, b. is composed of 75% inorganic material and 25% organic material; a portion of osseous tissue of definite shape and size, forming a part of the animal skeleton; in man there are 200 distinct ossa in the skeleton, not including the ossicula auditus of the tympanic cavity or the ossa sesamoidea other than the two patellae. Bone consists of a dense outer layer of compact substance or cortical substance covered by the periosteum, and an inner loose, spongy substance; the central portion of a long bone is filled with marrow. **2.** For defini-

tions of bones as part of the animal skeleton, see
os. For definitions of bones as part of the animal
skelton, see Os. SYN os [NA]. [A.S. *bān*]

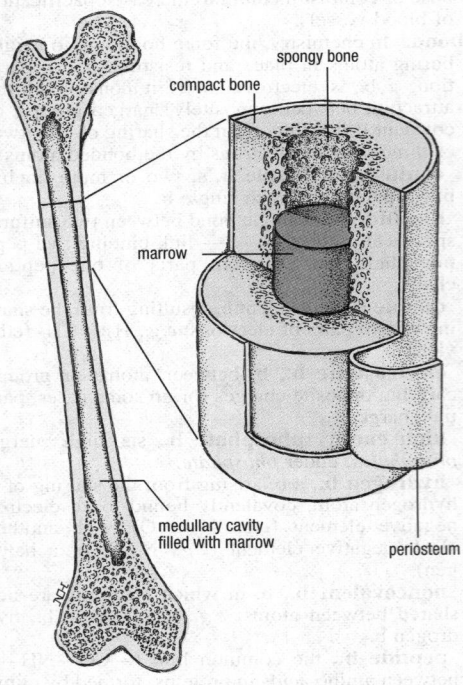

compact bone

spongy bone

marrow

medullary cavity
filled with marrow

periosteum

bone

ankle b., SYN talus.
breast b., SYN sternum.
brittle b.'s, SYN *osteogenesis* imperfecta.
calf b., SYN fibula. [O.N. *kalfi,* fibula]
cancellous b., SYN *substantia* spongiosa.
capitate b., SYN capitate (1).
carpal b.'s, eight bones arranged in two rows
that articulate proximally with the radius and indirectly with the ulna, and distally with the five
metacarpal bones. SYN carpus (2) [NA].
   cartilage b., SYN endochondral b.
   collar b., SYN clavicle.
   compact b., the compact, noncancellous portion of bone that consists largely of concentric
lamellar osteons and interstitial lamellae. SYN
substantia compacta [NA], compact substance.
   cortical b., the superficial thin layer of compact
bone. SYN substantia corticalis [NA], cortical substance.
   cranial b.'s, SYN b.'s of skull.
   cuboid b., the lateral bone of the distal row of
the tarsus, articulating with the calcaneus, lateral
cuneiform, navicular (occasionally), and fourth
and fifth metatarsal bones.
   cuneiform b., SEE triquetral b.
   b.'s of digits, the phalanges and sesamoid
bones of the fingers and toes.
   ear b.'s, SYN auditory *ossicles,* under *ossicle.*

elbow b., SYN olecranon.
endochondral b., a b. that develops in a cartilage environment after the latter is partially or
entirely destroyed by calcification and subsequent resorption. SYN cartilage b.
   ethmoid b., an irregularly shaped bone lying
between the orbital plates of the frontal and anterior to the sphenoid bone; it consists of two lateral masses of thin plates enclosing air cells, attached above to a perforated horizontal lamina,
the cribriform plate, from which descends a median vertical or perpendicular plate in the interval
between the two lateral masses; the bone articulates with the sphenoid, frontal, maxillary, lacrimal, and palatine bones, the inferior nasal concha, and the vomer; it enters into the formation of
the anterior cranial fossa, the orbits, and the nasal
cavity.
   facial b.'s, the bones surrounding the mouth
and nose and contributing to the orbits; they are
the paired maxillae, zygomatic, nasal, lacrimal,
palatine, and inferior nasal conchae; and the unpaired ethmoid, vomer, mandible, and hyoid.
   flat b., a type of bone characterized by its thin,
flattened shape, such as the scapula or certain of
the cranial bones.
   frontal b., the large single bone forming the
forehead and the upper margin and roof of the
orbit on either side; it articulates with the parietal,
nasal, ethmoid, maxillary, and zygomatic bones,
and with the lesser wings of the sphenoid.
   greater multangular b., SYN trapezium.
   hamate b., the bone on the medial (ulnar) side
of the distal row of the carpus; it articulates with
the fourth and fifth metacarpal, triquetral, lunate,
and capitate. SYN unciform b.
   heel b., SYN calcaneus (1).
   hip b., a large flat bone formed by the fusion of
the ilium, ischium, and pubis (in the adult), constituting the lateral half of the pelvis; it articulates
with its fellow anteriorly, with the sacrum posteriorly, and with the femur laterally. SYN coxa (1),
innominate b.
   hollow b., SYN pneumatic b.
   hyoid b., a U-shaped bone lying between the
mandible and the larynx, suspended from the styloid processes by slender stylohyoid ligaments.
   iliac b., SYN ilium.
   incisive b., SYN *os* incisivum.
   innominate b., SYN hip b.
   intermaxillary b., SYN *os* incisivum.
   intermediate cuneiform b., a bone of the distal row of the tarsus; it articulates with the medial
and lateral cuneiform, navicular, and second metatarsal bones. SYN wedge b.
   irregular b., one of a group of bones having
peculiar or complex forms, *e.g.,* vertebrae, many
of the skull bones.
   ischial b., SYN ischium.
   jaw b., SYN mandible.
   jugal b., SYN zygomatic b.
   lacrimal b., an irregularly rectangular thin
plate, forming part of the medial wall of the orbit
behind the frontal process of the maxilla; it articulates with the inferior nasal concha, ethmoid,
frontal, and maxillary bones.
   lamellar b., the normal type of adult mamma-

lian b., whether cancellous or compact, composed of parallel lamellae in the former and concentric lamellae in the latter.

lateral cuneiform b., a bone of the distal row of the tarsus; it articulates with the intermediate cuneiform, cuboid, navicular, and second, third, and fourth metatarsal bones. SYN wedge b.

long b., one of the elongated bones of the extremities, consisting of a tubular shaft (diaphysis) and two extremities (epiphyses) usually wider than the shaft; the shaft is composed of compact bone surrounding a central medullary cavity. Cf. short b.

lunate b., one of the proximal row in the carpus between the scaphoid and triquetral; it articulates with the radius, scaphoid, triquetral, hamate, and capitate.

malar b., SYN zygomatic b.

mastoid b., SYN mastoid *process*.

medial cuneiform b., the largest of the three cuneiform bones, the medial bone of the distal row of the tarsus, articulating with the intermediate cuneiform, navicular, and first and second metatarsal bones. SYN wedge b.

membrane b., a b. that develops embryologically within a membrane of vascularized primitive mesenchymal tissue without prior formation of cartilage.

metacarpal b., one of the metacarpal bones, five long bones (numbered I to V, beginning with the bone on the radial or thumb side) forming the skeleton of the metacarpus or palm; they articulate with the bones of the distal row of the carpus and with the five proximal phalanges.

metatarsal b., one of the metatarsal bones; the five long bones numbered I to V beginning with the bone on the medial side forming the skeleton of the anterior portion of the foot, articulating posteriorly with the three cuneiform and the cuboid bones, anteriorly with the five proximal phalanges.

multangular b., SEE trapezium, trapezoid b.

nasal b., an elongated rectangular bone which, with its fellow, forms the bridge of the nose; it articulates with the frontal bone superiorly, the ethmoid and the frontal process of the maxilla posteriorly, and its fellow medially.

navicular b., a bone of the tarsus on the medial side of the foot articulating with the head of the talus, the three cuneiform bones, and occasionally the cuboid.

nonlamellar b., SYN woven b.

occipital b., a bone at the lower and posterior part of the skull, consisting of three parts (basilar, condylar, and squamous), enclosing a large oval hole, the foramen magnum; it articulates with the parietal and temporal bones on either side, the sphenoid anteriorly, and the atlas below.

palatine b., an irregularly shaped bone posterior to the maxilla, which enters into the formation of the nasal cavity, the orbit, and the hard palate; it articulates with the maxilla, inferior nasal concha, sphenoid, and ethmoid bones, the vomer and its fellow of the opposite side.

parietal b., a flat, curved bone of irregular quadrangular shape, at either side of the vault of the cranium; it articulates, with its fellow medially,

with the frontal anteriorly, the occipital posteriorly, and the temporal and sphenoid inferiorly.

perichondral b., in the development of a long b. a collar or cuff of osseous tissue forms in the perichondrium of the cartilage model; the connective tissue membrane of this perichondral b. then becomes periosteum.

pisiform b., a small bone resembling a pea in size and shape, in the proximal row of the carpus, lying on the anterior surface of the triquetral, with which it articulates; it gives insertion to the tendon of the flexor carpi ulnaris muscle.

pneumatic b., a bone that is hollow or contains many air cells, such as the mastoid process of the temporal bone. SYN hollow b.

premaxillary b., SYN os incisivum.

pubic b., the anteroinferior portion of the hip bone, distinct at birth but later becoming fused with the ilium and ischium; it consists of a body, which articulates with its fellow at the symphysis pubis, and two rami; the superior ramus enters into the formation of the acetabulum, and the inferior ramus fuses with the ramus of the ischium to form the ischiopubic ramus.

pyramidal b., SYN triquetral b.

reticulated b., SYN woven b.

rider's b., heterotopic bone ossification of the tendon of the adductor longus muscle from strain in horseback riding.

scaphoid b., the largest bone of the proximal row of the carpus on the lateral (radial) side, articulating with the radius, lunate, capitate, trapezium, and trapezoid.

semilunar b., obsolete term for lunate b.

sesamoid b., a bone formed after birth in a tendon where it passes over a joint, *e.g.,* the patella.

shin b., SYN tibia.

short b., one whose dimensions are approximately equal; it consists of a layer of cortical substance enclosing spongy substance and marrow. Cf. long b.

b.'s of skull, the paired inferior nasal concha, lacrimal, maxilla, nasal, palatine, parietal, temporal, and zygomatic; and the unpaired ethmoid, frontal, occipital, sphenoid, and vomer. SYN cranial b.'s.

sphenoid b., a bone of most irregular shape occupying the base of the skull; it is described as consisting of a central portion, or body, and six processes: two greater wings, two lesser wings and two pterygoid processes; it articulates with the occipital, frontal, ethmoid, and vomer, and with the paired temporal, parietal, zygomatic, palatine and sphenoidal concha bones. SYN sphenoid (2).

spongy b., (1) SYN *substantia* spongiosa. (2) a turbinated bone.

sutural b.'s, small irregular bones found along the sutures of the cranium, particularly related to the parietal bone. SYN wormian b.'s.

tarsal b.'s, the seven bones of the instep: talus, calcaneus, navicular, three cuneiform (wedge), and cuboid bones.

temporal b., a large irregular bone situated in the base and side of the skull; it consists of three parts, squamous, tympanic, and petrous, which

bo

are distinct at birth; the petrous part contains the vestibulocochlear organ; the bone articulates with the sphenoid, parietal, occipital, and zygomatic bones, and by a synovial joint with the mandible.

thigh b., SYN femur.

trabecular b., SYN *substantia* spongiosa.

trapezium b., SYN trapezium.

trapezoid b., a bone in the distal row of the carpus; it articulates with the second metacarpal, trapezium, capitate, and scaphoid. SYN trapezoid (3).

triangular b., SYN *os* trigonum.

triquetral b., a bone on the medial (ulnar) side of the proximal row of the carpus, articulating with the lunate, pisiform, and hamate. SYN pyramidal b.

tympanic b., SYN tympanic ring.

unciform b., SYN hamate b.

wedge b., SYN intermediate cuneiform b., lateral cuneiform b., medial cuneiform b.

wormian b.'s, SYN sutural b.'s.

woven b., bony tissue characteristic of the embryonal skeleton, in which the collagen fibers of the matrix are arranged irregularly in the form of interlacing networks. SYN nonlamellar b., reticulated b.

zygomatic b., a quadrilateral bone which forms the prominence of the cheek; it articulates with the frontal, sphenoid, temporal, and maxillary bone. SYN jugal b., mala (2), malar b., zygoma (1).

bone•let (bōn′let). SYN ossicle.

BOOP *bronchiolitis* obliterans with organizing pneumonia, an idiopathic form of *bronchiolitis* obliterans.

boost•er. SEE booster *dose*.

bor•bo•ryg•mus, pl. **bor•bo•ryg•mi** (bōr-bō-rig′mŭs, -rig′mī). Rumbling or gurgling noises produced by movement of gas, fluid, or both in the alimentary canal, and audible at a distance. [G. *borborygmos,* rumbling in the bowels]

bor•der (bōr′der). The part of a surface that forms its outer boundary. SEE ALSO margin. SYN margo [NA].

anterior b. of tibia, the sharp subcutaneous ridge of the tibia that extends from the tuberosity to the anterior part of the medial malleolus. SYN shin (2).

brush b., the apical epithelial surface bearing closely packed microvilli about 2 μm long, such as occur on the cells of the proximal tubule of the nephron.

denture b., (1) the limit or boundary or circumferential margin of a denture base; **(2)** the margin of the denture base at the junction of the polished surface with the impression (tissue) surface; **(3)** the extreme edges of a denture base at the buccolabial, lingual, and posterior limits. SYN periphery (2).

striated b., the free surface of the columnar absorptive cells of the intestine formed by closely packed microvilli about 1 μm long, giving the appearance of parallel striations.

vermilion b., the red margin of the upper and lower lip that commences at the exterior edge of the intraoral labial mucosa ("moist line") and extends outward, terminating at the extraoral labial

cutaneous junction; a thinly keratinized type of stratified squamous epithelium deeply penetrated by well-vascularized dermal papillae which show through the translucent epidermis to impart the typical red appearance of the lips.

Bor•de•tel•la (bōr-dĕ-tel′ă). A genus of strictly aerobic bacteria (family Brucellaceae) containing minute Gram-negative coccobacilli. Motile and nonmotile species occur; motile cells are peritrichous. The metabolism of these organisms is respiratory. They require nicotinic acid, cysteine, and methionine; hemin (X factor) and coenzyme I (V factor) are not required. They are parasites and pathogens of the mammalian respiratory tract. The type species is *B. pertussis.* [J. *Bordet*]

B. pertus′sis, a species that causes whooping cough; it produces cell-destroying toxins and causes thick mucus to collect in the airway. The type species of the genus *B.*

bo•ron (B) (bōr′on). A nonmetallic trivalent element, atomic no. 5, atomic wt. 10.811; occurs as a hard crystalline mass or as a brown powder, and forms borates and boric acid. A nutritional need has been reported in pregnant women. [Pers. *Burah*]

Bor•rel•ia (bō-rē′lē-ă, bo-rel′ē-ă). A genus of bacteria containing cells with coarse, shallow, irregular spirals and tapered, finely filamented ends. These organisms are parasitic on many forms of animal life. [A. *Borrell*]

B. burgdor′feri, a species causing Lyme disease. The vector transmitting this spirochete to humans is the tick, *Ixodes dammini.*

bor•re•li•o•sis (bō-rē-lē-ō′sis). Disease caused by bacteria of the genus *Borrelia.*

boss (baws). **1.** A protuberance; a circumscribed rounded swelling. **2.** The prominence of a kyphosis. [M. E. *boce,* fr. O. Fr.]

bos•se•lat•ed (baws′ĕ-lā-ted). Marked by numerous bosses or rounded protuberances. [Fr. *bosseler,* to emboss]

bot•ry•oid (bot′rē-oyd). Having numerous rounded protuberances resembling a bunch of grapes. SYN staphyline, uviform. [G. *botryoeidēs,* like a bunch of grapes (*botrys*)]

bot•u•lism (bot′yū-lizm). Food poisoning caused by the ingestion of the neurotoxin produced by *Clostridium botulinum,* usually in improperly canned or preserved food; causes paralysis and can be fatal. SEE ALSO *Clostridium botulinum.* [L. *botulus,* sausage]

bou•bas (boo′bahs). SYN yaws. [native Brazilian]

bou•gie (boo′zhē). A cylindrical instrument, usually somewhat flexible and yielding, used for calibrating or dilating constricted areas in tubular organs, such as the urethra or esophagus; sometimes containing a medication for local application. [Fr. candle]

bulbous b., a b. with a bulb-shaped tip, some of which are shaped like an acorn or an olive.

Eder-Pustow b., a metal olive-shaped b. with a flexible metal dilating system (for esophageal stricture).

elbowed b., a b. with a sharply angulated bend near its tip.

filiform b., a very slender b. usually used for gentle exploration of strictures or sinus tracts of small diameter where false passages can be encountered or created; the trailing end usually consists of a threaded cylinder into which the screw tip of a following b. can be inserted.

following b., a flexible tapered b. with a screw tip which is attached to the trailing end of a filiform b., to allow progressive dilation without danger of creating false passages.

Savary b.'s, Silastic tapered-tip b.'s used over a guide wire in esophageal dilatation.

bou·gie·nage (bū-zhē-nahzh'). Examination or treatment of the interior of any canal by the passage of a bougie or cannula.

boundaries (bown'dar-'es). Limits of one's personal space, including physical, psychosocial, or interpersonal domains.

bou·ton (bū-ton'). A button, pustule, or knob-like swelling. [Fr. button]

terminal b.'s, b.'s terminaux, SYN axon *terminals*, under *terminal*.

Bovie. An instrument used for electrosurgical dissection and hemostasis. Frequently used as a verb, *i.e.,* to Bovie something is to dissect or cauterize it with the Bovie instrument.

bo·vine (bō'vīn, -vin). Relating to cattle. [L. *bos* (*bov-*), ox]

bow·el. SYN intestinum (1). [through the Fr. from L. *botulus*, sausage]

bow·leg, bow-b. (bō'leg). SYN *genu varum.*

BP. avoirdupois *weight.*

BPF bronchopleural *fistula.*

BPH benign prostatic *hyperplasia.*

Br bromine.

brace (brās). An orthosis or orthopedic appliance that supports or holds in correct position any movable part of the body and that allows motion of the part, in contrast to a splint, which prevents motion of the part. [M. E., fr. O. Fr., fr. L. *bracchium,* arm, fr. G. *brachion*]

brac·es (brā'sez). Colloquialism for orthodontic appliances.

bra·chia (brā'kē-ă). Plural of brachium.

brach·i·al (brā'kē-ăl). Relating to the arm.

bra·chi·al·gia (brā-kē-al'jē-ă). Pain in the arm. [L. *brachium,* arm, + *algos,* pain]

◇**brachio-.** **1.** SYN arm (1). **2.** SYN radial. [L. *brachium*]

bra·chi·o·ce·phal·ic (brā'kē-ō-se-fal'ik). Relating to both arm and head.

bra·chi·o·cru·ral (brā'kē-ō-krū'răl). Relating to both arm and thigh.

bra·chi·o·cu·bi·tal (brā'kē-ō-kyū'bi-tăl). Relating to both arm and elbow or to both arm and forearm.

bra·chi·um, pl. **bra·chia** (brā'kē-ŭm, brak'; -ă) [NA]. **1.** SYN arm (1). **2.** An anatomical structure resembling an arm. [L. arm, prob. akin to G. *brachiōn*]

b. of inferior colliculus, a fiber bundle passing from the inferior colliculus on either side of the brainstem along the lateral border of the superior colliculus to the posterior part of the thalamus where it enters the medial geniculate body. It forms part of the major ascending auditory pathway.

b. of superior colliculus, a band of fibers of the optic tract bypassing the lateral geniculate

body to terminate in the superior colliculus and pretectal region.

◇**brachy-.** Short. [G. *brachys,* short]

brach·y·ba·sia (brak-ē-bā'sē-ă). The shuffling gait of pyramidal tract disease. [brachy- + G. *basis,* a stepping]

brach·y·ba·so·camp·to·dac·ty·ly (brak-ē-bā' sō-kamp-tō-dak'ti-lē). Disproportionate shortness and crookedness of the fingers. [brachy- + G. *basis,* base, + *campylos,* curved, + *daktylos,* finger]

brach·y·ba·so·pha·lan·gia (brak-ē-bā'sō-fă-lan' jē-ă). Abnormal shortness of the proximal phalanges. [brachy- + G. *basis,* base, + phalanx]

brach·y·car·dia (brak-ē-kar'dē-ă). SYN bradycardia.

brach·y·chei·lia, brach·y·chi·lia (brak'ē-kī'lē-ă). Abnormal shortness of the lips. [brachy- + G. *cheilos,* lip]

brach·y·dac·ty·ly (brak-ē-dak'ti-lē). Abnormal shortness of the fingers. [brachy- + G. *daktylos,* finger]

bra·chyg·na·thia (brak-ig-nā'thē-ă). Abnormal shortness or recession of the mandible. SEE ALSO micrognathia. [brachy- + G. *gnathos,* jaw]

brach·y·me·lia (brak-ē-mē'lē-ă). Disproportionate shortness of the limbs. [brachy- + G. *melos,* limb]

brach·y·me·so·pha·lan·gia (brak-ē-mes'ō-fă-lan'jē-ă). Abnormal shortness of the middle phalanges. [brachy- + G. *mesos,* middle, + phalanx]

brach·y·met·a·car·pia (brak'ē-met-ă-car'pē-ă). Abnormal shortness of the metacarpals, especially the fourth and fifth.

brach·y·met·a·tar·sia (brak'ē-met-ă-tar'sē-ă). Abnormal shortness of the metatarsals.

brach·y·o·nych·ia (brak'ē-ō-nik'ē-ă). Short nails, in which the width of the nail plate and nail bed is greater than the length. [G. *brachys,* short + *onyx, onychos,* nail, + suffix *-ia,* condition]

brach·y·pha·lan·gia (brak'ē-fă-lan'jē-ă). Abnormal shortness of the phalanges. [brachy- + phalanx]

brach·y·syn·dac·ty·ly (brak'ē-sin-dak'ti-lē). Abnormal shortness of fingers or toes combined with a webbing between the adjacent digits. [brachy- + syndactyly]

brach·y·te·le·pha·lan·gia (brak-ē-tel'ē-fă-lan'jē-ă). Abnormal shortness of the distal phalanges. [brachy- + G. *telos,* end, + phalanx]

brach·y·ther·a·py (brak-ē-thār'ă-pē). Radiotherapy in which the source of irradiation is placed close to the surface of the body or within a body cavity; *e.g.,* application of radium to the cervix.

◇**brady-.** Slow. [G. *bradys,* slow]

bra·dy·ar·rhyth·mia (brad'ē-ă-rith'mē-ă). Any disturbance of the heart's rhythm resulting in a rate under 60 beats per minute. [brady- + G. *a-* priv. + *rhythmos,* rhythm]

bra·dy·arth·ria (brad-ē-arth're-ă). A form of dysarthria characterized by an abnormal slowness or deliberateness of speech. SYN bradyglossia (2), bradylalia, bradylogia. [brady- + G. *arthroō,* to utter distinctly, fr. *arthron,* a joint]

bra·dy·car·dia (brad-ē-kar'dē-ă). Slowness of the heartbeat, usually a rate under 60 beats per minute. SYN brachycardia. [brady- + G. *kardia*, heart]

brad·y·car·di·ac (brad-ē-kar'dē-ak). Relating to or characterized by bradycardia. SYN bradycardic.

bra·dy·car·dic (brad-ē-kar'dik). SYN bradycardiac.

bra·dy·di·as·to·le (brad-ē-dī-as'tō-lē). Prolongation of the diastole of the heart.

bra·dy·es·the·sia (brad-ē-es-thē'zē-ă). Slow sensory perception. [brady- + G. *aisthēsis*, sensation]

bra·dy·glos·sia (brad-ē-glos'ē-ă). 1. Slow or difficult tongue movement. 2. SYN bradyarthria. [brady- + G. *glōssa*, tongue]

bra·dy·ki·ne·sia (brad-ē-kin-ē'zē-ă). A decrease in spontaneity and movement. One of the features of extrapyramidal disorders, such as Parkinson's disease. [brady- + G. *kinēsis*, movement]

bra·dy·ki·net·ic (brad-ē-ki-net'ik). Characterized by or pertaining to slow movement.

bra·dy·ki·nin (brad-ē-kī'nin). The nonapeptide Arg-Pro-Pro-Gly-Phe-Ser-Pro-Phe-Arg, normally present in blood in an inactive form; one of the plasma kinins, a potent vasodilator and mediator of anaphylaxis. [brady- + G. *kineō*, to move]

bra·dy·la·lia (brad-ē-lā'lē-ă). SYN bradyarthria. [brady- + G. *lalia*, speech]

bra·dy·lex·ia (brad-ē-lek'sē-ă). Abnormal slowness in reading. [brady- + G. *lexis*, word]

bra·dy·lo·gia (brad-ē-lō'jē-ă). SYN bradyarthria. [brady- + G. *logos*, word]

bra·dyp·nea (brad-ip-nē'ă). Abnormal slowness of respiration, specifically a low respiratory frequency. [brady- + G. *pnoē*, breathing]

bra·dy·sper·ma·tism (brad-ē-sper'mă-tizm). Absence of ejaculatory force, so that the semen trickles away slowly. [brady, + G. *sperma* (*spermat-*), seed, + ism]

bra·dy·sphyg·mia (brad-ē-sfig'mē-ă). Slowness of the pulse; can occur without bradycardia, as in ventricular bigeminy when every other beat may fail to produce a peripheral pulse. [brady- + G. *sphygmos*, pulse]

bra·dy·stal·sis (brad-ē-stahl'sis). Slow bowel motion. [G. *bradys*, slow, + (*peri*) *stalsis*, contracting around]

bra·dy·to·cia (brad-ē-tō'sē-ă). Tedious labor; slow delivery. [brady- + G. *tokos*, childbirth]

bra·dy·u·ria (brad-ē-yū'rē-ă). Slow micturition. [brady- + G. *ouron*, urine]

Brain, W. Russell, Lord, English physician, 1895–1966. SEE B.'s *reflex*.

▪ brain (brān). That part of the central nervous system contained within the cranium. SEE ALSO encephalon. Cf. cerebrum, cerebellum. [A.S. *braegen*]

brain·case (brān'kās). SYN neurocranium.

brain·stem, brain stem (brān'stem). Originally, the entire unpaired subdivision of the brain, composed of the rhombencephalon, mesencephalon, and diencephalon as distinguished from the brain's only paired subdivision, the telencephalon. More recently, the term's connotation has undergone several arbitrary modifications: some use it to denote no more than rhombencephalon plus mesencephalon, distinguishing that complex from the prosencephalon (diencephalon plus telencephalon); others restrict it even further to refer

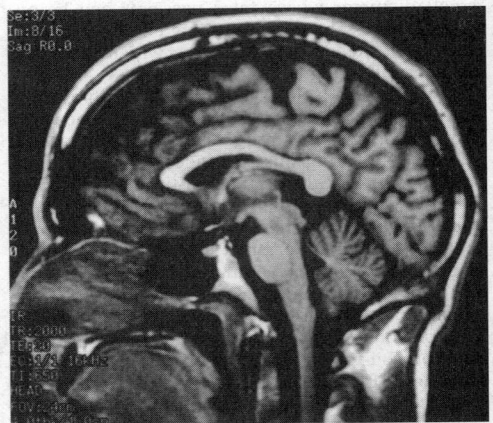

brain: magnetic resonance imaging (MRI) of a normal brain

exclusively to the rhombencephalon. From both developmental and architectural viewpoints, the original interpretation seems preferable.

brain·wash·ing (brān'wash'ing). Inducing a person to modify his attitudes and behavior in certain directions through various forms of psychological pressure or torture.

branch. An offshoot; in anatomy, one of the primary divisions of a nerve or blood vessel. A branch. SEE ramus, artery, nerve, vein. SYN ramus (1) [NA]. [Fr. *branche*, related to L. *branchium*, arm]

anastomotic b., a blood vessel that interconnects two neighboring vessels. It should not be used for the nervous system, because there is no analogy between a vascular anastomosing branch and a connection between nerves or their subdivisions.

ascending b. of the inferior mesenteric artery, b. of the left colic artery (from inferior mesenteric artery) that passes anteriorly to the left kidney into the transverse mesocolon, where it anastomoses with the middle colic artery. It thus forms an anastomosis between superior and inferior mesenteric arteries, and is a component of the marginal artery (Drummond) of the colon.

basal tentorial b. of internal carotid artery, a small b. from the cavernous part of the internal carotid artery to the base of the tentorium.

cavernous sinus b. of internal carotid artery, a number of small b.'s of the cavernous part of the internal carotid artery. SEE ganglionic b. of internal carotid artery, basal tentorial b. of internal carotid artery, marginal tentorial b. of internal carotid artery.

communicating b., a bundle of nerve fibers passing from one named nerve to join another. The term "communicating branch" is used in the nervous system to replace the inadequate "anastomosing branch" used for vascular systems.

ganglionic b.'s of maxillary nerve, the ganglionic branches, two short sensory branches of the maxillary nerve in the pterygopalatine fossa, the fibers of which pass through the pterygopalatine ganglion without synapse. SYN nervi pterygo-palatini.

ganglionic b. of internal carotid artery, b. to trigeminal ganglion; a small b. of the cavernous part of the internal carotid artery to the trigeminal ganglion.

marginal tentorial b. of internal carotid artery, a small b. from the cavernous part of the internal carotid artery to the free margin of the tentorium.

branch·ing. Dividing into parts; sending out offshoots; bifurcating.

Bran·ha·mel·la (bran-hă-mel′ă). A subgenus of aerobic, nonmotile, non–spore-forming bacteria containing Gram-negative cocci that occur in pairs with adjacent sides flattened. They are found in the mucous membranes of the upper respiratory tract and occasionally cause respiratory infections and otitis media. [Sara *Branham*]

bran·ny (bran′ē). Denoting desquamation of small husk-like scales. [M.E. *bran,* broken coat of cereal grain]

brawny (brahw′nē). Thickened (lichenified) and dusky (a darkened hue), as of a swelling. [M.E. fleshy]

breast (brest). 1. The pectoral surface of the thorax. 2. The organ of milk secretion; one of two hemispheric projections situated in the subcutaneous layer over the pectoralis major muscle on either side of the chest of the mature female; it is rudimentary in the male. SYN mamma [NA], teat (2). [A.S. *breōst*]
  chicken b., SYN *pectus* carinatum.
  funnel b., SYN *pectus* excavatum.
  pigeon b., SYN *pectus* carinatum.

breath (breth). 1. The respired air. 2. An inspiration. [A.S. *braeth*]

breath·ing (brēdh′ing). Inhalation and exhalation of air or gaseous mixtures.
  apneustic b., pauses in the respiratory cycle at full inspiration, caused by damage of the respiratory control centers in the pons.
  Biot's b., SYN Biot's *respiration.*
  continuous positive pressure b. (CPPB), SYN controlled mechanical *ventilation.*
  glossopharyngeal b., respiration unaided by the usual primary muscles of respiration; the air is forced into the lungs by use of the tongue and muscles of the pharynx.
  intermittent positive pressure b. (IPPB), SYN controlled mechanical *ventilation.*
  positive-negative pressure b. (PNPB), inflation of the lungs with positive pressure and deflation with negative pressure by an automatic ventilator.
  shallow b., a type of b. with abnormally low tidal volume.
  work of b., the total expenditure of energy necessary to accomplish the act of b. It may be computed in terms of the pulmonary pressure multiplied by the change in pulmonary volume, or in terms of the oxygen cost of breathing (*i.e.,* the O_2 consumption above basal metabolic O_2 utilization attributable to b.).

breech (brēch). SYN buttocks. [A.S. *brēc*]

breg·ma (breg′mă) [NA]. The point on the skull

corresponding to the junction of the coronal and sagittal sutures. [G. the forepart of the head]

breg·mat·ic (breg-mat′ik). Relating to the bregma.

brev·i·col·lis (brev-ē-kol′is). Abnormal shortness of the neck. [L. *brevis,* short, + *collum,* neck]

bre·vis (brev′is). Brief, short. [L. short]

bridge (bridj). 1. The upper part of the ridge of the nose formed by the nasal bones. 2. One of the threads of protoplasm that appear to pass from one cell to another. 3. SYN fixed partial *denture.*
  cantilever b., a fixed partial b. denture in which the pontic is retained only on one side by an abutment tooth.
  cell b.'s, SYN intercellular b.'s.
  cytoplasmic b.'s, SYN intercellular b.'s.
  dentin b., a deposit of reparative dentin or other calcific substances which forms across and reseals exposed tooth pulp tissue.
  intercellular b.'s, slender cytoplasmic strands connecting adjacent cells; in histological sections the b.'s are shrinkage artifacts; true b.'s with cytoplasmic confluence exist between incompletely divided germ cells. SYN cell b.'s, cytoplasmic b.'s.
  removable b., SYN removable partial *denture.*

bridge·work (bridj′wŏrk). SYN partial *denture.*

brim. The upper edge or rim of a hollow structure.

broach (brōch). A dental instrument for removing the pulp of a tooth or exploring the canal.

△**brom-, bromo-.** Prefixes that indicate bromine or a foul odor. [G. *brōmos,* a stench]

bro·mate (brō′māt). Salt or anion of bromic acid.

bro·mat·ed (brō′māt-ĕd). Combined or saturated with bromine or any of its compounds. SYN brominated.

brom·hi·dro·sis (brom-hi-drō′sis). SYN bromidrosis.

bro·mide (brō′mīd). The anion Br⁻; salt of hydrogen bromide (HBr); several salts formerly used as sedatives, hypnotics, and anticonvulsants.

bro·mi·dro·sis (brōm-i-drō′sis). Fetid or foul-smelling perspiration. SYN bromhidrosis, osmidrosis. [G. *brōmos,* a stench, + *hidrōs,* perspiration]

bro·min·at·ed (brō′min-āt-ĕd). SYN bromated.

bro·mine (Br) (brō′mēn, -min). A nonmetallic, reddish, volatile, liquid element; atomic no. 35, atomic wt. 79.904; valences 1 to 7, inclusive; it unites with hydrogen to form hydrobromic acid, and this reacts with many metals to form bromides, some of which are used in medicine. [Fr. *brome,* bromine, fr. G. *bromos,* stench]

bro·mism, bro·min·ism (brō′mizm, -min-izm). Chronic bromide intoxication, characterized by headache, drowsiness, confusion and occasionally violent delirium, muscular weakness, cardiac depression, an acneform eruption, foul breath, anorexia, and gastric distress.

△**bromo-.** SEE brom-.

bro·mo·der·ma (brō-mō-der′mă). An acneform or granulomatous eruption due to hypersensitivity to bromide. [bromide + G. *derma,* skin]

△**bronch-.** SEE broncho-.

bron·chi (brong′kī). Plural of bronchus.

△**bronchi-.** SEE broncho-.

bron•chia (brong′kē-ă). The smaller divisions of the bronchi. SEE ALSO bronchus, bronchiole. [G. pl. of *bronchion,* dim. of *bronchos,* trachea]

bron•chi•al (brong′kē-ăl). Relating to the bronchi.

bronchial provocation. a procedure for identifying and characterizing hyperresponsive airways by having the subject inhale an agent known to cause (or suspected of causing) a decrease in pulmonary function.

bron•chi•ec•ta•sis (brong-kē-ek′tă-sis). Chronic dilation of bronchi or bronchioles as a sequel of inflammatory disease or obstruction. [bronchi- + G. *ektasis,* a stretching]

bron•chi•ec•tat•ic (brong-kē-ek-tat′ik). Relating to bronchiectasis.

bron•chil•o•quy (brong-kil′ō-kwē). Rarely used term for bronchophony [bronchi- + L. *loquor,* to speak]

bron•chi•o•gen•ic (brong-kē-ō-jen′ik). SYN bronchogenic.

ℹ️ **bron•chi•ole** (brong′kē-ōl). One of approximately six generations of increasingly finer subdivisions of the bronchi, all less than 1 mm in diameter, and having no cartilage in its wall, but relatively abundant smooth muscle and elastic fibers. SYN bronchiolus [NA].

   respiratory b.'s, the smallest bronchioles (0.5 mm in diameter), which connect the terminal bronchioles to alveolar ducts; alveoli arise from part of the wall.

   terminal b., the end of the nonrespiratory conducting airway; the lining is simple columnar or cuboidal epithelium without mucous goblet cells; most of the cells are ciliated, but a few nonciliated serous secreting cells occur.

bron•chi•o•lec•ta•sis (brong′kē-ō-lek′tă-sis). Bronchiectasis involving the bronchioles. [bronchiole + G. *ektasis,* a stretching]

bron•chi•o•li (brong-kē′ō-lī). Plural of bronchiolus.

bron•chi•ol•i•tis (brong-kē-ō-lī′tis). Inflammation of the bronchioles, often associated with bronchopneumonia. [bronchiole + -*itis,* inflammation]

   constrictive b., obliteration of bronchioles by scarring following b. obliterans.

   b. fibro′sa oblit′erans, obstruction of bronchioles and alveolar ducts by fibrous granulation tissue induced by mucosal ulceration; the condition may follow inhalation of irritant gases (see silo-filler's *lung*) or may complicate pneumonia (see BOOP); associated with obstructive findings (see unilateral hyperlucent *lung,* Swyer-James *syndrome*). SYN b. obliterans.

   b. oblit′erans, SYN b. fibrosa obliterans.

   b. obliterans with organizing pneumonia (BOOP), b. fibrosa obliterans complicated by pneumonia with organization.

△**bronchiolo-.** Bronchiole. [L. *bronchiolus*]
bron•chi•o•lus, pl. **bron•chi•o•li** (brong-kē′ō-lŭs, -ō-lī) [NA]. SYN bronchiole. [Mod. L. dim. of *bronchus*]

bron•chi•o•ste•no•sis (brong′kē-ō-sten-ō′sis). Narrowing of the lumen of a bronchial tube.

bron•chit•ic (brong-kit′ik). Relating to bronchitis.

bron•chi•tis (brong-kī′tis). Inflammation of the mucous membrane of the bronchial tubes.

   chronic b., a condition of the bronchial tree characterized by cough, hypersecretion of mucus, and expectoration of sputum over a long period of time, associated with frequent bronchial infections; usually due to smoking.

   fibrinous b., inflammation of the bronchial mucous membrane, accompanied by a fibrinous exudation, with obstruction of air flow. SYN pseudomembranous b.

   obliterative b., b. oblit′erans, fibrinous b. in which the exudate is not expectorated but becomes organized, obliterating the affected portion of the bronchial tubes with consequent permanent collapse of affected portions of the lung.

   pseudomembranous b., SYN fibrinous b.

△**broncho-, bronch-, bronchi-.** Bronchus. [G. *bronchos,* windpipe]

bron•cho•al•ve•o•lar (brong′kō-al-vē′ō-lăr). SYN bronchovesicular.

bron•cho•cav•ern•ous (brong-kō-kav′er-nŭs). Relating to a bronchus or bronchial tube and a pathologic pulmonary cavity.

bron•cho•cele (brong′kō-sēl). A circumscribed dilation of a bronchus. [broncho- + G. *kēlē,* hernia]

bron•cho•con•stric•tor (brong-kō-kon-strik′ter, -tōr). **1.** Causing a reduction in caliber of a bronchus or bronchial tube. **2.** An agent that possesses this action (*e.g.,* histamine).

bron•cho•di•la•ta•tion (brong′kō-dil-ă-tā′shŭn). Increase in caliber of the bronchi and bronchioles in response to pharmacologically active substances or autonomic nervous activity.

bron•cho•di•la•tor (brong-kō-dī-lā′ter, -tōr). **1.** Causing an increase in caliber of a bronchus or bronchial tube. **2.** An agent that possesses this power (*e.g.,* epinephrine).

   adrenergic b.'s, a class of sympathomimetic antiasthma drugs which act by stimulating receptors in the bronchi and other organs; they are classified into three groups: α-adrenergic, β₁-adrenergic, and β₂-adrenergic b.'s.

bron•cho•e•soph•a•gol•o•gy (brong′kō-ē-sof-ă-gol′ō-jē). The specialty concerned with the diagnosis and treatment of diseases of the tracheobronchial tree and esophagus by endoscope and other means. [broncho- + G. *oisophagos,* esophagus, + *logos,* study]

bron•cho•e•soph•a•gos•co•py (brong′kō-ē-sof-ă-gos′kŏ-pē). Examination of the tracheobronchial tree and esophagus with appropriate endoscopes.

bron•cho•fi•ber•scope (brong-kō-fī′ber-skōp). A fiberoptic endoscope adapted for visualization of the trachea and bronchi.

bron•cho•gen•ic (brong-kō-jen′ik). Of bronchial origin; emanating from the bronchi. SYN bronchiogenic.

ℹ️ **bron•cho•gram** (brong′kō-gram). A radiograph obtained by bronchography; radiographic visualization of a bronchus. [broncho- + G. *gramma,* a writing]

   air b., radiographic appearance of an air-filled bronchus surrounded by fluid-filled airspaces.

bron•cho•lith (brong′kō-lith). A hard concretion

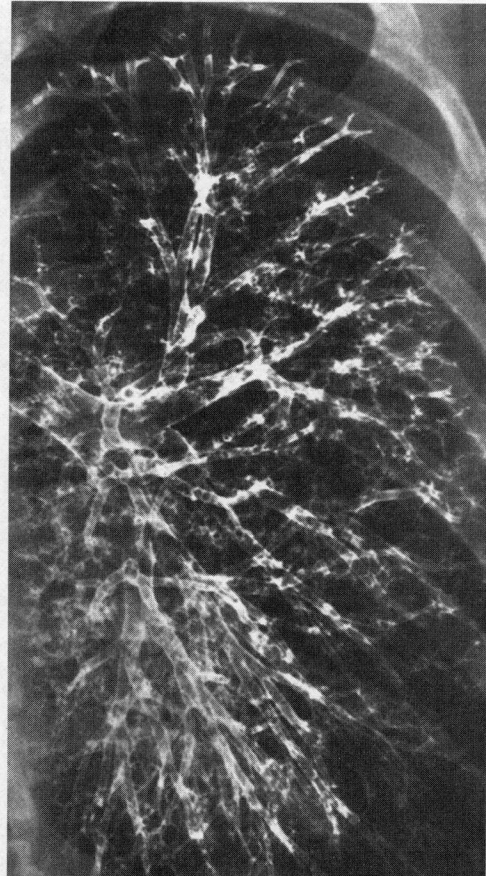

bronchogram: of the left lung

in a bronchus or bronchial tube. [broncho- + G. *lithos*, stone]

bron•cho•li•thi•a•sis (brong′kō-li-thī′ă-sis). Bronchial inflammation or obstruction caused by broncholiths.

bron•cho•ma•la•cia (brong′kō-mă-lā′shē-ă). Degeneration of elastic and connective tissue of bronchi and trachea. [broncho- + G. *malakia*, a softening]

bron•cho•my•co•sis (brong′kō-mī-kō′sis). Any fungus disease of the bronchial tubes or bronchi. [broncho- + G. *mykēs*, fungus]

bron•choph•o•ny (brong-kof′ō-nē). Increased intensity and clarity of voice sounds heard over a bronchus surrounded by consolidated lung tissue. SEE ALSO tracheophony. [broncho- + G. *phōnē*, voice]

bron•cho•plas•ty (brong′kō-plas-tē). Surgical alteration of the configuration of a bronchus. [broncho- + G. *plastos*, formed]

bron•cho•pneu•mo•nia (brong′ko-nu-mo′nĭ-ă). Acute inflammation of the walls of the smaller bronchial tubes, with varying amounts of pulmonary consolidation due to spread of the inflammation into peribronchiolar alveoli and the alveolar ducts; may become confluent or may be hemorrhagic. SYN bronchial pneumonia.

bron•cho•pul•mo•nary (brong-kō-pul′mō-nār-ē). Relating to the bronchi and the lungs.

bron•chor•rha•phy (brong-kōr′ă-fē). Suture of a wound of the bronchus. [broncho- + G. *rhaphē*, a seam]

bron•chor•rhea (brong′kō-rē′ă). Excessive secretion of mucus from the bronchial mucous membrane. [broncho- + G. *rhoia*, a flow]

bron•cho•scope (brong′kō-skōp). An endoscope for inspecting the interior of the tracheobronchial tree. [broncho- + G. *skopeō*, to view]

bron•chos•co•py (brong-kos′kŏ-pē). Inspection of the interior of the tracheobronchial tree through a bronchoscope.

bron•cho•spasm (brong′kō-spazm). Contraction of smooth muscle in the walls of the bronchi and bronchioles, causing narrowing of the lumen.

exercise-induced b., SYN exercise-induced *asthma.*

bron•cho•spi•rog•ra•phy (brong′kō-spī-rog′ră-fē). Use of a single-lumen endobronchial tube for measurement of ventilatory function of one lung. [broncho- + L. *spiro*, to breathe, + G. *graphō*, to write]

bron•cho•spi•rom•e•ter (brong′kō-spī-rom′ĕ-ter). A device for measurement of rates and volumes of airflow into each lung separately, using a double-lumen endobronchial tube. [broncho- + L. *spiro*, to breathe, + G. *metron*, measure]

bron•cho•spi•rom•e•try (brong′kō-spī-rom′ĕ-trē). Use of a bronchospirometer to measure ventilatory function of each lung separately.

bron•cho•stax•is (brong′kō-stak′sis). Hemorrhage from the bronchi. [broncho- + G. *staxis*, a dripping]

bron•cho•ste•no•sis (brong-kō-sten-ō′sis). Chronic narrowing of a bronchus.

bron•chos•to•my (brong-kos′tō-mē). Surgical formation of a new opening into a bronchus. [broncho- + G. *stoma*, mouth]

bron•chot•o•my (brong-kot′ō-mē). Incision of a bronchus.

bron•cho•tra•che•al (brong-kō-trā′kē-ăl). Relating to the trachea and bronchi.

bron•cho•ve•sic•u•lar (brong′kō-vĕ-sik′yū-lăr). Relating to the bronchioles and alveoli in the lungs. SYN bronchoalveolar.

bron•chus, pl. **bron•chi** (brong′kŭs, brong′kī) [NA]. One of the two subdivisions of the trachea serving to convey air to and from the lungs. The trachea divides into right and left main bronchi, which in turn form lobar, segmental, and subsegmental bronchi. In structure, the intrapulmonary bronchi have a lining of pseudostratified ciliated columnar epithelium, and a lamina propria with abundant longitudinal networks of elastic fibers; there are spirally arranged bundles of smooth muscle, abundant mucoserous glands, and, in the outer part of the wall, irregular plates of hyaline cartilage. [Mod. L., fr. G. *bronchos*, windpipe]

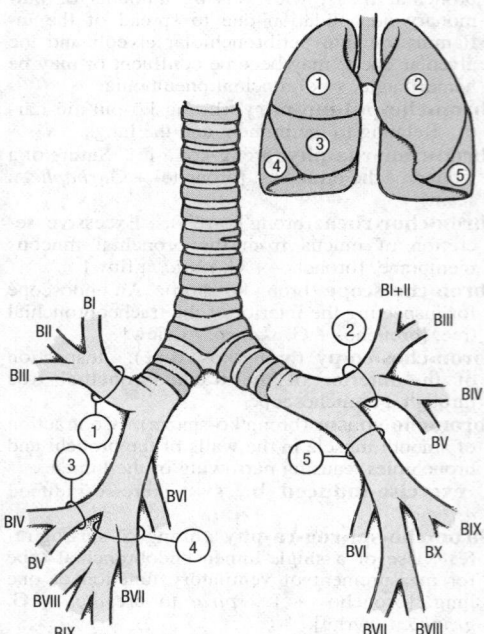

segmental bronchi: right lung: (BI) apical, (BII) posterior, (BIV) lateral, (BV) medial; left lung: (BI + II) apicoposterior, (BIV) superior lingular, (BV) inferior lingular; both lungs: (BIII) anterior, (BVI) superior, (BVII) medial basal, (BVIII) anterior basal, (BIX) lateral basal, (BX) posterior basal; lobes of lungs supplied: (1) right superior, (2) left superior, (3) right middle, (4) right inferior, (5) left inferior

brow. **1.** The eyebrow. SEE eyebrow. **2.** SYN forehead. [A.S. *brū*]

brow·lift. Operation to elevate the eyebrows.

Bru·cel·la (brū-sel′lă). A genus of encapsulated, nonmotile bacteria containing short, rod-shaped to coccoid, Gram-negative cells. These organisms are parasitic, invading all animal tissues and causing infection of the genital organs, the mammary gland, and the respiratory and intestinal tracts, and are pathogenic for humans and various species of domestic animals.

B. abor′tus, a species that causes undulant fever. SYN Bang's bacillus.

B. meliten′sis, a species that causes brucellosis in humans; it is the type species of the genus *B.*

B. su′is, a species causing brucellosis in humans; may also infect horses, dogs, cows, monkeys, goats, and laboratory animals.

Bru·cel·la·ce·ae (brū-sel-ā′sē-ē). A family of bacteria containing small, coccoid to rod-shaped, Gram-negative cells which occur singly, in pairs, in short chains, or in groups. The cells may not show bipolar staining. Motile and nonmotile species occur. These organisms are parasites and pathogens that affect warm-blooded animals, including humans. The type genus is *Brucella.*

bru·cel·lo·sis (brū-sel-ō′sis). An infectious disease caused by *Brucella,* characterized by fever, sweating, weakness, and aching, and transmitted to humans by direct contact with diseased animals or through ingestion of infected meat or milk. SYN undulant fever.

bruise (brūz). An injury producing a hematoma or diffuse extravasation of blood without rupture of the skin. [M.E. *bruisen,* fr. O.Fr., fr. Germanic]

bru·it (brū-ē′). A harsh or musical intermittent auscultatory sound, especially an abnormal one. [Fr.]

aneurysmal b., blowing murmur heard over an aneurysm.

carotid b., a systolic murmur heard in the neck but not at the aortic area; any b. produced by blood flow in a carotid artery.

b. de tambour (brū-ē′ dĕ tăm-bur′), reverberating, musical tone heard as the second heart sound over the aortic area, associated with syphilitic aortic valvular disease. [Fr. sound of drum]

thyroid b., vascular murmur heard over hyperactive thyroid gland, due to increased blood flow.

brux·ism (brŭk′sizm). A clenching of the teeth, associated with forceful lateral or protrusive jaw movements, resulting in rubbing, gritting, or grinding together of the teeth, usually during sleep; sometimes a pathologic condition. [G. *bruchō,* to grind the teeth]

BSA (body surface area) bovine serum *albumin.*

BSER brainstem evoked response. SEE brainstem evoked response *audiometry.*

BTPS Symbol indicating that a gas volume has been expressed as if it were *s*aturated with water vapor at *b*ody *t*emperature (37°C) and at the ambient barometric *p*ressure; used for measurements of lung volumes.

BTU British thermal *unit.*

bu·ba mad·re (bū′bă mah′dre). SYN mother *yaw.*

bu·bas (bū′bahs). SYN yaws.

bu·bo (bū′bō). Inflammatory swelling of one or more lymph nodes, usually in the groin. [G. *boubōn,* the groin, a swelling in the groin]

indolent b., a painless, chronic enlargement of an inguinal node.

malignant b., the enlarged lymph node associated with bubonic plague.

tropical b., SYN lymphogranuloma venereum.

venereal b., an enlarged gland in the groin associated with any sexually transmitted disease, especially chancroid.

bu·bon·al·gia (bū′bon-al′jē-ă). Rarely used term for pain in the groin. [G. *boubōn,* groin, + *algos,* pain]

bu·bon·ic (bū-bon′ik). Relating in any way to a bubo.

buc·ca, gen. and pl. **buc·cae** (bŭk′ă, bŭk′sē) [NA]. SYN cheek. [L.]

buc·cal (bŭk′ăl). Pertaining to, adjacent to, or in the direction of the cheek.

△**bucco-.** Cheek. [L. *bucca*]

buc·co·gin·gi·val (bŭk-ō-jin′ji-văl). Relating to the cheek and the gum.

buc·co·la·bi·al (bŭk-ō-lā′bē-ăl). **1.** Relating to both cheek and lip. **2.** DENTISTRY referring to that aspect of the dental arch or those surfaces of the teeth in contact with the mucosa of lip and cheek.

buc·co·lin·gual (bŭk-ō-ling′wăl). **1.** Pertaining to the cheek and the tongue. **2.** DENTISTRY referring to that aspect of the dental arch or those surfaces of the teeth in contact with the mucosa of the lip or cheek and the tongue.

buc·co·pha·ryn·ge·al (bŭk′ō-fă-rin′jē-ăl). Relating to both cheek or mouth and pharynx.

buc·co·ver·sion (bŭk′ō-ver-zhŭn). Malposition of a posterior tooth from the normal line of occlusion toward the cheek.

bud (bŭd). **1.** An outgrowth that resembles the b. of a plant, usually pluripotential, and capable of differentiating and growing into a definitive structure. **2.** To give rise to such an outgrowth. SEE ALSO gemmation. **3.** a small outgrowth from a parent cell; a form of asexual reproduction.

  end b., SYN tail b.

  limb b., an ectodermally covered mesenchymal outgrowth on the embryonic flank giving rise to either the forelimb or hindlimb.

  periosteal b., a vascular connective tissue bud from the perichondrium that invades the ossification center of the cartilaginous model of a developing long bone.

  tail b., the rapidly proliferating mass of cells at the caudal extremity of the embryo; remnant of the primitive node. SYN end b.

  taste b., one of a number of flask-shaped cell nests located in the epithelium of vallate, fungiform, and foliate papillae of the tongue and also in the soft palate, epiglottis, and posterior wall of the pharynx; it consists of sustentacular, gustatory, and basal cells between which the intragemmal sensory nerve fibers terminate.

  tooth b., the primordial structures from which a tooth is formed; the enamel organ, the dental papilla, and the dental sac enclosing them.

bud·ding (bŭd′ing). SYN gemmation.

buff·er (bŭf′er). **1.** A mixture of an acid and its conjugate base (salt), such as H_2CO_3/HCO_3^-; $H_2PO_4^-/HPO_4^{2-}$, which, when present in a solution, resists changes in pH that would otherwise occur in the solution when acid or alkali is added to it. SEE ALSO conjugate acid-base *pair*. **2.** To add a b. to a solution and thus give it the property of resisting a change in pH.

bulb (bŭlb). **1.** Any globular or fusiform structure. SYN bulbus [NA]. **2.** A short, vertical underground stem of plants, as of onion and garlic. [L. *bulbus*, a bulbous root]

  aortic b., the dilated first part of the aorta containing the aortic semilunar valves and the aortic sinuses. SYN bulbus aortae [NA].

  b. of corpus spongiosum, SYN b. of penis.

  dental b., the papilla, derived from mesoderm, that forms the part of the primordium of a tooth that is situated within the cup-shaped enamel organ.

  end b., one of the oval or rounded bodies in which the sensory nerve fibers terminate in mucous membrane.

  b. of eye, SYN eyeball.

  b. of hair, hair bulb, the lower expanded extremity of the hair follicle that fits like a cap over the papilla pili.

  Krause's end b.'s, nerve terminals in skin, mouth, conjunctiva, and other parts, consisting of a laminated capsule of connective tissue enclosing the terminal, branched, convoluted ending of an afferent nerve fiber; generally believed to be sensitive to cold.

  olfactory b., the grayish expanded rostral extremity of the olfactory tract, lying on the cribriform plate of the ethmoid and receiving the olfactory filaments. SYN bulbus olfactorius [NA].

  b. of penis, the expanded posterior part of the corpus spongiosum of the penis lying in the interval between the crura of the penis. SYN bulbus penis [NA], b. of corpus spongiosum, b. of urethra.

  speech b., a prosthetic speech aid; a restoration used to close a cleft or other opening in the hard or soft palate, or to replace absent tissue necessary for the production of good speech.

  b. of urethra, SYN b. of penis.

  b. of vestibule, a mass of erectile tissue on either side of the vagina united anterior to the urethra by the commissura bulborum.

bul·bar (bŭl′bar). **1.** Relating to a bulb. **2.** Relating to the rhombencephalon (hindbrain). **3.** Bulbshaped; resembling a bulb.

bul·bi (bŭl′bī). Plural of bulbus.

bul·bi·tis (bŭl-bī′tis). Inflammation of the bulbous portion of the urethra.

△**bulbo-.** Bulb; bulbus [L. *bulbus*]

bul·boid (bŭl′boyd). Bulb-shaped. [bulbo- + G. *eidos*, resemblance]

bul·bo·spi·nal (bŭl-bō-spī′năl). Relating to the medulla oblongata and spinal cord, particularly to nerve fibers interconnecting the two. SYN spinobulbar.

bul·bo·u·re·thral (bŭl′bō-yū-rē′thrăl). Relating to the bulbus penis and the urethra. SYN urethrobulbar.

bul·bus, gen. and pl. **bul·bi** (bŭl′bŭs, -bī) [NA]. SYN bulb (1). [L. a plant bulb]

  b. aor′tae [NA], SYN aortic *bulb.*

  b. oc′uli [NA], SYN eyeball.

  b. olfacto′rius [NA], SYN olfactory *bulb.*

  b. pe′nis [NA], SYN *bulb* of penis.

bu·lim·ia (bū-lim′ē-ă). SYN b. nervosa. [G. *bous*, ox, + *limos*, hunger]

  b. nervo′sa, a chronic morbid disorder involving repeated and secretive episodic bouts of eating characterized by uncontrolled rapid ingestion of large quantities of food over a short period of time (binge eating), followed by self-induced vomiting, use of laxatives or diuretics, fasting, or vigorous exercise in order to prevent weight gain; often accompanied by feelings of guilt, depression, or self-disgust. SYN bulimia.

bu·lim·ic (bū-lim′ik). Relating to, or suffering from, bulimia nervosa.

🄳**bul·la,** gen. and pl. **bul·lae** (bul′ă, -ē). **1.** A large blister appearing as a circumscribed area of separation of the epidermis from subepidermal structures or as a circumscribed area of separation of epidermal cells caused by the presence of serum, or an injected substance. **2** [NA]. A bubblelike structure. [L. bubble]

bul·lec·to·my (bul-ek′tō-mē). Resection of a bulla; helpful in treating some forms of bullous emphysema, in which giant bullae compress functioning lung tissue.

bul·lous (bul'ŭs). Relating to, of the nature of, or marked by, bullae.

BUN blood urea *nitrogen.*

bun·dle (bŭn'dl). A structure composed of a group of fibers, muscular or nervous; a fasciculus.

atrioventricular b., the bundle of modified cardiac muscle fibers that begins at the atrioventricular node as the trunk of the atrioventricular bundle and passes through the right atrioventricular fibrous ring to the membranous part of the interventricular septum where the trunk divides into two branches, the right crus of the atrioventricular b. and the left crus of the atrioventricular b.; the two crura ramify in the subendocardium of their respective ventricles. SYN ventriculonector.

ground b.'s, SYN *fasciculi* proprii, under *fasciculus.*

medial forebrain b., a fiber system coursing longitudinally through the lateral zone of the hypothalamus, connecting the latter reciprocally with the midbrain tegmentum and with various components of the limbic system; it also carries fibers from norepinephrine-containing and serotonin-containing cell groups in the brainstem to the hypothalamus and cerebral cortex, as well as dopamine-carrying fibers from the substantia nigra to the caudate nucleus and putamen.

bun·ion (bŭn'yŭn). A localized swelling at either the medial or dorsal aspect of the first metatarsophalangeal joint, caused by bursal inflammation and fibrosis; a medial b. is usually associated with hallux valgus. [O.F. *buigne,* bump on the head]

bun·ion·ec·to·my (bŭn-yŭn-ek'tō-mē). Excision of a bunion.

Bunsen burn·er. A gas lamp supplied with openings admitting sufficient air that carbon is completely burned, giving a hot but only slightly luminous flame. [R.W. Bunsen]

buph·thal·mia, buph·thal·mus, buph·thal·mos (būf-thal'mē-ă, -thal'mŭs, -thal'mos). An affection of infancy, marked by an increase of intraocular pressure with enlargement of the eyeball. SYN congenital glaucoma. [G. *bous,* ox, + *ophthalmos,* eye]

bur (bŭr). A rotary cutting instrument, used in dentistry, consisting of a small metal shaft and a head designed in various shapes; used at various rotational velocities for excavating decay, shaping cavity forms, and for reduction of tooth structure. SEE ALSO burr.

bu·ret, bu·rette (bū-ret'). A graduated glass tube with a tap at its lower end; used for measuring liquids in volumetric chemical analyses. [Fr.]

burn (bern). **1.** To cause a lesion by heat or any other agent, similar to that caused by heat. **2.** To suffer pain caused by excessive heat, or similar pain from any cause. **3.** A lesion caused by heat or any cauterizing agent, including friction, electricity, and electromagnetic energy. [A.S. *baernan*]

bur·nish·er (bŭr'nish-er). An instrument for smoothing and polishing the surface or edge of a dental restoration. [O. F. *burnir,* to polish]

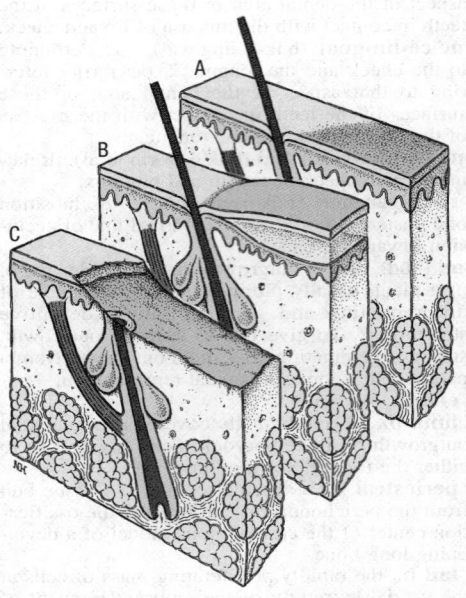

burns: (A) first degree, (B) partial thickness, (C) full thickness

burr (bŭr). A drilling tool for enlarging a trephine hole in the cranium. SEE ALSO bur.

bur·sa, pl. **bur·sae** (ber'să, ber'sē) [NA]. A closed sac or envelope lined with synovial membrane and containing fluid, usually found or formed in areas subject to friction; *e.g.,* over an exposed or prominent part or where a tendon passes over a bone. [Mediev. L., a purse]

anserine b., the b. between the tibial collateral ligament of the knee joint and the tendons of the sartorius, gracilis, and semitendinosus muscles.

Calori's b., a b. between the arch of the aorta and the trachea.

infraspinatus b., the b. located between the tendon of the infraspinatus and the capsule of the shoulder joint.

ischial b., the b. between the gluteus maximus muscle and the tuberosity of the ischium.

omental b., an isolated portion of the peritoneal cavity lying dorsal to the stomach and extending craniad to the liver and diaphragm and caudad into the greater omentum; it opens into the general peritoneal cavity at the epiploic foramen.

pharyngeal b., a cystic notochordal remnant found inconstantly in the posterior wall of the nasopharynx at the lower end of the pharyngeal tonsil.

prepatellar b., a b. between the skin and the lower part of the patella.

retrohyoid b., a b. between the posterior surface of the body of the hyoid bone and the thyrohyoid membrane.

subacromial b., between the acromion and the capsule of the shoulder joint.

subdeltoid b., the b. between the deltoid muscle and the capsule of the shoulder joint. It may be combined with the subacromial b.

subtendinous b. of gastrocnemius muscle, consists of a lateral and a medial (Brodie's b. (1)) b. between the heads of the gastrocnemius and capsule of the knee joint.

subtendinous b. of the tibialis anterior muscle, the small b. between the medial surface of the medial cuneiform bone and the tendon of the tibialis anterior.

subtendinous iliac b., the b. at the attachment of the iliopsoas muscle into the lesser trochanter.

suprapatellar b., a large b. between the lower part of the femur and the tendon of the quadriceps femoris muscle. It usually communicates with the cavity of the knee joint.

synovial b., a sac containing synovial fluid which occurs at sites of friction, as between a tendon and a bone over which it plays, or subcutaneously over a bony prominence. The NA lists the following types: subcutaneous synovial b., b. synovialis subcutanea [NA]; submuscular synovial b., b. synovialis submuscularis [NA]; subfascial synovial b., b. synovialis subfascialis [NA]; and subtendinous synovial b., b. synovialis subtendinea [NA].

b. of tendo calca′neus, b. between the tendo calcaneus and the upper part of the posterior surface of the calcaneum.

bur•sae (ber′sē).

bur•sal (ber′săl). Relating to a bursa.

bur•sec•to•my (ber-sek′tō-mē). Surgical removal of a bursa. [bursa + G. *ektomē,* excision]

bur•si•tis (ber-sī′tis). Inflammation of a bursa. SYN bursal synovitis.

bur•so•lith (ber′sō-lith). A calculus formed in a bursa. [bursa + G. *lithos,* stone]

bur•sop•a•thy (ber-sop′ă-thē). Any disease of a bursa.

bur•sot•o•my (ber-sot′ō-mē). Incision through the wall of a bursa. [bursa + G. *tome,* a cutting]

bu•tane (byū′tān). C_4H_{10}; A gaseous hydrocarbon present in natural gas.

bu•tan•o•yl (byū′tan-ō-il). $CH_3(CH_2)_2 COO^-$; the radical of butanoic acid. SYN butyryl.

but•ter (bŭt′er). **1.** A coherent mass of milk fat, obtained by churning or shaking cream until the separate fat globules run together, leaving a liquid residue, buttermilk. **2.** A soft solid having more or less the consistency of b. [L. *butyrum,* G. *boutyros,* prob. fr. *bous,* cow, + *tyros,* cheese]

but•ter•fly (bŭt′er-flī). **1.** Any structure or apparatus resembling in shape a butterfly with outstretched wings. **2.** A scaling erythematous lesion on each cheek, joined by a narrow band across the nose; seen in lupus erythematosus and seborrheic dermatitis.

but•tocks (bŭt′oks). The buttocks; the prominence formed by the gluteal muscles on either side. SYN clunes [NA], nates [NA], breech.

but•ton (bŭt′ŏn). A structure, lesion, or device of knob shape. [M.E., fr. O.Fr. *bouton,* fr. *bouter,* to thrust, fr. Germanic]

stoma b., short plastic tube with collar inserted into a tracheal stoma to maintain or enlarge it.

but•ton•hole (bŭt′ŏn-hōl). **1.** A short straight cut made through the wall of a cavity or canal. **2.** The contraction of an orifice down to a narrow slit; *i.e.,* the so-called mitral b. in extreme mitral stenosis.

bu•tyl (byū′til). $CH_3(CH_2)_3$—; a radical of *n*-butane.

bu•ty•ra•ce•ous (byū-tir-ā′shĭ-us). Buttery in consistency.

bu•ty•rate (byū′ti-rāt). A salt or ester of butyric acid.

bu•tyr•ic ac•id (byū-tir′ik). An acid of unpleasant odor occurring in butter, cod liver oil, sweat, and many other substances.

bu•ty•roid (byū′ti-royd). **1.** Buttery. **2.** Resembling butter.

bu•tyr•ous (byū′ti-rŭs). Denoting a tissue or bacterial growth of butter-like consistency.

bu•tyr•yl (byū′ti-ril). SYN butanoyl.

by•pass (bī′pas). **1.** A shunt or auxiliary flow. **2.** To create new flow from one structure to another through a diversionary channel. SEE ALSO shunt.

aortoiliac b., an operation in which a vascular prosthesis is united with the aorta and iliac artery to relieve obstruction of the lower abdominal aorta, its bifurcation, and the proximal iliac branches.

aortorenal b., insertion of a graft of autogenous artery, saphenous vein, or synthetic material between the aorta and the distal renal artery, to circumvent an obstruction of the renal artery.

bowel b., SYN jejunoileal b.

cardiopulmonary b., diversion of the blood flow returning to the heart through a pump oxygenator (heart-lung machine) and then returning it to the arterial side of the circulation; used in operations upon the heart to maintain extracorporeal circulation.

coronary b., vein grafts or other conduits shunting blood from the aorta to branches of the coronary arteries, to increase the flow beyond the local obstruction.

gastric b., high division of the stomach, anastomosis of the small upper pouch of the stomach to the jejunum, and closure of the distal part of the stomach that is retained; used for treatment of morbid obesity.

jejunoileal b., anastomosis of the upper jejunum to the terminal ileum for treatment of morbid obesity. SYN bowel b., jejunoileal shunt.

left heart b., any procedure that shunts blood returning from the pulmonary circulation to the systemic circulation without passing through the left heart. This is used during cardiac surgery and in severe left heart failure or cardiogenic shock.

right heart b., introduction of a circuit shunting blood from the venae cavae around the right atrium and ventricle and directly into the pulmonary artery.

bys•si•no•sis (bis-i-nō′sis). Obstructive airway disease in people who work with unprocessed cotton, flax, or hemp; caused by reaction to material in the dust. [G. *byssos,* flax, + *-osis,* condition]

C

C **1.** large *calorie*; carbon; cathodal; cathode; Celsius; cervical vertebra (C1 to C7); closure (of an electrical circuit); congius (gallon); contraction; coulomb; curie; cylinder; cylindrical *lens*; cytidine; cysteine; cytosine; *component* of complement (C1 1/N C9); third substrate in a multisubstrate enzyme-catalyzed reaction. **2.** When followed by subscript letters, *e.g.*, C_{In}, indicates renal clearance of a substance (*e.g.*, inulin). When followed by subscript numbers, *e.g.*, C_{19}, indicates the number of carbon atoms in a molecule.

c **1.** centi-; small *calorie*; centum; concentration; speed of light in a vacuum; circumference; curie. **2.** As a subscript, refers to blood *capillary*.

CA carcinoma; cardiac *arrest*; cancer; chronologic *age*; *cytosine* arabinoside.

CA-125. cancer antigen 125 *test*.

^{47}Ca calcium-47.

△**cac-.** SEE caco-.

ca·chec·tic (kă-kek′tik). Relating to or suffering from cachexia.

cac·hec·tin (kak-hek′tin). A polypeptide hormone, produced by endotoxin-activated macrophages, which has the ability to modulate adipocyte metabolism, lyse tumor cells *in vitro*, and induce hemorrhagic necrosis of certain transplantable tumors *in vivo*. [G. *kakos*, bad, + *hexis*, condition of body]

ca·chex·ia (kă-kek′sē-ă). A general weight loss and wasting occurring in the course of a chronic disease or emotional disturbance. [G. *kakos*, bad, + *hexis*, condition of body]

  c. hypophys′eopri′va, a condition following total removal of the hypophysis cerebri resulting in panhypopituitarism marked by a fall of body temperature, electrolyte imbalance, and hypoglycemia, followed by coma and death.

  hypophysial c., SYN Simmonds' *disease*, panhypopituitarism.

  pituitary c., SYN Simmonds' *disease*.

  c. strumipri′va, SYN c. thyropriva.

  c. thyropri′va, signs and symptoms of hypothyroidism (with or without myxedema) resulting from the loss of thyroid tissue, either from surgery, radiotherapy, or disease. SYN c. strumipriva.

cach·in·na·tion (kak-i-nā′shŭn). Laughter without apparent cause, often observed in schizophrenia. [L. *cachinno*, to laugh immoderately and loudly]

△**caco-, cac-, caci-.** Bad; ill. Cf. mal-. [G. *kakos*]

cac·o·geu·sia (kak-ō-gū′sē-ă). A bad taste. [caco- + G. *geusis*, taste]

cac·o·me·lia (kak-ō-mē′lē-ă). Congenital deformity of one or more limbs. [caco- + G. *melos*, limb]

ca·cos·mia (kă-koz′mē-ă). A subjective perception of nonexistent disagreeable odors. [G. *kakosmia*, a bad smell, fr. *kakos*, bad, + *osmē*, the sense of smell]

cac·u·men, pl. **cac·u·mi·na** (kak-yū′men, -mi-nă). The top or apex of a plant or an anatomical structure. [L. summit]

ca·dav·er (kă-dav′er). A dead body. SYN corpse. [L. fr. *cado*, to fall]

ca·dav·er·ic (kă-dav′er-ik). Relating to a dead body.

ca·dav·er·ine (kă-dav′er-in). A foul-smelling diamine formed by bacterial decarboxylation of lysine; poisonous and irritating to the skin.

ca·dav·er·ous (kă-dav′er-ŭs). Having the pallor and appearance of a corpse.

cad·mi·um (Cd) (kad′mē-ŭm). A metallic element, atomic no. 48, atomic wt. 112.411; its salts are poisonous and little used in medicine. Various compounds of c. are used commercially in metallurgy, photography, electrochemistry, etc.; a few have been used as ascaricides, antiseptics, and fungicides. [L. *cadmia*, fr. G. *kadmeia* or *kadmia*, an ore of zinc, calamine]

ca·du·ce·us (kă-dū′sē-ŭs). A staff with two oppositely twined serpents and surmounted by two wings; emblem of the U.S. Army Medical Corps. SEE ALSO staff of Aesculapius. [L. the staff of Mercury; G. *kēryx* herald, the staff of Hermes]

△**cae-.** For words so beginning, see under ce-.

caf·feine (kaf′ēn). An alkaloid obtained from the dried leaves of *Thea sinensis*, tea, or the dried seeds of *Coffea arabica*, coffee; used as a central nervous system stimulant, diuretic, circulatory and respiratory stimulant, and as an adjunct in the treatment of headaches.

caf·fein·ism (kaf′ēn-izm). Caffeine intoxication characterized by restlessness, tremulousness, excitement, insomnia, flushed face, diuresis, and gastrointestinal complaints, brought on by the ingestion of substances containing caffeine.

cage (kāj). **1.** An enclosure made partly or completely of open work and commonly used to house animals. **2.** A structure resembling such an enclosure. [M.E., fr. O.Fr., fr. L. *cavea*, hollow, stall]

  thoracic c., the skeleton of the thorax consisting of the thoracic vertebrae, ribs, costal cartilages, and sternum.

Cal large *calorie*.

cal small *calorie*.

cal·a·mus (kal′ă-mŭs). **1.** The dried, unpeeled rhizome of *Acorus calamus*, a carminative and anthelmintic. **2.** A reed-shaped structure. [L. reed, a pen]

  c. scripto′rius, inferior part of the rhomboid fossa; the narrow lower end of the fourth ventricle between the two clavae. [L. writing pen]

cal·ca·ne·al, cal·ca·ne·an (kal-kā′nē-al, kal-kā′nē-an). Relating to the calcaneus or heel bone.

△**calcaneo-.** The calcaneus. [L. *calcaneum*, heel]

cal·ca·ne·o·a·poph·y·si·tis (kal-kā′nē-ō-ă-pof-i-sī′tis). Inflammation at the posterior part of the os calcis, at the insertion of the Achilles tendon.

cal·ca·ne·o·as·trag·a·loid (kal-kā′nē-ō-as-trag′ă-loyd). Relating to the calcaneus, or os calcis, and the talus, or astragalus.

cal·ca·ne·o·cu·boid (kal-kā′nē-ō-kyū′boyd). Relating to the calcaneus and the cuboid bone.

cal·can·e·o·dyn·ia (kal-kā′nē-ō-din′ē-ă). SYN painful *heel*. [calcaneo- + G. *odynē*, pain]

cal·ca·ne·o·na·vic·u·lar (kal-kā′nē-ō-na-vik′yū-lăr). Relating to the calcaneus and the navicular bone.

cal·ca·ne·o·tib·i·al (kal-kā′nē-ō-tib′ē-ăl). Relating to the calcaneus and the tibia.

cal·ca·ne·um (kal-kā′nē-ŭm). SYN calcaneus (1). [L. the heel]

cal·ca·ne·us, gen. and pl. **cal·ca·nei** (kal-kā′nē-ŭs, -kā′nē-ī). 1 [NA]. The largest of the tarsal bones; it forms the heel and articulates with the cuboid anteriorly and the talus above. SYN calcaneum, heel bone. 2. SYN *talipes* calcaneus. [L. the heel (another form of *calcaneum*)]

cal·car (kal′kar). 1. A small projection from any structure; internal spurs (septa) at the level of division of arteries and confluence of veins when branches or roots form an acute angle. 2. A dull spine or projection from a bone. SYN spur. [L. spur, cock's spur]

cal·car·e·ous (kal-kā′rē-ŭs). Chalky; relating to or containing lime or calcium, or calcific material. [L. *calcarius,* pertaining to lime, fr. *calx,* lime]

cal·ca·rine (kal′kă-rēn). 1. Relating to a calcar. 2. Spur-shaped.

cal·car·i·u·ria (kal-kar-ē-yū′rē-ă). Excretion of calcium (lime) salts in the urine. [L. *calcarius,* of lime, + G. *ouron,* urine]

cal·ces (kal′sēz). Plural of calx.

cal·ci·co·sis (kal-si-kō′sis). Pneumoconiosis from the inhalation of limestone dust.

cal·ci·di·ol (kal-sĭ-dī′ol). 25-hydroxycholecalciferol (a 3,25-diol); the first step in the biological conversion of vitamin D₃ to the more active form, calcitriol; it is more potent than vitamin D₃.

cal·cif·er·ol (kal-sif′er-ol). SYN ergocalciferol.

cal·ci·fi·ca·tion (kal′si-fi-kā′shŭn). 1. Deposition of lime or other insoluble calcium salts. 2. A process in which tissue or noncellular material in the body becomes hardened as the result of precipitates or larger deposits of insoluble salts of calcium. SYN calcareous infiltration. [L. *calx,* lime, + *facio,* to make]

dystrophic c., c. occurring in degenerated or necrotic tissue, as in hyalinized scars, degenerated foci in leiomyomas, and caseous nodules.

eggshell c., a thin layer of c. around an intrathoracic lymph node, usually in silicosis, seen on a chest radiograph.

metastatic c., c. occurring in nonosseous, viable tissue in hypercalcemia.

pathologic c., c. occurring in excretory or secretory passages as calculi, and in tissues other than bone and teeth.

cal·ci·fy (kal′si-fī). To deposit or lay down calcium salts, as in the formation of bone.

cal·ci·no·sis (kal-si-nō′sis). A condition characterized by the deposition of calcium salts in nodular foci in various tissues. [calcium + *-osis,* condition]

c. circumscrip′ta, localized deposits of calcium salts in the skin and subcutaneous tissues, usually surrounded by a zone of granulomatous inflammation; clinically, the lesions resemble the tophi of gout.

reversible c., a form of c. sometimes observed in patients who ingest large quantities of milk and

alkaline medicines, as in the treatment of peptic ulcer.

c. universa′lis, diffuse deposits of calcium salts in the skin and subcutaneous tissues, connective tissue, and other sites; may be associated with dermatomyositis, occurs more frequently in young persons, and is often fatal; serum levels of calcium and phosphorus are generally within normal limits.

cal·ci·phil·ia (kal-si-fil′ē-ă). A condition in which the tissues manifest an unusual affinity for calcium salts. [calcium + G. *phileō,* to love]

cal·ci·phy·lax·is (kal′si-fī-lak′sis). A condition of induced systemic hypersensitivity in which tissues respond to appropriate challenging agents with a sudden, but sometimes evanescent, local calcification.

cal·ci·priv·ic (kal-si-priv′ik). Deprived of calcium.

cal·ci·to·nin (kal-si-tō′nin). A peptide hormone, of which eight forms are known; produced by the parathyroid, thyroid, and thymus glands; its action is opposite to that of parathyroid hormone in that c. increases deposition of calcium and phosphate in bone and lowers the level of calcium in the blood. [calci- + G. *tonos,* stretching, + -in]

cal·ci·um, gen. **cal′cii** (kal′sē-ŭm, -sē-ī). A metallic bivalent element; atomic no. 20, atomic wt. 40.078, density 1.55, melting point 842°C. Many c. salts have crucial uses in metabolism and in medicine. C. salts are responsible for the radiopacity of bone, calcified cartilage, and arteriosclerotic plaques in arteries. [Mod. L. fr. L. *calx,* lime]

cal·ci·um-47 (⁴⁷Ca). A radioisotope of calcium with a half-life of 4.54 days, used in the diagnosis of disorders of calcium metabolism.

cal·ci·um group. The metals of the alkaline earths: beryllium, magnesium, calcium, strontium, barium, and radium.

cal·ci·u·ria (kal-sē-yū′rē-ă). The urinary excretion of calcium; sometimes used as a synonym for hypercalciuria.

cal·co·dyn·ia (kal-kō-din′ē-ă). SYN painful *heel.* [L. *calx,* heel, + G. *odynē,* pain]

cal·co·sphe·rite (kal-kō-sfēr′īt). A tiny, spheroidal, concentrically laminated body containing deposits of calcium salts; found in papillary carcinoma of the thyroid and ovary and in meningioma. SYN psammoma bodies (3). [L. *calx,* lime, + G. *sphaira,* sphere]

cal·cu·li (kal′kyū-lī). Plural of calculus.

cal·cu·li (-lī).

cal·cu·lo·sis (kal-kyū-lō′sis). The tendency or disposition to form calculi or stones. [L. *calculus,* small stone, + G. *-osis,* condition]

cal·cu·lus, gen. and pl. **cal·cu·li** (kal′kyū-lŭs, -lī). A concretion formed in any part of the body, most commonly in the passages of the biliary and urinary tracts; usually composed of salts of inorganic or organic acids, or of other material such as cholesterol. SYN stone (1). [L. a pebble, a calculus]

apatite c., a c. in which the crystalloid component consists of calcium fluorophosphate.

cystine c., a c. composed of cystine, soft and faintly radiopaque.

dental c., (1) calcified deposits formed around the teeth; may appear as subgingival or supragingival c.; **(2)** SYN tartar (2).

encysted c., a urinary c. enclosed in a sac developed from the wall of the bladder. SYN pocketed c.

fibrin c., a urinary c. formed largely from fibrinogen in blood.

matrix c., a yellowish-white to light tan urinary c. containing calcium salts in an organic matrix and usually associated with chronic infection.

oxalate c., a urinary c. of calcium oxalate.

pancreatic c., a concretion, usually multiple, in the pancreatic duct, associated with chronic pancreatitis.

pocketed c., SYN encysted c.

preputial c., a c. occurring beneath the foreskin.

prostatic c., a concretion formed in the prostate gland, composed chiefly of calcium carbonate and phosphate (corpora amylacea).

renal c., a c. occurring within the kidney collecting system.

staghorn c., a c. occurring in the renal pelvis, with branches extending into the infundibula and calices.

urinary c., a c. in the kidney, ureter, bladder, or urethra.

uterine c., a calcified myoma of the uterus.

vesical c., a urinary c. formed or retained in the bladder.

cal·e·fa·cient (kal-ĕ-fā'shent). **1.** Making warm or hot. **2.** An agent causing a sense of warmth in the part to which it is applied. [L. *calefacio,* fr. *caleo,* to be warm, + *facio,* to make]

calf, pl. **calves** (kaf, kavz). SYN sural *region.* [Gael. *kalpa*]

cal·i·ber (kal'i-ber). The diameter of a hollow tubular structure. [Fr. *calibre,* of uncert. etym.]

cal·i·brate (kal'i-brāt). **1.** To graduate or standardize any measuring instrument. **2.** To measure the diameter of a tubular structure.

cal·i·bra·tor (kal'ĭ-brā-ter, -tōr). A standard or reference material or substance used to standardize or calibrate an instrument or laboratory procedure.

cal·i·ce·al (kal'i-se'al). Relating to the calix.

cal·i·cec·to·my (kal-i-sek'tō-mē). SYN calicotomy. [calix, + G. *ektomē,* excision]

ca·li·ces (kal'i-sēz). Plural of calix.

Cal·i·ci·vi·ri·dae (kal'i-sē-vī'ră-dē). A family of RNA viruses associated with epidemic viral gastroenteritis and certain forms of hepatitis.

cal·i·cot·o·my (kal-ĭ-sot'ō-mē). Incision into a calix, usually for removal of a calculus. SYN calicectomy. [calix, + G. *tomē,* a cutting]

ca·lic·u·lus, pl. **ca·lic·u·li** (kă-lik'yū-lŭs, lī). A bud-shaped or cup-shaped structure, resembling the closed calyx of a flower. [L. dim. from G. *kalyx,* the cup of a flower]

ca·li·ec·ta·sis (kā-lē-ek'tă-sis). Dilation of the calices, usually due to obstruction or infection.

cal·i·for·ni·um (Cf) (kal-i-fōr'nē-ŭm). An artificial transuranium element, symbol Cf, atomic no. 98, atomic wt. 251.08. [*California,* state and university where first prepared]

ca·li·o·plas·ty (kā'lē-ō-plas-tē). Surgical recon-

struction of a calix, usually designed to increase its lumen at the infundibulum.

ca·li·or·rha·phy (kā'lē-ōr-a-fē). **1.** Suturing of a calix. **2.** Plastic surgery of a dilated or obstructed calix to improve urinary drainage, often requiring combination of two or more calices or the massive movement of renal pelvic mucosa to rebuild the caliceal drainage system. [calix, + G. *rhaphē,* suture, seam]

cal·i·pers (kal'i-perz). An instrument used for measuring diameters. [a corruption of *caliber*]

cal·is·then·ics (kal-is-then'iks). Systematic practice of various exercises with the object of preserving health and increasing physical strength. [G. *kalos,* beautiful, + *sthenos,* strength]

ca·lix, pl. **ca·li·ces** (kā'liks, kal'i-sēz) [NA]. A flower-shaped or funnel-shaped structure; specifically one of the branches or recesses of the pelvis of the kidney into which the orifices of the malpighian renal pyramids project. SYN calyx. [L. fr. G. *kalyx,* the cup of a flower]

cal·lo·sal (ka-lō'săl). Relating to the corpus callosum.

cal·los·i·ty (ka-los'i-tē). A circumscribed thickening of the keratin layer of the epidermis as a result of repeated friction or intermittent pressure. SYN callus (1), keratoma (1), poroma (1), tyloma. [L. fr. *callosus,* thick-skinned]

cal·lous (kal'ŭs). Relating to a callus or callosity.

cal·lus (kal'ŭs). **1.** SYN callosity. **2.** A composite mass of tissue that forms at a fracture site to establish continuity between the bone ends; it is composed initially of uncallused fibrous tissue and cartilage, and ultimately of bone. [L. hard skin]

cal·mod·u·lin (kal-mod'yū-lin). A protein that binds calcium ions, thereby becoming the agent for many of the cellular effects long ascribed to calcium ions. [calcium + modulate]

ca·lor (kā'lōr). Heat, as one of the four signs of inflammation (c., rubor, tumor, dolor) enunciated by Celsus. [L.]

ca·lor·ic (kă-lōr'ik). **1.** Relating to a calorie. **2.** Relating to heat. [L. *calor,* heat]

cal·o·rie (kal'ō-rē). A unit of heat content or energy. The amount of heat necessary to raise 1 g of water from 14.5°C to 15.5°C (small c.). Calorie is being replaced by joule, the SI unit equal to 0.239 calorie. SEE ALSO British thermal *unit.* [L. *calor,* heat]

gram c., SYN small c.

kilogram c. (kcal), SYN large c.

large c. (Cal, C), the quantity of energy required to raise the temperature of 1 kg of water from 14.5° to 15.5°C; it is 1000 times the value of the small c. SYN kilocalorie, kilogram c.

mean c., one hundredth of the energy required to raise the temperature of 1 g of water from 0°C to 100°C.

small c. (cal, c), the quantity of energy required to raise the temperature of 1 g of water from 14.5°C to 15.5°C. SYN gram c.

ca·lor·i·gen·ic (kă-lōr-i-jen'ik). **1.** Capable of generating heat. **2.** Stimulating metabolic production of heat. SYN thermogenetic (2), thermogenic. [L. *calor,* heat, + G. *genesis,* production]

cal·o·rim·e·ter (kal-ō-rim'ĕ-ter). An apparatus

for measuring the amount of heat liberated in a chemical reaction. [L. *calor,* heat, + G. *metron,* measure]

▪ bomb c., an instrument for determining the potential energy of organic substances, including those in foods. In consists of a hollow steel container, lined with platinum and filled with pure oxygen, into which a weighed quantity of substance is placed and ignited with an electric fuse; the heat produced is absorbed by water surrounding the bomb and, from the rise in temperature, the calories liberated are calculated.

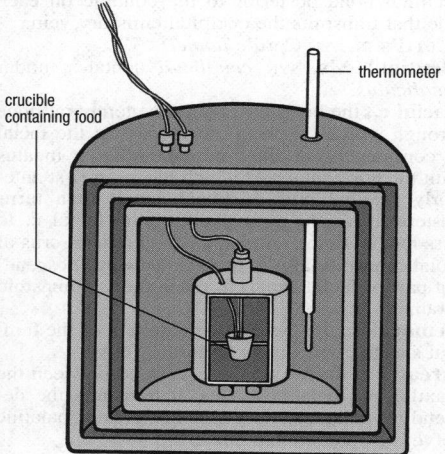

bomb calorimeter: measures heat produced by complete combustion of food sample

▪ human c., a device to measure the heat output of the human body during various levels of physical exertion. It consists of a chamber with closed air circulation and a means of comparing the temperature of water entering a coil completely surrounding the subject with the temperature of water leaving the coil.

cal·o·ri·met·ric (kă′lōr-i-met′rik). Relating to calorimetry.

cal·o·rim·e·try (kal-ō-rim′ĕ-trē). Measurement of the amount of heat given off by a reaction or group of reactions (as by an organism).

   direct c., measurement of the heat produced by a reaction, as distinguished from measurement of something other than heat production.

   indirect c., determination of heat production of an oxidation reaction by measuring uptake of oxygen and/or liberation of carbon dioxide and nitrogen excretion.

cal·var·ia, pl. **cal·var·i·ae** (kal-vā′rē-ă, -vā′rē-ē) [NA]. The upper domelike portion of the skull. SYN skullcap. [L. a skull]

cal·var·i·um (kal-vār′ē-ŭm). Incorrectly used for calvaria.

calx, gen. **cal·cis,** pl. **cal·ces** (kalks, kal′sis, kal-sēs). **1.** SYN lime (1). [L. limestone] **2.** The posterior rounded extremity of the foot. SYN heel (1). [L. heel]

ca·ly·ces (kal′i-sēz). Plural of calyx.

Ca·lym·ma·to·bac·te·ri·um (kă-lim′mă-tō-bak-tēr′ē-ŭm). A genus of nonmotile bacteria containing Gram-negative, pleomorphic rods with single or bipolar condensations of chromatin; cells occur singly and in clusters. The organisms are pathogenic only for man. The type species is *C. granulomatis;* this species causes *granuloma* inguinale. [G. *kalymma,* hood, veil, + *baktērion,* rod]

ca·lyx, pl. **ca·ly·ces** (kā′liks, kal′i-sēz). SYN calix. [G. cup of a flower]

CAM cell adhesion *molecule.*

cam·era, pl. **cam·er·ae, cam·er·as** (kam′er-ă, -ē). **1.** A closed box; especially one containing a lens, shutter, and light-sensitive film or plates for photography. **2** [NA]. In anatomy, any chamber or cavity, such as one of the chambers of the heart, or eye. [L. a vault]

   c. ante′rior bul′bi [NA], SYN anterior *chamber* of eye.

   gamma c., any one of several scintigraphic cameras that record simultaneously counts from the entire operative field of view. SYN scintillation c.

   multiformat c., photographic or laser printer for recording a variable number of video images on a sheet of film, as in computed tomography or ultrasound.

   c. oculi, SEE anterior *chamber* of eye, posterior *chamber* of eye.

   scintillation c., SYN gamma c.

cAMP adenosine 3′,5′-cyclic monophosphate (cyclic AMP).

cam·pim·e·ter (kam-pim′ĕ-ter). A small tangent screen used to measure central visual field. [L. *campus,* field, + G. *metron,* measure]

camp·to·cor·mia (kamp-tō-kōr′mē-ă). Static, often marked forward flexion of the trunk; usually manifestation of conversion reaction. SYN camptospasm. [G. *kamptos,* bent, + *kormos,* trunk of a tree]

camp·to·dac·ty·ly, camp·to·dac·tyl·ia (kamp-tō-dak′ti-lē, -dak-til′ē-ă). Permanent flexion of

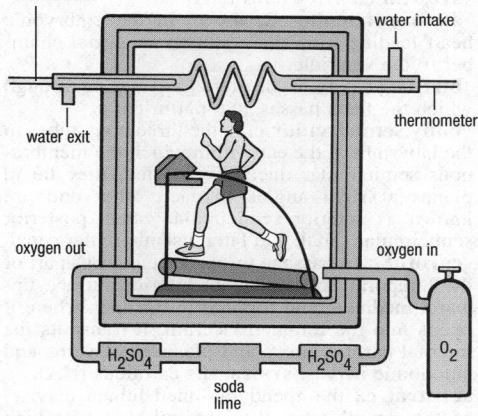

human calorimeter

one or both interphalangeal joints of one or more fingers, usually the little finger; often congenital in origin. [G. *kamptos,* bent, + *daktylos,* finger]

camp•to•me•lia (kamp-tō-mē'lē-ă). A skeletal dysplasia characterized by a bending of the long bones of the extremities, resulting in a permanent bowing or curvature of the affected part. [G. *kamptos,* bent, + *melos,* limb]

camp•to•mel•ic (kamp-tō-mel'ik). Denoting or characteristic of camptomelia.

camp•to•spasm (kamp'tō-spazm). SYN campto-cormia.

Cam•py•lo•bac•ter (kam'pi-lō-bak'ter). A genus of bacteria containing Gram-negative, non-spore-forming, spirally curved rods with a single polar flagellum at one or both ends of the cell; they are motile with a characteristic corkscrew-like motion. The type species, *C. fetus,* contins various subspecies, particularly *C. jejuni,* that can cause acute bacterial gastroenteritis. [G. *campylos,* curved, + *baktron,* staff or rod]

   C. jejuni, a species that causes an acute gastroenteritis of sudden onset with constitutional symptoms (malaise, myalgia, arthralgia, and headache) and cramping abdominal pain; potential sources of human infection include poultry, cattle, sheep, pigs, and dogs.

cam•py•lo•bac•ter•i•o•sis (kam'pi-lō-bak'ter-ē-ō'sis). Infection caused by microaerophilic bacteria of the genus *Campylobacter.*

ca•nal (kă-nal'). A duct or channel; a tubular structure. SEE ALSO canal, duct. SYN canalis [NA]. [L. *canalis*]

   adductor c., the space in middle third of the thigh between the vastus medialis and adductor muscles, converted into a canal by the overlying sartorius muscle. It gives passage to the femoral vessels and saphenous nerve, ending at the adductor hiatus. SYN canalis adductorius [NA], Hunter's c.

   Alcock's c., SYN pudendal c.

   alimentary c., SYN digestive *tract.*

   anal c., the terminal portion of the alimentary canal; it extends from the pelvic diaphragm to the anal orifice. SYN canalis analis [NA].

   arterial c., SYN *ductus* arteriosus.

   atrioventricular c., the c. in the embryonic heart leading from the common sinuatrial chamber to the ventricle.

   birth c., cavity of the uterus and vagina through which the fetus passes. SYN parturient c.

   bony semicircular c.'s, the three bony tubes in the labyrinth of the ear within which the membranous semicircular ducts are located; they lie in planes at right angles to each other and are known as anterior semicircular canal, posterior semicircular canal, and lateral semicircular canal.

   carotid c., a passage through the petrous part of the temporal bone from its inferior surface upward, medially, and forward to the apex where it opens into the foramen lacerum. It transmits the internal carotid artery and plexuses of veins and autonomic nerves. SYN canalis caroticus [NA].

   central c., the ependyma-lined lumen (cavity) of the neural tube, the cerebral part of which remains patent to form the ventricles of the brain, while the spinal part in the adult often is reduced

to a solid strand of modified ependyma. SYN syringocele (1).

   cervical c., a fusiform canal extending from the isthmus of the uterus to the opening of the uterus into the vagina. SYN canalis cervicis uteri [NA].

   cochlear c., the winding tube of the bony labyrinth which makes two and a half turns about the modiolus of the cochlea; it is divided incompletely into two compartments by a winding shelf of bone, the bony spiral lamina. SYN canalis spiralis cochleae [NA].

   condylar c., the inconstant opening through the occipital bone posterior to the condyle on each side that transmits the occipital emissary vein.

   Corti's c., SYN Corti's *tunnel.*

   dentinal c.'s, SYN *canaliculi* dentales, under *canaliculus.*

   facial c., the bony passage in the temporal bone through which the facial nerve passes; the facial c. commences at the internal auditory meatus with the horizontal part which passes at first anteriorly (medial crus of facial canal) then turns posteriorly at the geniculum of the facial c. to pass medial to the tympanic cavity (lateral crus of facial canal); finally, it turns downward (descending part of facial canal) to reach the stylomastoid foramen.

   femoral c., the medial compartment of the femoral sheath. SYN canalis femoralis [NA].

   greater palatine c., the c. formed between the maxilla and palatine bones; it transmits the descending palatine artery and the greater palatine nerve. SYN pterygopalatine c.

   haversian c.'s, vascular c.'s that run longitudinally in the center of haversian systems of compact osseous tissue.

   Hunter's c., SYN adductor c.

   hypoglossal c., the canal through which the hypoglossal nerve emerges from the skull. SYN canalis hypoglossalis [NA], anterior condyloid foramen.

   incisive c., incisor c., one of several bony canals leading from the floor of the nasal cavity into the incisive fossa on the palatal surface of the maxilla; they convey the nasopalatine nerves and branches of the greater palatine arteries which anastomose with the septal branch of the sphenopalatine artery. SYN canalis incisivus [NA].

   infraorbital c., a canal running beneath the orbital margin of the maxilla from the infraorbital groove, in the floor of the orbit, to the infraorbital foramen; it transmits the infraorbital artery and nerve. SYN canalis infraorbitalis [NA].

   inguinal c., the obliquely directed passage through the layers of the lower abdominal wall that transmits the spermatic cord in the male and the round ligament in the female. SYN canalis inguinalis [NA].

   interdental c.'s, c.'s that extend vertically through alveolar bone between roots of mandibular and maxillary incisor and maxillary bicuspid teeth.

   interfacial c.'s, intercellular spaces occurring in relation to intercellular attachments by desmosomes in stratified squamous epithelium, generally resulting from shrinkage of an artifact of fixation.

c.'s for lesser palatine nerves, c.'s located in the posterior part of the palatine bone.

musculotubal c., a canal beginning at the anterior border of the petrous portion of the temporal bone near its junction with the squamous portion, and passing to the tympanic cavity; it is divided by the cochleariform process into two semicanals: one for the auditory (eustachian) tube, the other for the tensor tympani muscle. SYN canalis musculotubarius [NA].

nasolacrimal c., the bony canal formed by the maxilla, lacrimal bone, and inferior concha that transmits the nasolacrimal duct from the orbit to the inferior meatus of the nose. SYN canalis nasolacrimalis [NA].

nutrient c., a canal in the shaft of a long bone or in other locations in irregular bones through which the nutrient artery enters a bone. SYN canalis nutricius [NA].

obturator c., the opening in the superior part of the obturator membrane through which the obturator nerve and vessels pass from the pelvic cavity into the thigh. SYN canalis obturatorius [NA].

optic c., the short canal through the lesser wing of the sphenoid bone at the apex of the orbit that gives passage to the optic nerve and the ophthalmic artery. SYN canalis opticus [NA], optic foramen.

parturient c., SYN birth c.

portal c.'s, connective tissue spaces in the substance of the liver that are occupied by preterminal ramifications of the bile ducts, portal vein, and hepatic artery, as well as nerves and lymphatics.

pterygoid c., an opening through the base of the medial pterygoid process of the sphenoid bone through which pass the artery, vein, and nerve of the pterygoid canal. SYN canalis pterygoideus [NA].

pterygopalatine c., SYN greater palatine c.

pudendal c., the space within the obturator internus fascia lining the lateral wall of the ischiorectal fossa that transmits the pudendal vessels and nerves. SYN canalis pudendalis [NA], Alcock's c.

pulp c., SYN root c. of tooth.

pyloric c., the segment of the stomach that succeeds the antrum and ends at the gastroduodenal junction. SYN canalis pyloricus [NA].

root c. of tooth, the chamber of the dental pulp lying within the root portion of a tooth. SYN canalis radicis dentis [NA], pulp c.

sacral c., the continuation of the vertebral canal in the sacrum. SYN canalis sacralis [NA].

Schlemm's c., SYN sinus venosus sclerae.

spinal c., SYN vertebral c.

spiral c. of modiolus, the space in the modiolus in which the spiral ganglion of the cochlear nerve lies. SYN canalis spiralis modioli [NA].

urogenital c., SYN urethra.

vertebral c., the canal that contains the spinal cord, spinal meninges, and related structures. It is formed by the vertebral foramina of successive vertebrae of the articulated vertebral column. SYN canalis vertebralis [NA], spinal c.

vestibular c., SYN scala vestibuli.

Wirsung's c., SYN pancreatic duct.

ca·na·les (kă-nā′lēz). Plural of canalis.

can·a·lic·u·lar (kan-ă-lik′yū-lăr). Relating to a canaliculus. [L. canaliculus, small channel, dim. fr. canalis, canal, + suffix -ar, pertaining to]

can·a·lic·u·li (-lī)

can·a·lic·u·li (kan-ă-lik′yū-lī). Plural of canaliculus.

can·a·lic·u·li·tis (kan′ă-lik-yū-lī′tis). Inflammation of the lacrimal canaliculus. [canaliculus + G. -itis, inflammation]

can·a·lic·u·li·za·tion (kan-ă-lik′yū-lī-zā′shŭn). The formation of canaliculi, or small canals, in any tissue.

can·a·lic·u·lus, pl. **can·a·lic·u·li** (kan-ă-lik′yū-lŭs, -lī) [NA]. A small canal or channel. SEE ALSO iter. [L. dim. fr. canalis, canal]

    biliary c., one of the intercellular channels, about 1 μm or less in diameter, that occur between liver cells forming the first portion of the bile system.

    bone c., c. connecting bone lacunae with one another or with a haversian canal; contains the interconnecting cytoplasmic processes of osteocytes.

    canalic′uli denta′les [NA], minute, wavy, branching tubes or canals in the dentin; they contain the long cytoplasmic processes of odontoblasts and extend radially from the pulp to the dentoenamel junction. SYN dentinal canals, dentinal tubules.

    cochlear c., a minute canal in the temporal bone that passes from the cochlea inferiorly to open in front of the medial side of the jugular fossa. It contains the perilymphatic duct.

    intercellular c., one of the fine channels between adjoining secretory cells, such as those between serous cells in salivary glands.

    intracellular c., a fine canal formed by invagination of the cell membrane into the cytoplasm of a cell, such as those of the parietal cells of the stomach.

    lacrimal c., a curved canal beginning at the lacrimal punctum in the margin of each eyelid near the medial commissure and running transversely medially to empty with its fellow into the lacrimal sac.

    mastoid c., the canal that extends from the jugular fossa laterally through the mastoid process. It transmits the auricular branch of the vagus.

    tympanic c., a minute canal passing from the inferior surface of the petrous portion of the temporal bone between the jugular fossa and carotid canal to the floor of the tympanic cavity. Located in the wedge of bone separating the jugular canal and carotid canal, it transmits the tympanic branch of the glossopharyngeal nerve.

ca·na·lis, pl. **ca·na·les** (ka-nā′lis, -lēz) [NA]. SYN canal. [L.]

    c. adductor′ius [NA], SYN adductor canal.

    c. ana′lis [NA], SYN anal canal.

    c. carot′icus [NA], SYN carotid canal.

    c. car′pi [NA], SYN carpal tunnel.

    c. cerv′icis u′teri [NA], SYN cervical canal.

    c. femora′lis [NA], SYN femoral canal.

    c. hypoglossa′lis [NA], SYN hypoglossal canal.

    c. incisi′vus [NA], SYN incisive canal.

    c. infraorbita′lis [NA], SYN infraorbital canal.

ca

c. **inguina′lis** [NA], SYN inguinal *canal.*
c. **musculotuba′rius** [NA], SYN musculotubal *canal.*
c. **nasolacrima′lis** [NA], SYN nasolacrimal *canal.*
c. **nutri′cius** [NA], SYN nutrient *canal.*
c. **obturato′rius** [NA], SYN obturator *canal.*
c. **op′ticus** [NA], SYN optic *canal.*
c. **pterygoi′deus** [NA], SYN pterygoid *canal.*
c. **pudenda′lis** [NA], SYN pudendal *canal.*
c. **pylor′icus** [NA], SYN pyloric *canal.*
c. **rad′icis den′tis** [NA], SYN root *canal* of tooth.
c. **sacra′lis** [NA], SYN sacral *canal.*
c. **spira′lis coch′leae** [NA], SYN cochlear *canal.*
c. **spira′lis modi′oli** [NA], SYN spiral *canal* of modiolus.
c. **vertebra′lis** [NA], SYN vertebral *canal.*
can·a·li·za·tion (kan-ăl-ī-zā′shŭn). The formation of canals or channels in a tissue.
can·cel·lat·ed (kan′sĕ-lā-ted). SYN cancellous. [L. *cancello,* to make a lattice work]
can·cel·lous (kan′sĕ-lŭs). Denoting bone that has a lattice-like or spongy structure. SYN cancelled.
can·cel·lus, pl. **can·cel·li** (kan-sel′ŭs, -lī). A lattice-like structure, as in spongy bone. [L. a grating, lattice]
can·cer (CA) (kan′ser). General term for malignant neoplasms; carcinoma or sarcoma, especially the former. [L. a crab, a cancer]
   stump c., carcinoma of the stomach developing after gastroenterostomy or gastric resection for benign disease.
can·cer·o·pho·bia (kan′ser-ō-fō′bē-ă). A morbid fear of acquiring a malignant growth. SYN carcinophobia. [cancer + G. *phobos,* fear]
can·cer·ous (kan′ser-ŭs). Relating to or pertaining to a malignant neoplasm, or being afflicted with such a process.
can·cra (kang′krä). Plural of cancrum.
can·cri·form (kang′kri-fōrm). Resembling cancer.
can·crum, pl. **can·cra** (kang′krŭm, -krä). A gangrenous, ulcerative, inflammatory lesion. [Mod. L., fr. L. *cancer,* crab]
can·de·la (cd) (kan′de-lă). The SI unit of luminous intensity, 1 lumen per m^2; the luminous intensity, in a given direction, of a source that emits monochromatic radiation of frequency 540 × 10^{12} hertz and that has a radiant intensity in that direction of 1/683 watt per steradian (solid angle). [L.]
Can·di·da (kan′did-ă). A genus of yeastlike fungi found in nature; a few species are isolated from the skin, feces, and vaginal and pharyngeal tissue, but the gastrointestinal tract is the source of the single most important species, *C. albicans.* [L. *candidus,* dazzling white]
can·di·de·mia (kan-di-dē′mē-ă). Presence of cells of *Candida* species in the peripheral blood. [*Candida* + G. *haima,* blood]
can·di·di·a·sis (kan-di-dī′ă-sis). Infection with, or disease caused by, *Candida,* especially *C. albicans.* This disease usually results from debilitation (as in immunosuppression and especially AIDS), physiologic change, prolonged adminis-

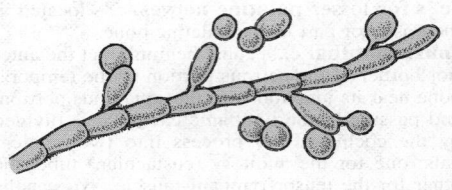

Candida

tration of antibiotics, and barrier breakage. SYN candidosis, moniliasis.
can·di·do·sis (kan-di-dō′sis). SYN candidiasis.
can·dle·me·ter (kan′dl-mē′ter). SYN lux.
ca·nine (kā′nīn). **1.** Relating to a dog. **2.** Relating to the c. teeth. **3.** SYN canine *tooth.* **4.** Referring to the cuspid tooth. [L. *caninus*]
ca·ni·ti·es (kă-nish′ē-ēz). Graying of hair. [L., fr. *canus,* hoary, gray]
   rapid c., whitening of hair overnight or over a few days; in the latter case, may be seen in alopecia areata, when surviving pigmented hairs are preferentially shed from gray hair.
can·ker (kang′ker). **1.** In cats and dogs, acute inflammation of the external ear and auditory canal. SEE aphtha. **2.** An outmoded term for aphthae. [L. *cancer,* crab, malignant growth]
can·nab·i·noids (ka-nab′i-noydz). Organic substances present in *Cannabis sativa,* having a variety of pharmacologic properties.
can·na·bis (kan′ă-bis). The dried flowering tops of the pistillate plants of *Cannabis sativa* (family Moraceae) containing isomeric tetrahydrocannabinols, cannabinol, and cannabidiol. Preparations of c. are smoked or ingested by members of various cultures and subcultures to induce psychotomimetic effects such as euphoria, hallucinations, drowsiness, and other mental changes. C. was formerly used as a sedative and analgesic; now available for restricted use in management of iatrogenic anorexia, especially that associated with oncologic chemotherapy and radiation therapy. Known by many colloquial or slang terms such as marijuana; marihuana; pot; grass; bhang; charas; ganja; hashish. [L., fr. G. *kannabis,* hemp]
can·na·bism (kan′ă-bizm). Poisoning by preparations of cannabis.
can·nu·la (kan′yū-lă). A tube which can be inserted into a cavity, usually by means of a trocar filling its lumen; after insertion of the c., the trocar is withdrawn and the c. remains as a channel for the transport of fluid. [L. dim. of *canna,* reed]
   Hasson c., a laparoscopic instrument for open (rather than blind needle insufflation) placement of the initial port. The Hasson has a blunt-tipped obturator instead of a sharp trocar and a balloon on the distal portion of the sheath to hold it in place.
can·nu·la·tion, can·nu·li·za·tion (kan-yū-lā′shŭn, -yū-lī-zā′shŭn). Insertion of a cannula.
CANS central auditory nervous *system.*
can·thal (kan′thăl). Relating to a canthus.
can·thec·to·my (kan-thek′tō-mē). Excision of a

palpebral canthus. [G. *kanthos,* canthus, + *ektomē,* excision]

can·thi (kan'thī). Plural of canthus.

can·thi·tis (kan-thī'tis). Inflammation of a canthus.

can·thol·y·sis (kan-thol'i-sis). SYN canthoplasty (1). [G. *kanthos,* canthus, + *lysis,* loosening]

can·tho·plas·ty (kan'thō-plas-tē). **1.** An operation for lengthening the palpebral fissure by incision through the lateral canthus. SYN cantholysis. **2.** An operation for restoration of the canthus. [G. *kanthos,* canthus, + *plassō,* to form]

can·thor·rha·phy (kan-thōr'ă-fē). Suture of the eyelids at either canthus. [G. *kanthos,* canthus, + *rhaphē,* suture]

can·thot·o·my (kan-thot'ō-mē). Slitting of the canthus. [G. *kanthos,* canthus, + *tomē,* incision]

can·thus, pl. **can·'thi** (kan'thŭs, -thī). The angle of the eye. [G. *kanthos,* corner of the eye]

CAP catabolite (gene) activator *protein.*

cap (kap). **1.** Any anatomical structure that resembles a c. or cover. **2.** A protective covering for an incomplete tooth. **3.** Colloquialism for restoration of the coronal part of a natural tooth by means of an artificial crown. **4.** The nucleotide structure found at the 5′ terminus of many eukaryotic messenger RNAs.

  acrosomal c., a collapsed membranous vesicle that covers the anterior part of the nucleus of the spermatozoon, derived from the acrosomal granule. SYN head c.

  apical c., a curved shadow at the apex of one or both hemithoraces on chest x-ray; caused by pleural and pulmonary fibrosis.

  cradle c., colloquialism for seborrheic dermatitis of the scalp of the newborn.

  duodenal c., the first portion of the duodenum, as seen in a roentgenogram or by fluoroscopy.

  enamel c., the enamel covering the crown of a tooth.

  head c., SYN acrosomal c.

  pyloric c., archaic term for duodenal c.

ca·pac·i·ta·tion (kă-pas'i-tā'shŭn). A process whereby the glycoprotein coat and seminal proteins are removed from the sperm's acrosome. Once c. has occurred, perforation of the acrosome can occur. [L. *capacitas,* fr. *capax,* capable of]

ca·pac·i·tor (kă-pas'i-ter, -tōr). A device for holding a charge of electricity. SYN condenser (4).

ca·pac·i·ty (kă-pas'i-tē). **1.** The potential cubic contents of a cavity or receptacle. **2.** Power to do. SEE ALSO volume. [L. *capax,* able to contain; fr. *capio,* to take]

  diffusing c. (symbol, D, followed by subscripts indicating location and chemical species), the amount of oxygen taken up by pulmonary capillary blood per minute per unit average oxygen pressure gradient between alveolar gas and pulmonary capillary blood; units are: ml/min/mm Hg; also applied to other gases such as carbon monoxide.

  forced vital c. (FVC), vital c. measured with the subject exhaling as rapidly as possible.

  functional residual c. (FRC), the volume of gas remaining in the lungs at the end of a normal expiration; it is the sum of expiratory reserve volume and residual volume. SYN functional residual air.

  heat c., the quantity of heat required to raise the temperature of a system 1°C. SYN thermal c.

  inspiratory c., the volume of air that can be inspired after a normal expiration; it is the sum of the tidal volume and the inspiratory reserve volume. SYN complementary air.

  maximum breathing c. (MBC), SYN maximum voluntary *ventilation.*

  oxygen c., the maximum quantity of oxygen that will combine chemically with the hemoglobin in a unit volume of blood; normally it amounts to 1.34 ml of O_2 per gm of Hb or 20 ml of O_2 per 100 ml of blood.

  residual c., SYN residual *volume.*

  respiratory c., SYN vital c.

  thermal c., SYN heat c.

  total iron binding c. (TIBC), an indirect method of determining the transferrin level in serum. Transferrin is saturated by the addition of iron to a serum specimen. Excess iron is removed and the specimen is analyzed for iron content. The result is the total amount of iron that can be bound by transferrin. This result is helpful in differentiating anemias. A high TIBC is associated with iron deficiency; low TIBC is associated with excess iron.

  total lung c. (TLC), the inspiratory c. plus the functional residual c.; *i.e.,* the volume of air contained in the lungs at the end of a maximal inspiration; also equals vital c. plus residual volume.

  vital c. (VC), the greatest volume of air that can be exhaled from the lungs after a maximum inspiration. SYN respiratory c.

cap·ac·tins (kap-ak'tinz). A class of proteins capping the ends of actin filaments.

CAPD continuous ambulatory peritoneal *dialysis.*

cap·il·lar·i·o·mo·tor (kap-i-lār'ē-ō-mō'tŏr). Vasomotor, with special reference to the capillaries.

cap·il·lar·i·tis (kap'i-lar-ī'tis). Inflammation of a capillary or capillaries.

cap·il·lar·i·ty (kap-i-lar'i-tē). The rise of liquids in narrow tubes or through the pores of a loose material, as a result of surface tension.

cap·il·la·rop·a·thy (kap'i-lă-rop'ă-thē). Any disease of the capillaries, often applied to vascular changes in diabetes mellitus. SYN microangiopathy. [capillary + G. *pathos,* disease]

cap·il·lary (kap'i-lār-ē). **1.** Resembling a hair; fine; minute. **2.** A capillary vessel; *e.g.,* blood c., lymph c. **3.** Relating to a blood or lymphatic c. vessel. [L. *capillaris,* relating to hair]

  arterial c., a c. opening from an arteriole or metarteriole.

  blood c. (symbol c, as a subscript), a vessel whose wall consists of endothelium and its basement membrane; its diameter, when the c. is open, is about 8 μm; with the electron microscope, fenestrated c.'s and continuous c.'s are distinguished.

  continuous c., a c. in which small vesicles (caveolae) are numerous and pores are absent.

  fenestrated c., a c., found in renal glomeruli, intestinal villi, and some glands, in which ultramicroscopic pores of variable size occur.

  lymph c., the beginning of the lymphatic sys-

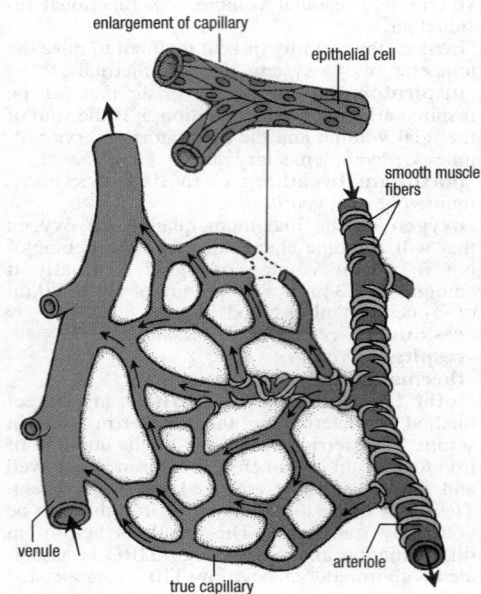

enlargement of capillary

epithelial cell

smooth muscle fibers

venule

true capillary

arteriole

capillary bed

tem of vessels; it is lined with a highly attenuated endothelium with poorly developed basement membrane and a lumen of variable caliber. SEE lacteal (2).

venous c., a c. opening into a venule.
ca·pi·ta (kap′i-tă). Plural of caput.
cap·i·tate (kap′i-tāt). **1.** The largest of the carpal bones; located in the distal row. SYN capitate bone. **2.** Head-shaped; having a rounded extremity. [L. *caput* (*capit-*), head]
capitation (kap′i-tā′shun). Payment system that fixes the amount paid by a managed-care plan to a health care provider for services to each managed-care subscriber, regardless of the actual services rendered. SEE ALSO managed *care*.
cap·i·tel·lum (kap-i-tel′ŭm). **1.** SYN capitulum (1). **2.** SYN *capitulum* of humerus. [L. dim. of *caput*, head]
ca·pit·u·la (kă-pit′yū-lă). Plural of capitulum.
ca·pit·u·lar (kă-pit′yū-lăr). Relating to a capitulum.
ca·pit·u·lum, pl. **ca·pit·u·la** (kă-pit′yū-lŭm, -lă). **1** [NA]. A small head or rounded articular extremity of a bone. SYN capitellum (1). SEE ALSO caput. **2.** The bloodsucking, probing, sensing, and holdfast mouthparts of a tick, including the basal supporting structure; relative size and shape of mouthparts forming the c. are characteristic for the genera of hard ticks. [L. dim. of *caput*, head]
c. of humerus, the small rounded eminence on the lateral half of the distal end of the humerus for articulation with the radius. SYN capitellum (2).
Cap·no·cy·to·pha·ga (kap′nō-sī-tŏf′a-ga). A genus of Gram-negative, fusiform-shaped bacteria associated with human periodontal disease.

cap·no·gram (kap′nō-gram). A continuous record of the carbon dioxide content of expired air. [G. *kapnos,* smoke, + *gramma,* something written]
cap·no·graph (kap′nō-graf). Instrument by which a continuous graph of the carbon dioxide content of expired air is obtained.
capnometer (kap-nom′ĕ-ter). An instrument which measures the carbon dioxide concentration of exhaled air. SYN CO_2 analyzer. [G. *kapnos,* smoke, + *metron,* a measure]
capnometry (kap-nom′ĕ-trē). The process of measuring and recording the carbon dioxide concentration of exhaled air at the patient's airway using a capnometer.
cap·rate (kap′rāt). A salt or ester of capric acid.
n-cap·ric ac·id (kap′rik). A fatty acid found among the hydrolysis products of fat in goat's milk, cow's milk, and other substances. Cf. *n*-caproic acid, caprylic acid.
n-ca·pro·ic ac·id (kap-rō′ik). A fatty acid found among the hydrolysis products of fat in butter, coconut oil, and some other substances.
cap·ro·yl (kap′rō-il). The acyl radical of caproic acid.
cap·ro·y·late (kap′rō-i-lāt). A salt or ester of caproic acid.
cap·ry·late (kap′ri-lāt). A salt or ester of caprylic acid.
ca·pryl·ic ac·id (kap-ril′ik). A fatty acid found among the hydrolysis products of fat in butter, coconut oil, and other substances.
cap·sid (kap′sid). SEE virion.
cap·su·la, gen. and pl. **cap·su·lae** (kap′sū-lă, -lē) [NA]. **1.** A membranous structure, usually dense collagenous connective tissue, that envelops an organ, a joint, or any other part. **2.** An anatomical structure resembling a capsule or envelope. SYN capsule (1). [L. dim. of *capsa,* a chest or box]
c. articula′ris [NA], SYN articular *capsule*.
c. exter′na [NA], SYN external *capsule*.
c. inter′na [NA], SYN internal *capsule*.
cap·su·lar (kap′sū-lăr). Relating to any capsule.
cap·sule (kap′sūl). **1.** SYN capsula. **2.** A fibrous tissue layer enveloping an organ or a tumor, especially if benign. **3.** A solid dosage form in which the drug is enclosed in either a hard or soft soluble container or "shell" of a suitable form of gelatin. **4.** A hyaline glycosaminoglycan sheath on the wall of a fungus cell, blastoconidium, or spore. [L. *capsula,* dim. of *capsa,* box]
articular c., a sac enclosing a joint, formed by an outer fibrous articular c. and an inner synovial membrane. SYN capsula articularis [NA], joint c.
auditory c., the cartilage that, in the embryo, surrounds the developing auditory vesicle and develops into the bony labyrinth of the inner ear.
bacterial c., a layer of slime of variable composition which covers the surface of some bacteria; capsulated cells of pathogenic bacteria are usually more virulent than cells without capsules because the former are more resistant to phagocytic action.
cartilage c., the more intensely basophilic matrix in hyaline cartilage surrounding the lacunae

in which the cartilage cells lie. SYN territorial matrix.

external c., a thin lamina of white substance separating the claustrum from the putamen. It joins the internal c. at either extremity of the putamen, forming a c. of white matter external to the lenticular nucleus. SYN capsula externa [NA].

fibrous c., any fibrous envelope of a part; the fibrous capsule of an organ.

fibrous articular c., the outer fibrous part of the capsule of a synovial joint, which may in places be thickened to form capsular ligaments.

fibrous c. of kidney, a fibrous membrane ensheathing the kidney.

fibrous c. of liver, (1) a layer of connective tissue ensheathing the hepatic artery, portal vein, and bile ducts as these ramify within the liver; **(2)** connective tissue c. surrounding the outer surface of the liver, but continuous with septae of some animals which divide parenchyme into lobule, and with the perivascular fibrous c. at the porta hepatis.

glomerular c., the expanded beginning of a nephron composed of an inner and outer layer: the visceral layer consists of podocytes which surround a tuft of capillaries (glomerulus); the parietal layer is simple squamous epithelium which becomes cuboidal at the tubular pole. SYN malpighian c. (1).

internal c., a massive layer (8 to 10 mm thick) of white matter separating the caudate nucleus and thalamus (medial) from the more laterally situated lentiform nucleus (globus pallidus and putamen). It consists of 1) fibers ascending from the thalamus to the cerebral cortex that compose, among others, the visual, auditory, and somatic sensory radiations, and 2) fibers descending from the cerebral cortex to the thalamus, subthalamic region, midbrain, hindbrain, and spinal cord. The internal c. is the major route by which the cerebral cortex is connected with the brainstem and spinal cord. Laterally and superiorly it is continuous with the corona radiata which forms a major part of the cerebral hemisphere's white matter; caudally and medially it continues, much reduced in size, as the crus cerebri which contains, among others, the pyramidal tract. On horizontal section it appears in the form of a V opening out laterally; the V's obtuse angle is called genu (knee); its anterior and posterior limbs, respectively, the crus anterior and crus posterior. SYN capsula interna [NA].

joint c., SYN articular c.

lens c., the capsule enclosing the lens of the eye.

malpighian c., (1) SYN glomerular c. **(2)** a thin fibrous membrane enveloping the spleen and continued over the vessels entering at the hilus.

nasal c., the cartilage around the developing nasal cavity of the embryo.

optic c., the concentrated zone of mesenchyme around the developing optic cup; the primordium of the sclera of the eye.

otic c., the cartilage c. surrounding the inner ear mechanism; in the embryo it is cartilaginous at first but later becomes bony.

cap•su•li•tis (kap′sū-lī′tis). Inflammation of the

capsule of an organ or part, as of the liver or the lens of the eye.

adhesive c., a condition in which there is limitation of motion in a joint due to inflammatory thickening of the capsule, a common cause of stiffness in the shoulder.

cap•su•lo•len•tic•u•lar (kap′sū-lō-len-tik′yū-lăr). Referring to the lens of the eye and its capsule.

cap•su•lo•plas•ty (kap′sū-lō-plas-tē). Plastic surgery of a capsule; more specifically, the capsule of a joint. [L. *capsula,* capsule, + G. *plastos,* formed]

cap•su•lor•rha•phy (kap-sū-lōr′ă-fē). Suture of a tear in any capsule; specifically, suture of a joint capsule to prevent recurring dislocation of the articulation. [L. *capsula,* capsule, + *rhaphē,* suture]

cap•su•lot•o•my (kap-sū-lot′ō-mē). **1.** Division of a capsule as around a breast implant. **2.** Creation of an opening through a capsule; *e.g.,* of a scar around a foreign body. **3.** Incision of the capsule of the lens in the extracapsular cataract operation. [L. *capsula,* capsule, + G. *tomē,* a cutting]

cap•ture (kap′chūr). Catching and holding a particle or an electrical impulse originating elsewhere. [L. *capio,* pp. *-tus,* to take, seize]

ca•put, gen. **ca•pi•tis,** pl. **ca•pi•ta** (kap′ut, ka′put; kap′i-tis; kap′ĭ-tă). **1** [NA]. The upper or anterior extremity of the animal body, containing the brain and the organs of sight, hearing, taste, and smell. **2** [NA]. The upper, anterior, or larger extremity, expanded or rounded, of any body, organ, or other anatomical structure. **3.** The rounded extremity of a bone. **4.** That end of a muscle which is attached to the less movable part of the skeleton. SYN head. [L.]

c. medu′sae, (1) varicose veins radiating from the umbilicus, seen in the Cruveilhier-Baumgarten syndrome; **(2)** dilated ciliary arteries girdling the corneoscleral limbus in rubeosis iridis. SYN Medusa head. [*Medusa,* G. myth. char.]

c. succeda′neum, an edematous swelling formed on the presenting portion of the scalp of an infant during birth.

△**carb-, carbo-.** Prefixes indicating carbon, especially the attachment of a group containing a carbon atom. [L. *carbo,* charcoal]

car•ba•mate (kar′bă-māt). **1.** A salt or ester of carbamic acid forming the basis of urethane hypnotics. **2.** A group of cholinesterase-inhibiting insecticides resembling organophosphates. SYN carbamoate.

car•bam•ic ac•id (kar-bam′ik). A hypothetical acid, NH_2-COOH, forming carbamates; the acyl radical is carbamoyl.

carb•a•mi•no•he•mo•glo•bin (kar-bam′i-nō-hē-mō-glō′bin). Carbon dioxide bound to hemoglobin by means of a reactive amino group on the latter; approximately 20% of the total carbon dioxide in blood is combined with hemoglobin in this manner.

car•bam•o•ate (kar′ba-mōt). SYN carbamate.

car•bam•o•yl (kar′bă-mō-il). The acyl radical, NH_2-CO-, the transfer of which plays an important role in certain biochemical reactions. SYN carbamyl.

car·bam·o·yl·trans·fer·as·es (kar′bă-mō-il-trans′fer-ās-ĕz) [EC group 2.1.3]. Enzymes transferring carbamoyl groups from one compound to another. SYN transcarbamoylases.

car·bam·o·yl·u·rea (kar′bă-mō-il-yū-rē′ă). SYN biuret.

car·ba·myl (kar′bă-mil). SYN carbamoyl.

△**carbo-.** SEE carb-.

car·bo·hy·drates (kar-bō-hī′drāts). Class name for the aldehydic or ketonic derivatives of polyhydric alcohols. Most such compounds have formulas that may be written $C_n(H_2O)_n$, although they are not true hydrates. The group includes simple sugars (monosaccharides, disaccharides, etc.), as well as macromolecular (polymeric) substances such as starch, glycogen, and cellulose polysaccharides. SEE ALSO saccharides.

car·bo·hy·drat·u·ria (kar′bō-hī-dră-tū′rē-ă). Excretion of one or more carbohydrates in the urine.

car·bo·lu·ria (kar-bō-lū′rē-ă). The presence of phenol (carbolic acid) in the urine. [carbolic acid + G. *ouron*, urine]

car·bon (C) (kar′bŏn). A nonmetallic tetravalent element, atomic no. 6, atomic wt. 12.011; the major bioelement. It has two natural isotopes, ^{12}C and ^{13}C (the former, set at 12.00000, being the standard for all molecular weights), and two artificial, radioactive isotopes of interest, ^{11}C and ^{14}C. The element occurs in diamond, graphite, charcoal, coke, and soot, and in the atmosphere as CO_2. Its compounds are found in all living tissues, and the study of its vast number of compounds constitutes most of organic chemistry. [L. *carbo*, coal]

  c. dioxide, CO_2; the product of the combustion of c. with an excess of air; in concentrations not less than 99.0% by volume of CO_2, used as a respiratory stimulant.

  c. monoxide (CO), a colorless, practically odorless, and poisonous gas formed by the incomplete combustion of c.; its toxic action is due to its strong affinity for hemoglobin, myoglobin, and the cytochromes, reducing oxygen transport and blocking oxygen utilization.

car·bon·ate (kar′bŏn-āt). **1.** A salt of carbonic acid. **2.** The ion $CO_3^=$.

carbon dioxide production ($\overset{v}{V}CO_2$). The volume of carbon dioxide produced by the body in one minute; it is reported in liters or ml per minute at STPD.

car·bon·yl (kar′bŏn-il). The characteristic group, —CO—, of the ketones, aldehydes, and organic acids.

△**carboxy-.** Combining form indicating addition of CO or CO_2.

car·box·y·he·mo·glo·bin (kar-bok′sē-hē-mō-glō′bin). A stable union of carbon monoxide with hemoglobin. The formation of c. prevents the normal transfer of carbon dioxide and oxygen during the circulation of blood; thus, increasing levels of c. result in various degrees of asphyxiation, including death. SYN carbon monoxide hemoglobin.

car·box·y·he·mo·glo·bi·ne·mia (kar-bok′sē-hē′mō-glō-bi-nē′mē-ă). Presence of carboxyhemoglobin in the blood, as in carbon monoxide poisoning.

car·box·yl (kar-bok′sil). The characterizing group (—COOH) of organic acids.

car·box·yl·ase (kar-bok′sil-ās). One of several carboxy-lyases catalyzing the addition of CO_2 to another molecule to create an additional —COOH group.

car·box·yl·a·tion (kar-bok-si-lā′shŭn). Addition of CO_2 to an organic acceptor to yield a —COOH group; catalyzed by carboxylases.

car·box·yl·trans·fer·as·es (kar-bok-sil-trans′fer-ās-ez) [EC group 2.1.3]. Enzymes transferring carboxyl groups from one compound to another. SYN transcarboxylases.

car·box·y·pep·ti·dase (kar-bok-sē-pep′ti-dās). A hydrolase that removes the amino acid at the free carboxyl end of a polypeptide chain; an exopeptidase.

car·bun·cle (kar′bŭng-kl). **1.** Deep-seated pyogenic infection of the skin and subcutaneous tissues, usually arising in several contiguous hair follicles, with formation of connecting sinuses. **2.** SYN anthrax. [L. *carbunculus,* dim. of *carbo,* a live coal, a carbuncle]

car·bun·cu·lar (kar-bŭng′kyū-lăr). Relating to a carbuncle.

car·bun·cu·lo·sis (kar-bŭng-kyū-lō′sis). A condition marked by the occurrence of several carbuncles simultaneously or within a short period of time.

△**carcino-, carcin-.** Cancer; crab. [G. *karkinos,* crab, cancer]

car·ci·no·em·bry·on·ic (kar′si-nō-em-brē-on′ik). Pertaining to a substance found in embryonic tissue but absent from adult tissue except in certain carcinomas of the lung, digestive tract, and pancreas.

car·cin·o·gen (kar-sin′ō-jen, kar′si-nō-jen). Any cancer-producing substance or organism, such as polycyclic aromatic hydrocarbons, or agents such as certain types of irradiation. [carcino- + G, -*gen*, producing]

  complete c., a chemical c. that is able to induce cancer without provocation by a tumor-promoting agent introduced during therapy.

car·ci·no·gen·e·sis (kar′si-nō-jen′ĕ-sis). The origin, production, or development of cancer, including carcinomas and other malignant neoplasms. [carcino- + G. *genesis,* generation]

car·ci·no·gen·ic (kar′si-nō-jen′ik). Causing cancer.

car·ci·no·lyt·ic (kar′si-nō-lit′ik). Destructive to the cells of carcinoma. [carcino- + G. *lytikos,* causing a solution]

car·ci·no·ma (CA), pl. **car·ci·no·mas, car·ci·no·ma·ta** (kar-si-nō′mă, -măz, -nō′mă-tă). Any of the various types of malignant neoplasm derived from epithelial tissue, occurring more frequently in the skin and large intestine in both sexes, the lung and prostate gland in men, and the lung and breast in women. Carcinomas are identified histologically on the basis of invasiveness and the changes that indicate anaplasia, *i.e.,* loss of polarity of nuclei, loss of orderly maturation of cells (especially in squamous cell type), variation in the size and shape of cells, hyperchromatism of nuclei (with clumping of chromatin), and increase in the nuclear-cytoplasmic ratio. Carcinomas may be undifferentiated, or the neoplastic tissue may resemble (to varying degree) one of the types of normal epithelium. [G. *karkinōma,* fr. *karkinos,* cancer, + *-oma,* tumor]

adenoid cystic c., a histologic type of c. characterized by round, glandlike spaces or cysts bordered by layers of epithelial cells without intervening stroma, forming a pattern like a slice of Swiss cheese; perineural invasion and hematogenous metastasis are common; occurs most commonly in salivary glands. SYN cylindromatous c.

adenoid squamous cell c., SYN adenoacanthoma.

alveolar cell c., SYN bronchiolar c.

apocrine c., (1) a c. composed predominantly of cells with abundant eosinophilic granular cytoplasm, occurring in the breast; **(2)** a c. of the apocrine glands.

basal cell c., a slow-growing, invasive, but usually non-metastasizing neoplasm of the epidermis or hair follicles, most commonly arising in sun-damaged skin of the elderly and fair-skinned. SYN basal cell epithelioma.

basosquamous c., basisquamous c., a c. of the skin which in structure and behavior is considered transitional between basal cell and squamous cell c.

bronchiolar c., a c., thought to be derived from epithelium of terminal bronchioles, in which the neoplastic tissue extends along the alveolar walls and grows in small masses within the alveoli; may be diffuse, nodular, or lobular; the neoplastic cells are cuboidal or columnar and form papillary structures; metastases are infrequent. SYN alveolar cell c., bronchiolo-alveolar c.

bronchiolo-alveolar c., SYN bronchiolar c.

bronchogenic c., squamous cell or oat cell c. that arises in the mucosa of the large bronchi; local growth causes bronchial obstruction and is observed radiologically as an enlarging lung mass; malignant tumor cells can be detected in the sputum, and they metastasize early to the thoracic lymph nodes and to the brain, adrenal glands, and other organs via the bloodstream.

colloid c., SYN mucinous c.

cylindromatous c., SYN adenoid cystic c.

embryonal c., a malignant neoplasm of the testis, composed of large anaplastic cells with indistinct cellular borders; embryonal carcinomas may be malignant teratomas without differentiated elements.

endometrioid c., adenocarcinoma of the ovary or prostate resembling endometrial adenocarcinoma, possibly arising from ovarian foci of endometriosis.

epidermoid c., squamous cell c. of the skin.

fibrolamellar liver cell c., primary hepatic c. in which malignant hepatocytes are intersected by fibrous lamellated bands. SYN oncocytic hepatocellular tumor.

giant cell c., a malignant epithelial neoplasm characterized by unusually large anaplastic cells.

hepatocellular c., SYN malignant *hepatoma.*

Hürthle cell c., SYN Hürthle cell *tumor.*

inflammatory c., c. of the breast presenting

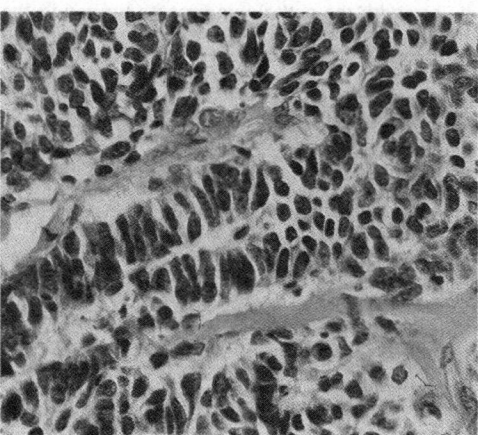

bronchogenic carcinoma: small cell

with edema, hyperemia, tenderness, and rapid enlargment of the breast; microscopically, there is extensive invasion of dermal lymphatics by the c.

large cell c., an anaplastic c., particularly bronchogenic, composed of cells which are much larger than those in oat cell c. of the lung.

medullary c., a malignant neoplasm, comparatively soft and brainlike in consistency, that consists chiefly of neoplastic epithelial cells, with only a scant amount of fibrous stroma.

melanotic c., obsolete term for melanoma.

mesometanephric c., SYN mesonephroma.

metaplastic c., a c. in which some of the tumor cells are spindle shaped, suggesting a sarcoma, or in which the stroma shows foci of bone or cartilage.

mucinous c., a variety of adenocarcinoma in which the neoplastic cells secrete conspicuous quantities of mucin; the neoplasms are glistening, sticky, and gelatinoid in consistency. SYN colloid c.

oat cell c., an anaplastic, highly malignant, and usually bronchogenic c. composed of small ovoid cells with very scanty cytoplasm; this c. and small round cell carcinomas comprise over one-third of carcinomas of the lung. SYN small cell c. (2).

papillary c., a malignant neoplasm characterized by the formation of numerous irregular finger-like projections of fibrous stroma covered with a layer of neoplastic epithelial cells.

scar c., c. of the lung, usually adenocarcinoma, arising from a peripheral lung scar or associated with interstitial fibrosis in a honeycomb lung.

scirrhous c., a hard c., fibrous in nature, resulting from a desmoplastic reaction by the stromal tissue. SYN fibrocarcinoma.

secretory c., c. of the breast with pale-staining cells showing prominent secretory activity, as seen in pregnancy and lactation, but found mostly in children.

c. in si′tu (CIS), a lesion characterized by cytologic changes of the type associated with invasive c., but with the pathologic process limited to the lining epithelium and without histologic evidence of extension to adjacent structures. The lesion is presumed to be the precursor of invasive c., *i.e.*, a localized and curable phase of c.

small cell c., (1) an anaplastic c. composed of small cells; (2) SYN oat cell c.

spindle cell c., a c. composed of elongated cells, frequently a poorly differentiated squamous cell c. which may be difficult to distinguish from a sarcoma.

◼**squamous cell c.,** a malignant neoplasm derived from stratified squamous epithelium, which may also occur in sites where only glandular or columnar epithelium is normally present.

sweat gland c., usually a solitary tumor, nodular and fixed to the skin and underlying structures, having slow growth for long periods followed by rapid growth and dissemination.

transitional cell c., a malignant neoplasm derived from transitional epithelium, occurring chiefly in the urinary bladder, ureters, or renal pelves.

tubular c., a well-differentiated form of ductal breast c. with invasion of the stroma by small epithelial tubules.

villous c., a form of c. in which there are numerous closely packed papillary projections of neoplastic epithelial tissue.

car·ci·no·ma·ta (kar-si-nō′mă-tă). Alternative plural of carcinoma.

car·ci·no·ma·to·sis (kar′si-nō-mă-tō′sis). Widespread dissemination of carcinoma in various organs or tissues of the body. SYN carcinosis.

car·ci·nom·a·tous (kar-si-nom′ă-tŭs). Pertaining to or manifesting the properties of carcinoma.

car·ci·no·pho·bia (kar′sin-ō-fō′bē-ă). SYN cancerophobia.

car·ci·no·sar·co·ma (kar′si-nō-sar-kō′mă). A malignant neoplasm that contains elements of carcinoma and sarcoma so extensively intermixed as to indicate neoplasia of epithelial and mesenchymal tissue.

car·ci·no·sis (kar-si-nō′sis). SYN carcinomatosis.

△**cardi-.** SEE cardio-.

car·di·ec·ta·sia (kar′dē-ek-tā′zē-ă). Dilation of the heart. [cardi- + G. *ektasis*, a stretching]

△**cardio-, cardi-.** The heart. [G. *kardia*, heart]

car·di·o·ac·cel·er·a·tor (kar′dē-ō-ak-sel′er-ā-ter). Accelerator of the heart beat.

car·di·o·ac·tive (kar′dē-ō-ak′tiv). Influencing the heart.

car·di·o·a·or·tic (kar′dē-ō-ā-ōr′tik). Relating to the heart and the aorta.

car·di·o·ar·te·ri·al (kar′dē-ō-ar-tēr′ē-ăl). Relating to the heart and the arteries.

Car·di·o·bac·te·ri·um (kar′d-ō-bak-tē′rē-um). A genus of nonmotile, pleomorphic, Gram-negative, facultatively anaerobic, rod-shaped bacteria found in the nasal flora and associated with endocarditis in humans.

***C. hom′inis*,** a species that causes endocarditis in humans. The type species of *Cardiobacterium*. SEE HACEK *group*.

car·di·o·cele (kar′dē-ō-sēl). A herniation or protrusion of the heart through an opening in the diaphragm, or through a wound. [cardio- + G. *kēlē*, hernia]

car·di·o·cha·la·sia (kar′dē-ō-kă-lā′zē-ă). Achalasia of the cardia.

car·di·o·dy·nam·ics (kar′dē-ō-dī-nam′iks). The mechanics of the heart's action, including its movement and the forces generated thereby.

car·di·o·dyn·ia (kar′dē-ō-din′ē-ă). Pain in the heart. [cardio- + G. *odynē*, pain]

car·di·o·e·soph·a·ge·al (kar′dē-ō-ē-sof-ă-jē′ăl). Denoting the junction of the esophagus and cardiac part of the stomach.

car·di·o·gen·ic (kar′dē-ō-jen′ik). Of cardiac origin.

car·di·o·gram (kar′dē-ō-gram). 1. The graphic tracing made by the stylet of a cardiograph. 2. Any recording derived from the heart, with such prefixes as apex-, echo-, electro-, phono-, or vector- being understood. [cardio- + G. *gramma*, a diagram]

car·di·o·graph (kar′dē-ō-graf). An instrument for recording graphically the movements of the heart, constructed on the principle of the sphygmograph. [cardio- + G. *graphō*, to write]

car·di·og·ra·phy (kar-dē-og′ră-fē). The use of the cardiograph.

ultrasound c., SYN echocardiography.

vector c., the integration of scalar electrocardiographic recordings on two or three planes to produce a vector cardiogram consisting of loops for all the waves of the electrocardiogram.

car·di·o·he·pat·ic (kar′dē-ō-hĕ-pat′ik). Relating to the heart and the liver.

car·di·o·ky·mo·gram (kar′dē-ō-kī′mō-gram). Record made by a cardiokymograph.

car·di·o·ky·mo·graph (kar′dē-ō-kī′mō-graf). Device placed on the chest to record anterior left ventricle segmental wall motion; consists of a plate transducer with recording probe; changes in wall motion affect the magnetic field and thus the oscillatory frequency, which is recorded on a waveform polygraph.

car·di·o·ky·mog·ra·phy (kar′dē-ō-kī-mog′ră-fē). Use of a cardiokymograph.

car·di·o·lip·in (kar′dē-ō-lip′in). A 1,3-bis-(phosphatidyl)glycerol found in many biomembranes with immunological properties; used in serological diagnosis of syphilis.

car·di·ol·o·gist (kar-dē-ol′ō-jist). Physician specializing in cardiology.

car·di·ol·o·gy (kar-dē-ol′ō-jē). The medical specialty concerned with the diagnosis and treatment of heart disease. [cardio- + G. *logos*, study]

car·di·o·ma·la·cia (kar′dē-ō-mă-lā′shē-ă). Softening of the walls of the heart. [cardio- + G. *malakia*, softness]

car·di·o·meg·a·ly (kar-dē-ō-meg′ă-lē). Enlargement of the heart. SYN macrocardia, megalocardia. [cardio- + G. *megas*, large]

car·di·o·mo·til·i·ty (kar′dē-ō-mō-til′ĭ-tē). Movements of the heart.

car·di·o·mus·cu·lar (kar′dē-ō-mŭs′kyū-lăr). Pertaining to the cardiac musculature.

car·di·o·my·o·li·po·sis (kar′dē-ō-mī′ō-li-pō′sis). Fatty degeneration of the myocardium. [cardio- + G. *mys*, muscle, + *lipos*, fat, + -*osis*, condition]

car·di·o·my·op·a·thy (kar′dē-ō-mī-op′ă-thē).

Disease of the myocardium; a primary disease of heart muscle in the absence of a known underlying etiology. SYN myocardiopathy. [cardio- + G. *mys,* muscle, + *pathos,* disease]

   familial hypertrophic c., familial form of hypertrophic c.

   hypertrophic c., cardiac hypertrophy of unknown cause, possibly genetic, with impairment of left ventricular filling, emptying, or both. SEE ALSO sudden *death.*

car·di·o·my·o·plas·ty (kar′dē-ō-mī′ō-plas-tē). An operation that uses latissimus dorsi muscle to assist cardiac function. The muscle is moved into the thorax through the bed of the resected second or third rib, wrapped around the left and right ventricles, and stimulated to contract during cardiac systole by means of an implanted burst-stimulator.

car·di·o·neph·ric (kar′dē-ō-nef′rik). SYN cardiorenal.

car·di·o·neu·ral (kar′dē-ō-nūr′ăl). Relating to the nervous control of the heart. [cardio- + G. *neuron,* nerve]

car·di·o·neu·ro·sis (kar′dē-ō-nū-rō′sis). SYN cardiac *neurosis.*

car·di·o·o·men·to·pexy (kar′dē-ō-ō-men′tō-pek-sē). Operation for the attachment of omentum to the heart with the object of improving its blood supply. [cardio- + omentum, + G. *pēxis,* fixation]

car·di·op·a·thy (kar-dē-op′ă-thē). Any disease of the heart. [cardio- + G. *pathos,* disease]

car·di·o·per·i·car·di·o·pexy (kar′dē-ō-pār-i-kar′ dē-ō-pek-sē). An operation to increase the blood supply to the myocardium; magnesium silicate is spread within the pericardial sac, or the sac is mechanically abraded, to cause an adhesive pericarditis and an increase in blood supply to develop. [cardio- + pericardium, + G. *pēxis,* fixation]

car·di·o·pho·bia (kar′dē-ō-fō′bē-ă). Morbid fear of heart disease.

car·di·o·plas·ty (kar′dē-ō-plas-tē). An operation on the cardia of the stomach. SYN esophagogastroplasty. [cardio- (2) + G. *plastos,* formed]

car·di·o·ple·gia (kar′dē-ō-plē′jē-ă). **1.** Paralysis of the heart. **2.** An elective stopping of cardiac activity temporarily by injection of chemicals, selective hypothermia, or electrical stimuli. [cardio- + G. *plēgē,* stroke]

car·di·o·ple·gic (kar-dē-ō-plē′jik). Relating to cardioplegia.

car·di·op·to·sia (kar′dē-op-tō′sē-ă). A condition in which the heart is unduly movable and displaced downward, as distinguished from bathycardia. [cardio- + G. *ptōsis,* a falling]

car·di·o·pul·mo·nary (kar′dē-ō-pŭl′mo-nār-ē). Relating to the heart and lungs. SYN pneumocardial.

car·di·o·py·lo·ric (kar′dē-ō-pī-lōr′ik, -pi-lōr′ik). Relating to the cardiac and pyloric extremities of the stomach.

car·di·o·re·nal (kar′dē-ō-rē′năl). Relating to the heart and the kidney. SYN cardionephric, nephrocardiac.

car·di·or·rha·phy (kar-dē-ōr′ă-fē). Suture of the heart wall. [cardio- + G. *rhaphē,* suture]

car·di·or·rhex·is (kar-dē-ō-rek′sis). Rupture of the heart wall. [cardio- + G. *rhēxis,* rupture]

car·di·o·se·lec·tive (kar′dē-ō-sĕ-lek′tiv). Denoting or having the properties of cardioselectivity.

car·di·o·se·lec·tiv·i·ty (kar′dē-ō-sĕ-lek-tiv′i-tē). The relatively predominant cardiovascular pharmacologic effect of a drug with multipharmacologic effects; used especially when describing beta-blocking agents.

car·di·o·spasm (kar′dē-ō-spazm). SYN esophageal *achalasia.*

car·di·o·sphyg·mo·graph (kar′dē-ō-sfig′mō-graf). An instrument for recording graphically the movements of the heart and the radial pulse. [cardio- + G. *sphygmos,* pulse, + *graphō,* to write]

car·di·o·ta·chom·e·ter (kar′dē-ō-tă-kom′ĕ-ter). An instrument for measuring heart rate. [cardio- + G. *tachos,* rapidity, + *metron,* measure]

car·di·ot·o·my (kar′dē-ot′ō-mē). **1.** Incision of a heart wall. **2.** Incision of the cardiac part of the stomach. [cardio- + G. *tomē,* incision]

car·di·o·ton·ic (kar′dē-ō-ton′ik). Exerting a favorable, so-called tonic effect upon the action of the heart; usually intended to indicate increased force of contraction. [cardio- + G. *tonos,* tension]

car·di·o·tox·ic (kar′dē-ō-tok′sik). Having a deleterious effect upon the action of the heart, due to poisoning of the cardiac muscle or of its conducting system. [cardio- + G. *toxikon,* poison]

car·di·o·val·vu·li·tis (kar′dē-ō-val-vyū-lī′tis). Inflammation of the heart valves.

car·di·o·vas·cu·lar (kar′dē-ō-vas′kyū-lăr). Relating to the heart and the blood vessels or the circulation. [cardio- + L. *vasculum,* vessel]

car·di·o·ver·sion (kar′dē-ō-ver′zhŭn). Restoration of the heart's rhythm to normal by electrical countershock. [cardio- + con*version*]

car·di·o·ver·ter (kar′dē-ō-ver′ter). A machine used to perform cardioversion.

car·di·tis (kar-dī′tis). Inflammation of the heart.

care (kār). In medicine and public health, a general term for the application of knowledge to the benefit of a community or individual.

   ambulatory c., medical or surgical health c. provided during an episode of c. that lasts less than 24 hours and from which the patient goes home; outpatient rather than inpatient c.

   managed c., an arrangement whereby a third-party payer (*e.g.,* insurance company, federal government, or corporation) mediates between physicians and patients, negotiating fees for service and overseeing the types of treatment given. The third-party payer requires second opinions and precertification review for patients requiring hospital admission, negotiates wholesale prices with physicians, and carries out cost-containment measures, including auditing hospitals and reviewing claims. SEE health maintenance organization. SEE ALSO capitation.

   pharmaceutical c., the responsible provision of drug therapy for the purpose of achieving definite outcomes that improve a patient's quality of life.

   primary c., health care services such as family practice, internal medicine, obstetrics/gynecology, or pediatrics that are the first point of health care for a patient in an ambulatory setting.

respiratory c., a life-supporting, life-enhancing health c. profession which includes cardiopulmonary diagnostic testing, therapeutics, monitoring, emergency procedures, patient transport, and rehabilitation practiced under qualified medical direction provided in all health care settings and the home.

Carey Coombs mur•mur. See under murmur.

car•ies (kăr′ēz). Microbial destruction or necrosis of teeth. [L. dry rot]

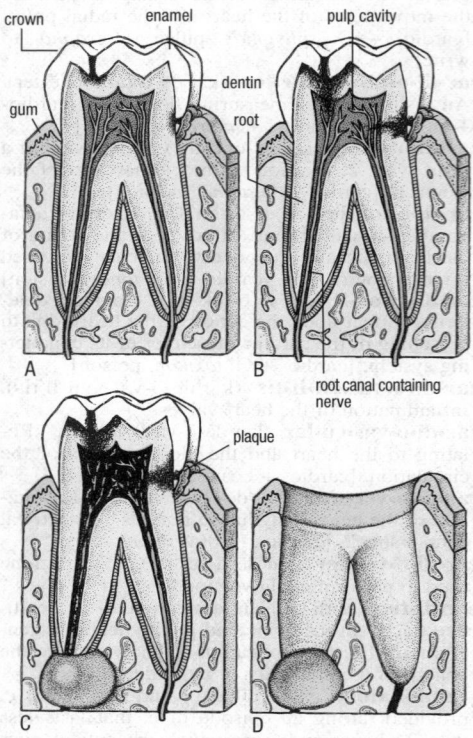

caries: (A) acid, enzymes, or both produced by oral bacteria break down enamel to form cavities; (B) bacteria penetrate dentin to invade pulp cavity; (C) infection destroys pulp and extends through left root canal to cause periapical disease; (D) tooth has been lost, leaving periapical cyst on the left

ca•ri•na, pl. **ca•ri•nae** (kă-rī′nă, -rī′nē). A term applied to anatomical structures forming a projecting central ridge. [L. the keel of a boat]

car•i•nate (kar′i-nāt). Shaped like a keel; relating to or resembling a carina.

cario-. Caries. [L. *caries*]

car•i•o•gen•e•sis (ka′rē-ō-jen′ĕ-sis). The process of producing caries; the mechanism of caries production.

car•i•o•gen•ic (ka′rē-ō-jen′ik). Producing caries; usually said of diets.

car•i•o•ge•nic•i•ty (ka′rē-ō-jĕ-nis′i-tē). Potential for caries production.

car•i•ol•o•gy (ka-rē-ol′ō-jē). The study of dental caries and cariogenesis.

car•i•ous (kār′ē-ŭs). Relating to or affected with caries.

Carlen's tube. See under tube.

car•min•a•tive (kar-min′ă-tiv). **1.** Preventing the formation or causing the expulsion of flatus. **2.** An agent that relieves flatulence. [L. *carmino,* pp. *-atus,* to card wool; special Mod. L. usage, to expel wind]

car•mine (kar′min, kar′mēn) [C.I. 75470]. Red coloring matter derived from cochineal. [Mediev. L. *carminus,* contr. fr. *carmisinus,* fr. Ar. *qirmizē,* the cochineal insect]

car•min•o•phil, car•min•o•phile, car•mi•noph•i•lous (kar-min′ō-fil, -fīl, kar-mi-nof′i-lŭs). Staining readily with carmine dyes. [G. *phileō,* to love]

car•ni•tine (kar′ni-tēn). The L-isomer is a thyroid inhibitor found in muscle, liver, and meat extracts; L-c. is an acyl carrier with respect to the mitochondrial membrane; it thus stimulates fatty acid oxidation. [L. *caro, carn-,* flesh, + ine]

car•o•tene (kar′ō-tēn). Yellow-red pigments (lipochromes) widely distributed in plants and animals, notably in carrots, and closely related in structure to the xanthophylls and lycopenes and to the open-chain squalene; they include precursors of the vitamins A (provitamin A carotenoids).

β-car•o•tene 15,15′-di•ox•y•gen•ase (bā′ta-kar′ō-tēn dī-oks′ē-jen-āz). An enzyme catalyzing the reaction of β-carotene plus O_2 producing two retinals.

car•o•ten•e•mia (kar′ō-te-nē′mē-ă). Carotene in the blood, especially pertaining to increased quantities, which sometimes cause a pale yellow-red pigmentation of the skin that may resemble icterus. SYN xanthemia.

car•o•ten•o•der•ma (ka-rot′en-ō-der-mă). SYN carotenosis cutis. [carotene + G. *derma,* skin]

ca•rot•e•noid (ka-rot′e-noyd). **1.** Resembling carotene; having a yellow color. **2.** One of the carotenoids.

ca•rot•e•noids (ka-rot′e-noydz). Generic term for a class of carotenes and their oxygenated derivatives (xanthophylls). Many c.'s have anticancer activities.

car•o•te•no•sis cu•tis (kar-ō-te-nō′sis kyū′tis). A harmless reversible yellow coloration of the skin caused by an increase in carotene content. SYN carotenoderma.

ca•rot•i•co•tym•pan•ic (ka-rot′i-kō-tim-pan′ik). Relating to the carotid canal and the tympanum.

ca•rot•id (ka-rot′id). Pertaining to any c. structure. [G. *karōtides,* the carotid arteries, fr. *karoō,* to put to sleep (because compression of the c. artery results in unconsciousness)]

ca•rot•o•dyn•ia (kă-rot′ō-din′ē-ă). Pain caused by pressure on the carotid artery. [G. *odynē,* pain]

car•pal (kar′păl). Relating to the carpus.

car•pec•to•my (kar-pek′tō-mē). Excision of a portion or all of the carpus. [G. *karpos,* wrist, + *ektomē,* excision]

car•po•met•a•car•pal (kar′pō-met-ă-kar′păl). Relating to both carpus and metacarpus.

car•po•ped•al (kar′pō-ped′ăl). Relating to the

wrist and the foot, or the hands and feet; denoting especially c. spasm. [G. *karpos,* wrist, + L. *pes* (*ped-*), foot]

car·pus, gen. and pl. **car·pi** (kar'pŭs, kar'pī) [NA]. **1.** SYN wrist. **2.** SYN carpal *bones,* under *bone.* [Mod. L. fr. Gr. *karpos*]

car·ri·er (ka'rē-er). **1.** A person or animal that harbors a specific infectious agent in the absence of discernible clinical disease and serves as a potential source of infection. **2.** Any chemical capable of accepting an atom, radical, or subatomic particle from one compound, then passing it to another. **3.** A substance which, by having chemical properties closely related to or indistinguishable from those of a radioactive tracer, is able to carry the tracer through a precipitation or similar chemical procedure. SEE ALSO label, tracer. **4.** A large immunogen which when coupled to a hapten will facilitate an immune response to the hapten.

latent c., a person, typically a prospective parent, bearing the appropriate genotype of a trait (homozygous for recessive, homozygous or heterozygous for dominant, hemizygous or homozygous for X-linked) that manifests the trait only under certain conditions, *e.g.,* age, an environmental insult, etc.

car·ti·lage (kar'ti-lij). A connective tissue characterized by its nonvascularity and firm consistency; consists of cells (chondrocytes), an interstitial matrix of fibers (collagen), and a ground substance (proteoglycans). There are three kinds of c.: hyaline c., elastic c., and fibrocartilage. Nonvascular, resilient, flexible connective tissue found primarily in joints, the walls of the thorax, and tubular structures such as the larynx, air passages, and ears; comprises most of the skeleton in early fetal life, but is slowly replaced by bone. For gross anatomical description, see cartilago and its subentries. SYN cartilago [NA], gristle. [L. *cartilago (cartilagin-),* gristle]

articular c., the cartilage covering the articular surfaces of the bones participating in a synovial joint.

arytenoid c., one of a pair of small triangular pyramidal laryngeal cartilages that articulate with the lamina of the cricoid cartilage. It gives attachment at its anteriorly directed vocal process to the posterior part of the corresponding vocal ligament and to several muscles at its laterally-directed muscular process. SYN cartilago arytenoidea [NA].

auricular c., the cartilage of the auricle. SYN cartilago auriculae [NA].

connecting c., the c. in a cartilaginous joint such as the symphysis pubis. SYN interosseous c.

corniculate c., a conical nodule of elastic cartilage surmounting the apex of each arytenoid cartilage. SYN cartilago corniculata [NA].

costal c., the cartilage forming the anterior continuation of a rib, providing the means by which it reaches and articulates with the sternum. SYN cartilago costalis [NA].

cricoid c., the lowermost of the laryngeal cartilages; it is shaped like a signet ring, being expanded into a nearly quadrilateral plate (lamina)

posteriorly; the anterior portion is called the arch (arcus). SYN cartilago cricoidea [NA].

cuneiform c., a small nonarticulating rod of elastic cartilage in the aryepiglottic fold anterolateral and somewhat superior to the corniculate cartilage. SYN cartilago cuneiformis [NA].

elastic c., a c. in which the cells are surrounded by a territorial capsular matrix outside of which is an interterritorial matrix containing elastic fiber networks in addition to the collagen fibers and ground substance. SYN yellow c.

epiglottic c., a thin lamina of elastic cartilage forming the central portion of the epiglottis. SYN cartilago epiglottica [NA].

epiphysial c., SYN epiphysial *plate.*

floating c., a loose piece of c. within a joint cavity, detached from the articular c. or from a meniscus.

greater alar c., one of a pair of cartilages that form the tip of the nose. It consists of a medial crus that extends into the nasal septum with its fellow of the opposite side, and a lateral crus that forms the anterior part of the wing of the nose.

hyaline c., c. having a frosted-glass appearance, with interstitial substance containing fine collagen fibers.

interosseous c., SYN connecting c.

lateral c. of nose, the cartilage located in the lateral wall of the nose above the alar cartilage. SYN cartilago nasi lateralis [NA].

lesser alar c.'s, the two to four cartilaginous plates of the wing of the nose posterior to the greater alar cartilage.

mandibular c., a c. bar in the mandibular arch that forms a temporary supporting structure in the embryonic mandible; the cartilaginous primordia of the malleus and incus develop from its proximal end, and it also gives rise to the sphenomandibular and anterior malleolar ligaments.

nasal septal c., a thin cartilaginous plate located between vomer, perpendicular plate of the ethmoid, and nasal bones, and completing the nasal septum anteriorly.

permanent c., c. that is not replaced by bone.

precursory c., SYN temporary c.

semilunar c., one of the articular menisci of the knee joint.

slipping rib c., subluxation of rib c. at the costo-chondral junction, causing pain and audible click.

temporary c., a c. that is normally replaced by bone, to form a part of the skeleton. SYN precursory c.

thyroid c., the largest of the cartilages of the larynx; it is formed of two approximately quadrilateral plates joined anteriorly at an angle of from 90° to 120°, the prominence so formed constituting the laryngeal prominence (Adam's apple). SYN cartilago thyroidea [NA].

tracheal c.'s, the 16 to 20 incomplete rings of hyaline cartilage forming the skeleton of the trachea; the rings are deficient posteriorly for from one-fifth to one-third of their circumference. SYN cartilagines tracheales [NA].

vomerine c., vomeronasal c., SYN *cartilago* vomeronasalis.

xiphoid c., SYN xiphoid *process.*

Y c., Y-shaped c., the connecting c. for the ilium, ischium, and pubis; it extends through the acetabulum.

yellow c., SYN elastic c.

car·ti·la·gi·nes (kar-ti-laj′i-nĕz). Plural of cartilago.

car·ti·lag·i·noid (kar-ti-laj′i-noyd).   SYN chondroid (1).

car·ti·lag·i·nous (kar-ti-laj′i-nŭs). Relating to or consisting of cartilage. SYN chondral.

car·ti·la·go, pl. **car·ti·la·gi·nes** (kar-ti-lā′gō, -laj′i-nēs) [NA].   SYN cartilage. [L. gristle]

c. arytenoi′dea [NA], SYN arytenoid *cartilage*.

c. auric′ulae [NA], SYN auricular *cartilage*.

c. cornicula′ta [NA], SYN corniculate *cartilage*.

c. costa′lis [NA], SYN costal *cartilage*.

c. cricoi′dea [NA], SYN cricoid *cartilage*.

c. cuneifor′mis [NA], SYN cuneiform *cartilage*.

c. epiglot′tica [NA], SYN epiglottic *cartilage*.

c. epiphysia′lis [NA], SYN epiphysial *plate*.

c. na′si latera′lis [NA], SYN lateral *cartilage* of nose.

c. thyroid′ea [NA], SYN thyroid *cartilage*.

cartila′gines trachea′les [NA], SYN tracheal *cartilages*, under *cartilage*.

c. vomeronasa′lis [NA], a narrow strip of cartilage located between the lower edge of the cartilage of the nasal septum and the vomer. SYN vomerine cartilage, vomeronasal cartilage.

ca·run·cle (kar′ŭng-kl). SYN caruncula.

lacrimal c., a small reddish body at the medial angle of the eye, containing modified sebaceous and sweat glands.

urethral c., a small, fleshy, sometimes painful protrusion of the mucous membrane at the meatus of the female urethra.

ca·run·cu·la, pl. **ca·run·cu·lae** (kă-rŭng′kyū-lă, -lē).   [NA] A small, fleshy protuberance. SYN caruncle. [L. a small fleshy mass, fr. *caro,* flesh]

△**caryo-.**   Nucleus. SEE karyo-. [G. *karyon,* nut, kernel]

cas·cade (kas-kād′).   **1.** A series of sequential interactions, as of a physiological process, which once initiated continues to the final one; each interaction is activated by the preceding one, sometimes with cumulative effect. **2.** To spill over, especially rapidly. [Fr., fr. It. *cascare,* to fall]

case (kās).   **1.** An instance of disease with its attendant circumstances. Cf. patient. **2.** A box or container. [L. *casus,* an occurrence]

index c., SYN proband.

c. mix, the relative numbers of various types of patients being treated as categorized by DRG, severity of illness, and other indicators; used as a tool for managing and planning health care services.

ca·se·a·tion (kā-sē-ā′shŭn).   A form of coagulation necrosis in which the necrotic tissue resembles cheese and contains a mixture of protein and fat that is absorbed very slowly; occurs particularly in tuberculosis. SEE ALSO caseous *necrosis.* [L. *caseus,* cheese]

ca·sein (cā′sē-in, kā′sēn).   The principal protein of cow's milk and the chief constituent of cheese.

ca·se·ous (kā′sē-ŭs).   Pertaining to or manifesting the features of tissue affected by caseation.

cassette (ka-set′).   Lightproof carrying case for radiographic film and intensifying screens. SEE ALSO screen, film.

cast (kast).   **1.** An object formed by the solidification of a liquid poured into a mold. **2.** Rigid encasement of a part, as with plaster or a plastic, for purposes of immobilization. **3.** An elongated or cylindrical mold formed in a tubular structure (*e.g.,* renal tubule, bronchiole) that may be observed in histologic sections or in material such as urine or sputum; results from inspissation of fluid material secreted or excreted in the tubular structures. **4.** Restraint of a large animal, usually a horse, with ropes and harnesses in a recumbent position. **5.** In dentistry, a positive reproduction of the form of the tissues of the upper or lower jaw, which is made by the solidification of plaster, metal, etc., poured into an impression, and over which denture bases or other dental restorations may be fabricated. [M.E. *kasten,* fr. O.Norse *kasta*]

false c., an elongated, ribbon-like mucous thread with poorly defined edges and pointed or split ends, often confused with a true urinary c. SYN pseudocast.

cast brace (kast brās).   A specially designed plaster or plastic cast incorporating hinges and other brace components; used in the treatment of fractures to promote early activity and early joint motion.

cas·trate (kas′trāt).   To remove the testicles or the ovaries. [L. *castro,* pp. *-atus,* to deprive of generative power (male or female)]

cas·tra·tion (kas-trā′shŭn).   **1.** Removal of the testicles or ovaries. **2.** SEE castration *complex.* [see castrate]

CAT Abbreviation for computerized axial *tomography; chloramphenicol* acetyl transferase.

△**cata-.**   Down; opposite of ana-. SEE ALSO kata-. Cf. de-. [G. *kata,* down]

cat·a·bi·ot·ic (kat′ă-bī-ot′ik).   Used up in the carrying on of the vital processes other than growth, or in the performance of function, referring to the energy derived from food. [cata- + G. *biōtikos,* relating to life]

cat·a·bol·ic (kat-ă-bol′ik).   Relating to or promoting catabolism.

ca·tab·o·lism (kă-tab′ō-lizm).   **1.** The breaking down in the body of complex chemical compounds into simpler ones, often accompanied by the liberation of energy. **2.** The sum of all degradative processes. Cf. anabolism, metabolism. [G. *katabolē,* a casting down]

ca·tab·o·lite (kă-tab′ō-līt).   Any product of catabolism.

cat·a·chron·o·bi·ol·o·gy (kat′ă-kron′ō-bī-ol′ō-jē).   The study of the deleterious effects of time on a living system. [cata- + G. *chronos,* time, + biology]

cat·a·crot·ic (kat-ă-krot′ik).   Denoting a pulse tracing in which the downstroke is interrupted by one or more upward waves.

ca·tac·ro·tism (kă-tak′rō-tizm).   A condition of the pulse in which there are one or more secondary expansions of the artery following the main beat, producing secondary upward waves on the downstroke of the pulse tracing. [cata- + G. *krotos,* beat]

cat•a•di•crot•ic (kat′ă-dī-krot′ik). Denoting a pulse tracing in which there are two minor elevations interrupting the downstroke.

cat•a•di•cro•tism (kat-ă-dī′krō-tizm). A condition of the pulse marked by two minor expansions of the artery following the main beat, producing two secondary upward waves on the downstroke of the pulse tracing. [cata + G. *di-,* two, + *krotos,* beat]

cat•a•gen (kat′ă-jen). A regressing phase of the hair growth cycle during which cell proliferation ceases, the hair follicle shortens, and an anchored club hair is produced.

cat•a•gen•e•sis (kat-ă-jen′ĕ-sis). SYN involution. [cata- + G. *genesis,* origin]

cat•a•lase (kat′ă-lās). A hemoprotein catalyzing the decomposition of hydrogen peroxide to water and oxygen ($2H_2O_2 \rightarrow O_2 + 2H_2O$).

cat•a•lep•sy (kat′ă-lep-sē). A morbid condition characterized by waxy rigidity of the limbs, lack of response to stimuli, mutism and inactivity; occurs with some psychoses, especially catatonic schizophrenia. [G. *katalēpsis,* a seizing, catalepsy, fr. *kata,* down, + *lēpsis,* a seizure]

cat•a•lep•tic (kat-ă-lep′tik). Relating to, or suffering from, catalepsy.

cat•a•lep•toid (kat-ă-lep′toyd). Simulating or resembling catalepsy.

ca•tal•y•sis (kă-tal′i-sis). The effect that a catalyst exerts upon a chemical reaction. [G. *katalysis,* dissolution]

cat•a•lyst (kat′ă-list). A substance that accelerates a chemical reaction but is not consumed or changed permanently thereby.

cat•a•lyt•ic (kat-ă-lit′ik). Relating to or effecting catalysis.

cat•a•lyze (kat′ă-līz). To act as a catalyst.

cat•am•ne•sis (kat-am-nē′sis). The medical history of a patient after an illness; the follow-up history. [cata- + G *mnēmē,* memory]

cat•am•nes•tic (kat-am-nes′tik). Related to catamnesis.

cat•a•pha•sia (kat-ă-fā′zē-ă). SYN verbigeration. [cata- + G. *phasis,* a saying]

ca•taph•o•ra (kă-taf′ō-ră). Semicoma or somnolence interrupted by intervals of partial consciousness. [G. a falling down]

cat•a•pla•sia, cat•a•pla•sis (kat-ă-plā′sē-ă, -plā′sis). A degenerative change in cells or tissues that is the reverse of constructive or developmental change; a return to an earlier or embryonic stage. SYN retrogression. [cata- + G. *plasis,* a molding]

cat•a•plec•tic (kat-ă-plek′tik). **1.** Developing suddenly. **2.** Pertaining to cataplexy.

cat•a•plexy (kat′ă-plek-sē). A transient attack of extreme generalized muscular weakness, often precipitated by an emotional state such as laughing, surprise, fear, or anger. [cata- + G. *plēxis,* a blow, stroke]

cat•a•ract (kat′ă-rakt). Loss of transparency of the lens of the eye, or of its capsule. [L. *cataracta,* fr. G. *katarrhaktēs,* a downrushing, a waterfall, fr. *kata- rrhēgnymi,* to break down, rush down]

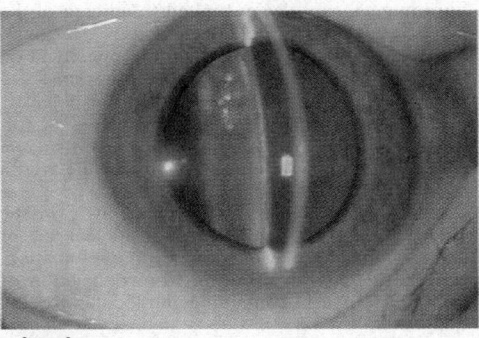
cataract

annular c., congenital c. in which a central white membrane replaces the nucleus.

atopic c., a c. associated with atopic dermatitis.

black c., a c. in which the lens is hardened and of a dark brown color.

blue c., coronary c. of bluish color.

capsular c., a c. in which the opacity affects the capsule only.

capsulolenticular c., a c. in which both the lens and its capsule are involved. SEE ALSO membranous c.

coronary c., peripheral cortical developmental c. occurring just after puberty; transmitted as a hereditary dominant characteristic.

cortical c., a c. in which the opacity affects the cortex of the lens.

cupuliform c., a common form of senile c. often confined to a region just within the posterior capsule.

embryopathic c., congenital c. as a result of intrauterine infection, *e.g.,* rubella.

fibroid c., fibrinous c., a sclerotic hardening of the capsule of the lens, following exudative iridocyclitis.

galactose c., a neonatal c. associated with intralenticular accumulation of galactose alcohol. SEE galactosemia.

glaucomatous c., a nuclear opacity usually seen in absolute glaucoma.

gray c., a c. of gray color, usually seen in senile, mature, or cortical c.

hypermature c., a c. in which the lens cortex becomes liquid, with the nucleus gravitating within the capsule (Morgagni's c.).

immature c., a stage of partial lens opacification.

juvenile c., a soft c. occurring in a child or young adult.

lamellar c., a c. in which the opacity is limited to the cortex. SYN zonular c.

mature c., a c. in which both the nucleus and cortex are opaque.

membranous c., a secondary c. composed of the remains of the thickened capsule and degenerated lens fibers.

Morgagni's c., a hypermature c. in which the nucleus gravitates within the capsule.

nuclear c., a c. involving the nucleus.

polar c., a capsular c. limited to an area of the anterior or posterior pole of the lens.

progressive c., a c. in which the opacification process progresses to involve the entire lens.

pyramidal c., a cone-shaped, anterior polar c.

secondary c., (1) a c. that accompanies or follows some other eye disease such as uveitis; **(2)** a c. occurring in the retained lens or capsule after a c. extraction.

senile c., a c. occurring spontaneously in the elderly; mainly a cuneiform c., nuclear c., or posterior subcapsular c., alone or in combination.

siderotic c., a c. resulting from deposition of iron from an iron-containing intraocular foreign body.

subcapsular c., a c. in which the opacities are concentrated beneath the capsule.

vascular c., congenital c. in which the degenerated lens is replaced with mesodermal tissue.

zonular c., SYN lamellar c.

cat•a•rac•to•gen•ic (kat′ă-rak-tō-jen′ik). Cataract-producing.

cat•a•rac•tous (kat-ă-rak′tŭs). Relating to a cataract.

ca•tarrh (kă-tahr′). Inflammation of a mucous membrane with increased flow of mucus or exudate. [G. *katarrheō,* to flow down]

ca•tarrh•al (kă-tah′răl). Relating to or affected with catarrh.

cat•a•stal•sis (kat-ă-stal′sis). A contraction wave resembling ordinary peristalsis but not preceded by a zone of inhibition. [G. *kata-stellō,* to put in order, check]

cat•a•stal•tic (kat-ă-stal′tik). **1.** Inhibitory, restricting, or restraining. **2.** An inhibitory or checking agent, such as an astringent or antispasmodic. [cata- + G. *staltos,* contracted, fr. *stellō,* to contract]

cat•a•to•nia (kat-ă-tō′nē-ă). A syndrome of psychomotor disturbances characterized by periods of physical rigidity, negativism, or stupor; may occur in schizophrenia, mood disorders, or organic mental disorders. [G. *katatonos,* stretching down, depressed, fr. *kata,* down, + *tonos,* tone]

cat•a•ton•ic, cat•a•to•ni•ac (kat-ă-ton′ik, -tō′nē-ak). Relating to, or characterized by, catatonia.

cat•a•tri•crot•ic (kat′ă-trī-krot′ik). Denoting a pulse tracing with three minor elevations interrupting the downstroke.

cat•a•tri•cro•tism (kat-ă-trī′krō-tizm). A condition of the pulse marked by three minor expansions of the artery following the main beat, producing three secondary upward waves on the downstroke of the pulse tracing. [cata- + G. *tri-,* three, + *krotos,* beat]

cat•e•chol•a•mines (kat-ĕ-kol′ă-mēnz). Pyrocatechols with an alkylamine side chain; examples of biochemical interest are epinephrine, norepinephrine, and L-dopa. C.'s are major elements in responses to stress.

cat•en•ate (kat′e-nāt). To connect in a series of links like a chain. [L. *catenatus,* chained together, fr. *catena,* chain]

cat•gut (kat′gŭt). An absorbable surgical suture material made from the collagenous fibers of the submucosa of certain animals, usually sheep or cows. [probably from *kit,* a small violin, through confusion with *kit,* a small cat]

ca•thar•sis (kă-thar′sis). **1.** SYN purgation. **2.** The release or discharge of emotional tension or anxiety by psychoanalytically guided emotional reliving of past, especially repressed, events. [G. *katharsis,* purification, fr. *katharos,* pure]

ca•thar•tic (kă-thar′tik). **1.** Relating to catharsis. **2.** An agent having purgative action.

ca•thec•tic (kă-thek′tik). Pertaining to cathexis.

cath•e•ter (kath′ĕ-ter). **1.** A tubular instrument to allow passage of fluid from or into a body cavity. SEE ALSO line (4). **2.** Especially a c. designed to be passed through the urethra into the bladder to drain it of urine. [G. *kathetēr,* fr. *kathiēmi,* to send down]

angiography c., a thin-walled tube suitable for percutaneous puncture and injection of contrast media for radiography.

balloon-tip c., (1) a tube with a balloon at its tip that can be inflated or deflated without removal after installation; the balloon may be inflated to facilitate passage of the tube through a blood vessel (propelled by the bloodstream) or to occlude the vessel in which the tube alone would allow free flow; such c.'s are used to enter the pulmonary artery to facilitate hemodynamic measurements or to enter arteries and then remove them while inflated to withdraw clots (embolectomy catheter); SEE ALSO Swan-Ganz c. **(2)** SYN Fogarty c.

Bozeman-Fritsch c., a slightly curved double-channel uterine c. with several openings at the tip.

brush c., a ureteral c. with a finely bristled brush tip that is endoscopically passed into the ureter or renal pelvis and by gentle to-and-fro movement brushes cells from the surface of suspected tumors.

cardiac c., SYN intracardiac c.

central venous c., a c. passed through a peripheral or central vein, ending in the thoracic vena cava or right atrium, for measurement of venous pressure or for infusion of concentrated solutions; the peripheral end may connect to a subcutaneous chamber for percutaneous injections given over periods of months or may exit from the skin at a distance from the vein.

double-channel c., a c. with two lumens, allowing irrigation and aspiration. SYN two-way c.

female c., a short, nearly straight c. for passage into the female bladder.

Fogarty c., a c. with an inflatable balloon near its tip; used to remove arterial emboli and thrombi from major veins and to remove stones from the biliary ducts. SYN balloon-tip c. (2).

Foley c., a urethral c. with a retaining balloon.

Gouley's c., a solid curved steel instrument grooved on its inferior surface so that it can be passed over a guide through a urethral stricture.

indwelling c., a c. left in place in the bladder, usually a balloon c.

intracardiac c., a c. that can be passed into the heart through a vein or artery, to withdraw samples of blood, measure pressures within the heart's chambers or great vessels, and inject contrast media; used mainly in the diagnosis and

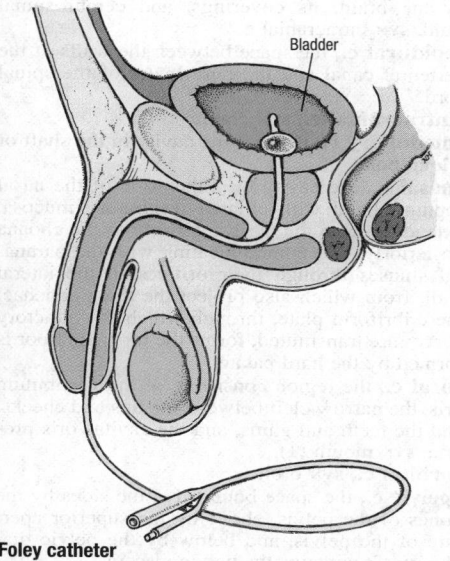

Bladder

Foley catheter

evaluation of congenital, rheumatic, and coronary artery lesions and to evaluate systolic and diastolic cardiac function. SYN cardiac c.

pacing c., a cardiac c. with one or more electrodes at its tip which can be used to artificially pace the heart.

pigtail c., an angiographic c. with a tightly curled end to reduce the impact of the injectant on the vessel wall.

self-retaining c., a c. so constructed that it remains in urethra and bladder until removed, *e.g.,* indwelling c.; Foley c.

suction c., a c. used to remove mucus and other secretions from the upper airway, trachea, and main bronchi.

Swan-Ganz c., a thin (5 Fr), flexible, flow-directed venous c. using a balloon to carry it through the heart to a pulmonary artery; when it is positioned in a small arterial branch, pulmonary wedge pressure is measured in front of the temporarily inflated and wedged balloon.

two-way c., SYN double-channel c.

vertebrated c., a c. made of several segments moving on each other like the links of a chain.

winged c., a soft rubber c. with little flaps at each side of the beak to retain it in the bladder.

cath•e•ter•i•za•tion (kath′ĕ-ter-ī-zā′shŭn). Passage of a catheter.

ca•thex•is (kă-thek′sis). A conscious or unconscious attachment of psychic energy to an idea, object, or person. [G. *kathexis,* a holding in, retention]

cath•o•dal (C) (kath′ō-dăl). Of, pertaining to, or emanating from a cathode.

cath•ode (C) (kath′ōd). 1. The negative pole of a galvanic battery or the electrode connected with it; the electrode to which positively charged ions (cations) migrate. Cf. anode. 2. negatively charged part of the x-ray tube head; it contains

the tungsten filament. SYN negative electrode. [G. *kathodos,* a way down, fr. *kata,* down, + *hodos,* a way]

cat•i•on (kat′ī-on). An ion carrying a charge of positive electricity, therefore going to the negatively charged cathode. [G. *katiōn,* going down]

cat•i•on ex•change. The process by which a cation in a liquid phase exchanges with another cation present as the counter-ion of a negatively charged solid polymer (cation exchanger). Cation exchange may be used chromatographically, to separate cations, and medicinally, to remove a cation. SEE ALSO *anion* exchange.

cau•da, pl. **cau•dae** (kaw′dă, kaw′dē) [NA]. SYN tail. [L. a tail]

   c. equi′na [NA], the bundle of spinal nerve roots arising from the lumbosacral enlargement and medullary cone and running through the lumbar cistern (subarachnoid space) within the vertebral canal below the first lumbar vertebra; it comprises the roots of all the spinal nerves below the first lumbar. [L. horse tail]

cau•dad (kaw′dad). 1. In a direction toward the tail. 2. Situated nearer the tail in relation to a specific reference point; opposite of craniad. SEE ALSO inferior.

cau•dal (kaw′dăl). Pertaining to the tail. [Mod. L. *caudalis*]

caul, cowl (kawl). 1. The amnion, either as a piece of membrane capping the baby's head at birth or the whole membrane when delivered unruptured with the baby. SYN galea (4), veil (2), velum (2). 2. SYN greater *omentum.* [Gaelic, *call,* a veil]

cau•mes•the•sia (kaw-mes-thē′zē-ă). Subjective heat sensation of uncomfortably high temperature; a type of thermal dysesthesia. [G. *kauma,* heat, + *aisthēsis,* sensation]

cau•sal•gia (kaw-zal′jē-ă). Persistent severe burning sensation, usually following partial injury of a peripheral nerve, accompanied by trophic changes (thinning of skin, loss of sweat glands and hair follicles). [G. *kausis,* burning, + *algos,* pain]

caus•tic (kaws′tik). 1. Exerting an effect resembling a burn. 2. An agent producing this effect. 3. Denoting a solution of a strong alkali; *e.g.,* caustic soda, NaOH. [G. *kaustikos,* fr. *kaiō,* to burn]

cau•ter•i•za•tion (kaw-ter-ī-zā′shŭn). The act of cauterizing. SEE ALSO cautery.

cau•ter•ize (kaw′ter-īz). To apply a cautery; to burn with a cautery.

cau•tery (kaw′ter-ē). 1. An agent or device used for scarring, burning, or cutting the skin or other tissues by means of heat, cold, electric current, or caustic chemicals. 2. Use of a cautery. [G. *kautēr-ion,* a branding iron]

   actual c., a c. acting directly through heat and not by chemical means.

   BICAP c., a form of bipolar electrocoagulation frequently used to arrest gastrointestinal bleeding.

   bipolar c., electrocautery by high frequency electrical current passed through tissue from an active to a passive electrode; used for hemostasis.

   monopolar c., electrocautery by high frequency electrical current passed from a single

ca

electrode, where the cauterization occurs, the patient's body serving as a ground.

ca·va (kā'vă). SEE inferior *vena* cava, superior *vena* cava.

ca·va·gram (kā'vă-gram). SYN cavogram.

ca·val (kā'văl). Relating to a vena cava.

cave (kāv). A hollow or enclosed space or cavity. SEE ALSO cavern, cavity.

　trigeminal c., the cleft in the meningeal layer of dura of the middle cranial fossa near the tip of the petrous part of the temporal bone; it encloses the roots of the trigeminal nerve and the trigeminal ganglion.

cav·e·o·la, pl. **cav·e·o·lae** (kav-ē-ō'lă, -lē). A small pocket, vesicle, cave, or recess communicating with the outside of a cell and extending inward, indenting the cytoplasm and the cell membrane. Caveolae are considered to be sites of uptake of materials into the cell, expulsion of materials from the cell, or addition or removal of cell (unit) membrane to or from the cell surface. [L.]

cav·ern (kav'ern). An anatomical cavity with many interconnecting chambers. SEE ALSO cave, cavity.

cav·er·nil·o·quy (kav-er-nil'ō-kwē). Low-pitched resonant pectoriloquy heard over a lung cavity. [L. *caverna,* cavern, + *loquor,* to talk]

cav·er·ni·tis (kav-er-nī'tis). Inflammation of the corpus cavernosum penis. SYN cavernositis.

cav·er·no·si·tis (kav'er-nō-sī'tis). SYN cavernitis.

cav·ern·ous (kav'er-nŭs). Relating to a cavern or a cavity; containing many cavities.

cav·i·tary (kav'i-tā-rē). Relating to a cavity or having a cavity or cavities.

cav·i·tas, pl. **cav·i·ta·tes** (kav'i-tas, -tā'tēs). SYN cavity. [Mod. L.]

cav·i·ta·tion (kav-i-tā'shŭn). **1.** Formation of a cavity, as in the lung in tuberculosis. **2.** The production of small vapor-containing bubbles or cavities in a liquid by ultrasound.

ca·vi·tis (kā-vī'tis). SYN celophlebitis.

cav·i·ty (kav'i-tē). **1.** A hollow space. A hollow, hole, or cavity. SEE ALSO cave, cavern. **2.** Lay term for the loss of tooth structure due to dental caries. SYN cavum [NA], cavitas. [L. *cavus,* hollow]

　abdominal c., the space bounded by the abdominal walls, the diaphragm, and the pelvis; it usually is arbitrarily separated from the pelvic cavity by a plane across the superior aperture of the pelvis; however, it may include the pelvis with the abdomen (see abdominopelvic c.); within the c. lie the greater part of the organs of digestion, the spleen, the kidneys, and the suprarenal glands. SYN enterocele (2).

　amniotic c., the fluid-filled c. inside the amnion which contains the developing embryo.

　axillary c., SYN axilla.

　body c., the collective visceral c. of the trunk (thoracic c. plus abdominopelvic c.), bounded by the superior thoracic aperture above, the pelvic floor below, and the body walls (parietes) in between. SYN celom (2), celoma.

　cleavage c., SYN blastocele.

　cotyloid c., SYN acetabulum.

　cranial c., the space within the skull occupied by the brain, its coverings, and cerebrospinal fluid. SYN intracranial c.

　epidural c., the space between the walls of the vertebral canal and the dura mater of the spinal cord.

　intracranial c., SYN cranial c.

　medullary c., the marrow cavity in the shaft of a long bone.

　nasal c., the cavity on either side of the nasal septum, lined with ciliated respiratory mucosa, extending from the naris anteriorly to the choana posteriorly, and communicating with the paranasal sinuses through their orifices in the lateral wall, from which also project the three conchae; the cribriform plate, through which the olfactory nerves are transmitted, forms the roof; the floor is formed by the hard palate.

　oral c., the region consisting of the vestibulum oris, the narrow cleft between the lips and cheeks, and the teeth and gums, and the cavitas oris propria. SYN mouth (1).

　orbital c., SYN orbit.

　pelvic c., the space bounded at the sides by the bones of the pelvis, above by the superior aperture of the pelvis, and below by the pelvic diaphragm; it contains the pelvic viscera.

　pericardial c., (1) the potential space between the parietal and the visceral layers of the serous pericardium; **(2)** in the embryo, that part of the primary celom containing the heart; originally it is in open communication with the pericardioperitoneal c.'s and indirectly, through them, with the peritoneal part of the celom.

　peritoneal c., the interior of the peritoneal sac, normally only a potential space between the parietal and visceral layers of the peritoneum.

　pleural c., the potential space between the parietal and visceral layers of the pleura. SYN pleural space.

　pulp c., the central hollow of a tooth consisting of the crown cavity and the root canal; it contains the fibrovascular dental pulp and is lined throughout by odontoblasts.

　segmentation c., SYN blastocele.

　thoracic c., the space within the thoracic walls, bounded below by the diaphragm and above by the neck.

　tympanic c., an air chamber in the temporal bone containing the ossicles; it is lined with mucous membrane and is continuous with the auditory tube anteriorly and the tympanic antrum and mastoid air cells posteriorly.

　uterine c., c. of uterus, the space within the uterus extending from the cervical canal to the openings of the uterine tubes.

ca·vo·gram (kā'vō-gram). An angiogram of a vena cava. SYN cavagram. [(vena) cava + G. *gramma,* a writing]

ca·vog·ra·phy (kā-vog'ră-fē). SYN venacavography.

ca·vo·sur·face (kā-vō-sŭr'făs). Relating to a cavity and the surface of a tooth.

ca·vum, pl. **ca·va** (ka'vŭm, -vă) [NA]. SYN cavity. [L. ntr. of adj. *cavus,* hollow]

CBC complete *blood count.*

CBG corticosteroid-binding *globulin.*

C.C. chief complaint, as recorded on a patient's medical history.

cc, c.c. cubic *centimeter.*

CCK cholecystokinin.

CCU coronary care *unit*; critical care *unit*.

CD curative *dose*; circular *dichroism*; cluster of differentiation.

CD2 *cluster of differentiation* 2.

CD3 *cluster of differentiation* 3.

CD4 *cluster of differentiation* 4.

CD8 *cluster of differentiation* 8.

Cd cadmium.

cd candela.

CDC Centers for Disease *Control*; previously known as the Communicable Disease Center.

CD4/CD8 count. The ratio of the number of helper-inducer T lymphocytes to cytotoxic-suppressor T lymphocytes, as measured by monoclonal antibodies to the CD4 surface antigen found on helper-inducer T cells, and the CD8 surface antigen found on cytotoxic-suppressor T cells. In healthy individuals, the H/S ratio ranges between 1.6 and 2.2. The CD4/CD8 count is used to monitor for signs of organ rejection after transplants, and to assess the relative condition of HIV patients.

cDNA complementary DNA.

CDP cytidine 5′-diphosphate.

Ce cerium.

CEA carcinoembryonic *antigen.*

⚠**cec-.** SEE ceco-.

ce•ca (sē′kă). Plural of cecum.

ce•ca (sē′kă).

ce•cal (sē′kăl). **1.** Relating to the cecum. **2.** Ending blindly in a cul-de-sac.

ce•cec•to•my (sē-sek′tō-mē). Excision of the cecum. SYN typhlectomy. [ceco- + G. *ektomē*, excision]

ce•ci•tis (sē-sī′tis). Inflammation of the cecum. SYN typhlenteritis, typhlitis, typhloenteritis.

⚠**ceco-, cec-.** The cecum. SEE ALSO typhlo- (1). Cf. typhlo-. [L. *caecum*, cecum, blind]

ce•co•co•los•to•my (sē′kō-kō-los′tō-mē). Formation of an anastomosis between cecum and colon.

ce•co•il•e•os•to•my (sē′kō-il-ē-os′tō-mē). SYN ileocecostomy.

ce•co•pexy (sē′kō-pek-sē). Operative anchoring of a movable cecum. SYN typhlopexy, typhlopexia. [ceco- + G. *pexis*, fixation]

ce•co•pli•ca•tion (sē′kō-pli-kā′shŭn). Operative reduction in size of a dilated cecum by the formation of folds or tucks in its wall. [ceco- + L. *plico*, pp. *-atus*, to fold]

ce•cor•rha•phy (sē-kōr′ă-fē). Suture of the cecum. SYN typhlorrhaphy. [ceco- + G. *rhaphē*, suture]

ce•co•sig•moid•os•to•my (sē′kō-sig-moy-dos′tō-mē). Formation of a communication between the cecum and the sigmoid colon.

ce•cos•to•my (sē-kos′tō-mē). Operative formation of a cecal fistula. SYN typhlostomy. [ceco- + G. *stoma*, mouth]

ce•cot•o•my (sē-kot′ō-mē). Incision into the cecum. SYN typhlotomy. [ceco- + G. *tomē*, incision]

ce•cum, pl. **ce•ca** (sē′kŭm, sē′kă) [NA]. **1.** The cul-de-sac, about 6 cm in depth, lying below the

terminal ileum forming the first part of the large intestine. **2.** Any similar structure ending in a cul-de-sac. [L. ntr. of *caecus*, blind]

  cupular c. of the cochlear duct, the upper blind extremity of the cochlear duct. SYN lagena (1).

⚠**-cele.** Swelling; hernia. [G. *kēlē*, tumor]

ce•li•ac (sē′lē-ak). Relating to the abdominal cavity. [G. *koilia*, belly]

⚠**celio-.** The abdomen. SEE ALSO celo- (3). [G. *koilia*, belly]

ce•li•o•cen•te•sis (sē′lē-ō-sen-tē′sis). Rarely used term for paracentesis of the abdomen. [celio- + G. *kentēsis*, puncture]

ce•li•or•rha•phy (sē-lē-ōr′ă-fē). Suture of a wound in the abdominal wall. SYN laparorrhaphy. [celio- + G. *rhaphē*, seam]

ce•li•os•co•py (sē-lē-os′kŏ-pē). SYN peritoneoscopy. [celio- + G. *skopeō*, to view]

ce•li•ot•o•my (sē-lē-ot′ō-mē). Transabdominal incision into the peritoneal cavity. SYN abdominal section, laparotomy (2), ventrotomy. [celio- + G. *tomē*, incision]

  vaginal c., opening the peritoneal cavity through the vagina.

ce•li•tis (sē-lī′tis). Any inflammation of the abdomen. [G. *koilia*, belly, + *-itis*, inflammation]

cell (sel). **1.** The smallest unit of living structure capable of independent existence, composed of a membrane-enclosed mass of protoplasm and containing a nucleus or nucleoid. C.'s are highly variable and specialized in both structure and function, though all must at some stage replicate proteins and nucleic acids, utilize energy, and reproduce themselves. **2.** A small closed or partly closed cavity; a compartment or hollow receptacle. **3.** A container of glass, ceramic, or other solid material within which chemical reactions generating electricity take place. [L. *cella*, a storeroom, a chamber]

  A c.'s, alpha c.'s of pancreas or of anterior lobe of hypophysis. SYN alpha c.'s (3).

  acid c., SYN parietal c.

  acinar c., any secreting c. lining an acinus, especially applied to the c.'s of the pancreas that furnish pancreatic juice and enzymes to distinguish them from the c.'s of ducts and the islets of Langerhans. SYN acinous c.

  acinous c., SYN acinar c.

  adipose c., SYN fat c.

  adventitial c., SYN pericyte.

  air c.'s, (1) SYN pulmonary *alveolus*. **(2)** air-containing spaces in the skull.

  alpha c.'s, (1) acidophil c.'s that constitute about 35% of the c.'s of the anterior lobe of the hypophysis; there are two varieties: one elaborates somatotropic hormone; the other mammotropic hormone; **(2)** c.'s of the islets of Langerhans that secrete glucagon. **(3)** SYN A c.'s.

  alveolar c., any of the c.'s lining the alveoli of the lung, including the squamous alveolar c.'s, the great alveolar c.'s, and the alveolar macrophages.

  ameboid c., a c. such as a leukocyte, having ameboid movements, with a power of locomotion. SYN wandering c.

  anaplastic c., (1) a c. that has reverted to an

embryonal state; (2) an undifferentiated c., characteristic of malignant neoplasms.

Anitschkow c., SYN cardiac *histiocyte.*

antigen-sensitive c., a small lymphocyte that, although not itself an immunologically activated c., responds to antigenic (immunogenic) stimulus by a process of division and differentiation that results in the production of immunologically activated cells.

APUD c.'s, SEE APUD.

argentaffin c.'s, c.'s that contain granules which precipitate silver from an ammoniacal silver nitrate solution. SEE ALSO enteroendocrine c.'s.

auditory receptor c.'s, columnar c.'s in the epithelium of the organ of Corti, having hairs (stereocilia) on their apical ends.

B c.'s, SYN beta c.'s (1).

band c., any c. of the granulocytic (leukocytic) series that has a nucleus that could be described as a curved or coiled band, no matter how marked the indentation, if it does not completely segment the nucleus into lobes connected by a filament. SYN stab c., staff c.

basal c., a c. of the deepest layer of stratified epithelium.

basket c., (1) a neuron enmeshing the cell body of another neuron with its terminal axon ramifications; (2) SYN smudge c.'s. (3) a myoepithelial c. with branching processes that occurs basal to the secretory c.'s of certain salivary gland and lacrimal gland alveoli.

beaker c., SYN goblet c.

beta c.'s, (1) basophil c.'s of the anterior lobe of the hypophysis that contain basophil granules and are believed to produce gonadotropic hormones; SYN B c.'s. (2) the predominant c.'s of the islets of Langerhans, which produce insulin.

Betz c.'s, large pyramidal c.'s in the motor area of the precentral gyrus of the cerebral cortex.

bipolar c., a neuron having two processes, such as those of the retina or the spiral and vestibular ganglia of the eighth nerve.

blast c., an immature precursor c.; *e.g.,* erythroblast, lymphoblast, neuroblast. SEE ALSO -blast.

bronchic c.'s, SYN pulmonary *alveolus.*

castration c.'s, altered basophilic c.'s of the anterior lobe of the pituitary that develop following castration; the body of the c. is occupied by a large vacuole that displaces the nucleus to the periphery, giving the c. a resemblance to a signet ring. SYN signet ring c.'s.

centroacinar c., a c. of the pancreatic ductule that occupies the lumen of an acinus; it secretes bicarbonate and water, providing an alkaline pH necessary for enzyme activity in the intestine.

chief c., the predominant cell type of a gland.

chromaffin c., a c. that stains with chromic salts, in adrenal medulla and paraganglia of the sympathetic nervous system.

chromophobe c.'s, c.'s in the adenohypophysis without stainable cytoplasmic granules.

clear c., (1) a c. in which the cytoplasm appears empty with the light microscope, as occurs in certain secretory c.'s of eccrine sweat glands and in the parathyroid glands when the glycogen is unstained; (2) any c., particularly a neoplastic one, containing abundant glycogen or other material that is not stained by hematoxylin or eosin, so that the c. cytoplasm is very pale in routinely stained sections.

cone c., one of the two types of visual receptor c.'s of the retina, essential for visual acuity and color vision; the second type is the rod c.

daughter c., one of the two or more c.'s formed in the division of a parent c.

decidual c., an enlarged, ovoid connective tissue c. appearing in the endometrium of pregnancy.

delta c., (1) a variety of c. in the anterior lobe of the hypophysis that has basophilic granules; (2) a c. of the islets of Langerhans, with fine granules that stain with aniline blue.

dendritic c.'s, in embryonic ectoderm, c.'s of neural crest origin with extensive processes; they develop melanin early.

Downey c., the atypical lymphocyte of infectious mononucleosis.

dust c., SYN alveolar *macrophage.*

enteroendocrine c.'s, c.'s with granules that may be either argentaffinic or argyrophilic; the c.'s, scattered throughout the digestive tract, are of several varieties and are believed to produce at least 20 different gastrointestinal hormones and neurotransmitters.

ependymal c., a c. lining the central canal of the spinal cord (those of pyramidal shape) or one of the brain ventricles (those of cuboidal shape).

epithelioid c., (1) a nonepithelial c. having certain characteristics of epithelium; (2) large mononuclear histiocytes having certain epithelial characteristics, particularly in tubercles where they are polygonal and have eosinophilic cytoplasm.

ethmoid air c.'s, the numerous small air-filled cells of the ethmoidal labyrinth.

fagot c., a neoplastic promyelocyte with bundles of Auer rods, found in hypergranular promyelocytic leukemia (M3).

fat c., a connective tissue c. distended with one or more fat globules, the cytoplasm usually being compressed into a thin envelope, with the nucleus at one point in the periphery. SYN adipocyte, adipose c.

fat-storing c., a multilocular fat-filled c. present in the perisinusoidal space in the liver. SYN lipocyte.

foam c.'s, c.'s with abundant, pale-staining, finely vacuolated cytoplasm, usually histiocytes that have ingested or accumulated material that dissolves during tissue preparation, especially lipids. SEE ALSO lipophage.

follicular c., an epithelial c. lining a follicle, such as that of the thyroid or ovary.

G c.'s, enteroendocrine c.'s that secrete gastrin, found primarily in the mucosa of the pyloric antrum of the stomach.

ganglion c., a neuron the c. body of which is located outside the limits of the brain and spinal cord, hence forming part of the peripheral nervous system; ganglion c.'s are either 1) the pseudounipolar c.'s of the sensory spinal and cranial nerves (sensory ganglia), or 2) the peripheral multipolar motor neurons innervating the viscera (visceral or autonomic ganglia). SYN gangliocyte.

Gaucher c.'s, large, finely and uniformly vacuolated c.'s derived from the reticuloendothelial system, and found especially in the spleen, lymph nodes, liver, and bone marrow of patients with Gaucher's disease; Gaucher c.'s contain kerasin (a cerebroside), which accumulates as a result of a genetically determined absence of the enzyme glucosylceramidase.

germ c., SYN sex c.

germinal c., a c. from which other c.'s proliferate.

ghost c., (1) a dead c. in which the outline remains visible, but without other cytoplasmic structures or stainable nucleus; (2) an erythrocyte after loss of its hemoglobin.

giant c., a c. of large size, often with many nuclei.

glia c.'s, SEE neuroglia.

glomerulosa c., a c. of the zona glomerulosa of the adrenal cortex that is the source of aldosterone; the c.'s are arranged in spherical or oval groups.

goblet c., an epithelial c. that becomes distended with a large accumulation of mucous secretory granules at its apical end, giving it the appearance of a goblet. SYN beaker c.

granule c.'s, (1) small nerve cell bodies in the external and internal granular layers of the cerebral cortex; (2) small nerve cell bodies in the granular layer of the cerebellar cortex.

granulosa c., a c. of the membrana granulosa lining the vesicular ovarian follicle that becomes a luteal c. of the corpus luteum after ovulation.

gustatory c.'s, SYN taste c.'s.

hair c.'s, sensory epithelial c.'s present in the organ of Corti, in the maculae and cristae of the membranous labyrinth of the ear, and in taste buds; they are characterized by having long stereocilia or kinocilia (or both) which, with the light microscope, appear as fine hairs. SEE ALSO taste c.'s.

hairy c.'s, medium-sized leukocytes that have features of reticuloendothelial c.'s and multiple cytoplasmic projections (hairs) on the c. surface, but which may be a variety of B lymphocyte; they are found in hairy cell leukemia.

HeLa c.'s, the first continuously cultured human malignant c.'s, derived from a cervical carcinoma of Henrietta Lacks; used in the cultivation of viruses.

helper c., a subset of T lymphocytes that acts in cooperation with B lymphocytes to permit antibody formation.

Hensen's c., one of the supporting c.'s in the organ of Corti, immediately to the outer side of the c.'s of Deiters.

hilus c.'s, c.'s in the hilus of the ovary that produce androgens; they are thought to be the ovarian counterpart of the interstitial c.'s of the testis.

hobnail c.'s, c.'s characteristic of a mesonephroma; a round expansion of clear cytoplasm projects into the lumen of neoplastic tubules, but the basal part of the c. containing the nucleus is narrow.

Hortega c.'s, SYN microglia.

I c., a cultured skin fibroblast containing membrane-bound inclusions; characteristic of mucolipidosis II. SEE ALSO immunocyte. SYN inclusion c.

inclusion c., SYN I c.

interstitial c.'s, (1) c.'s between the seminiferous tubules of the testis that secrete testosterone; (2) c.'s derived from the theca interna of atretic follicles of the ovary; they resemble luteal c.'s and are an important source of estrogens; (3) pineal c.'s similar to glial c.'s with long processes.

islet c., one of the c.'s of the pancreatic islets.

juvenile c., SYN metamyelocyte.

juxtaglomerular c.'s, c.'s located at the vascular pole of the renal corpuscle that secrete renin and form a component of the juxtaglomerular complex; they are modified smooth muscle c.'s primarily of the afferent arteriole of the renal glomerulus.

K c.'s, SYN killer c.'s.

killer c.'s, cytotoxic c.'s involved in antibody-dependent c.-mediated immune responses. SYN K c.'s, null c.'s (1), T cytotoxic c.'s.

Kupffer c.'s, phagocytic c.'s of the mononuclear phagocyte series found on the luminal surface of the hepatic sinusoids.

LE c., a polymorphonuclear leukocyte containing an amorphous round body; formed *in vitro* in the blood of patients with systemic lupus erythematosus, or by the action of the patient's serum on normal leukocytes. SYN lupus erythematosus c.

lupus erythematosus c., SYN LE c.

luteal c., lutein c., a c. of the corpus luteum of the ovary that is derived from the granulosa cells of the preovulatory follicle; it secretes progesterone and estrogen.

mast c., a connective tissue c. that contains coarse, basophilic, metachromatic granules; the c. is believed to contain heparin and histamine. SYN mastocyte.

mastoid air c.'s, numerous small intercommunicating cavities in the mastoid process of the temporal bone that empty into the mastoid or tympanic antrum.

mesoglial c.'s, SYN mesoglia.

Mexican hat c., SYN target c.

mirror-image c., (1) a c. whose nuclei have identical features and are placed in the cytoplasm in similar fashion; (2) a binucleate form of Reed-Sternberg c. often found in Hodgkin's disease; the twin nuclei are disposed in relation to an imaginary plane between them like a single nucleus together with its image in a mirror.

monocytoid c., a c. having morphological characteristics of a monocyte but which is nonphagocytic.

mother c., a c. which, by division, gives rise to two or more daughter c.'s. SYN metrocyte.

mucoserous c.'s, glandular c.'s intermediate in histologic characteristics between serous and mucous c.'s.

mucous c., a c. secreting mucus; *e.g.,* a goblet c.

multipolar c., a nerve c. with a number of dendrites arising from the c. body.

myoid c.'s, flattened smooth muscle-like c.'s of mesodermal origin that lie just outside the basal lamina of the seminiferous tubule. SYN peritubular contractile c.'s.

natural killer c.'s, large granular lymphocytes which do not express markers of either T or B c. lineage. These c.'s kill target c.'s using antibody-dependent cell-mediated cytotoxicity. NK c.'s can also use perforin to kill c.'s in the absence of antibody. Killing may occur without previous sensitization. SYN NK c.'s.

neurilemma c.'s, SYN Schwann c.'s.

neurolemma c.'s, SYN Schwann c.'s.

nevus c., the c. of a pigmented cutaneous nevus that differs from a normal melanocyte in that it lacks dendrites.

Niemann-Pick c., SYN Pick c.

NK c.'s, SYN natural killer c.'s.

null c.'s, (1) SYN killer c.'s. **(2)** large granular lymphocytes that lack surface markers or membrane-associated proteins of either B or T lymphocytes.

oat c., a short, bluntly spindle-shaped c. that contains a relatively large, hyperchromatic nucleus, frequently observed in undifferentiated bronchogenic carcinoma.

OKT c.'s, c.'s recognized by monoclonal antibodies to T lymphocyte antigens. Current usage favors CD designations. [*Ortho-Kung T* cell]

olfactory receptor c.'s, very slender nerve c.'s, with large nuclei and surmounted by six to eight long, sensitive cilia in the olfactory epithelium at the roof of the nose; they are the receptors for smell.

osteoprogenitor c., a mesenchymal c. that differentiates into an osteoblast. SYN preosteoblast.

oxyntic c., SYN parietal c.

oxyphil c.'s, c.'s of the parathyroid gland that increase in number with age; the cytoplasm contains numerous mitochondria and stains with eosin. Similar c.'s, and tumors composed of them, are found in salivary glands and the thyroid; in the latter, also called Hürthle c.'s.

pagetoid c.'s, atypical melanocytes resembling Paget's c.'s, found in some cutaneous melanomas.

parafollicular c.'s, c.'s present between follicles or interspersed among follicular c.'s; they are rich in mitochondria and are believed to be the source of thyrocalcitonin.

parietal c., one of the c.'s of the gastric glands; it lies upon the basement membrane, covered by the chief c.'s, and secretes hydrochloric acid that reaches the lumen of the gland through fine intracellular and intercellular canals (canaliculi). SYN acid c., oxyntic c.

peptic c., SYN zymogenic c.

peritubular contractile c.'s, SYN myoid c.'s.

photoreceptor c.'s, rod and cone c.'s of the retina.

Pick c., a relatively large mononuclear c. with foamlike cytoplasm that contains numerous droplets of sphingomyelin; such c.'s are widely distributed in the spleen and other tissues in patients with Niemann-Pick disease. SYN Niemann-Pick c.

plasma c., an ovoid c. with an eccentric nucleus having chromatin arranged like a clock face or spokes of a wheel; the cytoplasm is strongly basophilic because of the abundant RNA in its endoplasmic reticulum; plasma c.'s are derived from B lymphocytes and are active in the formation of antibodies. SYN plasmacyte.

polychromatic c., a primitive erythrocyte in bone marrow, with basophilic material as well as hemoglobin (acidophilic) in the cytoplasm. SYN polychromatophil c.

polychromatophil c., SYN polychromatic c.

prickle c., one of the c.'s of the stratum spinosum of the epidermis; so called because of shrinkage artifacts that occur in histological preparations, resulting in intercellular bridges at points of desmosomal adhesion.

pyramidal c.'s, neurons of the cerebral cortex which, in sections perpendicular to the cortical surface, exhibit a triangular shape with a long apical dendrite directed toward the surface of the cortex.

red blood c. (rbc, RBC), SYN erythrocyte.

Rieder c.'s, abnormal myeloblasts in which the nucleus may be widely and deeply indented or may actually be a bi- or multi-lobate structure; such c.'s are frequently observed in acute leukemia.

rod c., SYN rod (2).

Schwann c.'s, c.'s of ectodermal (neural crest) origin that compose a continuous envelope around each nerve fiber of peripheral nerves. SYN neurilemma c.'s, neurolemma c.'s.

segmented c., a polymorphonuclear leukocyte matured beyond the band c. so that two or more lobes of the nucleus occur.

sensitized c., (1) a c. that has combined with antibody to form a complex capable of reacting with complement components; **(2)** a small, "committed," c. derived, by division and differentiation, from a transformed lymphocyte; **(3)** a c. that has been either exposed to antigen or opsonized with antibodies and/or complement.

serous c., a c., especially of the salivary gland, that secretes a watery or thin albuminous fluid, as opposed to a mucous c.

sex c., a spermatozoon or an ovum. SYN germ c.

Sézary c., an atypical mononuclear c. seen in the peripheral blood in the Sézary syndrome; it has a large, convoluted nucleus and scanty cytoplasm containing PAS-positive vacuoles.

sickle c., an abnormal, crescentic erythrocyte that is characteristic of sickle c. anemia, resulting from an inherited abnormality of hemoglobin (hemoglobin S) causing decreased solubility at low oxygen tension. SEE ALSO sicklemia, sickling. SYN drepanocyte.

signet ring c.'s, SYN castration c.'s.

smudge c.'s, immature leukocytes of any type that have undergone partial breakdown during preparation of a stained smear or tissue section, because of their greater fragility; smudge c.'s are seen in largest numbers in chronic lymphocytic leukemia. SYN basket c. (2).

somatic c.'s, the c.'s of an organism other than the germ c.'s.

spindle c., a fusiform c., such as those in the deeper layers of the cerebral cortex.

squamous c., a flat scale-like epithelial c.

stab c., SYN band c.

staff c., SYN band c.

stellate c., a star-shaped c., such as an astrocyte or Kupffer c., that has many filaments extending radially.

stem c., (1) any precursor cell; **(2)** a c. whose daughter c.'s may differentiate into other c. types.

strap c., an elongated tumor c. of uniform width that may show cross-striations; found in rhabdomyosarcoma.

T c., SYN T *lymphocyte.*

T cytotoxic c.'s (Tc), SYN killer c.'s.

target c., (1) an erythrocyte in target c. anemia, with a dark center surrounded by a light band that again is encircled by a darker ring; it thus resembles a shooting target; such c.'s also appear after splenectomy; **(2)** a c. lysed by cytotoxic T lymphocytes, as in graft rejection. SYN leptocyte, Mexican hat c.

tart c., a monocyte with an engulfed nucleus in which the structure is still well preserved.

taste c.'s, darkly staining c.'s in a taste bud that have long hair-like microvilli. SYN gustatory c.'s.

teardrop c., SYN dacryocyte.

tendon c.'s, elongated fibroblastic c.'s arranged in rows between the collagenous tendon fibers.

T helper c.'s (Th), a subset of lymphocytes that secrete various cytokines that regulate the immune response.

Touton giant c., a xanthoma c. in which the multiple nuclei are grouped around a small island of nonfoamy cytoplasm.

transducer c., any c. responding to a mechanical, thermal, photic, or chemical stimulus by generating an electrical impulse synaptically transmitted to a sensory neuron in contact with the c.

tufted c., a particular type of c. in the olfactory bulb comparable to the bulb's mitral c. with respect to afferent and efferent relationships, but smaller and more superficially located.

vasoformative c., SYN angioblast (1).

virus-transformed c., a c. that has been genetically changed to a tumor c., the change being subsequently transmitted to all descendent c.'s; c.'s transformed by oncornaviruses continue to produce virus in high concentration without being killed; DNA tumor virus-transformed c.'s develop (along with other changes) tumor-associated antigens and rarely produce virus.

visual receptor c.'s, the rod and cone c.'s of the retina.

wandering c., SYN ameboid c.

white blood c. (WBC), SYN leukocyte.

zymogenic c., a c. that secretes an enzyme; specifically a chief c. of a gastric gland or an acinar c. of the pancreas. SYN peptic c.

cel·lu·la, gen. and pl. **cel·lu·lae** (sel'yū-lă, -lē). **1** [NA]. In gross anatomy, a small but macroscopic compartment. SYN cellule. **2.** In histology, a cell. [L. a small chamber, dim. of *cella*]

cel·lu·lar (sel'yū-lăr). **1.** Relating to, derived from, or composed of cells. **2.** Having numerous compartments or interstices. [L. *cellula,* dim. of *cella,* storeroom]

cel·lu·lar·i·ty (sel-yū-lar'i-tē). The degree, quality, or condition of cells that are present.

cel·lu·lase (sel'yū-lās). Endo-1,4-β-glucase; an enzyme catalyzing the hydrolysis of 1,4-β-glucoside links in cellulose. Used to produce digestive

tablets and in the removal of cellulose from foods for special diets.

cel·lule (sel'yūl). SYN cellula (1).

cel·lu·li·ci·dal (sel'yū-li-sī'dăl). Destructive to cells. [cellula + L. *caedo,* to kill]

cel·lu·lif·u·gal (sel-yū-lif'yū-găl). Moving from, or extending in a direction away from, a cell or cell body. [cellula + L. *fugio,* to flee]

cel·lu·lip·e·tal (sel-yū-lip'ĕ-tăl). Moving toward, or extending in a direction toward, a cell or cell body. [cellula + L. *peto,* to seek]

cel·lu·lite (sel'yū-līt). **1.** Colloquial term for deposits of fat and fibrous tissue causing dimpling of the overlying skin. **2.** SYN lipoedema.

cel·lu·li·tis (sel-yū-lī'tis). Inflammation of cellular or connective tissue.

dissecting c., a chronic dissecting folliculitis of the scalp.

pelvic c., SYN parametritis.

△**celo-. 1.** The celom. [G. *koilōma,* hollow (celom)] **2.** Hernia. [G. *kēlē,* hernia] **3.** The abdomen. SEE ALSO celio-. [G. *koilia,* belly]

ce·lom, ce·lo·ma (sē'lom, sē-lō'mă). **1.** The cavity between the splanchnic and somatic mesoderm in the embryo. **2.** SYN body *cavity.* [G. *koilōma,* a hollow]

ce·lom·ic (sē-lom'ik). Relating to the body *cavity.*

ce·lo·phle·bi·tis (sē-lō-flĕ-bī'tis). Inflammation of a vena cava. SYN cavitis. [G. *koilos,* hollow, + phlebitis]

Cel·si·us (C). SEE Celsius *scale.*

ce·ment (se-ment'). **1.** SYN cementum. **2.** In dentistry, a nonmetallic material used for luting, filling, or permanent or temporary restorative purposes, made by mixing components into a plastic mass that sets, or as an adherent sealer in attaching various dental restorations in or on the tooth. [see cementum]

glass ionomer c., a dental c. produced by mixing calcium aluminosilicate glass with an aqueous solution of polyacrylic acid. [ion + -mer (1)]

resin c., a monomer or monomer/polymer system used as a dental luting agent; used in cementation of restorations or orthodontic brackets to the teeth.

ce·ment·i·cle (se-men'ti-kl). A calcified spherical body, composed of cementum lying free within the periodontal membrane, attached to the cementum or imbedded within it.

ce·ment·o·blast (se-men'tō-blast). One of the cells concerned with the formation of the layer of cementum on the roots of teeth. [L. *cementum,* cement, + G. *blastos,* germ]

ce·ment·o·blas·to·ma (se-men'tō-blas-tō'mă). A benign odontogenic tumor of functional cementoblasts; it appears as a mixed radiolucent-radiopaque lesion attached to a tooth root.

ce·ment·o·cla·sia (se-men-tō-klā'zē-ă). Destruction of cementum by cementoclasts. [L. *cementum,* cement, + G. *klasis,* fracture]

ce·ment·o·clast (se-men'tō-klast). One of the multinucleated giant cells, identical with osteoclasts, that are associated with the resorption of cementum. [L. *cementum,* cement, + G. *klastos,* broken]

ce·ment·o·cyte (se-men'tō-sīt). An osteocyte-like cell with numerous processes, trapped in a lacuna in the cementum of the tooth. [L. *cementum,* cement, + G. *kytos,* cell]

ce·men·to·ma (se-men-tō'mă). Any benign cementum-producing tumor; four types are recognized: 1) periapical cemental dysplasia, 2) central ossifying fibroma, 3) cementoblastoma, 4) sclerotic cemental mass. When the type is not specified, c. usually refers to periapical cemental *dysplasia.* [L. *cementum,* cement, + G. *-ōma,* tumor]

ce·men·tum (se-men'tŭm) [NA]. A layer of bone-like mineralized tissue covering the dentin of the root and neck of a tooth that blends with the fibers of the periodontal ligament. SYN cement (1). [L. *caementum,* rough quarry stone, fr. *caedo,* to cut]

ce·nes·the·sia (sē-nes-thē'zē-ă). The general sense of bodily existence; the sensation caused by the functioning of the internal organs. [G. *koinos,* common, + *aisthēsis,* sensation]

ce·nes·the·sic, ce·nes·thet·ic (sē-nes-thē'zik, -sik; -thet'ik). Relating to cenesthesia.

△**ceno-.** **1.** Shared in common. [G. *koinos,* common] **2.** New, fresh. [G. *kainos,* new] **3.** Emptiness (rare). SEE ALSO coeno-. [G. *kenos,* empty]

cen·o·site (sē'nō-sīt). A facultative commensal organism that can sustain itself apart from its usual host. SYN coinosite. [G. *koinos,* common, + *sitos,* food]

cen·sor (sen'sōr). PSYCHOANALYTIC THEORY the psychic barrier that prevents certain unconscious thoughts and wishes from coming to consciousness. [L. a judge, critic, fr. *censeo,* to value, judge]

cen·sus (sen'sus). An enumeration of a population, originally for taxation and military purposes, now with many other purposes; basic facts about all persons—age, sex, occupation, nature of residence, etc.— are recorded in the census, which often also includes some information about health status. [L., fr. *censeo,* to count]

cen·ter (sen'ter). **1.** The middle point of a body; loosely, the interior of a body. A center of any kind, especially an anatomical center. **2.** A group of nerve cells governing a specific function. SYN centrum [NA]. [L. *centrum;* G. *kentron*]

   Broca's c., the posterior part of the inferior frontal gyrus of the left or dominant hemisphere; an essential component of the motor mechanisms governing articulated speech. SYN Broca's area, motor speech c.

   chondrification c., a site of earliest cartilage formation in the body.

   ciliospinal c., the preganglionic motor neurons in the first thoracic segment of the spinal cord which give rise to the sympathetic innervation of the dilator muscle of the pupil.

   epiotic c., the c. of ossification of the petrous part of the temporal bone that appears posterior to the posterior semicircular canal.

   motor speech c., SYN Broca's c.

   ossific c., SYN c. of ossification.

   c. of ossification, the site of earliest bone formation via accumulation of osteoblasts within connective tissue (membranous ossification) or of earliest destruction of cartilage prior to onset of

ossification (endochondral ossification). SYN ossific c., point of ossification.

   respiratory c., the region in the medulla oblongata concerned with integrating afferent information to determine the signals to the respiratory muscles; the inspiratory and expiratory c.'s considered together.

   sensory speech c., SYN Wernicke's c.

   speech c.'s, areas of the cerebral cortex centrally involved in speech function; one is in the left inferior frontal gyrus, a second one in the supramarginal, angular, and first and second temporal gyri. SEE ALSO Broca's c., Wernicke's c.

   Wernicke's c., the region of the cerebral cortex thought to be essential for understanding and formulating coherent, propositional speech; it encompasses a large region of the parietal and temporal lobes of the left cerebral hemisphere. SYN sensory speech c., Wernicke's area.

cen·te·sis (sen-tē'sis). Puncture, especially when used as a suffix, as in paracentesis. [G. *kentēsis,* puncture, fr. *kenteō,* to prick, pierce]

△**centi- (c).** Prefix used in the SI and metric systems to signify one hundredth (10^{-2}). [L. *centum,* one hundred]

cen·ti·grade (C) (sen'ti-grād). **1.** Basis of the former temperature scale in which 100 degrees separated the melting and boiling points of water. SEE Celsius *scale.* **2.** One hundredth of a circle, equal to 3.6° of the astronomical circle. [L. *centum,* one hundred, + *gradus,* step, degree]

cen·ti·gram (sen'ti-gram). One hundredth of a gram.

cen·tile (sen'til). One-hundredth. [L. *centum,* one hundred, + *-ilis,* adj. suffix]

cen·ti·li·ter (sen'ti-lē-ter). 10 milliliters; one hundredth of a liter; 162.3073 minims (U.S.).

cen·ti·me·ter (cm) (sen'ti-mē-ter). One hundredth of a meter; 0.3937008 inch.

   cubic c. (cc, c.c.), one thousandth of a liter; 1 milliliter.

cen·ti·mor·gan (cM) (sen'ti-mōr-găn). SEE morgan.

cen·ti·nor·mal (sen-ti-nōr'măl). One-hundredth normal; denoting the concentration of a solution.

cen·ti·poise (sen'ti-poyz). One hundredth of a poise.

cen·tra (sen'tră). Plural of centrum.

cen·trad (sen'trad). **1.** Toward the center. **2.** A unit of measurement of the refracting strength of a prism; it corresponds to the deviation of a ray of light, the arc of which is $1/100$ of the radius of the circle, or 0.57°.

cen·tren·ce·phal·ic (sen'tren-se-fal'ik). Relating to the center of the encephalon.

△**centric** (sen'trik). Having a center (of a specific kind or number) or having a specific thing as its center (of interest, focus, etc.). [G. *kentron,* center]

cen·tric·i·put (sen-tris'i-put). The central portion of the upper surface of the skull, between the occiput and the sinciput. [L. *centrum,* center, + *caput,* head]

cen·trif·u·gal (sen-trif'yū-găl). **1.** Denoting the direction of the force pulling an object outward (away) from an axis of rotation. **2.** Sometimes, by analogy, extended to describe any movement away from a center. Cf. eccentric (2). [L. *centrum,* center, + *fugio,* to flee]

cen·trif·u·ga·tion (sen-trif-yū-gā′shŭn). Sedimentation, by means of a centrifuge, of solids suspended in a fluid.

cen·tri·fuge (sen′tri-fūj). **1.** An apparatus by means of which particles in suspension in a fluid are separated by spinning the fluid, the centrifugal force throwing the particles to the periphery of the rotated vessel. **2.** To submit to rapid rotary action, as in a c.

cen·tri·lob·u·lar (sen-tri-lob′yū-lăr). At or near the center of a lobule, *e.g.,* of the liver.

cen·tri·ole (sen′trē-ōl). Tubular structures usually seen as paired organelles lying in the cytocentrum; c.'s may be multiple and numerous in some cells, such as the giant cells of bone marrow. [G. *kentron,* a point, center]

cen·trip·e·tal (sen-trip′e-tăl). **1.** SYN afferent. **2.** Denoting the direction of the force pulling an object toward an axis of rotation. SYN axipetal. [L. *centrum,* center, + *peto,* to seek]

△**centro-.** Combining form denoting center. [G. *kentron*]

cen·tro·ki·ne·sia (sen′trō-ki-nē′sē-ă). Movement excited by a stimulus of central origin. [centro- + G. *kinēsis,* movement]

cen·tro·ki·net·ic (sen′trō-ki-net′ik). **1.** Relating to centrokinesia. **2.** SYN excitomotor.

cen·tro·mere (sen′trō-mēr). The nonstaining primary constriction of a chromosome; the c. divides the chromosome into two arms, and its position is constant for a specific chromosome: near one end (acrocentric), near the center (metacentric), or between (submetacentric). [centro- + G. *meros,* part]

cen·tro·some (sen′trō-sōm). SYN cytocentrum. [centro- + G. *sōma,* body]

cen·tro·sphere (sen′trō-sfēr). The specialized cytoplasm of the cytocentrum. Contains the centrioles from which the astral fibers (microtubules) extend during mitosis. [centro- + G. *sphaira,* a ball, sphere]

cen·tro·stal·tic (sen-trō-stal′tik). Relating to the center of motion. [centro- + G. *stallein,* set forth, fetch]

cen·trum, pl. **cen·tra** (sen′trŭm, sen′tră) [NA]. SYN center. [L. fr. G. *kentron*]

cen·tum (c) (sĕn′tŭm). L. hundred [L. one hundred]

△**cephal-.** SEE cephalo-.

ceph·a·lad (sef′ă-lad). In a direction toward the head. SEE ALSO cranial (1).

ceph·a·lal·gia (sef′al-al′jē-ă). SYN headache. [cephal- + G. *algos,* pain]

ceph·al·e·de·ma (sef′al-ĕ-dē′mă). Edema of the head.

ceph·al·he·ma·to·cele (sef′al-hē-mat′ō-sēl). A cephalhematoma under the pericranium communicating with the dural sinuses. SYN cephalohematocele. [cephal- + G. *haima,* blood, + *kēlē,* tumor]

ceph·al·he·ma·to·ma (sef′ăl-hē-mă-tō′mă). An effusion of blood beneath the periosteum frequently in a newborn as a result of birth trauma; contrasted with caput succedaneum, in which the effusion overlies the periosteum and consists of

serum. SYN cephalohematoma. [cephal- + G. *haima,* blood, + -*ōma,* tumor]

ceph·al·hy·dro·cele (sef-ăl-hī′drō-sēl). An accumulation of serous or watery fluid under the pericranium. [cephal- + G. *hydōr,* water, + *kēlē,* tumor]

ce·phal·ic (se-fal′ik). SYN cranial (1).

ceph·a·li·tis (sef-ă-lī′tis). SYN encephalitis.

△**cephalo-, cephal-.** The head. [G. *kephalē*]

ceph·a·lo·cele (sef′ă-lō-sēl). Protrusion of part of the cranial contents, *e.g.,* meningocele, encephalocele. SEE ALSO encephalocele.

ceph·a·lo·cen·te·sis (sef′ă-lō-sen-tē′sis). Passage of a hollow needle or trocar into the brain to drain or aspirate an abscess or the fluid of a hydrocephalus. [cephalo- + G. *kentēsis,* puncture]

ceph·a·lo·dyn·ia (sef′ă-lō-din′ē-ă). Headache. [cephalo- + G. *odynē,* pain]

ceph·a·lo·gy·ric (sef′ă-lō-jī′rik). Relating to rotation of the head. [cephalo- + G. *gyros,* a circle]

ceph·a·lo·he·ma·to·cele (sef′ă-lō-hē-mat′ō-sēl). SYN cephalhematocele.

ceph·a·lo·he·ma·to·ma (sef′ă-lō-hē-mă-tō′mă). SYN cephalhematoma.

ceph·a·lo·meg·a·ly (sef′ă-lō-meg′ă-lē). Enlargement of the head. [cephalo- + G. *megas,* great]

ceph·a·lom·e·ter (sef-ă-lom′ĕ-ter). An instrument used to position the head to produce oriented, reproducible lateral and posterior-anterior head films. SYN cephalostat. [cephalo- + G. *metron,* measure]

ceph·a·lo·met·rics (sef-ă-lō-met′riks). ORAL SURGERY, ORTHODONTICS **1.** The scientific measurement of the bones of the cranium and face, utilizing a fixed, reproducible position for lateral radiographic exposure of skull and facial bones. **2.** A scientific study of the measurements of the head with relation to specific reference points; used for evaluation of facial growth and development, including soft tissue profile. [cephalo- + G. *metron,* measure]

ceph·a·lom·e·try (sef-ă-lom′ĕ-trē). Measurements on the living head, or head without removal of the soft parts. SEE ALSO cephalometrics. [cephalo- + G. *metron,* measure]

ceph·a·lo·mo·tor (sef′ă-lō-mō′ter). Relating to movements of the head.

ceph·a·lop·a·thy (sef-ă-lop′ă-thē). SYN encephalopathy. [cephalo- + G. *pathos,* suffering]

ceph·a·lo·pel·vic (sef′ă-lō-pel′vik). Pertaining to the size of the fetal head in relation to the maternal pelvis.

ceph·a·lo·pel·vim·e·try (sef′ă-lō-pel-vim′ĕ-trē). Roentgenographic measurement of the dimensions of the pelvis and the fetal head. [cephalo- + pelvimetry]

ceph·a·lo·stat (sef′ă-lō-stat). SYN cephalometer. [cephalo- + G. *statos,* stationary]

ceph·a·lo·tho·rac·ic (sef′ă-lō-thō-ras′ik). Relating to the head and the chest.

△**-ceptor.** Combining form denoting taker, receiver. [L. *capio,* pp. *captus,* to take]

cer·am·i·dase (ser-am′i-dās). An enzyme that hydrolyzes ceramides into sphingosine and a fatty acid. A deficiency of this enzyme is associated with Farber's disease.

cer·a·mide (ser′ă-mīd). Generic term for a class

of sphingolipid, *N*-acyl (fatty acid) derivatives of a long chain base or sphingoid such as sphingenine or sphingosine. C.'s accumulate in individuals with Farber's disease.

⚠**cerat-.** SEE kerat-.

⚠**cerato-.** SEE kerato-.

cer·car·ia, pl. **cer·car·i·ae** (ser-kā′rē-ă, -rē-ē). The free-swimming trematode larva that emerges from its host snail; it may penetrate the skin of a final host, encyst on vegetation, in or on fish, or penetrate and encyst in various arthropod hosts. Body and tail are greatly varied in form, and specialized function is adapted to the particular life cycle demands of each species. SEE ALSO sporocyst (1). [G. *kerkos,* tail]

cer·ci (ser′sī). Plural of cercus.

cer·clage (sair-klazh′). **1.** Bringing into close opposition and binding together the ends of an obliquely fractured bone or the fragments of a broken patella by a ring or by an encircling, tightly drawn wire loop. **2.** Operation for retinal detachment in which the choroid and retinal pigment epithelium are brought in contact with the detached sensory retina by a band encircling the sclera posterior. **3.** The placing of a nonabsorbable suture around an incompetent cervical os. SYN tiring. [Fr. an encircling, hooping, banding]

cer·co·cys·tis (ser-kō-sis′tis). A form of tapeworm larva that develops within the vertebrate host villus rather than in an invertebrate host. SEE ALSO cysticercus. [G. *kerkos,* tail, + *kystis,* bladder]

cer·cus, gen. and pl. **cer·ci** (ser′kŭs, -sē). A stiff hairlike structure. [Mod. L., fr. G. *kerkos,* tail]

ce·rea flex·i·bil·i·tas (sē′rē-ă flek-si-bil′i-tas). "Waxy flexibility," in which the limb remains where placed; often seen in catatonia. [L.]

cer·e·bel·lar (ser-e-bel′ar). Relating to the cerebellum.

cer·e·bel·li·tis (ser-ĕ-bel-ī′tis). Inflammation of the cerebellum.

⚠**cerebello-.** The cerebellum. [L. *cerebrum,* brain, + *-ellum,* dim. suff.]

cer·e·bel·lum, pl. **ce·re·bel·la** (ser-e-bel′ŭm, -bel′ă) [NA]. The large posterior brain mass lying dorsal to the pons and medulla and ventral to the posterior portion of the cerebrum; it consists of two lateral hemispheres united by a narrow middle portion, the vermis. [L. dim. of *cerebrum,* brain]

⚠**cerebr-.** SEE cerebro-.

ce·re·bra (sĕ-rē′bră). Plural of cerebrum.

ce·re·bral (ser′ĕ-brăl, sĕ-rē′brăl). Relating to the cerebrum.

cer·e·bra·tion (ser-ĕ-brā′shŭn). Activity of the mental processes; thinking. SEE ALSO cognition.

⚠**cerebri-.** SEE cerebro-.

cer·e·bri·form (se-rē′bri-fōrm). Resembling the external fissures and convolutions of the brain. [cerebri- + L. *forma,* shape, appearance, nature]

cer·e·bri·tis (ser-ĕ-brī′tis). Focal inflammatory infiltrates in the brain parenchyma.

⚠**cerebro-, cerebr-, cerebri-.** The cerebrum. SEE ALSO encephalo-. [L. *cerebrum,* brain]

cer·e·bro·ma. SYN encephaloma.

cer·e·bro·ma·la·cia (ser′ĕ-brō-mă-lā′shē-ă). SYN encephalomalacia.

cer·e·bro·men·in·gi·tis (ser′ĕ-brō-men-in-jī′tis). SYN meningoencephalitis.

cer·e·brop·a·thy (ser-ĕ-brop′ă-thē). SYN encephalopathy.

cer·e·bro·scle·ro·sis (ser′ĕ-brō-sklēr-ō′sis). Encephalosclerosis, hardening of the cerebral hemispheres. [cerebro- + G. *sklērōsis,* hardening]

cer·e·bro·side (ser′ĕ-brō-sīd). A class of glycosphingolipid; c.'s are found in the myelin sheath of nerve tissue.

cer·e·bro·spi·nal (ser′ĕ-brō-spī′năl, sĕ-rē′brō-). Relating to the brain and the spinal cord.

cer·e·brot·o·my (ser-ĕ-brot′ō-mē). Incision of the brain. [cerebro- + G. *tomē,* incision]

cer·e·bro·vas·cu·lar (ser′ĕ-brō-vas′kyū-lăr). Relating to the blood supply to the brain, particularly with reference to pathologic changes.

cer·e·brum, pl. **ce·re·bra, cer·e·brums** (ser′ĕ-brŭm, sĕ-rē′brŭm; -bră; -brŭmz) [NA]. Originally referred to the largest portion of the brain; it now usually refers only to the parts derived from the telencephalon and includes mainly the cerebral hemispheres (cerebral cortex and basal ganglia). [L., brain]

ce·ri·um (Ce) (sēr′ē-ŭm). A metallic element, atomic no. 58, atomic wt. 140.115. [fr. *Ceres,* the planetoid]

cer·ti·fi·a·ble (ser-ti-fī′ă-bl). Denoting a person showing disordered behavior of sufficient gravity to justify involuntary mental hospitalization.

cer·ti·fi·ca·tion (ser′ti-fi-kā′shŭn). **1.** The attainment of board certification in a specialty. **2.** The court procedure by which a patient is committed to a mental institution. **3.** Involuntary mental hospitalization.

cer·ti·fied nurse-mid·wife. A registered n.-m. with at least a master's degree in nursing and advanced education in the management of maternity. Certification is achieved through an organized program of study and national testing by the American College of Nurse-Midwives.

ce·ru·lo·plas·min (sĕ-rū′lō-plaz-min). A blue copper-containing α-globulin of blood plasma; involved in copper transport and regulation, and can reduce O_2 directly without known intermediates. C. is absent in congenital Wilson's disease. [L. *caeruleus,* dark blue]

ce·ru·men (sĕ-rū′men). The soft, brownish yellow, waxy secretion (a modified sebum) of the ceruminous glands of the external auditory meatus. [L. *cera,* wax]

ce·ru·mi·nal (se-rū′mi-năl). Relating to cerumen.

ce·ru·mi·no·lyt·ic (sĕ-rū′mi-nō-lit′ik). Any substance instilled into the external auditory canal to soften wax. [cerumen, + G. *lysis,* a loosening]

ce·ru·mi·no·sis (se-rū-mi-nō′sis). Excessive formation of cerumen.

ce·ru·mi·nous (sĕ-rū′mi-nŭs). Relating to cerumen.

cer·vi·cal (ser′vĭ-kal). Relating to a neck, or cervix, in any sense. [L. *cervix (cervic-),* neck]

cer·vi·cec·to·my (ser-vi-sek′tō-mē). Excision of the cervix uteri. SYN trachelectomy. [cervix + G. *ektomē,* excision]

cer·vi·ces (-sēz).

cer·vi·ces (ser′vi-sēz). Plural of cervix.

cer·vi·cis (ser′vi-sis).

cer·vi·ci·tis (ser-vi-sī′tis). Inflammation of the mucous membrane, frequently involving also the deeper structures, of the cervix uteri. SYN trachelitis.

△**cervico-**. A cervix, or neck, in any sense. [L. *cervix*, neck]

cer·vi·co·brach·i·al (ser′vi-kō-brā′kē-ăl). Relating to the neck and the arm.

cer·vi·co·dyn·ia (ser′vi-kō-din′ē-ă). Neck pain. SYN trachelodynia. [cervico- + G. *odynē*, pain]

cer·vi·co·fa·cial (ser′vi-kō-fā′shăl). Relating to the neck and the face.

cer·vi·cog·ra·phy (ser-vi-kog′ră-fē). Technique, equivalent to colposcopy, for photographing part or all of the uterine cervix. [cervix + G. *graphō*, to write]

cer·vi·co·oc·cip·i·tal (ser′vi-kō-ok-sip′i-tăl). Relating to the neck and the occiput.

cer·vi·co·plas·ty (ser′vi-kō-plas-tē). Plastic surgery on the cervix uteri or on the neck.

cer·vi·co·tho·rac·ic (ser′vi-kō-thōr-as′ik). Relating to: **1.** The neck and thorax; **2.** The transition between the neck and thorax; **3.** The fusion of these vertebrae.

cer·vi·cot·o·my (ser-vi-kot′ō-mē). Incision into the cervix uteri. SYN trachelotomy. [cervico- + G. *tomē*, incision]

cer·vi·co·ves·i·cal (ser′vi-kō-ves′i-kăl). Relating to the cervix of the uterus and the bladder.

cer·vix, gen. **cer·vi·cis**, pl. **cer·vi·ces** (ser′viks, ser′vi-sis, -sēz) [NA]. **1.** SYN collum. **2.** Any necklike structure. **3.** SYN c. of uterus. [L. neck]

   c. of uterus, the lower part of the uterus extending from the isthmus of the uterus into the vagina. It is divided into supravaginal and vaginal parts by its passage through the vaginal wall. SYN cervix (3) [NA].

ce·si·um (Cs) (sē′zē-ŭm). A metallic element, atomic no. 55, atomic wt. 132.90543; a member of the alkali metal group. ^{137}Cs (half-life equal to 30.1 years) is used in treatment of certain malignancies. [L. *caesius*, bluish gray]

Ces·to·da (ses-tō′dă). A subclass of tapeworms including the segmented tapeworms that parasitize humans and domestic animals. [G. *kestos*, girdle]

ces·tode, ces·toid (ses′tōd, -toyd). Common name for tapeworms of the class Cestoidea or its subclasses, Cestoda and Cestodaria.

Ces·toi·dea (ses-toy′dē-ă). The tapeworms, a class of platyhelminth flatworms characterized by lack of an alimentary canal and a segmented body with a scolex or holdfast organ at one end; adult worms are vertebrate parasites, usually found in the small intestine. [G. *kestos*, girdle, + *eidos*, form]

ce·tyl (sē′til). The univalent radical $C_{16}H_{33}-$ of cetyl alcohol.

CF citrovorum *factor*; coupling factor.

Cf californium.

CFU colony-forming *unit*.

CGS, cgs centimeter-gram-second. SEE centimeter-gram-second *system*.

chafe (chāf). To cause irritation of the skin by friction. [Fr. *chauffer*, to heat, fr. L. *calefacio*, to make warm]

cha·go·ma (sha-gō′mă). The skin lesion in acute Chagas' disease.

chain (chān). **1.** In chemistry, a series of atoms held together by one or more covalent bonds. **2.** In bacteriology, a linear arrangement of living cells that have divided in one plane and remain attached to each other. [L. *catena*]

   A c., **(1)** a polypeptide component of insulin containing 21 amino acyl residues; insulin is formed by the linkage of an A c. to a B c.; **(2)** in general, one of the polypeptides in a multiprotein complex.

   B c., a polypeptide component of insulin containing 30 amino acyl residues; insulin is formed by the linkage of a B c. to an A c.

   heavy c., a polypeptide c. of high molecular weight determining the class and subclass of an immunoglobulin.

   J c., a glycopeptide disulfide that is bonded to polymeric IgA and IgM; its function is to ensure correct polymerization of the subunits of IgA and IgM. [*joining*]

   kinematic c., a combination of several joints linking several limb segments together during a specific movement or posture.

   light c., a polypeptide c. with low molecular weight, as the κ or λ c.'s in immunoglobulin.

   side c., **(1)** a c. of noncyclic atoms linked to a benzene ring, or to any cyclic c. compound; **(2)** the atoms of an α-amino acid other than the α-carboxyl group, the α-amino group, the α-carbon, and the hydrogen attached to the α-carbon.

cha·la·sia, cha·la·sis (kă-lā′zē-ă, -lā′sis). Inhibition and relaxation of any previously sustained contraction of muscle, usually of a synergic group of muscles. [G. *chalaō*, to loosen]

cha·la·zi·on, pl. **cha·la·zia** (ka-lā′zē-on, -zē-ă). A chronic inflammatory granuloma of a meibomian gland. SYN meibomian cyst, tarsal cyst. [G. dim. of *chalaza*, a sty]

chal·i·co·sis (kal-i-kō′sis). Pneumoconiosis caused by the inhalation of dust incident to the occupation of stone cutting. [G. *chalix*, gravel]

cha·lone (kā′lōn). Any of a number of mitotic inhibitors elaborated by a tissue and active only on that type of tissue, regardless of species; a reversible tissue-specific mitotic inhibitor. [G. + *chalaō*, to relax, + *-one*]

cham·ber (chăm′ber). A compartment or enclosed space. SEE ALSO camera. [L. *camera*]

   anechoic c., a soundproof environment in which reverberation is largely eliminated, for the performance of audiologic testing and research.

   anterior c. of eye, the space between the cornea anteriorly and the iris/pupil posteriorly, filled with a watery fluid (aqueous humor) and communicating through the pupil with the posterior chamber. SYN camera anterior bulbi [NA].

   aqueous c.'s, the combined anterior and posterior c.'s of the eye containing the aqueous humor.

   counting c., a standardized ruled-glass slide used for counting cells (especially erythrocytes and leukocytes) and other particulate material in a measured volume of fluid; such slides are frequently known as hemocytometers.

   hyperbaric c., a c. providing pressures greater

ch

than atmospheric, commonly used to treat decompression sickness and to provide hyperbaric oxygenation.

ionization c., a c. for detecting ionization of the enclosed gas; used for determining intensity of ionizing radiation.

posterior c. of eye, the ringlike space, filled with aqueous humor, between the iris/pupil anteriorly and the lens and ciliary body posteriorly.

pulp c., that portion of the pulp cavity which is contained in the crown or body of the tooth.

chan•cre (shang′ker). The primary lesion of syphilis, which begins at the site of infection after an interval of 10 to 30 days as a papule or area of infiltration, of dull red color, hard, and insensitive; the center usually becomes eroded or breaks down into an ulcer that heals slowly after 4 to 6 weeks. SYN hard c., hard ulcer. [Fr. indirectly from L. *cancer*]

    hard c., SYN chancre.

    soft c., SYN chancroid.

chan•cri•form (shang′kri-fōrm). Resembling chancre.

chan•croid (shang′kroyd). An infectious, painful, ragged venereal ulcer at the site of infection by *Haemophilus ducreyi,* beginning after an incubation period of 3 to 5 days; seen more commonly in men. SYN soft chancre, soft ulcer, venereal ulcer. [chancre + G. *eidos,* resemblance]

chan•croi•dal (shang-kroy′dăl). Relating to or of the nature of chancroid.

chan•crous (shang′krŭs). Characterized by having a chancre.

change (chanj). An alteration; in pathology, structural alteration of which the cause and significance is uncertain. SYN shift.

    Crooke's hyaline c., replacement of cytoplasmic granules of basophil cells of the anterior pituitary by homogeneous hyaline material; a characteristic finding in Cushing's syndrome, but usually not present in the cells of a basophil adenoma.

chapped (chapt). Having or pertaining to skin, especially of the hands, that is dry, scaly, and fissured, owing to the action of cold or to the excess rate of evaporation of moisture from the skin surface. [M.E. *chap,* to chop, split]

char•ac•ter (kar′ak-ter). An attribute in individuals that is amenable to formal and logical analysis and may be used as the basis of generalizations about classes and other statements that transcend individuality. SYN characteristic (1). [G. *charakter,* stamp, mark, fr. *charassō,* to engrave]

    acquired c., a c. developed in a plant or animal as a result of environmental influences during the individual's life.

    dominant c., an inherited c. expressed in either the homozygous or heterozygous state. SEE phenotype.

    inherited c., a single attribute of an animal or plant that is transmitted at one locus from generation to generation in accordance with Mendel's law. SEE gene.

    primary sex c.'s, the sex glands, testes or ovaries, and the accessory sex organs.

    recessive c., an inherited c. expressed in the homozygous state only.

    secondary sex c.'s, those c.'s peculiar to the male or female that develop at puberty, *e.g.,* men's beards and women's breasts.

    sex-linked c., an inherited c. determined by a gene on a gonosome. SEE gene.

char•ac•ter•is•tic (kar′ak-ter-is′tik). **1.** SYN character. **2.** Typical or distinctive of a particular disorder.

char•coal (char′kōl). Carbon obtained by heating or burning wood with restricted access of air.

char•la•tan (shar′lă-tan). A medical fraud claiming to cure disease by useless procedures, secret remedies, and worthless diagnostic and therapeutic machines. SYN quack. [Fr., fr. It. *ciarlare,* to prattle]

char•la•tan•ism (shar′lă-tan-izm). A fraudulent claim to medical knowledge; treating the sick without knowledge of medicine or authority to practice medicine.

char•ley horse (char′lē hōrs). Localized pain or muscle stiffness following a strain or contusion of a muscle. [slang]

chart. 1. A recording of clinical data relating to a patient's case. **2.** SYN curve (2). **3.** In optics, symbols of graduated size for measuring visual acuity, or test types for determining far or near vision. [L. *charta,* sheet of papyrus]

    color c., an assembly of chromatic samples used in checking color vision.

    Tanner growth c., a series of c.'s showing distribution of parameters of physical development, such as stature, growth curves, and skinfold thickness, for children by sex, age, and stages of puberty.

cheek (chēk). The side of the face forming the lateral wall of the mouth. SYN bucca [NA], gena, mala (1). [A. S. *ceáce*].

△**cheil-.** SEE cheilo-.

chei•lec•to•my, chi•lec•to•my (kī-lek′tō-mē). **1.** Excision of a portion of the lip. **2.** Chiseling away bony irregularities at osteochondral margin of a joint cavity that interfere with movements of the joint. [cheil- + G. *ektomē,* excision]

cheil•ec•tro•pi•on, chil•ec•tro•pi•on (kī-lek-trō′pē-on). Eversion of the lips or a lip. [cheil- + G. *ektropos,* a turning out]

chei•li•tis, chi•li•tis (kī-lī′tis). Inflammation of the lips or of a lip. SEE ALSO cheilosis. [cheil- + G. *-itis,* inflammation]

    angular c., inflammation and fissuring radiating from the commissures of the mouth. SYN angular stomatitis.

    contact c., inflammation of the lips resulting from contact with a primary irritant or specific allergen, including ingredients of lipsticks.

    solar c., mucosal atrophy with drying, crusting, and fissuring of the vermilion border of the lower lip, resulting from chronic exposure to sunlight; dysplastic (premalignant) changes are noted microscopically.

△**cheilo-, cheil-.** Lips. SEE ALSO chilo-, labio-. [G. *cheilos,* lip]

chei•lo•plas•ty, chi•lo•plas•ty (kī′lō-plas-tē). Plastic surgery of the lips. SYN chiloplasty. [cheilo- + G. *plastos,* formed]

chei•lor•rha•phy, chi•lor•rha•phy (kī-lōr′ă-fē). Suturing of the lip. [cheilo- + G. *rhaphē,* suture]

chei·lo·sis, chi·lo·sis (kī-lō′sis). A condition characterized by dry scaling and fissuring of the lips. SEE ALSO cheilitis. [cheil- + G. *-osis*, condition]

chei·lot·o·my, chi·lot·o·my (kī-lot′ō-mē). Incision into the lip. SYN chilotomy. [cheilo- + G. *tomē*, incision]

△**cheir-.** SEE cheiro-.

△**cheiro-, cheir-.** Hand. SEE ALSO chiro-. [G. *cheir*, a hand]

chei·rog·nos·tic, chi·rog·nos·tic (kī′rog-nos′tik). Able to distinguish between right and left, as of the hands or of which side of the body is touched. [cheiro- + G. *gnostikos*, perceptive]

chei·ro·kin·es·the·sia (kī′rō-kin-es-thē′zē-ă). The subjective sensation of movement of the hands. [cheiro- + G. *kinēsis*, movement, + *aisthēsis*, sensation]

chei·ro·kin·es·thet·ic (kī′rō-kin-es-thet′ik). Relating to cheirokinesthesia.

chei·ro·plas·ty, chi·ro·plas·ty (kī′rō-plas-tē). Rarely used term for plastic surgery of the hand. [cheiro- + G. *plastos*, formed]

chei·ro·po·dal·gia, chi·ro·po·dal·gia (kī′rō-pō-dal′jē-ă). Pain in the hands and in the feet. SYN chiropodalgia. [cheiro- + G. *pous*, foot, + *algos*, pain]

chei·ro·pom·pho·lyx, chi·ro·pom·pho·lyx (kī-rō-pom′fō-liks). SYN dyshidrosis. [cheiro- + G. *pompholyx*, a bubble, fr. *pomphos*, a blister]

chei·ro·spasm, chi·ro·spasm (kī′rō-spazm). Spasm of the muscles of the hand, as in writers' cramp. [cheiro- + G. *spasmos*, spasm]

che·late (kē′lāt). **1.** To effect chelation. **2.** Pertaining to chelation. **3.** A complex formed through chelation.

che·la·tion (kē-lā′shŭn). Complex formation involving a metal ion and two or more polar groupings of a single molecule; can be used to remove an ion from participation in biological reactions, as in the c. of Ca^{2+} of blood by EDTA, which thus acts as an anticoagulant *in vitro*. [G. *chēlē*, claw]

△**chem-.** SEE chemo-.

chem·ex·fo·li·a·tion (kem′eks-fō-lē-ā′shŭn). A chemosurgical technique to remove acne scars or treat chronic skin changes caused by sunlight.

chem·i·cal (kem′i-kăl). Relating to chemistry.

chem·i·lu·mi·nes·cence (kē′mō-loom-in-ess′ens). Light produced by chemical action usually at, or below, room temperature.

chem·ist (kem′ist). **1.** A specialist or expert in chemistry. **2.** Pharmacist (British).

chem·is·try (kem′is-trē). **1.** The science concerned with the atomic composition of substances, the elements and their interreactions, and the formation, decomposition, and properties of molecules. **2.** The chemical properties of a substance. **3.** Chemical processes. [G. *chēmeia*, alchemy]

  inorganic c., the science concerned with compounds not involving carbon-containing molecules.

  organic c., that branch of c. concerned with covalently linked atoms, centering around carbon compounds of this type; originally, and still including, the c. of natural products.

△**chemo-, chem-.** Chemistry. [G. *chēmeia*, alchemy]

che·mo·au·to·troph (kem′ō-aw′tō-trōf, kē′mō-). An organism that depends on inorganic chemicals for its energy and principally on carbon dioxide for its carbon. SYN chemolithotroph. [chemo- + G. *autos*, self, + *trophikos*, nourishing]

che·mo·au·to·tro·phic (kem′ō-aw-tō-trof′ik, kē′mo-). Pertaining to a chemoautotroph. SYN chemolithotrophic.

che·mo·cau·tery (kem′ō-kaw-ter-ē, kē′mō-). Destruction of tissue by application of a chemical substance.

che·mo·dec·to·ma (kem′ō-dek-tō′mă, kē′mō-). A relatively rare, usually benign neoplasm originating in the chemoreceptor tissue of the carotid body, glomus jugulare, and aortic bodies. Cf. paraganglioma. SYN glomus jugulare tumor. [chemo- + G. *dektēs*, receiver, fr. *dechomai*, to receive, + *-oma*, tumor]

che·mo·dec·to·ma·to·sis (kem′ō-dek-tō-mă-to′sis, kē′mō-). Multiple tumors of perivascular tissue of chemoreceptor type, which have been reported in the lungs as minute neoplasms.

che·mo·ki·ne·sis (kem′ō-ki-nē′sis, kē′mō-). Stimulation of an organism by a chemical. [chemo- + G. *kinēsis*, movement]

che·mo·ki·net·ic (kem′-ō-ki-net′ik, kē′mo-). Referring to chemokinesis.

che·mo·lith·o·troph (kem′ō-lith′ō-trōf, kē′mō-). SYN chemoautotroph.

che·mo·lith·o·tro·phic (kem′ō-lith-ō-trof′ik, kē′mō-). SYN chemoautotrophic.

che·mo·nu·cle·ol·y·sis (kem′ō-nū-klē-ol′i-sis, kē′mō-). Injection of chymopapain into the herniated nucleus pulposus of an intervertebral disc.

che·mo·or·ga·no·troph (kem′ō-ōr′gă-nō-trōf, kē′mō-). An organism that depends on organic chemicals for its energy and carbon. [chemo- + G. *organon*, organ, + *trophē*, nourishment]

che·mo·or·ga·no·tro·phic (kem′ō-ōr-gă-nō-trof′ik, kē′mō-). Pertaining to a chemoorganotroph.

che·mo·pro·phy·lax·is (kem′ō-pro′fi-lak′sis, kē′mō-). Prevention of disease by the use of chemicals or drugs.

che·mo·re·cep·tor (kem′ō-rē-sep′tŏr, kē′mō-). Any cell that is activated by a change in its chemical milieu and results in a nerve impulse. Such cells can be either 1) "transducer" cells innervated by sensory nerve fibers (*e.g.*, the gustatory cells of the taste buds); or 2) nerve cells proper, such as the olfactory receptor cells of the olfactory mucosa.

che·mo·sen·si·tive (kem-ō-sen′si-tiv, kē-mō-). Capable of perceiving changes in the chemical composition of the environment.

che·mo·sis (kē-mō′sis). Edema of the bulbar conjunctiva, forming a swelling around the cornea. [G. *chēmē*, a yawning, the cockle (from its gaping shell)]

che·mo·sur·gery (kem′ō-ser-jer-ē, kē′mō-). Excision of diseased tissue after it has been fixed *in situ* by chemical means.

  Mohs' c., a technique for removal of skin tumors by excision and microscopic examination of frozen section of thin horizontal layers of tissue, until all of the tumor is removed.

ch

che•mo•tac•tic (kem-ō-tak′tik, kē-mō-). Relating to chemotaxis.

che•mo•tax•is (kem-ō-tak′sis, kē-mo-). Movement of cells or organisms in response to chemicals. SYN chemotropism. [chemo- + G. *taxis*, orderly arrangement]

che•mo•ther•a•peu•tic (kem′ō-thār-ă-pyū′tik, kē′mō-). Relating to chemotherapy.

che•mo•ther•a•py (kem′ō-thār-ă-pē, kē′mō-). Treatment of disease by means of chemical substances or drugs; usually used in reference to neoplastic disease. SEE ALSO pharmacotherapy.

che•mot•ic (kē-mot′ic). Relating to chemosis.

che•mot•ro•pism (kĕ-mot′rōp′izm). SYN chemotaxis. [chemo- + G. *tropos*, direction, turn]

che•rub•ism (chār′ŭb-izm) [MIM*118480]. Hereditary giant cell lesions of the jaws beginning in early childhood; multilocular radiolucencies and progressive symmetric painless swelling of the jaws. [Hebr. *kerubh,* cherub]

chest. The anterior wall of the chest or thorax; the breast. SEE ALSO thorax. SYN pectus [NA]. [A.S. *cest,* a box]

    barrel c., a c. with increased anteroposterior diameter, seen in emphysema.

    flail c., flapping chest wall; condition in which three or more consecutive ribs on the same side of the chest have been fractured in at least two places, with resulting instability of the chest wall, paradoxical respiratory movements of the injured segment, and loss of respiratory efficiency.

    flat c., a c. in which the anteroposterior diameter is shorter than the average.

    funnel c., SYN *pectus* excavatum.

chi (kī). **1.** The 22nd letter of the Greek alphabet, χ. **2.** In chemistry, denotes the 22nd in a series. **3.** Symbol for the dihedral angle between the α-carbon and the side-chains of amino acids in peptides and proteins.

chi•asm (kī′azm). **1.** The crossing of intertwined chromosomes during prophase. **2.** SYN chiasma. [G. *chiasma*]

    optic c., a flattened quadrangular body in front of the tuber cinereum and infundibulum, the point of crossing or decussation of the fibers of the optic nerves; most of the fibers cross to the opposite side, some run directly forward on each side without crossing, some pass transversely on the posterior surface between the two optic tracts and others pass transversely on the anterior surface between the two optic nerves. SYN optic decussation.

chi•as•ma, pl. **chi•as•ma•ta** (kī-az′mă, kī-az′mă-tă) [NA]. **1.** A decussation or crossing of two tracts, such as tendons or nerves; **2.** A site at which two homologous chromosomes appear to have exchanged material during meiosis. SYN chiasm (2). [G. *chiasma,* two crossing lines, fr. the letter *chi,* 3]

chick•en•pox (chik′en-poks). SYN varicella.

chig•ger (chig′er). The six-legged larva of *Trombicula* species; a bloodsucking stage of mites that includes the vectors of scrub typhus.

chig•oe (chig′ō). Common name for *Tunga penetrans.*

△**chil-.** SEE chilo-.

chil•blain (chil′blān). Erythema, itching, and burning, especially of the dorsa of the fingers and toes, and of the heels, nose, and ears caused by vascular constriction on exposure to extreme cold (usually associated with high humidity); lesions can be single or multiple, and can become blistered and ulcerated. SYN erythema pernio. [chill + A.S. *blegen,* a blain]

child•bear•ing (chīld′bār-ing). Pregnancy and parturition.

child•birth (chīld′berth). The process of labor and delivery in the birth of a child. SEE ALSO birth. SYN parturition.

child•hood (chīld′hud). The period of life between infancy and puberty.

chill. 1. A sensation of cold. **2.** A feeling of cold with shivering and pallor, accompanied by an elevation of temperature in the interior of the body; usually a prodromal symptom of an infectious disease due to the presence in the blood of foreign protein or toxins. SYN rigor (2). [A.S. *cele,* cold]

△**chilo-, chil-.** Lips. SEE ALSO cheilo-. [G. *cheilos,* lip]

chi•lo•plas•ty (kī′lō-plas-tē). SYN cheiloplasty.

chi•lor•rha•phy. SEE cheilorrhaphy.

chi•lot•o•my (kī-lot′ō-mē). SYN cheilotomy.

chi•me•ra (kī-mēr′ă, ki-). **1.** The individual produced by grafting an embryonic part of one animal on to the embryo of another, either of the same or of another species. **2.** An organism that has received a transplant of genetically and immunologically different tissue, such as bone marrow. **3.** Dizygotic twins that have immunologically distinct types of erythrocytes. **4.** Sometimes used as a synonym for mosaic. Chimeric antibodies may have the Fab fragment from one species fused with the Fc fragment from another. **5.** A protein fusion in which two different proteins, usually from different species, are linked via peptide bonds; usually genetically engineered. **6.** Any macromolecule fusion formed by two or more macromolecules from different species or from different genes. [L. *Chimaera,* G. *Chimaira,* mythic monster, (lit. a she-goat)]

chi•mer•ic (kī-mēr′ik). **1.** Relating to a chimera. Cf. chimera (5). **2.** Composed of parts that are of different origin and are seemingly incompatible.

chin. The prominence formed by the anterior projection of the mandible, or lower jaw. The chin. SYN mentum [NA]. [A.S. *cin*]

chi•ral•i•ty (kī-ral′i-tē). The property of nonidentity of an object with its mirror image; used in chemistry with respect to stereochemical isomers. [G. *cheir,* hand]

△**chiro-, chir-.** The hand. SEE ALSO cheiro-. [G. *cheir,* hand]

chi•rog•nos•tic. SEE cheirognostic.

chi•ro•po•dal•gia (kī′rō-pō-dal′jē-ă). SYN cheiropodalgia.

chi•rop•o•dist (kī-rop′ō-dist). SYN podiatrist. [chiro- + G. *pous,* foot]

chi•rop•o•dy (kī-rop′ō-dē). SYN podiatry.

chi•ro•pom•pho•lyx (kī-rō-pom′fō-liks). SYN dyshidrosis.

chi•ro•prac•tic (kī-rō-prak′tik). The system that in theory uses the recuperative powers of the body and the relationship between the musculo-skeletal structures and functions of the body, particularly of the spinal column and the nervous system, in the restoration and maintenance of health. [chiro- + G. *praktikos,* efficient]

chi·ro·prac·tor (kī-rō-prak'tŏr). One who is licensed and certified to practice chiropractic.

chi·ro·spasm. SEE cheirospasm.

chi·tin (kī'tin). A polymer of *N*-acetyl-D-glucosamine similar in structure to cellulose and the second most abundant polysaccharide in nature, comprising the horny substance in the exoskeleton of beetles, crabs, certain microorganisms, etc.

chi·tin·ous (kī'tin-ŭs). Of or relating to chitin.

Chla·myd·ia (kla-mid'ē-ă). The single genus of the family Chlamydiaceae, including all the agents of the psittacosis-lymphogranuloma-trachoma disease groups. [G. *chlamys,* cloak]

C. pneumo'niae, a species that causes pneumonia and upper and lower respiratory disease.

C. psi'ttaci, organisms that resemble *C. trachomatis,* but which do not produce glycogen and are not susceptible to sulfadiazine. Various strains of this species cause psittacosis in humans and ornithosis in birds.

C. tracho'matis, spherical nonmotile organisms that accumulate glycogen and are susceptible to sulfadiazine and tetracycline; various strains of this species cause trachoma, inclusion and neonatal conjunctivitis, lymphogranuloma venereum, nonspecific urethritis, epididymitis, cervicitis, salpingitis, proctitis, and pneumonia; chief agent of bacterial sexually transmitted diseases in the U.S.; the type species of the genus *C.*

chla·myd·ia, pl. **chla·myd·i·ae** (kla-mid'ē-ă, -mid'ē-ē). A vernacular term used to refer to any member of the genus *Chlamydia.*

Chlam·y·di·a·ce·ae (kla-mid'ē-ā'sē-ē). A family of the order Chlamydiales (formerly included in the order Rickettsiales) that includes the agents of the psittacosis-lymphogranuloma-trachoma group. The family contains small, coccoid, Gram-negative bacteria that resemble rickettsiae but differ from them by possessing a unique, obligately intracellular developmental cycle; intracytoplasmic microcolonies give rise to infectious forms by division.

chla·myd·i·al (kla-mid'ē-ăl). Relating to or caused by any bacterium of the genus *Chlamydia.*

chla·myd·i·o·sis (klă-mid-ē-ō'sis). General term for diseases caused by *Chlamydia* species. SEE ALSO ornithosis, psittacosis.

chlo·as·ma (klō-az'mă). Melanoderma or melasma characterized by brown patches of irregular shape and size on the face and elsewhere; if confluent, facial patches are called the mask of pregnancy, and are associated most commonly with pregnancy and use of oral contraceptives. [G. *chloazō,* to become green]

chlor-, chloro-. 1. Green. 2. Chlorine. [G. *chloros,* green]

chlor·ac·ne (klōr-ak'nē). An occupational acne-like eruption due to prolonged contact with certain chlorinated compounds. SYN chlorine acne.

chlor·am·phen·i·col (klōr-am-fen'i-kol). D-(-)-*threo*-2,2-Dichloro-*N*-[β-hydroxy-α-(hydroxymethyl)-*p*-nitrophenethyl]acetamide; an antibiotic originally obtained from *Streptomyces venezuelae.* It is effective against a number of pathogenic microorganisms including *Staphylococcus aureus, Brucella abortus,* Friedländer's bacillus, and the organisms of typhoid, typhus, and Rocky Mountain spotted fever; active by mouth. A serious reaction resulting in marrow damage with agranulocytosis or aplastic anemia may occur.

c. acetyl transferase (CAT), a bacterial enzyme often used as a marker for examining the control of eucaryotic gene expression.

chlo·rate (klōr'āt). A salt of chloric acid.

chlor·hy·dria (klōr-hī'drē-ă). SYN hyperchlorhydria.

chlo·ride (klōr'īd). A compound containing chlorine, at a valence of −1, as in the salts of hydrochloric acid.

chlor·i·du·ria (klōr-i-dū'rē-ă). SYN chloruresis.

chlo·ri·nat·ed (klōr'in-āt-ĕd). Having been treated with chlorine.

chlo·rine (Cl) (klōr'ēn). 1. A greenish, toxic, gaseous element; atomic no. 17, atomic wt. 35.4527; a halogen used as a disinfectant and bleaching agent in the form of hypochlorite or of c. water, because of its oxidizing power. One of the bioelements. 2. The molecular form of c. (1), Cl_2. [G. *chloros,* greenish yellow]

c. group, the halogens.

chlo·rine group. See under chlorine.

chlo·rite (klōr'īt). A salt of chlorous acid; the radical ClO_2^-.

chloro-. SEE chlor-.

chlo·ro·form·ism (klōr'ō-fōrm-izm). Habitual chloroform inhalation, or the symptoms caused thereby.

chlo·ro·leu·ke·mia (klōr'ō-lū-kē'mē-ă). SYN chloroma. [chloro- + G. *leukos,* white, + *haima,* blood]

chlo·ro·ma (klō-rō'mă). A condition characterized by green masses of abnormal cells (in most instances, myeloblasts), especially in relation to the periosteum of the skull, spine, and ribs; the clinical course is similar to that of acute myeloid leukemia. SEE ALSO granulocytic *sarcoma.* SYN chloroleukemia, chloromyeloma. [chloro- + G. *-ōma,* tumor]

chlo·ro·my·e·lo·ma (klōr'ō-mī-ĕ-lō'mă). SYN chloroma. [chloro- + G. *myelos,* marrow, + *-ōma,* tumor]

chlo·ro·phyll (klōr'ō-fil). A complex of light-absorbing green pigments that, in living plants, convert light energy into oxidizing and reducing power, thus fixing CO_2 and evolving O_2; the naturally occurring forms are c. *a, b, c,* and *d.*

chlo·rop·sia (klo-rop'sē-ă). A condition in which objects appear to be colored green, as may occur in digitalis intoxication. [chloro- + G. *opsis,* eyesight]

chlo·rot·ic (klo-rot'ik). Pertaining to or having the characteristic features of chlorosis.

chlor·u·re·sis (klōr-yū-rē'sis). The excretion of chloride in the urine. SYN chloriduria, chloruria.

chlor·u·ret·ic (klōr-yū-ret'ik). Increasing the excretion of chloride in the urine.

chlor·u·ria (klōr-yū'rē-ă). SYN chloruresis.

cho·a·na, pl. **cho·a·nae** (kō-an-ă, kō'an-ē) [NA]. The opening into the nasopharynx of the nasal cavity on either side. [Mod. L. fr. G. *choane*, a funnel]

choke (chōk). To prevent respiration by compression or obstruction of the larynx or trachea. [M.E. *choken*, fr. O.E. *āceōcian*]

chokes (chōks). A manifestation of decompression sickness or altitude sickness characterized by dyspnea, coughing, and choking.

△**chol-.** SEE chole-.

cho·la·gog·ic (kō-lă-goj´ĭk). SYN chalagogue (2).

cho·la·gogue (kō´lă-gog). **1.** An agent that promotes the flow of bile into the intestine, especially as a result of contraction of the gallbladder. **2.** Relating to such an agent or effect. SYN chalagogic. [chol- + G. *agōgos*, drawing forth]

cho·lan·ge·i·tis (kō´lan-jē-ī´tis). SYN cholangitis.

chol·an·gi·ec·ta·sis (kō-lan-jē-ek´tă-sis). Dilation of the bile ducts, usually as a sequel to obstruction. [chol- + G. *angeion*, vessel, + *ektasis*, a stretching]

chol·an·gi·o·car·ci·no·ma (kō-lan´jē-ō-kar-si-nō´mă). An adenocarcinoma, primarily in intrahepatic bile ducts, composed of ducts lined by cuboidal or columnar cells that do not contain bile, with abundant fibrous stroma.

chol·an·gi·o·en·ter·os·to·my (kō-lan´jē-ō-en-ter-os´tō-mē). Surgical anastomosis of bile duct to intestine.

chol·an·gi·o·fi·bro·sis (kō-lan´jē-ō-fī-brō´sis). Fibrosis of the bile ducts. [chol- + G. *angeion*, vessel, + fibrosis]

chol·an·gi·o·gas·tros·to·my (kō-lan´jē-ō-gas-tros´tō-mē). Formation of a communication between a bile duct and the stomach. [chol- + G. *angeion*, vessel, + *gastēr*, belly, + *stoma*, mouth]

chol·an·gi·o·gram (kō-lan´jē-ō-gram). The radiographic record of the bile ducts obtained by cholangiography.

chol·an·gi·og·ra·phy (kō-lan-jē-og´ră-fē). Radiographic examination of the bile ducts. [chol- + G. *angeion*, vessel, + *graphō*, to write]

 intravenous c., c. of bile ducts opacified by hepatic secretion of an intravenously injected contrast medium.

 percutaneous transhepatic c. (PTHC), contrast radiographic examination of biliary system performed by injection through a percutaneously placed needle inserted into an intrahepatic bile duct.

chol·an·gi·ole (kō-lan´jē-ōl). A ductule occurring between a bile canaliculus and an interlobular bile duct. [chol- + G. *angeion*, vessel, + *-ole*, small]

chol·an·gi·o·li·tis (kō-lan´jē-ō-lī´tis). Inflammation of the small bile radicles or cholangioles.

chol·an·gi·o·ma (kō-lan´jē-ō´mă). A neoplasm of bile duct origin, especially within the liver; may be either benign or malignant (cholangiocarcinoma). [chol- + G. *angeion*, vessel, + *-oma*, tumor]

chol·an·gi·o·pan·cre·a·tog·ra·phy (kō-lan´jē-ō-pan-krē-ă-tog´ră-fē). Radiographic examination of the bile ducts and pancreas.

 endoscopic retrograde c. (ERCP), a method of c. using an endoscope to inspect and cannulate the ampulla of Vater, with injection of contrast

medium for radiographic examination of the pancreatic, hepatic, and common bile ducts.

chol·an·gi·os·co·py (kō-lan-jē-os´kŏ-pē). Visual examination of bile ducts utilizing a fiberoptic endoscope. [chol- + G. *angeion*, vessel, + *skopeō*, to examine]

chol·an·gi·os·to·my (kō-lan-jē-os´tō-mē). Formation of a fistula into a bile duct. [chol- + G. *angeion*, vessel, + *stoma*, mouth]

chol·an·gi·ot·o·my (kō-lan-jǐ-ot´o-mǐ). Incision into a bile duct. [chol- + G. *angeion*, vessel, + *tomē*, incision]

chol·an·gi·tis (kō-lan-jī´tis). Inflammation of a bile duct or the entire biliary tree. SYN cholangeitis. [chol- + G. *angeion*, vessel, + *-itis*, inflammation]

cho·lan·o·poi·e·sis (kō´lan-ō-poy-ē´sis). Synthesis by the liver of cholic acid or its conjugates, or of natural bile salts. [chol- + G. *anō*, upward, + *poiēsis*, making]

cho·lan·o·poi·et·ic (kō´lan-ō-poy-et´ik). Pertaining to or promoting cholanopoiesis.

cho·late (kō´lāt). A salt or ester of a cholic acid.

△**chole-, chol-, cholo-.** Bile. Cf. bili-. [G. *cholē*]

cho·le·cal·cif·er·ol (kō´lē-kal-sif´er-ol). Probably the vitamin D of animal origin found in the skin, fur, and feathers of animals and birds exposed to sunlight, and also in butter, brain, fish oils, and egg yolk. SYN vitamin D$_3$.

cho·le·cyst (kō´le-sist). SYN gallbladder.

cho·le·cys·ta·gog·ic (kō´lē-sis-tă-goj´ik). Stimulating activity of the gallbladder.

cho·le·cys·ta·gogue (kō-lē-sis´tă-gog). A substance that stimulates activity of the gallbladder. [chole- + G. *kystis*, bladder, + *agōgos*, leader]

cho·le·cys·tec·ta·sia (kō´lē-sis-tek-tā´zē-ă). Rarely used term for dilation of the gallbladder. [chole- + G. *kystis*, bladder, + *ektasis*, extension]

cho·le·cys·tec·to·my (kō´lē-sis-tek´tō-mē). Surgical removal of the gallbladder. [chole- + G. *kystis*, bladder, + *ektomē*, excision]

cho·le·cyst·en·ter·os·to·my (kō´lē-sist-en-ter-os´tō-mē). Formation of a direct communication between the gallbladder and the intestine. [chole- + G. *kystis*, bladder, + *enteron*, intestine, + *stoma*, mouth]

cho·le·cys·tic (kō-lē-sis´tik). Relating to the cholecyst, or gallbladder.

cho·le·cys·tis (kō-lē-sis´tis). SYN gallbladder. [chole- + G. *kystis*, bladder]

cho·le·cys·ti·tis (kō´lē-sis-tī´tis). Inflammation of the gallbladder. [chole- + G. *kystis*, bladder, + *-itis*, inflammation]

cho·le·cys·to·co·los·to·my (kō´lē-sis´tō-kō-los´tō-mē). Establishment of a communication between the gallbladder and the colon. SYN cholocholecystostomy. [chole- + G. *kystis*, bladder, + *kōlon*, colon, + *stoma*, mouth]

cho·le·cys·to·du·o·de·nos·to·my (kō-lē-sis´tō-dū-ō-dē-nos´tō-mē). Establishment of a direct communication between the gallbladder and the duodenum. SYN duodenocholecystostomy, duodenocystostomy (1). [chole- + G. *kystis*, bladder, + L. *duodenum* + G. *stoma*, mouth]

cho·le·cys·to·gas·tros·to·my (kō-lē-sis´tō-gas-tros´tō-mē). Establishment of a communication between the gallbladder and the stomach. [chole-

+ G. *kystis,* bladder, + *gastēr,* stomach, + *stoma,* mouth]

cho•le•cys•to•gram (kō-lē-sis'tō-gram). The radiographic record of the gallbladder obtained by cholecystography.

cho•le•cys•tog•ra•phy (kō-lē-sis-tog'ră-fē). Radiographic study of the gallbladder after oral administration of a cholecystopaque; or scintigraphic imaging of the gallbladder and central bile ducts after administration of a radiopharmaceutical secreted by the liver. [chole- + G. *kystis,* bladder, + *grapho,* to write]

cho•le•cys•to•il•e•os•to•my (kō-lē-sis'tō-il-ē-os'tō-mē). Establishment of a communication between the gallbladder and the ileum. [chole- + G. *kystis,* bladder, + ileum + G. *stoma,* mouth]

cho•le•cys•to•je•ju•nos•to•my (kō-lē-sis'tō-jē-jū-nos'tō-mē). Establishment of a communication between the gallbladder and the jejunum. [chole- + G. *kystis,* bladder, + jejunum, + G. *stoma,* mouth]

cho•le•cys•to•ki•net•ic (kō'lē-sis'tō-ki-net'ik). Promoting emptying of the gallbladder.

cho•le•cys•to•ki•nin (CCK) (kō'lē-sis-tō-kī'nin). A polypeptide hormone liberated by the upper intestinal mucosa on contact with gastric contents; stimulates contraction of the gallbladder and secretion of pancreatic juice.

cho•le•cys•to•li•thi•a•sis (kō-lē-sis'tō-li-thī'ă-sis). Presence of one or more gallstones in the gallbladder. [chole- + G. *kystis,* bladder, + *lithos,* stone]

cho•le•cys•top•a•thy (kō'lē-sis-top'ă-thē). Disease of the gallbladder.

cho•le•cys•to•pexy (kō-lē-sis'tō-pek-sē). Suture of the gallbladder to the abdominal wall. [chole- + G. *kystis,* bladder, + *pēxis,* fixation]

cho•le•cys•tor•rha•phy (kō'lē-sis-tōr'ă-fē). Suture of an incised or ruptured gallbladder. [chole- + G. *kystis,* bladder, + *rhaphē,* sewing]

cho•le•cys•to•so•nog•ra•phy (kō-lē-sis'tō-sō-nog'ră-fē). Ultrasonic examination of the gallbladder. [cholecysto- + sonography]

cho•le•cys•tos•to•my (kō-lē-sis-tos'tō-mē). Establishment of a fistula into the gallbladder. [chole- + G. *kystis,* bladder, + *stoma,* mouth]

cho•le•cys•tot•o•my (kō'lē-sis-tot'ō-mē). Incision into the gallbladder. [chole- + G. *kystis,* bladder, + *tomē,* incision]

laparoscopic c., minimally invasive surgical technique for removal of the gallbladder that uses a laparoscope for visualization of the gallbladder and placement of instruments into the abdominal cavity through trocars.

choledoch-. SEE choledocho-.

cho•le•doch•al (kō-lē-dok'ăl, kō-led'ō-kal). Relating to the common bile duct.

cho•led•o•chec•to•my (kō-led-ō-kek'tō-mē). Surgical removal of a portion of the common bile duct. [choledoch- + G. *ektomē,* excision]

cho•led•o•chi•tis (kō-led-ō-kī'tis). Inflammation of the common bile duct. [choledoch- + G. *-itis,* inflammation]

choledocho-, choledoch-. The ductus choledochus (the common bile duct). [G. *cholēdochos,* containing bile, fr. *cholē,* bile, + *dechomai,* to receive]

cho•led•o•cho•du•o•de•nos•to•my (kō-led'ō-kō-dū'ō-dē-nos'tō-mē). Formation of a communication, other than the natural one, between the common bile duct and the duodenum. [choledocho- + duodenum + G. *stoma,* mouth]

cho•led•o•cho•en•ter•os•tomy (kō-led'ō-kō-en-ter-os'tō-mē). Establishment of a communication, other than the natural one, between the common bile duct and any part of the intestine. [choledocho- + G. *enteron,* intestine, + *stoma,* mouth]

cho•led•o•cho•je•ju•nos•to•my (kō-led'ō-kō-jĕ-jū-nos'tō-mē). Anastomosis between the common bile duct and the jejunum. [choledocho- + jejuno- + G. *stoma,* mouth]

cho•led•o•cho•li•thi•a•sis (kō-led'ō-kō-lith-ī'ă-sis). Presence of a gallstone in the common bile duct.

cho•led•o•cho•li•thot•o•my (kō-led'ō-kō-li-thot'ō-mē). Incision of the common bile duct for the extraction of an impacted gallstone. [choledocho- + G. *lithos,* stone, + *tomē,* incision]

cho•led•o•cho•plas•ty (kō-led'ō-kō-plas-tē). Plastic surgery of the common bile duct. [choledocho- + G. *plastos,* formed]

cho•led•o•chor•rha•phy (kō-led-ō-kōr'ră-fē). Suturing together the divided ends of the common bile duct. [choledocho- + G. *rhaphē,* suture]

cho•led•o•chos•to•my (kō-led-ō-kos'tō-mē). Establishment of a fistula into the common bile duct. [choledocho- + G. *stoma,* mouth]

cho•led•o•chot•o•my (kō-led-ō-kot'ō-mē). Incision into the common bile duct. [choledocho- + G. *tomē,* incision]

cho•led•o•chous (kō-led'ō-kŭs). Containing or conveying bile.

cho•le•ic (kō-lē'ik). SYN cholic.

cho•le•ic ac•ids. Compounds of bile acids and sterols.

cho•le•lith (kō'lē-lith). SYN gallstone. [chole- + G. *lithos,* stone]

cho•le•li•thi•a•sis (kō'lē-li-thī'ă-sis). Presence of concretions in the gallbladder or bile ducts.

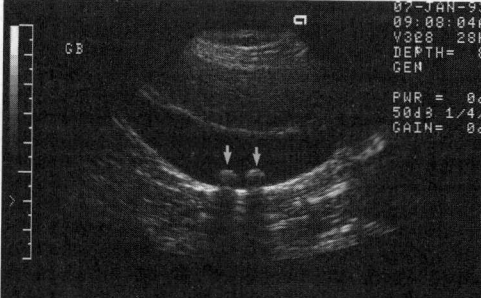

cholelithiasis: sonogram of two stones present in the gallbladder

cho•le•li•thot•o•my (kō'lē-li-thot'ō-mē). Operative removal of a gallstone. [chole- + G. *lithos,* stone, + *tomē,* incision]

cho•le•lith•o•trip•sy (kō-lē-lith'ō-trip-sē). The crushing of a gallstone. [chole- + G. *lithos,* stone, + *tripsis,* a rubbing]

cho·lem·e·sis (kō-lem′ĕ-sis). Vomiting of bile. [chole- + G. *emesis,* vomiting]

cho·le·mia (kō-lē′mē-ă). The presence of bile salts in the circulating blood. [chole- + G. *haima,* blood]

cho·lem·ic (kō-lē′mik). Relating to cholemia.

cho·le·per·i·to·ne·um (kō′lē-pār-i-tō-nē′ŭm). Bile in the peritoneum, which may lead to bile peritonitis.

cho·le·poi·e·sis (kō′lē-poy-ē′sis). Formation of bile. [chole- + G. *poiēsis,* making]

cho·le·poi·et·ic (kō′lē-poy-et′ik). Relating to the formation of bile.

chol·era (kol′er-ă). An acute epidemic infectious disease caused by the bacterium *Vibrio cholerae,* occurring primarily in Asia. A toxin elaborated by the bacterium activates the adenylate cyclase of the mucosa, causing active secretion of an isotonic fluid resulting in watery diarrhea, loss of fluid and electrolytes, and dehydration and collapse, but no gross morphologic change in the intestinal mucosa. [L. a bilious disease, fr. G. *cholē,* bile]

chol·er·a·ic (kol′er-ā′ik). Relating to cholera.

cho·le·re·sis (kō-ler-ē′sis). The secretion of bile, as opposed to the expulsion of bile, by the gallbladder. [chole- + G. *hairesis,* a taking]

cho·le·ret·ic (kol-er-et′ik). **1.** Relating to choleresis. **2.** An agent, usually a drug, that stimulates the liver to increase bile output.

chol·er·ic (kol′er-ik). SYN bilious (3).

chol·er·i·form (kol′er-i-fōrm). Resembling cholera. SYN choleroid.

chol·er·ine (kol′er-ēn). A mild form of diarrhea seen during epidemics of Asiatic cholera.

chol·er·oid (kol′er-oyd). SYN choleriform.

cho·ler·rha·gic (kō-lē-raj′ik). Referring to the flow of bile.

cho·le·sta·sia, cho·le·sta·sis (kō-les-tā′sē-ă, -les′tă-sis). An arrest in the flow of bile. [chole- + G. *stasis,* a standing still]

cho·le·stat·ic (kō-les-tat′ik). Tending to diminish or stop the flow of bile.

cho·les·te·a·to·ma (kō-les-tē-ă-tō′mă). **1.** A mass of keratinizing squamous epithelium and cholesterol in the middle ear, usually resulting from chronic otitis media, with squamous metaplasia or extension of squamous epithelium inward to line an expanding cystic cavity that may involve the mastoid and erode surrounding bone. **2.** An epidermoid cyst arising in the central nervous system in man or animals. [cholesterol + G. *stear (steat-),* tallow, + *-ōma,* tumor]

cho·les·ter·e·mia (kō-les-ter-ē′mē-ă). The presence of excessive cholesterol in the blood. SYN cholesterolemia. [cholesterol + G. *haima,* blood]

cho·les·ter·ol (kō-les′ter-ol). 5-Cholesten-3β-ol; the most abundant steroid in animal tissues; circulates in the plasma complexed to proteins of various densities and plays an important role in the pathogenesis of atheroma formation in arteries.

cho·les·ter·ol·e·mia (kō-les′ter-ol-ē′mē-ă). SYN cholesteremia. [cholesterol + G. *haima,* blood]

cho·les·ter·ol·o·sis (kō-les′ter-ol-ō′sis). **1.** A condition resulting from a disturbance in metabolism of lipids, characterized by deposits of cho-

lesterol in tissue. **2.** Cholesterol crystals in the anterior chamber of the eye, as in aphakia with associated retinal separation. SYN cholesterosis.

cho·les·ter·ol·u·ria (kō-les′ter-ol-ū′rē-ă). The excretion of cholesterol in the urine.

cho·les·ter·o·sis (kō′les-ter-ō′sis). SYN cholesterolosis.

cho·le·u·ria (kō-lē-yū′rē-ă). SYN biliuria.

cho·lic (kō′lik). Relating to the bile. SYN choleic.

cho·lic ac·id. A family of steroids comprising the bile acids (or salts), generally in conjugated form (*e.g.,* glycocholic and taurocholic acids); c. a.'s are derived from cholesterol.

cho·line (kō′lēn). Found in most animal tissues. It is included in the vitamin B complex; as acetylcholine it is essential for synaptic transmission. Several salts of choline are used in medicine.

    c. acetyltransferase, an enzyme catalyzing the condensation of choline and acetyl-coenzyme A, forming *O*-acetylcholine and coenzyme A.

    c. kinase, an enzyme that catalyzes the formation of *O*-phosphocholine and ADP from choline and ATP.

cho·lin·er·gic (kol-in-er′jik). Relating to nerve cells or fibers that employ acetylcholine as their neurotransmitter. Cf. adrenergic. [choline + G. *ergon,* work]

cho·lin·es·ter·ase (kō-lin-es′ter-ās). One of a family of enzymes capable of catalyzing the hydrolysis of acylcholines and a few other compounds. Found in cobra venom.

cho·lin·o·cep·tive (kō′lin-ō-sep′tiv). Referring to chemical sites in effector cells with which acetylcholine unites to exert its actions. Cf. adrenoceptive. [acetylcholine + L. *capio,* to take]

cho·li·no·lyt·ic (kō′lin-ō-lit′ik). Preventing the action of acetylcholine. [acetylcholine + G. *lysis,* loosening]

chol·i·no·mi·met·ic (kol′i-nō-mi-met′ik). Having an action similar to that of acetylcholine; term proposed to replace the less accurate term, parasympathomimetic. Cf. adrenomimetic. [acetylcholine + G. *mimētikos,* imitating]

cho·lin·o·re·ac·tive (kō′lin-ō-rē-ak′tiv). Responding to acetylcholine and related compounds.

chol·i·no·re·cep·tors (kol′i-nō-rē-sep′terz, -tōrz). SEE cholinergic *receptors,* under *receptor.*

cholo-. SEE chole-.

cho·lo·yl (kō′lō-il). The radical of cholic acid or cholate.

chol·ur·ia (kō-lū′rē-ă). SYN biliuria. [G. *cholē,* bile, + *ouron,* urine]

chon·dral (kon′drăl). SYN cartilaginous. [G. *chondros,* cartilage]

chon·dral·gia (kon-dral′jē-ă). SYN chondrodynia. [G. *chondros,* cartilage, + *algos,* pain]

chon·drec·to·my (kon-drek′tō-mē). Excision of cartilage. [G. *chondros,* cartilage, + *ektomē,* excision]

chon·dri·fi·ca·tion (kon′dri-fi-kā′shŭn). Conversion into cartilage. [G. *chondros,* cartilage, + L. *facio,* to make]

chondrio-. SEE chondro-.

chon·dri·tis (kon-drī′tis). Inflammation of cartilage. [G. *chondros,* cartilage, + *-itis,* inflammation]

chondro-, chondrio-. **1.** Cartilage or cartilaginous. **2.** Granular or gritty substance. [G. *chondrion*, dim. of *chondros*, groats (coarsely ground grain), grit, gristle, cartilage]

chon·dro·blast (kon′drō-blast). A dividing cell of growing cartilage tissue. SYN chondroplast. [chondro- + G. *blastos*, germ]

chon·dro·blas·to·ma (kon′drō-blas-tō′mǎ). A benign tumor arising in the epiphyses of long bones, consisting of highly cellular tissue resembling fetal cartilage.

chon·dro·cal·ci·no·sis (kon′drō-kal-si-nō′sis). Calcification of cartilage. [chondro- + calcium + G. -*osis*, condition]

chon·dro·clast (kon′drō-klast). A multinucleated giant cell involved in the resorption of calcified cartilage; morphologically identical to osteoblasts. [chondro- + G. *klastos*, broken in pieces]

chon·dro·cos·tal (kon-drō-kos′tăl). SYN costochondral. [chondro- + L. *costa*, rib]

chon·dro·cra·ni·um (kon-drō-krā′nē-ŭm). A cartilaginous skull; the cartilaginous parts of the developing skull. [chondro- + G. *kranion*, skull]

chon·dro·cyte (kon′drō-sīt). A nondividing cartilage cell; occupies a lacuna within the cartilage matrix. [chondro- + G. *kytos*, a hollow (cell)]

chon·dro·dyn·ia (kon-drō-din′ē-ǎ). Pain in cartilage. SYN chondralgia. [chondro- + G. *odynē*, pain]

chon·dro·dys·pla·sia (kon′drō-dis-plā′zē-ǎ). SYN chondrodystrophy. [chondro- + G. *dys*, bad, + *plasis*, a molding]

chon·dro·dys·tro·phia (kon′drō-dis-trō′fē-ǎ). SYN chondrodystrophy.

chon·dro·dys·tro·phy (kon-drō-dis′trō-fē) [MIM*215150]. A disturbance in the development of the cartilage of the long bones, especially of the epiphysial plates, resulting in arrested growth and dwarfism in which the extremities are abnormally short, but the head and trunk are essentially normal. SYN chondrodysplasia, chondrodystrophia. [chondro- + G. *dys*, bad, + *trophē* nourishment]

chon·dro·fi·bro·ma (kon′drō-fī-brō′mǎ). SYN chondromyxoid *fibroma*.

chon·dro·gen·e·sis (kon-drō-jen′ĕ-sis). Formation of cartilage. SYN chondrosis. [chondro- + G. *genesis*, origin]

chon·droid (kon′droyd). **1.** Resembling cartilage. SYN cartilaginoid. **2.** Uncharacteristically developed cartilage, primarily cellular with a basophilic matrix and thin or nonexistent capsules. [chondro- + G. *eidos*, resemblance]

chon·drol·y·sis (kon-drol′i-sis). Disappearance of articular cartilage as the result of disintegration or dissolution of the cartilage matrix and cells.

chon·dro·ma (kon-drō′mǎ). A benign neoplasm derived from mesodermal cells that form cartilage. [chondro- + G. -*ōma*, tumor]

chon·dro·ma·la·cia (kon′drō-mǎ-lā′shē-ǎ). Softening of any cartilage. [chondro- + G. *malakia*, softness]

c. patellae (kŏn-drō-mǎ-lā′shē-ǎ pǎ-tĕl′ē), degenerative condition in the articular cartilage of the c. caused by abnormal compression or shearing forces at the knee joint. SEE ALSO articular *cartilage.*

c. patel′lae, degenerative condition in the articular cartilage of the patella caused by abnormal compression or shearing forces at the knee joint; may cause patellalgia.

chon·dro·ma·to·sis (kon′drō-mǎ-tō′sis). Presence of multiple tumorlike foci of cartilage.

chon·dro·ma·tous (kon-drō′mǎ-tŭs). Pertaining to or manifesting the features of a chondroma.

chon·dro·mere (kon′drō-mēr). A cartilage unit of the fetal axial skeleton; a primordial cartilaginous vertebra together with its costal component. [chondro- + G. *meros*, part]

chon·dro·myx·o·ma (kon′drō-mik-sō′mǎ). SYN chondromyxoid *fibroma.*

chon·dro·os·se·ous (kon-drō-os′ē-ŭs). Relating to cartilage and bone.

chon·dro·os·te·o·dys·tro·phy (kon′drō-os′tē-ō-dis′trō-fē). Term used for a group of disorders of bone and cartilage which includes Morquio syndrome and similar conditions. SYN osteochondrodystrophy.

chon·drop·a·thy (kon-drop′ǎ-the). Any disease of cartilage. [chondro- + G. *pathos*, suffering]

chon·dro·phyte (kon′drō-fīt). An abnormal cartilaginous mass that develops at the articular surface of a bone. [chondro- + G. *phytos*, a growth]

chon·dro·plast (kon′drō-plast). SYN chondroblast. [chondro- + G. *plastos*, formed]

chon·dro·plas·ty (kon′drō-plas-tē). Reparative or plastic surgery of cartilage. [chondro- + G. *plastos*, formed]

chon·dro·po·ro·sis (kon′drō-pōr-ō′sis). Condition of cartilage in which spaces appear, either normal (in the process of ossification) or pathologic. [chondro- + L. *porosus*, porous]

chon·dro·sar·co·ma (kon′drō-sar-kō′mǎ). A malignant neoplasm derived from cartilage cells.

chon·dro·sis (kon-drō′sis). SYN chondrogenesis.

chon·dro·ster·nal (kon-drō-ster′năl). **1.** Relating to a sternal cartilage. **2.** Relating to the costal cartilages and the sternum.

chon·dro·ster·no·plas·ty (kon-drō-ster′nō-plas-tē). Surgical correction of malformations of the sternum.

chon·drot·o·my (kon-drot′ō-mē). Division of cartilage. [chondro- + G. *tomē*, a cutting]

chon·dro·xi·phoid (kon-drō-zif′oyd). Relating to the xiphoid or ensiform cartilage. [chondro- + G. *xiphos*, sword, + *eidos*, appearance]

chord-. Cord. SEE ALSO cord-. [G. *chordē*]

chor·da, pl. **chor·dae** (kōr′dă, -dē) [NA]. A tendinous or a cord-like structure. SEE ALSO cord. [L., cord]

chor′dae tendin′eae [NA], the tendinous strands running from the papillary muscles to the atrioventricular valves (mitral and tricuspid). SYN tendinous cords.

c. tym′pani [NA], a nerve given off from the facial nerve in the facial canal which passes through the posterior canaliculus of the c. tympani into the tympanic cavity, crosses over the tympanic membrane and handle of the malleus, and passes out through the anterior canaliculus of the c. tympani in the petrotympanic fissure to join the lingual branch of the mandibular nerve in the infratemporal fossa; it conveys taste sensation from the anterior two-thirds of the tongue and carries parasympathetic preganglionic fibers to the submandibular ganglion, for innervation of the submandibular and sublingual salivary glands.

chord•al (kōr′dăl). Relating to any chorda or cord, especially to the notochord.

Chor•da•ta (kor-dā′tă). The phylum that includes the vertebrates, defined by possession of: 1) a single dorsal nerve cord (the brain and spinal cord of mammals); 2) a cartilaginous rod, the notochord, which forms dorsal to the primitive gut in the early embryo, and is surrounded and replaced by the vertebral column in the subphylum vertebrata; 3) by presence at some stage in development of gill slits in the pharynx or throat. [L. *chorda*, fr. G. *chordē*, a string]

chor•date (kōr′dāt). An animal of the phylum *Chordata*.

chor•dee (kōr-dē′). **1.** Painful erection of the penis in gonorrhea or Peyronie's disease, with curvature resulting from lack of distensibility of the corpus cavernosum urethrae. **2.** Ventral curvature of the penis, most apparent on erection, as seen in hypospadias due to congenital shortness of the ventral skin and, on rare occasions, in patients with a normally situated meatus. [Fr. corded]

chor•di•tis (kōr-dī′tis). Inflammation of a cord; usually a vocal cord. [G. *chordē*, cord, + *-itis*, inflammation]

chor•do•ma (kōr-dō′mă). A rare neoplasm of skeletal tissue in adults, derived from persistent portions of the notochord. [(noto)chord + G. *-oma*, tumor]

chor•do•skel•e•ton (kōr-dō-skel′ĕ-tŏn). The part of the embryonic skeleton that develops in conjunction with the notochord.

chor•dot•o•my (kōr-dot′ō-mē). SYN cordotomy.

cho•rea (kōr-ē′ă). **1.** Irregular, spasmodic, involuntary movements of the limbs or facial muscles, often accompanied by hypotonia. **2.** SYN Sydenham's c. [L. fr. G. *choreia*, a choral dance, fr. *choros*, a dance]

   hereditary c., SYN Huntington's c.

   Huntington's c., a hereditary progressive disorder usually beginning by middle age, consisting of choreoathetosis and dementia. SYN hereditary c., Huntington's disease.

   Sydenham's c., a postinfectious c. appearing after streptococcal infection with subsequent rheumatic fever. SYN chorea (2).

cho•re•al (kōr-ē′ăl). Relating to chorea.

cho•re•ic (kōr-ē′ik). Relating to or of the nature of chorea.

cho•re•i•form (kōr-ē′i-fŏrm). SYN choreoid.

△**choreo-.** Chorea.

cho•re•o•ath•e•toid (kōr′ē-ō-ath′ĕ-toyd). Pertaining to or characterized by choreoathetosis.

cho•re•o•ath•e•to•sis (kōr′ē-ō-ath-ĕ-tō′sis). Abnormal movements of body of combined choreic and athetoid pattern. [choreo- + G. *athetos*, unfixed, + *-ōsis*, condition]

cho•re•oid (kōr′ē-oyd). Resembling chorea. SYN choreiform.

cho•re•o•phra•sia (kōr′ē-ō-frā′zē-ă). Continual repetition of meaningless phrases. [choreo- + G. *phrasis*, speaking]

△**chorio-.** Any membrane, especially that enclosing the fetus. [G. *chorion*, membrane]

cho•ri•o•ad•e•no•ma (kō′rē-ō-ad-ĕ-nō′mă). A benign neoplasm of chorion, especially with hydatidiform mole formation.

cho•ri•o•al•lan•to•ic (kō′rē-ō-al-an-tō′ik). Pertaining to the chorioallantois.

cho•ri•o•al•lan•to•is (kō′rē-ō-ă-lan′tō-is). Extraembryonic membrane formed by the fusion of the allantois with the serosa or false chorion. In mammals it forms the fetal portion of the placenta; in avian embryos it is fused with the shell.

cho•ri•o•am•ni•o•ni•tis (kō′rē-ō-am′nē-ō-nī′tis). Infection involving the chorion, amnion, and amniotic fluid; usually the placental villi and decidua are also involved.

cho•ri•o•an•gi•o•ma (kō′rē-ō-an-jē-ō′mă). Benign tumor of placental blood vessels, usually of no clinical significance. SEE ALSO chorioangiosis. [chorion + angioma]

cho•ri•o•an•gi•o•sis (kō′rē-ō-an-jē-ō′sis). An abnormal increase in the number of vascular channels in placental villi; severe c. is associated with a high incidence of neonatal death and major congenital malformations. [chorio- + G. *angeion*, vessel, + *-osis*, condition]

cho•ri•o•cap•il•la•ris (kō′rē-ō-kap-i-lā′ris). SYN choriocapillary layer.

cho•ri•o•car•ci•no•ma (kō′rē-ō-kar-si-nō′mă). A highly malignant neoplasm derived from placental syncytial trophoblasts and cytotrophoblasts; villi are not formed; neoplastic cells invade blood vessels. Hemorrhagic metastases are found in the lungs, liver, brain, and vagina; c. may follow any type of pregnancy, especially hydatidiform mole, and occasionally originates in teratoid neoplasms of the ovaries or testes. SYN chorioepithelioma.

cho•ri•o•cele (kō′rē-ō-sēl). A hernia of the choroid coat of the eye through a defect in the sclera. [chorio- + G. *kēlē*, hernia]

cho•ri•o•ep•i•the•li•o•ma (kō′rē-ō-ep-i-thē-lē-ō′mă). SYN choriocarcinoma.

△**chorioid-, chorioido-.** For words beginning thus and not found here, see choroid-, choroido-.

cho•ri•o•men•in•gi•tis (kō-rē-ō-men-in-jī′tis). A cerebral meningitis in which there is a more or less marked cellular infiltration of the meninges, often with a lymphocytic infiltration of the choroid plexuses.

   lymphocytic c., meningitis that usually occurs in young adults during the fall and winter months. Caused by a virus carried by the common house mouse. SEE ALSO lymphocytic choriomeningitis *virus*.

cho•ri•on (kō′rē-on). The multilayered, outermost fetal membrane consisting of extraembryonic somatic mesoderm, trophoblast, and, on the maternal surface, villi bathed by maternal blood; as pregnancy progresses, part of the c. becomes the definitive fetal placenta. SYN membrana serosa (1). [G. *chorion*, membrane enclosing the fetus]

cho•ri•on•ic (kō-rē-on′ik). Relating to the chorion.

cho•ri•o•ret•i•nal (kō-rē-ō-ret′i-năl). Relating to the choroid coat of the eye and the retina. SYN retinochoroid.

cho·ri·o·ret·i·ni·tis (kō'rē-ō-ret-i-nī'tis). SYN retinochoroiditis.

cho·ri·o·ret·i·nop·a·thy (kō'rē-ō-ret-i-nop'ă-thē). A primary abnormality of the choroid with extension to the retina. SEE ALSO choroidopathy.

cho·ris·ta (kō-ris'tă). A focus of tissue that is histologically normal per se, but is not normally found in the organ or structure in which it is located. Cf. choristoma. [G. *chōristos,* separated]

cho·ris·to·ma (kō-ris-tō'mă). A mass formed by maldevelopment of tissue of a type not normally found at that site. [G. *chōristos,* separated, + -ōma]

cho·roid (ko'royd). The middle vascular tunic of the eye lying between the retina and the sclera. SYN choroidea [NA]. [G. *choroeidēs,* a false reading for *chorioeidēs,* like a membrane]

cho·roi·dal (kō-roy'dăl). Relating to the choroid (choroidea).

cho·roi·dea (kō-royd'ē-ă) [NA]. SYN choroid. [SEE *choroid*]

cho·roid·i·tis (kō-roy-dī'tis). Inflammation of the choroid. Cf. choroidopathy, chorioretinopathy.

△**choroido-.** The choroid.

cho·roid·o·cy·cli·tis (kō-roy'dō-sī-klī'tis). Inflammation of the choroid coat and the ciliary body. [choroido- + G. *kyklos,* circle]

cho·roi·dop·a·thy (kō-roy-dop'ă-thē). Noninflammatory degeneration of the choroid.

cho·roid·o·ret·i·ni·tis (kō-roy'dō-ret-i-nī'tis). SYN retinochoroiditis.

△**chrom-, chromat-, chromato-, chromo-.** Color. [G. *chrōma*]

chro·maf·fin (krō'maf-in). Giving a brownish yellow reaction with chromic salts; denoting certain cells in the medulla of the adrenal glands and in paraganglia. SYN chromatophil (3), chromophil (3), chromophile, pheochrome (1). [chrom- + L. *affinis,* affinity]

chro·maf·fin·o·ma (krō-maf-in-ō'mă). A neoplasm composed of chromaffin cells occurring in the adrenal medullae, the organs of Zuckerkandl, or the paraganglia of the thoracolumbar sympathetic chain; some c.'s secrete catecholamines. SEE ALSO pheochromocytoma. SYN chromaffin tumor.

chro·maf·fin·op·a·thy (krō'maf-in-op'ă-thē). Any pathologic condition of chromaffin tissue, as in the adrenal medullae or the organs of Zuckerkandl. [chromaffin + G. *pathos,* suffering]

△**chromat-.** SEE chrom-.

chro·mat·ic (krō-mat'ik). Of or pertaining to color or colors; produced by, or made in, a color or colors.

chro·ma·tid (krō'mă-tid). Each of the two strands formed by longitudinal duplication of a chromosome that becomes visible during prophase of mitosis or meiosis; the two c.'s are joined by the still undivided centromere; after the centromere has divided at metaphase and the two c.'s have separated, each c. becomes a chromosome. [G. *chrōma,* color, + -id (2),]

chro·ma·tin (krō'ma-tin). The genetic material of the nucleus, consisting of deoxyribonucleoprotein. During mitotic division the c. condenses into chromosomes. [G. *chrōma,* color]

sex c., a small condensed mass of the inactivated X-chromosome usually located just inside the nuclear membrane of the interphase nucleus; the number of sex c. bodies per nucleus is one less than the number of X-chromosomes, hence normal males have none and normal females have one. For technical reasons only about half the cells in a preparation show typical masses. SEE ALSO Lyon *hypothesis.* SYN Barr chromatin body.

chro·ma·tism (krō'mă-tizm). **1.** Abnormal pigmentation. **2.** SYN chromatic aberration. [G. *chrōma,* color]

△**chromato-.** SEE chrom-.

chro·ma·tog·e·nous (krō-mă-toj'ĕ-nŭs). Producing color; causing pigmentation. [chromato- + -gen, producing]

chro·mat·o·gram (krō-mat'ō-gram). The graphic record produced by chromatography.

chro·mat·o·graph·ic (krō'mat-ō-graf'ik). Pertaining to chromatography.

chro·ma·tog·ra·phy (krō-mă-tog'ră-fē). The separation of chemical substances and particles by differential movement through a two-phase system. SYN absorption c. [chromato- + G. *graphō,* to write]

absorption c., SYN chromatography.

column c., a form of partition, adsorption, ion exchange, or affinity c. in which one phase is liquid (aqueous) flowing down a column packed with the second phase, a solid.

gas c., a chromatographic procedure in which the mobile phase is a mixture of gases or vapors, which are separated by their differential adsorption on a stationary phase.

gas-liquid c. (GLC), gas c., with the stationary phase being liquid rather than solid.

high-performance liquid c. (HPLC), a chromatographic technology used to separate and quantitate mixtures of substances in solution. The technique is used to measure organic compounds including steroid hormones, pesticides and poisons, toxic and carcinogenic compounds, and drugs. SYN high-pressure liquid c.

high-pressure liquid c. (HPLC), SYN high-performance liquid c.

ion exchange c., c. in which cations or anions in the mobile phase are separated by electrostatic interactions with the stationary phase. SEE ALSO *anion* exchange, cation exchange.

liquid-liquid c., c. in which both the moving phase and the stationary (or reverse-moving) phase are liquids, as in countercurrent distribution.

paper c., partition c. in which the moving phase is a liquid and the stationary phase is paper.

partition c., the separation of similar substances by repeated divisions between two immiscible liquids, so that the substances, in effect, cross the partition between the liquids in opposite directions.

thin-layer c. (TLC), c. through a thin layer of cellulose or similar inert material supported on a glass or plastic plate.

chro·ma·tol·y·sis (krō-mă-tol'i-sis). The disintegration of the granules of chromophil substance (Nissl bodies) in a nerve cell body which may occur after exhaustion of the cell or damage to its peripheral process. SYN chromolysis. [chromato- + G. *lysis,* dissolution]

chro·mat·o·lyt·ic (krō-mă-tō-lit′ik). Relating to chromatolysis.

chro·mat·o·phil (krō-mat′ō-fil). **1.** SYN chromophilic. **2.** SYN chromophil (2). **3.** SYN chromaffin.

chro·mat·o·phil·ia (krō′mă-tō-fil′ē-ă). SYN chromophilia.

chro·mat·o·phil·ic, chro·ma·toph·i·lous (krō-mă-tō-fil′ik, -tof′i-lŭs). SYN chromophilic.

chro·mat·o·pho·bia (krō′mă-tō-fō′bē-ă). SYN chromophobia.

chro·mat·o·phore (krō-mat′ō-fōr). **1.** A colored plastid, due to the presence of chlorophyll or other pigments, found in certain forms of protozoa. **2.** Melanophage; a pigment-bearing phagocyte found chiefly in the skin, mucous membrane, and choroid coat of the eye, and also in melanomas. **3.** SYN chromophore. **4.** A colored plastid in plants; *e.g.,* chloroplasts, leukoplasts, etc. [chromato- + G. *phoros,* bearing]

chro·ma·top·sia (krō-mă-top′sē-ă). A condition in which objects appear to be abnormally colored or tinged with color. SYN chromatic vision, colored vision. Cf. dyschromatopsia. [chromato- + G. *opsis,* vision]

chro·ma·tu·ria (krō-mă-tū′rē-ă). Abnormal coloration of the urine. [chromato- + G. *ouron,* urine]

chrome (krōm). Chromium, especially as a source of pigment.

chro·mes·the·sia (krō-mes-thē′zē-ă). **1.** The color sense. **2.** A condition in which non-visual stimuli, such as taste or smell, cause the perception of color. [G. *chrōma,* color, + *aisthēsis,* sensation]

chrom·hi·dro·sis (krōm-hī-drō′sis). A rare condition characterized by the excretion of sweat containing pigment. [chrom- + G. *hidros,* sweat]

apocrine c., excretion of colored sweat, usually black, from apocrine glands of the face; due to an abnormal lipochrome content of the secretion.

chro·mi·um (Cr) (krō′mē-ŭm). A metallic element, atomic no. 24, atomic wt. 51.9961. A dietary essential bioelement. ^{51}Cr (half-life of 27.70 days) is used as a diagnostic aid in many disorders (*e.g.,* gastrointestinal protein loss). [G. *chroma,* color]

△**chromo-.** SEE chrom-.

chro·mo·blast (krō′mō-blast). An embryonic cell with the potentiality of developing into a pigment cell. [chromo- + G. *blastos,* germ]

chro·mo·blas·to·my·co·sis (krō′mō-blas′tō-mī-kō′sis). A localized chronic mycosis of the skin and subcutaneous tissues characterized by skin lesions so rough and irregular as to present a cauliflower-like appearance; caused by dematiaceous fungi such as *Phialophora verrucosa, P. dermatitidis, Fonsecaea pedrosoi, F. compacta,* and *Cladosporium carrionii;* fungal cells resembling copper pennies form rounded sclerotic bodies in tissue, with epidermal hyperplasia and intraepidermal microabscesses. SYN chromomycosis. [chromo- + G. *blastos,* germ, + *mykē,* fungus, + *-osis,* condition]

chro·mo·cys·tos·co·py (krō′mō-sis-tos′kŏ-pē).

SYN cystochromoscopy. [chromo- + G. *kystis,* bladder, + *skopeō,* to view]

chro·mo·cyte (krō′mō-sīt). Any pigmented cell, such as a red blood corpuscle. [chromo- + G. *kytos,* cell]

chro·mo·gen (krō′mō-jen). **1.** A substance, itself without definite color, that may be transformed into a pigment. **2.** A microorganism that produces pigment.

chro·mo·gen·e·sis (krō-mō-jen′ĕ-sis). Production of coloring matter or pigment. [chromo- + G. *genesis,* production]

chro·mo·gen·ic (krō-mō-jen′ik). **1.** Denoting a chromogen. **2.** Relating to chromogenesis.

chro·mol·y·sis (krō-mol′i-sis). SYN chromatolysis.

chro·mo·mere (krō′mō-mēr). **1.** A condensed segment of a chromonema; densely staining bands visible in chromosomes under certain conditions. **2.** SYN granulomere. [chromo- + G. *meros,* a part]

chro·mo·my·co·sis (krō′mō-mī-kō′sis). SYN chromoblastomycosis. [chromo- + G. *mykēs,* fungus, + *-osis,* condition]

chro·mo·ne·ma, pl. chro·mo·ne·ma·ta (krō-mō-nē′mă, -ma-tă). The coiled filament in which the genes are located, which extends the entire length of a chromosome. [chromo- + G. *nēma,* thread]

chro·mo·phil, chro·mo·phile (krō′mō-fil, krō′mō-fīl). **1.** SYN chromophilic. **2.** A cell or any histologic element that stains readily. SYN chromatophil (2). **3.** SYN chromaffin. [chromo- + G. *phileō,* to love]

chro·mo·phil·ia (krō-mō-fil′ē-ă). The property possessed by most cells of staining readily with appropriate dyes. SYN chromatophilia. [chromo- + G. *phileō,* to love]

chro·mo·phil·ic, chro·moph·i·lous (krō-mō-fil′ik, -mof′i-lŭs). Staining readily; denoting certain cells and histologic structures. SYN chromatophil (1), chromatophilic, chromatophilous, chromophil (1), chromophile.

chro·mo·phobe (krō′mō-fōb). Resistant to stains, staining with difficulty or not at all; denoting certain degranulated cells in the anterior lobe of the pituitary gland. SYN chromophobic. [chromo- + G. *phobos,* fear]

chro·mo·pho·bia (krō-mō-fō′bē-ă). **1.** Resistance to stains on the part of cells and tissues. **2.** A morbid dislike of colors. SYN chromatophobia. [chromo- + G. *phobos,* fear]

chro·mo·pho·bic (krō-mō-fō′bik). SYN chromophobe. [chromo- + *phobos,* fear]

chro·mo·phore (krō′mō-fōr). The atomic grouping upon which the color of a substance depends. SYN chromatophore (3). [chromo- + G. *phoros,* bearing]

chro·mo·phor·ic, chro·moph·o·rous (krō-mō-fōr′ik, -mof′ŏr-ŭs). **1.** Relating to a chromophore. **2.** Producing or carrying color; denoting certain microorganisms.

chro·mo·som·al (krō′mō-sō′măl). Pertaining to chromosomes.

chro·mo·som·al map. A formal, stylized representation of the karyotype and of the positioning and ordering on it of those loci that have been localized by any of several mapping methods.

chro·mo·some (krō'mō-sōm). One of the bodies (normally 46 in humans) in the cell nucleus that is the bearer of genes, has the form of a delicate chromatin filament during interphase, contracts to form a compact cylinder segmented into two arms by the centromere during metaphase and anaphase stages of cell division, and is capable of reproducing its physical and chemical structure through successive cell divisions. [chromo- + G. *sōma*, body]

   acrocentric c., a c. with the centromere placed very close to one end so that the short arm is very small, often with a satellite.

   bivalent c.'s, a pair of c.'s temporarily united.

   fragile X c., an X c. with a fragile site near the end of the long arm, resulting in the appearance of an almost detached fragment; frequently associated with X-linked mental retardation.

   heterotypical c., SYN allosome.

   Philadelphia c., an abnormal minute c. Formed by a rearrangement of c.'s 9 and 22; found in cultured leukocytes of many patients with chronic granulocytic leukemia.

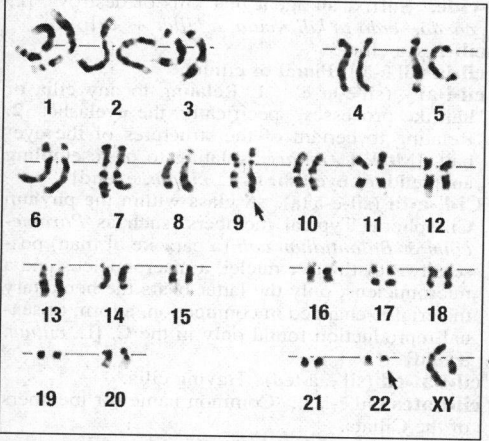

Philadelphia chromosome translocation: karyotype from a patient with CML showing the Philadelphia chromosome translocation, t(9;22)(q34;q11); the Philadelphia chromosome is chromosome number 22

   homologous c.'s, members of a single pair of c.'s.

   metacentric c., a c. with a centrally placed centromere that divides the c. into two arms of approximately equal length.

   mitochondrial c., the DNA component of mitochondria, the chief function of which is synthesis of adenosine triphosphate and the management of cellular energy.

   ring c., a c. with ends joined to form a circular structure. The ring form is abnormal in humans but the normal form of the c. in certain bacteria.

   sex c.'s, the pair of c.'s responsible for sex determination. In humans and most animals, the sex c.'s are designated X and Y; females have two X c.'s, males have one X and one Y c.

   X c., Y c., SEE sex c.'s.

chro·mo·some map·ping. The process of determining the position of loci on specific chromosomes and constructing a diagram of each chromosome showing the relative positions of loci; techniques include family studies with linkage analysis, somatic cell hybridization, and chromosome deletion mapping.

chro·mo·some walk·ing. A process of extending a genetic map by successive hybridization steps.

chro·nax·ie (krō'nak-sē). A measurement of excitability of nervous or muscular tissue; the shortest duration of an effective electrical stimulus having a strength equal to twice the minimum strength required for excitation. [G. *chronos*, time, + *axia*, value]

chron·ic (kron'ik). **1.** Referring to a health-related state, lasting a long time. **2.** Referring to exposure, prolonged or long-term, sometimes meaning also low-intensity. **3.** The U.S. National Center for Health Statistics defines a chronic condition as one of three months' duration or longer. [G. *chronos*, time]

chrono-. Time. [G. *chronos*]

chro·no·bi·ol·o·gy (kron'ō-bī-ol'ō-jē). That aspect of biology concerned with the timing of biological events, especially repetitive or cyclic phenomena. [chrono- + G. *bios*, life, + *logos*, study]

chron·o·on·col·o·gy (kron'ō-on-kol'ō-jē). The study of the influence of biological rhythms on neoplastic growth. [G. *chronos*, time, + oncology]

chro·no·tro·pic (kron'ō-trop'ik). Affecting the rate of rhythmic movements such as the heartbeat.

chro·not·ro·pism (kron-ot'rō-pizm). Modification of the rate of a periodic movement, *e.g.*, the heartbeat, through some external influence. [chrono- + G. *tropē*, turn, change]

chrys-, chryso-. Gold; corresponds to L. *auro-*. [G. *chrysos*]

chry·si·a·sis (kri-sī'ă-sis). A permanent slate-gray discoloration of the skin and sclera resulting from deposition of gold in the connective tissue of the skin and eye together with increased melanin formation after administration of gold. SYN chrysoderma. [G. *chrysos*, gold]

chrys·o·der·ma (kris-ō-der'mă). SYN chrysiasis. [G. *chrysos*, gold, + *derma*, skin]

Chrys·ops (kris'ops). The deerfly, a genus of biting flies with about 80 North American species; *C. discalis* is a vector of *Francisella tularensis* in the U.S.; *C. dimidiatus* and *C. silaceus* are the principal vectors of *Loa loa* in west Africa. [G. *chrysos*, gold, + *ōps*, eye]

chrys·o·ther·a·py (kris-ō-thār'ă-pē). Treatment of disease by the administration of gold salts. [G. *chrysos*, gold]

chyl-. SEE chylo-, chyle. [G. *chylos*, juice, chyle]

chy·lan·gi·o·ma (kī-lan-jē-ō'mă). A mass of prominent, dilated lacteals and larger intestinal lymphatic vessels. [chyl- + G. *angeion*, vessel, + *-ōma*, tumor]

chyle (kīl). A turbid white or pale yellow fluid

taken up by the lacteals from the intestine during digestion and carried by the lymphatic system via the thoracic duct into the circulation. [G. *chylos,* juice]

chy·le·mia (kī-lē′mē-ă). The presence of chyle in the circulating blood. [chyl- + G. *haima,* blood]

chy·li·fac·tion (kī-li-fak′shŭn). SYN chylopoiesis. [chyl- + L. *facio,* to make]

chy·li·fac·tive (kī-li-fak′tiv). SYN chylopoietic.

chy·lif·er·ous (kī-lif′er-ŭs). Conveying chyle. SYN chylophoric. [chyl- + L. *fero,* to carry]

chy·li·fi·ca·tion (kī′li-fi-kā′shŭn). SYN chylopoiesis.

chy·li·form (kī′li-fōrm). Resembling chyle.

⌂**chylo-, chyl-.** Chyle. [G. *chylos,* juice.]

chy·lo·cele (kī′lō-sēl). A cystlike lesion resulting from the effusion of chyle into the tunica vaginalis propria and cavity of the tunica vaginalis testis. [chylo- + G. *kēlē,* tumor]

chy·lo·der·ma (kī-lō-der′mă). SYN *elephantiasis scroti.* [chylo- + G. *derma,* skin]

chy·lo·me·di·as·ti·num (kī′lō-mē-dē-as-tī′nŭm). Abnormal presence of chyle in the mediastinum.

chy·lo·mi·cron, pl. **chy·lo·mi·cra, chy·lo·mi·crons** (kī-lō-mi′kron, -mī′kră, -mi′kronz). A droplet of reprocessed lipid synthesized in epithelial cells of the small intestine; the least dense of the plasma lipoproteins. [chylo- + G. *micros,* small]

chy·lo·mi·cro·ne·mia (kī′lō-mī-krō-nē′mē-ă). The presence of chylomicrons, especially an increased number, in the circulating blood, as in type I familial hyperlipoproteinemia.

chy·lo·per·i·car·di·um (kī′lō-pār-i-kar′dē-ŭm). A milky pericardial effusion resulting from obstruction of the thoracic duct, from trauma, or of idiopathic origin.

chy·lo·per·i·to·ne·um (kī′lō-pār-i-tō-nē′ŭm). SYN chylous *ascites.*

chy·lo·phor·ic (kī-lō-fōr′ik). SYN chyliferous. [chylo- + G. *phoros,* bearing]

chy·lo·pneu·mo·tho·rax (kī′lō-nū-mō-thōr′aks). Free chyle and air in the pleural space.

chy·lo·poi·e·sis (kī′lō-poy-ē′sis). Formation of chyle in the intestine. SYN chylifaction, chylification. [chylo- + G. *poiesis,* a making]

chy·lo·poi·et·ic (kī′lō-poy-et′ik). Relating to chylopoiesis. SYN chylifactive.

chy·lo·sis (kī-lō′sis). The formation of chyle from the food in the intestine, its digestion and absorption by the intestinal mucosa, and its mixture with the blood and conveyance to the tissues.

chy·lo·tho·rax (kī-lō-thōr′aks). An accumulation of milky chylous fluid in the pleural space, usually on the left.

chy·lous (kī′lŭs). Relating to chyle.

chy·lu·ria (kī-lū′rē-ă). The passage of chyle in the urine; a form of albiduria. [chyl- + G. *ouron,* urine]

chyme (kīm). The semifluid mass of partly digested food passed from the stomach into the duodenum. SYN pulp (3). [G. *chymos,* juice]

chy·mi·fi·ca·tion (kī-mi-fi-kā′shŭn). SYN chymopoiesis. [G. *chymos,* juice, + L. *facio,* to make]

chy·mo·poi·e·sis (kī′mō-poy-ē′sis). The production of chyme; the physical state of food (semi-

fluid) brought about by digestion in the stomach. SYN chymification. [G. *chymos,* juice, chyme, + *poiesis,* a making]

chy·mo·sin (kī′mō-sin). A proteinase structurally homologous with pepsin; the milk-curdling enzyme obtained from the stomach of the calf. SYN rennin.

chy·mo·tryp·sin (kī-mō-trip′sin). A serine proteinase of the gastrointestinal tract, synthesized in the pancreas as chymotrypsinogen; used in the treatment of inflammation and edema associated with trauma and to facilitate intracapsular cataract extraction.

chy·mo·tryp·sin·o·gen (kī′mō-trip-sin′ō-jen). The precursor of chymotrypsin. Converted to π-chymotrypsin by the action of trypsin.

Ci curie.

cic·a·trec·to·my (sik-ă-trek′tō-mē). Excision of a scar. [L. *cicatrix,* scar, + G. *ektomē,* excision]

cic·a·tri·ces (si-kā′tri-sēz). Plural of cicatrix.

cic·a·tri·cial (sik-ă-trish′ăl). Relating to a scar.

cic·a·trix, pl. **cic·a·tri·ces** (sik′ă-triks, si-kā′triks; sik-ă-trī′sēz). A scar. [L.]

cic·a·tri·za·tion (sik′ă-tri-zā′shŭn). **1.** The process of scar formation. **2.** The healing of a wound otherwise than by first intention.

-cide. Suffix: an agent that kills or destroys. [L. *caedo, -cido* to kill, *-cida, a killer + -al*]

⌂**cili-.** SEE cilio-.

cil·ia (sil′ē-ă). Plural of cilium.

cil·i·ary (sil′ē-ar-ē). **1.** Relating to any cilia or hairlike processes, specifically, the eyelashes. **2.** Relating to certain of the structures of the eyeball. [Mod. L. *ciliaris,* relating to or resembling an eyelid, or eyelash, fr. L. *cilium,* eyelid]

Ci·li·a·ta (sil-ē-ā′tă). A class within the phylum Ciliophora. Typical members, such as *Paramecium* or *Balantidium coli* (a parasite of man) possess two distinctive nuclei, a macronucleus and a micronucleus; only the latter bears the hereditary material exchanged in conjugation, a form of sexual reproduction found only in the C. [L. *cilium,* eyelid]

cil·i·at·ed (sil′ē-ā-ted). Having cilia.

cil·i·ates (sil′ē-āts). Common name for members of the Ciliata.

cil·i·ec·to·my (sil-ē-ek′tō-mē). SYN cyclectomy.

⌂**cilio-, cili-.** Cilia or ciliary, in any sense; eyelashes. [L. *cilium,* eyelid (eyelash)]

cil·i·o·ret·i·nal (sil′ē-ō-ret′i-năl). Pertaining to the ciliary body and the retina.

cil·i·o·scle·ral (sil′ē-ō-sklē′răl). Relating to the ciliary body and the sclera.

cil·i·o·spi·nal (sil′ē-ō-spī′nal). Relating to the ciliary body and the spinal cord; denoting in particular the ciliospinal *center.*

cil·i·um, pl. **cil·ia** (sil′ē-ŭm, -ă). **1** [NA]. SYN eyelash. **2.** A motile extension of a cell surface, *e.g.,* of certain epithelial cells, containing nine longitudinal double microtubules arranged in a peripheral ring, together with a central pair. [L. an eyelid]

Ci·mex lec·tu·lar·i·us (sī′meks lek-tyū-lār-ē-ŭs). Member of the family Cimicidae, with a flat, reddish-brown wingless body, prominent lateral eyes, and a three-jointed beak; it produces a characteristic pungent odor from thoracic stink glands and is an abundant pest in human abodes, especially in the tropics under poor sanitary conditions. Although the bedbug's bite produces characteristic linear groups of pruritic wheals with a central hemorrhagic punctum, human disease has not been proved to be transmitted by it, with the possible exception of hepatitis B. SYN bedbug. [L. *cimex,* bug, L. *lectulus,* a bed]

CIN cervical intraepithelial *neoplasia.*

△**cin-.** SEE cine-.

△**cine-, cin-.** Movement, usually relating to motion pictures. [G. *kineō,* to move]

cin•e•an•gi•o•car•di•og•ra•phy (sin'ē-an'jē-ō-kar-dē-og'ră-fē). Motion pictures of the passage of a contrast medium through chambers of the heart and great vessels.

cin•e•flu•o•rog•ra•phy (sin'ĕ-flūr-og'ră-fē). SYN cineradiography.

cin•e•plas•tics (sin-ĕ-plas'tiks). SYN cineplastic *amputation.*

cin•e•ra•di•og•ra•phy (sin'ĕ-rā-dē-og'ră-fē). Radiography of an organ in motion, *e.g.,* the heart, the gastrointestinal tract. SYN cinefluorography.

ci•ne•rea (si-nē'rē-ă). The gray matter of the brain and other parts of the nervous system. [L. fem. of *cinereus,* ashy, fr. *cinis,* ashes]

ci•ne•re•al (si-nē'rē-ăl). Relating to the gray matter of the nervous system.

cin•gu•late (sin'gyū-lāt). Relating to a cingulum.

cin•gu•lec•to•my (sin-gyū-lek'tō-mē). SYN cingulotomy. [cingulum + G. *ektomē,* excision]

cin•gu•lot•o•my (sin-gyū-lot'ō-mē). Electrolytic destruction of the anterior cingulate gyrus and callosum. SYN cingulectomy. [cingulum + G. *tomē,* a cutting]

cin•gu•lum, gen. **cin•'gu•li,** pl. **cin•gu•la** (sin' gyū-lŭm, -lē, -lă) [NA]. **1.** SYN girdle. **2.** A well-marked fiber bundle passing longitudinally in the white matter of the cingulate gyrus; the bundle extends from the region of the anterior perforated substance back over the dorsal surface of the corpus callosum; behind the latter's splenium it curves down and then forward in the white matter of the parahippocampal gyrus; composed largely of fibers from the anterior thalamic nucleus to the cingulate and parahippocampal gyri, it also contains association fibers connecting these gyri with the frontal cortex, and their various subdivisions with each other. [L. girdle, fr. *cingo,* to surround]

cir•ca•di•an (ser-kā'dē-ăn). Relating to biologic variations or rhythms with a cycle of about 24 hours. Cf. infradian, ultradian. [L. *circa,* about, + *dies,* day]

cir•ci•nate (ser'si-nāt). Circular; ring-shaped. [L. *circinatus,* made round, pp. of *circino,* to make round, fr. *circinus,* a pair of compasses]

cir•cle (ser'kl). **1.** A ring-shaped structure or group of structures. **2.** A line or process with every point equidistant from the center. [L. *circulus*]

  arterial c. of cerebrum, an anastomotic "circle" of arteries (roughly pentagonal in outline) at the base of the brain, formed, sequentially and in anterior to posterior direction, by the anterior communicating artery, the two anterior cerebral, the two internal carotid, the two posterior com-

municating, and the two posterior cerebral arteries.

  Haller's c., (1) SYN vascular c. of optic nerve. **(2)** SYN areolar venous *plexus.*

  vascular c. of optic nerve, a network of branches of the short ciliary arteries on the sclera around the point of entrance of the optic nerve. SYN Haller's c. (1).

  vicious c., (1) the mutually accelerating action of two independent diseases or phenomena, or of a primary and secondary affection; **(2)** the passage of food, after a gastroenterostomy, from the artificial opening through the intestinal loop by antiperistaltic action and back into the stomach again by the pyloric orifice, or the reverse.

cir•cu•la•tion (ser-kyū-lā'shŭn). Movements in a circle, or through a circular course, or through a course which leads back to the same point; usually referring to blood c. unless otherwise specified. [L. *circulatio*]

  collateral c., c. maintained in small anastomosing vessels when the main vessel is obstructed.

  compensatory c., c. established in dilated collateral vessels when the main vessel of the part is obstructed.

  enterohepatic c., c. of substances such as bile salts which are absorbed from the intestine and carried to the liver, where they are secreted into the bile and again enter the intestine.

  extracorporeal c., the c. of blood outside of the body through a machine that temporarily assumes an organ's functions, *e.g.,* through a heart-lung machine or artificial kidney.

  placental c., the c. of blood through the placenta during intrauterine life, serving the needs of the fetus for aeration, absorption, and excretion; also, maternal circulation through the intervillous space of the placenta.

  portal c., (1) c. of blood to the liver from the small intestine, the right half of the colon, and the spleen via the portal vein; sometimes specified as the hepatic portal c.; **(2)** more generally, any part of the systemic circulation in which blood draining from the capillary bed of one structure flows through a larger vessel(s) to supply the capillary bed of another structure before returning to the heart; *e.g.,* the hypothalamohypophysial portal system.

  portal hypophysial c., a capillary network that carries hormones from the hypothalamus to their sites of action in the anterior hypophysis. SEE portal c., hypophysis, hypothalamus. SYN hypothalamohypophysial portal system.

  ▮**pulmonary c.,** the passage of blood from the right ventricle through the pulmonary artery to the lungs and back through the pulmonary veins to the left atrium.

  systemic c., the c. of blood through the arteries, capillaries, and veins of the general system, from the left ventricle to the right atrium.

cir•cu•la•to•ry (ser'kyū-lă-tō-rē). **1.** Relating to the circulation. **2.** SYN sanguiferous.

cir•cu•lus, gen. and pl. **cir•cu•li** (ser'kyū-lŭs, -lī). **1** [NA]. Any ringlike structure. **2.** A circle formed by connecting arteries, veins, or nerves. [L. dim. of *circus,* circle]

△**circum-.** A circular movement, or a position sur-

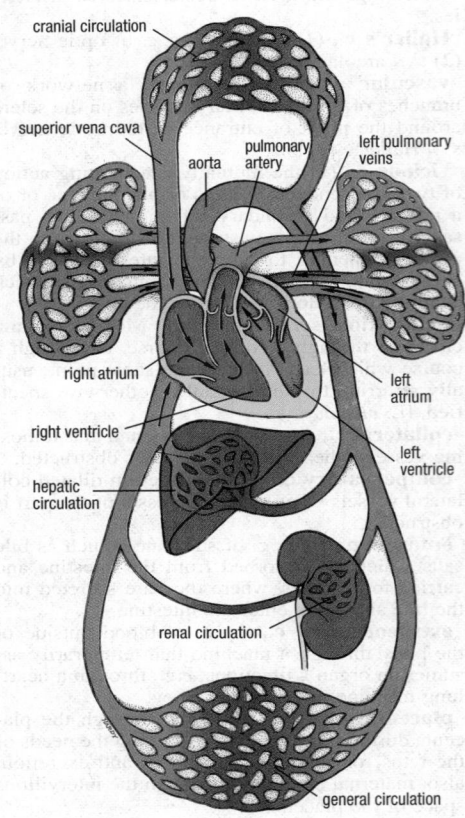

cranial circulation

superior vena cava

pulmonary artery

aorta

left pulmonary veins

right atrium

left atrium

right ventricle

left ventricle

hepatic circulation

renal circulation

general circulation

pulmonary circulation: through the lungs, from the right ventricle to the left atrium

systemic circulation: through the body, from the left ventricle to the right atrium

rounding the part indicated by the word to which it is joined. SEE ALSO peri-. [L. around]

cir·cum·ar·tic·u·lar (ser′kŭm-ar-tik′yū-lăr). Surrounding a joint. [circum- + L. *articulus,* joint]

cir·cum·ax·il·lary (ser-kŭm-ak′si-lār-ē). Around the axilla.

cir·cum·cise (ser′kŭm-sīz). To perform circumcision, especially of the prepuce.

cir·cum·ci·sion (ser-kŭm-sizh′ŭn). **1.** Operation to remove part or all of the prepuce. SYN peritomy (2). **2.** Cutting around an anatomical part (*e.g.,* the areola of the breast). SYN peritectomy (2). [L. *circumcido,* to cut around, fr. *circum,* around, + *caedo,* to cut]

cir·cum·duc·tion (ser-kŭm-dŭk′shŭn). **1.** Movement of a part, *e.g.,* an extremity, in a circular direction. **2.** SYN cycloduction. [circum- + L. *duco,* pp. *ductus,* to draw]

cir·cum·fer·ence (c) (ser-kŭm′fer-ens). The

outer boundary, especially of a circular area. [L. *circumferentia, a bearing around*]

cir·cum·flex (ser′kŭm-fleks). Describing an arc of a circle or that which winds around something; denotes several anatomical structures: arteries, veins, nerves, and muscles. [circum- + L. *flexus,* to bend]

cir·cum·or·bit·al (ser-kŭm-ōr′bi-tăl). Around the orbit. SYN periorbital (2).

cir·cum·scribed (ser′kŭm-skrībd). Bounded by a line; limited or confined. [circum- + L. *scribo,* to write]

cir·cum·stan·ti·al·i·ty (ser′kŭm-stan-shē-al′i-tē). A disturbance in the thought process in which one gives an excessive amount of detail that is often tangential, elaborate, and irrelevant, to avoid making a direct statement or answer to a question; observed in schizophrenia and in obsessional disorders. Cf. tangentiality. [L. *circum-sto,* pr. p. *-stans,* to stand around]

cir·cum·val·late (ser-kŭm-val′āt). Denoting a structure surrounded by a wall, as the c. (vallate) papillae of the tongue. [circum- + L. *vallum,* wall]

cir·cum·vo·lute (ser-kŭm-vol′ūt). Twisted around; rolled about. [L. *circum-volvo,* pp. *-volutus,* to roll around]

cir·rho·sis (sir-rō′sis). Progressive disease of the liver characterized by diffuse damage to hepatic parenchymal cells, with nodular regeneration, fibrosis, and disturbance of normal architecture; associated with failure in the function of hepatic cells and interference with blood flow in the liver, frequently resulting in jaundice, portal hypertension, ascites, and ultimately hepatic failure. [G. *kirrhos,* yellow (liver), + *-osis,* condition]

alcoholic c., c. that frequently develops in chronic alcoholism, characterized in an early stage by enlargement of the liver due to fatty change with mild fibrosis, and later by Laënnec's c. with contraction of the liver.

biliary c., c. due to biliary obstruction, which may be a primary intrahepatic disease or secondary to obstruction of extrahepatic bile ducts; the latter may lead to cholestasis and proliferation in small bile ducts with fibrosis, but marked disturbance of the lobular pattern is infrequent.

cardiac c., an extensive fibrotic reaction within the liver as a result of chronic constrictive pericarditis or prolonged congestive heart failure; true c. with fibrous bridging of lobules is unusual.

cholangiolitic c., a form of c. in which there is diffuse inflammation of the cholangioles, with inflammation, fibrosis, and regeneration; characterized by chronicity, relapses, and febrile episodes.

fatty c., early nutritional c., especially in alcoholics, in which the liver is enlarged by fatty change, with mild fibrosis.

Laënnec's c., c. in which normal liver lobules are replaced by small regeneration nodules, sometimes containing fat, separated by a fairly regular framework of fine fibrous tissue strands (hob-nail liver); usually due to chronic alcoholism. Can progress to severe impairment of liver function, portal hypertension with ascites and esophageal varices, and life-threatening complications.

necrotic c., SYN postnecrotic c.

posthepatitic c., SYN active chronic *hepatitis.*

postnecrotic c., post-necrotic c., c. characterized by necrosis involving whole hepatic lobules, with collapse of the reticular framework to form large scars; regeneration nodules are also large; may follow viral or toxic necrosis, or develop as a result of ischemic necrosis. SYN necrotic c.

toxic c., c. of the liver resulting from chronic poisoning or carbon tetrachloride.

cir·rhot·ic (sir-rot′ik). Relating to or affected with cirrhosis or advanced fibrosis.

CIS *carcinoma in situ.*

△**cis-.** **1.** Prefix meaning on this side, on the near side; opposite of trans-. **2.** GENETICS a prefix denoting the location of two or more genes on the same chromosome of a homologous pair, in coupling. **3.** ORGANIC CHEMISTRY a form of geometric isomerism in which similar functional groups are attached on the same side of the plane that includes two adjacent, fixed carbon atoms in a ring structure. **4.** ORGANIC CHEMISTRY a form of geometric isomerism with regard to carbon-carbon double bonds. Identical functional groups on the same side of the double bond are cis-. When the four moieties attached to the carbons of the double bond are all different, then the E/Z nomenclature has to be followed. [L.]

cis·tern (sis′tern). SYN cisterna. [L. *cisterna*]

cis·ter·na, gen. and pl. **cis·ter·nae** (sis-ter′nă, -ter′nē). **1** [NA]. Any cavity or enclosed space serving as a reservoir, especially for chyle, lymph, or cerebrospinal fluid. **2.** An ultramicroscopic space occurring between the membranes of the flattened sacs of the endoplasmic reticulum, the Golgi complex, or the two membranes of the nuclear envelope. SYN cistern. [L. an underground cistern for water, fr. *cista,* a box]

cis·ter·nal (sis-ter′năl). Relating to a cisterna.

cis·tern·og·ra·phy (sis′tern-og′ră-fē). The radiographic study of the basal cisterns of the brain after the subarachnoid introduction of contrast medium, or a radiopharmaceutical with a suitable detector. [cisterna + G. *graphō,* to write]

cis·tron (sis′tron). **1.** The smallest functional unit of heritability; a length of chromosomal DNA associated with a single biochemical function. In modern molecular biology, the c. is essentially equivalent to the structural gene. **2.** The genetic unit defined by the *cis/trans* test. [*cis tr*-ans + -on]

cit·rate (sit′rāt, sī′trāt). A salt or ester of citric acid; used as anticoagulants because they bind calcium ions.

cit·ric ac·id (sit′rik). The acid of citrus fruits, widely distributed in nature and a key intermediate in intermediary metabolism.

ci·trul·line (sit′rul-ēn). An amino acid formed from L-ornithine in the course of the urea cycle as well as a product in nitric oxide biosynthesis; also found in watermelon (*Citrullus vulgaris*) and in casein. Elevated in individuals with a deficiency of argininosuccinate synthetase or argininosuccinate lyase.

cit·rul·li·nu·ria (sit′rŭl-i-nū′rē-ă). Enhanced urinary excretion of citrulline; a manifestation of citrullinemia.

Cl chlorine.

clad·o·spo·ri·o·sis (klad′ō-spō-rē-ō′sis). Infection with a fungus of the genus *Cladosporium.*

Clad·o·spo·ri·um (klad-ō-spōr′i-ŭm). A genus of fungi having dematiaceous or dark-colored conidiophores with oval or round spores, commonly isolated in soil or plant residues. [G. *klados,* a branch, + *sporos,* seed]

clair·voy·ance (klār-voy′ans). Perception of objective events (past, present, or future) not ordinarily discernible by the senses; a type of extrasensory perception. [Fr.]

clamp (klamp). An instrument for compression of a structure. Cf. forceps. [M.E., fr. Middle Dutch *klampe*]

cla·rif·i·cant (kla-rif′i-kant). An agent that makes a turbid liquid clear. [L. *clarus,* clear, + *facio,* to make]

clasp. 1. A part of a removable partial denture that acts as a direct retainer and/or stabilizer for the denture by partially surrounding or contacting an abutment tooth. **2.** A direct retainer of a removable partial denture, usually consisting of two arms joined by a body which connects with an occlusal rest; at least one arm of a clasp usually terminates in the infrabulge (gingival convergence) area of the tooth enclosed.

class (klas). In biologic classification, the next division below the phylum (or subphylum) and above the order. [L. *classis,* a class, division]

clas·si·fi·ca·tion (klas′i-fi-kā′shŭn). A systematic arrangement into classes or groups based on perceived common characteristics; a means of giving order to a group of disconnected facts.

adansonian c., the c. of organisms based on giving equal weight to every character of the organism; this principle has its greatest application in numerical taxonomy. [M. *Adanson*]

Angle's c. of malocclusion, a c. of different types of malocclusion, based on the mesiodistal relationship of the permanent molars upon their eruption and locking, and composed of three classes; *Class I:* normal relationship of the jaws, wherein the mesiobuccal cusp of the maxillary first molar occludes in the buccal groove of the mandibular first permanent molar; *Class II:* distal relationship of the mandible, wherein the distobuccal cusp of the maxillary first permanent molar occludes in the buccal groove of the mandibular first molar, and further classified as Division 1, labioversion of maxillary incisor teeth, and Division 2, linguoversion of maxillary central incisors, both of which may be unilateral conditions; *Class III:* mesial relationship of the mandible, wherein the mesiobuccal cusp of the maxillary first molar occludes in the embrasure between the mandibular first and second permanent molars, further classified as a unilateral condition.

Caldwell-Moloy c., a c. of the variations in the female pelvis; namely gynecoid, android, anthropoid, and platypelloid pelvis, based on the type of the posterior and anterior segments of the inlet.

Fredrickson's c., a c. system of hyperlipoproteinemia that uses plasma appearance, triglyceride values and total cholesterol values. There are five types: I, II, III, IV, V. SEE ALSO hyperlipoproteinemia.

French-American-British c. system (FAB), a c. and nomenclature system for acute leukemias based on morphologic characteristics and cytochemical stain reactions. The acute myeloid leukemias are subdivided into eight FAB groups: M0, M1, M2, M3, M4, M5, M6, M7. The acute lymphoid leukemias are subdivided into three groups: L1, L2, L3. The myelodysplastic syndromes have also been subdivided by the FAB group into five subgroups: RA, RARS, RAEB, RAEB-T, CMML. SEE ALSO myelodysplastic *syndrome*.

Kiel c., c. of non-Hodgkin's lymphoma into low-grade malignancy (lymphocytic, lymphoplasmacytoid, centrocytic, and centroblastic-centrocytic types) and high-grade malignancy (centroblastic, lymphoblastic of Burkitt's or convoluted cell, and immunoblastic types).

Lancefield c., a serologic c. dividing hemolytic streptococci into groups (A to O) based on precipitation tests for group-specific carbohydrate substances. Group A contains strains pathogenic for humans.

New York Heart Association c., a functional c. to assess cardiovascular disability. Class I: cardiac disease without limitation of physical activity. Ordinary activity does not cause symptoms. Class II: cardiac disease with slight limitation of activity; comfortable at rest. Ordinary physical activity results in fatigue, palpitations, dyspnea or angina. Class III: cardiac disease producing marked limitation of activity: comfortable at rest. Less than ordinary physical activity causes symptoms. Class IV: cardiac disease resulting in inability to carry on any physical activity without discomfort. Symptoms may be present even at rest.

clas·tic (klas'tik). Breaking up into pieces, or exhibiting a tendency so to break or divide. [G. *klastos,* broken]

clas·to·gen·ic (klas-tō-jen'ik). Relating to the action of a clastogen.

clas·to·thrix (klas'tō-thriks). SYN *trichorrhexis nodosa.* [G. *klastos,* broken, + *thrix,* hair]

clath·rate (klath'rāt). A type of inclusion compound in which small molecules are trapped in the cage-like lattice of macromolecules. [L. *clathrare,* pp. *-atus,* to furnish with a lattice]

clau·di·ca·tion (klaw-di-kā'shŭn). Limping, usually referring to intermittent c. [L. *claudicatio,* fr. *claudico,* to limp]

intermittent c., a condition caused by ischemia of the muscles; characterized by attacks of lameness and pain, brought on by walking, chiefly in the calf muscles; however, the condition may occur in other muscle groups. SYN Charcot's syndrome, myasthenia angiosclerotica.

clau·di·ca·tory (klaw'di-kă-tōr-ē). Relating to claudication, especially intermittent claudication.

claus·tra (klaws'tră). Plural of claustrum.

claus·tral (klaws'trăl). Relating to the claustrum.

claus·tro·pho·bia (klaw-strō-fō'bē-ă). A morbid fear of being in a confined place. [L. *claustrum,* an enclosed space, + G. *phobos,* fear]

claus·tro·pho·bic (klaw-strō-fō'bik). Relating to or suffering from claustrophobia.

claus·trum, pl. **claus·tra** (klaws'trŭm, klaws'tră). 1. One of several anatomical structures bearing a resemblance to a barrier. 2 [NA]. A thin, vertically placed lamina of gray matter lying close to the putamen, from which it is separated by the external capsule. Cells of the c. have reciprocal connections with sensory areas of the cerebral cortex. [L. barrier]

cla·vi (klā'vī). Plural of clavus.

clav·i·cle (klav'i-kl). A doubly curved long bone that forms part of the shoulder girdle. Its medial end articulates with the manubrium sterni at the sternoclavicular joint, its lateral end with the acromion of the scapula at the acromioclavicular joint. SYN clavicula [NA], collar bone.

cla·vic·u·la, pl. **cla·vic'·u·lae** (klă-vik'yū-lă, -lē) [NA]. SYN clavicle. [L. *clavicula,* a small key, fr. *clavis,* key]

cla·vic·u·lar (kla-vik'yū-lăr). Relating to the clavicle.

cla·vus, pl. **cla·vi** (klā'vŭs, -vī). A small conical callosity caused by pressure over a bony prominence, usually on a toe. SYN corn, heloma. [L. a nail, wart, corn]

claw·foot (klaw'fut). A condition of the foot characterized by hyperextension at the metatarsophalangeal joint and flexion at the interphalangeal joints, as a fixed contracture.

claw·hand (klaw'hand). Atrophy of the interosseous muscles of the hand with hyperextension of the metacarpophalangeal joints and flexion of the interphalangeal joints.

clear·ance (klēr'ans). 1. (C with a subscript indicating the substance removed). Removal of a substance from the blood, *e.g.,* by renal excretion, expressed in terms of the volume flow of arterial blood or plasma that would contain the amount of substance removed per unit time; measured in ml/min. 2. A condition in which bodies may pass each other without hindrance, or the distance between bodies. 3. Removal of something from some place; *e.g.,* "esophageal acid c." refers to removal from the esophagus of some acid that has refluxed into it from the stomach, evaluated by the time taken for restoration of a normal pH in the esophagus.

creatinine c., a mathematical calculation of the total amount of creatinine excreted in the urine over a period of time. It tests renal function. The calculation is: creatinine c. (ml/min) = urine creatinine concentration (ml/dl) × volume of urine (ml/24 hour) ÷ plasma creatinine concentration (mg/dl) x 1440 min/24 hour.

inulin c., an accurate measure of the rate of filtration through the renal glomeruli, because inulin filters freely with water and is neither excreted nor reabsorbed through tubule walls. Inulin is not a normal constituent of plasma and must be infused continously to maintain a steady plasma concentration and a steady rate of urinary excretion during the measurement.

urea c., the volume of plasma (or blood) that would be completely cleared of urea by one minute's excretion of urine.

cleav·age (klēv'ij). 1. Series of mitotic cell divisions occurring in the ovum immediately following its fertilization. SEE ALSO cleavage *division*. **2.** Splitting of a complex molecule into two or more simpler molecules. SYN scission (2). **3.** Linear clefts in the skin indicating the direction of the fibers in the dermis. SEE ALSO cleavage *lines*, under *line*. **4.** Midline depression or furrow between mature female breasts (common).

cleft (kleft). A fissure.

    branchial c.'s, The branchial ectodermal grooves of mammalian embryos, which are imperforate, rudimentary homologues of gill clefts in fishes.

    pudendal c., the cleft between the labia majora.

    synaptic c., the space about 20 nm wide between the axolemma and the postsynaptic surface. SEE ALSO synapse.

    visceral c., any c. between two branchial (visceral) arches in the embryo.

cleid-. SEE cleido-.

clei·dal (klī′dăl). Relating to the clavicle. SYN clidal.

cleido-, cleid-. The clavicle; also spelled clido-, clid-. [G. *kleis,* bar, bolt]

clei·do·cos·tal (klī-dō-kos′tăl). Relating to the clavicle and a rib. SYN clidocostal. [cleido- + L. *costa,* rib]

clei·do·cra·ni·al (klī′dō-krā′nē-ăl). Relating to the clavicle and the cranium. SYN clidocranial. [G. *kleis,* clavicle, + *kranion,* cranium]

-cleisis. Closure. [G. *kleisis,* a closing]

CLIA ′67 Clinical Laboratory Improvement Act of 1967.

CLIA ′88 Clinical Laboratory Improvement Amendments of 1988.

click (klik). A slight, sharp sound.

clid-. SEE clido-.

cli·dal (klī′dăl). SYN cleidal.

clido-, clid-. The clavicle. SEE ALSO cleido-. [G. *kleis,* bar, bolt]

cli·do·cos·tal (klī-dō-kos′tăl). SYN cleidocostal.

cli·do·cra·ni·al (klī-dō-krā′nē-ăl). SYN cleidocranial.

cli·mac·ter·ic (klī-mak′ter-ik, klī-mak-ter′ik). **1.** The period of endocrinal, somatic, and transitory psychologic changes occurring in the menopause. **2.** A critical period of life. [G. *klimaktēr,* the rung of a ladder]

cli·max (klī′maks). **1.** The height or acme of a disease; its stage of greatest severity. **2.** SYN orgasm. [G. *klimax,* staircase]

clin·i·cal (klin′i-kl). **1.** Relating to the bedside of a patient. **2.** Denoting the symptoms and course of a disease, as distinguished from the laboratory findings of anatomical changes. **3.** Relating to a clinic.

Clinical Laboratory Improvement Act of 1967 (CLIA ′67). Federal law (Public Law 90-174) regulating medical laboratories that process more than 100 specimens per year in interstate commerce. Usually affects only large, independent laboratories. SEE ALSO Clinical Laboratory Improvement Amendments of 1988.

Clinical Laboratory Improvement Amendments of 1988 (CLIA ′88). Amendments enacted by U.S. Congress in 1988 (Public Law 100-578) to revise and expand the Clinical Laboratory

Improvement Act of 1967 and Medicare and Medicaid provisions. The amendments classify and regulate laboratories based on the complexity of procedures being performed and establishes personnel qualifications. These rules apply to all testing sites, but several procedures and tests have waivers from these regulations. SEE ALSO Clinical Laboratory Improvement Act of 1967.

cli·ni·cian (klin-ish′ŭn). A health professional engaged in the care of patients, as distinguished from one working in other areas.

clin·i·co·path·o·log·ic (klin′i-kō-path-ō-loj′ik). Pertaining to the signs and symptoms manifested by a patient, and also the results of laboratory studies, as they relate to the findings in the gross and histologic examination of tissue by means of biopsy or autopsy, or both.

clino-. A slope (inclination or declination) or bend. [G. *klinō,* to slope, incline, or bend]

cli·no·ceph·a·ly (klī′nō-sef′ă-lē). Craniosynostosis in which the upper surface of the skull is concave, presenting a saddle-shaped appearance in profile. SYN saddle head. [clino- + G. *kephalē,* head]

cli·no·dac·ty·ly (klī′nō-dak′ti-lē). Permanent deflection of one or more fingers. [clino- + G. *daktylos,* finger]

CLIP corticotropin-like intermediate-lobe *peptide.*

clip (klip′). A fastener used to hold a part or thing together with another.

    wound c., a metal clasp or device for surgical approximation of skin incisions.

clith·ro·pho·bia (klīth-rō-fō′bē-ă). Morbid fear of being locked in. [G. *kleithron,* a bolt, + *phobos,* fear]

clit·o·ri·dec·to·my (klit′ō-ri-dek′tō-mē). Removal of the clitoris. [clitoris + G. *ektomē,* excision]

clit·o·ri·di·tis (klit′ō-ri-dī′tis). Inflammation of the clitoris. SYN clitoritis. [clitoris + G. *-itis,* inflammation]

clit·o·ris, pl. **cli·to·ri·des** (klit′ō-ris, -tōr′i-dēz; klī′tō-ris) [NA]. A cylindric, erectile body, rarely exceeding 2 cm in length, situated at the most anterior portion of the vulva and projecting between the branched limbs or laminae of the labia minora, which form its prepuce and frenulum. It consists of a glans, a corpus, and two crura. [G. *kleitoris*]

clit·o·rism (klit′ō-rizm). Prolonged and usually painful erection of the clitoris; the analogue of priapism.

clit·o·ri·tis (klit-ō-rī′tis). SYN clitoriditis.

clit·or·o·meg·a·ly (klit′ōr-ō-meg′ă-lē). An enlarged clitoris. [clitoris + G. *megas,* great]

cli·vus, pl. **cli·vi** (klī′vŭs, -vē). **1.** A downward sloping surface. **2** [NA]. The sloping surface from the dorsum sellae to the foramen magnum composed of part of the body of the sphenoid and part of the basal part of the occipital bone. [L. slope]

clo·a·ca (klō-ā′kă). **1.** In early embryos, the endodermally lined chamber into which the hindgut and allantois empty. **2.** In birds and monotremes, the common chamber into which open the hindgut, bladder, and genital ducts. [L. sewer]

persistent c., a condition in which the urorectal fold has failed to divide the c. of the embryo into rectal and urogenital portions.

clo·a·cal (klō-ā′kăl). Pertaining to the cloaca.

clo·nal (klō′năl). Pertaining to a clone.

clone (klōn). **1.** A colony of organisms or cells cells derived from a single organism or cell by asexual reproduction, all having identical genetic constitutions. **2.** To produce such a colony or individual. **3.** A short section of DNA which has been copied by means of gene cloning. SEE cloning. [G. *klōn,* slip, cutting used for propagation]

clo·nic (klon′ik). Relating to or characterized by clonus.

clon·ic·i·ty (klon-is′i-tē). The state of being clonic.

clon·i·co·ton·ic (klon′i-kō-ton′ik). Both clonic and tonic; said of certain forms of muscular spasm.

clon·ing (klōn′ing). **1.** Growing a colony of genetically identical cells or organisms in vitro. **2.** Transplantation of a nucleus from a somatic cell to an ovum, which then develops into an embryo; many identical embryos can thus be generated by asexual reproduction. **3.** With blastocysts, dividing a cluster of cells through microsurgery and transferring one half the cells to a zona pellucida that has been emptied of its contents. The resulting embryos, genetically identical, may be implanted in an animal for gestation. **4.** A recombinant DNA technique used to produce millions of copies of a DNA fragment. The fragment is spliced into a cloning vehicle (*i.e.,* plasmid, bacteriophage, or animal virus). The cloning vehicle penetrates a bacterial cell or yeast (the host), which is then grown in vitro or in an animal host. In some cases, as in the production of genetically engineered drugs, the inserted DNA becomes activated and alters the chemical functioning of the host cell.

clo·nism (klon′izm). A long continued state of clonic spasms.

clo·no·gen·ic (klō-nō-jen′ik). Arising from or consisting of a clone.

clo·nor·chi·a·sis (klō-nōr-kī′ă-sis). A disease caused by the fluke *Clonorchis sinensis,* affecting the distal bile ducts after ingestion of raw, smoked, or undercooked fish or raw crayfish; repeated or chronic infection induces an intense proliferative and granulomatous condition.

Clo·nor·chis si·nen·sis (klō-nōr′kis sī-nen′sis). The Chinese liver fluke, a species of trematodes that in the Far East infects the bile passages; fish serve as second intermediate hosts and snails as the first intermediate hosts.

clon·o·spasm (klon′ō-spazm). SYN clonus.

clo·nus (klō′nŭs). A form of movement marked by contractions and relaxations of a muscle, occurring in rapid succession seen with, among other conditions, spasticity and some seizure disorders. SEE ALSO contraction. SYN clonospasm. [G. *klonos,* a tumult]

clos·trid·i·al (klos-trid′ē-ăl). Relating to any bacterium of the genus *Clostridium.*

Clos·trid·i·um (klos-trid′ē-ŭm). A genus of anaerobic (or anaerobic, aerotolerant), sporeforming, motile (occasionally nonmotile) bacteria con-

taining Gram-positive rods. Exotoxins are sometimes produced by these organisms. They may cause disease in man and other animals. They are generally found in soil and in the intestinal tract of man and other animals. The type species is *C. butyricum.* [G. *klōstēr,* a spindle]

C. bifermen′tans, a species found in putrid meat and gaseous gangrene; also commonly in soil, feces, and sewage. Its pathogenicity varies from strain to strain.

C. botuli′num, a species that occurs widely in nature and is a frequent cause of food poisoning (botulism) from preserved meats, fruits, or vegetables that have not been properly sterilized before canning.

C. histoly′ticum, a species found in war wounds, where it induces necrosis of tissue; it produces a cytolytic exotoxin that causes local necrosis and sloughing on injection; it is not toxic on feeding; it is pathogenic for small laboratory animals.

C. no′vyi, a species causing gaseous gangrene and necrotic hepatitis.

C. parabotuli′num, a species that produces a powerful exotoxin and is pathogenic for man and other animals.

C. perfrin′gens, a species that is the chief causative agent of gas gangrene; it may also be involved in causing enteritis, appendicitis, and puerperal fever; it is one of the most common causes of food poisoning in the U.S. SYN *C. welchii,* gas bacillus.

C. tet′ani, a species that causes tetanus; it produces a potent exotoxin (neurotoxin) that is intensely toxic for humans and other animals when formed in tissues or injected, but not when ingested.

C. welch′ii, SYN *C. perfringens.*

clos·trid·i·um, pl. **clos·trid·ia** (klos-trid′ē-ŭm, -ă). A vernacular term used to refer to any member of the genus *Clostridium.*

clo·sure (klō′zhŭr). **1.** The completion of a reflex pathway. **2.** The place of coupling between stimuli in the establishment of conditioned learning. **3.** To achieve or experience a sense of completion in a mental task. **4.** Definitive repair of an open wound, traumatic or surgical.

visual c., identification of forms or objects from incomplete presentation.

clot (klot). **1.** To coagulate, said especially of blood. **2.** A soft, nonrigid, insoluble mass formed when a liquid (*e.g.,* blood or lymph) gels. [O.E. *klott,* lump]

chicken fat c., c. formed *in vitro* or postmortem from leukocytes and plasma of sedimented blood.

currant jelly c., a jelly-like mass of red blood cells and fibrin formed by the *in vitro* or postmortem clotting of whole or sedimented blood.

laminated c., a c. formed in a succession of layers such as occurs in an aneurysm.

passive c., a c. formed in an aneurysmal sac consequent to cessation or slowing of circulation.

club·bing (klŭb′ing). A condition affecting the fingers and toes in which proliferation of distal tissues, especially the nail beds, results in thickening and widening of the extremities of the digits; the nails are abnormally curved and shiny.

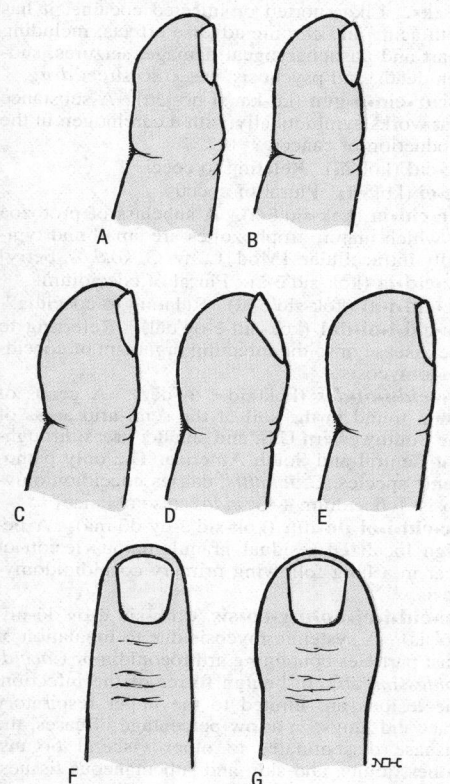

varieties of digital clubbing: (A) normal, (B) increased curvature of nail, (C) mild clubbing, (D) parrot's beak type, (E) watch glass type, (F) normal, (G) drumstick type

hereditary c., simple hereditary c. of the digits without associated pulmonary or other progressive disease.

club·foot (klŭb′fut). SYN *talipes* equinovarus.

club·hand (klŭb′hand). Congenital or acquired angulation deformity of the hand associated with partial or complete absence of radius or ulna; usually with intrinsic deformities in the hand in congenital variants.

clump·ing (klŭmp′ing). The massing together of bacteria or other cells or particles suspended in a fluid.

clu·ne·al (klū′nē-ăl). Pertaining to the clunes.

clu·nes (klū′nēz) [NA]. SYN buttocks. [pl. of L. *clunis*, buttock]

clus·ter of dif·fer·en·ti·a·tion (CD). Cell membrane molecules that are used to classify leukocytes into subsets. CD molecules are classified by monoclonal antibodies.

  c. of d. 2 (CD2), a glycoprotein that is expressed on all peripheral T cells, large granular lymphocytes and most, but not all, thymocytes.

CD2 is involved in signal transduction and cell adhesion.

  c. of d. 3 (CD3), a complex of 5 polypeptides associated with the T cell receptor and is involved in signal transduction.

  c. of d. 4 (CD4), a glycoprotein found on various subsets of T cells, *i.e.,* usually on helper and some T cytotoxic cells.

  c. of d. 8 (CD8), membrane glycoprotein found on subsets of T lymphocytes. CD8 is expressed on T cytotoxic cells and T suppressor cells.

cluttering (klut′er-ing). Speech disorder characterized by rapid, jerky utterances with many omissions and transpositions of speech sounds; sometimes confused with stuttering. SEE stuttering.

cly·sis (klī′sis). **1.** An infusion of fluid, usually subcutaneously, for therapeutic purposes. **2.** Formerly, a fluid enema; later, the washing out of material from any body space or cavity by fluids. [G. *klysis*, a drenching by a clyster]

Cm curium.

cM centimorgan.

cm centimeter; cm^2 for square centimeter; cm^3 for cubic *centimeter.*

CMA Certified Medical Assistant.

cmc critical micelle *concentration.*

CMI cell-mediated *immunity.*

CML cell-mediated lymphocytotoxicity.

CMP cytidine 5′-monophosphate (secondarily, any cytidine monophosphate).

CMT Certified Medical Transcriptionist. SEE medical transcriptionist.

CMV 1. Controlled mechanical *ventilation;* cytomegalovirus. **2.** A cancer drug combination treatment consisting of cisplatin, methotrexate, and vinblastine, used in the treatment of bladder and other malignancies.

CNS 1. central nervous *system.* **2.** Symbol for the thiocyanate radical, CNS^- or —CNS.

CO Symbol for *carbon* monoxide.

Co cobalt; coccygeal.

co-. SEE con-.

CoA coenzyme A.

co·ad·ap·ta·tion (kō′ad-ap-tā′shŭn). GENETICS The operation of selection jointly on two or more loci.

co·ag·glu·ti·nin (kō-ă-glū′ti-nin). A substance that does not agglutinate an antigen, but does result in agglutination of antigen that is coated with univalent antibody. SEE ALSO conglutination.

co·ag·u·la (kō-ag′yū-lă). Plural of coagulum.

co·ag·u·la·ble (kō-ag′yū-lă-bl). Capable of being coagulated or clotted.

co·ag·u·lant (kō-ag′yū-lant). **1.** An agent that causes, stimulates, or accelerates coagulation, especially with reference to blood. **2.** SYN coagulative.

co·ag·u·late (kō-ag′yū-lāt). **1.** To convert a fluid or a substance in solution into a solid or gel. **2.** To clot; to curdle; to change from a liquid to a solid or gel. [L. *coagulo*, pp. -atus, to curdle]

co·ag·u·la·tion (kō-ag-yū-lā′shŭn). **1.** Clotting; the process of changing from a liquid to a solid, said especially of blood. **2.** A clot or coagulum. **3.** Transformation of a sol into a gel or semisolid mass.

disseminated intravascular c. (DIC), a hemorrhagic syndrome that occurs following the uncontrolled activation of clotting factors and fibrinolytic enzymes throughout small blood vessels; fibrin is deposited, platelets and clotting factors are consumed, and fibrin degradation products inhibit fibrin polymerization, resulting in tissue necrosis and bleeding. SEE ALSO consumption *coagulopathy.*

co·ag·u·la·tive (kō-ag′yū-lă-tiv). Causing coagulation. SYN coagulant (2).

co·ag·u·lop·a·thy (kō-ag-yū-lop′ă-thē). A disease affecting the coagulability of the blood.

consumption c., a disorder in which marked reductions develop in blood concentrations of platelets with exhaustion of the coagulation factors in the peripheral blood as a result of disseminated intravascular coagulation.

co·ag·u·lum, pl. **co·ag·u·la** (kō-ag′yū-lŭm, -lă). A clot or a curd; a soft, nonrigid, insoluble mass formed when a sol undergoes coagulation. [L. a means of coagulating, rennet]

co·a·les·cence (kō-ă-les′ens). Fusion of originally separate parts. SYN concrescence (1).

co·ap·ta·tion (kō-ap-tā′shŭn). Joining or fitting together of two surfaces; *e.g.,* the lips of a wound or the ends of a broken bone. [L. *co-apto,* pp. *-aptatus,* to fit together]

co·arct (kō-arkt′). To restrict or press together. SYN coarctate (1). [L. *co-arcto,* pp. *-arctatus,* to press together]

co·arc·tate (kō-ark′tāt). 1. SYN coarct. 2. Pressed together.

co·arc·ta·tion (kō-ark-tā′shŭn). A constriction, stricture, or stenosis, usually of the aorta.

reversed c., aortic arch syndrome in which blood pressure in the arms is lower than in the legs.

coat (kōt). 1. The outer covering or envelope of an organ or part. 2. One of the layers of membranous or other tissues forming the wall of a canal or hollow organ. SEE tunic.

buffy c., the light-colored layer of blood that is seen when anticoagulated blood is centrifuged or allowed to stand. It appears as a layer between the plasma and red cells and is composed of leukocytes and platelets.

muscular c., the muscular, usually middle, layer of a tubular structure; for most of the gastrointestinal tract, it consists of an outer longitudinal layer of muscle and an inner circular layer.

co·bal·a·min (kō-bal′ă-min). General term for compounds containing the dimethylbenzimidazolylcobamide nucleus of vitamin B_{12}.

co·balt (Co) (kō′bawlt). A steel-gray metallic element, atomic no. 27, atomic wt. 58.93320; a bioelement and a constituent of vitamin B_{12}; certain of its compounds are pigments, *e.g.,* c. blue. [Ger. *kobalt,* goblin or evil spirit]

co·caine (kō-kān′). Benzoylmethylecgonine; an alkaloid obtained from the leaves of *Erythroxylon coca,* or by synthesis from ecgonine or its derivatives; it has moderate vasoconstrictor activity and pronounced psychotropic effects; its salts are used as a topical anesthetic.

crack c., a derivative of cocaine, usually smoked, producing brief, intense euphoria. Crack

c. is relatively inexpensive and extremely addictive; dependency can develop in less than 2 weeks. Like snorted or injected cocaine, it has both acute and chronic adverse effects, including heart and nasopharyngeal damage, seizures, sudden death, and psychosis. SEE ALSO street *drug.*

co·car·cin·o·gen (kō-kar′si-nō-jen). A substance that works symbiotically with a carcinogen in the production of cancer.

coc·cal (kok′ăl). Relating to cocci.

coc·ci (kok′sī). Plural of coccus.

Coc·cid·i·a (kok-sid′ē-ă). A subclass of protozoa in which mature trophozoites are small and typically intracellular. [Mod. L., fr. G. *kokkos,* berry]

coc·cid·i·a (kok-sid′ē-ă). Plural of coccidium.

coc·cid·i·al (kok-sid′ē-ăl). Relating to coccidia.

coc·cid·i·oi·dal (kok-sid-ē-oy′dăl). Referring to the disease or to the infecting organism of coccidioidomycosis.

Coc·cid·i·oi·des (kok-sid-ē-oy′dēz). A genus of fungi found in the soil of the semi-arid areas of the Southwestern U.S. and smaller areas throughout Central and South America. The only pathogenic species, *C. immitis,* causes coccidioidomycosis. [coccidium + G. *eidos,* resemblance]

coc·cid·i·oi·do·ma (kok-sid′ē-oy-dō′mă). A benign localized residual granulomatous lesion or scar in a lung following primary coccidioidomycosis.

coc·cid·i·oi·do·my·co·sis (kok-sid-ē-oy′dō-mī-kō′sis). A systemic mycosis due to inhalation of dust particles containing arthroconidia of *Coccidioides immitis.* In benign forms of the infection, the lesions are limited to the upper respiratory tract and lungs; in a low percentage of cases, the disease disseminates to other visceral organs, bones, joints, and skin and subcutaneous tissues. [coccidioides + G. *mykēs,* fungus, + *-osis,* condition]

coc·cid·i·o·sis (kok-sid-ē-ō′sis). Group name for diseases due to any species of coccidia; a common disease of many species of domestic animals and birds; both intestinal and pulmonary c. have been reported in human individuals with AIDS.

coc·cid·i·um, pl. **coc·cid·ia** (kok-sid′ē-ŭm, -ē-ă). Common name given to protozoan parasites in which schizogony occurs within epithelial cells, generally in the intestine. Coccidia are parasitic in domestic and wild birds and mammals, occasionally in humans; the majority are nonpathogenic. SEE *Isospora.* [Mod. L. dim. of G. *kokkos,* berry]

coc·co·bac·il·lary (kok′ō-bas′i-lār-ē). Relating to a coccobacillus.

coc·co·ba·cil·lus (kok′ō-bă-sil′ŭs). A short, thick bacterial rod of the shape of an oval or slightly elongated coccus. [G. *kokkos,* berry]

coc·coid (kok′oyd). Resembling a coccus. [G. *kokkos,* berry, + *eidos,* resemblance]

coc·cus, pl. **coc·ci** (kok′ŭs, kok′sī). 1. A bacterium of round, spheroidal, or ovoid form. 2. SYN cochineal. [G. *kokkos,* berry]

coc·cy·al·gia (kok-sē-al′jē-ă). SYN coccygodynia. [coccyx + G. *algos,* pain]

coc·cy·dyn·ia (kok-sē-din′ē-ă). SYN coccygodynia. [coccyx + G. *ōdyne,* pain]

coc•cyg•eal (Co) (kok-sij′ē-ăl). Relating to the coccyx.

coc•cy•gec•to•my (kok-sē-jek′tō-mē). Removal of the coccyx. [coccyx + G. *ektomē*, excision]

coc•cy•go•dyn•ia (kok′si-gō-din′ē-ă). Pain in the coccygeal region. SYN coccyalgia, coccydynia, coccyodynia. [coccyx + G. *odynē*, pain]

coc•cy•got•o•my (kok-sē-got′ō-mē). Operation for freeing the coccyx from its attachments. [coccyx + G. *tomē*, a cutting]

coc•cy•o•dyn•ia (kok′sē-ō-din′ē-ă). SYN coccygodynia.

coc•cyx, gen. **coc•cy•gis,** pl. **coc•cy•ges** (kok′ siks, -si-jis, -si-jēs). The small bone at the end of the vertebral column in man, formed by the fusion of four rudimentary vertebrae; it articulates above with the sacrum. [G. *kokkyx*, a cuckoo, the coccyx]

coch•i•neal (kotch′i-nēl) [C.I. 75470]. The dried female insects, *Coccus cacti*, enclosing the young larvae, or the dried female insect, *Dactylopius coccus*, containing eggs and larvae, from which coccinellin is obtained; used as a red coloring agent and a stain. SEE carmine. SYN coccus (2). [O.Sp. *cochinilla*, wood louse, fr. G. *kokkinos*, berry]

co•chlea, pl. **co•chle•ae** (kok′lē-ă, lē-ē) [NA]. A cone-shaped cavity in the petrous portion of the temporal bone, forming one of the divisions of the labyrinth or internal ear. It consists of a spiral canal making two and a half turns around a central core of spongy bone, the modiolus; this spiral canal of the cochlea contains the membranous cochlea, or cochlear duct, in which is the spiral organ (Corti). [L. snail shell]

co•chle•ar (kok′lē-ăr). Relating to the cochlea.

co•chle•o•ves•tib•u•lar (kok′lē-ō-ves-tib′yū-lăr). Relating to the cochlea and the vestibule of the ear.

cock•tail (kok′tāl). A mixture that includes several ingredients or drugs.

  Brompton c., a c. of morphine and cocaine usually used for analgesia in terminal cancer patients; the formulations vary, but typically it contains 15 mg of morphine hydrochoride and 10 mg of cocaine hydrochloride per 10 ml of the c. [*Brompton* Chest Hospital, London, England, where developed]

cocontraction. OCCUPATIONAL THERAPY Simultaneous contraction of both the agonist and the antagonist around a joint to hold a stable position. SYN coinnervation.

code (kōd). **1.** A set of rules, principles, or ethics. **2.** Any system devised to convey information or facilitate communication. **3.** Term used in hospitals to describe an emergency situation requiring trained members of the staff, such as a cardiopulmonary resuscitation team, or the signal to summon such a team. **4.** A numerical system for ordering and classifying information, *e.g.,* about diagnostic categories. [L. *codex*, book]

  genetic c., the genetic information carried by the specific DNA molecules of the chromosomes; specifically, the system whereby particular combinations of three consecutive nucleotides in a DNA molecule control the insertion of one particular amino acid in equivalent places in a protein molecule.

coding (kō′ding). Assigning a number to a disease process, surgical procedure, or other type of health care service for the purpose of reimbursement, health care planning, and research.

co•dom•i•nant (kō-dom′i-nant). In genetics, denoting an equal degree of dominance of two genes, both being expressed in the phenotype of the individual; *e.g.,* genes A and B of the ABO blood group are codominant; individuals with both are type AB.

co•don (kō′don). A set of three consecutive nucleotides in a strand of DNA or RNA that provides the genetic information to code for a specific amino acid which will be incorporated into a protein chain or serve as a termination signal. SYN triplet (3). [code + -on]

  amber c., the termination codon UAG.

  initiation c., a specific mRNA sequence (usually AUG, but sometimes GUG) that is the signal for the addition of fMet-tRNA and the beginning of translation.

  ochre c., the termination c. UAA.

  opal c., SYN umber c.

  umber c., the termination c. UGA. SYN opal c.

△**coe-.** For words so beginning, and not found here, see ce-.

co•ef•fi•cient (kō-ĕ-fish′ĕnt). **1.** The expression of the amount or degree of any quality possessed by a substance, or of the degree of physical or chemical change normally occurring in that substance under stated conditions. **2.** The ratio or factor that relates a quantity observed under one

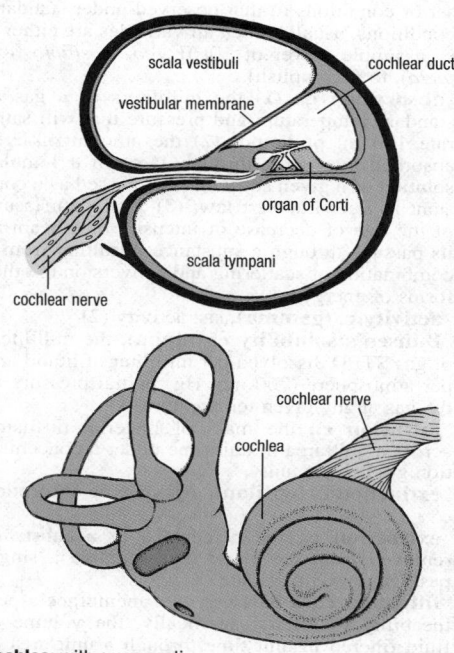

cochlea: with cross section

(labels: scala vestibuli, cochlear duct, vestibular membrane, organ of Corti, scala tympani, cochlear nerve, cochlea)

CO

set of conditions to that observed under standard conditions, usually when all variables are either 1 or a simple power of 10. [L. *co-* + *efficio* (*ex-facio*), to accomplish]

absorption c., (1) the milliliters of a gas at standard temperature and pressure that will saturate 100 ml of liquid; (2) the amount of light absorbed in passing through 1 cm of a 1 molar solution of a given substance, expressed as a constant in Beer-Lambert law; (3) X-RAY a measure of the rate of decrease of intensity of a beam in its passage through a substance, resulting from a combination of scattering and conversion to other forms of energy.

activity c. (gamma), SEE activity (2).

Bunsen's solubility c. (alpha), the milliliters of gas STPD dissolved per milliliter of liquid and per atmosphere (760 mm Hg) partial pressure of the gas at any given temperature.

diffusion c., the mass of material diffusing across a unit area in unit time under a concentration gradient of unity.

extinction c. (epsilon), SYN specific absorption c.

extraction c., the percentage of a substance removed from the blood or plasma in a single passage through a tissue.

filtration c., a measure of a membrane's permeability to water; specifically, the volume of fluid filtered in unit time through a unit area of membrane per unit pressure difference, taking into account both hydraulic and osmotic pressures.

molar absorption c. (epsilon), absorbance (of light) per unit path length (usually the centimeter) and per unit of concentration (moles per liter); a fundamental unit in spectrophotometry. SYN absorbancy index (2), absorptivity (2).

Ostwald's solubility c. (lambda), the milliliters of gas dissolved per milliliter of liquid and per atmosphere (760 mm of Hg) partial pressure of the gas at any given temperature. This differs from Bunsen's solubility c. (α) in that the amount of dissolved gas is expressed in terms of its volume at the temperature of the experiment, instead of STPD.

permeability c., a c. associated with simple diffusion through a membrane that is proportional to the partition coefficient and the diffusion coefficient and inversely proportional to membrane thickness.

phenol c., SYN Rideal-Walker c.

reflection c. (σ), a measure of the relative permeability of a particular membrane to a particular solute; calculated as the ratio of observed osmotic pressure to that calculated from van't Hoff's law.

Rideal-Walker c., a figure expressing the disinfecting power of any substance; it is obtained by dividing the figure indicating the degree of dilution of the disinfectant that kills a microorganism in a given time by that indicating the degree of dilution of phenol which kills the organism in the same space of time under similar conditions. SYN phenol c.

sedimentation c. (s), SYN sedimentation *constant*.

selection c. (s), the proportion of progeny or potential progeny not surviving to sexual maturity; usually defined artificially by expressing the fitness of a phenotype as a fraction of the mean or optimal fitness to give the relative fitness, and subtracting this fraction from unity. If the mean size of family in the population is 3.2 and that for a particular genotype is 2.4 then the fitness of the phenotype is $2.4/3.2 = 0.75$ and the selection coefficient $=1-0.75 =.25 = 5$

specific absorption c. (*a*), absorbance (of light) per unit path length (usually the centimeter) and per unit of mass concentration. Cf. molar absorption c. SYN absorbancy index (1), absorptivity (1), extinction c., specific extinction.

c. of variation (CV), a unitless number used to describe dispersion of data. It allows comparison of standard deviations of test results expressed in different units. It is calculated from the standard deviation (s) and mean (x). $CV = 100s \div x$.

Coe·len·ter·a·ta (sē-len-tĕ-rā'tă). One of the major phyla of invertebrates, to which such forms as jellyfish belong.

coe·len·ter·ate (sē-len'ter-at). Common name for members of the Coelenterata.

△**coeno-**. Shared in common. SEE ALSO ceno-. [G. *koinos*, common]

co·en·zyme (kō-en'zīm). A substance (excluding solo metal ions) that enhances or is necessary for the action of enzymes; c.'s are of smaller molecular size than the enzymes themselves; several vitamins are c. precursors. SYN cofactor (1).

co·en·zyme A (CoA). A coenzyme containing pantothenic acid, adenosine 3'-phosphate 5'-pyrophosphate, and cysteamine; involved in the transfer of acyl groups, notably in transacetylations.

co·en·zyme Q (Q). Quinones with isoprenoid side chains (specifically, ubiquinones) that mediate electron transfer between cytochrome *b* and cytochrome *c*.

coeur (kūr). SYN heart. [Fr.]

c. en sabot (awn sah-bo'), the radiographic configuration of the heart in the tetralogy of Fallot; the elevated apex gives a silhouette like that of a wooden shoe.

co·fac·tor (kō'fak'ter, tōr). 1. SYN coenzyme. 2. An atom or molecule essential for the action of a large molecule; *e.g.,* heme in hemoglobin, magnesium in chlorophyll.

COG center of *gravity*.

cog·ni·tion (kog-ni'shŭn). 1. The mental activities associated with thinking, learning, and memory. 2. Any process whereby one acquires knowledge. [L. *cognitio*]

cog·ni·tive (kog'ni-tiv). Pertaining to cognition.

co·he·sion (kō-hē'zhŭn). The attraction between molecules or masses that holds them together. [L. *co-haereo*, pp. *-haesus*, to stick together]

co·hort (kō'hōrt). 1. Component of the population born during a particular period and identified by period of birth so that its characteristics can be ascertained as it enters successive time and age periods. 2. Any designated group followed or traced over a period, as in an epidemiological cohort study. [L. *cohors*, retinue, military unit]

coil (kōil). 1. A spiral or series of loops. 2. An object made of wire wound in a spiral configuration, used in electronic applications, or a loop of wire used as an antenna.

detector c., a c. used in magnetic resonance imaging as an antenna to record radiofrequency emissions of stimulated nuclei, *e.g.,* body coil, head coil.

surface c., a detector c. applied directly to a body part for high resolution imaging; often a single loop of metal.

co•in•ner•va•tion (kō′in-ner-vā′shun). SYN cocontraction.

coin•o•site (koyn′ō-sīt). SYN cenosite.

co•i•tal (ko′i-tăl). Pertaining to coitus.

co•i•tion (kō-ish′ŭn). SYN coitus. [L. *co-eo,* pp. *-itus,* to come together]

co•i•tus (kō′i-tŭs). Sexual union between male and female. SYN coition, copulation (1), pareunia, sexual intercourse. [L.]

c. interrup′tus, sexual intercourse that is interrupted before the male ejaculates.

c. reserva′tus, c. in which ejaculation is postponed or suppressed.

col (kol). A crater-like area of the interproximal oral mucosa joining the lingual and buccal interdental papillae.

cold (kōld). **1.** A low temperature; the sensation produced by a temperature notably below an accustomed norm or a comfortable level. **2.** Popular term for a virus infection involving the upper respiratory tract and characterized by congestion of the mucosa, watery nasal discharge, and general malaise, with a duration of 3 to 5 days. SEE ALSO rhinitis. SYN frigid (1).

col•ec•to•my (kō-lek′tō-mē). Excision of a segment or all of the colon. [G. *kolon,* colon, + *ektomē,* excision]

COLG center of *gravity.*

co•li•bac•il•lo•sis (kō′li-bas-i-lō′sis). Diarrheal disease caused by the bacterium *Escherichia coli.* Often called enteric c.

col•ic (kol′ik). **1.** Relating to the colon. **2.** Spasmodic pains in the abdomen. **3.** In young infants, paroxysms of gastrointestinal pain, with crying and irritability, due to a variety of causes, such as swallowing of air, emotional upset, or overfeeding. [G. *kōlikos,* relating to the colon]

col•i•cin (kol′i-sin). Bacteriocin produced by strains of *Escherichia coli* and other enterobacteria. [(*Escherichia*) *coli* + bacteriocin]

col•icky (kol′i-kē). Denoting or resembling the pain of colic.

co•li•pase (kō′lip-ās). A small protein in pancreatic juice that is essential for the efficient action of pancreatic lipase. [co- + lipase]

co•li•phage (kō′li-fāj, kol′i-). A bacteriophage with an affinity for one or another strain of *Escherichia coli.* [(*Escherichia*) *coli* + bacteriophage]

co•li•tis (kō-lī′tis). Inflammation of the colon. [G. *kōlon,* colon, + *-itis,* inflammation]

amebic c., inflammation of the colon in amebiasis.

collagenous c., c. occurring mostly in middle-aged women and characterized by persistent watery diarrhea and a deposit of a band of collagen beneath the basement membrane of colon surface epithelium.

granulomatous c., changes, identical to those of regional enteritis, involving the colon.

hemorrhagic c., abdominal cramps and bloody diarrhea, without fever, attributed to a self-limited infection by a strain of *Escherichia coli.*

mucous c., an affection of the mucous membrane of the colon characterized by colicky pain, constipation or diarrhea (sometimes alternating), and passage of mucous or slimy pseudomembranous shreds and patches. SYN myxomembranous c.

myxomembranous c., SYN mucous c.

pseudomembranous c., SYN pseudomembranous *enterocolitis.*

⊞**ulcerative c.,** a chronic disease of unknown cause characterized by ulceration of the colon and rectum, with rectal bleeding, mucosal crypt abscesses, inflammatory pseudopolyps, abdominal pain, and diarrhea; frequently causes anemia, hypoproteinemia, and electrolyte imbalance, and is sometimes complicated by peritonitis, toxic megacolon, or carcinoma of the colon.

col•la (kol′ă). Plural of collum.

col•la•gen (kol′lă-jen). The major protein of the white fibers of connective tissue, cartilage, and bone; insoluble in water but can be altered to easily digestible, soluble gelatins by boiling in water, dilute acids, or alkalies. SEE ALSO collagen *fiber.* SYN ossein, osseine, ostein, osteine. [G. *koila,* glue, + *-gen,* producing]

col•la•gen•ase (kol-ă′jě-nās). A proteolytic enzyme that acts on one or more of the collagens.

col•la•gen•ic (kol-ă-jen′ik). SYN collagenous.

col•lag•e•ni•za•tion (ko-laj′ě-ni-zā′shŭn). **1.** Replacement of tissues or fibrin by collagen. **2.** Synthesis of collagen by fibroblasts.

col•lag•e•no•lyt•ic (ko-laj′ě-nō-lit′ik). Causing the lysis of collagen, gelatin, and other proteins containing proline. [collagen + G. *lysis,* dissolving]

col•lag•e•nous (ko-laj′ě-nŭs). Producing or containing collagen. SYN collagenic.

col•lapse (kō-laps′). **1.** A condition of extreme prostration. **2.** A state of profound physical depression. **3.** A falling together of the walls of a structure or the failure of a physiological system. [L. *col-labor,* pp. *-lapsus,* to fall together]

col•lat•er•al (kol-lat′er-ăl). **1.** Indirect, subsidiary, or accessory to the main thing; side by side. **2.** A side branch of a nerve axon or blood vessel.

col•lic•u•lec•to•my (ko-lik-yū-lek′tō-mē). Excision of the colliculus seminalis.

col•lic•u•li•tis (ko-lik-yū-lī′tis). Inflammation of the urethra in the region of the colliculus seminalis.

col•lic•u•lus, pl. **col•lic•u•li** (ko-lik′yū-lŭs, -lī) [NA]. A small elevation above the surrounding parts. [L. mound, dim. of *collis,* hill]

seminal c., an elevated portion of the urethral crest upon which open the two ejaculatory ducts and the prostatic utricle.

col•li•ma•tion (kol-i-mā′shŭn). The process, in x-ray, of restricting and confining the x-ray beam to a given area and, in nuclear medicine, of restricting the detection of emitted radiations from

CO

a given area of interest. [L. *collineo,* to direct in a straight line]

col·li·qua·tion (kol-i-kwā'shŭn). **1.** Excessive discharge of fluid. **2.** Liquefaction in the process of necrosis. [L. *col-,* together, + *liquo,* pp. *liquatus,* to cause to melt]

col·liq·ua·tive (ko-lik'wă-tiv). Denoting or characteristic of colliquation.

col·loid (kol'oyd). **1.** Aggregates of atoms or molecules in a finely divided state (submicroscopic), dispersed in a gaseous, liquid, or solid medium, and resisting sedimentation, diffusion, and filtration, thus differing from precipitates. SEE ALSO hydrocolloid. **2.** Gluelike. **3.** A translucent, yellowish, homogeneous material of the consistency of glue, less fluid than mucoid or mucinoid, found in the cells and tissues in a state of c. degeneration. SYN colloidin. **4.** The stored secretion within follicles of the thyroid gland. [G. *kolla,* glue, + *eidos,* appearance]

  c. pseudomilium, SYN colloid *milium.*

col·loi·dal (ko-loyd'ăl). Denoting or characteristic of a colloid.

col·loi·din (ko-loy'din). SYN colloid (3).

col·lum, pl. **col·la** (kol'ŭm, kol'ă). **1** [NA]. The part between the shoulders or thorax and the head. **2.** A constricted or necklike portion of any organ or other anatomical structure. SYN cervix (1) [NA]. [L.]

col·lyr·i·um (ko-lir'ē-ŭm). Originally, any preparation for the eye; now, an eyewash. [G. *kollyrion,* poultice, eye salve]

△**colo-.** The colon. [G. *kolon*]

col·o·bo·ma (kol-ō-bō'mă). Any defect, congenital, pathologic, or artificial, especially of the eye. [G. *kolobōma,* lit., the part taken away in mutilation, fr. *koloboō,* to dock, mutilate]

co·lo·cen·te·sis (kō'lō-sen-tē'sis). Puncture of the colon with a trochar or scalpel to relieve distention. SYN colopuncture. [colo- + G. *kentēsis,* a puncture]

co·lo·cho·le·cys·tos·to·my (kō'lō-kō-lē-sis-tos'tō-mē). SYN cholecystocolostomy.

co·lo·co·los·to·my (kō'lō-kō-los'tō-mē). Establishment of a communication between two noncontinuous segments of the colon. [colo- + colo- + G. *stoma,* mouth]

co·lo·en·ter·i·tis (kō'lō-en-ter-ī'tis). SYN enterocolitis.

co·lon (kō'lon) [NA]. The division of the large intestine extending from the cecum to the rectum. [G. *kolon*]

  ascending c., the portion of the c. between the ileocecal orifice and the right colic flexure.

  descending c., the part of the c. extending from the left colic flexure to the pelvic brim.

  iliac c., that portion of the descending c. which occupies the left iliac fossa, between the crest of the left ilium and the pelvic brim.

  irritable c., tendency to colonic hyperperistalsis, sometimes with colicky pains and diarrhea.

  sigmoid c., the part of the c. describing an S-shaped curve between the pelvic brim and the third sacral segment; it is continuous with the rectum.

  transverse c., the part of the c. between the right and left colic flexures. It may extend some-

what transversely across the abdomen, but more often sags cent ally, frequently to subumbilical levels.

co·lon·ic (ko-lon'ik). Relating to the colon.

co·lon·op·a·thy (kō-lŏ-nop'ă-thē). Rarely used term for any disordered condition of the colon. SYN colopathy.

▣co·lon·o·scope (kō-lon'ō-skōp). An elongated endoscope, usually fiberoptic.

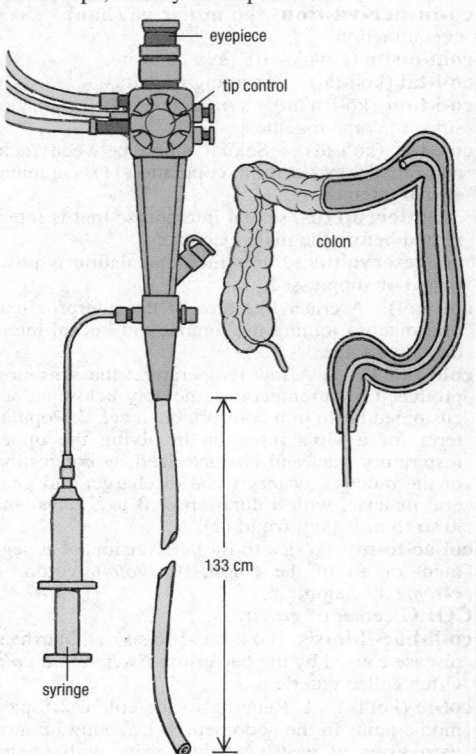

colonoscope: eyepiece — tip control — colon — 133 cm — syringe

colonoscope: with fiberoptics

co·lon·os·co·py (kō-lon-os'kŏ-pē). Visual examination of the inner surface of the colon by means of a colonoscope. SYN coloscopy. [colon + G. *skopeō,* to view]

col·o·ny (kol'ŏ-nē). **1.** A group of cells growing on a solid nutrient surface, each arising from the multiplication of an individual cell; a clone. **2.** A group of people with similar interests, living in a particular location or area. [L. *colonia,* a colony]

co·lop·a·thy (kō-lop'ă-thē). SYN colonopathy.

col·o·pexy (kol'ō-pek-sē). Attachment of a portion of the colon to the abdominal wall. [colo- + G. *pēxis,* fixation]

co·lo·pli·ca·tion (kō'lō-pli-kā'shŭn). Reduction of the lumen of a dilated colon by making folds or tucks in its walls. [colo- + Mod. L. *plica,* fold]

co·lo·proc·ti·tis (kō'lō-prok-tī'tis). Inflammation of both colon and rectum. SYN colorectitis. [colo- + G. *prōktos,* anus (rectum), + *-itis,* inflammation]

co·lo·proc·tos·to·my (kō'lō-prok-tos'tō-mē). Establishment of a communication between the rectum and a discontinuous segment of the colon. SYN colorectostomy. [colo- + G. *prōktos*, anus (rectum), + *stoma*, mouth]

co·lop·to·sis, co·lop·to·sia (kō-lop-tō'sis, -tō'sē-ă). Downward displacement, or prolapse, of the colon, especially of the transverse portion. [colo- + G. *ptōsis*, a falling]

co·lo·punc·ture (kō-lō-pŭnk'chūr). SYN colocentesis.

col·or (kŭl'ŏr). **1.** That aspect of the appearance of objects and light sources that may be specified as to hue, lightness (brightness), and saturation. **2.** That portion of the visible (370-760 nm) electromagnetic spectrum specified as to wavelength, luminosity, and purity. [L.]
   saturated c., a c. containing a minimum amount of whiteness.

co·lo·rec·tal (kol'ō-rek'tăl). Relating to the colon and rectum, or to the entire large bowel.

co·lo·rec·ti·tis (kō'lō-rek-tī'tis). SYN coloproctitis.

co·lo·rec·tos·to·my (kō'lō-rek-tos'tō-mē). SYN coloproctostomy.

col·or·i·met·ric (kŏl-er-i-met'rik). Relating to colorimetry.

col·or·im·e·try (kol-er-im'ĕ-trē). A procedure for quantitative chemical analysis, based on comparison of the color developed in a solution of the test material with that in a standard solution; the two solutions are observed simultaneously in a colorimeter, and quantitated on the basis of the absorption of light.

co·lor·rha·gia (kō-lō-rā'jē-ă). An abnormal discharge from the colon. [colo- + G. *rhēgnymi*, to burst forth]

co·lor·rha·phy (kō-lōr'ă-fē). Suture of the colon. [colo- + G. *rhaphē*, suture]

co·los·co·py (kō-los'kŏ-pē). SYN colonoscopy. [colo- + G. *skopeō*, to view]

co·lo·sig·moi·dos·to·my (kō'lō-sig-moy-dos'tō-mē). Establishment of an anastomosis between any other part of the colon and the sigmoid colon.

co·los·to·my (kō-los'tō-mē). Establishment of an artificial cutaneous opening into the colon. [colo- + G. *stoma*, mouth]

co·los·tric (kō-los'trik). Relating to the colostrum.

co·los·tror·rhea (kō-los-trōr-rē'ă). Abnormally profuse secretion of colostrum. [colostrum, + G. *rhoia*, flow]

co·los·trum (kō-los'trŭm). A thin white opalescent fluid, the first milk secreted at the termination of pregnancy; it differs from the milk secreted later by containing more lactalbumin and lactoprotein; c. is also rich in antibodies which confer passive immunity to the newborn. SYN foremilk. [L.]

co·lot·o·my (kō-lot'ō-mē). Incision into the colon. [colo- + G. *tomē*, incision]

Col·our In·dex. A publication concerned with the chemistry of dyes, with each listed dye identified by a five-digit C.I. number, *e.g.,* methylene blue is C.I. 52015.

colp-. SEE colpo-.

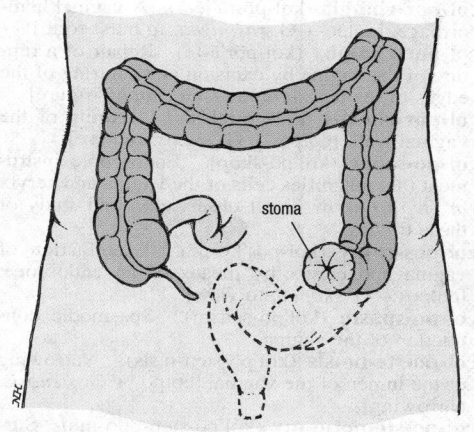

colostomy

col·pa·tre·sia (kol-pa-trē'zē-ă). SYN vaginal *atresia*. [colp- + G. *atrētos*, imperforate]

col·pec·ta·sis, col·pec·ta·sia (kol-pek'tă-sis, -pek-tā'si-ă). Distention of the vagina. [colp- + G. *aktasis*, stretching]

col·pec·to·my (kol-pek'tō-mē). SYN vaginectomy. [colp- + G. *ektomē*, excision]

△**colpo-, colp-.** The vagina. SEE ALSO vagino-. [G. *kolpos*, fold or hollow]

col·po·cele (kol'pō-sēl). **1.** A hernia projecting into the vagina. SYN vaginocele. **2.** SYN colpoptosis. [colpo- + G. *kēlē*, hernia]

col·po·clei·sis (kol-pō-klī'sis). Operation for obliterating the lumen of the vagina. [colpo- + G. *kleisis*, closure]

col·po·cys·to·cele (kol-pō-sis'tō-sēl). SYN cystocele. [colpo- + G. *kystis*, bladder, + *kēlē*, hernia]

col·po·cys·to·plas·ty (kol-pō-sis'tō-plas-tē). Plastic surgery to repair the vesicovaginal wall. [colpo- + G. *kystis*, bladder, + *plastos*, formed]

col·po·dyn·ia (kol-pō-din'ē-ă). SYN vaginodynia. [colpo- + G. *odynē*, pain]

col·po·mi·cros·co·py (kol'pō-mī-kros'kŏ-pē). Direct observation and study of cells in the vagina and cervix magnified *in vivo*, in the undisturbed tissue, by means of a colpomicroscope.

col·po·per·i·ne·o·plas·ty (kol'pō-pār-i-nē'ō-plas-tē). SYN vaginoperineoplasty. [colpo- + perineum, + G. *plastos*, formed]

col·po·per·i·ne·or·rha·phy (kol'pō-pār-i-nē-ōr'ă-fē). SYN vaginoperineorrhaphy. [colpo- + perineum, + G. *rhaphē*, sewing]

col·po·pexy (kol'pō-pek-sē). SYN vaginofixation. [colpo- + G. *pēxis*, fixation]

col·po·plas·ty (kol'pō-plas-tē). SYN vaginoplasty. [colpo- + G. *plastos*, formed]

col·po·poi·e·sis (kol'pō-poy-ē'sis). Surgical construction of a vagina. [colpo- + G. *poiēsis*, a making]

col·po·pto·sis, col·po·pto·sia (kol-pō-tō'sis, -tō'sē-ă; kol-pop-tō'sis). Prolapse of the vaginal walls. SYN colpocele (2). [colpo- + G. *ptōsis*, a falling]

col·por·rha·gia (kol-pō-rā′jē-ă). A vaginal hemorrhage. [colpo-+ G. *rhēgnymi,* to burst forth]

col·por·rha·phy (kol-pōr′ă-fē). Repair of a rupture of the vagina by excision and suturing of the edges of the tear. [colpo- + G. *rhaphē,* suture]

col·por·rhex·is (kol-pō-rek′sis). Tearing of the vaginal wall. [colpo- + G. *rhēxis,* rupture]

col·po·scope (kol′pō-skōp). Endoscopic instrument that magnifies cells of the vagina and cervix *in vivo* to allow direct observation and study of these tissues.

col·pos·co·py (kol-pos′kŏ-pē). Examination of vagina and cervix by means of an endoscope. [colpo- + G. *skopeō,* to view]

col·po·spasm (kol′pō-spazm). Spasmodic contraction of the vagina.

col·po·ste·no·sis (kol′pō-sten-ō′sis). Narrowing of the lumen of the vagina. [colpo- + G. *stenōsis,* narrowing]

col·po·ste·not·o·my (kol′pō-sten-ot′ō-mē). Surgical correction of a colpostenosis. [colpo- + G. *stenōsis,* narrowing, + *tomē,* incision]

col·pot·o·my (kol-pot′ō-mē). SYN vaginotomy. [colpo- + G. *tomē,* incision]

col·po·xe·ro·sis (kol-pō-zē-rō′sis). Abnormal dryness of the vaginal mucous membrane. [colpo- + G. *xērōsis,* dryness]

col·u·mel·la, pl. **col·u·mel·lae** (kol-ū-mel′ă, -mel′ē). **1.** A small column. SYN columnella. **2.** In fungi, a sterile invagination of a sporangium, as in Zygomycetes. [L. dim. of *columna,* column]

col·umn (kol′ŭm). **1.** An anatomical part or structure in the form of a pillar or cylindric funiculus. SEE ALSO fascicle. **2.** A vertical object (usually cylindrical), mass, or formation. SYN columna [NA]. [L. *columna*]

anal c.'s, a number of anatomical vertical ridges in the mucous membrane of the upper half of the anal canal formed as the caliber of the canal is sharply reduced from that of the rectal ampulla. SYN columnae anales [NA], rectal c.'s.

anterior c., the pronounced, ventrally oriented ridge of gray matter in each half of the spinal cord; it corresponds to the anterior or ventral horn appearing in transverse sections of the cord, and contains the motor neurons innervating the skeletal musculature of the trunk, neck, and extremities. SEE ALSO gray c.'s.

c. of fornix, that part of the fornix that curves down in front of the thalamus and the interventricular foramen of Monro, then continues through the hypothalamus to the mamillary body; consisting primarily of fibers originating in the hippocampus and subiculum, the c. of fornix is the direct continuation of the body of the fornix.

gray c.'s, the three somewhat ridge-shaped masses of gray matter (anterior, posterior, and lateral c.'s) that extend longitudinally through the center of each lateral half of the spinal cord; in transverse sections these c.'s appear as gray horns and are therefore commonly called ventral or anterior, dorsal or posterior, and lateral horn, respectively. SYN columnae griseae [NA].

lateral c., a slight protrusion of the gray matter of the spinal cord into the lateral funiculus of either side, especially marked in the thoracic region where it encloses preganglionic motor neu-

rons of the sympathetic division of the autonomic nervous system; it corresponds to the lateral horn appearing in transverse sections of the spinal cord. SEE ALSO gray c.'s.

posterior c., the pronounced, dorsolaterally oriented ridge of gray matter in each lateral half of the spinal cord, corresponding to the posterior or dorsal horn appearing in transverse sections of the cord. SYN posterior c. of spinal cord (1).

posterior c. of spinal cord, (1) SYN posterior c. **(2)** in clinical parlance, the term often refers to the posterior funiculus of the spinal cord.

rectal c.'s, SYN anal c.'s.

renal c.'s, the prolongations of cortical substance separating the pyramids of the kidney. SYN columnae renales [NA].

spinal c., SYN vertebral c.

vertebral c., the series of vertebrae that extend from the cranium to the coccyx, providing support and forming a flexible bony case for the spinal cord. SYN columna vertebralis [NA], backbone, rachis, spina (1), spina (2), spinal c., spine (2).

co·lum·na, gen. and pl. **co·lum·nae** (ko-lŭm′nă, -nē) [NA]. SYN column, column. [L.]

colum′nae ana′les [NA], SYN anal *columns,* under *column.*

colum′nae gris′eae [NA], SYN gray *columns,* under *column.*

colum′nae rena′les [NA], SYN renal *columns,* under *column.*

c. vertebra′lis [NA], SYN vertebral *column.*

co·lum·nel·la, pl. **col·um·nel·lae** (ko-lŭm-nel′ă, -nel′ē). SYN columella (1). [L. dim. of *columna,* a column; another form of *columella*]

△**com-.** SEE con-.

co·ma (kō′mă). **1.** A state of profound unconsciousness from which one cannot be roused. [G. *kōma,* deep sleep, trance] **2.** An aberration of spherical lenses; occurring in cases of oblique incidence (*e.g.,* the image of a point becomes comet-shaped). [G. *kome,* hair]

diabetic c., c. that develops in severe and inadequately treated diabetes mellitus and is commonly fatal, unless appropriate therapy is instituted promptly; results from reduced oxidative metabolism of the central nervous system that, in turn, stems from severe ketoacidosis and possibly also from the histotoxic action of the ketone bodies and disturbances in water and electrolyte balance. SYN Kussmaul's c.

hepatic c., c. that occurs with advanced hepatic insufficiency and portal-systemic shunts, caused by elevated blood ammonia levels; characteristic findings include asterixis in the precoma stage and paroxysms of bilaterally synchronous triphasic waves on EEG examination.

hyperosmolar (hyperglycemic) nonketotic c., a complication seen in *diabetes* mellitus in which marked hyperglycemia occurs (such as levels over 800 mg/dL),causing osmotic shifts in water in brain cells and resulting in coma. It can be fatal or lead to permanent neurologic damage. Ketoacidosis does not occur.

hypoglycemic c., a metabolic encephalopathy caused by hypoglycemia; usually seen in diabetics, and due to exogenous insulin excess.

Kussmaul's c., SYN diabetic c.

metabolic c., coma resulting from diffuse failure of neuronal metabolism, caused by such abnormalities as intrinsic disorders of neuron or glial cell metabolism, or extracerebral disorders that produce intoxication or electrolyte imbalances.

uremic c., a metabolic encephalopathy caused by renal failure.

co•ma•tose (kō'mǎ-tōs). In a state of coma.

com•bus•ti•ble (kom-bus'ti-bl). Capable of combustion.

com•bus•tion (kom-bǔs'chǔn). Burning, the rapid oxidation of any substance accompanied by the production of heat and light. [L. *comburo,* pp. *-bustus,* to burn up]

com•e•do, pl. **com•e•dos, com•e•do•nes** (kom'ē-dō, kō-mē'dō; kom'ē-dōz; kom-ē-dō'nēz). A dilated hair follicle infundibulum filled with keratin squamae, bacteria, particularly *Propionibacterium acnes,* and sebum; the primary lesion of acne vulgaris. [L. a glutton, fr. *com-edo,* to eat up]

   closed c., a c. with a narrow or obstructed opening on the skin surface; closed c.'s may rupture, producing a low-grade dermal inflammatory reaction. SYN whitehead (2).

   open c., a c. with a wide opening on the skin surface capped with a melanin-containing blackened mass of epithelial debris. SYN blackhead (1).

com•e•do•car•ci•no•ma (kō-mē'dō-kar-si-nō'mǎ). Form of carcinoma of the breast or other organ in which plugs of necrotic malignant cells may be expressed from the ducts.

com•e•do•gen•ic (kom'ē-dō-jen'ik). Tending to promote the formation of comedones. [comedo + G. *genesis,* production]

co•mes, pl. **com•i•tes** (kō'mēz, kom'i-tēz). A blood vessel accompanying another vessel or a nerve; the veins accompanying an artery, often two in number, are called venae comitantes or venae comites. [L. a companion, fr. *com-,* together, + *eo,* pp. *itus,* to go]

com•men•sal (kǒ-men'sǎl). **1.** Pertaining to or characterized by commensalism. **2.** An organism participating in commensalism.

com•men•sal•ism (kǒ-men'sǎl-izm). A symbiotic relationship in which one species derives benefit and the other is unharmed. Cf. metabiosis, mutualism, parasitism. [L. *con-,* with, together, + *mensa,* table]

com•mi•nut•ed (kom'i-nū-ted). Broken into several pieces; denoting especially a fractured bone. [L. *com-minuo,* pp. *-minutus,* to make smaller, break into pieces, fr. *minor,* less]

com•mi•nu•tion (kom-i-nū'shǔn). A breaking into several pieces.

com•mis•su•ra, gen. and pl. **com•mis•su•rae** (kom-i-syūr'ǎ, -syūr'ē) [NA]. SYN commissure. [L. a joining together, seam, fr. *com- mitto,* to send together, combine]

   c. poste'rior cer'ebri [NA], SYN posterior cerebral *commissure.*

   commissu'rae supraop'ticae [NA], the commissural fibers that lie above and behind the optic chiasm. SYN supraoptic commissures.

com•mis•sur•al (kom-i-syūr'ǎl). Relating to a commissure.

com•mis•sure (kom'i-syūr). **1.** Angle or corner of the eye, lips, or labia. **2.** A bundle of nerve fibers passing from one side to the other in the brain or spinal cord. SYN commissura [NA].

   anterior c., a round bundle of nerve fibers that crosses the midline of the brain near the anterior limit of the third ventricle. It consists of a smaller anterior part, the fibers of which pass in part to the olfactory bulbs, and a larger posterior part, which interconnects the left and right temporal lobes.

   posterior cerebral c., a thin band of white matter, crossing from side to side beneath the habenula of the pineal body and over the aditus ad aqueductum cerebri; it is largely composed of fibers interconnecting the left and right pretectal region and related cell groups of the midbrain; dorsally, it marks the junction of the diencephalon and mesencephalon. SYN commissura posterior cerebri [NA].

   posterior labial c., a slight fold uniting the labia majora posteriorly in front of the anus.

   supraoptic c.'s, SYN *commissurae* supraopticae, under *commissura.*

com•mis•sur•ot•o•my (kom'i-syūr-ot'ō-mē). **1.** Surgical division of any commissure, fibrous band, or ring via surgery or a balloon catheter technique. **2.** SYN midline *myelotomy.*

com•mu•ni•ca•ble (kǒ-myūn'i-kǎ-bl). Capable of being communicated or transmitted; said especially of disease.

com•mu•ni•ca•tion (kǒ-myū-ni-kā'shǔn). **1.** An opening or connecting passage between two structures. **2.** ANATOMY a joining or connecting; said of fibrous, solid structures, *e.g.,* tendons and nerves. **3.** The exchange of information between individuals using symbol systems such as spoken language or writing but also including elements such as icons, gestures, tone of voice, and facial expression. [L. *communicatio*]

   augmentative and alternative c. (AAC), (1) any type of compensation for impaired use of verbal language, including techniques such as gesture systems and devices such as voice amplifiers, picture boards, and computerized instrumentation; SEE ALSO communication board. **(2)** the clinical practice of determining appropriate compensatory techniques for inadequate verbal communication, and providing training in the use of those techniques. SYN nonoral c., nonverbal c.

   facilitated c., method in which individuals who are unable to communicate effectively are aided by a "facilitator" who physically assists them to use augmentative c. systems such as a c. board or typewriter. SEE augmentative and alternative c. SEE ALSO communication board.

   nonoral c., SYN augmentative and alternative c.

   nonverbal c., SYN augmentative and alternative c.

   total c., habilitation of individuals who are deaf or hearing impaired using any or all appropriate methods to enhance c.; particularly, the combination of manual and oral techniques.

communication board. any arrangement of letters, words, symbols, or pictures designed to aid

CO

an individual whose expressive language ability is inadequate. SEE augmentative and alternative *communication.* SYN conversation board, language board.

com·mu·ni·ty men·tal health cen·ter. A mental health treatment center located in a neighborhood catchment area close to the homes of patients, introduced in the 1960's via new federal legislation designed to replace the large state hospitals, which usually were located in remote rural areas; features include offering a series of comprehensive services by one or more members of the four mental health professions, provision of continuity of care, participation of consumers in the centers, community location to provide accessibility, a combination of indirect or preventive and direct services, the use of program-centered as well as case-centered consultation, a requirement for program evaluation, and various linkages to a variety of health and human services.

co·mor·bid·i·ty (kō-mōr-bid′i-tē). A concomitant but unrelated pathologic or disease process; usually used in epidemiology to indicate the coexistence of two or more disease processes. [co- + L. *morbidus,* diseased]

com·pen·sa·tion (kom-pen-sā′shŭn). **1.** A process in which a tendency for a change in a given direction is counteracted by another change so that the original change is not evident. **2.** An unconscious mechanism by which one tries to make up for fancied or real deficiencies. [L. *com-penso,* pp. *-atus,* to weigh together, counterbalance]

gene dosage c., the putative mechanism that adjusts the X-linked phenotypes of males and females to compensate for the haploid state in males and the diploid state in females. It is now largely ascribed to lyonization which compensates the mean of the dose but not its variance, which is greater in females.

com·pen·sa·to·ry (kom-pen′să-tōr-ē). Providing compensation; making up for a deficiency or loss.

com·pe·tence (kom′pĕ-tens). **1.** The quality of being competent or capable of performing an allotted function. **2.** The normal tight closure of a cardiac valve. **3.** The ability of a group of embryonic cells to respond to an organizer. **4.** The ability of a (bacterial) cell to take up free DNA, which may lead to transformation. **5.** PSYCHIATRY the ability to distinguish right from wrong and to manage one's own affairs, or to assist one's defense in a legal proceeding. [Fr. *competence,* fr. L.L. *competentia,* congruity]

com·plaint (kom-plānt′). A disorder, disease, or symptom, or the description of it. [O. Fr. *complainte,* fr. L. *complango,* to lament]

chief c., the primary symptom that a patient states as the reason for seeking medical care.

com·ple·ment (kom′plĕ-ment). A serum protein complex comprising at least 20 distinct proteins, the activity of which is affected by a series of enzymatic cleavages and which can follow one or the other of at least two pathways. In immune hemolysis (classical pathway), the complex comprises nine components (designated C1 through C9) which react in a definite sequence and the activation of which is effected by the antigen-

antibody complex; only the first seven components are involved in chemotaxis, and only the first four are involved in immune adherence or phagocytosis. An alternative pathway (see properdin *system*) is activated by factors other than antigen-antibody complexes and involves components other than C1, C4, and C2 in the activation of C3. SEE ALSO *component* of complement. [L. *complementum,* that which completes, fr. *com-pleo,* to fill up]

com·ple·men·tar·i·ty (kom-plĕ-men-tār′i-tē). **1.** The degree of base-pairing between two sequences of DNA and/or RNA molecules. **2.** The degree of affinity, or fit, of antigen and antibody combining sites.

com·ple·men·ta·tion (kom′plĕ-men-tā′shŭn). **1.** Interaction between two defective viruses permitting replication under conditions inhibitory to the single virus. **2.** Interaction between two genetic units, one or both of which are defective, permitting the organism containing these units to function normally, whereas it could not do so if either unit were absent.

com·plex (kom′pleks). **1.** An organized constellation of feelings, thoughts, perceptions, and memories that may be in part unconscious and may strongly influence associations and attitudes. **2.** CHEMISTRY the relatively stable combination of two or more compounds into a larger molecule without covalent binding. **3.** A composite of chemical or immunological structures. **4.** A structural anatomical entity made up of three or more interrelated parts. **5.** An informal term used to denote a group of individual structures known or believed to be anatomically, embryologically, or physiologically related. [L. *complexus,* woven together]

anomalous c., a c. in the electrocardiogram differing significantly from the physiologic type in the same lead.

atrial c., p wave in the electrocardiogram.

avian leukosis-sarcoma c., avian leukemia-sarcoma c., (1) a group of transmissible virus-induced diseases of chickens; the agents are closely related viruses (avian leukosis-sarcoma virus) causing proliferation of immature erythroid, myeloid, or lymphoid cells; (2) a division of the RNA tumor viruses causing the avian leukosis-sarcoma c. of diseases. SYN avian leukosis-sarcoma virus.

Cain c., extreme envy or jealousy of a brother, leading to hatred. [*Cain,* biblical personage]

castration c., (1) a child's fear of injury to the genitals by the parent of the same sex as punishment for unconscious guilt over oedipal feelings; (2) fantasied loss of the penis by a female or fear of its actual loss by a male; (3) unconscious fear of injury from those in authority.

Diana c., ideas leading to the adoption of masculine traits and behavior in a female. [*Diana,* L. myth. char.]

Eisenmenger's c., the combination of ventricular septal defect with pulmonary hypertension and consequent right-to-left shunt through the defect, with or without an associated overriding aorta.

Electra c., unresolved conflicts during childhood toward the father which subsequently influence a woman's relationships with men. [*Electra,* daughter of Agamemnon]

femininity c., PSYCHOANALYSIS the unconscious fear, in boys and men, of castration at the hands of the mother with resultant identification with the aggressor and envious desire for breasts and vagina.

histocompatibility c., a family of fifty or more genes on the sixth human chromosome that code for cell surface proteins and play a role in the immune response. Histocompatibility genes control the production of proteins on the outer membranes of tissue and blood cells, especially lymphocytes, and are vital elements in cell-cell recognition. The proteins also determine the level and type of immune response, and may serve other biochemical or immunologic functions. In the case of allografts, it is necessary to determine whether donor and recipient possess compatible sets of proteins (histocompatibility antigens), to minimize the likelihood of rejection. Histocompatibility testing (HLA tissue typing) provides this information.

HLA c., the major histocompatibility c. in humans. SEE ALSO human lymphocyte *antigens,* under *antigen.*

immune c., antigen combined with specific antibody, to which complement may also be fixed, and which may precipitate or remain in solution. Frequently associated with autoimmune disease.

inferiority c., a sense of inadequacy which is expressed in extreme shyness, diffidence, or timidity, or as a compensatory reaction in exhibitionism or aggressiveness.

Jocasta c., a mother's libidinous fixation on a son. [*Jocasta,* mother and wife of Oedipus]

knee c., the knee joint, the patellofemoral joint, and related musculature and connective tissue. SEE ALSO patellofemoral *joint.*

Lear c., a father's libidinous fixation on a daughter. [*Lear,* Shakespearean character]

major histocompatibility c. (MHC), a group of linked loci, collectively termed H-2 c. in the mouse and HLA c. in humans, that codes for cell-surface histocompatibility antigens and is the principal determinant of tissue type and transplant compatibility. SEE ALSO human lymphocyte *antigens,* under *antigen.*

Oedipus c., a group of associated ideas, aims, instinctual drives, and fears in male children 3 to 6 years old: at the peak of the phallic phase of psychosexual development, the child's sexual interest is attached primarily to the parent of the opposite sex and is accompanied by aggressive feelings toward the parent of the same sex; in psychoanalytic theory, it is replaced by the castration c. [*Oedipus,* G. myth. char.]

primary c., the typical lesions of primary pulmonary tuberculosis, consisting of a small peripheral focus of infection, with hilar or paratracheal lymph node involvement.

QRS c., portion of electrocardiogram corresponding to the depolarization of ventricular myocardium.

shoulder c., (1) the sternoclavicular, acromioclavicular, glenohumeral, and scapulothoracic joints, together with associated muscle and connective tissues; **(2)** the shoulder and the pectoral girdle. **(3)** SYN shoulder *girdle.*

sicca c., dryness of the mucous membranes, as of the eyes and mouth, in the absence of a connective tissue disease such as rheumatoid arthritis.

spike and wave c., a generalized, synchronous pattern seen on the electroencephalogram, consisting of a sharply contoured fast wave followed by a slow wave; particularly found in patients with generalized epilepsies.

superiority c., term sometimes given to the compensatory behavior, *e.g.,* aggressiveness, self-assertion, associated with inferiority c.

symptom c., (1) SEE syndrome. **(2)** SEE complex (1).

synaptinemal c., a submicroscopic structure interposed between the homologous chromosome pairs during synapsis.

ventricular c., the continuous QRST waves of each beat in the electrocardiogram.

com•plex•ion (kom-plek′shŭn). The color, texture, and general appearance of the skin of the face. [L. *complexio,* a combination, (later) physical condition]

com•pli•ance (kom-plī′ans). **1.** A measure of the distensibility of a chamber expressed as a change in volume per unit change in pressure. **2.** The consistency and accuracy with which a patient follows the regimen prescribed by a physician or other health professional. Cf. adherence (2), maintenance. **3.** PHYSIOLOGY a measure of the ease with which a hollow viscus (*e.g.,* lung, urinary bladder, gallbladder) may be distended, *i.e.,* the volume change resulting from the application of a unit pressure differential between the inside and outside of the viscus; the reciprocal of elastance. [M.E. fr. O. Fr., fr. L. *compleo,* to fulfill]

respiratory c., the extent to which the lungs expand for each unit increase in transpulmonary pressure, defined as the volume change in the lung per unit of pressure change. Units are measured in liters per centimeter of water.

com•pli•ca•tion (kom-pli-kā′shŭn). A morbid process or event occurring during a disease that is not an essential part of the disease, although it may result from it or from independent causes.

com•po•nent (kom-pō′nent). An element forming a part of the whole. [L. *com-pono,* pp. *-positus,* to place together]

c. of complement (C), any one of the nine distinct protein units (designated C1 through C9) that effect the immunological activities associated with complement.

com•pos men•tis (kom′pos men′tis). Of sound mind; usually used in its opposite form, *non compos mentis.* [L. possessed of one's mind; *compos,* having control, + *mens (ment-),* mind]

com•pound (kom′pownd). **1.** CHEMISTRY a substance formed by the covalent or electrostatic union of two or more elements, generally differing entirely in physical characteristics from any of its components. **2.** PHARMACY a preparation containing several ingredients. [through O. Fr., fr. L. *compono*]

CO

acyclic c., an organic c. in which the chain does not form a ring. SYN open chain c.

aromatic c., SEE cyclic c.

carbamino c., any carbamic acid derivative formed by the combination of carbon dioxide with a free amino group to form an *N*-carboxyl group.

closed chain c., SYN cyclic c.

cyclic c., any c. in which the constituent atoms, or any part of them, form a ring. Used mainly in organic chemistry. SYN closed chain c.

inorganic c., a c. in which the atoms or radicals consist of elements other than carbon and are typically held together by electrostatic forces rather than by covalent bonds; often are capable of dissociation into ions in polar solvents (*e.g.,* H_2O). Cf. organic c.

open chain c., SYN acyclic c.

organic c., a c. composed of atoms (some of which are carbon) held together by covalent (shared electron) bonds. Cf. inorganic c.

com·pre·hen·sion (kom-prē-hen′shŭn). Knowledge or understanding of an object, situation, event, or verbal statement.

com·press (kom′pres). A pad of gauze or other material applied for local pressure. [L. *com-primo,* pp. *-pressus,* to press together]

com·pres·sion (kom-presh′ŭn). A squeezing together; the exertion of pressure on a body in such a way as to tend to increase its density; the decrease in a dimension of a body under the action of two external forces directed toward one another.

intermittent c., (1) a neurodevelopmental treatment technique to facilitate contraction by applying pressure directly to the muscles surrounding a joint requiring better stabilization; SYN pressure tapping. **(2)** a treatment procedure that employs intermittent external pressure to reduce edema in the extremities.

com·pres·sor (kom-pres′er, -ōr). **1.** A muscle, contraction of which causes compression of any structure. **2.** An instrument for making pressure on a part, especially on an artery to prevent loss of blood.

com·pul·sion (kom-pŭl′shŭn). Uncontrollable impulses to perform an act, often repetitively, as an unconscious mechanism to avoid unacceptable ideas and desires which, by themselves, arouse anxiety; the anxiety becomes fully manifest if performance of the compulsive act is prevented; may be associated with obsessive thoughts. [L. *com-pello* pp. *-pulsus,* to drive together, compel]

com·pul·sive (kom-pŭl′siv). Influenced by compulsion; of a compelling and irresistible nature.

Computer-Based Patient Record Institute (CPRI). Institution supporting development of the computer-based patient record by facilitating dialogue on a national level with regard to issues such as technology, standardization of data definitions, and confidentiality. SEE ALSO computer-based patient *record.*

⚠con-. With, together, in association; appears as com- before p, b, or m, as col- before l, and as co- before a vowel; corresponds to G. *syn-.* [L. *cum,* with, together]

conA, con A concanavalin A.

co·nar·i·um (kō-nā′rē-ŭm). SYN pineal *body.* [G. *kōnarion* (dim. of *kōnos,* cone), the pineal body]

co·na·tion (kō-nā′shŭn). The conscious tendency to act, usually an aspect of mental process; historically aligned with cognition and affection, but more recently used in the wider sense of impulse, desire, purposeful striving. [L. *conātio,* an undertaking, effort]

co·na·tive (kon′ă-tiv). Pertaining to, or characterized by, conation.

con·ca·nav·a·lin A (conA, con A) (kon-kă-nav′ă-lin). A phytomitogen, extracted from the jack bean (*Canavalia ensiformis*) that agglutinates the blood of mammals and reacts with glucosans; like other phytohemagglutinins, con A stimulates T lymphocytes more vigorously than it does B lymphocytes.

con·cave (kon′kāv). Having a depressed or hollowed surface. [L. *concavus,* arched or vaulted]

con·cav·i·ty (kon-kav′i-tē). A hollow or depression, with more or less evenly curved sides, on any surface.

con·ca·vo·con·cave (kon-kā′vō-kon′kāv). SYN biconcave.

con·ca·vo·con·vex (kon-kā′vō-kon′veks). Concave on one surface and convex on the opposite surface.

con·cen·tra·tion (c) (kon-sen-trā′shŭn). **1.** A preparation made by extracting a crude drug, precipitating from the solution, and drying. **2.** Increasing the amount of solute in a given volume of solution by evaporation of the solvent. **3.** The quantity of a substance per unit volume or weight. In renal physiology, symbol U for urinary c., P for plasma c.; in respiratory physiology, symbol C for amount per unit volume in blood, F for fractional c. (mole fraction or volume per volume) in dried gas; subscripts indicate location and chemical species. [L. *con-,* together, + *centrum,* center]

critical micelle c. (cmc), the c. at which an amphipathic molecule (*e.g.,* a phospholipid) will form a micelle.

mean corpuscular hemoglobin c. (MCHC), Hgb/Hct; the average hemoglobin c. in a given volume of packed red cells, calculated from the hemoglobin therein and the hematocrit, in erythrocyte indices.

normal c. (N), SEE normal (3).

concentrator (kon′sen-trā′tōr). A device for making a substance stronger or purer.

oxygen concentrator, an electrically powered device for oxygen delivery in the home; it uses a filtering mechanism to purify entrained ambient air.

con·cen·tric (kon-sen′trik). Having a common center; said of two or more circles or spheres having a common center.

con·cept (kon′sept). **1.** An abstract idea or notion. **2.** An explanatory variable or principle in a scientific system. SYN conception (1). [L. *conceptum,* something understood, pp. ntr. of *concipio,* to receive, apprehend]

self c., an assessment of one's own status with respect to one or several traits, using societal or personal norms as criteria.

con·cep·ti (kon-sep′tī). Plural of conceptus.

con·cep·tion (kon-sep′shŭn). **1.** SYN concept. **2.** Act of forming a general idea or notion. **3.** Act of conceiving, or becoming pregnant; fertilization of the oocyte (ovum) by a spermatozoon to form a viable zygote. [L. *conceptio;* see concept]

con·cep·tu·al (kon-sep′chŭ-ăl). Relating to the formation of ideas, usually higher order abstractions, to mental conceptions.

con·cep·tus, pl. **con·cep·ti** (kon-sep′tŭs, -sep′tī). The product of conception, *i.e.,* embryo and membranes.

con·cha, pl. **con·chae** (kon′kă, kon′kē) [NA]. In anatomy, a structure comparable to a shell in shape, as the auricle or pinna of the ear or a turbinated bone in the nose. [L. a shell]

  c. of ear, the large hollow, or floor of the auricle, between the anterior portion of the helix and the antihelix; it is divided by the crus of the helix into the cymba above and the cavum below.

  inferior nasal c., (1) a thin, spongy, bony plate with curved margins, on the lateral wall of the nasal cavity, separating the middle from the inferior meatus; it articulates with the ethmoid, lacrimal, maxilla, and palate bones; (2) the above bony plate and its thick mucoperiosteum containing an extensive cavernous vascular bed for heat exchange.

  middle nasal c., (1) the middle thin, spongy, bony plate with curved margins, part of the ethmoidal labyrinth, projecting from the lateral wall of the nasal cavity and separating the superior meatus from the middle meatus; (2) the above bony plate and its thick mucoperiosteum containing a cavernous vascular bed for heat exchange.

  sphenoidal conchae, paired ossicles of pyramidal shape, the spines of which are in contact with the medial pterygoid lamina, the bases forming the roof of the nasal cavity.

  superior nasal c., (1) the upper thin, spongy, bony plate with curved margins, part of the ethmoidal labyrinth, projecting from the lateral wall of the nasal cavity and separating the superior meatus from the sphenoethmoidal recess; (2) the above bony plate and its thick mucoperiosteum, which is less vascular than that of the middle and inferior conchae.

  supreme nasal c., a small c. frequently present on the posterosuperior part of the lateral nasal wall; it overlies the supreme nasal meatus.

con·chae (kon′kē).

con·cor·dance (kon-kōr′dans). Agreement in the types of data that occur in natural pairs. [L. *concordia,* agreeing, harmony]

con·cor·dant (kon-kōr′dant). Denoting or exhibiting concordance.

con·cres·cence (kon-kres′ens). **1.** SYN coalescence. **2.** DENTISTRY the union of the roots of two adjacent teeth by cementum.

con·cre·tio cor·dis (kon-krē′shē-ō kōr′dis). Extensive adhesion between parietal and visceral layers of the pericardium with partial or complete obliteration of the pericardial cavity. SYN internal adhesive pericarditis.

con·cre·tion (kon-krē′shŭn). Formation of solid material by the aggregation of discrete units or particles. [L. *cum,* together, + *crescere,* to grow]

con·cus·sion (kon-kŭsh′ŭn). **1.** A violent shaking or jarring. **2.** An injury of a soft structure, as the brain, resulting from a blow or violent shaking. [L. *concussio,* fr. *con- cutio,* pp. *-cussus,* to shake violently]

  brain c., a clinical syndrome due to mechanical, usually traumatic, forces; characterized by immediate and transient impairment of neural function, such as alteration of consciousness, disturbance of vision and equilibrium, etc.

  spinal cord c., injury to the spinal cord due to a blow to the vertebral column with transient or prolonged dysfunction below the level of the lesion.

con·den·sa·tion (kon-den-sā′shŭn). **1.** Making more solid or dense. **2.** The change of a gas to a liquid, or of a liquid to a solid. **3.** PSYCHOANALYSIS an unconscious mental process in which one symbol stands for a number of others. **4.** DENTISTRY the process of packing a filling material into a cavity, using such force and direction that no voids result. [L. *con- denso,* pp. *-atus,* to make thick, condense]

con·dens·er (kon-den′ser). **1.** An apparatus for cooling a gas to a liquid, or a liquid to a solid. **2.** DENTISTRY a manual or powered instrument used for packing a plastic or unset material into a cavity of a tooth; variation in sizes and shapes allows conformation of the mass to the cavity outline. **3.** The simple or compound lens on a microscope that is used to focus the illumination. **4.** SYN capacitor.

con·di·tion (kon-dish′ŭn). **1.** To train; to undergo conditioning. **2.** A certain response elicited by a specifiable stimulus or emitted in the presence of certain stimuli with reward of the response during prior occurrence. **3.** Referring to several classes of learning in the behavioristic branch of psychology. [L. *conditio,* fr. *condico,* to agree]

con·di·tion·ing (kon-dish′ŭn-ing). The process of acquiring, developing, educating, establishing, learning, or training new responses in an individual; a change in the frequency or form of behavior as a result of the influence of the environment.

con·dom (kon′dom). Sheath or cover for the penis or vagina, for use in the prevention of conception or infection during coitus.

con·duc·tance (kon-dŭk′tans). **1.** A measure of conductivity; the ratio of the current flowing through a conductor to the difference in potential between the ends of the conductor; the c. of a circuit is the reciprocal of its resistance. **2.** The ease with which a fluid or gas enters and flows through a conduit, air passage, or respiratory tract; the flow per unit pressure difference.

con·duc·tion (kon-dŭk′shŭn). **1.** The act of transmitting or conveying certain forms of energy, such as heat, sound, or electricity, from one point to another, without evident movement in the conducting body. **2.** The transmission of stimuli of various sorts by living protoplasm. [L. *con- duco,* pp. *ductus,* to lead, conduct]

  air c., in relation to hearing, the transmission of sound to the inner ear through the external auditory canal and the structures of the middle ear.

  bone c., in relation to hearing, the transmission of sound to the inner ear through vibrations applied to the bones of the skull.

intra-atrial c., c. of the cardiac impulse through the atrial myocardium, represented by the P wave in the electrocardiogram.

intraventricular c., c. of the cardiac impulse through the ventricular myocardium, represented by the QRS complex in the electrocardiogram. SYN ventricular c.

nerve c., the transmission of an impulse along a nerve fiber.

saltatory c., nerve c. in which the impulse jumps from one node of Ranvier to the next.

synaptic c., the c. of a nerve impulse across a synapse.

ventricular c., SYN intraventricular c.

con·duc·tiv·i·ty (kon-dŭk-tiv′i-tē). **1.** The power of transmission or conveyance of certain forms of energy, as heat, sound, and electricity, without perceptible motion in the conducting body. **2.** The property, inherent in living protoplasm, of transmitting a state of excitation; *e.g.,* in muscle or nerve.

con·duc·tor (kon-dŭk′ter, -tōr). **1.** A probe or sound with a groove along which a knife is passed in slitting open a sinus or fistula; a grooved director. **2.** Any substance possessing conductivity.

con·duit (kon′dū-it). A channel.

con·du·pli·cate (kon-dū′pli-kāt). Folded upon itself lengthwise. [L. *con-,* with, + *duplico,* pp. *-atus*]

con·dy·lar (kon′di-lăr). Relating to a condyle.

con·dy·lar·thro·sis (kon′di-lar-thrō′sis). A joint, like that of the knee, formed by condylar surfaces. [G. *kondylos,* condyle, + *arthrōsis,* a jointing]

con·dyle (kon′dīl). A rounded articular surface at the extremity of a bone. SYN condylus [NA].

balancing side c., DENTISTRY the mandibular c. on the side away from which the mandible moves in a lateral excursion.

con·dy·lec·to·my (kon-di-lek′tō-mē). Excision of a condyle. [G. *kondylos,* condyle, + *ektomē,* excision]

con·dy·loid (kon′di-loyd). Relating to or resembling a condyle. [G. *kondylōdēs,* like a knuckle, fr. *kondylos,* condyle, + *eidos,* resemblance]

con·dy·lo·ma, pl. **con·dy·lo·ma·ta** (kon-di-lō′mă, -mah′tă). A wartlike excrescence on the skin of the genitals, perineum, or anus. [G. *kondylōma,* a knob]

⎵c. acumina′tum, a warty growth on the external genitals or at the anus, consisting of fibrous overgrowths covered by thickened epithelium showing koilocytosis, due to sexually transmitted infection with human papilloma virus; malignant change is associated with particular types of the virus. SYN genital wart, venereal wart.

flat c., (1) SYN c. latum. (2) a c. of the uterine cervix or other site caused by human papilloma virus infection and characterized histologically by koilocytosis without papillomatosis.

giant c., a large type of c. acuminatum found in the anus, vulva, or preputial sac of the penis of middle-aged, uncircumcised men; it tends to extend deeply and recur.

c. la′tum, a secondary syphilitic eruption of flat-topped papules, found at the anus and wher-

ever contiguous folds of skin produce heat and moisture. SYN flat c. (1).

con·dy·lom·a·tous (kon-di-lō′mă-tŭs). Relating to a condyloma.

con·dy·lot·o·my (kon-di-lot′ō-mē). Division, without removal, of a condyle. [G. *kondylos,* condyle, + *tomē,* incision]

con·dy·lus (kon′di-lŭs) [NA]. SYN condyle. [L. fr. G. *kondylos,* knuckle, the knuckle of any joint]

cone (kōn). **1.** A figure having a circular base with sides inclined so as to meet at a point above. **2.** The photosensitive, outward-directed, conical process of a c. cell essential for sharp vision and color vision; c.'s are the only photoreceptor in the fovea centralis and become interspersed with increasing numbers of rods toward the periphery of the retina. **3.** Metallic cylinder or c. used to confine a beam of x-rays. SYN conus (1). [G. *kōnos,* cone]

arterial c., the left or anterosuperior, smooth-walled portion of the cavity of the right ventricle of the heart, which begins at the supraventricular crest and terminates in the pulmonary trunk. SYN conus arteriosus [NA], infundibulum (4)✲.

c. down, to narrow a beam of x-rays to a region of interest using a collimator or c. (3); colloq., to delimit one's attention or activities.

c. of light, SYN *pyramid* of light.

medullary c., the tapering lower extremity of the spinal cord. SYN conus medullaris [NA].

◁-cone. The cusp of a tooth in the upper jaw.

con·fab·u·la·tion (kon′fab-yū-lā′shŭn). The making of bizarre and incorrect responses, and a readiness to give a fluent but tangential answer, with no regard whatever to facts, to any question put; seen in amnesia, presbyophrenia, and Wernicke-Korsakoff syndrome. [L. *con-fabulor,* pp. *-fabulatus,* to talk together, fr. *fabula,* narrative]

con·fec·tion (kon-fek′shŭn). A pharmaceutical preparation consisting of a drug mixed with honey or syrup; a soft solid, sometimes used as an excipient for pill masses. SYN electuary. [L. *confectio*]

con·fi·den·ti·al·i·ty (kon′fi-den-shē-al′i-tē). The statutorily protected right and duty of health professionals not to disclose information acquired during consultation with a patient. [L. *con-fido,* to trust, be assured]

con·fig·u·ra·tion (kon-fig-yū-rā′shŭn). **1.** The general form of a body and its parts. **2.** CHEMISTRY the spatial arrangement of atoms in a molecule. The c. of a compound (*e.g.,* a sugar) is the unique spatial arrangement of its atoms such that no other arrangement of these atoms is superimposable thereon with complete correspondence. Cf. conformation.

con·fine·ment (kon-fīn′ment). Lying-in; giving birth to a child. [L. *confine* (ntr.), a boundary, confine, fr. *con-* + *finis,* boundary]

con·flict (kon′flikt). Tension or stress experienced by an organism when satisfaction of a need, drive, motive, or wish is thwarted by the presence of other attractive or unattractive needs, drives, or motives.

c. of interest, a c. between the personal interests and professional responsibilities of a health provider toward a patient or other consumer.

con·flu·ence (kon'flū-ĕns). A flowing together; a joining of two or more streams. [L. *confluens*]

con·flu·ent (kon'flū-ent). **1.** Joining; running together; denoting certain skin lesions which become merged, forming a patch; denoting a disease characterized by lesions which are not discrete, or distinct one from the other. **2.** Denoting a bone formed by the blending together of two originally distinct bones. [L. *con-fluo,* to flow together]

con·for·ma·tion (kon-fōr-mā'shŭn). The spatial arrangement of a molecule achieved by rotation of groups about single covalent bonds, without breaking any covalent bonds. Cf. configuration.

con·found·ing (kon-fown'ding). **1.** A situation in which the effects of two or more processes are not separated; the distortion of the apparent effect of an exposure on risk, brought about by the association with other factors that can influence the outcome. **2.** A relationship between the effects of two or more causal factors observed in a set of data, such that it is not logically possible to separate the contribution of any single causal factor to the observed effects.

con·fu·sion (kon-fyū'zhŭn). A mental state in which reactions to environmental stimuli are inappropriate because the subject is bewildered, perplexed, or disoriented. [L. *confusio,* a confounding]

con·ge·ner (kon'jē-ner). **1.** One of two or more things of the same kind, as of animal or plant with respect to classification. **2.** One of two or more muscles with the same function. [L. *con-,* with, + *genus,* race]

con·gen·i·tal (kon-jen'i-tăl). Existing at birth, referring to mental or physical traits, anomalies, malformations, or diseases, which may be either hereditary or due to an influence occurring during gestation up to the moment of birth. [L. *congenitus,* born with]

con·gest·ed (kon-jes'ted). Containing an abnormal amount of blood; in a state of congestion.

con·ges·tion (kon-jes'chŭn). Presence of an abnormal amount of fluid in the vessels or passages of a part or organ; especially, of blood due either to increased influx or to an obstruction to the return flow. SEE ALSO hyperemia. [L. *congestio,* a bringing together, a heap, fr. *con-gero,* pp. *-gestus,* to bring together]

  active c., c. due to an increased flow of arterial blood to a part.

  functional c., hyperemia occurring during functional activity of an organ. SYN physiologic c.

  hypostatic c., c. due to pooling of venous blood in a dependent part. SYN hypostasis (2).

  passive c., c. caused by obstruction or slowing of the venous drainage, resulting in partial stagnation of blood in the capillaries and venules.

  physiologic c., SYN functional c.

con·ges·tive (kon-jes'tiv). Relating to congestion.

con·glo·bate (kon-glō'bāt). Formed in a single rounded mass. [L. *con-globo,* pp. *-atus,* to gather into a *globus,* ball]

con·glom·er·ate (kon-glom'ĕ-rāt). Composed of

several parts aggregated into one mass. [L. *conglomero,* pp. *-atus,* to roll together, fr. *glomus,* a ball]

con·glu·ti·nant (kon-glū'ti-nant). Adhesive, promoting the union of a wound. [L. *con-glutino,* pp. *-atus,* to glue together, fr. *gluten,* glue]

con·glu·ti·na·tion (kon-glū-ti-nā'shŭn). **1.** SYN adhesion (1). **2.** Agglutination of antigen-(erythrocyte)-antibody-complement complex by normal bovine serum (and certain other colloidal materials); the procedure provides a means of detecting the presence of nonagglutinating antibody.

con·go·phil·ic (kon-gō-fil'ik). Denoting any substance that takes a Congo red stain.

Con·go red (kong'gō) [C.I. 22120]. An acid direct cotton dye, used as an indicator (pH 3.0, blue-violet, to pH 5.0, red) in testing for free hydrochloric acid in gastric contents; the dye is absorbed by amyloid and induces green fluorescence in amyloid in polarized light; used as a laboratory aid in the diagnosis of amyloidosis and as a histologic stain.

co·ni (kō'nī). Plural of conus.

△**-conid.** The cusp of a tooth in the lower jaw.

co·ni·o·fi·bro·sis (kō'nē-ō-fī-brō'sis). Fibrosis produced by dust, especially of the lungs by inhaled dust. [G. *konis,* dust, + fibrosis]

co·ni·o·phage (kō'nē-ō-fāj). SYN alveolar *macrophage.* [G. *konis,* dust, + *phagō,* to eat]

co·ni·o·sis (kō-nē-ō'sis). Any disease or morbid condition caused by dust. [G. *konis,* dust]

con·i·za·tion (kō-nī-zā'shŭn). Excision of a cone of tissue, *e.g.,* mucosa of the cervix uteri.

con·ju·gant (kon'jū-gant). A member of a mating pair of organisms or gametes undergoing conjugation. [L. *con-jugo,* to join]

con·ju·ga·ta (kon-jū-gā'tă) [NA]. Conjugate diameters of the pelvis. SEE conjugate. [L. fem. of *conjugatus,* pp. of *con-jugo,* to join together]

con·ju·gate (kon'jū-gāt). **1.** Joined or paired. SYN conjugated. **2.** Conjugate diameters of the pelvis. The distance between any two specified points on the periphery of the pelvic canal. [L. *conjugatus,* joined together. See conjugata]

  diagonal c., the anteroposterior dimension of the inlet; the clinical distance from the promontory of the sacrum to the lower margin of the symphysis pubica. SYN false c. (1).

  effective c., the internal c. measured from the nearest lumbar vertebra to the symphysis, in spondylolisthesis. SYN false c. (2).

  external c., the distance in a straight line between the depression under the last spinous process of the lumbar vertebrae and the upper edge of the pubic symphysis.

  false c., (1) SYN diagonal c. **(2)** SYN effective c.

  obstetric c., the shortest diameter through which the head must pass in descending into the superior strait and measures; as measured by x-ray, the distance from the promontory of the sacrum to a point on the inner surface of the symphysis a few millimeters below its upper margin.

  c. of pelvic inlet, distance from the promontory of the sacrum to the upper posterior edge of the pubic symphysis.

con·ju·gat·ed (kon'jū-gāt-ed). SYN conjugate (1).

CO

con•ju•ga•tion (kon-jŭ-gā'shŭn). **1.** The union of two unicellular organisms or of the male and female gametes of multicellular forms followed by partition of the chromatin and the production of two new cells. **2.** Bacterial c., effected by simple contact, through which transfer genes and other genes of the plasmid are transferred to recipient bacteria. **3.** Sexual reproduction among protozoan ciliates, during which two individuals of appropriate mating types fuse along part of their lengths; their macronuclei degenerate and the micronuclei in each macronucleus divide several times (including a meiotic division); one of the resulting haploid pronuclei passes from each conjugant into the other and fuses with the remaining haploid nucleus in each conjugant; the organisms then separate (becoming exconjugants), undergo nuclear reorganization, and subsequently divide by asexual mitosis. **4.** The combination, especially in the liver, of certain toxic substances formed in the intestine, drugs, or steroid hormones with glucuronic or sulfuric acid; a means by which the biological activity of certain chemical substances is terminated and the substances made ready for excretion. **5.** The formation of glycyl or tauryl derivatives of the bile acids. [L. con-jugo, pp. -jugatus, to join together]

con•junc•ti•va, pl. **con•junc•ti•vae** (kon-jŭnk-tī'vă, -vē). The mucous membrane investing the anterior surface of the eyeball and the posterior surface of the lids. [L. fem. of conjunctivus, from conjungo, pp. -junctus, to bind together]

con•junc•ti•val (kon-jŭnk-tī'văl). Relating to the conjunctiva.

con•junc•ti•vi•tis (kon-jŭnk-ti-vī'tis). Inflammation of the conjunctiva.

   acute contagious c., acute c. marked by intense hyperemia and profuse mucopurulent discharge. SYN pinkeye (1).

   acute hemorrhagic c., specific acute endemic c. with eyelid swelling, tearing, conjunctival hemorrhages, and follicles; usually caused by *Enterovirus* type 70.

   allergic c., SYN vernal c.

   gonococcal c., a type of hyperacute, purulent c.

   granular c., SYN trachomatous c.

   inclusion c., a follicular c. caused by *Chlamydia trachomatis.*

   infantile purulent c., SYN *ophthalmia* neonatorum.

   spring c., SYN vernal c.

   swimming pool c., c. in a swimmer, which can be caused by pool chlorination, adenovirus, and rarely, *Chlamydia.*

   trachomatous c., a chronic infection of the conjunctiva due to *Chlamydia trachomatis*, characterized by conjunctival follicles and subsequent cicatrization. SEE ALSO trachoma. SYN granular c.

   vernal c., a chronic, bilateral conjunctival inflammation with photophobia and intense itching that recurs seasonally during warm weather; characterized in the palpebral form by cobblestone papillae in the upper palpebral conjunctiva and in the bulbar form by gelatinous nodules adjacent to the corneoscleral limbus. SYN allergic c., spring c.

con•junc•ti•vo•plas•ty (kon-jŭnk-tī'vō-plas-tē,

kon-jŭngk'ti-vō-). Plastic surgery on the conjunctiva.

con•nec•tion (kŏ-nek'shŭn). A union of elements or things; a connecting structure.

con•san•guin•e•ous (kon-sang-gwin'ē-ŭs). Denoting consanguinity. [L. *cum,* with, + *sanguis,* blood: *consanguineus*]

con•san•guin•i•ty (kon-sang-gwin'i-tē). Kinship because of common ancestry. SYN blood relationship. [L. *consanguinitas,* blood relationship]

con•scious (con'shŭs). **1.** Aware; having present knowledge or perception of oneself, one's acts and surroundings. **2.** Denoting something occurring with the perceptive attention of the individual, as a c. act or idea, distinguished from automatic or instinctive. [L. *conscius,* knowing]

con•scious•ness (con'shŭs-nes). The state of being aware, or perceiving physical facts or mental concepts; a state of general wakefulness and responsiveness to environment; a functioning sensorium. [L. *con-scio,* to know, to be aware of]

con•sen•su•al (kon-sen'shū-ăl). Denoting what something is by the fact of agreement between the perceiving of several persons. SYN reflex (3). [L. *con-,* with, + *sensus,* sensation]

con•ser•va•tive (kon-ser'vă-tiv). Denoting treatment by gradual, limited, or well-established procedures, as opposed to radical.

con•sol•i•da•tion (kon-sol-i-dā'shŭn). Solidification into a firm dense mass; applied especially to inflammatory induration of a normally aerated lung due to the presence of cellular exudate in the pulmonary alveoli. [L. *consolido,* to make thick, condense, fr. *solidus,* solid]

con•spi•cu•i•ty (kon-spi-kyū'i-tē). The visibility of a structure of interest on a radiograph, a function of the inherent contrast of the structure and the complexity (noise) of the surrounding image.

con•stan•cy (kon'stan-sē). The quality of being constant. [L. *constantia,* fr. *consto,* to stand still]

   form c., recognition of forms and objects as the same although they appear in various environments, positions, and sizes.

con•stant (kon'stănt). A quantity that, under stated conditions, does not vary with changes in the environment.

   Avogadro's c., SYN Avogadro's *number.*

   decay c., the fractional change in the number of atoms of a radionuclide which occurs in unit time; the constant l in the equation for the fraction (DN/N) of the number of atoms (N) of a radionuclide disintegrating in time Dt, $DN/N = -lDt$. SYN radioactive c.

   flotation c. (S_f), characteristic sedimentation behavior of a lipoprotein fraction of plasma in a centrifugal field in a medium of appropriate density, achieved by adding a salt or D_2O to the plasma. SYN Svedberg of flotation.

   Michaelis c., (1) the true dissociation constant for the enzyme-substrate binary complex in a single-substrate rapid equilibrium enzyme-catalyzed reaction (usually symbolized by K_s); **(2)** the concentration of the substrate at which half the true maximum velocity of an enzyme-catalyzed reaction is achieved.

   Newtonian c. of gravitation (G), a universal c. relating the gravitational force, *f*, attracting two masses, m_1 and m_2, toward each other when they are separated by a distance, r, in the equation: $f = G(m_1m_2/r^2)$; it has the value of 6.67259×10^{-8} dyne cm^2 g^{-2} = 6.67259×10^{-11} m^3 kg^{-1} s^{-2} in SI units.

permeability c., a measure of the ease with which an ion can cross a unit area of membrane driven by a 1.0 M difference in concentration; usually expressed in centimeters per second. Cf. permeability *coefficient*.

Planck's c. (*h*), a c., $6.6260755 \times 10^{-34}$ J · s (joule-seconds) or $6.6260755 \times 10^{-27}$ erg-seconds = $6.6260755 \times 10^{-34}$ J Hz^{-1} (joule per hertz).

radioactive c. (lambda), SYN decay c.

rate c.'s (*k*), proportionality c.'s equal to the initial rate of a reaction divided by the concentration of the reactant(s); *e.g.*, in the reaction A → B + C, the rate of the reaction equals −d[A]/dt = k_1[A]. The rate c. k_1 is a unimolecular rate c. since there is only one molecular species reacting and has units of reciprocal time (*e.g.*, sec^{-1}). For the reverse reaction, B + C → A, the rate equals −d[B]/dt = d[A]/dt = k_2[B][C]. The rate c. k_2 is a bimolecular rate c. and has units of reciprocal concentration-time (*e.g.*, M^{-1} sec^{-1}).

sedimentation c., the c. *s* in Svedberg's equation for estimating the molecular weight of a protein from the rate of movement in a centrifugal field. The Svedberg unit (S) is arbitrarily set at 1 × 10^{-13} second and is very often used to describe the sedimentation rate of macromolecules; *e.g.*, 4 S RNA. SYN sedimentation coefficient.

con•sti•pate (kon'sti-pāt). To cause constipation.

con•sti•pat•ed (kon'sti-pāt-ed). Suffering from constipation.

con•sti•pa•tion (kon-sti-pā'shŭn). A condition in which bowel movements are infrequent or incomplete. [L. *con-stipo,* pp. *-atus,* to press together]

con•sti•tu•tion (kon-sti-tū'shŭn). **1.** The physical makeup of a body, including the mode of performance of its functions, the activity of its metabolic processes, the manner and degree of its reactions to stimuli, and its power of resistance to the attack of pathogenic organisms. **2.** CHEMISTRY the number and kind of atoms in the molecule and the relation they bear to each other. [L. *constitutio,* constitution, disposition, fr. *constituo,* pp. *-stitutus,* to establish, fr. *statuo,* to set up]

con•sti•tu•tion•al (kon-sti-tū'shŭn-ăl). **1.** Relating to a body's constitution. **2.** General; relating to the system as a whole; not local.

con•stric•tion (kon-strik'shŭn). **1.** A normally or pathologically constricted or narrowed portion of a luminal structure. SEE ALSO stricture, stenosis. **2.** The act or process of binding or contracting, becoming narrowed; the condition of being constricted. squeezed. **3.** A subjective sensation of pressure or tightness, as if the body or any part were tightly bound or squeezed. [L. *con-stringo,* pp. *-strictus,* to draw together]

pyloric c., a prominent fold of mucous membrane at the gastroduodenal junction overlying the pyloric sphincter.

con•stric•tor (kon-strik'ter, -tōr). **1.** Anything that binds or squeezes a part. **2.** A muscle, the action of which is to narrow a canal; a sphincter. [L. fr. *constringo,* to draw together]

con•sul•tant (kon-sŭl'tant). **1.** A physician or surgeon who does not take full responsibility for a patient, but acts in an advisory capacity, deliberating with and counseling the attending physician or surgeon. **2.** A member of a hospital staff who has no active service but stands ready to advise in any case, at the request of the attending physician or surgeon. [L. *consulto,* pp. *-atus,* to deliberate, ask advice]

con•sul•ta•tion (kon-sŭl-tā'shŭn). Meeting of two or more physicians or surgeons to evaluate the nature and progress of disease in a particular patient and to establish diagnosis, prognosis, and/or therapy.

con•sump•tion (kon-sŭmp'shŭn). The using up of something, especially the rate at which it is used. [L. *con-sumo,* pp. *-sumptus,* to take up wholly, use up, waste]

oxygen c. (VO₂), the volume of oxygen consumed by the body in one minute; it is reported in liters or ml per minute at STPD.

con•tact (kon'takt). **1.** The touching or apposition of two bodies. **2.** A person who has been exposed to a contagious disease. [L. *con- tingo,* pp. *-tactus,* to touch, seize, fr. *tango,* to touch]

c. with reality, correctly interpreting external phenomena in relation to the norms of one's social or cultural milieu.

con•tac•tant (kon-tak'tănt). Any allergen that elicits manifestations of hypersensitivity by direct contact with skin or mucosa.

con•ta•gion (kon-tā'jŭn). **1.** SYN contagium. **2.** Transmission of infection by direct contact, droplet spread, or contaminated fomites. **3.** Production via suggestion or imitation of a neurosis or psychosis in several or more members of a group. [L. *contagio;* fr. *contingo,* to touch closely]

con•ta•gious (kon-tā'jŭs). Relating to contagion; communicable or transmissible by contact with the sick or their fresh secretions or excretions.

con•ta•gious•ness (kon-tā'jŭs-nes). The quality of being contagious.

con•ta•gium (kon-tā'jē-ŭm). The agent of an infectious disease. SYN contagion (1). [L. a touching]

con•tam•i•nant (kon-tam'i-nant). An impurity; any extraneous material associated with a chemical, a pharmaceutical preparation, a physiologic principle, or an infectious agent.

con•tam•i•nate (kon-tam'i-nāt). To cause or result in contamination. [L. *con-tamino,* to mingle, corrupt]

con•tam•i•na•tion (kon-tam-i-nā'shŭn). **1.** The presence of an infectious agent on a body surface; also on or in clothes, bedding, toys, surgical instruments or dressings, or other inanimate articles or substances including water, milk and food or that infectious agent itself. **2.** EPIDEMIOLOGY the situation that exists when a population being studied for one condition or factor also possesses other conditions or factors that modify results of the study. **3.** Freudian term for a fusion and condensation of words. [L. *contamino,* pp. *-atus,* to stain, defile]

con•tent (kon'tent). **1.** That which is contained within something else, usually in this sense in the plural form, contents. **2.** In psychology, the form of a dream as presented to consciousness. **3.** Ambiguous usage for concentration (3); *e.g.,* blood hemoglobin c. could mean either its concentration or the product of its concentration and the blood volume. [L. *contentus,* fr. *con- tineo,* pp. *-tentus,* to hold together, contain]

latent c., the hidden, unconscious meaning of thoughts or actions, especially in dreams or fantasies.

manifest c., those elements of fantasy and dreams which are consciously available and reportable.

oxygen c., the total amount of oxygen carried in the blood; it is equal to the amount of oxygen carried by the hemoglobin in the red blood cells plus the amount of oxygen dissolved in the plasma.

con•ti•gu•i•ty (kon-ti-gyū'i-tē). **1.** Contact without actual continuity, *e.g.,* the contact of the bones entering into the formation of a cranial suture. Cf. continuity. **2.** Occurrence of two or more objects, events, or mental impressions together in space or time. [L. *contiguus,* touching, fr. *contingo,* to touch]

con•tig•u•ous (kon-tig'ū-ŭs). Adjacent or in actual contact.

con•ti•nence (kon'ti-nens). **1.** Moderation, temperance, or self-restraint in respect to the appetites, especially to sexual intercourse. **2.** The ability to retain urine and/or feces until a proper time for their discharge. [L. *continentia,* fr. *con- tineo,* to hold back]

con•ti•nu•i•ty (kon-ti-nu'i-tē). Absence of interruption, a succession of parts intimately united, *e.g.,* the unbroken conjunction of cells and structures that make up a single bone of the skull. Cf. contiguity. [L. *continuus,* continued]

con•tour (kon'tūr). **1.** The outline of a part; the surface configuration. **2.** DENTISTRY to restore the normal outlines of a broken or otherwise misshapen tooth, or to create the external shape or form of a prosthesis. [L. *con-* (intens.), + *torno,* to turn (in a lathe), fr. *tornus,* a lathe]

height of c., SEE *height* of contour.

△**contra-.** Opposed, against. SEE ALSO counter-. Cf. anti-. [L.]

con•tra•ap•er•ture (kon'tră-ap'er-chūr). SYN counteropening.

con•tra•cep•tion (kon-tră-sep'shŭn). Prevention of conception or impregnation.

con•tra•cep•tive (kon-tră-sep'tiv). **1.** An agent for the prevention of conception. **2.** Relating to any measure or agent designed to prevent conception. [L. *contra,* against, + conceptive]

barrier c., a mechanical device designed to prevent spermatozoa from penetrating the cervical os; usually used in combination with a spermicidal agent, *i.e.,* vaginal diaphragm.

oral c., any orally effective preparation designed to prevent conception.

con•tract (kon-trakt'). **1.** To shorten; to become reduced in size; in the case of muscle, either to shorten or to undergo an increase in tension. **2.** To acquire by contagion or infection. **3** (kon' trakt). An explicit bilateral commitment by psychotherapist and patient to a defined course of

action to attain the goal of the psychotherapy. [L. *con-traho,* pp. *-tractus,* to draw together]

con•trac•tile (kon-trak'tīl). Having the property of contracting.

con•trac•til•i•ty (kon-trak-til'i-tē). The ability or property of a substance, especially of muscle, of shortening, or becoming reduced in size, or developing increased tension.

con•trac•tion (C) (kon-trak'shŭn). **1.** A shortening or increase in tension; denoting the normal function of muscular tissue. **2.** A shrinkage or reduction in size. **3.** Heart beat, as in premature c. SEE ALSO beat. [L. *contractio,* a drawing together]

carpopedal c., SYN carpopedal *spasm.*

concentric c., a shortening c. in which a muscle's attachments are drawn toward one another as the muscle contracts and overcomes an external resistance.

eccentric c., a lengthening action in which a muscle's attachments are drawn away from one another by an external resistance, even though the muscle is activated.

fibrillary c.'s, c.'s occurring spontaneously in individual muscle fibers.

hourglass c., constriction of the middle portion of a hollow organ, such as the stomach or the gravid uterus.

hunger c.'s, strong c.'s of the stomach associated with hunger pains.

idiomuscular c., SYN myoedema.

isometric c., force development at constant length. Cf. isotonic c.

isotonic c., shortening at constant force development. Cf. isometric c.

myotatic c., a reflex c. of a skeletal muscle that occurs as a result of stimulation of the stretch receptors in the muscle, *i.e.,* as part of a myotatic reflex.

paradoxical c., a tonic c. of the anterior tibial muscles when a sudden passive dorsal flexion of the foot is made.

postural c., maintenance of muscular tension (usually isometric) sufficient to maintain posture.

tonic c., sustained contraction of a muscle, as employed in the maintenance of posture.

uterine c., rhythmic activity of the myometrium associated with menstruation, pregnancy, or labor.

con•trac•ture (kon-trak'chūr). Static muscle shortening due to tonic spasm or fibrosis of muscle or supporting tissues resulting from paralysis or ischemia. [L. *contractura,* fr. *con-traho,* to draw together]

Dupuytren's c., a disease of the palmar fascia resulting in thickening and shortening of fibrous bands on the palmar surface of the hand and fingers.

ischemic c. of the left ventricle, irreversible contraction of the left ventricle of the heart as a complication seen in the early period of cardiopulmonary bypass and now avoided by appropriate cardioplegic solutions. SYN stone heart.

organic c., c., usually due to fibrosis within the muscle that persists whether the subject is conscious or unconscious.

con•tra•fis•sura (kon'tră-fi-shūr'ă). Fracture of a bone, as in the skull, at a point opposite that where the blow was received. [L. *contra,* against, counter, + *fissura,* fissure]

con·tra·in·di·ca·tion (kon-tră-in-di-kā′shŭn). Any special symptom or circumstance that renders the use of a remedy or the carrying out of a procedure inadvisable, usually because of risk.

con·tra·lat·er·al (kon-tră-lat′er-ăl). Relating to the opposite side, as when pain is felt or paralysis occurs on the side opposite to that of the lesion. SYN heterolateral. [L. *contra,* opposite, + *latus,* side]

con·trast (kon′trast). **1.** A comparison in which differences are demonstrated or enhanced. **2.** RADIOLOGY the difference between the image densities of two areas. [L. *contra,* against, + *sto,* pp. *status,* to stand]

 radiographic c., the variation of the light and dark areas on a radiograph.

con·tre·coup (kawn-tr-kū′). Denoting the manner of a contrafissura, as in the skull, at a point opposite that at which the blow was received. SEE ALSO contrecoup *injury* of brain. [Fr. counterblow]

con·trol (kon-trōl′). **1.** (v.) To regulate, restrain, correct, restore to normal. **2.** (n. or adj.) Ongoing operations or programs aimed at reducing or eliminating a disease. **3.** (n.) Person(s) in a comparison group that differs in disease experience or allocation to a regimen from the subjects of a study. **4.** (v.) STATISTICS to adjust or take into account extraneous influences. [Mediev. L. *contrarotulum,* a counterroll for checking accounts, fr. L. *rotula,* dim. of *rota,* a wheel]

 birth c., (1) restriction of the number of offspring by means of contraceptive measures; (2) projects, programs, or methods to control reproduction, by either improving or diminishing fertility.

 Centers for Disease C. (CDC), The federal facility for disease eradication, epidemiology, and education headquartered in Atlanta, Georgia, which encompasses the Center for Infectious Diseases, Center for Environmental Health, Center for Health Promotion and Education, Center for Prevention Services, Center for Professional Development and Training, and Center for Occupational Safety and Health. Formerly named Center for Disease Control (1970), Communicable Disease Center (1946).

 quality c., the c. of laboratory analytical error by monitoring analytical performance with control sera and maintaining error within established limits around the mean control values, most commonly ±2 SD.

 stimulus c., the use of conditioning techniques to bring the target behavior of an individual under environmental c.

Con·trol of Com·mun·i·ca·ble Dis·eases in Man. The internationally recognized authoritative manual, now in the 16th (1995) edition, published by the American Public Health Association.

con·tu·sion (kon-tū′shŭn). Any mechanical injury (usually caused by a blow) resulting in hemorrhage beneath unbroken skin. SEE ALSO bruise. [L. *contusio,* a bruising]

Co·nus (kō′nŭs). A genus of shellfish that inhab-

its the shores of some South Pacific islands. Several species are poisonous, their sting or spine causing acute pain, edema, numbness, spreading paralysis, and sometimes coma and death.

co·nus, pl. **co·ni** (kō′nŭs, -nī). **1** [NA]. SYN cone. **2.** Posterior staphyloma in myopic choroidopathy. [L. fr. G. *kōnos,* cone]

 c. arterio′sus [NA], SYN arterial *cone.*

 c. medulla′ris [NA], SYN medullary *cone.*

con·va·les·cence (kon-vă-les′ens). A period between the end of a disease and the patient's restoration to complete health. [L. *con-valesco,* to grow strong, fr. *valeo,* to be strong]

con·va·les·cent (kon-vă-les′ent). **1.** Getting well or one who is getting well. **2.** Denoting the period of convalescence.

con·vec·tion (kon-vek′shŭn). Conveyance of heat in liquids or gases by movement of the heated particles, as when the layer of water at the bottom of a heated pot rises or the warm air of a room ascends to the ceiling. [L. *con-veho,* pp. *-vectus,* to carry or bring together]

con·ver·gence (kon-ver′jens). **1.** The tending of two or more objects toward a common point. **2.** The direction of the visual lines to a near point. [L. *con-vergere,* to incline together]

 angle of c., the angle that the visual axis makes with the median line when a near object is viewed.

 negative c., the slight divergence of the visual axes when c. is at rest, as when observing the far point or during sleep.

 positive c., inward deviation of the visual axes even when c. is at rest, as in cases of convergent squint.

con·ver·gent (kon-ver′jent). Tending toward a common point.

conversation board. SYN communication board.

con·ver·sion (kon-ver′zhŭn). **1.** SYN transmutation. **2.** An unconscious defense mechanism by which the anxiety which stems from an unconscious conflict is converted and expressed symbolically as a physical symptom; transformation of an emotion into a physical manifestation, as in c. hysteria. SEE conversion *hysteria.* **3.** VIROLOGY the acquisition by bacteria of a new property associated with presence of a prophage. SEE ALSO lysogeny. [L. *con-verto,* pp. *-versus,* to turn around, to change]

con·ver·tase (kon′ver-tās). Proteases of complement that convert one component into another. SEE *component* of complement.

con·ver·tin (kon-ver′tin). Active form of factor VII designated VIIa.

con·vex (kon′veks, kŏn-veks′). Applied to a surface that is evenly curved outward, the segment of a sphere. [L. *convexus,* vaulted, arched, convex, fr. *con-veho,* to bring together]

con·vex·o·con·cave (kon-vek′sō-kon′kāv). Convex on one surface and concave on the opposite surface.

con·vex·o·con·vex (kon-vek′sō-kon′veks). SYN biconvex.

con·vo·lu·tion (kon-vō-lū′shŭn). **1.** A coiling or rolling of an organ. **2.** Specifically, a gyrus of the cerebral or cerebellar cortex. [L. *convolutio*]

con·vul·sion (kon-vŭl′shŭn). **1.** A violent spasm

or series of jerkings of the face, trunk, or extremities. **2.** SYN seizure (2). [L. *convulsio,* fr. *con-vello,* pp. *-vulsus,* to tear up]

clonic c., a c. in which the contractions are intermittent, the muscles alternately contracting and relaxing.

febrile c., a brief seizure, lasting less than 15 minutes, seen in a neurologically normal infant or young child, associated with fever.

tonic c., a c. in which muscle contraction is sustained.

con·vul·sive (kon-vŭl′siv). Relating to convulsions; marked by or producing convulsions.

co·or·di·na·tion (kō-ōr′di-nā′shun). The harmonious working together, especially of several muscles or muscle groups in the execution of complicated movements. [L. *co-,* together, + *ordino,* pp. *-atus,* to arrange, fr. *ordo* (*ordin-*), arrangement, order]

bilateral c., the ability to coordinate the two sides of the body.

co-oximeter (ko-ok-sim-ter). A laboratory instrument capable of measuring the concentration of oxyhemoglobin, reduced hemoglobin, carboxyhemoglobin, and methemoglobin in a sample of blood. SYN hemoximeter.

COPD chronic obstructive pulmonary *disease.*

cope (kōp). **1.** The upper half of a flask in the casting art; hence applicable to the upper or cavity side of a denture flask. **2.** An act that enables one to adjust to the environmental circumstances.

cop·per (Cu) (kop′er). A metallic element, atomic no. 29, atomic wt. 63.546; several of its salts are used in medicine. A bioelement found in a number of proteins. [L. *cuprum,* orig. *Cyprium,* fr. Cyprus, where it was mined]

cop·rem·e·sis (kop-rem′ē-sis). SYN fecal *vomiting.* [G. *kopros,* dung, + emesis]

△**copro-.** Filth, dung, usually used in referring to feces. SEE ALSO scato-, sterco-. [G. *kopros,* dung]

cop·ro·an·ti·bod·ies (kop′rō-an′ti-bod-ēz). Antibodies found in the intestine and in feces; they probably are formed by plasma cells in the intestinal mucosa and consist chiefly of the IgA class.

cop·ro·lag·nia (kop-rō-lag′nē-ă). A form of sexual perversion in which the thought or sight of excrement causes pleasurable sensation. [copro- + G. *lagneia,* lust]

cop·ro·la·lia (kop-rō-lā′lē-ă). Involuntary utterances of vulgar or obscene words; seen in Gilles de la Tourette's syndrome. [copro- + G. *lalia,* talk]

cop·ro·lith (kop′rō-lith). A hard mass consisting of inspissated feces. SYN fecalith, stercolith. [copro- + G. *lithos,* stone]

co·prol·o·gy (kop-rol′ō-jē). SYN scatology (1). [copro- + G. *logos,* study]

cop·ro·ma (kop-rō′mă). An accumulation of inspissated feces in the colon or rectum giving the appearance of an abdominal tumor. SYN fecaloma, stercoroma. [copro- + G. *-ōma,* tumor]

cop·ro·pha·gia (kop′rō-fā′jya). The eating of excrement.

cop·ro·phil, cop·ro·phil·ic (kop′rō-fil, -fil′ik). **1.** Denoting microorganisms occurring in fecal matter. **2.** Relating to coprophilia. [see coprophilia]

cop·ro·phil·ia (kop-rō-fil′ē-ă). **1.** Attraction of microorganisms to fecal matter. **2.** PSYCHIATRY a morbid attraction to, and interest in (with a sexual element) fecal matter. [copro- + G. *philos,* fond]

cop·ro·pho·bia (kop-rō-fō′bē-ă). Morbid fear of defecation and feces. [copro- + G. *phobos,* fear]

cop·ro·por·phyr·ia (kop′rō-pōr-fir′ē-ă). Presence of coproporphyrins in the urine, as in variegate porphyria.

cop·ro·por·phy·rin (kop-rō-pōr′fi-rin). One of two porphyrin compounds found normally in feces as a decomposition product of bilirubin (hence, from hemoglobin); certain c.'s are elevated in certain porphyrias. SEE ALSO porphyrinogens.

cop·u·la (kop′yū-lă). **1.** ANATOMY a narrow part connecting two structures, *e.g.,* the body of the hyoid bone. **2.** A swelling that is formed during the early development of the tongue by the medial portion of the second branchial arch; it is overgrown by the hypobranchial eminence and is not present in the adult tongue. [L. a bond, tie]

cop·u·la·tion (kop-yū-lā′shŭn). **1.** SYN coitus. **2.** In protozoology, conjugation between two cells that do not fuse but separate after mutual fertilization; observed in the ciliophora, as in *Paramecium.* [L. *copulatio,* a joining]

cor, gen. **cor·dis** (kōr, kōr′dis) [NA]. SYN heart. [L.]

c. adipo′sum, SYN fatty *heart* (2).

c. bilocula′re, a heart in which the interatrial and interventricular septa are absent or incomplete.

c. pulmona′le, chronic c. p. is characterized by hypertrophy of the right ventricle resulting from disease of the lungs; acute c. p. is characterized by dilation and failure of the right side of the heart due to pulmonary embolism. In both types, characteristic electrocardiogram changes occur, and in later stages there is usually right-sided cardiac failure.

c. triatria′tum, a heart with three atrial chambers, the left atrium being subdivided by a transverse septum with a single small opening which separates the openings of the pulmonary veins from the mitral valve.

c. trilocula′re, three-chambered heart due to absence of the interatrial or the interventricular septum.

cor·a·co·a·cro·mi·al (kōr′ă-kō-ă-krō′mē-ăl). Relating to the coracoid and acromial processes. SYN acromiocoracoid.

cor·a·co·cla·vic·u·lar (kōr′ă-kō-kla-vik′yū-lăr). Relating to the coracoid process and the clavicle. SYN scapuloclavicular (2).

cor·a·co·hu·mer·al (kōr′ă-kō-hyū′mer-ăl). Relating to the coracoid process and the humerus.

cor·a·coid (kōr′ă-koyd). Shaped like a crow's beak; denoting a process of the scapula. [G. *korakōdēs,* like a crow's beak, fr. *korax,* raven, + *eidos,* appearance]

cord (kōrd). **1.** In anatomy, any long ropelike structure. A small, cordlike structure composed of several to many longitudinally oriented fibers, vessels, ducts, or combinations thereof. SEE ALSO chorda. **2.** In histopathology, a line of tumor cells only one cell in width. SYN funiculus [NA], funicle. [L. *chorda,* a string]

false vocal c., SYN vestibular *fold.*

genital c., one of a pair of mesenchymal ridges bulging into the caudal part of the celom of a young embryo and containing the mesonephric and paramesonephric duct.

gonadal c.'s, columns of germinal and follicle cells penetrating centripetally into the embryonic ovarian or testicular cortex.

lateral c. of brachial plexus, in the brachial plexus, the bundle of nerve fibers formed by the anterior divisions of the superior and middle trunks which is located lateral to the axillary artery. This cord gives off the lateral pectoral nerve and terminates by dividing into the musculocutaneous nerve and the lateral root of the median nerve.

medial c. of brachial plexus, in the brachial plexus, the bundle of nerve fibers formed by the anterior division of the inferior trunk which lies medial to the axillary artery; it gives off the medial pectoral nerve, the medial brachial cutaneous, and medial antebrachial cutaneous nerves and end by dividing into the medial root of the median nerves and the ulnar nerve.

posterior c. of brachial plexus, in the brachial plexus, the bundle of nerve fibers formed by the posterior divisions of the upper, middle and lower trunks which lies posterior to the axillary artery; it gives rise to the upper and lower subscapular and thoracodorsal nerves, terminates by dividing into the axillary, and radial nerves.

spermatic c., the cord formed by the ductus deferens and its associated structures extending from the deep inguinal ring through the inguinal canal into the scrotum. SYN funiculus spermaticus [NA], testicular c.

spinal c., the elongated cylindrical portion of the cerebrospinal axis, or central nervous system, which is contained in the spinal or vertebral canal. SYN medulla spinalis [NA].

tendinous c.'s, SYN *chordae* tendineae, under *chorda.*

testicular c., SYN spermatic c.

true vocal c., SYN vocal *fold.*

umbilical c., the definitive connecting stalk between the embryo or fetus and the placenta; at birth it is primarily composed of Wharton's jelly in which the umbilical vessels are embedded. SYN funiculus umbilicalis [NA], funis (1).

cord-. SEE chord-.

cor•date (kōr′dāt). Heart-shaped.

cor•dec•to•my (kōr-dek′tō-mē). Excision of a part or whole of a cord. [G. *chordē,* cord, + *ektomē,* excision]

cor•di•form (kōr′di-fōrm). Heart-shaped. [L. *cor* (*cord*-), heart, + *forma,* shape]

cor•do•cen•te•sis (cor-dō-cen-tē′sis). Transabdominal blood sampling of the fetal umbilical cord, performed under ultrasound guidance. SYN funipuncture. [cord + G. *kentēsis,* puncture]

cor•do•pexy (kōr′dō-pek-sē). **1.** Operative fixation of any displaced anatomical cord. **2.** Lateral fixation of one or both vocal cords to correct glottic stenosis. [G. *chordē,* cord, + *pēxis,* fixation]

cor•dot•o•my (kōr-dot′ō-mē). **1.** Any operation on the spinal cord. **2.** Division of tracts of the spinal cord, which may be performed percutaneously (stereotactic c.) or after laminectomy (open c.) by various techniques such as incision or radio frequency coagulation. **3.** Incision through the membranous vocal fold to widen the posterior glottis in bilateral vocal paralysis. SYN chordotomy. [G. *chordē,* cord, + *tomē,* a cutting]

△**core-, coreo-, coro-.** The pupil (of the eye). [G. *korē,* pupil]

cor•ec•to•pia (kōr-ek-tō′pē-ă). Eccentric location of the pupil so that it is not in the center of the iris. [G. *korē,* pupil, + *ektopos,* out of place]

co•rel•y•sis (kō-rē-lī′sis). A rarely used term for freeing of adhesions between lens capsule and the iris. [G. *korē,* pupil, + *lysis,* a loosening]

△**coreo-.** SEE core-.

cor•e•o•plas•ty (kōr′ē-ō-plas-tē). The procedure to correct a misshapen, miotic, or occluded pupil. [G. *korē,* pupil, + *plassō,* to form]

cor•e•pexy (kōr′ĕ-peks-ē). A suturing of the iris to modify the shape or size of the pupil.

cor•e•praxy (kōr-e-prak′sē). A procedure designed to widen a small pupil. [G. *korē,* pupil, + *praxis,* action]

co•re•pres•sor (kō-rē-pres′ŏr). A molecule, usually a product of a specific metabolic pathway, that combines with and activates a repressor produced by a regulator gene. The repressor then attaches to an operator gene site and inhibits activity of the structural genes. This homeostatic mechanism regulates enzyme production in repressible enzyme systems.

co•ri•um, pl. **co•ria** (kō′rē-ŭm, -rē-ă) [NA]. SYN dermis. [L. skin, hide, leather]

corn (kōrn). SYN clavus. [L. *cornu,* horn, hoof]

hard c., the usual form of c. over a toe joint. SYN heloma durum.

soft c., a c. formed by pressure between two toes, the surface being macerated and yellowish in color. SYN heloma molle.

cor•nea (kōr′nē-ă) [NA]. The transparent tissue constituting the anterior sixth of the outer wall of the eye, with a 7.7 mm radius of curvature as contrasted with the 13.5 mm of the sclera; it consists of stratified squamous epithelium continuous with that of the conjunctiva, a substantia propria, regularly arranged collagen imbedded in mucopolysaccharide, and an inner layer of endothelium. It is the chief refractory structure of the eye. [L. fem. of *corneus,* horny]

conical c., SYN keratoconus.

cor•ne•al (kōr′nē-ăl). Relating to the cornea.

cor•ne•o•sclera (kōr′nē-ō-sklēr′ă). The combined cornea and sclera when considered as forming the external coat of the eyeball.

cor•ne•o•scler•al (kōr′nē-ō-sklēr′ăl). Pertaining to the cornea and sclera.

cor•ne•ous (kōr′nē-ŭs). SYN horny. [L. *corneus,* fr. *cornu,* horn]

cor•nic•u•late (kōr-nik′yū-lāt). **1.** Resembling a horn. **2.** Having horns or horn-shaped appendages. [L. *corniculatus,* horned]

cor•nic•u•lum (kōr-nik′yū-lŭm). A cornu of small size. [L. dim. of *cornu,* horn]

CO

cor·ni·fi·ca·tion (kōr-ni-fi-kā'shŭn). SYN keratin-ization. [L. *cornu,* horn, + *facio,* to make]

cor·nu, gen. **cor·nus,** pl. **cor·nua** (kōr'nū, -nŭs, -nū-ă). 1 [NA]. SYN horn. 2. Any structure composed of horny substance. 3. One of the coronal extensions of the dental pulp underlying a cusp or lobe. 4. The major subdivisions of the lateral ventricle in the cerebral hemisphere (the frontal horn, occipital horn, and temporal horn). SEE ALSO lateral *ventricle.* [L. horn]

  c. ammo'nis, SYN Ammon's *horn.*

  c. ante'rius [NA], SYN anterior *horn.*

  c. posterius, SYN posterior *horn.*

cor·nua (kōr'nū-ă). Plural of cornua.

cor·nu·al (kōr'nū-ăl). Relating to a cornu.

△**coro-.** SEE core-.

co·ro·na, pl. **co·ro·nae** (kō-rō'nă, -nē) [NA]. SYN crown. [L. garland, crown, fr. G. *korōnē*]

  c. of glans penis, the prominent posterior border of the glans penis.

  c. radia'ta, (1) [NA], a fan-shaped fiber mass on the white matter of the cerebral cortex, composed of the widely radiating fibers of the internal capsule; **(2)** a single layer of columnar cells derived from the cumulus oophorus, which anchor on the pellucid zone of the oocyte in a secondary follicle. SYN radiate crown.

cor·o·nad (kōr'ŏ-nad). In a direction toward any corona.

cor·o·nal (kōr'ŏ-năl). Relating to a corona or the coronal plane.

cor·o·na·ri·tis (kōr'ō-nă-rī'tis). Inflammation of coronary artery or arteries.

cor·o·nary (kōr'o-năr-ē). 1. Relating to or resembling a crown. 2. Encircling; denoting various anatomical structures, *e.g.,* nerves, blood vessels, ligaments. 3. Specifically, denoting the c. blood vessels of the heart and, colloquially, c. thrombosis. [L. *coronarius;* fr. *corona,* a crown]

Co·ro·na·vir·i·dae (kō-rō'nă-vir'i-dē). A family of single-stranded RNA-containing viruses, some of which cause upper respiratory tract infections in man similar to the "common cold." [L. *corona,* garland, crown]

Co·ro·na·vi·rus (kō-rō'nă-vī'rŭs). A genus in the family Coronaviridae that is associated with upper respiratory tract infections and possibly gastroenteritis in man.

co·ro·na·vi·rus (kō-rō'nă-vī'rŭs). Any virus of the family Coronaviridae.

cor·o·ner (kōr'on-er). An official whose duty it is to investigate sudden, suspicious, or violent death to determine the cause; in some communities, the office has been replaced by that of medical examiner. [L. *corona,* a crown]

cor·o·noi·dec·to·my (kōr'ŏ-noy-dek'tō-mē). Surgical removal of the coronoid process of the mandible. [coronoid + G. *ektomē,* excision]

cor·po·ra (kōr'pōr-ă). Plural of corpus.

cor·po·re·al (kōr-pō'rē-ăl). Pertaining to the body, or to a corpus.

corpse (kōrps). SYN cadaver. [L. *corpus,* body]

cor·pu·lence, cor·pu·len·cy (kōr'pyū-lens, -len-sē). SYN obesity. [L. *corpulentia,* magnification of *corpus,* body]

cor·pu·lent (kōr'pyū-lent). SYN obese.

cor·pus, gen. **cor·po·ris,** pl. **cor·po·ra** (kōr'pŭs, -pōr-is, -pōr-ă) [NA]. 1. SYN body. 2. Any body or mass. 3. The main part of an organ or other anatomical structure, as distinguished from the head or tail. SEE ALSO body, shaft, soma. [L. body]

  c. al'bicans [NA], a retrogressed c. luteum characterized by increasing cicatrization and shrinkage of the cicatricial core with an amorphous, convoluted, completely hyalinized lutein zone surrounding the central plug of scar tissue. SYN albicans (2).

  c. amyla'ceum, pl. **cor'pora amyla'cea,** one of a number of small ovoid or rounded, sometimes laminated, bodies resembling a grain of starch and found in nervous tissue, in the prostate, and in pulmonary alveoli.

  cor'pora arena'cea, small calcareous concretions in the stroma of the pineal and other central nervous system tissues. SYN psammoma bodies (2).

  c. callo'sum [NA], the great commissural plate of nerve fibers interconnecting the cortical hemispheres (with the exception of most of the temporal lobes which are interconnected by the anterior commissure). Lying at the floor of the longitudinal fissure, and covered on each side by the cingulate gyrus, it is arched from behind forward and is thick at each extremity (splenium and genu) but thinner in its long central portion (truncus); it curves back underneath itself at the genu to form the rostrum of the c. callosum.

  c. caverno'sum clitor'idis [NA], one of the two parallel columns of erectile tissue forming the body of the clitoris; they diverge at the root to form the crura of the clitoris.

  c. caverno'sum pe'nis [NA], one of two parallel columns of erectile tissue forming the dorsal part of the body of the penis; they are separated posteriorly, forming the crura of the penis.

  c. cilia're [NA], SYN ciliary *body.*

  c. fimbria'tum, (1) SYN *fimbria* hippocampi. **(2)** the outer, ovarian extremity of the oviduct.

  c. genicula'tum latera'le [NA], SYN lateral geniculate *body.*

  c. genicula'tum media'le [NA], SYN medial geniculate *body.*

  c. hemorrhag'icum, a hematoma with a lining formed by the thinned-out bright yellow lutein zone; gradual resorption of the blood elements leaves a cavity filled with a clear fluid, *i.e.,* a c. luteum cyst.

  c. lu'teum [NA], the yellow endocrine body formed in the ovary at the site of a ruptured ovarian follicle; there is a stage of proliferation and vascularization before full maturity; later, there is a festooned and bright yellowish lutein zone traversed by trabeculae of theca interna containing numerous blood vessels; the c. luteum secretes estrogen, as did the follicle, and also secretes progesterone. If pregnancy does not occur, it is called a **c. luteum spurium,** which undergoes progressive retrogression to a c. albicans. If pregnancy does occur, it is called a **c. luteum verum,** which increases in size, persisting to the fifth or sixth month of pregnancy before retrogression.

c. mamilla're [NA], SYN mamillary *body*.

c. oliva're, SYN oliva.

corpora para-aortica, [NA] SYN aortic *body*.

c. pinea'le [NA], SYN pineal *body*.

c. spongio'sum pe'nis [NA], the median column of erectile tissue located between and ventral to the two corpora cavernosa penis; posteriorly it expands into the bulbus penis and anteriorly it terminates as the enlarged glans penis; it is traversed by the urethra.

c. spongio'sum ure'thrae mulie'bris, the submucous coat of the female urethra, containing a venous network that insinuates itself between the muscular layers, giving to them an erectile nature.

c. stria'tum [NA], SYN striate *body*.

c. vit'reum [NA], SYN vitreous *body*. SEE ALSO vitreous.

cor•pus•cle (kōr'pŭs-l). **1.** A small mass or body. **2.** A blood cell. SYN corpusculum [NA]. [L. *corpusculum,* dim. of *corpus,* body]

articular c.'s, encapsulated nerve terminations within joint capsules. SYN corpuscula articularia [NA].

corneal c.'s, connective tissue cells found between the laminae of fibrous tissue in the cornea.

genital c.'s, special encapsulated nerve endings found in the skin of the genitalia and nipple. SYN corpuscula genitalia [NA].

ghost c., SYN achromocyte.

Golgi-Mazzoni c., an encapsulated sensory nerve ending similar to a pacinian c. but simpler in structure.

lamellated c.'s, small oval bodies in the skin of the fingers, in the mesentery, tendons, and elsewhere, formed of concentric layers of connective tissue with a soft core in which the axon of a nerve fiber runs, splitting up into a number of fibrils that terminate in bulbous enlargements; they are sensitive to pressure. SYN corpuscula lamellosa [NA], pacinian c.'s.

lymph c., lymphatic c., lymphoid c., a mononuclear type of leukocyte formed in lymph nodes and other lymphoid tissue, and also in the blood.

Meissner's c., SYN tactile c.

pacinian c.'s, SYN lamellated c.'s.

phantom c., SYN achromocyte.

red c., SYN erythrocyte.

renal c., the tuft of glomerular capillaries and the capsula glomeruli that encloses it. SYN corpusculum renis [NA].

tactile c., one of numerous oval bodies found in the papillae of the skin, especially those of the fingers and toes; they consist of a connective tissue capsule in which the axon fibrils terminate around and between a pile of wedge-shaped epithelioid cells. SYN Meissner's c.

thymic c., small spherical bodies of keratinized and usually squamous epithelial cells arranged in a concentric pattern around clusters of degenerating lymphocytes, eosinophils, and macrophages; found in the medulla of the lobules of the thymus.

white c., any type of leukocyte.

cor•pus•cu•lar (kōr-pŭs'kyū-lăr). Relating to a corpuscle.

cor•pus•cu•lum, pl. **cor•pus•cu•la** (kōr-pŭs'kyū-lŭm, -kyū-lă) [NA]. SYN corpuscle.

corpus'cula articula'ria [NA], SYN articular *corpuscles,* under *corpuscle.*

corpus'cula genita'lia [NA], SYN genital *corpuscles,* under *corpuscle.*

corpus'cula lamello'sa [NA], SYN lamellated *corpuscles,* under *corpuscle.*

c. re'nis, pl. **corpus'cula re'nis** [NA], SYN renal *corpuscle.*

cor•rec•tive (kō-rek'tiv). **1.** Counteracting, modifying, or changing what is injurious. **2.** A drug that modifies or corrects an undesirable or injurious effect of another drug. [L. *cor-rigo (conr-),* pp. *-rectus,* to set right, fr. *rego,* to keep straight]

cor•re•spon•dence (kōr-ĕ-spon'dens). OPTICS those points on each retina that have the same visual direction.

anomalous c., abnormal c., a condition, frequent in strabismus, in which corresponding retinal points do not have the same visual direction; the fovea of one eye corresponds to an extrafoveal area of the fellow eye.

dysharmonious c., a type of anomalous retinal c. in which the angle of the visual direction of the two retinas is different from the objective angle of the strabismus.

harmonious c., a type of anomalous retinal c. in which the angle of the visual direction of the two retinas is equal to the objective angle of strabismus.

cor•rin (kōr'in). The cyclic system of four pyrrole rings forming corrinoids, which are the central structure of the vitamins B_{12} and related compounds. [fr. *core* (of vitamin B_{12} molecule)]

cor•ro•sive (kŏ-rō'siv). **1.** Causing corrosion. **2.** An agent that produces corrosion; *e.g.,* a strong acid or alkali.

cor•ru•ga•tor (kōr'ŭ-gā-ter, -tōr). A muscle that draws together the skin, causing it to wrinkle. [L. *cor-rugo (conr-),* pp. *-atus,* to wrinkle, fr. *ruga,* a wrinkle]

cor•tex, gen. **cor•ti•cis,** pl. **cor•ti•ces** (kōr'teks, -ti-sis, -ti-sēz) [NA]. The outer portion of an organ, such as the kidney, as distinguished from the inner, or medullary, portion. [L. bark]

association c., generic term denoting the large expanses of the cerebral c. that are not sensory or motor in the customary sense, but are involved in advanced stages of sensory information processing, multisensory integration, or sensorimotor integration. SEE ALSO cerebral c. SYN association areas.

auditory c., the region of the cerebral c. that receives the auditory radiation from the medial geniculate body, a thalamic cell group receiving auditory input from the cochlear nuclei in the rhombencephalon. SYN auditory area.

cerebellar c., the thin gray surface layer of the cerebellum, consisting of an outer molecular layer or stratum moleculare, a single layer of Purkinje cells (the ganglionic layer), and an inner granular layer or stratum granulosum.

cerebral c., the gray cellular mantle (1 to 4 mm thick) covering the entire surface of the cerebral hemisphere of mammals; characterized by a laminar organization of cellular and fibrous components such that its nerve cells are stacked in defined layers varying in number from one, as in the archicortex of the hippocampus, to five or six in the larger neocortex; the outermost (molecular or plexiform) layer contains very few cell bodies and is composed largely of the distal ramifications of the long apical dendrites issued perpendicularly to the surface by pyramidal and fusiform cells in deeper layers. From the surface inward, the layers as classified in K. Brodmann's parcellation are: 1) molecular or plexiform layer; 2) outer granular layer; 3) pyramidal cell layer; 4) inner granular layer; 5) inner pyramidal layer (ganglionic layer); and 6) multiform cell layer, many of which are fusiform. This multilaminate organization is typical of the neocortex (homotypic c.; isocortex in O. Vogt's terminology), which in humans covers the largest part by far of the cerebral hemisphere. The more primordial heterotypic c. or allocortex (Vogt) has fewer cell layers. A form of c. intermediate between isocortex and allocortex, called juxtallocortex (Vogt) covers the ventral part of the cingulate gyrus and the entorhinal area of the parahippocampal gyrus.

On the basis of local differences in the arrangement of nerve cells (cytoarchitecture), Brodmann outlined 47 areas in the cerebral cortex which, in functional terms, can be classified into three categories: motor c. (areas 4 and 6), characterized by a poorly developed inner granular layer (agranular c.) and prominent pyramidal cell layers; sensory c., characterized by a prominent inner granular layer (granular c. or koniocortex) and comprising the somatic sensory c. (areas 1 to 3), the auditory c. (areas 41 and 42), and the visual c. (areas 17 to 19); and association c., the vast remaining expanses of the cerebral c.

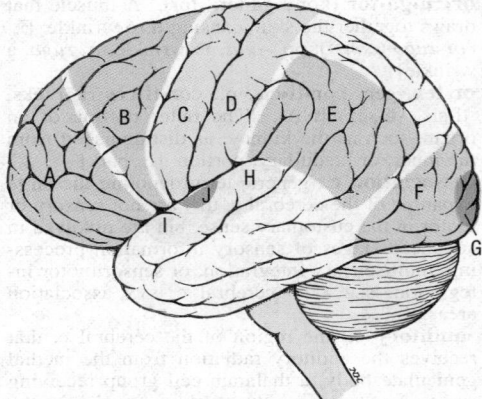

cerebral cortex: major functional areas: (A) biological intelligence, (B) premotor, (C) somatomotor, (D) somatosensory, (E) bodily awareness, (F) visual psychic, (G) visual sensory, (H) speech understanding, (I) auditory psychic, (J) auditory sensory

frontal c., c. of the frontal lobe of the cerebral hemisphere. SYN frontal area.

granular c., SEE cerebral c.

heterotypic c., SYN allocortex.

motor c., the region of the cerebral c. most immediately influencing movements of the face, neck, trunk, arms, and leg; its effects upon the motor neurons innervating the skeletal musculature are mediated by the pyramidal tract. SYN excitable area, motor area, Rolando's area.

c. of ovary, the layer of the ovarian stroma lying immediately beneath the tunica albuginea, composed of connective tissue cells and fibers, among which are scattered primary and secondary (antral) follicles in various stages of development; the c. varies in thickness according to the age of the individual, becoming thinner with advancing years.

renal c., the part of the kidney consisting of renal lobules in the outer zone beneath the capsule and also the lobules of the renal columns that are extensions inward between the pyramids; contains the renal corpuscles and the proximal and distal convoluted tubules.

sensory c., formerly denoting specifically the somatic sensory c., but now used to refer collectively to the somatic sensory, auditory, visual, and olfactory regions of the cerebral c.

somatic sensory c., somatosensory c., the region of the cerebral c. receiving the somatic sensory radiation from the ventrobasal nucleus of the thalamus; it represents the primary cortical processing mechanism for sensory information originating at the body surfaces (touch) and in deeper tissues such as muscle, tendons, and joint capsules (position sense).

suprarenal c., the outer part of the adrenal gland, consisting of three zones from without inward: zona glomerulosa, zona fasciculata, and zona reticularis; this part of the adrenal c. yields steroid hormones such as corticosterone, deoxycorticosterone, and estrone.

visual c., the region of the cerebral c. occupying the entire surface of the occipital lobe, and composed of Brodmann's areas 17 to 19. Area 17 (which is also called striate c. or area because the line of Gennari is grossly visible on its surface) is the primary visual c., receiving the visual radiation from the lateral geniculate body of the thalamus. The surrounding areas 18 (parastriate c. or area) and 19 (peristriate c. or area) are probably involved in subsequent steps of visual information processing; area 18 is referred to as the secondary visual c. SYN visual area.

cor·ti·cal (kōr′ti-kăl). Relating to a cortex.

cor·ti·ces (kōr′ti-sēz). Plural of cortex.

cor·ti·cif·u·gal (kōr-ti-sif′yū-găl). Passing in a direction away from the outer surface; denoting especially nerve fibers conveying impulses away from the cerebral cortex. SYN corticofugal. [L. *cortex,* rind, bark, + *fugio,* to flee]

cor·ti·cip·e·tal (kōr-ti-sip′e-tăl). Passing in a direction toward the outer surface; denoting nerve fibers conveying impulses toward the cerebral cortex. [L. *cortex,* rind, bark, + *peto,* to seek]

cor·ti·co·bul·bar (kōr-ti-kō-bŭl′bar). Corticofugal fibers projecting to the rhombencephalon that terminate 1) directly on some motor cranial nerve nuclei, 2) in the reticular formation, and 3) on sensory relay nuclei, such as the cuneate nucleus and gracile nucleus and the spinal trigeminal nucleus.

cor•ti•cof•u•gal (kōr'ti-kō-fyū'găl). SYN corticifugal.

cor•ti•coid (kōr'ti-koyd). **1.** Having an action similar to that of a hormone of the adrenal cortex. **2.** Any substance exhibiting this action. **3.** SYN corticosteroid.

cor•ti•co•lib•er•in (kōr'ti-kō-lib'er-in). SYN corticotropin releasing *hormone*. [corticosteroid + L. *libero*, to free, + -in]

cor•ti•co•ste•roid (kōr'ti-kō-stēr'oyd). A steroid produced by the adrenal cortex (*i.e.,* adrenal corticoid); a corticoid containing a steroid. SYN corticoid (3).

cor•ti•co•troph (kōr'ti-kō-trof). A cell of the adenohypophysis that produces adrenocorticotropic hormone (ACTH).

cor•ti•co•tro•pin (kōr'ti-kō-trō'pin). **1.** SYN adrenocorticotropic *hormone*. **2.** SYN β-corticotropin. [G. *tropē*, a turning]

β-cor•ti•co•tro•pin. Acid- or pepsin-degraded β-corticotropin. SYN corticotropin (2).

cor•ti•sol (kōr'ti-sol). SYN hydrocortisone.

cor•ti•sone (kōr'ti-sōn). A glucocorticoid not normally secreted in significant quantities by the human adrenal cortex. It exhibits no biological activity until converted to hydrocortisone (cortisol); it acts upon carbohydrate metabolism and influences the nutrition and growth of connective (collagenous) tissues.

co•rym•bi•form (kŏ-rim'bi-fōrm). Denoting the flower-like clustering configuration of skin lesions in granulomatous diseases (*e.g.,* syphilis, tuberculosis). [L. *corymbus,* cluster, garland]

Cor•y•ne•bac•te•ri•um (kŏ-rī'nē-bak-tēr'ē-ŭm). A genus of nonmotile (except for some plant pathogens), aerobic to anaerobic bacteria (family Corynebacteriaceae) containing irregularly staining, Gram-positive, straight to slightly curved, often club-shaped rods which, as a result of snapping division, show a picket fence arrangement. These organisms are widely distributed in nature. The best known species are parasites and pathogens of humans and domestic animals. The type species is *C. diphtheriae.* [G. *coryne,* a club, + *bacterium,* a small rod]

 C. diphthe'riae, type species of the genus *Corynebacterium,* the cause of diphtheria. It induces a severe membranous pharyngitis and produces an exotoxin that damages myocardium and other tissues; may also infect superficial wounds; an asymptomatic carrier state is common.

cor•y•ne•bac•te•ri•um, pl. **cor•y•ne•bac•te•ria** (kŏ-rī'nē-bak-tēr'ē-ŭm, -ă). A vernacular term used to refer to any member of the genus *Corynebacterium.*

co•ry•za (kŏ-rī'ză). SYN acute *rhinitis.* [G.]

Co•ry•za•vi•rus (kŏ-rī'ză-vī'rŭs). Former name for *Rhinovirus.*

cos•me•sis (koz-mē'sis). A concern in therapeutics, especially in surgical operations, for the appearance of the patient. [G. *kosmēsis,* an adorning, fr. *kosmeō,* to order, arrange, adorn, fr. *kosmos,* order]

cos•met•ic (koz-met'ik). **1.** Relating to cosmesis. **2.** Relating to the use of cosmetics.

cos•met•ics (koz-met'iks). Composite term for a variety of adornments and camouflages applied to the skin, lips, hair, and nails in accordance with cultural dictates.

cos•mo•pol•i•tan (koz-mō-pol'i-tan). BIOLOGICAL SCIENCES a term denoting worldwide distribution. [G. *kosmos,* universe, + *polis,* city-state]

cos•ta, gen. and pl. **cos•tae** (kos'tă, -tē). **1** [NA]. SYN Rib. **2.** A rodlike internal supporting organelle that runs along the base of the undulating membrane of certain flagellate parasites such as *Trichomonas.* SYN basal rod. [L.]

 c. cervica'lis [NA], SYN cervical *rib.*

 cos'tae fluitan'tes [NA], SYN floating *ribs,* under *rib.*

 cos'tae spu'riae [NA], SYN false *ribs,* under *rib.*

 cos'tae ve'rae [NA], SYN true *ribs,* under *rib.*

cos•tal (kos'tăl). Relating to a rib.

cos•tal•gia (kos-tal'jē-ă). SYN pleurodynia. [L. *costa,* rib, + G. *algos,* pain]

cos•tec•to•my (kos-tek'tō-mē). Excision of a rib. [L. *costa,* rib, + G. *ektomē,* excision]

△**costo-.** The ribs. [L. *costa,* rib]

cos•to•chon•dral (kos-tō-kon'drăl). Relating to the costal cartilages. SYN chondrocostal.

cos•to•chon•dri•tis (kos'tō-kon-drī'tis). Inflammation of one or more costal cartilages, characterized by local tenderness and pain of the anterior chest wall that may radiate, but without the local swelling typical of Tietze's syndrome. [costo- + G. *chondros,* cartilage, + -*itis,* inflammation]

cos•to•cla•vic•u•lar (kos-tō-klă-vik'yū-lăr). Relating to the ribs and the clavicle.

cos•to•cor•a•coid (kos-tō-kōr'ă-koyd). Relating to the ribs and the coracoid process of the scapula.

cos•to•gen•ic (kos-tō-jen'ik). Arising from a rib.

cos•to•scap•u•lar (kos-tō-skap'yū-lăr). Relating to the ribs and the scapula.

cos•to•ster•nal (kos-tō-ster'năl). Pertaining to the ribs and the sternum.

cos•to•ster•no•plas•ty (kos-tō-ster'nō-plas-tē). Operation to correct a malformation of the anterior chest wall. [costo- + G. *sternon,* chest, + *plastos,* formed]

cos•tot•o•my (kos-tot'ō-mē). Division of a rib. [costo- + G. *tomē,* a cutting]

cos•to•trans•verse (kos-tō-trans-vers'). Relating to the ribs and the transverse processes of the vertebrae articulating with them.

cos•to•trans•ver•sec•to•my (kos'tō-tranz-ver-sek'tō-mē). Excision of a proximal portion of a rib and the articulating transverse process.

cos•to•ver•te•bral (kos-tō-ver'tĕ-brăl). Relating to the ribs and the bodies of the thoracic vertebrae with which they articulate. SYN vertebrocostal (1).

cos•to•xi•phoid (kos-tō-zī'foyd). Relating to the ribs and the xiphoid cartilage of the sternum.

cothromboplastin (ko-throm-bo-plas-tin). SYN *factor* VII.

co•trans•port (kō-trans'pōrt). The transport of one substance across a membrane, coupled with the simultaneous transport of another substance across the same membrane in the same direction.

CO

cot·y·le·don (kot-i-lē′don). **1.** In plants, a seed leaf, the first leaf to grow from a seed. **2.** A placental unit. [G. *kotylēdon,* any cup-shaped hollow]

cot·y·loid (kot′i-loyd). **1.** Cup-shaped; cuplike. **2.** Relating to the cotyloid cavity or acetabulum. [G. *kotylē,* a small cup, + *eidos,* appearance]

cough (kawf). **1.** A sudden expulsion of air through the glottis, occurring immediately on opening the previously closed glottis, and excited by mechanical or chemical irritation of the trachea or bronchi, or by pressure from adjacent structures. **2.** To force air through the glottis by a series of expiratory efforts. [echoic]

   dry c., a c. not accompanied by expectoration; a nonproductive c.

   productive c., a c. accompanied by expectoration.

   reflex c., a c. excited reflexly by irritation in some distant part, as the ear or the stomach.

   whooping c., SYN pertussis.

cou·lomb (C, Q) (kū-lom′). The unit of electrical charge, equal to 3×10^9 electrostatic units; the quantity of electricity delivered by a current of 1 ampere in 1 second; equal to 1/96,485 faraday. [C. A. de *Coulomb,* Fr. physicist, 1736–1806]

coulometry (kū-lŏm′ĕt-rē). A titration technique in which the titrant is electrochemically generated. The Ag^+ titrant in the chloridometer is commonly used to determine the concentration of chloride in the sample. [coulomb + -metry]

count (kownt). **1.** A tally of instruments and materials performed at the beginning of a surgical operation and again before the incision is closed, to ensure that no foreign object remains in the patient. **2.** To enumerate or score. **3.** A tally of instruments and materials performed at the beginning of a surgical operation and again before the incision is closed, to ensure that no foreign object remains in the patient.

   Arneth c., the percentage distribution of polymorphonuclear neutrophils, based on the number of lobes in the nuclei (from 1 to 5). SEE ALSO Arneth *index.*

   blood c., SEE blood count.

   complete c. (CBC), a combination of the following determinations: red blood cell count, white blood cell count, erythrocyte indices, hematocrit, and differential blood count.

   Schilling's c., a method of counting blood in which the polymorphonuclear neutrophils are separated into four groups according to the number and arrangement of the nuclear masses in these cells.

count·er (kown′ter). A device that counts.

   automated differential leukocyte c., an instrument using digital imaging or cytochemical techniques to differentiate leukocytes.

   electronic cell c., an automatic blood cell c. in which cells passing through an aperture alter resistance and are counted as voltage pulses, or in which cells passing through a flow cell deflect light; some types of c. are capable of multiple simultaneous measurements on each blood sample; *e.g.,* leukocyte count, red cell count, hemoglobin, hematocrit, and red cell indices.

   scintillation c., an instrument used for the detection and measurement of radioactivity.

   whole-body c., shielding and instrumentation, usually involving more than one detector, designed to evaluate the total-body burden of various gamma-emitting nuclides.

△**counter-.** Opposite, opposed, against. SEE ALSO contra-. [L. *contra,* against]

count·er·con·di·tion·ing (kown′ter-kon-dish′ŭn-ing). Any behavior therapy in which a second conditioned response (*e.g.,* approaching or even touching a snake) is introduced for the purpose of counteracting or nullifying a previously conditioned or learned response (*e.g.,* fear and avoidance of snakes).

count·er·ex·ten·sion (kown′ter-eks-ten′shŭn). SYN countertraction.

count·er·im·mu·no·e·lec·tro·pho·re·sis (kown′ter-im′yū-nō-ē-lek′trō-fōr-ē′sis). Immunoelectrophoresis in which antigen is placed in wells cut in the sheet of agar gel toward the cathode, and antiserum is placed in wells toward the anode; antigen and antibody, moving in opposite directions, form precipitates in the area between the cells where they meet in concentrations of optimal proportions.

count·er·in·ci·sion (kown′ter-in-sizh′ŭn). A second incision adjacent to a primary incision.

count·er·ir·ri·tant (kown-ter-ir′i-tant). **1.** An agent that causes irritation or a mild inflammation of the skin in order to relieve symptoms of a deep-seated inflammatory process. **2.** Relating to or producing counterirritation.

count·er·ir·ri·ta·tion (kown′ter-ir-i-tā′shŭn). Irritation or mild inflammation (redness, vesication, or pustulation) of the skin excited for the purpose of relieving symptoms of an inflammation of the deeper structures. SYN revulsion (1).

count·er·o·pen·ing (kown′ter-ō-pen-ing). A second opening made at the dependent part of an abscess or other cavity containing fluid, which is not draining satisfactorily through an opening previously made. SYN contra-aperture, counterpuncture.

count·er·pul·sa·tion (kown′ter-pŭl-sā′shŭn). A means of assisting the failing heart by automatically removing arterial blood just before and during ventricular ejection and returning it to the circulation during diastole; a balloon catheter is inserted into the aorta and activated by an automatic mechanism triggered by the ECG.

count·er·punc·ture (kown′ter-pŭnk-chūr). SYN counteropening.

count·er·shock (kown′ter-shok). An electric shock applied to the heart to terminate a disturbance of its rhythm.

count·er·stain (kown′ter-stān). A second stain of a different color, having affinity for tissues, cells, or parts of cells other than those taking the primary stain, used to render more distinct the parts taking the first stain.

count·er·trac·tion (kown-ter-trak′shŭn). The resistance, or back-pull, made to traction or pulling on a limb; *e.g.,* in the case of traction made on the leg, c. may be effected by raising the foot of the bed so that the weight of the body pulls against the weight attached to the limb. SYN counterextension.

count·er·trans·fer·ence (kown'ter-trans-fer'ens). PSYCHOANALYSIS the analyst's transference (often unconscious) toward the patient of his emotional needs and feelings, with personal involvement to the detriment of the desired objective analyst-patient relationship.

count·er·trans·port (kown-ter-tranz'pōrt). The transport of one substance across a membrane, coupled with the simultaneous transport of another substance across the same membrane in the opposite direction.

coup de glotte. SYN glottal *attack.*

cou·ple (kŭ'pl). To copulate; to perform coitus; said especially of the lower animals.

cou·pling (kŭp'ling). **1.** The repeated pairing of a normal sinus beat with a ventricular extrasystole. **2.** A condition in which one or more products of a reaction are the subsequent reactants (or substrates) of a second reaction.

cou·vade (kū-vahd'). A primitive custom in certain cultures in which a man develops labor pains while his wife is in labor and then submits to the same postpartum purification rites and taboos. [Fr. *couver,* to hatch]

co·va·lent (kō-vāl'ent). Denoting an interatomic bond characterized by the sharing of 2, 4, or 6 electrons.

cov·er·age (kov'er-ej). A measure of the extent to which the services rendered cover the potential need for these services in a community; applied specifically to such services as immunization in developing countries.

cowl. SEE caul.

cow·per·i·an (kow-pēr'ē-an). Relating to or described by Cowper.

cow·per·i·tis (kow-per-ī'tis). Inflammation of Cowper's gland.

coxa, gen. and pl. **cox·ae** (kok'să, -sē). **1.** SYN hip *bone.* **2.** SYN hip *joint.* [L]

  c. mag'na, enlargement, and often deformation of the femoral head; usually refers to a sequela of Legg-Calve é-Perthes disease or osteoarthritis.

  c. val'ga, alteration of the angle made by the axis of the femoral neck to the axis of the femoral shaft, so that the angle exceeds 135°; the femoral neck is in more of a straight-line relationship to the shaft of the femur.

  c. va'ra, alteration of the angle made by the axis of the femoral neck to the axis of the femoral shaft so that the angle is less than 135°; the femoral neck becomes more horizontal.

cox·al·gia (koks-al'jē-ă). SYN coxodynia. [L. *coxa,* hip, + G. *algos,* pain]

Cox·i·el·la (kok-sē-el'ă). A genus of filterable bacteria (order Rickettsiales) containing small, pleomorphic, rod-shaped or coccoid, Gram-negative cells which occur intracellularly in the cytoplasm of infected cells and possibly extracellularly in infected ticks. These organisms have not been cultivated in cell-free media; they are parasitic on man and other animals. The type species is *C. burnetii.* [H. R. *Cox,* U.S. bacteriologist, *1907]

  C. burnet'ii, a species that causes Q fever in man; it is more resistant than other rickettsiae and

may be passed via aerosols as well as living vectors. Acute pneumonia and chronic endocarditis are also associated with this species. The type species of the genus *Coxiella.*

cox·o·dyn·ia (koks-ō-din'ē-ă). Pain in the hip joint. SYN coxalgia. [L. *coxa,* hip, + G. *odynē,* pain]

cox·o·fem·o·ral (kok-sō-fem'ŏ-răl). Relating to the hip bone and the femur.

cox·o·tu·ber·cu·lo·sis (koks'ō-tū-ber-kyū-lō'sis). Tuberculous hip-joint disease.

Cox·sack·ie·vi·rus (kok-sak'ē-vī'rŭs). A group of picornaviruses causing myositis, paralysis, and death in young mice, and responsible for a variety of diseases in man, although inapparent infections are common. They are divided antigenically into two groups, A and B, each of which includes a number of serological types. Type A viruses cause herpangina and hand-foot-and-mouth disease; type B viruses cause epidemic pleurodynia; both type viruses may cause aseptic meningitis, myocarditis and pericarditis, and acute onset juvenile diabetes. [*Coxsackie,* N.Y., where first isolated]

CPAP continuous positive airway *pressure.*

CPPB continuous positive pressure *breathing.*

CPR (computer-based patient record) cardiopulmonary *resuscitation.*

CPRI Computer-Based Patient Record Institute.

cps cycles per second.

CPT Current Procedural Terminology.

CR conditioned *reflex;* crown-rump *length.*

Cr 1. chromium. **2.** creatinine.

crack. SEE crack *cocaine.* [slang]

crac·kle (krak'l). Short, sharp, or rough sounds heard with a stethoscope over the chest. Most often heard in pleurisy with fibrinous exudate. [echoic]

cra·dle (krā'dl). A frame used to keep bedclothes from coming in contact with a patient. [M.E. *cradel*]

cramp (kramp). **1.** A painful muscle spasm caused by prolonged tetanic contraction. **2.** A localized muscle spasm related to occupational use, qualified according to the occupation of the sufferer; *e.g.,* writer's c. [M.E. *crampe,* fr. O. Fr., fr. Germanic]

  heat c.'s, painful muscle spasms resulting from excessive water and electrolyte loss. SEE hyperthermia. SEE ALSO dehydration.

  intermittent c., (1) SYN tetany. (2) SYN benign *tetanus.*

△**crani-.** SEE cranio-.

cra·nia (krā'nē-ă). Plural of cranium.

cra·ni·ad (krā'nē-ad). Situated nearer the head in relation to a specific reference point; opposite of caudad. SEE ALSO superior.

cra·ni·al (krā'nē-ăl). **1.** Relating to the cranium or head. SYN cephalic. SEE ALSO cephalad. **2.** SYN superior (2).

cra·ni·ec·to·my (krā'nē-ek'tō-mē). Excision of a portion of the skull. [G. *kranion,* skull, + *ektomē,* excision]

△**cranio-, crani-.** The cranium. Cf. cerebro-. [G. *kranion,* skull]

cra·ni·o·cele (krā'nē-ō-sēl). SYN encephalocele. [cranio- + G. *kēlē,* hernia]

cra·ni·o·ce·re·bral (krā'nē-ō-ser'ē-brăl). Relating to the skull and the brain.

cra·ni·o·fa·cial (krā'nē-ō-fā'shăl). Relating to both the face and the cranium.

cra·ni·o·fe·nes·tria (krā'nē-ō-fe-nes'trē-ă). SYN craniolacunia. [cranio- + L. *fenestra,* window]

cra·ni·o·la·cu·nia (krā'nē-ō-lă-kū'nē-ă). Incomplete formation of the bones of the vault of the fetal skull so that there are nonossified areas in the calvaria. SYN craniofenestria. [cranio- + L. *lacuna,* cleft]

cra·ni·o·ma·la·cia (krā'nē-ō-mă-lā'shē-ă). Softening of the bones of the skull. [cranio- + G. *malakia,* softness]

cra·ni·op·a·thy (krā-nē-op'ă-thē). Any pathological condition of the cranial bones. [cranio- + G. *pathos,* suffering]

metabolic c., SYN Morgagni's *syndrome.*

cra·ni·o·pha·ryn·ge·al (krā'nē-ō-fă-rin'jē-ăl). Relating to the skull and to the pharynx.

cra·ni·o·pha·ryn·gi·o·ma (krā'nē-ō-fă-rin-jē-ō'mă). A suprasellar neoplasm that develops from Rathke's pouch; the histologic pattern consists of nesting of squamous epithelium bordered by radially arranged cells. [cranio- + pharyngio- + -oma]

cra·ni·o·plas·ty (krā'nē-ō-plas-tē). Plastic surgery of the skull; a surgical correction of a skull defect. [cranio- + G. *plastos,* formed]

cra·ni·o·punc·ture (krā'nē-ō-pŭnk'chūr). Puncture of the brain for exploratory purposes.

cra·ni·or·rha·chis·chi·sis (krā'nē-ō-ră-kis'ki-sis). Severe congenital malformation in which there is incomplete closure of the skull and spinal column. [cranio- + G. *rhachis,* spine, + *schisis,* a cleaving]

cra·ni·o·sa·cral (krā'nē-ō-sā'krăl). Denoting the cranial and sacral origins of the parasympathetic division of the autonomic nervous system.

cra·ni·os·chi·sis (krā-nē-os'ki-sis). Congenital malformation in which there is incomplete closure of the skull. Usually accompanied by grossly defective development of the brain. [cranio- + G. *schisis,* a cleavage]

cra·ni·o·scle·ro·sis (krā'nē-ō-skler-ō'sis). Thickening of the skull. [cranio- + G. *sklēros,* hard, + -*osis,* condition]

cra·ni·o·spi·nal (krā'nē-ō-spī'năl). Relating to the cranium and spinal column.

cra·ni·o·ste·no·sis (krā'nē-ō-sten-ō'sis). Premature closure of cranial sutures resulting in malformation of the skull. [cranio- + G. *stenōsis,* a narrowing]

cra·ni·o·syn·os·to·sis (krā'nē-ō-sin'os-tō'sis). Premature ossification of the skull and obliteration of the sutures.

cra·ni·o·tabes (krā'nē-ō-tā'bēz). A disease marked by areas of thinning and softening in the bones of the skull and widening of the sutures and fontanelles. Usually of syphilitic or rachitic origin. [cranio- + L. *tabes,* a wasting]

cra·ni·ot·o·my (krā-nē-ot'ō-mē). Opening into the skull, either by attached or detached c. or by trephination. [cranio- + G. *tomē,* incision]

cra·ni·o·tym·pan·ic (krā'nē-ō-tim-pan'ik). Relating to the skull and the middle ear.

cra·ni·um, pl. **cra·nia** (krā'nē-ŭm, -ă) [NA]. SYN skull. [Mediev. L. fr. G. *kranion*]

crash cart. A movable collection of emergency equipment and supplies meant to be readily available for resuscitative effort. It includes medication as well as the equipment for defibrillation, intubation, intravenous medication, and passage of central lines.

cream (krēm). **1.** The upper fatty layer which forms in milk on standing or which is separated from it by centrifugation; it contains about the same amount of sugar and protein as milk, but from 12 to 40% more fat. **2.** Any whitish viscid fluid resembling c. **3.** A semisolid emulsion of either the oil-in-water or the water-in-oil type, ordinarily intended for topical use. [L. *cremor,* thick juice, broth]

crease (krēs). A line or linear depression as produced by a fold. SEE ALSO fold, groove, line.

digital c., one of the grooves on the palmar surface of a finger, at the level of an interphalangeal joint.

ear lobe c., a diagonal c. found on one or both earlobes with a possible connection to coronary heart disease in males.

cre·a·ti·nase (krē'ă-tī-nās). An enzyme catalyzing the hydrolysis of creatine to sarcosine and urea.

cre·a·tine (krē'ă-tēn, -tin). Ours in urine, sometimes as such, but generally as creatinine, and in muscle, generally as phosphocreatine. Elevated in urine in muscular dystrophy.

c. kinase, an enzyme catalyzing the reversible transfer of phosphate from phosphocreatine to ADP, forming creatine and ATP; of importance in muscle contraction. Certain isozymes are elevated in plasma following myocardial infarctions. Three isoenzyme forms can be readily separated: CK-BB (brain type), CK-MB (hybrid type), and CK-MM (muscle type). The major form in healthy individuals is CK-MM. CK-MB is derived from myocardium and is considered the most specific indicator of myocardial infarction if increased in the blood.

c. phosphate, SYN phosphocreatine.

cre·a·ti·ne·mia (krē'ă-ti-nē'mē-ă). The presence of abnormal concentrations of creatine in peripheral blood. [creatine + G. *haima,* blood]

cre·at·i·nin·ase (krē-at'i-nin-ās). An amidohydrolase catalyzing the conversion of creatine to creatinine.

cre·at·i·nine (Cr) (krē-at'i-nēn, -nin). A component of urine and the final product of creatine catabolism; formed by the nonenzymatic dephosphorylative cyclization of phosphocreatine to form the internal anhydride of creatine.

cre·a·tin·u·ria (krē'ă-ti-nū'rē-ă). The urinary excretion of increased amounts of creatine. [creatine + G. *ouron,* urine]

cre·mas·ter (krē-mas'ter). SEE cremaster *muscle.* [G. *kremastēr,* a suspender, in pl. the muscles by which the testicles are retracted, fr. *kremannymi,* to hang]

crem·as·ter·ic (krē-mas-ter'ik). Relating to the cremaster.

crem·no·cele (krem'nō-sēl). A protrusion of intestine into the labium majus. [G. *krēmnos,* overhanging cliff, labium pudendi, + *kēlē,* hernia]

cre·na, pl. **cre·nae** (krē'nă, krē'nē). A V-shaped

cut or the space created by such a cut; one of the notches into which the opposing projections fit in the cranial sutures. [L. a notch]

cre•nate, cre•nat•ed (krē′nāt, -nā-ted). Indented; denoting the outline of a shriveled red blood cell, as observed in a hypertonic solution. [L. *crena,* a notch]

creno•cyte (krē′nō-sīt). A red blood cell with serrated, notched edges. [L. *crena,* a notch, + G. *kytos,* a hollow (cell)]

crep•i•tant (krep′i-tant). **1.** Relating to or characterized by crepitation. **2.** Denoting a fine bubbling noise (rale) produced by air entering fluid in lung tissue; heard in pneumonia and in certain other conditions. **3.** The sensation imparted to the palpating finger by gas or air in the subcutaneous tissues.

crep•i•ta•tion (krep-i-tā′shŭn). **1.** Crackling; the quality of a fine bubbling sound (rale) that resembles noise heard on rubbing hair between the fingers. **2.** The sensation felt on placing the hand over the seat of a fracture when the broken ends of the bone are moved, or over tissue, in which gas gangrene is present. **3.** Noise or vibration produced by rubbing bone or irregular cartilage surfaces together as by movement of patella against femoral condyles in arthritis and other conditions. SYN crepitus (1). [see crepitus]

crep•i•tus (krep′i-tŭs). **1.** SYN crepitation. **2.** A noisy discharge of gas from the intestine. [L. fr. *crepo,* to rattle]

cres•cent (kres′ent). **1.** Any figure of the shape of the moon in its first quarter. **2.** The figure made by the gray columns or cornua on cross-section of the spinal cord. **3.** SYN malarial c. [L. *cresco,* pp. *cretus,* to grow]

  malarial c., the male or female gametocyte(s) of *Plasmodium falciparum,* whose presence in human red blood cells is diagnostic of falciparum malaria. SYN crescent (3).

  myopic c., a white or grayish white crescentic area in the fundus of the eye located on the temporal side of the optic disk; caused by atrophy of the choroid, permitting the sclera to become visible.

cres•cen•tic (kres-sen′tik). Shaped like a crescent.

cre•sol red (krē′sol). An acid-base indicator with a pK value of 8.3; yellow at pH values below 7.4, red above 9.0.

CREST Acronym for *c*alcinosis, *R*aynaud's phenomenon, *e*sophageal motility disorders, *s*clerodactyly, and *t*elangiectasia. SEE CREST *syndrome.*

crest (krest). A ridge, especially a bony ridge. **2.** The ridge of the neck of a male animal, especially of a stallion or bull. **3.** Feathers on the top of a bird's head, or fin rays on the top of a fish's head. SYN crista [NA]. [L. *crista*]

  ampullary c., an elevation on the inner surface of the ampulla of each semicircular duct; filaments of the vestibular nerve pass through the c. to reach hair cells on its surface; the hair cells are capped by the cupula, a gelatinous protein-polysaccharide mass.

  anterior lacrimal c., a vertical ridge on the

lateral surface of the frontal process of the maxilla that forms part of the medial rim of the orbit.

  c. of palatine bone, palatine c., a transverse ridge near the posterior border of the bony palate, located on the inferior surface of the horizontal plate of the palatine bone.

  ethmoidal c., bony ridge which articulates with, or provides attachment for, any part of the ethmoid bone, especially the middle nasal concha.

  external occipital c., a ridge extending from the external occipital protuberance to the border of the foramen magnum.

  frontal c., a ridge arising at the termination of the sagittal sulcus on the cerebral surface of the frontal bone and ending at the foramen caecum.

  c. of head of rib, the ridge that separates the superior and inferior articular surfaces of the head of a rib.

  iliac c., the long, curved upper border of the wing of the ilium.

  infratemporal c., a rough ridge marking the angle of union of the temporal and infratemporal surfaces of the greater wing of the sphenoid bone.

  internal occipital c., a ridge running from the internal occipital protuberance to the posterior margin of the foramen magnum, giving attachment to the falx cerebelli.

  intertrochanteric c., the rounded ridge that connects the greater and lesser trochanters of the femur posteriorly and marks the junction of the neck and shaft of the bone.

  lateral sacral c.'s, c.'s which are rough ridges lying lateral to the sacral foramina; they represent the fused transverse processes of sacral vertebrae.

  median sacral c., an unpaired c. formed by the fused spinous processes of the upper four sacral vertebrae.

  nasal c., the midline ridge in the floor of the nasal cavity, formed by the union of the paired maxillae and palatine bones; the vomer attaches to the crest.

  neural c., a band of neuroectodermal cells along either side of the line of closure of the embryonic neural groove; with the formation of the neural tube, these bands come to lie dorsolateral to the developing spinal cord and lateral to the brainstem, where they separate into clusters of cells that develop into, for example, dorsalroot ganglion cells, autonomic ganglion cells, the chromaffin cells of the adrenal medulla, Schwann cells, sensory ganglia of cranial nerves, 5, 7, 8, 9, and 10, part of the meninges, or integumentary pigment cells.

  obturator c., a ridge that extends from the pubic tubercle to the acetabular notch, giving attachment to the pubofemoral ligament of the hip joint.

  posterior lacrimal c., a vertical ridge on the orbital surface of the lacrimal bone which, together with the anterior lacrimal crest, bounds the fossa for the lacrimal sac.

  pubic c., the rough anterior border of the body of the pubis, continuous laterally with the pubic tubercle.

  sacral c., one of three rough irregular ridges on

the posterior surface of the sacrum; median sacral c.; lateral sacral c.'s.

sphenoid c., a vertical ridge in the midline of the anterior surface of the sphenoid bone that articulates with the perpendicular plate of the ethmoid bone.

supramastoid c., the ridge that forms the posterior root of the zygomatic process of the temporal bone.

supraventricular c., the internal muscular ridge that separates the conus arteriosus from the remaining part of the cavity of the right ventricle of the heart.

urethral c., longitudinal mucosal fold in the dorsal wall of the urethra.

vestibular c., c. of vestibule, an oblique ridge on the inner wall of the vestibule of the labyrinth, bounding the spherical recess above and posteriorly.

cre•tin (krē'tin). An individual exhibiting cretinism. [Fr. *crétin*]

cre•tin•ism (krē'tin-izm). Obsolete term for congenital *hypothyroidism*. SEE infantile *hypothyroidism*.

cre•tin•oid (krē'tin-oyd). Resembling a cretin; presenting symptoms similar to those of cretinism.

cre•tin•ous (krē'tin-ŭs). Relating to cretinism or a cretin; affected with cretinism.

crev•ice (krev'is). A crack or small fissure, especially in a solid substance. [Fr. *crevasse*]

cre•vic•u•lar (krĕ-vik'yū-lăr). **1.** Relating to any crevice. **2.** DENTISTRY relating especially to the gingival crevice or sulcus.

CRF corticotropin releasing *factor*.

CRH corticotropin releasing *hormone*.

crib-bit•ing (krib-bīt'ing). A behavior disorder of horses in which the animal grasps the edge of a convenient fixture and presses down, raising the floor of its mouth, forcing the soft palate open, and sometimes swallowing air. SEE aerophagia.

cri•bra (krī'bră, krib'ră). Plural of cribrum.

crib•rate (krib'rāt). SYN cribriform.

cri•bra•tion (kri-brā'shŭn). **1.** Sifting; passing through a sieve. **2.** The condition of being cribrate or numerously pitted or punctured.

crib•ri•form (krib'ri-fōrm). Sievelike; containing many perforations. SYN cribrate, polyporous. [L. *cribrum,* a sieve, + *forma,* form]

cri•brum, pl. **cri•bra** (krī'brŭm, krib'rŭm; -bră, -ra). SYN cribriform *plate* of ethmoid bone. [L. a sieve]

cri•co•ar•y•te•noid (krī'kō-ar-i-tē'noyd). Relating to the cricoid and arytenoid cartilages.

cri•coid (krī'koyd). Ring-shaped; denoting the cricoid cartilage. [L. *cricoideus,* fr. G. *krikos,* a ring, + *eidos,* form]

cri•co•pha•ryn•ge•al (krī'kō-fă-rin'jē-ăl). Relating to the cricoid cartilage and the pharynx; a part of the inferior constrictor muscle of the pharynx. SEE inferior constrictor *muscle* of pharynx.

cri•co•thy•roid (krī-kō-thī'royd). Relating to the cricoid and thyroid cartilages.

cri•co•thy•rot•o•my (krī'kō-thī-rot'ō-mē). Incision through the skin and cricothyroid membrane for relief of respiratory obstruction; used prior to or in place of tracheotomy in certain emergency respiratory obstructions. SYN intercricothyrotomy. [cricoid + thyroid + G. *tomē,* incision]

cri•cot•o•my (krī-kot'ō-mē). Division of the cricoid cartilage, as in cricoid split, to enlarge the subglottic airway. [cricoid + G. *tomē,* incision]

crin•o•gen•ic (krin-ō-jen'ik). Causing secretion; stimulating a gland to increased function. [G. *krinō,* to separate, + *-gen,* to produce]

crin•oph•a•gy (krin-of'ă-jē). Disposal of excess secretory granules by lysosomes.

cri•sis, pl. **cri•ses** (krī'sis, -sēz). **1.** A sudden change, usually for the better, in the course of an acute disease, in contrast to gradual improvement by lysis. **2.** A paroxysmal pain in an organ or circumscribed region of the body occurring in the course of tabetic neurosyphilis. **3.** A convulsive attack. [G. *krisis,* a separation, crisis]

addisonian c., SYN acute adrenocortical *insufficiency*.

adrenal c., SYN acute adrenocortical *insufficiency*.

Dietl's c., intermittent pain, sometimes with nausea and emesis, caused by intermittent proximal obstruction of ureter.

identity c., a disorientation concerning one's sense of self, values, and role in society, often of acute onset and related to a particular and significant event in one's life.

midlife c., a point in a sequence of events during the middle years of life at which certain trends of prior and subsequent events in one's life are pondered, generally involving an aggregate of personal, career, or sexual dissatisfactions.

sickle cell c., SEE sickle cell *anemia*.

therapeutic c., a turning point leading to positive or negative change in psychiatric treatment.

thyrotoxic c., thyroid c., the exacerbation of symptoms that occurs in severe thyrotoxicosis; marked by rapid pulse, nausea, diarrhea, fever, loss of weight, and extreme restlessness; coma and death may occur. SYN thyroid storm.

cris•ta, pl. **cris•tae** (kris'tă, -tē) [NA]. SYN crest. [L. crest]

c. gal•li [NA], the triangular midline process of the ethmoid bone extending superiorly from the cribriform plate; it gives anterior attachment to the falx cerebri.

CRL crown-rump *length*.

cRNA. complementary ribonucleic acid.

cross•bite (kros'bīt). An abnormal relation of one or more teeth of one arch to the opposing tooth or teeth of the other arch due to labial, buccal, or lingual deviation of tooth position, or to abnormal jaw position.

cross-dress•ing (kros'dres'ing). Clothing oneself in attire generally associated with the opposite sex. SEE transvestism.

cross-eye (kros'ī). Alternative spelling for crossed *eyes,* under *eye*.

cross•ing-over, cross•over (kros-ing-ō'ver, kros'ō-ver). Reciprocal exchange of material between two paired chromosomes during meiosis, resulting in the transfer of a block of genes from each chromosome to its homologue.

somatic c.-o., c.-o. that occurs during the mitosis of somatic cells, in contrast to that which occurs in meiosis.

cross-match·ing (kros′match-ing). **1.** A test for incompatibility between donor and recipient blood, carried out before transfusion to avoid hemolytic reactions between the donor's red blood cells and antibodies in the recipient's plasma, or the reverse; performed by mixing a sample of red blood cells of the donor with plasma of the recipient (*major crossmatch*) and the red blood cells of the recipient with the plasma of the donor (*minor crossmatch*). Incompatibility is indicated by clumping of red blood cells and contraindicates use of the donor's blood. **2.** In allotransplantation of solid organs (*e.g.,* kidney), a test for identification of antibody in the serum of potential allograft recipients which reacts directly with the lymphocytes or other cells of a potential allograft donor; presence of these antibodies usually, if not always, contraindicates the performance of the transplantation because virtually all such grafts will be subject to a hyperacute type of rejection.

croup (krūp). **1.** Laryngotracheobronchitis in infants and young children caused by parainfluenza viruses 1 and 2. **2.** Any affection of the larynx in children, characterized by difficult and noisy respiration and a hoarse cough. [Scots, probably from A.S. *kropan,* to cry aloud]

croup·ous (krū′pŭs). Relating to croup; marked by a fibrinous exudation.

crowd·ing (krowd′ing). A condition in which the teeth are crowded, assuming altered positions such as bunching, overlapping, displacement in various directions, torsiversion, etc.

crown (krown). **1.** Any structure, normal or pathologic, resembling or suggesting a crown or a wreath. **2.** DENTISTRY that part of a tooth that is covered with enamel, or an artificial substitute for that part. SYN corona [NA]. [L. *corona*]

  radiate c., SYN *corona* radiata.

crown·ing (krown′ing). **1.** Preparation of the natural crown of a tooth and covering the prepared crown with a veneer of suitable dental material (gold or non-precious metal casting, porcelain, plastic, or combinations). **2.** That stage of childbirth when the fetal head has negotiated the pelvic outlet and the largest diameter of the head is encircled by the vulvar ring.

CRP cAMP receptor *protein*; C-reactive *protein*.

CRT circuit resistance *training*.

cru·ces (krū′sēz). Plural of crux.

cru·ci·ate (krū′shē-āt). Shaped like, or resembling, a cross. [L. *cruciatus*]

cru·ra (krū′ră). Plural of crus.

cru·ral (krū′răl). Relating to the leg or thigh, or to any crus.

cru·ris (krū′ris).

crus, gen. **cru·ris,** pl. **cru·ra** (krūs, krū′ris, -ră) [NA]. **1.** SYN leg. **2.** Any anatomical structure resembling a leg; usually (in the plural) a pair of diverging bands or elongated masses. SEE ALSO limb. [L.]

  c. cer′ebri [NA], specifically, the massive bundle of corticofugal nerve fibers passing longitudinally on the ventral surface of the midbrain on each side of the midline; it consists of fibers descending from the cortex to the tegmentum of the brainstem, pontine gray matter, and spinal cord. SEE ALSO cerebral *peduncle*.

  c. of clitoris, the continuation on each side of the corpus cavernosum of the clitoris which diverges from the body posteriorly and is attached to the pubic arch.

  crura of the diaphragm, the muscular origins of the diaphragm from the bodies of the upper lumbar vertebrae that pass the aorta upward to the central tendon. SYN crura diaphragmatis.

  crura diaphragmatis, [NA] SYN crura of the diaphragm.

  c. for′nicis [NA], that part of the fornix that rises in a forward curve behind the thalamus to continue forward as the body for fornix ventral to the corpus callosum.

  c. of penis, the posterior, tapering portion of the corpus cavernosum penis which diverges from its contralateral partner to be attached to the ischiopubic ramus.

crust (krŭst). **1.** A hard outer layer or covering; cutaneous crusts are often formed by dried serum or pus on the surface of a ruptured blister or pustule. **2.** A scab. SYN crusta. [L. *crusta*]

  milk c., SYN *crusta* lactea.

crus·ta, pl. **crus·tae** (krŭs′tă, -tē). SYN crust. [L.]

  crusta lac′tea, seborrhea of the scalp in an infant. SYN milk crust.

crutch (krŭtch). A device used singly or in pairs to assist in walking when the act is impaired by a lower extremity (or trunk) disability; it transfers all or part of weight-bearing to the upper extremity. [A. S. *cryce*]

crux, pl. **cru·ces** (krŭks, krū′sēz). A junction or crossing. [L.]

  cru′ces pilo′rum [NA], crosslike figures formed by hairs growing from two directions that meet and then separate in a direction perpendicular to the original orientation.

cry-. SEE cryo-.

cry·al·ge·sia (krī-al-jē′zē-ă). Pain caused by cold. SYN crymodynia. [G. *kryos,* cold, + *algos,* pain]

cry·an·es·the·sia (krī′an-es-thē′zē-ă). Inability to perceive cold. [G. *kryos,* cold, + *an-* priv. + *aisthēsis,* sensation]

cry·es·the·sia (krī-es-thē′zē-ă). **1.** A subjective sensation of cold. **2.** Sensitiveness to cold. [G. *kryos,* cold, + *aisthēsis,* sensation]

cry for help. Telephone calls, notes left in conspicuous places, and other behaviors that communicate extreme distress and possible consideration of suicide.

crymo-. Cold. SEE ALSO cryo-, psychro-. [G. *krymos,*]

cry·mo·dyn·ia (krī-mō-din′ē-ă). SYN cryalgesia. [crymo- + G. *odynē,* pain]

cry·mo·phil·ic (krī-mō-fil′ik). Preferring cold; denoting microorganisms which thrive best at low temperatures. SYN cryophilic. [crymo- + G. *philos,* fond]

cry·mo·phy·lac·tic (krī′mō-fi-lak′tik). Resistant to cold, said of certain microorganisms that are not destroyed even by freezing temperatures. SYN cryophylactic. [crymo- + G. *phylaxis,* a guarding against]

⌂**cryo-, cry-.** Cold. SEE ALSO crymo-, psychro-. [G. *kryos,*]

cry·o·an·es·the·sia (krī′ō-an-es-thē′zē-ă). Localized application of cold as a means of producing regional anesthesia. SYN refrigeration anesthesia.

cry·o·cau·tery (krī-ō-kaw′ter-ē). Any substance, such as liquid air or carbon dioxide snow, or a low temperature instrument, the application of which causes destruction of tissue by freezing.

cry·o·ex·trac·tion (krī′ō-ek-strak′shŭn). Removal of cataracts by the adhesion of a freezing probe to the lens; now rarely done.

cry·o·fi·brin·o·gen (krī′ō-fī-brin′ō-jen). An abnormal type of fibrinogen very rarely found in human plasma; it is precipitated upon cooling, but redissolves when warmed to room temperature.

cry·o·fi·brin·o·gen·e·mia (krī′ō-fī-brin′ō-je-nē′mē-ă). The presence in the blood of cryofibrinogens.

cry·o·gen·ic (krī-ō-jen′ik). **1.** Denoting or characteristic of a cryogen. **2.** Relating to cryogenics.

cry·o·glob·u·lin·e·mia (krī′ō-glob′yū-li-nē′mē-ă). The presence of abnormal quantities of cryoglobulin in the blood plasma.

cry·o·glob·u·lins (krī-ō-glob′yū-linz). Abnormal plasma proteins characterized by precipitating, gelling, or crystallizing when serum or solutions of them are cooled; they may appear in patients with multiple myeloma.

cryokinetics (krī-ō-kĭ-nĕt′iks). Application of cold before an exercise session. SEE ALSO cryotherapy. SYN cold therapy. [cryo- + kinetics]

cry·ol·y·sis (krī-ol′i-sis). Destruction by cold. [cryo- + G. *lysis,* dissolution]

cry·op·a·thy (krī-op′ă-thē). A morbid condition in which exposure to cold is an important factor. [cryo- + G. *pathos,* suffering]

cry·o·pexy (krī′ō-pek-sē). In retinal detachment surgery, sealing the sensory retina to the pigment epithelium and choroid by a freezing probe applied to the sclera. [cryo- + G. *pēxis,* a fixing in place]

cry·o·phil·ic (krī-ō-fil′ik). SYN crymophilic. [cryo- + G. *philos,* fond]

cry·o·phy·lac·tic (krī′ō-fī-lak′tik). SYN crymophylactic.

cry·o·pre·cip·i·tate (krī′ō-prē-sip′i-tāt). Precipitate that forms when soluble material is cooled, especially with reference to the precipitate that forms in normal blood plasma which has been subjected to cold precipitation and which is rich in factor VIII.

cry·o·pres·er·va·tion (krī′ō-pres-er-vā′shŭn). Maintenance of the viability of excised tissues or organs at extremely low temperatures.

cry·o·probe (krī′ō-prōb). An instrument used in cryosurgery to apply extreme cold to a selected area. [cryo- + L. *probo,* to test]

cry·o·pro·tein (krī-ō-prō′tēn). A protein that precipitates from solution when cooled and redissolves upon warming.

cry·os·co·py (krī-os′kŏ-pē). The determination of the freezing point of a fluid, usually blood or urine, compared with that of distilled water. [cryo- + G. *skopeō,* to examine]

cry·o·sur·gery (krī-ō-ser′jer-ē). An operation using freezing temperature (achieved by liquid nitrogen or carbon dioxide) to destroy tissue.

cry·o·ther·a·py (krī′ō-thār′ă-pē). The use of cold in the treatment of disease.

cry·o·tol·er·ant (krī-ō-tol′er-ant). Tolerant of very low temperatures.

crypt (kript). A pitlike depression or tubular recess.

> **dental c.,** the space filled by the dental follicle.
> **enamel c.,** the narrow, mesenchyme-filled space between the dental ledge and an enamel organ.
> **synovial c.,** a diverticulum of the synovial membrane of a joint.
> **tonsillar c.,** one of the variable number of deep recesses that extend into the palatine and pharyngeal tonsils from the free surface where they open at the tonsillar fossa.

⌂**crypt-.** SEE crypto-.

cryp·tec·to·my (krip-tek′tō-mē). Excision of a tonsillar or other crypt. [crypt + G. *ektomē,* excision]

cryp·tic (krip′tik). Hidden; occult; larvate. [G. *kryptikos*]

cryp·ti·tis (krip-tī′tis). Inflammation of a follicle or glandular tubule, particularly in the rectum.

⌂**crypto-, crypt-.** Hidden, obscure; without apparent cause. [G. *kryptos,* hidden, concealed]

cryp·to·coc·co·sis (krip′tō-kok-ō′sis). Infection by *Cryptococcus neoformans,* causing a pulmonary, disseminated, or meningeal mycosis. The most familiar and readily recognized form involves the central nervous system, with subacute or chronic meningitis. SYN Busse-Buschke disease.

Cryp·to·coc·cus (krip-tō-kok′ŭs). A genus of yeastlike fungi that reproduce by budding. [crypto- + G. *kokkos,* berry]

cryp·to·gen·ic (krip-tō-jen′ik). Of obscure, indeterminate etiology or origin, in contrast to phanerogenic. [crypto- + G. *genesis,* origin]

cryp·to·lith (krip′tō-lith). A concretion in a gland follicle. [crypto- + G. *lithos,* stone]

cryp·to·men·or·rhea (krip′tō-men-ō-rē′ă). Occurrence each month of the general symptoms of the menses without any flow of blood, as in cases of imperforate hymen. [crypto- + G. *mēn,* month, + *rhoia,* flow]

cryp·to·po·dia (krip-tō-pō′dē-ă). A swelling of the lower part of the leg and the foot, in such a manner that there is great distortion and the sole seems to be a flattened pad. [crypto- + G. *pous,* foot]

cryptorchidectomy (kript-or-ki-dek′tō-mē). Surgical removal of an undescended testis. [crypto- + G. *orchis,* orchid-, testis, + *ektome,* excision + -y]

cryp·tor·chi·dism (krip-tōr′ki-dizm). SYN cryptorchism.

cryp·tor·chi·do·pexy (krip-tōr′ki-dō-pek′sē). SYN orchiopexy. [crypto- + G. *orchis,* testis, + *pēxis,* fixation]

cryp·tor·chism (krip-tōr′kizm). Failure of one or both of the testes to descend. SYN cryptorchidism.

cryp·to·spo·rid·i·o·sis (krip′tō-spō-rid-ē-ō′sis). An enteric disease caused by waterborne protozoan parasites of the genus *Cryptosporidium;*

disease in immunocompetent persons is manifest as a self-limiting diarrhea, whereas in immunocompromised persons it is manifest as a prolonged severe diarrhea that can be fatal.

Cryp·to·spo·rid·i·um (krip′tō-spō-rid′ē-ŭm). A genus of coccidian sporozoans that are important pathogens of domestic animals, and common opportunistic parasites of humans with compromised immune function.

cryp·to·zy·gous (krip-toz′i-gŭs, -tō-zī′gŭs). Having a narrow face as compared with the width of the cranium, so that, when the skull is viewed from above, the zygomatic arches are not visible. [crypto- + G. *zygon*, yoke]

crys·tal (kris′tăl). A solid of regular shape and, for a given compound, characteristic angles, formed when an element or compound solidifies slowly enough, as a result either of freezing from the liquid form or of precipitating out of solution, to allow the individual molecules to take up regular positions with respect to one another. [G. *krystallos*, clear ice, crystal]

   Charcot-Leyden c.'s, c.'s in the shape of elongated double pyramids, formed from eosinophils, found in the sputum in bronchial asthma.

crys·tal·lin (kris′tă-lin). A type of protein found in the lens of the eye.

crys·tal·line (kris′tă-lēn). **1.** Clear; transparent. **2.** Relating to a crystal or crystals.

crys·tal·li·za·tion (kris′tăl-i-zā′shŭn). Assumption of a crystalline form when a vapor or liquid becomes solidified, or a solute precipitates from solution.

crys·tal·loid (kris′tăl-oyd). **1.** Resembling a crystal, or being such. **2.** A body that in solution can pass through a semipermeable membrane, as distinguished from a colloid, which cannot do so.

crys·tal·lu·ria (kris-tă-lū′rē-ă). The excretion of crystalline materials in the urine.

Cs cesium.

C-sec·tion. SEE cesarean *section.*

CSF cerebrospinal *fluid*; colony-stimulating *factors*, under *factor.*

CT computed *tomography.*

CTD cumulative trauma *disorders*, under *disorder.*

Cteno·ce·phal·i·des (tē-nō-se-fal′i-dēz). A genus of fleas. *C. canis* (dog flea) and *C. felis* (cat flea) are nearly universal ectoparasites of household pets; will attack humans when starving owing to absence of pets. [G. *ktenōdēs*, like a cockle, + *kephalē*, head]

CTP cytidine 5′-triphosphate.

Cu copper.

cu·bi·tal (kyū′bi-tăl). Relating to the elbow or to the ulna.

cu·bi·tus, gen. and pl. **cu·bi·ti** (kyū′bi-tŭs, -tī) [NA]. **1.** SYN elbow (1). **2.** SYN ulna. [L. elbow]

   c. val′gus, deviation of the extended forearm to the outer (radial) side of the axis of the limb.

   c. va′rus, deviation of the extended forearm to the inward (ulnar) side of the axis of the limb.

cu·boid, cu·boi·dal (kyū′boyd, kyū-boy′dăl). **1.** Resembling a cube in shape. **2.** Relating to the os cuboideum. [G. *kybos*, cube, + *eidos*, resemblance]

cuff (kŭf). Any structure shaped like a c.

rotator c. of shoulder, the upper half of the capsule of the shoulder joint reinforced by the tendons of insertion of the supraspinatus, infraspinatus, teres minor, and subscapularis muscles.

cul-de-sac, pl. **culs-de-sac** (kŭl-de-sak′). **1.** A blind pouch or tubular cavity closed at one end; *e.g.,* diverticulum; cecum. **2.** SYN rectouterine *pouch.* [Fr. bottom of a sack]

cul·do·cen·te·sis (kŭl′dō-sen-tē′sis). Aspiration of fluid from the cul-de-sac by puncture of the vaginal vault near the midline between the uterosacral ligaments. [cul-de-sac + G. *kentēsis,* puncture]

cul·do·plas·ty (kŭl′dō-plas-tē). Plastic surgery to remedy relaxation of the posterior fornix of the vagina. [cul-de-sac + G. *plastos,* formed]

cul·do·scope (kŭl′dō-skōp). Endoscopic instrument used in culdoscopy.

cul·dos·co·py (kŭl-dos′kŏ-pē). Introduction of an endoscope through the posterior vaginal wall for viewing the rectovaginal pouch and pelvic viscera. [cul-de-sac + G. *skopeō,* to view]

Cu·lex (kyū′leks). A genus of mosquitoes including over 2,000 species. Largely tropical but worldwide in distribution; they are vectors for a number of diseases of man and of domestic and wild animals and birds. [L. gnat]

cu·li·ci·dal (kyū-li-sī′dăl). Destructive to mosquitoes. [L. *culex,* gnat, + *caedo,* to kill]

cu·li·cide (kyū′li-sīd). An agent that destroys mosquitoes.

Cu·li·coi·des (kyū-li-koy′dēz). A genus of minute biting gnats or midges, vectors of several nonpathogenic human filariae (*Mansonella, Dipetalonema*). [L. *culex,* gnat]

cul·ti·va·tion (kŭl-ti-vā′shŭn). SYN culture. [Mediev. L. *cultivo,* pp. *-atus,* fr. L. *colo,* pp. *cultus,* to till]

cul·tur·al di·ver·si·ty (kul′chū-ral dĭ-ver′sĭ-tē). The inevitable variety in customs, attitudes, practices, and behavior that exists among groups of individuals from different ethnic, racial, or national backgrounds who come into contact.

cul·ture (kŭl′chŭr). **1.** The propagation of microorganisms on or in media of various kinds. **2.** A mass of microorganisms on or in a medium. **3.** The propagation of mammalian cells, *i.e.,* cell culture. SEE cell c. SYN cultivation. [L. *cultura,* tillage, fr. *colo,* pp. *cultus,* to till]

   cell c., the maintenance or growth of dispersed cells after removal from the body, commonly on a glass surface immersed in nutrient fluid.

   mixed lymphocyte c., SEE mixed lymphocyte culture *test.*

   organ c., the maintenance or growth of tissues, organ primordia, or the parts or whole of an organ *in vitro* in such a way as to allow differentiation or preservation of the architecture or function.

   pure c., in the ordinary bacteriologic sense, a c. consisting of the descendants of a single cell.

   slant c., a c. made on the slanting surface of a medium which has been solidified in a test tube inclined from the perpendicular so as to give a greater area than that of the lumen of the tube.

   smear c., a c. obtained by spreading material

presumed to be infected on the surface of a solidified medium.

stab c., a c. produced by inserting an inoculating needle with inoculum down the center of a solid medium contained in a test tube.

stock c., a c. of a microorganism maintained solely for the purpose of keeping the microorganism in a viable condition by subculture, as necessary, into fresh medium.

streak c., a c. produced by lightly stroking an inoculating needle or loop with inoculum over the surface of a solid medium.

tissue c., the maintenance of live tissue after removal from the body, by placing in a vessel with a sterile nutritive medium.

type c., a type strain of microorganism preserved in a c. collection as the standard.

cu•mu•la•tive (kyū′myū-lă-tiv). Tending to accumulate or pile up, as with certain drugs that may have a c. effect.

cu•ne•ate (kyū′nē-āt). Wedge-shaped. [L. *cuneus,* wedge]

cu•ne•o•cu•boid (kyū′nē-ō-kyū′boyd). Relating to the lateral cuneiform and the cuboid bones.

cu•ne•o•na•vic•u•lar (kyū-nē-ō-na-vik′yū-lăr). Relating to the cuneiform and the navicular bones.

cu•ne•us, pl. **cu•nei** (kyū′nē-ŭs, kū′nē-ī) [NA]. That region of the medial aspect of the occipital lobe of each cerebral hemisphere bounded by the parietooccipital fissure and the calcarine fissure. [L. wedge]

cu•nic•u•lus, pl. **cu•nic•u•li** (kyū-nik′yū-lŭs -lī). The burrow of the scabies mite in the epidermis. [L. a rabbit; an underground passage]

cun•ni•lin•gus (kŭn-i-ling′gŭs). Oral stimulation of the vulva or clitoris; contrasted with fellatio, which is the oral stimulation of the penis. [L. *cunnus,* pudendum, + *lingo,* to lick]

cup (kŭp). **1.** An excavated or cup-shaped structure, either anatomical or pathologic. **2.** SYN cupping *glass.* [A.S. *cuppe*]

eye c., a small oval receptacle used to apply a liquid to the external eye.

glaucomatous c., a deep depression of the optic disk combined with optic atrophy; caused by glaucoma. SYN glaucomatous excavation.

optic c., the double-walled c. formed by the invagination of the embryonic optic vesicle; its inner component becomes the sensory layer of the retina, its outer layer, the pigment layer.

cu•po•la (kū′pŏ-lă, kyū′). SYN cupula.

cup•ping (kŭp′ing). **1.** Formation of a hollow, or cup-shaped excavation. **2.** Application of a c. glass. SEE ALSO cup.

cu•pu•la, pl. **cu•pu•lae** (kū′pū-lă, -lē; kyū′pyū-lă) [NA]. A cup-shaped or domelike structure. SYN cupula. [L. dim. of *cupa,* a tub]

cu•pu•lo•gram (kū′pū-lō-gram). A graphic representation of vestibular function relative to normal performance.

cur•a•tive (kyūr′ă-tiv). **1.** That which heals or cures. **2.** Tending to heal or cure.

cure (kyūr). **1.** To heal; to make well. **2.** A restoration to health. **3.** A special method or course of treatment. [L. *curo,* to care for]

cu•ret. SEE curette.

cu•ret•ment (kyū-ret′ment, kū-). SYN curettage.

cu•ret•tage (kyū-rĕ-tahzh′, kū-). A scraping, usually of the interior of a cavity or tract, for the removal of new growths or other abnormal tissues, or to obtain material for tissue diagnosis. SYN curetment, curettement.

periapical c., (1) removal of a cyst or granuloma from its pathologic bony crypt, utilizing a curette; **(2)** the removal of tooth fragments and debris from sockets at the time of extraction or of bone sequestra subsequently.

subgingival c., removal of subgingival calculus, ulcerated epithelial and granulation tissues found in periodontal pockets.

cu•rette, cu•ret (kyū-ret′, kū-). Instrument in the form of a loop, ring, or scoop with sharpened edges attached to a rod-shaped handle, used for curettage. [Fr.]

cu•rette•ment (kyū-ret′ment, kū-). SYN curettage.

cu•rie (c, C, Ci) (kyū′rē). A unit of measurement of radioactivity, 3.70×10^{10} disintegrations per second; superseded by the S.I. unit, the becquerel (1 disintegration per second). [Marie (1867–1934) and Pierre (1859–1906) *Curie,* French chemists and physicists and Nobel laureates]

cu•ri•um (Cm) (kyū′rē-ŭm). An element, atomic no. 96, atomic wt. 247.07, not occurring naturally on earth, but first formed artificially in 1944 by bombarding ^{239}Pu with alpha particles; the most stable of the c. isotopes is ^{247}Cm, with a half-life of 15.6 million years. [see curie]

cur•rent (ker′rĕnt). A stream or flow of fluid, air, or electricity. [L. *currens,* pres. p. of *curro,* to run]

action c., an electrical c. induced in muscle fibers when they are effectively stimulated; normally it is followed by contraction.

alternating c. (AC), electric c. that reverses direction (positive-negative polarity) many times each second (with each rotation of the armature of the dynamo generating the c.

axial c., the central rapidly moving portion of the bloodstream in an artery.

direct c. (DC), a c. that flows only in one direction; *e.g.,* that derived from a battery; sometimes referred to as galvanic c.

Current Procedural Terminology (CPT). A coding system for all medical procedures and services, published by the American Medical Association (as *Physicians' Current Procedural Terminology*) and revised annually.

cur•va•ture (ker′vă-chūr). A bending or flexure. SEE angulation. [L. *curvatura,* fr. *curvo,* pp. *-atus,* to bend, curve]

angular c., a gibbous deformity, *i.e.,* a sharp angulation of the spine, occurring in Pott's disease.

greater c. of stomach, the border of the stomach to which the greater omentum is attached.

lesser c. of stomach, the right border of the stomach to which the lesser omentum is attached.

spinal c., SEE kyphosis, lordosis, scoliosis.

curve (kerv). **1.** A nonangular continuous bend or line. **2.** A chart or graphic representation, by means of a continuous line connecting individual observations, of the course of a physiological activity, of the number of cases of a disease in a given period, or of any entity that might be otherwise presented by a table of figures. SYN chart (2). [L. *curvo,* to bend]

alignment c., the line passing through the center of the teeth laterally in the direction of the c. of the dental arch.

bell-shaped c., SYN gaussian *distribution.*

Frank-Starling c., SYN Starling's c.

Friedman c., a graph on which hours of labor are plotted against cervical dilation in centimeters.

c. of occlusion, (1) a curved surface which makes simultaneous contact with the major portion of the incisal and occlusal prominences of the existing teeth; **(2)** the c. of a dentition on which the occlusal surfaces lie.

oxyhemoglobin dissociation c., a graphic illustration of the relationship between oxygen saturation of hemoglobin and the partial pressure of arterial oxygen (PaO_2); the position and overall shape of this sigmoidal curve are affected by the hydrogen ion concentration (pH), body temperature, carbon dioxide concentration (PCO_2), and organic phosphates.

Price-Jones c., a distribution c. of the measured diameters of red blood cells.

Starling's c., a graph in which cardiac output or stroke volume is plotted against mean atrial or ventricular end-diastolic pressure; with increasing venous return and atrial pressure the output proportionately increases until further increments overload the heart and the output falls. SYN Frank-Starling c.

tension c., the direction of the trabeculae in cancellous bone tissue adapted to resist stress.

Traube-Hering c.'s, slow oscillations in blood pressure usually extending over several respiratory cycles; related to variations in vasomotor tone; rhythmical variations in blood pressure. SYN Traube-Hering waves.

cush·ing·oid (kush'ing-oyd). Resembling the signs and symptoms of Cushing's disease or syndrome: buffalo hump obesity, striations, adiposity, hypertension, diabetes, and osteoporosis, usually due to exogenous corticosteroids.

cush·ion (kush'ŭn). ANATOMY any structure resembling a pad or c.

atrioventricular canal c.'s, a pair of mounds of embryonic connective tissue covered by endothelium, bulging into the embryonic atrioventricular canal; located one dorsally and one ventrally, they grow together and fuse with each other and with the lower edge of the septum primum, dividing the originally single canal into right and left atrioventricular orifices.

Passavant's c., a prominence on the posterior wall of the naso-pharynx formed by contraction of the superior constrictor of the pharynx during swallowing.

cusp (kŭsp). **1.** DENTISTRY a conical elevation arising on the surface of a tooth from an independent calcification center. **2.** A leaflet of one of the heart's valves. [L. *cuspis,* point]

cus·pal (kŭs'păl). Pertaining to a cusp.

cus·pid (kŭs'pid). **1.** Having but one cusp. SYN cuspidate. **2.** SYN canine *tooth.* [L. *cuspis,* point]

cus·pi·date (kŭs'pi-dāt). SYN cuspid (1).

cu·ta·ne·ous (kyū-tā'nē-ŭs). Relating to the skin. [L. *cutis,* skin]

cut·down (kŭt'down). Dissection of a vein for insertion of a cannula or needle for the administration of intravenous fluids or medication. SYN venostomy.

cu·ti·cle (kyū'ti-kl). **1.** An outer thin layer, usually horny in nature. **2.** The layer, chitinous in some invertebrates, which occurs on the surface of epithelial cells. **3.** SYN epidermis. [L. *cuticula,* dim. of *cutis,* skin]

cu·ti·re·ac·tion (kyū'ti-rē-ak'shŭn). The inflammatory reaction to a skin test in a sensitive (allergic) subject. [L. *cutis,* skin, + reaction]

cu·tis (kyū'tis) [NA]. SYN skin. [L.]

c. anseri'na, contraction of the arrectores pilorum produced by cold, fear, or other stimulus, causing the follicular orifices to become prominent.

c. lax'a [MIM*123700], a congenital or acquired condition characterized by deficient elastic fibers of the skin, which may hang in folds; vascular anomalies may be present. SYN pachydermatocele.

c. marmora'ta, a normal, physiologic, pink, marble-like mottling of the skin in infants, persisting abnormally in some children on exposure to cold.

c. rhomboida'lis nu'chae, geometric furrowed configurations of the skin of the back of the neck as a result of prolonged exposure to sunlight with solar elastosis.

c. ve'ra, SYN dermis.

CV *coefficient* of variation.

CVA cerebrovascular *accident.*

CVP central venous *pressure.*

△**cyan-.** SEE cyano-.

cy·a·nide (sī'an-īd). **1.** The radical –CN or ion $(CN)^-$. The ion is extremely poisonous, forming hydrocyanic acid in water; inhibits respiratory enzymes. **2.** A salt of HCN or a cyano-containing molecule.

cy·an·met·he·mo·glo·bin (sī'an-met-hē'mō-glō-bin). A relatively nontoxic compound of cyanide with methemoglobin, which is formed when methylene blue is administered in cases of cyanide poisoning.

△**cyano-, cyan-. 1.** blue. **2.** Chemical prefix frequently used in naming compounds that contain the cyanide group, CN. [G. *kyanos,* a dark blue substance]

Cy·a·no·bac·te·ria (sī'ă-nō-bak-tēr'ē-ă). A division of the kingdom Prokaryotae consisting of unicellular or filamentous bacteria that are either nonmotile or possess a gliding motility, reproduce by binary fission, and perform photosynthesis with the production of oxygen. SYN Cyanophyceae.

cy·a·no·co·bal·a·min (sī'an-ō-kō-bal'ă-min). A complex of cyanide and cobalamin, as in vitamin B_{12}.

cy·an·o·phil, cy·an·o·phile (sī'an-ō-fil, -fīl). A cell or element that is differentially colored blue by a staining procedure. [cyano- + G. *philos,* fond]

cy·a·noph·i·lous (sī-ă-nof'i-lŭs). Readily stainable with a blue dye.

Cy·a·no·phy·ce·ae (sī'ă-nō-fī'sē-ē). SYN Cyanobacteria. [cyano- + G. *phykos,* seaweed]

cy·a·nop·sia (sī-ă-nop'sē-ă). A condition in which all objects appear blue; may temporarily follow cataract extraction. [cyano- + G. *opsis,* vision]

cy·a·nosed (sī'ă-nōst). SYN cyanotic.

cy·a·nose tar·dive (sē-ă-nōs' tar-dēv'). Cyanosis developing in congenital heart disease only after the heart begins to fail. SYN tardive cyanosis. [F. delayed cyanosis]

cy·a·no·sis (sī-ă-nō'sis). A dark bluish or purplish coloration of the skin and mucous membrane due to deficient oxygenation of the blood, evident when reduced hemoglobin in the blood exceeds 5 g per 100 ml. [G. dark blue color, fr. *kyanos,* blue substance]

    compression c., c. accompanied by edema and petechial hemorrhages over the head, neck, and upper part of the chest, as a venous reflex resulting from severe compression of the thorax or abdomen; the conjunctiva and retinas are similarly affected.

    enterogenous c., apparent c. caused by the absorption of nitrites or other toxic materials from the intestine with the formation of methemoglobin or sulfhemoglobin; the skin color change is due to the chocolate color of methemoglobin.

    tardive c., SYN cyanose tardive.

cy·a·not·ic (sī-ă-not'ik). Relating to or marked by cyanosis. SYN cyanosed.

cy·ber·net·ics (sī-ber-net'iks). 1. The comparative study of electronic calculators and the human nervous system, with intent to explain the functioning of the brain. 2. The science of control and communication in both living and nonliving systems; characteristically, control is governed by feedback, that is, by communication within the system concerning the difference between the actual and the desired result, action then being modified so as to minimize this difference. SEE ALSO feedback. [G. *kybernētica,* things pertaining to control or piloting]

△**cycl-.** SEE cyclo-.

cy·clar·thro·di·al (sī-klar-thrō'dē-ăl). Relating to a cyclarthrosis.

cy·clar·thro·sis (sī-klar-thrō'sis). A joint capable of rotation. [cyclo- + G. *arthrōsis,* articulation]

cy·clase (sī'klās). Descriptive name applied to an enzyme that forms a cyclic compound; *e.g.,* adenylate cyclase.

cy·cle (sī'kl). 1. A recurrent series of events. 2. A recurring period of time. 3. One successive compression and rarefaction of a wave, as of a sound wave. [G. *kyklos,* circle]

    carbon dioxide c., carbon c., the circulation of carbon as CO_2 from the expired air of animals and decaying organic matter to plant life where it is synthesized (through photosynthesis) to carbohydrate material, from which, as a result of catabolic processes in all life, it is again ultimately released to the atmosphere as CO_2.

    cardiac c., the complete round of cardiac systole and diastole with the intervals between, commencing with any event in the heart's action and ending when same event is repeated.

    cell c., the periodic biochemical and structural

events occurring during proliferation of cells such as in tissue culture.

    citric acid c., SYN tricarboxylic acid c.

    Cori c., the phases in the metabolism of carbohydrate: 1) glycogenolysis in the liver; 2) passage of glucose into the circulation; 3) deposition of glucose in the muscles as glycogen; 4) glycogenolysis during muscular activity and conversion to lactate, which is converted to glycogen in the liver.

    dicarboxylic acid c., (1) that portion of the tricarboxylic acid c. involving the dicarboxylic acids (succinic, fumaric, malic, and oxaloacetic acids); **(2)** a cyclic scheme in which certain steps of the tricarboxylic acid c. are used with the glyoxylate c.; important in the utilization of glyoxylic acid in microorganisms.

    duty c. (t_i/t_{tot}), the ratio of inspiratory (t_i) time to total-breathing-cycle time (t_{tot}).

    estrous c., the series of cyclic uterine, ovarian, and other changes that occur in higher animals.

    fatty acid oxidation c., a series of reactions involving acyl-coenzyme A compounds; the major pathway of fatty acid catabolism in living tissue.

    Krebs c., SYN tricarboxylic acid c.

    Krebs-Henseleit c., Krebs ornithine c., Krebs urea c., SYN urea c.

    menstrual c., the period in which an ovum matures, is ovulated, and enters the uterine lumen via the uterine tube; ovarian hormonal secretions effect endometrial changes such that, if fertilization occurs, nidation will be possible; in the absence of fertilization, ovarian secretions wane, the endometrium sloughs, and menstruation begins; this c. lasts an average of 28 days, with day 1 of the c. designated as that day on which menstrual flow begins.

    nitrogen c., the series of events in which the nitrogen of the atmosphere is fixed, thus made available for plant and animal life, and is then returned to the atmosphere: nitrifying bacteria convert N_2 and O_2 to NO_2^- and NO_3^-, the latter being absorbed by plants and converted to protein; if plants decay, the nitrogen is in part given up to the atmosphere and the remainder is converted by microorganisms to ammonia, nitrites, and nitrates; if the plants are eaten, the animals' excreta or bacterial decay return the nitrogen to the soil and air.

    ovarian c., the normal sex c. which includes development of an ovarian (graafian) follicle, rupture of the follicle with discharge of the ovum, and formation and regression of a corpus luteum.

    reproductive c., the c. which begins with conception and extends through gestation and parturition.

    tricarboxylic acid c., together with oxidative phosphorylation, the main source of energy in the mammalian body and the end toward which carbohydrate, fat, and protein metabolism are directed; a series of reactions, beginning and ending with oxaloacetic acid, during the course of which a two-carbon fragment is completely oxidized to carbon dioxide and water with the production of 12 high-energy phosphate bonds. SYN citric acid c., Krebs c.

urea c., the sequence of chemical reactions, occurring primarily in the liver, that results in the production of urea. SYN Krebs-Henseleit c., Krebs ornithine c., Krebs urea c.

cy·clec·to·my (sī-klek'tō-mē, sik-lek'tō-mē). Excision of a portion of the ciliary body. SYN ciliectomy. [cyclo- + G. *ektomē,* excision]

cy·clen·ceph·a·ly, cy·clen·ce·pha·lia (sī-klen-sef'ă-lē, -se-fā'lē-ă). Condition in a malformed fetus characterized by poor development and a varying degree of fusion of the two cerebral hemispheres. SYN cyclocephaly, cyclocephalia. [cyclo- + G. *enkephalos,* brain]

cy·cles per sec·ond (cps). The number of successive compressions and rarefactions per second of a sound wave. The preferred designation for this unit of frequency is hertz.

cy·clic (sī'klik, sik'lik). **1.** Pertaining to, or characteristic of, a cycle; occurring periodically, denoting the course of the symptoms in certain diseases or disorders. **2.** CHEMISTRY pertaining to a molecule containing a ring of atoms; denoting a c. compound.

cy·clic AMP. SYN adenosine 3′,5′-cyclic monophosphate.

3′,5′-cy·clic AMP syn·the·tase. SYN *adenylate cyclase.*

cy·cli·tis (sī-klī'tis). Inflammation of the ciliary body. [G. *kyklos,* circle (ciliary body), + *-itis,* inflammation]

△**cyclo-, cycl-.** **1.** A circle or cycle; the ciliary body. **2.** CHEMISTRY a molecule consisting of atoms in a ring. [G. *kyklos,* circle]

cy·clo·ceph·a·ly, cy·clo·ce·pha·lia (sī-klō-sef'ă-lē, -sĕ-fā'lē-ă). SYN cyclencephaly. [cyclo- + G. *kephalē,* head]

cy·clo·cho·roid·i·tis (sī'klō-kō-roy-dī'tis). Inflammation of the ciliary body and the choroid.

cy·clo·cry·o·ther·a·py (sī'klō-krī'ō-thār'ă-pē). Transscleral freezing of the ciliary body in the treatment of glaucoma.

cy·clo·di·al·y·sis (sī'klō-dī-al'i-sis). Establishment of a communication between the anterior chamber and the suprachoroidal space in order to reduce intraocular pressure in glaucoma. [cyclo- + G. *dialysis,* separation]

cy·clo·di·a·ther·my (sī'klō-dī-ă-ther'mē). Diathermy applied to the sclera adjacent to the ciliary body in the treatment of glaucoma.

cy·clo·duc·tion (sī-klō-dŭk'shŭn). Rotation of the eye around its visual axis. SYN circumduction (2). [cyclo- + L. *duco,* pp. *ductus,* to draw]

cy·clo·pep·tide (sī-klō-pep'tīd). A polypeptide lacking terminal —NH₂ and —COOH groups by virtue of their combination to form another peptide link, forming a ring.

cy·clo·pho·ras·es (sī-klō-fōr'ās-ez). The group of enzymes in mitochondria that catalyze the complete oxidation of pyruvic acid to carbon dioxide and water; essentially, those enzymes and coenzymes involved in the tricarboxylic acid cycle.

cy·clo·pho·ria (sī-klō-fō'rē-ă). Abnormal tendency for each eye to rotate around its anteroposterior axis, the rotation being prevented by visual fusional impulses. [cyclo- + G. *phora,* movement]

cy·clo·pho·to·co·ag·u·la·tion (sī'klō-fō'tō-kō-ag-yū-lā'shŭn). Photocoagulation of the ciliary processes to reduce the secretion of aqueous humor in glaucoma. [cyclo- + photocoagulation]

cy·clo·pia (sī-klō'pē-ă). A congenital defect in which the two orbits merge to form a single cavity containing one eye, its origin evidenced by fusion of the right and left optic primordia, and in which the nose is absent; usually combined with cyclencephaly. SYN synophthalmia. [G. *Kyklōps,* fr. *kyklos,* circle, + *ōps,* eye]

cy·clo·pi·an (sī-klō'pē-an). Denoting or relating to cyclopia.

cy·clo·ple·gia (sī-klō-plē'jē-ă). Loss of power in the ciliary muscle of the eye; may be by denervation or by pharmacologic action. [cyclo- + G. *plēgē,* stroke]

cy·clo·ple·gic (sī-klō-plē'jik). **1.** Relating to cycloplegia. **2.** A drug that paralyzes the ciliary muscle and thus the power of accommodation.

cy·clo·thy·mia (sī-klō-thī'mē-ă). A mental disorder characterized by marked swings of mood from depression to hypomania but not to the degree that occurs in bipolar disorder. [cyclo- + G. *thymos,* rage]

cy·clot·o·my (sī-klot'ō-mē). Operation of cutting the ciliary muscle. [cyclo- + G. *tomē,* incision]

cy·clo·tro·pia (sī-klō-trō'pē-ă). A disparity of ocular position in which one eye is rotated around its visual axis, with respect to the other eye. [cyclo- + G. *tropē,* a turn, turning]

Cyd Symbol for cytidine.

cyl·in·der (C) (sil'in-der). **1.** A cylindrical *lens.* **2.** A cylindrical or rodlike renal cast. **3.** A cylindrical metal container for gases stored under high pressure. [G. *kylindros,* a roll]

cyl·in·dro·ad·e·no·ma (sil'in-drō-ad-ĕ-nō'mă). SYN cylindroma.

cyl·in·dro·ma (sil-in-drō'mă). A histologic type of epithelial neoplasm, frequently malignant, characterized by islands of neoplastic cells embedded in a hyalinized stroma; may form from ducts of glands, especially in salivary glands, skin, and bronchi. SYN cylindroadenoma. [G. *kylindros,* cylinder, *-oma,* tumor]

cyl·in·dru·ria (sil-in-drū'rē-ă). The presence of renal cylinders or casts in the urine.

cym·bo·ce·phal·ic, cym·bo·ceph·a·lous (sim-bō-se-fal'ik, -sef'ă-lŭs). Relating to cymbocephaly.

cym·bo·ceph·a·ly. SYN scaphocephaly. [G. *kymbē,* the hollow of a vessel, a boat-shaped structure, *kephalē,* head]

cy·no·ceph·a·ly (sī-nō-sef'ă-lē). Craniostenosis in which the skull slopes back from the orbits, producing a resemblance to the head of a dog. [G. *kyōn,* dog, + *kephalē,* head]

cy·no·pho·bia (sī-nō-fō'bē-ă). Morbid fear of dogs. [G. *kyōn,* dog, + *phobos,* fear]

Cys Symbol for cysteine (half-cystine) or its mono- or diradical.

cyst (sist). **1.** A bladder. **2.** An abnormal sac containing gas, fluid, or a semisolid material, with a membranous lining. SEE ALSO pseudocyst. [G. *kystis,* bladder]

adventitious c., SYN pseudocyst (1).

aneurysmal bone c., a solitary benign osteolytic lesion expanding a long bone or within a vertebra, consisting of blood-filled spaces, and separated by fibrous tissue containing multinucleated giant cells; such c.'s cause swelling, pain, and tenderness.

◼ **apical periodontal c.,** an inflammatory odontogenic c. derived histogenetically from Malassez's epithelial rests surrounding the root apex of a nonvital tooth.

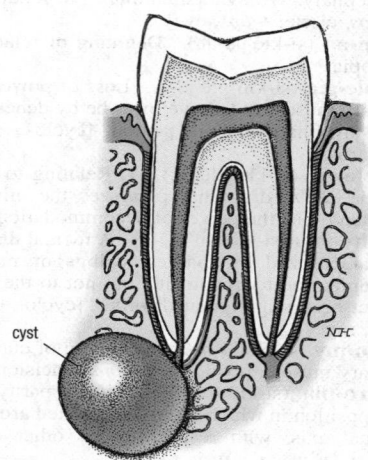

cyst

apical periodontal cyst

arachnoid c., a fluid-filled c. lined with arachnoid membrane, frequently situated near the lateral aspect of the fissure of Sylvius; usually congenital in origin.

Baker's c., a collection of synovial fluid which has escaped from the knee joint or a bursa and formed a new synovial-lined sac in the popliteal space; seen in degenerative or other joint diseases.

Bartholin's c., a c. arising from the major vestibular gland or its ducts.

blood c., SYN hemorrhagic c.

blue dome c., (1) one of a number of small dark blue nodules or c.'s in the vaginal fornix due to retained menstrual blood in endometriosis affecting this region; (2) a benign retention c. of the mammary gland in fibrocystic disease, containing a pale slightly yellow fluid which gives a blue color to the c. when seen through the surrounding fibrous tissue.

bronchogenic c., a c. lined by ciliated columnar epithelium believed to represent bronchial differentiation; smooth muscle and mucous glands may be present.

calcifying and keratinizing odontogenic c., SYN calcifying odontogenic c.

calcifying odontogenic c., a mixed radiolucent-radiopaque lesion of the jaws with features of both a c. and a solid neoplasm; characterized by ghost cell keratinization, dentinoid, and calcification. SYN calcifying and keratinizing odontogenic c.

chocolate c., c. of the ovary with intracavitary hemorrhage and formation of a hematoma containing old brown blood; often seen with endometriosis of the ovary but occasionally with other types of c.'s.

choledochal c., c. originating from common bile duct; usually becomes apparent early in life as a right upper abdominal mass in association with jaundice.

daughter c., a secondary c., usually multiple, derived from a mother c.

dentigerous c., an odontogenic c. derived from the reduced enamel epithelium surrounding the crown of an impacted or embedded tooth. SYN follicular c. (2).

dentinal lamina c., a small keratin-filled c., usually multiple, on the alveolar ridge of newborn infants; it is derived from remnants of the dental lamina.

dermoid c., a tumor consisting of displaced ectodermal structures along lines of embryonic fusion, the wall being formed of epithelium-lined connective tissue, including skin appendages and containing keratin, sebum, and hair. SYN dermoid tumor, dermoid (2).

echinococcus c., SYN hydatid c.

enterogenous c.'s, mediastinal cysts derived from cells sequestered from the primitive foregut; may be classified histologically as bronchogenic, esophageal, or gastric.

epidermal c., a c. formed of a mass of epidermal cells which, as a result of trauma, has been pushed beneath the epidermis; the c. is lined with stratified squamous epithelium and contains concentric layers of keratin.

epidermoid c., a spherical, unilocular c. of the dermis, composed of encysted keratin and sebum; the c. is lined by a keratinizing epithelium resembling the epidermis derived from the follicular infundibulum.

exudation c., a c. resulting from distention of a closed cavity, such as a bursa, by an excessive secretion of its normal fluid contents.

follicular c., (1) a cystic graafian follicle; **(2)** SYN dentigerous c.

ganglion c., collection of fluid or benign tumor mass within tendons of the wrist or ankle, most commonly on the dorsal aspect of the wrist.

granddaughter c., a tertiary c. sometimes developed within a daughter c., as in the hydatid cyst of *Echinococcus*.

hemorrhagic c., a c. containing blood or resulting from the encapsulation of a hematoma. SYN blood c., hematocele (1), hematocyst.

hydatid c., a c. formed in the liver by the larval stage of *Echinococcus*, chiefly in ruminants; two morphological forms caused by *Echinococcus granulosus* are found in humans: the unilocular hydatid c. and the osseous hydatid c.; a third form in humans is the alveolar hydatid c., caused by *Echinococcus multilocularis*. SYN echinococcus c., hydatid (1).

incisive canal c., a c. in or near the incisive canal, arising from proliferation of epithelial remnants of the nasopalatine duct; the most common maxillary development c.

keratinous c., an epithelial c. containing keratin.

meibomian c., SYN chalazion.

mother c., a hydatid c. from the inner, or germinal, layer, from which secondary c.'s containing scoleces (daughter c.'s) are developed; occurs most frequently in the liver, but may be found in other organs and tissue. SYN parent c.

mucous c., a retention c. resulting from obstruction in the duct of a mucous gland.

multilocular c., a c. containing several compartments formed by membranous septa.

myxoid c., SYN ganglion (2).

nabothian c., a retention c. that develops when a mucous gland of the cervix uteri is obstructed; of no pathologic significance. SYN nabothian follicle.

neurenteric c.'s, paravertebral c.'s commonly connected to the meninges or a portion of the gastrointestinal tract that develop due to incomplete separation of endoderm from the notochord during early fetal life; often symptomatic.

odontogenic c., a c. derived from odontogenic epithelium. [odont- + G. *genos*, birth, origin, + suffix *-ic*, pertaining to]

osseous hydatid c., a morphological form of hydatid c. caused by *Echinococcus granulosus* and found in the long bones or the pelvic arch of humans if the embryo is filtered out in bony tissue; in this site no limiting membrane forms and the c. grows in an uncontrolled fashion, producing cancellous structures and inducing fracture, followed by spread to new sites.

ovarian c., a cystic tumor of the ovary, either non-neoplastic (follicle, lutein, germinal inclusion, or endometrial) or neoplastic.

parasitic c., a c. formed by the larva of a metazoan parasite, such as a hydatid or trichinal c.

parent c., SYN mother c.

pilar c., a common c. of the skin and subcutis which contains sebum and keratin, and is lined by pale-staining stratified epithelial cells derived from follicular trichilemma.

retention c., a c. resulting from some obstruction to the excretory duct of a gland.

sebaceous c., a common c. of the skin and subcutis containing sebum and keratin, and lined by epithelium derived from the pilosebaceous follicle. SEE epidermoid c., pilar c.

serous c., a c. containing clear serous fluid, such as a hygroma.

solitary bone c., a unilocular c. containing serous fluid and lined with a thin layer of connective tissue, occurring usually in the shaft of a long bone in a child. SYN osteocystoma, unicameral bone c.

sterile c., a hydatid c. without brood capsules or viable scoleces.

sublingual c., SYN ranula (2).

synovial c., SYN ganglion (2).

tarry c., a c. or collection of old blood having a tarry or black, sticky appearance; usually due to endometriosis.

tarsal c., SYN chalazion.

tubular c., SYN tubulocyst.

unicameral bone c., SYN solitary bone c.

unilocular c., a c. having a single sac.

vitellointestinal c., a small red sessile or pedunculated tumor at the umbilicus in an infant; it is due to the persistence of a segment of the vitellointestinal duct.

wolffian c., a c. lying in the broad ligaments of the uterus and arising from any mesonephric structures.

△**cyst-.** SEE cysto-.

cyst·ad·e·no·car·ci·no·ma (sist-ad′en-ō-kar-si-nō′mă). A malignant neoplasm derived from glandular epithelium, in which cystic accumulations of retained secretions are formed; the neoplastic cells manifest varying degrees of anaplasia and invasiveness, and local extension and metastases occur; c.'s develop frequently in the ovaries, where pseudomucinous and serous types are recognized.

cyst·ad·e·no·ma (sist′ad-ĕ-nō′mă). A histologically benign neoplasm derived from glandular epithelium, in which cystic accumulations of retained secretions are formed. SYN cystoadenoma.

cyst·al·gia (sist-al′jē-ă). Pain in a bladder, especially the urinary bladder. [cyst- + G. *algos,* pain]

cys·ta·thi·o·nase (sis-tă-thī′ō-nās). SYN cystathionine γ-lyase.

cys·ta·thi·o·nine (sis-tă-thī′ō-nēn). An intermediate in the conversion of L-methionine to L-cysteine; cleaved by cystathionases.

cys·ta·thi·o·nine γ-ly·ase. A liver enzyme that catalyzes the hydrolysis of L-cystathionine to L-cysteine and 2-ketobutyrate. A deficiency of this enzyme results in cystathioninuria. A step in methionine catabolism and in cysteine biosynthesis. SYN cystathionase.

cys·tec·ta·sia, cys·tec·ta·sy (sis-tek-tā′zē-ă, sis-tek′tă-sē). Dilation of the bladder. [cyst- + G. *ektasis,* a stretching]

cys·tec·to·my (sis-tek′tō-mē). **1.** Excision of the the urinary bladder. **2.** Excision of the gallbladder (cholecystectomy). **3.** Removal of a cyst. [cyst- + G. *ektomē,* excision]

cys·te·ic ac·id (sis-tā′ik). An oxidation product of cysteine, and a precursor of taurine and isethionic acid.

cys·te·ine (C, Cys) (sis′ta-ēn). An amino acid found in most proteins; especially abundant in keratin.

△**cysti-.** SEE cysto-.

cys·tic (sis′tik). **1.** Relating to the urinary bladder or gallbladder. **2.** Relating to a cyst. **3.** Containing cysts.

cys·ti·cer·co·sis (sis′ti-ser-kō′sis). **1.** Disease caused by encystment of cysticercus larvae (*e.g.,* *Taenia solium* or *T. saginata*) in subcutaneous, muscle, or central nervous system tissues; c. is typically developed in swine and cattle, producing measly pork and beef. In humans, it results from the hatching of the eggs of *Taenia solium* in the intestines or by accidental ingestion of eggs from human feces; encystment in the brain may cause serious nervous damage, and encystment in the eye (usually the rear chamber) may cause ophthalmic damage. **2.** Larval infections in animals with other taeniid tapeworm larvae.

Cys·ti·cer·cus (sis-ti-ser′kŭs). The encysted larva of taenioid tapeworms. SEE cysticercus. [G. *kystis,* bladder, + *kerkos,* tail]

cys·ti·cer·cus, pl. **cys·ti·cer·ci** (sis-ti-ser′kŭs, -ser′sī). The larval form of certain *Taenia* species, typically found in muscles of mammalian intermediate hosts; it consists of a fluid-filled bladder in which the invaginated cestode scolex develops. SEE ALSO *Taenia saginata, Taenia solium.* [G. *kystis,* bladder, + *kerkos,* tail]

cys·ti·form (sis′ti-fōrm). SYN cystoid (1).

cys·tine (sis′tīn). The disulfide product of two cysteines in which two –SH groups become one –S–S– group; sometimes occurs as a deposit in the urine, or forming a vesical calculus.

cys·ti·ne·mia (sis-ti-nē′mē-ă). The presence of cystine in the blood. [cystine + G. *haima,* blood]

cys·ti·nu·ria (sis-ti-nū′rē-ă) [MIM*220100]. Excessive urinary excretion of cystine, along with lysine, arginine, and ornithine, arising from defective transport systems for these acids in the kidney and intestine; renal function is sometimes compromised by cystine crystalluria and nephrolithiasis; occurs in certain heritable diseases, such as Fanconi's syndrome (cystinosis) and hepatolenticular degeneration. [cystine + G. *ouron,* urine]

cys·ti·tis (sis-tī′tis). Inflammation of the urinary bladder. [cyst- + G. *-itis,* inflammation]

  c. cys′tica, c. glandularis with the formation of cysts.

  follicular c., chronic c. characterized by small mucosal nodules due to lymphocytic infiltration.

  c. glandula′ris, chronic c. with glandlike metaplasia of transitional epithelium.

  hemorrhagic c., bladder inflammation with macroscopic hematuria. Generally the result of a chemical or other traumatic insult to the bladder (chemotherapy, radiation therapy).

  interstitial c., a chronic inflammatory condition of unknown etiology involving the mucosa and muscularis of the bladder, resulting in reduced bladder capacity, pain relieved by voiding, and severe bladder irritative symptoms. SEE ALSO Hunner's *ulcer.*

△**cysto-, cysti-, cyst-.** Combining forms relating to: **1.** The bladder. **2.** The cystic duct. **3.** A cyst. Cf. vesico-. [G. *kystis,* bladder, pouch]

cys·to·ad·e·no·ma (sis′tō-ad-ĕ-nō′mă). SYN cystadenoma.

cys·to·car·ci·no·ma (sis′tō-kar-si-nō′mă). A carcinoma in which cystic degeneration has occurred; sometimes used incorrectly as a term for cystadenocarcinoma. SYN cystoepithelioma.

cys·to·cele (sis′tō-sēl). Hernia of the bladder usually into the vagina and introitus. SYN colpocystocele, vesicocele. [cysto- + G. *kēlē,* hernia]

cys·to·chro·mos·co·py (sis′tō-krō-mos′kŏ-pē). Examination of the interior of the bladder after administration of a dye to aid in the identification or study of the function of the ureteral orifices. SYN chromocystoscopy. [cysto- + G. *chrōma,* color + *skopeō,* to view]

cys·to·du·o·de·nos·to·my (sis′tō-dū′ō-dē-nos′tō-mē). Drainage of a cyst, usually pancreatic pseudocyst, into duodenum. SYN duodenocystostomy (2). [cysto- + duodenum, + G. *stoma,* mouth]

  pancreatic c., surgical or endoscopic drainage of pancreatic pseudocyst into duodenum. SYN duodenocystostomy (3).

cys·to·ep·i·the·li·o·ma (sis′tō-ep-i-thē-lē-ō′mă). SYN cystocarcinoma.

cys·to·fi·bro·ma (sis′tō-fī-brō′mă). A fibroma in which cysts or cystlike foci have formed.

cys·to·gram (sis′tō-gram). Radiographic demonstration of the bladder filled with contrast medium.

  voiding c., SYN cystourethrogram.

cys·tog·ra·phy (sis-tog′ră-fē). Radiography of the bladder following injection of a radiopaque substance. [cysto- + G. *graphō,* to write]

cys·toid (sis′toyd). **1.** Bladder-like, resembling a cyst. SYN cystiform, cystomorphous. **2.** A tumor resembling a cyst, with fluid, granular, or pulpy contents, but without a capsule. [cysto- + G. *eidos,* appearance]

cys·to·li·thi·a·sis (sis′tō-li-thī′ă-sis). The presence of a vesical calculus. [cysto- + G. *lithos,* stone, + *-iasis,* condition]

cys·to·lith·ic (sis-tō-lith′ik). Relating to a vesical calculus.

cys·to·li·thot·o·my (sis′tō-li-thot′ō-mē). Removal of a stone from the bladder through an incision in its wall. [cysto- + G. *lithos,* stone, + *tomē,* incision]

cys·to·ma (sis-tō′mă). A cystic tumor; a new growth containing cysts. [cyst- + G. *-oma,* tumor]

cys·tom·e·ter (sis-tom′ĕ-ter). A device for studying bladder function by measuring capacity, sensation, intravesical pressure, and residual urine. [cysto- + G. *metron,* measure]

cys·to·met·ro·gram (sis-tō-met′rō-gram). A graphic recording of urinary bladder pressure at various volumes. [cysto- + G. *metron,* measure, + *gramma,* a writing]

cys·to·me·trog·ra·phy (sis′tō-mĕ-trog′ră-fē). SYN cystometry.

cys·tom·e·try (sis-tom′ĕ-trē). A method for measurement of the pressure/volume relationship of the bladder. SEE cystometer. SYN cystometrography.

cys·to·mor·phous (sis-tō-mōr′fŭs). SYN cystoid (1). [cysto- + G. *morphē,* form]

cys·to·pan·en·dos·co·py (sis′tō-pan-en-dos′kŏ-pē). Inspection of the interior of the bladder and urethra by means of specially designed endoscopes introduced in retrograde fashion through the urethra and into the bladder. [cysto- + panendoscope]

cys·to·pa·ral·y·sis (sis-tō-pă-ral′i-sis). SYN cystoplegia.

cys·to·pexy (sis′tō-pek-sē). Surgical attachment of the gallbladder or of the urinary bladder to the abdominal wall or to other supporting structures. [cysto- + G. *pēxis,* fixation]

cys·to·plas·ty (sis′tō-plas-tē). Any reconstructive operation on the urinary bladder. Cf. ileocystoplasty. [cysto- + G. *plastos,* formed]

cys·to·ple·gia (sis-tō-plē′jē-ă). Paralysis of the bladder. SYN cystoparalysis. [cysto- + G. *plēgē,* a stroke]

cystoptosis (-to-ze-a). Prolapse of the vesical mucous membrane into the urethra. [cysto- + G. *ptosis,* a falling + -ia]

cys·to·py·e·li·tis (sis′tō-pī-el-ī′tis). Inflammation of both the bladder and the pelvis of the kidney.

[cysto- + G. *pyelos,* trough (pelvis), + *-itis,* inflammation]

cys•to•py•e•lo•ne•phri•tis (sis-tō-pī′el-ō-nef-rī′tis). Inflammation of the bladder, the pelvis of the kidney, and the kidney parenchyma. [cysto- + G. *pyelos,* trough (pelvis), + *nephros,* kidney, + *-itis,* inflammation]

cystorectostomy (sis-to-rek-tos-to-me). SYN vesicorectostomy. [cysto + rectum + -o- + G. *stoma,* the mouth, + -y]

cys•tor•rha•phy (sis-tōr′ă-fē). Suture of a wound or defect in the urinary bladder. [cysto- + G. *rhaphē,* a sewing]

cys•tor•rhea (sis′tō-rē-ă). A mucous discharge from the bladder. [cysto- + G. *rhoia,* a flow]

cys•to•sar•co•ma (sis′tō-sar-kō′mă). A sarcoma in which the formation of cysts or cystlike foci has occurred.

cys•to•scope (sis′tō-skōp). A lighted tubular endoscope for examining the interior of the bladder. [cysto- + G. *skopeō,* to examine]

cys•tos•co•py (sis-tos′kŏ-pē). The inspection of the interior of the bladder by means of a cystoscope.

cys•tos•to•my (sis-tos′tō-mē). Creation of an opening into the urinary bladder. SYN vesicostomy. [cysto- + G. *stoma,* mouth]

cys•to•tome (sis′tō-tōm). **1.** An instrument for incising the urinary bladder or gallbladder. **2.** A surgical instrument used for incising the capsule of a lens.

cys•tot•o•my (sis-tot′ō-mē). Incision into urinary bladder or gallbladder. SYN vesicotomy. [cysto- + G. *tomē,* incision]

   suprapubic c., opening into the bladder through an incision or puncture above the symphysis pubis.

cys•to•u•re•ter•i•tis (sis′tō-yū-rē-ter-ī′tis). Inflammation of the bladder and of one or both ureters.

cys•to•u•re•ter•o•gram (sis′tō-yū-rē′ter-ō-gram). Radiographic demonstration of the bladder and ureters.

cys•to•u•re•ter•og•ra•phy (sis′tō-ū-rē′ter-og′ră-fē). Radiography of the bladder and ureters.

cys•to•u•re•thri•tis (sis′tō-yū-rē-thrī′tis). Inflammation of the bladder and of the urethra.

cys•to•u•re•thro•gram (sis-tō-yū-rēth′rō-gram). An x-ray image made during voiding and with the bladder and urethra filled with contrast medium to demonstrate the urethra. SYN voiding cystogram.

cys•to•u•re•throg•ra•phy (sis′tō-yū′rē-throg′ră-fē). Radiography of the bladder and urethra during voiding, following filling of the bladder with a radiopaque contrast medium either by intravenous injection or retrograde catheterization.

cys•to•u•re•thro•scope (sis-tō-yū-rē′thrō-skōp). An instrument combining the uses of a cystoscope and a urethroscope, whereby both the bladder and urethra can be visually inspected.

Cyt cytosine.

⌂**cyt-.** SEE cyto-.

cy•ta•pher•e•sis (sī′tă-fĕ-rē′sis). A procedure in which various blood cells can be separated and retained, with the plasma and other formed elements retransfused into the donor. [cyt- + G. *aphairesis,* a withdrawal]

⌂**-cyte.** cell. [G. *kyton,* a hollow (cell)]

cyt•i•dine (C, Cyd) (sī′ti-dēn). A major component of ribonucleic acids. SYN cytosine ribonucleoside.

cyt•i•dine 5′-di•phos•phate (CDP). An ester, at the 5′ position, between cytidine and diphosphoric acid.

cyt•i•dine 5′-tri•phos•phate (CTP). An ester, at the 5′ position, between cytidine and triphosphoric acid.

cyt•i•dyl•ic ac•id (sī-ti-dil′ik). Cytidine monophosphate (five are possible, depending on the site of attachment of the phosphate to the ribosyl OH's); a constituent of ribonucleic acids.

⌂**cyto-, cyt-.** A cell. [G. *kytos,* a hollow (cell)]

cy•to•ar•chi•tec•ture (sī′tō-ar′ki-tek-chŭr). The arrangement of cells in a tissue; the term commonly refers to the arrangement of nerve-cell bodies in the brain, especially the cerebral cortex.

cy•to•cen•trum (sī-tō-sen′trŭm). A zone of cytoplasm containing one or two centrioles but devoid of other organelles; usually located near the nucleus of a cell. SYN centrosome, microcentrum. [cyto- + G. *kentron,* center]

cy•to•chem•is•try (sī′tō-kem′is-trē). The study of intracellular distribution of chemicals, reaction sites, enzymes, etc., often by means of staining reactions, radioactive isotope uptake, selective metal distribution in electron microscopy, or other methods. SYN histochemistry.

cy•to•chrome (sī′tō-krōm). A class of hemoprotein whose principal biological function is electron and/or hydrogen transport by virtue of a reversible valency change of the heme iron. Many variants exist, particularly among bacteria and in green plants and algae, one being a variant of the *c* type cytochrome called cytochrome *f.* The mitochondrial system of c.'s provides electron transport through cytochrome *c* oxidase to molecular oxygen as the terminal electron acceptor (respiration). [cyto- + G. *chrōma,* color]

cy•toc•i•dal (sī-tō-sī′dăl). Causing the death of cells. [cyto- + L. *caedo,* to kill]

cy•to•cide (sī′tō-sīd). An agent that is destructive to cells. [cyto- + L. *caedo,* to kill]

cy•toc•la•sis (sī-tok′lă-sis). Fragmentation of cells. [cyto- + G. *klasis,* a breaking]

cy•to•clas•tic (sī-tō-klas′tik). Relating to cytoclasis.

cy•to•di•ag•no•sis (sī′tō-dī-ag-nō′sis). Diagnosis of a pathologic process by means of microscopic study of cells.

cy•to•gen•e•sis (sī-tō-jen′ĕ-sis). The origin and development of cells. [cyto- + G. *genesis,* origin]

cy•to•ge•net•i•cist (sī′tō-jĕ-net′i-sist). A specialist in cytogenetics.

cy•to•ge•net•ics (sī′tō-jĕ-net′iks). The branch of genetics concerned with the structure and function of the cell, especially the chromosomes. Modern molecular cytogenetics involves the microscopic study of chromosomes that have been arranged as karyotypes. Individuals can be classified according to characteristic banding patterns that appear when the karyotypes are exposed to certain dyes. In addition, DNA probes may be applied to locate specific gene sequences. Cytogenetic techniques are used to test for inborn errors of metabolism, for disorders such as Down syndrome, and to determine sex in cases where anatomy is inconclusive.

cy•to•gen•ic (sī-tō-jen′ik). Relating to cytogenesis.

cy•tog•e•nous (sī-toj′ĕ-nŭs). Cell-forming.

cy•to•glu•co•pe•nia (sī′tō-glū-kō-pē′nē-ă). An intracellular deficiency of glucose. [cyto- + glucose + G. *penia*, poverty]

cy•toid (sī′toyd). Resembling a cell. [cyto- + G. *eidos*, resemblance]

cy•to•kine (sī′tō-kīn). Hormone-like proteins, secreted by many cell types, which regulate the intensity and duration of immune responses and are involved in cell-to-cell communication. SEE ALSO interferon, interleukin, lymphokines. [cyto- + G. *kinēsis*, movement]

cy•to•ki•ne•sis (sī′tō-ki-nē′sis). Changes occurring in the protoplasm of the cell outside the nucleus during cell division. [cyto- + G. *kinēsis*, movement]

cy•to•log•ic (sī-tō-loj′ik). Relating to cytology.

cy•tol•o•gist (sī-tol′ō-jist). One who specializes in cytology.

cy•tol•o•gy (sī-tol′ō-jē). The study of the anatomy, physiology, pathology, and chemistry of the cell. SYN cellular biology. [cyto- + G. *logos*, study]

   exfoliative c., the examination, for diagnostic purposes, of cells denuded from a neoplasm or an epithelial surface, recovered from exudate, secretions, or washings from tissue (*e.g.*, sputum, vaginal secretion, gastric washings, urine). SYN cytopathology (2).

cy•tol•y•sin (sī-tol′i-sin). A substance *i.e.*, an antibody that effects partial or complete destruction of an animal cell; may require complement. SEE ALSO perforin.

cy•tol•y•sis (sī-tol′i-sis). The dissolution of a cell. [cyto- + G. *lysis*, loosening]

cy•to•ly•so•some (sī-tō-lī′sō-sōm). A variety of secondary lysosome that contains the remnants of mitochondria, ribosomes, or other organelles.

cy•to•lyt•ic (sī-tō-lit′ik). Pertaining to cytolysis; possessing a solvent or destructive action on cells.

cy•to•meg•a•lo•vi•rus (CMV) (sī-tō-meg′ă-lō-vī′rŭs). A group of herpesviruses infecting humans and other animals, many having special affinity for salivary glands, and causing development of characteristic inclusions in the cytoplasm or nucleus. Most infections are asymptomatic, but if symptoms are present, they manifest as mononucleosis-like illness. Congenital infection may cause malformation or fetal death; infection in immunocompromised persons may be life-threatening. SYN human herpesvirus 5. [cyto- + G. *megas*, big]

cy•to•met•a•pla•sia (sī′tō-met-ă-plā′zē-ă). Change of form or function of a cell, other than that related to neoplasia. [cyto- + G. *metaplasis*, transformation]

cy•tom•e•ter (sī-tom′ĕ-ter). A device used to count and measure cells, especially blood cells, either visually (with a microscope) or automati-

cally (as in flow cytometry). [cyto- + G. *metron*, measure]

cy•tom•e•try (sī-tom′ĕ-trē). The counting of cells, especially blood cells, using a cytometer or hemocytometer.

   flow c., a method of measuring fluorescence from stained cells that are in suspension and flowing through a narrow orifice, usually with one or two lasers to activate the dyes; used to measure cell size, number, viability, and nucleic acid content.

cy•to•mor•phol•o•gy (sī′tō-mōr-fol′ō-jē). The study of the structure of cells.

cy•to•mor•pho•sis (sī′tō-mōr-fō′sis). Changes that the cell undergoes during the various stages of its existence. SEE ALSO prosoplasia. [cyto- + G. *morphōsis*, a shaping]

cy•to•path•ic (sī-tō-path′ik). Pertaining to or exhibiting cytopathy.

cy•to•path•o•gen•ic (sī′tō-path-ō-jen′ik). Pertaining to an agent or substance that causes a diseased condition in cells, in contrast to histologic changes; used especially with reference to effects observed in cells in tissue cultures.

cy•to•path•o•log•ic, cy•to•path•o•log•i•cal (sī′tō-pa-thō-loj′ik, -loj′i-kăl). **1.** Denoting cellular changes in disease. **2.** Relating to cytopathology.

cy•to•pa•thol•o•gist (sī′tō-pa-thol′ō-jist). A physician specially trained and experienced in cytopathology.

cy•to•pa•thol•o•gy (sī′tō-pa-thol′ō-jē). **1.** The study of disease changes within individual cells or cell types. **2.** SYN exfoliative *cytology*.

cy•top•a•thy (sī-top′ă-thē). Any disorder of a cell or anomaly of any of its constituents. [cyto- + G. *pathos*, disease]

cy•to•pe•nia (sī-tō-pē′nē-ă). A reduction, *i.e.*, hypocytosis, or a lack of cellular elements in the circulating blood. [cyto- + G. *penia*, poverty]

cy•toph•a•gous (sī-tof′ă-gŭs). Devouring, or destructive to, cells.

cy•toph•a•gy (sī-tof′ă-jē). Devouring of other cells by phagocytes. [cyto- + G. *phagō*, to devour]

cy•to•phil•ic (sī-tō-fil′ik). SYN cytotropic. [cyto- + G. *philos*, fond]

cy•to•pho•tom•e•try (sī′tō-fō-tom′ĕ-trē). A method of measuring the absorption of monochromatic light by stained microscopic structures (*e.g.*, chromosomes, nuclei, whole cells) with the aid of a photoelectric cell; also used to measure emitted light from such objects by fluorescence in combination with selected fluorochrome dyes. [cyto- + G. *phōs*, light + *metron*, measure]

cy•to•phy•lac•tic (sī′tō-fī-lak′tik). Relating to cytophylaxis.

cy•to•phy•lax•is (sī′tō-fī-lak′sis). Protection of cells against lytic agents. [cyto- + G. *phylaxis*, a guarding]

cy•to•plasm (sī′tō-plazm). The substance of a cell, exclusive of the nucleus, which contains various organelles and inclusions within a colloidal protoplasm. SEE ALSO protoplasm, hyaloplasm, cytosol. [cyto- + G. *plasma*, thing formed]

cy•to•plas•mic (sī-tō-plaz′mik). Relating to the cytoplasm.

cy•to•plast (sī′tō-plast). The living intact cytoplasm that remains following cell enucleation. [cyto- + G. *plastos,* formed]

cy•to•sine (Cyt) (sī'tō-sēn). A pyrimidine found in nucleic acids.

   c. arabinoside (CA), (1) a synthetic nucleoside used as an antimetabolite in the treatment of neoplasms. **(2)** incorrect term for arabinosylcytosine.

   c. ribonucleoside, SYN cytidine.

cy•to•sis (sī-tō'sis). **1.** A condition in which there is more than the usual number of cells, as in the spinal fluid in meningitis. **2.** Frequently used with a prefixed combining form as a means of describing certain features pertaining to cells; *e.g.,* isocytosis, equality in size; polycytosis, abnormal increase in number. [cyto- + G. *-osis,* condition]

cy•to•skel•e•ton (sī-tō-skel'ĕ-ton). The tonofilaments, keratin, desmin, neurofilaments, or other intermediate filaments serving as supportive cytoplasmic elements to stiffen cells or to organize intracellular organelles.

cy•to•sol (sī'tō-sol). Cytoplasm exclusive of the mitochondria, endoplasmic reticulum, and other membranous components. [cyto- + "sol," abbrev. of soluble]

cy•to•sol•ic (sī-tō-sol'ik). Relating to or contained in the cytosol.

cy•to•some (sī'tō-sōm). **1.** The cell body exclusive of the nucleus. **2.** One of the osmiophilic bodies that are 1 μm or less in diameter, have concentric lamellae, and occur in the great alveolar cells of the lung. SYN multilamellar body. [cyto- + G. *sōma,* body]

cy•tos•ta•sis (sī-tos'tă-sis). The slowing of movement and accumulation of blood cells, especially polymorphonuclear leukocytes, in the capillaries, as in a region of inflammation; obstruction of a capillary as the result of accumulated leukocytes. [cyto- + G. *stasis,* standing]

cy•to•stat•ic (sī-tō-stat'ik). Characterized by cytostasis.

cy•to•tac•tic (sī-tō-tak'tik). Relating to cytotaxis.

cy•to•tax•is, cy•to•tax•ia (sī-tō-tak'sis, -tak'sē-ă). The attraction (**positive c.**) or repulsion (**negative c.**) of cells for one another. [cyto- + G. *taxis,* arrangement]

cy•to•the•sis (sī-toth'ĕ-sis). The repair of injury in a cell; the restoration of cells. [cyto- + G. *thesis,* a placing]

cy•to•tox•ic (sī-tō-tok'sik). Detrimental or destructive to cells; pertaining to the effect of noncytophilic antibody on specific antigen, frequently, but not always, mediating the action of complement.

cy•to•tox•ic•i•ty (sī'tō-tok-sis'i-tē). The quality or state of being cytotoxic.

cy•to•tox•in (sī-tō-tok'sin). A specific substance, which may or may not be antibody, that inhibits or prevents the functions of cells, causes destruction of cells, or both. [cyto- + G. *toxikon,* poison]

cy•to•tro•pho•blast (sī-tō-trof'ō-blast). The inner layer of the trophoblast.

cy•to•tro•pic (sī-tō-trop'ik). Having an affinity for cells. SYN cytophilic.

cy•tot•ro•pism (sī-tot'rō-pizm). **1.** Affinity for cells. **2.** Affinity for specific cells, especially the ability of viruses to localize in and damage specific cells. [cyto- + G. *tropos,* a turning]

cy•tu•ria (sī-tū'rē-ă). The passage of cells in unusual numbers in the urine. [G. *kytos,* cell, + *ouron,* urine]

D

Δ, δ. delta. SEE delta.

d deci-; *dexter* [L], right; diameter; day.

Ⓒd-. Prefix indicating a chemical compound to be dextrorotatory; should be avoided when (+) or (−) could be used. Cf. L-.

ⒸD-. Prefix indicating that a chemical compound is sterically related to D-glyceraldehyde, the basis of stereochemical nomenclature. Cf. lambda.

Ⓒ-d. Suffix indicating the presence of deuterium in a compound in concentrations above normal, thus labelling the compound; subscripts (d_2, d_3, etc.) indicate the number of such atoms so fortified.

DA developmental *age* (2).

Da dalton.

dA, dAdo deoxyadenosine.

da deca-.

Ⓒdacry-. SEE dacryo-.

Ⓒdacryo-, dacry-. Tears; lacrimal sac or duct. [G. *dakryon*, tear]

dac·ry·o·ad·e·ni·tis (dak-rē-ō-ad-ĕ-nī'tis). Inflammation of the lacrimal gland. [dacryo- + G. *adēn*, gland, + *-itis*, inflammation]

dac·ry·o·blen·nor·rhea (dak-rē-ō-blen-ō-rē'ă). A chronic discharge of mucus from a lacrimal sac. [dacryo- + G. *blenna*, mucus, + *rhoia*, flow]

dac·ry·o·cele (dak'rē-ō-sēl). SYN dacryocystocele.

dac·ry·o·cyst (dak'rē-ō-sist). SYN lacrimal *sac.* [dacryo- + G. *kystis*, sac]

dac·ry·o·cys·tal·gia (dak'rē-ō-sis-tal'jē-ă). Pain in the lacrimal sac. [dacryocyst + G. *algos*, pain]

dac·ry·o·cys·tec·to·my (dak'rē-ō-sis-tek'tō-mē). Surgical removal of the lacrimal sac. [dacryocyst + G. *ektomē*, excision]

dac·ry·o·cys·to·cele (dak'rē-ō-sis'tō-sēl). Enlargement of the lacrimal sac with fluid. SYN dacryocele. [dacryocyst + G. *kēlē*, hernia]

dac·ry·o·cys·tog·ra·phy (DCG) (dak'rē-ō-sis-tog'ra-fē). Radiography of the lacrimal drainage system by introduction of a contrast agent. [dacryocyst + -o- + G. *graphō*, to scratch, to write]

dac·ry·o·cys·to·rhi·nos·to·my (dak'rē-ō-sis'tō-rī-nos'tō-mē). An operation providing an anastomosis between the lacrimal sac and the nasal mucosa through an opening in the lacrimal bone. [dacryocyst + G. *rhis* (rhin-), nose, + *stoma*, mouth]

dac·ry·o·cys·tot·o·my (dak'rē-ō-sis-tot'ō-mē). Incision of the lacrimal sac. [dacryocyst + G. *tomē*, incision]

dacryocyte (dăk'rē-ō-sīt). An abnormally shaped red cell with a single point or elongation; also called a teardrop. This form of poikilocyte is associated with myelofibrosis with myeloid metaplasia. SYN teardrop cell. [dacryo- + -cyte]

dac·ry·o·hem·or·rhea (dak'rē-ō-hem-ō-rē'ă). Bloody tears. [dacryo- + G. *haima*, blood, + *rhoia*, flow]

dac·ry·o·lith (dak'rē-ō-lith). A concretion in the lacrimal apparatus. SYN ophthalmolith, tear stone. [dacryo- + G. *lithos*, stone]

dac·ry·o·li·thi·a·sis (dak'rē-ō-li-thī'ă-sis). The formation and presence of dacryoliths.

dac·ry·ops (dak'rē-ops). **1.** Excess of tears in the eye. **2.** A cyst of a duct of the lacrimal gland. [dacryo- + G. *ōps*, eye]

dac·ry·o·py·or·rhea (dak'rē-ō-pī-ō-rē'ă). The discharge of tears containing leukocytes. [dacryo- + G. *pyon*, pus, + *rhoia*, flow]

dac·ry·or·rhea (dak'rē-ō-rē'ă). An excessive secretion of tears. [dacryo- + G. *rhoia*, flow]

dac·ry·o·ste·no·sis (dak'rē-ō-ste-nō'sis). Stricture of a lacrimal or nasal duct. [dacryo- + G. *stenōsis*, narrowing]

dac·tyl (dak'til). SYN digit. [G. *daktylos*]

Ⓒdactyl-. SEE dactylo-.

dac·ty·li·tis (dak-ti-lī'tis). Inflammation of one or more fingers.

   blistering distal d., infection of the volar fat pad of the distal phalanx of the finger by group A β-hemolytic streptococci.

Ⓒdactylo-, dactyl-. The fingers, and (less often) toes. See entries under digit. [G. *daktylos*, finger]

dac·ty·lo·camp·sis (dak'ti-lō-kamp'sis). Permanent flexion of the fingers. [dactylo- + G. *kampsis*, bending]

dac·ty·lo·gry·po·sis (dak'ti-lō-gri-pō'sis). Permanent curvature or deformity of the fingers. [dactylo- + G. *grypōsis*, a crooking]

dac·tyl·o·meg·a·ly (dak'til-ō-meg'ă-lē). SYN megadactyly. [dactylo- + G. *megas*, large]

dac·ty·lus, pl. **dac·ty·li** (dak'ti-lŭs, -lī). SYN digit. [G. *daktylos*]

Dalton, John, English chemist, mathematician, and natural philosopher, 1766–1844. SEE D.'s *law.*

dal·ton (Da) (dawl'tŏn). Term unofficially used to indicate a unit of mass equal to $^1/_{12}$ the mass of a carbon-12 atom, 1.0000 in the atomic mass scale; numerically, but not dimensionally, equal to molecular or particle weight (atomic mass units). [J. *Dalton*]

dam. **1.** Any barrier to the flow of fluid. **2.** SURGERY, DENTISTRY A sheet of thin rubber arranged so as to shut off the part operated upon from the access of fluid. [A.S. *fordemman*, to stop up]

dAMP deoxyadenylic acid.

damp. **1.** Humid; moist. **2.** Atmospheric moisture. **3.** Foul air in a mine; air charged with carbon oxides (black or choke d.) or with various explosive hydrocarbon vapors (firedamp).

dan·der. **1.** A fine scaling of the skin and scalp. SEE ALSO dandruff. **2.** A normal effluvium of animal hair or coat capable of causing allergic responses in atopic persons.

dan·druff (dan'drŭf). The presence, in varying amounts, of white or gray scales in the hair of the scalp, due to exfoliation of the epidermis. SEE ALSO seborrheic *dermatitis.* SYN scurf, seborrhea sicca (2).

DANS 1-dimethylaminonaphthalene-5-sulfonic acid; a green fluorescing compound used in immunohistochemistry to detect antigens.

dan·syl (Dns, DNS) (dan'sil). The 5-dimethylaminonaphthalene-1-sulfonyl radical; a blocking agent for NH_2 groups, used in peptide synthesis.

Darrow red. A basic oxazin dye, $C_{18}H_{14}N_3O_2Cl$,

used as a substitute for cresyl violet acetate in the staining of Nissl substance. [Mary A. *Darrow,* U.S. stain technologist, 1894–1973]

dar·win·i·an (dar-win'ē-an). Relating to or ascribed to Darwin.

DAS developmental *apraxia* of speech.

da·ta. Facts (usually established by observation, measurement, or experiment) used as a basis for inference, testing, models, etc. The word is plural and takes a plural verb.

data dictionary, standardized set of definitions of all data elements collected in a given health care facility.

da·tum (dā'tŭm). An individual piece of information used in a scholarly field. [L., *given,* fr. *do,* pp. *datum,* to give]

dau·no·ru·bi·cin (daw'nō-roo'bĭ-sin). SYN rubidomycin.

dB, db decibel.

DC direct *current.*

D & C dilation and curettage.

DCG (dac·ry·o·cys·tog·ra·phy). dacryocystography.

dCMP deoxycytidylic acid.

D & E dilation and evacuation.

◁**de-.** **1.** Away from, cessation, without; sometimes has an intensive force. **2.** For names with this prefix not found here, see under the principal part of the name. [L. *de,* from, away]

de·ac·yl·ase (dē-as'il-ās). **1.** A member of the subclass of hydrolases (EC class 3), especially of that subclass of esterases, lipases, lactonases, and hydrolases (EC subclass 3.1). **2.** Any enzyme catalyzing the hydrolytic cleavage of an acyl group (R-CO-) in an ester linkage; also includes enzymes cleaving amide linkages (EC subclass 3.5) and similar acyl compounds.

deaf (def). Unable to hear; hearing indistinctly; hard of hearing. [A.S. *deáf*]

de·af·fer·en·ta·tion (dē-af'er-en-tā'shŭn). A loss of the sensory input from a portion of the body, usually caused by interruption of the peripheral sensory fibers. [L. *de,* from, + afferent]

deaf·mut·ism (def-myū'tizm). Inability to speak, due to congenital or early acquired profound deafness.

deaf·ness (def'nes). General term for loss of the ability to hear, without designation of the degree or cause of the loss.

  acoustic trauma d., sensorineural hearing loss due to overexposure to high intensity noise.

  Alexander's d. [MIM*203500], high frequency d. due to membranous cochlear dysplasia.

  central d., d. due to disorder of the auditory system of the brainstem or cerebral cortex.

  conductive d., hearing impairment caused by interference with sound or transmission through the external canal, middle ear, or ossicles.

  cortical d., d. resulting from bilateral lesions of the primary receptive area of the temporal lobe.

  functional d., SYN psychogenic d.

  psychogenic d., hearing loss without evidence of organic cause or malingering; often follows severe psychic shock. SYN functional d.

  sensorineural d., hearing impairment due to disorders of the cochlear division of the 9th cranial nerve (auditory nerve), the cochlea, or the

retrocochlear nerve tracts, as opposed to conductive d.

de·al·co·hol·i·za·tion (dē-al'kō-hol-i-zā'shun). The removal of alcohol from a fluid; in histologic technique, the removal of alcohol from a specimen that has been previously immersed in this fluid.

de·am·i·das·es (dē-am'i-dā-sez). SYN amidohydrolases.

de·am·i·da·tion, de·am·i·di·za·tion (dē-am-i-dā'shun, dē-am'i-di-zā'shun). The hydrolytic removal of an amide group.

de·am·i·nas·es (dē-am'i-nā-sez) [EC group 3.5.4]. Enzymes catalyzing simple hydrolysis of C—NH_2 bonds of purines, pyrimidines, and pterins. SYN deaminating enzymes.

de·am·i·na·tion, de·am·i·ni·za·tion (dē-am-i-nā'shun, dē-am'i-ni-zā'shun). Removal, usually by hydrolysis, of the NH_2 group from an amino compound.

de·ar·te·ri·al·i·za·tion (dē-ar-tēr'ē-ăl-i-zā'shun). Changing the character of arterial blood to that of venous blood; *i.e.,* deoxygenation of blood.

death (deth). The cessation of life. In higher organisms, a cessation of integrated tissue and organ functions; in humans, manifested by the loss of heartbeat, the absence of spontaneous breathing, and cerebral d. SYN mors. [A.S. *dēath*]

  black d., term applied to the worldwide epidemic of the 14th century, of which some 60 million persons are said to have died; the descriptions indicate that it was pneumonic plague.

  cerebral d., a clinical syndrome characterized by the permanent loss of cerebral and brain stem function, manifested by absence of responsiveness to external stimuli, absence of cephalic reflexes, and apnea. An isoelectric electroencephalogram for at least 30 minutes in the absence of hypothermia and poisoning by central nervous system depressants supports the diagnosis.

  crib d., SYN sudden infant death *syndrome.*

  fetal d., d. prior to the complete expulsion or extraction from the mother of a product of conception, irrespective of the duration of pregnancy. Fetal death is considered *early* if it takes place in the first 20 weeks of gestation; *middle* (intermediate) if it takes place from 21 to 28 weeks of gestation, and *late* if it takes place after 28 weeks.

  local d., d. of a part of the body or of a tissue by necrosis.

  somatic d., systemic d., d. of the entire body, as distinguished from local d.

  sudden d., **(1)** an arrhythmogenic d. in aortic stenosis, coronary disease, mesothelioma of the AV node, or single coronary artery. **(2)** unexpected d. occurring within one hour of onset of symptoms; most often used to describe death caused by cardiac failure. SEE ALSO hypertrophic *cardiomyopathy.*

de·band·ing (dē-band'ing). The removal of fixed orthodontic appliances.

de·bil·i·tat·ing (dĕ-bil'i-tāt-ing). Denoting or characteristic of a morbid process that causes weakness.

debt (det). A deficit; a liability. [L. *debitum,* debt]

  oxygen d., the extra oxygen, taken in by the

body during recovery from exercise, beyond the resting needs of the body; sometimes used as if synonymous with oxygen deficit.

⚠**deca- (da).** Prefix used in the SI and metric systems to signify 10. Also spelled deka-. [G. *deka,* ten]

de·cal·ci·fi·ca·tion (dē′kal-si-fi-kā′shŭn). **1.** Removal of calcium salts from bones and teeth, either *in vitro* or as a result of a pathologic process. **2.** Precipitation of calcium from blood as by oxalate or fluoride, or the conversion of blood calcium to an un-ionized form as by citrate, thus preventing or delaying coagulation. [L. *de-,* away, + *calx* (*calc-*), lime, + *facio,* to make]

de·cal·ci·fy·ing (dē-kal′si-fī-ing). Denoting an agent, measure, or process that causes decalcification.

de·ca·pac·i·ta·tion (dē′kă-pas-i-tā′shŭn). Prevention of spermatozoa from undergoing capacitation and thus from becoming able to fertilize ova.

de·cap·i·ta·tion (dē-kap-i-tā′shŭn). Removal of a head.

de·cap·su·la·tion (dē-kap-sū-lā′shŭn). Incision and removal of a capsule or enveloping membrane.

de·car·box·yl·ase (dē-kar-boks′ē-lās). Any enzyme (EC subclass 4.1.1) that removes a molecule of carbon dioxide from a carboxylic group.

de·car·box·yl·a·tion (dē′kar-boks-ē-lā′shŭn). A reaction involving the removal of a molecule of carbon dioxide from a carboxylic acid.

de·cay (dē-kā′). **1.** Destruction of an organic substance by slow combustion or gradual oxidation. **2.** SYN putrefaction. **3.** To deteriorate; to undergo slow combustion or putrefaction. **4.** DENTISTRY caries. **5.** PSYCHOLOGY Loss of information registered by the senses and processed into short-term memory. SEE ALSO memory. **6.** Loss of radioactivity with time; spontaneous emission of radiation or charged particles or both from an unstable nucleus. [L. *de,* down, + *cado,* to fall]

   free induction d. (FID), in magnetic resonance imaging, the d. curve that is detected by the radiofrequency coil after the application of an excitation pulse, without additional pulses (free).

de·cer·e·brate (dē-ser′ĕ-brāt). **1.** To cause decerebration. **2.** Denoting an animal so prepared, or a patient whose brain has suffered an injury causing neurologic impairment comparable to that of a decerebrate animal.

de·cer·e·bra·tion (dē-ser′ĕ-brā′shŭn). Removal of the brain above the lower border of the corpora quadrigemina, or a complete section of the brain at this level or somewhat below.

de·cho·les·ter·ol·i·za·tion (dē′kō-les′ter-ol-i-zā′shŭn). Therapeutic reduction of the cholesterol concentration of the blood.

⚠**deci- (d).** Prefix used in the SI and metric system to signify one-tenth (10^-). [L. *decimus,* tenth]

dec·i·bel (dB, db) (des′i-bel). One-tenth of a bel; unit for expressing the relative loudness of sound on a logarithmic scale. [L. *decimus,* tenth, + bel]

de·cid·ua (dē-sid′yū-ă). SYN deciduous *membrane.* [L. *deciduus,* falling off (qualifying *membrana,* membrane, understood)]

   d. basa′lis [NA], the area of endometrium between the implanted chorionic vesicle and the myometrium, which develops into the maternal part of the placenta. SYN d. serotina.

   d. capsula′ris [NA], the layer of endometrium overlying the implanted chorionic vesicle; it becomes progressively attenuated as the chorionic vesicle enlarges and, by the fourth month, is squeezed against the d. parietalis and thereafter undergoes rapid regression. SYN d. reflexa, membrana adventitia (2).

   d. menstrua′lis, the succulent mucous membrane of the nonpregnant uterus at the menstrual period.

   d. parieta′lis [NA], the altered mucous membrane lining the main cavity of the pregnant uterus other than at the site of attachment of the chorionic vesicle. SYN d. vera.

   d. polypo′sa, d. parietalis showing polypoid projections of the endometrial surface.

   d. reflex′a, SYN d. capsularis.

   d. seroti′na, SYN d. basalis.

   d. spongio′sa, the portion of the d. basalis attached to the myometrium.

   d. ve′ra, SYN d. parietalis.

de·cid·u·al (dē-sid′yū-ăl). Relating to the decidua.

de·cid·u·a·tion (dē-sid-yū-ā′shŭn). Shedding of endometrial tissue during menstruation. [L. *deciduus,* falling off]

de·cid·u·i·tis (dē-sid-yū-ī′tis). Inflammation of the decidua.

de·cid·u·o·ma (dē-sid-yū-ō′mă). An intrauterine mass of decidual tissue, probably the result of hyperplasia of decidual cells retained in the uterus. SYN placentoma.

de·cid·u·ous (dē-sid′yū-ŭs). **1.** Not permanent; denoting that which eventually falls off. **2.** DENTISTRY often used to designate the first or primary dentition. SEE deciduous *tooth.* [L. *deciduus,* falling off]

dec·li·na·tion (dek-li-nā′shŭn). A bending, sloping, or other deviation from a normal vertical position. [L. *declinatio,* a bending aside]

de·clive (dē-klīv′) [NA]. The posterior sloping portion of the monticulus of the vermis of the cerebellum; vermal lobule caudal to the primary fissure. SYN declivis. [L. *declivis,* sloping downward, fr. *clivus,* a slope]

de·cli·vis (dē-klī′vis). SYN declive.

de·com·pen·sa·tion (de′kom-pen-sā′shŭn). **1.** A failure of compensation in heart disease. **2.** The appearance or exacerbation of a mental disorder due to failure of defense mechanisms.

de·com·po·si·tion (dē′kom-pō-zish′ŭn). SYN putrefaction.

de·com·pres·sion (dē′kom-presh-ŭn). Removal of pressure. [L. *de-,* from, down, + *com-primo,* pp. *-pressus,* to press together]

   cardiac d., incision into the pericardium or aspiration of fluid from pericardium to relieve pressure due to blood or other fluid in the pericardial sac. SYN pericardial d.

   cerebral d., removal of a piece of the cranium, usually in the subtemporal region, with incision of the dura, to relieve intracranial pressure.

   nerve d., release of pressure on a nerve trunk

by the surgical excision of constricting bands or widening of a bony canal.

   pericardial d., SYN cardiac d.

   spinal d., the removal of pressure upon the spinal cord as created by a tumor, cyst, hematoma, herniated nucleus pulposus, abscess, or bone.

de·con·ges·tant (dē-kon-jes′tant). **1.** SYN decongestive. **2.** An agent that possesses this action.

de·con·ges·tive (dē-kon-jes′tiv). Having the property of reducing congestion. SYN decongestant (1).

de·con·tam·i·na·tion (dē′kon-tam-i-nā′shŭn). Removal or neutralization of poisonous gas or other injurious agents from the environment.

de·cor·ti·ca·tion (dē-kōr-ti-kā′shŭn). **1.** Removal of the cortex, or external layer, beneath the capsule from any organ or structure. **2.** An operation for removal of the clot and scar tissue that form after a hemothorax or neglected empyema. [L. *decortico,* pp. *-atus,* to deprive of bark, fr. *de,* from, + *cortex,* rind, bark]

de·cru·des·cence (dē-krū-des′ens). Abatement of the symptoms of disease. [L. *de,* from, + *crudesco,* to become worse, fr. *crudus,* crude]

de·cu·bi·tal (dē-kyū′bi-tăl). Relating to a decubitus ulcer.

de·cu·bi·tus (dē-kyū′bi-tŭs). **1.** The position of the patient in bed; *e.g.,* dorsal d., lateral d. SEE ALSO decubitus *film.* **2.** Sometimes used in referring to a decubitus ulcer. [L. *decumbo,* to lie down]

de·cus·sate (dē′kŭ-sāt, dē-kŭs′āt). **1.** To cross. **2.** Crossed like the arms of an X. [L. *decusso,* pp. *-atus,* to make in the form of an X, fr. *decussis,* a large, bronze Roman coin marked with an X to indicate its denomination]

de·cus·sa·tio, pl. **de·cus·sa·ti·o·nes** (dē-kŭ-sā′shē-ō, -ō′nēz) [NA]. **1.** In general, any crossing over or intersection of parts. **2.** The intercrossing of two homonymous fiber bundles as each crosses over to the opposite side of the brain in the course of its ascent or descent through the brainstem or spinal cord. SYN decussation. [L. (see decussate)]

   d. lemnisco′rum [NA], SYN *decussation* of medial lemniscus.

   d. pyram′idum [NA], SYN pyramidal *decussation.*

   decussatio′nes tegmen′ti [NA], SYN tegmental *decussations,* under *decussation.*

de·cus·sa·tion (dē-kŭ-sā′shŭn). SYN decussatio. [L. *decussatio*]

   Forel's d., SEE tegmental d.'s (2).

   fountain d., SEE tegmental d.'s (1).

   d. of medial lemniscus, the intercrossing of the fibers of the left and right medial lemniscus ascending from the gracile and cuneate nuclei, immediately rostral to the level of the decussation of the pyramidal tracts in the medulla oblongata. SYN decussatio lemniscorum [NA].

   Meynert's d., SEE tegmental d.'s (1).

   motor d., SYN pyramidal d.

   optic d., SYN optic *chiasm.*

   pyramidal d., the intercrossing of the bundles of the pyramidal tracts at the lower border region

of the medulla oblongata. SYN decussatio pyramidum [NA], motor d.

   rubrospinal d., SEE tegmental d.'s (2).

   d. of superior cerebellar peduncles, the decussation of the left and right superior cerebellar peduncles in the tegmentum of the caudal mesencephalon.

   tegmental d.'s, (1) the dorsal tegmental decussation (fountain or Meynert's decussation, d. fontinalis) of the left and right tectospinal and tectobulbar tracts; **(2)** the ventral tegmental d. (rubrospinal or Forel's d.) of the left and right rubrospinal and rubrobulbar tracts; both are located in the mesencephalon. SYN decussationes tegmenti [NA].

de·dif·fer·en·ti·a·tion (dē-dif′er-en-shē-ā′shŭn). **1.** The return of parts to a more homogeneous state. **2.** SYN anaplasia.

de·duc·tion (dē-duk′shun). The logical derivation of a conclusion from certain premises. The conclusion will be true if the premises are true and the deductive argument is valid. Cf. induction (9).

de·ep·i·car·di·al·i·za·tion (dē-ep-i-kar′dē-al-i-zā′shŭn). Surgical destruction of the epicardium, usually by the application of phenol, designed to promote collateral circulation to the myocardium.

def, DEF decayed, extracted, or filled tooth.

def·e·cate (def′ě-kāt). To perform defecation.

def·e·ca·tion (def-ě-kā′shŭn). The discharge of feces from the rectum. SYN movement (3). [L. *defaeco,* pp. *-atus,* to remove the dregs, purify]

de·fec·og·ra·phy (de-fě-kog′ră-fē). Radiographic examination of the act of defecation of a radiopaque stool. [defecation + G. *graphō,* to write]

de·fect (dē′fekt). An imperfection, malformation, dysfunction, or absence; an attribute of quality, in contrast with deficiency, which is an attribute of quantity. [L. *deficio,* pp. *-fectus,* to fail, to lack]

   atrial septal d., a congenital d. in the interatrial septum between the atria of the heart, due to failure of the foramen primum or secundum to close normally.

   congenital ectodermal d., incomplete development of the epidermis and skin appendages; the skin is smooth and hairless, the facies abnormal, and the teeth and nails may be affected; sweating may be deficient. SYN congenital ectodermal dysplasia.

   fibrous cortical d., a common 1 to 3 cm d. in the cortex of a bone, most commonly the lower femoral shaft of a child, filled with fibrous tissue. Nonosteogenic or nonossifying fibroma by convention refers to lesions greater than 3 cm in diameter. SYN nonosteogenic fibroma.

   filling d., displacement of contrast medium by a space-occupying lesion in a radiographic study of a contrast-filled hollow viscus, such as a polyp on a barium enema; also applied to defects in the otherwise uniform distribution of radionuclide in an organ, such as a metastasis in the liver on a ^{99m}Tc-sulfur colloid scan.

   obstructive ventilatory d., slowing of airflow during forced ventilatory maneuvers, generally expiratory.

   restrictive ventilatory d., reduction in lung

volumes not explainable by obstruction of the airways. It is most commonly characterized physiologically by a reduction in total lung capacity (TLC).

ventricular septal d., a congenital d. in the septum between the cardiac ventricles, usually resulting from failure of the spiral septum to close the interventricular foramen.

de·fec·tive (dē-fek′tiv). Denoting or exhibiting a defect; imperfect; a failure of quality.

de·fense (dē-fens′). The psychological mechanisms used to control anxiety, *e.g.,* rationalization, projection. [L. *defendo,* to ward off]

ur-d.'s, SEE ur-defenses. [Ger. *ur-*, primitive, earliest, + defenses]

de·fen·sins (dē-fen′sinz). A class of basic antibiotic peptides, found in neutrophils, that apparently kill bacteria by causing membrane damage. [L. *de-fendo,* pp. *de-fensum,* to repel, avert, + -in]

defensiveness (dē-fen′-siv-nes). Excessive reaction to sensory stimuli.

auditory d., excessive reaction to sound (*e.g.,* because of its volume or novelty).

oral d., overreaction to the tastes or textures of things placed in one's mouth.

tactile d., a sensory integrative dysfunction resulting in excessive reactions to tactile stimulation.

def·er·ent (def′er-ent). Carrying away. [L. *deferens,* pres. p. of *defero,* to carry away]

def·er·en·tec·to·my (def′er-en-tek′tō-mē). SYN vasectomy. [(ductus) deferens, + G. *ektomē,* excision]

def·er·en·tial (def-er-en′shăl). Relating to the ductus deferens.

def·er·en·ti·tis (def′er-en-tī′tis). Inflammation of the ductus deferens. SYN vasitis.

de·fer·ves·cence (def-er-ves′ens). Falling of an elevated temperature; abatement of fever. [L. *defervesco,* to cease boiling, fr. *de-* neg. + *fervesco,* to begin to boil]

de·fi·bril·la·tion (dē-fib-ri-lā′shŭn). The arrest of fibrillation of the cardiac muscle (atrial or ventricular) with restoration of the normal rhythm.

de·fi·bril·la·tor (dē-fib′ri-lā-ter). **1.** Any agent or measure, *e.g.,* an electric shock, that arrests fibrillation of the ventricular muscle and restores the normal beat. **2.** The machine designed to administer a defibrillating electric shock.

de·fi·bri·na·tion (dē-fī-bri-nā′shŭn). Removal of fibrin from the blood, usually by means of constant agitation while the blood is collected in a container with glass beads or chips.

de·fi·cien·cy (dē-fish′en-sē). An insufficient quantity of some substance (as in dietary d., hemoglobin d. as in marrow aplasia), organization (as in mental d.), activity (as in enzyme d. or reduced oxygen-carrying capacity of the blood), etc., of which the amount present is of normal quality. SEE ALSO deficiency *disease.* [L. *deficio,* to fail, fr. *facio,* to do]

adult lactase d., onset of lactase d., with resulting milk intolerance and malabsorption, in adulthood. Inherited forms may not be manifested until adulthood; any process that damages the intestinal lining cells can cause lactase d. in adults.

antitrypsin d., d. of α_1-antitrypsin, a glycopro-

tein of human serum. The severe form is often associated with familial emphysema or hepatic cirrhosis.

glucose-6-phosphate dehydrogenase d., congenital d. of glucose-6-phosphate dehydrogenase, an enzyme important for maintaining cellular concentrations of reduced nucleotides. It can cause a variety of anemias including favism, primaquine sensitivity and other drug sensitivity anemias, anemia of the newborn, and chronic nonspherocytic hemolytic anemia.

β-*d*-glucuronidase d., a rare d. of β-*d*-glucuronidase; an autosomal recessive disorder with several allelic forms, characterized by abnormal mucopolysaccharide metabolism leading to progressive mental deterioration, splenic and hepatic enlargement, and dysostosis multiplex.

LCAT d., a rare condition characterized by corneal opacities, hemolytic anemia, proteinuria, renal insufficiency, and premature atherosclerosis, and very low levels of lecithin cholesterol acyltransferase (LCAT) activity; results in accumulation of unesterfied cholesterol in plasma and tissues.

leukocyte adhesion d. (LAD), an inherited disorder in which there is a defective CD18 adherence complex that disturbs d. chemotaxis. It is characterized by recurrent bacterial infections and impaired wound healing.

def·i·cit (def′i-sit). The result of consuming or losing something faster than it is being replenished or replaced. [L. *deficio,* to fail]

base d., a decrease in the total concentration of blood buffer base, indicative of metabolic acidosis or compensated respiratory alkalosis.

oxygen d., the difference between oxygen uptake of the body during early stages of exercise and during a similar duration in a steady state of exercise; sometimes considered as the formation of the oxygen debt.

pulse d., (1) the absence of palpable pulse waves in a peripheral artery for one or more heart beats, as is often seen in atrial fibrillation; **(2)** the number of such missing pulse waves (usually expressed as heart rate minus pulse rate per minute).

de·flec·tion (dē-flek′shŭn). **1.** A moving to one side. **2.** In the electrocardiogram, a deviation of the curve from the isoelectric base line; any wave or complex of the electrocardiogram. [L. *deflecto,* pp. *-flexus,* to bend aside]

de·flex·ion (dē′fleks-shŭn). Term used to describe the position of the fetal head in relation to the maternal pelvis in which the head is descending in a nonflexed or extended attitude. [de- + L. *flexio,* a bending, fr. *flecto,* pp. *flexum,* to bend]

de·flu·vi·um (dē-flū′vē-ŭm). SYN defluxion. [L., fr. *de-fluo,* pp. *-fluxus,* to flow down]

de·flux·ion (dē-flŭk′shŭn). **1.** A falling down or out, as of the hair. SEE ALSO effluvium. **2.** A flowing down or discharge of fluid. SYN defluvium. [L. *defluxio, de-fluo,* pp. *-fluxus,* to flow down]

de·for·ma·tion (dē-fōr-mā′shŭn). **1.** Deviation of form from the normal; specifically, an alteration in shape and/or structure of a previously normally formed part. It occurs after organogenesis and often involves the musculoskeletal system (*e.g.*, clubfoot). **2.** SYN deformity. **3.** RHEOLOGY The change in the physical shape of a mass by applied stress. [L. *de-formo,* pp. *-atus,* to deform, fr. *forma,* form]

de•for•mi•ty (dē-fōr′mi-tē). A permanent structural deviation from the normal shape or size, resulting in disfigurement; may be congenital or acquired. SYN deformation (2).

    Akerlund d., indentation (incisura) with niche of duodenal cap as seen radiologically.

    boutonnière d. (bū-tawn-yār′), rupture of the central slip of a digital extensor tendon at the middle phalanx, marked by extension of the metacarpopophalangeal and distal interphalangeal joints and flexion of the proximal interphalangeal joint. [Fr., buttonhole]

    gunstock d., a form of cubitus varus resulting from condylar fracture at the elbow in which the axis of the extended forearm is not continuous with that of the arm but is displaced toward midline.

    Madelung's d., a distal radioulnar subluxation due to a relative deficiency of axial growth of the medial side of the distal radius, which, as a consequence, is abnormally inclined proximally and ulnarwards.

    reduction d., congenital absence or attenuation of one or more body parts; usually of the limbs or limb components.

    silver-fork d., the d. resembling the curve of the back of a fork seen in Colles' fractures.

    torsional d., ORTHOPEDICS a d. caused by rotation of a portion of an extremity with relationship to the long axis of the entire extremity.

de•gen•er•ate. **1** (dē-jen′er-āt). To pass to a lower level of mental, physical, or moral state; to fall below the normal or acceptable type or state. **2** (dē-jen′ĕ-răt). Below the normal or acceptable; that which has passed to a lower level.

de•gen•er•a•tion (dē-jen-er-ā′shŭn). **1.** Degeneration; passing from a higher to a lower level or type. **2.** A worsening of mental, physical, or moral qualities. **3.** A retrogressive pathologic change in cells or tissues, in consequence of which their functions often are impaired or destroyed; sometimes reversible. [L. *degeneratio*]

    adipose d., SYN fatty d.

    amyloid d., infiltration of amyloid between cells and fibers of tissues and organs. SYN waxy d. (1).

    ascending d., (1) retrograde d. of an injured nerve fiber; *i.e.,* toward the nerve cell of the fiber; **(2)** d. cephalad to a spinal cord lesion.

    atheromatous d., focal accumulation of lipid material (atheroma) in the intima and subintimal portion of arteries, eventually resulting in fibrous thickening or calcification.

    calcareous d., in a precise sense, not a degenerative process *per se,* but the deposition of insoluble calcium salts in tissue that has degenerated and become necrotic, as in dystrophic calcification.

    caseous d., SYN caseous *necrosis.*

    colloid d., a d. similar to mucoid d., in which the material is inspissated.

    descending d., (1) orthograde (wallerian) d. of

an injured nerve fiber; *i.e.,* distal to the lesion; **(2)** d. caudal to the level of a spinal cord lesion.

    disciform d., subretinal neovascularization with retinal separation and hemorrhage leading finally to a circular mass of fibrous tissue with marked loss of visual acuity.

    elastoid d., (1) SYN elastosis (2). **(2)** hyaline d. of the elastic tissue of the arterial wall, seen during involution of the uterus.

    elastotic d., SYN elastosis (2).

    familial pseudoinflammatory macular d. [MIM*136900], macular d. that occurs during the fifth decade of life, with sudden development of a central scotoma in one eye followed rapidly by a similar lesion in the opposite eye.

    fascicular d., muscular d. due to loss of motor neurons in the spinal cord or brainstem.

    fatty d., abnormal formation of microscopically visible droplets of fat in the cytoplasm of cells, as a result of injury. SYN adipose d., steatosis (2).

    fibrinoid d., fibrinous d., a process resulting in acidophilic refractile deposits with staining reactions that resemble fibrin, occurring in connective tissue, blood vessel walls, and other sites.

    fibrous d., not a d. *per se,* but rather a reparative process; cells and foci of tissue previously affected with degenerative processes, and necrosis, are replaced by cellular fibrous tissue.

    gray d., d. of the white substance of the spinal cord, the fibers of which lose their myelin sheaths and become darker in color.

    hepatolenticular d., (1) a familial disorder characterized by copper deposition in the liver, causing chronic hepatitis and eventually cirrhosis; d. of the lenticular (pallidal and putaminal) nuclei, and marked hyperplasia of astrocytes in the cerebral cortex, cerebellum, basal ganglia, and brainstem nuclei; plasma levels of ceruloplasmins and copper are decreased, urinary excretion of copper is increased, and the amounts of copper in the liver, brain, and kidneys is high; clinical features include deposition of golden brown pigment in the cornea (Kayser-Fleischer rings), dysphasia and dysarthria, rigidity, and a coarse resting tremor, which increases when the limbs are outstretched ("wing-beating" tremor). **(2)** SYN Wilson's *disease* (1).

    hyaline d., a group of degenerative processes that affect various cells and tissues, resulting in rounded masses ("droplets") or broad bands of substances that are homogeneous, translucent, refractile, and acidophilic; may occur in the collagen of old fibrous tissue, smooth muscle of arterioles or the uterus, and as droplets in parenchymal cells. SYN hyalinosis.

    hydropic d., SYN cloudy *swelling.*

    mucoid d., a conversion of any of the connective tissues into a gelatinous or mucoid substance. SYN myxomatosis (1).

    orthograde d., SYN wallerian d.

    parenchymatous d., SYN cloudy *swelling.*

    reticular d., severe epidermal edema resulting in multilocular bullae.

    secondary d., SYN wallerian d.

    subacute combined d. of the spinal cord, a disorder of the spinal cord, such as that occurring in vitamin B_{12} deficiency, characterized by glio-

de

sis with spongiform degeneration of the posterior and lateral columns. SYN Putnam-Dana syndrome, vitamin B_{12} neuropathy.

transsynaptic d., an atrophy of nerve cells following damage to the axons that make synaptic connection with them; noted especially in the lateral geniculate body.

wallerian d., the degenerative changes observed in the distal segment of a peripheral nerve fiber (axon and myelin) when its continuity with its cell body is interrupted by a focal lesion. SYN orthograde d., secondary d.

waxy d., (1) SYN amyloid d. (2) SYN Zenker's d.

Zenker's d., a form of severe hyaline d. or necrosis in skeletal muscle, occurring in severe infections. SYN waxy d. (2).

de·gen·er·a·tive (dē-jen′er-ă-tiv). Relating to degeneration.

de·glov·ing (dē-glov′ing). **1.** Intraoral surgical exposure of the anterior mandible used in various orthognathic surgical operations such as genioplasty or mandibular alveolar surgery. **2.** SEE degloving injury.

de·glu·ti·tion (dē-glū-tish′ŭn). The act of swallowing. [L. de-glutio, to swallow]

deg·ra·da·tion (deg-ră-dā′shŭn). The change of a chemical compound into a less complex compound. [L. degradatus, degrade]

de·gree (dĕ-grē′). **1.** One of the divisions on the scale of a measuring instrument such as a thermometer, barometer, etc. See Comparative Temperature Scales appendix. SEE scale. **2.** The 360th part of the circumference of a circle. **3.** A position or rank within a graded series. **4.** A measure of damage to tissue. [Fr. degré; L. gradus, a step]

de·gus·ta·tion (dē-gŭs-tā′shŭn). **1.** The act of tasting. **2.** The sense of taste. [L. degustatio, fr. de-gusto, pp. -atus, to taste]

de·his·cence (dē-his′ens). A bursting open, splitting, or gaping along natural or sutured lines. [L. dehisco, to split apart or open]

de·hy·drase (dē-hī′drās). Former name for dehydratase.

de·hy·dra·tase (dē-hī′dră-tās). A subclass (EC 4.2.1) of lyases (hydro-lyases) that remove H and OH as H_2O from a substrate, leaving a double bond, or add a group to a double bond by the elimination of water from two substances to form a third.

de·hy·dra·tion (dē-hī-drā′shŭn). **1.** Deprivation of water. SYN anhydration. **2.** Reduction of water content. **3.** SYN exsiccation (2). **4.** SYN desiccation.

△**dehydro-.** Prefix used in the names of chemical compounds that differ from more familiar compounds in the absence of two hydrogen atoms; e.g., dehydroascorbic acid, which resembles ascorbic acid in all structural features except for its lack of two hydrogen atoms that are present in the ascorbic acid molecule. In systematic nomenclature, didehydro- is preferred as being more exact.

11-de·hy·dro·cor·ti·co·ster·one (dē-hī′drō-kōr-ti-kos′ter-ōn). A metabolite of corticosterone, found in the adrenal cortex.

de·hy·dro·gen·ase (dē-hī′drō-jen-ās). Class

name for those enzymes that oxidize substrates by catalyzing removal of hydrogen from metabolites (hydrogen donors) and transferring it to other substances (hydrogen acceptors).

de·hy·dro·gen·a·tion (dē-hī′drō-jen-ā′shŭn). Removal of a pair of hydrogen atoms from a compound by the action of enzymes (dehydrogenases) or other catalysts.

de·in·sti·tu·tion·al·i·za·tion (dē′in-sti-tū′shŭn-ăl-i-zā-shŭn). The discharge of institutionalized patients from a mental hospital into treatment programs in half-way houses and other community-based programs.

de·jec·tion (dē-jek′shŭn). **1.** SYN depression (4). **2.** The discharge of excrementitious matter. **3.** The matter so discharged. [L. dejectio, fr. dejicio, pp. -jectus, to cast down]

△**deka-.** SEE deca-.

de·lam·i·na·tion (dē-lam-i-nā′shŭn). Division into separate layers. [L. de, from, + lamina, a thin plate]

delayed onset muscle soreness (DOMS). residual muscle d. o. m. s. that appears within 24 hours and may last for several days following unaccustomed heavy muscular activity, particularly with eccentric muscle actions; related to actual muscle cell damage.

de-lead (dē-led′). To cause the mobilization and excretion of lead deposited in the bones and other tissues, as by the administration of a chelating agent.

del·e·te·ri·ous (del-ĕ-tēr′ē-ŭs). Injurious; noxious; harmful. [G. dēlētērios, fr. dēleomai, to injure]

de·le·tion (dĕ-lē′shŭn). In genetics, any spontaneous elimination of part of the normal genetic complement, whether cytogenetically visible (chromosomal d.) or inferred from phenotypic evidence (point d.). [L. deletio, destruction]

chromosomal d., a microscopically evident loss of part of a chromosome. SEE ALSO monosomy.

del·i·ques·cence (del-i-kwes′ens). Becoming damp or liquid by absorption of water from the atmosphere; a property of certain salts, such as $CaCl_2$. [L. de-liquesco, to melt or become liquid]

de·li·ria (dē-lir′ē-ă). Plural of delirium.

de·lir·i·ous (dē-lir′ē-ŭs). In a state of delirium.

de·lir·i·um, pl. **de·li·ria** (dē-lir′ē-ŭm, dē-lir′ē-ă). An altered state of consciousness, consisting of confusion, distractibility, disorientation, disordered thinking and memory, defective perception (illusions and hallucinations), prominent hyperactivity, agitation and autonomic nervous system overactivity; caused by a number of toxic structural and metabolic disorders. [L. fr. deliro, to be crazy, fr. de- + lira, a furrow (i.e., go out of the furrow)]

posttraumatic d., d. caused by a structural traumatic brain injury.

d. tre′mens (DT), a severe, sometimes fatal, form of d. due to alcoholic withdrawal following a period of sustained intoxication. [L. pres. p. of tremo, to tremble]

de·liv·er (dē-liv′er). **1.** To assist a woman in childbirth. **2.** To extract from an enclosed place, as the fetus from the womb, an object or foreign body, *e.g.,* a tumor from its capsule or surroundings, or the lens of the eye in cases of cataract. [fr. O. Fr. fr. L. *de-* + *liber,* free]

de·liv·ery (dē-liv′er-ē). Passage of the fetus and the placenta from the genital canal into the external world.

   forceps d., assisted birth of the child by an instrument designed to grasp the fetal head.

   outlet forceps d., d. by forceps applied to the fetal head when it has reached the perineal floor and is visible between contractions.

   postmortem d., extraction of the fetus after the death of its mother.

   premature d., birth of a fetus before its proper time. SEE ALSO premature *birth.*

del·le (del′eh). The central lighter-colored portion of the erythrocyte, as observed in a stained film of blood. [Ger. *Delle,* low ground, pit]

del·len (del′en). Shallow, saucer-like, clearly defined excavations at the margin of the cornea, about 1.5 by 2 mm, due to localized dehydration; also called Fuchs' dellen. [Ger. pl. of *Delle,* low ground, pit]

delta (Δ, δ) (del′tă). **1.** Fourth letter of the Greek alphabet. **2.** CHEMISTRY A double bond, usually with a superscript to indicate position in a chain (Δ^5); application of heat in a reaction ($A \xrightarrow{\Delta} B$); absence of heat treatment ($\overset{\triangle}{\triangle}$); distance between two atoms in a molecule, or position of a substituent located on the fourth atom from the carboxyl or other primary functional group (δ); change (Δ); thickness (δ); chemical shift in NMR (δ). **3.** ANATOMY a triangular surface.

del·ta check. A comparison of consecutive values for a given test in a patient's laboratory file used to detect abrupt changes, usually generated as a part of computer-based quality control programs.

del·toid (del′toyd). **1.** Resembling the Greek letter delta (Δ); triangular. **2.** SYN deltoid *muscle.* [G. *deltoeidēs,* shaped like the letter *delta*]

de·lu·sion (dē-lū′zhŭn). A false belief or wrong judgment held with conviction despite incontrovertible evidence to the contrary. [L. *de-ludo,* pp. *-lusus,* to play false, deceive, fr. *ludo,* to play]

   d. of grandeur, a d. in which one believes oneself possessed of great wealth, intellect, importance, power, etc.

   d. of negation, a d. in which one imagines that the world and all that relates to it have ceased to exist.

   organic d.'s, false beliefs experienced in the delirium associated with injury to the brain, organic change in the brain such as in Alzheimer's syndrome, or cocaine or other drug intoxication.

   d. of persecution, persecutory d., a false notion that one is being persecuted; characteristic symptom of paranoid schizophrenia.

   somatic d., a d. having reference to a nonexistent lesion or alteration of some organ or part of the body; sometimes indistinguishable from hypochondriasis.

   systematized d., a d. that is logically constructed from a false premise and embraces a specific sector of the patient's life.

   unsystematized d., one of a group of apparently discrete, disconnected d.'s.

de·lu·sion·al (dē-lū′zhŭn-ăl). Relating to a delusion.

de·mat·i·a·ceous (dē-mat-ē-ā′shŭs). Denoting dark conidia and/or hyphae, usually brown or black; used frequently to denote dark-colored fungi.

de·men·tia (dē-men′shē-ă). The loss, usually progressive, of cognitive and intellectual functions, without impairment of perception or consciousness; caused by a variety of disorders, most commonly structural brain disease. Characterized by disorientation, impaired memory, judgment, and intellect, and a shallow labile affect. SYN amentia (2). [L. fr. *de-* priv. + *mens,* mind]

   Alzheimer's d., SYN Alzheimer's *disease.*

   dialysis d., SYN dialysis encephalopathy *syndrome.*

   paralytic d., d. and paralysis resulting from a chronic syphilitic meningoencephalitis.

   posttraumatic d., d. caused by traumatic brain injury.

   presenile d., d. preseni′lis, (1) d. of Alzheimer's disease developing before age 65; **(2)** SYN Alzheimer's *disease.*

   primary d., d. occurring independently as a mental disorder.

   primary senile d., SYN Alzheimer's *disease.*

   secondary d., chronic d. following and due to a psychosis or some other underlying disease process.

   senile d., d. of Alzheimer's disease developing after age 65.

   vascular d., a step-like deterioration in intellectual functions with focal neurological signs, as the result of multiple infarctions of the cerebral hemispheres.

△**demi-.** Half, lesser. SEE ALSO hemi-, semi-. [Fr. fr. L. *dimidius,* half]

dem·i·lune (dem′ē-lūn). **1.** A small body with a form similar to that of a half-moon or a crescent. **2.** The gametocyte of *Plasmodium falciparum.* [Fr. half-moon]

de·min·er·al·i·za·tion (dē-min′er-ăl-ī-zā′shŭn). A loss or decrease of the mineral constituents of the body or individual tissues, especially of bone.

Dem·o·dex (dem′ō-deks). A genus of minute mites that inhabit the skin and are usually found in the sebaceous glands and hair follicles. [G. *dēmos,* tallow, + *dēx,* a woodworm]

de·mog·ra·phy (dē-mog′ră-fē). The study of populations, especially with reference to size, density, fertility, mortality, growth rate, age distribution, migration, and vital statistics. [G. *demos,* people, + *graphō,* to write]

de·mul·cent (de-mŭl′sent). **1.** Soothing; relieving irritation. **2.** An agent, such as a mucilage or oil, that soothes and relieves irritation, especially of the mucous surfaces. [L. *de-mulceo,* pp. *-mulctus,* to stroke lightly, to soften]

de·my·e·li·na·tion, de·my·e·lin·i·za·tion (dē-mī′ĕ-li-nā′shŭn, dē-mī′ĕ-lin-i-za′shŭn). Loss of myelin with preservation of the axons or fiber tracts. Central demyelination occurs within the central nervous system (*e.g.,* the demyelination seen with multiple sclerosis); peripheral demyelination affects the peripheral nervous system (*e.g.,* the demyelination seen with Guillain-Barré syndrome.

de·na·tur·a·tion (dē-na-tyū-rā′shŭn). The process of becoming denatured.

de·na·tured (dē-nā′tyūrd). **1.** Made unnatural or changed from the normal; often applied to proteins or nucleic acids heated or otherwise treated to the point where tertiary structural characteristics are altered. **2.** Adulterated, as by addition of methanol to ethanol.

den·dri·form (den′dri-fōrm). Tree-shaped, or branching. SYN arborescent, dendritic (1), dendroid. [G. *dendron*, tree, + L. *forma*, form]

den·drite (den′drīt). **1.** One of the two types of branching protoplasmic processes of the nerve cell (the other being the axon). SYN dendritic process, dendron, neurodendrite. **2.** A crystalline treelike structure formed during the freezing of an alloy. [G. *dendritēs*, relating to a tree]

den·drit·ic (den-drit′ik). **1.** SYN dendriform. **2.** Relating to the dendrites of nerve cells.

den·droid (den′droyd). SYN dendriform. [G. *dendron*, tree, + *eidos*, appearance]

den·dron. SYN dendrite (1). [G. a tree]

de·ner·vate (dē-ner′vāt). To cause denervation.

de·ner·va·tion (dē-ner-vā′shŭn). Loss of nerve supply.

den·gue (den′gā). A disease of tropical and subtropical regions, caused by dengue virus and transmitted by a mosquito of the genus *Aedes*. Four grades of severity are recognized: grade I, fever and constitutional symptoms; grade II, spontaneous bleeding (of skin, gums, or gastrointestinal tract); grade III, agitation and circulatory failure; grade IV, profound shock. SYN dengue fever, dengue hemorrhagic fever. [Sp. corruption of "dandy" fever]

de·ni·al (dē-nī′ăl). An unconscious defense mechanism used to allay anxiety by denying the existence of important conflicts or troublesome impulses. SYN negation. [M.E., fr, O. Fr., fr. L. *denegare*, to say no]

den·i·da·tion (den-i-dā′shŭn). Exfoliation of the superficial portion of the mucous membrane of the uterus; stripping off of the menstrual decidua. [L. *de*, from, + *nidus*, nest]

dens, pl. **den·tes** (denz, den′tēz) [NA]. **1.** SYN tooth. **2.** A strong toothlike process projecting upward from the body of the axis, or epistropheus, around which the atlas rotates. SYN odontoid process of epistropheus. [L.]

  d. cani′nus, pl. **den′tes cani′ni** [NA], SYN canine *tooth*.

  d. decid′uus, pl. **den′tes deci′dui** [NA], SYN deciduous *tooth*.

  d. in den′te, a developmental disturbance in tooth formation resulting from invagination of the epithelium associated with crown development into the area destined to become pulp space; after calcification there is an invagination of enamel and dentin into the pulp space, giving the radiographic appearance of a "tooth within a tooth."

  d. incisi′vus, pl. **den′tes incisi′vi** [NA], SYN incisor *tooth*.

  d. molaris, pl. **den′tes mola′res** [NA], SYN molar *tooth*. SEE ALSO molar.

  d. per′manens, pl. **den′tes permanen′tes** [NA], SYN permanent *tooth*.

  d. premola′ris, pl. **den′tes premola′res** [NA], SYN premolar *tooth*.

  d. seroti′nus [NA], SYN third *molar*.

den·sim·e·ter (den-sim′ĕ-ter). SYN densitometer (1). [L. *densitas*, density, + G. *metron*, measure]

den·si·tom·e·ter (den-si-tom′ĕ-ter). **1.** An instrument for measuring the density of a fluid. SYN densimeter. **2.** An instrument for measuring, by virtue of relative turbidity, the growth of bacteria in broth; useful in microbiologic assay of nutrients and antibiotics, phage studies, etc. **3.** An instrument for measuring the density of components (*e.g.*, protein fractions) separated by electrophoresis or chromatography, utilizing light absorption or reflection. **4.** An electronic instrument for measuring the blackening of radiographic film by x-ray exposure; used for film sensitometry, bone densitometry, measurement of line spread function (microdensitometer). [L. *densitas*, density, + G. *metron*, measure]

den·si·tom·e·try (den-si-tom′ĕ-trē). A procedure utilizing a densitometer.

den·si·ty (den′si-tē). **1.** The compactness of a substance; the ratio of mass to unit volume, usually expressed as g/cm^3 (kg/m^3 in the SI system). **2.** The quantity of electricity on a given surface or in a given time per unit of volume. **3.** In radiological physics, the opacity to light of an exposed radiographic or photographic film; the darker the film, the greater the measured d. **4.** In clinical radiology, a less-exposed area on a film, corresponding to a region of greater x-ray attenuation (radiopacity) in the subject; the more light transmitted by the film, the greater the d. of the subject; this is not actually the opposite of the prior definition, since one concerns film d. and the other subject d. [L. *densitas*, fr. *densus*, thick]

  optical d. (OD), SYN absorbance.

  radiographic d., the amount of blackening on an x-ray film produced by the interaction of silver halide crystals with developing agents.

  spin d., the number of nuclear dipoles per unit volume.

△**dent-, denti-, dento-.** Teeth; dental. SEE ALSO odonto-. [L. *dens*, tooth]

den·tal (den′tăl). Relating to the teeth. [L. *dens*, tooth]

den·tal·gia (den-tal′jē-ă). SYN toothache. [L. *dens*, tooth, + G. *algos*, pain]

den·tate (den′tāt). Notched; toothed; cogged. [L. *dentatus*, toothed]

den·tes (den′tēz). Plural of dens. [L.]

△**denti-.** SEE dent-.

den·ti·cle (den′ti-kl). **1.** SYN endolith. **2.** A toothlike projection from a hard surface. [L. *denticulus*, a small tooth]

den·ti·frice (den′ti-fris). Any preparation used in the cleansing of the teeth, *e.g.*, a tooth powder, toothpaste, or tooth wash. [L. *dentifricium*, fr. *dens*, tooth, + *frico*, pp. *frictus*, to rub]

den·tig·er·ous (den-tij′er-ŭs). Arising from or associated with teeth, as a d. cyst. [denti- + L. *gero*, to bear]

den·ti·la·bi·al (den′ti-lā′bē-ăl). Relating to the teeth and lips. [denti- + L. *labium*, lip]

den•ti•lin•gual (den-ti-ling′gwăl). Relating to the teeth and tongue. [denti- + L. *lingua,* tongue]

den•tin (den′tin). The ivory forming the mass of the tooth. Calcified tissue that is not as hard as enamel but harder than cementum. About 20% is organic matrix, mostly collagen, with some elastin and a small amount of mucopolysaccharide; the inorganic fraction (70%) is mainly hydroxyapatite, with some carbonate, magnesium, and fluoride. The d. is traversed by a large number of fine tubules running from the pulp cavity outward; within the tubules are processes from the odontoblasts. SYN dentinum [NA]. [L. *dens,* tooth]

   interglobular d., imperfectly calcified matrix of d. situated between the calcified globules near the dentinal periphery.

   irregular d., irritation d., SYN tertiary d.

   opalescent d., d. usually associated with dentinogenesis imperfecta. It gives an unusual opalescent or translucent appearance to the teeth.

   primary d., d. which forms until the root is completed.

   reparative d., SYN tertiary d.

   sclerotic d., d. characterized by calcification of the dentinal tubules as a result of injury or normal aging. SYN transparent d.

   secondary d., d. formed by normal pulp function after root end formation is complete.

   tertiary d., morphologically irregular d. formed in response to an irritant. SYN irregular d., irritation d., reparative d.

   transparent d., SYN sclerotic d.

den•ti•nal (den′ti-năl). Relating to dentin.

den•ti•nal•gia (den-ti-nal′jē-ă). Dentinal sensitivity or pain. [dentin + G. *algos,* pain]

den•tin•o•ce•ment•al (den′ti-nō-se-men′tăl). Relating to the dentin and cementum of teeth.

den•tin•o•e•nam•el (den′ti-nō-ē-nam′ĕl). Relating to the dentin and enamel of teeth. SYN amelodentinal.

den•tin•o•gen•e•sis (den′ti-nō-jen′ĕ-sis). The process of dentin formation in the development of teeth. [dentin + G. *genesis,* production]

   d. imperfec′ta [MIM*125490 & MIM*125500], a hereditary disorder of the teeth characterized by translucent gray to yellow-brown teeth involving both primary and permanent dentition; the enamel fractures easily, leaving exposed dentin which undergoes rapid attrition; radiographically, the pulp chambers and canals appear obliterated and the roots are short and blunted; sometimes occurs in association with osteogenesis imperfecta.

den•ti•noid (den′ti-noyd). **1.** Resembling dentin. **2.** SYN dentinoma. [dentin + G. *eidos,* resembling]

den•ti•no•ma (den′ti-nō′mă). A rare benign odontogenic tumor consisting microscopically of dysplastic dentin and strands of epithelium within a fibrous stroma. SYN dentinoid (2). [dentin + G. -*oma,* tumor]

den•ti•num (den′ti-nŭm) [NA]. SYN dentin. [L. *dens,* tooth]

den•tip•a•rous (den-tip′ă-rŭs). Tooth-bearing. [denti- + L. *pario,* to bear]

den•tist. A legally qualified practitioner of dentistry.

den•tis•try (den′tis-trē). The healing science and art concerned with the embryology, anatomy, physiology, and pathology of the oral-facial complex, and with the prevention, diagnosis, and treatment of deformities, pathoses, and traumatic injuries thereof. SYN odontology.

   forensic d., (1) the relation and application of dental facts to legal problems, as in using the teeth for identifying the dead; **(2)** the law in its bearing on the practice of dentistry.

   preventive d., a philosophy and method of dental practice which seeks to prevent the initiation, progression, and recurrence of dental caries.

   restorative d., individual restoration of teeth by means of amalgam, synthetic porcelainlike materials, resins, or inlays. SEE ALSO oral *surgery,* implant.

den•ti•tion (den-tish′ŭn). The natural teeth, as considered collectively, in the dental arch; may be deciduous, permanent, or mixed. [L. *dentitio,* teething]

   deciduous d., SYN deciduous *tooth.*

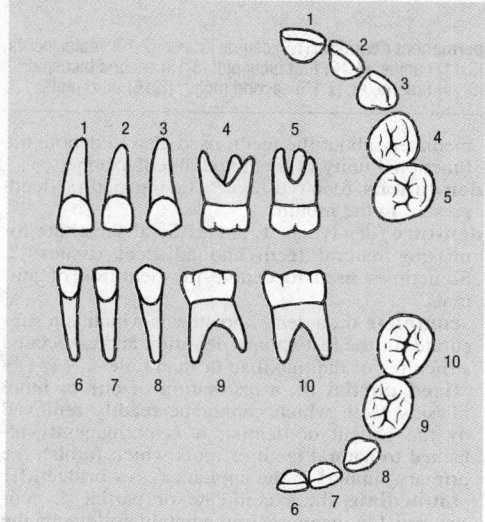

deciduous dentition: (1,6) central incisor; (2,7) lateral incisor; (3, 8) canine; (4,9) first molar; (5,10) second molar

   delayed d., delayed eruption of the teeth.

   permanent d., the adult d. of 32 teeth, consisting in each quadrant of two incisors, one canine, two bicuspids, and three molars, in that order from the midline.

   primary d., SYN deciduous *tooth.*

   retarded d., d. in which calcification, elongation, and eruption occur later than normal as a result of some systemic metabolic dysfunction (*e.g.,* hypothyroidism).

   secondary d., SYN permanent *tooth.*

△**dento-.** SEE dent-.

den•to•al•ve•o•lar (den′to-al-vē′ō-lăr). Usually, denoting that portion of the alveolar bone im-

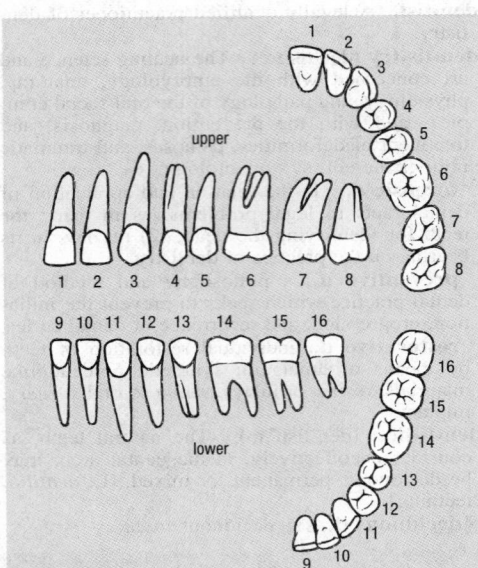

permanent dentition: (1,9) central incisor; (2,10) lateral incisor; (3,11) canine; (4,12) first bicuspid; (5,13) second bicuspid; (6,14) first molar; (7,15) second molar; (8,16) third molar

mediately about the teeth; used also to denote the functional unity of teeth and alveolar bone.

den·tu·lous (den′tyū-lŭs). Having natural teeth present in the mouth.

den·ture (den′tyūr). **1.** An artificial substitute for missing natural teeth and adjacent tissues. **2.** Sometimes used to denote the dentition of animals.

   complete d., a dental prosthesis which is a substitute for the lost natural dentition and associated structures of the maxillae or mandible.

   fixed partial d., a restoration of one or more missing teeth which cannot be readily removed by the patient or dentist; it is permanently attached to natural teeth or roots which furnish the primary support to the appliance. SYN bridge (3).

   immediate d., a complete or partial d. constructed for insertion immediately following the removal of natural teeth.

   implant d., a d. that receives its stability and retention from a substructure which is partially or wholly implanted under the soft tissues of the d. basal seat.

   interim d., a dental prosthesis to be used for a short time for reasons of esthetics, mastication, occlusal support, or convenience, or to condition the patient to accept an artificial substitute for missing natural teeth until more definite prosthetic dental treatment can be provided. SYN temporary d.

   overlay d., a complete d. that is supported by both soft tissue and natural teeth that have been altered so as to permit the d. to fit over them. The altered teeth may have been fitted with short or long copings, locking devices, or connecting bars. SYN overdenture.

   partial d., a dental prosthesis which restores one or more, but not all, of the natural teeth and/or associated parts, and is supported by the teeth and/or the mucosa; it may be removable or fixed. SYN bridgework.

   removable partial d., a partial d. which supplies teeth and associated structures on a partially edentulous jaw, and which can be readily removed from the mouth. SYN removable bridge.

   temporary d., SYN interim d.

   transitional d., a partial d. which is to serve as a temporary prosthesis to which teeth will be added as more teeth are lost, and which will be replaced after postextraction tissue changes have occurred; a transitional d. may become an interim d. when all of the teeth have been removed from the dental arch.

   trial d., a setup of artificial teeth so fabricated that it may be placed in the patient's mouth to verify esthetics, for the making of records, or for any other operation deemed necessary before final completion of the d.

de·nu·cle·at·ed (dē-nū′klē-ā-ted). Deprived of a nucleus.

de·nu·da·tion (den-yū-dā′shŭn). Depriving of a covering or protecting layer; the act of laying bare, as in the removal of the epithelium from an underlying surface. [L. *de-nudo,* to lay bare, fr. *de,* from, + *nudus,* naked]

de·nude (dē′nūd). To perform denudation.

de·o·dor·ant (dē-ō′der-ant). **1.** Eliminating or masking a smell, especially an unpleasant one. **2.** An agent having such an action; especially a cosmetic combined with an antiperspirant. SYN deodorizer. [L. *de-* priv. + *odoro,* pp. *-atus,* to give an odor to, fr. *odor,* a smell]

de·o·dor·iz·er (dē-ō′der-īz-er). SYN deodorant (2).

de·os·si·fi·ca·tion (dē-os′i-fi-kā′shŭn). Removal of the mineral constituents of bone. [L. *de,* from, + *os,* bone, + *facio,* to make]

de·ox·y·a·den·o·sine (dA, dAdo) (dē-oks′ē-ă-den′ō-sēn). 2′-Deoxyribosyladenine, one of the four major nucleosides of DNA (the others being deoxycytidine, deoxyguanosine, and thymidine). The 5′ derivative is also an important component of one form of vitamin B_{12}. D. accumulates in individuals with severe combined immunodeficiency disease.

de·ox·y·ad·e·nyl·ic ac·id (dAMP) (dē-oks′ē-aden-il′ik). Deoxyadenosine monophosphate, a hydrolysis product of DNA, differing from adenylic acid in containing deoxyribose in place of ribose. SYN adenine deoxyribonucleotide.

de·ox·y·cho·late (dē-oks-ē-kō′lāt). A salt or ester of deoxycholic acid.

de·ox·y·cho·lic ac·id (dē-oks-ē-kō′lik). A bile acid and choleretic; used in biochemical preparations as a detergent.

de·ox·y·cor·ti·cos·ter·one (dē-oks′ē-kōr-ti-kos′ter-ōn). An adrenocortical steroid, principally a biosynthetic precursor of corticosterone and possibly aldosterone, that rarely appears in adrenocortical secretions; a potent mineralocorticoid with no appreciable glucocorticoid activity. SYN 21-hydroxyprogesterone.

de·ox·y·cyt·i·dine (dē-oks-ē-sī′ti-dēn). 2′-Deoxyribosylcytosine, one of the four major nucleosides of DNA (the others being deoxyadenosine, deoxyguanosine, and thymidine).

de·ox·y·cyt·i·dyl·ic ac·id (dCMP) (dē-oks′ē-sī-ti-dil′ik). Deoxycytidine monophosphate, a hydrolysis product of DNA.

de·ox·y·gua·no·sine (dē-oks-ē-gwan′ō-sēn). One of the four major nucleosides of DNA (the others being deoxyadenosine, deoxycytidine, and thymidine). Found to accumulate in individuals with purine nucleoside phosphorylase deficiency.

de·ox·y·gua·nyl·ic ac·id (dGMP) (dē-oks-ē-gwan-il′ik). Deoxyguanosine monophosphate, a hydrolysis product of DNA. SYN guanine deoxyribonucleotide.

de·ox·y·ri·bo·nu·cle·ase (DNAse, DNAase, DNase) (de-oks′ē-rī-bō-nū′klē-ās). Any enzyme (phosphodiesterase) hydrolyzing phosphodiester bonds in DNA. SEE ALSO endonuclease, nuclease.

de·ox·y·ri·bo·nu·cle·ic ac·id (DNA) (dē-oks′ē-rī′bō-nū-klē′ik). The type of nucleic acid containing deoxyribose as the sugar component, found principally in the nuclei (chromatin, chromosomes) and mitochondria of animal and vegetable cells, usually loosely bound to protein (hence the term deoxyribonucleoprotein); the autoreproducing component of chromosomes and of many viruses, and the repository of hereditary characteristics. Chromosomes are composed of double-stranded DNA; mitochondrial DNA is circular.

    blunt-ended DNA, double-stranded DNA in which at least one of the ends has no unpaired bases.

    complementary DNA (cDNA), (1) single-stranded DNA that is complementary to messenger RNA; **(2)** DNA that has been synthesized from mRNA by the action of reverse transcriptase.

    junk DNA, that portion of DNA which is not transcribed and expressed, comprising about 90% of the 3 billion base pairs of the human genome; its function is not known.

    recombinant DNA, SEE recombinant DNA.

    sticky-ended DNA, double-stranded DNA in which one of the strands extends beyond the other strand (*i.e.,* has a number of unpaired bases) at one end or both.

    Z-DNA, a form of DNA in which the helix is left-handed, and the overall appearance is elongated and slim.

de·ox·y·ri·bo·nu·cle·o·pro·tein (dē-oks′ē-rī-bō-nū′klē-ō-prō′tēn). The complex of DNA and protein in which DNA is usually found upon cell disruption and isolation.

de·ox·y·ri·bo·nu·cle·o·side (dē-oks′ē-rī-bō-nū′klē-ō-sīd). A nucleoside component of DNA containing 2-deoxy-D-ribose; the condensation product of deoxy-D-ribose with purines or pyrimidines.

de·ox·y·ri·bo·nu·cle·o·tide (dē-oks′ē-rī-bō-nū′klē-ō-tīd). A nucleotide component of DNA containing 2-deoxy-D-ribose; the phosphoric ester of deoxyribonucleoside; formed in nucleotide biosynthesis.

de·ox·y·ri·bose (dē-oks-ē-rī′bōs). A deoxypentose, 2-deoxy-D-ribose being the most common

example, occurring in DNA and responsible for its name.

de·ox·y·thy·mi·dine (dT) (dē-oks′ē-thi′mi-dēn). SYN thymidine.

de·ox·y·thy·mi·dyl·ic ac·id (dTMP) (dē-oks′ē-thī-mi-dil′ik). A component of DNA; originally and properly called thymidylic acid, but use of deoxy- is less ambiguous, as ribothymidylic acid is now known to exist.

de·pen·dence (dē-pen′dens). The quality or condition of relying upon, being influenced by, or being subservient to a person or object reflecting a particular need. [L. *dependeo,* to hang from]

    substance d., a pattern of behavioral, physiologic, and cognitive symptoms due to substance use or abuse; usually indicated by tolerance to the effects of the substance and withdrawal symptoms when use of the substance is terminated.

de·per·son·al·i·za·tion (dē-per′sŏn-ăl-i-zā′shŭn). A state in which a person loses the feeling of his own identity in relation to others in his family or peer group, or loses the feeling of his own reality.

de·phas·ing (dē-fāz′ing). MAGNETIC RESONANCE the gradual loss of orientation of the magnetic atomic nuclei due to random molecular energy transfer or relaxation following alignment by a radiofrequency pulse.

de·pig·men·ta·tion (dē-pig-men-tā′shŭn). Loss of pigment which may be partial or complete. SEE ALSO achromia (1).

dep·i·late (dep′i-lāt). To remove hair by any means. Cf. epilate. [L. *de-pilo,* pp. *-atus,* to deprive of hair, fr. *de-* neg. + *pilo,* to grow hair]

dep·i·la·tion (dep-i-lā′shŭn). SYN epilation.

de·pil·a·to·ry (dē-pil′ă-tō-rē). **1.** SYN epilatory (1). **2.** An agent that causes the falling out of hair. SYN epilatory (2).

de·po·lar·i·za·tion (dē-pō′lăr-i-zā′shŭn). The destruction, neutralization, or change in direction of polarity.

de·pol·y·mer·ase (dē-pol′i-mer-ās). An enzyme catalyzing the hydrolysis of a macromolecule to simpler components. SEE nuclease.

de·pres·sant (dē-pres′ănt). **1.** Diminishing functional tone or activity. **2.** An agent that reduces nervous or functional activity, such as a sedative or anesthetic. [L. *de-primo,* pp. *-pressus,* to press down]

de·pressed (dē-prest′). **1.** Flattened from above downward. **2.** Below the normal level or the level of the surrounding parts. **3.** Below the normal functional level. **4.** Dejected; low in spirits.

de·pres·sion (dē-presh′ŭn). **1.** Reduction of the level of functioning. **2.** A hollow or sunken area. **3.** Displacement of a part downward or inward. **4.** A temporary mental state or chronic mental disorder characterized by feelings of sadness, loneliness, despair, low self-esteem, and self-reproach; accompanying signs include psychomotor retardation or less frequently agitation, withdrawal from social contact, and vegetative states such as loss of appetite and insomnia. SYN dejection (1). [L. *depressio,* fr. *deprimo,* to press down]

    agitated d., d. with excitement and restlessness.

    anaclitic d., impairment of an infant's physical, social, and intellectual development following separation from its mother or from a mothering surrogate; characterized by listlessness, withdrawal, and anorexia.

endogenous d., endogenomorphic d., a descriptive syndrome for a cluster of symptoms and features occurring in the absence of external precipitants and believed to have a biologic origin; *e.g.,* anhedonia, psychomotor agitation or retardation, diurnal mood variation with increased severity in the morning, early morning awakening and insomnia in the middle of the night, weight loss, self-reproach or guilt, and lack of reactivity to one's environment.

exogenous d., similar signs and symptoms as endogenous d. but the precipitating factors are social or environmental and outside the individual.

involutional d., depression or psychosis first occurring in the involutional years (40 to 55 for women, 50 to 65 for men).

reactive d., a psychological state occasioned directly by an intensely sad external situation (frequently loss of a loved person), relieved by the removal of the external situation (*e.g.,* reunion with a loved person).

de•pres•sor (dē-pres′ŏr). **1.** A muscle that flattens or lowers a part. **2.** Anything that depresses or retards functional activity. **3.** An instrument or device used to push certain structures out of the way during an operation or examination. **4.** An agent that decreases blood pressure. [L. *de-primo,* pp. *-pressus,* to press down]

dep•ri•va•tion (dep′ri-vā′shŭn). Absence, loss, or withholding of something needed.

emotional d., lack of adequate and appropriate interpersonal or environmental experiences, or both, usually in the early developmental years.

sensory d., diminution or absence of usual external stimuli or perceptual experiences, commonly resulting in psychological distress and aberrant functioning if continued too long.

depth. Distance from the surface downward.

anesthetic d., the degree of central nervous system depression produced by a general anesthetic agent; a function of potency of the anesthetic and the concentration in which it is administered.

focal d., d. of focus, the greatest distance through which an object point can be moved while remaining in focus.

de•range•ment (dē-rānj′ment). **1.** A disturbance of the regular order or arrangement. **2.** Rarely used term for a mental disturbance or disorder. [Fr.]

de•re•al•i•za•tion (dē-rē′ă-li-zā′shŭn). An alteration in one's perception of the environment such that things that are ordinarily familiar seem strange, unreal, or two-dimensional.

de•re•ism (dē′rē-izm). Mental activity in fantasy in contrast to reality. [L. *de,* away, + *res,* thing]

de•re•is•tic (dē-rē-is′tik). Living in imagination or fantasy with thoughts that are incongruent with logic or experience.

der•en•ceph•a•ly (dār-en-sef′ă-lē). Cervical rachischisis and anencephaly, a malformation involving an open cranial vault with a rudimentary brain usually crowded back toward bifid cervical vertebrae. [G. *derē,* neck, + *enkephalos,* brain]

de•re•pres•sion (dē-rē-presh′ŭn). A homeostatic mechanism for regulating enzyme production in an inducible enzyme system: an inducer, usually a substrate of a specific enzyme pathway, by combining with an active repressor (produced by a regulator gene) deactivates it.

der•i•va•tion (dār-i-vā′shŭn). **1.** The drawing of blood or the body fluids to one part to relieve congestion in another. SYN revulsion (2). **2.** The source or process of an evolution. [L. *derivatio,* fr. *derivo,* pp. *-atus,* to draw off, fr. *rivus,* a stream]

de•riv•a•tive (dě-riv′ă-tiv). **1.** Relating to or producing derivation. **2.** Something produced by modification of something preexisting. **3.** Specifically, a chemical compound that may be produced from another compound of similar structure in one or more steps, as in replacement of H by an alkyl, acyl, or amino group.

△**derm-, derma-.** The skin; corresponds to the L. *cut-.* See entries under cut. [G. *derma*]

der•ma•brad•er (derm′ă-brād-er). A motordriven device used in dermabrasion.

der•ma•bra•sion (der-mă-brā′zhŭn). Operative procedure used to remove acne scars or pits performed with sandpaper, rotating wire brushes, or other abrasive materials. SYN planing.

Der•ma•cen•tor (der-mă-sen′ter). An ornate, characteristically marked genus of hard ticks whose members commonly attack dogs, humans, and other mammals. [derm- + G. *kentōr,* a goader]

D. anderso′ni, the wood tick; vector of Rocky Mountain spotted fever; also transmits tularemia and causes tick paralysis.

D. varia′bilis, the American dog tick, a common pest of dogs along the eastern seaboard of the U.S., a vector of tularemia, and a principal vector of *Rickettsia rickettsii* which causes Rocky Mountain spotted fever in the central and eastern U.S.; may also cause tick paralysis.

der•mal (der′măl). Relating to the skin. SYN dermatic, dermatoid (2), dermic.

△**dermat-.** The skin. SEE ALSO derm-, dermato-, dermo-. [G. *derma*]

der•mat•ic (der-mat′ik). SYN dermal.

der•ma•tit•i•des (-tit′i-dēz).

der•ma•ti•tis, pl. **der•ma•tit•i•des** (der-mă-tī′tis, -tit′i-dēz). Inflammation of the skin. [derm- + G. *-itis,* inflammation]

actinic d., SYN photodermatitis.

allergic contact d., a delayed type IV allergic reaction of the skin with varying degrees of erythema, edema, and vesiculation resulting from cutaneous contact with a specific allergen. SYN contact allergy.

atopic d., d. characterized by the distinctive phenomena of atopy, including infantile and flexural eczema.

berloque d., berlock d., a type of photosensitization resulting in deep brown pigmentation on exposure to sunlight after application of bergamot oil and other essential oils in perfume.

bubble gum d., allergic contact d. developing about the lips in children who chew bubble gum; caused by plastics in the gum.

chemical d., allergic contact d. or primary irritation d. due to application of chemicals; usually characterized by erythema, edema, and vesiculation.

🔲**contact d.,** d. resulting from cutaneous contact with a specific allergen (allergic contact d.) or irritant (irritant contact d.).

contact-type d., d. resembling contact d. or eczema, but caused by an ingested or injected allergen, usually a drug, and with a widespread or generalized distribution.

diaper d., colloquially referred to as diaper, ammonia, or napkin rash; d. of thighs and buttocks resulting from exposure to urine and feces in infants' diapers. Formerly attributed to ammonia formation; moisture, bacterial growth, and alkalinity may all induce lesions. SYN diaper rash.

d. exfoliati′va infan′tum, d. exfoliati′va ne-onato′rum, a generalized pyoderma accompanied by exfoliative d., with constitutional symptoms, affecting young infants, which may result from atopic d., Leiner's disease, or staphylococcal scalded skin syndrome. SYN impetigo neonatorum (1).

exfoliative d., generalized exfoliation with scaling of the skin and usually with erythema (erythroderma); may be a drug reaction or associated with various benign dermatoses, lupus erythematosus, lymphomas, or of undetermined cause. SYN pityriasis rubra, Wilson's disease (2).

d. gangreno′sa infan′tum, a bullous or pustular eruption, of uncertain origin, followed by necrotic ulcers or extensive gangrene in children under 2 years of age; if untreated, death may result from hematogenous infection, such as liver abscess. SYN pemphigus gangrenosus (1).

🔲**d. herpetifor′mis,** a chronic disease of the skin marked by a symmetric itching eruption of vesicles and papules that occur in groups; relapses are common; associated with gluten-sensitive enteropathy and IgA immune complexes beneath the epidermis of lesioned and normal-appearing skin. SYN Duhring's disease.

infectious eczematoid d., an inflammatory reaction of skin adjacent to the site of a pyogenic infection; thought to be due to a local sensitization to the resident organisms.

irritant contact d., skin reactions ranging from erythema and scaling to necrotic burns resulting from nonimmunologic damage by chemicals in contact with the skin immediately or repeatedly.

livedoid d., a reddish blue mottled condition of the skin due to affection of the cutaneous vascular apparatus.

meadow d., meadow grass d., a photoallergic reaction to contact with a plant containing furocoumarin; often occurs after sunbathing. SYN phytophlyctodermatitis.

d. medicamento′sa, SYN drug eruption.

d. papilla′ris capillit′ii, SYN acne keloid.

d. re′pens, SYN pustulosis palmaris et plantaris. [L. creeping]

schistosomal d., a sensitization response to repeated cutaneous invasion by cercariae of bird, mammal, or human schistosomes. SYN swimmer's itch (2), water itch (2).

seborrheic d., d. seborrhe′ica, a common scaly macular eruption that occurs primarily on the face, scalp (dandruff), and other areas of increased sebaceous gland secretion; the lesions are covered with a slightly adherent oily scale. SYN dyssebacia, dyssebacea, seborrheic dermatosis.

stasis d., erythema and scaling of the lower extremities due to impaired venous circulation, seen commonly in older women or secondary to deep vein thrombosis.

△**dermato-.** SEE derm-. [G. derma, skin]

der·mat·o·fi·bro·ma (der′mă-tō-fī-brō′mă). A slowly growing benign skin nodule consisting of poorly demarcated cellular fibrous tissue enclosing collapsed capillaries, with scattered hemosiderin-pigmented and lipid macrophages. The following terms are considered by some to be synonymous with, and by others to be varieties of, d.: sclerosing hemangioma, fibrous histiocytoma, nodular subepidermal fibrosis.

der·mat·o·glyph·ics (der′mă-tō-glif′iks). **1.** The configurations of the characteristic ridge patterns of the volar surfaces of the skin; in the human hand, the distal segment of each digit has three types of configurations: whorl, loop, and arch. SEE ALSO fingerprint. **2.** The science or study of these configurations or patterns. [dermato- + glyphē, carved work]

der·ma·tog·ra·phism (der-mă-tog′ră-fizm). A form of urticaria in which whealing occurs in the site and in the configuration of application of stroking (pressure, friction) of the skin. SYN dermographia, dermographism, dermography. [dermato- + G. graphō, to write]

der·ma·toid (der′mă-toyd). **1.** Resembling skin. SYN dermoid (1). **2.** SYN dermal.

der·ma·tol·o·gist (der-mă-tol′ō-jist). A physician who specializes in the diagnosis and treatment of cutaneous diseases and related systemic diseases.

der·ma·tol·o·gy (der-mă-tol′ō-jē). The branch of medicine concerned with the study of the skin, diseases of the skin, and the relationship of cutaneous lesions to systemic disease. [dermato- + G. logos, study]

der·ma·tol·y·sis (der-mă-tol′i-sis). Loosening of the skin or atrophy of the skin by disease; erroneously used as a synonym for cutis laxa. [dermato- + G. lysis, a loosening]

der·ma·to·ma (der-mă-tō′mă). A circumscribed thickening or hypertrophy of the skin. [dermato- + G. -oma, tumor]

🔲**der·ma·tome** (der′mă-tōm). **1.** An instrument for cutting thin slices of skin for grafting, or excising small lesions. **2.** The dorsolateral part of an embryonic somite. SYN cutis plate. **3.** The area of skin supplied by cutaneous branches from a single spinal nerve; neighboring d.'s may overlap. [dermato- + G. tomē, a cutting]

der·mat·o·meg·a·ly (der′mă-tō-meg′ă-lē). Congenital or acquired defect in which the skin hangs in folds. [dermato- + G. megas, large]

der·ma·to·mere (der′mă-tō-mēr). A metameric area of the embryonic integument. [dermato- + G. meros, part]

der·mat·o·my·co·sis (der′mă-tō-mī-kō′sis). Fungus infection of the skin caused by dermato-

de

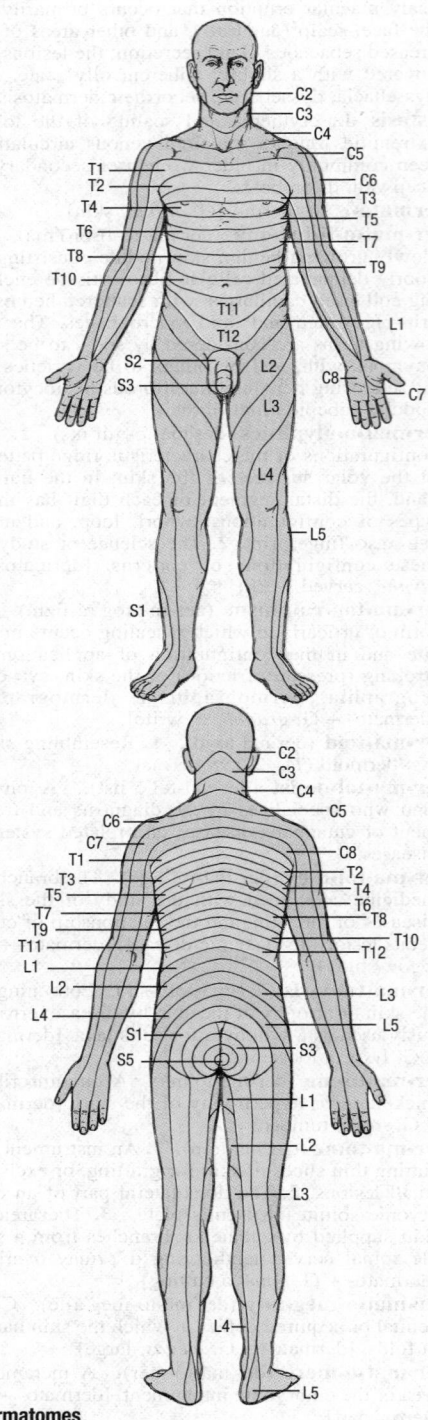

dermatomes

phytes, yeasts, and other fungi. Cf. dermatophytosis.

der·mat·o·my·o·ma (der′mă-tō-mī-ō′mă). SYN *leiomyoma* cutis. [dermato- + G. *mys,* muscle, + *-oma,* tumor]

der·mat·o·my·o·si·tis (der′mă-tō-mī-ō-sī′tis). A progressive condition characterized by symmetric proximal muscular weakness with elevated muscle enzyme levels and a skin rash, typically a purplish-red or heliotrope erythema on the face, and edema of the eyelids and periorbital tissue; affected muscle tissue shows degeneration of fibers with a chronic inflammatory reaction; occurs in children and adults, and in the latter may be associated with visceral cancer. [dermato- + G. *mys,* muscle, + *-itis,* inflammation]

der·mat·o·neu·ro·sis (der′mă-tō-nū-ro′sis). Any cutaneous eruption due to emotional stimuli.

der·mat·o·pa·thol·o·gy (der′mă-tō-pa-thol′ō-jē). Histopathology of the skin and subcutis, and study of the causes of skin disease.

der·ma·top·a·thy (der′mă-top′ă-thē). Any disease of the skin. SYN dermopathy. [dermato- + G. *pathos,* suffering]

Der·ma·toph·a·goi·des pter·o·nys·si·nus (der-mă-tof-ă-goy′dēz ter-ō-ni-sī′nŭs). A species of mites found in house dust and a common cause of atopic asthma. [dermato- + G. *phagō,* to eat; ptero- + G. *nyssō,* to prick, stab]

der·mat·o·phy·lax·is (der′mă-tō-fī-lak′sis). Protection of the skin against potentially harmful agents; *e.g.,* infection, excessive sunlight, noxious agents. [dermato- + G. *phylaxis,* protection]

der·mat·o·phyte (der′mă-tō-fīt). A fungus that causes superficial infections of the skin, hair, and/or nails, *i.e.,* keratinized tissues. Species of *Epidermophyton, Microsporum,* and *Trichophyton* are regarded as dermatophytes, but causative agents of tinea versicolor, tinea nigra, and cutaneous candidiasis are not so classified. [dermato- + G. *phyton,* plant]

der·mat·o·phy·tid (der-mă-tof′i-tid). An allergic manifestation of dermatophytosis at a site distant from that of the primary fungous infection. The lesions, usually small vesicles on the hands and/or arms, are devoid of the fungus and may become extensive, covering wide areas of the body and causing extreme discomfort to the patient. SEE ALSO -id (1).

der·mat·o·phy·to·sis (der′mă-tō-fī-tō′sis). An infection of the hair, skin, or nails caused by any one of the dermatophytes. The lesions are characterized by erythema, small papular vesicles, fissures, and scaling. Common sites of infection are the feet (tinea pedis), nails (onychomycosis), and scalp (tinea capitis). Cf. dermatomycosis.

der·mat·o·plas·ty (der′ma-tō-plas-tē). Plastic surgery of the skin, as by skin grafting. SYN dermoplasty. [dermato- + G. *plastos,* formed]

der·mat·o·pol·y·neu·ri·tis (der′mă-tō-pol′ē-nū-rī′tis). SYN acrodynia (2).

der·mat·o·scle·ro·sis (der′mă-tō-skler-ō′sis). SYN scleroderma. [dermato- + G. *sklēroō,* to harden]

der·ma·to·sis, pl. **der·ma·to·ses** (der-mă-tō′sis, -sēz). Nonspecific term used to denote any cutaneous abnormality or eruption. [dermato- + G. *-osis,* condition]

lichenoid d., any chronic skin eruption, characterized by induration and thickening of the skin with accentuation of skin markings.

d. medicamento′sa, SYN drug *eruption.*

radiation d., skin changes at the site of ionizing radiation, particularly erythema in the acute stage, temporary or permanent epilation, and chronic changes in the epidermis and dermis resembling actinic keratosis.

seborrheic d., SYN seborrheic *dermatitis.*

transient acantholytic d., a pruritic papular eruption of the chest, with scattered lesions of the back and lateral aspects of the extremities, lasting from weeks to months; seen predominantly in males over 40.

der·mat·o·ther·a·py (der′mă-tō-thār′ă-pē). Treatment of skin diseases.

der·mat·o·tro·pic (der′mă-tō-trop′ik). Having an affinity for the skin. SYN dermotropic. [dermato- + G. *trōpe,* a turning]

der·mic (der′mik). SYN dermal.

der·mis (der′mis) [NA]. A layer of skin composed of a superficial thin layer that interdigitates with the epidermis, the stratum papillare, and the stratum reticulare; it contains blood and lymphatic vessels, nerves and nerve endings, glands, and, except for glabrous skin, hair follicles. SYN corium [NA], cutis vera. [G. *derma,* skin]

dermo-. SEE derm-. [G. *derma,* skin]

der·mo·blast (der′mō-blast). One of the mesodermal cells from which the corium is developed. [dermo- + G. *blastos,* germ]

der·mo·graph·ia, der·mog·ra·phism, der·-mog·ra·phy (der-mō-graf′ē-ă, -mog′ră-fizm, -mog′ră-fē). SYN dermatographism.

der·moid (der′moyd). **1.** SYN dermatoid (1). **2.** SYN dermoid *cyst.* [dermo- + G. *eidos,* resemblance]

der·mop·a·thy (der-mop′ă-thē). SYN dermatopathy.

diabetic d., small macules and papules of the extensor surfaces of the extremities, most commonly the shins of diabetics, which become atrophic, hyperpigmented, and occasionally undergo ulceration with scarring; may be a manifestation of microangiopathy.

der·mo·plas·ty (der′mō-plas-tē). SYN dermatoplasty.

der·mo·tro·p·ic (der-mō-trop′ik). SYN dermatotropic.

der·mo·vas·cu·lar (der-mō-vas′kyū-lăr). Pertaining to the blood vessels of the skin. [dermo- + L. *vasculum,* small vessel]

de·ro·ta·tion (dē-rō-tā′shŭn). **1.** A turning back. **2.** ORTHOPEDICS the correction of a rotation deformity by turning or rotating the deformed structure toward a normal position. [L. *de,* away, + *rotatio,* turning]

des-. CHEMISTRY a prefix indicating absence of some component of the principal part of the name; largely replaced by de- (*e.g.,* deoxyribonucleic acid, dehydro-).

de·sat·u·ra·tion (dē′sat-yū-rā′shŭn). The act, or the result of the act, of making something less completely saturated; more specifically, the per-

centage of total binding sites remaining unfilled, *e.g.,* when hemoglobin is 70% saturated with oxygen and nothing else, its d. is 30%. Cf. saturation (5).

des·ce·me·ti·tis (des′ĕ-mĕ-tī′tis). Inflammation of Descemet's membrane.

des·ce·met·o·cele (des-ĕ-met′ō-sēl). A bulging forward of Descemet's membrane caused by the destruction of the substance of the cornea by infection.

de·scen·sus (dē-sen′sŭs). A falling away from a higher position. SEE ALSO ptosis, procidentia. SYN descent (1). [L.]

d. tes′tis [NA], descent of the testis from the abdomen into the scrotum during the seventh and eighth months of intrauterine life.

de·scent (dē-sent′). **1.** SYN descensus. **2.** OBSTETRICS The passage of the presenting part of the fetus into and through the birth canal. [L. descensus]

de·sen·si·tiz·a·tion (dē-sen′si-ti-zā′shŭn). **1.** The reduction or abolition of allergic sensitivity or reactions to the specific antigen (allergen). SYN antianaphylaxis. **2.** The act of removing an emotional complex.

de·sen·si·tize (dē-sen′si-tīz). **1.** To reduce or remove any form of sensitivity. **2.** To effect desensitization (1). **3.** DENTISTRY To eliminate or subdue the painful response of exposed, vital dentin to irritative agents or thermal changes.

des·e·tope (dē′se-tōp). That part of the Class II major histocompatibility molecule that interacts with the antigen. [*determinant selection* + -tope]

des·flu·rane (dés′flūr′ān). An inhalation anesthetic with physical characteristics that provide rapid induction of and recovery from anesthesia.

des·ic·cant (des′i-kant). **1.** Drying; causing or promoting dryness. SYN desiccative. **2.** An agent that absorbs moisture; a drying agent. SYN exsiccant. [L. *de-sicco,* pp. *-siccatus,* to dry up]

des·ic·cate (des′i-kāt). To dry thoroughly; to render free from moisture. SYN exsiccate.

des·ic·ca·tion (des-i-kā′shŭn). The process of being desiccated. SYN dehydration (4), exsiccation (1).

des·ic·ca·tive (des-i-kā′tiv). SYN desiccant (1).

desm-. SEE desmo-.

des·mi·tis (dez-mī′tis). Inflammation of a ligament. [desm- + G. *-itis,* inflammation]

desmo-, desm-. Fibrous connection; ligament. [G. *desmos,* a band]

des·mo·cra·ni·um (dez-mō-krā′nē-ŭm). The mesenchymal primordium of the cranium.

des·mog·e·nous (dez-moj′ĕ-nŭs). Of connective tissue or ligamentous origin or causation; *e.g.,* denoting a deformity due to contraction of ligaments, fascia, or a scar. [desmo- + G. *-gen,* producing]

des·moid (dez′moyd). **1.** Fibrous or ligamentous. **2.** A nodule or mass of firm scarlike connective tissue resulting from active proliferation of fibroblasts, occurring most frequently in the abdominal muscles of women who have borne children. SYN desmoid tumor. [desmo- + G. *eidos,* appearance, form]

des·mo·las·es (dez′mō-lā′sez). Enzymes catalyzing reactions other than those involving hydroly-

de

sis; *e.g.,* those involving oxidation and reduction, isomerization, the breaking of carbon-carbon bonds.

des·mop·a·thy (dez-mop′ă-thē). Any disease of the ligaments. [desmo- + G. *pathos,* suffering]

des·mo·pla·sia (dez-mō-plā′zē-ă). Hyperplasia of fibroblasts and disproportionate formation of fibrous connective tissue, especially in the stroma of a carcinoma. [desmo- + G. *plasis,* a molding]

des·mo·plas·tic (des-mō-plas′tik). 1. Causing or forming adhesions. 2. Causing fibrosis in the vascular stroma of a neoplasm.

des·mo·pres·sin (des-mō-pres′in). An analog of vasopressin (antidiuretic hormone, ADH) possessing powerful antidiuretic activity.

des·mo·some (dez′mō-sōm). A site of adhesion between two epithelial cells, consisting of a dense attachment plaque separated from a similar structure in the other cell by a thin layer of extracellular material. SYN macula adherens. [desmo- + G. *sōma,* body]

de·spe·ci·a·tion (dē-spē′shē-ā′shŭn). 1. Alteration or loss of species characteristics. 2. Removal of species-specific antigenic properties from a foreign protein.

des·qua·ma·tion (des-kwă-mā′shŭn). The shedding of the cuticle in scales or of the outer layer of any surface.

des·qua·ma·tive (des-kwam′ă-tiv). Relating to or marked by desquamation.

de·sulf·hy·dras·es (dē′sulf-hī′dră-sez). Enzymes or groups of enzymes catalyzing the removal of a molecule of H_2S or substituted H_2S from a compound, as in the conversion of cysteine to pyruvic acid by cysteine desulfhydrase (cystathionine γ-lyase).

de·tach·ment (dē-tach′ment). 1. A voluntary or involuntary feeling or emotion that accompanies a sense of separation from normal associations or environment. 2. Separation of a structure from its support.

▣ **retinal d., d. of retina,** loss of apposition between the sensory retina and the retinal pigment epithelium. SYN detached retina.

vitreous d., separation of the peripheral vitreous humor from the retina.

de·tec·tor (dē-tek′ter, -tōr). The component of a laboratory instrument which detects the chemical or physical signal indicating the presence or quantity of the substance of interest.

de·ter·gent (dē-ter′jent). 1. Cleansing. 2. A cleansing or purging agent, usually salts of long-chain aliphatic bases or acids which, through a surface action that depends on their possessing both hydrophilic and hydrophobic properties, exert cleansing (oil-dissolving) and antibacterial effects. [L. *de-tergeo,* pp. *-tersus,* to wipe off]

de·te·ri·o·ra·tion (dē-tēr′i-ō-rā′shŭn). The process or condition of becoming worse. [L. *deterior,* worse]

de·ter·mi·nant (dē-ter′mi-nănt). The factor that contributes to the generation of a trait. [L. *determans,* determining, limiting]

antigenic d., the particular chemical group of a molecule that determines immunological specificity.

disease d.'s, any variables that directly or indirectly influence the frequency of occurrence and/or the distribution of any given disease; they include specific disease agents, host characteristics, and environmental factors.

genetic d., any antigenic d. or identifying characteristic, particularly those of allotypes.

de·ter·mi·na·tion (dē-ter-mi-nā′shŭn). 1. A change, for the better or for the worse, in the course of a disease. 2. A general move toward a given point. 3. The measurement or estimation of any quantity or quality in scientific or laboratory investigation. 4. Discernment of a state or category (*e.g.,* in diagnosis). 5. A process, both necessary and sufficient, whereby an effect is caused. [L. *de-termino,* pp. *-atus,* to limit, determine, fr. *terminus,* a boundary]

sex d., d. of the sex of a fetus *in utero* by identification of fetal chromosomes.

de·ter·mi·nism (dē-ter′mi-nizm). The proposition that all behavior is caused exclusively by genetic and environmental influences with no random components, and independent of free will. [L. *determino,* to limit, fr. *terminus,* boundary + -ism]

de·tox·i·cate (dē-tok′si-kāt). To diminish or remove the poisonous quality of any substance; to lessen the virulence of any pathogenic organism. SYN detoxify. [L. *de,* from, + *toxicum,* poison]

de·tox·i·ca·tion (dē-tok-si-kā′shŭn). 1. Recovery from the toxic effects of a drug. 2. Removal of the toxic properties from a poison. 3. Metabolic conversion of pharmacologically active principles to pharmacologically less active principles. SYN detoxification.

de·tox·i·fi·ca·tion (dē-tok′si-fi-kā′shŭn). SYN detoxication.

de·tox·i·fy (dē-tok′si-fī). SYN detoxicate.

detraining. SYN reversibility *principle.*

de·tri·tion (dē-trish′ŭn). A wearing away by use or friction. [L. *de-tero,* pp. *-tritus,* to rub off]

de·tri·tus (dē-trī′tŭs). Any broken-down material, carious or gangrenous matter, gravel, etc. [L. (see detrition)]

de·tru·sor (dē-trū′ser, -sōr). A muscle that has the action of expelling a substance. [L. *detrudo,* to drive away]

de·tu·mes·cence (dē-tū-mes′ens). Subsidence of a swelling. [L. *de,* from, + *tumesco,* to swell up, fr. *tumeo,* to swell]

⌂ **deut-.** SEE deutero-.

deu·ter·an·o·pia (dū′ter-ă-nō′pē-ă). A congenital abnormality of the retina in which there are two rather than three retinal cone pigments (dichromatism) and complete insensitivity to middle wavelengths (green). [G. *deuteros,* second, + anopia]

⌂ **deuterio-.** Prefix indicating "containing deuterium."

deu·te·ri·um (dū-tēr′ē-ŭm). SYN hydrogen-2. [G. *deuteros,* second]

⌂ **deutero-, deut-, deuto-.** Two, or second (in a series); secondary. [G. *deuteros,* second]

deu·ter·o·my·ce·tes (du′ter-ō-mī-sē′tēz). Members of the class Deuteromycetes or the phylum Deuteromycota.

deu·ter·o·path·ic (dū′ter-ō-path′ik). Relating to a deuteropathy.

deu·ter·op·a·thy (dū-ter-op′ă-thē). A secondary disease or symptom. [deutero- + G. *pathos,* suffering]

deu·ter·o·plasm (dū′ter-ō-plazm). SYN deutoplasm. [deutero- + G. *plasma,* thing formed]

deuto-. SEE deutero-.

deu·to·plasm (dū′tō-plazm). The yolk of a meroblastic egg; the nonliving material in the cytoplasm, especially that stored in the ovum as food for the developing embryo, the commonest types being lipoid droplets and yolk granules. SYN deuteroplasm. [deuto- + G. *plasma,* thing formed]

de·vas·cu·lar·i·za·tion (dē-vas′kyū-lăr-i-zā′shŭn). Occlusion of all or most of the blood vessels to any part or organ. [L. *de,* away, + *vasculum,* small vessel, + G. *izo,* to cause]

de·vel·op·er (dē-vel′ŏp-er). 1. An individual or procedure that develops. 2. SYN eluent. 3. The chemicals used to develop film by reducing the light-activated silver halide molecules to atomic silver.

de·vel·op·ment (dē-vel′ŏp-ment). 1. The act or process of natural progression in physical and psychological maturation from a previous, lower, or embryonic stage to a later, more complex, or adult stage. 2. The process of chromatography.

  life-span d., development and mastery (or loss) of differing biologic, intellectual, behavioral, and social skills in different epochs of the life-span from the prenatal through the gerontological periods of growth.

  psychosexual d., maturation and development of the psychic and behavioral phases of sexuality from birth to adult life through the oral, anal, phallic, latency, and genital phases.

de·vel·op·men·tal mile·stones. a stage in the neuromuscular, mental, or social maturation of an infant or young child, generally marked by the attainment of a capacity or skill, such as rolling over, sitting with good head control, smiling spontaneously, laughing, and following moving objects with the eyes; all of these occur by the age of 2–4 months in the normal infant.

de·vi·ance (dē′vē-ans). SYN deviation (3).

de·vi·ant (dē′vē-ant). 1. Denoting or indicative of deviation. 2. An individual exhibiting deviation, especially sexual.

de·vi·a·tion (dē-vē-ā′shŭn). 1. A turning away or aside from the normal point or course. 2. An abnormality. 3. PSYCHIATRY, BEHAVIORAL SCIENCES a departure from an accepted norm, role, or rule. SYN deviance. 4. A statistical measure representing the difference between an individual value in a set of values and the mean value in that set. [L. *devio,* to turn from the straight path, fr. *de,* from, + *via,* way]

  axis d., deflection of the electrical axis of the heart to the right or left of the normal. SEE ALSO axis. SYN axis shift.

  conjugate d. of the eyes, (1) rotation of the eyes equally and simultaneously in the same direction, as occurs normally; **(2)** a condition in which both eyes are turned to the same side as a result of either paralysis or muscular spasm.

  primary d., the ocular deviation seen in paralysis of an ocular muscle when the nonparalyzed eye is used for fixation.

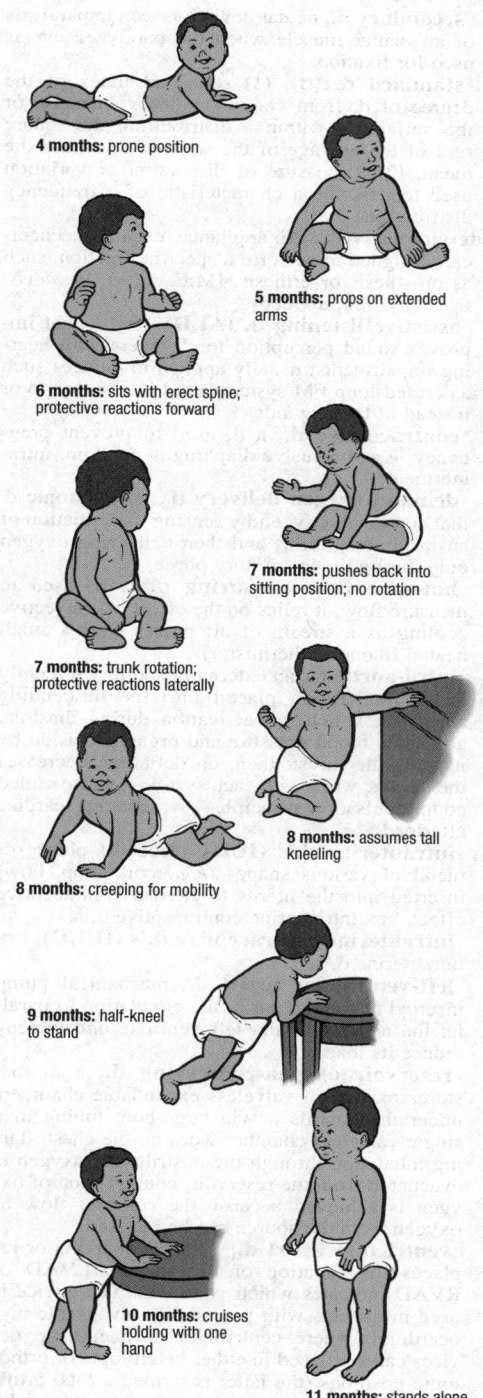

4 months: prone position

5 months: props on extended arms

6 months: sits with erect spine; protective reactions forward

7 months: pushes back into sitting position; no rotation

7 months: trunk rotation; protective reactions laterally

8 months: assumes tall kneeling

8 months: creeping for mobility

9 months: half-kneel to stand

10 months: cruises holding with one hand

11 months: stands alone

developmental milestones

de

secondary d., ocular deviation seen in paralysis of an ocular muscle when the paralyzed eye is used for fixation.

standard d. (σ), (1) statistical index of the degree of d. from central tendency, namely, of the variability within a distribution; the square root of the average of the squared d.'s from the mean. **(2)** a measure of dispersion or variation used to describe a characteristic of a frequency distribution.

de•vice (dē-vīs′). An appliance, usually mechanical, designed to perform a specific function, such as prosthesis or orthesis. [M.E., fr. O. Fr. *devis*, fr. L. *divisum*, divided]

assistive listening d. (ALD), any d. that improves sound perception for listeners with hearing impairments; usually applied to devices such as closed-loop FM systems used in addition to or instead of hearing aids.

contraceptive d., a d. used to prevent pregnancy; *e.g.,* occlusive diaphragm, condom, intrauterine d.

demand oxygen delivery d., an electronic d. that conserves oxygen by sensing the initiation of an inspiratory effort and then delivering oxygen only during the inspiratory phase.

hot-wire flow-measuring d., a d. used to measure flow; it relies on the effect of convective cooling as a stream of air passes over a small heated filament (thermistor).

intra-aortic d., an externally and intermittently inflatable balloon placed into the descending aorta and which, on activation during diastole, augments blood pressure and organ perfusion by its pulsatile thrust; then, on deflation, decreases the cardiac work with each systole—the so-called counterpulsation principle—by reducing cardiac afterload.

intrauterine d.'s (IUD), pieces of plastic or metal of various shapes (*e.g.,* coil, loop, bow) inserted into the uterus to exert a contraceptive effect. SYN intrauterine contraceptive d.'s.

intrauterine contraceptive d.'s (IUCD), SYN intrauterine d.'s.

left-ventricular assist d., mechanical pump inserted at some point in the circulation to parallel the activity of the left ventricle and thereby reduce its load.

reservoir oxygen-conserving d., a d. that stores oxygen in valveless expandable chambers under the nostrils or via large-bore tubing in a single valveless chamber worn on the chest; during inhalation through the nostrils, the oxygen is evacuated from the reservoir; conservation of oxygen is achieved because the constant flow of oxygen from the source can be reduced.

ventricular assist d., a d. that supports or replaces the function of a ventricle (LVAD or RVAD indicates which ventricle). The device is used in patients with potentially salvageable myocardium, where centrifugal or pneumatic devices can be placed in either heterotopic or orthotopic positions (the latter is termed a total artificial heart). The function of either the left, right, or both ventricles can thus be supported for days to weeks. Either recovery of heart function or need for transplantation then becomes apparent.

de•vi•om•e•ter (dē-vē-om′ĕ-ter). A form of strabismometer.

de•vi•tal•ized (dē-vī′tăl-īzd). Devoid of life; dead.

dex•ter (deks′ter) [NA]. Located on or relating to the right side. [L. fr. *dextra*, neut. *dextrum*]

△**dextr-.** SEE dextro-.

dex•trad (deks′trad). Toward the right side. [L. *dexter*, right, + *ad*, to]

dex•tral (deks′trăl). SYN right-handed.

dex•tral•i•ty (deks-tral′i-tē). Right-handedness; preference for the right hand in performing manual tasks.

dex•tran•ase (deks′tran-ās). An enzyme hydrolyzing 1,6-α-D-glucosidic linkages in dextran; used in the prevention of caries.

dex•trase (deks′trās). Nonspecific term for the complex of enzymes that converts dextrose (D-glucose) into lactic acid.

dex•tri•nase (deks′tri-nās). Any of the enzymes catalyzing the hydrolysis of dextrins; *e.g.,* amylo-1,6-glucosidase, dextrin dextranase.

dex•trin dex•tran•ase (deks′trin deks′tran-āz). A glucosyltransferase transferring 1,4-α-D-glucosyl residues, thus catalyzing the synthesis of dextrans from dextrins by glucose transfer.

α-dex•trin en•do-1,6-α-glu•co•si•dase. An enzyme with action similar to that of isoamylase; it cleaves 1,6-α-glucosidic linkages in pullalan, amylopectin, and glycogen, and in α- and β-amylase limit-dextrins of amylopectin and glycogen. Cf. isoamylase.

dex•tri•no•sis (deks-trin-ō′sis). SYN glycogenosis.

dex•tri•nu•ria (deks-tri-nū′rē-ă). The passage of dextrin in the urine.

△**dextro-, dextr-. 1.** Right, toward, or on the right side. **2.** Dextrorotatory. [L. *dexter*, on the right-hand side]

dex•tro•am•phet•a•mine sul•fate (deks′trō-am-fet′ă-mēn sul′fāt). (+)-α-Methylphenethylamine sulfate; similar in action to racemic amphetamine sulfate, but more stimulating to the central nervous system; sympathomimetic and appetite depressant.

dex•tro•car•dia (deks′trō-kar′dē-ă). Displacement of the heart to the right, either as dextroposition, with simple displacement to the right, or as cardiac heterotaxia, with complete transposition of the right and left chambers, resulting in a heart that is the mirror image of a normal heart. [dextro- + G. *kardia*, heart]

d. with si′tus inver′sus, displacement of the heart to the right side of the chest with mirror transposition of the cardiac chambers together with transposition of the abdominal viscera.

dex•tro•gas•tria (deks′trō-gas′trē-ă). Condition in which the stomach is displaced to the right; may represent either simple displacement or situs inversus. Usually associated with dextrocardia. [dextro- + G. *gastēr*, stomach]

dex•tro•gy•ra•tion (deks′trō-jī-rā′shŭn). A twisting to the right. [dextro- + L. *gyro*, pp. -*atus,* to turn in a circle, fr. *gyrus,* circle]

dex•trop•e•dal (deks-trop′ĕ-dăl). Denoting one who uses the right leg in preference to the left. SYN right-footed. [dextro- + L. *pes (ped-),* foot]

dex•tro•po•si•tion (deks'trō-pō-zi'shŭn). Abnormal right-sided location or origin of a normally left-sided structure, *e.g.*, origin of the aorta from the right ventricle.

d. of the heart, SEE dextrocardia.

dex•tro•ro•ta•to•ry (deks-trō-rō'tă-tōr-ē). Denoting dextrorotation, or certain crystals or solutions capable of such action; as a chemical prefix, usually abbreviated *d-*. Cf. levorotatory.

dex•trose (deks'trōs). SEE glucose.

dex•tro•si•nis•tral (deks'trō-si-nis'trăl). In a direction from right to left. [dextro- + L. *sinister,* left]

dex•tro•tor•sion (deks-trō-tōr'shŭn). **1.** A twisting to the right. **2.** OPHTHALMOLOGY A conjugate rotation of the upper pole of both corneas to the right. [dextro- + L. *torsio,* a twisting]

dex•tro•tro•p•ic (dek-trō-trop'ik). Turning to the right. [dextro- + G. *tropos,* a turn]

dex•tro•ver•sion (deks'trō-ver'zhŭn). **1.** Version toward the right. **2.** In ophthalmology, a conjugate rotation of both eyes to the right. [dextro- + L. *verto,* pp. *versus,* to turn]

df, DF decayed and filled teeth.

dGMP deoxyguanylic acid.

di-. **1.** Two, twice. **2.** CHEMISTRY Often used in place of bis- when not likely to be confusing; *e.g.,* dichloro- compounds. Cf. bi-, bis-. [G. *dis,* two]

dia-. Through, throughout, completely. [G. *dia,* through]

di•a•be•tes (dī-ă-bē'tēz). Either d. insipidus or d. mellitus, diseases having in common the symptom polyuria; when used without qualification, refers to d. mellitus. [G. *diabētēs,* a compass, a siphon, diabetes]

adult-onset d., non–insulin-dependent d. mellitus.

brittle d., d. mellitus in which there are marked fluctuations in blood glucose concentrations that are difficult to control.

bronze d., d. mellitus associated with hemochromatosis, with iron deposits in the skin, liver, pancreas, and other viscera, often with severe liver damage and glycosuria. SEE ALSO hemochromatosis. SYN bronzed disease.

chemical d., SYN latent d.

gestational d., carbohydrate intolerance during pregnancy usually resolving after delivery.

growth-onset d., SYN insulin-dependent d. mellitus.

d. insip'idus, chronic excretion of very large amounts of pale urine of low specific gravity, causing dehydration and extreme thirst; ordinarily results from inadequate output of pituitary antidiuretic hormone. SEE ALSO nephrogenic d. insipidus.

insulin-dependent d. mellitus (IDDM), severe d. mellitus, often brittle, usually of abrupt onset during the first two decades of life but can develop at any age; characterized by polydipsia, polyuria, increased appetite, weight loss, low plasma insulin levels, and episodic ketoacidosis; immune-mediated destruction of pancreatic B cells; insulin therapy and dietary regulation are necessary. SYN growth-onset d., juvenile-onset d., type I d.

d. intermit'tens, d. mellitus in which there are periods of relatively normal carbohydrate metabolism followed by relapses to the previous diabetic state.

juvenile-onset d., SYN insulin-dependent d. mellitus.

latent d., a mild form of d. mellitus in which the patient has no overt symptoms, but displays abnormal responses to certain diagnostic procedures, such as an elevated fasting blood glucose concentration or reduced glucose tolerance. SYN chemical d.

maturity-onset d., non-insulin-dependent d. mellitus.

d. melli'tus (DM), a metabolic disease in which carbohydrate utilization is reduced and that of lipid and protein enhanced; it is caused by an absolute or relative deficiency of insulin and is characterized, in more severe cases, by chronic hyperglycemia, glycosuria, water and electrolyte loss, ketoacidosis, and coma; long-term complications include development of neuropathy, retinopathy, nephropathy, generalized degenerative changes in large and small blood vessels, and increased susceptibility to infection. SEE ALSO insulin-dependent d. mellitus, non-insulin-dependent d. mellitus. [L. sweetened with honey]

nephrogenic d. insipidus [MIM*304800], d. insipidus due to inherited inability of the kidney tubules to respond to antidiuretic hormone.

non-insulin-dependent d. mellitus (NIDDM), an often mild form of d. mellitus of gradual onset, usually in obese individuals over age 35; absolute plasma insulin levels are normal to high, but relatively low in relation to plasma glucose levels; ketoacidosis is rare, but hyperosmolar coma can occur; responds well to dietary regulation and/or oral hypoglycemic agents, but diabetic complications and degenerative changes can develop.

phosphate d., excessive secretion of phosphate in the urine due to a defect in tubular reabsorption; usually part of a more generalized abnormality, such as Fanconi syndrome.

starvation d., after prolonged fasting, glycosuria following the ingestion of carbohydrate or glucose because of reduced output of insulin and/or reduced rate of glucose metabolism with a reduced ability to form glycogen.

subclinical d., a form of d. mellitus that is clinically evident only under certain circumstances, such as pregnancy or extreme stress; persons so afflicted may, in time, manifest more severe forms of the disease.

type I d., SYN insulin-dependent d. mellitus.

type II d., non-insulin-dependent d. mellitus.

di•a•bet•ic (dī-ă-bet'ik). **1.** Relating to or suffering from diabetes. **2.** One who suffers from diabetes.

di•a•be•to•gen•ic (dī'ă-bet-ō-jen'ik, -bē-tō-jen' ik). Causing diabetes.

di•a•be•tog•en•ous (dī'ă-bĕ-toj'en-ŭs). Caused by diabetes.

di•a•be•tol•o•gy (dī'ă-be-tol'ō-jē). The field of medicine concerned with diabetes.

di•a•ce•tic ac•id (dī-ă-sē'tik, -set'ik). SYN acetoacetic acid.

di

di·a·ce·tyl·mon·ox·ime (dī-as′ĕ-til-mon-ok′sīm). A 2-oxo-oxime that can reactivate phosphorylated acetylcholinesterase *in vitro* and *in vivo;* it penetrates the blood-brain barrier.

di·a·chron·ic (dī-ă-kron′ik). Systematically observed over time in the same subjects throughout as opposed to synchronic or cross-sectional. [dia- + G. *chronos,* time]

di·a·crit·ic, di·a·crit·i·cal (dī-ă-krit′ik, -krit′i-kăl). Distinguishing; diagnostic; allowing for distinction. [G. *diakritikos,* able to distinguish]

di·ad (dī′ad). **1.** The transverse tubule and a cisterna in cardiac muscle fibers. **2.** SYN dyad (1).

di·ad·o·cho·ki·ne·sia, di·ad·o·cho·ki·ne·sis (dī-ad′ō-kō-ki-nē′zē-ă, -ki-nē′sis). The normal power of alternately bringing a limb into opposite positions, as of flexion and extension or of pronation and supination. [G. *diadochos,* working in turn, + *kinēsis,* movement]

di·ad·o·cho·ki·net·ic (dī-ad′ō-kō-ki-net′ik). Relating to diadochokinesia.

di·ag·nose (dī-ag-nōs′). To make a diagnosis.

di·ag·no·sis (dī-ag-nō′sis). The determination of the nature of a disease. [G. *diagnōsis,* a deciding]

  clinical d., a d. made from a study of the signs and symptoms of a disease.

  differential d., the determination of which of two or more diseases with similar symptoms is the one from which the patient is suffering, by a systematic comparison and contrasting of the clinical findings. SYN differentiation (2).

  d. by exclusion, a d. made by excluding those diseases to which only some of the patient's symptoms might belong, leaving one disease as the most likely d., although no definitive tests or findings establish that d.

  laboratory d., a d. made by a chemical, microscopic, microbiologic, immunologic, or pathologic study of secretions, discharges, blood, or tissue.

  neonatal d., systematic evaluation of the newborn for evidence of disease or malformations, and the conclusion reached.

  physical d., a d. made by means of physical examination of the patient, or the process of a physical examination.

  prenatal d., d. utilizing procedures available for the recognition of diseases and malformations *in utero,* and the conclusion reached.

  principal d., d. found, after testing and study, to be the main reason for the patient's need for health care services.

di·ag·no·sis-re·lat·ed group (DRG). A classification of patients by diagnosis or surgical procedure (sometimes including age) into major diagnostic categories (each containing specific diseases, disorders, or procedures) for the purpose of determining payment of hospitalization charges, based on the premise that treatment of similar medical diagnoses generates similar costs. See Diagnosis-Related Groups appendix for individual groups.

di·ag·nos·tic (dī-ag-nos′tik). **1.** Relating to or aiding in diagnosis. **2.** Establishing or confirming a diagnosis.

di·ag·nos·ti·cian (dī′ag-nos-tish′ăn). One who is skilled in making diagnoses.

Diagnostic and Statistical Manual. An American Psychiatric Association publication that classifies mental illnesses. Currently in its fourth edition (DSM-IV), the manual provides health practitioners with a comprehensive system for diagnosing mental illnesses based on specific ideational and behavioral symptoms.

di·a·ki·ne·sis (dī′ă-ki-nē′sis). Final stage of prophase in meiosis I, in which the chromosomes continue to shorten and the nucleolus and nuclear membrane disappear. [G. *dia,* through, + *kinēsis,* movement]

di·al·y·sance (dī-al′i-sans). The number of milliliters of blood completely cleared of any substance by an artificial kidney or by peritoneal dialysis in a unit of time; conventional clearance formulas are expressed as mm/min. [fr. dialysis]

di·al·y·sate (dī-al′i-sāt). That part of a mixture that passes through a dialyzing membrane. SYN diffusate.

di·al·y·sis (dī-al′i-sis). A form of filtration to separate crystalloid from colloid substances (or smaller molecules from larger ones) in a solution by interposing a semipermeable membrane between the solution and water; the crystalloid (smaller) substances pass through the membrane into the water on the other side, the colloids do not. SYN diffusion (2). [G. a separation, fr. *dialyo,* to separate]

  continuous ambulatory peritoneal d. (CAPD), method of peritoneal d. performed in ambulatory patients with influx and efflux of dialysate during normal activities.

  equilibrium d., IMMUNOLOGY a method for determination of association constants for hapten-antibody reactions in a system in which the hapten (dialyzable) and antibody (nondialyzable) solutions are separated by semipermeable membranes.

  peritoneal d., removal from the body of soluble substances and water by transfer across the peritoneum, utilizing a d. solution which is intermittently introduced into and removed from the peritoneal cavity.

  d. ret′inae, congenital or traumatic separation of the peripheral sensory retina from the retinal pigment epithelium at the ora serrata, often causing a retinal detachment.

di·a·lyz·er (dī′ă-lī-zer). The apparatus for performing dialysis; a membrane used in dialysis.

di·a·me·lia (dī-ă-mē′lē-ă). Absence of two limbs.

di·am·e·ter (dī-am′ĕ-ter). **1.** A straight line connecting two opposite points on the surface of a more or less spherical or cylindrical body, or at the boundary of an opening or foramen, passing through the center of such body or opening. **2.** The distance measured along such a line. [G *diametros,* fr. *dia,* through, + *metron,* measure]

  biparietal d., the d. of the fetal head between the two parietal eminences.

  oblique d., a measurement across the pelvic inlet from the sacroiliac joint of one side to the opposite iliopectineal eminence.

  occipitofrontal d., the d. of the fetal head from the external occipital protuberance to the most prominent point of the frontal bone in the mid line.

occipitomental d., the d. of the fetal head from the external occipital protuberance to the midpoint of the chin.

posterior sagittal d., distance from the sacrococcygeal junction to the middle of an imaginary line running between the left and right ischial tuberosities.

suboccipitobregmatic d., the d. of the fetal head from the lowest posterior point of the occipital bone to the center of the anterior fontanelle.

total end-diastolic d., cross sectional d. of the left ventricle including the septum and posterior wall thicknesses in diastole.

total end-systolic d., cross sectional d. of the left ventricle including the septum and posterior wall thicknesses in systole.

trachelobregmatic d., the d. of the fetal head from the middle of the anterior fontanelle to the neck.

transverse d., the breadth d. of the pelvic inlet, measured between the terminal lines.

di•a•pause (dī′ă-pawz). A period of biological quiescence or dormancy with decreased metabolism; an interval in which development is arrested or greatly slowed. [dia- + G. *pausis*, pause]

di•a•pe•de•sis (dī′ă-pĕ-dē′sis). The passage of blood, or any of its formed elements, through the intact walls of blood vessels. SYN migration (2). [G. *dia*, through, + *pēdēsis*, a leaping]

di•aph•a•nos•cope (dī-af′ă-nō-skōp). An instrument for illuminating the interior of a cavity to determine the translucency of its walls. [G. *diaphanēs*, transparent, + *skopeō*, to examine]

di•aph•a•nos•co•py (dī-af-ă-nos′kŏ-pē). Examination of a cavity with a diaphanoscope.

di•a•phe•met•ric (dī′ă-fĕ-met′rik). Relating to the determination of the degree of tactile sensibility. [G. *dia*, through, + *haphē*, touch, + *metron*, measure]

di•a•pho•re•sis (dī′ă-fō-rē′sis). SYN perspiration (1). [G. *diaphorēsis*, fr. *dia*, through, + *phoreō*, to carry]

di•a•pho•ret•ic (dī-ă-fō-ret′ik). 1. Relating to, or causing, perspiration. 2. An agent that increases perspiration.

di•a•phragm (dī′ă-fram). 1. The musculomembranous partition between the abdominal and thoracic cavities. SYN midriff. 2. A thin disk pierced with an opening, used in a microscope, camera, or other optical instrument in order to shut out the marginal rays of light, thus giving a more direct illumination. 3. A flexible ring covered with a dome-shaped sheet of elastic material used in the vagina to prevent pregnancy. 4. In radiography, a grid (2). [G. *diaphragma*]

Bucky d., in radiography, a d. with a moving grid that avoids grid shadows. SYN Potter-Bucky d.

pelvic d., d. of pelvis, the paired levator ani and coccygeus muscles together with the fascia above and below them.

Potter-Bucky d., SYN Bucky d.

urogenital d., a triangular sheet of muscle between the ischiopubic rami; composed of the sphincter urethrae, and the deep transverse perineal muscles.

di•a•phrag•mat•ic (dī′ă-frag-mat′ik). Relating to a diaphragm. SYN phrenic (1).

di•a•phy•sec•to•my (dī′ă-fi-sek′tō-mē). Partial or complete removal of the shaft of a long bone. [diaphysis + G. *ektomē*, excision]

di•a•phys•i•al (dī-ă-fiz′ē-ăl). Relating to a diaphysis.

di•aph•y•sis, pl. **di•aph•y•ses** (dī-af′i-sis, -sēz) [NA]. SYN shaft. [G. a growing between]

di•a•pi•re•sis (dī′ă-pī-rē′sis). Passage of colloidal or other small particles of suspended matter through the unruptured walls of the blood vessels. SEE ALSO diapedesis. [G. *diapeirō*, to drive through, fr. *peirō*, to pierce]

di•ar•rhea (dī-ă-rē′ă). An abnormally frequent discharge of semisolid or fluid fecal matter from the bowel. [G. *diarrhoia*, fr. *dia*, through, + *rhoia*, a flow, a flux]

choleraic d., SYN summer d.

lienteric d., d. in which undigested food appears in the stools.

summer d., d. of infants in hot weather, usually an acute gastroenteritis due to *Shigella* or *Salmonella*. SYN choleraic d.

traveler's d., d. of sudden onset, often accompanied by abdominal cramps, vomiting, and fever, occurring sporadically in travelers usually during the first week of a trip; most commonly caused by strains of enterotoxigenic *Escherichia coli*. SYN turista.

tropical d., SYN tropical *sprue*.

di•ar•rhe•al, di•ar•rhe•ic (dī-ă-rē′ăl, -rē′ik). Relating to diarrhea.

di•ar•thric (dī-ar′thrik). Relating to two joints. SYN biarticular, diarticular. [G. *di-*, two, + *arthron*, joint]

di•ar•thro•sis, pl. **di•ar•thro•ses** (dī-ar-thrō′sis, -sēz). SYN synovial *joint*. [G. articulation]

di•ar•tic•u•lar (dī-ar-tik′yū-lăr). SYN diarthric.

di•as•chi•sis (dī-as′ki-sis). A sudden inhibition of function produced by an acute focal disturbance in a portion of the brain at a distance from the original seat of injury, but anatomically connected with it through fiber tracts. [G. a splitting]

di•a•scope (dī′ă-skōp). A flat glass plate through which one can examine superficial skin lesions by means of pressure. [G. *dia*, through, + *skopeō*, to view]

di•as•co•py (dī-as′kŏ-pē). Examination of superficial skin lesions with a diascope. [G. *dia*, through, + *skopeō*, to see]

di•a•stal•sis (dī-ă-stal′sis). The type of peristalsis in which a region of inhibition precedes the wave of contraction, as seen in the intestinal tract. [G. an arrangement]

di•a•stal•tic (dī-ă-stal′tik). Pertaining to diastalsis.

di•as•ta•sis (dī-as′tă-sis). 1. Any simple separation of normally joined parts. SYN divarication. 2. The mid-portion of diastole when the blood enters the ventricle slowly or ceases to enter prior to atrial systole. Diastasis duration is in inverse proportion to heart rate and is absent at very high heart rates. [G. a separation]

di•as•tas•u•ria (dī-as-tās-yū′rē-ă). SYN amylasuria.

di•a•stat•ic (dī-ă-stat′ik). Relating to a diastasis.

di•a•ste•ma, pl. **di•a•ste•ma•ta** (dī′ă-stē′mă, -stē′ mă-tă). **1.** Fissure or abnormal opening in any part, especially if congenital. **2** [NA]. Space between two adjacent teeth in the same dental arch. **3.** Cleft or space between the maxillary lateral incisor and canine teeth, into which the lower canine is received when the jaws are closed; abnormal in man but normal in dogs and many other animals. [G. *diastēma,* an interval]

di•a•ste•ma•to•cra•nia (dī-ă-stē′mă-tō-krā′nē-ă). Congenital sagittal fissure of the skull. [G. *diastēma,* an interval, + *kranion,* skull]

di•a•ste•ma•to•my•e•lia (dī-ă-stē′mă-tō-mī-e′lē-ă). Complete or incomplete sagittal division of the spinal cord by an osseous or fibrocartilaginous septum. [G. *diastēma,* interval, + *myelon,* marrow]

di•as•to•le (dī-as′tō-lē). Normal postsystolic dilation of the heart cavities, during which they fill with blood; d. of the atria precedes that of the ventricles; d. of either chamber alternates rhythmically with systole or contraction of that chamber. [G. *diastolē,* dilation]
  electrical d., period from end of T wave to beginning of next Q wave.

di•a•stol•ic (dī-ă-stol′ik). Relating to diastole.

di•a•tax•ia (dī′ă-tak′sē-ă). Ataxia affecting both sides of the body.

di•a•ther•mal (dī-ă-ther′mal). SYN diathermic. [G. *dia,* through, + *thermē,* heat]

di•a•ther•ma•nous (dī-ă-ther′man-ŭs). Permeable by heat rays. SYN transcalent. [G. *diathermaino,* to heat through, fr. *thermos,* hot]

di•a•ther•mic (dī-ă-ther′mik). Relating to, characterized by, or affected by diathermy. SYN diathermal.

di•a•ther•my (dī′ă-ther-mē). Local elevation of temperature within the tissues, produced by high frequency current, ultrasonic waves, or microwave radiation. [G. *dia,* through, + *thermē,* heat]
  medical d., d. of mild degree causing no destruction of tissue.
  surgical d., electrocoagulation with a high frequency electrocautery, resulting in local tissue destruction; usually used to seal blood vessels and arrest bleeding.
  ultrashortwave d., shortwave d. in which the wavelength is under 10 meters.

di•ath•e•sis (dī-ath′ĕ-sis). The constitutional or inborn state disposing to a disease, group of diseases, or metabolic or structural anomaly. [G. arrangement, condition]

di•a•thet•ic (dī-ă-thet′ik). Relating to a diathesis.

di•a•tom•ic (dī-ă-tom′ik). **1.** Denoting a compound with a molecule made up of two atoms. **2.** Denoting any ion or atomic grouping composed of two atoms only.

⚘**diazo-.** Prefix denoting a compound containing the ≡C–N=N–X grouping, where X is not carbon (except for CN), or the grouping N_2 attached by one atom to carbon. Cf. azo-. [G. *di-,* two, + Fr. *azote,* nitrogen]

di•ba•sic (dī-bā′sik). Having two replaceable hydrogen atoms, denoting an acid with two ionizable hydrogen atoms.

di•bu•caine num•ber (DN) (dī-bū′kăn num′ber). A test for differentiation of one of several forms of atypical pseudocholinesterases that are unable to inactivate succinylcholine at normal rates; based upon percent inhibition of the enzymes by dibucaine. SEE ALSO fluoride number.

DIC disseminated intravascular *coagulation.*

di•cen•tric (dī-sen′trik). Having two centromeres, an abnormal state.

di•cho•ri•al, di•cho•ri•on•ic (dī-kō′rē-ăl, dī-kō-rē-on′ik). Showing evidence of two chorions. [G. *di-,* two, + chorion]

di•chro•ic (dī-krō′ik). Relating to dichroism.

di•chro•ism (dī′krō-izm). The property of seeming to be differently colored when viewed from emitted light and from transmitted light. [G. *di-,* two, + *chrōa,* color]
  circular d. (CD), the change from circular polarization to elliptical polarization of monochromatic, circularly polarized light in the immediate vicinity of the absorption band of the substance through which the light passes.

di•chro•mate (dī-krō′māt). A compound containing the radical $Cr_2O_7^{=}$.

di•chro•mat•ic (dī-krō-mat′ik). **1.** Having or exhibiting two colors. **2.** Relating to dichromatism (2).

di•chro•ma•tism (dī-krō′mă-tizm). **1.** The state of being dichromatic (1). **2.** The abnormality of color vision in which only two of the three retinal cone pigments are present, as in protanopia, deuteranopia, and tritanopia. SYN dichromatopsia. [G. *di-,* two, + *chrōma,* color]

di•chro•ma•top•sia (dī-krō-mă-top′sē-ă). SYN dichromatism (2). [G. *di-,* two, + *chrōma,* color, + *opsis,* vision]

di•co•ria (dī-kō′rē-ă). SYN diplocoria. [G. *di-,* two, + *korē,* pupil]

di•crot•ic (dī-krot′ik). Relating to dicrotism. [G. *dikrotos,* double-beating]

di•cro•tism (dī′krō-tizm). That form of the pulse in which a double beat can be appreciated at any arterial pulse for each beat of the heart; due to accentuation of the dicrotic wave. [G. *di-,* two, + *krotos,* a beat]

dicta- (dik′ta). Two hundred. [G.]

dic•ty•o•ma (dik-tē-ō′mă). A benign tumor of the ciliary epithelium with a net-like structure resembling embryonic retina. [G. *dikyton,* net (retina), + *-oma,* tumor]

di•dac•tic (dī-dak′tik). Instructive; denoting medical teaching by lectures or textbooks, as distinguished from clinical demonstrations with patients or laboratory exercises. [G. *didaktikos,* fr. *didaskō,* to teach]

di•dac•ty•lism (dī-dak′ti-lizm). Congenital condition of having two fingers on a hand or two toes on a foot. [G. *di-,* two, + *daktylos,* finger or toe]

di•del•phic (dī-del′fik). Having or relating to a double uterus. [G. *di-,* two, + *delphys,* womb]

⚘**didym-, didymo-.** The didymus, testis. [G. *didymos,* twin]

did•y•mus (did′ĕ-mŭs). SYN testis. [G. *didymos,* a twin, pl. *didymoi,* testes]

⚘**-didymus.** A conjoined twin, with the first element of the complete word designating fused parts. SEE ALSO -dymus, -pagus. [G. *didymos,* twin]

di•e•cious (dī-ē′shŭs). Denoting animals or plants

that are sexually distinct, the individuals being of one or the other sex. [G. *di-*, two, + *oikia*, house]

di·en·ceph·a·lon, pl. **di·en·ceph·a·la** (dī-en-sef′ă-lon, -sef′ă-lă) [NA]. That part of the prosencephalon composed of the epithalamus, dorsal thalamus, subthalamus, and hypothalamus. [G. *dia*, through, + *enkephalos*, brain]

Di·ent·a·moe·ba frag·i·lis (dī-ent-ă-mē′bă fraj′i-lis). A species of small ameba-like flagellates related to *Trichomonas*, parasitic in the large intestine of humans and certain monkeys; usually nonpathogenic, but sometimes causing low-grade inflammation with mucous diarrhea.

di·er·e·sis (dī-er′ĕ-sis). SYN *solution* of continuity. [G. *diairesis*, a division]

di·es·trous (dī-es′trŭs). Pertaining to diestrus.

di·es·trus (dī-es′trŭs). A period of sexual quiescence intervening between two periods of estrus. [G. *dia*, between, + *oistros*, desire]

di·et (dī′et). **1.** Food and drink in general. **2.** A prescribed course of eating and drinking in which the amount and kind of food, as well as the times at which it is to be taken, are regulated for therapeutic purposes. **3.** Reduction of caloric intake so as to lose weight. **4.** To follow any prescribed or specific d. [G. *diaita*, a way of life; a diet]

acid-ash d., SYN alkaline-ash d.

alkaline-ash d., a d. consisting mainly of fruits, vegetables, and milk which, when catabolized, leave an alkaline residue to be excreted in the urine. SYN acid-ash d.

balanced d., a d. containing the essential nutrients with a reasonable ration of all the major food groups.

bland d., a regular d. omitting foods that mechanically or chemically irritate the gastrointestinal tract.

challenge d., a d. in which one or more specific substances are included for the purpose of determining whether an abnormal reaction occurs.

diabetic d., a dietary adjustment for patients with *diabetes* mellitus intended to decrease the need for insulin or oral diabetic agents and control weight by adjusting caloric and carbohydrate intake.

elimination d., a d. designed to detect what component of the diet causes allergic manifestations in the patient; food items to which the patient may be sensitive are withdrawn separately and successively from the d. until that which causes the symptoms is discovered.

gluten-free d., elimination of all wheat, rye, barley, and oat gluten from the d.; treatment for gluten-sensitive enteropathy (celiac disease). SEE celiac *disease*.

high-fiber d., a d. high in the nondigestible part of plants, which is fiber. Fiber is found in fruits, vegetables, whole grains, and legumes. Insoluble fiber increases stool bulk, decreases transit time of food in the bowel, and decreases constipation and the risk of colon cancer. Soluble fiber delays absorption of glucose, which helps to control blood sugar in diabetes mellitus, and delays absorption of lipids, which helps to control hyperlipidemia. Recommended in treatment of diverticular disease of the colon.

ketogenic d., a high-fat, low-carbohydrate, and normal protein d. causing ketosis.

low purine d., a d. low in precursors of purines (such as tissues rich in cells with abundant nuclei, as in liver, glandular meats, etc.) to minimize formation of uric acid. Useful in treatment of patients with gout or urate-containing renal calculi.

low salt d., a d. with restricted amounts of sodium chloride, and other sodium salts, necessary in the treatment of some cases of hypertension, heart failure, and other syndromes characterized by fluid retention and/or edema formation.

macrobiotic d., a d. claimed to promote longevity, often by promoting an emphasis on natural foods and restrictions on noncereal foods, as well as liquids.

smooth d., a d. containing little roughage; used primarily in diseases of the colon.

soft d., a normal d. limited to soft foods for those who have difficulty chewing or swallowing; there are no restrictions on seasoning or method of food preparation.

di·e·tary (dī′ĕ-tār-ē). Relating to the diet.

di·e·tet·ic (dī-ĕ-tet′ik). **1.** Relating to the diet. **2.** Descriptive of food that, naturally or through processing, has a low caloric content.

di·e·tet·ics (dī-ĕ-tet′iks). The practical application of diet in the prophylaxis and treatment of disease.

di·eth·yl·stil·bes·trol (dī-eth′il-stil-bes′trol). A synthetic nonsteroidal estrogenic compound. Sometimes used as a postcoital antipregnancy agent to prevent implantation of the fertilized ovum. The first demonstrated transplacental carcinogen responsible for a delayed clear cell vaginal carcinoma in female offspring of mothers who took the drug during pregnancy when the drug was erroneously thought to prevent threatened abortion.

di·e·ti·tian (dī-ĕ-tish′ŭn). An expert in dietetics.

dif-. (L.) Prefix: separation, taking apart, in two, reversal, not, un-.

dif·fer·ence (dif′er-ens). The magnitude or degree by which one quality or quantity differs from another of the same kind.

A-aO$_2$ d., the d. or gradient between the partial pressure of oxygen in the alveolar spaces and that in arterial blood. Normally less than 10 mmHg, it is increased with large right-to-left cardiac or vascular shunts. SEE alveolar air *equation*. SYN alveolar-arterial oxygen tension d.

alveolar-arterial oxygen d., the gradient between the partial pressure of oxygen in the alveolar spaces and the arterial blood: $P_{(A-a)}O_2$. Normally in young adults this value is less than 20 mm Hg.

alveolar-arterial oxygen tension d., SYN A-aO$_2$ d.

arteriovenous carbon dioxide d., the d. in carbon dioxide content (in ml per 100 ml blood) between arterial and venous blood.

arteriovenous oxygen d., the d. in the oxygen content (in ml per 100 ml blood) between arterial and venous blood.

standard error of d., a statistical index of the

di

probability that a d. between two sample means is greater than zero.

dif·fer·en·ti·a·tion (dif'er-en-shē-ā'shŭn). **1.** The acquisition or possession of one or more characteristics or functions different from that of the original type. SYN specialization (2). **2.** SYN differential *diagnosis.* **3.** Partial removal of a stain from a histologic section to accentuate the staining differences of tissue components.

dif·frac·tion (di-frak'shŭn). Deflection of the rays of light from a straight line in passing by the edge of an opaque body or in passing an obstacle of about the size of the wavelength of the light. [L. *dif- fringo,* pp. *-fractus,* to break in pieces]

dif·fu·sate (di-fyū'zāt). SYN dialysate. [L. *dif-fundo,* pp. *-fusus,* to pour in different directions]

dif·fuse (di-fyūs). **1** (di-fyūz'). To disseminate; to spread about. **2** (di-fyūs'). Disseminated; spread about; not restricted. [L. *dif-fundo,* pp. *-fusus,* to pour in different directions]

dif·fus·i·ble (di-fyūz'i-bl). Capable of diffusing.

dif·fu·sion (di-fyū'zhŭn). **1.** The random movement of molecules or ions or small particles in solution or suspension toward a uniform distribution throughout the available volume. **2.** SYN dialysis.

di·gas·tric (dī-gas'trik). **1.** Having two bellies; denoting especially a muscle with two fleshy parts separated by an intervening tendinous part. SYN biventral. SEE digastric *muscle.* **2.** Relating to the d. muscle; denoting a fossa or groove with which it is in relation and a nerve supplying its posterior belly. [G. *di-,* two, + *gastēr,* belly]

di·gen·e·sis (dī-jen'ĕ-sis). Reproduction in distinctive patterns in alternate generations, as seen in the nonsexual (invertebrate) and the sexual (vertebrate) cycles of digenetic trematode parasites. [G. *di-,* two, + G. *genesis,* generation]

di·ge·net·ic (dī-jĕ-net'ik). **1.** Pertaining to or characterized by digenesis. SYN heteroxenous. **2.** Pertaining to the digenetic fluke.

di·gest. **1** (di-jest', dī-). To soften by moisture and heat. **2** (di-jest', dī-). To hydrolyze or break up into simpler chemical compounds by means of hydrolyzing enzymes or chemical action. **3** (dī'jest). The materials resulting from digestion or hydrolysis. [L. *digero,* pp. *-gestus,* to force apart, divide, dissolve]

di·ges·tant (di-jes'tănt, dī-). **1.** Aiding digestion. **2.** An agent that favors or assists the process of digestion. SYN digestive (2).

di·ges·tion (di-jes'chŭn, dī-). **1.** The process of making a digest. **2.** The mechanical, chemical, and enzymatic process whereby ingested food is converted into material suitable for assimilation for synthesis of tissues or liberation of energy. [L. *digestio.* See digest]

  gastric d., that part of d., chiefly of the proteins, carried on in the stomach by the enzymes of the gastric juice. SYN peptic d.

  intestinal d., that part of d. carried on in the intestine; it affects all the foodstuffs: starches, fats, and proteins.

  pancreatic d., d. in the intestine by the enzymes of the pancreatic juice.

  peptic d., SYN gastric d.

  primary d., d. in the alimentary tract.

  salivary d., the conversion of starch into sugar by the action of salivary amylase.

  secondary d., the change in the chyle effected by the action of the cells of the body, whereby the final products of d. are assimilated in the process of metabolism.

di·ges·tive (di-jes'tiv, dī-). **1.** Relating to digestion. **2.** SYN digestant (2).

dig·it (dij'it). A finger or toe. SYN digitus [NA], dactyl, dactylus. [L. *digitus*]

  binary d., (1) The smallest unit of digital information expressed in the binary system of notation (either 0 or 1). (2) The signal in computing.

  clubbed d.'s, SEE clubbing.

dig·i·tal (dij'i-tăl). Relating to or resembling a digit or digits or an impression made by them; based on numerical methodology.

dig·i·tal·i·za·tion (dij'i-tal-i-zā'shŭn). Administration of digitalis until sufficient amounts are present in the body to produce the desired therapeutic effects.

dig·i·tate (dij'i-tāt). Marked by a number of finger-like processes or impressions. [L. *digitatus,* having fingers, fr. *digitus,* finger]

dig·i·ta·tion (dij-i-tā'shŭn). A process resembling a finger. [Mod. L. *digitatio*]

di·gi·ti (dij'i-tī). Plural of digitus. [L.]

dig·i·tus, pl. **di·gi·ti** (dij'i-tŭs, -tī) [NA]. SYN digit. [L.]

di·glos·sia (dī-glos'ē-ă). A developmental condition that results in a longitudinal split in the tongue. SEE ALSO bifid *tongue.* [G. *di-,* two, + *glōssa,* tongue]

di·het·er·o·zy·gote (dī-het'er-ō-zī'gōt). An individual heterozygous at two loci of interest, especially in genetic linkage analysis.

di·hy·drate (dī-hī'drāt). A compound with two molecules of water of crystallization.

⟐**dihydro-.** Prefix indicating the addition of two hydrogen atoms. [G. *di,* two + *hydōr,* water]

7,8-di·hy·dro·fo·lic ac·id (dī-hī-drō-fō'lik). Intermediate between folic acid and 5,6,7,8-tetrahydrofolic acid.

di·hy·dro·lip·o·am·ide ace·tyl·trans·fer·ase (dī-hī'drō-lip-ō-am'id ă-sē-til-trans'fer-āz). An enzyme transferring acetyl from S^6-acetyldihydrolipoamide to coenzyme A. A part of many enzyme complexes (*e.g.,* pyruvate dehydrogenase complex). SYN lipoate acetyltransferase, thioltransacetylase A.

di·hy·dro·or·o·tate (dī-hī'drō-ōr-ō'tāt). L-5,6-dihydroorotate; an intermediate in the biosynthesis of pyrimidines.

di·hy·dro·pte·ro·ic ac·id (dī-hī'drō-te-rō'ik). An intermediate in the formation of folic acid; a compound of 6-hydroxymethylpterin and *p*-aminobenzoic acid, the combining of which is inhibited by sulfonamides.

di·hy·dro·ur·i·dine (dī-hī-drō-yūr'i-dēn). Uridine in which the 5,6- double bond has been saturated by addition of two hydrogen atoms; a rare constituent of transfer ribonucleic acids.

⟐**dihydroxy-.** Prefix denoting addition of two hydroxyl groups; as a suffix, becomes -diol.

di·hy·drox·y·ac·e·tone (dī'hī-drok-sē-as'e-tōn). the simplest ketose.

di•i•o•dide (dī-ī′ō-dīd). A compound containing two atoms of iodine per molecule.

diiodo-. Prefix indicating two atoms of iodine. [G. *di,* + *ioeidēs,* violet flower color]

di•i•o•do•ty•ro•sine (DIT) (dī′ī-ō-dō-tī′rō-sēn). An intermediate in the biosynthesis of thyroid hormone.

di•ke•tone (dī-kē′tōn). A molecule containing two carbonyl groups; *e.g.,* acetylacetone ($CH_3COCH_2COCH_3$).

di•ke•to•pi•per•a•zines (dī-kē′tō-pī-per′ă-zēnz). A class of organic compounds with a closed ring structure formed from two α-amino acids by the joining of the α-amino group of each to the carboxyl group of the other.

di•lac•er•a•tion (dī-las-er-ā′shŭn). Displacement of some portion of a developing tooth which is then further developed in its new relation, resulting in a tooth with sharply angulated root(s). [L. *di-lacero,* pp. *laceratus,* to tear in pieces, fr. *lacer,* mangled]

dil•a•ta•tion (dil-ă-tā′shŭn). SYN dilation.

dil•a•ta•tor (dil′ă-tā-tĕr, -tōr). SYN dilator.

di•late (dī′lāt). To perform or undergo dilation.

di•la•tion (dī-lā′shŭn). **1.** Physiologic or artificial enlargement of a hollow structure or opening. **2.** The act of stretching or enlarging an opening or the lumen of a hollow structure. SYN dilatation. [L. *dilato,* pp. *dilatatus,* to spread out, dilate]

di•la•tion and cu•ret•tage (D & C). Dilation of the cervix and curettement of the endometrium.

di•la•tion and evac•u•a•tion (D & E). Dilation of the cervix and removal of the products of conception.

di•la•tor (dī′lā-tĕr). **1.** An instrument designed for enlarging a hollow structure or opening. **2.** A muscle that pulls open an orifice. **3.** A substance that causes dilation or enlargement of an opening or the lumen of a hollow structure. SYN dilatator.

dil•u•ent. **1.** Ingredient in a medicinal preparation which lacks pharmacological activity but is pharmaceutically necessary or desirable. May be a liquid for the dissolution of drugs to be injected, ingested, or inhaled. **2.** Diluting; denoting that which dilutes.

di•lute (dī-lūt′). **1.** To reduce the concentration, strength, quality, or purity of a solution or mixture. **2.** Diluted; denoting a solution or mixture so altered. [L. *di-luo,* to wash away, dilute]

di•lu•tion (dī-lū′shŭn). **1.** The act of being diluted. **2.** A diluted solution or mixture. **3.** MICRO-BIOLOGY a method for counting the number of viable cells in a suspension; a sample is diluted to the point where an aliquot, when plated, yields a countable number of separate colonies.

closed-circuit helium d., a gas d. technique for measuring the functional residual capacity (FRC); the subject rebreathes helium from a spirometer while oxygen is added and carbon dioxide is removed to maintain a constant system volume.

serial d., a series of d.'s in which each subsequent d. is made from the previous d. The concentration of each d. is calculated by multiplying the ratios of solute to solution in each d. preceding and up to the dilution of interest. This type of d. is used to titer antibodies or to make very dilute solutions from a more concentrated solution.

di•me•lia (dī-mē′lē-ă). Congenital duplication of the whole or a part of a limb. [G. *di-,* two, + *melos,* limb]

di•men•sion (di-men′shŭn). Scope, size, magnitude; denoting, in the plural, linear measurements of length, width, and height.

di•mer (dī′mer). A compound or unit produced by the combination of two like molecules; in the strictest sense, without loss of atoms, but usually by elimination of H_2O or a similar small molecule; higher orders of complexity are called trimers, tetramers, oligomers, and polymers. [G. *di-,* two, + -mer]

di•mer•ic (dī′mer-ik). Having the characteristics of a dimer.

di•meth•yl sulf•ox•ide (dī-meth′il). Me_2SO; Methyl sulfoxide; a penetrating solvent, enhancing absorption of therapeutic agents from the skin; an industrial solvent that has been proposed as an effective analgesic and anti-inflammatory agent in arthritis and bursitis.

di•mor•phic (dī-mōr′fik). **1.** In fungi, a term referring to growth and reproduction in two forms: mold and yeast. SYN dimorphous (2). **2.** SYN dimorphous (1).

di•mor•phism (dī-mōr′fizm). Existence in two shapes or forms; denoting a difference of crystalline form exhibited by the same substance, or a difference in form or outward appearance between individuals of the same species. [G. *di-,* two, + *morphē,* shape]

sexual d., the somatic differences within species between male and female individuals that arise as a consequence of sexual maturation; inclusive of, but not restricted to, the secondary sexual characters.

di•mor•phous (dī-mōr′fŭs). **1.** Having the property of dimorphism. SYN dimorphic (2). **2.** SYN dimorphic (1).

dim•ple (dim′pl). **1.** A natural indentation, usually circular and of small area, in the chin, cheek, or sacral region. **2.** A depression of similar appearance to a d., resulting from trauma or the contraction of scar tissue. **3.** To cause d.'s.

dimp•ling (dim′pling). **1.** Causing dimples. **2.** A condition marked by the formation of dimples, natural or artificial.

-diol (dī′ol). **1.** Suffix form of the prefix dihydroxy. **2.** A member of a class of compounds containing two hydroxyl groups.

di•op•ter (dī-op′ter). The unit of refracting power of lenses, denoting the reciprocal of the focal length expressed in meters. [G. *dioptra,* a leveling instrument]

prism d., the unit of measurement of the deviation of light in passing through a prism, being a deflection of 1 cm at a distance of 1 m.

di•op•trics (dī-op′triks). The branch of optics concerned with the refraction of light.

di•ov•u•lar (dī′ov-yū-lar). Relating to two ova. SYN biovular. [di- + Mod. L. *ovulum,* dim. of L. *ovum,* egg]

di•ov•u•la•to•ry (dī-ō′vyū-lă-tō′rē). Releasing two ova in one ovarian cycle.

di·ox·ide (dī-oks′īd). A molecule containing two atoms of oxygen; *e.g.,* carbon dioxide, CO_2.

di·ox·in (dī-oks′in) **1.** A ring consisting of two oxygen atoms, four CH groups, and two double bonds; the positions of the oxygen atoms are specified by prefixes, as in 1,4-dioxin. **2.** Abbreviation for dibenzo[*b,e*][1,4]dioxin. **3.** 2,3,7,8-Tetrachlorodibenzo[*b,e*][1,4]dioxin; a contaminant in the herbicide, 2,4,5-T; its potential toxicity, carcinogenicity, and teratogenicity are controversial.

di·ox·y·gen·ase (dī-oks′ē-jen-ās). An oxidoreductase that incorporates two atoms of oxygen (from one molecule of O_2) into the (reduced) substrate.

dip. 1. A downward inclination or slope. **2.** A preparation for coating a surface by submersion, as for the destruction of skin parasites. [M.E. *dippen*]

di·pep·ti·dase (dī-pep′ti-dās) [EC 3.4.13.11.]. A hydrolase catalyzing the hydrolysis of a dipeptide to its constituent amino acids.

di·pep·tide (dī-pep′tīd). A combination of two amino acids by means of a peptide (–CO–NH–) link.

di·pep·ti·dyl pep·ti·dase (dī-pep-tī′dil pep′ti-dāz). A hydrolase occurring in two forms: **dipeptidyl peptidase I,** dipeptidyl transferase, cleaving dipeptides from the amino end of polypeptides; **dipeptidyl peptidase II,** with properties similar to those of I, has a different specificity.

di·pep·ti·dyl trans·fer·ase (dī-pep-tī′dil trans′fer-āz). Cleaving dipeptides from the amino end of polypeptides. SEE dipeptidyl peptidase.

di·phal·lus (dī-fal′ŭs). Congenital duplication, partial or complete, of the penis. May also be associated with exstrophy of the urinary bladder. [G. *di-,* two, + *phallos,* penis]

di·pha·sic (dī-fā′zik). Occurring in or characterized by two phases or stages.

di·phen·yl (dī-fen′il). Phenylbenzene; colorless liquid; used as heat transfer agent, frequently as polychlorinated biphenyls (PCBs); as fungistat for oranges and in organic syntheses. Produces convulsions and central nervous system depression. SYN biphenyl.

2,5-di·phen·yl·ox·a·zole (PPO) (dī′fen-il-oks′ă-zōl). A scintillator used in radioactivity measurements by scintillation counting.

1,3-di·phos·pho·glyc·er·ate (dī-fos′fō-glis′er-āt). An intermediate in glycolysis which enzymatically reacts with ADP to generate ATP and 3-phosphoglycerate.

2,3-di·phos·pho·glyc·er·ate. An intermediate in the Rapoport-Luebering shunt, formed between 1,3-P$_2$Gri and 3-phosphoglycerate; an important regulator of the affinity of hemoglobin for oxygen; an intermediate of phosphoglycerate mutase.

diph·the·ria (dif-thēr′ē-ă). A specific infectious disease due to *Corynebacterium diphtheriae* and its highly potent toxin; marked by severe inflammation with formation of a thick membranous coating of the pharynx, the nose, and sometimes the tracheobronchial tree; the toxin produces degeneration in peripheral nerves, heart muscle, and other tissues. Had a high fatality rate, especially in children; now rare due to an effective toxoid. [G. *diphthera,* leather]

diph·the·ri·al, diph·the·rit·ic (dif-thēr′ē-ăl, dif-thĕ-rit′ik). Relating to diphtheria, or the membranous exudate characteristic of this disease.

diph·the·roid (dif′thĕ-royd). **1.** One of a group of local infections suggesting diphtheria, but caused by microorganisms other than *Corynebacterium diphtheriae.* SYN pseudodiphtheria. **2.** Any microorganism resembling *Corynebacterium diphtheriae.* [diphtheria + G. *eidos,* resemblance]

di·phyl·lo·both·ri·a·sis (dī-fil′ō-both-rī′ă-sis). Infection with the cestode *Diphyllobothrium latum;* human infection is caused by ingestion of raw or inadequately cooked fish infected with the plerocercoid larva. Leukocytosis and eosinophilia may occur; if the worm is high enough in the alimentary canal, it may preempt the supply of vitamin B_{12} or alter its absorption, leading to hyperchromic macrocytic anemia.

Di·phyl·lo·both·ri·um (dī-fil-lō-both′rē-ŭm). A large genus of tapeworms. Several species are found in humans, although only one, *D. latum,* is of widespread importance. [G. *di-,* two, + *phyllon,* leaf, + *bothrion,* little ditch]

di·phy·o·dont (dif′ē-ō-dont). Developing two successive sets of teeth, as occurs in humans and most other mammals. [G. *di-,* two, + *phyō,* to produce, + *odous* (*odont*-), tooth]

dip·la·cu·sis (dip-lă-kū′sis). Abnormal perception of sound, either in time or in pitch, so that one sound is heard as two. [G. *diplous,* double, + *akousis,* a hearing]

  binaural d., a d. in which the same sound is heard differently by the two ears.

di·ple·gia (dī-plē′jē-ă). Paralysis of corresponding parts on both sides of the body. [G. *di-,* two, + *plēgē,* a stroke]

△**diplo-.** Double, twofold. SEE haplo-. [G. *diploos,* double]

dip·lo·ba·cil·lus (dip′lō-bă-sil′ŭs). Two rod-shaped bacterial cells linked end to end. [diplo- + bacillus]

dip·lo·bac·te·ria (dip′lō-bak-tēr′ē-ă). Bacterial cells linked together in pairs.

dip·lo·blas·tic (dip-lō-blas′tik). Formed of two germ layers. [diplo- + G. *blastos,* germ]

dip·lo·car·dia (dip-lō-kar′dē-ă). An anomaly in which the two lateral halves of the heart are separated to varying degrees by a central fissure. [diplo- + G. *kardia,* heart]

dip·lo·coc·ci (dip′lō-kok′sī). Plural of diplococcus.

dip·lo·coc·cus, pl. **dip·lo·coc·ci** (dip′lō-kok′ŭs, -kok′sī). Spherical or ovoid bacterial cells joined together in pairs. [diplo- + G. *kokkos,* berry]

dip·lo·co·ria (dip-lō-kō′rē-ă). The occurrence of two pupils in the eye. SYN dicoria. [diplo- + G. *korē,* pupil]

dip·lo·gen·e·sis (dip-lō-jen′ē-sis). Production of a double fetus or of one with some parts doubled. [diplo- + G. *genesis,* production]

dip·loid (dip′loyd). Denoting the state of a cell containing two haploid sets derived from the father and from the mother respectively; the normal chromosome complement of somatic cells (in humans, 46 chromosomes). [diplo- + G. *eidos* resemblance]

dip·lo·my·e·lia (dip-lō-mī-ē′lē-ă). Complete or incomplete doubling of the spinal cord; may be accompanied by a bony septum of the vertebral canal. [diplo- + G. *myelon,* marrow]

dip·lo·ne·ma (dip-lō-nē′mă). The doubled form of the chromosome strand visible at the diplotene stage of meiosis. [diplo- + G. *nēma,* thread]

dip·lop·a·gus (dip-lop′ă-gŭs). General term for conjoined twins, each with fairly complete bodies, although one or more internal organs may be in common. SEE conjoined *twins,* under *twin.* [diplo- + G. *pagos,* something fixed]

diplophonia (dĭp-lō-fō′nē-ă). Vibration of both the ventricular folds and the vocal folds, producing two simultaneous voice tones. [diplo- + -phonia]

dip·lo·pia (di-plō′pē-ă). The condition in which a single object is perceived as two objects. SYN double vision. [diplo- + G. *ōps,* eye]
   crossed d., d. in which the image seen by the right eye is to the left of the image seen by the left eye.
   monocular d., a double image or an extra ghost image produced in one eye, almost always by an aberration of the ocular media.

dip·lo·some (dip′lō-sōm). Paired allosomes; the pair of centrioles of mammalian cells. [diplo- + G. *sōma,* body]

dip·lo·so·mia (dip-lō-sō′mē-ă). Condition in which twins who seem functionally independent are joined at one or more points. SEE conjoined *twins,* under *twin.* [diplo- + G. *sōma,* body]

dip·lo·tene (dip′lō-tēn). The late stage of prophase in meiosis in which the paired homologous chromosomes begin to repel each other and move apart. [diplo- + G. *tainia,* band]

dip·se·sis (dip-sē′sis). An abnormal or excessive thirst, or a craving for unusual forms of drink. SYN dipsosis. [G. *dipseō,* to thirst]

dip·so·ma·nia (dip-sō-mā′nē-ă). A recurring compulsion to drink alcoholic beverages to excess. SEE alcoholism. [G. *dipsa,* thirst, + *mania,* madness]

dip·so·sis (dip-sō′sis). SYN dipsesis. [G. *dipsa,* thirst, + *-osis,* condition]

dip·so·ther·a·py (dip′sō-thār′ă-pē). Treatment of certain diseases by abstention, as far as possible, from liquids.

dip·stick. A strip of plastic or paper bearing one or more dots or squares of reagent, used to perform qualitative or semiquantitative tests on urine; results of tests are read as color changes.

Dip·tera (dip′ter-ă). An important order of insects (the two-wing flies and gnats), including many significant disease vectors such as the mosquito, tsetse fly, sandfly, and biting midge. [G. *di-,* two, + *pteron,* wing]

dip·ter·an (dip′ter-an). Denoting insects of the order Diptera.

dip·ter·ous (dip′ter-ŭs). Relating to or characteristic of the order Diptera.

dip·y·li·di·a·sis (dip′i-li-dī′ă-sis). Infection of carnivores and man with the cestode *Dipylidium caninum.*

Dip·y·lid·i·um ca·ni·num (dip-ĭ-lid′ē-ŭm kā-nī′

nŭm). The commonest species of dog tapeworm, the double-pored tapeworm, the larvae of which are harbored by dog fleas or lice; the worm occasionally infects humans. [G. *dipylos,* with two entrances; L. ntr. of *caninus,* pertaining to *canis,* dog]

di·rec·tor (di-rek′ter, -tōr, dī-). **1.** A smoothly grooved instrument used with a knife to limit the incision of tissues. SYN staff (2). **2.** The head of a service or specialty division. [L. *dirigo,* pp. *-rectus,* to arrange, set in order]

dir. prop. Abbreviation for L. *direction propria,* with proper direction.

dirt-eat·ing. SYN geophagia.

△**dis-.** In two, apart; un-, not; very. Cf. dys-. [L. separation]

dis·a·bil·i·ty.(dis-ă-bil′i-tē). **1.** Any restriction or lack of ability to perform an activity in a manner or within the range considered normal for a human being. **2.** An impairment or defect of one or more organs or members.
   developmental d., loss of function brought on by prenatal and postnatal events in which the predominant disturbance is in the acquisition of cognitive, language, motor, or social skills; *e.g.,* mental retardation, autistic disorder, learning disorder, and attention-deficit hyperactivity disorder.
   learning d., a disorder in one or more of the basic cognitive and psychological processes involved in understanding or using written or spoken language; may be manifested in age-related impairment in the ability to read, write, spell, speak, or perform mathematical calculations.

di·sac·cha·ride (dī-sak′ă-rīd). A condensation product of two monosaccharides by elimination of water.

dis·ag·gre·ga·tion (dis′ag-grĕ-gā′shŭn). **1.** A breaking up into component parts. **2.** An inability to coordinate various sensations and failure to comprehend their mutual relations. [L. *dis-,* separating, + *ag- grego* (adg-), pp. *-gregatus,* to add to something]

dis·ar·tic·u·la·tion (dis-ar-tik-yū-lā′shŭn). Amputation of a limb through a joint, without cutting of bone. SYN exarticulation. [L. *dis-,* apart, + *articulus,* joint]

dis·as·so·ci·a·tion (dis′ă-sō-sē-ā′shŭn). SYN dissociation (1).

disc (disk). **1.** A round, flat plate; any approximately flat circular structure. **2.** SYN lamella (2).
   articular d., a plate or ring of fibrocartilage attached to the joint capsule and separating the articular surfaces of the bones for a varying distance, sometimes completely; it serves to adapt two articular surfaces that are not entirely congruent.
   intervertebral d., a disk interposed between the bodies of adjacent vertebrae. It is composed of an outer fibrous part (annulus fibrosus) that surrounds a central gelatinous mass (nucleus pulposus).

△**disc-.** SEE disco-.

disc·ec·to·my (dis-ek′tō-mē). Excision, in part or whole, of an intervertebral disk. SYN discotomy. [disco- + G. *ektomē,* excision]

dis·charge (dis′charj). **1.** That which is emitted

or evacuated, as an excretion or a secretion. **2.**
The activation or firing of a neuron.

dis·chro·na·tion (dis-krō-nā'shŭn). A disturbance in the consciousness of time. [L. *dis*-,
apart, + G. *chronos*, time]

dis·ci (dis'kī). Plural of discus.

dis·ci·form (dis'i-fōrm). Disk-shaped.

dis·cis·sion (di-sish'ŭn). **1.** Incision or cutting
through a part. **2.** OPHTHALMOLOGY Opening of the
capsule and breaking up of the cortex of the lens
with a needle knife or laser. [L. *di- scindo*, pp.
-*scissus*, to tear asunder]

dis·ci·tis (dis-kī'tis). Nonbacterial inflammation
of an intervertebral disk or disk space. SYN diski-
tis.

disco-, disc-. A disk; disk-shaped. [G. *diskos*]

dis·co·gen·ic (dis'kō-gen'ik). Denoting a disorder originating in or from an intervertebral disk.
[disco- + G. *genesis*, origin]

dis·coid (dis'koyd). **1.** Resembling a disk. **2.** DEN-
TISTRY An excavating or carving instrument hav-
ing a circular blade with a cutting edge around
the periphery. [disco- + G. *eidos*, appearance]

dis·cop·a·thy (dis-kop'ă-thē). Disease of a disk,
particularly of an invertebral disk. [disco- + G.
pathos, disease]

 traumatic d., an injury characterized by fissu-
ration, laceration or fragmentation of the disc or
surrounding ligaments, with or without displacement of fragments against spinal cord, nerve
roots, or ligaments.

dis·co·pla·cen·ta (dis-kō-pla-sen'tă). A placenta
of discoid shape.

dis·cor·dance (dis-kōr'dans). Dissociation of
two characteristics in the members of a sample
from a population; used as a measure of dependence. Cf. concordance.

dis·cot·o·my (dis-kot'ō-mē). SYN discectomy.
[disco- + G. *tomē*, incision]

dis·crete (dis-krēt'). Separate; distinct; not joined
to or incorporated with another; denoting especially certain lesions of the skin. [L. *dis- cerno*,
pp. -*cretus*, to separate]

dis·crim·i·na·tion (dis'krim-i-nā'shŭn). The capacity or act of distinguishing between different
things; the ability to perceive different things as
different, or to repond to them differently. [L.
discrimino, pp. -*atus*, to separate]

 right-left d., the process of identifying one side
of the body as distinct from the other.

dis·cus, pl. **dis·ci** (dis'kŭs, -kī) [NA]. SYN lamella
(2). [L. fr. G. *diskos*, a quoit, disk]

 d. ner'vi op'tici [NA], SYN optic *disk.*

dis·ease (di-zēz'). **1.** An interruption, cessation,
or disorder of body functions, systems, or organs.
SYN illness, morbus, sickness. **2.** A morbid entity
characterized usually by at least two of these
criteria: recognized etiologic agent(s), identifiable group of signs and symptoms, or consistent
anatomical alterations. SEE ALSO syndrome. **3.** Literally, dis-ease, the opposite of ease, when something is wrong with a bodily function. [Eng. *dis*-
priv. + ease]

 ABO hemolytic d. of the newborn, erythroblastosis fetalis due to maternal-fetal incompatibility with respect to an antigen of the ABO
blood group; the fetus possesses A or B antigen

which is lacking in the mother, and the mother
produces immune antibody which causes hemolysis of fetal erythrocytes.

 Acosta's d., SYN altitude *sickness.*

 Adams-Stokes d., SYN Adams-Stokes *syndrome.*

 Addison's d., SYN chronic adrenocortical *insufficiency.*

 akamushi d. (ak-kǎ-mū'shē), SYN tsutsugamushi d.

 Almeida's d., SYN paracoccidioidomycosis.

 Alzheimer's d., progressive mental deterioration manifested by loss of memory, ability to
calculate, and visual-spatial orientation; confusion; disorientation. Begins in late middle life and
results in death in 5–10 years. The brain is
atrophic; histologically, there is distortion of the
intracellular neurofibrils (neurofibrillary tangles)
and senile plaques composed of granular or filamentous argentophilic masses with an amyloid
core; the most common degenerative brain disorder. SYN Alzheimer's dementia, presenile dementia (2), dementia presenilis, primary senile dementia.

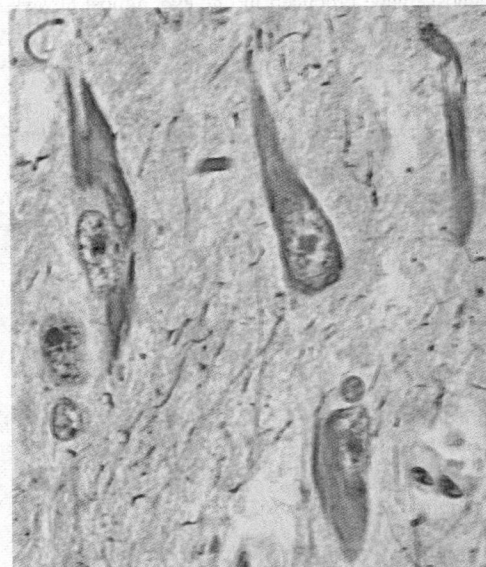

Alzheimer's disease: neurofibrillary tangles in the distended
cytoplasm of pyramidal neurons impregnated with silver

 aortoiliac occlusive d., obstruction of the abdominal aorta and its main branches by atherosclerosis.

 Aran-Duchenne d., SYN amyotrophic lateral
sclerosis.

 Australian X d., SYN Murray Valley *encephalitis.*

 autoimmune d., any disorder in which loss of
function or destruction of normal tissue arises
from humoral or cellular immune responses of
the individual to his own tissue constituents; may

be systemic, as systemic lupus erythematosus, or organ specific, as thyroiditis.

Ayerza's d., SYN Ayerza's *syndrome*.

Bamberger-Marie d., SYN hypertrophic pulmonary *osteoarthropathy*.

Bannister's d., SYN angioedema.

Barlow's d., SYN infantile *scurvy*.

Bayle's d., SYN paresis (2).

Bechterew's d., SYN *spondylitis* deformans.

Berger's d., SYN focal *glomerulonephritis*.

Bernhardt's d., SYN *meralgia* paraesthetica.

Besnier-Boeck-Schaumann d., SYN sarcoidosis.

Binswanger's d., one of the causes of multi-infarct dementia, in which there are many infarcts and lacunae in the white matter, with relative sparing of the cortex and basal ganglia. SYN Binswanger's encephalopathy.

Blocq's d., SYN astasia-abasia.

Blount's d., tibia vara; nonrachitic bowlegs in children.

Bornholm d., SYN epidemic *pleurodynia*. [*Bornholm,* Danish island in the Baltic where the d. was first described]

Bowen's d., a form of intraepidermal carcinoma characterized by the development of pinkish or brownish papules covered with a thickened horny layer; microscopically, there is dyskeratosis with large round epidermal cells with large nuclei and pale-staining cytoplasm which are scattered through all levels of the epidermis.

brancher glycogen storage d., type of glycogen storage d., due to deficiency of amylo-1,4-1,6-transglucosidase (brancher enzyme).

Brill's d., SYN Brill-Zinsser d.

Brill-Zinsser d., an endogenous reinfection in persons who previously had epidemic typhus fever; it is mild and may be mistaken for endemic (murine) typhus. SYN Brill's d., recrudescent typhus.

Briquet's d., hysterical neurosis, conversion type.

bronzed d., SYN bronze *diabetes*. SEE hemochromatosis.

Buerger's d., SYN *thromboangiitis* obliterans.

Busse-Buschke d., SYN cryptococcosis.

caisson d. (kā'son), SYN decompression *sickness.* [Fr. *caisson* (fr. *caisse,* a chest) a watertight box or cylinder containing air under high pressure used in sinking structural pilings underwater]

cat-scratch d., a chronic benign adenopathy, especially in children and young adults, commonly associated with a recent cat scratch or bite and caused by bacteria including *Rochalimaea henselae* and *Afipia felis;* the lymphadenopathy usually resolves spontaneously within a period of several months, but complications involving central nervous system, liver, spleen, lung, and skin have been seen. SYN benign inoculation lymphoreticulosis, benign inoculation reticulosis, cat-scratch fever, regional granulomatous lymphadenitis.

celiac d., a disease occurring in children and adults characterized by sensitivity to gluten, with chronic inflammation and atrophy of the mucosa of the upper small intestine; manifestations include diarrhea, malabsorption, steatorrhea, and nutritional and vitamin deficiencies. SYN gluten enteropathy.

Chagas-Cruz d., SYN South American *trypanosomiasis*.

Charcot-Marie-Tooth d., SYN peroneal muscular *atrophy*.

Charcot's d., SYN amyotrophic lateral *sclerosis*.

Christmas d., SYN *hemophilia* B.

chronic granulomatous d., a congenital defect in the killing of phagocytosed bacteria by polymorphonuclear leukocytes. As a result there is an increased susceptibility to severe infection.

chronic obstructive pulmonary d. (COPD), general term used for those diseases with permanent or temporary narrowing of small bronchi, in which forced expiratory flow is slowed, especially when no etiologic or other more specific term can be applied.

collagen d.'s, collagen-vascular d.'s, a group of generalized d.'s affecting connective tissue and frequently characterized by fibrinoid necrosis or vasculitis; in some collagen d.'s, auto-immunization, particularly antinuclear antibodies, has been shown and circulating immune complexes are found. The term is not entirely acceptable because there is no evidence that collagen is primarily involved.

communicable d., any d. that is transmissible by infection or contagion directly or through the agency of a vector.

contagious d., an infectious d. transmissible by direct or indirect contact; now used synonymously with communicable d.

Cori's d., SYN type 3 *glycogenosis*.

Creutzfeldt-Jakob d., a type of subacute spongiform encephalopathy caused by a transmissible agent termed a prion. Affects adults, especially older adults, and is characterized by progressive dementia, myoclonic jerks, ataxia, and dysarthria; rapidly progressive and invariably fatal, usually within one year of onset. Pathologically, nerve cell degeneration and loss with associated astroglial proliferation are confined primarily to the cerebral and cerebellar cortices.

Crigler-Najjar d., SYN Crigler-Najjar *syndrome*.

Crohn's d., SYN regional *enteritis*.

Cruveilhier's d., SYN amyotrophic lateral *sclerosis*.

Cushing's d., adrenal hyperplasia (Cushing's syndrome) caused by an ACTH-secreting basophil adenoma of the pituitary.

cystic d. of the breast, fibrocystic condition of the breasts.

cytomegalic inclusion d., the presence of inclusion bodies within the cytoplasm and nuclei of enlarged cells of various organs of newborn infants dying with jaundice, hepatomegaly, splenomegaly, purpura, thrombocytopenia, and fever; the condition also occurs, at all ages, as a complication of other d.'s in which immune mechanisms are severely depressed, and has been found incidentally in salivary gland epithelium, apparently as a localized or mild infection (salivary gland virus d.). SYN cytomegalovirus d., inclusion body d.

cytomegalovirus d., SYN cytomegalic inclusion d.

Darling's d., SYN histoplasmosis.

deficiency d., any d. resulting from undernutrition or an inadequacy of calories, proteins, essential amino acids, fatty acids, vitamins, or trace minerals.

degenerative joint d., SYN osteoarthritis.

Dejerine-Sottas d., a familial type of demyelinating sensorimotor polyneuropathy that begins in early childhood and is slowly progressive; clinically characterized by foot pain and paresthesias, followed by symmetrical weakness and wasting of the distal limbs; one of the causes of stork legs; patients are wheelchair-bound at an early age; peripheral nerves are palpably enlarged and non-tender; pathologically, onion bulb formation is seen in the nerves: whorls of overlapping, intertwined Schwann cell processes that encircle bare axons; usually autosomal recessive inheritance. SYN progressive hypertrophic polyneuropathy.

demyelinating d., generic term for a group of d.'s, of unknown cause, in which there is extensive loss of the myelin in the central nervous system, as in multiple sclerosis.

de Quervain's d., fibrosis of the sheath of a tendon of the thumb.

Devic's d., SYN neuromyelitis optica.

Dubois' d., SYN Dubois' abscesses, under abscess.

Duchenne-Aran d., SYN amyotrophic lateral sclerosis.

Duhring's d., SYN dermatitis herpetiformis.

Ebstein's d., SYN Ebstein's anomaly.

endemic d., continued prevalence of a d. in a specific population or area. SEE ALSO endemic.

epidemic d., marked increase in prevalence of a d. in a specific population or area, usually with an environmental cause, such as an infectious or toxic agent.

extramammary Paget d., an intraepidermal form of mucinous adenocarcinoma, most commonly in the anogenital region. SYN Paget's d. (3).

extrapyramidal d., a general term for a number of disorders caused by abnormalities of the basal ganglia or certain brain stem or thalamic nuclei; characterized by motor deficits, loss of postural reflexes, bradykinesia, tremor, rigidity, and various involuntary movements.

fifth d., SYN erythema infectiosum. [after scarlatina, morbilli, rubella, and fourth d.]

Filatov-Dukes' d., an exanthem-producing infectious disease of childhood of unknown etiology. SYN fourth d., scarlatinoid (2).

Fothergill's d., (1) SYN trigeminal neuralgia. (2) SYN anginose scarlatina.

fourth d., SYN Filatov-Dukes' d.

Freiberg's d., avascular necrosis affecting the second metatarsal head; most commonly seen in adolescents. SEE ALSO avascular necrosis.

functional d., SYN functional disorder.

gastroesophageal reflux d. (GERD), a syndrome of chronic or recurrent epigastric or retro-sternal pain, accompanied by varying degrees of belching, nausea, cough, or hoarseness, due to reflux of acid gastric juice into the lower esophagus; results from malfunction of the lower esophageal sphincter (LES) and disordered gastric motility; may lead to peptic esophagitis, ulceration, stricture, or Barrett's esophagus.

Gaucher's d., a lysosomal storage d. resulting from glycocerebroside accumulation due to a genetic deficiency of glucocerebrosidase; may occur in adults but occurs most severely in infants; marked by hepatosplenomegaly, regression of neurological maturation, and characteristic histiocytes (Gaucher cells) in the viscera.

Gierke's d., SYN type 1 glycogenosis.

Glanzmann's d., SYN Glanzmann's thrombasthenia.

Goldflam d., SYN myasthenia gravis.

graft versus host d., an incompatibility reaction (which may be fatal) in a subject (host) of low immunological competence (deficient lymphoid tissue) who has been the recipient of immunologically competent lymphoid tissue from a donor who lacks at least one antigen possessed by the recipient host; the reaction, or disease, is the result of action of the transplanted cells against those host tissues that possess the antigen not possessed by the donor.

Graves' d., (1) toxic goiter characterized by diffuse hyperplasia of the thyroid gland, a form of hyperthyroidism; exophthalmos is a common, but not invariable, concomitant; (2) thyroid dysfunction and all or any of its clinical associations; (3) an organ-specific autoimmune disease of the thyroid gland. SEE thyrotoxicosis, Hashimoto's thyroiditis, goiter, myxedema.

Hamman's d., SYN Hamman's syndrome.

hand-foot-and-mouth d., an exanthematous eruption of small, pearl-gray vesicles of the fingers, toes, palms, and soles, accompanied by painful vesicles and ulceration of the buccal mucous membrane and the tongue and by slight fever; the d. lasts 4 to 7 days, and is usually caused by Coxsackie virus type A-16, but other types have been identified.

Hand-Schüller-Christian d., the chronic disseminated form of Langerhans cell histiocytosis. The classic triad of signs consists of diabetes insipidus, exopthalmus, and bony lesions composed of histiocytes.

Hansen's d., chronic granulomatous infection caused by Mycobacterium leprae (Hansen's bacillus) and affecting various parts of the body including the skin. SYN leprosy (2).

Hartnup d. [MIM*234500], a congenital metabolic disorder consisting of aminoaciduria due to a defect in renal tubular absorption of neutral α-amino acids and urinary excretion of tryptophan derivatives, because defective intestinal absorption leads to bacterial degradation of unabsorbed tryptophan in the gut; characterized by a pellagra-like, light-sensitive skin rash with temporary cerebellar ataxia. SYN Hartnup syndrome.

Hashimoto's d., SYN Hashimoto's thyroiditis.

heavy chain d., a term used for a group of d.'s, the paraproteinemias, characterized by production of homogeneous immunoglobulins or fragments, and associated with malignant disorders of the plasmacytic and lymphoid cell series.

hemolytic d. of newborn, SYN *erythroblastosis* fetalis.

hemorrhagic d. of the newborn, a syndrome characterized by spontaneous internal or external bleeding accompanied by hypoprothrombinemia, slightly decreased platelets, and markedly elevated bleeding and clotting times, usually occurring between the third and sixth days of life and effectively treated with vitamin K.

Hirschsprung's d., SYN congenital *megacolon.*

Hodgkin's d., a d. marked by chronic enlargement of the lymph nodes, often local at the onset and later generalized, together with enlargement of the spleen and often of the liver, no pronounced leukocytosis, and commonly anemia and continuous or remittent (Pel-Ebstein) fever; considered to be a malignant neoplasm of lymphoid cells of uncertain origin (Reed-Sternberg cells), associated with inflammatory infiltration of lymphocytes and eosinophilic leukocytes and fibrosis; can be classified into lymphocytic predominant, nodular sclerosing, mixed cellularity, and lymphocytic depletion type.

Hodgson's d., dilation of the arch of the aorta associated with insufficiency of the aortic valve.

hookworm d., SEE ancylostomiasis, necatoriasis.

Huntington's d. [MIM*143100], SYN Huntington's *chorea.*

Hutchinson-Gilford d., SYN progeria.

hydatid d., infection with larvae of the tapeworm *Echinococcus.*

hyperendemic d. (hī′per-en-dem′ik), a d. that is constantly present at a high incidence and/or prevalence rate and affects all age groups equally.

Iceland d., SYN epidemic *neuromyasthenia.*

immune complex d., an immunologic category of d.'s evoked by the deposition of antigen-antibody or antigen-antibody-complement complexes on cell surfaces, with subsequent development of vasculitis; nephritis is common. Most of the connective tissue d.'s, may belong in this immunologic category; immune complex d.'s can also occur during a variety of d.'s of known etiology, such as subacute bacterial endocarditis. SEE ALSO autoimmune d.

inclusion body d., SYN cytomegalic inclusion d.

industrial d., a morbid condition resulting from exposure to an agent discharged by a commercial enterprise into the environment. Cf. occupational d.

infectious d., infective d., a d. resulting from the presence and activity of a microbial agent.

interstitial d., a d. occurring chiefly in the connective-tissue framework of an organ, the parenchyma suffering secondarily.

iron-storage d., the storage of excess iron in the parenchyma of many organs, as in idiopathic hemochromatosis or transfusion hemosiderosis.

Jensen's d., SYN *retinochoroiditis* juxtapapillaris.

jumping d., jumper d., one of the pathological startle syndromes found in isolated parts of the world, characterized by greatly exaggerated responses, such as jumping, flinging the arms and yelling, to minimal stimuli.

Kimmelstiel-Wilson d., SYN Kimmelstiel-Wilson *syndrome.*

Kussmaul's d., SYN *polyarteritis* nodosa.

Larson-Johansson d., inflammation or partial avulsion of the lower pole of the patella due to traction forces. SEE ALSO Osgood-Schlatter d.

Legg-Calvé-Perthes d., Legg's d., Legg-Perthes d., epiphysial aseptic necrosis of the upper end of the femur.

Legionnaire's d., an acute infectious d., caused by *Legionella pneumophila,* with prodromal influenza-like symptoms and a rapidly rising high fever, followed by severe pneumonia and production of usually nonpurulent sputum, mental confusion, hepatic fatty changes, and renal tubular degeneration. It has a high case-fatality rate. Acquired from water systems rather than person to person. [American *Legion* convention, 1976, at which many delegates were so affected]

Leiner's d., SYN *erythroderma* desquamativum.

Lou Gehrig's d., SYN amyotrophic lateral *sclerosis.*

Lutz-Splendore-Almeida d., SYN paracoccidioidomycosis.

⊞Lyme d., an inflammatory disorder typically occurring during the summer months and caused by *Borrelia burgdorferi,* a spirochete transmitted by *Ixodes dammini* in the eastern U.S. and *I. pacificus* in the western U.S.; the characteristic skin lesion, erythema chronicum migrans, usually is preceded or accompanied by fever, malaise, fatigue, headache, and stiff neck; neurologic or cardiac manifestations, or arthritis (Lyme arthritis) may occur weeks to months later. Dogs, horses, and cattle are also affected. [Lyme, CT, where first observed]

lysosomal d., a d. due to inadequate functioning of a lysosomal enzyme; most such d.'s are associated with a storage d.

Manson's d., SYN *schistosomiasis* mansoni.

Marburg d., infection with an unusual rhabdovirus composed of RNA and lipid, tentatively assigned to the family of Filoviridae. Virus is "pantropic" and affects most organ systems. The disease is characterized by a prominent rash and hemorrhages in many organs and is often fatal. First seen among laboratory workers in Marburg, Germany, exposed to African green monkeys. Some person-to-person spread has been observed. Attempts to isolate virus should be done only in high-security laboratories. SYN Marburg virus d.

Marburg virus d., SYN Marburg d.

Marchiafava-Bignami d., a disorder characterized by demyelination of the corpus callosum and cortical laminar necrosis involving the frontal and temporal lobes. Occurs predominantly in chronic alcoholics, particularly wine drinkers.

McArdle's d., SYN type 5 *glycogenosis.*

McArdle-Schmid-Pearson d., SYN type 5 *glycogenosis.*

Ménétrier's d., gastric mucosal hyperplasia, either mucoid or glandular; the latter type may be associated with the Zollinger-Ellison syndrome.

Ménière's d., an affection characterized clinically by vertigo, nausea, vomiting, tinnitus, and

di

progressive deafness due to swelling of the endo-lymphatic duct. SYN auditory vertigo, labyrinthine vertigo.

mental d., SEE mental *illness*.

Minamata d., a neurologic disorder caused by methyl mercury intoxication; first described in the inhabitants of Minamata Bay, Japan, resulting from their eating fish contaminated with mercury industrial waste. Characterized by peripheral sensory loss, tremors, dysarthria, ataxia, and both hearing and visual loss.

Mitchell's d., SYN erythromelalgia.

mixed connective-tissue d., d. with overlapping features of various systemic connective-tissue d.'s and with serum antibodies to nuclear ribonucleoprotein.

molecular d., a d. in which the manifestations are due to alterations in molecular structure and function.

Mondor's d., thrombophlebitis of the thoraco-epigastric vein of the breast and chest wall.

Monge's d., SYN chronic mountain *sickness*.

Morgagni's d., SYN Adams-Stokes *syndrome*.

Morvan's d., SYN syringomyelia.

motor neuron d., a general term including progressive spinal muscular atrophy (infantile, juvenile, and adult), amyotrophic lateral sclerosis, progressive bulbar paralysis, and primary lateral sclerosis; frequently a familial d.

notifiable d., a d. that, by statutory requirements, must be reported to public health or veterinary authorities. SYN reportable d.

occupational d., a morbid condition resulting from exposure to an agent during the usual performance of one's occupation. Cf. industrial d.

Oppenheim's d., SYN amyotonia congenita (1).

organic d., a d. in which there are anatomical or pathophysiological changes in some bodily tissue or organ, in contrast to a disorder of psychogenic origin.

orphan d., a d. for which no treatment has been developed because of its rarity. SEE ALSO orphan *products*, under *product*.

Osgood-Schlatter d., epiphysial aseptic necrosis of the tibial tubercle.

Osler's d., (1) SYN polycythemia vera.

Osler-Vaquez d., SYN polycythemia vera.

Otto's d., a d. characterized by an inward bulging of the acetabulum into the pelvic cavity, resulting from arthritis of the hip joints, usually due to rheumatoid arthritis.

Paget's d., (1) a generalized skeletal disease, frequently familial, of older persons in which bone resorption and formation are both increased, leading to thickening and softening of bones (*e.g.,* the skull), and bending of weight-bearing bones; SYN osteitis deformans. **(2)** a d. of elderly women, characterized by an infiltrated, somewhat eczematous lesion surrounding and involving the nipple and areola, and associated with subjacent intraductal cancer of the breast and infiltration of the lower epidermis by malignant cells; **(3)** SYN extramammary Paget d.

paper mill worker's d., extrinsic allergic alveolitis caused by moldy wood pulp containing spores of *Alternaria* fungi.

Parkinson's d., SYN parkinsonism (1).

Pel-Ebstein d., SYN Pel-Ebstein *fever*.

Pellegrini's d., a calcific density in the medial collateral ligament and/or bony growth at the internal condyle of the femur.

pelvic inflammatory d. (PID), acute or chronic inflammation in the organs of the female pelvic cavity, particular suppurative lesions of the upper genital tract; most commonly due to infection by *Chlamydia trachomatis* or *Neisseria gonorrhoeae*, which have ascended into the uterus, uterine tubes, or ovaries from the lower genital tract as a result of childbirth or surgical procedures. The chief symptoms are pelvic pain and fever; complications include abscess formation and generalized peritonitis. Scarring may cause tubal infertility and raise the risk of ectopic pregnancy.

periodic d., any condition or d. in which episodes tend to recur at regular intervals; many such cases are manifestations of familial Mediterranean fever; the cause of the periodicity is usually unknown.

Peyronie's d., a d. of unknown cause in which plaques of dense fibrous tissue surround the corpus cavernosum of the penis, causing deformity and painful erection; sometimes associated with Dupuytren's contracture.

pink d., SYN acrodynia (2).

polycystic d. of kidneys, SYN polycystic *kidney*.

Pompe's d., SYN type 2 *glycogenosis*.

Pott's d., SYN tuberculous *spondylitis*.

primary d., a d. that arises spontaneously and is not associated with or caused by a previous disease, injury, or event, but which may lead to a secondary d.

pulseless d., SYN Takayasu's *arteritis*.

Raynaud's d., SYN Raynaud's *syndrome*.

reactive airways d., SYN asthma.

Recklinghausen's d. of bone, SYN osteitis fibrosa cystica.

Reiter's d., SYN Reiter's *syndrome*.

reportable d., SYN notifiable d.

rheumatic heart d., d. of the heart resulting from rheumatic fever, chiefly manifested by abnormalities of the valves.

Roger's d., a congenital cardiac anomaly consisting of a small, isolated, asymptomatic defect of the interventricular septum.

Rokitansky's d., SYN acute yellow atrophy of the liver.

salivary gland d., disorder of salivary glands; *i.e.,* Sjögren's *syndrome*.

Scheuermann's d., epiphysial aseptic necrosis of vertebral bodies.

Schilder's d., term used to describe at least two separate disorders described by Schilder: 1) Diffuse sclerosis or encephalitis periaxialis diffusa; a nonfamilial disorder affecting primarily children and young adults and characterized by progressive dementia, visual disturbances, deafness, pseudobulbar palsy, and hemiplegia or quadriplegia. 2) The leukodystrophies. SYN encephalitis periaxialis diffusa.

secondary d., (1) a d. that follows and results from an earlier disease, injury, or event; **(2)** a wasting disorder that follows successful transplantation of bone marrow into a lethally irradiated host; frequently severe and usually associated with fever, anorexia, diarrhea, dermatitis, and desquamation. SEE ALSO graft versus host d.

serum d., SYN serum *sickness.*

Sever's d., a traction-type injury or osteochondrosis of the calcaneal apophysis seen in young adolescents. SEE apophysitis. SEE ALSO Osgood-Schlatter d., Larson-Johansson d.

sexually transmitted d. (STD), any contagious d. acquired during sexual contact; *e.g.,* syphilis, gonorrhea, chancroid, genital warts, AIDS. SYN venereal d.

sickle cell d., SYN sickle cell *anemia.*

sickle cell C d. [MIM*141900], a d. resulting from abnormal sickle-shaped erythrocytes (containing hemoglobin C and S) which appear in response to a lowering of the partial pressure of oxygen; characterized by anemia, crises due to hemolysis or vascular occlusion, chronic leg ulcers and bone deformities, and infarcts of bone or of the spleen.

Simmonds' d., anterior pituitary insufficiency due to trauma, vascular lesions, or tumors; usually developing postpartum as a result of pituitary necrosis caused by ischemia during a hypotensive episode during delivery; characterized clinically by asthenia, loss of weight and body hair, arterial hypotension, and manifestations of thyroid, adrenal, and gonadal hypofunction. SYN hypophysial cachexia, pituitary cachexia.

sixth d., SYN *exanthema* subitum.

slow virus d., a d. that follows a slow, progressive course spanning months to years, frequently involving the central nervous system, and ultimately leading to death, such as subacute sclerosing panencephalitis, seemingly caused by the measles virus; spongiform encephalopathies including kuru of humans and scrapie of sheep may also be classified under slow virus d. but their respective etiologic agents have not been adequately characterized.

Still's d., a form of juvenile chronic arthritis (formerly juvenile rheumatoid arthritis) characterized by high fever and signs of systemic illness that can exist for months before the onset of arthritis.

storage d., any accumulation of a specific substance within tissues, generally because of congenital deficiency of an enzyme necessary for further metabolism of the substance; *e.g.,* glycogen-storage d.'s.

Swift's d., SYN acrodynia (2).

Takayasu's d., SYN Takayasu's *arteritis.*

Tay-Sachs d., a lysosomal storage disease, resulting from hexosaminidase A deficiency. The monosialoganglioside is stored in central and peripheral neuronal cells. Infants present with hyperacusis and irritability, hypotonia, and failure to develop motor skills. Blindness with macular cherry red spots and seizures are evident in the first year.

third d., SYN rubella.

thyrocardiac d., heart d. resulting from hyperthyroidism.

tropical d.'s, infectious and parasitic d.'s endemic in tropical and subtropical zones, including Chagas' disease, leishmaniasis, leprosy, malaria, onchocerciasis, schistosomiasis, sleeping sickness, yellow fever, and others; often water- or insect-borne.

tsutsugamushi d. (sū′sū-gă-mū′shē), an acute infectious disease, caused by *Rickettsia tsutsugamushi* and transmitted by *Trombicula akamushi* and *T. deliensis*, that occurs in harvesters of hemp in some parts of Japan; characterized by fever, painful swelling of the lymphatic glands, a small blackish scab on the genitals, neck, or axilla, and an eruption of large dark red papules. SYN akamushi d., mite typhus, scrub typhus, tropical typhus.

vagabond's d., SYN parasitic *melanoderma.*

vagrant's d., SYN parasitic *melanoderma.*

venereal d., SYN sexually transmitted d.

veno-occlusive d. of the liver, obliterating endophlebitis of small hepatic vein radicles, described in Jamaican children, associated with ingestion of toxic plant substances in bush tea; causes ascites, which may progress to cirrhosis.

Vincent's d., SYN necrotizing ulcerative *gingivitis.*

von Gierke's d., SYN type 1 *glycogenosis.*

von Willebrand's d. [MIM*193400], a hereditary hemorrhagic diathesis characterized by tendency to bleed primarily from mucous membranes, prolonged bleeding time, normal platelet count, normal clot retraction, partial and variable deficiency of factor VIIIR, and possibly a morphologic defect of platelets.

Weil's d., a form of leptospirosis generally caused by *Leptospira interrogans* serogroup *icterohaemorrhagiae*, believed to be acquired by contact with the urine of infected rats; characterized clinically by fever, jaundice, muscular pains, conjunctival congestion, and albuminuria; agglutinins regularly appear in the serum.

Wernicke's d., SYN Wernicke's *syndrome.*

Westphal-Strümpell d., SYN Wilson's d. (1).

Wilson's d., (1) hereditary disorder (autosomal recessive) characterized by hepatic cirrhosis, degeneration in the basal ganglia of the brain, and deposition of green pigment in the periphery of the cornea; plasma levels of ceruloplasmin and copper are decreased, urinary excretion of copper is increased, and the amounts of copper in the liver, brain, kidneys, and lenticular nucleus are unusually high. SYN hepatolenticular degeneration (2), Westphal-Strümpell d. SEE ALSO Kayser-Fleischer *ring.* [S.A.K. Wilson] **(2)** SYN exfoliative *dermatitis.* [Sir W.J.E. Wilson]

dis·en·gage·ment (dis-en-gāj′ment). **1.** The act of setting free or extricating; in childbirth, the emergence of the head from the vulva. **2.** Ascent of the presenting part from the pelvis after the inlet has been negotiated. [Fr.]

dis·e·qui·lib·ri·um (dis-ē′kwi-lib′rē-ŭm). A disturbance or absence of equilibrium.

linkage d., a state involving two loci in which the probability of a joint gamete is not equal to the product of the probabilities of the constituent genes. The difference between these quantities is the increase of the d.; there are many causes of the d.

disfluency. SYN dysfluency.

dis•ger•mi•no•ma (dis-jer-mi-nō'mă). SYN dysgerminoma.

dis•im•pac•tion (dis'im-pak'shŭn). **1.** Separation of impaction in a fractured bone. **2.** Removal of impacted feces, usually manually.

dis•in•fect (dis-in-fekt'). To destroy pathogenic microorganisms in or on any substance or to inhibit their growth and vital activity.

dis•in•fec•tant (dis-in-fek'tănt). **1.** Capable of destroying pathogenic microorganisms or inhibiting their growth. **2.** An agent that possesses this property.

dis•in•fec•tion (dis-in-fek'shŭn). Destruction of pathogenic microorganisms or their toxins or vectors by direct exposure to chemical or physical agents.

  concurrent d., application of disinfective measures as soon as possible after discharge of infectious material from the body of an infected person, or after soiling of articles with such infectious discharges.

  terminal d., application of disinfective measures after the patient has been removed, *e.g.,* by death, or has ceased to be a source of infection.

dis•in•te•gra•tion (dis-in-tĕ-grā'shŭn). **1.** Loss or separation of the component parts of a substance, as in catabolism or decay. **2.** Disorganization of psychic and behavioral processes. [dis- + L. *integer,* whole, intact]

dis•junc•tion (dis-jŭnk'shŭn). The normal separation of pairs of chromosomes at the anaphase stage of meiosis I or II. [dis- + L. *junctio,* a joining, fr. *jungo,* pp. *junctum,* to join]

disk. 1. SYN lamella (2). **2.** In dentistry, a circular piece of thin paper or other material, coated with an abrasive substance, used for cutting and polishing teeth and fillings. **3.** SEE disc. [L. *discus;* G. *diskos,* a quoit, disk]

  blood d., SYN platelet.

  choked d., SYN papilledema.

  ciliary d., SYN orbiculus ciliaris.

  germinal d., germ d., the point in a teloleci-thal ovum where the embryo begins to be formed.

  herniated d., protrusion of a degenerated or fragmented intervertebral d. into the intervertebral foramen with potential compression of a nerve root or into the spinal canal with potential compression of the cauda equina in the lumbar region or the spinal cord at higher levels. SYN protruded d., ruptured d.

  intercalated d., a specialized intercellular attachment of cardiac muscle comprising gap junctions, fascia adherens, and occasionally desmosomes.

  optic d., an oval area of the ocular fundus devoid of light receptors where the axons of the retinal ganglion cell converge to form the optic nerve head. SYN discus nervi optici [NA], blind spot (3), optic papilla.

  protruded d., SYN herniated d.

  ruptured d., SYN herniated d.

dis•ki•tis (dis-kī'tis). SYN discitis.

△**disko-.** SEE disco-.

dis•lo•cate (dis'lō-kāt). To luxate; to put out of joint.

⊞**dis•lo•ca•tion** (dis-lō-kā'shŭn). Displacement of an organ or any part; specifically a disturbance or

disarrangement of the normal relation of the bones entering into the formation of a joint. SYN luxation (1). [L. *dislocatio,* fr. *dis-,* apart, + *locatio,* a placing]

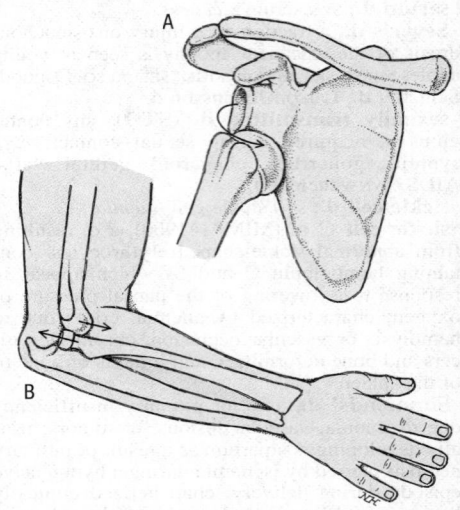

dislocations: (A) subglenoid dislocation of shoulder, (B) dislocation of elbow

  closed d., a d. not complicated by an external wound. SYN simple d.

  compound d., SYN open d.

  open d., a d. complicated by a wound opening from the surface down to the affected joint. SYN compound d.

  simple d., SYN closed d.

dis•mem•ber (dis-mem'ber). To amputate an arm or leg.

dis•mu•tase (dis'myū-tās). Generic name for enzymes catalyzing the reaction of two identical molecules to produce two molecules in differing states of oxidation or phosphorylation.

dis•or•der (dis-ōr'der). A disturbance of function, structure, or both, resulting from a genetic or embryologic failure in development or from exogenous factors such as poison, trauma, or disease.

  adjustment d.'s, (1) a class of mental and behavioral d.'s in which the development of symptoms is related to the presence of some environmental stressor or life event and is expected to remit when the stress ceases; **(2)** a d. whose essential feature is a maladaptive reaction to an identifiable psychological stress, or stressors, that occurs within weeks of the onset of the stressors and persists for up to six months.

  affective d.'s, a class of mental d.'s characterized by a disturbance in mood.

  antisocial personality d., a personality d. characterized by a history of continuous and chronic antisocial behavior with disregard for and violation of the rights of others, beginning before the age of 15; early childhood signs include chronic lying, stealing, fighting, and truancy; in adolescence there may be unusually early or aggressive sexual behavior, excessive drinking, and use of illicit drugs, such behavior continuing in adulthood.

anxiety d.'s, a category of interrelated mental illnesses involving anxiety reactions in response to stress. The types include: 1) generalized anxiety, by far the most prevalent condition, which strikes slightly more females than males, mostly in the 20–35 age group; 2) panic d., in which a person suffers repeated panic attacks. Some 2–5 percent of Americans are subject to this ailment, about twice as many women as men; 3) obsessive-compulsive d., afflicting 2–3 percent of the U.S. population. About two-thirds of these patients go on to experience a major depressive episode; 4) posttraumatic stress disorder, most frequent among combat veterans or survivors of major physical trauma; and 5) the phobias (*e.g.,* fear of snakes, crowds, confinement, heights, etc.), which on a minor scale affect about one in eight people in the U.S. Drugs that have proven effective against anxiety d.'s are beta-blockers, which act on adrenaline receptors; anxiolytics; antidepressants; and serotonergic drugs. Regular exercise has also proved beneficial.

attention deficit d., a d. of attention and impulse control with specific DSM criteria, appearing in childhood and sometimes persisting to adulthood. Hyperactivity may be a feature, but is not necessary for the diagnosis. SEE ALSO attention deficit hyperactivity d.

attention deficit hyperactivity d., a disorder of childhood and adolescence manifested at home, in school, and in social situations by developmentally inappropriate degrees of inattention, impulsiveness, and hyperactivity; also called hyperactivity or hyperactive child syndrome. SEE ALSO attention deficit d.

behavior d., general term used to denote mental illness or psychological dysfunction, specifically those mental, emotional, or behavioral subclasses for which organic correlates do not exist. SEE ALSO antisocial personality d.

bipolar d., an affective d. characterized by the occurrence of alternating periods of euphoria (mania) and depression. SYN manic-depressive psychosis.

borderline personality d., a mental d. in which the symptoms are not continually psychotic yet are not strictly neurotic: may include impulsivity and unpredictability, unstable interpersonal relationships, inappropriate or uncontrolled anger, identity disturbances, rapid shifts of mood, suicidal acts, self-mutilations, job and marital instability, chronic feelings of emptiness or boredom, and intolerance of being alone.

character d., a term referring to a group of behavioral d.'s, now replaced by a more general term, personality d., of which character d.'s are now a subclass.

communication d., any impairment of hearing, language, or speech that interferes with the ability to transmit or receive linguistic information. SYN communicative d.

communicative d., SYN communication d.

conduct d., a mental d. of childhood or adolescence characterized by a persistent pattern of violating societal norms and the rights of others; children with the d. may exhibit physical aggression, cruelty to animals, vandalism and robbery, along with truancy, cheating, and lying. SEE borderline personality d.

conversion d., a mental d. in which an unconscious emotional conflict is expressed as an alteration or loss of physical functioning, usually controlled by the voluntary nervous system.

cumulative trauma d.'s (CTD), chronic d.'s involving tendon, muscle, joint, and nerve damage, often resulting from work-related physical activities. CTDs, including repetitive motion d.'s and carpal tunnel syndrome, result when the body is subjected to direct pressure, vibration, or repetitive movements for prolonged periods.

cyclothymic d., an affective d. characterized by mood swings including periods of hypomania and depression; a form of depressive disorder.

dysthymic d., a chronic disturbance of mood characterized by mild depression or loss of interest in usual activities. SEE depression.

emotional d., SEE mental *illness*, behavior d.

functional d., a physical d. with no known or detectable organic basis to explain the symptoms. SEE behavior d., neurosis. SYN functional disease.

generalized anxiety d., chronic, repeated episodes of anxiety or dread accompanied by autonomic changes. SEE ALSO anxiety.

identity d., a mental d. of childhood or adolescence in which one suffers severe distress regarding one's ability to reconcile aspects of the self into a coherent acceptable sense of self.

immunoproliferative d.'s, d.'s in which there is a continuing proliferation of cells of the immunocyte complex associated with autoallergic disturbances and immunoglobulin abnormalities, such as in chronic lymphocytic leukemia, "macroglobulinemias," and multiple myeloma.

impulse control d., a class of mental d.'s characterized by failure to resist an impulse to perform some act harmful to oneself or to others; includes pathological gambling, pedophilia, kleptomania, pyromania, trichotillomania, intermittent and isolated explosive d.'s.

intermittent explosive d., an uncommon disorder that begins in early childhood, characterized by repeated acts of violent, aggressive behavior in otherwise normal persons that is markedly out of proportion to the event that provokes it.

isolated explosive d., a d. of impulse control characterized by a single episode of failure to resist a violent, externally directed act that has a harmful impact on others.

mental d., a psychological syndrome or behavioral pattern that is associated with either subjective distress or objective impairment. SEE ALSO mental *illness*, behavior d.

neuropsychologic d., a disturbance of mental function due to brain trauma, associated with one or more of the following: neurocognitive, psychotic, neurotic, behavioral, or psychophysiologic manifestations, or mental impairment. SEE ALSO mental *illness*.

obsessive-compulsive d., a type of anxiety d. whose essential feature is recurrent obsessions, persistent, intrusive ideas, thoughts, impulses or images, or compulsions (repetitive, purposeful, and intentional behaviors performed in response to an obsession) sufficiently severe to cause marked distress, be time-consuming, or interfere significantly with the individual's normal routine, occupational functioning, or usual social activities or relationships with others.
oppositional d., a mental d. of childhood or adolescence marked by a pattern of disobedient, negativistic, and provocative opposition to authority figures.
organic mental d., a psychological, cognitive, or behavioral abnormality associated with transient or permanent dysfunction of the brain, usually characterized by the presence of an organic mental syndrome.
overanxious d., a mental d. of childhood or adolescence marked by excessive worrying and fearful behavior not related specifically to separation or due to recent stress.
panic d., recurrent panic attacks that occur unpredictably. SEE generalized anxiety d.
personality d., general term for a group of behavioral d.'s characterized by usually lifelong, ingrained, maladaptive patterns of deviant behavior, life style, and social adjustment that are different in quality from psychotic and neurotic symptoms; former designations for individuals with these personality d.'s were psychopath and sociopath. SEE ALSO antisocial personality d.
pervasive developmental d., a class of mental disorders of infancy, childhood, or adolescence characterized by distortions in the development of the multiple basic psychological functions involved in the development of social skills and language.
posttraumatic stress d., development of characteristic symptoms following a psychologically traumatic event that is generally outside the range of usual human experience; symptoms include numbed responsiveness to environmental stimuli, a variety of autonomic and cognitive dysfunctions, and dysphoria.
psychogenic pain d., a d. in which the principal complaint is pain that is out of proportion to objective findings and that is related to psychological factors.
psychosomatic d., psychophysiologic d., a d. characterized by physical symptoms of psychic origin, usually involving a single organ system innervated by the autonomic nervous system; physiological and organic changes stem from a sustained disturbance.
regulatory d., a d. that is first evident in infancy and early childhood and is characterized by a distinct behavioral pattern that presents with a sensory, sensorimotor, or organizational processing difficulty that interferes with the child's ability to maintain positive interaction and relationships and to make daily adaptation.
seasonal affective d. (SAD), a depressive mood disorder that occurs at approximately the same time year after year and spontaneously remits at the same time each year. The most com-

mon type is winter depression, characterized by morning hypersomnia, low energy, increased appetite, weight gain, and carbohydrate craving, all of which remit in the spring.
somatization d., a mental d. characterized by presentation of a complicated medical history and of physical symptoms referring to a variety of organ systems, but without a detectable or known organic basis. SEE ALSO conversion, hysteria.
substance abuse d.'s, a class of mental d.'s in which behavioral and biological changes are associated with regular use of alcohol, drugs, and related substances that affect the central nervous system and personal and social functioning.
dis•or•ga•ni•za•tion (dis-ōr′gan-i-zā′shŭn). Destruction of an organ or tissue with consequent loss of function.
dis•o•ri•en•ta•tion (dis′ōr-ē-en-tā′shŭn). Loss of the sense of familiarity with one's surroundings (time, place, and person); loss of one's bearings.
dis•pen•sa•ry (dis-pen′ser-ē). 1. A physician's office, especially the office of one who dispenses medicines. 2. The office of a hospital pharmacist, where medicines are given out on physicians' orders. 3. An outpatient department of a hospital. [L. *dis-penso,* pp. *-atus,* to distribute by weight, fr. *penso,* to weigh]
Dis•pen•sa•to•ry (dis-pen′să-tō-rē). A work originally intended as a commentary on the Pharmacopeia, but now more of a supplement to that work, which contains an account of the sources, mode of preparation, physiologic action, and therapeutic uses of most of the agents, official and nonofficial, used in the treatment of disease. [L. *dispensator,* a manager, steward; see dispensary]
dis•pense (dis-pens′). To give out medicine and other necessities to the sick; to fill a medical prescription.
dis•perse (dis-pers′). To dissipate, to cause disappearance of, to scatter, to dilute.
dis•per•sion (dis-per′zhŭn). 1. The act of dispersing or of being dispersed. 2. Incorporation of the particles of one substance into the mass of another, including solutions, suspensions, and colloidal dispersions (solutions). 3. Specifically, what is usually called a colloidal *solution.* [L. *dispersio*]
di•spi•reme (dī-spī′rēm). The double chromatin skein in the telophase of mitosis. [G. *di-,* twice, + *speirēma,* coil, convolution]
dis•place•ment (dis-plās′ment). 1. Removal from the normal location or position. 2. The adding to a fluid (particularly a gas) in an open vessel one of greater density whereby the first is expelled. 3. CHEMISTRY A change in which one element, radical, or molecule is replaced by another, or in which one element exchanges electric charges with another by reduction or oxidation. 4. PSYCHIATRY The transfer of impulses from one expression to another, as from fighting to talking.
disposition. Follow-up list detailed in the health care record, after initial episode of care, of services and treatments to be provided to the patient.
dis•sect (di-sekt′, dī-). 1. To cut apart or separate the tissues of the body for study. 2. In an operation, to separate the different structures along nat-

ural lines by dividing the connective tissue framework. [L. *dis-seco,* pp. *-sectus,* to cut asunder]

dis•sec•tion (di-sek′shŭn, dī-). The act of dissecting. SYN anatomy (3), necrotomy (1).

aortic d., a pathologic process, characterized by splitting of the media layer of the aorta, which leads to formation of a dissecting aneurysm.

dis•sem•i•nat•ed (di-sem′i-nā-ted). Widely scattered throughout an organ, tissue, or the body. [L. *dis-semino,* pp. *-atus,* to scatter seed, fr. *semen* (*-min-*), seed]

dis•sim•u•la•tion (di-sim-yū-lā′shŭn). Concealment of the truth about a situation, especially about a state of health or during a mental status examination, as by a malingerer or someone with a factitious disorder. [L. *dissimulatio,* fr. *dissimulo,* to feign, fr. *dis,* apart, + *similis,* same]

dis•so•ci•a•tion (di-sō-sē-ā′shŭn, -shē-ā′shŭn). **1.** Separation, or a dissolution of relations. SYN disassociation. **2.** The change of a complex chemical compound into a simpler one by any lytic reaction or by ionization. **3.** An unconscious separation of a group of mental processes from the rest of the thinking processes, resulting in an independent functioning of these processes and a loss of the usual associations, *e.g.,* a separation of affect from cognition. SEE multiple *personality.* [L. *dis-socio,* pp. *-atus,* to disjoin, separate, fr. *socius,* partner, ally]

atrial d., mutually independent beating of the two atria or of parts of the atria.

atrioventricular d., A-V d., (1) any situation in which atria and ventricles are activated and contract independently, as in complete A-V block; (2) more specifically, the d. between atria and ventricles that results from slowing of the atrial pacemaker or acceleration of the ventricular pacemaker at nearly equal (rarely equal) rates, each depolarizing its own chamber, thus interfering with depolarization by the other (interference-dissociation).

electromechanical d., persistence of electrical activity in the heart without associated mechanical contraction; often a sign of cardiac rupture.

longitudinal d., d. between parallel chambers of the heart, as between one atrium and the other or between one ventricle and the other, in contrast to d. between atria and ventricles.

dis•solve (di-zolv′). To change or cause to change from a solid to a dispersed form by immersion in a fluid of suitable properties. [L. *dissolvo,* pp. *-solutus,* to loose asunder, to dissolve]

dis•so•nance (di′sō-nans). SOCIAL PSYCHOLOGY An aversive state which arises when an individual is minimally aware of internal inconsistency or conflict. [L. *dissonus,* discordant, confused]

cognitive d., a motivational state which exists when a person's attitudes, perceptions, and related d. state are inconsistent with each other, *e.g.,* hating African Americans as a group but admiring Martin Luther King, Jr.

dis•tad (dis′tad). Toward the periphery; in a distal direction.

dis•tal (dis′tăl). **1.** Situated away from the center of the body, or from the point of origin; specifically applied to the extremity or distant part of a

limb or organ. **2.** DENTISTRY Away from the median sagittal plane of the face, following the curvature of the dental arch. SYN distalis [NA]. [L. *distalis*]

dis•ta•lis (dis-tā′lis) [NA]. SYN distal.

dis•tance (dis′tans). The measure of space between two objects. [L. *distantia,* fr. *di-sto,* to stand apart, be distant]

focal d., the d. from the center of a lens to its focus.

focal-film d. (FFD), the d. from the source of radiation (the focal spot of the x-ray tube) to the film or other image-receptor. SYN source-to-image-receptor d.

infinite d., the limit of distant vision, the rays entering the eyes from an object at that point being practically parallel.

interarch d., (1) the vertical d. between the maxillary and mandibular arches under conditions of vertical dimensions which must be specified; (2) the vertical d. between maxillary and mandibular ridges.

interocclusal d., (1) the vertical d. between the opposing occlusal surfaces, assuming rest relation unless otherwise designated; (2) SYN freeway *space.*

pupillary d., the d. between the center of each pupil; the major reference points in measuring for fitting of spectacle frames and lenses.

source-to-image-receptor d. (SIRD), SYN focal-film d.

dis•ten•tion, dis•ten•sion (dis-ten′shŭn). The act or state of being distended or stretched. SEE ALSO dilation. [L. *dis-tendo,* to stretch apart]

dis•til•late (dis′ti-lāt). The product of distillation.

dis•til•la•tion (dis-ti-lā′shŭn). Volatilization of a liquid by heat and subsequent condensation of the vapor; a means of separating the volatile from the nonvolatile, or the more volatile from the less volatile, part of a liquid mixture. [L. *de-(di-)stillo,* pp. *-atus,* to drop down]

dis•to•buc•cal (dis-tō-bŭk′kăl). Relating to the distal and buccal surfaces of a tooth; denoting the angle formed by their junction.

dis•to•buc•co•oc•clu•sal (dis′tō-bŭk′ŏ-ō-klū′săl). Relating to the distal, buccal, and occlusal surfaces of a bicuspid or molar tooth; denoting especially the angle formed by the junction of these surfaces.

dis•to•buc•co•pul•pal (dis′tō-bŭk′ŏ-pŭl′păl). Relating to the point (trihedral) angle formed by the junction of a distal, buccal, and pulpal wall of a cavity.

dis•to•cer•vi•cal (dis-tō-ser′vi-kăl). Relating to the line angle formed by the junction of the distal and cervical (gingival) walls of a class V cavity.

dis•to•clu•sal (dis-tō-klū′săl). **1.** Relating to or characterized by distoclusion. **2.** Denoting a compound cavity or restoration involving the distal and occlusal surfaces of a tooth. **3.** Denoting the line angle formed by the distal and occlusal walls of a class V cavity.

dis•to•clu•sion (dis-tō-klū′zhŭn). A malocclusion in which the mandibular arch articulates with the maxillary arch in a position distal to normal; in Angle's classification, a Class II malocclusion. SYN distal occlusion (2).

di

dis·to·gin·gi·val (dis-tō-jin′ji-văl). Relating to the junction of the distal surface with the gingival line of a tooth.

dis·to·in·ci·sal (dis′tō-in-sī′zăl). Relating to the line (dihedral) angle formed by the junction of the distal and incisal walls of a class V cavity in an anterior tooth.

dis·to·la·bi·al (dis-tō-lā′bē-ăl). Relating to the distal and labial surfaces of a tooth; denoting the angle formed by their junction.

dis·to·la·bi·o·pul·pal (dis′tō-lā′bē-ō-pŭl′păl). Relating to the point (trihedral) angle formed by the junction of distal, labial and pulpal walls of the incisal part of a class IV (mesioincisal) cavity.

dis·to·lin·gual (dis-tō-ling′gwăl). Relating to the distal and lingual surfaces of a tooth; denoting the angle formed by their junction.

dis·to·lin·guo·oc·clu·sal (dis′tō-ling′gwō-ŏ-klū′zăl). Relating to the distal, lingual, and occlusal surfaces of a bicuspid or molar tooth; denoting especially the angle formed by the junction of these surfaces.

dis·to·mo·lar (dis-tō-mō′lăr). A supernumerary tooth located in the region posterior to the third molar tooth.

dis·to·pul·pal (dis-tō-pŭl′păl). Relating to the line (dihedral) angle formed by the junction of the distal and pulpal walls of a cavity.

dis·tor·tion (dis-tōr′shŭn). **1.** PSYCHIATRY A defense mechanism that helps to repress or disguise unacceptable thoughts. **2.** In dental impressions, the permanent deformation of the impression material after the registration of an imprint. **3.** A twisting out of normal shape or form. [L. *distortio,* fr. *dis-torqueo,* to wrench apart]

parataxic d., an attitude toward another person based on a distorted evaluation, usually because of too close an identification of that person with emotionally significant figures in the patient's past life.

radiologic d., misrepresentation of the true size and shape of an object being radiographed (as in magnification, elongation, and foreshortening).

dis·to·ver·sion (dis′tō-ver-zhŭn). Malposition of a tooth distal to normal, in a posterior direction following the curvature of the dental arch.

dis·trac·tion (dis-trak′shŭn). **1.** Difficulty or impossibility of concentration or fixation of the mind. **2.** Manipulation or traction of a limb to separate bony fragments or joint surfaces. [L. *dis-traho,* pp. *-tractus,* to pull in different directions]

dis·tress (dis-tres′). Mental or physical suffering or anguish. [L. *distringo,* to draw asunder]

dis·tri·bu·tion (dis-tri-byū′shŭn). **1.** The passage of the branches of arteries or nerves to the tissues and organs. **2.** The area in which the branches of an artery or a nerve terminate, or the area supplied by such an artery or nerve. **3.** The relative numbers of individuals in each of various categories or populations, such as in different age, sex, or occupational samples. [L. *dis-tribuo,* pp. *-tributus,* to distribute, fr. *tribus,* a tribe]

gaussian d., the statistical d. of members of a population around the population mean. In a gaussian d., 68.2% of values fall within ± 1 standard deviation (SD); 95.4% fall within ± 2 SD of the mean; and 99.7% fall within ± 3 SD of the mean. SYN bell-shaped curve, normal d.

normal d., SYN gaussian d.

dis·trix (dis′triks). Splitting of the hairs at their ends. [G. *dis,* twice, + *thrix,* hair]

di·sul·fate (dī-sŭl′fāt). A molecule containing two sulfates.

di·sul·fide (dī-sŭl′fīd). **1.** A molecule containing two atoms of sulfur to one of the reference element, *e.g.,* CS_2, carbon disulfide. **2.** A compound containing the –S–S– group, *e.g.,* cystine.

DIT diiodotyrosine.

di·ter·penes (dī-ter′pēnz). Hydrocarbons or their derivatives containing 4 isoprene units, hence containing 20 carbon atoms and 4 branched methyl groups; *e.g.,* vitamin A, retinene, aconitine.

di·u·re·sis (dī-yū-rē′sis). Excretion of urine; commonly denotes production of unusually large volumes of urine. [G. *dia,* throughout, completely, + *ourēsis,* urination]

di·u·ret·ic (dī-yū-ret′ik). **1.** Promoting the excretion of urine. **2.** An agent that increases the amount of urine excreted.

loop d., a class of d. agents (*e.g.,* furosemide, ethacrynic acid) that act by inhibiting reabsorption of sodium and chloride, not only in the proximal and distal tubules but also in Henle's loop.

osmotic d.'s, drugs, such as mannitol, which by their osmotic effects promote the elimination of water and electrolytes in the urine.

potassium sparing d.'s, d. agents that retain potassium; examples are triamterene and amiloride. Used in hypertension and in congestive heart failure.

di·ur·nal (dī-er′năl). **1.** Pertaining to the daylight hours; opposite of nocturnal. **2.** Repeating once each 24 hours, *e.g.,* a d. variation or a d. rhythm. Cf. circadian. [L. *diurnus,* of the day]

di·va·lence, di·va·len·cy (dī-vā′lens, dī-vā′len-sē). SYN bivalence.

di·va·lent (dī-vā′lent, div′ă-). SYN bivalent (1).

di·var·i·ca·tion (dī′var-i-kā′shŭn). SYN diastasis (1). [L. *divaricare,* to spread asunder]

di·ver·gence (dī-ver′jens). **1.** A moving or spreading apart or in different directions. **2.** The spreading of branches of the neuron to form synapses with several other neurons. [L. *di-,* apart, + *vergo,* to incline]

di·ver·gent (dī-ver′jent). Moving in different directions; radiating.

di·ver·tic·u·la (dī-ver-tik′yū-lă). Plural of diverticulum.

di·ver·tic·u·lar (dī-ver-tik′yū-lăr). Relating to a diverticulum.

di·ver·tic·u·lec·to·my (dī′ver-tik-yū-lek′tō-mē). Excision of a diverticulum.

di·ver·tic·u·li·tis (dī′ver-tik-yū-lī′tis). Inflammation of a diverticulum, especially of the small pockets in the wall of the colon which fill with stagnant fecal material and become inflamed; rarely, they may cause obstruction, perforation, or bleeding.

di·ver·tic·u·lo·ma (dī′ver-tik-yū-lō′mă). Development of a granulomatous mass in the wall of the colon. [diverticulum + G. *-oma,* tumor]

di·ver·tic·u·lo·sis (dī′ver-tik-yū-lō′sis). Presence of a number of diverticula of the intestine, common in middle age; the lesions are acquired pulsion diverticula.

di·ver·tic·u·lum, pl. **di·ver·tic·u·la** (dī-ver-tik′ yū-lŭm, yū-lă) [NA]. A pouch or sac opening from a tubular or saccular organ, such as the gut or bladder. [L. *deverticulum* (or *di*-), a by-road, fr. *de-verto,* to turn aside]

diverticula of colon, diverticula, which are herniations of mucosa and submucosa between fibers of the major muscle layer (muscularis propria) of the colon. Can cause bleeding and episodes of severe inflammation.

false d., a d. of the intestine that passes through a defect in the muscular wall of the gut and thus does not include a layer of muscle in its wall.

hypopharyngeal d., SYN pharyngoesophageal d.

Meckel's d., the remains of the yolk stalk of the embryo, which, when persisting abnormally as a blind sac or pouch in the adult, is located on the ileum a short distance above the cecum; it may be attached to the umbilicus and, if the lining includes gastric mucosa, peptic ulceration and bleeding may result.

pharyngoesophageal d., most common d. of the esophagus; arises between the inferior pharyngeal constrictor and the crico-pharyngeus muscle. SYN hypopharyngeal d., Zenker's d.

pituitary d., a tubular outgrowth of ectoderm from the stomodeum of the embryo; it grows dorsad toward the infundibular process of the diencephalon, around which it forms a cup-like mass, giving rise to the pars distalis and pars juxtaneuralis of the hypophysis. SYN Rathke's pouch.

pulsion d., a d. formed by pressure from within, frequently causing herniation of mucosa through the muscularis.

traction d., a d. formed by the pulling force of contracting bands of adhesion, occurring mainly in the distal esophagus, from tuberculous hilar or mediastinal lymphadenitis.

true d., a term denoting a d. that includes all the layers of the wall from which it protrudes.

vesical d., a d. of the bladder wall; may be either true or false type.

Zenker's d., SYN pharyngoesophageal d.

di·vi·sion (di-vizh′ŭn). A separating into two or more parts.

cleavage d., the rapid mitotic d. of the zygote with decrease in size of individual cells or blastomeres and the formation of a morula. SEE ALSO cleavage (1).

direct nuclear d., SYN amitosis.

indirect nuclear d., SYN mitosis.

multiplicative d., reproduction by simultaneous d. of a mother cell into a number of daughter cells. If the process occurs without fertilization of the mother cell, or encystment, the daughter cells are called merozoites; if they develop within a cyst, and usually after fertilization, they are called sporozoites.

di·vul·sion (di-vŭl′shŭn). **1.** Removal of a part by tearing. **2.** Forcible dilation of the walls of a cavity or canal.

di·vul·sor (di-vŭl′sĕr, -sōr). An instrument for forcible dilation of the urethra or other canal or cavity.

di·zy·got·ic, di·zy·gous (dī′zī-got′ik, dī-zī′gŭs). Relating to twins derived from two separate zygotes but sharing a common intrauterine environment. [G. *di-,* two, + *zygotos,* yoked together]

diz·zi·ness (diz′i-nes). Imprecise term commonly used by patients in an attempt to describe various symptoms such as faintness, vertigo, disequilibrium, or unsteadiness. SEE ALSO vertigo. [A. S. *dyzig,* foolish]

DL-. Prefix (in small capital letters) denoting a substance consisting of equal quantities of the two enantiomorphs, D and L; replaces the older *dl-* (in lower case italics) as a more exact definition of structure.

DM adamsite; *diabetes* mellitus; diastolic *murmur*; dopamine.

dmf, DMF decayed, missing, or filled teeth. SEE ALSO dmfs caries *index.*

dmfs, DMFS decayed or missing teeth and filled surfaces. SEE ALSO dmfs caries *index.*

DN dibucaine number.

DNA deoxyribonucleic acid.

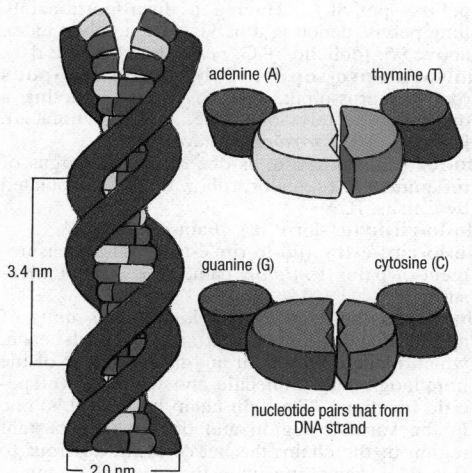

adenine (A) thymine (T)

3.4 nm guanine (G) cytosine (C)

2.0 nm

nucleotide pairs that form DNA strand

DNA (deoxyribonucleic acid)

DNA fin·ger·print·ing. See under fingerprint.

DNA markers. Segments of chromosomal DNA known to be linked with heritable traits or diseases. Although the markers themselves do not produce the conditions, they exist in concert with the genes responsible and are passed on with them. Certain markers, restriction fragment length polymorphisms, consist of segments of DNA that can be identified on autoradiographs (produced after digestion of the DNA by restriction enzymes and segregation of the resulting fragments through gel electrophoresis).

DNAse, DNAase, DNase deoxyribonuclease.

DNR Do not resuscitate.

Dns, DNS dansyl.

DOA dead on arrival.

doc·tor (dok'ter). **1.** A title conferred by a university on one who has followed a prescribed course of study, or given as a title of distinction; as d. of medicine, laws, philosophy, etc. **2.** A physician, especially one upon whom has been conferred the degree of M.D. by a university or medical school. [L. a teacher, fr. *doceo,* pp. *doctus,* to teach]

dol (dōl). A unit measure of pain. [L. *dolor,* pain]

△**dolicho-.** Long. [G. *dolichos*]

dol·i·cho·ce·phal·ic, dol·i·cho·ceph·a·lous (dol-i-kō-sĕ-fal'ik, -sef'ă-lŭs). Having a disproportionately long head; denoting a skull with a cephalic index below 75. [dolicho- + G. *kephalē,* head]

dol·i·cho·fa·cial (dol-i-kō-fā'shăl). SYN dolichoprosopic.

dol·i·chol (dol'i-kol). Polyisoprenes in which the terminal member is saturated and oxidized to an alcohol, usually phosphorylated and often glycosylated; found in endoplasmic reticulum, but not in mitochondrial or plasma membranes; urinary levels are elevated in disorders exhibiting abnormal skin, rectal, or brain profiles in electron microscopy of biopsies.

dol·i·cho·pel·lic, dol·i·cho·pel·vic (dol-i-kō-pel'ik, -pel'vik). Having a disproportionately long pelvis; denoting a pelvis with a pelvic index above 95. [dolicho- + G. *pellis,* bowl (pelvis)]

dol·i·cho·pro·sop·ic, dol·i·cho·pro·so·pous (dol-i-kō-pros-ō'pik, -kō-pros'ō-pŭs). Having a disproportionately long face. SYN dolichofacial. [dolicho- + G. *prosōpikos,* facial]

do·lor (dō'lōr). Pain, as one of the four signs of inflammation (d., calor, rubor, tumor) enunciated by Celsus. [L.]

do·lor·if·ic (dō-lōr-if'ik). Pain-producing.

do·lo·rim·e·try (dō-lō-rim'ě-trē). The measurement of pain. [L. *dolor,* pain, + G. *metron,* measure]

do·mains (dō-mānz'). **1.** Homologous units of approximately 110 to 120 amino acids each, which make up the light and heavy chains of the immunoglobulin molecule and which serve specific functions. The light chain has two d.'s, one in the variable region and one in the constant region of the chain; the heavy chain has four to five d.'s, depending upon the class of immunoglobulin, one in the variable region and the remaining ones in the constant region. **2.** A region of a protein having some distinctive physical feature or role. [Fr. *domaine,* fr. L. *dominium,* property, dominion]

do·mes·tic vi·o·lence. Intentionally inflicted injury perpetrated by and on family member(s); varieties include spouse abuse, child abuse, and sexual abuse, including incest. Various kinds of abuse, such as sexual abuse, also happen outside of the family unit.

dom·i·cil·i·at·ed (dō-mi-sil'ē-āt-ed). A state of close association of an organism within human abodes or activities, such that partial domestication results, leading to the organism's dependence on continued association with the human environment; this frequently results in the d. organism becoming a noxious pest, a vector, or an intermediate host of human disease. [L. *domicilium,* a dwelling]

dom·i·nance (dom'i-nans). The state of being dominant.

cerebral d., the fact that one hemisphere is dominant over the other and will exercise greater influence over certain functions; the left cerebral hemisphere is usually dominant in the control of speech, language and analytical processing, and mathematics, while the right hemisphere (usually nondominant) processes spatial concepts and language as related to certain types of visual images; handedness (right-handed people have left cerebral d.) is considered a general example of cerebral d.

dom·i·nant (dom'i-nant). **1.** Ruling or controlling. **2.** In genetics, denoting an allele possessed by one of the parents of a hybrid which is expressed in the latter to the exclusion of a contrasting allele (the recessive) from the other parent. [L. *dominans,* pres. p. of *dominor,* to rule, fr. *dominus,* lord, master, fr. *domus,* house]

DOMS delayed onset muscle soreness.

Don Juan (don hwahn). PSYCHIATRY A term used to denote males with compulsive sexual or romantic overactivity, usually with a succession of female partners. [legendary Spanish nobleman]

do·nor (dō'ner). **1.** An individual from whom blood, tissue, or an organ is taken for transplantation. **2.** A compound that will transfer an atom or a radical to an acceptor. **3.** An atom that readily yields electrons to an acceptor. [L. *dono,* pp. *donatus,* to donate, to give]

hydrogen d., a metabolite from which hydrogen is removed (by a dehydrogenase system) and transferred by a hydrogen carrier to another metabolite, which is thus reduced.

universal d., in blood grouping, a person belonging to group O; *i.e.,* one whose erythrocytes do not contain either agglutinogen A or B and are, therefore, not agglutinated by plasma containing either of the ordinary isoagglutinins, alpha or beta.

don·o·va·no·sis (don'ō-vă-nō'sis). SYN *granuloma* inguinale.

do·pa, DO·PA, Do·pa (dō'pă). An intermediate in the catabolism of L-phenylalanine and L-tyrosine, and in the biosynthesis of norepinephrine, epinephrine, and melanin; the L form, levodopa, is biologically active.

do·pa·mine (DM) (dō'pă-mēn). 3,4-dihydroxyphenylethylamine; an intermediate in tyrosine metabolism and precursor of norepinephrine and epinephrine.

dope (dōp). **1.** Any drug, either stimulating or depressing, administered for its temporary effect, or taken habitually or addictively. **2.** To administer or take such a drug. [Dutch, *doop,* sauce]

doping (dōp'ing). The administration of foreign substances to an individual; often used in reference to athletes who try to stimulate physical and psychological strength.

blood doping, infusion of red blood cells, usually freeze-preserved autologous blood, to increase hematocrit and hemoglobin levels; used by endurance athletes to increase blood's oxygen-carrying capacity and thus enhance endurance performance. SYN blood boosting, induced erythrocythemia.

Doppler, Christian J., Austrian mathematician and physicist in U.S., 1803–1853. SEE D. *echocardiography, effect, shift, ultrasonography*.

Dop·pler. A diagnostic instrument that emits an ultrasonic beam into the body; the ultrasound reflected from moving structures changes its frequency (Doppler effect). Of diagnostic value in peripheral vascular and cardiac disease.

dor·sa (dōr'să). Plural of dorsum.

dor·sad (dor'sad). Toward or in the direction of the back. [L. *dorsum,* back, + *ad,* to]

dor·sal (dōr'săl). **1.** Pertaining to the back or any dorsum. **2.** SYN posterior (2). [Mediev. L. *dorsalis,* fr. *dorsum,* back]

dor·sal·gia (dōr-sal'jē-ă). Pain in the upper back. [L. *dorsum,* back, + G. *algos,* pain]

dor·si·flex·ion (dor-si-flek'shŭn). Turning upward of the foot or toes or of the hand or fingers.

dor·si·spi·nal (dōr'si-spī'năl). Relating to the vertebral column, especially to its dorsal aspect.

dor·so·ceph·a·lad (dōr'sō-sef'ă-lad). Toward the occiput, or back of the head. [L. *dorsum,* back, + G. *kephalē,* head, + L. *ad,* to]

dor·so·lat·er·al (dōr-sō-lat'er-ăl). Relating to the back and the side.

dor·so·lum·bar (dōr-sō-lŭm'bar). Referring to the back in the region of the lower thoracic and upper lumbar vertebrae.

dor·so·ven·trad (dōr-sō-ven'trad). In a direction from the dorsal to the ventral aspect.

dor·sum, gen. **dor·si,** pl. **dor·sa** (dōr'sŭm, -sī, -să) [NA]. **1.** The back of the body. **2.** The upper or posterior surface, or the back, of any part. [L. back]

dos·age (dō'sij). **1.** The giving of medicine or other therapeutic agent in prescribed amounts. **2.** The size, frequency, and number of doses of medicine to be given (sometimes incorrectly used for dose). Cf. dose.

dose (dōs). The quantity of a drug or other remedy to be taken or applied all at one time or in fractional amounts within a given period. Cf. dosage (2). [G. *dosis,* a giving]

absorbed d., the amount of energy absorbed per unit mass of irradiated material at the target site; RADIATION THERAPY the former unit for absorbed d. is the rad; the current (S.I.) unit is the gray.

booster d., a d. given at some time after an initial d. to enhance the effect, said usually of antigens for the production of antibodies.

curative d. (CD), (1) the quantity of any substance required to effect the cure of a disease or that will correct the manifestations of a deficiency of a particular factor in the diet; **(2)** effective d. used with therapeutically applied compounds.

effective d., (1) the d. that produces the desired effect; when followed by a subscript (generally "ED_{50}"), it denotes the d. having such an effect on a certain percentage (*e.g.,* 50%) of the test animals; ED_{50} is the median effective dose; **(2)** in radiation protection, the sum of the equivalent d.'s in all tissues and organs of the body weighted for tissue effects of radiation. The unit of effective d. is the sievert (Sv).

erythema d., the minimum d. of x-rays or other form of radiation sufficient to produce erythema.

exposure d., the radiation d., expressed in roentgens, delivered at a point in free air.

L d.'s, a group of terms that indicate the relative activity or potency of diphtheria toxin; the L d.'s are different from the minimal lethal d. and minimal reacting d., inasmuch as the latter two represent the direct effects of toxin, whereas the L d.'s pertain to the combining power of toxin with specific antitoxin. ["L" for L. *limes,* limit, boundary]

lethal d., the d. of a chemical or biologic preparation (*e.g.,* a bacterial exotoxin or a suspension of bacteria) that is likely to cause death; it varies in relation to the type of animal and the route of administration; when followed by a subscript (generally "LD_{50}" or median lethal d.), it denotes the d. likely to cause death in a certain percentage (*e.g.,* 50%) of the test animals; median lethal d. is LD_{50}, absolute lethal d. is LD_{100}, and minimal lethal d. is LD_{05}.

Lr d., L_r d., the limes reacting d. of diphtheria toxin, *i.e.,* the smallest amount of toxin that, when mixed with one unit of antitoxin and injected intracutaneously in the shaved skin of a susceptible guinea pig, yields a minimal, positive reaction and inflammation localized to the region of the injection; the L_rd. closely approximates the L_0d., as would be expected, inasmuch as a slight excess of unneutralized toxin results in a reaction.

maximal d., the largest amount of a drug or physical procedure that an adult can take with safety.

maximum permissible d. (MPD), defined by the International Commission on Radiological Protection as the greatest d. of radiation which, in the light of present knowledge, is not expected to cause detectable bodily injury to a person at any time during his lifetime. This d. has been reduced with each Commission report. The MPD is given in terms of acute or chronic exposure of the whole body or of organs, systems, or regions of the body, and differs for persons who are occupationally exposed versus the public at large.

median effective d. (ED_{50}), SEE effective d.

minimal d., the smallest amount of a drug or physical procedure that will produce a desired physiologic effect in an adult.

· **minimal infecting d. (M.I.D.),** the smallest quantity of infectious material regularly producing infection; usually expressed as $I.D._{50}$, the quantity causing infection in 50% of a suitable series of animals or cells (cell cultures).

minimal lethal d. (MLD, mld), (1) the minimal d. of a toxic substance or infectious agent that is lethal, as assayed in various experimental animals; when followed by a subscript (generally "MLD_{50}"), denotes the minimal dose that is lethal to a certain percentage (*e.g.,* 50%) of animals so assayed; **(2)** LD_{05}. SEE lethal d.

minimal reacting d. (MRD, mrd), the minimal d. of a toxic substance causing a reaction, as manifested in the skin of a series of susceptible test animals; the assay is based on the development of a characteristic, minimal but definite, "standard," focal inflammation.

optimum d., the d. of a drug or radiation that will produce the desired effect with minimum likelihood of undesirable symptoms.

skin d., the quantity of radiation delivered to the skin surface.

tolerance d., the largest d. of a remedy that can be accepted without the production of injurious symptoms.

dos·im·e·ter (dō-sim′ĕ-ter). **1.** A device for measuring radiation, especially x-rays. **2.** In pulmonary function testing, a device, which can be triggered automatically by a sensor near the subject's mouth or manually by a technician, that allows for the delivery of a reproducible dose from a nebulizer. [G. *dosis*, dose, + *metron*, measure]

pocket d., small ionization chamber that provides an immediate reading of radiation exposure. SEE ALSO film badge.

thermoluminescent d. (TLD), device resembling a film badge but that uses lithium fluoride crystals instead of film to record radiation exposure. SEE ALSO film badge.

do·sim·e·try (dō-sim′ĕ-trē). Measurement of radiation exposure, especially x-rays or gamma rays; calculation of radiation dose from internally administered radionuclides.

dot. A small spot.

Horner-Trantas d.'s, evanescent white cellular infiltrates occurring in the bulbar form of vernal keratoconjunctivitis.

dot·age (dō′tij). The deterioration of previously intact mental powers, common in old age.

dou·blet (dŭb′let). A combination of two lenses designed to correct the chromatic and spherical aberration.

douche (dūsh). **1.** A current of water, gas, or vapor directed against a surface or projected into a cavity. **2.** An instrument for giving a d. **3.** To apply a d. [Fr. fr. *doucher*, to pour]

dox·a·cu·ri·um chlo·ride (doks′a-kū′rē-um). A nondepolarizing neuromuscular blocking drug similar to pancuronium but without cardiovascular side effects.

DPN diphosphopyridine *nucleotide*.

DPN⁺ oxidized diphosphopyridine nucleotide.

DPT. diphtheria-pertussis-tetanus (vaccine).

DR *reaction* of degeneration.

drachm (dram). SYN dram. [G. *drachmē*, an ancient Greek weight, equivalent to about 60 gr]

dra·cun·cu·li·a·sis, dra·cun·cu·lo·sis (dra-kŭng-kyū-lī′ă-sis, -kyū-lō′sis). Infection with *Dracunculus medinensis*.

Dra·cun·cu·lus (dra-kŭng′kyū-lŭs). A genus of nematodes that have some resemblances to true filarial worms; however, adults are larger and the intermediate host is a freshwater crustacean rather than an insect. [L. dim. of *draco*, serpent]

draft. 1. A current of air in a confined space. **2.** A quantity of liquid medicine ordered as a single dose.

drain (drān). **1.** To draw off fluid from a cavity as it forms. **2.** A device, usually in the shape of a tube or wick, for removing fluid as it collects in a cavity, especially a wound cavity. [A. S. *drehnian*, to draw off]

cigarette d., a wick of gauze wrapped in rubber tissue, providing capillary drainage.

Penrose d., a soft tube-shaped rubber drain.

stab d., a d. passed into a cavity through a puncture made at a dependent part away from the wound of operation, so placed to prevent infection of the wound.

sump d., a d. consisting of an outer tube with a smaller tube within it which is attached to a suction pump; the outer tube has multiple perforations that allow fluid and air to pass into its interior and be carried away through the suction tube.

drain·age (drān′ij). Continuous flow or withdrawal of fluids from a wound or other cavity.

capillary d., d. by means of a wick of gauze or other material.

closed d., d. of a body cavity via a water- or air-tight system.

dependent d., d. from the lowest part and into a receptacle at a level lower than the structure being drained.

infusion-aspiration d., a type of d. in which antibiotics are continuously infused into a cavity at the same time fluid is being drained (aspirated) from the cavity.

open d., d. allowing air to enter.

postural d., d. used in bronchiectasis and lung abscess. The patient's body is positioned so that the trachea is inclined downward and below the affected chest area.

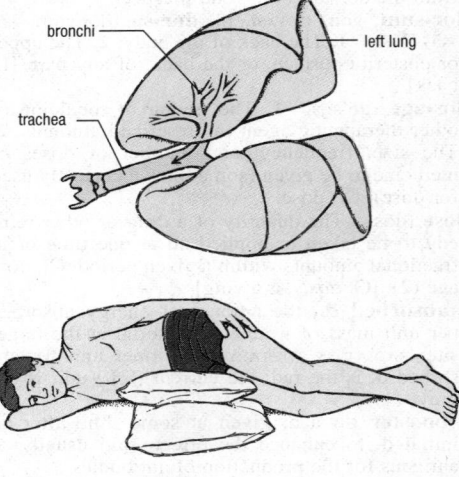

postural drainage of left lung

suction d., closed drainage of a cavity, with a suction apparatus attached to the drainage tube.

through d., d. obtained by the passage of a perforated tube, open at both extremities, through a cavity; in addition, the cavity can be washed out by a solution passed through the tube.

tidal d., d. of the urinary bladder by means of an intermittent filling and emptying apparatus.

dram. A unit of weight: $^1/_8$ oz.; 60 gr, apothecaries' weight; $^1/_{16}$ oz., avoirdupois weight. SYN drachm. [see drachm]

drape (drāp). **1.** To cover parts of the body other than those to be examined or operated upon. **2.** The cloth or materials used for such cover. [M.E., fr. L.L. *drappus,* cloth]

dream (drēm). Mental activity during sleep in which events, thought, emotions, and images are experienced as real.

drep·a·no·cyte (drep′ă-nō-sīt). SYN sickle *cell.* [G. *drepanē,* sickle, + *kytos,* a hollow (cell)]

drep·a·no·cyt·ic (drep′ă-nō-sit′ik). Relating to or resembling a sickle cell.

dress·ing (dres′ing). The material applied, or the application itself of material, to a wound for protection, absorbance, drainage, etc.

    adhesive absorbent d., a sterile individual d. consisting of a plain absorbent compress affixed to a film of fabric coated with a pressure-sensitive adhesive.

    antiseptic d., a sterile d. of gauze impregnated with an antiseptic.

    occlusive d., a d. that hermetically seals a wound.

    pressure d., a d. by which pressure is exerted on the area covered to prevent the collection of fluids in the underlying tissues; most commonly used after skin grafting and in the treatment of burns.

DRG diagnosis-related group.

drift. 1. A gradual movement, as from an original position. **2.** A gradual change in the value of a random variable over time as a result of various factors, some random and some systematic effects of trend, manipulation, etc.

    antigenic d., the process of "evolutionary" changes in molecular structure of DNA/RNA in microorganisms during their passage from one host to another; it may be due to recombination, deletion, or insertion of genes, point mutations or combinations of these events; it leads to alteration (usually slow and progressive) in the antigenic composition, and therefore in the immunologic responses of individuals and populations to exposure to the microorganism concerned.

drip. 1. To flow a drop at a time. **2.** A flowing in drops.

    intravenous d., the slow but continuous introduction of solutions intravenously, a drop at a time.

    Murphy d., SYN proctoclysis.

    postnasal d., term sometimes used to describe sensation of excessive mucoid or mucopurulent discharge from the posterior nares.

drive. 1. A basic compelling urge. **2.** PSYCHOLOGY Classified as either innate (*e.g.,* hunger) or learned (*e.g.,* hoarding) and appetitive (*e.g.,* hunger, thirst, sex) or aversive (*e.g.,* fear, pain, grief). SEE ALSO motive.

    acquired d.'s, SYN secondary d.'s.

    learned d., SYN motive (1).

    physiological d.'s, those d.'s such as hunger and thirst which stem from the biological needs of an organism.

    secondary d.'s, those d.'s not directly related to biological needs; a secondary d. can be learned as an offshoot of a primary d., in which case it is often referred to as a motive. SYN acquired d.'s.

driv·ing (drīv′ing). The induction of a frequency

in the electroencephalogram by sensory stimulation at this frequency.

    photic d., a normal EEG phenomenon whereby the frequency of the activity recorded over the parieto-occipital regions is time-locked to the flash frequency during photic stimulation.

drom·o·graph (drom′ō-graf). An instrument for recording the rapidity of the blood circulation. [G. *dromos,* a running, + *graphō,* to record]

drom·o·ma·nia (drom-ō-mā′nē-ă). An uncontrollable impulse to wander or travel. [G. *dromos,* a running, + *mania,* insanity]

dro·mo·tro·pic (drō-mō-trop′ik). Influencing the velocity of conduction of excitation, as in nerve or cardiac muscle fibers. [G. *dromos,* a running, + *tropē,* a turn]

drop. 1. To fall, or to be dispensed or poured in globules. **2.** A liquid globule. **3.** A volume of liquid regarded as a unit of dosage, equivalent in the case of water to about 1 minim. **4.** A solid confection in globular form, usually intended to be allowed to dissolve in the mouth. [A.S. *droppan*]

drop·let (drop′let). A diminutive drop, such as a particle of moisture discharged from the mouth during coughing, sneezing, or speaking; these may transmit infections to others by their airborne passage. [drop + -*let,* dim. suffix]

drown·ing. Death from suffocation induced by immersion in water or other fluid, with filling of pulmonary air spaces and passages with fluid to the detriment of gas exchange. [M.E. *drounen*]

drows·i·ness (drow′zē-nes). A state of impaired awareness associated with a desire or inclination to sleep.

drug (drŭg). **1.** Therapeutic agent; any substance, other than food, used in the prevention, diagnosis, alleviation, treatment, or cure of disease. For types or classifications of d.'s, see the specific name. SEE ALSO agent. **2.** To administer or take a d., usually implying an overly large quantity or a narcotic. **3.** General term for any substance, stimulating or depressing, that can be habituating or addictive, especially a narcotic. [M.E. *drogge*]

    d. holidays, intervals when a chronically medicated patient temporarily stops taking the medication; used to allow some recuperation of normal functions and/or to maintain sensitivity to the drug(s).

    nonsteroidal anti-inflammatory d.'s, d.'s exerting anti-inflammatory (and also usually analgesic and antipyretic) actions; examples include aspirin, diclofenac, ibuprofen, and naproxen. A contrast is made with steroidal compounds (such as hydrocortisone or prednisone) exerting anti-inflammatory activity.

    orphan d.'s, SYN orphan *products,* under *product.*

    street d., a controlled substance taken for non-medical purposes. Street d.'s comprise various amphetamines, anesthetics, barbiturates, opiates, and psychoactive drugs, and many are derived from natural sources (*e.g.,* the plants *Papaver somniferum, Cannibis sativa, Amanita pantherina, Lophophora williamsii*). Slang names include acid (lysergic acid diethylamide), angel dust (phencyclidine), coke (cocaine), downers (barbiturates), grass (marijuana), hash (concentrated tetrahydrocannibinol), magic mushrooms (psilocybin), and speed (amphetamines). During the 1980s, a new class of "designer drugs" arose, mostly analogs of psychoactive substances intended to escape regulation under the Controlled Substances Act. Also, crack cocaine, a potent, smokable form of cocaine, emerged as a major public health problem. In the U.S., illicit use of drugs such as cocaine, marijuana, and heroin historically has occurred in cycles.

therapeutic d., prescription or over-the-counter medication used to treat an injury or illness.

drug-fast. Pertaining to microorganisms that resist or become tolerant to an antibacterial agent.

drug in·ter·ac·tions. The pharmacological result, either desirable or undesirable, of drugs interacting with other drugs, with endogenous physiologic chemical agents (*e.g.,* MAOI with epinephrine), with components of the diet, and with chemicals used in diagnostic tests or the results of such tests.

drug use evaluation. SYN Drug Use Review.

Drug Use Review (DUR). A program that reviews, analyzes, and interprets rates, costs, and appropriateness of drug usage within specific health care environments. SYN drug use evaluation.

drum, drum·head (drŭm, drŭm′hed). SYN tympanic *membrane.*

drunk·en·ness (drŭnk′en-nes). Intoxication, usually alcoholic. SEE ALSO acute *alcoholism.*

dru·sen (drū′sen). Small bright structures seen in the retina and in the optic disc. [Ger. pl. of *Druse,* stony nodule, geode]

DRVVT (dilute Russell's viper venom test) dilute Russell's viper venom *test.*

DSA digital subtraction *angiography.*

DT *delirium* tremens; duration *tetany.*

dT deoxythymidine.

dTDP thymidine 5′-diphosphate.

dThd thymidine.

dTMP deoxythymidylic acid.

DTR deep tendon reflex.

du·al·ism (dū′ăl-izm). **1.** CHEMISTRY theory that every compound, no matter how many elements enter into it, is composed of two parts, one electrically negative, the other positive; applicable to polar compounds but not to nonpolar compounds. **2.** HEMATOLOGY The concept that blood cells have two origins, *i.e.,* lymphogenous and myelogenous. **3.** The theory that the mind and body are two distinct systems, independent and different in nature. [L. *dualis,* relating to two, fr. *duo,* two]

duct (dŭkt). A tubular structure giving exit to the secretion of a gland, or conducting any fluid. SEE ALSO canal. SYN ductus [NA]. [L. *duco,* pp. *ductus,* to lead]

accessory pancreatic d., the excretory duct of the head of the pancreas, one branch of which joins the pancreatic duct, the other opening independently into the duodenum at the lesser duodenal papilla. SYN Santorini's d.

alveolar d., **(1)** the part of the respiratory passages distal to the respiratory bronchiole; from it arise alveolar sacs and alveoli; **(2)** the smallest of the intralobular d.'s in the mammary gland, into which the secretory alveoli open. SYN ductulus alveolaris [NA].

anal d.'s, short d.'s lined with simple columnar to stratified columnar epithelium that extend from the valvulae anales to the sinus anales.

arterial d., SYN *ductus* arteriosus.

bile d., any of the d.'s conveying bile between the liver and the intestine, including hepatic, cystic, and common bile d. SYN biliary d.

biliary d., SYN bile d.

Botallo's d., SYN *ductus* arteriosus.

cochlear d., a spirally arranged membranous tube suspended within the cochlea, occupying the lower portion of the scala vestibuli; it begins by a blind extremity, the vestibular cecum, in the cochlear recess of the vestibule, terminating in another blind extremity, the cecum cupulare or lagena, at the cupola of the cochlea; it contains endolymph and communicates with the sacculus by the ductus reuniens; the spiral organ (of Corti), the neuroepithelial receptor organ for hearing, occupies the floor of the duct. SYN scala media.

common bile d., a duct formed by the union of the hepatic and cystic ducts; it discharges at the duodenal papilla.

common hepatic d., the part of the biliary duct system that is formed by the confluence of right and left hepatic ducts. At the porta hepatis it is joined by the cystic duct to become the common bile duct.

cystic d., cystic gall d., the d. leading from the gallbladder; it joins the hepatic duct to form the common bile duct.

deferent d., SYN *ductus* deferens.

ejaculatory d., the duct formed by the union of the deferent duct and the excretory duct of the seminal vesicle, which opens into the prostatic urethra. SYN spermiduct (2).

endolymphatic d., a small membranous canal, connecting with both saccule and utricle of the membranous labyrinth, passing through the aqueduct of vestibule, and terminating in a dilated blind extremity, the endolymphatic sac, on the posterior surface of the petrous portion of the temporal bone beneath the dura mater.

excretory d., a d. carrying the secretion from a gland or a fluid from any reservoir.

excretory d.'s of lacrimal gland, the multiple (6 to 10) excretory ducts of the lacrimal gland that open into the superior fornix of the conjunctival sac.

galactophorous d.'s, SYN lactiferous d.'s.

hepatic d., SEE common hepatic d.

intercalated d.'s, the minute d.'s of glands, such as the salivary and the pancreas, that lead from the acini; they are lined by low cuboidal cells.

interlobar d., a d. draining the secretion of the lobe of a gland and formed by the junction of a number of interlobular d.'s.

interlobular d., any d. leading from a lobule of a gland and formed by the junction of the fine d.'s draining the acini.

intralobular d., a d. that lies within a lobule of a gland.

lactiferous d.'s, the ducts, numbering 15 or 20, which drain the lobes of the mammary gland; they open at the nipple. SYN galactophore, galactophorous d.'s, mamillary d.'s, milk d.'s.

left hepatic d., the duct that drains bile from the left half of the liver, including the quadrate lobe and the left part of the caudate lobe.

lymphatic d., one of the two large lymph channels, right lymphatic duct or thoracic d.

major sublingual d., the duct that drains the anterior portion of the sublingual gland; it opens at the sublingual papilla.

mamillary d.'s, SYN lactiferous d.'s.

mesonephric d., a duct in the embryo draining the mesonephric tubules; in the male it becomes the ductus deferens; in the female it becomes vestigial. SYN wolffian d.

metanephric d., the slender tubular portion of the metanephric diverticulum; the primordium of the epithelial lining of the ureter.

milk d.'s, SYN lactiferous d.'s.

minor sublingual d.'s, from 8 to 20 small ducts of the sublingual salivary gland that open into the mouth on the surface of the sublingual fold; a few join the submandibular ducts.

nasolacrimal d., the passage leading downward from the lacrimal sac on each side to the anterior portion of the inferior meatus of the nose, through which tears are conducted into the nasal cavity.

omphalomesenteric d., SYN yolk *stalk.*

pancreatic d., the excretory duct of the pancreas that extends through the gland from tail to head, where it empties into the duodenum at the greater duodenal papilla. SYN Wirsung's canal.

papillary d.'s, the largest straight excretory d.'s in the kidney medulla and papillae whose openings form the area cribrosa; they are a continuation of the collecting tubules.

paramesonephric d., either of the two paired embryonic tubes extending along the mesonephros roughly parallel to the mesonephric duct and emptying into the cloaca; in the female, the upper parts of the ducts form the uterine tubes, while the lower fuse to form the uterus and part of the vagina; in the male, vestiges of the ducts form the vagina masculina and the appendix testis.

paraurethral d.'s, inconstant ducts along the side of the female urethra that convey the mucoid secretion of Skene's glands to the vestibule.

parotid d., the duct of the parotid gland opening from the cheek into the vestibule of the mouth opposite the neck of the superior second molar tooth. SYN Stensen's d., Steno's d.

perilymphatic d., a fine canal connecting the perilymphatic space of the cochlea with the subarachnoid space. SYN aqueductus cochleae.

prostatic d.'s, SYN prostatic *ductules,* under *ductule.*

right hepatic d., the duct that transmits bile to the common hepatic duct from the right half of the liver and the right part of the caudate lobe.

right lymphatic d., one of the two terminal lymph vessels, a short trunk, about 2 cm in length, formed by the union of the right jugular lymphatic vessel and vessels from the lymph nodes of the right superior limb, thoracic wall,

and both lungs; it lies on the right side of the root of the neck and empties into the right brachiocephalic vein.

Santorini's d., SYN accessory pancreatic d.

semicircular d.'s, three small membranous tubes in the bony semicircular canals that lie within the bony labyrinth and form loops of about two-thirds of a circle. The three (anterior semicircular d., lateral semicircular d., and posterior semicircular d.) lie in planes at right angles to each other and open into the vestibule by five openings of which one is common to the anterior and lateral ducts. Each duct has an ampulla at one end within which filaments of the vestibular nerve terminate.

seminal d., any one of the d.'s conveying semen from the epididymis to the urethra, ductus deferens, or ejaculatory d. SYN gonaduct (1).

spermatic d., SYN *ductus* deferens.

d. of common bile duct, smooth muscle sphincter of the common bile duct immediately proximal to the hepatopancreatic ampulla; it is this sphincter that controls the flow of bile in the duodenum. SYN musculus sphincter ductus choledochi [NA].

d. of pancreatic duct, smooth muscle sphincter of the main pancreatic duct immediately proximal to the hepatoduodenal ampulla. SYN musculus sphincter ductus pancreatici.

Stensen's d., Steno's d., SYN parotid d.

striated d., a type of intralobular d. found in some salivary glands that modifies the secretory product; it derives its name from extensive infolding of the basal membrane.

submandibular d., the duct of the submandibular salivary gland; it opens at the sublingual papilla near the frenulum of the tongue. SYN Wharton's d.

thoracic d., the largest lymph vessel in the body, beginning at the cisterna chyli at about the level of the second lumbar vertebra; the abdominal part extends superiorly to pass through the aortic opening of the diaphragm, where it becomes the thoracic part and crosses the posterior mediastinum to form the arch of the thoracic duct and discharge into the left venous angle (origin of the brachiocephalic vein).

Wharton's d., SYN submandibular d.

wolffian d., SYN mesonephric d.

duc·tal (dŭk′tăl). Relating to a duct.

duc·tile (dŭk′tĭl). Denoting the property of a material that allows it to be bent, drawn out (as a wire), or otherwise deformed without breaking. [L. *ductilis,* capable of being led or drawn]

duct·less (dŭkt′les). Having no duct; denoting certain glands having only an internal secretion.

duc·tu·lar (dŭk′tū-lăr). Relating to a ductule.

duc·tule (dŭk′tūl). A minute duct. SYN ductulus [NA].

biliary d.'s, the excretory ducts of the liver that connect the interlobular ductules to the right (or left) hepatic duct. SYN ductuli biliferi [NA].

efferent d.'s of testis, one of 12 to 14 small seminal ducts leading from the testis to the head of the epididymis. SYN vas efferens (3) [NA].

prostatic d.'s, about 20 minute canals that receive the prostatic secretion from the glandular tubules and discharge it through openings on either side of the urethral crest in the posterior wall of the urethra. SYN ductuli prostatici [NA], prostatic ducts.

duc•tu•lus, pl. **duc•tu•li** (dŭk'tū-lŭs, -tū-lī) [NA]. SYN ductule. [Mod. L. dim. of L. *ductus*, duct]

d. alveola'ris, pl. **duc'tuli alveola'res** [NA], SYN alveolar *duct*.

duc'tuli bilif'eri [NA], SYN biliary *ductules*, under *ductule*.

duc'tuli prostat'ici [NA], SYN prostatic *ductules*, under *ductule*.

duc•tus, gen. and pl. **duc•tus** (dŭk'tŭs) [NA]. SYN duct. [L. a leading, fr. *duco*, pp. *ductus*, to lead]

d. arterio'sus [NA], a fetal vessel connecting the left pulmonary artery with the descending aorta; in the first two months after birth, it normally changes into a fibrous cord, the ligamentum arteriosum; occasional postnatal failure to close causes a surgically correctable cardiovascular handicap. SYN arterial canal, arterial duct, Botallo's duct.

d. def'erens [NA], the secretory duct of the testicle, running from the epididymis, of which it is the continuation, to the prostatic urethra where it terminates as the ejaculatory duct. SYN deferent duct, spermatic duct, spermiduct (1), vas deferens.

d. veno'sus [NA], in the fetus, continuation of the left umbilical vein through the liver to the vena cava inferior; after birth, its lumen becomes obliterated, forming the ligamentum venosum.

dull (dŭl). Not sharp or acute, in any sense; qualifying a surgical instrument, the action of the mind, pain, a sound (especially the percussion note), etc. [M.E. *dul*]

dump•ing (dŭmp'ing). SEE dumping *syndrome*.

du•o•de•nal (dū'ō-dē'năl, dū-od'ĕ-năl). Relating to the duodenum.

du•o•de•nec•to•my (dū-ō-dĕ-nek'tō-mē). Excision of the duodenum. [duodenum + G. *ektomē*, excision]

du•o•de•ni•tis (dū-od-ĕ-nī'tis). Inflammation of the duodenum.

⚠**duodeno-**. Combining form relating to the duodenum. [L. *duodenum (digitorum)*, breadth of 12 fingers]

du•o•de•no•cho•lan•gi•tis (dū-ō-dē'nō-kō-lan-jī'tis). Inflammation of the duodenum and common bile duct. [duodeno- + G. *cholē*, bile, + *angeion*, vessel, + *-itis*, inflammation]

du•o•de•no•cho•le•cys•tos•to•my (dū-ō-dē'nō-kō-lē-sis-tos'tō-mē). SYN cholecystoduodenostomy. [duodeno- + G. *cholē*, bile, + *kystis*, bladder, + *stoma*, mouth]

du•o•de•no•cho•led•o•chot•o•my (dū-ō-dē'nō-kō-led-ō-kot'ō-mē). Incision into the common bile duct and the adjacent portion of the duodenum. [duodeno- + G. *choledochus*, bile duct, + *tomē*, incision]

du•o•de•no•cys•tos•to•my (dū-ō-dē'nō-sis-tos'tō-mē). **1.** SYN cholecystoduodenostomy. **2.** SYN cystoduodenostomy. **3.** SYN pancreatic *cystoduodenostomy*.

du•o•de•no•en•ter•os•to•my (dū-ō-dē'nō-en-ter-os'tō-mē). Establishment of communication between the duodenum and another part of the intestinal tract. [duodeno- + G. *enteron*, intestine, + *stoma*, mouth]

du•o•de•no•je•ju•nos•to•my (dū-ō-dē'nō-jĕ-jū-nos'tō-mē). Operative formation of an artificial communication between the duodenum and the jejunum. [duodeno- + jejunum, + G. *stoma*, mouth]

du•o•de•nol•y•sis (dū-ō-dĕ-nol'i-sis). Incision of adhesions to the duodenum. [duodeno- + G. *lysis*, a freeing]

du•o•de•nor•rha•phy (dū-ō-dĕ-nōr'ă-fē). Suture of a tear or incision in the duodenum. [duodeno- + G. *rhaphē*, a seam]

du•o•de•nos•co•py (dū-ō-dĕ-nos'kŏ-pē). Inspection of the interior of the duodenum through an endoscope. [duodeno- + G. *skopeō*, to examine]

du•o•de•nos•to•my (dū-ō-dĕ-nos'tō-mē). Establishment of a fistula into the duodenum. [duodeno- + G. *stoma*, mouth]

du•o•de•not•o•my (dū-ō-dĕ-not'ō-mē). Incision of the duodenum. [duodeno- + G. *tomē*, incision]

du•o•de•num, gen. **du•o•de•ni**, pl. **du•o•de•na** (dū-ō-dē'nŭm, dū-od'ĕ-nŭm; -od'ĕ-nă, -dē'nă) [NA]. The first division of the small intestine, about 25 cm in length, extending from the pylorus to the junction with the jejunum at the level of the first or second lumbar vertebra on the left side. It is divided into the superior part, the first part of which is the duodenal cap, the descending part, into which the bile and pancreatic ducts open, the horizontal (inferior) part and the ascending part, terminating at the duodenojejunal junction. [Mediev. L. fr. L. *duodeni*, twelve]

du•pli•ca•tion (dū-pli-kā'shŭn). **1.** A doubling. SEE ALSO reduplication. **2.** Inclusion of two copies of the same genetic material in a genome; an important step in diversification of genomes; as in the evolution of the (non-allelic) hemoglobin chains from a common ancestor. [L. *duplicatio*, a doubling, fr. *duplico*, to double]

d. of chromosomes, a chromosome aberration resulting from unequal crossing over or exchange of segments between two homologous chromosomes; one chromosome of the pair loses a small segment, while the other gains this segment; the chromosome gaining the segment has undergone d. while its homologue has undergone deletion.

DUR Drug Use Review.

du•ra (dū'ră). SYN dura mater. [L. fem. of *durus*, hard]

durable power of attorney. SYN advance directive.

du•ral (dū'răl). Relating to the dura mater.

du•ra mat•er (dū'ră mā'ter). Pachymeninx (as distinguished from leptomeninx, the combined pia mater and arachnoid); a tough, fibrous membrane forming the outer covering of the central nervous system. SYN dura. [L. hard mother, mistransl. of Ar. *umm al-jāfīyah*, tough protector or covering]

du•ra•tion (dū-rā'shŭn). A continuous period of time.

dwarf (dwōrf). An abnormally undersized person with disproportion among the bodily parts. SEE dwarfism. [A.S. *dweorh*]

dwarf·ism (dwôrf′izm). The condition of being abnormally undersized.

   achondroplastic d., SEE achondroplasia.

   asexual d., d. in which adult sexual development is deficient.

   camptomelic d., d. with shortening of the lower limbs due to anterior bending of the femur and tibia.

   chondrodystrophic d., SEE chondrodystrophy.

   Laron type d., d. associated with deficiency of somatomedin C (insulin-like growth factor I) or abnormalities in receptor activity.

   mesomelic d., d. with shortness of the forearms and lower legs.

   micromelic d., d. with abnormally short or small limbs.

   pituitary d., a rare form of d. caused by the absence of a functional anterior pituitary gland; may be present at birth or develop during early childhood.

Dy dysprosium.

dy·ad (dī′ad). **1.** A pair. SYN diad (2). **2.** CHEMISTRY A bivalent element. **3.** A pair of persons in an interactional situation, *e.g.,* patient and therapist, husband and wife. **4.** The double chromosome resulting from the splitting of a tetrad during meiosis. [G. *dyas,* the number two, duality]

dye (dī). A stain or coloring matter; a compound consisting of chromophore and auxochrome groups attached to one or more benzene rings, its color being due to the chromophore and its dyeing affinities to the auxochrome. D.'s are used for intravital coloration of living cells, staining tissues and microorganisms, as antiseptics and germicides, and some as stimulants of epithelial growth. For individual d.'s, see the specific names. Commonly used for radiographic contrast medium. [A.S. *deah, deag*]

   acidic d.'s, d.'s which ionize in solution to produce negatively charged ions or anions; they consist of sodium salts of phenols and carboxylic acid dyes; their solutions tend to be neutral or slightly alkaline; examples are eosin and aniline blue.

   basic d.'s, d.'s which ionize in solution to give positively charged ions or cations; the auxochrome group is an amine which can form a salt with an acid; solutions are usually slightly acidic.

   natural d.'s, d.'s obtained from animals or plants.

   nitro d.'s, d.'s in which the chromophore is -NO$_2$, which is so acidic that all dyes in this group are of the acid type.

   oxazin d.'s, similar to azin d.'s except that one of the connecting N atoms is replaced by O.

   synthetic d.'s, organic d. compounds originally derived from coal-tar derivatives; presently produced by synthesis from benzene and its derivatives.

   thiazin d.'s, similar to azin d.'s except that one of the connecting N atoms is replaced by S; includes many important biological stains, especially in hematology.

   xanthene d.'s, derivatives of the compound xanthene.

△**-dymus. 1.** Suffix to be combined with number roots; *e.g.,* didymus, tridymus, tetradymus. **2.** Occasionally used for -didymus. [G. *-dymos,* fold]

dy·nam·ics (dī-nam′iks). **1.** The science of motion in response to forces. **2.** PSYCHIATRY The determination of how emotional and mental disorders develop. **3.** BEHAVIORAL SCIENCES Any of the numerous intrapersonal and interpersonal influences or phenomena associated with personality development and interpersonal processes. [G. *dynamis,* force]

△**dynamo-.** Combining form, force, energy. [G. *dynamis,* power]

dy·na·mo·gen·e·sis (dī′nă-mō-jen′ĕ-sis). The production of force, especially of muscular or nervous energy. [dynamo- + G. *genesis,* production]

dy·na·mo·gen·ic (dī′nă-mō-jen′ik). Producing power or force, especially nervous or muscular power or activity.

dy·nam·o·graph (dī-nam′ō-graf). An instrument for recording the degree of muscular power. [dynamo- + G. *graphō,* to write]

dy·na·mom·e·ter (dī-nă-mom′ĕ-ter). An instrument for measuring the degree of muscular power. SYN ergometer. [dynamo- + G. *metron,* measure]

dyne (dīn). The unit of force in the CGS system, replaced in the SI system by the newton (1 newton = 10^5 dynes), that gives a body of 1 g mass an acceleration of 1 cm/sec^2; expressed as F (dynes) = m (grams) × a (cm/sec^2). [G. *dynamis,* force]

dyn·ein (dīn′ēn). A protein associated with motile structures, exhibiting adenosine triphosphatase activity; it forms "arms" on the outer tubules of cilia and flagella. SEE ALSO tubulin. [dyne + protein]

△**dys-.** Bad, difficult, un-, mis-; opposite of eu-. Cf. dis-. [G.]

dys·a·cou·sia, dys·a·cu·sia (dis-ă-kū′sē-ă). SYN dysacusis.

dys·a·cu·sis (dis-ă-kū′sis). **1.** Any impairment of hearing involving difficulty in processing details of sound as opposed to any loss of sensitivity to sound. **2.** Pain or discomfort in the ear from exposure to sound. SYN dysacousia, dysacusia. [dys- + G. *akousis,* hearing]

dys·a·phia (dis-ā′fē-ă, dis-af′ē-ă). Impairment of the sense of touch. [dys- + G. *haphē,* touch]

dys·ar·te·ri·ot·o·ny (dis-ar-tēr-ē-ot′ō-nē). Abnormal blood pressure, either too high or too low. [dys- + G. *artēria,* artery, + *tonos,* tension]

dys·ar·thria (dis-ar′thrē-ă). A disturbance of speech and language due to emotional stress, to brain injury or to paralysis, incoordination, or spasticity of the muscles used for speaking. SYN dysarthrosis (1). [dys- + G. *arthroō,* to articulate]

   ataxic d., d. associated with damage to the cerebellar system, characterized by imprecise consonants, excess and equal stress, inconsistent articulatory errors, and monotony of pitch and volume. SEE ataxia.

   flaccid d., d. associated with peripheral muscle weakness usually due to lower motor neuron disorders, causing hypernasality, imprecise consonants, breathy voice, and monotony of pitch. SEE hypernasality.

hyperkinetic d., d. associated with disorders of the extrapyramidal motor system resulting in involuntary movements of the articulatory and respiratory systems that cause variations in voice loudness and rate, and interruptions in ongoing speech. SEE ALSO extrapyramidal motor *system*, myoclonus, athetosis, Gilles de la Tourette's *syndrome*.

hypokinetic d., d. associated with disorders of the extrapyramidal motor system resulting in reduction and rigidity of movement, causing monotony of pitch and loudness, reduced stress, and imprecise enunciation of consonants. SEE ALSO extrapyramidal motor *system*, parkinsonian d.

parkinsonian d., a hypokinetic d. associated with Parkinson's disease, characterized by rigidity and reduced range of articulatory movements, monotony of pitch and loudness, reduced loudness, short rushes of speech, and rapid rate. SEE parkinsonism.

spastic d., d. associated with upper motor neuron disorders causing excess tone and limited range in muscle movements, characterized by imprecise consonants, monotony of pitch and reduced stress, and a labored voice quality. SEE pseudobulbar *palsy*.

dys•ar•thric (dis-ar′thrik). Relating to dysarthria.

dys•ar•thro•sis (dis-ar-thrō′sis). **1.** SYN dysarthria. **2.** Malformation of a joint. **3.** A false joint. [dys- + G. *arthrōsis,* joint]

dys•au•to•no•mia (dis′aw-tō-nō′mē-ă). Abnormal functioning of the autonomic nervous system. [dys- + G. *autonomia,* self-government]

familial d. [MIM*223900], a congenital syndrome with aberrations in autonomic nervous system function such as indifference to pain, diminished lacrimation, poor vasomotor homeostasis, motor incoordination, labile cardiovascular reactions, hyporeflexia, frequent attacks of bronchial pneumonia, hypersalivation with aspiration and difficulty in swallowing, hyperemesis, emotional instability, and an intolerance for anesthetics.

dys•ba•rism (dis′bar-izm). General term for the symptom complex resulting from exposure to decreased or changing barometric pressure, including all physiologic effects resulting from such changes with the exception of hypoxia, and including the effects of rapid decompression. [dys- + G. *baros,* weight]

dys•ba•sia (dis-bā′zē-ă). **1.** Difficulty in walking. **2.** The difficult or distorted walking that occurs in persons with certain mental disorders. [dys- + G. *basis,* a step]

dys•bu•lia (dis-bū′lē-ă). Weakness and uncertainty of volition. [dys- + G. *boulē,* will]

dys•bu•lic (dis-bū′lik). Relating to, or characterized by, dysbulia.

dys•cal•cu•lia (dis-kal-kyū′lē-ă). Difficulty in performing simple mathematical problems; commonly seen in parietal lobe lesions. [dys- + L. *calculo,* to compute, fr. *calculus,* pebble, counter]

dys•ce•pha•lia (dis-sĕ-fā′lē-ă). Malformation of the head and face. [dys- + G. *kephalē,* head]

dys•chei•ral, dys•chi•ral (dis-kī′răl). Relating to dyscheiria.

dys•che•zia (dis-kē′zē-ă). Difficulty in defecation. [dys- + G. *chezō,* to defecate]

dys•chon•dro•gen•e•sis (dis-kon-drō-jen′ĕ-sis). Abnormal development of cartilage. [dys- + G. *chondros,* cartilage, + *genesis,* production]

dys•chon•dro•pla•sia (dis-kon-drō-plā′zē-ă). SYN enchondromatosis. [dys- + G. *chondros,* cartilage, + *plasis,* a forming]

dys•chro•ma•top•sia (dis′krō-mă-top′sē-ă). A condition in which the ability to perceive colors is not fully normal. Cf. dichromatism, monochromatism, chromatopsia. [dys- + G. *chrōma,* color, + *opsis,* vision]

dys•chro•mia (dis-krō′mē-ă). Any abnormality in the color of the skin.

dys•co•ria (dis-kō′rē-ă). Abnormality in the shape of the pupil. [dys- + G. *korē,* pupil of eye]

dys•cra•sia (dis-krā′zē-ă). **1.** A morbid general state resulting from the presence of abnormal material in the blood, usually applied to diseases affecting blood cells or platelets. **2.** Old term indicating disease. [G. bad temperament, fr. dys- + *krasis,* a mixing]

blood d., a diseased state of the blood; usually refers to abnormal cellular elements of a permanent character.

dys•cra•sic, dys•crat•ic (dis-krā′sik, krat′ik). Pertaining to or affected with dyscrasia.

dys•en•ter•ic (dis-en-tār′ik). Relating to or suffering from dysentery.

dys•en•tery (dis-en-tār-ē). A disease marked by frequent watery stools, often with blood and mucus, and characterized clinically by pain, tenesmus, fever, and dehydration. [G. *dysenteria,* fr. *dys-,* bad, + *entera,* bowels]

amebic d., diarrhea resulting from ulcerative inflammation of the colon, caused chiefly by infection with *Entamoeba histolytica;* may be associated with amebic infection of other organs.

bacillary d., infection with *Shigella dysenteriae, S. flexneri,* or other organisms.

bilharzial d., d. due to infection with *Schistosoma mansoni, S. haematobium,* or *S. japonicum.*

viral d., profuse watery diarrhea due to, or thought to be due to, infection by a virus.

dys•er•e•thism (dis-er′ĕ-thizm). A condition of slow response to stimuli. [dys- + G. *erethismos,* irritation]

dys•er•gia (dis-er′jē-ă). Lack of harmonious action between the muscles concerned in executing any definite voluntary movement. [dys- + G. *ergon,* work]

dys•es•the•sia (dis-es-thē′zē-ă). **1.** Impairment of sensation short of anesthesia. **2.** A condition in which a disagreeable sensation is produced by ordinary stimuli; caused by lesions of the sensory pathways, peripheral or central. **3.** Abnormal sensations experienced in the absence of stimulation. [G. *dysaisthēsia,* fr. *dys-,* hard, difficult, + *aisthēsis,* sensation]

dys•fi•brin•o•ge•ne•mia (dis′fī-brin′ō-jĕ-nē′mē-ă) [MIM*134820]. An autosomal dominant disorder of qualitatively abnormal fibrinogens of various types, resulting in abnormalities of coagulation tests (bleeding time, clotting time, thrombin time); symptoms vary from none to abnormal bleeding and excessive clotting.

dysfluency (dĭs-flū-ĕn-sē). Speech interrupted in its forward flow by hesitations, repetitions, or prolongations of sounds. Although dysfluencies are the common manifestation of a stuttering disorder, they are also present in normal speech, particularly during speech development in young children. SEE stuttering. SYN disfluency, nonfluency.

dys·func·tion (dis-fŭnk′shŭn). Difficult or abnormal function.

minimal brain d., SEE attention deficit *disorder.*

psychosexual d., sexual d., a disturbance of sexual functioning, *e.g.,* impotence, premature ejaculation, anorgasmia, presumed to be of psychological rather than physical etiology.

temporomandibular joint d. (TMJ), chronic or impaired function of the temporomandibular articulation. SEE myofacial pain-dysfunction *syndrome.*

dys·gam·ma·glob·u·lin·e·mia (dis-gam′ă-glob′yū-li-nē′mē-ă) [MIM*308230]. An immunoglobulin abnormality, especially a disturbance of the percentage distribution of γ-globulins.

dys·gen·e·sis (dis-jen′ĕ-sis). Defective development. [dys- + G. *genesis,* generation]

gonadal d., defective gonadal development, varying types and degrees of which have been identified, including gonadal aplasia or agenesis, rudimentary gonads, congenitally defective gonads, and true hermaphroditism.

seminiferous tubule d., a disorder in which the seminiferous tubules exhibit an abnormal cytoarchitecture and extensive hyalinization; the testes are small, and few spermatozoa are formed; the body habitus may be eunuchoid, and gynecomastia may be present; urinary gonadotropin output is usually high, and the incidence of mental deficiency and illness increased; sex chromatin may be male or female, and androgen secretion ranges from subnormal to normal. It is a constant feature of (and is often used synonymously with) Klinefelter's *syndrome.*

dys·gen·ic (dis-jen′ik). Applying to factors that have a detrimental effect upon hereditary qualities, physical or mental.

dys·ger·mi·no·ma (dis-jer-mi-nō′mă). A rare malignant neoplasm of the ovary composed of undifferentiated gonadal germinal cells and occurring more frequently in patients less than 20 years of age. The neoplasms contain foci of necrosis and hemorrhage, and tend to be encapsulated; characteristically, they spread by way of lymphatic vessels, but widespread metastases also occur. SYN disgerminoma. [dys- + L. *germen,* a bud or sprout, + G. *-ōma,* tumor]

dys·geu·sia (dis-gū′sē-ă). Impairment or perversion of the gustatory sense. [dys- + G. *geusis,* taste]

dys·gna·thia (dis-nath′ē-ă). Any abnormality that extends beyond the teeth and includes the maxilla or mandible, or both. [dys- + G. *gnathos,* jaw]

dys·gnath·ic (dis-nath′ik). Pertaining to or characterized by abnormality of the maxilla and mandible.

dys·gno·sia (dis-nō′sē-ă). Any cognitive disorder, *i.e.,* any mental illness. [G. *dysgnōsia,* difficulty of knowing]

dys·hem·a·to·poi·e·sis (dis-hē′mă-tō-poy-ē′sis). Defective formation of the blood. SYN dyshemopoiesis. [dys- + G. *haima (haimat-),* blood, + *poiēsis,* making]

dys·hem·a·to·poi·et·ic (dis-hē′mă-tō-poy-et′ik). Pertaining to or characterized by dyshematopoiesis. SYN dyshemopoietic.

dys·he·mo·poi·e·sis (dis-hē′mō-poy-ē′sis). SYN dyshematopoiesis.

dys·he·mo·poi·et·ic (dis-hē′mō-poy-et′ik). SYN dyshematopoietic.

dys·hi·dro·sis (dis-i-drō′sis). A vesicular or vesicopustular eruption of multiple causes that occurs primarily on the volar surfaces of the hands and feet; the lesions spread peripherally but have a tendency to central clearing. SYN cheiropompholyx, chiropompholyx, chiropompholyx. [dys- + G. *hidrōs,* sweat]

dys·kar·y·o·sis (dis-kar-ē-ō′sis). Abnormal maturation seen in exfoliated cells that have normal cytoplasm but hyperchromatic nuclei, or irregular chromatin distribution; may be followed by the development of a malignant neoplasm. [dys- + G. *karyon,* nucleus, + *-ōsis,* condition]

dys·kar·y·ot·ic (dis-kar-ē-ot′ik). Pertaining to or characterized by dyskaryosis.

dys·ker·a·to·ma (dis-ker-ă-tō′mă). A skin tumor exhibiting dyskeratosis. [dys- + G. *keras,* horn, + *-oma,* tumor]

dys·ker·a·to·sis (dis′ker-ă-tō′sis). **1.** Premature keratinization in individual epithelial cells that have not reached the keratinizing surface layer; dyskeratotic cells generally become rounded, and they may break away from adjacent cells and fall off. **2.** Epidermalization of the conjunctival and corneal epithelium. **3.** A disorder of keratinization. [dys- + G. *keras,* horn, + *-osis,* condition]

malignant d., d. that may occur in precancerous or malignant lesions.

dys·ker·a·tot·ic (dis′ker-a-tot′ik). Relating to or characterized by dyskeratosis.

dys·ki·ne·sia (dis-ki-nē′zē-ă). Difficulty in performing voluntary movements. Term usually used in relation to various extrapyramidal disorders. [dys- + G. *kinēsis,* movement]

d. al′gera, a hysterical condition in which active movement causes pain.

extrapyramidal d.'s, abnormal involuntary movements attributed to pathological states of one or more parts of the striate body and characterized by insuppressible, stereotyped, automatic movements that cease only during sleep; *e.g.,* Parkinson's disease; chorea; athetosis; hemiballism.

d. intermit′tens, intermittent disability of the limbs due to impairment of circulation.

dys·ki·net·ic (dis-ki-net′ik). Denoting or characteristic of dyskinesia.

dys·lex·ia (dis-lek′sē-ă). Impaired reading ability with a competence level below that expected on the basis of the individual's level of intelligence, and in the presence of normal vision and letter recognition and normal recognition of the meaning of pictures and objects. [dys- + G. *lexis,* word, phrase]

dys·lex·ic (dis-lek′sik). Relating to, or characterized by, dyslexia.

dys·lo·gia (dis-lō′jē-ă). Impairment of speech and reasoning as the result of a mental disorder. [dys- + G. *logos*, speaking, reason]

dys·ma·ture (dis′mă-tyūr). **1.** Denoting faulty development or ripening; often connoting structural and/or functional abnormalities. **2.** OBSTETRICS Denoting an infant whose birth weight is inappropriately low for its gestational age. **3.** Immature development of the placenta so that normal function does not occur.

dys·ma·tu·ri·ty (dis′mă-chūr-i-tē). Syndrome of an infant born with relative absence of subcutaneous fat, wrinkling of the skin, prominent finger and toe nails, and meconium staining of skin and placental membranes; often associated with postmaturity or placental insufficiency.

dys·me·lia (dis-mē′lē-ă). Congenital abnormality characterized by missing or foreshortened limbs, sometimes with associated spine abnormalities; caused by metabolic disturbance at the time of primordial limb development. SEE amelia, phocomelia. [dys- + G. *melos*, limb]

dys·men·or·rhea (dis-men-ōr-ē′ă). Difficult and painful menstruation. SYN menorrhalgia. [dys- + G. *mēn*, month, + *rhoia*, a flow]

  essential d., SYN primary d.

  functional d., SYN primary d.

  intrinsic d., SYN primary d.

  mechanical d., d. due to obstruction of discharge of menstrual blood, as in cervical stenosis. SYN obstructive d.

  membranous d., d. accompanied by an exfoliation of the menstrual decidua.

  obstructive d., SYN mechanical d.

  primary d., d. due to a functional disturbance and not due to inflammation, new growths, or anatomic factors. SYN essential d., functional d., intrinsic d.

  secondary d., d. due to inflammation, infection, tumor, or anatomical factors.

  spasmodic d., d. accompanied by painful contractions of the uterus.

dys·met·ria (dis-mē′trē-ă, -met′rē-ă). An aspect of ataxia, in which the ability to control the distance, power, and speed of an act is impaired. Usually used to describe abnormalities of movement caused by cerebellar disorders. SEE ALSO hypermetria, hypometria. [dys- + G. *metron*, measure]

dys·mor·phism (dis-mōr′fizm). Abnormality of shape. [G. *dysmorphia*, badness of form]

dys·mor·pho·gen·e·sis (dis′mōr-fō-jen′ĕ-sis). The process of abnormal tissue formation. [dys- + G. *morphē*, form, + *genesis*, production]

dys·mor·phol·o·gy (dis-mōr-fol′ō-jē). General term for the study of, or the subject of, abnormal development of tissue form. A branch of clinical genetics. [dys- + G. *morphē*, form, + *logos*, study]

dys·my·o·to·nia (dis-mī-ō-tō′nē-ă). Abnormal muscular tonicity (either hyper- or hypo-). SEE dystonia. [dys- + G. *mys*, muscle, + *tonos*, tension, tone]

dys·o·don·ti·a·sis (dis′ō-don-tī′ă-sis). Difficulty or irregularity in the eruption of the teeth. [dys- + G. *odous*, tooth, + *-iasis*, condition]

dys·on·to·gen·e·sis (dis′on-tō-jen′ĕ-sis). Defective embryonic development. [dys- + G. *ōn*, being, + *genesis*, origin]

dys·on·to·ge·net·ic (dis′on-tō-jĕ-net′ik). Characterized by dysontogenesis.

dys·o·rex·ia (dis-ō-rek′sē-ă). Diminished or perverted appetite. [dys- + G. *orexis*, appetite]

dys·os·mia (dis-oz′mē-ă). Altered sense of smell. [dys- + G. *osmē*, smell]

dys·os·te·o·gen·e·sis (dis′os-tē-ō-jen′ĕ-sis). Defective bone formation. SYN dysostosis. [dys- + G. *osteon*, bone, + *genesis*, production]

dys·os·to·sis (dis-os-tō′sis). SYN dysosteogenesis. [dys- + G. *osteon*, bone, + *-osis*, condition]

  metaphysial d., a rare developmental abnormality of the skeleton in which metaphyses of tubular bones are expanded by deposits of cartilage.

dys·pa·reu·nia (dis-pa-rū′nē-ă). Occurrence of pain during sexual intercourse. [dys- + G. *pareunos*, lying beside, fr. *para*, beside, + *eunē*, a bed]

dys·pep·sia (dis-pep′sē-ă). Impaired gastric function or "upset stomach" due to some disorder of the stomach; characterized by epigastric pain, sometimes burning, nausea, and gaseous eructation. SYN gastric indigestion. [dys- + G. *pepsis*, digestion]

dys·pep·tic (dis-pep′tik). Relating to or suffering from dyspepsia.

dys·pha·gia, dys·pha·gy (dis-fā′jē-ă, dis′fă-jē). Difficulty in swallowing. SYN aglutition. [dys- + G. *phagō*, to eat]

dys·pha·sia (dis-fā′zē-ă). SYN aphasia. [dys- + G. *phasis*, speaking]

dys·pha·sic (dis-fā′zic). SYN aphasiac.

dys·phe·mia (dis-fē′mē-ă). Disordered phonation, articulation, or hearing due to emotional or mental deficits. [dys- + G. *phēmē*, speech]

dys·pho·nia (dis-fō′nē-ă). Any disorder of phonation affecting voice quality or ability to produce voice. SEE aphonia. [dys- + G. *phōnē*, voice]

  spasmodic d., repeated disruptions of phonation due to sudden over- or underadduction of the vocal folds. SYN spastic d.

  spastic d., SYN spasmodic d.

dys·pho·ria (dis-fōr′ē-ă). A mood of general dissatisfaction, restlessness, depression, and anxiety; a feeling of unpleasantness or discomfort. [dys- + G. *phora*, a bearing]

dys·phra·sia (dis-frā′zē-ă). SYN aphasia. [dys- + G. *phrasis*, speaking]

dys·pig·men·ta·tion (dis′pig-men-tā′shŭn). Any abnormality in the formation or distribution of pigment, especially in the skin; usually applied to an abnormal reduction in pigmentation (depigmentation).

dys·pla·sia (dis-plā′zē-ă). Abnormal tissue development. SEE ALSO heteroplasia. [dys- + G. *plasis*, a molding]

  bronchopulmonary d., chronic pulmonary insufficiency arising from long-term artificial pulmonary ventilation; seen more frequently in premature infants than in mature infants.

  cerebral d., abnormal development of the telencephalon.

chondroectodermal d. [MIM*225500], triad of chondrodysplasia, ectodermal d., and polydactyly, with congenital heart defects in over half of patients; autosomal recessive inheritance.

congenital ectodermal d., SYN congenital ectodermal *defect*.

dentin d., a hereditary disorder of the teeth, involving both primary and permanent dentition, in which the clinical morphology and color of the teeth are normal, but the teeth radiographically exhibit short roots [MIM125400], obliteration of the pulp chambers and canals, and mobility and premature exfoliation.

fibrous d. of bone, a disturbance in which bone undergoing physiologic lysis is replaced by abnormal fibrous tissue, resulting in asymmetric distortion and expansion of bone; may be confined to a single bone (monostotic fibrous d.) or involve multiple bones (polyostotic fibrous d.).

mandibuloacral d., an autosomal recessive disorder characterized by dental crowding, acroosteolysis, stiff joints, and atrophy of the skin of the hands and feet; clavicles are hypoplastic, cranial sutures are wide, and multiple wormian bones are present.

metaphysial d., an abnormality that occurs when new bone at the metaphyses of long bones fails to undergo remodeling to the normal tubular structure; the ends of long bones appear to be expanded and porotic, with thin cortex; there may be an associated overgrowth of cranial bones (craniometaphysial d.).

Mondini d., congenital anomaly of osseus and membranous labyrinth characterized by aplastic cochlea, and deformity of the vestibule and semicircular canals with partial or complete loss of auditory and vestibular function; may be associated with spontaneous cerebrospinal fluid otorrhoea resulting in meningitis.

multiple epiphysial d., a dominantly inherited abnormality of epiphyses [MIM*132400] characterized by difficulty in walking, pain and stiffness of joints, stubby fingers, and often dwarfism of short-limb type; on x-ray examination, the epiphyses are mottled and irregular; ossification centers are late in appearance and may be multiple, but the vertebrae are normal. There is also an autosomal recessive form [MIM *226900].

periapical cemental d., a benign, painless, non-neoplastic condition of the jaws which occurs almost exclusively in middle-aged black females; lesions are usually multiple, most frequently involve vital mandibular anterior teeth, surround the root apices, and are initially radiolucent (becoming more opaque as they mature).

septo-optic d., congenital optic nerve hypoplasia associated with midline cerebral anomalies.

dys•plas•tic (dis-plas'tik). Pertaining to or marked by dysplasia.

dysp•nea (disp-nē'ă). Shortness of breath, a subjective difficulty or distress in breathing, usually associated with disease of the heart or lungs; occurs normally during intense physical exertion or at high altitude. [G. *dyspnoia,* fr. *dys-,* bad, + *pnoē,* breathing]

paroxysmal nocturnal d., acute d. appearing suddenly at night, usually waking the patient after an hour or two of sleep; caused by pulmonary congestion that results from left-sided heart failure.

dysp•ne•ic (disp-nē'ik). Out of breath; relating to or suffering from dyspnea.

dys•prax•ia (dis-prak'sē-ă). Impaired or painful functioning in any organ. [dys- + G. *praxis,* a doing]

developmental d. of speech, SYN developmental *apraxia* of speech.

d. of speech, SYN verbal *apraxia*.

verbal d., SYN verbal *apraxia*.

dys•pro•si•um (Dy) (dis-prō'sē-ŭm). A metallic element of the lanthanide (rare earth) series, atomic no. 66, atomic wt. 162.50. [G. *dysprositos,* hard to get at]

dys•pro•tein•e•mia (dis-prō'tēn-ē'mē-ă). An abnormality in plasma proteins, usually in immunoglobulins.

dys•pro•tein•e•mic (dis-prō-tēn-ē'mik). Relating to dysproteinemia.

dys•ra•phism, dys•raph•ia (dis'ră-fizm, dis-raf'ē-ă). Defective fusion, especially of the neural folds, resulting in status dysraphicus. [dys- + G. *rhaphē,* suture]

dys•rhyth•mia (dis-rith'mē-ă). Defective rhythm. See also entries under rhythm. Cf. arrhythmia. [dys- + G. *rhythmos,* rhythm]

cardiac d., any abnormality in the rate, regularity, or sequence of cardiac activation.

electroencephalographic d., a diffusely irregular brain wave tracing.

dys•se•ba•cia, dys•se•ba•cea (dis-sĕ-bā'shē-ă, dis'sē-bă'shē-ă). SYN seborrheic *dermatitis*. [dys- + L. *sebum,* grease]

dys•som•nia (dis-som'nē-ă). Disturbance of normal sleep or rhythm pattern.

dys•sta•sia (dis-stā'sē-ă). Difficulty in standing. [dys- + G. *stasis,* standing]

dys•stat•ic (dis-tat'ik). Marked by difficulty in standing.

dys•syn•er•gia (dis-in-er'jē-ă). An aspect of ataxia, in which an act is not performed smoothly or accurately because of lack of harmonious association of its various components; usually used to describe abnormalities of movement caused by cerebellar disorders. [dys- + G. *syn,* with, + *ergon,* work]

d. cerebellaris myoclonica, a familial disorder beginning in late childhood, characterized by progressive cerebellar ataxia, action myoclonus and preserved intellect. Probably due to multiple causes, mitochondrial abnormalities being one.

dys•thy•mia (dis-thī'mē-ă). A chronic mood disorder manifested as depression for most of the day, more days than not, accompanied by some of the following symptoms: poor appetite or overeating, insomnia or hypersomnia, low energy or fatigue, low self-esteem, poor concentration, difficulty making decisions, and feelings of hopelessness. SEE endogenous *depression,* exogenous *depression.* [dys- + G. *thymos,* mind, emotion]

dys•thy•mic (dis-thī'mik). Relating to dysthymia.

dys•to•cia (dis-tō'sē-ă). Difficult childbirth. [G. *dystokia,* fr. *dys-,* difficult, + *tokos,* childbirth]

fetal d., d. due to an abnormality of the fetus.

maternal d., d. caused by an abnormality or physical problem in the mother.

placental d., retention or difficult delivery of the placenta.

dys•to•nia (dis-tō′nē-ă). A state of abnormal (either hypo- or hyper-) tonicity in any of the tissues. SYN torsion spasm. [dys- + G. *tonos,* tension]

d. musculo′rum defor′mans, a genetic, environmental, or idiopathic disorder, usually beginning in childhood or adolescence, marked by muscular contractions that distort the spine, limbs, hips, and sometimes the cranial-innervated muscles. The abnormal movements are increased by excitement and, at least initially, abolished by sleep. The musculature is hypertonic when in action, hypotonic when at rest.

dys•ton•ic (dis-ton′ik). Pertaining to dystonia.

dys•to•pia (dis-tō′pē-ă). Faulty or abnormal position of a part or organ. SYN malposition. [dys- + G. *topos,* place]

dys•top•ic (dis-top′ik). Pertaining to, or characterized by, dystopia. SEE ALSO ectopic.

dys•tro•phia (dis-trō′fē-ă). SYN dystrophy. [L. fr. G. *dys-,* bad, + *trophē,* nourishment]

d. adipo′sogenita′lis, a disorder characterized primarily by obesity and hypogonadotrophic hypogonadism in adolescent boys; dwarfism is rare, and when present is thought to reflect hypothyroidism. Visual loss, behavioral abnormalities, and diabetes insipidus may occur. The most common causes are pituitary and hypothalamic neoplasms. SYN adiposogenital dystrophy, hypophysial syndrome.

d. epithelialis corneae, a corneal dystrophy causing stromal edema and epithelial bullae, erosions, and scarring. SYN Fuchs epithelial dystrophy.

d. un′guium, dystrophy of the nails.

dys•tro•phic (dis-trof′ik). Relating to dystrophy.

dys•tro•phin (dis-trō′fin). A protein found in the sarcolemma of normal muscle; it is missing in individuals with pseudohypertrophic muscular dystrophy and in other forms of muscular dystrophy.

dys•tro•phy (dis′trō-fē). Progressive changes that may result from defective nutrition of a tissue or organ. SYN dystrophia. [dys- + G. *trophē,* nourishment]

adiposogenital d., SYN *dystrophia* adiposogenitalis.

adult pseudohypertrophic muscular d. [MIM*310200.0002], muscular d. of late onset, often in the second or third decade, with relatively mild course.

Duchenne d., the most common childhood muscular d., with onset usually before age 6. Characterized by symmetrical weakness and wasting of first the pelvic and crural muscles and then the pectoral and proximal upper extremity muscles; pseudohypertrophy of some muscles, especially the calf; heart involvement; sometimes mild mental retardation; progressive course and early death, usually in adolescence. X-linked inheritance (affects males and transmitted by females).

endothelial d. of cornea, spontaneous loss of corneal endothelium leading to edema of the corneal stroma and epithelium.

epithelial d., corneal d. affecting primarily the epithelium and its basement membrane.

gutter d. of cornea, a marginal furrow usually inferiorly about 1 mm from the limbus; and sometimes bilateral. SYN keratoleptynsis (1).

infantile neuroaxonal d., a rare, familial disorder of early childhood manifested as progressive psychomotor deterioration, increased reflexes, Babinski sign, hypotonia and progressive blindness.

limb-girdle muscular d. [MIM*253600], one of the less well-defined types of muscular d. Characterized by weakness and wasting, usually symmetrical, of the pelvic girdle muscles, the shoulder girdle muscles, or both, but not the facial muscles. Muscle pseudohypertrophy, heart involvement, and mental retardation are absent. Variable inheritance.

macular d., a group of disorders involving predominantly the posterior portion of the ocular fundus, due to degeneration in the sensory layer of the retina, retinal pigment epithelium, Bruch's membrane, choroid, or a combination of these tissues.

muscular d., a general term for a number of hereditary, progressive degenerative disorders affecting skeletal muscles, and often other organ systems as well. SYN myodystrophy, myodystrophia.

oculopharyngeal d., a dominantly inherited form of chronic progressive external *ophthalmoplegia* usually presenting in middle life or old age with chronic ptosis and/or difficulty swallowing. Many sufferers have French-Canadian ancestry.

reflex sympathetic d. (RSD), diffuse persistent pain usually in an extremity often associated with vasomotor disturbances, trophic changes, and limitation or immobility of joints; frequently follows local injury. SEE ALSO causalgia.

reticular d. of cornea, bilateral, progressive, superficial degeneration of the corneal epithelium and adjacent Bowman's membrane.

dys•u•ria (dis-yū′rē-ă). Difficulty or pain in urination. [dys- + G. *ouron,* urine]

dys•u•ric (dis-yū′rik). Relating to or suffering from dysuria.

dys•ver•sion (dis-ver′zhŭn). A turning in any direction, less than inversion; particularly d. of the optic nerve head (situs inversus of the optic disk). [dys- + L. *verto,* to turn]

E

ε. epsilon. SEE epsilon.

E 1. exa-; extraction *ratio*; glutamic acid; energy; electromotive *force*; glutamyl; internal *energy*. **2.** As a subscript, refers to expired *gas*.

E entgegen.

e elementary charge; base of natural logarithms (2.71828...).

ear (ēr). The organ of hearing: composed of the **external e.**, which includes the auricle and the external acoustic, or auditory, meatus; the **middle e.**, or the tympanic cavity with its ossicles; and the **internal e.** or **inner e.**, or labyrinth, which includes the semicircular canals, vestibule, and cochlea. SEE ALSO auricle. SYN auris [NA]. [A.S. *eáre*]

   Blainville e.'s, asymmetry in size or shape of the auricles.

   Cagot e. (kă-gō′), an auricle having no lobulus. [a people in the Pyrenees among whom physical stigmata are common]

   cauliflower e., thickening and induration of the e. with distortion of contours following extravasation of blood within its tissues; a chronic deformity following (usually) repeated trauma.

   external e., SEE ALSO auricle, pinna.

   internal e., SEE ALSO labyrinth.

   middle e., SEE ALSO tympanic *cavity*.

   swimmer's e., infection that occurs in the external auditory canal; often develops in persons who swim frequently and get water trapped in their e.'s. SYN otitis externa.

ear·ache (ēr′āk). Pain in the ear. SYN otalgia, otodynia.

ear·drum (ēr′drŭm). SYN tympanic *membrane*.

earth (erth). **1.** Soil; the soft material of the land, as opposed to rock and sand. **2.** An easily pulverized mineral. **3.** An insoluble oxide of aluminum or of certain other elements characterized by a high melting point. [A.S. *eorthe*]

   alkaline e.'s, SEE alkaline earth *elements*, under *element*.

   diatomaceous e., a powder made of desiccated diatom material; used as a filtering agent, adsorbent, and abrasive in many chemical operations.

   fuller's e., (1) an amorphous variety of kaolin of varying composition, containing an aluminum magnesium silicate. (2) a refined clay sometimes used as a dusting powder or applied moistened with water as a form of poultice. Used as decolorizer for oils and other liquids, filtering medium, filler for rubber, and in agricultural formulations. [fr. *fulling*, an old process of cleaning wool with earth or clay]

   rare e.'s, SEE lanthanides.

eb·ur·na·tion (ē-bŭr-nā′shŭn). A change in exposed subchondral bone in degenerative joint disease in which it is converted into a dense substance with a smooth surface like ivory. [L. *eburneus,* of ivory]

ebur·ni·tis (ē-bŭr-nī′tis). Increased density and hardness of dentin, which may occur after the dentin is exposed. [L. *eburneus,* of ivory, + G. -itis, inflammation]

EBV Epstein-Barr *virus.*

ec-. Out of, away from. [G.]

ec·cen·tric (ek-sen′trik). **1.** Abnormal or peculiar in ideas or behavior. **2.** Proceeding from a center.

ec

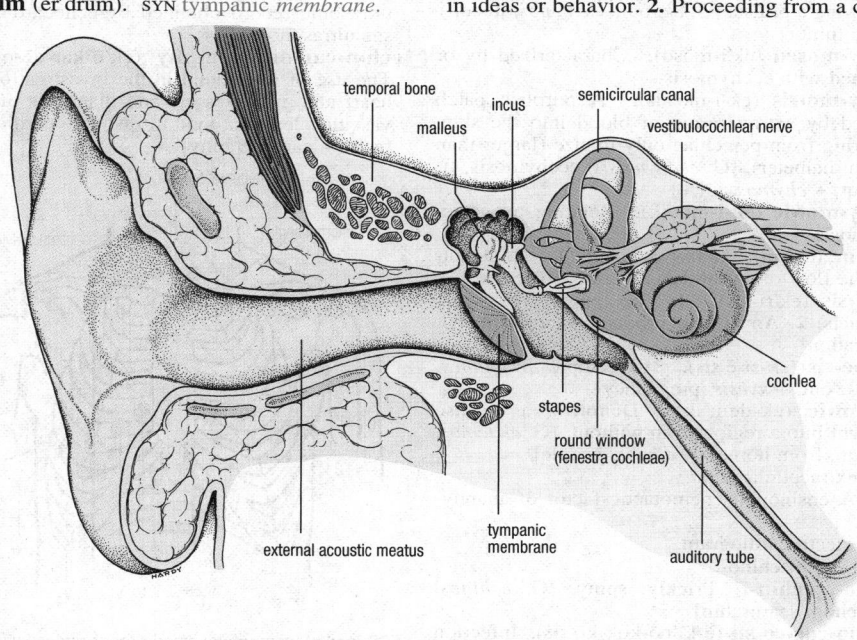

temporal bone   incus   semicircular canal

malleus   vestibulocochlear nerve

cochlea

stapes

round window (fenestra cochleae)

external acoustic meatus

tympanic membrane

auditory tube

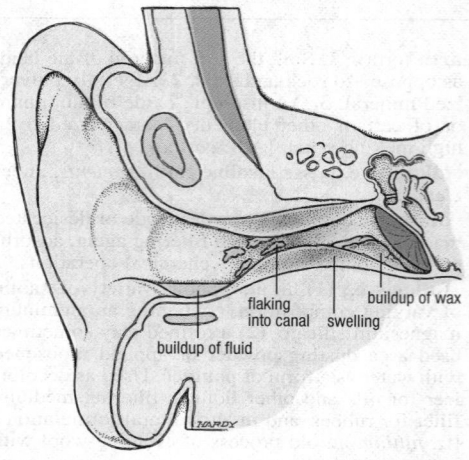

swimmer's ear

Cf. centrifugal (2). **3.** SYN peripheral. [G. *ek*, out, + *kentron*, center]

ec·chon·dro·ma (ek-kon-drō′mă). **1.** A neoplasm arising from cartilage as a mass protruding from the articular surface of a bone. **2.** An enchondroma which has burst through the shaft of a bone and become pedunculated. SYN ecchondrosis. [G. *ek*, from, + *chondros*, cartilage, + *-oma*, tumor]

ec·chon·dro·sis (ek-kon-drō′sis). SYN ecchondroma.

ec·chy·mo·ma (ek-i-mō′mă). A slight hematoma following a bruise. [G. *ek*, out, + *chymos*, juice, + *-oma*, tumor]

ec·chy·mosed (ek′i-mōsd). Characterized by or affected with ecchymosis.

ec·chy·mo·sis (ek-i-mō′sis). A purplish patch caused by extravasation of blood into the skin, differing from petechiae only in size (larger than 3 mm diameter). [G. *ekchymōsis*, ecchymosis, fr. *ek*, out, + *chymos*, juice]

ec·chy·mot·ic (ek-i-mot′ik). Relating to an ecchymosis.

ec·crine (ek′rin). **1.** SYN exocrine (1). **2.** Denoting the flow of sweat. [G. *ek-krino*, to secrete]

ec·cri·sis (ek′ri-sis). **1.** The removal of waste products. **2.** Any waste product; excrement. [G. separation]

ec·cy·e·sis (ek-sī-ē′sis). SYN ectopic *pregnancy*. [G. *ek*, out, + *kyēsis*, pregnancy]

ec·dem·ic (ek-dem′ik). Denoting a disease brought into a region from without. [G. *ekdēmos*, foreign, from home, fr. *dēmos*, people]

ECF extracellular *fluid*.

ECF-A eosinophil chemotactic factor of anaphylaxis.

ECG electrocardiogram.

echin-. SEE echino-.

echino-, echin-. Prickly, spiny. [G. *echinos*, hedgehog, sea urchin]

echi·no·coc·co·sis (ĕ-kī′nō-kok-kō′sis). Infection with *Echinococcus*; larval infection is called hydatid *disease*.

Echi·no·coc·cus (ĕ-kī′nō-kok′ŭs). A genus of very small tapeworms; adults are found in various carnivores but not in humans; larvae, in the form of hydatid cysts, are found in the liver and other organs of ruminants, pigs, horses, rodents, and, under certain epidemiological circumstances, humans. [echino- + G. *kokkos*, a berry]

ech·o (ek′ō). **1.** A reverberating sound sometimes heard during auscultation of the chest. **2.** ULTRASONOGRAPHY The acoustic signal received from scattering or reflecting structures or the corresponding pattern of light on a CRT or ultrasonogram. **3.** MAGNETIC RESONANCE IMAGING The signal detected following an inverting pulse. [G.]

Kemp e., phenomenon noted by David Kemp in 1978, *i.e.,* that otoacoustic emissions are generated in the normal cochlea either spontaneously or in response to acoustic stimulation. SEE ALSO otoacoustic *emissions*, under *emission*.

e. planar, a method of magnetic resonance imaging that allows rapid image acquisition during free induction decay, using rapidly oscillating radiofrequency gradients.

spin e., a commonly used technique to recover T^2 relaxation signals in magnetic resonance imaging, by using a 180° inverting pulse in the pulse sequence to compensate for loss of transverse magnetization caused by magnetic field inhomogeneities.

ech·o·a·cou·sia (ek′ō-ă-kū′zē-ă). A subjective disturbance of hearing in which a sound appears to be repeated. [echo + G. *akouō*, to hear]

ech·o·a·or·tog·ra·phy (ek′ō-ā-ōr-tog′ră-fē). Application of ultrasound techniques to the diagnosis and study of the aorta. [echo + aortography]

ech·o·car·di·o·gram (ek-ō-kar′dē-ō-gram). The ultrasonic record obtained by echocardiography. SEE ultrasonography.

ech·o·car·di·og·ra·phy (ek′ō-kar-dē-og′ră-fē). The use of ultrasound in the investigation of the heart and great vessels and diagnosis of cardiovascular lesions. SYN ultrasound cardiography. [echo + cardiography]

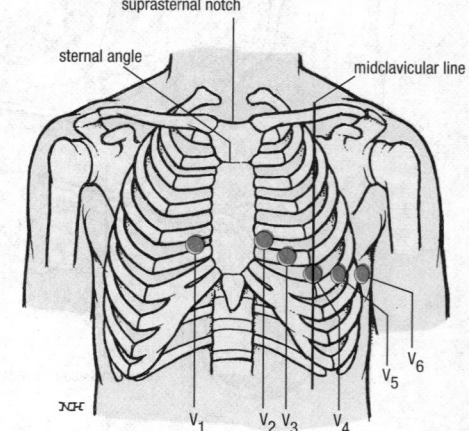

ECG lead placement: landmarks for chest lead placement

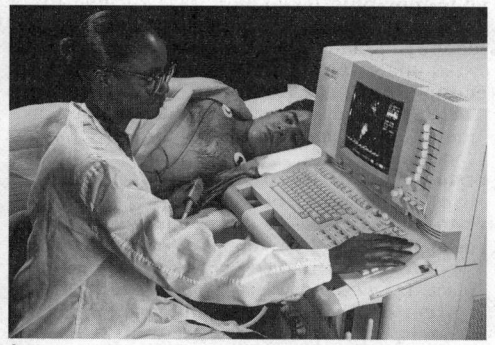

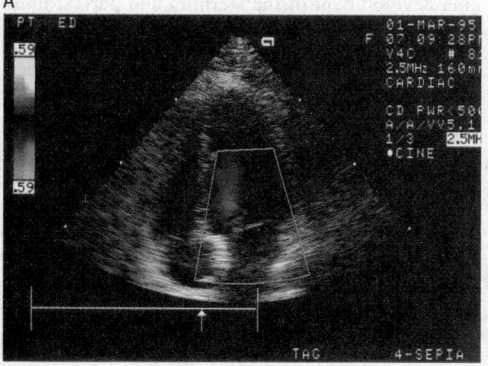

echocardiography: (A) technique; (B) echocardiogram, normal two dimensional, apical four chamber view

Doppler e., use of Doppler ultrasonography techniques to augment two-dimensional e. by allowing velocities to be registered within the echocardiographic image. SEE ALSO duplex *ultrasonography*, Doppler *ultrasonography*.

transesophageal e., recording of the echocardiogram from a swallowed transducer.

two-dimensional e., e. in which an image is reconstructed from the echoes stimulated and detected by a linear array or moving transducers.

ech•o•en•ceph•a•log•ra•phy (ek′ō-en-sef-ă-log′ră-fē). The use of reflected ultrasound in the diagnosis of intracranial processes. [echo + encephalography]

ech•o•gen•ic (ek-ō-jen′ik). Pertaining to a structure or medium (*e.g.,* tissue) that is capable of producing echoes. Contrast with the terms hypoechoic, hyperechoic, and anechoic, which refer to the paucity, abundance, and absence of echoes displayed on the image.

ech•o•gram (ek′ō-gram). A record obtained using high frequency acoustic reflection techniques in any one of the various display modes, especially an echocardiogram. SEE ALSO ultrasonogram. [echo + G. *gramma,* a diagram]

echog•ra•phy (e-kog′ră-fē). SYN ultrasonography. [echo + G. *graphō,* to write]

ech•o•la•lia (ek-ō-lā′lē-ă). Involuntary parrot-like repetition of a word or sentence just spoken by another person. Usually seen with schizophrenia. SYN echophrasia. [echo + G. *lalia,* a form of speech]

ech•o•mim•ia (ek-ō-mim′ē-ă). SYN echopathy. [echo + G. *mimēsis,* imitation]

ech•o•mo•tism (ek′ō-mō′tizm). SYN echopraxia. [echo + L. *motio,* motion]

e•chop•a•thy (ĕ-kop′ă-thē). A form of psychopathology, usually associated with schizophrenia, in which the words (echolalia) or actions (echopraxia) of another are imitated and repeated. SYN echomimia. [echo + G. *pathos,* suffering]

ech•o•phra•sia (ek-ō-frā′zē-ă). SYN echolalia. [echo + *phrasis,* speech]

ech•o•prax•ia (ek′ō-prak′sē-ă). Involuntary imitation of movements made by another. SEE echopathy. SYN echomotism. [echo + G. *praxis,* action]

ech•o•vi•rus (ek′ō-vī-rŭs). SYN ECHO *virus.*

ec•la•bi•um (ek-lā′bē-ŭm). Eversion of a lip. [G. *ek,* out, + L. *labium,* lip]

ec•lamp•sia (ek-lamp′sē-ă). Occurrence of one or more convulsions, not attributable to other cerebral conditions such as epilepsy or cerebral hemorrhage, in a patient with preeclampsia. [G. *eklampsis,* a shining forth]

  puerperal e., convulsions and coma associated with hypertension, edema, or proteinuria occurring in a woman following delivery.

ec•lamp•tic (ek-lamp′tik). Relating to eclampsia.

ec•lamp•to•gen•ic, ec•lamp•tog•e•nous (ek-lamp-tō-jen′ik, -tog′ĕ-nŭs). Causing eclampsia.

ECMO extracorporeal-membrane *oxygenation.*

△**eco-.** The environment. [G. *oikos,* house, household, habitation]

e•col•o•gy (ē-kol′ō-jē). The branch of biology concerned with interrelationships among living organisms, encompassing the relations of organisms to each other, to the environment, and to energy balance within a given ecosystem. [eco- + G. *logos,* study]

  e. of human performance, framework for understanding human performance as a transactional process through which the individual, the context, and performance of the task affect each other. Each transaction affects a person's future performance range and options.

ec•o•sys•tem (ē′kō-sis-tem). **1.** The fundamental unit in ecology, comprising the living organisms and the nonliving elements that interact in a defined region. **2.** A biocenosis (biotic community) and its biotope.

ec•o•tax•is (ē-kō-tak′sis). Migration of lymphocytes from the thymus and bone marrow into tissues possessing an appropriate microenvironment. [eco- + G. *taxis,* order, arrangement]

ec•phy•ma (ek-fī′mă). A warty growth or protuberance. [G. a pimply eruption]

ECS Abbreviation for electrocerebral silence.

ECT electroconvulsive *therapy.*

△**ect-.** SEE ecto-.

ec•tad (ek′tad). Outward. [G. *ektos,* outside, + L. *ad,* to]

ec•tal (ek′tăl). Outer; external. [G. *ektos,* outside]

ec•ta•sia, ec•ta•sis (ek-tā′zē-ă, ek′tă-sis). Dilation of a tubular structure. [G. *ektasis,* a stretching]

  annuloaortic e., supravalvular dilation of the

aorta involving both its wall and the valve ring, which, however, remains of smaller diameter than the more distal ectatic wall; many cases are related to Marfan's syndrome.

e. cor′dis, dilation of the heart.

hypostatic e., dilation of a blood vessel, usually a vein, in a dependent portion of the body, as in varicose veins of the leg.

mammary duct e., dilation of mammary ducts by lipid and cellular debris in older women; rupture of ducts may result in granulomatous inflammation and infiltration by plasma cells. SEE ALSO plasma cell *mastitis*.

△**-ectasia, -ectasis.** Dilation, expansion. [G. *ektasis,* a stretching]

ec·tat·ic (ek-tat′ik). Relating to, or marked by, ectasis.

ec·ten·tal (ek-ten′tăl). Relating to both ectoderm and endoderm; denoting the line where these two layers join. [G. *ektos,* outside, + *entos,* within]

ec·thy·ma (ek-thī′mă). A pyogenic infection of the skin initiated by β-hemolytic streptococci and characterized by adherent crusts beneath which ulceration occurs; the ulcers heal with scar formation. [G. a pustule]

△**ecto-, ect-.** Outer, on the outside. SEE ALSO exo-. [G. *ektos,* outside]

ec·to·an·ti·gen (ek-tō-an′ti-jen). Any toxin or other excitor of antibody formation, separate or separable from its source. SYN exoantigen.

ec·to·blast (ek′tō-blast). **1.** SYN ectoderm. **2.** As used by some experimental embryologists, the original outer cell layer from which the primary germ layers are formed; in this sense, synonymous with protoderm. **3.** A cell wall. [ecto- + G. *blastos,* germ]

ec·to·car·dia (ek-tō-kar′dē-ă). Congenital displacement of the heart. SYN exocardia. [ecto- + G. *kardia,* heart]

ec·to·cer·vi·cal (ek′tō-ser′vi-kăl). Pertaining to the pars vaginalis of the cervix uteri lined with stratified squamous epithelium.

ec·to·derm (ek′tō-derm). The outer layer of cells in the embryo, after establishment of the three primary germ layers (ectoderm, mesoderm, endoderm). SYN ectoblast (1). [ecto- + G. *derma,* skin]

ec·to·der·mal (ek-tō-der′măl). Relating to the ectoderm.

ec·to·en·tad (ek-tō-en′tad). From without inward.

ec·to·en·zyme (ek-tō-en′zīm). An enzyme that is excreted externally and that acts outside the organism.

ec·tog·e·nous (ek-toj′e-nŭs). SYN exogenous. [ecto- + G. *-gen,* producing]

ec·to·glob·u·lar (ek-tō-glob′yū-lăr). Not within a globular body; specifically not within a red blood cell.

ec·to·mere (ek′tō-mēr). One of the blastomeres involved in formation of ectoderm. [ecto- + G. *meros,* part]

ec·to·morph (ek′tō-mōrf). A constitutional body type or build (biotype or somatotype) in which tissues originating from the ectoderm predominate; from a morphological standpoint, the limbs predominate over the trunk. [ecto- + G. *morphē,* form]

ec·to·mor·phic (ek-tō-mōrf′ik). Relating to, or having the characteristics of, an ectomorph.

△**-ectomy.** Removal of an anatomical structure. SEE ALSO -tomy. [G. *ektomē,* a cutting out]

ec·top·a·gus (ek-top′ă-gŭs). Conjoined twins in which the bodies are joined laterally. SEE conjoined *twins,* under *twin.* [ecto- + G. *pagos,* something fixed]

ec·to·par·a·site (ek-tō-par′ă-sīt). A parasite that lives on the surface of the host body.

ec·to·pia (ek-tō′pē-ă). Congenital displacement or malposition of any organ or part of the body. SYN ectopy, heterotopia (1). [G. *ektopos,* out of place, fr. *ektos,* outside, + *topos,* place]

e. cor′dis, congenital condition in which the heart is exposed on the chest wall because of maldevelopment of the sternum and pericardium.

crossed renal e., ectopic kidney located on opposite (contralateral) side of midline from its ureteral insertion into bladder. In most instances, the two renal moieties are fused (crossed fused ectopia).

e. len′tis, displacement of the lens of the eye.

e. pupil′lae congen′ita, displacement of the pupil present at birth.

e. tes′tis, SYN testis e.

testis e., testis that is malpositioned other than along the normal path of descent. SYN e. testis, parorchidium.

ec·top·ic (ek-top′ik). **1.** Out of place; said of an organ not in its proper position, or of a pregnancy occurring elsewhere than in the cavity of the uterus. SYN aberrant (3), heterotopic (1), imperforate anus (2). **2.** CARDIOGRAPHY Denoting a heartbeat that has its origin in some abnormal focus; developing from a focus other than the sinoatrial node. [see ectopia]

ec·to·py (ek′tō-pē). SYN ectopia.

ec·tos·te·al (ek-tos′tē-ăl). Relating to the external surface of a bone. [ecto- + G. *osteon,* bone]

ec·tos·to·sis (ek-tos-tō′sis). Ossification in cartilage beneath the perichondrium, or formation of bone beneath the periosteum. [ecto- + G. *osteon,* bone, + *-osis,* condition]

ec·to·thrix (ek′tō-thriks). A sheath of spores (conidia) on the outside of a hair. [ecto- + G. *thrix,* hair]

△**ectro-.** Congenital absence of a part. [G. *ektrōsis,* miscarriage]

ec·tro·dac·ty·ly, ec·tro·dac·tyl·ia, ec·tro·dac·tyl·ism (ek-trō-dak′ti-lē, -dak-til′i-ă, -dak′ti-lizm). Congenital absence of all or part of one or more fingers or toes. Known also as split-hand/foot deformity, lobster claw. There are several varieties and the pattern of inheritance is usually somewhat irregular. [ectro- + G. *daktylos,* finger]

ec·tro·gen·ic (ek-trō-jen′ik). Relating to ectrogeny.

ec·trog·e·ny (ek-troj′ĕ-nē). Congenital absence or defect of any bodily part. [ectro- + G. *-gen,* producing]

ec·tro·me·lia (ek-trō-mē′lē-ă). **1.** Congenital hypoplasia or aplasia of one or more limbs. **2.** A disease of mice caused by the ectromelia virus; characterized by gangrenous loss of feet and necrotic areas in the internal organs; in laboratory mouse colonies, it usually results in high mortality rates. [ectro- + G. *melos,* limb]

ec•tro•mel•ic (ek-trō-mel'ik). Pertaining to, or characterized by, ectromelia.

ec•tro•pi•on, ec•tro•pi•um (ek-trō'pē-on, -pē-ŭm). A rolling outward of the margin of a part, *e.g.,* of an eyelid. [G. *ek,* out, + *tropē,* a turning]
e. u'veae, eversion of the pigmented posterior epithelium of the iris at the pupillary margin.

ec•trop•o•dy (ek-trop'ō-dē). Total or partial absence of a foot. [ectro- + G. *pous,* foot]

ec•tro•syn•dac•ty•ly (ek'trō-sin-dak'ti-lē). Congenital deformity marked by the absence of one or more digits and the fusion of others. [ectro- + G. *syn,* together, + *daktylos,* finger]

ec•ze•ma (ek'zĕ-mă, eg'zĕ-mă, eg-zē'mă). Generic term for inflammatory conditions of the skin, particularly with vesiculation in the acute stage, typically erythematous, edematous, papular, and crusting; followed often by lichenification and scaling and occasionally by duskiness of the erythema and, infrequently, hyperpigmentation; often accompanied by sensations of itching and burning; the vesicles form by intraepidermal spongiosis. Sometimes referred to colloquially as tetter, dry tetter, scaly tetter. [G. fr. *ekzeō,* to boil over]
allergic e., macular, papular, or vesicular eruption due to an allergic reaction.
e. herpet'icum, a febrile condition caused by cutaneous dissemination of herpesvirus type 1, occurring most commonly in children, consisting of a widespread eruption of vesicles rapidly becoming umbilicated pustules.
infantile e., e. in infants; the clinical appearance varies according to the dominant causative mechanism, *e.g.,* contact-type hypersensitivity, candidiasis, atopy, seborrhea, or a combination including intertrigo and diaper dermatitis.
e. margina'tum, SYN *tinea* cruris.
nummular e., discrete, coin-shaped patches of e.
stasis e., eczematous eruption on legs due to or aggravated by venous stasis.

ec•ze•ma•toid (ek-zem'ă-toyd). Resembling eczema in appearance.

ec•ze•ma•tous (ek-zem'ă-tŭs). Marked by or resembling eczema.

ED₅₀ median effective *dose.*

ede•ma (e-dē'mă). An accumulation of an excessive amount of watery fluid in cells, tissues, or serous cavities. [G. *oidēma,* a swelling]
angioneurotic e., SYN angioedema.
brawny e., SYN nonpitting e.
cardiac e., e. resulting from congestive heart failure.
cerebral e., brain swelling due to increased volume of the extravascular compartment from the uptake of water in the neuropile and white matter. SEE ALSO brain *swelling.*
dependent e., a clinically detectable increase in extracellular fluid volume localized in a dependent area, as of a limb, characterized by swelling or pitting.
gestational e., a generalized and excessive accumulation of fluid in the tissues of greater than 1+ pitting after 12 hours' bed rest, or of a weight

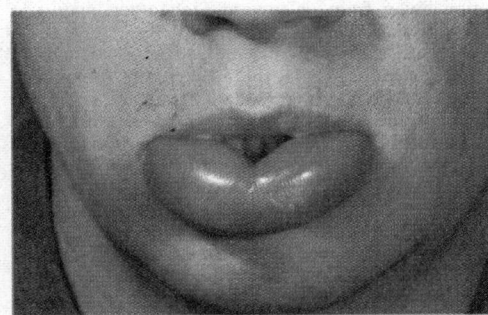
angioneurotic edema: of the lower lip

gain of 5 pounds or more in 1 week due to the influence of pregnancy.
nonpitting e., swelling of subcutaneous tissues which cannot be indented easily by compression. Usually due to metabolic abnormality, such as increased glycosaminoglycan content, like that which occurs in Graves' disease (pretibial myxedema) or in early phase of scleroderma. SYN brawny e.
pitting e., e. that retains for a time the indentation produced by pressure.
pulmonary e., e. of lungs usually resulting from mitral stenosis or left ventricular failure.

edem•a•tous (e-dem'ă-tŭs). Marked by edema.

eden•tate (ē-den'tāt). SYN edentulous. [L. *edentatus*]

eden•tu•lous (ē-den'tyū-lŭs). Toothless, having lost the natural teeth. SYN edentate. [L. *edentulus,* toothless]

ed•e•tate (ed'ĕ-tāt). USAN-approved contraction for ethylenediaminetetraacetate.

EEG electroencephalogram; electroencephalography.

EENT eye, ear, nose, and throat. See also ENT.

effacement. In obstetrics, the progressive obliteration of the endocervical canal during delivery.

ef•fect (e-fekt'). The result or consequence of an action. [L. *ef-ficio,* pp. *effectus,* to accomplish, fr. *facio,* to do]
abscopal e., a reaction produced following irradiation but occurring outside the zone of actual radiation absorption.
additive e., an e. wherein two or more substances or actions used in combination produce a total e. the same as the arithmetic sum of the individual e.'s.
Bohr e., the e. of H⁺ concentration on the affinity of hemoglobin for oxygen. As the H⁺ concentration increases, the oxygen affinity decreases, causing a release of more oxygen to the tissue. One of the most important buffer systems in the body.
cumulative e., the condition in which repeated administration of a drug may produce e.'s that are more pronounced than those produced by the first dose. SYN cumulative action.
Doppler e., a change in frequency observed when the sound and observer are in relative mo-

ef

tion away from or toward each other. SEE ALSO Doppler *shift*.

Edison e., SYN thermionic *emission.*

experimenter e.'s, the influence of the experimenter's behavior, personality traits, or expectancies on the results of that person's own research.

Haldane e., the promotion of carbon dioxide dissociation by oxygenation of hemoglobin.

halo e., (1) the e. (usually beneficial) that the manner, attention, and caring of a provider have on a patient during a medical encounter, regardless of what medical procedure or services the encounter involves; (2) the influence upon an observation of the observer's perception of the characteristics of the individual observed (other than the characteristics under study) or the influence of the observer's recollection or knowledge of findings on a previous occasion.

Mach e., the appearance of a light or dark line on a radiograph where there is a concave or convex interface in the subject, a physiological optical form of edge enhancement.

position e., a change in the phenotypic expression of one or more genes due to a change in its physical location with respect to other genes; may result from change in chromosome structure or from crossing-over.

Somogyi e., in diabetes, a rebound phenomenon of reactive hyperglycemia in response to a preceding period of relative hypoglycemia that has increased secretion of hyperglycemic agents (epinephrine, norepinephrine, glucagon, cortisol, and growth hormone); described in diabetic patients given too much insulin who developed unrecognized nocturnal hypoglycemia that made them hyperglycemic (suggesting insufficient insulin) when tested the next morning.

ef·fec·tor (ē-fek′tŏr, -tōr). **1.** A peripheral tissue that receives nerve impulses and reacts by contraction (muscle), secretion (gland), or a discharge of electricity (electric organ of certain bony fishes). **2.** A small metabolic molecule that by combining with a repressor gene depresses the activity of an operon. **3.** A small molecule that binds to a protein and, in so doing, alters the activity of that protein. **4.** A substance, technique, procedure, or individual that causes an effect. [L. producer]

ef·fem·i·na·tion (e-fem-i-nā′shŭn). Acquisition of feminine characteristics, either physiologically as part of female maturation, or pathologically by individuals of either sex. [L. *ef-femino,* pp. *-atus,* to make feminine, fr. *ex,* out, + *femina,* woman]

ef·fer·ent (ef′er-ent). Conducting (fluid or a nerve impulse) outward from a given organ or part thereof; *e.g.,* the efferent connections of a group of nerve cells, efferent blood vessels, or the excretory duct of an organ. [L. *efferens,* fr. *effero,* to bring out]

ef·fi·cien·cy (ĕ-fish′en-sē). **1.** The production of the desired effects or results with minimum waste of time, effort, or skill. **2.** A measure of effectiveness; specifically, the useful work output divided by the energy input.

ef·fleu·rage (e-fler-ahz′). A stroking movement in massage. [Fr. *effleurer,* to touch lightly]

ef·flo·resce (e-flōr-es′). To become powdery by losing the water of crystallization on exposure to a dry atmosphere. [L. *ef-floresco* (*exf-*), to blossom, fr. *flos* (*flor-*), flower]

ef·flu·vi·um, pl. **ef·flu·via** (e-flū′vē-ŭm, -ē-ă). Shedding of hair. SEE ALSO defluxion (1). [L. a flowing out, fr. *ef-fluo,* to flow out]

anagen e., sudden diffuse hair shedding with cancer chemotherapy or radiation, usually reversible when treatment ends.

telogen e., increased transient shedding of normal club hairs by premature development of telogen in anagen follicles, resulting from various kinds of stress, *e.g.,* childbirth, shock, drug intake or cessation of an oral contraceptive, fever, and dieting with marked weight loss.

ef·fu·sion (e-fū′zhŭn). **1.** The escape of fluid from the blood vessels or lymphatics into the tissues or a cavity. **2.** The fluid effused. [L. *effusio,* a pouring out]

joint e., increased fluid in synovial cavity of a joint.

pericardial e., increased amounts of fluid within the pericardial sac, usually due to inflammation.

pleural e., increased amounts of fluid within the pleural cavity, usually due to inflammation.

EGD esophagogastroduodenoscopy.

eges·ta (ē-jes′tă). Unabsorbed food residues that are discharged from the digestive tract. [L. *e-gero,* pp. *-gestus,* to carry out, discharge]

egg (eg). The female sexual cell or gamete. SEE ALSO oocyte, ovum. [A.S. *aeg*]

egg clus·ter. One of the clumps of cells resulting from the breaking up of the gonadal cords in the ovarian cortex; these clumps later develop into primary ovarian follicles.

e·go (ē′gō). PSYCHOANALYSIS One of the three components of the psychic apparatus in the freudian structural framework, the other two being the id and superego. The e. occupies a position between the primal instincts (pleasure principle) and the demands of the outer world (reality principle), and therefore mediates between the person and external reality by performing the important functions of perceiving the needs of the self, both physical and psychological, and the qualities and attitudes of the environment. It is also responsible for certain defensive functions to protect the person against the demands of the id and superego. [L. I]

ego·bron·choph·o·ny (ē′gō-brong-kof′ō-nē). Egophony with bronchophony. [G. *aix* (*aig-*), goat, + *bronchos,* bronchus, + *phōnē,* voice]

ego·cen·tric (ē-gō-sen′trik). Marked by extreme concentration of attention upon oneself, *i.e.,* self-centered. SYN egotropic. [ego + G. *kentron,* center]

ego-dys·ton·ic (ē′gō-dis-ton′ik). Repugnant to or at variance with the aims of the ego and related psychological needs of the individual (*e.g.,* an obsessive thought or compulsive behavior); the opposite of ego-syntonic. [ego + G. *dys,* bad, + *tonos,* tension]

ego·ma·nia (ē-gō-mā′nē-ă). Extreme self-centeredness, self-appreciation, or self-content. [ego + G. *mania,* frenzy]

ego·phon·ic (ē-gō-fon′ik). Relating to egophony.

egoph•o•ny (ē-gof′ō-nē). A peculiar broken quality of the voice sounds, like the bleating of a goat, heard about the upper level of the fluid in cases of pleurisy with effusion. [G. *aix* (*aig*-), goat, + *phōnē*, voice]

ego-syn•ton•ic (ē′gō-sin-ton′ik). Acceptable to the aims of the ego and the related psychological needs of the individual (*e.g.*, a delusion); the opposite of ego-dystonic. [ego + G. *syn*, together, + *tonos*, tension]

ego•tro•pic (ē-gō-trop′ik). SYN egocentric. [ego + G. *tropē*, a turning]

EHEC enterohemorrhagic *Escherichia coli.*

Ehr•lich•ia (er-lik′ē-ă). A genus of small, often pleomorphic, coccoid to ellipsoidal, nonmotile, Gram-negative bacteria (order Rickettsiales) that occur either singly or in compact inclusions in circulating mammalian leukocytes; species are the etiologic agents of ehrlichiosis and are transmitted by ticks. The type species is *E. canis.* [P. *Ehrlich*]

E. chaffee′nsis, a recently described species associated with human ehrlichiosis and carried by the tick vector, *Amblyomma americanum*, the Lone Star tick.

ehr•lich•i•o•sis (er-lik-ē-ō′sis). A tickborn infection of human beings and dogs, caused by bacteria of the genus *Ehrlichia*, which produces manifestations similar to those of Rocky Mountain spotted fever.

human granulocytic e., a febrile disease causing headache and myalgia and sometimes involving the respiratory, digestive, and central nervous systems; caused by *Ehrlichia phagocytophaga*, which is transmitted by ixodid ticks; laboratory findings include leukopenia, thrombocytopenia, and inclusion bodies (morulae) in neutrophils.

human monocytic e., a febrile disease caused by *Ehrlichia chaffeensia* and transmitted by the Lone Star tick (*Amblyomma americanum*); similar to human granulocytic e., except that inclusions are found in monocytes.

EIA enzyme *immunoassay.*

ei•co•sa•noids (ī′kō-să-noydz). The physiologically active substances derived from arachidonic acid, *i.e.,* the prostaglandins, leukotrienes, and thromboxanes; synthesized via a cascade pathway. [G. *eicosa-*, twenty, + *eidos*, form]

EIEC enteroinvasive *Escherichia coli.*

Ei•ken•el•la cor•ro•dens (ī-kĕ-nel′ă kōr-rō′denz). A species of nonmotile, rod-shaped, Gram-negative, facultatively anaerobic bacteria that is part of the normal flora of the adult human oral cavity but may be an opportunistic pathogen, especially in immunocompromised hosts. [M. *Eiken*, 1958]

ein•stein (īn′stīn). A unit of energy equal to 1 mol quantum, hence to 6.0221367×10^{23} quanta. The value of e., in kJ, is dependent upon the wavelength. [A. *Einstein*, German-born theoretical physicist and Nobel laureate in U.S., 1879–1955]

ein•stein•i•um (Es) (īn-stūn′ē-ŭm). An artificially prepared transuranium element, atomic no. 99, atomic wt. 254.0; it has many isotopes, all of which are radioactive (^{252}Es has the longest known half-life, 1.29 years).

ejac•u•late (ē-jak′yū-lāt). **1.** To expel suddenly, as of semen. **2.** Semen expelled in ejaculation. [see ejaculation]

ejac•u•la•tio (ē-jak-yū-lā′shē-ō). SYN ejaculation.

ejac•u•la•tion (ē-jak-yū-lā′shŭn). Emission of seminal fluid. SYN ejaculatio. [L. *e-iaculo*, pp. *-atus*, to shoot out]

premature e., during sexual intercourse, too rapid achievement of climax and e. in the male relative to his own or his partner's wishes.

ejac•u•la•to•ry (ē-jak′yū-lă-tōr-ē). Relating to an ejaculation.

ejec•ta (ē-jek′tă). SYN ejection (2). [L. ntr. pl. of *ejectus*, pp. of *ejicio*, to throw out]

ejec•tion (ē-jek′shŭn). **1.** The act of driving or throwing out by physical force from within. **2.** That which is ejected. SYN ejecta. [L. *ejectio*, from *ejicio*, to cast out]

△**eka-.** Prefix used to denote an undiscovered or just discovered element in the periodic system before a proper and official name is assigned by authorities; *e.g.*, eka-osmium, now plutonium. [Sanskrit *eka*, one]

EKG electrocardiogram.

elab•o•ra•tion (ē-lab′ōr-ā′shŭn). The process of working out in detail by labor and study. [L. *e-laborō*, pp. *-atus*, to labor, endeavor, fr. *labor*, toil, to work out]

elas•tance (ē-las′tans). A measure of the tendency of a structure to return to its original form after removal of a deforming force. In medicine and physiology, usually a measure of the tendency of a hollow viscus (*e.g.*, lung, urinary bladder, gallbladder) to recoil toward its original dimensions upon removal of a distending or compressing force.

elas•tase (ĕ-las′tās). A serine proteinase hydrolyzing elastin.

elas•tic (ĕ-las′tik). **1.** Having the property of returning to the original shape after being compressed, bent, or otherwise distorted. **2.** A rubber or plastic band used in orthodontics as either a primary or adjunctive source of force to move teeth. The term is generally modified by an adjective to describe the direction of the force or the location of the terminal connecting points. [G. *elastreō*, epic form of *elaunō*, drive, push]

elas•ti•cin (ĕ-las′ti-sin). SYN elastin.

elas•tic•i•ty (ĕ-las-tis′i-tē). The quality or condition of being elastic.

elas•tin (ĕ-las′tin). A yellow elastic fibrous mucoprotein that is the major connective tissue protein of elastic structures (large blood vessels, tendons, and ligaments). SYN elasticin.

elas•to•fi•bro•ma (ĕ-las′tō-fī-brō′mă). A nonencapsulated slow-growing mass of poorly cellular, collagenous, fibrous tissue and elastic tissue; occurs usually in subscapular adipose tissue of old persons. [G. *elastos*, beaten, + L. *fibra*, *-oma* tumor]

elas•to•ma (ĕ-las-tō′mă). A tumor-like deposit of elastic tissue.

elas•to•sis (ĕ-las-tō′sis). **1.** Degenerative change in elastic tissue. **2.** Degeneration of collagen fibers, with altered staining properties resembling elastic tissue, or formation by fibroblast-activated ultraviolet or mast cell mediators of abnormal

el

fibers. SYN elastoid degeneration (1), elastotic degeneration.

solar e., e. seen histologically in the sun-exposed skin of the elderly or in those who have chronic actinic damage.

el·bow (el′bō). **1.** The joint between the arm and the forearm. SYN cubitus (1) [NA]. **2.** An angular body resembling a flexed e. [A.S. *elnboga*]

Little League e., tension stress injury to the medial epicondyle, often seen in adolescents. SYN medial epicondylitis.

nursemaid's e., longitudinal subluxation of the radial head from the annular ligament. SYN Malgaigne's luxation.

tennis e., chronic inflammation at the origin of the extensor muscles of the forearm from the lateral epicondyle of the humerus, as a result of unusual strain (not necessarily from playing tennis). SYN lateral humeral epicondylitis.

⌂**electro-.** Electric, electricity. [G. *ēlektron*, amber (on which static electricity can be generated by friction)]

elec·tro·an·al·ge·sia (ē-lek′trō-an-ăl-jē′zē-ă). Analgesia induced by the passage of an electric current.

elec·tro·an·es·the·sia (ē-lek′trō-an-es-thē′zē-ă). Anesthesia produced by an electric current.

elec·tro·car·di·o·gram (ECG, EKG) (ē-lek-trō-kar′dē-ō-gram). Graphic record of the heart's integrated action currents obtained with the electrocardiograph. [electro- + G. *kardia*, heart, + *gramma*, a drawing]

elec·tro·car·di·o·graph (ē-lek-trō-kar′dē-ō-graf). An instrument for recording the potential of the electrical currents that traverse the heart and initiate its contraction.

elec·tro·car·di·og·ra·phy (ē-lek′trō-kar-dē-og′ră-fē). **1.** A method of recording the electrical activity of the heart: impulse formation and conduction, depolarization and repolarization of atria and ventricles. **2.** The study and interpretation of electrocardiograms.

elec·tro·cau·ter·i·za·tion (ē-lek′trō-caw′ter-i-zā′shŭn). Cauterization by passage of high frequency current through tissue or by metal that has been electrically heated.

elec·tro·cau·tery (ē-lek′trō-caw′ter-ē). **1.** An instrument for directing a high frequency current through a local area of tissue. **2.** A metal cauterizing instrument heated by an electric current.

elec·tro·ce·re·bral si·lence (ECS) (ē-lek′trō-ser-ē′brăl sī′lens). Flat or isoelectric encephalogram; an electroencephalogram with absence of cerebral activity from symmetrically placed electrode pairs; if such a record is present for 30 minutes in a clinically brain dead adult and if drug intoxication, hypothermia, and recent hypotension have been excluded, the diagnosis of ce-

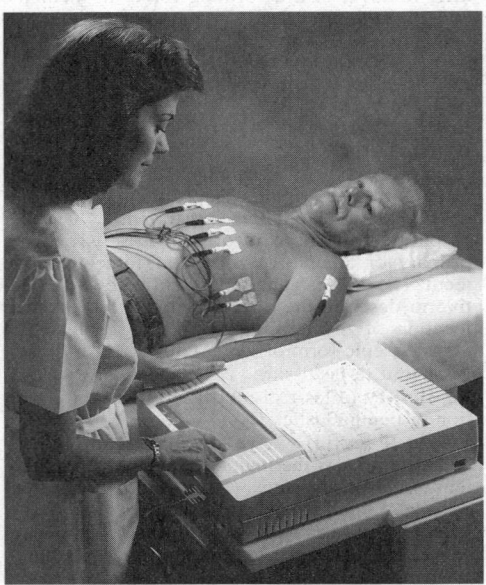

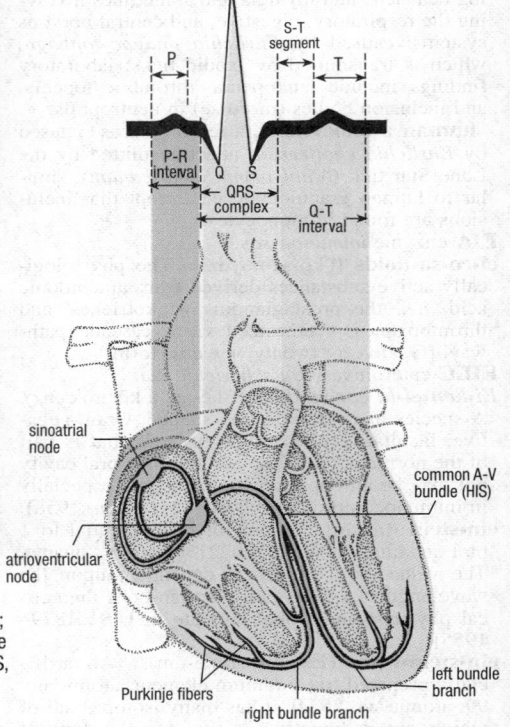

electrocardiography (ECG): (left) resting electrocardiogram; (right) an electrical picture of the heart is represented by positive and negative deflections on a graph labeled with the letters P,Q,R,S, and T, corresponding to the events of the cardiac cycle

rebral death is supported. SYN flat electroencephalogram.

elec·tro·chem·i·cal (ē-lek′trō-kem′i-kăl). Denoting chemical reactions involving electricity, and the mechanisms involved.

elec·tro·co·ag·u·la·tion (ē-lek′trō-kō-ag-yū-lā′shŭn). Coagulation produced by an electrocautery.

elec·tro·co·chle·o·gram (ē-lek′trō-kok′lē-ō-gram). The record obtained by electrocochleography.

elec·tro·co·chle·og·ra·phy (ē-lek′trō-kok-lē-og′ră-fē). A measurement of the electrical potentials generated in the inner ear as a result of sound stimulation. [electro- + L. *cochlea,* snail shell, + G. *graphō,* to write]

elec·tro·con·trac·til·i·ty (ē-lek′trō-kon-trak-til′i-tē). The power of contraction of muscular tissue in response to an electrical stimulus.

elec·tro·con·vul·sive (ē-lek′trō-kon-vŭl′siv). Denoting a convulsive response to an electrical stimulus. SEE electroshock *therapy.*

elec·tro·cor·ti·co·gram (ē-lek-trō-kōr′ti-kō-gram). A record of electrical activity derived directly from the cerebral cortex.

elec·tro·cor·ti·cog·ra·phy (ē-lek′trō-kōr-ti-kog′ră-fē). The technique of recording the electrical activity of the cerebral cortex by means of electrodes placed directly on it.

elec·trode (ē-lek′trōd). **1.** One of the two extremities of an electric circuit; one of the two poles of an electric battery or of the end of the conductors connected thereto. **2.** An electrical terminal specialized for a particular electrochemical reaction. [electro- + G. *hodos,* way]

  negative e., SYN cathode.

elec·tro·der·mal (ē-lek′trō-der′măl). Pertaining to electric properties of the skin, usually referring to altered resistance. [electro- + G. *derma,* skin]

elec·tro·des·ic·ca·tion (ē-lek′trō-des-i-kā′shŭn). Destruction of lesions or sealing off of blood vessels (usually of the skin, but also of available surfaces of mucous membrane) by monopolar high-frequency electric current. [electro- + L. *desicco,* to dry up]

elec·tro·di·ag·no·sis (ē-lek′trō-dī-ag-nō′sis). **1.** The use of electronic devices for diagnostic purposes. **2.** By convention, the studies performed in the EMG laboratory, *i.e.,* nerve conduction studies and needle electrode examination (EMG proper). SYN electroneurography. **3.** Determination of the nature of a disease through observation of changes in electrical activity.

elec·tro·di·al·y·sis (ē-lek′trō-dī-al′i-sis). In an electric field, the removal of ions from larger molecules and particles.

elec·tro·en·ceph·a·lo·gram (EEG) (ē-lek′trō-en-sef′ă-lō-gram). The record obtained by means of the electroencephalograph.

  flat e., SYN electrocerebral silence.

elec·tro·en·ceph·a·lo·graph (ē-lek′trō-en-sef′ă-lō-graf). A system for recording the electric potentials of the brain derived from electrodes attached to the scalp. [electro- + G. *encephalon,* brain, + *graphō,* to write]

elec·tro·en·ceph·a·log·ra·phy (EEG) (ēlek′trō-

en-sef′ă-log′ră-fē). Registration of the electrical potentials recorded by an electroencephalograph.

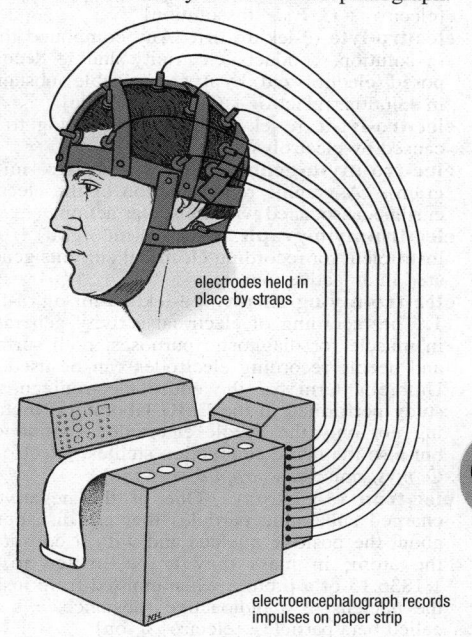

electrodes held in place by straps

electroencephalograph records impulses on paper strip

electroencephalography

elec·tro·en·dos·mo·sis (ē-lek′trō-en-dos-mō′sis). Endosmosis produced by means of an electric field.

elec·tro·gas·tro·gram (ē-lek′trō-gas′trō-gram). The record obtained with the electrogastrograph.

elec·tro·gas·tro·graph (ē-lek′trō-gas′trō-graf). An instrument used in electrogastrography. [electro- + G. *gastēr,* stomach, + *graphō,* to write]

elec·tro·gas·trog·ra·phy (ē-lek′trō-gas-trog′ră-fē). The recording of the electrical phenomena associated with gastric secretion and motility.

elec·tro·gram (ē-lek′trō-gram). **1.** Any record on paper or film made by an electrical event. **2.** ELECTROPHYSIOLOGY A recording taken directly from the surface by unipolar or bipolar leads.

  His bundle e. (HBE), an e. recorded from the His bundle, either in the experimental animal or in man during cardiac catheterization.

elec·tro·he·mo·sta·sis (ē-lek′trō-hē-mos′tă-sis, -hē-mō-stā′sis). Arrest of hemorrhage by means of an electrocautery. [electro- + G. *haima,* blood, + *stasis,* halt]

elec·tro·im·mu·no·dif·fu·sion (ē-lek′trō-im′yū-nō-di-fyū′zhŭn). An immunochemical method that combines electrophoretic separation with immunodiffusion by incorporating antibody into the support medium.

electrolarynx. SYN artificial *larynx.*

elec·trol·y·sis (ē-lek-trol′i-sis). **1.** Decomposition of a salt or other chemical compound by means of an electric current. **2.** Destruction of certain hair follicles by means of galvanic electricity. [electro- + G. *lysis,* dissolution]

elec·tro·lyte (ē-lek'trō-līt). Any compound that, in solution, conducts electricity and is decomposed (electrolyzed) by it; an ionizable substance in solution. [electro- + G. *lytos,* soluble]

elec·tro·lyt·ic (ē-lek-trō-lit'ik). Referring to or caused by electrolysis.

elec·tro·my·o·gram (EMG) (ē-lek-trō-mī'ō-gram). A graphic representation of the electric currents associated with muscular action.

elec·tro·my·o·graph (ē-lek-trō-mī'ō-graf). An instrument for recording electrical currents generated in an active muscle.

elec·tro·my·og·ra·phy (ē-lek'trō-mī-og'ră-fē). **1.** The recording of electrical activity generated in muscle for diagnostic purposes; both surface and needle recording electrodes can be used. **2.** Umbrella term for the entire electrodiagnostic study performed in the EMG laboratory, including not only the needle electrode examination, but also the nerve conduction studies. [electro- + G. *mys,* muscle, + *graphō,* to write]

elec·tron (ē-lek'tron). One of the negatively charged subatomic particles that are distributed about the positive nucleus and with it constitute the atom; in mass they are estimated to be 1/1836.15 of a proton; when emitted from inside the nucleus of a radioactive substance, e.'s are called beta particles. [electro- + -on]

elec·tro·nar·co·sis (ē-lek'trō-nar-kō'sis). Production of insensibility to pain by the use of electrical current.

elec·tro·neg·a·tive (ē-lek-trō-neg'ă-tiv). Relating to or charged with negative electricity; referring to an element whose uncharged atoms have a tendency to ionize by adding electrons, thus becoming anions (*e.g.,* oxygen, fluorine, chlorine).

elec·tro·neu·rog·ra·phy (ē-lek'trō-nū-rog'ră-fē). SYN electrodiagnosis (2).

elec·tro·neu·ro·my·og·ra·phy (ē-lek'trō-nūr'ō-mī-og'ră-fē). A method of measuring changes in a peripheral nerve by combining electromyography of a muscle with electrical stimulation of the nerve trunk carrying fibers to and from the muscle.

elec·tron-volt (eV, ev). The energy imparted to an electron by a potential of 1 volt; equal to 1.60218×10^{-12} erg in the CGS system, or 1.60218×10^{-19} joule in the SI system.

elec·tro·nys·tag·mog·ra·phy (ENG) (ē-lek'trō-nis'tag-mog'ră-fē). A method of nystagmography based on electro-oculography; skin electrodes are placed at outer canthi to register horizontal nystagmus or above and below each eye for vertical nystagmus. [electro- + nystagmus + G. *graphō,* to write]

elec·tro·oc·u·log·ra·phy (EOG) (ē-lek'trō-ok'yū-log'ră-fē). Oculography in which electrodes placed on the skin adjacent to the eyes measure changes in standing potential between the front and back of the eyeball as the eyes move; a sensitive electrical test for detection of retinal pigment epithelium dysfunction.

elec·tro·ol·fac·to·gram (EOG) (ē-lek'trō-ol-fak'tō-gram). An electronegative wave of potential

occurring on the surface of the olfactory epithelium in response to stimulation by an odor.

elec·tro·pher·o·gram (ē-lek-trō-fer'ō-gram). The densitometric or colorimetric pattern obtained from filter paper or similar porous strips on which substances have been separated by electrophoresis; may also refer to the strips themselves. SYN electrophoretogram.

elec·tro·phil, elec·tro·phile (ē-lek'trō-fil, -fīl). **1.** The electron-attracting atom or agent in an organic reaction. Cf. nucleophil. **2.** Relating to an electrophil. SYN electrophilic. [electro- + G. *philos,* fond]

elec·tro·phil·ic (ē-lek-trō-fil'ik). SYN electrophil (2).

elec·tro·pho·re·sis (ē-lek-trō-fōr'ē-sis). The movement of particles in an electric field toward anode or cathode. SEE ALSO electropherogram. SYN ionophoresis, phoresis (1). [electro- + G. *phorēsis,* a carrying]

  polyacrylamide gel e. (PAGE), separation of proteins or nucleic acids on the basis of both size and charge in a gel formed by cross-linking of acrylamide.

  pulse-field gel e., gel e. in which, after electrophoretic migration has begun, the current is briefly stopped and reapplied in a different orientation; allows for the purification of long DNA molecules.

elec·tro·pho·ret·ic (ē-lek'trō-phōr-et'ik). Relating to electrophoresis, as an e. separation. SYN ionophoretic.

elec·tro·pho·ret·o·gram (ē-lek'trō-fōr-et'ō-gram). SYN electropherogram.

elec·tro·ret·i·no·gram (ERG) (ē-lek'trō-ret'i-nō-gram). A record of the retinal action currents produced in the retina by an adequate light stimulus. [electro- + retina + G. *gramma,* something written]

elec·tro·ret·i·nog·ra·phy (ē-lek'trō-ret'i-nog'ră-fē). The recording and study of the retinal action currents.

elec·tro·scis·sion (ē-lek'trō-si-shŭn). Division of tissues by means of an electrocautery knife. [electro- + L. *scissio,* a splitting, fr. *scindo,* to split]

elec·tro·shock (ē-lek'trō-shok). SEE electroshock *therapy.*

elec·tro·sur·gery (ē-lek-trō-ser'jer-ē). Division of tissues by high frequency current applied locally with a metal instrument or needle. SEE ALSO electrocautery.

elec·tro·tax·is (ē-lek-trō-tak'sis). Reaction of plant or animal protoplasm to either an anode or a cathode. SEE ALSO tropism. SYN electrotropism. [electro- + G. *taxis,* orderly arrangement]

elec·tro·ther·a·peu·tics, elec·tro·ther·a·py (ē-lek'trō-thār-ă-pyū'tiks, -thār'ă-pē). Use of electricity in the treatment of disease.

elec·tro·ton·ic (ē-lek-trō-ton'ik). Relating to electrotonus.

elec·trot·o·nus (ē-lek-trot'ō-nŭs). Changes in excitability and conductivity in a nerve or muscle cell caused by the passage of a constant electric current. [electro- + G. *tonos,* tension]

elec·trot·ro·pism (ē-lek-trot'rō-pizm, ē-lek-trō-

trō'pizm). SYN electrotaxis. [electro- + G. *tropē,* a turning]

elec·tu·ar·y (ē-lek'chū-ā-rē). SYN confection. [G. *eleikton,* a medicine that melts in the mouth, fr. *ekleichō,* to lick up]

ele·i·din (ē-lē'ī-din). A refractile and weakly staining keratin present in the cells of the stratum lucidum of the palmar and plantar epidermis.

el·e·ment (el'ĕ-ment). **1.** A substance composed of atoms of only one kind, *i.e.,* of identical atomic (proton) number, that therefore cannot be decomposed into two or more e.'s, and that can lose its chemical properties only by union with some other e. or by a nuclear reaction changing the proton number. **2.** An indivisible structure or entity. **3.** A functional entity, frequently exogenous, within a bacterium, such as an extrachromosomal e. [L. *elementum,* a rudiment, beginning]

alkaline earth e.'s, those e.'s in the family Be, Mg, Ca, Sr, Ba, and Ra, the hydroxides of which are highly ionized and hence alkaline in water solution.

extrachromosomal e., extrachromosomal genetic e., SYN plasmid.

trace e.'s, e.'s present in minute amounts in the body, many of which are essential in metabolism or for the manufacture of essential compounds; *e.g.,* Zn, Se, V, Ni, Mg, Mn.

transposable e., a DNA sequence that can move from one location in the genome to another; the transposition event can involve both recombination and replication, producing two copies of the moving piece of DNA; the insertion of these DNA fragments can disrupt the integrity of the target gene, possibly causing activation of dormant genes, deletions, inversions, and a variety of chromosomal aberrations.

eleo-. Oil. SEE ALSO oleo-. [G. *elaion,* olive oil]

el·e·phan·ti·ac, el·e·phan·ti·as·ic (el-ĕ-fan'tē-ak, fan-tē-as'ik). Relating to elephantiasis.

el·e·phan·ti·a·sis (el-ĕ-fan-tī'ă-sis). Hypertrophy and fibrosis of the skin and subcutaneous tissue, especially of the lower extremities and genitalia, due to long-standing obstruction of lymphatic vessels, most commonly after years of infection by the filarial worms *Wuchereria bancrofti* or *Brugia malayi.* [G. fr. *elephas,* elephant]

e. scro'ti, brawny swelling of the scrotum as a result of chronic lymphatic obstruction. SYN chyloderma.

el·e·va·tor (el'ĕ-vā-tĕr). **1.** An instrument for prying up a sunken part, as the depressed fragment of bone in fracture of the skull, or for elevating tissues. **2.** A surgical instrument used to luxate and remove teeth and roots that cannot be engaged by the beaks of a forceps, or to loosen teeth and roots prior to forceps application. [L. fr. *e-levo,* pp. *-atus,* to lift up]

periosteal e., an instrument used for separating the periosteum from the bone. SYN rugine (1).

elim·i·na·tion (ē-lim-i-nā'shŭn). Expulsion; removal of waste material from the body; the getting rid of anything. [L. *elimino,* pp. *-atus,* to turn out of doors, fr. *limen,* threshold]

ELISA enzyme-linked immunosorbent *assay.*

elix·ir (ē-lik'ser). A clear, sweetened, hydroalco-

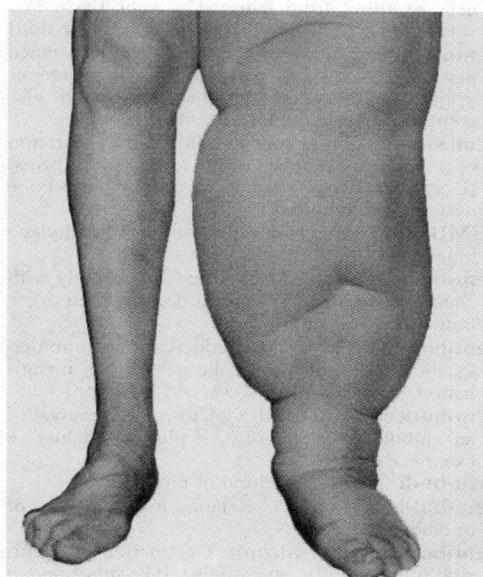

elephantiasis: lymphedema

holic liquid intended for oral use; e.'s contain flavoring substances and are used either as vehicles or for the therapeutic effect of the active medicinal agents. [Mediev. L., fr. Ar. *al- iksir,* the philosopher's stone]

el·lip·to·cyte (ē-lip'tō-sīt). An elliptical red blood corpuscle found normally in the lower vertebrates with the exception of Cyclostomata; in mammals it occurs normally only among the camels, hence cameloid cell. SYN ovalocyte. [G. *elleipsis,* a leaving out, an ellipse, + *kytos,* cell]

el·lip·to·cy·to·sis (ē-lip'tō-sī-tō'sis). A hereditary abnormality of hemopoiesis in which 50 to 90% of the red blood cells consist of rod forms and elliptocytes, often with an associated hemolytic anemia. SYN ovalocytosis.

elongation. RADIOLOGY Radiographic distortion where the image appears longer than the actual image. Caused by insufficient vertical angulation.

el·u·ant (el'yū-ant). The material that has been eluted.

el·u·ate (el'yū-āt). The solution emerging from a column or paper in chromatography. [see elution]

el·u·ent (el'yū-ent). The mobile phase in chromatography. SYN developer (2). [see elution]

elu·tion (ē-lū'shŭn). **1.** The separation, by washing, of one solid from another. **2.** The removal, by means of a suitable solvent, of one material from another that is insoluble in that solvent, as in column chromatography. **3.** The removal of antibodies absorbed onto the erythrocyte surface. [L. *e-luo,* pp. *lutus,* to wash out]

elytro-. The vagina. SEE ALSO colpo-, vagino-. [G. *elytron,* sheath (vagina)]

em-. SEE en-.

ema·ci·a·tion (ē-mā-sē-ā'shŭn). Abnormal thinness resulting from extreme loss of flesh. SYN wasting (1). [L. *e-macio,* pp. *-atus,* to make thin]

em·a·na·tion (em-ă-nā′shŭn). **1.** Any substance that flows out or is emitted from a source or origin. **2.** The radiation from a radioactive element. [L. *e- mano,* pp. *-atus,* to flow out]

emas·cu·la·tion (ē-mas-kyū-lā′shŭn). Castration of the male by removal of the testes and/or penis. [L. *emasculo,* pp. *-atus,* to castrate, fr. *e-* priv. + *masculus,* masculine]

EMB eosin-methylene blue. SEE eosin-methylene blue *agar.*

em·balm (em-bahlm′). To treat a dead body with chemicals to preserve it from decay. [L. *in,* in, + *balsamum,* balsam]

em·bo·le (em′bō-lē). **1.** Reduction of a limb dislocation. **2.** Formation of the gastrula by invagination. SYN emboly. [G. *embolē,* insertion]

em·bo·lec·to·my (em-bō-lek′tō-mē). Removal of an embolus. [G. *embolos,* a plug (embolus), + *ektomē,* excision]

em·bo·li (em′bō-lī). Plural of embolus.

em·bol·ic (em-bol′ik). Relating to an embolus or to embolism.

🛈 **em·bo·lism** (em′bō-lizm). Obstruction or occlusion of a vessel by an embolus. [G. *embolisma,* a piece or patch; lit. something thrust in]

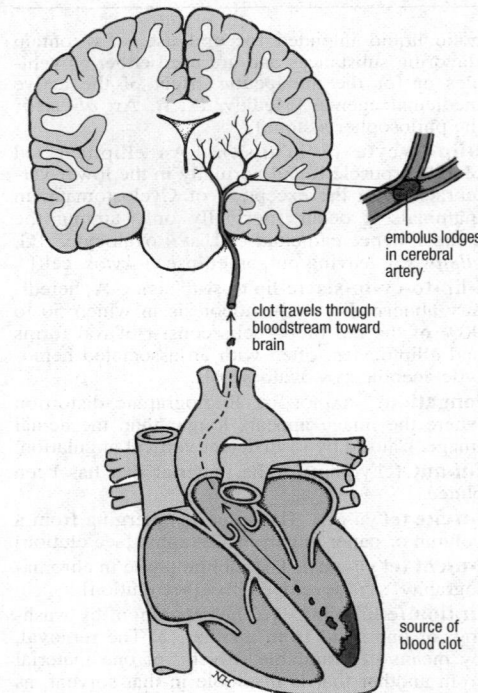

embolus lodges in cerebral artery

clot travels through bloodstream toward brain

source of blood clot

embolism

air e., e. that occurs when air enters veins as a result of trauma, surgery, or deliberate injection; a large air embolism may cause lethal derangement of cardiac function.

cholesterol e., e. of lipid debris from an ulcerated atheromatous deposit, generally from a large artery to small arterial branches; it is usually small and rarely causes infarction.

cotton-fiber e., e. by cotton fibers from sterile gauze used in intravenous medication or transfusion; may form as foreign body granulomas in small pulmonary arteries.

crossed e., (1) obstruction of a systemic artery by an embolus originating in the venous system which passes through a septal defect, patent foramen ovale, or other shunt to the arterial system; (2) obstruction by a minute embolism that passes through the pulmonary capillaries from the venous to the arterial system.

fat e., the occurrence of fat globules in the circulation following fractures of a long bone, in burns, in parturition, and in association with fatty degeneration of the liver; the emboli most commonly block pulmonary or cerebral vessels when symptoms referable to either or both of these regions appear.

infective e., SYN pyemic e.

miliary e., e. occurring simultaneously in a number of capillaries.

obturating e., complete closing of the lumen of a vessel by an embolism.

pulmonary e., e. of pulmonary arteries, most frequently by detached fragments of thrombus from a leg or pelvic vein, commonly when thrombosis has followed an operation or confinement to bed.

pyemic e., plugging of an artery by an embolus detached from a suppurating thrombus. SYN infective e.

retrograde e., e. of a vein by an embolus carried in a direction opposite to that of the normal blood current, after being diverted into a smaller vein.

em·bo·li·za·tion (em′bol-i-zā′shŭn). **1.** The formation and release of an embolus into the circulation. **2.** Therapeutic introduction of various substances into the circulation to occlude vessels, either to arrest or prevent hemorrhaging or to devitalize a structure or organ by occluding its blood supply.

em·bo·lo·la·lia (em′bō-lō-lā′lē-ă). Interjection of meaningless words into a sentence when speaking. SYN embolophrasia. [G. *embolos,* something thrown in, fr. *emballo,* to throw in, + *lalia,* speaking]

em·bo·lo·phra·sia (em′bō-lō-frā′zē-ă). SYN embolalia. [G. *embolos,* something thrown in, + *phrasis,* phrase]

em·bo·lo·ther·a·py (em-bō-lō-thăr′ă-pē). Occlusion of arteries by insertion of blood clots, Gelfoam, coils, balloons, etc., with an angiographic catheter; used for control of inoperable hemorrhage or preoperative management of highly vascular neoplasms. [G. *embolos,* plug, + *therapeia,* medical treatment]

em·bo·lus, pl. **em·bo·li** (em′bō-lŭs, -lī). **1.** A plug, composed of a detached thrombus or vegetation, mass of bacteria, or other foreign body, occluding a vessel. **2.** SYN emboliform *nucleus.* [G. *embolos,* a plug, wedge or stopper]

catheter e., coiled worm-shaped platelet and

fibrin aggregates produced during vascular catheterization, originating on the catheter or its guide wire; embolization of the catheter itself.

em•bo•ly (em′bō-lē). SYN embole (2).

em•bra•sure (em-brā′shūr). DENTISTRY An opening that widens outwardly or inwardly; specifically, that space adjacent to the interproximal contact area that spreads toward the facial, gingival, lingual, occlusal, or incisal aspect. [Fr. an opening in a wall for cannon]

em•bryo (em′brē-ō). 1. An organism in the early stages of development. 2. In humans, the developing organism from conception until approximately the end of the second month; developmental stages from this time to birth are commonly designated as fetal. 3. A primordial plant within a seed. [G. *embryon,* fr. *en,* in, + *bryō,* to be full, swell]

embryo-. The embryo. [G. *embryon,* a young one]

em•bry•o•blast (em′brē-ō-blast). The cells at the embryonic pole of the blastocyst concerned with formation of the body of the embryo *per se.* [embryo- + G. *blastos,* germ]

em•bry•o•car•dia (em′brē-ō-kar′dē-ă). A condition in which the cadence of the heart sounds resembles that of the fetus, the first and second sounds becoming alike and evenly spaced; a sign of serious myocardial disease. [embryo- + G. *kardia,* heart]

em•bry•o•gen•e•sis (em′brē-ō-jen′ē-sis). That phase of prenatal development involved in establishment of the characteristic configuration of the embryonic body; in humans, e. is usually regarded as extending from the end of the second week, when the embryonic disk is formed, to the end of the eighth week, after which the conceptus is usually spoken of as a fetus. [embryo- + G. *genesis,* origin]

em•bry•o•gen•ic, em•bry•o•ge•net•ic (em-brē-ō-jen′ik, -jĕ-net′ik). Producing an embryo; relating to the formation of an embryo.

em•bry•og•e•ny (em-brē-oj′ĕ-nē). The origin and growth of the embryo.

em•bry•ol•o•gist (em-brē-ol′ō-jist). One who specializes in embryology.

em•bry•ol•o•gy (em-brē-ol′ōjē). Science of the origin and development of the organism from fertilization of the ovum to the end of the eighth week. [embryo- + G. *logos,* study]

em•bry•o•ma (em-brē-ō′mă). SYN embryonal *tumor.*

em•bry•o•nal (em′brē-ō′năl). Relating to an embryo.

em•bry•on•i•za•tion (em′brē-on-i-zā′shŭn). Reversion of a cell or tissue to an embryonic form.

em•bry•o•noid (em′brē-ō-noyd). Resembling an embryo or a fetus. [embryo- + G. *eidos,* appearance]

em•bry•o•ny (em′brē-ō-nē). The forming of an embryo.

em•bry•op•a•thy (em-brē-op′ă-thē). A morbid condition in the embryo or fetus. SYN fetopathy. [embryo- + G. *pathos,* disease]

em•bry•o•plas•tic (em-brē-ō-plas′tik). 1. Producing an embryo. 2. Relating to the formation of an embryo. [embryo- + G. *plassō,* to form]

em•bry•ot•o•my (em-brē-ot′ō-mē). Any mutilating operation on the fetus to make possible its removal when delivery is impossible by natural means. [embryo- + G. *tomē,* cutting]

em•bry•o•tox•ic•i•ty (em′brē-ō-tok-sis′i-tē). Injury to the embryo, which may result in death or in abnormal development of a part, owing to substances that enter the placental circulation.

em•bry•o•tox•on (em′brē-ō-tok′son). Congenital opacity of the periphery of the cornea, a feature of osteogenesis imperfecta. [embryo- + G. *toxon,* bow]

anterior e., SYN *arcus* cornealis.

posterior e., a developmental abnormality marked by a prominent white ring of Schwalbe and iris strands that partially obscure the chamber angle.

em•bry•o•troph (em′brē-ō-trōf). 1. Nutritive material supplied to the embryo during development. Cf. hemotroph. 2. In the implantation stages of deciduate placental mammals, fluid adjacent to the blastodermic vesicle; a mixture of the secretion of the uterine glands, cellular debris resulting from the trophoblastic invasion of the endometrium, and exudated plasma. [embryo- + G. *trophē,* nourishment]

em•bry•o•tro•phic (em′brē-ō-trof′ik). Relating to any process or agency involved in the nourishment of the embryo.

em•bry•ot•ro•phy (em′brē-ot′rō-fē). The nutrition of the embryo. [embryo- + G. *trophē,* nourishment]

emed•ul•late (ē-med′yū-lāt). To extract any marrow. [L. *e-,* from, + *medulla,* marrow]

emei•o•cy•to•sis (ē′mē-ō-sī-tō′sis). SYN exocytosis (2). [L. *emitto,* to send forth, + G. *kytos,* cell, + *-osis,* condition]

em•e•sis (em′ĕ-sis). 1. SYN vomiting. 2. Combining form, used in the suffix position, for vomiting. [G. *emeō,* to vomit]

emet•ic (ĕ-met′ik). 1. Relating to or causing vomiting. 2. An agent that causes vomiting. [G. *emetikos,* producing vomiting, fr. *emeō,* to vomit]

em•e•to•ca•thar•tic (em′ĕ-tō-kă-thar′tik). 1. Both emetic and cathartic. 2. An agent that causes vomiting and purging of the lower intestines.

EMF electromotive *force.*

EMG electromyogram.

-emia. Blood. [G. *haima*]

em•i•gra•tion (em-i-grā′shŭn). The passage of white blood cells through the endothelium and wall of small blood vessels. [L. *e-migro,* pp. *-atus,* to emigrate]

em•i•nence (em′i-nens). A circumscribed area raised above the general level of the surrounding surface, particularly on a bone surface. SYN eminentia [NA]. [L. *eminentia*]

hypothenar e., the fleshy mass at the medial side of the palm. SYN hypothenar (1).

thenar e., the fleshy mass on the lateral side of the palm; the radial palm; the ball of the thumb. SYN thenar (1).

em•i•nen•tia, pl. **em•i•nen•ti•ae** (em-i-nen′shē-ă, -shē-ē) [NA]. SYN eminence. [L. prominence, fr. *e-mineo,* to stand out, project]

e. pyramida′lis [NA], a conical projection posterior to the vestibular window in the middle ear; it is hollow and contains the stapedius muscle.

em·i·o·cy·to·sis (ē'mē-ō-sī-tō'sis). SYN exocytosis (2). [L. *emitto*, to send forth, + G. *kytos*, cell, + *-osis*, condition]

em·is·sary (em'i-sār-ē). **1.** Relating to, or providing, an outlet or drain. **2.** SYN emissary *vein*. [see emissarium]

emis·sion (ē-mish'ŭn). A discharge; referring usually to a seminal discharge occurring during sleep (**nocturnal e.**). [L. *emissio*, fr. *e- mitto*, to send out]

    nasal e., SPEECH PATHOLOGY the sound of air forcefully flowing through the nose during speech (as opposed to nasal resonance), usually due to poor valving between the oral and nasal cavities, as in cleft palate. SEE hypernasality. SYN nasal escape, snorting.

    otoacoustic e.'s (OAE), sounds that issue from the external acoustic meatus as a result of vibrations originating within the cochlea. SEE ALSO Kemp *echo*.

    thermionic e., e. of free electrons by a filament that is heated by an electric current passing through it, as in an x-ray tube. SYN Edison effect.

EMIT enzyme-multiplied *immunoassay* technique.

em·men·ia (ĕ-men'ē-ă, ĕ-mē'nē-ă). SYN menses. [G. *emmēnos*, monthly]

em·men·ic (ĕ-men'ik). SYN menstrual.

em·men·i·op·a·thy (ĕ-men'ē-op'ă-thē). Any disorder of menstruation. [G. *emmēnos*, monthly, + *pathos*, suffering]

em·me·tro·pia (em-ĕ-trō'pē-ă). The state of refraction of the eye in which parallel rays, when the eye is at rest, are focused exactly on the retina. [G. *emmetros*, according to measure, + *ōps*, eye]

em·me·tro·pic (em-ĕ-trop'ik). Pertaining to or characterized by emmetropia.

emol·lient (ē-mol'ē-ent). **1.** Soothing to the skin or mucous membrane. **2.** An agent that softens the skin or soothes irritation in the skin or mucous membrane. [L. *emolliens*, pres. p. of *e- mollio*, *emollire*, to soften]

emo·tion (ē-mō'shŭn). A strong feeling, aroused mental state, or intense state of drive or unrest directed toward a definite object and evidenced in both behavior and in psychologic changes, with accompanying autonomic nervous system manifestations. [L. *e-moveo*, pp. *-motus*, to move out, agitate]

emo·tion·al (ē-mō'shŭn-ăl). Relating to or marked by an emotion.

em·path·ic (em-path'ik). Relating to or marked by empathy.

em·pa·thize (em'pă-thīz). To feel empathy in relation to another person; to put oneself in another's place.

em·pa·thy (em'pă-thē). **1.** The ability to intellectually and emotionally sense the emotions, feelings, and reactions that another person is experiencing and to effectively communicate that understanding to the individual. Cf. sympathy (3). **2.** The anthropomorphization or humanizing of objects and the feeling of oneself as being in

and part of them. [G. *en* (*em*), in, + *pathos*, feeling]

em·phy·se·ma (em-fi-sē'mă). **1.** Presence of air in the interstices of the connective tissue of a part. **2.** A condition of the lung characterized by increase beyond the normal in the size of air spaces distal to the terminal bronchiole (those parts containing alveoli), with destructive changes in their walls and reduction in their number. Clinical manifestations include dyspnea on exertion, "barrel chest," with prolonged expiration and increased residual volume; symptoms of chronic bronchitis often, but not necessarily, coexist. Two structural varieties are described: panlobular e. and centrilobular e. SYN pulmonary e. [G. inflation of stomach, etc. fr. *en*, in, + *physēma*, a blowing, fr. *physa*, bellows]

    bullous e., e. in which the enlarged airspaces are one to several cm in diameter, often visible on chest radiographs. Thin-walled air sacs under tension compress pulmonary tissue, either single or multiple.

    centrilobular e., e. affecting the lobules around their central bronchioles, causally related to bronchiolitis, and seen in coal-miner's pneumoconiosis.

    diffuse obstructive e., the major component of chronic obstructive lung disease.

    ectatic e., obstructive airway disease with areas of dilatation of alveoli acini. Seen primarily in association with inherited deficiency of alpha$_1$ protease inhibitor. SEE panlobular e.

    interlobular e., interstitial e. in the connective tissue septa between the pulmonary lobules.

    interstitial e., (1) presence of air in the pulmonary tissues consequent upon rupture of the air cells; **(2)** presence of air or gas in the connective tissue.

    intestinal e., SYN *pneumatosis* cystoides intestinalis.

    mediastinal e., deflection of air, usually from a ruptured emphysematous bleb in the lung, into the mediastinal tissue.

    panlobular e., e. affecting all parts of the lobules, in part, or usually the whole, of the lungs, and usually associated with α$_1$-antiprotease deficiency e.

    pulmonary e., SYN emphysema (2).

    subcutaneous e., the presence of air or gas in the subcutaneous tissues. SYN pneumoderma.

    surgical e., subcutaneous e. from air trapped in the tissues by an operation or injury.

    unilateral lobar e., a state in which the roentgenographic density of one lung (or one lobe) is markedly less than the density of the other(s) because of the presence of air trapped during expiration. SYN Swyer-James syndrome (1).

em·phy·sem·a·tous (em-fi-sem'ă-tŭs). Relating to or affected with emphysema.

em·pir·ic (em-pir'ik). **1.** SYN empirical. **2.** A member of a school of Graeco-Roman physicians who placed their confidence in and based their practice purely on experience, avoiding all speculation, theory, or abstract reasoning. **3.** Modern: testing a hypothesis by careful observation, hence rationally based on experience. [see empirical]

em·pir·i·cal (em-pir'i-kăl). **1.** Founded on practical experience, rather than on reasoning alone, but not proved scientifically, in contrast to rational (1). **2.** Relating to an empiric (2). **3.** Based on careful observational testing of a hypothesis; rational. SYN empiric (1). [G. *empeirikos;* fr. *empeiria,* experience, fr. *en,* in, + *peira,* a trial]

em•pros•thot•o•nos (em′pros-thot′ō-nŭs). A tetanic contraction of the flexor muscles, curving the back with concavity forward. [G. *emprosthen,* forward, + *tonos,* tension]

em•py•e•ma (em-pī-ē′mă, -pi-ē′mă). Pus in a body cavity; when used without qualification, refers specifically to pyothorax. [G. *empyēma,* suppuration, fr. *en,* in, + *pyon,* pus]

em•py•e•mic (em-pī-ē′mik). Relating to empyema.

em•py•e•sis (em-pī-ē′sis). A pustular eruption. [G. suppuration]

emul•si•fi•er (ē-mŭl′si-fī-er). An agent, such as gum arabic or the yolk of an egg, used to make an emulsion of a fixed oil. Soaps, detergents, steroids, and proteins can act as emulsifiers.

emul•sion (ē-mŭl′shŭn). A system containing two immiscible liquids in which one is dispersed, in the form of very small globules (internal phase), throughout the other (external phase). [Mod. L. fr. *e-mulgeo,* pp. *-mulsus,* to milk or drain out]

emul•soid (ē-mŭl′soyd). A colloidal dispersion in which the dispersed particles are more or less liquid and exert a certain attraction on and absorb a certain quantity of the fluid in which they are suspended.

en-. In; appears as em- before b, p, or m. [G.]

enam•el (ē-nam′ĕl). The hard glistening substance covering the exposed portion of the tooth. In its mature form, it is composed of an inorganic portion made up of 90% hydroxyapatite and 6-8% calcium carbonate, calcium fluoride, and magnesium carbonate, the remainder comprising an organic matrix of protein and glycoprotein; structurally, it is made up of oriented rods each of which consists of a stack of rodlets encased in an organic prism sheath. [M.E., fr. Fr. *enamailer,* to apply enamel, fr. *en,* on, + *amail,* enamel, fr. Germanic]

mottled e., alterations in e. structure due to excessive fluoride ingestion during tooth formation.

enam•el•o•gen•e•sis (ē-nam′ĕl-ō-jen′ĕ-sis). SYN amelogenesis.

enam•el•o•ma (ē-nam-ĕl-ō′mă). A developmental anomaly in which there is a small nodule of enamel below the cementoenamel junction, usually at the bifurcation of molar teeth.

en•an•them, en•an•the•ma (en-an′them, en-an-thē′mă). A mucous membrane eruption, especially one occurring in connection with one of the exanthemas. [G. *en,* in, + *anthēma,* bloom, eruption, fr. *antheō,* to bloom]

en•an•them•a•tous (en-an-them′ă-tŭs). Relating to an enanthem.

en•an•the•sis (en-an-thē′sis). The skin eruption of a general disease, such as scarlatina or typhoid fever. [G. *en,* in, + *anthēsis,* full bloom]

en•ar•thro•di•al (en-ar-thrō′dē-al). Relating to an enarthrosis.

en•ar•thro•sis (en-ar-thrō′sis). SYN ball-and-socket *joint.* [G. *en-arthrōsis,* a jointing where the ball is deep set in the socket]

en bloc (ăhn blok). In a lump; as a whole; used to refer to autopsy techniques in which visceral organs are removed in large blocks allowing the prosector to retain a continuity in organ architecture during the subsequent dissection. [Fr., in a lump]

en•cap•su•la•tion (en-kap-sū-lā′shŭn). Enclosure in a capsule or sheath. [L. *in* + capsula, dim. of *capsa,* box]

encephal-. SEE encephalo-.

en•ceph•a•lal•gia (en-sef-ă-lal′jē-ă). SYN headache. [encephalo- + G. *algos,* pain]

en•ceph•a•la•tro•phic (en-sef-ă-lă-trof′ik). Relating to encephalatrophy.

en•ceph•a•lat•ro•phy (en-sef-ă-lat′rō-fē). Atrophy of the brain. [encephalo- + G. *a-* priv. + *trophē,* nourishment]

en•ce•phal•ic (en′se-fal′ik). Relating to the brain, or to the structures within the cranium.

en•ceph•a•lit•ic (en-sef-ă-lit′ik). Relating to encephalitis.

en•ceph•a•lit•i•des (en-sef-ă-lit′i-dēz).

en•ceph•a•li•tis, pl. **en•ceph•a•lit•i•des** (en-sef-ă-lī′tis, en-sef-ă-lit′i-dēz). Inflammation of the brain. SYN cephalitis. [G. *enkephalos,* brain, + *-itis,* inflammation]

acute necrotizing e., an acute form of e., characterized by destruction of brain parenchyma.

bunyavirus e., e. of abrupt onset, with severe frontal headache and low-grade to moderate fever, caused by members of the genus *Bunyavirus.*

Coxsackie e., a viral e., seen mainly in infants and involving principally the gray matter of the medulla and cord, caused by *Enterovirus* Coxsackie B.

herpes simplex e., the most common acute encephalitis, caused by HSV-1; affects persons of any age; preferentially involves the inferomedial portions of the temporal lobe and the orbital portions of the frontal lobes; pathologically, severe hemorrhagic necrosis is present along with, in the acute stages, intranuclear eosinophilic inclusion bodies in the neurons and glial cells.

Japanese B e., an epidemic e. or encephalomyelitis of Japan, Siberian Russia, and other parts of Asia; due to the Japanese B e. virus (genus *Flavivirus*) and transmitted by mosquitoes; can occur as a symptomless, subclinical infection but may cause an acute meningoencephalomyelitis.

lead e., SYN lead *encephalopathy.*

Murray Valley e., a severe e. with a high mortality rate occurring in the Murray Valley of Australia; the disease is most severe in children and is characterized by headache, fever, malaise, drowsiness or convulsions, and rigidity of the neck; extensive brain damage may result; it is caused by the Murray Valley encephalitis virus (genus *Flavivirus*). SYN Australian X disease.

e. periaxialis diffusa, SYN Schilder's *disease.*

Powassan e., an acute disease of children varying clinically from undifferentiated febrile illness to e.; caused by the Powassan virus and transmitted by ixodid ticks.

secondary e., collective term for post-infectious, post-exanthem, and post-vaccinal encephalitides.

tick-borne e. (Eastern subtype), a severe form of e. caused by a flavivirus and transmitted by ticks (*Ixodes pertulcatus* and *I. ricinus*).

varicella e., e. occurring as a complication of chickenpox.

⌂**encephalo-, encephal-.** The brain. Cf. cerebro-. . [G. *enkephalos,* brain]

en·ceph·a·lo·cele (en-sef'ă-lō-sēl). A congenital gap in the skull with herniation of brain substance. SYN craniocele. [encephalo- + G. *kēlē,* hernia]

en·ceph·a·lo·gram (en-sef'ă-lō-gram). The record obtained by encephalography. [encephalo- + G. *gramma,* a drawing]

en·ceph·a·log·ra·phy (en-sef-ă-log'ră-fē). Radiographic representation of the brain. [encephalo- + G. *graphō,* to write]

en·ceph·a·loid (en-sef'ă-loyd). Resembling brain substance; denoting a carcinoma of soft, brainlike consistency. [encephalo- + G. *eidos,* resemblance]

en·ceph·a·lo·lith (en-sef'ă-lō-lith). A concretion in the brain or one of its ventricles. [encephalo- + G. *lithos,* stone]

en·ceph·a·lo·ma (en-sef-ă-lō'mă). Herniation of brain substance. SYN cerebroma.

en·ceph·a·lo·ma·la·cia (en-sef'ă-lō-mă-lā'shē-ă). Abnormal softness of the cerebral parenchyma often due to ischemia or infarction. SYN cerebromalacia. [encephalo- + G. *malakia,* softness]

en·ceph·a·lo·men·in·gi·tis (en-sef-ă-lō-men-in-jī'tis). SYN meningoencephalitis. [encephalo- + G. *mēninx,* membrane, + *-itis,* inflammation]

en·ceph·a·lo·me·nin·go·cele (en-sef'ă-lō-me-ning'gō-sēl). SYN meningoencephalocele. [encephalo- + G. *mēninx,* membrane, + *kēlē,* hernia]

en·ceph·a·lo·men·in·gop·a·thy (en-sef'ă-lō-men-in-gop'ă-thē). SYN meningoencephalopathy.

en·ceph·a·lo·mere (en-sef'ă-lō-mēr). A neuromere. [encephalo- + G. *meros,* a part]

en·ceph·a·lom·e·ter (en-sef-ă-lom'ě-ter). An apparatus for indicating on the skull the location of the cortical centers. [encephalo- + G. *metron,* measure]

en·ceph·a·lo·my·e·li·tis (en-sef-ă-lō-mī'ě-lī'tis). Inflammation of the brain and spinal cord. [encephalo- + G. *myelon,* marrow, + *-itis,* inflammation]

acute disseminated e., an acute demyelinating disorder of the central nervous system, in which focal demyelination is present throughout the brain and spinal cord. This process is common to postinfectious, postexanthem, and postvaccinal encephalomyelitis.

acute necrotizing hemorrhagic e., a fulminating demyelinating disorder of the central nervous system that affects mainly children and young adults. Almost always preceded by a respiratory infection, characterized by the abrupt onset of fever, headache, confusion, and nuchal rigidity, soon followed by focal seizures, hemiplegia, or quadriplegia, brainstem findings, and coma.

benign myalgic e., SYN epidemic *neuromyasthenia.*

granulomatous e., an e. in which granulomas occur.

postvaccinal e., a severe type of encephalomyelitis that can follow the rabies vaccination.

western equine e., an equine e. found in the western U.S. and parts of South America, transmitted by mosquitoes and caused by the western equine e. virus; the infection is similar to but milder than eastern equine e. in man and is, as a rule, inapparent, but some cases with central nervous system involvement have been fatal.

en·ceph·a·lo·my·e·lo·cele (en-sef'ă-lō-mī'ě-lō-sēl). Congenital defect usually in the occipital region (foramen magnum) and cervical vertebrae, with herniation of the meninges, medulla, and spinal cord. [G. *enkephalos,* brain, + *myelon,* marrow, + *kēlē,* hernia]

en·ceph·a·lo·my·e·lo·neu·rop·a·thy (en-sef'ă-lō-mī'ě-lō-nū-rop'ă-thē). A disease involving the brain, spinal cord, and peripheral nerves.

en·ceph·a·lo·my·e·lop·a·thy (en-sef'ă-lō-mī-ě-lop'ă-thē). Any disease of both brain and spinal cord. [G. *enkephalos,* brain, + *myelon,* marrow, + *pathos,* suffering]

paraneoplastic e., an encephalomyelopathy as a remote effect of carcinoma, most often oat cell carcinoma of the lung.

en·ceph·a·lo·my·e·lo·ra·dic·u·li·tis (en-sef'ă-lō-mī'ě-lō-ră-dik'yū-lī-tis). SYN encephalomyeloradiculopathy.

en·ceph·a·lo·my·e·lo·ra·dic·u·lop·a·thy (en-sef'ă-lō-mī'ě-lō-ră-dik'yū-lop-ă-thē). A disease process involving the brain, spinal cord, and spinal roots. SYN encephalomyeloradiculitis.

en·ceph·a·lo·my·o·car·di·tis (en-sef'ă-lō-mī'ō-kar-dī'tis). Associated encephalitis and myocarditis; often caused by a viral infection such as in polio myelitis.

en·ceph·a·lon, pl. **en·ceph·a·la** (en-sef'ă-lon, lă) [NA]. That portion of the cerebrospinal axis contained within the cranium, composed of the prosencephalon, mesencephalon, and rhombencephalon. [G. *enkephalos,* brain, fr. *en,* in, + *kephalē,* head]

en·ceph·a·lop·a·thy (en-sef'ă-lop'ă-thē). Any disorder of the brain. SYN cephalopathy, cerebropathy, encephalosis. [encephalo- + G. *pathos,* suffering]

bilirubin e., SYN kernicterus.

Binswanger's e., SYN Binswanger's *disease.*

hepatic e., (1) SYN portal-systemic e. **(2)** SYN Reye's *syndrome.*

hypernatremic e., subarachnoid and subdural effusions in infants with hypernatremic dehydration.

lead e., a metabolic e., caused by the ingestion of lead compounds and seen particularly in early childhood; it is characterized pathologically by extensive cerebral edema, status spongiosus, neurocytolysis, and some reactive inflammation; clinical manifestations include convulsions, delirium, and hallucinations. SEE ALSO lead *poisoning.* SYN lead encephalitis.

metabolic e., e. characterized by memory loss, vertigo, and generalized weakness, due to metabolic brain disease including hypoxia, ischemia, hypoglycemia, or secondary to other organ failure such as liver or kidney.

portal-systemic e., an e. associated with cirrhosis of the liver, attributed to the passage of toxic nitrogenous substances from the portal to the systemic circulation; cerebral manifestations may include coma. SYN hepatic e. (1).

spongiform e., an e. characterized by vacuolation within nerve and glial cells.

subacute spongiform e., a form of spongiform e. that is associated with a "slow virus", which to date has not been adequately described, is transmissible, and has a rapidly progressive, fatal course; e.g., Creutzfeldt-Jakob disease, kuru, Gerstmann-Sträussler syndrome, scrapie. SEE prion.

traumatic e., an e. resulting from structural brain injury.

"viral" spongiform e., progressive vacuolation in dendritic and axonal processes and in neuronal cell bodies, associated with slow virus infections.

Wernicke-Korsakoff e., SEE Wernicke's *syndrome*, Korsakoff's *syndrome*.

Wernicke's e., SYN Wernicke's *syndrome*.

en·ceph·a·los·chi·sis (en-sef-ă-los'ki-sis). Developmental failure of closure of the rostral part of the neural tube. [encephalo- + G. *schisis*, fissure]

en·ceph·a·lo·scle·ro·sis (en-sef'ă-lō-sklēr-o'sis). A sclerosis, or hardening, of the brain. SEE ALSO cerebrosclerosis. [encephalo- + G. *sklērōsis*, hardening]

en·ceph·a·lo·sis. SYN encephalopathy.

en·ceph·a·lot·o·my (en-sef-ă-lot'ŏ-mē). Dissection or incision of the brain. [encephalo- + G. *tomē*, incision]

en·chon·dro·ma (en-kon-drō'mă). A benign cartilaginous growth starting within the medullary cavity of a bone originally formed from cartilage; e.'s may distend the cortex, especially of small bones, and may be solitary or multiple (endochondromatosis). [Mod. L. fr. G. *en*, in, + *chondros*, cartilage, + *-oma*, tumor]

en·chon·dro·ma·to·sis (en-kon'drō-ma-tō'sis) [MIM*166000]. A rarely familial, and probably hamartomatous proliferation of cartilage in the metaphyses of several bones, most commonly of the hands and feet, causing distorted growth in length or pathological fractures; chondrosarcoma frequently develops. When combined with hemangiomas in the cutaneous or visceral regions, called Maffucci's syndrome. SYN dyschondroplasia.

en·chon·drom·a·tous (en-kon-drō'mă-tŭs). Relating to or having the elements of enchondroma.

en·clave (en-klāv, ahn-klahv'). An enclosure; a detached mass of tissue enclosed in tissue of another kind; seen especially in the case of isolated masses of gland tissue detached from the main gland. [Fr. fr. L. *clavis*, key]

en·cod·ing (en-kōd'ing). The first stage in the memory process, followed by storage and retrieval, involving processes associated with receiving or briefly registering stimuli through one or more of the senses and modifying that information.

en·cop·re·sis (en-kō-prē'sis). The repeated, generally involuntary passage of feces into inappropriate places (e.g., clothing); considered a mental disorder if it occurs in a child more than 4 years old. [G. *enkopros*, full of manure]

encounter. A health care contact between the patient and the provider who is responsible for diagnosing and treating the patient.

en·cyst·ed (en-sis'ted). Encapsulated by a membranous bag. [G. *kystis*, bladder]

end. An extremity, or the most remote point of an extremity.

distal e., the posterior extremity of a dental appliance. SYN heel (2).

⚠**end-.** SEE endo-.

end·an·ge·i·tis. SEE endangiitis.

end·an·gi·i·tis, end·an·ge·i·tis (end-an-jē-ī'tis). Inflammation of the intima of a blood vessel. SYN endovasculitis. [endo- + G. *angeion*, vessel, + *-itis*, inflammation]

end·a·or·ti·tis (end'ā-ōr-tī'tis). Inflammation of the intima of the aorta.

end·ar·ter·ec·to·my (end-ar-ter-ek'tō-mē). Excision of diseased endothelial and media or most of the media of an artery, and also of occluding atheromatous deposits, so as to leave a smooth lining, mostly consisting of adventitia. [endo- + artery + G. *ektomē*, excision]

end·ar·te·ri·tis (end'ar-ter-ī'tis). Inflammation of the intima of an artery. SYN endoarteritis.

bacterial e., implantation and growth of bacteria with formation of vegetations on the arterial wall, such as may occur in a patent ductus arteriosus or arteriovenous fistula.

e. oblit'erans, obliterating e., an extreme degree of e. proliferans closing the lumen of the artery. SYN arteritis obliterans, obliterating arteritis.

e. prolif'erans, proliferating e., chronic e. accompanied by a marked increase of fibrous tissue in the intima.

end·au·ral (end-aw'răl). Within the ear. [endo- + L. *auris*, ear]

end·brain. SYN telencephalon.

en·dem·ic (en-dem'ik). Present in a community or among a group of people; said of a disease prevailing continually in a region. Cf. epidemic, sporadic. [G. *endēmos*, native, fr. *en*, in, + *dēmos*, the people]

en·dem·o·ep·i·dem·ic (en-dem'ō-ep-i-dem'ik). Denoting a temporary large increase in the number of cases of an endemic disease.

end·er·gon·ic (en-der-gon'ik). Referring to a chemical reaction that takes place with absorption of energy from its surroundings (i.e., a positive change in Gibbs free energy). Cf. exergonic. [endo- + G. *ergon*, work]

end-feet. SYN axon *terminals*, under *terminal*.

end·ing (end'ing). **1.** A termination or conclusion. **2.** A nerve e.

free nerve e.'s, a form of peripheral ending of sensory nerve fibers in which the terminal filaments end freely in the tissue.

⚠**endo-, end-.** Prefixes indicating within, inner,

absorbing, or containing. SEE ALSO ento-. [G. *endon,* within]

en·do·an·eu·rys·mo·plas·ty (en'dō-an-yū-riz'mō-plas-tē). SYN aneurysmoplasty.

en·do·an·eu·rys·mor·rha·phy (en'dō-an-yū-riz-mōr'ă-fē). SYN aneurysmoplasty. [endo- + G. *aneurysma,* aneurysm, + *rhaphē,* suture]

en·do·ar·te·ri·tis (en'dō-ar-ter-ī'tis). SYN endarteritis.

en·do·blast (en'dō-blast). Entoderm. [endo- + G. *blastos,* germ]

en·do·car·dit·ic (en'dō-kar-dit'ik). Relating to endocarditis.

en·do·car·di·tis (en'dō-kar-dī'tis). Inflammation of the endocardium.

　atypical verrucous e., SYN Libman-Sacks e.

　bacterial e., e. caused by the direct invasion of bacteria and leading to deformity and destruction of the valve leaflets. Two types are acute bacterial endocarditis and subacute bacterial endocarditis.

　infectious e., infective e., e. due to infection by microorganisms.

　Libman-Sacks e., verrucous e. sometimes associated with disseminated lupus erythematosus. SYN atypical verrucous e., Libman-Sacks syndrome, nonbacterial verrucous e.

　mural e., inflammation of the endocardium involving the walls of the chambers of the heart.

　nonbacterial verrucous e., SYN Libman-Sacks e.

　rheumatic e., endocardial involvement as part of rheumatic heart disease, recognized clinically by valvular involvement; in the acute stage, there may be tiny fibrin vegetations along the lines of closure of the valve leaflets, with subsequent fibrous thickening and shortening of the leaflets.

　subacute bacterial e. (SBE), e. usually involving cardiac valves with congenital or acquired abnormalities and usually due to alpha-hemolytic streptococci.

　valvular e., inflammation confined to the endocardium of the valves.

　vegetative e., verrucous e., e. associated with the presence of fibrinous clots (vegetations) forming on the ulcerated surfaces of the valves.

en·do·car·di·um, pl. **en·do·car·dia** (en-dō-kar'dē-ŭm, -ē-ă) [NA]. The innermost tunic of the heart, which includes endothelium and subendothelial connective tissue; in the atrial wall, smooth muscle and numerous elastic fibers also occur. [endo- + G. *kardia,* heart]

en·do·cer·vi·cal (en'dō-ser'vi-kăl). 1. Within any cervix, specifically within the cervix uteri. 2. Relating to the endocervix.

en·do·cer·vi·ci·tis (en'dō-ser-vi-sī'tis). Inflammation of the mucous membrane of the cervix uteri. SYN endotrachelitis.

en·do·cer·vix (en-dō-ser'viks). The mucous membrane of the cervical canal.

en·do·co·li·tis (en'dō-kō-lī'tis). Simple catarrhal inflammation of the colon.

en·do·cra·ni·al (en-dō-krā'nē-ăl). 1. Within the cranium. 2. Relating to the endocranium.

en·do·cra·ni·um (en'dō-krā'nē-ŭm). The lining membrane of the cranium, or dura mater of the brain.

en·do·crine (en'dō-krin). 1. Secreting internally, most commonly into the systemic circulation; of or pertaining to such secretion. Cf. paracrine. 2. The internal or hormonal secretion of a ductless gland. 3. Denoting a gland that furnishes an internal secretion. [endo- + G. *krinō,* to separate]

en·do·cri·nol·o·gist (en'dō-kri-nol'ō-jist). One who specializes in endocrinology.

en·do·cri·nol·o·gy (en'dō-kri-nol'ō-jē). The science and medical specialty concerned with the internal or hormonal secretions and their physiologic and pathologic relations. [endocrine + G. *logos,* study]

en·do·cri·no·ma (en'dō-kri-nō'mă). A tumor with endocrine tissue that retains the function of the parent organ, usually to an excessive degree.

en·do·crin·o·path·ic (en'dō-kri-nō-path'ik). Relating to or suffering from an endocrinopathy.

en·do·cri·nop·a·thy (en'dō-kri-nop'ă-thē). A disorder in the function of an endocrine gland and the consequences thereof. [endocrine + G. *pathos,* disease]

en·do·cys·ti·tis (en'dō-sis-tī'tis). Inflammation of the mucous membrane of the bladder. [endo- + G. *kystis,* bladder, + *-itis,* inflammation]

en·do·cy·to·sis (en'dō-sī-tō'sis). Internalization of substances from the extracellular environment through the formation of vesicles formed from the plasma membrane. SEE ALSO phagocytosis. Cf. exocytosis (2). [endo- + G. *kytos,* cell, + *-osis,* condition]

en·do·derm (en'dō-derm). The innermost of the three primary germ layers of the embryo (ectoderm, mesoderm, endoderm); from it is derived the epithelial lining of the primitive gut tract and the epithelial component of the glands and other structures (*e.g.,* lower respiratory system) that developed as outgrowths from the gut tube. SYN entoderm, hypoblast. [endo- + G. *derma,* skin]

en·do·don·tia (en-dō-don'shē-ă). SYN endodontics.

en·do·don·tics (en-dō-don'tiks). A field of dentistry concerned with the diseases and injuries of the dental pulp and periapical tissues, and with the prevention, diagnosis, and treatment of diseases and injuries in these tissues. SYN endodontia, endodontology. [endo- + G. *odous,* tooth]

en·do·don·tist (en-dō-don'tist). One who specializes in the practice of endodontics.

en·do·don·tol·o·gy (en'dō-don-tol'ō-jē). SYN endodontics.

en·do·en·ter·i·tis (en'dō-en-ter-ī'tis). Inflammation of the intestinal mucous membrane. [endo- + G. *enteron,* intestine, *-itis,* inflammation]

en·dog·a·my (en-dog'ă-mē). Reproduction by conjugation between sister cells, the descendants of one original cell. [endo- + G. *gamos,* marriage]

en·dog·e·nous (en-doj'ĕ-nŭs). Originating or produced within the organism or one of its parts. [endo- + G. *-gen,* production]

en·do·in·tox·i·ca·tion (en'dō-in-tok-si-kā'shŭn). Poisoning by an endogenous toxin.

en·do·lith (en'dō-lith). A calcified body found in the pulp chamber of a tooth; may be composed of irregular dentin (true denticle) or due to ectopic calcification of pulp tissue (false denticle). SYN denticle (1). [endo- + G. *lithos,* stone]

en·do·lymph (en′dō-limf). The fluid contained within the membranous labyrinth of the inner ear. SYN Scarpa's fluid.

en·do·lym·phic (en-dō-lim′fik). Relating to the endolymph.

en·do·me·tria (en-dō-mē′trē-ă). Plural of endometrium.

en·do·me·tri·al (en-dō-mē′trē-ăl). Relating to or composed of endometrium.

en·do·me·tri·oid (en-dō-mē′trē-oyd). Microscopically resembling endometrial tissue.

en·do·me·tri·o·ma (en′dō-mē-trē-ō′mă). Circumscribed mass of ectopic endometrial tissue in endometriosis. [endometrium + -oma, tumor]

en·do·me·tri·o·sis (en′dō-mē-trē-ō′sis). Ectopic occurrence of endometrial tissue, frequently forming cysts containing altered blood. [endometrium + -osis, condition]

en·do·me·tri·tis (en′dō-mē-trī′tis). Inflammation of the endometrium. [endometrium + -itis, inflammation]

en·do·me·tri·um, pl. **en·do·me·tria** (en′dō-mē′trē-ŭm, -trē-ă) [NA]. The mucous membrane comprising the inner layer of the uterine wall; it consists of a simple columnar epithelium and a lamina propria that contains simple tubular uterine glands. The structure, thickness, and state of the endometrium undergo marked change with the menstrual cycle. [endo- + G. *mētra*, uterus]

en·do·mi·to·sis (en′dō-mī-tō′sis). SYN endopolyploidy.

en·do·morph (en′dō-mōrf). A constitutional body type or build (biotype or somatotype) in which tissues that originated in the endoderm prevail; from a morphological standpoint, the trunk predominates over the limbs. [endo- + G. *morphē*, form]

en·do·mor·phic (en′dō-mōr′fik). Relating to, or having the characteristics of, an endomorph.

En·do·my·ce·ta·les (en′dō-mī-sē-tā′lēz). An order of Ascomycota that includes the yeasts.

en·do·my·o·car·di·al (en′dō-mī-ō-kar′dē-ăl). Relating to the endocardium and the myocardium.

en·do·my·o·car·di·tis (en-dō-mī′ō-kar-dī′tis). Inflammation of both endocardium and myocardium.

en·do·my·o·me·tri·tis (en′dō-mī-ō-mē-trī′tis). Sepsis involving the tissues of the uterus. [endo- + G. *mys*, muscle, + *mētra*, uterus, + -itis, inflammation]

en·do·mys·i·um (en′dō-miz′ē-ŭm, -mis′ē-ŭm). The fine connective tissue sheath surrounding a muscle fiber. [endo- + G. *mys*, muscle]

en·do·neu·ri·um (en-dō-nū′rē-ŭm). The innermost connective tissue supportive structure present in peripheral nerve trunks, found within the fascicles. With the perineurium and epineurium, composes the peripheral nerve stroma. SYN Henle's sheath. [endo- + G. *neuron*, nerve]

en·do·nu·cle·ase (en-dō-nū′klē-ās). A nuclease (phosphodiesterase) that cleaves polynucleotides (nucleic acids) at interior bonds, thus producing poly- or oligonucleotide fragments of varying size. Cf. exonuclease.

restriction e., one of many e.'s isolated from bacteria that hydrolyze (cut) double-stranded DNA chains at specific sequences, thus inactivating a foreign (viral or other) DNA and restricting its activity; standard laboratory devices for making specific cuts in DNA as a first step in deducing sequences. SYN restriction enzyme.

en·do·par·a·site (en-dō-par′ă-sīt). A parasite living within the body of its host.

en·do·pep·ti·dase (en-dō-pep′ti-dās). An enzyme catalyzing the hydrolysis of a peptide chain at points well within the chain, not near termini; *e.g.*, pepsin, trypsin. Cf. exopeptidase.

en·do·per·i·car·di·tis (en′dō-pār′i-kar-dī′tis). Simultaneous inflammation of the endocardium and pericardium. [endo- + G. *peri*, around, + *kardia*, heart, + -itis, inflammation]

en·do·per·i·my·o·car·di·tis (en′dō-pār′i-mī′ō-kar-dī′tis). Simultaneous inflammation of the heart muscle and of the endocardium and pericardium. [endo- + G. *peri*, around, + *mys*, muscle, + *kardia*, heart, + -itis, inflammation]

en·do·per·i·to·ni·tis (en′dō-pār′i-tō-nī′tis). Superficial inflammation of the peritoneum.

en·do·phle·bi·tis (en′dō-fle-bī′tis). Inflammation of the intima of a vein. [endo- + G. *phleps* (*phleb-*), vein, + -itis, inflammation]

en·doph·thal·mi·tis (en-dof-thal-mī′tis). Inflammation of the tissues within the eyeball. [endo- + G. *ophthalmos*, eye, + -itis, inflammation]

en·do·plasm (en′dō-plazm). The inner or medullary part of the cytoplasm, as opposed to the ectoplasm, containing the cell organelles.

en·do·pol·y·ploid (en-dō-pol′ē-ployd). Relating to endopolyploidy.

en·do·pol·y·ploi·dy (en-dō-pol′ē-ploy-dē). The process or state of duplication of the chromosomes without accompanying spindle formation or cytokinesis, resulting in a polyploid nucleus. SYN endomitosis. [endo- + polyploidy]

en·do·re·du·pli·ca·tion (en′dō-rē-dū′pli-kā′shŭn). A form of polyploidy or polysomy by redoubling of chromosomes, giving rise to four-stranded chromosomes at prophase and metaphase.

end or·gan. See under organ.

en·dor·phin·er·gic (en′dōr-fin-er′jik). Relating to nerve cells or fibers that employ an endorphin as their neurotransmitter. [endorphin + G. *ergon*, work]

en·do·sac (en′dō-sak). A sac or bag used in laparoscopic surgery in which tissue is placed to facilitate removal or morcellation.

en·do·sal·pin·gi·tis (en′dō-sal-pin-jī′tis). Inflammation of the lining membrane of the eustachian or the fallopian tube. [endo- + G. *salpinx* (*salping-*), tube, + -itis, inflammation]

en·do·scope (en′dō-skōp). An instrument for the examination of the interior of a tubular or hollow organ. [endo- + G. *skopeō*, to examine]

en·dos·co·pist (en-dos′kŏ-pist). A specialist trained in the use of an endoscope.

en·dos·co·py (en-dos′kŏ-pē). Examination of the interior of a canal or hollow viscus by means of a special instrument, such as an endoscope. [see endoscope]

en·do·skel·e·ton (en-dō-skel′ĕ-tŏn). The internal bony framework of the body; the skeleton in its usual context as distinguished from exoskeleton.

en·do·so·nos·co·py (en-dō-son′ŏ-skŏ-pē). A sonographic study carried out by transducers inserted into the body as miniature probes in the esophagus, urethra, bladder, vagina, or rectum.

en·do·spore (en′dō-spōr). **1.** A body formed within the vegetative cells of some bacteria, particularly those belonging to the genera *Bacillus* and *Clostridium*. **2.** A fungus spore borne within a cell or within the tubular end of a sporophore as in the spherule of *Coccidioides immitis.* [endo- + G. *sporos,* seed]

en·dos·te·al (en-dos′tē-ăl). Relating to the endosteum.

en·dos·te·i·tis, en·dos·ti·tis (en′dos-tē-ī′tis, en′dos-tī′tis). Inflammation of the endosteum or of the medullary cavity of a bone. SYN central osteitis (2), perimyelitis. [endo- + G. *osteon,* bone, + *-itis,* inflammation]

en·dos·te·o·ma (en-dos′tē-ō′mă). A benign neoplasm of bone tissue in the medullary cavity of a bone. SYN endostoma. [endo- + G. *osteon,* bone, + *-ōma,* tumor]

en·dos·te·um (en-dos′tē-ŭm) [NA]. A layer of cells lining the inner surface of bone in the central medullary cavity. SYN medullary membrane. [endo- + G. *osteon,* bone]

en·dos·to·ma (en-dō-stō′mă). SYN endosteoma.

en·do·ten·din·e·um (en′dō-ten-din′ē-ŭm). The fine connective tissue surrounding secondary fascicles of a tendon. [endo- + L. *tendon,* tendon, + *-eus,* adj.; the whole, in its neuter form, used substantively]

en·do·the·li·a (en-dō-thē′lē-ă). Plural of endothelium.

en·do·the·li·al (en-dō-thē′lē-ăl). Relating to the endothelium.

en·do·the·li·oid (en-dō-thē′lē-oyd). Resembling endothelium.

en·do·the·li·o·ma (en′dō-thē-lē-ō′mă). Generic term for a group of neoplasms, particularly benign tumors, derived from the endothelial tissue of blood vessels or lymphatic channels; e.'s may be benign or malignant. [endothelium + *-oma,* tumor]

en·do·the·li·o·sis (en′dō-thē-lē-ō′sis). Proliferation of endothelium.

en·do·the·li·um, pl. **en·do·the·li·a** (en-dō-thē′lē-ŭm, -lē-ă). A layer of flat cells lining especially blood and lymphatic vessels and the heart. [endo- + G. *thēlē,* nipple]

en·do·ther·mic (en-dō-ther′mik). Denoting a chemical reaction during which heat (enthalpy) is absorbed. Cf. exothermic (1). [endo- + G. *thermē,* heat]

en·do·thrix (en′dō-thriks). Fungal spores (conidia) invading the interior of a hair shaft; there is no conspicuous external sheath of spores, as there is with ectothrix. [endo- + G. *thrix,* hair]

en·do·tox·e·mia (en′dō-tok-sē′mē-ă). Presence in the blood of endotoxins, which, if derived from Gram-negative rod-shaped bacteria, may cause a generalized Shwartzman phenomenon with shock.

en·do·tox·ic (en-dō-tok′sik). Denoting an endotoxin.

en·do·tox·i·co·sis (en′dō-tok-si-kō′sis). Poisoning by an endotoxin.

en·do·tox·in (en-dō-tok′sin). **1.** A bacterial toxin not freely liberated into the surrounding medium, in contrast to exotoxin. **2.** The complex phospholipid-polysaccharide macromolecules which form an integral part of the cell wall of strains of Gram-negative bacteria. The toxins may cause a state of shock accompanied by severe diarrhea, and, in smaller doses, fever and leukopenia followed by leukocytosis. SYN intracellular toxin.

en·do·tra·che·al (en′dō-trā′kē-ăl). Within the trachea.

en·do·tra·che·li·tis (en′dō-trak-el-ī′tis). SYN endocervicitis.

en·do·vas·cu·li·tis (en′dō-vas′kyū-lī′tis). SYN endangiitis.

   hemorrhagic e., endothelial and medial hyperplasia of placental blood vessels with thrombosis, fragmentation, and diapedesis of red blood cells resulting in stillbirth or fetal developmental disorders.

end-piece. The terminal part of the tail of a spermatozoon consisting of the axoneme and the flagellar membrane.

end·plate, end-plate (end′plāt). The ending of a motor nerve fiber in relation to a skeletal muscle fiber.

   motor e., the large and complex end-formation by which the axon of a motor neuron establishes synaptic contact with a striated muscle fiber (cell).

end-tid·al (end-tī′dăl). At the end of a normal expiration.

en·dur·ance. Sustaining of cardiac, pulmonary, and musculoskeletal exertion over time.

   muscular e., ability of muscles to exert tension over an extended period.

△**-ene.** Suffix applied to a chemical name indicating the presence of a carbon-carbon double bond; *e.g.,* propene (unsaturated propane, CH_3—CH= CH_2). [G. *enos,* origin]

en·e·ma (en′ĕ-mă). A rectal injection to clear out the bowel or to administer drugs or food. [G.]

   air contrast e., a double contrast e. in which air is introduced after coating of the colon with a dense barium suspension for radiographic study. SYN double contrast e.

   analeptic e., an e. of a pint of lukewarm water with one-half teaspoonful of table salt.

□**barium e. (BE),** a type of contrast enema; administration of barium, a radiopaque medium, for radiographic and fluoroscopic study of the lower intestinal tract.

   double contrast e., SYN air contrast e.

   high e., an e. instilled high up into the colon. SYN enteroclysis (1).

en·er·gy (en′er-jē). The exertion of power; the capacity to do work, taking the forms of kinetic e., potential e., chemical e., electrical e., etc. [G. *energeia,* fr. *en,* in, + *ergon,* work]

   chemical e., e. liberated or absorbed by a chemical reaction, *e.g.,* oxidation of carbon, or absorbed in the formation of a chemical compound.

   free e. (F), a thermodynamic function symbolized as F, or G (Gibbs free e.), $= H - TS$, where H is the enthalpy of a system, T the absolute temperature, and S the entropy; chemical reac-

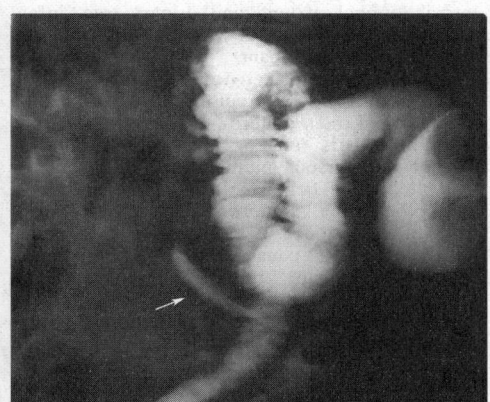

barium enema: radiograph of colon showing ruptured diverticulum (arrow)

tions proceed spontaneously in the direction that involves a net decrease in the free e. of the system (*i.e.*, $\Delta G < 0$).

Helmholtz e. (A), e. equivalent to the internal energy minus the entropy contribution (TS).

internal e. (U), e. of a system measured by the heat absorbed from the system's surroundings and the amount of work done on the system by its surroundings.

kinetic e., the e. of motion.

potential e., the e., existing in a body by virtue of its position or state of existence, which is not being exerted at the time.

en·er·va·tion (en-er-vā′shŭn). Failure of nerve force; weakening. [L. *enervo,* pp. *-atus,* to enervate, fr. *e-* priv. + *nervus,* nerve]

ENG electronystagmography.

en·gage·ment (en-gāj′ment). OBSTETRICS The mechanism by which the biparietal diameter of the fetal head enters the plane of the inlet.

en·gorged (en-gōrjd′). Absolutely filled; distended with fluid. SEE ALSO congested, hyperemic. [O. Fr. fr. Mediev. L. *gorgia,* throat, narrow passage, fr. L. *gurges,* a whirlpool]

en·gram (en′gram). In the mnemic hypothesis, a physical habit or memory trace made on the protoplasm of an organism by the repetition of stimuli. [G. *en,* in, + *gramma,* mark]

en·graph·ia (en-graf′ē-ă). The formation of engrams.

en·hanc·ers. Genetic elements important in the function of a specific promoter. [M.E. *enhauncen,* raise, increase, fr. O. Fr. *enhaucier,* fr. L.L. *inalto,* fr. *altus,* high, + *-er,* agent suffix]

en·keph·a·lin·er·gic (en-kef′ă-lin-er′jik). Relating to nerve cells or fibers that employ an enkephalin as their neurotransmitter. [enkephalin + G. *ergon,* work]

en·large·ment (en-larj′ment). **1.** An increase in size; an anatomical swelling, enlargement, or prominence. **2.** An intumescence or swelling. SYN intumescence (1).

-enoic. Suffix indicating an unsaturated acid. [-ene + -ic]

enol (ē′nol). A compound possessing a hydroxyl group (alcohol) attached to a doubly bonded (ethylenic) carbon atom (–CH=CH(OH)–). [-ene + -ol]

eno·lase (ē′nol-ās). An enzyme catalyzing the reversible dehydration of 2-phospho-D-glycerate to phospho*enol*pyruvate and water.

en·oph·thal·mos (en′of-thal′mos). Recession of the eyeball within the orbit. [G. *en,* in, + *ophthalmos,* eye]

en·os·to·sis (en-os-tō′sis). A mass of proliferating bone tissue within a bone. [G. *en,* in, + *osteon,* bone, + *-osis,* condition]

en·o·yl (ēn′ō-il). The acyl radical of an unsaturated aliphatic acid. [-ene + -oyl]

en·si·form (en′si-fōrm). SYN xiphoid. [L. *ensis,* sword, + *forma,* appearance]

ENT ears, nose, and throat. SEE otorhinolaryngology.

△**ent-.** SEE ento-.

en·tad. Toward the interior. [G. *entos,* within, + L. *ad,* to]

en·tal (en′tăl). Relating to the interior; inside. [G. *entos,* within]

ent·am·e·bi·a·sis (ent-ă-mē-bī′ă-sis). Infection with *Entamoeba histolytica.* SEE amebiasis, amebic *dysentery.*

ℹ*Ent·a·moe·ba* (ent-ă-mē′bă). A genus of ameba parasitic in the cecum and large bowel; with the exception of *E. histolytica,* members of the genus appear to be relatively harmless. [G. *entos,* within + *amoibē,* change]

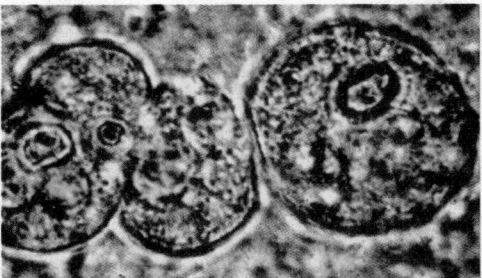

Entamoeba histolytica: trophozoites in stool

△**enter-.** SEE entero-.

en·ter·al (en′ter-ăl). Within, or by way of, the intestine or gastrointestinal tract, especially as distinguished from parenteral. A term used to describe tube feedings. [G. *enteron,* intestine]

en·ter·al·gia (en-ter-al′jē-ă). Enterdynia; severe abdominal pain accompanying spasm of the bowel. SYN enterodynia. [entero- + G. *algos,* pain]

en·ter·ec·ta·sis (en-ter-ek′tă-sis). Dilation of the bowel. [entero- + G. *ektasis,* a stretching]

en·ter·ec·to·my (en-ter-ek′tō-mē). Resection of a segment of the intestine. [entero- + G. *ektomē,* excision]

en·ter·el·co·sis (en-ter-el-kō′sis). Ulceration of the bowel. [entero- + G. *helkos,* ulcer]

en·ter·ic (en-ter′ik). Relating to the intestine. [G. *enterikos,* from *entera,* bowels]

en·ter·i·tis (en-ter-ī′tis). Inflammation of the intestine, especially of the small intestine. [entero- + G. -itis, inflammation]

granulomatous e., SYN regional e.

mucomembranous e., a disorder of the intestinal mucous membrane characterized by constipation or diarrhea (sometimes alternating), colic, and the passage of pseudomembranous shreds or incomplete casts of the intestine. SYN mucoenteritis (2).

e. necrot′icans, e. with necrosis of the bowel wall caused by *Clostridium welchii*.

pseudomembranous e., SYN pseudomembranous *enterocolitis*.

regional e., a chronic e., of unknown cause, involving the terminal ileum and less frequently other parts of the gastrointestinal tract; characterized by patchy deep ulcers that may cause fistulas, and narrowing and thickening of the bowel by fibrosis and lymphocytic infiltration, with noncaseating tuberculoid granulomas that also may be found in regional lymph nodes; symptoms include fever, diarrhea, cramping abdominal pain, and weight loss. SYN Crohn's disease, distal ileitis, regional ileitis, terminal ileitis, granulomatous e.

tuberculous e., enteric tuberculosis that may occur in the absence of obvious pulmonary t.; may be caused by bovine tuberculosis contracted through drinking of unpasteurized milk or swallowing of tubercle bacilli expectorated from cavitary lesions in the lung.

△**entero-, enter-.** The intestines. [G. *enteron*, intestine]

en·ter·o·a·nas·to·mo·sis (en′ter-ō-an-as-tō-mō′sis). SYN enteroenterostomy.

en·ter·o·bi·a·sis (en′ter-ō-bī′ă-sis). Infection with *Enterobius vermicularis*, the human pinworm.

En·te·ro·bi·us (en-ter-ō′bī-ŭs). A genus of nematode worms which includes the pinworms (*E. vermicularis*). [entero- + G. *bios*, life]

en·ter·o·cele (en′ter-o-sēl). **1.** A hernial protrusion through a defect in the rectovaginal or vesicovaginal pouch. [entero- + G. *kēlē*, hernia] **2.** SYN abdominal *cavity*. [entero- + G. *koilia*, a hollow] **3.** An intestinal hernia. [see 1]

en·ter·o·cen·te·sis (en′ter-ō-sen-tē′sis). Puncture of the intestine with a hollow needle (trocar and cannula) to withdraw substances. [entero- + G. *kentēsis*, puncture]

en·ter·o·clei·sis (en-ter-ō-klī′sis). Occlusion of the lumen of the alimentary canal. [entero- + G. *kleisis*, a closing]

en·ter·oc·ly·sis (en-ter-ok′li-sis). **1.** SYN high *enema*. **2.** In radiography of the small intestine, filling by introduction of contrast medium through a catheter advanced into the duodenum or jejunum from above. [entero- + G. *klysis*, a washing out]

radiological e., method of imaging the duodenum and small intestine by intubation of the duodenum and instillation of dilute barium; also known as small bowel enema.

En·ter·o·coc·cus. Genus of facultatively anaerobic, generally nonmotile, non–spore-forming, Gram-positive bacteria. Found in the intestinal tract of humans and animals, enterococci cause intraabdominal, wound and urinary tract infections. Type species is *E. faecalis*. *E. faecium* is also clinically significant.

en·ter·o·coc·cus, pl. **en·ter·o·coc·ci** (en′ter-ō-kok′ŭs, -kok′sī). A streptococcus that inhabits the intestinal tract. [entero- + G. *kokkos*, a berry]

en·ter·o·co·li·tis (en′ter-ō-kō-lī′tis). Inflammation of the mucous membrane of a greater or lesser extent of both small and large intestines. SYN coloenteritis. [entero- + G. *kolon*, colon, + -*itis*, inflammation]

antibiotic e., e. caused by oral administration of broad spectrum antibiotics, resulting from overgrowth of antibiotic-resistant staphylococci or yeasts and fungi, when the normal fecal Gram-negative organisms are suppressed, resulting in diarrhea or pseudomembranous disease.

necrotizing e., extensive ulceration and necrosis of the ileum and colon in premature infants.

pseudomembranous e., e. with the formation and passage of pseudomembranous material, due to infection by *Clostridium difficile;* it is commonly a sequel to prolonged antibiotic therapy. SYN pseudomembranous colitis, pseudomembranous enteritis.

en·ter·o·co·los·to·my (en′ter-ō-kō-los′tō-mē). Establishment of an artificial opening between the small intestine and the colon. [entero- + G. *kōlon*, colon, + *stoma*, mouth]

en·ter·o·cyst (en′ter-ō-sist). A cyst of the wall of the intestine. SYN enterocystoma. [entero- + G. *kystis*, bladder]

en·ter·o·cys·to·cele (en′ter-ō-sis′tō-sēl). A hernia of both intestine and bladder wall. [entero- + G. *kystis*, bladder, + *kēlē*, hernia]

en·ter·o·cys·to·ma (en′ter-ō-sis-tō′mă). SYN enterocyst.

en·ter·o·dyn·ia (en′ter-ō-din′ē-ă). SYN enteralgia. [entero- + G. *odynē*, pain]

en·ter·o·en·ter·os·to·my (en′ter-ō-en-ter-os′tō-mē). Establishment of a new communication between two segments of intestine. SYN enteroanastomosis, intestinal anastomosis.

en·ter·o·gas·tri·tis (en′ter-ō-gas-trī′tis). SYN gastroenteritis. [entero- + G. *gastēr*, belly, + -*itis*, inflammation]

en·ter·o·gas·trone (en′ter-ō-gas′trōn). A hormone, obtained from intestinal mucosa, that inhibits gastric secretion and motility; secretion of e. is stimulated by exposure of duodenal mucosa to dietary lipids.

en·ter·og·e·nous (en-ter-oj′ĕ-nŭs). Of intestinal origin. [entero- + G. -*gen*, producing]

en·ter·o·hep·a·ti·tis (en′ter-ō-hep-ă-tī′tis). Inflammation of both the intestine and the liver. [entero- + G. *hēpar* (*hēpat-*), liver, + -*itis*, inflammation]

en·ter·o·hep·a·to·cele (en′ter-ō-hep′ă-tō-sēl). Congenital umbilical hernia containing intestine and liver. SEE omphalocele. [entero- + G. *hēpar* (*hēpat-*), liver, + *kēlē*, hernia]

en·ter·o·ki·ne·sis (en′ter-ō-ki-nē′sis). Muscular contraction of the alimentary canal. SEE ALSO peristalsis. [entero- + G. *kinēsis*, movement]

en·ter·o·ki·net·ic (en′ter-ō-ki-net′ik). Relating to, or producing, enterokinesis.

en·ter·o·lith (en′ter-ō-lith). An intestinal calculus formed of layers of soaps and earthy phosphates surrounding a nucleus of some hard body such as a swallowed fruit stone or other indigestible substance. [entero- + G. *lithos*, stone]

en•ter•o•li•thi•a•sis (en′ter-ō-li-thī′ă-sis). Presence of calculi in the intestine.

en•ter•ol•o•gy (en-ter-ol′ō-jē). The branch of medical science concerned especially with the intestinal tract. [entero- + G. *logos*, study]

en•ter•ol•y•sis (en-ter-ol′i-sis). Division of intestinal adhesions. [entero- + G. *lysis*, dissolution]

en•ter•o•meg•a•ly, en•ter•o•me•ga•lia (en′ter-ō-meg′ă-lē,; -ō-me-gā′lē-ă). SYN megaloenteron. [entero- + G. *megas*, great]

en•ter•o•my•co•sis (en′ter-ō-mī-kō′sis). An intestinal disease of fungal origin. [entero- + G. *mykēs*, fungus, + *-osis*, condition]

en•ter•o•pa•re•sis (en′ter-ō-pă-rē′sis, -par′i-sis). Rarely used term for a state of diminished or absent peristalsis with flaccidity of the muscles of the intestinal walls. [entero- + G. *paresis*, slackening, relaxation]

en•ter•o•path•o•gen (en′ter-ō-path′ō-jen). An organism capable of producing disease in the intestinal tract.

en•ter•o•path•o•gen•ic (en′ter-ō-path-ō-jen′ik). Capable of producing disease in the intestinal tract.

en•ter•op•a•thy (en-ter-op′ă-thē). An intestinal disease. [entero- + G. *pathos*, suffering]
  gluten e., SYN celiac *disease.*
  protein-losing e., increased fecal loss of serum protein, especially albumin, causing hypoproteinemia.

en•ter•o•pep•ti•dase (en′ter-ō-pep′ti-dās). An intestinal proteolytic glycoenzyme from the duodenal mucosa that converts trypsinogen into trypsin (removes a hexapeptide from trypsinogen).

en•ter•o•pex•y (en′ter-ō-pek-sē). Fixation of a segment of the intestine to the abdominal wall. [entero- + G. *pēxis*, fixation]

en•ter•op•to•sis, en•ter•op•to•sia (en′ter-ō-tō′sis, -tō′sē-ă). Abnormal descent of the intestines in the abdominal cavity, usually associated with falling of the other viscera. [entero- + G. *ptōsis*, a falling]

en•ter•op•tot•ic (en′ter-ō-tot′ik). Relating to or suffering from enteroptosis.

en•ter•or•rha•gia (en-ter-ō-rā′jē-ă). Bleeding within the intestinal tract. [entero- + G. *rhēgnymi*, to burst forth]

en•ter•or•rha•phy (en-ter-ōr′ă-fē). Suture of the intestine. [entero- + G. *rhaphē*, suture]

en•ter•o•sep•sis (en′ter-ō-sep′sis). Sepsis occurring in or derived from the alimentary canal. [entero- + G. *sēpsis*, putrefaction]

en•ter•o•spasm (en′ter-ō-spazm). Increased, irregular, and painful peristalsis. [entero- + G. *spasmos*, spasm]

en•ter•o•sta•sis (en-ter-os′tă-sis). Intestinal stasis; a retardation or arrest of the passage of the intestinal contents. [entero- + G. *stasis*, a standing]

en•ter•o•ste•no•sis (en′ter-ō-sten-ō′sis). Narrowing of the lumen of the intestine. [entero- + G. *stenōsis*, narrowing]

en•ter•os•to•my (en-ter-os′tō-mē). An artificial anus or fistula into the intestine through the abdominal wall. [entero- + G. *stoma*, mouth]

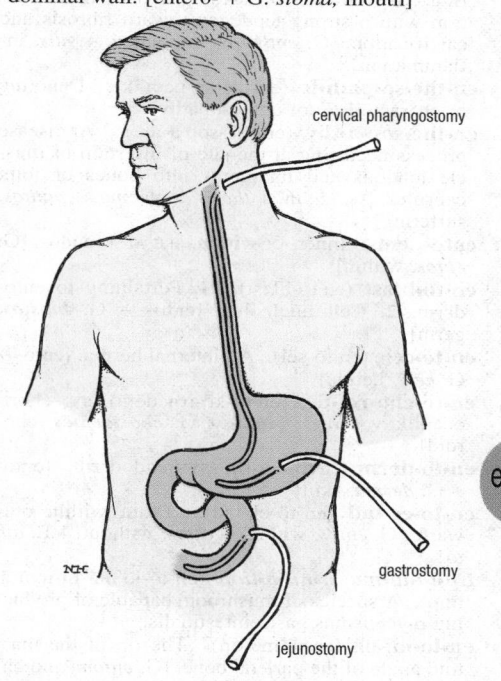

cervical pharyngostomy

gastrostomy

jejunostomy

enterostomy

en•ter•ot•o•my (en-ter-ot′ō-mē). Incision into the intestine.

en•ter•o•tox•i•gen•ic (en′ter-ō-tok-si-jen′ik). Denoting an organism containing or producing a toxin specific for cells of the intestinal mucosa.

en•ter•o•tox•in (en′ter-ō-tok′sin). A cytotoxin specific for the cells of the intestinal mucosa.

en•ter•o•tro•pic (en′ter-ō-trop′ik). Attracted by or affecting the intestine. [entero- + G. *tropikos*, turning]

En•te•ro•vi•rus (en′ter-ō-vī′rŭs). A large and diverse group of viruses that includes poliovirus types 1 to 3, Coxsackievirus A and B, echoviruses, and the enteroviruses identified since 1969 and assigned type numbers.

en•ter•o•zo•ic (en′ter-ō-zō′ik). Relating to an enterozoon.

en•ter•o•zo•on (en′ter-ō-zō′on). An animal parasite in the intestine. [entero- + G. *zōon*, animal]

ent•ge•gen (E) (ent′ge-gen). Term used when the two higher ranking groups, attached to different carbon atoms in a carbon-carbon double bond, are on opposite sides of the double bond (hence, analogous to trans-). [Ger. opposite]

en•thal•py (H) (en′thal-pē). Heat content, symbolized as H; a thermodynamic function, defined as $E + PV$, where E is the internal energy of a system, P the pressure, and V the volume; the heat of a reaction, measured at constant pressure, is ΔH. SYN heat (3). [G. *enthalpō*, to warm in]

en•the•si•tis (en-thĕ-sī′tis). Traumatic disease occurring at the insertion of muscles where recurring concentration of stress provokes inflammation with a strong tendency toward fibrosis and calcification. [G. *enthetos*, implanted, + *-itis*, inflammation]

en·the·so·path·ic (en-thē-sō-path′ik). Denoting or characteristic of enthesopathy.

en·the·sop·a·thy (en-thē-sop′ă-thē). A disease process occurring at the site of insertion of muscle tendons and ligaments into bones or joint capsules. [G. *en*, in, + *thesis*, a placing, + *pathos*, suffering]

△**ento-, ent-**. Inner, or within. SEE ALSO endo-. [G. *entos*, within]

en·to·blast (en′tō-blast). **1.** Pertaining to entoderm. **2.** Cell nucleolus. [ento- + G. *blastos*, germ]

en·to·cele (en′tō-sēl). An internal hernia. [ento- + G. *kēlē*, hernia]

en·to·cho·roi·dea (en′tō-kō-roy′dē-ă). SYN choriocapillary *layer*. [ento- + G. *chorioeidēs*, choroid]

en·to·derm (en′tō-derm). SYN endoderm. [ento- + G. *derma*, skin]

en·to·ec·tad (en-tō-ek′tad). From within outward. [G. *entos*, within, + *ektos*, without, + L. *ad*, to]

En·to·lo·ma si·nu·a·tum (en-tō-lō′mă sī-nyū-ā′tum). A species of mushroom capable of producing mycetismus gastrointestinalis.

en·to·mi·on (en-tō′mē-on). The tip of the mastoid angle of the parietal bone. [G. *entomē*, notch]

en·to·mol·o·gy (en-tō-mol′ō-jē). The science concerned with the study of insects. [G. *entomon*, insect, + *logos*, study]

en·to·moph·tho·ra·my·co·sis (en-tō-mof′thō-ră-mī-kō′sis). A disease caused by fungi of the genera *Basidiobolus* or *Conidiobolus;* tissues are invaded by broad nonseptate hyphae that become surrounded by eosinophilic material. A form of zygomycosis. SEE zygomycosis. [Entomophthorales (order name) + G. *mykēs*, fungus + -osis, condition]

en·top·ic (ent-op′ik). Placed within; occurring or situated in the normal place; opposed to ectopic. [G. *en*, within, + *topos*, place]

ent·op·tic (en-top′tik). Within the eyeball. Often used to describe visual phenomena generated by mechanical or electrical stimulations of the retina. [ento- + G. *optikos*, relating to vision]

en·to·ret·i·na (en-tō-ret′i-nă). The layers of the retina from the outer plexiform to the nerve fiber layer inclusive.

en·to·zo·al (en-tō-zō′ăl). Relating to entozoa.

en·to·zo·on, pl. **en·to·zoa** (en-tō-zō′on, -ă). An animal parasite whose habitat is any of the internal organs or tissues. [ento- + G. *zōon*, animal]

en·tro·pi·on, en·tro·pi·um (en-trō′pē-on, -pē-ŭm). **1.** Inversion or turning inward of a part. **2.** The infolding of the margin of an eyelid. [G. *en*, in, + *tropē*, a turning]

en·tro·py (en′trō-pē). That fraction of heat (energy) content not available for the performance of work, usually because (in a chemical reaction) it has been used to increase the random motion of the atoms or molecules in the system; thus, e. is a measure of randomness or disorder. [G. *entropia*, a turning towards]

en·ty·py (en′ti-pē). A type of gastrulation seen in some early mammalian embryos in which the endoderm covers the embryonic and amniotic ectoderm; part of the preplacental trophoblast may also be covered. [G. *entypē*, pattern]

enu·cle·ate (ē-nū′klē-āt). To remove entirely; to shell like a nut, as in the removal of an eye from its capsule or a tumor from its enveloping capsule.

enu·cle·a·tion (ē-nū-klē-ā′shŭn). **1.** Removal of an entire structure (such as an eyeball or tumor), without rupture, as one shells the kernel of a nut. **2.** Removal or destruction of the nucleus of a cell. [L. *enucleo*, to remove the kernel, fr. *e*, out, + *nucleus*, nut, kernel]

en·u·re·sis (en-yū-rē′sis). Urinary incontinence; may be intentional or involuntary but not due to a physical disorder. [G. *en-oureō*, to urinate in]

nocturnal e., urinary incontinence during sleep. SYN bed-wetting.

en·ve·lope (en′vĕ-lōp). In anatomy, a structure that encloses or covers.

corneocyte e., an electron-dense layer of highly cross-linked protein on the cytoplasmic surface of the cell membrane of epidermal corneocytes.

nuclear e., the double membrane at the boundary of the nucleoplasm; it has regularly spaced pores covered by a disklike nuclear pore complex and a space or cisterna about 150 Å wide between the two layers; the outer membrane is continuous at intervals with the endoplasmic reticulum. SYN nuclear membrane.

viral e., the outer structure that encloses the nucleocapsids of some viruses; may contain host material.

en·ven·om·a·tion (en-ven-ō-mā′shŭn). The act of injecting a poisonous material (venom) by sting, spine, bite, or other venom apparatus.

en·vi·ron·ment (en-vī′ron-ment). The milieu; the aggregate of all of the external conditions and influences affecting the life and development of an organism. [Fr. *environ*, around]

en·zo·ot·ic (en-zō-ot′ik). Denoting a temporal pattern of disease occurrence in an animal population in which the disease occurs with predictable regularity with only relatively minor fluctuations in its frequency over time. SEE epizootic, sporadic. Cf. epizootic, sporadic. [G. *en*, in, + *zōon*, animal]

en·zy·got·ic (en-zī-got′ik). Derived from a single fertilized ovum; denoting twins so derived. [G. *eis* (*en*), one, + *zygote*]

en·zy·mat·ic (en-zī-mat′ik). Relating to an enzyme.

en·zyme (en′zīm). A protein that acts as a catalyst to induce chemical changes in other substances, itself remaining apparently unchanged by the process. E.'s, with the exception of those discovered long ago (*e.g.*, pepsin, emulsin), are generally named by adding -ase to the name of the substrate on which the e. acts (*e.g.*, glucosidase), the substance activated (*e.g.*, hydrogenase), and/or the type of reaction (*e.g.*, oxidoreductase, transferase, hydrolase, lyase, isomerase, ligase or synthetase. For individual enzymes not listed below, see the specific name. [G. + L. *en*, in, + *zymē*, leaven]

acetyl-activating e., SYN *acetyl-CoA* ligase.

1,4-α-D-glucan branching e., amylo-(1,4→1,6)-transglucosylase or transglucosidase; an enzyme in muscle and in plants (Q enzyme) that cleaves α-1,4 linkages in glycogen or starch, transferring the fragments into α-1,6 linkages, creating branches in the polysaccharide molecules; in plants, it converts amylose to amylopectin; this enzyme is deficient in individuals with glycogen storage disease type IV.

angiotensin-converting e., a hydrolase responsible for the conversion of angiotensin I to the vasoactive angiotensin II by removal of a dipeptide (histidylleucine) from angiotensin I. Drugs that inhibit ACE are used to treat hypertension and congestive heart failure.

autolytic e., an e. capable of causing lysis of the cell forming it.

deamidizing e.'s, SYN amidohydrolases.

deaminating e.'s, SYN deaminases.

debranching e.'s, e.'s that bring about destruction of branches in glycogen; a mixture of transferases and hydrolases.

extracellular e., an e. performing its functions outside a cell; *e.g.*, the various digestive e.'s. SYN exoenzyme.

induced e., inducible e., an e. that can be detected in a growing culture of a microorganism, after the addition of a particular substance (inducer) to the culture medium, but not prior to the addition.

repressible e., an e. that is produced continuously unless production is repressed by excess of an inhibitor (corepressor). SEE ALSO inactive *repressor*.

respiratory e., a tissue e. that is part of an oxidation-reduction system accomplishing the conversion of substrates to CO_2 and H_2O and the transfer of the electrons removed to O_2.

restriction e., SYN restriction *endonuclease*.

en·zy·mol·o·gy (en-zī-mol′ō-jē). The branch of chemistry concerned with the properties and actions of enzymes. [enzyme + G. *logos*, study]

en·zy·mol·y·sis (en-zī-mol′i-sis). **1.** The splitting or cleavage of a substance into smaller parts by means of enzymatic action. **2.** Lysis by the action of an enzyme. [enzyme + G. *lysis*, dissolution]

en·zy·mop·a·thy (en-zī-mop′ă-thē). Any disturbance of enzyme function, including genetic deficiency or defect in specific enzymes. [enzyme + G. *pathos*, disease]

EOG electro-oculography; electro-olfactogram.

eo·sin (ē′ō-sin). A fluorescent acid dye used for cytoplasmic stains and counterstains in histology and in Romanovsky-type blood stains. [G. *ēōs*, dawn]

e. B, the disodium salt of 4′,5′-dibromo-2′,7′-dinitrofluorescein. SYN e. I bluish. [C.I. 45400]

e. I bluish, SYN e. B.

e. y, e. Ys, the disodium salt of 2′,4′,5′,7′-tetrabromofluorescein. SYN e. yellowish. [C.I. 45380]

e. yellowish, SYN e. y.

eo·sin·o·pe·nia (ē′ō-sin-ō-pē′nē-ă). An abnormally small number of eosinophils in the peripheral bloodstream. [eosino(phil) + G. *penia*, poverty]

eo·sin·o·phil, eo·sin·o·phile (ē-ō-sin′ō-fil, -fīl). SYN eosinophilic *leukocyte*. [eosin + G. *philos*, fond]

eo·sin·o·phil·ia (ē′ō-sin-ō-fil′ē-ă). SYN eosinophilic *leukocytosis*.

tropical e., e. associated with cough and asthma, caused by occult filarial infection without evidence of microfilaremia, occurring most frequently in India and Southeast Asia.

eo·sin·o·phil·ic (ē-ō-sin-ō-fil′ik). Staining readily with eosin dyes; denoting such cell or tissue elements.

eo·sin·o·phil·u·ria (ē-ō-sin′ō-fil-yū′rē-ă). Presence of eosinophils in the urine.

EP endogenous *pyrogens*.

ep·ax·i·al (ep-ak′sē-ăl). Above or behind any axis, such as the spinal axis or the axis of a limb. [G. *epi*, upon, + L. *axis*, axis]

EPEC. enteropathogenic *Escherichia coli*.

ep·en·dy·ma (ep-en′di-mă) [NA]. The cellular membrane lining the central canal of the spinal cord and the brain ventricles. [G. *ependyma*, an upper garment]

ep·en·dy·mal (ep-en′di-măl). Relating to the ependyma.

ep·en·dy·mi·tis (ep-en-di-mī′tis). Inflammation of the ependyma.

ep·en·dy·mo·blast (ep-en′di-mō-blast). An embryonic ependymal cell. [ependyma + G. *blastos*, germ]

ep·en·dy·mo·cyte (ep-en′di-mō-sīt). An ependymal cell. [ependyma + G. *kytos*, cell]

ep·en·dy·mo·ma (ep-en-di-mō′mă). A glioma derived from relatively undifferentiated ependymal cells; e.'s may originate from the lining of any of the ventricles or, more commonly, from the central canal of the spinal cord.

myxopapillary e., a slow-growing e. of the filum terminale, occurring most often in young adults, consisting of cuboidal cells in papillary arrangement around a mucinous vascular core.

eph·apse (ef′aps). A place where two or more nerve cell processes (axons, dendrites) touch without forming a typical synaptic contact; some form of neural transmission may occur at such nonsynaptic contact sites. [G. *ephapsis*, contact]

eph·ap·tic (e-fap′tik). Relating to an ephapse.

ephe·bic (ĕ-fē′bik). Rarely used term relating to the period of puberty or to a youth. [G. *ephēbikos*, relating to youth, fr. *hēbē*, youth]

ephe·lis, pl. **ephe·li·des** (ef-ē′lis, ef-ē′li-dēz). SYN freckle. [G.]

epi-. Upon, following, or subsequent to. [G.]

ep·i·an·dros·ter·one (ep′i-an-dros′ter-ōn). Inactive isomer of androsterone; found in urine and in testicular and ovarian tissue.

ep·i·blast (ep′i-blast). Gives rise to ectoderm and mesoderm. The mesoderm then displaces the hypoblast cells and forms the entodermal cell layer on its inner surface. [epi- + G. *blastos*, germ]

ep·i·blas·tic (ep-i-blas′tik). Relating to epiblast.

ep·i·bleph·a·ron (ep′i-blef′ă-ron). A congenital horizontal skin fold near the margin of the eyelid, caused by abnormal insertion of muscle fibers. In the upper lid, it simulates blepharochalasis; in the lower lid, it causes a turning inward of the lashes. [epi- + G. *blepharon*, eyelid]

ep·ib·o·ly, epib·o·le (ē-pib'ō-lē). **1.** A process involved in gastrulation of telolecithal eggs in which, as a result of differential growth, some of the cells of the protoderm move over the surface toward the lips of the blastopore. **2.** Growth of epithelium in an organ culture to surround the underlying mesenchymal tissue. [G. *epibolē*, a throwing or laying on]

ep·i·bul·bar (ep-i-bŭl'bar). Upon a bulb of any kind; specifically, upon the eyeball.

ep·i·car·dia (ep-i-kar'dē-ă). The portion of the esophagus from where it passes through the diaphragm to the stomach. [epi- + G. *kardia*, heart]

ep·i·car·di·al (ep-i-kar'dē-ăl). **1.** Relating to the epicardia. **2.** Relating to the epicardium.

ep·i·con·dy·lal·gia (ep'i-kon-di-lal'jē-ă). Pain in an epicondyle of the humerus or in the tendons or muscles originating therefrom. [epicondyle + G. *algos*, pain]

ep·i·con·dyle (ep-i-kon'dīl). A projection from a long bone near the articular extremity above or upon the condyle. SYN epicondylus [NA]. [epi- + G. *kondylos*, a knuckle]

ep·i·con·dy·li·tis (ep'i-kon-di-lī'tis). Infection or inflammation of an epicondyle.

lateral humeral e., SYN tennis *elbow.*
medial e., SYN Little League *elbow.*

ep·i·con·dy·lus, pl. **ep·i·con·dy·li** (ep-i-kon'di-lŭs, -lī) [NA]. SYN epicondyle. [L.]

ep·i·cra·ni·um (ep-i-krā'nē-ŭm). The muscle, aponeurosis, and skin covering the cranium. [epi- + G. *kranion*, skull]

ep·i·cri·sis (ep-i-krī'sis). A secondary crisis; a crisis terminating a recrudescence of morbid symptoms following a primary crisis.

ep·i·crit·ic (ep-i-krit'ik). That aspect of somatic sensation which permits the discrimination and the topographical localization of the finer degrees of touch and temperature stimuli. Cf. protopathic. [G. *epikritikos*, adjudicatory, fr. *epi*, on, + *krinō*, to separate, judge]

ep·i·cys·ti·tis (ep'i-sis-tī'tis). Inflammation of the cellular tissue around the bladder. [epi- + G. *kystis*, bladder, + *-itis*, inflammation]

ep·i·dem·ic (ep-i-dem'ik). The occurrence in a community or region of cases of an illness, specific health-related behavior, or other health-related events clearly in excess of normal expectancy. Cf. endemic, sporadic. [epi- + G. *dēmos*, the people]

behavioral e., an e. originating in behavioral patterns (in contrast to invading microorganisms); examples include medieval dancing mania, episodes of crowd panic.

point e., an e. where a pronounced clustering of cases of disease occurs within a very short period of time (within a few days or even hours) due to exposure of persons or animals to a common source of infection such as food or water.

ep·i·dem·ic·i·ty (ep'i-dem-is'i-tē). The state of prevailing disease in epidemic form.

ep·i·de·mi·ol·o·gist (ep-i-dē-mē-ol'ō-jist). An investigator who studies the occurrence of disease or other health-related conditions, states, or events in specified populations; one who prac-

tices epidemiology; the control of disease usually is also considered a task of the epidemiologist.

ep·i·de·mi·ol·o·gy (ep-i-dē-mē-ol'ō-jē). The study of the distribution and determinants of health-related states or events in specified populations, and the application of this study to control of health problems. [G. *epidēmios*, epidemic, + *logos*, study]

ep·i·der·mal, ep·i·der·mat·ic (ep-i-der'măl, -der-mat'ik). Relating to the epidermis. SYN epidermic.

ep·i·der·mal·i·za·tion (ep-i-der'mal-i-zā'shŭn). SYN squamous *metaplasia.*

ep·i·der·mic (ep-i-der'mik). SYN epidermal.

ep·i·der·mis, pl. **ep·i·derm·i·des** (ep-i-derm'is, -derm'i-dēz) [NA]. **1.** The superficial epithelial portion of the skin (cutis). The e. of the palms and soles has the following strata: stratum corneum (horny layer), stratum lucidum (clear layer), stratum granulosum (granular layer), stratum spinosum (prickle cell layer), and stratum basale (basal cell layer); in other parts of the body, the stratum lucidum may be absent. **2.** BOTANY The outermost layer of cells in leaves and the young parts of plants. SYN cuticle (3). [G. *epidermis*, the outer skin, fr. *epi*, on, + *derma*, skin]

ep·i·der·mi·tis (ep-i-der-mī'tis). Inflammation of the epidermis or superficial layers of the skin.

ep·i·der·mo·dys·pla·sia (ep-i-der'mō-dis-plā'zē-ă). Faulty growth or development of the epidermis. [epidermis + G. *dys-*, bad, + *plasis*, a molding]

ep·i·der·moid (ep-i-der'moyd). **1.** Resembling epidermis. **2.** A cholesteatoma or other cystic tumor arising from aberrant epidermal cells. [epidermis + G. *eidos*, appearance]

ep·i·der·mol·y·sis (ep'i-der-mol'i-sis). A condition in which the epidermis is loosely attached to the corium, readily exfoliating or forming blisters. [epidermis + G. *lysis*, loosening]

e. bullo'sa [MIM*131800], a group of inherited chronic noninflammatory skin diseases in which large bullae and erosions result from slight mechanical trauma; a form limited to the hands and feet is also called Weber-Cockayne syndrome.

Ep·i·der·mo·phy·ton (ep'i-der-mof'i-ton, -der'mō-fī'ton). A genus of fungi whose macroconidia are clavate and smooth-walled. The only species, *E. floccosum*, is a common cause of tinea pedis and tinea cruris. [epidermis + G. *phyton*, plant]

ep·i·der·mot·ro·pism (ep-i-der-mot'rō-pizm). Movement towards the epidermis, as in the migration of T lymphocytes into the epidermis in mycosis fungoides. [epidermis + G. *tropē*, a turning]

ep·i·did·y·mal (ep-i-did'i-măl). Relating to the epididymis.

ep·i·did·y·mec·to·my (ep'i-did-i-mek'tō-mē). Operative removal of the epididymis. [epididymis + G. *ektomē*, excision]

ep·i·did·y·mis, gen. **ep·i·did·y·mi·dis**, pl. **ep·i·did·y·mi·des** (ep-i-did'i-mis, -di-dim'i-dis, -di-dim'i-dēz) [NA]. An elongated structure connected to the posterior surface of the testis, consisting of the head of the epididymis, body of epididymis, and tail of epididymis, which turns sharply upon itself to become the ductus deferens; the main component is the very convoluted duct of the epididymis which in the tail and the beginning of the ductus deferens is a reservoir for spermatozoa. The e. transports, stores, and matures spermatozoa between testis and ductus deferens (vas deferens). [Mod. L. fr. G. *epididymis*, fr. *epi*, on, + *didymos*, twin, in pl. testes]

ep·i·did·y·mi·tis (ep-i-did-i-mī'tis). Inflammation of the epididymis.

ep·i·did·y·mo-or·chi·tis (ep-i-did'i-mō-ōr-kī'tis). Simultaneous inflammation of both epididymis and testis. [epididymis + G. *orchis*, testis]

ep·i·did·y·mo·plas·ty (ep-i-did'i-mō-plas-tē). Surgical repair of the epididymis. [epididymis + G. *plastos*, formed]

ep·i·did·y·mot·o·my (ep'i-did-i-mot'ō-mē). Incision into the epididymis, as in preparation for epididymovasostomy or for drainage of purulent material. [epididymis + G. *tomē*, a cutting]

ep·i·did·y·mo·vas·ec·to·my (ep-i-did'i-mō-va-sek'tō-mē). Surgical removal of the epididymis and vas deferens. [epididymis + vasectomy]

ep·i·did·y·mo·va·sos·to·my (ep-i-did'i-mō-va-sos'tō-mē). Surgical anastomosis of the vas deferens to the epididymis. [epididymis + vasostomy]

ep·i·du·ral (ep-i-dū'răl). Upon (or outside) the dura mater.

ep·i·du·rog·ra·phy (ep-i-dū-rog'ră-fē). Radiographic visualization of the epidural space following the regional instillation of a radiopaque contrast medium.

ep·i·es·tri·ol (ep-i-es'trē-ol). SEE estriol.

ep·i·gas·tral·gia (ep'i-gas-tral'jē-ă). Pain in the epigastric region. [epigastrium + G. *algos*, pain]

ep·i·gas·tric (ep-i-gas'trik). Relating to the epigastrium.

ep·i·gen·e·sis (ep-i-jen'ĕ-sis). **1.** Development of offspring from a zygote. **2.** Regulation of the expression of gene activity without alteration of genetic structure. [epi- + G. *genesis*, creation]

ep·i·ge·net·ic (ep'i-jĕ-net'ik). Relating to epigenesis.

ep·i·glot·tic, ep·i·glot·tid·e·an (ep-i-glot'ik, ep-i-glo-tid'ē-an). Relating to the epiglottis.

ep·i·glot·ti·dec·to·my (ep'i-glot-i-dek'tō-mē). Excision of the epiglottis. [epiglottis + G. *ektomē*, excision]

ep·i·glot·ti·di·tis (ep'i-glot-i-dī'tis). SYN epiglottitis.

ep·i·glot·tis (ep-i-glot'is) [NA]. A leaf-shaped plate of elastic cartilage, covered with mucous membrane, at the root of the tongue, which serves as a diverter valve over the superior aperture of the larynx during the act of swallowing; it stands erect when liquids are being swallowed, but is passively bent over the aperture by solid foods being swallowed. [G. *epiglōttis*, fr. *epi*, on, + *glōttis*, the mouth of the windpipe]

ep·i·glot·ti·tis (ep-i-glot-ī'tis). Inflammation of the epiglottis, which may cause respiratory obstruction, especially in children; frequently due to infection by *Haemophilus influenzae* type b. SYN epiglottiditis.

ep·i·ker·a·to·phak·ia (ep'i-ker'ă-tō-phak'ē-ă). Modification of refractive error by application of a donor cornea to the anterior surface of the patient's cornea from which epithelium has been removed. [epi- + G. *keras*, horn, + *phakos*, lens]

ep·i·late (ep'i-lāt). To extract a hair; to remove the hair from a part by forcible extraction, electrolysis, or loosening at the root by chemical means. Cf. depilate. [L. *e*, out, + *pilus*, a hair]

ep·i·la·tion (ep-i-lā'shŭn). The act or result of removing hair. SYN depilation.

epil·a·to·ry (e-pil'ă-tō-rē). **1.** Having the property of removing hair; relating to epilation. SYN depilatory (1). **2.** SYN depilatory (2).

ep·i·lem·ma (ep-i-lem'ă). The connective tissue sheath of nerve fibers near their termination. [epi- + G. *lemma*, husk]

ep·i·lep·sy (ep'i-lep'sē). A chronic disorder characterized by paroxysmal brain dysfunction due to excessive neuronal discharge, and usually associated with some alteration of consciousness. The clinical manifestations of the attack may vary from complex abnormalities of behavior including generalized or focal convulsions to momentary spells of impaired consciousness. These clinical states have been subjected to a variety of classifications, none universally accepted to date and, accordingly, the terminologies used to describe the different types of attacks remain purely descriptive and nonstandardized; they are variously based on 1) the clinical manifestations of the seizure (motor, sensory, reflex, psychic or vegetative), 2) the pathological substrate (hereditary, inflammatory, degenerative, neoplastic, traumatic, or cryptogenic), 3) the location of the epileptogenic lesion (rolandic, temporal, diencephalic regions), and 4) the time of life at which the attacks occur (nocturnal, diurnal, menstrual, etc.). SYN fit (3). [G. *epilēpsia*, seizure]

anosognosic e., epilepsy characterized by attacks of which the person is unaware.

childhood absence e., a generalized e. syndrome characterized by the onset of absence seizures in childhood, typically at age six or seven years. There is a strong genetic predisposition and girls are affected more often than boys. EEG reveals generalized 3 Hz spike-wave activity on a normal background. Prognosis for remission is good if the patient does not also have generalized tonic-clonic seizures. SEE ALSO absence.

complex precipitated e., a form of reflex e. initiated by specialized sensory stimuli, *e.g.*, certain visual patterns.

eating e., epileptic seizures provoked by eating; a type of reflex e.

focal e., e. of various etiologies characterized by focal seizures or secondarily generalized tonic-clonic seizures. Ictal symptoms are often related to the brain region where the seizure begins focally.

frontal lobe e., e. with seizures originating in the frontal lobe. Frontal lobe epilepsies have been divided into several specific syndromes including the syndrome of supplementary motor seizures, cingulate seizures, anterior frontal polar region seizures, orbital frontal seizures, dorsolateral seizures, opercular seizures, and seizures of the motor cortex.

ep

generalized tonic-clonic e., SYN generalized tonic-clonic *seizure.*

jacksonian e., SYN jacksonian *seizure.*

juvenile myoclonic e., an inherited e. syndrome typically beginning in early adolescence, and characterized by early morning myoclonic jerks that may progress into a generalized tonic-clonic seizure.

myoclonic astatic e., a petit mal variant characterized by atonic (drop attacks) and tonic or tonic-clonic attacks in neurologically disabled (hemiplegic, ataxic, etc.) children with mental retardation; usually progresses in spite of medication.

myoclonus e. [MIM*159800], a clinically diverse group of epilepsy syndromes, some benign, some progressive. Many are hereditary and all are characterized by the occurrence of myoclonus. Specific syndromes include cherry red spot myoclonus syndrome, ceroid lipofuscinosis, myoclonic e. with ragged red fibers, and Baltic myoclonus.

occipital lobe e., a localization-related e. where seizures originate from the occipital lobe. Symptoms commonly include visual abnormalities during seizures.

pattern sensitive e., a form of reflex e. precipitated by viewing certain patterns.

photogenic e., a form of reflex e. precipitated by light.

posttraumatic e., a convulsive state following and causally related to head injury, with brain damage either manifested clinically or ascertained by special examinations such as computed tomography.

procursive e., a psychomotor attack initiated by whirling or running.

psychomotor e., attacks with elaborate and multiple sensory, motor, and/or psychic components, the common feature being a clouding or loss of consciousness and amnesia for the event; clinical manifestations may take the form of automatisms, emotional outbursts, or motor or psychic disturbances. SEE ALSO procursive e. SYN psychomotor seizure.

reflex e., seizures which are induced by peripheral stimulation; *e.g.,* audiogenic, laryngeal, photogenic, or other stimulation.

rolandic e., a benign, autosomal dominant form of e. occurring in children, characterized clinically by arrest of speech, by muscular contractions of the side of the face and arm, and by epileptic discharges electroencephalographically. [Luigi *Rolando*]

sensory e., focal e. initiated by a somatosensory phenomenon.

startle e., a form of reflex e. precipitated by sudden noises.

temporal lobe e., e. with seizures originating from the temporal lobe, most commonly the mesial temporal lobe.

tonic e., an attack in which the body is rigid.

ep·i·lep·tic (ep-i-lep′tik). Relating to, characterized by, or suffering from epilepsy.

ep·i·lep·ti·form (ep-i-lep′ti-fōrm). SYN epileptoid.

ep·i·lep·to·gen·ic, ep·i·lep·tog·e·nous (ep-i-lep-tō-jen′ik, ep-i-lep-toj′ĕ-nŭs). Causing epilepsy.

ep·i·lep·toid (ep-i-lep′toyd). Resembling epilepsy; denoting certain convulsions, especially of functional nature. SYN epileptiform. [G. *epilēpsia,* seizure, epilepsy, + *eidos,* resemblance]

ep·i·man·dib·u·lar (ep-i-man-dib′yū-lăr). Upon the lower jaw. [epi- + L. *mandibulum,* mandible]

ep·i·men·or·rha·gia (ep-i-men-ō-rā′jē-ă). Prolonged and profuse menstruation occurring at any time, but most frequently at the beginning and end of menstrual life.

ep·i·men·or·rhea (ep-i-men-ō-rē′ă). Too frequent menstruation, occurring at any time, but particularly at the beginning and end of menstrual life.

ep·i·mer (ep′i-mer). One of two molecules (having more than one chiral center) differing only in the spatial arrangement about a single chiral atom. SEE sugars. Cf. anomer. [epi- + G. *meros,* part]

ep·i·mer·ase (ep′i-mer-ās) [EC 5.1]. A class of enzymes catalyzing epimeric changes.

ep·i·mere (ep′i-mēr). The dorsal part of the myotome. SEE myotome (3). [epi- + G. *meros,* part]

ep·i·mor·pho·sis (ep′i-mōr-fō′sis). Regeneration of a part of an organism by growth at the cut surface. [epi- + G. *morphē,* shape]

ep·i·mys·i·ot·o·my (ep′i-mis-ē-ot′ō-mē). Incision of the sheath of a muscle. [epimysium + G. *tomē,* a cutting]

ep·i·mys·i·um (ep-i-mis′ē-ŭm). The fibrous connective tissue envelope surrounding a skeletal muscle. [epi- + G. *mys,* muscle]

ep·i·neph·rine (ep′i-nef′rin). A catecholamine that is the chief neurohormone of the adrenal medulla. The L-isomer is the most potent stimulant (sympathomimetic) of adrenergic α- and β-receptors, resulting in increased heart rate and force of contraction, vasoconstriction or vasodilation, relaxation of bronchiolar and intestinal smooth muscle, glycogenolysis, lipolysis, and other metabolic effects; used in the treatment of bronchial asthma, acute allergic disorders, open-angle glaucoma, and heart block, and as a topical and local vasoconstrictor. SYN adrenaline. [epi- + G. *nephros,* kidney, + -ine]

ep·i·neph·ros (ep-i-nef′ros). SYN suprarenal *gland.* [epi- + G. *nephros,* kidney]

ep·i·neu·ral (ep-i-nū′răl). On a neural arch of a vertebra.

ep·i·neu·ri·al (ep-i-nū′rē-ăl). Relating to the epineurium.

ep·i·neu·ri·um (ep-i-nū′rē-ŭm). The outermost supporting structure of peripheral nerve trunks, consisting of a condensation of areolar connective tissue; subdivided into those layers that surround the whole nerve trunk (epifascicular e.), and those layers which extend between the nerve fascicles (interfascicular e.). With the endoneurium and perineurium, the e. composes the peripheral nerve stroma. [epi- + G. *neuron,* nerve]

ep·i·phar·ynx (ep′i-far′ingks). SYN nasopharynx. [G. *epi,* on, over, + *pharynx*]

ep·i·phe·nom·e·non (ep′i-fĕ-nom′ĕ-non). A symptom appearing during the course of a disease, not of usual occurrence, and not necessarily associated with the disease.

epiph·o·ra (ē-pif'ō-ră). An overflow of tears upon the cheek, due to imperfect drainage by the tear-conducting passages. SYN tearing. [G. a sudden flow, fr. *epi*, on, + *pherō*, to bear]

epiph·y·si·ol·y·sis (ep-i-fiz-ē-ol'i-sis). **1.** Loosening or separation, either partial or complete, of an epiphysis from the shaft of a bone. **2.** Arrest of growth by ablation of the growth plate cartilage. [epiphysis + G. *lysis*, loosening]

epiph·y·sis, pl. **epiph·y·ses** (e-pif'i-sis, -sēz) [NA]. A part of a long bone developed from a center of ossification distinct from that of the shaft and separated at first from the latter by a layer of cartilage. [G. an excrescence, fr. *epi*, upon, + *physis*, growth]

 pressure e., a secondary center of ossification in the articular end of a long bone.

 traction e., a secondary center of ossification at the site of attachment of a tendon.

epiph·y·si·tis (e-pif-i-sī'tis). Inflammation of an epiphysis.

ep·i·pi·al (ep'i-pī'ăl). On the pia mater.

epiplo-. Omentum. SEE ALSO omento-. [G. *epiploon*]

ep·i·plo·ic (ep'i-plō'ik). SYN omental.

ep·i·scle·ra (ep'i-sklēr'ă). The connective tissue between the sclera and the conjunctiva. [epi- + sclera]

ep·i·scle·ral (ep-i-sklēr'ăl). **1.** Upon the sclera. **2.** Relating to the episclera.

ep·i·scle·ri·tis (ep-i-skle-rī'tis). Inflammation of the episcleral connective tissue. SEE ALSO scleritis.

episio-. The vulva. SEE ALSO vulvo-. [G. *episeion*, pubic region]

ep·i·si·o·per·i·ne·or·rha·phy (e-piz'ē-ō-per'i-nē-ōr'ă-fē, e-pis'). Repair of an incised or a ruptured perineum and lacerated vulva or repair of a surgical incision of the vulva and perineum. [episio- + G. *perinaion*, perineum, + *rhaphē*, a stitching]

ep·i·si·o·plas·ty (e-piz'ē-ō-plas-tē, e-pis'). Plastic surgery of the vulva. [episio- + G. *plastos*, formed]

ep·i·si·or·rha·phy (e-piz-i-ōr'ră-fē, e-pis-). Repair of a lacerated vulva or an episiotomy. [episio- + G. *rhaphē*, a stitching]

ep·i·si·o·ste·no·sis (e-piz'ē-i-ō-stē-nō'sis, e-pis'). Narrowing of the vulvar orifice. [episio- + G. *stenōsis*, narrowing]

ep·i·si·ot·o·my (e-piz-ē-ot'ō-mē, e-pis-). Surgical incision of the vulva to prevent laceration at the time of delivery or to facilitate vaginal surgery. [episio- + G. *tomē*, incision]

ep·i·so·de (ep'i-sōd). An important event or series of events taking place in the course of continuous events, *e.g.*, an episode of depression.

 manic e., manifestation of a major mood disorder in which there is a distinct period during which the predominant mood of the individual is either elevated, expansive, or irritable, and there are associated symptoms of the excited or manic phase of the bipolar disorder. SEE affective *disorders*, under *disorder*, endogenous *depression*.

ep·i·some (ep'i-sōm). An extrachromosomal element (plasmid) that may either integrate into the bacterial chromosome of the host or replicate and function stably when physically separated from the chromosome. [epi- + G. *sōma*, body (chromosome)]

ep·i·spa·di·as (ep-i-spā'dē-ăs). A malformation in which the urethra opens on the dorsum of the penis; frequently associated with exstrophy of the bladder. [epi- + G. *spaō*, to tear or gouge]

ep·i·sple·ni·tis (ep-i-splē-nī'tis). Inflammation of the capsule of the spleen.

epis·ta·sis (e-pis'tă-sis). **1.** The formation of a pellicle or scum on the surface of a liquid, especially as on standing urine. **2.** Phenotypic interaction of non-allelic genes. **3.** A form of gene interaction whereby one gene masks or interferes with the phenotypic expression of one or more genes at other loci; the gene whose phenotype is expressed is said to be "epistatic," while the phenotype altered or suppressed is then said to be "hypostatic". [G. scum; epi- + G. *stasis*, a standing]

ep·i·stat·ic (ep-is-tat'ik). Relating to epistasis.

ep·i·stax·is (ep'i-stak'sis). Profuse bleeding from the nose. SYN nosebleed. [G. fr. *epistazō*, to bleed at the nose, fr. *epi*, on, + *stazō*, to fall in drops]

ep·i·ster·nal (ep-i-ster'năl). **1.** Over or on the sternum. **2.** Relating to the episternum.

ep·i·stro·phe·us (ep-i-strō'fē-ŭs). SYN axis (5). [G. the pivot]

ep·i·ten·din·e·um (ep'i-ten-din'ē-ŭm). The white fibrous sheath surrounding a tendon. [L.]

ep·i·thal·a·mus (ep'i-thal'ă-mŭs) [NA]. A small dorsomedial area of the thalamus corresponding to the habenula and its associated structures, the medullary stria, pineal body, and habenular commissure. [epi- + thalamus]

ep·i·the·lia (ep-i-thē'lē-ă). Plural of epithelium.

ep·i·the·li·al (ep-i-thē'lē-ăl). Relating to or consisting of epithelium.

ep·i·the·li·al·i·za·tion (ep-i-thē'lē-ăl-i-zā'shŭn). Formation of epithelium over a denuded surface. SYN epithelization.

ep·i·the·li·oid (ep-i-thē'lē-oyd). Resembling or having some of the characteristics of epithelium. [epithelium + G. *eidos*, resemblance]

ep·i·the·li·o·lyt·ic (ep-i-thē'lē-ō-lit'ik). Destructive to epithelium.

ep·i·the·li·o·ma (ep'i-thē-lē-ō'mă). **1.** An epithelial neoplasm or hamartoma of the skin, especially of skin appendage origin. **2.** A carcinoma of the skin derived from squamous, basal, or adnexal cells. [epithelium + G. *-ōma*, tumor]

 basal cell e., SYN basal cell *carcinoma*.

 chorionic e., obsolete term for choriocarcinoma.

 malignant ciliary e., malignant hyperplasia of ciliary epithelium with frequent involvement of the pigmented layer.

 sebaceous e., a benign tumor of the sebaceous gland epithelium in which small basaloid or germinative cells predominate.

ep·i·the·li·om·a·tous (ep-i-thē-lē-ō'mă-tŭs). Pertaining to epithelioma.

ep·i·the·li·um, pl. **ep·i·the·lia** (ep-i-thē'lē-ŭm, -ă) [NA]. The purely cellular avascular layer covering all the free surfaces, cutaneous, mucous, and serous, including the glands and other structures derived therefrom. [G. *epi*, upon, + *thēlē*, nipple, a term applied originally to the thin skin covering the nipples and the papillary layer of the border of the lips]

ciliated e., any e. having motile cilia on the free surface.

columnar e., e. formed of a single layer of prismatic cells taller than they are wide.

cuboidal e., simple e. with cells appearing as cubes in a vertical section but as polyhedra in surface view.

germinal e., a cuboidal layer of peritoneal e. covering the gonads, once thought to be the source of germ cells.

glandular e., e. composed of secretory cells.

junctional e., a collar of epithelial cells attached to the tooth surface and subepithelial connective tissue found at the base of the gingival crevice.

laminated e., SYN stratified e.

olfactory e., an e. of the pseudostratified type that contains olfactory, receptor, nerve cells whose axons extend to the olfactory bulb of the brain.

pseudostratified e., an e. that gives a superficial appearance of being stratified because the cell nuclei are at different levels, but in which all cells reach the basement membrane,.

seminiferous e., the e. lining the convoluted tubules of the testis where spermatogenesis and spermiogenesis occur.

simple e., an e. having one layer of cells.

simple squamous e., e. composed of a single layer of flattened scalelike cells, such as mesothelium, endothelium, and that in the pulmonary alveoli.

squamous e., e. consisting of a single layer of cells.

stratified e., a type of e. composed of a series of layers, the cells of each varying in size and shape. It is named more specifically according to the type of cells at the surface, *e.g.,* stratified squamous e., stratified columnar e., stratified ciliated columnar e. SYN laminated e.

surface e., (1) a layer of celomic epithelial cells covering the gonadal ridges as they are formed on the medial border of the mesonephroi near the root of the mesentery; (2) the mesothelial covering of the definitive ovary.

transitional e., a highly distensible pseudostratified e. with large polyploid superficial cells that are cuboidal in the relaxed state but broad and squamous in the distended state; occurs in the kidney, ureter, and bladder.

ep·i·the·li·za·tion (ep-i-thē-li-zā'shŭn). SYN epithelialization.

ep·i·tope (ep'i-tōp). The simplest form of an antigenic determinant, on a complex antigenic molecule, which can combine with antibody or T cell receptor. [epi- + -tope]

ep·i·trich·i·um (ep-i-trik'ē-ŭm). SYN periderm. [epi- + G. *trichion,* dim. of *thrix,* (*trich-*), hair]

ep·i·tym·pan·ic (ep-i-tim-pan'ik). Above, or in the upper part of, the tympanic cavity or membrane.

ep·i·zo·ic (ep-i-zō'ik). Living as a parasite on the skin surface.

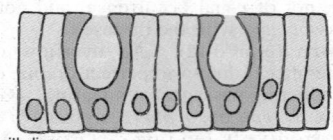

columnar epithelium of intestines

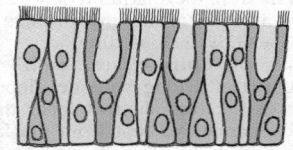

pseudostratified ciliated columnar epithelium

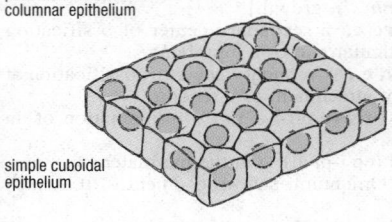

simple cuboidal epithelium

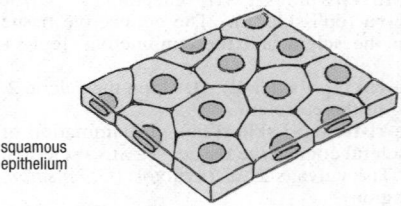

squamous epithelium

types of epithelium

ep·i·zo·ol·o·gy (ep'i-zō-ol'ō-jē). SYN epizootiology. [epi- + G. *zōon,* animal, + *logos,* study]

ep·i·zo·on, pl. **ep·i·zoa** (ep-i-zō'on, -zō'ă). An animal parasite living on the body surface. [epi- + G. *zōon,* animal]

ep·i·zo·ot·ic (ep'i-zō-ot'ik). **1.** Disease occurrence in an animal population with a frequency clearly in excess of the expected. **2.** An outbreak (epidemic) of disease in an animal population; often with the implication that it may also affect human populations. [epi- + G. *zōon,* animal]

ep·i·zo·ot·i·ol·o·gy (ep'i-zō-ot'ē-ol'ō-jē). Epidemiology of disease in animal populations. SYN epizoology. [epi- + G. *zōon,* animal, + *logos,* study]

ep·o·nych·ia (ep-ō-nik'ē-ă). Infection involving the proximal nail fold.

ep·o·nych·i·um (ep-ō-nik'ē-ŭm). **1.** The thin, condensed, eleidin-rich layer of epidermis that precedes and initially covers the nail plate in the embryo. It normally degenerates by the eighth month except at the nail base, where it remains as the cuticle of the nail. **2** [NA]. The corneal layer of epidermis overlapping and in direct contact with the nail root proximally or the sides of the nail plate laterally, forming the undersurface of the nail wall or nail folds of the nail. SYN perionychium. **3.** The thin skin adherent to the nail at its proximal portion. [G. *epi,* upon, + *onyx* (*onych-*), nail]

ep•o•nym (ep′ō-nim). The name of a disease, structure, operation, or procedure, usually derived from the name of the person who first discovered or described it. [G. *epōnymos,* named after]

ep•o•nym•ic (ep-ō-nim′ik). **1.** Relating to an eponym. **2.** An eponym.

ep•ox•y (ē-pok′sē). Chemical term describing an oxygen atom bound to two linked carbon atoms Generally, any cyclic ether, but commonly applied to a 3-membered ring. E.'s are important chemical intermediates, and the basis of e. resins (polymers) formed from e. monomers.

ep•sil•on (ε) (ep′sil-on). **1.** Fifth letter of the Greek alphabet. **2.** Molar absorption *coefficient* or extinction *coefficient.* For terms beginning with this prefix, see the specific term. **3.** CHEMISTRY a position of a substituent located on the fifth atom from the carboxyl or other primary functional group. For terms with the prefix ε, see the specific term.

epu•lis (ep-yū′lis). A nonspecific exophytic gingival mass. [G. *epoulis,* a gumboil]

ep•u•loid (ep′yū-loyd). A gingival mass that resembles an epulis.

equa•tion (ē-kwā′zhŭn). A statement expressing the equality of two things, usually with the use of mathematical or chemical symbols. [L. *aequare,* to make equal]

  alveolar air e., an e. that calculates an approximation of alveolar oxygen tension if the fractional concentration of inspired oxygen, arterial carbon dioxide tension, and respiratory exchange ratio (that is, carbon dioxide production divided by oxygen consumption) are known.

  energy balance e., e. stating that body mass remains constant when caloric intake equals caloric expenditure. Any chronic imbalance on either side of the e. causes body mass to change.

  Henderson-Hasselbalch e., a formula relating the pH value of a solution to the pK_a value of the acid in the solution and the ratio of the acid and the conjugate base concentrations: $pH = pK_a + \log ([A^-]/[HA])$ where $[A^-]$ is the concentration of the conjugate base and $[HA]$ is the concentration of the protonated acid.

  Hill's e., the e.,$y(1-y) = [S]^n/K_d$, where y is the fractional degree of saturation, $[S]$ is the binding ligand concentration, n is the Hill coefficient, and K_d is the dissociation constant for the ligand. The Hill coefficient is a measure of the cooperativity of the protein; the larger the value, the higher the cooperativity.

  personal e., a slight error in judgment, perceptual response, or action peculiar to the individual and so constant that it is usually possible to allow for it in accepting the person's statements or conclusions, thus arriving at approximate exactness.

equi•ax•i•al (ē′kwi-ak′sē-ăl). Having axes of equal length.

equi•i•bra•tion (ē′kwi-li-brā′shŭn, e-kwil-ĭ-). **1.** The act of maintaining an equilibrium or balance. **2.** The act of exposing a liquid, *e.g.,* blood or plasma, to a gas at a certain partial pressure until the partial pressures of the gas within and without

the liquid are equal. **3.** DENTISTRY Modification of occlusal forms of the teeth by grinding, with the intent of equalizing occlusal stress, producing simultaneous occlusal contacts, or harmonizing cuspal relations. **4.** CHROMATOGRAPHY The saturation of the stationary phase with the vapor of the elution solvent to be used.

  occlusal e., the modification of occlusal forms of teeth by grinding with the intent of equalizing occlusal stress, or producing simultaneous occlusal contacts, or of harmonizing cuspal relations.

equi•lib•ri•um (ē-kwi-lib′rē-ŭm). **1.** The condition of being evenly balanced; a state of repose between two or more antagonistic forces that exactly counteract each other. **2.** CHEMISTRY A state of apparent repose created by two reactions proceeding in opposite directions at equal speed; in chemical equations, sometimes indicated by two opposing arrows (↔) or (⇄). SYN dynamic e. [L. *aequilibrium,* a horizontal position, fr. *aequus,* equal, + *libra,* a balance]

  dynamic e., SYN equilibrium (2).

  nutritive e., condition in which there is a perfect balance between intake and excretion of nutritive material, so that there is no increase or loss in weight.

e•quine (ē′kwīn). Relating to, derived from, or resembling the horse, mule, ass, or other members of the genus *Equus.* [L. *equinus,* fr. *equus,* horse]

equi•no•val•gus (ē-kwī-nō-val′gŭs, ek′wi-nō-). SYN *talipes* equinovalgus.

equi•no•var•us (ē-kwī-nō-vā′rŭs, ek′wi-nō-). SYN *talipes* equinovarus.

equi•tox•ic (ē-kwi-tok′sik). Of equivalent toxicity.

equiv•a•lence, equiv•a•len•cy (ē-kwiv′ă-lens, -len-sē). The property of an element or radical of combining with or displacing, in definite and fixed proportion, another element or radical in a compound. [L. *aequus,* equal, + *valentia,* strength (valence)]

equiv•a•lent (ē-kwiv′ă-lent). **1.** Equal in any respect. **2.** That which is equal in size, weight, force, or any other quality to something else. [see equivalence]

  gram e., (1) the weight in grams of an element that combines with or replaces 1 gram of hydrogen; (2) the atomic or molecular weight in grams of an atom or group of atoms involved in a chemical reaction divided by the number of electrons donated, taken up, or shared by the atom or group of atoms in the course of that reaction; **(3)** the weight of a substance contained in 1 liter of 1 normal solution; a variant of (1).

  Joule's e. (J), the dynamic e. of heat; the amount of work converted to heat that will raise the temperature of 1 pound of water 1°F is 778 foot-pounds; in metric units, 1 calorie, which raises 1 gram of water 1°C, equals 4.184×10^7 dyne-centimeters, which equals 4.184 joules.

  metabolic e. (MET), the oxygen cost of energy expenditure measured at supine rest (1 MET = 3.5 ml O_2 per kg of body weight per minute); multiples of MET are used to estimate the oxygen cost of activity.

  nitrogen e., the nitrogen content of protein;

used in calculating the protein breakdown in the body from the nitrogen excreted in the urine, 1 g of nitrogen considered as having originated in 6.25 g of protein catabolized.

ER endoplasmic *reticulum*; emergency room.

Er erbium.

ERBF effective renal blood *flow*.

er·bi·um (Er) (er'bē-ŭm). A rare earth (lanthanide) element, atomic no. 68, atomic wt. 167.26. [from Ytterby, a village in Sweden]

ERCP endoscopic retrograde *cholangiopancreatography*.

erec·tile (ē-rek'tīl). Capable of erection.

erec·tion (ē-rek'shŭn). The condition of erectile tissue when filled with blood, which then becomes hard and unyielding; denoting especially this state of the penis. [L. *erectio,* fr. *erigo,* pp. *erectus,* to set up]

erec·tor (ērek'tŏr, -tōr). **1.** One who or that which raises or makes erect. **2.** Denoting specifically certain muscles having such action. SYN arrector. [Mod. L.]

er·e·thism (er'ĕ-thizm). An abnormal state of excitement or irritation, either general or local. [G. *erethismos,* irritation]

er·e·this·mic, er·e·this·tic, er·e·thit·ic (er-ĕ-thiz'mik, -this'tik, -thit'ik). Excited; marked by or causing erethism; irritable.

ERG Abbreviation for electroretinogram.

erg. The unit of work in the CGS system; the amount of work done by 1 dyne acting through 1 cm, 1 g cm^2 s^{-2}; in the SI system, 1 erg equals 10^{-7} joule. [G. *ergon,* work]

er·ga·sia (er-gā'zē-ă). **1.** Any form of activity, especially mental. **2.** The total of functions and reactions of an individual. [G. work]

er·gas·to·plasm (er-gas'tō-plazm). SYN granular endoplasmic *reticulum.* [G. *ergastēr,* a workman, + *plasma,* something formed]

ergo-. Work. [G. *ergon*]

er·go·cal·cif·er·ol (er'gō-kal-sif'er-ol). Activated ergosterol, the vitamin D of plant origin; it arises from ultraviolet irradiation of ergosterol; used in prophylaxis and treatment of vitamin D deficiency. SYN calciferol, vitamin D$_2$.

er·go·graph (er'gō-graf). An instrument for recording the amount of work done by muscular contractions, or the amplitude of contraction. [ergo- + G. *graphō,* to write]

er·go·graph·ic (er-gō-graf'ik). Relating to the ergograph and the record made by it.

er·gom·e·ter (er-gom'ĕ-ter). SYN dynamometer. [ergo- + G. *metron,* measure]

er·go·nom·ics (er-gō-nom'iks). A branch of ecology concerned with human factors in the design and operation of machines and the physical environment. [ergo- + G. *nomos,* law]

er·gos·ter·ol (er-gos'ter-ol). The most important of the provitamins D$_2$; ultraviolet irradiation converts it to lumisterol, tachysterol, and ergocalciferol; main sterol in yeast.

er·got (er'got). The resistant, overwintering stage of the parasitic ascomycetous fungus *Claviceps purpurea,* a pathogen of rye grass that transforms the seed of rye into a compact spurlike mass of fungal pseudotissue (the sclerotium) containing five or more optically isomeric pairs of alkaloids.

The levorotary isomers induce uterine contractions, control bleeding, and alleviate certain localized vascular disorders (migraine headaches). [O. Fr. *argot,* cock's spur]

er·got·ism (er'got-izm). Poisoning by a toxic substance contained in the sclerotia of the fungus, *Claviceps purpura,* growing on rye grass; characterized by necrosis of the extremities (gangrene) due to contraction of the peripheral vascular bed.

erode (ē-rōd'). **1.** To cause, or to be affected by, erosion. **2.** To remove by ulceration. [L. *erodo,* to gnaw away]

erog·e·nous (ĕ-roj'ĕ-nŭs). Capable of producing sexual excitement when stimulated. [G. *eros,* love, + *genos,* birth]

eros (ē'ros, ār'os). PSYCHOANALYSIS The life principle representing all instinctual tendencies toward procreation and life. See also entries under instinct. [G. love]

ero·sion (ē-rō'zhŭn). **1.** A wearing away or a state of being worn away, as by friction or pressure. **2.** A shallow ulcer; in the stomach and intestine, an ulcer limited to the mucosa, with no penetration of the muscularis mucosae. **3.** The wearing away of a tooth by chemical action or abrasive; when the cause is unknown, it is referred to as idiopathic e. SYN odontolysis. [L. *erosio,* fr. *erodo,* to gnaw away]

ero·sive (ē-rō'siv). **1.** Having the property of eroding or wearing away. **2.** An eroding agent.

erot·ic (ĕ-rot'ik). Lustful; relating to sexual passion; having the quality to produce sexual arousal. [G. *erōtikos,* relating to love, fr. *erōs,* love]

ero·to·gen·ic (er'ō-tō-jen'ik). Capable of causing sexual excitement or arousal. [G. *erōs,* love, + *-gen,* production]

ero·to·ma·nia (er'ō-tō-mā'nē-ă). **1.** Excessive or morbid inclination to erotic thoughts and behavior. **2.** The delusional belief that one is involved in a relationship with another, generally of higher socioeconomic status. [G. *erōs,* love, + *mania,* frenzy]

ero·to·path·ic (er'ō-tō-path'ik). Relating to erotopathy.

er·o·top·a·thy (er-ō-top'ă-thē). Any abnormality of the sexual impulse. [G. *erōs,* love, + *pathos,* suffering]

ero·to·pho·bia (er'ō-tō-fō'bē-ă). Morbid aversion to the thought of sexual love and to its physical expression. [G. *erōs,* love, + *phobos,* fear]

ERPF effective renal plasma *flow.*

er·ror (er'ōr). **1.** A defect in structure or function. **2.** BIOSTATISTICS 1) A mistaken decision, as in hypothesis testing or classification by a discriminant function; 2) the difference between the true value and the observed value of a variate, ascribed to randomness or misreading by an observer. **3.** A false or mistaken belief; in biomedical and other sciences, there are many varieties of e., for example due to bias, inaccurate measurements, or faulty instruments.

   experimental e., the total e. of measurement ascribed to the conduct of an empirical observation. It is commonly expressed as the standard deviation of replicated experiments. There may be many components, including those in the sampling procedure, the measurements, injudicious choice of a model, observer bias, etc.

inborn e.'s of metabolism, a group of disorders, each of which involves a disorder of a single unique enzyme, genetic in origin and operating from birth; effects are ascribable to accumulation of the substrate on which the enzyme normally acts (*e.g.,* phenylketonuria), to deficiency of the product of the enzyme (*e.g.,* albinism), or to forcing metabolism through an auxiliary pathway (*e.g.,* oxaluria).

interobserver e., the differences in interpretation by two or more individuals making observations of the same phenomenon.

intraobserver e., the differences in interpretation by an individual making observations of the same phenomenon at different times.

eruc·ta·tion (ē-rŭk-tā′shŭn). The voiding of gas or of a small quantity of acid fluid from the stomach through the mouth. SYN belching. [L. *eructo,* pp. *-atus,* to belch]

erup·tion (ē-rŭp′shŭn). **1.** A breaking out, especially the appearance of lesions on the skin. **2.** A rapidly developing dermatosis of the skin or mucous membranes, especially when appearing as a local manifestation of one of the exanthemata; an e. is characterized, according to the nature of the lesion, as macular, papular, vesicular, pustular, bullous, nodular, erythematous, etc. **3.** The passage of a tooth through the alveolar process and perforation of the gums. [L. *e-rumpo,* pp. *-ruptus,* to break out]

drug e., any e. caused by the ingestion, injection, or inhalation of a drug, most often the result of allergic sensitization; reactions to drugs applied to the cutaneous surface are not generally designated as drug e., but as contact-type dermatitis. SYN dermatitis medicamentosa, dermatosis medicamentosa, drug rash.

fixed drug e., a type of drug e. that recurs at a fixed site (or sites) following the administration of a particular drug.

polymorphous light e., a common pruritic papular e. appearing in a few hours and lasting up to several days on skin exposed to shortwave ultraviolet light; subepidermal edema and deep perivascular lymphocytic infiltration is seen microscopically.

erup·tive (ē-rŭp′tiv). Characterized by eruption.

ERV Abbreviation for expiratory reserve *volume.*

er·y·sip·e·las (er-i-sip′ĕ-las). A specific, acute, cutaneous inflammatory disease caused by β-hemolytic streptococci and characterized by hot, red, edematous, brawny, and sharply defined eruptions; usually accompanied by severe constitutional symptoms. [G., fr. *erythros,* red + *pella,* skin]

er·y·si·pel·a·tous (er′i-si-pel′ă-tŭs). Relating to erysipelas.

er·y·sip·e·loid (er-i-sip′ĕ-loyd). A specific, usually self-limiting, cellulitis of the hand caused by *Erysipelothrix rhusiopathiae;* appears as a dusky erythema with diamondlike configuration of the skin at the site of a wound sustained in handling fish or meat and may become generalized, with plaques of erythema and bullae, and occasionally,

severe toxemia. [G. *erysipelas* + *eidos,* resemblance]

Er·y·sip·e·lo·thrix (ār-i-sip′ĕ-lō-thriks, -si-pel′ō-thriks). A genus of bacteria containing nonmotile, Gram-positive, rod-shaped organisms which have a tendency to form long filaments. Members of this genus are parasitic on mammals, birds, and fish. The type species is *E. rhusiopathiae.* [erysipelas + G. *thrix,* hair]

er·y·the·ma (er-i-thē′mă). Redness of the skin due to capillary dilatation. [G. *erythēma,* flush]

e. ab ig′ne, SYN e. caloricum.

e. annula′re, rounded or ringed lesions.

e. annula′re centrif′ugum, a chronic recurring erythematous eruption consisting of small and large annular lesions, with a scant marginal scale, usually of unknown cause.

e. arthrit′icum epidem′icum, SYN Haverhill *fever.*

e. calor′icum, a reticulated, pigmented, macular eruption that occurs, mostly on the shins, of bakers, stokers, and others exposed to radiant heat. SYN e. ab igne.

e. chron′icum mi′grans, a raised erythematous ring with advancing indurated borders and central clearing, radiating from the site of a tick bite such as that by *Ixodes dammini;* the characteristic skin lesion of Lyme disease; due to the spirochete *Borrelia burgdorferi.*

e. indura′tum, recurrent hard subcutaneous nodules that frequently break down and form necrotic ulcers, usually on the calves and less frequently on the thighs or arms of middle-aged women; probably a form of nodular vasculitis.

e. infectio′sum, a mild infectious exanthema of childhood characterized by an erythematous maculopapular eruption, resulting in a lacelike facial rash or "slapped cheek" appearance. Fever and arthritis may also accompany infection; caused by Parvovirus B 19. SYN fifth disease.

e. i′ris, concentric rings of e. varying in intensity, characteristic of e. multiforme. SYN herpes iris (1).

e. margina′tum, a variant of e. multiforme seen in rheumatic fever.

e. mi′grans, e. mi′grans ling′uae, SYN geographic *tongue.*

e. multifor′me, an acute eruption of macules, papules, or subdermal vesicles presenting a multiform appearance, the characteristic lesion being the target or iris lesion over the dorsal aspect of the hands and forearms; its origin may be allergic, seasonal, or from drug sensitivity, and the eruption, although usually self-limited, may be recurrent or may run a severe course, sometimes with fatal termination (Stevens-Johnson syndrome). SYN herpes iris (2).

e. nodo′sum, a panniculitis marked by the sudden formation of painful nodes on the extensor surfaces of the lower extremities, with lesions that are self-limiting but tend to recur; associated with arthralgia and fever; may be the result of drug sensitivity or associated with sarcoidosis and various infections. Deep biopsies show a septal panniculitis with infiltration by lymphocytes and scattered multinucleated giant cells.

e. per′nio, SYN chilblain.

e. tox′icum, flushing of the skin due to allergic reaction to some toxic substance.

e. tox′icum neonato′rum, a common transient idiopathic eruption of erythema, small papules, and occasionally pustules filled with eosinophilic leukocytes overlying hair follicles of the newborn.

er•y•them•a•tous (er-i-them′ă-tŭs, -thē′mă-tŭs). Relating to or marked by erythema.

er•y•the•ma•to•ve•sic•u•lar (er-i-thē′mă-tō-ve-sik′yū-lăr). Denoting a condition characterized by erythema and vesiculation, as in allergic contact dermatitis.

△**erythr-.** SEE erythro-.

er•y•thral•gia (ār-i-thral′jē-ă). Painful redness of the skin. SEE ALSO erythromelalgia. [erythro- + G. *algos,* pain]

ery•thras•ma (er-i-thraz′mă). An eruption of well-circumscribed reddish brown patches, in the axillae and groins especially, due to the presence of *Corynebacterium minutissimum* in the stratum corneum. [G. *erythrainō,* to redden]

eryth•re•de•ma (ĕ-rith-rē-dē′mă). SYN acrodynia (2). [erythro- + G. *oidēma,* swelling]

er•y•thre•mia (er-i-thrē′mē-ă). SYN *polycythemia* vera. [erythro- + G. *haima,* blood]

er•y•thrism (er′i-thrizm, ĕ-rith′rizm). Redness of the hair with a ruddy, freckled complexion. [G. *erythros,* red]

er•y•thris•tic (er-i-thris′tik). Relating to or marked by erythrism; having a ruddy complexion and reddish hair. SYN rufous.

△**erythro-, erythr-. 1.** Combining form denoting red or red blood cell; corresponds to L. *rub-.* **2.** Indicates the structure of erythrose in a larger sugar; used as such, it is italicized (*e.g.,* 2-deoxy-D-*erythro*-pentose). [G. *erythros,* red]

eryth•ro•blast (ĕ-rith′rō-blast). The first generation of cells in the red blood cell series that can be distinguished from precursor endothelial cells. In normal maturation four stages of development can be recognized: 1) pronormoblast, 2) basophilic normoblast, 3) polychromatic normoblast, and 4) orthochromatic normoblast. [erythro- + G. *blastos,* germ]

eryth•ro•blas•te•mia (ĕ-rith′rō-blas-tē′mē-ă). The presence of nucleated red cells in the peripheral blood. [erythroblast + G. *haima,* blood]

eryth•ro•blas•to•pe•nia (ĕ-rith′rō-blas-tō-pē′nē-ă). A primary deficiency of erythroblasts in bone marrow, seen in aplastic anemia. [erythroblast + G. *penia,* poverty]

eryth•ro•blas•to•sis (ĕ-rith′rō-blas-tō′sis). The presence of erythroblasts in considerable number in the blood. [erythroblast + -*osis,* condition]

e. feta′lis, a grave hemolytic anemia that, in most instances, results from development in the mother of anti-Rh antibody in response to the Rh factor in the (Rh-positive) fetal blood; it is characterized by many erythroblasts in the circulation, and often generalized edema (hydrops fetalis) and enlargement of the liver and spleen; the disease is sometimes caused by antibodies for antigens other than Rh. SYN congenital anemia, hemolytic disease of newborn, neonatal anemia.

eryth•ro•blas•tot•ic (ĕ-rith′rō-blas-tot′ik). Per-taining to erythroblastosis, especially erythroblastosis fetalis.

eryth•ro•cla•sis (er-i-throk′lă-sis). Fragmentation of the red blood cells. [erythro- + G. *klasis,* breaking]

eryth•ro•clas•tic (ĕ-rith′rō-klas′tik). Pertaining to erythroclasis; destructive to red blood cells.

eryth•ro•cy•a•no•sis (ĕ-rith′rō-sī-ă-nō′sis). A condition seen in girls and young women in which exposure of the limbs to cold causes them to become swollen and dusky red; it results from direct exposure to cold, but not freezing, temperatures. [erythro- + G. *kyanos,* blue, + -*osis,* condition]

■ **eryth•ro•cyte** (ĕ-rith′rō-sīt). A mature red blood cell. SYN red blood cell, red corpuscle. [erythro- + G. *kytos,* cell]

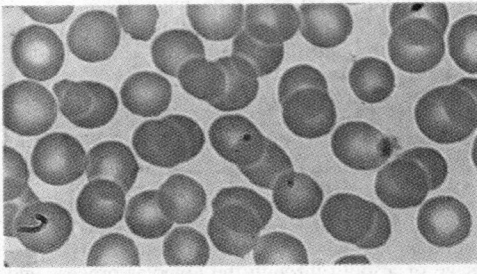

erythrocytes: in blood smear

eryth•ro•cy•the•mia (ĕ-rith′rō-sī-thē′mē-ă). SYN polycythemia. [erythro- + G. *kytos,* cell, + *haima,* blood]

induced e., SYN blood *doping.*

eryth•ro•cyt•ic (ĕ-rith-rō-sit′ik). Pertaining to an erythrocyte.

eryth•ro•cy•tol•y•sin (ĕ-rith′rō-sī-tol′i-sin). SYN hemolysin (1).

eryth•ro•cy•tol•y•sis (ĕ-rith′rō-sī-tol′i-sis). SYN hemolysis. [erythrocyte + G. *lysis,* loosening]

eryth•ro•cy•tor•rhex•is (ĕ-rith′rō-sī-tō-rek′sis). A partial erythrocytolysis in which particles of protoplasm escape from the red blood cells, which then become crenated and deformed. SYN erythrorrhexis. [erythrocyte + G. *rhēxis,* rupture]

eryth•ro•cy•tos•chi•sis (ĕ-rith′rō-sī-tos′ki-sis). A breaking up of the red blood cells into small particles that morphologically resemble platelets. [erythrocyte + G. *schisis,* a splitting]

eryth•ro•cy•to•sis (ĕ-rith′rō-sī-tō′sis). Polycythemia, especially that which occurs in response to some known stimulus.

eryth•ro•de•gen•er•a•tive (ĕ-rith′rō-de-jen′er-a-tiv). Pertaining to or characterized by degeneration of the red blood cells.

eryth•ro•der•ma (ĕ-rith-rō-der′mă). A nonspecific designation for intense and usually widespread reddening of the skin from dilatation of blood vessels, often preceding, or associated with exfoliation. SYN erythrodermatitis. [erythro- + G. *derma,* skin]

bullous congenital ichthyosiform e. (ik-thē-os′ē-form), diffusely red, eroded skin at birth, with subsequent scaling, tending to improve in later life, characterized by generalized epidermolytic hyperkeratosis.

congenital ichthyosiform e., a genodermatosis characterized by diffuse chronic erythema and scale formation which may be separated into bullous and nonbullous forms. SYN ichthyosiform e.

e. desquamati′vum, severe, extensive seborrheic dermatitis with exfoliative dermatitis, generalized lymphadenopathy, and diarrhea in the newborn; frequently occurs in undernourished, cachectic children. SYN Leiner's disease.

ichthyosiform e., SYN congenital ichthyosiform e.

e. psoriat′icum, extensive exfoliative dermatitis simulating psoriasis.

eryth·ro·der·ma·ti·tis (ĕ-rith′rō-der-mă-tī′tis). SYN erythroderma.

eryth·ro·don·tia (ĕ-rith-rō-don′shē-ă). Reddish discoloration of the teeth, as may occur in porphyria. [erythro- + G. *odous,* tooth]

eryth·ro·gen·ic (ĕ-rith-rō-jen′ik). **1.** Producing red, as causing an eruption or a red color sensation. **2.** Pertaining to the formation of red blood cells. [erythro- + -*gen,* producing]

er·y·throid (er′i-throyd, ĕ-rith′royd). Reddish in color.

eryth·ro·ki·net·ics (ĕ-rith′rō-ki-net′iks). The kinetics of erythrocytes from their generation to destruction. [erythro- + G. *kinēsis,* movement]

eryth·ro·leu·ke·mia (ĕ-rith′rō-lū-kē′mē-ă). Simultaneous neoplastic proliferation of erythroblastic and leukoblastic tissues.

eryth·ro·leu·ko·sis (ĕ-rith′rō-lū-kō′sis). A condition resembling leukemia in which the erythropoietic tissue is affected in addition to the leukopoietic tissue.

er·y·throl·y·sin (er-i-throl′i-sin). SYN hemolysin (1).

er·y·throl·y·sis (er-i-throl′i-sis). SYN hemolysis.

eryth·ro·mel·al·gia (ĕ-rith′rō-mel-al′jē-ă). **1.** Paroxysmal throbbing and burning pain in the skin often precipitated by exertion or heat, affecting the hands and feet, accompanied by a dusky mottled redness of the parts with increased skin temperature; may be associated with myeloproliferative disorders. **2.** A rare disorder of middle age, characterized by paroxysmal attacks of severe burning pain, reddening, hyperalgesia and sweating, involving one or more extremities, usually both feet; the attacks can be triggered by warmth, and are usually relieved by cold and limb elevation. SYN Mitchell's disease, red neuralgia. [erythro- + G. *melos,* limb, + *algos,* pain]

er·y·thron (er′i-thron). The total mass of circulating red blood cells, and that part of the hematopoietic tissue from which they are derived.

eryth·ro·ne·o·cy·to·sis (ĕ-rith′rō-nē-ō-sī-tō′sis). The presence in the peripheral circulation of regenerative forms of red blood cells. [erythrocyte + G. *neos,* new, + *kytos,* cell, + -*osis,* condition]

eryth·ro·pe·nia (ĕ-rith-rō-pē′nē-ă). Deficiency in the number of red blood cells. [erythrocyte + G. *penia,* poverty]

eryth·ro·pha·gia (ĕ-rith-rō-fā′jē-ă). Phagocytic destruction of red blood cells. [erythrocyte + G. *phagō,* to eat, + -ia]

eryth·ro·phag·o·cy·to·sis (ĕ-rith′rō-fag′ō-sī-tō′sis). Phagocytosis of erythrocytes.

eryth·ro·phil (ĕ-rith′rō-fil). **1.** Staining readily with red dyes. SYN erythrophilic. **2.** A cell or tissue element that stains red. [erythro- + G. *philos,* fond]

eryth·ro·phil·ic (ĕ-rith-rō-fil′ik). SYN erythrophil (1).

eryth·ro·pla·kia (ĕ-rith-rō-plā′kē-ă). A red, velvety, plaquelike lesion of mucous membrane which often represents malignant change. [erythro- + G. *plax,* plate]

eryth·ro·pla·sia (ĕ-rith-rō-plā′zē-ă). Erythema and dysplasia of the epithelium. [erythro- + G. *plassō,* to form]

e. of Queyrat, carcinoma *in situ* of the glans penis.

eryth·ro·poi·e·sis (ĕ-rith′rō-poy-ē′sis). The formation of red blood cells. [erythrocyte + G. *poiēsis,* a making]

eryth·ro·poi·et·ic (ĕ-rith′rō-poy-et′ik). Pertaining to or characterized by erythropoiesis.

eryth·ro·poi·e·tin (ĕ-rith-rō-poy′ĕ-tin). A protein that enhances erythropoiesis by stimulating formation of proerythroblasts and release of reticulocytes from bone marrow; it is secreted by the kidney and possibly by other tissues.

eryth·ro·pros·o·pal·gia (ĕ-rith′rō-pros-ō-pal′jē-ă). A disorder similar to erythromelalgia, but with the pain and redness occurring in the face. [erythro- + G. *prosōpon,* face, + *algos,* pain]

eryth·rop·sia (ĕ-rith-rop′sē-ă). An abnormality of vision in which all objects appear to be tinged with red. [erythro- + G. *ōps,* eye]

er·y·thror·rhex·is (er′i-thrō-rek′sis, ĕ-rith-rō-rek′sis). SYN erythrocytorrhexis. [erythrocyte + G. *rhēxis,* rupture]

er·y·thru·ria (er-i-thrū′rē-ă). The passage of red urine. [erythro- + G. *ouron,* urine]

Es einsteinium.

es·cape (es-kāp′). CARDIOLOGY term used to describe the situation when a higher pacemaker defaults or A-V conduction fails and a lower pacemaker assumes the function of pacemaking for one or more beats.

nasal e., SYN nasal *emission.*

ventricular e., e. with an ectopic ventricular focus as pacemaker.

es·char (es′kar). A thick, coagulated crust or slough which develops following a thermal burn or chemical or physical cauterization of the skin. [G. *eschara,* a fireplace, a scab caused by burning]

es·cha·rot·ic (es-kă-rot′ik). Caustic or corrosive. [G. *escharōtikos*]

es·cha·rot·o·my (es-kă-rot′ō-mē). Surgical incision in an eschar to lessen constriction, as might be done following a burn. [eschar + G. *tomē,* incision]

Esch·e·rich·ia (esh-ĕ-rik′ē-ă). A genus of aerobic, facultatively anaerobic bacteria containing short, motile or nonmotile, Gram-negative rods. Motile cells are peritrichous. Glucose and lactose are fermented with the production of acid and gas. These organisms are found in feces; some are pathogenic to man, causing enteritis, peritonitis, cystitis, etc. It is the type genus of the family

es

Enterobacteriaceae. The type species is *E. coli*. [T. *Escherich*, German pediatrician and bacteriologist, 1857–1911]

enterohemorrhagic *E. coli* (EHEC), enterohemorrhagic strains of *E. coli*, usually of the serotype 0157:H7; produces a toxin resembling that produced by *Shigella;* associated with damage to the epithelium, ischemia of the bowel, and necrosis of the colon. Apparently responsible for a hemorrhagic form of colitis without fever, which can be very severe, spread primarily by contaminated beef. May also cause microangiopathic hemolytic anemia, renal failure, and the hemolytic uremic syndrome.

enteroinvasive *E. coli* (EIEC), enteroinvasive strain of *E. coli* that penetrates gut mucosa and multiplies in colon epithelial cells, resulting in shigellosis-like changes of the mucosa. This strain produces a severe diarrheal illness that can resemble shigellosis except for the absence of vomiting and shorter duration of illness.

enteropathogenic *E. coli* (EPEC), enteropathogenic strain of *E. coli;* organisms adhere to small bowel mucosa and produce characteristic changes in the microvilli. This strain produces symptomatic, sometimes serious, gastrointestinal illnesses, especially severe in neonates and young children; typically it produces toxins.

enterotoxigenic *E. coli* (ETEC), enterotoxigenic strain of *E. coli;* attaches to the duodenum or proximal small intestine mucosa, where it forms heat-stable and heat-labile toxins that activate adenylate cyclase, causing wasting diarrhea. Responsible for 40–70% of traveler's diarrhea; chiefly water-borne via human feces.

E. co'li, a species that occurs normally in the intestines of man and other vertebrates, is widely distributed in nature, and is a frequent cause of infections of the urogenital tract and of diarrhea in infants; enteropathogenic strains (serovars) of *E. coli* cause diarrhea due to enterotoxin, the production of which seems to be associated with a transferable episome; the type species of the genus.

esoph·a·ge·al (ē-sof′ă-jē′ăl, ē′-sŏ-faj′ē-ăl). Relating to the esophagus.

esoph·a·gec·ta·sis, esoph·a·gec·ta·sia (ē-sof-ă-jek′tă-sis, -jek-tā′zē-ă). Dilation of the esophagus. [esophagus + G. *ektasis,* a stretching]

e·soph·a·gec·to·my (ē-sof-ă-jek′tō-mē). Excision of any part of the esophagus. [esophagus + G. *ektomē,* excision]

transhiatal e., resection of the esophagus by blunt dissection from a cervical incision from above and transhiatal approach through an abdominal incision.

transthoracic e., resection of the esophagus through a thoracotomy incision.

esoph·a·gi (ē-sof′ă-jī, -gī). Plural of esophagus.

esoph·a·gism (ē-sof′ă-jizm). Esophageal spasm causing dysphagia.

esoph·a·gi·tis (ē-sof-ă-jī′tis). Inflammation of the esophagus.

reflux e., peptic e., inflammation of the lower esophagus from regurgitation of acid gastric contents, usually due to malfunction of the lower esophageal sphincter; symptoms include substernal pain, heartburn, and regurgitation of acid juice.

esoph·a·go·car·di·o·plas·ty (ē-sof′ă-gō-kar′dē-ō-plas-tē). Plastic surgery of the esophagus and cardiac end of the stomach.

esoph·a·go·cele (ē-sof′ă-gō-sēl). Protrusion of the mucous membrane of the esophagus through a tear in the muscular coat. [esophagus + G. *kēlē,* hernia]

esoph·a·go·en·ter·os·to·my (ē-sof′ă-gō-en-ter-os′tō-mē). Surgical formation of a direct communication between the esophagus and intestine. [esophagus + G. *enteron,* intestine, + *stoma,* mouth]

esoph·a·go·gas·trec·to·my (ē-sof′ă-gō-gas-trek′tō-mē). Removal of a portion of the lower esophagus and proximal stomach for treatment of neoplasms or strictures of those organs, especially those lesions located at or near the cardioesophageal junction.

esoph·a·go·gas·tro·a·nas·to·mo·sis (ē-sof′ă-gō-gas′trō-ă-nas-tō-mō′sis). SYN esophagogastrostomy.

esoph·a·go·gas·tro·du·o·de·nos·co·py (EGD) (ĕ-sof′ă-gō-gas′trō-dū′ō-den-os-kō-pē). Endoscopic examination of the esophagus, stomach and duodenum usually performed using a fiberoptic instrument.

esoph·a·go·gas·tro·plas·ty (ē-sof′ă-gō-gas′trō-plas-tē). SYN cardioplasty.

esoph·a·go·gas·tros·to·my (ē-sof′ă-gō-gas-tros′tō-mē). Anastomosis of esophagus to stomach, usually following esophagogastrectomy. SYN esophagogastroanastomosis, gastroesophagostomy. [esophagus + G. *gastēr,* stomach, + *stoma,* mouth]

esoph·a·go·gram (e-sof′ă-gō-gram). A roentgenogram of the esophagus.

esoph·a·gog·ra·phy (ē-sof-ă-gog′ră-fē). Radiography of the esophagus using swallowed or injected radiopaque contrast media; the technique of obtaining an esophagogram. [esophagus + G. *graphō,* to write]

esoph·a·go·ma·la·cia (ē-sof′ă-gō-mă-lā′shē-ă). Softening of the walls of the esophagus. [esophagus + G. *malakia,* softness]

esoph·a·go·my·ot·o·my (ē-sof′ă-gō-mī-ot′ō-mē). Treatment of esophageal achalasia by longitudinal division of the lowest part of the esophageal muscle down to the submucosal layer; some muscle fibers of the cardia may also be divided. [esophagus + G. *mys,* muscle, + *tomē,* incision]

esoph·a·go·plas·ty (ē-sof′ă-gō-plas-tē). Plastic surgery of the wall of the esophagus. [esophagus + G. *plastos,* formed]

esoph·a·go·pli·ca·tion (ē-sof′ă-gō-pli-kā′shŭn). Reduction in size of a dilated esophagus or of a pouch in it by making longitudinal folds or tucks in its wall. [esophagus + L. *plico,* to fold]

esoph·a·go·pto·sis, esoph·a·go·pto·sia (ē-sof′ă-gō-tō′sis, -tō′sē-ă). Relaxation and downward displacement of the walls of the esophagus. [esophagus + G. *ptōsis,* a falling]

esoph·a·go·scope (ē-sof′ă-gō-skōp). An endoscope for inspecting the interior of the esophagus. [esophagus + G. *skopeō,* to examine]

esoph·a·gos·co·py (ē-sof-ă-gos′kŏ-pē). Inspection of the interior of the esophagus by means of an endoscope. [esophagus + G. *skopeō*, to examine]

esoph•a•go•spasm (ē-sof′ă-gō-spazm). Spasm of the walls of the esophagus.

esoph•a•go•ste•no•sis (ē-sof′ă-gō-stĕ-nō′sis). Stricture or a general narrowing of the esophagus. [esophagus + G. *stenōsis*, a narrowing]

esoph•a•gos•to•my (ē-sof-ă-gos′tō-mē). Surgical formation of an opening directly into the esophagus from without. [esophagus + G. *stoma*, mouth]

esoph•a•got•o•my (ē-sof-ă-got′ō-mē). An incision through the wall of the esophagus. [esophagus + G. *tomē*, an incision]

esoph•a•gus, pl. **esoph•a•gi** (ē-sof′ă-gŭs, -gī; -jī) [NA]. The portion of the digestive canal between the pharynx and stomach. It is about 25 cm long and consists of three parts: the cervical part, from the cricoid cartilage to the thoracic inlet; the thoracic part, from the thoracic inlet to the diaphragm; and the abdominal part, below the diaphragm to the cardiac opening of the stomach. [G. *oisophagos*, gullet]

 Barrett's e., columnar metaplasia of the lower esophagus, seen particularly in gastroesophageal reflux disease; sometimes evolves into adenocarcinoma.

es•o•pho•ria (es-ō-fō′rē-ă). A tendency for the eyes to turn inward, prevented by binocular vision. [G. *esō*, inward, + *phora*, a carrying]

es•o•phor•ic (es-ō-fōr′ik). Relating to or marked by esophoria.

es•o•tro•pia (es-ō-trō′pē-ă). The form of strabismus in which the visual axes converge; may be paralytic or concomitant, monocular or alternating, accommodative or nonaccommodative. SYN convergent strabismus. [G. *esō*, inward, + *tropē*, turn]

es•o•tro•pic (es-ō-trop′ik). Relating to or marked by esotropia.

ESP extrasensory *perception*.

es•pun•dia (es-pūn′dē-ă). A type of American leishmaniasis caused by *Leishmania braziliensis* that affects the mucous membranes, particularly in the nasal and oral region, resulting in grossly destructive changes; may develop metastatically from sores originally found elsewhere on the body. [Sp., fr. L. *spongia*, sponge]

ESR erythrocyte sedimentation *rate*; electron spin resonance.

es•sen•tial (ĕ-sen′shăl). **1.** Necessary, indispensable, (*e.g.*, e. amino acids, e. fatty acids). **2.** Characteristic of. **3.** Determining. **4.** Of unknown etiology. **5.** Relating to an essence (*e.g.*, e. oil). **6.** SYN intrinsic.

EST. electroshock *therapy*.

es•ter (es′ter). An organic compound containing the grouping, –X(O)–O–R (X = carbon, sulfur, phosphorus, etc.; R = radical of an alcohol), formed by the elimination of H_2O between the –OH of an acid group and the –OH of an alcohol group.

es•ter•ase (es′ter-ās). A generic term for enzymes that catalyze the hydrolysis of esters.

es•ter•i•fi•ca•tion (es′ter′i-fi-kā′shŭn). The process of forming an ester, as in the reaction of ethanol and acetic acid to form ethyl acetate.

△**esthesio-**. **1.** Sensation, perception. [G. *aesthēsis*, sense perception]

es•the•si•od•ic (es-thē-zē-od′ik). Conveying sensory impressions. SYN esthesodic. [esthesio- + G. *hodos*, way]

es•the•si•o•gen•e•sis (es-thē′zē-ō-jen′ĕ-sis). The production of sensation, especially of nervous erethism. [esthesio- + G. *genesis*, origin]

es•the•si•o•gen•ic (es-thē-zē-ō-jen′ik). Producing a sensation.

es•the•si•om•e•ter (es-thē-zē-om′ĕ-ter). An instrument for determining the state of tactile and other forms of sensibility. SYN tactometer. [esthesio- + G. *metron*, measure]

es•the•si•om•e•try (es-thē-zē-om′ĕ-trē). Measurement of the degree of tactile or other sensibility.

es•the•si•o•phys•i•ol•o•gy (es-thē′zē-ō-fiz-ē-ol′ō-jē). The physiology of sensation and the sense organs.

es•the•sod•ic (es′thē-zod′ik). SYN esthesiodic.

es•thet•ic (es-thet′ik). **1.** Pertaining to the sensations. **2.** Pertaining to esthetics (*i.e.*, beauty). [G. *aisthēsis*, sensation]

es•thet•ics (es-thet′iks). The branch of philosophy concerned with art and beauty, especially with the components thereof.

es•ti•val (es′ti-văl). Relating to or occurring in the summer. [L. *aestivus*, summer (adj.)]

es•ti•vo•au•tum•nal (es′ti-vō-aw-tŭm′năl). Relating to or occurring in summer and autumn. [L. *aestivus*, summer (adj.), + *autumnalis*, autumnal]

es•tra•di•ol (es-tră-dī′ol). The most potent naturally occurring estrogen, formed by the ovary, placenta, testis, and possibly the adrenal cortex.

es•tri•ol (es′trē-ol). An estrogenic metabolite of estradiol, usually the predominant estrogenic metabolite found in urine (especially during pregnancy).

es•tro•gen (es′trō-jen). Generic term for any substance, natural or synthetic, that exerts biological effects characteristic of estrogenic hormones. E.'s are formed by the ovary, placenta, testes, and possibly the adrenal cortex, as well as by certain plants; stimulate secondary sexual characteristics, and exert systemic effects, such as growth and maturation of long bones; given after menopause or oophorectomy to lower the risk of heart attack and prevent osteoporosis; also used to prevent or stop lactation, suppress ovulation, and palliate carcinoma of the breast and prostate. [G. *oistrus*, estrus, + *-gen*, producing]

es•tro•gen•ic (es-trō-jen′ik). **1.** Causing estrus in animals. **2.** Having an action similar to that of an estrogen.

es•trone (es′trōn). A metabolite of 17β-estradiol, commonly found in urine, ovaries, and placenta; with considerably less biological activity than the parent hormone.

es•trus (es′trŭs). That portion or phase of the sexual cycle of female animals characterized by willingness to permit coitus; readily detectable behavioral and other signs are exhibited by animals during this period. SYN heat (2). [G. *oistros*, mad desire]

ESWL electrohydraulic shock wave *lithotripsy*; extracorporeal shock wave *lithotripsy*

ES

Et ethyl.

eta (āt′a). The seventh letter of the Greek alphabet. **1.** CHEMISTRY Denotes the position seven atoms from the carboxyl group or other primary functional group. **2.** Symbol for viscosity.

ETEC. enterotoxigenic *Escherichia coli.*

eth•a•nol (eth′an-ol). SYN alcohol (2).

eth•en•yl (eth′en-il). SYN vinyl.

ether (ē′ther). **1.** Any organic compound in which two carbon atoms are independently linked to a common oxygen atom, thus containing the group –C–O–C–. SEE ALSO epoxy. **2.** Loosely used to refer to diethyl e. For individual e.'s, see the specific name. [G. *aithēr,* the pure upper air]

ethe•re•al (ē-thēr′ē-ăl). Relating to or containing ether. [G. *aitherios,* etherial, fr. *aithēr,* the upper air]

eth•i•cal (eth′i-kăl). Relating to ethics; in conformity with the rules governing personal and professional conduct.

eth•ics (eth′iks). The branch of philosophy that deals with the distinction between right and wrong, with the moral consequences of human actions. [G. *ethikos,* arising from custom, fr. *ethos,* custom]

△**ethmo-.** **1.** Ethmoid. **2.** The ethmoid bone. [G. *ēthmos,* sieve]

eth•moid (eth′moyd). **1.** Resembling a sieve. **2.** Relating to the e. bone. SYN ethmoidal. [G. *ēthmos,* sieve, + *eidos,* resemblance]

eth•moi•dal (eth-moy′dăl). SYN ethmoid.

eth•moi•dec•to•my (eth-moy-dek′tō-mē). Removal of all or part of the mucosal lining and bony partitions between the ethmoid sinuses. [ethmo- + G. *ektomē,* excision]

eth•moid•i•tis (eth-moy-dī′tis). Inflammation of the ethmoid sinuses.

eth•mo•tur•bi•nals (eth-mō-ter′bi-nalz). The conchae of the ethmoid bone; the superior and middle conchae; occasionally a third, the supreme concha, exists.

eth•nic group (eth′nik). A social group characterized by a distinctive social and cultural tradition maintained from generation to generation, a common history and origin and a sense of identification with the group.

eth•no•cen•trism (eth-nō-sen′trizm). The tendency to evaluate other groups according to the values and standards of one's own ethnic group, especially with the conviction that one's own ethnic group is superior to the other groups. [G. *ethnos,* race, tribe, + *kentron,* center of a circle]

eth•o•phar•ma•col•o•gy (eth′ō-far-mă-kol′ō-jē). The study of drug effects on behavior, relying on observation and description of species-specific elements (acts and postures during social encounters). [G. *ethos,* character, habit, + pharmacology]

eth•oxy (e-thok′sē). The monovalent radical, $CH_3CH_2O–$.

eth•yl (Et) (eth′il). The hydrocarbon radical, $CH_3CH_2–$.

 e. alcohol, SYN alcohol (2).

eth•yl•ate (eth′i-lāt). A compound in which the hydrogen of the hydroxyl group of ethanol is replaced by a metallic atom, usually sodium or potassium; *e.g.,* C_2H_5ONa, sodium ethylate.

eth•yl•di•chlo•ro•ar•sine (eth′il-dī-klōr-ō-ar′

sēn). $C_2H_5AsCl_2$; a blister agent used in World War I; irritating to the respiratory tract.

eth•yl•i•dene (eth-il′i-dēn). The radical $CH_3CH=$.

eth•yl•i•dyne (eth-il′i-dīn). The radical $CH_3C\equiv$.

eti•o•la•tion (ē-tē-ō-lā′shŭn). **1.** Pallor resulting from absence of light, as in persons confined because of illness or imprisonment, or in plants bleached by being deprived of light. **2.** The process of blanching, bleaching, or making pale by withholding light. [Fr. *étioler,* to blanch]

eti•o•log•ic (ē′tē-ō-loj′ik). Relating to etiology.

eti•ol•o•gy (ē-tē-ol′ō-jē). **1.** The science and study of the causes of disease and their mode of operation. Cf. pathogenesis. **2.** The science of causes, causality; in common usage, cause. [G. *aitia,* cause, + *logos,* treatise, discourse]

Eu europium.

△**eu-.** Good, well; opposite of dys-, caco-. [G.]

Eu•bac•te•ri•um (yū′bak-tēr′ē-ŭm). A genus of anaerobic, nonsporeforming, nonmotile bacteria containing straight or curved Gram-positive rods which usually occur singly, in pairs, or in short chains. Usually these organisms attack carbohydrates. They may be pathogenic. Rarely associated with intraabdominal sepsis in humans. The type species is *E. limosum.*

eu•chlor•hy•dria (yū-klōr-hi′drē-ă). A condition in which free hydrochloric acid exists in normal amount in the gastric juice. [eu- + cholohydric (acid) + -ia]

eu•cho•lia (yū-kō′lē-ă). A normal state of the bile as regards quantity and quality. [eu- + G. *cholē,* bile]

eu•chro•ma•tin (yū-krō′mă-tin). The parts of chromosomes that, during interphase, are uncoiled dispersed threads and not stained by ordinary dyes; metabolically active, in contrast to the inert heterochromatin.

eu•di•a•pho•re•sis (yū-dī′ă-fō-rē′sis). Normal free sweating. [eu- + G. *diaphorēsis,* perspiration]

eu•gen•ic (yū-jen′ik). Relating to eugenics.

eu•gen•ics (yū-jen′iks). **1.** Practices and policies, as of mate selection or of sterilization, that tend to better the innate qualities of progeny and human stock. **2.** Practices and genetic counseling directed to anticipating genetic disability and disease. [G. *eugeneia,* nobility of birth, fr. *eu,* well, + *genesis,* production]

eu•glob•u•lin (yū-glob′yū-lin). That fraction of the serum globulin less soluble in $(NH_4)_2SO_4$ solution than the pseudoglobulin fraction.

eu•gly•ce•mia (yū-glī-sē′mē-ă). A normal blood glucose concentration. SYN normoglycemia. [eu- + G. *glykys,* sweet, + *haima,* blood]

eu•gly•ce•mic (yū-glī-sē′mik). Denoting, characteristic of, or promoting euglycemia. SYN normoglycemic.

eu•gna•thia (yū-nā′thē-ă, -nath′ē-ă). An abnormality that is limited to the teeth and their immediate alveolar supports. [eu- + G. *gnathos,* jaw]

eu•gon•ic (yū-gon′ik). A term used to indicate that the growth of a bacterial culture is rapid and relatively luxuriant; used especially in reference to the growth of cultures of the human tubercle bacillus (*Mycobacterium tuberculosis*). [G. *eugo-*

nos, productive, fr. *eu,* well, + *gonos,* seed, off-spring]

Eu·kar·y·o·tae, Eu·car·y·o·tae (yū-kar-ē-ō'tē). A superkingdom of organisms characterized by eukaryotic cells; acellular members (kingdom Protoctista) are characterized by a single eukaryotic unit; more complex (multicellular) members have been assigned to the kingdoms Fungi, Plantae, and Animalia.

eu·kar·y·ote (yū-kar'ē-ōt). **1.** A cell containing a membrane-bound nucleus with chromosomes of DNA, RNA, and proteins, with cell division involving a form of mitosis in which mitotic spindles (or some microtubule arrangement) are involved; mitochondria are present, and, in photosynthetic species, plastids are found. Possession of a e. type of cell characterizes the four kingdoms above the Monera or prokaryote level of complexity: Protoctista, Fungi, Plantae, and Animalia, combined into the superkingdom Eukaryotae. **2.** Common name for members of the Eukaryotae. [eu- + G. *karyon,* kernel, nut]

eu·kar·y·ot·ic (yū'kar-ē-ot'ik). Pertaining to or characteristic of a eukaryote.

eu·me·tria (yū-mē'trē-ă). Graduation of the strength of nerve impulses to match the need. [G. moderation, goodness of meter]

eu·nuch (yū'nŭk). A male whose testes have been removed or have never developed. [G. *eunouchos,* chamberlain, fr. *eunē,* bed, + *echō,* to have]

eu·nuch·oid (yū'nŭ-koyd). Resembling, or having the general characteristics of, a eunuch; usually indicating the physical habitus of a male in whom hypogonadism occurred before puberty. [G. *eunouchos,* eunuch, + *eidos,* resembling]

eu·nuch·oid·ism (yū'nŭ-koyd-izm). A state in which testes are present but fail to function normally; may be of gonadal or pituitary origin.

hypergonadotropic e., e. of gonadal origin, commonly accompanied by enhanced levels of pituitary gonadotropins in the blood and urine, as in Klinefelter's *syndrome.*

eu·pep·sia (yū-pep'sē-ă). Good digestion. [G., fr. *eu,* well, + *pepsis,* digestion]

eu·pep·tic (yū-pep'tik). Digesting well; having a good digestion.

eu·pep·tide (yū-pep'tīd). A peptide containing normal peptide bonds (between α-carboxyl groups and α-amino groups). Cf. peptide. [G. *eu-,* normal, usual + peptide]

eu·pho·ret·ic (yū-fō-ret'ik). SYN euphoriant.

eu·pho·ria (yū-fōr'ē-ă). A feeling of well-being, commonly exaggerated and not necessarily well founded. [eu- + G. *pherō,* to bear]

eu·pho·ri·ant (yū-fōr'ē-ant). **1.** Having the capability to produce a sense of well-being. **2.** An agent with such a capability. SYN euphoretic.

eu·ploid (yū'ployd). Relating to euploidy.

eu·ploidy (yū'ploy-dē). The state of a cell containing whole haploid sets. [eu- + G. *-ploos,* -fold]

eup·nea (yūp-nē'ă). Easy, free respiration; the type observed in a normal individual under resting conditions. [G. *eupnoia,* fr. *eu,* well, + *pnoia,* breath]

eu·prax·ia (yū-prak'sē-ă). Normal ability to per-form coordinated movements. [eu- + G. *praxis,* a doing]

eu·rhyth·mia (yū-rith'mē-ă). Harmonious body relationships of the separate organs. [eu- + G. *rhythmos,* rhythm]

eu·ro·pi·um (Eu) (yū-rō'pē-ŭm). An element of the rare earth (lanthanide) group, atomic no. 63, atomic wt. 151.965. [L. *Europa,* Europe]

△**eury-.** Broad, wide; opposite of steno-. [G. *eurys,* wide]

eu·ry·ce·phal·ic, eu·ry·ceph·a·lous (yū'rē-se-fal'ik, -sef'ă-lŭs). Having an abnormally broad head; sometimes used in reference to a brachycephalic head. [eury- + G. *kephalē,* head]

eu·ryg·nath·ic (yū-rig-nath'ik). Having a wide jaw.

eu·ry·on (yū'rē-on). The extremity, on either side, of the greatest transverse diameter of the head; a point used in craniometry. [G. *eurys,* broad]

eu·sta·chi·an (yū-stā'shŭn, yū-stā'kē-ăn). Described by or attributed to Bartolomeo Eustachio (1524–1574); usually referring to the auditory tube.

eu·sys·to·le (yū-sis'tō-lē). A condition in which the cardiac systole is normal in force and time. [eu- + systole]

eu·sys·tol·ic (yū-sis-tol'ik). Relating to eusystole.

eu·tha·na·sia (yū-thă-nā'zē-ă). **1.** The intentional putting to death of a person with an incurable or painful disease, intended as an act of mercy. **2.** A quiet, painless death. [eu- + G. *thanatos,* death]

eu·then·ics (yū-then'iks). The science concerned with establishing optimum living conditions for plants, animals, or humans, especially through proper provisioning and environment. [G. *eutheneō,* to thrive]

eu·ther·mic (yū-ther'mik). At an optimal temperature. [eu- + G. *thermos,* warm]

eu·ton·ic (yū-ton'ik). SYN normotonic (1). [eu- + G. *tonos,* tone]

eu·tro·phia (yū-trō'fē-ă). A state of normal nourishment and growth. [G. fr. *eu,* well, + *trophē,* nourishment]

eu·tro·phic (yū-trof'ik). Relating to, characterized by, or promoting eutrophia.

eV, ev electron-volt.

evac·u·ant (ē-vak'yū-ant). **1.** Promoting an excretion, especially of the bowels. **2.** An agent that increases excretion, especially a cathartic.

evac·u·a·tion (ē-vak-yū-ā'shŭn). **1.** Removal of material, especially wastes from the bowels by defecation. **2.** SYN stool (2). **3.** Removal of air from a closed vessel; production of a vacuum.

evac·u·a·tor (ē-vak'yū-ā-tŏr). A mechanical evacuant; an instrument for the removal of fluid or small particles from a body cavity, or of impacted feces from the rectum.

evag·i·na·tion (ē-vaj-i-nā'shŭn). Protrusion of some part or organ from its normal position. [L. *e,* out, + *vagina,* sheath]

ev·a·nes·cent (ev-ă-nes'ent). Of short duration. [L. *e,* out, + *vanesco,* to vanish]

Evans blue [C.I. 23860]. A diazo dye used for the determination of the blood volume on the basis of the dilution of a standard solution of the

Ev

dye in the plasma after its intravenous injection; it binds to proteins and is also used as a vital stain for following diffusion through blood vessel walls.

e•vap•o•rate (ē-vap′ōr-āt). To cause or undergo evaporation.

evap•o•ra•tion (ē-vap-ŏ-ra′shŭn). **1.** A change from liquid to vapor form. **2.** Loss of volume of a liquid by conversion into vapor. SYN volatilization. [L. *e*, out, + *vaporo*, to emit vapor]

event. An incident or occurrence; anything that happens.

    adverse drug e., SYN adverse drug *reaction.*

even•tra•tion (ē′ven-trā′shŭn). **1.** Protrusion of omentum and/or intestine through an opening in the abdominal wall. SYN evisceration (3). **2.** Removal of the contents of the abdominal cavity. [L. *e*, out, + *venter*, belly]

    e. of the diaphragm, extreme elevation of a half or part of the diaphragm, which is usually atrophic and abnormally thin.

ever•sion (ē-ver′zhŭn). A turning outward, as of the eyelid or foot. [L. *e-everto*, pp. *-versus*, to overturn]

evert (ē-vert′). To turn outward. [L. *e-verto*, to overturn]

evis•cer•a•tion (ē-vis-er-ā′shŭn). **1.** SYN exenteration. **2.** Removal of the contents of the eyeball, leaving the sclera and sometimes the cornea. **3.** SYN eventration (1). [L. *eviscero*, to disembowel]

evo•ca•tion (ev-ō-kā′shŭn, ē-vō-kā′shŭn). Induction of a particular tissue produced by the action of an evocator during embryogenesis. [L. *evoco*, pp. *evocatus*, to call forth, evoke]

evo•ca•tor (ev′ō-kā-ter, -tōr). A factor in the control of morphogenesis in the early embryo.

ev•o•lu•tion (ev-ō-lū′shŭn). **1.** A continuing process of change from one state, condition or form to another. **2.** A progressive distancing between the genotype and the phenotype in a line of descent. [L. *e-volvo*, pp. *-volutus*, to roll out]

    biologic e., the doctrine that all forms of animal or plant life have been derived by gradual changes from simpler forms and ultimately unicellular organisms. SYN organic e.

    convergent e., the evolutionary development of similar structures in two or more species, often widely separated phylogenetically, in response to similarities of environment; for example, the wings in insects, birds, and flying mammals.

    Darwinian e., the proposition that the phylogeny of all species is wholly ascribable to random variation (mutation) in genotypes and the operation of preferential survival of those resulting phenotypes most suited to survive in the contemporary environment.

    organic e., SYN biologic e.

    saltatory e., the theory that e. of a new species from an older one may occur as a large jump, such as a major repatterning of chromosomes, rather than by gradual accumulation of small steps or mutations.

evul•sion (ē-vŭl′shŭn). A forcible pulling out or extraction. Cf. avulsion. [L. *evulsio*, fr. *e-vello*, pp. *-vulsus*, to pluck out]

△**ex-.** Out of, from, away from. [L. and G. out of]

△**exa- (E).** Prefix used in the SI and metric systems to signify one quintillion (10^{18}).

ex•ac•er•ba•tion (eg-zas-er-bā′shŭn, -ek-sas-). An increase in the severity of a disease or any of its signs or symptoms. [L. *ex- acerbo*, pp. *-atus*, to exasperate, increase, fr. *acerbus*, sour]

ex•am•i•na•tion (eg-zam-i-nā′shŭn). Any investigation or inspection made for the purpose of diagnosis; usually qualified by the method used.

    fiberoptic endoscopic e. of swallowing (FEES), a diagnostic technique for evaluation of deviant swallowing patterns, using a transnasal fiberoptic endoscope to visualize the larynx and pharynx. SEE ALSO fiberoptics, endoscope.

ex•an•them (eg-zan′them). SYN exanthema.

ex•an•the•ma (eg-zan-thē′mă). A skin eruption occurring as a symptom of an acute viral or coccal disease, as in scarlet fever or measles. SYN exanthem. [G. efflorescence, an eruption, fr. *anthos*, flower]

    keratoid e., a symptom occurring in the secondary stage of yaws: patches of fine, light colored, furfuraceous desquamation, scattered irregularly over limbs and trunk.

    e. sub′itum, a disease due to herpes virus-6 of infants and young children, marked by sudden onset with fever lasting several days (sometimes with convulsions) and followed by a fine macular (sometimes maculopapular) rash that appears within a few hours to a day after the fever has subsided. SYN roseola infantilis, roseola infantum, sixth disease.

ex•an•them•a•tous (eg-zan-them′ă-tŭs). Relating to an exanthema.

ex•ar•tic•u•la•tion (eks-ar-tik-yū-lā′shŭn). SYN disarticulation. [L. *ex*, out, + *articulus*, joint]

ex•cal•a•tion (eks-kă-lā′shŭn). Absence, suppression, or failure of development of one of a series of structures, as of a digit or vertebra. [G. *ex*, from, + *chalaō*, to abate, release]

ex•ca•va•tio (eks-kă-vā′shē-ō) [NA]. SYN excavation (1). [L. fr. *ex-cavo*, pp. *-cavatus*, to hollow out, fr. *ex*, out, + *cavus*, hollow]

    e. rectouteri′na [NA], SYN rectouterine *pouch.*

    e. rectovesica′lis [NA], SYN rectovesical *pouch.*

ex•ca•va•tion (eks-kă-vā′shŭn). **1.** A natural cavity, pouch, or recess. SYN excavatio [NA]. **2.** A cavity formed artificially or as the result of a pathologic process.

    atrophic e., an exaggeration of the normal or physiologic cupping of the optic disk caused by atrophy of the optic nerve.

    glaucomatous e., SYN glaucomatous *cup.*

    e. of optic disc, the normally occurring depression or pit in the center of the optic disc.

ex•ca•va•tor (eks′că-vā-tŏr, -tŏr). **1.** An instrument like a large sharp spoon or scoop, used in scraping out pathologic tissue. **2.** DENTISTRY An instrument, generally a small spoon or curette, for cleaning out and shaping a carious cavity preparatory to filling.

ex•ce•men•to•sis (ek′sē-men-tō′sis). A nodular outgrowth of cementum on the root surface of a tooth.

ex•cen•tric (ek-sen′trik). Alternative spelling for eccentric (2, 3).

ex•cess (ek'ses). That which is more than the usual or specified amount.

   antibody e., in a precipitation test, the presence of antibody in an amount greater than that required to combine with all of the antigen present.

   antigen e., (1) in a precipitation test, the presence of uncombined antigen above that required to combine with all of the antibody; (2) *in vivo* the resultant antigen-antibody interaction in such an antigen e. may give rise to immune complexes, which have a potential to induce cellular damage.

   base e., a measure of metabolic alkalosis; the amount of strong acid that would have to be added per unit volume of whole blood to titrate it to pH 7.4 while at 37°C and at a carbon dioxide pressure of 40 mm Hg.

   convergence e., that condition in which an esophoria or esotropia is greater for near vision than for far vision.

   negative base e., a measure of metabolic acidosis; the amount of strong alkali that would have to be added per unit volume of whole blood to titrate it to pH 7.4 while at 37°C and at a carbon dioxide pressure of 40 mm Hg.

ex•change (eks-chānj'). To substitute one thing for another, or the act of such substitution.

ex•cip•i•ent (ek-sip'ē-ent). A more or less inert substance added in a prescription as a diluent or vehicle or to give form or consistency when the remedy is given in pill form. [L. *excipiens;* pres. p. of *ex- cipio,* to take out]

ex•cise (ek-sīz'). To cut out. SEE ALSO resect.

ex•ci•sion (ek-sizh'ŭn). 1. The act of cutting out; the surgical removal of part or all of a structure or organ. SYN resection (2). SEE ALSO resection. 2. MOLECULAR BIOLOGY A recombination event in which a genetic element is removed. SYN exeresis. [L. *excido,* to cut out]

   loop e., a diagnostic and therapeutic gynecological surgical technique for removing dysplastic cells from the cervix with a small wire loop.

ex•cit•a•bil•i•ty (ek-sī'tă-bil'i-tē). Having the capability of being excited.

   supranormal e., at the end of phase three of the cardiac action potential, the successful stimulation threshold falls below (*i.e.,* less negative than) the level necessary to produce excitation during the rest of the phase of diastole, so that an ordinary subthreshold stimulus becomes effective.

ex•cit•a•ble (ek-sī'tă-bl). 1. Capable of quick response to a stimulus; having potentiality for emotional arousal. Cf. irritable. 2. NEUROPHYSIOLOGY Referring to a tissue, cell, or membrane capable of undergoing excitation in response to an adequate stimulus.

ex•ci•ta•tion (ek-sī-tā'shŭn). 1. The act of increasing the rapidity or intensity of physical or mental processes. 2. NEUROPHYSIOLOGY The complete all-or-none response of a nerve or muscle to an adequate stimulus, ordinarily including propagation of e. along the membranes of the cell or cells involved. SEE ALSO stimulation.

ex•cite•ment (ek-sīt'ment). An emotional state sometimes characterized by its potential for impulsive or poorly controlled activity.

ex•ci•to•mo•tor (ek-sī'tō-mō'ter). Causing or increasing the rapidity of motion. SYN centrokinetic (2).

ex•clave (eks-klāv'). An outlying, detached portion of a gland or other part, such as the thyroid or pancreas; an accessory gland. [L. *ex,* out, + -*clave* (in enclave)]

ex•clu•sion (eks-klū'zhŭn). A shutting out; disconnection from the main portion. [L. *ex- cludo,* pp. -*clusus,* to shut out]

ex•co•ri•ate (eks-kō'rē-āt). To scratch or otherwise denude the skin by physical means.

ex•co•ri•a•tion (eks-kō'rē-ā'shŭn). A scratch mark; a linear break in the skin surface, usually covered with blood or serous crusts. [L. *excorio,* to skin, strip, fr. *corium,* skin, hide]

ex•cre•ment (eks'krĕ-ment). Waste matter or any excretion cast out of the body; *e.g.,* feces. [L. *excerno,* pp. -*cretus,* to separate]

ex•cre•men•ti•tious (eks'krē-men-tish'ŭs). Relating to any excrement.

ex•cres•cence (eks-kres'ens). Any outgrowth from a surface. [L. *ex- cresco,* pp. -*cretus,* to grow forth]

ex•cre•ta (eks-krē'tă). SYN excretion (2). [L. neut. pl. of *excretus,* pp. of *ex-cerno,* to separate]

ex•crete (eks-krēt'). To separate from the blood and cast out; to perform excretion.

ex•cre•tion (eks-krē'shŭn). 1. The process whereby the undigested residue of food and the waste products of metabolism are eliminated, material is removed to regulate the composition of body fluids and tissues, or substances are expelled to perform functions on an exterior surface. 2. The product of a tissue or organ that is material to be passed out of the body. SYN excreta. Cf. secretion. [see excrement]

ex•cre•to•ry (eks'krē-tō-rē). Relating to excretion.

ex•cy•clo•pho•ria (ek-sī-klō-fō'rē-ă). A cyclophoria in which the upper poles of each cornea tend to rotate laterally. [ex- + cyclo- + G. *phora,* a carrying]

ex•cys•ta•tion (ek-sis-tā'shŭn). The action of an encysted organism in escaping from its envelope.

ex•e•mia (ek-sē'mē-ă). A condition, as in shock, in which a considerable portion of the blood is removed from the main circulation but remains within blood vessels in certain areas where it is stagnant. [G. *ex,* out of, + *haima,* blood]

ex•en•ce•phal•ic (eks'en-se-fal'ik). Relating to exencephaly.

ex•en•ceph•a•ly (eks-en-sef'ă-lē). Condition in which the skull is defective with the brain exposed or extruding. [G. *ex,* out, + *enkephalos,* brain]

ex•en•ter•a•tion (eks-en-ter-ā'shŭn). Removal of internal organs and tissues, usually radical removal of the contents of a body cavity. SYN evisceration (1). [G. *ex,* out, + *enteron,* bowel]

ex•en•ter•i•tis (eks-en-ter-ī'tis). Inflammation of the peritoneal covering of the intestine. [G. *exō,* on the outside, + enteritis]

ex•er•cise (ek'ser-sīz). 1. *Active:* bodily exertion for the sake of restoring the organs and functions to a healthy state or keeping them healthy. 2.

Passive: motion of limbs without effort by the patient.

isometric e., e. consisting of muscular contractions without movement of the involved parts of the body.

progressive-resistance e. (PRE), the practical application of the overload principle in order to improve muscular strength and size. Resistance is gradually and continually increased to keep pace with strength gains as training progresses.

ex·er·e·sis (ek-ser′ĕ-sis). SYN excision. [G. *exairesis,* a taking out, fr. *haireō,* to take, grasp]

ex·er·gon·ic (ek-ser-gon′ik). Referring to a chemical reaction that takes place with release of Gibbs free energy to its surroundings. Cf. endergonic. [exo- + G. *ergon,* work]

ex·fo·li·a·tion (eks-fō-lē-ā′shŭn). **1.** Detachment and shedding of superficial cells from any tissue surface. **2.** Scaling or desquamation of the horny layer of epidermis. **3.** Loss of deciduous teeth following physiological loss of root structure. [Mod. L. fr. L. *ex,* out, + *folium,* leaf]

ex·fo·li·a·tive (eks-fō′lē-ā-tiv). Marked by exfoliation, desquamation, or profuse scaling. [Mod. L. *exfoliativus*]

ex·ha·la·tion (eks-hă-lā′shŭn). **1.** Breathing out. SYN expiration (1). **2.** The giving forth of gas or vapor. **3.** Any exhaled or emitted gas or vapor. [L. *ex-halo,* pp. *-halatus,* to breathe out]

ex·hale (eks′hāl). **1.** To breathe out. SYN expire (1). **2.** To emit a gas, vapor, or odor.

ex·haus·tion (eg-zos′chŭn). **1.** Extreme fatigue; inability to respond to stimuli. **2.** Removal of contents; using up of a supply of anything. **3.** Extraction of the active constituents of a drug by treating with water, alcohol, or other solvent. [L. *ex-haurio,* pp. *-haustus,* to draw out, empty]

heat e., a form of reaction to heat, marked by prostration, weakness, and collapse, resulting from severe dehydration.

ex·hi·bi·tion·ism (ek-si-bish′ŭn-izm). A morbid compulsion to expose a part of the body, especially the genitals, with the intent of provoking sexual interest in the viewer.

ex·hi·bi·tion·ist (ek-si-bish′ŭn-ist). One who engages in exhibitionism.

△**exo-.** Exterior, external, or outward. SEE ALSO ecto-. [G. *exō,* outside]

ex·o·an·ti·gen (ek-sō-an′ti-jen). SYN ectoantigen.

ex·o·car·dia (ek-sō-kar′dē-ă). SYN ectocardia.

ex·o·crine (ek′sō-krin). **1.** Denoting glandular secretion delivered to an apical or luminal surface. SYN eccrine (1). **2.** Denoting a gland that secretes outwardly through excretory ducts. [exo- + G. *krinō,* to separate]

ex·o·cy·to·sis (ek′sō-sī-to′sis). **1.** The appearance of migrating inflammatory cells in the epidermis. **2.** The process whereby secretory granules or droplets are released from a cell; the membrane around the granule fuses with the cell membrane, which ruptures, and the secretion is discharged. SYN emeiocytosis, emiocytosis. Cf. endocytosis. [exo- + G. *kytos,* cell, + *-osis,* condition]

ex·o·de·vi·a·tion (ek′sō-dē-vē-ā′shŭn). **1.** SYN exophoria. **2.** SYN exotropia.

ex·o·don·tia (ek-sō-don′shē-ă). The branch of dental practice concerned with the extraction of teeth. [exo- + G. *odous,* tooth]

ex·o·don·tist (ek-sō-don′tist). One who specializes in the extraction of teeth.

ex·o·en·zyme (ek-sō-en′zīm). SYN extracellular *enzyme.*

ex·og·a·my (ek-sog′ă-mē). Sexual reproduction by means of conjugation of two gametes of different ancestry, as in certain protozoan species. [exo- + G. *gamos,* marriage]

ex·o·gas·tru·la (eks-ō-gas′trū-lă). An abnormal embryo in which the primitive gut has been everted.

ex·og·e·nous (eks-oj′ĕ-nŭs). Originating or produced outside of the organism. SYN ectogenous. [exo- + G. *-gen,* production]

ex·om·pha·los (eks-om′fă-lŭs). **1.** Protrusion of the umbilicus. SYN exumbilication (1). **2.** SYN umbilical *hernia.* **3.** SYN omphalocele. [G. *ex,* out, + *omphalos,* umbilicus]

ex·on (ek′son). A portion of a DNA that codes for a section of the mature messenger RNA from that DNA, and is therefore expressed ("translated" into protein) at the ribosome. [ex- + on]

ex·o·nu·cle·ase (ek-sō-nū′klē-ās). A nuclease that releases one nucleotide at a time, serially, beginning at one end of a polynucleotide (nucleic acid). Cf. endonuclease.

ex·o·pep·ti·dase (ek-sō-pep′ti-dās). An enzyme that catalyzes the hydrolysis of the terminal amino acid of a peptide chain; *e.g.,* carboxypeptidase. Cf. endopeptidase.

Ex·o·phi·a·la (ek-sō-fī′ă-lă). A genus of pathogenic fungi having dematiaceous conidiophores. They cause mycetoma or phaeohyphomycosis; in cases of mycetoma, black granules develop in subcutaneous abscesses; in cases of phaeohyphomycosis, sclerotic bodies are found in tissues. [*exo* + G. *phialē,* a broad flat vessel]

E. jeansel′mei, a species found in cases of mycetoma or phaeohyphomycosis.

E. wernec′kii, a species that causes tinea nigra.

ex·o·pho·ria (ek′so-fō′rē-ă). Tendency of the eyes to deviate outward when fusion is suspended. SYN exodeviation (1). [exo- + G. *phora,* a carrying]

ex·o·phor·ic (ek-sō-fōr′ik). Relating to exophoria.

ex·oph·thal·mic (ek-sof-thal′mik). Relating to exophthalmos; marked by prominence of the eyeball.

ex·oph·thal·mom·e·ter (ek-sof-thal-mom′ĕ-ter). An instrument to measure the distance between the anterior pole of the eye and a fixed reference point, often the zygomatic bone. [exophthalmos + G. *metron,* measure]

ex·oph·thal·mos, ex·oph·thal·mus (ek-sof-thal′mos). Protrusion of one or both eyeballs; can be congenital and familial, or due to pathology, such as a retro-orbital tumor (usually unilateral) or thyroid disease (usually bilateral). SYN proptosis. [G. *ex,* out, + *ophthalmos,* eye]

ex·o·phyte (ek′sō-fīt). An exterior or external plant parasite. [exo- + G. *phyton,* plant]

ex·o·phyt·ic (ek-sō-fit′ik). **1.** Pertaining to an exophyte. **2.** Denoting a neoplasm or lesion that grows outward from an epithelial surface.

ex•o•se•ro•sis (ek′sō-se-rō′sis). Serous exudation from the skin surface, as in eczema or abrasions.

ex•o•skel•e•ton (ek-sō-skel′ĕ-tŏn). **1.** All hard parts, such as hair, teeth, nails, feathers, dermal plates, scales, etc., developed from the ectoderm or somatic mesoderm in vertebrates. **2.** Outer chitinous envelope of an insect, certain Crustacea, and other invertebrates.

ex•os•to•sis, pl. **ex•os•to•ses** (eks-os-tō′sis, -sēz). A cartilage-capped bony projection arising from any bone that develops from cartilage. SEE ALSO osteochondroma. SYN hyperostosis (2), poroma (2). [exo- + G. *osteon*, bone, + *-osis*, condition]

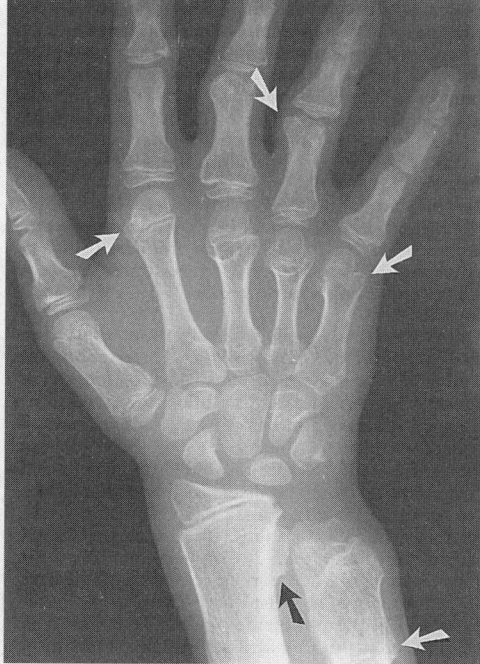

exostosis: multiple small osteochondromas (arrows)

ex•o•ter•ic (ek-sō-tār′ik). Of external origin; arising outside the organism. [G. *exōterikos*, outer]

ex•o•ther•mic (ek-sō-ther′mik). **1.** Denoting a chemical reaction during which heat (*i.e.*, enthalpy) is emitted. Cf. endothermic. **2.** Relating to the external warmth of the body. [exo- + G. *thermē*, heat]

ex•o•tox•ic (ek-sō-tok′sik). **1.** Relating to an exotoxin. **2.** Relating to the introduction of an exogenous poison or toxin.

ex•o•tox•in (ek-sō-tok′sin). A specific, soluble, antigenic, usually heat labile, injurious substance elaborated by certain bacteria; it is formed within the cell, but is released into the environment where it is rapidly active in extremely small amounts; most e.'s are protein in nature. SYN extracellular toxin.

ex•o•tro•pia (ek-sō-trō′pē-ă). That type of strabismus in which the visual axes diverge; may be paralytic or concomitant, monocular or alternating, constant or intermittent. SYN divergent strabismus, exodeviation (2), wall-eye (1). [exo- + G. *tropē*, turn]

ex•pan•sion (eks-pan′shŭn). **1.** An increase in size as of chest or lungs. **2.** The spreading out of any structure, as a tendon. **3.** An expanse; a wide area. [L. *ex-pando*, pp. *-pansus*, to spread out]

ex•pec•to•rant (ek-spek′tō-rănt). **1.** Promoting secretion from the mucous membrane of the air passages or facilitating its expulsion. **2.** An agent that increases bronchial secretion and facilitates its expulsion. [L. *ex*, out, + *pectus*, chest]

ex•pec•to•rate (ek-spek′tō-rāt). To spit; to eject saliva, mucus, or other fluid from the mouth.

ex•pec•to•ra•tion (ek-spek-tō-rā′shŭn). **1.** Mucus and other fluids formed in the air passages and upper food passages (the mouth), and expelled by coughing. SEE ALSO sputum (1). **2.** The act of spitting; the expelling from the mouth of saliva, mucus, and other material from the air or upper food passages.

ex•pe•ri•ence (ek-spēr′ē-ens). The feeling of emotions and sensations, as opposed to thinking; involvement in what is happening rather than abstract reflection on an event or interpersonal encounter. [L. *experientia*, fr. *experior*, to try]

ex•per•i•ment (eks-per′i-ment). **1.** A study in which the investigator intentionally alters one or more factors under controlled conditions in order to study the effects of doing so. **2.** MAGNETIC RESONANCE The term applied to a pulse sequence. [L. *experimentum*, fr. *experior*, to test, try]

  control e., an e. used to check another, to verify the result, or to demonstrate what would have occurred had the factor under study been omitted. SEE ALSO control.

  double blind e., an e. conducted with neither experimenter nor subjects knowing which e. is the control; prevents bias in recording results. SEE ALSO double-masked e.

  double-masked e., a double-blind study conducted so that neither the subject nor the observer knows the identity of the control or variable.

  factorial e.'s, an experimental design in which two or more series of treatments are tried in all combinations.

ex•pi•ra•tion (eks-pi-rā′shŭn). **1.** SYN exhalation (1). **2.** Death. [L. *expiro* or *ex-spiro*, pp. *-atus*, to breathe out]

ex•pi•ra•to•ry (ek-spī′ră-tō-rē). Relating to expiration.

ex•pire (ek-spīr′). **1.** SYN exhale (1). **2.** To die.

ex•plant (eks′plant). Living tissue transferred from an organism to an artificial medium for culture.

ex•plo•ra•tion (eks-plōr-ā′shŭn). An active examination, usually involving endoscopy or a surgical procedure, to ascertain conditions present as an aid in diagnosis. [L. *ex-ploro*, pp. *-ploratus*, to explore]

ex•plor•a•to•ry (eks-plōr′ă-tōr-ē). Relating to, or with a view to, exploration.

ex•plor•er (ek′splōr′er). A sharp pointed probe used to investigate natural or restored tooth surfaces in order to detect caries or other defects.

ex•press (eks-pres′). To press or squeeze out. [L. *ex-premo,* pp. *-pressus,* to press out]

ex•pres•sion (eks-presh′ŭn). **1.** Squeezing out; expelling by pressure. **2.** Mobility of the features giving a particular emotional significance to the face. SYN facies (3). **3.** Any act by an individual. **4.** Something that manifests something else.

gene e., (1) the detectable effect of a gene. (2) appearance of an inherited trait; for many reasons, a gene may not be expressed at all.

ex•pul•sive (eks-pŭl′siv). Tending to expel. [L. *ex-pello,* pp. *-pulsus,* to drive out]

ex•qui•site (eks-kwiz′it). Extremely intense, keen, sharp; said of pain or tenderness. [L. *exquiro,* pp. *exquisitus,* to search out]

ex•san•gui•nate (ek-sang′gwi-nāt). **1.** To remove or withdraw the circulating blood; to make bloodless. **2.** SYN exsanguine. [L. *ex,* out, + *sanguis* (*-guin*), blood]

ex•san•gui•na•tion (ek-sang′gwi-nā′shŭn). Removal of blood; making exsanguine.

ex•san•guine (ek-sang′gwin). Deprived of blood. SYN exsanguinate (2).

ex•sic•cant (ek-sik′ant). SYN desiccant.

ex•sic•cate (ek′si-kāt). SYN desiccate.

ex•sic•ca•tion (ek-si-kā′shŭn). **1.** SYN desiccation. **2.** The removal of water of crystallization. SYN dehydration (3). [L. *ex sicco,* pp. *siccatus,* to dry up]

ex•sorp•tion (ek-sōrp′shŭn). Movement of substances from the blood into the lumen of the gut. [L. *ex,* out, + *sorbeo,* to suck]

ex•stro•phy (ek′strō-fē). Congenital eversion of a hollow organ. [G. *ex,* out, + *strophē,* a turning]

e. of the bladder, a congenital gap in the anterior wall of the bladder and the abdominal wall in front of it, the posterior wall of the bladder being exposed.

ex•tend (eks-tend′). To straighten a limb, to diminish or extinguish the angle formed by flexion; to place the distal segment of a limb in such a position that its axis is continuous with that of the proximal segment. [L. *ex- tendo,* pp. *-tensus,* to stretch out]

ex•ten•sion (eks-ten′shŭn). **1.** The act of bringing the distal portion of a joint in continuity with the long axis of the proximal portion. **2.** A pulling or dragging force exerted on a limb in a distal direction. [L. *extensio,* a stretching out]

Buck's e., apparatus for applying longitudinal skin traction on the leg through contact between the skin and adhesive tape.

joint e., SYN close pack *position.*

skeletal e., SYN skeletal *traction.*

ex•ten•sor (eks-ten′ser, -sōr) [NA]. A muscle the contraction of which causes movement at a joint with the consequence that the limb or body assumes a more straight line, or so that the distance between the parts proximal and distal to the joint is increased or extended; the antagonist of a flexor. SEE muscle. [L. one who stretches, fr. *extendo,* to stretch out]

ex•te•ri•or•ize (eks-tēr′ē-ōr-īz). **1.** To direct interests, thoughts, or feelings into a channel leading outside the self, to some definite aim or object. **2.** To expose an organ temporarily for observation, or permanently for purposes of physiologic experiment.

ex•tern (eks′tern). An advanced student or recent graduate who assists in the medical or surgical care of hospital patients. [F. *externe,* outside, a day scholar]

ex•ter•nal (eks-ter′năl). On the outside or farther from the center; often incorrectly used to mean lateral. [L. *externus*]

ex•ter•o•cep•tive (eks′ter-ō-sep′tiv). Relating to the exteroceptors; denoting the surface of the body containing the end organs adapted to receive impressions or stimuli from without. [L. *exterus,* outside, + *capio,* to take]

ex•ter•o•cep•tor (eks′ter-ō-sep′ter, -tōr). One of the peripheral end organs of the afferent nerves in the skin or mucous membrane, which respond to stimulation by external agents. [L. *exterus,* external, + *receptor,* receiver]

ex•ter•o•fec•tive (eks′ter-ō-fek′tiv). Pertaining to the response of the nervous system to external stimuli. [L. *extero,* from outside, + *affectus,* affected]

ex•tinc•tion (eks-tingk′shŭn). **1.** In behavior modification or classical or operant conditioning, a progressive decrease in the frequency of a response that is not positively reinforced. SEE conditioning. **2.** SYN absorbance. [L. *extinguo,* to quench]

specific e., SYN specific absorption *coefficient.*

ex•tin•guish (eks-ting′gwish). **1.** To abolish; to quench, as a flame; to cause loss of identity; to destroy. **2.** PSYCHOLOGY To abolish a conditioned response. SEE conditioning. [L. *extinguo,* to quench]

ex•tir•pa•tion (eks-tir-pā′shŭn). Complete removal of an organ or diseased tissue. [L. *extirpo,* to root out, fr. *stirps,* a stalk, root]

ex•tor•sion (eks-tōr′shŭn). **1.** Outward rotation of a limb or of an organ. **2.** Conjugate rotation of the upper poles of each cornea outward. [L. *extorsio,* fr. *ex- torqueo,* to twist out]

△**ex•tra-.** Without, outside of. [L.]

ex•tra•cel•lu•lar (eks-tră-sel′yū-lăr). Outside the cells.

ex•tra•cor•po•re•al (eks′tră-kōr-pō′rē-ăl). Outside of, or unrelated to, the body or any anatomical "corpus."

ex•tract. **1** (ek′strakt). A concentrated preparation of a drug obtained by removing the active constituents with suitable solvents, evaporating all or nearly all of the solvent, and adjusting the residual mass or powder to the prescribed standard. **2** (ek-strakt′). To remove part of a mixture with a solvent. **3.** To perform extraction. [L. *extraho,* pp. *-tractus,* to draw out]

allergenic e., e. (usually containing protein) from various sources, *e.g.,* food, bacteria, pollen, and the like, suspected of in stimulating manifestations of allergy; may be used for skin testing or desensitization. SYN allergic e.

allergic e., SYN allergenic e.

ex•trac•tion (ek-strak′shŭn). **1.** Luxation and removal of a tooth from its alveolus. **2.** Partitioning of material (solute) into a solvent. **3.** The active portion of a drug; the making of an extract. **4.** Surgical removal by pulling out. **5.** Removal of the fetus from the uterus or vagina at or near the end of pregnancy, either manually or with instruments. **6.** Removal by suction of the product of conception before a menstrual period has been missed. [L. *ex-traho,* pp. *-tractus,* to draw out]

   serial e., selective e. of certain teeth during the early years of dental development, usually with the eventual e. of the first, or occasionally the second, premolars, to relieve crowding of anterior teeth.

ex·trac·tives (ek-strak′tivs). Substances present in vegetable or animal tissue that can be separated by successive treatment with solvents and recovered by evaporation of the solution.

ex·trac·tor (ek-strak′ter, tōr). Instrument for use in drawing or pulling out any natural part, as a tooth, or a foreign body.

ex·tra·cys·tic (eks-tră-sis′tik). Outside of, or unrelated to, the gallbladder or urinary bladder or any cystic tumor.

ex·tra·em·bry·on·ic (eks′tră-em-brē-on′ik). Outside the embryonic body; *e.g.,* those membranes involved with the embryo's protection and nutrition which are discarded at birth without being incorporated in its body.

ex·tra·phys·i·o·log·ic (eks′tră-fiz-ē-ō-loj′ik). Outside of the domain of physiology; more than physiologic, therefore pathologic.

ex·tra·sen·so·ry (eks-tră-sen′sōr-ē). Outside or beyond the ordinary senses; not limited to the senses, as in extrasensory *perception.*

ex·tra·sys·to·le (eks′tră-sis′tō-lē). An ectopic beat from any source in the heart. SYN premature systole.

   atrial e., a premature contraction of the heart arising from an ectopic atrial focus.

   atrioventricular e., A-V e., an e. arising from the "junctional" tissues, either the A-V node or A-V bundle.

   atrioventricular nodal e., A-V nodal e., a premature beat arising from the A-V junction and leading to a simultaneous or almost simultaneous contraction of atria and ventricles.

   infranodal e., SYN ventricular e.

   interpolated e., a ventricular e. which, instead of being followed by a compensatory pause, is sandwiched between two consecutive sinus cycles.

   return e., a form of reciprocal rhythm in which the impulse having arisen in the ventricle ascends toward the atria, but before reaching the atria is reflected to the ventricles to produce a second ventricular contraction.

   ventricular e., a premature contraction of the ventricle. SYN infranodal e.

ex·trav·a·sate (eks-trav′ă-sāt). **1.** To exude from or pass out of a vessel into the tissues, said of blood, lymph, or urine. **2.** The substance thus exuded. SYN extravasation (2), suffusion (4). [L. *extra,* out of, + *vas,* vessel]

ex·trav·a·sa·tion (eks-trav′ă-sā′shŭn). **1.** The act of extravasating. **2.** SYN extravasate (2). [extra- + L. *vas,* vessel]

ex·tra·ver·sion (eks-tră-ver′zhŭn, -shŭn). SYN extroversion.

ex·trem·i·tas (eks-trem′i-tas) [NA]. SYN extremity. SEE limb. [L. fr. *extremus,* last, outermost]

ex·trem·i·ty (eks-trem′i-tē). One of the ends of an elongated or pointed structure. Incorrectly used to mean limb. SYN extremitas [NA].

   lower e., SYN lower *limb.*

   upper e., SYN upper *limb.*

ex·trin·sic (eks-trin′sik). Originating outside of the part where found or upon which it acts; denoting especially a muscle, such as extrinsic muscles of hand. [L. *extrinsecus,* from without]

ex·tro·ver·sion (eks′trō-ver′zhŭn, -shŭn). **1.** A turning outward. **2.** A trait involving social intercourse, as practiced by an extrovert. Cf. introversion. SYN extraversion. [incorrectly formed fr. L. *extra,* outside, + *verto,* pp. *versus,* to turn]

ex·tro·vert, ex·tra·vert (eks′trō-vert). A gregarious person whose chief interests lie outside the self, and who is socially self-confident and involved in the affairs of others. Cf. introvert.

ex·trude (eks-trūd′). To thrust, force, or press out.

ex·tru·sion (eks-trū′zhŭn). **1.** A thrusting or forcing out of a normal position. **2.** The overeruption or migration of a tooth beyond its normal occlusal position.

ex·tu·ba·tion (eks′tū-bā′shŭn). Removal of a tube from an organ, structure, or orifice. [L. *ex,* out, + *tuba,* tube]

ex·u·ber·ant (ek-zū′ber-ănt). Denoting excessive proliferation or growth, as of granulation tissue. [L. *exubero,* to abound, be abundant]

ex·u·date (eks′ū-dāt). Any fluid that has exuded out of a tissue or its capillaries because of injury or inflammation. Cf. transudate. SYN exudation (2). [L. *ex,* out, + *sudo,* to sweat]

ex·u·da·tion (eks-ū-dā′shŭn). **1.** The act or process of exuding. **2.** SYN exudate.

ex·ud·a·tive (eks-ū′dă-tiv). Relating to the process of exudation or to an exudate.

ex·ude (ek-zūd′). In general, to ooze or pass gradually out of a body structure or tissue. [L. *ex,* out, + *sudo,* to sweat]

ex·um·bil·i·ca·tion (eks′ŭm-bil-i-kā′shŭn). **1.** SYN exomphalos (1). **2.** SYN umbilical *hernia.* **3.** SYN omphalocele. [L. *ex,* out, + *umbilicus,* navel]

eye (ī). **1.** The organ of vision that consists of the eyeball and the optic nerve; SYN oculus [NA]. **2.** The area of the eye, including lids and other accessory organs of the eye; the contents of the orbit (common). [A.S. *eage*]

   aphakic e., the e. from which the lens is absent.

   black e., ecchymosis of the lids and their surroundings.

   crossed e.'s, SYN strabismus.

   dark-adapted e., an e. that has been in darkness or semidarkness and has undergone regeneration of rhodopsin (visual purple), which renders it more sensitive to reduced illumination. SYN scotopic e.

   dominant e., the e. that is customarily used for monocular tasks.

   exciting e., the injured e. in sympathetic ophthalmia.

   light-adapted e., an e. that has been exposed to light, with bleaching of rhodopsin (visual purple) and insensitivity to low illumination. SYN photopic e.

   phakic e., an e. containing the natural lens.

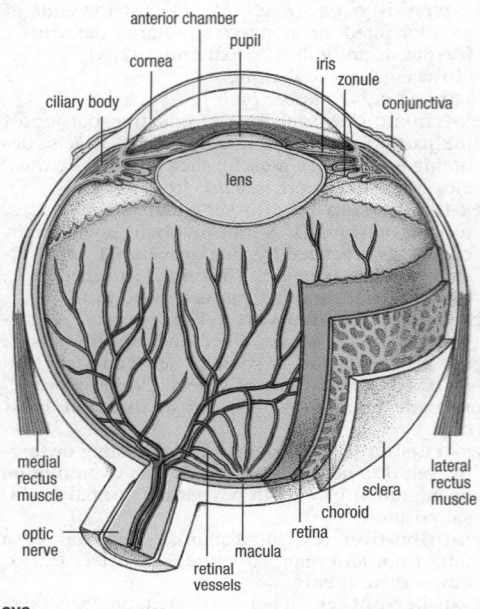

anterior chamber
pupil
cornea
iris
zonule
ciliary body
conjunctiva
lens
medial
rectus
muscle
lateral
rectus
muscle
sclera
choroid
optic
nerve
retina
macula
retinal
vessels

eye

---

photopic e., SYN light-adapted e.

raccoon e.'s, descriptive term for the appearance produced by bilateral periorbital or infraorbital ecchymoses.

scotopic e., SYN dark-adapted e.

eye·ball (ī'bawl). The eye proper without the appendages. SYN bulbus oculi [NA], bulb of eye.

eye bank. A place where corneas of eyes removed after death are preserved for subsequent keratoplasty.

eye·brow. The crescentic line of hairs at the superior edge of the orbit. SYN supercilium (1) [NA].

eye·glass·es. SYN spectacles.

eye·grounds (ī'growndz). The fundus of the eye as seen with the ophthalmoscope.

eye·lash. One of the stiff hairs projecting from the margin of the eyelid. SYN cilium (1).

piebald e., an isolated bundle of white e.'s among normally pigmented e.'s.

eye·lid. One of the two movable folds covering the front of the eyeball when closed; formed of a fibrous core (tarsal plate) and the palpebral portions of the orbicularis oculi muscle covered with skin on the superficial, anterior surface and lined with conjunctiva on the deep, posterior surface; they each have fixed (orbital) and free margins, the latter separated centrally by the palpebral fissure, united at the lateral and medial palpebral commissures, and bearing eyelashes, the openings of tarsal and ciliary glands and (medially) the lacrimal puncta. SYN palpebra [NA].

eye·piece (ī'pēs). The compound lens at the end of the microscope tube nearest the eye; it magnifies the image made by the objective.

eye·strain. SYN asthenopia.

F

F **1.** fractional concentration, followed by subscripts indicating location and chemical species; free *energy*; farad; faraday; Fahrenheit; visual *field*; fluorine; force; filial *generation*, followed by subscript numerals indicating indicating specified matings; phenylalanine. **2.** focus (1).

F0 fundamental *frequency*.

F1.2 (prothrombin fragment 1.2) prothrombin *fragment* 1.2.

f femto-; respiratory *frequency*; fugacity; formyl.

FAB SEE French-American-British *classification* system.

Fab. SEE Fab *fragment*.

fa·bel·la (fa-bel′lă). A sesamoid bone in the tendon of the lateral head of the gastrocnemius muscle. [Mod. L. dim. of *faba,* bean]

face (fās). **1.** The front portion of the head; the visage including eyes, nose, mouth, forehead, cheeks, and chin; excludes ears. SYN facies (1). **2.** SYN surface.

 hippocratic f., SYN hippocratic *facies.*

 masklike f., SYN Parkinson's *facies.*

 moon f., the round, usually red face, with large jowls, seen in Cushing's disease or in exogenous hyperadrenocorticalism.

face-bow. A caliperlike device used to record the relationship of the jaws to the temporomandibular joints; the record may then be used to orient a cast or model of the maxilla to the opening and closing axis of the articulator.

face-lift. SEE rhytidectomy.

fac·et, fa·cette (fas′et, fă-set′). **1.** A small smooth area on a bone or other firm structure. **2.** A worn spot on a tooth, produced by chewing or grinding. [Fr. *facette*]

fac·e·tec·to·my (fas-ĕ-tek′tō-mē). Excision of a facet. [facet + G. *ektomē,* excision]

fa·cial (fā′shăl). Relating to the face.

-facient. Causing; one who or that which brings about. [L. *facio,* to make]

fa·ci·es, pl. **fa·ci·es** (fā′shē-ēz, fash′ē-ēz). **1** [NA]. SYN face (1). **2** [NA]. SYN surface. **3.** SYN expression (2). [L.]

 adenoid f., the open-mouthed and often dull appearance in children with adenoid hypertrophy, associated with a pinched nose.

 Corvisart's f., the characteristic f. seen in cardiac insufficiency or aortic regurgitation; a swollen, purplish, cyanotic face with shiny eyes and puffy eyelids.

 hippocratic f., f. hippocra′tica, a pinched expression of the face, with sunken eyes, concavity of cheeks and temples, relaxed lips, and leaden complexion; observed in one close to death after severe and prolonged illness. SYN hippocratic face.

 Hutchinson's f., the peculiar facial expression produced by the drooping eyelids and motionless eyes in external ophthalmoplegia.

 leonine f., SYN leontiasis.

 myasthenic f., the facial expression in myasthenia gravis, caused by drooping of the eyelids and corners of the mouth, and weakness of the muscles of the face.

 Parkinson's f., the expressionless or masklike f. characteristic of parkinsonism (1). SYN masklike face.

fa·cil·i·ta·tion (fă-sil′i-tā′shŭn). Enhancement or reinforcement of a reflex or other nervous activity by the arrival at the reflex center of other excitatory impulses. [L. *facilitas,* fr. *facilis,* easy]

 proprioceptive neuromuscular f. (PNF), form of exercise that stimulates proprioceptors in muscles, tendons, and joints to improve flexibility and strength.

fac·ing (fās′ing). A tooth-colored material (usually plastic or porcelain) used to hide the buccal or labial surface of a metal crown to give the outward appearance of a natural tooth.

facio-. The face. SEE ALSO prosopo-. [L. *facies*]

fa·ci·o·plas·ty (fā′shē-ō-plas-tē). Plastic surgery involving the face. [facio- + G. *plastos,* formed]

fa·ci·o·ple·gia (fā′shē-ō-plē′jē-ă). SYN facial *paralysis.* [facio- + G. *plēgē,* a stroke]

F.A.C.N.M. the American College of Nuclear Medicine.

F.A.C.N.P. Abbreviation for Fellow of the American College of Nuclear Physicians.

FACS fluorescence-activated cell sorter.

F-ac·tin. See under actin.

fac·ti·tious (fak-tish′ŭs). Artificial; self-induced; not naturally occurring. [L. *factitius,* made by art, fr. *facio,* to make]

fac·tor (fak′ter). **1.** One of the contributing causes in any action. **2.** One of the components that by multiplication makes up a number or expression. **3.** SYN gene. **4.** A vitamin or other essential element. **5.** An event, characteristic, or other definable entity that brings about a change in a health condition. **6.** A categorical independent variable, used to identify, by means of numerical codes, membership in a qualitatively identifiable group; for example, "overcrowding is a factor in disease transmission." [L. maker, causer, fr. *facio,* to make]

 accelerator f., SYN f. V.

 adrenocorticotropic releasing f., hormone produced by the hypothalamus that causes the pituitary to secrete adrenocorticotropic hormone.

 angiogenesis f., a substance of 2000 to 20,000 MW which is secreted by macrophages and stimulates neovascularization in healing wounds or in the stroma of tumors.

 antihemophilic f. A (AHF), SYN f. VIII.

 antinuclear f. (ANF), a f., usually antibodies, present in serum with strong affinity for nuclei and detected by fluorescent antibody technique; present in lupus erythematosus, rheumatoid arthritis, and certain other autoimmune conditions; may also be present at lower levels in normal individuals.

 Castle's intrinsic f., SYN intrinsic f.

 Christmas f., SYN f. IX.

 citrovorum f. (CF), SYN folinic acid.

 clearing f.'s, lipoprotein lipases that appear in plasma during lipemia and catalyze hydrolysis of triglycerides only when the latter are bound to protein and when an acceptor (*e.g.*, serum albumin) is present, thus "clearing" the plasma.

clotting f., any of the various plasma components involved in the clotting process.

colony-stimulating f.'s (CSF), a group of glycoprotein growth f.'s regulating differentiation in myeloid cell lines.

complement chemotactic f., the activated complex of the fifth, sixth, and seventh components of complement (C567) which induces chemotaxis of polymorphonuclear leukocytes.

corticotropin releasing f. (CRF), SYN corticotropin releasing *hormone*.

coupling f.'s, proteins that restore phosphorylating ability to mitochondria that have lost it.

elongation f., proteins that catalyze the elongation of peptide chains during protein biosynthesis. SYN transfer f. (3).

eosinophil chemotactic f. of anaphylaxis, a peptide that is chemotactic for eosinophilic leukocytes and is released from disrupted mast cells.

extrinsic f., dietary vitamin B_{12}.

F f., SYN F *plasmid*.

Fletcher f., SYN prekallikrein.

follicle-stimulating hormone-releasing f., SYN folliberin.

glycotropic f., a principle in extracts of the anterior lobe of the hypophysis that raises the blood sugar and antagonizes the action of insulin; purified pituitary growth hormone produces an identical effect. SYN insulin-antagonizing f.

gonadotropin-releasing f., SYN gonadoliberin (1).

granulocyte colony-stimulating f. (G-CSF), glycoproteins that are synthesized by a variety of cells and are involved in growth and differentiation of hematopoietic stem cells. SEE ALSO colony-stimulating f.'s.

granulocyte-macrophage colony-stimulating f. (GM-CSF), a glycoprotein secreted by macrophages or bone stromal cells that functions as a growth factor for myeloid progenitor cells such as granulocytes, macrophages, and eosinophils. SEE ALSO colony-stimulating f.'s.

growth hormone-releasing f. (GHRF, GH-RF), SYN somatoliberin.

Hageman f., SYN f. XII.

hematopoietic growth f. (HGF), any of several glycoproteins that regulate the survival, self-renewal, proliferation, and differentiation of hematopoietic progenitor cells. There are two nomenclature groups: interleukins (IL) and colony-stimulating factors (CSF).

human antihemophilic f., a lyophilized concentrate of f. VIII, obtained from fresh normal human plasma; used as a hemostatic agent in hemophilia.

f. I, in the clotting of blood a f. that is converted to fibrin through the action of thrombin. SEE ALSO fibrinogen.

f. III, in the clotting of blood, tissue f. or thromboplastin; it initiates the extrinsic pathway by reacting with f. VII and calcium to form f. VIIa. SEE thromboplastin.

initiation f. (IF), one of several soluble proteins involved in the initiation of protein or RNA synthesis.

insulin-antagonizing f., SYN glycotropic f.

insulin-like growth f.'s (IGF), peptides whose formation is stimulated by growth hormone. These peptides bring about peripheral tissue effects of that hormone and have high (about 70%) homology to human insulin.

intrinsic f. (IF), a relatively small mucoprotein secreted by the neck cell of the gastric glands and required for adequate absorption of vitamin B_{12}; deficiency results in pernicious anemia. SYN Castle's intrinsic f.

f. IV, in the clotting of blood, calcium ions.

f. IX, in the clotting of blood, also known as: Christmas f., plasma thromboplastin component, and antihemophilic globulin B, F. IX is required for the formation of intrinsic blood thromboplastin; deficiency causes hemophilia B. SYN antihemophilic globulin B, Christmas f.

Laki-Lorand f., SYN f. XIII.

lethal f., SEE genetic *lethal*.

luteinizing hormone/follicle-stimulating hormone-releasing f., SYN gonadoliberin (2).

luteinizing hormone-releasing f., former name for luteinizing *hormone*-releasing *hormone*.

lymph node permeability f. (LNPF), a substance, released by lymphocytes when stimulated or damaged, that increases capillary permeability and the accumulation of mononuclear cells.

macrophage colony-stimulating f. (M-CSF), a glycoprotein growth f. that causes the committed cell line to proliferate and mature into macrophages. SEE ALSO colony-stimulating f.'s.

melanotropin-releasing f., SYN melanoliberin.

myocardial depressant f. (MDF), a toxic f. in shock that impairs cardiac contractility.

osteoclast activating f., a lymphokine that stimulates bone resorption and inhibits bone-collagen synthesis.

Passavoy f. (pas-a-voy), a clotting f. of which congenital deficiency causes a moderate bleeding diathesis in which the activated partial thromboplastin time (APTT) is prolonged.

platelet f. 3, a blood coagulation factor derived from platelets; chemically, a phospholipid lipoprotein that acts with certain plasma thromboplastin f.'s to convert prothrombin to thrombin.

platelet f. 4 (PF), a cationic polypeptide synthesized by megakaryocytes and contained in platelet alpha granules; these granules, released when platelets are activated, neutralize the anticoagulant activity of heparin.

platelet-activating f., SYN platelet-aggregating f.

platelet-aggregating f., phospholipid mediator of platelet aggregation, inflammation, and anaphylaxis. Produced in response to specific stimuli by a variety of cell types, including neutrophils, basophils, platelets, and endothelial cells. Several molecular species of PAF have been identified which vary in the length of the *O*-alkyl side chain. It is an important mediator of bronchoconstriction. SYN platelet-activating f.

platelet tissue f., SYN thromboplastin.

prolactin-inhibiting f. (PIF), SYN prolactostatin.

prolactin-releasing f. (PRF), SYN prolactoliberin.

properdin f. A, a component of the properdin system; a hydrazine-sensitive β_1-globulin now known to be C3 (third component of complement).

properdin f. B, a normal serum protein and a component of the properdin system.

properdin f. D, a normal serum α-globulin required in the properdin system.

properdin f. E, a serum protein required for activation of C3 (third component of complement) by cobra venom factor. SEE ALSO properdin *system.*

recognition f.'s, f.'s which effect "recognition" of target antigens by polymorphonuclear leukocytes; apparently the Fc portion of antibody molecules and the activated third component of complement (C3), for both of which phagocytes have receptor sites.

releasing f., (1) substances, usually of hypothalamic origin, capable of accelerating the rate of secretion of a given hormone by the anterior pituitary gland; **(2)** f.'s required in the termination phase of either RNA biosynthesis or protein biosynthesis. SYN liberins, releasing hormone.

resistance-transfer f., the transfer gene of the resistance plasmid.

rheumatoid f.'s, antibodies in the serum of individuals with rheumatoid arthritis that react with antigenic determinants or immunoglobulins that enhance agglutination of suspended particles coated with pooled human γ-globulin. Rheumatoid f.'s also occur in other autoimmune and certain infectious diseases.

somatotropin release-inhibiting f., SYN somatostatin.

somatotropin-releasing f., SYN somatoliberin.

Stuart f., Stuart-Prower f., SYN f. X.

sun protection f. (SPF), the ratio of the minimal ultraviolet dose required to produce erythema with and without a sunscreen; useful sunscreens have an SPF of at least 15.

transfer f., (1) the transfer gene of a conjugative plasmid, especially of the resistance plasmid; **(2)** a dialyzable extract that is obtained from the leukocytes of a person with a delayed-type sensitivity and that, following injection into the skin of a nonsensitive person, transfers the specific sensitivity to the recipient; **(3)** SYN elongation f.

transforming f., the DNA responsible for bacterial transformation.

tumor angiogenic f. (TAF), a substance released by solid tumors which induces formation of new blood vessels to supply the tumor.

f. V, a plasma factor in blood coagulation. F. V does not have enzymatic action but participates in the common pathway of coagulation by binding f. Xa to platelet surfaces. Deficiency of this f. leads to a rare hemorrhagic tendency known as parahemophilia or hypoproaccelerinemia. SYN accelerator f., plasma accelerator globulin, proaccelerin, prothrombin accelerator.

f. VII, a plasma factor in blood coagulation. F. VII forms a complex with tissue thromboplastin and calcium to activate f. X. It accelerates the conversion of prothrombin to thrombin, in the presence of tissue thromboplastin, calcium, and f. V. SYN cothromboplastin, proconvertin, serum ac-

celerator, serum prothrombin conversion accelerator.

f. VIII, a plasma factor in blood coagulation. F. VIII participates in the clotting of the blood by forming a complex with f. IXa, platelets, and calcium and enzymatically catalyzing the activation of f. X. Deficiency of f. VIII is associated with classic hemophilia A. **F. VIII:C** is the coagulant component of f. VIII, which circulates in the plasma complexed with **f. VIIIR** (von Willebrand f.), a glycoprotein that is synthesized by endothelial cells and megakaryocytes, and binds to arteries that have lost their endothelial cell linings, creating a surface to which platelets adhere. Disorders involving f. VIIIR form a heterogenous group of abnormalities called von Willebrand's disease. SYN antihemophilic f. A, antihemophilic globulin A, proserum prothrombin conversion accelerator.

f. X, a plasma coagulation factor that assists in the conversion of prothrombin to thrombin. A deficiency of f. X will lead to impaired blood coagulation. SYN prothrombinase, Stuart f., Stuart-Prower f.

f. Xa, the active form of f. X; it is formed from f. X by limited proteolysis via f. VIIa and tissue f. (extrinsic pathway) or f. IXa, VIIIa (intrinsic pathway). F. Xa forms a complex with factor Va, phospholipid, and calcium to convert.

f. XI, a plasma coagulation factor; a component of the contact system which is absorbed from plasma and serum by glass and similar surfaces. Deficiency of f. XI results in a hemorrhagic tendency. SYN plasma thromboplastin antecedent.

f. XII, a plasma coagulation factor. When activated by glass or otherwise to its active form, f. XIIa (EC 3.4.21.38), a serine proteinase, it activates f.'s VII and XI and converts f. XI to its active form, f. XIa. Deficiency of f. XII results in great prolongation of the clotting time of venous blood, but only rarely in a hemorrhagic tendency. SYN Hageman f.

f. XIII, a plasma coagulation factor catalyzed by thrombin into its active form, f. XIIIa, which cross-links subunits of the fibrin clot to form insoluble fibrin. SYN Laki-Lorand f.

fac•ul•ta•tive (fak-ŭl-tā′tiv). Able to live under more than one specific set of environmental conditions; possessing an alternative pathway.

fac•ul•ty (fak′ŭl-tē). A natural or specialized power of a living organism.

FAD *flavin* adenine dinucleotide.

fail•ure (fāl′yūr). The state of insufficiency or nonperformance.

acute respiratory f. (ARF), loss of pulmonary function either acute or chronic that results in hypoxemia or hypercarbia.

backward heart f., a concept that maintains that the phenomena of congestive heart f. result from passive engorgement of the veins caused by a "backward" rise in pressure proximal to the failing cardiac chambers. Cf. forward heart f.

congestive heart f., SYN heart f. (1).

coronary f., acute coronary insufficiency.

electrical f., f. in which the cardiac inadequacy is secondary to disturbance of the electrical impulse.

forward heart f., a concept that maintains that the phenomena of congestive heart f. result from the inadequate cardiac output, and especially from the consequent inadequacy of renal blood flow with resulting retention of sodium and water. Cf. backward heart f.

heart f., (1) inadequacy of the heart so that as a pump it fails to maintain the circulation of blood, with the result that congestion and edema develop in the tissues; SYN cardiac insufficiency, congestive heart f., myocardial insufficiency. SEE ALSO forward heart f., backward heart f., right ventricular f., left ventricular f. (2) resulting clinical syndromes including shortness of breath, pitting edema, enlarged tender liver, engorged neck veins, and pulmonary rales in various combinations.

left ventricular f., congestive heart f. manifested by signs of pulmonary congestion and edema.

right ventricular f., congestive heart f. manifested by distention of the neck veins, enlargement of the liver, and dependent edema due to pump f. of the right ventricle.

f. to thrive, a condition in which an infant's weight gain and growth are far below usual levels for age.

faint (fānt). **1.** Extremely weak; threatened with syncope. **2.** An episode of syncope. SEE ALSO syncope. [M.E., fr. O. Fr. *feindre*, to feign]

fal•cate (fal′kāt). SYN falciform.

fal•ces (fal′sēz). Plural of falx.

fal•ci•form (fal′si-fōrm). Having a crescentic or sickle shape. SYN falcate. [L. *falx*, sickle, + *forma*, form]

fal•cu•la (fal′kyū-lă). SYN *falx* cerebelli. [L. dim. of *falx*]

fal•cu•lar (fal′kyū-lăr). **1.** Resembling a sickle or falx. **2.** Relating to the falx cerebelli or cerebri.

fal•lo•pi•an (fa-lō′pē-an). Described by or attributed to Gabriele Fallopio (1523–1562); usually referring to the uterine tube.

false neg•a•tive (fawls neg′ă-tiv). **1.** A test result which erroneously excludes an individual from a specific diagnostic or reference group. **2.** An individual excluded by erroneous test results from a particular diagnostic group. **3.** A false-negative *result*.

false pos•i•tive (fawls pos′i-tiv). **1.** A test result which erroneously assigns an individual to a specific diagnostic or reference group. **2.** An individual included by erroneous test results in a particular diagnostic group. **3.** A false-positive *result*.

falsetto (fahl-sĕt′ō). High-pitched voice produced by vibration of the anterior third of the vocal folds while the posterior folds are tightly adducted. SEE ALSO voice. [Ital., unnatural voice, fr. *falso*, false, + *-etto*, dim. suff.]

fal•si•fi•ca•tion (fawl′si-fi-kā′shŭn). The deliberate act of misrepresentation so as to deceive. [L. *falsus*, false, + *facio*, to make]

retrospective f., unconscious distortion of past experience to conform to present psychological needs.

falx, pl. **fal•ces** (falks, fal′sēz) [NA]. A sickle-shaped structure. [L. sickle]

f. cerebel′li [NA], a short process of dura mater projecting forward from the internal occipital crest below the tentorium; it occupies the posterior cerebellar notch and the vallecula, and bifurcates below into two diverging limbs passing to either side of the foramen magnum. SYN falcula.

f. cer′ebri [NA], the scythe-shaped fold of dura mater in the longitudinal fissure between the two cerebral hemispheres; it is attached anteriorly to the crista galli of the ethmoid bone and caudally to the upper surface of the tentorium.

fa•mil•i•al (fa-mil′ē-ăl). Affecting more members of the same family than can be accounted for by chance, usually within a single sibship; commonly but incorrectly used to mean genetic. [L. *familia,* family]

fam•i•ly (fam′ĭ-lē). **1.** A group of two or more persons united by blood, adoptive or marital ties, or the common law equivalent. **2.** In biologic classification, a taxonomic grouping at the level intermediate between the order and the tribe or genus. [L. *familia*]

cancer f., a group of blood relatives of whom several have had cancer.

nuclear f., in genetics, two parents and their progeny in common.

fan•ta•sy (fan′tă-sē). Imagery that is more or less coherent, as in dreams and daydreams, yet unrestricted by reality. SYN phantasia. [G. *phantasia*, idea, image]

far•ad (F) (fa′rad). A practical unit of electrical capacity; the capacity of a condenser having a charge of 1 coulomb under an electromotive force of 1 volt. [M. *Faraday*]

Faraday, Michael, English physicist and chemist, 1791–1867. SEE farad; faraday.

far•a•day (F), Fa•ra•day (fa′ră-dā). 96,485.309 coulombs per mole, the amount of electricity required to reduce one equivalent of a monovalent ion. [M. *Faraday*]

far′del (far′del). The total measurable penalty that is incurred as a result of the occurrence of a genetic disease in one individual; one of two major quantitative considerations in the prognostic aspects of genetic counseling, the other being risk of occurrence. [M.E., fr. O. Fr., fr. Ar. *fardah*, bundle]

far•sight•ed•ness (far′sīt′ed-nes). SYN hyperopia.

fas•cia, pl. **fas•ci•ae, fas•ci•as** (fash′ē-ă, -ē-ē) [NA]. A sheet of fibrous tissue that envelops the body beneath the skin; it also encloses muscles and groups of muscles, and separates their several layers or groups. [L. a band or fillet]

f. adhe′rens, a broad intercellular junction in the intercalated disk of cardiac muscle that anchors actin filaments.

deep f., a thin fibrous membrane, devoid of fat, that invests the muscles, separating the several groups and the individual muscles, forms sheaths for the nerves and vessels, becomes specialized around the joints to form or strengthen ligaments, envelops various organs and glands, and binds all the structures together into a firm compact mass.

deep f. of thigh, the strong deep f. of the thigh, enveloping the muscles of the thigh and thickened laterally as the iliotibial track.

endothoracic f., the extrapleural f. that lines

the wall of the thorax; it extends over the cupula of the pleura as the suprapleural membrane and also forms a thin layer between the diaphragm and pleura (phrenicopleura f.)

extraperitoneal f., the thin layer of f. and adipose tissue between the peritoneum and f. transversalis. SYN f. subperitonealis [NA].

pelvic f., it includes parietal and visceral components: fascia pelvis parietalis and fascia pelvis visceralis.

f. perine′i superficia′lis [NA], SYN superficial f. of perineum.

phrenicopleural f., the thin layer of endothoracic f. intervening between the diaphragmatic pleura and the diaphragm.

renal f., the condensation of the fibroareolar tissue and fat surrounding the kidney to form a sheath for the organ.

Scarpa's f., the deeper, membranous or lamellar part of the subcutaneous tissue of the lower abdominal wall; it is continuous with the superficial perineal (Colles') f.

f. subperitonea′lis [NA], SYN extraperitoneal f.

superficial f., a loose fibrous envelope beneath the skin, containing fat in its meshes (panniculus adiposus) or fasciculi of muscular tissue (panniculus carnosus); it contains the cutaneous vessels and nerves and is in relation by its undersurface with the deep fascia. SYN tela subcutanea [NA], hypodermis.

superficial f. of perineum, the membranous layer of the subcutaneous tissue in the urogenital region attaching posteriorly to the border of the urogenital diaphragm, at the sides to the ischiopubic rami, and continuing anteriorly onto the abdominal wall. SYN f. perinei superficialis [NA].

thoracolumbar f., the f. which covers the deep muscles of the back; it is attached to the angles of the ribs and to the spines of the thoracic, lumbar, and sacral vertebrae, to the transverse processes of the lumbar vertebrae, to the lower border of the twelfth rib and to the iliac crest, as well as to the lumbocostal, iliolumbar, intertransverse, and supraspinous ligaments.

transversalis f., the lining f. of the abdominal cavity, between the inner surface of the abdominal musculature and the peritoneum.

fas·cial (fash′ē-ăl). Relating to any fascia.

fas·ci·as. SEE fascia.

fas·ci·cle (fas′i-kl). A band or bundle of fibers, usually of muscle or nerve fibers; a nerve fiber tract. SYN fasciculus [NA].

fas·cic·u·lar (fa-sik′yū-lăr). Relating to a fasciculus; arranged in the form of a bundle or collection of rods.

fas·cic·u·la·tion (fa-sik-yū-lā′shŭn). **1.** An arrangement in the form of fasciculi. **2.** Involuntary contractions, or twitchings, of groups (fasciculi) of muscle fibers, a coarser form of muscular contraction than fibrillation.

fas·cic·u·li (fa-sik′yū-lī). Plural of fasciculus.

fas·cic·u·lus, gen. and pl. **fas·cic·u·li** (fă-sik′yū-lŭs, fă-sik′yū-lī) [NA]. SYN fascicle. [L. dim. of *fascis,* bundle]

cuneate f., the larger lateral subdivision of the posterior funiculus. SYN cuneate funiculus.

dorsolateral f., a longitudinal bundle of thin, unmyelinated and poorly myelinated fibers capping the apex of the posterior horn of the spinal gray matter, composed of posterior root fibers and short association fibers that interconnect neighboring segments of the posterior horn.

gracile f., the smaller medial subdivision of the posterior funiculus.

inferior longitudinal f., a well-marked bundle of long association fibers running the whole length of the occipital and temporal lobes of the cerebrum, in part parallel with the inferior horn of the lateral ventricle. SYN f. longitudinalis inferior [NA].

f. longitudina′lis infe′rior [NA], SYN inferior longitudinal f.

f. longitudina′lis media′lis [NA], SYN medial longitudinal f.

f. longitudina′lis supe′rior [NA], SYN superior longitudinal f.

longitudinal pontine fasciculi, the massive bundles of corticofugal fibers passing longitudinally through the ventral part of pons; they are composed of corticopontine, corticobulbar, and corticospinal fibers.

mamillothalamic f., a compact, thick bundle of nerve fibers that passes dorsalward from the mamillary body on either side to terminate in the anterior nucleus of the thalamus.

medial longitudinal f., a longitudinal bundle of fibers extending from the upper border of the mesencephalon into the cervical segments of the spinal cord, located close to the midline and ventral to the central gray matter; it is composed largely of fibers from the vestibular nuclei ascending to the motor neurons innervating the external eye muscles (abducens, trochlear, and oculomotor nuclei), and descending to spinal cord segments innervating the musculature of the neck. SYN f. longitudinalis medialis [NA].

fascic′uli pro′prii [NA], Flechsig's fasciculi or ground bundles (f. anterior proprius and f. lateralis proprius or lateral ground bundle); intersegmental fasciculi; ascending and descending association fiber systems of the spinal cord which lie deep in the anterior, lateral, and posterior funiculi adjacent to the gray matter. SYN ground bundles.

superior longitudinal f., long association fiber bundle lateral to the centrum ovale of the cerebral hemisphere, connecting the frontal, occipital, and temporal lobes; the fibers pass from the frontal lobe through the operculum to the posterior end of the lateral sulcus where many fibers radiate into the occipital lobe and others turn downward and forward around the putamen and pass to anterior portions of the temporal lobe. SYN f. longitudinalis superior [NA].

unciform f., uncinate f., a band of long association fibers reciprocally connecting the frontal and temporal lobes of the cerebrum, running caudally through the white matter of the frontal lobe, sharply curving ventrally under the stem of the sylvian fissure, and then fanning out to the cortex of the anterior half of the superior and middle temporal gyri.

uncinate f.,

fas·ci·ec·to·my (fash-ē-ek′tō-mē). Excision of strips of fascia. [fascia + G. *ektomē,* excision]

fas•ci•i•tis (fas-ē-ī′tis, fash-). **1.** Inflammation in fascia. **2.** Reactive proliferation of fibroblasts in fascia.

    group A streptococcal necrotizing f., a complication of infection with GAS (group A streptococci) in which the bacteria attack and destroy muscle tissue.

△**fascio-.** A fascia. [L. *fascia,* a band or fillet]

fas•ci•od•e•sis (fas-ē-od′ĕ-sis, fas-). Surgical attachment of a fascia to another fascia or a tendon. [fascio- + G. *desis,* a binding together]

fas•ci•o•la, pl. **fas•ci•o•lae** (fa-sē′ō-lă, fa-sī′ō-lă; -ō-lē). A small band or group of fibers. [L. dim. of *fascia,* band, fillet]

fas•ci•o•lar (fa-sē′ō-lăr, fa-sī′). Relating to the gyrus fasciolaris.

fas•ci•o•plas•ty (fash′ē-ō-plas-tē). Plastic surgery of a fascia. [fascia + G. *plastos,* formed]

fas•ci•or•rha•phy (fash-ē-ōr′ă-fē). Suture of a fascia or aponeurosis. SYN aponeurorrhaphy. [fascio- + G. *rhaphē,* suture]

fas•ci•ot•o•my (fash-ē-ot′ō-mē). Incision through a fascia; used in the treatment of certain vascular disorders and injuries when marked swelling is anticipated which could compromise blood flow; f. may be combined with embolectomy in the treatment of acute arterial embolism. [fascio- + G. *tomē,* incision]

fast. 1. Durable; resistant to change; applied to stained microorganisms which cannot be decolorized. SEE ALSO acid-fast. **2.** Not eating. [A.S. *foest,* firm, fixed]

fas•tid•i•ous (fas-tid′ē-ŭs). In bacteriology, having complex nutritional requirements.

fas•tig•i•um (fas-tij′ē-ŭm). **1.** Apex of the roof of the fourth ventricle of the brain, an angle formed by the anterior and posterior medullary vela extending into the substance of the vermis. **2.** The acme or period of full development of a disease. [L. top, as of a gable; a pointed extremity]

fat. 1. SYN adipose *tissue.* **2.** Common term for obese. **3.** A greasy, soft-solid material, found in animal tissues and many plants, composed of a mixture of glycerol esters; together with oils they make up the homolipids. **4.** SYN triacylglycerol. [A.S. *faet*]

fa•tal (fā′tăl). Pertaining to or causing death; denoting especially inevitability or inescapability of death. [L. *fatalis,* of or belonging to fate]

fat•i•ga•bil•i•ty (fat′i-gă-bil′i-tē). A condition in which fatigue is easily induced.

fa•tigue (fă-tēg′). **1.** That state, following a period of mental or bodily activity, characterized by a lessened capacity for work and reduced efficiency of accomplishment, usually accompanied by a feeling of weariness, sleepiness, or irritability; may also supervene when, from any cause, energy expenditure outstrips restorative processes and may be confined to a single organ. **2.** Sensation of boredom and lassitude due to absence of stimulation, monotony, or lack of interest in one's surroundings. [Fr., fr. L. *fatigo,* to tire]

    battle f., a term used to denote psychiatric illness consequent to the stresses of battle. SEE ALSO war *neurosis.* SYN shell shock.

fat-pad. An accumulation of somewhat encapsulated adipose tissue.

fat•ty (fat′ē). Oily or greasy; relating in any sense to fat.

fat•ty ac•id. Any acid derived from fats by hydrolysis (*e.g.,* oleic, palmitic, or stearic acids); any long-chain monobasic organic acid; they accumulate in disorders associated with the peroxisomes.

    saturated f. a., a f. a., the carbon chain of which contains no ethylenic or other unsaturated linkages between carbon atoms (*e.g.,* stearic acid and palmitic acid); called saturated because it is incapable of absorbing any more hydrogen.

    unsaturated f. a., a f. a., the carbon chain of which possesses one or more double or triple bonds (*e.g.,* oleic acid, with one double bond in the molecule, and linoleic acid, with two); called unsaturated because it is capable of absorbing additional hydrogen.

fau•ces, gen. **fau•ci•um** (faw′sēz, faw′sē-ŭm) [NA]. The space between the cavity of the mouth and the pharynx, bounded by the soft palate and the base of the tongue. SEE ALSO *isthmus* of fauces. [L. the throat]

fau•cial (faw′shăl). Relating to the fauces.

fau•na (faw′nă). The animal forms of a continent, district, locality, or habitat. [Mod. L. application of *Fauna,* sister of *Faunus,* a rural deity]

fa•ve•o•late (fā-vē′ō-lāt). Pitted.

fa•ve•o•lus, pl. **fa•ve•o•li** (fā-vē′ō-lŭs, -ō-lī). A small pit or depression. [Mod. L. dim. of *favus,* honeycomb]

fa•vid (fā′vid). An allergic reaction in the skin observed in patients who have favus.

fa•vism (fā′vizm). An acute condition seen following the ingestion of certain species of beans, *e.g., Vicia faba,* or inhalation of the pollen of its flower, in individuals with genetic erythrocytic deficiency of glucose 6-phosphate dehydrogenase; characterized by fever, headache, abdominal pain, severe anemia, prostration, and coma. [Ital. *favismo,* from *fava,* bean]

fa•vus (fā′vŭs, fah′vŭs). A severe type of chronic ringworm of the scalp and nails; it occurs more frequently in the Mediterranean countries, southeastern Europe, southern Asia, and northern Africa. Differences in severity are related to hygiene. [L. honeycomb]

Fc. SEE Fc *fragment.*

F.C.C.P. Fellow of the College of Chest Physicians.

FDA Food and Drug Administration of the United States Department of Health and Human Services.

Fe iron. [L. *ferrum,* iron]

fear (fēr). Apprehension; dread; alarm; by having an identifiable stimulus, f. is differentiated from anxiety, which has no easily identifiable stimulus. [A.S. *faer*]

fe•brif•u•gal (fē-brif′yū-găl). SYN antipyretic (1).

feb•ri•fuge (feb′ri-fyūj). SYN antipyretic (2). [L. *febris,* fever, + *fugo,* to put to flight]

feb•rile (feb′ril, fē′brīl). Denoting or relating to fever. SYN feverish (1), pyretic.

fe•cal (fē′kăl). Relating to feces.

fe•ca•lith (fē′kă-lith). SYN coprolith. [L. *faeces,* feces, + G. *lithos,* stone]

fe·cal·oid (fē'kă-loyd). Resembling feces. [L. *faeces*, feces, + G. *eidos*, resemblance]

fe·ca·lo·ma (fē'kă-lō-mă). SYN coproma.

fe·ca·lu·ria (fē-kă-lū'rē-ă). The commingling of feces with urine passed from the urethra in persons with a fistula connecting the intestinal tract and bladder. [L. *faeces*, feces, + G. *ouron*, urine]

fe·ces (fē'sēz). The matter discharged from the bowel during defecation, consisting of the undigested residue of the food, epithelium, the intestinal mucus, bacteria, and waste material from the food. SYN stercus. [L., pl. of *faex* (*faec*-), dregs]

fec·u·lent (fek'yū-lent). Foul. [L. *faeculentus*, full of excrement, fr. *faeces*, dregs, feces]

fe·cund (fē'kŭnd, fek'ŭnd). SYN fertile (1). [L. *fecundus*, fruitful]

fec·un·da·tion (fē-kŭn-dā'shŭn). The act of rendering fertile. SEE ALSO fertilization.

fe·cun·di·ty (fē-kŭn'di-tē). The ability to produce live offspring.

feed·back (fēd'bak). **1.** In a given system, the return, as input, of some of the output, as a regulatory mechanism; *e.g.*, regulation of a furnace by a thermostat. **2.** An explanation for the learning of motor skills: sensory stimuli set up by muscle contractions modulate the activity of the motor system. **3.** The feeling evoked by another person's reaction to oneself. SEE biofeedback.

feed·ing (fēd'ing). Giving food or nourishment.
  forced f., forcible f., (1) giving liquid food through a nasal tube passed into the stomach; **(2)** forcing a person to eat more food than desired.
  gastric f., giving of nutriment directly into the stomach by means of a tube inserted via the nasopharynx and esophagus or directly through the abdominal wall.

fee-for-service. Payment made at the time of health care service; the amount varies according to the provider's estimate of the costs involved.

FEES fiberoptic endoscopic *examination* of swallowing.

FEF forced expiratory *flow*.

fel·la·tio (fĕ-lā'shē-ō). Oral stimulation of the penis. [L.]

fel·on (fel'ŏn). A purulent infection or abscess involving the bulbous distal end of a finger. SYN whitlow. [M.E. *feloun*, malignant]

felt·work. **1.** A fibrous network. **2.** A close plexus of nerve fibrils. SEE neuropil.

fe·male (fē'māl). ZOOLOGY Denoting the sex that bears the young or the ovum.
  genetic f., (1) an individual with a normal female karyotype, including two X chromosomes; **(2)** an individual whose cell nuclei contain Barr sex chromatin bodies, which are normally absent in males.

fem·i·ni·za·tion (fem'i-ni-zā'shŭn). Development of what are superficially external female characteristics by a male.

fem·o·ral (fem'ŏ-răl). Relating to the femur or thigh.

fem·o·ro·cele (fem'ŏ-rō-sēl). SYN femoral *hernia*. [L. *femur*, thigh, + G. *kēlē*, hernia]

fem·o·ro·tib·i·al (fem'ŏ-rō-tib'ē-ăl). Relating to the femur and the tibia.

femto- (f). SI and metric systems to signify one-quadrillionth (10^{-15}). [Danish and Norwegian *femten*, fifteen]

fe·mur, gen. **fe·mo·ris**, pl. **fem·o·ra** (fē'mŭr, fem'ŏ-ris, -ă) [NA]. **1.** The thigh. **2.** The long bone of the thigh, articulating with the hip bone proximally and the tibia and patella distally. SYN thigh bone. [L. thigh]

fe·nes·tra, pl. **fe·nes·trae** (fe-nes'tră, -trē). **1** [NA]. An anatomical aperture, often closed by a membrane. **2.** An opening left in a plaster of Paris cast or other form of fixed dressing in order to permit access to a wound or inspection of the part. **3.** The opening in one of the blades of an obstetrical forceps. **4.** A lateral opening in the sheath of an endoscopic instrument that allows lateral viewing or operative maneuvering through the sheath. **5.** Openings in the wall of a tube, catheter, or trocar designed to promote better flow of air or fluids. SYN window. [L. window]
  f. coch'leae [NA], an opening on the medial wall of the middle ear leading into the cochlea, closed in life by the secondary tympanic membrane. SYN round window.
  f. vestib'uli [NA], an oval opening on the medial wall of the tympanic cavity leading into the vestibule, closed in life by the foot of the stapes. SYN oval window.

fen·es·trat·ed (fen'es-trā'ted). Having fenestrae or window-like openings.

fen·es·tra·tion (fen-es-trā'shŭn). **1.** The presence of openings or fenestrae in a part. **2.** Making openings in a dressing to allow inspection of the parts. **3.** DENTISTRY A surgical perforation of the mucoperiosteum and alveolar process to expose the root tip of a tooth to permit drainage of tissue exudate.

fer·ment (fer-ment'). To cause or to undergo fermentation. [L. *fermentum*, leaven]

fer·men·ta·tion (fer-men-tā'shŭn). **1.** A chemical change induced in a complex organic compound by the action of an enzyme, whereby the substance is split into simpler compounds. **2.** BACTERIOLOGY The anaerobic dissimilation of substrates with the production of energy and reduced compounds; the mechanism of f. does not involve a respiratory chain or cytochrome, hence oxygen is not the final electron acceptor as it is in oxidation. [L. *fermento*, pp. *-atus*, to ferment, from L. *fermentum*, yeast]

fer·ment·a·tive (fer-ment'ă-tiv). Causing or having the ability to cause fermentation.

fer·mi·um (Fm) (fer'mē-ŭm). Radioactive element, artificially prepared in 1955, atomic no. 100, atomic wt. 257.095; ^{257}Fm has the longest known half-life (100.5 days). [E. *Fermi*, It.-U.S. physicist and Nobel laureate, 1901–1954]

fern·ing. A term used to describe the pattern of arborization produced by a thin film of cervical mucus, secreted at midcycle, upon drying, which resembles somewhat a fern or a palm leaf.

fer·re·dox·ins (fer-ĕ-dok'sinz). Proteins containing iron and (labile) sulfur in equal amounts, displaying electron-carrier activity but no classical enzyme function. F. are found in green plants, algae, and anaerobic bacteria, and are involved in several oxidation-reduction reactions in living organisms (*e.g.*, nitrogen fixation).

fe

△**ferri-.** Prefix designating the presence of a ferric ion in a compound. [L. *ferrum,* iron]

fer·ric (fer'ik). Relating to iron, especially denoting a salt containing iron in its higher (triad) valence, Fe^{3+}.

fer·ri·heme (fe'rī-hēm, fer'ē-). SYN hematin.

fer·ri·tin (fer'ĭ-tin, fer'ă-). An iron protein complex, containing up to 23% iron, formed by the union of ferric iron with apoferritin; it is found in the intestinal mucosa, spleen, bone marrow, reticulocytes, and liver, and regulates iron storage and transport from the intestinal lumen to plasma.

△**ferro-.** Prefix designating the presence of metallic iron or of the divalent ion Fe^{2+}. [L. *ferrum,* iron]

fer·ro·ki·net·ics (fār-ō-ki-net'iks). The study of iron metabolism using radioactive iron. [L. *ferrum,* iron, + G. *kinēsis,* movement]

fer·ro·pro·teins (fār-ō-prō'tēnz). Proteins containing iron in a prosthetic group; *e.g.,* heme, cytochrome.

fer·rous (fār'ŭs). Relating to iron, especially denoting a salt containing iron in its lowest valence state, Fe^{2+}. [L. *ferreus,* made of iron]

fer·ru·gi·na·tion (fe-rū'ji-nā'shŭn). Deposition of mineral including iron in the walls of small blood vessels and at the site of a dead neuron. [L. *ferrugo,* iron-rust]

fer·ru·gi·nous (fe-rū'ji-nŭs). **1.** Iron-bearing; associated with or containing iron. **2.** Of the color of iron rust. [L. *ferrugineus,* iron rust, rust-colored]

fer·tile (fer'til). **1.** Fruitful; capable of conceiving and bearing young. SYN fecund. **2.** Impregnated; fertilized. [L. *fertilis,* fr. *fero,* to bear]

fer·til·i·ty (fer-til'i-tē). The actual production of live offspring, *i.e.,* does not include stillbirths.

fer·til·i·za·tion (fer'til-i-zā'shŭn). The process beginning with penetration of the secondary oocyte by the spermatozoon and completed by fusion of the male and female pronuclei.

in vivo **f.,** f. of a ripe egg within the distal uterine tube of a fertile donor female (rather than in an artificial medium), for subsequent nonsurgical transfer to an infertile recipient.

fes·ter. 1. To form pus or putrefy. **2.** To make inflamed. [L. *fistula*]

fes·ti·nant (fes'ti-nant). Rapid; hastening; accelerating. [L. *festino,* to hasten]

fes·ti·na·tion (fes-ti-nā'shŭn). SYN festinating *gait.* [L. *festino,* to hasten]

fes·toon (fes-tūn'). **1.** A carving in the base material of a denture that simulates the contours of the natural tissue that is being replaced by the denture. **2.** A distinguishing characteristic of certain hard tick species, consisting of small rectangular areas separated by grooves along the posterior margin of the dorsum of both males and females. [thr. Fr. fr. L. *festum,* festival, hence festive decorations]

fes·toon·ing (fes-tūn'ing). Undulating, like the pattern of dermal papillae beneath a subepidermal blister.

FET forced expiratory *time.*

fe·tal (fē'tăl). **1.** Relating to a fetus; **2.** In utero development after the eighth week.

fe·ti·cide (fē'ti-sīd). Destruction of the embryo or fetus in the uterus. [L. *fetus* + *caedo,* to kill]

fet·id (fet'id, fē'tid). Foul-smelling. [L. *foetidus*]

fet·ish (fet'ish, fē'tish). An inanimate object or nonsexual body part that is regarded as endowed with magic or erotic qualities. [Fr. *fétiche,* fr. L. *factitius,* made by art, artificial]

fet·ish·ism (fet'ish-izm, fē'tish-). The act of worshipping or using for sexual arousal and gratification that which is regarded as a fetish.

fe·to·glob·u·lins (fē-tō-glob'yū-linz). One of a number of proteins found in fetal blood, of unknown function. α-F. occurs in normal adults and in larger amounts in the fetus and pregnant mother, especially in the second trimester; elevated levels are also detected in patients with liver disease and neoplasms.

fe·tol·o·gy (fē-tol'ō-jē). SYN fetal *medicine.* [L. *fetus* + G. *logos,* study]

fe·tom·e·try (fē-tom'ĕ-trē). Estimation of the size of the fetus, especially of its head, prior to delivery. [L. *fetus* + G. *metron,* measure]

fe·top·a·thy (fē-top'ă-thē). SYN embryopathy. [L. *fetus* + G. *pathos,* suffering, disease]

fe·to·pla·cen·tal (fē'tō-pla-sen'tăl). Relating to the fetus and its placenta.

fe·to·pro·teins (fē-tō-prō'tēnz). Fetal proteins found in small amounts in adults in the following forms: α-**f.** (AFP) increases in maternal blood during pregnancy and, when detected by amniocentesis, is an important indicator of open neural tube defects and is also used as a tumor marker in adults with hepatocellular carcinoma; β-**f.,** although a fetal liver protein, has been detected in adult patients with liver disease; γ-**f.** occurs in various neoplasms. SEE ALSO fetoglobulins.

fe·tor (fē'tōr). A very offensive odor. [L. an offensive smell, fr. *feteo,* to stink]

f. hepat'icus, a peculiar odor to the breath in persons with severe liver disease; caused by volatile aromatic substances that accumulate in the blood and urine due to defective hepatic metabolism.

fe·to·scope (fē'tō-skōp). **1.** A fiberoptic endoscope used in fetology. **2.** A stethoscope designed for listening to fetal heart sounds.

fe·tos·co·py (fē-tos'kŏ-pē). Use of a fiberoptic endoscope to view the fetus and the fetal surface of the placenta transabdominally, and also for collection of fetal blood from the umbilical vein for antenatal diagnosis of fetal disorders.

fe·tus, pl. **fe·tus·es** (fē'tŭs, fē'tŭs-ez). **1.** The unborn young of a viviparous animal after it has taken form in the uterus. **2** [NA]. In humans, the product of conception from the end of the eighth week to the moment of birth. [L. offspring]

f. **fe'tus,** a species that contains various subspecies which can cause human infections as well as abortion in sheep and cattle; it is the type species of the genus *f.*

harlequin f., a severe form of collodion baby in a newborn, usually premature; a form of ichthyosiform erythroderma characterized by encasement of the body in grayish brown, often fissured plaques resembling plates of armor, and by grotesque deformity of the face, hands, and feet; usually fatal within a few days.

impacted f., a f. which, because of its large size or narrowing of the pelvic canal, has become wedged and incapable of spontaneous advance or recession.

f. papyra′ceus, one of twin f.'s that has died and been pressed flat against the uterine wall by the growth of the living f.

FEV forced expiratory *volume,* with subscript indicating time interval in seconds.

fe•ver (fē′ver). A complex physiologic response to disease mediated by pyrogenic cytokines and characterized by a rise in core temperature, generation of acute phase reactants and activation of immunologic systems. SYN pyrexia. [A.S. *fefer*].

blackwater f., hemoglobinuria resulting from severe hemolysis occurring in falciparum malaria.

boutonneuse f., tick-borne infection with *Rickettsia conorii* seen in Africa, Europe, the Middle East, and India. SYN tick typhus.

brass founder's f., an occupational disease, characterized by malaria-like symptoms, due to inhalation of particles and fumes of metallic oxides. Fumes are formed by evaporation at very high temperature and condensation in air into fine particles.

camp f., (1) SYN typhus. **(2)** any epidemic febrile illness affecting troops in an encampment.

cat-scratch f., SYN cat-scratch *disease.*

childbed f., SYN puerperal f.

Colorado tick f., an infection caused by Colorado tick f. virus and transmitted to humans by *Dermacentor andersoni;* the symptoms are mild, there is no rash, fever is not excessive, and the disease is rarely fatal. SYN tick f. (5).

dengue f., SYN dengue.

dengue hemorrhagic f., SYN dengue.

elephantoid f., lymphangitis and an elevation of temperature marking the beginning of endemic elephantiasis (filariasis).

enteric f., (1) SYN typhoid f. **(2)** the group of typhoid and paratyphoid f.'s.

entericoid f., a f., neither paratyphoid nor typhoid, resembling the latter.

epidemic hemorrhagic f., a condition characterized by acute onset of headache, chills and high f., sweating, thirst, photophobia, coryza, cough, myalgia, arthralgia, and abdominal pain with nausea and vomiting; this phase lasts from three to six days and is followed by capillary and renal interstitial hemorrhages, edema, oliguria, azotemia, and shock; most varieties are caused by viruses and are are rodent-borne. SYN hemorrhagic f. with renal syndrome.

Fort Bragg f., SYN pretibial f.

Haverhill f., an infection by *Streptobacillus moniliformis* marked by initial chills and high f. (gradually subsiding), by arthritis usually in the larger joints and spine, and by a rash occurring chiefly over the joints and on the extensor surfaces of the extremities. SYN erythema arthriticum epidemicum. [*Haverhill,* MA, where an epidemic occurred in 1926]

hay f., a form of atopy characterized by an acute irritative inflammation of the mucous membranes of the eyes and upper respiratory passages accompanied by itching and profuse watery secretion, followed occasionally by bronchitis and asthma; the episode recurs annually at the same or nearly the same time of the year, in spring, summer, or late summer and autumn, caused by an allergic reaction to the pollen of trees, grasses, weeds, flowers, etc.

hemorrhagic f., a syndrome that occurs in infections by a number of different viruses. Some types of hemorrhagic f. are tick-borne, others mosquito-borne, and some seem to be zoonoses; clinical manifestations are high f., scattered petechiae, gastrointestinal tract and other organ bleeding, hypotension, and shock; kidney damage may be severe, especially in Korean hemorrhagic f. and neurologic signs may appear, especially in the Argentinean-Bolivian types. Four types of hemorrhagic f. are transmissible person-to-person: Lassa f., Ebola f., Marburg virus disease, and Crimean-Congo hemorrhagic f. SEE ALSO epidemic hemorrhagic f.

hemorrhagic f. with renal syndrome, SYN epidemic hemorrhagic f.

icterohemorrhagic f., infection with the variety of *Leptospira interrogans* serotype known as icterohemorrhagiae, characterized by fever, jaundice, hemorrhagic lesions, azotemia, and central nervous system manifestations.

Korean hemorrhagic f., a form of epidemic hemorrhagic f. caused by the Hantaan virus.

Lassa f., a severe form of epidemic hemorrhagic f. which is highly fatal. It was first recognized in Lassa, Nigeria, is caused by the Lassa virus, a member of the Arenaviridae family, and is characterized by high f., sore throat, severe muscle aches, skin rash with hemorrhages, headache, abdominal pain, vomiting, and diarrhea; the multimammate rat *Mastomys natalensis* serves as reservoir, but person-to-person transmission also is common.

Mediterranean exanthematous f., an affection occurring sporadically in the Mediterranean littoral marked by a severe chill with abrupt rise of temperature, pains in the joints, tonsillitis, diarrhea, vomiting, and, on the third to fifth day, a rash of elevated nonconfluent macules beginning on the thighs and spreading to the entire body; lasts from ten days to two weeks and then disappears by rapid lysis without desquamation; probably caused by *Rickettsia conorii,* like Boutonneuse fever.

miliary f., (1) an infectious disease characterized by profuse sweating and the production of sudamina, occurring formerly in severe epidemics; **(2)** SYN miliaria.

milk f., (1) a slight elevation of temperature following childbirth, said to be due to the establishment of the secretion of milk, but probably the same as absorption f.; **(2)** an afebrile metabolic disease, occurring shortly after parturition in dairy cattle, characterized by hypocalcemia and manifested by loss of consciousness and general paralysis.

mud f., a leptospirosis caused by the *grippotyphosa* serovar of *Leptospira interrogans.*

Oroya f., a generalized, acute, febrile, endemic, and systemic form of bartonellosis; marked by high fever, rheumatic pains, progressive, severe anemia, and albuminuria.

paratyphoid f., an acute infectious disease with symptoms and lesions resembling those of typhoid f., though milder in character; associated with the presence of the paratyphoid organism of which at least three varieties (types A, B, and C) have been described. SYN paratyphoid.

parenteric f., one of a group of f.'s clinically resembling typhoid and paratyphoid A and B, but caused by bacteria differing specifically from those of either of these diseases.

parrot f., SYN psittacosis.

Pel-Ebstein f., the remittent fever common in Hodgkin's disease. SYN Pel-Ebstein disease.

pharyngoconjunctival f., a disease characterized by fever, pharyngitis, and conjunctivitis, and caused by adenoviruses, often type 3 but occasionally other types.

pretibial f., a mild disease first observed among military personnel at Fort Bragg, North Carolina, characterized by f., moderate prostration, splenomegaly, and a rash on the anterior aspects of the legs; due to the *autumnalis* serovar of *Leptospira interrogans*. SYN Fort Bragg f.

puerperal f., postpartum sepsis with a rise in temperature after the first 24 hours following delivery, but before the eleventh postpartum day. SYN childbed f.

Q f., a febrile disease characterized by headache and myalgia and sometimes pneumonitis or hepatitis; caused by *Coxiella burnetii;* the organism propagates in sheep and cattle, where it produces no symptoms; human infections occur as a result of contact not only with such animals but also with other infected humans, air and dust, wild reservoir hosts, and other sources. [*Q*, for "query," so named because etiologic agent was unknown]

rat-bite f., a single designation for two bacterial diseases associated with rat bites, one caused by *Streptobacillus moniliformis* (Haverhill f.), the other by *Spirillum minus* (sodoku); both diseases are characterized by relapsing f., chills, headache, arthralgia, lymphadenopathy, and a maculopapular rash on the extremities.

relapsing f., an acute infectious disease caused by any one of a number of strains of *Borrelia*, marked by febrile attacks lasting about six days and separated from each other by apyretic intervals of about the same length; the microorganism is found in the blood during the febrile periods but not during the intervals. There are two epidemiologic varieties: 1) the louse-borne variety, occurring chiefly in Europe, northern Africa, and India, and caused by strains of *B. recurrentis;* 2) the tick-borne variety, occurring in Africa, Asia, and North and South America, caused by various species of *Borrelia*, each of which is transmitted by a different species of the soft tick, *Ornithodoros*.

rheumatic f., f. following infection of the throat with group A streptococci, occurring primarily in children and young adults, and inducing an immunopathy variably associated with acute migratory polyarthritis, Sydenham's chorea, subcutaneous nodules over bony prominences, myo-

carditis with formation of Aschoff bodies which may cause acute cardiac failure, and endocarditis (frequently followed by scarring of valves, causing stenosis or incompetence); relapses are common if repeated streptococcal infections occur.

Rocky Mountain spotted f., an acute infectious disease of high mortality, characterized by frontal and occipital headache, intense lumbar pain, malaise, a moderately high continuous f., and a rash on wrists, palms, ankles, and soles from the second to the fifth day, later spreading to all parts of the body; it occurs in the spring of the year primarily in the southeast U.S. and the Rocky Mountain region, although it is also endemic elsewhere in the U.S., in parts of Canada, in Mexico, and in South America; the pathogenic organism is *Rickettsia rickettsii*, transmitted by two or more tick species of the genus *Dermacentor;* in the U.S. it is spread by *D. andersoni* in the western states and *D. variabilis* (a dog tick) in the eastern states. SYN tick f. (4).

scarlet f., SYN scarlatina.

septic f., SYN septicemia.

Sindbis f., a febrile illness of humans in Africa, Australia, and other countries, characterized by arthralgia, rash, and malaise; caused by the Sindbis virus, a member of the family Togaviridae, and transmitted by culicine mosquitoes.

South African tick-bite f., a typhus-like f. of South Africa caused by *Rickettsia rickettsii* and usually characterized by primary eschar and regional adenitis, rigors, and maculopapular rash on the fifth day, often with severe central nervous system symptoms.

spotted f., tick typhus caused by *Rickettsia rickettsii* in North and South America and Siberia.

swamp f., (1) SYN equine infectious *anemia*. (2) SYN malaria.

tick f., (1) any infectious disease of man or the lower animals caused by a protozoan blood parasite, a bacterium, a rickettsia, or a virus, and transmitted by a tick; (2) the tick-borne variety of relapsing f.; (3) SYN bovine *babesiosis*. (4) SYN Rocky Mountain spotted f. (5) SYN Colorado tick f.

trench f., an uncommon rickettsial f. caused by *Rochalimaea quintana* and transmitted by the louse *Pediculus humanus*, first appearing as an epidemic during the trench warfare of World War I; characterized by the sudden onset of chills and f., myalgia (especially of the back and legs), headache, and general malaise that typically lasts five days but may recur.

typhoid f., an acute infectious disease caused by *Salmonella typhi* and characterized by a continued f., severe physical and mental depression, an eruption of rose-colored spots on the chest and abdomen, tympanites, often diarrhea, and sometimes intestinal hemorrhage or perforation of the bowel; average duration is four weeks, although aborted forms and relapses are not uncommon; the lesions are located chiefly in the lymph follicles of the intestines (Peyer's patches), the mesenteric glands, and the spleen; antibody titer of the Widal test rises during the infection, and early positive blood and urine cultures become negative. SYN enteric f. (1), typhoid (2).

undifferentiated type f.'s, a term applied to illnesses resulting from infection by any one of the arboviruses pathogenic for man, in which the only constant manifestation is f.; rash, lymphadenopathy, or arthralgia (alone or in combination) may occur in some individuals but not in others; some arboviruses may induce infections in which undifferentiated type f. is the only manifestation, whereas other arboviruses may induce in some persons only undifferentiated f., and in other persons similar f. followed by secondary manifestations, *e.g.,* a hemorrhagic f. or encephalitis.

undulant f., SYN brucellosis. [referring to the wavy appearance of the long temperature curve]

f. of unknown origin (FUO), a sustained elevation of temperature, lasting two weeks or longer, for which no explanation can be found despite vigorous diagnostic evaluation. SYN pyrexia of unknown origin.

uveoparotid f., chronic enlargement of the parotid glands and inflammation of the uveal tract accompanied by a long-continued f. of low degree; a form of sarcoidosis.

yellow f., a tropical mosquito-borne viral hepatitis, due to yellow f. virus, with an urban form transmitted by *Aedes aegypti*, and a rural, jungle, or sylvatic form from tree-dwelling mammals by various mosquitoes of the *Haemagogus* species complex; characterized clinically by fever, slow pulse, albuminuria, jaundice, congestion of the face, and hemorrhages, especially hematemesis; immunity to reinfection accompanies recovery.

fe•ver•ish (fē′ver-ish). **1.** SYN febrile. **2.** Having a fever.

FF filtration *fraction*.

FFD focal-film *distance*.

FFM fat-free body *mass*.

F.F.R. Fellow of the Faculty of Radiologists.

FIA (fluoroimmunoassay) feline infectious *anemia*.

fi•ber (fī′ber). A slender thread or filament. **1.** Extracellular filamentous structures such as collagenic or elastic connective tissue f.'s. **2.** The nerve cell axon with its glial envelope. **3.** Elongated, hence threadlike, cells such as muscle cells and the epithelial cells composing the major part of the eye lens. SYN fibra [NA]. [L. *fibra*]

A f.'s, myelinated nerve f.'s in somatic nerves, measuring 1 to 22 μm in diameter, conducting nerve impulses at a rate of 6 to 120 m/sec.

accelerator f.'s, postganglionic sympathetic nerve f.'s originating in the superior, middle, and inferior cervical ganglia of the sympathetic trunk, conveying nervous impulses to the heart that increase the rapidity and force of the cardiac pulsations.

adrenergic f.'s, nerve f.'s that transmit nervous impulses to other nerve cells (or smooth muscle or gland cells) by the medium of the adrenaline-like transmitter substance norepinephrine (noradrenaline).

afferent f.'s, those that convey impulses to a ganglion or to a nerve center in the brain or spinal cord.

alpha f.'s, large somatic motor or propriocep-

tive nerve f.'s conducting impulses at rates near 100 m/sec.

arcuate f.'s, nervous or tendinous f.'s passing in the form of an arch from one part to another.

association f.'s, nerve f.'s interconnecting subdivisions of the cerebral cortex of the same hemisphere or different segments of the spinal cord on the same side.

B f.'s, myelinated f.'s autonomic nerves, with a diameter of 2 μm or less, conducting at a rate of 3 to 15 m/sec.

beta f.'s, nerve f.'s having conduction velocities of about 40 m/sec.

C f.'s, unmyelinated f.'s, 0.4 to 1.2 μm in diameter, conducting nerve impulses at a velocity of 0.7 to 2.3 m/sec.

cholinergic f.'s, nerve f.'s that transmit impulses to other nerve cells, muscle fibers, or gland cells by the medium of the transmitter substance acetylcholine.

collagen f., collagenous f., an individual f. that varies in diameter from less than 1 μm to about 12 μm and is composed of fibrils; the f.'s, which are usually arranged in bundles, undergo some branching and are of indefinite length; chemically the f. is a glycoprotein, collagen, which yields gelatin upon boiling; they make up the principal element of irregular connective tissue, tendons, aponeuroses, and most ligaments, and occur in the matrix of cartilage and osseous tissue. SYN white f. (2).

commissural f.'s, nerve f.'s crossing the midline and connecting two corresponding parts or regions of the nervous system.

depressor f.'s, sensory nerve f.'s having pressure-sensitive endings in the wall of certain arteries capable of activating blood pressure-lowering brainstem mechanisms when stimulated by an increase in intra-arterial pressure.

dietary f., the plant polysaccharides and lignin that are resistant to hydrolysis by the digestive enzymes in humans.

elastic f.'s, f.'s that are 0.2 to 2 μm in diameter but may be larger in some ligaments; they branch and anastomose to form networks and fuse to form fenestrated membranes; the f.'s and membranes consist of microfibrils about 10 nm wide and an amorphous substance containing elastin. SYN yellow f.'s.

exogenous f.'s, nerve f.'s by which a given region of the central nervous system is connected with other regions; the term applies to both afferent and efferent fiber connections.

gamma f.'s, nerve f.'s that have a conduction rate of about 20 m/sec.

gray f.'s, SYN unmyelinated f.'s.

inhibitory f.'s, nerve f.'s that inhibit the activity of the nerve cells with which they have synaptic connections, or of the effector tissue (smooth muscle, heart muscle, glands) in which they terminate.

intrafusal f.'s, muscle f.'s present within a neuromuscular spindle.

motor f.'s, nerve f.'s that transmit impulses that activate effector cells, *e.g.,* in muscle or gland tissue.

nonmedullated f.'s, SYN unmyelinated f.'s.

osteogenetic f.'s, the f.'s in the osteogenetic layer of the periosteum.

perforating f.'s, bundles of collagenous f.'s that pass into the outer circumferential lamellae of bone or the cementum of teeth.

precollagenous f.'s, immature, argyrophilic f.'s.

pressor f.'s, sensory nerve f.'s whose stimulation causes vasoconstriction and rise of blood pressure.

projection f.'s, nerve f.'s connecting the cerebral cortex with other centers in the brain or spinal cord; fibers arising from cells in the central nervous system that pass to distant loci.

reticular f.'s, the collagen (type III) f.'s forming the distinctive loose connective tissue stroma of embryonic tissues, mesenchyme, red pulp of the spleen, cortex and medulla of lymph nodes, and the hematopoietic compartments of bone marrow and accounting for a substantial portion of the collagen f.'s of the skin, blood vessels, synovial membrane, uterine tissue, and granulation tissue; characterized by its organization as a reticular meshwork of fine filaments and an affinity for silver and for periodic acid-Schiff stains.

sudomotor f.'s, postganglionic and cholinergic sympathetic nerve f.'s that innervate the sweat glands.

tautomeric f.'s, nerve f.'s of the spinal cord that do not extend beyond the limits of the spinal cord segment in which they originate.

unmyelinated f.'s, a f. having no myelin covering (CNS); a naked axon; in the PNS represented by all axons lying in troughs in a single Schwann cell (Schwann cell unit); a slow conducting f. SYN gray f.'s, nonmedullated f.'s.

white f., (1) white mammalian muscle f.'s; larger in diameter than red f.'s they have less myoglobin, sarcoplasm, and mitochondria, and contract more quickly; **(2)** SYN collagen f.

yellow f.'s, SYN elastic f.'s.

fi·ber·op·tic (fī-ber-op′tik). Pertaining to fiberoptics.

fi·ber·op·tics (fī-ber-op′tiks). An optical system in which the image is conveyed by a compact bundle of small diameter, flexible, glass or plastic fibers.

fi·ber·scope (fī′ber-skōp). An optical instrument that transmits light and carries images back to the observer through a flexible bundle of small glass or plastic fibers. It is used to inspect interior portions of the body. SEE ALSO fiberoptics.

△**fibr-.** SEE fibro-.

fi·bra, pl. **fi·brae** (fī′brǎ, fī′brē) [NA]. SYN fiber, fiber. [L.]

fi·bre·mia (fī-brē′mē-ǎ). Presence of formed fibrin in the blood, causing thrombosis or embolism. SYN inosemia (2). [fibrin + G. *haima,* blood]

fi·bril (fī′bril). A minute fiber or component of a fiber. SYN fibrilla. [Mod. L. *fibrilla*]

fi·bril·la, pl. **fi·bril·lae** (fī-bril′ǎ, -ē). SYN fibril. [Mod. L. dim. of L. *fibra,* a fiber]

fi·bril·lar, fi·bril·lary (fī′bril-lǎr, -lar-ē). **1.** Relating to a fibril. **2.** Denoting the fine rapid contractions or twitchings of fibers or of small

groups of fibers in skeletal or cardiac muscle. SYN filar (1).

fi·bril·late (fī′bri-lāt). **1.** To make or to become fibrillar. **2.** SYN fibrillated. **3.** To be in a state of fibrillation (3).

fi·bril·lat·ed (fī′bri-lā-ted). Composed of fibrils. SYN fibrillate (2).

fi·bril·la·tion (fī-bri-lā′shŭn, fib-rĭ-). **1.** The condition of being fibrillated. **2.** The formation of fibrils. **3.** Exceedingly rapid contractions or twitching of muscular fibrils, but not of the muscle as a whole. **4.** Vermicular twitching, usually slow, of individual muscular fibers; commonly occurs in atria or ventricles of the heart as well as in recently denervated skeletal muscle fibers.

atrial f., auricular f., f. in which the normal rhythmical contractions of the cardiac atria are replaced by rapid irregular twitchings of the muscular wall; the ventricles respond irregularly to the dysrhythmic bombardment from the atria.

ventricular f., coarse or fine, rapid, fibrillary movements of the ventricular muscle that replace the normal contraction.

fi·bril·lo·gen·e·sis (fī′bril-ō-jen′ĕ-sis). The development of fine fibrils (as seen with the electron microscope) normally present in collagenous fibers of connective tissue.

fi·brin (fī′brin). An elastic filamentous protein derived from fibrinogen by the action of thrombin, which releases fibrinopeptides A and B from fibrinogen in coagulation of the blood; a component of thrombi, vegetations, and acute inflammatory exudates such as in diphtheria and lobar pneumonia. [L. *fibra,* fiber]

fi·brin·ase (fī′brin-ās). **1.** Former term for *factor XIII.* **2.** SYN plasmin.

△**fibrino-.** Fibrin. [L. *fibra,* fiber]

fi·bri·no·cel·lu·lar (fī′bri-nō-sel′yū-lǎr). Composed of fibrin and cells, as in certain types of exudates resulting from acute inflammation.

fi·brin·o·gen (fī-brin′ō-jen). A globulin of the blood plasma that is converted into fibrin by the action of thrombin in the presence of ionized calcium to produce coagulation of the blood; the only coagulable protein in the blood plasma of vertebrates; it is absent in afibrinogenemia and is defective in dysfibrinogenemia.

fi·brin·o·ge·ne·mia (fī-brin′ō-jĕ-nē′mē-ǎ). SYN hyperfibrinogenemia.

fi·bri·no·gen·e·sis (fī′bri-nō-jen′ĕ-sis). Formation or production of fibrin.

fi·bri·no·gen·ic, fi·bri·nog·e·nous (fī′brin-ō-jen′ik, fī′bri-noj′ĕ-nŭs). **1.** Pertaining to fibrinogen. **2.** Producing fibrin.

fi·brin·o·gen·ol·y·sis (fī-brin′ō-jen-ol′i-sis). The inactivation or dissolution of fibrinogen in the blood. [fibrinogen + G. *lysis,* dissolution]

fi·brin·o·gen·o·pe·nia (fī-brin′ō-jen-ō-pē′nē-ǎ). A concentration of fibrinogen in the blood that is less than the normal. [fibrinogen + G. *penia,* poverty]

fi·brin·oid (fī′bri-noyd). **1.** Resembling fibrin. **2.** A deeply or brilliantly acidophilic, homogeneous, refractile, proteinaceous material that: 1) is frequently formed in the walls of blood vessels and in connective tissue of patients with such diseases as disseminated lupus erythematosus, polyarteritis nodosa, scleroderma, dermatomyositis, and rheumatic fever; 2) is sometimes observed in healing wounds, chronic peptic ulcers, the placenta, necrotic arterioles of malignant hypertension, and other unrelated conditions. [fibrin + G. *eidos,* resemblance]

fi•bri•nol•y•sin (fī-brin-ō-lī′sin). SYN plasmin.

fi•bri•nol•y•sis (fī-bri-nol′i-sis). Hydrolysis of fibrin. [fibrino- + G. *lysis,* dissolution]

fi•bri•no•lyt•ic (fī-brin-ō-lit′ik). Denoting, characterized by, or causing fibrinolysis.

fi•brin•o•pep•tide (fī′brin-ō-pep′tīd). One of two pairs of peptides (A and B) released from the amino-terminal ends of 2α- and 2β-chains of fibrinogen by the action of thrombin to form fibrin; they have a vasoconstrictive effect.

fi•bri•no•pu•ru•lent (fī′bri-nō-pyū′rū-lent). Pertaining to pus or suppurative exudate that contains a relatively large amount of fibrin.

fi•brin•ous (fī′brin-ŭs). Pertaining to or composed of fibrin.

fi•bri•nu•ria (fī-bri-nū′rē-ă). The passage of urine that contains fibrin. [fibrin + G. *ouron,* urine]

⌂**fibro-, fibr-.** Fiber. [L. *fibra*]

fi•bro•ad•e•no•ma (fī′brō-ad-ĕ-nō′mă). A benign neoplasm derived from glandular epithelium, in which there is a conspicuous stroma of proliferating fibroblasts and connective tissue elements; commonly occurs in breast tissue. SYN fibroid adenoma, adenoma fibrosum.

fi•bro•ad•i•pose (fī-brō-ad′i-pōz). Relating to or containing both fibrous and fatty structures.

fi•bro•a•re•o•lar (fī′brō-ă-rē′ō-lăr). Denoting connective tissue that is both fibrous and areolar in character.

fi•bro•blast (fī′brō-blast). A stellate or spindle-shaped cell with cytoplasmic processes present in connective tissue, capable of forming collagen fibers; an inactive f. is sometimes called a fibrocyte.

fi•bro•blas•tic (fī-brō-blas′tik). Relating to fibroblasts.

fi•bro•car•ci•no•ma (fī′brō-kar-si-nō′mă). SYN scirrhous *carcinoma.*

fi•bro•car•ti•lage (fī-brō-kar′ti-lij). A variety of cartilage that contains visible type I collagen fibers; appears as a transition between tendons or ligaments or bones.

    circumferential f., a ring of f. around the articular end of a bone, serving to deepen the joint cavity.

    semilunar f., SEE lateral *meniscus,* medial *meniscus.*

fi•bro•car•ti•lag•i•nous (fī′brō-kar-ti-laj′i-nŭs). Relating to or composed of fibrocartilage.

fi•bro•cel•lu•lar (fī-brō-sel′yū-lăr). Both fibrous and cellular.

fi•bro•chon•dri•tis (fī′brō-kon-drī′tis). Inflammation of a fibrocartilage.

fi•bro•chon•dro•ma (fī′brō-kon-drō′mă). A benign neoplasm of cartilaginous tissue, in which there is a relatively unusual amount of fibrous stroma.

fi•bro•cyst (fī′brō-sist). Any cystic lesion circumscribed by or situated within a conspicuous amount of fibrous connective tissue.

fi•bro•cys•tic (fī-brō-sis′tik). Pertaining to or characterized by the presence of fibrocysts.

fi•bro•cys•to•ma (fī′brō-sis-tō′mă). A benign neoplasm, usually derived from glandular epithelium, characterized by cysts within a conspicuous fibrous stroma.

fi•bro•e•las•tic (fī′brō-ē-las′tik). Composed of collagen and elastic fibers.

fi•broid (fī′broyd). **1.** Resembling or composed of fibers or fibrous tissue. **2.** Old term for certain types of leiomyoma, especially those occurring in the uterus. **3.** SYN fibroleiomyoma. [fibro- + G. *eidos,* released form]

fi•broid•ec•to•my (fī-broy-dek′tō-mē). Removal of a fibroid tumor. [fibroid + G. *ektomē,* excision]

fi•bro•lei•o•my•o•ma (fī′brō-lī′ō-mī-ō′mă). A leiomyoma containing non-neoplastic collagenous fibrous tissue, which may make the tumor hard; f. usually arises in the myometrium, and the proportion of fibrous tissue increases with age. SYN fibroid (3), leiomyofibroma.

fi•bro•li•po•ma (fī′brō-li-pō′mă). A lipoma with an abundant stroma of fibrous tissue.

fi•bro•ma (fī-brō′mă). A benign neoplasm derived from fibrous connective tissue. [fibro- + G. *-oma,* tumor]

    ameloblastic f., a benign mixed odontogenic tumor characterized by neoplastic proliferation of both epithelial and mesenchymal components of the tooth bud without the production of dental hard tissue; presents clinically as a slow-growing painless radiolucency occurring most commonly in the mandible of children and adolescents.

    aponeurotic f., a calcifying recurrent non-metastasizing but infiltrating f. seen most frequently on the palms of young people as a small firm nodule not attached to the overlying skin.

    central ossifying f., a painless, slow-growing, expansile, sharply circumscribed benign fibro-osseus tumor of the jaws that is derived from cells of the periodontal ligament; presents initially as a radiolucency that becomes progressively more opaque as it matures.

    chondromyxoid f., an uncommon benign bone tumor, occurring most frequently in the tibia of adolescents and young adults, composed of lobulated myxoid tissue with scanty chondroid foci. SYN chondrofibroma, chondromyxoma.

    desmoplastic f., a benign fibrous tumor of bone affecting children and young adults; cortical destruction may result.

    giant cell f., a tumor of the oral mucosa composed of fibrous connective tissue with large stellate and multinucleate fibroblasts.

    irritation f., a slow-growing nodule on the oral mucosa, composed of fibrous tissue covered by epithelium, resulting from mechanical irritation by dentures, fillings, cheek biting, etc.

    nonosteogenic f., SYN fibrous cortical *defect.*

    peripheral ossifying f., a reactive focal gingival overgrowth derived histogenetically from cells of the periodontal ligament and usually developing in response to local irritants (plaque and calculus) on associated teeth; consists microscopically of a hyperplastic cellular fibrous stroma supporting deposits of bone, cementum, or dystrophic calcification.

telangiectatic f., a benign neoplasm of fibrous tissue in which there are numerous small and large, frequently dilated vascular channels. SYN angiofibroma.

fi·bro·ma·toid (fī-brō′mă-toyd). A focus, nodule, or mass of proliferating fibroblasts that resembles a fibroma but is not regarded as neoplastic.

fi·bro·ma·to·sis (fī′brō-mă-tō′sis). **1.** A condition characterized by the occurrence of multiple fibromas, with a relatively large distribution. **2.** Abnormal hyperplasia of fibrous tissue.

plantar f., nodular fibroblastic proliferation in plantar fascia of one or both feet; rarely associated with contracture.

fi·bro·ma·tous (fī-brō′mă-tŭs). Pertaining to, or of the nature of, a fibroma.

fi·bro·mus·cu·lar (fī′brō-mŭs′kyū-lăr). Both fibrous and muscular; relating to both fibrous and muscular tissues.

fi·bro·my·ec·to·my (fī′brō-mī-ek′tō-mē). Excision of a fibromyoma.

fi·bro·my·o·ma (fī′brō-mī-ō′mă). A leiomyoma that contains a relatively abundant amount of fibrous tissue.

fi·bro·my·o·si·tis (fī′brō-mī-ō-sī′tis). Chronic inflammation of a muscle with an overgrowth, or hyperplasia, of the connective tissue. [fibro- + G. *mys,* muscle, + -*itis,* inflammation]

fi·bro·myx·o·ma (fī′brō-mik-sō′mă). A myxoma that contains a relatively abundant amount of mature fibroblasts and connective tissue. [fibro- + G. *myxa,* mucus, + -*ōma,* tumor]

fi·bro·nec·tins (fī-brō-nek′tins). Glycoproteins found on cell membranes and in blood and other body fluids, which are thought to function as adhesive ligand-like molecules. Possible roles in other processes include transformation to malignancy. Deficiency of fibronectin is associated with Ehlers-Danlos syndrome. [L. *fibra,* fiber, + *nexus,* interconnection]

plasma f., a circulating α_2-glycoprotein that functions as an opsonin, mediating reticuloendothelial and macrophage clearance of fibrin microaggregates, collagen debris, and bacterial particulates, protecting microvascular perfusion and lymphatic drainage.

fi·bro·neu·ro·ma (fī′brō-nū-rō′mă). SYN neurofibroma.

fi·bro·pap·il·lo·ma (fī′brō-pap-i-lō′mă). A papilloma characterized by a conspicuous amount of fibrous connective tissue at the base and forming the cores upon which the neoplastic epithelial cells are massed.

fi·bro·pla·sia (fī-brō-plā′zē-ă). Production of fibrous tissue, usually implying an abnormal increase of non-neoplastic fibrous tissue. [fibro- + G. *plasis,* a molding]

fi·bro·plas·tic (fī-brō-plas′tik). Producing fibrous tissue. [fibro- + G. *plastos,* formed]

fi·bro·re·tic·u·late (fī′brō-re-tik′yū-lāt). Relating to or consisting of a network of fibrous tissue.

fi·bro·sar·co·ma (fī′brō-sar-kō′mă). A malignant neoplasm derived from deep fibrous tissue, characterized by bundles of immature proliferating fibroblasts arranged in a distinctive herringbone pattern with variable collagen formation,

which tends to invade locally and metastasize by the bloodstream.

ameloblastic f., a rapidly growing, painful, destructive, radiolucent odontogenic tumor that usually arises through malignant change in the mesenchymal component of a pre-existing ameloblastic fibroma. SYN ameloblastic sarcoma.

fi·bro·se·rous (fī-brō-sē′rŭs). Composed of fibrous tissue with a serous surface; denoting any serous membrane.

fi·bro·sis (fī-brō′sis). Formation of fibrous tissue as a reparative or reactive process, as opposed to formation of fibrous tissue as a normal constituent of an organ or tissue.

cystic f., cystic f. of the pancreas [MIM* 219700], a congenital metabolic disorder, inherited as an autosomal trait, in which secretions of exocrine glands are abnormal; excessively viscid mucus causes obstruction of passageways (including pancreatic and bile ducts, intestines, and bronchi), and the sodium and chloride content of sweat are increased throughout the patient's life; symptoms usually appear in childhood and include meconium ileus, poor growth despite good appetite, malabsorption and foul bulky stools, chronic bronchitis with cough, recurrent pneumonia, bronchiectasis, emphysema, clubbing of the fingers, and salt depletion in hot weather. Detailed genetic mapping and molecular biology have been accomplished by the methods of reverse genetics.

endomyocardial f., thickening of the ventricular endocardium by f., involving the subendocardial myocardium, and sometimes the atrioventricular valves, with mural thrombosis, leading to progressive right and left ventricular failure with mitral and tricuspid insufficiency; occurs in adults and is endemic in parts of Africa.

idiopathic pulmonary f. (IPF), subacute form also called Hamman-Rich syndrome; an acute to chronic inflammatory process of the lungs, the healing stage of diffuse alveolar damage or acute interstitial pneumonia, either idiopathic or associated with collagen-vascular diseases.

mediastinal f., f. that may obstruct the superior vena cava, pulmonary arteries, veins, or bronchi; most common cause is histoplasmosis; less commonly tuberculosis or unknown.

retroperitoneal f., f. of retroperitoneal structures commonly involving and often obstructing the ureters; the cause is usually unknown.

fi·bro·si·tis (fī-brō-sī′tis). **1.** Inflammation of fibrous tissue. **2.** Term used to denote aching, soreness, or stiffness, with multiple tender foci (trigger points); unknown etiology; thought by some to be due to a sleep disturbance preventing normal muscle relaxation. [fibro- + G. -*itis,* inflammation]

fi·brot·ic (fī-brot′ik). Pertaining to or characterized by fibrosis.

fi·brous (fī′brŭs). Composed of or containing fibroblasts, and also the fibrils and fibers of connective tissue formed by such cells.

fib·u·la (fib′yū-lă) [NA]. The lateral and smaller of the two bones of the leg; it is not-weight bearing and articulates with the tibia above and the tibia and talus below. SYN calf bone. [L. *fibula* (contr. fr. *figibula*), that which fastens, a clasp, buckle, fr. *figo*, to fix, fasten]

fib·u·lar (fib′yū-lăr). Relating to the fibula. [L. *fibularis*]

fib·u·lo·cal·ca·ne·al (fib′yū-lō-kal-kā′nē-ăl). Relating to the fibula and the calcaneus.

FID free induction *decay*.

field (fēld). A definite area of plane surface, considered in relation to some specific object. [A.S. *feld*]

　auditory f., the space included within the limits of hearing of a definite sound, as of a tuning fork.

　individuation f., the f. within which an organizer can bring about the rearrangement of primordial tissues in such a manner that a complete embryo is formed.

　visual f. (F), the area simultaneously visible to one eye without movement; often measured by means of a bowl perimeter located 330 mm from the eye.

FIGLU formiminoglutamic acid.

fig·ure (fig′yūr). 1. A form or shape. 2. A person representing the essential aspects of a particular role. 3. A form, shape, outline, or representation of an object or person. [L. *figura*, fr *fingo*, to shape, fashion]

　authority f., a real or projected person in a position of power; one's parents, police, and boss are authority figures to some people; during the transference phase of psychoanalysis, the psychoanalyst becomes an authority f.

　mitotic f., the microscopic appearance of a cell undergoing mitosis; a cell of which the chromosomes are visible by the light microscope.

fig·ure and ground. That aspect of perception wherein the perceived is separated into at least two parts, each with different attributes but influencing one another. Figure is the most distinct; ground the least formed; *e.g.,* a bird or tree (figure) seen against the sky (ground).

fi·la (fī′lă). Plural of filum. [L.]

fi·la·ceous (fī-lā′shŭs). SYN filamentous. [L. *filum*, a thread]

fil·a·ment (fil′ă-ment). 1. SYN filamentum. 2. BACTERIOLOGY A fine threadlike form, unsegmented or segmented without constrictions. [L. *filamentum*, fr. *filum*, a thread]

　actin f., one of the contractile elements in muscular fibers and other cells; in skeletal muscle, the actin f.'s are about 5 nm wide and 100 μm long, and attach to the transverse Z f.'s.

　axial f., the central f. of a flagellum or cilium; with the electron microscope is seen as a complex of nine peripheral diplomicrotubules and a central pair of microtubules. SYN axoneme (2).

　myosin f., one of the contractile elements in skeletal, cardiac, and smooth muscle fibers; in skeletal muscle, the f. is about 10 nm thick and 1.5 μm long.

　Z f., the thin zig-zag structure at the Z line of striated muscle fibers to which the actin f.'s attach.

fil·a·men·tous (fil-ă-men′tŭs). 1. Threadlike in structure. SYN filiform (1). 2. Composed of filaments or threadlike structures. SYN filaceous, filar (2).

fil·a·men·tum, pl. **fil·a·men·ta** (fil-ă-men′tŭm, -tă). A fibril, fine fiber, or threadlike structure. SYN filament (1). [L.]

fi·lar (fī′lăr). 1. SYN fibrillar. 2. SYN filamentous. [L. *filum*, a thread]

Fi·lar·ia (fī-lar′ē-ă). Nematodes classified in several genera of the family Onchocercidae; *e.g.,* *Wuchereria bancrofti*, *Brugia malayi*, *Onchocerca volvulus*, *Mansonella perstans*, *M. streptocerca*, *M. ozzardi*, *Loa loa*, and *Dracunculus medinensis*. SEE ALSO filaria.

fi·lar·ia, pl. **fi·lar·i·ae** (fī-lar′ē-ă, -ē-ē). Common name for nematodes of the family Onchocercidae, which live as adults in the blood, tissue fluids, tissues, or body cavities of many vertebrates. The females lay partially embryonated eggs, the embryos uncoil and circulate in blood or tissue fluids as microfilariae; if ingested by an appropriate bloodsucking arthropod, larval stages develop; later, infective larvae may be deposited on another vertebrate host's skin when the arthropod seeks another blood meal. [L. *filum*, a thread]

fi·lar·i·al (fi-lā′rē-ăl). Pertaining to a filaria (or filariae), including the microfilaria stage.

fil·a·ri·a·sis (fil-ă-rī′ă-sis). Presence of filariae in the tissues of the body or in blood (microfilaremia) or tissue fluids (microfilariasis), occurring in tropical and subtropical regions; living worms cause minimal tissue reaction, which may be asymptomatic, but death of the adult worms leads to granulomatous inflammation and permanent fibrosis causing obstruction of the lymphatic channels from dense hyalinized scars in the subcutaneous tissues; the most serious consequence is elephantiasis or pachyderma.

fi·lar·i·ci·dal (fi-lar-i-sī′dăl). Fatal to filariae.

fi·lar·i·cide (fi-lar′i-sīd). An agent that kills filariae. [filaria + L. *caedo*, to kill]

fi·lar·i·form (fi-lar′i-fōrm). 1. Resembling filariae or other types of small nematode worms. 2. Thin or hairlike.

fil·i·al (fil′ē-ăl). Denoting the relationship of offspring to parents. SEE filial *generation*. [L. *filialis*, fr. *filius*, son, *filia*, daughter]

fi·li·form (fil′i-fōrm). 1. SYN filamentous (1). 2. BACTERIOLOGY Denoting an even growth along the line of inoculation, either stroke or stab. [L. *filum*, thread]

fil·let (fil′et). 1. SYN lemniscus. 2. A skein, loop of cord, or tape used for making traction on a part of the fetus. [Fr. *filet*, a band]

fill·ing (fil′ing). Lay term for a dental restoration.

　capillary f., the return of a normal pink color to an area of skin, or a nail bed, after cutaneous capillaries have been emptied of blood by firm digital pressure; the promptness of return is a rough measure of general and vascular competence.

film. 1. A thin sheet of flexible material coated with a light-sensitive or x-ray-sensitive substance used in taking photographs or radiographs. 2. A thin layer or coating. 3. A radiograph (colloq.).

　absorbable gelatin f., a sterile, nonantigenic, absorbable, water-insoluble sheet of gelatin prepared by drying a gelatin-formaldehyde solution on plates; used in the closure and repair of defects in membranes such as the dura mater or the pleura; it undergoes absorption over a period of 1 to 6 months.

bitewing f., a special packaging of radiographic f. that allows appendage of the f. package to be held between the occlusal surfaces of the teeth.

  decubitus f., a radiograph exposed with the subject in the decubitus position; named for the side that is dependent.

occlusal f., intraoral projection taken to provide a wider view of either the maxilla and palate or the mandible and floor of the mouth.

panoramic x-ray f., DENTISTRY a radiograph taken to give a panoramic view of the entire upper and lower dental arch as well as the temporomandibular joints.

periapical f., intraoral radiographic projection taken to include tooth apices and surrounding alveolar bone. F. sizes 0–2 may be utilized. SEE periapical *radiograph.*

  plain f., a radiograph made without use of a contrast medium.

  scout f., a radiograph exposed before contrast medium is given, such as the preliminary film for

an angiogram, urogram, or barium contrast gastrointestinal examination.

film badge. Small packet of x-ray film and filters worn by radiation workers to monitor exposure to radiation on a monthly basis. SEE ALSO pocket *dosimeter,* thermoluminescent *dosimeter.*

fi·lo·pres·sure (fī-lō-presh′ŭr). Temporary pressure on a blood vessel by a ligature, which is removed when the flow of blood has ceased. [L. *filum,* thread]

fil·ter (fil′ter). **1.** A porous substance through which a liquid or gas is passed in order to separate it from contained particulate matter or impurities. **2.** To use or to subject to the action of a f. **3.** RADIOLOGY a device, used in both diagnostic and therapeutic radiology, that permits passage of useful x-rays and absorbs those that have a lower and less desirable energy. **4.** A device used in spectrophotometric analysis to isolate a segment of the spectrum. **5.** A mathematical algorithm applied to image data for the purpose of enhancing image quality, usually by suppression of high

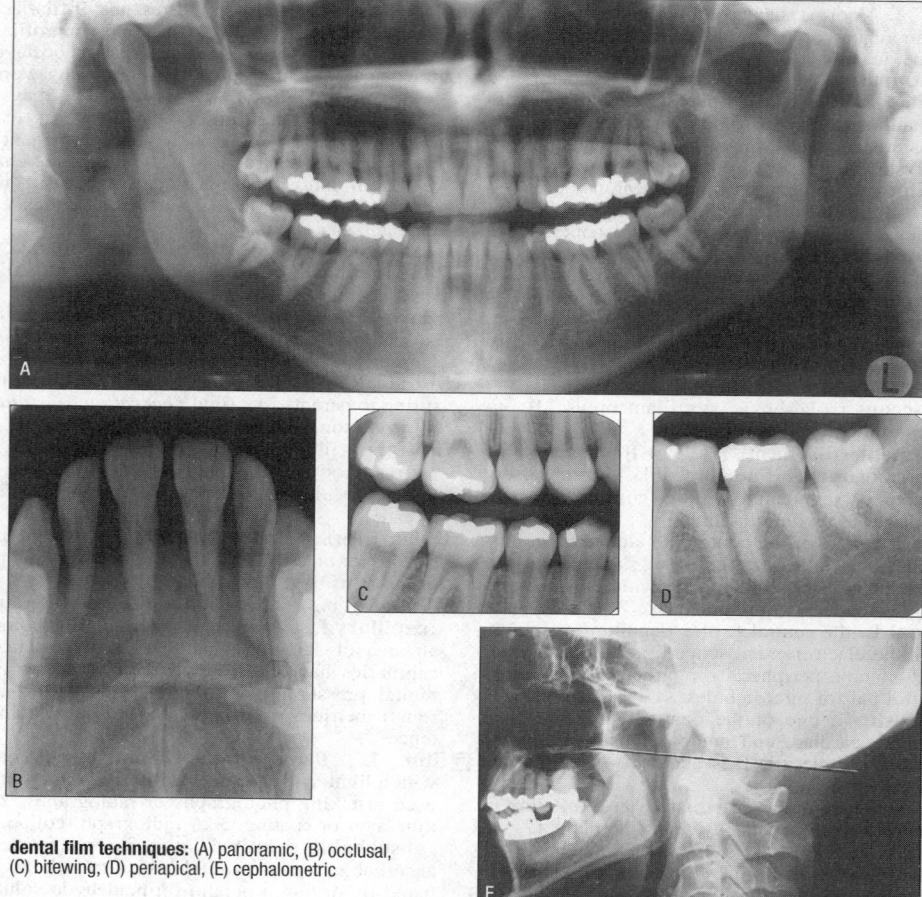

dental film techniques: (A) panoramic, (B) occlusal, (C) bitewing, (D) periapical, (E) cephalometric

spatial frequency noise. [Mediev. L. *filtro,* pp. *-atus,* to strain through felt, fr. *filtrum,* felt]

Greenfield f., a multistrutted spring-styled filter usually placed in the inferior vena cava to prevent venous emboli from reaching the pulmonary circulation from the lower extremity.

fil·tra·ble, fil·ter·a·ble (fil′tră-bl, fil′ter-ă-bl). Capable of passing a filter; frequently applied to smaller viruses and some bacteria.

fil·trate (fil′trāt). That which has passed through a filter.

fil·tra·tion (fil-trā′shŭn). **1.** The process of passing a liquid or gas through a filter. **2.** RADIOLOGY The process of attenuating and hardening a beam of x-rays or gamma rays by interposing a filter (3) between the radiation source and the object being irradiated; inherent f. is that which is caused by the apparatus itself, such as the glass of an x-ray tube, without addition of a filter. SYN percolation (1).

fi·lum, pl. **fi·la** (fī′lŭm, -lă) [NA]. A structure of filamentous or threadlike appearance. [L. thread]

radicular fi′la, the small, individual fiber fascicles into which the roots of all of the spinal nerves and several cranial nerves (hypoglossus, vagus, oculomotorius) divide in fanlike fashion before entering or leaving the spinal cord or brainstem; the spinal dorsal root may divide into 8 to 12 such rootlets.

f. of spinal dura mater, the thread-like termination of the spinal dura mater, surrounding and fused to the f. terminale of the cord, and attached to the deep dorsal sacrococcygeal ligament; extends from S_{2-3} to Co_2 vertebral levels.

terminal f., a long, slender connective tissue (pia mater) strand extending from the extremity of the medullary cone to the internal aspect of the spinal dural sac (f. terminale internum); stout strands of connective tissue attaching the spinal dural sac to the coccyx (f. terminale externum), commonly called the coccygeal ligament.

fim·bria, pl. **fim·bri·ae** (fim′brē-ă, -brē-ē). **1** [NA]. Any fringelike structure. **2.** SYN pilus (2). [L. fringe]

f. hippocam′pi [NA], a narrow sharp-edged crest of white fiber matter, continuous with the alveus hippocampi, attached to the medial border of the hippocampus; composed of efferent fibers of the hippocampus that form the fornix, fibers of the hippocampal commissure, and septohippocampal fibers. SYN corpus fimbriatum (1).

fim′briae of uterine tube, the irregularly branched or fringed processes surrounding the ampulla at the abdominal opening of the uterine tube; most of the lining epithelial cells have cilia that beat toward the uterus.

fim·bri·ate, fim·bri·at·ed (fim′brē-āt, -ā-ted). Having fimbriae.

fim·bri·o·cele (fim′brē-ō-sēl). Hernia of the corpus fimbriatum of the oviduct. [L. *fimbria,* fringe, + G. *kēlē,* hernia]

fin·ger (fing′ger). One of the digits of the hand. [A.S.]

baseball f., an avulsion, partial or complete, of the long finger extensor from the base of the distal phalanx. SYN mallet f. (2).

clubbed f.'s, SEE clubbing.

hippocratic f.'s, SEE clubbing.

index f., the second f. (the thumb being counted as the first). SYN index (1).

jersey f. (jŭr′zē), avulsion of the flexor digitorum profundus tendon from the distal phalanx due to abrupt passive extension of the actively flexed f.

mallet f., (1) flexion deformity of a distal phalanx due to avulsion of the extensor tendon by forceful passive flexion of the phalanx **(2)** SYN baseball f.

ring f., fourth finger.

webbed f.'s, two or more f.'s united and enclosed in a common sheath of skin.

fin·ger·print (fing′ger-print′). **1.** An impression of the inked bulb of the distal phalanx of a finger, showing the configuration of the surface ridges, used as a means of identification. SEE ALSO dermatoglyphics. **2.** Any analytical method capable of making fine distinctions between similar compounds or gel patterns; *e.g.,* the pattern of an infrared absorption curve or of a two-dimensional paper chromatograph. **3.** GENETICS The analysis of DNA fragments to determine the identity of an individual or the paternity of a child.

DNA fingerprinting, a technique used to compare individuals by molecular genotyping. DNA is isolated from a specific individual, digested, and fractionated according to size. A Southern hybridization with a radiolabeled repetitive DNA probe provides an autoradiographic pattern unique to the individual. DNA f. offers a statistical basis for evaluating the probability that samples of blood, hair, semen, or tissue have originated from a given individual.

fingerspelling. Method of communication using specific finger and hand movements, representing letters of the alphabet, to spell words. SEE ALSO American Manual Alphabet.

first aid. Immediate assistance administered in the case of injury or sudden illness by a bystander or other lay person, before the arrival of trained medical personnel.

FISH fluorescence in situ *hybridization.*

fis·sion (fish′ŭn). **1.** The act of splitting, *e.g.,* amitotic division of a cell or its nucleus. **2.** Splitting of the nucleus of an atom. [L. *fissio,* a cleaving, fr. *findo,* pp. *fissus,* to cleave]

binary f., simple f. in which the two new cells are approximately equal in size.

multiple f., division of the nucleus into a number of daughter nuclei, followed by division of the cell body into an equal number of daughter cells, each containing a nucleus.

simple f., division of the nucleus and then the cell body into two parts. SEE ALSO binary f.

fis·si·par·i·ty (fis-i-par′i-tē). SYN schizogenesis. [L. *fissio,* cleaving, fr. *findo,* to cleave, + *pario,* to bring forth]

fis·sip·a·rous (fi-sip′ă-rŭs). Reproducing or propagating by fission. [L. *findo,* pp. *fissus,* split, + *pario,* to produce]

fis·su·ra, pl. **fis·su·rae** (fi-sū′ră, -sū′rē) [NA]. **1.** SYN fissure. **2.** NEUROANATOMY A particularly deep sulcus of the surface of the brain or spinal cord. [L. fr. *findo,* to cleave]

fissu′rae cerebel′li [NA], SYN cerebellar *fissures*, under *fissure*.

fis•sure (fish′ŭr). **1.** A deep furrow, cleft, or slit. (For most of the brain fissures, see entries under sulcus). **2.** In dentistry, a developmental break or fault in the tooth enamel. SYN fissura (1) [NA]. [L. *fissura*]

abdominal f., congenital failure of the ventral body wall to close. SEE ALSO gastroschisis.

anal f., a crack or slit in the mucous membrane of the anus.

Bichat's f., the nearly circular f. corresponding to the medial margin of the cerebral (pallial) mantle, marking the hilus of the cerebral hemisphere, consisting of the callosomarginal f. and choroidal f. along the hippocampus, both of which are continuous with the stem of the f. of Sylvius at the anterior extremity of the temporal lobe.

caudal transverse f., SYN *porta* hepatis.

cerebellar f.'s, the deep furrows which divide the lobules of the cerebellum. SYN fissurae cerebelli [NA].

glaserian f., SYN petrotympanic f.

horizontal f. of cerebellum, horizontal f. that divides the ansiform lobule into its major parts, crus I (superior semilunar lobule) and crus II (inferior semilunar lobule).

f. of ligamentum venosum, a deep cleft extending from the porta hepatis and the inferior vena cava between the left lobe and the caudate lobe; it lodges the ligamentum venosum and is thus a vestige of the fossa of the ductus venosus.

f. of round ligament of liver, a cleft on the inferior surface of the liver, running from the inferior border to the left extremity of the porta hepatis; it lodges the round ligament of the liver.

palpebral f., SYN *rima* palpebrarum.

paracentral f., a curved f. (sulcus) on the medial surface of the cerebral hemisphere, bounding the paracentral gyrus and separating it from the precuneus and the cingulate gyrus.

petro-occipital f., a fissure between the petrous part of the temporal bone and the basilar part of the occipital bone that extends anteromedially from the jugular foramen; includes the jugular foramen (at its posterior end).

petrotympanic f., a fissure between the tympanic and petrous portions of the temporal bone; it transmits the chorda tympani nerve through a small patent portion, the anterior canaliculus of the chorda tympani. SYN glaserian f.

portal f., SYN *porta* hepatis.

primary f. of cerebellum, the deepest f. of the cerebellum; demarcates the division of anterior and posterior lobes of the cerebellum; second to appear embryologically.

superior orbital f., a cleft between the greater and the lesser wings of the sphenoid establishing a channel of communication between the middle cranial fossa and the orbit, through which pass the oculomotor and trochlear nerves, the ophthalmic division of the trigeminal nerve, the abducens nerve, and the ophthalmic veins.

tympanomastoid f., a fissure separating the tympanic portion from the mastoid portion of the temporal bone; it transmits the auricular branch of the vagus nerve.

fis•tu•la, pl. **fis•tu•lae, fis•tu•las** (fis′tyū-lă, -tyū-lē, -tyū-lăs). An abnormal passage from one epithelialized surface to another; congenital, caused by disease or injury, or created surgically. [L. a pipe, a tube]

amphibolic f., amphibolous f., a complete anal f. opening both externally and internally.

anal f., a f. opening at or near the anus; usually, but not always, opening into the rectum above the internal sphincter.

arteriovenous f., an abnormal communication between an artery and a vein, usually resulting in the formation of an arteriovenous aneurysm.

blind f., a f. that ends in a cul-de-sac, being open at one extremity only. SYN incomplete f.

bronchopleural f. (BPF), communication between a bronchus and the pleural cavity; usually caused by necrotizing pneumonia or empyema; also may follow pulmonary surgery or irradiation.

carotid-cavernous f., a fistulous communication, of spontaneous or traumatic origin, between the cavernous sinus and the traversing internal carotid artery; a pulsating unilateral exophthalmos and a detectable cranial bruit are common manifestations.

complete f., a f. that is open at both ends.

Eck f., transposition of the portal circulation to the systemic by making an anastomosis between the vena cava and portal vein and then ligating the latter close to the liver.

external f., a f. between a hollow viscus and the skin.

fecal f., SYN intestinal f.

gastric f., a fistulous tract from the stomach to the abdominal wall.

horseshoe f., an anal f. partially encircling the anus and opening at both extremities on the cutaneous surface.

incomplete f., SYN blind f.

internal f., a f. between hollow viscera.

intestinal f., a tract leading from the lumen of the small intestine to the exterior. SYN fecal f.

parietal f., a f., either blind or complete, opening on the wall of the thorax or abdomen.

reverse Eck f., side-to-side anastomosis of the portal vein with the inferior vena cava and ligation of the latter above the anastomosis but below the hepatic veins; the blood from the lower part of the body is thus directed through the hepatic circulation.

salivary f., a pathologic communication between a salivary duct or gland and the cutaneous surface or the oral mucus.

urethrovaginal f., a f. between the urethra and the vagina.

vesicouterine f., a f. between the bladder and the uterus.

fis•tu•la•tion, fis•tu•li•za•tion (fis-tyū-lā′shŭn, -tyū-li-zā′shŭn). Formation of a fistula in a part; becoming fistulous.

fis•tu•lec•to•my (fis-tyū-lek′tō-mē). Excision of a fistula. SYN syringectomy. [fistula + G. *ektomē,* excision]

fis•tu•lot•o•my (fis-tyū-lot′ō-mē). Incision or

surgical enlargement of a fistula. SYN syringotomy. [fistula + G. *tomē*, incision]

fis•tu•lous (fis′tyū-lŭs). Relating to or containing a fistula.

fit. 1. An attack of an acute disease or the sudden appearance of some symptom, such as coughing. **2.** A convulsion. **3.** SYN epilepsy. **4.** DENTISTRY The adaptation of any dental restoration, *e.g.,* of an inlay to the cavity preparation in a tooth, or of a denture to its basal seat. [A.S. *fitt*]

FITC fluorescein isothiocyanate.

fit•ness (fit′nes). **1.** Well-being. **2.** Suitability. **3.** POPULATION GENETICS A measure of the relative survival and reproductive success of a given individual or phenotype, or of a population subgroup. **4.** A set of attributes, primarily respiratory and cardiovascular, relating to ability to perform tasks requiring expenditure of energy.

   clinical f., absence of frank disease or of subclinical precursors.

   evolutionary f., the probability that the line of descent from an individual with a specific trait will not eventually die out.

   genetic f., in a phenotype, the mean number of surviving offspring that it generates in its lifetime, usually expressed as a fraction or percentage of the average genetic f. of the population.

   health-related physical f., components of physical f. (most commonly, aerobic f., body composition, abdominal muscular strength and endurance, and lower back and hamstring flexibility) that are associated with some aspect of overall good health or disease prevention. h

   physical f., a set of attributes relating to one's ability to perform physical activity. SEE health-related physical f.

fix•a•tion (fik-sā′shŭn). **1.** The condition of being firmly attached or set. **2.** HISTOLOGY The rapid killing of tissue elements and their preservation and hardening to retain as nearly as possible the same relations they had in the living body. SYN fixing. **3.** CHEMISTRY The conversion of a gas into solid or liquid form by chemical reactions, with or without the help of living tissue. **4.** PSYCHOANALYSIS The quality of being firmly attached to a particular person or object or period in one's development. **5.** PHYSIOLOGICAL OPTICS The coordinated positioning and accommodation of both eyes that results in bringing or maintaining a sharp image of a stationary or moving object on the fovea of each eye. [L. *figo,* pp. *fixus,* to fix, fasten]

   complement f., f. of complement in a serum by an antigen-antibody combination whereby it is rendered unavailable to complete a reaction in a second antigen-antibody combination for which complement is necessary; the second system usually serves as an indicator (red blood cells plus specific hemolysin); if complement is fixed with the first antigen-antibody union, hemolysis does not occur, but, if complement is not so removed, it causes hemolysis in the second system.

   external f., f. of fractured bones by splints, plastic dressings, or transfixion pins.

   internal f., stabilization of fractured bony parts by direct f. to one another with surgical wires, screws, pins, rods, plates, or methylmethacrylate.

fix•a•tive (fik′să-tiv). **1.** Serving to fix, bind, or make firm or stable. **2.** A substance used for the preservation of gross and histologic specimens of tissue, or individual cells, usually by denaturing and precipitating or cross-linking the protein constituents. SEE ALSO fluid, solution.

fix•a•tor (fik-sā′ter). A device providing rigid immobilization through external skeletal fixation by means of rods (f.'s) attached to pins which are placed in or through the bone.

fix•ing (fik′sing). SYN fixation (2).

flac•cid (flak′sid, flas′id). Relaxed, flabby, or without tone. [L. *flaccidus*]

flac•cid•i•ty (flă-sid′i-tē). The condition or state of being flaccid.

fla•gel•la (flă-jel′ă). Plural of flagellum.

fla•gel•lar (fla-jel′ăr). Relating to a flagellum or to the extremity of a protozoan.

flag•el•late (flaj′ĕ-lāt). **1.** Possessing one or more flagella. **2.** A member of the class Mastigophora.

flag•el•lat•ed (flaj′ĕ-lā-ted). Possessing one or more flagella.

flag•el•la•tion (flaj′ĕ-lā′shŭn). **1.** Whipping either one's self or another as a means of arousing or heightening sexual feeling. **2.** The pattern of formation of flagella. [L. *flagellatus,* fr. *flagello,* to whip or scourge]

flag•el•lo•sis (flaj′ĕ-lō′sis). Infection with flagellated protozoa in the intestinal or genital tract, *e.g.,* trichomoniasis.

fla•gel•lum, pl. **fla•gel•la** (flă-jel′ŭm, -ă). A whiplike locomotory organelle of constant structural arrangement consisting of nine double peripheral microtubules and two single central microtubules; it arises from a deeply staining basal granule, often connected to the nucleus by a fiber, the rhizoplast. [L. dim. of *flagrum,* a whip]

flange (flanj). That part of the denture base which extends from the cervical ends of the teeth to the border of the denture.

flank. SYN latus.

flap. 1. Mass or tongue of tissue for transplantation, vascularized by a pedicle or stem; specifically, a pedicle f. **2.** An uncontrolled movement, as of the hands. SEE asterixis. [M.E. *flappe*]

   advancement f., SYN sliding f.

   axial pattern f., a f. that includes a direct specific artery within its longitudinal axis.

   buried f., a f. denuded of both surface epithelium and superficial dermis and transferred into the subcutaneous tissues.

   caterpillar f., a tubed f. transferred end-over-end (in stages) from the donor area to a distant recipient area. SYN waltzed f.

   composite f., compound f., a f. of 2 or more elements incorporating underlying muscle, bone, or cartilage.

   cross f., a skin f. transferred from one part of the body to a corresponding part, as from one arm to the other.

   delayed f., a f. raised in its donor area in two or more stages to increase its chances of survival after transfer.

   direct f., a f. raised completely and transferred at the same stage. SYN immediate f.

   distant f., a f. in which the donor site is distant from the recipient area.

fl

Filatov f., SYN tubed f.

Filatov-Gillies f., SYN tubed f.

flat f., a f. in which during transfer the pedicle is left flat or open, *i.e.,* untubed. SYN open f.

free f., island f. in which the donor vessels are severed proximally, the f. is transported as a free object to the recipient area, and the f. is revascularized by anastomosing its supplying vessels to vessels there.

hinged f., a turnover f. transferred by lifting it over on its pedicle as if the pedicle were a hinge.

immediate f., SYN direct f.

island f., a f. in which the pedicle consists solely of the supplying artery and vein(s), sometimes including a nerve.

jump f., a distant f. transferred in stages via an intermediate carrier; *e.g.,* an abdominal f. is attached to the wrist, then at a later stage the wrist is brought to the face.

local f., a f. transferred to an adjacent area.

open f., SYN flat f.

partial-thickness f., SYN split-thickness f.

pedicle f., (**1**) a skin f. sustained by a blood-carrying stem from the donor site during transfer; (**2**) PERIODONTAL SURGERY a f. used to increase the width of attached gingiva, or to cover a root surface, by moving the attached gingiva, which remains joined at one side, to an adjacent position and suturing the free end.

pharyngeal f., f. of tissue placed to reduce the size of the opening between the oral and nasal cavities, to mitigate insufficient velar closure. SEE ALSO hypernasality, cleft *palate.*

random pattern f., a f. in which the pedicle blood supply is derived randomly from the network of vessels in the area, rather than from a single longitudinal artery as in an axial pattern f.

rotation f., a pedicle f. that is rotated from the donor site to an adjacent recipient area, usually as a direct f.

sliding f., a rectangular f. raised in an elastic area, with its free end adjacent to a defect; the defect is covered by stretching the f. longitudinally until the end comes over it. SYN advancement f.

split-thickness f., a f. of a portion of the skin, *i.e.,* the epidermis and part of the dermis, or of part of the mucosa and submucosa, but not including the periosteum. SYN partial-thickness f.

subcutaneous f., a pedicle f. in which the pedicle is denuded of epithelium and buried in the subcutaneous tissue of the recipient area.

tubed f., a f. in which the sides of the pedicle are sutured together to create a tube, with the entire surface covered by skin. SYN Filatov f., Filatov-Gillies f.

waltzed f., SYN caterpillar f.

flare (flār). **1.** A gradual tapering or spreading outward. **2.** A diffuse redness of the skin extending beyond the local reaction to the application of an irritant; it is due to dilation of the arterioles and capillaries; depends upon an axon reflex set up by the liberation of a histamine-like substance in skin when injured. SEE ALSO triple *response.*

flash. 1. A sudden and brief burst of light or heat. **2.** Excess material extruded between the sections of a flask in the process of molding denture bases or other dental restorations.

hot f., colloquialism for one of the vasomotor symptoms of the climacteric that may involve the whole body as a f. of heat; also used interchangeably with hot *flush.*

flash•back. An involuntary recurrence of some aspect of a hallucinatory experience or perceptual distortion occurring some time after ingestion of the hallucinogen that produced the original effect and without subsequent ingestion of the substance.

flat•foot (flat′fut). SYN *talipes* planus.

flat•u•lence (flat′yū-lens). Presence of an excessive amount of gas in the stomach and intestines. [Mod. L. *flatulentus,* fr. L. *flatus,* a blowing, fr. *flo,* pp. *flatus,* to blow]

flat•u•lent (flat′yū-lent). Relating to or suffering from flatulence.

fla•tus (flā′tŭs). Gas or air in the gastrointestinal tract which may be expelled through the anus. [L. a blowing]

flat•worm (flat′werm). A member of the phylum Platyhelminthes, including the parasitic tapeworms and flukes.

fla•vin, fla•vine (flā′vin, -vēn, flav′in, -ēn). A yellow acridine dye, preparations of which are used as antiseptics. [L. *flavus,* yellow]

f. adenine dinucleotide (FAD), a condensation product of riboflavin and adenosine 5′-diphosphate; the coenzyme of various aerobic dehydrogenases, *e.g.,* D-amino-acid oxidase and aldehyde dehydrogenase; strictly speaking, FAD is not a dinucleotide since it contains a sugar alcohol.

f. mononucleotide (FMN), riboflavin 5′-phosphate; the coenzyme of a number of oxidation-reduction enzymes; *e.g.,* NADH dehydrogenase and L-amino acid oxidase. Strictly speaking, FMN is not a nucleotide since it contains a sugar alcohol instead of a sugar.

Fla•vi•vi•rus (flā′vi-vī-rŭs). A genus in the family Flaviviridae that includes yellow fever, dengue, and St. Louis encephalitis viruses. [L. *flavus,* yellow, + virus]

Fla•vo•bac•te•ri•um (flā-vō-bak-tēr′ē-ŭm). A genus of aerobic to facultatively anaerobic, nonsporeforming, motile and nonmotile bacteria containing Gram-negative rods. These organisms characteristically produce yellow, orange, red, or yellow-brown pigments. They are found in soil and fresh and salt water. Some species are pathogenic. [L. *flavus,* yellow]

fla•vo•en•zyme (flā-vō-en′zīm). Any enzyme that possesses a flavin nucleotide as coenzyme; *e.g.,* xanthine oxidase, succinate dehydrogenase.

fla•vo•pro•tein (flā′vō-prō′tēn). A compound protein possessing a flavin as prosthetic group. Cf. flavoenzyme.

flea (flē). An insect of the order Siphonaptera, marked by lateral compression, sucking mouthparts, extraordinary jumping powers, and ectoparasitic adult life in the hair and feathers of warm-blooded animals.

flesh. 1. The meat of animals used for food. **2.** SYN muscular *tissue.* [A.S. *flaesc*]

proud f., exuberant granulation tissue on the surface of a wound.

flex (fleks). To bend; to move a joint in such a direction as to approximate the two parts which it connects. [L. *flecto,* pp. *flexus,* to bend]

flex·i·bil·i·tas ce·rea (flek-si-bil'i-tas sē'rē-ă). The rigidity of catalepsy which may be overcome by slight external force, but which returns at once, holding the limb firmly in the new position. [L. waxy flexibility]

flexibility. Total range of motion at a joint dependent on normal joint mechanics, mobility of soft tissues, and muscle extensibility. SEE range of motion.

flex·ion (flek'shŭn). **1.** The act of flexing or bending, *e.g.,* bending of a joint so as to approximate the parts it connects; bending of the spine so that the concavity of the curve looks forward. **2.** The condition of being flexed or bent. SYN open-packed position (2). [L. *flecto,* pp. *flexus,* to bend]

flex·or (flek'ser, -sōr). A muscle the action of which is to flex a joint.

flex·u·ra, pl. **flex·u·'rae** (flek-shyūr'ă, -shyūr'ē) [NA]. SYN flexure. [L. a bending]
  f. co'li dex'tra [NA], SYN right colic *flexure.*
  f. co'li sinis'tra [NA], SYN left colic *flexure.*
  f. duode'nojejuna'lis [NA], SYN duodenojejunal *flexure.*

flex·ur·al (flek'sher-ăl). Relating to a flexure.

flex·ure (flek'sher). A bend, as in an organ or structure. SYN flexura [NA]. [L. *flexura*]
  basicranial f., SYN pontine f.
  caudal f., the bend in the lumbosacral region of the embryo. SYN sacral f.
  cephalic f., the sharp, ventrally concave bend in the developing midbrain of the embryo. SYN cranial f., mesencephalic f.
  cervical f., the ventrally concave bend at the juncture of the brainstem and spinal cord in the embryo.
  cranial f., SYN cephalic f.
  dorsal f., a f. in the mid-dorsal region in the embryo.
  duodenojejunal f., an abrupt bend in the small intestine at the junction of the duodenum and jejunum. SYN flexura duodenojejunalis [NA].
  hepatic f., SYN right colic f.
  left colic f., the bend at the junction of the transverse and descending colon. SYN flexura coli sinistra [NA], splenic f.
  lumbar f., the normal ventral curve of the vertebral column in the lumbar region.
  mesencephalic f., SYN cephalic f.
  pontine f., the dorsally concave curvature of the rhombencephalon in the embryo; appearance indicates division of rhombencephalon into myelencephalon and metencephalon. SYN basicranial f., transverse rhombencephalic f.
  right colic f., the bend of the colon at the juncture of its ascending and transverse portions. SYN flexura coli dextra [NA], hepatic f.
  sacral f., SYN caudal f.
  sacral f. of rectum, the anteroposterior curve with concavity anteriorward of the first portion of the rectum.
  splenic f., SYN left colic f.

telencephalic f., a f. appearing in the embryonic forebrain region.
  transverse rhombencephalic f., SYN pontine f.

flight in·to dis·ease. Gain through falling ill or assuming the sick role. SEE primary *gain,* secondary *gain.*

flight in·to health. DYNAMIC PSYCHOTHERAPY The early but often only temporary disappearance of the symptoms that ostensibly brought the patient into therapy; a defense against the anxiety engendered by the prospect of further psychoanalytic exploration of the patient's conflicts.

float·er (flōt'er). An object in the field of vision that originates in the vitreous body. SEE ALSO muscae volitantes.

float·ing (flōt'ing). **1.** Free or unattached. **2.** Unduly movable; out of the normal position; denoting an occasional abnormal condition of certain organs, such as the kidneys, liver, and spleen.

floc·cil·la·tion (flok-si-lā'shŭn). An aimless plucking at the bedclothes, as if one were picking off threads or tufts of cotton. [Mod. L. *flocculus*]

floc·cose (flok'ōs). BACTERIOLOGY Applied to a growth of short, curving filaments or chains closely but irregularly disposed. [L. *floccus,* a flock of wool]

floc·cu·lar (flok'yū-lăr). Relating to a flocculus of any sort; specifically to the flocculus of the cerebellum.

floc·cu·late (flok'yū-lāt). To become flocculent.

floc·cu·la·tion (flok-yū-lā'shŭn). Precipitation from solution in the form of fleecy masses; the process of becoming flocculent.

floc·cu·lent (flok'yū-lent). **1.** Resembling tufts of cotton or wool; denoting a fluid, such as the urine, containing numerous shreds or fluffy particles of gray-white or white mucus or other material. **2.** BACTERIOLOGY Denoting a fluid culture in which there are numerous colonies either floating in the fluid medium or loosely deposited at the bottom.

floc·cu·lus, pl. **floc·cu·li** (flok'yū-lŭs, -lī). **1.** A tuft or shred of cotton or wool or anything resembling it. **2** [NA]. A small lobe of the cerebellum at the posterior border of the middle cerebellar peduncle anterior to the biventer lobule; it is associated with the nodulus of the vermis; together, these two structures compose the vestibular part of the cerebellum. [Mod. L. dim. of L. *floccus,* a tuft of wool]

flood (flŭd). **1.** To bleed profusely from the uterus, as after childbirth or in cases of menorrhagia. **2.** Colloquialism for a profuse menstrual discharge. [A.S. *flōd*]

flood·ing (flŭd'ing). **1.** Bleeding profusely from the uterus, especially after childbirth or in severe cases of menorrhagia. **2.** A type of behavior therapy; a therapeutic strategy at the beginning of therapy, in which the patients imagine the most anxiety-producing scene and fully immerse (flood) themselves in it.

flo·ra (flō'ră). **1.** Plant life, usually of a certain locality or district. **2.** The population of microorganisms inhabiting the internal and external surfaces of healthy conventional animals. [L. *Flora,* goddess of flowers, fr. *flos* (*flor-*), a flower]

flor·id (flōr′id). **1.** Of a bright red color; denoting certain cutaneous lesions. **2.** Fully developed. [L. *floridus,* flowery]

flo·ta·tion (flō-tā′shŭn). A process for separating solids by their tendency to float upon or sink into a liquid.

flow (flō) **1.** To bleed from the uterus less profusely than in flooding. **2.** The menstrual discharge. **3.** Movement of a liquid or gas; specifically, the volume of liquid or gas passing a given point per unit of time. **4.** RHEOLOGY A permanent deformation of a body which proceeds with time. [A.S. *flōwan*]

Doppler color f., a computer-generated color image produced by Doppler ultrasonography in which different directions of f. are represented by different hues. SEE Doppler *ultrasonography.*

effective renal blood f. (ERBF), the amount of blood flowing to the parts of the kidney that are involved with production of constituents of urine.

effective renal plasma f. (ERPF), the amount of plasma flowing to the parts of the kidney that have a function in the production of constituents of urine; the clearance of substances such as iodopyracet and *p*-aminohippuric acid, assuming that the extraction ratio in the peritubular capillaries is 100%.

forced expiratory f. (FEF), expiratory f. during measurement of forced vital capacity; subscripts specify the exact parameter measured.

laminar f., the relative motion of elements of a fluid along smooth parallel paths, which occurs at lower values of Reynolds number.

peak expiratory f., the maximum f. at the outset of forced expiration, which is reduced in proportion to the severity of airway obstruction, as in asthma.

turbulent f., the f. of gas that is characterized by a rough and tumble pattern; all molecules proceed at the same velocity, and resistance to f. is increased when compared to laminar f.

flow·ers (flow′erz). A mineral substance in a powdery state after sublimation.

flow·me·ter (flō′mē-ter). A device for measuring velocity or volume of flow of liquids or gases.

peak f. (PEFR), a portable device for measuring and displaying the highest expiratory flow produced by a patient; it is commonly used to monitor pulmonary function in patients with a reversible disease of the airways.

flu (flū). SYN influenza.

fluc·tu·ate (flŭk′tyū-āt). **1.** To move in waves. **2.** To vary, to change from time to time, as in referring to any quantity or quality (blood pressure, concentration of substance in urine or blood, secretory activity). [L. *fluctuo,* pp. *-atus,* to flow in waves]

flu·ence (flū′ens). A measure of the quantity of x-radiation in a beam in diagnostic radiology, either particle f., the number of photons entering a sphere of unit cross-sectional area, or energy f., the sum of the energies of the photons passing through a unit area. Cf. flux. [L. *fluentia,* a flowing, fr. *fluo,* to flow]

flu·id (flū′id). **1.** Consisting of particles or distinct entities that can readily change their relative

positions; *i.e.,* tending to move or capable of flowing. **2.** A nonsolid substance, such as a liquid or gas, that tends to flow or conform to the shape of the container. [L. *fluidus,* fr. *fluo,* to flow]

allantoic f., the f. within the allantoic cavity.

amniotic f., a liquid within the amnion that surrounds the fetus and protects it from mechanical injury.

cerebrospinal f. (CSF), a fluid largely secreted by the choroid plexuses of the ventricles of the brain, filling the ventricles and the subarachnoid cavities of the brain and spinal cord.

extracellular f. (ECF), (1) the interstitial f. and the plasma, constituting about 20% of the weight of the body; **(2)** sometimes used to mean all f. outside of cells, usually excluding transcellular f.

extravascular f., all f. outside the blood vessels, *i.e.,* intracellular, interstitial, and transcellular f.'s; it constitutes about 48 to 58% of the body weight.

interstitial f., the f. in spaces between the tissue cells, constituting about 16% of the weight of the body; closely similar in composition to lymph.

intracellular f. (ICF), the f. within the tissue cells, constituting about 30 to 40% of the body weight.

pleural f., the thin film of f. between the visceral and parietal pleurae.

prostatic f., succus prostaticus; a whitish secretion that is one of the constituents of the semen.

Scarpa's f., SYN endolymph.

seminal f., SYN semen (1).

synovial f., a clear thixotropic fluid, the main function of which is to serve as a lubricant in a joint, tendon sheath, or bursa; consists mainly of mucin with some albumin, fat, epithelium, and leukocytes; synovial f. also helps to nourish the avascular articular cartilage. SYN synovia [NA].

transcellular f.'s, the f.'s that are not inside cells, but are separated from plasma and interstitial f. by cellular barriers; *e.g.,* cerebrospinal f., synovial f., pleural f.

flu·id·ex·tract (flū-id-eks′trakt). Pharmacopeial liquid preparation of vegetable drugs, made by percolation, containing alcohol as a solvent or as a preservative, or both, and so made that each milliliter contains the therapeutic constituents of 1 g of the standard drug that it represents.

flu·id·ounce (flū′id-owns′). A measure of capacity: 8 fluidrams. The imperial f. is a measure containing 1 avoirdupois ounce, 437.5 grains, of distilled water at 15.6°C, and equals 28.4 ml; the U.S. f. is $^1/_{128}$ gallon, contains 454.6 grains of distilled water at 25°C, and equals 29.57 ml.

flu·i·drachm, flu·i·dram (flū′i-dram′). A measure of capacity: $^1/_8$ of a fluidounce; a teaspoonful. The imperial f. contains 54.8 grains of distilled water, and equals 3.55 ml; the U.S. f. contains 57.1 grains of distilled water and equals 3.70 ml.

fluke (flūk). Common name for members of the class Trematoda. All f.'s of mammals (subclass Digenea) are internal parasites in the adult stage and are characterized by complex digenetic life cycles involving a snail initial host, in which larval multiplication occurs, and the release of swimming larvae (cercariae) which directly penetrate the skin of the final host (as in schistosomes), encyst on vegetation (as in *Fasciola*), or encyst in or on another intermediate host (as in *Clonorchis* and other fish-borne f.'s). Blood f.'s live in the mesenteric-portal bloodstream and associated vesical and pelvic venous plexuses; they include *Schistosoma haematobium* (the vesical blood f.), *S. mansoni* (Manson's intestinal blood f.), and *S. japonicum* (the Oriental blood f.). Other important f.'s are *Paragonimus westermani* (bronchial or lung f.), *Opisthorchis felineus* (cat liver f.), *Clonorchis sinensis* (Chinese liver or Oriental f.), *Heterophyes heterophyes* (Egyptian or small intestinal f.), *Fasciolopsis buski* (large intestinal f.), *Dicrocoelium dendriticum* (lancet f.), *Fasciola hepatica* (liver or sheep liver f.), and *Paramphistomum* (rumen f.). [A.S. *flōc*, flatfish]

flu·men, pl. **flu·mi·na** (flū′men, flū′min-ă). A flowing, or stream. [L.]

fluor-, fluoro-. Fluorine.

flu·o·res·ce·in (flūr-es′ē-in) [C.I. 45350]. An orange-red crystalline powder that yields a bright green fluorescence in solution, and is reduced to fluorescin; a nontoxic, water-soluble indicator used diagnostically to trace water flow and to visualize corneal abrasions or ulcers.

flu·o·res·ce·in iso·thi·o·cy·a·nate (FITC) (ī′sō-thī-ō-sī′ă-nāt). A fluorochrome dye frequently coupled to antibodies which are used to locate and identify specific antigens.

flu·o·res·cence (flūr-es′ens). Emission of a longer wavelength radiation by a substance as a consequence of absorption of energy from a shorter wavelength radiation, continuing only as long as the stimulus is present; distinguished from phosphorescence in that, in the latter, emission persists for a perceptible period of time after the stimulus has been removed. [*fluor*spar + -*escence*, inchoative suffix]

flu·o·res·cence-ac·ti·vat·ed cell sort·er (FACS) (flūr-es′ens). A machine that can separate and analyze cells, such as lymphocytes, which are labeled with fluorochrome-conjugated antibody, by their fluorescence and light scattering patterns.

flu·o·res·cent (flūr-es′ent). Possessing the quality of fluorescence.

flu·o·ri·da·tion (flūr′i-dā′shŭn). Addition of fluorides to a community water supply, usually 1 ppm, to reduce incidence of dental decay.

flu·o·ride (flūr′īd). A compound of fluorine with a metal, a nonmetal, or an organic radical; the anion of fluorine; inhibits enolase; found in bone and tooth apatite; f. has a cariostatic effect; high levels are toxic.

flu·o·ride num·ber. The percent inhibition of pseudocholinesterase produced by fluorides; used to differentiate normal from atypical pseudocholinesterases. SEE ALSO dibucaine number.

flu·o·ri·di·za·tion (flūr′i-di-zā′shŭn). Therapeutic use of fluorides to reduce the incidence of dental decay; sometimes used to refer to the topical application of fluoride agents to the teeth.

flu·o·rine (F) (flūr′ēn). A gaseous chemical element, atomic no. 9, atomic weight 18.9984032; ^{18}F (half-life of 1.83 hours) is used as a diagnostic aid in various tissue scans. [L. *fluere*, flow]

fluoro-. SEE fluor-.

flu·o·ro·chrome (flūr′ō-krōm). Any fluorescent dye used to label or stain.

flu·o·rog·ra·phy (flūr-og′ră-fē). SYN photofluorography.

fluoroimmunoassay (flur-o-im-yu-no-as-a). An immunoassay that has antigen or antibody labeled with a fluorophore.

flu·o·rom·e·ter (flūr-om′ĕ-ter). A device employing an ultraviolet source, monochromators for selection of wavelength, and a detector of visible light; used in fluorometry.

flu·o·rom·e·try (flūr-om′ĕ-trē). An analytic method for detecting fluorescent compounds, using a beam of ultraviolet light that excites the compounds and causes them to emit visible light. [fluoro- + G. *metron*, measure]

flu·o·ro·pho·tom·e·try (flūr′ō-fō-tom′ĕ-trē). Photomultiplier tube measurement of fluorescence emitted from the interior of the eye after intravenous administration of fluorescein; used to measure the rate of formation of aqueous humor or integrity of the retinal vasculature.

flu·o·ro·scope (flūr′ō-skōp). An apparatus for rendering visible the patterns of x-rays which have passed through a body under examination, by interposing a glass plate coated with fluorescent materials, such as calcium tungstate; to examine a patient by fluoroscopy. [fluorescence + G. *skopeō*, to examine]

flu·o·ro·scop·ic (flūr-ō-skop′ik). Relating to or effected by means of fluoroscopy.

flu·o·ros·co·py (flūr-os′kŏ-pē). Examination of the tissues and deep structures of the body by x-ray, using the fluoroscope.

flu·o·ro·sis (flūr-ō′sis). A condition caused by an excessive intake of fluorides (2 or more p.p.m. in drinking water), characterized mainly by mottling, staining, or hypoplasia of the enamel of the teeth, although the skeletal bones are also affected.

flush (flŭsh). **1.** To wash out with a full stream of fluid. **2.** A transient erythema due to heat, exertion, stress, or disease. **3.** Flat, or even with another surface, as a f. stoma.

    hot f., colloquialism for a vasomotor symptom of the climacteric characterized by sudden vasodilation with a sensation of heat, usually involving the face and neck, and upper part of the chest. Cf. hot *flash*.

    promontory f., SYN Schwartze *sign*.

flut·ter (flŭt′er). Agitation; tremulousness. [A.S. *floterian*, to float about]

    atrial f., auricular f., rapid regular atrial contractions occurring usually at rates between 250 and 350 per minute and often producing "sawtooth" waves in the electrocardiogram, particularly leads II, III, and aVF.

    diaphragmatic f., rapid rhythmical contractions (average, 150 per minute) of the diaphragm, simulating atrial f. clinically and sometimes electrocardiographically.

    impure f., mixture of atrial flutter (FF) waves

and fibrillation (ff) waves in the electrocardiogram. SYN flutter-fibrillation.

ventricular f., a form of rapid ventricular tachycardia in which the electrocardiographic complexes assume a regular undulating pattern without distinct QRS and T waves.

flut·ter-fi·bril·la·tion. SYN impure *flutter.*

flux (flŭks). **1.** The discharge of a fluid material in large amount from a cavity or surface of the body. SEE ALSO diarrhea. **2.** Material discharged from the bowels. **3.** A material used to remove oxides from the surface of molten metal and to protect it when casting; serves a similar purpose in soldering operations. Also, an ingredient in dental porcelain that by its lower melting temperature helps to bond the silica particles. **4** (*J*). The moles of a substance crossing through a unit area of a boundary layer or membrane per unit of time. **5.** Bidirectional movement of a substance at a membrane or surface. **6.** DIAGNOSTIC RADIOLOGY Photon fluence per unit time. [L. *fluxus,* a flow]

fly (flī). A two-winged insect in the order Diptera. Typical flies of the housefly type and similar forms are in the family Muscidae. Important f.'s include *Simulium* (black f.), *Calliphora* (bluebottle f.), *Chrysops* (deer f.), *Cochliomyia hominivorax* (primary screw-worm f.) and *C. macellaria* (secondary screw-worm f.), *Glossina* (tsetse f.), and members of the insect order Trichoptera. [A.S. *fleóge*]

Fm fermium.

FMN *flavin* mononucleotide.

FNA fine needle aspiration biopsy.

fo·cal (fō'kăl). **1.** Denoting a focus. **2.** Relating to a localized area.

fo·cus, pl. **fo·ci** (fō'kŭs, fō'sī). **1** (**F**). The point at which the light rays meet after passing through a convex lens. **2.** The center, or the starting point, of a disease process. [L. a hearth]

Ghon's f., SYN Ghon's *tubercle.*

fog·ging (fog'ing). A method of refraction in which accommodation is relaxed by overcorrection with a convex spherical lens.

fo·late (fō'lāt). A salt or ester of folic acid.

fold (fōld). **1.** A ridge or margin apparently formed by the doubling back of a lamina. SEE ALSO plica. **2.** In the embryo, a transient elevation or reduplication of tissue in the form of a lamina.

amniotic f., a f. of amniotic membrane enclosing the yolk stalk and extending from the point of insertion of the umbilical cord to the yolk sac.

aryepiglottic f., arytenoepiglottidean f., a prominent fold of mucous membrane stretching between the lateral margin of the epiglottis and the arytenoid cartilage on either side; it encloses the aryepiglottic muscle. SYN plica aryepiglottica [NA].

circular f.'s, SYN *plicae* circulares, under *plica.*

epicanthal f., a fold of skin extending from the root of the nose to the medial termination of the eyebrow, overlapping the medial angle of the eye; its presence is normal in fetal life and in Asians.

gluteal f., a prominent f. that marks the upper limit of the thigh and the lower limit of the buttock; it coincides with the lower border of the gluteus maximus muscle. SYN gluteal furrow.

head f., a ventral folding of the cephalic extremity in the embryonic disk, so that the brain lies rostrad to the mouth and pericardium.

interureteric f., a fold of mucous membrane extending from the orifice of the ureter of one side to that of the other side. SYN plica interureterica [NA], Mercier's bar.

lacrimal f., a fold of mucous membrane guarding the lower opening of the nasolacrimal duct. SYN plica lacrimalis [NA].

lateral f.'s, ventral foldings of the lateral margins of the embryonic disk, the development of which establishes the definitive embryonic body form.

mammary f., SYN mammary *ridge.*

mesonephric f., SYN mesonephric *ridge.*

nail f., the fold of skin overlapping the lateral and proximal margins of the nail.

neural f.'s, the elevated margins of the neural groove.

palmate f.'s, the two longitudinal ridges, anterior and posterior, in the mucous membrane lining the cervix uteri, from which numerous secondary folds, or rugae, branch off. SYN plicae palmatae [NA].

sacrouterine f., a fold of peritoneum, containing the rectouterine muscle, passing from the sacrum to the base of the broad ligament on either side, forming the lateral boundary of the rectouterine (Douglas') pouch.

semilunar conjunctival f., SYN *plica* semilunaris conjunctivae.

spiral f. of cystic duct, a series of crescentic folds of mucous membrane in the upper part of the cystic duct, arranged in a somewhat spiral manner. SYN plica spiralis ductus cystici [NA].

tail f., the ventral folding of the caudal extremity of the embryonic disk.

transverse rectal f.'s, the three or four crescentic f.'s placed horizontally in the rectal mucous membrane; the superior rectal f. is situated near the beginning of the rectum on the left side; the middle rectal f. (Nélaton's f.) is most prominent and consistent and projects from the right side about 8 cm above the anus (approximately the level of the floor of the rectouterine or rectovesical pouch); the inferior rectal f. is on the left side about 5 cm above the anus. h

ventricular f., SYN vestibular f.

vestibular f., one of the pair of folds of mucous membrane stretching across the laryngeal cavity from the angle of the thyroid cartilage to the arytenoid cartilage; they enclose a space called the rima vestibuli or false glottis. SYN plica vestibularis [NA], false vocal cord, ventricular band of larynx, ventricular f.

vocal f., one of Ferrein's cords; the sharp edge of a fold of mucous membrane overlying the vocal ligament and stretching along either wall of the larynx from the angle between the laminae of the thyroid cartilage to the vocal process of the arytenoid cartilage; the vocal folds are the agents concerned in voice production. SYN plica vocalis [NA], true vocal cord.

fo·lia (fō'lē-ă). Plural of folium.

fo·lic ac·id (fō'lik). **1.** Collective term for pteroylglutamic acids and their oligoglutamic acid conjugates. **2.** Pteroylmonoglutamic acid, a member of the vitamin B complex necessary for the normal production of red blood cells. It is a hemopoietic vitamin present in liver, green vegetables, and yeast; used to treat folate deficiency and megaloblastic anemia.

fo•lie (fō-lē′). Old term for madness or insanity. [Fr. folly]

f. du doute (du-dūt), an excessive doubting about all the affairs of life and a morbid scrupulousness concerning minutiae. [Fr. from doubt]

fo•li•nate (fō′li-nāt). A salt or ester of folinic acid.

fo•lin•ic ac•id (fō-lin′ik). The active form of folic acid which acts as a formyl group carrier in transformylation reactions; the calcium salt, leucovorin calcium, has therapeutic use. SYN citrovorum factor.

fo•li•um, pl. **fo•lia** (fō′lē-ŭm, -lē-ă) [NA]. A broad, thin, leaflike structure. [L. a leaf]

fol•lib•er•in (fol-lib′er-in). A decapeptide of hypothalamic origin capable of accelerating pituitary secretion of follitropin. SYN follicle-stimulating hormone-releasing factor, follicle-stimulating hormone-releasing hormone. [follicle-stimulating hormone + L. *libero*, to free, + -in]

fol•li•cle (fol′i-kl). **1.** A more or less spherical mass of cells usually containing a cavity. **2.** A crypt or minute cul-de-sac or lacuna, such as the depression in the skin from which the hair emerges. SYN folliculus [NA]. [L. *folliculus*, a small sac, dim. of *follis*, a pair of bellows]

dental f., the dental sac with its enclosed odontogenic organ and developing tooth.

graafian f., SYN vesicular ovarian f.

hair f., a tube-like invagination of the epidermis from which the hair shaft develops and into which the sebaceous glands open; the follicle is lined by a cellular inner and outer root sheath of epidermal origin and is invested with a fibrous sheath derived from the dermis. SYN folliculus pili [NA].

intestinal f.'s, SYN intestinal *glands,* under *gland.*

lingual f.'s, SYN *folliculi* linguales, under *folliculus.*

lymph f., lymphatic f., one of the spherical masses of lymphoid cells, frequently having a more lightly staining center. SYN folliculus lymphaticus, lymph nodule, nodulus lymphaticus.

nabothian f., SYN nabothian *cyst.*

ovarian f., one of the spheroidal cell aggregations in the ovary containing an ovum.

primary ovarian f., an ovarian f. before the appearance of an antrum; marked by developmental changes in the oocyte and follicular cells so that the latter form one or more layers of cuboidal or columnar cells; the f. becomes surrounded by a sheath of stroma, the theca.

primordial ovarian f., a f. in which the primordial oocyte is surrounded by a single layer of flattened follicular cells.

sebaceous f.'s, SYN sebaceous *glands,* under *gland.*

secondary f., SYN vesicular ovarian f.

solitary lymphatic f.'s, minute collections of lymphoid tissue in the mucosa of the small and large intestines, being especially numerous in the cecum and appendix.

splenic lymph f.'s, small nodular masses of lymphoid tissue attached to the sides of the smaller arterial branches. SYN folliculi lymphatici lienales [NA], malpighian bodies.

vesicular ovarian f., a f. in which the oocyte attains its full size and is surrounded by an extracellular glycoprotein layer (zona pellucida) that separates it from a peripheral layer of follicular cells permeated by one or more fluid-filled antra; the theca of the f. develops into internal and external layers. SYN graafian f., secondary f.

fol•lic•u•li (fō-lik′yū-lī). Plural of folliculus.

fol•lic•u•li•tis (fō-lik-yū-lī′tis). An inflammatory reaction in hair follicles; the lesions may be papules or pustules.

f. bar′bae, SYN *tinea* barbae.

f. decal′vans, a papular or pustular inflammation of the hair follicles of the scalp seen mostly in men, resulting in scarring and loss of hair in the affected area.

eosinophilic pustular f., a dermatosis characterized by sterile pruritic papules and pustules that coalesce to form plaques with papulovesicular borders; spontaneous exacerbations and remissions may be accompanied by peripheral leukocytosis, eosinophilia, or both, and may result in eventual destruction of hair follicles and formation of eosinophilic abscesses. The disease has been reported in AIDS, and a possibly separate form of eosinophilic pustular f. occurs in infants.

f. keloida′lis, SYN acne *keloid.*

f. ulerythemato′sa reticula′ta, erythematous "ice-pick" or pitted scars on the cheeks; a scarring type of folliculitis, associated with keratosis pilaris.

fol•lic•u•lo•ma (fō-lik-yū-lō′mă). **1.** SYN granulosa cell *tumor.* **2.** Cystic enlargement of a graafian follicle.

fol•lic•u•lo•sis (fō-lik-yū-lō′sis). Presence of lymph follicles in abnormally great numbers.

fol•lic•u•lus, pl. **fol•lic•u•li** (fō-lik′yū-lŭs, -yū-lī) [NA]. SYN follicle. [L. a small sac, dim. of *follis,* bellows]

follic′uli glan′dulae thyroi′deae, the small spherical vesicular components of the thyroid gland lined with epithelium and containing colloid in varying amounts; the colloid serves for storage of the thyroid hormone precursor, thyroglobulin.

follic′uli lingua′les, collections of lymphoid tissue in the mucosa of the pharyngeal part of the tongue posterior to the terminal sulcus collectively forming the lingual tonsil. SYN lingual follicles.

follic′uli lymphat′ici liena′les [NA], SYN splenic lymph *follicles,* under *follicle.*

f. lymphat′icus, SYN lymph *follicle.*

f. pi′li [NA], SYN hair *follicle.*

fol•li•tro•pin (fol-i-trō′pin). An acidic glycoprotein hormone of the anterior pituitary that stimulates the graafian follicles of the ovary and assists subsequently in follicular maturation and the secretion of estradiol; in the male, it stimulates the epithelium of the seminiferous tubules and is partially responsible for inducing spermatogenesis.

SYN follicle-stimulating hormone. [follicle + G. *tropē*, a turning, + -in]

fo•men•ta•tion (fō-men-tā′shŭn). **1.** A warm application. SEE ALSO poultice. **2.** Application of warmth and moisture in the treatment of disease. [L. *fomento*, pp. *-atus*, to foment, fr. *fomentum*, a poultice, fr. *foveo*, to keep warm]

fo•mes, pl. **fom•i•tes** (fō′mēz, fōm′i-tēz). Objects such as clothing, towels, and utensils that harbor a disease agent and are capable of transmitting it; usually used in the plural. SYN fomite. [L. tinder, fr. *foveo*, to keep warm]

fo•mite (fō′mīt). SYN fomes.

fom•i•tes (fō′mi-tēz). Plural of fomes.

fon•ta•nel, fon•ta•nelle (fon′tă-nel′). One of several membranous intervals at the angles of the cranial bones in the infant. SYN fonticulus [NA]. [Fr. dim. of *fontaine*, fountain, spring]

fon•tic•u•lus, pl. **fon•tic•u•li** (fon-tik′yū-lŭs, -lī) [NA]. SYN fontanel. [L. dim. of *fons (font-)*, fountain, spring]

food (fūd). That which is eaten to supply necessary nutritive elements. [A.S. *fōda*]

foot (fut). **1.** The lower, pedal, podalic, extremity of the leg. SYN pes (1). **2.** A unit of length, containing 12 inches, equal to 30.48 cm. [A.S. *fōt*]

athlete's f., SYN *tinea* pedis.

claw f., SEE clawfoot.

club f., SEE *talipes* equinovarus.

drop f., SEE foot-drop.

f. of hippocampus, the anterior thickened extremity of the hippocampus.

immersion f., a condition resulting from prolonged exposure to damp and cold; the extremity is initially cold and anesthetic, but on rewarming becomes hyperemic, paresthetic, and hyperhidrotic; recovery is often slow.

foot•can•dle (fut′kan-dl). Illumination or brightness equivalent to 1 lumen per square foot; replaced in the SI system by the candela.

foot-drop (fut′drop). Paralysis or weakness of the dorsiflexor muscles of the foot, as a consequence of which the foot falls, the toes dragging on the ground in walking; many causes, both central and peripheral.

foot•plate, foot-plate (fut′plāt). **1.** SYN *base* of stapes. **2.** SYN pedicel.

foot-pound (fut′pownd). Energy expended, or work done, in raising a mass of 1 pound a height of 1 foot vertically against gravitational force.

foot-pound•al (fut′pownd-ăl). Energy exerted, or work done, when a force of 1 poundal displaces a body 1 foot in the direction of the force; equal to about 0.01 calorie.

fo•ra•men, pl. **fo•ram•i•na** (fō-rā′men, fō-ram′i-nă) [NA]. An aperture or perforation through a bone or a membranous structure. [L. an aperture, fr. *foro*, to pierce]

anterior condyloid f., SYN hypoglossal *canal*.

apical f. of tooth, the opening at the apex of the root of a tooth that gives passage to the nerve and blood vessels.

f. ce′cum medul′lae oblonga′tae, a small triangular depression at the lower boundary of the pons that marks the upper limit of the median fissure of the medulla oblongata.

conjugate f., a f. formed by the notches of two bones in apposition.

epiploic f., the passage, below and behind the portal hepatis, connecting the two sacs of the peritoneum; it is bounded anteriorly by the hepatoduodenal ligament and posteriorly by a peritoneal fold over the inferior vena cava.

ethmoidal f., either of two foramina formed by grooves on either edge of the ethmoidal notch of the frontal bone, and completed by similar grooves on the ethmoid bone: anterior ethmoidal f., located in an anterior position; posterior ethmoidal f. located in a posterior position.

great f., SYN f. magnum.

greater palatine f., an opening in the posterolateral corner of the hard palate opposite the last molar tooth, marking the lower end of the pterygopalatine canal.

incisive f., one of several (usually four) openings of the incisive canals into the incisive fossa.

infraorbital f., the external opening of the infraorbital canal, on the anterior surface of the body of the maxilla.

interventricular f., the short, often slitlike passage that, on both the left and right side, connects the third brain ventricle (of the diencephalon) with the lateral ventricles (of the cerebral hemispheres); the passage is bounded anteriomedially by the column of fornix and posterolaterally by the anterior pole of the thalamus. SYN porta (2).

jugular f., a passage between the petrous portion of the temporal bone and the jugular process of the occipital, sometimes divided into two by the intrajugular processes; it contains the internal jugular vein, inferior petrosal sinus, the glossopharyngeal, vagus, and accessory nerves, and meningeal branches of the ascending pharyngeal and occipital arteries.

lesser palatine foramina, openings on the hard palate of palatine canals passing vertically through the tuberosity of the palatine bone and transmitting the smaller palatine nerves and vessels. SYN foramina palatina minora [NA].

f. mag′num [NA], the large opening in the basal part of the occipital bone through which the spinal cord becomes continuous with the medulla oblongata. SYN great f.

mastoid f., an opening at the posterior portion of the mastoid process, transmitting the mastoid branch of the occipital artery to the dura and an emissary vein to the sigmoid sinus.

mental f., the anterior opening of the mandibular canal on the body of the mandible lateral to and above the mental tubercle giving passage to the mental artery and nerve.

nutrient f., the external opening of the nutrient canal in a bone.

obturator f., a large, oval or irregularly triangular aperture in the hip bone, the margins of which are formed by the pubis and the ischium; it is closed in the natural state by the obturator membrane, except for a small opening for the passage of the obturator vessels and nerve.

olfactory f., one of the openings in the cribriform plate of the ethmoid bone, transmitting the olfactory nerves.

optic f., SYN optic *canal*.

f. ova′le, oval f., (1) [NA] in the fetal heart, the oval opening in the septum secundum; the persistent part of the septum primum acts as a valve for this interatrial communication during fetal life and normally postnatally becomes fused to the septum secundum to close it; **(2)** [NA] a large oval opening in the base of the greater wing of the sphenoid bone, transmitting the mandibular nerve and a small meningeal artery; **(3)** valvular incompetence of the f. ovale of the heart; a condition contrasting with probe patency of the f. ovale in that the valvula foraminis ovalis has abnormal perforations in it, or is of insufficient size to afford adequate valvular action at the f. ovale prenatally, or effect a complete closure postnatally.

foram′ina palati′na mino′ra [NA], SYN lesser palatine foramina.

parietal f., an inconstant f. in the parietal bone occasionally found bilaterally near the sagittal margin posteriorly; when present it transmits an emissary vein to the superior sagittal sinus.

f. rotun′dum [NA], an opening in the base of the greater wing of the sphenoid bone, transmitting the maxillary nerve.

sacral f., one of the openings between the fused sacral vertebrae transmitting the sacral nerves. The anterior sacral foramina transmit ventral primary rami of the sacral nerves. The posterior sacral foramina give passage to dorsal primary rami of the sacral nerves.

sciatic f., either of two foramina formed by the sacrospinous and sacrotuberous ligaments crossing the sciatic notches of the hip bone: greater sciatic f. and lesser sciatic f.

sphenopalatine f., the f. formed from the sphenopalatine notch of the palatine bone in articulation with the sphenoid bone; it transmits the sphenopalatine artery and accompanying nerves.

f. spino′sum [NA], an opening in the base of the greater wing of the sphenoid bone, anterior to the spine of the sphenoid, transmitting the middle meningeal artery.

stylomastoid f., the distal or external opening of the facial canal on the inferior surface of the petrous portion of the temporal bone, between the styloid and mastoid processes; it transmits the facial nerve and stylomastoid artery.

supraorbital f., a f. in the supraorbital margin of the frontal bone at the junction of the medial and intermediate thirds.

transverse f., f. processus transversus. SYN vertebroarterial f.

vertebral f., the f. formed by the union of the vertebral arch with the body; in the articulated vertebral column, the vertebral foramina collectively form the vertebral column.

vertebroarterial f., SYN transverse f.

Weitbrecht's f., an opening in the articular capsule of the shoulder joint, communicating with the subtendinous bursa of the subscapularis muscle.

zygomaticofacial f., the opening on the lateral surface of the zygomatic bone below the orbital margin that transmits the zygomaticofacial nerve.

zygomatico-orbital f., the common opening on the orbital surface of the zygomatic bone of the canals transmitting the zygomaticofacial and zygomaticotemporal nerves; sometimes each of these canals has a separate opening on the orbital surface.

zygomaticotemporal f., the opening, on the temporal surface of the zygomatic bone, of the canal that gives passage to the zygomaticotemporal nerve.

fo·ram·i·na (fō-ram′i-nă). Plural of foramen.

force (F) (fōrs). That which tends to produce motion in a body. [L. *fortis,* strong]

electromotive f. (EMF), the f. (measured in volts) that causes the flow of electricity from one point to another.

f. of mastication, the f. created by the action of the muscles during mastication. SYN masticatory f.

masticatory f., SYN f. of mastication.

occlusal f., the result of muscular f. applied on opposing teeth.

reciprocal f.'s, in dentistry, f.'s whereby the resistance of one or more teeth is utilized to move one or more opposing teeth.

reserve f., the energy residing in the organism or any of its parts above that required for its normal functioning.

for·ceps (fōr′seps). 1. An instrument for seizing a structure, and making compression or traction. Cf. clamp. 2 [NA]. Bands of white fibers in the brain, major f. and minor f. [L. a pair of tongs]

alligator f., a long f. with a small hinged jaw on the end.

arterial f., a locking f. with sloping blades for grasping the end of a blood vessel until a ligature is applied.

axis-traction f., obstetrical f. provided with a second handle so attached that traction can be made in the line in which the head must move in the axis of the pelvis.

bayonet f., f. with offset blades, such as those for use through an otoscope.

bone f., a strong f. used for seizing or removing fragments of bone.

bulldog f., a f. for occluding a blood vessel.

bullet f., a f. with thin curved blades with serrated grasping surfaces, for extracting a bullet from tissues.

capsule f., f. used for removing the capsule of the lens in extracapsular extraction of a cataract.

clamp f., a f. with pronged jaws designed to engage the jaws of a rubber dam clamp so that they may be separated to pass over the widest buccolingual contour of a tooth. SYN rubber dam clamp f.

clip f., a small f. with spring catch to hold a bleeding vessel.

cup biopsy f., a slender flexible f. with movable cup-shaped jaws, used to obtain biopsy specimens through an endoscope.

dental f., f. used to luxate teeth and remove them from the alveolus. SYN extracting f.

dressing f., a f. for general use in dressing wounds, removing fragments of necrotic tissue, small foreign bodies, etc.

extracting f., SYN dental f.

hemostatic f., a f. with a catch for locking the

blades, used for seizing the end of a blood vessel to control hemorrhage.

mouse-tooth f., a f. with one or two fine points at the tip of each blade, fitting into hollows between the points on the opposite blade.

needle f., SYN needle-holder.

nonfenestrated f., obstetrical f. without openings in the blades, thus facilitating rotation of the head.

obstetrical f., f. used for grasping and applying traction to or for rotation of the fetal head; the blades are introduced separately into the genital canal, permitting the fetal head to be grasped firmly but with minimal compression, and are articulated after being placed in position.

rubber dam clamp f., SYN clamp f.

speculum f., a tubular f. for use through a speculum.

tenaculum f., a f. with jaws armed each with a sharp, straight hook like a tenaculum.

thumb f., a spring f. used by compression with thumb and forefinger.

tubular f., a long slender f. intended for use through a cannula or other tubular instrument.

vulsella f., vulsellum f., a f. with hooks at the tip of each blade. SYN vulsella, vulsellum.

for·ci·pres·sure (fōr'si-presh-ŭr). A method of arresting hemorrhage by compressing a blood vessel with forceps.

fore·arm (fōr'arm). The segment of the upper limb between the elbow and the wrist. SYN antebrachium [NA].

fore·brain (fōr'brān). SYN prosencephalon.

fore·con·scious (fōr'kon-shŭs). Denoting memories, not at present in the consciousness, which can be evoked from time to time, or an unconscious mental process which becomes conscious only on the fulfillment of certain conditions. Cf. preconscious.

fore·gut (fōr'gŭt). The cephalic portion of the primitive digestive tube in the embryo. From its endoderm arises the epithelial lining of the pharynx, trachea, lungs, esophagus, and stomach, the first part and cranial half of the second part of the duodenum, and the parenchyma of the liver, gallbladder, and pancreas.

fore·head (fōr'ed, fōr'hed). The part of the face between the eyebrows and the hairy scalp. SYN frons [NA], brow (2).

fore·milk (fōr'milk). SYN colostrum.

fo·ren·sic (fō-ren'sik). Pertaining or applicable to personal injury, murder, and other legal proceedings. [L. *forensis,* of a forum]

fore·play (fōr'plā). Stimulative sexual activity preceding sexual intercourse.

foreshortening. RADIOLOGY Radiographic distortion occurring where the image appears shorter than the actual image. Caused by excessive vertical angulation.

fore·skin (fōr'skin). SYN prepuce.

fore·wa·ters (fōr'wah-terz). Colloquialism for the bulging fluid-filled amniotic membrane presenting in front of the fetal head.

fork. 1. a pronged instrument used for holding or lifting; **2.** an instrument resembling a fork in that it has tines or prongs.

tuning f. (TF), steel or magnesium-alloy in-

strument roughly resembling a two-pronged f., the vibrations of the prongs of which, when struck, give a musical tone of restricted bandwidth; used to test the hearing and vibratory sensation.

form (fōrm). Shape; mold. [L. *forma*]

replicative f., (1) an intermediate stage in the replication of either DNA or RNA viral genomes that is usually double stranded; **(2)** the altered, double-stranded f. to which single-stranded coliphage DNA is converted after infection of a susceptible bacterium, formation of the complementary ("minus") strand being mediated by enzymes that were present in the bacterium before entrance of the viral ("plus") strand.

⚠-**form.** In the form, shape of; equivalent to -oid. SEE morpho-. [L. *-formis*]

for·mam·i·dase (fōr-mam'i-dās). An enzyme catalyzing the hydrolysis of N-formyl-L-kynurenine to L-kynurenine and formate, a reaction of significance in L-tryptophan catabolism. SYN formylase.

for·mate (fōr'māt). A salt or ester of formic acid; *i.e.,* the monovalent radical HCOO– or the anion HCOO⁻.

for·ma·tio, pl. **for·ma·ti·o·nes** (fōr-mā'shē-ō, -ō'nēz) [NA]. **1.** SYN formation. **2.** A structure of definite shape or cellular arrangement. [L. fr. *formo,* pp. *-atus,* to form]

f. reticula'ris [NA], SYN reticular *formation.*

for·ma·tion (fōr-mā'shŭn). **1.** A formation; a structure of definite shape or cellular arrangement. **2.** That which is formed. **3.** The act of giving form and shape. SYN formatio (1) [NA].

concept f., PSYCHOLOGY The learning to conceive and respond in terms of abstract ideas based upon an action or object.

personality f., the life history associated with the development of individual patterns and of one's individuality.

reaction f., in psychoanalysis, a postulated defense mechanism in which attitudes and behaviors that are adopted are the opposites of that which the individual would ordinarily be expected to express and actually feel at an unconscious level.

reticular f., a massive but vaguely delimited neural apparatus composed of gray and white matter extending throughout the central core of the brainstem into the diencephalon; the term refers to the large neuronal population of the brainstem that does not compose motoneuronal cell groups or cell groups forming part of specific sensory conduction systems; its neurons generally have long dendrites and heterogeneous afferent connections; the reticular f. has complex, largely polysynaptic ascending and descending connections that play a role in the central control of autonomic (respiration, blood pressure, thermoregulation, etc.) and endocrine functions, as well as in bodily posture, skeletomuscular reflex activity, and general behavioral states such as alertness and sleep. SYN formatio reticularis [NA], reticular substance (2).

rouleaux f., the arrangement of red blood cells in fluid blood (or in diluted suspensions) with their biconcave surfaces in apposition, thereby forming groups that resemble stacks of coins. [Fr. pl. of *rouleau,* a roll]

forme fruste, pl. **formes frustes** (fōrm′ frūst′). A partial, arrested, or inapparent form of disease. [Fr. unfinished form]

for•mic ac•id. HCOOH; the smallest carboxylic acid; a strong caustic, used as an astringent and counterirritant.

for•mi•ca•tion (fŏr-mi-kā′shŭn). A form of paresthesia or tactile hallucination; a sensation as if small insects were creeping under the skin. [L. *formica,* ant]

for•mim•i•no•glu•tam•ic ac•id (FIGLU) (fŏr-mim′i-nō-glū-tam′ik). An intermediate metabolite in L-histidine catabolism in the conversion of L-histidine to L-glutamic acid, with the formimino group being transferred to tetrahydrofolic acid; it may appear in the urine of patients with folic acid or vitamin B_{12} deficiency, or liver disease.

for•mu•la, pl. **for•mu•las, for•mu•lae** (fōr′myū-lă, -lăz, -lē). **1.** A recipe or prescription containing directions for the compounding of a medicinal preparation. **2.** CHEMISTRY A symbol or collection of symbols expressing the number of atoms of the element or elements forming one molecule of a substance, together with, on occasion, information concerning the arrangement of the atoms within the molecule, their electronic structure, their charge, the nature of the bonds within the molecule, etc. **3.** An expression by symbols and numbers of the normal order or arrangement of parts or structures. [L. dim. of *forma,* form]

   dental f., a statement in tabular form of the number of each kind of teeth in the jaw.

   empirical f., CHEMISTRY A f. indicating the kind and number of atoms in the molecules of a substance, or its composition, but not the relation of the atoms to each other or the intimate structure of the molecule.

   official f., a f. contained in the Pharmacopeia or the National Formulary.

   rational f., CHEMISTRY A f. that indicates the constitution as well as the composition of a substance.

   stereochemical f., a chemical f. in which the arrangement of the atoms or atomic groupings in space is indicated.

   structural f., a f. in which the connections of the atoms and groups of atoms, as well as their kind and number, are indicated.

   vertebral f., a f. indicating the number of vertebrae in each segment of the spinal column; for man it is C. 7, T. 12, L. 5, S. 5, Co. 4 = 33, the letters standing for cervical, thoracic, lumbar, sacral, and coccygeal.

for•mu•lary (fōr′myū-lā-rē). A collection of formulas for the compounding of medicinal preparations. SEE National Formulary, Pharmacopeia.

   hospital f., a continually revised compilation of approved pharmaceuticals that reflects the current clinical judgment of the institution's medical staff.

for•myl (f) (fōr′mil). The radical, HCO–.

for•my•lase (fōr′mi-lās). SYN formamidase.

for•ni•cate (fōr′ni-kāt). **1.** Vaulted or arched; resembling a fornix. [L. *fornicatus,* arched, fr. *for-*

nix, vault, arch] **2.** To have sexual intercourse. [see fornication]

for•ni•ca•tion (fŏr-ni-kā′shŭn). Sexual intercourse, especially between unmarried partners. [L. *fornicatio,* an arched or vaulted basement (brothel)]

for•nix, gen. **for•ni•cis,** pl. **for•ni•ces** (fōr′niks, -ni-sis, -ni-sēz). **1** [NA]. In general, an arch-shaped structure; often the arch-shaped roof (or roof portion) of an anatomical space. **2** [NA]. The compact, white fiber bundle by which the hippocampus of each cerebral hemisphere projects to the contralateral hippocampus and to the septum, anterior nucleus of the thalamus, and mamillary body. Arising from pyramidal cells of Ammon's horn, the fibers of the f. form the alveus hippocampi and the fimbria hippocampi, and in their further course compose, sequentially, the crus fornicis, body of fornix, commissura fornicis, and column of fornix; the f. fibers to the septum issue from the upper part of the column of fornix, passing in part anterior to the anterior commissure as the precommissural f., while all others follow the compact postcommissural f. bundle to the anterior thalamic nucleus and mamillary body. [L. arch, vault]

fos•sa, gen. and pl. **fos•sae** (fos′ă, fos′ē) [NA]. A depression usually more or less longitudinal in shape below the level of the surface of a part. [L. a trench or ditch]

   acetabular f., a depressed area in the floor of the acetabulum superior to the acetabular notch.

   adipose fossae, subcutaneous spaces containing accumulations of fat in the breast.

   condylar f., a depression behind the condyle of the occipital bone in which the posterior margin of the superior facet of the atlas lies in extension.

   digastric f., a hollow on the posterior surface of the base of the mandible, on either side of the median plane, giving attachment to the anterior belly of the digastric muscle.

   epigastric f., the slight depression in the midline just inferior to the xiphoid process of the sternum.

   f. for gallbladder, a depression on the visceral surface of the liver anteriorly, between the quadrate and the right lobes, lodging the gallbladder.

   glenoid f., (1) the hollow in the head of the scapula that receives the head of the humerus to make the shoulder joint; **(2)** SYN mandibular f.

   hyaloid f., a depression on the anterior surface of the vitreous body in which lies the lens.

   hypophysial f., f. of the sphenoid bone housing the pituitary gland. SEE ALSO *sella* turcica.

   infraclavicular f., a triangular depression bounded by the clavicle and the adjacent borders of the deltoid and pectoralis major muscles.

   infratemporal f., the cavity on the side of the skull bounded laterally by the zygomatic arch and ramus of the mandible, medially by the lateral pterygoid plate, anteriorly by the zygomatic process of the maxilla, posteriorly by the articular tubercle of the temporal bone and the posterior border of the lateral pterygoid plate, and above by the squama of the temporal bone and the infratemporal crest on the greater wing of the sphenoid bone.

fo

interpeduncular f., deep depression on the inferior surface of the mesencephalon, between the crura cerebri, the floor of which is formed by the posterior perforated substance.

jugular f., an oval depression near the posterior border of the petrous portion of the temporal bone, medial to the styloid process, in which lies the beginning of the internal jugular vein (jugular bulb);

lacrimal f., a hollow in the orbital plate of the frontal bone, formed by the overhanging margin and zygomatic process, lodging the lacrimal gland.

mandibular f., a deep hollow in the squamous portion of the temporal bone at the root of the zygoma, in which rests the condyle of the mandible. SYN glenoid f. (2).

navicular f. of urethra, the terminal dilated portion of the urethra in the glans penis.

f. ova′lis, (1) [NA], an oval depression on the lower part of the septum of the right atrium; it is a vestige of the foramen ovale, and its floor corresponds to the septum primum of the fetal heart; **(2)** SYN saphenous *opening.*

ovarian f., a depression in the parietal peritoneum of the pelvis; it is bounded in front by the obliterated umbilical artery, and behind by the ureter and the uterine vessels; it lodges the ovary.

popliteal f., the diamond-shaped space posterior to the knee joint bounded superficially by the diverging biceps femoris and semimembranosus muscles above and inferiorly by the two heads of the gastrocnemius muscle; deeply, the f. is bound superiorly by the diverging supracondylar lines of the femur and the soleal line of the tibia inferiorly. Contents: tibial nerve, popliteal artery, vein, fat.

rhomboid f., the floor of the fourth ventricle of the brain, formed by the ventricular surface of the rhombencephalon.

subarcuate f., an irregular depression on the posterior surface of the petrous portion of the temporal bone just below its crest and above and lateral to the internal acoustic meatus. In the fetus, the flocculus of the cerebellum rests here; in the adult, a small vein enters the bone here.

sublingual f., a shallow depression on either side of the mental spine, on the inner surface of the body of the mandible, superior to the mylohyoid line, lodging the sublingual gland.

submandibular f., the depression on the medial surface of the body of the mandible inferior to the mylohyoid line in which the submandibular gland is lodged.

temporal f., the space on the side of the cranium bounded by the temporal lines and terminating below at the level of the zygomatic arch.

tonsillar f., the depression between the palatoglossal and palatopharyngeal arches occupied by the palatine tonsil.

f. of vestibule of vagina, the portion of the vestibule of the vagina between the frenulum of the labia minora and the posterior labial commissure of the vulva.

fos•sette (fo-set′). **1.** SYN fossula. **2.** A seldom-used term for corneal ulcer of small diameter. [Fr. dim. of *fosse,* a ditch]

fos•su•la, pl. **fos•su•lae** (fos′yū-lă, -lē). **1** [NA]. A small fossa. **2.** A minor fissure or slight depression on the surface of the cerebrum. SYN fossette (1). [L. dim. of *fossa,* ditch]

Foster frame. See under frame.

fou•lage (fū-lahzh′). Kneading and pressure of the muscles, constituting a form of massage. [Fr. impression]

foun•da•tion (fown-dā′shŭn). A base; a supporting structure.

denture f., that portion of the oral structures which is available to support a denture.

Fou•ri•er transform. a mathematical technique to express a time-varying function or signal into components at different frequencies, giving the phase and amplitude of each; used in computed tomography and magnetic resonance image reconstruction transformation.

fo•vea, pl. **fo•ve•ae** (fō′vē-ă, fō′vē-ē) [NA]. A relatively small cup-shaped depression or pit. [L. a pit]

central retinal f., a depression in the center of the macula retinae containing only cones and lacking blood vessels.

fo•ve•ate, fo•ve•at•ed (fō′-vē-āt, -ā-ted). Pitted; having foveas or depressions on the surface.

fo•ve•a•tion (fō-vē-ā′shŭn). Pitted scar formation, as in chickenpox. [L. *fovea,* a pit]

fo•ve•o•la, pl. **fo•ve•o•lae** (fō-vē′ō-lă, -lē) [NA]. A minute fovea or pit. [Mod. L. dim. of L. *fovea,* pit]

fo•ve•o•lar (fō-vē′ō-lăr). Pertaining to a foveola.

fo•ve•o•late (fō′vē-ō-lāt, fō-vē′ō-lāt). Having minute pits (foveolae) or small depressions on the surface.

FPS, fps foot-pound-second. SEE foot-pound-second *system,* foot-pound-second *unit.*

Fr 1. francium. **2.** French *scale.*

frac•tion (frak′shŭn). **1.** The quotient of two quantities. **2.** An aliquot portion or any portion.

blood plasma f.'s, portions of the blood plasma as separated by electrophoresis or other technique.

filtration f. (FF), the f. of the plasma entering the kidney that filters into the lumen of the renal tubules, determined by dividing the glomerular filtration rate by the renal plasma flow; normally, it is around 0.17.

human plasma protein f., a sterile solution of selected proteins derived from the blood plasma of adult human donors, containing 4.5 to 5.5 g of protein per 100 ml, of which 83 to 90% is albumin and the remainder is α- and β-globulins; used as a blood volume supporter.

frac•tion•a•tion (frak-shŭn-ā′shŭn). **1.** Separation of the components of a mixture. **2.** The administration of a course of therapeutic radiation of a neoplasm in a planned series of fractions of the total dose, most often once a day for several weeks, in order to minimize radiation damage of contiguous normal tissues.

fracture (frak′chūr). **1.** To break. **2.** A break, especially the breaking of a bone or cartilage. [L. *fractura,* a break]

avulsion f., a f. that occurs when a joint capsule, ligament, or muscle insertion of origin is pulled from the bone as a result of a sprain,

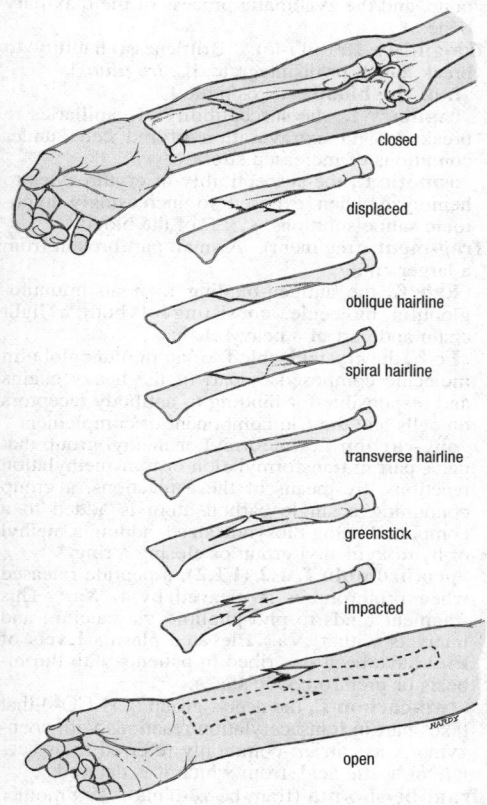

closed

displaced

oblique hairline

spiral hairline

transverse hairline

greenstick

impacted

open

types of fractures

dislocation, or strong contracture of the muscle against resistance; as the soft tissue is pulled away from the bone, a fragment or fragments of the bone may come away with it.

Barton's f., f. of the distal radius with dislocation of the radiocarpal joint.

bending f., an injury in which a long bone or bones, usually the radius and ulna, are bent due to multiple microfractures, none of which can be seen by x-ray imaging.

Bennett's f., f. dislocation of the first metacarpal bone at the carpal-metacarpal joint.

bimalleolar f. (bī-mă-lē'ō-lar), f. of both medial and lateral malleoli. SEE ALSO malleolus.

blow-out f., a f. of the floor of the orbit, without a fracture of the rim, produced by a blow on the globe with the force being transmitted via the globe to the orbital floor.

boxer's f., f. of the neck of a metacarpal bone (most often the fifth) with volar displacement of the head of the bone. SYN f. of fifth metacarpal.

capillary f., SYN hairline f.

chondral f., f. involving the articular cartilage of a joint. SEE ALSO articular *cartilage*.

closed f., a f. in which skin is intact at site of f. SYN simple f.

Colles' f., a f. of the distal radius and ulna with dorsal displacement of the distal segment.

comminuted f., a f. in which the bone is broken into pieces.

compound f., SYN open f.

compression f., a f. causing loss of height of the vertebral body either by trauma or by pathology; it occurs most commonly in thoracic and lumbar spines. A common sequela of osteoporosis.

f. by contrecoup, skull f. at a point distant from the site of impact.

craniofacial dysjunction f., a complex f. in which the facial bones are separated from the cranial bones.

depressed skull f., a f. with inward displacement of a part of the calvarium; may or may not be associated with disruption of the underlying dura or cerebral cortex.

direct f., a f., especially of the skull, occurring at the point of injury.

dislocation f., a f. of a bone near an articulation with its concomitant dislocation from that joint.

displaced f., a f. in which the fragments are separated and are not in alignment.

epiphyseal f., injury to the growth plate of a long bone in children and adolescents.

expressed skull f., a f. with outward displacement of a part of the cranium.

f. of fifth metacarpal, SYN boxer's f.

fissured f., SYN linear f.

greenstick f., the bending of a bone with incomplete f. involving the convex side of the curve only.

gutter f., a long, narrow, depressed f. of the skull.

hairline f., a f. without separation of the fragments, the line of break being hairlike, as seen sometimes in the skull. SYN capillary f.

hangman's f., a f. of the cervical spine through the pedicles of C_2; may be associated with an anterior dislocation of the C_2 vertebral body with respect to C_3.

horizontal maxillary f., a horizontal f. at the base of the maxillae above the apices of the teeth. SYN Lefort I f.

impacted f., a f. in which one of the fragments is driven into the cancellous tissue of the other fragment.

indirect f., a f., especially of the skull, that occurs at a point not at the site of impact.

intrauterine f., a f. of one or more bones of a fetus occurring before birth.

Jones' f., transverse stress f. of the proximal shaft of the fifth metatarsal.

Lefort I f., SYN horizontal maxillary f.

linear f., a f. running parallel with the long axis of the bone. SYN fissured f.

longitudinal f., a f. involving the bone in the line of its axis.

march f., a stress f. in the shaft of a metatarsal bone, often due to prolonged marching in military recruits unaccustomed to such activity.

multiple f., (1) f. at two or more places in a bone; (2) f. of several bones occurring simultaneously.

fr

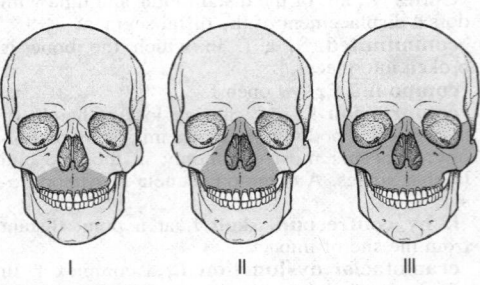

LeFort fractures

oblique f., a f. the line of which runs obliquely to the axis of the bone.

occult f., a condition in which there are clinical signs of f. but no x-ray evidence; after 3 or 4 weeks x-ray imaging shows new bone formation.

open f., f. in which the skin is perforated and there is an open wound down to the f. SYN compound f.

pathologic f., a f. occurring at a site weakened by preexisting disease, especially neoplasm or necrosis, of the bone.

Pott's f., f. of the lower part of the fibula and of the malleolus of the tibia, with outward displacement of the foot.

pyramidal f., a f. of the midfacial skeleton with the principal f. lines meeting at an apex at or near the superior aspect of the nasal bones.

segmental f., a f. in two parts of the same bone.

silver-fork f., a Colles' f. of the wrist in which the deformity has the appearance of a fork in profile.

simple f., SYN closed f.

Smith's f., reversed Colles' f.; f. of the radius near its lower articular surface with displacement of the fragment toward the palmar (volar) aspect.

spiral f., a f. the line of which is helical in the bone.

sprain f., an avulsion f. in which a small portion of adjacent bone has been pulled or pushed off.

stellate f., a f. in which the lines of break radiate from a central point.

strain f., the tearing off, by a sudden force, of a piece of bone attached to a tendon, ligament, or capsule.

stress f., a fatigue f. caused by repetitive, relatively low-magnitude local stress on a bone, as in marching or running, rather than by a single violent injury.

torsion f., a f. resulting from twisting of the limb.

torus f., a deformity in children consisting of a local bulging caused by the longitudinal compression of the soft bone; it occurs commonly in the radius or ulna or both.

transverse f., a f. the line of which forms a right angle with the axis of the bone.

tripod f., a facial f. involving the three supports of the malar prominence, the arch of the zygomatic bone, the zygomatic process of the frontal bone, and the zygomatic process of the maxillary bone.

fra•gil•i•ty (fră-jil′i-tē). Brittleness; liability to break, burst, or disintegrate. [L. *fragilitas*]

f. of the blood, SYN osmotic f.

capillary f., the susceptibility of capillaries to breakage and extravasation of red cells under conditions of increased stress.

osmotic f., the susceptibility of erythrocytes to hemolyze when exposed to increasingly hypotonic saline solutions. SYN f. of the blood.

frag•ment (frag′ment). A small part broken from a larger entity.

Fab f., the antigen-binding f. of an immunoglobulin molecule, consisting of both a light chain and part of a heavy chain.

Fc f., the crystallizable f. of an immunoglobulin molecule composed of part of the heavy chains and responsible for binding to antibody receptors on cells and the Clq component of complement.

one-carbon f., the formyl or methyl group that takes part in transformylation or transmethylation reactions; by means of these reactions, a group containing a single carbon atom is added to a compound being biosynthesized, adding a methyl or hydroxymethyl group or closing a ring.

prothrombin f. 1.2 (F1.2), a peptide released when prothrombin is cleaved by f. Xa. This fragment binds to phospholipid via calcium and interacts with f. Va. Elevated plasma levels of F1.2 have been described in patients with thrombosis or prethrombotic states.

two-carbon f., the acetyl group (CH_3CO-) that takes part in transacetylation reactions with coenzyme A as carrier; commonly referred to as acetate or acetic acid, from which it is derived.

fram•be•si•o•ma (fram-bē-zē-ō′mă). SYN mother *yaw*. [frambesia + *-oma*, tumor]

frame (frām). A supporting or integrating structure made of parts fitted together.

Balkan f., an overhead f., supported on uprights attached to the bedposts or to a separate stand, from which a splinted limb is slung in the treatment of fracture or joint disease. SYN Balkan splint.

biomechanical f. of reference, (1) an intervention approach used when a person cannot maintain posture through appropriate involuntary muscle activity because of neuromuscular or musculoskeletal dysfunction; artificial supports are provided, temporarily or permanently; (2) a therapeutic technique in which strength, endurance, and range of motion are increased in patients who have dysfunction in the peripheral nervous system or the musculoskeletal, integumentary, or cardiopulmonary systems.

Bradford f., an oblong rectangular f. made of pipe, over which are stretched transversely two strips of canvas; permits trunk and lower extremities of a bed-ridden patient to move as a unit.

Foster f., a reversible bed similar to a Stryker f.

Stryker f., a f. that holds the patient and permits turning in various planes without individual motion of parts.

trial f., a type of spectacle f. with variable adjustments, for holding trial lenses during refraction.

Francisella (fran′si-sel′lă). A genus of nonmotile, nonsporeforming, aerobic bacteria that contain small, Gram-negative cocci and rods. Capsules are rarely produced and the cells may show bipolar staining. These organisms are highly pleomorphic; they do not grow on plain agar or in liquid media without special enrichment; they are pathogenic and cause tularemia in humans. The type species is *F. tularensis.*

F. tularen′sis, a species that causes tularemia in man, transmitted to man from wild animals by bloodsucking insects or by contact with infected animals such as ticks; main sources of infection are rabbits and ticks; it can penetrate unbroken skin to cause infection; it is the type species of the genus *F.*

fran·ci·um (Fr) (fran′sē-ŭm). Radioactive element of the alkali metal series; atomic no. 87; half-life of most stable known isotope, ^{223}Fr, is 21.8 minutes. [*France,* native country of Mlle. M. Perey, the discoverer]

Frank, Otto, German physiologist, 1865–1944. SEE F.-Starling *curve.*

frank. Unmistakable; manifest; clinically evident.

FRC functional residual *capacity.*

freck·le (frek′l). Yellowish or brownish macules developing on the exposed parts of the skin, especially in persons of light complexion; the lesions increase in number on exposure to the sun; the epidermis is microscopically normal except for increased melanin. SEE ALSO lentigo. SYN ephelis. [O. E. *freken*]

freeze-dry·ing (frēz′drī-ing). SYN lyophilization.

freez·ing (frē′zing). Congealing, stiffening, or hardening by exposure to cold.

frem·i·tus (frem′i-tŭs). A vibration imparted to the hand resting on the chest or other part of the body. SEE ALSO thrill. [L. a dull roaring sound, fr. *fremo,* pp. -*itus,* to roar, resound]

hydatid f., SYN hydatid *thrill.*

pericardial f., vibration in the chest wall produced by the friction of opposing roughened surfaces of the pericardium.

pleural f., vibration in the chest wall produced by the rubbing together of inflamed opposing surfaces of the pleura.

rhonchal f., f. produced by vibrations from the passage of air in bronchial tubes partially obstructed by mucous secretion.

tactile f., vibration felt with the hand on the chest during vocal f.

tussive f., a form of f. similar to the vocal, produced by a cough.

vocal f., the vibration in the chest wall, felt on palpation, produced by the spoken voice.

fre·na (frē′nă). Plural of frenum.

fre·nal (frē′năl). Relating to any frenum.

fre·nec·to·my (frē-nek′tō-mē). Removal of any frenum. [frenum + G. *ektomē,* excision]

fre·no·plas·ty (frē′nō-plas-tē). Correction of an abnormally attached frenum by surgically repositioning it. [frenum + G. *plastos,* formed]

fre·not·o·my (frē-not′ō-mē). Division of any frenum or frenulum, especially that of the tongue. [frenum + G. *tomē,* a cutting]

fren·u·lum, pl. **fren·u·la** (fren′yū-lŭm, -lă)

[NA]. A small frenum or bridle. SYN habenula (1). [Mod. L. dim. of L. *frenum,* bridle]

f. of clitoris, the line of union of the inner-laminae portions of the labia minora on the undersurface of the glans clitoridis.

f. of the labia minora, the fold connecting the two labia minora posteriorly.

lingual f., a fold of mucous membrane extending from the floor of the mouth to the midline of the undersurface of the tongue.

f. of lower lip, f. of upper lip, f. labii inferioris et superioris; f. of the lower lip; f. of the upper lip; the folds of mucous membrane extending from the gingiva to the midline of the lower and upper lips, respectively.

f. of prepuce, a fold of mucous membrane passing from the undersurface of the glans penis to the deep surface of the prepuce.

f. of upper lip,

fre·num, pl. **fre·na, fre·nums** (frē′nŭm, -nă, -nŭmz). **1.** A narrow reflection or fold of mucous membrane passing from a more fixed to a movable part, serving to check undue movement of the part. **2.** An anatomical structure resembling such a fold. [L. a bridle, curb]

fre·quen·cy (ν) (frē′kwen-sē). **1.** The number of regular recurrences in a given time, *e.g.,* heartbeats, sound vibrations. **2.** ACOUSTICS the number of cycles of compression and rarefaction of a sound wave that occur in one second, expressed in hertz (Hz). **3.** The rate of vocal fold vibration (*i.e.,* the number of times the glottis opens and closes in one second) during phonation; perceived as voice pitch. [L. *frequens,* repeated, often, constant]

fundamental f. (F0), (1) ACOUSTICS the basic frequency of a vibrating object or sound as opposed to its harmonics, or the principal component of a complex sound wave; **(2)** the frequency of vocal fold vibration at the glottis, unaffected by resonance. SEE ALSO optimal *pitch.*

modal f., SYN habitual *pitch.*

resonant f., the f. at which individual magnetic nuclei absorb or emit radiofrequency energy in magnetic resonance studies. SYN resonance (6).

respiratory f. (f), the number of breaths per minute.

speech f.'s, acoustic sound wave f. range in which most speech sounds occur, generally 500–3000 Hz. SEE frequency.

fret·ting (fret′ing). Abrasive polishing and wear of two metallic surfaces at their interface due to repetitive motion. [M.E., fr. O.E. *fretan,* to devour]

freud·i·an (froyd′ē-ăn). Relating to or described by Sigmund Freud (1856-1939).

f. slip, A mistake in speech or deed which presumably suggests some underlying motive, often sexual or aggressive in nature.

FRH. follitropin-releasing hormone.

fri·a·ble (frī′ă-bl). **1.** Easily reduced to powder. **2.** BACTERIOLOGY Denoting a dry and brittle culture falling into powder when touched or shaken. **3.** Said of tissue that readily tears, fragments, or bleeds when gently palpated or manipulated. [L. *friabilis,* fr. *frio,* to crumble]

fric·tion (frik′shŭn). **1.** The act of rubbing the

surface of an object against that of another; especially rubbing the limbs of the body to aid the circulation. **2.** The force required for relative motion of two bodies that are in contact. [L. *frictio,* fr. *frico,* to rub]

frig·id (frij'id). **1.** SYN cold. **2.** Temperamentally, especially sexually, unresponsive. [L. *frigidus,* cold]

fri·gid·i·ty (fri-jid'i-tē). **1.** Inability in the female to achieve orgasm or any other satisfactory level of sexual response. **2.** The state of being frigid (2).

frons, gen. **fron·tis** (fronz, fron'tis) [NA]. SYN forehead. [L.]

front·ad (frŭn'tad). Toward the front.

fron·tal (frŭn'tăl). **1.** In front; relating to the anterior part of a body. **2.** Referring to the frontal (coronal) plane or to the frontal bone or forehead. SYN frontalis [NA].

fron·ta·lis (frŭn-tā'lis) [NA]. SYN frontal. [L.]

fron·to·ma·lar (frŭn'tō-mā'lăr). SYN frontozygomatic.

fron·to·max·il·lary (frŭn'tō-mak'si-lā-rē). Relating to the frontal and the maxillary bones.

fron·to·na·sal (frŭn'tō-nā'zăl). Relating to the frontal and the nasal bones.

fron·to·oc·cip·i·tal (frŭn'tō-ok-sip'i-tăl). Relating to the frontal and the occipital bones, or to the forehead and the occiput.

fron·to·pa·ri·e·tal (frŭn'tō-pa-rī'ĕ-tăl). Relating to the frontal and the parietal bones.

fron·to·tem·po·ral (frŭn-tō-tem'pŏ-răl). Relating to the frontal and the temporal bones.

fron·to·zy·go·mat·ic (frŭn'tō-zī'gō-mat'ik). Relating to the frontal and zygomatic bones. SYN frontomalar.

Frost, Albert D., U.S. ophthalmologist, 1889–1945. SEE F. *suture.*

Frost, William A., English ophthalmologist, 1853–1935.

frost. A deposit resembling that of frozen vapor or dew.

urea f., uremic f., powdery deposits on the skin, especially the face, of urea and uric acid salts due to excretion of nitrogenous compounds in the sweat; seen in severe uremia.

frost·bite (frost'bīt). Local tissue destruction resulting from exposure to extreme cold; in mild cases, it results in superficial, reversible freezing followed by erythema and slight pain; in severe cases, it can be painless or paresthetic and result in blistering, persistent edema, and gangrene.

frot·tage (frō-tahzh'). **1.** The rubbing movement in massage. **2.** Production of sexual excitement by rubbing against someone. [F. a rubbing]

⌂**fructo-.** Chemical prefix denoting the fructose configuration. [L. *fructus,* fruit]

fruc·to·fu·ra·nose (frŭk-tō-fūr'ă-nōs, fruk-). Fructose in furanose form.

β-**fruc·to·fu·ran·o·sid·ase** (frŭk'tō-fūr-ă-nō-sīd'ās, fruk-). β-*h*-Fructosidase; an enzyme hydrolyzing β-D-fructofuranosides and releasing free D-fructose; if the substrate is sucrose, the product is D-glucose plus D-fructose (invert sugar); invert sugar is more easily digestible than sucrose.

fruc·to·ki·nase (frŭk-tō-kī'nās, fruk-). A liver enzyme that catalyzes the reaction of ATP and D-

fructose to form fructose 6-phosphate and ADP; deficient in individuals with essential fructosuria (hepatic f. deficiency).

fruc·tose (frŭk'tōs, fruk-). D-*arabino*-2-Hexulose; the D-isomer (also referred to as fruit sugar, levoglucose, levulose, and D-*arabino*-2-hexulose, is a 2-ketohexose that in D form is physiologically the most important of the ketohexoses and one of the two products of sucrose hydrolysis, and is metabolized or converted to glycogen in the absence of insulin. [L. *fructus,* fruit, + -ose]

fruc·to·se·mia (frŭk-tō-sē'mē-ă, fruk-). Presence of fructose in the circulating blood.

fruc·to·side (frŭk'tō-sīd, fruk'). Fructose in -C-O- linkage where the -C-O- group is the original 2 group of the fructose.

fruc·to·su·ria (frŭk-tō-sū'rē-ă, fruk-). Excretion of fructose in the urine. [fructose + G. *ouron,* urine]

⌂**fructosyl-.** Chemical prefix indicating fructose in -C-R- (not -C-O-R-) linkage through its carbon-2 (R usually C).

frus·tra·tion (frŭs'trā'shŭn). The thwarting of or inability to gratify a desire or to satisfy an urge or need. [L. *frustro,* pp. -*atus,* to deceive, disappoint, fr. *frustra* (adv.), in vain]

FTA-ABS. fluorescent treponemal antibody absorption. SEE fluorescent treponemal antibody-absorption *test.*

fuch·sin (fuk'sin). A nonspecific term referring to any of several red rosanilin dyes used as stains in histology and bacteriology. [Leonhard *Fuchs,* German botantist, 1501–1506]

acid f. [C.I. 42685], a mixture of sulfonated salts of rosanilin and pararosanilin; used as an indicator dye and for staining of cytoplasm and collagen.

basic f. [C.I. 42500], a triphenylmethane dye whose dominant component is pararosanilin; an important stain in histology, histochemistry, and bacteriology.

fuch·sin·o·phil (fuk'si-nō-fil). **1.** Staining readily with fuchsin dyes. SYN fuchsinophilic. **2.** A cell or histologic element that stains readily with fuchsin. [fuchsin + G. *philos,* fond]

fuch·sin·o·phil·ic (fuk'si-nō-fil'ik). SYN fuchsinophil (1).

fu·cose (fyū'kōs). 6-Deoxygalactose; a methylpentose, the L-configuration of which occurs in the mucopolysaccharides of the blood group substances, in human milk (as a polysaccharide), and elsewhere in nature. The D-configuration has been found in certain antibiotics.

fu·gac·i·ty (f) (fū-gas'i-tē). The tendency of the molecules in a fluid, as a result of all forces acting on them, to leave a given site in the body; the escaping tendency of a fluid, as in diffusion, evaporation, etc. [L. *fuga,* flight]

⌂**-fugal.** Movement away from the part indicated by the main portion of the word. [L. *fugio,* to flee]

⌂**-fuge.** Flight, denoting the place from which flight takes place or that which is put to flight. [L. *fuga* a running away]

fugue (fyūg). A condition in which an individual suddenly abandons a present activity or lifestyle and starts a new and different one, often in a different city; afterward, the individual alleges amnesia for events occurring during the f. period, although earlier events are remembered and habits and skills are usually unaffected. [Fr. fr. L. *fuga*, flight]

ful·crum, pl. **ful·cra, ful·crums** (ful'krŭm, -kră, -krŭmz). A support or the point thereon on which a lever turns. [L. a bedpost, fr. *fulcio*, to prop up]

ful·gu·rant (ful'gŭ-rănt). Sharp and piercing. Cf. fulminant. SYN fulgurating (1). [L. *fulgur*, flashing lightning]

ful·gu·rat·ing (ful'gŭ-rā-ting). 1. SYN fulgurant. 2. Relating to fulguration.

ful·gu·ra·tion (ful-gŭ-rā'shŭn). Destruction of tissue by means of a high-frequency electric current: **direct f.** utilizes an insulated electrode with a metal point, which is connected to the uniterminal of the high-frequency apparatus, from which a spark of electricity is allowed to impinge on the area to be treated; **indirect f.** involves directly connecting the patient by a metal contact to the uniterminal and utilizing an active electrode to complete an arc from the patient. [L. *fulgur*, lightning stroke]

ful·mi·nant (ful'mi-nănt). Occurring suddenly, with lightning-like rapidity, and with great intensity or severity. Cf. fulgurant. [L. *fulmino*, pp. *-atus*, to hurl lightning, fr. *fulmen*, lightning]

ful·mi·nat·ing (ful'mi-nā'ting). Running a speedy course, with rapid worsening.

fu·ma·rate hy·dra·tase (fyŭ'mă-rāt hī'dră-tāz). An enzyme catalyzing the reversible interconversion of fumaric acid and water to malic acid, a reaction of importance in the tricarboxylic acid cycle. Deficiency leads to mental retardation.

fu·mar·ic ac·id (fyū-mar'ik). *Trans*-Butanedioic acid; an unsaturated dicarboxylic acid occurring as an intermediate in the tricarboxylic acid cycle.

fu·mi·gant (fyū'mi-gănt). A substance utilized in fumigation.

fu·mi·gate (fyū'mi-gāt). To expose to the action of smoke or of fumes of any kind as a means of disinfection or eradication. [L. *fumigo* pp. *-atus*, to fumigate, fr. *fumus*, smoke, + *ago*, to drive]

fu·mi·ga·tion (fyū-mi-gā'shŭn). The act of fumigating; the use of a fumigant.

fum·ing (fyūm'ing). Giving forth a visible vapor, a property of concentrated nitric, sulfuric, and hydrochloric acids, and certain other substances. [L. *fumus*, smoke]

func·tio lae·sa (fŭngk'shē-ō lē'să). Impaired function; a fifth sign of inflammation added by Galen to those enunciated by Celsus (rubor, tumor, calor, and dolor). [L.]

func·tion (fŭngk'shŭn). 1. The special action or physiologic property of an organ or other part of the body. 2. To perform its special work or office, said of an organ or other part of the body. 3. The general properties of any substance, depending on its chemical character and relation to other substances, according to which it may be grouped among acids, bases, alcohols, esters, etc. 4. A particular reactive grouping in a molecule; *e.g.*, a functional group, such as the –OH group of an alcohol. 5. A quality, trait, or fact that is so related to another as to be dependent upon and to

vary with this other. [L. *functio*, fr. *fungor*, pp. *functus*, to perform]

func·tion·al (fŭnk'shŭn-ăl). 1. Relating to a function. 2. Not organic in origin; denoting a disorder with no known or detectable organic basis to explain the symptoms. SEE neurosis.

fun·dec·to·my (fŭn-dek'tō-mē). SYN fundusectomy. [fundus + G. *ektomē*, excision]

fun·dic (fŭn'dik). Relating to a fundus.

fun·di·form (fŭn'di-fōrm). Looped; sling-shaped. [L. *funda*, a sling, + *forma*, shape]

fun·do·pli·ca·tion (fŭn'dō-pli-kā'shŭn). Suture of the fundus of the stomach around the esophagus to prevent reflux in repair of hiatal hernia. [fundus + L. *plico*, to fold]

fun·dus, pl. **fun·di** (fŭn'dŭs, dī) [NA]. The bottom or lowest part of a sac or hollow organ; that part farthest removed from the opening or exit; occasionally a broad cul-de-sac. [L. bottom]

f. of gallbladder, the wide closed end of the gallbladder situated at the inferior border of the liver.

f. oc·uli, the portion of the interior of the eyeball around the posterior pole, visible through the ophthalmoscope. SEE eyegrounds. SYN f. of eye.

f. of eye, SYN f. oculi.

f. of stomach, the portion of the stomach that lies above the cardiac notch. SYN f. ventriculi*.

tessellated f., a normal f. to which a deeply pigmented choroid gives the appearance of dark polygonal areas between the choroidal vessels, especially in the periphery.

f. of urinary bladder, the f. is formed by the posterior wall which is somewhat convex. SYN f. vesicae urinariae [NA].

f. of uterus, the upper rounded extremity of the uterus above the openings of the uterine (fallopian) tubes.

f. ventric'uli, *official alternate term for f. of stomach.

f. vesi'cae urina'riae [NA], SYN f. of urinary bladder.

fun·du·sec·to·my (fŭn-dŭ-sek'tō-mē). Excision of the fundus of an organ. SYN fundectomy. [L. *fundus*, + G. *ektomē*, excision]

fun·gal (fŭng'găl). SYN fungous.

fun·gate (fŭng'gāt). To grow exuberantly like a fungus.

fun·ge·mia (fŭn-jē'mē-ă). Fungal infection disseminated by way of the bloodstream.

Fun·gi (fŭn'jī). A division of eukaryotic organisms that grow in irregular masses, without roots, stems, or leaves, and are devoid of chlorophyll or other pigments capable of photosynthesis. Each organism (thallus) is unicellular to filamentous, and possesses branched somatic structures (hyphae) surrounded by cell walls containing cellulose or chitin or both, and containing true nuclei. They reproduce sexually or asexually (spore formation), and may obtain nutrition from other living organisms as parasites or from dead organic matter as saprobes (saprophytes). [L. *fungus*, a mushroom]

fun·gi (fŭn'jī). Plural of fungus.

fun·gi·ci·dal (fŭn-ji-sī'dăl). Having a killing action on fungi. [fungus + L. *caedo*, to kill]

fun·gi·cide (fŭn′ji-sīd). Any substance that has a destructive killing action upon fungi.

fun·gi·form (fŭn′ji-fōrm). Shaped like a fungus or mushroom; applied to any structure with a broad, often branched, free portion and a narrower base.

Fun·gi Im·per·fec·ti (fŭn′jī im-per-fek′tī). A phylum of fungi in which sexual reproduction is not known or in which one of the mating types has not yet been discovered.

fun·gi·stat·ic (fŭn-ji-stat′ik). Having an inhibiting action upon the growth of fungi. [fungus + G. *statos,* standing]

fun·gi·tox·ic (fŭn-ji-tok′sik). Poisonous or in any way deleterious to the growth of fungi.

fun·goid (fŭng′goyd). Resembling a fungus; denoting an exuberant morbid growth on the surface of the body.

fun·gos·i·ty (fŭng-gos′i-tē). A fungoid growth.

fun·gous (fŭng′gŭs). Relating to a fungus. SYN fungal.

fun·gus, pl. **fun·gi** (fŭng′gŭs, fŭn′jī). A general term used to encompass the diverse morphological forms of yeasts and molds. Originally classified as primitive plants without chlorophyll, the fungi are placed in the kingdom Fungi and some in the kingdom Protista, along with algae, protozoa, and slime molds. Fungi share with bacteria the ability to break down complex organic substances and are essential to the recycling of carbon and other elements. Fungi are important as foods and to the fermentation process in the development of substances of industrial and medical importance, including alcohol, the antibiotics, other drugs, and antitoxins. Relatively few fungi are pathogenic for humans, whereas most plant diseases are caused by fungi. [L. *fungus,* a mushroom]

    dematiaceous fungi (de-măt′ē-ā-cē-ous), dark f. that form melanin. [Mod. L. *Dematium* (genus name), fr. g. *demation,* fine strand, fr. *dema,* band, fr. *deō,* to bind + suffix *-aceous,* characterized by]

    imperfect f., a f. in which the means of sexual reproduction is not yet recognized; these fungi generally reproduce by means of conidia.

    perfect f., a f. possessing both sexual and asexual means of reproduction, and in which both mating forms are recognized.

fu·nic (few′nik). Relating to the funis, or umbilical cord. SYN funicular (2).

fu·ni·cle (fyū′ni-kl). SYN cord.

fu·nic·u·lar (fyū-nik′yū-lăr). 1. Relating to a funiculus. 2. SYN funic.

fu·nic·u·li·tis (fyū-nik′yū-lī′tis). 1. Inflammation of a funiculus, especially of the spermatic cord. 2. Inflammation of the umbilical cord usually associated with chorioamnionitis. [funiculus + G. *-itis,* inflammation]

fu·nic·u·lo·pexy (fyū-nik′yū-lō-pek-sē). Suturing of the spermatic cord to the surrounding tissue in the correction of an undescended testicle. [funiculus + G. *pēxis,* a fixing]

fu·nic·u·lus, pl. **fu·nic·u·li** (fyū-nik′yū-lŭs, -lī) [NA]. SYN cord. [L. dim. of *funis,* cord]

    anterior f., anterior white column of spinal cord, a column or bundle of white matter on either side of the anterior median fissure, between that and the anterolateral sulcus.

    cuneate f., SYN cuneate *fasciculus.*

    lateral f., the lateral white column of the spinal cord between the lines of exit and entrance of the anterior and posterior nerve roots.

    posterior f., posterior white column of the spinal cord, the large wedge-shaped fiber bundle lying between the posterior gray column and the posterior median septum, and composed largely of dorsal root fibers.

    f. spermat′icus [NA], SYN spermatic *cord.*

    f. umbilica′lis [NA], SYN umbilical *cord.*

fu·ni·form (fyū′ni-fōrm). Ropelike. [L. *funis,* cord, + *forma,* shape]

fu·ni·punc·ture (fyū-nē-pŭnk-chŭr). SYN cordocentesis. [L. *funis,* cord, + puncture]

fu·nis (fyū′nis). 1. SYN umbilical *cord.* 2. A cordlike structure. [L. a rope, cord]

FUO *fever* of unknown origin.

fu·ra·nose (fyūr′ă-nōs). A saccharide unit or molecule containing the furan grouping. [furan + -ose(1)]

fur·cal (fer′kăl). Forked.

fur·ca·tion (fŭr-kā′shŭn). 1. A forking, or a forklike part or branch. 2. DENTAL HISTOLOGY the region of a multirooted tooth at which the roots divide. [L. *furca,* fork]

fur·fu·ra·ceous (fer-fyū-rā′shŭs). Branny, or composed of small scales; denoting a form of desquamation. SYN pityroid. [L. *furfuraceus,* fr. *furfur,* bran]

fu·ror ep·i·lep·ti·cus (fyū′rōr ep-i-lep′ti-kŭs). Attacks of anger to which epileptic individuals are occasionally subject, occurring without apparent provocation and without disturbance of consciousness.

fur·row (fer′rō). A groove or sulcus. [A.S. *furh*]

    genital f., a groove on the genital tubercle in the embryo, appearing toward the end of the second month.

    gluteal f., SYN gluteal *fold.*

fu·run·cle (fyū′rŭng-kl). A localized pyogenic infection, most frequently by *Staphylococcus aureus,* originating deep in a hair follicle. SYN boil, furunculus. [L. *furunculus,* a petty thief]

fu·run·cu·lar (fyū-rŭng′kyū-lăr). Relating to a furuncle. SYN furunculous.

fu·run·cu·loid (fyū-rŭng′kyū-loyd). Resembling a furuncle. [furunculus + G. *eidos,* resemblance]

fu·run·cu·lo·sis (fyū-rŭng-kyū-lō′sis). A condition marked by the presence of furuncles, often chronic and recurrent.

fu·run·cu·lous (fyū-rŭng′kyū-lŭs). SYN furuncular.

fu·run·cu·lus, pl. **fu·run·cu·li** (fyū-rŭng′kyū-lŭs, -lī). SYN furuncle. [L. a petty thief, a boil, dim. of *fur,* a thief]

Fu·sar·i·um (fyū-zā′rē-ŭm). A genus of rapidly growing fungi producing characteristic sickle-shaped, multiseptate macroconidia which can be mistaken for those produced by some dermatophytes. A few species can produce corneal ulcers; some are common colonizers of burned skin and some may cause disseminated hyalohyphomycosis. [L. *fusus,* spindle]

fu·si·form (fyū′zi-fōrm, fyū′si-). Spindle-shaped;

tapering at both ends. [L. *fusus,* a spindle, + *forma,* form]

fu·si·mo·tor (fyū'zē-mō'ter). Pertaining to the efferent innervation of intrafusal muscle fibers by gamma motor neurons. SEE ALSO neuromuscular *spindle.* [L. *fusus,* spindle, + *moveo,* to move]

fu·sion (fyū'zhŭn). **1.** Liquefaction, as by melting by heat. **2.** Union, as by joining together. **3.** The blending of slightly different images from each eye into a single perception. **4.** The joining of two or more adjacent teeth during their development by a dentinal union. SEE ALSO concrescence. **5.** Joining of two genes, often neighboring genes. [L. *fusio,* a pouring, fr. *fundo,* pp. *fusus,* to pour]

  cell f., the merging of the contents of two cells by artificial means without the destruction of either, resulting in a heterokaryon that, for at least a few generations, will reproduce its kind; an important method in assignment of loci to chromosomes.

  centric f., SYN robertsonian *translocation.*

  spinal f., spine f., a surgical procedure to accomplish bony ankylosis between two or more vertebrae. SYN spondylosyndesis.

Fu·so·bac·te·ri·um (fyū'zō-bak-tēr'ē-ŭm). A genus of bacteria containing Gram-negative, non–spore-forming, obligately anaerobic rods which produce butyric acid as a major metabolic product. These organisms are found in cavities of humans and other animals; some species are pathogenic. [L. *fusus,* a spindle, + bacterium]

fu·so·cel·lu·lar (fyū'zō-sel'yū-lăr). Spindle-celled.

fu·so·spi·ro·chet·al (fyū-zō-spī-rō-kē'tăl). Referring to the associated fusiform and spirochetal organisms found in the lesions of Vincent's angina.

Futcher's line. See under line.

FVC forced vital *capacity.*

G

γ. gamma. SEE gamma.

G Newtonian *constant* of gravitation, gap (3); gauss; giga-; D-glucose, as in UDPG; guanosine, as in GDP; glycine; guanine.

G G_{act} or $G^{‡}$.

g gram.

g. Unit of acceleration based on the acceleration produced by the earth's gravitational attraction, where 1 g = 980.621 cm/sec^2 (about 32.1725 ft/sec^2) at sea level and 45° latitude. At 30° latitude, g equals 979.329 cm/sec^2.

Ga gallium.

G-ac·tin. See under actin.

gad·o·lin·i·um (Gd) (gad-ō-lin′ē-ŭm). An element of the lanthanide group, atomic no. 64, atomic wt. 157.25. The magnetic properties of this element are used in contrast media for magnetic resonance imaging. [mineral, gadolinite, from Johan *Gadolin,* Finnish chemist, 1760–1852]

gag. 1. To retch; to cause to retch or heave. **2.** To prevent from talking. **3.** An instrument adjusted between the teeth to keep the mouth from closing during operations in the mouth or throat.

gain (gān). **1.** Profit; advantage. **2.** The ratio of output to input of an amplifying system, generally expressed in decibels. [M.E. *gayne,* booty, fr. O.Fr., fr. Germanic]

  primary g., interpersonal, social, or financial advantages from the conversion of emotional stress directly into illness (*e.g.,* hysterical blindness or paralysis). Cf. secondary g.

  secondary g., interpersonal or social advantages (*e.g.,* assistance, attention, sympathy) gained indirectly from illness. Cf. primary g.

gait (gāt). Manner of walking.

  antalgic g. (ant-al′jik), a limping walk used to avoid pain. [G. *anti-,* against, + *algos,* pain]

  ataxic g., SYN cerebellar g.

  cerebellar g., wide-based gait with lateral veering, unsteadiness, and irregularity of steps; often with a tendency to fall to one side, forward, or backward. SYN ataxic g.

  festinating g., g. in which the trunk is flexed, legs are flexed at the knees and hips, but stiff, while the steps are short and progressively more rapid; characteristically seen with parkinsonism (1) and other neurologic diseases. SYN festination.

  helicopod g., a g., seen in some conversion reactions or hysterical disorders, in which the feet describe half circles. SYN helicopodia.

  hemiplegic g., g. in which the leg is stiff, without flexion at knee and ankle, and with each step is rotated away from the body, then towards it, forming a semicircle. SYN spastic g.

  high steppage g., a g. in which the foot is raised high and brought down suddenly in a flapping manner; often seen in peroneal nerve palsy and tabes.

  spastic g., SYN hemiplegic g.

  steppage g., a g. in which the advancing foot is lifted higher than usual so that it can clear the ground, because it cannot be dorsiflexed. Seen with peroneal neuropathies and other disorders causing foot dorsiflexion weakness. SEE high steppage g.

Gal galactose.

△**galact-.** SEE galacto-.

ga·lac·ta·cra·sia (gă-lak′tă-krā′zē-ă). Abnormal composition of mother's milk. [galact- + G. *akrasia,* bad mixture, fr. *a-* priv. + *krasis,* a mixing]

ga·lac·ta·gogue (gă-lak′tă-gog). An agent that promotes the secretion and flow of milk. [galact- + G. *agōgos,* leading]

ga·lac·tic (gă-lak′tik). Pertaining to milk; promoting the flow of milk.

△**galacto-, galact-.** Milk. Cf. lact-. [G. *gala*]

ga·lac·to·cele (gă-lak′tō-sēl). Retention cyst caused by occlusion of a lactiferous duct. SYN lactocele. [galacto- + G. *kēlē,* tumor]

ga·lac·to·ki·nase (gă-lak-tō-kī′nās). An enzyme (phosphotransferase) that, in the presence of ATP, catalyzes the phosphorylation of D-galactose to D-galactose 1-phosphate, the first step in the metabolism of D-galactose; g. is deficient in one form of galactosemia.

ga·lac·to·phore (gă-lak′tō-fōr). SYN lactiferous *ducts,* under *duct.* [galacto- + G. *phoros,* bearing]

ga·lac·to·pho·ri·tis (gă-lak′tō-fō-rī′tis). Inflammation of the milk ducts. [galacto- + G. *phoros,* carrying, + -itis, inflammation]

gal·ac·toph·o·rous (gal-ak-tof′ŏ-rŭs). Conveying milk.

ga·lac·to·poi·e·sis (gă-lak′tō-poy-ē′sis). Milk production. [galacto- + G. *poiēsis,* forming]

ga·lac·to·poi·et·ic (gă-lak′tō-poy-et′ik). Pertaining to galactopoiesis.

ga·lac·tor·rhea (gă-lak-tō-rē′ă). **1.** A flow of milk from the breasts other than normal lactation. **2.** Any white discharge from a nipple. SYN lactorrhea. [galacto- + G. *rhoia,* a flow]

ga·lac·tos·a·mine (gă-lak-tō-sam′ēn). The 2-amino-2-deoxy derivative of galactose, in which the NH_2 replaces the 2-OH group; the D-isomer occurs in various mucopolysaccharides, notably of chondroitin sulfuric acid and of B blood group substance; usually found as the *N*-acetyl derivative.

ga·lac·tos·am·i·no·gly·can (gă-lak′tōs-am-i-nō-glī′kan). SEE mucopolysaccharide.

ga·lac·tose (Gal) (gă-lak′tōs). An aldohexose found (in D form) as a constituent of lactose, cerebrosides, gangliosides, mucoproteins, etc., in galactoside or galactosyl combination; an epimer of D-glucose.

ga·lac·to·se·mia (gă-lak-tō-sē′mē-ă) [MIM* 230400]. An inborn error of galactose metabolism due to congenital deficiency of the enzyme galactosyl-1-phosphate uridyltransferase, resulting in tissue accumulation of galactose 1-phosphate; manifested by nutritional failure, hepatosplenomegaly with cirrhosis, cataracts, mental retardation, galactosuria, aminoaciduria, and albuminuria, which regress or disappear if galactose is removed from the diet. [galactose + G. *haima,* blood]

α-D-**ga·lac·to·sid·ase** (gă-lak-tō-sīd′ās). An enzyme catalyzing the hydrolysis of α-D-galacto-sides to release free D-galactose. A deficiency of type A α-D-galactosidase is associated with Fabry's disease.

β·D·ga·lac·to·sid·ase. A sugar-splitting enzyme that catalyzes the hydrolysis of lactose into D-glucose and D-galactose, and that of other β-D-galactosides; it also catalyzes galactotransferase reactions; a deficiency of β-D -galactosidase leads to problems in the intestinal digestion of lactose; used in the production of milk products for adults who do not have the intestinal enzyme; a defect of one isozyme of β-D-galactosidase is associated with Morquio's syndrome type B. SYN lactase.

ga·lac·to·side (gă-lak'tō-sīd). A compound in which the H of the OH group on carbon-1 of galactose is replaced by an organic radical.

ga·lac·to·sis (gal-ak-tō'sis). Formation of milk by the lacteal glands. [galacto- + G. -osis, condition]

ga·lac·tos·u·ria (gă-lak-tō-sū'rē-ă). The excretion of galactose in the urine. [galactose + G. ouron, urine]

ga·lac·to·syl (gă-lak'tō-sil). A compound in which the –OH attached to carbon-1 of galactose is replaced by an organic radical.

ga·lac·to·ther·a·py (gă-lak'tō-thār'ă-pē). Treatment of disease by means of an exclusive or nearly exclusive milk diet. SYN lactotherapy.

ga·lea (gā'lē-ă). 1 [NA]. A structure shaped like a helmet. 2. SYN epicranial *aponeurosis*. 3. A form of bandage covering the head. 4. SYN caul (1). [L. a helmet]

ga·len·i·cals (gā-len'i-kălz). 1. Herbs and other vegetable drugs, as distinguished from the mineral or chemical remedies. 2. Crude drugs and the tinctures, decoctions, and other preparations made from them, as distinguished from the alkaloids and other active principles. 3. Remedies prepared according to an official formula. [Claudius *Galen*]

gall·blad·der (gawl'blad-er). A pear-shaped receptacle on the inferior surface of the liver, in a hollow between the right lobe and the quadrate lobe; it serves as a storage reservoir for bile. SYN vesica biliaris [NA], cholecyst, cholecystis.

  Courvoisier's g., an enlarged, often palpable g. in a patient with carcinoma of the head of the pancreas. It is associated with jaundice due to obstruction of the common bile duct.

gal·li·um (Ga) (gal'ē-ŭm). A rare metal, atomic no. 31, atomic wt. 69.723. [L. *Gallia,* France]

gal·li·um-67. A cyclotron-produced radionuclide with a half-life of 3.260 days and major gamma ray emissions; as a tumor- and inflammation-localizing radiotracer.

gal·li·um-68. A positron emitter with a radioactive half-life of 1.130 hours.

gal·lon (găl'ŭn). A measure of U.S. liquid capacity containing 4 quarts, 231 cubic inches, or 8.3293 pounds of distilled water at 20° C; it is the equivalent of 3.785412 liters. The British imperial g. contains 277.4194 cubic inches. [O.Fr. *galon*]

gal·lop (gal'op). A triple cadence to the heart sounds due to an abnormal third or fourth heart sound being added in addition to the first and second sounds; sometimes indicative of serious disease. SYN cantering rhythm, gallop rhythm.

  presystolic g., g. rhythm in which the g. sound is an audible fourth heart sound due to forceful ventricular filling.

  protodiastolic g., g. rhythm in which the g. sound is an abnormal third heart sound.

  summation g., g. rhythm in which the g. sound is due to superimposition of third and fourth heart sounds; sometimes heard in normal subjects with tachycardia, but usually indicative of myocardial disease.

gall·stone (gal'stōn). A concretion in the gallbladder or a bile duct, composed chiefly of a mixture of cholesterol, calcium bilirubinate, and calcium carbonate, occasionally as a pure stone composed of just one of these substances. SYN cholelith.

gam·ete (gam'ēt). 1. One of two haploid cells undergoing karyogamy. 2. Any germ cell, whether ovum or spermatozoon. [G. *gametēs,* husband; *gametē,* wife]

△**gameto-.** A gamete. [G. *gametēs,* husband, *gametē,* wife, fr. *gameō,* to marry]

ga·me·to·cide (gă-mē'tō-sīd). An agent destructive of gametes, specifically the malarial gametocytes. [gameto- + L. *caedo,* to kill]

ga·me·to·cyte (gă-mē'tō-sīt). A cell capable of dividing to produce gametes, *e.g.,* a spermatocyte or oocyte. [gameto- + G. *kytos,* cell]

ga·me·to·gen·e·sis (gam'ĕ-tō-jen'ĕ-sis). The process of formation and development of gametes. [gameto- + G. *genesis,* production]

gamma (γ) (gă'mă) **1.** Third letter in the Greek alphabet. **2.** CHEMISTRY the third in a series, the fourth carbon in an aliphatic acid, or position 2 removed from the α position in the benzene ring. **3.** Symbol for 10^{-4} gauss; surface *tension;* activity *coefficient.* **4.** photon. For terms with the prefix γ, see the specific term.

gam·mop·a·thy (gă-mop'ă-thē). A primary disturbance in immunoglobulin synthesis.

  polyclonal g., a g. in which there is a heterogeneous increase in immunoglobulins involving more than one cell line; may be caused by any of a variety of inflammatory, infectious, or neoplastic disorders.

gam·o·gen·e·sis (gam-ō-jen'ĕ-sis). SYN sexual *reproduction.* [G. *gamos,* marriage, + *genesis,* production]

gan·glia (gang'glē-ă). Plural of ganglion.

gan·gli·al (gang'glē-ăl). SYN ganglionic.

gan·gli·ate, gan·gli·at·ed (gang'glē-āt, gang'glē-ā-ted). Having ganglia. SYN ganglionated.

gan·gli·ec·to·my (gang-glē-ek'tō-mē). SYN ganglionectomy.

gan·gli·form (gang'glē-fōrm). Having the form or appearance of a ganglion. SYN ganglioform.

gan·gli·i·tis (gang-glē-ī'tis). SYN ganglionitis.

gan·gli·o·blast (gang'glē-ō-blast). An embryonic cell from which develop ganglion cells. [ganglion + G. *blastos,* germ]

gan·gli·o·cyte (gang'glē-ō-sīt). SYN ganglion *cell.*

gan·gli·o·cy·to·ma (gang'glē-ō-sī-tō'mă). A rare lesion that contains neuronal (ganglion) cells in a sparse glial stoma. SYN central ganglioneuroma. [ganglion + G. *kytos*, cell, + *-oma*, tumor]

gan·gli·o·form (gang'glē-ō-fōrm). SYN ganglioform.

gan·gli·o·gli·o·ma (gang'glē-ō-glē-ō'mă). A rare tumor consisting of a glioma component and an atypical neuronal (ganglion) cell component; in younger patients often associated with seizures.

gan·gli·ol·y·sis (gang-glē-ol'i-sis). The dissolution or breaking up of a ganglion.

gan·gli·o·ma (gang-glē-ō'mă). SYN ganglioneuroma.

gan·gli·on, pl. **gan·glia, gan·gli·ons** (gang'glē-on, -glē-ă, -glē-onz). **1** [NA]. Originally, any group of nerve cell bodies in the central or peripheral nervous system; currently, an aggregation of nerve cell bodies located in the peripheral nervous system. SYN neuroganglion. **2.** A cyst containing mucopolysaccharide-rich fluid within fibrous tissue or, occasionally, muscle bone or a semilunar cartilage; usually attached to a tendon sheath in the hand, wrist, or foot, or connected with the underlying joint. SYN myxoid cyst, synovial cyst. [G. a swelling or knot]

Acrel's g., (1) pseudoganglion on the posterior interosseous nerve on the dorsal aspect of the wrist joint; **(2)** a cyst on a tendon of an extensor muscle at the level of the wrist.

autonomic ganglia, visceral ganglia. SEE autonomic nervous *system*.

ganglia of autonomic plexuses, autonomic ganglia lying in plexuses of autonomic fibers, *e.g.,* the celiac and inferior mesenteric ganglia of the sympathetic, and the small parasympathetic ganglia of the myenteric plexus. SYN ganglia plexuum autonomicorum [NA].

basal ganglia, large masses of gray matter at the base of the cerebral hemisphere: the striate body (caudate and lentiform nuclei) and cell groups associated with the striate body, such as the subthalamic nucleus and substantia nigra.

cardiac ganglia, parasympathetic ganglia of the cardiac plexus lying between the arch of the aorta and the bifurcation of the pulmonary artery.

carotid g., a small ganglionic swelling on filaments from the internal carotid plexus, lying on the undersurface of the carotid artery in the cavernous sinus.

celiac ganglia, the largest and highest group of prevertebral sympathetic ganglia, located on the superior part of the abdominal aorta, on either side of the origin of the celiac artery; contains sympathetic neurons whose unmyelinated postganglionic axons innervate the stomach, liver, gallbladder, spleen, kidney, small intestine, and ascending and transverse colon. h

cervicothoracic g., a sympathetic trunk g. lying behind the subclavian artery near the origin of the vertebral artery, it is formed by the fusion of the inferior cervical ganglion, at the level of the seventh cervical vertebra, with the first thoracic g.

g. cer'vicothora'cicum [NA], a sympathetic trunk g. lying behind the subclavian artery near the origin of the vertebral artery, at the level of the seventh cervical vertebra, close to the first thoracic g. with which it is usually fused.

ciliary g., a small parasympathetic g. lying in the orbit between the optic nerve and the lateral rectus muscle; it receives preganglionic innervation from the Edinger-Westphal nucleus by way of the oculomotor nerve, and in turn gives rise to postganglionic fibers that innervate the ciliary muscle and the sphincter of the iris (sphincter pupillae muscle).

coccygeal g., SYN g. impar.

geniculate g., a g. of the nervus intermedius fibers conveyed by the facial nerve, located within the facial canal at the genu of the canal and containing the sensory neurons innervating the taste buds on the anterior two-thirds of the tongue and a small area on the external ear.

g. im'par [NA], the most inferior, unpaired g. of the sympathetic trunk; inconstant. SYN coccygeal g.

inferior g. of glossopharyngeal nerve, the lower of two sensory g.'s on the glossopharyngeal nerve as it traverses the jugular foramen.

Ludwig's g., a small collection of parasympathetic nerve cells in the interatrial septum.

otic g., an autonomic g. situated below the foramen ovale medial to the mandibular nerve; its postganglionic, parasympathetic fibers are distributed to the parotid gland.

parasympathetic ganglia, those ganglia of the autonomic nervous system composed of cholinergic neurons receiving afferent fibers from preganglionic visceral motor neurons in either the brainstem or the middle sacral spinal segments (S2 to S4); on the basis of their location with respect to the organs they innervate, most parasympathetic ganglia, at least outside the head, can be categorized as juxtamural or intramural ganglia. SEE ALSO autonomic nervous *system*.

paravertebral ganglia, SYN ganglia of sympathetic trunk.

pelvic ganglia, the parasympathetic ganglia scattered through the pelvic plexus on either side.

phrenic ganglia, several small autonomic ganglia contained in the plexuses accompanying the inferior phrenic arteries.

gang'lia plex'uum autonomico'rum [NA], SYN ganglia of autonomic plexuses.

prevertebral ganglia, the sympathetic ganglia (celiac, aorticorenal, superior and inferior mesenteric) lying in front of the vertebral column, as distinguished from the ganglia of the sympathetic trunk (paravertebral ganglia); these ganglia occur mostly around the origin of the major branches of the abdominal aorta; all are in the abdominopelvic cavity, concerned with innervation of abdomino-pelvic viscera.

pterygopalatine g., a small parasympathetic g. in the upper part of the pterygopalatine fossa whose postsynaptic fibers supply the lacrimal, nasal, palatine and pharyngeal glands.

renal ganglia, small scattered sympathetic ganglia along the renal plexus.

sensory g., a cluster of primary sensory neurons forming a usually visible swelling in the course of a peripheral nerve or its dorsal root; such nerve cells establish the sole afferent neural connection between the sensory periphery (skin, mucous membranes of the oral and nasal cavities, muscle tissue, tendons, joint capsules, special sense organs, blood vessel walls, tissues of the internal organs) and the central nervous system; they are the cells of origin of all sensory fibers of the peripheral nervous system.

spinal g., the g. of the posterior root of each spinal segmental nerve; contains the cell bodies of the pseudounipolar primary sensory neurons whose peripheral axonal branches become part of the mixed segmental nerve, while the central axonal branches enter the spinal cord as a component of the sensory posterior root.

spiral g. of cochlea, an elongated g. of bipolar sensory nerve cell bodies on the cochlear part of the vestibulocochlear nerve in the spiral canal of the modiolus; each g. cell gives rise to a peripheral process that passes between the layers of the bony spiral lamina to the organ of Corti, and a central axon that enters the hindbrain as a component of the inferior (cochlear) root of the eighth nerve.

splanchnic g., a small sympathetic g. often present in the course of the greater splanchnic nerve.

submandibular g., a small parasympathetic g. suspended from the lingual nerve; its postganglionic branches go to the submandibular and sublingual glands; its preganglionic fibers come from the superior salivatory nucleus by way of the chorda tympani.

superior g. of glossopharyngeal nerve, the upper and smaller of two ganglia on the glossopharyngeal nerve as it traverses the jugular foramen.

superior g. of vagus nerve, a small sensory g. on the vagus as it traverses the jugular foramen.

sympathetic ganglia, those ganglia of the autonomic nervous system that receive efferent fibers originating from preganglionic visceral motor neurons in the intermediolateral cell column of thoracic and upper lumbar spinal segments (T1–L2). On the basis of their location, the sympathetic ganglia can be classified as paravertebral ganglia (ganglia trunci sympathici) and prevertebral ganglia (ganglia celiaca). SEE ALSO autonomic nervous *system.*

ganglia of sympathetic trunk, the clusters of postganglionic neurons located at intervals along the sympathetic trunks, including the superior cervical, middle cervical, and cervicothoracic (stellate) g., the thoracic, lumbar, and sacral ganglia, and the g. impar. SYN ganglia trunci sympathici [NA], paravertebral ganglia.

trigeminal g., the large flattened sensory g. of the trigeminal nerve lying close to the cavernous sinus along the medial part of the middle cranial fossa in the trigeminal cavity of the dura mater.

gang′lia trun′ci sympath′ici [NA], SYN ganglia of sympathetic trunk.

tympanic g., a small g. on the tympanic nerve during its passage through the petrous portion of the temporal bone.

vestibular g., a collection of bipolar nerve cell bodies forming a swelling on the vestibular part of the eighth nerve in the internal acoustic meatus; consists of a superior part and an inferior part connected by a narrow isthmus.

gan·gli·on·at·ed (gang′glē-ō-nā′ted). SYN gangliate.

gan·gli·on·ec·to·my (gang′glē-ō-nek′tō-mē). Excision of a ganglion. SYN gangliectomy. [ganglion + G. *ektomē,* excision]

gan·glio·neu·ro·ma (gang′glē-ō-nū-rō′mă). A benign neoplasm composed of mature ganglionic neurons, in varying numbers, scattered singly or in clumps within a relatively abundant and dense stroma of neurofibrils and collagenous fibers; usually found in the posterior mediastinum and retroperitoneum, sometimes in relation to the adrenal glands. SYN ganglioma. [ganglion + G. *neuron,* nerve, + -*oma,* tumor]

    central g., SYN gangliocytoma.

gan·gli·on·ic (gang-glē-on′ik). Relating to a ganglion. SYN ganglial.

gan·gli·on·i·tis (gang′glē-ō-nī′tis). **1.** Inflammation of a lymphatic ganglion. **2.** Inflammation of a nerve ganglion. SYN gangliitis.

gan·gli·o·nos·to·my (gang′glē-ō-nos′tō-mē). Making an opening into a ganglion (2). [ganglion + G. *stoma,* mouth]

gan·gli·o·ple·gic (gang′glē-ō-plē′jik). A pharmacologic compound that paralyzes an autonomic ganglion, usually for a relatively short period of time. [ganglion + G. *plēgē,* stroke, shock]

gan·gli·o·side (gang′glē-ō-sīd). A glycosphingolipid chemically similar to cerebrosides but containing one or more sialic acid residues; found principally in nerve tissue, spleen, and thymus; G_{M1} accumulates in generalized gangliosidosis; G_{M2} accumulates in Tay-Sachs disease.

gan·gli·o·si·do·sis (gang′glē-ō-si-dō′sis). Any disease characterized, in part, by the abnormal accumulation within the nervous system of specific gangliosides, *e.g.,* G_{M2} gangliosidosis, Tay-Sachs disease, caused by hexosaminidase A enzyme deficiency with accumulation of G_{M2} ganglioside.

    G_{M1} **g.,** three forms exist: infantile, generalized; juvenile; and adult; g. characterized by accumulation of a specific monosialoganglioside, G_{M1}; due to deficiency of G_{M1}-β-galactosidase.

    G_{M2} **g.,** one of the hereditary metabolic disorders; several forms exist, including Tay-Sachs disease, Sandhoff's disease, AV variant and adult onset; characterized by accumulation of a specific metabolite, G_{M2} ganglioside, due to deficiency of hexosaminidase A or B, or G_{M2} activator factor.

gan·grene (gang′grēn). **1.** Necrosis due to obstruction, loss, or diminution of blood supply; it may be localized to a small area or involve an entire extremity or organ (such as the bowel), and may be wet or dry. SYN mortification. **2.** Extensive necrosis from any cause, *e.g.,* gas g. [G. *gangraina,* an eating sore, fr. *graō,* to gnaw]

    dry g., a form of g. in which the involved part is dry and shriveled. SYN mummification (1).

    gas g., g. occurring in a wound infected with various anaerobic sporeforming bacteria, especially *Clostridium perfringens* and *C. novyi,* which cause crepitation of the surrounding tissues, due to gas liberated by bacterial fermentation, and constitutional septic symptoms.

    moist g., SYN wet g.

    spontaneous g. of newborn, g. due to vascu-

ga

lar occlusion of unknown cause, usually in marasmic or dehydrated infants.

symmetrical g., g. affecting the extremities of both sides of the body; it is seen particularly in severe arteriosclerosis, myocardial infarction, and ball-valve thrombus.

wet g., ischemic necrosis of an extremity with bacterial infection, producing cellulitis adjacent to the necrotic areas. SYN moist g.

white g., death of a part accompanied by the formation of grayish white sloughs.

gan·gre·nous (gang'grĕ-nŭs). Relating to or affected with gangrene. SYN mortified.

gap. 1. A hiatus or opening in a structure. **2.** An interval or discontinuity in any series or sequence. **3 (G).** A period in the cell cycle.

g. 1, in the somatic cell cycle, the g. that follows mitosis and is followed by synthesis in preparation for the next cycle.

g. 2, in the somatic cell cycle, a pause between completion of synthesis and the onset of cell division.

air-bone g., an abnormal condition in which the auditory threshold for an air-conducted test tone is higher than that for a bone-conducted test tone of the same frequency. SEE ALSO conductive *hearing loss.*

anion g., the arithmetical difference between the concentrations of routinely measured cations (Na^+ + K^+) and of routinely measured anions (Cl^- + HCO_3^-) in plasma or serum; unmeasured anions (phosphate, sulfate, protein, other organic ions) account for the g., which is increased in metabolic acidosis due to diabetic ketosis, renal failure, or extraneous substances (methanol, salicylate).

auscultatory g., the period during which Korotkoff sounds indicating true systolic pressure fade away and reappear at a lower pressure point; responsible for errors made in recording falsely low systolic blood pressure, especially in hypertensive patients, of up to 25 mm Hg, and avoided by pumping the cuff 30 mm Hg above palpable systolic pressure.

Gard·ner·el·la (gărd'ner-el'ă). A genus of facultatively anaerobic, oxidase- and catalase-negative, non–spore-forming, nonencapsulated, non-motile, pleomorphic bacteria with Gram-variable rods.

G. vaginalis, a species that is the etiologic agent of bacterial vaginosis.

gar·gle (gar'gl). **1.** To rinse the fauces with fluid in the mouth through which expired breath is forced to produce a bubbling effect while the head is held far back. **2.** A medicated fluid used for gargling; a throat wash. [O. Fr. fr. L. *gurgulio,* gullet, windpipe]

gas. 1. fluid, like air, capable of indefinite expansion but convertible by compression and cold into a liquid and, eventually, a solid. **2.** In clinical practice, a liquid entirely in its vapor phase at 1 atmosphere of pressure because ambient temperature is above its boiling point. [coined by J.B. van Helmont, Flemish chemist, 1577–1644]

alveolar g. (symbol subscript A), the g. in the pulmonary alveoli, where O_2-CO_2 exchange with pulmonary capillary blood occurs. SYN alveolar air.

anesthetic g., SEE inhalation *anesthetic.*

blood g.'s, a clinical expression for the determination of the partial pressures of oxygen and carbon dioxide in blood.

expired g., (1) any g. that has been expired from the lungs; **(2)** often used synonymously with mixed expired g.

inert g.'s, SYN noble g.'s.

inspired g. (I) (symbol subscript I), **(1)** any g. that is being inhaled; **(2)** specifically, that g. after it has been humidified at body temperature.

mixed expired g., one or more complete breaths of expired g. coming thoroughly mixed from the dead space and the alveoli.

noble g.'s, elements in the zero group in the periodic series: helium, neon, argon, krypton, xenon, and radon. SYN inert g.'s.

tear g., a g., such as acetone, benzene bromide, and xylol, that causes irritation of the conjunctiva and profuse lacrimation. SEE ALSO lacrimator.

gas·e·ous (gas'ē-ŭs). Of the nature of gas.

gas·o·met·ric (gas-ō-met'rik). Relating to gasometry.

gas·om·e·try (gas-om'ĕ-trē). Measurement of gases; determination of the relative proportion of gases in a mixture.

Gasser (Gasserio), Johann L., Austrian anatomist, 1723–1765. SEE gasserian.

gas·ser·i·an (ga-ser'ē-an). Relating to or described by Johann L. Gasser.

gas·sing (gas'ing). Poisoning by irrespirable or otherwise noxious gases.

gas·ter (gas'ter) [NA]. SYN stomach. [G. *gastēr,* belly]

gastr-. SEE gastro-.

gas·trad·e·ni·tis (gas'trad-ĕ-nī'tis). Inflammation of the glands of the stomach. [gastr- + G. *adēn,* gland, + *-itis,* inflammation]

gas·trec·ta·sis, gas·trec·ta·sia (gas-trek'tă-sis, gas-trek-tā'zē-ă). Dilation of the stomach. [gastr- + G. *ektasis,* extension]

gas·trec·to·my (gas-trek'tō-mē). Excision of a part or all of the stomach. [gastr- + G. *ektomē,* excision]

gas·tric (gas'trik). Relating to the stomach.

gas·trin·o·ma (gas-tri-nō'mă). A gastrin-secreting tumor associated with the Zollinger-Ellison syndrome.

gas·trins (gas'trinz). Hormones secreted in the pyloric-antral mucosa of the mammalian stomach that stimulate secretion of HCl by the parietal cells of the gastric glands; a competitive inhibitor of g. is cholecystokinin. [G. *gastēr,* stomach, + -in]

gas·tri·tis (gas-trī'tis). Inflammation, especially mucosal, of the stomach. [gastr- + G. *-itis,* inflammation]

atrophic g., chronic g. with atrophy of the mucous membrane and destruction of the peptic glands, sometimes associated with pernicious anemia or gastric carcinoma; also applied to gastric atrophy without inflammatory changes.

catarrhal g., g. with excessive secretion of mucus.

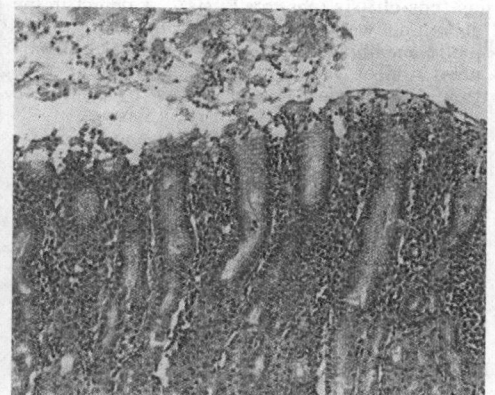

acute gastritis: with epithelial damage and inflammation of the peptic glands

exfoliative g., g. with excessive shedding of mucosal epithelial cells.

interstitial g., inflammation of the stomach involving the submucosa and muscle coats.

pseudomembranous g., g. characterized by the formation of a false membrane.

gastro-, gastr-. The stomach, abdomen. [G. *gastēr,* the belly]

gas·tro·a·nas·to·mo·sis (gas′trō-an-as-tō-mō′sis). Anastomosis of the cardiac and antral segments of the stomach, for relief from marked hour-glass contraction of the stomach. SYN gastrogastrostomy.

gas·tro·car·di·ac (gas′trō-kar′dē-ak). Relating to both the stomach and the heart.

gas·tro·cele (gas′trō-sēl). Hernia of a portion of the stomach. [gastro- + G. *kēlē,* hernia]

gas·troc·ne·mi·us (gas-trok-nē′mē-ŭs). SYN gastrocnemius *muscle.* [G. *gastroknēmia,* calf of the leg, fr. *gaster* (*gastr*-), belly, + *knēmē,* leg]

gas·tro·col·ic (gas′trō-kol′ik). Relating to the stomach and the colon.

gas·tro·co·li·tis (gas′trō-kō-lī′tis). Inflammation of both stomach and colon.

gas·tro·co·los·to·my (gas′trō-kō-los′tō-mē). Establishment of a communication between stomach and colon. [gastro- + G. *kōlon,* colon, + *stoma,* mouth]

gas·tro·du·o·de·nal (gas′trō-dū′ō-dē′năl, -dū-od′ĕ-nal). Relating to the stomach and duodenum.

gas·tro·du·o·de·ni·tis (gas′trō-dū-ō-dē-nī′tis). Inflammation of both stomach and duodenum.

gas·tro·du·o·de·nos·co·py (gas′trō-dū-ō-dĕ-nos′kŏ-pē). Visualization of the interior of the stomach and duodenum by a gastroscope. [gastro- + duodenum, + G. *skopeō,* to view]

gas·tro·du·o·de·nos·to·my (gas′trō-dū-ō-dĕ-nos′tō-mē). Establishment of a communication between the stomach and the duodenum. [gastro- + duodenum + G. *stoma,* mouth]

gas·tro·en·ter·ic (gas′trō-en-ter′ik). SYN gastrointestinal.

gas·tro·en·ter·i·tis (gas′trō-en-ter-ī′tis). Inflammation of the mucous membrane of both stomach and intestine. SYN enterogastritis. [gastro- + G. *enteron,* intestine, + *-itis,* inflammation]

gas·tro·en·ter·o·co·li·tis (gas′trō-en′ter-ō-kō-lī′tis). Inflammatory disease involving the stomach and intestines. [gastro- + G. *enteron,* intestine, + *kōlon,* colon, + *-itis,* inflammation]

gas·tro·en·ter·ol·o·gist (gas′trō-en-ter-ol′ō-jist). A specialist in gastroenterology.

gas·tro·en·ter·ol·o·gy (gas′trō-en-ter-ol′ō-jē). The medical specialty concerned with the function and disorders of the gastrointestinal tract, including stomach, intestines, and associated organs. [gastro- + G. *enteron,* intestine, + *logos,* study]

gas·tro·en·ter·op·a·thy (gas′trō-en-ter-op′ă-thē). Any disorder of the alimentary canal. [gastro- + G. *enteron,* intestine, + *pathos,* suffering]

gas·tro·en·ter·o·plas·ty (gas′trō-en-ter-ō-plas′tē). Operative repair of defects in the stomach and intestine. [gastro- + G. *enteron,* intestine, + *plassō,* to form]

gas·tro·en·ter·op·to·sis (gas′trō-en-ter-ō-tō′sis). Downward displacement of the stomach and a portion of the intestine. [gastro- + G. *enteron,* intestine, + *ptōsis,* a falling]

gas·tro·en·ter·os·to·my (gas′trō-en-ter-os′tō-mē). Establishment of a new opening between the stomach and the intestine, either anterior or posterior to the transverse colon. [gastro- + G. *enteron,* intestine, + *stoma,* mouth]

gas·tro·en·ter·ot·o·my (gas′trō-en-ter-ot′ō-mē). Section into both stomach and intestine. [gastro- + G. *enteron,* intestine, + *tomē,* incision]

gas·tro·ep·i·plo·ic (gas′trō-ep′i-plō′ik). Relating to the stomach and the greater omentum (epiploon).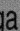

gas·tro·e·soph·a·ge·al (gas′trō-ē-sof′ă-jē′ăl). Relating to both stomach and esophagus. [gastro- + G. *oisophagos,* gullet (esophagus)]

gas·tro·e·soph·a·gi·tis (gas′trō-ē-sof-ă-jī′tis). Inflammation of the stomach and esophagus.

gas·tro·e·soph·a·gos·to·my (gas′trō-ē-sof-ă-gos′tō-mē). SYN esophagogastrostomy. [gastro- + G. *oisophagos,* gullet (esophagus), + *stoma,* mouth]

gas·tro·gas·tros·to·my (gas′trō-gas-tros′tō-mē). SYN gastroanastomosis.

gas·tro·ga·vage (gas-trō-gă-vahzh′). SYN gavage (1).

gas·tro·gen·ic (gas-trō-jen′ik). Deriving from or caused by the stomach.

gas·tro·he·pat·ic (gas′trō-he-pat′ik). Relating to the stomach and the liver. [gastro- + G. *hēpar* (*hēpat*-), liver]

gas·tro·il·e·i·tis (gas′trō-il-ē-ī′tis). Inflammation of the alimentary canal in which the stomach and ileum are primarily involved.

gas·tro·il·e·os·to·my (gas′trō-il-ē-os′tō-mē). A surgical joining of stomach to ileum; a technical error in which the ileum instead of jejunum is selected for the site of a gastrojejunostomy.

gas·tro·in·tes·ti·nal (GI) (gas′trō-in-tes′tin-ăl). Relating to the stomach and intestines. SYN gastroenteric.

gas·tro·je·ju·no·co·lic (gas′trō-jē-jū′nō-kol′ik). Referring to the stomach, jejunum, and colon.

gas·tro·je·ju·nos·to·my (gas′trō-jē-jū-nos′tō-mē). Establishment of a direct communication between the stomach and the jejunum. [gastro- + jejunum G. *stoma,* mouth]

gas•tro•li•e•nal (gas-trō-lī′ē-năl). SYN gastrosplenic. [gastro- + L. *lien,* spleen]

gas•tro•lith (gas′trō-lith). A concretion in the stomach. [gastro- + G. *lithos,* stone]

gas•tro•li•thi•a•sis (gas′trō-li-thī′ă-sis). Presence of one or more calculi in the stomach. [gastro- + G. *lithos,* stone + *-iasis,* condition]

gas•trol•y•sis (gas-trol′i-sis). Division of perigastric adhesions. [gastro- + G. *lysis,* loosening]

gas•tro•ma•la•cia (gas′trō-mă-lā′shē-ă). Softening of the walls of the stomach. [gastro- + G. *malakia,* softness]

gas•tro•meg•a•ly (gas′trō-meg′ă-lē). 1. Enlargement of the stomach. 2. Enlargement of the abdomen. [gastro- + G. *megas* (*megal-*), large]

gas•tro•myx•or•rhea (gas′trō-mik-sō-rē′ă). Excessive secretion of mucus in the stomach. [gastro- + G. *myxa,* mucus, + *rhoia,* a flow]

gas•tro•pa•ral•y•sis (gas′trō-pă-ral′i-sis). Paralysis of the muscular coat of the stomach.

gas•tro•pa•re•sis (gas-trō-pă-rē′sis, -par′ĕ-sis). A slight degree of gastroparalysis. [gastro- + G. *paresis,* a letting go, paralysis]

gas•tro•path•ic (gas-trō-path′ik). Denoting gastropathy.

gas•trop•a•thy (gas-trop′ă-thē). Any disease of the stomach. [gastro- + G. *pathos,* disease]

gas•tro•pex•y (gas′trō-pek-sē). Attachment of the stomach to the abdominal wall or diaphragm. [gastro- + G. *pēxis,* fixation]

gas•tro•phren•ic (gas′trō-fren′ik). Relating to the stomach and the diaphragm. [gastro- + G. *phrēn,* diaphragm]

gas•tro•plas•ty (gas′trō-plas-tē). Operative treatment of a defect in the stomach or lower esophagus which utilizes the stomach wall for the reconstruction. [gastro- + G. *plastos,* formed]

▪ vertical banded g., a g. for treatment of morbid obesity in which an upper gastric pouch is formed by a vertical staple line, with a cloth band applied to prevent dilation at the outlet into the main pouch.

gas•tro•pli•ca•tion (gas′trō-pli-kā′shŭn). An operation for reducing the size of the stomach by suturing a longitudinal fold with the peritoneal surfaces in apposition. SYN gastrorrhaphy (2). [gastro- + L. *plico,* to fold]

gas•trop•to•sis, gas•trop•to•sia (gas-trō-tō′sis, -tō′sē-ă). Downward displacement of the stomach. [gastro- + G. *ptosis,* a falling]

gas•tro•pul•mo•nary (gas-trō-pŭl′mo-nar-ē). SYN pneumogastric.

gas•tro•py•lor•ec•to•my (gas′trō-pī-lor-ek′tō-mē). SYN pylorectomy.

gas•tro•py•lor•ic (gas′trō-pī-lōr′ik). Relating to the stomach as a whole and to the pylorus.

gas•tror•rha•gia (gas′trō-rā′jē-ă). Hemorrhage from the stomach. [gastro- + G. *rhēgnymi,* to burst forth]

gas•tror•rha•phy (gas-trōr′ă-fē). 1. Suture of a perforation of the stomach. 2. SYN gastroplication. [gastro- + G. *rhaphē,* a stitching]

gas•tror•rhea (gas-trō-rē′ă). Excessive secretion of gastric juice or of mucus (gastromyxorrhea) by the stomach. [gastro- + G. *rhoia,* a flow]

gas•tros•chi•sis (gas-tros′ki-sis). A defect in the abdominal wall resulting from rupture of the amniotic membrane during physiological gut-loop herniation or, later, owing to delayed umbilical ring closure; usually accompanied by protrusion of viscera. [gastro- + G. *schisis,* a fissure]

gas•tro•scope (gas′trō-skōp). An endoscope for inspecting the inner surface of the stomach. [gastro- + G. *skopeō,* to examine]

gas•tro•scop•ic (gas-trō-skop′ik). Relating to gastroscopy.

gas•tros•co•py (gas-tros′kŏ-pē). Inspection of the inner surface of the stomach through an endoscope.

gas•tro•spasm (gas′trō-spazm). Spasmodic contraction of the walls of the stomach.

gas•tro•splen•ic (gas-trō-splen′ik). Relating to the stomach and the spleen. SYN gastrolienal.

gas•tro•stax•is (gas′trō-stak′sis). Oozing of blood from the mucous membrane of the stomach. [gastro- + G. *staxis,* trickling]

gas•tro•ste•no•sis (gas-trō-ste-nō′sis). Diminution in size of the cavity of the stomach. [gastro- + G. *stenōsis,* narrowing]

gas•tros•to•la•vage (gas-tros′tō-lă-vahzh′). Lavage of the stomach through a gastric fistula.

gas•tros•to•my (gas-tros′tō-mē). Establishment of a new opening into the stomach. [gastro- + G. *stoma,* mouth]

gas•trot•o•my (gas-trot′ō-mē). Incision into the stomach. [gastro- + G. *tomē,* incision]

gas•tro•to•nom•e•try (gas′trō-tō-nom′ĕ-trē). The measurement of intragastric pressure. [gastro- + G. *tonos,* tension, + *metron,* measure]

gas•tro•tro•pic (gas-trō-trop′ik). Affecting the stomach. [gastro- + G. *tropikos,* turning]

gas•tru•la (gas′trū-lă). The embryo in the stage of development following the blastula; in the human embryo, the absence of yolk allows for a rapid, direct "putting in place" of the germ layers (ectoderm and endoderm), which are derived from the pluripotential embryonic disc. [Mod. L. dim. of G. *gastēr,* belly]

gas•tru•la•tion (gas-trū-lā′shŭn). Transformation of the blastula into the gastrula; the development and invagination of the embryonic germ layers.

gate•keep•er (gāt′kēp-er). A health professional, typically a physician or nurse, who has the first encounter with a patient and who thus controls the patient's entry into the health care system.

gat•ing (gāt′ing). 1. In a biological membrane, the opening and closing of a channel, believed to be associated with changes in integral membrane proteins. 2. A process in which electrical signals are selected by a gate, which passes such signals only when the gate pulse is present to act as a control signal, or passes only the signals that have certain characteristics.

cardiac gating, using an electronic signal from the cardiac cycle to trigger an event, such as in imaging separate phases of cardiac contraction.

gauge (gāj). A measuring device.

Bourdon g., a type of flow-regulating device used in the delivery of medical gas.

Gauss, Johann K.F., German physicist, 1777–1855. SEE gauss.

gauss (G) (gows). A unit of magnetic field intensity, equal to 10^{-4} tesla. [J.K.F. *Gauss*]

gaus·si·an (gows'ē-ăn). Relating to or described by Johann K.F. Gauss.

gauze (gawz). A bleached cotton cloth of plain weave, used for dressings, bandages, and absorbent sponges; petrolatum g. is saturated with petrolatum. [Fr. *gaze*, fr. Ar. *gazz*, raw silk]

ga·vage (gă-vahzh'). **1.** Forced feeding by stomach tube. SYN gastrogavage. **2.** Therapeutic use of a high-potency diet administered by stomach tube. [Fr. *gaver*, to gorge fowls]

gay (gā). **1.** A homosexual, especially male. **2.** Denoting a homosexual individual or the male homosexual lifestyle. SEE ALSO lesbian.

gaze (gāz). The act of looking steadily at an object.

G-CSF granulocyte colony-stimulating *factor*.

Gd Symbol for gadolinium.

Ge Symbol for germanium.

gel (jel). **1.** A jelly, or the solid or semisolid phase of a colloidal solution. **2.** To form a g. or jelly; to convert a sol into a g. [Mod. L. *gelatum*]

   colloidal g., a colloid that has developed resistance to flow because of chemical or thermal change.

   pharmacopeial g., a suspension, in a water medium, of an insoluble drug in hydrated form wherein the particle size approaches or attains colloidal dimensions.

gel·a·tin (jel'ă-tin). A derived protein formed from the collagen of tissues by boiling in water; it swells up when put in cold water, but dissolves only in hot water; used as a hemostat, plasma substitute, and protein food adjunct in malnutrition. [L. *gelo*, pp. *gelatus*, to freeze, congeal]

ge·lat·i·nize (jĕ-lat'i-nīz). **1.** To convert into gelatin. **2.** To become gelatinous.

ge·lat·i·nous (jĕ-lat'i-nŭs). **1.** Pertaining to or characteristic of gelatin. **2.** Jellylike or resembling gelatin.

ge·la·tion (jĕ-lā'shŭn). COLLOIDAL CHEMISTRY The transformation of a sol into a gel.

gem·i·nate (jem'i-nāt). Occurring in pairs. [L. *gemino*, pp. *-atus*, to double, fr. *geminus*, twin]

gem·i·na·tion (jem-i-nā'shŭn). Embryologic partial division of a primordium. For example, g. of a single tooth germ results in two partially or completely separated crowns on a single root. [L. *geminatio*, a doubling]

gem·ma·tion (jem-ā'shŭn). A form of fission in which the parent cell does not divide, but puts out a small budlike process (daughter cell) with its proportionate amount of chromatin; the daughter cell then separates to begin independent existence. SYN budding. [L. *gemma*, a bud]

gem·mule (jem'yūl). **1.** A small bud that projects from the parent cell, and finally becomes detached, forming a cell of a new generation. **2.** SYN dendritic *spines*, under *spine*. [L. *gemmula*, dim. of *gemma*, bud]

gen-. Being born, producing, coming to be. [G. *genos*, birth]

-gen. Suffix denoting "precursor of." SEE ALSO pro- (2).

ge·na (jē'nă). SYN cheek. [L.]

ge·nal (jē'năl). Relating to the gena, or cheek.

gen·der (jen'der). Category to which an individual is assigned by self or others, on the basis of sex. Cf. sex, gender *role*.

gene (jēn). A functional unit of heredity which occupies a specific place (locus) on a chromosome, is capable of reproducing itself exactly at each cell division, and directs the formation of an enzyme or other protein. The g. as a functional unit consists of a discrete segment of a giant DNA molecule containing purine and pyrimidine bases in the correct sequence to code the sequence of amino acids of a specific peptide. Protein synthesis is mediated by molecules of messenger-RNA formed on the chromosome with the g. acting as template. G.'s normally occur in pairs in all cells except gametes. SYN factor (3). [G. *genos*, birth]

   allelic g., SEE allele, dominance of *traits*, under *trait*.

   autosomal g., a g. located on any chromosome other than the sex chromosomes (X or Y).

   BCR/ABL g., a fusion g. produced when a segment of the Abelson protooncogene, ABL, from chromosome 9, translocates to the major breakpoint cluster region (M-BCR) on chromosome 22. The fusion g. produces a specific protein, P210. This fusion g. is found in chronic myelocytic leukemia (CML).

   dominant g., SEE dominance of *traits*, under *trait*.

   holandric g., SYN Y-linked g.

   immune response g.'s, g.'s in the HLA-D region of the histocompatibility complex of human chromosome 6 which control the immune response to specific antigens.

   lethal g., a g. that produces a genotype that leads to death of the organism before reproduction is possible or that precludes reproduction; for a recessive g. the homozygous or hemizygous state is lethal.

   mutant g., a g. that has been changed from an ancestral type, not necessarily in the current generation. SEE ALSO mutant, mutation.

   operator g., a g. with the function of activating the production of messenger RNA by one or more adjacent structural loci; part of the feedback system for determining the rate of production of an enzyme.

   pleiotropic g., a g. that has multiple, apparently unrelated, phenotypic manifestations. SYN polyphenic g.

   polyphenic g., SYN pleiotropic g.

   regulator g., a g. that produces a repressor substance that inhibits an operator g. when combined with it. It thus prevents production of a specific enzyme. When the enzyme is again in demand, a specific regulatory metabolite inhibits the repressor substance.

   repressor g., a g. that prevents a nonallele from being transcribed.

   structural g., a g. that codes for a specific protein or peptide.

   tumor suppressor g., (1) a g. whose function is to suppress cellular proliferation. Also known as an antioncogene because it suppresses neoplastic transformation. Loss of a tumor suppressor g. through chromosomal aberration leads to height-

ge

ened susceptibility to neoplasia. **(2)** SYN antioncogene.

X-linked g., a g. located on an X chromosome.
Y-linked g., a g. located on a Y chromosome. SYN holandric g.

ge·ne·al·o·gy (jē-nē-awl′ō-jē). **1.** Heredity. **2.** The explicit assembly of the descent of a person or family; it may be of any length. [G. *genea,* descent, + *logos,* study]

gen·era (jen′er-ă). Plural of genus.

gen·er·al·ist (jen′er-ăl-ist). A general physician or family physician; a physician trained to take care of the majority of nonsurgical diseases, sometimes including obstetrics.

gen·er·al·ized (jen′er-ă-līzd). Involving the whole of an organ, as opposed to a focal or regional process.

gen·er·a·tion (jen-er-ā′shŭn). **1.** SYN reproduction (2). **2.** A discrete stage in succession of descent; *e.g.,* father, son, and grandson are three g.'s. It may not be a unique designation, *e.g.,* the offspring of an uncle-niece marriage is in the third generation in the paternal line but the fourth in the maternal line. [L. *generatio,* fr. *genero,* pp. *-atus,* to beget]

asexual g., reproduction by fission, gemmation, or in any other way without union of the male and female cell, or conjugation. SEE ALSO parthenogenesis. SYN heterogenesis (2), nonsexual g.

filial g. (F), the offspring of a genetically specified mating: first filial g. (symbol F_1), the offspring of parents of contrasting genotypes; second filial g. (F_2), the offspring of two F_1 individuals; third filial g. (F_3), fourth filial g. (F_4), etc., the offspring in succeeding g.'s of continued inbreeding of F_1 descendents.

nonsexual g., SYN asexual g.

parental g. (P_1), the parents of a mating, commonly experimental, involving contrasting genotypes; the original mating of a genetic experiment; parents of the F_1 g.

sexual g., reproduction by conjugation, or the union of male and female cells, as opposed to asexual g.

spontaneous g., the false concept according to which living matter can arise by the vitalization of nonliving matter. SEE ALSO biogenesis. SYN heterogenesis (3).

gen·er·a·tive (jen′er-ă-tiv). Pertaining to the process of generating.

gen·er·a·tor (jen′er-ā-ter). An apparatus for conversion of chemical, mechanical, atomic, or other forms of energy into electricity. [*generator,* a begetter, producer]

aerosol g., a device for producing airborne suspensions of small particles for inhalation therapy or experimental work.

pulse g., a device that produces an electrical discharge with a regular or rhythmic wave form in which the electromotive force varies in a specific pattern in relation to time; *e.g.,* in an electronic pacemaker, it produces an electric discharge at regular intervals, and these intervals may be modified by a sensory circuit which can reset the time-base for subsequent discharge on the basis of other electrical activity, such as that produced by spontaneous cardiac beating.

ge·ner·ic (jĕ-nār′ik). **1.** Relating to or denoting a genus. **2.** General. **3.** Characteristic or distinctive. [L. *genus (gener-),* birth]

ge·ner·ic name. **1.** CHEMISTRY A noun that indicates the class or type of a single compound; *e.g.,* salt, saccharide (sugar), hexose, alcohol, aldehyde, lactone, acid, amine, alkane, steroid, vitamin. "Class" is more appropriate and more often used than is "generic." **2.** In the pharmaceutical and commercial fields, a misnomer for nonproprietary name. **3.** In the biologic sciences, the first part of the scientific name (Latin binary combination or binomial) of an organism; written with an initial capital letter and in italics. In bacteriology, the species name consists of two parts (comprising one name): the g. n. and the specific epithet; in other biologic disciplines, the species name is regarded as being composed of two names: the g. n. and the specific name.

gen·e·sis (jen′ĕ-sis). An origin or beginning process; also used as combining form in suffix position. [G.]

gene splic·ing. SYN splicing (1).

ge·net·ic (jĕ-net′ik). Pertaining to genetics; genetical.

ge·net·i·cist (jĕ-net′i-sist). A specialist in genetics.

ge·net·ics (jĕ-net′iks). The branch of science concerned with the means and consequences of transmission and generation of the components of biological inheritance. [G. *genesis,* origin or production]

behavioral g., the study of heritable factors in behavioral patterns, as by pedigree analysis, biochemical abnormality, or karyotypic analysis.

clinical g., g. applied to the diagnosis, prognosis, management, and prevention of genetic diseases. Cf. medical g.

epidemiological g., the study of g. as a phenomenon of defined populations by the criteria, methods, and objectives of epidemiology rather than of population g.

human g., the study of the genetic aspects of humans as a species. Cf. medical g.

medical g., the study of the etiology, pathogenesis, and natural history of human diseases which are at least partially genetic in origin. Cf. clinical g., human g.

population g., the study of genetic influences on the components of cause and effect in the somatic characteristics of populations.

ge·net·o·tro·phic (jĕ-net-ō-trof′ik). Relating to inherited individual distinctions in nutritional requirements. [G. *genesis,* origin, + *trophē,* nourishment]

ge·ni·al, ge·ni·an (jĕ-nī′ăl, -nī′an). SYN mental (2). [G. *geneion,* chin]

△ **-genic.** Producing, forming; produced, formed by. [G. *genos,* birth]

ge·nic·u·la (je-nik′yū-lă). Plural of geniculum.

ge·nic·u·lar (je-nik′yū-lăr). Commonly used to mean genual.

ge·nic·u·late (je-nik′yū-lāt). **1.** Bent like a knee. **2.** Referring to the geniculum of the facial nerve, denoting the ganglion there present. **3.** Denoting the lateral or medial geniculate body. [L. *geniculo,* pp. *-atus,* to bend the knee, fr. *genu,* knee]

ge·nic·u·lum, pl. **ge·nic·u·la** (je-nik′yū-lŭm, -lă). **1** [NA]. A small genu or angular kneelike structure. **2.** A knotlike structure. [L. dim. of *genu*, knee]

ge·ni·on (jĕ-nī′on). The tip of the mental spine, a point in craniometry. [G. *geneion*, chin]

ge·ni·o·plas·ty (jĕ′nī-ō-plas-tē). SYN mentoplasty. [G. *geneion*, chin, cheek, + *plastos*, formed]

gen·i·tal (jen′i-tăl). **1.** Relating to reproduction or generation. **2.** Relating to the primary female or male sex organs or genitals. **3.** Relating to or characterized by genitality. [L. *genitalis*, pertaining to reproduction, fr. *gigno*, to bring forth]

gen·i·ta·lia (jen′i-tā′lē-ă). SYN genital *organs*, under *organ*. [L. neut. pl. of *genitalis*, genital]

  ambiguous external g., external g. not clearly of either sex; most commonly designates external g. that are incompletely masculinized.

  external g., the vulva in the female, and the penis and scrotum in the male.

gen·i·tal·i·ty (jen-i-tal′i-tē). PSYCHOANALYSIS A term referring to the genital components of sexuality (*i.e.*, the penis and vagina), as opposed, for example, to orality and anality.

gen·i·tals (jen′i-tălz). SYN genital *organs*, under *organ*. [see genitalia]

gen·i·to·fem·o·ral (jen′i-tō-fem′ŏ-răl). Relating to the genitalia and the thigh; denoting the g. nerve.

gen·i·to·u·ri·nary (GU) (jen′i-tō-yū′ri-nar-ē). Relating to the organs of reproduction and urination. SYN urogenital.

gen·o·copy (jen′ō-kop-e). A genotype at one locus that produces a phenotype which at some levels of resolution is indistinguishable from that produced by another genotype; *e.g.*, two types of elliptocytosis that are g.'s of each other, but are distinguished by the fact that one is linked to the Rh blood group locus and the other is not.

ge·no·der·ma·to·sis (jen′ō-der-mă-tō′sis). A skin condition of genetic origin.

ge·nome (je′nōm, -nom). **1.** A complete set of chromosomes derived from one parent, the haploid number of a gamete. **2.** The total gene complement of a set of chromosomes found in higher life forms (the haploid set in a eukaryotic cell), or the functionally similar but simpler linear arrangements found in bacteria and viruses. SEE ALSO Human Genome Project. [gene + chromosome]

ge·nom·ic (jĕ-nom′ik). Relating to a genome.

ge·no·spe·cies (jē′nō-spē-sēz, jen′). A group of organisms in which interbreeding is possible, as evidenced by genetic transfer and recombination.

ge·note (jē′nōt). MICROBIAL GENETICS An element of recombination in which one of the pair is not a complete chromosome; commonly used as a suffix (*e.g.*, endogenote, exogenote, F genote). [gene + G. *-ōtēs*, toponymic suffix]

ge·no·tox·ic (jē-nō-toks′ik). Denoting a substance that by damaging DNA may cause mutation or cancer. [gene + toxic]

gen·o·type (jen′ō-tīp). **1.** The genetic constitution of an individual. **2.** Gene combination at one specific locus or any specified combination of loci. For specific blood group genotypes, see Blood Groups appendix. [G. *genos*, birth, descent, + *typos*, type]

gen·o·typ·i·cal (jen-ō-tip′i-kăl). Relating to the genotype.

gen·tian·o·phil, gen·tian·o·phile (jen′shŭn-o-fil, -fīl). Staining readily with gentian violet. [gentian + G. *philos*, fond]

gen·tian·o·pho·bic (jen′shŭn-ō-fō′bik). Not taking a gentian violet stain, or taking it poorly. [gentian + G. *phobos*, fear]

gen·tian vi·o·let. An unstandardized dye mixture of violet rosanilins.

genu, gen. **ge·′nus**, pl. **gen·ua** (jē′nū, jē′nŭs, jen′ū-ă) [NA]. **1.** The place of articulation between the thigh and the leg. SYN knee (1). SEE ALSO knee *joint*, geniculum. **2.** Any structure of angular shape resembling a flexed knee. [L.]

  g. recurva′tum, hyperextension of the knee, the lower extremity having a forward curvature.

  g. val′gum, a deformity marked by lateral angulation of the leg in relation to the thigh. SYN knock-knee, tibia valga.

  g. va′rum, a deformity marked by medial angulation of the leg in relation to the thigh; an outward bowing of the legs. SYN bowleg, bow-leg, tibia vara.

gen·u·al (jen′yū-ăl). Relating to the knee. [L. *genu*, knee]

ge·nus, pl. **gen·era** (jē′nŭs, jen′er-ă). In natural history classification, the taxonomic level of division between the family, or tribe, and the species; a group of species alike in the broad features of their organization but different in detail, and incapable of fertile mating. [L. birth, descent]

△**geo-**. The earth, soil. [G. *gē*, earth]

ge·ode (jē′ōd). A cystlike space (or spaces) with or without an epithelial lining, observed radiologically in subarticular bone, usually in arthritic disorders. [Fr., fr. L. *geodes*, precious stone, fr. G. *gē*, earth, + *-ōdēs*, appearance]

geometric unsharpness. SYN penumbra.

ge·o·pha·gia, ge·oph·a·gism, ge·oph·a·gy (jē-ō-fā′jē-ă, jē-of′ă-jizm, -of′ă-jē). The practice of eating dirt or clay. SYN dirt-eating. [geo- + G. *phagō*, to eat]

ge·ot·ri·cho·sis (jē′ō-tri-kō′sis). An opportunistic systemic hyalohyphomycosis caused by *Geotrichum candidum;* ascribed symptoms are diverse and suggestive of secondary or mixed infections. [geo- + G. *thrix*, hair, + *-osis*, condition]

GERD gastroesophageal reflux *disease.*

ger·i·at·ric (jār-ē-at′rik). Relating to old age or to geriatrics.

ger·i·at·rics (jār-ē-at′riks). The branch of medicine concerned with the medical problems and care of the aged. [G. *gēras*, old age, + *iatrikos*, healing]

  dental g., treatment of dental problems peculiar to advanced age. SYN gerodontics, gerodontology.

germ (jerm). **1.** A microbe; a microorganism. **2.** A primordium; the earliest trace of a structure within an embryo. [L. *germen*, sprout, bud, germ]

  enamel g., the enamel organ of a developing tooth; one of a series of knoblike projections from the dental lamina, later becoming bell-shaped and receiving in its hollow the dental papilla.

ge

tooth g., the enamel organ and dentin papilla, constituting the developing tooth.

ger·ma·ni·um (Ge) (jer-mān'ē-ŭm). A metallic element, atomic no. 32, atomic wt. 72.61. [L. *Germania,* Germany]

ger·mi·ci·dal (jer-mi-sī'dăl). SYN germicide (1).

ger·mi·cide (jer'mi-sīd). **1.** Destructive to germs or microbes. SYN germicidal. **2.** An agent with this action. [germ + L. *caedo,* to kill]

ger·mi·nal (jer'mi-năl). Relating to a germ or, in botany, to germination.

ger·mi·no·ma (jer-mi-nō'mă). A neoplasm of the germinal tissue of gonads, mediastinum, or pineal region such as seminoma. [L. *germen,* bud, + *-oma,* tumor]

△**gero-, geront-, geronto-.** Old age. SEE ALSO presby-. [G. *gerōn,* old man]

ger·o·der·ma (jār-ō-der'mă). **1.** The atrophic skin of the aged. **2.** Any condition in which the skin is thinned and wrinkled, resembling the integument of old age. [gero- + G. *derma,* skin]

ger·o·don·tics, ger·o·don·tol·o·gy (jār-ō-don'tiks, -don-tol'ō-jē). SYN dental *geriatrics.* [gero- + G. *odous,* tooth]

ge·ron·tal (jār-on'tăl). Relating to old age.

△**geronto-.** SEE gero-.

ger·on·tol·o·gist (jār-on-tol'ō-jist). One who specializes in gerontology.

ger·on·tol·o·gy (jār-on-tol'ō-jē). The scientific study of the process and problems of aging. [geronto- + G. *logos,* study]

ger·on·tox·on (jār'on-tok'son). SYN *arcus* cornealis. [geronto- + G. *toxon,* bow]

ges·ta·gen (jes'tă-jen). Any of several gestagenic substances, which are usually steroid hormones.

ge·stalt (ge-stahlt). A perceived entity so integrated as to constitute a functional unit with properties not derivable from its parts. SEE ALSO gestaltism. [Ger. shape]

ge·stalt·ism (ge-stahlt'izm). The theory in psychology that the objects of mind come as complete forms or configurations which cannot be split into parts; *e.g.,* a square is perceived as such rather than as four discrete lines. [see gestalt]

ges·ta·tion (jes-tā'shŭn). SYN pregnancy. [L. *gestatio,* from *gesto,* pp. *gestatus,* to bear]

ges·to·sis, pl. **ges·to·ses** (jes-tō'sis, -sēz). Any disorder of pregnancy. [L. *gesto,* to carry, to bear, + G. *-osis,* condition]

GFR glomerular filtration *rate.*

GH growth *hormone.*

GHRF, GH-RF growth hormone-releasing *factor.*

GHRH, GH-RH Abbreviation for growth *hormone*-releasing *hormone.*

GHz gigahertz, equal to one billion (10^9) hertz; used in ultrasound.

GI gastrointestinal; Gingival Index.

gi·ant·ism (jī'an-tizm). SYN gigantism.

Gi·ar·dia (jē-ar'dē-ă). A genus of parasitic flagellates that parasitize the small intestine of many mammals, including most domestic animals and humans. [Alfred *Giard,* Fr. biologist, 1846–1908]

gi·ar·di·a·sis (jē-ar-dī'ă-sis). Infection with the protozoan parasite *Giardia; Giardia lamblia* may cause diarrhea, dyspepsia, and occasionally malabsorption in humans.

gib·bous (gib'ŭs). Humped; humpbacked; denoting a sharp angle in the flexion of the spine. [L. *gibbosus*]

gib·bus (gib'ŭs). Extreme kyphosis, hump, or hunch; a deformity of spine in which there is a sharply angulated segment, the apex of the angle being posterior. [L. a hump]

△**giga- (G).** Prefix used in the SI and metric systems to signify one billion (10^9). [G. *gigas,* giant]

gi·gan·tism (jī'gan-tizm). A condition of abnormal size or overgrowth of the entire body or of any of its parts. SYN giantism. [G. *gigas,* giant]

cerebral g., a syndrome characterized by increased birth weight and length (above 90th percentile), accelerated growth rate for the first 4 or 5 years without elevation of serum growth hormone levels, and then reversion to normal growth rate; characteristic facies include prognathism, hypertelorism, antimongoloid slant, and dolichocephalic skull; moderate mental retardation and impaired coordination are also associated.

eunuchoid g., g. with deficient development of sexual organs; may be of pituitary or gonadal origin; g. accompanied by body proportions typical of hypogonadism during adolescence.

pituitary g., a form of g. caused by hypersecretion of pituitary growth hormone; a rare disorder commonly the result of a pituitary adenoma.

△**giganto-.** Huge, gigantic. [G. *gigas,* one of the race of giants]

gi·gan·to·mas·tia (jī-gan'tō-mas'tē-ă). Massive hypertrophy of the breast. [giganto- + G. *mastos,* breast]

GIH growth *hormone*-inhibiting *hormone.*

gin·gi·va, gen. and pl. **gin·gi·vae** (jin'ji-vă, -vē) [NA]. The dense fibrous tissue, covered by mucous membrane, that envelops the alveolar processes of the upper and lower jaws and surrounds the necks of the teeth. SYN gum (2). [L.]

alveolar g., gingival tissue applied to the alveolar bone.

attached g., that part of the oral mucosa which is firmly bound to the tooth and alveolar process.

free g., that portion of the g. that surrounds the tooth and is not directly attached to the tooth surface; the outer wall of the gingival sulcus.

gin·gi·val (jin'ji-văl). Relating to the gums.

Gin·gi·val In·dex (GI). An index of periodontal disease based upon the severity and location of the lesion.

Gin·gi·val-Per·i·o·don·tal In·dex (GPI). An index of gingivitis, gingival irritation, and advanced periodontal disease.

gin·gi·vec·to·my (jin-ji-vek'tō-mē). Surgical resection of unsupported gingival tissue. SYN gum resection. [gingiva + G. *ektomē,* excision]

gin·gi·vi·tis (jin-ji-vī'tis). Inflammation of the gingiva as a response to bacterial plaque on adjacent teeth; characterized by erythema, edema, and fibrous enlargement of the gingiva without resorption of the underlying alveolar bone. [gingiva + G. *-itis,* inflammation]

acute necrotizing ulcerative g. (ANUG), SEE necrotizing ulcerative g.

chronic desquamative g., a gingival condition of unknown etiology in middle-aged and older women, characterized by erythema, mucosal atrophy, and desquamation, and usually accompanied by a burning sensation and pain; diagnosis is usually made by biopsy and direct immunofluorescence. SYN gingivosis.

fusospirochetal g., SYN necrotizing ulcerative g.

hyperplastic g., g. of long-standing duration in which the gingiva becomes enlarged and firm due to proliferation of fibrous connective tissue.

necrotizing ulcerative g. (NUG), an acute or recurrent g. of young and middle-aged adults characterized clinically by gingival erythema and pain, fetid odor, and necrosis and sloughing of interdental papillae and marginal gingiva which gives rise to a gray pseudomembrane; fever, regional lymphadenopathy, and other systemic manifestations also may be present. A fusiform bacillus and *Treponema vincentii* can be isolated from the gingival tissues in large numbers and are felt to play a significant but poorly defined role in the pathogenesis. SYN fusospirochetal g., trench mouth, ulceromembranous g., Vincent's disease.

suppurative g., g. in which a purulent exudate can be expressed from the gingival surface.

ulceromembranous g., SYN necrotizing ulcerative g.

gingivo-. The gingivae, the gums of the mouth. [L. *gingiva*]

gin·gi·vo·glos·si·tis (jin′ji-vō-glos-sī′tis). Inflammation of both the tongue and gingival tissues. SEE ALSO stomatitis.

gin·gi·vo·lin·guo·ax·i·al (jin′ji-vō-ling′gwō-ak′sē-ăl). Referring to the point angle formed by the gingival, lingual, and axial walls of a cavity.

gin·gi·vo·os·se·ous (jin′ji-vō-os′ē-ŭs). Referring to the gingiva and its underlying bone.

gin·gi·vo·plas·ty (jin′ji-vō-plas-tē). A surgical procedure that reshapes and recontours the gingival tissue in order to attain esthetic, physiologic, and functional form.

gin·gi·vo·sis (jin-ji-vō′sis). SYN chronic desquamative *gingivitis.*

gin·gi·vo·sto·ma·ti·tis (jin′ji-vō-stō′mă-tī′tis). Inflammation of the gingiva and other oral mucous membranes. [gingivo- + G. *stoma,* mouth, + -*itis,* inflammation]

gin·gly·form (jing′gli-fōrm, ging-). SYN ginglymoid. [G. *ginglymos,* a hinge joint, + L. *forma,* form]

gin·glym·o·ar·thro·di·al (jing′gli-mō-ar-thrō′dē-ăl, ging-). Denoting a joint having the form of both ginglymus and arthrodia, or hinge joint and sliding joint.

gin·gly·moid (jing′gli-moyd, ging-). Relating to or resembling a hinge joint. SYN ginglyform. [G. *ginglymos,* a hinge joint, + *eidos,* resembling]

gin·gly·mus (jing′gli-mŭs, ging-) [NA]. SYN hinge joint. [G. *ginglymos*]

GIP gastric inhibitory *polypeptide;* gastric inhibitory *peptide.*

gir·dle (ger′dl). A belt; a zone. A structure that has the form of a belt or girdle. SYN cingulum (1) [NA]. [A.S. *gyrdel*]

pectoral g., SYN shoulder g.

pelvic g., the bony ring formed by the hip bones and the sacrum, to which the lower limbs are attached.

shoulder g., the bony ring, incomplete behind, that serves for the attachment and support of the upper limbs. It is formed by the manubrium sterni, the clavicles, and the scapulae. SYN pectoral g., shoulder complex (3).

gla·bel·la (glă-bel′ă). **1** [NA]. A smooth prominence, most marked in the male, on the frontal bone above the root of the nose. **2.** The most forward projecting point of the forehead in the midline at the level of the supraorbital ridges. SYN mesophryon. SEE ALSO antinion. SYN intercilium. [L. *glabellus,* hairless, smooth, dim. of *glaber*]

gla·brous, gla·brate (glā′brŭs, glā′brāt). Smooth or hairless; denoting areas of the body where hair does not normally grow, *i.e.,* palms or soles. [L. *glaber,* smooth]

gland. An organized aggregation of cells functioning as a secretory or excretory organ. SYN glandula (1). [L. *glans,* acorn]

accessory g., a small mass of glandular structure, detached from but lying near another and larger g., to which it is similar in structure and probably in function.

acinotubular g., SYN tubuloacinar g.

acinous g., a g. in which the secretory unit(s) has a grapelike shape and a very small lumen; *e.g.,* the exocrine part of the pancreas.

adrenal g., SYN suprarenal g.

alveolar g., a g. in which the secretory unit(s) has a saclike form and an obvious lumen; *e.g.,* the active mammary gland.

anterior lingual g., one of the small mixed glands deeply placed near the apex of the tongue on each side of the frenulum. SYN apical g.

apical g., SYN anterior lingual g.

apocrine g., a g. whose secretory product includes an apical portion of the secretory cell such as the secretion of lipid droplets in lactation.

areolar g.'s, a number of small mammary glands forming small rounded projections from the surface of the areola of the breast; they enlarge with pregnancy and during lactation secrete a substance presumed to resist chapping.

Bartholin's g., SYN greater vestibular g.

bronchial g.'s, (1) SYN bronchopulmonary *lymph nodes,* under *lymph node.* **(2)** mucous and seromucous glands whose secretory units lie outside the muscle of the bronchi.

buccal g.'s, numerous racemose, mucous, or serous glands in the submucous tissue of the cheeks. SYN genal g.'s.

bulbourethral g., one of two small compound racemose glands, that produce a mucoid secretion, lying side by side along the membranous urethra just above the bulb of the corpus spongiosum; they discharge through a small duct into the spongy portion of the urethra. SYN Cowper's g.

cardiac g., a coiled tubular g. located in the cardiac region of the stomach; secretes primarily mucus.

ceruminous g.'s, apocrine sudoriferous glands in the external acoustic meatus. SYN glandulae ceruminosae (1) [NA].

cervical g.'s, branched mucus-secreting glands in the mucosa of the cervix.

ciliary g.'s, a number of modified apocrine su-

gl

doriferous glands in the eyelids, with ducts that usually open into the follicles of the eyelashes.

circumanal g.'s, large apocrine sweat glands surrounding the anus.

compound g., a g. whose larger excretory ducts branch repeatedly into smaller ducts, which ultimately drain secretory units.

Cowper's g., SYN bulbourethral g.

ductless g.'s, SYN endocrine g.'s.

duodenal g.'s, small, branched, coiled tubular glands that occur mostly in the submucosa of the first third of the duodenum; they secrete an alkaline mucoid substance that serves to neutralize gastric juice.

eccrine g., a coiled tubular sweat g. (other than apocrine g.'s) that occurs in the skin on almost all parts of the body.

endocrine g.'s, glands that have no ducts, their secretions being absorbed directly into the blood. SYN ductless g.'s.

excretory g., a g. separating excrementitious or waste material from the blood.

exocrine g., a g. from which secretions reach a free surface of the body by ducts.

g.'s of the female urethra, numerous mucous g.'s in the wall of the female urethra.

gastric g.'s, branched tubular glands lying in the mucosa of the fundus and body of the stomach; such glands contain parietal cells that secrete hydrochloric acid, zymogen cells that produce pepsin, and mucous cells.

genal g.'s, SYN buccal g.'s.

greater vestibular g., one of two mucoid-secreting tubuloalveolar glands on either side of the lower part of the vagina, the equivalent of the bulbourethral glands in the male; ensheathed with vestibular bulbs by ischiocavernosus muscles. Thus erection and muscle contraction cause secretion into vestibule of vagina. SYN Bartholin's g.

hematopoietic g., a blood-forming organ, such as the spleen.

holocrine g., a g. whose secretion consists of disintegrated cells of the g. itself, *e.g.,* a sebaceous g., in contrast to a merocrine g.

intestinal g.'s, the tubular glands in the mucous membrane of the small and large intestines. SYN intestinal follicles.

jugular g., SYN signal *node.*

lacrimal g., the gland that secretes tears; it consists of 6 to 12 separate compound tubuloalveolar serous glands, located in the upper lateral part of the orbit, and is partially divided into a smaller palpebral part and a larger orbital part by the aponeurosis of the levator palpebrae muscle.

lesser vestibular g.'s, a number of minute mucous glands opening on the surface of the vestibule between the orifices of the vagina and urethra.

lymph g., SYN lymph node.

major salivary g.'s, a category of salivary g.'s that includes the three largest g.'s of the oral cavity that also secrete most of the saliva: the parotid, submandibular, and sublingual g.'s.

g.'s of the male urethra, numerous mucous glands in the wall of the penile urethra.

mammary g., the compound alveolar apocrine secretory gland that forms the breast. It consists of 15 to 24 lobes, each consisting of many lobules, separated by adipose tissue and fibrous septa; the parenchyma of the resting gland consists of ducts; the alveoli develop only during pregnancy.

master g., SYN hypophysis.

maxillary g., SYN submandibular g.

meibomian g.'s, SYN tarsal g.'s.

merocrine g., a g. that releases only an acellular secretory product, in contrast to a holocrine g.

minor salivary g.'s, the smaller, largely mucous-secreting, exocrine g.'s of the oral cavity, consisting of the labial, buccal, molar, lingual, and palatine g.'s.

mixed g., (1) a g. that contains both serous and mucous secretory units; **(2)** a g. that is both exocrine and endocrine, *e.g.,* the pancreas.

mucous g., a gland that secretes mucus.

mucous g.'s of auditory tube, glands located principally near the pharyngeal end of the auditory tube.

olfactory g.'s, branched tubuloalveolar serous secreting glands (of Bowman) in the mucous membrane of the olfactory region of the nasal cavity.

parathyroid g., one of Gley's glands or Sandström's bodies; one of two small paired endocrine glands, superior and inferior, usually found embedded in the connective tissue capsule on the posterior surface of the thyroid gland; they secrete parathyroid hormone that regulates the metabolism of calcium and phosphorus. The parenchyma is composed of chief and oxyphilic cells arranged in anastomosing cords. Inadvertent removal of all parathyroid g.'s, as during thyroidectomy, produces tetany and death. SYN parathyroid (2).

parotid g., the largest of the salivary glands, one of two compound acinous glands situated inferior and anterior to the ear, on either side, extending from the angle of the jaw to the zygomatic arch and posteriorly to the sternocleidomastoid muscle; it is subdivided into a superficial part and a deep part by emerging branches of the facial nerve, and discharges through the parotid duct.

pileous g., a sebaceous g. emptying into the hair follicle.

pineal g., SYN pineal *body.*

pituitary g., SYN hypophysis.

preputial g.'s, sebaceous glands of the corona glandis and inner surface of the prepuce, which produce an odoriferous substance called smegma.

prostate g., SYN prostate.

pyloric g.'s, the coiled, tubular glands of the pylorus whose cells secrete mucus.

racemose g., a g. that has the appearance of a bunch of grapes if viewed as a three-dimensional reconstruction; *e.g.,* a compound acinous or alveolar g.

saccular g., a single alveolar g.

sebaceous g.'s, numerous holocrine glands in the dermis that usually open into the hair follicles and secrete an oily semifluid sebum. SYN sebaceous follicles.

seminal g., SYN seminal *vesicle.*

HUMAN ANATOMY

CONTENTS

INDEX

A

Anatomical images provided by:

A.D.A.M.
Software, Inc.
1600 RiverEdge Parkway
Suite 800
Atlanta, GA 30328
(770) 980-0888
www.adam.com

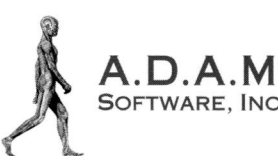

A.D.A.M.
SOFTWARE, INC.

Bringing Multimedia To Life

ANATOMY

medial, A19, A20
mediate, A20

D

Diaphragm, A23, A24
urogenital, A26
Duct
ejaculatory, A26
parotid, A5
Ductus deferens, A26
Duodenum, A24
Dura mater, A6

E

Edge, falciform, of saphenoid hiatus, A12
Epicondyle
lateral, A15
lateral, of humerus, A18
medial, A15
Epididymis, A26
Epiglottis, A6
Esophagus, A24

F

Fascia
deep, A12
deep, of penis, A12
external spermatic, A12
thoracolumbar, A14
Femur, A13, A19, A20
Fibers, intercrural, of external abdominal oblique muscle
aponeurosis, A12
Fibula, A13, A19, A20
Fissure
horizontal, of right lung, A23
oblique, of left lung, A23
oblique, of right lung, A23
Fold
salpingopalatine, A6
salpingopharyngeal, A6
vestibular, A6
vocal, A6, A23
Foramen
infraorbital, A1
mental, A1
posterior sacral, A8
supraorbital, A1
Fornix, A6
anterior, of vagina, A26
posterior, of vagina, A26
Fossa
coronoid, A15
iliac, A19, A20
incisive, A6
navicular, A26
Fundus, A26

G

Gallbladder, A24
Glabella, A1, A2
Gland
parotid, A5
pituitary, A6
prostate, A26
submandibular, A5
Glans penis, A26
Groove, intertubercular, A15
Gyrus
angular, A7
inferior frontal, A7
middle frontal, A7
middle temporal, A7

postcentral, A7
precentral, A7
superior frontal, A7
superior temporal, A7
supramarginal, A7

H

Head
lateral, of triceps brachii muscle, A18
long, of biceps brachii muscle, A18
long, of biceps femoris muscle, A22
medial, of gastrocnemius muscle, A22
short, of biceps femoris muscle, A22
Head of femur, A19, A20
Head of fibula, A19
Hiatus of deltopectoral triangle, A12
Humerus, A13, A15, A17
Hypophysis, A6

I

Ileum, A24
Ilium, A13
Intestine
large, A24
small, A24
Ischium, A13, A19, A20

J

Jejunum, A24
Joint(s)
acromioclavicular, A15
ankle, A19, A20
calcaneocuboid, A19, A20
carpometacarpal, A15
carpometacarpal, of thumb, A15
distal radioulnar, A15
distal tibiofibular, A19, A20
elbow, A15
hip, A19, A20
humeroradial, A15
humeroulnar, A15
interphalangeal, A19, A20
knee, A19, A20
metacarpophalangeal, A15
proximal interphalangeal, A15
proximal radioulnar, A15
proximal tibiofibular, A19, A20
radiocarpal, A15
sacroiliac, A19, A20
shoulder, A15
sternoclavicular, A15
tarsometatarsal, A19, A20
temporomandibular, A2

L

Labium majus, A26
Labium minus, A26
Lamina, quadrigeminal, A6
Lamina terminalis, A6
Laryngopharynx, A23, A24
Larynx, A6, A23, A24
Ligament
falciform, of liver, A24
inguinal, A9, A12
median umbilical, A26
patellar, A22
posterior longitudinal, A6
sacrospinous, A22
suspensory, of penis, A12, A26
Ligaments, suspensory, A12
Ligamentum, nuchae, A6
Linea alba, A12

ANATOMY

M

N

ANATOMY

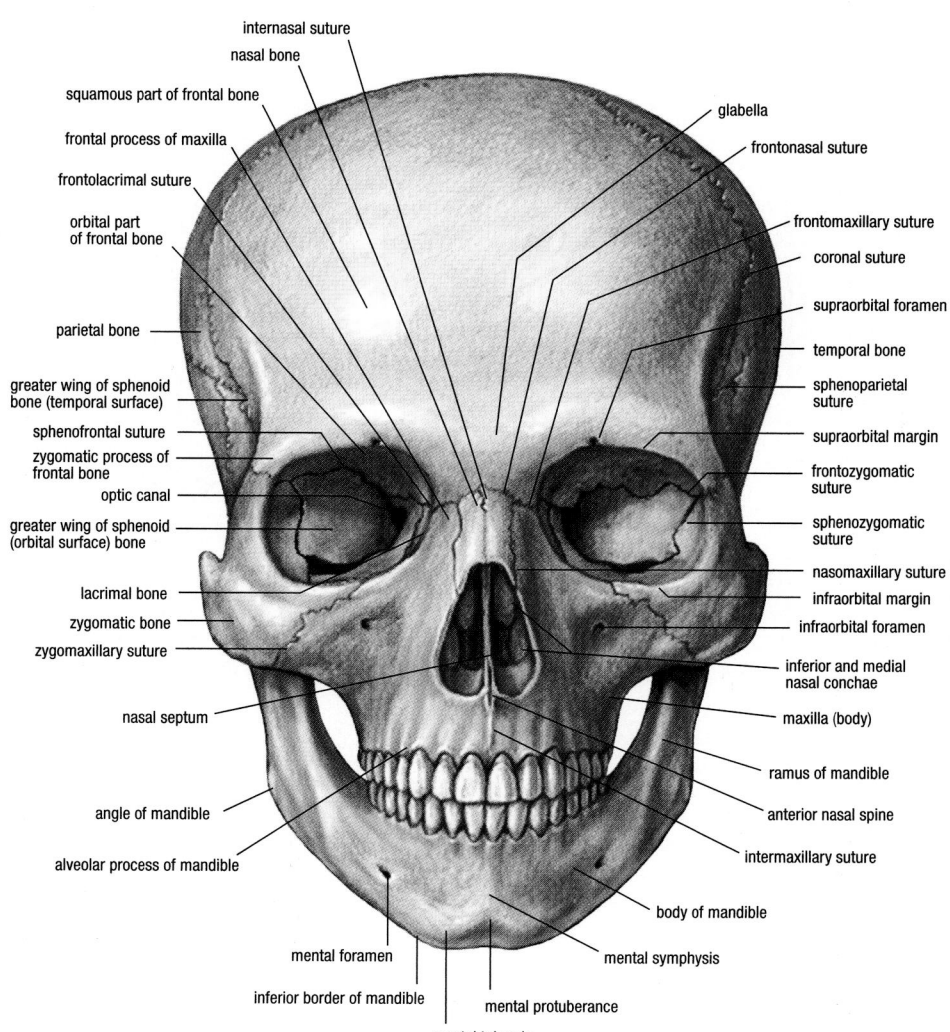

internasal suture

nasal bone

squamous part of frontal bone

frontal process of maxilla

frontolacrimal suture

orbital part
of frontal bone

parietal bone

greater wing of sphenoid
bone (temporal surface)

sphenofrontal suture

zygomatic process of
frontal bone

optic canal

greater wing of sphenoid
(orbital surface) bone

lacrimal bone

zygomatic bone

zygomaxillary suture

nasal septum

angle of mandible

alveolar process of mandible

mental foramen

inferior border of mandible

mental tubercle

mental protuberance

mental symphysis

body of mandible

intermaxillary suture

anterior nasal spine

ramus of mandible

maxilla (body)

inferior and medial
nasal conchae

infraorbital foramen

infraorbital margin

nasomaxillary suture

sphenozygomatic
suture

frontozygomatic
suture

supraorbital margin

sphenoparietal
suture

temporal bone

supraorbital foramen

coronal suture

frontomaxillary suture

frontonasal suture

glabella

ANATOMY

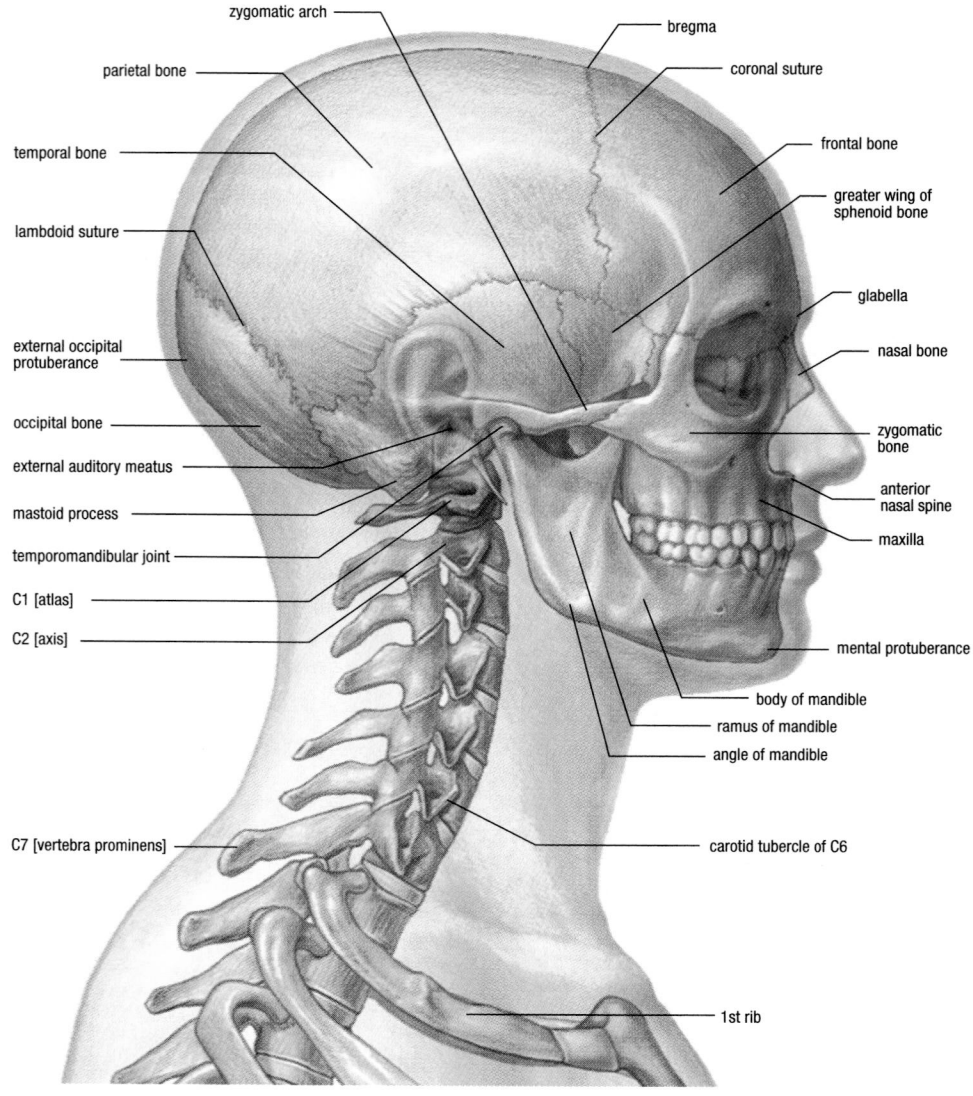

zygomatic arch

bregma

parietal bone

coronal suture

temporal bone

frontal bone

greater wing of
sphenoid bone

lambdoid suture

glabella

external occipital
protuberance

nasal bone

occipital bone

zygomatic
bone

external auditory meatus

anterior
nasal spine

mastoid process

maxilla

temporomandibular joint

C1 [atlas]

C2 [axis]

mental protuberance

body of mandible

ramus of mandible

angle of mandible

C7 [vertebra prominens]

carotid tubercle of C6

1st rib

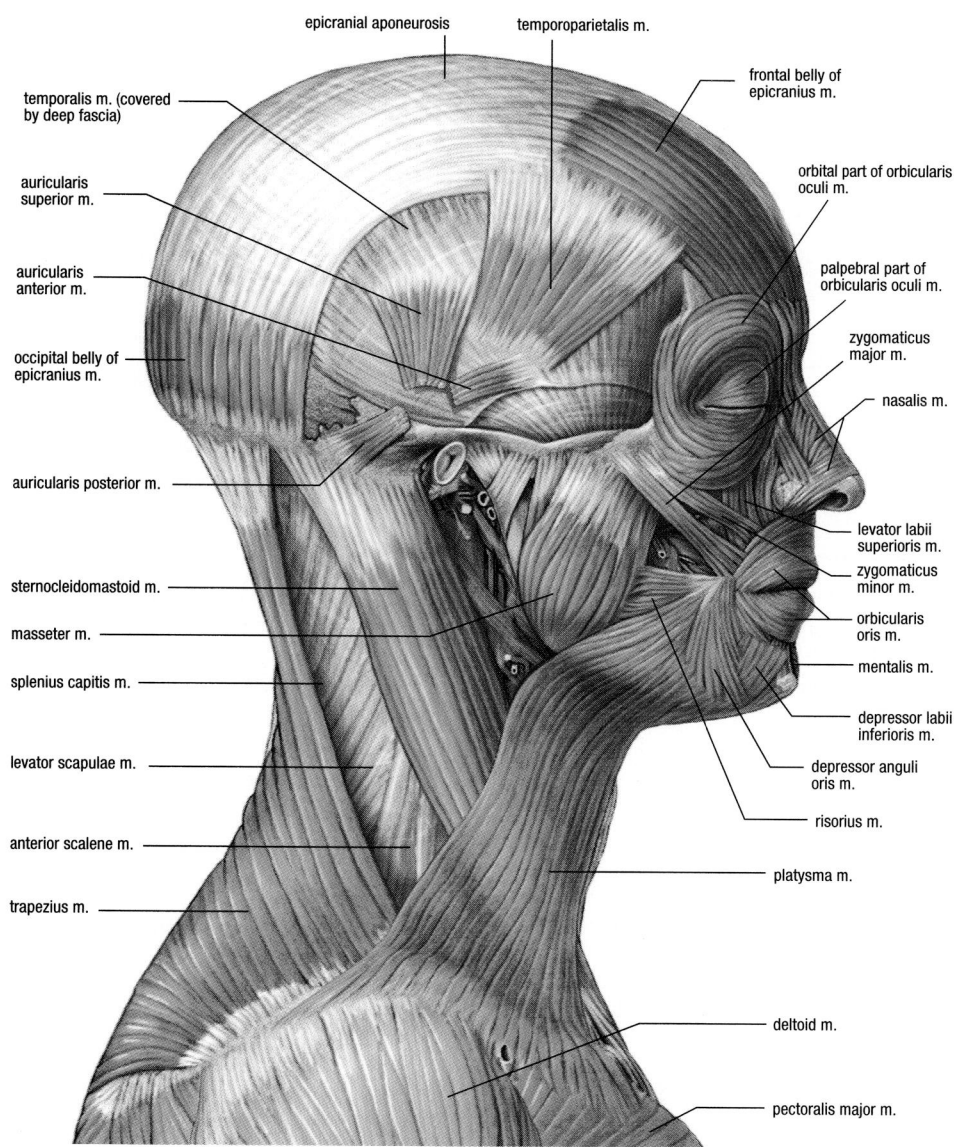

epicranial aponeurosis

temporoparietalis m.

frontal belly of
epicranius m.

temporalis m. (covered
by deep fascia)

orbital part of orbicularis
oculi m.

auricularis
superior m.

palpebral part of
orbicularis oculi m.

auricularis
anterior m.

zygomaticus
major m.

occipital belly of
epicranius m.

nasalis m.

auricularis posterior m.

levator labii
superioris m.

zygomaticus
minor m.

sternocleidomastoid m.

orbicularis
oris m.

masseter m.

mentalis m.

splenius capitis m.

depressor labii
inferioris m.

levator scapulae m.

depressor anguli
oris m.

anterior scalene m.

risorius m.

trapezius m.

platysma m.

deltoid m.

pectoralis major m.

ANATOMY

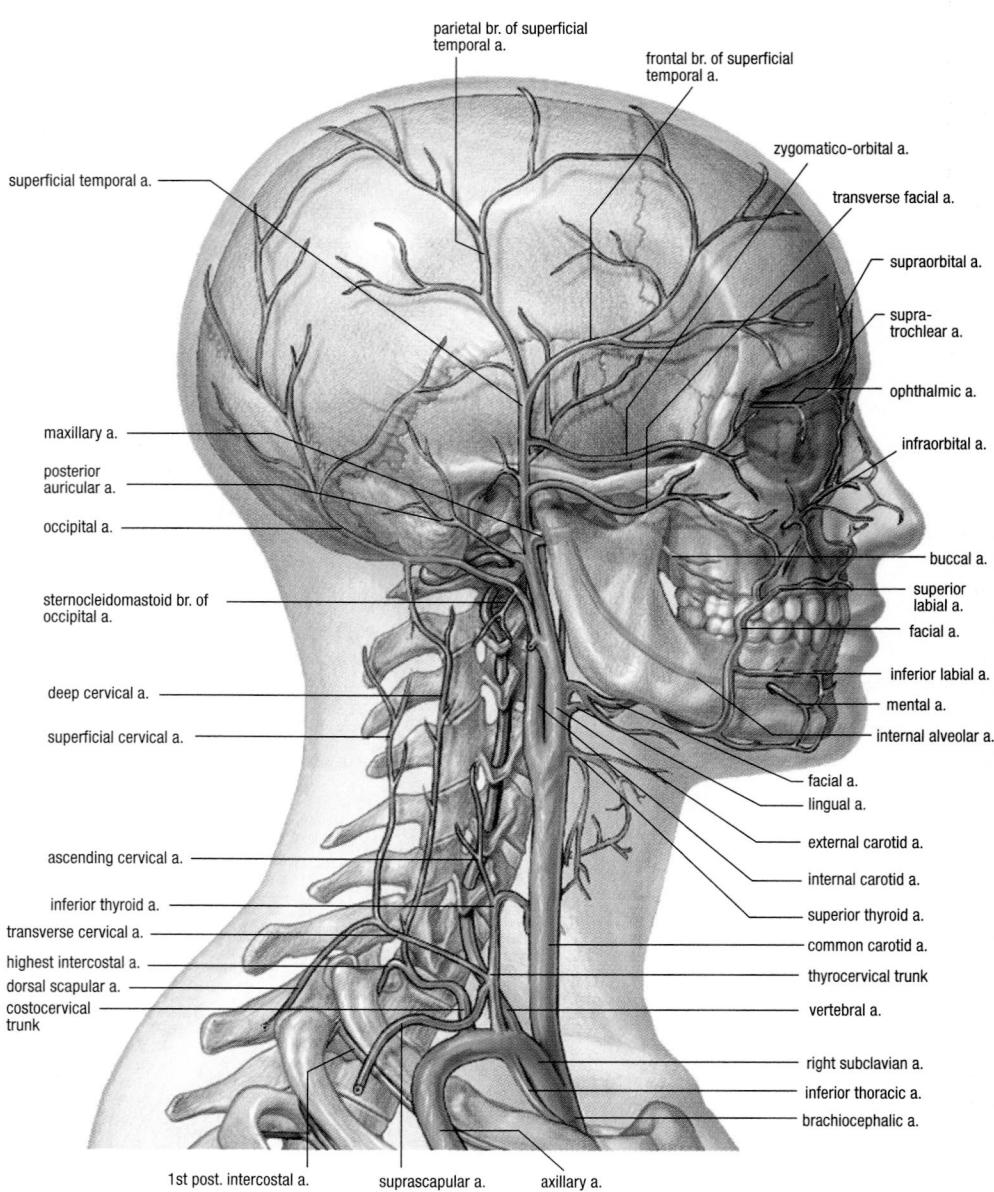

parietal br. of superficial temporal a.

frontal br. of superficial temporal a.

zygomatico-orbital a.

transverse facial a.

superficial temporal a.

supraorbital a.

supra-trochlear a.

ophthalmic a.

maxillary a.

infraorbital a.

posterior auricular a.

occipital a.

buccal a.

superior labial a.

facial a.

sternocleidomastoid br. of occipital a.

inferior labial a.

mental a.

deep cervical a.

internal alveolar a.

superficial cervical a.

facial a.

lingual a.

external carotid a.

internal carotid a.

ascending cervical a.

superior thyroid a.

inferior thyroid a.

common carotid a.

transverse cervical a.

thyrocervical trunk

highest intercostal a.

vertebral a.

dorsal scapular a.

costocervical trunk

right subclavian a.

inferior thoracic a.

brachiocephalic a.

1st post. intercostal a.

suprascapular a.

axillary a.

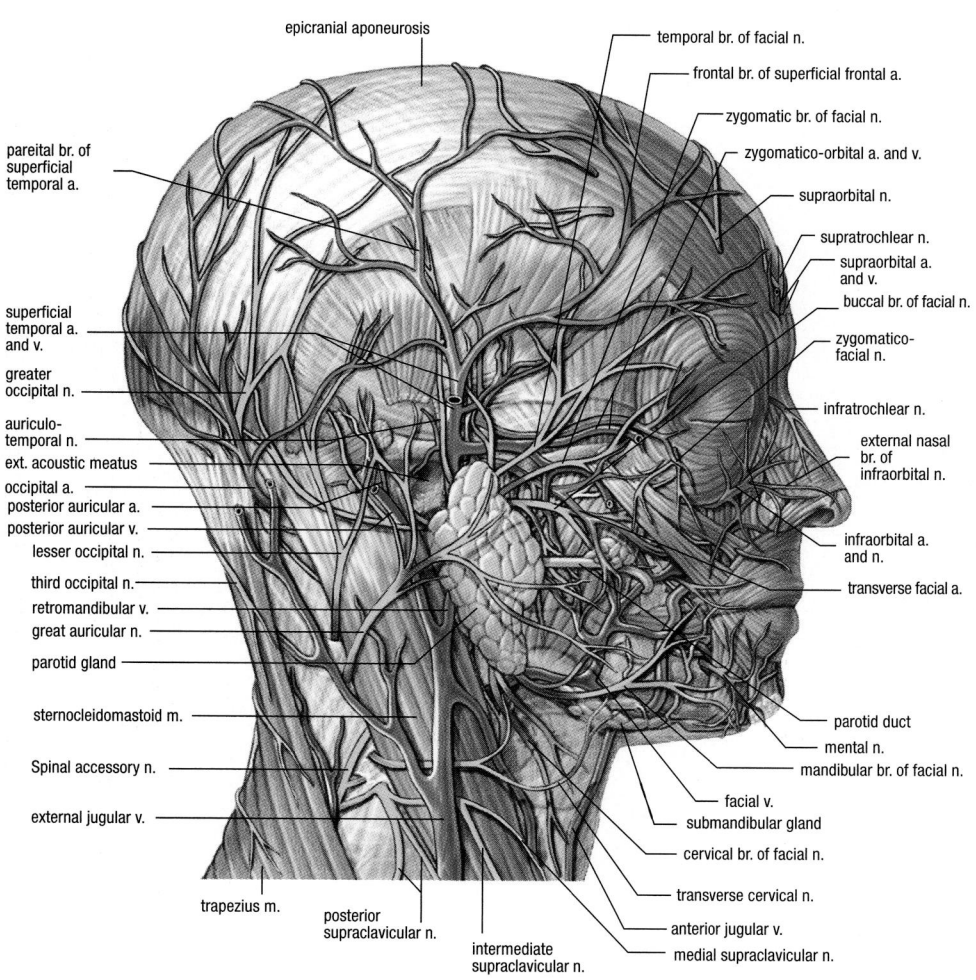

epicranial aponeurosis

temporal br. of facial n.

frontal br. of superficial frontal a.

zygomatic br. of facial n.

zygomatico-orbital a. and v.

supraorbital n.

pareital br. of superficial temporal a.

supratrochlear n.

supraorbital a. and v.

buccal br. of facial n.

superficial temporal a. and v.

zygomatico-facial n.

greater occipital n.

infratrochlear n.

auriculo-temporal n.

external nasal br. of infraorbital n.

ext. acoustic meatus

occipital a.

posterior auricular a.

posterior auricular v.

infraorbital a. and n.

lesser occipital n.

third occipital n.

transverse facial a.

retromandibular v.

great auricular n.

parotid gland

sternocleidomastoid m.

parotid duct

mental n.

Spinal accessory n.

mandibular br. of facial n.

external jugular v.

facial v.

submandibular gland

cervical br. of facial n.

transverse cervical n.

trapezius m.

posterior supraclavicular n.

anterior jugular v.

medial supraclavicular n.

intermediate supraclavicular n.

ANATOMY

A5

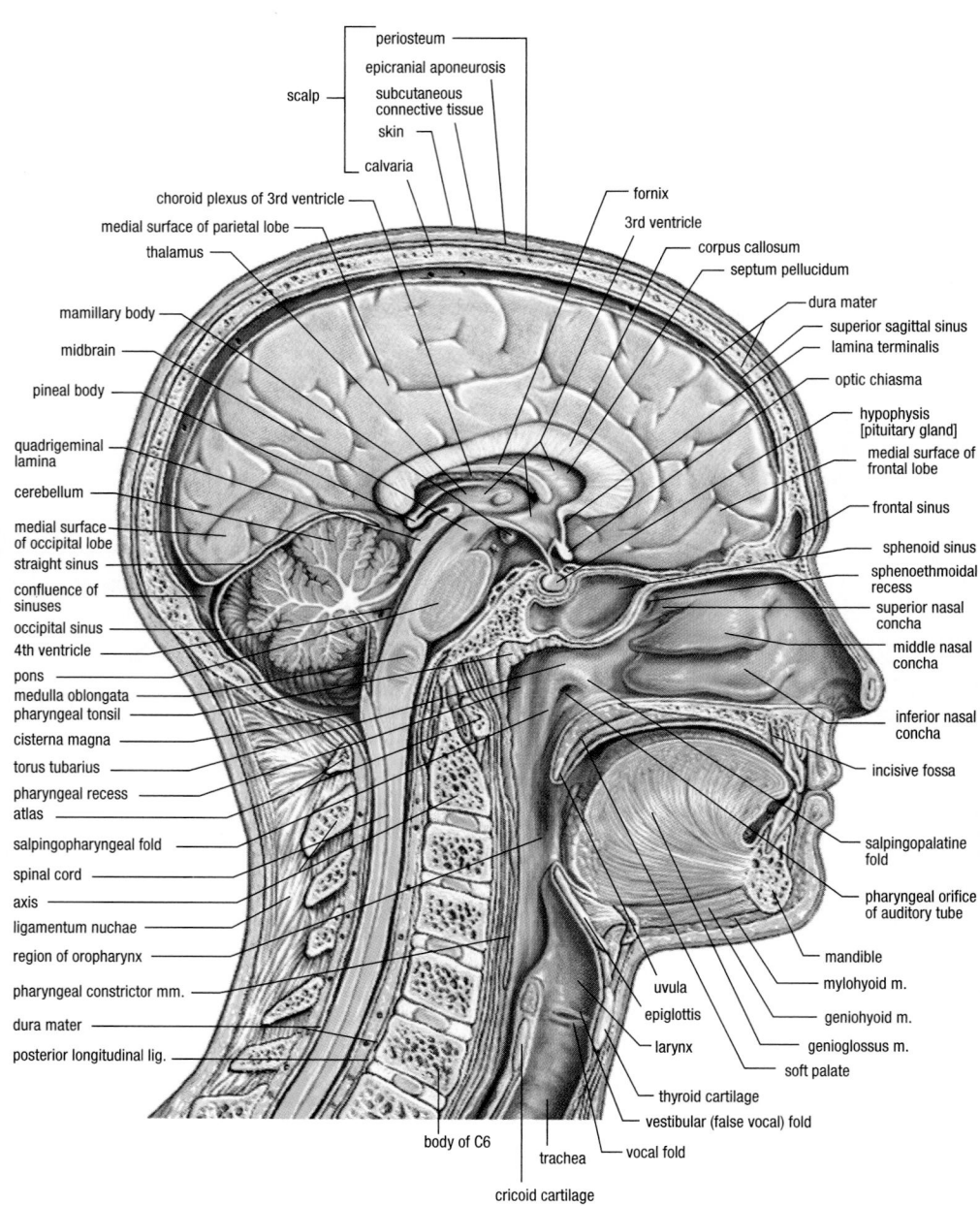

periosteum
epicranial aponeurosis
scalp
subcutaneous connective tissue
skin
calvaria
fornix
3rd ventricle
choroid plexus of 3rd ventricle
corpus callosum
medial surface of parietal lobe
septum pellucidum
thalamus
dura mater
superior sagittal sinus
mamillary body
lamina terminalis
midbrain
optic chiasma
pineal body
hypophysis [pituitary gland]
quadrigeminal lamina
medial surface of frontal lobe
cerebellum
frontal sinus
medial surface of occipital lobe
sphenoid sinus
straight sinus
sphenoethmoidal recess
confluence of sinuses
superior nasal concha
occipital sinus
4th ventricle
middle nasal concha
pons
medulla oblongata
pharyngeal tonsil
inferior nasal concha
cisterna magna
torus tubarius
incisive fossa
pharyngeal recess
atlas
salpingopharyngeal fold
salpingopalatine fold
spinal cord
axis
pharyngeal orifice of auditory tube
ligamentum nuchae
region of oropharynx
mandible
pharyngeal constrictor mm.
mylohyoid m.
uvula
dura mater
geniohyoid m.
epiglottis
posterior longitudinal lig.
larynx
genioglossus m.
soft palate
thyroid cartilage
vestibular (false vocal) fold
body of C6
vocal fold
trachea
cricoid cartilage

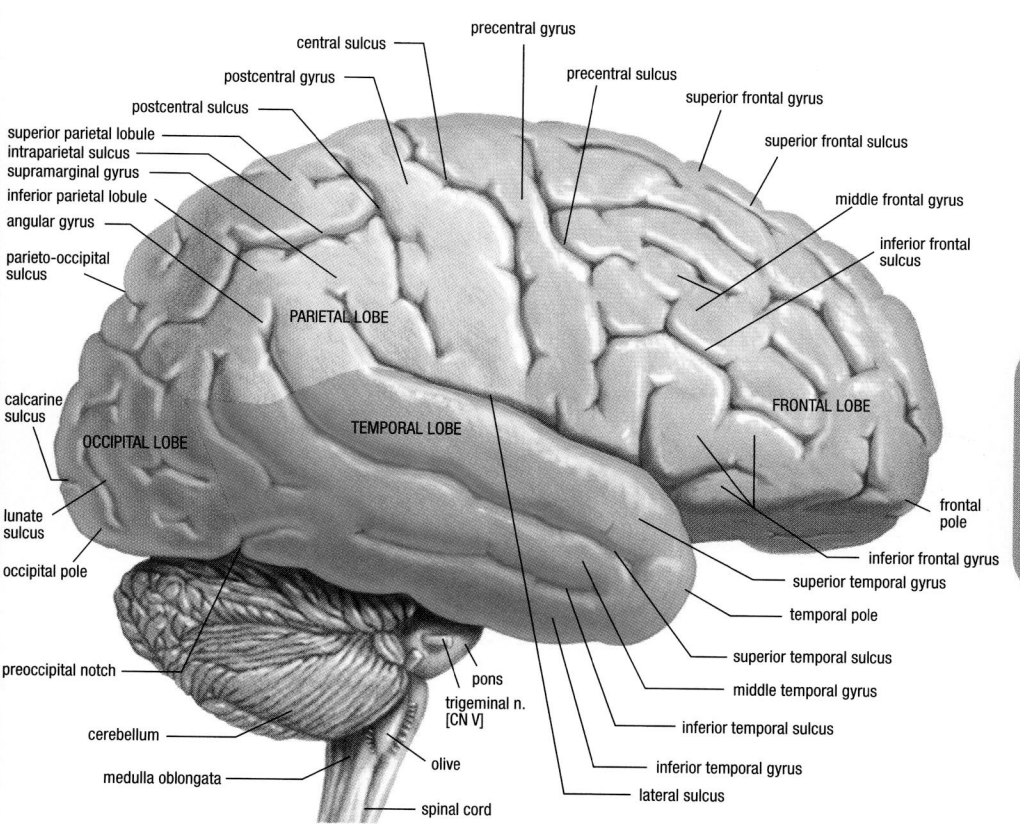

central sulcus
precentral gyrus
postcentral gyrus
precentral sulcus
postcentral sulcus
superior frontal gyrus
superior parietal lobule
superior frontal sulcus
intraparietal sulcus
supramarginal gyrus
middle frontal gyrus
inferior parietal lobule
angular gyrus
inferior frontal sulcus
parieto-occipital sulcus
PARIETAL LOBE
calcarine sulcus
FRONTAL LOBE
OCCIPITAL LOBE
TEMPORAL LOBE
lunate sulcus
frontal pole
occipital pole
inferior frontal gyrus
superior temporal gyrus
preoccipital notch
temporal pole
pons
trigeminal n. [CN V]
superior temporal sulcus
cerebellum
middle temporal gyrus
olive
inferior temporal sulcus
medulla oblongata
inferior temporal gyrus
spinal cord
lateral sulcus

ANATOMY

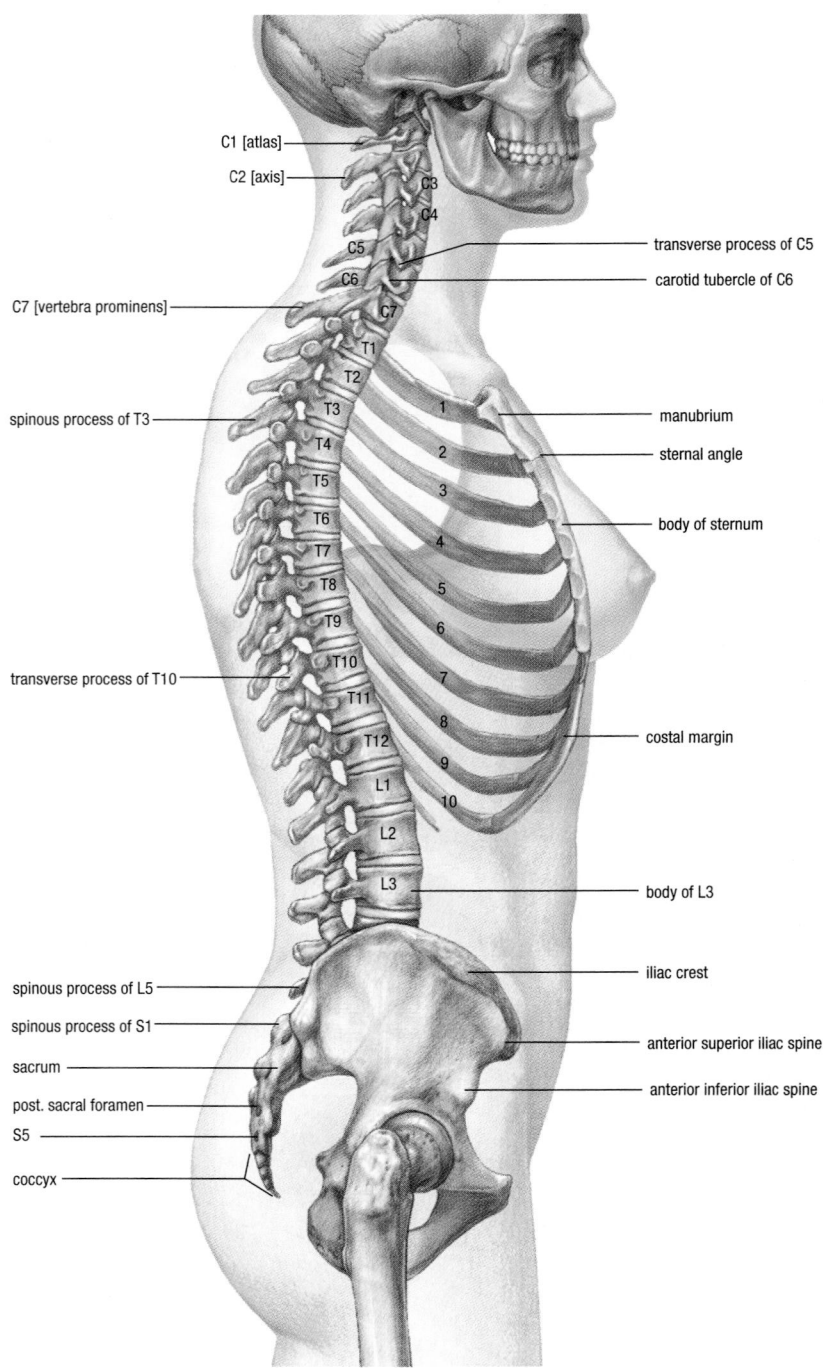

C1 [atlas]

C2 [axis]

C3

C4

C5 — transverse process of C5

C6 — carotid tubercle of C6

C7 [vertebra prominens]

C7

T1

T2

T3

spinous process of T3 — T3 — manubrium

T4 — sternal angle

T5

T6 — body of sternum

T7

T8

T9

transverse process of T10 — T10

T11

T12 — costal margin

L1

L2

L3 — body of L3

iliac crest

spinous process of L5

spinous process of S1 — anterior superior iliac spine

sacrum — anterior inferior iliac spine

post. sacral foramen

S5

coccyx

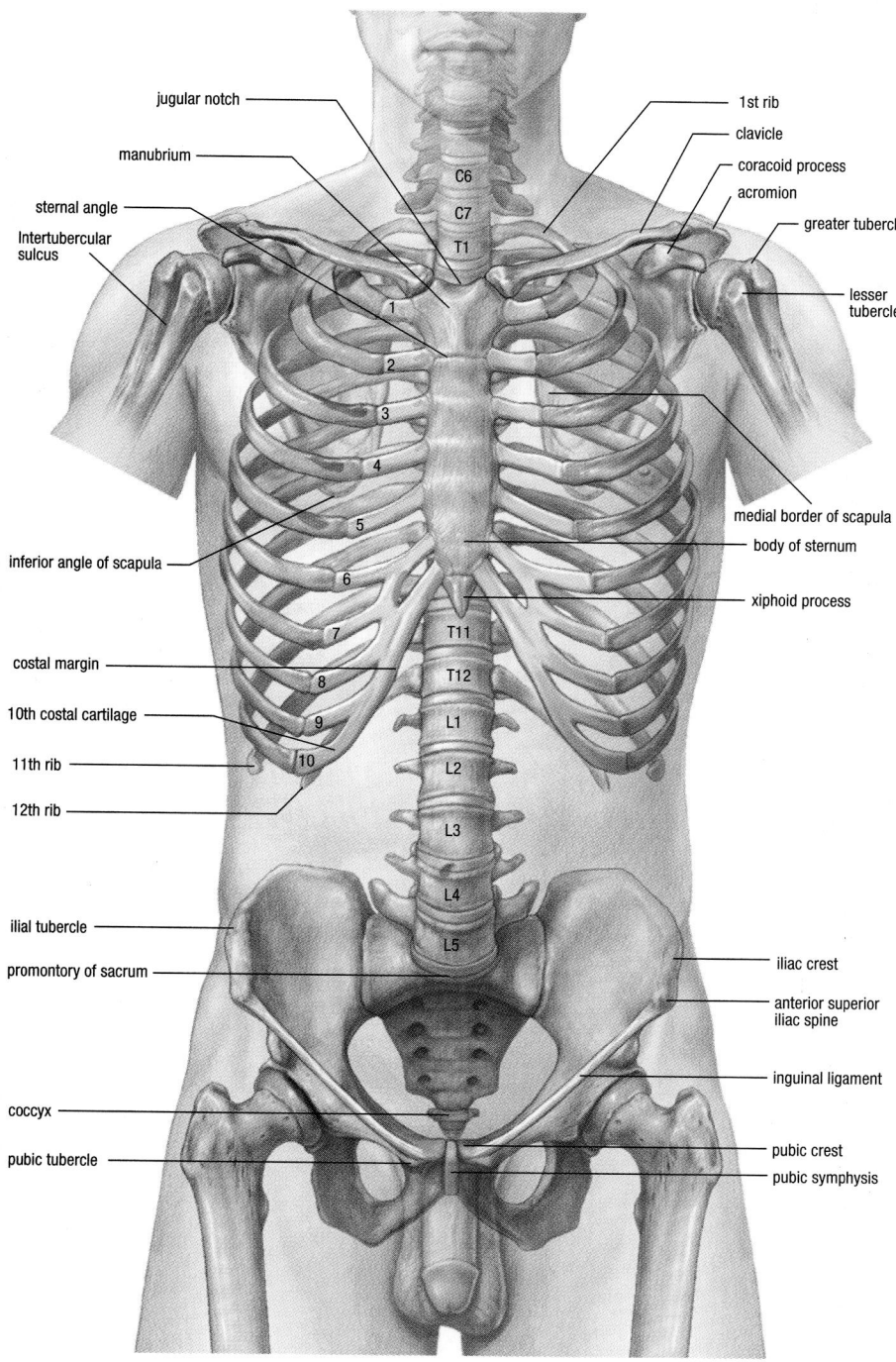

jugular notch

manubrium

sternal angle

Intertubercular
sulcus

C6

C7

T1

1

2

3

4

5

6

7

8

9

10

1st rib

clavicle

coracoid process

acromion

greater tubercle

lesser
tubercle

medial border of scapula

body of sternum

xiphoid process

inferior angle of scapula

costal margin

10th costal cartilage

11th rib

12th rib

T11

T12

L1

L2

L3

L4

L5

ilial tubercle

promontory of sacrum

coccyx

pubic tubercle

iliac crest

anterior superior
iliac spine

inguinal ligament

pubic crest

pubic symphysis

ANATOMY

Imagery © 1996 A.D.A.M. Software, Inc.

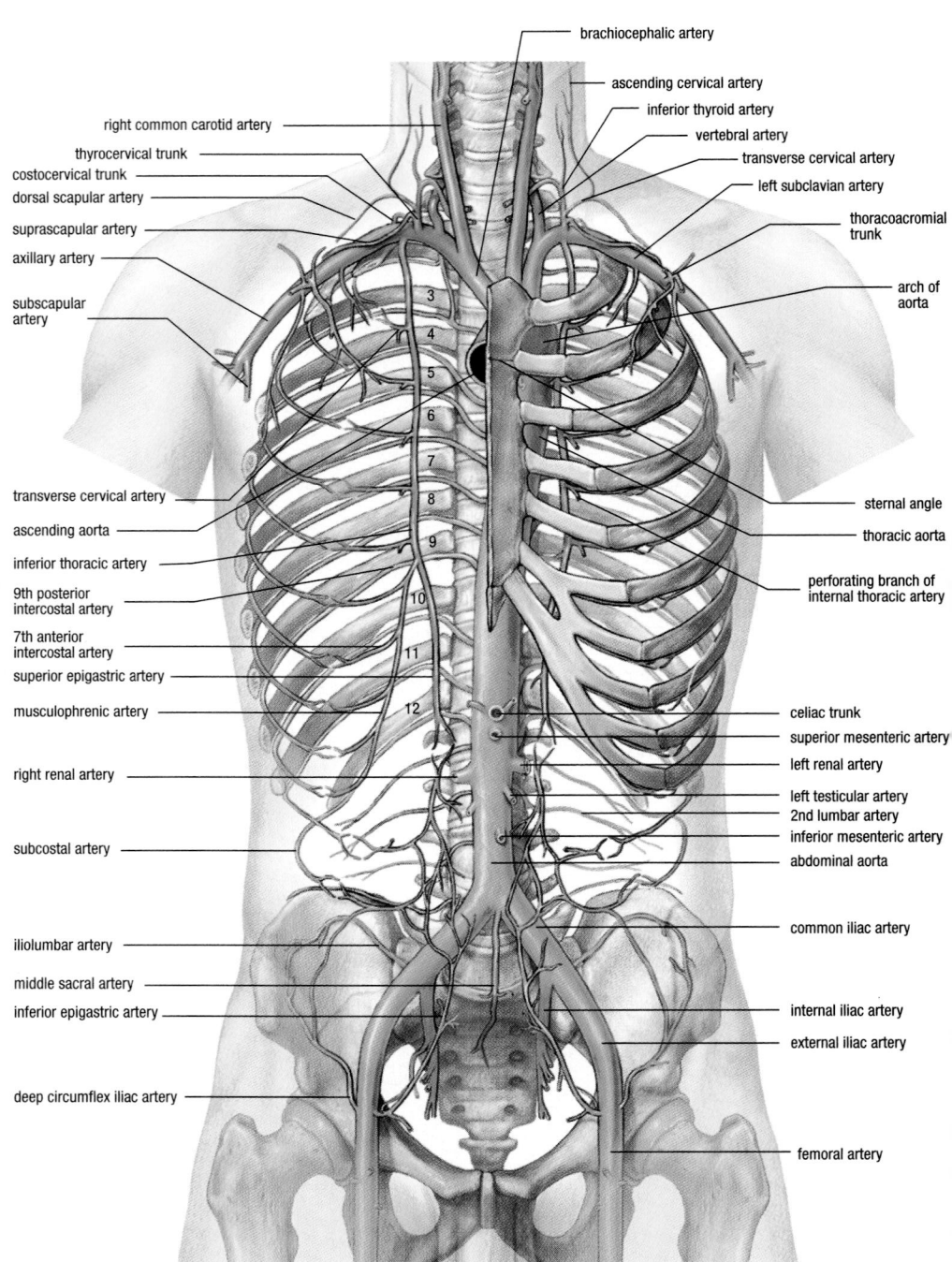

brachiocephalic artery

ascending cervical artery

inferior thyroid artery

vertebral artery

transverse cervical artery

left subclavian artery

right common carotid artery

thyrocervical trunk

costocervical trunk

dorsal scapular artery

suprascapular artery

axillary artery

thoracoacromial trunk

subscapular artery

arch of aorta

sternal angle

thoracic aorta

perforating branch of internal thoracic artery

transverse cervical artery

ascending aorta

inferior thoracic artery

9th posterior intercostal artery

7th anterior intercostal artery

superior epigastric artery

musculophrenic artery

celiac trunk

superior mesenteric artery

left renal artery

right renal artery

left testicular artery

2nd lumbar artery

inferior mesenteric artery

abdominal aorta

subcostal artery

iliolumbar artery

common iliac artery

middle sacral artery

inferior epigastric artery

internal iliac artery

external iliac artery

deep circumflex iliac artery

femoral artery

Imagery © 1996 A.D.A.M. Software, Inc.

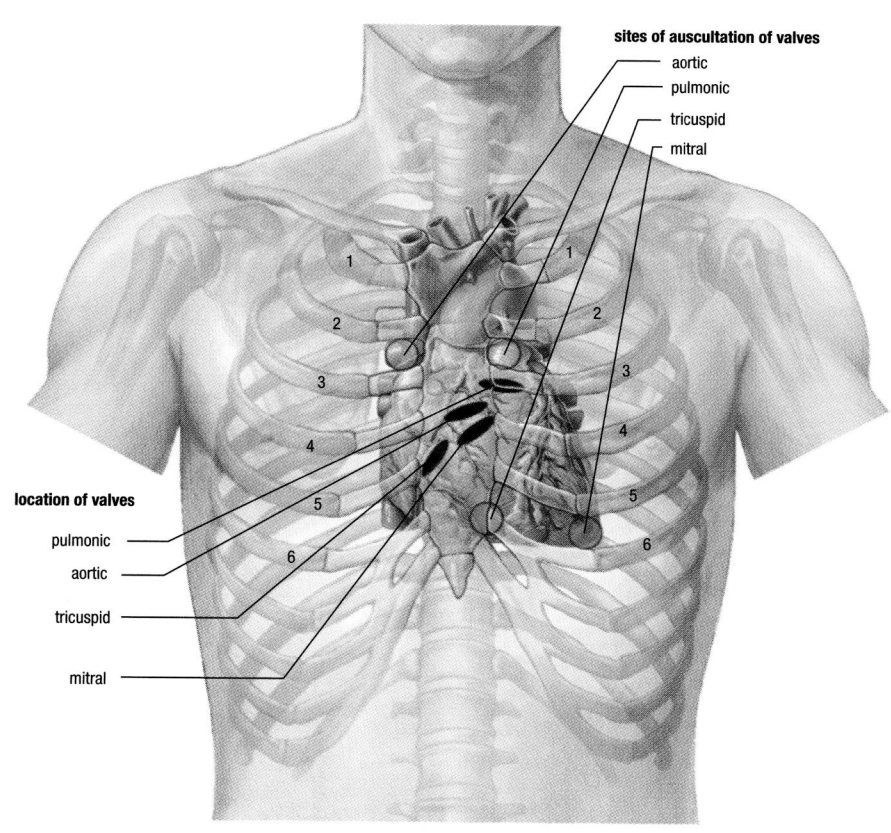

sites of auscultation of valves
- aortic
- pulmonic
- tricuspid
- mitral

location of valves
- pulmonic
- aortic
- tricuspid
- mitral

ANATOMY

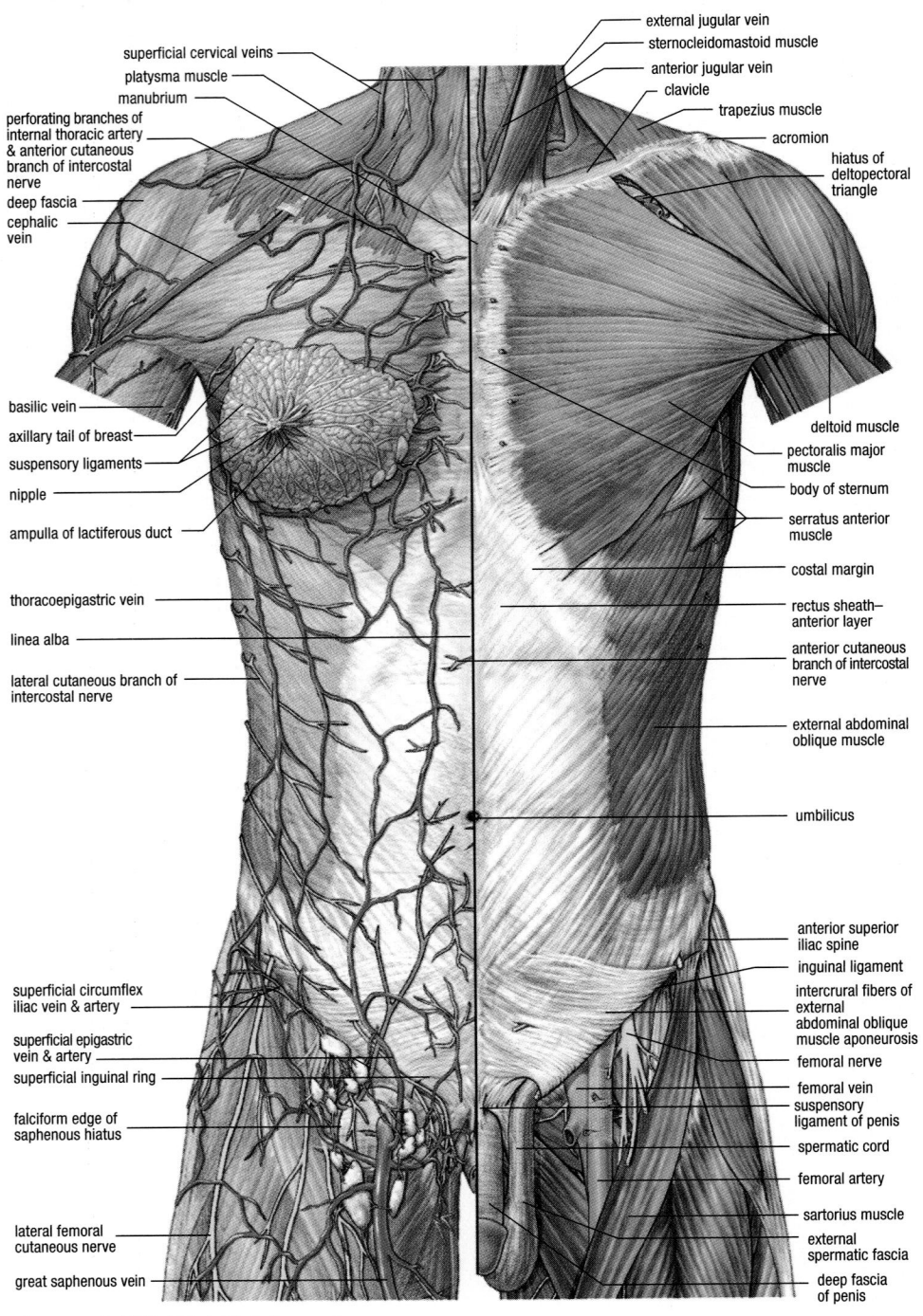

Imagery © 1996 A.D.A.M. Software, Inc.

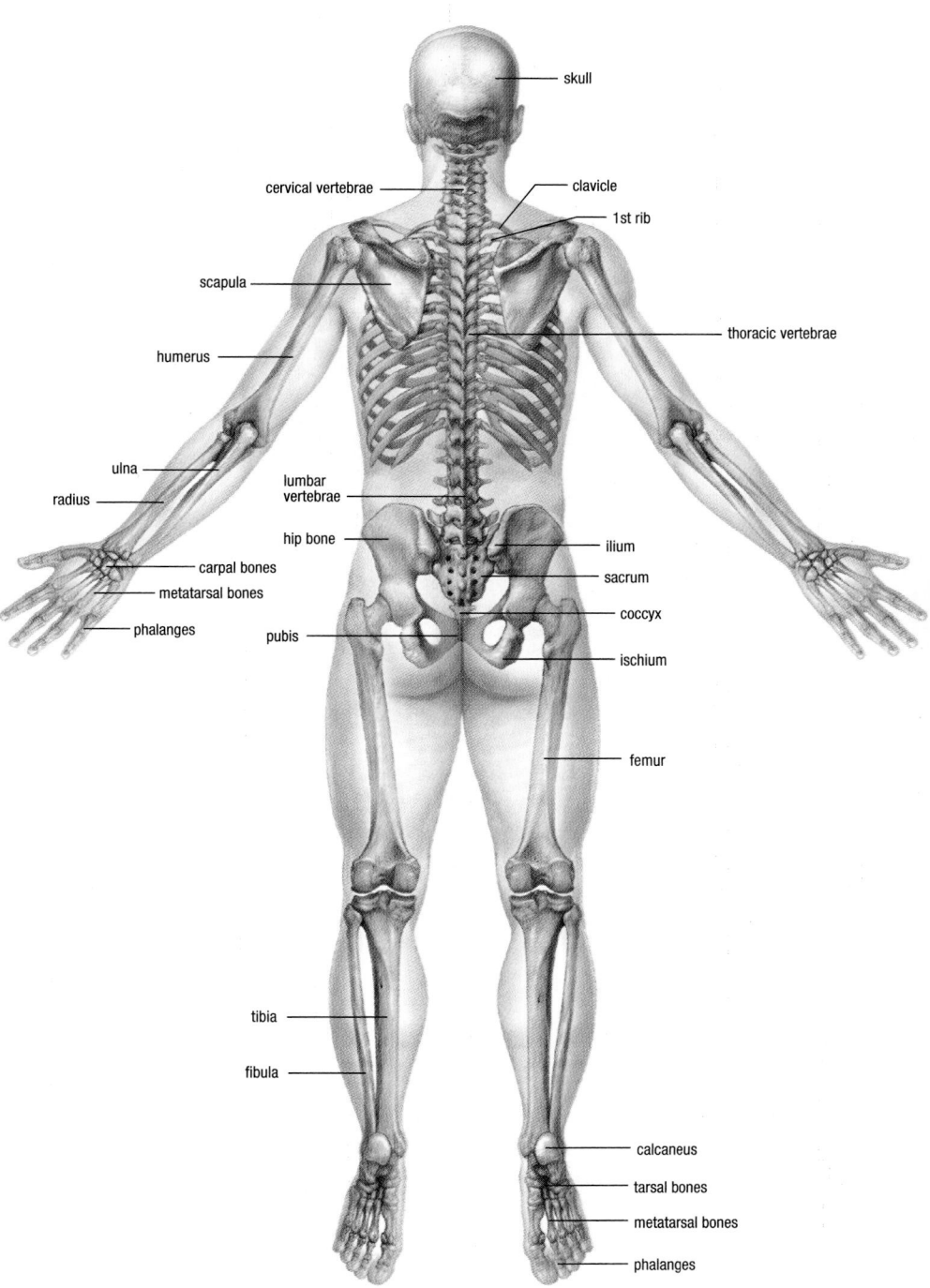

skull

cervical vertebrae

clavicle

1st rib

scapula

thoracic vertebrae

humerus

ulna

radius

lumbar vertebrae

hip bone

ilium

sacrum

carpal bones

metatarsal bones

coccyx

phalanges

pubis

ischium

femur

tibia

fibula

calcaneus

tarsal bones

metatarsal bones

phalanges

ANATOMY

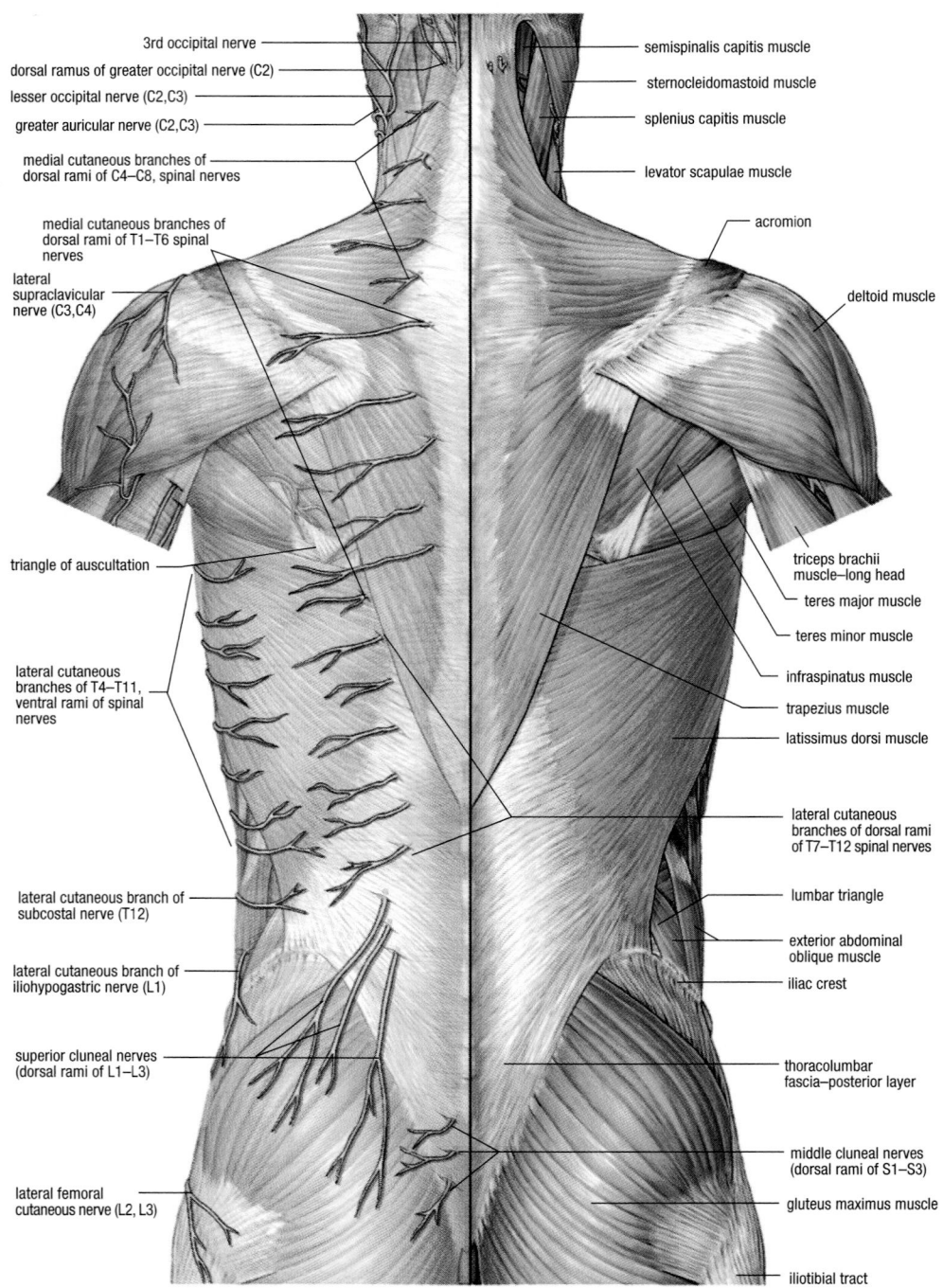

3rd occipital nerve

dorsal ramus of greater occipital nerve (C2)

lesser occipital nerve (C2,C3)

greater auricular nerve (C2,C3)

medial cutaneous branches of dorsal rami of C4–C8, spinal nerves

medial cutaneous branches of dorsal rami of T1–T6 spinal nerves

lateral supraclavicular nerve (C3,C4)

triangle of auscultation

lateral cutaneous branches of T4–T11, ventral rami of spinal nerves

lateral cutaneous branch of subcostal nerve (T12)

lateral cutaneous branch of iliohypogastric nerve (L1)

superior cluneal nerves (dorsal rami of L1–L3)

lateral femoral cutaneous nerve (L2, L3)

semispinalis capitis muscle

sternocleidomastoid muscle

splenius capitis muscle

levator scapulae muscle

acromion

deltoid muscle

triceps brachii muscle–long head

teres major muscle

teres minor muscle

infraspinatus muscle

trapezius muscle

latissimus dorsi muscle

lateral cutaneous branches of dorsal rami of T7–T12 spinal nerves

lumbar triangle

exterior abdominal oblique muscle

iliac crest

thoracolumbar fascia–posterior layer

middle cluneal nerves (dorsal rami of S1–S3)

gluteus maximus muscle

iliotibial tract

Imagery © 1996 A.D.A.M. Software, Inc.

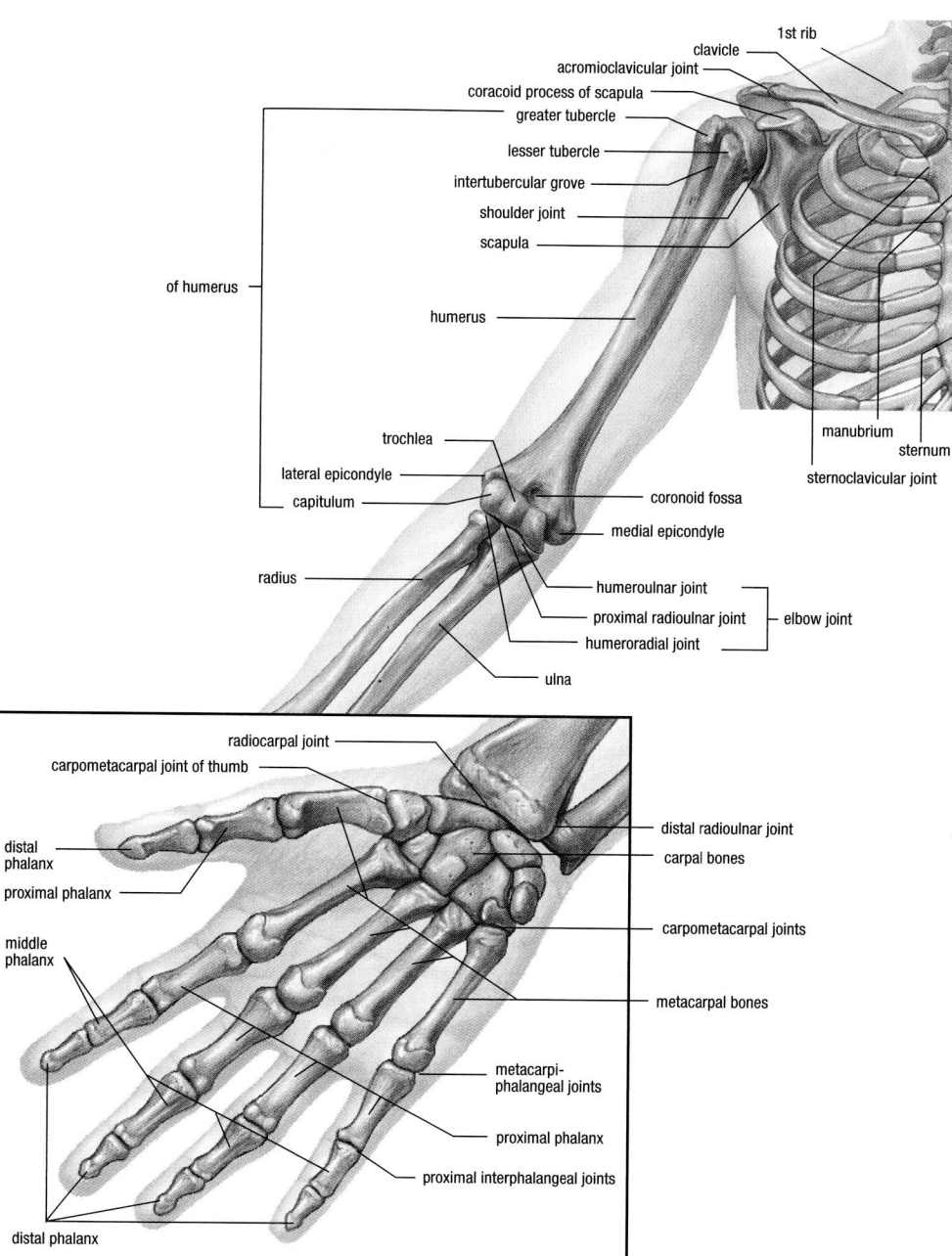

1st rib
clavicle
acromioclavicular joint
coracoid process of scapula
greater tubercle
lesser tubercle
intertubercular grove
shoulder joint
scapula
of humerus
humerus
trochlea
lateral epicondyle
capitulum
coronoid fossa
medial epicondyle
radius
humeroulnar joint
proximal radioulnar joint — elbow joint
humeroradial joint
ulna
manubrium
sternum
sternoclavicular joint

radiocarpal joint
carpometacarpal joint of thumb
distal phalanx
proximal phalanx
middle phalanx
distal radioulnar joint
carpal bones
carpometacarpal joints
metacarpal bones
metacarpi-phalangeal joints
proximal phalanx
proximal interphalangeal joints
distal phalanx

Imagery © 1996 A.D.A.M. Software, Inc.

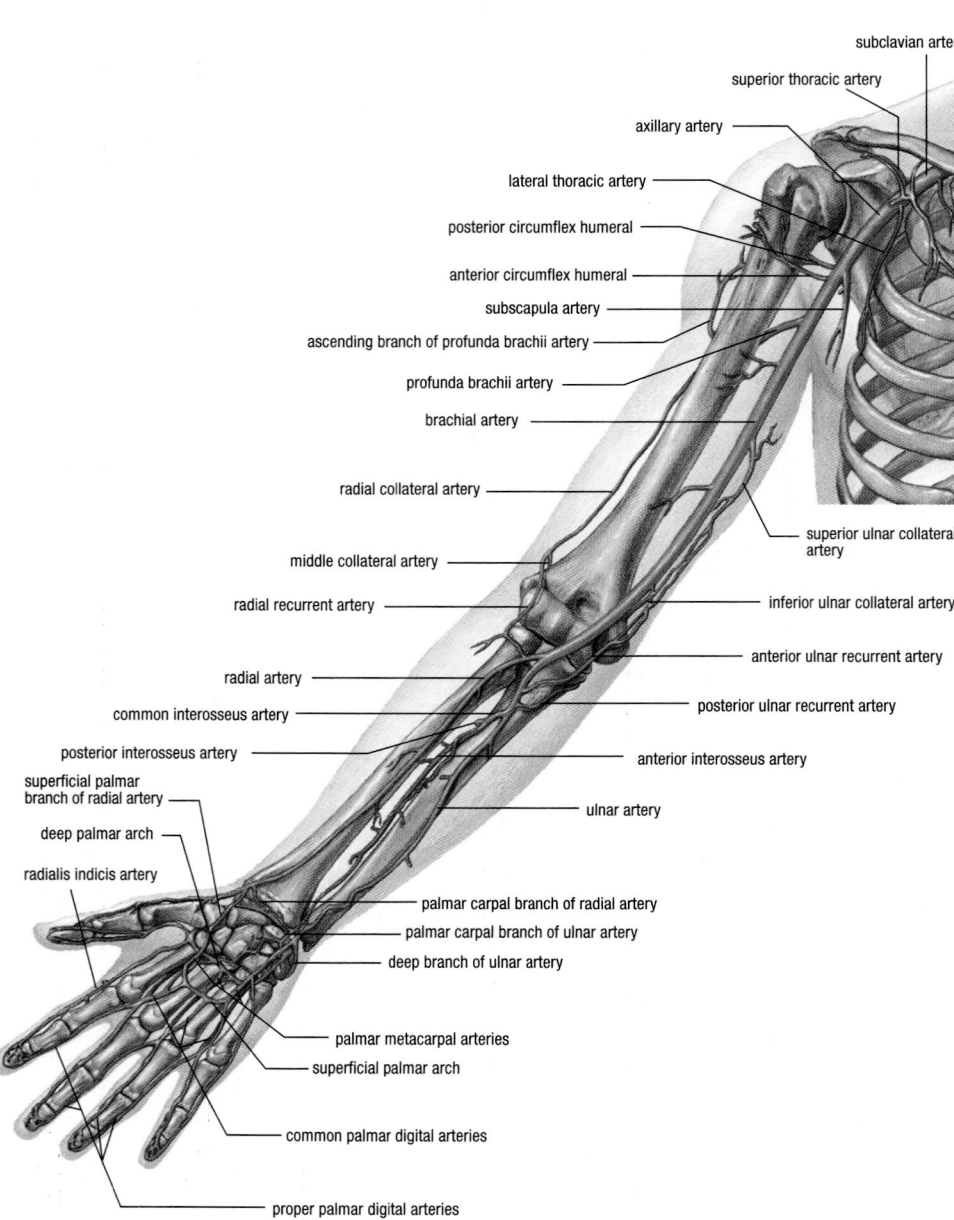

subclavian artery

superior thoracic artery

axillary artery

lateral thoracic artery

posterior circumflex humeral

anterior circumflex humeral

subscapula artery

ascending branch of profunda brachii artery

profunda brachii artery

brachial artery

radial collateral artery

middle collateral artery

radial recurrent artery

radial artery

common interosseus artery

posterior interosseus artery

superficial palmar branch of radial artery

deep palmar arch

radialis indicis artery

superior ulnar collateral artery

inferior ulnar collateral artery

anterior ulnar recurrent artery

posterior ulnar recurrent artery

anterior interosseus artery

ulnar artery

palmar carpal branch of radial artery

palmar carpal branch of ulnar artery

deep branch of ulnar artery

palmar metacarpal arteries

superficial palmar arch

common palmar digital arteries

proper palmar digital arteries

Imagery © 1996 A.D.A.M. Software, Inc.

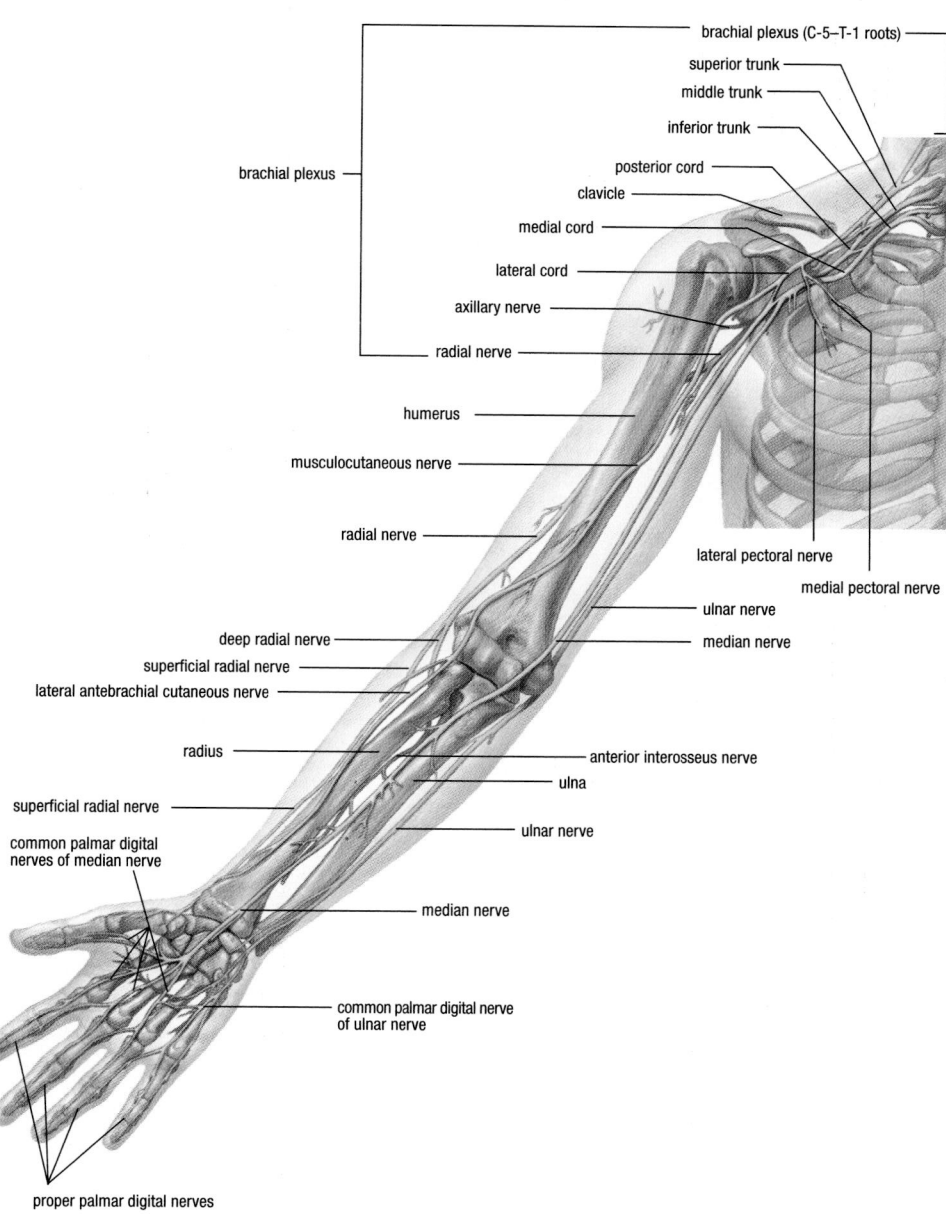

brachial plexus (C-5–T-1 roots)

superior trunk

middle trunk

inferior trunk

brachial plexus

posterior cord

clavicle

medial cord

lateral cord

axillary nerve

radial nerve

humerus

musculocutaneous nerve

radial nerve

lateral pectoral nerve

medial pectoral nerve

ulnar nerve

median nerve

deep radial nerve

superficial radial nerve

lateral antebrachial cutaneous nerve

radius

anterior interosseus nerve

ulna

superficial radial nerve

ulnar nerve

common palmar digital
nerves of median nerve

median nerve

common palmar digital nerve
of ulnar nerve

proper palmar digital nerves

ANATOMY

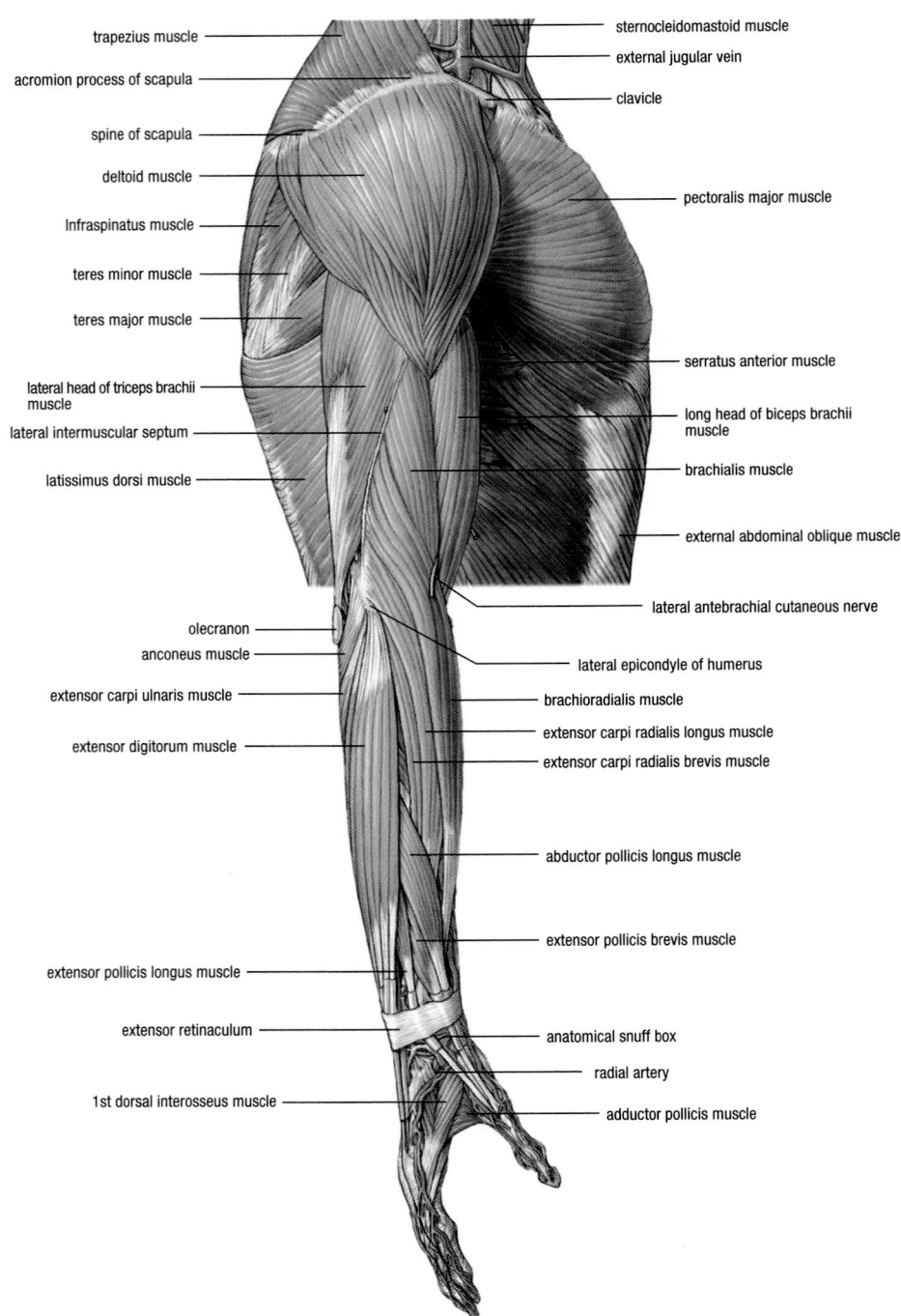

trapezius muscle

acromion process of scapula

spine of scapula

deltoid muscle

Infraspinatus muscle

teres minor muscle

teres major muscle

lateral head of triceps brachii muscle

lateral intermuscular septum

latissimus dorsi muscle

olecranon

anconeus muscle

extensor carpi ulnaris muscle

extensor digitorum muscle

extensor pollicis longus muscle

extensor retinaculum

1st dorsal interosseus muscle

sternocleidomastoid muscle

external jugular vein

clavicle

pectoralis major muscle

serratus anterior muscle

long head of biceps brachii muscle

brachialis muscle

external abdominal oblique muscle

lateral antebrachial cutaneous nerve

lateral epicondyle of humerus

brachioradialis muscle

extensor carpi radialis longus muscle

extensor carpi radialis brevis muscle

abductor pollicis longus muscle

extensor pollicis brevis muscle

anatomical snuff box

radial artery

adductor pollicis muscle

Imagery © 1996 A.D.A.M. Software, Inc.

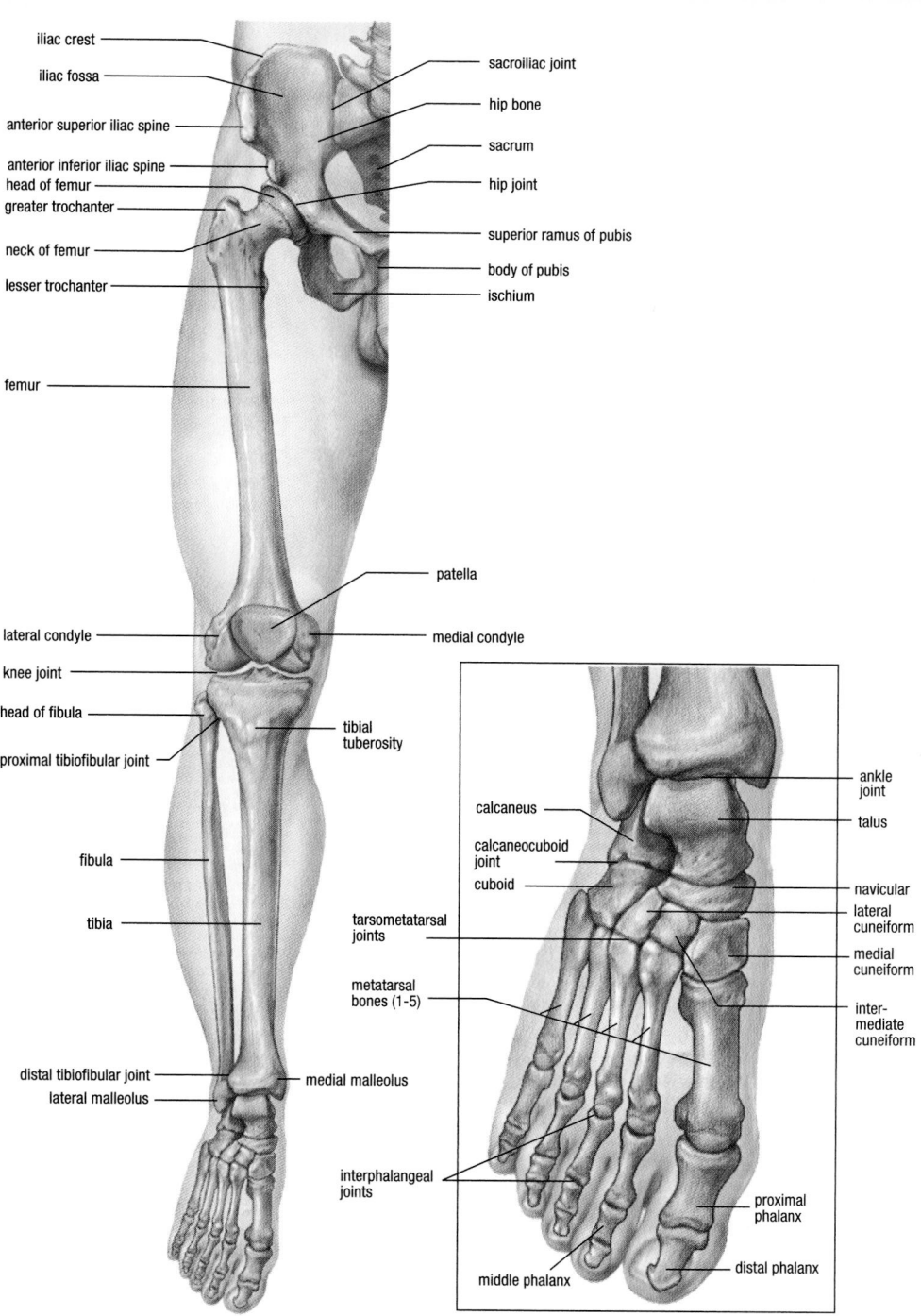

iliac crest

iliac fossa

anterior superior iliac spine

anterior inferior iliac spine

head of femur

greater trochanter

neck of femur

lesser trochanter

femur

lateral condyle

knee joint

head of fibula

proximal tibiofibular joint

fibula

tibia

distal tibiofibular joint

lateral malleolus

sacroiliac joint

hip bone

sacrum

hip joint

superior ramus of pubis

body of pubis

ischium

patella

medial condyle

tibial tuberosity

tarsometatarsal joints

metatarsal bones (1-5)

interphalangeal joints

medial malleolus

calcaneus

calcaneocuboid joint

cuboid

middle phalanx

ankle joint

talus

navicular

lateral cuneiform

medial cuneiform

intermediate cuneiform

proximal phalanx

distal phalanx

ANATOMY

Imagery © 1996 A.D.A.M. Software, Inc.

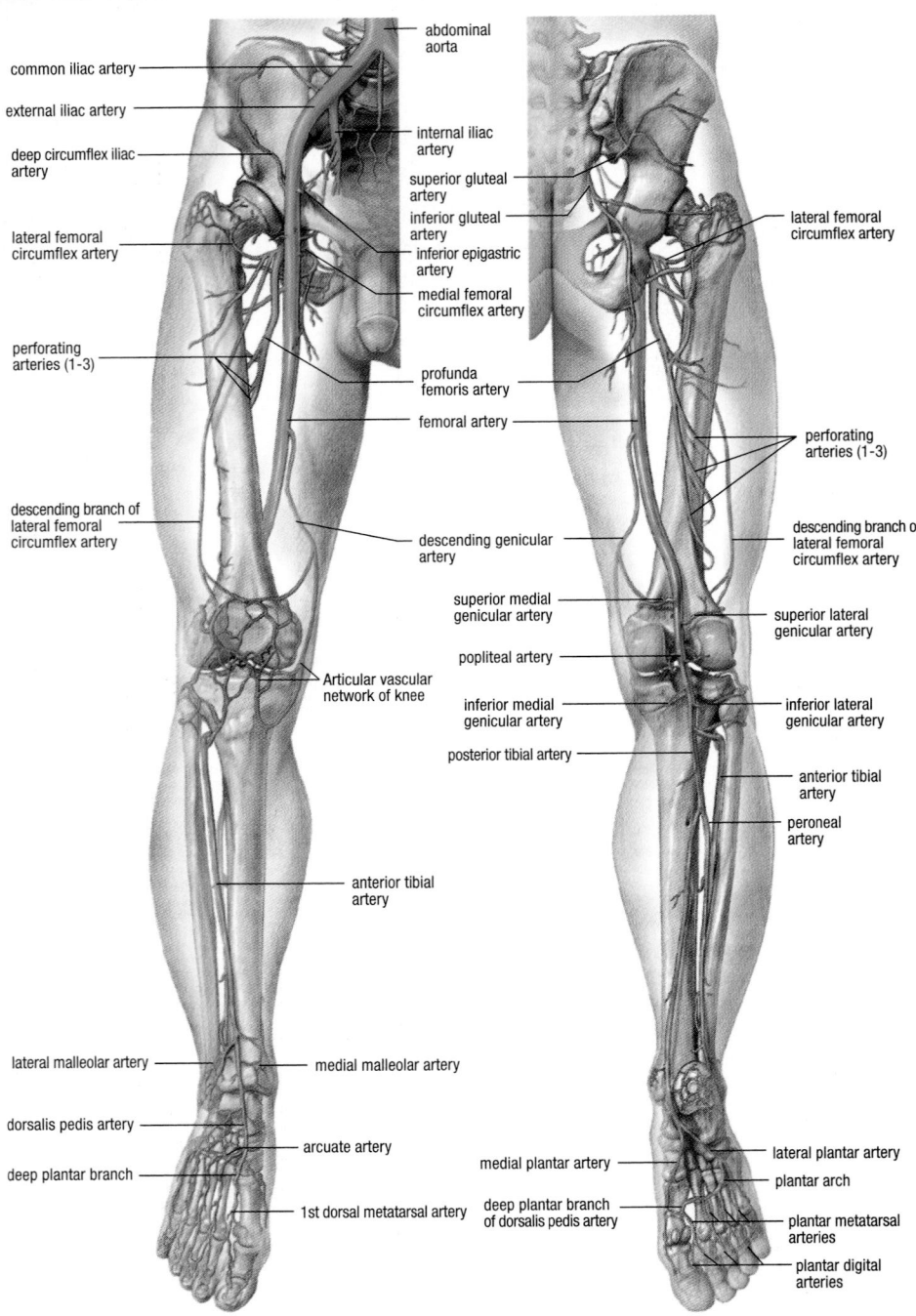

abdominal aorta

common iliac artery

external iliac artery

deep circumflex iliac artery

internal iliac artery

superior gluteal artery

inferior gluteal artery

inferior epigastric artery

lateral femoral circumflex artery

medial femoral circumflex artery

lateral femoral circumflex artery

perforating arteries (1-3)

profunda femoris artery

femoral artery

perforating arteries (1-3)

descending branch of lateral femoral circumflex artery

descending genicular artery

descending branch of lateral femoral circumflex artery

superior medial genicular artery

superior lateral genicular artery

popliteal artery

Articular vascular network of knee

inferior medial genicular artery

inferior lateral genicular artery

posterior tibial artery

anterior tibial artery

peroneal artery

anterior tibial artery

lateral malleolar artery

medial malleolar artery

dorsalis pedis artery

arcuate artery

deep plantar branch

medial plantar artery

lateral plantar artery

plantar arch

1st dorsal metatarsal artery

deep plantar branch of dorsalis pedis artery

plantar metatarsal arteries

plantar digital arteries

Imagery © 1996 A.D.A.M. Software, Inc.

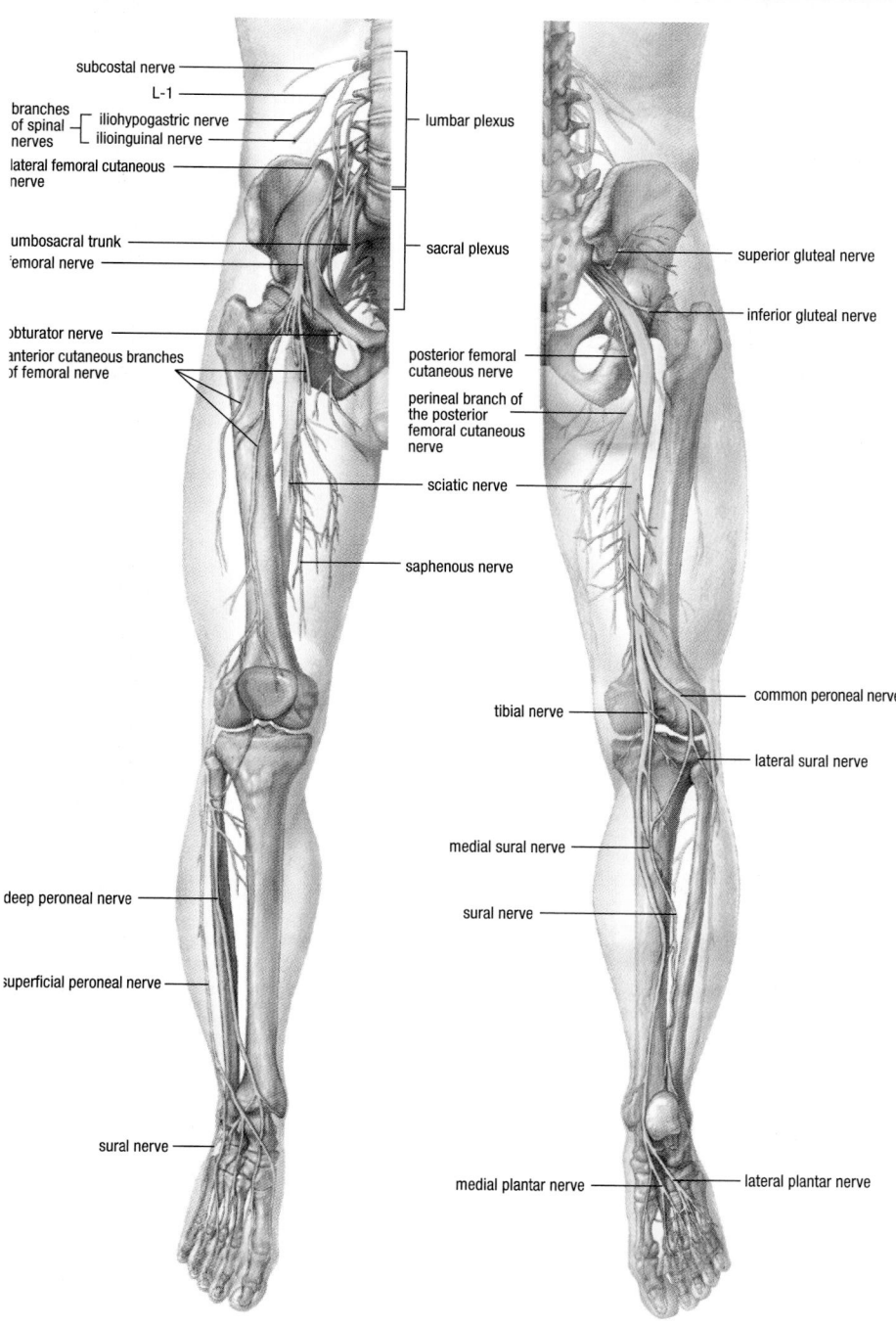

subcostal nerve

L-1

branches of spinal nerves
— iliohypogastric nerve
— ilioinguinal nerve

lateral femoral cutaneous nerve

lumbar plexus

lumbosacral trunk

femoral nerve

sacral plexus

superior gluteal nerve

inferior gluteal nerve

obturator nerve

anterior cutaneous branches of femoral nerve

posterior femoral cutaneous nerve

perineal branch of the posterior femoral cutaneous nerve

sciatic nerve

saphenous nerve

common peroneal nerve

tibial nerve

lateral sural nerve

medial sural nerve

deep peroneal nerve

sural nerve

superficial peroneal nerve

sural nerve

medial plantar nerve

lateral plantar nerve

ANATOMY

Imagery © 1996 A.D.A.M. Software, Inc.

PLATE 22: MUSCULATURE OF LOWER LIMB, LATERAL AND MEDIAL VIEWS

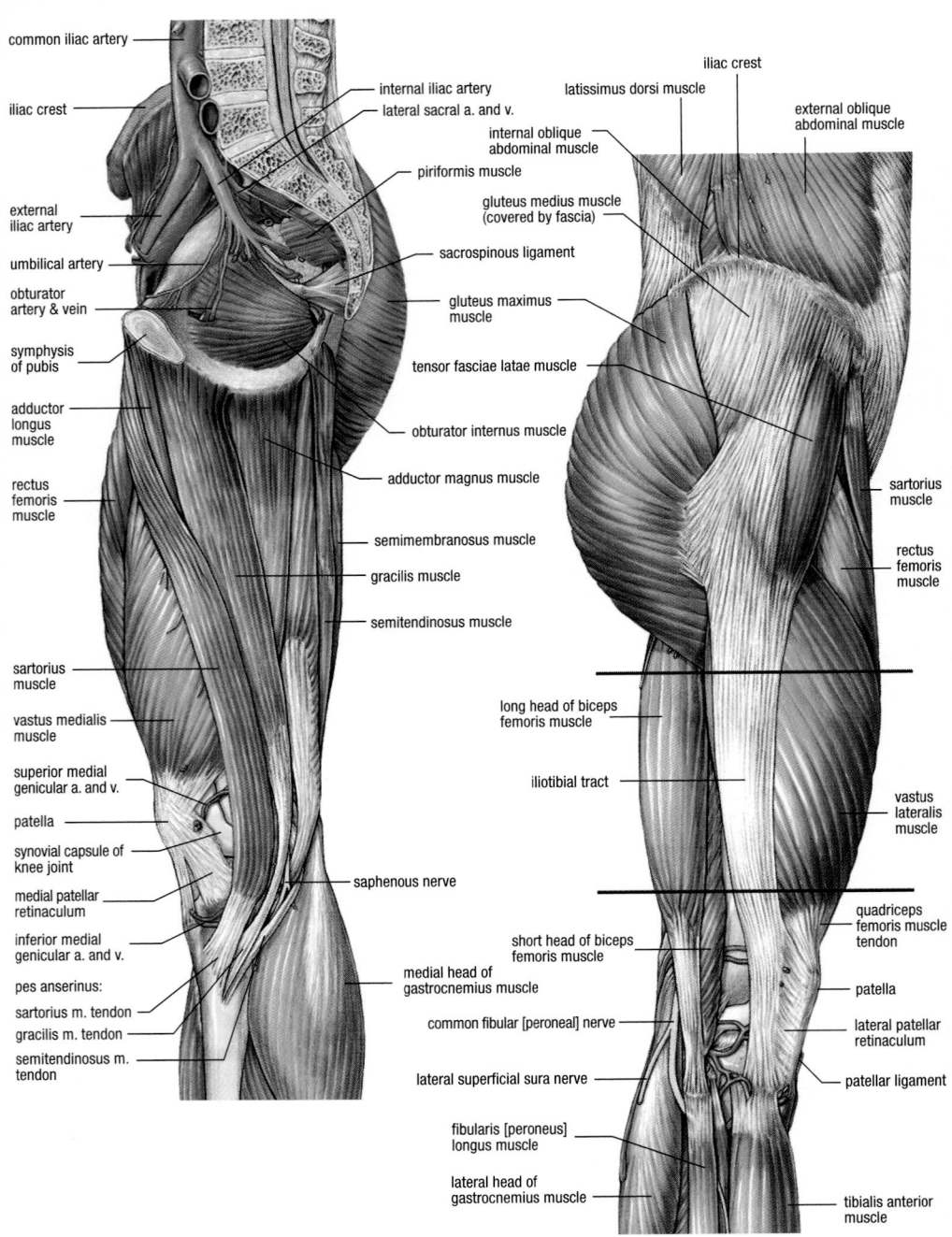

common iliac artery

iliac crest

external iliac artery

umbilical artery

obturator artery & vein

symphysis of pubis

adductor longus muscle

rectus femoris muscle

sartorius muscle

vastus medialis muscle

superior medial genicular a. and v.

patella

synovial capsule of knee joint

medial patellar retinaculum

inferior medial genicular a. and v.

pes anserinus:

sartorius m. tendon

gracilis m. tendon

semitendinosus m. tendon

internal iliac artery

lateral sacral a. and v.

internal oblique abdominal muscle

piriformis muscle

gluteus medius muscle (covered by fascia)

sacrospinous ligament

gluteus maximus muscle

tensor fasciae latae muscle

obturator internus muscle

adductor magnus muscle

semimembranosus muscle

gracilis muscle

semitendinosus muscle

saphenous nerve

long head of biceps femoris muscle

iliotibial tract

short head of biceps femoris muscle

medial head of gastrocnemius muscle

common fibular [peroneal] nerve

lateral superficial sura nerve

fibularis [peroneus] longus muscle

lateral head of gastrocnemius muscle

latissimus dorsi muscle

iliac crest

external oblique abdominal muscle

sartorius muscle

rectus femoris muscle

vastus lateralis muscle

quadriceps femoris muscle tendon

patella

lateral patellar retinaculum

patellar ligament

tibialis anterior muscle

Imagery © 1996 A.D.A.M. Software, Inc.

A22

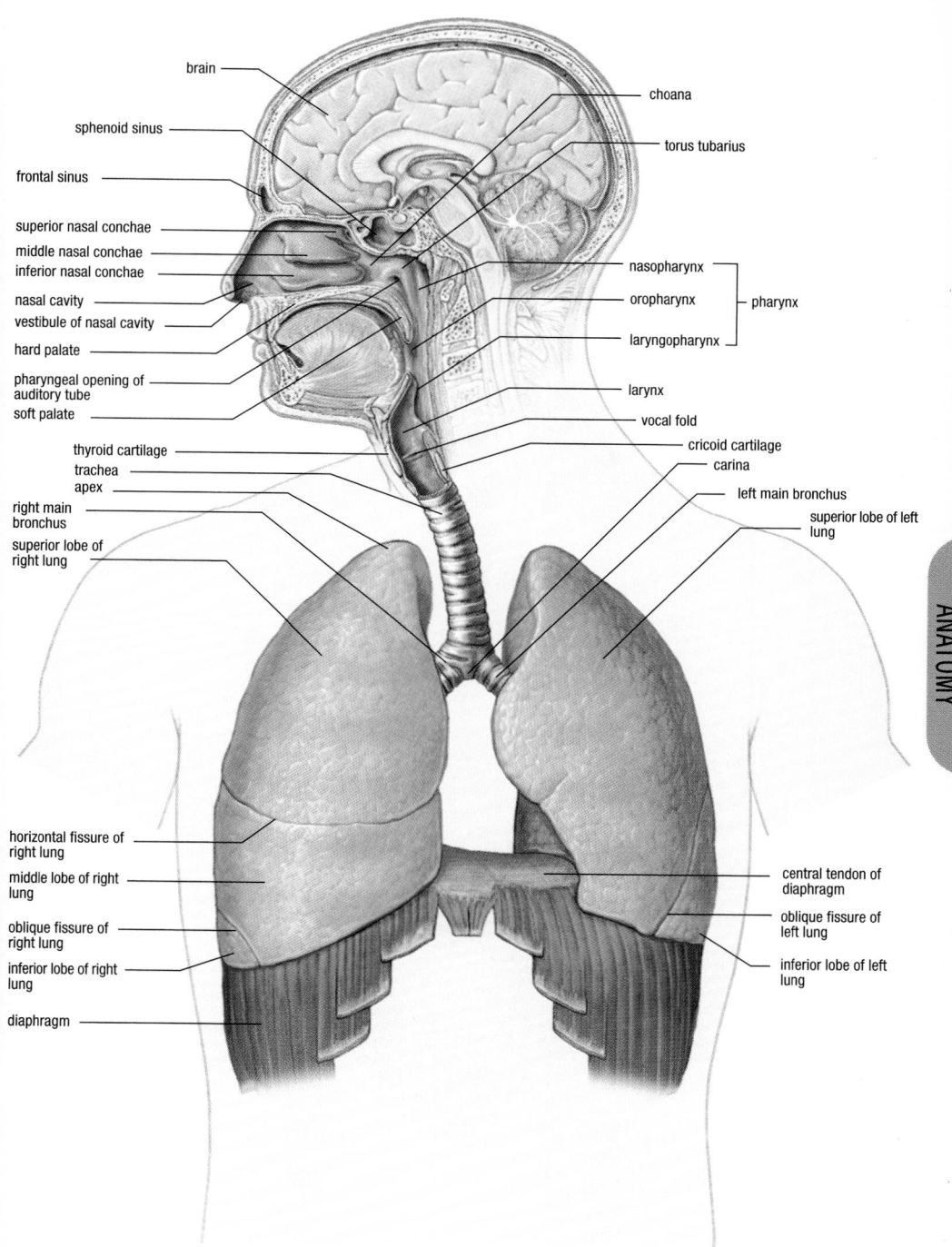

brain

choana

sphenoid sinus

torus tubarius

frontal sinus

superior nasal conchae

middle nasal conchae

nasopharynx

inferior nasal conchae

oropharynx

pharynx

nasal cavity

laryngopharynx

vestibule of nasal cavity

hard palate

pharyngeal opening of auditory tube

larynx

soft palate

vocal fold

thyroid cartilage

cricoid cartilage

trachea

carina

apex

left main bronchus

right main bronchus

superior lobe of left lung

superior lobe of right lung

horizontal fissure of right lung

middle lobe of right lung

central tendon of diaphragm

oblique fissure of right lung

oblique fissure of left lung

inferior lobe of right lung

inferior lobe of left lung

diaphragm

ANATOMY

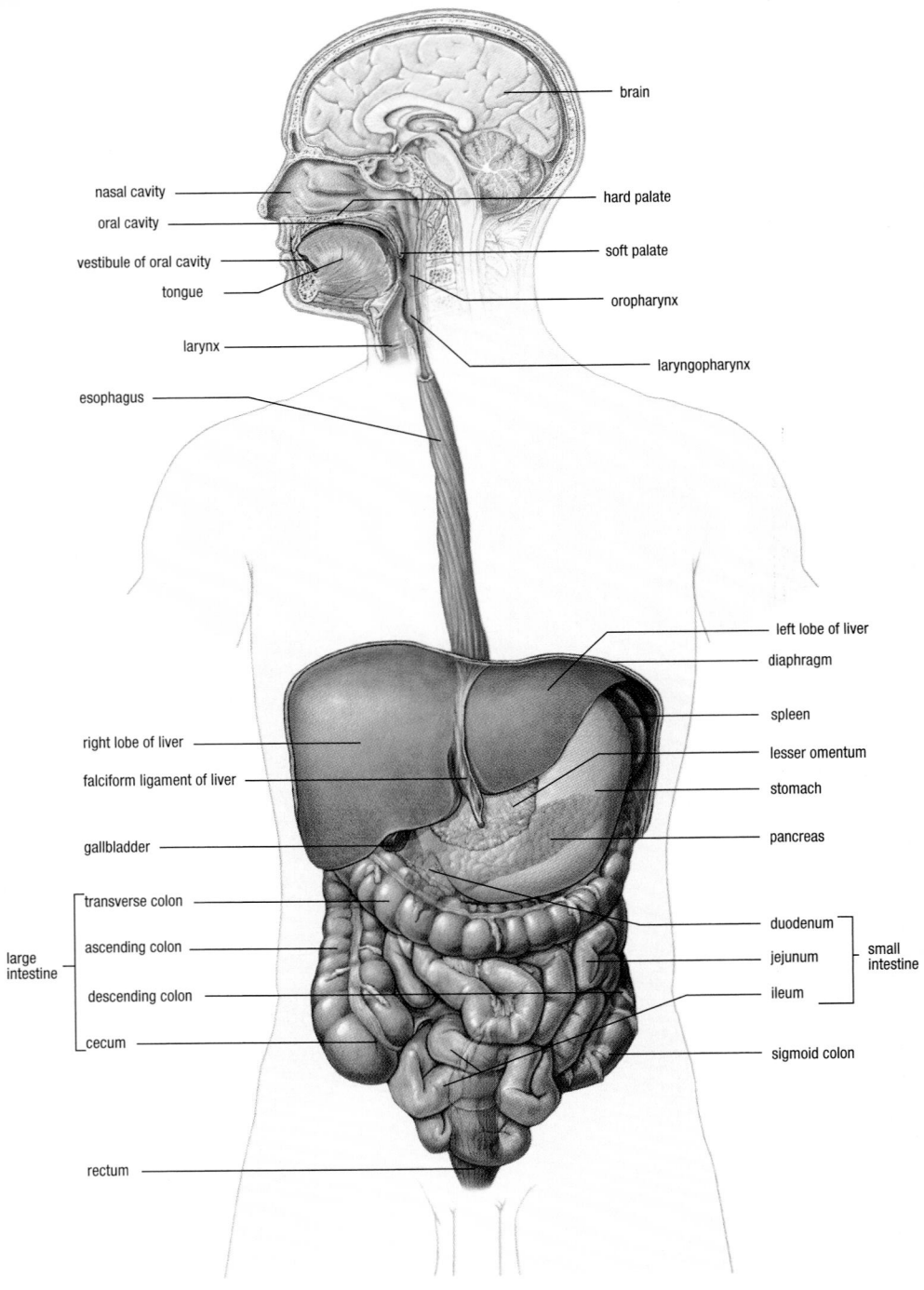

brain

nasal cavity

hard palate

oral cavity

soft palate

vestibule of oral cavity

tongue

oropharynx

larynx

laryngopharynx

esophagus

left lobe of liver

diaphragm

spleen

right lobe of liver

lesser omentum

falciform ligament of liver

stomach

pancreas

gallbladder

transverse colon

duodenum

ascending colon

jejunum

small intestine

large intestine

descending colon

ileum

cecum

sigmoid colon

rectum

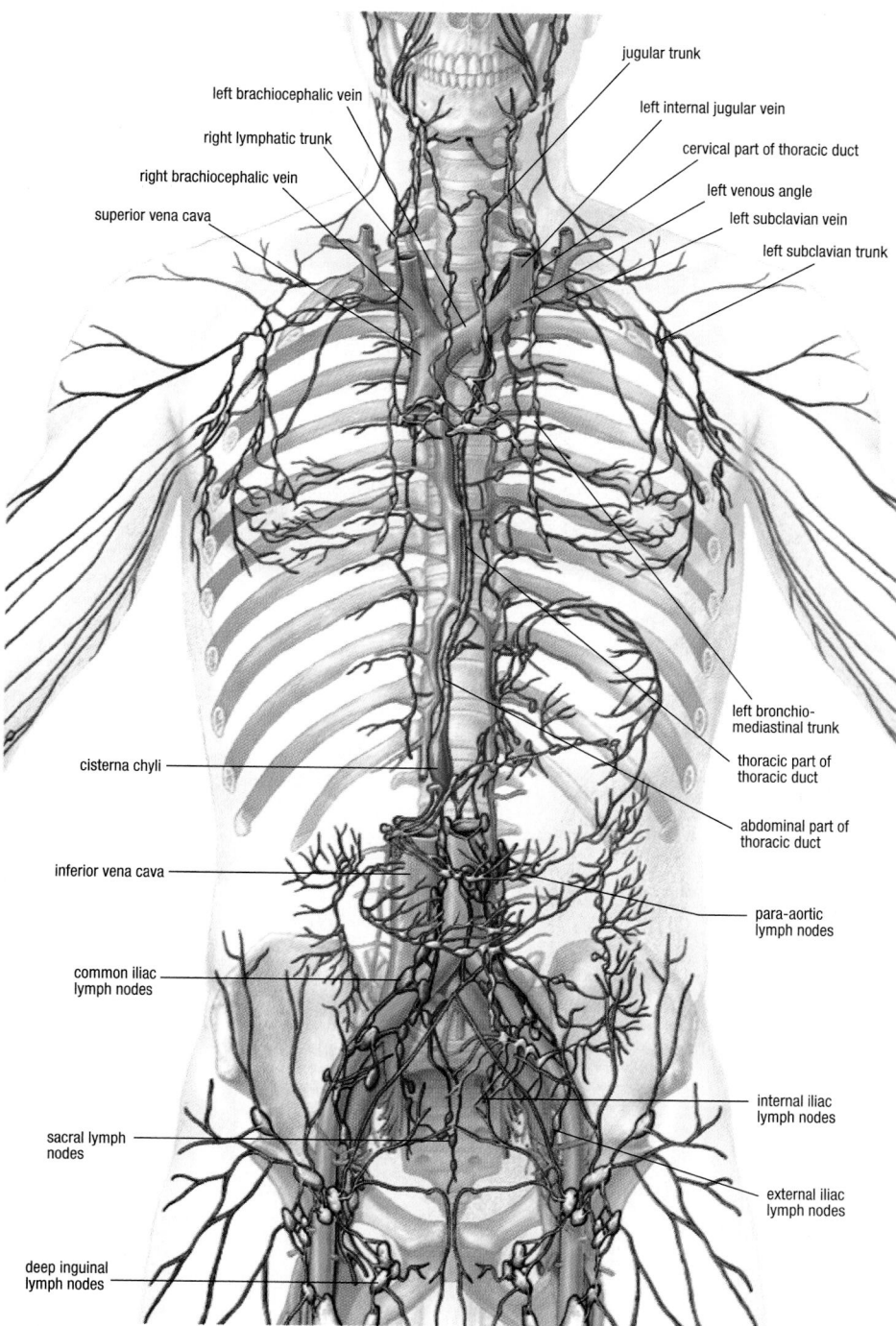

jugular trunk

left brachiocephalic vein

left internal jugular vein

right lymphatic trunk

cervical part of thoracic duct

right brachiocephalic vein

left venous angle

superior vena cava

left subclavian vein

left subclavian trunk

left bronchio-mediastinal trunk

cisterna chyli

thoracic part of thoracic duct

abdominal part of thoracic duct

inferior vena cava

para-aortic lymph nodes

common iliac lymph nodes

internal iliac lymph nodes

sacral lymph nodes

external iliac lymph nodes

deep inguinal lymph nodes

ANATOMY

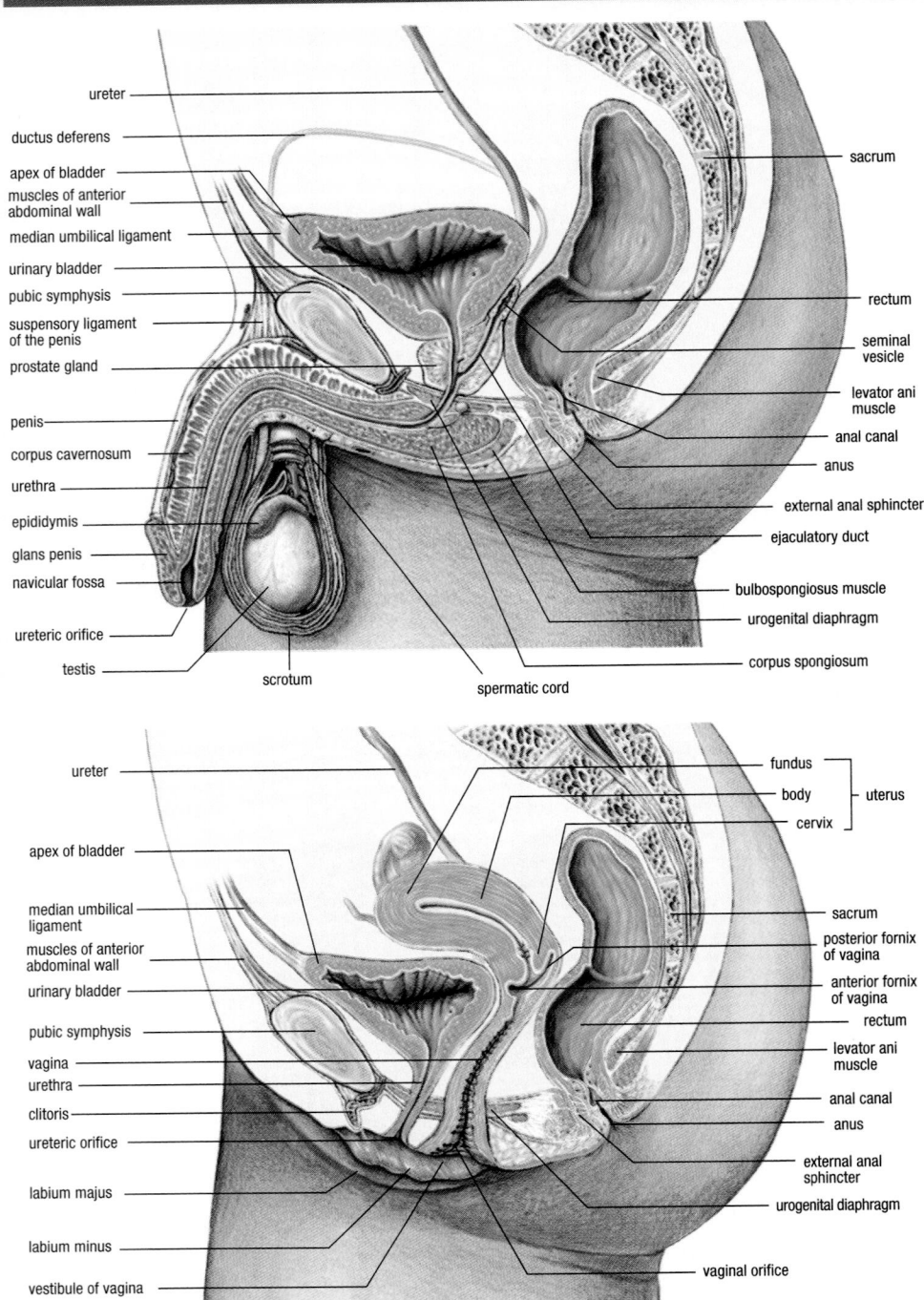

ureter

ductus deferens

apex of bladder

muscles of anterior abdominal wall

median umbilical ligament

urinary bladder

pubic symphysis

suspensory ligament of the penis

prostate gland

penis

corpus cavernosum

urethra

epididymis

glans penis

navicular fossa

ureteric orifice

testis

scrotum

spermatic cord

sacrum

rectum

seminal vesicle

levator ani muscle

anal canal

anus

external anal sphincter

ejaculatory duct

bulbospongiosus muscle

urogenital diaphragm

corpus spongiosum

ureter

apex of bladder

median umbilical ligament

muscles of anterior abdominal wall

urinary bladder

pubic symphysis

vagina

urethra

clitoris

ureteric orifice

labium majus

labium minus

vestibule of vagina

fundus

body — uterus

cervix

sacrum

posterior fornix of vagina

anterior fornix of vagina

rectum

levator ani muscle

anal canal

anus

external anal sphincter

urogenital diaphragm

vaginal orifice

sentinel g., a single enlarged lymph node in the omentum that may be an indication of an ulcer opposite to it in the greater or lesser curvature of the stomach.

seromucous g., (1) a gland in which some of the secretory cells are serous and some mucous; **(2)** a gland whose cells secrete a fluid intermediate between a watery and a viscous mucoid substance.

serous g., a gland that secretes a watery substance that may or may not contain an enzyme.

sublingual g., one of two salivary glands in the floor of the mouth beneath the tongue, discharging through the sublingual ducts; most of the secretory units in the human gland are mucus-secreting with serous demilunes.

submandibular g., one of two salivary glands in the neck, located in the space bounded by the two bellies of the digastric muscle and the angle of the mandible; it discharges through the submandibular duct; the secretory units are predominantly serous although a few mucous alveoli, some with serous demilunes, occur. SYN maxillary g.

suprarenal g., a flattened, roughly triangular body resting upon the upper end of each kidney; it is one of the ductless glands furnishing internal secretions (epinephrine and norepinephrine from the medulla and steroid hormones from the cortex). SYN adrenal g., epinephros, paranephros.

sweat g.'s, the coil glands of the skin that secrete the sweat.

target g., the effector that functions when stimulated by the internal secretion of another gland or by some other stimulus.

tarsal g.'s, sebaceous glands embedded in the tarsal plate of each eyelid, discharging at the edge of the lid near the posterior border. Their secretions create a lipid barrier along the margin of the eyelids which contains the normal secretions in the conjunctival sac by preventing the watery fluid from spilling over the barrier when the eye is open. SYN meibomian g.'s.

thymus g., SYN thymus.

thyroid g., a ductless gland, consisting of irregularly spheroidal follicles, lying in front and to the sides of the upper part of the trachea, and of horseshoe shape, with two lateral lobes connected by a narrow central portion, the isthmus; occasionally an elongated offshoot, the pyramidal lobe, passes upward from the isthmus in front of the trachea. It is supplied by branches from the external carotid and subclavian arteries, and its nerves are derived from the middle cervical and cervicothoracic ganglia of the sympathetic system. It secretes thyroid hormone and calcitonin.

tubular g., a g. composed of one or more tubules ending in a blind extremity.

tubuloacinar g., a g. whose secretory elements are elongated acini. SYN acinotubular g.

unicellular g., a single secretory cell such as a mucous goblet cell.

urethral g.'s, SEE g.'s of the female urethra, g.'s of the male urethra.

uterine g.'s, numerous simple tubular glands in the uterine mucosa that secrete a glycogen-rich

mucous fluid during the luteal phase of the menstrual cycle.

vaginal g., one of the mucous g.'s in the mucous membrane of the vagina.

glan·des (glan'dēz). Plural of glans.

glan·di·lem·ma (glan-di-lem'ă). The capsule of a gland. [L. *glandula,* gland, + G. *lemma,* sheath]

glan·du·la, pl. **glan·du·lae** (glan-dū-lă, -lē). **1** [NA]. SYN gland. **2.** SYN glandule. [L. gland, dim. of *glans,* acorn]

glan′dulae cerumino′sae [NA], **(1)** SYN ceruminous glands, under gland. **(2)** tubuloalveolar glands of the external auditory meatus believed to be modified apocrine sweat glands; they secrete cerumen.

glan·du·lar (glan'dū-lăr). Relating to a gland. SYN glandulous.

glan·dule (glan'dūl). A small gland. SYN glandula (2). [L. *glandula*]

glan·du·lous (glan'dū-lŭs). SYN glandular.

glans, pl. **glan·des** (glanz, glan'dēz) [NA]. A conical acorn-shaped structure. [L. acorn]

g. of clitoris, a small mass of highly-sensitized erectile tissue capping the body of the clitoris.

g. pe′nis [NA], the conical expansion of the corpus spongiosum which forms the head of the penis.

gla·se·ri·an (gla-ser'ē-an). Relating to or described by Johann H. Glaser.

glass. A transparent substance composed of silica and oxides of various bases. [A.S. *glaes*]

cupping g., a g. vessel, from which the air has been exhausted by heat or a special suction apparatus, formerly applied to the skin in order to draw blood to the surface. SEE ALSO cupping, cup. SYN cup (2).

glass·es (glas'ez). **1.** SYN spectacles. **2.** Lenses for correcting refractive errors in the eyes.

glau·co·ma (glaw-kō'mă). A disease of the eye characterized by increased intraocular pressure and excavation and atrophy of the optic nerve; produces defects in the visual field and may result in blindness. [G. *glaukōma,* opacity of the crystalline lens, fr. *glaukos,* bluish green]

angle-closure g., primary g. in which contact of the iris with the peripheral cornea excludes aqueous humor from the trabecular drainage meshwork. SYN narrow-angle g.

combined g., g. with angle-closure and open-angle mechanisms in the same eye.

congenital g., SYN buphthalmia.

narrow-angle g., SYN angle-closure g.

open-angle g., primary g. in which the aqueous humor has free access to the trabecular meshwork. SYN simple g., g. simplex.

phacogenic g., SYN phacomorphic g.

phacomorphic g., secondary g. caused by either excessive size or spherical shape of the lens. SYN phacogenic g.

secondary g., g. occurring as a sequel of preexisting ocular disease or injury.

simple g., g. sim′plex, SYN open-angle g.

glau·co·ma·tous (glaw-kō'mă-tŭs). Relating to glaucoma.

GLC gas-liquid *chromatography.*

Glc, GlcA, GlcN, GlcNAc, GlcUA. Symbols for the radicals of D-glucose, gluconic and glucu-

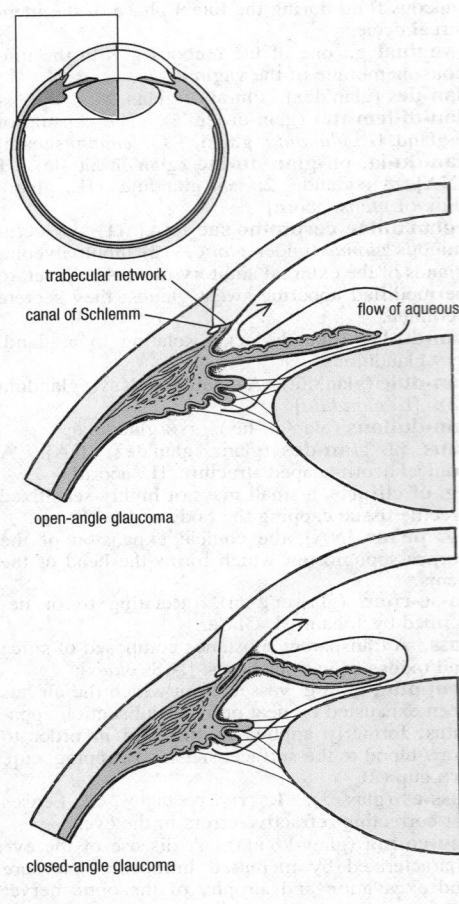

trabecular network

canal of Schlemm

flow of aqueous

open-angle glaucoma

closed-angle glaucoma

glaucoma

ronic acid, glucosamine, *N*-acetylglucosamine, and glucuronic acid, respectively.

gle·no·hu·mer·al (glē′nō-hyū′mer-ăl). Relating to the glenoid cavity and the humerus.

gle·noid (glē′noyd, glen′oyd). Resembling a socket; denoting the articular depression of the scapula entering into the formation of the shoulder joint. [G. *glēnoeidēs,* fr. *glēnē,* pupil of eye, socket of joint, honeycomb, + *eidos,* appearance]

glia (glī′ă). SYN neuroglia. [G. glue]

gli·a·cyte (glī′ă-sīt). A neuroglia cell. SEE neuroglia. [G. *glia,* glue, + *kytos,* cell]

gli·a·din (glī′ă-din). A class of protein, separable from wheat and rye glutens, that contains up to 40% L-glutamine; a member of the prolamins, which are insoluble in water, absolute alcohol, and neutral solvents, but soluble in 50 to 90% alcohol.

gli·al (glī′ăl). Pertaining to glia or neuroglia.

△**glio-**. Glue, gluelike (relating specifically to the neuroglia). [G. *glia,* glue]

gli·o·blast (glī′ō-blast). An early neural cell developing, like the neuroblast, from the early ep-

endymal cell of the neural tube; gives rise to neuroglial and ependymal cells, astrocytes, and oligodendrocytes. SEE ALSO spongioblast. [glio- + G. *blastos,* germ]

gli·o·blas·to·ma multiforme (glī′ō-blas-tō′mă). A glioma consisting chiefly of undifferentiated anaplastic cells of glial origin that show marked nuclear pleomorphism, necrosis, and vascular endothelial proliferation; frequently, tumor cells are arranged radially about an irregular focus of necrosis; these neoplasms grow rapidly, invade extensively, and occur most frequently in the cerebrum of adults. SYN grade IV astrocytoma. [G. *glia,* glue, + *blastos,* germ, + *-oma,* tumor]

gli·o·ma (glī-ō′mă). Any neoplasm derived from one of the various types of cells that form the interstitial tissue of the brain, spinal cord, pineal gland, posterior pituitary gland, and retina. [G. *glia,* glue, + *-oma,* tumor]

gli·o·ma·to·sis (glī-ō-mă-tō′sis). Neoplastic growth of neuroglial cells in the brain or spinal cord; the term is used especially with reference to a relatively large neoplasm or to multiple foci. SYN neurogliomatosis.

gli·o·ma·tous (glī-ō′mă-tŭs). Pertaining to or characterized by a glioma.

gli·o·neu·ro·ma (glī′ō-nū-rō′mă). A ganglioneuroma derived from neurons, with numerous glial cells and fibers in the matrix.

gli·o·sar·co·ma (glī′ō-sar-kō′mă). A glioblastoma multiforme with an associated malignant mesenchymal component. Sometimes used as a term for a malignant neoplasm derived from connective tissue (*e.g.,* that associated with blood vessels in the brain) in which there are proliferating glial cells.

gli·o·sis (glī-ō′sis). Overgrowth of the astrocytes in an area of damage in the brain or spinal cord.

Gln glutamine or its acyl radical, glutaminyl.

glob·al (glō′băl). Complete, generalized, overall, or total.

glo·bi (glō′bī). **1.** Plural of globus. **2.** Brown bodies sometimes found in the granulomatous lesions of leprosy.

glo·bin (glō′bin). The protein of hemoglobin; α-g. and β-g. represent the two types of chains found in adult hemoglobin. SYN hematohiston.

glo·bo·side (glō′bō-sīd). A glycosphingolipid isolated from kidney and erythrocytes; accumulates in individuals with Sandhoff's disease.

glob·ule (glob′yūl). **1.** A small spherical body of any kind. **2.** A fat droplet in milk. [L. *globulus,* dim. of *globus,* a ball]

glob·u·lin (glob′yū-lin). Name for a family of proteins precipitated from plasma by ammonium sulfate. G.'s may be further fractionated by solubility, electrophoresis, ultracentrifugation, and other separation methods into many subgroups, the main groups being α-, β-, and γ-g.; these differ with respect to their content of physiologically important factors. Among the latter are immunoglobulins, lipoproteins, gluco- or mucoproteins, and metal-binding and metal-transporting proteins. [L. *globulus,* globule]

accelerator g. (AcG, ac-g) [MIM*227300], g. in serum that promotes the conversion of prothrombin to thrombin in the presence of thromboplastin and ionized calcium. SEE *factor* V, serum accelerator g.

    antihemophilic g. A, SYN *factor* VIII.

    antihemophilic g. B, SYN *factor* IX.

    antihuman g., serum from a rabbit or other animal previously immunized with purified human g. to prepare antibodies directed against IgG and complement; used in the direct and indirect Coombs' tests. SYN Coombs' serum.

    β_{1C} **g.,** the third component (C3) of complement. SEE *component* of complement.

    β_{1E} **g.,** the fourth component (C4) of complement. SEE *component* of complement.

    β_{1F} **g.,** the fifth component (C5) of complement. SEE *component* of complement.

    corticosteroid-binding g. (CBG), SYN transcortin.

    hepatitis B immune g. (HBIG), a high-titer passive immune g. directed against type B hepatitis virus. Passive immunity to type B hepatitis can be conferred by administration of this immune serum g. It is recommended for those exposed to fluids from persons infected with HBV.

    human gamma g., a preparation of the proteins of liquid human plasma, containing the antibodies of normal adults; it is obtained from pooled liquid human plasma from a number of donors.

    plasma accelerator g., SYN *factor* V.

    Rh-immune g. (RhIG), a concentrated solution of IgG anti-D that is administered to an Rh-negative person who has been exposed to Rh-positive red cells, particularly a woman who may be carrying an Rh-positive fetus, or has delivered or aborted an Rh-negative baby, to counteract the immunizing effect of the cells.

    serum accelerator g., a substance in serum that accelerates the conversion of prothrombin to thrombin in the presence of thromboplastin and calcium.

glob·u·li·nu·ria (glob′yū-li-nū′rē-ă). The excretion of globulin in the urine, usually, if not always, in association with serum albumin.

glo·bus, pl. **glo·bi** (glō′bŭs, -bī). **1** [NA]. A round body; ball. **2.** SEE globi. [L.]

    g. hyster′icus, difficulty in swallowing; a sensation as of a ball in the throat or as if the throat were compressed; a symptom of conversion *disorder.*

    g. pal′lidus [NA], the inner and lighter gray portion of the lentiform nucleus. SEE ALSO paleostriatum. SYN pallidum.

glo·mal (glō′măl). Relating to or involving a glomus.

glo·man·gi·o·ma (glō-man-jē-ō′mă). A variant of glomus *tumor,* characterized by multiple tumors resembling cavernous hemangioma.

glo·man·gi·o·sis (glō-man-jē-ō′sis). The occurrence of multiple complexes of small vascular channels, each resembling a glomus.

glo·mec·to·my (glō-mek′tō-mē). Excision of a glomus tumor. [L. *glomus* + G. *ektomē,* cutting out]

glom·era (glom′er-ă). Plural of glomus.

glo·mer·u·lar (glō-mār′yū-lăr). Relating to or affecting a glomerulus or the glomeruli.

glom·er·ule (glom′er-yūl). SYN glomerulus.

glo·mer·u·li·tis (glō-mār′yū-lī′tis). Inflammation of a glomerulus, specifically of the renal glomeruli, as in glomerulonephritis.

glo·mer·u·lo·ne·phri·tis (glō-mār′yū-lō-nef-rī′tis). Renal disease characterized by inflammatory changes in glomeruli which are not the result of infection of the kidneys. SYN glomerular nephritis. [glomerulus + G. *nephros,* kidney, + -*itis,* inflammation]

    anti-basement membrane g., g. resulting from anti-basement membrane antibodies, characterized by smooth linear deposits of IgG and C3 along glomerular capillary walls; includes rapidly progressive g. and g. in Goodpasture's syndrome.

    focal g., g. affecting a small proportion of renal glomeruli which commonly presents with hematuria and may be associated with acute upper respiratory infection in young males, not usually due to streptococci; associated with IgA deposits in the glomerular mesangium and may also be associated with systemic disease, as in Henoch-Schönlein purpura. SYN Berger's disease.

    lobular g., SYN membranoproliferative g.

    membranoproliferative g., chronic g. characterized by mesangial cell proliferation, increased lobular separation of glomeruli, thickening of glomerular capillary walls and increased mesangial matrix, and low serum levels of complement; occurs mainly in older children, with a variably slow progressive course, episodes of hematuria or edema, and hypertension. SYN lobular g.

    membranous g., g. characterized by diffuse thickening of glomerular capillary basement membranes, due in part to subepithelial deposits of immunoglobulins separated by spikes of basement membrane material, and clinically by an insidious onset of the nephrotic syndrome and failure of disappearance of proteinuria; the disease is most commonly idiopathic but may be secondary to malignant tumors, drugs, infections, or systemic lupus erythematosus.

    mesangial proliferative g., g. characterized clinically by the nephrotic syndrome and histologically by diffuse glomerular increases in endocapillary and mesangial cells and in mesangial matrix; in some cases, there are mesangial deposits of IgM and complement.

glo·mer·u·lop·a·thy (glō-mār-yū-lop′ă-thē). Glomerular disease of any type. [glomerulus + G. *pathos,* suffering]

glo·mer·u·lo·scle·ro·sis (glō-mār′yū-lō-sklĕ-rō′sis). Hyaline deposits or scarring within the renal glomeruli, a degenerative process occurring in association with renal arteriosclerosis or diabetes. [glomerulus + G. *sklērōsis,* hardness]

    diabetic g., rounded hyaline or laminated nodules in the periphery of the glomeruli with capillary basement membrane thickening and increased mesangial matrix occurring in long-standing diabetes, proteinuria, and ultimately renal failure. SYN intercapillary g.

    focal segmental g., segmental collapse of glomerular capillaries with thickened basement membranes and increased mesangial matrix; seen in some glomeruli of patients with nephrotic syndrome or mesangial proliferative glomerulonephritis.

intercapillary g., SYN diabetic g.

glo•mer•u•lus, pl. **glo•mer•u•li** (glō-mār′yū-lŭs, -yū-lī) [NA]. **1.** A plexus of capillaries. **2.** A tuft formed of capillary loops at the beginning of each nephric tubule in the kidney; this tuft with its capsule (Bowman's capsule) constitutes the corpusculum renis (malpighian body). **3.** The twisted secretory portion of a sweat gland. **4.** A cluster of dendritic ramifications and axon terminals forming a complex synaptic relationship and surrounded by a glial sheath. SYN glomerule. [Mod. L. dim. of L. *glomus,* a ball of yarn]

glo•mus, pl. **glom•era** (glō′mŭs, glom′er-ă). **1** [NA]. A small globular body. **2.** A highly organized arteriolovenular anastomosis forming a tiny nodular focus in the nailbed, pads of the fingers and toes, ears, hands, and feet and many other organs of the body. The afferent arteriole enters the connective tissue capsule of the g., becomes devoid of an internal elastic membrane, and develops a relatively thick epithelioid muscular wall and small lumen; the anastomosis may be branched and convoluted, richly innervated with sympathetic and myelinated nerves, and connected with a short, thin-walled vein that drains into a periglomic vein and then into one of the veins of the skin. The g. functions as a shunt- or bypass-regulating mechanism in the flow of blood, temperature, and conservation of heat in the part as well as in the indirect control of the blood pressure and other functions of the circulatory system. [L. *glomus,* a ball]

   g. aorticum, SYN aortic *body.*

   choroid g., a marked enlargement of the choroid plexus of the lateral ventricle at the junction of the central part with the inferior horn.

   jugular g., a microscopic collection of chemoreceptor tissue in the adventitia of the jugular bulb; a tumor of this g. may cause paralysis of the vocal cords, attacks of dizziness, blackouts, and nystagmus.

△**gloss-.** SEE glosso-.

glos•sa (glos′ă). SYN tongue (1). [G.]

glos•sal (glos′ăl). SYN lingual (1).

glos•sal•gia (glos-al′jē-ă). SYN glossodynia. [gloss- + G. *algos,* pain]

glos•sec•to•my (glo-sek′tō-mē). Resection or amputation of the tongue. SYN lingulectomy (1). [gloss- + G. *ektomē,* excision]

Glos•si•na (glo-sī′nă). A genus of bloodsucking Diptera (tsetse flies) confined to Africa; they serve as vectors of the trypanosomes that cause African sleeping sickness. [G. *glōssa,* tongue]

glos•si•tis (glo-sī′tis). Inflammation of the tongue. [gloss- + G. *-itis,* inflammation]

   g. area′ta exfoliati′va, SYN geographic *tongue.*

   median rhomboid g., an asymptomatic, ovoid or rhomboid, macular or mamillated, erythematous lesion with papillary atrophy on the dorsum of the tongue just anterior to the circumvallate papillae; thought to represent a persistent tuberculum impar.

△**glosso-, gloss-.** Language; corresponds to L. *linguo-.* Cf. linguo-. [G. *glōssa,* tongue]

glos•so•cele (glos′ō-sēl). Protrusion of the tongue from the mouth, owing to its excessive size. SEE ALSO macroglossia. [glosso- + G. *kēlē,* tumor, hernia]

glos•so•dyn•ia (glos′ō-din′ē-ă). A condition characterized by burning or painful tongue. SYN glossalgia. [glosso- + G. *odynē,* pain]

glos•so•ep•i•glot•tic, glos•so•ep•i•glot•tid•e•an (glos′ō-ep-i-glot′ik, glos′ō-ep-i-glo-tid′ē-an). Relating to the tongue and the epiglottis.

glos•so•hy•al (glos-ō-hī′ăl). SYN hyoglossal.

glos•so•la•lia (glos-ō-lā′lē-ă). Rarely used term for unintelligible jargon or babbling. [glosso- + G. *lalia,* talk, chat]

glos•sop•a•thy (glos-op′ă-thē). A disease of the tongue. [glosso- + G. *pathos,* suffering]

glos•so•pha•ryn•ge•al (glos′ō-fă-rin′jē-ăl). Relating to the tongue and the pharynx.

glos•so•plas•ty (glos′ō-plas-tē). Plastic surgery of the tongue. [glosso- + G. *plastos,* formed]

glos•sor•rha•phy (glo-sōr′ă-fē). Suture of a wound of the tongue. [glosso- + G. *rhaphē,* suture]

glos•so•spasm (glos′ō-spazm). Spasmodic contraction of the tongue.

glos•sot•o•my (glo-sot′ō-mē). Any cutting operation on the tongue, usually to obtain access to further reaches of the pharynx. [glosso- + G. *tomē,* incision]

glos•so•trich•ia (glos-ō-trik′ē-ă). SYN hairy *tongue.* [glosso- + G. *thrix,* hair]

glot•tal (glot′ăl). Relating to the glottis.

glottal fry. vocal fold vibration in the lowest part of the pitch range, characterized by a creaky, pulsed type of phonation. SYN gravel voice, vocal fry.

glot•tic (glot′ik). Relating to (1) the tongue or (2) the glottis.

glot•tis, pl. **glot•ti•des** (glot′is, glot′i-dēz) [NA]. The vocal apparatus of the larynx, consisting of the vocal folds of mucous membrane investing the vocal ligament and vocal muscle on each side, the free edges of which are the vocal cords, and of a median fissure, the rima glottidis. [G. *glōttis,* aperture of the larynx]

glot•ti•tis (glo-tī′tis). Inflammation of the glottic portion of the larynx.

Glu glutamic acid or its acyl radical, glutamyl.

glu•ca•gon (glū′kă-gon). A hormone produced by pancreatic alpha cells. Parenteral administration of 0.5 to 1 mg results in prompt mobilization of hepatic glycogen, thus elevating blood glucose concentration. It is used in the treatment of glycogen storage disease (von Gierke's) and hypoglycemia, particularly hypoglycemic coma due to exogenously administered insulin. [glucose + G. *agō,* to lead]

glu•ca•gon•o•ma (glū′kă-gon-ō′mă). A glucagon-secreting tumor, usually derived from pancreatic islet cells.

glu•can (glū′kan). A polyglucose; *e.g.,* callose, cellulose, starch amylose, glycogen amylose.

1,4-α-D-glu•can 6-α-D-glu•co•syl•trans•fer•ase. A glucosyltransferase that transfers an α-glucosyl residue in a 1,4-α-glucan to the primary hydroxyl group of glucose in a 1,4-α-glucan.

4-α-Dβ-glucanotransferase. A 4-glycosyltransferase which converts maltodextrins into amylose and glucose by transferring parts of 1,4-glucan chains to new 4-positions on glucose or other 1,4-glucans.

gluco-. glucose. SEE ALSO glyco-. [G. *gleukos,* sweet new wine, sweetness]

glu•co•cer•e•bro•side (glū-kō-ser′ĕ-brō-sīd). SYN glucosylceramide.

glu•co•cor•ti•coid (glū-kō-kōr′ti-koyd). **1.** Any steroid-like compound capable of promoting hepatic glycogen deposition and of exerting a clinically useful anti-inflammatory effect. Cortisol is the most potent of the naturally occurring g.'s; most semisynthetic g.'s are cortisol derivatives. **2.** Denoting this type of biological activity. SYN glycocorticoid.

glu•co•fu•ra•nose (glū-kō-fūr′ă-nōs). Glucose in furanose form.

glu•co•gen•e•sis (glū-kō-jen′ĕ-sis). Formation of glucose. [gluco- + G. *genesis,* production]

glu•co•gen•ic (glū-kō-jen′ik). Giving rise to or producing glucose.

glu•co•ki•nase (glū-kō-kī′nās). Phosphotransferase that catalyzes the conversion of D-glucose and ATP D-glucose 6-phosphate and ADP; the liver enzyme has a higher K_m value for D-glucose than does hexokinase.

glu•co•ki•net•ic (glū′kō-ki-net′ik). Tending to mobilize glucose; usually evidenced by a reduction of the glycogen stores in the tissues to produce an increase in the concentration of glucose circulating in the blood.

glu•co•lip•ids (glū-kō-lip′idz). Glycosphingolipids that contain D-glucose.

glu•co•ne•o•gen•e•sis (glū′kō-nē-ō-jen′ĕ-sis). The formation of glucose from noncarbohydrates, such as protein or fat. Cf. glyconeogenesis.

glu•con•ic ac•id (glū-kon′ik). The hexonic (aldonic) acid derived from glucose by oxidation of the –CHO group to –COOH.

glu•co•pro•tein (glū-kō-prō′tēn). A glycoprotein in which the sugar is glucose.

glu•co•pyr•a•nose (glū-kō-pir′ă-nōs). Glucose in its pyranose form.

glu•co•sans (glū′kō-sanz). Polysaccharides yielding glucose upon hydrolysis; *e.g.,* cellulose, glycogen, starch, dextrins.

glu•cose (glū′kōs). A dextrorotatory monosaccharide found in the free form in fruits and other parts of plants, and in combination in glucosides, glycogen, disaccharides, and polysaccharides (starch cellulose); the chief source of energy in human metabolism, the final product of carbohydrate digestion, and the principal sugar of the blood; insulin is required for the use of glucose by cells; in diabetes mellitus the level of glucose in the blood is excessive, and it also appears in the urine. SYN D-glucose.

D-glu•cose (G, Glc) (glū′kōs). SYN glucose.

glu•cose 6-phos•phate. An ester of glucose with phosphoric acid; made in the course of glucose metabolism by mammalian and other cells; a normal constituent of resting muscle.

glu•co•si•das•es (glū′kō-sid-ās-ez). Enzymes that hydrolyze glucosides.

glu•co•side (glū′kō-sīd). A compound of glucose with an alcohol or other R–OH compound involving loss of the H atom of the 1-OH (hemiace-tal) group of the glucose, yielding a –C–O–R link from the C-1 of the glucose; a glycoside of glucose.

glu•cos•u•ria (glū-kō-sū′rē-ă). The urinary excretion of glucose, usually in enhanced quantities. SYN glycosuria (1), glycuresis (1). [glucose + G. *ouron,* urine]

glu•co•syl•cer•a•mide (glū′kō-sil-ser′ă-mīd). A neutral glycolipid containing equimolar amounts of fatty acid, glucose, and sphingosine (or a derivative thereof); accumulates in individuals with Gaucher disease. SYN glucocerebroside.

glu•co•syl•trans•fer•ase (glū′kō-sil-trans′fer-ās). Any enzyme transferring glucosyl groups from one compound to another.

glu•cu•ro•nate (glū-kūr′ō-nāt). A salt or ester of glucuronic acid.

glu•cu•ron•ic ac•id (glū-kū-ron′ik). The uronic acid of glucose in which C-6 is oxidized to a carboxyl group; the D-isomer detoxicates or inactivates various substances (*e.g.,* benzoic acid, phenol, camphor, and the female sex hormones), the glucuronides so formed being excreted in the urine.

β-D-glu•cu•ron•i•dase (glū-kū-ron′i-dās). An enzyme catalyzing the hydrolysis of various β-D-glucuronides, liberating free D-glucuronic acid and an alcohol; a deficiency of this enzyme is associated with Sly syndrome.

glu•cu•ro•nide (glū-kū′ron-īd). A glycoside of glucuronic acid; many foreign chemicals, as well as catabolic products of normal body constituents (*e.g.,* steroid hormones), are commonly excreted in the urine as D-g.'s, the conjugation taking place in the liver.

glue-sniff•ing (glū′snif-ing). Inhalation of fumes from plastic cements; the solvents, which include toluene, xylene, and benzene, induce central nervous system stimulation followed by depression.

glu•ta•mate (glū′tă-māt). A salt or ester of glutamic acid.

glu•tam•ic ac•id (E, Glu) (glū-tam′ik). An amino acid that occurs in proteins; the sodium salt is monosodium glutamate. Cf. glutamate.

glu•tam•ic-ox•a•lo•ace•tic trans•am•i•nase (GOT). SYN *aspartate* aminotransferase.

glu•tam•ic-py•ru•vic trans•am•i•nase (GPT). SYN alanine aminotransferase.

glu•ta•min•ase (glū-tam′in-ās). An enzyme in kidney and other tissues that catalyzes the hydrolysis of L-glutamine to ammonia and L-glutamic acid; an important enzyme for urinary ammonia formation.

glu•ta•mine (Gln, Q) (glū′tă-mēn, -tă-min, glū-tam′in). The δ-amide of glutamic acid, derived by oxidation from proline in the liver or by the combination of glutamic acid with ammonia; the L-isomer is present in proteins and in blood and other tissues, and is an important source of urinary ammonia.

glu•tam•i•nyl (Gln, Q) (glū-tam′i-nil). The acyl radical of glutamine.

glu•tam•o•yl (glū-tam′ō-il). The radical of glutamic acid from which both α- and δ-hydroxyl groups have been removed.

glu•tam•yl (E, Glu) (glū-tam′il, glū′tă-mil). The

radical of glutamic acid from which either the α- or the δ-hydroxyl group has been removed.

glutaraldehyde. High-level disinfectant. EPA-registered as a sterilant/disinfectant chemical.

glu·tar·ic ac·id (glū-tar′ik). An intermediate in tryptophan catabolism; accumulates in glutaric acidemia.

glu·ta·thi·one (GSH) (glū-tă-thī′ōn). **1.** γ-L-Glutamyl-L-cysteinylglycine; G. has a wide variety of roles in a cell. A deficiency of g. can cause hemolysis with oxidative stress. **2.** The principal low molecular weight thiol compound of living plant cells; used in the course of intermediary metabolism as a donor of thiol (SH) groups; essential for detoxification of acetaminophen.

glu·te·al (glū′tē-ăl). Relating to the buttocks. [G. *gloutos,* buttock]

glu·ten (glū′těn). The insoluble protein (prolamines) constituent of wheat and other grains; a mixture of gliadin, glutenin, and other proteins; the presence of g. allows flour to rise. [L. *gluten,* glue]

glu·te·o·fem·o·ral (glū′tē-ō-fem′ō-răl). Relating to the buttock and the thigh.

glu·ti·nous (glū′tin-ŭs). Sticky.

glu·ti·tis (glū-tī′tis). Inflammation of the muscles of the buttock. [G. *gloutos,* buttock, + *-itis,* inflammation]

Gly glycine or its acyl radical, glycyl.

gly·can (glī′kan). SYN polysaccharide.

gly·ce·mia (glī-sē′mē-ă). The presence of glucose in the blood. [G. *glykys,* sweet, + *haima,* blood]

glyc·er·al·de·hyde (glis-er-al′dě-hīd). A triose and the simplest optically active aldose; the dextrorotatory isomer is taken as the structural reference point for all D compounds, the levorotatory isomer for all L compounds.

gly·cer·ic ac·id (gli-ser′ik, glis′er-ik). The fatty acid analog of glycerol; occurs particularly in the form of phosphorylated derivatives, as an intermediate in glycolysis.

L-gly·cer·ic ac·i·du·ria. Excretion of L-glyceric acid in the urine; a primary metabolic error due to deficiency of D-glyceric dehydrogenase resulting in excretion of L-glyceric and oxalic acids, leading to the clinical syndrome of oxalosis with frequent formation of oxalate renal calculi.

glyc·er·i·das·es (glis′er-ĭ-dās-ez). General term for enzymes catalyzing the hydrolysis of glycerol esters (glycerides); *e.g.,* triacylglycerol lipase.

glyc·er·ide (glis′er-id, -īd). An ester of glycerol.

glyc·er·in (glis′er-in). SYN glycerol.

glyc·er·ol (glis′er-ol). A sweet oily fluid obtained by the saponification of fats and fixed oils; used as a solvent, as a skin emollient, by injection or in the form of suppository for constipation, orally to reduce ocular tension, and as a vehicle and sweetening agent. SYN glycerin.

glyc·er·yl (glis′er-il). The trivalent radical, $C_3H_5^{\equiv}$, of glycerol; often used in error for glycero- or glycerol.

gly·cine (G, Gly) (glī′sēn). $^+NH_3-CH_2-COO^-$; the simplest amino acid; a major component of gelatin and silk fibroin; used as a nutrient and dietary supplement, and in solution for irrigation; used in the treatment of sweaty feet syndrome.

g. amidinotransferase, an enzyme catalyzing the transfer of an amidine group from L-arginine to glycine, forming guanidinoacetate and L-ornithine; an important reaction in creatine synthesis; it can also act on canavanine.

gly·ci·nu·ria (glī-si-nū′rē-ă). The excretion of glycine in the urine. [glycine + G. *ouron,* urine]

△**glyco-.** Combining form denoting relationship to sugars (*e.g.,* glycogen), or to glycine (*e.g.,* glycocholate). SEE ALSO gluco-. [G. *glykys,* sweet]

gly·co·ca·lyx (glī-kō-kā′liks). A PAS-positive filamentous coating on the apical surface of certain epithelial cells, composed of carbohydrate moieties of proteins that protrude from the free surface of the plasma membrane. [glyco- + G. *kalyx,* husk, shell]

gly·co·cho·late (glī-kō-kō′lāt). A salt or ester of glycocholic acid.

gly·co·cho·lic ac·id (glī-kō-kō′lik). N-Cholylglycine; one of the major bile acid conjugates, formed by condensation of the —COOH group of cholic acid and the amino group of glycine; water-soluble and a powerful detergent.

gly·co·cor·ti·coid (glī′kō-kōr′ti-koyd). SYN glucocorticoid.

gly·co·gen (glī′kō-jen). A glucosan of high molecular weight, resembling amylopectin in structure (with α(1,4 linkages) but even more highly branched (α(1,6 linkages), found in most of the tissues of the body, especially those of the liver and muscle; as the principal carbohydrate reserve, it is readily converted into glucose.

gly·co·gen·e·sis (glī-kō-jen′ě-sis). Formation of glycogen from D-glucose by means of glycogen synthase and dextrin dextranase; the first enzyme catalyzes formation of a polyglucose with α-1,4 links from UDP glucose, the second cleaves fragments from one chain and transfers them to an α-1,6 linkage in another. [glyco- + G. *genesis,* production]

gly·co·ge·net·ic (glī′kō-jě-net′ik). Glycogenic (2); relating to glycogenesis.

gly·co·gen·ol·y·sis (glī′kō-jě-nol′i-sis). The hydrolysis of glycogen to glucose.

gly·co·ge·no·sis (glī′kō-jě-nō′sis). Any glycogen deposition disease characterized by accumulation of glycogen of normal or abnormal chemical structure in tissue; there may be enlargement of the liver, heart, or striated muscle, including the tongue, with progressive muscular weakness. SYN dextrinosis.

type 1 g., g. due to glucose 6-phosphatase deficiency, resulting in accumulation of excessive amounts of glycogen of normal chemical structure, particularly in liver and kidney. SYN Gierke's disease, von Gierke's disease.

type 2 g., g. due to lysosomal α-1,4-glucosidase deficiency, resulting in accumulation of excessive amounts of glycogen of normal chemical structure in heart, muscle, liver, and nervous system. SYN Pompe's disease.

type 3 g., g. due to amylo-1,6-glucosidase deficiency, resulting in accumulation of abnormal glycogen with short outer chains in liver and muscle. SYN Cori's disease.

type 5 g., g. due to muscle glycogen phosphorylase deficiency, resulting in accumulation of glycogen of normal chemical structure in muscle. SYN McArdle's disease, McArdle-Schmid-Pearson disease.

type 6 g., g. due to hepatic glycogen phosphorylase deficiency, resulting in accumulation of glycogen of normal chemical structure in liver and leukocytes.

glycohemoglobin (gli-ko-he-mo-glo-bin). Any one of four hemoglobin A fractions to which glucose and related monosaccharides bind; concentrations are increased in the erythrocytes of patients with diabetes mellitus. The glycohemoglobin levels change slowly and can be used as a retrospective index of glucose control over the previous 8-10 weeks in such patients.

gly·col·al·de·hyde (glī-kol-al′dě-hīd). The simplest (2-carbon) sugar; the aerobic deamination product of ethanolamine.

gly·col·ic ac·id (glī-kol′ik). An intermediate in the interconversion of glycine and ethanolamine.

gly·col·ic ac·i·du·ria. Excessive excretion of glycolic acid in the urine; a primary metabolic defect due to deficiency of 2-hydroxy-3-oxoadipate carboxylase, resulting in excretion of glycolic and oxalic acids, leading to the clinical syndrome of oxalosis.

gly·co·lip·id (glī-kō-lip′id). A lipid with one or more covalently attached sugars.

gly·co·lyl (glī′kō-lil). The acyl radical of glycolic acid, replacing acetyl in some sialic acids; the products are called *N*-glycolylneuraminic acids.

gly·col·y·sis (glī-kol′ĭ-sis). The energy-yielding conversion of D-glucose to lactic acid (instead of pyruvate oxidation products) in various tissues, notably muscle, when sufficient oxygen is not available; since molecular oxygen is not consumed in the process, this is frequently referred to as "anaerobic g." [glyco- + G. *lysis*, a loosening]

gly·co·lyt·ic (glī-kō-lit′ik). Relating to glycolysis.

gly·co·ne·o·gen·e·sis (glī′kō-nē-ō-jen′ě-sis). The formation of glycogen from noncarbohydrates, such as protein or fat, by conversion of the latter to D-glucose. SEE ALSO glycogenesis. Cf. gluconeogenesis. [glyco- + G. *neos*, new, + *genesis*, production]

gly·co·pe·nia (glī-kō-pē′nē-ă). A deficiency of any or all sugars in an organ or tissue. [glyco- + G. *penia*, poverty]

gly·co·pep·tide (glī-kō-pep′tīd). A compound containing sugar(s) linked to amino acids (or peptides), with the latter preponderant, as in bacterial cell walls. Cf. peptidoglycan.

gly·co·phil·ia (glī-kō-fil′ē-ă). A condition in which there is a distinct tendency to develop hyperglycemia, even after the ingestion of a relatively small quantity of glucose. [glyko- + G. *phileō*, to love]

gly·co·pro·tein (glī-kō-prō′tēn). **1.** One of a group of protein-carbohydrate compounds (conjugated proteins), among which the most important are the mucins, mucoid, and amyloid. **2.** Sometimes restricted to proteins containing small amounts of carbohydrate, in contrast to mucoids or mucoproteins. SEE ALSO mucoprotein.

gly·co·pty·a·lism (glī-kō-tī′ă-lizm). SYN glycosialia. [glyco- + G. *ptyalon*, saliva]

gly·cor·rha·chia (glī-kō-rā′kē-ă, -rak-ē-ă). Presence of sugar in the cerebrospinal fluid. [glyco- + G. *rhachis*, spine]

gly·cor·rhea (glī-kō-rē′ă). A discharge of sugar from the body, as in glucosuria, especially in unusually large quantities. [glyco- + G. *rhoia*, a flow]

gly·co·se·cre·to·ry (glī′kō-sē-krē′tō-rē). Causing or involved in the secretion of glycogen.

gly·co·si·a·lia (glī′kō-sī-al′ē-ă, -ā′lē-ă). The presence of sugar in the saliva. SYN glycoptyalism. [glyco- + G. *sialon*, saliva]

gly·co·si·a·lor·rhea (glī′kō-sī′ă-lō-rē′ă). An excessive secretion of saliva that contains sugar. [glyco- + G. *sialon*, saliva, + *rhoia*, a flow]

gly·co·side (glī′kō-sīd). Condensation product of a sugar with any other radical involving the loss of the H of the hemiacetal or hemiketal OH of the sugar, leaving the O of this OH as the link.

gly·co·sphin·go·lip·id (glī′kō-sfing-gō-lip′id). A ceramide linked to one or more sugars via the terminal OH group; included as g.'s are cerebrosides, gangliosides, and ceramide oligosaccharides (oligoglycosylceramides). The prefix glyc-may be replaced by gluc-, galact-, lact-, etc.

gly·co·stat·ic (glī-kō-stat′ik). Indicating the property of certain extracts of the anterior hypophysis that permits the body to maintain its glycogen stores in muscle, liver, and other tissues.

gly·cos·ur·ia (glī-kō-sū′rē-ă). **1.** SYN glucosuria. **2.** Urinary excretion of carbohydrates. SYN glycuresis (2). [glyco- + G. *ouron*, urine]

alimentary g., g. developing after the ingestion of a moderate amount of sugar or starch because the rate of intestinal absorption exceeds the capacity of the liver and the other tissues to remove the glucose, thus allowing blood glucose levels to become high enough for renal excretion to occur.

phlorizin g., phloridzin g., the presence of sugar in the urine after the experimental administration of phlorizin, which results in a lower renal threshold for glucose reabsorption of glucose.

renal g., the recurring or persistent excretion of glucose in the urine, in association with blood glucose levels that are in the normal range; results from the failure of proximal renal tubules to reabsorb glucose at a normal rate from the glomerular filtrate (low renal threshold); defect in the glucose carrier in the nephron.

gly·co·syl (glī′kō-sil). The radical resulting from detachment of the OH of the hemiacetal or hemiketal of a saccharide. Cf. glycoside.

gly·co·sy·la·tion (glī′kō-sī-lā′shŭn). Formation of linkages with glycosyl groups, as between D-glucose and the hemoglobin chain to form the fraction hemoglobin A_{Ic}, whose level rises in association with the raised blood D-glucose concentration in poorly controlled or uncontrolled diabetes mellitus. SEE ALSO glycosylated *hemoglobin*.

gly·co·syl·trans·fer·ase (glī′kō-sil-trans′fer-ās). Any enzyme (EC subclass 2.4) transferring glycosyl groups from one compound to another.

glyc·u·re·sis (glī-kū-rē′sis). **1.** SYN glucosuria. **2.** SYN glycosuria (2). [glyco- + G. *ourēsis*, urination]

gly·cu·ron·ate (glī-kūr'on-āt). A salt or ester of a glycuronic acid.

gly·cyl (Gly) (glī'sil). The acyl radical of glycine.

GM-CSF granulocyte-macrophage colony-stimulating *factor*.

GMP guanylic acid.

gnat (nat). A midge; general term applied to several species of minute insects, including species of *Simulium* (buffalo g.) and *Hippelates* (eye g.). [A.S. *gnaet*]

△**gnath-.** SEE gnatho-.

gnath·ic (nath'ik). Relating to the jaw or alveolar process. [G. *gnathos,* jaw]

gnath·i·on (nath'ē-on) [NA]. The most inferior point of the mandible in the midline. In cephalometrics, it is the midpoint between the most anterior and inferior point on the bony chin, measured at the intersection of the mandibular baseline and the nasion-pogonion line. [G. *gnathos,* jaw]

△**gnatho-, gnath-.** The jaw. [G. *gnathos*]

gnath·o·dy·nam·ics (nath'ō-dī-nam'iks). The study of the relationship of the magnitude and direction of the forces developed by and upon the components of the masticatory system during function. [gnatho- + G. *dynamis,* power]

gnath·o·dy·na·mom·e·ter (nath'ō-dī-nă-mom'ĕ-ter). A device for measuring biting pressure. [gnatho- + dynamometer]

gnath·o·log·ic·al (nath-ō-loj'i-kăl). Pertaining to gnathodynamics.

gnath·o·plas·ty (nath'ō-plas-tē). Plastic surgery of the jaw. [gnatho- + G. *plastos,* formed]

gno·sia (nō'sē-ă). The perceptive faculty enabling one to recognize the form and the nature of persons and things; the faculty of perceiving and recognizing. [G. *gnōsis,* knowledge]

gno·to·bi·ol·o·gy (nō'tō-bī-ol'ō-jē). The study of animals in the absence of contaminating microorganisms; *i.e.,* of "germ-free" animals. [G. *gnotos,* known, + *bios,* life, + *logos,* study]

gno·to·bi·o·ta (nō'tō-bī-ō'tă). Living colonies or species, assembled from pure isolates. [G. *gnotos,* known, + Mod. L. *biota,* fr. G. *bios,* life]

gno·to·bi·ot·ic (nō'tō-bī-ot'ik). Denoting germ-free or formerly germ-free organisms in which the composition of any associated microbial flora, if present, is fully defined. [see gnotobiota]

GnRH gonadotropin-releasing *hormone*.

goi·ter (goy'ter). A chronic enlargement of the thyroid gland, not due to a neoplasm, occurring endemically in certain localities, especially mountainous regions, and sporadically elsewhere. SYN struma. [Fr. from L. *guttur,* throat]

aberrant g., enlargement of a supernumerary thyroid gland.

adenomatous g., an enlargement of the thyroid gland due to the growth of one or more encapsulated adenomas or multiple nonencapsulated colloid nodules within its substance.

colloid g., a form of g. in which the contents of the follicles increase greatly, causing pressure atrophy of the epithelium so that the gelatinous matter predominates in the tumor.

cystic g., an enlargement in the thyroid region due to the presence of one or more cysts within the gland.

diving g., a freely movable g. that is sometimes above and sometimes below the sternal notch. SYN wandering g.

exophthalmic g., any of the various forms of hyperthyroidism in which the thyroid gland is enlarged and exophthalmos is present.

familial g., a group of heritable thyroid disorders in which g. is commonly apparent first during childhood; often associated with skeletal and/or mental retardation, and with other signs of hypothyroidism that may develop with age.

fibrous g., a firm hyperplasia of the thyroid and its capsule.

follicular g., SYN parenchymatous g.

lingual g., a tumor of thyroid tissue involving the embryonic rudiment at the base of the tongue.

multinodular g., adenomatous g. with several colloid nodules.

nontoxic g., g. not accompanied by hyperthyroidism.

parenchymatous g., a form of g. in which there is a great increase in the follicles with proliferation of the epithelium. SYN follicular g.

simple g., thyroid enlargement unaccompanied by constitutional effects, *e.g.,* hypo- or hyperthyroidism, commonly caused by inadequate dietary intake of iodine.

substernal g., enlargement of the thyroid gland, chiefly of the lower part of the isthmus, palpable with difficulty or not at all.

suffocative g., a g. that by pressure causes extreme dyspnea.

toxic g., a g. that forms an excessive secretion, causing signs and symptoms of hyperthyroidism.

wandering g., SYN diving g.

goi·tro·gen·ic (goy-trō-jen'ik). Causing goiter.

goi·trous (goy'trŭs). Denoting or characteristic of a goiter.

gold (Au). A yellow metallic element, atomic no. 79, atomic wt. 196.96654; ^{198}Au (half-life of 2.694 days) is used in the treatment of certain tumors and in imaging. SYN aurum.

gom·i·to·li (gō-mē'tō-lē). Intricately coiled and looped capillary vessels present largely in the upper infundibular stem of the stalk of the pituitary gland; they make up a portion of the pituitary portal circulation. [It. *gomitolo,* coil]

gom·pho·sis (gom-fō'sis) [NA]. A form of fibrous joint in which a peglike process fits into a hole, as the root of a tooth into the socket in the alveolus. [G. *gomphos,* bolt, nail, + *-osis,* condition]

go·nad (gō'nad). An organ that produces sex cells; a testis or an ovary. [Mod. L. fr. G. *gonē,* seed]

indifferent g., the primordial organ in an embryo before its differentiation into testis or ovary.

△**gonad-.** SEE gonado-.

go·nad·al (gō-nad'ăl). Relating to a gonad.

go·nad·ec·to·my (gō-nad-ek'tō-mē). Excision of ovary or testis. [gonado- + G. *ektomē,* excision]

△**gonado-, gonad-.** The gonads. [G. *gonē,* seed]

go·nad·o·crins (gō-nad'ō-krinz). Peptides that stimulate release of both follicle-stimulating hormone and luteinizing hormone from the pituitary;

found in ovarian follicular fluid in rats. [gonad + G. *krinō*, to secrete]

go•nad•o•lib•er•in (gō′nad-ō-lib′er-in). **1.** A hypothalamic substance causing the release of gonadotropin. SYN gonadotropin-releasing factor, gonadotropin-releasing hormone. **2.** A decapeptide from pig hypothalami that induces release of both lutropin and follitropin in constant proportions and thus acts as both luliberin and folliberin. SYN luteinizing hormone/follicle-stimulating hormone-releasing factor. [gonad + L. *libero*, to free, + -in]

gon•a•dop•athy (gon-ă-dop′ă-thē). Disease affecting the gonads. [gonado- + G. *pathos*, suffering]

go•nad•o•rel•in hy•dro•chlo•ride (gō-nad-ō-rel′in). A gonadotropin-releasing hormone obtained from sheep, pigs, or other animals and used to evaluate the functional capacity of the gonadotrophs of the anterior pituitary. [*gonado*tropin-*rel*easing + -in]

go•nad•o•troph (gō-nad′ō-trōf, -gon′ă-dō-). An endocrine cell of the adenohypophysis that affects certain cells of the ovary or testis.

go•nad•o•tro•phic (gō′nad-o-trōf′ik, gon′ă-dō-). SYN gonadotropic. [gonado- + G. *trophē*, nourishment]

go•nad•o•tro•phin (gō′nad-ō-trō′fin, gon′ă-dō-). SYN gonadotropin. [for gonadotrophin, fr. gonad + G. *trophē*, nourishment]

  human chorionic g., SEE chorionic *gonadotropin*.

go•nad•o•tro•pic (gō′nad-ō-trōp′ik, gon′ă-dō-). **1.** Descriptive of or relating to the actions of a gonadotropin. **2.** Promoting the growth and/or function of the gonads. SYN gonadotrophic. [gonado- + G. *tropē*, a turning]

go•nad•o•tro•pin (gō′nad-ō-trō′pin, gon′ă-dō-). A hormone capable of promoting gonadal growth and function; such effects, as exerted by a single hormone, usually are limited to discrete functions or histological components of a gonad, such as stimulation of follicular growth or of androgen formation; most g.'s exert their effects in both sexes, although the effect of a given g. will differ in males and females. SYN gonadotrophin, gonadotropic hormone.

  anterior pituitary g., any g. of hypophysial origin. SYN pituitary gonadotropic hormone.

  chorionic g., a glycoprotein with a carbohydrate fraction composed of D-galactose and hexosamine, produced by the placental trophoblastic cells; its most important role appears to be stimulation, during the first trimester, of ovarian secretion of the estrogen and progesterone required for the integrity of the conceptus; it appears to play no significant role in the last two trimesters of pregnancy, as the estrogen and progesterone are then formed by the placenta. Testing for the beta fraction of human chorionic g. is the basis for most serum and urine pregnancy tests. SYN anterior pituitary-like hormone, chorionic gonadotropic hormone, chorionic gonadotrophic hormone.

  human menopausal g., a hormone of pituitary originally obtained from the urine of postmenopausal women now produced synthetically; used to induce ovulation. SEE ALSO menotropins.

gon•a•duct (gon′ă-dŭkt). **1.** SYN seminal *duct*. **2.** SYN uterine *tube*. [gonado- + duct]

go•nal•gia (gō-nal′jē-ă). Pain in the knee. [G. *gony*, knee, + *algos*, pain]

gonangiectomy (gon-an-je-ek-to-me). SYN vasectomy. [G. *gonē*, seed. + *angeion*, vessel, + *ektome*, excision, + -y]

gon•ar•thri•tis (gon-ar-thrī′tis). Inflammation of the knee joint. [G. *gony*, knee, + *arthron*, joint, + -*itis*, inflammation]

gon•ar•throt•o•my (gon-ar-throt′ō-mē). Incision into the knee joint. [G. *gony*, knee, + *arthron*, joint, + *tomē*, incision]

gon•e•cyst, gon•e•cys•tis (gon′ĕ-sist, gon-ĕ-sis′tis). SYN seminal *vesicle*. [G. *gonē*, seed, + *kystis*, bladder]

go•nia (gō′nē-ă). Plural of gonion.

△**gonio-.** Angle. [G. *gōnia*]

go•ni•om•e•ter (gō-nē-om′ĕ-ter). **1.** An instrument for measuring angles. **2.** An appliance for the static test of labyrinthine disease, which consists of a plank, one end of which may be raised to any desired height; as one end of the plank is gradually raised, the point at which a patient loses balance is noted. **3.** A calibrated device designed to measure the arc or range of motion of a joint. SYN arthrometer. [G. *gōnia*, angle, + *metron*, measure]

go•ni•on, pl. **go•nia** (gō′nē-on, gō′nē-ă) [NA]. The lowest posterior and most outward point of the angle of the mandible. In cephalometrics, it is measured by bisecting the angle formed by the tangents to the lower and the posterior borders of the mandible; when the angles of both sides of the mandible appear on the lateral radiograph, a point midway between the right and left side is used. [G. *gōnia*, an angle]

go•ni•o•punc•ture (gō′nē-ō-pŭnk-chūr). An operation for congenital glaucoma in which a puncture is made in the filtration angle of the anterior chamber.

go•ni•o•scope (gō′nē-ō-skōp). A lens designed to study the angle of the anterior chamber of the eye. [G. *gōnia*, angle, + *skopeō*, to examine]

go•ni•os•co•py (gō-nē-os′kŏ-pē). Examination of the angle of the anterior chamber of the eye with a gonioscope or with a contact prism lens.

go•ni•o•syn•ech•ia (gō′nē-ō-si-nek′ē-ă). Adhesion of the iris to the posterior surface of the cornea in the angle of the anterior chamber; associated with angle-closure glaucoma. [G. *gōnia*, angle, + *synechis*, holding together]

go•ni•ot•o•my (gō-nē-ot′ō-mē). Surgical opening of the trabecular meshwork in congenital glaucoma. [G. *gōnia*, angle, + *tomē*, incision]

gon•o•cele (gon′ō-sēl). A cystic lesion of the epididymis or rete testis, resulting from obstruction and containing secretions from the testis. [G. *gonē*, seed, + *kēlē*, tumor]

gon•o•coc•cal (gon′ō-kok′ăl). Relating to the gonococcus. SYN gonococcic.

gon•o•coc•ce•mia (gon′ō-kok-sē′mē-ă). The presence of gonococci in the circulating blood. [gonococcus + G. *haima*, blood]

gon•o•coc•ci (gon-ō-kok′sī). Plural of gonococcus.

gon•o•coc•cic (gon′ō-kok′sik). SYN gonococcal.

⊠ gon·o·coc·cus, pl. **gon·o·coc·ci** (gon-ō-kok′ŭs, -sī). SYN *Neisseria gonorrhoeae.* [G. *gonē,* seed, + *kokkos,* berry]

gon·o·phore, gon·oph·o·rus (gon′ŏ-fōr, gō-nof′ ŏ-rŭs). Any structure serving to store up or conduct the sexual cells; oviduct, spermatic duct, uterus, or seminal vesicle; an accessory generative organ. [G. *gonē,* seed, + *phoros,* bearing]

gon·or·rhea (gon-ō-rē′ă). A contagious catarrhal inflammation of the genital mucous membrane, transmitted chiefly by coitus and due to *Neisseria gonorrhoeae;* may involve the lower or upper genital tract, especially the urethra, endocervix, and uterine tubes, or spread to the peritoneum and rarely to the heart, joints, or other structures by way of the bloodstream. [G. *gonorrhoia,* fr. *gonē,* seed, + *rhoia,* a flow]

gon·or·rhe·al (gon-ō-rē′ăl). Relating to gonorrhea.

go·ny·camp·sis (gon-ē-kamp′sis). Ankylosis or any abnormal curvature of the knee. [G. *gony,* knee, + *kampsis,* a bending or curving]

gor·get (gōr′jet). A director or guide with wide groove for use in lithotomy.

GOT glutamic-oxaloacetic transaminase.

gouge (gowj). A strong, curved chisel used in operations on bone.

gout (gowt). A disorder of purine metabolism, occurring especially in men, characterized by a raised but variable blood uric acid level and severe recurrent acute arthritis of sudden onset resulting from deposition of crystals of sodium urate in connective tissues and articular cartilage; most cases are inherited, resulting from a variety of abnormalities of purine metabolism. [L. *gutta,* drop]

   latent g., hyperuricemia without symptoms of gout. Often used synonymously with interval g.

   secondary g., g. resulting from increased serum uric acid levels as a result of an antecedent disease, such as a proliferative disease of the blood and bone marrow, lead poisoning, or prolonged chronic renal failure (on dialysis).

   tophaceous g., g. in which deposits of uric acid and urates occur as gouty tophi.

gouty (gow′tē). Relating to or characteristic of gout.

GPI Gingival-Periodontal Index.

GPT glutamic-pyruvic transaminase.

grad. L. *gradatim,* by degrees, gradually.

gra·di·ent (grā′dē-ent). Rate of change of temperature, pressure, or other variable as a function of distance, time, etc.

grad·u·at·ed (grad′yū-āt′ed). **1.** Marked by lines or in other ways to denote capacity, degrees, percentages, etc. **2.** Divided or arranged in levels, grades, or successive steps.

graft. 1. Any free (unattached) tissue or organ for transplantation. **2.** To transplant such structures. SEE ALSO flap, implant, transplant. [A.S. *graef*]

   accordion g., a skin g. in which multiple slits have been made, so it can be stretched to cover a large area.

   allogeneic g., SYN allograft.

   autodermic g., a skin autograft.

   autogeneic g., SYN autograft.

   autologous g., SYN autograft.

   autoplastic g., SYN autograft.

   Blair-Brown g., a split-thickness g. of intermediate thickness.

   cable g., a multiple strand nerve g. arranged as a pathway for regeneration of axons.

   chip g., a g. consisting of small pieces of cartilage or bone which are packed into a bone defect.

   composite g., a g. composed of several structures, such as skin and cartilage or a full-thickness segment of the ear.

   corneal g., SYN keratoplasty.

   delayed g., application of a skin g. after waiting several days for healthy granulations to form.

   dermal g., a g. of dermis, made from skin by cutting away a thin split-thickness g.

   Esser g., SYN inlay g.

   fascia g., a g. of fibrous tissue, usually the fascia lata.

   fascicular g., a nerve g. in which each bundle of fibers is approximated and sutured separately.

   free g., a g. transplanted without its normal attachments, or a pedicle, from one site to another.

   full-thickness g., a g. of the full thickness of mucosa and submucosa or of skin and subcutaneous tissue.

   funicular g., a nerve g. in which each funiculus (composed of two or more fasciculi) is approximated and sutured separately.

   heterologous g., SYN xenograft.

   homologous g., SYN allograft.

   homoplastic g., SYN allograft.

   inlay g., a skin g. wrapped (raw side out) around a bolus of dental compound and inserted into a prepared surgical pocket. SYN Esser g.

   isogeneic g., SYN syngraft.

   isologous g., SYN syngraft.

   isoplastic g., SYN syngraft.

   Ollier g., a thin split-thickness g., usually in small pieces. SYN Ollier-Thiersch g.

   Ollier-Thiersch g., SYN Ollier g.

   omental g., a segment of omentum, with its supplying blood vessels, transplanted as a free flap to a distant area and revascularized by arterial and venous anastomoses.

   partial-thickness g., SYN split-thickness g.

   periosteal g., a g. of periosteum, usually placed on bare bone.

   Phemister g., an autogenous onlay bone graft used in treating delayed union of fractures.

   pinch g., small bits of skin, of partial or full thickness, removed from a healthy area and seeded in a site to be covered.

   punch g.'s, small full-thickness g.'s of the scalp, removed with a circular punch and transplanted to a bald area to grow hair.

   split-thickness g., a g. of portions of the skin, *i.e.,* the epidermis and part of the dermis, or of part of the mucosa and submucosa, but not including the periosteum. SYN partial-thickness g.

   vascularized g., the state of a g. after the recipient vasculature has been connected with the vessels in the g.

   white g., rejection of a skin allograft so acute that vascularization never occurs.

   Wolfe g., a full-thickness skin g. without any subcutaneous fat.

grain (grān). **1.** Cereal plants, such as corn, wheat, or rye, or a seed of one of them. **2.** A minute, hard particle of any substance, as of sand. **3.** A unit of weight, $\frac{1}{60}$ dram (apoth. or troy), $\frac{1}{437.5}$ avoirdupois ounce, $\frac{1}{480}$ troy ounce, $\frac{1}{5760}$ troy pound, $\frac{1}{7000}$ avoirdupois pound; the equivalent of 0.064799 g. [L. *granum*]

Gram, Hans C.J., Danish bacteriologist, 1853–1938. SEE G.'s *stain*.

gram (g). A unit of weight in the metric or centesimal system, the equivalent of 15.432358 grains or 0.03527 avoirdupois ounce.

-gram. A recording, usually by an instrument. Cf. -graph. [G. *gramma*, character, mark]

gram•cen•ti•me•ter. The energy exerted, or work done, when a mass of 1 g is raised a height of 1 cm; equal to 9.807×10^{-5} joules or newton-meters.

gram-i•on. The weight in grams of an ion that is equal to the sum of the atomic weights of the atoms making up the ion.

gram-me•ter. A unit of energy equal to 100 gram-centimeters.

gram-mol•e•cule. See under molecule.

Gram-neg•a•tive. Refers to the inability of a bacterium to resist decolorization with alcohol after being treated with Gram's crystal violet. However, following decolorization, these bacteria can be readily counterstained with safranin, imparting a pink or red color to the bacterium when viewed by light microscopy. SEE Gram's *stain*.

Gram-pos•i•tive. Refers to the ability of a bacterium to resist decolorization with alcohol after being treated with Gram's crystal violet stain, imparting a violet color to the bacterium when viewed by light microscopy. SEE Gram's *stain*.

gran•u•lar (gran′yū-lăr). **1.** Composed of or resembling granules or granulations. **2.** Particles with strong affinity for nuclear stains, seen in many bacterial species.

gra•nu•la•tio, pl. **gran•u•la•ti•o•nes** (gran-yū-lā′shē-ō, -shē-o′nēz). SYN granulation. [L.]

    granulatio′nes arachnoidea′les [NA], SYN arachnoid *granulations,* under *granulation.* SEE ALSO arachnoid *villi,* under *villus.*

gran•u•la•tion (gran′yū-lā′shŭn). **1.** Formation into grains or granules; the state of being granular. **2.** A granular mass in or on the surface of any organ or membrane; or one of the individual granules forming the mass. **3.** The formation of minute, rounded, fleshy connective tissue projections on the surface of a wound, ulcer, or inflamed tissue surface in the process of healing; one of the fleshy granules composing this surface. SEE ALSO granulation *tissue.* **4.** PHARMACY The formation of crystals by constant agitation of a supersaturated solution of a salt. SYN granulatio. [L. *granulatio*]

    arachnoid g.'s, tufted prolongations of pia-arachnoid, composed of numerous arachnoid villi that penetrate dural venous sinuses and effect transfer of cerebrospinal fluid to the venous system. SYN granulationes arachnoideales [NA], pacchionian bodies.

gran•ule (gran′yūl). **1.** A grain-like particle; a granulation; a minute discrete mass. **2.** A very small pill, usually gelatin-coated or sugar-coated,

containing a drug to be given in a small dose. **3.** A colony of the bacterium or fungus causing a disease or simply colonizing the tissues of the patient. In compromised patients the differentiation is difficult. [L. *granulum,* dim. of *granum,* grain]

    acrosomal g., the single glycoprotein rich g. within an acrosomal vesicle, which results from the coalescence of proacrosomal g.'s.

    alpha g., a g. of an alpha cell that was named as the first of several kinds or because it was acidophilic.

    basal g., SYN basal *body.*

    beta g., a g. of a beta cell.

    cone g., nucleus of a retinal cell connecting with one of the cones.

    delta g., a g. of a delta cell.

    elementary g., a particle of blood dust, or hemoconia.

    glycogen g., glycogen occurring in cells as beta g.'s which average about 300 Å in diameter, or as alpha g.'s which are aggregates measuring 900 Å of smaller particles.

    juxtaglomerular g.'s, osmophilic secretory g.'s present in the juxtaglomerular cells, thought to contain renin.

    keratohyalin g.'s, irregularly shaped basophilic g.'s in the cells of the stratum granulosum of the epidermis.

    membrane-coating g., SYN keratinosome.

    Nissl g.'s, SYN Nissl *substance.*

    proacrosomal g.'s, small carbohydrate-rich g.'s appearing in vesicles of the Golgi apparatus of spermatids; they coalesce into a single acrosomal g. contained within an acrosomal vesicle.

    rod g., the nucleus of a retinal cell connecting with one of the rods.

    seminal g., one of the minute granular bodies present in the semen.

granulo-. Granular, granules. [L. *granulum,* a small grain.]

gran•u•lo•cyte (gran′yū-lō-sīt). A mature granular leukocyte, including neutrophilic, acidophilic, and basophilic types of polymorphonuclear leukocytes, *i.e.,* respectively, neutrophils, eosinophils, and basophils. [granulo- + G. *kytos,* cell]

gran•u•lo•cy•to•pe•nia (gran′yū-lō-sī-tō-pē′nē-ă). Less than the normal number of granular leukocytes in the blood. SYN granulopenia. [granulocyte + G. *penia,* poverty]

gran•u•lo•cy•to•poi•e•sis (gran′yū-lō-sī′tō-poy-ē′sis). SYN granulopoiesis.

gran•u•lo•cy•to•poi•et•ic (gran′yū-lō-sī′tō-poy-et′ik). SYN granulopoietic. [granulocyte + G. *poieō,* to make]

gran•u•lo•cy•to•sis (gran′yū-lō-sī-tō′sis). A condition characterized by more than the normal number of granulocytes in the circulating blood or in the tissues.

gran•u•lo•ma (gran-yū-lō′mă). Indefinite term applied to nodular inflammatory lesions, usually small or granular, firm, persistent, and containing compactly grouped mononuclear phagocytes. SEE ALSO granulomatosis. [granulo- + G. *-oma,* tumor]

    actinic g., an annular eruption on sun-exposed skin which microscopically shows phagocytosis of dermal elastic fibers by giant cells and histiocytes.

amebic g., SYN ameboma.

apical g., SYN periapical g.

dental g., SYN periapical g.

eosinophilic g., a lesion observed more frequently in children and adolescents, occasionally in young adults, which occurs chiefly as a solitary focus in one bone, although multiple involvement is sometimes observed and similar foci may develop in the lung; characterized by numerous Langerhans cells and eosinophils, and occasional foci of necrosis; may be related to Hand-Schüller-Christian disease, possibly representing a benign form.

foreign body g., a g. caused by the presence of foreign particulate material in tissue, characterized by a histiocytic reaction with foreign body giant cells.

giant cell g., a non-neoplastic lesion characterized by a proliferation of granulation tissue containing numerous multinucleated giant cells; it occurs on the gingiva and alveolar mucosa (occasionally on other soft tissues) where it presents as a soft red-blue hemorrhagic nodular swelling; it also occurs within the mandible or maxilla as a unilocular or multilocular radiolucency. Identical bony lesions may be seen in hyperparathyroidism and cherubism. SEE ALSO giant cell *tumor* of bone.

g. inguina′le, a specific g., classified as a sexually transmitted disease and caused by *Calymmatobacterium granulomatis* observed in macrophages as Donovan bodies; the ulcerating granulomatous lesions occur in the inguinal regions and on the genitalia. SYN donovanosis, g. venereum, ulcerating g. of pudenda.

lethal midline g., destruction of the nasal septum, hard palate, lateral nasal walls, paranasal sinuses, skin of the face, orbit and nasopharynx by an inflammatory infiltrate with atypical lymphocytic and histiocytic cells; presumably a form of lymphoma in most cases. SYN malignant g.

lipoid g., g. characterized by aggregates or accumulations of fairly large mononuclear phagocytes that contain lipid.

malignant g., SYN lethal midline g.

g. multifor′me, a chronic granulomatous annular eruption of the skin on the upper body in older adults in central Africa; of unknown cause.

paracoccidioidal g., SYN paracoccidioidomycosis.

periapical g., a proliferation of granulation tissue surrounding the apex of a nonvital tooth and arising in response to pulpal necrosis. SYN apical g., dental g.

⊞pyogenic g., g. pyogen′icum, an acquired small rounded mass of highly vascular granulation tissue, frequently with an ulcerated surface, projecting from the skin or mucosa; histologically, the mass resembles a capillary hemangioma.

sarcoidal g., a non-necrotizing epithelioid cell g. similar to those seen in sarcoidosis.

g. trop′icum, SYN yaws.

ulcerating g. of pudenda, SYN g. inguinale.

g. vene′reum, SYN g. inguinale.

gran·u·lo·ma·to·sis (gran′yū-lō-mă-tō′sis). Any condition characterized by multiple granulomas.

bronchocentric g., a severe form of allergic bronchopulmonary aspergillosis.

lipid g., lipoid g., SYN xanthomatosis.

Wegener's g., a disease, occurring mainly in the fourth and fifth decades, characterized by necrotizing granulomas and ulceration of the upper respiratory tract, with purulent rhinorrhea, nasal obstruction, and sometimes with otorrhea, hemoptysis, pulmonary infiltration and cavitation, and fever; exophthalmos, involvement of the larynx and pharynx, and glomerulonephritis may occur; the underlying condition is a vasculitis affecting small vessels, and is possibly due to an immune disorder.

gran·u·lom·a·tous (gran-yū-lom′ă-tŭs). Having the characteristics of a granuloma.

gran·u·lo·mere (gran′yū-lō-mēr). The central part of a blood platelet. SYN chromomere (2). [granulo- + G. *meros,* a part]

gran·u·lo·pe·nia (gran′yū-lō-pē′nē-ă). SYN granulocytopenia.

gran·u·lo·plas·tic (gran′yū-lō-plas′tik). Forming granules.

gran·u·lo·poi·e·sis (gran′yū-lō-poy-ē′sis). Production of granulocytes. In adults, granulocytes are produced chiefly in the red bone marrow of flat bones. SYN granulocytopoiesis. [granulo-(cyte) + G. *poiēsis,* a making]

gran·u·lo·poi·et·ic (gran′yū-lō-poy-et′ik). Pertaining to granulopoiesis. SYN granulocytopoietic.

gran·u·lo·sis (gran-yū-lō′sis). A mass of minute granules of any character.

△-graph. 1. Something written, as in monograph, radiograph. **2.** The instrument for making a recording, as in kymograph. Cf. -gram. [G. *graphō,* to write]

graph·an·es·the·sia (graf′an-es-thē′zē-ă). Tactual inability to recognize figures or letters written on the skin; may be due to spinal cord or brain disease. [G. *graphē,* writing + *anaisthēsia,* fr. *an-* priv. + *aisthēsis,* perception]

graph·or·rhea (graf-ō-rē′ă). Rarely used term for the writing of long lists of meaningless words, associated with a schizophrenic disorder. [grapho- + G. *rhoia,* flow]

△-graphy. A writing, a description. [G. *graphō,* to write]

grat·tage (gră-tazh′). Scraping or brushing an ulcer or surface with sluggish granulations to stimulate the healing process. [Fr. scraping]

grave (grāv). Denoting symptoms of a serious or dangerous character. [L. *gravis,* heavy, grave]

grav·el (grav′l). Small concretions, usually of uric acid, calcium oxalate, or phosphates, formed in the kidney and passed through the ureter, bladder, and urethra. [M.E., fr. O.Fr.]

grav·id. SYN pregnant.

grav·i·da (grav′i-dă). A pregnant woman. Gravida followed by a roman numeral or preceded by a Latin prefix (primi-, secundi-, etc.) designates the number of pregnancies; *e.g.,* **g. I,** primigravida: a woman in her first pregnancy; **g. II,** secundigravida: a woman in her second pregnancy. Also, gravida (or G) 1, 2, etc. Cf. para. [L. *gravidus* (adj.), fem. *gravida,* fr. *gravis,* heavy]

gra·vid·ic (grav-id′ik). Relating to pregnancy or a pregnant woman.

gra·vid·i·ty (gră-vid′i-tē). The number of pregnancies (complete or incomplete) experienced by a woman. [L. *graviditas,* pregnancy]

grav·i·met·ric (grav-i-met′rik). Relating to or determined by weight.

grav·i·re·cep·tors (grav′i-rē-sep′terz). Highly specialized receptor organs and nerve endings in the inner ear, joints, tendons, and muscles that give the brain information about body position, equilibrium, direction of gravitational forces, and the sensation of "down" or "up." [L. *gravis,* heavy, + receptor]

grav·i·ty (grav′i-tē). The attraction toward the earth that makes any mass exert downward force or have weight. [L. *gravitas*]

 center of g. (COG, COLG), the point on a body or system where, if pressure equal to the weight of the object is applied, forces acting on the object will be in equilibrium; the location of the COG in a human being in the anatomical position is just anterior to the second sacral vertebra.

 specific g., the weight of any body compared with that of another body of equal volume regarded as the unit; usually the weight of a liquid compared with that of distilled water.

gray (Gy) (grā). The SI unit of absorbed dose of ionizing radiation, equivalent to 1 J/kg of tissue; 1 Gy = 100 rad. [Louis H. *Gray,* British radiologist, 1905–1965]

grid. 1. A chart with horizontal and perpendicular lines for plotting curves. **2.** X-RAY IMAGING A device formed of lead strips for preventing scattered radiation from reaching the x-ray film. [M.E. *gridel,* fr. L. *craticula,* lattice]

grief (grēf). A normal emotional response to an external loss; distinguished from a depressive disorder since it usually subsides after a reasonable time.

grind·ing (grīnd′ing). SYN abrasion (3).

grind·ing-in. A term used to denote the act of correcting occlusal disharmonies by grinding the natural or artificial teeth.

grip. SYN influenza.

 devil's g., SYN epidemic *pleurodynia.*

grippe (grip). SYN influenza. [Fr. *gripper,* to seize]

gris·tle (gris′l). SYN cartilage. [A.S.]

groin (groyn). **1.** SYN inguinal *region.* **2.** Sometimes used to indicate just the crease in the junction of the thigh with the trunk.

groove (grūt). A narrow elongated depression or furrow on any surface. SEE ALSO sulcus.

 coronary g., a groove on the outer surface of the heart marking the division between the atria and the ventricles.

 developmental g.'s, fine lines found in the enamel of a tooth that mark the junction of the lobes of the crown in its development. SYN developmental lines.

 Harrison's g., a deformity of the ribs which results from the pull of the diaphragm on ribs weakened by rickets or other softening of the bone.

 median g. of tongue, median groove or me-

dian longitudinal raphe of tongue; raphe linguae; a slight longitudinal depression running forward on the dorsal surface of the tongue from the foramen cecum.

 g. of nail matrix, SYN *sulcus* matricis unguis.

 neural g., the gutter-like g. formed in the midline of the embryo's dorsal surface by the progressive elevation of the lateral margins of the neural plate; the ultimate dorsal fusion of the margins results in the formation of the neural tube.

 pontomedullary g., the transverse g. on the ventral aspect of the brainstem that demarcates the pons from the medulla oblongata; from its bottom the sixth, seventh, and eighth cranial nerves emerge.

 popliteal g., a g. on the lateral condyle of the femur between the epicondyle and the articular margin. Its anterior end gives origin to the popliteus muscle; its posterior end lodges the tendon of the muscle when the knee is fully flexed.

 primitive g., the median depression in the primitive streak flanked by the primitive ridges.

 urethral g., the g. on the ventral surface of the embryonic penis which ultimately is closed to form the penile portion of the urethra.

gross. Coarse or large; large enough to be visible to the naked eye.

group (grūp). **1.** A number of similar or related objects. **2.** CHEMISTRY A radical. For individual chemical groups, see the specific name.

 activity g., a group designed to assist individuals who share common concerns or problems related to the acquisition or maintenance of performance components and occupational skills.

 ambulatory patient g. (APG), a classification of patients by surgical procedure into categories for the purpose of determining reimbursement of health care costs, based on the premise that treatment of similar procedures would generate similar costs.

 blood g., SEE blood group.

 characterizing g., a g. of atoms in a molecule that distinguishes the class of substances in which it occurs from all other classes; thus carbonyl (CO) is the characterizing g. of ketones; COOH, of organic acids, etc.

 control g., a g. of subjects participating in the same experiment as another g. of subjects, but which is not exposed to the variable under investigation. SEE ALSO experimental g.

 diagnosis related g., a scheme for billing for medical and especially hospital services by combining diseases into g.'s according to the resources needed for care, arranged by diagnostic category. A dollar value is assigned to each g. as the basis of payment for all cases in that group, without regard to the actual cost of care or duration of hospitalization of any individual case, as a mechanism to motivate health-care providers to economize.

 encounter g., a form of psychological sensitivity training that emphasizes the experiencing of individual relationships within the g. and minimizes intellectual and didactic input; the g. focuses on the present rather than concerning itself with the past or outside problems of its members.

gr

experimental g., a g. of subjects exposed to the variable of an experiment, as opposed to the control g.

HACEK g., a group of Gram-negative bacteria that includes *Haemophilus* spp., *Actinobacillus actinomycetemcomitans*, *Cardiobacterium hominis*, *Eikenella corrodens*, and *Kingella kingae*. Bacteria in this group have in common a culture requirement of an enhanced carbon dioxide atmosphere and ability to infect human heart valves.

matched g.'s, a method of experimental control in which subjects in one g. are matched on a one-to-one basis with subjects in other g.'s concerning all organism variables (*e.g.,* age, sex, height, weight) which the experimenter believes could influence the variable being investigated.

prosthetic g., a non-amino acid compound attached to a protein, often in a reversible fashion, that confers new properties upon the conjugated protein thus produced. SEE ALSO coenzyme.

training g., any g. emphasizing training in self-awareness and group dynamics.

growth (grōth). The increase in size of a living being or any of its parts occurring in the process of development.

accretionary g., g. by an increase of intercellular material.

appositional g., g. accomplished by the addition of new layers on those previously formed; *e.g.,* the addition of lamellae in the formation of bone; it is the characteristic method of g. when rigid materials are involved.

interstitial g., g. from a number of different centers within an area; in contrast with appositional g., it can occur only when the materials involved are nonrigid.

gru•mous (grū′mŭs). Thick and lumpy, as clotting blood. [L. *grumus,* a little heap]

gry•po•sis (gri-pō′sis). An abnormal curvature. [G. *grypos,* hooked, + *-osis,* condition]

GSH glutathione.

GSR galvanic skin *response.*

GSSG glutathione disulfide.

GTP guanosine 5′-triphosphate.

GU genitourinary.

gua•nase (gwahn′ās). SYN *guanine* deaminase.

gua•nine (G) (gwahn′ēn, -in). One of the two major purines (the other being adenine) occurring in all nucleic acids.

g. deaminase, a deaminase of the liver that catalyzes the hydrolysis of guanine into xanthine and ammonia; the first step in purine degradation. SYN guanase.

g. deoxyribonucleotide, SYN deoxyguanylic acid.

g. ribonucleotide, SYN guanylic acid.

gua•no•sine (G, Guo) (gwahn′ō-sēn, -sin). A major constituent of RNA and of guanine nucleotides.

gua•no•sine 5′-tri•phos•phate (GTP). An immediate precursor of guanine nucleotides in RNA; similar to ATP; has a crucial role in microtubule formation.

gua•nyl•ic ac•id (GMP) (gwă-nil′ik). A major component of ribonucleic acids. SYN guanine ribonucleotide.

guard•ing (gard′ing). A spasm of muscles to minimize motion or agitation of sites affected by injury or disease.

abdominal g., a spasm of abdominal wall muscles, detected on palpation, to protect inflamed abdominal viscera from pressure; usually a result of inflammation of the peritoneal surface as in appendicitis, diverticulitis, or generalized peritonitis.

gu•ber•nac•u•lum (gū′ber-nak′yū-lŭm). A fibrous cord connecting two structures. A mesenchymal column of tissue that connects the fetal testis to the developing scrotum; it appears to play a role in testicular descent. SYN g. testis [NA]. [L. a helm]

g. den′tis, a connective tissue band uniting the tooth sac with the gum.

g. tes′tis [NA], SYN gubernaculum.

guide (gīd). **1.** To lead in a set course. **2.** Any device or instrument by which another is led into its proper course, *e.g.,* a grooved director, a catheter g. [M.E., fr. O.Fr. *guier,* to show the way, fr. Germanic]

guide•wire (gīd′wīr). A long and flexible fine spring used to introduce and position an intravascular angiographic catheter (see Seldinger technique).

guil•lo•tine (gil′ŏ-tēn, gē′ō-tēn). An instrument in the shape of a metal ring through which runs a sliding knifeblade, used in cutting off an enlarged tonsil. [Fr. an instrument for execution by decapitation]

gul•let (gŭl′et). SYN throat (1). [L. *gula,* throat]

gum (gŭm). **1.** The dried exuded sap from a number of trees and shrubs, forming an amorphous brittle mass; it usually forms a mucilaginous solution in water. [L. *gummi*] **2.** SYN gingiva. [A.S. *goma,* jaw]

gum•ma, pl. **gum•ma•ta**, **gum•mas** (gŭm′ă, ă-tă, -ž). An infectious granuloma that is characteristic of tertiary syphilis. Gummas are characterized by an irregular central portion that is firm, sometimes partially hyalinized, and consisting of coagulative necrosis in which "ghosts" of structures may be recognized; a poorly defined middle zone of epithelioid cells, with occasional multinucleated giant cells; and a peripheral zone of fibroblasts and numerous capillaries, with infiltrated lymphocytes and plasma cells. SYN syphiloma. [L. *gummi,* gum, fr. G. *kommi*]

gum•ma•tous (gŭm′ă-tŭs). Pertaining to or characterized by the features of a gumma.

Guo guanosine.

gur•ney (gŭr′nē). A stretcher or cot with wheels used to transport hospital patients. [Scottish *gurn,* to grimace in pain; Sir Goldsworthy *Gurney,* British physician and inventor, 1793–1875]

gus•ta•tion (gŭs-tā′shŭn). **1.** The act of tasting. **2.** The sense of taste. [L. *gustatio,* fr. *gusto,* pp. *-atus,* to taste]

gus•ta•to•ry (gŭs′tă-tōr-ē). Relating to gustation, or taste.

gut. **1.** SYN intestinum. **2.** Embryonic digestive tube. **3.** Abbreviated term for catgut. SEE ALSO suture.

primitive g., a flat sheet of intraembryonic endoderm that will change into a tubular g. due to

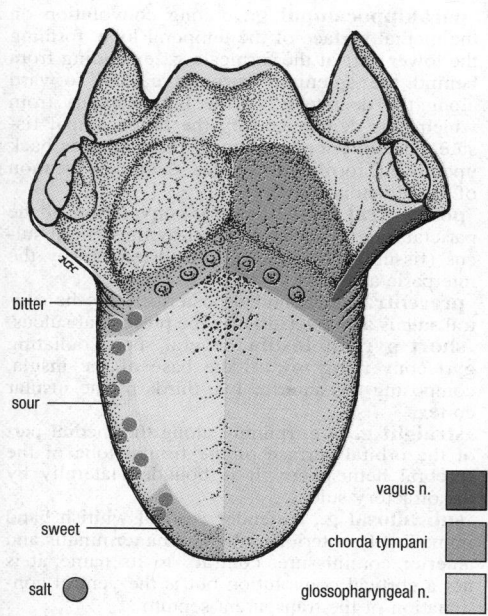

bitter

sour

sweet

salt

vagus n.

chorda tympani

glossopharyngeal n.

gustation: regions of taste perception and their gustatory nerves

the folding of embryonic body—head, tail and lateral body folds.

gut·ta-per·cha (gŭt′ă-per′chă). The coagulated, purified, dried, milky juice of trees of the genera *Palaguium* and *Payena* (family Sapotaceae); used as a filling material in dentistry, and in the manufacture of splints and electrical insulators; a solution is used as a substitute for collodion, as a protective, and to seal incised wounds. Solid at room temperature and soft and plastic when heated.

gut·tate (gŭt′tāt). Of the shape of, or resembling, a drop, characterizing certain cutaneous lesions.

gut·tur·al (gŭt′er-ăl). Relating to the throat.

GVHR graft versus host *reaction.*

GXT graded exercise *test.*

Gy gray (unit of absorbed radiation).

GYN gynecology.

gyn-, gyne-, gyneco-, gyno-. Female. [G. *gynē,* woman]

gy·nan·drism (ji-nan′drizm, gī′nan-drizm). A developmental abnormality characterized by hypertrophy of the clitoris and union of the labia majora, simulating in appearance the penis and scrotum. SEE hermaphroditism. [gyn- + G. *anēr* (*andr-*), man]

gy·nan·dro·blas·to·ma (ji-nan′drō-blas-tō′mă, gī-). **1.** SYN arrhenoblastoma. **2.** A rare variety of arrhenoblastoma of the ovary, containing granulosa or theca cell elements and producing simultaneous androgenic and estrogenic effects.

gy·nan·droid (gī-nan′droyd, jī-). An individual exhibiting gynandrism. [gyn- + G. *anēr* (*andr-*), man, + *eidos,* resemblance]

gy·nan·dro·mor·phism (gī-nan-drō-mōr′fizm, jī-). **1.** An abnormal combination of male and female characteristics. **2.** The presence of male and female sex chromosome complements in different tissues; sex chromosome mosaicism. [gyn- + G. *anēr* (*andr-*), a male human, + *morphē,* form]

gy·nan·dro·mor·phous (gī-nan-drō-mōr′fŭs, jī-). Having both male and female characteristics.

gyne-. SEE gyn-.

gy·ne·cic (gī-nē′sik, jī-). Pertaining to or associated with women.

gy·ne·coid (gī′nĕ-koyd, jin′ĕ-). **1.** Resembling a woman in form and structure. **2.** OBSTETRICS Referring to the shape of the normal female pelvis. [gyneco- + G. *eidos,* resemblance]

gy·ne·co·log·ic, gy·ne·co·log·i·cal (gī′nĕ-kō-loj′ik, jin′ĕ-; -loj′i-kăl). Relating to gynecology.

gy·ne·col·o·gist (gī-nĕ-kol′ō-jist, jī-nĕ-). A physician specializing in gynecology.

gy·ne·col·o·gy (GYN) (gī-nĕ-kol′ō-jē, jin-ĕ-). The medical specialty concerned with diseases of the female genital tract, as well as endocrinology and reproductive physiology of the female. [gyneco- + G. *logos,* study]

gy·ne·co·ma·stia, gy·ne·co·mas·ty (gī′nĕ-kō-mas′tē-ă, jin′ĕ-; -mas′tē). Excessive development of the male mammary glands, due mainly to ductal proliferation with periductal edema; frequently secondary to increased estrogen levels, but mild g. may occur in normal adolescence. [gyneco- + G. *mastos,* breast]

gy·ne·pho·bia (gī-nĕ-fō′bē-ă, jin-ĕ-). Morbid fear of women or of the female sex. [gyne- + G. *phobos,* fear]

gyno-. SEE gyn-.

gy·no·gen·e·sis (gī-nō-jen′ĕ-sis, jin-ō-). Egg development activated by a spermatozoon, but to which the male gamete contributes no genetic material. [gyno- + G. *genesis,* production]

gy·rate (jī′rāt). **1.** Of a convoluted or ring shape. **2.** To revolve. [L. *gyro,* pp. *gyratus,* to turn round in a circle, *gyrus*]

gy·rec·to·my (jī-rek′tō-mē). Excision of a cerebral gyrus. [G. *gyros,* ring, + *ektomē,* excision]

gy·ri (jī′rī). Plural of gyrus. [L.]

Gy·ro·mi·tra es·cu·len·ta (gī-rō-mē′tră es-kyū-len′tă). A species of mushroom that may produce a monomethylhydrazine toxin which causes nausea, diarrhea, and other symptoms; in severe cases death may occur.

gy·rose (jī′rōs). Marked by irregular curved lines like the surface of a cerebral hemisphere. [G. *gyros,* circle]

gy·ro·spasm (jī′rō-spazm). Spasmodic rotary movements of the head. [G. *gyros,* circle, + *spasmos,* spasm]

gy·rus, gen. and pl. **gy·ri** (jī′rŭs, -rī) [NA]. One of the prominent rounded elevations that form the cerebral hemispheres, each consisting of an exposed superficial portion and a portion hidden from view in the wall and floor of the sulcus. [L. fr. G. *gyros,* circle]

angular g., a folded convolution in the inferior parietal lobule formed by the union of the

gy

posterior ends of the superior and middle temporal gyri.

central gyri, the precentral and postcentral gyri.

cingulate g., a long, curved convolution of the medial surface of the cortical hemisphere, arched over the corpus callosum from which it is separated by the deep sulcus of corpus callosum; together with the parahippocampal g., with which it is continuous behind the corpus callosum, it forms the fornicate g.

dentate g., one of the two interlocking gyri composing the hippocampus, the other one being the Ammon's horn.

fornicate g., the horseshoe-shaped cortical convolution bordering the hilus of the cerebral hemisphere; its upper limb is formed by the cingulate g., its lower by the parahippocampal g.; SYN g. fornicatus (1).

g. fornica′tus, (1) SYN fornicate g. **(2)** used previously to refer to the entire limbic system.

fusiform g., an extremely long convolution extending lengthwise over the inferior aspect of the temporal and occipital lobes, demarcated medially by the collateral sulcus from the lingual g. and the anterior part of the parahippocampal g., laterally by the inferior temporal sulcus from the inferior temporal g.

insular gyri, the short gyri of insula and long g. of insula.

lingual g., a relatively short horizontal convolution on the inferomedial aspect of the occipital and temporal lobes, demarcated from the lateral occipitotemporal or fusiform g. by the deep collateral sulcus, from the cuneus by the calcarine sulcus; its anterior extreme abuts the isthmus of the parahippocampal g.; the medial or upper strip of the g. forming the lower bank of the calcarine sulcus corresponds to the inferior half of the striate area or primary visual cortex and represents the contralateral upper quadrant of the binocular field of vision.

long g. of insula, the most posterior and longest of the slender straight gyri that compose the insula.

orbital gyri, a number of small, irregular convolutions occupying the concave inferior surface of each frontal lobe of the cerebrum.

parahippocampal g., a long convolution on the medial surface of the temporal lobe, forming the lower part of the fornicate g., extending from behind the splenium corporis callosi forward along the dentate g. of the hippocampus from which it is demarcated by the hippocampal fissure. The anterior extreme of the g. curves back upon itself, forming the uncus, the major location of the olfactory cortex.

postcentral g., the anterior convolution of the parietal lobe, bounded in front by the central sulcus (fissure of Rolando) and posteriorly by the interparietal sulcus.

precentral g., bounded posteriorly by the central sulcus and anteriorly by the precentral sulcus.

short gyri of insula, several short, radiating gyri converging toward the base of the insula, composing the anterior two-thirds of the insular cortex.

straight g., a g. running along the medial part of the orbital surface of the frontal lobe of the cerebral hemisphere. It is bounded laterally by the olfactory sulcus.

subcallosal g., a slender vertical whitish band immediately anterior to the lamina terminalis and anterior commissure; contrary to its name, it is not a cortical convolution but is the ventral continuation of the transparent septum.

superior frontal g., a broad convolution running in an anteroposterior direction on the medial edge of the convex surface and of each frontal lobe.

supramarginal g., a folded convolution capping the posterior extremity of the lateral (sylvian) sulcus; together with the angular g., it forms the inferior half of the parietal lobe.

transitional g., a small convolution connecting two lobes or two main gyri in the depth of a sulcus.

transverse temporal gyri, two or three convolutions running transversely on the upper surface of the temporal lobe bordering on the lateral (sylvian) fissure, separated from each other by the transverse temporal sulci.

uncinate g., SYN uncus (2).

H

H hyperopia or hyperopic; horizontal; Hauch; Holzknecht *unit*; henry, unit of electrical inductance; hydrogen; the Fraunhofer line at λ 3968 due to calcium; histidine; magnetic field strength; heroin.

H^+ hydrogen *ion*, the proton.

^1H hydrogen-1.

^2H hydrogen-2.

H enthalpy, heat content, in the equation for free energy.

h hecto-; height; hour.

h Planck's *constant*; $h = h/2\pi$.

ha·be·na, pl. **ha·be·nae** (hă-bē′nă, -bē′nē). **1.** A frenum or restricting fibrous band. **2.** A restraining bandage. **3.** SYN habenula (2). [L. strap]

hab·e·nal, ha·be·nar (hab′ĕ-năl, hă-bē′năr). Relating to a habena.

ha·ben·u·la, pl. **ha·ben·u·lae** (ha-ben′yū-lă, -lē). **1.** SYN frenulum. **2** [NA]. NEUROANATOMY A circumscript cell mass in the dorsomedial thalamus, embedded in the posterior end of the medullary stria from which it receives most of its afferent fibers. By way of the retroflex fasciculus (habenulointerpeduncular tract) it projects to the interpeduncular nucleus and other paramedian cell groups of the midbrain tegmentum. Despite its proximity to the pineal stalk, no habenulopineal fiber connection is known to exist. It is a part of the epithalamus. SYN habena (3). [L.]

ha·ben·u·lar (hă-ben′yū-lăr). Relating to a habenula, especially the stalk of the pineal body.

hab·it. 1. An act, behavioral response, practice, or custom established in one's repertoire by frequent repetition of the same act. SEE ALSO addiction. **2.** A basic variable in the study of conditioning and learning used to designate a new response learned either by association or by being followed by a reward or reinforced event. SEE conditioning, learning. [L. *habeo*, pp. *habitus*, to have]

ha·bit·u·a·tion (ha-bit-chū-ā′shŭn). **1.** The process of forming a habit, referring generally to psychological dependence on the continued use of a drug to maintain a sense of well-being, which can result in drug addiction. **2.** The method by which the nervous system reduces or inhibits responsiveness during repeated stimulation.

hab·i·tus (hab′i-tŭs). The physical characteristics of a person. [L. habit]

haem-. SEE hem-.

Hae·moph·i·lus (hē-mof′i-lŭs). A genus of aerobic to facultatively anaerobic, nonmotile bacteria containing minute, Gram-negative, rod-shaped cells which sometimes form threads and are pleomorphic. These organisms are strictly parasitic, growing best, or only, on media containing blood. They may or may not be pathogenic. They occur in various lesions and secretions, as well as in normal respiratory tracts, of vertebrates. The type species is *H. influenzae*. [G. *haima*, blood, + *philos*, fond]

  H. aegyp′ticus, a species that causes acute or subacute infectious conjunctivitis in warm climates. SYN Koch-Weeks bacillus.

  H. ducrey′i, a species which causes soft chancre (chancroid). SYN Ducrey's bacillus.

  H. influen′zae, a species found in the respiratory tract that causes acute respiratory infections including pneumonia, acute conjunctivitis, bacterial meningitis, and purulent meningitis in children, rarely in adults; originally considered to be the cause of influenza, it is the type species of the genus *H.* SYN Pfeiffer's bacillus.

haf·ni·um (Hf) (haf′nē-ŭm). A rare chemical element, atomic no. 72, atomic wt. 178.49. [L. *Hafnia,* Copenhagen]

hahn·i·um (hahn′ē-ŭm). Name proposed for the artificially made element 105. [Otto *Hahn,* Ger. physical chemist and Nobel laureate, 1879–1968]

hair (hār). **1.** SYN pilus (1). **2.** One of the fine hairlike processes of the auditory cells of the labyrinth, and of other sensory cells, called auditory h.'s, sensory h.'s, etc. SYN thrix. [A.S. *haer*]

  auditory h.'s, cilia on the free surface of the auditory cells.

  bamboo h., h. with regularly spaced nodules along the shaft caused by intermittent fractures with invagination of the distal h. into the proximal portion, with intervening lengths of normal h., giving the appearance of bamboo; seen in Netherton's syndrome. SYN trichorrhexis invaginata.

  bayonet h., a spindle-shaped developmental defect occurring at the tapered end of the h.

  beaded h., SYN monilethrix.

  club h., a h. in resting state, prior to shedding, in which the bulb has become a club-shaped mass.

  ingrown h.'s, h.'s that grow at more acute angles than is normal, and in all directions; they incompletely clear the follicle, turn back in, and cause pseudofolliculitis.

  lanugo h., SYN lanugo.

  moniliform h., SYN monilethrix.

  scalp h., a hair of the head.

  stellate h., h. split in several strands at the free end.

  taste h.'s, hairlike projections of gustatory cells of taste buds; electron micrographs show them to be clusters of microvilli.

  terminal h., a mature pigmented, coarse h.

  twisted h.'s, SYN *pili torti,* under *pilus.*

hairy (hār′ē). **1.** Of or resembling hair. **2.** Covered with hair. SEE ALSO hirsutism. SYN pilar, pilary, pileous, pilose.

ha·la·tion (hă-lā′shŭn). Blurring of the visual image by glare.

half-life (haf′līf). The period in which the radioactivity or number of atoms of a radioactive substance decreases by half; similarly applied to any substance whose quantity decreases exponentially with time. Time required for the serum concentration of a drug to decline by 50%. Cf. half-time.

half-time (haf′tīm). The time, in a first-order chemical (or enzymic) reaction, for half of the substance (substrate) to be converted or to disappear. Cf. half-life.

half·way house (haf′wā hows). A facility for

individuals who no longer require the complete facilities of a hospital or institution but are not yet prepared to return to independent living.

hal·ide (hal'īd). A salt of a halogen.

hal·i·to·sis (hal-i-tō'sis). A foul odor of the breath. [L. *halitus*, breath, + G. *-osis*, condition]

hal·i·tus (hal'i-tŭs). Any exhalation, as of a breath or vapor. [L., fr. *halo*, to breathe]

hal·lu·cal (hal'ū-kăl). Relating to the hallux.

hal·lu·ci·na·tion (ha-lū'si-nā'shŭn). The subjective perception of an object or event when no such stimulus or situation is present; may be visual, auditory, olfactory, gustatory, or tactile. [L. *alucinor*, to wander in mind]

 hypnagogic h., a common symptom in narcolepsy characterized by vivid, dreamlike perceptions occurring with sleep onset. Often these perceptions involve fearful situations that are described as realistic and include visual, tactile, and auditory h.'s.

 hypnopompic h., vivid hallucinations that occur when wakening from sleep; occurs with narcolepsy, but grouped with hypnagogic hallucination.

 mood-congruent h., h. in which the content is mood appropriate.

 mood-incongruent h., h. that is not consistent with external stimuli; content is not consistent with either manic or depressed mood.

hal·lu·ci·no·gen (ha-lū'si-nō-jen). A mind-altering chemical, drug, or agent, specifically a chemical whose most prominent pharmacologic action is on the central nervous system; in normal subjects, it elicits optical or auditory hallucinations, depersonalization, perceptual disturbances, and disturbances of thought processes. [L. *alucinor*, to wander in mind, + G. *-gen*, producing]

hal·lu·ci·no·gen·ic (ha-lū'si-nō-jen'ik). SYN psychodelic.

hal·lu·ci·no·sis (ha-lū-si-nō'sis). A syndrome, usually of organic origin (*e.g.*, alcoholic h. characterized by more or less persistent hallucinations).

hal·lux, pl. **hal·lu·ces** (hal'ŭks, hal'yū-sēz) [NA]. The great toe; the first digit of the foot. [a Mod. L. form for L. *hallex* (*hallic-*), great toe]

 h. doloro'sus, a condition, usually associated with flatfoot, in which walking causes severe pain in the metatarsophalangeal joint of the great toe.

 h. flex'us, hammer toe involving the first toe.

 h. rig'idus, a condition in which there is stiffness in the first metatarsophalangeal joint; the joint may be the site of osteoarthritis.

 h. val'gus, a deviation of the tip of the great toe, or main axis of the toe, toward the outer or lateral side of the foot.

 h. va'rus, deviation of the main axis of the great toe to the inner side of the foot away from its neighbor.

ha·lo (hā'lō). **1.** A reddish yellow ring surrounding the optic disk, due to a widening of the scleral ring making the deeper structures visible. **2.** An annular flare of light surrounding a luminous body or a depigmented ring around a mole. SEE halo *nevus.* **3.** SYN areola (4). **4.** A circular metal band used in a h. cast or h. brace, attached to the skull with pins. [G. *halōs,* threshing floor on which oxen trod a circle; the halo round the sun or moon]

 anemic h., pale, relatively avascular areas in the skin seen around vascular spiders, cherry angiomas, and sometimes in acute macular eruptions.

 glaucomatous h., (**1**) a yellowish white ring surrounding the optic disk, indicating atrophy of the choroid in glaucoma; (**2**) a h. surrounding lights, caused by corneal edema in glaucoma.

hal·o·gen (hal'ō-jen). One of the chlorine group (fluorine, chlorine, bromine, iodine, astatine) of elements; h.'s form monobasic acids with hydrogen, and their hydroxides (fluorine forms none) are also monobasic acids. [G. *hals,* salt, + *-gen,* producing]

hal·o·gen·o·der·ma (hal-ō-gen'ō-der-mă). Dermatosis caused by ingestion or injection of halogens, most notably bromides and iodides. [halogen + G. *derma,* skin]

ha·lom·e·ter (hal-om'ĕ-ter). An instrument used to measure the diffraction halo of a red blood cell; based on the premise that the halo of the large erythrocyte of pernicious anemia is smaller than that of the normal cell; the hazy colorless halo of normal size is characteristic of secondary anemia.

hal·o·phil, hal·o·phile (hal'ō-fil, -fīl). A microorganism whose growth is enhanced by or dependent on a high salt concentration. [G. *hals,* salt, + *philos,* fond]

hal·o·phil·ic (hal-ō-fil'ik). Requiring a high concentration of salt for growth.

ha·mar·tia (ham-ar'shē-ă). A localized developmental disturbance characterized by abnormal arrangement and/or combinations of the tissues normally present in the area. [G. *hamartion,* a bodily defect]

ham·ar·to·blas·to·ma (hă-mar'tō-blas-tō'mă). A malignant neoplasm of undifferentiated anaplastic cells thought to be derived from a hamartoma. [hamartoma + blastoma]

ham·ar·to·ma (ham-ar-tō'mă). A focal malformation that resembles a neoplasm, grossly and even microscopically, but results from faulty development in an organ; composed of an abnormal mixture of tissue elements, or an abnormal proportion of a single element, normally present in that site, which develop and grow at virtually the same rate as normal components, and are not likely to result in compression of adjacent tissue (in contrast to a neoplasm). [G. *hamartion,* a bodily defect, + *-oma,* tumor]

 pulmonary h., h. of the lung, producing a coin lesion composed primarily of cartilage and bronchial epithelium. SYN adenochondroma.

ham·ar·tom·a·tous (ham-ar-tō'mă-tŭs). Relating to hamartoma.

ham·mer (ham'er). SYN malleus.

ham·string. One of the tendons bounding the popliteal space on either side; the **medial h.** comprises the tendons of the semimembranosus and semitendinosus, gracilis, and sartorius muscles; the **lateral h.** is the tendon of the biceps femoris muscle. H. muscles (a) have origin from the ischial tuberosity, (b) act across (at) both the hip and knee joints (producing extension and flexion, respectively), and (c) are innervated by the tibial portion of the sciatic nerve. The medial h. contributes to medial rotation of the leg at the flexed knee joint, while the lateral h. contributes to lateral rotation.

ham•u•lar (ham′yū-lăr). Hook-shaped; unciform. [L. *hamulus, q.v.*]

ham•u•lus, gen. and pl. **ham•u•li** (ham′yū-lŭs, -lī) [NA]. Any hooklike structure. [L. dim. of *hamus,* hook]

▌hand. The portion of the upper limb distal to the radiocarpal joint, comprising the wrist, palm, and fingers. SYN manus [NA]. [A.S.]

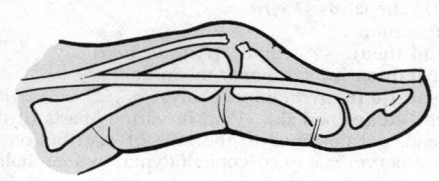

boutonnière deformity

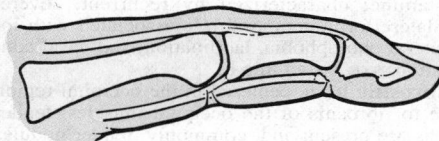

jersey finger

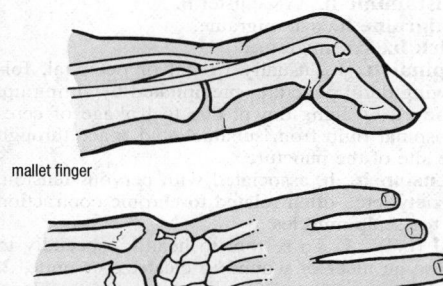

mallet finger

Colles' fracture

hand deformities and fractures

accoucheur's h., position of the h. in tetany or in muscular dystrophy; the fingers are flexed at the metacarpophalangeal joints and extended at the phalangeal joints, with the thumb flexed and adducted into the palm; in resemblance to the position of the physician's hand in making a vaginal examination. SYN obstetrical h.

claw h., SEE clawhand.

cleft h., a congenital deformity in which the division between the fingers, especially between the third and fourth, extends into the metacarpal region. SYN split h.

club h., congenital or acquired angulation deformity of h. associated with partial or complete absence of radius or ulna; usually with intrinsic deformities of the h. in congenital variants.

drop h., SYN *wrist*-drop.

obstetrical h., SYN accoucheur's h.

split h., SYN cleft h.

writing h., a contraction of the h. muscles in parkinsonism, bringing the fingers somewhat into the position of holding a pen.

hand•ed•ness (hand′ed-nes). Preference for the use of one hand, most commonly the right, associated with dominance of the opposite cerebral hemisphere; may also be the result of training or habit.

hand•i•cap (hand′i-kap). **1.** A physical, mental, or emotional condition that interferes with an individual's normal functioning. **2.** Reduction in a person's capacity to fulfill a social role as a consequence of an impairment, inadequate training for the role, or other circumstances. SEE ALSO disability. [fr. *hand in cap* (game)]

handling. Use of the therapist's hands in a trained manner on parts of the patient's body to decrease the frequency of abnormal patterns of movement and to increase the occurrence of automatic normal movement.

hang•nail (hang′nāl). A loose triangular tag of skin attached at the proximal portion in the medial or lateral nail fold.

Han•ta•vi•rus (han′tā-vā-rŭs). A genus of Bunyaviridae responsible for pneumonia and hemorrhagic fevers. Four members of the genus are recognized thus far: Hantaan, Puumala, Seoul, and Prospect Hill. The first three of these are known human pathogens; Hantaan virus causes Korean hemorrhagic fever. Various rodent species are the asymptomatic carriers of these viruses, which are shed in saliva, urine, and feces. Human infection is direct, or by the respiratory route from contaminated specimens; person-to-person spread has not been demonstrated. In 1992 this virus was isolated from patients in Arizona and New Mexico. Affected persons may have a mild to fatal course. The most seriously ill have hemorrhagic fevers accompanied by renal failure and sometimes respiratory collapse.

haph•al•ge•sia (haf-al-jē′zē-ă). Pain or an extremely disagreeable sensation caused by the merest touch. [G. *haphē,* touch, + *algēsis,* sense of pain]

△**haplo-.** Simple, single. [G. *haplous*]

hap•loid (hap′loyd). Denoting the number of chromosomes in sperm or ova, which is half the number in somatic (diploid) cells; the h. number in normal human beings is 23. [G. *haplos,* simple, + *eidos,* appearance]

hap•lo•pro•tein (hap-lō-prō′tēn). The functional complex between an apoprotein and the prosthetic group that together are responsible for biological activity.

hap•lo•scop•ic (hap-lō-skop′ik). Relating to a haploscope.

hap•lo•type (hap′lō-tīp). **1.** The genetic constitution of an individual with respect to one member of a pair of allelic genes; individuals are of the same h. (but of different genotypes) if alike with

ha

respect to one allele of a pair but different with respect to the other allele of a pair. **2.** IMMUNOGE-NETICS That portion of the phenotype determined by a set of closely linked genes inherited from one parent (*i.e.,* genes located on one of the pair of chromosomes). The human major histocompatability complex comprises 4 recognized loci (A, B, C, and D) for which there are more than 50 alleles. Similarly, the allotypic markers (antigens) of the immunoglobulin subclasses IgG1, IgG2, IgG3, and IgA2 occur in combinations and are inherited as units almost always unchanged in transmission; the alleles that control these various h.'s are not linked to those controlling the antigens of the κ type L chains. [haplo- + G. *typos,* impression, model]

hap•ten. A molecule that is incapable, alone, of causing the production of antibodies but can, however, combine with a larger antigenic molecule called a carrier. SYN incomplete antigen, partial antigen. [G. *haptō,* to fasten, bind]

  conjugated h., a h. that may cause the production of antibodies when it has been covalently linked to protein. SYN conjugated antigen.

hap•tics (hap′tiks). The science concerned with the tactile sense. [G. *haptō,* to grasp, touch]

hap•to•glo•bin (hap-tō-glō′bin) [MIM*140100 &]. A group of α_2-globulins in human serum, so called because of their ability to combine with hemoglobin; variant types form a polymorphic system, with α- and β-polypeptide chains controlled by separate genetic loci. [G. *haptō,* to grasp, + hemoglobin]

hare•lip (hār′lip). SYN cleft *lip.*

har•vest. To obtain cells or tissues for grafting or transplantation, from either a donor or the patient.

hash•ish (hash′ish). A form of cannabis that consists largely of resin from the flowering tops and sprouts of cultivated female hemp plants of the species *Cannabis sativa;* contains the highest concentration of cannabinols among the preparations derived from cannabis. [Ar. hay]

Hauch (H) (howkh). A term used to designate the flagellar antigen of bacteria. SEE ALSO H *antigen.* [Ger. breath]

haus•tra (haw′strǎ). Plural of haustrum. [L.]

haus•tral (haw′strǎl). Relating to a haustrum.

haus•tra•tion (haw-strǎ′shŭn). **1.** The process of formation of a haustrum. **2.** An increase in prominence of the haustra.

haus•trum, pl. **haus•tra** (haw′strŭm, haw′strǎ). One of a series of saccules or pouches, so called because of a fancied resemblance to the buckets on a water wheel. [L. a machine for drawing water, fr. *haurio,* pp. *haustus,* to draw up, drink up]

HAV hepatitis A *virus.*

ha•ver•si•an (ha-ver′shan). Relating to Clopton Havers and the various osseous structures described by him.

Hb hemoglobin.

Hb A *hemoglobin A.*

HB$_c$Ab antibody to the hepatitis B core *antigen.*

HB$_c$Ag hepatitis B core *antigen.*

HB$_s$Ag hepatitis B surface *antigen.*

Hb C *hemoglobin C.*

HBE His bundle *electrogram.*

HBe, HB$_e$Ag hepatitis B e *antigen.*

Hb F *hemoglobin F.*

HBIG hepatitis B immune *globulin.*

Hb S sickle cell *hemoglobin.*

Hb S *hemoglobin S.*

HBV hepatitis B *virus.*

HCFA (Health Care Financing Administration) Health Care Financing Administration.

HCS Abbreviation for human chorionic somatomammotropic *hormone;* human chorionic *somatomammotropin.*

Hct hematocrit.

HCV hepatitis C *virus.*

HDL high density lipoprotein. SEE lipoprotein.

HDV hepatitis D *virus.*

He helium.

head (hed). SYN caput. [A.S. *heáfod*]

  Medusa h., SYN *caput* medusae.

  saddle h., SYN clinocephaly.

head•ache (hed′āk). Pain in various parts of the head, not confined to the area of distribution of any nerve. SEE ALSO cephalodynia. SYN cephalalgia, encephalalgia.

  cluster h., possibly due to a hypersensitivity to histamine; characterized by recurrent, severe, unilateral orbitotemporal h.'s associated with ipsilateral photophobia, lacrimation, and nasal congestion. SYN histaminic h.

  fibrositic h., h. centered in the occipital region due to fibrositis of the occipital muscles; tender areas are present and, commonly, tender nodules are found in the scalp in the lower occipital region.

  histaminic h., SYN cluster h.

  migraine h., SEE migraine.

  sick h., SYN migraine.

  spinal h., h., usually frontal or occipital, following dural puncture; precipitated by sitting up, relieved by lying down; due to leakage of cerebrospinal fluid from subarachnoid space through the site of the puncture.

  tension h., h. associated with nervous tension, anxiety, etc., often related to chronic contraction of the scalp muscles.

heal (hēl). **1.** To restore to health, especially to cause an ulcer or wound to cicatrize or unite. **2.** To become well, to be cured; to cicatrize or close, said of an ulcer or wound. [A.S. *healan*]

heal•ing (hēl′ing). **1.** Restoring to health; promoting the closure of wounds and ulcers. **2.** The process of a return to health. **3.** Closing of a wound. SEE ALSO union.

  h. by first intention, h. by fibrous adhesion, without suppuration or granulation tissue formation. SYN primary adhesion, primary union.

  h. by second intention, delayed closure of two granulating surfaces. SYN secondary adhesion, secondary union.

  h. by third intention, the slow filling of a wound cavity or ulcer by granulations, with subsequent cicatrization.

health (helth). **1.** The state of the organism when it functions optimally without evidence of disease or abnormality. **2.** A state of dynamic balance in which an individual's or a group's capacity to cope with all the circumstances of living is at an optimum level. **3.** A state characterized by anatomical, physiological, and psychological integrity, ability to perform personally valued family, work, and community roles; ability to deal with physical, biological, psychological and social stress; a feeling of well-being; and freedom from the risk of disease and untimely death. **4.** Complete physical, mental, and social well-being, not just the absence of disease, as defined by the World Health Organization. [A.S. *haelth*]

mental h., emotional, behavioral, and social maturity or normality; the absence of a mental or behavioral disorder; a state of psychological well-being in which the individual has achieved a satisfactory integration of instinctual drives acceptable to both self and social milieu; an appropriate balance of love, work, and leisure pursuits.

public h., the art and science of community health, concerned with statistics, epidemiology, hygiene, and the prevention and eradication of epidemic diseases; an effort organized by society to promote, protect, and restore the people's health; public h. is a social institution, a service, and a practice.

Health Care Financing Administration. Agency of the U.S. Department of Health and Human Services that manages the federal health care programs of Medicare and Medicaid.

health care provider. General term for any institution or member of the health care team providing health care. SEE ALSO doctor, physician, nurse.

health information management (HIM). collection and analysis of health care data in order to provide information for health care decisions involving patient care, institutional management, health care policies and planning, and research; formerly known as medical records management. SEE ALSO record.

health main·te·nance or·ga·ni·za·tion (HMO). A comprehensive prepaid system of health care with emphasis on the prevention and early detection of disease, and continuity of care. HMOs may be nonprofit or profit-making ventures, and along with preferred provider organizations (PPOs) and managed care plans have begun to dominate the health care market. HMOs generally offer a package of services; however, the choice of physician is frequently limited to those working within the HMO. SEE ALSO managed *care*, preferred provider *organization*.

group model HMO, HMO that contracts with a physician practice group to be sole providers to that HMO's subscribers.

independent practice association HMO, arrangement by which physician providers are paid by the HMO on a fee-for-service basis for each patient seen, as negotiated with the HMO

network model HMO, arrangement by which an HMO contracts with group practice physicians to be providers for HMO subscribers, with the physicians retaining the option to see other patients.

staff model HMO, arrangement under which physician providers are salaried employees of an HMO.

health risk ap·prais·al. A method of describing an individual's chance of falling ill or dying of a specified condition, based on actuarial calculations that allow for known exposure to risk; expressed as expected age at which death or disease will occur, and intended as a way of drawing an individual's attention to the probable consequences of risk behavior.

healthy (helth'ē). Well; in a state of normal functioning; free from disease.

hear·ing (hēr'ing). The ability to perceive sound; the sensation of sound as opposed to vibration. SYN -acousis (2), audition.

h. aid (hēr'ing ād), An electronic amplifying device designed to bring sound more effectively into the ear; it consists of a microphone, amplifier, and receiver.

color h., a subjective perception of color produced by certain sounds. SYN pseudochromesthesia (2).

H. Handicap Inventory for the Elderly (HHIE-S), Screening test that uses a communication scale to determine if older adults have difficulty hearing and understanding speech.

hear·ing loss, hear·ing im·pair·ment. A reduction in the ability to perceive sound; may range from slight to complete deafness. SEE ALSO deafness.

conductive h. l., h. l. caused by an obstruction or lesion in the outer ear, middle ear, or both. SEE ALSO air-bone *gap*.

heart (hart). A hollow muscular organ which receives the blood from the veins and propels it into the arteries. It is divided by a musculomembranous septum into two halves—right or venous and left or arterial—each of which consists of a receiving chamber (atrium) and an ejecting chamber (ventricle). SYN cor [NA], coeur. [A.S. *heorte*]

artificial h., a mechanical pump used to replace the function of a damaged heart, either temporarily or as a permanent prosthesis.

athlete's h., nonpathological enlarged heart in athletes reflecting specific adaptation to prolonged training. Manifestations in response to resistance training are thickened left ventricular wall and concentric hypertrophy, and in response to endurance training are enlarged left ventricular cavity and eccentric hypertrophy. SEE hypertrophy.

fatty h., (1) fatty degeneration of the myocardium; **(2)** accumulation of adipose tissue on the external surface of the h. with occasional infiltration of fat between the muscle bundles of the h. wall. SYN adiposis cardiaca, cor adiposum.

horizontal h., description of the h.'s electrical position; recognized in the electrocardiogram when the electrical axis lies between −30° and +30°.

intermediate h., description of the h.'s electrical axis when this is directed at approximately between +30° and +60°.

Jarvik artificial h., a pneumatic artificial heart.

left h., the left atrium and left ventricle.

he

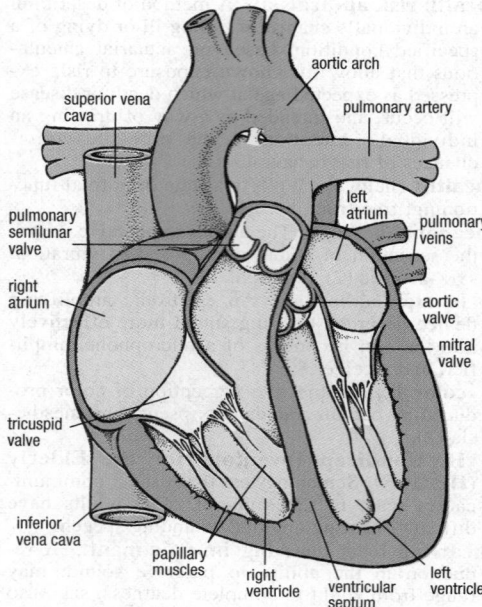

heart: frontal view showing chambers

Labels on figure: aortic arch · superior vena cava · pulmonary artery · left atrium · pulmonary veins · pulmonary semilunar valve · aortic valve · mitral valve · right atrium · tricuspid valve · inferior vena cava · papillary muscles · right ventricle · ventricular septum · left ventricle

ox h., a very large h., usually due to chronic hypertension or, more often, to aortic valve disease.

right h., the right atrium and right ventricle.

round h., abnormally smooth arcuate contours of the heart due either to disease of the ventricles or to a false cardiac appearance produced by excessive pericardial fluid.

semihorizontal h., refers to the h.'s electrical axis when this is directed at approximately 0°.

semivertical h., descriptive of the h.'s electrical axis when this is directed at approximately +60°.

stone h., SYN ischemic *contracture* of the left ventricle.

tobacco h., cardiac irritability marked by irregular action, palpitation, and sometimes pain, believed to occur as a result of the heavy use of tobacco.

vertical h., descriptive of the h. electrical axis when this is directed at approximately +90°.

heart•beat (hart′bēt). A single complete cycle of contraction and dilation of heart muscle.

heart•burn (hart′bern). SYN pyrosis.

heat (hēt). **1.** A high temperature; the sensation produced by proximity to fire or an incandescent object, as opposed to cold. The basis of h. is the kinetic energy of atoms and molecules, which becomes zero at absolute zero. **2.** SYN estrus. **3.** SYN enthalpy. [A.S. *haete*]

conductive h., h. transmitted by direct contact, as by an electric pad or hot-water bottle.

convective h., h. conveyed by a warm medium, such as air or water, in motion from its source.

conversive h., h. produced in a body by the absorption of waves that are not in themselves hot, such as the sun's rays or infrared radiation.

prickly h., SYN *miliaria* rubra.

heat-la•bile (hēt′lā′bl). Destroyed or altered by heat.

heat•stroke (hēt′strōk). A severe and often fatal illness produced by exposure to excessively high temperatures, especially when accompanied by marked exertion; characterized by headache, vertigo, confusion, hot dry skin, and a slight rise in body temperature; in severe cases, very high fever, vascular collapse, and coma develop.

he•be•phre•nia (hē-bĕ-frē′nē-ă, heb′ē-). A syndrome characterized by shallow and inappropriate affect, giggling, and silly, regressive behavior and mannerisms; a subtype of schizophrenia now renamed disorganized *schizophrenia*. [G. *hēbē*, puberty, + *phrēn*, the mind]

he•be•phren•ic (hē-bĕ-frēn′ik, heb-ē-). Relating to or characterized by hebephrenia.

he•bet•ic (hē-bet′ik). Pertaining to youth. [G. *hēbētikos*, youthful, fr. *hēbē*, youth]

he•bi•at•rics (hē-bē-at′riks). SYN adolescent *medicine*. [G. *hēbē*, youth, + *iatrikos*, relating to medicine]

hec•a•ter•o•mer•ic (hek′ă-ter-ō-mer′ik). Denoting a spinal neuron whose axon divides and gives off processes to both sides of the cord; usually the same as a heteromeric neuron. [G. *hekateros*, each of two, + *meros*, part]

⬦**hecto-** (**h**). Prefix used in the SI and metric systems to signify one hundred (10^2). [G. *hekaton*, one hundred]

hed•ro•cele (hed′rō-sēl). Prolapse of the intestine through the anus. [G. *hedra*, a seat, the fundament, + *kēlē*, hernia]

heel (hēl). **1.** SYN calx (2). **2.** SYN distal *end*. [A.S. *hēla*]

cracked h., SYN *keratoderma* plantare sulcatum.

painful h., a condition in which bearing weight on the h. causes pain of varying severity. SYN calcaneodynia, calcodynia.

prominent h., a condition marked by a tender swelling on the os calcis due to a thickening of the periosteum or fibrous tissue covering the back of the os calcis.

height (**h**) (hīt). Vertical measurement.

h. of contour, the line encircling a tooth or other structure at its greatest bulge or diameter with respect to a selected path of insertion.

cusp h., (**1**) the shortest distance between the tip of a cusp and its base plane; (**2**) the shortest distance between the deepest part of the central fossa of a posterior tooth and a line connecting the points of the cusps of the tooth.

HeLa (hē′la). Referring to cells of the first continuously cultured (human cervical) carcinoma strain. [*Henrietta La*cks (d. 1951), whose cervical carcinoma was the source of the cell line]

hel•i•cal (hel′i-kăl). **1.** Relating to a helix. SYN helicine (2). **2.** SYN helicoid. [G. *helix*, a coil]

hel•i•ces (hel′i-sēz). Plural of helix.

hel•i•cine (hel′i-sēn). **1.** Coiled. **2.** SYN helical (1). [G. *helix*, a coil]

Hel•i•co•bac•ter (hel′ĭ-kō-bak′ter). A genus of helical, curved, or straight microaerophilic bacteria with rounded ends and multiple sheathed flagella (unipolar or bipolar and lateral) with terminal bulbs. Found in gastric mucosa; some species are associated with gastric and peptic ulcers.

H. pylo'ri, a recently identified species that produces urease and is associated with several gastroduodenal diseases including gastritis and peptic ulcer. The type species of the genus *Helicobacter.*

hel·i·coid (hel'i-koyd). Resembling a helix. SYN helical (2). [G. *helix*, a coil, + *eidos*, resemblance]

hel·i·co·po·dia (hel'i-kō-pō'dē-ă). SYN helicopod *gait*. [G. *helix*, a coil, + *pous*, foot]

hel·i·co·tre·ma (hel'i-kō-trē'mă) [NA]. A semilunar opening at the apex of the cochlea through which the scala vestibuli and the scala tympani of the cochlea communicate with one another. [G. *helix*, a spiral, + *trēma*, a hole]

he·li·en·ceph·a·li·tis (hē-lē-en-sef-ă-lī'tis). Inflammation of the brain following sunstroke. [G. *helios*, sun, + *enkephalos*, brain, + *-itis*, inflammation]

he·li·um (He) (hē'lē-ŭm). A gaseous element present in minute amounts in the atmosphere (0.000524% of dry volume); atomic no. 2, atomic wt. 4.002602; used as a diluent of medicinal gases, particularly oxygen [G. *hēlios*, the sun]

he·lix, pl. **hel·i·ces** (hē'liks, hel'i-sēz). 1 [NA]. The margin of the auricle; a folded rim of cartilage forming the upper part of the anterior, the superior, and the greater part of the posterior edges of the auricle. 2. A line in the shape of a coil (or a spring, or the threads on a bolt), each point being equidistant from a straight line that is the axis of the cylinder in which each point of the h. lies; often, mistakenly, applied to a spiral (the threads on a screw). [L. fr. G. *helix*, a coil]

     DNA h., SYN Watson-Crick h.

     double h., SYN Watson-Crick h.

     Watson-Crick h., the helical structure assumed by two strands of deoxyribonucleic acid, held together throughout their length by hydrogen bonds between bases on opposite strands, referred to as Watson-Crick base pairing. SEE base *pair*. SYN DNA h., double h.

hel·minth. An intestinal vermiform parasite, primarily nematodes, cestodes, trematodes, and acanthocephalans. [G. *helmins*, worm]

hel·min·tha·gogue (hel-minth'ă-gog). SYN anthelmintic (1). [G. *helmins*, worm, + *agōgos*, leading]

hel·min·them·e·sis (hel-min-them'ĕ-sis). The vomiting or expulsion through the mouth of intestinal worms. [G. *helmins*, a worm, + *emesis*, vomiting]

hel·min·thi·a·sis (hel-min-thī'ă-sis). The condition of having intestinal vermiform parasites.

hel·min·tho·ma (hel-min-thō'mă). A discrete nodule of granulomatous inflammation (including the healed stage) caused by a helminth or its products. [G. *helmins*, worm, + *-oma*, tumor]

Hel·min·tho·spo·ri·um (hel-min-thō-spōr'ē-ŭm). A saprobic fungus, often isolated in clinical laboratories.

he·lo·ma (hē-lō'mă). SYN clavus. [G. *hēlos*, nail, + *-oma*, tumor]

     h. dur'um, SYN hard *corn*.

     h. mol'le, SYN soft *corn*.

he·lot·o·my (hē-lot'ŏ-mē). Surgical treatment of corns. [heloma + G. *tomē*, cutting]

△**hem-, hema-.** Blood. SEE ALSO hemat-, hemato-, hemo-. [G. *haima*]

he·ma·cy·tom·e·ter (hē'mă-sī-tom'ĕ-ter, hem'ă-). SYN hemocytometer.

he·mad·sorp·tion (hē'mad-sōrp-shŭn, hem'ad-). A phenomenon manifested by an agent or substance adhering to or being adsorbed on the surface of a red blood cell.

he·mag·glu·ti·na·tion (hē-mă-glū'ti-nā'shŭn). The agglutination of red blood cells; may be immune (as a result of specific antibody to red blood cell antigens or other antigens which coat the red blood cells), or nonimmune (as in h. caused by viruses or other microbes).

     passive h., agglutination in which erythrocytes, usually modified by treatment with chemicals, adsorb soluble antigen and then agglutinate in the presence of antiserum specific for the adsorbed antigen. SYN indirect hemagglutination test.

     reverse passive h., a diagnostic technique for virus infection using agglutination by viruses of red blood cells that previously have been coated with antibody specific to the virus.

     viral h., the nonimmune agglutination of suspended red blood cells by certain of a wide range of otherwise unrelated viruses, usually by the virion itself but in some instances by products of viral growth, the species of erythrocyte agglutinated differing with the different viruses.

he·mag·glu·ti·nin (hē'mă-glū'ti-nin, hem-). A substance, antibody or other, that causes hemagglutination.

he·ma·gog·ic (hē-mă-goj'ik, hem-ă-). Promoting a flow of blood.

he·mal (hē'măl). 1. Relating to the blood or blood vessels. 2. Referring to the ventral side of the vertebral bodies or their precursors, where the heart and great vessels are located, as opposed to neural (2). [G. *haima*, blood]

he·mal·um (hē-mal'ŭm, hem-). A solution of hematoxylin and alum used as a nuclear stain in histology, especially with eosin as a counterstain.

he·ma·nal·y·sis (hē-mă-nal'ĭ-sis, hem-). Analysis of the blood; an examination of blood, especially with reference to chemical methods. [G. *haima*, blood, + analysis]

△**hemangi-.** blood vessel. [G. *haima*, blood + *angeion*, vessel]

he·man·gi·ec·ta·sis, he·man·gi·ec·ta·sia (hē-man-jē-ek'tăsis, hem-an-; -ek-tā'zē-ă). Dilation of blood vessels. [G. *haima*, blood, + *angeion*, vessel, + *ektasis*, a stretching]

△**hemangio-.** The blood vessels. [G. *haima*, blood, + *angeion*, vessel]

he·man·gi·o·blast (he-man'jē-ō-blast). A primitive embryonic cell of mesodermal origin producing cells from which are derived vascular endothelium, reticuloendothelial elements, and blood-forming cells of all types. [hemangio- + G. *blastos*, germ]

he·man·gi·o·blas·to·ma (he-man'jē-ō-blas-tō'mă). A benign cerebellar neoplasm composed of capillary vessel-forming endothelial cells and

       he

stromal cells; a slowly growing tumor that affects, primarily, middle-aged individuals; increased incidence in von Hippel-Lindau disease. SYN angioblastoma.

he·man·gi·o·en·do·the·li·o·blas·to·ma (hē-man'jē-ō-en-dō-thē'-lē-ō-blas-tō'mă). Hemangioendothelioma in which the endothelial cells seem to be especially immature forms. [hemangio- + endothelium + G. *blastos*, germ, + *-oma*, tumor]

he·man·gi·o·en·do·the·li·o·ma (he-man'jē-ō-en-dō-thē-lē-ō'mă). A neoplasm derived from blood vessels, characterized by numerous prominent endothelial cells that occur singly, in aggregates, and as the lining of congeries of vascular tubes or channels; in the elderly, may be malignant (angiosarcoma or hemangiosarcoma), but in children are benign and probably represent a growing stage of capillary hemangioma. [hemangio- + endothelium + G. *-oma*, tumor]

he·man·gi·o·fi·bro·ma (he-man'jē-ō-fī-brō'mă). A hemangioma with an abundant fibrous tissue framework.

he·man·gi·o·ma (he-man'jē-ō'mă). A congenital anomaly, in which proliferation of blood vessels leads to a mass that resembles a neoplasm; it can occur anywhere in the body but is most frequently noticed in the skin and subcutaneous tissues. SEE ALSO nevus. [hemangio- + G. *-oma*, tumor]

   capillary h., an overgrowth of capillary blood vessels, seen most commonly in the skin, at or soon after birth, as a soft bright red to purple nodule or plaque that usually disappears by the fifth year. The most common type of h. SYN nevus vascularis, nevus vasculosus.

   cavernous h., a vascular malformation containing large blood-filled spaces, due apparently to dilation and thickening of the walls of the capillary loops; in the skin, extends more deeply than a capillary h. and is less likely to regress spontaneously.

   sclerosing h., a benign lung or bronchial lesion, often subpleural, sometimes multiple, which forms hyalinized connective tissue.

   senile h., a red papule due to weakening of the capillary wall, seen mostly in persons over 30 years of age. SYN cherry angioma.

   strawberry h., hyperproliferation of immature capillary vessels, usually on the head and neck, present at birth or within the first 2 to 3 months postnatally, which commonly regresses without scar formation.

   verrucous h., a variant of the angiomatous nevus, appearing at birth or in early childhood, situated on the lower extremities with bluish-red nodules and warty surface; they enlarge and sometimes have satellite lesions.

he·man·gi·o·ma·to·sis (he-man'jē-ō-mă-tō'sis). A condition in which there are numerous hemangiomas.

he·man·gi·o·per·i·cy·to·ma (he-man'jē-ō-per'i-sī-tō'mă). An uncommon vascular, usually benign, neoplasm composed of round and spindle cells that are derived from the pericytes and surround endothelium-lined vessels. [hemangio- + pericyte + G. *-oma*, tumor]

he·man·gi·o·sar·co·ma (he-man'jē-ō-sar-kō'

mă). A rare malignant neoplasm characterized by rapidly proliferating, extensively infiltrating, anaplastic cells derived from blood vessels and lining irregular blood-filled or lumpy spaces.

he·mar·thro·sis (hē'mar-thrō'sis, hem'ar-). Blood in a joint. [G. *haima*, blood, + *arthron*, joint]

△**hemat-.** Blood. SEE ALSO hem-, hemato-, hemo-. [G. *haima* (*haimat-*)]

he·ma·tem·e·sis (hē-mă-tem'ĕ-sis, hem-ă-). Vomiting of blood. [hemat- + G. *emesis*, vomiting]

he·mat·en·ceph·a·lon (hē'mat-en-sef'ă-lon, hem' at-). SYN cerebral *hemorrhage*. [hemat- + G. *enkephalos*, brain]

he·mat·ic (hē-mat'ik). **1.** Relating to blood. SYN hemic. **2.** SYN hematinic (2).

he·ma·ti·dro·sis (hē'mat-i-drō'sis, hem'at-). Excretion of blood or blood pigment in the sweat; an extremely rare disorder. SYN hemidrosis (1). [hemat- + G. *hidrōs*, sweat]

hem·a·tin (hē'mă-tin, hem'ă-). Heme in which the iron is Fe(III) (Fe^{3+}); the prosthetic group of methemoglobin. SYN ferriheme, oxyheme, oxyhemochromogen.

   h. chloride, SYN hemin.

   reduced h., SYN heme.

he·ma·ti·ne·mia (hē'mă-ti-nē'mē-ă, hem'ă-). The presence of heme in the circulating blood. [hematin + G. *haima*, blood]

hem·a·tin·ic (hē-mă-tin'ik, hem-a-). **1.** Improving the condition of the blood. **2.** An agent that improves the quality of blood by increasing the number of erythrocytes and/or the hemoglobin concentration. SYN hematic (2).

△**hemato-.** Combining form denoting blood. SEE ALSO hem-, hemat-, hemo-. [G. *haima* (*haimat-*)]

he·ma·to·blast (hē'mă-tō-blast, hem'ă-). A primitive, undifferentiated form of blood cell from which erythroblasts, lymphoblasts, myeloblasts, and other immature blood cells are derived; in normal bone marrow, present only in small numbers and difficult to identify in smears, inasmuch as h.'s are fragile and easily disintegrated. [hemato- + G. *blastos*, germ]

he·ma·to·cele (hē'mă-tō-sēl, hem'ă-). **1.** SYN hemorrhagic *cyst*. **2.** Effusion of blood into a canal or a cavity of the body. **3.** Swelling due to effusion of blood into the tunica vaginalis testis. [hemato- + G. *kēlē*, tumor]

hem·a·to·ceph·a·ly (hē'mă-tō-sef'ă-lē, hem'ă-). Intracranial effusion of blood, commonly in a fetus. [hemato- + G. *kephalē*, head]

he·ma·to·che·zia (hē'mă-tō-kē'zē-ă, hem'ă-). Passage of bloody stools, in contradistinction to melena, or tarry stools. [hemato- + G. *chezō*, to go to stool]

he·ma·to·chy·lu·ria (hē'mă-tō-kī-lū're-ă, hem' a-). Presence of blood as well as chyle in the urine. [hemato- + G. *chylos*, juice, + *ouron*, urine]

he·ma·to·col·po·me·tra (hē'mă-tō-kol'pō-mē'tră). Accumulation of blood in the uterus and vagina resulting from an imperforate hymen or other lower vaginal obstruction. [hemato- + G. *kolpos*, vagina, + *mētra*, womb]

he·ma·to·col·pos (hē'mă-tō-kol'pos, hem'ă-). An

accumulation of menstrual blood in the vagina in consequence of imperforate hymen or other obstruction. SYN retained menstruation. [hemato- + G. *kolpos,* vagina]

he·mat·o·crit (Hct) (hē′mă-tō-krit, hem′ă-). Percentage of the volume of a blood sample occupied by cells. Cf. plasmacrit. [hemato- + G. *krinō,* to separate]

he·ma·to·cyst (hē′mă-tō-sist, hem′ă-). SYN hemorrhagic *cyst.*

he·ma·to·cys·tis (hē′mă-tō-sis′tis, hem′ă-). An effusion of blood into the bladder. [hemato- + G. *kystis,* bladder]

he·ma·to·gen·e·sis (hē′mă-tō-jen′ĕ-sis, hem′ă-). SYN hemopoiesis. [hemato- + G. *genesis,* production]

he·ma·to·gen·ic, he·ma·tog·e·nous (hē′mă-tō-jen′ik, hem′ă-; hem-ă-toj′en-ŭs). **1.** SYN hemopoietic. **2.** Pertaining to anything produced from, derived from, or transported by the blood.

he·ma·to·his·ton (hē′mă-tō-his′tŏn, hem′ă-). SYN globin.

he·ma·toid (hē′mă-toyd, hem′ă-). Resembling blood. [hemato- + G. *eidos,* resemblance]

he·ma·toi·din (hē-mă-toy′din). A pigment derived from hemoglobin which contains no iron but is closely related to or similar to bilirubin. H. is formed intracellularly, presumably within reticuloendothelial cells, but is often found extracellularly after 5 to 7 days in foci of previous hemorrhage. [hemato- + G. *eidos,* resemblance, + -in]

he·ma·tol·o·gist (hē-mă-tol′ō-jist, hem-ă-). A physician trained and experienced in hematology, *i.e.,* skilled in performing diagnostic examinations of blood and bone marrow, or in treatment of such diseases, or both.

he·ma·tol·o·gy (hē-mă-tol′ō-jē, hem-ă-). The medical specialty that pertains to the anatomy, physiology, pathology, symptomatology, and therapeutics related to the blood and blood-forming tissues. [hemato- + G. *logos,* study]

he·ma·to·lymph·an·gi·o·ma (hē′mă-tō-limf′an-jē-ō′-mă, hem′ă-). A congenital anomaly consisting of numerous, closely packed, variably sized lymphatic vessels and larger channels, in association with a moderate number of blood vessels of a similar type.

he·ma·tol·y·sis (hē-mă-tol′ĭ-sis, hem-ă-). SYN hemolysis.

he·ma·to·lyt·ic (hē′ma-tō-lit′ik, hem′ă). SYN hemolytic.

he·ma·to·ma (hē-mă-tō′mă, hem-ă-). A localized mass of extravasated blood that is relatively or completely confined within an organ or tissue, a space, or a potential space; the blood is usually clotted, and, depending on how long it has been there, may manifest various degrees of organization and decolorization. [hemato- + G. *-oma,* tumor]

auricle h., hematoma between the perichondrium and cartilage of the outer ear.

epidural h., SYN extradural *hemorrhage.*

intramural h., a h. in the wall of a structure, such as the bowel or bladder, usually resulting from trauma.

subdural h., SYN subdural *hemorrhage.*

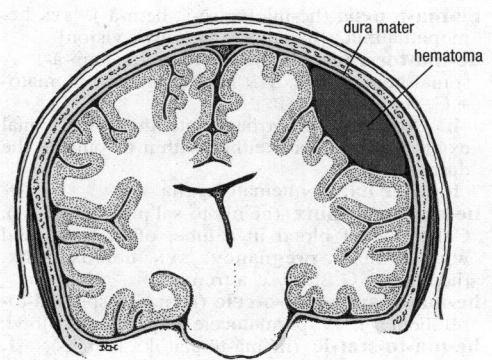

subdural hematoma: showing frontal section of brain

subungual h., collection of blood beneath a fingernail or toenail, usually due to trauma.

he·ma·to·me·tra (hē′mă-tō-mē′tră, hem′ă-). A collection or retention of blood in the uterine cavity. SYN hemometra. [hemato- + G. *mētra,* uterus]

he·ma·tom·e·try (hē-mă-tom′ĕ-trē, hem-ă). Examination of the blood in order to determine any or all of the following: 1) the total number, types, and relative proportions of various blood cells; 2) the number or proportion of other formed elements; 3) the percentage of hemoglobin. In some instances, h. is used to include a determination of blood pressure. [hemato- + G. *metron,* measure]

he·mat·om·pha·lo·cele (hē′mat-om-fal′ō-sēl, hem′at-). Umbilical hernia into which an effusion of blood has taken place. [hemato- + G. *omphalos,* umbilicus, + *kēlē,* hernia]

he·ma·to·my·e·lia (hē′mă-tō-mē′lē-ă). Hemorrhage into the substance of the spinal cord; it is usually a posttraumatic lesion but may also be encountered in instances of spinal cord capillary telangiectases. SYN hematorrhachis interna, myelapoplexy, myelorrhagia. [hemato- + G. *myelos,* marrow]

he·ma·to·my·e·lo·pore (hē′mă-tō-mī′ĕ-lō-por). Formation of porosities in the spinal cord as a result of hemorrhages. [hemato- + G. *myelos,* marrow, + *poros,* a pore]

he·ma·to·pa·thol·o·gy (hē′mă-tō-path-ol′ō-jē, hem′ă-). The division of pathology concerned with diseases of the blood and of hemopoietic and lymphoid tissues. SYN hemopathology. [hemato- + G. *pathos,* suffering, + *logos,* study]

he·ma·to·plas·tic (hē′mă-tō-plas′tik, hem′ă). SYN hemopoietic. [hemato- + G. *plassō,* to form]

he·ma·to·poi·e·sis (hē′mă-tō-poy-ē′sis, hem′ă-). SYN hemopoiesis.

he·ma·to·poi·et·ic (hē′mă-tō-poy-et′ik). SYN hemopoietic.

he·ma·to·por·phy·rin (hē′mă-tō-pōr′fi-rin, hem′ă-). A porphyrin resulting from the decomposition of hemoglobin; chemical composition is that of heme with the iron removed and the two vinyl groups hydrated to hydroxyethyl. SYN hemoporphyrin.

he

he·ma·top·sia (hē-mă-top'sē-ă, hem-ă-). SYN hemophthalmia. [hemato- + G. *opsis,* vision]

he·ma·tor·rha·chis (hē-mă-tōr'ă-kis, hem-ă-). A spinal hemorrhage. SYN hemorrhachis. [hemato- + G. *rhachis,* spine]

   h. exter′na, hemorrhage into the spinal canal external to the cord, either within or outside the dura.

   h. inter′na, SYN hematomyelia.

he·ma·to·sal·pinx (hē'mă-tō-sal'pinks, hem'ă-). Collection of blood in a tube, often associated with a tubal pregnancy. SYN hemosalpinx. [hemato- + G. *salpinx,* a trumpet]

he·ma·to·sper·mat·o·cele (hē'mă-tō-sper'mă-tō-sēl, hem'ă-). A spermatocele that contains blood.

he·ma·to·stat·ic (hē'mă-tō-stat'ik, hem'ă-). **1.** Variant of hemostatic. **2.** Due to stagnation or arrest of blood in the vessels of the part.

he·ma·to·stax·is (hē'mă-tō-stak'sis, hem'ă-). Spontaneous bleeding due to a disease of the blood. [hemato- + G. *staxis,* a dripping]

he·ma·tos·te·on (hē-mă-tos'tē-on, hem-ă). Bleeding in the medullary cavity of a bone. [hemato- + G. *osteon,* bone]

he·ma·to·tox·in (hē'mă-tō-toks'in, hem'ă-). SYN hemotoxin.

he·ma·to·tro·pic (hē'mă-tō-trop'ik, hem'ă-). SYN hemotropic.

he·ma·tox·y·lin (hē-mă-toks'i-lin, hem-ă-) [C.I. 75290]. A crystalline compound containing the coloring matter of *Haematoxylon campechianum* (logwood), from which it is obtained by extraction with ether. It is used as a dye in histology, especially for cell nuclei and chromosomes, muscle cross-striations, and enterochromaffin cells, and as an indicator (red to yellow at pH 0.0 to 1.0, yellow to violet at pH 5.0 to 6.0).

   phosphotungstic acid h. (PTAH), a stain with broad application in cytology and histology; nuclei, mitochrondria, fibrin, neuroglial fibrils, and cross-striations of skeletal and cardiac muscle stain blue; cartilage ground substance, bone reticulum, and elastin appear in shades of yellow-orange and brownish red; also useful for demonstrating abnormal or diseased astrocytes, often in combination with periodic acid-Schiff stain and Luxol fast blue.

he·ma·tu·ria (hē-mă-tū'-rē-ă, hem-ă-). Any condition in which the urine contains blood or red blood cells. [hemato- + G. *ouron,* urine]

   endemic h., SYN *schistosomiasis* haematobium.

   false h., SYN pseudohematuria.

   renal h., h. resulting from extravasation of blood into the glomerular spaces, tubules, or pelves of the kidneys.

   urethral h., h. in which the site of bleeding is in the urethra.

   vesical h., h. in which the site of bleeding is in the urinary bladder.

heme (hēm). **1.** The porphyrin chelate of iron in which the iron is Fe(II) (Fe^{2+}); the oxygen-carrying, color-furnishing, prosthetic group of hemoglobin. **2.** Iron complexed with nonporphyrins but related tetrapyrrole structures (*e.g.,* biliverdin heme). SYN reduced hematin. [G. *haima,* blood]

hem·er·a·lo·pia (hem'er-al-ō'pē-ă). Inability to see as distinctly in a bright light as in reduced illumination; seen in patients with impaired cone function. SYN day blindness. [G. *hēmera,* day, + *alaos,* obscure, + *ōps,* eye]

△**hemi-.** One-half. Cf. semi-. [G.]

hem·i·ac·e·tal (hem'ē-as'e-tăl). RCH(OH)OR′, a product of the addition of an alcohol to an aldehyde (an acetal is formed by the addition of an alcohol to a hemiacetal). In the aldose sugars, the h. formation is internal and labile, brought about by the 4-OH or 5-OH attack on the carbonyl O, yielding the furanose or pyranose structures; the h. forms of the sugars are involved in all polysaccharides, as glycosyls or glycosides. SEE ALSO hemiketal, acetal.

hem·i·a·geu·sia (hem'ē-ă-gū'sē-ă). Loss of taste from one side of the tongue. [hemi- + G. *a-* priv. + *geusis,* taste]

hem·i·an·al·ge·sia (hem'ē-an'al-jē'zē-ă). Analgesia affecting one side of the body.

hem·i·an·en·ceph·a·ly (hem'ē-an-en-sef'ă-lē). Anencephaly on one side only, or involving one side much more extensively than the other.

hem·i·an·es·the·sia (hem'ē-an-es-thē'-zē-ă). Anesthesia on one side of the body. SYN unilateral anesthesia.

hem·i·a·no·pia (hem'ē-ă-nō'pē-ă). Loss of vision for one half of the visual field of one or both eyes.

hem·i·an·os·mia (hem'ē-an-oz'mē-ă). Loss of the sense of smell on one side. [hemi- + G. *an-* priv. + *osmē,* smell]

hem·i·a·prax·ia (hem'ē-ă-prak'sē-ă). Apraxia affecting one side of the body.

hem·i·a·tax·ia (hem'ē-ă-tak'sē-ă). Ataxia affecting one side of the body.

hem·i·ath·e·to·sis (hem'ē-ath'ĕ-tō'sis). Athetosis affecting one hand, or one hand and foot, only.

hem·i·at·ro·phy (hem-ē-at'rō-fē). Atrophy of one lateral half of a part or of an organ, as the face or tongue.

hem·i·bal·lis·mus (hem-ē-bal-iz'mŭs). Ballism involving one side of the body. [hemi- + G. *ballismos,* jumping about]

hem·i·block (hem'ē-blok). Arrest of the impulse in one of the two main divisions of the left branch of the bundle of His; *i.e.,* in either the anterior (superior) division or the posterior (inferior) division.

he·mic (hē'mik). SYN hematic (1).

hem·i·car·dia (hem-ē-kar'dē-ă). **1.** Either lateral half, including atrium and ventricle, of the heart. **2.** A congenital malformation of the heart in which only two of the usual four chambers are formed. [hemi- + G. *kardia,* heart]

hem·i·cen·trum (hem'ē-sen'trŭm). One of the two lateral halves of the body of the vertebra. [hemi- + G. *kentron,* center]

hem·i·ceph·a·lal·gia (hem'ē-sef'ă-lal'jē-ă). The unilateral headache characteristic of migraine. SYN hemicrania (2). [hemi- + G. *kephalē,* head, + *algos,* pain]

hem·i·ce·pha·lia (hem-ē-se-fā'lē-ă). Congenital failure of the cerebrum to develop normally; usually the cerebellum and basal ganglia are represented at least in rudimentary form. [hemi- + G. *kephalē,* head]

hem·i·cho·rea (hem′ē-kōr-ē′ă). Chorea involving the muscles on one side only.

hem·i·col·ec·to·my (hem′ē-kō-lek′tō-mē). Removal of the right or left side of the colon. [hemi- + G. *kolon,* colon, + *ektomē,* excision]

hem·i·cor·po·rec·to·my (hem′ē-kōr-pō-rek′tō-mē). Surgical removal of the lower half of the body, including the lower extremities, bony pelvis, genitalia, and various of the pelvic contents including the lower part of the rectum to the anus. [hemi- + L. *corpus,* body, + G. *ektomē,* excision]

hem·i·cra·nia (hem-ē-krā′nē-ă). **1.** SYN migraine. **2.** SYN hemicephalalgia. [hemi- + G. *kranion,* skull]

hem·i·cra·ni·o·sis (hem′ē-krā-nē-ō′sis). Enlargement of one side of the cranium.

hem·i·des·mo·somes (hem-ē-des′mō-sōmz). Half desmosomes that occur on the basal surface of the stratum basalis of stratified squamous epithelium.

hem·i·di·a·pho·re·sis (hem′ē-dī-ă-fō-rē′sis). Diaphoresis, or sweating, on one side of the body. SYN hemidrosis (2), hemihidrosis.

hem·i·dro·sis (hem-i-drō′sis). **1.** SYN hematidrosis. **2.** SYN hemidiaphoresis.

hem·i·dys·es·the·sia (hem′ē-dis-es-thē′-zē-ă). Dysesthesia affecting one side of the body.

hem·i·dys·tro·phy (hem-ē-dis′trō-fē). Underdevelopment of one lateral half of the body. [hemi- + G. *dys-,* ill, + *trophē,* nourishment, growth]

hem·i·ec·tro·me·lia (hem′ē-ek-trō-mē′lē-ă). Defective development of the limbs on one side of the body. [hemi- + ectromelia]

hem·i·fa·cial (hem-ē-fā′shăl). Pertaining to one side of the face.

hem·i·gas·trec·to·my (hem′ē-gas-trek-tō-mē). Excision of the distal one-half of the stomach.

hem·i·glos·sec·to·my (hem′ē-glos-ek′tō-mē). Surgical removal of one-half of the tongue. [hemi- + G. *glōssa,* tongue, + *ektomē,* excision]

hem·i·glos·si·tis (hem′ē-glos-ī′tis). A vesicular eruption on one side of the tongue and the corresponding inner surface of the cheek, probably herpetic. [hemi- + G. *glōssa,* tongue, + *-itis,* inflammation]

hem·i·gna·thia (hem-ē-nath′ē-ă). Defective development of one side of the mandible. [hemi- + G. *gnathos,* jaw]

hem·i·hi·dro·sis (hem′ē-hī-drō′sis). SYN hemidiaphoresis.

hem·i·hyp·al·ge·sia (hem′ē-hī-pal-je′zē-ă). Hypalgesia affecting one side of the body.

hem·i·hy·per·es·the·sia (hem′ē-hī′per-es-thē′zē-ă). Hyperesthesia, or increased tactile and painful sensibility, affecting one side of the body.

hem·i·hy·per·i·dro·sis (hem′ē-hī-per-i-drō′sis). Hemihyperhidrosis.

hem·i·hy·per·to·nia (hem′ē-hī-per-tō′nē-ă). Exaggerated muscular tonicity on one side of the body. [hemi- + G. *hyper,* over, + *tonos,* tone]

hem·i·hy·per·tro·phy (hem′ē-hī-per′trō-fē). Muscular or osseous hypertrophy of one side of the face or body.

hem·i·hyp·es·the·sia (hem′ē-hī-pes-thē′zē-ă). Diminished sensibility in one side of the body. [hemi- + G. *hypo,* under, + *aesthēses,* sensation]

hem·i·hy·po·to·nia (hem′ē-hī-pō-tō′nē-ă). Partial loss of muscular tonicity on one side of the body. [hemi- + G. *hypo,* under, + *tonos,* tone]

hem·i·ke·tal (hem′ē-kē-tăl). RC(R′)(OH)OR″, a product of the addition of an alcohol to a ketone. In the ketose sugars, the h. formation is from an attack by an internal OH on the ketone carbonyl leading to intramolecular cyclization (furanose or pyranose); the h. forms of the sugars are involved in polysaccharide formation, as glycosyls or glycosides. SEE ALSO hemiacetal, ketal.

hem·i·lam·i·nec·to·my (hem′ē-lam-i-nek′tō-mē). Removal of a portion of a vertebral lamina, usually performed for exploration of, access to, or decompression of the intraspinal contents. [hemi- + L. *lamina,* layer, + G. *ektomē,* excision]

hem·i·lar·yn·gec·to·my (hem′ē-lar-in-jek′tō-mē). Excision of one lateral half of the larynx. [hemi- + G. *larynx (laryng-),* larynx, + *ektomē,* excision]

hem·i·lat·er·al (hem-ē-lat′er-ăl). Relating to one lateral half.

he·min (hēm′in). Chloride of heme in which Fe^{2+} has become Fe^{3+}. H. crystals are called Teichmann's crystals. SYN hematin chloride.

hem·i·pa·re·sis (hem-ē-pa-rē′sis, -par′ĕ-sis). Weakness affecting one side of the body.

hem·i·pel·vec·to·my (hem′ē-pel-vek′tō-mē). Amputation of an entire leg together with the os coxae. SYN interpelviabdominal amputation. [hemi- + L. *pelvis,* basin (pelvis), + G. *ektomē,* excision]

hem·i·ple·gia (hem-ē-plē′jē-ă). Paralysis of one side of the body. [hemi- + G. *plēgē,* a stroke]

  contralateral h., paralysis occurring on the side opposite to the causal central lesion.

  facial h., paralysis of one side of the face, the muscles of the extremities being unaffected.

  spastic h., a h. with increased tone in the antigravity muscles of the affected side.

hem·i·ple·gic (hem-ē-plē′jik). Relating to hemiplegia.

hem·i·sen·so·ry (hem′ē-sen′sōr-ē). Loss of sensation on one side of the body. Cf. hemianesthesia.

hem·i·spasm (hem′ē-spazm). A spasm affecting one or more muscles of one side of the face or body.

hem·i·sphere (hem′i-sfēr). Half of a spherical structure. SYN cerebral h. (1). [hemi- + G. *sphaira,* ball, globe]

  cerebellar h., the large part of the cerebellum lateral to the vermis cerebelli.

  cerebral h., (1) SYN hemisphere. **(2)** the large mass of the telencephalon, on either side of the midline, consisting of the cerebral cortex and its associated fiber systems, together with the deeper-lying subcortical telencephalic nuclei (*i.e.,* basal ganglia [nuclei]).

  dominant h., that cerebral hemisphere containing the representation of speech and controlling the arm and leg used preferentially in skilled movements; usually the left hemisphere.

hem·i·sys·to·le (hem-ē-sis′tō-lē). Contraction of the left ventricle following every second atrial contraction only, so that there is but one pulse beat to every two heart beats.

hem·i·tho·rax (hem-ē-thō′raks). One side of the thorax.

hem·i·trun·cus (hem′ē-trunk′us). A variant truncus arteriosus in which only one pulmonary artery originates from the truncal artery.

hem·i·ver·te·bra (hem-ē-ver′tĕ-bră). A congenital defect of the spine in which one side of a vertebra fails to develop completely.

hem·i·zy·gos·i·ty (hem′i-zī-gos′i-tē). The state of being hemizygous.

hem·i·zy·gote (hem-i-zī′gōt). An individual hemizygous with respect to one or more specified loci; *e.g.*, a normal male is a h. with respect to the gene for all X-linked or Y-linked genes in his genome. [hemi- + G. *zygōtos*, yoked]

hem·i·zy·got·ic (hem′i-zī-got′ik). SYN hemizygous.

hem·i·zy·gous (hem-i-zī′gŭs). Having unpaired genes in an otherwise diploid cell; males are normally h. for genes on both sex chromosomes. SYN hemizygotic.

△**hemo-**. Combining form denoting blood. SEE ALSO hem-, hemat-, hemato-. [G. *haima*]

he·mo·blast (hēm′ō-blast). SYN hemocytoblast.

he·mo·blas·to·sis (hē′mō-blas-tō′sis). A proliferative condition of the hematopoietic tissues in general.

he·mo·cath·e·re·sis (hē′mō-kath-e-rē′sis). Destruction of the blood cells, especially of erythrocytes (hemocytocatheresis). [hemo- + G. *kathairesis*, destruction]

he·mo·cath·e·re·tic (hē′mō-kath-ĕ-ret′ik). Pertaining to or characterized by hemocatheresis.

he·mo·chro·ma·to·sis (hē′mō-krō-mă-tō′sis). A disorder of iron metabolism characterized by excessive absorption of ingested iron, saturation of iron-binding protein, and deposition of hemosiderin in tissue, particularly in the liver, pancreas, and skin; cirrhosis of the liver, diabetes (bronze diabetes), bronze pigmentation of the skin, and, eventually heart failure may occur; also can result from administration of large amounts of iron orally, by injection, or in forms of blood transfusion therapy. [hemo- + G. *chrōma*, color, + *-osis*, condition]

    primary h. [MIM*235200], a specific inherited metabolic defect with increased absorption and accumulation of iron on a normal diet.

    secondary h., increased intake and accumulation of iron secondary to known cause, such as oral iron therapy or multiple transfusions.

he·moc·la·sis, he·mo·cla·sia (hē-mok′lă-sis, hē′mō-klā′zē-ă). Rupture, dissolution (hemolysis), or other type of destruction of red blood cells. [hemo- + G. *klasis*, a breaking]

he·mo·clas·tic (hē′mō-klas′tik). Pertaining to hemoclasis.

he·mo·con·cen·tra·tion (hē′mō-kon-sen-trā′shŭn). Decrease in the volume of plasma in relation to the number of red blood cells; increase in the concentration of red blood cells in the circulating blood.

he·mo·co·nia (hē-mō-kō′nē-ă). Small refractive particles in the circulating blood, probably lipid material associated with fragmented stroma from red blood cells. [hemo- + G. *konis*, dust]

he·mo·co·ni·o·sis (hē′mō-kō-nē-ō′sis). A condition in which there is an abnormal concentration of hemoconia in the blood.

he·mo·cyte (hē′mō-sīt). Any cell or formed element of the blood. [hemo- + G. *kytos*, a hollow (cell)]

he·mo·cy·to·blast (hē′mō-sī′tō-blast). A blood cell derived from embryonic mesenchyme, characterized by basophilic cytoplasm and a relatively large nucleus with a spongy, loose network of chromatin and several nucleoli; mitochondria are extremely fine and delicate. H.'s represent the primitive stem cells of the monophyletic theory of the origin of blood and have the potentiality of developing into erythroblasts, young forms of the granulocytic series, megakaryocytes, etc. SYN hemoblast. [hemo- + G. *kytos*, cell, + *blastos*, germ]

he·mo·cy·to·ca·ther·e·sis (hē′mō-sī′tō-kă-ther′ē-sis). Hemolysis, or other type of destruction of red blood cells. [hemo- + G. *kytos*, a hollow (cell), + *kathairesis*, destruction]

he·mo·cy·tol·y·sis (hē′mō-sī-tol′i-sis). The dissolution of blood cells, including hemolysis. [hemo- + G. *kytos*, cell, + *lysis*, dissolution]

he·mo·cy·tom·e·ter (hē′mō-sī-tom′ĕ-ter). An apparatus for estimating the number of blood cells in a quantitatively measured volume of blood; it consists of a glass pipette with an ampulla for collecting and diluting the blood, and a counting chamber marked in squares. SYN hemacytometer. [hemo- + G. *kytos*, cell, + *metron*, measure]

he·mo·cy·tom·e·try (hē′mō-sī-tom′ĕ-trē). The counting of red blood cells.

he·mo·cy·to·trip·sis (hē′mō-sī-tō-trip′sis). Fragmentation or disintegration of blood cells by means of mechanical trauma, *e.g.,* compression between hard surfaces. [hemo- + G. *kytos*, + *tripsis*, a grinding]

he·mo·di·ag·no·sis (hē′mō-dī-ag-nō′sis). Diagnosis by means of examination of the blood.

he·mo·di·al·y·sis (hē′mō-dī-al′i-sis). Dialysis of soluble substances and water from the blood by diffusion through a semipermeable membrane; separation of cellular elements and colloids from soluble substances is achieved by pore size in the membrane and rates of diffusion.

he·mo·di·a·lyz·er (hē-mō-dī′ă-lī-zer). A machine for hemodialysis in acute or chronic renal failure; toxic substances in the blood are removed by exposure to dialyzing fluid across a semipermeable membrane. SYN artificial kidney.

he·mo·di·lu·tion (hē′mō-di-lū′shŭn). Increase in the volume of plasma in relation to red blood cells; reduced concentration of red blood cells in the circulation.

he·mo·dy·nam·ic (hē′mō-dī-nam′ik). Relating to the physical aspects of the blood circulation.

he·mo·dy·nam·ics (hē′mō-dī-nam′iks). The study of the dynamics of the blood circulation. [hemo- + G. *dynamis*, power]

he·mo·fil·tra·tion (hē′mō-fil-trā′shŭn). A process, similar to hemodialysis, by which blood is dialyzed using ultrafiltration and simultaneous reinfusion of physiologic saline solution.

he·mo·flag·el·lates (hē-mō-flaj′ĕ-lāts). Protozoan flagellates that are parasitic in the blood;

they include the genera *Leishmania* and *Trypano-soma*, several species of which are important pathogens. [hemo- + L. *flagellum,* dim. of *flagrum,* a whip]

he•mo•fus•cin (hē-mō-fŭs'in). A brown pigment derived from hemoglobin that occurs in urine occasionally along with hemosiderin, usually indicative of increased red blood cell destruction; occurs also in the liver with hemosiderin in cases of hemochromatosis.

he•mo•gen•e•sis (hē-mō-jen'ĕ-sis). SYN hemopoiesis.

he•mo•gen•ic (hē-mō-jen'ik). SYN hemopoietic.

he•mo•glo•bin (Hb) (hē-mō-glō'bin) [MIM* 141800 to 142310]. The red respiratory protein of erythrocytes, consisting of approximately 3.8% heme and 96.2% globin, with a molecular weight of 64,450, which as oxyhemoglobin (HbO_2) transports oxygen from the lungs to the tissues where the oxygen is readily released and HbO_2 becomes Hb. When Hb is exposed to certain chemicals, its normal respiratory function is blocked; *e.g.,* the oxygen in HbO_2 is easily displaced by carbon monoxide, thereby resulting in the formation of fairly stable carboxyhemoglobin (HbCO), as in asphyxiation resulting from inhalation of exhaust fumes from gasoline engines. When the iron in Hb is oxidized from the ferrous to ferric state, as in poisoning with nitrates and certain other chemicals, a nonrespiratory compound, methemoglobin (MetHb), is formed.

In humans there are five kinds of normal Hb: two embryonic Hb's (Hb Gower-1, Hb Gower-2), fetal (Hb F), and two adult types (Hb A, Hb A_2). There are two α globin chains containing 141 amino acid residues, and two of another kind (β, γ, δ, ε, or ζ), each containing 146 amino acid residues in four of the Hb's. Hb Gower-1 has two ζ chains and two ε chains. The production of each kind of globin chain is controlled by a structural gene of similar Greek letter designation; normal individuals are homozygous for the normal allele at each locus. Substitution of one amino acid for another in the polypeptide chain can occur at any codon in any of the five loci and have resulted in the production of many hundreds of abnormal Hb types, most of no known clinical significance. In addition, deletions of one or more amino acid residues are known, as well as gene rearrangements due to unequal crossing over between homologous chromosomes.

The Hb types below are the main abnormal types known to be of clinical significance. Newly discovered abnormal Hb types are first assigned a name, usually the location where discovered, and a molecular formula is added when determined. The formula consists of Greek letters to designate the basic chains, with subscript 2 if there are two identical chains; a superscript letter (^{A} if normal for adult Hb, etc.) is added, or the superscript may designate the site of amino acid substitution (numbering amino acid residues from the N terminus of the polypeptide) and specifying the change, using standard abbreviations for the amino acids. There is an exhaustive listing of variant h.'s in MIM where a composite numbering system is used.

carbon monoxide h., SYN carboxyhemoglobin.

glycosylated h., any one of four h. A fractions (A_{Ia1}, A_{Ia2}, A_{Ib}, or A_{Ic}) to which D-glucose and related monosaccharides bind; concentrations are increased in the erythrocytes of patients with diabetes mellitus and can be used as a retrospective index of glucose control over time in such patients.

h. A (Hb A) [MIM*141800], normal adult h., consisting of two variants, designated Hb A (by far the more prevalent) and Hb A_2.

h. C (Hb C) [MIM*141900-0038], an abnormal h. that affects the physical properties of erythrocytes, causing hemolytic anemia; often found in persons also having sickle cell disease or thalassemia.

h. F (Hb F) [MIM*142200], normal fetal h.; production is greatly reduced after infancy except in certain congenital or acquired hematologic disorders.

h. S (Hb S) [MIM*141900], an abnormal h. that renders erythrocytes subject to sickling and hemolysis at reduced oxygen tension; makes up 70–100% of h. in persons with sickle cell anemia. SYN sickle cell h.

mean corpuscular h. (MCH), the h. content of the average red cell, calculated from the h. therein and the red cell count, in erythrocyte indices.

muscle h., SYN myoglobin.

reduced h., the form of Hb in red blood cells after the oxygen of oxyhemoglobin is released in the tissues.

sickle cell h. (Hb S), SYN h. S.

he•mo•glo•bi•ne•mia (hē'mō-glo-bi-nē'mē-ă). The presence of free hemoglobin in the blood plasma, as when intravascular hemolysis occurs.

he•mo•glo•bi•nol•y•sis (hē'mō-glō-bi-nol'i-sis). Destruction or chemical splitting of hemoglobin. [hemoglobin + G. *lysis,* dissolution]

he•mo•glo•bi•nop•a•thy (hē'mō-glō-bi-nop'ă-thē). A disorder or disease caused by or associated with the presence of hemoglobins in the blood. [hemoglobin + G. *pathos,* disease]

he•mo•glo•bi•no•phil•ic (hē'mō-glō'bi-nō-fil'ik). Denoting certain microorganisms that cannot be cultured except in the presence of hemoglobin. [hemoglobin + G. *phileō,* to love]

he•mo•glo•bi•nu•ria (hē'mō-glō-bi-nū'rē-ă). The presence of hemoglobin in the urine, including certain closely related pigments formed from slight alteration of the hemoglobin molecule; indicative of intravascular hemolysis or of bleeding into the urinary tract, with hemolysis there. The urine may be reddish yellow to dark red. [hemoglobin + G. *ouron,* urine]

epidemic h., the presence of hemoglobin in the urine of young infants, attended with cyanosis, jaundice, and other conditions; may be due to secondary methemoglobinemia; also called Winckel's disease.

march h., a form occurring after marathon races, protracted marching, or heavy physical exercise.

paroxysmal cold h. (PCH), an autoimmune hemolytic anemia characterized by hemolysis and subsequent hemoglobinuria upon exposure to

he

cold. The hemolysis is caused by the Donath-Landsteiner antibody, which attaches to the red cell at temperatures below 15°C. Upon warming, the antibody dissociates from the cell, but the terminal complement components are activated, causing cell injury and hemolysis. SEE ALSO Donath-Landsteiner *antibody*.

paroxysmal nocturnal h. (PNH), a hemolytic anemia in which the red cell membrane is abnormal, rendering the cell more susceptible to hemolysis by complement. The membrane defects include a lack of decay-accelerating factor (DAF) and C8 binding protein (C8bp) due to lack of glycosyl phosphatidyl inositol (GPI). GPI is a membrane glycolipid that attaches proteins to the cell membrane. Hemolysis is intravascular and intermittent, characterized by passage of reddish urine.

toxic h., h. occurring after the ingestion of various poisons, in certain blood diseases, and in certain infections.

he·mo·glo·bi·nu·ric (hē′mō-glō-bi-nū′rik). Relating to or marked by hemoglobinuria.

he·mo·gram (hē′mō-gram). A complete detailed record of the findings in a thorough examination of the blood, especially with reference to the numbers, proportions, and morphologic features of the formed elements. [hemo- + G. *gramma*, a drawing]

he·mo·his·ti·o·blast (hē′mō-his′tē-ō-blast). A primitive mesenchymal cell believed to be capable of developing into all types of blood cells, including monocytes, and into histiocytes. [hemo- + G. *histion*, web, + *blastos*, germ]

he·mo·lith (hē′mō-lith). A concretion in the wall of a blood vessel. [hemo- + G. *lithos*, stone]

he·mol·y·sate (hē-mol′i-sāt). Preparation resulting from the lysis of erythrocytes.

he·mo·ly·sin (hē-mol′i-sin). **1.** Any substance elaborated by a living agent and capable of causing lysis of red blood cells and liberation of their hemoglobin. SYN erythrocytolysin, erythrolysin. **2.** A sensitizing that combines with red blood cells of the antigenic type that stimulated formation of the h., so that complement fixes with the antibody-cell union and causes dissolution of the cells.

he·mo·ly·sin·o·gen (hē′mō-lī-sin′ō-jen). The antigenic material in red blood cells that stimulates the formation of hemolysin.

he·mol·y·sis (hē-mol′i-sis). Alteration, dissolution, or destruction of red blood cells in such a manner that hemoglobin is liberated into the medium in which the cells are suspended. SYN erythrocytolysis, erythrolysis, hematolysis. [hemo- + G. *lysis*, destruction]

phenylhydrazine h. (fen′il-hī′-dră-zin), an *in vitro* test for G6PD deficiency; h. resulting from *in vitro* addition of phenylhydrazine to blood with red cells which are deficient in glucose-6-phosphate dehydrogenase (G6PD), with the appearance of Heinz-Ehrlich bodies.

he·mo·lyt·ic (hē-mō-lit′ik). Destructive to blood cells, resulting in liberation of hemoglobin. SYN hematolytic, hemotoxic (2), hematotoxic, hematoxic.

he·mo·lyze (hē′mō-līz). To produce hemolysis or liberation of the hemoglobin from red blood cells.

he·mo·me·di·as·ti·num (hē′mō-mē-dē-ă-stī′nŭm). Blood in the mediastinum.

he·mo·me·tra (hē-mō-mē′tră). SYN hematometra.

he·mo·pa·thol·o·gy (hē′mō-pa-thol′ō-jē). SYN hematopathology.

he·mop·a·thy (hē-mop′ă-thē). Any abnormal condition or disease of the blood or hemopoietic tissues. [hemo- + G. *pathos*, suffering]

he·mo·per·fu·sion (hē′mō-per-fyū′zhŭn). Passage of blood through columns of adsorptive material, such as activated charcoal, to remove toxic substances from the blood. [hemo- + L. *perfusio*, to pass through]

he·mo·per·i·car·di·um (hē′mō-pār′-i-kar′dē-ŭm). Blood in the pericardial sac.

he·mo·per·i·to·ne·um (hē′mō-pār-i-tō-nē′ŭm). Blood in the peritoneal cavity.

he·mo·pex·in (hēm-ō-peks′in). A serum protein related to β-globulins, important in binding heme and porphyrins, preventing excretion, and perhaps regulating heme in drug metabolism. [hemo- + G. *pēxis*, fixation, + -in]

he·mo·phil, he·mo·phile (hē′mō-fil, -fīl). A microorganism growing preferably in media containing blood. [hemo- + G. *philos*, fond]

he·mo·phil·ia (hē-mō-fil′ē-ă). An inherited disorder of blood coagulation characterized by a permanent tendency to hemorrhages, spontaneous or traumatic, due to a defect in the blood coagulating mechanism. [hemo- + G. *philos*, fond]

h. A [MIM*306900-various], h. due to deficiency of factor VIII, occurring almost exclusively in males, and characterized by prolonged clotting time, decreased formation of thromboplastin, and diminished conversion of prothrombin.

h. B [MIM*306900-various], a clotting disorder resembling h. A, caused by hereditary deficiency of factor IX. SYN Christmas disease.

he·mo·phil·i·ac (hē-mō-fil′ē-ak). A person suffering from hemophilia.

he·mo·phil·ic (hē-mō-fil′ik). Relating to hemophilia.

he·mo·pho·re·sis (hē′mō-fō-rē′sis). Blood convection or irrigation of tissues. [hemo- + G. *phoreō*, to bear]

he·moph·thal·mia, he·moph·thal·mus (hē-mof-thal′mē-ah, -mof-thal′mŭs). A blood-filled eye. SYN hematopsia. [hemo- + G. *ophthalmos*, eye]

he·mo·plas·tic (hē-mō-plas′tik). SYN hemopoietic.

he·mo·pneu·mo·per·i·car·di·um (hē′mō-nū′mō-pār-i-kar′dē-ŭm). The occurrence of blood and air in the pericardium. SYN pneumohemopericardium. [hemo- + G. *pneuma*, air, + pericardium]

he·mo·pneu·mo·tho·rax (hē′mō-nū-mō-thō′raks). Accumulation of air and blood in the pleural cavity. SYN pneumohemothorax. [hemo- + G. *pneuma*, air, + thorax]

he·mo·poi·e·sis (hē′mō-poy-ē′sis). The process of formation and development of the various types of blood cells and other formed elements.

SYN hematogenesis, hematopoiesis, hemogenesis, sanguification. [hemo- + G. *poiēsis,* a making]

he·mo·poi·et·ic (hē′mō-poy-et′ik). Pertaining to or related to the formation of blood cells. SYN hematogenic (1), hematogenous, hematoplastic, hematopoietic, hemogenic, hemoplastic, sanguifacient.

he·mo·por·phy·rin (hē-mō-pōr′fi-rin). SYN hematoporphyrin.

he·mo·pre·cip·i·tin (hē′mō-prē-sip′i-tin). An antibody that combines with and precipitates soluble antigenic material from erythrocytes.

he·mo·pro·tein (hē-mō-prō′tēn). Protein linked to a metal-porphyrin compound (*e.g.,* cytochromes, myoglobin, catalase).

he·mop·ty·sis (hē-mop′ti-sis). The spitting of blood derived from the lungs or bronchial tubes as a result of pulmonary or bronchial hemorrhage. [hemo- + G. *ptysis,* a spitting]

he·mor·rha·chis (hē-mōr′ă-kis). SYN hematorrhachis.

hem·or·rhage (hem′ŏ-rij). **1.** An escape of blood through ruptured or unruptured vessel walls. **2.** To bleed. [G. *haimorrhagia,* fr. *haima,* blood, + *rhēgnymi,* to burst forth]

ℹ **cerebral h.,** h. into the substance of the cerebrum, usually in the region of the internal capsule by the rupture of the lenticulostriate artery. SYN hematencephalon.

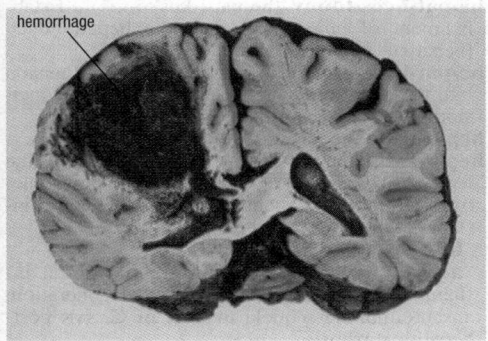
hemorrhage

cerebral hemorrhage: left cerebral hemisphere, including lateral ventricle

concealed h., SYN internal h.

extradural h., an accumulation of blood between the skull and the dura mater. SYN epidural hematoma.

internal h., bleeding into organs or cavities of the body. SYN concealed h.

intracranial h., escape of blood within the cranium due to loss of integrity of vascular channels, frequently forming a hematoma.

intrapartum h., h. occurring in the course of normal labor and delivery.

parenchymatous h., bleeding into the substance of an organ.

petechial h., capillary h. into the skin that forms petechiae. SYN punctate h.

postpartum h., h. from the birth canal in excess of 500 ml after a vaginal delivery or 1000 ml

after a cesarean delivery during the first 24 hours after birth.

primary h., h. immediately after an injury or operation, as distinguished from intermediate or secondary h.

punctate h., SYN petechial h.

secondary h., h. at an interval after an injury or an operation.

splinter h.'s, multiple tiny longitudinal subungual h.'s typically seen in but not diagnostic of bacterial endocarditis and trichinelliasis.

subdural h., extravasation of blood between the dural and arachnoidal membranes; acute and chronic forms occur; chronic hematomas may become encapsulated by neomembranes. SYN subdural hematoma.

hem·or·rhag·ic (hem-ŏ-raj′ik). Relating to or marked by hemorrhage.

hem·or·rhag·ins (hem-ŏ-raj′inz, -rā′jins). Toxins found in certain venoms and poisonous material from some plants, *e.g.,* rattlesnake venom and ricin; h. cause degeneration and lysis of endothelial cells in capillaries and small vessels, thereby resulting in numerous small hemorrhages in the tissues. [hemorrhage + -in]

hem·or·rhoid (hem′ŏ-royd). One of the tumors or varices constituting hemorrhoids.

hem·or·rhoi·dal (hem-ŏ-roy′dăl). Relating to hemorrhoids.

hem·or·rhoid·ec·to·my (hem′ŏ-roy-dek′tō-mē). Surgical removal of hemorrhoids; usually accomplished by excision of hemorrhoidal tissues by sharp dissection, or by application of elastic ligature at the base of the hemorrhoidal bundles to produce ischemic necrosis and ultimate ablation of the h. [hemorrhoids + G. *ektomē,* excision]

hem·or·rhoids (hem′ŏ-roydz). A varicose condition of the external or internal rectal veins causing painful swellings at the anus. SYN piles. [G. *haimorrhois,* pl. *haimorrhoides,* veins likely to bleed, fr. *haima,* blood, + *rhoia,* a flow]

he·mo·sal·pinx (hē′mō-sal′pinks). SYN hematosalpinx.

he·mo·sid·er·in (hē-mō-sid′er-in). A yellow or brown protein produced by phagocytic digestion of hematin; found in most tissues, especially in the liver; but with a higher content, as stains blue with Perl's Prussian blue stain. [hemo- + G. *sidēros,* iron, + -in]

he·mo·sid·er·o·sis (hē′mō-sid-er-ō′sis). Accumulation of hemosiderin in tissue, particularly in liver and spleen. SEE hemochromatosis. [hemosiderin + -osis, condition]

he·mo·sper·mia (hē′mō-sper′mē-ă). The presence of blood in the seminal fluid. [hemo- + G. *sperma,* seed]

he·mo·sta·sis (hē′mō-stā-sis, hē-mos′tă-sis). **1.** The arrest of bleeding. **2.** The arrest of circulation in a part. **3.** Stagnation of blood. [hemo- + G. *stasis,* a standing]

he·mo·stat (hē′mō-stat). **1.** Any agent that arrests, chemically or mechanically, the flow of blood from an open vessel. **2.** An instrument for arresting hemorrhage by compression of the bleeding vessel.

he·mo·stat·ic (hē-mō-stat′ik). **1.** Arresting the

flow of blood within the vessels. **2.** SYN antihemorrhagic.

he•mo•ther•a•py, he•mo•ther•a•peu•tics (hē′mō-thār′ă-pē, thār-ă-pyū′tiks). Treatment of disease by the use of blood or blood derivatives, as in transfusion.

he•mo•tho•rax (hē-mō-thōr′aks). Blood in the pleural cavity.

he•mo•tox•ic, he•ma•to•tox•ic, he•ma•tox•ic (hē-mō-tok′sik; hē′mă-tō-toks′ik, hem′ă-; hē-mă-toks′ik, hem-ă-). **1.** Causing blood poisoning. **2.** SYN hemolytic.

he•mo•tox•in (hē-mō-tok′sin). Any substance that causes destruction of red blood cells, including various hemolysins; usually used with reference to substances of biologic origin, in contrast to chemicals. SYN hematotoxin.

he•mo•troph, he•mot•ro•phe (hēm′ō-trof). The nutritive materials supplied to the embryos of placental mammals through the maternal bloodstream. Cf. embryotroph. [hemo- + G. *trophē,* food]

he•mo•tro•pic (hē-mō-trop′ik). Pertaining to the mechanism by which a substance in or on blood cells, especially the erythrocytes, attracts phagocytic cells; the latter change direction and migrate toward the h. cells. SYN hematotropic. [hemo- + G. *tropos,* direction (or *tropē,* a turning)]

he•mo•tym•pa•num (hē′mō-tim′pă-nŭm). The presence of blood in the middle ear.

hemoximeter (hem-ok-sim-e-ter). SYN co-oximeter.

hemoximetry (hem-ok-sim-e-tre). Spectrophotometric analysis of blood for determination of the saturation of oxyhemoglobin and of dyshemoglobins (for example, carboxyhemoglobin and methemoglobin).

Hen•der•so•nu•la to•ru•loi•dea (hen-der-sō-nyū′lă tōr-yū-loy′dē-ă). A species of black yeast capable of producing chronic infections of the nails as well as of the skin of the feet.

Henry, William, British chemist, 1775–1837. SEE H.'s *law.*

hen•ry (H) (hen′rē). The unit of electrical inductance, when 1 volt is induced by a change in current of 1 ampere/sec. [Joseph *Henry*]

He•pad•na•vi•ri•dae (hē-pa′dnă-vī′rā-dā). A family of DNA-containing viruses. The principal genus *Hepadnavirus* is associated with hepatitis B. [*hepa*titis + DNA + virus]

he•par, gen. **hep•a•tis** (hē′par, hē′pah-tis) [NA]. SYN liver, liver. [L. borrowed fr. G. *hēpar,* gen. *hēpatos,* the liver]

hep•a•rin (hep′ă-rin). An anticoagulant that is a component of various tissues (especially liver and lung) and mast cells. Its principal active constituent is a glycosaminoglycan composed of D-glucuronic acid and D-glucosamine. In conjunction with a serum protein cofactor (the so-called heparin cofactor), h. acts as an antithrombin and an antiprothrombin by preventing platelet agglutination and consequent thrombus formation.

hep•a•rin•ize (hep′ă-rin-īz). To perform therapeutic administration of heparin.

△**hepat-, hepatico-, hepato-.** The liver. [G. *hēpar* (*hēpat-*)]

hep•a•ta•tro•phia, hep•a•tat•ro•phy (hep′ă-tă-trō′fē-ă, hep-ă-tat′rō-fē). Atrophy of the liver.

hep•a•tec•to•my (hep-ă-tek′tō-mē). Removal of the liver, whole or in part. [hepat- + G. *ektomē,* excision]

he•pa•tic (he-pat′ik). Relating to the liver. [G. *hēpatikos*]

△**hepatico-.** SEE hepat-.

he•pat•i•co•do•chot•o•my (he-pat′i-kō-dō-kot′ō-mē). Combined hepaticotomy and choledochotomy.

he•pat•i•co•du•o•de•nos•to•my (he-pat′i-kō-dū′ō-de-nos′tō-mē). Establishment of a communication between the hepatic ducts and the duodenum. [hepatico- + duodenostomy]

he•pat•i•co•en•ter•os•to•my (he-pat′i-kō-en-ter-os′tō-mē). Establishment of a communication between the hepatic ducts and the intestine. [hepatico- + enterostomy]

he•pat•i•co•gas•tros•to•my (he-pat′i-kō-gas-tros′tō-mē). Establishment of a communication between the hepatic duct and the stomach. [hepatico- + gastrostomy]

he•pat•i•co•li•thot•o•my (he-pat′i-kō-li-thot′ō-mē). Removal of a stone from a hepatic duct. [hepatico- + G. *lithos,* stone, + *tomē,* a cutting]

he•pat•i•co•lith•o•trip•sy (he-pat′i-kō-lith′ō-trip-sē). The crushing or fragmentation of a biliary calculus in the hepatic duct. [hepatico- + G. *lithos,* stone, + *tripsis,* a rubbing]

he•pat•i•cos•to•my (he-pat-i-kos′tō-mē). Establishment of an opening into the hepatic duct. [hepatico- + G. *stoma,* mouth]

he•pat•i•cot•o•my (he-pat-i-kot′ō-mē). Incision into the hepatic duct. [hepatico- + G. *tomē,* incision]

hep•a•tit•ic (hep-ă-tit′ik). Relating to hepatitis.

hep•a•ti•tis (hep-ă-tī′tis). Inflammation of the liver; usually from a viral infection, but sometimes from toxic agents. [hepat- + G. *-itis,* inflammation]

 h. A, SYN viral h. type A.

 active chronic h., h. with chronic portal inflammation and progressive hepatic degeneration; an autoimmune sequela to h. B or C. SYN post-hepatitic cirrhosis.

 anicteric virus h., a relatively mild h., without jaundice.

 h. B, SYN viral h. type B.

 h. C, a viral h., usually mild but often progressing to a chronic stage; the most prevalent type of post-transfusion h.

 cholangiolitic h., h. with inflammatory changes around small bile ducts, producing mainly obstructive jaundice; may be due to viral infection or bacterial infection ascending biliary tree because of obstruction.

 delta h., SYN viral h. type D.

 h. E, a viral h. occurring chiefly in the tropics; transmitted by the fecal-oral route, it does not become chronic or lead to a carrier state, but has a higher mortality than hepatitis A, particularly in pregnancy.

 lupoid h., jaundice with evidence of liver cell damage and positive antinuclear antibody or LE cell tests, but without evidence of systemic lupus erythematosus.

neonatal h., h. in the neonatal period due to a variety of causes, chiefly viral.

persistent chronic h., a benign chronic h. that may follow acute viral h. B or C or complicate bowel diseases; rarely progresses to cirrhosis, portal hypertension, or liver failure.

viral h., (1) h. caused by any one of at least five immunologically unrelated viruses: h. A virus, h. B virus, h. C virus, h. D virus, h. E virus; **(2)** h. caused by a viral infection, including that by Epstein-Barr virus and cytomegalovirus.

viral h. type A, a virus disease with a short incubation period (usually 15 to 50 days), caused by h. A virus, a member of the family Picornaviridae, often transmitted by fecal-oral route; may be inapparent, mild, severe, or occasionally fatal and occurs sporadically or in epidemics, commonly in school-age children and young adults; necrosis of periportal liver cells with lymphocytic and plasma cell infiltration is characteristic and jaundice is a common symptom. SYN h. A.

viral h. type B, a virus disease with a long incubation period (usually 50 to 160 days), caused by hepatitis B virus; transmitted by blood or blood products, contaminated needles or instruments, or sexually; differs from h. A in having a higher mortality and in the possibility of progression to a chronic disease, a carrier state, or both. SYN h. B.

viral h. type D, acute or chronic h. caused by the h. delta virus, a defective RNA virus requiring HBV for replication. The acute type occurs in two forms: 1) coinfection, the simultaneous occurrence of h. B virus and h. delta virus infections; 2) superinfection, the appearance of h. delta virus infection in a h. B virus carrier. SYN delta h.

hep•a•ti•za•tion (hep′ă-ti-zā′shŭn). Conversion of a loose tissue into a firm mass like the substance of the liver macroscopically, denoting especially such a change in the lungs in the consolidation of pneumonia.

gray h., the second stage of h. in pneumonia, when the exudate is beginning to degenerate prior to breaking down; the color is a yellowish gray or mottled.

red h., the first stage of h. in which the exudate is blood-stained.

yellow h., the final stage of h. in which the exudate is becoming purulent.

△**hepato-.** SEE hepat-.

he•pa•to•blas•to•ma (hep′ă-tō-blas-tō′mă). A malignant neoplasm occurring in young children, primarily in the liver, composed of tissue resembling embryonal or fetal hepatic epithelium, or mixed epithelial and mesenchymal tissues.

he•pa•to•car•ci•no•ma (hep′ă-tō-kar-si-nō′mă). SYN malignant *hepatoma.*

he•pa•to•cele (hep′ă-tō-sēl, he-pat′ō-sēl). Protrusion of part of the liver through the abdominal wall or the diaphragm. [hepato- + G. *kēlē,* hernia]

he•pa•to•chol•an•gi•o•je•ju•nos•to•my (hep′ă-tō-kō-lan′jē-ō-jē-jū-nos′tō-mē). Union of the hepatic duct to the jejunum. [hepato- + G. *cholē,* bile, + *angeion,* vessel, + jejunostomy]

he•pa•to•chol•an•gi•os•to•my (hep′ă-tō-kō-lan-

jē-os′tō-mē). Creation of an opening into the common bile duct to establish drainage.

he•pa•to•chol•an•gi•tis (hep′ă-tō-kō-lan-jī′tis). Inflammation of the liver and biliary tree.

he•pa•to•cys•tic (hep′ă-tō-sis′tik). Relating to the gallbladder, or to both liver and gallbladder. [hepato- + G. *kystis,* bladder]

he•pa•to•cyte (hep′ă-tō-sīt). A parenchymal liver cell.

he•pa•to•en•ter•ic (hep′ă-tō-en-těr′ik). Relating to the liver and the intestine. [hepato- + G. *enteron,* intestine]

hep•a•to•fu•gal (hep′ă-tō-fyū′găl). Away from the liver, usually referring to portal blood flow.

he•pa•to•gas•tric (hep′ă-tō-gas′trik). Relating to the liver and the stomach.

he•pa•to•gen•ic, he•pa•tog•e•nous (hep-ă-tō-jen′ik, -toj′en-ŭs). Of hepatic origin; formed in the liver.

he•pa•tog•ra•phy (hep-ă-tog′ră-fē). Radiography of the liver. [hepato- + G. *graphē,* a writing]

he•pa•toid (hep′ă-toyd). Resembling or like the liver. [hepato- + G. *eidos,* resemblance]

he•pa•to•lith (hep′ă-tō-lith). A concretion in the liver. [hepato- + G. *lithos,* stone]

he•pa•to•li•thec•to•my (hep′ă-tō-li-thek′tō-mē). Removal of a calculus from the liver. [hepato- + G. *lithos,* stone, + *ektomē,* excision]

he•pa•to•li•thi•a•sis (hep′ă-tō-li-thī′ă-sis). Presence of calculi in the liver. [hepato- + G. *lithiasis,* presence of a calculus]

he•pa•tol•o•gy (hep-ă-tol′ō-jē). The branch of medicine concerned with diseases of the liver. [hepato- + G. *logos,* study]

he•pa•tol•y•sin (hep-ă-tol′i-sin). A cytolysin that destroys parenchymal cells of the liver.

he•pa•to•ma (hep-ă-tō′mă). SEE malignant h. [hepato- + G. *-oma,* tumor]

malignant h., a carcinoma derived from parenchymal cells of the liver. SYN hepatocarcinoma, hepatocellular carcinoma.

he•pa•to•meg•a•ly, he•pa•to•me•ga•lia (hep′ă-tō-meg′ă-lē, -mě-gā′lē-ă). Enlargement of the liver. SYN megalohepatia. [hepato- + G. *megas,* large]

he•pa•to•mel•a•no•sis (hep′ă-tō-mel′ă-nō′sis). Heavy pigmentation of the liver. [hepato- + G. *melas,* black, + *-osis,* condition]

he•pa•tom•pha•lo•cele (hep′ă-tom-fal′ō-sēl, hep-ă-tom′fă-lō-sēl). Umbilical hernia with involvement of the liver. [hepato- + omphalocele]

he•pa•to•neph•ric (hep′ă-tō-nef′rik). SYN hepatorenal.

he•pa•to•path•ic (hep′ă-tō-path′ik). Damaging the liver.

he•pa•top•a•thy (hep-ă-top′ă-thē). Disease of the liver. [hepato- + G. *pathos,* suffering]

hep•a•to•pet•al (hep′ă-tō-pet′al). Toward the liver, usually referring to the normal direction of portal blood flow.

he•pa•to•pex•y (hep′ă-tō-pek-sē). Anchoring of the liver to the abdominal wall. [hepato- + G. *pēxis,* fixation]

he•pa•to•pneu•mon•ic (hep′ă-tō-nū-mon′ik). Relating to the liver and the lungs. SYN hepatopulmonary. [hepato- + G. *pneumonikos,* pulmonary]

he

he·pa·to·por·tal (hep′ă-tō-pōr′tăl). Relating to the portal system of the liver.

he·pa·to·pul·mo·nary (hep′ă-tō-pŭl′mō-nār′ē). SYN hepatopneumonic.

he·pa·to·re·nal (hep-ă-tō-rē′năl). Relating to the liver and the kidney. SYN hepatonephric. [hepato- + L. *renalis*, renal, fr. *renes*, kidneys]

he·pa·tor·rha·phy (hep-ă-tōr′ă-fē). Suture of a wound of the liver. [hepato- + G. *rhaphē*, a suture]

he·pa·tor·rhex·is (hep′ă-tō-rek′sis). Rupture of the liver. [hepato- + G. *rhēxis*, rupture]

he·pa·tos·co·py (hep-ă-tos′kŏ-pē). Examination of the liver. [hepato- + G. *skopeō*, to examine]

he·pa·to·sple·ni·tis (hep′ă-tō-splē-nī′tis). Inflammation of the liver and spleen.

he·pa·to·sple·nog·ra·phy (hep′ă-tō-splē-nog′ră-fē). The use of a contrast medium to outline or depict the liver and spleen radiographically.

he·pa·to·splen·o·meg·a·ly (hep′ă-tō-splē-nō-meg′ă-lē). Enlargement of the liver and spleen. [hepato- + G. *splēn*, spleen, + *megas*, large]

he·pa·to·sple·nop·a·thy (hep′ă-tō-splē-nop′ă-thē). Disease of the liver and spleen.

he·pa·tot·o·my (hep-ă-tot′ō-mē). Incision into the liver. [hepato- + G. *tomē*, incision]

he·pa·to·tox·e·mia (hep′ă-tō-tok-sē′mē-ă). Autointoxication assumed to be due to improper functioning of the liver. [hepato- + G. *toxikon*, poison, + *haima*, blood]

he·pa·to·tox·ic (hep′ă-tō-tok′sik). Relating to an agent that damages the liver, or pertaining to any such action.

he·pa·to·tox·in (hep′ă-tō-tok′sin). A toxin that is destructive to parenchymal cells of the liver.

hept-. Seven. [G. *hepta*, seven]

△**hepta-.** Prefix denoting seven. Cf. septi-, sept-. [G. *hepta*]

hep·tose (hep′tōs). A sugar with seven carbon atoms in its molecule; *e.g.*, sedoheptulose.

herd. A group of people or animals in a given area. [O.E. *heord*]

he·red·i·tary (hĕ-red′i-ter-ē). Transmissible from parent to offspring by information encoded in the parental germ cell. [L. *hereditarius;* fr. *heres* (*hered*-), an heir]

he·red·i·ty (hĕ-red′i-tē). **1.** The transmission of characters from parent to offspring by information encoded in the parental germ cells. **2.** Genealogy. [L. *hereditas*, inheritance, fr. *heres* (*hered*-), heir]

△**heredo-.** Heredity. [L. *heres*, an heir]

her·i·ta·bil·i·ty (her′i-ta-bil′i-tē). **1.** PSYCHOMETRICS A statistical term used to denote the extent of variance of an individual's total score or response which is attributable to a presumed genetic component, in contrast to an acquired component. **2.** GENETICS A statistical term used to denote the proportion of phenotypic variance due to variance in genotypes that is genetically determined, denoted by the traditional symbol h^2. [see heredity]

her·maph·ro·dite (her-maf′rō-dīt). An individual with hermaphroditism. [G. *Hermaphroditos*, the son of *Hermēs*, Mercury, + *Aphroditē*, Venus]

her·maph·ro·dit·ism (her-maf′rō-dīt-izm). The presence in one individual of both ovarian and testicular tissue; *i.e.*, true h.

bilateral h., true h. with an ovotestis on both sides.

false h., SYN pseudohermaphroditism.

lateral h., a form in which a testis is present on one side and an ovary on the other.

transverse h., pseudohermaphroditism in which the external genitalia are characteristic of one sex and the gonads are characteristic of the other sex.

unilateral h., h. in which the doubling of sex characteristics occurs on one side only: ovotestis on one side and either ovary or testis on the other.

her·met·ic (her-met′ik). Airtight; denoting a vessel closed or sealed in such a way that air can neither enter it nor issue from it.

her·nia (her′nē-ă). Protrusion of a part or structure through the tissues normally containing it. SYN rupture (1). [L. rupture]

abdominal h., a h. protruding through or into any part of the abdominal wall. SYN laparocele.

Barth's h., a loop of intestine between a persistent vitelline duct and the abdominal wall.

Bochdalek's h., SYN congenital diaphragmatic h.

cerebral h., protrusion of brain substance through a defect in the skull.

Cloquet's h., a femoral h. perforating the aponeurosis of the pectineus and insinuating itself between this aponeurosis and the muscle, lying therefore behind the femoral vessels.

complete h., an indirect inguinal h. in which the contents extend into the tunica vaginalis.

congenital diaphragmatic h., absence of the pleuroperitoneal membrane (usually on the left) or an enlarged Morgagni's foramen which allows protrusion of abdominal viscera into the chest. SYN Bochdalek's h.

crural h., SYN femoral h.

▪**diaphragmatic h.,** protrusion of abdominal contents into the chest through a weakness in the respiratory diaphragm; a common type is the hiatal h.

epigastric h., h. through the linea alba above the navel.

extrasaccular h., SYN sliding h.

fatty h., SYN pannicular h.

femoral h., h. through the femoral ring. SYN crural h., femorocele.

gastroesophageal h., a hiatal h. into the thorax.

Hesselbach's h., h. with diverticula through the cribriform fascia, presenting a lobular outline.

hiatal h., hiatus h., h. of a part of the stomach through the esophageal hiatus of the diaphragm.

Holthouse's h., inguinal h. with extension of the loop of intestine along Poupart's ligament.

incarcerated h., SYN irreducible h.

incisional h., h. occurring through a surgical incision or scar.

▪**inguinal h.,** a h. at the inguinal region: direct inguinal hernia involves the abdominal wall between the deep epigastric artery and the edge of the rectus muscle; indirect inguinal hernia involves the internal inguinal ring and passes into the inguinal canal.

interstitial h., a h. in which the protrusion is

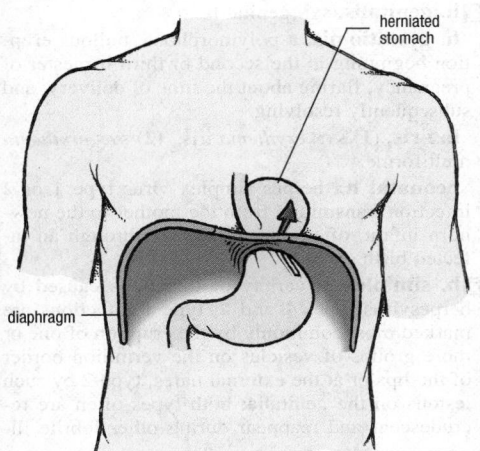

diaphragmatic hernia

between any two of the layers of the abdominal wall.

irreducible h., a h. that cannot be reduced without operation. SYN incarcerated h.

ischiatic h., a h. through the sacrosciatic foramen.

labial h., h. through the canal of Nuck.

Littré's h., (1) SYN parietal h. **(2)** h. of Meckel's diverticulum.

lumbar h., a protrusion between the last rib and the iliac crest where the aponeurosis of the transversus muscle is covered only by the latissimus dorsi.

obturator h., h. through the obturator foramen.

pannicular h., the escape of subcutaneous fat through a gap in a fascia or an aponeurosis. SYN fatty h.

pantaloon h., an inguinal h. that involves both an indirect and a direct component.

paraperitoneal h., a vesical h. in which only a part of the protruded organ is covered by the peritoneum of the sac.

parietal h., a h. in which only a portion of the wall of the intestine is engaged. SYN Littré's h. (1), Richter's h.

perineal h., a h. protruding through the pelvic diaphragm.

reducible h., a h. in which the contents of the sac can be returned to their normal location.

retrograde h., a double loop h. the central loop of which lies in the abdominal cavity.

Richter's h., SYN parietal h.

sciatic h., protrusion of intestine through the great sacrosciatic foramen. SYN ischiocele.

scrotal h., complete inguinal h., located in the scrotum.

sliding h., a h. in which an abdominal viscus forms part of the sac. SYN extrasaccular h., slipped h.

slipped h., SYN sliding h.

strangulated h., an irreducible h. in which the circulation is arrested; gangrene occurs unless relief is prompt.

synovial h., protrusion of a fold of the stratum synoviale through a rent in the stratum fibrosum of a joint capsule.

umbilical h., a h. in which bowel or omentum protrudes through the abdominal wall under the skin at the umbilicus. SEE ALSO omphalocele. SYN exomphalos (2), exumbilication (2).

vesicle h., protrusion of a segment of the bladder through the abdominal wall or into the inguinal canal and into the scrotum.

vitreous h., prolapse of the vitreous humor into the anterior chamber; may follow removal or displacement of the lens from the lenticular space.

her·nial (her'nē-ăl). Relating to hernia.

her·ni·at·ed (her'nē-ā-ted). Denoting any structure protruded through a hernial opening.

her·ni·a·tion (her-nē-ā'shŭn). Formation of a protrusion.

△**hernio-.** A hernia. [L. *hernia*, rupture]

her·ni·oid (her'nē-oyd). Resembling hernia. [hernio- + G. *eidos*, resemblance]

her·ni·o·plas·ty (her'nē-ō-plas-tē). SYN herniorrhaphy. [hernio- + G. *plastos*, formed]

her·ni·or·rha·phy (her'nē-ōr'ă-fē). Surgical repair of a hernia. SYN hernioplasty. [hernio- + G. *rhaphē*, a seam]

her·ni·ot·o·my (her-nē-ot'ō-mē). Surgical division of the constriction or strangulation of a hernia, often followed by herniorrhaphy. [hernio- + G. *tomē*, a cutting]

he·ro·ic (hē-rō'ik). Denoting an aggressive, daring procedure in a dangerously ill patient which may endanger the patient but which also has a possibility of being successful, whereas lesser action would result in failure. [G. *hērōikos*, pertaining to a hero]

her·o·in (H) (her'ō-in). An alkaloid prepared

he

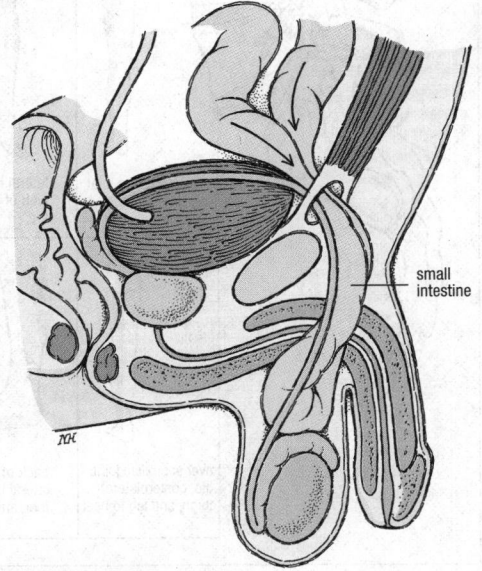

Indirect inguinal hernia

from morphine by acetylation; formerly used for the relief of cough. Except for research, its use in the United States is prohibited by federal law because of its potential for abuse.

her·pan·gi·na (her-pan′ji-nă, herp-an-jī′nă). A disease caused by types of coxsackievirus and marked by vesiculopapular lesions around the fauces that break down to form grayish yellow ulcers. [G. *herpēs*, vesicular eruption, + L. *angina*, quinsy, fr. *ango*, to strangle]

her·pes (her′pēz). An inflammatory skin disease caused by herpesvirus; an eruption of groups of deep-seated vesicles on erythematous bases. SYN serpigo (2). [G. *herpēs*, a spreading skin eruption, shingles, fr. *herpō*, to creep]

genital h., herpetic lesions on the penis of the male or on the cervix, perineum, vagina, or vulva of the female, caused by herpesvirus (h. simplex virus) type 2. SYN h. genitalis.

h. genitalis, SYN genital h.

h. gestatio′nis, a polymorphous, bullous eruption beginning in the second or third trimester of pregnancy, flaring about the time of delivery, and subsequently resolving.

h. i′ris, (1) SYN *erythema* iris. (2) SYN *erythema* multiforme.

neonatal h., herpes simplex virus type 1 or 2 infection transmitted from the mother to the newborn infant, often during passage through an infected birth canal.

h. sim′plex, a variety of infections caused by herpesvirus types 1 and 2; type 1 infections are marked most commonly by the eruption of one or more groups of vesicles on the vermilion border of the lips or at the external nares, type 2 by such lesions on the genitalia; both types often are recrudescent and reappear during other febrile ill-

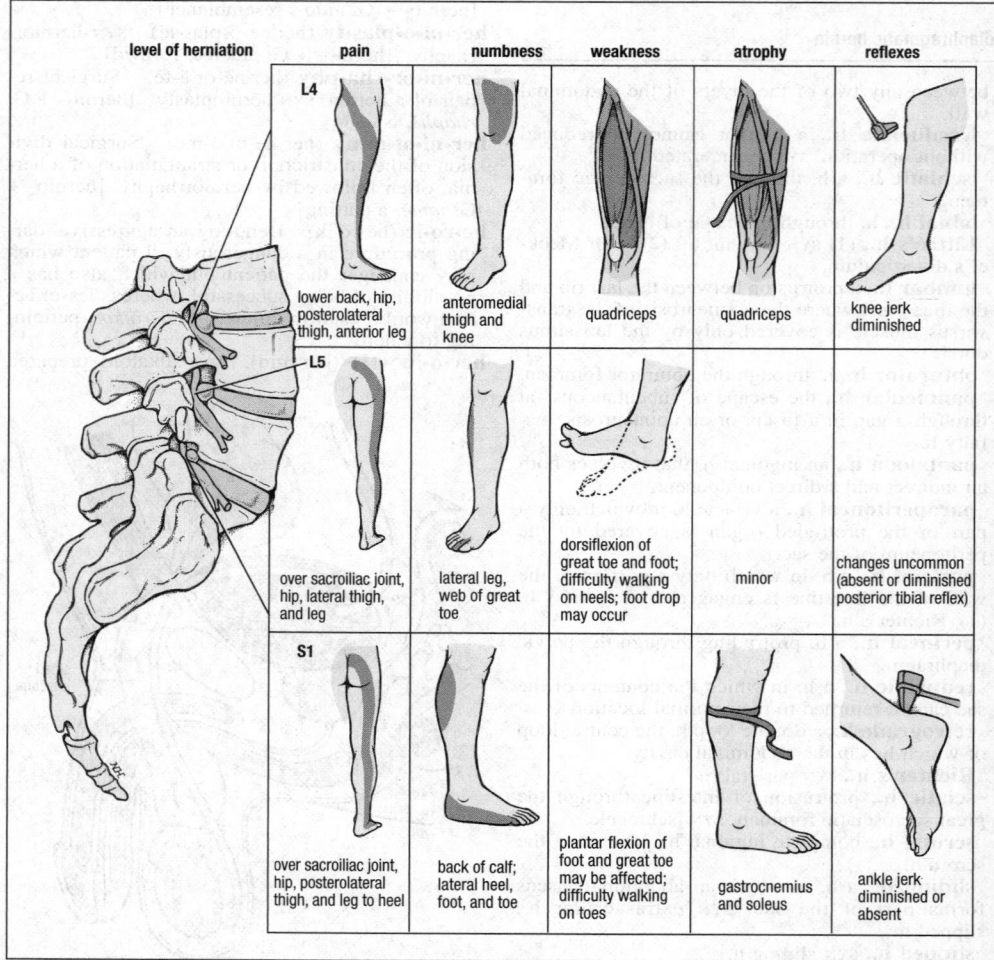

level of herniation	pain	numbness	weakness	atrophy	reflexes
L4	lower back, hip, posterolateral thigh, anterior leg	anteromedial thigh and knee	quadriceps	quadriceps	knee jerk diminished
L5	over sacroiliac joint, hip, lateral thigh, and leg	lateral leg, web of great toe	dorsiflexion of great toe and foot; difficulty walking on heels; foot drop may occur	minor	changes uncommon (absent or diminished posterior tibial reflex)
S1	over sacroiliac joint, hip, posterolateral thigh, and leg to heel	back of calf; lateral heel, foot, and toe	plantar flexion of foot and great toe may be affected; difficulty walking on toes	gastrocnemius and soleus	ankle jerk diminished or absent

intervertebral disc herniation

nesses or even physiologic states such as menstruation.

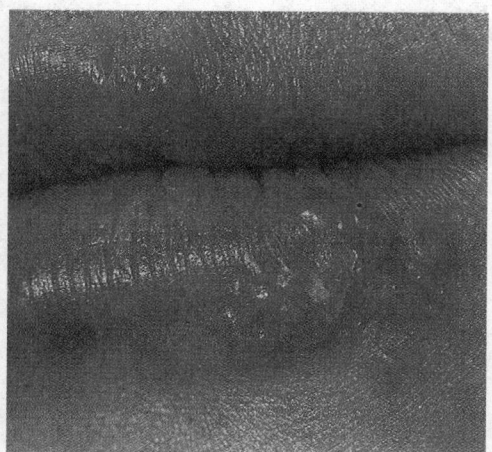

herpes simplex: of the lip

h. zos′ter, an infection caused by varicella-zoster virus, characterized by an eruption of groups of vesicles on one side of the body following the course of a nerve, due to inflammation of ganglia and dorsal nerve roots; the condition is self-limited but may be accompanied by or followed by severe postherpetic pain. SYN shingles, zona (2), zoster.

h. zos′ter o′ticus, a painful varicella virus infection presenting with a vesicular eruption on the pinna, with or without facial nerve paralysis. SYN Ramsay Hunt's syndrome (2).

her•pes•vi•rus (her′pēz-vī′rŭs). Any virus belonging to the family Herpesviridae.

human h. 1, herpes simplex virus, type 1. SEE *herpes* simplex.

human h. 2, herpes simplex virus, type 2. SEE *herpes* simplex.

human h. 3, SYN varicella-zoster *virus*.

human h. 4, SYN Epstein-Barr *virus*.

human h. 5, SYN cytomegalovirus.

human h. 6, a herpesvirus found in certain lymphoproliferative disorders, and associated with roseola (exanthema subitum).

her•pet•ic (her-pet′ik). **1.** Relating to or characterized by herpes. **2.** Relating to or caused by a herpetovirus or herpesvirus.

her•pet•i•form (her-pet′i-fŏrm). Resembling herpes.

her•sage (ār-sahzh′). Separating the individual fibers of a nerve trunk. [Fr. (from L. *hirpex,* a large rake), a harrowing]

Hertz, Heinrich R., German physicist, 1857–1894. SEE hertz.

hertz (Hz) (herts). A unit of frequency equivalent to 1 cycle per second. [H.R. *Hertz*]

hes•i•tan•cy (hez′i-tăn-sē). An involuntary delay or inability in starting the urinary stream.

△**heter-.** SEE hetero-.

het•er•ax•i•al (het-er-ak′sē-ăl). Having mutually perpendicular axes of unequal length.

het•er•e•cious (het-er-ē′shŭs). Having more than one host; said of a parasite passing different stages of its life cycle in different animals. [heter- + G. *oikion,* home]

het•er•e•cism (het′er-ē-sizm). The occurrence, in a parasite, of two cycles of development passed in two different hosts. [heter- + G. *oikion,* home]

het•er•es•the•sia (het-er-es-thē′zē-ă). A change occurring in the degree (either plus or minus) of the sensory response to a cutaneous stimulus as the latter crosses a certain line on the surface. [heter- + G. *aisthēsis,* sensation]

△**hetero-, heter-.** The other, different; opposite of homo- [G. *heteros,* other]

het•er•o•ag•glu•ti•nin (het′er-ō-ă-glū′ti-nin). A form of hemagglutinin, one that agglutinates the red blood cells of species other than that in which the h. occurs. SEE ALSO hemagglutinin.

het•er•o•an•ti•body (het′er-ō-an′ti-bod-ē). Antibody that is heterologous with respect to antigen, in contradistinction to isoantibody.

het•er•o•an•ti•se•rum (het′er-ō-an′ti-sē-rŭm). Antiserum developed in one animal species against antigens or cells of another species.

het•er•o•blas•tic (het-er-ō-blas′tik). Developing from more than a single type of tissue. [hetero- + G. *blastos,* germ]

het•er•o•cel•lu•lar (het′er-ō-sel′yū-lăr). Formed of cells of different kinds.

het•er•o•chro•ma•tin (het′er-ō-krō′mă-tin). The part of the chromonema that remains tightly coiled and condensed during interphase and thus stains readily.

het•er•o•chro•mia (het′er-ō-krō′mē-ă). A difference in coloration in two structures which are normally alike in color. [hetero- + G. *chrōma,* color]

het•er•o•chro•mo•some (het′er-ō-krō′mō-sōm). SYN allosome.

het•er•o•chro•mous (het′er-ō-krō′mŭs). Having an abnormal difference in coloration.

het•er•o•chro•nia (het-er-ō-krō′nē-ă). Origin or development of tissues or organs at an unusual time or out of the regular sequence. Cf. synchronia. [hetero- + G. *chronos,* time]

het•er•o•chron•ic (het-er-ō-kron′ik). SYN heterochronous.

het•er•och•ro•nous (het-er-ok′rō-nŭs). Relating to heterochronia. SYN heterochronic.

het•er•o•crine (het′er-ō-krin). Denoting the secretion of two or more kinds of material. [hetero- + G. *krinō,* to separate]

het•er•o•cy•to•tro•pic (het′er-ō-sī′tō-trop′ik). Having an affinity for cells of a different species. [hetero- + G. *kytos,* cell, + *tropē,* a turning toward]

het•er•od•ro•mous (het-er-ōd′rŏ-mŭs). Moving in the opposite direction. [hetero- + G. *dromos,* running]

het•er•o•e•rot•ic (het′er-ō-ĕ-rot′ik). SYN alloerotic.

het•er•o•er•o•tism (het′er-ō-ār′ō-tizm). SYN alloerotism.

het•er•o•ga•met•ic (het′er-ō-gă-met′ik). Having sex gametes of contrasting types; human males are h. [hetero- + G. *gametikos,* connubial]

he

het•er•og•a•mous (het-er-og′ă-mŭs). Relating to heterogamy.

het•er•og•a•my (het-er-og′ă-mē). **1.** Conjugation of unlike gametes. **2.** Bearing different types of flowers. **3.** Reproduction by indirect methods of pollination. [hetero- + G. *gamos,* marriage]

het•er•o•ge•ne•i•ty (het′er-ō-jĕ-nē′i-tē). Heterogeneous state or quality.

het•er•o•ge•neous (het′er-ō-jē′nē-ŭs). Comprising elements with various and dissimilar properties.

het•er•o•gen•e•sis (het′er-ō-jen′ĕ-sis). **1.** Alternation of generations. **2.** SYN asexual *generation.* **3.** SYN spontaneous *generation.* [hetero- + G. *genesis,* production]

het•er•o•ge•net•ic (het′er-ō-jĕ-net′ik). Relating to heterogenesis.

het•er•o•gen•ic, het•er•o•ge•ne•ic (het′er-ō-jen′ik, -jĕ-nē′ik). Having different gene constitutions, especially in diverse species.

het•er•og•e•nous (het-er-oj′ĕ-nŭs). Of foreign origin. Commonly confused with heterogeneous.

het•er•o•graft (het′er-ō-graft). SYN xenograft.

het•er•o•ki•ne•sis (het′er-ō-ki-nē′sis). Differential distribution of X and Y chromosomes during meiotic cell division. [hetero- + G. *kinēsis,* movement hetero- + G. *kinēsis,* movement]

het•er•o•la•lia (het′er-ō-lā′lē-ă). The habitual substitution of meaningless or inappropriate words for those intended; a form of aphasia. SYN heterophemia, heterophemy. [hetero- + G. *lalia,* speech]

het•er•o•lat•er•al (het′er-ō-lat′er-ăl). SYN contralateral. [hetero- + L. *latus,* side]

het•er•ol•o•gous (het-er-ol′ō-gŭs). **1.** Pertaining to cytologic or histologic elements occurring where they are not normally found. SEE ALSO xenogeneic. **2.** Derived from an animal of a different species, as the serum of a horse is h. for a rabbit. [hetero- + G. *logos,* ratio, relation]

het•er•ol•y•sis (het-er-ol′i-sis). Dissolution or digestion of cells or protein components from one species by a lytic agent from a different species. [hetero- + G. *lysis,* a loosening]

het•er•o•lyt•ic (het′er-ō-lit′ik). Pertaining to heterolysis or to the effect of a heterolysin.

het•er•o•mer•ic (het′er-ō-mār′ik). **1.** Having a different chemical composition. **2.** Denoting spinal neurons that have processes passing over to the opposite side of the cord. [hetero- + G. *meros,* part]

het•er•o•met•a•pla•sia (het′er-ō-met-ă-plā′zē-ă). Tissue transformation resulting in production of a tissue foreign to the part where produced.

het•er•o•me•tro•pia (het′er-ō-me-trō′pē-ă). A condition in which the refraction is different in the two eyes. [hetero- + G. *metron,* measure, + ōps, eye]

het•er•o•mor•pho•sis (het′er-ō-mōr-fō′sis). **1.** Development of one tissue from a tissue of another kind or type. **2.** Embryonic development of tissue or an organ inappropriate to its site. [hetero- + G. *morphōsis,* a molding]

het•er•o•mor•phous (het′er-ō-mōr′fŭs). Differing from the normal form.

het•er•on•o•mous (het-er-on′ō-mŭs). **1.** Different from the type; abnormal. **2.** Subject to the direction or control of another; not self-governing. [hetero- + G. *nomos,* law]

het•er•on•o•my (het-er-on′ō-mē). The condition or state of being heteronomous. [hetero- + G. *nomos,* law]

het•er•op•a•thy (het′er-op′ă-thē). **1.** Abnormal sensitivity to stimuli. **2.** SYN allopathy. [hetero- + G. *pathos,* suffering]

het•er•oph•a•gy (het-er-of′ă-jē). Digestion within a cell of an exogenous substance phagocytosed from the cell's environment. [hetero- + G. *phagō,* to eat]

het•er•o•phe•mia, het•er•o•phe•my (het′er-ō-fē′mē-ă, het-er-of′ĕ-mē). SYN heterolalia. [hetero- + G. *phēmē,* a speech]

het•er•o•phil, het•er•o•phile (het′er-ō-fil, -fīl). **1.** The neutrophilic leukocyte. **2.** Pertaining to heterogenetic antigens occurring in different species or to antibodies directed against such antigens. [hetero- + G. *philos,* fond]

het•er•o•pho•nia (het′er-ō-fō′nē-ă). **1.** The change of voice at puberty. **2.** Any abnormality in the voice sounds. [hetero- + G. *phōnē,* voice]

het•er•o•pho•ria (het′er-ō-fō′rē-ă). A tendency for deviation of the eyes from parallelism, prevented by binocular vision. [hetero- + G. *phora,* movement]

het•er•oph•thal•mus (het-er-of-thal′mŭs). A seldom-used term for a difference in the appearance of the two eyes, usually due to heterochromia iridis. [hetero- + G. *ophthalmos,* eye]

het•er•o•phy•i•a•sis (het′er-ō-fī-ī′ă-sis). Infection with a heterophyid trematode, particularly *Heterophyes heterophyes.*

het•er•o•pla•sia (het′er-ō-plā′zē-ă). **1.** Development of cytologic and histologic elements that are not normal for the organ or part in question, as the growth of bone in a site where there is normally fibrous connective tissue. **2.** Malposition of tissue or a part that is otherwise normal, as a ureter that develops at the lower pole of a kidney. [hetero- + G. *plasis,* a forming]

het•er•o•plas•tic (het′er-ō-plas′tik). **1.** Pertaining to or manifesting heteroplasia. **2.** Relating to heteroplasty.

het•er•o•ploid (het′er-ō-ployd). Relating to heteroploidy.

het•er•o•ploi•dy (het′er-ō-ploy′dē). The state of a cell possessing some number of complete haploid sets other than the normal. [hetero- + G. *ploides,* in form]

het•er•o•pyk•no•sis (het′er-ō-pik-nō′sis). Any state of variable density or condensation, usually in different chromosomes or between different regions of the same chromosome; a region may be attentuated (negative h.) or accentuated (positive h.). [hetero- + G. *pyknos,* dense]

het•er•o•pyk•not•ic (het′er-ō-pik-not′ik). Relating to or characterized by heteropyknosis.

het•er•o•sex•u•al (het′er-ō-sek′shū-ăl). **1.** A person whose sexual orientation is toward persons of the opposite sex. **2.** Relating to or characteristic of heterosexuality. **3.** One whose interests and behavior are characteristic of heterosexuality.

het•er•o•sex•u•al•i•ty (het′er-ō-sek-shū-al′i-tē). Erotic attraction, predisposition, or activity, including sexual congress between persons of the opposite sex.

het·er·o·sug·ges·tion (het′er-ō-sŭg-jes′chŭn). Hypnotic suggestion received from another person; opposed to autosuggestion.

het·er·o·tax·ia (het′er-ō-taks′ē-ă). Abnormal arrangement of organs or parts of the body in relation to each other. [hetero- + G. *taxis,* arrangement]

het·er·o·tax·ic (het-er-ō-taks′ik). Abnormally placed or arranged.

het·er·o·to·nia (het′er-ō-tō′nē-ă). Abnormality or variation in tension or tonus. [hetero- + G. *tonos,* tension]

het·er·o·to·pia (het-er-ō-tō′pē-ă). 1. SYN ectopia. 2. NEUROPATHOLOGY Displacement of gray matter, typically into the deep cerebral white matter. [hetero- + G. *topos,* place]

het·er·o·top·ic (het-er-ō-top′ik). 1. SYN ectopic (1). 2. Relating to heterotopia (2). [hetero- + *topos,* place, + suffix -*ic,* pertaining to]

het·er·ot·o·pous (het-er-ot′ō-pŭs). Heterotopic, especially in reference to teratomas composed of tissues that are out of place in the region where found.

het·er·o·trans·plan·ta·tion (het′er-ō-tranz-plan-tā′shŭn). Transfer of a heterograft (xenograft).

het·er·o·tri·cho·sis (het′er-ō-tri-kō′sis). A condition characterized by hair growth of variegated color. [hetero- + G. *trichōsis,* growth of hair]

het·er·o·troph (het′er-ō-trof, -trōf). A microorganism that obtains its carbon, as well as its energy, from organic compounds. SEE ALSO autotroph. [hetero- + G. *trophē,* nourishment]

het·er·o·tro·phic (het′er-ō-tro-fik). 1. Relating to or exhibiting the properties of heterotrophy. 2. Relating to a heterotroph.

het·er·o·tro·pia, het·er·ot·ro·py (het′er-ō-trō′pē-ă, het-er-ot′rō-pē). SYN strabismus. [hetero- + G. *tropē,* a turning]

het·er·o·typ·ic (het′er-ō-tip′ik). Of a different or unusual type or form.

het·er·o·xan·thine (het′er-ō-zan′thin). 7-Methylxanthine; one of the alloxuric bases in urine, representing end products of purine metabolism.

het·er·ox·e·nous (het-er-oks′ĕ-nŭs). SYN digenetic (1). [hetero- + G. *xenos,* stranger]

het·er·o·zy·gos·i·ty, het·er·o·zy·go·sis (het′er-ō-zī-gos′i-tē, -zī-gō′sis). The state of being heterozygous. [hetero- + G. *zygon,* a yoke]

het·er·o·zy·gote (het′er-ō-zī′gōt). A heterozygous individual. [hetero- + G. *zygotos,* yoked]

 compound h., MEDICAL GENETICS The presence of two different mutant alleles at the same loci.

 manifesting h., an organism heterozygous for what is ordinarily a recessive condition which, as a result of special mechanisms (such as lyonization, allelic exclusion, or a deletion in the homologous chromosome), has phenotypic manifestations.

het·er·o·zy·gous (het′er-ō-zī′gŭs). Having different allelic genes at one locus or (by extension) many loci; heterotic.

 doubly h., denoting that genotype in which a parent is h. at both loci, the state that on average

contains the maximum information about the linkage.

HEV hepatitis E *virus.*

△**hexa-, hex-.** six. [G. *hex*]

hex·ad (heks′ad). A sexivalent element or radical.

hex·a·dac·ty·ly, hex·a·dac·tyl·ism (hek′să-dak′ti-lē, -lizm). The presence of six fingers or six toes on one or both hands or feet. [hexa- + G. *daktylos,* finger]

Hex·ad·no·vi·rus (hecks′-ad-nō-vī-rŭs). A genus in the family Hepadnaviridae, which is the cause of hepatitis B.

hex·a·mer (hek′să-mer). 1. SEE virion. 2. A complex or compound containing six subunits or moieties. [hexa- + G. *meros,* part]

hex·ane (hek′sān). A saturated hydrocarbon, C_6H_{14}, of the paraffin series.

hex·a·ploi·dy (heks′ă-ploy-dē). SEE polyploidy.

hex·i·tol (heks′i-tol). The polyol (sugar alcohol) obtained on the reduction of a hexose (*e.g.,* D-sorbitol).

hex·o·ki·nase (heks-ō-kī′nās). A phosphotransferase present in yeast, muscle, brain, and other tissues that catalyzes the phosphorylation of D-glucose and other hexoses to form D-glucose 6-phosphate (or other hexose 6-phosphate) (phosphate is transferred from ATP, which is converted to ADP); the first step in glycolysis; a deficiency of h. can result in hemolytic anemia and impaired glycolysis.

hex·os·a·mine (hek′sō-sam′ēn). The amine derivative (NH_2 replacing OH) of a hexose; *e.g.,* glucosamine.

hex·os·a·min·i·dase (hek′sō-sa-min′i-dās). General term for enzymes cleaving *N*-acetylhexose residues from ganglioside-like oligosaccharides.

hex·o·sans (hek′sō-sanz). Polysaccharides with the general formula ($C_6H_{10}O_5$)$_x$ which, on hydrolysis, yield hexoses; included are glucosans (glucans), mannans, galactans, and fructosans (fructans).

hex·ose (hek′sōs). A monosaccharide containing six carbon atoms in the molecule ($C_6H_{12}O_6$); D-glucose is the principal h. in nature.

hex·ose phos·pha·tase. An enzyme catalyzing the hydrolysis of a hexose phosphate to a hexose (*e.g.,* glucose-6-phosphatase).

hex·u·lose (hek′syū-lōs). SYN ketohexose.

hex·yl (hek′sil). The radical of hexane, $CH_3(CH_2)_4CH_2^-$.

Hf hafnium.

HFV high-frequency *ventilation.*

Hg mercury (hydrargyrum).

HGF hematopoietic growth *factor.*

HHIE-S *Hearing* Handicap Inventory for the Elderly.

hi·a·tal (hī-ā′tăl). Relating to a hiatus.

hi·a·tus, pl. **hi·a·tus** (hī-ā′tŭs) [NA]. An aperture, opening, or foramen. [L. an aperture, fr. *hio, pp. hiatus,* to yawn]

 aortic h., the opening in the diaphragm bounded by the two crura, the vertebral column, and the median arcuate ligament, through which pass the aorta and thoracic duct.

 h. of canal of lesser petrosal nerve, the small opening in the petrous bone lateral to the h. of facial canal that gives passage to the lesser petrosal nerve.

esophageal h., the opening in the right crus of the diaphragm, between the central tendon and the h. aorticus, through which pass the esophagus and the two vagus nerves.

semilunar h., a deep, narrow groove in the lateral wall of the middle meatus of the nasal cavity, into which the maxillary sinus, the frontonasal duct, and the middle ethmoid cells open.

hi•ber•no•ma (hī′ber-nō′mă). A rare benign neoplasm consisting of brown fat that resembles the fat in certain hibernating animals. [L. *hibernus,* pertaining to winter, + G. *-ōma,* tumor]

hic•cup, hic•cough (hik′ŭp). A diaphragmatic spasm causing a sudden inhalation which is interrupted by a spasmodic closure of the glottis, producing a noise.

⌂**hidr-.** SEE hidro-.

hi•drad•e•ni•tis (hī-drad′ĕ-nī′tis). Inflammation of the sweat glands. [G. *hidrōs,* sweat, + *adēn,* gland, + *-itis,* inflammation]

h. suppurati′va, chronic suppurative folliculitis of apocrine sweat-gland–bearing skin producing abscesses or sinuses with scarring.

hi•drad•e•no•ma (hī-drad-ĕ-nō′mă). A benign neoplasm derived from epithelial cells of sweat glands. [G. *hidrōs,* sweat, + *adēn,* gland, + *-oma,* tumor]

papillary h., a solitary benign tumor occurring in women usually in the labia majora, cystic and papillary, and composed of epithelium resembling that of apocrine glands. SYN apocrine adenoma.

⌂**hidro-, hidr-.** Sweat, sweat glands. Cf. sudor-. [G. *hidrōs*]

hi•dro•cys•to•ma (hī′drō-sis-tō′mă). A cystic form of hidradenoma, usually apocrine. SYN syringocystoma. [hidro- + G. *kystis,* bladder, + *-ōma,* tumor]

hi•dro•poi•e•sis (hī′drō-poy-ē′sis, hid′rō-). The formation of sweat. [hidro- + G. *poiēsis,* formation]

hi•dros•che•sis (hī-dros′kē-sis, hid-ros′). Suppression of sweating. [hidro- + G. *schesis,* a checking]

hi•dro•sis (hi-drō′sis, hī-). The production and excretion of sweat. [G. *hidrōs,* sweat, + *-osis,* condition]

hi•drot•ic (hi-drot′ik, hī-). Relating to or causing hidrosis.

high risk register (HRR). AUDIOLOGY checklist of conditions known to exhibit a higher-than-normal prevalence of hearing loss. Conditions include: familial history of hearing loss, congenital infections, craniofacial anomalies, low birth weight, hyperbilirubinemia, ototoxic medications, bacterial meningitis, severe CNS depression at birth. SEE screening.

hi•la (hī′lă). Plural of hilum.

hi•lar (hī′lăr). Pertaining to a hilum.

hi•li•tis (hī-lī′tis). Inflammation of the lining membrane of any hilus.

hil•lock (hil′lok). ANATOMY Any small elevation or prominence.

axon h., the conical area of origin of the axon from the nerve cell body; it contains parallel ar-

rays of microtubules and is devoid of Nissl substance.

hi•lum, pl. **hi•la** (hī′lŭm, hī′lă) [NA]. **1.** The part of an organ where the nerves and vessels enter and leave. SYN porta (1). **2.** A depression or slit resembling the h. in the olivary nucleus of the brain. [L. a small bit or trifle]

hi•lus (hī′lŭs). hilum. [an Eng. variant of L. *hilum*]

HIM health information management.

hind•brain (hīnd′brān). SYN rhombencephalon.

hind•gut (hīnd′gŭt). **1.** The caudal or terminal part of the embryonic gut. **2.** Descending and sigmoid colon, rectum and anal canal; some include entire large intestine.

hind•wa•ter (hīnd′wah-ter). Colloquialism for amniotic fluid *in utero* behind the presenting part of the fetus.

hip. 1. The lateral prominence of the pelvis from the waist to the thigh. **2.** Head, neck and greater trochanter of femur. It is this sense that is intended in the common phrases "hip fracture" or "hip replacement." **3.** More strictly, the hip joint. [A.S. *hype*]

hip bone. See under bone.

hip•po•cam•pal (hip-ō-kam′păl). Relating to the hippocampus.

hip•po•cam•pus (hip-ō-kam′pŭs) [NA]. The complex, internally convoluted structure that forms the medial margin of the cerebral hemisphere, bordering the choroid fissure of the lateral ventricle, and composed of two gyri (Ammon's horn and the dentate gyrus), together with their white matter, the alveus and fimbria hippocampi. In humans the h. is confined to the temporal lobe by the massive development of the corpus callosum. The h. forms part of the limbic system. Its major afferent connections are with the entorhinal area of the parahippocampal gyrus, and transparent septum; by way of the fornix it projects to the septum, anterior nucleus of the thalamus, and mamillary body. [G. *hippocampos,* seahorse]

hip•po•crat•ic (hip-ŏ-krat′ik). Relating to, described by, or attributed to Hippocrates.

Hip•po•crat•ic Oath. An oath taken by physicians about to enter the practice of their profession, which, though usually attributed to Hippocrates of Cos, is probably an ancient oath of the Asclepiads.

hip•pus (hip′ŭs). Intermittent pupillary dilation and constriction, independent of illumination, convergence, or psychic stimuli. [G. *hippos,* horse, from a fancied suggestion of galloping movements]

hir•cus, gen. and pl. **hir•ci** (her′kŭs, her′sī). **1.** The odor of the axillae. **2** [NA]. One of the hairs growing in the axillae. **3.** SYN tragus (1). [L. hegoat]

hir•sute (her-sūt′). Relating to or characterized by hirsutism. [L. *hirsutus,* shaggy]

hir•sut•ism (her′sū-tizm). Presence of excessive bodily and facial terminal hair, in a male pattern, especially in women; may be present in normal adults as an expression of an ethnic characteristic or may develop in children or adults as the result of androgen excess due to tumors or drugs, or nonandrogenic drugs. [L. *hirsutus,* shaggy]

hir·u·di·cide (hi-rū′di-sīd). An agent that kills leeches. [L. *hirudo,* leech, + *caedo,* to kill]

hir·u·din (hir′yū-din). An antithrombin substance extracted from the salivary glands of the leech that has the property of preventing coagulation of the blood. [L. *hirudo,* leech]

Hir·u·din·ea (hir′ū-din′ē-ă). The leeches, a class of worms with flat, segmented bodies, a sucker at the posterior end, and often a smaller sucker at the anterior end; they are predatory on invertebrate tissues, or feed on blood and tissue exudates of vertebrates. [L. *hirudo,* leech]

Hir·u·do (hi-rū′dō). A genus of leeches; previously used in medicine. [L. leech]

His, Wilhelm, Jr., German physician, 1863–1934. SEE H. bundle *electrogram.*

His, Wilhelm, Sr., Swiss anatomist and embryologist in Germany, 1831–1904. SEE H.'s *line.*

His- Histidyl.

-His Histidino.

His. Histidine.

his·ta·mine (his′tă-mēn). A depressor amine derived from histidine and present in ergot and in animal tissues. It is a powerful stimulant of gastric secretion, a constrictor of bronchial smooth muscle and a vasodilator (capillaries and arterioles) that causes a fall in blood pressure. H. is liberated in the skin as a result of injury. When pricked into the skin in high dilution, it causes the triple response.

his·ta·mine-fast. Indicating the absence of the normal response to histamine, especially in speaking of true gastric anacidity.

his·ta·mi·ne·mia (his′tă-mi-nē′mē-ă). The presence of histamine in the circulating blood. [histamine + G. *haima,* blood]

his·ta·mi·nu·ria (his′tă-mi-nū′rē-ă). The excretion of histamine in the urine. [histidine + G. *ouron,* urine]

his·ti·dase (his′ti-dās). SYN *histidine* ammonia-lyase.

his·ti·dine (His, H) (his′ti-dēn). The L-isomer is a basic amino acid found in most proteins.

  h. ammonia-lyase, an enzyme catalyzing deamination of L-histidine; this enzyme is absent or deficient in individuals with histidinemia. SYN histidase.

  h. decarboxylase, an enzyme catalyzing the decarboxylation of L-histidine to histamine and CO_2; it plays a role in constriction of bronchial smooth muscle.

his·ti·dino (-His) (his′ti-din-ō). The radical of histidine produced by removal of a hydrogen from a nitrogen atom.

his·ti·di·nu·ria (his′ti-di-nū′rē-ă). Excretion of considerable amounts of histidine in the urine; frequently observed in later months of pregnancy, and in histidinemia.

his·ti·dyl (His-) (his′ti-dil). The acyl radical of histidine.

histio-. Tissue, especially connective tissue. [G. *histion,* web]

his·ti·o·blast (his′tē-ō-blast). A tissue-forming cell. SYN histoblast. [histio- + G. *blastos,* germ]

his·ti·o·cyte (his′tē-ō-sīt). A macrophage present in connective tissue. SYN histocyte. [histio- + G. *kytos,* cell]

cardiac h., a large mononuclear cell found in connective tissue of the heart wall in inflammatory conditions, especially in the Aschoff body. SYN Anitschkow cell, Anitschkow myocyte.

his·ti·o·cy·to·ma (his′tē-ō-sī-tō′mă). A tumor composed of histiocytes. [histio- + G. *kytos,* cell, + -*ōma,* tumor]

  malignant fibrous h., a deeply situated tumor, especially on the extremities of adults, frequently recurring after surgery and metastasizing to the lungs; shows partial fibroblastic and histiocytic differentiation with a variable storiform pattern, myxoid areas, and giant cells.

his·ti·o·cy·to·sis (his′tē-ō-sī-tō′sis). A generalized multiplication of histiocytes. SYN histocytosis.

  malignant h., a rapidly fatal form of lymphoma, characterized by fever, jaundice, pancytopenia, and enlargement of the liver, spleen, and lymph nodes; the affected organs show focal necrosis and hemorrhage, with proliferation of histiocytes and phagocytosis of red blood cells.

  h. X, proliferation of Langerhans cells of undetermined clinical type, possibly Hand-Schüller-Christian d., Letterer-Siwe disease, and eosinophilic granuloma.

his·ti·o·gen·ic (his′tē-ō-jen′ik). SYN histogenous.

histo-. Tissue. [G. *histos,* web (tissue)]

his·to·blast (his′tō-blast). SYN histioblast.

his·to·chem·is·try (his′tō-kem′is-trē). SYN cytochemistry.

his·to·com·pat·i·bil·i·ty (his′tō-kom-pat-i-bil′i-tē). A state of immunologic similarity (or identity) that permits successful homograft transplantation.

his·to·com·pat·i·bil·i·ty test·ing. See under testing.

his·to·cyte (his′tō-sīt). SYN histiocyte.

his·to·cy·to·sis (his′tō-sī-tō′sis). SYN histiocytosis.

his·to·dif·fer·en·ti·a·tion (his′tō-dif-er-en-shē-ā′shŭn). The morphologic appearance of tissue characteristics during development.

his·to·gen·e·sis (his-tō-jen′ĕ-sis). The origin of a tissue; the formation and development of the tissues of the body. [histo- + G. *genesis,* origin]

his·to·ge·net·ic (his-tō-jĕ-net′ik). Relating to histogenesis.

his·tog·e·nous (his-toj′ĕ-nŭs). Formed by the tissues; *e.g.,* the h. cells in an exudate arising from proliferation of the fixed tissue cells. SYN histiogenic. [histo- + G. -*gen,* producing]

his·toid (his′toyd). **1.** Resembling in structure one of the tissues of the body. **2.** The histologic structure of a neoplasm derived from and consisting of a single, relatively simple type of neoplastic tissue that closely resembles the normal. [histo- + G. *eidos,* resemblance]

his·to·in·com·pat·i·bil·i·ty (his′tō-in′kom-pat-i-bil′i-tē). A state of immunologic dissimilarity of tissues sufficient to cause rejection of a homograft when tissue is transplanted from one individual to another; implies a difference in histocompatibility genes in donor and recipient.

his·to·log·ic, his·to·log·i·cal (his-tō-loj′ik, i-kăl). Pertaining to histology.

his·tol·o·gist (his-tol'ō-jist). One who specializes in the science of histology. SYN microanatomist.

his·tol·o·gy (his-tol'ō-jē). The science concerned with the minute structure of cells, tissues, and organs in relation to their function. SEE ALSO microscopic *anatomy*. SYN microanatomy. [histo- + G. *logos*, study]

his·tol·y·sis (his-tol'i-sis). Disintegration of tissue. [histo- + G. *lysis*, dissolution]

his·to·ma (his-tō'mă). A benign neoplasm in which the cytologic and histologic elements are closely similar to those of normal tissue from which the neoplastic cells are derived. [histo- + G. *-oma*, tumor]

his·to·met·a·plas·tic (his'tō-met-ă-plas'tik). Exciting tissue metaplasia.

his·tom·o·ni·a·sis (hi-stom'ō-nī'ă-sis). A disease chiefly affecting turkeys, caused by *Histomonas meleagridis* and characterized by ulcerative and necrotic lesions of the liver and cecum, acute onset, and a high mortality rate. It is transmitted inside the eggs of the nematode *Heterakis gallinae*, which is primarily responsible for maintaining and spreading the infection. SYN blackhead (2).

his·tone (his'tōn). One of a number of simple proteins (often found in the cell nucleus) that contains a high proportion of basic amino acids, are soluble in water, dilute acids, and alkalies, and are not coagulable by heat.

his·to·nu·ria (his-tō-nū'rē-ă). The excretion of histone in the urine, as observed in certain instances of leukemia, febrile illnesses, and wasting diseases. [histone + G. *ouron*, urine]

his·to·path·o·gen·e·sis (his'tō-path-ō-jen'ĕ-sis). Abnormal embryonic development or growth of tissue. [histogenesis + pathogenesis]

his·to·pa·thol·o·gy (his'tō-pa-thol'ō-jē). The science or study dealing with the cytologic and histologic structure of abnormal or diseased tissue.

his·to·phys·i·ol·o·gy (his'tō-fiz-ē-ol'ō-jē). The microscopic study of tissues in relation to their functions.

His·to·plas·ma cap·su·la·tum (his-tō-plaz'mă kap-sū-lā'tŭm). A dimorphic fungus species that causes histoplasmosis; its ascomycetous state is *Ajellomyces capsulatum*. The organism's natural habitat is soil fertilized with bird and bat droppings, where it grows as a mold, fragments of which, following inhalation, produce the primary pulmonary infection; within the mammalian host, inhaled mycelial fragments grow as uninuclear yeasts that reproduce by budding. [histo- + G. *plasma*, something formed]

his·to·plas·min (his'tō-plas'min). An antigenic extract of *Histoplasma capsulatum*, used in immunological tests for the diagnosis of histoplasmosis; also used in skin test surveys of populations to determine the geographic distribution of the fungus and to predict those that are endemic for histoplasmosis.

his·to·plas·mo·ma (his'tō-plaz-mō'mă). An infectious granuloma caused by *Histoplasma capsulatum*.

his·to·plas·mo·sis (his'tō-plaz-mō'sis). A widely distributed infectious disease caused by *Histoplasma capsulatum* and occurring frequently in epidemics; usually acquired by inhalation of spores of the fungus in soil dust and manifested by a primary benign pneumonitis; occasionally, the primary disease progresses to produce localized lesions in lung, such as pulmonary cavitation, or the typical disseminated disease of the reticuloendothelial system which is manifested by fever, emaciation, splenomegaly, and leukopenia. SYN Darling's disease.

   presumed ocular h., subretinal neovascularization in the macular region associated with chorioretinal atrophy and pigment proliferation adjacent to the optic disk, and peripheral chorioretinal atrophy ("histo-spots").

his·tor·rhex·is (his-tō-rek'sis). Breakdown of tissue by some agency other than infection. [histo- + G. *rhēxis*, rupture]

his·to·tome (his'tō-tōm). SYN microtome. [histo- + G. *tomē*, cut]

his·tot·o·my (his-tot'ō-mē). SYN microtomy.

his·to·tope (his'tō-tōp). That part of the Class II major histocompatibility molecule that interacts with the T cell receptor. [histo- + -tope]

his·to·tox·ic (his-tō-tok'sik). Relating to poisoning of the respiratory enzyme system of the tissues.

his·to·tro·phic (his-tō-trof'ik). Providing nourishment for or favoring the formation of tissue. [histo- + G. *trophē*, nourishment]

his·to·tro·pic (his-tō-trop'ik). Attracted toward the tissues; denoting certain parasites, stains, and chemical compounds. [histo- + G. *tropikos*, turning]

HIV human immunodeficiency *virus*.

hives (hīvz). **1.** SYN urticaria. **2.** SYN wheal.

HLA human lymphocyte *antigens*, under *antigen*.

HLA typ·ing. Tests done in order to determine if a patient has antibodies against a potential donor's HLA antigens. The presence of antibodies means that a graft will be rejected.

HMO hypothetical mean *organism*; health maintenance organization.

HMWK. high molecular weight *kininogen*.

Ho holmium.

hoarse (hōrs). Having a rough, harsh voice. [A.S. *hās*]

hol·an·dric (hol-an'drik). Related to genes located on the Y chromosome. [G. *holos*, entire, + *aner*, human male]

ho·lism (hō'lizm). **1.** The principle that an organism, or one of its actions, is not equal to merely the sum of its parts but must be perceived or studied as a whole. **2.** The approach to the study of a psychological phenomenon through the analysis of a phenomenon as a complete entity in itself. [G. *holos*, entire]

ho·lis·tic (hō-lis'tik). Pertaining to the characteristics of holism or h. psychologies.

hol·mi·um (Ho) (hol'mē-ŭm). An element of the lanthanide group, atomic no. 67, atomic wt. 164.93032. [L. *Holmia*, for Stockholm]

△holo-. Whole, entire, complete. [G. *holos*]

hol·o·blas·tic (hol-ō-blas'tik). Denoting the involvement of the entire ovum in cleavage. [holo- + G. *blastos*, germ]

hol·o·cord (hol'ō-kōrd). Relating to the entire

spinal cord, extending from the cervico-medullary junction to the conus medullaris.

hol•o•crine (hol'ō-krin). SEE holocrine *gland*. [holo- + G. *krinō*, to separate]

hol•o•di•a•stol•ic (hol'ō-dī-ă-stol'ik). Relating to or occupying the entire diastolic period.

hol•o•en•dem•ic (hol'ō-en-dem'ik). Endemic in the entire population.

hol•o•en•zyme (hol-ō-en'zīm). A complete enzyme, *i.e.*, apoenzyme plus coenzyme, cofactor, metal ion, and/or prosthetic group.

hol•o•gram (hol'ō-gram). A three-dimensional image produced by wavefront reconstruction and recorded on a photographic plate. [holo- + G. *gramma*, something written]

hol•o•gyn•ic (hol-ō-jin'ik). Related to characters manifest only in females. [holo- + G. *gynē*, woman]

hol•o•pros•en•ceph•a•ly (hol'ō-pros-en-sef'ă-lē). Failure of the forebrain or prosencephalon to divide into hemispheres or lobes; cyclopia occurs in the severest form. It is often accompanied by a deficit in midline facial development. [holo- + G. *prosō*, forward, + *enkephalos*, brain]

hol•o•ra•chis•chi•sis (hol'ō-ră-kis'ki-sis). Spina bifida of the entire spinal column. [holo- + G. *rhachis*, spine, + *schisis*, fissure]

hol•o•sys•tol•ic (hol'ō-sis-tol'ik). SYN pansystolic.

hom•ax•i•al (hō-mak'sē-ăl). Having all the axes alike, as a sphere. [G. *homos*, the same, + *axis*]

homeo-. The same, alike. SEE ALSO homo- (1). [G. *homoios*, similar]

ho•me•o•mor•phous (hō'mē-ō-mōr'fŭs). Of similar shape, but not necessarily of the same composition. [homeo- + G. *morphē*, shape]

ho•me•o•path (hō'mē-ō-path). SYN homeopathist.

ho•me•o•path•ic (hō'mē-ō-path'ik). **1.** Relating to homeopathy. SYN homeotherapeutic (1). **2.** Denoting an extremely small dose of a pharmacological agent, such as might be used in homeopathy; more generally, a dose believed to be too small to produce the effect usually expected from that agent. Cf. pharmacologic (2), physiologic (4). [homeo- + G. *pathos*, disease]

ho•me•op•a•thist (hō-mē-op'ă-thist). A medical practitioner of homeopathy. SYN homeopath.

ho•me•op•a•thy (hō-mē-op'ă-thē). A system of therapy developed by Samuel Hahnemann based on the "law of infinitesimal doses" in *similia similibus curantur* (likes are cured by likes), which holds that a medicinal substance that can evoke certain symptoms in healthy individuals may be effective in the treatment of illnesses having symptoms closely resembling those produced by the substance. [homeo- + G. *pathos*, suffering]

ho•me•o•pla•sia (hō'mē-ō-plā'zē-ă). The formation of new tissue of the same character as that already existing in the part. [homeo- + G. *plasis*, a molding]

ho•me•o•plas•tic (hō'mē-ō-plas'tik). Relating to or characterized by homeoplasia.

ho•me•o•sta•sis (hō'mē-ō-stā'sis, -os'tă-sis). **1.** The state of equilibrium (balance between opposing pressures) in the body with respect to various functions and to the chemical compositions of the fluids and tissues. **2.** The processes through which such bodily equilibrium is maintained. [homeo- + G. *stasis*, a standing]

Bernard-Cannon h., the set of mechanisms responsible for the cybernetic adjustment of physiological and biochemical states in postnatal life.

ho•me•o•stat•ic (hō'mē-ō-stat'ik). Relating to homeostasis.

ho•me•o•ther•a•peu•tic (hō'mē-ō-thār-ă-pyū'tik). **1.** SYN homeopathic (1). **2.** Relating to homeotherapy.

ho•me•o•ther•a•py, ho•me•o•ther•a•peu•tics (hō'mē-ō-thār'ă-pē, -thār-ă-pyū'tiks). Treatment or prevention of a disease using the principles of homeopathy.

homo-. **1.** Combining form meaning the same, alike; opposite of hetero-. SEE ALSO homeo-. **2.** CHEMISTRY Prefix used to indicate insertion of one more carbon atom in a chain. [G. *homos*, the same]

ho•mo•bi•o•tin (hō-mō-bī'ō-tin). A compound resembling biotin except for the substitution of an oxygen atom for the sulfur and the presence of an additional CH_2 group in the side chain; an active biotin antagonist.

ho•mo•blas•tic (hō-mō-blas'tik). Developing from a single type of tissue. [homo- + G. *blastos*, germ]

ho•mo•car•no•sine (hō-mō-kar'nō-sēn). A constituent of the brain formed from L-histidine and γ-aminobutyric acid.

ho•mo•car•no•sin•o•sis (hō-mō-kar'nō-sēn-ō-sis). An inborn error in metabolism in which homocarnosine levels are elevated, particularly in the cerebral spinal fluid.

ho•mo•cit•rul•li•nu•ria (hō-mō-sit'ru-lēn-ūr'ē-ă). An inherited disorder associated with elevated urinary levels of homocitrulline.

ho•mo•cys•te•ine (hō-mō-sis'tē-ēn). A homolog of cysteine, produced by the demethylation of methionine, and an intermediate in the biosynthesis of L-cysteine from L-methionine via L-cystathionine.

ho•mo•cys•tine (hō-mō-sis'tēn). The disulfide resulting from the mild oxidation of homocysteine; an analog of cystine.

ho•mo•cys•ti•ne•mia (hō'mō-sis-ti-nē'mē-ă). Presence of an excess of homocystine in the plasma, as in homocystinuria.

ho•mo•cy•to•tro•pic (hō'mō-sī'tō-trop'ik). Having an affinity for cells of the same or a closely related species. [homo- + G. *kytos*, cell, + *tropē*, a turning toward]

ho•mo•ga•met•ic (hō'mō-gă-met'ik). Producing only one type of gamete with respect to sex chromosomes; in humans and most animals, the female is h. SYN monogametic. [homo- + G. *gametikos*, connubial]

ho•mog•a•my (hō-mog'ă-mē). Similarity of husband and wife in a specific trait. [homo- + G. *gamos*, marriage]

ho•mo•ge•neous (hō-mō-jē'nē-ŭs). Of uniform structure or composition throughout. [homo- + G. *genos*, race]

ho•mo•gen•e•sis (hō-mō-jen'ĕ-sis). Production of

ho

offspring similar to the parents, in contrast to heterogenesis. [homo- + G. *genesis,* production]

ho·mog·e·nous (hō-moj′ĕ-nŭs). Having a structural similarity because of descent from a common ancestor. Commonly confused with homogeneous. [homo- + G. *genos,* family, kind]

ho·mo·gen·tis·ic ac·id (hō′mō-jen-tis′ik). An intermediate in L-phenylalanine and L-tyrosine catabolism; if made alkaline, it oxidizes rapidly in air to a quinone that polymerizes to a melanin-like material; elevated levels are observed in individuals having alcaptonuria. SYN alcapton, alkapton.

ho·mo·graft (hō′mō-graft). SYN allograft *rejection.*

ho·mo·lat·er·al (hō-mō-lat′er-ăl). SYN ipsilateral. [homo- + L. *latus,* side]

ho·mol·o·gous (hō-mol′ō-gŭs). Corresponding or alike in certain critical attributes. **1.** BIOLOGY Denoting organs or parts corresponding in evolutionary origin and similar to some extent in structure, but not necessarily similar in function. **2.** CHEMISTRY Denoting a single chemical series, differing by fixed increments. **3.** GENETICS Denoting chromosomes or chromosome parts identical with respect to their construction and genetic content. **4.** IMMUNOLOGY Denoting serum or tissue derived from members of a single species, or an antibody with respect to the antigen that produced it. [see homologue]

ho·mol·y·sin (hō-mol′i-sin). A sensitizing hemolytic antibody (hemolysin) formed as the result of stimulation by an antigen derived from an animal of the same species. [homo- + hemolysin]

ho·mol·y·sis (hō-mol′i-sis). Lysis of red blood cells by a homolysin and complement.

ho·mo·mor·phic (hō-mō-mōr′fik). Denoting two or more structures of similar size and shape. [homo- + G. *morphē,* shape, appearance]

ho·mon·o·mous (hō-mon′ō-mŭs). Denoting parts, having similar form and structure, arranged in a series, as the fingers or toes. [G. *homonomos,* under the same laws, fr. *homos,* same, + *nomos,* law]

ho·mon·y·mous (hō-mon′i-mŭs). Having the same name or expressed in the same terms, *e.g.,* the corresponding halves (right or left, superior or inferior) of the retinas. [G. *homōnymous,* of the same name, fr. *onyma,* name]

ho·mo·phil (hō′mō-fil). Denoting an antibody that reacts only with the specific antigen which induced its formation. [homo- + G. *philos,* fond]

ho·mo·plas·tic (hō-mō-plas′tik). Similar in form and structure, but not in origin. [homo- + G. *plastos,* formed]

ho·mo·plas·ty (hō′mō-plas′tē). Repair of a defect by a homograft.

ho·mo·pol·y·mer (hō-mō-pol′i-mer). A polymer composed of a series of identical radicals; *e.g.,* polylysine, poly(adenylic acid), polyglucose.

hom·or·gan·ic (hom-ōr-gan′ik). Produced by the same organs, or by homologous organs.

ho·mo·ser·ine (hō-mō-ser′ēn). A hydroxyamino acid differing from serine in the possession of an additional CH_2 group; formed in the conversion of L-methionine to L-cysteine.

ho·mo·sex·u·al (hō-mō-sek′shū-ăl). **1.** Relating to or characteristic of homosexuality. **2.** One whose interests and behavior are characteristic of homosexuality. SEE gay, lesbian.

ho·mo·sex·u·al·i·ty (hō′mō-sek-shū-al′i-tē). Erotic attraction, predisposition, or activity, including sexual congress, between individuals of the same sex, especially past puberty.

ego-dystonic h., a psychological or psychiatric disorder in which an individual experiences persistent distress associated with same-sex preference and a strong need to change the behavior or, at least, to alleviate the distress associated with the h.

overt h., homosexual inclinations consciously experienced and expressed in actual homosexual behavior.

ho·mo·ton·ic (hō-mō-ton′ik). Of uniform tension or tonus.

ho·mo·top·ic (hō-mō-top′ik). Pertaining to or occurring at the same place or part of the body. [homo- + G. *topos,* place]

ho·mo·type (hō′mō-tīp). Any part or organ of the same structure or function as another, especially as one on the opposite side of the body. [homo- + G. *typos,* type]

ho·mo·typ·ic, ho·mo·typ·i·cal (hō-mō-tip′ik, i-kăl). Of the same type or form; corresponding to the other one of two paired organs or parts.

ho·mo·va·nil·lic ac·id (HVA) (hō′mō-vă-nil′ik). A phenol found in human urine; produced through the methylation of homoprotocatechuic acid on the *meta*-OH group.

ho·mo·zy·gos·i·ty, ho·mo·zy·go·sis (hō′mō-zī-gos′i-tē, -zī-gō′sis). The state of being homozygous. [homo- + G. *zygon,* yoke]

ho·mo·zy·gote (hō-mō-zī′gōt). A homozygous individual. [homo- + G. *zygōtos,* yoke]

ho·mo·zy·gous (hō-mō-zī′gŭs). Having identical genes at one or more loci.

ho·mo·zy·gous by de·scent. Possessing two genes at a given locus that are descended from a single source, as may occur in consanguineous mating.

ho·mun·cu·lus (hō-mŭngk′yū-lŭs). The figure of a human sometimes superimposed on pictures of the surface of the brain to represent the motor or sensory regions of the body represented there. [L. dim. of *homo,* man]

hook·worm (huk′werm). Common name for bloodsucking nematodes, chiefly members of the genera *Ancylostoma* (the Old World hookworm), *Necator,* and *Uncinaria,* and including the species *A. caninum* (dog h.) and *N. americanus* (New World h.).

hor·de·o·lum (hōr-dē′ō-lŭm). A suppurative inflammation of a gland of the eyelid. [Mod. L. *hordeolus,* a sty in the eye, dim. of *hordeum,* barley]

h. exter′num, inflammation of the sebaceous gland of an eyelash. SYN sty, stye.

hor·mo·nal (hōr-mōn′ăl). Pertaining to hormones.

hor·mone (hōr′mōn). A chemical substance, formed in one organ or part of the body and carried in the blood to another organ or part; depending on the specificity of their effects, h.'s can alter the functional activity, and sometimes the structure, of just one organ or of various numbers of them. A number of h.'s are formed by ductless glands, but secretin and pancreozymin, formed in the gastrointestinal tract, by definition are also h.'s. For h.'s not listed below, see specific names. [G. *hormōn*, pres. part. of *hormaō*, to rouse or set in motion]

adipokinetic h., SYN adipokinin.

adrenal androgen-stimulating h. (AASH), a putative pituitary h. that may be responsible for increased secretion of adrenal androgens at the time of puberty.

adrenocorticotropic h. (ACTH), the h. of the anterior lobe of the hypophysis which governs the nutrition and growth of the adrenal cortex, stimulates it to functional activity, and also possesses extraadrenal adipokinetic activity. SYN adrenotropin, corticotropin (1).

adrenomedullary h.'s, h.'s produced by the adrenal medulla, particularly the catecholamines epinephrine and norepinephrine.

anterior pituitary-like h., SYN chorionic *gonadotropin*.

antidiuretic h., SYN vasopressin.

chorionic gonadotropic h., chorionic gonadotrophic h., SYN chorionic *gonadotropin*.

chorionic "growth h.-prolactin", SYN human placental *lactogen*.

corpus luteum h., SYN progesterone.

cortical h.'s, steroid h.'s produced by the adrenal cortex.

corticotropin releasing h. (CRH), a factor secreted by the hypothalamus that stimulates the pituitary to release adrenocorticotropic h. SYN corticoliberin, corticotropin releasing factor.

follicle-stimulating h., SYN follitropin.

follicle-stimulating h.-releasing h., SYN folliberin.

gonadotropic h., SYN gonadotropin.

gonadotropin-releasing h. (GnRH), SYN gonadoliberin (1).

growth h. (GH), SYN somatotropin.

growth h.-inhibiting h. (GIH), SYN somatostatin.

growth h.-releasing h. (GHRH, GH-RH), SYN somatoliberin.

human chorionic somatomammotropic h. (HCS), SYN human placental *lactogen*.

interstitial cell-stimulating h., SYN lutropin.

lactogenic h., SYN prolactin.

lipotropic h., lipotropic pituitary h., SYN lipotropin.

lipotropic pituitary h.,

luteinizing h., SYN lutropin.

luteinizing h.-releasing h., SYN luliberin.

luteotropic h., SYN luteotropin.

melanocyte-stimulating h., SYN melanotropin.

melanotropin release-inhibiting h. (MIH), SYN melanostatin.

melanotropin-releasing h. (MRH), SYN melanoliberin.

parathyroid h., a peptide h. formed by the parathyroid glands; it maintains the serum calcium level by promoting intestinal absorption and renal tubular reabsorption of calcium, and release of calcium from bone to extracellular fluid.

pituitary gonadotropic h., SYN anterior pituitary *gonadotropin*.

pituitary growth h., SYN somatotropin.

placental growth h., SYN human placental *lactogen*.

progestational h., SYN progesterone.

prolactin-inhibiting h. (PIH), SYN prolactostatin.

prolactin-releasing h., SYN prolactoliberin.

proparathyroid h., the immediate precursor of parathyroid h.

releasing h., SYN releasing *factors*.

sex h.'s, a general term covering those steroid h.'s that are formed by testicular, ovarian, and adrenocortical tissues, and that are androgens or estrogens.

somatotropic h., SYN somatotropin.

somatotropin release-inhibiting h. (SIH), SYN somatostatin.

somatotropin-releasing h. (SRH), SYN somatoliberin.

steroid h.'s, those h.'s possessing the steroid ring system; *e.g.*, androgens, estrogens, adrenocortical h.'s.

thyroid-stimulating h., SYN thyrotropin.

thyrotropin-releasing h., SYN thyroliberin.

hor•mo•no•gen•e•sis (hōr′mō-nō-jen′ĕ-sis). The formation of hormones. SYN hormonopoiesis.

hor•mo•no•gen•ic (hōr′mō-nō-jen′ik). Pertaining to the formation of a hormone. SYN hormonopoietic.

hor•mo•no•poi•e•sis (hōr′mō-nō-poy-ē′sis). SYN hormonogenesis. [hormone + G. *poiēsis*, production]

hor•mo•no•poi•et•ic (hōr′mō-nō-poy-et′ik). SYN hormonogenic.

horn (hōrn). Any structure resembling a horn in shape. SYN cornu (1). [A.S.]

Ammon's h., one of the two interlocking gyri composing the hippocampus, the other being the dentate gyrus. SYN cornu ammonis. [G. *Ammōn*, the Egyptian deity *Amūn*]

anterior h., (1) the anterior or frontal division of the lateral ventricle of the brain, extending forward from Monro's interventricular foramen; SEE lateral *ventricle*. (2) the anterior or ventral gray column of the spinal cord as appearing in cross section. SEE ALSO gray *columns*, under *column*. SYN cornu anterius [NA], ventral h.

cutaneous h., a protruding keratotic growth of the skin; the base may show changes of actinic keratosis or carcinoma.

posterior h., the posterior or occipital division of the lateral ventricle of the brain, extending backward into the occipital lobe; the posterior gray column of the spinal cord as appearing in cross section. SYN cornu posterius.

pulp h., a prolongation of the pulp extending toward the cusp of a tooth.

ventral h., SYN anterior h.

horny (hōrn′ē). Of the nature or structure of horn. SYN corneous, keratic, keratinous (2), keratoid (1), keroid.

ho•rop•ter (hō-rop′ter). The sum of the points in space, the images of which for a given fixation point fall on corresponding retinal points. [G.

horos, limit, + *optēr,* spy, scout, fr. *oraō,* fut. *opsomai,* to see]

hose. Thin, form-fitting leg covering; in medicine, used in the treatment of circulatory problems.

TED h., elastic stockings that compress the superficial veins in the lower extremities; used in postoperative patients and others immobilized by illness, to prevent thrombophlebitis by shunting blood through the deep veins of the calves and thighs. TED is an abbreviation for thromboembolic disease.

hos•pice (hos′pis). An institution that provides a centralized program of palliative and supportive services to dying persons and their families, in the form of physical, psychological, social, and spiritual care; such services are provided by an interdisciplinary team of professionals and volunteers who are available at home and in specialized inpatient settings. [L. *hospitium,* hospitality, lodging, fr. *hospes,* guest]

hos•pi•tal (hos′pi-tăl). An institution for the treatment, care, and cure of the sick and wounded, for the study of disease, and for the training of physicians, nurses, and allied health personnel. [L. *hospitalis,* for a guest, fr. *hospes* (*hospit-*), a host, a guest]

acute care h., a h. where inpatients have an average length of stay of 30 days or less.

closed h., a h. that restricts membership on its attending or consulting staff, and thereby limits who may admit and treat patients.

open h., a h. where all physicians, not members of the regular staff, are permitted to send their patients and control their treatment.

private h., (1) a h. similar to a group h. except that it is controlled by a single practitioner or by the practitioner and the associates in his or her office; **(2)** a h. operated for profit.

teaching h., a h. that also functions as a formal center of learning for the training of physicians, nurses, and allied health personnel.

hos•pi•tal•i•za•tion (hos′pi-tăl-i-zā′shŭn). Confinement in a hospital as a patient for diagnostic study and treatment.

host. The organism in or on which a parasite lives, deriving its body substance or energy from the h. [L. *hospes,* a host]

dead-end h., a h. from which infectious agents are not transmitted to other susceptible h.'s.

definitive h., one in which a parasite reaches the adult or sexually mature stage.

intermediate h., intermediary h., (1) one in which larval or developmental stages occur; **(2)** a host through which a microorganism can pass or which contains an asexual stage of a parasite.

reservoir h., the h. of an infection in which the infectious agent multiplies and/or develops, and upon which the agent is dependent for survival in nature.

house of•fi•cer. An intern or resident employed by a hospital to provide service to patients while receiving training in a medical specialty.

HPLC high-pressure liquid *chromatography;* high-performance liquid *chromatography.*

HPV human papilloma *virus.*

HRCT high-resolution computed *tomography.*

HRR high risk register.

HSV herpes simplex *virus.*

5-HT 5-hydroxytryptamine.

Ht total *hyperopia.*

HTLV human T-cell lymphoma/leukemia *virus.*

HTLV-I T-cell lymphotrophic virus type I; human lymphotropic virus, type 1.

HTLV-II T-cell lymphotrophic virus type II; human lymphotropic virus, type 2.

HTLV-III human T-cell lymphotropic virus type III. SEE human immunodeficiency *virus.*

hum (hŭm). A low continuous murmur. [echoic]

venous h., brief or continuous noise originating from the neck veins that may be confused with cardiac murmurs, particularly with the continuous murmur of patent ductus arteriosus.

Human Genome Project. A comprehensive effort by molecular biologists worldwide to map the human genome, which consists of about 100,000 genes, or 3 billion DNA base pairs. The wholesale sequencing of the genome would not be possible without the automated method of gene sequencing, invented by Leroy Hood.

hu•mer•al (hyū′mer-ăl). Relating to the humerus.

hu•mer•o•ra•di•al (hyū′mer-ō-rā′dē-ăl). Relating to both humerus and radius; denoting especially the ratio of length of one to the other.

hu•mer•o•scap•u•lar (hyū′mer-ō-skap′yū-lăr). Relating to both humerus and scapula.

hu•mer•o•ul•nar (hyū′mer-ō-ŭl′năr). Relating to both humerus and ulna; denoting especially the ratio of length of one to the other.

hu•mer•us, gen. and pl. **hu•meri** (hyū′mer-ŭs, -ī) [NA]. The bone of the arm, articulating with the scapula above and the radius and ulna below. [L. shoulder]

humidifier. A device to increase the moisture of air.

bubble-through humidifier, a device that humidifies therapeutic gas (e.g., oxygen) by bubbling the gas through water.

hu•mid•i•ty (hyū-mid′i-tē). Moisture or dampness, as of the air. [L. *humiditas,* dampness]

absolute h., the mass of water vapor actually present per unit volume of gas or air.

relative h., the actual amount of water vapor present in the air or in a gas, divided by the amount necessary for saturation at the same temperature and pressure; expressed as a percentage.

hu•mor, gen. **hu•mor•is** (hyū′mor, hyū-mōr′is). **1** [NA]. Any clear fluid or semifluid hyaline anatomical substance. **2.** One of the elemental body fluids that were the basis of the physiologic and pathologic teachings of the hippocratic school: blood, yellow bile, black bile, and phlegm. [L. correctly, *umor,* liquid]

aqueous h., the watery fluid that fills the anterior and posterior chambers of the eye. It is secreted by the ciliary processes within the posterior chambers and passes through the the pupil into the anterior chamber where it filters through the trabecular meshwork and is reabsorbed into the venous system at the iridocorneal angle by way of the sinus venosus of the sclera;

ocular h., one of the two humors of the eye: aqueous and vitreous.

vitreous h., the fluid component of the vitreous body, with which it is often erroneously equated.

hu·mor·al (hyū′mōr-ăl). Relating to a humor in any sense.

hump (hŭmp). A rounded protuberance or bulge.

dowager's h., postmenopausal cervical kyphosis of older women.

hump·back (hŭmp′bak). Nonmedical term for kyphosis or gibbus.

hun·ger (hŭn′ger). **1.** A desire or need for food. **2.** Any appetite, strong desire, or craving. [A.S.]

HVA homovanillic acid.

HVL half-value *layer*.

hyal-. SEE hyalo-.

hy·a·lin (hī′ă-lin). A clear, eosinophilic, homogeneous substance occurring in degeneration; *e.g.,* in arteriolar walls in arteriolar sclerosis and in glomerular tufts in diabetic glomerulosclerosis. [G. *hyalos,* glass]

hy·a·line (hī′ă-lin, -lēn). Transparent or colorless. SYN hyaloid. [G. *hyalos,* glass]

hy·a·lin·i·za·tion (hī′ă-lin-i-zā′shŭn). The formation of hyalin.

hy·a·li·no·sis (hī′ă-li-li-nō′sis). SYN hyaline *degeneration.*

hy·a·li·nu·ria (hī′ă-li-nū′rē-ă). The excretion of hyalin or casts of hyaline material in the urine. [hyalin + G. *ouron,* urine]

hy·a·li·tis (hī′ă-lī′tis). SYN vitreitis.

suppurative h., purulent vitreous humor due to exudation from adjacent structures, as in panophthalmitis.

hyalo-, hyal-. Glassy, hyalin; vitreous. Cf. vitreo-. [G. *hyalos,* glass]

hy·al·o·gens (hī-al′ō-jenz). Substances similar to mucoids that are found in many animal structures (*e.g.,* cartilage, vitreous humor, hydatid cysts) and yield sugars on hydrolysis.

hy·a·lo·hy·pho·my·co·sis (hī′ă-lō-hī′fō-mī-kō′sis). An infection caused by a fungus with hyaline (colorless) mycelia in tissue, usually with a decrease in body resistance due to surgery, indwelling catheters, steroid therapy, or immunosuppressive drugs or cytotoxins. [hyalo- + G. *hyphē,* web, + *mykēs,* fungus, + *-osis,* condition]

hy·a·loid (hī′ă-loyd). SYN hyaline. [hyalo- + G. *eidos,* resemblance]

hy·al·o·mere (hī′ă-lō-mēr). The clear periphery of a blood platelet. [hyalo- + G. *meros,* part]

hy·a·lo·pha·gia, hy·a·loph·a·gy (hī′ă-lō-fā′jē-ă, hī-ă-lof′ă-jē). The eating or chewing of glass. [hyalo- + G. *phagō,* to eat]

hy·al·o·plasm, hy·a·lo·plas·ma (hī′ă-lō-plazm, -plaz′mă). The protoplasmic fluid substance of a cell. [hyalo- + G. *plasma,* thing formed]

hy·a·lo·sis (hī-ă-lō′sis). Degenerative changes in the vitreous body. [hyalo- + G. *-osis,* condition]

asteroid h., numerous small spherical bodies ("snowball" opacities) in the corpus vitreum, visible ophthalmoscopically; an age change, usually unilateral, and not affecting vision.

punctate h., a condition marked by minute opacities in the vitreous.

hy·al·o·some (hī-al′ō-sōm). An oval or round structure within a cell nucleus that stains faintly but otherwise resembles a nucleolus. [hyalo- + G. *sōma,* body]

hy·al·u·ro·nate (hī-ă-lū′ron-āt). A salt or ester of hyaluronic acid.

hy·al·u·ron·ic ac·id (hī′ă-lū-ron′ik). A mucopolysaccharide forming a gelatinous material in the tissue spaces and acting as a lubricant and shock absorbant; it is hydrolyzed by hyaluronidase.

hy·brid (hī′brid). **1.** An individual (plant or animal) whose parents are different varieties of the same species or belong to different but closely allied species. **2.** Fused tissue culture cells, as in a hybridoma. [L. *hybrida,* offspring of a tame sow and a wild boar, fr. G. *hybris,* violation, wantonness]

DNA-RNA h., double-stranded polynucleic acids in which one strand is DNA and the other strand is the complementary RNA; formed during transcription and during multiplication of oncogenic RNA viruses.

hy·brid·i·za·tion (hī′brid-i-zā′shŭn). **1.** The process of breeding a hybrid. **2.** Crossing over between related but nonallelic genes. **3.** The specific reassociation of complementary strands of polynucleic acids; *e.g.,* the formation of a DNA-RNA hybrid.

fluorescence in situ h. (FISH), molecular diagnostic laboratory method in which whole chromosomes are hybridized to complementary nucleotide probes and examined microscopically

in situ h., a technique for annealing nucleic acid probes to cellular DNA for detection by autoradiography. In situ h. constitutes a key step in DNA fingerprinting.

hy·brid·o·ma (hī-brid-ō′mă). A tumor of hybrid cells used in the production *in vitro* of specific monoclonal antibodies; produced by fusion of an established tissue culture line of lymphocyte tumor cells and specific antibody-producing cells. [G. *hybris,* violation, wantonness, + *-ōma,* tumor]

hy·dan·to·in (hī-dan′tō-in). A crystalline heterocyclic compound derived from urea or from allantoin; the NH–CH₂–CO group is prototypical of α-amino acids.

hy·da·tid (hī′da-tid). **1.** SYN hydatid *cyst.* **2.** A vesicular structure resembling an *Echinococcus* cyst. [G. *hydatis,* a drop of water, a hyatid]

hy·da·tid·i·form (hī-da-tid′i-form). Having the form or appearance of a hydatid.

hy·da·tid·o·cele (hī-da-tid′ō-sēl). A cystic mass composed of one or more hydatids formed in the scrotum. [hydatid + G. *kēlē,* tumor]

hy·da·ti·do·ma (hī′da-ti-dō′mă). A benign neoplasm in which there is prominent formation of hydatids. [hydatid + G. *-oma,* tumor]

hy·da·tid·o·sis (hī′da-ti-dō′sis). The morbid state caused by the presence of hydatid cysts.

hy·da·ti·dos·to·my (hī′da-ti-dos′tō-mē). Surgical evacuation of a hydatid cyst. [hydatid + G. *stoma,* mouth]

hydr-. SEE hydro-.

hy·dram·ni·on, hy·dram·ni·os (hī-dram′nē-on, -nē-os). Presence of an excessive amount of amniotic fluid. [G. *hydōr,* water, + amnion]

hy·dran·en·ceph·a·ly (hī′dran-en-sef′ă-lē). Absence of cerebral hemispheres, which have been replaced by fluid-filled sacs, lined by leptomenin-

hy

ges. The skull and its brain cavities are normal. [hydr- + G. *an-* priv. + *enkephalos,* brain]

hy·drar·gyr·ia, hy·drar·gy·rism (hī-drar-jir'ē-ă, hī-drar'jir-izm). SYN mercury *poisoning.* [L. *hydrargyrum,* mercury]

hy·drar·thro·di·al (hī-drar-thrō'dē-ăl). Relating to hydrarthrosis.

hy·drar·thro·sis (hī-drar-thrō'sis). Effusion of a serous fluid into a joint cavity. [hydr- + G. *arthron,* joint]

hy·drase (hī'drās). Former name for hydratase.

hy·dra·tase (hī'drǎ-tās). Certain hydro-lyases (EC class 4.2.1) catalyzing hydration-dehydration.

hy·drate (hī'drāt). An aqueous solvate (in older terminology, a hydroxide); a compound crystallizing with one or more molecules of water.

hy·dra·tion (hī-drā'shŭn). **1.** Chemically, the addition of water; differentiated from hydrolysis, where the union with water is accompanied by a splitting of the original molecule and the water molecule. **2.** Clinically, the taking in of water; used commonly in the sense of reduced h. or dehydration.

hy·dre·mia (hī-drē'mē-ă). A condition in which the blood volume is increased as a result of an increase in the water content of plasma. [hydr- + G. *haima,* blood]

hy·dren·ceph·a·lo·cele (hī-dren-sef'ă-lō-sēl). Protrusion, through a cleft in the skull, of brain substance expanded into a sac containing fluid. SYN hydrocephalocele, hydroencephalocele. [hydr- + G. *enkephalos,* brain, + *kēlē,* tumor]

hy·dren·ceph·a·lo·me·nin·go·cele (hī'dren-sef'ă-lō-me-ning'gō-sēl). Protrusion, through a defect in the skull, of a sac containing meninges, brain substance, and cerebrospinal fluid.

hy·dric (hī'drik). Relating to hydrogen in chemical combination.

hy·dride (hī'drīd). A negatively charged hydrogen (*i.e.,* H:⁻) or a compound of hydrogen in which it assumes a formal negative charge.

△**hydro-, hydr-.** **1.** Water, watery. **2.** Containing or combined with hydrogen. **3.** A hydatid. [G. *hydōr,* water]

hy·droa (hī-drō'ă). Any bullous eruption. [hydro + G. *ōon,* egg]

h. vaccinifor'me, a recurrent eruption of erythema evolving to umbilicated bullae, occurring on exposure to the sun and affecting chiefly male children with resolution before adult life.

hy·dro·cal·y·co·sis (hī'drō-kal-i-kō'sis). A usually symptomless anomaly of the renal calix that is dilated from obstruction of the infundibulum; usually discovered incidentally at pyelography or autopsy; may become infected. [hydro- + G. *kalyx,* cup of a flower]

hy·dro·car·bon (hī-drō-kar'bŏn). A compound containing only hydrogen and carbon.

hy·dro·cele (hī'drō-sēl). A collection of serous fluid in a sacculated cavity; specifically, such a collection in the tunica vaginalis testis, or in a separate pocket along the spermatic cord. [hydro- + G. *kēlē,* hernia]

hy·dro·ce·lec·to·my (hī'drō-sē-lek'tō-mē). Excision of a hydrocele. [hydrocele + G. *ektomē,* excision]

hy·dro·ce·phal·ic (hī'drō-se-fal'ik). Relating to or suffering from hydrocephalus.

hy·dro·ceph·a·lo·cele (hī-drō-sef'ă-lō-sēl). SYN hydrencephalocele.

hy·dro·ceph·a·loid (hī-drō-sef'ă-loyd). **1.** Resembling hydrocephalus. **2.** A condition in infants suffering from diarrhea or other debilitating disease, in which there is dehydration and general symptoms resembling those of hydrocephalus without, however, any abnormal accumulation of cerebrospinal fluid.

hy·dro·ceph·a·lus (hī-drō-sef'ă-lŭs). A condition marked by an excessive accumulation of fluid resulting in dilation of the cerebral ventricles and raised intracranial pressure; may also result in enlargement of the cranium and atrophy of the brain. SYN hydrocephaly. [hydro- + G. *kephalē,* head]

communicating h., type of h. in which there is an abnormality in cerebrospinal fluid absorption; there is no obstruction to cerebrospinal fluid flow in the ventricular system or where the cerebrospinal fluid passes into the spinal canal.

double compartment h., independent supra- and infra-tentorial h. usually due to a veil occlusion of the aqueduct of Sylvius.

h. ex vac'uo, h. due to loss or atrophy of brain tissue; less commonly associated with raised intracranial pressure.

noncommunicating h., SYN obstructive h.

normal pressure h., a type of h. developing usually in older people, due to failure of cerebrospinal fluid to be absorbed by the pacchionian granulations, and characterized clinically by progressive dementia, unsteady gait, urinary incontinence, and usually, a normal spinal fluid pressure.

obstructive h., h. secondary to a block in cerebrospinal fluid flow in the ventricular system or between the ventricular system and spinal canal. SYN noncommunicating h.

hy·dro·ceph·a·ly (hī-drō-sef'ă-lē). SYN hydrocephalus.

hy·dro·chlo·ric ac·id (hī-drō-klōr'ik). HCl; the acid of gastric juice. The gas and the concentrated solution are strong irritants.

hy·dro·chlo·ride (hī-drō-klōr'īd). A compound formed by the addition of a hydrochloric acid molecule to an amine or related substance.

hy·dro·cho·le·re·sis (hī'drō-kō-ler-ē'sis, -kol-er-). Increased output of a watery bile of low specific gravity, viscosity, and solid content. [hydro- + G. *cholē,* bile, + *hairesis,* a taking]

hy·dro·cho·le·ret·ic (hī'drō-kō-ler-et'ik). Pertaining to hydrocholeresis.

hy·dro·col·loid (hī-drō-kol'oyd). A gelatinous colloid in unstable equilibrium with its contained water, useful in dentistry for impressions because of its dimensional stability under controlled conditions.

hy·dro·col·po·cele, hy·dro·col·pos (hī-drō-kol'pō-sēl, -kol'pos). Accumulation of mucus or other nonsanguineous fluid in the vagina. [hydro- + G. *kolpos,* bosom (vagina)]

hy·dro·cor·ti·sone (hī-drō-kōr'ti-sōn). A steroid hormone secreted by the adrenal cortex and the most potent of the naturally occurring glucocorticoids in humans. SYN cortisol.

hy·dro·cyst (hī′drō-sist). A cyst with clear, watery contents. [hydro- + G. *kystis,* bladder]

hy·dro·en·ceph·a·lo·cele (hī′drō-en-sef′ă-lō-sēl). SYN hydrencephalocele.

hy·dro·gel (hī′drō-jel). A colloid in which the particles are in the external or dispersion phase and water in the internal or dispersed phase.

hy·dro·gen (H) (hī′drō-jen). **1.** A gaseous element, atomic no. 1, atomic wt. 1.00794. **2.** The molecular form of the element, H_2. [hydro- + G. -*gen,* producing]

   h. chloride, HCl; a very soluble gas which, in solution, forms hydrochloric acid.

hy·dro·gen-1 (^{1}H). The common h.-1 isotope, making up 99.985% of the h.-1 atoms occurring in nature.

hy·dro·gen-2 (^{2}H). The isotope of h.-2 of atomic weight 2; the less common stable isotope of h.-2 making up 0.015% of the h.-2 atoms occurring in nature. SYN deuterium.

hy·dro·gen-3. A hydrogen isotope of atomic weight 3; weakly radioactive, emitting beta particles to become the stable helium-3; half-life, 12.32 years. SYN tritium.

hy·dro·gen·ase (hī′drō-je-nās, hī-droj′ĕ-nās). Any enzyme that removes a hydride ion (or H:⁻) from NADH (or NADPH) or adds hydrogen to ferricytochrome or to ferredoxin.

hy·dro·gen·a·tion (hī′drō-jĕ-nā′shŭn, hī-droj′ĕ-nā-shŭn). Addition of hydrogen to a compound, especially to an unsaturated fat or fatty acid; thus, soft fats or oils are solidified or "hardened."

hy·dro·gen ex·po·nent. The logarithm of the hydrogen ion concentration in blood or other fluid; its negative is the pH of that fluid.

hy·dro·ki·net·ic (hī′drō-ki-net′ik). Pertaining to the motion of fluids and the forces giving rise to such motion.

hy·dro·las·es (hī′drō-lās-ez). Enzymes (EC class 3) cleaving substrates with addition of H_2O at the point of cleavage.

hy·dro·ly·as·es (hī-drō-lī′ās-ĕz). A class of lyases (EC class 4.2.1) comprising enzymes removing H and OH as water, leading to formation of new double bonds within the affected molecule.

hy·drol·y·sate (hī-drol′i-sāt). A solution containing the products of hydrolysis.

hy·drol·y·sis (hī-drol′i-sis). A chemical process whereby a compound is cleaved into two or more simpler compounds with the uptake of the H and OH parts of a water molecule on either side of the chemical bond cleaved; h. is effected by the action of acids, alkalies, or enzymes. Cf. hydration. [hydro- + G. *lysis,* dissolution]

hy·dro·lyt·ic (hī-drō-lit′ik). Referring to or causing hydrolysis.

hy·dro·ma (hī-drō′mă). SYN hygroma.

hy·dro·me·nin·go·cele (hī′drō-men-ing′gō-sēl). Protrusion of the meninges of brain or spinal cord through a defect in the bony wall, the sac so formed containing cerebrospinal fluid. [hydro- + G. *mēninx,* membrane, + *kēlē,* hernia]

hy·drom·e·ter (hī-drom′e-ter). An instrument for determining the specific gravity of a liquid. [hydro- + G. *mēron,* measure]

hy·dro·me·tra (hī-drō-mē′tră). Accumulation of thin mucus or other watery fluid in the cavity of the uterus. [hydro- + G. *mētra,* uterus]

hy·dro·met·ric (hī-drō-met′rik). Relating to hydrometry or the hydrometer.

hy·dro·me·tro·col·pos (hī′drō-mē-trō-kol′pos). Distention of uterus and vagina by fluid other than blood or pus. [hydro- + G. *mētra,* uterus, + *kolpos,* bosom (vagina)]

hy·drom·e·try (hī-drom′ĕ-trē). Determination of the specific gravity of a fluid by means of a hydrometer.

hy·dro·mi·cro·ceph·a·ly (hī′drō-mī-krō-sef′ă-lē). Microcephaly associated with an increased amount of cerebrospinal fluid.

hy·dro·my·e·lia (hī-drō-mī-ē′lē-ă). An increase of fluid in the dilated central canal of the spinal cord, or in congenital cavities elsewhere in the cord substance. [hydro- + G. *myelos,* marrow]

hy·dro·my·e·lo·cele (hī-drō-mī′ĕ-lō-sēl). Protrusion of a portion of cord, thinned out into a sac distended with cerebrospinal fluid, through a spina bifida. [hydro- + G. *myelos,* marrow, + *kēlē,* tumor, hernia]

hy·dro·my·o·ma (hī′drō-mī-ō′mă). A leiomyoma that contains cystlike foci of proteinaceous fluid; h.'s occur more frequently in leiomyomas of the uterus, as a result of degenerative changes. [hydro- + G. *mys,* muscle, + -*oma,* tumor]

hy·dro·ne·phro·sis (hī′drō-ne-frō′sis). Dilation of the pelvis and calices of one or both kidneys resulting from obstruction to the flow of urine. SYN uronephrosis. [hydro- + G. *nephros,* kidney, + -*osis,* condition]

hy·dro·ne·phrot·ic (hī′drō-ne-frot′ik). Relating to hydronephrosis.

hy·dro·per·i·car·di·tis (hī′drō-pār-i-kar-dī′tis). Pericarditis with a large serous effusion.

hy·dro·per·i·car·di·um (hī′drō-pār-i-kar′dē-ŭm). A noninflammatory accumulation of fluid in the pericardial sac.

hy·dro·per·i·to·ne·um, hy·dro·per·i·to·nia (hī′drō-pār-i-tō-nē′ŭm, -tō′nē-ă). SYN ascites. [hydro- + peritoneum]

hy·dro·phil·ia (hī-drō-fil′ē-ă). A tendency of the blood and tissues to absorb fluid. [hydro- + G. *philos,* fond]

hy·dro·phil·ic (hī-drō-fil′ik). Denoting the property of attracting or associating with water molecules, possessed by polar radicals or ions, as opposed to hydrophobic (2).

hy·dro·pho·bia (hī-drō-fō′bē-ă). SYN rabies. [hydro- + G. *phobos,* fear]

hy·dro·pho·bic (hī-drō-fōb′ik). **1.** Relating to or suffering from hydrophobia. **2.** Lacking an affinity for water molecules, as opposed to hydrophilic.

hy·dro·pneu·ma·to·sis (hī-drō-nū-mă-tō′sis). Combined emphysema and edema; the presence of liquid and gas in tissues. [hydro- + G. *pneuma,* breath, spirit]

hy·dro·pneu·mo·go·ny (hī′drō-nū-mō′gō-nē). Injection of air into a joint to determine the amount of effusion. [hydro- + G. *pneuma,* air, + *gony,* knee]

hy·dro·pneu·mo·per·i·car·di·um (hī-drō-nū′mō-per-i-kar′dē-ŭm). The presence of a serous

hy

effusion and of gas in the pericardial sac. SYN pneumohydropericardium. [hydro- + G. *pneuma,* air, + pericardium]

hy·dro·pneu·mo·per·i·to·ne·um (hī-drō-nū′mō-pār-i-tō-nē′ŭm). The presence of gas and serous fluid in the peritoneal cavity. SYN pneumohydroperitoneum. [hydro- + G. *pneuma,* air, + peritoneum]

hy·dro·pneu·mo·tho·rax (hī′drō-nū-mō-thōr′aks). The presence of both gas and fluids in the pleural cavity. SYN pneumohydrothorax. [hydro- + G. *pneuma,* air, + thorax]

hy·drops (hī′drops). An excessive accumulation of clear, watery fluid in any of the tissues or cavities of the body; synonymous, according to its character and location, with ascites, anasarca, edema, etc. [G. *hydrōps*]

   fetal h., h. fetal′is, abnormal accumulation of serous fluid in the fetal tissues, as in erythroblastosis fetalis.

hy·dro·py·o·ne·phro·sis (hī′drō-pī′ō-ne-frō′sis). Presence of purulent urine in the pelvis and calices of the kidney following obstruction of the ureter. [hydro- + G. *pyon,* pus, + nephrosis]

hy·dror·rhea (hī-drō-rē′ă). A profuse discharge of watery fluid from any part of the body. [hydro- + G. *rhoia,* flow]

hy·dro·sal·pinx (hī-drō-sal′pinks). Accumulation of serous fluid in the uterine tube, often an end result of pyosalpinx. [hydro- + G. *salpinx,* trumpet]

hy·dro·sar·co·cele (hī-drō-sar′kō-sēl). A chronic swelling of the testis complicated with hydrocele. [hydro- + G. *sarx,* flesh, + *kēlē,* tumor]

hy·dro·stat·ic (hī-drō-stat′ik). Relating to the pressure of fluids or to their properties when in equilibrium.

hydrostatic weighing. SYN underwater weighing.

hy·dro·sy·rin·go·my·e·lia (hī′drō-sǐ-rin′gō-mī-ē′lē-ă). SYN syringomyelia. [hydro- + G. *hydōr,* water, + *syrinx,* a tube, + *myelos,* marrow]

hy·dro·tax·is (hī-drō-tak′sis). The movement of cells or organisms in relation to water. [hydro- + G. *taxis,* arrangement]

hy·dro·thi·o·ne·mia (hī′drō-thī-ō-nē′mē-ă). The presence of hydrogen sulfide in the circulating blood. [hydro- + G. *theion,* sulfur, + *haima,* blood]

hy·dro·thi·o·nu·ria (hī′drō-thī-ō-nū′rē-ă). The excretion of hydrogen sulfide in the urine. [hydro- + G. *theion,* sulfur, + *ouron,* urine]

hy·dro·tho·rax (hī-drō-thōr′aks). Presence of fluid in one or both pleural cavities, usually resulting from cardiac failure.

hy·drot·ro·pism (hī-drot′rō-pizm, hī-drō-trō′pizm). The property in growing organisms of turning toward a moist surface (**positive h.**) or away from a moist surface (**negative h.**). [hydro- + G. *tropos,* a turning]

hy·dro·tu·ba·tion (hī′drō-tū-bā′shŭn). Injection of a liquid medication or saline solution through the cervix into the uterine cavity and uterine tubes for dilation and/or treatment of the tubes.

hy·dro·u·re·ter (hī′drō-yū-rē′ter, -yūr′ē-ter). Distention of the ureter with urine, due to blockage from any cause.

hy·dro·va·ri·um (hī-drō-vā′rē-ŭm). A collection of fluid in the ovary.

hy·drox·ide (hī-drok′sīd). A compound containing a potentially ionizable hydroxyl group; particularly a compound that liberates OH⁻ upon dissolving in water.

△**hydroxy-.** Prefix indicating addition or substitution of the –OH group to or in the compound whose name follows. SEE ALSO oxa-, oxo-, oxy-.

hy·drox·y·ap·a·tite (hī-drok′sē-ap-ă-tīt). $Ca_{10}(PO_4)_6(OH)_2$; a natural mineral structure resembling the crystal lattice of bones and teeth; used in chromatography of nucleic acids; also found in pathologic calcifications.

hy·drox·yl (hī-drok′sil). The radical, –OH.

hy·drox·y·las·es (hī-drok′si-lā-sez). Enzymes catalyzing formation of hydroxyl groups by addition of an oxygen atom, hence oxidizing the substrate.

hy·drox·y·phen·yl·u·ria (hī-drok′sē-fen-il-ū′rē-ă). Urinary excretion of tyrosine and phenylalanine, as a result of ascorbic acid deficiency; occurs notably in those premature infants who lack this vitamin.

21-hy·drox·y·pro·ges·ter·one. SYN deoxycorticosterone.

5-hy·drox·y·tryp·ta·mine (5-HT) (hī-drok-sē-trip′tă-mēn). SYN serotonin.

hy·giene (hī′jēn). **1.** The science of health and its maintenance. **2.** Cleanliness that promotes health and well being, especially of a personal nature. [G. *hygieinos,* healthful, fr. *hygiēs,* healthy]

   bronchial h., those activities contributing to the removal of bronchial secretions and the maintenance of clear airways.

   industrial h., practices adopted by an industrial concern to minimize occupation-related disease and/or injury.

   mental h., the science and practice of maintaining and restoring mental health; a branch of early twentieth century psychiatry that has become an interdisciplinary field including subspecialities in psychology, nursing, social work, law, and other professions.

   oral h., the cleaning of the mouth by means of brushing, flossing, irrigating, massaging, or the use of other devices.

hy·gien·ic (hī-jen′ik, hī-jē-en′ik). Healthful; relating to hygiene; tending to maintain health.

hy·gien·ist (hī-jē′nist, hī′jē-en-ist). One who is skilled in the science of health and its maintenance.

   dental h., a licensed, professional auxiliary in dentistry who is both an oral health educator and clinician, and who uses preventive, therapeutic, and educational methods for the control of oral diseases.

△**hygr-.** SEE hygro-.

△**hygro-, hygr-.** Moisture, humidity; opposite of xero-. [G. *hygros,* moist]

hy·gro·ma (hī-grō′mă). A cystic swelling containing a serous fluid. SYN hydroma. [hygro- + G. *-oma,* tumor]

hy·grom·e·try (hī-grom′ĕ-trē). SYN psychrometry.

hy·gro·scop·ic (hī-grō-skop′ik). Denoting a substance capable of readily absorbing and retaining moisture; *e.g.*, NaOH, CaCl$_2$.

hy·men (hī'men) [NA]. A thin membranous fold, highly variable in appearance, which partly occludes the ostium of the vagina prior to its rupture, which may occur for a variety of reasons. It is frequently absent, even in virgins, although remnants are commonly present as hymenal tags (caruncula). [G. *hymēn*, membrane]

hy·men·al (hī'men-ăl). Relating to the hymen.

hy·me·nec·to·my (hī-me-nek'tō-mē). Excision of the hymen. [G. *hymēn*, membrane, + *ektomē*, excision]

hy·me·ni·tis (hī-me-nī'tis). Inflammation of the hymen.

hy·me·nol·o·gy (hī-mĕ-nol'ō-jē). The branch of anatomy and physiology concerned with the membranes of the body. [G. *hymēn*, membrane, + *logos*, study]

hy·men·ot·o·my (hī-me-not'ō-mē). Surgical division of a hymen. [G. *hymēn*, membrane, + *tomē*, incision]

hy·o·ep·i·glot·tic (hī'ō-ep-i-glot'ik). Relating to the hyoid bone and the epiglottis; denoting the elastic h. ligament connecting the two structures.

hy·o·glos·sal (hī'ō-glos'ăl). Relating to the hyoid bone and the tongue. SYN glossohyal.

hy·oid (hī'oyd). U-shaped or V-shaped; denoting the os hyoideum and the apparatus hyoideus. [G. *hyoeidēs*, shaped like the letter upsilon, υ]

hyp-. Variation of the prefix hypo-, often used before a vowel. Cf. sub-.

hyp·a·cu·sis (hī'pă-kū'sis, hip'ă-). Hearing impairment of a conductive or neurosensory nature. SYN hypoacusis. [hypo- + G. *akousis*, hearing]

hyp·al·bu·mi·ne·mia (hī'pal-byū-mi-nē'mē-ă, hip'al-). SYN hypoalbuminemia. [G. *hypo*, under, + albuminemia]

hyp·al·ge·sia (hī'pal-jē'zē-ă, hīp'al-). Decreased sensibility to pain. SYN hypoalgesia. [G. *hypo*, under, + *algēsis*, sense of pain]

hyp·al·ge·sic, hyp·al·get·ic (hī'pal-jē'sik, hip'al-; -jet'ik). Relating to hypalgesia; having diminished sensitiveness to pain.

hyper-. Excessive, above normal; opposite of hypo-. [G. *hyper*, above, over]

hy·per·a·cid·i·ty (hī'per-a-sid'i-tē). An abnormally high degree of acidity, as of the gastric juice.

hy·per·ac·tiv·i·ty (hī'per-ak-tiv'i-tē). 1. SYN superactivity. 2. General restlessness or excessive movement such as that characterizing children with attention deficit disorder or hyperkinesis.

hy·per·a·cu·sis, hy·per·a·cu·sia (hī'per-ă-kū'sis, -kū'sē-ă). Abnormal acuteness of hearing due to increased irritability of the auditory apparatus. [hyper- + G. *akousis*, a hearing]

hy·per·ad·e·no·sis (hī'per-ad-ĕ-nō'sis). Glandular enlargement, especially of the lymphatic glands. [hyper- + G. *adēn*, gland, + *-ōsis*, condition]

hy·per·ad·i·po·sis, hy·per·ad·i·pos·i·ty (hī'per-ad-i-pō'sis, -pos'i-tē). An extreme degree of adiposis or fatness.

hy·per·al·do·ste·ron·ism (hī'per-al-dos'ter-on-izm). SYN aldosteronism.

hy·per·al·ge·sia (hī-per-al-jē'zē-ă). Extreme sensitivity to painful stimuli. [hyper- + G. *algos*, pain]

hy·per·al·ge·sic, hy·per·al·get·ic (hī'per-al-jē'sik, -jet'ik). Relating to hyperalgesia.

hy·per·al·i·men·ta·tion (hī'per-al'i-men-tā'shŭn). Administration or consumption of nutrients beyond minimum normal requirements, in an attempt to replace nutritional deficiencies.

hy·per·am·y·la·se·mia (hī'per-am'i-lā-sē'mē-ă). Elevated serum amylase, usually seen as one of the manifestations of acute pancreatitis. [hyper- + amylase, + G. *haima*, blood]

hy·per·an·a·ki·ne·sia, hy·per·an·a·ki·ne·sis (hī'per-an-ă-ki-nē'zē-ă, -ki-nē'sis). Excessive to-and-fro movement, *e.g.*, of the stomach or intestine. [hyper- + G. *anakinēsis*, to-and-fro movement]

hy·per·a·phia (hī'per-ā'fē-ă). Extreme sensitivity to touch. [hyper- + G. *haphē*, touch]

hy·per·aph·ic (hī-per-af'ik). Marked by hyperaphia.

hy·per·bar·ic (hī-per-bar'ik). 1. Pertaining to pressure of ambient gases greater than 1 atmosphere. 2. Concerning solutions, more dense than the diluent or medium; *e.g.*, in spinal anesthesia, a h. solution has a density greater than that of spinal fluid. [hyper- + G. *baros*, weight]

hy·per·bar·ism (hī-per-bar'izm). Disturbances in the body resulting from the pressure of ambient gases at greater than 1 atmosphere; *e.g.*, nitrogen narcosis, oxygen toxicity, bends. [hyper- + G. *baros*, weight]

hy·per·bil·i·ru·bi·ne·mia (hī'per-bil'i-rū-bi-nē'mē-ă). An abnormally large amount of bilirubin in the circulating blood, resulting in clinically apparent icterus or jaundice when the concentration is sufficient.

   neonatal h., serum bilirubin greater than 12.9 mg/dl (220 μmol/L) or rising at a rate greater than 5 mg/dl per day; also applied to a nonphysiologic pattern of h., *i.e.*, jaundice in the first 24 hours of life or extending beyond the first week of life in term infants.

hy·per·cal·ce·mia (hī'per-kal-sē'mē-ă). An elevated concentration of calcium ions in the blood.

   idiopathic h. of infants, persistent h. of unknown cause in very young children, associated with osteosclerosis, renal insufficiency, and sometimes hypertension.

hy·per·cal·ci·u·ria (hī'per-kal-sē-yu're-ă). Excretion of abnormally large amounts of calcium in the urine.

hy·per·cap·nia (hī-per-kap'nē-ă). Abnormally increased arterial carbon dioxide tension. SYN hypercarbia. [hyper- + G. *kapnos*, smoke, vapor]

hy·per·car·bia (hī-per-kar'bē-ă). SYN hypercapnia.

hy·per·ce·men·to·sis (hī'per-sē-men-tō'sis). Excessive deposition of secondary cementum on the root of a tooth, which may be caused by localized trauma or inflammation, excessive tooth eruption, or osteitis deformans, or may occur idiopathically. [hyper- + L. *caementum*, a rough quarry stone, + *-osis*, condition]

hy·per·chlor·e·mia (hī'per-klō-rē'mē-ă). An abnormally large concentration of chloride ions in the circulating blood.

hy·per·chlor·hy·dria (hī′per-klōr-hī′drē-ă). Presence of an excessive amount of hydrochloric acid in the stomach. SYN chlorhydria. [hyper- + chlorhydric (acid)]

hy·per·cho·les·ter·e·mia (hī′per-kō-les′ter-ē′mē-ă). SYN hypercholesterolemia.

hy·per·cho·les·ter·ol·e·mia (hī′per-kō-les′ter-ol-ē′mē-ă). The presence of an abnormally large amount of cholesterol in the blood. SYN hypercholesteremia.

   familial h., SYN type II familial *hyperlipoproteinemia.*

   familial h. with hyperlipemia, SYN type III familial *hyperlipoproteinemia.*

hy·per·cho·lia (hī-per-kō′lē-ă). A condition in which an abnormally large amount of bile is formed in the liver. [hyper- + G. *cholē*, bile]

hy·per·chro·ma·sia (hī′per-krō-mā′zē-ă). SYN hyperchromatism.

hy·per·chro·mat·ic (hī′per-krō-mat′ik). **1.** Abnormally highly colored, excessively stained, or overpigmented. SYN hyperchromic (1). **2.** Showing increased chromatin. [hyper- + G. *chrōma*, color]

hy·per·chro·ma·tism (hī′per-krō′mă-tizm). **1.** Excessive pigmentation. **2.** Increased staining capacity, especially of cell nuclei for hematoxylin. **3.** An increase in chromatin in cell nuclei. SYN hyperchromasia, hyperchromia. [hyper- + G. *chrōma*, color]

hy·per·chro·mia (hī-per-krō′mē-ă). SYN hyperchromatism.

hy·per·chro·mic (hī-per-krōm′ik). **1.** SYN hyperchromatic (1). **2.** Denoting increased light absorption.

hy·per·chy·lia (hī-per-kī′lē-ă). Excessive secretion of gastric juice. [hyper- + G. *chylos*, juice]

hy·per·chy·lo·mi·cro·ne·mia (hī′per-kī′lō-mī-krō-nē′mē-ă). Increased plasma concentrations of chylomicrons.

   familial h., SYN type I familial *hyperlipoproteinemia.*

hy·per·cor·ti·coid·ism (hī′per-kōr′ti-koyd-izm). Excessive secretion of one or more steroid hormones of the adrenal cortex; sometimes used also to designate the state produced by therapeutic administration of large quantities of steroids having glucocorticoid activity, *e.g.,* hydrocortisone. SEE ALSO Cushing's *syndrome.*

hy·per·cry·al·ge·sia (hī′per-krī-al-jē′zē-ă). SYN hypercryesthesia. [hyper- + G. *kryos*, cold, + *algēsis,* the sense of pain]

hy·per·cry·es·the·sia (hī′per-krī-es-thē′zē-ă). Extreme sensibility to cold. SYN hypercryalgesia. [hyper- + G. *kryos*, cold, + *aisthēsis,* sensation]

hy·per·cu·pre·mia (hī′per-kū-prē′mē-ă). An abnormally high level of plasma copper. [hyper- + L. *cuprum,* copper, + G. *haima,* blood]

hy·per·cy·a·not·ic (hī′per-sī-ă-not′ik). Marked by extreme cyanosis.

hy·per·cy·the·mia (hī′per-sī-thē′mē-ă). The presence of an abnormally high number of red blood cells in the circulating blood. SYN hypererythrocythemia. [hyper- + G. *kytos*, cell, + *haima,* blood]

hy·per·cy·to·sis (hī′per-sī-tō′sis). Any condition in which there is an abnormal increase in the number of cells in the circulating blood or the tissues; frequently used synonymously with leukocytosis.

hy·per·di·crot·ic (hī′per-dī-krot′ik). Pronouncedly dicrotic.

hy·per·em·e·sis (hī-per-em′ĕ-sis). Excessive vomiting. [hyper- + G. *emesis,* vomiting]

hy·per·e·met·ic (hī′per-ĕ-met′ik). Marked by excessive vomiting.

hy·per·e·mia (hī-per-ē′mē-ă). The presence of an increased amount of blood in a part or organ. SEE ALSO congestion. [hyper- + G. *haima,* blood]

   active h., h. due to an increased afflux of arterial blood into dilated capillaries. SYN fluxionary h.

   collateral h., increased blood flow through abundant collateral channels when the circulation through the main artery to a part is arrested.

   fluxionary h., SYN active h.

   passive h., h. due to an obstruction in the flow of blood from the affected part, the venous radicles becoming distended. SYN venous h.

   reactive h., h. following the arrest and subsequent restoration of the blood supply to a part.

   venous h., SYN passive h.

hy·per·e·mic (hī-per-ē′mik). Denoting hyperemia.

hy·per·en·ceph·a·ly (hī′per-en-sef′ă-lē). A fetal developmental deficiency of the vault of the cranium, exposing the poorly formed brain. [hyper- + G. *enkephalos,* brain]

hy·per·e·o·sin·o·phil·ia (hī′per-ē-ō-sin-ō-fil′ē-ă). A greater degree of increase in the number of eosinophilic granulocytes in the circulating blood or the tissues than would be expected in the disease or condition causing the increase.

hy·per·er·ga·sia (hī-per-er-gā′zē-ă). Increased or excessive functional activity. [hyper- + G. *ergasia,* work]

hy·per·er·gia (hī′per-er′jē-ă). An allergic hypersensitivity. SYN hypergia.

hy·per·er·gic (hī-per-er′jik). Relating to hyperergia. SYN hypergic.

hy·per·e·ryth·ro·cy·the·mia (hī′per-ē-rith′rō-sī-thē′mē-ă). SYN hypercythemia.

hy·per·es·o·pho·ria (hī′per-es-ō-fō′rē-ă). A tendency of one eye to deviate upward and inward, prevented by binocular vision. [hyper- + G. *esō,* inward, + *phora,* movement]

hy·per·es·the·sia (hī′per-es-thē′zē-ă). Abnormal acuteness of sensitivity to touch, pain, or other sensory stimuli. SYN oxyesthesia. [hyper- + G. *aisthēsis,* sensation]

hy·per·es·thet·ic (hī-per-es-thet′ik). Marked by hyperesthesia.

hy·per·ex·o·pho·ria (hī′per-ek-sō-fō′rē-ă). A tendency of one eye to deviate upward and outward, prevented by binocular vision. [hyper- + G. *exō,* outward, + *phora,* movement]

hy·per·ex·ten·sion (hī′per-eks-ten′shŭn). Extension of a limb or part beyond the normal limit.

hy·per·fer·re·mia (hī′per-fer-ē′mē-ă). High serum iron level; found in hemochromatosis.

hy·per·fi·brin·o·ge·ne·mia (hī′per-fī-brin′ō-jĕ-nē′mē-ă). An increased level of fibrinogen in the blood. SYN fibrinogenemia.

hy·per·fi·bri·nol·y·sis (hī′per-fī-brin-ol′i-sis).

Markedly increased fibrinolysis, as in subdural hematomas.

hy·per·flex·ion (hī-per-flek'shŭn). Flexion of a limb or part beyond the normal limit.

hy·per·gal·ac·to·sis (hī'per-ga-lak-tō'sis). Excessive secretion of milk. [hyper- + G. *gala,* milk, + *-ōsis,* condition]

hy·per·gam·ma·glob·u·lin·e·mia (hī'per-gam-ă-glob'yū-li-nē'mē-ă). An increased concentration of γ-globulins in the plasma.

hy·per·gen·e·sis (hī-per-jen'ĕ-sis). Excessive development or redundant production of parts or organs of the body. [hyper- + G. *genesis,* production]

hy·per·ge·net·ic (hī-per-jĕ-net'ik). Relating to hypergenesis.

hy·per·gen·i·tal·ism (hī-per-jen'i-tăl-izm). Abnormal overdevelopment of genitalia.

hy·per·geu·sia (hī-per-gū'sē-ă, -jū'sē-ă). Abnormal acuteness of the sense of taste. SYN oxygeusia. [hyper- + G. *geusis,* taste]

hy·per·gia (hī-per'jē-ă). SYN hyperergia.

hy·per·gic (hī-per'jik). SYN hyperergic.

hy·per·glan·du·lar (hī-per-glan'dyŭ-lăr). Characterized by overactivity or increased size of a gland.

hy·per·glob·u·lin·e·mia (hī'per-glob'yū-lin-ē'mē-ă). An abnormally high concentration of globulins in the circulating blood plasma.

hy·per·glyc·er·i·de·mia (hī'per-glis'er-i-dē'mē-ă). Elevated plasma concentration of glycerides; normal if transiently present after absorption of a meal containing lipids, abnormal if a persistent state.

  endogenous h., type IV familial hyperlipoproteinemia or, more commonly, a nonfamilial sporadic variety.

  exogenous h., persistent h. due to retarded rate of removal from plasma of chylomicrons of dietary origin.

hy·per·gly·ci·ne·mia (hī'per-glī-si-nē'mē-ă). Elevated plasma glycine concentration.

hy·per·gly·ci·nu·ria (hī'per-glī-si-nū'rē-ă). Enhanced urinary excretion of glycine.

hy·per·gly·co·gen·ol·y·sis (hī'per-glī'kŏ-jĕ-nol'i-sis). Excessive glycogenolysis. [hyper- + glycogen + G. *lysis,* loosening]

hy·per·gly·cor·rha·chia (hī'per-glī-kō-rak'ē-ă). Excessive sugar in the cerebrospinal fluid. [hyper- + G. *glykys,* sweet, + *rhachis,* spine]

hy·per·gly·co·su·ria (hī'per-glī-kō-sū'rē-ă). Persistent excretion of unusually large amounts of glucose in the urine.

hy·per·go·nad·ism (hī-per-gō'nad-izm). A clinical state resulting from enhanced secretion of gonadal hormones.

hy·per·go·nad·o·tro·pic (hī'per-gō'nă-dō-trop'ik). Indicating an increased production or excretion of gonadotropic hormones.

hy·per·he·mo·glo·bi·ne·mia (hī'per-hē'mō-glō-bi-nē'mē-ă). An unusually large amount of hemoglobin in the circulating blood plasma.

hy·per·hi·dro·sis (hī'per-hī-drō'sis). Excessive or profuse sweating. SYN hyperidrosis, polyhidrosis, polyidrosis. [hyper- + hidrosis]

  gustatory h., excessive sweating of the lips, nose, and forehead after eating certain foods.

hy·per·hy·dra·tion (hī'per-hī-drā'shŭn). Excess water content of the body.

hy·per·i·dro·sis (hī'per-i-drō'sis). SYN hyperhidrosis.

hy·per·in·fec·tion (hī'per-in-fek'shŭn). Infection by very large numbers of organisms as a result of immunologic deficiency.

hy·per·in·su·lin·ism (hī'per-in'sū-lin-izm). Increased levels of insulin in the plasma due to increased secretion of insulin by the beta cells of the pancreatic islets.

  alimentary h., elevated levels of insulin in the plasma following ingestion of meals by individuals with abnormally rapid gastric emptying.

hy·per·in·vo·lu·tion (hī'per-in'vō-lū'shŭn). SYN superinvolution.

hy·per·i·so·ton·ic (hī'per-ī-sō-ton'ik). SYN hypertonic.

hy·per·ka·le·mia (hī'per-kă-lē'mē-ă). A greater than normal concentration of potassium ions in the circulating blood. SYN hyperpotassemia. [hyper- + Mod. L. *kalium,* potash, + G. *haima,* blood]

hy·per·ker·a·tin·i·za·tion (hī'per-ker'at-i-ni-zā'shŭn). SYN hyperkeratosis.

hy·per·ker·a·to·sis (hī'per-ker-ă-tō'sis). Thickening of the horny layer of the epidermis or mucous membrane. SEE ALSO keratoderma, keratosis. SYN hyperkeratinization.

hy·per·ke·to·ne·mia (hī'per-kē'tō-nē'mē-ă). Elevated concentrations of ketone bodies in the blood.

hy·per·ke·ton·u·ria (hī'per-kē'tō-nū'rē-ă). Increased urinary excretion of ketonic compounds.

hy·per·ki·ne·mia (hī'per-ki-nē'mē-ă). Increased circulation rate; increased volume flow through the circulation; supernormal cardiac output. [hyper- + G. *kineō,* to move, + *haima,* blood]

hy·per·ki·ne·sis, hy·per·ki·ne·sia (hī'per-ki-nē'sis, -nē'zē-ă). **1.** Excessive motility. **2.** Excessive muscular activity. SYN supermotility. [hyper- + G. *kinēsis,* motion]

hy·per·ki·net·ic (hī-per-ki-net'ik). Pertaining to or characterized by hyperkinesia.

hy·per·leu·ko·cy·to·sis (hī'per-lū'kō-sī-tō'sis). An increase in the number and proportion of leukocytes in the circulating blood or the tissues greater than that ordinarily observed in most instances of leukocytosis.

hy·per·li·pe·mia (hī'per-li-pē'mē-ă). H. is associated with a deficiency of δ-aminoadipic semialdehyde synthase. SEE ALSO lipemia. [hyper- + G. *lipos,* fat, + *haima,* blood]

  familial fat-induced h., SYN type I familial *hyperlipoproteinemia.*

hy·per·lip·id·e·mia (hī'per-lip-i-dē'mē-ă). SYN lipemia.

hy·per·lip·oi·de·mia (hī'per-lip-oy-dē'mē-ă). SYN lipemia.

hy·per·lip·o·pro·tein·e·mia (hī'per-lip'ō-prō'tē-in-ē'mē-ă, -prō'tēn-). An increase in the lipoprotein concentration of the blood.

  acquired h., nonfamilial h. that develops as a consequence of some primary disease, such as thyroid deficiency.

  type I familial h. [MIM*238600], h. characterized by the presence of large amounts of chylo-

hy

microns and triglycerides in the plasma when the patient has a normal diet, and their disappearance on a fat-free diet. It is accompanied by bouts of abdominal pain, hepatosplenomegaly, pancreatitis, and eruptive xanthomas; autosomal recessive inheritance. SYN familial fat-induced hyperlipemia, familial hyperchylomicronemia, familial hypertriglyceridemia (1).

type II familial h. [MIM*144400], h. characterized by increased plasma levels of β-lipoproteins, cholesterol, and phospholipids, but normal triglycerides. Homozygotes have xanthomatosis and frank clinical atherosclerosis as young adults. The primary defect is a deficiency of apoprotein of VLDL. SYN familial hypercholesterolemia.

type III familial h. [MIM*107741], h. characterized by increased plasma levels of LDL, β-lipoproteins, pre-β-lipoproteins, cholesterol, phospholipids, and triglycerides; frequent eruptive xanthomas and atheromatosis, particularly coronary artery disease; biochemical defect lies in apolipoproteins. SYN familial hypercholesterolemia with hyperlipidemia.

type IV familial h. [MIM*144600], plasma levels of VLDL, pre-β-lipoproteins and triglycerides are increased on a normal diet, but β-lipoproteins, cholesterol, and phospholipids are normal; may be accompanied by abnormal glucose tolerance and susceptibility to ischemic heart disease. SYN familial hypertriglyceridemia (2).

type V familial h. [MIM*144650], h. characterized by increased plasma levels of chylomicrons, VLDL, pre-β-lipoproteins, and triglycerides; may be accompanied by bouts of abdominal pain, hepatosplenomegaly, susceptibility to atherosclerosis, and abnormal glucose tolerance.

hy·per·li·thu·ria (hī′per-li-thu′rē-ă). An excessive excretion of uric (lithic) acid in the urine.

hy·per·lu·cent (hī′-per-lū′sent). A region on a chest film showing greater than normal film blackening from increased transmission of x-rays. [hyper- + L. *lucens*, shining, fr. *luceo*, to shine]

hy·per·ly·si·nu·ria (hī′per-lī-si-nū′rē-ă). The presence of abnormally high concentrations of lysine in the urine; a form of aminoaciduria that occurs in cystinuria, hepatolenticular degeneration, and the Fanconi syndrome.

hy·per·mag·ne·se·mia (hī′per-mag-nĕ-sē′mē-ă). An abnormally large concentration of magnesium in the blood serum.

hy·per·mas·tia (hī-per-mas′tē-ă). **1.** SYN polymastia. **2.** Excessively large mammary glands. [hyper- + G. *mastos*, breast]

hy·per·men·or·rhea (hī′per-men-ō-rē′ă). Excessively prolonged or profuse menses. SYN menorrhagia, menostaxis. [hyper- + G. *mēn*, month, + *rhoia*, flow]

hy·per·me·tab·o·lism (hī′per-me-tab′ŏ-lizm). Heat production by the body above normal, as in thyrotoxicosis.

hy·per·me·tria (hī-per-mē′trē-ă). Ataxia characterized by overreaching a desired object or goal; usually seen with cerebellar disorders. Cf. hypometria. [hyper- + G. *metron*, measure]

hy·per·me·tro·pia (hī′per-me-trō′pē-ă). SYN hyperopia. [hyper- + G. *metron*, measure, + *ōps*, eye]

hy·per·my·o·to·nia (hī′per-mī-ō-tō′nē-ă). Extreme muscular tonus. [hyper- + G. *mys*, muscle, + *tonos*, tension]

hy·per·my·ot·ro·phy (hī′per-mī-ot′rō-fē). Muscular hypertrophy. [hyper- + G. *mys*, muscle, + *trophē*, nourishment]

hypernasality. Speech produced with excessive resonance in the nasal cavity, often due to dysfunction of the soft palate. SYN hyperrhinophonia.

hy·per·na·tre·mia (hī′per-nă-trē′mē-ă). An abnormally high plasma concentration of sodium ions. [hyper- + natrium, + G. *haima*, blood]

hy·per·ne·o·cy·to·sis (hī′per-nē′ō-sī-tō′sis). Hyperleukocytosis in which there are considerable numbers of immature and young cells (especially in the granulocytic series). [hyper- + G. *neos*, new, + *kytos*, cell, + *-osis*, condition]

hy·per·on·cot·ic (hī′per-on-kot′ik). Indicating an oncotic pressure higher than normal, *e.g.*, of blood plasma.

hy·per·o·nych·ia (hī′per-ō-nik′ē-ă). Hypertrophy of the nails. [hyper- + G. *onyx*, (onych-), nail]

hy·per·o·pia (H) (hī-per-ō′pē-ă). Longsightedness; that optical condition in which only convergent rays can be brought to focus on the retina. SYN farsightedness, hypermetropia. [hyper- + G. *ōps*, eye]

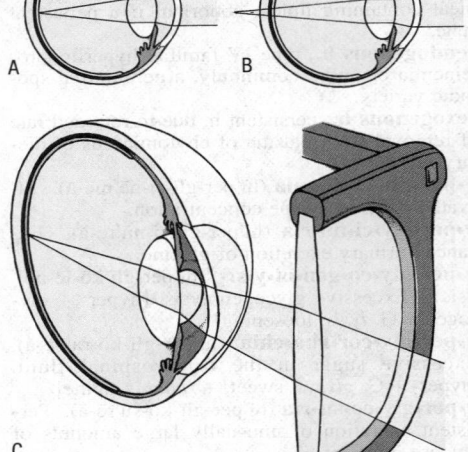

hyperopia: (A) normal (20/20) vision, light rays focus sharply on retina; (B) hyperopic (farsighted) vision, light rays from close objects come to sharp focus behind the retina; (C) hyperopia corrected by eyeglasses with convex lenses

absolute h., manifest h. that cannot be overcome by an effort of accommodation.

axial h., h. due to shortening of the anteroposterior diameter of the globe of the eye.

curvature h., h. due to decreased refraction of the anterior ocular segment.

facultative h., SYN manifest h.

latent h., the difference between total and manifest h.

manifest h., h. that can be compensated by accommodation. SYN facultative h.

total h. (Ht), that which can be determined after complete paralysis of accommodation by means of a cycloplegic.

hy·per·o·pic (H) (hī-per-ō′pik). Pertaining to hyperopia.

hy·per·or·chi·dism (hī-per-ōr′ki-dizm). Increased size or functioning of the testes. [hyper- + G. *orchis,* testis]

hy·per·or·tho·cy·to·sis (hī-per-ōr′thō-sī-tō′sis). Hyperleukocytosis in which the relative percentages of the various types of white blood cells are within the normal range. [hyper- + G. *orthos,* correct, + *kytos,* cell, + -*osis,* condition]

hy·per·os·mia (hī-per-oz′mē-ă). An exaggerated or abnormally acute sense of smell. [hyper- + G. *osmē,* sense of smell]

hy·per·os·mo·lal·i·ty (hī′per-oz-mō-lal′i-tē). Increased concentration of a solution expressed as osmoles of solute per kilogram of serum water.

hy·per·os·mo·lar·i·ty (hī′per-oz-mō-lar′i-tē). An increase in the osmotic concentration of a solution expressed as osmoles of solute per liter of solution.

hy·per·os·mot·ic (hī′per-oz-mot′ik). **1.** Having an osmolality greater than another fluid, ordinarily assumed to be plasma or extracellular fluid. **2.** Relating to increased osmosis.

hy·per·os·te·oi·do·sis (hī′per-os-tē-oy-dō′sis). Excessive formation of osteoid, as seen in rickets and osteomalacia.

hy·per·os·to·sis (hī′per-os-tō′sis). **1.** Hypertrophy of bone. **2.** SYN exostosis. [hyper- + G. *osteon,* bone, + -*ōsis,* condition]

diffuse idiopathic skeletal h., a generalized spinal and extraspinal articular disorder characterized by calcification and ossification of ligaments, particularly of the anterior longitudinal ligament; distinct from ankylosing spondylitis or degenerative joint disease.

hy·per·o·var·i·an·ism (hī′per-ō-vā′rē-an-izm). Sexual precocity in young girls due to premature development of ovaries accompanied by the secretion of ovarian hormones.

hy·per·ox·al·u·ria (hī′per-ok-să-lū′rē-ă). Presence of an unusually large amount of oxalic acid or oxalates in the urine. SYN oxaluria.

hy·per·ox·ia (hī-per-ok′sē-ă). **1.** An increased amount of oxygen in tissues and organs. **2.** A greater oxygen tension than normal.

hy·per·par·a·sit·ism (hī-per-par′ă-sīt-izm). A condition in which a secondary parasite develops within a previously existing parasite.

hy·per·par·a·thy·roid·ism (hī′per-par-ă-thī′royd-izm). A condition due to an increase in the secretion of the parathyroids, causing elevated serum calcium, decreased serum phosphorus, and increased excretion of both calcium and phosphorus, calcium stones and sometimes generalized osteitis fibrosa cystica.

hy·per·pep·sin·ia (hī′per-pep-sin′ē-ă). An excess of pepsin in the gastric juice.

hy·per·per·i·stal·sis (hī′per-per-i-stal′sis). Excessive rapidity of the passage of food through the stomach and intestine.

hy·per·phen·yl·al·a·ni·ne·mia (hī′per-fen′il-al-ă-ni-nē′mē-ă). The presence of abnormally high blood levels of phenylalanine in newborn infants associated with phenylketonuria, maternal phenylketonuria, or transient deficiency of phenylalanine hydroxylase or *p*-hydroxyphenylpyruvic acid oxidase.

hy·per·pho·ne·sis (hī′per-fō-nē′sis). An increase in the percussion sound or of the voice sound in auscultation. [hyper- + G. *phōnēsis,* a sounding]

hy·per·pho·ria (hī-per-fō′rē-ă). A tendency of the visual axis of one eye to deviate upward, prevented by binocular vision. [hyper- + G. *phora,* motion]

hy·per·phos·pha·te·mia (hī′per-fos-fă-tē′mē-ă). Abnormally high concentration of phosphates in the circulating blood.

hy·per·phos·pha·tu·ria (hī′per-fos-fă-tū′rē-ă). An increased excretion of phosphates in the urine.

hy·per·pig·men·ta·tion (hī′per-pig-men-tā′shŭn). An excess of pigment in a tissue or part.

hy·per·pi·tu·i·ta·rism (hī′per-pi-tū′i-tă-rizm). Excessive production of anterior pituitary hormones, especially growth hormone; may result in gigantism or acromegaly.

hy·per·pla·sia (hī-per-plā′zē-ă). An increase in number of cells in a tissue or organ, excluding tumor formation, whereby the bulk of the part or organ may be increased. SEE ALSO hypertrophy. [hyper- + G. *plasis,* a molding]

benign prostatic h. (BPH), progressive enlargement of the prostate due to h. of both glandular and stromal components, typically beginning in the fifth decade and sometimes causing obstructive or irritative symptoms or both; does not evolve into cancer.

congenital virilizing adrenal h., any inborn error of metabolism causing h. of the adrenal cortex and overproduction of virilizing hormones. Most forms are due to partial or complete 21-hydroxylase deficiency, leading to increased ACTH production by the pituitary, stimulating adrenal growth and function. Clinical features include ambiguous genitalia, virilization, and salt-wasting.

inflammatory papillary h., closely arranged papules of the palatal mucosa underlying an ill-fitting denture.

hy·per·plas·tic (hī-per-plas′tik). Relating to hyperplasia.

hy·per·pnea (hī-per-nē′ă, hī-perp′nē-ă). Breathing that is deeper and more rapid than is normal at rest. [hyper- + G. *pnoē,* breathing]

hy·per·po·lar·i·za·tion (hī′per-pō′lăr-i-zā′shŭn). An increase in polarization of membranes of nerves or muscle cells; the reverse change from that associated with excitatory action.

hy·per·po·ne·sis (hī′per-pō-nē′sis). Exaggerated activity within the motor portion of the nervous system. [hyper- + G. *ponos,* toil]

hy·per·po·tas·se·mia (hī′per-pō-tas-ē′mē-ă). SYN hyperkalemia.

hy·per·pre·be·ta·lip·o·pro·tein·e·mia (hī′per-

hy

prē-bā′tă-lip-ō-prō′tēn-ē′mē-ă). Increased concentrations of pre-β-lipoproteins in the blood.

hy·per·pro·in·su·li·ne·mia (hī′per-prō-in′sŭl-i-nē′mē-ă). Elevated plasma levels of proinsulin or proinsulin-like material.

hy·per·pro·lac·ti·ne·mia (hī′per-prō-lak-ti-nē′mē-ă). Elevated levels of prolactin in the blood; a normal physiological reaction during lactation, but pathological otherwise; often due to physical or emotional stress or rapid weight loss, sometimes to pituitary adenoma; amenorrhea is usually present.

hy·per·pro·tein·e·mia (hī′per-prō′tē-in-ē′mē-ă, -prō′tēn-). An abnormally large concentration of protein in plasma.

hy·per·pro·te·o·sis (hī′per-prō-tē-ō′sis). The condition due to an excessive amount of protein in the diet.

hy·per·py·ret·ic (hī′per-pī-ret′ik). Relating to hyperpyrexia. SYN hyperpyrexial.

hy·per·py·rex·ia (hī′per-pī-rek′sē-ă). Extremely high fever. [hyper- + G. *pyrexis*, feverishness]

hy·per·py·rex·i·al (hī′per-pī-rek′sē-ăl). SYN hyperpyretic.

hy·per·re·flex·ia (hī′per-rē-flek′sē-ă). A condition in which the deep tendon reflexes are exaggerated.

hy·per·res·o·nance (hī-per-rez′ō-nans). **1.** An extreme degree of resonance. **2.** Resonance increased above the normal, and often of lower pitch, on percussion of an area of the body; occurs in the chest due to overinflation of the lung as in emphysema or pneumothorax and in the abdomen over a distended bowel.

hyperrhinophonia. SYN hypernasality.

hy·per·sal·i·va·tion (hī′per-sal-i-vā′shŭn). Increased salivation.

hy·per·sen·si·tiv·i·ty (hī′per-sen-si-tiv′i-tē). Abnormal sensitivity, a condition in which there is an exaggerated response by the body to the stimulus of a foreign agent. SEE allergy.

hy·per·sen·si·ti·za·tion (hī′per-sen′si-ti-zā′shŭn). The immunological process by which hypersensitivity is induced.

hy·per·som·nia (hī-per-som′nē-ă). A condition in which sleep periods are excessively long, but the person responds normally in the intervals; distinguished from somnolence. [hyper- + L. *somnus*, sleep]

hy·per·splen·ism (hī-per-splēn′izm). Any condition in which the cellular components of the blood or platelets are removed at an abnormally high rate by the spleen.

hy·per·sthe·nia (hī-per-sthē′nē-ă). Excessive tension or strength. [hyper- + G. *sthenos*, strength]

hy·per·sthen·ic (hī-per-sthen′ik). Pertaining to or marked by hypersthenia.

hy·per·sthen·u·ria (hī′per-sthen-yū′rē-ă). Excretion of urine of unusually high specific gravity and concentration of solutes, resulting from loss or deprivation of water. [hyper- + G. *sthenos*, strength, + *ouron*, urine]

hy·per·tel·or·ism (hī-per-tel′ōr-izm). Abnormal distance between two paired organs. [hyper- + G. *tēle*, far off, + *horizō*, to separate, fr. *horos*, a boundary]

ocular h. [MIM*145400], increased width between the eyes due to an enlarged sphenoid bone; other congenital deformities and mental retardation may be associated.

hy·per·ten·sion (hī′per-ten′shŭn). High blood pressure. Despite many discrete and inherited but rare forms that have been identified, the evidence is that for the most part blood pressure is a multifactorial, perhaps galtonian trait. Its strong cybernetic properties may also be largely inherited but would not be reflected in measurements of heritability. The definition of what is "high" or "low" blood pressure is then entirely arbitrary, but extreme cases are undoubtedly dysgenic. [hyper- + L. *tensio*, tension]

  adrenal h., h. due to an adrenal medullary pheochromocytoma or to hyperactivity or functioning tumor of the adrenal cortex.

  benign h., h. that runs a relatively long and symptomless course.

  essential h., h. without known cause.

  Goldblatt h., increased blood pressure following obstruction of blood flow to one kidney.

  malignant h., severe h. that runs a rapid course, causing necrosis of arteriolar walls in kidney and retina, hemorrhages, and death most frequently due to uremia or rupture of a cerebral vessel.

  portal h., h. in the portal system as seen in cirrhosis of the liver and other conditions causing obstruction to the portal vein.

  pulmonary h., h. in the pulmonary circuit; may be primary, or secondary to pulmonary or cardiac disease, *e.g.*, fibrosis of the lung or mitral stenosis.

  renal h., h. secondary to renal disease.

  renovascular h., h. produced by renal arterial obstruction.

hy·per·ten·sive (hī-per-ten′siv). **1.** Marked by an increased blood pressure. **2.** Denoting a person suffering from high blood pressure.

hy·per·ten·sor (hī-per-ten′ser, -sōr). SYN pressor.

hy·per·the·co·sis (hī′per-thē-kō′sis). Diffuse hyperplasia of the theca cells of the graafian follicles.

hy·per·the·lia (hī-per-thē′lē-ă). SYN polythelia. [hyper- + G. *thēlē*, nipple]

hy·per·ther·mal·ge·sia (hī′per-ther-măl-jē′zē-ă). Extreme sensitiveness to heat. [hyper- + G. *thermē*, heat, + *algēsis*, pain]

hy·per·ther·mia (hī-per-ther′mē-ă). Therapeutically induced hyperpyrexia. [hyper- + G. *thermē*, heat]

  malignant h., rapid onset of extremely high fever with muscle rigidity, precipitated by exogenous agents in genetically susceptible persons, especially by halothane or succinylcholine.

hy·per·throm·bi·ne·mia (hī′per-throm-bi-nē′mē-ă). An abnormal increase of thrombin in the blood, frequently resulting in a tendency to intravascular coagulation.

hy·per·thy·mic (hī-per-thī′mik). **1.** Pertaining to hyperthymia. **2.** Pertaining to hyperthymism.

hy·per·thy·roid·ism (hī-per-thī′royd-izm). An abnormality of the thyroid gland in which secretion of thyroid hormone is usually increased and is no longer under regulatory control of hypothalamic-pituitary centers; characterized by a hypermetabolic state, usually with weight loss, tremulousness, elevated plasma levels of thyroxin and/or triiodothyronine; often associated with exophthalmos (Graves' disease).

hy·per·thy·rox·i·ne·mia (hī′per-thī-rok-si-nē′mē-ă). An elevated thyroxine concentration in the blood.

hy·per·to·nia (hī-per-tō′nē-ă). Extreme tension of the muscles or arteries. SYN hypertonicity (1). [hyper- + G. *tonos*, tension]

hy·per·ton·ic (hī-per-ton′ik). **1.** Having a greater degree of tension. SYN spastic (1). **2.** Having a greater osmotic pressure than a reference solution, which is ordinarily assumed to be blood plasma or interstitial fluid; more specifically, refers to a fluid in which cells shrink. SYN hyperisotonic.

hy·per·to·nic·i·ty (hī′per-tō-nis′i-tē). **1.** SYN hypertonia. **2.** An increased effective osmotic pressure of body fluids.

hy·per·tri·cho·sis (hī′per-tri-kō′sis). Growth of hair in excess of the normal. SEE ALSO hirsutism. [hyper- + G. *trichōsis*, being hairy]

hy·per·tri·glyc·er·i·de·mia (hī′per-trī-glis′er-i-dē′mē-ă). Elevated triglyceride concentration in the blood.

    familial h., (1) SYN type I familial *hyperlipoproteinemia.* **(2)** SYN type IV familial *hyperlipoproteinemia.*

hy·per·tro·phic (hī-per-trof′ik). Relating to or characterized by hypertrophy.

hy·per·tro·phy (hī-per′trō-fē). General increase in bulk of a part or organ, due to increase in size, but not in number, of the individual tissue elements. SEE ALSO hyperplasia. [hyper- + G. *trophē*, nourishment]

    adaptive h., thickening of the walls of a hollow organ, like the urinary bladder, when there is obstruction to outflow.

    compensatory h., increase in size of an organ or part of an organ or tissue, when called upon to do additional work or perform the work of destroyed tissue or of a paired organ.

    complementary h., increase in size or expansion of part of an organ or tissue to fill the space left by the destruction of another portion of the same organ or tissue.

    concentric h., thickening of the walls of the heart or any cavity with apparent diminution of the capacity of the cavity.

    eccentric h., thickening of the wall of the heart or other cavity, with dilation.

    physiologic h., temporary increase in size of an organ or part to provide for a natural increase of function.

    vicarious h., h. of an organ following failure of another organ because of a functional relationship between them; *e.g.,* enlargement of the pituitary gland, after destruction of the thyroid.

hy·per·tro·pia (hī′per-trō′pē-ă). An ocular deviation with one eye higher than the other. [hyper- + G. *trope*, a turn]

hy·per·u·ri·ce·mia (hī′per-yū-rē-sē′mē-ă). Enhanced blood concentrations of uric acid.

hy·per·u·ri·ce·mic (hī′per-yū-ri-sē′mik). Relating to or characterized by hyperuricemia.

hy·per·val·i·ne·mia (hī′per-val-i-nē′mē-ă). Abnormally high plasma concentrations of valine, a common finding in maple syrup urine disease.

hy·per·vas·cu·lar (hī′per-vas′kyū-ler). Abnormally vascular; containing an excessive number of blood vessels. [hyper- + L. *vas,* a vessel]

hy·per·ven·ti·la·tion (hī′per-ven-ti-lā′shŭn). Increased alveolar ventilation relative to metabolic carbon dioxide production, so that alveolar carbon dioxide pressure decreases to below normal.

hy·per·vi·ta·min·o·sis (hī′per-vī′tă-mi-nō′sis). A condition resulting from the ingestion of an excessive amount of a vitamin preparation, symptoms varying according to the particular vitamin.

hy·per·vo·le·mia (hī′per-vō-lē′mē-ă). Abnormally increased volume of blood. SYN plethora (1), repletion (1). [hyper- + L. *volumen*, volume, + G. *haima,* blood]

hy·per·vo·le·mic (hī′per-vō-lē′mik). Pertaining to or characterized by hypervolemia.

hyp·es·the·sia (hī-pes-thē′zē-ă). Diminished sensitivity to stimulation. SYN hypoesthesia. [G. *hypo,* under, + *aisthēsis,* feeling]

hy·pha, pl. **hy·phae** (hī′fă, hī′fē). A branching tubular cell characteristic of the filamentous fungi (molds). Intercommunicating hyphae constitute a mycelium, the visible colony on natural substrates or artificial laboratory media. [G. *hyphē,* a web]

hyp·he·do·nia (hīp-hē-dō′nē-ă). A habitually lessened or attenuated degree of pleasure from that which should normally give great pleasure. [G. *hypo,* under, + *hēdonē,* pleasure]

hy·phe·ma (hī-fē′mă). Blood in the anterior chamber of the eye. [G. *hyphaimos,* suffused with blood]

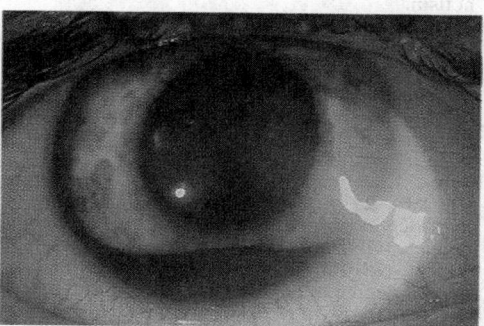
hyphema

hy·phe·mia (hī-fē′mē-ă). SYN hypovolemia. [hypo- + G. *haima,* blood]

hypn-. SEE hypno-.

hyp·na·gog·ic (hip-nă-goj′ik). Denoting a transitional state, related to the hypnoidal, preceding sleep; applied also to various hallucinations that may manifest themselves at that time. SEE ALSO hypnoidal. [hypno- + G. *agōgos,* leading]

hyp·na·gogue (hip′nă-gog). An agent that induces sleep. [hypno- + G. *agōgos,* leading]

hyp·nap·a·gog·ic (hip-nap-ă-goj′ik). Denoting a state similar to the hypnagogic, through which the mind passes in coming out of sleep; denoting also hallucinations experienced at such time. [hypno- + G. *apo,* from, + *agōgos,* leading]

⚠**hypno-, hypn-.** Sleep, hypnosis. [G. *hypnos,*]

hyp·no·a·nal·y·sis (hip′nō-ă-nal′ĭ-sis). Psychoanalysis or other psychotherapy which employs hypnosis as an adjunctive technique.

hyp·no·gen·e·sis (hip-nō-jen′ĕ-sis). The induction of sleep or of the hypnotic state. [hypno- + G. *genesis,* production]

hyp·no·gen·ic, hyp·nog·e·nous (hip-nō-jen′ik, -nŏj′ĕ-nŭs). 1. Relating to hypnogenesis. 2. An agent capable of inducing a hypnotic state. SEE hypnosis.

hyp·noi·dal (hip-noy′dăl). Resembling hypnosis; denoting the subwaking state, a mental condition intermediate between sleeping and waking. SEE ALSO hypnagogic. [hypno- + G. *eidos,* resemblance]

hyp·no·sis (hip-nō′sis). An artificially induced trancelike state, resembling somnambulism, in which the subject is highly susceptible to suggestion and responds readily to the commands of the hypnotist. SEE ALSO mesmerism. [G. *hypnos,* sleep, + *-osis,* condition]

hyp·no·ther·a·py (hip-nō-thār′ă-pē). 1. Psychotherapeutic treatment by means of hypnotism. 2. Treatment of disease by inducing a trance-like sleep.

hyp·not·ic (hip-not′ik). 1. Causing sleep. 2. An agent that promotes sleep. 3. Relating to hypnotism. [G. *hypnōtikos,* causing one to sleep]

hyp·no·tism (hip′nō-tizm). 1. The process or act of inducing hypnosis. SYN somnipathy (2). 2. The practice or study of hypnosis. SEE mesmerism. [G. *hypnos,* sleep]

hyp·no·tist (hip′nō-tist). One who practices hypnotism.

hyp·no·tize (hip′nō-tīz). To induct one into hypnosis.

hyp·no·zo·ite (hip-nō-zō′ĭt). Exoerythrocytic schizozoite of *Plasmodium vivax* or *P. ovale* in the human liver, characterized by delayed primary development; thought to be responsible for malarial relapse.

⚠**hypo-.** 1. Deficient, below normal. SEE ALSO hyp-. Cf. sub-. 2. CHEMISTRY Denoting the lowest, or least rich in oxygen, of a series of chemical compounds. [G. *hypo,* under]

hy·po·a·cid·i·ty (hī′pō-a-sid′i-tē). A lower than normal degree of acidity, as of the gastric juice.

hy·po·a·cu·sis (hī′pō-ă-kū′sis). SYN hypacusis.

hy·po·a·dre·nal·ism (hī′pō-ă-drē′năl-izm). Reduced adrenocortical function.

hy·po·al·bu·mi·ne·mia (hī′pō-al-bū-mi-nē′mē-ă). An abnormally low concentration of albumin in the blood. SYN hypalbuminemia.

hy·po·al·do·ster·on·u·ria (hī′pō-al-dos′ter-on-ū′rē-ă). Abnormally low levels of aldosterone in the urine.

hy·po·al·ge·sia (hī-pō-al-jē′zē-ă). SYN hypalgesia. [hypo- + G. *algēsis,* a sense of pain]

hy·po·az·o·tu·ria (hī′pō-az-ō-tū′rē-ă). Excretion of abnormally small quantities of nonprotein nitrogenous material (especially urea) in the urine. [hypo- + Fr. *azote,* nitrogen, + G. *ouron,* urine]

hy·po·bar·ic (hī-pō-bar′ik). 1. Pertaining to pressure of ambient gases below 1 atmosphere. 2.

With respect to solutions, less dense than the diluent or medium; *e.g.,* in spinal anesthesia, a h. solution has a density lower than that of spinal fluid. [hypo- + G. *baros,* weight]

hy·po·bar·ism (hī-pō-bar′izm). Dysbarism resulting from decreasing barometric pressure on the body without hypoxia; gas in body cavities tends to expand, and gases dissolved in body fluids tend to come out of solution as bubbles. Cf. decompression *sickness.*

hy·po·ba·rop·a·thy (hī′pō-ba-rop′ă-thē). Sickness produced by reduced barometric pressure. [hypo- + G. *baros,* weight, + *pathos,* suffering]

hy·po·be·ta·lip·o·pro·tein·e·mia (hī′pō-bā′tă-lip′ō-prō′tēn-ē′mē-ă) [MIM*107730]. Abnormally low levels of β-lipoproteins in the plasma occasionally with acanthocytosis and neurological signs. SEE ALSO abetalipoproteinemia.

hy·po·blast (hī′pō-blast). SYN endoderm. [hypo- + G. *blastos,* germ]

hy·po·blas·tic (hī-pō-blas′tik). Relating to or derived from the hypoblast.

hy·po·cal·ce·mia (hī′pō-kal-sē′mē-ă). Abnormally low levels of calcium in the circulating blood; commonly denotes subnormal concentrations of calcium ions.

hy·po·cal·ci·fi·ca·tion (hī′pō-kal-si-fi-kā′shŭn). Deficient calcification of bone or teeth.

hy·po·cap·nia (hī-pō-kap′nē-ă). Abnormally decreased arterial carbon dioxide tension. SYN hypocarbia. [hypo- + G. *kapnos,* smoke, vapor]

hy·po·car·bia (hī-pō-kar′bē-ă). SYN hypocapnia.

hy·po·chlor·e·mia (hī′pō-klō-rē′mē-ă). An abnormally low level of chloride ions in the circulating blood.

hy·po·chlor·hy·dria (hī′pō-klōr-hī′drē-ă, -hid′rī-ah). Presence of an abnormally small amount of hydrochloric acid in the stomach.

hy·po·chlor·u·ria (hī′pō-klōr-yū′rē-ă). Excretion of abnormally small quantities of chloride ions in the urine.

hy·po·cho·les·ter·ol·e·mia (hī′pō-kō-les′ter-ol-ē′mē-ă). The presence of abnormally small amounts of cholesterol in the circulating blood.

hy·po·chon·dria (hī-pō-kon′drē-ă). SYN hypochondriasis.

hy·po·chon·dri·ac (hī-pō-kon′drē-ak). 1. A person with a somatic overconcern, including morbid attention to the details of bodily functioning and exaggeration of any symptoms no matter how insignificant. 2. A person manifesting hypochondriasis. 3. Beneath the ribs; relating to the hypochondrium.

hy·po·chon·dri·a·cal (hī′pō-kon-drī′ă-kăl). Relating to or suffering from hypochondriasis.

hy·po·chon·dri·a·sis (hī′pō-kon-drī′ă-sis). A morbid concern about one's own health and exaggerated attention to any unusual bodily or mental sensations; a delusion that one is suffering from some disease for which no physical basis is evident. SYN hypochondria. [fr. hypochondrium, regarded as the site of hypochondria, + G. *-iasis,* condition]

hy·po·chon·dro·pla·sia (hī′pō-kon-drō-plā′zē-ă) [MIM*146000]. Dwarfism similar to achondroplasia, not evident until mid-childhood; the skull and facies are normal. [hypo- + G. *chondros*, cartilage, + *plasis*, a molding]

hy•po•chro•ma•sia (hī′pō-krō-mā′zē-ă). SYN hypochromia.

hy•po•chro•mat•ic (hī′-pō-krō-mat′ik). Containing a small amount of pigment, or less than the normal amount for the individual tissue. SYN hypochromic (1). [hypo- + G. *chrōma*, color]

hy•po•chro•ma•tism (hī-pō-krō′mă-tizm). **1.** The condition of being hypochromatic. **2.** SYN hypochromia.

hy•po•chro•mia (hī-pō-krō′mē-ă). An anemic condition in which the percentage of hemoglobin in the red blood cells is less than the normal range. SYN hypochromasia, hypochromatism (2). [hypo- + G. *chrōma*, color]

hy•po•chro•mic (hī-pō-krō′mik). **1.** SYN hypochromatic. **2.** Denoting decrease in light absorption with a shift in λ inferior to a lower wavelength.

hy•po•cor•ti•coid•ism (hī-pō-kōr′ti-koyd-izm). SYN adrenocortical *insufficiency*.

hy•po•cu•pre•mia (hī′pō-kū-prē′mē-ă). Reduced copper content of the blood; found in Wilson's disease because ceruloplasmin is depressed, even though serum albumin-attached copper is increased. [hypo- + L. *cuprum*, copper, + G. *haima*, blood]

hy•po•cy•cloi•dal (hī′-pō-sī-kloy′dăl). A tricyclic motion used by mechanical tomography units to optimize blurring and reduce artifacts. [hypo- + G. *kuklos*, circle, + *-oeidēs*, appearance]

hy•po•cy•the•mia (hī′pō-sī-thē′mē-ă). Hypocytosis of the circulating blood, such as that observed in aplastic anemia. [hypo- + G. *kytos*, cell, + *haima*, blood]

hy•po•dac•ty•ly, hy•po•dac•tyl•ia, hy•po•dac•tyl•ism (hī′pō-dak′ti-lē, -dak-til′ē-ă, -dak′til-izm). Less than the full normal complement of digits. [hypo- + G. *daktylos*, finger]

hy•po•der•mic (hī′pō-der′mik). SYN subcutaneous. **3.** SYN hypodermic *syringe*.

hy•po•der•mis (hī-pō-der′mis). SYN superficial *fascia*.

hy•po•der•moc•ly•sis (hī′pō-der-mok′li-sis). Subcutaneous injection of a saline or other solution. [hypo- + G. *derma*, skin, + *klysis*, a washing out]

hy•po•dip•sia (hī-pō-dip′sē-ă). A reduced sese of thirst; a physiologic condition, perhaps caused by hypertonicity of body fluids; loosely, oligodipsia. [hypo- + G. *dipsa*, thirst]

hy•po•don•tia (hī-pō-don′shē-ă). A condition of having fewer than the normal complement of teeth, either congenital or acquired. SYN oligodontia. [hypo- + G. *odous*, tooth]

hy•po•dy•nam•ic (hī′pō-dī-nam′ik). Possessing or exhibiting subnormal power or force.

hy•po•ec•cri•sis (hī′pō-ek′ri-sis). Reduced excretion of waste matter. [hypo- + G. *eccrisis*, separation]

hy•po•ec•crit•ic (hī′pō-ě-krit′ik). Characterized by hypoeccrisis.

hy•po•ech•o•ic (hī′pō-ē-kō′ik). Pertaining to a region in an ultrasound image in which the echoes are weaker or fewer than normal or in the surrounding regions. [hypo- + echo + -ic]

hy•po•es•o•pho•ria (hī′pō-es-ō-fō′rē-ă). A tendency of the visual axis of one eye to deviate downward and inward, prevented by binocular vision. [hypo- + G. *esō*, within, + *phoros*, bearing]

hy•po•es•the•sia (hī′pō-es-thē′zē-ă). SYN hypesthesia.

hy•po•ex•o•pho•ria (hī′pō-ek-sō-fō′rē-ă). A tendency of the visual axis of one eye to deviate downward and outward, prevented by binocular vision. [hypo- + G. *exō*, without, + *phoros*, bearing]

hy•po•fer•re•mia (hī′pō-fer-ē′mē-ă). A deficiency of iron in the circulating blood.

hy•po•fi•brin•o•ge•ne•mia (hī′pō-fī-brin′ō-jě-nē′mē-ă). Abnormally low concentration of fibrinogen in the circulating blood plasma.

hy•po•func•tion (hī′pō-fŭnk-shŭn). Reduced, low, or inadequate function.

hy•po•ga•lac•tia (hī′pō-ga-lak′shē-ă). Less than normal milk secretion. [hypo- + G. *gala*, milk]

hy•po•ga•lac•tous (hī′pō-ga-lak′tŭs). Producing or secreting a less than normal amount of milk.

hy•po•gam•ma•glob•u•lin•e•mia (hī′pō-gam′ă-glob′yū-li-nē′mē-ă). Decreased gamma fraction of serum globulin; associated with increased susceptibility to pyogenic infections.

transient h. of infancy, a type of primary immunodeficiency that occurs in infants, probably resulting from immaturity of lymphoid tissue.

X-linked h., X-linked infantile h. [MIM* 300300], a congenital, X-linked recessive, primary immunodeficiency characterized by decreased numbers (or absence) of circulating B-lymphocytes with corresponding decrease in immunoglobulins; associated with marked susceptibility to infection by pyogenic bacteria after loss of maternal antibodies.

hy•po•gan•gli•o•no•sis (hī′pō-gang-lē-on-ō′sis). A reduction in the number of ganglionic nerve cells.

hy•po•gas•tric (hī-pō-gas′trik). Relating to the hypogastrium.

hy•po•gas•tros•chi•sis (hī′pō-gas-tros′ki-sis). Congenital fissure of the abdominal wall in the hypogastric region. [hypogastrium + G. *schisis*, cleaving]

hy•po•gen•e•sis (hī′pō-jen′ĕ-sis). Congenital defect of growth with underdevelopment of parts or organs of the body. [hypo- + G. *genesis*, origin]

hy•po•ge•net•ic (hī′pō-jě-net′ik). Relating to hypogenesis.

hy•po•gen•i•tal•ism (hī-pō-jen′i-tăl-izm). Partial or complete failure of maturation of the genitalia; commonly, a consequence of hypogonadism.

hy•po•geu•sia (hī-pō-gū′sē-ă). Blunting of the sense of taste. [hypo- + G. *geusis*, taste]

hy•po•glos•sal (hī-pō-glos′ăl). **1.** Below the tongue. **2.** Relating to the twelfth cranial nerve, nervus hypoglossus. [L. *hypoglossus* fr. hypo- + *glossus*, tongue]

hy•po•glot•tis (hī′pō-glot′is). The undersurface of the tongue. [G. *hypoglōssis*, or -*glōttis*, undersurface of tongue, fr. *hypo*, under, + *glōssa*, tongue]

hy•po•gly•ce•mia (hī′pō-glī-sē′mē-ă). An abnor-

hy

mally small concentration of glucose in the circulating blood.

hy·po·gly·ce·mic (hī′pō-glī-sē′mik). Pertaining to or characterized by hypoglycemia.

hy·po·gly·co·gen·ol·y·sis (hī′pō-glī′kō-jĕ-nol′i-sis). Deficient glycogenolysis.

hy·po·gly·cor·rha·chia (hī′pō-glī-kō-rak′ē-ă). Depressed concentration of glucose in the cerebrospinal fluid; a characteristic of bacterial, fungal, and tuberculous meningitis. [hypo- + G. *glykys*, sweet, + *rhachis*, spine]

hy·pog·na·thous (hī′pō-nath′ŭs, hī-pog′na-thŭs). Having a congenitally defective lower jaw. [hypo- + G. *gnathos*, jaw]

hy·po·go·nad·ism (hī′pō-gō′nad-izm). Inadequate gonadal function, as manifested by deficiencies in gametogenesis and/or the secretion of gonadal hormones.

hy·po·go·nad·o·tro·pic (hī′pō-gon′ă-dō-trop′ik). Indicating inadequate secretion of gonadotropins and its consequences.

hy·po·hi·dro·sis (hī′pō-hī-drō′sis). Diminished perspiration.

hy·po·hi·drot·ic (hī′pō-hi-drot′ik). Characterized by diminished sweating.

hy·po·ka·le·mia (hī′pō-ka-lē′mē-ă). The presence of an abnormally small concentration of potassium ions in the circulating blood; occurs in familial periodic paralysis and in potassium depletion due to excessive loss from the gastrointestinal tract or kidneys. The changes of h. may include vacuolation of renal tubular epithelial cytoplasm with impairment of urinary concentrating power and acidification, flattening of the T wave of the electrocardiogram, and muscle weakness. SYN hypopotassemia. [hypo- + Mod. L. *kalium*, potassium, + G. *haima*, blood]

hy·po·ki·ne·sis, hy·po·ki·ne·sia (hī′pō-ki-nē′sis, -nē′zē-ă). Diminished or slow movement. SYN hypomotility. [hypo- + G. *kinēsis*, movement]

hy·po·ki·net·ic (hī′pō-ki-net′ik). Relating to or characterized by hypokinesis.

hy·po·ley·dig·ism (hī-pō-lī′dig-izm). Subnormal secretion of androgens by the interstitial (Leydig's) cells of the testes.

hy·po·mag·ne·se·mia (hī′pō-mag-nē-sē′mē-ă). Subnormal blood serum concentration of magnesium.

hy·po·mas·tia (hī′pō-mas′tē-ă). Atrophy or congenital smallness of the breasts. [hypo- + G. *mastos*, breast]

hy·po·me·lia (hī-pō-mē′lē-ă). General term for hypoplasia of some or all parts of one or more limbs. [hypo- + G. *melos*, limb]

hy·po·men·or·rhea (hī′pō-men-ō-rē′ă). Diminution of the flow or a shortening of the duration of menstruation. [hypo- + G. *mēn*, month, + *rhoia*, flow]

hy·po·mere (hī′pō-mēr). **1.** The portion of the myotome that extends ventrolaterally to form body-wall muscle, innervated by the primary ventral ramus of a spinal nerve. **2.** Somatic and splanchnic layers of the lateral mesoderm which give rise to the lining of the celom. [hypo- + G. *meros*, part]

hy·po·me·tab·o·lism (hī′pō-me-tab′ō-lizm). Reduced metabolism.

hy·po·met·ria (hī-pō-mē′trē-ă). Ataxia characterized by underreaching an object or goal; seen with cerebellar disease. Cf. hypermetria. [hypo- + G. *metron*, measure]

hy·pom·ne·sia (hī-pō-nē′zē-ă). Impaired memory. [hypo- + G. *mnēmē*, memory]

hy·po·morph (hī′pō-mōrf). **1.** A person whose standing height is short in proportion to the sitting height, owing to shortness of the limbs. Cf. endomorph. **2.** A mutant gene that causes a partial decrease in the activity controlled by the gene. [hypo- + G. *morphē*, form]

hy·po·mo·til·i·ty (hī′pō-mō-til′i-tē). SYN hypokinesis.

hy·po·my·e·li·na·tion, hy·po·my·e·lin·o·gen·e·sis (hī′pō-mī′ĕ-lin-ā-shun, -ō-jen′ĕ-sis). Defective formation of myelin in the spinal cord and brain; the basis for a number of demyelinating diseases.

hy·po·my·o·to·nia (hī′pō-mī-ō-tō′nē-ă). A condition of diminished muscular tonus. [hypo- + G. *mys (myo-)* muscle, + *tonos*, tension]

hy·po·myx·ia (hī′pō-mik′sē-ă). A condition in which the secretion of mucus is diminished. [hypo- + G. *myxa*, mucus]

hyponasality. Insufficient nasal resonance during speech, usually due to obstruction of the nasal tract. SYN hyporhinophonia.

hy·po·na·tre·mia (hī′pō-nă-trē′mē-ă). Abnormally low concentrations of sodium ions in the circulating blood. [hypo- + natrium, + G. *haima*, blood]

hy·po·ne·o·cy·to·sis (hī′pō-nē′ō-sī-tō′sis). Leukopenia associated with the presence of immature and young leukocytes (especially in the granulocytic series). [hypo- + G. *neos*, new, + *kytos*, cell, + *-osis*, condition]

hy·po·nych·i·al (hī′pō-nik′ē-ăl). **1.** SYN subungual. **2.** Relating to the hyponychium.

hy·po·nych·i·um (hī′pō-nik′ē-ŭm) [NA]. The epithelium of the nail bed, particularly its proximal part in the region of the nailroot and lunula, forming the nail matrix. [hypo- + G. *onyx*, nail]

hy·pon·y·chon (hī-pon′i-kon). An ecchymosis beneath a fingernail or toenail. [hypo- + G. *onyx*, nail]

hy·po·or·tho·cy·to·sis (hī′pō-ōr′thō-sī-tō′sis). Leukopenia in which the relative numbers of the various types of white blood cells are within the normal ranges. [hypo- + G. *orthos*, correct, + *kytos*, cell, + *-osis*, condition]

hy·po·pan·cre·a·tism (hī′pō-pan′krē-ă-tizm). A condition of diminished activity of digestive enzyme secretion by the pancreas.

hy·po·par·a·thy·roid·ism (hī′pō-par-ă-thī′roydizm). A condition due to diminution or absence of the secretion of the parathyroid hormones, with low serum calcium, tetany, and sometimes increased bone density. SEE ALSO pseudohypoparathyroidism.

hy·po·pha·lan·gism (hī′pō-fă-lan′jizm). Congenital absence of one or more of the phalanges of a finger or toe.

hy·po·phar·ynx (hī′pō-far′inks). SYN laryngopharynx.

hy·po·pho·ne·sis (hī′pō-fō-nē′sis). In percussion or auscultation, a sound that is diminished or fainter than usual. [hypo- + G. *phōnēsis*, a sounding]

hy·po·pho·ria (hī′pō-fō′rē-ă). A tendency of the visual axis of one eye to deviate downward, prevented by binocular vision. [hypo- + G. *phora*, motion]

hy·po·phos·pha·ta·sia (hī′pō-fos′fă-tā′zē-ă). An abnormally low content of alkaline phosphatase in the circulating blood.

hy·po·phos·pha·te·mia (hī′pō-fos-fă-tē′mē-ă). Abnormally low concentrations of phosphates in the circulating blood.

hy·po·phos·pha·tu·ria (hī′pō-fos′fă-tū′rē-ă). Reduced urinary excretion of phosphates.

hy·poph·y·sec·to·my (hī′pof-i-sek′tō-mē). Surgical removal of the hypophysis or pituitary gland.

hy·po·phys·e·o·priv·ic (hī′pō-fiz′ē-ō-priv′ik). SYN hypophysioprivic.

hy·po·phys·e·o·tro·pic (hī′pō-fiz′ē-ō-trop′ik). SYN hypophysiotropic.

hy·po·phy·si·al (hī′pō-fiz′ē-ăl). Relating to a hypophysis.

hy·po·phys·i·o·priv·ic (hī′pō-fiz′ē-ō-priv′ik). Pertaining to absence or depressed function of the pituitary gland. SYN hypophyseoprivic. [hypophysis + L. *privus*, deprived of]

hy·po·phys·i·o·tro·pic (hī′pō-fiz′ē-ō-trop′ik). Denoting a stimulatory hormone that acts on the pituitary gland (hypophysis). SYN hypophyseotropic.

hy·poph·y·sis (hī-pof′i-sis) [NA]. An unpaired compound gland suspended from the base of the hypothalamus by a short extension of the infundibulum, the infundibular or pituitary stalk. The h. consists of two major subdivisions: 1) the neurohypophysis, comprising the infundibulum and its bulbous termination, the neural part or infundibular process (posterior lobe), which is composed of neuroglia-like pituicytes, blood vessels, and unmyelinated nerve fibers of the hypothalamohypophyseal tract whose cell bodies reside in the supraoptic and paraventricular nuclei of the hypothalamus, and convey to the lobe for storage and release the neurosecretory hormones oxytocin and antidiuretic hormone; 2) the adenohypophysis, comprising the larger distal part, a sleevelike extension of this lobe (infundibular part) which invests the infundibular stalk, and a thin intermediate part (poorly developed in humans) between the anterior and posterior lobes; the anterior lobe consists of cords of cells of several different types interspersed with capillaries of the hypothalamohypophysial portal system; secretion of somatotropins, prolactin, thyroid-stimulating hormone, gonadotropins, adrenal corticotropin, and other related peptides in the adenohypophysis is regulated by releasing and inhibiting factors elaborated by neurons in the hypothalamus which are taken up by a primary plexus of capillaries in the median eminence and transported via portal vessels in the infundibular part and infundibular stem to a secondary plexus of capillaries in the distal part. SEE ALSO hypothalamus. SYN master gland, pituitary gland. [G. an undergrowth]

hy·poph·y·si·tis (hī-pof-i-sī′tis). Inflammation of the hypophysis.

 lymphocytic h., an acute anterior pituitary lymphocytic reaction characterized clinically by signs and symptoms of anterior pituitary insufficiency; probably an autoimmune disorder because antipituitary antibodies are present in the serum.

hy·po·pi·e·sis (hī′pō-pī-ē′sis). SYN hypotension (1). [hypo- + G. *piesis*, pressure]

hy·po·pi·tu·i·ta·rism (hī′pō-pi-tū′i-tă-rizm). A condition due to diminished activity of the anterior lobe of the hypophysis, with inadequate secretion of one or more anterior pituitary hormones.

hy·po·pla·sia (hī′pō-plā′zē-ă). **1.** Underdevelopment of a tissue or organ, usually due to a decrease in the number of cells. **2.** Atrophy due to destruction of some of the elements and not merely to their general reduction in size. [hypo- + G. *plasis*, a molding]

 renal h., an abnormally small kidney that is morphologically normal but has either a reduced number of nephrons or smaller nephrons.

hy·po·plas·tic (hī′pō-plas′tik). Pertaining to or characterized by hypoplasia.

hy·po·pnea (hī-pop′nē-ă). Breathing that is shallower, and/or slower, than normal. SYN oligopnea. [hypo- + G. *pnoē*, breathing]

hy·po·po·sia (hī′pō-pō′sē-ă). Hypodipsia, with emphasis on reduced tendency to drink rather than on the reduced sensation of thirst. [hypo- + G. *posis*, drinking]

hy·po·po·tas·se·mia (hī′pō-pō-ta-sē′mē-ă). SYN hypokalemia.

hy·po·prax·ia (hī-pō-prak′sē-ă). Deficient activity. [hypo- + G. *praxis*, action, + *-ia*, condition]

hy·po·pro·tein·e·mia (hī′pō-prō′tē-in-ē′mē-ă, -prō-tēn-). Abnormally small amounts of total protein in the blood.

hy·po·pro·throm·bin·e·mia (hī′pō-prō-throm′bin-ē′mē-ă). Abnormally small amounts of prothrombin in the circulating blood.

hy·pop·ty·a·lism (hī′pō-tī′ă-lizm). SYN hyposalivation. [hypo- + G. *ptyalon*, saliva]

hy·po·py·on (hī-pō′pi-on). The presence of leukocytes in the anterior chamber of the eye. [hypo- + G. *pyon*, pus]

hy·po·re·flex·ia (hī′pō-rē-flek′sē-ă). A condition in which the deep tendon reflexes are weakened.

hy·po·ren·i·ne·mia (hī′pō-ren-i-nē′mē-ă). Low levels of renin in the circulating blood.

hy·po·ren·i·nem·ic (hī′pō-ren-i-nē′mik). Denoting or characterized by hyporeninemia.

hyporhinophonia. SYN hyponasality.

hy·po·ri·bo·fla·vin·o·sis (hī′pō-rī′bō-flā-vi-nō′sis). NUTRITION a condition produced by a deficiency of riboflavin in the diet, characterized by cheilosis and magenta tongue and usually associated with other manifestations of B vitamin deficiency. A more correct term than the more commonly used ariboflavinosis.

hy·po·sal·i·va·tion (hī′pō-sal′i-vā′shŭn). Reduced salivation. SYN hypoptyalism.

hy

hy·po·scle·ral (hī-pō-sklēr′ăl). Beneath the sclerotic coat of the eyeball.

hy·po·sen·si·tiv·i·ty (hī′pō-sen-si-tiv′i-tē). A condition of subnormal sensitivity, in which the response to a stimulus is unusually delayed or lessened in degree.

hy·pos·mia (hī-poz′mē-ă). Diminished sense of smell. [hypo- + G. osmē, smell]

hy·po·so·ma·to·tro·pism (hī′pō-sō′mă-tō-trō′pizm). A state characterized by deficient secretion of pituitary growth hormone (somatotropin).

hy·po·spa·di·ac (hī′pō-spā′dē-ak). Relating to hypospadias.

hy·po·spa·di·as (hī′pō-spā′dē-ăs). A developmental anomaly characterized by a defect on the ventral surface of the penis so that the urethral meatus is more proximal than its normal glandular location; may be associated with chordee; also a similar defect in the female in which the urethra opens into the vagina. Cf. epispadias. [hypo- + G. spaō, to tear or gouge]

hy·po·splen·ism (hī′pō-splēn′izm). Absent or reduced splenic function, usually due to surgical removal, congenital aplasia, tumor replacement, or splenic vascular accident.

hy·pos·ta·sis (hi-pos′tă-sis). **1.** Formation of a sediment at the bottom of a liquid. **2.** SYN hypostatic *congestion*. **3.** The phenomenon whereby the phenotype that would ordinarily be manifested at one locus is obscured by the genotype at another epistatic locus. [G. *hypo-stasis*, a standing under, sediment]

hy·po·stat·ic (hī-pō-stat′ik). **1.** Sedimentary; resulting from a dependent position. **2.** Relating to hypostasis.

hy·po·sthe·nia (hī′pos-thē′nē-ă). Weakness. SEE asthenia. [hypo- + G. sthenos, strength]

hy·po·sthen·ic (hī-pos-then′ik). Weak.

hy·pos·the·nu·ria (hī′pos-thē-nū′rē-ă). Excretion of urine of low specific gravity, due to inability of the renal tubules to produce concentrated urine; also occurs following excessive water ingestion in diabetes insipidus. [hypo- + G. sthenos, strength, + ouron, urine]

hy·po·sto·mia (hī′pō-stō′mē-ă). A form of microstomia in which the oral opening is a small vertical slit. [hypo- + G. stoma, mouth]

hy·po·tel·or·ism (hī-pō-tel′ŏr-izm). Abnormal closeness of eyes. [hypo- + G. tēle, far off, + horizō, to separate, fr. horos, boundary]

hy·po·ten·sion (hī′pō-ten′shŭn). **1.** Subnormal arterial blood pressure. SYN hypopiesis. **2.** Reduced pressure or tension of any kind. [hypo- + L. tensio, a stretching]

  induced h., controlled h., deliberate acute reduction of arterial blood pressure to reduce operative blood loss by pharmacologic means during anesthesia and surgery.

  orthostatic h., a form of low blood pressure that occurs in a standing posture.

hy·po·ten·sive (hī′pō-ten′siv). Characterized by low blood pressure or causing reduction in blood pressure.

hy·po·thal·a·mus (hī′pō-thal′ă-mŭs) [NA]. The ventral and medial region of the diencephalon forming the walls of the ventral half of the third ventricle; it is delineated from the thalamus by the hypothalamic sulcus, lying medial to the internal capsule and subthalamus, continuous with the precommissural septum anteriorly and with the mesencephalic tegmentum and central gray substance posteriorly. Its ventral surface is marked by, from before backward, the optic chiasma, the unpaired infundibulum that extends by way of the infundibular stalk into the posterior lobe of the hypophysis, and the paired mamillary bodies. The nerve cells of the h. are grouped into the supraoptic paraventricular, lateral preoptic, lateral hypothalamic, tuberal, anterior hypothalamic, ventromedial, dorsomedial, arcuate, posterior hypothalamic, and premamillary nuclei and the mamillary body. It has afferent fiber connections with the mesencephalon, limbic system, cerebellum, and efferent fiber connections with the same structures and with the posterior lobe of the hypophysis; its functional connection with the anterior lobe of the hypophysis is established by the hypothalamohypophysial portal system. The h. is prominently involved in the functions of the autonomic nervous system and, through its vascular link with the anterior lobe of the hypophysis, in endocrine mechanisms; it also appears to play a role in neural mechanisms underlying moods and motivational states. SEE ALSO hypophysis. [hypo- + thalamus]

hy·po·the·nar (hī′pō-thē′nar, hī-poth′ĕ-nar). **1** [NA]. SYN hypothenar *eminence*. **2.** Denoting any structure in relation with the hypothenar eminence or its underlying collective components. [hypo- + G. thenar, the palm]

hy·po·ther·mal (hī-pō-ther′măl). Denoting hypothermia.

hy·po·ther·mia (hī′pō-ther′mē-ă). A body temperature significantly below 98.6°F (37°C). [hypo- + G. thermē, heat]

  accidental h., unintentional decrease in body temperature, especially in the newborn, infants, and elderly, particularly during operations.

  regional h., reduction of the temperature of an extremity or organ by external cold or perfusion with cold blood or solutions.

  total body h., the deliberate reduction of total body temperature, in order to reduce tissue metabolism.

hy·poth·e·sis (hī-poth′ĕ-sis). A conjecture cast in a form that is amenable to confirmation or refutation by experiment and the assembly of data; not to be confused with assumption, postulation, or unfocused speculation. SEE ALSO postulate, theory. [G. foundation, assumption fr. hypotithēmi, to lay down]

  autocrine h., that tumor cells containing viral oncogenes may have encoded a growth factor, normally produced by other cell types, and thereby produce the factor autonomously, leading to uncontrolled proliferation.

  Lyon h., SYN lyonization.

  Michaelis-Menten h., that a complex is formed between an enzyme and its substrate (the O'Sullivan-Tompson h.), which complex then decomposes to yield free enzyme and the reaction products (Brown h.), the latter rate determining the overall rate of substrate-product conversion.

  null h., the statistical hypothesis that one variable has no association with another, or that experimental results do not differ from those that might be expected by the operation of chance alone.

Starling's h., the principle that net filtration through capillary membranes is proportional to the transmembrane hydrostatic pressure difference minus the transmembrane oncotic pressure difference.

zwitter h., that an amphoteric molecule (*e.g.,* an amino acid) has, at its isoelectric point, equal numbers of positive and negative charges, thus becoming a zwitterion.

hy·po·throm·bi·ne·mia (hī′pō-throm-bin-ē′mē-ă). Abnormally small amounts of thrombin in the circulating blood.

hy·po·thy·mia (hī′pō-thī′mē-ă). Depression of spirits; the "blues." [hypo- + G. *thymos,* mind, soul]

hy·po·thy·roid (hī′pō-thī′royd). Marked by reduced thyroid function.

hy·po·thy·roid·ism (hī′pō-thī′royd-izm). Diminished production of thyroid hormone, leading to clinical manifestations of thyroid insufficiency, including low metabolic rate, tendency to weight gain, somnolence and sometimes myxedema. [hypo- + G. *thyreoeidēs,* thyroid]

  congenital h., lack of thyroid secretion. SEE infantile h.

  infantile h., can be due to endemic congenital goiter, nonendemic cases are usually due to defective thyroidal embryogenesis, defective hypothalamic-pituitary function, congenital defects in thyroid hormone synthesis or action, or intrauterine exposure to goitrogenic agents.

hy·po·to·nia (hī′pō-tō′nē-ă). **1.** Reduced tension in any part, as in the eyeball. **2.** Relaxation of the arteries. **3.** A condition in which there is a diminution or loss of muscular tonicity, in consequence of which the muscles may be stretched beyond their normal limits. SYN hypotonicity (1). [hypo- + G. *tonos,* tone]

hy·po·ton·ic (hī-pō-ton′ik). **1.** Having a lesser degree of tension. **2.** Having a lesser osmotic pressure than a reference solution, ordinarily plasma or interstitial fluid.

hy·po·to·nic·i·ty (hī′pō-tō-nis′i-tē). **1.** SYN hypotonia. **2.** A decreased effective osmotic pressure.

hy·po·tri·cho·sis (hī′pō-tri-kō′sis). A less than normal amount of hair on the head and/or body. [hypo- + G. *trichōsis,* hairiness]

hy·po·tro·pia (hī-pō-trō′pē-ă). An ocular deviation with one eye lower than the other. [hypo- + G. *tropē,* turn]

hy·po·tym·pa·not·o·my (hī′pō-tim-pă-not′ō-mē). Surgical extirpation, without sacrifice of hearing, of small tumors confined to the lower tympanic cavity. [hypo- + G. *tympanon,* tympanum, + *tomē,* incision]

hy·po·tym·pa·num (hī′pō-tim′pă-nŭm). The lower part of the tympanic cavity.

hy·po·u·ri·ce·mia (hī′pō-yū-ri-sē′mē-ă). Reduced blood concentration of uric acid.

hy·po·u·ri·cu·ria (hī′pō-yū′ri-kyū′rē-ă). Reduced excretion of uric acid in the urine.

hy·po·ven·ti·la·tion (hī′pō-ven-ti-lā′shŭn). Reduced alveolar ventilation relative to metabolic

carbon dioxide production, so that alveolar carbon dioxide pressure increases above normal.

hy·po·vi·ta·min·o·sis (hī′pō-vī′tă-min-ō′sis). Insufficiency of one or more vitamins in the diet; manifested first by depletion of tissue levels, then by functional changes, and finally by appearance of morphologic lesions. Cf. avitaminosis.

hy·po·vo·le·mia (hī′pō-vō-lē′mē-ă). A decreased amount of blood in the body. SYN hyphemia. [hypo- + L. *volumen,* volume, + G. *haima,* blood]

hy·po·vo·le·mic (hī′pō-vō-lē′mik). Pertaining to or characterized by hypovolemia.

hy·po·vo·lia (hī-pō-vō′lē-ă). Diminished water content or volume of a given compartment; *e.g.,* extracellular h. [hypo- + L. *volumen,* volume]

hy·po·xan·thine (hī-pō-zan′thin). A purine present in the muscles and other tissues, formed during purine catabolism by deamination of adenine; elevated in molybdenum-cofactor deficiency.

hy·pox·e·mia (hī-pok-sē′mē-ă). Subnormal oxygenation of arterial blood, short of anoxia. [hypo- + oxygen, + G. *haima,* blood]

hy·pox·ia (hī-pok′sē-ă). Decrease below normal levels of oxygen in inspired gases, arterial blood, or tissue, short of anoxia. [hypo- + oxygen]

  anemic h., h. resulting from a decreased concentration of functional hemoglobin or a reduced number of erythrocytes.

  diffusion h., decrease in alveolar oxygen tension when room air is inhaled at the conclusion of nitrous oxide anesthesia, because nitrous oxide diffusing out of the blood dilutes the alveolar oxygen.

  hypoxic h., h. resulting from a defective mechanism of oxygenation in the lungs.

  ischemic h., tissue h. characterized by tissue oligemia and caused by arterial or arteriolar obstruction or vasoconstriction.

  oxygen affinity h., h. due to reduced ability of hemoglobin to release oxygen.

hy·pox·ic (hī-pok′sik). Denoting or characterized by hypoxia.

hyp·sa·rhyth·mia, hyp·sar·rhyth·mia (hip′să-rith′mē-ă). The abnormal and characteristically chaotic electroencephalogram in patients with infantile spasms. [G. *hypsi,* high, + *a-* priv. + *rhythmos,* rhythm]

⌂ **hyster-.** SEE hystero-.

hys·ter·al·gia (his′ter-al′jē-ă). Pain in the uterus. SYN hysterodynia, metrodynia. [hystero- + G. *algos,* pain]

hys·ter·a·tre·sia (his′ter-ă-trē′zē-ă). Atresia of the uterine cavity, usually resulting from inflammatory endocervical adhesions.

hys·ter·ec·to·my (his-ter-ek′tō-mē). Removal of the uterus; unless otherwise specified, usually denotes complete removal of the uterus (corpus and cervix). [hystero- + G. *ektomē,* excision]

  abdominal h., removal of the uterus through an incision in the abdominal wall. SYN abdomino-hysterectomy.

  cesarean h., cesarean section followed by h.

  radical h., complete removal of the uterus, upper vagina, and parametrium.

  supracervical h., removal of the fundus of the uterus, leaving the cervix.

vaginal h., removal of the uterus through the vagina.

hys·ter·e·sis (his-ter-ē'sis). **1.** Failure of either one of two related phenomena to keep pace with the other; or any situation in which the value of one depends upon whether the other has been increasing or decreasing. Cf. allosterism. **2.** The lag of a magnetic effect behind its cause. **3.** The temperature differential that exists when a substance melts at one temperature and solidifies at another. **4.** A type of cooperativity in enzyme-catalyzed reactions in which the degree of cooperativity is associated with a slow conformational change of the enzyme. Cf. allosterism. [G. *hysterēsis,* a coming later]

hys·ter·eu·ry·sis (his-ter-yū'rē-sis). Dilation of the lower segment and cervical canal of the uterus. [hystero- + G. *eurynō,* to dilate, fr. *eurys,* wide]

hys·te·ria (his-ter'ē-ă, his-tēr'). A somatoform disorder in which there is an alteration or loss of physical functioning that suggests a physical disorder such as paralysis of an arm or disturbance of vision, but that is instead apparently an expression of a psychological conflict or need. [G. *hystera,* womb, from the original notion of womb-related disturbances in women]

anxiety h., h. characterized by manifest anxiety.

conversion h., h. characterized by the substitution of physical signs or symptoms such as blindness, deafness, and paralysis for anxiety. SYN conversion hysteria neurosis, conversion reaction.

mass h., (1) simultaneous identical physical and/or emotional symptoms among a group of individuals; **(2)** a socially contagious frenzy of irrational behavior in a group of people as a reaction to an event.

minor h., a mild form of h. characterized chiefly by subjective pains, nervousness, undue sensitiveness, and sometimes episodes of emotional excitement, but without paralysis or other such symptoms.

hys·ter·i·cal, hys·ter·ic (his-ter'ē-kăl, -ter'ik). Relating to or characterized by hysteria.

hys·ter·ics (his-ter'iks). An expression of emotion accompanied often by crying, laughing, and screaming.

hystero-, hyster-. 1. The uterus. SEE ALSO metr-, utero-. [G. *hystera,* womb (uterus)] **2.** Hysteria. [G. *hystera,* womb (uterus)] **3.** Later, following. [G. *hysteros,* later]

hys·ter·o·cat·a·lep·sy (his'ter-ō-kat'ă-lep-sē). Hysteria with cataleptic manifestations.

hys·ter·o·cele (his'ter-ō-sēl). **1.** An abdominal or perineal hernia containing part or all of the uterus. **2.** Protrusion of uterine contents into a weakened, bulging area of uterine wall. [hystero- + G. *kēlē,* hernia]

hys·ter·o·clei·sis (his'ter-ō-klī'sis). Operative occlusion of the uterus. [hystero- + G. *kleisis,* closure]

hys·ter·o·dyn·ia (his'ter-ō-din'ē-ă). SYN hysteralgia. [hystero- + G. *odynē,* pain]

hys·ter·o·ep·i·lep·sy (his'ter-ō-ep'i-lep-sē). Hysterical convulsions.

hys·ter·o·gen·ic, hys·ter·og·en·ous (his-ter-ō-jen'ik, his-ter-oj'ĕ-nŭs). Causing hysterical symptoms or reactions. [hysteria + G. *-gen,* producing]

hys·ter·o·gram (his'ter-ō-gram). **1.** X-ray examination of the uterus, usually using a contrast medium. **2.** A recording of the strength of uterine contractions.

hys·ter·o·graph (his'ter-ō-graf). Apparatus for recording the strength of uterine contractions.

hys·ter·og·ra·phy (his'ter-og'ră-fē). **1.** Radiographic examination of the uterine cavity filled with a contrast medium. **2.** Graphic procedure used to record uterine contractions. [hystero- + G. *graphō,* to write]

hys·ter·oid (his'ter-oyd). Resembling or simulating hysteria. [hystero- + G. *eidos,* resemblance]

hys·ter·ol·y·sis (his-ter-ol'i-sis). Breaking up of adhesions between the uterus and neighboring parts. [hystero- + G. *lysis,* dissolution]

hys·ter·om·e·ter (his-ter-om'ĕ-ter). A graduated sound for measuring the depth of the uterine cavity. SYN uterometer. [hystero- + G. *metron,* measure]

hys·ter·o·my·o·ma (his'ter-ō-mī-ō'mă). A myoma of the uterus. [hystero- + G. *mys,* muscle, + *-oma,* tumor]

hys·ter·o·my·o·mec·to·my (his'ter-ō-mī-ō-mek'tō-mē). Operative removal of a uterine myoma. [hysteromyoma + G. *ektomē,* excision]

hys·ter·o·my·ot·o·my (his'ter-ō-mī-ot'ō-mē). Incision into the muscles of the uterus. [hystero- + G. *mys,* muscle, + *tomē,* incision]

hys·ter·o·o·oph·o·rec·to·my (his'ter-ō-ō'of-ō-rek'tō-mē). Surgical removal of the uterus and ovaries. [hystero- + G. *ōon,* egg, + *phoros,* bearing, + *ektomē,* excision]

hys·ter·op·a·thy (his-ter-op'ă-thē). Any disease of the uterus. [hystero- + G. *pathos,* suffering]

hys·ter·o·pex·y (his'ter-ō-pek-sē). Fixation of a displaced or abnormally movable uterus. SYN uterofixation, uteropexy. [hystero- + G. *pēxis,* fixation]

hys·ter·o·plas·ty (his'ter-ō-plas-tē). SYN uteroplasty.

hys·ter·or·rha·phy (his'ter-ōr'ă-fē). Sutural repair of a lacerated uterus. [hystero- + G. *rhaphē,* suture]

hys·ter·or·rhex·is (his'ter-ō-rek'sis). Rupture of the uterus. [hystero- + G. *rhēxis,* rupture]

hys·ter·o·sal·pin·gec·to·my (his'ter-ō-sal-pin-jek'tō-mē). Operation for the removal of the uterus and one or both uterine tubes. [hystero- + G. *salpinx,* a trumpet, + *ektomē,* excision]

hys·ter·o·sal·pin·gog·ra·phy (his'ter-ō-sal-ping-gog'ră-fē). Radiography of the uterus and uterine tubes after the injection of radiopaque material. SYN hysterotubography, metrosalpingography, uterosalpingography, uterotubography. [hystero- + G. *salpinx,* a trumpet, + *graphō,* to write]

hys·ter·o·sal·pin·go·o·oph·o·rec·to·my (his'ter-ō-sal-ping'gō-ō-of-ō-rek'tō-mē). Excision of the uterus, oviducts, and ovaries. [hystero- + G. *salpinx,* trumpet, + *ōon,* egg, + *phoros,* bearing, + *ektomē,* excision]

hys·ter·o·sal·pin·gos·to·my (his'ter-ō-sal-ping-gos'tō-mē). Operation to restore patency of a uterine tube. [hystero- + G. *salpinx,* trumpet, + *stoma,* mouth]

hys·ter·o·scope (his′ter-ō-skōp). An endoscope used in direct visual examination of the uterine cavity. SYN metroscope, uteroscope. [hystero- + G. *skopeō,* to view]

hys·ter·os·co·py (his-ter-os′kŏ-pē). Visual instrumental inspection of the uterine cavity. SYN uteroscopy.

hys·ter·o·spasm (his′ter-ō-spazm). Spasm of the uterus.

hys·ter·ot·o·my (his-ter-ot′ō-mē). Incision of the uterus. SYN uterotomy. [hystero- + G. *tomē,* incision]

  abdominal h., transabdominal incision into the uterus. Also called abdominohysterotomy; celiohysterotomy; laparohysterotomy; laparouterotomy. SYN abdominohysterotomy.

  vaginal h., incision into the uterus via the vagina.

hys·ter·o·trach·e·lec·to·my (his′ter-ō-trak-el-ek′tō-mē). Removal of the cervix uteri. [hystero- + G. *trachēlos,* neck, + *ektomē,* excision]

hys·ter·o·trach·e·lo·plas·ty (his′ter-ō-trak′ĕ-lō-plas-tē). Plastic surgery of the cervix uteri. [hystero- + G. *trachēlos,* neck, + *plastos,* formed, shaped]

hys·ter·o·tra·che·lor·rha·phy (his′ter-ō-trak-ĕ-lōr′ă-fē). Sutural repair of a lacerated cervix uteri. [hystero- + G. *trachēlos,* neck, + *rhaphē,* a seam]

hys·ter·o·trach·e·lot·o·my (his′ter-ō-trak-ĕ-lot′ō-mē). Incision of the cervix uteri. [hystero- + G. *trachēlos,* neck, + *tomē,* incision]

hys·ter·o·tu·bog·ra·phy (his′ter-ō-tū-bog′ră-fē). SYN hysterosalpingography.

Hz hertz.

I

ι (ī-ō′ta) iota. SEE iota.

I 1. iodine; luminous *intensity* or radiant *intensity*; ionic *strength* (in mol/L); isoleucine; inosine. **2.** intensity of electrical current, expressed in amperes. **3.** As a subscript, symbol for inspired *gas.* **4.** Designation for I blood group (see Blood Groups appendix).

△**-ia.** Condition, used in formation of names of many diseases. Cf. -ism. [G. *-ia,* an ancient noun-forming suffix]

IAP intermittent acute *porphyria.*

△**-iasis.** A condition or state, especially an unhealthy one. [G. suffix forming nouns from verbs]

iat·ric (ī-at′rik). Pertaining to medicine or to a physician or healer. [G. *iatros,* physician]

△**iatro-.** Physicians, medicine, treatment. Cf. medico-. [G. *iatros,* physician]

iat·ro·gen·ic (ī-at-rō-jen′ik). Denoting response to medical or surgical treatment, induced by the treatment itself; usually used for unfavorable responses. [iatro- + G. *-gen,* producing]

△**-ic. 1.** Suffix denoting of, pertaining to. **2.** Chemical suffix denoting an element in a compound in one of its highest valencies. Cf. -ous (1). **3.** Suffix indicating an acid. [L. *-icus,* fr. G. *-ikos*]

ICD *International Classification of Diseases.*

ICDA *International Classification of Diseases, Adapted for Use in the United States.*

ICF 1. intracellular *fluid.* **2.** intermediate care facility **3.** intermediate care nursing facility

ichor (ī′kōr). Rarely used term for a thin watery discharge from an ulcer or unhealthy wound. [G. *ichōr,* serum]

icho·roid (ī′kō-royd). Denoting a thin purulent discharge. [G. *ichōr,* serum, + *eidos,* resemblance]

ichor·ous (ī′kōr-ŭs). Relating to or resembling ichor.

ichor·rhea (ī′kō-rē′ă). A profuse ichorous discharge. [G. *ichōr,* serum, + *rhoia,* a flow]

ich·thy·ism (ik′thi-izm). Poisoning by eating stale or otherwise unfit fish. [G. *ichthys,* fish]

△**ichthyo-.** Fish. [G. *ichthys*]

ich·thy·oid (ik′thē-oyd). Fish-shaped. [ichthyo- + G. *eidos,* resemblance]

ich·thy·o·sis (ik-thē-ō′sis). Congenital disorders of keratinization characterized by noninflammatory dryness and scaling of the skin, often associated with other defects and with abnormalities of lipid metabolism; distinguishable genetically, clinically, microscopically, and by epidermal cell kinetics. [ichthyo- + G. *-osis,* condition]

ich·thy·ot·ic (ik-thē-ot′ik). Relating to ichthyosis.

ich·thy·o·tox·ism (ik′thē-ō-tok′sizm). Poisoning by fish. [ichthyo- + G. *toxikon,* poison]

ICP intracranial *pressure.*

ICRP International Commission on Radiological Protection.

△**-ics.** Organized knowledge, practice, treatment. [-ic + -s]

ICSH interstitial cell-stimulating hormone.

ic·tal (ik′tăl). Relating to or caused by a stroke or seizure. [L. *ictus,* a stroke]

ic·ter·ic (ik-ter′ik). Relating to or marked by jaundice. [G. *ikterikos,* jaundiced]

△**ictero-.** Icterus. [G. *ikteros,* jaundice]

ic·ter·o·gen·ic (ik′ter-ō-jen′ik). Causing jaundice. [ictero- + G. *-gen,* producing]

ic·ter·o·hep·a·ti·tis (ik′ter-ō-hep-ă-tī′tis). Inflammation of the liver with jaundice as a prominent symptom. [ictero- + G. *hēpar,* liver, + *-itis,* inflammation]

ic·ter·oid (ik′ter-oyd). Yellow-hued, or seemingly jaundiced. [ictero- + G. *eidos,* resemblance]

ic·ter·us (ik′ter-ŭs). SYN jaundice. [G. *ikteros*]

 i. gra′vis, jaundice associated with high fever and delirium; seen in severe hepatitis and other diseases of the liver with severe functional failure. SYN malignant jaundice.

 i. neonato′rum, i. in the newborn, which can be accentuated by excessive hemolysis, sepsis, neonatal hepatitis, or congenital atresia of the biliary system. SYN physiologic i. SYN jaundice of the newborn, physiologic jaundice.

 physiologic i., SYN i. neonatorum.

ic·tus (ik′tŭs). **1.** A stroke or attack. **2.** A beat. [L.]

ICU intensive care *unit.*

id. 1. PSYCHOANALYSIS One of three components of the psychic apparatus in the freudian structural framework, the other two being the ego and superego. It is completely in the unconscious realm, is unorganized, and is the reservoir of psychic energy or libido, and is under the influence of the primary processes. **2.** The total of all psychic energy available from the innate biologic hungers, appetites, bodily needs, drives and impulses, in a newborn infant. [L. *id,* that]

△**-id. 1.** A state of sensitivity of the skin in which a part remote from the primary lesion reacts ("-id reaction") to the pathogen, giving rise to a secondary inflammatory lesion; the lesion manifesting the reaction is designated by the use of -id as a suffix. [G. *-eidēs,* resembling, through Fr. *-id*] **2.** Small, young specimen. [G. *-idion,* a diminutive ending]

IDDM insulin-dependent *diabetes* mellitus.

△**-ide. 1.** Suffix denoting the more electronegative element in a binary chemical compound. **2.** Suffix (in a sugar name) indicating substitution for the H of the hemiacetal OH; *e.g.,* glycoside.

IDEA Individuals with Disabilities Education Act.

idea (ī-dē′ă). Any mental image or concept. [G. semblance]

 autochthonous i.'s, thoughts that suddenly burst into awareness as if they are vitally important, often as if they have come from an outside source.

 compulsive i., a fixed and repetitively recurring i.

 dominant i., an i. that governs all one's actions and thoughts.

 fixed i., (1) an exaggerated notion, belief, or delusion that persists, despite evidence to the contrary, and controls the mind; **(2)** the obstinate conviction of a psychotic person regarding the correctness of a delusion.

flight of i.'s, an uncontrollable symptom of the manic phase of a bipolar depressive disorder in which streams of unrelated words and i.'s occur to the patient at a rate that is impossible to vocalize despite a marked increase in the individual's overall output of words. SEE ALSO mania.

i. of reference, the misinterpretation that other people's statements or acts or neutral objects in the environment are directed toward one's self when, in fact, they are not.

ide·al (ī-dēl′). A standard of perfection.

ego i., the part of the personality that comprises the goals, aspirations, and aims of the self, usually growing out of the emulation of a significant person with whom one has identified.

ide·a·tion (ī-dē-ā′shŭn). The formation of ideas or thoughts.

ide·a·tion·al (ī-dē-ā′shŭn-ăl). Relating to ideation.

iden·ti·fi·ca·tion (ī-den′ti-fi-kā′shŭn). A sense of oneness with another person or group; a defense mechanism whereby anxiety regarding one's personal identity or worth is dissipated by perceiving oneself as having characteristics in common with a person in the public eye, or (in childhood) identifying with a more powerful person such as a parent. [Mediev. L. *identicus,* fr. L. *idem,* the same, + *facio,* to make]

iden·ti·ty (ī-den′ti-tē). The sum of characteristics by which a person is recognized (by self and others).

ego i., the ego's sense of its own identity.

gender i., the sex role adopted by an individual; the degree to which an individual acts out a stereotypical masculine or feminine role in everyday behavior. Cf. gender *role,* sex *role.*

ideo-. Ideas; ideation Cf. idio-. [G. *idea,* form, notion]

ide·ol·o·gy (ī-dē-ol′ō-jē, id-ē-). The composite system of ideas, beliefs, and attitudes that constitutes an individual's or group's organized view of others. [ideo- + G. *logos,* study]

idio-. Private, distinctive, peculiar to. Cf. ideo-. [G. *idios,* one's own]

id·i·o·gram (id′ē-ō-gram). **1.** SYN karyotype. **2.** Diagrammatic representation of chromosome morphology characteristic of a species or population. [idio- + G. *gramma,* something written]

id·i·o·het·er·o·ag·glu·ti·nin (id′ē-ō-het′er-ō-ă-glū′tin-in). An idioagglutinin occurring in the blood of one animal, but capable of combining with the antigenic material from another species. [idio- + G. *heteros,* another, + agglutinin]

id·i·o·het·er·o·ly·sin (id′ē-ō-het-er-ol′i-sin). An idiolysin occurring in the blood of one species, but capable of hemolyzing red blood cells of another species.

id·i·o·i·so·ag·glu·ti·nin (id′ē-ō-ī′sō-ă-glū′tin-in). An idioagglutinin occurring in the blood of a certain species, capable of agglutinating cells from animals of the same species. [idio- + G. *isos,* equal, + agglutinin]

id·i·o·i·sol·y·sin (id′ē-ō-ī-sol′y-sin). An idiolysin occurring in the blood of an animal of a certain species, capable of hemolyzing red blood cells from animals of the same species.

id·i·ol·y·sin (id-ē-ol′i-sin). A lysin that occurs naturally in the blood of a person or an animal, without the injection of a stimulating antigen or the passive transfer of antibody.

id·i·o·path·ic (id′ē-ō-path′ik). Denoting a disease of unknown cause. SYN agnogenic. [idio- + G. *pathos,* suffering]

id·i·op·a·thy (id-ē-op′ă-thē). An idiopathic disease. [idio- + G. *pathos,* suffering]

id·i·o·phren·ic (id′ē-ō-fren′ik). Relating to, or originating in, the mind or brain alone, not reflex or secondary. [idio- + G. *phrēn,* mind]

id·i·o·syn·cra·sy (id′ē-ō-sin′kră-sē). **1.** An individual mental, behavioral, or physical characteristic or peculiarity. **2.** PHARMACOLOGY An abnormal reaction to a drug, sometimes specified as genetically determined. [G. *idiosynkrasia,* fr. *idios,* one's own, + *synkrasis,* a mixing together]

id·i·o·syn·crat·ic (id′ē-ō-sin-krat′ik). Relating to or marked by an idiosyncrasy.

id·i·ot-sa·vant (ē-dē-ō′ sah-vahn′). A person of low general intelligence who possesses an unusual facility in performing certain mental tasks of which most normal persons are incapable. [Fr.]

id·i·o·type (id′ē-ō-tīp). A determinant that confers on an immunoglobulin molecule an antigenic "individuality" and is frequently a unique attribute of a given antibody in a given animal. [idio- + G. *typos,* model]

id·i·o·ven·tric·u·lar (id-ē-ō-ven-trik′yū-lăr). Pertaining to or associated with the cardiac ventricles alone.

IEP individualized education *program.*

IF initiation *factor*; intrinsic *factor.*

IFN interferon.

Ig immunoglobulin.

IgA immunoglobulin A.

IgD immunoglobulin D.

IgE immunoglobulin E.

IGF insulin-like growth *factors,* under *factor.*

IgG immunoglobulin G.

IgM immunoglobulin M.

ig·ni·punc·ture (ig′ni-pŭngk-chūr). The original procedure of closing a retinal separation by transfixation with cautery. [L. *ignis,* fire, + puncture]

IL interleukin.

IL-3 interleukin-3.

IL-4 interleukin-4.

IL-5 interleukin-5.

IL-6 interleukin-6.

IL-7 interleukin-7.

IL-8 interleukin-8.

IL-9 interleukin-9.

IL-10 interleukin-10.

IL-11 interleukin-11.

IL-12 interleukin-12.

IL-13 interleukin-13.

IL-14 interleukin-14.

IL-15 interleukin-15.

ILA insulin-like *activity.*

il·e·ac (il′ē-ak). **1.** Relating to ileus. **2.** Relating to the ileum.

il·e·al (il′ē-ăl). Of or pertaining to the ileum.

il·e·ec·to·my (il-ē-ek′tō-mē). Removal of the ileum. [ileum + G. *ektomē,* excision]

il·e·i·tis (il-ē-ī′tis). Inflammation of the ileum.
distal i., regional i., terminal i., SYN regional *enteritis.*

△**ileo-.** The ileum; bottom of the small intestine. [New L. *ileum,* groin]

il·e·o·ce·cal (il′ē-ō-sē′kăl). Relating to both ileum and cecum.

il·e·o·ce·cos·to·my (il′ē-ō-sē-kos′tŏ′mē). Anastomosis of the ileum to the cecum. SYN cecoileostomy.

il·e·o·co·lic (il′ē-ō-kol′ik). Relating to the ileum and the colon.

il·e·o·co·li·tis (il′ē-ō-kō-lī′tis). Inflammation of both ileum and colon.

il·e·o·co·los·to·my (il′ē-ō-kō-los′tō-mē). Establishment of a new communication between the ileum and the colon. [ileo- + colostomy]

il·e·o·cys·to·plas·ty (il′ē-ō-sis′tō-plas-tē). Surgical reconstruction of the bladder involving the use of an isolated intestinal segment to augment bladder capacity. [ileo- + G. *kystis,* bladder, + *plastos,* formed]

il·e·o·il·e·os·to·my (il′ē-ō-il-ē-os′tō-mē). 1. Establishment of a communication between two segments of the ileum. 2. The opening so established. [ileum + ileum + G. *stoma,* mouth]

il·e·o·je·ju·ni·tis (il′ē-ō-je-jū-nī′tis). A chronic inflammatory condition involving the jejunum and the ileum.

il·e·o·pexy (il′ē-ō-pek′sē). Surgical fixation of ileum. [ileo- + G. *pēxis,* fixation]

il·e·o·proc·tos·to·my (il′ē-ō-prok-tos′tō-mē). Establishment of a communication between the ileum and the rectum. [ileo- + G. *prōktos,* anus (rectum), + *stoma,* mouth]

il·e·or·rha·phy (il′ē-ōr′ă-fē). Suturing the ileum. [ileo- + G. *rhaphē,* suture]

il·e·o·sig·moid·os·to·my (il′ē-ō-sig′moyd-os′tō-mē). Establishment of a communication between the ileum and the sigmoid colon. [ileo- + sigmoid, + G. *stoma,* mouth]

▊**il·e·os·to·my** (il′ē-os′tō-mē). Establishment of a fistula through which the ileum discharges directly to the outside of the body. [ileo- + G. *stoma,* mouth]

il·e·ot·o·my (il′ē-ot′ō-mē). Incision into the ileum. [ileo- + G. *tomē,* incision]

il·e·um (il′ē-ŭm) [NA]. The third portion of the small intestine, about 3.6 m (12 ft) in length, extending from the jejunum to the ileocecal opening. [L. fr. G. *eileō,* to roll up, twist]

il·e·us (il′ē-ŭs). Mechanical, dynamic, or adynamic obstruction of the bowel; may be accompanied by severe colicky pain, abdominal distention, vomiting, absence of passage of stool, and often fever and dehydration. [G. *eileos,* intestinal colic, from *eilō,* to roll up tight]
adynamic i., obstruction of the bowel due to paralysis of the bowel wall, usually as a result of localized or generalized peritonitis or shock. SYN paralytic i.
dynamic i., intestinal obstruction due to spastic contraction of a segment of the bowel. SYN spastic i.
mechanical i., obstruction of the bowel due to some mechanical cause, *e.g.,* volvulus, gallstone, adhesions.

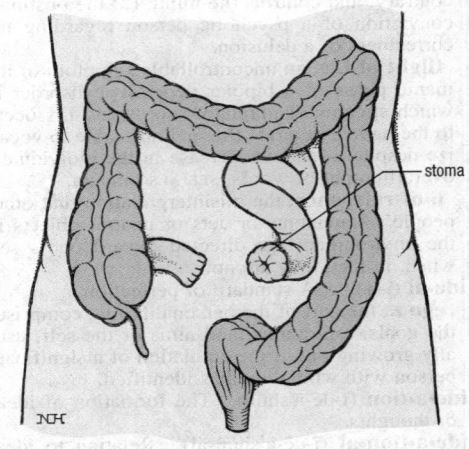
— stoma

ileostomy

meconium i., intestinal obstruction in the fetus and newborn following inspissation of meconium and caused by lack of trypsin; associated with cystic fibrosis.
occlusive i., complete mechanical blocking of the intestinal lumen.
paralytic i., SYN adynamic i.
spastic i., SYN dynamic i.
i. subpar′ta, obstruction of the large bowel by pressure of the pregnant uterus.

il·i·ac (il′ē-ak). Relating to the ilium.

△**ilio-.** The ilium; top of hip bone. [L. *ilium*]

il·i·o·coc·cyg·e·al (il′ē-ō-kok-sij′ē-ăl). Relating to the ilium and the coccyx.

il·i·o·fem·o·ral (il′ē-ō-fem′ŏ-răl). Relating to the ilium and the femur.

il·i·o·in·gui·nal (il′ē-ō-ing′gwi-năl). Relating to the iliac region and the groin.

il·i·o·lum·bar (il-ē-ō-lŭm′băr). Relating to the iliac and the lumbar regions.

il·i·o·pec·tin·e·al (il′ē-ō-pek-tin′ē-ăl). Relating to the ilium and the pubis.

il·i·o·tro·chan·ter·ic (il′ē-ō-trō-kan-ter′ik). Relating to the ilium and the great trochanter of the femur.

il·i·um, pl. **il·ia** (il′ē-ŭm, il′ē-ă). The broad, flaring portion of the hip bone, distinct at birth but later becoming fused with the ischium and pubis; it consists of a body, which joins the pubis and ischium to form the acetabulum and a broad thin portion, called the ala or wing. SYN iliac bone. [L. groin, flank]

ill·ness (il′nes). SYN disease (1).
mental i., (1) a broadly inclusive term, generally denoting one or all of the following: 1) a disease of the brain, with predominant behavioral symptoms; 2) a disease of the "mind" or personality, evidenced by abnormal behavior, as in hysteria or schizophrenia; **(2)** any psychiatric illness listed in *Current Medical Information and Terminology* of the American Medical Association or in the *Diagnostic and Statistical Manual of Men-*

tal Disorders of the American Psychiatric Association. SEE ALSO behavior *disorder*.

il·lu·sion (i-lū′zhŭn). A false perception; the mistaking of something for what it is not. [L. *illusio*, fr. *il- ludo*, pp. *-lusus*, to play at, mock]

il·lu·sion·al (i-lū′zhŭn-ăl). Relating to or of the nature of an illusion.

IM internal *medicine*.

im·age (im′ij). **1.** Representation of an object made by the rays of light emanating or reflected from it. **2.** Representation produced by x-rays, ultrasound, tomography, thermography, radioisotopes, etc. **3.** To produce such a representation. [L. *imago*, likeness]

body i., **(1)** the cerebral representation of all body sensation organized in the parietal cortex; **(2)** personal conception of one's own body as distinct from one's actual body or the conception other persons have of it.

false i., the i. in the deviating eye in strabismus.

homonymous i.'s, double i.'s produced by stimuli arising from points proximal to the horopter.

latent i., the undeveloped i. on an exposed x-ray film; it becomes visible after chemical processing.

mental i., a picture of an object not present, produced in the mind by memory or imagination.

motor i., the i. of body movements.

optical i., an i. formed by the refraction or reflection of light.

phase i., a magnetic resonance i. showing only phase shift information, to detect motion.

sensory i., an i. based on one or more types of sensation.

tactile i., an i. of an object as perceived by the sense of touch.

im·ag·e·ry (im′ij-rē). A technique in behavior therapy in which the client or patient is conditioned to substitute pleasant fantasies to counter the unpleasant feelings associated with anxiety.

imag·ing (im′ă-jing). Radiological production of a clinical image using x-rays, ultrasound, computed tomography, magnetic resonance, radionuclide scanning, or thermography; especially, cross-sectional imaging, such as ultrasonography, CT, or MRI. [see image]

blood pool i., nuclear medicine study using a radionuclide that is confined to the vascular compartment.

⚫ magnetic resonance i. (MRI), a diagnostic modality in which the magnetic nuclei (especially protons) of a patient are aligned in a strong, uniform magnetic field, absorb energy from tuned radiofrequency pulses, and emit radiofrequency signals as their excitation decays. These signals, which vary in intensity according to nuclear abundance and molecular chemical environment, are converted into sets of tomographic images by using field gradients in the magnetic field, which permits 3-dimensional localization of the point sources of the signals. Unlike conventional radiography or CT, MRI does not expose patients to ionizing radiation.

ima·go, pl. **imag·ines** (i-mā′gō, i-maj′i-nēz). **1.** The last stage of an insect after it has completed all its metamorphoses through the egg, larva, and

pupa; the adult insect form. **2.** SYN archetype (2). [L. image]

im·bal·ance (im-bal′ans). **1.** Lack of equality between opposing forces. **2.** Lack of equality in some aspect of binocular vision, such as muscle balance or image size. [L. *in-* neg. + *bi-lanx* (*-lanc-*), having two scales, fr. *bis*, twice, + *lanx*, dish, scale of a balance]

autonomic i., a lack of balance between sympathetic and parasympathetic nervous systems, especially in relation to vasomotor disturbances. SYN vasomotor i.

occlusal i., an inharmonious relationship between the teeth of the maxilla and mandible during closing or functional movements of the jaw.

vasomotor i., SYN autonomic i.

im·bi·bi·tion (im-bi-bish′ŭn). **1.** Absorption of fluid by a solid body without resultant chemical change in either. **2.** Taking up of water by a gel. [L. *im-bibo*, to drink in (*in* + *bibo*)]

im·bri·cate, im·bri·cat·ed (im′bri-kāt, im′bri-kā-ted). Overlapping like shingles. [L. *imbricatus*, covered with tiles]

im·id·a·zole (im-id-az′ōl). A five-membered heterocyclic compound occurring in L-histidine and other biologically important compounds.

im·ide (im′īd). The radical or group, =NH, attached to two –CO– groups.

△imido-. Prefix denoting the radical of an imide, formed by the loss of the H of the =NH group.

im·i·dole (im′i-dōl). SYN pyrrole.

△-imine. Suffix denoting the group =NH.

△imino-. Prefix denoting the group =NH.

im·i·no ac·ids (im′i-nō, i-mē′nō). Compounds with molecules containing both an acid group and an imino group.

im·mer·sion (i-mer′zhŭn). **1.** The placing of a body under water or other liquid. **2.** MICROSCOPY Filling the space between the objective lens and the top of the cover glass with a fluid, such as water or oil, to reduce spherical aberration and increase effective numerical aperture. [L. *immergo*, pp. *-mersus*, to dip in (*in* + *mergo*)]

im·mis·ci·ble (i-mis′i-bl). Incapable of mutual solution; *e.g.,* oil and water. [L. *immisceo*, to mix in (*in* + *misceo*)]

im·mit·tance (i-mit′ans). AUDIOLOGY A general term describing measurements of tympanic membrane impedance, compliance, or admittance. [L. *immitto*, to send in]

im·mo·bi·lize (i-mō′bi-līz). To render fixed or incapable of moving. [L. *in-* neg. + *mobilis*, movable]

im·mor·tal·i·za·tion (i-mōr′tăl-i-zā′shŭn). Conferring on normal cells cultured *in vitro* the property of an infinite lifespan, as from spontaneous mutation, by exposure to chemical carcinogens, or by viral infection.

im·mune (i-myūn′). **1.** Free from the possibility of acquiring a given infectious disease; resistant to an infectious disease. **2.** Pertaining to cell-mediated or humoral immunity, whereby an organism is so altered by previous contact with an antigen that it responds quickly and upon specifically subsequent contact; also to reactions *in vitro* with antibody-containing serum from such sensi-

im

tized organisms. [L. *immunis,* free from service, fr. *in,* neg., + *munus* (*muner-*), service]

im·mu·ni·fa·cient (im'yū-ni-fā'shent). Making immune after a specific disease. [L. *immunis,* exempt, + *faciens,* making, pr. part. of *facio*]

im·mu·ni·ty (i-myū'ni-tē). The status or quality of being immune (1). SYN insusceptibility. [L. *immunitas* (see immune)]

  acquired i., resistance resulting from previous exposure of the individual in question to an infectious agent or antigen; it may be *active,* as a result of naturally acquired infection or vaccination; or *passive,* being acquired from transfer of antibodies from another person or from an animal, either from mother to fetus or by inoculation.

  active i., SEE acquired i.

  cell-mediated i. (CMI), cellular i., immune responses which are initiated by T lymphocytes and mediated by T lymphocytes, macrophages, or both (*e.g.,* graft rejection, delayed-type hypersensitivity).

  general i., i. associated with widely diffused mechanisms that tend to protect the body as a whole, as compared with local i.

  herd i., the resistance to invasion and spread of an infectious agent in a group or community, based on the resistance to infection of a high proportion of individual members of the group.

  humoral i., i. associated with circulating antibodies, in contradistinction to cellular i.

  infection i., the paradoxical immune status in which resistance to reinfection coincides with the persistence of the original infection.

  innate i., resistance manifested by an organism that has not been sensitized by previous infection or vaccination; innate i. is nonspecific and is not stimulated by specific antigens. SEE ALSO self. SYN natural i., nonspecific i.

  local i., a natural or acquired i. to certain infectious agents, as manifested by an organ or a tissue, as a whole or in part.

  natural i., nonspecific i., SYN innate i.

  passive i., SEE acquired i.

  specific i., the immune status in which there is an altered reactivity directed solely against the antigenic determinants (infectious agent or other) that stimulated it. SEE acquired i.

im·mu·ni·za·tion. Protection of susceptible individuals from communicable diseases by administration of a living modified agent, a suspension of killed organisms, or an inactivated toxin. SEE ALSO vaccination.

im·mu·nize (im'yū-nīz). To render immune.

△**immuno-.** Immune, immunity. [L. *immunis,* immune]

im·mu·no·ad·ju·vant (im'yū-nō-ad'jū-vant). SEE adjuvant (2).

im·mu·no·as·say (im'yū-nō-as'ā). Detection and assay of substances by serological (immunological) methods. SEE ALSO radioimmunoassay, radioimmunoelectrophoresis, immunologic pregnancy *test.* SYN immunochemical assay.

  chemiluminescence i., an i. technique in which the antigen or antibody is labeled with a molecule capable of emitting light during a

chemical reaction; this light is used to measure the formation of the antigen-antibody complex.

  enzyme i. (EIA), assay using antibodies to detect the analyte of interest and an enzyme linked to the antigen-antibody complex. The enzyme reacts with a substrate to produce a product that is measured to quantitate the amount of antigenantibody formed. SEE ALSO enzyme-linked immunosorbent *assay,* enzyme-multiplied i. technique.

  enzyme-multiplied i. technique (EMIT), a type of i. in which the ligand is labeled with an enzyme. SEE ALSO competitive binding *assay,* enzyme-linked immunosorbent *assay.*

im·mu·no·blast (im'yū-nō-blast). An antigenically stimulated lymphocyte; a large cell with well-defined basophilic cytoplasm, a large nucleus with prominent nuclear membrane, distinct nucleoli, and clumped chromatin. [immuno- + G. *blastos,* germ]

im·mu·no·blot, im·mu·no·blot·ting (i'mū-nōblot'). Process by which antigens can be separated by electrophoresis and blotted to nitrocellulose sheets, where they bind and are subsequently identified by staining with labeled antibodies. SEE ALSO Western blot *analysis.*

im·mu·no·blot·ting. SEE immunoblot.

im·mu·no·com·pe·tence (im'yū-nō-kom'pĕtens). The ability to produce a normal immune response.

im·mu·no·com·pe·tent (im'yū-nō-kom'pĕ-tent). Possessing the ability to mount a normal immune response.

im·mu·no·com·pro·mised (im'yū-nō-kom'promīzd). Denoting an individual whose immunologic mechanism is deficient either because of an immunodeficiency disorder or because it has been rendered so by immunosuppressive agents.

im·mu·no·con·glu·ti·nin (im'yū-nō-kon-glū'ti-nin). An autoantibody-like immunoglobulin (IgM) formed by an organism against its own complement, following injection of complement-containing complexes or sensitized bacteria.

im·mu·no·cyte (im'yū-nō-sīt). An immunologically competent leukocyte capable of producing antibodies or reacting in cell-mediated immunity reactions. SEE ALSO I *cell.* [immuno- + G. *kytos,* cell]

im·mu·no·cy·to·ad·her·ence (im'ū-nō-sī'tō-adher'ens). A method for determining cell surface properties, in which immunoglobulin or receptors on the surface of one cell population cause cells with corresponding molecular configurations on their surface to adhere in rosettes around the cells.

im·mu·no·cy·to·chem·is·try (im'yū-nō-sī-tō-kem'is-trē). The study of cell constituents by immunologic methods, such as the use of fluorescent antibodies.

im·mu·no·de·fi·cien·cy (im'yū-nō-dē-fish'en-sē). A condition resulting from a defective immune mechanism; may be *primary* (due to a defect in the immune mechanism itself) or *secondary* (dependent upon another disease process).

  cellular i. with abnormal immunoglobulin synthesis, a group of disorders of unknown cause, associated with recurrent bacterial, fungal, protozoal, and viral infections; there is thymic hypoplasia with depressed cellular (T-lymphocyte) immunity combined with defective humoral (B-lymphocyte) immunity.

combined i., i. of both the B-lymphocytes and T-lymphocytes.

im·mu·no·de·fi·cient (im′yū-nō-dē-fish′ent). Lacking in some essential function of the immune system.

im·mu·no·dif·fu·sion (im′yū-nō-di-fyū′zhŭn, i-myū′nō-). A technique of study of antigen-antibody reactions by observing precipitates formed by combination of specific antigen and antibodies which have diffused in a gel in which they have been separately placed.

im·mu·no·e·lec·tro·pho·re·sis (im′yū-nō-ē-lek′trō-fō-rē′sis). A kind of precipitin test in which the components of one group of immunological reactants are first separated on the basis of electrophoretic mobility, the separated components then being identified on the basis of precipitates formed by reaction with components of the other group of reactants.

im·mu·no·en·hance·ment (im′yū-nō-en-hans′ment). IMMUNOLOGY The potentiating effect of specific antibody in establishing and in delaying rejection of a tumor allograft.

im·mu·no·en·hanc·er (im′yū-nō-en-hans′er). Any specific or nonspecific substance that increases the degree of the immune response.

im·mu·no·flu·o·res·cence (im′yū-nō-flūr-es′ens, i-myū′nō-). An immunohistochemical technique using labeling of antibodies by fluorescent dyes to identify bacterial, viral, or other antigenic material specific for the labeled antibody; the binding of antibody can be determined microscopically by the application of ultraviolet rays to the preparation. SEE ALSO fluorescent antibody *technique*.

im·mu·no·gen (i-myū′nō-jen). SYN antigen.

behavioral i., not smoking, regular exercise, and related health-enhancing personal habits and lifestyle of an individual which are associated with a decreased risk of physical illness and dysfunction, and with greater longevity.

im·mu·no·ge·net·ics (im′yū-nō-jĕ-net′iks). The study of the genetics of transplantation and tissue rejection, histochemical loci, immunologic response, immunoglobulin structure, and immunosuppression.

im·mu·no·gen·ic (im′yū-nō-jen′ik). SYN antigenic.

im·mu·no·ge·nic·i·ty (im′yū-nō-jĕ-nis′i-tē). SYN antigenicity.

im·mu·no·glob·u·lin (Ig) (im′yū-nō-glob′yū-lin) [MIM*146880-146910]. One of a class of structurally related proteins, each consisting of two pairs of polypeptide chains, one pair of light (L) [low molecular weight] chains (κ or λ), and one pair of heavy (H) chains (γ, α, δ, and ε), all four linked together by disulfide bonds. On the basis of the structural and antigenic properties of the H chains, Ig's are classified (in order of relative amounts present in normal human serum) as IgG (7 S in size, 80%), IgA (10 to 15%), IgM (19 S, a pentamer of the basic unit, 5 to 10%), IgD (less than 0.1%), and IgE (less than 0.01%). All of these classes are homogeneous and susceptible to

amino acid sequence analysis. Each class of H chain can associate with either κ or λ L chains. Subclasses of Ig's, based on differences in the H chains, are referred to as IgG1, etc.

When split by papain, IgG yields three pieces: the Fc piece, consisting of the C-terminal portion of the H chains, with no antibody activity but capable of fixing complement, and crystallizable; and two identical Fab pieces, carrying the antigen-binding sites and each consisting of an L chain bound to the remainder of an H chain.

Antibodies are Ig's, and all Ig's probably function as antibodies. However, Ig refers not only to the usual antibodies, but also to a great number of pathological proteins classified as myeloma proteins, which appear in multiple myeloma along with Bence Jones proteins, myeloma globulins, and Ig fragments.

From the amino acid sequences of Bence Jones proteins, it is known that all L chains are divided into a region of variable sequence (V_L) and one of constant sequence (C_L), each comprising about half the length of the L chain. The constant regions of all human L chains of the same type (κ or λ) are identical except for a single amino acid substitution, under genetic controls. H chains are similarly divided, although the V_H region, while similar in length to the V_L region, is only one-third or one-fourth the length of the C_H region. Binding sites are a combination of V_L and V_H protein regions. The large number of possible combinations of L and H chains make up the "libraries" of antibodies of each individual.

i. domains, structural units of i. heavy or light chains that are composed of approximately 110 amino acids. Light chains of an i. are composed of one constant domain and one variable domain. Heavy chains are composed of either three or four constant domains and one variable domain.

monoclonal i., a homogeneous i. resulting from the proliferation of a single clone of plasma cells and which, during electrophoresis of serum, appears as a narrow band or "spike"; it is characterized by heavy chains of a single class and subclass, and light chains of a single type. SYN paraprotein (2).

thyroid-stimulating i.'s (TSI), in Graves' disease, the antibodies to TSH receptors in the thyroid gland. These antibodies are produced by B-lymphocytes and stimulate the receptors, causing hyperthyroidism.

im·mu·no·his·to·chem·is·try (im′yū-nō-his′tō-kem′is-trē). Demonstration of specific antigens in tissues by the use of markers that are either fluorescent dyes or enzymes.

im·mu·nol·o·gist (im-yū-nol′ō-jist). A specialist in the science of immunology.

im·mu·nol·o·gy (im′yū-nol′ō-jē). **1.** The science concerned with the various phenomena of immunity, induced sensitivity, and allergy. **2.** Study of the structure and function of the immune system. [immuno- + G. *logos,* study]

im·mu·no·mod·u·la·to·ry (im′yū-nō-mod′ū-la-to-rē). **1.** Capable of modifying or regulating one or more immune functions. **2.** An immunological adjustment, regulation, or potentiation.

im

im·mu·no·po·ten·ti·a·tion (im′yū-nō-pō-ten-shē-ā′shŭn). Enhancement of the immune response by increasing its rate or prolonging its duration.

im·mu·no·po·ten·ti·a·tor (im′yū-nō-pō-ten′shē-ā-tŏr). Any substance which on inoculation enhances or augments an immune response.

im·mu·no·re·ac·tive (im′yū-nō-rē-ak′tiv). Denoting or exhibiting immunoreaction.

im·mu·no·sor·bent (im′yū-nō-sōr′bent). An antibody (or antigen) used to remove specific antigen (or antibody) from solution or suspension.

im·mu·no·sup·pres·sant (im′yū-nō-sŭ-pres′ant). An agent that induces immunosuppression. SYN immunosuppressive (2).

im·mu·no·sup·pres·sion (im′yū-nō-sŭ-presh′ŭn). Prevention or interference with the development of immunologic response; may reflect natural immunologic unresponsiveness (tolerance), may be artificially induced by chemical, biological, or physical agents, or may be caused by disease.

im·mu·no·sup·pres·sive (im′yū-nō-sŭ-pres′iv). **1.** Denoting or inducing immunosuppression. **2.** SYN immunosuppressant.

im·mu·no·sur·veil·lance (im′ū-nō-ser-vā′lance). Theory that holds that the immune system eliminates tumor cells that arise spontaneously.

im·mu·no·ther·a·py (im′yū-nō-thār′ă-pē). Therapeutic administration of serum or gamma globulin containing preformed antibodies produced by another individual as well as nonspecific systemic stimulation, adjuvants, active specific i., and adoptive i. New forms of immunotherapy include the use of monoclonal antibodies. Immunotherapy aims to boost immune system function, as with the administration of interferons and interleukin-2, or to attack cancerous cells directly, as with the injection of monoclonal antibodies.

adoptive i., passive transfer of immunity from an immune donor through inoculation of sensitized lymphocytes, transfer factor, immune RNA, or antibodies in serum or gamma globulin.

im·mu·no·trans·fu·sion (im′yū-nō-trans-fyū′zhŭn, i-myū′nō-). An indirect transfusion in which the donor is first immunized by injections of antigen from microorganisms isolated from the recipient; later, the donor's blood is collected, defibrinated, and then administered to the patient; the latter is thus passively immunized by antibody formed in the donor,.

IMP inosine 5′-monophosphate.

im·pact·ed (im-pak′ted). Wedged or pressed closely so as to be immovable.

im·pair·ment (im-pār′ment). Any loss or abnormality of psychological, physiological or anatomical structure or function.

im·ped·ance (im-pē′dăns). **1.** Opposition to flow of gases, liquids, or electrical current. **2.** Resistance of an acoustic system to being set in motion.

im·per·fo·rate (im-per′fōr-āt). SYN atretic.

im·per·fo·ra·tion (im-per-fōr-ā′shŭn). Condition of being atretic, occluded, or closed; indicated in compound words by the prefix atreto- or the suffix -atresia. [L. im- neg. + per-foro, pp. -atus, to bore through]

im·per·me·a·ble (im-per′mē-ă-bl). Not permitting the passage of liquids, gases, or heat through a membrane or other structure. [L. impermeabilis, not to be passed through]

im·pe·tig·i·nous (im-pe-tij′i-nŭs). Relating to impetigo.

◨im·pe·ti·go (im-pe-tī′gō). A contagious superficial pyoderma, caused by Staphylococcus aureus or Group A streptococci, that begins with a superficial flaccid vesicle which ruptures and forms a thick yellowish crust, most commonly occurring on the faces of children. SYN i. contagiosa, i. vulgaris. [L. a scabby eruption, fr. im-peto (inp-), to rush upon, attack]

bullous i. of newborn, disseminated bullous lesions appearing soon after birth, caused by infection with Staphylococcus aureus. SYN i. neonatorum (2), pemphigus gangrenosus (2).

i. contagio′sa, SYN impetigo.

i. herpetifor′mis, a rare pyoderma, occurring most commonly in the third trimester of pregnancy as an eruption of small closely aggregated pustules accompanied by severe constitutional symptoms and fetal death.

i. neonato′rum, (1) SYN dermatitis exfoliativa infantum. **(2)** SYN bullous i. of newborn.

i. vulga′ris, SYN impetigo.

im·plant. **1** (im-plant′). To graft or insert. **2** (im′plant). Material inserted or grafted into tissues. SEE ALSO graft, transplant. **3.** DENTISTRY A graft or insert set in or onto the alveolar recess prepared for its insertion. SEE ALSO implant denture. **4.** ORTHOPAEDICS A metallic or plastic device employed in joint reconstruction. [L. im-, in, + planto, pp. -atus, to plant, fr. planta, a sprout, shoot]

cochlear i., amplification device surgically implanted with its stimulating electrodes inserted directly into the nonfunctioning cochlea. SEE hearing aid. SEE ALSO amplification.

◨dental i.'s, crowns, bridges, or dentures attached permanently to the jaw by means of metal anchors, most frequently titanium posts.

im·plan·ta·tion (im-plan-tā′shŭn). **1.** Attachment of the fertilized ovum (blastocyst) to the endometrium, and its subsequent embedding in the compact layer. **2.** Insertion of a natural tooth into an artificially constructed alveolus. **3.** Tissue grafting. SEE ALSO transplantation.

im·plo·sion (im-plō′shŭn). **1.** A sudden collapse, as of an evacuated vessel, in which there is a bursting inward rather than outward as in explosion. **2.** A type of behavior therapy, similar to flooding, during which the patient is given massive exposure to extreme anxiety-arousing stimuli.

im·po·tence, im·po·ten·cy (im′pŏ-tens, -ten-sē). **1.** Weakness; lack of power. **2.** Inability of the male to achieve and/or maintain penile erection and thus engage in copulation; a manifestation of neurological, vascular, or psychological dysfunction. [L. impotentia, inability, fr. in- neg. + potentia, power]

im·preg·nate (im-preg′nāt). **1.** To fecundate; to cause to conceive. **2.** To diffuse or permeate with another substance. SEE ALSO saturate. [L. im-, in, + praegnans, with child]

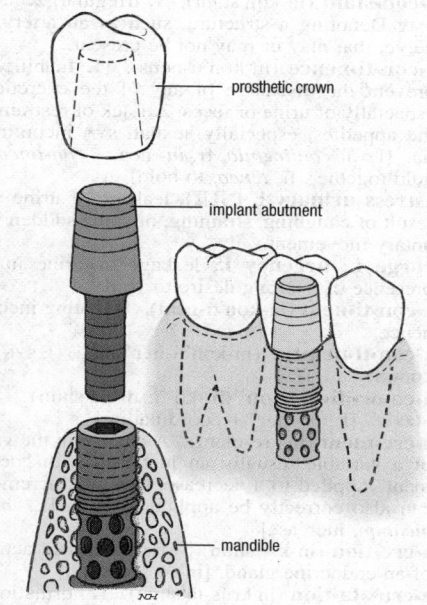

prosthetic crown

implant abutment

mandible

dental implant

im·pres·sion (im-presh'ŭn). **1.** A mark made by pressure of one structure or organ on another. See also *groove* for the various impressions of the lungs. **2.** An effect produced upon the mind by some external object acting through the organs of sense. **3.** An imprint or negative likeness; especially, the negative form of the teeth and/or other tissues of the oral cavity, made in a plastic material in order to reproduce a positive form or cast of the recorded tissues. [L. *impressio,* fr. *imprimo,* pp. *-pressus,* to press upon]

im·print·ing. A kind of learning characterized by its occurrence in the first few hours of life, and which determines species-recognition behavior.

im·pulse (im'pŭls). **1.** A sudden pushing or driving force. **2.** A sudden, often unreasoning, determination to perform some act. **3.** The action potential of a nerve fiber. [L. *im-pello,* pp. *-pulsus,* to push against, impel (inp-)]

im·pul·sion (im-pŭl'shŭn). An abnormal urge to perform a certain activity.

im·pul·sive (im-pŭl'siv). Relating to or actuated by an impulse, rather than controlled by reason or careful deliberation.

IMV intermittent mandatory *ventilation.*

In indium; inulin.

in-. **1.** Not, akin to G. *a-,* *an-* or Eng. *un-.* **2.** In, within, inside. **3.** Very; appears as im- before b, p, or m. [L.]

in·ac·ti·vate (in-ak'ti-vāt). To destroy the biological activity or the effects of an agent or substance.

in·an·i·mate (in-an'i-māt). Not alive. [L. *in-* neg. + *anima,* breath, soul]

in·a·ni·tion (in'ă-nish'ŭn). Severe weakness and

wasting as occurs from lack of food, defect in assimilation, or neoplastic disease. [L. *inanis,* empty]

in·ap·pe·tence (in-ap'ĕ-tens). Lack of desire or of craving. [L. *in-* neg. + *ap-peto,* pp. *-petitus,* to strive after, long for *(adp-)*]

in·ar·tic·u·late (in-ar-tik'yū-lit). **1.** Not articulate in the form of intelligible speech. **2.** Unable to satisfactorily express oneself in words.

in·as·sim·i·la·ble (in-ă-sim'il-ă-bl). Not assimilable; not capable of undergoing assimilation. SEE assimilation.

in·born (in'bōrn). Implanted during development *in utero.* In the specific context of i. error of metabolism, it connotes a genetic disruption of an enzyme. SEE inborn *errors* of metabolism, under *error.* SYN innate.

in·bred. Denoting populations (groups, genetic lines, etc.) descended over several generations almost exclusively from a small set of ancestors, and hence having a high rate of consanguinity.

in·breed·ing (in'brēd-ing). **1.** Mating between organisms that are genetically more closely related than organisms selected at random from the population. **2.** A practice of mating animals that are closely related.

in·car·cer·at·ed (in-kar'ser-ā-ted). Confined; imprisoned; trapped. [L. *in,* in, + *carcero,* pp. *-atus,* to imprison, fr. *carcer,* prison]

in·cest (in'sest). **1.** Sexual relations between persons closely related by blood, especially between parents and their children, and between siblings. **2.** The crime of sexual relations between persons related by blood, where such cohabitation is prohibited by law. [L. *incestus,* unchaste, fr. *in-,* not, + *castus,* chaste]

in·ces·tu·ous (in-ses'chū-ŭs). **1.** Pertaining to incest. **2.** Guilty of incest.

in·ci·dence (in'si-dens). **1.** The number of specified new events, *e.g.,* persons falling ill with a specified disease, during a specified period in a specified population. **2.** OPTICS Intersection of a ray of light with a surface. [L. *incido,* to fall into or upon, to happen]

in·ci·dent·a·lo·ma (in'sĭ-den-tă-lō'mă). Mass lesion, usually of the adrenal gland, noted fortuitously during computerized tomographic examinations performed for other reasons. [incidental + *-oma,* tumor]

in·ci·sal (in-sī'zăl). Cutting; relating to the cutting edges of the incisor and cuspid teeth. [L. *incido,* pp. *-cisus,* to cut into]

in·cise (in-sīz'). To cut with a knife.

in·ci·sion (in-sizh'ŭn). A cut; a surgical wound; a division of the soft parts made with a knife. [L. *incisio*]

in·ci·sive (in-sī'siv). **1.** Cutting; having the power to cut. **2.** Relating to the incisor teeth.

in·ci·sor (in-sī'zŏr). One of the cutting teeth, i. teeth, four in number in each jaw at the apex of the dental arch. [L. *incido,* to cut into]

in·ci·sure (in-sī'zhŭr). SYN notch. [L. *incisura*]

   Schmidt-Lanterman i.'s, funnel-shaped interruptions in the regular structure of the myelin sheath of nerve fibers.

in·cli·na·tion (in-kli-nā'shŭn). **1.** A leaning or sloping. **2.** DENTISTRY Deviation of the long axis

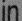

in

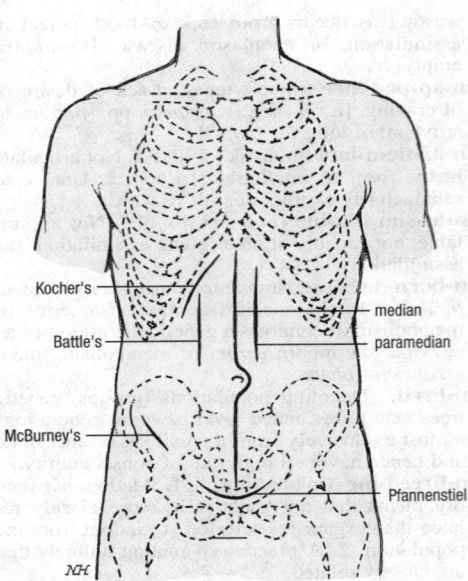

Kocher's

Battle's

McBurney's

median

paramedian

Pfannenstiel

NH

surgical incisions

of a tooth from the perpendicular. SYN version (3). [L. *inclinatio,* a leaning]

in·clu·sion (in-klū′zhŭn). **1.** Any foreign or heterogeneous substance contained in a cell or in any tissue or organ, not introduced as a result of trauma. **2.** The process by which a foreign or heterogeneous structure is misplaced in another tissue. [L. *inclusio,* a shutting in, fr. *in-cludo,* pp. *-clusis,* to close in]

cell i.'s, (1) the residual elements of the cytoplasm that are metabolic products of the cell, *e.g.,* pigment granules or crystals; SYN metaplasm. **(2)** storage materials such as glycogen or fat; **(3)** engulfed material such as carbon or other foreign substances. SEE ALSO inclusion *bodies,* under *body.*

in·com·pat·i·ble (in-kom-pat′i-bl). **1.** Not suitable to be combined or mixed with another substance. **2.** Denoting persons who are unable to associate with one another without anxiety and conflict. **3.** Having genotypes that put progeny at high risk of severe recessive disorders or that promote harmful maternal-fetal reaction. [L. *in-* neg., + *con-,* with, + *patior,* pp. *passus,* to suffer, tolerate]

in·com·pe·tence, in·com·pe·ten·cy (in-kom′pe-tens, in-kom′pĕ-ten-sē). **1.** The quality of being incompetent or incapable of performing the allotted function, especially failure of cardiac or venous valves to close completely. SYN insufficiency (2). **2.** FORENSIC PSYCHIATRY The inability to distinguish right from wrong or to manage one's affairs. [L. *in-,* neg. + *com-peto,* strive after together]

cardiac valvular i., failure of a valve to close its aperture completely and prevent regurgitation of blood.

in·con·stant (in-kon′stant). **1.** Irregular. **2.** ANATOMY Denoting a structure, such as an artery, or nerve, that may or may not be present.

in·con·ti·nence (in-kon′ti-nens). **1.** Inability to prevent the discharge of any of the excretions, especially of urine or feces. **2.** Lack of restraint of the appetites, especially sexual. SYN incontinentia. [L. *in-continentia,* fr. *in-* neg. + *con-tineo,* to hold together, fr. *teneo,* to hold]

stress urinary i. (SUI), leakage of urine as a result of coughing, straining, or some sudden voluntary movement.

urge i., urgency i., leakage of urine in the presence of a strong desire to void.

in·con·ti·nent (in-kon′ti-nent). Denoting incontinence.

in·con·ti·nen·tia (in-kon′ti-nen′shē-ă). SYN incontinence. [L.]

in·co·or·di·na·tion (in-kō-ōr-di-nā′shŭn). SYN ataxia. [L. *in-* neg. + coordination]

in·cre·ment (in′kre-ment). A change in the value of a variable; usually an increase, with "decrement" applied to a decrease, though "increment" can also correctly be applied to both. [L. *incrementum,* increase]

in·cre·tion (in-krē′shŭn). The functional activity of an endocrine gland. [in- + secretion]

in·crus·ta·tion (in′krŭs-tā′shŭn). **1.** Formation of a crust or a scab. **2.** A coating of some adventitious material or an exudate; a scab. [L. *in-crusto,* pp. *-atus,* to incrust, fr. *crusta,* crust]

in·cu·ba·tion (in′kyū-bā′shŭn). **1.** Maintaining controlled environmental conditions to favor growth or development of microbial or tissue cultures. **2.** Maintenance of an artificial environment for an infant, usually a premature or hypoxic one, by providing proper temperature, humidity, and, usually, oxygen. **3.** The development, without sign or symptom, of an infection from the time the infectious agent gains entry until the appearance of the first signs or symptoms. [L. *incubo,* to lie on]

in·cu·ba·tor (in′kyū-bā′tōr). **1.** A container in which controlled environmental conditions may be maintained; *e.g.,* for culturing microorganisms. **2.** An apparatus for maintaining an infant (usually premature) in an environment of proper oxygenation, humidity, and temperature.

in·cu·bus (in′kū-bŭs). **1.** Originally, an evil spirit that lay upon and oppressed sleeping persons; especially, a male spirit that copulated with sleeping women. Cf. succubus. **2.** SYN nightmare. [L. fr. *incubo,* to lie on]

in·cu·dal (in′kū-dăl). Relating to the incus.

in·cu·dec·to·my (in-kū-dek′tō-mē). Removal of the incus of the tympanum. [incus + G. *ektomē,* excision]

in·cu·des (in-kū′dēz). Plural of incus. [L.]

in·cu·do·sta·pe·di·al (in-kū′dō-stā-pē′dē-ăl). Relating to the incus and the stapes; denoting the articulation between the incus and the stapes in the middle ear.

in·cur·va·tion (in′ker-vā′shŭn). An inward curvature; a bending inward.

in·cus, gen. **in·cu·dis,** pl. **in·cu·des** (ing′kŭs, in-kū′dis, in-kū′dēz) [NA]. The middle of the three ossicles in the middle ear; it has a body and two limbs or processes (long crus and short crus); at the tip of the long crus is a small knob, the lenticular process which articulates with the head of the stapes. SYN anvil. [L. anvil]

in·cy·clo·duc·tion (in-sī-klō-dŭk′shŭn). A cycloduction in which the upper pole of the cornea is rotated inward (medially). [in- + cyclo- + L. *duco*, pp. *ductus*, to lead]

in·cy·clo·pho·ria (in-sī′klō-fō′rē-ă). A cyclophoria in which the 12 o'clock position in the iris tends to twist medially. [L. in- + cyclo- + G. *phora*, a carrying]

in·cy·clo·tro·pia (in-sī-klō-trō′pē-ă). A cyclotropia in which the upper poles of the corneas are rotated inward (medially) to each other. [in- + cyclo- + G. *trope*, a turning]

in·dex, gen. **in·di·cis**, pl. **in·di·ces**, **in·dex·es** (in′deks, -di-sis, -di-sēz, -dek-sĕz). **1** [NA]. SYN index *finger*. **2.** A guide, standard, indicator, symbol, or number denoting the relation in respect to size, capacity, or function, of one part or thing to another. SEE ALSO quotient, ratio. **3.** A core or mold used to record or maintain the relative position of a tooth or teeth to one another and/or to a cast. **4.** A guide, usually made of plaster, used to reposition teeth, casts, or parts. **5.** In epidemiology, a rating scale. **6.** A numerical or alphabetical list. [L. one that points out, an informer, the forefinger, an index, fr. *in-dico*, pp. *-atus*, to declare]

absorbancy i., (1) SYN specific absorption *coefficient.* **(2)** SYN molar absorption *coefficient.*

anesthetic i., ratio of the number of units of anesthetic required for anesthesia to the number of units of anesthetic required to produce respiratory or cardiovascular failure.

Arneth i., an expression based on adding the percentages of polymorphonuclear neutrophils with 1 or 2 lobes in their nuclei, plus one-half the percentage with 3 lobes; the normal value is 60%. SEE ALSO Arneth *count.*

body mass i. (BMI), an anthropometric measure of body mass, defined as weight in kilograms divided by height in meters squared; a method of determining caloric nutritional status.

cardiac i., the amount of blood ejected by the heart in a unit of time divided by the body surface area; usually expressed in liters per minute per square meter.

dmfs caries i., DMFS caries i., an i. of past caries experience based upon the number of decayed, missing, and filled surfaces of deciduous (indicated by lowercase letters) or permanent (indicated by uppercase letters) teeth.

erythrocyte indices, calculations for determining the average size, hemoglobin content, and concentration of hemoglobin in red blood cells, specifically mean cell volume, mean cell hemoglobin, and mean cell hemoglobin concentration.

heat stress i., measure of environment's potential to cause heat injury; based on ambient air temperature and relative humidity

leukopenic i., a significant decrease in the white blood count after ingestion of food to which a patient is hypersensitive, a count made during the normal fasting state being used as the basis for evaluation of the postprandial count.

master patient i. (MPI), database of all patients ever treated at a health care facility.

maturation i., an i. indicating the degree of maturation attained by the vaginal epithelium as adjudged by the cell types being exfoliated; serves as an objective means of evaluating hormonal secretion or response; represents the percentage of parabasal cells/intermediate cells-/superficialis, in that order; "shift to the left" indicates more immature cells on the surface (atrophy), while "shift to the right" indicates more mature epithelium.

opsonic i., a value that indicates the relative content of opsonin in the blood of a person with an infectious disease, as evaluated *in vitro* in comparison with presumably normal blood; the opsonic i. is calculated from the following equation: phagocytic i. of normal serum ÷ phagocytic i. of test serum = $1 ÷ x$, where x represents the opsonic i.

Periodontal I. (PI), An index for the epidemiological classification of periodontal disease.

phagocytic i., the average number of bacteria observed in the cytoplasm of polymorphonuclear leukocytes after mixing and incubating, at 37°C, 1) a suspension of washed, presumably normal leukocytes, 2) the serum to be tested for opsonin, and 3) a young culture of microorganisms that are causing disease in the patient.

pressure-volume i., method of evaluating the cerebrospinal fluid hydrodynamics.

refractive i. (*n*), the relative velocity of light in another medium compared to the velocity in air.

reticulocyte production i. (RPI), a calculated value that serves as an indicator of the bone marrow response in anemia. It is calculated as patient's hematocrit ÷ 0.45 L/L × reticulocyte count (%) × 1 ÷ maturation time of shift reticulocytes.

Robinson i., an i. used to calculate heart work load. SEE ALSO double *product.*

root caries i., the ratio of the number of teeth with carious lesions of the root, and/or restorations of the root, to the number of teeth with exposed root surfaces.

saturation i., an indication of the relative concentration of hemoglobin in the red blood cells, calculated as: grams of hemoglobin per 100 ml (expressed as percent of normal) ÷ hematocrit value (expressed as percent of normal) = saturation i.

small increment sensitivity i., SEE SISI *test.*

stroke work i., a measure of the work done by the heart with each contraction, adjusted for body surface area; equal to the stroke volume of the heart multiplied by the arterial pressure and divided by body surface area.

therapeutic i., the ratio of LD_{50} to ED_{50}, used in quantitative comparison of drugs.

vital i., the ratio of births to deaths within a population during a given time.

volume i., an indication of the relative size (*e.g.,* volume) of erythrocytes, calculated as follows: hematocrit value, expressed as per cent of normal ÷ red blood cell count, expressed as per cent of normal = volume i.

windchill i., measure of environment's poten-

in

tial to cause cold injury, based on ambient air temperature and wind velocity.

in·di·can·i·dro·sis (in′di-kan-i-drō′sis). Excretion of indican in the sweat. [indican + G. *hidrōs,* sweat]

in·di·can·u·ria (in′di-kan-yū′rē-ă). An increased urinary excretion of indican, a derivative of indol formed chiefly in the intestine when protein is putrefied; indol is also formed during the putrefaction of protein in other sites.

in·di·ca·tion (in-di-kā′shŭn). The basis or rationale for using a particular treatment or diagnostic test; may be furnished by a knowledge of the cause (**causal i.**), by the symptoms present (**symptomatic i.**), or by the nature of the disease (**specific i.**). [L. fr. *in-dico,* pp. *-atus,* to point out, fr. *dico,* to proclaim]

in·di·ca·tor (in′di-kā-ter, -tōr). In chemical analysis, a substance that changes color within a certain definite range of pH or oxidation potential, or in any way renders visible the completion of a chemical reaction. [L. one that points out]

    biologic i., a preparation of nonpathogenic microorganisms, usually bacterial spores, carried by an ampoule or specially impregnated paper enclosed within a package during sterilization and subsequently incubated to verify that the spores were killed by the sterilization process.

in·di·ces (in′di-sēz). Alternative plural of index.

in·di·ges·tion (in-di-jes′chŭn). Nonspecific term for a variety of symptoms resulting from a failure of proper digestion and absorption of food in the alimentary tract.

    acid i., i. resulting from hyperchlorhydria; often used by the laity as a synonym for pyrosis.

    gastric i., SYN dyspepsia.

    nervous i., i. caused by emotional upsets or stress.

in·di·um (In) (in′dē-ŭm). A metallic element, atomic no. 49, atomic wt. 114.82. [*indigo,* because of its blue line in the spectrum]

Individuals with Disabilities Education Act (IDEA). Federal law (Public Law 94-142, enacted in 1975 and subsequently amended) guaranteeing all students with disabilities, ages 3 through 21, the right to a free and appropriate public education designed to meet their individual needs. SEE ALSO individualized education *program.*

in·di·vid·u·a·tion (in′di-vid-yū-ā′shŭn). **1.** Development of the individual from the specific. **2.** JUNGIAN PSYCHOLOGY The process by which one's personality is differentiated, developed, and expressed. **3.** Regional activity in an embryo as a response to an organizer.

in·do·cy·a·nine green (in-dō-sī′ă-nēn). A tricarbocyanine dye that binds to serum albumin and is used in blood volume determinations and in liver function tests.

in·dol·ac·e·tu·ria (in′dōl-as-ĕ-tū′rē-ă). Excretion of an appreciable amount of indoleacetic acid in the urine; a manifestation of Hartnup disease.

in·dol·a·mine (in-dol′ă-mēn). An indole or indole derivative containing a primary, secondary, or tertiary amine group.

in·dole (in′dōl). **1.** 2,3-Benzopyrrole; basis of many biologically active substances (*e.g.,* seroto-

nin, tryptophan); formed in degradation of tryptophan. SYN ketole. **2.** Any of many alkaloids containing the i. (1) structure.

in·do·lent (in′dō-lent). Inactive; sluggish; painless or nearly so, said of a morbid process. [L. in-neg. + *doleo,* pr. p. *dolens* (*-ent-*), to feel pain]

in·dol·ic ac·ids (in-dōl′ik). Metabolites of L-tryptophan formed within the body or by intestinal microorganisms.

in·dox·yl (in-dok′sil). The radical of 3-hydroxyindole; a product of intestinal bacterial degradation of indoleacetic acid; increased amounts are excreted in in the urine in phenylketonuria.

in·dox·yl·u·ria (in-dok-sil-yū′rē-ă). The excretion of indoxyl, especially indoxyl sulfate, in the urine; i. may be associated with indicanuria, inasmuch as hydrolysis of indican results in formation of indoxyl.

in·duc·er (in-dūs′er). A molecule, usually a substrate of a specific enzyme pathway, that combines with and deactivates an active repressor (produced by a regulator gene); this allows an operator gene previously repressed to activate the structural genes controlled by it to resume enzyme production.

in·duc·tance (in-dŭk′tans). The coefficient of electromagnetic induction; the unit of inductance is the henry. [see induction]

in·duc·tion (in-dŭk′shŭn). **1.** Production or causation. **2.** Production of an electric current or magnetic state in a body by electricity or magnetism in another body close to the first body. **3.** The period from the start of anesthesia to the establishment of a depth of anesthesia adequate for a surgical procedure. **4.** EMBRYOLOGY The influence exerted by an organizer or evocator on the differentiation of adjacent cells or on the development of an embryonic structure. **5.** A modification imposed on the offspring by the action of environment on the germ cells of one or both parents. **6.** MICROBIOLOGY The change from probacteriophage to vegetative phage that may occur spontaneously or after stimulation by certain physical and chemical agents. **7.** ENZYMOLOGY The process of increasing the amount or the activity of a protein. SEE ALSO inducer. **8.** A stage in the process of hypnosis. **9.** Causal analysis; a method of reasoning in which an inference is made from one or more specific observations to a more general statement. Cf. deduction. [L. *inductio,* a leading in]

in·duc·tor (in-dŭk′ter, -tōr). **1.** That which brings about induction. **2.** EMBRYOLOGY An evocator or an organizer.

in·du·rat·ed (in′dū-rāt-ed). Hardened, usually used with reference to soft tissues becoming extremely firm but not as hard as bone. [L. *in-duro,* pp. *-duratus,* to harden, fr. *durus,* hard]

in·du·ra·tion (in-dū-rā′shŭn). **1.** The process of becoming extremely firm or hard, or having such physical features. **2.** A focus or region of indurated tissue. SYN sclerosis (1). [L. *induratio* (see indurated)]

    brown i. of the lung, fibrosis and hemosiderin pigmentation of the lungs due to long-standing pulmonary congestion.

    cyanotic i., i. related to persistent, chronic venous congestion in an organ or tissue, frequently resulting in fibrous thickening of the walls of the veins and eventual fibrosis of adjacent tissue.

gray i., a condition occurring in lungs during and after pneumonic processes in which there is failure of resolution; there is an increase in fibrous tissue but usually not a prominent degree of pigmentation, unless chronic passive congestion is also present.

red i., a condition observed in lungs in which there is an advanced degree of acute passive congestion, or acute pneumonitis (sometimes termed interstitial pneumonia), or a similar pathologic process.

in•du•ra•tive (in′dū-ră-tiv). Pertaining to, causing, or characterized by induration.

in•du•si•um, pl. **in•du•sia** (in-dū′zē-ŭm, -zē-ă). 1. A membranous layer or covering. 2. The amnion. [L. a woman's undergarment, fr. *induo,* to put on]

i. gris′eum [NA], a thin layer of gray matter on the dorsal surface of the corpus callosum in which the medial and lateral longitudinal striae lie embedded. The i. griseum is a rudimentary component of the hippocampus, continuous caudally around the splenium of the corpus callosum with the fasciolar gyrus, a slender convolution in turn continuous with the dentate gyrus of the hippocampus; rostrally the i. griseum curves around the genu and rostrum of the corpus callosum and extends ventralward to the olfactory trigone as the tenia tecta or rudimentum hippocampi, hidden in the depth of the posterior parolfactory sulcus that marks the anterior border of the subcallosal gyrus or precommissural septum.

in•e•bri•ant (in-ē′brē-ant). 1. Making drunk; intoxicating. 2. An intoxicant, such as alcohol. SEE inebriation.

in•e•bri•a•tion (in-ē-brē-ā′shŭn). Intoxication, especially by alcohol. SEE inebriant. [L. *in-,* intensive + *ebrietas,* drunkenness]

in•ert (in-ert′). 1. Slow in action; sluggish; inactive. 2. Devoid of active chemical properties, as the inert gases. 3. Denoting a drug or agent having no pharmacologic or therapeutic action. [L. *iners,* unskillful, sluggish, fr. *in,* neg. + *ars,* art]

in•er•tia (in-er′shē-ă, in-er′shăh). 1. The tendency of a physical body to oppose any force tending to move it from a position of rest or to change its uniform motion. 2. Denoting inactivity or lack of force, lack of mental or physical vigor, or sluggishness of thought or action. [L. want of skill, laziness]

in ex•tre•mis (in eks-trē′mis). At the point of death. [L. *extremus,* last]

in•fan•cy (in′fan-sē). Babyhood; the earliest period of extrauterine life; roughly, the first year of life.

in•fant. A child under the age of 1 year; more specifically, a newborn baby. [L. *infans,* not speaking]

liveborn i., the product of a live birth; an i. who shows evidence of life after birth.

postmature i., a baby born after over 42 weeks of gestation, which puts the child at risk because of inadequate placental function. The infant usu-

ally shows wrinkled skin, sometimes more serious abnormalities.

post-term i., an i. with a gestational age of 42 completed weeks or more (294 days or more).

preterm i., an i. with gestational age of less than 37 completed weeks (259 completed days).

stillborn i., an i. who shows no evidence of life after birth. Cf. liveborn i.

in•fan•ti•cide (in-fan′ti-sīd). 1. The killing of an infant. 2. One who murders an infant. [infant + L. *caedo,* to kill]

in•fan•tile (in′făn-tīl). 1. Relating to, or characteristic of, infants or infancy. 2. Denoting childish behavior.

in•fan•ti•lism (in-fan′ti-lizm). 1. A state marked by slow development of mind and body. 2. Childishness, as characterized by a temper tantrum of an adolescent or adult. 3. Underdevelopment of the sexual organs.

sexual i., failure to develop secondary sexual characteristics after the normal time of puberty.

in•farct (in′farkt). An area of necrosis resulting from a sudden insufficiency of arterial or venous blood supply. SYN infarction (2). [L. *in-farcio,* pp. *-fartus* (*-ctus,* an incorrect form), to stuff into]

anemic i., an i. in which little or no bleeding into tissue spaces occurs when the blood supply is obstructed. SYN white i. (1).

hemorrhagic i., an i. red in color from infiltration of blood from collateral vessels into the necrotic area.

septic i., an area of necrosis resulting from vascular obstruction due to emboli composed of clumps of bacteria or infected material.

white i., (1) SYN anemic i. (2) in the placenta, intervillous fibrin with ischemic necrosis of villi.

in•farc•tion (in-fark′shŭn). 1. Sudden insufficiency of arterial or venous blood supply due to emboli, thrombi, vascular torsion, or pressure that produces a macroscopic area of necrosis; the heart, brain, spleen, kidney, intestine, lung, and testes are likely to be affected, as are tumors, especially of the ovary or uterus. 2. SYN infarct.

myocardial i. (MI), i. of an area of the heart muscle, usually as a result of occlusion of a coronary artery.

silent myocardial i., i. that produces none of the characteristic symptoms and signs of myocardial i.

watershed i., cortical i. in an area where the distribution of major cerebral arteries meet or overlap.

in•fect (in-fekt′). 1. To enter, invade, or inhabit another organism, causing infection or contamination. 2. To dwell internally, endoparasitically, as opposed to externally (infest). [L. *in-ficio,* pp. *-fectus,* to dip into, dye, corrupt, infect, fr. *in* + *facio,* to make]

in•fec•tion (in-fek′shŭn). Multiplication of parasitic organisms within the body; multiplication of usual bacterial flora of the intestinal tract is not usually viewed as i.

cross i., i. spread from one source to another, person to person, animal to person, person to animal, animal to animal.

droplet i., i. acquired through the inhalation of droplets or aerosols of saliva or sputum containing virus or other microorganisms expelled by another person during sneezing, coughing, laughing, or talking.

endogenous i., i. caused by an infectious agent already present in the body, the previous i. having been inapparent.

focal i., local i. that can serve as a source of disseminated or metastatic i.

terminal i., an acute i., commonly pneumonic or septic, occurring toward the end of any disease and often the cause of death.

urinary tract i. (UTI), microbial i., usually bacterial, of any part of the urinary tract.

in•fec•tious (in-fek′shŭs). **1.** Capable of being transmitted by infection, with or without actual contact. **2.** SYN infective. **3.** Denoting a disease due to the action of a microorganism.

in•fec•tious•ness (in-fek′shŭs-nes). The state or quality of being infectious.

in•fec•tive (in-fek′tiv). Capable of transmitting an infection. SYN infectious (2).

in•fec•tiv•i•ty (in-fek-tiv′i-tē). **1.** The characteristic of a disease agent that embodies capability of entering, surviving in, and multiplying in a susceptible host. **2.** The proportion of exposures in defined circumstances that result in infection.

in•fe•ri•or (in-fē′rē-ōr). **1.** Situated below or directed downward. **2** [NA]. ANATOMY Situated nearer the soles of the feet in relation to a specific reference point; opposite of superior. **3.** Less useful or of poorer quality. [L. lower]

in•fe•ri•or•i•ty (in-fēr-ē-ōr′i-tē). The condition or state of being or feeling inadequate or inferior, especially relative to one's peers or to others similarly situated.

in•fer•til•i•ty (in-fer-til′i-tē). Diminished or absent ability to produce offspring; does not imply sterility. [L. in- neg. + fertilis, fruitful]

in•fest (in-fest′). To dwell on or in a host as a parasite. [L. infesto, pp. -atus, to attack]

in•fes•ta•tion. Parasitization of a host; usually refers to multicellular parasites (worms, arthropods).

in•fil•trate (in-fil′trāt). **1.** To perform or undergo infiltration. **2.** SYN infiltration (2). **3.** Infiltration (1) in the lung as inferred from appearance of a localized, ill-defined opacity on a chest radiograph. [L. in + Mediev. L. filtro, pp. -atus, to strain through felt, fr. filtrum, felt]

in•fil•tra•tion (in′fil-trā′shŭn). **1.** The act of permeating or penetrating into a substance, cell, or tissue; said of gases, fluids, or matter held in solution. **2.** The gas, fluid, or dissolved matter that has entered any substance, cell, or tissue. SYN infiltrate (2). **3.** Injection of solution into tissues, as in infiltration anesthesia. **4.** Extravasation of solutions intended for intravascular injection.

adipose i., growth of normal adult fat cells in sites where they are not usually present.

calcareous i., SYN calcification.

cellular i., migration of cells from their sources of origin, or direct extension of cells as a result of unusual growth and multiplication; used especially with reference to such changes associated with inflammations and certain types of malignant neoplasms.

fatty i., abnormal accumulation of fat droplets

in the cytoplasm of cells, particularly of fat derived from outside the cells. SEE ALSO fatty *degeneration.*

lipomatous i., nonencapsulated adipose tissue forming a lipoma-like mass, usually in the cardiac interatrial septum where it may cause arrhythmia and sudden death.

in•firm (in-ferm′). Weak or feeble because of old age or disease. [L. *in-firmus,* fr. *in-* neg. + *firmus,* strong]

in•fir•ma•ry (in-fer′mă-rē). A clinic or small hospital, especially in a school or college. [L. *infirmarium;* see infirm]

in•fir•mi•ty (in-fer′mi-tē). A weakness; an abnormal, more or less disabling, condition of mind or body. [see infirm]

in•flam•ma•tion (in-flă-mā′shŭn). A fundamental, stereotyped complex of cytologic and chemical reactions that occur in affected blood vessels and adjacent tissues in response to an injury or abnormal stimulation caused by a physical, chemical, or biologic agent. [L. *inflammo,* pp. *-atus,* fr. *in,* in, + *flamma,* flame]

acute i., any i. that has a fairly rapid onset, quickly becomes severe, usually manifested for only a few days; characterized histopathologically by edema, hyperemia, and infiltrates of polymorphonuclear leukocytes.

catarrhal i., an inflammatory process that may occur in any mucous membrane, and is characterized by hyperemia of the mucosal vessels, edema of the interstitial tissue, enlargement of the secretory epithelial cells, and an irregular layer of viscous, mucinous material on the surface.

chronic i., an i. that may begin with a relatively rapid onset or in a slow, insidious, and even unnoticed manner, tends to persist for several weeks, months, or years and has a vague and indefinite termination; characterized histopathologically by infiltrates of small, round cells (lymphocytes), fibrosis, and granuloma formation.

exudative i., i. in which the conspicuous or distinguishing feature is an exudate, which may be chiefly serous, serofibrinous, fibrinous, or mucous, or may be characterized by relatively large numbers of cells.

fibrinous i., an exudative i. in which there is a disproportionately large amount of fibrin.

granulomatous i., a form of proliferative i. SEE ALSO granuloma.

necrotic i., necrotizing i., an acute inflammatory reaction in which the predominant histologic change is rapid necrosis that occurs diffusely or extensively throughout the affected tissue.

proliferative i., an inflammatory reaction in which the distinguishing feature is an increase in the number of tissue cells, especially the reticuloendothelial macrophages, rather than of cells exuded from blood vessels.

pseudomembranous i., a form of exudative i. that involves mucous and serous membranes; large quantities of fibrin in the exudate result in a tenacious membrane-like covering that is adherent to the underlying acutely inflamed tissue.

purulent i., an acute exudative i. in which polymorphonuclear leukocytes cause liquefaction of the affected tissues, focally or diffusely; the purulent exudate is frequently termed pus. SYN suppurative i.

serous i., an exudative i. in which the exudate is predominantly fluid; relatively few cells are observed.

subacute i., an i. that is intermediate in duration between that of an acute i. and that of a chronic i., usually persisting longer than 3 or 4 weeks.

suppurative i., SYN purulent i.

in·flam·ma·to·ry (in-flam′ă-tōr-ē). Pertaining to, characterized by, causing, resulting from, or becoming affected by inflammation.

in·fla·tion (in-flā′shŭn). Distention by a fluid or gas. SYN vesiculation (2). [L. *inflatio,* fr. *in-flo,* pp. *-flatus,* to blow into, inflate]

in·flec·tion, in·flex·ion (in-flek′shŭn). An inward bending. [L. *in-flecto,* pp. *-flexus,* to bend]

in·flu·en·za (in-flū-en′ză). An acute infectious respiratory disease, caused by influenza viruses, which attacks the respiratory epithelial cells and produces a catarrhal inflammation; characterized by sudden onset, chills, fever of short duration, severe prostration, headache, muscle aches, and a cough that usually is dry until secondary infection occurs. The disease commonly occurs in epidemics, sometimes in pandemics; strain-specific immunity develops, but mutations in the virus are frequent, and the immunity usually does not protect against antigenically different strains. SYN flu, grip, grippe. [It. influence (of planets or stars), fr. L. *influentia,* fr. *in-fluo,* to flow in]

Hong Kong i., influenza caused by a serotype of influenza virus type A and first identified in Hong Kong.

Spanish i., i. that caused several waves of pandemic in 1918–1919, resulting in more than 20 million deaths worldwide.

in·flu·en·zal (in-flū-en′zăl). Relating to, marked by, or resulting from influenza.

In·flu·en·za·vi·rus (in-flū-en′ză-vī-rŭs). The genus of Orthomyxoviridae that comprises influenza viruses types A and B.

in·formed con·sent. Voluntary consent given by a person or a responsible proxy (*e.g.,* a parent) for participation in a study, immunization program, or treatment regimen, after being informed of the purpose, methods, procedures, benefits, and risks. The essential criteria of i. c. are that the subject has both knowledge and comprehension, that consent is freely given without duress or undue influence, and that the right of withdrawal at any time is clearly communicated to the subject.

in·for·mo·fers (in-fōr′mō-fers). Name suggested for the protein particles that appear when RNA is removed from nucleoprotein particles. [*informa-tion* + -fer]

in·for·mo·somes (in-fōr′mō-sōmz). Name suggested for the bodies composed of messenger (informational) RNA and protein that are found in the cytoplasm of animal cells. [*inform*ation + G. *sōma,* body]

infra-. A position below the part denoted by the word to which it is joined. [L. below]

in·fra·bulge (in′fră-bŭlj). **1.** That portion of the crown of a tooth gingival to the height of contour. **2.** That area of a tooth where the retentive portion

of a clasp of a removable partial denture is placed.

in·fra·clu·sion (in-fră-klū′zhŭn). The state wherein a tooth has failed to erupt to the maxillomandibular plane of interdigitation. SYN infraocclusion, infraversion (3).

in·frac·tion (in-frak′shŭn). A fracture; especially one without displacement. [L. *infractio,* a breaking, fr. *infringere,* to break]

in·fra·di·an (in-frā′dē-ăn). Relating to biologic variations or rhythms occurring in cycles less frequent than every 24 hours. Cf. circadian, ultradian. [infra- + L. *dies,* day]

in·fra·mam·il·lary (in-fră-mam′ĭ-lār-ē). Relating to that which is situated below a nipple.

in·fra·mar·gin·al (in-fră-mar′ji-năl). Below any margin or edge.

in·fra·max·il·lary (in-fră-mak′si-lā-rē). SYN mandibular.

in·fra·oc·clu·sion (in′fră-ŏ-klū′zhŭn). SYN infraclusion.

in·fra·psy·chic (in-fră-sī′kik). Denoting ideas or actions originating below the level of consciousness.

in·fra·red (in′fră-red). That portion of the electromagnetic spectrum with wavelengths between 770 and 1000 nm.

in·fra·son·ic (in′fră-son′ik). Denoting those frequencies that lie below the range of human hearing. [infra- + L. *sonus,* sound]

in·fra·ver·sion (in′fră-ver′shŭn). **1.** A turning (version) downward. **2.** PHYSIOLOGICAL OPTICS Rotation of both eyes downward. **3.** SYN infraclusion.

in·fun·dib·u·la (in-fŭn-dib′yū-lă). Plural of infundibulum.

in·fun·dib·u·lar (in-fŭn-dib′yū-lăr). Relating to an infundibulum.

in·fun·dib·u·lec·to·my (in′fŭn-dib′yū-lek′tō-mē). Excision of an infundibulum, especially of hypertrophied ventricular septal myocardium encroaching on the ventricular outflow tract. [infundibulum + G. *ektomē,* excision]

in·fun·dib·u·lo·fol·lic·u·li·tis (in-fŭn-dib′yū-lō-fo-lik′yū-lī′tis). Inflammation of the follicular infundibulum, the superficial part of the hair follicle above the opening of the sebaceous gland.

in·fun·dib·u·lo·ma (in-fŭn-dib′yū-lō′mă). A pilocytic astrocytoma arising in the neurohypophysis of the pituitary. [infundibulum + G. *-oma,* tumor]

in·fun·dib·u·lum, pl. **in·fun·dib·u·la** (in-fŭn-dib′yū-lŭm, -yū-lă). **1** [NA]. A funnel or funnel-shaped structure or passage. **2.** SYN i. of uterine tube. **3.** The expanding portion of a calix as it opens into the pelvis of the kidney. **4** [NA]. SYN arterial cone. **5.** Termination of a bronchiole in the alveolus. **6.** Termination of the cochlear canal beneath the cupola. **7** [NA]. The funnel-shaped, unpaired prominence of the base of the hypothalamus behind the optic chiasm, enclosing the infundibular recess of the third ventricle and continuous below with the stalk of the hypophysis. **8.** The contact surface indentation in the incisor and cheek teeth of a horse. SYN mark (2). [L. a funnel]

ethmoidal i., a passage from the middle meatus

in

of the nose communicating with the anterior eth-moidal cells and frontal sinus.

hypothalamic i., the apical portion of the tuber cinereum extending into the stalk of the hypophysis.

i. of uterine tube, the funnel-like expansion of the abdominal extremity of the uterine (fallopian) tube. SYN infundibulum (2).

in·fu·sion (in-fyū′zhŭn). **1.** The process of steeping a substance in water, either cold or hot (below the boiling point), in order to extract its soluble principles. **2.** A medicinal preparation obtained by steeping the crude drug in water. **3.** The introduction of fluid other than blood, *e.g.,* saline solution, into a vein. [L. *infusio,* fr. *in-fundo,* pp. *-fusus,* to pour in]

in·ges·ta (in-jes′tă). Solid or liquid nutrients taken into the body. [pl. of L. *ingestum,* ntr. pp. of *in-gero, -gestus,* to carry in]

in·ges·tion (in-jes′chŭn). **1.** Introduction of food and drink into the stomach. **2.** Incorporation of particles into the cytoplasm of a phagocytic cell by invagination of a portion of the cell membrane as a vacuole. [L. *in-gero,* to carry in]

in·ges·tive (in-jes′tiv). Relating to ingestion.

in·gra·ves·cent (in-gră-ves′ent). Increasing in severity. [L. *ingravesco,* to grow heavier, fr. *gravis,* heavy]

in·gui·nal (ing′gwi-năl). Relating to the groin.

in·gui·no·cru·ral (ing′gwi-nō-krū′răl). Relating to the groin and the thigh.

in·gui·no·dyn·ia (ing′gwi-nō-din′ē-ă). Rarely used term for pain in the groin. [L. *inguen (inguin-),* groin, + G. *odynē,* pain]

in·gui·no·la·bi·al (ing′gwi-nō-lā′bē-ăl). Relating to the groin and the labium.

in·gui·no·per·i·to·ne·al (ing′gwi-nō-per′i-tō-nē′ăl). Relating to the groin and the peritoneum.

in·gui·no·scro·tal (ing′gwi-nō-skrō′tăl). Relating to the groin and the scrotum.

INH isonicotinic acid hydrazide.

in·hal·ant (in-hā′lant). **1.** That which is inhaled; a remedy given by inhalation. **2.** A drug (or combination of drugs) with high vapor pressure, carried by an air current into the nasal passage, where it produces its effect. **3.** Group of products consisting of finely powdered or liquid drugs that are carried to the respiratory passages by the use of special devices such as low pressure aerosol containers. SYN insufflation (2). SEE ALSO inhalation, aerosol. [see inhalation]

in·ha·la·tion (in-hă-lā′shŭn). **1.** The act of drawing in the breath. SYN inspiration. **2.** Drawing a medicated vapor in with the breath. **3.** A solution of a drug or combination of drugs for administration as a nebulized mist intended to reach the respiratory tree. [L. *in-halo,* pp. *-halatus,* to breathe at or in]

in·hale (in-hāl′). To draw in the breath. SYN inspire.

in·hal·er (in-hāl′er). **1.** SYN respirator (1). **2.** An apparatus for administering pharmacologically active agents by inhalation.

▣ **metered-dose i. (MDI),** a device consisting of a canister, propellant, drug, and mouthpiece (or other patient adjunct) that delivers a known dose of drug as an aerosol with each actuation.

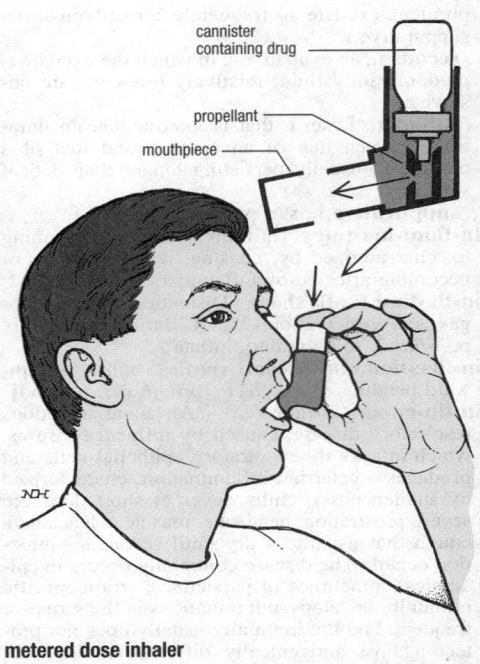

cannister containing drug

propellant

mouthpiece

metered dose inhaler

in·her·ent (in-her′ent). Occurring as a natural part or consequence; intrinsic. [L. *inhaerens,* sticking to, adhering]

in·her·i·tance (in-her′i-tans). **1.** Characters or qualities that are transmitted from parent to offspring by coded cytological data; that which is inherited. **2.** Cultural or legal endowment. **3.** The act of inheriting. [L. *heredito,* inherit, fr. *heres (hered-),* an heir]

codominant i., i. in which two alleles are individually expressed in the presence of each other.

collateral i., the appearance of characters in collateral members of a family group, as when an uncle and a niece show the same character inherited from a common ancestor.

cytoplasmic i., transmission of characters dependent on self-perpetuating elements not nuclear in origin (*e.g.,* mitochondrial DNA).

dominant i., SEE dominance of *traits,* under *trait.*

extrachromosomal i., transmission of characters dependent on some factor not connected with the chromosomes.

mendelian i., i. in which stable and undecomposable characters controlled entirely or overwhelmingly by a single genetic locus are transmitted over many generations. SEE *law* of segregation, *law* of independent assortment.

mosaic i., i. in which the paternal influence is dominant in one group of cells and the maternal in another. Cf. lyonization.

multifactorial i., i. involving many factors, of which at least one is genetic but none is of overwhelming importance, as in the causation of a disease by multiple genetic and environmental factors.

recessive i., SEE dominance of *traits*, under *trait*.

sex-influenced i., i. that is autosomal but has a different intensity of expression in the two sexes, *e.g.,* male pattern baldness.

sex-limited i., i. of a trait that can be expressed in one sex only, *e.g.,* testicular feminization.

sex-linked i., the pattern of inheritance that may result from a mutant gene located on either the X or Y chromosome.

in·her·it·ed (in-her´it-ed). Derived from a preformed genetic code present in the parents. Contrast with acquired.

in·hib·it (in-hib´it). To curb or restrain.

in·hi·bi·tion (in-hi-bish´ŭn). **1.** Depression or arrest of a function. SEE ALSO inhibitor. **2.** PSYCHOANALYSIS The restraining of instinctual or unconscious drives or tendencies, especially if they conflict with one's conscience or with societal demands. **3.** PSYCHOLOGY The gradual attenuation, masking, and extinction of a previously conditioned response. [L. *in-hibeo,* pp. *-hibitus,* to keep back, fr. *habeo,* to have]

competitive i., blocking of the action of an enzyme by a compound that binds to the free enzyme, preventing the substrate from binding and thus prevents the enzyme from acting on that substrate. SYN selective i.

contact i., cessation of replication of dividing cells that come into contact, as in the center of a healing wound.

feedback i., i. of activity by an end product of the pathway of which that activity is a part. SYN feedback mechanism.

noncompetitive i., a type of enzyme i. in which the inhibiting compound does not compete with the natural substrate for the active site on the enzyme, but inhibits the reaction by combining with the enzyme-substrate complex, once the latter has been formed, and with the free enzyme.

reflex i., a situation in which sensory stimuli decrease reflex activity.

selective i., SYN competitive i.

in·hib·i·tor (in-hib´i-ter, -tōr). **1.** An agent that restrains or retards physiologic, chemical, or enzymatic action. **2.** A nerve, stimulation of which represses activity. SEE ALSO inhibition.

angiotensin-converting enzyme i.'s, a class of drugs used in the treatment of hypertension; they produce a reduction of peripheral arterial resistance, although the exact mechanism of action has not been fully determined; they block the conversion of angiotensin I to angiotensin II, a powerful vasoconstrictor.

cholinesterase i., a drug, such as neostigmine, which, by inhibiting biodegradation of acetylcholine, restores myoneural function in myasthenia gravis or after nondepolarizing neuromuscular relaxants have been administered.

glucosidase i.'s, agents such as acarbose which reduce gastrointestinal absorption of carbohydrates. This group of drugs has been known popularly as "starch blockers." They lower plasma glucose levels and tend to cause weight loss. A limiting side effect is flatulence.

HMG-CoA reductase i.'s, class of antilipemic drugs used to lower serum cholesterol.

β-lactamase i.'s, drugs such as clavulanic acid, which are used to inhibit bacterial β-lactamases; often used with a penicillin or cephalosporin to overcome drug resistance.

monoamine oxidase i., any of the hydrazine and hydrazide derivatives that inhibit several enzymes and raise the brain norepinephrine and 5-hydroxytryptamine levels; used as antidepressant and hypotensive agents.

selective serotonin reuptake i. (SSRI), a class of drugs that selectively prevent the reuptake of serotonin and are used for the treatment of depression, *e.g.,* fluoxetine, sertraline.

in·hib·i·to·ry (in-hib´i-tōr-ē). Restraining; tending to inhibit.

in·i·on (in´ē-on) [NA]. A point located on the external occipital protuberance at the intersection of the midline with a line drawn tangent to the uppermost convexity of the right and left superior nuchal lines. [G. nape of the neck]

in·i·ti·a·tion (i-ni-shē-ā´shŭn). **1.** The first stage of tumor induction by a carcinogen; subtle alteration of cells by exposure to a carcinogenic agent so that they are likely to form a tumor upon subsequent exposure to a promoting agent (promotion). **2.** Starting point of replication or translation in macromolecule biosynthesis. **3.** Start of chemical or enzymatic reaction.

in·i·tis (in-ī´tis). **1.** Inflammation of fibrous tissue. **2.** SYN myositis. [G. *is* (*in-*), fiber, + *-itis,* inflammation]

in·ject (in-jekt´). To introduce into the body; denoting a fluid forced beneath the skin or into a blood vessel. [L. *injicio,* to throw in]

in·ject·ed (in-jek´ted). **1.** Denoting a fluid introduced into the body. **2.** Denoting a surface whose blood vessels are visibly dilated.

injection. 1. Introduction of a medicinal substance or nutrient material into the subcutaneous tissue (subcutaneous or hypodermic i.), the muscular tissue (intramuscular i.), a vein (intravenous i.), an artery (intraarterial i.), the rectum (rectal i. or enema), the vagina (vaginal i. or douche), the urethra, or other canals or cavities of the body. **2.** An injectable pharmaceutical preparation. **3.** Congestion or hyperemia. [L. *injectio,* a throwing in, fr. *in-jicio,* to throw in]

intradermal i., an i. into the corium, or substance of the skin.

in·ju·ry (in´jer-ē). The damage or wound of trauma. [L. *injuria,* fr. *in-* neg. + *jus* (*jur-*), right]

blast i., tearing of lung tissue or rupture of abdominal viscera without external i., as by the force of an explosion.

closed head i., a head i. in which continuity of the scalp and mucous membranes is maintained.

contrecoup i., i. occurring at a site other than that at which a blow is received, due to indirect transmission of force.

contrecoup i. of brain, an i. occurring beneath the skull opposite to the area of impact.

coup i. of brain, an i. occurring directly beneath the skull at the area of impact.

degloving i., avulsion of the skin of the hand (or foot) in which the part is skeletonized by

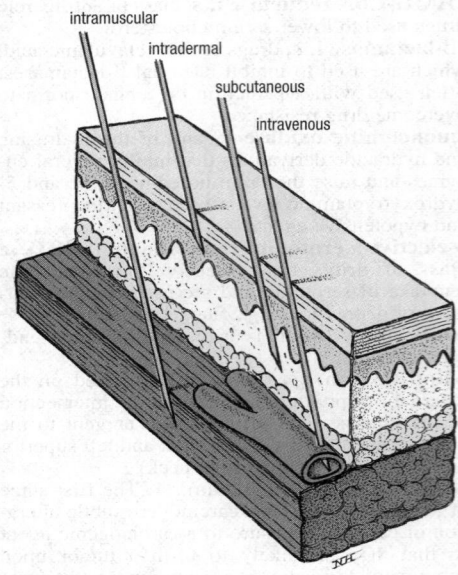

intramuscular
intradermal
subcutaneous
intravenous

injection

removal of most or all of the skin and subcutaneous tissue.

diffuse i.'s, i. over a large body area usually resulting from encounters with low velocity-high mass forces.

focal i., i. to a small, concentrated area, usually caused by high velocity-low mass forces.

hyperextension-hyperflexion i., violence to the body causing the unsupported head to hyperextend and hyperflex the neck rapidly.

open head i., a head i. in which there is a loss of continuity of scalp or mucous membranes; the term is sometimes used to indicate a communication between the exterior and the intracranial cavity. SEE ALSO penetrating *wound.*

whiplash i., popular term for hyperextension-hyperflexion i.

in•lay (in′lā). **1.** DENTISTRY A prefabricated restoration sealed in the cavity with cement. **2.** A graft of bone into a bone cavity. **3.** A graft of skin into a wound cavity for epithelialization. **4.** ORTHOPAEDICS An orthomechanical device inserted into a shoe; commonly called an "arch support."

in•let. A passage leading into a cavity. SYN aditus [NA].

in•nate (i′nāt, i-nāt′). SYN inborn. [L. *in-nascor,* pp. *-natus,* to be born in, pp. as adj. inborn, innate]

in•ner•va•tion (in′er-vā′shŭn). The supply of nerve fibers functionally connected with a part. [L. *in,* in, + *nervus,* nerve]

in•nid•i•a•tion (i-nid-ē-ā′shŭn). The growth and multiplication of abnormal cells in location to which they have been transported by means of lymph or the blood stream, or both. SEE ALSO metastasis. [L. *in,* in, + *nidus,* nest]

in•no•cent (in′ō-sent). **1.** Not apparently harmful.

2. Free from moral wrong. [L. *innocens (-ent-),* fr. *in,* neg., + *noceo,* to injure]

in•noc•u•ous (i-nok′yū-ŭs). Harmless. [L. *innocuus*]

in•nom•i•nate (i-nom′i-nāt). SYN anonyma. [L. *innominatus,* fr. *in-* neg. + *nomen (nomin-),* name]

Ino inosine.

in•oc•u•la•bil•i•ty (i-nok′yū-lă-bil′i-tē). The quality of being inoculable.

in•oc•u•la•ble (i-nok′yū-lă-bl). **1.** Transmissible by inoculation. **2.** Susceptible to a disease transmissible by inoculation.

in•oc•u•late (i-nok′yū-lāt). **1.** To introduce the agent of a disease or other antigenic material into the subcutaneous tissue or a blood vessel, or through an abraded or absorbing surface for preventive, curative, or experimental purposes. **2.** To implant microorganisms or infectious material into or upon culture media. **3.** To communicate a disease by transferring its virus. [L. *inoculo,* pp. *-atus,* to ingraft]

in•oc•u•la•tion (i-nok-yū-lā′shŭn). Introduction into the body of the causative organism of a disease.

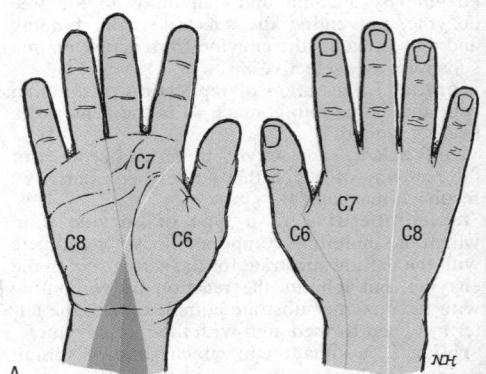

A

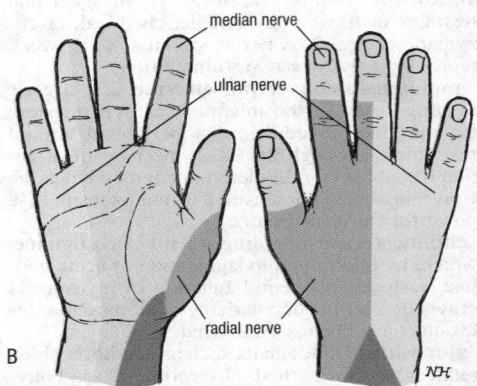

median nerve
ulnar nerve
radial nerve

B

innervation of the hand and wrist: (A) segmental dermatomes, (B) cutaneous nerve distribution

in·oc·u·lum (i-nok′yū-lŭm). The microorganism or other material introduced by inoculation.

in·op·er·a·ble (in-op′er-ă-bl). Denoting that which cannot be operated upon, or cannot be corrected or removed by an operation.

in·or·gan·ic (in-ōr-gan′ik). **1.** Not organic; not formed by living organisms. **2.** SEE inorganic *compound*. **3.** Not containing carbon.

in·os·a·mine (in-ōs′ă-mēn). An inositol in which an –OH group is replaced by an –NH₂ group.

in·os·co·py (in-os′kŏ-pē). The microscopic examination of biologic materials (*e.g.,* tissue, sputum, clotted blood) after dissecting or chemically digesting the fibrillary elements and strands of fibrin. [ino- + G. *skopeō,* to look at]

in·o·se·mia (in-ō-sē′mē-ă). **1.** The presence of inositol in the circulating blood. **2.** SYN fibremia. [inose + G. *haima,* blood]

in·o·sine (I, Ino) (in′ō-sēn). A nucleoside formed by the deamination of adenosine.

  i. 5′-monophosphate (IMP), SYN inosinic acid.

  i. 5′-triphosphate (ITP), inosine with triphosphoric acid esterified at its 5′ position; participates in a number of enzyme-catalyzed reactions.

in·o·sin·ic ac·id (in-ō-sin′ik). A mononucleotide found in muscle and other tissues; a key intermediate in purine biosynthesis; also produced in relatively high levels in muscle. SYN inosine 5′-monophosphate.

in·o·si·tol (in-ō′si-tōl, -tol). A member of the vitamin B complex.

  myo-**i.,** A constituent of various phosphatidylinositols and the most widely distributed form of i. found in microorganisms, higher plants, and animals.

in·o·si·tu·ria (in′ō-sī-tū′rē-ă). The excretion of inositol in the urine. [inositol + G. *ouron,* urine]

in·o·tro·pic (in-ō-trop′ik). Influencing the contractility of muscular tissue. [ino- + G. *tropos,* a turning]

inpatient. Patient who receives food and is assigned a bed in a health care facility while undergoing diagnosis and treatment.

in·quest (in′kwest). A legal inquiry into the cause of sudden, violent, or mysterious death. [L. *in,* in, + *quaero,* pp. *quaesitus,* to seek]

in·sane (in-sān′). **1.** Of unsound mind; severely mentally impaired; deranged; crazy. **2.** Relating to insanity. [L. *in*- neg. + *sanus,* sound, sane]

in·san·i·tary (in-san′i-tār-ē). Injurious to health, usually in reference to an unclean or contaminated environment. SYN unsanitary. [L. *in*- neg. + *sanus,* sound]

in·san·i·ty (in-san′i-tē). **1.** A nonmedical term referring to severe mental illness or psychosis. **2.** LAW That degree of mental illness which negates the individual's legal responsibility or capacity. [L. *in*- neg. + *sanus,* sound]

in·scrip·tion (in-skrip′shŭn). **1.** The main part of a prescription; that which indicates the drugs and the quantity of each to be used in the mixture. **2.** A mark, band, or line. [L. *inscriptio*]

in·sec·ti·cide (in-sek′ti-sīd). An agent that kills insects. [insect + L. *caedō,* to kill]

in·se·cu·ri·ty (in-sē-kyūr′i-tē). A feeling of unprotectedness and helplessness.

  gravitational i., overreaction to changes in head position in relation to gravity; fear or strong emotional response to situations that normally require only a balance reaction.

in·sem·i·na·tion (in-sem-i-nā′shŭn). Deposit of seminal fluid within the vagina, normally during coitus. SYN semination. [L. *in-semino,* pp. *-atus,* to sow or plant in, fr. *semen,* seed]

  artificial i., the introduction of semen into the vagina other than by coitus.

in·se·nes·cence (in-sē-nes′ens). The process of growing old. [L. *insenesco,* to begin to grow old]

in·sen·si·ble (in-sen′si-bl). **1.** SYN unconscious. **2.** Not appreciable by the senses. [L. *in-sensibilis,* fr. *in,* neg. + *sentio,* pp. *sensus,* to feel]

in·ser·tion (in-ser′shŭn). **1.** A putting in. **2.** The attachment of a muscle to the more movable part of the skeleton, as distinguished from origin. **3.** DENTISTRY The intraoral placing of a dental prosthesis. **4.** Intrusion of fragments of any size from molecular to cytogenetic into the normal genome. [L. *insertio,* a planting in, fr. *insero, -sertus,* to plant in]

in·sid·i·ous (in-sid′ē-ŭs). Treacherous; stealthy; denoting a disease that progresses gradually with inapparent symptoms. [L. *insidiosus,* cunning, fr. *insidiae* (pl.), an ambush]

in·sight (in′sīt). Self-understanding as to the motives and reasons behind one's own actions or those of another's.

in si·tu (in sī′tū). In position, not extending beyond the focus or level of origin. [L. *in,* in, + *situs,* site]

in·sol·u·ble (in-sol′yū-bl). Not soluble.

in·som·ni·a (in-som′nē-ă). Inability to sleep, in the absence of external impediments, such as noise, a bright light, etc., during the period when sleep should normally occur; may vary in degree from restlessness or disturbed slumber to a curtailment of the normal length of sleep or to absolute wakefulness. [L. fr. *in-* priv. + *somnus,* sleep]

in·som·ni·ac (in-som′nē-ak). **1.** A sufferer from insomnia. **2.** Exhibiting, tending toward, or producing insomnia.

in·sorp·tion (in-sōrp′shŭn). Movement of substances from the lumen of the gut into the blood. [L. *in,* in, + *sorbeo,* to suck]

in·sper·sion (in-sper′shŭn, -zhŭn). Sprinkling with a fluid or a powder. [L. *inspersio,* fr. *in-spergo,* pp. *-spersus,* to scatter upon, fr. *spargo,* to scatter]

in·spi·ra·tion (in-spi-rā′shŭn). SYN inhalation (1). [L. *inspiratio,* fr. *in-spiro,* pp. *-atus,* to breathe in]

in·spi·ra·to·ry (in-spī′ră-tō-rē). Relating to or timed during inhalation.

in·spire (in-spīr′). SYN inhale.

in·spis·sate (in-spis′āt). To perform or undergo inspissation.

in·spis·sa·tion (in-spi-sā′shŭn). **1.** The act of thickening or condensing, as by evaporation or absorption of fluid. **2.** An increased thickening or diminished fluidity. [L. *in,* intensive, + *spisso,* pp. *-atus,* to thicken]

in·sta·bil·i·ty (in-stă-bil′i-tē). **1.** The state of being unstable, or lacking stability. **2.** The abnormal tendency of a joint to subluxate or dislocate with normal activities and stresses. SEE ALSO laxity.

spinal i., the inability of the spinal column, under physiologic loads, to maintain its normal configuration; may result in damage to the spinal cord or nerve roots or lead to the development of a painful spinal deformity.

in·star (in′stahr). Any of the successive nymphal or larval stages in the metamorphosis of insects. [L. form]

in·step. The arch, or highest part of the dorsum of the foot. SEE ALSO tarsus.

in·stil·la·tion (in-sti-lā′shŭn). Dropping of a liquid on or into a part. [L. *instillatio,* fr. *in-stillo,* pp. *-atus,* to pour in by drops, fr. *stilla,* a drop]

in·stinct (in′stinkt). **1.** An enduring disposition or tendency to act in an organized and biologically adaptive manner. **2.** The unreasoning impulse to perform some purposive action without an immediate consciousness of the end to which that action may lead. **3.** PSYCHOANALYTIC THEORY The forces assumed to exist behind the tension caused by the needs of the id. [L. *instinctus,* impulse]

death i., the i. of all living creatures toward self-destruction, death, or a return to the inorganic lifelessness from which they arose.

herd i., tendency or inclination to band together with and share the customs of others of a group, and to conform to the opinions and adopt the views of the group.

life i., the i. of self-preservation and sexual procreation; the basic urge toward preservation of the species.

in·stinc·tive, in·stinc·tu·al (in-stink′tiv, -stink′ chū-ăl). Relating to instinct.

in·stru·ment (in′strū-ment). A tool or implement. [L. *instrumentum*]

purse-string i., an intestinal clamp with jaws at an angle to the handle; when closed across the bowel, large grooved interdigitating serrations allow passage of a straight needle and suture through each side to form a purse-string suture.

stereotactic i., stereotaxic i., an apparatus attached to the head, used to localize precisely an area in the brain by means of coordinates related to intracerebral structures.

in·stru·men·tar·i·um (in′strū-men-tār′ē-ŭm). A collection of instruments and other equipment for an operation or for a medical procedure.

in·su·date (in′sū-dāt). Fluid swelling within an arterial wall (ordinarily serous), differing from an exudate in that it does not come to lie extramurally. [L. *in,* in, + *sudo,* pp. *-atus,* to sweat]

in·suf·fi·cien·cy (in-sŭ-fish′en-sē). **1.** Lack of completeness of function or power. **2.** SYN incompetence (1). [L. *in-,* neg. + *sufficientia,* fr. *sufficio* to suffice]

acute adrenocortical i., severe adrenocortical i. when an illness or trauma causes an increased demand for adrenocortical hormones in a patient with adrenal insufficiency. SYN addisonian crisis, adrenal crisis.

adrenocortical i., loss, to varying degrees, of adrenocortical function. SYN hypocorticoidism.

aortic i., SEE valvular *regurgitation.*

cardiac i., SYN heart *failure* (1).

chronic adrenocortical i., adrenocortical i. usually as the result of idiopathic atrophy or destruction of both adrenal glands by tuberculosis, an autoimmune process, or other diseases. SYN Addison's disease.

convergence i., that condition in which an esophoria or esotropia is more marked for far vision than for near vision.

coronary i., inadequate coronary circulation leading to anginal pain.

divergence i., that condition in which an exophoria or exotropia is more marked for near vision than for far vision.

mitral i., SEE valvular *regurgitation.*

myocardial i., SYN heart *failure* (1).

primary adrenocortical i., adrenocortical i. caused by disease, destruction, or surgical removal of the adrenal cortices.

pulmonary i., SEE valvular *regurgitation.*

secondary adrenocortical i., adrenocortical i. caused by failure of ACTH secretion resulting from anterior pituitary disease or inhibition of ACTH production resulting from exogenous steroid therapy.

tricuspid i., SEE valvular *regurgitation.*

valvular i., SYN valvular *regurgitation.*

velopharyngeal i., anatomical or functional deficiency in the soft palate or superior constrictor muscle, resulting in the inability to achieve velopharyngeal closure.

venous i., inadequate drainage of venous blood from a part, resulting in edema or dermatosis.

in·suf·flate (in-sŭf′lāt). To blow air, gas, or fine powder into a cavity. [L. *in-sufflo,* to blow on or into]

in·suf·fla·tion (in-sŭf-lā′shŭn). **1.** The act or process of insufflating. **2.** SYN inhalant (3).

in·su·la, gen. and pl. **in·su·lae** (in′sū-lă, -lē). **1** [NA]. An oval region of the cerebral cortex overlying the extreme capsule, lateral to the lenticular nucleus, buried in the depth of the fissura lateralis cerebri (sylvian fissure). SYN island of Reil. **2.** SYN island. **3.** Any circumscribed body or patch on the skin. [L. island]

in·su·lar (in′sū-lăr). Relating to any insula, especially the island of Reil.

in·su·lin (in′sŭ-lin). A polypeptide hormone, secreted by beta cells in the islets of Langerhans, that promotes glucose utilization, protein synthesis, and the formation and storage of neutral lipids; obtained from various animals and available in a variety of preparations, i. is used parenterally in the treatment of diabetes mellitus. [L. *insula,* island, + -in]

human i., a protein that has the normal structure of i. produced by the human pancreas, prepared by recombinant DNA techniques and by semisynthetic processes.

isophane i., a modified form of i. composed of i., protamine, and zinc; an intermediately acting preparation used for the treatment of diabetes mellitus.

in·su·lin·o·gen·e·sis (in′sŭ-lin-ō-jen′ĕ-sis). Production of insulin. [insulin + G. *genesis,* production]

in·su·lin·o·gen·ic, in·su·lo·gen·ic (in′sŭ-lin-ō-jen′ik, in′su̇-lō-jen′ik). Relating to insulinogenesis.

in·su·li·no·ma (in′su̇-li-nō′mă). An islet cell adenoma that secretes insulin. SYN insuloma.

in·su·li·tis (in′su̇-lī′tis). Inflammation of the islands of Langerhans, with lymphocytic infiltration which may result from viral infection and be the initial lesion of insulin-dependent diabetes mellitus. [L. *insula*, island, + *-itis*, inflammation]

in·su·lo·ma (in-su̇-lō′mă). SYN insulinoma. [L. *insula*, island, + *-oma*, tumor]

in·sult (in′sŭlt). An injury, attack, or trauma. [LL. *insultus*, fr L. *insulto*, to spring upon]

in·sus·cep·ti·bil·i·ty (in′su̇-sep′ti-bil′i-tē). SYN immunity. [L. *suscipio*, pp. *-ceptus*, to take upon one, fr. *sub*, under, + *capio*, to take]

in·te·gra·tion (in-tĕ-grā′shŭn). **1.** The state of being combined, or the process of combining, into a complete and harmonious whole. **2.** PHYSIOLOGY The process of building up, as by accretion, anabolism, etc. **3.** MATHEMATICS The process of ascertaining a function from its differential. **4.** MOLECULAR BIOLOGY A recombination event in which a genetic element is inserted. [L. *integro*, pp. *-atus*, to make whole, fr. *integer*, whole]
  sensory i., the process of organizing sensory information in the brain in order to make an adaptive response.

in·teg·ri·ty (in-teg′ri-tē). Soundness or completeness of structure; a sound or unimpaired condition.

in·teg·u·ment (in-teg′yū-ment). **1.** The enveloping membrane of the body; includes, in addition to the epidermis and dermis, all of the derivatives of the epidermis, *e.g.,* hairs, nails, sudoriferous and sebaceous glands, and mammary glands. **2.** The rind, capsule, or covering of any body or part. SYN tegument (2). SYN integumentum commune [NA], tegument (1). [L. *integumentum,* a covering, fr. *in-tego,* to cover]

in·teg·u·men·ta·ry (in-teg-yū-men′tă-rē). Relating to the integument. SEE ALSO cutaneous, dermal.

in·teg·u·men·tum com·mune (in-teg-yū-men′ tŭm kō-mū′nē) [NA]. SYN integument.

in·tel·lec·tu·al·i·za·tion (in-te-lek′chū-ăl-i-zā′ shŭn). An unconscious defense mechanism in which reasoning, logic, or focusing on and verbalizing intellectual minutiae is used in an attempt to avoid confrontation with an objectionable impulse, affect, or interpersonal situation. [L. *intellectus*, perception, discernment]

in·tel·li·gence (in-tel′i-jens). **1.** An individual's aggregate capacity to act purposefully, think rationally, and deal effectively with the environment, especially in meeting challenges and solving problems. **2.** PSYCHOLOGY An individual's relative standing on two quantitative indices, measured i. and effectiveness of adaptive behavior; a quantitative score or similar index on both indices constitutes the operational definition of i. [L. *intelligentia*]

in·ten·si·ty (in-ten′si-tē). Marked tension; great activity; often used simply to denote a measure of the degree or amount of some quality. [L. *intendo*, pp. *-tensus*, to stretch out]

luminous i. (I), the luminous flux per unit solid angle in a given direction. SYN radiant i.
  radiant i. (I), SYN luminous i.

in·ten·tion (in-ten′shŭn). **1.** An objective. **2.** SURGERY A process or operation. [L. *intentio*, a stretching out; intention]

△**inter-.** Among, between. [L. *inter,* between]

in·ter·ac·tion (int′er-ak′shŭn). **1.** The reciprocal action between two entities in a common environment, as in chemical i., ecological i., and social i. **2.** The effects when two entities concur that would not be observed with either in isolation. **3.** STATISTICS, PHARMACOLOGY, QUANTITATIVE GENETICS The phenomenon that the combined effects of two causes differ from the sum of the effects separately (as in synergism and antagonism). **4.** Independent operation of two or more causes to produce or prevent an effect. **5.** STATISTICS The necessity for a product term in a linear model.

in·ter·bod·y (in′ter-bod′ē). Between the bodies of two adjacent vertebrae.

in·ter·ca·dence (in-ter-kā′dens). The occurrence of an extra beat between two regular pulse beats. [inter- + L. *cado*, pr. p. *cadens (-ent-)*, to fall]

in·ter·ca·dent (in-ter-kā′dent). Irregular in rhythm; characterized by intercadence.

in·ter·ca·lary (in-ter′kă-ler-ē, in-ter-kal′er-ē). **1.** Occurring between two others; as in a pulse tracing, an upstroke interposed between two normal pulse beats. **2.** In fungi, located in a hypha or between hyphal segments, not at a hyphal terminus. [L. *intercalarius*, concerning an insertion]

in·ter·ca·lat·ed (in-ter′kă-lā-ted). Interposed; inserted between two others. [L. *intercalatus*]

in·ter·cil·i·um (in-ter-sil′ē-ŭm). SYN glabella. [inter- + L. *cilium*, eyelid]

in·ter·course (in′ter-kōrs). Communication or dealings between or among people. [L. *intercursus,* a running between]
  sexual i., SYN coitus.

in·ter·cri·co·thy·rot·o·my (in-ter-krī′kō-thī-rot′ ō-mē). SYN cricothyrotomy.

in·ter·cross (in′ter-kros). A mating between two individuals both heterozygous at a specified locus or loci.

in·ter·cur·rent (in-ter-ker′ent). Intervening; said of a disease attacking a person who already has another disease. [inter- + L. *curro,* pr. p. *currens (-ent-)*, to run]

in·ter·cus·pa·tion (in′ter-kŭs-pā′shŭn). **1.** The cusp-to-fossa relation of the maxillary and mandibular posterior teeth to each other. **2.** The interlocking or fitting together of the cusps of opposing teeth. SYN interdigitation (4).

in·ter·den·tal (in-ter-den′tăl). **1.** Between the teeth. **2.** Denoting the relationship between the proximal surfaces of the teeth of the same arch. [inter- + L. *dens,* tooth]

in·ter·den·ti·um (in-ter-den′shē-ŭm). The interval between any two contiguous teeth.

in·ter·dig·it (in-ter-dij′it). That part of the hand or foot lying between any two adjacent fingers or toes.

in·ter·dig·i·ta·tion (in′ter-dij-i-tā′shŭn). **1.** The mutual interlocking of toothed or tonguelike processes. **2.** The processes thus interlocked. **3.** Infoldings or plicae of adjacent cell or plasma membranes. **4.** SYN intercuspation (2). [inter- + L. *digitus,* finger]

in·ter·dis·ci·pli·nary (in-ter-dis′i-pli-nār-ē). Denoting the overlapping interests of different fields of medicine and science. [inter- + L. *disciplina,* instruction, teaching]

in·ter·face (in′ter-fās). **1.** A surface that forms a common boundary of two bodies. **2.** The boundary between regions of different radiopacity, acoustic, or magnetic resonance properties; the projection of the i. between tissues of different such properties on an image.

in·ter·fer·ence (in-ter-fēr′ens). **1.** The coming together of waves in various media in such a way that the crests of one series correspond to the hollows of the other, the two thus neutralizing each other; or so that the crests of the two series correspond, thus increasing the excursions of the waves. **2.** Collision within the myocardium of two waves of excitation at the junction of territories controlled by each, as is seen in A-V dissociation. **3.** Also, in A-V dissociation, the disturbance of the regular rhythm of the ventricles by a conducted impulse from the atria, *e.g.,* by a ventricular capture (interference beat). **4.** The condition in which infection of a cell by one virus prevents superinfection by another virus, or in which superinfection prevents effects which would result from infection by either virus alone, even though both viruses persist. [inter- + L. *ferio,* to strike]

in·ter·fer·on (IFN) (in-ter-fēr′on). A class of small glycoproteins that exert antiviral activity at least in homologous cells through cellular metabolic processes involving synthesis of double-stranded RNA. [interfere + -on]

in·ter·ic·tal (in-ter-ik′tăl). The period between convulsions. [inter- + L. *ictus,* stroke]

in·ter·ki·ne·sis (in′ter-ki-nē′sis). Period between the first and second divisions of meiosis; comparable to interphase of mitosis. [inter- + G. *kinēsis,* movement]

in·ter·leukin (IL) (in-ter-loo′kin). The name given to cytokines once their amino acid structure is known. SEE ALSO lymphokines, cytokine. [inter- + *leuk*ocyte + -in]

in·ter·leu·kin-1. A cytokine, derived primarily from mononuclear phagocytes, which enhances the proliferation of T helper cells and growth and differentiation of B cells.

in·ter·leu·kin-2. A cytokine derived from T helper lymphocytes that causes proliferation of T lymphocytes and activated B lymphocytes.

in·ter·leu·kin-3 (IL-3). A cytokine derived from monocytes, fibroblasts, and endothelial cells that increases production of monocytes.

in·ter·leu·kin-4 (IL-4). A cytokine derived from T4 lymphocytes that causes differentiation of B lymphocytes.

in·ter·leu·kin-5 (IL-5). A cytokine derived from T lymphocytes that causes activation of B lymphocytes and differentiation of eosinophils.

in·ter·leu·kin-6 (IL-6). A cytokine derived from fibroblasts, macrophages, and tumor cells that increases synthesis and secretion of immunoglobulins by B lymphocytes.

in·ter·leu·kin-7 (IL-7). A cytokine derived from bone marrow cells that causes proliferation of B and T lymphocytes.

in·ter·leu·kin-8 (IL-8). A cytokine derived from endothelial cells, fibroblasts, keratinocytes, macrophages, and monocytes which causes chemotaxis of neutrophils and T cell lymphocytes.

in·ter·leu·kin-9 (IL-9). A cytokine derived from T cells which causes growth and proliferation of T cells.

in·ter·leu·kin-10 (IL-10). A cytokine derived from helper T cell lymphocytes, B cell lymphocytes, and monocytes that inhibits gamma-interferon (IFNγ) secretion by T cell lymphocytes and it inhibits mononuclear cell inflammation.

in·ter·leu·kin-11 (IL-11). A cytokine derived from bone marrow stromal cells (endothelial cells, macrophages, and preadipocytes) which stimulates increased plasma concentrations of acute phase proteins.

in·ter·leu·kin-12 (IL-12). A cytokine derived from B lymphocytes, T lymphocytes, and macrophages that induces gamma-interferon (IFNγ) gene expression in T lymphocytes and NK cells.

in·ter·leu·kin-13 (IL-13). A cytokine derived from helper T cell lymphocytes that inhibits mononuclear cell inflammation.

in·ter·leu·kin-14 (IL-14). A cytokine derived from T cells which stimulates B cell proliferation and inhibits Ig secretion.

in·ter·leu·kin-15 (IL-15). A cytokine derived from T cells which stimulates T cell proliferation and NK cell activation.

in·ter·lo·bi·tis (in′ter-lō-bī′tis). Inflammation of the pleura separating two pulmonary lobes.

in·ter·me·di·ate (in′ter-mē′dē-it). **1.** Between two extremes; interposed; intervening. **2.** A substance formed in the course of chemical reactions that then proceeds to participate rapidly in further reactions, so that at any given moment it is present in minute concentrations only; such substances, when appearing in the course of the reactions involved in metabolism, are metabolic i.'s. **3.** DENTISTRY A cement base. **4.** An element or organ between right and left (or lateral and medial) structures. SYN intermedius [NA].

intermediate care facility (ICF). institutional setting where services are provided that do not require the level of care provided in a hospital or skilled-nursing facility. SEE nursing facility.

intermediate care nursing facility (ICF). nursing facility providing 24-hour supervision and nursing care as needed.

in·ter·me·di·us (in-ter-mē′dē-ŭs) [NA]. SYN intermediate. [L.]

in·ter·mit·tent (in-ter-mit′ent). Marked by intervals of complete quietude between two periods of activity.

in·tern (in′tern). An advanced student or recent graduate undertaking further education by assisting in the medical or surgical care of hospital patients, with supervision and instruction; formerly, one who resided within the institution. [F. *interne,* inside]

in·ter·nal (in-ter′năl). Away from the surface; often incorrectly used to mean medial. [L. *internus*]

in·ter·nal·i·za·tion (in-ter′năl-i-zā′shŭn). Adopting as one's own the standards and values of another person or society.

In·ter·na·tion·al Clas·si·fi·ca·tion of Dis··eases. The classification of specific conditions and groups of conditions determined by an internationally representative expert committee that advises the World Health Organization, which publishes the complete list in a periodically revised book, the *Manual of the International Statistical Classification of Diseases, Injuries and Causes of Death.* The 10th revision of the ICD came into use in 1992. The *International Classification of Diseases, Adapted for Use in the United States* (ICDA) is an adaptation of the ICD that includes a classification of surgical operations and other therapeutic and diagnostic procedures.

In·ter·na·tion·al Clas·si·fi·ca·tion of Health Prob·lems in Pri·ma·ry Care. A classification of diseases, conditions and problems arranged for use in primary care where diagnostic precision is seldom possible.

In·ter·na·tion·al Clas·si·fi·ca·tion of Impair·ments, Dis·a·bil·i·ties and Hand·i·caps. A WHO-sponsored numerical taxonomy of the impairments, disabilities and handicaps consequent upon injury and disease.

International Phonetic Alphabet (IPA). System of orthographic symbols devised for representing speech sounds; can be used for any language or to represent the sounds of disordered speech.

In·ter·na·tion·al Sys·tem of Units (SI). A system of measurements, based on the metric system, adopted at the 11th General Conference on Weights and Measures of the International Organization for Standardization (1960) to cover both the coherent units (basic, supplementary, and derived units) and the decimal multiples and submultiples of these units formed by use of prefixes proposed for general international scientific and technological use. SI proposes seven basic units: meter (m), kilogram (kg), second (s), ampere (A), Kelvin (K), candela (cd), and mole (mol) for the basic quantities of length, mass, time, electric current, temperature, luminous intensity, and amount of substance; supplementary units proposed include the radian (rad) for plane angle and steradian (sr) for solid angle; derived units (*e.g.,* force, power, frequency) are stated in terms of the basic units (*e.g.,* velocity is in meters per second, m/s^{-1}). Multiples (prefixes) in descending order are: exa- (E, 10^{18}), peta- (P, 10^{15}), tera- (T, 10^{12}), giga- (G, 10^{9}), mega- (M, 10^{6}), kilo- (k, 10^{3}), hecto- (h, 10^{2}), deca- (da, 10^{1}), deci- (d, 10^{-1}), centi- (c, 10^{-2}), milli- (m, 10^{-3}), micro- (μ, 10^{-6}), nano- (n, 10^{-9}), pico- (p, 10^{-12}), femto- (f, 10^{-15}), atto- (a, 10^{-18}). The prefix zepto (z) has been proposed for 10^{-21}. Those involving a multiple of 10^{3} are recommended; compounds of these are not recommended (*e.g.,* mμ for n). [Fr. *Système International d'Unités*]

in·ter·neu·rons (in′ter-nū′ronz). Combinations or groups of neurons between sensory and motor neurons that govern coordinated activity.

in·tern·ist (in-ter′nist, in′ter-nist). A physician trained in internal medicine.

in·ter·node (in′ter-nōd). SYN internodal *segment.*

in·ter·nu·cle·ar (in-ter-nū′klē-ăr). Between nerve cell groups in the brain or retina.

in·ter·nun·ci·al (in-ter-nun′sē-ăl). **1.** Indicating a neuron functionally interposed between two or more other neurons. **2.** Acting as a medium of communication between two organs. [L. *inter-nuntius* (or *-nuncius*), a messenger between two parties, fr. *inter,* between, + *nuncius,* a messenger]

in·ter·o·cep·tive (in′ter-ō-sep′tiv). Relating to the sensory nerve cells innervating the viscera (thoracic, abdominal and pelvic organs, and the cardiovascular system), their sensory end organs, or the information they convey to the spinal cord and the brain. [inter- + L. *capio,* to take]

in·ter·o·cep·tor (in′ter-ō-sep′ter). One of the various forms of small sensory end organs (receptors) situated within the walls of the respiratory and gastrointestinal tracts or in other viscera. [inter- + L. *capio,* to take]

in·ter·par·ox·ys·mal (in′ter-par-ok-siz′măl). Occurring between successive paroxysms of a disease.

in·ter·pha·lan·ge·al (in′ter-fă-lan′jē-ăl). Between two phalanges; denoting the finger or toe joints.

in·ter·phase (in′ter-fāz). The stage between two successive divisions of a cell nucleus in which the biochemical and physiologic functions of the cell are performed and replication of chromatin occurs.

in·ter·phy·let·ic (in′ter-fī-let′ik). Denoting the transitional forms between two kinds of cells during the course of metaplasia. [inter- + G. *phylē,* tribe]

in·ter·pre·ta·tion (in-ter-pre-tā′shŭn). **1.** PSYCHO-ANALYSIS The characteristic therapeutic intervention of the analyst. **2.** CLINICAL PSYCHOLOGY Drawing inferences and formulating the meaning in terms of the psychological dynamics inherent in an individual's responses to psychological tests or during psychotherapy.

in·ter·prox·i·mal (in-ter-prok′si-măl). Between adjoining surfaces.

in·ter·space (in′ter-spās). Any space between two similar objects, such as a costal i. or interval between two ribs.

in·ter·stice, pl. **in·ter·stic·es** (in-ter′stis, -sti-siz). SYN interstitium. [L. *interstitium,* fr. *sisto,* to stand]

in·ter·sti·tial (in-ter-stish′ăl). **1.** Relating to spaces or interstices in any structure. **2.** Relating to spaces within a tissue or organ, but excluding such spaces as body cavities or potential space. Cf. intracavitary.

in·ter·stit·i·um (in-ter-stish′ē-ŭm). A small area, space, or gap in the substance of an organ or tissue. SEE ALSO connective *tissue.* SYN interstice. [L.]

in·ter·tar·sal (in-ter-tar′săl). Denoting the articulations of the tarsal bones with each other.

in·ter·tri·go (in-ter-trī′gō). Irritant dermatitis occurring between folds or juxtaposed surfaces of the skin, as between the scrotum and the thigh, caused by friction, sweat retention, moisture, warmth, and concomitant overgrowth of resident microorganisms. [L. a galling of the skin, fr. *inter,* between, + *tero,* to rub]

in·ter·val (in′ter-văl). A time or space between two periods or objects; a break in continuity. [L. *inter-vallum,* space between breastworks in a camp, an interval, fr. *vallum,* a rampart, wall]

A-V i., the time from the beginning of atrial systole to the beginning of ventricular systole as measured the electrocardiogram.

P-R i., in the electrocardiogram, the time elapsing between the beginning of the P wave and the beginning of the next QRS complex; it corresponds to the a-c i. of the venous pulse and is normally 0.12-0.20 sec.

Q-T i., time from electrocardiogram Q wave to the end of the T wave corresponding to electrical systole.

sphygmic i., the period in the cardiac cycle when the semilunar valves are open and blood is being ejected from the ventricles into the arterial system. SYN ejection period.

in·ter·ven·tion (in-ter-ven′shŭn). An action or ministration that produces an effect or that is intended to alter the course of a pathologic process. [L. *inter-ventio,* a coming between, fr *intervenio,* to come between]

in·tes·ti·nal (in-tes′ti-năl). Relating to the intestine.

in·tes·tine (in-tes′tin). SYN intestinum (1). [L. *intestinum*]

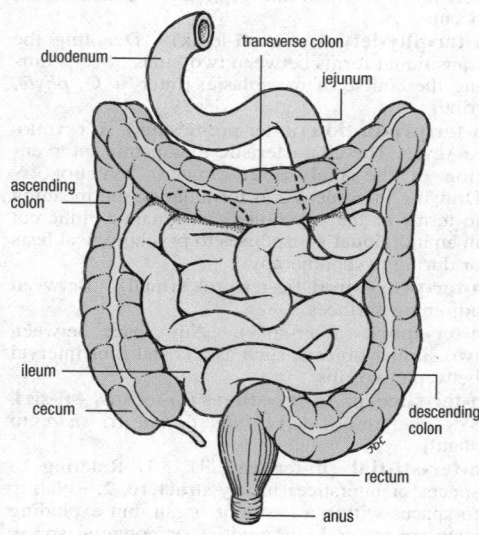

duodenum — transverse colon — jejunum — ascending colon — ileum — cecum — descending colon — rectum — anus

intestines

large i., the portion of the digestive tube extending from the ileocecal valve to the anus; it comprises the cecum, colon, rectum, and anal canal.

small i., the portion of the digestive tube between the stomach and the cecum or beginning of the large intestine; it consists of three portions: duodenum, jejunum, and ileum.

in·tes·ti·num, pl. **in·tes·ti·na** (in-tes-tī′nŭm, -nă). **1** [NA]. The digestive tube passing from the stomach to the anus. It is divided primarily into the i. tenue (small intestine) and the i. crassum (large intestine). SYN bowel, intestine. **2.** Inward; inner. [neuter of *intestinus*] SYN gut (1). [L. *intestinus,* internal, ntr. as noun, the entrails, fr. *intus,* within]

in·ti·ma (in′ti-mă). Innermost. SEE *tunica* intima. [L. fem. of *intimus,* inmost]

in·ti·mal (in′ti-măl). Relating to the intima or inner coat of a vessel.

in·ti·mi·tis (in-ti-mī′tis). Inflammation of an intima, as in endangiitis. [intima + G. -*itis,* inflammation]

in·toe (in′tō). Medial deviation of the axis of the foot. SYN *metatarsus* varus.

in·tol·er·ance (in-tol′er-ăns). Abnormal metabolism, excretion, or other disposition of a given substance; term often used to indicate impaired utilization or disposal of dietary constituents.

in·tor·sion (in-tōr′shŭn). Conjugate rotation of the upper poles of each cornea inward. [L. *intorqueo,* pp. *tortus,* to twist]

in·tor·tor (in-tōr′tŏr). A muscle that turns a part medialward. SEE ALSO invertor.

in·tox·a·tion (in-tok-sā′shŭn). Poisoning, especially by the toxic products of bacteria or poisonous animals, other than alcohol. [see intoxication]

in·tox·i·cant (in-tok′si-kant). **1.** Having the power to intoxicate. **2.** An intoxicating agent, such as alcohol.

in·tox·i·ca·tion (in-tok-si-kā′shŭn). **1.** SYN poisoning. **2.** SYN acute *alcoholism.* [L. *in,* in, + G. *toxikon,* poison]

△**intra-.** Inside, within; opposite of extra-. SEE ALSO endo-, ento-. [L. within]

in·tra·cath·e·ter (in′tră-kath′e-ter). A plastic tube, usually attached to the puncturing needle, inserted into a blood vessel for infusion, injection, or pressure monitoring.

in·tra·cav·i·tary (in′tră-cav′i-tār-ē). Within an organ or body cavity.

in·tra·cor·po·re·al (in′tră-kōr-po′rē-ăl). **1.** Within the body. **2.** Within any structure anatomically styled a corpus. [intra- + L. *corpus,* body]

in·trac·ta·ble (in′trak′tă-bl). **1.** SYN refractory (1). **2.** SYN obstinate (1). [L. *in-tractabilis,* fr. in-neg. + *tracto,* to draw, haul]

in·trad (in′trăd). Toward the inner part.

in·tra·em·bry·on·ic (in′tră-em-brē-on′ik). Within the embryonic body, the portion of the umbilical vein within the embryo. Cf. extraembryonic.

in·tra·fi·lar (in′tră-fī′lăr). Lying within the meshes of a network. [intra- + L. *filum,* thread]

in·tra·fu·sal (in′tră-fyū′săl). Applied to structures within the muscle spindle.

in·tra·par·tum (in′tră-par′tŭm). During labor and delivery or childbirth. Cf. antepartum, postpartum. [intra- + L. *partus,* childbirth]

in·tra·psy·chic (in′tră-sī′kik). Denoting the psychological dynamics that occur inside the mind without reference to the individual's exchanges with other persons or events.

in·tra vi·tam (in′tră vī′tăm). During life. [L. *vita,* life]

in·trin·sic (in-trin′sik). **1.** Belonging entirely to a part. **2.** ANATOMY Denoting those muscles whose origin and insertion are both within the structure under consideration, distinguished from the extrinsic muscles which have their origin outside of the structure under consideration; applied especially to the limbs but also to the ciliary muscle as distinguished from the recti and other orbital muscles which are outside the eyeball. SYN essential (6). [L. *intrinsecus,* on the inside]

intro-.   Inwardly, into; opposite of extra-. Cf. intra-. [L. *intro,* into]

in·tro·duc·er (in-trō-dūs′er).   An instrument, such as a catheter, needle, or endotracheal tube, for introduction of a flexible device. [L. *intro-duco,* to lead into, introduce]

in·tro·flec·tion, in·tro·flex·ion (in′trō-flek′shŭn). A bending inward. [intro- + L. *flecto,* pp. *flectus,* to bend]

in·tro·i·tus (in-trō′i-tŭs). The entrance into a canal or hollow organ, as the vagina. [L. entrance, fr. *intro-eo,* to go into]

in·tro·jec·tion (in-trō-jek′shŭn). A psychological defense mechanism involving appropriation of an external happening and its assimilation by the personality, making it a part of the self. [intro- + L. *jacto,* to throw]

in·tro·mis·sion (in-trō-mish′ŭn). The insertion or introduction of one part into another. [intro- + L. *mitto,* to send]

in·tro·mit·tent (in-trō-mit′ent). Conveying or sending into a body or cavity.

in·tron (in′tron). A portion of DNA that lies between two exons, is transcribed into RNA, but does not appear in that RNA after maturation, and so is not expressed (as protein) in protein synthesis. [inter- + -on]

in·tro·spec·tion (in-trō-spek′shŭn). Looking inward; self-scrutinizing; contemplating one's own mental processes. [intro- + L. *specto,* to look at, inspect]

in·tro·spec·tive (in-trō-spek′tiv). Relating to introspection.

in·tro·sus·cep·tion (in′trō-sŭs-sep′shŭn). SYN intussusception.

in·tro·ver·sion (in-trō-ver′zhŭn). **1.** The turning of a structure into itself. SEE ALSO intussusception, invagination. **2.** A trait of preoccupation with oneself, as practiced by an introvert. Cf. extraversion. [intro- + L. *verto,* pp. *versus,* to turn]

in·tro·vert. **1** (in′trō-vert). One who tends to be unusually shy, introspective, self-centered, and avoids becoming concerned with or involved in the affairs of others. Cf. extrovert. **2** (in-trō-vert′). To turn a structure into itself.

in·tu·bate (in′tū-bāt). To perform intubation.

in·tu·ba·tion (in-tū-bā′shŭn). Insertion of a tubular device into a canal, hollow organ, or cavity; specifically, passage of an oro- or nasotracheal tube for anesthesia or for control of pulmonary ventilation. [L. *in,* in, + *tuba,* tube]

   endotracheal i., passage of a tube through the nose or mouth into the trachea for maintenance of the airway during anesthesia or for maintenance of an imperiled airway.

in·tu·mesce (in-tū-mes′). To swell up; to enlarge. [L. *in-tumesco,* to swell up, fr. *tumeo,* to swell]

in·tu·mes·cence (in-tū-mes′ens). **1.** SYN enlarge-

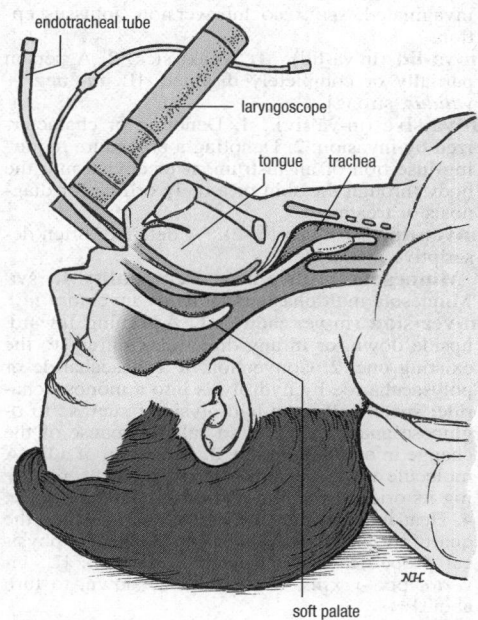

intubation

ment. **2.** The process of enlarging or swelling; used to describe the spinal enlargements.

in·tu·mes·cent (in-tū-mes′ent). Enlarging; becoming enlarged or swollen.

in·tus·sus·cep·tion (in′tŭs-sŭ-sep′shŭn). **1.** The taking up or receiving of one part within another, especially the enfolding of one segment of the intestine within another. SEE ALSO introversion, invagination. **2.** The incorporation of new material in the growth of the cell wall. SYN introsusception. [L. *intus,* within, + *sus-cipio,* to take up, fr. *sub + capio,* to take]

in·tus·sus·cep·tive (in′tŭs-sŭ-sep′tiv). Relating to or characterized by intussusception.

in·tus·sus·cep·tum (in′tŭs-sŭ-sep′tŭm). The inner segment in an intussusception; that part of the bowel which is received within the other part.

in·tus·sus·cip·i·ens (in′tŭs-sŭ-sip′ē-enz). The portion of the bowel, in intussusception, which receives the other portion. [L. *intus,* within, + *suscipiens,* pr. p. of *suscipio,* to take up]

in·u·lin (In) (in′yū-lin). A fructose polysaccharide from the rhizome of *Inula* and other plants; used by intravenous injection to determine the rate of glomerular filtration. Cf. inulin *clearance.*

in·unc·tion (in-ŭngk′shŭn). Administration of a drug in ointment form by rubbing to cause absorption of the active ingredient. [L. *inunctio,* an anointing, fr. *inunguo,* pp. *-unctus,* to smear on]

in·vag·i·nate (in-vaj′i-nāt). To ensheathe, infold, or insert a structure within itself or another. [L. *in,* in, + *vagina,* a sheath]

in·vag·i·na·tion (in-vaj′i-nā′shŭn). **1.** The ensheathing, enfolding, or insertion of a structure within itself or another. **2.** The state of being

in

invaginated. SEE ALSO introversion, intussusception.

in•va•lid (in′vă-lid). **1.** Weak; sick. **2.** A person partially or completely disabled. [L. *in*- neg. + *validus,* strong]

in•va•sive (in-vā′siv). **1.** Denoting or characterized by invasion. **2.** Denoting a procedure requiring insertion of an instrument or device into the body through the skin or a body orifice for diagnosis or treatment.

in•ven•to•ry (in′ven-tōr-ē). A detailed, often descriptive, list of items.

Minnesota Multiphasic Personality I., SYN Minnesota multiphasic personality inventory *test.*

in•ver•sion (in-ver′zhŭn). **1.** A turning inward, upside down, or in any direction contrary to the existing one. **2.** Conversion of a disaccharide or polysaccharide by hydrolysis into a monosaccharide; specifically, the hydrolysis of sucrose to D-glucose and D-fructose; so called because of the change in optical rotation. **3.** Alteration of a DNA molecule made by removing a fragment, reversing its orientation, and putting it back into place. **4.** Heat-induced transition of silica, in which the quartz tridymite or cristobalite changes its physical properties as to thermal expansion. [L. *inverto,* pp. *-versus,* to turn upside down, to turn about]

  i. of the uterus, a turning of the uterus inside out, usually following childbirth.

in•ver•te•brate (in-ver′tĕ-brāt). **1.** Not possessed of a spinal or vertebral column. **2.** Any animal that has no spinal column.

in•ver•tor (in-ver′ter, -tōr). A muscle that inverts or causes inversion or turns a part, such as the foot, inward. [see inversion]

in•vet•er•ate (in-vet′er-āt). Long seated; firmly established; said of a disease or of confirmed habits. [L. *in-vetero,* pp. *-atus,* to render old, fr. *vetus,* old]

in•vis•ca•tion (in-vis-kā′shŭn). **1.** Smearing with mucilaginous matter. **2.** The mixing of the food, during mastication, with the buccal secretions. [L. *in,* in, on, + *viscum,* birdlime]

in vit•ro (in vē′trō). In an artificial environment, referring to a process or reaction occurring therein, as in a test tube or culture media. Cf. *in vivo.* [L. in glass]

in vi•vo (in vī′vō). In the living body, referring to a process or reaction occurring therein. Cf. *in vitro.* [L. in the living being]

in•vo•lu•crum, pl. **in•vo•lu•cra** (in-vō-lū′krŭm, -lū′kră). **1.** An enveloping membrane, *e.g.,* a sheath or sac. **2.** The sheath of new bone that forms around a sequestrum. [L. a wrapper, fr. *involvo,* to roll up]

in•vol•un•tary (in-vol′ŭn-tār-ē). **1.** Independent of the will; not volitional. **2.** Contrary to the will. [L. *in-* neg. + *voluntarius,* willing, fr. *volo,* to wish]

in•vo•lu•tion (in-vō-lū′shŭn). **1.** Return of an enlarged organ to normal size. **2.** Turning inward of the edges of a part. **3.** PSYCHIATRY Mental decline associated with advanced age. SYN catagenesis. [L. *in-volvo,* pp. *-volutus,* to roll up]

in•vo•lu•tion•al (in-vō-lū′shŭn-ăl). Relating to involution.

io•dide (ī′ō-dīd). The negative ion of iodine, I⁻.

io•di•nate (ī′ō-di-nāt). To treat or combine with iodine.

io•dine (I) (ī′ō-dīn, -dēn). A nonmetallic chemical element, atomic no. 53, atomic wt. 126.90447; used as a catalyst, reagent, tracer, constituent of radiographic contrast media, topical antiseptic, therapy in thyroid disease, antidote for alkaloidal poisons, and in certain stains and solutions. [G. *iōdēs,* violet-like, fr. *ion,* a violet, + *eidos,* form]

io•dine-fast. Denoting hyperthyroidism unresponsive to iodine therapy, which develops frequently in most cases so treated.

io•din•o•phil, io•din•o•phile (ī-ō-din′ō-fil, -fīl). **1.** Staining readily with iodine. SYN iodinophilous. **2.** Any histologic element that stains readily with iodine. [iodine + G. *philos,* fond]

io•din•oph•i•lous (ī-ō-din-of′i-lŭs). SYN iodinophil (1).

io•dism (ī′ō-dizm). A condition marked by coryza, an acneform eruption, weakness, salivation, and foul breath, caused by the continuous administration of iodine or one of the iodides.

io•dize (ī′ō-dīz). To treat or impregnate with iodine.

io•do•der•ma (ī-ō′dō-der′mă). An eruption of follicular papules and pustules, or a granulomatous lesion, caused by iodine toxicity or sensitivity.

io•do•met•ric (ī-ō′dō-met′rik). Relating to iodometry.

io•dom•e•try (ī-ō-dom′ĕ-trē). Analytical techniques involving titrations in which iodine is either formed or consumed, the sudden appearance or disappearance of iodine marking the end point. [iodine + G. *metron,* measure]

io•do•phil•ia (ī-ō′dō-fil′ē-ă). An affinity for iodine, as manifested by some leukocytes in certain conditions. [iodine + G. *phileō,* to love]

iodophor (ī-ō′dō-for). Any compound in which iodine is combined with an organic carrier; an intermediate-level disinfectant registered with the EPA as hospital disinfectant with tuberculocidal action. Available in topical antiseptics and hard-surface disinfectant form. [io- + G. *phoros,* carrying]

io•dop•sin (ī-ō-dop′sin). A visual pigment, composed of 11-*cis*-retinal bound to an opsin, found in the cones of the retina. SYN visual violet. [G. *ion,* violet, + *ōps,* eye, + -in]

io•do•ther•a•py (ī′ō-dō-thār′ă-pē). Treatment with iodine.

io•du•ria (ī-ō-dū′rē-ă). Urinary excretion of iodine.

ion (ī′on). An atom or group of atoms carrying an electric charge by virtue of having gained or lost one or more electrons. I.'s charged with negative electricity (anions) travel toward a positive pole (anode); those charged with positive electricity (cations) travel toward a negative pole (cathode). I.'s may exist in solid, liquid, or gaseous environments, although those in liquid (electrolytes) are more common and familiar. [G. *iōn,* going]

  dipolar i.'s, i.'s possessing both a negative charge and a positive charge, each localized at a different point in the molecule, which thus has both positive and negative "poles." SYN zwitteri-ons.

gram-i., SEE gram-ion.

hydrogen i. (H^+), a hydrogen atom minus its electron and therefore carrying a unit positive charge (*i.e.*, a proton); in water, it combines with a water molecule to form hydronium i., H_3O^+.

ion ex·change (ī'on eks-chanj'). SEE *anion* exchange, cation exchange, ion exchange *chromatography*.

ion·ic (ī-on'ik). Relating to an ion.

ion·i·za·tion (ī'on-i-zā'shŭn). **1.** Dissociation into ions, occurring when an electrolyte is dissolved in water or certain liquids or when molecules are subjected to electrical discharge or ionizing radiation. **2.** Production of ions as a result of interaction of radiation with matter. **3.** SYN iontophoresis.

ion·ize (ī'on-īz). To separate into ions; to dissociate atoms or molecules into electrically charged atoms or radicals.

ion·o·phore (ī-on'ō-fōr). A compound or substance that forms a complex with an ion and transports it across a membrane. [ion + G. *phore*, a bearer]

ion·o·pho·re·sis (ī-on'ō-fōr-ē'sis). SYN electrophoresis. [ion + G. *phorēsis*, a carrying]

ion·o·pho·ret·ic (ī-on'ō-fōr-et'ik). SYN electrophoretic.

ion·to·pho·re·sis (ī-on'tō-fōr-ē'sis). The introduction into the tissues, by means of an electric current, of the ions of a chosen medicament. SYN ionization (3). [ion + G. *phorēsis*, a carrying]

ion·to·pho·ret·ic (ī-on'tō-fōr-et'ik). Relating to iontophoresis.

io·pro·mide (ī-ō'prō-mid). A monomeric, nonionic, water-soluble, low osmolar radiographic contrast medium for intravenous urography or angiography.

i·o·ta (ι) (ī-ōt'a). **1.** The ninth letter in the Greek alphabet. **2.** CHEMISTRY denotes the ninth in a series, or the ninth atom from a carboxyl group or other functional group. **3.** A tiny or minute amount.

IPA International Phonetic Alphabet.

ip·e·cac·u·a·nha (ip-ē-kak-yū-an'ă). The dried root of *Uragoga (Cephaelis) ipecacuanha* (family Rubiaceae), a shrub of Brazil and other parts of South America; contains emetine, cephaeline, emetamine, ipecacuanhic acid, psychotrine, and methylpsychotrine; has expectorant, emetic, and antidysenteric properties. [native Brazilian word]

IPF idiopathic pulmonary *fibrosis*.

ipo·date. A radiographic contrast medium, given orally as the sodium or, more often, the calcium salt, for opacification of the gallbladder and central biliary tree.

IPPB intermittent positive pressure *breathing*.

IPPV intermittent positive pressure *ventilation*.

ip·si·lat·er·al (ip-si-lat'er-ăl). On the same side, with reference to a given point, *e.g.*, a dilated pupil on the same side as an extradural hematoma with contralateral limbs being paretic. SYN homolateral. [L. *ipse*, same, + *latus* (*later-*), side]

IQ intelligence *quotient*.

IR infrared.

Ir iridium.

△irid-. SEE irido-.

ir·i·dal (ī'ri-dăl, ir'i-dăl). Relating to the iris. SYN iridial, iridian, iridic.

ir·i·dec·to·my (ir'i-dek'tō-mē). **1.** Excision of a portion of the iris. **2.** The hole in the iris produced by a surgical iridectomy. [irido- + G. *ektomē*, excision]

ir·i·den·clei·sis (ir'i-den-klī'sis). The incarceration of a portion of the iris by corneoscleral incision in glaucoma to effect filtration between the anterior chamber and subconjunctival space. [irido- + G. *enkleiō*, to shut in]

ir·i·der·e·mia (ir'i-der-ē'mē'ă, ī'rid-). Condition wherein the iris is so rudimentary as to appear to be absent. Cf. aniridia. [irido- + G. *erēmia*, absence]

ir·i·des (ir'i-dēz). Plural of iris. [G.]

irid·e·sis (i-rid'ĕ-sis, ī-ri-dē'sis). Ligature of a portion of the iris brought out through an incision in the cornea. [irido- + G. *desis*, a binding together]

irid·i·al, irid·i·an, irid·ic (ī-rid'ē-al; ī-rid'ē-an; ī-rid'ik, i-rid'-). SYN iridal.

irid·i·um (Ir) (i-rid'ē-ŭm). A white, silvery metallic element, atomic no. 77, atomic wt. 192.22; ^{192}Ir is a radioisotope that has been used in the interstitial treatment of certain tumors. [L. *iris*, rainbow]

△irido-, irid-. The iris. [G. *iris* (*irid-*), rainbow]

ir·i·do·a·vul·sion (ir'i-dō-ă-vŭl'shŭn). Avulsion, or tearing away, of the iris.

ir·i·do·cele (ir'i-dō-sēl). Herniation of a portion of the iris through a corneal defect. [irido- + G. *kēlē*, hernia]

ir·i·do·cho·roid·i·tis (ir'i-dō-kō-roy-dī'tis). Inflammation of both iris and choroid.

ir·i·do·col·o·bo·ma (ir'i-dō-ko-lō-bō'mă). A coloboma or congenital defect of the iris. [irido- + G. *kolobōma*, coloboma]

ir·i·do·cy·clec·to·my (ir'i-dō-sī-klek'tō-mē). Removal of the iris and ciliary body for excision of a tumor. [irido- + G. *kyklos*, circle (ciliary body), + *ektomē*, excision]

ir·i·do·cy·cli·tis (ir'i-dō-sī-klī'tis). Inflammation of both iris and ciliary body. SEE ALSO iritis, uveitis. [irido- + G. *kyklos*, circle (ciliary body), + *-itis*, inflammation]

ir·i·do·cy·clo·cho·roid·i·tis (ir'i-dō-sī'klō-kō-royd-ī'tis). Inflammation of the iris, involving the ciliary body and the choroid.

ir·i·do·cys·tec·to·my (ir'i-dō-sis-tek'tō-mē). An operation for making an artificial pupil when posterior synechiae follow extracapsular extraction of cataract. [irido- + G. *kystis*, bladder (capsule), + *ektomē*, excision]

ir·i·do·di·al·y·sis (ir'i-dō-dī-al'i-sis). A colobomatous defect of the iris caused by its separation from the scleral spur. [irido- + G. *dialysis*, loosening]

ir·i·do·di·la·tor (ir'i-dō-dī-lā'ter). Causing dilation of the pupil; applied to the musculus dilator pupillae.

ir·i·do·do·ne·sis (ir'i-dō-dō-nē'sis). Agitated motion of the iris. [irido- + G. *doneō*, to shake to and fro]

ir·i·do·ki·net·ic (ir′i-dō-ki-net′ik). Relating to the movements of the iris. SYN iridomotor.

ir·i·do·ma·la·cia (ir′i-dō-mă-lā′shē-ă). Degenerative softening of the iris. [irido- + G. *malakia*, softness]

ir·i·do·mes·o·di·al·y·sis (ir′i-dō-mes′ō-dī-al′i-sis). Separation of adhesions around the inner margin of the iris. [irido- + G. *mesos*, middle, + *dialysis*, loosening]

ir·i·do·mo·tor (ir′i-dō-mō′tŏr). SYN iridokinetic.

ir·i·do·pa·ral·y·sis (ir′i-dō-pă-ral′i-sis). SYN iridoplegia.

ir·i·dop·a·thy (ir-i-dop′ă-thē). Pathologic lesions in the iris.

ir·i·do·ple·gia (ir′i-dō-plē′jē-ă). Paralysis of the musculus sphincter iridis. SYN iridoparalysis. [irido- + G. *plēgē*, stroke]

ir·i·dop·to·sis (ir′i-dop-tō′sis). Prolapse of the iris. [irido- + G. *ptōsis*, a falling]

ir·i·dor·rhex·is (ir′i-dō-rek′sis). Deliberate, surgical tearing of the iris from the scleral spur in order to increase the breadth of a coloboma. [irido- + G. *rhēxis*, rupture]

ir·i·dos·chi·sis (ir-i-dos′ki-sis). Separation of the anterior layer of the iris from the posterior layer; ruptured anterior fibers float in the aqueous humor. [irido- + G. *schisma*, cleft]

ir·i·do·scle·rot·o·my (ir′i-dō-skle-rot′ō-mē). An incision involving both sclera and iris. [irido- + sclera, + G. *tomē*, incision]

ir·i·dot·o·my (ir-i-dot′ō-mē). Transverse division of some of the fibers of the iris, forming an artificial pupil. [irido- + G. *tomē*, incision]

iris, pl. **ir·i·des** (ī′ris, ir′i-dēz) [NA]. The anterior division of the vascular tunic of the eye, a diaphragm, perforated in the center (the pupil), attached peripherally to the scleral spur; it is composed of stroma and a double layer of pigmented retinal epithelium from which are derived the sphincter and dilator muscles of the pupil. [G. rainbow, the iris of the eye]

irit·ic (ī-rit′ik). Relating to iritis.

iri·tis (ī-rī′tis). Inflammation of the iris. SEE ALSO iridocyclitis, uveitis.

IRMA immunoradiometric *assay*.

iron (Fe) (ī′ern, ī′rŭn). A metallic element, atomic no. 26, atomic wt. 55.847, that occurs in the heme of hemoglobin, myoglobin, transferrin, ferritin, and iron-containing porphyrins, and is an essential component of enzymes such as catalase, peroxidase, and the various cytochromes; its salts are used medicinally. [A.S. *iren*]

iron-59. An iron isotope; a gamma and beta emitter with a half-life of 44.51 days; used as tracer in study of iron metabolism, determination of blood volume, and in blood transfusion studies.

ir·ra·di·ate (i-rā′dē-āt). To apply radiation from a source to a structure or organism. [see irradiation]

ir·ra·di·a·tion (i-rā-dē-ā′shŭn). 1. The subjective enlargement of a bright object seen against a dark background. 2. Exposure to the action of electromagnetic radiation (*e.g.*, heat, light, x-rays). 3. The spreading of nervous impulses from one area in the brain or cord, or from a tract, to another

tract. SEE ALSO radiation. [L. *ir-radio, (in-r),* pp. *-radi-atus,* to beam forth]

ir·ra·tion·al (i-rash′ŭn-ăl). Not rational; unreasonable (contrary to reason) or unreasoning (not exercising reason). [L. *irrationalis*, without reason]

ir·re·duc·i·ble (ir-rē-dū′si-bl, i-rē-). 1. Not reducible; incapable of being made smaller. 2. CHEMISTRY Incapable of being made simpler, or of being replaced, hydrogenated, or reduced in positive charge.

ir·re·sus·ci·ta·ble (ir′rē-sŭs′i-tă-bl). Incapable of being revived.

ir·ri·gate (ir′i-gāt). To perform irrigation. [L. *ir-rigo,* pp. *-atus,* to irrigate, fr. *in,* on, + *rigo,* to water]

ir·ri·ta·bil·i·ty (ir′i-tă-bil′i-tē). The property inherent in protoplasm of reacting to a stimulus. [L. *irritabilitas,* fr. *irrito,* pp. *-atus,* to excite]
  myotatic i., the ability of a muscle to contract in response to the stimulus produced by a sudden stretching.

ir·ri·ta·ble (ir′i-tă-bl). 1. Capable of reacting to a stimulus. 2. Tending to react immoderately to a stimulus. Cf. excitable.

ir·ri·tant (ir′i-tant). 1. Irritating; causing irritation. 2. Any agent with this action.

ir·ri·ta·tion (ir-i-tā′shŭn). 1. Inflammatory reaction of the tissues to an injury. 2. The normal response of nerve or muscle to a stimulus. 3. The evocation of a normal or exaggerated reaction in the tissues by the application of a stimulus. [L. *irritatio*]

ir·ri·ta·tive (ir-i-tā′tiv). Causing irritation.

ir·rup·tion (i-rŭp′shŭn). Act or process of breaking through to a surface. [L. *irruptio,* fr. *irrumpo,* to break in]

IRV inspiratory reserve *volume.*

is·aux·e·sis (ī-sawk-zē′sis). Growth of parts at the same rate as growth of the whole. [G. *isos,* even, + *auxēsis,* increase]

is·che·mia (is-kē′mē-ă). Local anemia due to mechanical obstruction (mainly arterial narrowing) of the blood supply. [G. *ischō,* to keep back, + *haima,* blood]

is·che·mic (is-kē′mik). Relating to or affected by ischemia.

is·chia (is′kē-ă). Plural of ischium.

is·chi·ad·ic (is-kē-ad′ik). SYN sciatic (1).

is·chi·al (is′kē-ăl). SYN sciatic (1).

is·chi·al·gia (is-kē-al′jē-ă). 1. Pain in the hip; specifically, the ischium. SYN ischiodynia. 2. Rarely used term for sciatica. [G. *ischion,* hip, + *algos,* pain]

is·chi·at·ic (is-kē-at′ik). SYN sciatic (1).

ischio-. Ischium. [G. *ischion,* a hip-joint, haunch (ischium)]

is·chi·o·cap·su·lar (is-kē-ō-kap′sū-lăr). Relating to the ischium and the capsule of the hip joint; denoting that part of the capsule which is attached to the ischium.

is·chi·o·cele (is′kē-ō-sēl). SYN sciatic *hernia.* [ischio- + G. *kēlē,* hernia]

is·chi·o·coc·cyg·e·al (is-kē-ō-kok-sij′ē-ăl). Relating to the ischium and the coccyx.

is·chi·o·dyn·ia (is′kē-ō-din′ē-ă). SYN ischialgia (1). [ischio- + G. *odynē,* pain]

is·chi·o·fem·o·ral (is-kē-ō-fem′ŏ-răl). Relating to the ischium, or hip bone, and the femur, or thigh bone.

is·chi·o·fib·u·lar (is′kē-ō-fib′yū-lăr). Relating to or connecting the ischium and the fibula.

is·chi·o·ni·tis (is′kē-ō-nī′tis). Inflammation of the ischium.

is·chi·o·tib·i·al (is′kē-ō-tib′ē-ăl). Relating to or connecting the ischium and the tibia.

is·chi·o·ver·te·bral (is-kē-ō-ver′tĕ-brăl). Relating to the ischium and the vertebral column.

is·chi·um, gen. **is·chii**, pl. **is·chia** (is′kē-ŭm, -ī, -ă). The lower and posterior part of the hip bone, distinct at birth but later becoming fused with the ilium and pubis; it consists of a body, where it joins the ilium and superior ramus of the pubis to form the acetabulum, and a ramus joining the inferior ramus of the pubis. SYN ischial bone. [Mod. L. fr. G. *ischion*, hip]

is·chu·ria (is-kū′rē-ă). Retention or suppression of urine. [G. *ischō*, to keep back, + *ouron*, urine]

is·land (ī′land). ANATOMY Any isolated part, separated from the surrounding tissues by a groove, or marked by a difference in structure. SYN insula (2). [A.S. *īgland*]

    i. of Reil, SYN insula (1).

is·let (ī′let). A small island.

■ i.'s of Langerhans, cellular masses varying from a few to hundreds of cells lying in the interstitial tissue of the pancreas; they are the source of insulin and glucagon.

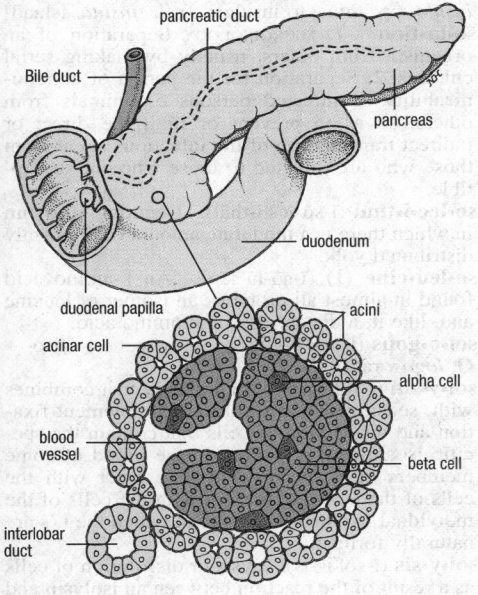

pancreatic duct

Bile duct

pancreas

duodenum

duodenal papilla

acini

acinar cell

alpha cell

blood vessel

beta cell

interlobar duct

islet of Langerhans

◌-ism. **1.** A medical condition or a disease resulting from or involving some specified thing. **2.** A practice, doctrine. Cf. -ia, -ismus. [G. *-isma*, *-ismos*, noun-forming suffix]

◌-ismus. L. for -ism; customarily used to imply

spasm, contraction. [L. fr. G. *-ismos*, suffix forming nouns of action]

◌iso-. **1.** Prefix meaning equal, like. **2.** CHEMISTRY Prefix indicating "isomer of" (isomerism); *e.g.*, isocyanate vs. cyanate. **3.** IMMUNOLOGY Prefix designating sameness with respect to species; in recent years, the meaning has shifted to sameness with respect to genetic constitution of individuals. [G. *isos*, equal]

iso·ag·glu·ti·na·tion (ī′sō-ă-glū-ti-nā′shŭn). Agglutination of red blood cells as a result of the reaction between an isoagglutinin and specific antigen in or on the cells. SYN isohemagglutination. [iso- + L. *ad*, to, + *gluten*, glue]

iso·ag·glu·ti·nin (ī′sō-ă-glū′ti-nin). An isoantibody that causes agglutination of cells of genetically different members of the same species. SYN isohemagglutinin.

iso·ag·glu·tin·o·gen (ī′sō-ă-glū-tin′ō-jen). An isoantigen that induces agglutination of the cells to which it is attached upon exposure to its specific isoantibody.

iso·am·y·lase (ī-sō-am′il-ās). A hydrolase that cleaves 1,6-α-D-glucosidic branch linkages in glycogen, amylopectin, and their β-limit dextrins; part of the complex known as debranching enzyme.

iso·an·ti·body (ī′sō-an′ti-bod-ē). **1.** An antibody that occurs only in some individuals of a species and reacts specifically with a particular foreign isoantigen. For specific i.'s of blood groups, see the Blood Groups appendix. **2.** Sometimes used as a synonym of alloantibody. [G. *isos*, equal]

iso·an·ti·gen (ī′sō-an′ti-jen). **1.** An antigenic substance that occurs only in some individuals of a species, such as the blood group antigens of humans. For specific i.'s of blood groups, see the Blood Groups appendix. **2.** Sometimes used as a synonym of alloantigen.

iso·bar (ī′sō-bar). **1.** One of two or more nuclides having the same total number of protons plus neutrons, but with different distribution. **2.** The line on a map connecting points of equal barometric pressure. [iso- + G. *baros*, weight]

iso·bar·ic (ī-sō-bar′ik). **1.** Having equal weights or pressures. **2.** With respect to solutions, having the same density as the diluent or medium.

iso·cap·nia (ī-sō-kap′nē-ă). A state in which the arterial carbon dioxide pressure remains constant or unchanged. [iso- + G. *kapnos*, vapor]

iso·cel·lu·lar (ī′sō-sel′yū-lăr). Composed of cells of equal size or of similar character. [iso- + L. *cellula*, dim. of *cella*, a storeroom]

iso·chro·mat·ic (ī-sō-krō-mat′ik). **1.** Of uniform color. **2.** Denoting two objects of the same color. [iso- + G. *chrōma*, color]

iso·chro·mat·o·phil, iso·chro·mat·o·phile (ī′sō-krō-mat′ō-fil, fīl). Having an equal affinity for the same dye; said of cells or tissues. [iso- + G. *chrōma*, color, + *philos*, fond]

iso·chro·mo·some (ī′sō-krō′mō-sōm). A chromosomal aberration that arises as a result of transverse rather than longitudinal division of the centromere during meiosis; two daughter chromosomes are formed, each lacking one chromosome arm but with the other doubled.

iso·chro·nia (ī-sō-krō′nē-ă). **1.** The state of having the same chronaxie. **2.** Agreement, with respect to time, rate, or frequency, between processes. [iso- + G. *chronos*, time]

isoch•ro•nous (ī-sok′rŏ-nŭs). Occurring during the same time.

iso•ci•trate (ī-sō-sit′rāt). (ī-sīt′rāt) A salt or ester of isocitric acid.

   i. dehydrogenase, one of two enzymes that catalyze the conversion of *threo*-D$_s$-isocitrate to α-ketoglutarate (2-oxoglutarate) and CO$_2$.

iso•cit•ric ac•id (ī-sō-sit′rik). An intermediate in the tricarboxylic acid cycle.

iso•co•ria (ī-sō-kō′rē-ă). Equality in the size of the two pupils. [iso- + G. *korē*, pupil]

iso•cor•tex (ī-sō-kōr′teks). O. and C. Vogt's term for the larger part of the mammalian cerebral cortex, distinguished from the allocortex by being composed of a larger number of nerve cells arranged in six layers. SEE ALSO cerebral *cortex*.

iso•cy•tol•y•sin (ī′sō-sī-tol′i-sin). A cytolysin that reacts with the cells of certain other animals of the same species, but not with the cells of the individual that formed the i.

iso•dense (ī′sō-dens). Denoting a tissue having a radiopacity (radiodensity) similar to that of another or adjacent tissue.

iso•dy•nam•ic (ī′sō-dī-nam′ik). **1.** Of equal force or strength. **2.** Relating to foods or other materials that liberate the same amount of energy on combustion. [iso- + G. *dynamis*, force]

iso•en•er•get•ic (ī′sō-en-er-jet′ik). Exerting equal force; equally active.

iso•en•zyme (ī-sō-en′zīm). One of a group of enzymes that catalyze the same reaction but may be differentiated by variations in physical properties, such as isoelectric point, electrophoretic mobility, kinetic parameters, or modes of regulation. SYN isozyme.

   creatine kinase i.'s, the isoenzymes of creatine kinase: CK-MM, the predominant form, found primarily in skeletal muscle; CK-MB, found in cardiac muscle, tongue, diaphragm, and in small amounts in skeletal muscle; and CK-BB found in the brain, smooth muscle, thyroid, lungs, and prostate. Elevations can help in the differential diagnosis of a variety of states, with CK-MB elevations as an important marker following myocardial infarctions, elevations in CK-MM an indicator of muscle disease, and elevations in CK-BB an occasional finding following brain infarcts, bowel infarcts, or in the presence of certain malignancies.

iso•e•ryth•rol•y•sis (ī′sō-ĕ-rith-rol′i-sis). Destruction of erythrocytes by isoantibodies. [iso- + erythrocyte = G. *lysis*, dissolution]

iso•ga•mete (ī-sō-gam′ēt). **1.** One of two or more similar cells that conjugate or fuse and subsequently divide, resulting in reproduction. **2.** A gamete of the same size as the gamete with which it unites. [iso- + G. *gametēs* or *gametē*, husband or wife]

isog•a•my (ī-sog′ă-mē). Conjugation between two equal gametes or two individual cells alike in all respects. [iso- + G. *gamos*, marriage]

iso•ge•ne•ic, iso•gen•ic (ī′sō-jĕ-nē′ik, -jen′ik). SYN syngeneic.

isog•e•nous (ī-soj′ĕ-nŭs). Of the same origin, as

in development from the same tissue or cell. [iso- + G. *genos*, family, kind]

iso•graft (ī′sō-graft). SYN syngraft.

iso•he•mag•glu•ti•na•tion (ī′sō-hē′mă-glū′ti-nā′shŭn). SYN isoagglutination. [iso- + G. *haima*, blood, + L. *ad*, to, + *gluten*, glue]

iso•he•mag•glu•ti•nin (ī′sō-hē′mă-glū′ti-nin). SYN isoagglutinin.

iso•he•mo•ly•sin (ī′sō-hē-mol′i-sin). An isolysin that reacts with red blood cells.

iso•he•mol•y•sis (ī′sō-hē-mol′i-sis). Dissolution of red blood cells as a result of the reaction between an isolysin (isohemolysin) and specific antigen in or on the cells. [iso- + G. *haima*, blood, + *lysis*, dissolution]

iso•im•mu•ni•za•tion (ī′sō-im′yū-nī-zā′shŭn). Development of a significant titer of specific antibody as a result of antigenic stimulation with material contained on or in the red blood cells of another individual of the same species.

iso•late (ī′sō-lāt). **1.** To separate, to set apart from others; that which is so treated. **2.** To free of chemical contaminants. **3.** PSYCHOANALYSIS To separate experiences or memories from the affects pertaining to them. **4.** GROUP PSYCHOTHERAPY An individual who is not responded to by others in the group. **5.** Viable organisms separated on a single occasion from a field sample in experimental hosts, culture systems, or stabilates. **6.** A population that for geographic, linguistic, cultural, social, religious, or other reasons is subject to little or no gene flow. [It. *isolare*; Mediev. L. *insulo*, pp. *-atus*, to insulate, fr. L. *insula*, island]

iso•la•tion. **1.** MICROBIOLOGY Separation of an organism from others, usually by making serial cultures. **2.** Separation for the period of communicability of infected persons or animals from others, so as to prevent or limit the direct or indirect transmission of the infectious agent from those who are infected to those who are susceptible.

iso•lec•i•thal (ī-sō-les′i-thăl). Denoting an ovum in which there is a moderate amount of uniformly distributed yolk.

iso•leu•cine (I) (ī-sō-lū′sēn). An L-amino acid found in almost all proteins; an isomer of leucine and, like it, a dietary essential amino acid.

isol•o•gous (lī-sol′ō-gŭs). SYN syngeneic. [iso- + G. *logos*, ratio]

isol•y•sin (ī-sol′i-sin). An antibody that combines with, sensitizes, and results in complement-fixation and dissolution of cells that contain the specific isoantigen; i.'s occur in the blood of some members of a species and they react with the cells of that species, but not with the cells of the individual (or the same type) in which the i.'s are naturally formed.

isol•y•sis (ī-sol′i-sis). Lysis or dissolution of cells as a result of the reaction between an isolysin and specific antigen in or on the cells. SEE ALSO isohemolysis. [iso- + G. *lysis*, dissolution]

iso•lyt•ic (ī-sō-lit′ik). Pertaining to, characterized by, or causing isolysis.

iso•malt•ose (ī-sō-mal′tōs). A disaccharide in which two glucose molecules are attached by an α1,6 link, rather than an α1,4 link as in maltose.

iso•mer (ī′sō-mer). **1.** One of two or more substances displaying isomerism. Cf. stereoisomer. **2.** One of two or more nuclides having the same atomic and mass numbers but differing in energy states for a finite period of time. [iso- + G. *meros,* part]

isom·er·ase (ī-som′er-ās). A class of enzymes (EC class 5) catalyzing the conversion of a substance to an isomeric form.

iso·mer·ic (ī-sō-mār′ik). Relating to or characterized by isomerism.

isom·er·ism (ī-som′er-izm). The existence of a chemical compound in two or more forms that are identical with respect to percentage composition but differ as to the positions of one or more atoms within the molecules, and also in physical and chemical properties.

    geometric i., a form of i. displayed by unsaturated or ring compounds where free rotation about a bond (usually a carbon-carbon bond) is restricted. Cf. cis-, trans-.

    optical i., stereoisomerism involving the arrangement of substituents about an asymmetric atom or atoms (usually carbon) so that there is a difference in the behavior of the various isomers with regard to the extent of their rotation of the plane of polarized light. Cf. stereoisomerism.

    structural i., i. involving the same atoms in different arrangements.

isom·er·i·za·tion (ī-som′er-ī-zā′shŭn). A process in which one isomer is formed from another, as in the action of isomerases.

iso·met·ric (ī-sō-met′rik). **1.** Of equal dimensions. **2.** PHYSIOLOGY Denoting the condition when the ends of a contracting muscle are held fixed so that contraction produces increased tension at a constant overall length. Cf. auxotonic, isotonic (3), isovolumic. [iso- + G. *metron,* measure]

iso·me·tro·pia (ī′sō-me-trō′pē-ă). Equality in refraction in the two eyes. [iso- + G. *metron,* measure, + *ōps* (*ōp-*), eye]

iso·mor·phic (ī-sō-mōr′fik). SYN isomorphous.

iso·mor·phism (ī-sō-mōr′fizm). Similarity of form between two or more organisms or between parts of the body. [iso- + G. *morphē,* shape]

iso·mor·phous (ī-sō-mōr′fŭs). Having the same form or shape, or being morphologically equal. SYN isomorphic.

isop·a·thy (ī-sop′ă-thē). Treatment of disease by means of the causal agent or a product of the same disease; or treatment of a diseased organ by an extract of a similar organ from a healthy animal. SEE ALSO homeopathy. [iso- + G. *pathos,* suffering]

isoph·a·gy (ī-sof′ă-jē). SYN autolysis. [iso- + G. *phagō,* to eat]

iso·plas·tic (ī-sō-plas′tik). SYN syngeneic. [iso- + G. *plassō,* to form]

iso·pre·cip·i·tin (ī′sō-prē-sip′i-tin). An antibody that combines with and precipitates soluble antigenic material in the plasma or serum, or in an extract of the cells, from another member, but not all members, of the same species. [iso- + precipitin]

iso·prene (ī′sō-prēn). An unsaturated five-carbon hydrocarbon with a branched chain, the basis for the formation of isoprenoids (terpenes, carote-

noids, and rubber). Fat-soluble vitamins either are isoprenoid or have isoprenoid side chains; steroids are synthesized via isoprenoid intermediates.

iso·pre·noids (ī-sō-prēn′oydz). Polymers whose carbon skeletons consist in whole or in large part of isoprene units joined end to end.

isop·ter (ī-sop′ter). A line of equal retinal sensitivity in the visual field. [iso- + G. *optēr,* observer]

isor·rhea (ī-sō-rē′ă). Equality of intake and output of water; maintenance of water equilibrium. [iso- + G. *rhoia,* a flow]

iso·sex·u·al (ī-sō-sek′shū-ăl). **1.** Relating to the existence of characteristics or feelings of both sexes in one person. **2.** Descriptive of an individual's somatic characteristics, or of internal processes, that are consonant with the sex of that individual.

is·os·mot·ic (ī′sos-mot′ik). Having the same total osmotic pressure or osmolality as another fluid (ordinarily intracellular fluid); such a fluid is not isosmotic if it includes solutes that freely permeate cell membranes.

Isos·po·ra (ī-sos′pō-ră). A genus of coccidia parasitizing chiefly mammals. [iso- + G. *sporos,* seed]

isos·po·ri·a·sis (ī-sos-pō-rī′ă-sis). Disease caused by infection with a species of *Isospora,* such as *I. belli* of humans; human disease usually is mild except in cases of immunosuppression, as in AIDS, where it may cause an intractable diarrhea.

isos·the·nu·ria (ī-sos′thē-nū′rē-ă, ī′sō-sthē-). A state in chronic renal disease in which the kidney cannot form urine with a higher or a lower specific gravity than that of protein-free plasma; specific gravity of the urine becomes fixed around 1.010, irrespective of the fluid intake. [iso- + G. *sthenos,* strength, + *ouron,* urine]

iso·ther·mal (ī-sō-ther′măl). Having the same temperature. [iso- + G. *thermē,* heat]

iso·tone (ī′sō-tōn). One of several nuclides having the same number of neutrons in their nuclei. [iso- + G. *tonos,* stretching, tension]

iso·to·nia (ī-sō-tō′nē-ă). A condition of tonic equality in which tension or osmotic pressure in two substances or solutions is the same. [iso- + G. *tonos,* tension]

iso·ton·ic (ī-sō-ton′ik). **1.** Relating to isotonicity or isotonia. **2.** Having equal tension; denoting solutions possessing the same osmotic pressure; more specifically, limited to solutions in which cells neither swell nor shrink. Thus, a solution that is isosmotic with intracellular fluid will not be i. if it includes solute, such as urea, that freely permeates cell membranes. **3.** PHYSIOLOGY Denoting the condition when a contracting muscle shortens against a constant load, as when lifting a weight. Cf. auxotonic, isometric (2).

iso·to·nic·i·ty (ī-sō-tō-nis′i-tē). **1.** The quality of possessing and maintaining a uniform tone or tension. **2.** The property of a solution in being isotonic.

iso·tope (ī′sō-tōp). One of two or more nuclides that are chemically identical, having the same number of protons, yet differ in mass number,

is

since their nuclei contain different numbers of neutrons; individual i.'s are named with the inclusion of their mass number in the superior position (^{12}C) and the atomic number (nuclear protons) in the inferior position ($_6$C). [iso- + G. *topos*, part, place]

radioactive i., an i. with an unstable nuclear composition; such nuclei decompose spontaneously by emission of a nuclear electron (β particle) or helium nucleus (α particle) and radiation (γ rays), thus achieving a stable nuclear composition; used as tracers, and as radiation and energy sources. SEE half-life.

stable i., a nonradioactive nuclide; an i. that shows no tendency to undergo radioactive decomposition.

iso•to•pic (ī-sō-top'ik).   Of identical chemical composition but differing in some physical property, such as atomic weight.

iso•tro•pic, isot•ro•pous (ī-sō-trop'ik, ī-sot'rō-pŭs). Having properties that are the same in all directions. [iso- + G. *tropē,* a turn]

iso•type (ī'sō-tīp).   An antigenic determinant (marker) that occurs in all members of a subclass of an immunoglobulin class. [iso- + G. *typos,* model]

iso•typ•ic (ī-sō-tip'ik).   Pertaining to an isotype.

iso•vol•u•mic (ī'sō-vol-yū'mik).   Occurring without an associated alteration in volume, as when, in early ventricular systole, the muscle fibers initially increase their tension without shortening so that ventricular volume remains unaltered. SEE ALSO isometric.

iso•zyme (ī'sō-zīm).   SYN isoenzyme.

isth•mec•to•my (is-mek'tō-mē).   Excision of the midportion of the thyroid. [G. *isthmos,* isthmus, + *ektomē,* excision]

isth•mic, isth•mi•an (is'mik, is'mē-an).   Denoting an anatomical isthmus.

isth•mo•pa•ral•y•sis (is'mō-pă-ral'i-sis). Paralysis of the velum pendulum palati and the muscles forming the anterior pillars of the fauces. SYN isthmoplegia. [G. *isthmos,* isthmus, + paralysis]

isth•mo•ple•gia (is'mō-plē'jē-ă).   SYN isthmoparalysis. [G. *isthmos,* isthmus, + *plēgē,* stroke]

isth•mus, pl. **isth•mi, isth•mus•es** (is'mŭs, -mī, -mŭs-ez). **1.** A constriction connecting two larger parts of an organ or other anatomical structure. **2.** A narrow passage connecting two larger cavities. **3.** The narrowest portion of the brainstem at the junction between midbrain and hindbrain. [G. *isthmos*]

i. of auditory tube, the narrowest portion of the auditory tube at the junction of the cartilaginous and bony portions. SYN i. of eustachian tube.

i. of eustachian tube, SYN i. of auditory tube.

i. of fauces, the constricted and short space which establishes the connection between the cavity of the mouth and the oro-pharynx, bounded anteriorly by the palatoglossal folds and posteriorly by the palatopharyngeal folds; the lateral well is the tonsillar fossa.

rhombencephalic i., (1) a constriction in the embryonic neural tube delineating the mesen-

cephalon from the rhombencephalon; **(2)** the anterior portion of the rhombencephalon connecting with the mesencephalon.

i. of thyroid, the central part of the thyroid gland joining the two lateral lobes.

i. of uterine tube, the narrow portion of the uterine tube adjoining the uterus.

i. of uterus, an elongated constriction at the junction of the body and cervix of the uterus.

itch. 1. A peculiar irritating sensation in the skin that arouses the desire to scratch. SYN pruritus (2). **2.** Common name for scabies. [A.S. *gikkan*]

bath i., SYN bath *pruritus.*

jock i., SYN *tinea* cruris.

straw i., straw-bed i., an urticarial eruption caused by the mite, *Pyemotes ventricosus,* which can infest straw used in mattresses.

swimmer's i., (1) SYN cutaneous *ancylostomiasis.* **(2)** SYN schistosomal *dermatitis.*

water i., (1) SYN cutaneous *ancylostomiasis.* **(2)** SYN schistosomal *dermatitis.*

itch•ing. An uncomfortable sensation of irritation of the skin or mucous membranes which causes scratching or rubbing of the affected parts. SYN pruritus (1).

△**-ite. 1.** Of the nature of, resembling. **2.** A salt of an acid that has the termination -ous. **3.** COMPARATIVE ANATOMY A suffix denoting an essential portion of the part to the name of which it is attached. SEE ALSO -ites. [G. *-itēs,* fem. *-itis*]

iter (ī'ter).   A passage leading from one anatomical part to another. SEE ALSO canaliculus. [L. *iter* (*itiner-*), a way, journey]

iter•al (ī'ter-ăl).   Relating to an iter.

△**-ites.** Adjectival suffix to nouns, corresponding to L. *-alis, -ale,* or *-inus, -inum,* or Eng. -y, -like, or the hyphenated nouns; the adjective so formed is used without the qualified noun. SEE ALSO -ite. [G. *itēs,* m., or *-ites,* n.]

△**-itides.** Plural of -itis.

△**-itis.** SEE -ites. [G. fem. of *-ites*]

ITP idiopathic thrombocytopenic *purpura; inosine* 5′-triphosphate.

IUCD intrauterine contraceptive *devices,* under *device.*

IUD intrauterine *devices,* under *device.*

IVC Abbreviation for inferior *vena* cava.

IVU intravenous urogram; preferred to IVP. SEE intravenous *urography.*

Ix•o•des (ik-sō'dēz).   A genus of hard ticks, many species of which are parasitic on man; these include vectors of Lyme disease and agents of tick paralysis. [G. *ixōdēs,* sticky, like birdlime, fr. *ixos,* mistletoe, + *eidos,* form]

I. damm'ini, a species that is a vector of Lyme disease (*Borrelia burgdorferi*) and human babesiosis (*Babesia microti*) in the U.S. Bites causing Lyme disease in humans are from nymphal ticks about the size of a pencil point, infected with *B. burgdorferi* from white-footed field mice. Adult ticks complete their two-year life cycle feeding on deer.

ix•o•di•a•sis (ik-sō-dī'ă-sis).   Skin lesions caused by the bites of certain ixodid ticks.

ix•od•ic (ik-sod′ik). Relating to or caused by ticks.

ix•o•did (ik′sō-did). Common name for members of the family Ixodidae.

Ix•od•i•dae (ik-sod′i-dē). A family of ticks, the so-called hard ticks, genera of which transmit many important human and animal diseases and cause tick paralysis.

J

J joule; electric current density.

J flux (4).

jack·et (jak′et). **1.** A fixed bandage applied around the body in order to immobilize the spine. **2.** DENTISTRY An artificial crown composed of fired porcelain or acrylic resin. [M.E., fr. O.Fr. *jaquet*, dim. of *jaque*, tunic, fr. *Jacques*, nickname of Fr. peasants.]

jac·ti·ta·tion (jak-ti-tā′shŭn). Extreme restlessness or tossing about from side to side. [L. *jactatio*, a tossing, fr. *jacto*, pp. *-atus*, to throw]

jan·i·ceps (jan′i-seps). Conjoined twins having their two heads fused together, with the faces looking in opposite directions. SEE conjoined twins, under *twin*. [L. *Janus*, a Roman diety having two faces, + *caput*, head]

Janus green B [C.I. 11050]. diethyl-safraninazodimethylaniline chloride; A basic dye used in histology and to stain mitochondria supravitally.

jar·gon (jar′gŏn). **1.** Language or terminology peculiar to a specific field, profession, or group. **2.** SYN paraphasia. [Fr. gibberish]

jaun·dice (jawn′dis). A yellowish staining of the integument, sclerae, and deeper tissues and the excretions with bile pigments, which are increased in the plasma. SYN icterus. [Fr. *jaune*, yellow]

    acholuric j., j. with excessive amounts of unconjugated bilirubin in the plasma and without bile pigments in the urine.

    cholestatic j., j. produced by inspissated bile or bile plugs in small biliary passages in the liver.

    familial j., SYN hereditary *spherocytosis*.

    familial nonhemolytic j. [MIM*143500], mild j. due to increased amounts of unconjugated bilirubin in the plasma without evidence of liver damage, biliary obstruction, or hemolysis; thought to be due to an inborn error of metabolism in which the excretion of bilirubin by the liver is defective.

    hematogenous j., SYN hemolytic j.

    hemolytic j., j. resulting from increased production of bilirubin from hemoglobin as a result of any process (toxic, genetic, or immune) causing increased destruction of erythrocytes. SYN hematogenous j.

    hepatocellular j., j. resulting from diffuse injury or inflammation or failure of function of the liver cells, usually referring to viral or toxic hepatitis.

    hepatogenous j., j. resulting from disease of the liver, as distinguished from that due to blood changes.

    leptospiral j., j. associated with infection by various species of *Leptospira*.

    malignant j., SYN icterus gravis.

    mechanical j., SYN obstructive j.

    j. of the newborn, SYN icterus neonatorum.

    nonobstructive j., any j. in which the main biliary passages are not obstructed.

    nuclear j., SYN kernicterus.

    obstructive j., j. resulting from obstruction to the flow of bile into the duodenum, whether intra- or extrahepatic. SYN mechanical j.

    physiologic j., SYN *icterus* neonatorum.

    regurgitation j., j. due to biliary obstruction, the bile pigment having been conjugated and secreted by the hepatic cells and then reabsorbed into the bloodstream.

    retention j., j. due to insufficiency of liver function or to an excess of bile pigment production; the bilirubin is unconjugated because it has not passed through the liver cells; van den Bergh test is indirect.

jaw. 1. One of the two bony structures, in which the teeth are set, forming the framework of the mouth. **2.** Common name for either the maxillae or the mandible. [A.S. *ceōwan*, to chew]

    j. winking, a paradoxical movement of eyelids associated with movements of the jaw.

JCAHO Joint Commission on Accreditation of Healthcare *Organizations*.

△**jejun-.** SEE jejuno-.

je·ju·nal (je-jū′năl). Relating to the jejunum.

je·ju·nec·to·my (je-jū-nek′tō-mē). Excision of all or a part of the jejunum. [jejunum + G. *ektomē*, excision]

je·ju·ni·tis (je-jū-nī′tis). Inflammation of the jejunum.

△**jejuno-, jejun-.** The jejunum, jejunal. [L. *jejunus*, empty]

je·ju·no·co·los·to·my (je-jū-nō-kō-los′tō-mē). Establishment of a communication between the jejunum and the colon. [jejuno- + colon + G. *stoma*, mouth]

je·ju·no·il·e·al (je-jū′nō-il′ē-ăl). Relating to the jejunum and the ileum.

je·ju·no·il·e·i·tis (je-jū′nō-il-ē-ī′tis). Inflammation of the jejunum and ileum.

je·ju·no·il·e·os·to·my (je-jū′nō-il-ē-os′tō-mē). Establishment of a new communication between the jejunum and the ileum. [jejuno- + ileum + G. *stoma*, mouth]

je·ju·no·je·ju·nos·to·my (je-jū′nō-jĕ-jū-nos′tō-mē). An anastomosis between two portions of jejunum. [jejuno- + jejuno- + G. *stoma*, mouth]

je·ju·no·plas·ty (je-jū′nō-plas-tē). A corrective surgical procedure on the jejunum. [jejuno- + G. *plastos*, molded]

je·ju·nos·to·my (je-jū-nos′tō-mē). Operative establishment of an opening from the abdominal wall into the jejunum, usually with creation of a stoma on the abdominal wall. [jejuno- + G. *stoma*, mouth]

je·ju·not·o·my (je-jū-not′ō-mē). Incision into the jejunum. [jejuno- + G. *tomē*, incision]

je·ju·num (jĕ-jū′nŭm) [NA]. The portion of small intestine, about 8 feet in length, between the duodenum and the ileum. The jejunum is distinct from the ileum in being more proximal, of larger diameter with a thicker wall, having larger, more highly developed plicae circulares, being more vascular (redder in appearance), with the jejunal arteries forming fewer tiers of arterial arcades and longer vasa recta. [L. *jejunus*, empty]

jel·ly (jel′ē). A semisolid tremulous compound

usually containing some form of gelatin in aqueous solution. [L. *gelo*, to freeze]

cardiac j., The gelatinous, noncellular material between the endothelial lining and the myocardial layer of the heart in very young embryos; later in development it serves as a substratum for cardiac mesenchyme.

interlaminar j., The gelatinous material between ectoderm and endoderm that serves as the substrate on which mesenchymal cells migrate.

Wharton's j., the mucous connective tissue of the umbilical cord.

jel·ly·fish (jel'ē-fish). Marine coelenterates, including some poisonous species; toxin is injected into the skin by nematocysts on the tentacles, causing linear wheals.

jerk. 1. A sudden pull. **2.** SYN deep *reflex.*

jet. A region of very high blood velocity immediately downstream of a vessel stenosis.

jet lag. An imbalance of the normal circadian rhythm resulting from subsonic or supersonic travel through a number of time zones and leading to fatigue, irritability, and functional disturbances.

jig·ger. Common name for *Tunga penetrans.* SEE ALSO chigoe.

joint (joynt). In anatomy, the place of union, usually more or less movable, between two or more bones. J.'s between skeletal elements exhibit a great variety of form and function, and are classified into three general morphological types: fibrous j.'s; cartilaginous j.'s; and synovial j.'s. SYN articulatio [NA], arthrosis (1), articulation (1), junctura (1). [L. *junctura;* fr. *jungo,* pp. *junctus,* to join]

acromioclavicular j., a plane synovial joint between the acromial end of the clavicle and the medial margin of the acromion.

ankle j., a hinge synovial joint between the tibia and fibula above and the talus below. SYN ankle (1), mortise j., talocrural j.

arthrodial j., SYN plane j.

ball-and-socket j., a multiaxial synovial joint in which a more or less extensive sphere on the head of one bone fits into a rounded cavity in the other bone. SYN cotyloid j., enarthrodial j., enarthrosis, spheroid j.

biaxial j., one in which there are two principal axes of movement situated at right angles to each other; *e.g.,* saddle j.'s.

bicondylar j., a synovial joint in which two distinct rounded surfaces of one bone articulate with shallow depressions on another bone.

bilocular j., one in which the intra-articular disk is complete, dividing the j. into two distinct cavities.

carpal j.'s, (1) SYN intercarpal j.'s. **(2)** SYN wrist j.

carpometacarpal j.'s, the synovial joints between the carpal and metacarpal bones; these are all plane joints except that of the thumb, which is saddle-shaped.

cartilaginous j., a joint in which the apposed bony surfaces are united by cartilage. SYN synarthrodial j. (2).

Charcot's j., SYN tabetic *arthropathy.*

Chopart's j., SYN transverse tarsal j.

cochlear j., a of hinge j. in which the elevation and depression, respectively, on the opposing articular surfaces form part of a spiral, flexion being accompanied by a certain amount of lateral deviation. SYN spiral j.

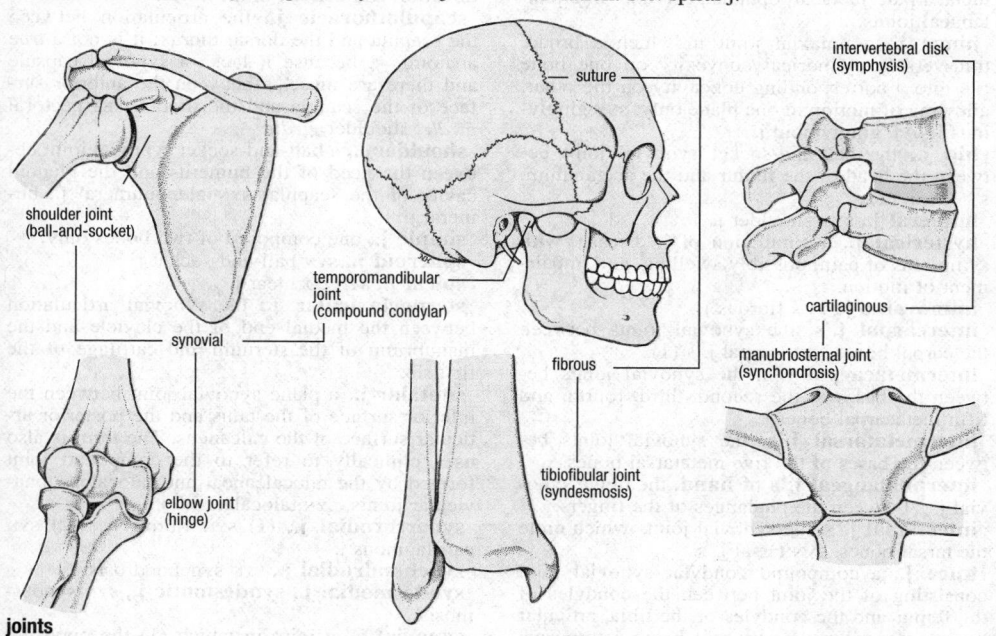

joints

compound j., a joint composed of three or more skeletal elements, or in which two anatomically separate joints function as a unit.

condylar j., SYN ellipsoidal j.

cotyloid j., SYN ball-and-socket j.

cubital j., SYN elbow j.

diarthrodial j., SYN synovial j.

dry j., a j. affected with atrophic desiccating changes.

elbow j., a compound hinge synovial joint between the humerus and the bones of the forearm; it consists of the j. humeroradialis and the j. humeroulnaris. SYN cubital j.

ellipsoidal j., a modified ball-and-socket synovial joint in which the joint surfaces are elongated or ellipsoidal; it is a biaxial joint, *i.e.,* two axes of motion at right angles to each other. SYN condylar j.

enarthrodial j., SYN ball-and-socket j.

false j., SYN pseudarthrosis.

fibrous j., a union of two bones by fibrous tissue such that there is no joint cavity and almost no motion possible; the types of fibrous joints are sutures, syndesmoses, and gomphoses. SYN immovable j., synarthrodia, synarthrodial j. (1).

flail j., a j. with loss of function caused by loss of ability to stabilize the j. in any plane within its normal range of motion.

j.'s of foot, j.'s including the talocrural, intertarsal, tarsometatarsal, intermetatarsal, metatarsophalangeal and interphalangeal joints.

ginglymoid j., SYN hinge j.

glenohumeral j., SYN shoulder j.

gliding j., SYN plane j.

j.'s of hand, these joints include the radiocarpal or wrist joint; intercarpal, carpometacarpal, intermetacarpal; metacarpophalangeal and interphalangeal joints.

hinge j., a uniaxial joint in which a broad, transversely cylindrical convexity on one bone fits into a corresponding concavity on the other, allowing of motion in one plane only. SYN ginglymus [NA], ginglymoid j.

hip j., the ball-and-socket synovial joint between the head of the femur and the acetabulum. SYN coxa (2).

humeral j., SYN shoulder j.

hysterical j., a simulation of j. disease, with symptoms of pain, possibly swelling, and impairment of motion.

immovable j., SYN fibrous j.

intercarpal j.'s, the synovial joints between the carpal bones. SYN carpal j.'s (1).

intermetacarpal j.'s, the synovial joints between the bases of the second, third, fourth, and fifth metacarpal bones.

intermetatarsal j.'s, the synovial joints between the bases of the five metatarsal bones.

interphalangeal j.'s of hand, the hinge synovial j.'s between the phalanges of the fingers.

intertarsal j.'s, the synovial joints which unite the tarsal bones. SYN tarsal j.'s.

knee j., a compound condylar synovial joint consisting of the joint between the condyles of the femur and the condyles of the tibia, articular menisci (semilunar cartilages) being interposed, and the articulation between femur and patella.

mandibular j., SYN temporomandibular j.

metacarpophalangeal j.'s, the spheroid synovial joints between the heads of the metacarpals and the bases of the proximal phalanges.

metatarsophalangeal j.'s, the spheroid synovial joints between the heads of the metatarsals and the bases of the proximal phalanges of the toes.

mortise j., SYN ankle j.

movable j., SYN synovial j.

multiaxial j., one in which movement occurs in a number of axes. SEE ball-and-socket j. SYN polyaxial j.

neuropathic j., j. disease caused by diminished proprioceptive sensation, with gradual destruction of the j. by repeated subliminal injury, commonly associated with tabes dorsalis or diabetic neuropathy. SYN neuropathic arthropathy.

patellofemoral j., the sliding articulation between the patella and the distal femur. SEE ALSO knee *complex.*

pivot j., a synovial joint in which a section of a cylinder of one bone fits into a corresponding cavity on the other. SYN rotary j., rotatory j., trochoid j.

plane j., a synovial joint in which the opposing surfaces are nearly planes and in which there is only a slight, gliding motion, as in the intermetacarpal joints. SYN arthrodia, arthrodial j., gliding j.

polyaxial j., SYN multiaxial j.

radiocarpal j., SYN wrist j.

rotary j., rotatory j., SYN pivot j.

saddle j., a biaxial synovial joint in which the double motion is effected by the opposition of two surfaces, each of which is concave in one direction and convex in the other.

scapulothoracic j., the articulation between the scapula and the dorsal thorax; it is not a true anatomic j. because it lacks a synovial capsule and there are muscles between the anterior surface of the scapula and the thorax. SEE pectoral *girdle,* shoulder *girdle.*

shoulder j., a ball-and-socket synovial joint between the head of the humerus and the glenoid cavity of the scapula. SYN glenohumeral j., humeral j.

simple j., one composed of two bones only.

spheroid j., SYN ball-and-socket j.

spiral j., SYN cochlear j.

sternoclavicular j., the synovial articulation between the medial end of the clavicle and the manubrium of the sternum and cartilage of the first rib.

subtalar j., a plane synovial joint between the inferior surface of the talus and the posterior articular surface of the calcaneus. The term is also used clinically to refer to the compound joint formed by the talocalcaneal and talocalcaneonavicular joints. SYN talocalcaneal j.

synarthrodial j., (1) SYN fibrous j. **(2)** SYN cartilaginous j.

synchondrodial j., SYN synchondrosis.

syndesmodial j., syndesmotic j., SYN syndesmosis.

synovial j., a joint in which (1) the opposing bony surfaces are covered with a layer of hyaline cartilage or fibrocartilage, (2) there is a joint cavity containing synovial fluid, lined with synovial membrane and reinforced by a fibrous capsule and ligaments, and (3) there is some degree of free movement possible. SYN diarthrodial j., diarthrosis, movable j.

talocalcaneal j., SYN subtalar j.

talocalcaneonavicular j., a ball-and-socket synovial joint, part of which participates in the transverse tarsal joint, formed by the head of the talus articulating with the navicular bone and the anterior part of the calcaneus.

talocrural j., SYN ankle j.

tarsal j.'s, SYN intertarsal j.'s.

tarsometatarsal j.'s, the three synovial joints between the tarsal and metatarsal bones, consisting of a medial joint between the first cuneiform and first metatarsal, an intermediate joint between the second and third cuneiforms and corresponding metatarsals, and a lateral joint between the cuboid and fourth and fifth metatarsals.

i temporomandibular j., the synovial articulation between the head of the mandible and the mandibular fossa and articular tubercle of the temporal bone. SYN mandibular j.

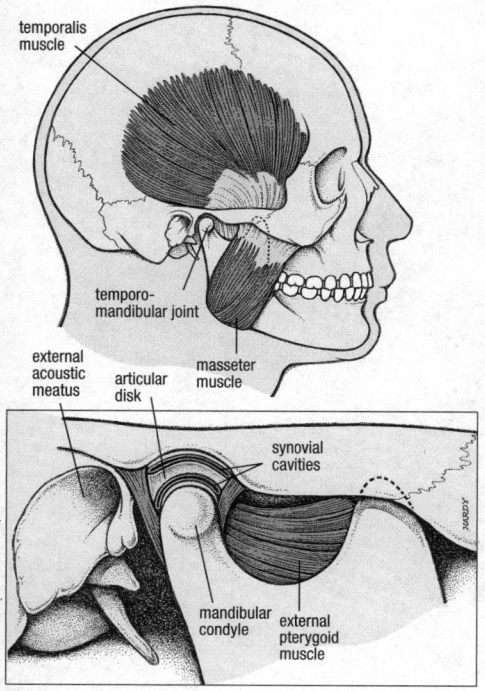

temporalis muscle

temporo-mandibular joint

external acoustic meatus

articular disk

masseter muscle

synovial cavities

mandibular condyle

external pterygoid muscle

temporomandibular joint

transverse tarsal j., the synovial joints between the talus and navicular bone medially and the calcaneus and navicular bones laterally which act as a unit in allowing the front of the foot to pivot relative to the back of the foot about the longitudinal axis of the foot, contributing to the total inversion and eversion movements. SYN Chopart's j.

trochoid j., SYN pivot j.

uniaxial j., one in which movement is around one axis only.

unilocular j., one in which an intra-articular disk is incomplete or absent, the j. having but a single cavity.

wedge-and-groove j., a form of fibrous joint in which the sharp edge of one bone is received in a cleft in the edge of the other. SYN schindylesis [NA], wedge-and-groove suture.

wrist j., the synovial joint between the distal end of the radius and its articular disk and the proximal row of carpal bones with the exception of the pisiform bone. SYN carpal j.'s (2), radiocarpal j.

Joule, James P., British physicist, 1818–1889. SEE joule.

joule (J) (jūl, jowl). A unit of energy; the heat generated, or energy expended, by an ampere flowing through an ohm for 1 second; equal to 10^7 ergs and to a newton-meter. It is an approved multiple of the SI fundamental unit of energy, the erg, and is intended to replace the calorie (4.184 J). [J.P. *Joule*]

judgment. Ability to evaluate the positive and negative aspects of a behavior or situation and act or react appropriately.

ju•ga (jū′gă). Plural of jugum.

ju•gal (jū′găl). **1.** Connecting; yoked. **2.** Relating to the zygomatic bone. [L. *jugalis,* yoked together, fr. *jugum,* a yoke]

ju•ga•le (jū-gā′lē). A craniometric point at the union of the temporal and frontal processes of the zygomatic bone. SYN jugal point.

jug•u•lar (jŭg′yū-lar). **1.** Relating to the throat or neck. **2.** Relating to the j. veins. **3.** A j. vein. [L. *jugulum,* throat]

ju•gum, pl. **ju•ga** (jū′gŭm, -gă). **1.** A ridge or furrow connecting two points. SYN yoke. **2.** A type of forceps. [L. a yoke]

juice (jūs). **1.** The interstitial fluid of a plant or animal. **2.** A digestive secretion. [L. *jus,* broth]

junc•tion (jŭngk′shŭn). SYN junctura (2).

cardioesophageal j., the abrupt transition from esophageal mucosa to that of the cardiac portion of stomach, demarcated internally in the living by the z-line, and approximated externally by the cardiac notch.

cementodentinal j., the surface at which the cementum and dentin of the root of a tooth are joined.

cementoenamel j., the surface at which the enamel of the crown and the cementum of the root of a tooth are joined. SEE ALSO cervical *line.*

dentinoenamel j., the surface at which the enamel and the dentin of the crown of a tooth are joined.

esophagogastric j., terminal end of esophagus and beginning of stomach at the cardiac orifice; site of the physiologic inferior esophageal sphincter.

gap j., (1) an intercellular j. having a 2-nm gap between apposed cell membranes; the gap contains subunits in the form of polygonal lattices; it occurs in epithelia, between certain nerve cells,

ju

and in smooth and cardiac muscle. SEE ALSO synapse. **(2)** areas of increased electrochemical communication between myometrial cells which aid in the propagation of the contractions of labor. SYN nexus.

mucocutaneous j., the site of transition from epidermis to the epithelium of a mucous membrane.

myoneural j., the synaptic connection of the axon of the motor neuron with a muscle fiber. SEE motor *endplate.*

tight j., an intercellular j. between epithelial cells in which the outer leaflets of lateral cell membranes fuse to form a variable number of parallel interweaving strands that greatly reduce transepithelial permeability to macromolecules, solutes, and water via the paracellular route.

ureteropelvic j. (UPJ), site of origin of the ureter from the renal pelvis, a common location for congenital or acquired obstruction.

junc•tu•ra, pl. **junc•tu•rae** (jŭngk-tū′ră, -rē). **1.** SYN joint. **2.** The point, line, or surface of union of two parts, mainly bones or cartilages. SYN junction, juncture. [L. a joining]

junc•ture (jŭngk′chūr). SYN junctura (2).

jung•i•an (yung′ē-an). The psychological system or the psychoanalytic form of treatment deriving from it; developed by Carl Gustav Jung.

jux•ta•crine (juks′tă-krin). A mode of hormone action that requires the cell producing the effector to be in direct contact with the cell containing the appropriate receptor. [L. *juxta,* close to, + G. *krinō,* to separate]

jux•ta•ep•i•phys•i•al (jŭks′tă-ep-i-fiz′ē-ăl). Close to or adjoining an epiphysis.

jux•ta•glo•mer•u•lar (jŭks′tă-glŏ-mer′yū-lăr). Close to or adjoining a renal glomerulus.

jux•tal•lo•cor•tex (jŭks′tă-lō-kōr′teks). Collective term for regions of the cerebral cortex between the isocortex and the allocortex.

jux•ta•po•si•tion (jŭks-tă-pō-zish′ŭn). A position side by side. SEE ALSO apposition, contiguity. [L. *juxta,* near to, + *positio,* a placing, fr. *pono,* pp. *positus,* to place]

K

κ kappa. SEE kappa.

K 1. potassium (kalium); phylloquinone; kelvin; lysine. **2.** OPTICS The coefficient of scleral rigidity. **3.** In contact lens fitting, the radius of curvature of the flattest meridian of the apical cornea.

k kilo-.

k rate *constants,* under *constant.*

△**kak-, kako-.** SEE caco-.

△**kal-, kali-.** Potassium; sometimes improperly written as *kalio-.* [L. *kalium,* potassium]

ka·la azar (kah′lah ah-zahr′). SYN visceral *leishmaniasis.* [Hind. *kala,* black, + *azar,* poison]

ka·le·mia (kă-lē′mē-ă). The presence of potassium in the blood.

ka·li·o·pe·nia (kā′lē-ō-pē′nē-ă). Insufficiency of potassium in the body. [Mod. L. *kalium,* potassium, + G. *penia,* poverty]

ka·li·o·pe·nic (kā′lē-ō-pē′nik). Relating to kaliopenia.

ka·li·um (K) (kā′lē-ŭm). SYN potassium. [Mod. L. fr. Ar. *qali,* potash]

ka·li·u·re·sis (kā′lē-yū-rē′sis). SYN kaluresis.

ka·li·u·ret·ic (kā′lē-yū-ret′ik). SYN kaluretic.

kal·lak (kah-lak′). A pustular dermatitis observed among Eskimos. [Eskimo word meaning skin disease]

kal·li·kre·in (kal-i-krē′in). A group of enzymes (*e.g.,* plasma, tissue, pancreatic, urinary, submandibular k.) that can convert kininogen by proteolysis to bradykinin or kallidin; trypsin and plasmin can also effect the conversion; plasma k. activates the Hageman factor and acts on kininogen. SYN kininogenase, kininogenin.

kal·u·re·sis (kal-yū-rē′sis). The increased urinary excretion of potassium. SYN kaliuresis. [Mod. L. *kalium,* potassium, + G. *ourēsis,* urination]

kal·u·ret·ic (kal-yū-ret′ik). Relating to, causing, or characterized by kaluresis. SYN kaliuretic.

ka·od·ze·ra (kah′od-ze′rā). A disease prevalent in Zimbabwe (formerly Rhodesia), similar to sleeping sickness, caused by *Trypanosoma rhodesiense.* SEE ALSO Rhodesian *trypanosomiasis.*

ka·o·lin·o·sis (kā′ō-lin-ō′sis). Pneumoconiosis caused by the inhalation of clay dust.

kap·pa (κ) (kap′a). **1.** The 10th letter in the Greek alphabet. **2.** In chemistry, denotes the position of a substituent located on the 10th atom from the carboxyl or other functional group. **3.** A measure of the degree of nonrandom agreement between observers or measurements of the same categorical variable.

△**karyo-.** Nucleus. Cf. nucleo-. [G. *karyon,* nucleus]

kar·y·o·cyte (kar′ē-ō-sīt). A young, immature normoblast. [karyo- + G. *kytos,* cell]

kar·y·o·gam·ic (kar-ē-ō-gam′ik). Relating to or marked by karyogamy.

kar·y·og·a·my (kar-ē-og′ă-mē). Fusion of the nuclei of two cells, as occurs in fertilization or true conjugation. [karyo- + G. *gamos,* marriage]

kar·y·o·gen·e·sis (kar-ē-ō-jen′ě-sis). Formation of the nucleus of a cell. [karyo- + G. *genesis,* production]

kar·y·o·gen·ic (kar-ē-ō-jen′ik). Relating to karyogenesis; forming the nucleus.

kar·y·ol·o·gy (kar′ē-ol′o-jē). The branch of cytology that deals with the study of the cell nucleus, its organelles, structures, and functions. [karyo + -logy]

kar·y·ol·y·sis (kar-ē-ol′i-sis). Destruction of the nucleus of a cell by swelling, with the loss of affinity of its chromatin for basic dyes. [karyo- + G. *lysis,* dissolution]

kar·y·o·lyt·ic (kar′ē-ō-lit′ik). Relating to karyolysis.

kar·y·o·mor·phism (kar′ē-ō-mōr′fizm). **1.** Development of the nuclear shapes of a cell. **2.** Denoting the nuclear shapes of cells, especially leukocytes. [karyo- + G. *morphē,* form]

kar·y·on (kar′ē-on). SYN nucleus (1). [G. *karyon,* a nut, kernel]

kar·y·o·phage (kar′ē-ō-fāj). An intracellular parasite that feeds on the host nucleus. [karyo- + G. *phagō,* to devour]

kar·y·o·plast (kar′ē-ō-plast). A cell nucleus surrounded by a narrow band of cytoplasm and a plasma membrane. [karyo- + G. *plastos,* formed]

kar·y·o·pyk·no·sis (kar′ē-ō-pik-nō′sis). Cytologic characteristics of the superficial or cornified cells of stratified squamous epithelium in which there is shrinkage of the nuclei and condensation of the chromatin into structureless masses. [karyo- + G. *pyknos,* thick, crowded, + *-osis,* condition]

kar·y·or·rhex·is (kar-ē-ō-rak′sis). Fragmentation of the nucleus whereby its chromatin is distributed irregularly throughout the cytoplasm; a stage of necrosis usually followed by karyolysis. [karyo- + G. *rhexis,* rupture]

kar·y·o·some (kar′ē-ō-sōm). A mass of chromatin often found in the interphase cell nucleus representing a more condensed zone of chromatin filaments. [karyo- + G. *sōma,* body]

kar·y·o·type (kar′ē-ō-tīp). The chromosome characteristics of an individual cell or of a cell line, usually presented as a systematized array of metaphase chromosomes from a photomicrograph of a single cell nucleus arranged in pairs in descending order of size and according to the position of the centromere. SYN idiogram (1). [karyo- + G. *typos,* model]

kat katal.

△**kata-.** Alternative spelling for cata-; down. [G. *kata,* down]

kat·al (kat) (kat′ăl). Unit of catalytic activity equal to one mole of product formed (or substrate consumed) per second, as of the amount of enzyme that catalyzes transformation of one mole of substrate per second.

kc kilocycle.

kcal kilogram *calorie;* kilocalorie.

KCT (kaolin clotting time) kaolin clotting *time.*

■**ke·loid** (kē′loyd). A nodular, firm, often linear mass of hyperplastic scar tissue, consisting of irregularly distributed bands of collagen; occurs in the dermis, usually after trauma, surgery, a

ke

burn, or severe cutaneous disease. [G. *kēlē,* a tumor (or *kēlis,* a spot), + *eidos,* appearance]

acne k., a chronic eruption of fibrous papules which develop at the site of follicular lesions, usually on the back of the neck at the hairline. SYN dermatitis papillaris capillitii, folliculitis keloidalis.

ke·loi·do·sis (kē′loy-dō′sis). Multiple keloids.

ke·lo·plas·ty (kē′lō-plas-tē). Operative removal of a scar or keloid. [keloid + G. *plastos,* formed]

Kelvin, Lord William Thomson, Scottish physicist, 1824–1907. SEE kelvin; K. *scale.*

kel·vin (K). A unit of thermodynamic temperature equal to $\frac{1}{273.16}$ of the thermodynamic temperature of the triple point of water. SEE ALSO Kelvin *scale.* [Lord *Kelvin*]

Kendall. SEE Abell-Kendall *method.*

△**keno-.** SEE ceno- (3). [G. *kenos,* empty]

△**kerat-.** SEE kerato-.

ker·a·tan sul·fate (ker′ă-tan). A type of sulfated mucopolysaccharide found in cartilage, bone, connective tissue, the cornea, aorta, and in the intervertebral discs; accumulates in Morquio syndrome. SYN keratosulfate.

ker·a·tec·to·my (ker-ă-tek′tō-mē). An operation done to change the refraction of the cornea; a crescentic piece of corneal stroma is removed and the resultant corneal wound is sutured. This steepens the cornea and increases its power in that axis. [kerato- + G. *ektomē,* excision]

ke·rat·ic (ke-rat′ik). SYN horny. [G. *keras* (*kerat-*), horn]

ker·a·tin (ker′ă-tin). A scleroprotein or albuminoid present in hair and nails; it contains a relatively large amount of sulfur, is insoluble in gastric juice, and is sometimes used for coating tablets that are intended to be dissolved only in the intestine. [G. *keras* (*kerat-*), horn, + -in]

ker·a·tin·as·es (ker′ă-tin-ās-ez). Hydrolases catalyzing the hydrolysis of keratin.

ker·a·tin·i·za·tion (ker′ă-tin-i-zā′shŭn). Keratin formation or development of a horny layer; may also apply to premature formation of keratin. SYN cornification.

ke·rat·i·no·cyte (ke-rat′i-nō-sīt). A cell of the living epidermis and certain oral epithelium that produces keratin in the process of differentiating into the dead and fully keratinized cells of the stratum corneum.

ke·rat·i·no·some (ke-rat′i-nō-sōm). A granule located in the upper layers of the stratum spinosum of certain stratified squamous epithelia. SYN membrane-coating granule.

ke·rat·i·nous (ke-rat′i-nŭs). **1.** Relating to keratin. **2.** SYN horny.

ker·a·ti·tis (ker-ă-tī′tis). Inflammation of the cornea. SEE ALSO keratopathy. [kerato- + G. *-itis,* inflammation]

dendriform k., dendritic k., a form of herpetic k.

disciform k., large disk-shaped infiltration of the central or paracentral corneal stroma. This lesion is deep and nonsuppurative and is seen in virus infections, particularly herpetic.

exposure k., inflammation of the cornea resulting from irritation caused by inability to close the eyelids.

geographic k., k. with coalescence of superficial lesions in herpes keratitis.

herpetic k., inflammation of the cornea (or cornea and conjunctiva) due to herpes simplex virus. SYN herpetic keratoconjunctivitis.

interstitial k., an inflammation of the corneal stroma, often with neovascularization.

metaherpetic k., a postinfectious corneal inflammation in herpetic k. leading to epithelial erosion; not due to virus replication.

neuroparalytic k., SYN neurotrophic k.

neurotrophic k., inflammation of the cornea after corneal anesthesia. SYN neuroparalytic k.

phlyctenular k., an inflammation of the corneal conjunctiva with the formation of small red nodules of lymphoid tissue (phlyctenulae) near the corneoscleral limbus.

sclerosing k., inflammation of the cornea complicating scleritis; characterized by opacification of the corneal stroma.

trachomatous k., SEE pannus, corneal *pannus.*

△**kerato-, kerat-. 1.** The cornea. **2.** Horny tissue or cells. SEE ALSO cerat-, cerato-. [G. *keras,* horn]

▯**ker·a·to·ac·an·tho·ma** (ker′ă-tō-ak′an-thō′mă). A rapidly growing, umbilicated tumor, usually occurring on exposed areas of the skin, which invades the dermis but remains localized and usually resolves spontaneously. [kerato- + G. *akantha,* thorn, +-*oma,* tumor]

ker·a·to·cele (ker′ă-tō-sēl). Hernia of Descemet's membrane through a defect in the outer layers of the cornea. [kerato- + G. *kēlē,* hernia]

ker·a·to·con·junc·ti·vi·tis (ker′ă-tō-kon-jŭngk′-ti-vī′tis). Inflammation of the conjunctiva and of the cornea.

atopic k., a chronic papillary inflammation of the conjunctiva showing Trantas dots in a patient with a history of hypersensitivity.

epidemic k., follicular conjunctivitis followed by subepithelial corneal infiltrates; often caused by adenovirus type 8, less commonly by other types. SYN virus k.

herpetic k., SYN herpetic *keratitis.*

infectious bovine k., a disease of cattle caused by the bacterium *Moraxella bovis* and characterized by blepharospasm, conjunctivitis, lacrimation, and corneal opacity and ulceration. SYN pinkeye (2).

superior limbic k., inflammatory edema of the superior corneoscleral limbus.

ultraviolet k., acute k. resulting from exposure to intense ultraviolet irradiation.

virus k., SYN epidemic k.

ker·a·to·co·nus (ker′ă-tō-kō′nŭs). A conical protrusion of the cornea caused by thinning of the stroma; usually bilateral. SYN conical cornea. [kerato- + G. *kōnos,* cone]

ker·a·to·cyst (ker′ă-tō-sist). Odontogenic cyst derived from remnants of the dental lamina and appearing as a unilocular or multilocular radiolucency which may produce jaw expansion; associated with the bifid rib basal cell nevus syndrome.

odontogenic k. (ke-rā′tō-sist), a cyst of dental lamina origin with a high recurrence rate, a corrugated parakeratin surface, uniformly thin epithelium, and a palisaded basal layer. One manifestation of the basal cell nevus syndrome.

ker·a·to·cyte (ker'ă-tō-sīt). The fibroblastic stromal cell of the cornea.

ker·a·to·der·ma (ker'ă-tō-der'mă). **1.** Any horny superficial growth. **2.** A generalized thickening of the horny layer of the epidermis. [kerato- + G. *derma*, skin]

mutilating k. [MIM*124500], diffuse k. of the extremities, with the development during childhood of constricting fibrous bands around the middle phalanx of the fingers or toes which may lead to spontaneous amputation.

k. planta're sulca'tum, hyperkeratosis and fissure formation on the soles. SYN cracked heel.

ker·a·to·ec·ta·sia (ker'ă-tō-ek-tā'zē-ă). A bulging forward of the cornea.

ker·a·to·ep·i·the·li·o·plas·ty (ker'ă-tō-ep-i-the'lē-ō-plas-tē). A surgical procedure for the repair of persistent corneal epithelial defects. Corneal epithelium is removed and small pieces of donor cornea, with epithelium attached, are placed at the corneoscleral limbus. [kerato- + epithelio- + G. *plastos*, formed]

ker·a·tog·e·nous (ker-ă-toj'ĕ-nŭs). Causing a growth of cells that produce keratin and result in the formation of horny tissue, such as fingernails, scales, feathers, etc.

ker·a·to·glo·bus (ker-ă-tō-glō'bŭs). Congenital anomaly consisting of an enlarged anterior segment of the eye. SYN megalocornea. [kerato- + L. *globus*, ball]

ker·a·to·hy·a·lin (ker'ă-tō-hī'ă-lin). The substance in the large basophilic granules of the stratum granulosum of the epidermis. [kerato- + hyalin]

ker·a·toid (ker'ă-toyd). **1.** SYN horny. **2.** Resembling corneal tissue. [kerato- + G. *eidos*, resemblance]

ker·a·to·lep·tyn·sis (ker'ă-tō-lep-tin'sis). **1.** SYN gutter *dystrophy* of cornea. **2.** An operation for removing the surface of the cornea and replacement by bulbar conjunctiva for cosmetic reasons. [kerato- + G. *leptynsis*, a making thin]

ker·a·to·leu·ko·ma (ker'ă-tō-lū-kō'mă). A white corneal opacity. [kerato- + G. *leukos*, white, + *-ōma*, growth]

ker·a·tol·y·sis (ker-ă-tol'i-sis). **1.** Separation or loosening of the horny layer of the epidermis. **2.** A disease characterized by a shedding of the epidermis recurring at more or less regular intervals. [kerato- + G. *lysis*, loosening]

pitted k., noninflammatory Gram-positive bacterial infection of the plantar surfaces producing small depressions in the stratum corneum, associated frequently with humidity and hyperhidrosis.

ker·a·to·lyt·ic (ker'ă-tō-lit'ik). Relating to keratolysis.

ker·a·to·ma (ker-ă-tō'mă). **1.** SYN callosity. **2.** A horny tumor. [kerato- + G. *-oma*, tumor]

ker·a·to·ma·la·cia (ker-ă-tō-mă-lā'shē-ă). Dryness with ulceration and perforation of the cornea occurring in cachectic children; results from severe vitamin A deficiency. [kerato- + G. *malakia*, softness]

ker·a·tome (ker'ă-tōm). A knife used for incising the cornea. SYN keratotome.

ker·a·tom·e·ter (ker-ă-tom'ĕ-ter). An instrument for measuring the curvature of the anterior corneal surface. SYN ophthalmometer. [kerato- + G. *metron,* measure]

ker·a·tom·e·try (ker-ă-tom'ĕ-trē). Measurement of the radii of corneal curvature.

ker·a·to·mi·leu·sis (ker'ă-tō-mī-lū'sis). Surgical alteration of refractive error by changing the shape of a deep layer of the cornea: the anterior lamella is peeled back, frozen, and recurved on its back surface on a lathe; or, some of the corneal stroma can be removed from the bed with a laser or a knife. [coinage, prob. fr. G. *keras* (*kerat-*), horn, cornea, + *smileusis,* carving]

ker·a·top·a·thy (ker-ă-top'ă-thē). Any corneal disease, damage, dysfunction, or abnormality. [kerato- + G. *pathos,* suffering, disease]

band-shaped k., a horizontal, gray, interpalpebral opacity of the cornea in hypercalcemia, chronic iridocyclitis, and Still's disease.

bullous k., edema of the corneal stroma and epithelium; occurs in Fuchs' epithelial dystrophy, advanced glaucoma and iridocyclitis, and sometimes after intraocular lens implantation.

neuroparalytic k., corneal inflammation or ulceration associated with dysfunction of the ophthalmic branch of the trigeminal nerve.

ker·a·to·pha·kia (ker'ă-tō-fak'ē-ă). Implantation of a donor cornea or plastic lens within the corneal stroma to modify refractive error. [kerato- + G. *phakos,* lens]

ker·a·to·plas·ty (ker'ă-tō-plas-tē). Any surgical modification of the cornea; the removal of a portion of the cornea containing an opacity and the insertion in its place of a piece of cornea of the same size and shape removed from elsewhere. SYN corneal graft. [kerato- + G. *plassō,* to form]

optical k., transplantation of transparent corneal tissue to replace a leukoma or scar that impairs vision.

refractive k., any procedure in which the shape of the cornea is modified, with the intent of changing the refractive error of the eye; for example, if the cornea is flattened, the eye becomes less myopic. SEE keratophakia, keratomileusis, radial *keratotomy.*

tectonic k., grafting to replace lost corneal tissue.

ker·a·to·pros·the·sis (ker'ă-tō-pros-thē'sis). Replacement of the central area of an opacified cornea by plastic. [kerato- + G. *prosthesis,* addition]

ker·a·to·rhex·is, ker·a·tor·rhex·is (ker'ă-tō-rek'sis). Rupture of the cornea, due to trauma or perforating ulcer. [kerato- + G. *rhēxis,* a bursting]

ker·a·to·scle·ri·tis (ker'ă-tō-skle-rī'tis). Inflammation of both cornea and sclera.

ker·a·to·scope (ker'ă-tō-skōp). An instrument marked with lines or circles by means of which the corneal reflex can be observed. [kerato- + G. *skopeō,* to examine]

ker·a·tos·co·py (ker-ă-tos'kŏ-pē). **1.** Examination of the reflections from the anterior surface of the cornea in order to determine the character and amount of corneal astigmatism. **2.** A term first applied by Cuignet to his method of retinoscopy. [kerato- + G. *skopeō,* to examine]

ke

ker•a•tose (ker′ă-tōs). Keratotic, relating to or marked by keratosis.

ker•a•to•sis, pl. **ker•a•to•ses** (ker-ă-tō′sis, -sēz). Any lesion on the epidermis marked by the presence of circumscribed overgrowths of the horny layer. [kerato- + G. -osis, condition]

   actinic k., a premalignant warty lesion occurring on the sun-exposed skin of the face or hands in aged light-skinned persons; hyperkeratosis may form a cutaneous horn, and squamous cell carcinoma of low-grade malignancy may develop in a small proportion of untreated patients.

   k. follicula′ris [MIM*124200], a familial eruption, beginning usually in childhood, in which keratotic papules originating from both follicles and interfollicular epidermis of the trunk, face, scalp, and axillae become crusted and verrucous; often intensely pruritic.

   lichenoid k., a solitary benign papule or plaque, with microscopic features resembling lichen planus, occurring on sun-exposed or unexposed skin.

   seborrheic k., k. seborrhe′ica, superficial, benign, verrucous, often pigmented, greasy lesions consisting of proliferating epidermal cells, resembling basal cells, enclosing horn cysts; they usually occur after the third decade.

ker•a•to•sul•fate (ker′ă-tō-sŭl-fāt). SYN keratan sulfate.

ker•a•to•tome (ker′ă-tō-tōm). SYN keratome.

ker•a•tot•o•my (ker′ă-tot′ō-mē). **1.** Any incision through the cornea. **2.** An operation making a partial thickness incision into the cornea to flatten it and reduce its refractive power in that meridian. [kerato- + G. tomē, incision]

   radial k., a k. with radial incisions around a clear central zone. A form of refractive keratoplasty used in the treatment of myopia.

   refractive k., modification of corneal curvature by means of corneal incisions to minimize hyperopia, myopia, or astigmatism. In this type of radial keratotomy surgery, performed by excimer laser, pie-shaped pieces of cornea are removed under local anesthetic. The resulting scar tissue formation reshapes the cornea.

ke•ri•on (kē′rē-on). A granulomatous secondarily infected lesion complicating fungal infection of the hair; typically, a raised boggy lesion. [G. kērion, honeycomb; a skin disease, fr. kēros, beeswax]

ker•nic•ter•us (ker-nik′ter-ŭs). Yellow staining and degenerative lesions in basal ganglia associated with high levels of unconjugated bilirubin in infants; may occur with hemolytic disorder such as Rh or ABO erythroblastosis or G6PD deficiency as well as with neonatal sepsis or Crigler-Najjar syndrome; characterized by opisthotonus, high-pitched cry, lethargy, and poor sucking, as well as abnormal or absent Moro reflex, and loss of upward gaze; later consequences include deafness, cerebral palsy, other sensorineural deficits, and mental retardation. SYN bilirubin encephalopathy, nuclear jaundice. [Ger. Kern, kernel (nucleus), + Ikterus, jaundice]

ker•oid (ker′oyd). SYN horny. [G. keroeidēs, horn-like]

ke•tal (kē′tăl). a hydrated ketone in which both hydroxyl groups are esterified with alcohols.

△**keto-.** Combining form denoting a compound containing a ketone group; replaced by oxo- in systematic nomenclature. [Ger.]

ke•to ac•id (kē′tō). An acid containing a ketone group (–CO–) in addition to the acid group(s).

ke•to•ac•i•do•sis (kē′tō-as-i-dō′sis). Acidosis, as in diabetes or starvation, caused by the enhanced production of ketone bodies.

ke•to•ac•i•du•ria (kē′tō-as-i-dū′rē-ă). Excretion of urine having an elevated content of ketonic acids.

ke•to•gen•e•sis (kē-tō-jen′ĕ-sis). Metabolic production of ketones or ketone bodies.

ke•to•gen•ic (kē-tō-jen′ik). Giving rise to ketone bodies in metabolism.

ke•to•hep•tose (kē-tō-hep′tōs). A seven-carbon sugar possessing a ketone group.

ke•to•hex•ose (kē-tō-heks′ōs). A six-carbon sugar possessing a ketone group; e.g., fructose. SYN hexulose.

ke•tol (kē′tol). A ketone that has an OH group near the CO group.

ke•tole (kē′tōl). SYN indole (1).

ke•tole group. Carbons 1 and 2 of a 2-ketose (HOCH₂CO–). $(\text{HOCH}_2\text{CO}-)$.

ke•to•lyt•ic (kē-tō-lit′ik). Causing the dissolution of ketone or acetone substances, referring usually to oxidation products of glucose and allied substances.

ke•tone (kē′tōn). A substance with the carbonyl group linking two carbon atoms; the most important in medicine and the simplest in chemistry is dimethyl k. (acetone).

ke•to•ne•mia (kē-tō-nē′mē-ă). The presence of recognizable concentrations of ketone bodies in the plasma. [ketone + G. haima, blood]

ke•ton•u•ria (kē-tō-nū′rē-ă). Enhanced urinary excretion of ketone bodies.

ke•tose (kē′tōs). A carbohydrate containing the characteristic carbonyl group of the ketones.

ke•to•sis (kē-tō′sis). Enhanced production of ketone bodies, as in diabetes mellitus or starvation. [ketone + -osis, condition]

17-ke•to•ste•roids (kē-tō-stēr′oydz). Any steroid with a ketone group on C-17; commonly used to designate urinary metabolites of androgenic and adrenocortical hormones that possess this structural feature. SYN 17-oxosteroids.

ke•to•tic (kē′tot-ik). Pertaining to ketone bodies; presence of acidosis due to excess ketone body production such as occurs in uncontrolled insulin-dependent diabetes.

kg kilogram.

kid•ney (kid′nē). One of the two organs that excrete the urine. The k.'s are bean-shaped organs (about 11 cm long, 5 cm wide, and 3 cm thick) lying on either side of the vertebral column, posterior to the peritoneum, about opposite the twelfth thoracic and first three lumbar vertebrae. SYN ren [NA]. [A.S. cwith, womb, belly, + neere, kidney (L. ren, G. nephros)]

   amyloid k., a k. in which amyloidosis has occurred, usually in association with some chronic illness such as multiple myeloma, tuberculosis,

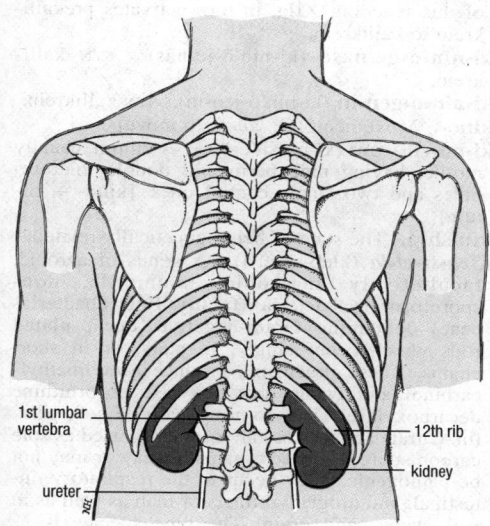

1st lumbar vertebra

12th rib

kidney

ureter

kidney: location

osteomyelitis, or other chronic suppurative inflammation. SYN waxy k.

artificial k., SYN hemodialyzer.

cake k., a solid, irregularly lobed organ of bizarre shape, usually situated in the pelvis toward the midline, produced by fusion of the renal anlagen.

contracted k., a diffusely scarred k. in which fibrous tissue and ischemic atrophy lead to reduction in the size of the organ.

duplex k., a k. in which two pelviocaliceal systems are present.

fatty k., a k. in which there is fatty metamorphosis of the parenchymal cells, especially fatty degeneration.

floating k., the abnormally mobile k. in nephroptosis. SYN wandering k.

fused k., a single, anomalous organ produced by fusion of the renal anlagen.

Goldblatt k., a k. whose arterial blood supply has been compromised, as a consequence of which arterial (renovascular) hypertension develops.

horseshoe k., union of the lower or occasionally the upper extremities of the two k.'s by a band of tissue extending across the midline.

medullary sponge k., cystic disease of the renal pyramids associated with calculus formation and hematuria; differs from cystic disease of the renal medulla in that renal failure does not usually develop.

pancake k., a disk-shaped organ produced by fusion of both poles of the contralateral k. anlagen.

polycystic k., a progressive disease characterized by formation of multiple cysts of varying size scattered diffusely throughout both k.'s, resulting in compression and destruction of k. parenchyma, usually with hypertension, gross he-

maturia, and uremia. SYN polycystic disease of kidneys.

wandering k., SYN floating k.

waxy k., SYN amyloid k.

Kiel clas·si·fi·ca·tion. See under classification.

kilo- (k). Prefix used in the SI and metric systems to signify one thousand (10^3). [French fr. G. *chilioi,* one thousand]

kil·o·cal·o·rie (kcal) (kil′ō-kal-ō-rē). SYN large *calorie.*

kil·o·cy·cle (kc) (kil′ō-sī-kl). One thousand cycles per second.

kil·o·gram (kg) (kil′ō-gram). The SI unit of mass, 1000 g; equivalent to 15,432.358 gr, 2.2046226 lb. avoirdupois, or 2.6792289 lb. troy.

kil·o·gram-me·ter. The energy exerted, or work done, when a mass of 1 kg is raised a height of 1 m; equal to 9.80665 J in the SI system.

kil·o·volt (kv) (kil′ō-vōlt). A unit of electrical potential, potential difference, or electromotive force, equal to 10^3 volts. [kilo + volt]

kin·an·es·the·sia (kin-an-es-thē′zē-ă). A disturbance of deep sensibility in which there is inability to perceive either direction or extent of movement, the result being ataxia. [G. *kinēsis,* motion, + *an-* priv. + *aisthēsis,* sensation]

ki·nase (kī′nās). **1.** An enzyme catalyzing the conversion of a proenzyme to an active enzyme. **2.** An enzyme catalyzing the transfer of phosphate groups to form triphosphates (*e.g.,* ATP). For individual k.'s, see specific name.

kin·dred. An aggregate of genetically related persons; distinguished from pedigree, which is a stylized representation of a k. [O.E. *kynrēde,* fr. *cyn,* kin, + *rēde,* condition]

kin·e·mat·ics (kin-ĕ-mat′iks). PHYSIOLOGY The science concerned with movements of the parts of the body. [G. *kinēmatica,* things that move]

kin·e·plas·tics (kin′ĕ-plas-tiks). SYN cineplastic *amputation.*

kin·e·sal·gia (kin-ĕ-sal′jē-ă). Pain caused by muscular movement. SYN kinesialgia. [G. *kinēsis,* motion, + *algos,* pain]

kinesi-, kinesio-, kineso-. Motion. [G. *kinēsis*]

ki·ne·sia (ki-nē′sē-ă, -nē′zē-). SYN motion *sickness.* [G. *kinēsis,* movement]

ki·ne·si·al·gia (ki-nē-sē-al′jē-ă). SYN kinesalgia.

ki·ne·si·at·rics (ki-nē′sē-at′riks). SYN kinesitherapy. [G. *kinēsis,* movement, + *iatrikos,* relating to medicine]

ki·ne·sics (ki-nē′siks). The study of nonverbal, bodily motion in communication.

kin·e·sim·e·ter (kin-ĕ-sim′ĕ-ter). An instrument for measuring the extent of a movement. SYN kinesiometer. [G. *kinēsis,* movement, + *metron,* measure]

kinesio-. SEE kinesi-.

ki·ne·si·ol·o·gy (ki-nē-sē-ol′ō-jē). The science or the study of movement, and the active and passive structures involved. [G. *kinēsis,* movement, + *-logos,* study]

ki·ne·si·om·e·ter (ki-nē-sē-om′ĕ-ter). SYN kinesimeter.

ki·ne·sis (ki-nē′sis). Motion. As a termination, used to denote movement or activation, particularly the kind induced by a stimulus. [G.]

ki·ne·si·ther·a·py (ki-nē-si-thār′ă-pē). Physical

ki

therapy involving motion and range of motion exercises. SEE movement. SYN kinesiatrics.

⚭**kineso-.** SEE kinesi-.

kin·es·the·sia (kin'es-thē'zē-ă). **1.** The sense perception of movement; the muscular sense. **2.** An illusion of moving in space. [G. *kinēsis,* motion, + *aisthēsis,* sensation]

kin·es·the·si·om·e·ter (kin'es-thē'zē-om'ĕ-ter). An instrument for determining the degree of muscular sensation. [kinesthesia, + G. *metron,* measure]

kin·es·thet·ic (kin-es-thet'ik). Relating to kinesthesia.

kinesthetic awareness. SYN body *scheme.*

ki·net·ic (ki-net'ik). Relating to motion or movement. [G. *kinētikos,* of motion, fr. *kinētos,* moving]

ki·net·ics (ki-net'iks). The study of motion, acceleration, or rate of change.

⚭**kineto-.** Motion. [G. *kinētos,* moving, movable]

ki·ne·to·car·di·o·gram (ki-nē'tō-kar'dē-ō-gram, ki-net'ō-). One type of graphic recording of the vibrations of the chest wall produced by cardiac activity.

ki·ne·to·car·di·o·graph (ki-nē'tō-kar'dē-ō-graf, ki-net'ō-). A device for recording precordial impulses due to cardiac movement; the absolute displacement of a point on the chest wall is recorded relative to a fixed reference point above the recumbent patient.

ki·ne·to·chore (ki-nē'tō-kōr, ki-net'ō-). The structural portion of the chromosome to which microtubules attach. Cf. centromere. [kineto- + G. *chōra,* space]

ki·ne·to·gen·ic (ki-nē-tō-jen'ik, ki-net-ō-). Causing or producing motion.

ki·ne·to·plast (ki-nē'tō-plast, ki-net'ō-). An intensely staining extranuclear DNA structure found in parasitic flagellates near the base of the flagellum. Electron micrographs show it to be part of a single giant mitochondrion filling most of the cytoplasm of amastigote flagellates. SEE ALSO parabasal *body.* [kineto- + G. *plastos,* formed]

Kin·gel·la (kin-jel'ah). Newly recognized member of the family Neisseriaceae; a Gram-negative coccus with a requirement of enhanced carbon dioxide for recovery in culture.

  K. indolog'enes, a species that causes eye infections or endocarditis (when prosthetic heart valves are present) in humans.

  K. kin'gae, a species that causes endocarditis in humans. SEE HACEK *group.*

ki·nin (kī'nin). One of a number of differing substances having pronounced physiological effects. Some are polypeptides, formed in blood in various pathological processes, that stimulate visceral smooth muscle but relax vascular smooth muscle, thus producing vasodilation. [G. *kineō,* to move, + -in]

ki·nin·o·gen (ki-nin'ō-jen). The globulin precursor of a (plasma) kinin.

  high molecular weight k. (HMWK), a plasma protein of 110,000 molecular weight that normally exists in plasma in a 1:1 complex with prekallikrein. The complex is a cofactor in the activation of coagulation factor XII. The product

of this reaction, XIIa, in turn activates prekallikrein to kallikrein.

ki·nin·o·ge·nase (ki-nin'ō-jĕ-nās). SYN kallikrein.

ki·nin·o·gen·in (ki-nin'ō-jen-in). SYN kallikrein.

⚭**kino-.** Movement. [G. *kineō,* to move]

ki·no·cil·i·um (kī-nō-sil'ē-ŭm). A cilium, usually motile, having nine peripheral double microtubules and two single central ones. [kino- + cilium]

kin·ship. The state of being genetically related.

Kleb·si·el·la (kleb-sē-el'ă). A genus of aerobic, facultatively anaerobic, nonmotile, nonsporeforming bacteria (family Enterobacteriaceae) containing Gram-negative, encapsulated rods which occur singly, in pairs, or in short chains. These organisms produce acetylmethylcarbinol and lysine decarboxylase or ornithine decarboxylase. They do not usually liquefy gelatin. Citrate and glucose are ordinarily used as sole carbon sources. These organisms may or may not be pathogenic. They occur in the respiratory, intestinal, and urogenital tracts of man as well as in soil, water, and grain. The type species is *K. pneumoniae.* [E. *Klebs*]

  K. pneumo'niae, a species found in soil and water, on grain, and in the intestinal tract of humans and other animals; it also occurs in association with several pathologic conditions, urinary tract infections, sputum, feces, and metritis in mares; capsular types 1, 2, and 3 of this organism may be causative agents in pneumonia; organisms previously identified as nonmotile strains of *Aerobacter aerogenes* are now placed in this species; it is the type species of *K.*

klep·to·ma·nia (klep-tō-mā'nē-ă). A disorder of impulse control characterized by a morbid tendency to steal. [G. *kleptō,* to steal, + *mania,* insanity]

klep·to·ma·ni·ac (klep-tō-mā'nē-ak). A person exhibiting kleptomania.

knee (nē). **1.** SYN genu (1). **2.** Any structure of angular shape resembling a flexed knee. [A.S. *cneōw*]

  housemaid's k., an adventitious occupational bursitis occurring over the tibial tuberosity, the area of contact when kneeling; not to be confused with infrapatellar bursitis.

  locked k., a condition in which the k. lacks full extension and flexion because of internal derangement, usually the result of a torn medial meniscus.

knee·cap (nē'kap). SYN patella.

knit·ting (nit'ing). Nonmedical term denoting the process of union of the fragments of a broken bone or of the edges of a wound. [M.E., *knitten,* to knot, fr. A.S. *cnyttan*]

knock-knee (nok'nē). SYN genu valgum.

knot (not). **1.** An intertwining of the ends of two cords, tapes, sutures, etc. in such a way that they cannot spontaneously become separated; or a similar twining or infolding of a cord in its continuity. **2.** ANATOMY, PATHOLOGY A node, ganglion, or circumscribed swelling suggestive of a k. [A.S. *cnotta*]

  granny k., a double k. in which the free ends of

the second loop are asymmetric and not in the same plane as the free ends of the first loop.

laparoscopic k., a k. placed intracorporally through a laparoscopic instrument. The k. itself may be tied extracorporally and passed into the body through a cannula or the k. may be both placed and tied intracorporally.

primitive k., SYN primitive *node.*

surgeon's k., the first loop of the k. has two throws rather than a single throw. The second loop has only one throw and that is placed in a square knot fashion leaving the free ends in the same plane as the first loop.

syncytial k., a localized aggregation of syncytiotrophoblastic nuclei in the villi of the placenta during early pregnancy.

knuck•le (nŭk′l). **1.** A joint of a finger when the fist is closed, especially a metacarpophalangeal joint. **2.** A kink or loop of intestine, as in a hernia. [M.E. *knokel*]

koi•lo•cyte (koy′lō-sīt). A squamous cell, often binucleated, showing a perinuclear halo; characteristic of condyloma acuminatum. [G. *koilos*, hollow, + *kytos*, cell]

koi•lo•cy•to•sis (koy′lō-sī-tō′sis). Perinuclear vacuolation. SEE ALSO koilocyte. [G. *koilos*, hollow, + *kytos*, cell, + *-osis*, condition]

koi•lo•nych•ia (koy-lō-nik′ē-ă). A malformation of the nails in which the outer surface is concave; often associated with iron deficiency or softening by occupational contact with oils. SYN spoon nail. [G. *koilos*, hollow, + *onyx* (*onych-*), nail]

kolp-. SEE colpo-.

ko•lyt•ic (kō-lit′ik). Denoting an inhibitory action. [G. *kolyō*, to hinder]

ko•ni•o•cor•tex (kō′nē-ō-kōr′teks). Regions of the cerebral cortex characterized by a particularly well developed inner granular layer (layer 4); this type of cerebral cortex is represented by the primary sensory area 17 of the visual cortex, areas 1 to 3 of the somatic sensory cortex, and area 41 of the auditory cortex. SEE ALSO cerebral *cortex.* [G. *konis*, dust, + L. *cortex*, bark]

kopro-. SEE copro-.

Kr krypton.

krau•ro•sis vul•vae (kraw-rō′sis vŭl′vē). Atrophy and shrinkage of the epithelium of the vagina and vulva, often accompanied by a chronic inflammatory reaction in the deeper tissues, as in lichen sclerosus. [G. *krauros*, dry, brittle]

krin•gle (krin′gle). A structural motif or domain seen in certain proteins in which a fold of large loops is stabilized by disulfide bonds; an important structural feature in blood coagulation factors. [Ger. *Kringel*, curl]

krymo-, kryo-. SEE crymo-, cryo-.

kryp•ton (Kr) (krip′ton). One of the inert gases, present in small amounts in the atmosphere (1.14 ppm by dry volume); atomic no. 36, atomic wt. 83.80; ^{85}Kr has been used in studies of cardiac abnormalities. [G. *kryptos*, concealed]

ku•ru (kū′rū). A progressive, fatal form of spongiform encephalopathy, endemic in New Guinea and caused by prions. Transmission is believed to occur through ritual cannibalism. SEE prion. [native dialect, to shiver from fear or cold]

kv kilovolt.

kVp (kilovolt peak) kilovolts peak, the highest instantaneous energy across an x-ray tube, corresponding to the highest energy x-rays emitted.

kwa•shi•or•kor (kwah-shē-ōr′kōr). A disease seen in African children one to three years old, due to dietary deficiency, particularly of protein; characterized by marked hypoalbuminemia, anemia, edema, pot belly, depigmentation of the skin, loss of hair or change in hair color to red, and bulky stools containing undigested food. [Native, red boy or displaced child]

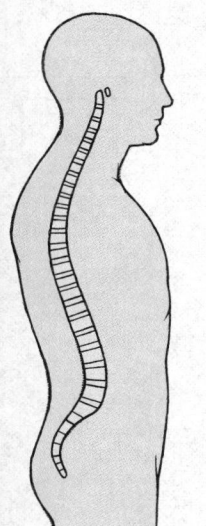
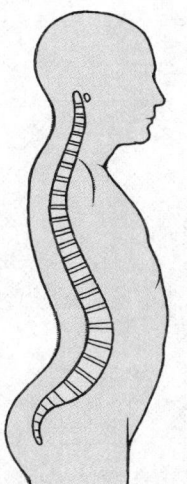
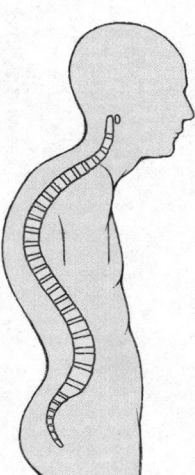
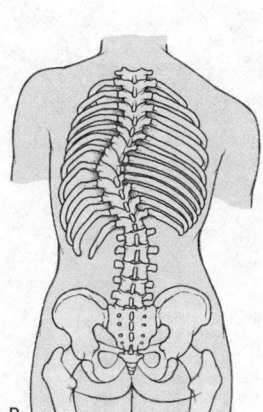

spinal curvatures: (A) normal, (B) lordosis, (C) kyphosis, (D) scoliosis

⚠️**ky-.** For words beginning thus and not found below, see cy-.

ky•ma•tism (kī′mă-tizm). SYN myokymia. [G. *kyma,* wave]

ky•mo•gram (kī′mō-gram). The graphic curve made by a kymograph.

ky•mo•graph (kī′mō-graf). An instrument for recording wavelike motions or modulation; it consists of a drum revolved by clockwork and covered smoked paper upon which the curve is inscribed by writing point. [G. *kyma,* wave, + *graphō,* to record]

ky•mog•ra•phy (kī-mog′ră-fē). Use of the kymograph.

kyn•u•ren•ic ac•id (kin-yū-rē′nik, -ren′ik). A product of the metabolism of L-tryptophan; appears in urine in pyridoxine deficiency.

kyn•u•ren•ine (kī-nū′rĕ-nēn, -nin). A product of the metabolism of L-tryptophan, excreted in the urine.

ky•phos (kī′fos). A hump, the convex prominence in kyphosis. [G.]

ky•pho•sco•li•o•sis (kī′fō-skō-lē-ō′sis). Kyphosis combined with scoliosis; congestive heart failure is a late complication.

ky•pho•sis (kī-fō′sis). A deformity of the spine characterized by extensive flexion. [G. *kyphōsis,* hump-back, fr. *kyphos,* bent, hump-backed]

ky•phot•ic (kī-fot′ik). Relating to or suffering from kyphosis.

⚠️**kyto-.** SEE cyto-.

L

λ. SEE Λ.

Λ, λ. lambda. SEE lambda.

l liter.

L-. Prefix indicating a chemical compound to be structurally (sterically) related to L-glyceraldehyde. Cf. D-.

l-. Levorotatory. Cf. d-. [L. *laevus,* on the left-hand side]

La lanthanum.

la·bel. 1. To incorporate into a compound a substance that is readily detected, such as a radionuclide, whereby its metabolism can be followed or its physical distribution detected. **2.** The substance so incorporated.

la belle in·dif·fér·ence (lah bel an-dif-er-ahns'). A naive, inappropriate lack of emotion or concern for the perceptions by others of one's disability, typically seen in persons with conversion hysteria. [Fr.]

la·bia (lā′bē-ă). Plural of labium.

la·bi·al (lā′bē-ăl). **1.** Relating to the lips or any labium. **2.** Toward a lip. **3.** One of the letters formed by means of the lips. [L. *labium,* lip]

la·bile (lā′bīl, -bil). Unstable; unsteady; not fixed; denoting: **1.** An adaptability to alteration or modification, *i.e.,* relatively easily changed or rearranged. **2.** Constituents of serum affected by increases in heat. **3.** An electrode that is kept moving over the surface during the passage of an electric current. **4.** PSYCHOLOGY Free and uncontrolled mood or behavioral expression of the emotions. **5.** Easily removable; *e.g.,* a l. hydrogen atom. [L. *labilis,* liable to slip, fr. *labor,* pp. *lapsus,* to slip]

la·bil·i·ty (lă-bil′i-tē). The state of being labile.

labio-. The lips. SEE ALSO cheilo-. [L. *labium,* lip]

la·bi·o·cer·vi·cal (lā′bē-ō-ser′vi-kăl). Relating to a lip and a neck; specifically, to the labial or buccal surface of the neck of a tooth. [labio- + L. *cervix,* neck]

la·bi·o·cho·rea (lā-bē-ō-kōr-ē′ă). A chronic spasm of the lips, interfering with speech. [labio- + G. *choreia,* dance]

la·bi·o·cli·na·tion (lā′bē-ō-kli-nā′shŭn). Inclination of position more toward the lips than is normal; said of a tooth.

la·bi·o·den·tal (lā-bē-ō-den′tăl). Relating to the lips and the teeth; denoting certain letters the sound of which is formed by both lips and teeth. [labio- + L. *dens,* tooth]

la·bi·o·gin·gi·val (lā′bē-ō-jin′ji-văl). Relating to the point of junction of the labial border and the gingival line on the distal or mesial surface of an incisor tooth.

la·bi·o·glos·so·la·ryn·ge·al (lā′bē-ō-glos′ō-lă-rin′jē-ăl). Relating to the lips, tongue, and larynx; describing bulbar paralysis in which these parts are involved. [labio- + G. *glōssa,* tongue, + larynx]

la·bi·o·glos·so·pha·ryn·ge·al (lā′bē-ō-glos′ō-fă-rin′jē-ăl). Relating to the lips, tongue, and pharynx; describing bulbar paralysis involving these parts. [labio- + G. *glōssa,* tongue, + pharynx]

la·bi·o·graph (lā′bē-ō-graf). An instrument for recording the movements of the lips in speaking. [labio- + G. *graphō,* to record]

la·bi·o·men·tal (lā′bē-ō-men′tăl). Relating to the lower lip and the chin. [labio- + L. *mentum,* chin]

la·bi·o·na·sal (lā′bē-ō-nā′săl). **1.** Relating to the upper lip and the nose, or to both lips and the nose. **2.** Denoting a letter which is both labial and nasal in the production of its sound.

la·bi·o·pal·a·tine (lā′bē-ō-pal′ă-tīn). Relating to the lips and the palate.

la·bi·o·place·ment (lā′bē-ō-plās′ment). Positioning (*e.g.,* of a tooth) more toward the lips than normal.

la·bi·o·plas·ty (lā′bē-ō-plas-tē). Plastic surgery of a lip. [labio- + G. *plastos,* formed]

la·bi·o·ver·sion (lā′bē-ō-ver-zhŭn). Malposition of an anterior tooth from the normal line of occlusion toward the lips.

la·bi·um, gen. **la·bii**, pl. **la·bia** (lā′bē-ŭm, -bē-ī, -bē-ă) [NA]. **1.** SYN lip. **2.** Any lip-shaped structure. [L.]

l. ma′jus, one of two rounded folds of integument forming the lateral boundaries of the pudendal cleft. The labia majora are the female homolog of the scrotum.

l. mi′nus, one of two narrow longitudinal folds of mucous membrane enclosed in the pudendal cleft within the labia majora; posteriorly, they gradually merge into the labia majora and join to form the frenulum labiorum pudendi (fourchette); anteriorly, each l. divides into two portions which unite with those of the opposite side in front of the glans clitoridis to form the prepuce.

la·bor (lā′bŏr). The process of expulsion of the fetus and the placenta from the uterus. The **stages of l.** are: **first stage,** beginning with the onset of uterine contractions through the period of dilation of the os uteri; **second stage,** the period of expulsive effort, beginning with complete dilation of the cervix and ending with expulsion of the infant; **third s.** or **placental stage,** the period beginning at the expulsion of the infant and ending with the completed expulsion of the placenta and membranes. [L. toil, suffering]

missed l., brief uterine contractions which do not lead to labor and expulsion of the infant, but which cease, resulting in the indefinite retention of the fetus (usually lifeless).

precipitate l., very rapid l. ending in delivery of the fetus.

premature l., onset of labor before the 37th completed week of pregnancy dated from the last normal menstrual period.

lab·o·ra·tory (lab′ŏ-ră-tō-rē, lab′ră-). A place equipped for the performance of tests, experiments, and investigative procedures and for the preparation of reagents, therapeutic chemical materials, and so on. [Mediev. L. *laboratorium,* a workplace, fr. L. *laboro,* pp. *-atus,* to labor]

physician office laboratory (POL), clinical laboratory located in a physician's office for on-site testing of specimens from patients seen by the physician.

la·bra (lā′bră). Plural of labrum. [L.]

la

la·brum, pl. **la·bra** (lā′brŭm, lā′bră) [NA]. **1.** A lip. **2.** A lip-shaped structure. [L.]

glenoid l., soft tissue lip around the periphery of the glenoid fossa that widens and deepens the shoulder joint to aid in the achievement of stability. SEE ALSO acetabulum.

lab·y·rinth (lab′i-rinth). Any of several anatomical structures with numerous intercommunicating cells or canals. **1.** The internal or inner ear, composed of the semicircular ducts, vestibule, and cochlea. **2.** Any group of communicating cavities, as in each lateral mass of the ethmoid bone. **3.** SYN convoluted *part* of kidney lobule. **4.** A group of upright test tubes terminating below in a base of communicating, alternately ∪-shaped and ∩-shaped tubes, used for isolating motile from nonmotile organisms in culture, or a motile from a less motile organism (as the typhoid from the colon bacillus), the former traveling faster and farther through the tubes than the latter.

bony l., a series of cavities (cochlea, vestibule, and semicircular canals) contained within the otic capsule of the petrous portion of the temporal bone; the bony labyrinth is filled with perilymph, in which the delicate, endolymph-filled membranous labyrinth is suspended.

ethmoidal l., a mass of air cells with thin bony walls forming part of the lateral wall of the nasal cavity; the cells are arranged in three groups, anterior, middle, and posterior, and are closed laterally by the orbital plate which forms part of the wall of the orbit.

membranous l., a complex arrangement of communicating membranous canaliculi and sacs, filled with endolymph and surrounded by perilymph, suspended within the cavity of the bony labyrinth; its chief divisions are the cochlear labyrinth and the vestibular labyrinth.

lab·y·rin·thec·to·my (lab-ĭ-rin-thek′tō-mē). Excision of the labyrinth; a destructive operation to destroy labyrinthine function. [labyrinth + G. *ektomē,* excision]

lab·y·rin·thine (lab-ĭ-rin′thin). Relating to any labyrinth.

lab·y·rin·thi·tis (lab′ĭ-rin-thī′tis). Inflammation of the labyrinth (the internal ear), sometimes accompanied by vertigo and deafness. SYN otitis interna.

lab·y·rin·thot·o·my (lab-ĭ-rin-thot′ō-mē). Incision into the labyrinth. [labyrinth + G. *tomē,* incision]

lac·er·at·ed (las′er-ā-ted). Torn; rent; having a ragged edge. [L. *lacero,* pp. *-atus,* to tear to pieces]

lac·er·a·tion (las-er-a′shŭn). **1.** A torn or jagged wound caused by blunt trauma; incorrectly applied to a cut. **2.** The process or act of tearing the tissues. [L. *lacero,* pp. *-atus,* to tear to pieces]

la·cer·tus (lă-ser′tŭs). **1.** The muscular part of the upper limb from shoulder to elbow. **2** [NA]. A fibrous band, bundle, or slip related to a muscle. [L.]

lac·ri·mal (lak′ri-măl). Relating to the tears, their secretion, the secretory glands, and the drainage apparatus. [L. *lacrima,* a tear]

lac·ri·ma·tion (lak′ri-mā′shŭn). The secretion of tears, especially in excess. [L. *lacrimatio*]

lac·ri·ma·tor (lak′ri-mā-ter). An agent (such as tear gas) that irritates the eyes and produces tears. [L. *lacrima,* tear]

lac·ri·ma·to·ry (lak′ri-mă-tō-rē). Causing lacrimation.

lac·ri·mot·o·my (lak-ri-mot′ō-mē). The operation of incising the lacrimal duct or sac. [L. *lacrima,* tear, + G. *tomē,* incision]

△**lact-, lacti-, lacto-.** Milk. SEE ALSO galacto-. [L. *lac, lactis*]

lac·tac·i·do·sis (lak-tas-i-dō′sis). Acidosis due to increased lactic acid.

lac·tam, lac·tim (lak′tam, -tim). Contractions of "lactoneamine" and "lactoneimine," and applied to the tautomeric forms –NH–CO– and –N=C(OH)–, respectively, observed in many purines, pyrimidines, and other substances.

β-lac·tam. A cyclical unit found in the molecular structure of penicillins and cephalosporins.

β-lac·ta·mase (lak′tă-mās). An enzyme that brings about the hydrolysis of a β-lactam (as penicillin to penicilloic acid); found in most staphylococcus strains that are naturally resistant to penicillin.

lac·tase (lak′tās). SYN β-D-galactosidase.

lac·tate (lak′tāt). **1.** A salt or ester of lactic acid. **2.** To produce milk in the mammary glands.

l. dehydrogenase (LDH), name for four enzymes. The first two transfer H to ferricytochrome *c;* the last two transfer it to NAD$^+$, in catalyzing the oxidation of lactate to pyruvate; the isozyme distribution of heart and muscle l. dehydrogenase is of diagnostic use in myocardial infarction.

lac·ta·tion (lak-tā′shŭn). **1.** Production of milk. **2.** Period following birth during which milk is secreted in the breasts. [L. *lactatio,* suckle]

lac·te·al (lak′tē-ăl). **1.** Relating to or resembling milk; milky. **2.** A lymphatic vessel that conveys chyle from the intestine. SYN chyle vessel, lacteal vessel.

△**lacti-.** SEE lact-.

lac·tic ac·id. A normal intermediate in the fermentation (oxidation, metabolism) of sugar.

lac·tif·er·ous (lak-tif′er-ŭs). Yielding milk. SYN lactigerous. [lacti- + L. *fero,* to bear]

lac·tig·e·nous (lak-tij′ĕ-nŭs). Producing milk. [lacti- + *-gen,* producing]

lac·tig·er·ous (lak-tij′er-ŭs). SYN lactiferous. [lacti- + L. *gero,* to carry]

lac·tim (-tim). SEE lactam.

△**lacto-.** SEE lact-.

Lac·to·ba·cil·lus (lak-tō-bă-sil′ŭs). A genus of microaerophilic or anaerobic, non–spore-forming, ordinarily nonmotile bacteria containing Gram-positive rods which vary from long and slender cells to short coccobacilli; chains are commonly produced. These organisms are found in dairy products, the effluents of grain and meat products, water, sewage, beer, wine, fruits and fruit juices, pickled vegetables, and in sourdough and mash, and are part of the normal flora of the mouth, intestinal tract, and vagina of many warm-blooded animals, including humans; rarely are they pathogenic. The type species is *L. delbrueckii.* [lacto- + bacillus]

lac·to·ba·cil·lus (lak-tō-bă-sil′ŭs). A vernacular

term used to refer to any member of the genus *Lactobacillus*.

lac•to•cele (lak′tō-sēl). SYN galactocele. [lacto- + G. *kēlē*, tumor]

lac•to•gen (lak′tō-jen). An agent that stimulates milk production or secretion. [lacto- + G. *-gen,* producing]

human placental l., l. isolated from human placentas; its biological activity mimics that of somatotropin and prolactin; secreted into maternal circulation; deficiency during pregnancy leads to abnormal intrauterine and postnatal growth. SYN chorionic "growth hormone-prolactin", human chorionic somatomammotropic hormone, human chorionic somatomammotropin, placental growth hormone.

lac•to•gen•e•sis (lak-tō-jen′ĕ-sis). Milk production. [lacto- + G. *genesis,* production]

lac•to•gen•ic (lak-tō-jen′ik). Pertaining to lactogenesis.

lac•to•glob•u•lin (lak-tō-glob′yū-lin). The globulin present in milk; it makes up 50 to 60% of bovine whey protein.

lac•tone (lak′tōn). An intramolecular organic anhydride formed from a hydroxyacid by the loss of water between an –OH and a –COOH group; a cyclic ester.

lac•tor•rhea (lak-tō-rē′ă). SYN galactorrhea. [lacto- + G. *rhoia,* a flow]

lac•tose (lak′tōs). A disaccharide present in milk, obtained from cow's milk and used in food for infants and convalescents and in pharmaceutical preparations; large doses act as an osmotic diuretic and as a laxative. SYN milk sugar.

lac•tos•u•ria (lak′tō-sū′rē-ă). Excretion of lactose (milk sugar) in the urine; a common finding during pregnancy and lactation, and in newborn, especially premature, babies. [lactose + G. *ouron,* urine, + -ia]

lac•to•ther•a•py (lak-tō-thār′ă-pē). SYN galactotherapy.

la•cu•na, pl. **la•cu•nae** (lă-kū′nă, -kū′nē). **1** [NA]. A small space, cavity, or depression. **2.** A gap or defect. **3.** An abnormal space between strata or between the cellular elements of the epidermis. **4.** SYN corneal *space.* [L. a pit, dim. of *lacus,* a hollow, a lake]

cartilage l., a cavity within the matrix of cartilage, occupied by a chondrocyte. SYN cartilage space.

Howship's lacunae, tiny depressions, pits, or irregular grooves in bone that is being resorbed by osteoclasts. SYN resorption lacunae.

intervillous l., one of the blood spaces in the placenta into which the chorionic villi project.

lateral venous lacunae, lateral expansions of the superior sagittal sinus of the dura mater, often increasing in width with advancing age until, in the very old, they may extend two cm lateral to the midline; the endothelium-lined lumen of the lacunae are usually reduced to a spongelike labyrinth by numerous arachnoid granulations and dural trabeculae. SYN parasinoidal sinuses.

l. mag′na, a recess on the roof of the fossa navicularis of the penis, formed by a fold of mucous membrane, the valve of the navicular fossa.

osseous l., a cavity in bony tissue occupied by an osteocyte.

resorption lacunae, SYN Howship's lacunae.

trophoblastic l., one of the spaces in the early syncytiotrophoblastic layer of the chorion before the formation of villi; in human embryos maternal blood enters these spaces by the 10th day; with the differentiation of the chorionic villi they become intervillous spaces, sometimes called intervillous lacunae.

vascular l., the medial compartment beneath the inguinal ligament, for the passage to the femoral vessels; it is separated from the muscular l. by the iliopectineal arch.

la•cu•nar (lă-kū′năr). Relating to a lacuna.

la•cu•nule (lă-kū′nūl). A very small lacuna. [Mod. L. *lacunula,* dim. of L. *lacuna*]

la•cus, pl. **la•cus** (lā′kŭs). A small collection of fluid. SYN lake (1). [L. lake]

l. lacrima′lis [NA], SYN lacrimal *lake.*

l. semina′lis, the vault of the vagina after insemination. SYN seminal lake.

LAD leukocyte adhesion *deficiency.*

la•e•trile (lā′ĕ-tril). An allegedly antineoplastic drug consisting chiefly of amygdalin derived from apricot pits; its antitumor effect is unproven.

△**laev-.** SEE levo-.

la•ge•na, pl. **la•ge•nae** (lă-jē′nă, -jē-nē). **1.** SYN cupular *cecum* of the cochlear duct. **2.** One of the three parts of the membranous labyrinth of the inner ear of lower vertebrates; in mammals, the l. becomes the cochlea. [L. flask]

lag•ging. Retarded or diminished ventilatory movement of the affected side of the chest due to pleural disease with muscle splinting or collapse of a lung.

lake (lāk). **1.** SYN lacus. **2.** To cause blood plasma to become red as a result of the release of hemoglobin from the erythrocytes, as when the latter are suspended in water. SEE ALSO lacuna. [A.S. *lacu,* fr. L. *lacus,* lake]

capillary l., the total mass of blood contained in capillary vessels.

lacrimal l., the small cistern-like area of the conjunctiva at the medial angle of the eye, in which the tears collect after bathing the anterior surface of the eyeball and the conjunctival sac. SYN lacus lacrimalis [NA].

seminal l., SYN lacus *seminalis.*

subchorial l., SYN subchorial *space.*

Laki-Lorand fac•tor. See under factor.

laky (lā′kē). Pertaining to the transparent bright red appearance of blood serum or plasma, developing as a result of hemoglobin being released from destroyed red blood cells.

lal•ling (lal′ing). A form of stammering in which the speech is almost unintelligible. [G. *laleō,* to chatter]

lal•o•che•zia (lal-ō-kē′zē-ă). Emotional discharge gained by uttering indecent or filthy words. [G. *lalia,* speech, + *chezō,* to relieve oneself]

la•lo•ple•gia (la-lō-plē′jē-ă). Paralysis of the muscles concerned in the mechanism of speech. [G. *lalia,* speech, + *plēgē,* a stroke]

lambda (Λ, λ) (lam′dă) **1.** The 11th letter of the Greek alphabet. **2.** Symbol (λ) for Avogadro's *number*; wavelength; radioactive *constant*; Ostwald's solubility *coefficient*; molar conductivity of an electrolyte (Λ). **3.** CHEMISTRY the position of a substituent located on the 11th atom from the carboxyl or other functional group (λ). **4.** The craniometric point at the junction of the sagittal and lambdoid sutures.

lamb·doid (lam′doyd). Resembling the Greek letter lambda, as does the lambdoid suture. [lambda + G. *eidos*, resemblance]

la·mel·la, pl. **la·mel·lae** (lă-mel′ă, -mel′ē). **1.** A thin sheet or layer, such as occurs in compact bone. **2.** A preparation in the form of a medicated gelatin disc, used as a means of making local applications to the conjunctiva in place of solutions. SYN discus [NA], disc (2), disk (1). [L. dim. of *lamina*, plate, leaf]

articular l., the compact layer of bone on its articular surface that is firmly attached to the overlying articular cartilage.

circumferential l., a bony l. that encircles the outer or inner surface of a bone.

concentric l., one of the concentric tubular layers of bone surrounding the central canal in an osteon. SYN haversian l.

elastic l., a thin sheet or membrane composed of elastic fibers.

ground l., SYN interstitial l.

haversian l., SYN concentric l.

interstitial l., one of the lamellae of partially resorbed osteons occurring between newer, complete osteons. SYN ground l.

vitreous l., SYN *lamina* basalis choroideae.

lam·el·lar (lam′ĕ-lăr, lă-mel′ăr). **1.** Arranged in thin plates or scales. **2.** Relating to lamellae.

la·mel·li·po·di·um, pl. **la·mel·li·po·dia** (lă-mel-i-pō′dē-ŭm, -ă). A cytoplasmic veil produced on all sides of migrating polymorphonuclear leukocytes.

lam·i·na, pl. **lam·i·nae** (lam′i-nă, lam′i-nē) [NA]. Thin plate or flat layer. SEE ALSO layer, stratum. [L]

anterior elastic l. of cornea, a homogeneous, acellular tissue layer just beneath the epithelium of the cornea. SYN Bowman's membrane, l. limitans anterior corneae.

l. ar′cus ver′tebrae [NA], SYN l. of vertebral arch.

basilar l., SYN basilar *membrane*.

basal l. of ciliary body, the inner layer of the ciliary body, continuous with the basal layer of the choroid and supporting the pigment epithelium of the ciliary retina.

basal l. of neural tube, the ventral division of the lateral walls of the neural tube in the embryo; it contains neuroblasts giving rise to somatic and visceral motor neurons.

l. basa′lis choroi′deae [NA], the transparent, nearly structureless inner layer of the choroid in contact with the pigmented layer of the retina. SYN basal layer of choroid, vitreous lamella, vitreous membrane (3).

l. choroidocapilla′ris [NA], SYN choriocapillary *layer*.

l. cribro′sa os′sis ethmoida′lis [NA], SYN cribriform *plate* of ethmoid bone.

l. cribro′sa scle′rae, the portion of the sclera through which pass the fibers of the optic nerve.

elastic laminae of arteries, 1) external: the layer of elastic connective tissue lying immediately outside the smooth muscle of the tunica media; 2) internal: a fenestrated layer of elastic tissue of the tunica intima. SYN elastic layers of arteries.

epithelial l., the layer of modified ependymal cells that forms the inner layer of the tela choroidea, facing the ventricle.

l. fusca of sclera, an exceedingly delicate layer of loose, pigmented connective tissue on the inner surface of the sclera, connecting it with the choroid.

l. of lens, one of a series of concentric layers composed of the lens fibers that make up the substance of the lens.

l. limitans anterior corneae, SYN anterior elastic l. of cornea.

l. limitans posterior corneae, SYN posterior elastic l. of cornea.

l. of mesencephalic tectum, the roofplate of the mesencephalon formed by the quadrigeminal bodies.

osseous spiral l., a double plate of bone winding spirally around the modiolus dividing the spiral canal of the cochlea incompletely into two, scala tympani and scala vestibuli; between the two plates of this l. the fibers of the cochlear nerve reach the spiral organ (of Corti).

posterior elastic l. of cornea, a delicate hyaline membrane lying between the substantia propria of the cornea and the corneal endothelium. SYN Descemet's membrane, l. limitans posterior corneae.

lamina l., the layer of connective tissue underlying the epithelium of a mucous membrane.

vascular l. of choroid, the outer portion of the choroid of the eye containing the largest blood vessels.

l. of vertebral arch, the flattened posterior portion of the vertebral arch extending between the pedicles and the midline, forming the dorsal wall of the vertebral foramen; the spinous process extends from the midline junction of right and left laminae. SYN l. arcus vertebrae [NA], neurapophysis.

l. viscera′lis [NA], SYN visceral *layer*.

lam·i·na·gram (lam′i-nă-gram). An image made by laminagraphy.

lam·i·na·graph (lam′i-nă-graf). A device for laminagraphy; a laminagram.

lam·i·nag·ra·phy, lami·nog·ra·phy (lam′i-nahg′ră-fē, lam′i-nog-ră-fē). Radiographic technique in which the images of tissues above and below the plane of interest are blurred out by movement of the x-ray tube and film holder, to show a specific area more clearly. SEE ALSO tomography. [lamina + G. *graphē*, a writing]

lam·i·nar (lam′i-nar). **1.** Arranged in plates or laminae. **2.** Relating to any lamina.

lam·i·nec·to·my (lam′i-nek′tō-mē). Excision of a vertebral lamina; commonly used to denote removal of the posterior arch. [L. *lamina*, layer, + G. *ektomē*, excision]

lam·i·ni·tis (lam-i-nī′tis). Inflammation of any lamina.

lami·nog·ra·phy (lam'i-nog-ră-fē). SEE laminagraphy.

lam·i·not·o·my (lam'i-not'ō-me). An operation on one or more vertebral laminae. SYN rachiotomy. [L. *lamina*, layer, + G. *tomē*, incision]

lamp. Illuminating device; source of light. SEE ALSO light.

    annealing l., an alcohol l. with a soot-free flame used in dentistry to drive off the protective NH$_3$ gas coating from the surface of cohesive gold foil.

    heat l., a l. that emits infrared light and produces heat; used to apply topical heat to the skin.

    hollow-cathode l., a l. consisting of a metal cathode and an inert gas that can emit a line spectrum of specific wavelength; used in atomic absorption spectrophotometry.

    slit l., a combination of a microscope and a narrow beam of collimated light, used to examine the eye.

    spirit l., a l., used mainly for heating in laboratory work, in which alcohol is burned.

    Wood's l., an ultraviolet l. with a nickel oxide filter that only passes light with a maximal wavelength of about 3660 Å; used to detect by fluorescence hairs infected with species of *Microsporum*.

lance (lans). **1.** To incise a part, as an abscess or boil. **2.** A lancet. [L. *lancea*, a slender spear]

lan·cet (lan'set). A surgical knife with a short, wide, sharp-pointed, two-edged blade. [Fr. *lancette*]

lan·ci·nat·ing (lan'si-nāt'ing). Denoting a sharp cutting or tearing pain. [L. *lancino*, pp. *-atus*, to tear]

Landau-Kleffner syn·drome. See under syndrome.

language board. SYN communication board.

lan·tha·nides (lan'thă-nīdz). Those elements with atomic numbers 57–71 which closely resemble one another chemically and were once difficult to separate from one another. [*lanthanum*, first element of the series]

lan·tha·num (La) (lan'thă-nŭm). A metallic element, atomic no. 57, atomic wt. 138.9055; first of the rare earth elements (lanthanides). [G. *lanthanō*, to lie hidden]

la·nu·gi·nous (lă-nū'ji-nŭs). Covered with lanugo.

la·nu·go (lă-nū'gō) [NA]. Fine, soft, lightly pigmented fetal hair with minute shafts and large papillae; it appears toward the end of the third month of gestation. SYN lanugo hair. [L. down, wooliness, from *lana*, wool]

LAO left anterior oblique projection, used in chest radiography, especially to assess the size of the left atrium and ventricle.

laparo-. The loins (less properly, the abdomen in general). [G. *lapara*, flank, loins]

lap·a·ro·cele (lap'ă-rō-sēl). SYN abdominal *hernia*. [laparo- + G. *kēlē*, hernia]

lap·a·ror·rha·phy (lap'ă-rōr'ă-fē). SYN celiorrhaphy.

lap·a·ro·scope (lap'ă-rō-skōp). An endoscope for examining the peritoneal cavity. SYN peritoneoscope. [laparo- + G. *skopeō*, to view]

lap·a·ros·co·py (lap'ă-ros'kŏ-pē). Examination of the contents of the peritoneum with a laparoscope. The abdomen is first inflated with carbon dioxide, and the laparoscope passed through a small incision in the abdominal wall. The device is frequently used to view the female reproductive organs, in particular where endometriosis or pelvic inflammatory disease is suspected. Fitted with grasping and cutting tools, the laparoscope can perform minor surgery and take tissue samples for biopsy. SEE ALSO peritoneoscopy.

lap·a·rot·o·my (lap'ă-rot'ō-me). **1.** Incision into the loin. **2.** SYN celiotomy. [laparo- + G. *tomē*, incision]

lap·i·ni·za·tion (lap'i-ni-zā'shŭn). Serial passage of a virus or vaccine in rabbits. [Fr. *lapin*, rabbit]

lap·i·nized (lap'i-nīzd). Denoting viruses which have been adapted to develop in rabbits by serial transfers in this species. [Fr. *lapin*, rabbit]

lard. SYN adeps (2). [L. *lardum*]

lar·va, pl. **lar·vae** (lar'vă, lar'vē). **1.** The worm-like developmental stage or stages of an insect or helminth. **2.** The second stage in the life cycle of a tick; the stage which hatches from the egg and, following engorgement, molts in the nymph. **3.** The young of fishes or amphibians which often differ in appearance from the adult. [L. a mask]

lar·va cur·rens (lar'vă kŭr'enz). Cutaneous larva migrans caused by rapidly moving larvae of *Strongyloides stercoralis* (up to 10 cm/hr), typically extending from the anal area down the upper thighs and observed as a rapidly progressing linear urticarial trail. [L. *larva*, mask + *currens*, racing]

lar·val (lar'văl). **1.** Relating to larvae. **2.** SYN larvate.

lar·va mi·grans (lar'vă mī'granz). A larval worm, typically a nematode, that wanders for a period in the host tissues but does not develop to the adult stage; this usually occurs in abnormal hosts that inhibit normal development of the parasite. [L. *larva*, mask, + *migro*, to transfer, migrate]

    cutaneous l. m., an advancing serpiginous or netlike tunneling in the skin, with marked pruritus, caused by wandering hookworm larvae not adapted to intestinal maturation in man; especially common in the eastern and southern coastal U.S. and other tropical and subtropical coastal areas; various hookworms of dogs and cats have been implicated, chiefly *Ancylostoma braziliense* in the U.S., but also *Ancylostoma caninum* of dogs, *Uncinaria stenocephalia*, the European dog hookworm, and *Bunostomum phlebotomum*, the cattle hookworm; *Strongyloides* species of animal origin may also contribute to human cutaneous l. m.

lar·vate (lar'văt). Masked or concealed; applied to a disease with undeveloped, absent, or atypical symptoms. SYN larval (2). [L. *larva*, mask]

lar·vi·cid·al (lar-vi-sī'dăl). Destructive to larvae.

lar·vi·cide (lar'vi-sīd). An agent that kills larvae. [larva + L. *caedo*, to kill]

laryng-. SEE laryngo-.

la·ryn·ge·al (lă-rin'jē-ăl). Relating in any way to the larynx.

la·ryn·gec·to·my (lar'in-jek'tō-me). Excision of the larynx. [laryngo- + G. *ektomē*, excision]

la·ryn·ges (lă-rin′jēz). Plural of larynx. [L.]

lar·yn·gis·mus (lar-in-jiz′mŭs). A spasmodic narrowing or closure of the rima glottidis. [L. fr. G. *larynx*, + -*ismos*, -ism]

   l. strid′ulus, a spasmodic closure of the glottis, lasting a few seconds, followed by a noisy inspiration. Cf. *laryngitis* stridulosa. SYN pseudocroup.

lar·yn·git·ic (lar-in-jit′ik). Relating to or caused by laryngitis.

lar·yn·gi·tis (lar-in-jī′tis). Inflammation of the mucous membrane of the larynx. [laryngo- + G. -*itis*, inflammation]

   membranous l., a form in which there is a pseudomembranous exudate on the vocal cords.

   l. stridulo′sa, catarrhal inflammation of the larynx in children, accompanied by night attacks of spasmodic closure of the glottis, causing inspiratory stridor.

△**laryngo-, laryng-.** The larynx. [G. *larynx*]

la·ryn·go·cele (lă-ring′gō-sēl). An air sac communicating with the larynx through the ventricle, often bulging outward into the tissue of the neck, especially during coughing. [laryngo- + G. *kēlē*, hernia]

la·ryn·go·fis·sure (lă-ring′gō-fish′er). Operative opening into the larynx, generally through the midline, commonly done for the excision of early carcinoma or the correction of laryngostenosis. SYN thyrotomy (2).

lar·yn·gol·o·gy (lar′ing-gol′ō-jē). The branch of medical science concerned with the larynx; the specialty of diseases of the larynx. [laryngo- + G. *logos*, study]

la·ryn·go·pa·ral·y·sis (lă-ring′gō-pă-ral′i-sis). Paralysis of the laryngeal muscles. SYN laryngoplegia.

la·ryn·go·pha·ryn·ge·al (lă-ring′gō-fă-rin′jē-ăl). Relating to both larynx and pharynx or to the laryngopharynx.

la·ryn·go·phar·yn·gec·to·my (lă-ring′gō-far′in-jek′tō-mē). Resection or excision of both larynx and pharynx.

la·ryn·go·phar·yn·gi·tis (lă-ring′gō-far-in-jī′tis). Inflammation of the larynx and pharynx.

la·ryn·go·phar·ynx (lă-ring′gō-far-ingks). The part of the pharynx lying below the aperture of the larynx and behind the larynx; it extends from the vestibule of the larynx to the esophagus at the level of the inferior border of the cricoid cartilage. SYN hypopharynx.

la·ryn·go·plas·ty (lă-ring′gō-plas-tē). Reparative or plastic surgery of the larynx. [laryngo- + G. *plassō*, to form]

la·ryn·go·ple·gia (lă-ring′gō-plē′jē-ă). SYN laryngoparalysis. [laryngo- + G. *plēgē*, stroke]

la·ryn·go·pto·sis (lă-ring′gō-tō′sis). An abnormally low position of the larynx at birth; does not impair the health of the neonate. Some degree of l. occurs with aging. [laryngo- + G. *ptōsis*, a falling]

la·ryn·go·scope (lă-ring′gō-skōp). Any of several types of hollow tubes, equipped with electrical lighting, used in examining or operating upon the interior of the larynx through the mouth. [laryngo- + G. *skopeō*, to inspect]

la·ryn·go·scop·ic (lă-ring′gō-skop′ik). Relating to laryngoscopy.

lar·yn·gos·co·py (lar′ing-gos′kŏ-pē). Inspection of the larynx by means of the laryngoscope.

   direct l., inspection of the larynx by means of either a rigid, hollow instrument or a fiberoptic cable.

   indirect l., inspection of the larynx by means of a reflected image on a mirror.

la·ryn·go·spasm (lă-ring′gō-spazm). Spasmodic closure of the glottic aperture.

la·ryn·go·ste·no·sis (lă-ring′gō-stĕ-nō′sis). Stricture or narrowing of the lumen of the larynx. [laryngo- + G. *stenōsis*, a narrowing]

lar·yn·gos·to·my (lar′ing-gos′tō-mē). The establishment of a permanent opening from the neck into the larynx. [laryngo- + G. *stoma*, mouth]

lar·yn·got·o·my (lar-ing-got′ō-mē). A surgical incision of the larynx. [laryngo- + G. *tomē*, incision]

la·ryn·go·tra·che·al (lă-ring′gō-trā′kē-ăl). Relating to both larynx and trachea.

la·ryn·go·tra·che·i·tis (lă-ring′gō-trā-kē-ī′tis). Inflammation of both larynx and trachea.

la·ryn·go·tra·che·o·bron·chi·tis (lă-ring′gō-trā-kē-ō-brong-kī′tis). An acute respiratory infection involving the larynx, trachea, and bronchi. SEE croup.

lar·ynx, pl. **la·ryn·ges** (lar′ingks, lă-rin′jēz) [NA]. The organ of voice production; the part of the respiratory tract between the pharynx and the trachea; it consists of a framework of cartilages and elastic membranes housing the vocal folds and the muscles which control the position and tension of these elements. [Mod. L. fr. G.]

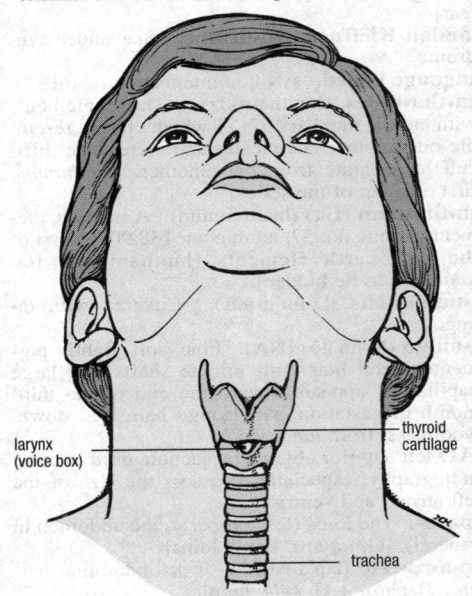

larynx (voice box)

thyroid cartilage

trachea

larynx

artificial l., mechanical device used to create alaryngeal speech. The most common types are battery powered and provide a buzzing sound source; the vibrating source is placed against the neck or in the oral cavity via a tube, and speech is articulated normally. Pneumatic assistive listening devices use expired air from the trachea to create vibration, which is relayed to the oral cavity by a tube. SYN electrolarynx.

lase (lāz). To cut, divide, or dissolve a substance, or to treat an anatomical structure, with a laser beam.

la·ser (lā′zer). 1. (noun) A device that concentrates high energies into an intense narrow beam of nondivergent monochromatic electromagnetic radiation; used in microsurgery, cauterization, and for a variety of diagnostic purposes. 2. (verb) To treat a structure with a laser beam. [acronym coined from *l*ight *a*mplification by *s*timulated *e*mission of *r*adiation]

las·si·tude (las′i-tūd). A sense of weariness. [L. *lassitudo,* fr. *lassus,* weary]

la·tah (lah′tah). One of the pathological startle syndromes. A culture-bound disorder characterized by an exaggerated physical response to being startled or to unexpected suggestion, the subjects involuntarily uttering cries or executing movements in response to command or in imitation of what they hear or see in others. SEE ALSO jumping *disease*. [Malay, ticklish]

la·ten·cy (lā′ten-sē). 1. The state of being latent. 2. In conditioning, or other behavioral experiments, the period of apparent inactivity between the time the stimulus is presented and the moment a response occurs. 3. PSYCHOANALYSIS The period of time from approximately age five to puberty.

la·tent (lā′tent). Not manifest, dormant, but potentially discernible. [L. *lateo,* pres. p. *latens* (-*ent*-), to lie hidden]

lat·er·ad (lat′er-ad). Toward the side. [L. *latus,* side, + *ad,* to]

lat·er·al (lat′er-ăl). 1. On the side. 2. Farther from the median or midsagittal plane. 3. DENTISTRY A position either right or left of the midsagittal plane. 4. A radiographic projection made with the film in the sagittal plane; especially, the second view of a chest series. [L. *lateralis,* lateral, fr. *latus,* side]

lat·er·al·i·ty (lat-er-al′i-tē). Referring to a side of the body or of a structure; specifically, the dominance of one side of the brain or the body.

latero-. Lateral, to one side. [L. *lateralis,* lateral, fr. *latus,* side]

lat·er·o·de·vi·a·tion (lat′er-ō-dē-vē-ā′shŭn). A bending or a displacement to one side. [latero- + L. *devio,* to turn aside, fr. *via,* a way]

lat·er·o·duc·tion (lat′er-ō-dŭk′shŭn). A drawing to one side; denoting a movement of a limb or turning of the eyeball away form the midline. [latero- + L. *duco,* pp. *ductus,* to lead]

lat·er·o·flex·ion, lat·er·o·flec·tion (lat′er-ō-flek′shŭn). A bending or curvature to one side. [latero- + L. *flecto,* pp. *flexus,* to bend]

lat·er·o·tor·sion (lat′er-ō-tōr′shŭn). A twisting to one side; denoting rotation of the eyeball around its anteroposterior axis, so that the top part of the cornea turns away from the sagittal plane. [latero- + L. *torsio,* a twisting]

lat·er·o·tru·sion (lat′er-ō-trū′zhŭn). The out-

ward thrust given by the muscles of mastication to the rotating mandibular condyle during movement of the mandible. [latero- + L. *trudo,* pp. *trusus,* to thrust]

lat·er·o·ver·sion (lat′er-ō-ver′zhŭn). Version to one side or the other, denoting especially a malposition of the uterus. [latero- + L. *verto,* pp. *versus,* to turn]

la·tex (lā′teks). 1. An emulsion or suspension produced by some seed plants; it contains suspended microscopic globules of natural rubber. 2. Similar synthetic materials such as polystyrene, polyvinyl chloride, etc. [L. liquid]

lath·y·rism (lath′i-rizm). A disease occurring in Ethiopia, Algeria, and India, characterized by various nervous manifestations, tremors, spastic paraplegia, and paresthesias; prevalent in districts where vetches, khasari (*Lathyrus sativus*), and allied species form the main food. [L. *lathyrus,* vetch]

lat·i·tude (la′ti-tūd). The range of light or x-ray exposure acceptable with a given photographic emulsion. [L. *latitudo,* width, fr. *latus,* wide]

La·tro·dec·tus (lat-rō-dek′tŭs). A genus of relatively small spiders, the widow spiders, capable of inflicting highly poisonous, neurotoxic, painful bites. [L. *latro,* servant, robber, + G. *dēktēs,* a biter]

LATS long-acting thyroid *stimulator.*

la·tus, gen. **la·te·ris,** pl. **la·te·ra** (lā′tŭs, lat′er-is, lat′er-ă). The side of the body between the pelvis and the ribs. SYN flank. [L. broad]

LAV lymphadenopathy-associated *virus.*

la·vage (lă-vahzh′). The washing out of a hollow cavity or organ by copious injections and rejections of fluid. [Fr. from L. *lavo,* to wash]

bronchoalveolar l., a procedure performed via fiberoptic bronchoscopy, during which a distal airway is occluded and liquid is then introduced into the airway and recovered for examination of cell types and microorganisms.

law. 1. A principle or rule. 2. A statement of a sequence or relation of phenomena that is invariable under the given conditions. SEE ALSO principle, rule, theorem. [A.S. *lagu*]

all or none l., SYN Bowditch's l.

Beer's l., the intensity of a color or of a light ray is inversely proportional to the depth of liquid through which it is transmitted; it is concluded that the absorption is dependent upon the number of molecules in the path of the ray.

Behring's l., parenteral administration of serum from an immunized person provides a relative, passive immunity to that disease (*i.e.,* prevents it, or favorably modifies its course) in a previously susceptible person.

Bell's l., the ventral spinal roots are motor, the dorsal are sensory.

Bernoulli's l., when friction is negligible, the velocity of flow of a gas or fluid through a tube is inversely related to its pressure against the side of the tube; *i.e.,* velocity is greatest and pressure lowest at a point of constriction.

Bowditch's l., consistently total response to any effective stimulus. SYN all or none l.

Boyle's l., at constant temperature the volume

of a given quantity of gas varies inversely with its absolute pressure.

Charles l., all gases expand equally on heating, namely, $\frac{1}{273.16}$ of their volume at 0°C for every degree Celsius.

l. of contiguity, when two ideas or psychologically perceived events have once occurred in close association they are likely to so occur again, the subsequent occurrence of one tending to elicit the other; this l. figures prominently in modern theories of conditioning and learning.

Dalton's l., each gas in a mixture of gases exerts a pressure proportionate to the percentage of the gas and independent of the presence of the other gases present. SYN l. of partial pressures.

Donders' l., the rotation of the eyeball is determined by the distance of the object from the median plane and the line of the horizon.

Einthoven's l., in the electrocardiogram the potential of any wave or complex in lead II is equal to the sum of the potentials of leads I and III.

l. of excitation, a motor nerve responds, not to the absolute value, but to the alteration of value from moment to moment, of the electric current; *i.e.,* rate of change of intensity of the current is a factor in determining its effectiveness.

Fechner-Weber l., SYN Weber-Fechner l.

Graham's l., the relative rapidity of diffusion of two gases varies inversely as the square root of their densities, *i.e.,* their molecular weights.

Hamburger's l., albumins and phosphates pass from red corpuscles to serum and chlorides pass from serum to cells when blood is acid; the reverse occurs when blood is alkaline.

Hardy-Weinberg l., if mating occurs at random with respect to any one autosomal locus in a population in which the gene frequencies are equal in the two sexes, and the factors tending to change gene frequencies (mutation, differential selection, migration) are either absent or negligible, then in one generation the probabilities of all possible genotypes will on average equal the same proportions as if the genes were assembled at random. The l. does not apply to two or more loci jointly, nor to X-linked traits where the initial gene frequencies differ in the two sexes.

l. of the heart, the energy liberated by the heart when it contracts is a function of the length of its muscle fibers at the end of diastole. SYN Starling's l.

Hellin's l., twins occur once in 89 births, triplets once in 89^2, and quadruplets once in 89^3.

Henry's l., at equilibrium, at a given temperature, the amount of gas dissolved in a given volume of liquid is directly proportional to the partial pressure of that gas in the gas phase (this only holds for gases that do not react chemically with the solvent).

Hilton's l., the nerve supplying a joint supplies also the muscles which move the joint and the skin covering the articular insertion of those muscles.

Hooke's l., the stress applied to stretch or compress a body is proportional to the strain, or change in length thus produced, so long as the limit of elasticity of the body is not exceeded.

l. of independent assortment, different hereditary factors assort independently when the gametes are formed; traits at linked loci are an exception.

Listing's l., when the eye leaves one object and fixes upon another, it revolves about an axis perpendicular to a plane cutting both the former and the present lines of vision.

Nasse's l., an early statement of the pattern of X-linked recessive inheritance: hemophilia affects only boys but is transmitted through mothers and sisters.

Nysten's l., rigor mortis affects first the muscles of the head and spreads toward the feet.

l. of partial pressures, SYN Dalton's l.

Pascal's l., fluids at rest transmit pressure equally in every direction.

Poiseuille's l., in laminar flow, the volume of a homogeneous fluid passing per unit time through a capillary tube is directly proportional to the pressure difference between its ends and to the fourth power of its internal radius, and inversely proportional to its length and to the viscosity of the fluid.

Raoult's l., the vapor pressure of a solution of a nonvolatile nonelectrolyte is that of the pure solvent multiplied by the mole-fraction of the solvent in the solution.

l. of recapitulation, SYN recapitulation *theory.*

l. of referred pain, pain arises only from irritation of nerves which are sensitive to those stimuli that produce pain when applied to the surface of the body.

l. of segregation, factors that affect development retain their individuality from generation to generation, do not become contaminated when mixed in a hybrid, and become sorted out from one another when the next generation of gametes is formed.

l. of similars, SEE similia similibus curantur.

Starling's l., SYN l. of the heart.

Weber-Fechner l., the intensity of a sensation varies by a series of equal increments (arithmetically) as the strength of the stimulus is increased geometrically; if a series of stimuli is applied and so adjusted in strength that each stimulus causes a just perceptible change in intensity of the sensation, then the strength of each stimulus differs from the preceding one by a constant fraction. SYN Fechner-Weber l.

Wolff's l., every change in the form and the function of a bone, or in its function alone, is followed by certain definite changes in its internal architecture and secondary alterations in its external conformation.

law·ren·ci·um (Lr) (law-ren′sē-ŭm). An artificial transplutonium element; atomic no. 103; atomic wt. 262.11. [E.O. *Lawrence,* U.S. physicist and Nobel laureate, 1901–1958]

lax·a·tive (lak′să-tiv). **1.** Mildly cathartic; having the action of loosening the bowels. **2.** A mild cathartic; a remedy that moves the bowels slightly without pain or violent action. [L. *laxativus,* fr. *laxo,* pp. *-atus,* to slacken, relax]

lax·i·ty (lăks′ĭ-tē). Looseness or freedom of movement in a joint, normal or excessive. SEE ALSO instability. [L. *laxitas,* looseness]

valgus l., abnormal flexibility on the medial side of a joint upon lateral movement of the distal segment.

varus l., abnormal flexibility on the lateral side of a joint upon medial movement of the distal segment.

lay•er (lā′er). A sheet of one substance lying on another and distinguished from it by a difference in texture or color or by not being continuous with it. SEE ALSO stratum, lamina.

ameloblastic l., the internal l. of the enamel organ. SYN enamel l.

anterior limiting l. of cornea, a transparent homogeneous acellular layer, 6 to 9 μm thick, lying between the basal l. of the outer layer of stratified epithelium and the substantia propria of the cornea; considered to be a basement membrane.

bacillary l., SYN l. of rods and cones.

basal l., SYN *stratum* basale (1).

basal l. of choroid, SYN *lamina* basalis choroideae.

choriocapillary l., the internal layer of the choroidea of the eye, composed of a very close capillary network. SYN lamina choroidocapillaris [NA], choriocapillaris, entochoroidea, Ruysch's membrane.

clear l. of epidermis, SYN *stratum* lucidum.

corneal l., SYN *stratum* corneum epidermidis.

elastic l.'s of arteries, SYN elastic *laminae* of arteries, under *lamina*.

enamel l., SYN ameloblastic l.

germ l., one of the three primordial cell l.'s (ectoderm, endoderm, mesoderm) established in an embryo during gastrulation and the immediately following stages.

half-value l. (HVL), the thickness of a specific absorber (*e.g.,* aluminum), that will reduce the intensity of a beam of radiation to one-half its initial value. SEE ALSO filter.

horny l., SYN *stratum* corneum epidermidis.

molecular l. of cerebellum, the outer lamina of the cortex, containing the cell bodies and dendrites of Purkinje cells, the axons of the granule cells, and the cell bodies, dendrites, and axons of basket cells.

odontoblastic l., a l. of connective tissue cells at the periphery of the dental pulp of the tooth.

osteogenetic l., the inner bone-forming l. of the periosteum.

piriform neuron l., the layer of Purkinje cells between the molecular and granular layers of the cerebellar cortex.

posterior limiting l. of cornea, a transparent homogeneous acellular layer between the substantia propria and the endothelial layer of the cornea; considered to be a highly developed basement membrane. SYN membrana vitrea [NA], vitreous membrane (1).

prickle cell l., SYN *stratum* spinosum epidermidis.

l. of rods and cones, the l. of the retina next to the pigment l. and containing the visual receptors. SEE ALSO retina. SYN bacillary l.

spinous l., SYN *stratum* spinosum epidermidis.

still l., the l. of the bloodstream in the capillary vessels, next to the wall of the vessel, that flows slowly and transports the white blood cells along the l. wall, while in the center the flow is rapid and transports the red blood cells. SYN Poiseuille's space.

subendocardial l., the loose connective tissue l. that joins the endocardium and myocardium; in the ventricles, it contains branches of the conducting system of the heart.

subendothelial l., the thin l. of connective tissue lying between the endothelium and elastic lamina in the intima of blood vessels.

visceral l., the inner l. of an enveloping sac or bursa which lines the outer surface of the enveloped structure, as opposed to the parietal layer which lines the walls of the occupied space or cavity. The visceral l. is usually thin, delicate and not apparent as being separate, but rather appears to be the outer surface of the structure itself. SYN lamina visceralis [NA].

visceral l. of serous pericardium, the inner part of the serous pericardium applied directly on the heart.

LDH *lactate* dehydrogenase.

LDL low density lipoprotein. See lipoprotein.

LE, L.E. left eye; *lupus* erythematosus.

leach•ing (lēch′ing). Removal of the soluble constituents of a substance by running water through it. SYN lixiviation. [A.S. *leccan,* to wet]

lead (lēd). **1.** An electrical conductor carrying current or intermittent signals between an organ or tissue and an electrical or electronic device. **2.** The tracing obtained from a particular combination of electrode positions.

bipolar l., a record obtained with two electrodes placed on different regions of the body, each electrode contributing significantly to the record; *e.g.,* a standard limb l.

chest l.'s, those in which the exploring electrode is on the chest overlying the heart or its vicinity. SYN precordial l.'s.

esophageal l., an electrocardiographic l. passed down the throat into the esophagus to record the electrocardiogram at various levels of the esophagus; especially useful for certain types of arrhythmias. Similarly, a transducer for echocardiography can be passed into the esophagus.

limb l., one of the three standard l.'s (l.'s I, II, III) or one of the unipolar limb l.'s (aVR, aVL, aVF).

pacemaker l., a wire transmitting impulses from an artificial pacemaker to the heart.

precordial l.'s, SYN chest l.'s.

unipolar l.'s, those in which the exploring electrode is on the chest in the vicinity of the heart or on one of the limbs, while the other or indifferent electrode is the central terminal.

lead (Pb) (led). A metallic element, atomic no. 82, atomic wt. 207.2; occurs in nature as an oxide or one of the salts, but chiefly as the sulfide, or galena; ^{210}Pb (half-life equal to 22.6 years) has been used in the treatment of certain eye conditions. SYN plumbum.

learned help•less•ness. A laboratory model of depression involving both classical (respondent) and instrumental (operant) conditioning techniques; application of unavoidable shock is fol-

le

lowed by failure to cope in situations where coping might otherwise be possible.

learn·ing (lern'ing). Generic term for the relatively permanent change in behavior that occurs as a result of practice. SEE ALSO conditioning, memory.

 latent l., that l. which is not evident to the observer at the time it occurs, but which is inferred from later performance in which l. is more rapid than would be expected without the earlier experience.

 rote l., the l. of arbitrary relationships, usually by repetition of the l. procedure through memorization and without an understanding of the relationships.

 state-dependent l., l. during a specific state of sleep or wakefulness, or during a chemically altered state, where retrieval of learned information cannot be demonstrated unless the subject is restored to the state that originally existed during l.

lec·i·thal (les'i-thăl). Having a yolk or pertaining to the yolk of any egg; used especially as a suffix. [G. *lekithos,* egg yolk]

lec·i·thin (les'i-thin). Traditional term for phospholipids that on hydrolysis yield two fatty acid molecules and a molecule each of glycerophosphoric acid and choline. L.'s are found in nervous tissue, especially in the myelin sheaths, in egg yolk, and as essential constituents of animal and vegetable cells. [G. *lekithos,* egg yolk]

lec·i·thi·nase (les'i-thi-nās). SYN phospholipase.

lec·i·tho·blast (les'i-thō-blast). One of the cells proliferating to form the yolk-sac endoderm. [G. *lekithos,* egg yolk, + *blastos,* germ]

lec·tin (lek'tin). A protein of primarily plant (usually seed) origin that binds to glycoproteins on the surface of cells causing agglutination, precipitation, or other phenomena resembling the action of specific antibody; l.'s include plant agglutinins (phytoagglutinins, phytohemagglutinins), plant precipitins, and perhaps certain animal proteins; some have mitogenic properties. [L. *lego,* pp. *lectum,* to select, + -in]

ledge (lej). In anatomy, a structure resembling a ledge. SEE ALSO lamina.

 dental l., a band of ectodermal cells growing from the epithelium of the embryonic jaws into the underlying mesenchyme; local buds from the l. give rise to the primordia of the enamel organs of the teeth.

leech (lēch). **1.** A bloodsucking aquatic annelid worm (genus *Hirudo*) formerly used in medicine for local withdrawal of blood. **2.** To treat medically by applying leeches. [A.S. *laece,* a physician; a leech, because of its therapeutic use]

LEEP loop electrocautery excision *procedure.*

left-foot·ed. SYN sinistropedal.

left-hand·ed. Denoting the habitual or more skillful use of the left hand for writing and for most manual operations. SYN sinistromanual.

leg. 1. The segment of the inferior limb between the knee and the ankle; commonly used to mean the entire inferior limb. **2.** A structure resembling a leg. SYN crus (1) [NA].

 bow-l., SEE *genu* varum.

△**-legia.** Reading, as distinguished from the G.

derivatives, *-lexis* and *-lexy,* which signify speech, from G. *legō,* to say. [L. *lego,* to read]

Le·gion·el·la (lē-jŭ-nel'lă). A genus of aerobic, motile, non-acid-fast, non-encapsulated, Gram-negative bacilli; they are water-dwelling and airborne-spread, and are pathogenic for humans. The type species is *L. pneumophila.*

 L. bozeman'ii, a species that causes human pneumonia.

 L. micda'dei, a species that causes Pittsburgh pneumonia, a variant of Legionnaires' disease. Accounts for approximately 60% of *Legionella* pneumonias other than those caused by *L. pneumophila.* SYN Pittsburgh pneumonia agent.

△**leio-.** Smooth. [G. *leios*]

lei·o·der·mia (lī-ō-der'mē-ă). Smooth, glossy skin. [leio- + G. *derma,* skin]

lei·o·my·o·fi·bro·ma (lī-ō-mī'ō-fī-brō'mă). SYN fibroleiomyoma.

lei·o·my·o·ma (lī'ō-mī-ō'mă). A benign neoplasm derived from smooth (nonstriated) muscle. [leio- + G. *mys,* muscle, + -*oma,* tumor]

 l. cu'tis, cutaneous eruption of multiple small painful nodules composed of smooth muscle fibers; derived from arrector muscles of hair. SYN dermatomyoma.

 vascular l., a markedly vascular l., apparently arising from the smooth muscle of blood vessels.

lei·o·my·o·sar·co·ma (lī'ō-mī'ō-sar-kō'mă). A malignant neoplasm derived from smooth (nonstriated) muscle. [leio- + myosarcoma]

Leish·man·ia (lēsh-man'ē-ă). A genus of digenetic, asexual, protozoan flagellates that occur as amastigotes in the macrophages of vertebrate hosts, and as promastigotes in invertebrate hosts and in cultures. [W. B. *Leishman*]

leish·man·i·a·sis (lēsh'mă-nī'ă-sis). Infection with a species of *Leishmania* resulting in a group of diseases traditionally divided into four major types: 1) visceral l. (kala azar); 2) Old World cutaneous l.; 3) New World cutaneous l.; 4) mucocutaneous l. SEE tropical *diseases,* under *disease.*

 American l., SYN mucocutaneous l.

 cutaneous l., infection with promastigotes (leptomonads) of *Leishmania tropica* and of *L. major* inoculated into the skin by the bite of an infected sandfly, *Phlebotomus* (commonly *P. papatasi*); it is endemic in parts of Asia Minor, northern Africa, and India. The ulcer begins as a papule that enlarges to a nodule and then breaks down into an ulcer. Two distinctive clinical and epidemiological diseases are recognized, the more common and widespread zoonotic rural disease with a moist acute form, caused by *L. major,* with reservoir rodent hosts; and an urban, anthroponotic, dry, chronic form of l. caused by *L. tropica,* without a reservoir host, and now largely controlled. SEE zoonotic cutaneous l. SYN Old World l., tropical sore.

 diffuse cutaneous l., l. caused by several New and Old World species and strains of *Leishmania.* The condition is associated with a suppressed cell-mediated immune response.

 mucocutaneous l., a grave disease caused by *Leishmania braziliensis braziliensis,* endemic in Mexico and Central and South America. The organism does not invade the viscera, and the disease is limited to the skin and mucous membranes, the lesions resembling the sores of cutaneous l. The sores heal after a time, but some months or years later, fungating and eroding forms of ulceration may appear on the tongue and buccal or nasal mucosa. SEE ALSO espundia. SYN American l., nasopharyngeal l., New World l.

nasopharyngeal l., SYN mucocutaneous l.

New World l., SYN mucocutaneous l.

Old World l., SYN cutaneous l.

visceral l., a chronic disease of the tropics caused by *Leishmania donovani* and transmitted by the bite of a species of sandfly of the genus *Phlebotomus* or *Lutzomyia;* the organisms grow and multiply in macrophages, eventually causing them to burst and liberate amastigote parasites which then invade other macrophages; proliferation of macrophages in the bone marrow causes crowding out of erythroid and myeloid elements, resulting in leukopenia, and anemia, splenomegaly, and hepatomegaly which are characteristic, along with enlargement of lymph nodes; fever, fatigue, malaise, and secondary infections also occur. SYN kala azar.

zoonotic cutaneous l., a form of cutaneous l. characterized by rural distribution of human cases near infected rodents, particularly communal ground squirrels; characterized by rapidly developing dermal lesions that become severely inflamed, with moist necrotizing sores or ulcers that heal in two to eight months (after a two- to four-month incubation period).

lem·mo·blast (lem′ō-blast). In an embryo, a cell of neural crest origin capable of forming a cell of the neurilemma sheath. [G. *lemma,* husk, + *blastos,* germ]

lem·mo·cyte (lem′ō-sīt). One of the cells of the neurolemma. [G. *lemma,* husk, + *kytos,* cell]

lem·nis·cus, pl. **lem·nis·ci** (lem-nis′kŭs, -nis′ī) [NA]. A bundle of nerve fibers ascending from sensory relay nuclei to the thalamus. SYN fillet (1). [L. from G. *lēmniskos,* ribbon or fillet]

length. Linear distance between two points.

crown-heel l., l. of an outstretched embryo or fetus from skull vertex to heel.

crown-rump l. (CR, CRL), a measurement from the skull vertex to the midpoint between the apices of the buttocks of an embryo or fetus, that permits approximation of embryonic or fetal age.

lens (lenz). **1.** A transparent material with one or both surfaces having a concave or convex curve; acts upon electromagnetic energy to cause convergence or divergence of light rays. **2** [NA]. The transparent biconvex cellular refractive structure lying between the iris and the vitreous humor, consisting of a soft outer part (cortex) with a denser part (nucleus), and surrounded by a basement membrane (capsule); the anterior surface has a cuboidal epithelium, and at the equator the cells elongate to become lens fibers. [L. a lentil]

achromatic l., a compound l. made of two or more l.'s having different indices of refraction, so correlated as to minimize chromatic aberration.

aplanatic l., a l. designed to correct spherical aberration and coma (*q.v.*).

astigmatic l., SYN cylindrical l.

biconcave l., a l. that is concave on two opposing surfaces. SYN concavoconcave l.

biconvex l., a l. with both surfaces convex. SYN convexoconvex l.

bifocal l., a l. used in cases of presbyopia, in which one portion is suited for distant vision, the other for reading and close work in general.

concave l., a diverging minus power lens.

concavoconcave l., SYN biconcave l.

concavoconvex l., a converging meniscus l. that is concave on one surface and convex on the opposite surface.

contact l., a l. that fits over the cornea and sclera or cornea only; used to correct refractive errors.

convex l., a converging l.

convexoconcave l., a minus power l. having one surface convex and the opposite surface concave, with the latter having the greater curvature.

convexoconvex l., SYN biconvex l.

cylindrical l. (C), a l. in which one of the surfaces is curved in one meridian and less curved in the opposite meridian; commonly used to correct the visual distortion resulting from astigmatism. SYN astigmatic l.

meniscus l., a l. having a spherical concave curve on one side and a spherical convex curve on the other. SYN meniscus (1).

multifocal l., a l. with segments providing two or more powers; commonly, a trifocal l.

omnifocal l., a l. for near and distant vision in which the reading portion is a continuously variable curve.

photochromic l., a light-sensitive spectacle l. that reduces light transmission in sunlight and increases transmission in reduced light.

planoconcave l., a l. that is flat on one side and concave on the other.

planoconvex l., a l. that is flat on one side and convex on the other.

safety l., a l. that meets government specifications of impact resistance; the increased impact resistance required for safety l.'s is obtained by tempering, by an ion-exchange process, or by using laminated or plastic lenses.

spherical l. (S), a l. in which all refracting surfaces are spherical; commonly used to correct refractive errors not compounded by astigmatism.

trial l.'s, a series of cylindrical and spherical l.'s used in testing vision.

trifocal l., a l. with segments of three focal powers: distant, intermediate, and near.

lens·ec·to·my (len-zek′tō-mē). Removal of the lens of the eye by an infusion-aspiration cutter; often done by puncture incision through the pars plana in the course of vitrectomy. [lens + G. *ektomē,* excision]

len·ti·co·nus (len-ti-kō′nŭs). Conical projection of the anterior or posterior surface of the lens of the eye, occurring as a developmental anomaly. [lens + L. *conus,* cone]

len·tic·u·lar (len-tik′yū′lăr). **1.** Relating to or resembling a lens of any kind. **2.** Of the shape of a lentil. [L. *lenticula,* a lentil]

len·tic·u·lo·pap·u·lar (len-tik′yū-lō-pap′yū-lăr). Indicating an eruption with dome-shaped or lens-shaped papules.

le

len·ti·form (len′ti-fōrm). Lens-shaped.

len·tig·i·no·sis (len-tij-i-nō′sis). Presence of lentigenes in very large numbers or in a distinctive configuration.

   generalized l., lentigines occurring singly or in groups from infancy onward.

len·ti·glo·bus (len-ti-glō′bŭs). Rare congenital anomaly with a spheroid elevation on the posterior surface of the lens of the eye. [lens + L. *globus,* sphere]

len·ti·go, pl. **len·tig·i·nes** (len-tī′gō, len-tij′i-nēz). A brown macule resembling a freckle except that the border is usually regular, and microscopic proliferation of rete ridges is present; scattered melanocytes are seen in the basal cell layer. SEE ALSO junction *nevus.* [L. fr. *lens* (*lent*-), a lentil]

   l. maligna, a brown or black mottled, irregularly outlined, slowly enlarging lesion resembling a l. in which there are increased numbers of scattered atypical melanocytes in the epidermis, usually occurring on the face of older persons; after many years the dermis may be invaded and the lesion is then termed l. maligna melanoma.

   senile l., a variably pigmented l. occurring on exposed skin of older Caucasians. SYN liver spot.

le·on·ti·a·sis (lē-on-tī′ă-sis). The ridges and furrows on the forehead and cheeks of patients with advanced lepromatous leprosy, giving a leonine appearance. SYN leonine facies. [G. *leōn* (*leont*-), lion]

lep·er (lep′er). A person who has leprosy. [G. *lepra*]

le·pid·ic (lĕ-pid′ik). Relating to scales or a scaly covering layer. [G. *lepis* (*lepid*-), scale, rind]

lep·o·thrix (lep′ō-thriks). SYN *trichomycosis* axillaris. [G. *lepos,* rind, husk, + *thrix,* hair]

lep·re·chaun·ism (lep′rĕ-kawn-izm) [MIM* 246200]. Congenital dwarfism characterized by extreme growth retardation, endocrine disorders, and emaciation, with elfin facies and large lowset ears. [Irish *leprechaun,* elf]

lep·rid. Early cutaneous lesion of leprosy. [G. *lepra,* leprosy, + *-id* (1)]

le·pro·ma (lĕ-prō′mă). A discrete focus of granulomatous inflammation, caused by *Mycobacterium leprae.* [G. *lepros,* scaly, + *-oma,* tumor]

lep·rom·a·tous (lep-rō′mă-tŭs). Pertaining to, or characterized by, the features of a leproma.

lep·ro·min (lep′rō-min). An extract of tissue infected with *Mycobacterium leprae* used in skin tests to classify the stage of leprosy. SEE ALSO test.

lep·ro·sar·i·um (lep′rō-sar′ē-ŭm). A hospital especially designed for the care of those suffering from leprosy, especially those who need expert care.

lep·ro·stat·ic (lep-rō-stat′ik). **1.** Inhibiting to the growth of *Mycobacterium leprae.* **2.** An agent having this action.

lep·ro·sy (lep′rō-sē). **1.** A name used in the Bible to describe various cutaneous diseases, especially those of a chronic or contagious nature, which probably included psoriasis and leukoderma. **2.** SYN Hansen's *disease.* [G. *lepra,* from *lepros,* scaly]

   anesthetic l., a form of l. chiefly affecting the nerves, marked by hyperesthesia succeeded by anesthesia, and by paralysis, ulceration, and various trophic disturbances, terminating in gangrene and mutilation. SYN trophoneurotic l.

   histoid l., a form of lepromatous l. with lesions microscopically resembling dermatofibromas or other spindle-celled tumors.

   lepromatous l., a form of l. in which nodular cutaneous lesions are infiltrated, have ill-defined borders, and are bacteriologically positive.

   macular l., a form of tuberculoid l. in which the lesions are small, hairless, and dry, and are erythematous in light skin and hypopigmented or copper-colored in dark skin.

   nodular l., SYN tuberculoid l.

   trophoneurotic l., SYN anesthetic l.

   tuberculoid l., a benign, stable, and resistant form of the disease in which the lepromin reaction is strongly positive and in which the lesions are erythematous, insensitive, infiltrated plaques with clear-cut edges. SYN nodular l.

△-lepsis, -lepsy. A seizure. [G. *lēpsis*]

△lepto-. Light, thin, frail. [G. *leptos,* slender, delicate, weak]

lep·to·ceph·a·lous (lep-tō-sef′ă-lŭs). Having an abnormally tall, narrow cranium. [lepto- + G. *kephalē,* head]

lep·to·ceph·a·ly (lep-tō-sef′ă-lē). A malformation characterized by an abnormally tall, narrow cranium. [lepto- + G. *kephalē,* head]

lep·to·cyte (lep′tō-sīt). SYN target *cell.* [lepto- + G. *kytos,* cell]

lep·to·cy·to·sis (lep′tō-sī-tō′sis). The presence of leptocytes in the circulating blood, as seen in thalassemia and after splenectomy.

lep·to·dac·ty·lous (lep-tō-dak′ti-lŭs). Having slender fingers. [lepto- + G. *daktylos,* finger]

lep·to·me·nin·ge·al (lep′tō-me-nin′jē-ăl). Pertaining to the leptomeninges.

lep·to·me·nin·ges, sing. **lep·to·me·ninx** (lep-tō-me-nin′jēz, lep′tō-mē′ninks). The two delicate layers of the meninges, the arachnoid mater and pia mater considered together. SEE ALSO arachnoid, pia mater. SYN pia-arachnoid, piarachnoid. [lepto- + G. *mēninx,* pl. *mēninges,* membrane]

lep·to·men·in·gi·tis (lep′tō-men-in-jī′tis). Inflammation of leptomeninges. SEE ALSO arachnoiditis. SYN pia-arachnitis.

lep·to·so·mat·ic, lep·to·som·ic (lep′tō-sō-mat′ik, -tō-sō′mik). Having a slender, light, or thin body. [lepto- + G. *sōma,* body]

Lep·to·spi·ra (lep′tō-spī′ră). A genus of aerobic bacteria containing thin, tightly coiled organisms 6 to 20 μm in length. Associated with icterohemorrhagic fever. [lepto- + G. *speira,* a coil]

lep·to·spi·ro·sis (lep′tō-spī-rō′sis). Infection with *Leptospira interrogans.*

lep·to·spi·ru·ria (lep′tō-spī-rū′rē-ă). Presence of species of the genus *Leptospira* in the urine, as a result of leptospirosis in the renal tubules.

lep·to·tene (lep′tō-tēn). Early stage of prophase in meiosis in which the chromosomes contract and become visible as long filaments well separated from each other. [lepto- + G. *tainia,* band, tape]

Lep·to·trich·ia (lep-tō-trik′ē-ă). A genus of anaerobic, nonmotile bacteria containing Gram-negative, straight or slightly curved rods, with one or both ends rounded or pointed. These organisms occur in the oral cavity of humans. The type species is *L. buccalis.* [lepto- + G. *thrix,* hair]

Lep·to·trom·bid·i·um (lep′tō-trom-bid′ē-ŭm). An important genus of trombiculid mites, which includes all of the vectors of scrub typhus (tsutsugamushi disease).

    L. akamu′shi, one of two species, the other being *L. deliensis* (*T. deliensis*), implicated in the transmission of *Rickettsia tsutsugamushi,* agent of tsutsugamushi disease in the Orient.

LES lower esophageal *sphincter.*

les·bi·an (lez′bē-ăn). **1.** A female homosexual or a female homosexual lifestyle. **2.** One who practices lesbianism. SEE ALSO gay.

les·bi·an·ism (lez′bē-ăn-izm). Homosexuality between women. SYN sapphism. [G. *lesbios,* relating to the island of Lesbos]

le·sion (lē′zhŭn). **1.** A wound or injury. **2.** A pathologic change in the tissues. **3.** One of the individual points or patches of a multifocal disease. [L. *laedo,* pp. *laesus,* to injure]

    Bankart's l., avulsion or damage to the anterior lip of the glenoid fossa as the humerus slides forward in an anterior dislocation.

    Ghon's primary l., SYN Ghon's *tubercle.*

    Hill-Sachs l., an articular cartilage defect on the posterior aspect of the humeral head, often caused by injury to the humeral head by the rim of the glenoid fossa after anterior glenohumeral dislocation.

    Janeway l., one of the stigmata of infectious endocarditis: irregular, erythematous, flat, painless macules on the palms, soles, thenar and hypothenar eminences of the hands, tips of the fingers, and plantar surfaces of the toes.

    Mallory-Weiss l., laceration of the gastric cardia, as seen in the Mallory-Weiss syndrome. SYN Mallory-Weiss tear.

Lesser's tri·an·gle. See under triangle.

LET leukocyte esterase *test.*

le·thal (lē′thăl). Pertaining to or causing death; denoting especially the causal agent. [L. *letalis,* fr. *letum,* death]

    clinical l., a disorder that culminates in premature death.

    genetic l., a disorder that prevents effective reproduction by those affected.

leth·ar·gy (leth′ar-jē). A state of deep and prolonged unconsciousness, resembling profound slumber, from which one can be aroused but into which one immediately relapses. [G. *lēthargis,* drowsiness]

LETS *large, external transformation-sensitive* fibronectin. SEE fibronectins.

leuc-, leuco-. White; white blood cell. SEE leuko-, leuk-. [G. *leukos,* white]

leu·cine (lū′sēn). The L-isomer is one of the amino acids of proteins; a nutritionally essential amino acid.

leu·cin·u·ria (lū-si-nū′rē-ă). The excretion of leucine in the urine.

leuk-. SEE leuko-.

leuk·a·phe·re·sis (lū′kă-fĕ-rē′sis). A procedure, analogous to plasmapheresis, in which leukocytes are removed from the withdrawn blood and the remainder of the blood is retransfused into the donor. [leuko- + G. *aphairesis,* a withdrawal]

leu·ke·mia (lū-kē′mē-ă). Progressive proliferation of abnormal leukocytes found in hemopoietic tissues, other organs, and usually in the blood in increased numbers. L. is classified by the dominant cell type, and by duration from onset to death. This occurs in *acute l.* within a few months in most cases, and is associated with acute symptoms including severe anemia, hemorrhages, and slight enlargement of lymph nodes or the spleen. The duration of *chronic l.* exceeds one year, with a gradual onset of symptoms of anemia or marked enlargement of spleen, liver, or lymph nodes. [leuko- + G. *haima,* blood]

    acute lymphocytic l. (ALL), SEE lymphocytic l.

    acute promyelocytic l., l. presenting as a severe bleeding disorder, with infiltration of the bone marrow by abnormal promyelocytes and myelocytes, a low plasma fibrinogen, and defective coagulation.

    adult T-cell l. (ATL), SYN adult T-cell *lymphoma.*

    aleukemic l., l. in which abnormal (or leukemic) cells are absent in the peripheral blood.

    basophilic l., basophilocytic l., a form of granulocytic l. in which there are unusually great numbers of basophilic granulocytes in the tissues and circulating blood. SYN mast cell l.

    l. cu′tis, yellow-brown, red, blue-red, or purple, sometimes nodular lesions associated with diffuse infiltration of leukemic cells in the skin.

    embryonal l., SYN stem cell l.

    eosinophilic l., eosinophilocytic l., a form of granulocytic l. in which there are conspicuous numbers of eosinophilic granulocytes in the tissues and circulating blood, or in which such cells are predominant.

    granulocytic l., a form of l. characterized by an uncontrolled proliferation of myelopoietic cells in the bone marrow and in extramedullary sites, and the presence of large numbers of immature and mature granulocytic forms in various tissues (and organs) and in the circulating blood. The predominant cell is usually of the neutrophilic series, but, in a few instances, eosinophilic or basophilic granulocytes, or even megakaryocytes, may represent the chief form. SYN myelocytic l., myelogenic l., myelogenous l., myeloid l.

    hairy cell l., a rare, usually chronic disorder characterized by proliferation of hairy cells in reticuloendothelial organs and blood.

    leukopenic l., a form of lymphocytic, granulocytic, or monocytic l. in which the number of white blood cells is in the normal range or slightly depressed.

    lymphatic l., SYN lymphocytic l.

    lymphoblastic l., acute lymphocytic l. in which the abnormal cells are chiefly (or almost totally) blast forms of the lymphocytic series, or in which unusually large numbers of the immature forms occur in association with adult lymphocytes.

    lymphocytic l., a variety of l. characterized by an uncontrolled proliferation and conspicuous enlargement of lymphoid tissue in various sites (*e.g.,* lymph nodes, spleen, bone marrow, lungs),

primary lesions

flat, discolored, nonpalpable changes in skin color

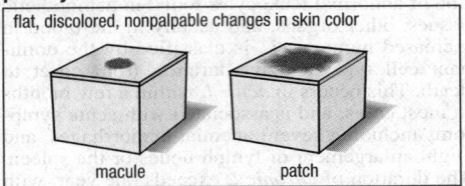

macule   patch

elevated, palpable solid masses

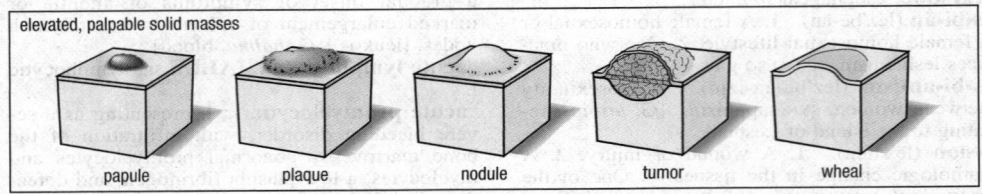

papule   plaque   nodule   tumor   wheal

elevation formed by fluid in a cavity

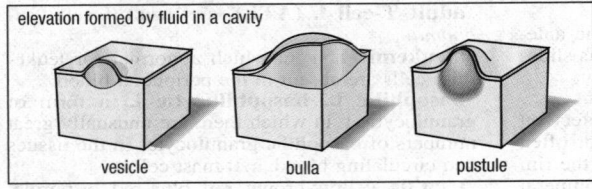

vesicle   bulla   pustule

secondary lesions

loss of skin surface

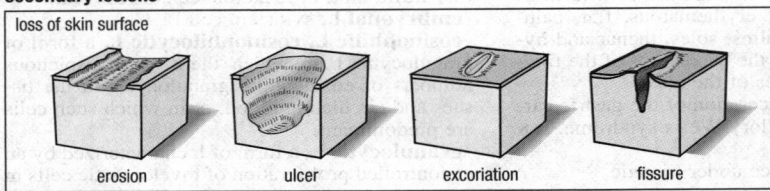

erosion   ulcer   excoriation   fissure

material on skin surface

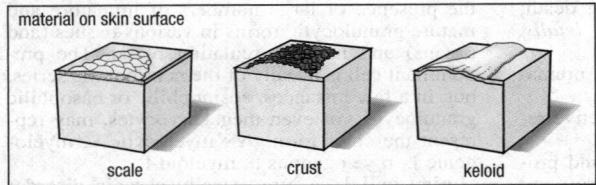

scale   crust   keloid

vascular lesions

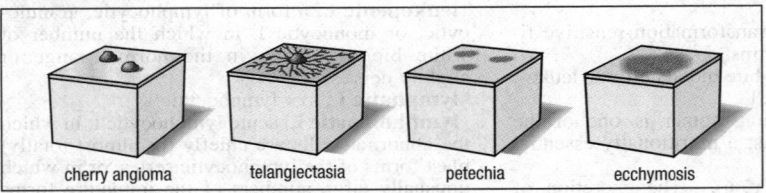

cherry angioma   telangiectasia   petechia   ecchymosis

lesions: types of primary, secondary, and vascular lesions

and the occurrence of increased numbers of cells of the lymphocytic series in the blood. SYN lymphatic l.

mast cell l., SYN basophilic l.

megakaryocytic l., an unusual form of myelopoietic disease that is characterized by uncontrolled proliferation of megakaryocytes in the bone marrow, and sometimes by the presence of megakaryocytes in the blood.

micromyeloblastic l., a form of myelocytic l. in which relatively large proportions of micromyeloblasts are found in the circulating blood and in bone marrow and other tissues.

mixed l., mixed cell l., granulocytic l. with occurrence in the blood of increased numbers of cells in the myeloid series (*i.e.,* neutrophilic, eosinophilic, and basophilic granulocytes).

monocytic l., a form of l. characterized by large numbers of cells that can be definitely identified as monocytes, in addition to larger, apparently related cells formed from the uncontrolled proliferation of the reticuloendothelial tissue. The disease runs an acute or subacute course in older persons, and is characterized by swelling of gums, oral ulceration, bleeding in skin or mucous membranes, secondary infection, and splenomegaly.

myeloblastic l., a form of granulocytic l. in which there are large numbers of myeloblasts in various tissues and in the blood. Used synonymously for acute granulocytic l.

myelocytic l., myelogenic l., myelogenous l., myeloid l., SYN granulocytic l.

plasma cell l., an unusual disease characterized by leukocytosis and other signs and symptoms that are suggestive of l., in association with diffuse infiltrations and aggregates of plasma cells in the spleen, liver, bone marrow, and lymph nodes, and plasma cells in the blood.

Rieder cell l., a special form of acute granulocytic l. in which affected tissues and the blood contain atypical myeloblasts (*i.e.,* Rieder cells) that have faintly granular, immature cytoplasm and a bizarre nucleus with deep indentations (suggestive of lobulation).

smoldering l., SYN myelodysplastic *syndrome.*

stem cell l., a form of l. in which the abnormal cells are thought to be the precursors of lymphoblasts, myeloblasts, or monoblasts. SYN embryonal l.

subleukemic l., a form of l. in which abnormal cells are present in the peripheral blood, but the total leukocyte count is not elevated.

leu•ke•mic (lū-kē'mik). Pertaining to, or having the characteristics of, any form of leukemia.

leu•ke•mid (lū-kem'id). Any nonspecific type of cutaneous lesion that is associated with leukemia but is not a localized accumulation of leukemic cells; *e.g.,* petechiae, vesicles, wheals, bullae, hematomas, and the lesions of exfoliative dermatitis and herpes zoster. [leuko- + G. *haima,* blood, + *id* (1)]

leu•ke•mo•gen (lū-kē'mō-jen). Any substance or entity considered to be a causal factor in the occurrence of leukemia.

leu•ke•mo•gen•e•sis (lū-kē-mō-jen'ĕ-sis). The causation (or induction), development, and pro-

gression of a leukemic disease. [leukemia + G. *genesis,* production]

leu•ke•mo•gen•ic (lū-kē-mō-jen'ik). Pertaining to the causation, induction, and development of leukemia; manifesting the ability to cause leukemia.

leu•ke•moid (lū-kē'moyd). Resembling leukemia in various signs and symptoms, especially with reference to changes in the circulating blood. SEE ALSO leukemoid reaction. [leukemia + G. *eidos,* resemblance]

leu•ke•moid re•ac•tion. Leukocytosis similar to that occurring in leukemia, but not the result of leukemic disease. l. r.'s are sometimes observed as a feature of infectious disease (tuberculosis, diphtheria), intoxication (eclampsia, mustard gas poisoning), malignant neoplasms, and acute hemorrhage or hemolysis.

△**leuko-, leuk-.** White; white blood cells. For some words beginning thus, see leuc- and leuco-. [G. *leukos,* white]

leu•ko•ag•glu•ti•nin (lū'kō-ă-glū'ti-nin). An antibody that agglutinates white blood cells.

leu•ko•blast (lū'kō-blast). An immature white blood cell that is transitional between the lymphoidocyte and the promyelocyte; the cytoplasm is polychromatophilic, the nuclear chromatin is thicker, and the nucleoli less distinct. [leuko- + G. *blastos,* germ]

leu•ko•blas•to•sis (lū'kō-blas-tō'sis). A general term for the abnormal proliferation of leukocytes, especially that occurring in myelocytic and lymphocytic leukemia.

leu•ko•ci•din (lū-kos'i-din, lū-kō-sī'din). A heat-labile substance that is elaborated by many strains of *Staphylococcus aureus, Streptococcus pyogenes,* and pneumococci and manifests a destructive action on leukocytes, with or without lysis of the cells. [leukocyte + L. *caedo,* to kill]

leu•ko•co•ria, leu•ko•ko•ria (lū-kō-kō're-ă, lū-kō-kō're-ă). Reflection from a white mass within the eye giving the appearance of a white pupil. SYN leukokoria. [leuko- white, + G. *korē,* pupil]

leu•ko•cyte (lū'kō-sīt). A type of cell formed in the myelopoietic, lymphoid, and reticular portions of the reticuloendothelial system in various parts of the body, and normally present in those sites and in the circulating blood (rarely in other tissues). Under various abnormal conditions, the total numbers or proportions, or both, may be characteristically increased, decreased, or not altered, and they may be present in other tissues and organs. L.'s represent three lines of development from primitive elements: myeloid, lymphoid, and monocytic series. On the basis of features observed with various methods of staining with polychromatic dyes (*e.g.,* Wright's stain, and others), cells of the myeloid series are frequently termed granular l.'s, or granulocytes; cells of the lymphoid and monocytic series also have granules in the cytoplasm but, owing to their tiny, inconspicuous size and different properties (frequently not clearly visualized with routine methods), lymphocytes and monocytes are sometimes termed nongranular or agranular l.'s. Granulocytes are commonly known as polymorphonuclear l.'s (also polynuclear or multinuclear l.'s), inasmuch as the mature nucleus is divided into two to five rounded or ovoid lobes that are connected with thin strands or small bands of chromatin; they consist of three distinct types: neutrophils, eosinophils, and basophils, named on the basis of the staining reactions of the cytoplasmic granules. Cells of the lymphocytic series occur as two, somewhat arbitrary, normal varieties: small and large lymphocytes; the former represent the ordinary forms and are conspicuously more numerous in the circulating blood and normal lymphoid tissue; the latter may be found in normal circulating blood, but are more easily observed in lymphoid tissue. The small lymphocytes have nuclei that are deeply or densely stained (the chromatin is coarse and bulky) and almost fill the cells, with only a slight rim of cytoplasm around the nuclei; the large lymphocytes have nuclei that are approximately the same size as, or only slightly larger than, those of the small forms, but there is a broader, easily visualized band of cytoplasm around the nuclei. Cells of the monocyte series are usually larger than the other l.'s, and are characterized by a relatively abundant, slightly opaque, pale blue or blue-gray cytoplasm that contains myriads of extremely fine reddish-blue granules. Monocytes are usually indented, reniform, or shaped similarly to a horseshoe, but are sometimes rounded or ovoid; their nuclei are usually large and centrally placed and, even when eccentrically located, are completely surrounded by at least a small band of cytoplasm. SYN white blood cell. [leuko- + G. *kytos,* cell]

basophilic l., a polymorphonuclear l. characterized by many large, coarse, metachromatic granules (dark purple or blue-black with Wright's stain) that usually fill the cytoplasm and may almost mask the nucleus; they usually do not occur in increased numbers as the result of acute infectious disease; the granules, which contain heparin and histamine, may degranulate in response to hypersensitivity reactions and can be of significance in general inflammation. SYN mast l.

endothelial l., old term for a monocyte, a type of l. thought to be derived from reticuloendothelial tissue.

eosinophilic l., a polymorphonuclear l. characterized by prominent cytoplasmic granules that are bright yellow-red or orange when treated with Wright's stain; the nuclei are usually larger than those of neutrophils and characteristically have two lobes; these l.'s are motile phagocytes with distinctive antiparasitic functions. SYN eosinophil, eosinophile, oxyphil (2), oxyphile, oxyphilic l.

granular l., any one of the polymorphonuclear l.'s, especially a neutrophilic l. SEE ALSO granulocyte, basophilic l., eosinophilic l.

mast l., SYN basophilic l.

neutrophilic l., a neutrophilic granulocyte, the most frequent of the polymorphonuclear l.'s, and also the most active phagocyte among the various types of white blood cells; when treated with Wright's stain the fairly abundant cytoplasm is faintly pink, and numerous tiny pink or violet-pink granules are recognizable in the cytoplasm; the deeply stained blue nucleus is sharply distin-

guished from the cytoplasm and is distinctly lobated, with thin strands of chromatin connecting the three to five lobes.

oxyphilic l., SYN eosinophilic l.

polymorphonuclear l., polynuclear l., common term for granulocyte or granulocytic l.; the term includes basophilic, eosinophilic, and neutrophilic l.'s, but is usually used especially with reference to the neutrophilic l.'s.

leu·ko·cyt·ic (lū-kō-sit′ik). Pertaining to or characterized by leukocytes.

leu·ko·cy·to·blast (lū-kō-sī′tō-blast). A nonspecific term for any immature cell from which a leukocyte develops, including lymphoblast, myeloblast, and the like. [leukocyte + G. *blastos,* germ]

leu·ko·cy·toc·la·sis (lū′kō-sī-tok′lă-sis). Karyorrhexis of leukocytes. [leuko- + G. *kytos,* cell, + *klasia,* a breaking]

leu·ko·cy·to·gen·e·sis (lū′kō-sī-tō-jen′ĕ-sis). The formation and development of leukocytes. [leukocyte + G. *genesis,* production]

leu·ko·cy·tol·y·sin (lū′kō-sī-tol′i-sin). Any substance (including lytic antibody) that causes dissolution of leukocytes. SYN leukolysin.

leu·ko·cy·tol·y·sis (lū′kō-sī-tol′i-sis). Dissolution or lysis of leukocytes. [leukocyte + G. *lysis,* dissolution]

leu·ko·cy·to·lyt·ic (lū′kō-sī-tō-lit′ik). Pertaining to, causing, or manifesting leukocytolysis.

leu·ko·cy·to·ma (lū′kō-sī-tō′mă). A fairly well circumscribed, nodular, dense accumulation of leukocytes. [leukocyte + G. *-oma,* tumor]

leu·ko·cy·to·pe·nia (lū′kō-sī-tō-pē′nē-ă). SYN leukopenia.

leu·ko·cy·to·pla·nia (lū′kō-sī-tō-plā′nē-ă). Movement of leukocytes from the lumens of blood vessels, through serous membranes, or in the tissues. [leukocyte + G. *planē,* a wandering]

leu·ko·cy·to·poi·e·sis (lū′kō-sī-tō-poy-ē′sis). SYN leukopoiesis. [leukocyte + G. *poiēsis,* a making]

leu·ko·cy·to·sis (lū′kō-sī-tō′sis). An abnormally large number of leukocytes; a white blood cell count of 10,000 or more per cu mm. Most examples of l. represent a disproportionate increase in the neutrophils, and the term is frequently synonymous with neutrophilia. [leukocyte + G. *-osis,* condition]

absolute l., an actual increase in the total number of leukocytes in the blood, as distinguished from a relative increase (such as that observed in dehydration).

eosinophilic l., a form of relative l. in which the greatest proportionate increase is in the eosinophils. SYN eosinophilia.

physiologic l., any form of l. that is associated with apparently normal situations and that is not directly related to a pathologic condition.

relative l., an increased proportion of one or more types of leukocytes in the circulating blood, without an actual increase in the total number of white blood cells.

leu·ko·cy·to·tac·tic (lū′kō-sī-tō-tak′tik). Pertaining to, characterized by, or causing leukocytotaxia. SYN leukotactic.

leu·ko·cy·to·tax·ia (lū-kō-sī-tō-tak′sē-ă). **1.** The

active ameboid movement of leukocytes, especially the neutrophilic granulocytes, either toward (**positive l.**) or away from (**negative l.**) certain microorganisms as well as various substances formed in inflamed tissue. **2.** The property of attracting or repelling leukocytes. SYN leukotaxia, leukotaxis. [leukocyte + G. *taxis,* arrangement]

leu·ko·cy·to·tox·in (lū′kō-sī-tō-tok′sin). Any substance that causes degeneration and necrosis of leukocytes, including leukolysin and leukocidin. SYN leukotoxin. [leukocyte + G. *toxikon,* poison]

leu·ko·cy·tu·ria (lū′kō-sī-tū′rē-ă). The presence of leukocytes in urine that is recently voided or collected by means of a catheter. [leukocyte + G. *ouron,* urine]

leu·ko·der·ma (lū-kō-der′mă). An absence of pigment, partial or total, in the skin. SYN leukopathia, leukopathy. [leuko- + G. *derma,* skin]

syphilitic l., a fading of the roseola of secondary syphilis, leaving reticulated depigmented and hyperpigmented areas located chiefly on the sides of the neck. SYN melanoleukoderma colli.

leu·ko·dys·tro·phy (lū-kō-dis′trō-fē). Term for a group of white matter diseases, some familial, characterized by progressive cerebral deterioration in early life and primary absence or degeneration of the myelin of the central and peripheral nervous systems; probably related to a defect in lipid metabolism; the adult type of Pelizaeus-Merzbacher disease is inherited as an autosomal dominant trait [MIM*169500]. [leuko- + G. *dys,* bad, + *trophē,* nourishment]

metachromatic l., a metabolic disorder, usually of infancy, characterized by myelin loss, accumulation of metachromatic lipids (galactosyl sulfatidates) in the white matter of the central and peripheral nervous systems, progressive paralysis, and mental retardation; psychosis and dementia are seen in adults.

leu·ko·e·de·ma (lū′kō-e-dē′mă). A bluish-white opalescence of the buccal mucosa which becomes the normal mucosal color on stretching the tissue; may be considered a normal anatomic variation.

leu·ko·en·ceph·a·li·tis (lū′kō-en-sef-ă-lī′tis). Encephalitis restricted to the white matter.

acute epidemic l., a disease characterized by acute onset of fever, followed by convulsions, delirium, and coma, and associated with perivascular demyelination and hemorrhagic foci in the central nervous system.

leu·ko·en·ceph·a·lop·a·thy (lū′kō-en-sef-ă-lop′ă-thē). White matter changes first described in children with leukemia, associated with radiation and chemotherapy injury, often associated with methotrexate; pathologically characterized by diffuse reactive astrocytosis with multiple areas of necrotic foci without inflammation. [leuko- + G. *enkephalos,* brain, + *pathos,* suffering]

progressive multifocal l. (PML), a rare, subacute, afebrile disease characterized by areas of demyelinization surrounded by markedly altered neuroglia, including inclusion bodies in glial cells; it occurs usually in individuals with AIDS, leukemia, lymphoma, or other debilitating diseases, or in those who have been receiving immu-

nosuppressive treatment. Caused by JC virus, a human polyoma virus.

leu·ko·e·ryth·ro·blas·to·sis (lū′kō-ě-rith′rō-blas-tō′sis). Any anemic condition resulting from space-occupying lesions in the bone marrow; the blood contains immature cells of the granulocytic series and nucleated red blood cells. SYN myelophthisic anemia, myelopathic anemia.

leu·ko·ko·ria (lū-kō-kō′rē-ă). SEE leukocoria.

leu·kol·y·sin (lū-kol′i-sin). SYN leukocytolysin.

leu·ko·ma (lū-kō′mă). A dense white opacity of the cornea. [G. whiteness, a white spot in the eye, fr. *leukos,* white]

leu·ko·ma·tous (lū-kō′mă-tŭs). Denoting leukoma.

leu·ko·my·e·lop·a·thy (lū′kō-mī′ě-lop′ă-thē). Any disease involving the white matter or the conducting tracts of the spinal cord. [leuko- + G. *myelos,* marrow, + *pathos,* suffering]

leu·ko·nych·ia (lū-kō-nik′ē-ă). The occurrence of white spots, streaks, or patches under the nails, due to the presence of air bubbles between the nail and its bed. [leuko- + G. *onyx* (*onych-*), nail]

leu·ko·path·ia, leu·kop·a·thy (lū-kō-path′ē-ă, lū-kop′ă-thē). SYN leukoderma. [leuko- + G. *pathos,* disease]

leu·ko·pe·de·sis (lū′kō-pē-dē′sis). The movement of white blood cells (especially polymorphonuclear leukocytes) through the walls of capillaries and into the tissues. [leuko- + G. *pēdēsis,* a leaping]

leu·ko·pe·nia (lū-kō-pē′nē-ă). Any condition in which the number of leukocytes in the circulating blood is less than normal, the lower limit of which is generally regarded as 4000–5000 per cu mm. SYN leukocytopenia. [leuko(cyte) + G. *penia,* poverty]

basophilic l., a decrease in the number of basophilic granulocytes in the circulating blood.

eosinophilic l., a decrease in the number of eosinophilic granulocytes normally present in the circulating blood.

leu·ko·pe·nic (lū-kō-pē′nik). Pertaining to leukopenia.

leu·ko·pla·kia (lū-kō-plā′kē-ă). A white patch of oral mucous membrane which cannot be wiped off and cannot be diagnosed clinically; biopsy may show malignant or premalignant changes. [leuko- + G. *plax,* plate]

hairy l., a white lesion appearing on the tongue or buccal mucosa of patients with AIDS; the lesion appears raised, with a corrugated or "hairy" surface. In otherwise healthy individuals, hairy l., caused by the Epstein-Barr virus, rarely becomes cancerous. However, among those with AIDS, the risk of malignant change is elevated.

l. vul′vae, a clinical term for hyperkeratotic white patches of the vulvar epithelium; biopsy is necessary for specific diagnosis.

leu·ko·poi·e·sis (lū′kō-poy-ē′sis). Formation and development of the various types of white blood cells. SYN leukocytopoiesis. [leuko- + G. *poiēsis,* a making]

leu·ko·poi·et·ic (lū′kō-poy-et′ik). Pertaining to or characterized by leukopoiesis, as manifested by portions of the bone marrow and reticuloendothelial and lymphoid tissues, which form (respec-

le

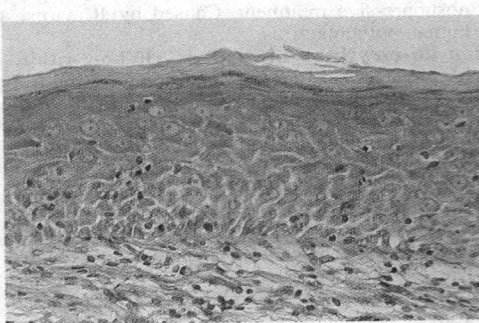

leukoplakia: of the oral mucosa

tively) the granulocytes, monocytes, and lymphocytes.

leu·kor·rha·gia (lū-kō-rā'jē-ă). SYN leukorrhea. [leuko- + G. *rhēgnymi,* to burst forth]

leu·kor·rhea (lū-kō-rē'ă). Discharge from the vagina of a white or yellowish viscid fluid. SYN leukorrhagia. [leuko- + G. *rhoia,* flow]

leu·ko·sis (lū-kō'sis). Abnormal proliferation of one or more of the leukopoietic tissues; the term includes myelosis, certain forms of reticuloendotheliosis, and lymphadenosis.

leu·ko·tac·tic (lū-kō-tak'tik). SYN leukocytotactic.

leu·ko·tax·ia (lū-kō-tak'sē-ă). SYN leukocytotaxia.

leu·ko·tax·ine (lū-kō-tak'sēn). A cell-free nitrogenous material prepared from injured, acutely degenerating tissue and from inflammatory exudates.

leu·ko·tax·is (lū-kō-tak'sis). SYN leukocytotaxia.

leu·kot·ic (lū-kot'ik). Pertaining to, characterized by, or manifesting leukosis.

leu·kot·o·my (lū-kot'ō-mē). Incision into the white matter of the frontal lobe of the brain. [leuko- + G. *tomē,* a cutting]

leu·ko·tox·in (lū-kō-tok'sin). SYN leukocytotoxin.

leu·ko·trich·ia (lū-kō-trik'ē-ă). Whiteness of the hair. [leuko- + G. *thrix,* hair]

leu·ko·tri·enes (LT) (lū-kō-trī'ēnz). Products of eicosanoid metabolism with physiologic roles in inflammation and allergic reactions.

le·va·tor (le-vā'ter, tōr). **1.** A surgical instrument for prying up the depressed part in a fracture of the skull. **2.** One of several muscles whose action is to raise the part into which it is inserted. [L. a lifter, fr. *levo,* pp. *-atus,* to lift, fr. *levis,* light]

lev·el (le'vel). Any rank, position, or status in a graded scale of values.

Clark's l., the l. of invasion of primary malignant melanoma of the skin; limited to the epidermis, I; into the underlying papillary dermis, II; to the junction of the papillary and reticular dermis, III; into the reticular dermis, IV; into the subcutaneous fat, V. The prognosis is worse with each successive deeper l. of invasion.

△**levo-.** Left, toward or on the left side. [L. *laevus*]

le·vo·car·dia (lē-vō-kar'dē-ă). Situs inversus of the other viscera but with the heart normally situ-

ated on the left; congenital cardiac lesions are commonly associated. [levo- + G. *kardia,* heart]

le·vo·duc·tion (lē-vō-dŭk'shŭn). Turning of one eye to the left. [levo- + L. *duco,* pp. *ductus,* to lead]

le·vo·ro·ta·tion (lē-vō-rō-tā'shŭn). **1.** A turning or twisting to the left; in particular, the counterclockwise twist given the plane of plane-polarized light by solutions of certain optically active substances. **2.** SYN sinistrotorsion. [levo- + L. *roto,* to turn]

le·vo·ro·ta·to·ry (lē-vō-rō'tă-tōr-ē). Denoting levorotation, or crystals or solutions capable of causing it; as a chemical prefix, usually abbreviated *l-* or (−). Cf. dextrorotatory.

le·vo·tor·sion (lē-vō-tōr'shŭn). **1.** SYN sinistrotorsion. **2.** Rotation of the upper pole of the cornea of one or both eyes to the left. [levo- + L. *torsio,* a twisting]

le·vo·ver·sion (lē'vō-ver'zhŭn). **1.** Version toward the left. **2.** Conjugate turning of both eyes to the left. [levo- + L. *verto,* pp. *versus,* to turn]

△**-lexis, -lexy.** Suffixes that properly relate to speech, although often confused with -legia (Latin *-lego,* to read) and thus erroneously employed to relate to reading. [G. *lexis,* word, speech, from *legō,* to say]

LFT Left frontotransverse *position;* liver function *test.*

Li lithium.

li·ber·ins (lib'er-ins). SYN releasing *factors.* [L. *libero,* to free, + -in]

li·bid·i·nous (li-bid'i-nŭs). Lascivious; invested with or arousing sexual desire or energy. [L. *libidinosus,* fr. *libido* (*libidin-*), pleasure, desire]

li·bi·do (li-bē'dō, -bī'dō). **1.** Conscious or unconscious sexual desire. **2.** Any passionate interest or form of life force. **3.** In jungian psychology, synonymous with psychic energy. [L. lust]

lice (līs). Plural of louse.

li·chen (lī'ken). A discrete flat papule or an aggregate of papules giving a patterned configuration resembling lichens growing on rocks. [G. *leichēn,* lichen; a lichen-like eruption]

l. myxedemato′sus, a lichenoid eruption of papules or plaques of mucinous edema due to deposit of glycosaminoglycans in the skin and fibroblast proliferation, in the absence of endocrine disease. SYN papular mucinosis.

l. pla′nus, eruption of flat-topped, shiny, violaceous papules on flexor surfaces, male genitalia, and buccal mucosa of unknown cause; may form linear groups. Spontaneous resolution is common after months to years. SYN l. ruber planus.

l. ru′ber pla′nus, SYN l. planus.

l. sclero′sus et atro′phicus, a chronic eruption, seen chiefly in the anogenital region, consisting of white atrophic papules which may be discrete or confluent and may contain a central depression or a black keratotic plug.

l. scrofuloso′rum, small asymptomatic l. papules on the trunk of children with tuberculosis. SYN papular tuberculid.

l. stria′tus, a self-limited papular eruption occurring primarily in children (more commonly in females); the lesions are arranged in linear groups and usually occur on one extremity.

tropical l., l. trop′icus, SYN *miliaria* rubra.

l. urtica′tus, SYN papular *urticaria.*

li·chen·i·fi·ca·tion (lī′ken-i-fi-kā′shŭn). Leathery induration and thickening of the skin with hyperkeratosis, caused by scratching in atopic or chronic contact dermatitis. [lichen + L. *facio,* to make]

li·chen·oid (lī′kĕ-noyd). **1.** Resembling lichen. **2.** Accentuation of normal skin markings observed in cases of chronic eczema. **3.** Microscopically resembling lichen planus.

lie (lī). Relationship of the long axis of the fetus to that of the mother.

    longitudinal l., that relationship in which the long axis of the fetus is longitudinal and roughly parallel to the long axis of the mother; the presenting part may be either the head or the breech.

    oblique l., that relationship in which the long axis of the fetus crosses the maternal axis at an angle other than a right angle.

    transverse l., that relationship in which the long axis of the fetus is transverse or at right angles to that of the mother.

lie de·tec·tor. SYN polygraph (2).

li·en (lī′en) [NA]. ✩official alternate term for spleen. [L.]

    l. accesso′rius, SYN accessory *spleen.*

    l. mo′bilis, SYN floating *spleen.*

lien-, lieno-. The spleen. SEE spleno-. [L. *lien*]

li·e·nal (lī′ĕ-năl). SYN splenic.

li·en·ter·ic (lī-en-ter′ik). Relating to, or marked by, lientery.

li·en·tery (lī′en-ter-ē). Passage of undigested food in the stools. [G. *leienteria,* fr. *leios,* smooth, + *enteron,* intestine]

life (līf). **1.** The essential condition of being alive; the state of existence characterized by such functions as metabolism, growth, reproduction, adaptation, and response to stimuli. **2.** Living organisms such as animals and plants. [A.S. *lif*]

    half-l., SEE half-life.

life e·vents. Occurrences in one's daily life, some of which act as stressors.

life-style. Habits and customs influenced by the lifelong process of socialization, including social use of alcohol and tobacco, dietary habits, and exercise, all of which have important implications for health.

lig·a·ment (lig′ă-ment). **1.** A band or sheet of fibrous tissue connecting two or more bones, cartilages, or other structures, or serving as support for fasciae or muscles. **2.** A fold of peritoneum supporting any of the abdominal viscera. **3.** Any structure resembling a l. though not performing the function of such. **4.** The cordlike remains of a fetal vessel or other structure that has lost its original lumen. SYN ligamentum [NA]. [L. *ligamentum,* a band, bandage]

    accessory l.'s, l.'s about a joint that are in addition to the articular capsule. They may lie within, or on the outside of the latter.

    alveolodental l., SYN periodontal l.

    annular l., one of a number of l.'s encircling various parts; the principal annular l.'s are those of the stapes, radius, and trachea.

    anterior cruciate l., the l. that extends from the anterior intercondylar area of the tibia to the

posterior part of the medial surface of the lateral condyle of the femur.

    broad l. of the uterus, the peritoneal fold passing from the lateral margin of the uterus to the wall of the pelvis on either side and ensheathing the ovaries and uterine tubes. SYN ligamentum latum uteri [NA].

    capsular l., thickened portions of the fibrous membrane of an articular capsule.

    cardinal l., a fibrous band attached to the uterine cervix and the vault of the lateral fornix of the vagina; continuous with the tissue ensheathing the pelvic vessels.

    coracoacromial l., the heavy arched fibrous band that passes between the coracoid process and the acromion above the shoulder joint; the osseofibrous arch thus formed prevents upward dislocation of the shoulder (glenohumeral) joint.

    coracoclavicular l., the strong l. that unites the clavicle to the coracoid process; it is subdivided into the conoid ligament and the trapezoid ligament. The free upper limb is passively suspended from the clavicular "strut" by the coracoclavicular l.; the l. also plays an important role in preventing dislocation of the acromioclavicular joint. SYN ligamentum coracoclaviculare [NA].

    costoclavicular l., the l. that connects the first rib and the clavicle near its sternal end; limits elevation of shoulder (at sternoclavicular joint). SYN ligamentum costoclaviculare [NA], rhomboid l.

    costotransverse l., the l. that connects the dorsal aspect of the neck of a rib to the ventral aspect of the corresponding transverse process. SYN ligamentum costotransversarium [NA].

    cruciate l.'s, major l.'s that crisscross the knee in the anteroposterior direction, providing stability in that plane. SEE ALSO Lachman *test.*

    cruciate l.'s of knee, the two l.'s which pass from the intercondylar area of the tibia to the intercondylar fossa of the femur.

    cystoduodenal l., a peritoneal fold that sometimes passes from the gallbladder to the first part of the duodenum.

    deltoid l., compound l. consisting of four component l.'s which pass downward from the medial malleolus of the tibia to the tarsal bones: 1) tibionavicular l. (pars tibionavicularis [NA]), 2) tibiocalcaneal l. (pars tibiocalcanea [NA]), 3) anterior tibiotalar l. (pars tibiotalaris anterior [NA]), and 4) posterior tibiotalar l. (pars tibiotalaris posterior [NA]). SYN ligamentum deltoideum✩.

    diaphragmatic l. of the mesonephros, the segment of the urogenital ridge that extends from the mesonephros to the diaphragm; becomes the suspensory l. of the ovary.

    dorsal radiocarpal l., the l. that extends from the distal end of the radius posteriorly to the proximal row of carpal bones.

    extracapsular l.'s, l.'s associated with a synovial joint but separate from and external to its articular capsule. SYN ligamenta extracapsularia [NA].

    falciform l., SYN falciform *process.*

    falciform l. of liver, a crescentic fold of peritoneum extending to the surface of the liver from the diaphragm and anterior abdominal wall; the round ligament lies in its free inferior border; remnant of embryonic ventral mesogastrium. SYN ligamentum falciforme hepatis [NA].

glenohumeral l.'s, three fibrous bands that reinforce the anterior part of the articular capsule of the shoulder joint; they are in continuity with the glenoid labrum at the supraglenoid tubercle of the scapula and blend with the fibrous capsule as it attaches to the anatomic neck of the humerus. SYN ligamenta glenohumeralia [NA].

l. of head of femur, a flattened l. that passes from the fovea in the head of the femur to the borders of the acetabular notch (transverse acetabular l.); the l. does not contribute to the integrity of the joint or control movements there. SYN ligamentum capitis femoris [NA], round l. of femur.

iliofemoral l., a triangular l. attached by its apex to the anterior inferior spine of the ilium and rim of the acetabulum, and by its base to the anterior intertrochanteric line of the femur; the strong medial band is attached to the lower part of the intertrochanteric line; the strong lateral part is fixed to the tubercle at the upper part of this line; the bands diverge, forming a Y-like figure with a weak area between; among the strongest of l.'s, it limits extension at the hip joint. SYN ligamentum iliofemorale [NA], Y-shaped l.

iliotrochanteric l., the lateral strong band of the Y-shaped iliofemoral l.; it is attached below to the tubercle at the upper part of the intertrochanteric line.

inguinal l., a fibrous band formed by the thickened inferior border of the aponeurosis of the external oblique muscle that extends from the anterior superior spine of the ilium to the pubic tubercle, bridging muscular and vascular lacunae; forms the floor of the inguinal canal; gives origin to the lowermost fibers of internal oblique and transversus abdominis muscles. SYN ligamentum inguinale [NA], Poupart's l.

intercarpal l.'s, three sets of short fibrous bands that bind together the two rows of carpal bones; according to their location they are named dorsal intercarpal l. (ligamentum intercarpalia dorsalia), interosseous intercarpal l. (ligamentum intercarpalia interossea), and palmar intercarpal l. (ligamentum intercarpalia palmaria).

intracapsular l.'s, ligaments located within and separate from the articular capsule of a synovial joint. SYN ligamenta intracapsularia [NA].

lacunar l., a curved fibrous band that passes horizontally backward from the medial end of the inguinal l. to the pectineal line; it forms the medial boundary of the femoral ring. SYN ligamentum lacunare [NA].

longitudinal l., one of two extensive fibrous bands running the length of the vertebral column: the anterior longitudinal l. and the posterior longitudinal l. SYN ligamentum longitudinale [NA].

lumbocostal l., a strong band that unites the twelfth rib with the tips of the transverse processes of the first and second lumbar vertebrae. SYN ligamentum lumbocostale [NA].

medial l., the bundle of fibers strengthening the medial part of the articular capsule of the temporomandibular joint.

medial collateral l., a broad, flat band attached superiorly to the medial condyle of the femur and inferiorly to the medial condyle of the tibia; stabilizes the knee joint medially, resisting valgus stress. SYN tibial collateral l.

nuchal l., SYN *ligamentum* nuchae.

palmar radiocarpal l., a strong l. that passes from the distal end of the radius to the proximal row of carpal bones on the anterior surface of the wrist joint.

palmar ulnocarpal l., the fibrous band that passes from the ulnar styloid process to the carpal bones.

patellar l., a strong flattened fibrous band passing from the apex and adjoining margins of the patella to the tuberosity of the tibia. SYN ligamentum patellae [NA].

pectineal l., a thick, strong fibrous band that passes laterally from the lacunar l. along the pectineal line of the pubis. SYN ligamentum pectineale [NA].

periodontal l., the connective tissue that surrounds the tooth root and attaches it to its bony socket; it consists of fibers anchored in the cementum and extending into the alveolar bone; the tissues that surround and support the teeth, including the gingivae, cementum, periodontal l., and alveolar and supporting bone. SYN periodontium [NA], alveolodental l., alveolodental membrane, peridental membrane, periodontal membrane.

phrenicocolic l., a triangular fold of peritoneum attached to the left flexure of the colon and to the diaphragm, on which rests the inferior pole or extremity of the spleen. SYN ligamentum phrenicocolicum [NA].

plantar calcaneonavicular l., a dense fibroelastic l. that extends from the sustentaculum tali to the plantar surface of the navicular bone; it supports the head of the talus.

posterior cruciate l., the strong fibrous cord that extends from the posterior intercondylar area of the tibia to the anterior part of the lateral surface of the medial condyle of the femur.

Poupart's l., SYN inguinal l.

pulmonary l., two-layered fold formed as the pleura of the mediastinum is reflected onto the lung inferior to the root of the lung. SYN ligamentum pulmonale [NA].

radiate l. of head of rib, the radiate, stellate, or anterior costovertebral l. connecting the head of each rib to the bodies of the two vertebrae with which it articulates.

reflected inguinal l., a triangular fibrous band extending from the aponeurosis of the external oblique to the pubic tubercle of the opposite side.

rhomboid l., SYN costoclavicular l.

round l. of femur, SYN l. of head of femur.

round l. of liver, the remains of the umbilical vein running within the free edge of the falciform l. from the umbilicus to the liver, where it continues within the fissure for the round l. to the origin of the left portal vein within the porta hepatis. SYN ligamentum teres hepatis [NA].

round l. of uterus, a fibromuscular band that is attached to the uterus on either side in front of and below the opening of the uterine tube; it passes through the inguinal canal to the labium majus. SYN ligamentum teres uteri [NA].

serous l., one of a number of peritoneal folds attaching certain of the viscera to the abdominal wall or to each other.

spiral l. of cochlea, the thickened periosteal lining of the bony cochlea forming the outer wall of the cochlear duct to which the basal lamina attaches.

splenorenal l., a peritoneal fold (portion of the greater omentum) which extends from the diaphragm and the anterior aspect of the left kidney to the hilar region of the spleen, conducting the splenic vessels from the posterior body wall to the spleen. SYN ligamentum splenorenale [NA].

suspensory l. of axilla, the continuation of the clavipectoral fascia downward to attach to the axillary fascia; it maintains the characteristic hollow of the armpit.

suspensory l.'s of breast, well developed retinacula cutis that extend from the fibrous stroma of the mammary gland to the overlying skin. SYN ligamenta suspensoria mammae [NA].

suspensory l. of eyeball, a thickening of the inferior part of the bulbar sheath which supports the eye within the orbit; it extends between the lateral and medial orbital margins and includes the medial and lateral check l.'s.

suspensory l. of lens, SYN ciliary *zonule.*

suspensory l. of ovary, a band of peritoneum that extends upward from the upper pole of the ovary; it contains the ovarian vessels and ovarian plexus of nerves. SYN ligamentum suspensorium ovarii [NA].

sutural l., a delicate membrane binding the bones at the cranial sutures.

synovial l., one of the large synovial folds in a joint.

tarsometatarsal l.'s, the ligaments that unite tarsal and metatarsal bones; they are arranged in dorsal, interosseous, and plantar sets.

tibial collateral l., SYN medial collateral l.

transverse carpal l., a strong fibrous band crossing the front of the carpus and binding down the flexor tendons of the digits and the flexor carpi radialis tendon and the median nerve; in so doing it creates the carpal tunnel.

transverse perineal l., the thickened anterior border of the urogenital diaphragm, formed by the fusion of its two fascial layers.

transverse l. of elbow, a bundle of fibers running from the olecranon to the coronoid process in association with the ulnar collateral l.

transverse l. of knee, a transverse band that passes between the lateral and medial menisci in the anterior part of the knee joint. SYN ligamentum transversum genus [NA].

trapezoid l., the lateral part of the coracoclavicular l. that attaches to the trapezoid line of the clavicle. SYN ligamentum trapezoideum [NA].

uterovesical l., a peritoneal fold extending from the uterus to the posterior portion of the bladder.

vocal l., the band that extends on either side from the thyroid cartilage to the vocal process of the arytenoid cartilage; it is the thickened, free upper border of the conus elasticus of the larynx. SYN ligamentum vocale [NA].

Y-shaped l., SYN iliofemoral l.

lig·a·men·to·pex·is, lig·a·men·to·pexy (lig'ă-men-tō-pek'sis, -pek'sē). Shortening of any ligament of the uterus. [ligament + G. *pēxis,* fixation]

lig·a·men·tous (lig'ă-men'tŭs). Relating to or of the form or structure of a ligament.

lig·a·men·tum, pl. **lig·a·men·ta** (lig'ă-men'tŭm, -men'tă) [NA]. SYN ligament. [L. a band, tie, fr. *ligo,* to bind]

l. cap'itis fem'oris [NA], SYN *ligament* of head of femur.

l. coracoclavicula're [NA], SYN coracoclavicular *ligament.*

l. costoclavicula're [NA], SYN costoclavicular *ligament.*

l. costotransversa'rium [NA], SYN costotransverse *ligament.*

l. deltoi'deum, ☆ official alternate term for deltoid *ligament.*

ligamen'ta extracapsula'ria [NA], SYN extracapsular *ligaments,* under *ligament.*

l. falcifor'me hep'atis [NA], SYN falciform *ligament* of liver.

ligamen'ta glenohumera'lia [NA], SYN glenohumeral *ligaments,* under *ligament.*

l. iliofemora'le [NA], SYN iliofemoral *ligament.*

l. inguina'le [NA], SYN inguinal *ligament.*

ligamen'ta intracapsula'ria [NA], SYN intracapsular *ligaments,* under *ligament.*

l. lacuna're [NA], SYN lacunar *ligament.*

l. la'tum u'teri [NA], SYN broad *ligament* of the uterus.

l. longitudina'le [NA], SYN longitudinal *ligament.*

l. lumbocosta'le [NA], SYN lumbocostal *ligament.*

l. nu'chae [NA], a sagittal ligamentous band at the back of the neck, formed of thickened supraspinous ligaments; it extends from the external occipital protuberance to the posterior border of the foramen magnum cranially, and to the seventh cervical spinous process caudally. SYN nuchal ligament.

l. patel'lae [NA], SYN patellar *ligament.*

l. pectinea'le [NA], SYN pectineal *ligament.*

l. phrenicocol'icum [NA], SYN phrenicocolic *ligament.*

l. pulmona'le [NA], SYN pulmonary *ligament.*

l. splenorena'le [NA], SYN splenorenal *ligament.*

ligamen'ta suspenso'ria mam'mae [NA], SYN suspensory *ligaments* of breast, under *ligament.*

l. suspenso'rium ova'rii [NA], SYN suspensory *ligament* of ovary.

l. te'res hep'atis [NA], SYN round *ligament* of liver.

l. te'res u'teri [NA], SYN round *ligament* of uterus.

l. transver'sum ge'nus [NA], SYN transverse *ligament* of knee.

l. trapezoi'deum [NA], SYN trapezoid *ligament.*

l. voca'le [NA], SYN vocal *ligament.*

lig·and (lig'and, li'gand). **1.** An organic molecule attached to a central metal ion by multiple coordi-

li

nate bonds. **2.** An organic molecule attached to a tracer element, *e.g.*, a radioisotope. **3.** A molecule that binds to a macromolecule, *e.g.*, a l. binding to a receptor. **4.** The analyte in competitive binding assays, such as radioimmunoassay. [L. *ligo*, to bind]

li•gase (lī′gās). Generic term for enzymes (EC class 6) catalyzing the joining of two molecules coupled with the breakdown of a pyrophosphate bond in ATP or a similar compound. SEE ALSO synthetase.

li•gate (lī′gāt). To apply a ligature. [L. *ligo*, pp. *-atus*, to bind]

li•ga•tion (lī-gā′shŭn). **1.** Application of a ligature. **2.** The act of binding or annealing. [L. *ligatio*, fr. *ligo*, to bind]

   tubal l., interruption of the continuity of the oviducts by cutting, cautery, or by a plastic or metal device to prevent future conception.

lig•a•ture (lig′ă-chūr). **1.** A thread, wire, fillet, or the like, tied tightly around a blood vessel, the pedicle of a tumor, or other structure to constrict it. **2.** ORTHODONTICS A wire or other material used to secure an orthodontic attachment or tooth to an archwire. [L. *ligatura*, a band or tie, fr. *ligo*, to tie]

   intravascular l., balloon occlusion of the feeding vessels of a cerebral arteriovenous malformation.

light (līt). That portion of electromagnetic radiation to which the retina is sensitive. SEE ALSO lamp. [A.S. *leōht*]

   polarized l., l. in which, as a result of reflection or transmission through certain media, the vibrations are all in one plane, transverse to the ray, instead of in all planes.

   stray l., radiant energy that reaches the detector of a spectrophotometer and consists of wavelengths other than those selected.

   Wood's l., ultraviolet l. produced by Wood's lamp.

light•en•ing (līt′en-ing). Sensation of decreased abdominal distention during the later weeks of pregnancy following the descent of the fetal head into the pelvic inlet.

limb (lim). **1.** An extremity; a member; an arm or leg. **2.** A segment of any jointed structure. SEE ALSO leg. [A.S. *lim*]

   lower l., the hip, thigh, leg, ankle, and foot. SYN lower extremity.

   phantom l., the sensation that an amputated l. is still present, often associated with painful paresthesia. SYN pseudesthesia (3).

   upper l., the shoulder, arm, forearm, wrist, and hand. SYN upper extremity.

lim•bic (lim′bik). **1.** Relating to a limbus. **2.** Relating to the limbic *system*.

lim•bus, pl. **lim•bi** (lim′bŭs, lim′bī) [NA]. The edge, border, or fringe of a part. [L. a border]

   l. of cornea, the margin of the cornea overlapped by the sclera.

lime (līm). **1.** CaO; an alkaline earth oxide occurring in grayish white masses (quicklime); on exposure to the atmosphere it becomes converted into calcium hydrate and calcium carbonate (airslaked l.); direct addition of water to calcium oxide produces calcium hydrate (slaked l.). SYN

calx (1). **2.** Fruit of the l. tree, *Citrus medica*, which is a source of ascorbic acid and acts as an antiscorbutic agent. [O.E. *līm*, birdlime]

li•men, pl. **li•mi•na** (lī′men, lim′i-nă) [NA]. Entrance; the external opening of a canal or space, such as l. insulae. SYN threshold (4). [L.]

   l. in′sulae [NA], the band of transition between the anterior portion of the gray matter of the insula and the anterior perforated substance; it is formed by a narrow strip of olfactory cortex along the lateral side of the lateral olfactory stria.

   l. na′si [NA], a ridge marking the boundary between the nasal cavity proper and the vestibule.

limes (lī′mēz). A boundary, limit, or threshold. SEE ALSO L *doses,* under *dose.* [L.]

lim•i•nal (lim′i-năl). **1.** Pertaining to a threshold. **2.** Pertaining to a stimulus just strong enough to excite a tissue, *e.g.*, nerve or muscle. [L. *limen (limin-)*, a threshold]

lim•it. A boundary or end. [L. *limes*, boundary]

   dose equivalent l.'s, radiation exposure l.'s for radiation workers. Will replace maximum permissible dose.

   short-term exposure l., the maximum concentration of a chemical to which workers may be exposed continuously for up to 15 minutes without danger to health or work efficiency and safety.

limp. A lame walk with a yielding step; asymmetrical gait. SEE ALSO claudication.

linc•ture, linc•tus (link′chŭr, link′tŭs). An electuary or a confection; originally a medical preparation taken by licking. [L. *lingo*, pp. *linctus*, to lick]

line (līn). **1.** A mark, strip, or streak. In anatomy, a long narrow mark, strip, or streak distinguished from the adjacent tissues by a color, texture, or elevation. SEE ALSO line. **2.** A unit of measurement used by histologists in the 19th century; it varied in different countries from $\frac{1}{10}$ to $\frac{1}{12}$ of an English inch. **3.** A laboratory derivative of a stock of organisms maintained under defined physical conditions. **4.** A section of tubing supplying fluid or conducting impulses for monitoring equipment; *e.g.*, intravenous l., arterial l. SYN linea [NA]. [L. *linea*, a linen thread, a string, line, fr *linum*, flax]

   absorption l.'s, the dark l.'s in the solar spectrum due to absorption by the solar and the earth's atmosphere.

   acanthomeatal l., an imaginary l. between the acanthion and the external auditory meatus; used for radiographic positioning of the skull.

   anocutaneous l., SYN pectinate l.

   arterial l., an intra-arterial catheter.

   base l., a l. approximating the base of the skull passing from the infraorbital ridge to the midline of the occiput, intersecting the superior margin or the external auditory meatus; the skull is in the anatomical position when the base line lies in the horizontal plane. SYN orbitomeatal l.

   bismuth l., a black zone on the free margin of gingiva, often the first sign of poisoning from prolonged parenteral administration of bismuth.

   blue l., a bluish l. along the free border of the gingiva, occurring in chronic heavy metal poisoning.

cell l., (1) in tissue culture, the cells growing in the first or later subculture from a primary culture. (2) a clone of cultured cells derived from an identified parental cell type.

cement l., the refractile boundary of an osteon or interstitial lamellar system in compact bone.

cervical l., a continuous anatomical irregular curved l. marking the cervical end of the crown of a tooth and the cementoenamel junction.

Clapton's l., a greenish discoloration of the marginal gingiva in cases of chronic copper poisoning.

cleavage l.'s, lines which can be extrapolated by connecting linear openings made when a round pin is driven into the skin of a cadaver, resulting from the principal axis of orientation of the subcutaneous connective tissue (collagen) fibers of the dermis; they vary in direction with the region of the body surface.

l. of demarcation, a zone of inflammatory reaction separating a gangrenous area from healthy tissue.

Dennie's l., an accentuated line or fold below the margin of the lower eyelid; characteristic in atopic dermatitis.

developmental l.'s, SYN developmental *grooves*, under *groove*.

epiphysial l., the line of junction of the epiphysis and diaphysis of a long bone where growth in length occurs. SYN linea epiphysialis [NA].

l. of fixation, a l. joining the object (or point of fixation) with the fovea.

Fleischner l.'s, coarse linear shadows on a chest radiograph, indicating bands of subsegmental atelectasis.

Futcher's l., a dorsoventral line of pigmentation occurring symmetrically and bilaterally for about 10 cm along the lateral edge of the biceps muscle; it is seen in some African Americans.

germ l., a collection of haploid cells derived from the specialized cells of the primitive gonad.

gum l., the position of the margin of the gingiva in relation to the teeth in the dental arch.

Hilton's white l., SYN white l. of anal canal.

His' l., a l. extending from the tip of the anterior nasal spine (acanthion) to the hindmost point on the posterior margin of the foramen magnum (opisthion), dividing the face into an upper and a lower, or dental part.

iliopectineal l., SYN *linea* terminalis.

inferior temporal l., the lower of two curved lines on the parietal bone; it marks the outer limit of attachment of the temporalis muscle.

intertrochanteric l., a rough line that separates the neck and shaft of the femur anteriorly; it passes downward and medially from the greater trochanter to the lesser trochanter and continues into the medial lip of the linea aspera. SYN linea intertrochanterica [NA].

isoelectric l., the baseline of the electrocardiogram.

Kerley B l.'s, fine peripheral septal l.'s.

M l., a fine l. in the center of the A band of the sarcomere of striated muscle myofibrils. SYN M band.

mamillary l., a vertical line passing through the nipple on either side. SYN nipple l.

mammary l., a transverse l. drawn between the two nipples.

milk l., SYN mammary *ridge*.

nipple l., SYN mamillary l.

orbitomeatal l. (OML), SYN base l.

pectinate l., the l. between the simple columnar epithelium of the rectum and the stratified epithelium of the anal canal. SYN linea anocutanea [NA], anocutaneous l.

Poupart's l., a vertical l. passing through the center of the inguinal ligament on either side; it marks off the hypochondriac, lumbar, and iliac from the epigastric, umbilical, and hypogastric regions, respectively.

Reid's base l., a l. drawn from the inferior margin of the orbit to the auricular point (center of the orifice of the external acoustic meatus) and extending backward to the center of the occipital bone. Used as the zero plane in computed tomography.

semilunar l., SYN *linea* semilunaris.

Shenton's l., a curved l. formed by the top of the obturator foramen and the inner side of the neck of the femur, seen on an anteroposterior frontal radiograph of a normal hip joint; it is disturbed in lesions of the joint such as dislocation or fracture.

sternal l., a vertical line corresponding to the lateral margin of the sternum. SYN linea sternalis [NA].

superior temporal l., the upper of two curved lines on the parietal bone; the temporal fascia is attached to it.

terminal l., SYN *linea* terminalis.

trapezoid l., the area on the inferior surface of the clavicle near its lateral extremity on which the trapezoid ligament attaches.

vibrating l., the imaginary l. across the posterior part of the palate, marking the division between the movable and immovable tissues.

white l., (1) SYN *linea* alba. (2) a pale streak appearing within 30 to 60 seconds after stroking the skin with a fingernail, and lasting for several minutes; regarded as a sign of diminished arterial tension.

white l. of anal canal, a bluish pink, narrow, wavy zone in the mucosa of the anal canal below the pectinate l. at the level of the interval between the subcutaneous part of the external sphincter and the lower border of the internal sphincter, said to be palpable. SYN Hilton's white l.

Z l., a cross-striation bisecting the I band of striated muscle myofibrils and serving as the anchoring point of actin filaments at either end of the sarcomere. SYN Z band.

lin•e•a, gen. and pl. **lin•e•ae** (lin′ē-ă, -ē-ē) [NA]. SYN line. [L.]

l. al′ba [NA], a fibrous band running vertically the entire length of the center of the anterior abdominal wall, receiving the attachments of the oblique and transverse abdominal muscles. SYN white line (1).

l. anocuta′nea [NA], SYN pectinate *line*.

lin′eae atroph′icae, SYN *striae* cutis distensae, under *stria*.

l. epiphysia′lis [NA], SYN epiphysial *line*.

li

l. intertrochanter´ica [NA], SYN intertrochanteric *line*.

l. ni´gra, the l. alba in pregnancy, which then becomes pigmented.

l. semiluna´ris [NA], the slight groove in the external abdominal wall parallel to the lateral edge of the rectus sheath. SYN semilunar line.

l. sterna´lis [NA], SYN sternal *line*.

l. termina´lis [NA], an oblique ridge on the inner surface of the ilium and continued on the pubis, which forms the lower boundary of the iliac fossa; it separates the true from the false pelvis. SYN iliopectineal line, terminal line.

lin·e·ar (lin´ē-ăr). Pertaining to or resembling a line.

lin·gua, gen. and pl. **lin·guae** (ling´gwă, ling´gwē) [NA]. **1.** SYN tongue (1). **2.** SYN tongue (2). [L. tongue]

l. geograph´ica, SYN geographic *tongue*.

l. ni´gra, SYN black *tongue*.

lin·gual (ling´gwăl). **1.** Relating to the tongue or any tongue-like part. SYN glossal. **2.** Next to or toward the tongue.

lin·gui·form (ling´gwi-fōrm). Tongue-shaped.

lin·gu·la, pl. **lin·gu·lae** (ling´gyū-lă, -lē) [NA]. **1.** A term applied to several tongue-shaped processes, particularly that of the cerebellum and of the upper lobe of the left lung. **2.** When not qualified, the l. of cerebellum. [L. dim. of *lingua,* tongue]

lin·gu·lar (ling´gyū-lăr). Pertaining to any lingula.

lin·gu·lec·to·my (ling´gyū-lek´tō-mē). **1.** SYN glossectomy. **2.** Excision of the lingular portion of the upper lobe of the left lung.

△**linguo-.** The tongue. [L. *lingua*]

lin·guo·clu·sion (ling-gwō-klū´zhŭn). Displacement of a tooth toward the interior of the dental arch, or toward the tongue.

lin·guo·pap·il·li·tis (ling´gwō-pap´i-lī´tis). Small painful ulcers involving the papillae on the tongue margins.

lin·guo·ver·sion (ling´gwō-ver-zhŭn). Malposition of a tooth lingual to the normal position.

lin·i·ment (lin´i-ment). A liquid preparation for external use; frequently applied by friction to the skin. [L., fr. *lino,* to smear]

li·ni·tis (li-nī´tis, lī-nī´tis). Inflammation of cellular tissue, specifically of the perivascular tissue of the stomach. [G. *linon,* flax, linen cloth, + *-itis,* inflammation]

l. plas´tica, infiltrating scirrhous carcinoma, causing extensive thickening of the wall of the stomach; often called leather-bottle stomach.

link·age (lingk´ij). **1.** A chemical covalent bond. **2.** The relationship between syntenic loci sufficiently close that the respective alleles are not inherited independently by the offspring; a characteristic of loci, not genes.

sex l., inheritance of a trait or a sex chromosome or gonosome. A man receives all his sex-linked genes from his mother and transmits them all to his daughters but not to his sons; a recessive sex-linked character is much more likely to be expressed in the male. SEE ALSO sex *chromosomes,* under *chromosome.*

linked. Said of two genetic loci that exhibit genetic linkage.

link·er. A fragment of synthetic DNA containing a restriction site that may be used for splicing genes.

lip. 1. One of the two muscular folds with an outer mucosa having a stratified squamous epithelial surface layer that bound the mouth anteriorly. **2.** Any liplike structure bounding a cavity or groove. SEE ALSO labium, labrum. SYN labium (1) [NA]. [A.S. *lippa*]

cleft l., a congenital facial deformity of the l. (usually the upper l.) due to failure of fusion of the medial and lateral nasal prominences and maxillary process; frequently but not necessarily associated with cleft alveolus and cleft palate. SYN harelip.

l.'s of mouth, lips of the mouth.

△**lip-.** SEE lipo-.

li·pase (lip´ās). Any fat-splitting or lipolytic enzyme; a carboxylesterase.

lip·ec·to·my (lip-ek´tō-mē). Surgical removal of fatty tissue, as in cases of adiposity. [lipo- + G. *ektomē,* excision]

lip·e·de·ma (lip´e-dē´mă). Chronic swelling, usually of the lower extremities, particularly in middle-aged women, caused by the widespread even distribution of subcutaneous fat and fluid. [lipo- + G. *oidēma,* swelling]

li·pe·mia (lip-ē´mē-ă). The presence of an abnormally high concentration of lipids in the circulating blood. SYN hyperlipidemia, hyperlipoidemia, lipidemia, lipoidemia. [lipid + G. *haima,* blood]

alimentary l., relatively transient l. occurring after the ingestion of foods with a large content of fat.

l. retina´lis, a creamy appearance of the retinal blood vessels that occurs when the lipids of the blood exceed 5%.

li·pe·mic (li-pē´mik). Relating to lipemia.

lip·id (lip´id). An operational term describing a solubility characteristic, not a chemical substance, *i.e.,* denoting substances extracted from animal or vegetable cells by nonpolar or "fat" solvents; included are fatty acids, glycerides and glyceryl ethers, phospholipids, sphingolipids, alcohols and waxes, terpenes, steroids, and "fat soluble" vitamins A, D, and E. [G. *lipos,* fat]

lip·i·de·mia (lip´i-dē´mē-ă). SYN lipemia.

lip·i·do·sis, pl. **lip·i·do·ses** (lip-i-dō´sis, -sēz). Hereditary abnormality of lipid metabolism that results in abnormal amounts of lipid deposition; classification is based on the responsible enzymatic deficiency and type of lipid involved. Such enzymatic activity takes place in the lysosomes and the abnormal products appear as lysosomal storage diseases. Sphingolipidoses make up the largest portion of recognized lipidoses, including abnormal metabolism of gangliosides, ceramides and cerebrosides. [lipid + G. *-ōsis,* condition]

△**lipo-, lip-.** Fatty, lipid. [G. *lipos,* fat]

lip·o·ar·thri·tis (lip´ō-ar-thrī´tis). Inflammation of the periarticular fatty tissues of the knee. [lipo- + arthritis]

lip·o·ate (lip´ō-āt). A salt or ester of lipoic acid.

l. acetyltransferase, SYN dihydrolipoamide acetyltransferase.

lip·o·at·ro·phy (lip-ō-at′rō-fē). Loss of subcutaneous fat, which may be total, congenital, and associated with hepatomegaly, excessive bone growth, and insulin-resistant diabetes. [G. *lipos*, fat, + *a-*, priv. + *trophē*, nourishment]

lip·o·blast (lip′ō-blast). An embryonic fat cell. [lipo- + G. *blastos*, germ]

lip·o·blas·to·ma (lip′ō-blas-tō′mă). 1. SYN liposarcoma. 2. A benign subcutaneous tumor composed of embryonal fat cells separated into distinct lobules, occurring usually in infants.

lip·o·blas·to·ma·to·sis (lip′ō-blas-tō-mă-tō′sis). A diffuse form of lipoblastoma that infiltrates locally but does not metastasize.

lip·o·cer·a·tous (lip-ō-ser′ă-tŭs). SYN adipoceratous.

lip·o·cere (lip′ō-sēr). SYN adipocere. [lipo- + L. *cera*, wax]

lip·o·chrome (lip′ō-krōm). 1. A pigmented lipid, *e.g.*, lutein, carotene. 2. More specifically, yellow pigments that seem to be identical to carotene and xanthophyll and are frequently found in the serum, skin, adrenal cortex, corpus luteum, and arteriosclerotic plaques, as well as in the liver, spleen, and adipose tissue. 3. The pigment produced by certain bacteria. [lipo- + G. *chroma*, color]

lip·o·crit (lip′ō-krit). An apparatus and procedure for separating and volumetrically analyzing the amount of lipid in blood or other body fluid. [lipo- + G. *krinō*, to separate]

lip·o·cyte (lip′ō-sīt). SYN fat-storing *cell*. [lipo- + G. *kytos*, cell]

lip·o·der·moid (lip-ō-der′moyd). Congenital, yellowish-white, fatty, benign tumor located subconjunctivally. [lipo- + dermoid]

lip·o·dys·tro·phy (lip-ō-dis′trō-fē) [MIM* 157660]. Defective metabolism of fat. [lipo- + G. *dys-*, bad, difficult, + *trophē*, nourishment]

lip·o·e·de·ma (lip′ō-e-dē′mă). Edema of subcutaneous fat, causing painful swellings, especially of the legs in women. SYN cellulite (2).

lip·o·fi·bro·ma (lip′ō-fī-brō′mă). A benign neoplasm of fibrous connective tissue, with conspicuous numbers of adipose cells.

lip·o·fus·cin (lip-ō-fyūs′in). Brown pigment granules representing lipid-containing residues of lysosomal digestion and considered one of the aging or "wear and tear" pigments; found in liver, kidney, heart muscle, adrenal, and ganglion cells.

lip·o·fus·ci·no·sis (lip′ō-fyūs-i-nō′sis). Abnormal storage of any one of a group of fatty pigments.

lip·o·gen·e·sis (lip-ō-jen′ĕ-sis). The production of fat, either fatty degeneration or fatty infiltration; also applied to the normal deposition of fat or to the conversion of carbohydrate or protein to fat. SYN adipogenesis. [lipo- + G. *genesis*, production]

lip·o·gen·ic (lip-ō-jen′ik). Relating to lipogenesis. SYN adipogenic, adipogenous, lipogenous.

li·pog·e·nous (li-poj′ĕ-nŭs). SYN lipogenic.

lip·o·gran·u·lo·ma (lip′ō-gran-yū-lō′mă). A nodule or focus of granulomatous inflammation (usually of the foreign-body type) in association with lipid material deposited in tissues, *e.g.*, after the injection of certain oils. SEE ALSO paraffinoma.

lip·o·gran·u·lo·ma·to·sis (lip′ō-gran′yū-lō-mă-tō′sis). 1. Presence of lipogranulomas. 2. Local inflammatory reaction to necrosis of adipose tissue.

lip·oid (lip′oyd). 1. Resembling fat. 2. Former term for lipid. SYN adipoid. [lipo- + G. *eidos*, appearance]

lip·oi·de·mia (lip-oy-dē′mē-ă). SYN lipemia.

lip·oi·do·sis (lip-oy-do′sis). Presence of anisotropic lipoids in the cells.

li·pol·y·sis (li-pol′i-sis). The splitting up (hydrolysis), or chemical decomposition, of fat. [lipo- + G. *lysis*, dissolution]

lip·o·lyt·ic (lip-ō-lit′ik). Relating to or causing lipolysis.

li·po·ma (li-pō′mă). A benign neoplasm of adipose tissue, composed of mature fat cells. [lipo- + G. *-oma*, tumor]

  atypical l., l., occurring primarily in older men on the posterior neck, shoulders, and back, which is benign but microscopically atypical, containing giant cells with multiple overlapping nuclei forming a circle. SYN pleomorphic l.

  pleomorphic l., SYN atypical l.

  spindle cell l., a microscopically distinctive form of l. in which adipose tissue is infiltrated by fibroblasts and collagen; usually found in the shoulder or neck of elderly men.

li·po·ma·toid (li-pō′mă-toyd). Resembling a lipoma, frequently said of accumulations of adipose tissue that is not thought to be neoplastic.

lip·o·ma·to·sis (lip′ō-mă-tō′sis). SYN adiposis.

li·po·ma·tous (li-pō′mă-tŭs). Pertaining to or manifesting the features of lipoma, or characterized by the presence of a lipoma (or lipomas).

lip·o·me·nin·go·cele (lip′ō-mĕ-ning′gō-sēl). An intraspinal cauda equinal lipoma associated with a spina bifida. [lipo- + G. *mēninx*, membrane, + *kēlē*, tumor]

lip·o·pe·nia (lip-ō-pē′nē-ă). An abnormally small amount, or a deficiency, of lipids in the body. [lipo- + G. *penia*, poverty]

lip·o·phage (lip′ō-fāj). A cell that ingests fat. [G. *lipos*, fat, + *phagō*, to eat]

lip·o·phag·ic (lip-ō-fā′jik). Relating to lipophagy.

lip·oph·a·gy (lip-of′ă-jē). Ingestion of fat by a lipophage. [lipo- + G. *phagō*, to eat]

lip·o·phil (lip′ō-fil). A substance with lipophilic (hydrophobic) properties. [lipo- + G. *philos*, fond of]

lip·o·phil·ic (lip-ō-fil′ik). Capable of dissolving, of being dissolved in, or of absorbing lipids.

lip·o·pol·y·sac·cha·ride (lip′ō-pol′ē-sak′ă-rīd). A compound or complex of lipid and carbohydrate; the l. (endotoxin) released from the cell walls of Gram-negative organisms that produces septic shock.

lip·o·pro·tein (lip-ō-prō′tēn). Complexes or compounds containing lipid and protein. Almost all the lipids in plasma are present as l.'s and are therefore transported as such. Plasma l.'s are characterized by their flotation constants as chylomicra, very low density (VLDL), intermediate density (IDL), low density (LD), high density

(HDL), very high density (VHDL). They range in molecular weight from 175,000 to 1×10^9. Levels of l.'s are important in assessing the risk of cardiovascular disease.

α_1**-lip·o·pro·tein.** A lipoprotein fraction of relatively low molecular weight, high density, rich in phospholipids, and found in the α_1-globulin fraction of human plasma.

β_1**-lip·o·pro·tein.** A lipoprotein fraction of relatively high molecular weight, low density, rich in cholesterol, and found in the β-globulin fraction of human plasma.

lip·o·pro·tein li·pase. An enzyme that hydrolyzes one fatty acid from a triacylglycerol; its activity is enhanced by heparin and inactivated by heparinase. SEE ALSO clearing *factors*, under *factor*.

lip·o·sar·co·ma (lip′ō-sar-kō′mă). A malignant neoplasm of adults that occurs especially in the retroperitoneal tissues and the thigh; planes composed of well-differentiated fat cells, or may be dedifferentiated, either myxoid, round celled, or pleomorphic; recurrences are common, and dedifferentiated l.'s metastasize to the lungs or serosal surfaces. SYN lipoblastoma (1). [lipo- + *sarx*, flesh, + *-oma*, tumor]

li·po·sis (li-pō′sis). **1.** SYN adiposis. **2.** Fatty infiltration, neutral fats being present in the cells. [lipo- + G. *-osis*, condition]

lip·o·sol·u·ble (lip-ō-sol′yū-bl). Fat-soluble.

lip·o·suc·tion·ing (lip′ō-sŭk′shŭn-ing). Removal of fat by high vacuum pressure; used in body contouring.

lip·o·tro·phic (lip-ō-trof′ik). Relating to lipotrophy.

li·pot·ro·phy (li-pot′rō-fē). An increase of fat in the body. [lipo- + G. *trophē*, nourishment]

lip·o·tro·pic (lip-ō-trop′ik). **1.** Pertaining to substances preventing or correcting excessive fat deposits in liver such as occurs in choline deficiency. **2.** Relating to lipotropy.

lip·o·tro·pin (lip-ō-trō′pin). A pituitary hormone mobilizing fat from adipose tissue. SYN lipotropic hormone, lipotropic pituitary hormone.

li·pot·ro·py (li-pot′rō-pē). **1.** Affinity of basic dyes for fatty tissue. **2.** Prevention of accumulation of fat in the liver. **3.** Affinity of nonpolar substances for each other. [lipo- + G. *tropē*, turning]

lip·o·vac·cine (lip′ō-vak-sēn). A vaccine having a vegetable oil as a solvent.

li·pox·i·dase (li-poks′i-dās). SYN lipoxygenase.

li·pox·y·ge·nase (li-poks′ē-jĕ-nās). An enzyme that catalyzes the oxidation of unsaturated fatty acids with O_2 to yield hydroperoxides of the fatty acids. SYN lipoxidase.

lip·ping (lip′ing). The formation of a liplike structure, as at the articular end of a bone in osteoarthritis.

li·pu·ria (li-pū′rē-ă). Presence of lipids in the urine. SYN adiposuria. [lipo- + G. *ouron*, urine]

li·pur·ic (li-pū′rik). Pertaining to lipuria.

liq·ue·fa·cient (lik′we-fā′shent). **1.** Making liquid; causing a solid to become liquid. **2.** Denoting a resolvent supposed to cause the resolution of a solid tumor by liquefying its contents. [L. *lique-*

facio, pres. p. *-faciens*, to make fluid, fr. *liqueo*, to be liquid]

liq·ue·fac·tion (lik-wĕ-fak′shŭn). The act of becoming liquid; change from a solid to a liquid form. [see liquefacient]

li·ques·cent (li-kwes′ent). Becoming or tending to become liquid. [L. *liquesco*, to become liquid]

liq·uid (lik′wid). **1.** An inelastic substance, like water, that is neither solid nor gaseous. **2.** Flowing like water. [L. *liquidus*]

li·quor, gen. **li·quor·is**, pl. **li·quo·res** (lik′er, lik′ wōr; -wōr-is; -wō′rēs). **1.** Any liquid or fluid. **2.** A term used for certain body fluids. **3.** The pharmacopeial term for any aqueous solution (not a decoction or infusion) of a nonvolatile substance and for aqueous solutions of gases. SEE ALSO solution. [L.]

lisp·ing. Mispronunciation of the sibilants *s* and *z*.

lis·sen·ce·pha·lia (lis′en-sĕ-fā′lē-ă). SYN agyria. [G. *lissos*, smooth, + *enkephalos*, brain]

lis·sen·ce·phal·ic (lis′en-sĕ-fal′ik). Pertaining to, or characterized by, lissencephalia.

lis·sive (lis′iv). Having the property of relieving muscle spasm without causing flaccidity. [G. *lissos*, smooth]

lis·so·sphinc·ter (lis′ō-sfingk′ter). A sphincter of smooth musculature. [G. *lissos*, smooth, + sphincter]

Lis·te·ria (lis-tēr-ē-ă). A genus of aerobic to microaerophilic, motile, bacteria (family Corynebacteriaceae) containing small, coccoid, Gram-positive rods; found in the feces of humans and other animals, on vegetation, and in silage, and parasitic on poikilothermic and warm-blooded animals, including humans. The type species is *L. monocytogenes*. [Joseph *Lister*]

lis·te·ri·o·sis (lis-tēr′ē-ō′sis). A sporadic disease of animals and humans, particularly those who are immunocompromised or pregnant, caused by the bacterium, *Listeria monocytogenes*. [fr. organism *Listeria*]

lis·ter·ism (lis′ter-izm). SYN Lister's *method*.

li·ter (l) (lē′ter). A measure of capacity of 1000 cubic centimeters or 1 cubic decimeter; equivalent to 1.056688 quarts (U.S., liquid). [Fr., fr. G. *litra*, a pound]

△**lith-.** SEE litho-.

lith·a·gogue (lith′ă-gog). Causing the dislodgment or expulsion of calculi, especially urinary calculi. [litho- + G. *agōgos*, drawing forth]

li·thec·to·my (li-thek′tō-mē). SYN lithotomy. [litho- + G. *ektomē*, excision]

li·thi·a·sis (li-thī′ă-sis). Formation of calculi of any kind, especially of biliary or urinary calculi. [litho- + G. *-iasis*, condition]

lith·i·um (Li) (lith′ē-ŭm). An element of the alkali metal group, atomic no. 3, atomic wt 6.941. Many salts have clinical applications. [Mod. L. fr. G. *lithos*, a stone]

△**litho-, lith-.** A stone, calculus, calcification. [G. *lithos*]

lith·o·clast (lith′ō-klast). SYN lithotrite. [litho- + G. *klastos*, broken]

lith·o·gen·e·sis, li·thog·e·ny (lith-ō-jen′ĕ-sis, lith-oj′ĕ-nē). Formation of calculi. [litho- + G. *genesis*, production]

lith·o·gen·ic (lith-ō-jen′ik). Promoting the formation of calculi.

lith·og·e·nous (lith-oj′ĕ-nŭs). Calculus-forming.

li·thol·a·paxy (li-thol′ă-pak-sē). The operation of crushing a stone in the bladder and washing out the fragments through a catheter. [litho- + G. *lapaxis,* an emptying out]

li·thol·y·sis (li-thol′i-sis). The dissolution of urinary calculi. [litho- + G. *lysis,* dissolution]

lith·o·lyt·ic (lith-ō-lit′ik). **1.** Tending to dissolve calculi. **2.** An agent having such properties. [litho- + G. *lysis,* dissolution]

lith·o·ne·phri·tis (lith′ō-ne-frī′tis). Interstitial nephritis associated with calculus formation.

lith·o·pe·di·on, lith·o·pe·di·um (lith-ō-pē′dē-on, -ŭm). A retained fetus, usually extrauterine, which has become calcified. [litho- + G. *paidion,* small child]

li·thot·o·my (li-thot′ō-mē). Cutting for stone; a cutting operation for the removal of a calculus, especially a vesical calculus. SYN lithectomy. [litho- + G. *tomē,* incision]

lith·o·trip·sy (lith′ō-trip-sē). The crushing of a stone in the renal pelvis, ureter, or bladder, by mechanical force or sound waves. SYN lithotrity. [litho- + G. *tripsis,* a rubbing]

  electrohydraulic shock wave l. (ESWL), destruction of calculi (urinary tract or other) by fragmentation using shock waves sent transcutaneously.

  extracorporeal shock wave l. (ESWL) (lith′ō-trip′sē), breaking up of renal or ureteral calculi by focused ultrasound energy.

lith·o·trip·tic (lith-ō-trip′tik). **1.** Relating to lithotripsy. **2.** An agent that effects the dissolution of a calculus.

lith·o·trip·tos·co·py (lith′ō-trip-tos′kŏ-pē). Crushing of a stone in the bladder under direct vision by use of a lithotriptoscope. [litho- + G. *tribō,* to rub, crush, + *skopeō,* to view]

lith·o·trite (lith′ō-trīt). A mechanical instrument used to crush a urinary calculus in lithotripsy. SYN lithoclast. [litho- + L. *tero,* pp. *tritus,* to rub]

li·thot·ri·ty (li-thot′ri-tē). SYN lithotripsy.

lith·u·re·sis (lith′yū-rē′sis). The passage of gravel in the urine. [litho- + G. *ourēsis,* urination]

lit·mus (lit′mŭs). A blue coloring matter obtained from *Roccella tinctorial* and other lichens, the principal component of which is azolitmin; used as an indicator (reddened by acids and turned blue again by alkalies). [Dutch *lakmoes*]

lit·ter (lit′er). **1.** A stretcher or portable couch for moving the sick or injured. **2.** A group of animals of the same parents, born at the same time. [Fr. *litière;* fr. *lit,* bed]

li·ve·do (li-vē′dō). A bluish discoloration of the skin, either in limited patches or general. [L. lividness, fr. *liveo,* to be black and blue]

  postmortem l., a purple coloration of dependent parts, except in areas of contact pressure, appearing within one half to two hours after death, as a result of gravitational movement of blood within the vessels. SYN postmortem lividity.

  l. reticula′ris, a persistent purplish network-patterned discoloration of the skin caused by dilation of capillaries and venules due to stasis or changes in underlying blood vessels including hyalinization.

liv·e·doid (liv′ĕ-doyd). Pertaining to or resembling livedo.

liv·er (liv′er). The largest gland of the body, lying beneath the diaphragm in the right hypochondrium and upper part of the epigastrium; it is of irregular shape and weighs from 1 to 2 kg, or about $\frac{1}{40}$ the weight of the body. It secretes the bile and is also of great importance in both carbohydrate and protein metabolism. SYN hepar [NA]. [A.S. *lifer*]

  fatty l., yellow discoloration of the l. due to fatty degeneration of l. parenchymal cells.

  frosted l., hyaloserositis of the liver.

  hobnail l., in Laënnec's cirrhosis, the contraction of scar tissue and hepatic cellular regeneration which causes a nodular appearance of the l.'s surface.

  polycystic l., gradual cystic dilation of intralobular bile ducts (Meyenburg's complexes) that fail to involute in embryonic development of the l.; associated with polycystic kidneys and occasionally with cystic involvement of the pancreas, lungs, and other organs.

liv·id. Having a black and blue or a leaden or ashy gray color, as in discoloration from a contusion, congestion, or cyanosis. [L. *lividus,* being black and blue]

li·vid·i·ty (li-vid′i-tē). The state of being livid.

  postmortem l., SYN postmortem *livedo.*

living will. Legal document used to indicate one's preference to die rather than be sustained artificially if sick or injured beyond the prospect of recovery. SEE advance directive.

li·vor (lī′vōr). The livid discoloration of the skin on the dependent parts of a corpse. [L. a black and blue spot]

lix·iv·i·a·tion (lik-siv-ē-ā′shŭn). SYN leaching. [L. *lixivius,* made into lye, fr. *lix,* lye]

LM licentiate in midwifery.

lm lumen (2).

LMA left mentoanterior position.

LMP left mentoposterior position.

LMT left mentotransverse position.

LNPF lymph node permeability *factor.*

load (lōd). A departure from normal body content, as of water, salt, or heat; positive l.'s are quantities in excess of the normal; negative l.'s are quantities in deficit.

  genetic l., the aggregate of more or less harmful genes that are carried, mostly hidden, in the genome and may be transmitted to descendants and cause disease.

load·ing (lōd′ing). Administration of a substance for the purpose of testing metabolic function or of rapidly achieving therapeutic levels of a drug.

  axial l., loading (application of weight or force) along the long axis of the body.

  carbohydrate l., combination of diet and exercise to significantly increase muscle and liver glycogen content. Frequently used by endurance athletes to enhance performance. SYN glycogen l.

  glycogen l., SYN carbohydrate l.

Loa loa (lō′ă lō′ă). The African eye worm, a species of the family Onchocercidae that is the causal agent of loiasis. Humans are the only known definitive host, and parasites are transmitted by *Chrysops* flies; infective larvae from the latter require 3 years or more to mature in humans, and the adult forms may persist in humans for as long as 17 years. SEE ALSO loiasis.

lo•bar (lō′bar). Relating to any lobe.

lo•bate (lō′bāt). **1.** Divided into lobes. **2.** Lobe-shaped; denoting a bacterial colony with a deeply undulate margin.

lobe (lōb). **1.** One of the subdivisions of an organ or other part, bounded by fissures, connective tissue, septa, or other structural demarcations. **2.** A rounded projecting part, as the l. of the ear. SEE ALSO lobule. **3.** One of the larger divisions of the crown of a tooth, formed from a distinct point of calcification. SYN lobus [NA]. [G. *lobos,* lobe]

   anterior l. of hypophysis, ☆official alternate term for adenohypophysis.

   az′ygos l. of lung, a small accessory l. sometimes found on the apex of the right lung; separated from the rest of the upper l. by a deep groove lodging the azygos vein.

   caudate l., SYN *lobus* caudatus.

   frontal l. of cerebrum, the portion of each cerebral hemisphere anterior to the central sulcus.

   left l. of liver, it is separated from the right lobe above and in front by the falciform ligament, and from the quadrate and caudate lobes by the fissure for the ligamentum teres and the fissure for the ligamentum venosum; the distribution of the portal vein, hepatic artery, and bile ducts does not correspond to the gross lobar divisions of the liver. It contains two segments, superior and inferior. SYN lobus hepatis sinister [NA].

   nervous l. of hypophysis, the bulbous part of the neurohypophysis attached to the hypothalamus by the infundibulum. It is composed of pituicytes, blood vessels, and terminals of nerve fibers from the supraoptic and paraventricular nuclei.

   occipital l. of cerebrum, the posterior, somewhat pyramid-shaped part of each cerebral hemisphere, demarcated by no distinct surface markings on the lateral convexity of the hemisphere from the parietal and temporal lobes, but sharply delineated from the parietal lobe by the parieto-occipital sulcus on the medial surface.

   parietal l. of cerebrum, the middle portion of each cerebral hemisphere, separated from the frontal lobe by the central sulcus, from the temporal lobe by the lateral sulcus in front and an imaginary line projected posteriorly, and from the occipital lobe only partially by the parieto-occipital sulcus on its medial aspect.

   posterior l. of hypophysis, SYN neurohypophysis.

   pyramidal l. of thyroid gland, an inconstant narrow lobe of the thyroid gland that arises from the upper border of the isthmus and extends upward, sometimes as far as the hyoid bone; it marks the point of continuity with the thyroglossal duct.

   quadrate l., (1) a lobe on the inferior surface of the liver located between the fossa for the gallbladder and the fissure for the ligamentum teres; **(2)** SYN quadrangular *lobule.* **(3)** SYN precuneus.

   Riedel's l., an occasional tongue-like process

extending downward from the right l. of the liver lateral to the gallbladder.

   right l. of liver, the largest lobe of the liver, separated from the left lobe above and in front by the falciform ligament and from the caudate and quadrate lobes by the sulcus for the vena cava and the fossa for the gallbladder; it contains two segments, anterior and posterior. SYN lobus hepatis dexter [NA].

   Spigelius' l., SYN *lobus* caudatus.

   temporal l., a long l., the lowest of the major subdivisions of the cortical mantle, forming the posterior two-thirds of the ventral surface of the cerebral hemisphere, separated from the frontal and parietal l.'s above it by the lateral sulcus arbitrarily delineated by an imaginary plane from the occipital l. with which it is continuous posteriorly. The temporal l. has a heterogeneous composition: in addition to a large neocortical component consisting of the superior, middle, and inferior temporal gyri and the lateral and medial occipitotemporal gyri, it includes the largely juxtallocortical parahippocampal gyrus with its paleocortical (olfactory) uncus and, beneath the latter, the amygdala. SYN lobus temporalis [NA].

lo•bec•to•my (lō-bek′tō-mē). Excision of a lobe of any organ or gland. [G. *lobos,* lobe, + *ektomē,* excision]

lo•bi (lō′bī). Plural of lobus. [L.]

lo•bi•tis (lō-bī′tis). Inflammation of a lobe.

lo•bot•o•my (lō-bot′ō-mē). **1.** Incision into a lobe. **2.** Division of one or more nerve tracts in a lobe of the cerebrum. [G. *lobos,* lobe, + *tomē,* cutting]

lob•u•lar (lob′yū-lăr). Relating to a lobule.

lob•u•late, lob•u•lat•ed (lob′yū-lāt, -ed). Divided into lobules.

lob•ule (lob′yūl). A small lobe or subdivision of a lobe. SYN lobulus [NA].

   cortical l.'s of kidney, one of the subdivisions of the kidney, consisting of a medullary ray and that portion of the convoluted port (renal corpuscles and convoluted tubules) associated with its collecting duct.

   l.'s of epididymis, the coiled portion of the efferent ductules that constitute the head of the epididymis; these join the ductus epididymidis. SYN lobuli epididymidis [NA].

   hepatic l., the conceptual polygonal histologic unit of the liver consisting of masses of liver cells arranged around a central vein, a terminal branch of one of the hepatic veins; at the periphery are located preterminal and terminal branches of the portal vein, hepatic artery, and bile duct. SYN lobulus hepatis [NA].

   portal l. of liver, a conceptual unit of the liver, emphasizing its exocrine function in bile secretion, which comprises a roughly triangular shaped cross-sectional area with a portal canal at its center and three or more venae centrales hepatis at its periphery.

   primary pulmonary l., SYN pulmonary *acinus.*

   quadrangular l., the main portion of the superior part of each hemisphere of the cerebellum, corresponding to the monticulus of the vermis; it is divided into two portions, the anterior and the posterior crescentic lobules, corresponding to the culmen and the decline of the vermis. SYN quadrate lobe (2).

lob•u•lus, gen. and pl. **lob•u•li** (lob′yū-lŭs, yū-lī) [NA]. SYN lobule. [Mod. L. dim. of *lobus,* lobe]

   lob′uli epididym′idis [NA], SYN *lobules* of epididymis, under *lobule.*

   l. hep′atis [NA], SYN hepatic *lobule.*

lo•bus, gen. and pl. **lo•bi** (lō′bŭs, lō′bī) [NA]. SYN lobe. [LL. fr. G. *lobos*]

   l. ante′rior hypophys′eos [NA], SYN adenohypophysis.

   l. cauda′tus [NA], a small lobe of the liver situated posteriorly between the sulcus for the vena cava and the fissure for the ligamentum venosum. SYN caudate lobe, Spigelius' lobe.

   l. hep′atis dex′ter [NA], SYN right *lobe* of liver.

   l. hep′atis sinis′ter [NA], SYN left *lobe* of liver.

   l. poste′rior hypophys′eos [NA], *official alternate term for neurohypophysis. SEE ALSO hypophysis.

   l. tempora′lis [NA], SYN temporal *lobe.*

lo•cal (lō′kăl). Having reference or confined to a limited part; not general or systemic. [L. *localis,* fr. *locus,* place]

lo•cal•i•za•tion (lō′kăl-i-zā′shŭn). **1.** Limitation to a definite area. **2.** The reference of a sensation to its point of origin. **3.** The determination of the location of a morbid process.

   cerebral l., the mapping of the cerebral cortex into areas and the correlation of the various areas with cerebral function, or determining the site of a brain lesion, based on the signs and symptoms manifested by the patient or by neuroimaging.

   germinal l., determination in very young embryos of the presumptive areas for specific organs or structures.

lo•cal•ized (lō′kăl-īzd). Restricted or limited to a definite part.

lo•ca•tor (lō′kā-ter, tōr). An instrument or apparatus for finding the position of a foreign object in tissue.

lo•chia (lō′kē-ă). Discharge from the vagina of mucus, blood, and tissue debris, following childbirth. [G. neut. pl. of *lochios,* relating to childbirth, fr. *lochos,* childbirth]

lo•chi•al (lō′kē-ăl). Relating to the lochia.

lo•chi•o•me•tra (lō-kē-ō-mē′tră). Distention of the uterus with retained lochia. [G. *mētra,* womb]

lo•chi•or•rha•gia (lō-kē-ō-rā′jē-ă). SYN lochiorrhea. [lochia + G. *rhēgnymi,* to burst forth]

lo•chi•or•rhea (lō-kē-ō-rē′ă). Profuse flow of the lochia. SYN lochiorrhagia. [lochia + G. *rhoia,* a flow]

lo•ci (lō′sī). Plural of locus.

lock (lŏk). **1.** An enclosing, fastening, or securing device. **2.** A mechanism which, when moved, permits or obstructs passage.

   heparin l., an indwelling venous catheter used when intravenous infusions or withdrawal of venous blood for testing must be performed repeatedly over an extended period; between uses it is filled with the anticoagulant heparin.

lock•jaw (lŏk′jaw). SYN trismus.

lo•co•mo•tor (lō-kō-mō′ter). Relating to locomotion, or movement from one place to another. [L. *locus,* place, + L. *moveo,* pp. *motus,* to move]

loc•u•lar (lok′yū-lăr). Relating to a loculus.

loc•u•late (lok′yū-lāt). Containing numerous loculi.

loc•u•la•tion (lok-yū-lā′shŭn). **1.** A loculate region in an organ or tissue, or a loculate structure formed between surfaces of organs or mucous or serous membranes. **2.** The process that results in the formation of a loculus or loculi.

loc•u•lus, pl. **loc•u•li** (lok′yū-lŭs, -lī). A small cavity or chamber. [L. dim. of *locus,* place]

lo•cus, pl. **lo•ci** (lō′kŭs, lō′sī). **1.** A place; usually, a specific site. **2.** The position that a gene occupies on a chromosome lod score. GENETICS The log of the odds ratio of observed to expected distribution of genetic markers. **3.** The position of a point, as defined by the coordinates on a graph. [L.]

   l. of control, a theoretical construct designed to assess a person's perceived control over personal behavior; classified as *internal* if the person feels in control of events, *external* if others are perceived to have that control.

lod score (lod skōr). A number used in genetic linkage studies; logarithm (base 10) of the odds in favor of genetic linkage. [*log*arithm + *od*ds]

△**log-.** SEE logo-.

log•ag•no•sia (log-ag-nō′sē-ă). SYN aphasia. [logo- + G. *agnosia,* ignorance]

log•a•graph•ia (log-ă-graf′ē-ă). SYN agraphia. [logo- + G. *a-* priv. + *graphō,* to write]

log•am•ne•sia (log-am-nē′zē-ă). SYN aphasia. [logo- + G. *amnēsia,* forgetfulness]

log•a•pha•sia (log-ă-fā′zē-ă). Aphasia of articulation. [logo- + G. *aphasia,* speechlessness]

log•as•the•nia (log-as-thē′nē-ă). SYN aphasia. [logo- + G. *astheneia,* weakness]

△**-logia. 1.** The study of the subject noted in the body of the word, or a treatise on the same; the Eng. equivalent is -logy, or, with a connecting vowel, -ology. [G. *logos,* discourse, treatise] **2.** Collecting or picking. [G. *legō,* to collect]

△**logo-, log-.** Speech, words. [G. *logos,* word, discourse]

log•o•ple•gia (log-ō-plē′jē-ă). Paralysis of the organs of speech. [logo- + G. *plēgē,* stroke]

log•or•rhea (log-ō-rē′ă). Rarely used term for abnormal or pathologic talkativeness or garrulousness. [logo- + G. *rhoia,* a flow]

△**-logy.** SEE -logia. [G. *logos,* treatise, discourse]

lo•i•a•sis (lō-ī′ă-sis). A chronic disease caused by the filarial nematode *Loa loa,* with symptoms first occurring three to four years after a bite by an infected tabanid fly. When the larvae mature, the adult worms move about through connective tissue, frequently becoming visible beneath the skin and mucous membranes. The worms provoke hyperemia and exudation of fluid; the patient is annoyed by the "creeping" in the tissues and intense itching, as well as occasional pain, especially when the swelling is in the region of tendons and joints.

loin (loyn). The part of the side and back between the ribs and the pelvis. SYN lumbus [NA]. [Fr. *longe;* E. *lumbus*]

lo•mus•tine (lō-mŭs′tēn). 1-(2-Chloroethyl)-3-cyclohexyl-1-nitrosourea; an antineoplastic agent.

lon·gev·i·ty (lon-jev'i-tē). Duration of a particular life beyond the norm for the species.

lon·gi·tu·di·nal (lon'ji-tū'di-năl). **1.** Running lengthwise; in the direction of the long axis of the body or any of its parts. **2.** Studied over a period of time, diachronic; contrast with cross-sectional or synchronic, which give equivalent results only under certain strict conditions of stability and equilibrium. [L. *longitudo,* length]

long-term care facility. SYN nursing facility.

loop (lūp). **1.** A sharp curve or complete bend in a vessel, cord, or other elongate body, forming an oval or circular ring. SEE ALSO ansa. **2.** A wire (usually of platinum or nichrome) fixed into a handle at one end and bent into a circle at the other, rendered sterile by flaming, and used to transfer microorganisms. [M.E. *loupe*]

  capillary l.'s, small blood vessels in the dermal papillae.

  cervical l., SYN *ansa cervicalis.*

  Henle's l., SYN nephronic l.

  lenticular l., the pallidal efferent fibers curving around the medial border of the internal capsule.

  nephronic l., the U-shaped part of the nephron extending from the proximal to the distal convoluted tubules, consisting of descending and ascending limbs, located in the medulla renalis and medullary ray. SYN Henle's l.

  l.'s of spinal nerves, loops of the spinal nerves, connecting ventral primary rami of the spinal nerves. SYN ansae nervorum spinalium.

loos·en·ing of as·so·ci·a·tions. A manifestation of a severe thought disorder characterized by the lack of an obvious connection between one thought or phrase and the next, or with the response to a question.

lor·do·sco·li·o·sis (lōr'dō-skō-lē-ō'sis). Combined backward and lateral curvature of the spine. [G. *lordos,* bent back, + *skoliōsis,* crookedness, fr. *skolios,* bent, aslant]

lor·do·sis (lōr-dō'sis). An abnormal extension deformity; anteroposterior curvature of the spine, generally lumbar with the convexity looking anteriorly. [G. *lordōsis,* a bending backward]

lor·dot·ic (lōr-dot'ik). Pertaining to or marked by lordosis.

LOT Left occipitotransverse position.

lo·tion (lō'shŭn). A class of liquid suspensions or dispersions intended for external application. [L. *lotio,* a washing, fr. *lavo,* to wash]

loupe (lūp). A magnifying lens. [Fr.]

louse, pl. **lice** (lows, līs). Common name for members of the ectoparasitic insect orders Anoplura (sucking lice) and Mallophaga (biting lice). [A.S. *lūs*]

lox·os·ce·lism (lok-sos'ĕ-lizm). Illness produced by the brown recluse spider, *Loxosceles reclusus;* characterized by gangrenous slough at the site of the bite, nausea, malaise, fever, hemolysis, and thrombocytopenia.

loz·enge (loz'enj). SYN troche. [Fr. *losange,* fr. *lozangé,* rhombic]

LPO left posterior oblique, a radiographic projection.

Lr, L_r SEE Lr *dose.*

Lr lawrencium.

LSA Left sacroanterior position.

LSP Left sacroposterior position.

LST Left sacrotransverse position.

LT leukotrienes, usually followed by another letter with a subscript number; *e.g.,* LTA_4, LTC_4.

LTM long-term *memory.*

Lu lutetium.

lu·cid·i·ty (lū-sid'i-tē). The quality or state of being lucid.

lu·cif·u·gal (lū-sif'yū-găl). Avoiding light. [L. *lux,* light, + *fugio,* to flee from]

lu·cip·e·tal (lū-sip'i-tăl). Seeking light. [L. *lux,* light, + *peto,* to seek]

lu·es (lū'ēz). A plague or pestilence; specifically, syphilis. [L. pestilence]

lu·et·ic (lū-et'ik). SYN syphilitic.

lu·lib·er·in (lū-lib'er-in). A decapeptide hormone from the hypothalamus that stimulates the anterior pituitary to release both follicle-stimulating hormone and luteinizing hormone. SYN luteinizing hormone-releasing hormone. [luteinizing hormone + L. *libero,* to free, + -in]

lum·ba·go (lŭm-bā'gō). Pain in mid and lower back; a descriptive term not specifying cause. SYN lumbar rheumatism. [L. fr. *lumbus,* loin]

lum·bar (lŭm'bar). Relating to the loins, or the part of the back and sides between the ribs and the pelvis. [L. *lumbus,* a loin]

lum·bar·i·za·tion (lŭm'bar-i-zā'shŭn). A congenital anomaly of the lumbosacral junction characterized by development of the first sacral vertebra as a lumbar vertebra; there are six lumbar vertebrae instead of five.

lum·bi (lŭm'bī). Plural of lumbus. [L.]

lum·bo·cos·tal (lŭm'bō-kos'tăl). **1.** Relating to the lumbar and the hypochondriac regions. **2.** Relating to the lumbar vertebrae and the ribs; denoting a ligament connecting the first lumbar vertebra with the neck of the twelfth rib. [L. *lumbus,* loin, + *costa,* rib]

lum·bo·in·gui·nal (lŭm'bō-ing'gwi-năl). Relating to the lumbar and the inguinal regions. [L. *lumbus,* loin, + *inguen* (inguin-), groin]

lum·bo·sa·cral (lŭm'bō-sā'krăl). Relating to the lumbar vertebrae and the sacrum. SYN sacrolumbar.

lum·bri·ci·dal (lŭm-bri-sī'dăl). Destructive to lumbricoid (intestinal) worms.

lum·bri·cide (lŭm'bri-sīd). An agent that kills lumbricoid (intestinal) worms. [L. *lumbricus,* worm, + *caedo,* to kill]

lum·bri·coid (lŭm'bri-koyd). Denoting or resembling a roundworm, especially *Ascaris lumbricoides.* SEE ALSO vermiform. [L. *lumbricus,* earthworm, + G. *eidos,* resemblance]

lum·bri·co·sis (lŭm'bri-kō'sis). Infection with round intestinal worms.

lum·bus, gen. and pl. **lum·bi** (lŭm'bŭs, -bī) [NA]. SYN loin. [L.]

lu·men, pl. **lu·mi·na, lu·mens** (lū'men, -min-ă, -menz). **1.** The space in the interior of a tubular structure, such as an artery or the intestine. **2 (lm).** The unit of luminous flux; the luminous flux emitted in a unit solid angle of 1 steradian by a uniform point source of light having a luminous intensity of 1 candela. [L. light, window]

lu·mi·nal (lū'mi-năl). Relating to the lumen of a blood vessel or other tubular structure.

lu·mi·nance (lū′mi-năns). The brightness of an object, expressed as the luminous flux per unit solid angle per unit projected area, measured in lamberts or in candelas per square meter. [L. *lumino*, to light up, fr. *lumen*, light]

lu·mi·nes·cence (lū-mi-nes′ens). Emission of light from a body as a result of a chemical reaction. [L. *lumen*, light]

lu·mi·nif·er·ous (lū-mi-nif′er-ŭs). Producing or conveying light. [L. *lumen*, light, + *fero*, to carry]

lu·mi·no·phore (lū′mi-nō-fōr). An atom or atomic grouping in an organic compound that increases its ability to emit light. [L. *lumen*, light, + G. *phoros*, bearing]

lu·mi·nous (lū′mi-nŭs). Emitting light, with or without accompanying heat. [L. *lumen*, light]

lu·mi·rho·dop·sin (lū′mi-rō-dop′sin). An intermediate between rhodopsin and all-*trans*-retinal plus opsin during bleaching of rhodopsin by light; formed from bathorhodopsin and converted to metarhodopsin. [L. *lumen*, light, + G. *rhodon*, rose, + *opsis*, vision]

lump·ec·to·my (lŭm-pek′tō-mē). Removal of either a benign or malignant lesion from the breast, with preservation of surrounding tissue. [lump + G. *ektomē*, excision]

lu·nar (lū′ner). **1.** Relating to the moon or to a month. **2.** Resembling the moon in shape, especially a half moon. SYN lunate (1), semilunar. SEE ALSO crescentic. **3.** Relating to silver (the moon was the symbol of silver in alchemy). [L. *luna*, moon]

lu·nate (lū′nāt). **1.** SYN lunar (2). **2.** Relating to the lunate bone.

lung (lŭng). One of a pair of viscera occupying the pulmonary cavities of the thorax, the organs of respiration in which aeration of the blood takes place. As a rule, the right l. is slightly larger than the left and is divided into three lobes (an upper, a middle, and a lower or basal), while the left has but two lobes (an upper and a lower or basal). Each l. is irregularly conical in shape, presenting a blunt upper extremity (the apex), a concave base following the curve of the diaphragm, an outer convex surface (costal surface), an inner or mediastinal surface (mediastinal surface), a thin and sharp anterior border, and a thick and rounded posterior border. SYN pulmo [NA]. [A.S. *lungen*]

air-conditioner l., an extrinsic allergic alveolitis caused by forced air contaminated by thermophilic actinomycetes and other organisms.

bird-breeder's l., bird-fancier's l., extrinsic allergic alveolitis caused by inhalation of particulate avian emanations.

black l., a form of pneumoconiosis, common in coal miners, characterized by deposit of carbon particles in the l. SYN miner's l. (2).

cheese worker's l., extrinsic allergic alveolitis caused by inhalation of spores of *Penicillium casei* from moldy cheese.

farmer's l., a hypersensitivity pneumonitis characterized by fever and dyspnea, caused by inhalation of organic dust from moldy hay containing spores of actinomycetes and certain true fungi, which thrive in the elevated temperatures of hay lofts and silos.

honeycomb l., the radiological and gross appearance of the l.'s resulting from interstitial fibrosis and cystic dilation of bronchioles and distal air spaces; a sequel of any of several diseases, including eosinophilic granuloma and sarcoidosis.

hyperlucent l., the radiographic finding that a l. or portion thereof is less dense than normal, as from air trapping by a bronchial foreign body, asymmetric emphysema, or decreasing blood flow.

iron l., SYN Drinker *respirator*.

miner's l., (1) SYN anthracosis. (2) SYN black l.

pump l., SYN shock l.

quiet l., the collapse of a l. during thoracic operations undertaken to facilitate surgical procedure through absence of l. movement.

shock l., in shock, the development of edema, impaired perfusion, and reduction in alveolar space so that the alveoli collapse. SYN pump l., wet l. (1), white l.

silo-filler's l., pulmonary *edema*, usually delayed for 1–4 hours, occurring in an individual exposed to silage, probably due to nitrogen dioxide; can progress to bronchiolitis obliterans.

unilateral hyperlucent l., chronic bronchiolitis obliterans predominating on one side. SEE unilateral lobar *emphysema*.

vanishing l., SEE vanishing lung *syndrome*.

wet l., white l., (1) SYN shock l. (2) SYN adult respiratory distress *syndrome*.

lung·worms (lŭng′wermz). Nematodes that inhabit the air passages of animals.

lu·nu·la, pl. **lu·nu·lae** (lū′nū-lă, -lē). **1** [NA]. The pale arched area at the proximal portion of the nail plate. **2.** A small semilunar structure. [L. dim. of *luna*, moon]

lu·pi·form (lū′pi-fōrm). SYN lupoid.

lu·poid (lū′poyd). Resembling lupus. SYN lupiform. [L. *lupus* + G. *eidos*, resemblance]

lu·pous (lū′pŭs). Relating to lupus.

lu·pus (lū′pŭs). A term originally used to depict erosion (as if gnawed) of the skin, now used with modifying terms designating the various diseases listed below. [L. wolf]

discoid l. erythemato′sus, a form of l. erythematosus in which cutaneous lesions appear on the face and and elsewhere; these are atrophic plaques with erythema, hyperkeratosis, follicular plugging, and telangiectasia.

disseminated l. erythemato′sus, SYN systemic l. erythematosus.

l. erythemato′sus (LE, L.E.), an illness which may be characterized by skin lesions alone or systemic (disseminated) with antinuclear antibodies present and usually involvement of vital structures. SEE ALSO discoid l. erythematosus, systemic l. erythematosus.

l. erythemato′sus profun′dus, a subcutaneous panniculitis with deep-seated, firm, rubbery nodules, usually of the face; may occur in systemic and localized l. erythematosus.

l. milia′ris dissemina′tus facie′i, a milletlike papular eruption of the face associated with a (histopathologically) tuberculoid perifollicular infiltration but probably related to rosacea rather than tuberculous infection.

lu

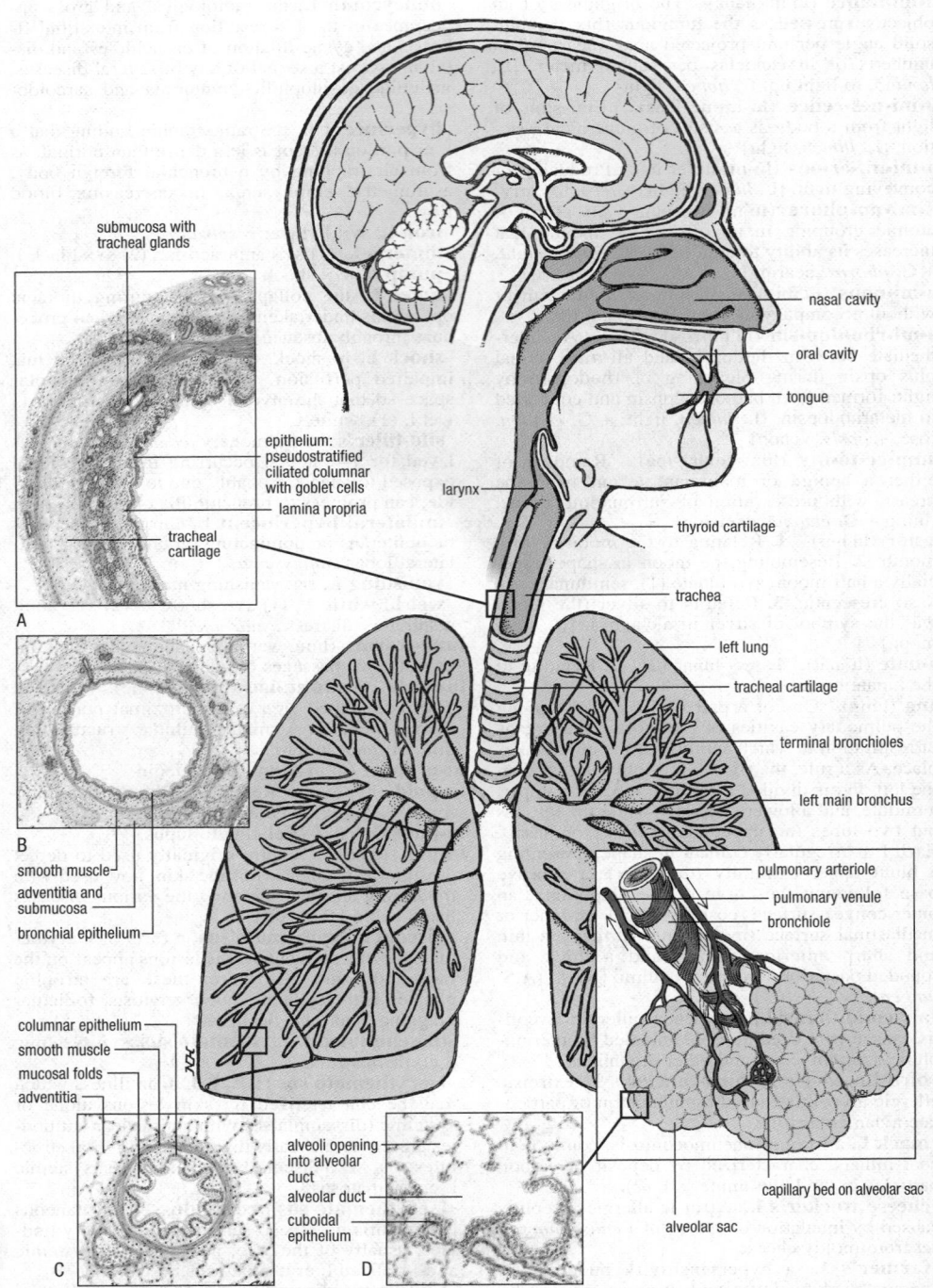

submucosa with
tracheal glands

epithelium:
pseudostratified
ciliated columnar
with goblet cells

lamina propria

tracheal
cartilage

nasal cavity

oral cavity

tongue

larynx

thyroid cartilage

trachea

left lung

tracheal cartilage

terminal bronchioles

left main bronchus

A

smooth muscle
adventitia and
submucosa
bronchial epithelium

B

pulmonary arteriole

pulmonary venule

bronchiole

columnar epithelium
smooth muscle
mucosal folds
adventitia

alveoli opening
into alveolar
duct

alveolar duct

cuboidal
epithelium

capillary bed on alveolar sac

alveolar sac

C

D

lungs and respiratory anatomy: (A) trachea (panoramic, transverse section); (B) intrapulmonary bronchus; (C) terminal bronchiole; (D) respiratory bronchiole with alveoli

l. per′nio, sarcoid lesions, clinically resembling frostbite and microscopically resembling l. vulgaris, involving ears, cheeks, nose, hands, and fingers.

systemic l. erythemato′sus (SLE), an inflammatory connective tissue disease with variable features including fever, weakness and fatigability, joint pains or arthritis resembling rheumatoid arthritis, diffuse erythematous skin lesions on the face, neck, or upper extremities, lymphadenopathy, pleurisy or pericarditis, glomerular lesions, anemia, hyperglobulinemia, and a positive LE cell test, with serum antibodies to double-stranded DNA and acidic nuclear protein (Sm). SYN disseminated l. erythematosus.

l. vulga′ris, cutaneous tuberculosis with characteristic nodular lesions on the face, particularly about the nose and ears.

LUQ left upper quadrant (of abdomen).

lu·te·al (lū′tē-ăl). Relating to the corpus luteum; l. cells, l. hormone, etc. [L. *luteus,* saffron-yellow]

lu·te·in (lū′tē-in). **1.** The yellow pigment in the corpus luteum, in the yolk of eggs, or any lipochrome. **2.** SYN xanthophyll. [L. *luteus,* saffron-yellow]

lu·te·in·i·za·tion (lū′tē-in-i-zā′shŭn). Transformation of the mature ovarian follicle and its theca interna into a corpus luteum after ovulation.

lu·te·o·hor·mone (lū′tē-ō-hōr′mōn). SYN progesterone.

lu·te·ol·y·sis (lū-tē-ol′i-sis). Degeneration or destruction of ovarian luteinized tissue.

lu·te·o·lyt·ic (lū-tē-ō-lit′ik). Promoting or characteristic of luteolysis.

lu·te·o·ma (lū-tē-ō′mă). An ovarian tumor of granulosa or theca-lutein cell origin, producing progesterone effects on the uterine mucosa.

lu·te·o·tro·pic, lu·te·o·tro·phic (lū′tē-ō-trop′ik, -trof′ik). Having a stimulating action on the development and function of the corpus luteum.

lu·te·o·tro·pin (lū′tē-ō-trō′pin). An anterior pituitary hormone whose action maintains the function of the corpus luteum. SYN luteotropic hormone.

lu·te·ti·um (Lu) (lū-tē′shē-ŭm). A rare earth element; atomic no. 71, atomic wt. 174.967. [L. *Lutetia,* Paris]

lu·tro·pin (lū′trō-pin). A glycoprotein hormone that stimulates the final ripening of the follicles and the secretion of progesterone by them, their rupture to release the egg, and the conversion of the ruptured follicle into the corpus luteum. SYN interstitial cell-stimulating hormone, luteinizing hormone.

lux (lŭks). A unit of light or illumination; the reception of a luminous flux of 1 lumen per square meter of surface. SYN candle-meter, meter-candle. [L. light]

lux·a·tion (lŭk-sā′shŭn). **1.** SYN dislocation. **2.** DENTISTRY The dislocation or displacement of the condyle in the temporomandibular fossa, or of a tooth from the alveolus. [L. *luxatio*]

Malgaigne's l., SYN nursemaid's *elbow.*

Lux·ol fast blue. Name for a group of closely related copper phthalocyanine dyes used as stains

(with PAS, PTAH, hematoxylin, silver nitrate, etc.) for myelin in nerve fibers.

LVET left ventricular ejection *time.*

ly·ase (lī′ās). Class name for enzymes removing groups nonhydrolytically (EC class 4); prefixes such as "hydro-," "ammonia-," etc., are used to indicate the type of reaction. Trivial names for lyases include synthases, decarboxylases, aldolases, dehydratases. Cf. synthase, synthetase.

ly·can·thro·py (lī-kan′thrō-pē). The morbid delusion that one is a wolf. [G. *lykos,* wolf, + *anthrōpos,* man]

ly·co·pene (lī′kō-pēn). Ψ,Ψ-Carotene; the red pigment of the tomato the parent substance from which all natural carotenoid pigments are derived.

ly·co·pe·ne·mia (lī′kō-pĕ-nē′mē-ă). A condition in which there is a high concentration of lycopene in the blood, producing carotenoid-like yellowish pigmentation of the skin; found in persons who consume excessive amounts of tomatoes or tomato juice, or lycopene-containing fruits and berries. [lycopene + G. *haima,* blood]

ly·co·per·do·no·sis (lī′kō-per-don-ō′sis). A persisting pneumonitis following inhalation of spores of the puffballs *Lycoperdon pyriforme* and *L. bovista.*

lymph (limf). A clear, transparent, sometimes faintly yellow and slightly opalescent fluid that is collected from the tissues throughout the body, flows in the lymphatic vessels (through the l. nodes), and is eventually added to the venous blood circulation. L. consists of a clear liquid portion, varying numbers of white blood cells (chiefly lymphocytes), and a few red blood cells. [L. *lympha,* clear spring water]

aplastic l., l. containing a relatively large number of leukocytes, but comparatively little fibrinogen; such l. does not form a good clot and manifests only a slight tendency to become organized.

euplastic l., l. that contains relatively few leukocytes, but a comparatively high concentration of fibrinogen; such l. clots fairly well and tends to become organized with fibrous tissue.

inflammatory l., a faintly yellow, usually coagulable fluid (*i.e.,* euplastic l.) that collects on the surface of an acutely inflamed membrane or cutaneous wound.

tissue l., true l., *i.e.,* l. derived chiefly from fluid in tissue spaces (in contrast to blood l.).

vaccine l., vaccinia l., that collected from the vesicles of vaccinia infection, and used for active immunization against smallpox.

△**lymph-.** SEE lympho-.

△**lymphaden-.** SEE lymphadeno-.

lym·phad·e·nec·to·my (lim-fad′ĕ-nek′tō-mē). Excision of lymph nodes. [lymphadeno- + G. *ektomē,* excision]

lym·phad·e·ni·tis (lim′-fad′ĕ-nī′tis). Inflammation of a lymph node or lymph nodes. [lymphadeno- + G. *-itis,* inflammation]

regional granulomatous l., SYN cat-scratch *disease.*

△**lymphadeno-, lymphaden-.** The lymph nodes. [L. *lympha,* spring water, + G. *adēn,* gland]

lym·phad·e·nog·ra·phy (lim-fad′ĕ-nog′ră-fē).

ly

Radiographic visualization of lymph nodes after injection of a contrast medium; lymphography. [lymphadeno- + G. *graphō*, to write]

lym·phad·e·noid (lim-fad′ĕ-noyd). Relating to, or resembling, or derived from a lymph node. [lymphadeno- + G. *eidos*, resemblance]

lym·phad·e·nop·a·thy (lim-fad-ĕ-nop′ă-thē). Any disease process affecting a lymph node or lymph nodes. [lymphadeno- + G. *pathos*, suffering]

    angioimmunoblastic l. with dysproteinemia, a lymphoproliferative disorder characterized by generalized l., hepatosplenomegaly, fever, sweats, weight loss, skin lesions, and pruritus with hypergammaglobulinemia; occurs primarily in older adults, often with fatal outcome. Proliferation of B cells, deficiency of T cells has been demonstrated.

lym·phad·e·no·sis (lim-fad′ĕ-nō′sis). The basic underlying proliferative process that results in enlargement of lymph nodes, as in lymphocytic leukemia and certain inflammations. [lymphadeno- + G. *-osis*, condition]

△**lymphangi-.** SEE lymphangio-.

lym·phan·gi·al (lim-fan′jē-ăl). Relating to a lymphatic vessel.

lym·phan·gi·ec·ta·sis, lym·phan·gi·ec·ta·sia (lim-fan′jē-ek′tă-sis, -ek-tā′zē-ă). Dilation of the lymphatic vessels, the basic process that may result in the formation of a lymphangioma. SYN lymphectasia. [lymphangio- + G. *ektasis*, a stretching]

lym·phan·gi·ec·tat·ic (lim-fan′jē-ek-tat′ik). Relating to or characterized by lymphangiectasis.

lym·phan·gi·ec·to·my (lim-fan′jē-ek′tō-mē). Excision of a lymph channel. [lymphangio- + G. *ektomē*, excision]

lym·phan·gi·i·tis (lim-fan′jē-ī′tis). SYN lymphangitis.

△**lymphangio-, lymphangi-.** The lymphatic vessels. [L. *lympha*, spring water, + G. *angeion*, vessel]

lym·phan·gi·o·en·do·the·li·o·ma (lim-fan′jē-ō-en′dō-thē-lē-ō′mă). A neoplasm consisting of irregular groups of endothelial cells, and intubate structures that are thought to be derived from lymphatic vessels. [lymphangio- + endothelium + *-oma*, tumor]

lym·phan·gi·og·ra·phy (lim-fan′jē-og′ră-fē). Radiographic demonstration of lymphatics and lymph nodes following the injection of a contrast medium; lymphography. [lymphangio- + G. *graphō*, to write]

lym·phan·gi·ol·o·gy (lim-fan-jē-ol′ō-jē). The branch of medical science concerned with the lymphatic vessels. SYN lymphology. [lymphangio- + G. *logos*, study]

lym·phan·gi·o·ma (lim-fan′jē-ō′mă). A well-circumscribed nodule of lymphatic vessels that are usually greatly dilated and are lined with normal endothelial cells; lymphoid tissue is usually present in the peripheral portions of the lesions, which are present at birth or shortly therafter, and probably represent anomalous development of lymphatic vessels (rather than true neoplasms); they occur most frequently in the neck and axilla. [lymphangio- + G. *-oma*, tumor]

lym·phan·gi·o·phle·bi·tis (lim-fan′jē-ō-flĕ-bī′tis). Inflammation of the lymphatic vessels and veins.

lym·phan·gi·o·plas·ty (lim-fan′jē-ō-plas-tē). Surgical alteration of lymphatic vessels. [lymphangio- + G. *plastos*, formed]

lym·phan·gi·o·sar·co·ma (lim-fan′jē-ō-sar-kō′mă). A malignant neoplasm derived from the endothelial cells of lymphatic vessels, usually developing in the arm several years after radical mastectomy.

lym·phan·gi·ot·o·my (lim-fan′jē-ot′ō-mē). Incision of lymphatic vessels. [lymphangio- + G. *tomē*, incision]

lym·phan·gi·tis (lim-fan-jī′tis). Inflammation of the lymphatic vessels. SYN lymphangiitis. [lymphangio- + G. *-itis*, inflammation]

lym·pha·phe·re·sis (lim′fă-fĕ-rē′sis). SYN lymphocytapheresis.

lym·phat·ic (lim-fat′ik). **1.** Pertaining to lymph. **2.** A vascular channel that transports lymph. **3.** Sometimes used to pertain to a sluggish or phlegmatic characteristic. [L. *lymphaticus*, frenzied; Mod. L. use, of or for lymph]

    afferent l., a l. vessel entering, or bringing lymph to, a node.

lym·phat·i·cos·to·my (lim-fat-i-kos′tō-mē). Making an opening into a lymphatic duct. [lymphatic + G. *stoma*, mouth]

lym·pha·ti·tis (lim-fă-tī′tis). Inflammation of the lymphatic vessels or lymph nodes. [lymphatic + G. *-itis*, inflammation]

lym·pha·tol·y·sis (lim′fă-tol′i-sis). Destruction of the lymphatic vessels or lymphoid tissue, or both. [lymphatic + G. *lysis*, dissolution]

lym·pha·to·lyt·ic (lim′fă-tō-lit′ik). Pertaining to or characterized by lymphatolysis.

lym·phec·ta·sia (lim-fek-tā′zē-ă). SYN lymphangiectasis. [lymph + G. *ektasis*, a stretching]

lymph·e·de·ma (limf′e-dē′mă). Swelling (especially in subcutaneous tissues) as a result of obstruction of lymphatic vessels or lymph nodes and the accumulation of large amounts of lymph in the affected region. [lymph + G. *oidēma*, a swelling]

lym·phe·mia (lim-fē′mē-ă). The presence of unusually large numbers of lymphocytes or their precursors, or both, in the circulating blood. [lymph(ocyte) + G. *haima*, blood]

lymph node. One of numerous round, oval, or bean-shaped bodies located along the course of lymphatic vessels, varying greatly in size (1 to 25 mm in diameter) and usually presenting a depressed area, the hilum, on one side through which blood vessels enter and efferent lymphatic vessels emerge. The structure consists of a fibrous capsule and internal trabeculae supporting lymphoid tissue and lymph sinuses; lymphoid tissue is arranged in nodules in the cortex and cords in the medulla of a node, with afferent vessels entering at many points of the periphery. SYN nodus lymphaticus [NA], lymph gland, lymphoglandula.

    axillary l. n.'s, numerous nodes around the axillary veins which receive the lymphatic drainage from the upper limb, scapular region and pectoral region (including mammary gland); they drain into the subclavian trunk.

bronchopulmonary l. n.'s, l. n.'s in the hilum of the lung that receive lymph from the pulmonary l. n.'s, and drain to the tracheobronchial nodes. SYN bronchial glands (1).

celiac l. n.'s, nodes located along the celiac trunk which drain lymph from the stomach, duodenum, pancreas, spleen, and biliary tract and drain to the cisterna chyli via the right and left intestinal lymphatic trunks.

cystic l. n., a l. n. at the neck of the gallbladder draining lymph into the hepatic nodes.

jugulo-omohyoid l. n., a l. n. of the lateral deep cervical group that lies above the intermediate tendon of the omohyoid muscle and anterior to the internal jugular vein; it receives lymphatic drainage from the submental, submandibular, and deep anterior cervical nodes; its efferent vessels go to other deep lateral cervical nodes.

jugulodigastric l. n., a prominent l. n. in the deep lateral cervical group lying below the digastric muscle and anterior to the internal jugular vein; it receives lymphatic drainage from the pharynx, palatine tonsil, and tongue.

juxta-esophageal pulmonary l. n.'s, juxta-esophageal l. n.'s, several nodes of the posterior mediastinal group located along either side of the esophagus; they receive lymph from both the esophagus and the lungs.

mandibular l. n., one of the facial l. n.'s located by the facial artery near the point it crosses the mandible.

l. n. of lymph node, the central portion of a node consisting of cordlike masses of lymphocytes, plasma cells, and macrophages in a stroma of reticular fibers separated by lymph sinuses; it reaches the surface of the node at the hilum.

middle rectal l. n., a l. n. along the middle rectal artery that receives afferents from the pararectal nodes and sends efferents to the internal iliac nodes.

nasolabial l. n., one of the facial l. n.'s located near the junction of the superior labial and facial arteries.

parietal l. n.'s, the l. n.'s draining the walls of the abdomen or of the pelvis.

retroauricular l. n.'s, two or three nodes in the region of the mastoid process; they receive afferent lymphatic vessels from the scalp and auricle and send efferent vessels to the superior deep cervical nodes.

visceral l. n.'s, the l. n.'s draining the viscera of the abdomen or of the pelvis.

lympho-, lymph-. Lymph. [L. *lympha*, spring water]

lym•pho•blast (lim′fō-blast). An immature cell that matures into a lymphocyte and is characterized by more abundant cytoplasm than in a lymphocyte, a nucleus in which the chromatin is finer than in a lymphocyte (but coarser than in a myeloblast), and one or two rather prominent nucleoli. SYN lymphocytoblast. [lympho- + G. *blastos*, germ]

lym•pho•blas•tic (lim-fō-blas′tik). Pertaining to the production of lymphocytes.

lym•pho•blas•to•ma (lim-fō-blas-tō′mă). A

form of malignant lymphoma in which the chief cells are lymphoblasts. [lymphoblast + G. *-oma*, tumor]

lym•pho•blas•to•sis (lim′fō-blas-tō′sis). The presence of lymphoblasts in the peripheral blood; sometimes used as a synonym for acute lymphocytic leukemia. [lymphoblast + G. *-osis*, condition]

lym•pho•cy•ta•phe•re•sis (lim′fō-sī-tă-fĕ-rē′sis). Separation and removal of lymphocytes from the withdrawn blood, with the remainder of the blood retransfused into the donor. SYN lymphapheresis. [lymphocyte + G. *aphairesis*, a withdrawal]

lym•pho•cyte (lim′fō-sīt). A white blood cell formed in lymphatic tissue (lymph nodes, spleen, thymus, tonsils, Peyer's patches, and sometimes in bone marrow), in normal adults comprising approximately 22 to 28% of the total number of leukocytes in the blood. L.'s are generally small (7 to 8 μm), but larger forms are frequent (10 to 20 μm); with Wright's stain, the nucleus is deeply colored, round, and eccentrically situated. [lympho- + G. *kytos*, call]

B l., a l. that resembles the bursa-derived l. of birds in that it is responsible for the production of immunoglobulins, *i.e.,* it is the precursor of the plasma cell and expresses immunoglobulins on its surface but does not release them. It does not play a direct role in cell-mediated immunity. SEE ALSO T l.

T l., a thymocyte-derived l. of immunological importance that is responsible for cell-mediated immunity. These cells have the characteristic T3 surface marker and may be further divided into subsets according to function, such as helper, suppressor, and cytotoxic. SEE ALSO B l. SYN T cell.

lym•pho•cy•the•mia (lim′fō-sī-thē′mē-ă). SYN lymphocytosis.

lym•pho•cyt•ic (lim-fō-sit′ik). Pertaining to or characterized by lymphocytes.

lym•pho•cy•to•blast (lim-fō-sī′tō-blast). SYN lymphoblast. [lymphocyte + G. *blastos*, germ]

lym•pho•cy•to•ma (lim′fō-sī-tō′mă). A circumscribed nodule or mass of mature lymphocytes, grossly resembling a neoplasm. [lymphocyte + G. *-oma*, tumor]

benign l. cutis, a soft red to violaceous skin nodule caused by dense infiltration of the dermis by lymphocytes and histiocytes.

lym•pho•cy•to•pe•nia (lim′fō-sī-tō-pē′nē-ă). SYN lymphopenia.

lym•pho•cy•to•poi•e•sis (lim′fō-sī-tō-poy-ē′sis). The formation of lymphocytes. [lymphocyte + G. *poiēsis*, a making]

lym•pho•cy•to•sis (lim′fō-sī-tō′sis). A form of leukocytosis in which there is an actual or relative increase in the number of lymphocytes. SYN lymphocythemia.

lym•pho•duct (lim′fō-dŭkt). A lymphatic vessel. [lympho- + L. *ductus*, a leading]

lym•pho•ep•i•the•li•o•ma (lim′fō-ep-i-thē-lē-ō′mă). A poorly differentiated radiosensitive squamous cell carcinoma involving lymphoid tissue in the region of the tonsils and nasopharynx; metastasizes early to cervical lymph nodes. [lympho- + epithelium + *-oma*, tumor]

lym·pho·gen·ic (lim-fō-jen'ik). SYN lymphoge-nous (1).

lym·phog·e·nous (lim-foj'ĕ-nŭs). **1.** Originating from lymph or the lymphatic system. SYN lymphogenic. **2.** Producing lymph.

lym·pho·glan·du·la (lim-fō-glan'dū-lă). SYN lymph node.

lym·phog·ra·phy (lim-fog'ră-fē). Visualization of lymphatics (lymphangiography), lymph nodes (lymphadenography), or both by radiography following the intra-lymphatic injection of a contrast medium, usually an iodized oil. [lympho- + graphō, to write]

lym·phoid (lim'foyd). **1.** Resembling lymph or lymphatic tissue, or pertaining to the lymphatic system. **2.** SYN adenoid (1). [lympho- + G. eidos, appearance]

lym·phoi·dec·to·my (lim-foy-dek'tō-mē). Excision of lymphoid tissue. [lymphoid + G. ektomē, excision]

lym·pho·kines (lim'fō-kīnz). Hormone-like peptides, released by activated lymphocytes that mediate immune responses. [lymphocyte + G. kineō, to set in motion]

lym·pho·ki·ne·sis (lim'fō-ki-nē'sis). **1.** Circulation of lymph in the lymphatic vessels and through the lymph nodes. **2.** Movement of endolymph in the semicircular canals of the inner ear. [lympho- + G. kinēsis, movement]

lym·phol·o·gy (lim-fol'ō-jē). SYN lymphangiology. [lympho- + G. logos, study]

▯**lym·pho·ma** (lim-fō'mă). Obsolete term for malignant l. [lympho- + G. -oma, tumor]

adult T-cell l. (ATL), an acute or subacute disease associated with a human T-cell virus, with lymphadenopathy, hepatosplenomegaly, skin lesions, peripheral blood involvement, and hypercalcemia. SYN adult T-cell leukemia.

Burkitt's l., a form of malignant l. reported in African children, involving facial bones, ovaries, and abdominal lymph nodes, which are infiltrated by undifferentiated stem cells with scattered pale macrophages; caused by Epstein-Barr virus.

follicular l., SYN nodular l.

large cell l., l. composed of large mononuclear cells of undetermined type.

lymphoblastic l., a diffuse l. in children, with supradiaphragmatic distribution and T lymphocytes having convoluted nuclei; many patients develop acute lymphoblastic leukemia.

malignant l., general term for malignant neoplasms of lymphoid and reticuloendothelial tissues which present as solid tumors composed of cells that appear primitive or resemble lymphocytes, plasma cells, or histiocytes. L.'s appear most frequently in lymph nodes, spleen, or other normal sites of lymphoreticular cells. L.'s are classified by cell type, degrees of differentiation, and nodular or diffuse pattern; Hodgkin's disease and Burkitt's l. are special forms.

nodular l., malignant l. arising from lymphoid follicular B cells which may be small or large, growing in a nodular pattern. SYN follicular l.

non-Hodgkin's l., a l. other than Hodgkin's disease, having either a nodular or diffuse tumor pattern; divided into those of low, intermediate, and high grade malignancy; and into subtypes reflecting cell of origin.

poorly differentiated lymphocytic l. (PDLL), a B-cell l. with nodular or diffuse lymph node or bone marrow involvement by large lymphoid cells.

well-differentiated lymphocytic l. (WDLL), essentially the same disease as chronic lymphocytic leukemia, except that lymphocytes are not increased in the peripheral blood; lymph nodes are enlarged and other lymphoid tissue or bone marrow is infiltrated by small lymphocytes.

lym·pho·ma·toid (lim-fō'mă-toyd). Resembling a lymphoma.

lym·pho·ma·to·sis (lim'fō-mă-to'sis). Any condition characterized by the occurrence of multiple, widely distributed sites of involvement with lymphoma.

lym·pho·ma·tous (lim-fō'mă-tŭs). Pertaining to or characterized by lymphoma.

lym·pho·myx·o·ma (lim'fō-mik-sō'mă). A soft nonmalignant neoplasm that contains lymphoid tissue in a matrix of loose, areolar connective tissue. [lympho- + G. myxa, mucus, + -oma, tumor]

lym·phop·a·thy (lim-fop'ă-thē). Any disease of the lymphatic vessels or lymph nodes. [lympho- + G. pathos, suffering]

lym·pho·pe·nia (lim-fō-pē'nē-ă). A reduction, relative or absolute, in the number of lymphocytes in the circulating blood. SYN lymphocytopenia. [lympho- + G. penia, poverty]

lym·pho·plas·ma·phe·re·sis (lim'fō-plaz'mă-fĕ-rē'sis). Separation and removal of lymphocytes and plasma from the withdrawn blood, with the remainder of the blood retransfused into the donor. [lymphocyte + plasma + G. aphairesis, a withdrawal]

lym·pho·poi·e·sis (lim-fō-poy-ē'sis). The formation of lymphatic tissue. [lympho- + G. poiēsis, a making]

lym·pho·poi·et·ic (lim-fō-poy-et'ik). Pertaining to or characterized by lymphopoiesis.

lym·pho·re·tic·u·lo·sis (lim'fō-rĕ-tik-yū-lō'sis). Proliferation of the reticuloendothelial cells (macrophages) of the lymph glands.

benign inoculation l., SYN cat-scratch disease.

lym·phor·rha·gia (lim-fō-rā'jē-ă). SYN lymphorrhea. [lympho- + G. rhēgnymi, to burst forth]

lym·phor·rhea (lim-fō-rē'ă). An escape of lymph on the surface from ruptured, torn, or cut lymphatic vessels. SYN lymphorrhagia. [lympho- + G. rhoia, a flow]

lym·phor·rhoid (lim'fō-royd). A dilation of a lymph channel, resembling a hemorrhoid. [lymph + -rrhoid, tending to leak, on the analogy of hemorrhoid]

lym·phos·ta·sis (lim-fos'tă-sis). Obstruction of the normal flow of lymph. [lympho- + G. stasis, a standing still]

lym·pho·tax·is (lim-fō-tak'sis). The exertion of an effect that attracts or repels lymphocytes. [lympho- + G. taxis, orderly arrangement]

lym·pho·tox·ic·i·ty (lim'fō-tok-sis'i-tē). Toxicity to lymphocytes.

lym·pho·tox·in (lim'fō-tok-sin). A lymphokine that lyses or damages many cell types.

lyo-. Dissolution. SEE ALSO lyso-. [G. *lyō,* to loosen, dissolve]

ly·on·i·za·tion (lī′on-i-zā′shŭn). The normal phenomenon that wherever there are two or more haploid sets of X-linked genes in each cell all but one of the genes are inactivated apparently at random and have no phenotypic expression. Its randomness explains the more variable expressivity of X-linked traits in women than in men. SEE ALSO gene dosage *compensation.* SYN Lyon hypothesis, X-inactivation. [M. *Lyon*]

ly·o·phil, ly·o·phile (lī′ō-fil, -fīl). A substance that is lyophilic.

ly·o·phil·ic (lī-ō-fil′ik). COLLOID CHEMISTRY Denoting a dispersed phase having a pronounced affinity for the dispersion medium; when the dispersed phase is l., the colloid is usually a reversible one. SYN lyotropic. [lyo- + G. *phileō,* to love]

ly·oph·i·li·za·tion (lī-of′i-li-zā′shŭn). The process of isolating a solid substance from solution by freezing the solution and evaporating the ice under vacuum. SYN freeze-drying.

ly·o·phobe (lī′ō-fōb). A substance that is lyophobic.

ly·o·pho·bic (lī-ō-fo′bik). COLLOID CHEMISTRY Denoting a dispersed phase having but slight affinity for the dispersion medium; when the dispersed phase is l., the colloid is usually an irreversible one. [lyo- + G. *phobos,* fear]

ly·o·tro·pic (lī-ō-trop′ik). SYN lyophilic. [lyo- + G. *tropē,* a turning]

Lys lysine, or its radicals in peptides.

lys-. SEE lyso-.

ly·sate (lī′sāt). Material produced by the destructive process of lysis.

lyse (līz). To break up, to disintegrate, to effect lysis. SYN lyze.

ly·se·mia (lī-sē′mē-ă). Disintegration or dissolution of red blood cells and the occurrence of hemoglobin in the circulating plasma and in the urine. [lyso- + G. *haima,* blood]

ly·sin (lī′sin). **1.** A complement-fixing antibody that acts destructively on cells and tissues; the various types are designated in accordance with the form of antigen that stimulates the production of the l., *e.g.,* hemolysin, bacteriolysin. **2.** Any substance that causes lysis.

ly·sine (K, Lys) (lī′sēn). A nutritionally essential α-amino acid found in many proteins; distinguished by an ε-amino group.

ly·sin·o·gen (lī-sin′ō-jen). An antigen that stimulates the formation of a specific lysin.

ly·si·no·gen·ic (lī′si-nō-jen′ik). Having the property of a lysinogen.

ly·sin·u·ria (lī-si-nū′rē-ă). The presence of lysine in the urine.

ly·sis (lī′sis). **1.** Gradual subsidence of fever and other symptoms of an acute disease, as distinguished from crisis. **2.** Destruction of red blood cells, bacteria, and other structures by a specific lysin, usually referred to by the structure destroyed (*e.g.,* hemolysis, bacteriolysis, nephrolysis); may be due to a direct toxin or an immune mechanism. [G. dissolution or loosening]

l. of adhesions, surgical division of postinflammatory or postoperative adhesions, particularly abdominal (peritoneal) adhesions.

lyso-, lys-. Lysis, dissolution. SEE ALSO lyo-. [G. *lysis,* a loosening]

ly·so·gen (lī′sō-jen). **1.** That which is capable of inducing lysis. **2.** A bacterium in the state of lysogeny. [lysin + G. *-gen,* producing]

ly·so·gen·e·sis (lī-sō-jen′ĕ-sis). The production of lysins.

ly·so·gen·ic (lī-sō-jen′ik). **1.** Causing or having the power to cause lysis, as the action of certain antibodies and chemical substances. **2.** Pertaining to bacteria in the state of lysogeny.

ly·so·ge·nic·i·ty (lī′sō-jĕ-nis′i-tē). The property of being lysogenic.

ly·sog·e·ny (lī-soj′ĕ-nē). The phenomenon by which a bacterium is infected by a temperate bacteriophage whose DNA is integrated into the bacterial genome and replicates along with the bacterial DNA but remains latent or unexpressed; triggering of the lytic cycle may occur spontaneously or by certain agents and will result in the production of bacteriophage and lysis of the bacterial cell.

ly·so·ki·nase (lī-sō-kī′nās). Term proposed for activator agents (*e.g.,* streptokinase, urokinase, staphylokinase) that produce plasmin by indirect or multiple-stage action on plasminogen.

ly·so·some (lī′sō-sōm). A cytoplasmic membrane-bound vesicle measuring 5–8 nm (primary l.) and containing a wide variety of glycoprotein hydrolytic enzymes active at an acid pH; serves to digest exogenous material, such as bacteria, as well as effete organelles of the cells. [lyso- + G. *soma,* body]

    primary l.'s, l.'s produced at the Golgi apparatus where hydrolytic enzymes are incorporated; they fuse with phagosomes or pinosomes to become secondary l.'s.

    secondary l.'s, l.'s in which lysis takes place, owing to the activity of hydrolytic enzymes; they are believed to eventually become residual bodies.

ly·so·type (li′so-typ). A type within a bacterial species determined by its reaction to specific phages. [lyso + type]

ly·so·zyme (lī′sō-zīm). An enzyme destructive to cell walls of certain bacteria; present in tears, egg white, and some plant tissues; used in the prevention of caries and in the treatment of infant formulas. SYN muramidase.

lys·sa (lis′ă). **1.** A cartilage in the tongue of the dog. SYN worm (2). **2.** Old term for rabies. [G. *madness*]

Lys·sa·vi·rus (lis′ă-vī-rŭs). A genus of viruses (family Rhabdoviridae) that includes the rabies virus group.

lyt·ic (lit′ik). Pertaining to lysis; used colloq. as an abbreviation for osteolytic.

lyze (līz). SYN lyse.

M

μ mu. SEE mu.
μμ micromicro-; micromicron.
μΩ microhm.
μC microcoulomb.
μCi microcurie.
μg microgram.
μl microliter.
μM micromolar.
μm micrometer.
μmol micromole.
μV microvolt.
M_r molecular weight *ratio* or relative molecular *mass*.
mμ millimicron.
mM millimolar (10^{-3} M).
M moles per liter (also written M or *M*).
△*m-* meta- (3).
MA mental *age*.
ma, mA milliampere.
mac·er·ate (mas′er-āt). To soften by steeping or soaking. [see maceration]
mac·er·a·tion (mas-er-ā′shŭn). 1. Softening by the action of a liquid. 2. Softening of tissues after death by nonputrefactive (sterile) autolysis; seen especially in the stillborn, with bullous separation of the epidermis. [L. *macero*, pp. *-atus*, to soften by soaking]
ma·chine (mă-shēn′). Any mechanical apparatus or device. [L. *machina*, contrivance]
   heart-lung m., a device incorporating a blood pump (artificial heart) and a blood oxygenator (artificial lung) to provide extracorporeal circulation and oxygenation of the blood during cardiac surgery.
△macr-. SEE macro-.
mac·ren·ceph·a·ly, mac·ren·ce·pha·lia (mak′ren-sef′ă-lē, -sě-fā′lē-ă). Hypertrophy of the brain; the condition of having a large brain. [macro- + G. *enkephalos*, brain]
△macro-, macr-. Large, long. SEE ALSO mega-, megalo-. [G. *makros*]
mac·ro·ad·e·no·ma (mak′rō-ad-ĕ-nō′mă). A pituitary adenoma larger than 10 mm in diameter.
mac·ro·am·y·lase (mak-rō-am′i-lās). A form of serum amylase in which the enzyme is joined to a globulin.
mac·ro·am·y·la·se·mia (mak′rō-am′i-lā-sē′mē-ă). A form of hyperamylasemia, in which a portion of serum amylase exists as macroamylase. [macroamylase + G. *haima*, blood]
mac·ro·bi·ot·ic (mak′rō-bī-ot′ik). 1. Long-lived. 2. Tending to prolong life.
mac·ro·blast (mak′rō-blast). A large erythroblast. [macro- + G. *blastos*, germ]
mac·ro·car·dia (mak-rō-kar′dē-ă). SYN cardiomegaly.
mac·ro·ce·phal·ic, mac·ro·ceph·a·lous (mak′rō-se-fal′ik, -sef′ă-lŭs). SYN megacephalic. [macro- + G. *kephalē*, head]
mac·ro·ceph·a·ly, mac·ro·ce·pha·lia (mak-rō-sef′ă-lē, -sě-fā′lē-ă). SYN megacephaly. [macro- + G. *kephalē*, head]
mac·ro·chei·lia, mac·ro·chi·lia (mak-rō-kī′lē-ă). 1. Abnormally enlarged lips. 2. Cavernous lymphangioma of the lip, a condition of permanent swelling resulting from the presence of greatly distended lymphatic spaces. [macro- + G. *cheilos,* lip]
mac·ro·chei·ria, mac·ro·chi·ria (mak-rō-kī′rē-ă). A condition characterized by abnormally large hands. SYN megalocheiria, megalochiria. [macro- + G. *cheir,* hand]
mac·ro·co·lon (mak′rō-kō′lon). A sigmoid colon of unusual length; a variety of megacolon.
mac·ro·cor·nea (mak-rō-kōr′nē-ă). An abnormally large cornea.
mac·ro·cra·ni·um (mak-rō-krā′nē-ŭm). An enlarged skull, especially the bones containing the brain, as seen in hydrocephalus; the face appears relatively small in comparison.
mac·ro·cry·o·glob·u·li·ne·mia (mak′rō-krī-ō-glob′yū-lin-ē′mē-ă). The presence of cold-precipitating macroglobulins in the peripheral blood; such macrocryoglobulins are often called cold hemagglutinins.
mac·ro·cyte (mak′rō-sīt). A large erythrocyte, such as those observed in pernicious anemia. [macro- + G. *kytos,* a hollow (cell)]
mac·ro·cy·the·mia (mak′rō-sī-thē′mē-ă). The occurrence of unusually large numbers of macrocytes in the circulating blood. SYN macrocytosis. [macrocyte + G. *haima,* blood]
ℹ mac·ro·cy·to·sis (mak′rō-sī-tō′sis). SYN macrocythemia. [macrocyte + G. *-osis,* condition]
mac·ro·don·tia, mac·ro·don·tism (mak-rō-don′shē-ă, -don′tizm). The state of having abnormally large teeth. SYN megadontism, megalodontia.
mac·ro·ele·ments (mak′rō-el′ĕ-ments). Inorganic nutrients needed in relatively high daily amounts (*i.e.,* more than 100 mg per day) *e.g.,* calcium, phosphorus, sodium, etc.
mac·ro·ga·mete (mak-rō-gam′ēt). The female element in anisogamy; it is the larger of the two sex cells, with more reserve material, and usually nonmotile. [macro- + G. *gametē,* wife]
mac·ro·ga·me·to·cyte (mak′rō-gă-mē′tō-sīt). The female gametocyte or mother cell producing the female or macrogamete among fungi or protozoa that undergo anisogamy.
mac·ro·gen·i·to·so·mia (mak′rō-jen′i-tō-sō′mē-ă). Excessive bodily and genital development. [macro- + L. *genitalis,* genital, + G. *sōma,* body]
ma·crog·lia (ma-krog′lē-ă). SYN astrocyte. [macro- + G. *glia,* glue]
mac·ro·glob·u·lin·e·mia (mak′rō-glob′yū-li-nē′mē-ă). Increased levels of macroglobulins in the blood.
mac·ro·glos·sia (mak-rō-glos′ē-ă). Enlargement of the tongue, either developmental or due to a neoplasm or vascular hamartoma. SYN megaloglossia. [macro- + G. *glōssa,* tongue]
mac·ro·gna·thia (mak-rō-nā′thē-ă). Enlargement or elongation of the jaw. [macro- + G. *gnathos,* jaw]
mac·ro·mas·tia, mac·ro·ma·zia (mak-rō-mas′tē-a, -mā′zē-ă). Abnormally large breasts. SEE

ALSO hypermastia (2). [macro- + G. *mastos,* breast]

mac·ro·me·lia (mak-rō-mē'lē-ă). Abnormal size of one or more of the limbs. SYN megalomelia. [macro- + G. *melos,* limb]

mac·ro·mol·e·cule (mak-rō-mol'ĕ-kyūl). A molecule of colloidal size; *e.g.,* proteins, polynucleic acids, polysaccharides.

mac·ro·mon·o·cyte (mak-rō-mon'ō-sīt). An unusually large monocyte.

mac·ro·my·e·lo·blast (mak-rō-mī'ĕ-lō-blast). An abnormally large myeloblast.

mac·ro·nor·mo·blast (mak-rō-nōr'mō-blast). **1.** A large normoblast. **2.** A large, incompletely hemoglobiniferous, nucleated red blood cell with a "cart-wheel" nucleus.

mac·ro·nu·cle·us (mak-rō-nū'klē-ŭs). **1.** A nucleus that occupies a relatively large portion of the cell, or the larger nucleus where two or more are present in a cell. **2.** The larger of the two nuclei in ciliates, which governs vegetative metabolic functions and not reproduction. SEE ALSO micronucleus (2).

mac·ro·nu·tri·ents (mak-rō-nū'trē-ents). Nutrients required in the greatest amount; *e.g.,* carbohydrates, protein, fats.

mac·ro·nych·ia (mak-rō-nik'ē-ă). Abnormally large fingernails or toenails. [macro- + G. *onyx,* nail]

mac·ro·pe·nis (mak-rō-pē'nis). An abnormally large penis.

mac·ro·phage (mak'rō-fāj). Any mononuclear, actively phagocytic cell arising from monocytic stem cells in the bone marrow; these cells are widely distributed in the body and vary in morphology and motility, though most are large, long-lived cells with a nearly round nucleus and abundant endocytic vacuoles, lysosomes, and phagolysosomes. Phagocytic activity is typically mediated by serum recognition factors, including certain immunoglobulins and components of the complement system, but also may be nonspecific for some inert materials and bacteria, as in the case of alveolar m.'s; m.'s also are involved in both the production of antibodies and in cell-mediated immune responses, participate in presenting antigens to lymphocytes, and secrete a variety of immunoregulatory molecules. [macro- + G. *phagō,* to eat]

   alveolar m., a vigorously phagocytic m. on the epithelial surface of lung alveoli where it ingests inhaled particulate matter. SYN coniophage, dust cell.

   fixed m., a relatively immotile m. found in connective tissue, lymph nodes, spleen, and bone marrow.

   free m., an actively motile m. typically found in sites of inflammation.

mac·ro·po·dia (mak-rō-pō'dē-ă). Abnormally large feet. SYN megalopodia. [macro- + G. *pous,* foot]

mac·ro·pol·y·cyte (mak-rō-pol'ē-sīt). An unusually large polymorphonuclear neutrophilic leukocyte that contains a multisegmented nucleus (*e.g.,* 8, 10, or more lobes); frequently observed pernicious anemia and certain other forms of anemia. [macro- + G. *polys,* many, + *kytos,* cell]

mac·ro·pro·so·pia (mak'rō-prō-sō'pē-ă). A condition in which the face is too large in proportion to the size of the cranial vault. [macro- + G. *prosōpon,* face]

mac·ro·rhin·ia (mak-rō-rin'ē-ă). Excessive size of the nose, either congenital or pathologic. [macro- + G. *rhis* (rhin-), nose]

mac·ro·scop·ic (mak-rō-skop'ik). **1.** Of a size visible with the naked eye or without the use of a microscope. **2.** Relating to macroscopy.

ma·cros·co·py (mă-kros'kŏ-pē). Examination of objects with the naked eye. [macro- + G. *skopeō,* to view]

mac·ro·sig·moid (mak-rō-sig'moyd). Enlargement or dilation of the sigmoid colon.

mac·ro·so·mia (mak-rō-sō'mē-ă). Abnormally large size of the body. [macro- + G. *sōma,* body]

mac·ro·sto·mia (mak-rō-stō'mē-ă). Abnormally large size of the mouth resulting from failure of fusion between the maxillary and mandibular processes of the embryonic face. [macro- + G. *stoma,* mouth]

mac·ro·tia (mak-rō'shē-ă). Congenital excessive enlargement of the auricle, particularly the pinna. [macro- + G. *ous,* ear]

mac·u·la, pl. **mac·u·lae** (mak'yū-lă, -yū-lē). **1** [NA]. A small spot, perceptibly different in color from the surrounding tissue. **2.** A small, discolored patch or spot on the skin, neither elevated above nor depressed below the skin's surface. SEE ALSO spot. SYN macule, spot (1). [L. a spot]

   mac'ulae acus'ticae, SEE m. of saccule, m. of utricle.

   m. adher'ens, SYN desmosome.

   m. atroph'ica, an atrophic glistening white spot on the skin.

   m. ceru'lea, a bluish stain on the skin caused by the bites of fleas or lice, seen especially in pediculosis pubis. SYN blue spot (1).

   m. cor'neae, a moderately dense opacity of the cornea.

   m. cribro'sa, pl. **mac'ulae cribro'sae** [NA], one of three areas on the wall of the vestibule of the labyrinth, marked by numerous foramina giving passage to nerve filaments supplying portions of the membranous labyrinth; **m. cribrosa inferior,** located in the posterior bony ampulla for passage of posterior ampullary nerve fibers; **m. cribrosa media,** area near the base of the cochlea through which the saccular nerve fibers pass; **m. cribrosa superior,** perforated area above the elliptical recess for passage of the utriculoampullary nerve fibers; **m. cribrosa quarta,** a name sometimes applied to the opening for the cochlear nerve.

   m. den'sa, a closely packed group of densely staining cells in the distal tubular epithelium of a nephron, in direct apposition to the juxtaglomerular cells; they may function as either chemoreceptors or as baroreceptors feeding information to the juxtaglomerular cells.

   m. fla'va, a yellowish spot at the anterior extremity of the rima glottidis where the two vocal folds join.

   m. ret'inae [NA], an oval area of the sensory retina, 3 by 5 mm, temporal to the optic disk corresponding to the posterior pole of the eye; at

ma

its center is the central fovea, which contains only retinal cones.

m. of saccule, the oval neuroepithelial sensory receptor in the anterior wall of the saccule; hair cells of the neuroepithelium support the statoconial membrane and have terminal arborizations of vestibular nerve fibers around their bodies.

m. of utricle, the neuroepithelial sensory receptor in the inferolateral wall of the utricle; hair cells of the neuroepithelium support the statoconial membrane and have terminal arborizations of vestibular nerve fibers around their bodies; sensitive to linear acceleration in the longitudinal axis of the body and to gravitational influences.

mac·u·lar, mac·u·late (mak′yū-lăr, -lāt). **1.** Relating to or marked by macules. **2.** Denoting the central retina, especially the macula retinae.

i mac·ule (mak′yūl). SYN· macula. [L. *macula,* spot]

mac·u·lo·ce·re·bral (mak′yū-lō-ser′ĕ-brăl). Relating to the macula lutea and the brain; denoting a type of nervous disease marked by degenerative lesions in both the retina and the brain.

mac·u·lo·er·y·the·ma·tous (mak′yū-lō-er-i-thē′mă-tŭs). Denoting lesions that are erythematous and macular, covering wide areas.

mac·u·lo·pap·ule (mak′yū-lō-pap′yŭl). A lesion with a flat base surrounding a papule in the center.

mac·u·lop·a·thy (mak-yū-lop′ă-thē). Any pathological condition of the macula lutea.

cystoid m., cystic degeneration of the central retina that may occur after cataract extraction, in senile macular degeneration, and in other retinal abnormalities.

mad·a·ro·sis. SYN *alopecia* adnata.

Mad·u·rel·la (mad′yū-rel′ă). A genus of fungi including a number of species that cause mycetoma. [*Madura,* India]

ma·du·ro·my·co·sis (mad′yū-rō-mī-kō′sis). SYN mycetoma (1). [*Madura,* India, + mycosis]

mag·got (mag′ot). A fly larva or grub.

mag·is·tral (maj′is-trăl). Denoting a preparation compounded according to a physician's prescription, in contrast to officinal (derived from a pharmacist's stock). [L. *magister,* master]

mag·ma (mag′mă). **1.** A soft mass left after extraction of the active principles. **2.** A salve or thick paste. [G. a soft mass or salve, fr. *massō,* to knead]

mag·ne·si·um (Mg) (mag-nē′zē-ŭm). An alkaline earth element, atomic no. 12, atomic wt. 24.3050, that oxidizes to magnesia; a bioelement; many salts have clinical applications. [Mod. L. fr. G. *Magnēsia,* a region in Thessaly]

m. oxide, used as an antacid and laxative.

mag·net. 1. A body that has the property of attracting particles of iron, cobalt, nickel, or any of various metallic alloys and that when freely suspended tends to assume a definite direction between the magnetic poles of the earth (magnetic polarity). h **2.** A bar or horseshoe-shaped piece of iron or steel that has been made magnetic by contact with another m. or, as in an electromagnet, by passage of electric current around a metallic (iron) core. **3.** An electromagnet built in a cylindrical configuration to accom-

modate a patient in its core, for magnetic resonance imaging. [G. *magnēs*]

superconducting m., a m. whose coils are cooled, usually with liquid helium, to a temperature at which the metal becomes superconducting, effectively removing all electrical resistance.

mag·ni·fi·ca·tion (mag′ni-fi-kā′shŭn). **1.** The seeming increase in size of an object viewed under the microscope; when written, this increased size is expressed by a figure preceded by ×, indicating the number of times its diameter is enlarged. **2.** The increased amplitude of a tracing, as of a muscular contraction, caused by the use of a lever with a long writing arm. [L. *magnifico,* pp. *-atus,* to magnify]

mag·no·cel·lu·lar (mag′nō-sel′yū-lăr). Composed of cells of large size. [L. *magnus,* large, + cellular]

MAI. *Mycobacterium avium-intracellulare.* SEE ALSO *Mycobacterium avium-intracellulare complex.*

mAi milliampere-impulse.

main·stream·ing (mān′strēm-ing). Providing the least restrictive environment (socially, physically, and educationally) for individuals with chronic disabilities by introducing them into the natural environment rather than. segregating them into homogeneous groups living in sheltered environments under constant supervision.

main·tain·er (mān-tā′ner). A device utilized to hold or keep teeth in a given position.

main·te·nance (mān′ten-ans). **1.** A therapeutic regimen intended to preserve benefit. Cf. compliance (2), adherence (2). **2.** The extent to which the patient continues good heath practices without supervision, incorporating them into a general life-style. Cf. compliance. [M.E., fr O.Fr., fr. Mediev. L. *manuteneo,* to hold in the hand]

mal (mahl). A disease or disorder. [Fr. fr. L. *malum,* an evil]

m. de mer, SYN seasickness.

grand m. (grahn), SYN generalized tonic-clonic *seizure.*

petit m. (pĕ-tē′), type of seizure. [Fr. small]

△**mal-.** Ill, bad; opposite of eu-. Cf. dys-, caco-. [L. *malus,* bad]

ma·la (mā′lă). **1.** SYN cheek. **2.** SYN zygomatic *bone.* [L. cheek bone]

mal·ab·sorp·tion (mal-ab-sōrp′shŭn). Imperfect, inadequate, or otherwise disordered gastrointestinal absorption.

ma·la·cia (mă-lā′shē-ă). A softening or loss of consistency and contiguity in any of the organs or tissues. Also used as a combining form in the suffix position. SYN mollities (2). SYN malacosis. [G. *malakia,* a softness]

mal·a·co·pla·kia, mal·a·ko·pla·kia (mal′ă-kō-plā′kē-ă, mal′a-kō-plā′kē-a). Rare lesion in the mucosa of the urinary bladder characterized by mottled yellow and gray soft nodules that consist of macrophages and calcospherites (Michaelis-Guttmann bodies). [malaco- + G. *plax,* plate, plaque]

mal·a·co·sis (mal′ă-kō′sis). SYN malacia.

mal·a·cot·ic (mal′ă-kot′ik). Pertaining to or characterized by malacia.

mal·ad·just·ment (mal-ad-jŭst′ment). In the

mental health professions, an inability to cope with the problems and challenges of everyday living. [mal- + *adjust,* fr. O.Fr. *adjuster,* fr. L.L. *adjuxto,* to put close to, + -ment]

mal•a•dy (mal′ă-dē). A disease or illness. [Fr. *maladie,* illness]

mal•aise (mă-lāz′). A feeling of general discomfort or uneasiness, an "out-of-sorts" feeling, often the first indication of an infection or other disease. [Fr. discomfort]

mal•a•lign•ment (mal-ă-līn′ment). Displacement of a tooth or teeth from a normal position in the dental arch.

ma•lar (mā′lăr). Relating to the mala, the cheek or cheek bones.

ma•lar•ia (mă-lār′ē-ă). A disease caused by the presence of the sporozoan *Plasmodium* in red blood cells, usually transmitted by the bite of an infected female mosquito of the genus *Anopheles* that previously sucked blood from a person with m. Human infection begins with the exoerythrocytic cycle in liver parenchyma cells, followed by a series of erythrocytic schizogenous cycles repeated at regular intervals; production of gametocytes in other red cells provides future gametes for another mosquito infection; characterized by episodic severe chills and high fever, prostration, occasionally fatal termination. SEE tropical *diseases,* under *disease.* SEE ALSO *Plasmodium.* SYN swamp fever (2). [It. *malo* (fem. *mala*), bad, + *aria,* air, referring to the old theory of the miasmatic origin of the disease]

 acute m., a form of m. consisting of a chill accompanied and followed by fever with its attendant general symptoms, and terminating in a sweating stage; the paroxysms, caused by release of merozoites from infected cells, recur every 48 hours in tertian (vivax or ovale) m., every 72 hours in quartan (malariae) m., and at indefinite but frequent intervals, usually about 48 hours, in malignant tertian (falciparum) m.

 chronic m., m. that develops after frequently repeated attacks of one of the acute forms, usually falciparum m.; it is characterized by profound anemia, enlargement of the spleen, emaciation, mental depression, sallow complexion, edema of ankles, feeble digestion, and muscular weakness.

 falciparum m., m. caused by *Plasmodium falciparum* and characterized by malarial paroxysms of severe form that occur every 48 hours with acute cerebral, renal, or gastrointestinal manifestations in severe cases, chiefly caused by the large number of red blood cells affected and the tendency for infected red cells to become sticky and clump, thus blocking capillaries. SYN malignant tertian m.

 malariae m., a malarial fever with paroxysms that recur every 72 hours or every fourth day, reckoning the day of the paroxysm as the first; due to the schizogony and release of merozoites from infected cells, with invasion of new red blood corpuscles by *Plasmodium malariae.* SYN quartan m.

 malignant tertian m., SYN falciparum m.
 quartan m., SYN malariae m.
 quotidian m., m. in which the paroxysms occur

daily; usually a double tertian m., in which there is an infection by two distinct groups of *Plasmodium vivax* parasites sporulating alternately every 48 hours.

 vivax m., a malarial fever with paroxysms that recur every 48 hours or every other day (every third day, reckoning the day of the paroxysm as the first); the fever is induced by release of merozoites and their invasion of new red blood corpuscles; causative agent is *Plasmodium vivax.*

ma•lar•i•al (mă-lār′ē-ăl). Pertaining to or affected with malaria.

Ma•las•sez•ia (mal-ă-sē′zē-ă). A genus of fungi of low pathogenicity; *M. furfur* causes tinea versicolor. [L. C. *Malassez*]

mal•as•sim•i•la•tion (mal′ă-sim-i-lā′shŭn). Rarely used term for incomplete or faulty assimilation; malabsorption.

ma•late (mal′āt). A salt or ester of malic acid.
 m. dehydrogenase, any enzyme that catalyzes the dehydrogenation of malate to oxaloacetate. At least six are known; one is an enzyme in the tricarboxylic acid cycle.

mal•ax•a•tion (mal′ak-sā′shŭn). **1.** Formation of ingredients into a mass for pills and plasters. **2.** A kneading process in massage. [L. *malaxo,* pp. *-atus,* to soften]

male (māl). **1.** ZOOLOGY Denoting the sex to which those belong that produce spermatozoa; an individual of that sex. **2.** SYN masculine. [L. *masculus,* fr. *mas,* male]

mal•e•rup•tion (mal-ē-rŭp′shŭn). Faulty eruption of teeth.

mal•for•ma•tion (mal-fōr-mā′shŭn). Failure of proper or normal development; more specifically, a primary structural defect that results from a localized error of morphogenesis; *e.g.,* cleft lip. Cf. deformation.

 Arnold-Chiari m., malformed posterior fossa structures resulting from caudad traction and displacement of the rhombencephalon caused by tethering of the spinal cord; may or may not be accompanied by spina bifida and associated anomalies such as meningomyelocele; weak evidence of autosomal recessive inheritance.

mal•func•tion (mal-fŭnk′shŭn). Disordered, inadequate, or abnormal function.

mal•ic ac•id (mal′ik, mā′lik). Hydroxysuccinic acid; found in apples and various other tart fruits; an intermediate in the tricarboxylic acid cycle, the glyoxylate cycle, and in a shuttle system.

ma•lig•nan•cy (mă-lig′nan-sē). The property or condition of being malignant.

ma•lig•nant (mă-lig′nănt). **1.** Resistant to treatment; occurring in severe form, and frequently fatal; tending to become worse. **2.** In reference to a neoplasm, having the property of locally invasive and destructive growth and metastasis. [L. *maligno,* pres. p. *-ans (ant-),* to do anything maliciously]

ma•lin•ger (mă-ling′ger). To engage in malingering.

ma•lin•ger•er (mă-ling′ger-er). One who engages in malingering.

mal•in•ter•dig•i•ta•tion (mal′in-ter-dij′i-tā′shŭn). Faulty intercuspation of teeth.

mal•le•a•ble (mal′ē-ă-bl). Capable of being

shaped by being beaten or by pressure; a property of certain metals such as gold and silver. [L. *malleus,* a hammer]

mal·le·o·in·cu·dal (mal′ē-ō-ing′kū-dăl). Relating to the malleus and the incus in the tympanum.

mal·le·o·lar (mă-lē′ō-lăr). Relating to one or both malleoli.

mal·le·o·lus, pl. **mal·le·o·li** (ma-lē′ō-lŭs, -lī) [NA]. A rounded bony prominence such as those on either side of the ankle joint. [L. dim. of *malleus,* hammer]

mal·le·ot·o·my (mal′ē-ot′ō-mē). **1.** Division of the malleus. [malleus + G. *tomē,* incision] **2.** Division of the ligaments holding the malleoli in apposition in order to permit their separation in certain cases of clubfoot. [malleolus + G. *tomē,* incision]

mal·le·us, gen. and pl. **mal·lei** (mal′ē-ŭs, mal′ē-ī) [NA]. The largest of the three auditory ossicles, resembling a club rather than a hammer; it is regarded as having a head, below which is the neck, and from this diverge the handle or manubrium, and the slender, anterior process; from the base of the manubrium the short lateral process arises. The manubrium and lateral process are firmly attached to the tympanic membrane, and the head articulates with a saddle-shaped surface on the body of the incus. SYN hammer. [L. a hammer]

mal·nu·tri·tion (mal-nū-trish′ŭn). Faulty nutrition resulting from malabsorption, poor diet, or overeating.

mal·oc·clu·sion (mal-ō-klū′zhŭn). **1.** Any deviation from a physiologically acceptable contact of opposing dentitions. **2.** Any deviation from a normal occlusion.

ma·lo·nic ac·id (mă-lō′nik, -lon′ik). A dicarboxylic acid of importance in intermediary metabolism; an inhibitor of succinate dehydrogenase.

mal·o·nyl-CoA. The condensation product of malonic acid and coenzyme A, an intermediate in fatty acid biosynthesis.

mal·pi·ghi·an (mahl-pig′ē-an). Described by or attributed to Marcello Malpighi.

mal·po·si·tion (mal-pō-zish′ŭn). SYN dystopia.

mal·prac·tice (mal-prak′tis). Mistreatment of a patient through ignorance, carelessness, neglect, or criminal intent.

mal·pre·sen·ta·tion (mal′prē-sen-tā′shŭn). Faulty presentation of the fetus; presentation of any part other than the occiput.

mal·ro·ta·tion (mal-rō-tā′shŭn). Failure during embryonic development of normal rotation of all or part of an organ or system such as gut tube or kidney.

mal·tose (mawl-tōs). A disaccharide formed in the hydrolysis of starch and consisting of two D-glucose residues.

ma·lum (mā′lŭm). A disease. [L. an evil]

△**mamil-, mamilli-.** The mamillae. SEE ALSO mammil-. Cf. thelo-. [L. *mamilla,* nipple]

ma·mil·la, pl. **ma·mil·lae** (mă-mil′ă, mă-mil′ē). **1.** A small rounded elevation resembling the female breast. **2.** SYN nipple. [L. nipple]

mam·il·lary (mam′i-lār-ē). Relating to or shaped like a nipple.

mam·il·late, mam·il·lat·ed (mam′i-lāt, -lāt′ed). Studded with nipple-like projections.

mam·il·la·tion (mam-i-lā′shŭn). **1.** A nipple-like projection. **2.** The condition of being mamillated.

ma·mil·li·form (mă-mil′i-fōrm). Nipple-shaped. [L. *mamilla,* nipple, + *forma,* form]

mam·ma, gen. and pl. **mam·mae** (mam′ă, mam′ē) [NA]. SYN breast. SEE ALSO mammary *gland.* [L.]

mam·mal·gia (mă-mal′jē-ă). SYN mastodynia. [L. *mamma,* breast, + G. *algos,* pain]

mam·ma·plas·ty (mam′ă-plas-tē). Plastic surgery of the breast to alter its shape, size, or position, or all of these. SYN mammoplasty, mastoplasty. [L. *mamma,* breast, + G. *plastos,* formed]

　augmentation m., plastic surgery to enlarge the breast, often by insertion of an implant.

　reconstructive m., the making of a simulated breast by plastic surgery, to replace the appearance of one that has been removed.

　reduction m., plastic surgery of the breast to reduce its size and (frequently) to improve its shape and position.

mam·ma·ry (mam′ă-rē). Relating to the breasts.

mam·mec·to·my (ma-mek′tō-mē). SYN mastectomy. [L. *mamma,* breast, + *ektomē,* excision]

mam·mi·form (mam′i-fōrm). Resembling a breast; breast-shaped. SYN mammose (1). [L. *mamma,* breast, + *forma,* form]

△**mammil-, mammilli-.** The mamillae. SEE ALSO mamil-. Cf. thelo-. [L. *mammilla (mamilla),* nipple]

mam·mil·la·plas·ty (ma-mil′ă-plas-tē). Plastic surgery of the nipple and areola. SYN theleplasty. [L. *mammilla,* nipple, + G. *plastos,* formed]

mam·mil·li·tis (mam-i-lī′tis). Inflammation of the nipple. [L., *mamilla,* nipple, + G. *-itis,* inflammation]

△**mammo-.** The breasts. Cf. masto-. [L. *mamma,* breast]

mam·mo·gram (mam′ō-gram). The record produced by mammography.

mam·mog·ra·phy (ma-mog′ră-fē). Imaging examination of the breast by means of x-rays, ultrasound, and nuclear magnetic resonance; used for screening and diagnosis of breast disease. [mammo- + G. *graphō,* to write]

mam·mo·plas·ty (mam′ō-plas-tē). SYN mammaplasty. [mammo- + G. *plastos,* formed]

mam·mose (mam′mōs). **1.** SYN mammiform. **2.** Having large breasts.

mam·mot·o·my (ma-mot′ō-mē). SYN mastotomy. [mammo- + G. *tomē,* incision]

mam·mo·tro·pic, mam·mo·tro·phic (mam-ō-trop′ik, -trof′ik). Having a stimulating effect upon the development, growth, or function of the mammary glands. [mammo- + G. *tropos,* a turning]

man·di·ble (man′di-bl). A U-shaped bone, forming the lower jaw, articulating by its upturned extremities with the temporal bone on either side. SYN mandibula [NA], jaw bone, submaxilla.

man·dib·u·la, pl. **man·dib·u·lae** (man-dib′yū-lă, -lē) [NA]. SYN mandible. [L. a jaw, fr. *mando,* pp. *mansus,* to chew]

man·dib·u·lar (man-dib′yū-lăr). Relating to the lower jaw. SYN inframaxillary, submaxillary (1).

man·dib·u·lo·fa·cial (man-dib′yū-lō-fā′shăl). Relating to the mandible and the face.

man·dib·u·lo·oc·u·lo·fa·cial (man-dib′yū-lō-ok′yū-lō-fā′shăl). Relating to the mandible and the orbital part of the face.

man·drel, man·dril. **1.** The shaft or spindle to which a tool is attached and by means of which it is rotated. **2.** SYN mandrin. **3.** DENTISTRY An instrument used in a handpiece to hold a disk, stone, or cup used for grinding, smoothing, or finishing. [G. *mandra,* a stable; the bed in which a ring's stone is set]

man·drin. A stiff wire or stylet inserted in the lumen of a soft catheter to give it shape and firmness while passing through a hollow tubular structure. SYN mandrel (2), mandril. [Fr. *mandrin,* mandrel]

ma·neu·ver (mă-nū′ver). A planned movement or procedure. [Fr. *manoeuvre,* fr. L. *manu operari,* to work by hand]

  Bracht m., delivery of a fetus in breech position by extension of the legs and trunk of the fetus over the symphysis pubis and abdomen of the mother; the fetal head is born spontaneously as the legs and trunk are lifted above the maternal pelvis, and as the body of the infant is extended by the operator.

  Brandt-Andrews m., the expression of the placenta by grasping the umbilical cord with one hand and placing the other hand on the abdomen, with the fingers over the anterior surface of the uterus at the junction of the lower uterine segment and the corpus uteri.

  Heimlich m., a procedure to expel an obstructing bolus of food from the throat by placing a fist on the abdomen between the navel and the costal margin, grasping the fist with the other hand, and thrusting it inward and upward so as to drive the diaphragm upward, forcing air up the trachea to dislodge the obstruction.

  key-in-lock m., a method by which obstetrical forceps are used to rotate the fetal head.

  Mauriceau's m., a method of assisted breech delivery in which the infant's body is astraddle the right forearm, and the middle finger of the right hand is in the fetal mouth to maintain flexion while traction is made upon the shoulders by the other hand.

  McRoberts m., m. to reduce a fetal shoulder dystocia by flexion of the maternal hips.

  Mendelsohn m., during a swallow, maintenance of the larynx for a few seconds at the highest position in the neck by voluntary muscular contraction. This laryngeal elevation results in wider and longer esophageal opening, and is a therapeutic technique for management of swallowing disorders.

  Pinard's m., in management of a frank breech presentation, pressure on the popliteal space is made by the index finger while the other three fingers flex the leg while sliding it along the other thigh as the foot of the flexed leg is brought down and out.

  Prague m., a technique for delivery of the fetus in breech position when the fetal occiput is posterior; one hand of the operator delivers the

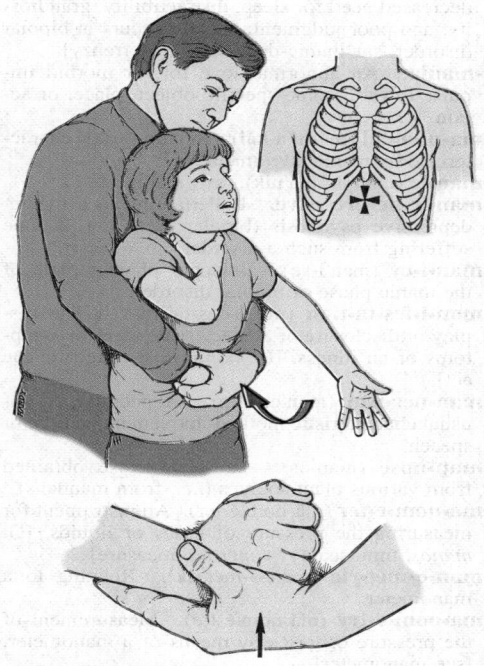

Heimlich maneuver

shoulders, while making pressure above the symphysis pubis with the other hand.

  Scanzoni's m., forceps rotation and traction in a spiral course, with reapplication of forceps for delivery.

  Sellick's m., pressure applied to the cricoid cartilage, to prevent regurgitation during tracheal intubation in the anesthetized patient.

  Toynbee m., action that accomplishes auditory (eustachian) tube opening when patient closes mouth, holds nose, and swallows. SEE ALSO Valsalva m., politzerization.

  Valsalva m., any forced expiratory effort ("strain") against a closed airway, whether at the nose and mouth or at the glottis; because high intrathoracic pressure impedes venous return to the right atrium, this m. is used to study cardiovascular effects of raised peripheral venous pressure and decreased cardiac filling and cardiac output.

man·ga·nese (Mn) (mang′gă-nēz). A metallic element resembling and often associated, in ores, with iron; atomic no. 25, atomic wt. 54.94; manganous salts are sometimes used in medicine. [Mod. L. *manganesium, manganum,* an altered form of *magnesium*]

mange (mānj). A cutaneous disease of domestic and wild animals caused by any one of several genera of skin-burrowing mites; in humans, mite infestations are usually referred to as scabies. [Fr. *manger,* to eat]

ma·nia (mā′nē-ă). An emotional disorder characterized by euphoria or irritability, increased psychomotor activity, rapid speech, flight of ideas, decreased need for sleep, distractibility, grandiosity, and poor judgment; usually occurs in bipolar disorder. SEE manic-depressive. [G. frenzy]

⚠-**mania.** An abnormal love for, or morbid impulse toward, some specific object, place, or action. [G. frenzy]

ma·ni·a·cal (mă-nī′ă-kăl). Relating to or characterized by mania. SYN manic.

man·ic (man′ik, mā′nik). SYN maniacal.

man·ic-de·pres·sive. 1. Pertaining to a manic-depressive psychosis (bipolar *disorder*). **2.** One suffering from such a disorder.

man·i·cy (man′i-sē). Behavior characteristic of the manic phase of bipolar disorder.

man·i·fes·ta·tion (man′i-fes-tā′shŭn). The display or disclosure of characteristic signs or symptoms of an illness. [L. *manifestus,* caught in the act]

man·ner·ism (man′er-izm). A peculiar or unusual characteristic mode of movement, action, or speech.

man·nose (man′ōs). An aldohexose obtained from various plant sources (*i.e.,* from mannans).

ma·nom·e·ter (mă-nom′ĕ-ter). An instrument for measuring the pressure of gases or liquids. [G. *manos,* thin, scanty, + *metron,* measure]

man·o·met·ric (man-ō-met′rik). Relating to a manometer.

ma·nom·e·try (mă-nom′ĕ-trē). Measurement of the pressure of gases by means of a manometer. [see manometer]

man. pr. Abbreviation for L. *mane primo,* early morning, first thing in the morning.

man·tle (man′tl). **1.** A covering layer. **2.** SYN pallium.

ma·nu·bri·um, pl. **ma·nu·bria** (mă-nū′brē-ŭm, -ă) [NA]. The portion of the sternum or of the malleus that represents the handle. [L. handle]

  m. of malleus, the handle of the malleus; the portion that extends downward, inward, and backward from the neck of the malleus; it is embedded throughout its length in the tympanic membrane.

  m. of sternum, the upper segment of the sternum, a flattened, roughly triangular bone, occasionally fused with the body of the sternum, forming with it a slight angle, the sternal angle.

ma·nus, gen. and pl. **ma·nus** (mā′nŭs) [NA]. SYN hand. [L.]

map. A representation of a region or structure; *e.g.,* of a stretch of DNA.

  contig m., a physical m. of a chromosome or stretch of DNA constructed from sets of overlapping and order clones (contig).

  physical m., a m. of a stretch of DNA with ordered landmarks a known distance from each other; the ultimate physical m. would be the base sequence of the entire chromosome.

map·ping func·tion. LINKAGE ANALYSIS A formula that converts the recombination fraction (which is on the probability scale) into map distance (in morgans).

ma·ran·tic (mă-ran′tik). SYN marasmic. [G. *marantikos,* wasting]

ma·ras·mic (mă-raz′mik). Relating to or suffering from marasmus. SYN marantic.

ma·ras·mus (mă-raz′mŭs). Cachexia, especially in young children, primarily due to prolonged dietary deficiency of protein and calories. [G. *marasmos,* withering]

mar·fan·oid (mar′fan-oyd). A term used of those whose phenotype bears a superficial resemblance to that of Marfan's syndrome.

mar·gin (mar′jin). A boundary, edge, or border, as of a surface or structure. SEE ALSO border. SYN margo [NA]. [L. *margo,* border, edge]

  gingival m., (**1**) the most coronal portion of the gingiva surrounding the tooth; (**2**) the edge of the free gingiva.

  m. of safety, the m. between the minimal therapeutic dose and the minimal toxic dose of a drug.

  supraorbital m., the superior half of the orbital rim, which constitutes the curved superior border of the orbital opening, formed by the frontal bone.

mar·gi·nal (mar′ji-năl). Relating to a margin.

mar·gin·a·tion (mar′ji-nā′shŭn). A phenomenon that occurs during the relatively early phases of inflammation; as a result of dilation of capillaries and slowing of the bloodstream, leukocytes tend to occupy the periphery of the cross-sectional lumen and adhere to the endothelial cells that line the vessels.

mar·gi·no·plas·ty (mar′ji-nō-plas-tē). Plastic surgery of the tarsal border of an eyelid.

mar·go, gen. **mar·gi·nis**, pl. **mar·gi·nes** (mar′gō, mar′ji-nis, -nēz) [NA]. SYN margin, border. [L.]

mar·i·hua·na (mar-i-wah′nă). Popular name for the dried flowering leaves of *Cannabis sativa,* which are smoked as cigarettes, "joints," or "reefers." In the U.S. m. includes any part of, or any extracts from, the female plant. Alternative spellings are mariguana, marijuana. SEE ALSO cannabis. [fr. Sp. *Maria-Juana,* Mary-Jane]

mark. 1. Any spot, line, or other figure on the cutaneous or mucocutaneous surface, visible through difference in color, elevation, or other peculiarity. **2.** SYN infundibulum (8). [A.S. *mearc*]

  port-wine m., SYN *nevus* flammeus.

  strawberry m., SYN strawberry *nevus.*

mark·er. 1. A device used to make a mark or to indicate measurement. **2.** A characteristic or factor by which a cell or molecule can be recognized or identified. **3.** A locus containing two or more alleles that, being harmless, are common and therefore yield high frequencies of heterozygotes which facilitate linkage analysis.

  linkage m., a locus at which there is a high probability of heterozygotes (indispensible state for linkage analysis), but in itself perhaps of no clinical interest.

  oncofetal m., a tumor m. produced by tumor tissue and by fetal tissue of the same type as the tumor, but not by normal adult tissue from which the tumor arises.

  tumor m., a substance, released into the circulation by tumor tissue, whose detection in the serum indicates the presence and specific type of tumor.

mar·mo·rat·ed (mar′mō-rā-ted). Denoting a condition in which the appearance of the skin is streaked like marble. SEE ALSO *cutis* marmorata. [L. *marmoratus,* marbled]

mar•row (mar'ō). **1.** A highly cellular hematopoietic connective tissue filling the medullary cavities and spongy epiphyses of bones that becomes predominantly fatty with age, particularly in the long bones of the limbs. **2.** Any soft gelatinous or fatty material resembling the m. of bone. SEE ALSO medulla. [A.S. *mearh*]

bone m., the tissue filling the cavities of bones, having a stroma of reticular fibers and cells.

mar•su•pi•al•i•za•tion (mar-sū'pē-ăl-i-zā'shŭn). Exteriorization of a cyst or other such enclosed cavity by resecting the anterior wall and suturing the cut edges of the remaining wall to adjacent edges of the skin, thereby creating a pouch. [L. *marsupium,* pouch]

Mar•y•land co•ma scale. SEE coma *scale.*

mA-s (milliampere-second) milliampere-second.

mas•cu•line (mas'kyū-lin). Relating to or marked by the characteristics of the male sex or gender. SYN male (2). [L. *masculus,* male, fr. *mas,* male]

mas•cu•lin•i•ty (mas-kyū-lin'i-tē). The qualities and characteristics of a male.

mas•cu•lin•i•za•tion (mas'kyū-lin-i-zā'shŭn). The condition marked by the attainment of male characteristics, such as facial hair, either physiologically as part of male maturation, or pathologically by individuals of either sex. [L. *masculus,* male]

mas•cu•li•nize (mas'kyū-li-nīz). To confer the qualities or characteristics peculiar to the male.

mask. 1. Any of a variety of disease states producing alteration or discoloration of the skin of the face. **2.** The expressionless appearance seen in certain diseases; *e.g.,* Parkinson's facies. **3.** A facial bandage. **4.** A shield designed to cover the mouth and nose for maintenance of aseptic conditions. **5.** A device designed to cover the mouth and nose for administration of inhalation anesthetics, oxygen, or other gases.

ecchymotic m., a dusky discoloration of the head and neck occurring when the trunk has been subjected to sudden and extreme compression, as in traumatic asphyxia.

Hutchinson's m., the sensation experienced in tabetic neurosyphilis as if the face were covered with a m. or with cobwebs.

luetic m., a dirty brownish yellow pigmentation, blotchy in character, resembling that of chloasma, occurring on the forehead, temples, and sometimes the cheeks in patients with tertiary syphilis.

partial rebreathing m., a face m. and a reservoir bag permitting a portion of the exhaled gas to enter the bag for mixing with source gas.

m. of pregnancy, SYN melasma.

Venturi m., a face m. designed to entrain atmospheric air in order to provide a constant fractional dilution of a pressurized gas, most commonly oxygen. [Giovanni Battista Venturi, Italian physicist, 1746–1822)]

mask•ing. 1. The use of noise of any kind to interfere with the audibility of another sound. For any given intensity, low pitched tones have a greater m. effect than those of a high pitch. **2.**

AUDIOLOGY The use of a noise applied to one ear while testing the hearing acuity of the other ear. **3.** The hiding of smaller rhythms in the brain wave record by larger and slower ones whose wave form they distort. **4.** DENTISTRY An opaque covering used to camouflage the metal parts of a prosthesis. **5.** RADIOGRAPHY Superimposition of an altered positive image on the original negative to produce an enhanced copy photographically.

mas•och•ism (mas'ō-kizm, maz'ō-). **1.** Passive algolagnia; a form of perversion, often sexual in nature, in which a person experiences pleasure in being abused, humiliated, or maltreated. Cf. sadism. **2.** A general orientation in life that personal suffering relieves guilt and leads to a reward. [Leopold von Sacher-*Masoch,* Austrian novelist, 1836–1895]

mas•och•ist (mas'ō-kist). The passive party in the practice of masochism.

MASS *m*itral valve prolapse, *a*ortic anomalies, *s*keletal changes, and *s*kin changes.

mass. 1. A lump or aggregation of coherent material. **2.** In pharmacy, a soft solid preparation containing an active medicinal agent, of such consistency that it can be divided into small pieces and rolled into pills. **3.** One of the seven fundamental quantities in the SI system; its unit is the kilogram, defined as the m. of the international prototype of the kilogram, which is made of platinum-iridium and kept at the International Bureau of Weights and Measures. SYN massa [NA]. [L. *massa,* a dough-like mass]

fat-free body m. (FFM), the body m. (weight) devoid of all extractable fat; includes muscle, bone, skin, organs, and water. (FFM = Body mass - Fat mass).

relative molecular m. (M_r), SYN molecular *weight.*

sclerotic cemental m., benign fibro-osseous jaw lesions of unknown etiology, which present as large painless radiopaque masses.

mas•sa, gen. and pl. **mas•sae** (mas'ă, mas'sē) [NA]. SYN mass. [L.]

mas•sage (mă-sahzh'). A method of manipulation of the body by rubbing, pinching, kneading, tapping, etc. [Fr. from G. *massō,* to knead]

🄸 closed chest m., rhythmic compression of the heart between sternum and spine by depressing the lower sternum with the heels of the hands, the patient lying supine.

gingival m., mechanical stimulation of the gingiva by rubbing or pressure.

heart m., rhythmic m. of the heart either in an open chest or through the chest wall to renew failed circulation during cardiac resuscitation.

open chest m., rhythmic manual compression of the ventricles of the heart with the hand inside the thoracic cavity.

prostatic m., (1) manual expression of prostatic secretions by digital rectal technique; **(2)** the emptying of prostatic sinuses and ducts by repeated downward compression maneuvers; used in the treatment of various congestive and inflammatory prostatic conditions.

mas•so•ther•a•py (mas-ō-thār'ă-pē). The therapeutic use of massage. [G. *massō,* to knead, + *therapeia,* treatment]

ma

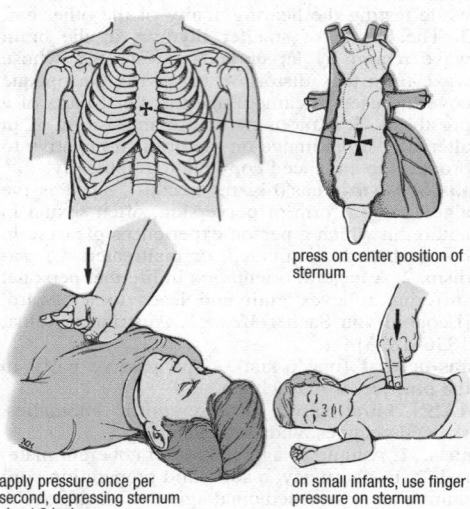

press on center position of sternum

apply pressure once per second, depressing sternum about 2 inches

on small infants, use finger pressure on sternum

closed chest massage

MAST military antishock trousers.

⌂**mast-.** SEE masto-.

mast•ad•e•ni•tis (mast′ad-ĕ-nī′tis). SYN mastitis. [masto- + G. *adēn,* gland, + *-itis,* inflammation]

mast•ad•e•no•ma (mast′ad-ĕ-nō′mă). An adenoma of the breast. [masto- + G. *adēn,* gland, + *-ōma,* tumor]

Mast•ad•e•no•vi•rus (mast-ad′ĕ-nō-vī′rŭs). A genus of adenoviruses with over 40 antigenic types (species) being infective for humans. They cause respiratory infections in children, epidemic acute respiratory disease in military recruits, acute follicular conjunctivitis in adults, and epidemic keratoconjunctivitis; many infections are inapparent. [G. *mastos,* breast, hence mammal, + adenovirus]

mas•tal•gia (mas-tal′jē-ă). SYN mastodynia. [masto- + G. *algos,* pain]

mas•tat•ro•phy, mas•ta•tro•phia (mas-tat′rō-fē, mast-ă-trō′fē-ă). Atrophy or wasting of the breasts. [masto- + atrophy]

mas•tec•to•my (mas-tek′tō-mē). Excision of the breast. SYN mammectomy. [masto- + G. *ektomē,* excision]

extended radical m., excision of the entire breast including the nipple, areola, and overlying skin, as well as the pectoral muscles and the lymphatic-bearing tissues of the axilla and chest wall and internal mammary chain of lymph nodes.

modified radical m., excision of the entire breast including the nipple, areola, and overlying skin, as well as the lymphatic-bearing tissue in the axilla with preservation of the pectoral muscles.

radical m., excision of the entire breast including the nipple, areola, and overlying skin, as well as the pectoral muscles, lymphatic-bearing tissue

in the axilla, and various other neighboring tissues. SYN Halsted's operation (2).

simple m., excision of the breast including the nipple, areola, and most of the overlying skin.

subcutaneous m., excision of the breast tissues, but sparing the skin, nipple, and areola; usually followed by implantation of a prosthesis.

mas•ti•cate (mas′ti-kāt). To chew; to perform mastication.

ℹ**mas•ti•ca•tion** (mas-ti-kā′shŭn). The process of chewing food in preparation for deglutition and digestion; the act of grinding or comminuting with the teeth. [L. *mastico,* pp. *-atus,* to chew]

mas•ti•ca•to•ry (mas′ti-kă-tō-rē). Relating to mastication.

mas•ti•gote (mas′ti-gōt). An individual flagellate. [G. *mastix,* a whip]

mas•ti•tis (mas-tī′tis). Inflammation of the breast. SYN mastadenitis. [masto- + G. *-itis,* inflammation]

plasma cell m., a condition of the breasts characterized by tumorlike indurated masses containing numerous plasma cells, usually resulting from mammary duct ectasia; although clinically resembling malignant disease (attachment to skin and enlargement of axillary lymph nodes), it is not neoplastic.

submammary m., inflammation of the tissues lying deep to the mammary gland.

⌂**masto-, mast-.** The breast; the mastoid. Cf. mammo-, mazo-. [G. *mastos*]

mas•to•cyte (mas′tō-sīt). SYN mast *cell.*

mas•to•cy•to•ma (mas′tō-sī-tō′mă). A fairly well-circumscribed accumulation or nodular focus of mast cells, grossly resembling a neoplasm. [mastocyte + G. *-oma,* tumor]

mas•to•cy•to•sis (mas′tō-sī-tō′sis). Abnormal proliferation of mast cells in a variety of tissues; may be systemic, involving a variety of organs, or cutaneous (urticaria pigmentosa). [mastocyte + G. *-osis,* condition]

diffuse cutaneous m., a benign process con-

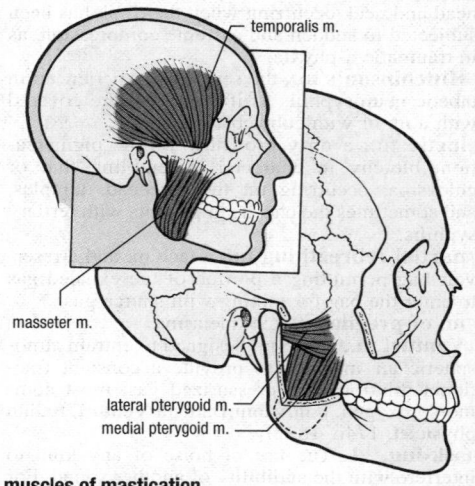

temporalis m.

masseter m.

lateral pterygoid m.

medial pterygoid m.

muscles of mastication

sisting of focal cutaneous infiltrates composed of mast cells; lesions are flat or slightly elevated, form wheals and itch when stroked; bone lesions may occur.

mas·to·dyn·ia (mas-tō-din′ē-ă).   Pain in the breast. SYN mammalgia, mastalgia. [masto- + G. *odynē,* pain]

mas·toid (mas′toyd).   **1.** Resembling a mamma; breast-shaped.   **2.** Relating to the m. process, antrum, cells, etc. [masto- + G. *eidos,* resemblance]

mas·toid·ec·to·my (mas′toy-dek′tō-mē).   Hollowing out of the mastoid process by curretting, gouging, drilling, or otherwise removing the bony partitions forming the mastoid cells. [mastoid (process) + G. *ektomē,* excision]

❚**mas·toid·i·tis** (mas-toy-dī′tis).   Inflammation of any part of the mastoid process.

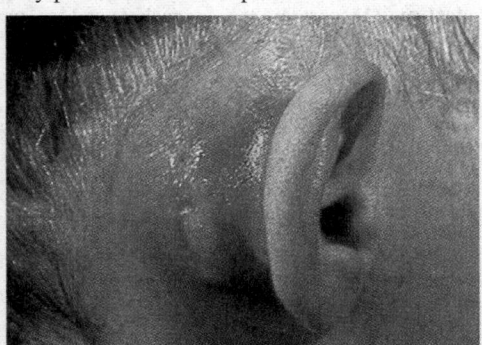

mastoiditis: ruptured retroauricular abscess

mas·ton·cus (mas-tong′kŭs).   A tumor or swelling of the breasts. [masto- + G. *onkos,* mass]

mas·to·oc·cip·i·tal (mas′tō-ok-sip′i-tăl).   Relating to the mastoid portion of the temporal bone and to the occipital bone, denoting the suture uniting them.

mas·to·pa·ri·e·tal (mas′tō-pa-rī′ĕ-tăl).   Relating to the mastoid portion of the temporal bone and to the parietal bone, denoting the suture uniting them.

mas·top·a·thy (mas-top′ă-thē).   Any disease of the breasts. [masto- + G. *pathos,* suffering]

mas·to·pexy (mas′tō-pek-sē).   Plastic surgery to affix sagging breasts in a more elevated and normal position, often with some improvement in shape. [masto- + G. *pēxis,* fixation]

mas·to·pla·sia (mas-tō-plā′zē-ă).   Enlargement of the breast. [masto- + G. *plasis,* a molding]

mas·to·plas·ty (mas′tō-plas-tē).   SYN mammaplasty. [masto- + G. *plastos,* formed]

mas·top·to·sis (mas-top-tō′sis).   Ptosis or sagging of the breast. [masto- + G. *ptōsis,* a falling]

mas·tor·rha·gia (mas-tō-rā′jē-ă).   Hemorrhage from a breast. [masto- + G. *rhēgnymi,* to burst forth]

mas·to·squa·mous (mas′tō-skwā′mŭs).   Relating to the mastoid and the squamous portions of the temporal bone.

mas·tot·o·my (mas-tot′ō-mē).   Incision of the breast. SYN mammotomy. [masto- + G. *tomē,* incision]

mas·tur·bate (mas′ter-bāt).   To practice masturbation. [L. *masturbari,* pp. *masturbatus*]

mas·tur·ba·tion.   Self-stimulation of the genitals for erotic pleasure, often resulting in orgasm.

match·ing.   The process of making a study group and a comparison group in an epidemiological study comparable with respect to extraneous or confounding factors such as age, sex, weight, etc.

ma·te·ria (mă-tē′rē-ă).   Substance or matter. [L. substance]

m. al′ba, accumulation or aggregation of microorganisms, desquamated epithelial cells, blood cells and food debris loosely adherent to surfaces of plaques, teeth, gingiva or dental appliances. [L. white matter]

m. med′ica, (1) that aspect of medical science concerned with the origin and preparation of drugs, their doses, and their mode of administration; **(2)** any agent used therapeutically. SEE ALSO pharmacognosy, pharmacology. [L. medical matter]

ma·ter·nal (mă-ter′năl).   Relating to or derived from the mother. [L. *maternus,* fr. *mater,* mother]

ma·ter·ni·ty (mă-ter′ni-tē).   Motherhood. [see maternal]

mat·ing (māt′ing).   The pairing of male and female for the purpose of reproduction.

assortative m., selection of a mate with preference for (or aversion to) a particular genotype, *i.e.,* nonrandom m.

random m., a practice of m. in a population in which at some specified locus m. patterns occur with expected frequencies predicted by the product of the frequencies of the genotypes in the population.

mat·ri·cal (mat′ri-kăl).   Relating to any matrix.

ma·tri·ces (mā′tri-sēz, mat′rĭ-sēz).   Plural of matrix. [L.]

mat·ri·cide (mat′ri-sīd).   **1.** The killing of one's mother.   **2.** One who commits such an act. [L. *mater,* mother, + *caedo,* to kill]

mat·ri·lin·e·al (mat-ri-lin′ē-ăl).   Denoting descent through the female line. [L. *mater,* mother, + *linea,* line]

ma·trix, pl. **ma·tri·ces** (mā′triks, mat′riks; mā′tri-sēz, mat′ri-sēz).   **1** [NA]. The formative portion of a tooth or a nail.   **2.** The intercellular substance of a tissue.   **3.** A surrounding substance within which something is contained or embedded.   **4.** A mold in which anything is cast or swaged; a counterdie; a specially shaped instrument, plastic material, or metal strip used for holding and shaping the material used in filling a tooth cavity.   **5.** A rectangular array of numbers or symbol quantities that simplify the execution of linear operations of tedious complexity; the theory of matrices is widely used in solving simultaneous equations and in population genetics. [L. womb; female breeding animal]

bone m., the intercellular substance of bone tissue consisting of collagen fibers, ground substance, and inorganic bone salts.

cartilage m., the intercellular substance of cartilage consisting of fibers and ground substance.

territorial m., SYN cartilage *capsule.*

m. un′guis [NA], SYN nail *bed.*

mat·ter. SYN substance. SEE ALSO substance. [L. *materies,* substance]

gray m., those regions of the brain and spinal cord which are made up primarily of the cell bodies and dendrites of nerve cells rather than myelinated axons. SYN substantia grisea [NA], gray substance.

white m., those regions of the brain and spinal cord that are largely or entirely composed of nerve fibers and contain few or no neuronal cell bodies or dendrites. SYN substantia alba [NA], alba, white substance.

mat·u·ra·tion (mat-yū-rā′shŭn). **1.** Achievement of full development or growth. **2.** Developmental changes that lead to maturity. **3.** Processing of a macromolecule; *e.g.,* posttranscriptional modification of RNA or posttranslational modification of proteins. [L. *maturatio,* a ripening, fr. *maturus,* ripe]

ma·ture (mă-chūr′, -tūr). **1.** Ripe; fully developed. **2.** To ripen; to become fully developed. [L. *maturus,* ripe]

ma·tu·ri·ty (mă-chūr′i-tē). A state of full development or completed growth.

max·il·la, gen. and pl. **max·il·lae** (mak-sil′ă, mak-sil′ē) [NA]. An irregularly shaped bone, supporting the superior teeth and taking part in the formation of the orbit, hard palate, and nasal cavity. [L. jawbone]

max·il·lary (mak′si-lār-ē). Relating to the maxilla, or upper jaw.

max·il·lo·den·tal (mak-sil′ō-den′tăl). Relating to the upper jaw and its associated teeth.

max·il·lo·fa·cial (mak-sil′ō-fā′shăl). Pertaining to the jaws and face, particularly with reference to specialized surgery of this region.

max·il·lo·man·dib·u·lar (mak-sil′ō-man-dib′yū-lăr). Relating to the upper and lower jaws.

max·il·lot·o·my (mak-si-lot′ō-mē). Surgical sectioning of the maxilla to allow movement of all or a part of the maxilla into the desired position. [maxilla + G. *tomē,* incision]

max·i·mum (mak′si-mŭm). The greatest amount, value, or degree attained or attainable. [L. neuter of *maximus,* greatest]

glucose transport m., the maximal rate of reabsorption of glucose from the glomerular filtrate; it amounts to approximately 320 mg/min in humans.

transport m. (Tm), the maximal rate of secretion or reabsorption of a substance by the renal tubules.

Mayo stand. a removable instrument tray set on a movable stand that is positioned over or adjacent to a surgical site; it provides a place for sterile instruments and supplies used during surgery.

⌂**mazo-.** The breast. SEE ALSO masto-. [G. *mazos*]

Mb Myoglobin.

MBC maximum breathing *capacity.*

MbCO Myoglobin in combination with CO.

MbO₂ oxymyoglobin.

mc for millicurie.

MCH mean corpuscular *hemoglobin.*

MCHC mean corpuscular hemoglobin *concentration.*

mCi millicurie.

MCP metacarpophalangeal.

M-CSF macrophage colony-stimulating *factor.*

MCV Abbreviation for mean corpuscular *volume.*

MD Abbreviation for methyldichloroarsine.

Md mendelevium.

MDF myocardial depressant *factor.*

MDI (metered-dose inhaler) metered-dose *inhaler.*

MDS minimum data *set.*

meal (mēl). **1.** The food consumed at regular intervals or at a specified time. **2.** Ground flour from a grain.

Boyden m., a m. consisting of three or four egg yolks, beaten up in milk, used to test the evacuation time of the gallbladder; two-thirds to three-quarters of the contents will normally be evacuated within 40 minutes.

test m., (1) toast and tea, or crackers and tea, or gruel or other bland food, given to stimulate gastric secretion before withdrawing gastric contents for analysis; **(2)** administration of food containing a substance thought to be responsible for symptoms, such as an allergic reaction.

mean (mēn). A statistical measurement of central tendency or average of a set of values, usually assumed to be the arithmetic m. unless otherwise specified. [M.E., *mene* fr. O.Fr., fr. L. *medianus,* in the middle]

arithmetic m., the m. calculated by adding a set of values and then dividing the sum by the number of values.

geometric m., the m. calculated as the antilogarithm of the arithmetic mean of the logarithms of the individual values; it can also be calculated as the *n*th root of the product of *n* values.

harmonic m., the m. calculated as the number of values being averaged, divided by the sum of their reciprocals.

mea·sles (mē′zlz). **1.** An acute exanthematous disease, caused by m. virus and marked by fever and other constitutional disturbances, a catarrhal inflammation of the respiratory mucous membranes, and a generalized maculopapular eruption of a dusky red color; the eruption occurs early on the buccal mucous membrane in the form of Koplik's spots; incubation period is from 10 to 12 days. SYN morbilli, rubeola. **2.** A disease of swine caused by the presence of *Cysticercus cellulosae,* the measle or larva of *Taenia solium,* the pork tapeworm. **3.** A disease of cattle caused by the presence of *Cysticercus bovis,* the measle or larva of *Taenia saginata,* the beef tapeworm of man. [D. *maselen*]

atypical m., unusual clinical manifestation of natural m. infection in persons with waning vaccination immunity, particularly in those who had received formaldehyde-inactivated vaccine; an accelerated allergic reaction characterized by high fever, absence of Koplik's spots, a shortened prodromal period, atypical rash, and pneumonia.

German m., SYN rubella.

hemorrhagic m., a severe form in which the eruption is dark in color due to effusion of blood into affected areas of the skin.

measurement. Determination of a dimension or quantity.

ℹ**skinfold m.'s,** determinations of the thickness

of a fold of skin using calipers. M.'s are used to assess body fat content. Standard tables are available relating skinfold thickness to body fat as a percentage of body weight according to age and sex.

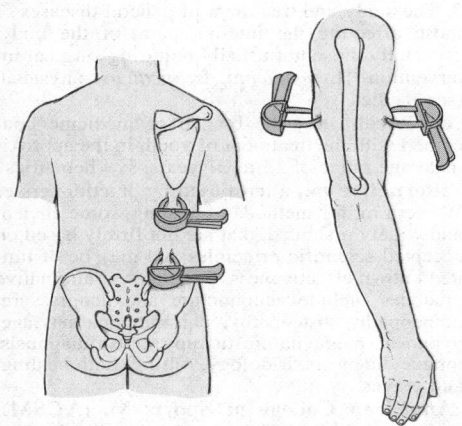

skin measurement: skinfold measurement with calipers at standard sites provides an accurate estimate of subcutaneous fat

me•a•tal (mē-ā′tăl). Relating to a meatus.

meato-. Meatus. [L. *meatus*, passage]

me•a•to•plas•ty (mē′ă-tō-plas-tē). Plastic surgery of a meatus or canal, *e.g.,* the external auditory meatus or the urethral meatus.

me•a•tor•rha•phy (mē-ă-tōr′ă-fē). Closing by suture the wound made by performing a meatotomy. [meato- + G. *rhaphē*, suture]

me•a•tos•co•py (mē-ă-tos′kŏ-pē). Inspection, usually instrumental, of any meatus, especially of the meatus of the urethra. [meato- + G. *skopeō*, to view]

me•a•tot•o•my (mē-ă-tot′ō-mē). An incision made to enlarge a meatus, *e.g.,* of the urethra or ureter. [meato- + G. *tomē*, incision]

me•a•tus, pl. **me•a•tus** (mē-ā′tŭs) [NA]. A passage or channel, especially the external opening of a canal. [L. a going, a passage, fr. *meo,* pp. *meatus,* to go, pass]

  acoustic m., (1) externus (NA): auditory canal; the passage leading inward through the tympanic portion of the temporal bone, from the auricle to the membrana tympani; (2) internus (NA): a canal running through the petrous portion of the temporal bone, giving passage to the facial and vestibulocochlear nerves and to the labyrinthine artery and veins. SYN m. acusticus.

  m. acusticus, [NA] SYN acoustic m.

  nasal m., the three passages (inferior, middle, superior) in the nasal cavity formed by the projection of the conchae. SYN m. nasi.

  m. nasi, [NA] SYN nasal m.

me•chan•i•cal (mĕ-kan′i-kăl). **1.** Performed by means of some apparatus, not manually. **2.** Explaining phenomena in terms of mechanics. **3.** Automatic. [G. *mechanikos,* relating to a machine, fr. *mēchanē,* a contrivance, machine]

me•chan•ics (mĕ-kan′iks). The science of the action of forces in promoting motion or equilibrium. [see mechanical]

mech•a•nism (mek′ă-nizm). **1.** An arrangement or grouping of the parts of anything that has a definite action. **2.** The means by which an effect is obtained. [G. *mēchanē,* a contrivance]

  countercurrent m., a system in the renal medulla that facilitates concentration of the urine as it passes through the renal tubules.

  defense m., (1) a psychological means of coping with conflict or anxiety, *e.g.,* conversion, denial, dissociation, rationalization, repression, sublimation; (2) the psychic structure underlying a coping strategy; (3) immunological m. vs. nonspecific defense m.

  feedback m., SYN feedback *inhibition.*

  gating m., (1) occurrence of the maximum refractory period among cardiac conducting cells approximately 2 mm proximal to the terminal Purkinje fibers in the ventricular muscle; gating m. may be a cause of ventricular aberration, bidirectional tachycardia, and concealed extrasystoles; (2) a m. by which painful impulses may be blocked from entering the spinal cord. Cf. gate-control *theory.*

  immunological m., the groups of cells (chiefly lymphocytes and cells of the reticuloendothelial system) that function in establishing active acquired immunity (induced sensitivity, allergy).

  proprioceptive m., the m. of sense of position and movement, by which muscular movements can be adjusted to a great degree of accuracy and equilibrium maintained.

  re-entrant m., the probable basis of most arrhythmias, requiring at least three criteria: 1. a loop circuit, 2. unidirectional block, 3. slowed conduction.

  speech m., peripheral structures involved in the normal production of speech, encompassing the organs of articulation, phonation, resonance, and respiration. SEE articulation, articulators, phonation, resonance, respiration.

mech•a•no•re•cep•tor (mek′ă-nō-rē-sep′tŏr). A receptor which responds to mechanical pressure or distortion; *e.g.,* receptors in the carotid sinuses, touch receptors in the skin.

me•co•ni•um (mē-kō′nē-ŭm). The first intestinal discharges of the newborn infant, greenish in color and consisting of epithelial cells, mucus, and bile. [L., fr. G. *mēkōnion,* dim. of *mēkōn,* poppy]

me•di•a (mē′dē-ă). **1.** SYN *tunica* media. **2.** Plural of medium. [L. fem. of *medius,* middle]

me•di•al (mē′dē-ăl). Relating to the middle or center; nearer to the median or midsagittal plane. [L. *medialis,* middle]

me•di•an (mē′dē-an). **1.** Central; middle; lying in the midline. **2.** The middle value in a set of measurements; like the mean, a measure of central tendency. [L. *medianus,* middle]

me•di•as•ti•nal (mē′dē-as-tī′năl). Relating to the mediastinum.

me•di•as•ti•ni•tis (mē′dē-as-ti-nī′tis). Inflammation of the cellular tissue of the mediastinum.

me•di•as•ti•nog•ra•phy (mē′dē-as-ti-nog′ră-fē).

me

Radiography of the mediastinum. [mediastinum + G. *graphō*, to write]

me·di·as·tin·o·per·i·car·di·tis (me'dē-as'tin-ō-per'i-kar-dī'tis). Inflammation of the pericardium and of the surrounding mediastinal cellular tissue.

me·di·as·tin·o·scope (mē-dē-as'tin'-ō-skōp). An endoscope for inspection of mediastinum through a suprasternal incision.

me·di·as·ti·nos·co·py (mē'dē-as-ti-nos'kŏ-pē). Exploration of the mediastinum through a suprasternal incision, for biopsy of paratracheal lymph nodes. [mediastinum + G. *skopeō*, to view]

me·di·as·ti·not·o·my (mē'dē-as-ti-not'ō-mē). Incision into the mediastinum. [mediastinum + G. *tomē*, incision]

me·di·as·ti·num (me'dē-as-tī'nŭm) [NA]. **1.** A septum between two parts of an organ or a cavity. **2.** The median partition of the thoracic cavity, covered by the mediastinal pleura and containing all the thoracic viscera and structures except the lungs. It is divided arbitrarily into five parts: anterior mediastinum, inferior mediastinum, middle mediastinum, posterior mediastinum, and superior mediastinum. SYN interpleural space, mediastinal space. [Mod. L. a middle septum, fr. Mediev. L. *mediastinus*, medial, fr. L. *mediastinus*, a lower servant, fr. *medius*, middle]

m. tes′tis [NA], a mass of fibrous tissue continuous with the tunica albuginea, projecting into the testis from its posterior border. SYN Highmore's body.

me·di·ate. **1** (mē'dē-it). Situated between; intermediate. **2** (mē'dē-āt). To effect something by means of an intermediary substance, as in complement-mediated phagocytosis. [L. *mediatus*, fr. *medio*, pp. *-atus*, to divide in the middle]

med·i·ca·ble (med'i-kă-bl). Treatable, with hope of a cure.

Medicaid. Program established under Title XIX of the Social Security Act, which provides health insurance to poor people; it is funded jointly by the state and federal governments. Formerly known as medical assistance. SEE ALSO Medicare.

med·i·cal (med'i-kăl). **1.** Relating to medicine or the practice of medicine. SYN medicinal (2). **2.** SYN medicinal (1). [L. *medicalis*, fr *medicus*, physician]

medical assistance. Former name of medical aid program now known as Medicaid. SEE Medicaid.

med·i·cal tran·scrip·tion·ist. An individual who performs machine transcription of physician-dictated medical records; a certified m. t. (CMT) has satisfied the requirements for certification by the American Association for Medical Transcription (AAMT).

Medicare. Federally managed health insurance plan covering Americans over age 65 and Americans under age 65 who have certain disabilities; established by a 1965 amendment to the Social Security Act. SEE ALSO Medicaid.

med·i·cate (med'i-kāt). **1.** To treat disease by the giving of drugs. **2.** To impregnate with a medicinal substance. [L. *medico*, pp. *-atus*, to heal]

med·i·ca·tion (med-i-kā'shŭn). **1.** The act of medicating. **2.** A medicinal substance, or medicament.

me·dic·i·nal (mĕ-dis'i-năl). **1.** Relating to medicine having curative properties. SYN medical (2). **2.** SYN medical (1).

med·i·cine (med'i-sin). **1.** A drug. **2.** The art of preventing, diagnosing, and treating disease; the science concerned with disease in all its relations. **3.** The study and treatment of general diseases or those affecting the internal parts of the body, especially those not usually requiring surgical intervention. [L. *medicina*, fr. *medicus*, physician (see medicus)]

adolescent m., the branch of medicine concerned with the treatment of youth in the approximate age range of 13 to 21 years. SYN hebiatrics.

alternative m., a term used by practitioners of Western m. for methods of healing, some ancient and widely practiced, that are not firmly based on accepted scientific principles and may be of limited known effectiveness. Examples of alternative practices include acupuncture and acupressure, homeopathy, osteopathy, chiropractic, massage, hypnosis, megavitamin therapy, pulse diagnosis, tongue diagnosis, iridology, rolfing, faith healing, and prayer.

American College of Sports M. (ACSM), national multidisciplinary professional and scientific society dedicated to the generation and dissemination of knowledge concerning the motivation, responses, adaptations, and health aspects of persons engaged in sports and exercise.

clinical m., the study and practice of m. in relation to the care of patients; the art of m. as distinguished from laboratory science.

defensive m., diagnostic or therapeutic measures conducted primarily as a safeguard against possible subsequent malpractice liability.

experimental m., the scientific investigation of medical problems by experimentation upon animals or by clinical research.

family m., the medical specialty concerned with providing continuous, comprehensive care to all age groups, from first patient contact to terminal care, with special emphasis on care of the family as a unit.

fetal m., study of the growth, development, care, and treatment of the fetus, and of environmental factors harmful to the fetus. SYN fetology.

folk m., treatment of ailments by nonphysicians with remedies and simple measures based upon experience and knowledge handed on from generation to generation.

forensic m., (1) the relation and application of medical facts to legal matters; **(2)** the law in its bearing on the practice of medicine. SYN legal m.

holistic m., an approach to medical care that emphasizes the study of all aspects of a person's health, especially that a person should be considered as a unit, including psychological as well as social and economic influences on health status.

internal m. (IM), the branch of m. concerned with nonsurgical diseases in adults, but not including diseases limited to the skin or to the nervous system.

legal m., SYN forensic m.

neonatal m., SYN neonatology.

nuclear m., the clinical discipline concerned with the diagnostic and therapeutic uses of radionuclides, excluding the therapeutic use of sealed radiation sources.

osteopathic m., SYN osteopathy (2).

patent m., a m., usually originally patented, advertised to the public.

perinatal m., SYN perinatology.

physical m., the study and treatment of disease mainly by mechanical and other physical methods. SYN physiatry.

podiatric m., SYN podiatry.

preventive m., the branch of medical science concerned with the prevention of disease and with promotion of physical and mental health, through study of the etiology and epidemiology of disease processes.

proprietary m., a medicinal compound the formula and mode of manufacture of which are the property of the maker.

psychosomatic m., the study and treatment of diseases, disorders, or abnormal states in which psychological processes resulting in physiological reactions are believed to play a prominent role.

socialized m., the organization and control of medical practice by a government agency, the practitioners being employed by the organization from which they receive standardized compensation for their services, and to which the public contributes, usually in the form of taxation rather than fee-for-service.

sports m., a field of m. that uses a holistic, comprehensive, and multidisciplinary approach to health care for those engaged in a sporting or recreational activity.

tropical m., the branch of m. concerned with diseases, mainly of parasitic origin, in areas having a tropical climate.

veterinary m., the field concerned with the diseases and health of all animal species other than humans.

⌂**medico-.** Medical. Cf. iatro-. [L. *medicus*, physician]

med·i·co·chi·rur·gi·cal (med′i-kō-kī-rŭr′ji-kăl). Relating to both medicine and surgery, or to both physicians and surgeons. [medico- G. *cheirourgia*, surgery]

med·i·co·le·gal (med′i-kō-lē′găl). Relating to both medicine and the law. SEE ALSO forensic *medicine*. [medico- + L. *legalis*, legal]

⌂**medio-, medi-.** Middle, median. [L. *medius*]

me·di·o·car·pal (mē′dē-ō-kar′păl). SYN midcarpal.

me·di·o·dor·sal (mē′dē-ō-dōr′săl). Relating to the median plane and the dorsal plane.

me·di·o·lat·er·al (mē′dē-ō-lat′er-ăl). Relating to the median plane and a side.

me·di·o·ne·cro·sis (mē′dē-ō-ne-krō′sis). Necrosis of a tunica media.

me·di·um, pl. **me·dia** (mē′dē-ŭm, -ă). **1.** A means; that through which an action is performed. **2.** A substance through which impulses or impressions are transmitted. **3.** SYN culture m. **4.** The liquid holding a substance in solution or suspension. [L. neuter of *medius*, middle]

contrast m., any internally administered substance that has a different opacity from soft tissue on radiography or computed tomography; used to opacify parts of the gastrointestinal tract, blood vessels, or the genitourinary tract.

culture m., a substance, either solid or liquid, used for the cultivation, isolation, identification, or storage of microorganisms. SYN medium (3).

dispersion m., SYN external *phase*.

Dorset's culture egg m., a m. for cultivating *Mycobacterium tuberculosis;* it consists of the whites and yolks of four fresh eggs and a solution of sodium chloride.

Mueller-Hinton m., an agar-based m. composed of beef infusion, casamino acids, and starch useful in the isolation of gonococci and meningococci; the recommended medium for antibacterial susceptibility tests for most common aerobic and facultatively anaerobic bacteria.

transport m., a m. for transporting clinical specimens to the laboratory for examination.

MEDLARS Medical Literature Analysis and Retrieval System, a computerized index system of the U.S. National Library of Medicine.

MEDLINE. [MEDLARS-on-line] A computer-based telephone linkage to MEDLARS for rapid provision of medical bibliographies.

me·dul·la, pl. **me·dul·lae** (me-dŭl′ă, me-dŭl′ē) [NA]. Any soft marrow-like structure, especially in the center of a part. SEE ALSO m. oblongata. SYN substantia medullaris (1). [L. marrow, fr. *medius*, middle]

m. of hair shaft, the central axis of some hairs, containing a column of large vacuolated and keratinized cells; the medullary portion is surrounded by the cortex.

m. oblonga′ta [NA], the most caudal subdivision of the brainstem, continuous with the spinal cord, extending from the lower border of the decussation of the pyramid to the pons; its ventral surface resembles that of the spinal cord except for the bilateral prominence of the inferior olive; the dorsal surface of its upper half forms part of the floor of the fourth ventricle. Motor nuclei of the m. oblongata include the hypoglossal nucleus, the dorsal motor nucleus, inferior salivatory nucleus, and the nucleus ambiguus; sensory nuclei include the nuclei of the posterior column (gracile and cuneate), the cochlear and vestibular nuclei, the mid and caudal portions of the spinal trigeminal nucleus, and the nucleus of the solitary tract. SEE ALSO medulla. SYN myelencephalon [NA], oblongata.

renal m., the inner, darker portion of the kidney parenchyma consisting of the renal pyramids.

m. spina′lis [NA], SYN spinal *cord*.

suprarenal m., it is composed principally of anastomosing cords of cells in the core of the gland; the cells display a chromaffin reaction because of the presence of epinephrine and norepinephrine in their granules.

me·dul·lar (med-yūl′ăr). SYN medullary.

med·ul·lar·y (med′ŭ-lār-ē, mĕ-dul′er-ē, med′yū-lār-ē). Relating to the medulla or marrow. SYN medullar.

med·ul·lat·ed (med′ŭ-lā-ted, med′yū-). **1.** Having a medulla or medullary substance. **2.** SYN myelinated.

med·ul·lec·to·my (med-ū-lek′tō-mē, med-yū-).

me

Excision of any medullary substance. [medulla + G. *ektomē*, excision]

med·ul·li·za·tion (med'ŭ-li-zā'shŭn, med'yū-). Enlargement of the medullary spaces in rarefying osteitis.

⚬**medullo-.** Medulla. Cf. myel-. [L. *medulla*]

me·dul·lo·ar·thri·tis (med-ŭ-lō-ar-thrī'tis). Inflammation of the cancellous articular extremity of a long bone.

me·dul·lo·blas·to·ma (med'ŭ-lō-blas-tō'mă). A tumor consisting of neoplastic cells that resemble the undifferentiated cells of the primitive medullary tube; m.'s are usually located in the vermis of the cerebellum, comprise approximately 3% of all intracranial neoplasms, and occur most frequently in children.

me·dul·lo·ep·i·the·li·o·ma (me'dŭ-lō-ep'ĭ-thē-lē-ō'mă). A rare, primitive, rapidly growing intracranial neoplasm thought to originate from the cells of the embryonic medullary canal. [medullo- + epithelium + -oma, tumor]

⚬**mega-.** 1. Large, oversize; opposite of micro-. SEE ALSO macro-, megalo-. 2. Prefix used in the SI and metric systems to signify one million (10⁶). [G. *megas*, big]

meg·a·bac·te·ri·um (meg'ă-bak-tēr'ē-ŭm). A bacterium of unusually large size.

megabladder (meg-a-blad-er). SYN megacystis.

meg·a·ce·phal·ic (meg'ă-se-fal'ik). Relating to or characterized by megacephaly. SYN macrocephalic, macrocephalous, megacephalous.

meg·a·ceph·a·lous (meg-ă-sef'ă-lŭs). SYN megacephalic.

meg·a·ceph·a·ly (meg-ă-sef'ă-lē). A condition, either congenital or acquired, in which the head is abnormally large; usually applied to an adult skull with a capacity of over 1450 ml. SYN macrocephaly, macrocephalia, megalocephaly, megalocephalia. [mega- + G. *kephalē*, head]

meg·a·co·lon (meg'ă-kō'lon). A condition of extreme dilation and hypertrophy of the colon.

congenital m., m. congen'itum, congenital dilation and hypertrophy of the colon due to absence (aganglionosis) or marked reduction (hypoganglionosis) in the number of ganglion cells of the myenteric plexus of the rectum and a varying but continuous length of gut above the rectum. SYN Hirschsprung's disease.

toxic m., acute nonobstructive dilation of the colon, seen in fulminating ulcerative colitis and Crohn's disease.

meg·a·cy·cle (meg'ă-sī-kl). One million cycles per second.

meg·a·cys·tis (meg'ă-sis-tis). Pathologically large bladder in children. SYN megabladder, megalocystis. [mega- + *kystis*, bladder]

meg·a·dac·ty·ly, meg·a·dac·tyl·ia, meg·a··dac·tyl·ism (meg-ă-dak'ti-le, -dak-til'ē-ă -dak'til-izm). Condition characterized by enlargement of one or more digits (fingers or toes). SYN dactylomegaly. [mega- + G. *daktylos*, digit]

meg·a·don·tism (meg-ă-don'tizm). SYN macrodontia.

meg·a·e·soph·a·gus (meg'ă-ē-sof'ă-gŭs, meg'ă-e-sof'). Great enlargement of the lower portion of the esophagus, as seen in patients with achalasia and Chagas' disease.

meg·a·hertz (MHz) (meg'ă-hertz). One million hertz.

meg·a·kar·y·o·blast (meg-ă-kar'ē-ō-blast). The precursor of a megakaryocyte.

meg·a·kar·y·o·cyte (meg-ă-kar'ē-ō-sīt). A large cell with a multilobed nucleus. m.'s are normally present in bone marrow, not in the circulating blood, and give rise to blood platelets. SYN megalokaryocyte. [mega- + G. *karyon*, nut (nucleus), + *kytos*, hollow vessel (cell)]

⚬**megal-.** SEE megalo-.

meg·al·gia (meg-al'jē-ă). Very severe pain. [mega- + G. *algos*, pain]

⚬**megalo-, megal-.** Large; opposite of micro-. SEE ALSO macro-, mega-. [G. *megas (megal-)*]

meg·a·lo·blast (meg'ă-lō-blast). A large, nucleated, embryonic type of cell that is a precursor of erythrocytes in an abnormal erythropoietic process observed in pernicious anemia; a m.'s four stages of development are as follows: 1) promegaloblast, 2) basophilic m., 3) polychromatic m., 4) orthochromatic m. SEE ALSO erythroblast. [megalo- + G. *blastos*, + germ, sprout]

meg·a·lo·car·dia (meg'ă-lō-kar'dē-ă). SYN cardiomegaly. [megalo- + G. *kardia*, heart]

meg·a·lo·ceph·a·ly, meg·a·lo·ce·pha·lia (meg'ă-lō-sef'ă-lē, -sě-fā'lē-ă). SYN megacephaly.

meg·a·lo·chei·ria, meg·a·lo·chi·ria (meg'ă-lō-kī'rē-ă). SYN macrocheiria. [megalo- + G. *cheir*, hand]

meg·a·lo·cor·nea (meg'ă-lō-kōr'nē-ă). SYN keratoglobus.

meg·a·lo·cys·tis (meg'ă-lō-sis'tis). SYN megacystis. [megalo- + G. *kystis*, bladder]

meg·a·lo·cyte (meg'ă-lō-sīt). A large (10 to 20 μm) nonnucleated red blood cell. [megalo- + G. *kytos*, cell]

meg·a·lo·don·tia (meg'ă-lō-don'shē-ă). SYN macrodontia.

meg·a·lo·en·ce·phal·ic (meg'ă-lō-en'sě-fal'ik). Denoting an abnormally large brain.

meg·a·lo·en·ceph·a·lon (meg'ă-lō-en-sef'ă-lon). An abnormally large brain. [megalo- + G. *enkephalos*, brain]

meg·a·lo·en·ceph·a·ly (meg'ă-lō-en-sef'ă-lē). Abnormal largeness of the brain. [megalo- + G. *enkephalon*, brain]

meg·a·lo·en·ter·on (meg'ă-lō-en'ter-on). Abnormal largeness of the intestine. SYN enteromegaly, enteromegalia. [megalo- + G. *enteron*, intestine]

meg·a·lo·gas·tria (meg'ă-lō-gas'trē-ă). Abnormally large size of the stomach. [megalo- + G. *gastēr*, stomach]

meg·a·lo·glos·sia (meg'ă-lō-glos'sē-ă). SYN macroglossia. [megalo- + G. *glōssa*, tongue]

meg·a·lo·he·pat·ia (meg'ă-lo-he-pat'ē-ă). SYN hepatomegaly.

meg·a·lo·kar·y·o·cyte (meg'ă-lō-kar'ē-ō-sīt). SYN megakaryocyte.

meg·a·lo·ma·nia (meg'ă-lō-mā'nē-ă). 1. A delusion of greatness; belief that one is Christ, God, Napoleon, a prince, ace athlete in all divisions of sport, etc. 2. Morbid verbalized overevaluation of oneself or of some aspect of oneself. [megalo- + G. *mania*, frenzy]

meg·a·lo·ma·ni·ac (meg'ă-lō-mā'nē-ak). A person exhibiting megalomania.

meg·a·lo·me·lia (meg'ă-lō-mē'lē-ă). SYN macromelia.

meg·a·loph·thal·mos (meg'ă-lof-thal'mŭs). Congenital large globe. [megalo- + G. *ophthalmos,* eye]

meg·a·lo·po·dia (meg'ă-lō-pō'dē-ă). SYN macropodia. [megalo- + G. *pous,* foot]

meg·a·lo·sple·nia (meg'ă-lō-splē'nē-ă). SYN splenomegaly.

meg·a·lo·syn·dac·ty·ly, meg·a·lo·syn·dac·tyl·ia (meg'ă-lō-sin-dak'ti-lē, -dak-til'ē-ă). Condition of webbed or fused fingers or toes of large size. [megalo- + G. *syn,* together, + *daktylos,* finger]

meg·a·lo·u·re·ter (meg'ă-lō-yū-rē'ter). An enlarged, dilated ureter.

△**-megaly.** Large. [G. *megas (megal-)*]

meg·a·rec·tum (meg-ă-rek'tŭm). Extreme dilation of the rectum.

meg·a·volt (meg'ă-vōlt). One million volts.

mei·bo·mi·an (mī-bō'mē-an). Attributed to or described by Meibom.

mei·bo·mi·tis, mei·bo·mi·a·ni·tis (mī'bō-mī'tis, mī-bō'mē-ă-nī'tis). Inflammation of the meibomian glands.

△**meio-.** For words beginning thus and not found here, see mio-.

mei·o·sis (mī-ō'sis). A special process of cell division comprising two nuclear divisions in rapid succession that result in four gametocytes, each containing half the number of chromosomes found in somatic cells. [G. *meiōsis,* a lessening]

mei·ot·ic (mī-ot'ik). Pertaining to meiosis.

△**mel-, melo-.** 1. Limb. [G. *melos*] 2. A cheek. [G. *mēlon*] 3. Honey, sugar. SEE ALSO meli-. [L. *mel, mellis,* G. *meli, melitos*] 4. Sheep. [G. *mēlon*]

me·lag·ra (mě-lag'ră). Rheumatic or myalgic pains in the arms or legs. [G. *melos,* limb, + *agra,* seizure]

me·lal·gia (mě-lal'jē-ă). Pain in a limb; specifically, burning pain in the feet extending up the leg and even to the thigh. [G. *melos,* a limb, + *algos,* pain]

△**melan-, melano-.** Black, extreme darkness of hue. [G. *melas*]

mel·an·cho·lia (mel-an-kō'lē-ă). 1. A severe form of depression marked by anhedonia, insomnia, psychomotor changes, and guilt. 2. A symptom occurring in other conditions, marked by depression of spirits and by a sluggish and painful process of thought. SYN melancholy. [melan- + G. *cholē,* bile. See humoral *doctrine*]

  hypochondriacal m., m. with many associated physical complaints, often with little basis in fact.

  involutional m., a depressive disorder of middle life, commonly associated with the climacteric.

mel·an·chol·ic (mel-an-kol'ik). 1. Relating to or characteristic of melancholia. 2. Denoting a temperament characterized by irritability and a pessimistic outlook. 3. A person who is exhibiting melancholia.

mel·an·choly (mel'an-kol-ē). SYN melancholia.

mel·an·e·de·ma (mel'an-e-dē'mă). SYN anthracosis. [melan- + G. *oidēma,* swelling]

mel·a·nif·er·ous (mel-ă-nif'er-ŭs). Containing melanin or other black pigment. [melan- (melanin) + L. *ferro,* to carry]

mel·a·nin (mel'ă-nin). Any of the dark brown to black pigments that occur in the skin, hair, pigmented coat of the retina, and medulla and zona reticularis of the adrenal gland. [G. *melas* (*melan-*), black]

mel·a·nism (mel'ă-nizm). Unusually marked, diffuse melanin pigmentation of body hair and skin (usually not affecting the iris). SEE ALSO melanosis.

△**melano-.** SEE melan-.

mel·a·no·ac·an·tho·ma (mel'ă-nō-ak-an-thō'mă). A seborrheic keratosis with melanin pigmentation associated with proliferation of intraepidermal melanocytes. [melano- + G. *akantha,* thorn, + suffix *-ōma,* tumor]

mel·a·no·blast (mel'ă-nō-blast). A cell derived from the neural crest; it migrates to various parts of the body early in embryonic life, and then becomes a mature melanocyte capable of forming melanin. [melano- + G. *blastos,* germ, sprout]

mel·a·no·cyte (mel'ă-nō-sīt). A pigment-producing cell located in the basal layer of the epidermis with branching processes by means of which melanosomes are transferred to epidermal cells, resulting in pigmentation of the epidermis. [melano- + G. *kytos,* cell]

mel·a·no·cy·to·ma (mel'ă-nō-sī-tō'mă). 1. A pigmented tumor of the uveal stroma. 2. Usually benign melanoma of the optic disk, appearing in markedly pigmented individuals as a small deeply pigmented tumor at the edge of the disk, sometimes extending into the retina and choroid. [megalo- + cyto- + G. *-oma;* tumor]

mel·a·no·der·ma (mel'ă-nō-der'mă). 1. An abnormal darkening of the skin by deposition of excess melanin. 2. Hyperpigmentation of the skin by melanin or deposition of dark metallic substances such as silver and iron. [melano- + G. *derma,* skin]

  parasitic m., excoriations and m. caused by scratching the bites of the body louse, *Pediculus corporis.* SYN vagabond's disease, vagrant's disease.

  senile m., cutaneous pigmentation occurring in the aged.

mel·a·no·der·ma·ti·tis (mel'ă-nō-der-mă-tī'tis). Excessive deposit of melanin in an area of dermatitis.

mel·a·no·der·mic (mel'ă-nō-der'mik). Relating to or marked by melanoderma.

me·la·no·gen (mě-lan'ō-jen, mel'ă-nō-jen). A colorless substance that may be converted into melanin. [melanin + G. *-gen,* producing]

mel·a·no·gen·e·sis (mel'ă-nō-jen'ě-sis). Formation of melanin. [melanin + G. *genesis,* production]

mel·a·no·glos·sia (mel'ă-nō-glos'ē-ă). SYN black tongue. [melano- + G. *glōssa,* tongue]

mel·a·noid (mel'ă-noyd). A dark pigment, resembling melanin, formed from glucosamines in chitin.

mel·a·no·leu·ko·der·ma (mel'ă-nō-lū-kō-der'mă). Marbled, or marmorated, skin. [melano- + G. *leukos,* white, + *derma,* skin]

  m. col'li, SYN syphilitic *leukoderma.*

me

mel·an·o·li·ber·in (mel'ă-nō-lib'er-in). A hexapeptide similar to oxytocin; it stimulates the release of melanotropin. SYN melanotropin-releasing factor, melanotropin-releasing hormone. [melanotropin + L. *libero*, to free, + -in]

mel·a·no·ma (mel'ă-nō'mă). A malignant neoplasm, derived from cells that are capable of forming melanin, arising most commonly in the skin or in the eye, and, rarely, in the mucous membranes of the genitalia, anus, oral cavity, or other sites; occurs mostly in adults and may originate *de novo* or from a pigmented nevus or lentigo maligna. M.'s frequently metastasize widely; regional lymph nodes, skin, liver, lungs, and brain are likely to be involved. SYN malignant m. [melano- + G. *-ōma*, tumor]

malignant m., SYN melanoma.

  malignant m. in situ, a m. limited to the epidermis and composed of nests of atypical melanocytes and scattered single cells extending into the upper epidermis; local excision is curative although the lesion, if untreated, may soon invade the dermis. Malignant lentigo may be considered a slowly progressive type of malignant m. in situ.

  subungual m., a m. beginning in the skin at the border of or beneath the nail.

mel·a·no·ma·to·sis (mel'ă-nō-mă-tō'sis). A condition characterized by numerous, widespread lesions of melanoma. [melanoma + G. *-osis*, condition]

mel·a·no·nych·ia (mel'ă-nō-nik'ē-ă). Black pigmentation of the nails. [melano- + G. *onyx* (*onych-*), nail]

mel·a·no·phage (mel'ă-nō-fāj, mě-lan'ō-fāj). A histiocyte that has phagocytized melanin. [melano- + G. *phagō*, to eat]

mel·a·no·pla·kia (mel'ă-nō-plā'kē-ă). The occurrence of pigmented patches on the tongue and buccal mucous membrane. [melano- + G. *plax*, plate, plaque]

mel·a·no·sis (mel-ă-nō'sis). Abnormal dark brown or brown-black pigmentation of various tissues or organs, as the result of melanin or substances that resemble it, which may occur in widespread metastatic melanoma, sunburn, and pregnancy. [melano- + G. *-osis*, condition]

  m. co'li, m. of the large intestinal mucosa due to accumulation of pigment of uncertain composition within macrophages in the lamina propria.

mel·a·no·some (mel'ă-nō-sōm). The generally oval pigment granule (0.2 by 0.6 μm) produced by melanocytes. [melano- + G. *sōma*, body]

mel·an·o·sta·tin. Inhibits synthesis and release of melanotropin. SYN melanotropin release-inhibiting hormone. [melanotropin + G. *states*, stationary, + -in]

mel·a·not·ic (mel'ă-not'ik). **1.** Pertaining to the presence, normal or pathologic, of melanin. **2.** Relating to or characterized by melanosis.

mel·a·no·troph (mel'ă-nō-trōf). A cell of the intermediate lobe of the hypophysis that produces melanotropin. [melano- + G. *trophē*, nourishment]

me·la·no·tro·pin (mel'ă-nō-trōp-in). A polypeptide hormone secreted by the intermediate lobe of the hypophysis in humans (in neurohypophysis in certain other species) which causes dispersion of

melanin by melanophores, resulting in darkening of the skin, presumably by promoting melanin synthesis; this effect is readily demonstated in some lower vertebrates, such as frogs and fish; α-m. is an *N*-acetylated peptide with 13 amino acids; β-m. has 22 amino acids. SYN melanocyte-stimulating hormone.

mel·a·nu·ria (mel-ă-nū'rē-ă). The excretion of urine of a dark color, resulting from the presence of melanin or other pigments or from the action of phenol and other coal tar derivatives. [melano- + G. *ouron*, urine]

mel·a·nu·ric (mel-ă-nū'rik). Pertaining to or characterized by melanuria.

me·las·ma (mě-laz'mă). A patchy or generalized pigmentation of the skin. SEE ALSO chloasma. SYN mask of pregnancy. [G. a black color, a black spot]

  m. gravida'rum, chloasma occurring in pregnancy.

mel·a·ton·in (mel-ă-tōn'in). A substance formed by the pineal gland that appears to depress gonadal function; a precursor is serotonin, m. is rapidly metabolized and is taken up by all tissues; it is involved in circadian rhythms. [melanophore + G. *tonos*, stretching, + -in]

me·le·na (me-lē'nă). Passage of dark-colored, tarry stools, due to the presence of blood altered by the intestinal juices. Cf. hematochezia. [G. *melaina*, fem. of *melas*, black]

meli-. Honey, sugar. SEE ALSO mel- (3). [G. *meli*]

me·li·tis (mē-lī'tis). Inflammation of the cheek. [G. *mēlon*, cheek, + *-itis*, inflammation]

melo-. SEE mel-.

mel·o·plas·ty (mel'ō-plas-tē). Plastic surgery of the cheek. [melo- + G. *plastos*, formed]

mel·o·rhe·os·to·sis (mel'ō-rē-os-tō'sis). Rheostosis confined to the long bones. [G. *melos*, limb, + *rheos*, stream, + *osteon*, bone, + *-ōsis*]

me·lo·tia (me-lō'shē-ă). Congenital displacement of the auricle onto the cheek. [G. *mēlon*, cheek, + *ous*, ear]

mem·ber. A limb. [L. *membrum*]

mem·bra (mem'bră) [NA]. Plural of membrum. [L.]

mem·bra·na, gen. and pl. **mem·bra·nae** (mem-brā'nă, -brā'nē) [NA]. SYN biomembrane. [L.]

  m. adventi'tia, (1) SYN adventitia. **(2)** SYN *decidua* capsularis.

  m. decid'ua [NA], SYN deciduous *membrane*.

  m. pupilla'ris [NA], SYN pupillary *membrane*.

  m. reticula'ris [NA], SYN reticular *membrane*.

  m. sero'sa, (1) SYN serosa, chorion. **(2)** SYN serosa (2).

  m. synovia'lis [NA], SYN synovial *membrane*.

  m. tecto'ria duc'tus cochlea'ris [NA], SYN tectorial *membrane* of cochlear duct.

  m. tym'pani [NA], SYN tympanic *membrane*.

  m. tym'pani secunda'ria [NA], SYN secondary tympanic *membrane*.

  m. vitelli'na, (1) the membrane enveloping the yolk; specifically, the thickened cell membrane of large-yolked ova; SYN ovular membrane, vitelline membrane. **(2)** sometimes used to designate the zona pellucida of a mammalian ovum. SYN yolk membrane.

m. vit′rea [NA], SYN posterior limiting *layer* of cornea.

mem·brane (mem′brān). **1.** A thin sheet or layer of pliable tissue, serving as a covering or envelope of a part, as the lining of a cavity, as a partition or septum, or to connect two structures. **2.** SYN biomembrane. [L. *membrana*, a skin or membrane that covers parts of the body, fr. *membrum*, a member]

allantoid m., SYN allantois.

alveolar-capillary m., the alveolar epithelium, interstitial space, and the capillary endothelium barrier that gases must cross in respiration; it is approximately 1 micron thick in healthy individuals and normally represents only a minimal obstacle to gas diffusion.

alveolodental m., SYN periodontal *ligament*.

arachnoid m., SYN arachnoid.

basement m., an amorphous extracellular layer closely applied to the basal surface of epithelium and also investing muscle cells, fat cells, and Schwann cells; thought to be a selective filter and to serve both structural and morphogenetic functions. It is composed of three successive layers (lamina lucida, lamina densa, and lamina fibroreticularis), a matrix of collagen, and several glycoproteins. SYN basilemma.

basilar m., the m. extending from the bony spiral m. to the basilar crest of the cochlea; it forms the greater part of the floor of the cochlear duct separating the latter from the scala tympani and it supports the organ of Corti. SYN basilar lamina.

Bichat's m., the inner elastic m. of arteries.

Bowman's m., SYN anterior elastic *lamina* of cornea.

Brunn's m., the epithelium of the olfactory region of the nose.

cell m., the protoplasmic boundary of all cells that controls permeability and may serve other functions through surface specializations; *e.g.,* active ion transport, absorption by formation of pinocytotic vesicles, and antigen recognition; its fine structure is trilaminar and consists of the electron-dense lamina externa and lamina interna with an electron-lucent lamina intermedia. SYN plasma m., plasmalemma.

cloacal m., a transitory m. in the caudal area of the ventral wall of the embryo, separating the endodermal from the ectodermal cloaca; it is divided into anal and genitourinary m.'s that break down during the eighth to ninth week to establish the external opening for the alimentary and genitourinary tracts.

Corti's m., SYN tectorial m. of cochlear duct.

croupous m., SYN false m.

deciduous m., the mucous m. of the pregnant uterus that has undergone changes, under the influence of the ovulation cycle, to fit it for the implantation and nutrition of the ovum; so-called because the m. is cast off after labor. SYN membrana decidua [NA], decidua.

Descemet's m., SYN posterior elastic *lamina* of cornea.

diphtheritic m., the false m. forming on the mucous surfaces in diphtheria.

drum m., SYN tympanic m.

egg m., the investing envelope of the ovum; a **primary egg m.** is produced from ovarian cytoplasm (*e.g.,* a vitelline m.); a **secondary egg m.** is the product of the ovarian follicle (*e.g.,* the zona pellucida); a **tertiary egg m.** is secreted by the lining of the oviduct (*e.g.,* a shell).

elastic m., a m. formed of elastic connective tissue, present as fenestrated lamellae in the coats of the arteries and elsewhere.

embryonic m., SYN fetal m.

enamel m., the internal layer of the enamel organ formed by the enamel cells.

false m., a thick, tough fibrinous exudate on the surface of a mucous m. or the skin, as seen in diphtheria. SYN croupous m., neomembrane, plica (2), pseudomembrane.

fenestrated m., an elastic m., as in elastic laminae of arteries.

fetal m., a structure or tissue that develops from the fertilized ovum but does not form part of the embryo proper. SYN embryonic m.

germ m., germinal m., SYN blastoderm.

glassy m., (1) the basement m. present between the stratum granulosum and the theca interna of a vesicular ovarian follicle; it becomes very prominent in large atretic follicles; **(2)** the basement m. and associated connective tissue of the hair follicle. SYN hyaline m. (2).

hyaline m., (1) the thin, clear basement m. beneath certain epithelia; **(2)** SYN glassy m. (2).

hyoglossal m., posterior widening of the lingual septum connecting the root of the tongue to the hyoid bone; the inferior fibers of the genioglossus are attached to it and by this means to the upper anterior body of the hyoid bone near the midline.

intercostal m.'s, the membranous layers between ribs.

Jackson's m., a thin vascular m. or veil-like adhesion, covering the anterior surface of the ascending colon from the cecum to the right flexure; it may cause obstruction by kinking of the bowel.

keratogenous m., SYN nail *bed*.

medullary m., SYN endosteum.

nuclear m., SYN nuclear *envelope*.

olfactory m., that part of the nasal mucosa having olfactory receptor cells and glands of Bowman.

ovular m., SYN *membrana* vitellina (1).

peridental m., SYN periodontal *ligament*.

periodontal m., SYN periodontal *ligament*.

placental m., the semipermeable layer of fetal tissue separating the maternal from the fetal blood in the placenta; composed of: 1) endothelium of the fetal vessels in the chorionic villi, 2) stromata of the villi, 3) cytotrophoblast (negligible after the fifth month of gestation), and 4) syncytial trophoblast covering the villi; the placental m. acts as a selective m. regulating passage of substances from the maternal to the fetal blood. SYN placental barrier.

plasma m., SYN cell m.

postsynaptic m., that part of the plasma m. of a neuron or muscle fiber with which an axon terminal forms a synaptic junction.

presynaptic m., that part of the plasma m. of

me

an axon terminal that faces the plasma m. of the neuron or muscle fiber with which the axon terminal establishes a synaptic junction. SEE ALSO synapse.

pupillary m., remnants of the central portion of the anterior layer of the iris stroma (the iridopupillary lamina) which occludes the pupil in fetal life, and normally atrophies about the seventh month of gestation. Failure to regress is a rare cause of congenital blindness. SYN membrana pupillaris [NA].

Reissner's m., SYN vestibular m.

reticular m., the m. formed by cuticular plates of the cells of the spiral organ of Corti; it appears netlike when viewed from above. SYN membrana reticularis [NA].

Ruysch's m., SYN choriocapillary *layer*.

Scarpa's m., SYN secondary tympanic m.

secondary tympanic m., the m. closing the fenestra cochleae or rotunda. SYN membrana tympani secundaria [NA], Scarpa's m.

serous m., SYN serosa.

synovial m., the connective tissue m. that lines the cavity of a synovial joint and produces the synovial fluid; it lines all internal surfaces of the cavity except for the articular cartilage of the bones. SYN membrana synovialis [NA], synovium.

tectorial m. of cochlear duct, a gelatinous m. that overlies the spiral organ (Corti) in the inner ear. SYN membrana tectoria ductus cochlearis [NA], Corti's m., tectorium (2).

tympanic m., a thin tense m. forming the greater part of the lateral wall of the tympanic cavity and separating it from the external acoustic meatus; it constitutes the boundary between the external and middle ear, is covered on both surfaces with epithelium, and in the tense part has an intermediate layer of outer radial and inner circular collagen fibers. SYN membrana tympani [NA], drum m., drum, drumhead, eardrum, myringa, myrinx.

undulating m., undulatory m., a locomotory organelle of certain flagellate (trypanosome and trichomonad) parasites, consisting of a finlike extension of the limiting m. with the flagellar sheath; wavelike rippling of the undulating m. produces a characteristic movement.

unit m., the trilaminar structure of the plasmalemma and other intercellular m.'s, when seen in cross-section with the electron microscope, composed of two electron-dense laminae separated by a less dense lamina.

vestibular m., the m. separating the cochlear duct from the vestibular canal; it consists of squamous epithelial cells with microvilli toward the ductus, a basement m., and a thin layer of connective tissue toward the scala. SYN Reissner's m.

vitelline m., SYN *membrana* vitellina (1).

vitreous m., (1) SYN posterior limiting *layer* of cornea. **(2)** a condensation of fine collagen fibers in places in the cortex of the vitreous body; formerly thought to form a m. or capsule at its periphery; **(3)** SYN *lamina* basalis choroideae.

yolk m., SYN *membrana* vitellina.

Zinn's m., the anterior layer of the iris.

mem•bra•ni•form (mem-brā'ni-fōrm). Of the

appearance or character of a membrane. SYN membranoid.

mem•bra•no•car•ti•lag•i•nous (mem'bră-nō-kar-ti-laj'i-nŭs). **1.** Partly membranous and partly cartilaginous. **2.** Derived from both a mesenchymal membrane and cartilage; denoting certain bones.

mem•bra•noid (mem'bră-noyd). SYN membraniform.

mem•bra•nous (mem'bră-nŭs). Relating to or of the form of a membrane.

mem•brum, pl. **mem•bra** (mem'brŭm, mem'bră) [NA]. A limb; a member. [L. member]

mem•o•ry (mem'ŏ-rē). **1.** General term for the recollection of that which was once experienced or learned. **2.** The mental information processing system that receives (registers), modifies, stores, and retrieves informational stimuli; composed of three stages: encoding, storage, and retrieval. [L. *memoria*]

long-term m. (LTM), that phase of the m. process considered the permanent storehouse of information which has been registered, encoded, passed into the short-term m., coded, rehearsed, and finally transferred and stored for future retrieval; material and information retained in LTM underlies cognitive abilities.

screen m., PSYCHOANALYSIS A consciously tolerable m. that unwittingly serves as a cover for another associated m. which would be emotionally painful if recalled.

short-term m. (STM), that phase of the m. process in which stimuli that have been recognized and registered are stored briefly; decay occurs rapidly, typically within seconds, but may be held indefinitely by using rehearsal as a holding process by which to recycle material over and over through STM.

visual m., retained m. of objects when the visual stimulus is no longer present.

men•ac•me (me-nak'mē). The period of menstrual activity in a woman's life. [G. *mēn,* month, + *akmē,* prime]

men•a•quin•one-6. Hexaprenylmenaquinone; prenylmenaquinone-6; 2-methyl-3-hexaprenyl-1,4-naphthoquinone; isolated from putrified fish meal; potency is about 60% of that of phylloquinone (vitamin K_1). SYN vitamin K_2, vitamin $K_2(30)$.

men•ar•che (me-nar'kē). Establishment of the menstrual function; the time of the first menstrual period. [G. *mēn,* month, + *arché,* beginning]

men•de•le•vi•um (Md) (men-dĕ-lē'vē-ŭm). An element, atomic no. 101, atomic wt. 258.1, prepared in 1955 by bombardment of einsteinium with alpha particles. [*D. Mendeléeff*]

men•de•li•an (men-dē'lē-ăn). Attributed to or described by Gregor Mendel; usually referring to the behavior and the mechanism of the genetic transmission of single-locus traits.

Men•de•li•an In•her•i•tance in Man. A standard, comprehensive, regularly updated reference source for traits in humans that have been shown to be mendelian or that are thought on reasonable grounds to be so. Each entry has a six-digit catalog number. Those securely established (by molecular biology or by extensive clinical studies) are marked with an asterisk.

△**mening-.** SEE meningo-.

me·nin·ge·al (mě-nin′jē-ăl, men′in-jē′ăl). Relating to the meninges.

me·nin·ge·or·rha·phy (mě-nin′jē-ōr′ă-fē). Suture of the cranial or spinal meninges or of any membrane. [G. *mēninx* (*mēning-*), membrane, + *rhaphē*, suture]

me·nin·ges (mě-nin′jēz). Plural of meninx.

me·nin·gi·o·ma (mě-nin′jē-ō′mă). A benign, encapsulated neoplasm of arachnoidal origin, occurring most frequently in adults; most frequent form consists of elongated, fusiform cells in whorls and pseudolobules with psammoma bodies frequently present; m.'s tend to occur along the superior sagittal sinus, along the sphenoid ridge, or in the vicinity of the optic chiasm; in addition to meningothelial m., angiomatous, chondromatous, osteomatous, lipomatous, melanotic, fibroblastic and transitional varieties are recognized. [mening- + G. *-oma*, tumor]

    psammomatous m., a firm cellular neoplasm derived from fibrous tissue of the meninges, choroid plexus, and certain other structures associated with the brain, characterized by the formation of multiple, discrete, concentrically laminated, calcareous bodies (psammoma bodies); most of these neoplasms are histologically benign, but may lead to severe symptoms as a result of compressing the brain.

me·nin·gism (men′in-jizm, mě-nin′jizm). A condition in which the symptoms simulate meningitis, but in which no actual inflammation of these membranes is present.

men·in·git·ic (men′in-jit′ik). Relating to or characterized by meningitis.

men·in·gi·tis, pl. **men·in·git·i·des** (men-in-jī′tis, -jit′i-dēz; -jit′i-dēz). Inflammation of the membranes of the brain or spinal cord. SEE ALSO arachnoiditis, leptomeningitis. SYN cerebrospinal m. [mening- + G. *itis*, inflammation]

    basilar m., m. at the base of the brain, due usually to tuberculosis, syphilis, or any low-grade chronic granulomatous process; may result in an internal hydrocephalus.

    cerebrospinal m., SYN meningitis.

    meningococcal m., an acute infectious disease affecting children and young adults, caused by *Neisseria meningitidis;* characterized by nasopharyngeal catarrh, headache, vomiting, convulsions, stiffness in the neck (nuchal rigidity), photophobia, constipation, cutaneous hyperesthesia, a purpuric or herpetic eruption, and the presence of Kernig's sign. Fulminant form may cause Waterhouse-Friderichsen syndrome.

    occlusive m., leptomeningitis causing occlusion of the spinal fluid pathways.

    otitic m., infection of the meninges secondary to mastoiditis or otitis media.

    serous m., acute m. with secondary external hydrocephalus.

    tuberculous m., inflammation of the cerebral leptomeninges marked by the presence of granulomatous inflammation; it is usually confined to the base of the brain (basilar m., internal hydrocephalus) and is accompanied in children by an accumulation of spinal fluid in the ventricles (acute hydrocephalus).

△**meningo-, mening-.** The meninges. [G. *mēninx*, membrane]

me·nin·go·cele (mě-ning′gō-sēl). Protrusion of the membranes of the brain or spinal cord through a defect in the skull or spinal column. [meningo- + G. *kēlē*, tumor]

me·nin·go·coc·ce·mia (mě-ning′gō-kok-sē′mē-ă). Presence of meningococci (*N. meningitidis*) in the circulating blood.

    acute fulminating m., rapidly systemic infection with *Neisseria meningitidis,* usually without meningitis, characterized by rash, usually petechial or purpuric, high fever, and hypotension. May lead to death within hours.

me·nin·go·coc·cus, pl. **me·nin·go·coc·ci** (mě-ning′gō-kok′ŭs, -kok′sī). SYN *Neisseria meningitidis.* [meningo- + G. *kokkos*, berry]

me·nin·go·cor·ti·cal (mě-ning′gō-kōr′ti-kăl). Relating to the meninges and the cortex of the brain.

me·nin·go·cyte (mě-ning′gō-sīt). A mesenchymal epithelial cell of the subarachnoid space; it may become a macrophage. [meningo- + G. *kytos*, cell]

me·nin·go·en·ceph·a·li·tis (mě-ning′gō-en-sef′ăl-ī′tis). An inflammation of the brain and its membranes. SYN cerebromeningitis, encephalomeningitis. [meningo- + G. *enkephalos*, brain, + *-itis*, inflammation]

me·nin·go·en·ceph·a·lo·cele (mě-ning′gō-en-sef′ă-lō-sēl). A protrusion of the meninges and brain through a congenital defect in the cranium, usually in the frontal or occipital region. SYN encephalomeningocele. [meningo- + G. *enkephalos*, brain, + *kēlē*, hernia]

me·nin·go·en·ceph·a·lo·my·e·li·tis (mě-ning′gō-en-sef′ă-lō-mī-ě-lī′tis). Inflammation of the brain and spinal cord together with their membranes. [meningo- + G. *enkephalos*, brain, + *myelos*, marrow, + *-itis*, inflammation]

me·nin·go·en·ceph·a·lop·a·thy (mě-ning′gō-en-sef-ă-lop′ă-thē). Disorder affecting the meninges and the brain. SYN encephalomeningopathy. [meningo- + G. *enkephalos*, brain, + *pathos*, suffering]

me·nin·go·my·e·li·tis (mě-ning′gō-mī′ě-lī′tis). Inflammation of the spinal cord and of its enveloping arachnoid and pia mater, and less commonly also of the dura mater. [meningo- + G. *myelos*, marrow, + *-itis*, inflammation]

me·nin·go·my·e·lo·cele (mě-ning′gō-mī′ě-lō-sēl). Protrusion of the spinal cord and its membranes through a defect in the vertebral column. SYN myelocystomeningocele, myelomeningocele. [meningo- + G. *myelos*, marrow, + *kēlē*, tumor]

me·nin·go·ra·dic·u·lar (mě-ning′gō-ra-dik′yū-lăr). Relating to the meninges covering cranial or spinal nerve roots. [meningo- + L. *radix*, root]

me·nin·go·ra·dic·u·li·tis (mě-ning′gō-ra-dik-yū-lī′tis). Inflammation of the meninges and roots of the nerves.

me·nin·gor·rha·chid·i·an (mě-ning′gō-ra-kid′ē-an). Relating to the spinal cord and its membranes. [meningo- + G. *rhachis*, spine]

me·nin·gor·rha·gia (mě-ning′gō-rā′jē-ă). Hem-

me

orrhage into or beneath the cerebral or spinal meninges. [meningo- + G. *rhēgnymi,* to burst forth]

men·in·go·sis (men'ing-gō'sis). Membranous union of bones, as in the skull of the newborn. [meningo- + G. *-ōsis,* condition]

me·nin·go·vas·cu·lar (mĕ-ning'gō-vas'kyū-lăr). Concerning the blood vessels in the meninges; or the meninges and blood vessels.

me·ninx, gen. **me·nin·gis,** pl. **me·nin·ges** (mē'ninks, -jēz; men'ingks; mĕ-nin'jes). Any membrane; specifically, one of the membranous coverings of the brain and spinal cord. SEE ALSO arachnoidea, dura mater, pia mater. [Mod. L. fr. G. *mēninx,* membrane]

men·is·cec·to·my (men'i-sek'tō-mē). Excision of a meniscus, usually from the knee joint. [G. *mēniskos,* crescent (meniscus) + *ektomē,* excision]

me·nis·ci (mĕ-nis'sī). Plural of meniscus.

men·is·ci·tis (men'i-sī'tis). Inflammation of a fibrocartilaginous meniscus. [G. *mēniskos,* crescent (meniscus), + *-itis,* inflammation]

me·nis·cus, pl. **me·nis·ci** (mĕ-nis'kŭs, mĕ-nis'sī). **1.** SYN meniscus *lens.* **2** [NA]. A crescent-shaped structure. **3.** A crescent-shaped fibrocartilaginous structure of the knee, the acromio- and sternoclavicular and the temporomandibular joints. [G. *mēniskos,* crescent]

  lateral m., attached to the lateral border of the upper articular surface of the tibia.

  medial m., attached to the medial border of the upper articular surface of the tibia.

  tactile m., a specialized tactile sensory nerve ending in the epidermis, characterized by a terminal cuplike expansion of an intraepidermal axon in contact with the base of a single modified keratinocyte.

⚠**meno-.** The menses, menstruation. [G. *mēn,* month]

men·o·me·tror·rha·gia (men'ō-mē-trō-rā'jē-ă). Irregular or excessive bleeding during menstruation and between menstrual periods. [meno- + G. *mētra,* uterus, + *rhēgnymi,* to burst forth]

men·o·pau·sal (men'ō-paw-zăl). Associated with or occasioned by the menopause.

men·o·pause (men'ō-pawz). Permanent cessation of the menses; termination of the menstrual life. [meno- + G. *pausis,* cessation]

men·or·rha·gia (men-ō-rā'jē-ă). SYN hypermenorrhea. [meno- + G. *rhēgnymi,* to burst forth]

men·or·rhal·gia (men-ō-ral'jē-ă). SYN dysmenorrhea. [meno- + G. *algos,* pain]

me·nos·che·sis (me-nos'ke-sis, men-ō-skē'sis). Suppression of menstruation. [meno- + G. *schesis,* retention]

men·o·stax·is (men-ō-stak'sis). SYN hypermenorrhea. [meno- + G. *staxis,* a dripping]

men·o·tro·pins (men-ō-trō'pinz). Extract of postmenopausal urine containing primarily the follicle-stimulating hormone. SEE ALSO human menopausal *gonadotropin,* urofollitropin.

men·ses (men'sēz). A periodic physiologic hemorrhage, occurring at approximately 4-week intervals, and having its source from the uterine mucous membrane; usually the bleeding is preceded by ovulation and predecidual changes in the en-

dometrium. SEE ALSO menstrual *cycle.* SYN emmenia, menstrual period. [L. pl. of *mensis,* month]

men·stru·al (men'strū-ăl). Relating to the menses. SYN emmenic. [L. *menstrualis*]

men·stru·ate (men'strū-āt). To undergo menstruation. [L. *menstruo,* pp. *-atus,* to be menstruant]

men·stru·a·tion (men-strū-ā'shŭn). Cyclic endometrial shedding and discharge of a bloody fluid from the uterus during the menstrual cycle. [see menstruate]

  anovular m., menstrual bleeding without recent ovulation; also occurs in subhuman primates.

  retained m., SYN hematocolpos.

  retrograde m., a flow of menstrual blood back through the fallopian tubes; it sometimes carries with it endometrial cells.

  vicarious m., bleeding from any surface other than the mucous membrane of the uterine cavity, occurring periodically at the time when the normal m. should take place.

men·stru·um, pl. **men·strua** (men'strū-ŭm, -strū-ă). Old term for solvent. [Mediev. L. menstrual fluid, thought to possess certain solvent properties, ntr. of L. *menstruus,* monthly]

men·tal. 1. Relating to the mind. [L. *mens (ment-),* mind] **2.** Relating to the chin. SYN genial, genian. [L. *mentum,* chin]

men·tal·i·ty (men-tal'i-tē). The functional attributes of the mind; mental activity.

men·to·plas·ty (men'tō-plas-tē). Plastic surgery of the chin, whereby its shape or size is altered. SYN genioplasty. [L. *mentum,* chin, + G. *plastos,* formed]

men·tum, gen. **men·ti** (men'tŭm, -tī) [NA]. SYN chin. [L.]

MEP (maximum expiratory pressure) maximum expiratory *pressure.*

me·phit·ic (me-fit'ik). Foul, poisonous, or noxious. [L. *mephitis,* a noxious exhalation]

mEq, meq milliequivalent.

⚠**-mer. 1.** Chemical suffix attached to a prefix such as mono-, di-, poly-, tri-, etc., to indicate the smallest unit of a repeating structure; *e.g.,* polymer. **2.** Suffix denoting a member of a particular group; *e.g.,* isomer, enantiomer.

me·ral·gia (me-ral'jē-ă). Pain in the thigh; specifically, m. paresthetica. [G. *mēros,* thigh, + *algos,* pain]

  m. paraesthet'ica, tingling, formication, itching, and other forms of paresthesia in the outer side of the lower part of the thigh in the area of distribution of the lateral femoral cutaneous nerve; there may be pain, but the skin is usually hypesthetic to the touch. SYN Bernhardt's disease.

mer·cap·tan (mer-kap'tan). **1.** A class of substances in which the oxygen of an alcohol has been replaced by sulfur (*e.g.,* cysteine). **2.** DENTISTRY A class of elastic impression compounds sometimes referred to as rubber base materials.

⚠**mercapto-.** Prefix indicating the presence of a thiol group, –SH.

mer·cap·tu·ric ac·id (mer-kap-tyūr'ik). A condensation product of L-cysteine with aromatic compounds, such as bromobenzene; formed in the liver and excreted in the urine.

mer·cu·ri·al (mer-kyū′rē-ăl). **1.** Relating to mercury. **2.** Any salt of mercury used medicinally. **3.** Having the characteristic of rapid, changing moods.

mer·cu·ri·a·lism (mer-kyū′rē-ă-lizm). SYN mercury *poisoning*.

mer·cu·ric (mer-kyū′rik). Denoting a salt of mercury in which the ion of the metal is bivalent.

mer·cu·rous (mer-kyū′rŭs, mer′kyū-rŭs). Denoting a salt of mercury in which the ion of the metal is univalent.

mer·cu·ry (Hg) (mer′kyū-rē). A dense liquid metallic element, atomic no. 80, atomic wt. 200.59; used in thermometers, barometers, manometers, and other scientific instruments; some salts and organic mercurials are used medicinally; ^{197}Hg (half-life of 2.672 days) and ^{203}Hg (half-life of 46.61 days) have been used in brain and renal scanning. [L. *Mercurius,* Mercury, the god of trade, messenger of the gods; in Mediev. L., quicksilver, mercury]

mere-, mero-. Part; also indicating one of a series of similar parts. SEE ALSO -mer. [G. *mēros,* share]

me·rid·i·an (mĕ-rid′-ē-an). **1.** A line encircling a globular body at right angles to its equator and touching both poles, or the half of such a circle extending from pole to pole. **2.** ACUPUNCTURE The lines connecting different anatomical sites. [L. *meridianus,* pertaining to midday, on the south side, southern]

me·rid·i·o·nal (mĕ-rid′ē-ŏ-năl). Relating to a meridian.

mero-. SEE mere-.

mer·o·di·a·stol·ic (mer′ō-dī-ă-stol′ik). Partially diastolic; relating to a part of the diastole of the heart. [mero- + diastole]

mer·o·gen·e·sis (mer-ō-jen′ĕ-sis). **1.** Reproduction by segmentation. **2.** Cleavage of an ovum. [mero- + G. *genesis,* origin]

mer·o·ge·net·ic, mer·o·gen·ic (mer-ō-jĕ-net′ik, -ō-jen′ik). Relating to merogenesis.

me·rog·o·ny (mĕ-rog′ō-nē). **1.** The incomplete development of an ovum that has been disorganized. **2.** A form of asexual schizogony, typical of sporozoan protozoa, in which the nucleus divides several times before the cytoplasm divides; the schizont divides to form merozoites in this asexual phase of the life cycle. [mero- + G. *gonē,* generation]

mer·o·me·lia (mer-ō-mē′lē-ă). Partial absence of a free limb (exclusive of girdle); *e.g.,* hemimelia, phocomelia. [mero- + G. *melos,* a limb]

mer·o·mi·cro·so·mia (mer′ō-mī′krō-sō′mē-ă). Abnormal smallness of some portion of the body; local dwarfism. [mero- + G. *mikros,* small, + *sōma,* body]

mer·o·my·o·sin (mer-ō-mī′ō-sin). A subunit of the tryptic digestion of myosin; two types are produced, H-m. and L-m.

me·ros·mia (me-roz′mē-ă). A condition in which the perception of certain odors is wanting; analogous to color blindness. [mero- + G. *osmē,* smell]

mer·o·sys·tol·ic (mer′ō-sis-tol′ik). Partially systolic; relating to a portion of the systole of the heart. [mero- + systole]

me·rot·o·my (me-rot′ō-mē). The procedure of cutting into parts, as the cutting of a cell into separate parts to study their capacity for survival and development. [mero- + G. *tomē,* incision]

mer·o·zo·ite (mer-ō-zō′īt). The motile infective stage of sporozoan protozoa that results from schizogony or a similar type of asexual reproduction. M.'s are responsible for the vast reproductive powers of sporozoan parasites. [mero- + G. *zōon,* animal]

me·ro·zy·gote (mē-rō-zī′gōt). MICROBIAL GENETICS An organism that, in addition to its own original genome (endogenote), contains a fragment (exogenote) of a genome from another organism; the relatively small size of the exogenote permits a diploid condition for only a limited region of the endogenote. [mero- + *zygotos,* yoked]

mes-. SEE meso-.

me·sad (mē′zad, mē′sad). Passing or extending toward the median plane of the body or of a part. SYN mesiad. [G. *mesos,* middle, + L. *ad,* to]

mes·an·gi·al (mes-an′jē-ăl). Referring to the mesangium.

mes·an·gi·um (mes-an′jē-ŭm). A central part of the renal glomerulus between capillaries; mesangial cells are phagocytic and for the most part separated from capillary lumina by endothelial cells. [mes- + G. *angeion,* vessel]

mes·a·or·ti·tis (mes-ā-ōr-tī′tis). Inflammation of the middle or muscular coat of the aorta. [mes- + aortitis]

mes·ar·ter·i·tis (mes-ar-ter-ī′tis). Inflammation of the middle (muscular) coat of an artery. [mes- + arteritis]

me·sat·i·pel·lic, me·sat·i·pel·vic (mĕ-sat′i-pel′ik, -pel′vik). Denoting an individual with a pelvic index between 90 and 95; the superior strait has a round appearance, with the transverse diameter longer than the anteroposterior by 1 cm or less. [G. *mesatos,* midmost, + *pellis,* a bowl (pelvis)]

mes·ax·on (mez-ak′son, mes-). The plasma membrane of the neurolemma that is folded in to surround a nerve axon. In electron micrographs this double layer resembles a mesentery in appearance.

mes·ec·to·derm (mez-ek′tō-derm). **1.** Cells in the area around the dorsal lip of the blastopore where mesoderm and ectoderm undergo a process of separation. **2.** That part of the mesenchyme derived from ectoderm, especially from the neural crest in the cephalic region in very young embryos. [mes- + ectoderm]

mes·en·ce·phal·ic (mez-en′se-fal′ik). Relating to the mesencephalon.

mes·en·ceph·a·li·tis (mez′en-sef′ă-lī′tis). Inflammation of the midbrain (mesencephalon).

mes·en·ceph·a·lon (mez-en-sef′ă-lon) [NA]. That part of the brainstem developing from the middle of the three primary cerebral vesicles of the embryo. In the adult, the m. is characterized by the unique conformation of its roof plate, the lamina of the mesencephalic tectum, composed of the bilaterally paired superior and inferior colliculi, and by the massive paired prominence of the crus cerebri at its ventral surface. Prominent cell groups of the m. include the motor nuclei of the trochlear and oculomotor nerves, the red nucleus, and the substantia nigra. SYN midbrain. [mes- + G. *enkephalos,* brain]

mes·en·ceph·a·lot·o·my (mez'en-sef'ă-lot'ō-mē). **1.** The sectioning of any structure in the midbrain, especially of the spinothalamic tracts for the relief of intractable pain or the cerebral peduncle for dyskinesias. **2.** A mesencephalic spinothalamic tractotomy. [mesencephalon + G. *tomē,* incision]

me·sen·chy·mal (mĕ-seng'ki-măl, mez-eng-kī' măl). Relating to the mesenchyme.

mes·en·chyme (mez'en-kīm). **1.** An aggregation of mesenchymal cells. **2.** Primordial embryonic connective tissue consisting of mesenchymal cells, usually stellate in form, supported in interlaminar jelly. [mes- + G. *enkyma,* infusion]

mes·en·chy·mo·ma (mez'en-kī-mō'mă). A neoplasm in which there is a mixture of mesenchymal derivatives, other than fibrous tissue. A **benign m.** may contain foci of vascular, muscular, adipose, osteoid, osseous, and cartilaginous tissue. A **malignant m.** may also occur as a similar mixture of two or more types of mesenchymal cells that are malignant.

mes·en·ter·ic (mez-en-ter'ik). Relating to the mesentery.

mes·en·ter·i·o·pexy (mes'en-ter-ē-ō-pek'sē). Fixation or attachment of a torn or incised mesentery. SYN mesopexy. [mesentery + G. *pēxis,* fixation]

mes·en·ter·i·or·rha·phy (mez'en-ter-ē-ōr'ă-fē). Suture of the mesentery. SYN mesorrhaphy. [mesentery + G. *rhaphē,* suture]

mes·en·ter·i·pli·ca·tion (mez'en-ter-i-pli-kā' shŭn). Reducing redundancy of a mesentery by making one or more tucks in it. [mesentery + L. *plico,* pp. *-atus,* to fold]

mes·en·ter·i·tis (mez'en-ter-ī'tis). Inflammation of the mesentery.

mes·en·te·ri·um (mez'en-ter'ē-ŭm) [NA]. SYN mesentery, mesentery. [Mod. L.]

mes·en·tery (mes'en-ter-ē). **1.** A double layer of peritoneum attached to the abdominal wall and enclosing in its fold a portion or all of one of the abdominal viscera, conveying to it its vessels and nerves. **2.** The fan-shaped fold of peritoneum encircling the greater part of the small intestines (jejunum and ileum) and attaching it to the posterior abdominal wall at the root of the m. (radix mesenterii). SYN mesenterium [NA]. [Mod. L. *mesenterium,* fr. G. *mesenterion,* fr. G. *mesos,* middle, + *enteron,* intestine]

me·si·ad (mē'zē-ad, mes'ē-ad). SYN mesad.

me·si·al (mē'zē-ăl, mes'ē-ăl). Toward the median plane following the curvature of the dental arch, in contrast to distal (2). SYN proximal (2). [G. *mesos,* middle]

△**mesio-.** Mesial (especially in dentistry). [G. *mesos,* middle]

me·si·o·buc·cal (mē'zē-ō-bŭk'ăl). Relating to the mesial and buccal surfaces of a tooth; denoting especially the angle formed by the junction of these two surfaces.

me·si·o·cer·vi·cal (mē'zē-ō-ser'vi-kăl). **1.** Relating to the line angle of a cavity preparation at the junction of the mesial and cervical walls. **2.** Per-

taining to the area of a tooth at the junction of the mesial surface and the cervical region.

me·si·o·clu·sion (mē'zē-ō-klū'zhŭn). A malocclusion in which the mandibular arch articulates with the maxillary arch in a position mesial to normal; in Angle's classification, a Class III malocclusion. SYN mesial occlusion (2).

me·si·o·dens (mē'zē-ō-denz). A supernumerary tooth located in the midline of the anterior maxillae, between the maxillary central incisor teeth. [mesio- + L. *dens,* tooth]

me·si·o·dis·tal (mē'zē-ō-dis'tăl). Denoting the plane or diameter of a tooth cutting its mesial and distal surfaces.

me·si·o·gin·gi·val (mē'zē-ō-jin'ji-văl). Relating to the angle formed by the junction of the mesial surface with the gingival line of a tooth.

me·si·o·la·bi·al (mē'zē-ō-lā'bē-ăl). Relating to the mesial and labial surfaces of a tooth; denoting especially the angle formed by their junction.

me·si·o·lin·gual (mē'zē-ō-ling'gwăl). Relating to the mesial and lingual surfaces of a tooth; denoting especially the angle formed by their junction.

me·si·o·lin·guo·oc·clu·sal (mē'zē-ō-ling'gwō-ŏ-klū'săl, -zăl). Denoting the angle formed by the junction of the mesial, lingual, and occlusal surfaces of a bicuspid or molar tooth.

me·si·o·lin·guo·pul·pal (mē'zē-ō-ling'gwō-pŭl' păl). Relating to the angle denoting the junction of the mesial, lingual, and pulpal surfaces in a tooth cavity preparation.

me·sio·oc·clu·sal (mē'zē-ō-ō-klū'săl, -zăl). Denoting the angle formed by the junction of the mesial and occlusal surfaces of a bicuspid or molar tooth.

me·sio·oc·clu·sion (mē'zē-ō-ō-klū'zhŭn). SYN mesial *occlusion* (1).

me·si·o·ver·sion (mē'zē-ō-ver-zhŭn). Malposition of a tooth mesial to normal, in an anterior direction following the curvature of the dental arch.

mes·mer·ism (mes'mer-izm). A system of therapeutics from which were developed hypnotism and therapeutic suggestion. [F.A. *Mesmer,* Austrian physician, 1734–1815]

△**meso-, mes-.** **1.** Middle, mean, intermediate. **2.** A mesentery, mesentery-like structure. **3.** A prefix denoting a compound, containing more than one chiral center, having an internal plane of symmetry; such compounds do not exhibit optical activity (*e.g., meso*-cystine). [G. *mesos*]

mes·o·ap·pen·dix (mez'ō-ă-pen'diks) [NA]. The short mesentery of the appendix lying behind the terminal ileum, in which the appendicular artery courses.

mes·o·bi·lane (mez-ō-bī'lān). A reduced mesobilirubin with no double bonds between the pyrrole rings and, consequently, colorless. SEE ALSO bilirubinoids. SYN mesobilirubinogen.

mes·o·bil·i·ru·bin (mez'ō-bil-i-rū'bin). A compound differing from bilirubin only in that the vinyl groups of bilirubin are reduced to ethyl groups. SEE ALSO bilirubinoids.

mes·o·bil·i·ru·bin·o·gen (mez'ō-bil-i-rū-bin'ō-jen). SYN mesobilane.

mes·o·blast (mez'ō-blast). SYN mesoderm. [meso- + G. *blastos,* germ]

mes·o·blas·te·ma (mez'ō-blas-tē'mă). All the cells collectively which constitute the early undifferentiated mesoderm. [meso- + G. *blastēma,* a sprout]

mes·o·blas·tem·ic (mez'ō-blas-tē'mik). Relating to or derived from the mesoblastema.

mes·o·blas·tic (mez'ō-blas'tik). Relating to or derived from the mesoderm.

mes·o·car·dia (mez'ō-kar'dē-ă). **1.** Atypical position of the heart in a central position in the chest, as in early embryonic life. **2.** Plural of mesocardium. [meso- + G. *kardia,* heart]

mes·o·car·di·um, pl. **mes·o·car·dia** (mez-ō-kar' dē-ŭm). The double layer of splanchnic mesoderm supporting the embryonic heart in the pericardial cavity. It disappears before birth. [meso- + G. *kardia,* heart]

mes·o·ce·cal (mez'ō-sē'kăl). Relating to the mesocecum.

mes·o·ce·cum (mez'ō-sē'kŭm). Part of the mesocolon, supporting the cecum, that occasionally persists when the ascending colon becomes retroperitoneal during fetal life. [meso- + cecum]

mes·o·col·ic (mez'ō-kol'ik). Relating to the mesocolon.

mes·o·co·lon (mez'ō-kō'lon) [NA]. The fold of peritoneum attaching the colon to the posterior abdominal wall; ascending m. (m. ascendens [NA]), transverse m. (m. transversum [NA]), descending m. (m. descendens [NA]), and sigmoid m. (m. sigmoideum [NA]) correspond to the respective divisions of the colon; the ascending and descending portions are usually fused to the peritoneum of the posterior abdominal wall, but can be mobilized. [meso- + *kolon,* colon]

mes·o·co·lo·pexy (mez'ō-kō'lō-pek-sē). An operation for shortening the mesocolon, for correction of undue mobility and ptosis. SYN mesocoloplication. [meso- + G. *kolon,* colon, + *pēxis,* fixation]

mes·o·co·lo·pli·ca·tion (mes'ō-kō'lō-pli-kā' shŭn). SYN mesocolopexy. [meso- + G. *kolon,* colon, + L. *plico,* pp. *-atus,* to fold]

mes·o·cord (mez'ō-kōrd). A fold of amnion that sometimes binds a segment of the umbilical cord to the placenta.

mes·o·derm (mez'ō-derm). The middle of the three primary germ layers of the embryo (the others being ectoderm and endoderm); m. is the origin of all connective tissues, all musculature, blood, cardiovascular and lymphatic systems, most of the urogenital system, and the lining of the pericardial, pleural, and peritoneal cavities. SYN mesoblast. [meso- + G. *derma,* skin]

mes·o·der·mic (mez-ō-der'mik). Relating to the mesoderm.

mes·o·du·o·de·nal (mez'ō-dū-ō-dē'năl). Relating to the mesoduodenum.

mes·o·du·o·de·num (mez'ō-dū'ō-dē'nŭm, -dū-od'ĕ-nŭm). The mesentery of the duodenum.

mes·o·ep·i·did·y·mis (mez-ō-ep-i-did'i-mis). An occasional fold of the tunica vaginalis binding the epididymis to the testis. [meso- + epididymis]

mes·o·gas·ter (mez-ō-gas'ter). SYN mesogastrium.

mes·o·gas·tric (mez-ō-gas'trik). Relating to the mesogastrium.

mes·o·gas·tri·um (mez-ō-gas'trē-ŭm). In the embryo, the mesentery of the dilated portion of the enteric canal that is the future stomach; it gives rise to the greater omentum and consequently is involved in the formation of the omental bursa. The spleen and body of the pancreas develop within it, and thus the splenorenal and gastrosplenic ligaments are derivatives of the (dorsal) mesogastrium. SYN mesogaster. [meso- + G. *gastēr* stomach]

mes·o·gen·ic (mez-ō-jen'ik). Denoting a virus capable of inducing lethal infection in embryonic hosts, after a short incubation period, and an inapparent infection in immature and adult hosts. [meso- + G. *-gen,* producing]

me·sog·li·a (me-sog'lē-ă). Neuroglial cells of mesodermal origin. SEE ALSO microglia. SYN mesoglial cells. [meso- + G. *glia,* glue]

mes·o·glu·te·al (mez'ō-glū'tē-ăl). Relating to the musculus gluteus medius.

mes·o·il·e·um (mez-ō-il'ē-ŭm). The mesentery of the ileum.

mes·o·je·ju·num (mez'ō-je-jū'nŭm). The mesentery of the jejunum.

mes·o·lym·pho·cyte (mez-ō-lim'fō-sīt). A mononuclear leukocyte of medium size, probably a lymphocyte, with a deeply staining nucleus of large size but relatively smaller than that in most lymphocytes. [meso- + lymphocyte]

mes·o·me·lia (mez-ō-mē'lē-ă). The condition of having abnormally short forearms and lower legs. [meso- + G. *melos,* limb]

mes·o·mere (mez'ō-mēr). **1.** A blastomere of a size intermediate between a macromere and a micromere. **2.** The zone between an epimere and a hypomere. [meso- + G. *meros,* part]

mes·o·me·tri·um (mez'ō-mē'trē-ŭm) [NA]. The broad ligament of the uterus, below the mesosalpinx. [meso- + G. *mētra,* uterus]

mes·o·morph (mez'ō-mōrf). A constitutional body type or build (biotype or somatotype) in which tissues that originate from the mesoderm prevail; from the morphological standpoint, there is a balance between trunk and limbs. SEE ALSO hypomorph, ectomorph, endomorph. [meso- + G. *morphē,* form]

mes·o·mor·phic (mez-ō-mōrf'ik). Relating to mesomorphs.

me·son (mez'on, mē'zon, mes'on). An elementary particle having a rest mass intermediate in value between the mass of an electron and that of a proton. [G. neuter of *mesos,* middle]

mes·o·neph·ric (mez-ō-nef'rik). Relating to the mesonephros.

mes·o·neph·roi (mez'ō-nef'roy). Plural of mesonephros.

mes·o·ne·phro·ma (mez'ō-ne-frō'mă). A rare malignant neoplasm of the ovary and corpus uteri, thought to originate in mesonephric structures that become misplaced in ovarian tissue during embryonic development. SYN mesometanephric carcinoma. [mesonephros + *-oma,* tumor]

mes·o·neph·ros, pl. **mes·o·neph·roi** (mez'ō-nef' ros, -roy) [NA]. One of three excretory organs appearing in the evolution of vertebrates; in life forms with a metanephros, the m. is located be-

me

tween the regressing pronephros and the metanephros, cephalic to the latter. In young mammalian embryos, the m. is well developed and briefly functional until establishment of the metanephros, the definitive kidney; in older embryos, the m. undergoes regression as an excretory organ, but its duct system is retained in the male as the epididymis and ductus deferens. SYN wolffian body. [meso- + G. *nephros*, kidney]

mes•o•neu•ri•tis (mez′ō-nū-rī′tis). Inflammation of a nerve or of its connective tissue without involvement of its sheath.

mes•o•pexy (mez′ō-pek-sē). SYN mesenteriopexy.

mes•o•phil, mes•o•phile (mez′ō-fil, -fīl). A microorganism with an optimum temperature between 25°C and 40°C, but growing within the limits of 10°C and 45°C. [meso- + G. *philos*, fond]

mes•o•phil•ic (mez′ō-fil′ik). Pertaining to a mesophil.

mes•o•phle•bi•tis (mez′ō-flē-bī′tis). Inflammation of the middle coat of a vein. [meso- + phlebitis]

me•soph•ry•on (mez-of′ri-on). SYN glabella (2). [meso- + Gr. *ophrys*, eyebrow]

mes•o•por•phy•rins (mez-ō-pōr′fi-rinz). Porphyrin compounds resembling the protoporphyrins except that the vinyl side chains of the latter are reduced to ethyl side chains; *e.g.*, mesobilane.

me•sor•chi•al (mez-ōr′kē-ăl). Relating to the mesorchium.

me•sor•chi•um (mez-ōr′kē-ŭm). **1.** In the fetus, a fold of tunica vaginalis testis supporting the mesonephros and the developing testis. **2.** In the adult, a fold of tunica vaginalis testis between the testis and epididymis. [meso- + G. *orchis*, testis]

mes•o•rec•tum (mez′ō-rek′tŭm). The peritoneal investment of the rectum, covering the upper part only.

mes•or•rha•phy (mez-ōr′ă-fē). SYN mesenteriorrhaphy.

mes•o•sal•pinx (mez′ō-sal′pinks) [NA]. The part of the broad ligament investing the uterine (fallopian) tube. [meso- + G. *salpinx*, trumpet]

mes•o•sig•moid (mez′ō-sig′moyd). Sigmoid mesocolon. SEE mesocolon.

mes•o•sig•moid•i•tis (mes′ō-sig-moy-dī′tis). Inflammation of the mesosigmoid.

mes•o•sig•moid•o•pexy (mez-ō-sig-moy′dō-pek-sē). Surgical fixation of the mesosigmoid.

mes•o•some (mes′ōsom). A convoluted membranous body formed by involution of the plasma membranes of certain bacteria; it functions in cellular respiration and septum formation. [meso + G. *soma*, body]

mes•o•ten•di•ne•um (mez′ō-ten-din′ē-ŭm) [NA]. SYN mesotendon.

mes•o•ten•don (mez′ō-ten′don). The synovial layers that pass from a tendon to the wall of a tendon sheath in certain places where tendons lie within osteofibrous canals. In most instances, the m. degenerates, leaving only the vincula. SYN mesotendineum [NA].

mes•o•the•li•a (mez-ō-thē′lē-ă). Plural of mesothelium.

mes•o•the•li•al (mez-ō-thē′lē-ăl). Relating to the mesothelium.

mes•o•the•li•o•ma (mez′ō-thē-lē-ō′mă). A rare malignant neoplasm, derived from the lining cells of the pleura and peritoneum, which grows as a thick sheet covering the viscera. [mesothelium + G. *-oma*, tumor]

mes•o•the•li•um, pl. **mes•o•the•li•a** (mez-ō-thē′lē-ŭm, -lē-ă). A single layer of flattened cells forming an epithelium that lines serous cavities; *e.g.*, peritoneum, pleura, pericardium. [meso- + epithelium]

mes•o•va•ri•um, pl. **mes•o•va•ri•a** (mez′ō-vā′rē-ŭm, -ă) [NA]. A short peritoneal fold connecting the anterior border of the ovary with the posterior layer of the broad ligament of the uterus. [meso- + L. *ovarium*, ovary]

mes•sen•ger RNA (mRNA). See under ribonucleic acid.

MET metabolic *equivalent*.

⚠ **meta-. 1.** After, subsequent to, behind, or hindmost. Cf. post-. **2.** CHEMISTRY An italicized prefix denoting joint, action sharing. **3** (*m-*). CHEMISTRY An italicized prefix denoting compound formed by two substitutions in the benzene ring separated by one carbon atom, *i.e.*, linked to the first and third, second and fourth, etc., carbon atoms of the ring. For terms beginning with *meta-*, or *m-*, see the specific name. [G. after, between, over]

met•a-anal•y•sis (met′ă-ă-nal′i-sis). Systematic process for finding, evaluating, and combining the results of sets of data from different scientific studies. SEE ALSO analysis.

me•tab•a•sis (mĕ-tab′ă-sis). Rarely used term for a change of any kind in symptoms or course of a disease. [G. a passing over, change, fr. *metabainō*, to pass over]

met•a•bi•o•sis (met′ă-bī-ō′sis). Dependence of one organism on another for its existence. SEE ALSO commensalism, mutualism, parasitism. [meta- + G. *biōsis*, way of life]

met•a•bol•ic (met-ă-bol′ik). Relating to metabolism.

me•tab•o•lism (mĕ-tab′ō-lizm). **1.** The sum of the chemical and physical changes occurring in tissue, consisting of anabolism, those reactions that convert small molecules into large, and catabolism, those reactions that convert large molecules into small, including both endogenous large molecules as well as biodegradation of xenobiotics. **2.** Often incorrectly used as a synonym for either anabolism or catabolism. [G. *metabolē*, change]

    protein m., decomposition and synthesis of protein in the tissues.

me•tab•o•lite (mĕ-tab′ō-līt). Any product (foodstuff, intermediate, waste product) of metabolism, especially of catabolism.

me•tab•o•lize (mĕ-tab′ō-līz). To undergo the chemical changes of metabolism.

met•a•car•pal (met′ă-kar′păl). **1.** Relating to the metacarpus. **2.** Any one of the metacarpal bones (I–V). SEE metacarpal *bone*.

met•a•car•pec•to•my (met′ă-kar-pek′tō-mē). Excision of one or all of the metacarpals. [metacarpus + G. *ektomē*, excision]

met•a•car•po•pha•lan•ge•al (MCP) (met′ă-kar′pō-fă-lan′jē-ăl). Relating to the metacarpus and the phalanges; denoting the articulations between them.

met·a·car·pus, pl. **met·a·car·pi** (met′ă-kar′pŭs, -kar′pī) [NA]. The five bones of the hand between the carpus and the phalanges. [meta- + G. *karpos*, wrist]

met·a·cen·tric (met-ă-sen′trik). Having the centromere about equidistant from the extremities, said of a chromosome. [meta- + G. *kentron*, circle]

met·a·cer·ca·ria, pl. **met·a·cer·ca·ri·ae** (met′ă-ser-kar′ē-ă, -ē). The post-cercarial encysted stage in the life history of a fluke, prior to transfer to the definitive host. Some cercariae attach themselves to vegetation, form m., and are ingested by herbivores; others encyst in muscles of fish or crayfish. [meta- + G. *kerkos*, tail]

met·a·chro·ma·sia (met′ă-krō-mā′zē-ă). **1.** The condition in which a cell or tissue component takes on a color different from the dye solution with which it is stained. SYN metachromatism (2). **2.** A change in the characteristic color of certain basic thiazine dyes, such as toluidine blue, when the dye molecules are bound to tissue polyanionic polymers. [meta- + G. *chrōma*, color]

met·a·chro·mat·ic (met′ă-krō-mat′ik). Denoting cells or dyes that exhibit metachromasia. SYN metachromophil, metachromophile.

met·a·chro·ma·tism (met-ă-krō′mă-tizm). **1.** Any color change, whether natural or produced by basic aniline dyes. **2.** SYN metachromasia (1). [meta- + G. *chrōma*, color]

met·a·chro·mo·phil, met·a·chro·mo·phile (met-ă-krō′mō-fil, -fīl). SYN metachromatic. [meta- + G. *chrōma*, color, + *philos*, fond]

met·a·ki·ne·sis, met·a·ki·ne·sia (met′ă-ki-nē′sis, -ki-nē′sē-ă). Moving apart; the separation of the two chromatids of each chromosome and their movement to opposite poles in the anaphase of mitosis. [meta- + G. *kinēsis*, movement]

met·al (met′ăl). One of the electropositive elements, either amphoteric or basic, characterized by luster, malleability, ductility, the ability to conduct electricity and heat, and the tendency to lose rather than gain electrons in chemical reactions. [L. *metallum*, a mine, a mineral, fr. G. *metallon*, a mine, pit]

   alkali m., an alkali of the family Li, Na, K, Rb, Cs, and Fr, all of which have highly ionized hydroxides. SYN alkali (3).

metallo-. Metal, metallic. [see metal]

me·tal·lo·en·zyme (mĕ-tal-ō-en′zīm). An enzyme containing a metal (ion) as an integral part of its active structure; *e.g.*, cytochromes (Fe, Cu), aldehyde oxidase (Mo), catechol oxidase (Cu), carbonic anhydrase (Zn).

me·tal·lo·por·phy·rin (mĕ-tal-ō-pōr′fi-rin). A combination of a porphyrin with a metal, *e.g.*, Fe (hematin), Mg (as in chlorophyll), Cu (in hemocyanin), Zn.

me·tal·lo·pro·tein (mĕ-tal-ō-prō′tēn). A protein with a tightly bound metal ion or ions; *e.g.*, hemoglobin.

me·tal·lo·thi·o·nein (mĕ-tal-ō-thī′ō-nēn). A small protein, rich in cysteinyl residues, that is synthesized in the liver and kidney in response to the presence of divalent ions (zinc, mercury, cadmium, copper, etc.) and that binds these ions tightly; of importance in ion transport and detoxification.

met·a·mer (met′ă-mer). An entity that is similar to, but ultimately differentiable from, another entity. [meta- + -mer]

met·a·mere (met′ă-mēr). One of a series of homologous segments in the body. SEE ALSO somite. [meta- + G. *meros*, part]

met·a·mer·ic (met-ă-mer′ik). Relating to or showing metamerism, or occurring in a metamere.

me·tam·er·ism (me-tam′er-izm). **1.** A pattern of anatomic structure exhibiting serially homologous metameres; in primitive forms, such as the annelids, the metameres are almost alike in structure; in vertebrates, specialization in the cephalic region masks the underlying m., which is still clearly evident in serially repeated vertebrae, ribs, intercostal muscles, and spinal nerves, and in young vertebrate embryos. **2.** CHEMISTRY Rarely used synonym for isomerism.

met·a·mor·phop·sia (met′ă-mōr-fop′sē-ă). Distortion of visual images. [meta- + G. *morphē*, shape, + *opsis*, vision]

met·a·mor·pho·sis (met-ă-mōr′fŏ-sis, -mōr-fō′sis). **1.** A change in form, structure, or function. **2.** Transition from one developmental stage to another. SYN transformation (1). [G. *meta*, beyond, over, + *morphē*, form]

   fatty m., the appearance of microscopically visible droplets of fat in the cytoplasm of cells. SEE ALSO fatty degeneration.

met·a·mor·phot·ic (met′ă-mōr-fot′ik). Relating to or marked by metamorphosis.

met·a·my·el·o·cyte (met-ă-mī′el-ō-sīt). A transitional form of myelocyte with nuclear construction that is intermediate between the mature myelocyte (myelocyte C of Sabin) and the two-lobed granular leukocyte. SYN juvenile cell. [meta- + G. *myelos*, marrow, + *kytos*, cell]

met·a·neph·ro·gen·ic, met·a·ne·phrog·e·nous (met′ă-nef-rō-jen′ik, -nĕ-froj′ĕ-nŭs). Applied to the more caudal part of the intermediate mesoderm which, under the inductive action of the metanephric diverticulum, has the potency to form metanephric tubules. [meta- + G. *nephros*, kidney, + *-gen*, producing]

met·a·neph·ros, pl. **met·a·neph·roi** (met-ă-nef′ros, -roy). The most caudally located of the three excretory organs appearing in the evolution of the vertebrates (the others being the pronephros and the mesonephros); in mammalian embryos, the m. develops caudal to the mesonephros during its regression, becoming the permanent kidney. [meta- + G. *nephros*, kidney]

met·a·phase (met′ă-fās). The stage of mitosis or meiosis in which the chromosomes become aligned on the equatorial plate of the cell separating the centromeres. In mitosis and in the second meiotic division, the centromeres of each chromosome divide and the two daughter centromeres are directed toward opposite poles of the cell; in the first division of meiosis, the centromeres do not divide but the centromeres of each pair of homologous chromosomes become directed toward opposite poles. [meta- + G. *phasis,* an appearance]

me·taph·y·sis, pl. **me·taph·y·ses** (mĕ-tafʹĭ-sis, -sēz) [NA]. A conical section of bone between the epiphysis and diaphysis of long bones. [meta- + G. *physis,* growth]

met·a·pla·sia (met-ă-plāʹzē-ă). Abnormal transformation of an adult, fully differentiated tissue of one kind into a differentiated tissue of another kind; an acquired condition, in contrast to heteroplasia. [G. *metaplasis,* transformation]

  apocrine m., alteration of acinar epithelium of breast tissue to resemble apocrine sweat glands; seen commonly in fibrocystic disease of the breasts.

  myeloid m., a syndrome characterized by anemia, enlargement of the spleen, nucleated red blood cells and immature granulocytes in the blood, and foci of extramedullary hemopoiesis in the spleen and liver; may develop in the course of polycythemia rubra vera; there is a high incidence of development of myeloid leukemia.

  squamous m., the transformation of glandular or mucosal epithelium into stratified squamous epithelium. SYN epidermalization.

  squamous m. of amnion, SYN *amnion* nodosum.

met·a·plasm (metʹă-plazm). SYN cell *inclusions* (1), under *inclusion.* [meta- + G. *plasma,* something formed]

met·a·plas·tic (met-ă-plasʹtik). Pertaining to metaplasia or metaplasis.

met·a·psy·chol·o·gy (metʹă-sī-kolʹō-jē). **1.** A systematic attempt to discern and describe what lies beyond the empirical facts and laws of psychology, such as the relations between body and mind, or concerning the place of the mind in the universe. **2.** PSYCHOANALYSIS Psychology concerning the fundamental assumptions of the freudian theory of the mind, which entail five points of view: 1) dynamic, concerning psychologic forces; 2) economic, concerning psychologic energy; 3) structural, concerning psychologic configurations; 4) genetic, concerning psychologic origins; 5) adaptive, concerning psychologic relations with the environment. [G. *meta,* beyond, transcending, + psychology]

met·ar·te·ri·ole (metʹar-tērʹē-ōl). One of the small peripheral blood vessels between the arterioles and the true capillaries that contain scattered groups of smooth muscle fibers in their walls. [meta- + arteriole]

met·a·ru·bri·cyte (met-ă-rūʹbri-sīt). Orthochromatic normoblast. SEE normoblast.

me·tas·ta·sis, pl. **me·tas·ta·ses** (mĕ-tasʹtă-sis, -sēz). **1.** The shifting of a disease or its local manifestations, from one part of the body to another, as in mumps when the symptoms referable to the parotid gland subside and the testis becomes affected. **2.** The spread of a disease process from one part of the body to another, as in the appearance of neoplasms in parts of the body remote from the site of the primary tumor; results from dissemination of tumor cells by the lymphatics or blood vessels or by direct extension through serous cavities or subarachnoid or other spaces. **3.** Transportation of bacteria from one part of the body to another, through the bloodstream (hematogenous m.) or through lymph channels (lymphogenous m.). [G. a removing, fr. *meta,* in the midst of, + *stasis,* a placing]

  hematogenous m., SEE metastasis.

  lymphogenous m., SEE metastasis.

me·tas·ta·size (mĕ-tasʹtă-sīz). To pass into or invade by metastasis.

met·a·stat·ic (met-ă-statʹik). Relating to metastasis.

met·a·tar·sal (metʹă-tarʹsăl). Relating to the metatarsus or to one of the metatarsal bones.

met·a·tar·sal·gia (metʹă-tar-salʹjē-ă). Pain in the forefoot in the region of the heads of the metatarsals. [meta- + G. *algos,* pain]

met·a·tar·sec·to·my (metʹă-tar-sekʹtō-mē). Excision of the metatarsus. [metarsus + G. *ektomē,* excision]

met·a·tar·so·pha·lan·ge·al (**MTP**) (metʹă-tarʹsō-fă-lanʹjē-ăl). Relating to the metatarsal bones and the phalanges; denoting the articulations between them.

met·a·tar·sus, pl. **me·ta·tar·si** (metʹă-tarʹsŭs, -sī) [NA]. The distal portion of the foot between the instep and the toes, having as its skeleton the five long bones (metatarsal bones) articulating posteriorly with the cuboid and cuneiform bones and distally with the phalanges. [meta- + G. *tarsos,* tarsus]

  m. laʹtus, deformity caused by sinking down of the transverse arch of the foot.

  m. vaʹrus, fixed deformity in which the forepart of the foot is rotated on the long axis of the foot, so that the plantar surface faces the midline of the body. SYN intoe.

met·a·thal·a·mus (metʹă-thalʹă-mŭs) [NA]. The most caudal and ventral part of the thalamus, composed of the medial and lateral geniculate bodies. [meta- + G. *thalamos,* thalamus]

me·tath·e·sis (me-tathʹĕ-sis). **1.** Transfer of a pathologic product (*e.g.,* a calculus) from one place to another where it causes less inconvenience or injury, when it is not possible or expedient to remove it from the body. **2.** CHEMISTRY A double decomposition, wherein a compound, A-B, reacts with another compound, C-D, to yield A-C + B-D, or A-D + B-C. [meta- + G. *thesis,* a placing]

met·a·tro·phic (met-ă-trofʹik). Denoting the ability to undertake anabolism or to obtain nourishment from varied sources, *i.e.,* both nitrogenous and carbonaceous organic matter. [meta- + G. *trophē,* nourishment]

Met·a·zoa (met-ă-zōʹă). A subkingdom of the kingdom Animalia, including all multicellular animal organisms in which the cells are differentiated and form tissues; distinguished from the subkingdom Protozoa, or unicellular animal organisms. [meta- + G. *zōon,* animal]

met·a·zo·o·no·sis (metʹă-zō-ō-nōʹsis). A zoonosis that requires both a vertebrate and an invertebrate host to complete the life cycle of the causative organism. [meta- + G. *zōon,* animal, + *nosos,* disease]

met·en·ce·phal·ic (metʹen-se-falʹik). Relating to the metencephalon.

met·en·ceph·a·lon (metʹen-sefʹă-lon) [NA]. The

anterior of the two major subdivisions of the rhombencephalon (the posterior being the myelencephalon or medulla oblongata), composed of the pons and the cerebellum. [meta- + G. *enkephalos*, brain]

me·te·or·ism (mē'tē-ŏ-rizm). SYN tympanites. [G. *meteōrismos*, a lifting up]

me·te·or·o·tro·pic (mē'tē-ōr-ō-trop'ik). Denoting diseases affected in their incidence by the weather. [G. *meteōra*, things high in the air, + G. *tropos*, a turning]

me·ter (mē'ter). **1.** The fundamental unit of length in the SI and metric systems, equivalent to 39.37007874 inches. Defined to be the length of path traveled by light in a vacuum in $\frac{1}{299792458}$ sec. **2.** A device for measuring the quantity of that which passes through it. [Fr. *metre*; G. *metron*, measure]

me·ter-can·dle (mē'ter-kan'dl). SYN lux.

met·es·trus, met·es·trum (met-es'trŭs, -trŭm). The period between estrus and diestrus in the estrous cycle. [meta- + estrus]

⚠**meth-, metho-.** Chemical prefixes usually denoting a methyl, methoxy group.

meth·ane (meth'ān). CH_4; an odorless gas produced by the decomposition of organic matter; explosive when mixed with 7 or 8 volumes of air, constituting then the firedamp in coal mines.

meth·an·o·gen (meth-an'ō-jen). Any methane-producing bacterium of the family Methanobacteriaceae.

meth·a·nol (meth'ă-nol). SYN *methyl* alcohol.

metHb methemoglobin.

met·hem·al·bu·min (met'hēm-al-bū'min, -hemal'bū-min). An abnormal compound formed in the blood as a result of heme combining with plasma albumin.

met·hem·al·bu·mi·ne·mia (met'hēm-al-bū-min-ē'mē-ă). The presence of methemalbumin in the circulating blood, indicative of hemoglobin breakdown; found in some patients with blackwater fever or paroxysmal nocturnal hemoglobinuria.

met·he·mo·glo·bin (metHb) (met-hē-mō-glō'bin). A transformation product of oxyhemoglobin because of the oxidation of the normal Fe^{2+} to Fe^{3+}, thus converting ferroprotoporphyrin to ferriprotoporphyrin; useless for respiration; found in sanguineous effusions and in the circulating blood after poisoning with acetanilid, potassium chlorate, and other substances.

met·he·mo·glo·bi·ne·mia (met-hē'mō-glō-bi-nē'mē-ă, meth'ĕ-mō-). The presence of methemoglobin in the circulating blood. [methemoglobin + G. *haima*, blood]

met·he·mo·glo·bi·nu·ria (met-hē'mō-glō-bi-nū're-ă, meth'ĕ-mō-). The presence of methemoglobin in the urine. [methemoglobin + G. *ouron*, urine].

me·thi·o·nine (me-thī'ō-nēn). A nutritionally essential amino acid and the most important natural source of "active methyl" groups in the body, hence usually involved in methylations *in vivo*.

⚠**metho-.** SEE meth-.

meth·od (meth'ŏd). The mode or manner or orderly sequence of events of a process or procedure. SEE ALSO fixative, operation, procedure,

stain, technique. [G. *methodos;* fr. *meta*, after, + *hodos*, way]

Abbott's m., a m. of treatment of scoliosis by use of a series of plaster jackets applied after partial correction of the curvature by external force.

Abell-Kendall m., a standard m. for estimation of total serum cholesterol that avoids interference by bilirubin, protein, and hemoglobin.

aristotelian m., a m. of study that stresses the relation between a general category and a particular object.

Bier's m., (1) SYN intravenous regional *anesthesia*. **(2)** treatment of various surgical conditions by reactive hyperemia.

closed circuit m., a m. for measuring oxygen consumption in which the subject rebreathes an initial quantity of oxygen through a carbon dioxide absorber and the decrease in the volume of oxygen being rebreathed is noted.

flash m., sterilization of milk by raising it rapidly to a temperature of 178°F, holding it there for a short time, and reducing it rapidly to 40°F.

flotation m., flotation of helminth eggs on the surface of a liquid of high specific gravity when eggs are difficult to find in direct examination.

glucose oxidase m., a highly specific m. for measurement of glucose in serum or plasma by reaction with glucose oxidase, in which gluconic acid and hydrogen peroxide are formed.

hexokinase m., the most specific m. for measuring glucose in serum or plasma, involving hexokinase, ATP, glucose 6-phosphate NADP, and glucose 6-phosphate dehydrogenase.

Lamaze m., a technique of psychoprophylactic preparation for childbirth, designed to minimize the pain of labor.

Lister's m., antiseptic surgery, as first advocated by Lister in 1867; the operation was performed under a cloud of diluted carbolic acid spray, the instruments were dipped in a carbolic solution before use, and the wound was dressed with a thick layer of carbolized gauze; from this was developed the present practice of aseptic surgery. SYN listerism.

micro-Astrup m., an interpolation technique for acid-base measurement, based on pH and the use of the Siggaard-Andersen nomogram.

open circuit m., a m. for measuring oxygen consumption and carbon dioxide production by collecting the expired gas over a known period of time and measuring its volume and composition.

Quick's m., SYN prothrombin *test.*

rhythm m., a natural contraceptive m. that spaces sexual intercourse to avoid the fertile period of the menstrual cycle. SYN rhythm (2).

Westergren m., a procedure for estimating the sedimentation rate in fluid blood by mixing venous blood with an aqueous solution of sodium citrate and allowing it to stand in an upright pipette; the fall of the red blood cells, in millimeters, is observed in 1 hour; the normal rate for men is 0 to 15 mm (average, 4 mm), and for women 0 to 20 mm (average, 5 mm).

⚠**methoxy-.** Chemical prefix denoting substitution of a methoxyl group.

me·thox·yl (me-thok'sil). The group, $-OCH_3$.

meth·yl (meth'il). The radical, –CH₃. [G. *methy,* wine, + *hylē,* wood]

  active m., a m. group attached to a quaternary ammonium ion or a tertiary sulfonium ion that can take part in transmethylation reactions.

  m. alcohol, CH₃OH; a flammable, toxic, mobile liquid, used as an industrial solvent, antifreeze, and in chemical manufacture; ingestion may result in severe acidosis, visual impairment, and other effects on the central nervous system. SYN methanol.

meth·yl·a·tion (meth-i-lā'shŭn). Addition of methyl groups; in histochemistry, used to esterify carboxyl groups and remove sulfate groups by treating tissue sections with hot methanol in the presence of hydrochloric acid; the net effect being to reduce tissue basophilia and abolish metachromasia.

meth·yl·di·chlo·ro·ar·sine (MD) (meth'il-dī-klōr-ō-ar'sēn). CH₃ASCl₂; a vesicant; irritating to the respiratory tract and will produce lung injury and eye injury; has been used in certain military operations.

meth·yl·ene (meth'i-lēn). The radical, –CH₂–.

meth·yl·ene blue [C.I. 52015]. A basic dye easily oxidized to azure, with dye mixtures; used in histology and microbiology, to stain intestinal protozoa in wet mount preparations, to track RNA and RNase in electrophoresis, and as an antidote for methemoglobinemia; its redox indicator properties are useful in milk bacteriology.

meth·yl green [C.I. 42585]. A basic triphenylmethane dye used as a chromatin stain and, in combination with pyronin, for differential staining of RNA (red) and DNA (green); also used as a tracking dye for DNA in electrophoresis.

meth·yl·ol (meth'i-lol). Hydroxymethyl; the radical, –CH₂OH.

meth·yl·pen·tose (meth-il-pen'tōs). A hexose (a 6-deoxyhexose) in which carbon-6 is part of a methyl group; *e.g.,* rhamnose, fucose.

meth·yl·trans·fer·ase (meth-il-trans'fer-ās). Any enzyme transferring methyl groups from one compound to another. SYN transmethylase.

metMb metmyoglobin.

met·my·o·glo·bin (metMb) (met'mī-ō-glō'bin). Myoglobin in which the ferrous ion of the heme prosthetic group is oxidized to ferric ion.

me·ton·y·my (mĕ-ton'i-mē). Imprecise or circumscribed labeling of objects or events, characteristic of the language disturbance of schizophrenics; *e.g.,* the patient speaks of having had a "menu" rather than a "meal." [meta- + G. *onyma,* name]

me·top·ic (me-tō'pik, me-top'ik). Relating to the forehead or anterior portion of the cranium. [G. *metōpon,* forehead]

met·o·po·plas·ty (met'ŏ-pō-plas-tē, me-top'ō-plas-tē). Plastic surgery of the skin or bone of the forehead. [G. *metōpon,* forehead, + *plastos,* formed]

⌂**metr-, metra-, metro-.** The uterus. SEE ALSO hystero- (1), utero-. [G. *mētra*]

me·tra (mē'tră). SYN uterus. [G. uterus]

me·tra·to·nia (mē-tră-tō'nē-ă). Atony of the uterine walls after childbirth. [metra- + G. *a*-priv. + *tonos,* tension]

me·trat·ro·phy, me·tra·tro·phia (mē-trat'rō-fē, mē-tră-trō'fē-ă). Uterine atrophy. [metra-atrophy]

me·tria (mē'trē-ă). Pelvic cellulitis or other inflammatory affection in the puerperal period. [G. *mētra,* uterus]

met·ric (met'rik). Quantitative; relating to measurement. SEE metric *system.* [G. *metrikos,* fr. *metron,* measure]

me·tri·tis (mē-trī'tis). Inflammation of the uterus. [G. *mētra,* uterus, + *-itis,* inflammation]

⌂**metro-.** SEE metr-. [G. *mētra,* uterus]

me·tro·cyte (mē'trō-sīt). SYN mother *cell.* [G. *mētēr,* mother, + *kytos,* a hollow (cell)]

me·tro·dyn·ia (mē-trō-dī'nē-ă). SYN hysteralgia. [metro- + G. *odynē,* pain]

me·tro·fi·bro·ma (mē'trō-fī-brō'mă). A fibroma of the uterus.

me·tro·lym·phan·gi·tis (mē'trō-lim-fan-jī'tis). Inflammation of the uterine lymphatics. [metro- + lymphangitis]

me·tro·par·al·y·sis (mē'trō-pă-ral'i-sis). Flaccidity or paralysis of the uterine muscle during or immediately after childbirth. [metro- + paralysis]

me·tro·path·ia (mē-trō-path'ē-ă). SYN metropathy. [L.]

  m. hemorrhag'ica, abnormal, excessive, often continuous uterine bleeding due to persistence and exaggeration of the follicular phase of the menstrual cycle; the endometrium is the seat of glandular hyperplasia with cyst formation.

me·tro·path·ic (me-trō-path'ik). Relating to or caused by uterine disease.

me·trop·a·thy (mē-trop'ă-thē). Any disease of the uterus, especially of the myometrium. SYN metropathia. [metro- + G. *pathos,* suffering]

me·tro·per·i·to·ni·tis (mē'trō-per-i-tō-nī'tis). Inflammation of the uterus involving the peritoneal covering. SYN perimetritis. [metro- + peritonitis]

me·tro·phle·bi·tis (mē'trō-flĕ-bī'tis). Inflammation of the uterine veins usually following childbirth. [metro- + G. *phleps,* vein, + *-itis,* inflammation]

met·ro·plas·ty (met'trō-plas-tē, mē'trō-). SYN uteroplasty.

me·tror·rha·gia (mē-trō-rā'jē-ă). Any irregular, acyclic bleeding from the uterus between periods. [metro- + G. *rhēgnymi,* to burst forth]

me·tror·rhea (mē'trō-rē'ă). Discharge of mucus or pus from the uterus. [metro- + G. *rhoia,* a flow]

me·tro·sal·pin·gi·tis (mē'trō-sal-pin-jī'tis). Inflammation of the uterus and of one or both fallopian tubes. [metro- + G. *salpinx,* trumpet (oviduct), + *-itis,* inflammation]

me·tro·sal·pin·gog·ra·phy (mē'trō-sal-pin-gog'ră-fē). SYN hysterosalpingography. [metro- + G. *salpinx,* tube, + *graphō,* to write]

me·tro·scope (mē'trō-skōp). SYN hysteroscope. [metro- + G. *skopeō,* to view]

me·tro·stax·is (mē-trō-stak'sis). Small but continuous hemorrhage of the uterine mucous membrane. [metro- + G. *staxis,* a dripping]

me·tro·ste·no·sis (mē'trō-ste-nō'sis). A narrowing of the uterine cavity. [metro- + G. *stenōsis,* a narrowing]

Mev 1 million electron-volts.

Mg magnesium.
mg milligram.
MHC major histocompatibility *complex*.
mho (mō). SYN siemens. [*ohm* reversed]
MHz megahertz.
MI myocardial *infarction*.
△**micr-**. SEE micro-.
mi·cra·cou·stic (mī′kră-kū′stik). **1.** Relating to faint sounds. **2.** Magnifying very faint sounds so as to make them audible. SYN microcoustic. [micro- + G. *akoustikos*, relating to hearing, fr. *akouō*, to hear]
mi·cren·ceph·a·ly (mī-kren-sef′ă-lē). Abnormal smallness of the brain. SYN microencephaly. [micro- + G. *enkephalos*, brain]
△**micro-, micr-**. **1.** Prefixes denoting smallness. **2** (μ). Prefix used in the SI and metric systems to signify one-millionth (10^{-6}) of such unit. **3.** CHEMISTRY Prefix to terms denoting chemical procedures or analyses that use minimal quantities of substance to be examined; specimen materials and reagents. **4.** Microscopic; opposite of macro-, megalo-. [G. *mikros*, small]
mi·cro·ab·scess (mī′krō-ab′ses). A very small circumscribed collection of leukocytes in solid tissues.
mi·cro·ad·e·no·ma (mī′krō-ad-ĕ-nō′mă). A pituitary adenoma less than 10 mm in diameter.
mi·cro·aer·o·phil, mi·cro·aer·o·phile (mī-krō-ār′ō-fil, -fīl). **1.** An aerobic bacterium that requires oxygen, but less than is present in the air, and grows best under modified atmospheric conditions. **2.** Relating to such an organism. SYN microaerophilic. [micro- + G. *aēr*, air, + *philos*, fond]
mi·cro·aer·o·phil·ic (mī′krō-ār-ō-fil′ik). SYN microaerophil (2).
microaggregate (mī′krō-ăg′rē-gāt, -gŭt). Small aggregates (20–120 microns) composed of fibrin, degenerating platelets, white cells, or cellular debris which form in blood stored in the refrigerator 5 or more days. Microaggregate filters can be used to filter out the microaggregates during administration of the blood unit.
mi·cro·a·nas·to·mo·sis (mī′krō-ă-nas-tō-mō′sis). Anastomosis of minute structures performed under a surgical microscope.
mi·cro·a·nat·o·mist (mī′krō-ă-nat′ŏ-mist). SYN histologist.
mi·cro·a·nat·o·my (mī′krō-ă-nat′ŏ-mē). SYN histology.
mi·cro·an·eu·rysm (mī′krō-an′yū-rizm). Focal dilation of retinal capillaries occurring in diabetes mellitus, retinal vein obstruction, and absolute glaucoma, or of arteriolocapillary junctions in many organs in thrombotic thrombocytopenic purpura.
mi·cro·an·gi·og·ra·phy (mī′krō-an-jē-og′ră-fē). Radiography of the finer vessels of an organ after the injection of a contrast medium and enlargement of the resulting radiograph. [micro- + angiography]
mi·cro·an·gi·op·a·thy (mī′krō-an-jē-op′ă-thē). SYN capillaropathy.
mi·crobe (mī′krōb). Any very minute organism, including both microscopic and ultramicroscopic organisms (spirochetes, bacteria, rickettsiae, and viruses). These organisms are considered to form a biologically distinctive group, in that the genetic material is not surrounded by a nuclear membrane, and mitosis does not occur during replication. [Fr., fr. G. *mikros*, small, + *bios*, life]
mi·cro·bi·al (mī-krō′bē-ăl). Relating to a microbe or to microbes.
mi·cro·bi·ci·dal (mī-krō′bi-sī′dăl). Destructive to microbes. SYN microbicide (1).
mi·cro·bi·cide (mī-krō′bi-sīd). **1.** SYN microbicidal. **2.** An agent destructive to microbes; a germicide; an antiseptic. [microbe + L. *caedo*, to kill]
mi·cro·bi·o·log·ic (mī′krō-bī-ō-loj′ik). Relating to microbiology.
mi·cro·bi·ol·o·gist (mī′krō-bī-ol′ō-jist). One who specializes in the science of microbiology.
mi·cro·bi·ol·o·gy (mī′krō-bī-ol′ō-jē). The science concerned with microorganisms, including fungi, protozoa, bacteria, and viruses. [Fr. *microbiologie*]
mi·cro·blast (mī′krō-blast). A small, nucleated red blood cell. [micro- + G. *blastos*, sprout, germ]
mi·cro·bleph·a·ron (-blef′ă-ron). Eyelids with abnormal vertical shortness. [micro + G. *blepharon*, eyelid + *ia*, condition]
mi·cro·body (mī′krō-bod-ē). SYN peroxisome.
mi·cro·bra·chia (mī-krō-brā′kē-ă). Abnormal smallness of the arms. [micro- + G. *brachiōn*, arm]
mi·cro·car·dia (mī-krō-kar′dē-ă). Abnormal smallness of the heart. [micro- + G. *kardia*, heart]
mi·cro·cen·trum (mī-krō-sen′trŭm). SYN cytocentrum. [micro- + G. *kentron*, center]
mi·cro·ce·phal·ic (mī-krō-sĕ-fal′ik). Having a small head. SYN nanocephalous, nanocephalic.
mi·cro·ceph·a·ly (mī-krō-sef′ă-lē). Abnormal smallness of the head; applied to a skull with a capacity below 1350 ml. Usually associated with mental retardation. SYN nanocephaly. [micro- + G. *kephalē*, head]
mi·cro·chei·lia, mi·cro·chi·lia (mī-krō-kī′lē-ă). Smallness of the lips. [micro- + G. *cheilos*, lip]
mi·cro·chei·ria, mi·cro·chi·ria (mī-krō-kī′rē-ă). Smallness of the hands. [micro- + G. *cheir*, hand]
mi·cro·chem·is·try (mī-krō-kem′is-trē). The use of chemical procedures involving minute quantities or reactions not visible to the unaided eye.
mi·cro·cin·e·ma·tog·ra·phy (mī′krō-sin-ĕ-mă-tog′ră-fē). The application of moving pictures taken through magnifying lenses to the study of an organ or system in motion; *e.g.*, the circulation in living embryos. [micro- + G. *kinēma*, movement, + *graphō*, to write]
mi·cro·cir·cu·la·tion (mī′krō-sir-kyū-lā′shŭn). Passage of blood in the smallest vessels, namely arterioles, capillaries, and venules.
Mi·cro·coc·ca·ce·ae (mī′krō-kok-ā′sē-ē). A family of bacteria containing Gram-positive spherical cells which occur singly or in pairs, tetrads, packets, irregular masses, or even chains. Free-living, saprophytic, parasitic, and pathogenic species occur. The type genus is *Micrococcus*.
mi·cro·coc·ci (mī′krō-kok′sī). Plural of micrococcus.

Mi·cro·coc·cus (mī′krō-kok-ŭs). A genus of Micrococcaceae) containing Gram-positive, spherical cells that occur in irregular masses, never in packets. Some species are motile or produce motile mutants. These organisms are saprophytic, facultatively parasitic, or parasitic but are not truly pathogenic. The type species is *M. luteus*. [micro- + G. *kokkos*, berry]

mi·cro·coc·cus, pl. **mi·cro·coc·ci** (mī′krō-kok′ ŭs, -kok′sī). A vernacular term used to refer to any member of the genus *Micrococcus*.

mi·cro·co·lon (mī′krō-kō-lon). A small-caliber unused colon, seen in the neonate on radiographic contrast enema; usually a consequence of intestinal atresia or meconium ileus.

mi·cro·co·ria (mī-krō-kō′rē-ă). A congenitally small pupil with an inability to dilate. [micro- + G. *korē*, pupil]

mi·cro·cor·nea (mī′krō-kōr′nē-ă). An abnormally small cornea.

mi·cro·cou·lomb (μC) (mī-krō-kū′lom). One-millionth of a coulomb.

mi·cro·cou·stic (mī′krō-kū′stik). SYN micracoustic.

mi·cro·cu·rie (μCi) (mī′krō-kyū′rē). One-millionth of a curie; a quantity of any radionuclide with 3.7×10^4 disintegrations per second.

mi·cro·cyst (mī′krō-sist). A tiny cyst, frequently of such dimensions that a magnifying lens or microscope is required for observation.

mi·cro·cyte (mī′krō-sīt). A small (5 μm or less) non-nucleated red blood cell. SYN microerythrocyte. [micro- + G. *kytos*, cell]

mi·cro·cy·the·mia (mī′krō-sī-thē′mē-ă). The presence of many microcytes in the circulating blood. SYN microcytosis. [microcyte + G. *haima*, blood]

🔲 mi·cro·cy·to·sis (mī′krō-sī-tō′sis). SYN microcythemia. [microcyte + G. *-osis*, condition]

mi·cro·dac·ty·ly (mī-krō-dak′ti-lē). Smallness or shortness of the fingers or toes. [micro- + G. *dactylos*, finger, toe]

mi·cro·dis·sec·tion (mī′krō-di-sek′shŭn). Dissection of tissues under a microscope or magnifying glass, usually done by teasing the tissues apart by means of needles.

mi·cro·don·tia, mi·cro·don·tism (mī-krō-don′ shē-ă, -don′tizm). A condition in which a single tooth, or pairs of teeth, or the whole dentition, may be disproportionately small. [micro- + G. *odous*, tooth]

mi·cro·en·ceph·a·ly (mī′krō-en-sef′ă-lē). SYN micrencephaly.

mi·cro·e·ryth·ro·cyte (mī′krō-ĕ-rith′rō-sīt). SYN microcyte.

mi·cro·fi·bril (mī-kro-fī′bril). A very small fibril having an average diameter of 13 nm; it may be a bundle of still smaller microfilaments.

mi·cro·fil·a·ment (mī-krō-fil′ă-ment). The finest filamentous element of the cytoskeleton, having a diameter of about 5 nm and consisting primarily of actin. SEE ALSO actin *filament*.

mi·cro·fil·a·re·mia (mī-krō-fil-ă-rē′mē-ă). Infection of the blood with microfilariae.

mi·cro·fi·lar·ia, pl. **mi·cro·fi·lar·i·ae** (mī′krō-fi-lar′ē-ă, -ē). Term for embryos of filarial nematodes in the family Onchocercidae. SEE *Filaria*.

mi·cro·ga·mete (mī-krō-gam′ēt). The male element in anisogamy, or conjugation of cells of unequal size; it is the smaller of the two cells and actively motile. [micro- + G. *gametēs*, husband]

mi·cro·ga·me·to·cyte (mī-krō-gam′ĕ-tō-sīt). The mother cell producing the microgametes, or male elements of sexual reproduction in sporozoan protozoans and fungi.

mi·cro·gas·tria (mī-krō-gas′trē-ă). Smallness of the stomach. [micro- + G. *gastēr*, stomach]

mi·cro·gen·ia (mī-krō-jēn′ē-ă). Abnormal smallness of the chin resulting from the underdevelopment of the mental symphysis. [micro- + G. *geneion*, chin]

mi·cro·gen·i·tal·ism (mī-krō-jen′i-tal-izm). Abnormal smallness of the external genital organs.

🔲 mi·cro·glia (mī-krog′lē-ă). Small neuroglial cells, possibly of mesodermal origin, which may become phagocytic, in areas of neural damage or inflammation. SYN Hortega cells. [micro- + G. *glia*, glue]

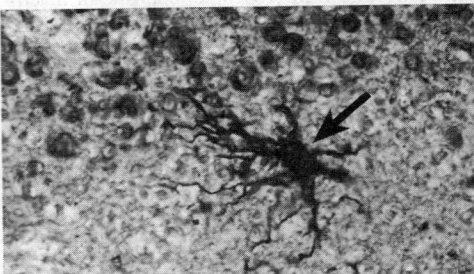

microglia: microglial cell (arrow) in gray and white matter of adult human spinal cord

mi·crog·li·a·cyte (mī-krŏg′lē-ă-sīt). A cell, especially an embryonic cell, of the microglia. [micro- + G. *glia*, glue, + *kytos*, cell]

mi·cro·glos·sia (mī-krō-glos′ē-ă). Smallness of the tongue. [micro- + G. *glōssa*, tongue]

mi·cro·gna·thia (mī-krō-nā′thē-ă, mī-krog-nath′ ē-ă). Abnormal smallness of the jaws, especially of the mandible. [micro- + G. *gnathos*, jaw]

mi·cro·gram (μg) (mī′krō-gram). One-millionth of a gram.

mi·cro·graph (mī′krō-graf). SYN photomicrograph. [micro- + G. *graphō*, to write]

mi·cro·gy·ria (mī-krō-jī′rē-ă). Abnormal narrowness of the cerebral convolutions. [micro- + G. *gyros*, convolution]

mi·cro·he·pat·ia (mī-krō-he-pat′ē-ă). Abnormal smallness of the liver. [micro- + G. *hepar* (*hepat*-), liver]

mi·crohm (μΩ) (mī′krōm). One-millionth of an ohm.

mi·cro·in·cis·ion (mī-krō-in-sizh′ŭn). An incision made with the aid of a microscope.

mi·cro·in·va·sion (mī′krō-in-vā′zhŭn). Invasion of tissue immediately adjacent to a carcinoma in situ, the earliest stage of malignant neoplastic invasion.

mi·cro·kat·al (mī′krō-kat′ăl). One-millionth of a katal.

mi·cro·li·ter (μl, λ) (mī′krō-lē-ter). One-millionth of a liter.

mi·cro·lith (mī′krō-lith). A minute calculus, usually multiple and constituting a coarse sand called gravel. [micro- + G. *lithos,* stone]

mi·cro·li·thi·a·sis (mī-krō-li-thī′ă-sis). The formation, presence, or discharge of minute concretions, or gravel.

  pulmonary alveolar m., microscopic granules of calcium or bone disseminated throughout the lungs.

mi·cro·ma·nip·u·la·tion (mī′krō-mă-nip′yū-lā′shŭn). Dissection, stimulation, and other mechanical operations performed on minute structures under the microscope.

mi·cro·me·lia (mī-krō-mē′lē-ă). Condition of having disproportionately short or small limbs. SEE ALSO achondroplasia. SYN nanomelia. [micro- + G. *melos,* limb]

mi·cro·mere (mī′krō-mēr). A blastomere of small size; for example, one of the blastomeres at the animal pole of an amphibian egg. [micro- + G. *meros,* a part]

mi·cro·me·tas·ta·sis (mī′krō-mĕ-tas′tă-sis). A stage of metastasis when the secondary tumors are too small to be clinically detected, as in micrometastatic disease.

mi·cro·met·a·stat·ic (mī′krō-met-ă-stat′ik). Denoting or characterized by micrometastasis, as in m. disease.

mi·crom·e·ter (μm) (mī-krom′ĕ-ter). **1.** One-millionth of a meter. **2.** A device for measuring various objects in an accurate and precise manner. In medicine and biology, the term is usually used with reference to a glass slide or lens that is accurately marked for measuring microscopic forms. [micro- + G. *metron,* measure]

mi·crom·e·try (mī-krom′ĕ-trē). Measurement of objects with some type of micrometer and a microscope.

micromicro- (μμ). Prefix formerly used to signify one-trillionth (10^{-12}); now pico-.

mi·cro·mi·cron (μμ) (mī-krō-mī′kron). Former term for picometer.

mi·cro·mo·lar (μM) (mī-krō-mō′lar). Denoting a concentration of 10^{-6} mole per liter (10^{-6} M or 1 μM).

mi·cro·mole (μmol) (mī′krō-mōl). One-millionth of a mole.

mi·cro·my·e·lia (mī′krō-mī-ē′lē-ă). Abnormal smallness or shortness of the spinal cord. [micro- + G. *myelos,* marrow]

mi·cro·my·el·o·blast (mī′krō-mī′el-ō-blast). A small myeloblast, often the predominating cell in myeloblastic leukemia.

mi·cron (μ) (mī′kron). Former term for micrometer.

mi·cro·nod·u·lar (mī′krō-nod′yū-lăr). Characterized by the presence of minute nodules; denoting a somewhat coarser appearance than that of a granular tissue or substance. [G. *mikros,* small]

mi·cro·nu·cle·us (mī-krō-nū′klē-ŭs). **1.** A small nucleus in a large cell, or the smaller nuclei in cells that have two or more such structures. **2.** The smaller of the two nuclei in ciliates dividing mitotically and bearing specific inheritable material. SEE ALSO macronucleus (2).

mi·cro·nu·tri·ents (mī-krō-nū′trē-ents). Essential food factors required in only small quantities by the body; *e.g.,* vitamins, trace minerals.

mi·cro·nych·ia (mī-krō-nik′ē-ă). Abnormal smallness of nails. [micro- + G. *onyx,* nail]

mi·cro·or·gan·ism (mī′krō-ōr′gan-izm). A microscopic organism (plant or animal).

mi·cro·pa·thol·o·gy (mī′krō-pa-thol′ō-jē). The microscopic study of disease changes. [micro- + G. *pathos,* suffering, + *logos,* study]

mi·cro·pe·nis (mī-krō-pē′nis). Abnormally small penis. SYN microphallus.

mi·cro·phage (mī′krō-fāj). A polymorphonuclear leukocyte that is phagocytic. SEE ALSO phagocyte. [micro- + phag(ocyte)]

mi·cro·phal·lus (mī-krō-fal′ŭs). SYN micropenis.

mi·cro·pho·to·graph (mī-krō-fō′tō-graf). A minute photograph of any object, as distinguished from a photomicrograph.

mi·croph·thal·mos (-thal′mos). Abnormal smallness of the eye. [micro + G. *ophthalmos,* eye]

mi·cro·pleth·ys·mog·ra·phy (mī′krō-pleth-iz-mog′ră-fē). The technique of measuring minute changes in the volume of a part as a result of blood flow into or out of it.

mi·cro·po·dia (mī-krō-pō′dē-ă). Abnormal smallness of the feet. [micro- + G. *pous,* foot]

mi·crop·sia (mī-krop′sē-ă). Perception of objects as smaller than they are. [micro- + G. *opsis,* sight]

mi·cro·punc·ture (mī′krō-pŭnk-chūr). A puncture made with the aid of a microscope.

mi·cro·re·frac·tom·e·ter (mī′krō-rē-frak-tom′ĕ-ter). A refractometer used in the study of blood cells.

mi·cro·res·pi·rom·e·ter (mī′krō-res-pi-rom′ĕ-ter). An apparatus for measuring the utilization of oxygen by small particles of isolated tissues or cells or particles of cells.

mi·cro·scope (mī′krō-skōp). An instrument that gives an enlarged image of an object or substance that is minute or not visible with the naked eye; usually the term denotes a compound m.; for low magnifications the term simple m., or magnifying glass, is used. [micro- + G. *skopeō,* to view]

  binocular m., a m. having two eyepieces; it may be a compound m. or a stereoscopic m.

  compound m., a m. having two or more magnifying lenses.

  confocal m., a m. that allows the observer to visualize objects in a single plane of focus, thereby creating a sharper image (usually the objects are fluorescent molecules); a refinement of this m. uses optical sectioning and a computer to record serial sections. This permits three-dimensional reconstruction.

  dark-field m., a m. that has a special condenser and objective with a diaphragm or stop that scatters light from the object observed, with the result that the object appears bright on a dark background.

  electron m., a visual and photographic m. in which electron beams with wavelengths thousands of times shorter than visible light are utilized in place of light, thereby allowing much greater resolution and magnification; in this technique, the electrons are transmitted through a very thin section of an embedded and dehydrated specimen maintained in a vacuum.

infrared m., a m. that is equipped with infrared transmitting optics and that measures the infrared absorption of minute samples with the aid of photoelectric cells; images may be observed with image converters or television.

operating m., SYN surgical m.

phase m., phase-contrast m., a specially constructed m. that has a special condenser and objective containing a phase-shifting ring whereby small differences in index of refraction are made visible as intensity or contrast differences in the image; particularly useful for examining structural details in transparent specimens such as living or unstained cells and tissues.

scanning electron m., a m. in which the object in a vacuum is scanned in a raster pattern by a slender electron beam, generating reflected and secondary electrons from the specimen surface that are used to modulate the image on a synchronously scanned cathode ray tube; with this method a three-dimensional image is obtained, with both high resolution and great depth of focus.

simple m., single m., a m. that has a single magnifying lens.

stereoscopic m., a m. having double eyepieces and objectives and thus independent light paths, giving a three-dimensional image.

stroboscopic m., a m. that has a light source that flashes at a constant rate so that an analysis of the motility of an object may be made; it may be used for high speed or low speed (time-lapse) cinephotomicrography.

surgical m., a binocular m. used to obtain good visualization of fine structures in the operating field; in the standing type of m., a motorized zoom lens system operated by hand or foot controls provides an adjustable working distance; in headborne models, interchangeable oculars provide the magnification needed. SYN operating m.

ultraviolet m., a m. having optics of quartz and fluorite that allow transmission of light waves shorter than those of the visible spectrum; the image is made visible by photography, fluorescence of special glasses, or television.

x-ray m., a m. in which images are obtained by using x-rays as an energy source that are recorded on a very fine-grained film, or the image is enlarged by projection; if film is used, it may be examined with the light m. at fairly high magnifications.

mi·cro·scop·ic, mi·cro·scop·i·cal (mī-krō-skop′ik, -i-kăl). **1.** Of minute size; visible only with the aid of the microscope. **2.** Relating to a microscope.

mi·cros·co·py (mī-kros′kŏ-pē). Investigation of minute objects by means of a microscope. SEE ALSO microscope.

fluorescence m., a procedure based on the fact that fluorescent materials emit visible light when they are irradiated with ultraviolet or violet-blue visible rays; some materials manifest this property naturally, whereas others may be treated with fluorescent solutions (somewhat analogous to staining).

immune electron m., electron m. of biological specimens to which specific antibody has been bound.

mi·cro·some (mī′krō-sōm). One of the small spherical vesicles derived from the endoplasmic reticulum after disruption of cells and ultracentrifugation. [micro- + G. *sōma,* body]

mi·cro·so·mia (mī-krō-sō′mē-ă). Abnormal smallness of body, as in dwarfism or as in a fetus. SYN nanocormia. [micro- + G. *sōma,* body]

mi·cro·spec·tro·pho·tom·e·try (mī′krō-spektrō-fō-tom′ĕ-trē). A technique for characterizing and quantitating nucleoproteins in single cells or cell organelles by their natural absorption spectra (ultraviolet) or after binding stoichiometrically in selective cytochemical staining reactions, as in the Feulgen stain for DNA.

mi·cro·spec·tro·scope (mī-krō-spek′trō-skōp). An instrument for observing the optical spectrum of microscopic objects.

mi·cro·sphe·ro·cy·to·sis (mī′krō-sfēr′ō-sī-tō′sis). A condition of the blood seen in hemolytic icterus in which small spherocytes are predominant; the red blood cells are smaller and more globular than normal.

mi·cro·sphyg·my (mī′krō-sfig′mē). A circumstance in which the pulse is difficult to discern manually. [micro- + G. *sphygmos,* pulse]

mi·cro·sple·nia (mī-krō-sple′nē-ă). Abnormal smallness of the spleen.

Mi·cros·po·rum (mī-kros′pŏ-rŭm, mī-krō-spō′rŭm). A genus of pathogenic fungi causing dermatophytosis. [micro- + G. *sporos,* seed]

mi·cro·steth·o·scope (mī-krō-steth′ō-skōp). A stethoscope that amplifies the sounds heard.

mi·cro·sto·mia (mī-krō-stō′mē-ă). Smallness of the oral aperture. [micro- + G. *stoma,* mouth]

mi·cro·sur·gery (mī-krō-ser′jer-ē). Surgical procedures performed under the magnification of a surgical microscope.

mi·cro·su·ture (mī-krō-sū′chūr). Tiny caliber suture material, often 9-0 or 10-0, with an attached needle of corresponding size, for use in microsurgery.

mi·cro·sy·ringe (mī′krō-si-rinj′). A hypodermic syringe that has a micrometer screw attached to the piston, whereby accurately measured minute quantities of fluid may be injected.

mi·cro·tia (mī-krō′shē-ă). Smallness of the auricle of the ear with a blind or absent external auditory meatus. [micro- + G. *ous,* ear]

mi·cro·tome (mī′krō-tōm). An instrument for making sections of biological tissue for examination under the microscope. SYN histotome.

mi·crot·o·my (mī-krot′ō-mē). The making of thin sections of tissues for examination under the microscope. SYN histotomy. [micro- + G. *tomē,* incision]

Mi·cro·trom·bid·i·um (mī′krō-trom-bid′ē-ŭm). A genus of chigger or harvest mites that cause severe itching from the presence of the larval stage (chigger) in the skin. [micro- + Mod. L. *trombidium,* a timid one]

mi·cro·tu·bule (mī-krō-tū′byūl). A cylindrical cytoplasmic element that occurs widely in the cytoskeleton of plant and animal cells; m.'s increase in number during mitosis and meiosis, where they may be related to movement of the chromosomes or chromatids on the nuclear spindle during nuclear division.

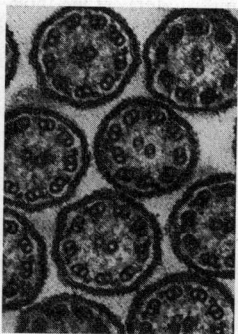 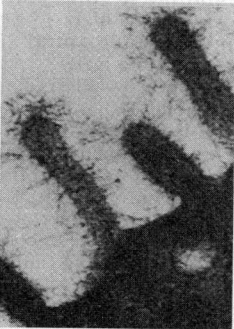

microtubules: (A) ciliated epithelium of mouse oviduct: cross-section showing characteristic arrangement; (B) microvilli: longitudinal section

mi·cro·vil·lus, pl. **mi·cro·vil·li** (mī-krō-vil'ŭs, -vil'ī). One of the minute projections of cell membranes greatly increasing surface area; microvilli form the striated or brush borders of certain cells.

mi·cro·volt (μV) (mī'krō-vōlt). One-millionth of a volt.

mi·cro·waves (mī'krō-wāvz). That portion of the radio wave spectrum of shortest wavelength, including the region with wavelengths of 1 mm to 30 cm (1000 to 300,000 megacycles per second).

mi·crox·y·phil (mī-krok'si-fil). A multinuclear oxyphil leukocyte. [micro- + G. *oxys*, acid, + *philos*, fond]

mi·cro·zo·on (mī-krō-zō'on). A microscopic form of the animal kingdom; a protozoon. [micro- + G. *zōon*, animal]

mi·crur·gi·cal (mī-krer'ji-kăl). Relating to procedures performed on minute structures under a microscope. [micro- + G. *ergon*, work]

mic·tion (mik'shŭn). SYN urination.

mic·tu·rate (mik'chū-rāt). SYN urinate. [see micturition]

mic·tu·ri·tion (mik-chū-rish'ŭn). **1.** SYN urination. **2.** The desire to urinate. **3.** Frequency of urination. [L. *micturio*, to desire to make water]

M.I.D. Abbreviation for minimal infecting *dose*.

mid-. Middle. [A.S. *mid, midd*]

mid·body (mid'bod'ē). A dense stalk of residual interzonal spindle fibers (microtubules) and actin-containing filaments that is formed during anaphase of mitosis and connects daughter cells during telophase; m.'s are frequently observed between spermatids.

mid·brain (mid'brān). SYN mesencephalon.

mid·car·pal (mid'kar-păl). **1.** Relating to the central part of the carpus. **2.** Denoting the articulation between the two rows of carpal bones. SYN mediocarpal.

mid·dle. Denoting an anatomical structure that is

between two other similar structures or that is midway in position.

mid·gut (mid'gŭt). **1.** The central portion of the digestive tube; the distal duodenum, small intestine, and proximal colon. **2.** The portion of the embryonic gut tract between the foregut and the hindgut which originally is open to the yolk sac.

mid·riff (mid'rif). SYN diaphragm (1). [A.S. *mid*, middle, + *hrif*, belly]

mid·tar·sal (mid'tar'săl). Relating to the middle of the tarsus.

mid·wife (mid'wīf). A person qualified to practice midwifery, having specialized training in obstetrics and child care. [A.S. *mid*, with, + *wif*, wife]

mid·wife·ry (mid'wīf'rē, mid-wif'ē-rē). Independent care of essentially normal, healthy women and infants by a midwife, antepartally, intrapartally, postpartally, and/or obstetrically in a hospital, birth center, or home setting, and including normal delivery of the infant, with medical consultation, collaborative management, and referral of cases in which abnormalities develop; strong emphasis is placed on educational preparation of parents for childbearing and childrearing, with an orientation toward childbirth as a normal physiological process requiring minimal intervention.

mi·graine (mī'grān, mi-grān'). A symptom complex occurring periodically and characterized by pain in the head (usually unilateral), vertigo, nausea and vomiting, photophobia, and scintillating appearances of light. Classified as classic m., common m., cluster headache, hemiplegic m., ophthalmoplegic m., and ophthalmic m. SYN hemicrania (1), sick headache. [through O. Fr., fr. G. *hēmi- krania*, pain on one side of the head, fr. *hēmi-*, half, + *kranion*, skull]

  classic m., a form of hemicrania m. preceded by a scintillating scotoma (teichopsia).

  common m., a form of m. headache without the visual prodrome, that is not limited on one side of the head but nevertheless is recognizable as m. because of the stereotyped course; the tendency to nausea, photophobia, and phonophobia; and the relief produced by sleep.

mi·gra·tion (mī-grā'shŭn). **1.** Passing from one part to another, said of certain morbid processes or symptoms. **2.** SYN diapedesis. **3.** Movement of a tooth or teeth out of normal position. **4.** Movement of molecules during electrophoresis. [L. *migro*, pp. *-atus*, to move from place to place]

MIH melanotropin release-inhibiting *hormone*.

mil·ia (mil'ē-ă). Plural of milium.

mil·i·a·ria (mil-ē-ā'rē-ă). An eruption of minute vesicles and papules due to retention of fluid at the orifices of sweat glands. SYN miliary fever (2). [L. *miliarius*, relating to millet, fr. *milium*, millet]

  m. ru'bra, an eruption of papules and vesicles at the orifices of sweat glands, accompanied by redness and inflammatory reaction of the skin. SYN heat rash, prickly heat, strophulus, tropical lichen, lichen tropicus.

mil·i·a·ry (mil'ē-ā-rē, mil'yă-rē). **1.** Resembling a millet seed in size (about 2 mm). **2.** Marked by the presence of nodules of millet seed size on any surface. [see miliaria]

mi·lieu (mē-lyū′). **1.** Surroundings; environment. **2.** PSYCHIATRY The social setting of the mental patient, *e.g.,* the family setting or a hospital unit. [Fr. *mi,* fr. L. *medius,* middle, + *lieu,* fr. L. *locus,* place]

mil·i·tar·y an·ti·shock trou·sers (MAST). SYN pneumatic antishock *garment.*

mil·i·um, pl. **mil·ia** (mil′ē-ŭm, -ē-ă). A small subepidermal keratin cyst, usually multiple and therefore commonly referred to in the plural. SYN whitehead (1). [L. millet]

   colloid m. (kol′loyd mil′ē-ŭm), Yellow papules developing in sun-damaged skin of the head and backs of the hands, composed of colloid material in the dermis resembling amyloid but with a different ultrastructure. SYN colloid acne, colloid pseudomilium. [L. *milium,* millet]

milk. **1.** A white liquid, containing proteins, sugar, and lipids, secreted by the mammary glands after childbirth, and serving for the nourishment of the infant. **2.** Any whitish milky fluid; *e.g.,* the juice of the coconut or a suspension of various metallic oxides. **3.** A pharmacopeial preparation that is a suspension of insoluble drugs in a water medium; distinguished from gels mainly in that the suspended particles of m. are larger. **4.** SYN strip (1). [A.S. *meolc*]

   certified m., cow's m. that does not have more than the maximal permissible limit of 10,000 bacteria per ml at any time prior to delivery to the consumer, and that must be cooled to 10°C or less and maintained at that temperature until delivery.

   certified pasteurized m., cow's m. in which the maximum permissible limit is 10,000 bacteria per ml before pasteurization and 500 bacteria per ml after pasteurization; it must be cooled to 7.2°C or less and maintained at that temperature until delivery.

   skim m., skimmed m., the aqueous (non-cream) part of m. from which casein is isolated.

   vitamin D m., cow's m. to which vitamin D has been added, to contain 400 USP units of vitamin D per quart.

   witch's m., a secretion of colostrum-like m. sometimes occurring in the glands of newborn infants of either sex 3 to 4 days after birth and lasting a week or two; due to endocrine stimulation from the mother before birth.

△**milli-.** Prefix used in the SI and metric systems to signify one-thousandth (10^{-3}). [L. *mille,* one thousand]

mil·li·am·pere (ma, mA) (mil′ē-am′pēr). One thousandth of an ampere.

milliampere-impulse (mAi). SYN milliampere-second.

milliampere-second (mA-s). A radiologic unit denoting the product of the number of electrons applied to the cathode of the X-ray tube multiplied by the exposure time in seconds; it directly determines the amount of X-ray energy produced. SYN milliampere-impulse.

mil·li·cu·rie (mc, mCi) (mil′i-kyū′rē). A unit of radioactivity equivalent to 3.7×10^7 disintegrations per second.

mil·li·e·quiv·a·lent (mEq, meq) (mil′i-ē-kwiv′ă-lent). One-thousandth equivalent; 10^{-3} mole divided by valence.

mil·li·gram (mg) (mil′i-gram). One-thousandth of a gram.

mil·li·li·ter (mL, ml) (mil′i-lē-ter). One-thousandth of a liter.

mil·li·me·ter (mm) (mil′i-mē-ter). One-thousandth of a meter.

△**millimicro-.** Prefix formerly used to signify one-billionth (10^{-9}); now nano-.

mil·li·mi·cron (mμ) (mil′i-mī-kron). Former term for nanometer.

mil·li·mole (mmol) (mil′i-mōl). One-thousandth of a gram-molecule.

mil·li·sec·ond (ms, msec) (mil′i-sek′ŏnd). One-thousandth of a second.

mil·li·volt (mV) (mil′i-vōlt). One thousandth of a volt.

mil·pho·sis (mil-fō′sis). Loss of eyelashes. [G. *milphōsis*]

MIM *Mendelian Inheritance in Man.*

mi·me·sis (mi-mē′sis, mī-). **1.** Hysterical simulation of organic disease. **2.** The symptomatic imitation of one organic disease by another. [G. *mimēsis,* imitation, fr. *mimeomai,* to mimic]

mi·met·ic (mi-met′ik, mī-). Relating to mimesis. [G. *mimētikos,* imitative]

mim·ic (mim′ik). To imitate or simulate. [G. *mimikos,* imitating, fr. *mimos,* a mimic]

mind. **1.** The organ or seat of consciousness and higher functions of the human brain, such as cognition, reasoning, willing, and emotion. **2.** The organized totality of all mental processes and psychic activities, with emphasis on the relatedness of the phenomena. [A.S. *gemynd*]

min·er·al (min′er-ăl). Any homogeneous inorganic material usually found in the earth's crust. [L. *mineralis,* pertaining to mines, fr. *mino,* to mine]

min·er·al·o·cor·ti·coid (min′er-al-ō-kōr′ti-koyd). One of the steroids of the adrenal cortex that influence salt (sodium and potassium) metabolism.

min·i·lap·a·rot·o·my (min′ē-lap-ă-rot′ō-mē). Technique for sterilization by surgical ligation of the uterine tubes, performed through a small suprapubic incision.

min·im. **1.** A fluid measure, $\frac{1}{60}$ of a fluidrachm; in the case of water about one drop. **2.** Smallest; least; the smallest of several similar structures. [L. *minimus,* least]

mi·nor (mī′ner). Smaller; lesser; denoting the smaller of two similar structures. [L.]

△**mio-.** Less. [G. *meiōn*]

mi·o·sis (mī-ō′sis). **1.** Contraction of the pupil. **2.** Incorrect alternative spelling for meiosis. [G. *meiōsis,* a lessening]

mi·o·sphyg·mia (mī′ō-sfig′mē-ă). Condition in which pulse beats are fewer than heart beats. [mio- + G. *sphygmos,* pulse]

mi·ot·ic (mī-ot′ik). **1.** Relating to or characterized by contraction of the pupil. **2.** An agent that causes the pupil to contract.

MIP maximum inspiratory *pressure.*

mire (mēr). One of the test objects in the ophthalmometer; its image (also called a m.), mirrored on the corneal surface, is measured to determine the radii of curvature of the cornea. [L. *miror,* pp. *-atus,* to wonder at]

mir•yach•it (mir-yach'it). A nervous affection observed in Siberia. SEE jumping *disease.*

mis•an•dry (mis'an-drē). Aversion to or hatred of men. [G. *miseō,* to hate, + *anēr, andros,* male]

mis•an•thro•py (mis-an'thrō-pē). Aversion to and hatred of human beings. [G. *miseō,* to hate, + *anthrōpos,* man]

mis•car•riage (mis-kar'ij). Spontaneous expulsion of the products of pregnancy before the middle of the second trimester.

mis•ce•ge•na•tion (mis'e-jĕ-nā'shŭn). Marriage or interbreeding of individuals of different races. [L. *misceo,* to mix, + *genus,* descent, race]

mis•ci•ble (mis'i-bl). Capable of being mixed and remaining so after the mixing process ceases. [L. *misceo,* to mix]

mis•di•ag•no•sis (mis'dī-ag-nō'sis). A wrong or mistaken diagnosis.

mi•sog•a•my (mi-sog'ă-mē). Aversion to marriage. [G. *miseō,* to hate, + *gamos,* marriage]

mi•sog•y•ny (mi-soj'i-nē). Aversion to or hatred of women. [G. *miseō,* to hate, + *gynē,* woman]

mis•o•pe•dia, mis•op•e•dy (mis-ō-pē'dē-ă, -op'ĕ-dē). Aversion to or hatred of children. [G. *miseō,* to hate, + *pais (paid-),* child]

mite (mīt). A minute arthropod of the order Acarina, a vast assemblage of parasitic and (primarily) free-living organisms. A few are of medical importance as vectors or intermediate hosts of pathogenic agents, by directly causing dermatitis or tissue damage, or by causing blood or tissue fluid loss. [A.S.]

mith•ri•da•tism (mith'ri-dā'tizm, mith-rid'ă-tizm). Immunity against the action of a poison produced by small and gradually increasing doses of the same. [*Mithridates,* King of Pontus (132–63 B.C.), supposedly an unsuccessful suicide (by poison) because of repeated small doses taken to become invulnerable to assassination by poison]

mi•ti•ci•dal (mī-ti-sī'dăl). Destructive to mites.

mi•ti•cide (mī'ti-sīd). An agent destructive to mites. [mite + L. *caedo,* to kill]

mit•i•gate (mit'i-gāt). SYN palliate. [L. *mitigo,* pp. *-atus,* to make mild or gentle, fr. *mitis,* mild, + *ago,* to do, make]

mi•to•chon•dria (mī-tō-kon'drē-ă). Plural of mitochondrion.

mi•to•chon•dri•al (mī-tō-kon'drē-ăl). Relating to mitochondria.

mi•to•chon•dri•on, pl. **mi•to•chon•dria** (mī-tō-kon'drē-on, mī-tō-kon'drē-ă). An organelle of the cell cytoplasm consisting of two sets of membranes, a smooth continuous outer coat and an inner membrane arranged in tubules or more often in folds that form platelike double membranes called cristae; mitochondria are the principal energy source of the cell and contain the cytochrome enzymes of terminal electron transport and the enzymes of the citric acid cycle, fatty acid oxidation, and oxidative phosphorylation. [G. *mitos,* thread, + *chondros,* granule, grits]

mi•to•gen (mī'tō-jen). A substance that stimulates mitosis and lymphocyte transformation; includes not only lectins such as phytohemagglu-

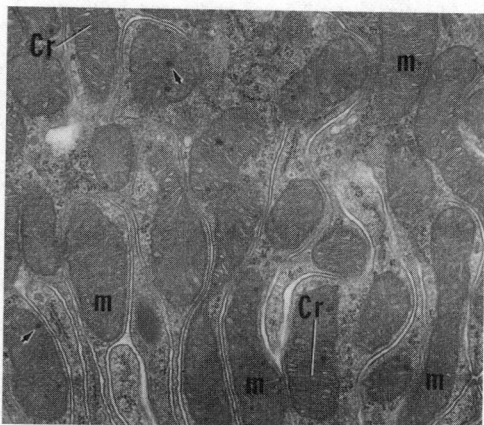

mitochondrion: in kidney of mouse, electron microscopy; (m) mitochondria, (Cr) cristae

tinins and concanavalin A, but also substances from streptococci (associated with streptolysin S) and from strains of α-toxin-producing staphylococci. [mitosis + G. *-gen,* producing]

mi•to•gen•e•sis (mī-tō-jen'ĕ-sis). The process of induction of mitosis in or transformation of a cell. [mitosis + G. *genesis,* origin]

mi•to•ge•net•ic (mī'tō-jĕ-net'ik). Pertaining to the factor or factors promoting cell mitosis.

mi•to•gen•ic (mī-tō-jen'ik). Causing mitosis or transformation.

mi•to•sis, pl. **mi•to•ses** (mī-tō'sis, -sēz). The usual process of somatic reproduction of cells consisting of a sequence of modifications of the nucleus (prophase, prometaphase, metaphase, anaphase, telophase) that result in the formation of two daughter cells with exactly the same chromosome and DNA content as that of the original cell. SEE ALSO cell *cycle.* SYN indirect nuclear division. [G. *mitos,* thread]

mi•tot•ic (mī-tot'ik). Relating to or marked by mitosis.

mi•tral (mī'trăl). **1.** Relating to the mitral or bicuspid valve. **2.** Shaped like a bishop's miter; denoting a structure resembling the shape of a headband or turban. [L. *mitra,* a coif or turban]

mi•tral•i•za•tion (mī'tră-li-zā'shŭn). Straightening of the left heart border on a chest radiograph due to prominence of the left atrial appendage or the pulmonary outflow tract; an unreliable indication of mitral valve disease.

mit•tel•schmerz (mit'el-shmārts). Abdominal pain occurring at the time of ovulation, resulting from irritation of the peritoneum by bleeding from the ovulation site. SYN intermenstrual pain (2). [Ger. Mittelschmerz, middle + pain]

mix•ture (miks'chŭr). **1.** A mutual incorporation of two or more substances, without chemical union, the physical characteristics of each of the components being retained. A **mechanical m.** is a m. of particles or masses distinguishable as such under the microscope or in other ways; a **physical m.** is a more intimate m. of molecules,

mi

as in the case of gases and many solutions. **2.** CHEMISTRY A mingling together of two or more substances without the occurrence of a reaction by which they would lose their individual properties, *i.e.,* without permanent gain or loss of electrons. **3.** PHARMACY A preparation, consisting of a liquid holding an insoluble medicinal substance in suspension by means of acacia, sugar, or some other viscid material. [L. *mixtura* or *mistura*]

Mi·ya·ga·wa·nel·la (mē'yă-gah'wă-nel'ă). Formerly considered a genus of Chlamydiaceae, but now synonymous with *Chlamydia.* [Y. *Miyagawa*]

mL, ml milliliter.

MLD, mld minimal lethal *dose.*

mm Abbreviation for millimeter.

M-mode. A diagnostic ultrasound presentation of the temporal changes in echoes in which the depth of echo-producing interfaces is displayed along one axis with time (T) along the second axis; motion (M) of the interfaces toward and away from the transducer is displayed.

mmol millimole.

Mn manganese.

mne·men·ic, mne·mic (nē-men'ik, nē'mik). Relating to memory.

mne·mon·ic (nē-mon'ik). SYN anamnestic (1).

mne·mon·ics (nē-mon'iks). The art of improving the memory; a system for aiding the memory. [G. *mnēmonikos,* mnemonic, pertaining to memory]

Mo molybdenum.

mo·bi·li·za·tion (mō'bi-li-zā'shŭn). **1.** Making movable; restoring the power of motion in a joint. **2.** The act or the result of the act of mobilizing; exciting a hitherto quiescent process into physiologic activity. [see mobilize]

   stapes m., an operation to remobilize the footplate of the stapes to relieve conductive hearing impairment caused by its immobilization through otosclerosis or middle ear disease.

mo·dal·i·ty (mō-dal'i-tē). **1.** A form of application or employment of a therapeutic agent or regimen. **2.** Various forms of sensation, *e.g.,* touch, vision, etc.. [Mediev. L. *modalitas,* fr. L. *modus,* a mode]

mode (mōd). In a set of measurements, that value which appears most frequently. [L. *modus,* a measure, quantity]

mod·el (mod'ĕl). **1.** A representation of something, often idealized or modified to make it conceptually easier to understand. **2.** Something to be imitated. **3.** DENTISTRY A cast. [It. *midello,* fr. L. *modus,* measure, standard]

   animal m., study in a population of laboratory animals that uses conditions of animals analogous to conditions of humans to simulate processes comparable to those that occur in human populations.

   biomedical m., a conceptual m. of illness that excludes psychological and social factors.

   biopsychosocial m., a conceptual m. that assumes that psychological and social factors must also be included along with the biological in understanding a person's medical illness or disorder.

   independent living m., service delivery m. that identifies the consumer as the decision maker

regarding health care and other daily living needs upon presentation of choices by health care providers.

mod·el·ing (mod'ĕl-ing). **1.** LEARNING THEORY The acquiring and learning of a new skill by observing and imitating that behavior being performed by another individual. **2.** BEHAVIOR MODIFICATION A treatment procedure whereby the therapist or another significant person presents (models) the target behavior which the learner is to imitate. **3.** A continuous process by which a bone is altered in size and shape during its growth by resorption and formation of bone at different sites and rates.

mod·i·fi·ca·tion (mod'i-fi-kā'shŭn). **1.** A nonhereditary change in an organism; *e.g.,* one that is acquired from its own activity or environment. **2.** A chemical or structural alteration in a molecule.

   behavior m., the systematic use of principles of conditioning and learning, especially operant or instrumental conditioning, to teach certain skills or to extinguish undesirable behaviors, attitudes, or phobias.

mo·di·o·lus, pl. **mo·di·o·li** (mō-dī'ō-lŭs, -ō-lī) [NA]. The central cone-shaped core of spongy bone about which turns the spiral canal of the cochlea. **2.** SYN m. labii. [L., the nave of a wheel]

   m. la'bii, a point near the corner of the mouth where several muscles of facial expression converge. SYN modiolus (2).

mod·u·la·tion (mod-yū-lā'shŭn). **1.** The functional and morphologic fluctuation of cells in response to changing environmental conditions. **2.** Systematic variation in a characteristic (*e.g.,* frequency, amplitude) of a sustained oscillation to code additional information. **3.** A change in the kinetics of an enzyme or metabolic pathway. **4.** The regulation of the rate of translation of mRNA by a modulating codon. [L. *modulor,* to measure off properly]

moi·e·ty (moy'i-tē). **1.** Originally a half; now, loosely, a portion of something. **2.** Functional group. [M.E. *moite,* a half]

mol mole (4).

mo·lal (mō'lăl). Denoting 1 mol of solute dissolved in 1000 g of solvent; such solutions provide a definite ratio of solute to solvent molecules. Cf. molar (4).

mo·lal·i·ty (mō-lal'i-tē). Moles of solute per kilogram of solvent; the molarity is equal to $m\rho/(1 + mM)$, where m is the molality, ρ is the density of the solution, and M is the molar mass of the solute. Cf. molarity.

mo·lar (mō'lăr). **1.** Denoting a grinding, abrading, or wearing away. [L. *molaris,* relating to a mill, millstone] **2.** SYN molar *tooth.* **3.** Massive; relating to a mass; not molecular. [L. *moles,* mass] **4.** Denoting a concentration of 1 grammolecular weight (1 mol) of solute per liter of solution, the common unit of concentration in chemistry. Cf. molal. **5.** Denoting specific quantity, *e.g.,* m. volume (volume of 1 mol).

   first m., first permanent m., sixth permanent tooth or fourth deciduous tooth in the maxilla and mandible on either side of the midsagittal plane of the head following the arch form.

   second m., seventh permanent or fifth deciduous tooth in the maxilla and mandible on either side of the midsagittal plane of the head following the arch form.

sixth-year m., the first permanent m. tooth.

third m., eighth permanent tooth in the maxilla and mandible on each side; the most posterior tooth in human dentition; usually erupts between the seventeenth and twenty-third years; the roots are often fused, the separation being marked only by grooves. SYN dens serotinus [NA], wisdom tooth.

twelfth-year m., the second permanent m. tooth.

mo·lar·i·ty (mō-lar′i-tē). Moles per liter of solution (mol/L). Cf. molality.

mold (mōld). **1.** A filamentous fungus, generally a circular colony that may be cottony, wooly, etc., or glabrous, but with filaments not organized into large fruiting bodies, such as mushrooms. **2.** A shaped receptacle into which wax is pressed or fluid plaster is poured in making a cast. **3.** To shape a mass of plastic material according to a definite pattern. **4.** To change in shape; denoting especially the adaptation of the fetal head to the pelvic canal. **5.** The term used to specify the shape of an artificial tooth (or teeth).

mole (mōl). **1.** SYN nevus (2). **2.** SYN *nevus* pigmentosus. [A.S. *māel* (L. *macula*), a spot] **3.** An intrauterine mass formed by the degeneration of the partly developed products of conception. [L. *moles,* mass] **4 (mol).** In the SI system, the unit of amount of substance, defined as that amount of a substance containing as many "elementary entities" as there are atoms in 0.0120 kg of carbon-12; "elementary entities" may be atoms, molecules, ions, or any describable entity or defined mixture of entities and must be specified when this term is used; in practical terms, the mole is 6.0221367×10^{23} "elementary entities." SEE ALSO Avogadro's *number.*

Breus m., an aborted ovum in which the fetal surface of the placenta presents numerous hematomata with an absence of blood vessels in the chorion and an ovum much smaller in size than normal in relation to the duration of the pregnancy.

hairy m., SYN *nevus* pilosus.

hydatidiform m., hydatid m., a vesicular or polycystic mass resulting from the proliferation of the trophoblast, with hydropic degeneration and avascularity of the chorionic villi.

mo·lec·u·lar (mō-lek′yū-lăr). Relating to molecules.

mol·e·cule (mol′ĕ-kyūl). The smallest possible quantity of a di-, tri-, or polyatomic substance that retains the chemical properties of the substance. [Mod. L. *molecula,* dim. of L. *moles,* mass]

accessory m.'s, cell surface adhesion m.'s on T cells that are involved in binding of one cell to another cell or in signal transduction.

adhesion m.'s, m.'s that are involved in T helper-accessory cell, T helper-B cell, and T cytotoxic-target cell interactions.

cell adhesion m. (CAM), proteins that hold cells together, *e.g.,* uvomorulin, and hold them to their substrates, *e.g.,* laminin.

gram-molecule, the amount of a substance with a mass in grams equal to its molecular weight; *e.g.,* a m. of hydrogen weighs 2.016 g, that of water 18.015 g.

mo·li·men, pl. **mo·lim·i·na** (mō-li′men, -lim′i-nă). An effort; laborious performance of a normal function. [L. an endeavor]

mol·li·ti·es (mō-lish′i-ēz). **1.** Characterized by a soft consistency. **2.** SYN malacia. [L. *mollis,* soft]

mol·lus·cous (mo-lŭs′kŭs). Relating to or resembling molluscum.

mol·lus·cum (mo-lŭs′kŭm). A disease marked by the occurrence of soft rounded tumors of the skin. [L. *molluscus,* soft]

m. contagio′sum, a contagious disease of the skin caused by intranuclear proliferation of a virus of the family Poxviridae and characterized by the appearance of small, pearly, umbilicated papular epidermal growths. In adults it typically occurs on or near the genitals and is sexually transmitted.

molt (mōlt). To cast off feathers, hair, or cuticle; to undergo ecdysis. [L. *muto,* to change]

mol wt molecular *weight.*

mo·lyb·den·ic, mo·lyb·de·nous (mō-lib′den-ik, -den-ŭs). Relating to molybdenum.

mo·lyb·de·num (Mo) (mō-lib′dĕ-nŭm). A silvery white metallic element, atomic no. 42, atomic wt. 95.94; a bioelement found in a number of proteins (*e.g.,* xanthine oxidase). SEE molybdenum target *tube.* [G. *molybdaina,* a piece of lead; a metal, prob. galena, fr. *molybdos,* lead]

△**mon-.** SEE mono-.

mo·nad (mō′nad, mon′ad). **1.** A univalent element or radical. **2.** A unicellular organism. **3.** In meiosis, the single chromosome derived from a tetrad after the first and second maturation divisions. [G. *monas,* the number one, unity]

mon·ar·thric (mon-ar′thrik). SYN monarticular.

mon·ar·thri·tis (mon-ar-thrī′tis). Arthritis of a single joint.

mon·ar·tic·u·lar (mon-ar-tik′yū-lăr). Relating to a single joint. SYN monarthric.

mon·as·ter (mon-as′ter). The single star figure at the end of prophase in mitosis. [mono- + G. *aster,* star]

mon·ath·e·to·sis (mon-ath-ĕ-tō′sis). Athetosis affecting one hand or foot.

mon·a·tom·ic (mon-ă-tom′ik). **1.** Relating to or containing a single atom. **2.** SYN monovalent (1).

mon·au·ral (mon-aw′răl). Pertaining to one ear. [mono- + L. *auris,* ear]

mon·es·thet·ic (mon-es-thet′ik). Relating to a single sense or sensation. [mono- + G. *aisthēsis,* sense perception]

mon·go·li·an (mon-gō′lē-ăn). Relating to a member of the Mongolian race.

mo·nil·e·thrix (mō-nil′ĕ-thriks). An inherited trichodystrophy in which brittle hairs show a series of constrictions, usually without a medulla. SYN beaded hair, moniliform hair. [L. *monile,* necklace, + G. *thrix,* hair]

Mo·nil·i·a (mo-nil′ē-ă). Generic term for a group of fungi that are commonly known as fruit molds; the sexual state is *Neurospora.* A few closely related pathogenic organisms formerly classified

mo

in this genus are now properly termed *Candida*. [L. *monile*, necklace]

mo·nil·i·al (mō-nil′ē-ăl). Pertaining to the genus *Candida* (formerly grouped with the genus *Monilia*).

mon·i·li·a·sis (mō-ni-lī′ă-sis). SYN candidiasis.

mo·nil·i·form (mō-nil′i-fōrm). Shaped like a string of beads or beaded necklace. [L. *monile*, necklace, + *forma*, appearance]

Mo·nil·i·for·mis (mō-nil-i-fōr′mis). A genus of thorny-headed worms. A few infections in humans have been reported. [L. *monile*, necklace, + *forma*, appearance]

mo·nil·i·id (mō-nil′ē-id). Minute macular or papular lesions occurring as an allergic reaction to monilial infection.

mon·i·tor (mon′i-ter, -tōr). A device that displays and/or records specified data for a given series of events, operations, or circumstances. [L., one who warns, fr. *moneo*, pp. *monitum*, to warn]

Holter m., a technique for long-term, continuous recording of electrocardiographic signals on magnetic tape for scanning and selection of significant but fleeting changes that might otherwise escape notice.

transcutaneous blood gas m., a device that uses miniature electrodes applied to the skin to estimate blood oxygen and carbon dioxide tension; the transcutaneous carbon dioxide tension ($tcPCO_2$) provides a relatively accurate estimate of arterial carbon dioxide ($PaCO_2$) in all age groups; the estimate of transcutaneous oxygen tension ($tcPO_2$) is more accurate in neonates and small children.

mono-, mon-. The participation or involvement of a single element or part. Cf. uni-. [G. *monos*, single]

mon·o·am·ide (mon-ō-am′īd, -id). A molecule containing one amide group.

mon·o·am·ine (mon-ō-am′īn, -in). A molecule containing one amine group.

mon·o·am·i·ner·gic (mon′ō-am-i-ner′jik). Referring to nerve cells or fibers that transmit nervous impulses by the medium of a catecholamine or indolamine. [monoamine + G. *ergon*, work]

mon·o·ba·sic (mon-ō-bā′sik). Denoting an acid with only one replaceable hydrogen atom, or only one replaced hydrogen atom.

mon·o·blast (mon′ō-blast). An immature cell that develops into a monocyte. [mono- + G. *blastos*, germ]

mon·o·cho·rea (mon′ō-kō-rē′ă). Chorea affecting the head alone or only one extremity.

mon·o·cho·ri·on·ic (mon′ō-kōr-ē-on′ik). Relating to or having a single chorion; denoting monovular twins.

mon·o·chro·mat·ic (mon′ō-krō-mat′ik). 1. Having but one color. 2. Indicating a light of a single wavelength. 3. Relating to or characterized by monochromatism.

mon·o·chro·ma·tism (mon-ō-krō′mă-tizm). 1. The state of having or exhibiting only one color. 2. SYN achromatopsia. [mono- + G. *chrōma*, color]

mon·o·chro·mat·o·phil, mon·o·chro·mat·o·phile (mon′ō-krō-mat′ō-fil, -fīl). 1. Taking only

one stain. 2. A cell or any histologic element staining with only one kind of dye. [mono- + G. *chrōma*, color, + *philos*, fond]

mon·o·clo·nal (mon-ō-klō′năl). IMMUNOCHEMISTRY Pertaining to a protein from a single clone of cells, all molecules of which are the same.

mon·o·crot·ic (mon′ō-krot′ik). Denoting a pulse the curve of which presents no notch or subsidiary wave in its descending line. [mono- + G. *krotos*, a beat]

mon·oc·ro·tism (mon-ok′rō-tizm). The state in which the pulse is monocrotic. [mono- + G. *krotos*, a beat]

mo·noc·u·lar (mon-ok′yū-lăr). Relating to, affecting, or visible by one eye only. [mono- + L. *oculus*, eye]

mon·o·cyte (mon′ō-sīt). A relatively large mononuclear leukocyte (16 to 22 μm in diameter), that normally constitutes 3 to 7% of the leukocytes of the circulating blood, and is normally found in lymph nodes, spleen, bone marrow, and loose connective tissue. In stained smears m.'s manifest an abundant pale blue or blue-gray cytoplasm that contains numerous fine red-blue granules and vacuoles; the nucleus is usually indented, or slightly folded. [mono- + G. *kytos*, cell]

mon·o·cy·to·pe·nia (mon′ō-sī-tō-pē′nē-ă). Diminution in the number of monocytes in the circulating blood. [mono- + G. *kytos*, cell, + *penia*, poverty]

mon·o·cy·to·sis (mon′ō-sī-tō′sis). An abnormal increase in the number of monocytes in the circulating blood.

mon·o·dac·ty·ly, mon·o·dac·tyl·ism (mon-ō-dak′ti-lē, -dak′-ti-lizm). The presence of a single finger on the hand, or a single toe on the foot. [mono- + G. *daktylos*, digit]

mon·o·ga·met·ic (mon′ō-gă-met′ik). SYN homogametic.

mo·nog·a·my (mon-og′ă-mē). The marriage or mating system in which each partner has but one mate. [mono- + G. *gamos*, marriage]

mon·o·gen·e·sis (mon-ō-jen′ĕ-sis). 1. The production of similar organisms in each generation. 2. The production of young by one parent only, as in nonsexual generation and parthenogenesis. 3. The process of parasitizing a single host, in which the entire life cycle of the parasite is passed. [mono- + G. *genesis*, origin, production]

mon·o·ge·net·ic (mon′ō-jĕ-net′ik). Relating to monogenesis. SYN monoxenous.

mon·o·gen·ic (mon-ō-jen′ik). Relating to a hereditary disease or syndrome, or to an inherited characteristic, controlled by alleles at a single genetic locus.

mo·nog·e·nous (mŏ-noj′ĕ-nŭs). Asexually produced, as by fission, gemmation, or sporulation.

mon·o·lay·ers (mon-ō-lā′erz). 1. Films, one molecule thick, formed on water by certain substances, such as proteins and fatty acids, characterized by molecules containing some atom groupings that are soluble in water and other atom groupings that are insoluble in water. 2. A confluent sheet of cells, one cell deep, growing on a surface in a cell culture.

mon·o·loc·u·lar (mon-ō-lok′yū-lăr). Having one

cavity or chamber. SYN unicameral, unicamerate. [mono- + L. *loculus,* a small place]

mon•o•ma•nia (mon-ō-mā′nē-ă). An obsession or abnormal enthusiasm for a single idea or subject; a psychosis marked by limitation of symptoms to a certain group, as the delusion in paranoia. [mono- + G. *mania,* frenzy]

mon•o•mel•ic (mon-ō-mel′ik). Relating to one limb. [mono- + G. *melos,* limb]

mon•o•mer (mon′ō-mer). 1. The molecular unit that, by repetition, constitutes a large structure or polymer. 2. The protein structural unit of a virion capsid. SEE virion. 3. The protein subunit of a protein composed of several loosely associated such units, usually noncovalently bound together. [mono- + -mer]

mon•o•mer•ic (mon-ō-mer′ik). 1. Consisting of a single component. 2. GENETICS Relating to a hereditary disease or characteristic controlled by genes at a single locus. 3. Consisting of monomers. [mono- + G. *meros,* part]

mon•o•mor•phic (mon-ō-mōr′fik). Of one shape; unchangeable in shape. [mono- + G. *morphē,* shape]

mon•o•my•o•ple•gia (mon′ō-mī′ō-plē′jē-ă). Paralysis limited to one muscle. [mono- + G. *mys,* muscle, + *plēgē,* a stroke]

mon•o•my•o•si•tis (mon′ō-mī-ō-sī′tis). Inflammation of a single muscle.

mon•o•neu•ral, mon•o•neu•ric (mon′ō-nū′răl, -nū′rik). 1. Having only one neuron. 2. Supplied by a single nerve.

mon•o•neu•ral•gia (mon′ō-nū-ral′jă). Pain along the course of one nerve.

mon•o•neu•ri•tis (mon′ō-nū-rī′tis). Inflammation of a single nerve.

mon•o•neu•rop•a•thy (mon′ō-nū-rop′ă-thē). Disorder involving a single nerve.

mon•o•nu•cle•ar (mon-ō-nū′klē-ăr). Having only one nucleus; used especially in reference to blood cells.

mon•o•nu•cle•o•sis (mon′ō-nū-klē-ō′sis). Presence of abnormally large numbers of mononuclear leukocytes in the circulating blood, especially with reference to forms that are not normal.

  infectious m., an acute febrile illness caused by the Epstein-Barr virus; frequently spread by saliva transfer; characterized by fever, sore throat, enlargement of lymph nodes and spleen, lymphocytosis with abnormal lymphocytes similar to monocytes, and heterophil antibody in serum.

mon•o•nu•cle•o•tide (mon-ō-nū′klē-ō-tīd). SYN nucleotide.

mon•o•ox•y•ge•na•ses (mon′ō-ok′si-jě-nā-sez). Oxidoreductases that induce the incorporation of one atom of oxygen from O_2 into the substance being oxidized.

mon•o•pa•re•sis (mon′o-pa-rē′sis, -par′ě-sis). Paresis affecting a single extremity or part of an extremity.

mon•o•par•es•the•sia (mon′ō-par-es-thē′zē-ă). Paresthesia affecting a single region only.

mon•o•path•ic (mon′ō-path′ik). Relating to a monopathy.

mo•nop•a•thy (mon-op′ă-thē). 1. A single uncomplicated disease. 2. A local disease affecting only one organ or part. [mono- + G. *pathos,* suffering]

mon•o•pha•sia (mon-ō-fā′zē-ă). Inability to speak other than a single word or sentence. [mono- + G. *phasis,* speech]

mon•o•pha•sic (mon-ō-fā′zik). 1. Marked by monophasia. 2. Occurring in or characterized by only one phase or stage. 3. Fluctuating from the baseline in one direction only.

mon•oph•thal•mos (mon-of-thal′mos). Failure of outgrowth of a primary optic vesicle with absence of ocular tissues; the remaining eye is often maldeveloped. [mono- + G. *ophthalmos,* eye]

mon•o•phy•let•ic (mon′ō-fī-let′ik). 1. Having a single cell type of origin; derived from one line of descent, in contrast to polyphyletic. 2. HEMATOLOGY Relating to monophyletism. [mono- + G. *phylē,* tribe]

mon•o•ple•gia (mon-ō-plē′jē-ă). Paralysis of one limb. [mono- + G. *plēgē,* a stroke]

mon•o•po•dia (mon-ō-pō′dē-ă). Malformation in which only one foot is externally recognizable. [mono- + G. *pous,* foot]

mon•or•chid•ic, mon•or•chid (mon-ōr-kid′ik, mon-ōr′kid). 1. Having only one testis. 2. Having apparently only one testis, the other being undescended.

mon•or•chism (mon′ōr-kizm). A condition in which only one testis is apparent, the other being absent or undescended. [mono- + G. *orchis,* testis]

mon•o•sac•cha•ride (mon-ō-sak′ă-rīd). A carbohydrate that cannot form any simpler sugar by simple hydrolysis; *e.g.,* pentoses, hexoses.

mon•o•so•mia (mon-ō-sō′mē-ă). In conjoined twins, a condition in which the trunks are completely merged although the heads remain separate. SEE conjoined *twins,* under *twin.* [mono- + G. *sōma,* body]

mon•o•so•mic (mon-ō-sō′mik). Relating to monosomy.

mon•o•so•my (mon′ō-sō-mē). Absence of one chromosome of a pair of homologous chromosomes. [see monosome]

mon•o•spasm (mon′ō-spazm). Spasm affecting only one muscle or group of muscles, or a single extremity.

mon•o•stot•ic (mon-os-tot′ik). Involving only one bone. [mono- + G. *osteon,* bone]

mon•o•stra•tal (mon-ō-strā′tăl). Composed of a single layer. [mono- + L. *stratum,* layer]

mon•o•symp•to•mat•ic (mon′ō-simp-tō-mat′ik). Denoting a disease or morbid condition manifested by only one marked symptom.

mon•o•sy•nap•tic (mon′ō-si-nap′tik). Referring to direct neural connections not involving an intermediary neuron.

mon•o•ther•mia (mon-ō-ther′mē-ă). Evenness of bodily temperature; absence of an evening rise in body temperature. [mono- + G. *thermē,* heat]

mo•not•ri•chous (mŏ-not′ri-kŭs). Denoting a microorganism possessing a single flagellum or cilium.

mon•o•va•lence, mon•o•va•len•cy (mon-ō-vā′lens, -vā′len-sē). A combining power (valence) equal to that of a hydrogen atom. SYN univalence, univalency.

mon•o•va•lent (mon-ō-vā′lent). **1.** Having the combining power (valence) of a hydrogen atom. SYN monatomic (2), univalent. **2.** Pertaining to a monovalent (specific) antiserum to a single antigen or organism.

mon•ox•e•nous (mon-oks′ĕ-nŭs). SYN monogenetic. [mono- + G. *xenos,* stranger]

mon•ox•ide (mon-ok′sīd). Any oxide having only one atom of oxygen; *e.g.,* CO.

mon•o•zy•got•ic, mon•o•zy•gous (mon-ō-zī-got′ik, -zī′gŭs). SYN unigerminal. SEE monozygotic *twins,* under *twin.* [mono- + G. *zygōtos,* yoked]

mons, gen. **mon•tis,** pl. **mon•tes** (monz, mon′tis, mon′tēz) [NA]. An anatomical prominence or slight elevation above the general level of the surface. [L. a mountain]

  m. pu′bis [NA], the prominence caused by a pad of fatty tissue over the symphysis pubis in the female.

mon•tic•u•lus, pl. **mon•tic•u•li** (mon-tik′yū-lŭs, -lī). **1.** Any slight rounded projection above a surface. **2.** The central portion of the superior vermis forming a projection on the surface of the cerebellum; its anterior and most prominent portion is called the culmen, its posterior sloping portion, the declive. [L. dim. of *mons,* mountain]

mood (mūd). The pervasive feeling, tone, and internal emotional state which, when impaired, can markedly influence virtually all aspects of a person's behavior or perception of external events.

mood swing. Oscillation of a person's emotional feeling tone between euphoria and depression.

Mor•ax•el•la (mōr′ak-sel′ă). A genus of obligately aerobic nonmotile bacteria containing Gram-negative coccoids or short rods which usually occur in pairs. They are parasitic on the mucous membranes of man and other mammals. [V. *Morax*]

mor•bid (mōr′bid). **1.** Diseased or pathologic. **2.** PSYCHOLOGY Abnormal or deviant. [L. *morbidus,* ill, fr. *morbus,* disease]

mor•bid•i•ty (mōr-bid′i-tē). **1.** A diseased state. **2.** The ratio of sick to well in a community. SEE ALSO morbidity *rate.* **3.** The frequency of the appearance of complications following a surgical procedure or other treatment.

mor•bif•ic (mōr-bif′ik). SYN pathogenic. [L. *morbus,* disease, + *facio,* to make]

mor•bil•li (mōr-bil′ī). SYN measles (1). [Mediev. L. *morbillus,* dim. of L. *morbus,* disease]

mor•bil•li•form (mōr-bil′i-fōrm). Resembling measles (1). [see morbilli]

Mor•bil•li•vi•rus (mōr-bil′i-vī′rŭs). A genus of the family Paramyxoviridae, including measles, canine distemper, and bovine rinderpest viruses.

mor•bus (mōr′bŭs). SYN disease (1). [L. disease]

mor•cel•la•tion (mōr-se-lā′shŭn). Division into and removal of small pieces, as of a tumor. [Fr. *morceler,* to subdivide]

mor•dant (mōr′dant). **1.** A substance capable of combining with a dye and the material to be dyed, thereby increasing the affinity or binding of the dye. **2.** To treat with a m. [L. *mordeo,* to bite]

Morgan, Harry de R., British physician, 1863–1931.

mor•gan (mōr′găn). The standard unit of genetic distance on the genetic map: the distance between two loci such that on average one crossing over will occur per meiosis; for working purposes, the centimorgan (0.01 M) is used. [T.H. *Morgan,* U.S. geneticist, 1866–1945]

Mor•gan•el•la (mōr′gan-el′ah). A genus of Gram-negative, facultatively anaerobic, chemoorganotrophic, straight rods that are motile by peritrichous flagella. Found in feces of human beings, other animals, and reptiles. Can cause opportunistic infections of the blood, respiratory tract, wounds, and urinary tract.

  M. morganii, type (and only) species of the genus *M.*

morgue (mōrg). **1.** A building where unidentified dead are kept pending identification before burial. **2.** A building or room in a hospital or other facility where the dead are kept pending autopsy, burial, or cremation. SYN mortuary (2). [Fr.]

mo•ria (mōr′ē-ă). **1.** Rarely used term denoting foolishness or dullness of comprehension. **2.** Rarely used term for a mental state marked by frivolity, joviality, an inveterate tendency to jest, and inability to take anything seriously.

mor•i•bund (mōr′i-bŭnd). Dying; at the point of death. [L. *moribundus,* dying, fr. *morior,* to die]

△**morph-.** SEE morpho-.

mor•phea (mōr-fē′ă). Cutaneous lesion(s) characterized by indurated, slightly depressed plaques of thickened dermal fibrous tissue, of a whitish or yellowish white color surrounded by a pinkish or purplish halo. SYN localized scleroderma. [G. *morphē,* form, figure]

mor•phine (mōr′fēn, mōr-fēn′). $C_{17}H_{19}NO_3$; the major phenanthrene alkaloid of opium, which contains 9–14% of anhydrous m. It produces a combination of depression and excitation in the central nervous system and some peripheral tissues; predominance of either central stimulation or depression depends upon the species and dose; repeated administration leads to the development of tolerance, physical dependence, and (if abused) psychic dependence. Used as an analgesic, sedative, and anxiolytic. [L. *Morpheus,* god of dreams or sleep]

  m. sulfate (MS), m. used for formulation of tablets as well as solutions for parenteral, epidural, or intrathecal injection to relieve pain.

△**morpho-, morph-.** Form, shape, structure. [G. *morphē*]

mor•pho•gen•e•sis (mōr-fō-jen′ĕ-sis). **1.** Differentiation of cells and tissues in the early embryo which establishes the form and structure of the various organs and parts of the body. **2.** The ability of a molecule or group of molecules (particularly macromolecules) to assume a certain shape. [morpho- + G. *genesis,* production]

mor•pho•ge•net•ic (mōr′fō-jĕ-net′ik). Relating to morphogenesis.

mor•pho•log•ic (mōr-fō-loj′ik). Relating to morphology.

mor•phol•o•gy (mōr-fol′ō-jē). The science concerned with the configuration or the structure of animals and plants. [morpho- + G. *logos,* study]

mor•pho•met•ric (mōr′fō-met′rik). Pertaining to morphometry.

mor·phom·e·try (mōr-fom'ĕ-trē). The measurement of the form of organisms or their parts. [morpho- + G. *metron*, measure]

mor·pho·sis (mōr-fō'sis). Mode of development of a part. [G. formation, act of forming]

mors, gen. **mor·tis** (mōrz, mōr'tis). SYN death. [L.]

mor·tal (mōr'tăl). **1.** Pertaining to or causing death. **2.** Destined to die. [L. *mortalis*, fr. *mors*, death]

mor·tal·i·ty (mōr-tal'i-tē). **1.** The state of being mortal. **2.** SYN death rate. **3.** A fatal outcome. [L. *mortalitas*, fr. *mors* (mort-), death]

mor·tar (mōr'tăr). A vessel with rounded interior in which crude drugs and other substances are crushed or bruised by means of a pestle. [L. *mortarium*]

mor·ti·fi·ca·tion (mōr'ti-fi-kā'shŭn). SYN gangrene (1). [L. *mors* (mort-), death, + *facio*, to make]

mor·ti·fied (mōr'ti-fīd). SYN gangrenous.

mor·tu·ary (mōr'tyū-ār-ē). **1.** Relating to death or to burial. **2.** SYN morgue. [L. *mortuus*, dead, part. adj. fr. *morior*, pp. *mortuus*, to die]

mor·u·la (mōr'ū-lă, mōr'yū-). The solid mass of blastomeres resulting from the early cleavage divisions of the zygote. [Mod. L. dim. of L. *morus*, mulberry]

mor·u·la·tion (mōr-ū-lā'shŭn, mōr-yū-). Formation of the morula.

mo·sa·ic (mō-zā'ik). **1.** Inlaid; resembling inlaid work. **2.** The juxtaposition in an organism of genetically different tissues; it may occur normally (as in lyonization, *q.v.*), or pathologically, as an occasional phenomenon. [Mod. L. *mosaicus*, *musaicus*, pertaining to the Muses, artistic]

mo·sa·i·cism (mō-zā'i-sizm). Condition of being mosaic (2).

mos·qui·to, pl. **mos·qui·toes** (mŭs-kē'tō, -tōs). A blood-sucking dipterous insect of the family Culicidae. *Aedes, Anopheles, Culex, Mansonia,* and *Stegomyia* are the genera containing most of the species involved in the transmission of protozoan and other disease-producing parasites. [Sp. dim. of *mosca*, fly, fr. L. *musca*, a fly]

mote (mōt). A small particle; a speck. [A.S. *mot*]

moth·er (mŭth'er). **1.** The female parent. **2.** Any cell or other structure from which other similar bodies are formed. [A.S. *mōdor*]

 surrogate m., a woman who has been contracted with to carry a pregnancy for another woman or couple.

mo·tile (mō'til). **1.** Having the power of spontaneous movement. **2.** Denoting the type of mental imagery in which one learns and recalls most readily that which has been felt. Cf. audile. **3.** A person having such mental imagery. [see motion]

mo·til·i·ty (mō-til'i-tē). The power of spontaneous movement.

mo·tive (mō'tiv). **1.** An acquired predisposition, need, or specific state of tension within an individual which arouses, maintains, and directs behavior toward a goal. SYN learned drive. **2.** The reason attributed to or given by an individual for a behavioral act. Cf. instinct. [L. *moveo*, to move, to set in motion]

mo·to·fa·cient (mō-tō-fā'shent). Causing mo-

tion; denoting the second phase of muscular activity in which actual movement is produced. [L. *motus*, motion, + *facio*, to make]

mo·to·neu·ron (mō'tō-nū'ron). SYN motor *neuron*.

mo·tor (mō'ter). **1.** ANATOMY, PHYSIOLOGY Denoting those neural structures which by the impulses generated and transmitted by them cause muscle fibers or pigment cells to contract, or glands to secrete. SEE ALSO motor *cortex*, motor *endplate*, motor *neuron*. **2.** PSYCHOLOGY Denoting the organism's overt reaction to a stimulus (motor response). [L. a mover, fr. *moveo*, to move]

mot·tling (mot'ling). An area of skin composed of macular lesions of varying shades or colors. [E. *motley*, variegated in color]

mound·ing (mownd'ing). SYN myoedema.

mount (mownt). **1.** To prepare for microscopic examination. **2.** To climb on for purposes of copulation.

mouth (mowth). **1.** SYN oral *cavity*. **2.** The opening, usually the external opening, of a cavity or canal. SEE os (2), ostium, orifice, stoma (2). [A.S. *mūth*]

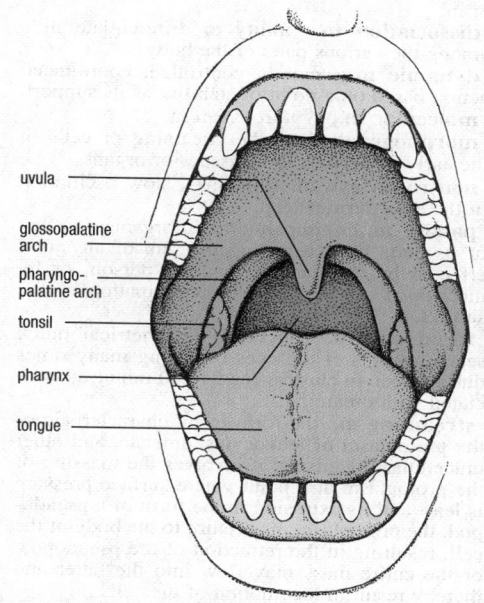

uvula

glossopalatine arch

pharyngo-palatine arch

tonsil

pharynx

tongue

mouth: and surrounding structures

 carp m., a m. like that of the carp, with downturning of the corners; observed in Cornelia de Lange syndrome and Silver-Russell dwarfism.

 tapir m., protrusion of the lips due to weakness of the orbicularis oris muscles; seen with some dystrophies.

 trench m., SYN necrotizing ulcerative *gingivitis*.

mouth·wash. A medicated liquid used for cleaning the mouth and treating diseased states of its mucous membranes.

move·ment (mūv'ment). **1.** The act of motion; said of the entire body or of one or more of its members or parts. **2.** SYN stool. **3.** SYN defecation. [L. *moveo,* pp. *motus,* to move]

ameboid m., a form of locomotion characteristic of leukocytes and protozoans with highly flexible cell membranes; involves extrusion of a pseudopod, into which the remaining cytoplasm of the cell flows. SEE ALSO streaming m.

brownian m., erratic, nondirectional, zigzag m. observed by microscope in suspensions of particles in fluid, resulting from the jostling or bumping of the larger particles by the molecules in the suspending medium. SYN molecular m., pedesis.

choreic m., an involuntary spasmodic twitching or jerking in groups of muscles not associated in the production of definite purposeful m.'s.

ciliary m., the rhythmic, sweeping m. of epithelial cell cilia, of ciliate protozoans, or the sculling m. of flagella, effected possibly by the alternate contraction and relaxation of contractile threads (myoids) on one side of the cilium or flagellum.

compensatory m., movement used habitually to achieve functional motor skills when a normal m. pattern has not been established or is unavailable, for example, hyperextension of the neck. It is influenced by abnormal postural tone, reflexes, or m.

dissociation m., ability to differentiate m.'s among the various parts of the body.

dynamic m., smooth, controlled, coordinated action based on a point of stability as its support.

molecular m., SYN brownian m.

morphogenetic m., the streaming of cells in the early embryo to form tissues or organs.

non-rapid eye m. (NREM), slow oscillation of the eyes during sleep.

passive m., m. imparted to an organism or any of its parts by external agency; m. of any joint effected by the hand of another person, or by mechanical means, without participation of the subject.

rapid eye m.'s (REM), symmetrical quick scanning m.'s of the eyes occurring many times during sleep in clusters for 5 to 60 minutes; associated with dreaming.

streaming m., the form of m. characteristic of the protoplasm of leukocytes, amebae, and other unicellular organisms; it involves the massing of the protoplasm at a point where surface pressure is least and its extrusion in the form of a pseudopod; the protoplasm may return to the body of the cell, resulting in the retraction of the pseudopod, or the entire mass may flow into the latter and thereby result in locomotion of the cell.

vermicular m., SYN peristalsis.

MPD maximum permissible *dose.*

MPI master patient *index.*

MRD, mrd minimal reacting *dose.*

MRF melanotropin-releasing *factor.*

MRH melanotropin-releasing *hormone.*

MRI magnetic resonance *imaging.*

mRNA messenger RNA. See entries under ribonucleic acid.

MS multiple *sclerosis*; *morphine* sulfate; mitral *stenosis*; and myasthenic *syndrome* (Lambert-Eaton syndrome).

ms millisecond.

msec millisecond.

MTP metatarsophalangeal.

mu (myū). **1.** Twelfth letter of the Greek alphabet (μ). **2.** micro- (2); micron; magnetic or electric dipole moment of a molecule; chemical *potential*; denotes the position of a substituent located on the 12th atom from the carboxyl or other functional group.

⌂**muci-.** Mucous, mucin. SEE ALSO muco-. [L. *mucus*]

mu·cif·er·ous (myū-sif′er-ŭs). SYN muciparous.

mu·ci·form (myū′si-fōrm). Resembling mucus. SYN blennoid, mucoid (2).

mu·ci·lage (myū′si-lij). A pharmacopeial preparation consisting of a solution in water of the mucilaginous principles of vegetable substances; used as a soothing application to the mucous membranes and in the preparation of official and extemporaneous mixtures. [L. *mucilago*]

mu·ci·lag·i·nous (myū-sĭ-laj′i-nŭs). **1.** Resembling mucilage; *i.e.,* adhesive, viscid, sticky. **2.** SYN muciparous.

mu·cin (myū′sin). A secretion containing carbohydrate-rich glycoproteins such as that from the goblet cells of the intestine, the submaxillary glands, and other mucous glandular cells; it is also present in the ground substance of connective tissue.

mu·cin·ase (myū′si-nās). Any enzyme that hydrolyzes mucopolysaccharide substances (mucins). SYN mucopolysaccharidase.

mu·cin·o·gen (myū′sin-ō-jen). A glycoprotein that forms mucin through the imbibition of water. [mucin + G. *-gen,* producing]

mu·ci·noid (myū′si-noyd). **1.** SYN mucoid (1). **2.** Resembling mucin.

mu·ci·no·sis (myū-si-nō′sis). A condition in which mucin is present in the skin in excessive amounts, or in abnormal distribution. Classified as metabolic m., secondary m., and localized m. [mucin + G. *-osis,* condition]

localized m., follicular, papular, plaque-like, focal, and myxoid or synovial cyst.

metabolic m., diffuse or pretibial myxedema, lichen myxedematosus, gargoylism.

papular m., SYN lichen myxedematosus.

secondary m., degeneration of m. in tumors.

mu·ci·nous (myū′si-nŭs). Relating to or containing mucin. SYN mucoid (3).

mu·cip·a·rous (myū-sip′ă-rŭs). Producing or secreting mucus. SYN blennogenic, blennogenous, muciferous, mucilaginous (2). [mucin + L. *pario,* to bring forth, bear]

⌂**muco-.** Mucous, mucous (mucous membrane). SEE ALSO muci-. [L. *mucus*]

mu·co·cele (myū′kō-sēl). A retention cyst of the salivary gland, lacrimal sac, paranasal sinuses, appendix, or gallbladder. Most common site is the lower lip lateral to the midline. [muco- + G. *kēlē,* tumor, hernia]

mucociliary (myū-kō-sĭl′ē-ār-e). Pertaining to ciliated columnar epithelium found in the bronchial tree to the level of the terminal bronchioles, and in the uterine tubes. SEE ciliary.

mu·co·cu·ta·ne·ous (myū′kō-kyū-tā′nē-ŭs). Relating to mucous membrane and skin; denoting the line of junction of the two at the nasal, oral, vaginal, and anal orifices.

mu·co·en·ter·i·tis (myū′kō-en-ter-ī′tis). **1.** Inflammation of the intestinal mucous membrane. **2.** SYN mucomembranous *enteritis.*

mu•co•ep•i•der•moid (myū′kō-ep-i-der′moyd). Denoting a mixture of mucus-secreting and epithelial cells, as in m. carcinoma.

mu•coid (myū′koyd). **1.** General term for a mucin, mucoprotein, or glycoprotein. SYN mucinoid (1). **2.** SYN muciform. **3.** SYN mucinous. [mucus + G. *eidos,* appearance]

mu•co•lyt•ic (myū-kō-lit′ik). Capable of dissolving, digesting, or liquefying mucus.

mu•co•mem•bra•nous (myū′kō-mem′bră-nŭs). Relating to a mucous membrane.

mu•co•per•i•os•te•al (myū′kō-per-ē-os′tē-ăl). Relating to mucoperiosteum.

mu•co•per•i•os•te•um (myū′kō-per-ē-os′tē-ŭm). Mucous membrane and periosteum so intimately united as to form practically a single membrane, as that covering the hard palate.

mu•co•pol•y•sac•cha•ri•dase (myū′kō-pol-ē-sak′ă-ri-dās). SYN mucinase.

mu•co•pol•y•sac•cha•ride (myū′kō-pol-ē-sak′ă-rīd). General term for a protein-polysaccharide complex obtained from proteoglycans and containing as much as 95% polysaccharide; m.'s include the blood group substances. A more modern term is glycosaminoglycan.

mu•co•pol•y•sac•cha•ri•du•ria (myū′kō-pol-ē-sak′ă-ri-dū′rē-ă). The excretion of mucopolysaccharides in the urine.

mu•co•pro•tein (myū-kō-prō′tēn). General term for a protein-polysaccharide complex, usually implying that the protein component is the major part of the complex. M.'s include the α₁- and α₂-globulins of serum.

   Tamm-Horsfall m., the matrix of urinary casts derived from the secretion of renal tubular cells.

mu•co•pu•ru•lent (myū-kō-pū′rū-lent). Pertaining to an exudate that is chiefly purulent (pus), but containing relatively conspicuous proportions of mucous material.

Mu•cor (myū′kōr). A genus of fungi (class Zygomycetes, family Mucoraceae), most species of which are saprobic; several are pathogenic and may cause zygomycosis in humans.

mu•cor•my•co•sis (myū′kōr-mī-kō′sis). SYN zygomycosis.

mu•co•sa (myū-kō′să). A mucous tissue lining various tubular structures, consisting of epithelium, lamina propria, and, in the digestive tract, a layer of smooth muscle. [L. fem. of *mucosus,* mucous]

mu•co•sal (myū-kō′săl). Relating to the mucosa or mucous membrane.

mu•co•san•guin•e•ous, mu•co•san•guin•o•lent (myū′kō-sang-gwin′ē-ŭs, -ŏ-lent). Pertaining to an exudate or other fluid material that has a relatively high content of blood and mucus. [muco- + L. *sanguis,* blood]

mu•co•sec•to•my (myū-kō-sek′tō-me). Excision of the mucosa, usually of the rectum prior to ileoanal anastomosis for treatment of ulcerative colitis. [mucosa + G. *ektomē,* excision]

mu•co•se•rous (myū-kō-sē′rŭs). Pertaining to an exudate or secretion that consists of both mucus and serum or a watery component.

mu•cous (myū′kŭs). Relating to mucus or a m. membrane. [L. *mucosus,* mucous, fr. *mucus*]

mu•cus (myū′kŭs). The clear viscid secretion of the mucous membranes, consisting of mucin, epithelial cells, leukocytes, and various inorganic salts suspended in water. [L.]

mu•li•e•bria (mū′lē-ē′brē-ă). The female genital organs. [L. neut pl. of *muliebris,* relating to *mulier,* a woman]

△**multi-.** Many. SEE ALSO pluri-. Cf. poly-. [L. *multus,* much]

mul•ti•ar•tic•u•lar (mŭl′tē-ar-tik′yū-lăr). Relating to or involving many joints. SYN polyarthric, polyarticular. [multi- + L. *articulus,* joint]

mul•ti•cus•pi•date (mŭl-tē-kŭs′pi-dăt). **1.** Having more than two cusps. **2.** A molar tooth with three or more cusps or projections on the crown.

mul•ti•fid (mŭl′tē-fid). Divided into many clefts or segments. [L. *multifidus,* fr. *multus,* much, + *findo,* to cleave]

mul•ti•fo•cal (mŭl-tē-fō′kăl). Relating to or arising from many foci.

mul•ti•form (mŭl′ti-fōrm). SYN polymorphic.

mul•ti•grav•i•da (mŭl-tē-grav′i-dă). A pregnant woman who has been pregnant one or more times previously. [multi- + L. *gravida,* pregnant]

mul•ti•in•fec•tion (mŭl′tē-in-fek′shŭn). Mixed infection with two or more varieties of microorganisms developing simultaneously.

mul•ti•lo•bar, mul•ti•lo•bate, mul•ti•lobed (mŭl-tē-lō′bar, -lō′bāt, -lōbd′). Having several lobes.

mul•ti•lob•u•lar (mŭl-tē-lob′yū-lăr). Having many lobules.

mul•ti•lo•cal (mŭl-tē-lō′kăl). Denoting traits with an etiology comprising effects of multiple genetic loci operating together and simultaneously.

mul•ti•loc•u•lar (mŭl-tē-lok′yū-lăr). Many-celled; having many compartments or loculi.

mul•ti•nod•u•lar, mul•ti•nod•u•late (mŭl-tē-nod′yū-lăr, -yū-lāt). Having many nodules.

mul•ti•nu•cle•ar, mul•ti•nu•cle•ate (mŭl-tē-nū′klē-ăr, -āt). Having two or more nuclei. SYN polynuclear, polynucleate.

mul•tip•a•ra (mŭl-tip′ă-ră). A woman who has given birth at least two times to an infant, live-born or not, weighing 500 g or more, or having an estimated length of gestation of at least 20 weeks. [multi- + L. *pario,* to bring forth, to bear]

mul•ti•par•i•ty (mŭl-tē-păr′i-tē). Condition of being a multipara.

mul•tip•a•rous (mŭl-tip′ă-rŭs). Relating to a multipara.

mul•ti•po•lar (mŭl-tē-pō′lăr). Having more than two poles; denoting a nerve cell in which the branches project from several points.

mul•ti•sy•nap•tic (mŭl′tē-si-nap′tik). SYN polysynaptic.

mul•ti•va•lence, mul•ti•va•len•cy (mŭl-tē-vā′lens, -vā′len-sē). The state of being multivalent.

mul•ti•va•lent (mŭl-tē-vā′lent). **1.** CHEMISTRY Having a combining power (valence) of more than one hydrogen atom. **2.** Efficacious in more than one direction. **3.** An antisera specific for more than one antigen or organism. SYN polyvalent (1).

mum•mi•fi•ca•tion (mŭm′i-fi-kā′shŭn). **1.** SYN

mu

dry *gangrene.* **2.** Shrivelling of a dead, retained fetus. **3.** DENTISTRY Treatment of inflamed dental pulp with fixative drugs (usually formaldehyde derivatives) in order to retain teeth so treated for relatively short periods; generally acceptable only for primary (deciduous) teeth. [mummy + L. *facio,* to make]

mumps (mŭmps). SYN epidemic *parotiditis.* [dialectic Eng. *mump,* a lump or bump]

mu•ral (myū′răl). Relating to the wall of any cavity. [L. *muralis;* fr. *murus,* wall]

mu•ram•i•dase (myū-ram′i-dās). SYN lysozyme.

mu•rine (myū′rīn, -rin, -rēn). Relating to animals of the family Muridae. [L. *murinus,* relating to mice, fr. *mus* (*mur-*), a mouse]

mur•mur (mer′mer). An abnormal, usually periodic sound heard on auscultation of the heart or blood vessels. [L.]

anemic m., a nonvalvular m. heard on auscultation of the heart and large blood vessels in cases of profound anemia associated mainly with turbulent blood flow due to decreased blood viscosity.

aortic m., a m. produced at the aortic orifice, either obstructive or regurgitant.

Austin Flint m., SYN Austin Flint *phenomenon,* Flint′s m.

cardiac m., a m. produced within the heart, at one of its valvular orifices or across ventricular septal defects.

cardiopulmonary m., an innocent extracardiac m., synchronous with the heart's beat but disappearing when the breath is held, believed due to movement of air in a segment of lung compressed by the contracting heart.

Carey Coombs m., a blubbering apical middiastolic m. occurring in the acute stage of rheumatic mitral valvulitis and disappearing as the valvulitis subsides.

continuous m., a m. that is heard without interruption throughout systole and into diastole.

crescendo m., a m. that increases in intensity and suddenly ceases; the presystolic m. of mitral stenosis is a common example.

Cruveilhier-Baumgarten m., a venous m. heard over collateral veins, connecting portal and caval venous systems, on the abdominal wall. SEE ALSO Cruveilhier-Baumgarten *sign.*

diastolic m. (DM), a m. heard during diastole.

ejection m., a diamond-shaped systolic m. produced by the ejection of blood into the aorta or pulmonary artery and ending by the time of the second heart sound component produced, respectively, by closing of the aortic or pulmonic valve.

Flint's m., a diastolic m., similar to that of mitral stenosis, heard best at the cardiac apex in some cases of free aortic insufficiency. SYN Austin Flint m.

functional m., a cardiac m. not associated with a significant heart lesion. SYN innocent m.

Gibson m., the typical continuous "machinery-like" m. of patent ductus arteriosus.

Graham Steell's m., an early diastolic m. of pulmonic insufficiency secondary to pulmonary hypertension, as in mitral stenosis and various congenital defects associated with pulmonary hypertension.

Hamman's m., a crunching precordial sound synchronous with the heart beat; heard in mediastinal emphysema.

hemic m., a cardiac or vascular m. heard in anemic persons who have no valvular lesion, probably due to the increased blood velocity and turbulence that characterizes anemia.

hourglass m., one in which there are two areas of maximum loudness decreasing to a point midway between the two.

innocent m., SYN functional m.

machinery m., the long "continuous" rumbling m. of patent ductus arteriosus.

mitral m., a m. produced at the mitral valve, either obstructive or regurgitant.

obstructive m., a m. caused by narrowing of one of the valvular orifices.

organic m., a m. caused by an organic lesion.

pansystolic m., a m. occupying the entire systolic interval, from first to second heart sounds.

pericardial m., a friction sound, synchronous with the heart movements, heard in certain cases of pericarditis.

presystolic m., a m. heard at the end of ventricular diastole (during atrial systole if in sinus rhythm), usually due to obstruction at one of the atrioventricular orifices.

pulmonary m., pulmonic m., a m. produced at the pulmonary orifice of the heart, either obstructive or regurgitant.

regurgitant m., a m. due to leakage or backward flow at one of the valvular orifices of the heart.

Roger's m., a loud pansystolic m. maximal at the left sternal border, caused by a small ventricular septal defect.

sea gull m., a m. imitating the cooing sound of a seagull; nearly always due to aortic stenosis or mitral regurgitation.

stenosal m., an arterial m. due to narrowing of the vessel from pressure or organic change.

Still's m., an innocent musical m. resembling the noise produced by a twanging string; almost exclusively in young children, of uncertain origin and ultimately disappearing.

systolic m., a m. heard during ventricular systole.

tricuspid m., a m. produced at the tricuspid orifice, either obstructive or regurgitant.

vesicular m., SYN vesicular *respiration.*

Mus•ca (mŭs′kă). A genus of flies that includes the common housefly, *M. domestica;* it breeds in filth and organic waste, and is involved in the mechanical transfer of numerous pathogens. [L. fly]

mus•cae vol•i•tan•tes (mŭs′sē, mŭs′kē vol-i-tan′tēs). Floaters; appearance of moving spots before the eyes, arising from remnants of the embryologic hyaloid vascular system in the vitreous humor. [L. pl. of *musca,* fly; pres. ppl. of *volito,* to fly to and fro]

mus•ca•rine (mŭs′kă-rēn, -rin). A toxin with neurologic effects, first isolated from *Amanita muscaria* (fly agaric) and also present in some species of *Hebeloma* and *Inocybe.* It is a cholinergic substance whose pharmacologic effects include cardiac inhibition, vasodilation, salivation, lacrimation, bronchoconstriction, and gastrointestinal stimulation.

mus·ca·rin·ic (mŭs-kă-rin'ik). **1.** Having a muscarine-like action, *i.e.*, producing effects that resemble postganglionic parasympathetic stimulation. **2.** An agent that stimulates the postganglionic parasympathetic receptor. SEE ALSO muscarine, nicotinic.

mus·cle (mŭs'ĕl). **1.** A primary tissue, consisting predominantly of highly specialized contractile cells, which may be classified as skeletal m., cardiac m., or smooth m.; microscopically, the latter is lacking in transverse striations characteristic of the other two types. For gross anatomical description, see musculus. **2.** One of the contractile organs of the body by which movements of the various organs and parts are effected; typical m. is a mass of m. fibers (venter or belly), attached at each extremity, by means of a tendon, to a bone or other structure; the more proximal or more fixed attachment is called the *origin*, the more distal or more movable attachment is the *insertion*. SYN musculus [NA]. [L. *musculus*]

abductor digiti minimi m. of foot, *origin*, lateral and medial processes of calcaneal tuberosity; *insertion*, lateral side of proximal phalanx of fifth toe; *action*, abducts and flexes little toe; *nerve supply*, lateral plantar nerve.

abductor digiti minimi m. of hand, *origin*, pisiform bone and pisohamate ligament; *insertion*, medial side of base of proximal phalanx of the little finger; *action*, abducts and flexes little finger; *nerve supply*, ulnar.

abductor hallucis m., *origin*, medial process of calcaneal tuberosity, flexor retinaculum, and plantar aponeurosis; *insertion*, medial side of proximal phalanx of great toe; *action*, abducts great toe; *nerve supply*, medial plantar. SYN musculus abductor hallucis [NA].

adductor brevis m., *origin*, superior ramus of pubis; *insertion*, upper third of medial lip of linea aspera; *action*, adducts thigh; *nerve supply*, obturator. SYN musculus adductor brevis [NA], short adductor m.

adductor hallucis m., *origin*, by two heads, the transverse head from the capsules of the lateral four metatarsophalangeal joints and the oblique head from the lateral cuneiform and bases of the third and fourth metatarsal bones; *insertion*, lateral side of base of proximal phalanx of great toe; *action*, adducts great toe; *nerve supply*, lateral plantar. SYN musculus adductor hallucis [NA].

adductor longus m., *origin*, symphysis and crest of pubis; *insertion*, middle third of medial lip of linea aspera; *action*, adducts thigh; *nerve supply*, obturator. SYN musculus adductor longus [NA], long adductor m.

adductor magnus m., *origin*, ischial tuberosity and ischiopubic ramus; *insertion*, linea aspera and adductor tubercle of femur; *action*, adducts and extends thigh; *nerve supply*, obturator and sciatic. SYN musculus adductor magnus [NA], great adductor m.

adductor pollicis m., *origin*, by two heads, the transverse head from the shaft of the third metacarpal and the oblique head from the front of the base of the second metacarpal, the trapezoid and capitate bones; *insertion*, medial side of base of proximal phalanx of thumb; *action*, adducts thumb; *nerve supply*, ulnar. SYN musculus adductor pollicis [NA].

anconeus m., *origin*, back of lateral condyle of humerus; *insertion*, olecranon process and posterior surface of ulna; *action*, extends forearm and abducts ulna in pronation of wrist; *nerve supply*, radial. SYN musculus anconeus [NA].

antagonistic m.'s, those having opposite functions, the contraction of one tending to "neutralize" that of the other.

anterior auricular m., *origin*, galea aponeurotica; *insertion*, cartilage of auricle; *action*, draws pinna of ear upward and forward; *nerve supply*, facial. Considered by some to be the anterior part of the temporoparietal m. SYN musculus attrahens aurem, musculus attrahens auriculam.

antitragicus m., a band of transverse muscular fibers on the outer surface of the antitragus, arising from the border of the intertragic notch and inserted into the anthelix and cauda helicis. SYN musculus antitragicus [NA].

appendicular m., one of the skeletal m.'s of the limbs.

articular m., a m. that inserts directly onto the capsule of a joint, acting to retract the capsule in certain movements.

arrector pili m.'s, bundles of smooth m. fibers, attached to the deep part of the hair follicles, passing outward alongside the sebaceous glands to the papillary layer of the corium; they act to pull the hairs erect, causing "goose bumps" or "goose flesh" (cutis anserina). SYN musculi arrectores pilorum [NA], erector m.'s of hairs.

articularis cubiti m., the name applied to a small slip of the medial head of the triceps that inserts into the capsule of the elbow joint. SYN musculus articularis cubiti [NA].

articularis genu m., *origin*, lower fourth of anterior surface of shaft of femur; *insertion*, suprapatellar bursa of knee joint; *action*, retracts suprapatellar bursa, during extension of knee; *nerve supply*, femoral. SYN musculus articularis genus [NA].

aryepiglottic m., the fibers of the oblique arytenoid m. that extend from the summit of the arytenoid cartilage to the side of the epiglottis; *action*, constricts the laryngeal aperture. SYN musculus aryepiglotticus [NA].

m.'s of auditory ossicles, the m. stapedius and m. tensor tympani.

axial m., one of the skeletal m.'s of the trunk or head.

Bell's m., a band of muscular fibers, forming a slight fold in the wall of the bladder, running from the uvula to the opening of the ureter on either side, bounding the trigonum.

biceps brachii m., *origin*, long head from supraglenoidal tuberosity of scapula, short head from coracoid process; *insertion*, tuberosity of radius; *action*, flexes and supinates forearm (it is the primary supinator of the forearm); *nerve supply*, musculocutaneous. SYN musculus biceps brachii [NA].

biceps femoris m., *origin*, long head (caput

mu

longum) from tuberosity of ischium, short head (caput breve) from lower half of lateral lip of linea aspera; *insertion*, head of fibula; *action*, flexes knee and rotates leg laterally; *nerve supply*, long head, tibial, short head, peroneal. SYN musculus biceps femoris [NA].

brachialis m., *origin*, lower two-thirds of anterior surface of humerus; *insertion*, coronoid process of ulna; *action*, flexes elbow; *nerve supply*, musculocutaneous, usually with a minor contribution from the radial. SYN musculus brachialis [NA].

brachioradialis m., *origin*, lateral supracondylar ridge of humerus; *insertion*, front of base of styloid process of radius; *action*, flexes elbow and assists slightly in supination; *nerve supply*, (common) radial. SYN musculus brachioradialis [NA].

bronchoesophageal m., muscular fascicles, arising from the wall of the left bronchus, which reinforce the musculature of the esophagus. SYN musculus bronchoesophageus [NA].

buccinator m., *origin*, posterior portion of alveolar portion of maxilla and mandible and pterygomandibular raphe; *insertion*, orbicularis oris at angle of mouth; *action*, flattens cheek, retracts angle of mouth; *nerve supply*, facial. Plays an important role in mastication, working with tongue to keep food between teeth; when it is paralyzed, food accumulates in the oral vestibule. SYN musculus buccinator [NA].

bulbocavernosus m., in the male: *origin*, the perineal membrane fascia on the dorsum of the bulb of the penis; *insertion*, central tendon of the perineum and the median raphe on the free surface of the bulb; *action*, constricts bulbous urethra when attempting to expel last drops following urination, or spasmodically with ejaculation to expel semen. In the female: *origin*, the dorsum of the clitoris, the corpus cavernosum, and the perineal membrane; *insertion*, central tendon of the perineum; *action*, acts as a weak sphincter of the vagina; when developed, is a part of "cross-member musculature" of pelvic floor which resists prolapse of pelvic viscera. *Nerve supply*, pudendal (deep perineal branch). SYN musculus bulbospongiosus [NA].

cardiac m., the m. comprising the myocardium, consisting of anastomosing transversely striated m. fibers formed of cells united at intercalated disks. SYN m. of heart.

ceratocricoid m., a fasciculus from the posterior cricoarytenoid m. inserted into the inferior horn of the thyroid cartilage. SYN musculus ceratocricoideus [NA].

ciliary m., the smooth m. of the ciliary body; it consists of circular fibers (Müller's m.) and radiating fibers (meridional fibers, or Brücke's m.); *action*, in contracting, its diameter is reduced (like a sphincter), reducing tensile (stretching) forces on lens, allowing it to thicken for near vision (accommodation). SYN musculus ciliaris [NA].

coccygeus m., *origin*, spine of ischium and sacrospinous ligament; *insertion*, sides of lower part of sacrum and upper part of coccyx; *action*, assists in support of pelvic floor, especially when

intra-abdominal pressures increase; *nerve supply*, third and fourth sacral. SYN musculus coccygeus [NA].

coracobrachialis m., *origin*, coracoid process of scapula; *insertion*, middle of medial border of humerus; *action*, adducts and flexes the arm; resists downward dislocation of shoulder joint; *nerve supply*, musculocutaneous. SYN musculus coracobrachialis [NA].

corrugator supercilii m., *origin*, from orbital portion of m. orbicularis oculi and nasal prominence; *insertion*, skin of eyebrow; *action*, draws medial end of eyebrow downward and wrinkles forehead vertically; *nerve supply*, facial. SYN musculus corrugator supercilii [NA].

cremaster m., *origin*, from internal oblique m. and inguinal ligament; *insertion*, cremasteric fascia (spermatic cord); *action*, raises testicle; *nerve supply*, genital branch of genitofemoral; in the male the muscle envelops the spermatic cord and testis; in the female, the round ligament of the uterus. SYN musculus cremaster [NA].

cricothyroid m., *origin*, anterior surface of arch of cricoid; *insertion*, the anterior or straight part passes upward to ala of thyroid; the posterior or oblique part passes more outward to inferior horn of thyroid; *action*, makes vocal folds tense, increasing the pitch of voice tone; *nerve supply*, external laryngeal branch of superior laryngeal nerve (from vagus). SYN musculus cricothyroideus [NA].

cruciate m., a general type of m. in which the m.'s or bundles of m. fibers cross in an X-shaped configuration; *e.g.*, the oblique arytenoid m.'s.

cutaneous m., a m. that lies in the subcutaneous tissue and attaches to the skin; it may or may not have a bony attachment. The m.'s of expression are the chief examples of cutaneous m.'s in the human.

deep transverse perineal m., *origin*, ramus of ischium; *insertion*, with its fellow in a median raphe; *action*, assists sphincter urethrae with some sphincteric action on vagina in female; *nerve supply*, pudendal (dorsal nerve of penis/clitoris). SYN musculus transversus perinei profundus [NA].

deltoid m., *origin*, lateral third of clavicle, lateral border of acromion process, lower border of spine of scapula; *insertion*, lateral side of shaft of humerus a little above its middle (deltoid tuberosity); *action*, abduction, flexion, extension, and rotation of arm; *nerve supply*, axillary from fifth and sixth cervical spinal cord segments through brachial plexus. SYN musculus deltoideus [NA], deltoid (2).

depressor anguli oris m., *origin*, lower border of mandible anteriorly; *insertion*, blends with other m.'s in lower lip near angle of mouth; *action*, pulls down corners of mouth; *nerve supply*, facial. SYN musculus depressor anguli oris [NA], triangular m. (2).

depressor labii inferioris m., *origin*, anterior portion of lower border of mandible; *insertion*, orbicularis oris m. and skin of lower lip; *action*, depresses lower lip; *nerve supply*, facial. SYN musculus depressor labii inferioris [NA].

depressor septi m., a vertical fasciculus from

the orbicularis oris m. passing upward along the median line of the upper lip, and inserted into the cartilaginous septum of the nose; *action*, depresses septum; *nerve supply*, facial. SYN musculus depressor septi [NA].

depressor supercilii m., fibers of the orbital part of the orbicularis oculi m. insert in the eyebrow; *action*, depresses eyebrow; *nerve supply*, facial. SYN musculus depressor supercilii [NA].

digastric m., (1) one of the suprahyoid group of m.'s consisting of two bellies united by a central tendon which is connected to the body of the hyoid bone; *origin*, by posterior belly from the digastric groove medial to the mastoid process; *insertion*, by anterior belly into lower border of mandible near midline; *action*, elevates the hyoid when mandible is fixed; depresses the mandible when hyoid is fixed; *nerve supply*, posterior belly from facial, anterior belly by nerve to the mylohyoid from the mandibular division of trigeminal; **(2)** a m. with two fleshy bellies separated by a fibrous insertion; SYN musculus digastricus [NA].

dilator m., a m. which opens an orifice or dilates the lumen of an organ; it is the dilating or opening component of a pylorus (the other component is the sphincter m.).

dilator pupillae m., the radial muscular fibers extending from the sphincter pupillae to the ciliary margin; some anatomists regard them as elastic, not muscular, in humans. SYN musculus dilator pupillae [NA].

elevator m. of scapula, SYN levator scapulae m.

elevator m. of soft palate, SYN levator veli palatini m.

elevator m. of upper eyelid, SYN levator palpebrae superioris m.

epicranius m., composed of the epicranial aponeurosis and the m.'s inserting into it, *i.e.,* the occipitofrontalis m. and temporoparietalis m. SYN musculus epicranius [NA].

erector m.'s of hairs, SYN arrector pili m.'s.

erector m. of spine, SYN erector spinae m.'s.

erector spinae m.'s, *origin*, from sacrum, ilium, and spines of lumbar vertebrae; it divides into three columns, iliocostalis m., longissimus m., and spinalis m., which insert into ribs and vertebrae with additional muscle slips joining the columns at successively higher levels; *action*, extends vertebral column; *nerve supply*, dorsal primary rami of spinal nerves. SYN musculus erector spinae [NA], erector m. of spine.

extensor carpi radialis brevis m., *origin*, lateral epicondyle of humerus; *insertion*, base of third metacarpal bone; *action*, extends and abducts wrist radialward; *nerve supply*, radial. SYN short radial extensor m. of wrist.

extensor carpi radialis longus m., *origin*, lateral supracondylar ridge of humerus; *insertion*, back of base of second metacarpal bone; *action*, extends and deviates wrist radialward; *nerve supply*, radial. SYN long radial extensor m. of wrist.

extensor carpi ulnaris m., *origin*, lateral epicondyle of humerus (humeral head) and oblique line and posterior border of ulna (ulnar head); *insertion*, base of fifth metacarpal bone; *action*, extends and abducts wrist ulnarward; *nerve sup-*ply, radial (posterior interosseous). SYN musculus extensor carpi ulnaris [NA], ulnar extensor m. of wrist.

extensor digiti minimi m., *origin*, lateral epicondyle of humerus; *insertion*, dorsum of proximal, middle, and distal phalanges of little finger; *action*, extends fingers; *nerve supply*, radial (posterior interosseous). SYN musculus extensor digiti minimi [NA], extensor m. of little finger.

extensor digitorum brevis m., *origin*, dorsal surface of calcaneus; *insertion*, by four tendons fusing with those of the extensor digitorum longus, and by a slip attached independently to the base of the proximal phalanx of the great toe; *action*, extends toes; *nerve supply*, deep peroneal. SYN musculus extensor digitorum brevis [NA], short extensor m. of toes.

extensor digitorum longus m., *origin*, lateral condyle of tibia, upper two-thirds of anterior margin of fibula; *insertion*, by four tendons to the dorsal surfaces of the bases of the proximal, middle, and distal phalanges of the second to fifth toes; *action*, extends the four lateral toes; *nerve supply*, deep branch of peroneal. SYN musculus extensor digitorum longus [NA], long extensor m. of toes.

extensor digitorum m., *origin*, lateral epicondyle of humerus; *insertion*, by four tendons into the base of the proximal and middle and base of the distal phalanges; *action*, extends fingers; *nerve supply*, radial (posterior interosseous). SYN musculus extensor digitorum [NA], extensor m. of fingers.

extensor hallucis brevis m., the medial belly of extensor digitorum brevis m., the tendon of which is inserted into the base of the proximal phalanx of the great toe. SYN musculus extensor hallucis brevis [NA], short extensor m. of great toe.

extensor hallucis longus m., *origin*, lateral surface of tibia and interosseous membrane; *insertion*, base of distal phalanx of great toe; *action*, extends the great toe; *nerve supply*, anterior tibial. SYN musculus extensor hallucis longus [NA].

extensor indicis m., *origin*, dorsal surface of ulna; *insertion*, dorsal extensor aponeurosis of index finger; *action*, assists in extending the forefinger; *nerve supply*, radial. SYN musculus extensor indicis [NA], index extensor m.

extensor m. of fingers, SYN extensor digitorum m.

extensor m. of little finger, SYN extensor digiti minimi m.

external oblique m., *origin*, fifth to twelfth ribs; *insertion*, anterior half of lateral lip of iliac crest, inguinal ligament, and anterior layer of the rectus sheath; *action*, diminishes capacity of abdomen, draws thorax downward; *nerve supply*, thoracoabdominal nerves. SYN musculus obliquus externus abdominis [NA].

external obturator m., SYN obturator externus m.

extraocular m.'s, the m.'s within the orbit including the four rectus muscles (superior, inferior, medial and lateral); two oblique muscles (su-

mu

perior and inferior), and the levator of the superior eyelid (levator palpebrae superioris).

■ **m. fiber,** classification of m. fiber based on contractile and metabolic characteristics. Slow-twitch (type I) fibers contract slowly and develop low tension; they display high oxidative and low glycolytic capacity associated with endurance performance. Fast-twitch (type II) fibers have rapid speed of activation and develop high tension; they display low oxidative and high glycolytic capacity associated with strength and power performance.

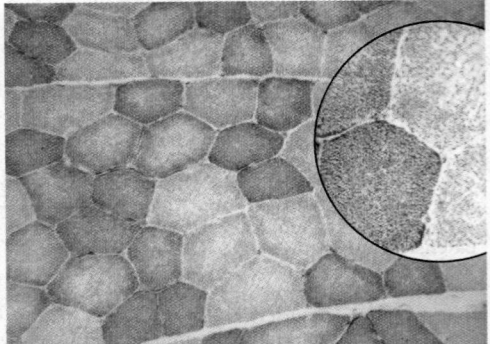

muscle fiber: cross-section of muscle fibers demonstrating two fiber types with the NADH-TR; the deeply stained, smaller muscle fibers are slow-twitch, Type I fibers; the lighter are fast-twitch, Type II fibers

fixator m., a m. that acts as a stabilizer of one part of the body during movement of another part.

flexor carpi radialis m., *origin*, common flexor origin of the medial condyle of humerus; *insertion*, anterior surface of the base of the second and most often sending a slip to that of the third metacarpal bone; *action*, flexes and abducts wrist radialward; *nerve supply*, median; its tendon travels in its own canal roofed by a layer of the transverse carpal ligament. SYN musculus flexor carpi radialis [NA], radial flexor m. of wrist.

flexor carpi ulnaris m., *origin*, humeral head from medial condyle of humerus, ulnar head from olecranon and upper three-fifths of posterior border of ulna; *insertion*, pisiform bone, but is continued to the fifth metacarpal bone via the pisometacarpal ligament; *action*, flexes and abducts wrist ulnarward; *nerve supply*, ulnar. SYN musculus flexor carpi ulnaris [NA], ulnar flexor m. of wrist.

flexor digiti minimi brevis m. of foot, *origin*, base of metatarsal bone of the little toe and sheath of m. peroneus longus; *insertion*, lateral surface of base of proximal phalanx of little toe; *action*, flexes the proximal phalanx of the little toe; *nerve supply*, lateral plantar. SYN musculus flexor digiti minimi brevis pedis [NA], short flexor m. of little toe.

flexor digiti minimi brevis m. of hand, *origin*, hamulus of hamate bone; *insertion*, medial side of proximal phalanx of little finger; *action*, flexes proximal phalanx of little finger; *nerve supply*, ulnar. SYN musculus flexor digiti minimi brevis manus [NA], short flexor m. of little finger.

flexor digitorum brevis m., *origin*, medial tubercle of calcaneus and central portion of plantar fascia; *insertion*, middle phalanges of four lateral toes by tendons perforated by those of the flexor longus; *action*, flexes lateral four toes; *nerve supply*, medial plantar. SYN musculus flexor digitorum brevis [NA], short flexor m. of toes.

flexor digitorum longus m., *origin*, middle third of posterior surface of tibia; *insertion*, by four tendons, perforating those of the flexor brevis, into bases of distal phalanges of four lateral toes; *action*, flexes second to fifth toes; *nerve supply*, tibial nerve. SYN musculus flexor digitorum longus [NA], long flexor m. of toes.

flexor digitorum profundus m., *origin*, anterior surface of upper third of ulna; *insertion*, by four tendons, piercing those of the superficialis, into base of distal phalanx of each finger; *action*, flexes distal interphalangeal joint of fingers; *nerve supply*, ulnar and median (anterior interosseous muscle). SYN musculus flexor digitorum profundus [NA].

flexor digitorum superficialis m., *origin*, humeroulnar head from the medial epicondyle of the humerus, the medial border of the coronoid process, and a tendinous arch between these points, radial head from the oblique line and middle third of the lateral border of the radius; *insertion*, by four split tendons, passing to either side of the profundus tendons, into sides of middle phalanx of each finger; *action*, flexes proximal interphalangeal joint of the fingers; *nerve supply*, median. SYN musculus flexor digitorum superficialis [NA], superficial flexor m. of fingers.

flexor hallucis brevis m., *origin*, medial surface of cuboid and middle and lateral cuneiform bones; *insertion*, by two tendons, embracing that of the flexor longus hallucis, into the sides of the base of the proximal phalanx of the great toe; *action*, flexes great toe; *nerve supply*, medial and lateral plantar. SYN short flexor m. of great toe.

flexor hallucis longus m., *origin*, lower two-thirds of posterior surface of fibula; *insertion*, base of distal phalanx of great toe; *action*, flexes great toe; *nerve supply*, medial plantar. SYN long flexor m. of great toe.

flexor pollicis brevis m., *origin*, superficial portion from flexor retinaculum of wrist, deep portion from ulnar side of first metacarpal bone; *insertion*, base of proximal phalanx of thumb; *action*, flexes proximal phalanx of thumb; *nerve supply*, median (superficial head) and deep branch of ulnar (deep head). Some authors consider the deep head to be the first in a series of four palmar interossei muscles of the hand. SYN short flexor m. of thumb.

flexor pollicis longus m., *origin*, anterior surface of middle third of radius; *insertion*, distal phalanx of thumb; *action*, flexes distal phalanx of thumb; *nerve supply*, median palmar interosseous. SYN long flexor m. of thumb.

gastrocnemius m., *origin,* by two heads (lateral and medial) from the lateral and medial condyles of the femur; *insertion,* with soleus by tendo calcaneus into lower half of posterior surface of calcaneus; *action,* plantar flexion of foot; *nerve supply,* tibial. SYN musculus gastrocnemius [NA], gastrocnemius.

Gavard's m., oblique fibers in the muscular coat of the stomach.

genioglossus m., one of the paired lingual m.'s; *origin,* mental spine of the mandible; *insertion,* lingual fascia beneath the mucous membrane and epiglottis; *action,* depresses and protrudes the tongue; *nerve supply,* hypoglossal. SYN musculus genioglossus [NA].

geniohyoid m., *origin,* mental spine of mandible; *insertion,* body of hyoid bone; *action,* draws hyoid forward, or depresses jaw when hyoid is fixed; *nerve supply,* fibers from ventral primary rami of first and second cervical spinal nerves accompanying hypoglossal. SYN musculus geniohyoideus [NA].

gluteus maximus m., *origin,* ilium behind posterior gluteal line, posterior surface of sacrum and coccyx, and sacrotuberous ligament; *insertion,* iliotibial band of fascia lata (superficial three-quarters) and gluteal ridge (deep inferior one-quarter) of femur; *action,* extends thigh, especially from the flexed position, as in climbing stairs or rising from a sitting position; *nerve supply,* inferior gluteal. SYN musculus gluteus maximus [NA].

gluteus medius m., *origin,* ilium between anterior and posterior gluteal lines; *insertion,* lateral surface of greater trochanter; *action,* abducts and rotates thigh; *nerve supply,* superior gluteal. SYN musculus gluteus medius [NA].

gluteus minimus m., *origin,* ilium between anterior and inferior gluteal lines; *insertion,* greater trochanter of femur; *action,* abducts thigh; *nerve supply,* superior gluteal. SYN musculus gluteus minimus [NA].

gracilis m., *origin,* ramus of pubis near symphysis; *insertion,* shaft of tibia below medial tuberosity (see *pes anserinus*); *action,* adducts thigh, flexes knee, rotates leg medially; *nerve supply,* obturator. SYN musculus gracilis [NA].

great adductor m., SYN adductor magnus m.

greater posterior rectus m. of head, SYN rectus capitis posterior major m.

hamstring m.'s, the m.'s at the back of the thigh, comprising the long head of biceps, the semitendinosus, and the semimembranosus m.

m.'s of head, the m.'s of expression, of mastication, and the suboccipital m.'s in general.

m. of heart, SYN cardiac m.

hyoglossal m., SYN hyoglossus m.

hyoglossus m., *origin,* body and greater horn of hyoid bone; *insertion,* side of the tongue; *action,* retracts and pulls down side of tongue; *nerve supply,* motor by hypoglossal, sensory by lingual. SYN musculus hyoglossus [NA], hyoglossal m.

iliac m., SYN iliacus m.

iliacus m., *origin,* iliac fossa; *insertion,* tendon of psoas, anterior surface of lesser trochanter, and capsule of hip joint; *action,* flexes thigh and rotates it medially; *nerve supply,* lumbar plexus. SYN musculus iliacus [NA], iliac m.

iliococcygeal m., SYN iliococcygeus m.

iliococcygeus m., the posterior part of the levator ani arising from the tendinous arch of the levator ani muscle and inserting on the anococcygeal ligament and coccyx. SYN musculus iliococcygeus [NA], iliococcygeal m.

iliocostal m., SYN iliocostalis m.

iliocostalis cervicis m., *origin,* angles of upper six ribs; *insertion,* transverse processes of middle cervical vertebrae; *action,* extends, abducts, and rotates cervical vertebrae; *nerve supply,* dorsal branches of upper thoracic nerves.

iliocostalis lumborum m., *origin,* with erector spinae; *insertion,* the angles of lower six ribs; *action,* extends, abducts, and rotates lumbar vertebrae; *nerve supply,* dorsal branches of thoracic and lumbar nerves. SYN lumbar iliocostal m.

iliocostalis m., the lateral division of the erector spinae, having three subdivisions: iliocostalis lumborum m., iliocostalis thoracis m., and iliocostalis cervicis m. SYN musculus iliocostalis [NA], iliocostal m.

iliopsoas m., a compound muscle, consisting of the iliacus m. and psoas major m. SYN musculus iliopsoas [NA].

index extensor m., SYN extensor indicis m.

inferior constrictor m. of pharynx, *origin,* outer surfaces of thyroid (thyropharyngeal part) and cricoid (cricopharyngeal part, musculus cricopharyngeus; superior or upper esophageal sphincter m.) cartilages; *insertion,* pharyngeal raphe in the posterior portion of wall of pharynx; *action,* narrows lower part of pharynx in swallowing, the cricopharyngeal part has a sphincteric function for the esophagus, allowing some voluntary control of eructation and reflux; *nerve supply,* pharyngeal plexus.

inferior gemellus m., *origin,* tuberosity of ischium; *insertion,* tendon of m. obturator internus; *action,* rotates thigh laterally; *nerve supply,* sacral plexus.

inferior oblique m., *origin,* orbital plate of maxilla lateral to the lacrimal groove; *insertion,* sclera between the superior and lateral recti; *action,* primary, extorsion; secondary, elevation and abduction; *nerve supply,* oculomotor (inferior branch). SYN musculus obliquus inferior [NA].

inferior rectus m., *origin,* inferior part of the common tendinous ring; *insertion,* inferior part of sclera of the eye; *action,* primary, depression; secondary, adduction and extorsion; *nerve supply,* oculomotor (inferior branch). SYN musculus rectus inferior [NA].

infraspinatus m., *origin,* infraspinous fossa of scapula; *insertion,* middle facet of greater tubercle of humerus; *action,* extends arm and rotates it laterally; *nerve supply,* suprascapular (from fifth to sixth cervical spinal nerves). SYN musculus infraspinatus [NA].

intermediate vastus m., SYN vastus intermedius m.

internal intercostal m., each arises from lower border of rib and passes obliquely downward and backward to be inserted into upper border of rib below; *action,* contract during expira-

mu

tion, also maintain tension in the intercostal spaces to resist mediolateral movement; *nerve supply*, intercostal.

internal oblique m., *origin*, iliac fascia deep to lateral part of inguinal ligament, anterior half of crest of ilium, and lumbar fascia; *insertion*, tenth to twelfth ribs and sheath of rectus; some of the fibers from inguinal ligament terminate in the conjoint tendon; *action*, diminishes capacity of abdomen, flexes lumbar vertebral column (bends thorax forward); *nerve supply*, lower thoracic. SYN musculus obliquus internus abdominis [NA].

internal obturator m., SYN obturator internus m.

interspinal m.'s, SYN interspinales m.'s.

interspinales m.'s, the paired m.'s between spinous processes of adjacent vertebrae; subdivided into cervical, thoracic, and lumbar m.'s. SYN musculi interspinales [NA], interspinal m.'s.

intertransverse m.'s, SYN intertransversarii m.'s.

intertransversarii m.'s, the paired m.'s between transverse processes of adjacent vertebrae; there are anterior and posterior m.'s in the cervical region; lateral and medial m.'s in the lumbar region; and single m.'s in the thoracic region. SYN musculi intertransversarii [NA], intertransverse m.'s.

involuntary m.'s, m.'s not ordinarily under control of the will; except in the case of the heart, they are smooth (nonstriated) m.'s, innervated by the autonomic nervous system.

ischiocavernous m., *origin*, ramus of ischium; *insertion*, corpus cavernosum penis (or clitoridis); *action*, compresses the crus of the penis (or clitoris) forcing blood in its sinuses into the distal part of the corpus cavernosum; *nerve supply*, perineal. SYN musculus ischiocavernosus [NA].

Kohlrausch's m., the longitudinal m.'s of the rectal wall.

m.'s of larynx, the intrinsic m.'s that regulate the length, position and tension of the vocal cords and adjust the size of the openings between the aryepiglottic folds, the ventricular folds, and the vocal folds. SYN musculi laryngis [NA].

lateral rectus m., *origin*, lateral part of the common tendinous ring that bridges superior orbital fissure; *insertion*, lateral part of sclera of eye; *action*, abduction; *nerve supply*, abducens. SYN musculus rectus lateralis [NA], abducens oculi.

lateral rectus m. of the head, SYN rectus capitis lateralis m.

lateral vastus m., SYN vastus lateralis m.

latissimus dorsi m., *origin*, spinous processes of lower five or six thoracic and the lumbar vertebrae, median ridge of sacrum, and outer lip of iliac crest; *insertion*, with teres major into posterior lip of bicipital groove of humerus; *action*, adducts arm, rotates it medially, and extends it; *nerve supply*, thoracodorsal. SYN musculus latissimus dorsi [NA].

levator anguli oris m., *origin*, canine fossa of maxilla; *insertion*, orbicularis oris and skin at angle of mouth; *action*, raises angle of mouth; *nerve supply*, facial. SYN musculus levator anguli oris [NA].

levator ani m., formed by pubococcygeus and iliococcygeus m.'s; *origin*, posterior body of pubis, tendinous arch of the levator ani, and spine of ischium; *insertion*, anococcygeal ligament, sides of the lower part of the sacrum and of coccyx; *action*, resists prolapsing forces and draws the anus upward following defecation; supports the pelvic viscera; *nerve supply*, nerve to levator ani (fourth sacral spinal nerve). SYN musculus levator ani [NA].

levator labii superioris alaeque nasi m., *origin*, root of nasal process of maxilla; *insertion*, wing of nose and orbicularis oris m. of upper lip; *action*, elevates upper lip and wing of nose; *nerve supply*, facial. SYN musculus levator labii superioris alaeque nasi [NA].

levator labii superioris m., *origin*, maxilla below infraorbital foramen; *insertion*, orbicularis oris of upper lip; *action*, elevates upper lip; *nerve supply*, facial. SYN musculus levator labii superioris [NA].

levator m. of thyroid gland, a fasciculus occasionally passing from the thyrohyoid m. to the isthmus of the thyroid gland. SYN musculus levator glandulae thyroideae [NA].

levator palpebrae superioris m., *origin*, orbital surface of the lesser wing of the sphenoid, above and anterior to the optic canal; *insertion*, skin of eyelid, tarsal plate, and orbital walls, by medial and lateral expansions of the aponeurosis of insertion; *action*, raises the upper eyelid; *nerve supply*, oculomotor. SYN musculus levator palpebrae superioris [NA], elevator m. of upper eyelid.

levator prostatae m., in the male, the most medial fibers of the levator ani (pubococcygeus) m. that extend from the pubis into the fascia of the prostate. SYN musculus levator prostatae [NA].

levator scapulae m., *origin*, from posterior tubercles of transverse processes of four upper cervical vertebrae; *insertion*, into superior angle of scapula; *action*, raises the scapula; *nerve supply*, dorsal scapular nerve. SYN musculus levator scapulae [NA], elevator m. of scapula.

levator veli palatini m., *origin*, apex of petrous portion of temporal bone and lower part of cartilaginous auditory (eustachian) tube; *insertion*, aponeurosis of soft palate; *action*, raises soft palate; through the expansion of its fleshy belly during contraction, it helps to "push" open the auditory tube; *nerve supply*, pharyngeal plexus (cranial root of accessory nerve). SYN musculus levator veli palatini [NA], elevator m. of soft palate.

long adductor m., SYN adductor longus m.

long extensor m. of toes, SYN extensor digitorum longus m.

long flexor m. of great toe, SYN flexor hallucis longus m.

long flexor m. of thumb, SYN flexor pollicis longus m.

long flexor m. of toes, SYN flexor digitorum longus m.

long m. of head, SYN longus capitis m.

longissimus capitis m., *origin*, from transverse processes of upper thoracic and transverse and articular processes of lower and middle cervical vertebrae; *insertion*, into mastoid process; *action*, keeps head erect, draws it backward or to one side; *nerve supply*, dorsal primary rami of cervical spinal nerves. SYN musculus longissimus capitis [NA].

longissimus cervicis m., *origin*, transverse processes of upper thoracic vertebrae; *insertion*, transverse processes of middle and upper cervical vertebrae; *action*, extends cervical vertebrae; *nerve supply*, dorsal primary rami of lower cervical and upper thoracic spinal nerves. SYN musculus longissimus cervicis [NA], musculus transversalis cervicis, musculus transversalis colli.

longissimus thoracis m., *origin*, with iliocostalis and from transverse processes of lower thoracic vertebrae; *insertion*, by lateral slips into most or all of the ribs between angles and tubercles and into tips of transverse processes of upper lumbar vertebrae, and by medial slips into accessory processes of upper lumbar and transverse processes of thoracic vertebrae; *action*, extends vertebral column; *nerve supply*, dorsal primary rami of thoracic and lumbar spinal nerves. SYN musculus longissimus thoracis [NA], thoracic longissimus m.

long levatores costarum m.'s, *insertion*, the second rib below their origin; *action*, raise ribs; *nerve supply*, intercostal.

long m. of neck, SYN longus colli m.

long radial extensor m. of wrist, SYN extensor carpi radialis longus m.

longus capitis m., *origin*, anterior tubercles of transverse processes of third to sixth cervical vertebrae; *insertion*, basilar process of occipital bone; *action*, twists or flexes neck anteriorly; *nerve supply*, cervical plexus. SYN musculus longus capitis [NA], long m. of head.

longus colli m., medial part: *origin*, the bodies of the third thoracic to the fifth cervical vertebrae; *insertion*, the bodies of the second to fourth cervical vertebrae; superolateral part: *origin*, the anterior tubercles of the transverse processes of the third to fifth cervical vertebrae; *insertion*, the anterior tubercle of the atlas; inferolateral part: *origin*, the bodies of the first to third thoracic vertebrae; *insertion*, the anterior tubercles of the transverse processes of the fifth and sixth cervical vertebrae; *action*, for all three parts, twist neck and flex neck anteriorly; *nerve supply*, for all three parts, ventral primary rami of cervical spinal nerves (cervical plexus). SYN musculus longus colli [NA], long m. of neck.

lumbar iliocostal m., SYN iliocostalis lumborum m.

lumbrical m.'s of foot, four intrinsic m.'s of the foot; *origin*, first: from tibial side of tendon to second toe of flexor digitorum longus; second, third, and fourth: from adjacent sides of all four tendons of this m.; *insertion*, tibial side of extensor tendon on dorsum of each of the four lateral toes; *action*, flex the proximal and extend the middle and distal phalanges; *nerve supply*, lateral (second to fourth lumbricals) and medial (first lumbrical) plantar. SYN musculus lumbricalis pedis [NA].

lumbrical m.'s of hand, four intrinsic muscles of the hand; *origin*, the two lateral: from the radial side of the tendons of the flexor digitorum profundus going to the index and middle fingers; the two medial: from the adjacent sides of the second and third, and third and fourth tendons; *insertion*, radial side of extensor tendon on dorsum of each of the four fingers; *action*, flexes metacarpophalangeal joint and extends the proximal and distal interphalangeal joint; *nerve supply*, the two radial m.'s by the median, the two ulnar m.'s by the ulnar. SYN musculus lumbricalis manus [NA].

Marcacci's m., a sheet of smooth m. fibers underlying the areola and nipple of the mammary gland.

masseter m., *origin*, superficial part: inferior border of the anterior two-thirds of the zygomatic arch; deep part: inferior border and medial surface of the zygomatic arch; *insertion*, lateral surface of ramus and coronoid process of the mandible; *action*, elevates mandible (closes jaw); *nerve supply*, masseteric branch of mandibular division of trigeminal. SYN musculus masseter [NA].

medial rectus m., *origin*, medial part of the anulus tendineus communis; *insertion*, medial part of sclera of the eye; *action*, adduction; *nerve supply*, oculomotor. SYN musculus rectus medialis [NA].

medial vastus m., SYN vastus medialis m.

mentalis m., *origin*, incisor fossa of mandible; *insertion*, skin of chin; *action*, raises and wrinkles skin of chin, thus elevating the lower lip; *nerve supply*, facial. SYN musculus mentalis [NA].

middle constrictor m. of pharynx, *origin*, stylohyoid ligament, lesser cornu of the hyoid bone (chondropharyngeal part) and greater cornu of the hyoid bone (ceratopharyngeal part); *insertion*, pharyngeal raphe in the posterior wall of the pharynx; *action*, narrows pharynx in the act of swallowing; *nerve supply*, pharyngeal plexus.

multifidus m., *origin*, from the sacrum, sacroiliac ligament, mamillary processes of the lumbar vertebrae, transverse processes of thoracic vertebrae, and articular processes of last four cervical vertebrae; *insertion*, into the spinous processes of all the vertebrae up to and including the axis; *action*, rotates vertebral column; *nerve supply*, dorsal primary rami of spinal nerves. SYN musculus multifidus [NA].

mylohyoid m., *origin*, mylohyoid line of mandible; *insertion*, upper border of hyoid bone and raphe separating m. from its fellow; *action*, elevates floor of mouth and the tongue, depresses jaw when hyoid is fixed; *nerve supply*, nerve to mylohyoid from mandibular division of trigeminal. SYN musculus mylohyoideus [NA].

nasal m., SYN nasalis m.

nasalis m., compound m. consisting of: a transverse part (pars transversa musculi nasalis [NA], musculus compressor naris) arising from the maxilla above the root of the canine tooth on each side and forming an aponeurosis across the bridge of the nose; and an alar part (pars alaris musculi nasalis [NA], musculus dilator naris) arising from the maxilla above the lateral incisor and attaching to the wing of the nose; the alar part dilates the nostril; *nerve supply*, facial. SYN musculus nasalis [NA], nasal m.

mu

obturator externus m., *origin,* lower half of margin of obturator foramen and adjacent part of external surface of obturator membrane; *insertion,* trochanteric fossa of greater trochanter; *action,* rotates thigh laterally; *nerve supply,* obturator. SYN musculus obturator externus [NA], external obturator m.

obturator internus m., *origin,* pelvic surface of obturator membrane and margin of obturator foramen; *insertion,* passes out of pelvis through lesser sciatic foramen, in so doing, making a 90° turn to insert into the medial surface of greater trochanter; *action,* rotates thigh laterally; *nerve supply,* nerve to obturator internus (sacral plexus). SYN musculus obturator internus [NA], internal obturator m.

occipitofrontal m., SYN occipitofrontalis m.

occipitofrontalis m., it is a part of m. epicranius; the occipital belly (occipitalis m.) arises from the occipital bone and inserts into the galea aponeurotica; the frontal belly (frontalis m.) arises from the galea and inserts into the skin of the eyebrow and nose; *action,* to move the scalp; *nerve supply,* facial. SYN musculus occipitofrontalis [NA], occipitofrontal m.

omohyoid m., formed of two bellies attached to intermediate tendon; *origin,* by inferior belly from upper border of scapula between superior angle and notch; *insertion,* by superior belly into hyoid bone; *action,* depresses hyoid; *nerve supply,* upper cervical spinal nerves through ansa cervicalis. SYN musculus omohyoideus [NA].

opponens digiti minimi m., *origin,* hamulus of the hamate bone and transverse carpal ligament; *insertion,* shaft of fifth metacarpal; *action,* "cups" palm, drawing ulnar side of hand toward center of palm; *nerve supply,* ulnar. SYN musculus opponens digiti minimi [NA].

opponens pollicis m., *origin,* ridge of trapezium and flexor retinaculum; *insertion,* anterior surface of the full length of the shaft of the first metacarpal bone; *action,* acts at carpometacarpal joint to "cup" palm, enabling one to oppose thumb to other fingers; *nerve supply,* median. SYN musculus opponens pollicis [NA].

orbicularis oculi m., consists of three portions: orbital part, or external portion, which arises from frontal process of maxilla and nasal process of frontal bone, encircles aperture of orbit, and is inserted near origin; palpebral part, or internal portion, which arises from medial palpebral ligament, passes through each eyelid, and is inserted into lateral palpebral raphe; lacrimal part (tensor tarsi muscle, Duverney's or Horner's muscle) arises from posterior lacrimal crest and passes across lacrimal sac to join palpebral portion; *action,* closes eye, wrinkles forehead vertically; *nerve supply,* facial. SYN musculus orbicularis oculi [NA].

orbicularis oris m., *origin,* by nasolabial band from septum of the nose, by superior incisive bundle from incisor fossa of maxilla, by inferior incisive bundle from lower jaw each side of symphysis; *insertion,* fibers surround mouth between skin and mucous membrane of lips and cheeks, and are blended with other m.'s; *action,* closes lips; *nerve supply,* facial. SYN musculus orbicularis oris [NA].

orbital m., SYN orbitalis m.

orbitalis m., a rudimentary nonstriated m., crossing the infraorbital groove and sphenomaxillary fissure, intimately united with the periosteum of the orbit. SYN musculus orbitalis [NA], orbital m.

palatoglossus m., forms anterior pillar of tonsillar fossa; *origin,* oral surface of soft palate; *insertion,* side of tongue; *action,* raises back of tongue and narrows fauces; *nerve supply,* pharyngeal plexus (cranial root of accessory nerve). SYN musculus palatoglossus [NA].

palatopharyngeal m., SYN palatopharyngeus m.

palatopharyngeus m., *origin,* soft palate; forms the posterior pillar of the fauces or tonsillar fossa; *insertion,* posterior border of thyroid cartilage and aponeurosis of pharynx; *action,* narrows fauces, depresses soft palate, elevates pharynx and larynx; *nerve supply,* pharyngeal plexus (cranial root of accessory nerve). SYN musculus palatopharyngeus [NA], palatopharyngeal m.

palmar interosseous m., three m.'s in the hand; *origin,* first: ulnar side of second metacarpal; second and third: radial sides of fourth and fifth metacarpals; *insertion,* first: into ulnar side of index; second and third: into radial sides of ring and little fingers; *action,* adducts fingers toward axis of middle finger; *nerve supply,* ulnar. SYN musculus interosseus palmaris [NA].

papillary m., one of the group of myocardial bundles which terminate in the chordae tendineae which attach to the cusps of the atrioventricular valves; each has an anterior and a posterior papillary muscle; the right ventricle sometimes has a septal papillary muscle. SYN musculus papillaris [NA].

pectinate m.'s, prominent ridges of atrial myocardium located on the inner surface of much of the right atrium and both auricles. SYN musculi pectinati [NA].

pectineal m., SYN pectineus m.

pectineus m., *origin,* crest of pubis; *insertion,* pectineal line of femur; *action,* adducts thigh and assists in flexion; *nerve supply,* obturator and femoral. SYN musculus pectineus [NA], pectineal m.

peroneus tertius m., *origin,* in common with m. extensor digitorum longus; *insertion,* dorsum of base of fifth metatarsal bone; *nerve supply,* deep branch of peroneal; *action,* assists in dorsiflexion and eversion of foot. SYN third peroneal m.

piriform m., SYN piriformis m.

piriformis m., *origin,* margins of pelvic sacral foramina and greater sciatic notch of ilium; *insertion,* upper border of greater trochanter; *action,* rotates thigh laterally; *nerve supply,* nerve to piriformis (sciatic plexus). SYN musculus piriformis [NA], piriform m.

plantar m., SYN plantaris m.

plantar interosseous m., three intrinsic m.'s of foot; *origin,* the medial side of the third, fourth, and fifth metatarsal bones; *insertion,* corresponding side of proximal phalanx of the same toes; *action*, adducts three lateral toes; *nerve supply*, lateral plantar. SYN musculus interosseus plantaris [NA].

plantaris m., *origin*, lateral supracondylar ridge; *insertion*, medial margin of tendo achilles and deep fascia of ankle; *action*, traditionally described as plantar flexion of foot; many investigators now believe the plantaris muscle to be primarily a proprioceptive organ; *nerve supply*, tibial nerve. SYN musculus plantaris [NA], plantar m.

platysma m., *origin*, subcutaneous layer and fascia covering pectoralis major and deltoid at level of first or second rib; *insertion*, lower border of mandible, risorius and platysma of opposite side; *action*, depresses lower lip, forms ridges in skin of neck and upper chest when jaws are "clenched", denoting stress, anger; *nerve supply*, cervical branch of facial.

pleuroesophageal m., muscular fasciculi, arising from the mediastinal pleura, which reinforce musculature of esophagus. SYN musculus pleuroesophageus [NA].

popliteal m., SYN popliteus m.

popliteus m., *origin*, lateral condyle of femur; *insertion*, posterior surface of tibia above oblique line; *action*, from the fully extended and "locked" position, rotates the femur medially, on the fixed (planted) tibial plateau about 5°, "unlocking" the knee to enable flexion to occur; *nerve supply*, tibial. SYN musculus popliteus [NA], popliteal m.

procerus m., *insertion*, into frontalis; *action*, assists frontalis; *origin*, from membrane covering bridge of nose; *nerve supply*, branch of facial. SYN musculus procerus [NA].

pronator quadratus m., *origin*, distal fourth of anterior surface of ulna; *insertion*, distal fourth of anterior surface of radius; *action*, pronates forearm; *nerve supply*, anterior interosseous. SYN musculus pronator quadratus [NA].

pronator teres m., *origin*, superficial (humeral) head (ulnar) from the common flexor origin on the medial epicondyle of the humerus, deep (ulnar) head from the medial side of the coronoid process of the ulna; *insertion*, middle of the lateral surface of the radius; *action*, pronates forearm; *nerve supply*, median. SYN musculus pronator teres [NA].

pubococcygeal m., SYN pubococcygeus m.

pubococcygeus m., fibers of the levator ani, arising from the pelvic surface of the body of the pubis and adjacent tendinous arch of obturator fascia, attaching to the coccyx. SYN musculus pubococcygeus [NA], pubococcygeal m.

puboprostatic m., smooth m. fibers within the puboprostatic ligament. SYN musculus puboprostaticus [NA].

puborectal m., SYN puborectalis m.

puborectalis m., the medial part of the m. levator ani (pubococcygeus muscle) that passes from the body of the pubis around the anus to form a muscular sling at the level of the anorectal junction; it contracts to increase the perineal flexure during a peristalsis to maintain fecal continence and relaxes to allow defecation. SYN musculus puborectalis [NA], puborectal m.

pubovaginal m., SYN pubovaginalis m.

pubovaginalis m., in the female, the most medial fibers of the levator ani (pubococcygeus) m. that extend from the pubis into the lateral walls of the vagina. SYN musculus pubovaginalis [NA], pubovaginal m.

pubovesical m., SYN pubovesicalis m.

pubovesicalis m., smooth m. fibers within the pubovesical ligament in the female. SYN musculus pubovesicalis [NA], pubovesical m.

pyramidal m., SYN pyramidalis m.

pyramidal auricular m., an occasional prolongation of the fibers of the tragicus to the spina helicis. SYN musculus pyramidalis auriculae [NA], pyramidal m. of auricle.

pyramidal m. of auricle, SYN pyramidal auricular m.

pyramidalis m., *origin*, crest of pubis; *insertion*, lower portion of linea alba; *action*, makes linea alba tense; *nerve supply*, subcostal. SYN musculus pyramidalis [NA], pyramidal m.

quadriceps m. of thigh, SYN quadriceps femoris m.

quadratus fem'oris m., *insertion*, intertrochanteric ridge; *origin*, lateral border of tuberosity of ischium; *action*, rotates thigh laterally; *nerve supply*, nerve to quadratus femoris (sacral plexus). SYN musculus quadratus femoris [NA].

quadratus lumborum m., *origin*, iliac crest, iliolumbar ligament, and transverse processes of lower lumbar vertebrae; *insertion*, twelfth rib and transverse processes of upper lumbar vertebrae; *action*, abducts trunk; *nerve supply*, ventral primary rami of upper lumbar spinal nerves. SYN musculus quadratus lumborum [NA].

quadratus plantae m., *origin*, by two heads from the lateral and medial borders of the inferior surface of the calcaneus; *insertion*, tendons of flexor digitorum longus; *action*, assists long flexor; *nerve supply*, lateral plantar. SYN musculus quadratus plantae [NA].

quadriceps fem'oris m., *origin*, by four heads: rectus femoris, vastus lateralis, vastus intermedius, and vastus medialis; *insertion*, patella, and thence by ligamentum patellae to tuberosity of tibia; *action*, extends leg; flexes thigh by action of rectus femoris; *nerve supply*, femoral. SYN musculus quadriceps femoris [NA], quadriceps m. of thigh.

radial flexor m. of wrist, SYN flexor carpi radialis m.

rectococcygeal m., SYN rectococcygeus m.

rectococcygeus m., a band of smooth m. fibers passing from the posterior surface of the rectum to the anterior surface of second or third coccygeal segment. SYN musculus rectococcygeus [NA], rectococcygeal m.

rectourethral m., SYN rectourethralis m.

rectourethralis m., smooth m. fibers that pass forward from the longitudinal m. layer of the rectum to the membranous urethra in the male. SYN musculus rectourethralis [NA], rectourethral m.

rectouterine m., a band of fibrous tissue and smooth muscle fibers passing between the cervix of the uterus and the rectum in the rectouterine fold, on either side. SYN musculus rectouterinus [NA].

mu

rectovesical m., SYN rectovesicalis m.

rectovesicalis m., smooth m. fibers in the sacrogenital fold in the male; they correspond to rectouterinus m. SYN musculus rectovesicalis [NA], rectovesical m.

rectus m. of abdomen, SYN rectus abdominis m.

rectus abdominis m., m. of ventral abdominal wall, flanking the linea alba, and characterized by tendinous intersections separating its length into multiple bellies; *origin*, crest and symphysis of the pubis; *insertion*, xiphoid process and fifth to seventh costal cartilages; *action*, flexes lumbar vertebral column, draws thorax downward toward pubis; *nerve supply*, thoracoabdominal nerves. SYN musculus rectus abdominis [NA], rectus m. of abdomen.

rectus capitis anterior m., *origin*, transverse process and lateral mass of atlas; *insertion*, basilar process of occipital bone; *action*, turns and inclines head forward; *nerve supply*, ventral primary ramus of first and second cervical spinal nerve. SYN musculus rectus capitis anterior [NA].

rectus capitis lateralis m., *origin*, transverse process of atlas; *insertion*, jugular process of occipital bone; *action*, inclines head to one side; *nerve supply*, ventral primary ramus of first cervical spinal nerve. SYN musculus rectus capitis lateralis [NA], lateral rectus m. of the head.

rectus capitis posterior major m., *origin*, spinous process of axis; *insertion*, middle of inferior nuchal line of occipital bone; *action*, rotates and draws head backward; *nerve supply*, dorsal branch of first cervical (suboccipital). SYN greater posterior rectus m. of head.

rectus capitis posterior minor m., *origin*, from posterior tubercle of atlas; *insertion*, medial third of inferior nuchal line of occipital bone; *action*, rotates head and draws it backward; *nerve supply*, dorsal branch of first cervical (suboccipital). SYN smaller posterior rectus m. of head.

rectus femoris m., *origin*, anterior inferior spine of ilium and upper margin of acetabulum; *insertion*, via common tendon of quadriceps femoris into patella, and via patellar ligament to tibial tuberosity. SYN musculus rectus femoris [NA], rectus m. of thigh.

rectus m. of thigh, SYN rectus femoris m.

red m., slow-twitch m. in which small dark "red" m. fibers predominate; myoglobin is abundant and great numbers of mitochondria occur, characterized by slow, sustained (tonic) contraction. Contrast with white m.

risorius m., *origin*, from platysma and fascia of masseter; *insertion*, orbicularis oris and skin at corner of mouth; *action*, draws angle of mouth laterally, lengthening rima oris; *nerve supply*, facial. SYN musculus risorius [NA].

rotator m.'s, SYN rotatores m.'s.

rotatores m.'s, deepest of the three layers of transversospinalis m.'s, chiefly developed in the thoracic region; they arise from the transverse process of one vertebra and are inserted into the root of the spinous process of the next two or three vertebrae above; *action*, traditionally described as a column, it is more likely that these m.'s, provided with a very high density of m.

spindles, are organs of proprioception; *nerve supply*, dorsal primary rami of the spinal nerves. SYN musculi rotatores [NA], rotator m.'s.

Ruysch's m., the muscular tissue of the fundus of the uterus.

salpingopharyngeal m., SYN salpingopharyngeus m.

salpingopharyngeus m., *origin*, medial lamina of cartilaginous part of auditory tube; *insertion*, longitudinal muscular layer of pharynx in association with m. palatopharyngeus; *action*, assists in elevating pharynx and, according to some, assists in opening the auditory tube during swallowing; *nerve supply*, pharyngeal plexus. SYN musculus salpingopharyngeus [NA], salpingopharyngeal m.

sartorius m., *origin*, anterior superior spine of ilium; *insertion*, medial border of tuberosity of tibia; *action*, flexes thigh and leg, rotates leg medially and thigh laterally; *nerve supply*, femoral. SYN musculus sartorius [NA].

scalenus medius m., *origin*, costotransverse lamellae of transverse processes of second to sixth cervical vertebrae; *insertion*, first rib posterior to subclavian artery; *action*, raises first rib; *nerve supply*, cervical plexus.

semimembranosus m., *origin*, tuberosity of ischium; *insertion*, medial condyle of tibia and by membrane to tibial collateral ligament of knee joint, popliteal fascia, and via its reflected tendon of insertion (oblique popliteal ligament) lateral condyle of femur; *action*, flexes knee and rotates leg medially when knee is flexed; and contributes to the stability of extended knee by making capsule of knee joint tense; *nerve supply*, tibial. SYN musculus semimembranosus [NA].

semispinalis capitis m., *origin*, transverse processes of five or six upper thoracic and articular processes of four lower cervical vertebrae; *insertion*, occipital bone between superior and inferior nuchal lines; *action*, rotates head and draws it backward; *nerve supply*, dorsal primary rami of cervical spinal nerves. SYN musculus semispinalis capitis [NA].

semispinalis cervicis m., continuous with m. semispinalis thoracis; *origin*, transverse processes of second to fifth thoracic vertebrae; *insertion*, spinous processes of axis and third to fifth cervical vertebrae; *action*, extends cervical spine; *nerve supply*, dorsal primary rami of cervical and thoracic spinal nerves. SYN musculus semispinalis cervicis [NA].

semispinalis thoracis m., *origin*, transverse processes of fifth to eleventh thoracic vertebrae; *insertion*, spinous processes of first four thoracic and fifth and seventh cervical vertebrae; *action*, extends vertebral column; *nerve supply*, dorsal primary rami of cervical and thoracic spinal nerves. SYN musculus semispinalis thoracis [NA].

semitendinosus m., *origin*, ischial tuberosity; *insertion*, medial surface of the upper fourth of shaft of tibia; *action*, extends thigh, flexes leg and rotates it medially; *nerve supply*, tibial. SYN musculus semitendinosus [NA].

serratus anterior m., *origin*, from center of lateral aspect of first eight to nine ribs; *insertion*, superior and inferior angles and intervening medial margin of scapula; *action*, rotates scapula and pulls it forward, elevates ribs; *nerve supply*, long thoracic from brachial plexus. SYN musculus serratus anterior [NA].

short adductor m., SYN adductor brevis m.

short extensor m. of great toe, SYN extensor hallucis brevis m.

short extensor m. of toes, SYN extensor digitorum brevis m.

short flexor m. of great toe, SYN flexor hallucis brevis m.

short flexor m. of little finger, SYN flexor digiti minimi brevis m. of hand.

short flexor m. of little toe, SYN flexor digiti minimi brevis m. of foot.

short flexor m. of thumb, SYN flexor pollicis brevis m.

short flexor m. of toes, SYN flexor digitorum brevis m.

short radial extensor m. of wrist, SYN extensor carpi radialis brevis m.

skeletal m., grossly, a collection of striated m. fibers connected at either or both extremities with the bony framework of the body; it may be an appendicular or an axial m.; histologically, a m. consisting of elongated, multinucleated, transversely striated skeletal m. fibers together with connective tissues, blood vessels, and nerves; individual m. fibers are surrounded by fine reticular and collagen fibers (endomysium); bundles (fascicles) of m. fibers are surrounded by irregular connective tissue (perimysium); the entire m. is surrounded, except at the m. tendon junction, by a dense connective tissue (epimysium).

smaller posterior rectus m. of head, SYN rectus capitis posterior minor m.

smooth m., one of the m. fibers of the internal organs, blood vessels, hair follicles, etc.; contractile elements are elongated, usually spindle-shaped cells with centrally located nuclei and a length from 20 to 200 μm, or even longer in the pregnant uterus; although transverse striations are lacking, both thick and thin myofibrils occur; smooth m. fibers are bound together into sheets or bundles by reticular fibers, and frequently elastic fiber nets are also abundant. SEE ALSO involuntary m.'s.

soleus m., *origin*, posterior surface of head and upper third of shaft of fibula, oblique line and middle third of medial margin of tibia, and a tendinous arch passing between tibia and fibula over the popliteal vessels; *insertion*, with gastrocnemius by tendo calcaneus (achilles) into tuberosity of calcaneus; *action*, plantar flexion of foot; *nerve supply*, tibial. SYN musculus soleus [NA].

sphincter m., SYN sphincter.

sphincter m. of pupil, SYN sphincter pupillae.

spinal m. of neck, SYN spinalis cervicis m.

spinalis capitis m., an inconstant extension of spinalis cervicis to the occipital bone, sometimes fusing with semispinalis capitis. SYN musculus spinalis capitis [NA].

spinalis cervicis m., an inconstant or rudimentary muscle; *origin*, spinous processes of sixth and seventh cervical vertebrae; *insertion*, spinous processes of axis and third cervical vertebra; *action*, extends cervical spine; *nerve supply*, dorsal primary rami of cervical. SYN musculus spinalis cervicis [NA], spinal m. of neck.

spinalis thoracis m., *origin*, spinous processes of upper lumbar and two lower thoracic vertebrae; *insertion*, spinous processes of middle and upper thoracic vertebrae; *action*, supports and extends vertebral column; *nerve supply*, dorsal primary rami of thoracic and upper lumbar. SYN musculus spinalis thoracis [NA].

splenius capitis m., *origin*, from ligamentum nuchae of last four cervical vertebrae and supraspinous ligament of first and second thoracic vertebrae; *insertion*, lateral half of superior nuchal line and mastoid process; *action*, rotates head and extends neck; *nerve supply*, dorsal primary rami of second to sixth cervical spinal nerves. SYN musculus splenius capitis [NA], splenius m. of head.

splenius cervicis m., *origin*, from supraspinous ligament and spinous processes of third to fifth thoracic vertebrae; *insertion*, posterior tubercles of transverse processes of first and second (sometimes third) cervical vertebrae; *action*, rotates and extends neck; *nerve supply*, dorsal primary rami of fourth to eighth cervical spinal nerves. SYN musculus splenius cervicis [NA], splenius m. of neck.

splenius m. of head, SYN splenius capitis m.

splenius m. of neck, SYN splenius cervicis m.

stapedius m., *origin*, internal walls of pyramidal eminence in tympanic cavity; *insertion*, neck of the stapes; *action*, dampens vibration of stapes by drawing head of stapes backward as a result of a protective reflex stimulated by loud noise; *nerve supply*, facial. SYN musculus stapedius [NA].

sternal m., SYN sternalis m.

sternalis m., an inconstant muscle, running parallel to the sternum across the costosternal origin of the pectoralis major, and usually connected with the sternocleidomastoid and rectus abdominis muscles due to their common development source. SYN musculus sternalis [NA], sternal m.

sternocleidomastoid m., *origin*, by two heads from anterior surface of manubrium of the sternum and sternal end of clavicle; *insertion*, mastoid process and lateral half of superior nuchal line; *action*, turns head obliquely to opposite side; when acting together, flex the neck and extend the head; *nerve supply*, motor by accessory, sensory by cervical plexus. SYN musculus sternocleidomastoideus [NA], sternomastoid m.

sternohyoid m., *origin*, posterior surface of manubrium sterni and first costal cartilage; *insertion*, body of hyoid bone; *action*, depresses hyoid bone; *nerve supply*, upper cervical via spinal nerves(ansa cervicalis). SYN musculus sternohyoideus [NA].

sternomastoid m., SYN sternocleidomastoid m.

sternothyroid m., *origin*, posterior surface of manubrium of sternum and first or second costal cartilage; *insertion*, oblique line of thyroid cartilage; *action*, depresses larynx; *nerve supply*, upper cervical via spinal nerves (ansa cervicalis). SYN musculus sternothyroideus [NA].

striated m., skeletal or voluntary m. in which

mu

cross striations occur in the fibers as a result of regular overlapping of thick and thin myofilaments; contrast with smooth muscle. Although cardiac muscle is also striated in appearance, the term "striated muscle" is commonly used as a synonym for voluntary, skeletal muscle.

styloglossus m., *action*, retracts tongue; *origin*, lower end of styloid process; *insertion*, side and undersurface of tongue; *nerve supply*, hypoglossal. SYN musculus styloglossus [NA].

stylohyoid m., *origin*, styloid process of temporal bone; *insertion*, hyoid bone by two slips on either side of intermediate tendon of digastric; *action*, elevates hyoid bone; *nerve supply*, facial. SYN musculus stylohyoideus [NA].

stylopharyngeal m., SYN stylopharyngeus m.

stylopharyngeus m., *origin*, root of styloid process; *insertion*, thyroid cartilage and wall of pharynx (becomes part of the longitudinal coat): *action*, elevates pharynx and larynx; *nerve supply*, glossopharyngeal. SYN musculus stylopharyngeus [NA], stylopharyngeal m.

subclavian m., SYN subclavius m.

subclavius m., *origin*, first costal cartilage; *insertion*, inferior surface of acromial end of clavicle; *action*, fixes clavicle or elevates first rib; *nerve supply*, subclavian from brachial plexus. SYN musculus subclavius [NA], subclavian m.

subcostal m., one of a number of inconstant muscles of the posterolateral thoracic wall having the same direction as the internal intercostal muscles but extending across (deep to) one or more ribs. SYN musculus subcostalis [NA].

subscapular m., SYN subscapularis m.

subscapularis m., *origin*, subscapular fossa; *insertion*, lesser tuberosity of humerus; *action*, rotates arm medially; *nerve supply*, upper and lower subscapular from posterior cord of brachial plexus (fifth and sixth cervical spinal nerves). SYN musculus subscapularis [NA], subscapular m.

superficial flexor m. of fingers, SYN flexor digitorum superficialis m.

superficial transverse perineal m., an inconstant muscle; *origin*, ramus of ischium; *insertion*, central tendon of perineum; *action*, draws back and fixes the central tendon of the perineum; *nerve supply*, pudendal (perineal). SYN musculus transversus perinei superficialis [NA].

superior auricular m., *origin*, galea aponeurotica; *insertion*, cartilage of auricle; *action* draws pinna of ear upward and backward; *nerve supply*, facial. Considered by some to be the posterior part of the temporoparietal muscle. SYN musculus attollens aurem, musculus attollens auriculam.

superior constrictor m. of pharynx, *origin*, medial pterygoid plate (pterygopharyngeal part), pterygomandibular raphe (buccopharyngeal part), mylohyoid line of mandible (myelopharyngeal part), and the mucous membrane of the floor of the mouth and the side of the tongue (glossopharyngeal part); *insertion*, pharyngeal raphe in the posterior wall of the pharynx; *action*, narrows pharynx; *nerve supply*, pharyngeal plexus.

superior gemellus m., *origin*, ischial spine and margin of lesser sciatic notch; *insertion*, tendon

of m. obturator internus; *action*, rotates thigh laterally; *nerve supply*, sacral plexus.

superior oblique m., *origin*, above the medial margin of the optic canal; *insertion*, by a tendon passing through the trochlea, or pulley, and then reflected backward, downward, and laterally to the sclera between the superior and lateral recti; *action*, primary, intorsion; secondary, depression and abduction; *nerve supply*, trochlear nerve. SYN musculus obliquus superior [NA].

superior rectus m., *origin*, superior part of common tendinous ring; *insertion*, superior part of sclera of the eye; *action*, primary, elevation; secondary, adduction and intorsion; *nerve supply*, oculomotor. SYN musculus rectus superior [NA].

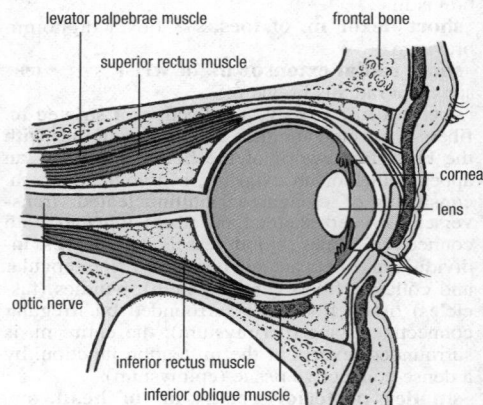

superior rectus muscle: with relationship to surrounding orbital anatomy

supinator m., *origin*, lateral epicondyle of humerus, radial collateral and anular ligaments, and supinator ridge of ulna; *insertion*, anterior and lateral surface of radius; *action*, supinates the forearm; *nerve supply*, radial (posterior interosseous). SYN musculus supinator [NA].

supraspinatus m., *origin*, supraspinous fossa of scapula; *insertion*, greater tuberosity of humerus; *action*, initiates abduction of arm; *nerve supply*, suprascapular from fifth and sixth cervical. SYN musculus supraspinatus [NA], supraspinous m.

supraspinous m., SYN supraspinatus m.

suspensory m. of duodenum, a broad flat band of smooth muscle and fibrous tissue attached to the right crus of the diaphragm and to the duodenum at its junction with the jejunum. SYN musculus suspensorius duodeni [NA].

synergistic m.'s, m.'s having a similar and mutually helpful function or action.

temporal m., SYN temporalis m.

temporalis m., *origin*, temporal fossa; *insertion*, coronoid process of mandible and anterior border of ramus; *action* elevates mandible (closes jaw); its posterior, nearly horizontally-oriented fibers are the primary retractors of the protruded mandible. *nerve supply*, deep temporal branches of mandibular division of trigeminal. SYN musculus temporalis [NA], temporal m.

temporoparietalis m., the part of epicranius m. that arises from the lateral part of the epicranial aponeurosis and inserts in the cartilage of the auricle. SYN musculus temporoparietalis [NA], temporoparietal m.

temporoparietal m., SYN temporoparietalis m.

tensor fasciae latae m., *origin*, anterior superior spine and adjacent lateral surface of the ilium; *insertion*, iliotibial band of fascia lata; *action*, tenses fascia lata; flexes, abducts and medially rotates thigh; *nerve supply*, superior gluteal. SYN musculus tensor fasciae latae [NA].

tensor m. of soft palate, SYN tensor veli palati m.

tensor m. of tympanic membrane, SYN tensor tympani m.

tensor tympani m., *origin*, the cartilaginous part of the auditory (eustachian) tube and the walls of its hemi-canal just above the bony portion of the auditory tube; *insertion*, handle of malleus; *action*, draws the handle of the malleus medialward tensing the tympanic membrane to protect it from excessive vibration by loud sounds. *nerve supply*, branches of trigeminal through the otic ganglion. SYN musculus tensor tympani [NA], tensor m. of tympanic membrane.

tensor veli palati m., tensor muscle of soft palate, m. tensor palati; m. palatosalpingeus; m. sphenosalpingostaphylinus; dilator tubae; *origin*, scaphoid fossa of sphenoid, cartilaginous and membranous part of auditory (eustachian) tube and spine of sphenoid; *insertion*, posterior border of hard palate and aponeurosis of soft palate; *action*, tenses the soft palate; contributes to opening of auditory tube; *nerve supply*, branches of trigeminal nerve through the otic ganglion. SYN musculus tensor veli palatini [NA], tensor m. of soft palate.

teres major m., *origin*, inferior angle and lower third of border of scapula; *insertion*, medial border of intertubercular groove of humerus; *action*, adducts and extends arm and rotates it medially; *nerve supply*, lower subscapular from posterior cord of brachial plexus (fifth and sixth cervical spinal nerves). SYN musculus teres major [NA].

teres minor m., *origin*, upper two-thirds of the lateral border of scapula; *insertion*, lower facet of greater tuberosity of humerus; *action*, adducts arm and rotates it laterally; *nerve supply*, axillary (fifth and sixth cervical spinal nerves). SYN musculus teres minor [NA].

third peroneal m., SYN peroneus tertius m.

thoracic longissimus m., SYN longissimus thoracis m.

thyroarytenoid m., *origin*, inner surface of thyroid cartilage; *insertion*, muscular process and outer surface of arytenoid; *action*, decreases tension on (relaxes) vocal cords lowering the pitch of the voice tone; *nerve supply*, recurrent laryngeal. SYN musculus thyroarytenoideus [NA].

thyroepiglottic m., thyroepiglottidean m., *origin*, inner surface of thyroid cartilage in common with m. thyroarytenoideus; *insertion*, aryepiglottic fold and margin of epiglottis; *action*, depresses base of epiglottis; *nerve supply*, recurrent laryngeal. SYN musculus thyroepiglotticus [NA].

thyrohyoid m., apparently a continuation of the sternothyroid; *origin*, oblique line of thyroid cartilage; *insertion*, body of hyoid bone; *action*, approximates hyoid bone to the larynx; *nerve supply*, upper cervical spinal nerves carried by hypoglossal. SYN musculus thyrohyoideus [NA].

trachealis m., the band of smooth muscular fibers in the fibrous membrane connecting posteriorly the ends of the tracheal rings. SYN musculus trachealis [NA].

m. of tragus, SYN tragicus m.

tragicus m., a band of vertical muscular fibers on the outer surface of the tragus of the ear. SYN musculus tragicus [NA], m. of tragus.

transverse m. of abdomen, SYN transversus abdominis m.

transverse m. of chin, SYN transversus menti m.

transverse m. of nape, SYN transversus nuchae m.

transverse m. of tongue, an intrinsic muscle of the tongue, the fibers of which arise from the septum and radiate to the dorsum and sides; *action*, decreases lateral dimension of the tongue; *nerve supply*, hypoglossal for motor, lingual for sensory. SYN musculus transversus linguae [NA].

transversospinal m., SYN transversospinalis m.

transversospinalis m., the group of muscles that originate from transverse processes of vertebrae and pass to spinous processes of higher vertebrae; they act as rotators and include the semispinalis (capitis, cervicis, thoracis), multifidus, and rotatores (cervicis, thoracis, lumborum) muscles. All are innervated by dorsal primary rami of spinal nerves. SYN musculus transversospinalis [NA], transversospinal m.

transversus abdominis m., *origin*, seventh to twelfth costal cartilages, lumbar fascia, iliac crest, and inguinal ligament; *insertion*, xiphoid cartilage and linea alba and, through the conjoint tendon, pubic tubercle and pecten; *action*, compresses abdominal contents; *nerve supply*, lower thoracic. SYN musculus transversus abdominis [NA], transverse m. of abdomen.

transversus menti m., inconstant fibers of the depressor anguli oris m. continue into the neck and cross to the opposite side inferior to the chin. SYN musculus transversus menti [NA], transverse m. of chin.

transversus nuchae m., an occasional muscle passing between the tendons of the trapezius and sternocleidomastoid, possibly a fasciculus of the posterior auricular muscle. SYN musculus transversus nuchae [NA], transverse m. of nape.

transversus thoracis m., *origin*, dorsal surface of xiphoid cartilage and lower portion of dorsal surface of body of sternum; *insertion*, second to sixth costal cartilages; *action*, contributes to depression of ribs, narrowing chest; *nerve supply*, intercostal. SYN musculus transversus thoracis [NA].

trapezius m., *origin*, medial third of superior nuchal line, external occipital protuberance, ligamentum nuchae, spinous processes of seventh

mu

cervical and the thoracic vertebrae and corresponding supraspinous ligaments; *insertion*, lateral third of posterior surface of clavicle, anterior side of acromion, and upper and medial border of the spine of the scapula; *action*, when scapulae are fixed, portions of muscle can act independently: cervical portion elevates scapula, thoracic portion contributes to depression of scapula; upper and lowermost portions act simultaneously to rotate glenoid fossa superiorly; when the entire muscle and especially middle part contracts, the scapulae retract; draws head to one side or backward; *nerve supply*, motor by accessory, sensory by cervical plexus. SYN musculus trapezius [NA], trapezius.

triangular m., (1) a muscle that is triangular in shape; (2) SYN depressor anguli oris m.

triceps m. of arm, SYN triceps brachii m.

triceps brachii m., *origin*, long or scapular head: lateral border of scapula below glenoid fossa, lateral head: lateral and posterior surface of humerus below greater tubercle, medial head: posterior surface of humerus below radial groove; *insertion*, olecranon of ulna; *action*, extends elbow; *nerve supply*, radial. SYN musculus triceps brachii [NA], triceps m. of arm.

triceps m. of calf, SYN triceps surae m.

triceps surae m., the two bellies of the gastrocnemius and soleus considered as one muscle. SYN musculus triceps surae [NA], triceps m. of calf.

ulnar extensor m. of wrist, SYN extensor carpi ulnaris m.

ulnar flexor m. of wrist, SYN flexor carpi ulnaris m.

m. of uvula, SYN uvular m.

uvular m., *origin*, posterior nasal spine; *insertion*, forms chief bulk of the uvula; *action*, raises the uvula; *nerve supply*, pharyngeal plexus. SYN musculus uvulae [NA], m. of uvula.

vastus intermedius m., *origin*, upper three-fourths of anterior surface of shaft of femur; *insertion*, tibial tuberosity by way of common tendon of quadriceps femoris and patellar ligament; *action*, extends leg; *nerve supply*, femoral. SYN intermediate vastus m.

vastus lateralis m., *origin*, lateral lip of linea aspera as far as great trochanter; *insertion*, tibial tuberosity by way of common tendon of quadriceps femoris and patellar ligament; *action*, extends leg; *nerve supply*, femoral. SYN lateral vastus m.

vastus medialis m., *origin*, medial lip of linea aspera; *insertion*, tibial tuberosity by way of common tendon of quadriceps femoris and ligamentum patellae; *action*, extends leg; *nerve supply*, femoral. SYN medial vastus m.

vertical m. of tongue, an intrinsic muscle of the tongue, consisting of fibers that pass from the aponeurosis of the dorsum to the aponeurosis of the inferior surface; *action*, decreases the superior to inferior dimension of (flattens) the tongue; *nerve supply*, hypoglossal for motor, lingual for sensory. SYN musculus verticalis linguae [NA].

vocal m., SYN vocalis m.

vocalis m., *origin*, depression between the two laminae of thyroid cartilage; *insertion*, portions of vocal process of arytenoid; *action*, shortens and relaxes vocal cords; *nerve supply*, recurrent laryngeal; a number of the deeper and finer fibers of the thyroarytenoid m. attached directly to the outer side of the true vocal cord. SYN musculus vocalis [NA], vocal m.

voluntary m., one whose action is under the control of the will; all the striated m.'s, except the heart, are voluntary m.'s.

white m., a rapid or fast-twitch m. in which pale large "white" fibers predominate; mitochondria and myoglobin are relatively sparse compared with red m.; involved in phasic contraction.

zygomaticus major m., *origin*, zygomatic bone anterior to temporozygomatic suture; *insertion*, muscles at angle of mouth; *action*, draws upper lip upward and laterally; *nerve supply*, facial. SYN musculus zygomaticus.

mus·cle-bound (mŭs′ĕl-bownd). Denoting a condition in which individual muscles are overdeveloped but dyssynergic in concerted action.

mus·cu·lar (mŭs′kyū-lăr). 1. Relating to a muscle or the muscles. 2. Having well developed musculature.

mus·cu·la·ris (mŭs-kyū-lā′ris). The muscular coat of a hollow organ or tubular structure. [Mod. L. muscular]

m. muco′sae, the thin layer of smooth muscle found in most parts of the digestive tube located outside the m. propria mucosae and adjacent to the tela submucosa.

mus·cu·lar·i·ty (mŭs′kyū-lar′i-tē). The state or condition of having well developed muscles.

mus·cu·la·ture (mŭs′kyū-lă-chūr). The arrangement of the muscles in a part or in the body as a whole.

mus·cu·lo·ap·o·neu·rot·ic (mŭs′kyū-lō-ap′ō-nū-rot′ik). Relating to muscular tissue and an aponeurosis of origin or insertion.

mus·cu·lo·cu·ta·ne·ous (mŭs′kyū-lō-kyū-tā′nē-ŭs). Relating to both muscle and skin. SYN myocutaneous.

mus·cu·lo·mem·bra·nous (mŭs′kyū-lō-mem′bră-nŭs). Relating to both muscular tissue and membrane; denoting certain muscles, such as the occipitofrontalis, that are largely membranous.

mus·cu·lo·skel·e·tal (mŭs′kyū-lō-skel′ĕ-tăl). Relating to muscles and to the skeleton, as, for example, the m. system.

mus·cu·lo·ten·di·nous (mŭs′kyū-lō-ten′di-nŭs). Relating to both muscular and tendinous tissues.

mus·cu·lo·tro·pic (mŭs′kyū-lō-trop′ik). Affecting, acting upon, or attracted to muscular tissue.

mus·cu·lus, gen. and pl. **mus·cu·li** (mŭs′kyū-lŭs, -kyū-lī) [NA]. SYN muscle. For histologic description, see muscle. [L. a little mouse, a muscle, fr. *mus* (*mur*-), a mouse]

m. abduc′tor hal′lucis [NA], SYN abductor hallucis *muscle*.

m. adduc′tor bre′vis [NA], SYN adductor brevis *muscle*.

m. adduc′tor hal′lucis [NA], SYN adductor hallucis *muscle*.

m. adduc′tor lon′gus [NA], SYN adductor longus *muscle*.

m. adduc′tor mag′nus [NA], SYN adductor magnus *muscle*.

m. adduc′tor pol′licis [NA], SYN adductor pollicis *muscle.*

m. anco′neus [NA], SYN anconeus *muscle.*

m. antitrag′icus [NA], SYN antitragicus *muscle.*

mus′culi arrecto′res pilo′rum [NA], SYN arrector pili *muscles,* under *muscle.*

m. articula′ris cu′biti [NA], SYN articularis cubiti *muscle.*

m. articula′ris ge′nus [NA], SYN articularis genu *muscle.*

m. aryepiglot′ticus [NA], SYN aryepiglottic *muscle.*

m. attol′lens au′rem, m. attol′lens auric′u-lam, SYN superior auricular *muscle.*

m. a′ttrahens au′rem, m. a′ttrahens auric′ulam, SYN anterior auricular *muscle.*

m. bi′ceps bra′chii [NA], SYN biceps brachii *muscle.*

m. bi′ceps fem′oris [NA], SYN biceps femoris *muscle.*

m. brachia′lis [NA], SYN brachialis *muscle.*

m. brachioradia′lis [NA], SYN brachioradialis *muscle.*

m. bronchoesopha′geus [NA], SYN bronchoesophageal *muscle.*

m. buccina′tor [NA], SYN buccinator *muscle.*

m. bulbospongio′sus [NA], SYN bulbocavernosus *muscle.*

m. ceratocricoi′deus [NA], SYN ceratocricoid *muscle.*

m. cilia′ris [NA], SYN ciliary *muscle.*

m. coccyg′eus [NA], SYN coccygeus *muscle.*

m. coracobrachia′lis [NA], SYN coracobrachialis *muscle.*

m. corruga′tor supercil′ii [NA], SYN corrugator supercilii *muscle.*

m. cremas′ter [NA], SYN cremaster *muscle.*

m. cricothyroi′deus [NA], SYN cricothyroid *muscle.*

m. deltoi′deus [NA], SYN deltoid *muscle.*

m. depres′sor an′guli o′ris [NA], SYN depressor anguli oris *muscle.*

m. depres′sor la′bii inferio′ris [NA], SYN depressor labii inferioris *muscle.*

m. depres′sor sep′ti [NA], SYN depressor septi *muscle.*

m. depres′sor supercil′ii [NA], SYN depressor supercilii *muscle.*

m. digas′tricus [NA], SYN digastric *muscle.*

m. dila′tor pupil′lae [NA], SYN dilator pupillae *muscle.*

m. dila′tor tu′bae, that portion of m. tensor veli palatini that attaches to the mucous membrane of the auditory tube; formerly described as a separate muscle.

m. epicra′nius [NA], SYN epicranius *muscle.*

m. erec′tor spi′nae [NA], SYN erector spinae *muscles,* under *muscle.*

m. exten′sor car′pi ulna′ris [NA], SYN extensor carpi ulnaris *muscle.*

m. exten′sor dig′iti min′imi [NA], SYN extensor digiti minimi *muscle.*

m. exten′sor digito′rum [NA], SYN extensor digitorum *muscle.*

m. exten′sor digito′rum bre′vis [NA], SYN extensor digitorum brevis *muscle.*

m. exten′sor digito′rum lon′gus [NA], SYN extensor digitorum longus *muscle.*

m. exten′sor hal′lucis bre′vis [NA], SYN extensor hallucis brevis *muscle.*

m. exten′sor hal′lucis lon′gus [NA], SYN extensor hallucis longus *muscle.*

m. exten′sor in′dicis [NA], SYN extensor indicis *muscle.*

m. flex′or car′pi radia′lis [NA], SYN flexor carpi radialis *muscle.*

m. flex′or car′pi ulna′ris [NA], SYN flexor carpi ulnaris *muscle.*

m. flex′or dig′iti min′imi brev′is ma′nus [NA], SYN flexor digiti minimi brevis *muscle* of hand.

m. flex′or dig′iti min′imi brev′is pe′dis [NA], SYN flexor digiti minimi brevis *muscle* of foot.

m. flex′or digito′rum bre′vis [NA], SYN flexor digitorum brevis *muscle.*

m. flex′or digito′rum lon′gus [NA], SYN flexor digitorum longus *muscle.*

m. flex′or digito′rum profun′dus [NA], SYN flexor digitorum profundus *muscle.*

m. flex′or digito′rum superficia′lis [NA], SYN flexor digitorum superficialis *muscle.*

m. gastrocne′mius [NA], SYN gastrocnemius *muscle.*

m. genioglos′sus [NA], SYN genioglossus *muscle.*

m. geniohyoi′deus [NA], SYN geniohyoid *muscle.*

m. glu′teus max′imus [NA], SYN gluteus maximus *muscle.*

m. glu′teus me′dius [NA], SYN gluteus medius *muscle.*

m. glu′teus min′imus [NA], SYN gluteus minimus *muscle.*

m. grac′ilis [NA], SYN gracilis *muscle.*

m. hyoglos′sus [NA], SYN hyoglossus *muscle.*

m. ili′acus [NA], SYN iliacus *muscle.*

m. il′iococcyg′eus [NA], SYN iliococcygeus *muscle.*

m. iliocosta′lis [NA], SYN iliocostalis *muscle.*

m. iliopso′as [NA], SYN iliopsoas *muscle.*

m. infraspina′tus [NA], SYN infraspinatus *muscle.*

m. interos′seus palma′ris, pl. **mus′culi interos′sei palma′res** [NA], SYN palmar interosseous *muscle.*

m. interos′seus planta′ris, pl. **mus′culi interos′sei planta′res** [NA], SYN plantar interosseous *muscle.*

mus′culi interspina′les [NA], SYN interspinales *muscles,* under *muscle.*

mus′culi intertransversa′rii [NA], SYN intertransversarii *muscles,* under *muscle.*

m. ischiocaverno′sus [NA], SYN ischiocavernosus *muscle.*

mus′culi laryn′gis [NA], SYN *muscles* of larynx, under *muscle.*

m. latis′simus dor′si [NA], SYN latissimus dorsi *muscle.*

m. leva′tor an′guli o′ris [NA], SYN levator anguli oris *muscle.*

m. leva′tor a′ni [NA], SYN levator ani *muscle.*

mu

m. leva′tor glan′dulae thyroi′deae [NA], SYN levator *muscle* of thyroid gland.

m. leva′tor la′bii superio′ris [NA], SYN levator labii superioris *muscle*.

m. leva′tor la′bii superio′ris alae′que na′si [NA], SYN levator labii superioris alaeque nasi *muscle*.

m. leva′tor pal′pebrae superio′ris [NA], SYN levator palpebrae superioris *muscle*.

m. leva′tor pro′statae [NA], SYN levator prostatae *muscle*.

m. leva′tor scap′ulae [NA], SYN levator scapulae *muscle*.

m. leva′tor ve′li palati′ni [NA], SYN levator veli palatini *muscle*.

m. longis′simus cap′itis [NA], SYN longissimus capitis *muscle*.

m. longis′simus cer′vicis [NA], SYN longissimus cervicis *muscle*.

m. longis′simus thora′cis [NA], SYN longissimus thoracis *muscle*.

m. lon′gus cap′itis [NA], SYN longus capitis *muscle*.

m. lon′gus col′li [NA], SYN longus colli *muscle*.

m. lumbrica′lis ma′nus, pl. **mus′culi lumbrica′les ma′nus** [NA], SYN lumbrical *muscles* of hand, under *muscle*.

m. lumbrica′lis pe′dis, pl. **mus′culi lumbrica′les pe′dis** [NA], SYN lumbrical *muscles* of foot, under *muscle*.

m. masse′ter [NA], SYN masseter *muscle*.

m. menta′lis [NA], SYN mentalis *muscle*.

m. multif′idus [NA], SYN multifidus *muscle*.

m. mylohyoi′deus [NA], SYN mylohyoid *muscle*.

m. nasa′lis [NA], SYN nasalis *muscle*.

m. obli′quus exter′nus abdom′inis [NA], SYN external oblique *muscle*.

m. obli′quus infe′rior [NA], SYN inferior oblique *muscle*.

m. obli′quus inter′nus abdom′inis [NA], SYN internal oblique *muscle*.

m. obli′quus supe′rior [NA], SYN superior oblique *muscle*.

m. obtura′tor exter′nus [NA], SYN obturator externus *muscle*.

m. obtura′tor inter′nus [NA], SYN obturator internus *muscle*.

m. occipitofronta′lis [NA], SYN occipitofrontalis *muscle*.

m. omohyoi′deus [NA], SYN omohyoid *muscle*.

m. oppo′nens dig′iti min′imi [NA], SYN opponens digiti minimi *muscle*.

m. oppo′nens pol′licis [NA], SYN opponens pollicis *muscle*.

m. orbicula′ris oc′uli [NA], SYN orbicularis oculi *muscle*.

m. orbicula′ris o′ris [NA], SYN orbicularis oris *muscle*.

m. orbita′lis [NA], SYN orbitalis *muscle*.

m. palatoglos′sus [NA], SYN palatoglossus *muscle*.

m. palatopharyn′geus [NA], SYN palatopharyngeus *muscle*.

m. papilla′ris [NA], SYN papillary *muscle*.

mus′culi pectina′ti [NA], SYN pectinate *muscles*, under *muscle*.

m. pectin′eus [NA], SYN pectineus *muscle*.

m. pirifor′mis [NA], SYN piriformis *muscle*.

m. planta′ris [NA], SYN plantaris *muscle*.

m. pleuroesopha′geus [NA], SYN pleuroesophageal *muscle*.

m. poplit′eus [NA], SYN popliteus *muscle*.

m. proce′rus [NA], SYN procerus *muscle*.

m. prona′tor quadra′tus [NA], SYN pronator quadratus *muscle*.

m. prona′tor te′res [NA], SYN pronator teres *muscle*.

m. pubococcyg′eus [NA], SYN pubococcygeus *muscle*.

m. puboprostat′icus [NA], SYN puboprostatic *muscle*.

m. puborecta′lis [NA], SYN puborectalis *muscle*.

m. pubovagina′lis [NA], SYN pubovaginalis *muscle*.

m. pubovesica′lis [NA], SYN pubovesicalis *muscle*.

m. pyramida′lis [NA], SYN pyramidalis *muscle*.

m. pyramida′lis auric′ulae [NA], SYN pyramidal auricular *muscle*.

m. quadra′tus fem′oris [NA], SYN quadratus femoris *muscle*.

m. quadra′tus la′bii superior′is, composed of three heads usually described as three separate muscles; they are the caput angulare or levator labii superioris alaeque nasi muscle; caput infraorbitale or levator labii superioris muscle; caput zygomaticum or zygomaticus minor muscle.

m. quadra′tus lumbo′rum [NA], SYN quadratus lumborum *muscle*.

m. quadra′tus plan′tae [NA], SYN quadratus plantae *muscle*.

m. quad′riceps fem′oris [NA], SYN quadriceps femoris *muscle*.

m. rectococcyg′eus [NA], SYN rectococcygeus *muscle*.

m. rectourethra′lis [NA], SYN rectourethralis *muscle*.

m. rectouteri′nus [NA], SYN rectouterine *muscle*.

m. rectovesica′lis [NA], SYN rectovesicalis *muscle*.

m. rec′tus abdom′inis [NA], SYN rectus abdominis *muscle*.

m. rec′tus cap′itis ante′rior [NA], SYN rectus capitis anterior *muscle*.

m. rec′tus cap′itis latera′lis [NA], SYN rectus capitis lateralis *muscle*.

m. rec′tus fem′oris [NA], SYN rectus femoris *muscle*.

m. rec′tus infe′rior [NA], SYN inferior rectus *muscle*.

m. rec′tus latera′lis [NA], SYN lateral rectus *muscle*.

m. rec′tus media′lis [NA], SYN medial rectus *muscle*.

m. rec′tus supe′rior [NA], SYN superior rectus *muscle*.

m. riso′rius [NA], SYN risorius *muscle*.

mus′culi rotato′res [NA], SYN rotatores *muscles*, under *muscle*.

m. salpingopharyn′geus [NA], SYN salpingopharyngeus *muscle.*

m. sarto′rius [NA], SYN sartorius *muscle.*

m. semimembrano′sus [NA], SYN semimembranosus *muscle.*

m. semispina′lis cap′itis [NA], SYN semispinalis capitis *muscle.*

m. semispina′lis cer′vicis [NA], SYN semispinalis cervicis *muscle.*

m. semispina′lis thora′cis [NA], SYN semispinalis thoracis *muscle.*

m. semitendino′sus [NA], SYN semitendinosus *muscle.*

m. serra′tus ante′rior [NA], SYN serratus anterior *muscle.*

m. sol′eus [NA], SYN soleus *muscle.*

m. sphinc′ter duc′tus choledo′chi [NA], SYN *sphincter* of common bile duct.

m. sphinc′ter duc′tus pancrea′tici, SYN *sphincter* of pancreatic duct.

m. sphinc′ter pupil′lae [NA], SYN *sphincter* pupillae.

m. sphinc′ter pylo′ri [NA], SYN pyloric *sphincter.*

m. sphinc′ter ure′thrae [NA], SYN *sphincter* urethrae.

m. sphinc′ter vesi′cae, SYN *sphincter* vesicae.

m. spina′lis cap′itis [NA], SYN spinalis capitis *muscle.*

m. spina′lis cer′vicis [NA], SYN spinalis cervicis *muscle.*

m. spina′lis thora′cis [NA], SYN spinalis thoracis *muscle.*

m. sple′nius cap′itis [NA], SYN splenius capitis *muscle.*

m. sple′nius cer′vicis [NA], SYN splenius cervicis *muscle.*

m. stape′dius [NA], SYN stapedius *muscle.*

m. sterna′lis [NA], SYN sternalis *muscle.*

m. sternocleidomastoi′deus [NA], SYN sternocleidomastoid *muscle.*

m. sternohyoi′deus [NA], SYN sternohyoid *muscle.*

m. sternothyroi′deus [NA], SYN sternothyroid *muscle.*

m. styloglos′sus [NA], SYN styloglossus *muscle.*

m. stylohyoi′deus [NA], SYN stylohyoid *muscle.*

m. stylopharyn′geus [NA], SYN stylopharyngeus *muscle.*

m. subcla′vius [NA], SYN subclavius *muscle.*

m. subcosta′lis, pl. **mus′culi subcosta′les** [NA], SYN subcostal *muscle.*

m. subscapula′ris [NA], SYN subscapularis *muscle.*

m. supina′tor [NA], SYN supinator *muscle.*

m. supraspina′tus [NA], SYN supraspinatus *muscle.*

m. suspenso′rius duode′ni [NA], SYN suspensory *muscle* of duodenum.

m. tempora′lis [NA], SYN temporalis *muscle.*

m. temporoparieta′lis [NA], SYN temporoparietalis *muscle.* SEE ALSO anterior auricular *muscle,* superior auricular *muscle.*

m. ten′sor fas′ciae la′tae [NA], SYN tensor fasciae latae *muscle.*

m. ten′sor tym′pani [NA], SYN tensor tympani *muscle.*

m. ten′sor ve′li palati′ni [NA], SYN tensor veli palati *muscle.*

m. te′res ma′jor [NA], SYN teres major *muscle.*

m. te′res mi′nor [NA], SYN teres minor *muscle.*

m. thyroarytenoi′deus [NA], SYN thyroarytenoid *muscle.*

m. thyroepiglot′ticus [NA], SYN thyroepiglottic *muscle.*

m. thyrohyoi′deus [NA], SYN thyrohyoid *muscle.*

m. tibiofascia′lis ante′rior, m. tibiofascia′lis anti′cus, separate fibers of the tibialis anterior inserted into the fascia of the dorsum of the foot.

m. trachea′lis [NA], SYN trachealis *muscle.*

m. tra′gicus [NA], SYN tragicus *muscle.*

m. transversa′lis cer′vicis, m. transversa′lis col′li, SYN longissimus cervicis *muscle.*

m. transversospina′lis [NA], SYN transversospinalis *muscle.*

m. transver′sus abdom′inis [NA], SYN transversus abdominis *muscle.*

m. transver′sus lin′guae [NA], SYN transverse *muscle* of tongue.

m. transver′sus men′ti [NA], SYN transversus menti *muscle.*

m. transver′sus nu′chae [NA], SYN transversus nuchae *muscle.*

m. transver′sus perine′i profun′dus [NA], SYN deep transverse perineal *muscle.*

m. transver′sus perine′i superficia′lis [NA], SYN superficial transverse perineal *muscle.*

m. transver′sus thora′cis [NA], SYN transversus thoracis *muscle.*

m. trape′zius [NA], SYN trapezius *muscle.*

m. tri′ceps bra′chii [NA], SYN triceps brachii *muscle.*

m. tri′ceps su′rae [NA], SYN triceps surae *muscle.*

m. u′vulae [NA], SYN uvular *muscle.*

m. vertica′lis lin′guae [NA], SYN vertical *muscle* of tongue.

m. voca′lis [NA], SYN vocalis *muscle.*

m. zygomat′icus, SYN zygomaticus major *muscle.*

mu·si·co·ther·a·py (myū′sik-ō-thār′ă-pē). An adjunctive treatment of mental disorders by means of music.

mus·si·ta·tion (mŭs-i-tā′shŭn). Movements of the lips as if speaking, but without sound; observed in delirium and in semicoma. [L. *mussito,* to murmur constantly, fr. *musso,* pp. *-atus,* to mutter]

mu·ta·gen (myū′tă-jen). Any agent that promotes a mutation or causes an increase in the rate of mutational events, *e.g.,* radioactive substances, x-rays, or certain chemicals. [L. *muto,* to change, + G. *-gen,* producing]

mu·ta·gen·e·sis (mū′tă-jen′ĕ-sis). Production of genetic alterations by using chemicals or radiation.

mu·ta·gen·e·sis (myū-tă-jen′ĕ-sis). Production of a mutation.

insertional m., mutation caused by insertion of new genetic material into a normal gene, particularly of retroviruses into chromosomal DNA.

mu

mu·ta·gen·ic (myū-tă-jen′ik). Promoting mutation.

mu·tant (myu′tant). **1.** A phenotype in which a mutation is manifested. **2.** A gene that is rare and usually harmful, in contrast to a wild-type gene, not necessarily generated recently.

mu·tase (myū′tās). Any enzyme that catalyzes the apparent migration of groups within one molecule; sometimes the transfer is from one molecule to another.

mu·ta·tion (myū-tā′shŭn). **1.** A change in the chemistry of a gene that is perpetuated in subsequent divisions of the cell in which it occurs; a change in the sequence of base pairs in the chromosomal molecule. **2.** The sudden production of a species, as distinguished from variation. [L. *muto*, pp. *-atus*, to change]

   lethal m., a mutant trait that leads to a phenotype incompatible with effective reproduction.

   missense m., a m. in which a base change or substitution results in a codon that causes insertion of a different amino acid into the growing polypeptide chain, giving rise to an altered protein. [mis-sense by analogy with non-sense]

   neutral m., a m. with a negligible impact on genetic fitness.

   point m., a m. that involves a single nucleotide; it may consist of loss of a nucleotide, substitution of one nucleotide for another, or the insertion of an additional nucleotide.

   somatic m., a m. occurring in the general body cells (as opposed to the germ cells) and hence not transmitted to progeny.

   spontaneous m., a m. that arises naturally and not as a result of exposure to mutagens.

   suppressor m., (1) A m. that alters the anticodon in a tRNA so that it is complementary to a termination codon, thus suppressing termination of the amino acid chain. **(2)** Genetic changes such that the effect of a m. in one place can be overcome by a second m. in another location. There are two types: intergenic suppression (occurring in a different gene) and intragenic suppression (occurring in the same gene but at a different site).

   transition m., a point m. involving substitution of one base-pair for another, *i.e.,* replacement of one purine for another and of one pyrimidine for another pyrimidine without change in the purine-pyrimidine orientation.

   transversion m., a point m. involving base substitution in which the orientation of purine and pyrimidine is reversed, in contradistinction to transition m.

mute (myūt). **1.** Unable or unwilling to speak. **2.** A person who does not have the faculty of speech. [L. *mutus*]

mu·tein (myū′tēn). A protein arising as a result of a mutation. [*mut*ation + prot*ein*]

mu·ti·la·tion (myū-ti-lā′shŭn). Disfigurement or injury by removal or destruction of any conspicuous or essential part of the body. [L. *mutilatio*, fr. *mutilo*, pp. *-atus*, to maim]

mut·ism (myū′tizm). **1.** The state of being silent. **2.** Organic or functional absence of the faculty of speech. [L. *mutus*, mute]

   akinetic m., subacute or chronic state of altered consciousness, in which the patient appears alert intermittently, but is not responsive, although the descending motor pathways appear intact; due to lesions of various cerebral structures.

   elective m., m. due to psychogenic causes.

mu·ton (myū′ton). GENETICS The smallest unit of a chromosome in which alteration can be effective in causing a mutation. [*mutation* + -on]

mu·tu·al·ism (myū′tyū-ăl-izm). Symbiotic relationship in which both species derive benefit. Cf. commensalism, metabiosis, parasitism.

mu·tu·al·ist (myū′tyū-ăl-ist). SYN symbion. [L. *mutuus*, in return, mutual]

mV millivolt.

MVV maximum voluntary *ventilation*.

MW molecular *weight*.

my·al·gia (mī-al′jē-ă). Muscular pain. SYN myodynia. [G. *mys*, muscle, + *algos*, pain]

   epidemic m., SYN epidemic *pleurodynia*.

my·as·the·nia (mī-as-thē′nē-ă). Muscular weakness. [G. *mys*, muscle, + *astheneia*, weakness]

   m. angiosclerot′ica, SYN intermittent *claudication*.

   m. gravis, disorder of neuromuscular transmission, marked by fluctuating weakness, especially of the oculofacial muscles and the proximal limb muscles; the weakness characteristically increases with activity; due to an immunological disorder. SYN Goldflam disease.

my·as·then·ic (mī′as-then′ik). Relating to myasthenia.

my·a·to·nia, my·at·o·ny (mī-ă-tō′nē-ă, mī-at′ō-nē). Abnormal extensibility of a muscle. [G. *mys*, muscle, + *a* priv. + *tonos*, tone]

   m. congen′ita, SYN *amyotonia* congenita (1).

my·ce·lia (mī-sē′lē-ă). Plural of mycelium.

my·ce·li·an (mī-sē′lē-an). Pertaining to a mycelium.

my·ce·li·um, pl. **my·ce·lia** (mī-sē′lē-ŭm, -ă). The mass of hyphae making up a colony of fungi. [G. *mykēs*, fungus, + *hēlos*, nail, wart, excrescence on animal or plant]

⌂**mycet-, myceto-.** Fungus. SEE ALSO myco-. [G. *mykēs*, fungus]

my·cete (mī′sēt). A fungus. [G. *mykēs*, fungus]

my·ce·tism, my·ce·tis·′mus (mī′sē-tizm, -tiz′ mŭs). Poisoning by certain species of mushrooms. [G. *mykēs*, fungus]

my·ce·to·ge·net·ic, my·ce·to·gen·ic (mī-sē′tō-jĕ-net′ik, mī′sē-tō-; -jen′ik). Caused by fungi. [G. *mykēs*, fungus, + *gennētos*, begotten]

my·ce·to·ma (mī-sē-tō′mă). **1.** A chronic infection involving the feet and characterized by the formation of localized lesions with tumefactions and multiple draining sinuses. The exudate contains granules that may be yellow, white, red, brown, or black, depending upon the causative agent. actinomycotic m. is caused by actinomycetes; eumycotic mycetoma is caused by true fungi. SYN Madura boil, maduromycosis. **2.** Any tumor with draining sinuses produced by filamentous fungi.

my·cid (mī′sid). An allergic reaction to a remote focus of mycotic infection. [G. *mykēs*, fungus, + -id]

⌂**myco-.** Fungus. SEE ALSO mycet-. [G. *mykēs*, fungus]

my·co·bac·te·ria (mī′kō-bak-tē′rē-ă). Organisms belonging to the genus *Mycobacterium*.

 atypical m., species of mycobacteria other than *M. tuberculosis* or *M. bovis* that can cause disease in immunocompromised humans.

my·co·bac·te·ri·o·sis (mī′kō-bak-tēr′ē-ō′sis). Infection with mycobacteria.

My·co·bac·te·ri·um (mī′kō-bak-tēr′ē-ŭm). A genus of aerobic, nonmotile bacteria (family Mycobacteriaceae) containing Gram-positive, acid-fast, slender, straight or slightly curved rods; slender filaments occasionally occur, but branched forms rarely are produced. Parasitic and saprophytic species occur. A number of species are associated with infections in immunocompromised persons, especially those with AIDS. The type species is *M. tuberculosis*. It is the type genus of the family Mycobacteriaceae. [myco- + bacterium]

 M. a′vium, a species causing tuberculosis in fowl and other birds. Recently linked to opportunistic infections in humans. SYN tubercle bacillus (3).

 M. avium-intracellulare complex, an opportunistic agent of infection in persons with AIDS. Difficult to treat because *Mycobacterium* is resistant to many antibiotics. May also cause chronic lower respiratory tract infections.

 M. bo′vis, a species that is the primary cause of tuberculosis in cattle; transmissible to humans and other animals, causing tuberculosis. SYN tubercle bacillus (2).

 M. chelo′nae, rapidly growing mycobacterium that cause sporadic infection following cardiothoracic surgery, peritoneal- and hemodialysis, augmentation mammaplasty, arthroplasty, and in immunocompromised patients.

 M. kansas′ii, a species causing a tuberculosis-like pulmonary disease; also found to cause infections (and usually lesions) in meninges, spleen, liver, pancreas, testes, hip joint, knee joint, finger, wrist, and lymph nodes.

 M. lep′rae, a species that causes Hansen's disease. SYN Hansen's bacillus.

 M. mari′num, a species causing spontaneous tuberculosis in saltwater fish; it also occurs in other cold-blooded animals, in some swimming pools in which it may cause human cutaneous infection, irrigation canals and ditches, and ocean beaches.

 M. scrofula′ceum, a species frequently associated with cervical adenitis in children.

 M. tuberculo′sis, a species which causes tuberculosis in humans;it is the type species of the genus *M.* SYN Koch's bacillus (1), tubercle bacillus (1).

my·co·der·ma·ti·tis (mī′kō-der-mă-tī′tis). A nonspecific term used to designate an eruption of mycotic (fungus, yeast, mold) origin.

my·col·o·gist (mī-kol′ŏ-jist). A person specializing in mycology.

my·col·o·gy (mī-kol′ō-jē). The study of fungi: their identification, classification, edibility, cultivation, and biology, including pathogenicity. [myco- + G. *logos,* study]

my·co·phage (mī′kō-fāj). A virus whose host is a fungus. SEE ALSO mycovirus. [myco- + G. *phagō,* to eat]

My·co·plas·ma (mī′kō-plaz-mă). A genus of aerobic to facultatively anaerobic bacteria containing Gram-negative cells that do not possess a true cell wall but are bounded by a three-layered membrane. The cells are pleomorphic, and in liquid media appear as coccoid bodies, rings, or filaments. These organisms are found in humans and other animals and are parasitic to pathogenic. [myco- + G. *plasma,* something formed (plasm)]

 M. hom′inis, a species that is an agent of pelvic inflammatory disease and other genitourinary tract infections; can also cause chorioamnionitis and postpartum fever.

 M. mycoi′des, a bacterial species of which subspecies cause contagious pleuropneumonia in cattle, sheep, and goats; it is the type species of the genus *M.*

 M. pharyn′gis, a species occurring as a commensal in the human oropharynx.

 M. pneumo′niae, a species causing primary atypical pneumonia in human beings. SYN Eaton agent.

my·co·plas·ma, pl. **my·co·plas·ma·ta** (as′ter-ō-kok′kŭs, -plaz′mah-tă). A vernacular term used to refer to any member of the genus *Mycoplasma.*

My·co·plas·ma·ta·les (mī′kō-plaz′mă-tā′lēz). An order of Gram-negative bacteria containing cells which are bounded by a three-layered membrane but which do not possess a true cell wall. Pathogenic and saprophytic species occur. These organisms reproduce through the breaking up of branched filaments into coccoid, filterable elementary bodies. The order includes the so-called pleuropneumonia-like *organisms,* under *organism* (PPLO).

my·co·sis, pl. **my·co·ses** (mī-kō′sis, -sēz). Any disease caused by a fungus (filamentous or yeast). [myco- + G. *-osis,* condition]

 m. fungoi′des, a chronic progressive lymphoma arising in the skin which initially simulates eczema or other inflammatory dermatoses; in advanced cases, ulcerated tumors and infiltrations of lymph nodes may occur.

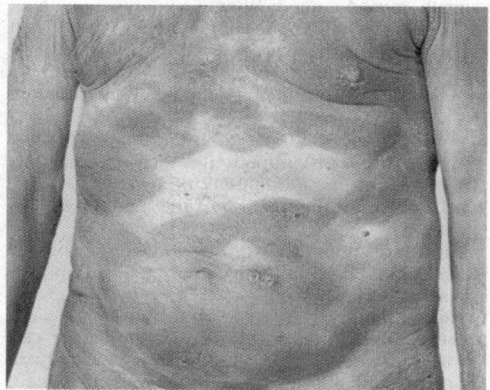

mycosis fungoides

my·cot·ic (mī-kot′ik). Relating to or caused by a fungus.

my·co·tox·i·co·sis (mī′kō-tok-si-kō′sis). Poisoning due to the ingestion of preformed substances produced by the action of certain fungi on particular foodstuffs or ingestion of the fungi themselves; *e.g.,* ergotism. [myco- + G. *toxikon,* poison, + *-osis,* condition]

my·co·tox·ins (mī′kō-tok-sinz). Toxic compounds produced by certain fungi, some of which are used for medicinal purposes; *e.g.,* muscarine, psilocybin.

my·co·vi·rus (mī′kō-vī-rŭs). A virus that infects fungi.

my·dri·a·sis (mi-drī′ă-sis). Dilation of the pupil. [G.]

myd·ri·at·ic (mi-drē-at′ik). **1.** Causing mydriasis or dilation of the pupil. **2.** An agent that dilates the pupil.

my·ec·to·my (mī-ek′tō-mē). Excision of all or part of a muscle. [G. *mys,* muscle, + *ektomē,* excision]

my·ec·to·py, my·ec·to·pia (mī-ek′tō-pē, mī-ek-tō′pē-ă). Rarely used term for dislocation of a muscle. [G. *mys,* muscle, + *ektopos,* out of place]

⌂**myel-, myelo-.** **1.** The bone marrow. **2.** The spinal cord and medulla oblongata. Cf. medullo-. **3.** The myelin sheath of nerve fibers. [G. *myelos,* medulla, marrow]

my·el·ap·o·plexy (mī′el-ap′ō-plek′sē). SYN hematomyelia. [myel- + G. *apoplēxia,* apoplexy]

my·el·a·te·lia (mī′el-ă-tē′lē-ă). Developmental defect of the spinal cord. [myel- + G. *ateleia,* incompleteness]

my·el·en·ceph·a·lon (mī′el-en-sef′ă-lon) [NA]. SYN *medulla* oblongata. [myel- + G. *enkephalos,* brain]

my·e·lin (mī′ĕ-lin). **1.** The lipoproteinaceous material of the myelin sheath, composed of alternating membranes of lipid and protein. **2.** Droplets of lipid formed during autolysis and postmortem decomposition.

my·e·li·nat·ed (mī′ĕ-li-nāt-ed). Having a myelin sheath. SYN medullated (2).

my·e·li·na·tion (mī′ĕ-li-nā′shŭn). The acquisition, development, or formation of a myelin sheath around a nerve fiber.

my·e·li·nol·y·sis (mī′ĕ-li-nol′i-sis). Dissolution of the myelin sheaths of nerve fibers. [myelin + G. *lysis,* dissolution]

my·e·lit·ic (mī-ĕ-lit′ik). Relating to or affected by myelitis.

my·e·li·tis (mī-ĕ-lī′tis). **1.** Inflammation of the spinal cord. **2.** Inflammation of the bone marrow. [myel- + G. *-itis,* inflammation]

   bulbar m., inflammation of the medulla oblongata.

   subacute necrotizing m., a disorder of the lower spinal cord in adult males resulting in progressive paraplegia.

⌂**myelo-.** SEE myel-.

my·e·lo·blast (mī′ĕ-lō-blast). An immature cell in the granulocytic series, occurring normally in bone marrow but not in the blood. When stained, the cytoplasm is light blue and variable in amount; the nucleus deep purple-blue with finely divided, punctate, threadlike chromatin. A few light blue nucleoli in the nucleus generally disappear as the m. matures into a promyelocyte and then a myelocyte. [myelo- + G. *blastos,* germ]

my·e·lo·blas·te·mia (mī′ĕ-lō-blas-tē′mē-ă). The presence of myeloblasts in the circulating blood. [myeloblast + G. *haima,* blood]

my·e·lo·blas·to·ma (mī′ĕ-lō-blas-tō′mă). A nodular focus or fairly well-circumscribed accumulation of myeloblasts, as sometimes observed in acute myeloblastic leukemia and chlorosis. [myeloblast + G. *-oma,* tumor]

my·e·lo·blas·to·sis (mī′ĕ-lō-blas-tō′sis). The presence of unusually large numbers of myeloblasts in the circulating blood, or tissues, or both (as in acute leukemia).

my·e·lo·cele (mī′ĕ-lō-sēl). **1.** Protrusion of the spinal cord in spina bifida. [myelo- + G. *kēlē,* hernia] **2.** The central canal of the spinal cord. [G. *myelos,* marrow, + *koilia,* a hollow]

my·e·lo·cyst (mī′ĕ-lō-sist). Any cyst (usually lined with columnar or cuboidal cells) that develops from a rudimentary medullary canal in the central nervous system. [myelo- + G. *kystis,* bladder]

my·e·lo·cyst·ic (mī′ĕ-lō-sist′ik). Pertaining to or characterized by the presence of a myelocyst.

my·e·lo·cys·to·cele (mī′ĕ-lō-sis′tō-sēl). Spina bifida containing spinal cord substance. [myelo- + G. *kystis,* bladder, + *kēlē,* tumor]

my·e·lo·cys·to·me·ning·o·cele (mī′ĕ-lō-sis′tō-mĕ-ning′gō-sēl). SYN meningomyelocele. [myelo- + G. *kystis,* bladder, + *mēninx (mēning-),* membrane, + *kēlē,* hernia]

my·e·lo·cyte (mī′ĕ-lō-sīt). **1.** A young cell of the granulocytic series, occurring normally in bone marrow, but not in circulating blood. When stained, the cytoplasm is distinctly basophilic and more abundant than in myeloblasts or promyelocytes; numerous cytoplasmic granules are present in the more mature forms. The nucleus is regular in contour (*i.e.,* not indented), and seems to be "buried" beneath the numerous cytoplasmic granules. **2.** A nerve cell of the gray matter of the brain or spinal cord. [myelo- + G. *kytos,* cell]

my·e·lo·cy·the·mia (mī′ĕ-lō-sī-thē′mē-ă). The presence of myelocytes in the circulating blood, especially in persistently large numbers (as in myelocytic leukemia). [myelocyte + G. *haima,* blood]

my·e·lo·cyt·ic (mī′ĕ-lō-sit′ik). Pertaining to or characterized by myelocytes.

my·e·lo·cy·to·ma (mī′ĕ-lō-sī-tō′mă). A nodular focus or fairly well-circumscribed, relatively dense accumulation of myelocytes, as in certain tissues of persons with myelocytic leukemia. [myelo- + G. *-oma,* tumor]

my·e·lo·cy·to·ma·to·sis (mī′ĕ-lō-sī′tō-mă-tō′sis). A form of tumor involving chiefly the myelocytes.

my·e·lo·cy·to·sis (mī′ĕ-lō-sī-tō′sis). The occurrence of abnormally large numbers of myelocytes in the circulating blood, or tissues, or both. [myelocyte + G. *-osis,* condition]

my·e·lo·dys·pla·sia (mī′ĕ-lō-dis-plā′zē-ă). **1.** An abnormality in development of the spinal cord, especially the lower part of the cord. **2.** A disorder within the bone marrow, characterized by the proliferation of abnormal stem cells, that has the potential of developing into a specific type of leukemia. [myelo- + G. *dys-*, difficult, + *plasis*, a molding]

my•e•lo•fi•bro•sis (mī′ĕ-lō-fī-brō′sis). Fibrosis of the bone marrow, especially generalized, associated with myeloid metaplasia of the spleen and other organs, leukoerythroblastic anemia, and thrombocytopenia, although the bone marrow often contains many megakaryocytes. SYN myelosclerosis.

my•e•lo•gen•e•sis (mī′ĕ-lō-jen′ĕ-sis). 1. Development of bone marrow. 2. Development of the central nervous system. 3. Formation of myelin around an axon.

my•e•lo•ge•net•ic, my•e•lo•gen•ic (mī′ĕ-lō-jĕ-net′ik, -jen′ik). 1. Relating to myelogenesis. 2. Produced by or originating in the bone marrow. SYN myelogenous.

my•e•log•e•nous (mī-ĕ-loj′ĕ-nŭs). SYN myelogenetic (2).

my•e•lo•gone, my•e•lo•go•ni•um (mī′ĕ-lō-gōn, mī′ĕ-lo-gō′nē-ŭm). An immature white blood cell of the myeloid series that is characterized by a large, deeply stained, reticulated nucleus and a scant amount of nongranular basophilic cytoplasm. [myelo- + G. *gonē*, seed]

my•e•lo•gram (mī′ĕ-lō-gram). Radiographic contrast study of the spinal subarachnoid space and its contents.

my•e•log•ra•phy (mī′ĕ-log′ră-fē). Radiography of the spinal cord and nerve roots after the injection of a contrast medium into the spinal subarachnoid space. [myelo- + G. *graphē*, a drawing]

my•e•loid (mī′ĕ-loyd). 1. Pertaining to, derived from, or manifesting certain features of the bone marrow. 2. Sometimes used with reference to the spinal cord. 3. Pertaining to certain characteristics of myelocytic forms, but not necessarily implying origin in the bone marrow. [myel- + -oid]

my•e•loi•do•sis (mī′ĕ-loy-dō′sis). General hyperplasia of myeloid tissue.

my•e•lo•li•po•ma (mī′ĕ-lō-li-pō′mă). Nodular foci that are not neoplasms, but probably represent localized proliferation of reticuloendothelial tissue in the adrenal glands; foci of bone marrow containing erythropoietic or myeloid cells.

my•e•lo•ma (mī-ĕ-lō′mă). 1. A tumor composed of cells derived from hemopoietic tissues of the bone marrow. 2. A plasma cell tumor. [myelo- + G. *-oma*, tumor]

   endothelial m., SYN Ewing's *tumor.*

   giant cell m., SYN giant cell *tumor* of bone.

   multiple m., m. mul′tiplex, an uncommon disease that occurs more frequently in men and is associated with anemia, hemorrhage, recurrent infections, and weakness. A malignant neoplasm that originates in bone marrow and involves chiefly the skeleton; characterized by numerous diffuse foci or nodular accumulations of abnormal or malignant plasma cells in the marrow of various bones and abnormal proteins in the serum and urine; the most frequent abnormalities in the metabolism of protein are Bence Jones proteinuria, an increase in monoclonal γ-globulin in the plasma, the formation of cryoglobulin, and a form of primary amyloidosis. SEE ALSO plasma cell m. SYN plasma cell m. (1).

   plasma cell m., (1) SYN multiple m. **(2)** plas-

macytoma of bone, which is usually a solitary lesion and not associated with the occurrence of Bence Jones protein or other disturbances in the metabolism of protein (as observed in multiple m.).

my•e•lo•ma•la•cia (mī′ĕ-lō-ma-lā′shē-ă). Softening of the spinal cord. [myelo- + G. *malakia*, a softness]

my•e•lo•ma•to•sis (mī′ĕ-lō-mă-tō′sis). A disease characterized by the occurrence of myeloma in various sites.

my•e•lo•me•ning•o•cele (mī′ĕ-lō-mĕ-ning′gō-sēl). SYN meningomyelocele. [myelo- + G. *mēninx*, membrane, + *kēlē*, hernia]

my•e•lo•mere (mī′ĕ-lō-mēr). Neuromere of the brain or spinal cord. [myelo- + G. *meros*, part]

my•e•lo•neu•ri•tis (mī′ĕ-lō-nū-rī′tis). SYN neuromyelitis.

my•e•lon•ic (mī-ĕ-lon′ik). Relating to the spinal cord. [G. *myelon*, fr. *myelos*, marrow]

my•e•lo•path•ic (mī′ĕ-lō-path′ik). Relating to myelopathy.

my•e•lop•a•thy (mī-ĕ-lop′ă-thē). 1. Disorder of the spinal cord. 2. A disease of the myelopoietic tissues. [myelo- + G. *pathos*, suffering]

my•e•lop•e•tal (mī-ĕ-lop′ĕ-tăl). Proceeding in a direction toward the spinal cord; said of different nerve impulses. [myelo- + L. *peto*, to seek]

my•e•lo•phthis•ic (mī′ĕ-lō-tiz′ik, -thiz′ik). Relating to or suffering from myelophthisis.

my•e•loph•thi•sis (mī′ĕ-lof′thi-sis, mī′ĕ-lō-tī′sis, -tē′sis). 1. Wasting or atrophy of the spinal cord as in tabes dorsalis. 2. Replacement of hemopoietic tissue in the bone marrow by abnormal tissue, usually fibrous tissue metastatic carcinomas. SYN panmyelophthisis. [myelo- + G. *phthisis*, a wasting away]

my•e•lo•plast (mī′ĕ-lō-plast). Any of the leukocytic series of cells in the bone marrow, especially young forms. [myelo- + G. *plastos*, formed]

my•e•lo•poi•e•sis (mī′ĕ-lō-poy-ē′sis). Formation of the tissue elements of bone marrow, or any of the types of blood cells derived from bone marrow; or both processes. [myelo- + G. *poiēsis*, a making]

my•e•lo•poi•et•ic (mī′ĕ-lō-poy-et′ik). Relating to myelopoiesis.

my•e•lo•pro•lif•er•a•tive (mī′ĕ-lō-prō-lif′er-ă-tiv). Pertaining to or characterized by unusual proliferation of myelopoietic tissue.

my•e•lo•ra•dic•u•li•tis (mī′ĕ-lō-ra-dik-yū-lī′tis). Inflammation of the spinal cord and nerve roots. [myelo- + L. *radicula,* root, + G. *-itis,* inflammation]

my•e•lo•ra•dic•u•lo•dys•pla•sia (mī′ĕ-lō-ra-dik′yū-lō-dis-plā-zē-ă). Congenital maldevelopment of the spinal cord and spinal nerve roots. [myelo- + L. *radicula,* root, + dysplasia]

my•e•lo•ra•dic•u•lop•a•thy (mī′ĕ-lō-ră-dik′yū-lop′ă-thē). Disease involving the spinal cord and nerve roots. SYN radiculomyelopathy. [myelo- + L. *radicula,* root, + G. *pathos,* disease]

my•e•lor•rha•gia (mī′ĕ-lō-rā′jē-ă). SYN hematomyelia. [myelo- + G. *rhēgnymi,* to burst forth]

my•e•lor•rha•phy (mī-ĕ-lōr′ă-fē). Suture of a

my

wound of the spinal cord. [myelo- + G. *rhaphē*, a seam]

my·e·lo·scle·ro·sis (mī'ĕ-lō-skle-rō'sis). SYN myelofibrosis. [myelo- + G. *sklērōsis*, induration]

my·e·lo·sis (mī-ĕ-lō'sis). **1.** A condition characterized by abnormal proliferation of tissue or cellular elements of bone marrow, *e.g.*, multiple myeloma, myelocytic leukemia, myelofibrosis. **2.** A condition in which there is abnormal proliferation of medullary tissue in the spinal cord, as in a glioma.

   chronic erythremic m., SYN myelodysplastic *syndrome.*

   erythremic m., a neoplastic process of erythropoietic tissue, characterized by anemia, irregular fever, splenomegaly, hepatomegaly, hemorrhagic disorders, and numerous erythroblasts in blood. Acute and chronic forms are recognized, but in the latter there is less prominence of the immature cells; the former is also called Di Guglielmo's disease and acute erythremia.

my·e·lot·o·my (mī-ĕ-lot'ō-mē). Incision of the spinal cord. [myelo- + G. *tomē*, incision]

   midline m., section of the midline transverse fibers of the spinal cord for the treatment of intractable pain. SYN commissurotomy (2).

my·e·lo·tox·ic (mī'ĕ-lō-tok'sik). **1.** Inhibitory, depressant, or destructive to one or more of the components of bone marrow. **2.** Pertaining to, derived from, or manifesting the features of diseased bone marrow.

my·en·ter·ic (mī-en-ter'ik). Relating to the myenteron.

my·en·ter·on (mī-en'ter-on). The muscular coat, or muscularis, of the intestine. [G. *mys*, muscle, + *enteron*, intestine]

my·es·the·sia (mī-es-thē'zē-ă). The sensation felt in muscle when it is contracting; awareness of movement or activity in muscles or joints; sense of position or movement mediated in large part by the posterior columns and medial lemniscus. SEE ALSO bathyesthesia. SYN kinesthetic sense, muscular sense. [G. *mys*, muscle, + *aisthēsis*, sensation]

my·i·a·sis (mī-ī'ă-sis). Any infection due to invasion of tissues or cavities of the body by larvae of dipterous insects. [G. *myia*, a fly]

my·lo·hy·oid (mī'lō-hī'oyd). Relating to the molar teeth, or posterior portion of the lower jaw, and to the hyoid bone; denoting various structures. SEE nerve, muscle, region, sulcus. [G. *mylē*, a mill, in pl. *mylai*, molar teeth]

△**myo-.** Muscle. [G. *mys*, muscle]

my·o·ar·chi·tec·ton·ic (mī'ō-ar'ki-tek-ton'ik). Relating to the structural arrangement of muscle or of fibers in general. [myo- + G. *architektonikos*, relating to construction]

my·o·blast (mī'ō-blast). A primitive muscle cell with the potentiality of developing into a muscle fiber. SYN sarcoblast. [myo- + G. *blastos*, germ]

my·o·blas·tic (mī-ō-blas'tik). Relating to a myoblast or to the mode of formation of muscle cells.

my·o·blas·to·ma (mī'ō-blas-tō'mă). A tumor of immature muscle cells. [myo- + G. *blastos*, germ, + *-oma*, tumor]

my·o·bra·dia (mī-ō-brā'dē-ă). Sluggish reaction

of muscle to stimulation. [myo- + G. *bradys*, slow]

my·o·car·di·al (mī-ō-kar'dē-ăl). Relating to the myocardium.

my·o·car·di·o·graph (mī'ō-kar'dē-ō-graf). An instrument composed of a tambour with recording lever attachment, by which a tracing is made of the movements of the heart muscle. [myo- + G. *kardia*, heart, + *graphō*, to record]

my·o·car·di·op·a·thy (mī'ō-kar-dē-op'ă-thē). SYN cardiomyopathy. [myocardium + G. *pathos*, suffering]

my·o·car·di·tis (mī'ō-kar-dī'tis). Inflammation of the muscular walls of the heart.

   acute isolated m., an acute interstitial m. of unknown cause, the endocardium and pericardium being unaffected.

my·o·car·di·um, pl. **my·o·car·dia** (mī-ō-kar'dē-ŭm, -kar'dē-ă) [NA]. The middle layer of the heart, consisting of cardiac muscle. [myo- + G. *kardia*, heart]

my·o·cele (mī'ō-sēl). **1.** Protrusion of muscle substance through a rent in its sheath. [myo- + G. *kēlē*, hernia] **2.** The small cavity that appears in somites. [myo- + G. *koilia*, a cavity]

my·o·cel·lu·li·tis (mī'ō-sel-yū-lī'tis). Inflammation of muscle and cellular tissue. [myo- + Mod. L. *cellularis*, cellular (tissue), + G. *-itis*, inflammation]

my·o·ce·ro·sis (mī'ō-sē-rō'sis). Waxy degeneration of the muscles. [myo- + G. *kēros*, wax]

my·o·clo·nia (mī'ō-klō'nē-ă). Any disorder characterized by myoclonus. [myo- + G. *klonos*, tumult]

my·o·clon·ic (mī-ō-klon'ik). Showing myoclonus.

my·oc·lo·nus (mī-ok'lō-nŭs, mī-ō-klo'nŭs). One or a series of shock like contractions of a group of muscles, of variable regularity, synchrony, and symmetry, generally due to a central nervous system lesion. [myo- + G. *klonos*, tumult]

   m. mul'tiplex, an ill-defined disorder marked by rapid and widespread muscle contractions. SYN polyclonia, polymyoclonus.

   nocturnal m., frequently repeated muscular jerks occurring at the moment of dropping off to sleep.

   stimulus sensitive m., m. induced by a variety of stimuli, *e.g.*, talking, calculation, loud noises, tapping, etc.

my·o·cu·ta·ne·ous (mī-ō-kyū-tā'nē-ŭs). SYN musculocutaneous. [myo- + L. *cutis*, skin]

my·o·cyte (mī'ō-sīt). A muscle cell. [myo- + G. *kytos*, cell]

   Anitschkow m., SYN cardiac histiocyte.

my·o·cy·tol·y·sis (mī-ō-sī-tol'i-sis). Dissolution of muscle fiber. [myo- + G. *kytos*, cell, + *lysis*, loosening]

my·o·cy·to·ma (mī'ō-sī-tō'mă). A benign neoplasm derived from muscle.

my·o·de·mia (mī-ō-dē'mē-ă). Fatty degeneration of muscle. [myo- + G. *dēmos*, tallow]

my·o·dyn·ia (mī'ō-din'ē-ă). SYN myalgia. [myo- + G. *odynē*, pain]

my·o·dys·to·ny (mī-ō-dis'tō-nē). A condition of slow relaxation, interrupted by a succession of slight contractions, following electrical stimulation of a muscle. [myo- + G. *dys-*, difficult, + *tonos*, tone, tension]

my•o•dys•tro•phy, my•o•dys•tro•phia (mī-ō-dis'trō-fē, mī'-ō-dis-trō'fē-ă). SYN muscular *dystrophy*. [myo- + G. *dys-*, difficult, poor, + *trophē*, nourishment]

my•o•e•de•ma (mī'ō-e-dē'mă). A localized contraction of a degenerating muscle, occurring at the point of a sharp blow, independent of the nerve supply. SYN idiomuscular contraction, mounding. [myo- + G. *oidēma*, swelling]

my•o•e•las•tic (mī'ō-e-las'tik). Pertaining to closely associated smooth muscle fibers and elastic connective tissue.

my•o•en•do•car•di•tis (mī-ō-en'dō-kar-dī'tis). Inflammation of the muscular wall and lining membrane of the heart. [myo- + G. *endon*, within, + *kardia*, heart, + *-itis*, inflammation]

my•o•ep•i•the•li•al (mī'ō-ep-i-thē'lē-ăl). Relating to myoepithelium.

my•o•ep•i•the•li•o•ma (mī'ō-ep-i-thē-lē-ō'mă). A benign tumor of myoepithelial cells. [myo- + epithelium, + G. *-ōma*, tumor]

my•o•ep•i•the•li•um (mī'ō-ep-i-thē'lē-ŭm). Spindle-shaped, contractile, smooth muscle-like cells of epithelial origin that are arranged longitudinally or obliquely around sweat glands and the secretory alveoli of the mammary gland; stellate myoepithelial cells occur around lacrimal and some salivary gland secretory units. [myo- + epithelium]

my•o•fas•ci•al (mī-ō-fash'ē-ăl). Of or relating to the fascia surrounding and separating muscle tissue.

my•o•fas•ci•tis (mī'ō-fă-sī'tis). SYN *myositis* fibrosa.

my•o•fi•bril (mī-ō-fī'bril). One of the fine longitudinal fibrils occurring in a skeletal or cardiac muscle fiber comprising many regularly overlapped ultramicroscopic thick and thin myofilaments. [myo- + Mod. L. *fibrilla*, fibril]

my•o•fi•bro•blast (mī-ō-fī'brō-blast). A cell thought to be responsible for contracture of wounds; such cells have some characteristics of smooth muscle, such as contractile properties and fibrils, and are also believed to produce, temporarily, type III collagen.

my•o•fi•bro•ma (mī'ō-fī-brō'mă). A benign neoplasm that consists chiefly of fibrous connective tissue, with variable numbers of muscle cells forming portions of the neoplasm.

my•o•fi•bro•sis (mī'ō-fī-brō'sis). Chronic myositis with diffuse hyperplasia of the interstitial connective tissue pressing upon and causing atrophy of the muscular tissue.

my•o•fi•bro•si•tis (mī'ō-fī-brō-sī'tis). Inflammation of the perimysium.

my•o•fil•a•ments (mī-ō-fil'ă-ments). The ultramicroscopic threads of filamentous proteins making up myofibrils in striated muscle. Thick ones contain myosin and thin ones actin; thick and thin m.'s also occur in smooth muscle fibers but are not regularly arranged in discrete myofibrils and thus do not impart a striated appearance to these cells.

my•o•gen•e•sis (mī-ō-jen'ĕ-sis). Embryonic for-

mation of muscle cells or fibers. [myo- + G. *genesis*, origin]

my•o•ge•net•ic, my•o•gen•ic (mī-ō-jĕ-net'ik, -jen'ik). **1.** Originating in or starting from muscle. **2.** Relating to the origin of muscle cells or fibers. SYN myogenous.

my•og•e•nous (mī-oj'ĕ-nŭs). SYN myogenetic.

my•o•glo•bin (MbO₂, Mb) (mī-ō-glō'bin). The oxygen-transporting and storage protein of muscle, resembling blood hemoglobin in function but with a molecular weight approximately one-quarter that of hemoglobin. Serum levels of this protein are often measured to assist in diagnosing an acute myocardial infarction; it is released into the circulation within 2–4 hours after myocardial infarction, peaks at about 8–12 hours, and returns to normal after 18–24 hours. SEE ALSO oxymyoglobin. SYN muscle hemoglobin. [myo- + hemoglobin]

my•o•glo•bi•nu•ria (mī'ō-glō-bi-nū'rē-ă). Excretion of myoglobin in the urine; results from muscle degeneration, which releases myoglobin into the blood; occurs in certain types of trauma (crush syndrome), advanced or protracted ischemia of muscle, or as a paroxysmal process of unknown etiology.

my•o•glob•u•lin (mī-ō-glob'yū-lin). Globulin present in muscle tissue.

my•o•glob•u•li•nu•ria (mī'ō-glob'yū-li-nū'rē-ă). The excretion of myoglobulin in the urine.

my•o•gram (mī'ō-gram). The tracing made by a myograph. [myo- + G. *gramma*, a drawing]

my•o•graph (mī'ō-graf). A recording instrument by which tracings are made of muscular contractions. [myo- + G. *graphō*, to write]

my•o•graph•ic (mī-ō-graf'ik). Relating to a myogram, or the record of a myograph.

my•og•ra•phy (mī-og'ră-fē). **1.** The recording of muscular movements by the myograph. **2.** A description of or treatise on the muscles.

my•oid (mī'oyd). **1.** Resembling muscle. **2.** One of the fine, contractile, threadlike protoplasmic elements found in certain epithelial cells in lower animals. [myo- + G. *eidos*, appearance]

my•o•kin•e•sim•e•ter (mī'ō-kin-ĕ-sim'ĕ-ter). A device for registering the exact time and extent of contraction of the larger muscles of the lower extremity in response to electric stimulation. [myo- + G. *kinesis*, movement, + *metron*, measure]

my•o•ky•mia (mī-ō-kī'mē-ă). Continuous involuntary quivering or rippling of muscles at rest, caused by spontaneous, repetitive firing of groups of motor unit potentials. SYN kymatism. [myo- + G. *kyma*, wave]

my•o•li•po•ma (mī'ō-li-pō'mă). A benign neoplasm that consists chiefly of fat cells (adipose tissue), with variable numbers of muscle cells forming portions of the neoplasm.

my•ol•o•gy (mī-ol'ō-jē). The branch of science concerned with the muscles and their accessory parts, tendons, aponeuroses, bursae, and fasciae. [myo- + G. *logos*, study]

my•ol•y•sis (mī-ol'i-sis). Dissolution or liquefaction of muscular tissue, frequently preceded by degenerative changes such as infiltration of fat, atrophy, and fatty degeneration. [myo- + G. *lysis*, dissolution]

my•o•ma (mī-ō′mă). A benign neoplasm of muscular tissue. SEE ALSO leiomyoma, rhabdomyoma. [myo- + G. *-oma*, tumor]

my•o•ma•la•cia (mī′ō-mă-lā′shē-ă). Pathologic softening of muscular tissue. [myo- + G. *malakia*, softness]

my•o•ma•tous (mī-ō′mă-tŭs). Pertaining to or characterized by the features of a myoma.

my•o•mec•to•my (mī-ō-mek′tō-mē). Operative removal of a myoma, specifically of a uterine myoma. [myoma + G. *ektomē*, excision]

my•o•mel•a•no•sis (mī′ō-melă-nō′sis). Abnormal dark pigmentation of muscular tissue. SEE ALSO melanosis. [myo- + G. *melanōsis*, becoming black]

my•o•mere (mī′ō-mēr). SYN myotome (4). [myo- + G. *meros*, a part]

my•om•e•ter (mī-om′ĕ-ter). An instrument for measuring the extent of a muscular contraction. [myo- + G. *metron*, measure]

my•o•me•tri•al (mī-ō-mē′trē-ăl). Relating to the myometrium.

my•o•me•tri•tis (mī′ō-mē-trī′tis). Inflammation of the muscular wall of the uterus. [myo- + G. *mētra*, uterus, + *-itis*, inflammation]

my•o•me•tri•um (mī′ō-mē′trē-ŭm) [NA]. The muscular wall of the uterus. [myo- + G. *mētra*, uterus]

my•o•ne•cro•sis (mī′ō-nĕ-krō′sis). Necrosis of muscle.

my•o•neme (mī′ō-nēm). **1.** A muscle fibril. **2.** One of the contractile fibrils of certain protozoans; thought to function in an analogous fashion to metazoan muscle fibers. [myo- + G. *nēma*, thread]

my•o•neu•ral (mī-ō-nū′răl). Relating to both muscle and nerve; denoting specifically the synapse of the motor neuron with striated muscle fibers: myoneural junction or motor endplate. SEE ALSO neuromuscular. [myo- + G. *neuron*, nerve]

my•o•pal•mus (mī-ō-pal′mŭs). Muscle twitching. [myo- + G. *palmos*, a quivering]

my•o•pa•ral•y•sis (mī-ō-pă-ral′i-sis). Muscular paralysis.

my•o•pa•re•sis (mī′ō-pă-rē′sis, -par′ē-sis). Slight muscular paralysis.

my•o•path•ic (mī-ō-path′ik). Denoting a disorder involving muscular tissue.

my•op•a•thy (mī-op′ă-thē). Any abnormal condition or disease of the muscular tissues; commonly designates a disorder involving skeletal muscle. [myo- + G. *pathos*, suffering]

my•o•per•i•car•di•tis (mī′ō-per-i-kar-dī′tis). Inflammation of the muscular wall of the heart and of the enveloping pericardium; also, perimyocarditis. [myo- + pericarditis]

▣ **my•o•pia** (mī-ō′pē-ă). That optical condition in which only rays from a finite distance from the eye focus on the retina. SYN nearsightedness, shortsightedness. [G. fr. *myo*, to shut, + *ōps*, eye]
  curvature m., m. due to refractive errors resulting from excessive corneal curvature.
  pathologic m., progressive m. marked by fundus changes, posterior staphyloma, and subnormal corrected acuity.

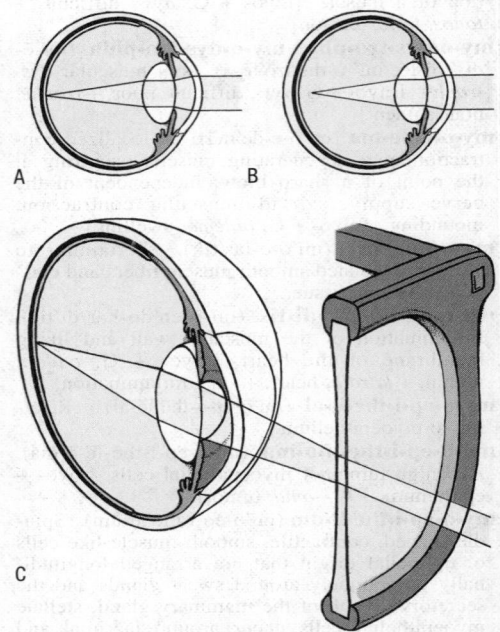

myopia: (A) normal (20/20) vision, light rays focus sharply on retina; (B) myopic (nearsighted) vision, light rays from a distance come to sharp focus in front of the retina; (C) myopia corrected by eyeglasses with concave lenses

my•o•pic (mī-op′ik, -ō′pik). Relating to or suffering from myopia.

my•o•plasm (mī′ō-plazm). The contractile portion of the muscle cell, as distinguished from the sarcoplasm. [myo- + G. *plasma*, a thing formed]

my•o•plas•tic (mī-ō-plas′tik). Relating to the plastic surgery of the muscles, or to the use of muscular tissue in correcting defects.

my•o•plas•ty (mī′ō-plas-tē). Plastic surgery of muscular tissue. [myo- + G. *plastos*, formed]

my•or•rha•phy (mī-ōr′ă-fē). Suture of a muscle. [myo- + G. *rhaphē*, seam]

my•or•rhex•is (mī-ō-rek′sis). Tearing of a muscle. [myo- + G. *rhēxis*, a rupture]

my•o•sal•pinx (mī′ō-sal′pingks). The muscular tunic of the uterine tube. [myo- + salpinx]

my•o•sar•co•ma (mī′ō-sar-kō′mă). A general term for a malignant neoplasm derived from muscular tissue. SEE ALSO leiomyosarcoma, rhabdomyosarcoma.

my•o•scle•ro•sis (mī′ō-skle-rō′sis). Chronic myositis with hyperplasia of the interstitial connective tissue.

my•o•sin (mī′ō-sin). A globulin present in muscle; in combination with actin, it forms actomyosin; m. forms the thick filaments in muscle.

my•o•sit•ic (mī-ō-sit′ik). Relating to myositis.

my•o•si•tis (mī-ō-sī′tis). Inflammation of a muscle. SYN initis (2). [myo- + G. *-itis*, inflammation]

epidemic m., m. epidem′ica acu′ta, SYN epidemic *pleurodynia*.

m. fibro′sa, induration of a muscle through an interstitial growth of fibrous tissue. SYN myofascitis.

multiple m., the occurrence of multiple foci of acute inflammation in the muscular tissue and overlying skin in various parts of the body, accompanied by fever and other signs of systemic infection. SEE ALSO dermatomyositis.

m. ossif′icans, ossification or deposit of bone in muscle with fibrosis, causing pain and swelling in muscles.

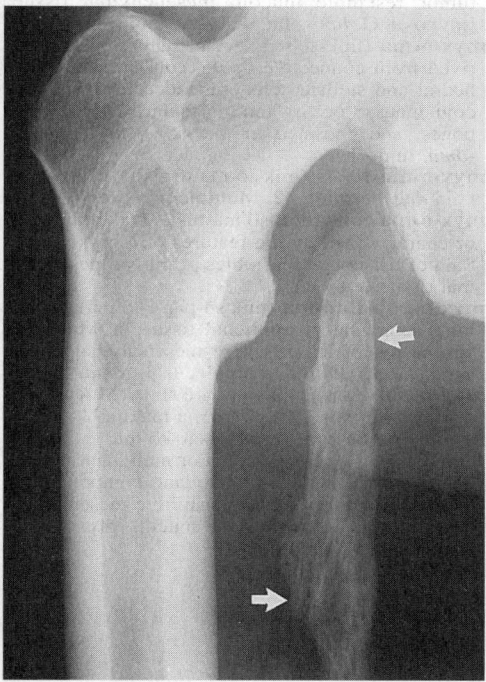

myositis ossificans: Prussian's disease; well-organized ossifying hematoma present in the adductor magnus muscle (arrows)

my·o·spasm, my·o·spas·mus (mī′ō-spazm, mī-ō-spaz′mŭs). Spasmodic muscular contraction.

my·o·tac·tic (mī-ō-tak′tik). Relating to the muscular sense. [myo- + L. *tactus,* a touching]

my·ot·a·sis (mī-ot′ă-sis). Stretching of a muscle. [myo- + G. *tasis,* a stretching]

my·o·tat·ic (mī-ō-tat′ik). Relating to myotasis.

my·o·ten·o·si·tis (mī′ō-te-nō-sī′tis). Inflammation of a muscle with its tendon. [myo- + G. *tenōn,* tendon, + *-itis,* inflammation]

my·o·te·not·o·my (mī′ō-te-not′ō-mē). Cutting through the principal tendon of a muscle, with division of the muscle itself in whole or in part. SYN tenomyotomy. [myo- + G. *tenōn,* tendon, + *tomē,* incision]

my·o·tome (mī′ō-tōm). 1. A knife for dividing muscle. 2. In embryos, that part of the somite that develops into skeletal muscle. SYN muscle plate.

3. All muscles derived from one somite and innervated by one segmental spinal nerve. **4.** In primitive vertebrates, the muscular part of a metamere. SYN myomere. [myo- + G. *tomos,* a cut]

my·ot·o·my (mī-ot′ō-mē). **1.** Anatomy or dissection of the muscles. **2.** Surgical division of a muscle. [myo- + G. *tomē,* excision]

my·o·to·nia (mī-ō-tō′nē-ă). Delayed relaxation of a muscle after a strong contraction, or prolonged contraction after mechanical stimulation (as by percussion) or brief electrical stimulation; due to abnormality of the muscle membrane, specifically the ion channels. [myo- + G. *tonos,* tension, stretching]

m. congen′ita [MIM*160800], a hereditary disease marked by momentary tonic spasms occurring when a voluntary movement is attempted.

my·o·ton·ic (mī-ō-ton′ik). Pertaining to or exhibiting myotonia.

my·ot·o·noid (mī-ot′ŏ-noyd). Denoting a muscular reaction, naturally or electrically excited, characterized by slow contraction and, especially, slow relaxation. [myo- + G. *tonos,* tone, tension, + *eidos,* resemblance]

my·ot·o·nus (mī-ot′ŏ-nŭs). A tonic spasm or temporary rigidity of a muscle or group of muscles. [myo- + G. *tonos,* tension, stretching]

my·ot·o·ny (mī-ot′ŏ-nē). Muscular tonus or tension. [myo- + G. *tonos,* tension]

my·ot·ro·phy (mī-ot′rō-fē). Nutrition of muscular tissue. [myo- + G. *trophē,* nourishment]

my·o·tube (mī′ō-tūb). A skeletal muscle fiber formed by the fusion of myoblasts during a developmental stage.

△**myring-.** SEE myringo-.

my·rin·ga (mi-ring′gă). SYN tympanic *membrane.* [Mod. L. drum membrane]

myr·in·gec·to·my (mir-in-jek′tō-mē). Excision of the tympanic membrane. [myring- + G. *ektomē,* excision]

myr·in·gi·tis (mir-in-jī′tis). Inflammation of the tympanic membrane. SYN tympanitis. [myring- + G. *-itis,* inflammation]

△**myringo-, myring-.** The membrana tympani. [Mod. L. *myringa*]

my·rin·go·plas·ty (mi-ring′gō-plas′tē). Operative repair of a damaged tympanic membrane. [myringo- + G. *plassō,* to form]

my·rin·go·sta·pe·di·o·pexy (mi-ring′gō-stā-pē′dē-ō-pek′sē). A technique of tympanoplasty in which the drum membrane or grafted drum membrane is brought into functional connection with the stapes. [*myringo-* + L. *stapes,* stirrup (stapes), + G. *pēxis,* fixation]

myr·in·got·o·my (mir-ing-got′ō-mē). Paracentesis of the tympanic membrane. SYN tympanostomy, tympanotomy. [myringo- + G. *tomē,* excision]

my·rinx (mī′ringks, mir′ringks). SYN tympanic *membrane.* [Mod. L. *myringa,* drum membrane]

myr·me·cia (mir-mē′shē-ă). A form of viral wart in which the lesion has a domed surface (*i.e.,* an ant hill configuration). [G. *murmex,* ant]

my·so·phil·ia (mī-sō-fil′ē-ă). Sexual interest in excretions. [G. *mysos,* defilement, + *philos,* fond]

my·so·pho·bia (mī-sō-fō′bē-ă). Morbid fear of

my

dirt or defilement from touching familiar objects. [G. *mysos*, defilement, + *phobos*, fear]

myx•ad•e•no•ma (mik-sad-ĕ-nō'mă). A benign neoplasm derived from glandular epithelial tissue.

myx•as•the•nia (mik-sas-thē'nē-ă). Faulty secretion of mucus. [myx- + G. *astheneia*, weakness]

myx•e•de•ma (mik-se-dē'mă). Hypothyroidism characterized by hard edema of subcutaneous tissue, somnolence, slow mentation, dryness and loss of hair, subnormal temperature, hoarseness, muscle weakness, and slow return of a muscle to the neutral position after a tendon jerk; usually caused by removal or loss of functioning thyroid tissue. [myx- + G. *oidēma*, swelling]

circumscribed m., nodules and plaques of mucoid edema of the skin, usually in the pretibial region, occurring in some patients with hyperthyroidism. SYN pretibial m.

pituitary m., m. resulting from inadequate secretion of the thyrotropic hormone; commonly occurs in association with inadequate secretion of other anterior pituitary hormones.

pretibial m., SYN circumscribed m.

myx•e•de•ma•toid (mik-sĕ-dem'ă-toyd). Resembling myxedema.

myx•e•dem•a•tous (mik-sĕ-dem'ă-tŭs). Relating to myxedema.

myx•o•chon•dro•fi•bro•sar•co•ma (mik'sō-kon'drō-fī'brō-sar-kō'mă). A malignant neoplasm derived from fibrous connective tissue in which there are foci of cartilaginous and myxomatous tissue. [myxo- + G. *chondros*, cartilage, + L. *fibra*, fiber, + G. *sarx*, flesh, + *-ōma*, tumor]

myx•o•chon•dro•ma (mik'sō-kon-drō'mă). A benign neoplasm of cartilaginous tissue in which the stroma resembles primitive mesenchymal tissue. [myxo- + G. *chondros*, cartilage, + *-ōma*, tumor]

myx•o•cyte (mik'sō-sīt). One of the stellate or polyhedral cells present in mucous tissue. [myxo- + G. *kytos*, cell]

myx•o•fi•bro•ma (mik'sō-fī-brō'mă). A benign neoplasm of fibrous connective tissue that resembles primitive mesenchymal tissue. [myxo- + L. *fibra*, fiber, + G. *-ōma*, tumor]

myx•o•fi•bro•sar•co•ma (mik'sō-fī'brō-sar-kō'mă). A malignant fibrous histiocytoma with a predominance of myxoid areas that resemble primitive mesenchymal tissue. [myxo- + L. *fibra*, fiber, + G. *sarx*, flesh, + *-ōma*, tumor]

myx•oid (mik'soyd). Resembling mucus. [myxo- + G. *eidos*, resemblance]

myx•o•li•po•ma (mik'sō-li-pō'mă). A benign neoplasm of adipose tissue in which portions of the tumor resemble mucoid mesenchymal tissue. [myxo- + G. *lipos*, fat, + *-ōma*, tumor]

myx•o•ma (mik-sō'mă). A benign neoplasm derived from connective tissue, consisting of polyhedral and stellate cells embedded in a soft mucoid matrix; occurs intramuscularly, in the jaw bones, and encysted in the skin. [myxo- + G. *-ōma*, tumor]

myx•o•ma•to•sis (mik'sō-mă-tō'sis). 1. SYN mucoid *degeneration*. 2. Multiple myxomas.

myx•o•ma•tous (mik-sō'mă-tŭs). 1. Pertaining to or characterized by the features of a myxoma. 2. Said of tissue that resembles primitive mesenchymal tissue.

myx•o•pap•il•lo•ma (mik'sō-pap-i-lō'mă). A benign neoplasm of epithelial tissue in which the stroma resembles primitive mesenchymal tissue. [myxo- + L. *papilla*, a nipple, + G. *-ōma*, tumor]

myx•o•poi•e•sis (mik'sō-poy-ē'sis). Mucus production. [myxo- + G. *poiēsis*, a making]

myx•o•sar•co•ma (mik'sō-sar-kō'mă). A sarcoma, usually a liposarcoma or malignant fibrous histiocytoma, with an abundant component of myxoid tissue resembling primitive mesenchyme containing connective tissue mucin. [myxo- + G. *sarx*, flesh, + *-ōma*, tumor]

ν nu. SEE nu.

N_A Avogadro's *number*.

n nano- (2); reaction order.

N normal *concentration*. SEE normal (3).

n. **1.** The number in a scientific study. Sample size. **2.** Symbol for refractive *index*.

NA Nomina Anatomica.

na·cre·ous (nā′krē-ŭs). Lustrous, like mother-of-pearl; descriptive term for bacterial colonies. [Fr. *nacre*, mother-of-pearl]

NAD nicotinamide adenine dinucleotide.

NAD⁺ nicotinamide adenine dinucleotide (oxidized form).

NADH nicotinamide adenine dinucleotide (reduced form).

NADP nicotinamide adenine dinucleotide phosphate.

NADP⁺ nicotinamide adenine dinucleotide phosphate (oxidized form).

NADPH nicotinamide adenine dinucleotide phosphate (reduced form).

nail (nāl). **1.** One of the thin, horny, translucent plates covering the dorsal surface of the distal end of each terminal phalanx of fingers and toes. A nail consists of corpus or body, the visible part, and radix or root at the proximal end concealed under a fold of skin. The under part of the nail is formed from the stratum germinativum of the epidermis, the free surface from the stratum lucidum, the thin cuticular fold overlapping the lunula representing the stratum corneum. **2.** A slender rod of metal, bone, or other solid substance, used in operations to fasten together the divided extremities of a broken bone. SYN unguis [NA], onyx. [A.S. *naegel*]

  azure lunules of n.'s, bluish nonblanching discoloration of the lunules of all the fingernails, in hepatolenticular degeneration.

  half and half n., division of the n. by a transverse line into a proximal dull white part and a distal pink or brown part; seen in uremia.

  hippocratic n.'s, the coarse curved n.'s capping clubbed digits (hippocratic fingers).

  ingrown n., a toenail, one edge of which is overgrown by the nailfold, producing a pyogenic granuloma; due to faulty trimming of the toenails or pressure from a tight shoe.

  pincer n., transverse overcurvature of the n. that increases distally, causing the lateral borders of the n. to pinch the soft tissue with resulting tenderness; may result from a developmental anomaly or subungual exostosis.

  shell n., nail dystrophy accompanying clubbing of digits in bronchiectasis, with excessive longitudinal curvature of the nail plate and atrophy of the nail bed and underlying bone.

  spoon n., SYN koilonychia.

nan·ism (nan′izm). dwarfism. [G. *nanos*; L. *nanus*, dwarf]

△**nano-.** **1.** dwarfism (nanism). **2 (n).** Prefix used in the SI and metric systems to signify one-billionth (10^{-9}). [G. *nanos*, dwarf]

nan·o·ceph·a·lous, nan·o·ce·phal·ic (nan-ō-sef′ă-lŭs, -se-fal′ik). SYN microcephalic.

nan·o·ceph·a·ly (nan-ō-sef′ă-lē). SYN microcephaly. [nano- + G. *kephalē*, head]

nan·o·cor·mia (nan-ō-kōr′mē-ă). SYN microsomia. [nano- + G. *kormos*, trunk]

nan·o·gram (ng) (nan′ō-gram). One-billionth of a gram (10^{-9} g).

nan·o·me·lia (nan-ō-mē′lē-ă). SYN micromelia. [nano- + G. *melos*, limb]

nan·o·me·ter (nm) (năn-om′ĕ-ter). One-billionth of a meter (10^{-9} m).

nape (nāp). SYN nucha.

naph·thol yel·low S [C.I. 10316]. An acid dye used as a stain for basic proteins in microspectrophotometry.

nar·cis·sism (nar-sis′izm, nar′si-sizm). **1.** Sexual attraction toward one's own person. **2.** A state in which the individual interprets and regards everything in relation to himself or herself and not to other persons or things. SYN self-love. [*Narkissos*, G. myth. char.]

△**narco-.** Stupor, narcosis. [G. *narkoō*, to benumb, deaden]

nar·co·a·nal·y·sis (nar′kō-ă-nal′i-sis). Psychotherapeutic treatment under light anesthesia. SYN narcosynthesis.

nar·co·hyp·nia (nar-kō-hip′nē-ă). A general numbness sometimes experienced at the moment of waking. [narco- + G. *hypnos*, sleep]

nar·co·hyp·no·sis (nar′kō-hip-nō′sis). Stupor or deep sleep induced by hypnosis. [narco- + G. *hypnos*, sleep]

nar·co·lep·sy (nar′kō-lep-sē). A sleep disorder that usually appears in young adulthood, consisting of recurring episodes of sleep during the day, and often disrupted nocturnal sleep; frequently accompanied by cataplexy, sleep paralysis, and hypnagogic hallucinations; a genetically determined disease. [narco- + G. *lēpsis*, seizure]

nar·co·sis (nar-kō′sis). General and nonspecific reversible depression of neuronal excitability, produced by a number of physical and chemical agents, usually resulting in stupor rather than in anesthesia (with which n. was once synonymous). [G. a benumbing]

  nitrogen n., (1) n. produced by nitrogenous materials such as occurs in certain forms of uremia and hepatic coma; (2) the stuporous condition characterized by disorientation and by loss of judgment and skill, attributed to an increased partial pressure of nitrogen in the inspired air of deepsea divers during underwater operations. Commonly referred to as "rapture of the deep."

nar·co·syn·the·sis (nar-kō-sin′thĕ-sis). SYN narcoanalysis.

nar·co·ther·a·py (nar-kō-thār′ă-pē). Psychotherapy conducted with the patient under the influence of a sedative or narcotic.

nar·cot·ic (nar-kot′ik). **1.** Any drug derived from opium or opium-like compounds with potent analgesic effects associated with both significant alteration of mood and behavior and potential for dependence and tolerance. **2.** Any drug, synthetic or naturally occurring, with effects similar to those of opium and opium derivatives. **3.** Capable of inducing a state of stuporous analgesia. [G. *narkōtikos,* benumbing]

na·ris, pl. **na·res** (nā′ris, -rēz) [NA]. SYN nostril. [L.]

na·sal (nā′zăl). Relating to the nose. SYN rhinal. [L. *nasus,* nose]

nas·cent (nas′ent, nā′sent). **1.** Beginning; being born or produced. **2.** Denoting the state of a chemical element at the moment it is set free from one of its compounds. [L. *nascor,* pres. p. *nascens,* to be born]

na·si·on (nā′zē-on) [NA]. A point on the skull corresponding to the middle of the nasofrontal suture. SYN nasal point. [L. *nasus,* nose]

⚠**naso-.** The nose. [L. *nasus*]

na·so·an·tral (nā′zō-an′trăl). Relating to the nose and the maxillary sinus.

na·so·fron·tal (nā-zō-frŭn′tăl). Relating to the nose and forehead, or to the nasal cavity and frontal sinuses.

na·so·gas·tric (nā-zō-gas′trik). Pertaining to or involving the nasal passages and the stomach, as in n. intubation.

na·so·la·bi·al (nā-zō-lā′bē-ăl). Relating to the nose and upper lip. [naso- + L. *labium,* lip]

na·so·lac·ri·mal (nā-zō-lak′ri-măl). Relating to the nasal and the lacrimal bones, or to the nasal cavity and the lacrimal ducts.

na·so·oral (nā-zō-ō′răl). Relating to the nose and mouth.

na·so·pal·a·tine (nā′zō-pal′ă-tēn, -tin). Relating to the nose and the palate.

na·so·pha·ryn·ge·al (nā′zō-fă-rin′jē-ăl). Relating to the nose or nasal cavity and the pharynx.

na·so·pha·ryn·go·la·ryn·go·scope (nā′zō-fa-ring′gō-lă-ring′gō-skōp). An instrument, often of fiberoptic type, used to visualize the upper airways and pharynx.

na·so·pha·ryn·gos·co·py (nā′zō-fa-ring-gos′kŏ-pē). Examination of the nasopharynx by flexible or rigid optical instruments, or with a mirror. [nasopharynx + G. *skopeō,* to view]

na·so·pha·rynx (nā′zō-far′ingks). The part of the pharynx that lies above the soft palate; anteriorly it opens into the nasal cavity; inferiorly, it communicates with the oropharynx via the pharyngeal isthmus; laterally it communicates with tympanic cavities via auditory tubes. SYN epipharynx.

na·so·si·nu·si·tis (nā′zō-sī-nŭ-sī′tis). Inflammation of the nasal cavities and of the accessory sinuses.

Nasse's law. See under law.

na·sus (nā′sŭs) [NA]. **1.** SYN external *nose.* **2.** SYN nose. [L.]

na·tal (nā′tăl). **1.** Relating to birth. [L. *natalis,* fr. *nascor,* pp. *natus,* to be born] **2.** Relating to the buttocks or nates. [L. *nates,* buttocks]

na·tal·i·ty (nā-tal′i-tē). The birth rate; the ratio of births to the general population. [see natal (1)]

na·tes (nā′tēz) [NA]. SYN buttocks. [L. pl. of *natis*]

na·ti·mor·tal·i·ty (nā′ti-mōr-tal′i-tē). The perinatal death rate; the proportion of fetal and neonatal deaths to the general natality. [L. *natus,* birth, + *mortalitas,* fr. *mors,* death]

Na·tion·al For·mu·lary. An official compendium formerly issued by the American Pharmaceutical Association but now published by the United States Pharmacopeial Convention for the purpose of providing standards and specifications that can be used to evaluate the quality of pharmaceuticals and therapeutic agents.

na·tre·mia, na·tri·e·mia (nā-trē′mē-ă, nā′trē-ē′mē-ă). The presence of sodium in the blood. [natrium, sodium, + G. *haima,* blood]

na·trif·er·ic (nā-trif′er-ik). Tending to increase sodium transport. [natrium + L. *fero,* to carry]

na·tri·um (nā′trē-ŭm). SYN sodium. [Ar. *natrūm,* fr. G. *nitron,* carbonate of soda]

na·tri·u·re·sis (nā′trē-yū-rē′sis). Urinary excretion of sodium; commonly designates enhanced sodium excretion, which may occur in certain diseases or as a result of the administration of diuretic drugs. [natrium + G. *ouron,* urine]

na·tri·u·ret·ic (nā′trē-yū-ret′ik). **1.** Pertaining to or characterized by natriuresis. **2.** A substance that increases urinary excretion of sodium, usually as a result of decreased tubular reabsorption of sodium ions from glomerular filtrate.

na·tur·o·path·ic (nā′chūr-ō-path′ik). Relating to or by means of naturopathy.

na·tur·op·a·thy (nā-chūr-op′ă-thē). A system of therapeutics in which neither surgical nor medicinal agents are used, dependence being placed only on natural (nonmedicinal) forces.

nau·sea (naw′zē-ă, -zhă). A feeling of being sick at the stomach; an inclination to vomit. [L. fr. G. *nausia,* seasickness, fr. *naus,* ship]

  n. gravida′rum, SYN morning *sickness.*

nau·se·ant (naw′zē-ănt). **1.** Nauseating; causing nausea. **2.** An agent that causes nausea.

nau·se·ate (naw′zē-āt). To cause an inclination to vomit.

nau·se·at·ed (naw′zē-ā-ted). Affected with nausea. SYN sick (2).

nau·seous (naw′zē-ŭs, naw′shŭs). Causing nausea.

na·vel (nā′vel). SYN umbilicus. [A.S. *nafela*]

na·vic·u·lar (nă-vik′yū-lăr). SYN scaphoid. [L. *navicularis,* relating to shipping]

Nb niobium.

Nd neodymium.

Ne neon.

near·sight·ed·ness (nēr′sīt-ed-nes). SYN myopia.

ne·ar·thro·sis (nē-ar-thrō′sis). A new joint; *e.g.,* a pseudarthrosis arising in an ununited fracture, or an artificial joint resulting from a total joint replacement operation. SYN neoarthrosis. [G. *neos,* new, + *arthrōsis,* a jointing]

neb·u·la, pl. **neb′·u·lae** (neb′yū-lă, -lē). **1.** A translucent foglike opacity of the cornea. **2.** A class of oily preparations, intended for application by atomization. SEE spray. **3.** A spray. [L. fog, cloud, mist]

neb·u·liz·er (neb′yū-līz-er). A device used to disperse liquid medication in a mist of extremely fine particles; useful in delivering medication to deeper parts of the respiratory tract. SEE ALSO atomizer, vaporizer.

  Babbington n., SYN hydrodynamic n.

  hydrodynamic n., a device used to create an aerosol by directing a high-pressure stream of gas so that it becomes perpendicular to a film of fluid coating a small sphere; the gas strikes the fluid film and breaks it into aerosolized particles; a second, smaller sphere is used as a baffle and removes the large particles from the aerosol. SYN Babbington n.

jet n., an atomizer that uses an air or gas stream to change a liquid into small particles.

ultrasonic n., a humidifier using high-frequency electricity to power a transducer that vibrates 1,350,000 times per second and churns water up into particles 0.5 to 3 μm in size in its nebulizing chamber; used in inhalation therapy.

Ne•ca•tor (nē-kā'tŏr). A genus of nematode hookworms. Species include *N. americanus*, the New World hookworm; the adults of this species attach to villi in the small intestine and suck blood, causing abdominal discomfort, diarrhea and cramps, anorexia, loss of weight, and hypochromic microcytic anemia. SEE ALSO *Ancylostoma*. [L. a murderer]

ne•ca•to•ri•a•sis (nē-kā-tō-rī'ă-sis). Hookworm disease caused by *Necator*, the resulting anemia being usually less severe than that from ancylostomiasis.

neck (nek). **1.** SYN *regions* of neck, under *region*. **2.** In anatomy, any constricted portion having a fancied resemblance to the n. of an animal. **3.** The germinative portion of an adult tapeworm which develops the segments or proglottids; the region of cestode segmentation behind the scolex. [A.S. *hnecca*]

buffalo n., combination of moderate kyphosis with thick heavy fat pad on the n., seen especially in persons with Cushing's disease or syndrome.

bull n., a heavy thick n. caused by hypertrophied muscles or enlarged cervical lymph nodes.

stiff n., nonspecific term for limited neck mobility, often due to muscle cramps and spasm accompanied by pain.

n. of urinary bladder, the lowest part of the bladder formed by the junction of the fundus and the inferolateral surfaces.

webbed n., the broad n. due to lateral folds of skin extending from the clavicle to the head but containing no muscles, bones, or other structures; occurs in Turner's and Noonan's syndromes.

wry n., SYN torticollis.

necr-. SEE necro-.

necro-, necr-. Death, necrosis. [G. *nekros*, corpse]

nec•ro•bi•o•sis (nek'rō-bī-ō'sis). **1.** Physiologic or normal death of cells or tissues as a result of changes associated with development, aging, or use. **2.** Necrosis of a small area of tissue. SYN bionecrosis. [necro- + G. *biŏs*, life]

n. lipoid'ica, n. lipoid'ica diabetico'rum, a condition often associated with diabetes, in which one or more yellow, atrophic lesions develop on the legs.

nec•ro•bi•ot•ic (nek'rō-bī-ot'ik). Pertaining to or characterized by necrobiosis.

nec•ro•cy•to•sis (nek'rō-sī-tō'sis). Abnormal death of cells [necro- + G. *kytos*, cell, + *-osis*, condition]

nec•ro•gen•ic (nek-rō-jen'ik). Relating to, living in, or having origin in dead matter. [necro- + G. *genesis*, origin]

ne•crol•o•gy (ně-krol'ō-jē). The science of the collection, classification, and interpretation of mortality statistics. [necro- + G. *logos*, study]

ne•crol•y•sis (ně-krol'i-sis). Necrosis and loosening of tissue. [necro- + G. *lysis*, loosening]

toxic epidermal n. (TEN), a syndrome in which a large portion of the skin becomes intensely erythematous, with epidermal necrosis and flaccid bullae, resulting from drug sensitivity or of unknown cause.

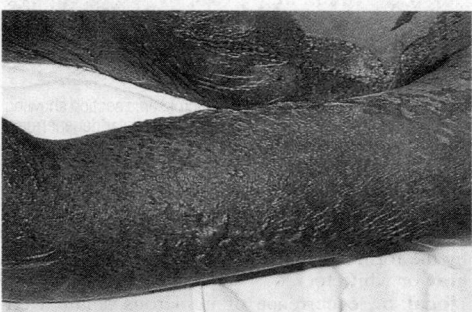

toxic epidermal necrolysis

nec•ro•ma•nia (nek-rō-mā'nē-ă). **1.** A morbid tendency to dwell with longing on death. **2.** A morbid attraction to dead bodies. [necro- + G. *mania*, frenzy]

ne•croph•a•gous (ně-krof'ă-gŭs). **1.** Living on carrion. **2.** SYN necrophilous. [necro- + G. *phagō*, to eat]

nec•ro•phil•ia, ne•croph•i•lism (nek-rō-fil'ē-ă, ně-krof'i-lizm). **1.** A morbid fondness for being in the presence of dead bodies. **2.** The impulse to have sexual contact, or the act of such contact, with a dead body, usually of males with female corpses. [necro- + G. *phileo*, to love]

ne•croph•i•lous (ně-krof'i-lŭs). Having a preference for dead tissue; denoting certain bacteria. SYN necrophagous (2). [necro- + G. *philos*, fond]

nec•ro•pho•bia (nek-rō-fō'bē-ă). Morbid fear of corpses. [necro- + G. *phobos*, fear]

nec•rop•sy (nek'rop-sē). SYN autopsy. [necro- + G. *opsis*, view]

ne•crose (ně-krōs'). **1.** To cause necrosis. **2.** To become the site of necrosis.

ne•cro•sis (ně-krō'sis). Pathologic death of one or more cells, or of a portion of tissue or organ, resulting from irreversible damage. [G. *nekrōsis*, death, fr. *nekroō*, to make dead]

aseptic n., death or decay of tissue due to local ischemia in the absence of infection. SYN avascular n.

avascular n., SYN aseptic n.

caseous n., caseation n., n. characteristic of certain inflammations (*e.g.,* tuberculosis, histoplasmosis); affected tissue manifests the friable, crumbly consistency and dull, opaque quality observed in cheese. SYN caseous degeneration.

central n., n. involving the deeper or inner portions of a tissue, or an organ or its units.

coagulation n., a type of n. in which the affected cells or tissue are converted into a dry, dull, homogeneous eosinophilic mass without nu-

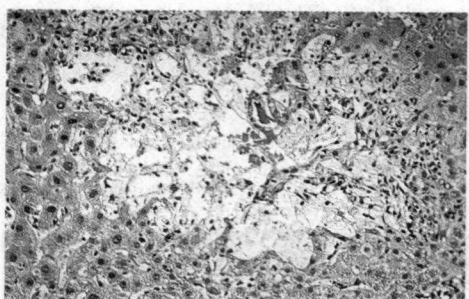

hepatic necrosis (centrilobular): microscopic section showing reticular transformation of cytoplasm, with cellular degeneration and fragmentation

clei, as a result of the coagulation of protein as occurs in an infarct.

   fat n., the death of adipose tissue, characterized by the formation of small (1–4 mm), dull, chalky, gray or white foci. SYN steatonecrosis.

   focal n., occurrence of numerous small, well-circumscribed zones of tissue that manifest coagulative, caseous, or gummatous n.

   ischemic n., n. caused by hypoxia resulting from local deprivation of blood supply, as by infarction.

   liquefactive n., a type of n. characterized by dull, opaque, partly or completely fluid remains of tissue. It is observed in abscesses and frequently in infarcts of the brain.

   zonal n., n. predominantly affecting or limited to an anatomical zone, especially parts of the hepatic lobules defined according to proximity to either the portal tracts or central (hepatic) veins.

nec•ro•sper•mia (nek-rō-sper′mē-ă). A condition in which there are dead or immobile spermatozoa in the semen. [necro- + G. *sperma,* seed]

ne•crot•ic (nĕ-krot′ik). Pertaining to or affected by necrosis.

ne•crot•o•my (ne-krot′ō-mē). **1.** SYN dissection. **2.** Operation for the removal of a necrosed portion of bone (sequestrum). [necro- + G. *tomē,* cutting]

nedocromil. A non-bronchodilator, anti-inflammatory, antiasthmatic drug that acts on the mast cells to inhibit the release of histamine.

nee•dle (nē′dl). **1.** A slender, usually sharp-pointed, instrument used for puncturing tissues, suturing, or passing a ligature around an artery. **2.** A hollow n. used for injection, aspiration, biopsy, or to guide introduction of a catheter into a vessel or other space. **3.** To separate the tissues by means of one or two n.'s, in the dissection of small parts. **4.** To perform discission of a cataract by means of a knife n. [M.E. *nedle,* fr. A.S. *nāedl*]

nee•dle-hold•er, nee•dle-car•ri•er, nee•dle-driv•er. An instrument for grasping a needle in suturing. SYN needle forceps.

nee•dling (nēd′ling). Discission of a soft or secondary cataract.

NEEP negative end-expiratory *pressure.*

ne•ga•tion (nĕ-gā′shŭn). SYN denial.

neg•a•tive (neg′ă-tiv). **1.** Not affirmative; refuta-

tive; not positive. **2.** MATHEMATICS Having a value less than zero. **3.** PHYSICS, CHEMISTRY Having an electric charge resulting from a gain or overabundance of electrons, hence able to donate (lose) electrons. **4.** MEDICINE Denoting a response to a diagnostic maneuver or laboratory study that indicates the absence of the disease or condition tested for. [L. *negativus,* fr. *nego,* to deny]

neg•a•tiv•ism (neg′ă-tiv-izm). A tendency to do the opposite of what one is requested to do, or to stubbornly resist for no apparent reason; seen in catatonic states and in toddlers.

neg•a•tron (neg′ă-tron). Term used for an electron to emphasize its negative charge in contradistinction to the positive charge carried by the otherwise similar positron.

Neis•se•ria (nī-sē′rē-ă). A genus of aerobic to facultatively anaerobic bacteria containing Gram-negative cocci which occur in pairs with the adjacent sides flattened. [A. *Neisser*]

   N. gonorrhoe′ae, a species that causes gonorrhea and other infections in humans; the type species of the genus *N.* SYN gonococcus.

   N. meningi′tidis, a species found in the nasopharynx; the causative agent of meningococcal meningitis; virulent organisms are strongly Gram-negative and occur singly or in pairs; in the latter case the cocci are elongated and are arranged with long axes parallel and facing sides kidney-shaped; groups characterized by serologically specific capsular polysaccharides are designated by capital letters (the main serogroups being A, B, C, and D). SYN meningococcus.

neis•se•ria, pl. **neis•se•ri•ae** (nī-sē′rē-ă, nī-sē′rē-ē). A vernacular term used to refer to any member of the genus *Neisseria.*

nem. A nutritional unit defined as 1 gram breast milk of specific nutritional components having a caloric value equivalent to ⅔ calorie. [Ger. *Nahrungseinheit Milch,* milk nutrition unit]

nem•a•to•cyst (nem′ă-tō-sist). A stinging cell of coelenterates consisting of a poison sac and a coiled barbed sting capable of being ejected and penetrating the skin of an animal on contact; of considerable consequence in large jellyfish and in the Portuguese man-of-war whose large numbers of these stinging cells can cause great pain and even death. [nemato- + G. *kystis,* bladder]

Nem•a•to•da (nem-ă-tō′dă). The roundworms, a large phylum that includes many of the helminths parasitic in man. Parasitic nematodes fall into two groups, the intestinal roundworms and the filarial roundworms of the blood, lymphatic tissues, and viscera. [nemat- + G. *eidos,* form]

nem•a•tode (nem′ă-tōd). A common name for any roundworm of the phylum Nematoda.

nem•a•to•di•a•sis (nem′ă-tō-dī′ă-sis). Infection with nematode parasites.

nem•a•toid (nem′ă-toyd). **1.** Resembling a thread. **2.** Relating to nematodes.

△**neo-.** New, recent. [G. *neos*]

ne•o•an•ti•gens (nē-ō-an′ti-jenz). SYN tumor *antigens,* under *antigen.*

ne•o•ar•thro•sis (nē-ō-ar-thrō′sis). SYN nearthrosis.

ne•o•blas•tic (nē-ō-blas′tik). Developing in or

characteristic of new tissue. [neo- + G. *blastos*, germ, offspring]

ne‧o‧cer‧e‧bel‧lum (nē′ō-ser-ĕ-bel′ŭm) [NA]. Phylogenetic term referring to the larger lateral portion of the cerebellar hemisphere receiving its dominant input from the pontine nuclei which, in turn, are dominated by afferent nerves originating from all parts of the cerebral cortex; phylogenetically, of more recent origin than the archicerebellum and paleocerebellum, *q.v.*, the n. reaches its largest development in humans and other primates.

ne‧o‧cys‧tos‧to‧my (nē′ō-sis-tos′tō-mē). An operation in which the ureter is implanted into the bladder. [neo- + G. *kystis*, bladder, + *stoma*, mouth]

neocyte (nē′ō-sīt). A new cell; cell recently released into the peripheral blood from the bone marrow. SEE reticulocyte. [neo- + -cyte]

ne‧o‧dym‧i‧um (Nd) (nē-ō-dim′ē-ŭm). One of the rare earth elements; atomic no. 60, atomic wt. 144.24. [*neo-*, new, + G. *didymos*, twin (of lanthanum)]

ne‧o‧gen‧e‧sis (nē-ō-jen′ĕ-sis). SYN regeneration (1). [neo- + G. *genesis*, origin]

ne‧o‧ge‧net‧ic (nē′ō-je-net′ik). Pertaining to or characterized by neogenesis.

ne‧o‧ki‧net‧ic (nē′ō-ki-net′ik). Denoting one of the divisions of the motor system, the function of which is the transmission of isolated synergic movements of voluntary origin; it represents a more highly specialized form of movement than the paleokinetic function. [neo- + G. *kinētikos*, relating to movement]

ne‧ol‧o‧gism (nē-ol′ō-jizm). A new word or phrase of the patient's own making often seen in schizophrenia (*e.g.*, headshoe to mean hat), or an existing word used in a new sense; in psychiatry, such usages may have meaning only to the patient or be indicative of the underlying condition. [neo- + G. *logos*, word]

ne‧o‧mem‧brane (nē-ō-mem′brān). SYN false membrane.

ne‧on (Ne) (nē′on). An inert gaseous element in the atmosphere; atomic no. 10, atomic wt. 20.1797. [G. *neos*, new]

ne‧o‧na‧tal (nē-ō-nā′tăl). Relating to the period immediately succeeding birth and continuing through the first 28 days of life. SYN newborn. [neo- + L. *natalis*, relating to birth]

ne‧o‧nate (nē′ō-nāt). A newborn infant. SYN newborn. [neo- + L. *natus*, born, fr. *nascor*, to be born]

ne‧o‧na‧tol‧o‧gist (nē′ō-nā-tol′ō-jist). One who specializes in neonatology.

ne‧o‧na‧tol‧o‧gy (nē′ō-nā-tol′ō-jē). The pediatric subspecialty concerned with disorders of the neonate. SYN neonatal medicine. [neo- + L. *natus*, pp. born, + G. *logos*, theory]

ne‧o‧pla‧sia (nē-ō-plā′zē-ă). The pathologic process that results in the formation and growth of a neoplasm. [neo- + G. *plasis*, a molding]

    cervical intraepithelial n. (CIN), dysplastic changes beginning at the squamocolumnar junction in the uterine cervix which may be precursors of squamous cell carcinoma: grade 1, mild dysplasia involving the lower one-third or less of the epithelial thickness; grade 2, moderate dysplasia with one-third to two-thirds involvement; grade 3, severe dysplasia or carcinoma in situ, with two-thirds to full-thickness involvement.

    prostatic intraepithelial n. (PIN), dysplastic changes involving glands and ducts of the prostate which may be a precursor of adenocarcinoma; low grade (PIN 1), mild dysplasia with variation in nuclear size and shape and irregular cell spacing; high grade (PIN 2 and 3), moderate to severe dysplasia with nucleomegaly, nucleolomegaly, and irregular cell spacing.

ne‧o‧plasm (nē′ō-plazm). An abnormal tissue that grows by cellular proliferation more rapidly than normal and continues to grow after the stimuli that initiated the new growth cease. N.'s show partial or complete lack of structural organization and functional coordination with the normal tissue, and usually form a distinct mass of tissue which may be either benign (benign *tumor*) or malignant (cancer). SYN tumor (2). [neo- + G. *plasma*, thing formed]

ne‧o‧plas‧tic (nē-ō-plas′tik). Pertaining to or characterized by neoplasia, or containing a neoplasm.

ne‧op‧ter‧in (nē-op′trin). A pteridine present in body fluids; elevated levels result from immune system activation, malignant disease, allograft rejection, and viral infections (especially as in AIDS). [neo- + G. *pteron*, wing, + -in]

ne‧o‧stri‧a‧tum (nē-ō-strī-ā′tŭm). The caudate nucleus and putamen considered as one and distinguished from the globus pallidus (paleostriatum).

ne‧o‧thal‧a‧mus (nē-ō-thal′ă-mŭs). The portion of the thalamus projecting to the neocortex.

ne‧o‧vas‧cu‧lar‧i‧za‧tion (nē′ō-vas′kyū-lar-i-zā′shŭn). Proliferation of blood vessels in tissue not normally containing them, or proliferation of blood vessels of a different kind than usual in tissue.

ne‧per (Np). A unit for comparing the magnitude of two powers, usually in electricity or acoustics; it is one half of the natural logarithm of the ratio of the two powers. [fr. *neperus*, latinized form of (John) *Napier*]

neph‧e‧lom‧e‧try (nef-ĕ-lom′ĕ-trē). Estimation of the number and size of particles in suspension by measurement of light scattered from a beam passed through the solution.

△**nephr-.** SEE nephro-.

ne‧phral‧gia (ne-fral′jē-ă). Pain in the kidney. [nephr- + G. *algos*, pain]

ne‧phrec‧to‧my (ne-frek′tō-mē). Removal of a kidney. [nephr- + G. *ektomē*, excision]

neph‧rel‧co‧sis (nef-rel-kō′sis). Ulceration of the mucous membrane of the pelvis or calices of the kidney. [nephr- + G. *helkōsis*, ulceration]

neph‧ric (nef′rik). Relating to the kidney. SYN renal.

ne‧phrit‧ic (ne-frit′ik). Relating to or suffering from nephritis.

ne‧phri‧tis, pl. **ne‧phrit‧i‧des** (ne-frī′tis, -frit′i-dēz). Inflammation of the kidneys. [nephr- + G. -*itis*, inflammation]

    glomerular n., SYN glomerulonephritis.

interstitial n., a form of n. in which the interstitial connective tissue is chiefly affected.

lupus n., glomerulonephritis occurring in some patients with systemic lupus erythematosus, characterized by hematuria and a progressive course culminating in renal failure.

mesangial n., glomerulonephritis with an increase in glomerular mesangial cells or matrix, or mesangial deposits.

salt-losing n., a rare disorder resulting from renal tubular damage of a variety of etiologies; mimics adrenocortical insufficiency in that abnormal renal loss of sodium chloride occurs, accompanied by hyponatremia, azotemia, acidosis, dehydration, and vascular collapse.

serum n., glomerulonephritis occurring in serum sickness or in animals injected with foreign serum protein.

suppurative n., focal glomerulonephritis with abscess formation in the kidney.

transfusion n., renal failure and tubular damage resulting from the transfusion of incompatible blood; the hemoglobin of the hemolyzed red cells is deposited as casts in the renal tubules.

tubulointerstitial n., n. affecting renal tubules and interstitial tissue, with infiltration by plasma cells and mononuclear cells; seen in lupus n., allograft rejection, and methicillin sensitization.

ne•phrit•o•gen•ic (nef'ri-tō-jen'ik). Causing nephritis; said of conditions or agents. [nephritis + G. *genesis,* production]

△**nephro-, nephr-.** The kidney. SEE ALSO reno-. [G. *nephros,* kidney]

neph•ro•cal•ci•no•sis (nef'rō-kal-si-nō'sis). A form of renal lithiasis characterized by diffusely scattered foci of calcification in the renal parenchyma; deposits of calcium phosphate, calcium oxalate monohydrate, and similar compounds are usually demonstrable radiologically. [nephro- + calcinosis]

neph•ro•car•di•ac (nef'rō-kar'dē-ak). SYN cardiorenal. [nephro- + G. *kardia,* heart]

neph•ro•cele (nef'rō-sēl). **1.** Hernial displacement of a kidney. [nephro- + G. *kēlē,* hernia] **2.** In lower vertebrates, the developmental cavity connecting the myocele with the celom. [nephro- + G. *koilōma,* a hollow (celom)]

neph•ro•cys•to•sis (nef'rō-sis-tō'sis). Formation of renal cysts. [nephro- + G. *kystis,* cyst, + *-osis,* condition]

neph•ro•ge•net•ic, neph•ro•gen•ic (nef'rō-jĕ-net'ik, -jen'ik). Developing into kidney tissue. [nephro- + G. *genesis,* origin]

ne•phrog•e•nous (ne-froj'ĕ-nŭs). Developing from kidney tissue.

neph•ro•gram (nef'rō-gram). Radiographic examination of the kidney after the intravenous injection of a water-soluble iodinated contrast material; also, the diffuse opacification of the renal parenchyma following such injection, an indication of renal blood flow and glomerular filtration. A persistent nephrogram indicates obstruction of kidney drainage.

ne•phrog•ra•phy (ne-frog'ră-fē). Radiography of the kidney. [nephro- + G. *graphō,* to write]

neph•roid (nef'royd). Kidney-shaped; resembling a kidney. SYN reniform. [nephro- + G. *eidos,* resemblance]

◨neph•ro•li•thi•a•sis (nef'rō-li-thī'ă-sis). Presence of renal calculi.

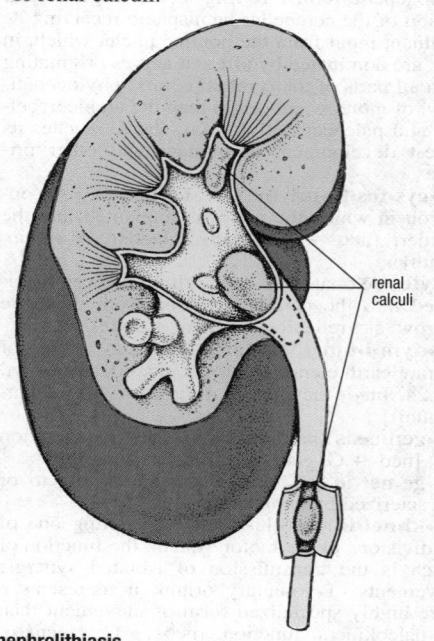

renal calculi

nephrolithiasis

neph•ro•li•thot•o•my (nef'rō-li-thot'ō-mē). Incision into the kidney for the removal of a renal calculus. [nephro- + G. *lithos,* stone, + *tomē,* incision]

ne•phrol•o•gy (ne-frol'ō-jē). The branch of medical science concerned with medical diseases of the kidneys. [nephro- + G. *logos,* study]

ne•phrol•y•sis (ne-frol'i-sis). **1.** Freeing of the kidney from inflammatory adhesions, with preservation of the capsule. **2.** Destruction of renal cells. [nephro- + G. *lysis,* dissolution]

neph•ro•lyt•ic (nef-rō-lit'ik). Pertaining to, characterized by, or causing nephrolysis. SYN nephrotoxic (2).

ne•phro•ma (ne-frō'mă). A tumor arising from renal tissue. [nephro- + G. *-oma,* tumor]

neph•ro•meg•a•ly (nef-rō-meg'ă-lē). Extreme hypertrophy of one or both kidneys. [nephro- + G. *megas,* great]

neph•ron (nef'ron). A long convoluted tubular structure in the kidney, consisting of the renal corpuscle, the proximal convoluted tubule, the nephronic loop, and the distal convoluted tubule. [G. *nephros,* kidney]

ne•phrop•a•thy (ne-frop'ă-thē). Any disease of the kidney. SYN nephrosis (1). [nephro- + G. *pathos,* suffering]

neph•ro•pexy (nef'rō-pek-sē). Operative fixation of a floating or mobile kidney. [nephro- + G. *pēxis,* fixation]

neph•roph•thi•sis (nef-rof'thī-sis, -tĭ-sis). **1.** Suppurative nephritis with wasting of the substance of the organ. **2.** Tuberculosis of the kidney. [nephro- + G. *phthisis,* a wasting]

neph·rop·to·sis, neph·rop·to·sia (nef-rop-tō′sis, -tō′sē-ă). Prolapse of the kidney. [nephro- + G. *ptōsis,* a falling]

neph·ro·py·o·sis (nef′rō-pī-ō′sis). SYN pyonephrosis. [nephro- + G. *pyōsis,* suppuration]

neph·ror·rha·phy (nef-rōr′ă-fē). Nephropexy by suturing the kidney. [nephro- + G. *rhaphē,* a suture]

neph·ro·scle·ro·sis (nef′rō-skle-rō′sis). Induration of the kidney from overgrowth and contraction of the interstitial connective tissue. [nephro- + G. *sklērōsis,* hardening]

   arterial n., patchy atrophic scarring of the kidney due to arteriosclerotic narrowing of the lumens of large branches of the renal artery, occurring in old or hypertensive persons and occasionally causing hypertension. SYN arterionephrosclerosis.

   arteriolar n., renal scarring due to arteriolar sclerosis resulting from longstanding hypertension; chronic renal failure develops infrequently. SYN arteriolonephrosclerosis.

   malignant n., the renal changes in malignant hypertension; subcapsular petechiae, necrosis in the walls of scattered afferent glomerular arterioles, and red blood cells and casts in the urine, with uremia as a common termination.

neph·ro·scle·rot·ic (nef′rō-skle-rot′ik). Pertaining to or causing nephrosclerosis.

neph·ro·scope (nef′rō-skōp). An endoscope passed into the renal pelvis to view it. Route of access may be percutaneous, through a surgically exposed kidney, or retrograde via the ureter.

ne·phro·sis (ne-frō′sis). **1.** SYN nephropathy. **2.** Degeneration of renal tubular epithelium. **3.** SYN nephrotic *syndrome.* [nephro- + G. *-osis,* condition]

   amyloid n., (1) SYN renal *amyloidosis.* (2) nephrotic syndrome due to deposition of amyloid in the kidney.

   hemoglobinuric n., acute oliguric renal failure associated with hemoglobinuria, due to massive intravascular hemolysis.

   hypoxic n., acute oliguric renal failure following hemorrhage, burns, shock, or other causes of hypovolemia and reduced renal blood flow;.

   lipoid n., idiopathic nephrotic syndrome occurring most commonly in children, in which glomeruli show minimal changes with no thickening of the basement membranes, fat vacuoles in the tubular epithelium, and fusion of glomerular foot processes.

   toxic n., acute oliguric renal failure due to chemical poisons, septicemia, or bacterial toxemia.

ne·phros·to·gram (ne-fros′tō-gram). A radiograph of the kidney after opacification of the renal pelvis by injecting a contrast agent through a nephrostomy tube. [nephrostomy + G. *gramma,* writing]

ne·phros·to·my (ne-fros′tō-mē). Establishment of an opening between the pelvis of the kidney through its cortex to the exterior of the body. [nephro- + G. *stoma,* mouth]

neph·rot·ic (nef-rot′ik). Relating to, caused by, or similar to nephrosis.

neph·ro·to·mo·gram (nef-rō-tō′mō-gram). A tomographic examination of the kidneys following the intravenous administration of water-soluble iodinated contrast material. [nephro- + G. *tomos,* a cutting + *gramma,* a writing]

neph·ro·to·mog·ra·phy (nef′rō-tō-mog′ră-fē). Tomographic examination of the kidney.

ne·phrot·o·my (ne-frot′ō-mē). Incision into the kidney. [nephro- + G. *tomē,* incision]

neph·ro·tox·ic (nef-rō-tok′sik). **1.** Pertaining to nephrotoxin; toxic to renal cells. **2.** SYN nephrolytic.

neph·ro·tox·ic·i·ty (nef′rō-tok-sis′i-tē). The quality or state of being toxic to kidney cells.

neph·ro·tox·in (nef-rō-tok′sin). A cytotoxin that is specific for cells of the kidney.

neph·ro·tro·phic (nef-rō-trof′ik). SYN renotrophic.

neph·ro·tro·pic (nef-rō-trop′ik). SYN renotropic.

neph·ro·tu·ber·cu·lo·sis (nef′rō-tū-ber-kyū-lō′sis). Tuberculosis of the kidney.

neph·ro·u·re·ter·ec·to·my (nef′rō-yū-rē′ter-ek′tō-mē). Surgical removal of a kidney and its ureter. SYN ureteronephrectomy. [nephro- + ureter + G. *ektomē,* excision]

neph·ro·u·re·ter·o·cys·tec·to·my (nef′rō-yū-rē′ter-ō-sis-tek′tō-mē). Removal of kidney, ureter, and part or all of the bladder. [nephro- + ureter + G. *kystis,* bladder, + *ektomē,* excision]

nep·tu·ni·um (Np) (nep-tū′nē-ŭm). A radioactive element; atomic no. 93; first element of the transuranian series (not found in nature); ^{237}Np has a half-life of 2.14×10^6 years. [planet, *Neptune*]

nerve (nerv). A whitish cordlike structure composed of one or more bundles (fascicles) of myelinated or unmyelinated n. fibers, or more often mixtures of both, coursing outside of the central nervous system, together with connective tissue within the fascicle and around the neurolemma of individual n. fibers (endoneurium), around each fascicle (perineurium), and around the entire n. and its nourishing blood vessels (epineurium), by which stimuli are transmitted from the central nervous system to a part of the body or the reverse. Nerve branches are given in the definition of the major nerve; many are also listed and defined under branch. SYN nervus [NA]. [L. *nervus*]

   abducent n., the sixth cranial nerve; a small motor nerve supplying the lateral rectus muscle of the eye; its origin is in the dorsal part of the tegmentum of the pons just below the surface of the rhomboid fossa, and it emerges from the brain in the fissure between the medulla oblongata and the posterior border of the pons; it enters the dura of the clivus and passes through the cavernous sinus, entering the orbit through the superior orbital fissure. SYN nervus abducens [NA], abducent (2).

   accelerator n.'s, certain of the cardiopulmonary splanchnic n.'s establishing the sympathetic innervation of the heart; originating from ganglion cells of the superior, middle, and inferior cervical ganglion of the sympathetic trunk, the unmyelinated efferent fibers of the accelerator n.'s stimulate an increase in the heart rate.

accessory n., the 11th cranial n.; arises by two sets of roots: cranial, emerging from the side of the medulla, and spinal, emerging from the ventrolateral part of the first five cervical segments of the spinal cord; these roots unite to form the accessory n. trunk, which divides into two branches, internal and external; the internal branch, carrying fibers of the cranial root, unites with the vagus in the jugular foramen and supplies the muscles of the pharynx, larynx, and soft palate; the external branch continues independently through the jugular foramen to supply the sternocleidomastoid and trapezius muscles. SYN nervus accessorius [NA].

accessory phrenic n.'s, accessory n. strands that arise from the fifth cervical n., often as branches of the n. to the subclavius, passing downward to join the phrenic n. SYN nervi phrenici accessorii [NA].

acoustic n., SYN vestibulocochlear n.

afferent n., a n. conveying impulses from the periphery to the central nervous system. SYN centripetal n.

anococcygeal n.'s, several small n.'s arising from the coccygeal plexus, supplying the skin over the coccyx. SYN nervi anococcygei [NA].

anterior auricular n.'s, branches of the auriculotemporal n. that supply the tragus and upper part of the auricle. SYN nervi auriculares anteriores [NA].

anterior interosseous n., a branch of the median n. arising in the elbow region, running on interosseous membrane, supplying the flexor pollicis longus, part of flexor digitorum profundus and the pronator quadratus muscles, as well as radiocarpal and intercarpal joints. SYN nervus interosseus anterior [NA].

articular n., a branch of a n. supplying a joint.

auditory n., SYN cochlear n.

auriculotemporal n., a branch of the mandibular, usually arising by two roots embracing the middle meningeal artery; it passes through the parotid gland conveying postsynaptic parasympathetic secretomotor fibers from the otic ganglion, and terminating in the skin of the temple and scalp; also sends branches to the external acoustic meatus, tympanic membrane, and auricle as well as a communicating branch to the facial n. SYN nervus auriculotemporalis [NA].

axillary n., arises from the posterior cord of the brachial plexus in the axilla, passes laterally and posteriorly through quadrangular space with the posterior circumflex artery, winding round the surgical neck of the humerus to supply the deltoid and teres minor muscles, terminating as the superior lateral brachial cutaneous n. SYN nervus axillaris [NA].

buccal n., a sensory branch of the mandibular division of the trigeminal n.; it passes downward emerging from beneath the ramus of the mandible to run forward on the buccinator muscle, piercing (but not supplying) it to innervate buccal mucous membrane and skin of the cheek near the angle of the mouth. SYN nervus buccalis [NA].

caroticotympanic n., one of two sympathetic branches from the internal carotid plexus to the tympanic plexus. SYN nervus caroticotympanicus [NA].

cavernous n.'s of clitoris, n.'s corresponding to the cavernous n.'s of penis in the male, arising from the vesicular portion of the pelvic plexus. SYN nervi cavernosi clitoridis [NA].

cavernous n.'s of penis, two n.'s, major and minor, derived from the prostatic portion of the pelvic plexus supplying sympathetic and parasympathetic fibers to the helicine arteries and arteriovenous anastomoses of the corpus cavernosum stimulating erection. SYN nervi cavernosi penis [NA].

centrifugal n., SYN efferent n.

centripetal n., SYN afferent n.

cervical n.'s, n.'s arising from the cervical segments of the spinal cord.

coccygeal n., a small n., the lowest of the spinal n.'s, entering into the formation of the coccygeal plexus. SYN nervus coccygeus [NA].

cochlear n., the part of the vestibulocochlear n. peripheral to the cochlear root; it is composed of fibers whose central n. processes arise from the bipolar neurons of the spiral ganglion and which have their peripheral processes on the four rows of neuroepithelial cells (hair cells) of the spiral organ. SYN auditory n.

▣**cranial n.'s,** those n.'s that emerge from, or enter, the cranium or skull, in contrast to the spinal n.'s, which emerge from the spine or vertebral column. The twelve paired cranial n.'s are the olfactory, optic, oculomotor, trochlear, trigeminal, abducent, facial, vestibulocochlear, glossopharyngeal, vagal, accessory, and hypoglossal n.'s. SYN nervi craniales [NA].

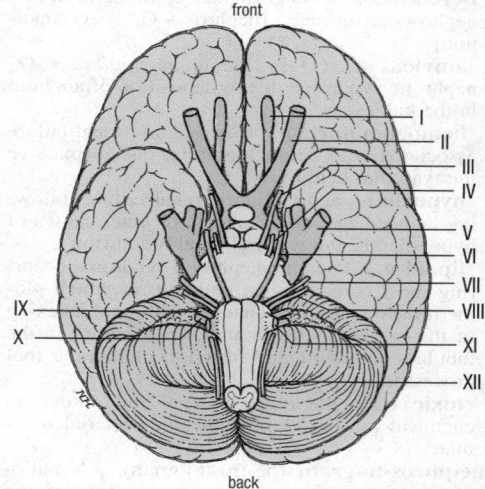

front

I
II
III
IV
V
VI
VII
VIII
IX
X
XI
XII

back

cranial nerves: (inferior view): (I) olfactory, (II) optic, (III) oculomotor, (IV) trochlear, (V) trigeminal, (VI) abducens, (VII) facial, (VIII) vestibulocochlear, (IX) glossopharyngeal, (X) vagus, (XI) accessory, (XII) hypoglossal

crural interosseous n., a n. given off from one

of the muscular branches of the tibial nerve which passes down over the posterior surface of the interosseous membrane supplying it and the two bones of the leg. SYN nervus interosseus cruris [NA].

cubital n., SYN ulnar n.

cutaneous n., a mixed n. supplying a region of the skin, including its sensory endings, blood vessels, smooth muscle and glands.

deep temporal n.'s, two branches, anterior and posterior, from the mandibular n., supplying the temporalis muscle and periosteum of the temporal fossa. SYN nervi temporales profundi [NA].

dorsal digital n.'s of foot, n.'s supplying the skin of the dorsal aspect of the proximal and middle phalanges of the toes. SYN nervi digitales dorsales pedis [NA].

dorsal digital n.'s of hand, terminal branches of the radial and ulnar n.'s in the hand supplying the skin of the dorsal surface of the proximal and middle phalanges of the fingers. SYN nervi digitales dorsales [NA].

dorsal n. of clitoris, the deep terminal branch of the pudendal, supplying especially the glans clitoridis after passing through the musculature of the urogenital diaphragm, to run along the dorsum of the clitoral shaft. SYN nervus dorsalis clitoridis [NA].

dorsal n. of penis, the deep terminal branch of the pudendal which runs through the urogenital diaphragm giving branches, then runs along the dorsum of the penis, supplying the skin of the penis, the prepuce, the corpora cavernosa, and the glans. SYN nervus dorsalis penis [NA].

dorsal scapular n., arises from ventral primary rami of the fifth to seventh cervical nerves and passes downward to supply the levator scapulae and the rhomboideus major and minor muscles. SYN nervus dorsalis scapulae [NA].

efferent n., a n. conveying impulses from the central nervous system to the periphery. SYN centrifugal n.

eighth cranial n., SYN central auditory nervous system.

excitor n., a n. conducting impulses that stimulate to increase function.

excitoreflex n., a visceral n. the special function of which is to cause reflex action.

external carotid n.'s, a number of sympathetic n. fibers conveyed via the cephalic arterial ramus of the sympathetic trunk which extends from the superior cervical ganglion to the external carotid artery, forming the external carotid plexus. SYN nervi carotici externi [NA].

■facial n., the seventh cranial n.; its origin is in the tegmentum of the lower portion of the pons, and it emerges from the brain at the posterior border of the pons; it leaves the cranial cavity through the internal acoustic meatus where it is joined by the intermediate n., traverses the facial canal in the petrous portion of the temporal bone, and makes its exit through the stylomastoid foramen; it passes through the parotid gland forming the intraparotid plexus, the various branches of which pass to the muscles of facial expression. SYN nervus facialis [NA].

femoral n., arises from the second, third, and

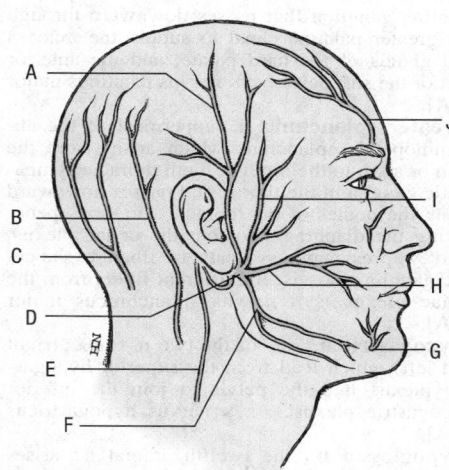

nerve supply to the head and neck: (A) auriculotemporal branch of facial nerve; (B) small occipital nerve; (C) great occipital nerve; (D) facial nerve; (E) great auricular nerve; (F) mandibular branch of facial nerve; (G) mental nerve; (H) buccal branch of facial nerve; (I) temporal branch of facial nerve; (J) supraorbital nerve

fourth lumbar n.'s in the substance of the psoas muscle and enters the thigh via the muscular lacuna beneath the inguinal ligament, lateral to the femoral vessels; it arborize within the femoral triangle into muscle branches to the sartorius, pectineus and quadriceps muscles and anterior femoral cutaneous n.'s to the skin of the anterior and medial region of the thigh; its terminal branch is the saphenous n. by which it supplies the skin of the medial leg and foot anterior region of the thigh. SYN nervus femoralis [NA].

frontal n., a branch of the ophthalmic n. which divides within the orbit into the supratrochlear and the supraorbital n.'s. SYN nervus frontalis [NA].

gangliated n., a sympathetic n.

genitofemoral n., arises from the first and second lumbar n.'s, passes distad along the anterior surface of psoas major muscle and divides into genital and femoral branches. SYN nervus genitofemoralis [NA].

glossopharyngeal n., the ninth cranial n.; it emerges from the rostral end of the medulla and passes through the jugular foramen to supply sensation to the pharynx and posterior third of the tongue; it also carries somatic motor fibers to the stylopharyngeus muscle and presynaptic parasympathetic fibers to the otic ganglion. SYN nervus glossopharyngeus [NA].

great auricular n., arises from the ventral primary rami of the second and third cervical spinal n.'s, supplies the skin of part of the auricle, adjacent portion of the scalp, and that overlying the angle of the jaw; it also innervates the parotid sheath, conveying from it the pain fibers stimulated by stretching of the sheath during parotitis (mumps). SYN nervus auricularis magnus [NA].

greater palatine n., a branch of the pterygopalatine ganglion that passes downward through the greater palatine canal to supply the mucosa and glands of the hard palate, and the anterior part of the soft palate. SYN nervus palatinus major [NA].

greater splanchnic n., uppermost of the abdominopelvic splanchnic which arises from the fifth or sixth to the ninth or tenth thoracic sympathetic ganglia in the thorax and passes downward along the bodies of the thoracic vertebrae, penetrating the diaphragm to join the celiac plexus; conveys presynaptic sympathetic fibers to the celiac ganglia, and visceral afferent fibers from the celiac plexus. SYN nervus splanchnicus major [NA].

hypogastric n., one of the two n. trunks (right and left) which lead from the superior hypogastric plexus into the pelvis to join the inferior hypogastric plexuses. SYN nervus hypogastricus [NA].

hypoglossal n., the twelfth cranial n.; arises from an oblong nucleus in the medulla and emerges by several root filaments between the pyramid and the olive; it passes through the hypoglossal canal, then courses downward and forward to supply the intrinsic and four of five extrinsic muscles of the tongue. SYN nervus hypoglossus [NA].

iliohypogastric n., arises from the first lumbar n.; it supplies the abdominal muscles and the skin of the lower part of the anterior abdominal wall. SYN nervus iliohypogastricus [NA].

ilioinguinal n., arises from the first lumbar n., passes through the inguinal canal and superficial inguinal ring to supply the skin of the upper medial thigh, mons pubis, and scrotum or labium majus. SYN nervus ilioinguinalis [NA].

inferior alveolar n., one of the terminal branches of the mandibular, it enters the mandibular canal to be distributed to the lower teeth, periosteum, and gingiva of the mandible; a branch, the mental n., passes through the mental foramen to supply the skin and mucosa of the lower lip and chin. SYN nervus alveolaris inferior [NA].

inferior rectal n.'s, several branches of the pudendal n. that pass to the external and sphincter anoderm and skin of the anal region. SYN nervi rectales inferiores [NA].

infraorbital n., the continuation of the maxillary n. after it has entered the orbit, via the infraorbital fissure, traversing the infraorbital canal to reach the face; it supplies the mucosa of the maxillary sinus, the upper incisors, canine and premolars, the upper gums, the inferior eyelid and conjunctiva, part of the nose and the superior lip. SYN nervus infraorbitalis [NA].

infratrochlear n., a terminal branch of the nasociliary n. running beneath the pulley of the superior oblique muscle to the front of the orbit, and supplying the skin of the eyelids and root of the nose. SYN nervus infratrochlearis [NA].

inhibitory n., a n. conveying impulses that diminish functional activity in a part.

intercostal n.'s, ventral primary rami of the thoracic n.'s. SYN nervi intercostales [NA].

intercostobrachial n.'s, lateral cutaneous branches of the second and third intercostal n.'s which pass to the skin of the medial side of the arm. SYN nervi intercostobrachiales [NA].

intermediary n., a root of the facial n. containing sensory fibers for taste from the anterior 2/3 of tongue whose cell bodies are located in the geniculate ganglion and presynaptic parasympathetic autonomic fibers whose cell bodies are located in the superior salivatory nucleus, i.e., the fibers eventually conveyed via the chorda tympani branch of the facial n. to the lingual n. SYN nervus intermedius [NA], intermediate n.

intermediate n., SYN intermediary n.

internal carotid n., the cephalic arterial ramus conveying postsynaptic sympathetic fibers from the superior cervical ganglion to the internal carotid artery to form the internal carotid plexus. SYN nervus caroticus internus [NA].

jugular n., a communicating branch between the superior cervical ganglion of the sympathetic n., the superior ganglion of the vagus n., and the inferior ganglion of the glossopharyngeal n. SYN nervus jugularis [NA].

lacrimal n., a branch of the ophthalmic n. supplying sensory fibers to the lateral part of the upper eyelid, conjunctiva, and lacrimal gland. The secretomotor fibers of the latter were conveyed to the lacrimal n. by the communicating branch of the zygomatic n. (a branch of the maxillary n.). SYN nervus lacrimalis [NA].

lesser palatine n.'s, usually two, these n.'s emerge through the lesser palatine foramina and supply the mucosa and glands of the soft palate and uvula; they are branches of the pterygopalatine ganglion and contain postsynaptic parasympathetic and sensory fibers of the maxillary n. SYN nervi palatini minores [NA].

lesser splanchnic n., one of the abdominopelvic splanchnic n.'s arising in the thorax from the last two thoracic sympathetic ganglia and passing through the diaphragm to the aorticorenal ganglion; conveys presynaptic sympathetic fibers and visceral afferent fibers. SYN nervus splanchnicus minor [NA].

lingual n., one of the branches of the mandibular n., passing medially to the lateral pterygoid muscle, between the medial pterygoid and the mandible, and beneath the mucous membrane of the floor of the mouth to the side of the tongue over the anterior two-thirds of which it is distributed; it supplies also the mucous membrane of the floor of the mouth. It passes close to the lingual side of the roots of the second and third lower molar teeth and is endangered during tooth extractions. SYN nervus lingualis [NA].

long thoracic n., arises from the fifth, sixth, and seventh cervical n.'s (roots of brachial plexus), descends the neck behind the brachial plexus, and is distributed to the serratus anterior muscle; it is somewhat unusual in that it courses on the superficial aspect of the muscle it supplies; its paralysis results in "winged scapula." SYN nervus thoracicus longus [NA].

lowest splanchnic n., one of the abdominopelvic splanchnic n.'s arising in the thorax and penetrating the diaphragm to supply presynaptic sympathetic fibers for the renal plexus; often combined with the lesser splanchnic n., but occasionally existing as an independent n. SYN nervus splanchnicus imus [NA].

lumbar n.'s, five bilaterally paired n.'s emerging from the lumbar portion of the spinal cord; the first four n.'s enter into the formation of the lumbar plexus, the fourth and fifth into that of the sacral plexus. SYN nervi lumbales [NA].

lumbar splanchnic n.'s, branches from the lumbar sympathetic trunks that pass anteriorly to convey presynaptic sympathetic fibers to, and visceral afferents from, the celiac, intermesenteric, aortic, and superior hypogastric plexuses. SYN nervi splanchnici lumbales [NA].

mandibular n., the third division of the trigeminal n. formed by the union of sensory fibers from the trigeminal ganglion and the motor root in the foramen ovale, through which the n. emerges; its branches are: meningeal, masseteric, deep temporal, lateral and medial pterygoid, buccal, auriculotemporal, lingual, and inferior alveolar; its sensory fibers are distributed to the auricle, external acoustic meatus, tympanic membrane, temporal region, cheek, skin overlying the mandible (except its angle), anterior 2/3 of tongue, floor of mouth, lower teeth and gingiva; its motor fibers innervate all the muscles of mastication plus the mylohyoid, anterior belly of the digestive and the tensores veli palati and tympani. SYN nervus mandibularis [NA].

masseteric n., a muscular branch of the mandibular n. passing through the mandibular notch to the medial surface of the masseter muscle; which it supplies, and the temporomandibular joint. SYN nervus massetericus [NA].

maxillary n., the second division of the trigeminal n., passing from the trigeminal ganglion through the foramen rotundum into the pterygopalatine fossa, where it gives off ganglionic branches to the pterygopalatine ganglion and continues forward to give off the zygomatic n. and enter the orbit, where it is named the infraorbital n. Its sensory fibers are distributed to the skin and conjunctiva of the lower eyelid, the skin and mucosa of the upper lip and cheek, the palate, upper teeth and gingiva, the maxillary sinus, wings of the nose and posterior/interior nasal cavity. SYN nervus maxillaris [NA].

median n., formed by the union of medial and lateral roots from the medial and lateral cords of the brachial plexus, respectively; it supplies all the muscles in the anterior compartment of the forearm with the exception of the flexor carpi ulnaris and ulnar half of the flexor digitorum profundus; it passes through the carpal tunnel to supply the thenar muscles (except adductor pollicis and the deep head of flexor pollicis brevis) via its recurrent thenar branch; its sensory fibers are distributed to the skin of the palmar and distal dorsal aspects of the radial 3 1/2 digits and adjacent palm. The median n. is most commonly injured through compression in carpal tunnel syndrome, resulting in a loss of ability to oppose the thumb ("ape hand") and loss of sensation over the radial portion of the hand. SYN nervus medianus [NA].

mental n., a branch of the inferior alveolar n., arising in the mandibular canal and passing through the mental foramen to the chin and lower lip. SYN nervus mentalis [NA].

mixed n., a n. containing both afferent and efferent fibers.

motor n., an efferent n. conveying an impulse that excites muscular contraction; motor n.'s in the autonomic nervous system also elicit secretions from glandular epithelia.

musculocutaneous n., arises from lateral cord of the brachial plexus, passes through the coracobrachialis muscle, and then downward between the brachialis and biceps, supplying these three muscles and being prolonged as the lateral cutaneous n. of the forearm. SYN nervus musculocutaneus [NA].

mylohyoid n., a small branch of the inferior alveolar n. given off posteriorly just before the n. enters the mandibular foramen, distributed to the anterior belly of the digastric muscle and to the mylohyoid muscle. SYN nervus mylohyoideus [NA].

nasociliary n., a branch of the ophthalmic n. in the superior orbital fissure, passing through the orbit, giving rise to the communicating branch to the ciliary ganglion, the long ciliary n.'s, and the posterior and anterior ethmoidal n.'s, and terminating as the infratrochlear and nasal branches, which supply the mucous membrane of the nose, the skin of the tip of the nose, and the conjunctiva. SYN nervus nasociliaris [NA].

nasopalatine n., a branch from the pterygopalatine ganglion, passing through the sphenopalatine foramen, crossing to and then down the nasal septum, and through the incisive foramen to supply the mucous membrane of the hard palate. SYN nervus nasopalatinus [NA].

obturator n., arises from the second, third, and fourth lumbar n.'s in the psoas muscle, crosses the brim of the pelvis, and enters the thigh through the obturator canal; it supplies muscles of the medial compartment of the thigh (adductors of thigh at the hip joint) and terminates as the cutaneous branch of the obturator n., supplying a small area of medial thigh above knee. SYN nervus obturatorius [NA].

oculomotor n., the third cranial n.; it supplies all the extrinsic muscles of the eye, except the lateral rectus and superior oblique; it also supplies the levator palpebrae superioris, and conveys presynaptic parasympathetic fibers to the ciliary ganglion for innervation of the ciliary muscle and sphincter pupillae; its origin is in the midbrain below the cerebral aqueduct; it emerges from the brain in the interpeduncular fossa, pierces the dura mater to the side of the posterior clinoid process, passes in the lateral wall of the cavernous sinus and enters the orbit through the superior orbital fissure. SYN nervus oculomotorius [NA].

olfactory n.'s, collective term denoting the numerous olfactory filaments: slender fascicles each composed of the thin, unmyelinated axons of 8 to 12 of the bipolar olfactory receptor cells in the olfactory portion of the nasal mucosa; the olfactory filaments pass through the cribriform plate of the ethmoid bone and enter the olfactory bulb, where they terminate in synaptic contact with mitral cells, tufted cells, and granule cells. SYN nervi olfactorii [NA].

ophthalmic n., a branch of the trigeminal n. that passes forward from the trigeminal ganglion in the lateral wall of the cavernous sinus, entering the orbit through the superior orbital fissure; through its branches, frontal, lacrimal, and naso-ciliary, it supplies sensation to the orbit and its contents, the anterior part of the nasal cavity, and the skin of the nose and forehead. SYN nervus ophthalmicus [NA].

optic n., the second cranial n.; originating from the ganglion cells of the retina, it passes out of the orbit through the optic canal to the chiasm, where part of the fibers cross to the opposite side and pass through the optic tract to the geniculate bodies, superior colliculus, and the pretectum. SYN nervus opticus [NA].

parasympathetic n., one of the n.'s of the parasympathetic nervous system.

perineal n.'s, the superficial terminal branches of the pudendal nerve, supplying most of the muscles of the perineum (deep branch) as well as the skin of that region (superficial branch). SYN nervi perineales [NA].

phrenic n., arises from the cervical plexus, chiefly from the fourth cervical n., passes down-ward in front of the anterior scalene muscle and enters the thorax between the subclavian artery and vein behind the sternoclavicular articulation; it then passes in front of the root of the lung to the diaphragm; it is mainly the motor n. of the diaphragm but sends sensory fibers to the medi-astinal parietal pleura, the pericardium, the dia-phragmatic pleura and peritoneum, and branches (phrenicoabdominales branches) that communi-cate with branches from the celiac plexus. SYN nervus phrenicus [NA].

pneumogastric n., SYN vagus n.

posterior auricular n., the first extracranial branch of the facial n., it passes behind the ear, supplying the posterior auricular muscle and in-trinsic muscles of the auricle and, through its occipital branch, innervating the occipital belly of the occipitofrontalis muscle. SYN nervus auricula-ris posterior [NA].

posterior interosseous n., the deep terminal branch of the radial n., arises in the cubital re-gion, penetrating and supplying the supinator and continuing with the posterior interosseous artery to supply all the extensor muscles in the forearm. SYN nervus interosseus posterior [NA].

pressor n., an afferent n., stimulation of which excites a reflex vasoconstriction, thereby raising the blood pressure.

pterygoid n., one of two motor branches, lat-eral and medial, of the mandibular n., supplying the lateral and medial pterygoid muscles with fibers of the motor root of the trigeninal n. SYN nervus pterygoideus [NA].

n. of pterygoid canal, the n. constituting the parasympathetic and sympathetic root of the pter-ygopalatine ganglion; it is formed in the region of the foramen lacerum by the union of the greater superficial petrosal and the deep petrosal n.'s, and runs through the pterygoid canal to the ptery-gopalatine fossa. SYN nervus canalis pterygoidei [NA].

pudendal n., formed by fibers from the ventral primary rami of the second, third, and fourth sa-cral spinal n.'s; it exits the pelvis via the greater sciatic foramen, passes posterior to the sacrospi-nous ligament, and accompanies the internal pu-dendal artery into the perineum via the lesser sciatic foramen; it gives off inferior rectal n.'s, then courses through the pudendal canal in the lateral wall of the ischiorectal fossa, terminating as the dorsal n. of the penis or of the clitoris. SYN nervus pudendus [NA].

radial n., arises from the posterior cord of the brachial plexus; it curves round the posterior sur-face of the humerus and passes down to the cubi-tal fossa where it divides into its two terminal branches, the superficial branch and the deep branch; it supplies muscular and cutaneous branches to the posterior compartments of the arm and forearm. The radial n. is most commonly injured by fractures of the middle third of the humerus, resulting in a loss of extension at the wrist ("wrist drop"). SYN nervus radialis [NA].

saccular n., a branch of the vestibular n. going to the macula of the sacculus. SYN nervus saccula-ris [NA].

sacral n.'s, five n.'s issuing from the sacral foramina on either side; the ventral branches of the first three enter into the formation of the sacral plexus, and the last two into the coccygeal plexus. SYN nervi sacrales [NA].

sacral splanchnic n.'s, branches from the sa-cral sympathetic trunk that pass to the inferior hypogastric plexus; part of the abdominopelvic (sympathetic) splanchnic n.'s, but their specific function is unclear. They tend to be confused with the pelvic splanchnic n.'s, which are much more significant structures. SYN nervi splanchnici sacrales [NA].

saphenous n., a branch of the femoral, extend-ing from the femoral triangle to the foot, becom-ing subcutaneous on the medial side of the knee; it supplies cutaneous branches to the skin of the leg and foot, by way of infrapatellar and medial crural branches. SYN nervus saphenus [NA].

sciatic n., arises from the sacral plexus, passes through the greater sciatic foramen and down the thigh, deep to the long head of biceps femoris n.; at the apex of the popliteal fossa it divides into the common peroneal and tibial n.'s, although the two may separate at higher levels. SYN nervus ischiadicus [NA].

secretory n., a n. conveying impulses that ex-cite functional activity in a gland.

sensory n., an afferent n. conveying impulses that are processed by the central nervous system so as to become part of the organism's perception of self and its environment.

somatic n., one of the n.'s of parietal sensation or voluntary motion, as distinguished from the visceral sensory, involuntary motor and secretory n.'s.

spinal n.'s, the n.'s emerging from the spinal cord; there are 31 pairs, each attached to the cord by two roots, anterior and posterior, or ventral and dorsal; the latter is provided with a circumscribed enlargement, the dorsal root (spinal) ganglion; the two roots unite in the intervertebral foramen, and the mixed spinal n. almost immediately divides again into ventral and dorsal primary rami, the former supplying the anterolateral trunk and the limbs, the latter the true muscles and overlying skin of the back. SYN nervi spinales [NA].

n. to stapedius muscle, a branch of the facial n. arising in the facial canal and innervating the stapedius muscle. SYN nervus stapedius [NA].

subclavian n., a branch from the superior trunk of the brachial plexus supplying the subclavius muscle. SYN nervus subclavius [NA].

subcostal n., the ventral ramus of the twelfth thoracic n.; it courses below the last rib, supplies parts of the abdominal muscles and gives off cutaneous branches to the skin of the lower-most ventrolateral abdominal wall and to the superolateral gluteal region. SYN nervus subcostalis [NA].

sublingual n., a branch of the lingual to the sublingual gland and mucous membrane of the floor of the mouth. SYN nervus sublingualis [NA].

suboccipital n., dorsal ramus of the first cervical n., passing through the suboccipital triangle and sending branches to the rectus capitis posterior major and minor, obliquus capitis superior and inferior, rectus capitis lateralis, and semispinalis capitis; the first cervical spinal n. is generally considered to have only motor fibers, but the suboccipital n. receives sensory fibers for proprioception via a communicating branch from the second cervical spinal n. SYN nervus suboccipitalis [NA].

superior alveolar n.'s, three branches (posterior, middle, and anterior) of the maxillary n. (or its continuation as the infraorbital n.) that enter the maxilla to supply the mucosa of the maxillary sinus, upper teeth and gingiva. SYN nervi alveolares superiores [NA].

supraorbital n., a branch of the frontal n. leaving the orbit through the supraorbital foramen or notch and dividing into branches distributed to the forehead and scalp, upper eyelid, and frontal sinus. SYN nervus supraorbitalis [NA].

suprascapular n., arises from the upper trunk of the brachial plexus (fifth and sixth cervical spinal n.'s), passes downward parallel to the cords of the brachial plexus, then through the scapular notch, supplying the supraspinatus and infraspinatus muscles, and also sending branches to the shoulder joint. It is vulnerable to injury in fractures of the middle 1/3 of the clavicle; a lesion of the suprascapular n. results in a loss of lateral rotation at the shoulder so that when relaxed the limb rotates medially (waiter's tip position); ability to initiate abduction is also affected. SYN nervus suprascapularis [NA].

supratrochlear n., a branch of the frontal n. supplying the medial part of the upper eyelid, the central part of the skin of the forehead, and the root of the nose. SYN nervus supratrochlearis [NA].

sural n., formed by the union of the medial sural cutaneous from the tibial and the peroneal communicating branch of the common peroneal n., usually about the middle of the calf, although this is highly variable; thence it accompanies the small saphenous vein around the lateral malleolus to the dorsum of the foot as the lateral dorsal cutaneous n. SYN nervus suralis [NA].

sympathetic n., one of the n.'s of the sympathetic nervous system.

temporomandibular n., SYN zygomatic n.

n. of tensor tympani muscle, a branch of the mandibular n. conveying fibers from the motor root of the trigeminal n. which pass through the otic ganglion without synapse to supply the tensor tympani muscle. SYN nervus tensoris tympani [NA].

n. of tensor veli palatini muscle, a branch of the mandibular n. conveying fibers from the motor root of the trigeminal n. which pass through the otic ganglion without synapse to supply the tensor veli palatini muscle. SYN nervus tensoris veli palatini [NA].

terminal n.'s, SYN *nervi* terminales, under *nervus.*

thoracic cardiac n.'s, part of the cardiopulmonary splanchnic n.'s from the second to fifth segments of the thoracic sympathetic trunk that pass medially and anteriorly to enter the cardiac plexus; they convey postsynaptic sympathetic fibers to, and visceral afferent (pain) fibers from, the heart. SYN nervi cardiaci thoracici [NA].

thoracic spinal n.'s, twelve n.'s on each side, mixed motor and sensory, supplying the muscles and skin of the thoracic and abdominal walls. SYN nervi thoracici [NA].

thoracodorsal n., arises from the posterior cord of the brachial plexus; it contains fibers from the sixth, seventh, and eighth cervical n.'s and supplies the latissimus dorsi muscle. SYN nervus thoracodorsalis [NA].

tibial n., one of the two major divisions of the sciatic n., it courses down the back of the leg to terminate as the medial and lateral plantar n.'s in the foot; it supplies the hamstring muscles, the muscles of the back of the leg (the dorsiflexors and invertors of the foot) and the plantar aspect of the foot, as well as the skin on the back of the leg and sole of the foot. SYN nervus tibialis [NA].

transverse cervical n., a branch of the cervical plexus that supplies the skin over the anterior triangle of the neck. SYN nervus transversus colli [NA].

trigeminal n., the fifth cranial n.; the chief sensory n. of the face and the motor n. of the muscles of mastication; its nuclei are in the mesencephalon and in the pons extending down into the cervical portion of the spinal cord; it emerges by two roots, sensory and motor, from the lateral portion of the surface of the pons, and enters a cavity of the dura mater, the trigeminal cave, at the apex of the petrous portion of the temporal bone, where the sensory root expands to form the trigeminal ganglion; from there the three divisions (ophthalmic, maxillary, and mandibular n.'s) arise. SYN nervus trigeminus [NA].

trochlear n., the fourth cranial n.; supplies the superior oblique muscle of the eye; its origin is in the midbrain below the cerebral aqueduct, its fibers decussate in the superior medullary velum, and emerge from the brain at the side of the frenulum, the only cranial n. to arise from the dorsal aspect of the brain stem; it therefore has the longest intracranial course, entering the dura in the free edge of the tentorium, close to the posterior clinoid process, and passing in the lateral wall of the cavernous sinus to enter the orbit through the superior orbital fissure. SYN nervus trochlearis [NA].

tympanic n., a n. from the inferior ganglion of the glossopharyngeal n., passing through the tympanic canaliculus to the tympanic cavity, forming there the tympanic plexus which supplies the mucous membrane of the tympanic cavity, mastoid cells, and auditory tube; presynaptic parasympathetic fibers also pass through the tympanic n. via the lesser superficial petrosal n. to the otic ganglion, where they synapse with postsynaptic fibers that continue to supply the parotid gland. SYN nervus tympanicus [NA].

ulnar n., arises from the medial cord of the brachial plexus and passes down the arm, behind the medial epicondyle of the humerus, and down the ulnar side of the anterior compartment of the forearm to the hand; it gives off muscular branches in the forearm to the flexor carpi ulnaris muscle and the ulnar portion of flexor digitorum profundus and supplies hypothenar, interosseous, medial lumbricals, adductor pollicis and deep head of flexor hallucis brevis; intrinsic muscles of the hand and the skin of the small finger and medial side of the ring finger and adjacent portions of the palm of the hand. The ulnar n. is most vulnerable to injury where it passes subcutaneously behind the medial epicondyle of the humerus. Mild injury here produces "crazy bone" sensation. An ulnar n. lesion here results in loss of flexion of metacarpophalangeal joints and of extension at the interphalangeal joints ("claw hand"). SYN nervus ulnaris [NA], cubital n.

utricular n., a branch of the utriculoampullar n., supplying the macula of the utricle. SYN nervus utricularis [NA].

utriculoampullar n., a division of the vestibular part of the eighth cranial n.; it gives off branches to the macula of the utricle (utricular n.) and to the cristae of the ampullae of the anterior and lateral semicircular ducts (anterior and lateral ampullary n.'s). SYN nervus utriculoampullaris [NA].

vaginal n.'s, several n.'s passing from the uterovaginal plexus to the vagina. SYN nervi vaginales [NA].

vagus n., the 10th cranial n.; a mixed n. that arises by numerous small roots from the side of the medulla oblongata, between the glossopharyngeal above and the accessory below; it leaves the cranial cavity by the jugular foramen and passes down to supply the pharynx; larynx, trachea, lungs, heart, and the gastrointestinal tract as far as the left colic (splenic) flexure. SYN nervus vagus [NA], pneumogastric n., vagus.

vascular n., a small n. filament that supplies the wall of a blood vessel.

vasomotor n., a motor n. effecting or inhibiting contraction of the blood vessels.

vertebral n., a branch from the stellate ganglion that ascends along the vertebral artery to the level of the axis or atlas, giving branches to the cervical n.'s and meninges. SYN nervus vertebralis [NA].

vestibular n., the part of the vestibulocochlear n. peripheral to the vestibular root; it is composed of the central processes of bipolar neurons which have their terminals of their peripheral processes on the hair cells in the ampullae of the semicircular ducts and the maculae of the saccule and utricle, and cell bodies of the vestibular ganglion.

vestibulocochlear n., the eighth cranial n.; a composite sensory n. innervating the receptor cells of the membranous labyrinth; it consists of two major, anatomically and functionally distinct components each of which have different central connections: the vestibular n. and cochlear n. SYN nervus vestibulocochlearis [NA], acoustic n.

zygomatic n., a branch of the maxillary n. in the inferior orbital fissure through which it passes; it gives rise to two sensory branches, the zygomaticotemporal and zygomaticofacial, which supply the skin of the temporal and zygomatic regions and is continued as the communicating branch of the lacrimal n. with the zygomatic n. SYN nervus zygomaticus [NA], temporomandibular n.

ner•vi (ner'vī) [NA]. Plural of nervus. [L.]

ner•vi•mo•tor (ner-vi-mō'ter). Relating to a motor nerve. SYN neurimotor.

ner•von•ic ac•id (ner-von'-ik). A 24-carbon straight-chain fatty acid unsaturated between C-15 and C-16; occurs in cerebrosides such as nervone.

ner•vous (ner'vŭs). **1.** Relating to a nerve or the nerves. **2.** Easily excited or agitated; suffering from mental or emotional instability; tense or anxious. **3.** Formerly, denoting a temperament characterized by excessive mental and physical alertness, rapid pulse, excitability, often volubility, but not always fixity of purpose. [L. nervosus]

ner•vous break•down. Nonmedical term for an emotional or mental illness; often a euphemism for a psychiatric disorder.

ner•vous•ness (ner'vŭs-nes). A condition of being nervous (2).

ner•vus, gen. and pl. **ner•vi** (ner'vŭs, -vī) [NA]. SYN nerve. [L.]

    n. abdu'cens [NA], SYN abducent nerve.

    n. accesso'rius [NA], SYN accessory nerve.

    ner'vi alveola'res superio'res [NA], SYN superior alveolar nerves, under nerve.

    n. alveola'ris infe'rior [NA], SYN inferior alveolar nerve.

    ner'vi anococcyg'ei [NA], SYN anococcygeal nerves, under nerve.

    ner'vi auricula'res anterio'res [NA], SYN anterior auricular nerves, under nerve.

    n. auricula'ris mag'nus [NA], SYN great auricular nerve.

    n. auricula'ris poste'rior [NA], SYN posterior auricular nerve.

    n. auriculotempora'lis [NA], SYN auriculotemporal nerve.

    n. axilla'ris [NA], SYN axillary nerve.

    n. bucca'lis [NA], SYN buccal nerve.

n. cana'lis pterygoi'dei [NA], SYN *nerve of* pterygoid canal.

ner'vi cardi'aci thora'cici [NA], SYN thoracic cardiac *nerves*, under *nerve*.

ner'vi carot'ici exter'ni [NA], SYN external carotid *nerves*, under *nerve*.

n. caroticotympan'icus, pl. **ner'vi caroticotympan'ici** [NA], SYN caroticotympanic *nerve*.

n. carot'icus inter'nus [NA], SYN internal carotid *nerve*.

ner'vi caverno'si clitor'idis [NA], SYN cavernous *nerves* of clitoris, under *nerve*.

ner'vi caverno'si pe'nis [NA], SYN cavernous *nerves* of penis, under *nerve*.

n. coccyg'eus [NA], SYN coccygeal *nerve*.

ner'vi crania'les [NA], SYN cranial *nerves*, under *nerve*.

ner'vi digita'les dorsa'les [NA], SYN dorsal digital *nerves* of hand, under *nerve*.

ner'vi digita'les dorsa'les pe'dis [NA], SYN dorsal digital *nerves* of foot, under *nerve*.

n. dorsa'lis clitor'idis [NA], SYN dorsal *nerve* of clitoris.

n. dorsa'lis pe'nis [NA], SYN dorsal *nerve* of penis.

n. dorsa'lis scap'ulae [NA], SYN dorsal scapular *nerve*.

n. facia'lis [NA], SYN facial *nerve*.

n. femora'lis [NA], SYN femoral *nerve*.

n. fronta'lis [NA], SYN frontal *nerve*.

n. genitofemora'lis [NA], SYN genitofemoral *nerve*.

n. glossopharyn'geus [NA], SYN glossopharyngeal *nerve*.

n. hypogas'tricus [NA], SYN hypogastric *nerve*.

n. hypoglos'sus [NA], SYN hypoglossal *nerve*.

n. iliohypogas'tricus [NA], SYN iliohypogastric *nerve*.

n. ilioinguina'lis [NA], SYN ilioinguinal *nerve*.

n. infraorbita'lis [NA], SYN infraorbital *nerve*.

n. infratrochlea'ris [NA], SYN infratrochlear *nerve*.

ner'vi intercosta'les [NA], SYN intercostal *nerves*, under *nerve*.

ner'vi intercostobrachia'les [NA], SYN intercostobrachial *nerves*, under *nerve*.

n. interme'dius [NA], SYN intermediary *nerve*.

n. interos'seus ante'rior [NA], SYN anterior interosseous *nerve*.

n. interos'seus cru'ris [NA], SYN crural interosseous *nerve*.

n. interos'seus poste'rior [NA], SYN posterior interosseous *nerve*.

n. ischia'dicus [NA], SYN sciatic *nerve*.

n. jugula'ris [NA], SYN jugular *nerve*.

n. lacrima'lis [NA], SYN lacrimal *nerve*.

n. lingua'lis [NA], SYN lingual *nerve*.

ner'vi lumba'les [NA], SYN lumbar *nerves*, under *nerve*.

n. mandibula'ris [NA], SYN mandibular *nerve*.

n. masseter'icus [NA], SYN masseteric *nerve*.

n. maxilla'ris [NA], SYN maxillary *nerve*.

n. media'nus [NA], SYN median *nerve*.

n. menta'lis [NA], SYN mental *nerve*.

n. musculocuta'neus [NA], SYN musculocutaneous *nerve*.

n. mylohyoi'deus [NA], SYN mylohyoid *nerve*.

n. nasocilia'ris [NA], SYN nasociliary *nerve*.

n. nasopalati'nus [NA], SYN nasopalatine *nerve*.

n. obturato'rius [NA], SYN obturator *nerve*.

n. oculomoto'rius [NA], SYN oculomotor *nerve*.

ner'vi olfacto'rii [NA], SYN olfactory *nerves*, under *nerve*.

n. ophthal'micus [NA], SYN ophthalmic *nerve*.

n. op'ticus [NA], SYN optic *nerve*.

ner'vi palati'ni mino'res [NA], SYN lesser palatine *nerves*, under *nerve*.

n. palati'nus ma'jor [NA], SYN greater palatine *nerve*.

ner'vi perinea'les [NA], SYN perineal *nerves*, under *nerve*.

ner'vi phren'ici accesso'rii [NA], SYN accessory phrenic *nerves*, under *nerve*.

n. phren'icus [NA], SYN phrenic *nerve*.

n. pterygoi'deus [NA], SYN pterygoid *nerve*.

ner'vi pterygopalati'ni, SYN ganglionic *branches* of maxillary nerve, under *branch*.

n. puden'dus [NA], SYN pudendal *nerve*.

n. radia'lis [NA], SYN radial *nerve*.

ner'vi recta'les inferio'res [NA], SYN inferior rectal *nerves*, under *nerve*.

n. saccula'ris [NA], SYN saccular *nerve*.

ner'vi sacra'les [NA], SYN sacral *nerves*, under *nerve*.

n. saphe'nus [NA], SYN saphenous *nerve*.

ner'vi spina'les [NA], SYN spinal *nerves*, under *nerve*.

ner'vi splanch'nici lumba'les [NA], SYN lumbar splanchnic *nerves*, under *nerve*.

ner'vi splanch'nici sacra'les [NA], SYN sacral splanchnic *nerves*, under *nerve*.

n. splanch'nicus i'mus [NA], SYN lowest splanchnic *nerve*.

n. splanch'nicus ma'jor [NA], SYN greater splanchnic *nerve*.

n. splanch'nicus mi'nor [NA], SYN lesser splanchnic *nerve*.

n. stape'dius [NA], SYN *nerve* to stapedius muscle.

n. subcla'vius [NA], SYN subclavian *nerve*.

n. subcosta'lis [NA], SYN subcostal *nerve*.

n. sublingua'lis [NA], SYN sublingual *nerve*.

n. suboccipita'lis [NA], SYN suboccipital *nerve*.

n. supraorbita'lis [NA], SYN supraorbital *nerve*.

n. suprascapula'ris [NA], SYN suprascapular *nerve*.

n. supratrochlea'ris [NA], SYN supratrochlear *nerve*.

n. sura'lis [NA], SYN sural *nerve*.

ner'vi tempora'les profun'di [NA], SYN deep temporal *nerves*, under *nerve*.

n. tenso'ris tym'pani [NA], SYN *nerve* of tensor tympani muscle.

n. tenso'ris ve'li palati'ni [NA], SYN *nerve* of tensor veli palatini muscle.

ner'vi termina'les [NA], delicate plexiform nerve strands passing parallel and medial to the olfactory tracts, distributing peripherally with the olfactory nerves and passing centrally into the anterior perforated substance; they are considered to have an autonomic function but the exact nature of this is unknown. SYN terminal nerves.

ner'vi thora'cici [NA], SYN thoracic spinal *nerves*, under *nerve*.

n. thora'cicus lon'gus [NA], SYN long thoracic *nerve*.

n. thoracodorsa'lis [NA], SYN thoracodorsal *nerve*.

n. tibia'lis [NA], SYN tibial *nerve*.

n. transver'sus col'li [NA], SYN transverse cervical *nerve*.

n. trigem'inus [NA], SYN trigeminal *nerve*.

n. trochlea'ris [NA], SYN trochlear *nerve*.

n. tympan'icus [NA], SYN tympanic *nerve*.

n. ulna'ris [NA], SYN ulnar *nerve*.

n. utricula'ris [NA], SYN utricular *nerve*.

n. utriculoampulla'ris [NA], SYN utriculoampullar *nerve*.

ner'vi vagina'les [NA], SYN vaginal *nerves*, under *nerve*.

n. va'gus [NA], SYN vagus *nerve*.

n. vertebra'lis [NA], SYN vertebral *nerve*.

n. vestibulocochlea'ris [NA], SYN vestibulocochlear *nerve*. See entries under radix.

n. zygomat'icus [NA], SYN zygomatic *nerve*.

net. SYN network (1).

net•work (net′werk). **1.** A structure bearing a resemblance to a woven fabric. A network of nerve fibers or small vessels. SYN rete (1) [NA], net. SEE ALSO reticulum. **2.** The persons in a patient's environment, especially as significant for the course of the illness.

   arteriolar n., a vascular network formed by anastomoses between minute arteries just before they become capillaries.

   articular vascular n. of elbow, vascular networks in the region of the elbow, composed of anastomoses between branches of the radial and middle collateral, superior and inferior ulnar collateral, radial recurrent, interosseous recurrent, and recurrent ulnar arteries.

△**neur-, neuri-, neuro-.** Nerve, nerve tissue, the nervous system. [G. *neuron*]

neu•ral (nūr′ăl). **1.** Relating to any structure composed of nerve cells or their processes, or that on further development will evolve into nerve cells. **2.** Referring to the dorsal side of the vertebral bodies or their precursors, where the spinal cord is located, as opposed to hemal (2). [G. *neuron*, nerve]

neu•ral•gia (nū-ral′jē-ă). Pain of a severe, throbbing, or stabbing character in the course or distribution of a nerve. SYN neurodynia. [neur- + G. *algos*, pain]

   n. facia'lis ve'ra, SYN geniculate n.

   Fothergill's n., SYN trigeminal n.

   geniculate n., a severe paroxysmal lancinating pain deep in the ear, on the anterior wall of the external meatus, and on a small area just in front of the pinna. SYN Hunt's n., n. facialis vera.

   Hunt's n., SYN geniculate n.

   idiopathic n., nerve pain not due to any apparent cause.

   Morton's n., n. of an interdigital nerve, usually the anastomotic branch between the medial and lateral plantar nerves, resulting from compression of the nerve by the metatarsophalangeal joint.

   red n., SYN erythromelalgia.

   trifacial n., SYN trigeminal n.

   trigeminal n., severe, paroxysmal bursts of pain in one or more branches of the trigeminal nerve; often induced by touching trigger points in or about the mouth. SYN Fothergill's disease (1), Fothergill's n., prosopalgia, prosoponeuralgia, tic douloureux, trifacial n.

neu•ral•gic (nū-ral′jik). Relating to, resembling, or of the character of, neuralgia.

neur•a•min•ic ac•id (nūr′ă-min′ik). An aldol product of D-mannosamine and pyruvic acid. The *N*- and *O*-acyl derivatives of n. a. are known as sialic acids and are constituents of gangliosides and of the polysaccharide components of muco- and glycoproteins from many tissues and secretions.

neur•an•a•gen•e•sis (nūr′an-ă-jen′ĕ-sis). Regeneration of a nerve. [neur- + G. *ana*, up, again, + *genesis*, origin]

neur•a•poph•y•sis (nūr-ă-pof′i-sis). SYN *lamina* of vertebral arch. [neur- + G. *apophysis*, offshoot]

neur•a•prax•ia (nūr-ă-prak′sē-ă). The mildest type of focal nerve lesion that produces clinical deficits; localized loss of conduction along a nerve without axon degeneration; caused by a focal lesion, usually demyelinating, and followed by a complete recovery. SEE ALSO axonotmesis. [neur- + G. a- priv. + *praxis*, action]

neur•as•the•nia (nūr-as-thē′nē-ă). An ill-defined condition, commonly accompanying or following depression, characterized by vague fatigue believed to be brought on by psychological factors. [neur- + G. *astheneia*, weakness]

neur•as•then•ic (nūr-as-then′ik). Relating to, or suffering from, neurasthenia.

neur•ax•is (nū-rak′sis). The axial, unpaired part of the central nervous system: spinal cord, rhombencephalon, mesencephalon, and diencephalon, in contrast to the paired cerebral hemisphere, or telencephalon.

neur•ec•ta•sis, neur•ec•ta•sia, neur•ec•ta•sy (nū-rek′tă-sis, nūr-ek-tā′zē-ă, -ek′tă-sē). The operation of stretching a nerve or nerve trunk. [neur- + G. *ektasis*, extension]

neu•rec•to•my (nū-rek′tō-mē). Excision of a segment of a nerve. [neur- + G. *ektomē*, excision]

   presacral n., cutting of the presacral nerve to relieve severe dysmenorrhea. SYN Cotte's operation, presacral sympathectomy.

neur•ec•to•pia, neur•ec•to•py (nūr-ek-tō′pē-ă, -ek′tō-pē). **1.** Dislocation of a nerve trunk. **2.** A condition in which a nerve follows an anomalous course. [neur- + G. *ektopos*, fr. *ek*, out of, + *topos*, place]

neu•rer•gic (nū-rer′jik). Relating to the activity of a nerve. [neur- + G. *ergon*, work]

neur•ex•er•e•sis (nūr-ek-ser′ĕ-sis). Tearing out or evulsion of a nerve. [neur- + G. *exairesis*, a taking out, fr. *haireō*, to grasp, take]

△**neuri-.** SEE neur-.

neu•ri•lem•ma (nūr-i-lem′ă). A cell that enfolds one or more axons of the peripheral nervous system; in myelinated fibers its plasma membrane forms the lamellae of myelin. SYN neurolemma, sheath of Schwann. [neuri + G. *lemma*, husk]

neu•ri•le•mo•ma (nūr′i-lē-mō′mă). SYN schwannoma. [neurilemma + G. *-oma*, tumor]

  acoustic n., schwannoma arising from cranial nerve eight.

neu•ri•mo•tor (nūr-i-mō′ter). SYN nervimotor.

neu•ri•no•ma (nūr-i-nō′mă). Obsolete term for schwannoma.

neu•rit•ic (nū-rit′ik). Relating to neuritis.

neu•ri•tis, pl. **neu•ri•ti•des** (nū-rī′tis, nū-rit′i-dēz). 1. Inflammation of a nerve. 2. SYN neuropathy. [neuri- + G. *-itis*, inflammation]

  adventitial n., inflammation of the sheath of a nerve. SEE ALSO perineuritis.

  endemic n., SYN beriberi.

  interstitial n., inflammation of the connective tissue framework of a nerve.

  multiple n., SYN polyneuropathy.

  optic n., inflammation of the optic nerve. SEE ALSO *neuromyelitis* optica, retrobulbar n., papillitis.

  parenchymatous n., inflammation of the nervous substance proper, the axons, and myelin.

  retrobulbar n., optic n. without swelling of the optic disk.

  segmental n., (1) inflammation occurring at several points along the course of a nerve; **(2)** segmental demyelinating neuropathy.

  toxic n., n. caused by an endogenous or exogenous toxin.

  traumatic n., nerve lesion following an injury.

neuro-. SEE neur-.

neu•ro•an•as•to•mo•sis (nūr′ō-an-as-tō-mō′sis). Surgical formation of a junction between nerves.

neu•ro•a•nat•o•my (nūr′ō-ă-nat′ō-mē). The anatomy of the nervous system, usually specific to the central nervous system.

neu•ro•ar•throp•a•thy (nūr′ō-ar-throp′ă-thē). A joint disorder caused by loss of joint sensation. SEE Charcot's *joint.* [neuro- + G. *arthron*, joint, + *pathos*, suffering, disease]

neu•ro•blast (nūr′ō-blast). An embryonic nerve cell. [neuro- + G. *blastos*, germ]

neu•ro•blas•to•ma (nūr′ō-blas-tō′mă). A malignant neoplasm characterized by immature nerve cells of embryonic type, *i.e.,* neuroblasts; the stroma is sparse and foci of necrosis and hemorrhage are not unusual. N.'s occur frequently in infants and children in the mediastinal and retroperitoneal regions; widespread metastases to the liver, lungs, lymph nodes, cranial cavity, and skeleton are very common.

neu•ro•car•di•ac (nūr-ō-kar′dē-ak). 1. Relating to the nerve supply of the heart. 2. Relating to a cardiac neurosis. [neuro- + G. *kardia*, heart]

neu•ro•chem•is•try (nūr-ō-kem′is-trē). The science concerned with the chemical aspects of nervous system structure and function.

neu•ro•cho•ri•o•ret•i•ni•tis (nūr-ō-kōr′ē-ō-ret-in-ī′tis). Inflammation of the choroid, the retina, and the optic nerve.

neu•ro•cho•roi•di•tis (nūr-ō-kō-roy-dī′tis). Inflammation of the choroid and the optic nerve.

neu•roc•la•dism (nū-rok′lă-dizm). The outgrowth of axons from the central stump to bridge the gap in a cut nerve. [neuro- + G. *klados*, a young branch]

neu•ro•cra•ni•um (nūr-ō-krā′nē-ŭm). Those bones of the skull enclosing the brain, as distinguished from the bones of the face. SYN braincase. [neuro- + G. *kranion*, skull]

neu•ro•cris•top•a•thy (nūr′ō-kris-top′ă-thē). Developmental anomaly of the neural crest manifested by abnormal development and tumors of the neural axis. [neuro- + L. *crista*, crest, + G. *pathos*, suffering]

neu•ro•cyte (nūr′o-sīt). SYN neuron. [neuro- + G. *kytos*, cell]

neu•ro•cy•tol•y•sis (nūr′ō-sī-tol′i-sis). Destruction of neurons. [neuro- + G. *kytos*, cell, + *lysis*, dissolution]

neu•ro•cy•to•ma (nūr′ō-sī-tō′mă). A tumor of neuronal differentiation usually intraventricular in location, consisting of sheets of cells with uniform nuclei and occasional perivascular pseudorosette formation. [neuro- + G. *kytos*, cell, + *-oma*, tumor]

neu•ro•den•drite (nūr-ō-den′drīt). SYN dendrite (1).

neu•ro•der•ma•ti•tis (nūr′ō-der-mă-tī′tis). A chronic lichenified skin lesion; loosely applied to atopic dermatitis. SYN neurodermatosis. [neuro- + G. *derma*, skin, + *-itis*, inflammation]

neu•ro•der•ma•to•sis (nūr′ō-der-mă-tō′sis). SYN neurodermatitis.

neu•ro•dy•nam•ic (nūr′ō-dī-nam′ik). Pertaining to nervous energy. [neuro- + G. *dynamis*, force]

neu•ro•dyn•ia (nūr-ō-din′ē-ă). SYN neuralgia. [neuro- + G. *odynē*, pain]

neu•ro•ec•to•derm (nūr-ō-ek′tō-derm). That central region of the early embryonic ectoderm which on further development forms the brain and spinal cord, and also evolves into the nerve cells and neurilemma or Schwann cells of the peripheral nervous system.

neu•ro•ec•to•der•mal (nūr′ō-ek-tō-der′măl). Relating to the neuroectoderm.

neu•ro•en•ceph•a•lo•my•e•lop•a•thy (nūr′ō-en-sef′ă-lō-mī-ĕ-op′ă-thē). Disease of the brain, spinal cord, and nerves.

neu•ro•en•do•crine (nūr-ō-en′dō-krin). 1. Pertaining to the anatomical and functional relationships between the nervous system and the endocrine apparatus. 2. Descriptive of cells that release a hormone into the circulating blood in response to a neural stimulus.

neu•ro•en•do•crin•ol•o•gy (nūr-ō-en′dō-krin-ol′ō-jē). The specialty concerned with the anatomical and functional relationships between the nervous system and the endocrine apparatus.

neu•ro•ep•i•the•li•al (nūr′ō-ep-i-thē′lē-ăl). Relating to the neuroepithelium.

neu•ro•ep•i•the•li•um (nūr′ō-ep-i-thē′lē-ŭm) [NA]. Epithelial cells specialized for the reception of external stimuli, such as the hair cells of the inner ear, the receptor cells of the taste buds and the rods and cones of the retina.

neu•ro•fi•bril (nūr-ō-fī′bril). A filamentous structure seen with the light microscope in the body, dendrites, axon, and sometimes synaptic endings of a nerve cell.

neu•ro•fi•bril•lar (nūr-ō-fī′bri-lĕr). Relating to neurofibrils.

neu•ro•fi•bro•ma (nūr′ō-fī-brō′mǎ). A benign, encapsulated tumor resulting from proliferation of Schwann cells. SYN fibroneuroma.

plexiform n., a type of n., representing an anomaly rather than a true neoplasm, in which the proliferation of Schwann cells occurs from the inner aspect of the nerve sheath; seen most frequently in neurofibromatosis. SYN plexiform neuroma.

neu•ro•fi•bro•ma•to•sis (nūr′ō-fī-brō-mǎ-tō′sis) [MIM*162200]. Two distinct major hereditary disorders called type 1 and type 2. Type 1 (peripheral) n., by far the more common, is characterized by patches of hyperpigmentation in both cutaneous and subcutaneous tumors. skin areas, present from birth, are called café-au-lait spots. The cutaneous and subcutaneous tumors, nerve sheath neoplasms called neurofibromas, can develop anywhere along the peripheral nerves. Neurofibromas can become quite large, causing disfigurement, eroding bone, and compressing peripheral nerves. SYN von Recklinghausen's disease. Type 2 (central) n. has few cutaneous manifestations, and consists primarily of acoustic neuromas, causing deafness, often accompanied by other intracranial/paraspinal neoplasms, such as meningiomas and gliomas.

neu•ro•fil•a•ment (nūr-ō-fil′ǎ-ment). A class of intermediate filaments found in neurons.

neu•ro•gang•li•on (nūr-ō-gang′lē-on). SYN ganglion (1).

neu•ro•gen•e•sis (nūr-ō-jen′ě-sis). Formation of the nervous system. [neuro- + G. *genesis,* production]

neu•ro•gen•ic, neu•ro•ge•net•ic (nūr-ō-jen′ik, -jě-net′ik). **1.** Originating in, starting from, or caused by, the nervous system or nerve impulses. SYN neurogenous. **2.** Relating to neurogenesis.

neu•rog•e•nous (nū-roj′ě-nŭs). SYN neurogenic (1).

neu•rog•lia (nū-rog′lē-ǎ). Non-neuronal cellular elements of the central and peripheral nervous system; thought to have important metabolic functions. In central nervous tissue they include oligodendroglia cells, astrocytes, ependymal cells, and microglia cells. SYN glia, reticulum (2). [neuro- + G. *glia,* glue]

neu•rog•li•a•cyte (nū-rog′lē-ă-sīt). A neuroglia cell. SEE neuroglia. [neuro- + G. *glia,* glue, + *kytos,* cell]

neu•rog•li•al, neu•rog•li•ar (nū-rog′lē-ăl, -lē-ăr). Relating to neuroglia.

neu•rog•li•o•ma•to•sis (nū-rog′lē-ō-mă-tō′sis). SYN gliomatosis.

neu•ro•gram (nūr′ō-gram). The imprint on the brain substance theoretically remaining after every mental experience, *i.e.,* the engram or physical register of the mental experience, stimulation of which retrieves and reproduces the original experience, thereby producing memory. [neuro- + G. *gramma,* something written]

neu•ro•his•tol•o•gy (nūr′ō-his-tol′ō-jē). The microscopic anatomy of the nervous system.

neu•ro•hor•mone (nūr-ō-hōr′mōn). A hormone

formed by neurosecretory cells and liberated by nerve impulses (*e.g.,* norepinephrine).

neu•ro•hy•po•phys•i•al (nūr′ō-hī-pō-fiz′ē-ăl). Relating to the neurohypophysis.

neu•ro•hy•poph•y•sis (nūr′ō-hī-pof′i-sis) [NA]. A neuroendocrine structure suspended from the base of the hypothalamus. It is composed of the infundibulum and the posterior lobe of the hypophysis. SEE ALSO hypophysis. SYN lobus posterior hypophyseos ☆ [NA], posterior lobe of hypophysis. [neuro- + hypophysis]

neu•roid (nūr′oyd). Resembling a nerve; nervelike. [neuro- + G. *eidos,* resemblance]

neu•ro•lem•ma (nūr-ō-lem′ǎ). SYN neurilemma. [neuro- + G. *lemma,* husk]

neu•ro•lept•an•al•ge•sia (nūr′ō-lept-an-ăl-jē′zē-ǎ). An intense analgesic and amnesic state produced by administration of narcotic analgesics and neuroleptic drugs; unconsciousness may or may not occur, and cardiorespiratory function may be altered.

neu•ro•lept•an•es•the•sia (nūr′ō-lept-an-es-thē′zē-ah). A technique of general anesthesia based upon intravenous administration of neuroleptic drugs, together with inhalation of a weak anesthetic with or without neuromuscular relaxants.

neu•ro•lep•tic (nūr-ō-lep′tik). **1.** Any of a class of psychotropic drugs used to treast psychosis, particularly schizophrenia; includes the phenothiazine, thioxanthene, and butyrophenone derivatives and the dihydroindolones. SYN neuroleptic agent. SEE ALSO antipsychotic *agent.* **2.** Denoting a condition similar to that produced by such an agent. [neuro- + G. *lēpsis,* taking hold]

neu•rol•o•gist (nū-rol′ō-jist). A specialist in the diagnosis and treatment of disorders of the neuromuscular system: the central, peripheral, and autonomic nervous systems, the neuromuscular junction, and muscle.

neu•rol•o•gy (nū-rol′ō-jē). The branch of medical science concerned with the various nervous systems (central, peripheral, and autonomic, plus the neuromuscular junction and muscle) and its disorders. [neuro- + G. *logos,* study]

neu•rol•y•sin (nū-rol′i-sin). An antibody causing destruction of ganglion and cortical cells, obtained by the injection of brain substance. SYN neurotoxin (1).

neu•rol•y•sis (nū-rol′i-sis). **1.** Destruction of nerve tissue. **2.** Freeing of a nerve from inflammatory adhesions. [neuro- + G. *lysis,* dissolution]

neu•ro•lyt•ic (nūr-ō-lit′ik). Relating to neurolysis.

neu•ro•ma (nū-ro′mǎ). General term for any neoplasm derived from cells of the nervous system, *e.g.,* ganglioneuroma, neurilemoma, pseudoneuroma, and others. [neuro- + G. *-oma,* tumor]

acoustic n., a benign tumor arising from Schwann cells of the auditory nerve (8th cranial nerve).

amputation n., SYN traumatic n.

n. cu′tis, neurofibroma of the skin.

false n., SYN traumatic n.

plexiform n., SYN plexiform *neurofibroma.*

n. telangiecto′des, a neurofibroma with a conspicuous number of blood vessels, some of which have unusually large lumens (in proportion to the thickness of the walls).

   traumatic n., the non-neoplastic proliferative mass of Schwann cells and neurites that may develop at the proximal end of a severed or injured nerve. SYN amputation n., false n.

neu•ro•ma•la•cia (nūr′ō-mă-lā′shē-ă). Pathologic softening of nervous tissue. [neuro- + G. *malakia,* softness]

neu•ro•ma•to•sis (nūr′ō-mă-tō′sis). The presence of multiple neuromas, as in neurofibromatosis.

neu•ro•mere (nūr′ō-mēr). Elevations in the wall of the developing neural tube, especially the rhombencephalon/rhombomeres; that segment of the developing spinal cord to which dorsal and ventral roots are attached. [neuro- + G. *meros,* part]

neu•ro•mus•cu•lar (nūr-ō-mŭs′kyū-lăr). Referring to the relationship between nerve and muscle, in particular to the motor innervation of skeletal muscles and its pathology (*e.g.,* neuromuscular disorders). SEE ALSO myoneural.

neu•ro•my•as•the•nia (nūr′ō-mī-as-thē′nē-ă). Obsolete term for muscular weakness due to a neurologic or psychologic disorder. [neuro- + G. *mys,* muscle, + *a-* priv. + *sthenos,* strength]

   epidemic n., an epidemic disease characterized by stiffness of the neck and back, headache, diarrhea, fever, and localized muscular weakness; probably viral in origin. SYN benign myalgic encephalomyelitis, Iceland disease.

neu•ro•my•e•li•tis (nūr′ō-mī-el-ī′tis). Neuritis combined with spinal cord inflammation. SYN myeloneuritis. [neuro- + G. *myelos,* marrow, + *-itis,* inflammation]

   n. op′tica, a demyelinating disorder consisting of a transverse myelopathy and optic neuritis. SYN Devic's disease.

neu•ro•my•op•a•thy (nūr′ō-mī-op′ă-thē). **1.** A disorder of muscle due to impairment of its nerve supply. **2.** Simultaneous disorders of nerve and muscles. [neuro- + G. *mys,* muscle, + *pathos,* disease]

neu•ron (nūr′on). The morphological and functional unit of the nervous system, consisting of the nerve cell body with its the dendrites and axon. SYN neurocyte. **2.** Obsolete term for axon. [G. *neuron,* a nerve]

   bipolar n., a n. that has two processes arising from opposite poles of the cell body.

   Golgi type I n., nerve cells whose long axons leave the gray matter of which they form a part.

   Golgi type II n., nerve cells with short axons which ramify in the gray matter.

   internuncial n., a n. interposed between and connecting two other n.'s.

   lower motor n., the final motor n.'s that innervate skeletal muscles; distinguished from upper motor n.'s of the motor cortex that contribute to the pyramidal or corticospinal tract. SEE ALSO motor n.

   motor n., a nerve cell in the spinal cord, rhombencephalon, or mesencephalon characterized by an axon that leaves the central nervous system to establish a functional connection with an effector (muscle or glandular) tissue; **somatic motor n.'s** directly synapse with striated muscle

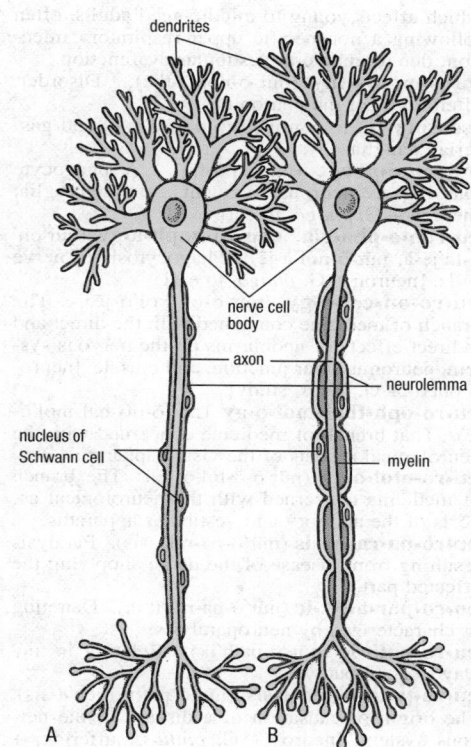

neuron: (A) unmyelinated, (B) myelinated

fibers by motor endplates; **visceral motor n.'s** or **autonomic motor n.'s** (preganglionic m. n.'s), by contrast, innervate smooth muscle fibers or glands only by the intermediary of a second, peripheral, n. (postganglionic or ganglionic m. n.) located in an autonomic ganglion. SEE ALSO motor *endplate,* autonomic nervous *system.* SYN motoneuron.

   multipolar n., a n. with several processes, usually an axon and three or more dendrites.

   unipolar n., a n. whose cell body gives off a single axonal process resulting from the fusion of two polar processes during development; at a variable distance from the cell body, the process divides into a peripheral axon branch extending outward as a peripheral afferent (sensory) nerve fiber, and a central axon branch that enters into synaptic contact with n.'s in the spinal cord or brainstem.

neu•ro•nal (nūr′ō-năl, nū-rō′năl). Pertaining to a neuron.

neu•ro•ne•vus (nūr-ō-nē′vŭs). A variety of intradermal nevus in adults in which nests of atrophic nevus cells in the lower dermis are hyalinized and resemble nerve bundles.

neu•ron•i•tis (nūr-ō-nī′tis). Inflammatory disorder of the neuron.

   vestibular n., a paroxysmal attack of severe vertigo, not accompanied by deafness or tinnitus, which affects young to middle-aged adults, often following a nonspecific upper respiratory infection; due to unilateral vestibular dysfunction.

neu•ro•nop•a•thy (nūr-ō-nop′ă-thē). Disorder, often toxic, of the neuron (1).

  sensory n., n. confined to dorsal root and gasserian ganglia.

neu•ron•o•phage (nū-ron′ō-fāj). A phagocyte that ingests neuronal elements. SEE microglia. [neuron + G. *phagō,* to eat]

neu•ron•o•pha•gia, neu•ro•noph•a•gy (nūr′on′ō-fā′jē-ă, nūr-ō-nof′ă-jē). Phagocytosis of nerve cells. [neuron + G. *phagō,* to eat]

neu•ro-on•col•o•gy (nūr′ō-on-kol′ō-jē). The branch of medicine concerned with the direct and indirect effects of neoplasms on the nervous system, neuromuscular junction, and muscle. [neuro- + onco- + G. *logos,* study]

neu•ro•oph•thal•mol•o•gy (nūr′ō-of-thal-mol′ō-jē). That branch of medicine concerned with the neurological aspects of the visual apparatus.

neu•ro-otol•o•gy (nūr′ō-ō-tol′ō-jē). The branch of medicine concerned with the neurological aspects of the auditory and vestibular apparatus.

neu•ro•pa•ral•y•sis (nūr′ō-pă-ral′i-sis). Paralysis resulting from disease of the nerve supplying the affected part.

neu•ro•par•a•lyt•ic (nūr′ō-pa-ră-lit′ik). Denoting or characterized by neuroparalysis.

neu•ro•path•ic (nūr-ō-path′ik). Relating in any way to neuropathy.

neu•ro•path•o•gen•e•sis (nūr′ō-path-ō-jen′ĕ-sis). The origin or causation of a disease of the nervous system. [neuro- + G. *pathos,* suffering, + *genesis,* origin]

neu•ro•pa•thol•o•gy (nūr′ō-pa-thol′ō-jē). **1.** Pathology of the nervous system. **2.** That branch of pathology concerned with the nervous system.

neu•rop•a•thy (nū-rop′ă-thē). **1.** Any disorder affecting the nervous system. **2.** In contemporary usage, a disease involving the cranial nerves, or the peripheral or autonomic nervous systems. SYN neuritis (2). [neuro- + G. *pathos,* suffering]

  compression n., a focal nerve lesion produced when sustained pressure is applied to a localized portion of the nerve, either from an external or internal source.

  diabetic n., a generic term for any diabetes mellitus-related disorder of the peripheral nervous system, autonomic nervous system, and some cranial nerves. This most commonly occurring of the chronic complications of diabetes takes two forms, peripheral (with dulling of the sensations of pain, temperature, and pressure, especially in the lower legs and feet), and autonomic (with alternating bouts of diarrhea and constipation, impotence, and reduced cardiac function).

  entrapment n., a focal nerve lesion produced by constriction or mechanical distortion of the nerve, within a fibrous or fibro-osseous tunnel, or by a fibrous band.

  familial amyloid n. [MIM*176300, various kinds], a disorder in which various peripheral nerves are infiltrated with amyloid and their functions disturbed, an abnormal prealbumin is also formed and is present in the blood; characteristi-

cally, it begins during mid-life and is found largely in persons of Portuguese descent; autosomal dominant inheritance. Other rare clinical types occur.

  giant axonal n., a rare disorder beginning at or after the third year of life, and presenting clinically with kinky hair, progressive clumsiness, muscle weakness and atrophy, sensory loss, and areflexia.

  vitamin B$_{12}$ n., SYN subacute combined *degeneration* of the spinal cord.

neu•ro•pep•tide (nūr-ō-pep′tīd). Any of a variety of peptides found in neural tissue; *e.g.,* endorphins, enkephalins.

neu•ro•phar•ma•col•o•gy (nūr′ō-far′mă-kol′ō-jē). The study of drugs that affect neuronal tissue.

neu•ro•phy•sins (nūr-ō-fiz′inz). A family of proteins synthesized in the hypothalamus as part of the large precursor protein that includes vasopressin and oxytocin in the neurosecretory granules; n. function as carriers in the transport and storage of neurohypophysial hormones.

neu•ro•phys•i•ol•o•gy (nūr′ō-fiz-ē-ol′ō-jē). Physiology of the nervous system.

neu•ro•pil, neu•ro•pile (nūr′ō-pil, -pīl). The complex, feltlike net of axonal, dendritic, and glial arborizations that forms the bulk of the central nervous system's gray matter, and in which the nerve cell bodies lie embedded. [neuro- + G. *pilos,* felt]

neu•ro•plasm (nūr′ō-plazm). The protoplasm of a nerve cell.

neu•ro•plas•ty (nūr′ō-plas-tē). Plastic surgery of the nerves. [neuro- + G. *plastos,* formed]

neu•ro•ple•gic (nūr-ō-plē′jik). Pertaining to paralysis due to nervous system disease. [neuro- + G. *plēgē,* a stroke]

neu•ro•po•dia (nūr-ō-pō′dē-ă). SYN axon *terminals,* under *terminal.* [pl. of *neuropodium* or *neuropodion,* fr. neuro- + G. *podion,* little foot]

neu•ro•pore (nūr′ō-pōr). An opening in the embryo leading from the central canal of the neural tube to the exterior of the tube. [neuro- + G. *poros,* pore]

neu•ro•psy•chi•a•try (nūr′ō-sī-kī′ă-trē). The specialty dealing with both organic and psychic disorders of the nervous system.

neu•ro•psy•chop•a•thy (nūr′ō-sī-kop′ă-thē). An emotional illness of neurologic and/or functional origin.

neu•ro•ra•di•ol•o•gy (nūr′rō-rā-dē-ol′ō-jē). The clinical subspecialty concerned with the diagnostic radiology of diseases of the central nervous system, head, and neck.

neu•ro•ret•i•ni•tis (nūr′ō-ret-i-nī′tis). An inflammation affecting the optic nerve head and the posterior pole of the retina, with cells in the nearby vitreous, usually producing a macular star. SYN papilloretinitis.

neu•ror•rha•phy (nūr-ōr′ă-fē). Joining together, usually by suture, of the two parts of a divided nerve. SYN neurosuture. [neuro- + G. *rhaphē,* suture]

neu•ro•sar•co•clei•sis (nūr′ō-sar-kō-klī′sis). An operation for the relief of neuralgia, consisting of resection of one of the walls of an osseous canal traversed by the nerve and transposition of the nerve into the soft tissues. [neuro- + G. *sarx*, flesh, + *kleisis*, closure]

neu•ro•sar•coid•o•sis (nūr′ō-sar-koy-dō′sis). A granulomatous disease of unknown etiology involving the central nervous system, usually with concomitant systemic involvement.

neu•ro•sci•enc•es (nūr-ō-sī′en-sez). The scientific disciplines concerned with the development, structure, function, chemistry, pharmacology, clinical assessments, and pathology of the nervous system.

neu•ro•se•cre•tion (nūr′ō-sē-krē′shŭn). The release of a secretory substance from the axon terminals of certain nerve cells in the brain into the circulating blood.

neu•ro•se•cre•to•ry (nūr′ō-sē′krě-tōr-ē, -sē-krē′ tōr-ē). Relating to neurosecretion.

neu•ro•sis, pl. **neu•ro•ses** (nū-rō′sis, -sēz). **1.** A psychological or behavioral disorder in which anxiety is the primary characteristic; defense mechanisms or any of the phobias are the adjustive techniques which an individual learns in order to cope with this underlying anxiety. In contrast to the psychoses, persons with a n. do not exhibit gross distortion of reality or disorganization of personality. **2.** A functional nervous disease, or one for which there is no evident lesion. **3.** A peculiar state of tension or irritability of the nervous system; any form of nervousness. SYN psychoneurosis. [neuro- + G. *-osis,* condition]

   anxiety n., chronic abnormal distress and worry to the point of panic followed by a tendency to avoid or run from the feared situation, associated with overaction of the sympathetic nervous system.

   battle n., SYN war n.

   cardiac n., anxiety concerning the state of the heart, as a result of palpitation, chest pain, or other symptoms not due to heart disease; a form of hypochondriasis. SYN cardioneurosis.

   character n., a subclass of personality disorders.

   compensation n., the development of symptoms of n. believed to be motivated by the desire for, and hope of, monetary or interpersonal gain.

   compulsive n., SYN obsessive-compulsive n.

   conversion hysteria n., SYN conversion *hysteria.*

   obsessive-compulsive n., a disorder characterized by the persistent and repetitive intrusion of unwanted thoughts, (obsessions) and irresistible urges to perform meaningless actions (compulsions); anxiety or distress is the underlying emotion or drive state, and the ritualistic behavior is a learned method of reducing the anxiety. SYN compulsive n.

   transference n., in psychoanalysis, the phenomenon of the patient's developing a strong emotional relationship with the analyst.

   traumatic n., any functional nervous disorder following an accident or injury. SEE posttraumatic stress *disorder.*

   war n., a stress condition or mental disorder induced by conditions existing in warfare. SEE ALSO battle *fatigue.* SYN battle n.

neu•ro•splanch•nic (nūr-ō-splangk′nik). SYN neurovisceral. [neuro- + G. *splanchnon,* a viscus]

Neu•ros•po•ra (nū-ros′pōr-ă). A genus of fungi grown in cultures and used in research in genetics and cellular biochemistry. [neuro- + G. *spora,* seed]

neu•ro•sur•geon (nūr-ō-ser′jŭn). A surgeon specializing in operations on the nervous system.

neu•ro•sur•gery (nūr-ō-ser′jer-ē). Surgery of the nervous system.

   functional n., destruction or chronic excitation of a part of the brain to treat disordered behavior or function.

neu•ro•su•ture (nūr-ō-sū′chūr). SYN neurorrhaphy.

neu•ro•syph•i•lis (nūr-ō-sif′i-lis). Infection of the central nervous system by *Treponema pallidum.*

   tabetic n., type of n. in which the posterior roots of the spinal cord, especially in the lumbosacral area, are the principal sites of infection, resulting in ataxia, hypotonia, impotence, constipation, hypotonic bladder, areflexia, and Romberg's sign; other findings include lancinating pains (most often in the legs), visceral crises, Argyll-Robertson pupils, optic atrophy, and Charcot joints; in most patients, the CSF is abnormal. SYN tabes dorsalis.

neu•ro•ten•di•nous (nūr-ō-ten′di-nŭs). Relating to both nerves and tendons.

neu•ro•ten•sin (nū-rō-ten′sin). A 13-amino acid peptide neurotransmitter found in synapsomes in the hypothalamus, amygdala, basal ganglia, and dorsal gray matter of the spinal cord.

neu•ro•the•ke•o•ma (nūr-ō-thē′kē-ō-mă). A benign myxoma of cutaneous nerve sheath origin. [neuro- + G. *thēkē,* box, sheath, + *-oma,* tumor]

neu•rot•ic (nū-rot′ik). Relating to or suffering from a neurosis. SEE neurosis.

neu•rot•i•za•tion (nūr′ō-ti-zā′shŭn). The acquisition of nervous substance; the regeneration of a nerve.

neu•rot•me•sis. A type of axon loss lesion resulting from focal peripheral nerve injury in which, at the lesion site, the nerve stroma is damaged to varying degrees, as well as the axon and myelin, which degenerate from that point distally. SEE axonotmesis, neurapraxia. [neuro- + G. *tmēsis,* a cutting]

neu•rot•o•my (nū-rot′ō-mē). Operative division of a nerve. [neuro- + G. *tomē,* a cutting]

neu•ro•ton•ic (nūr-ō-ton′ik). **1.** Relating to neurotony. **2.** Strengthening or stimulating impaired nervous action. **3.** An agent that improves the tone or force of the nervous system.

neu•ro•tox•ic (nūr-ō-tok′sik). Poisonous to nervous substance.

neu•ro•tox•in (nūr-ō-tok′sin). **1.** SYN neurolysin. **2.** Any toxin that acts specifically on nervous tissue.

neu•ro•trans•mit•ter (nūr′ō-trans-mit′er). Any specific chemical agent released by a presynaptic cell, upon excitation, that crosses the synapse to stimulate or inhibit the postsynaptic cell. [neuro- + L. *transmitto,* to send across]

neu·ro·trip·sy (nūr-ō-trip′sē). Operative crushing of a nerve. [neuro- + G. *tripsis,* a rubbing]

neu·ro·tro·phic (nūr-ō-trof′ik). Relating to neurotrophy.

neu·rot·ro·phy (nū-rot′rō-fē). Nutrition and metabolism of tissues under nervous influence. [neuro- + G. *trophē,* nourishment]

neu·ro·tro·pic (nūr-ō-trop′ik). Having an affinity for the nervous system.

neu·rot·ro·py, neu·rot·ro·pism (nū-rot′rō-pē, -pizm). **1.** Affinity of basic dyes for nervous tissue. **2.** The attraction of certain pathogenic microorganisms, poisons, and nutritive substances toward the nerve centers. [neuro- + G. *tropē,* a turning]

neu·ro·tu·bule (nūr′ō-tū-byūl). One of the microtubules, 10 to 20 nm in diameter, occurring in the cell body, dendrites, axon, and in some synaptic endings of neurons.

neu·ro·vac·cine (nūr-ō-vak′sēn). A fixed or standardized vaccine virus of definite strength, obtained by continued passage through the brain of rabbits.

neu·ro·vas·cu·lar (nūr-ō-vas′kyū-lăr). Relating to both nervous and vascular systems; relating to the nerves supplying the walls of the blood vessels, the vasomotor nerves.

neu·ro·vi·rus (nūr-ō-vī′rŭs). Vaccine virus modified by means of passage into and growth in nervous tissue.

neu·ro·vis·cer·al (nūr-ō-vis′er-ăl). Referring to the innervation of the internal organs by the autonomic nervous system. SYN neurosplanchnic. [neuro- + L. *viscera,* the internal organs]

neu·ru·la, pl. **neu·ru·lae** (nūr′ū-lă, -lē). Stage in embryonic development after the gastrula state, in which the prominent processes are the formation of the neural plate and the plate's closure to form the neural tube. [neur- + L. *-ulus,* small one]

neu·tral (nū′trăl). **1.** Exhibiting no positive properties; indifferent. **2.** CHEMISTRY Neither acid nor alkaline. [L. *neutralis,* fr. *neuter,* neither]

neu·tral·i·za·tion (nū′trăl-i-zā′shŭn). **1.** The change in reaction of a solution from acid or alkaline to neutral by the addition of just a sufficient amount of an alkaline or of an acid substance, respectively. **2.** The rendering ineffective of any action, process, or potential.

△**neutro-, neutr-.** Neutral. [L. *neutralis,* fr. *neuter,* neither]

neu·tro·clu·sion (nū-trō-klū′zhŭn). A malocclusion in which there is a normal anteroposterior relationship between the maxilla and mandible; in Angle's classification, a Class I malocclusion. SYN neutral occlusion (2). [neutro- + occlusion]

neu·tron (nū′tron). An electrically neutral particle in the nuclei of all atoms (except hydrogen-1) with a mass slightly larger than that of a proton; in isolation, it breaks down to a proton and an electron with a half-life of about 10.3 minutes. [L. *neuter,* neither]

neu·tro·pe·nia (nū-trō-pē′nē-ă). The presence of abnormally small numbers of neutrophils in the circulating blood. [neutrophil + G. *penia,* poverty]

    periodic n., n. recurring at regular intervals, in

association with various types of infectious diseases.

▣**neu·tro·phil, neu·tro·phile** (nū′trō-fil, -fīl). **1.** A mature white blood cell in the granulocytic series, formed by bone marrow and released into the circulating blood, where they normally represent from 54% to 65% of the total number of leukocytes. When stained, n.'s are characterized by: 1) a nucleus that is dark purple-blue and lobated; 2) a cytoplasm that is faintly pink and contains numerous fine pink or violet-pink granules. The precursors of n.'s' in order of increasing maturity, are: myeloblasts, promyelocytes, myelocytes, metamyelocytes, and band forms. SEE ALSO leukocyte, leukocytosis. **2.** Any cell or tissue that manifests no special affinity for acid or basic dyes, *i.e.,* the cytoplasm stains approximately equally with either type of dye. [neutro- + G. *philos,* fond]

neu·tro·phil·ia (nū-trō-fil′ē-ă). An increase of neutrophilic leukocytes in blood or tissues.

neu·tro·phil·ic (nū-trō-fil′ik). **1.** Pertaining to or characterized by neutrophils, such as an exudate in which the predominant cells are n. granulocytes. **2.** Characterized by a lack of affinity for acid or basic dyes, *i.e.,* staining approximately equally with either type.

neu·tro·tax·is (nū-trō-tak′sis). A phenomenon in which neutrophilic leukocytes are stimulated by a substance in such a manner that they are either attracted, and move toward it (**positive neutrotaxis**), or they are repelled, and move away from it (**negative neutrotaxis**). [neutrophil + G. *taxis,* arrangement]

ne·vi (nē′vī). Plural of nevus. [L.]

ne·void (nē′voyd). Resembling a nevus. SYN nevose (2), nevous. [L. *naevus,* mole (nevus), + G. *eidos,* resemblance]

ne·vose, ne·vous (nē′vōs, -vŭs). **1.** Marked with nevi. **2.** SYN nevoid.

ne·vus, pl. **ne·vi** (nē′vŭs, -vī). **1.** A circumscribed malformation of the skin, especially if colored by hyperpigmentation or increased vascularity; a n. may be predominantly epidermal, adnexal, melanocytic, vascular, or mesodermal, or a compound overgrowth of these tissues. **2.** A benign localized overgrowth of melanin-forming cells of the skin present at birth or appearing early in life. SYN mole (1). [L. *naevus,* mole, birthmark]

    acquired n., a melanocytic n. that is not visible at birth, but appears in childhood or adult life.

    basal cell n. [MIM*109400], a hereditary disease noted in infancy or childhood, characterized by lesions of the eyelids, nose, cheeks, neck, and axillae, appearing as flesh-colored papules histologically indistinguishable from basal cell epithelioma; the lesions usually remain benign, but in some cases malignant change occurs.

    bathing trunk n., a large hairy congenital pigmented n. with a predilection for the entire lower trunk; malignant melanoma may develop in childhood.

    blue n., a dark blue or blue-black n. covered by smooth skin and formed by heavily pigmented spindle-shaped or dendritic melanocytes in the reticular dermis.

    blue rubber-bleb nevi, a syndrome characterized by erectile, easily compressible, thin-walled hemangiomatous nodules, widely distributed in the skin and in the alimentary canal; lesions in the gut may perforate or cause hemorrhage.

n. comedon'icus, comedo n., congenital or childhood linear keratinous cystic invaginations of the epidermis, with failure of development of normal pilosebaceous follicles.

congenital n., a melanocytic n. that is visible at birth, is often larger than an acquired n., and more frequently involves deeper structures.

dysplastic n., SEE dysplastic nevus *syndrome.*

n. flam'meus, a large congenital vascular n. having a purplish color; it is usually found on the head and neck and persists throughout life. SYN port-wine mark, port-wine stain.

halo n., a benign, sometimes multiple, melanocytic n. in which involution occurs with a central brown mole surrounded by a uniformly depigmented zone or halo.

intradermal n., a n. in which nests of melanocytes are found in the dermis, but not at the epidermal-dermal junction; benign pigmented nevi in adults are most commonly intradermal.

junction n., a n. consisting of nests of melanocytes in the basal cell zone, at the junction of the epidermis and dermis, appearing as a slightly raised, small, flat, nonhairy pigmented (brown or black) tumor.

n. pigmento'sus, a benign pigmented melanocytic proliferation; raised or level with the skin, present at birth or arising early in life. SYN mole (2).

n. pilo'sus, a mole covered with an abundant growth of hair. SYN hairy mole.

spider n., SYN spider *angioma.*

n. spi'lus, a form of (flat) nevus pigmentosus.

Spitz n., a benign, slightly pigmented or red superficial small skin tumor composed of spindle-shaped, epithelioid, and multinucleated cells that may appear atypical; most common in children, but also appearing in adults.

strawberry n., a small n. vascularis (capillary hemangioma) resembling a strawberry in size, shape, and color; it usually disappears spontaneously in early childhood. SEE capillary *hemangioma.* SYN strawberry mark.

n. uni'us lat'eris, a congenital systematized linear n. limited to one side of the body or to portions of the extremities on one side; lesions are often extensive, forming wave-like bands on the trunk and spiraling streaks on the extremities.

n. vascula'ris, n. vasculo'sus, SYN capillary *hemangioma.*

verrucous n., a skin-colored or darker wartlike, often linear, lesion appearing at birth or early in childhood, and occurring in various sizes and locations, single or multiple.

new•born (nū'bōrn). SYN neonatal, neonate.

New Hamp•shire rule. See under rule.

Newton, Sir Isaac, English physicist, 1642–1727. SEE newton; Newtonian *constant* of gravitation.

new•ton (nū'tŏn). Derived unit of force in the SI system, expressed as meters-kilograms per second squared (m·kg·s^{-2}); equivalent to 10^5 dynes in the CGS system. [I. *Newton*]

new•ton-me•ter. A unit of the MKS system,

expressed as energy expended, or work done, by a force of 1 newton acting through a distance of 1 meter; equal to 1 joule = 10^7 ergs.

nex•us, pl. **nex•us** (nek'sŭs). SYN gap *junction.* [L. interconnection]

ng nanogram.

Ni nickel.

ni•a•cin (nī'ă-sin). SYN nicotinic acid.

ni•a•cin•a•mide (nī'ă-sin-am'īd). SYN nicotinamide.

nib. DENTISTRY The portion of a condensing instrument that comes into contact with the restorative material being condensed.

niche (nitch, nēsh). **1.** RADIOGRAPHY An eroded or ulcerated area, especially gastrointestinal or vascular, which can be detected when it fills with contrast medium. **2.** An ecological term for the position occupied by a species in a biotic community, particularly its relationships to various other competitor, predator, prey, and parasite species. [Fr.]

nick•el (Ni) (nik'l). A metallic bioelement, atomic no. 28, atomic wt. 58.6934, closely resembling cobalt and often associated with it. Protects ribosome structure against heat denaturation. A deficiency of n. causes changes in the ultrastructure of the liver. [abbrev. fr. Ger. *kupfer-nickel,* name of copper-colored ore from which nickel was first obtained; *nickel,* the Ger. word for a dwarfish imp]

nick•ing (nik'ing). Localized constrictions in retinal blood vessels.

nic•o•tin•a•mide (nik-ō-tin'ă-mīd). The biologically active amide of nicotinic acid, used in the prevention and treatment of pellagra. SYN niacinamide.

nic•o•tin•a•mide ad•e•nine di•nu•cle•o•tide (NAD). Ribosylnicotinamide 5'-phosphate (NMN) and adenosine 5'-phosphate (AMP) linked by the two phosphoric groups; binds as a coenzyme to proteins, serves in respiratory metabolism (hydrogen acceptor and donor). See also entries under NAD and NADP. SYN diphosphopyridine nucleotide.

nic•o•tin•a•mide ad•e•nine di•nu•cle•o•tide phos•phate (NADP). A coenzyme of many oxidases (dehydrogenases), in which the reaction $NADP^+ + 2H \leftrightarrow NADPH + H^+$ takes place; the third phosphoric group esterifies the 2'-hydroxyl of the adenosine moiety of NAD.

nic•o•tin•a•mide mon•o•nu•cle•o•tide (NMN). A condensation product of nicotinamide and ribose 5-phosphate, a precursor in the synthesis of NAD^+.

nic•o•tine (nik'ō-tēn). A poisonous volatile alkaloid derived from tobacco (*Nicotiana* spp.) and responsible for many of the effects of tobacco; it first stimulates (small doses), then depresses (large doses) at autonomic ganglia and myoneural junctions. N. is an important tool in physiologic and pharmacologic investigation and is used as an insecticide and fumigant.

nic•o•tin•ic (nik-ō-tin'ik). Relating to the stimulating action of acetylcholine and other nicotine-like agents on autonomic ganglia, adrenal medulla, and the motor end-plate of striated muscle.

nic•o•tin•ic ac•id. A part of the vitamin B complex; used in the prevention and treatment of pellagra, as a vasodilator, and as an HDL-raising agent. SYN niacin.

nic·ti·ta·tion (nik-ti-tā′shŭn). Winking. [L. *nicto,* pp. *-atus,* to wink, fr. *nico,* to beckon]

ni·dal (nī′dăl). Relating to a nidus, or nest.

ni·da·tion (nī-dā′shŭn). Embedding of the early embryo in the uterine endometrium. [L. *nidus,* nest]

NIDDM non-insulin-dependent *diabetes* mellitus.

ni·dus, pl. **ni·di** (nī′dŭs, nī′dī). **1.** A nest. **2.** The nucleus or central point of origin of a nerve. **3.** A focus of infection. **4.** The coalescence of molecules or small particles that is the beginning of a crystal or similar solid deposit. **5.** The focus of reduced density at the center of an osteoid osteoma, on bone radiographs. [L. nest]

    n. a′vis, a deep depression on each side of the inferior surface of the cerebellum, between the uvula and the biventral lobe, in which the tonsil rests. [L. bird's nest]

night·mare (nīt′mār). A terrifying dream, as in which one is unable to cry for help or to escape from a seemingly impending evil. SYN incubus (2). [*A.S. nyht,* night, + *mara,* a demon]

night·ter·rors (nīt′tār-erz). A disorder allied to nightmare, occurring in children, in which the child awakes screaming with fright, the distress persisting for a time during a state of semiconsciousness. SYN pavor nocturnus.

nig·ra (nī′gră). NEUROANATOMY The *substantia* nigra. [L. fr. *niger,* black]

ni·gri·ti·es (nī-grish′i-ēz). A black pigmentation. [L. blackness, fr. *niger,* black]

ni·gro·sin, ni·gro·sine (nī′grō-sin, -sēn) [C.I. 50420]. A mixture of blue-black aniline dyes used as a histologic stain for nervous tissue and as a negative stain for studying bacteria and spirochetes; also used to discriminate between live and dead cells in dye-exclusion staining.

ni·gro·stri·a·tal (nī′grō-strī-ā′tăl). Referring to the efferent connection of the substantia nigra with the striatum. SEE *substantia* nigra.

NIH National Institutes of Health (U.S. Public Health Service).

ni·hil·ism (nī′i-lizm, nī′hi-lizm). **1.** PSYCHIATRY The delusion of the nonexistence of everything, especially of the self or part of the self. **2.** Engagement in acts which are totally destructive to one's own purposes and those of one's group. [L. *nihil,* nothing]

nil per os. [L.] nothing by mouth.

nin·hy·drin (nin-hī′drin). Triketohydrindene, an analytic reagent that reacts with free amino acids to yield CO_2, NH_3, and an aldehyde, the NH_3 produced yielding a colored product. SEE ALSO ninhydrin *reaction.* [Ger. trade name, fr. the chemical name]

ni·o·bi·um (Nb) (nī-ō′bē-ŭm). A rare metallic element, atomic no. 41, atomic wt. 92.90638, usually found with tantalum. [*Niobe,* daughter of Tantalus]

nip·ple (nip′l). A wartlike projection at the apex of the breast on the surface of which the lactiferous ducts open; it is surrounded by a circular pigmented area, the areola. SYN mamilla (2), teat

(1), thelium (3). [dim. of A.S. *neb,* beak, nose (?)]

    aortic n., colloq. term for the radiographic appearance of the left superior intercostal or accessory hemiazygos vein as a bump on the aortic knob.

nit. 1. The ovum of a body, head, or crab louse; it is attached to human hair or clothing by a layer of chitin. **2.** A unit of luminance; a luminous intensity of 1 candela per square meter of orthogonally projected surface. [A.S. *knitu*]

ni·trate (nī′trāt). A salt of nitric acid.

ni·tric ac·id (nī′trik). HNO_3; a strong acid oxidant and corrosive.

ni·tric ox·ide (NO). A colorless, free-radical gas; it reacts rapidly with O_2 to form other nitrogen oxides (*e.g.,* $NO_2·$, N_2O_3, and N_2O_4) and ultimately is converted to nitrite (NO_2^-) and nitrate (NO_3^-). Physiologically, it is a naturally occurring vasodilator formed in endothelial cells, macrophages, neutrophils, and platelets, and a mediator of cell-to-cell communication formed in bone, brain, endothelium, granulocytes, pancreatic β-cells and peripheral nerves.

ni·trid·a·tion (nī-tri-dā′shŭn). Formation of nitrides; formation of nitrogen compounds through the action of ammonia (analogous to oxidation).

ni·tride (nī′trīd). A compound of nitrogen and one other element; *e.g.,* magnesium nitride, Mg_3N_2.

ni·tri·fi·ca·tion (nī′tri-fi-kā′shŭn). **1.** Bacterial conversion of nitrogenous matter into nitrates. **2.** Treatment of a material with nitric acid.

ni·trile (nī′tril). An alkyl cyanide. Individual n.'s are named for the acid formed on hydrolysis.

△**nitrilo-.** Prefix indicating a tervalent nitrogen atom attached to three identical groups; *e.g.,* nitrilotriacetic acid, $N(CH_2COOH)_3$.

ni·trite (nī′trīt). A salt of nitrous acid.

ni·tri·tu·ria (nī-tri-tū′rē-ă). The presence of nitrites in the urine, as a result of the action of *Escherichia coli, Proteus vulgaris,* and other microorganisms that may reduce nitrates.

△**nitro-.** Prefix denoting the group $-NO_2$. [G. *nitron,* sodium carbonate.]

ni·tro·fu·ran·to·in (nī′trō-fū-ran′tō-in). A nitrofuran compound (*O-*[5-nitrofurfurylideneamino]-hydantoin) with antimicrobial activity against a wide spectrum of Gram-positive and -negative bacteria.

ni·tro·gen (nī′trō-jen). **1.** A gaseous element, atomic no. 7, atomic wt. 14.00674; forms about 78.084% by volume of the dry atmosphere. **2.** The molecular form of n., N_2. **3.** Pharmaceutical grade N_2, containing not less than 99.0% by volume of N_2; used as a diluent for medicinal gases, and for air replacement in pharmaceutical preparations. [L. *nitrum,* niter, + *-gen,* to produce]

    blood urea n. (BUN), n., in the form of urea, in the blood; the most prevalent of nonprotein nitrogenous compounds in blood; blood normally contains 10 to 15 mg of urea/100 ml. SEE ALSO urea n.

    nonprotein n. (NPN), the n. content of other than protein bodies; *e.g.,* about one-half the nonprotein n. in the blood is contained in urea.

    undetermined n., the n. of blood, urine, etc.,

other than urea, uric acid, amino acids, etc., that can be directly estimated; in blood it amounts to about 25 mg per 100 ml.

urea n., the portion of n. in a biological sample, such as blood or urine, that derives from its content of urea. SEE ALSO blood urea n.

urinary n., n. excreted as urea, amino acids, uric acid, etc., in the urine; 1 g of urinary n. indicates the breakdown in the body of 6.25 g of protein. SEE ALSO nitrogen *equivalent*.

ni•tro•ge•nase (nī′trō-jĕ-nās). A term for enzyme systems that catalyze the reduction of molecular nitrogen to ammonia in nitrogen-fixing bacteria with reduced ferredoxin and ATP.

ni•tro•gen dis•tri•bu•tion. SYN nitrogen partition.

ni•tro•gen group. Five trivalent or quinquivalent elements whose hydrogen compounds are basic and whose oxyacids vary from monobasic to tetrabasic: nitrogen, phosphorus, arsenic, antimony, and bismuth.

ni•tro•gen lag. The length of time after the ingestion of a given protein before the amount of nitrogen equal to that in the protein has been excreted in the urine.

ni•trog•e•nous (nī-troj′ĕ-nŭs). Relating to or containing nitrogen.

ni•tro•gen par•ti•tion. Determination of the distribution of nitrogen in the urine among the various constituents. SYN nitrogen distribution.

nitroso-. Prefix denoting a compound containing nitrosyl. [L. *nitrosus*]

ni•tro•syl (nī′trō-sil). A univalent radical or atom group, –N=O, forming the nitroso compounds.

ni•trous (nī′trŭs). Denoting a nitrogen compound containing one less atom of oxygen than the nitric compounds; one in which the nitrogen is present in its trivalent state.

ni•trous ac•id. HNO_2; a standard biologic and clinical laboratory reagent.

ni•trous ox•ide. N_2O; a nonflammable, nonexplosive gas that will support combustion; widely used as a rapidly acting, rapidly reversible, nondepressant, and nontoxic inhalation analgesic to supplement other anesthetics and analgesics; its anesthetic potency is inadequate to provide surgical anesthesia.

ni•tryl (nī′tril). The radical $-NO_2$ of the nitro compounds.

nM nanomolar (10^{-9} M).

nm nanometer.

NMN nicotinamide mononucleotide.

NMR nuclear magnetic *resonance*.

NO nitric oxide.

No nobelium.

no•bel•i•um (No) (nō-bel′ē-ŭm). An unstable transuranium element, atomic no. 102, prepared by bombardment of curium with carbon-12 nuclei and similar heavy ions on other elements of the transuranium series. [*Nobel* Institute for Physics and A.B. Nobel, Swedish inventor, 1833–1896]

No•car•dia (nō-kar′dē-ă). A genus of aerobic nonmotile actinomycetes, transitional between bacteria and fungi, containing variably acid-fast, slender rods or filaments forming a mycelium. These organisms are mainly saprophytic but may produce disease in human beings. [E. *Nocard*]

N. asteroi′des, a species of aerobic, Gram-positive, partially acid-fast, branching organisms causing nocardiosis and possibly mycetoma in humans.

N. ca′viae, a species that causes mycetoma in humans.

N. farci′nica, a species causing bovine farcy; it is the type species of the genus *N.*

N. mediterra′nei, a species that produces rifamycin.

N. orienta′lis, a species that produces vancomycin.

no•car•dia, pl. **no•car•di•ae** (nō-kar′dē-ă, nō-kar′dē-ē). A vernacular term used to refer to any member of the genus *Nocardia*.

no•car•di•o•sis (nō-kar-dē-ō′sis). A generalized disease in humans and other animals caused by *Nocardia asteroides* and *N. brasiliensis* and characterized by primary pulmonary lesions which may be subclinical or chronic with hematogenous spread, and usually with involvement of the central nervous system.

noci-. Hurt, pain, injury. [L. *noceo*]

no•ci•cep•tive (nō-si-sep′tiv). Capable of appreciation or transmission of pain. [see nociceptor]

no•ci•cep•tor (nō-si-sep′ter, -tōr). A peripheral nerve organ or mechanism for the reception and transmission of painful or injurious stimuli. [noci- + L. *capio,* to take]

no•ci•fen•sor (nō-si-fen′ser). Denoting processes or mechanisms that act to protect the body from injury; specifically, a system of nerves in the skin and mucous membranes that react to adjacent injury by causing vasodilation. [noci- + L. *fendo* (only in compounds), to strike, ward off]

no•ci-in•flu•ence (nō′si-in′flū-ens). Injurious or harmful influence.

no•ci•per•cep•tion (nō′si-per-sep′shŭn). The appreciation of injurious influences, referring to nerve centers. [noci- + perception]

noct-. Nocturnal. SEE ALSO nycto-. [L. *nox,* night]

noc•tu•ria (nok-tū′rē-ă). Excessive urination at night. [noct- + G. *ouron,* urine]

noc•tur•nal (nok-ter′năl). Pertaining to the hours of darkness; opposite of diurnal (1). [L. *nocturnus,* of the night]

no•dal (nō′dăl). Relating to any node.

node (nōd). **1.** A knob or nodosity; a circumscribed swelling; in anatomy, a circumscribed mass of tissue. **2.** A circumscribed mass of differentiated tissue. **3.** A knuckle, or finger joint. SYN nodus [NA]. [L. *nodus,* a knot]

atrioventricular n., a small node of modified cardiac muscle fibers located near the ostium of the coronary sinus; it gives rise to the atrioventricular bundle of the conduction system of the heart.

n. of Cloquet, one of the deep inguinal lymph n.'s located in or adjacent to the femoral canal; sometimes mistaken for a femoral hernia when enlarged.

delphian n., a midline prelaryngeal lymph node, adjacent to the thyroid gland, enlargement of which is indicative of thyroid disease or early metastasis from the subglottic larynx.

Heberden's n.'s, exostoses about the size of a pea or smaller, found on the terminal phalanges of the fingers in osteoarthritis, which are enlargements of the tubercles at the articular extremities of the distal phalanges. SYN tuberculum arthriticum (1).

Hensen's n., SYN primitive n.

lymph n., SEE lymph node.

lymphatic n.,

Osler n., a small, tender, nodular cutaneous lesion in the pads of fingers or toes, probably of immunopathic origin, characteristic of subacute bacterial endocarditis. SYN Osler's sign.

primitive n., a local thickening of the blastoderm at the cephalic end of the primitive streak of the embryo. SYN Hensen's n., primitive knot.

Ranvier's n., a short interval in the myelin sheath of a nerve fiber, occurring between segments of the myelin sheath; at the n., the axon is invested only by short, finger-like cytoplasmic processes of the two neighboring Schwann cells or, in the central nervous system, oligodendroglia cells. SEE ALSO myelin *sheath.*

signal n., a firm supraclavicular lymph n., especially on the left side, sufficiently enlarged that it is palpable from the cutaneous surface; such a lymph n. is so termed because it may be the first evidence of a malignant neoplasm in one of the viscera. SYN jugular gland, Virchow's n.

sinuatrial n., the mass of specialized cardiac muscle fibers that normally acts as the "pacemaker" of the cardiac conduction system; it lies under the epicardium at the upper end of the sulcus terminalis.

Virchow's n., SYN signal n.

no·di (nō′dī). Plural of nodus. [L.]

no·dose (nō′dōs). Having nodes or knotlike swellings. SYN nodous, nodular, nodulate, nodulated, nodulous. [L. *nodosus*]

no·dos·i·ty (nō-dos′i-tē). **1.** A node; a knoblike or knotty swelling. **2.** The condition of being nodose. [L. *nodositas*]

no·dous, nod·u·lar, nod·u·late, nod·u·lat·ed (nō′dŭs, nod′yū-lăr, nod′yū-lāt, -lā′ted). SYN nodose.

nod·u·la·tion (nod-yū-lā′shŭn). The formation or the presence of nodules.

🔲**nod·ule** (nod′yūl). A small node. a small node. SEE ALSO nodule. SYN nodulus (1) [NA]. [L. *nodulus,* dim. of *nodus,* knot]

apple jelly n.'s, descriptive term for the papular lesions of lupus vulgaris, as they appear on diascopy.

cold n., a thyroid n. with a much lower uptake of radioactive iodine than the surrounding parenchyma; about one in four prove to be malignant.

hot n., a thyroid n. with a much higher uptake of radioactive iodine than the surrounding parenchyma; usually benign but sometimes causing hyperthyroidism.

Lisch n., iris hamartomas typically seen in type 1 neurofibromatosis.

lymph n., SYN lymph *follicle.*

rheumatoid n.'s, subcutaneous n.'s, occurring in some patients with rheumatoid arthritis.

n. of semilunar valve, a nodule at the center of the free border of each semilunar valve at the beginning of the pulmonary artery and aorta.

singer's n.'s, SYN vocal n.'s.

Sister Joseph's n., a malignant intra-abdominal neoplasm metastatic to the umbilicus.

speaker's n.'s, SYN vocal n.'s.

vocal n.'s, small, circumscribed, bilateral, beadlike enlargements on the vocal folds caused by overuse or abuse of the voice. SYN singer's n.'s, speaker's n.'s.

nod·u·lous (nod′yū-lŭs). SYN nodose.

no·du·lus, pl. **no·du·li** (nod′yū-lŭs, nod′yū-lī) [NA]. **1.** SYN nodule. **2.** The posterior extremity of the inferior vermis of the cerebellum, forming with the posterior medullary velum the central portion of the flocculonodular lobe. [L. dim. of *nodus*]

n. lymphat′icus, SYN lymph *follicle.*

no·dus, pl. **no·di** (nō′dŭs, -dī) [NA]. SYN node. [L. a knot]

no·dus lym·pha·ti·cus, pl. **no·di lym·pha·ti·ci** (nō′dŭs lim′fat′ē-kus, -nō′dī) [NA]. SYN lymph node. [lympho- + L. *nodus,* node]

noise (noyz). **1.** Unwanted additions to a signal not arising at its source; includes visual n. on imaging studies. SEE signal-to-noise *ratio.* **2.** Extraneous uncontrolled variables influencing the distribution of measurements in a set of data. [M.E., fr. O.Fr., fr. L.L. *nausea,* seasickness]

no·ma (nō′mă). A gangrenous stomatitis with conspicuous necrosis and sloughing of tissue. Several organisms are usually found in the necrotic material, but fusiform bacilli, *Borrelia* organisms, staphylococci, and anaerobic streptococci are most frequently observed. SYN stomatonecrosis. [G. *nomē,* a spreading (sore)]

no·men·cla·ture (nō′men-klă-chūr, nō-men′klă-chūr). A set system of names used in any science, as of anatomic structures, organisms, etc. [L. *nomenclatura,* a listing of names, fr. *nomen,* name, + *calo,* to proclaim]

Nom·i·na An·a·tom·i·ca (NA) (nom′i-nă an-ă-tom′i-kă, nō′mi-nă an′ă-tō′mi-kă). The modification of the Basle Nomina Anatomica or BNA system of anatomical terminology adopted in 1955 by the International Congress of Anatomists in Paris, France. The International Anatomical Nomenclature Committee is responsible for continued revisions of the NA which are reviewed and adopted by the International Congress of Anatomists meeting at five-year intervals since 1950.

🔲**nom·o·gram** (nōm′ō-gram). A form of line chart showing scales for the variables involved in a particular formula in such a way that corresponding values for each variable lie in a straight line intersecting all the scales. [G. *nomos,* law, + *gramma,* something written]

no·mo·top·ic (nō-mō-top′ik). Relating to, or occurring at, the usual or normal place. [G. *nomos,* law, custom, + *topos,* place]

non com·pos men·tis (non kom′pos men′tis). Not of sound mind; mentally incapable of managing one's affairs. [L. *non,* not, + *compos,* participating, competent, + *mens,* gen. *mentis,* mind]

non·dis·junc·tion (non-dis-jŭnk′shŭn). Failure of one or more pairs of chromosomes to separate at the meiotic stage of karyokinesis, with the result that both chromosomes are carried to the one daughter cell and none to the other.

primary n., n. occurring in a previously normal cell.

secondary n., n. occurring in an aneuploid cell that was the result of a primary n.

non·e·lec·tro·lyte (non-ē-lek′trō-līt). A substance with molecules that do not, in solution, dissociate to ions and therefore do not carry an electric current.

nonfluency. SYN dysfluency.

non·in·va·sive (non-in-vā′siv). Denoting a procedure that does not require insertion of an instrument or device through the skin or a body orifice for diagnosis or treatment.

non·ox·y·nol 9 (non′noks-ĭ-nol). A group of compounds which are surface acting agents, used in spermicidal preparations such as contraceptive foam and diaphragm jelly.

non·pen·e·trance (non-pen′ĕ-trans). The state in which a genetic trait, although present in the appropriate genotype, fails to manifest itself in the phenotype because of nongenetic mechanisms. Cf. hypostasis.

non·pro·pri·e·tary name (non-prō-prī′ĕ-tār-ē). A short name (often called a generic name) of a chemical, drug, or other substance that is not subject to trademark (proprietary) rights but is, in contrast to a trivial name, recognized or recommended by government agencies (*e.g.,* Federal Food and Drug Administration) and by quasi-official organizations (*e.g.,* U.S. Adopted Names Council) for general public use. Cf. trivial name, proprietary name, systematic name.

non·se·cre·tor (non-sē-krē′tŏr, -tōr). An individual whose saliva does not contain antigens of the ABO blood group. SEE ALSO secretor.

non·sense. As used in genetics, relating to a mutation that causes a sequence such that the growing peptide chain terminates, often after several incorrect amino acid residues are incorporated.

non·un·ion (non′yūn-yŭn). Failure of normal healing of a fractured bone.

non·va·lent (non-vā′lent). Having no valency; not capable of entering into chemical composition.

non·vi·a·ble (non-vī′ă-bl). **1.** Incapable of independent existence; often denoting a prematurely born fetus. **2.** Denoting a microorganism or parasite incapable of metabolic or reproductive activity.

△**nor-.** **1.** Chemical prefix denoting 1) elimination of one methylene group from a chain, the highest permissible locant being used; 2) contraction of a (steroid) ring by one CH_2 unit, the locant being the capital letter identifying the ring. Elimination of two methylene groups is denoted by the prefix dinor-; three groups, by trinor-, etc. **2.** Chemical prefix denoting "normal," *i.e.,* unbranched chain of carbon atoms in aliphatic compounds, as opposed to branched with the same number of carbon atoms; *e.g.,* norleucine, leucine.

nor·a·dren·a·line (nor-ă-dren′ă-lin). SYN norepinephrine.

nor·ep·i·neph·rine (nŏr′ep-i-nef′rin). A catecholamine hormone, the postganglionic adrenergic mediator, acting on alpha and beta receptors; it is stored in chromaffin granules in the adrenal medulla and secreted in response to hypotension and physical stress; used pharmacologically as a vasopressor. SYN noradrenaline.

nor·leu·cine (nŏr-lū′sin). α-Amino-*n*-caproic acid; 2-aminohexanoic acid; an α-amino acid, not found in proteins; a deamination product of L-lysine, to which it is linked in collagens.

nor·ma, pl. **nor·mae** (nŏr′mă, nŏr′mē) [NA]. SYN profile (1). [L. a carpenter's square]

nor·mal (nŏr′măl). **1.** Typical; usual; according to the rule or standard. **2.** BACTERIOLOGY Nonimmune; untreated; denoting an animal, or the serum or substance contained therein, that has not been experimentally immunized against any microorganism or its products. **3.** Denoting a solution containing 1 equivalent of replaceable hydrogen or hydroxyl per liter. **4.** PSYCHIATRY, PSYCHOLOGY Denoting a level of effective functioning which is satisfactory to both the patient and the patient's social milieu. [L. *normalis,* according to pattern]

△**normo-.** Normal, usual. [L. *normalis,* according to pattern]

nor·mo·blast (nŏr′mō-blast). A nucleated red blood cell, the immediate precursor of a normal erythrocyte in humans. Its four stages of development are: 1) pronormoblast, 2) basophilic n., 3) polychromatic n., and 4) orthochromatic n. SEE ALSO erythroblast. [normo- + G. *blastos,* sprout, germ]

nor·mo·cap·nia (nŏr-mō-kap′nē-ă). A state in which the arterial carbon dioxide pressure is normal, about 40 mm Hg. [normo- + G. *kapnos,* vapor]

nor·mo·chro·mia (nŏr-mō-krō′mē-ă). Normal color; referring to blood in which the amount of hemoglobin in the red blood cells is normal. [normo- + G. *chrōma,* color]

nor·mo·cy·to·sis (nŏr′mō-sī-tō′sis). A normal state of the blood with regard to its component formed elements.

nor·mo·gly·ce·mia (nŏr′mō-glī-sē′mē-ă). SYN euglycemia.

nor·mo·gly·ce·mic (nŏr′mō-glī-sē′mik). SYN euglycemic.

nor·mo·ka·le·mia, nor·mo·ka·li·e·mia (nŏr′mō-kă-lē′mē-ă, -ka-lē-ē′mē-ă). A normal level of potassium in the blood.

nor·mo·ten·sive (nŏr-mō-ten′siv). Indicating a normal arterial blood pressure. SYN normotonic (2).

nor·mo·ther·mia (nŏr-mō-ther′mē-ă). Environmental temperature that does not cause increased or depressed activity of body cells. [normo- + G. *thermē,* heat]

nor·mo·ton·ic (nŏr-mō-ton′ik). **1.** Relating to or characterized by normal muscular tone. SYN eutonic. **2.** SYN normotensive.

nor·mo·vol·e·mia (nŏr′mō-vol-ē′mē-ă). A normal blood volume. [normo- + volume, + G. *haima,* blood]

nose (nōz). That portion of the respiratory pathway above the hard palate; includes both the external nose and the nasal cavity. SYN nasus (2) [NA]. [A.S. *nosu*]

external n., the visible portion of the nose which forms a prominent feature of the face; it consists of a root, dorsum and apex from above downward and is perforated inferiorly by two nostrils separated by a septum. SYN nasus (1) [NA].

saddle n., a n. with markedly depressed bridge, seen in congenital syphilis or after injury from trauma or operation.

nose·bleed (nōs′blēd). SYN epistaxis.

nose·piece (nōs′pēs). A microscope attachment, consisting of several objectives surrounding a central pivot.

⚠ **noso-.** Disease. SEE ALSO path-. [G. *nosos*]

nos·o·co·mi·al (nos-ō-kō′mē-ăl). **1.** Relating to a hospital. **2.** Denoting a new disorder (not the patient's original condition) associated with being treated in a hospital, such as a hospital-acquired infection. [G. *nosokomeion,* hospital, fr. *nosos,* disease, + *komeō,* to take care of]

nos·o·gen·ic (nos-ō-jen′ik). SYN pathogenic.

nos·o·log·ic (nos-ō-loj′ik). Relating to nosology.

no·sol·o·gy (nō-sol′ō-jē). **1.** The science of classification of diseases. **2.** Classification of ill persons into groups, whatever the criteria for the classification, and agreement as to the boundaries of the groups. SYN nosonomy, nosotaxy. [noso- + G. *logos,* study]

nos·o·ma·nia (nos-ō-mā′nē-ă). An unfounded morbid belief that one is suffering from some special disease. [noso- + G. *mania,* insanity]

no·son·o·my (nō-son′ō-mē). SYN nosology. [noso- + G. *nomos,* law]

nos·o·phil·ia (nos-ō-fil′ē-ă). A morbid desire to be sick. [noso- + G. *phileō,* to love]

nos·o·pho·bia (nos-ō-fō′bē-ă). An inordinate dread and fear of disease. [noso- + G. *phobos,* fear]

nos·o·poi·et·ic (nos′ō-poy-et′ik). SYN pathogenic. [noso- + G. *poiēsis,* a making]

nos·o·taxy (nos′ō-tak-sē). SYN nosology. [noso- + G. *taxis,* arrangement]

nos·tal·gia (nos-tal′jē-ă). The longing to return home, to a former time in one's life, or to familiar people and surroundings. [G. *nostos,* a return (home), + *algos,* pain]

nos·tril. Anterior opening to either side of the nasal cavity. SYN naris [NA].

nos·trum (nos′trŭm). General term for a therapeutic agent, sometimes patented but usually of secret composition, offered to the general public as a specific remedy for any disease or class of diseases. [L. neuter of *noster,* our, "our own remedy"]

no·tal (nō′tăl). Relating to the back. [G. *nōtos,* the back]

no·tan·ce·pha·lia (nō′tan-se-fā′lē-ă). Fetal malformation characterized by a bony deficiency, *i.e.,* absence of the occipital bone of the cranium. [G. *nōtos,* back, + *an-* priv. + *kephalē,* head]

no·tan·en·ce·pha·lia (nō′tan-en-se-fā′lē-ă). Absence of the cerebellum. [G. *nōtos,* back, + *an-* priv. + *enkephalos,* brain]

notch. 1. An indentation at the edge of any structure. **2.** Any short, narrow, V-shaped deviation, whether positive or negative, in a linear tracing. SYN incisure.

antegonial n., the highest point of the n. or concavity of the lower border of the ramus where it joins the body of the mandible.

aortic n., the n. in a sphygmographic tracing caused by rebound following closure of the aortic valves.

cardiac n., a deep notch between the esophagus and fundus of the stomach.

Carhart n., isolated depression around 200 Hz in the bone-conduction audiogram of patients with otosclerosis. SEE air-bone *gap.* SEE ALSO otosclerosis.

dicrotic n. (dī-krot-ik), the acute drop in arterial pressure pulse curves following the systolic peak, corresponding to the incisura of the displacement pulse curve.

Hutchinson's crescentic n., the semilunar n. on the incisal edge of Hutchinson's teeth, encountered in congenital syphilis.

parotid n., the space between the ramus of the mandible and the mastoid process of the temporal bone.

no·ten·ceph·a·lo·cele (nō-ten-sef′ă-lō-sēl). Malformation in the occipital portion of the cranium with protrusion of brain substance. [G. *nōtos,* back, + *enkephalos,* brain, + *kēlē,* hernia]

no·to·chord (nō′tō-kōrd). **1.** In primitive vertebrates, the primary axial supporting structure of the body, derived from the notochordal or head process of the early embryo; an important organizer for determining the final form of the nervous system and related structures. **2.** In embryos, the axial fibrocellular cord about which the vertebral primordia develop; vestiges of it persist in the adult as the nuclei pulposi of the intervertebral discs. [G. *nōtos,* back, + *chordē,* cord, string]

no·to·chor·dal (nō-tō-kōr′dăl). Relating to the notochord.

nour·ish·ment (ner′ish-ment). A substance used to feed or to sustain life and growth of an organism.

nox·ious (nok′shŭs). Injurious; harmful. [L. *noxius,* injurious, fr. *noceo,* to injure]

Np 1. neptunium. **2.** neper.

NPN nonprotein *nitrogen.*

NPO (nil per os), n.p.o.. L. *non per os* or *nil per os,* nothing by mouth.

NREM non-rapid eye *movement.*

nRNA nuclear RNA.

nu (nū). **1.** Thirteenth letter of the Greek alphabet (ν). **2.** Symbol for kinematic *viscosity;* frequency; stoichiometric *number.* **3.** CHEMISTRY The position of a substituent located on the thirteenth atom from the carboxyl or other functional group.

nu·cha (nū′kă) [NA]. The back of the neck. SYN nape. [Fr. *nuque*]

nu·chal (nū′kăl). Relating to the nucha.

⚠ **nucl-.** SEE nucleo-.

nu·cle·ar (nū′klē-er). Relating to a nucleus, either cellular or atomic; in the latter sense, usually referring to radiation emanating from atomic nuclei (α, β, or γ) or to atomic fission.

nu·cle·ase (nū′klē-ās). General term for enzymes that catalyze the hydrolysis of nucleic acid into nucleotides or oligonucleotides. Cf. exonuclease, endonuclease.

nu·cle·ate (nū′klē-āt). A salt of a nucleic acid.

nu·cle·at·ed (nū′klē-ā-ted). Provided with a nucleus, a characteristic of all true cells.

nu·cle·a·tion (nū-klē-ā′shŭn). Process of forming a nidus (4).

nu·clei (nū′klē-ī). Plural of nucleus.

nu·cle·ic ac·id (nū-klē′ik, -klā′ik). A family of macromolecules found in the chromosomes, nucleoli, mitochondria, and cytoplasm of all cells, and in viruses; in complexes with proteins, they are called nucleoproteins.

nu·cle·i·form (nū′klē-i-fōrm). Shaped like or having the appearance of a nucleus. SYN nucleoid (1).

◊**nucleo-, nucl-.** Nucleus, nuclear. SEE ALSO karyo-, caryo-. [L. *nucleus*]

nu·cle·o·cap·sid (nū′klē-ō-kap′sid). SEE virion.

nu·cle·of·u·gal (nū-klē-of′yū-găl). **1.** Moving within the cell body in a direction away from the nucleus. **2.** Moving in a direction away from a nerve nucleus; said of nerve transmission. [nucleo- + L. *fugio*, to flee]

nu·cle·o·his·tone (nū′klē-ō-his′tōn). A complex of histone and deoxyribonucleic acid, the form in which the latter is usually found in the nuclei of cells.

nu·cle·oid (nū′klē-oyd). **1.** SYN nucleiform. **2.** A nuclear inclusion body. **3.** SYN nucleus (2). [nucleo- + G. *eidos*, resemblance]

nu·cle·o·lar (nū-klē′ō-lăr). Relating to a nucleolus.

nu·cle·o·li (nū-klē′ō-lī). Plural of nucleolus.

nu·cle·o·li·form (nū-klē′ō-le-fōrm). Resembling a nucleolus. SYN nucleoloid.

nu·cle·o·loid (nū-klē′ō-loyd). SYN nucleoliform. [nucleolus + G. *eidos*, resemblance]

nu·cle·o·lo·ne·ma (nū-klē′ō-lō-nē′mă). The irregular network or rows of fine ribonucleoprotein granules or microfilaments forming most of the nucleolus. [nucleolus + G. *nēma*, thread]

nu·cle·o·lus, pl. **nu·cle·o·li** (nū-klē′ō-lŭs, -lī). A small rounded mass within the cell nucleus where ribonucleoprotein is produced. [L. dim of *nucleus*, a nut, kernel]

nu·cle·on (nū′klē-on). **1.** One of the subatomic particles of the atomic nucleus; *i.e.,* either a proton or a neutron. **2.** Slang term for specialist in nuclear medicine. [nucleus + -on]

nu·cle·op·e·tal (nū-klē-op′ĕ-tăl). **1.** Moving in the cell body in a direction toward the nucleus. **2.** Moving in a direction toward a nerve nucleus; said of a nervous impulse. [nucleo- + L. *peto*, to seek]

nu·cle·o·phil, nu·cle·o·phile (nū′klē-ō-fil, -fīl). **1.** The electron pair donor atom in a chemical reaction in which a pair of electrons is picked up by an electrophil. **2.** Relating to a nucleophil. SYN nucleophilic (1). [nucleo- + G. *philos*, fond]

nu·cle·o·phil·ic (nū′klē-ō-fil′ik). **1.** SYN nucleophil (2). **2.** A reaction involving a nucleophile.

nu·cle·o·plasm (nū′klē-ō-plazm). The protoplasm of the nucleus of a cell.

nu·cle·o·pro·tein (nū′klē-ō-prō′tēn). A complex of protein and nucleic acid, the form in which essentially all nucleic acids exist in nature; chromosomes and viruses are largely n.

nu·cle·or·rhex·is (nū′klē-ō-rek′sis). Fragmenta-

tion of a cell nucleus. [nucleo- + G. *rhēxis*, rupture]

nu·cle·o·si·das·es (nū′klē-ō-sī′dās-ez). Enzymes that catalyze the hydrolysis or phosphorolysis of nucleosides, releasing the purine or pyrimidine base.

nu·cle·o·side (nū′klē-ō-sīd). A compound of a sugar (usually ribose or deoxyribose) with a purine or pyrimidine base.

nu·cle·o·some (nū′klē-ō-sōm). A localized aggregation of histone and DNA that is evident when chromatin is in the uncondensed stage. [nucleo- + G. *sōma*, body]

nu·cle·o·ti·da·ses (nū′klē-ō-tī-dās-ez). Enzymes that catalyze the hydrolysis of nucleotides into phosphoric acid and nucleosides.

nu·cle·o·tide (nū′klē-ō-tīd). A combination of a (nucleic acid) purine or pyrimidine, one sugar (usually ribose or deoxyribose), and a phosphoric group. SYN mononucleotide.

   diphosphopyridine n. (DPN) (dī′fos-fō-pir′i-dēn), SYN nicotinamide adenine dinucleotide.

   triphosphopyridine n. (TPN, TPNH) (trī-fos′fō-pir′i-dēn), Former name for nicotinamide adenine dinucleotide phosphate.

nu·cle·o·tid·yl·trans·fer·as·es (nū′klē-ō-tī′dil-trans′fer-ās-ez). Enzymes transferring nucleotide residues (nucleotidyls) from nucleoside di- or triphosphates into dimer or polymer forms.

nu·cle·o·tox·in (nū′klē-ō-tok′sin). A toxin acting upon the cell nuclei.

nu·cle·us, pl. **nu·clei** (nū′klē-ŭs, nū′klē-ī). **1.** In cytology, typically a rounded or oval mass of protoplasm within the cytoplasm of a plant or animal cell; it is surrounded by a nuclear envelope, which encloses euchromatin, heterochromatin, and one or more nucleoli, and undergoes mitosis during cell division. SYN karyon. **2.** By extension, because of similar function, the genome of microorganisms (microbes) that is relatively simple in structure, lacks a nuclear membrane, and does not undergo mitosis during replication. SYN nucleoid (3). SEE ALSO virion. **3** [NA]. In neuroanatomy, a group of nerve cells in the brain or spinal cord that can be demarcated from neighboring groups in cell type or the presence of a surrounding zone of nerve fibers or cell-poor neuropil. **4.** Any substance (*e.g.,* foreign body, mucus, crystal) around which a urinary or other calculus is formed. **5.** The central portion of an atom (composed of protons and neutrons) where most of the mass and all of the positive charge are concentrated. [L. a little nut, the kernel, stone of fruits, the inside of a thing, dim. of *nux*, nut]

   n. ambig′uus [NA], a very slender, longitudinal column of motor neurons in the ventrolateral medulla oblongata; its efferent fibers leave with the vagus and glossopharyngeal nerve and innervate the striated muscle fibers of the pharynx (including the musculus levator veli palatini) and the intrinsic muscles of the larynx.

   arcuate nuclei, a variable assembly of small cell groups, probably outlying components of the pontine nuclei, on the ventral and medial aspects of the pyramid in the medulla oblongata.

   branchiomotor nuclei, collective term for

those motoneuronal nuclei of the brainstem that develop from the branchiomotor column of the embryo and innervate striated muscle fibers.

caudate n., an elongated curved mass of gray matter, consisting of an anterior thick portion, the caput or head, which protrudes into the anterior horn of the lateral ventricle, a portion extending along the floor of the body of the lateral ventricle, known as the corpus or body, and an elongated curved thin portion, the cauda or tail, which curves downward, backward, and forward in the temporal lobe in the wall of the lateral ventricle.

centromedian n., a large, lentil-shaped cell group, the largest and most caudal of the intralaminar nuclei, located within the lamina medullaris interna of the thalamus between the mediodorsal n. and ventrobasal n.; so called by Luys because of its prominent appearance on frontal sections midway between the anterior and posterior pole of the human thalamus. The n. receives numerous fibers from the internal segment of the globus pallidus by way of the thalamic fasciculus, ansa lenticularis, and lenticular fasciculus as well as projections from area 4 of the motor cortex; its major efferent connection is with the putamen although collaterals reach broad areas of the cerebral cortex.

nu'clei cochlea'res [NA], the n. cochlearis dorsalis and n. cochlearis ventralis, located on the dorsal and lateral surface of the inferior cerebellar peduncle, in the floor of the lateral recess of the rhomboid fossa. They receive the incoming fibers of the cochlear part of the vestibulocochlear nerve and are the major source of origin of the lateral lemniscus or central auditory pathway.

cuneate n., the larger Burdach's n.; one of the three nuclei of the posterior column of the spinal cord; located near the dorsal surface of the medulla oblongata at and below the level of the obex, the n. receives posterior root fibers corresponding to the sensory innervation of the arm and hand of the same side; together with its medial companion, the gracile n., it is the major source of origin of the medial lemniscus.

dentate n. of cerebellum, the most lateral and largest of the cerebellar nuclei; it receives the axons of the Purkinje cells of the neocerebellum (lateral areas of cerebellar cortex); together with the more medially located globosus and emboliform nuclei it is the major source of fibers composing the massive superior cerebellar peduncle or brachium conjunctivum.

dorsal n. of vagus nerve, the visceral motor n. located in the vagal trigone (ala cinerea) of the floor of the fourth ventricle. It gives rise to the parasympathetic fibers of the vagus nerve innervating the heart muscle and the smooth musculature and glands of the respiratory and intestinal tracts.

emboliform n., a small wedge-shaped n. in the central white substance of the cerebellum just internal to the hilus of the dentate n.; receives axons of Purkinje cells of the intermediate area of the cerebellar cortex; axons of these cells exit the cerebellum via the superior cerebellar peduncle. SYN embolus (2).

fastigial n., the most medial of the cerebellar nuclei, lying medial to the interpositus n., near the midline, in the white matter underneath the vermis of the cerebellar cortex. It receives the axons of Purkinje cells from all parts of the vermis. Its major projection is to the vestibular nuclei and medullary reticular formation.

gracile n., the medial one of the three nuclei of the dorsal column, the remaining two being the cuneate n. and the accessory cuneate n., which corresponds to the clava; it receives dorsal-root fibers conveying sensory innervation of the leg, and lower trunk, and projects, by way of the medial lemniscus, to the ventral n. posterior n. of the thalamus.

hypoglossal n., the motor n. innervating the intrinsic and four of the five extrinsic muscles of the tongue; it is located in the medulla oblongata near the midline, immediately beneath the floor of the inferior recess of the rhomboid fossa.

inferior olivary n., a large aggregate of small densely packed nerve cells arranged in folded laminae shaped like a purse with the opening (hilum) directed medially. It corresponds in position to the oliva, projects to all parts of the contralateral half of the cerebellar cortex by way of the olivocerebellar tract, and is the only source of cerebellar climbing fibers. Its afferent connections include fibers from the spinal cord, the dentate nucleus and motor cortex, but its major input appears to be the central tegmental tract originating from multiple nuclei at midbrain levels.

intermediolateral n., the cell column that forms the lateral horn of the spinal cord's gray matter. Extending from the first thoracic through the second lumbar segment, the column contains the autonomic motor neurons that give rise to the preganglionic fibers of the sympathetic system.

intermediomedial n., a small group of scattered visceral motor neurons immediately ventral to the thoracic n. in the thoracic and upper two lumbar segments of the spinal cord; considered to receive visceral afferent fibers at all spinal levels.

interpeduncular n., a median, unpaired, ovoid cell group at the base of the midbrain tegmentum between the cerebral peduncles; it receives the retroflex fasciculus from the habenula, and projects to the raphe region (raphe nuclei) and periaqueductal gray substance of the midbrain.

lenticular n., lentiform n., the large cone-shaped mass of gray matter forming the central core of the cerebral hemisphere. The convex base of the cone, oriented laterally and rostrally, is formed by the putamen which together with the caudate nucleus composes the striatum; the apical part, oriented medially and caudally, consists of the two segments of the globus pallidus. The n. is ventral and lateral to the thalamus and caudate n., from which it is separated by the internal capsule, and together with the caudate n. composes the striate body.

lentiform n.,

oculomotor n., the composite group of motor neurons innervating all of the external eye muscles except the musculus rectus lateralis and musculus obliquus superior, and including the musculus levator palpebrae superioris; the most rostral component of the n. is the Edinger-Westphal n.

which innervates the musculi sphincter pupillae and ciliaris via the ciliary ganglion. The oculomotor n. lies in the rostral half of the midbrain, near the midline in the most ventral part of the central gray substance; fibers of the medial longitudinal fasciculus form its lateral borders.

Onuf's n., small somatic motor neurons in the ventral horn of the spinal cord at sacral 2 level which innervate the vesicorectal sphincters, that is, the external anal and the urethral sphincter; Onuf's n. has been identified in the cat, dog, and humans.

nuclei of origin, collections of motor neurons (forming a continuous column in the spinal cord, discontinuous in the medulla and pons) giving origin to the spinal and cranial motor nerves.

paraventricular n., a triangular group of large magnocellular neurons in the periventricular zone of the anterior half of the hypothalamus. The cells of the n. are similar to those of the supraoptic n.; the axons of about 20% of their number join in the formation of the supraopticohypophysial tract and are functionally associated with the posterior lobe of the hypophysis; they project fibers to the brainstem nuclei (dorsal motor n. and solitary n.) and to the intermediolateral cell column of the spinal cord at thoracic, lumbar, and spinal levels; similar descending autonomic fibers arise from the lateral and posterior hypothalamic nuclei.

pontine nuclei, the massive gray matter filling the basilar pons. The nuclei are of fairly homogeneous architecture and project to the cortex of the contralateral cerebellar hemisphere by way of the middle cerebellar peduncle. Their main afferents come from the entire extent of the cerebral neocortex by way of the longitudinal pontine bundles (corticopontine fibers); thus, the pontine nuclei form a major way-station in the impulse conduction from the cerebral cortex of one hemisphere to the posterior lobe of the opposite cerebellum.

raphe nuclei, collective term denoting a variety of unpaired nerve cell groups in and along the median plane of the mesencephalic and rhombencephalic tegmentum: the n. centralis tegmenti superior, and the n. raphes dorsalis, n. raphes pontis, n. raphes magnus, n. raphes pallidus, and n. raphes obscurus. These nuclei include neurons characterized by their containing the indolamine transmitter agent serotonin; their serotonin-carrying axons extend rostrally to the hypothalamus, septum, hippocampus, and cingulate gyrus and include projections to brainstem, cerebellum, and spinal cord.

red n., a large, well defined, somewhat elongated cell mass, of reddish-gray hue in the fresh brain, located in the rostral mesencephalic tegmentum. The n. receives a massive projection from the contralateral half of the cerebellum by way of the superior cerebellar peduncle, and an additional projection from the ipsilateral motor cortex. Projections from the anterior interposed n. and motor cortex to the red nucleus are somatopically organized. Its efferent connections are with the contralateral rhombencephalic reticular formation and spinal cord by way of the rubrobulbar

and rubrospinal tracts. Rubrospinal fibers have somatotopic origin.

n. of solitary tract, a slender cell column extending sagittally through the dorsal part of the medulla oblongata, beneath the floor of the rhomboid fossa, immediately lateral to the limiting sulcus. It is the visceral sensory (visceral afferent) n. of the brainstem, receiving the afferent fibers of the vagus, glossopharyngeal, and facial nerves by way of the solitary tract. The caudal two-thirds of the n. processes impulses originating in the pharynx, larynx, intestinal and respiratory tracts, and heart and large blood vessels; its rostral one-third receives impulses from the taste buds and is known as the rhombencephalic gustatory n.

somatic motor nuclei, collective term indicating the motor nuclei innervating the tongue musculature (hypoglossal n.) and the extraocular eye muscles (abducens n., trochlear n., and oculomotor n.).

subthalamic n., a circumscripta n., shaped like a biconvex lens, located in the ventral part of the subthalamus on the dorsal surface of the peduncular part of the internal capsule immediately rostral to the substantia nigra. The n. receives a massive topographic projection from the lateral segment of the globus pallidus, and a somatopically organized projection from the ipsilateral motor cortex; a smaller bundle of afferents from the centromedian n. of the thalamus terminate in the rostral part of the n. The subthalamic n. projects to both pallidal segments, to the pars reticulata of the substantia nigra, and in a small way to the ipsilateral pedunculopontine nucleus.

supraoptic n. of hypothalamus, a large-celled neurosecretory n. in the hypothalamus, located over the lateral border of the optic tract, from which the supraopticohypophysial tract arises; its neurons produce and transport vasopressin released into the general circulation from the axon terminals in the supraopticohypophysial tract.

tegmental nuclei, collective term for two small round cell groups in the caudal part of the midbrain (caudal pontine tegmental nucleus, nucleus tegmenti pontis caudalis and oral pontine tegmental nucleus, nucleus tegmenti pontis oralis), associated with the mamillary body by way of the mamillary peduncle and mamillotegmental tract.

terminal nuclei, nuclei termina′les, collective term indicating those nerve cell groups in the rhombencephalon and spinal cord in which the afferent fibers of the spinal and cranial nerves terminate.

nuclei termina′les,

thoracic n., a column of large neurons located in the base of the posterior gray column of the spinal cord, extending from the first thoracic through the second lumbar segment; it gives rise to the dorsal spinocerebellar tract of the same side.

vestibulocochlear nuclei, the combined cochlear and vestibular nuclei in the brainstem that receive the incoming fibers of the eighth cranial nerve.

nu•clide (nū′klīd). A particular (atomic) nuclear

species with defined atomic mass and number. SEE ALSO isotope.

NUG necrotizing ulcerative *gingivitis*.

nul·li·grav·i·da (nŭl-i-grav′i-dă). A woman who has never conceived a child. [L. *nullus,* none, + *gravida,* pregnant]

nul·lip·a·ra (nŭ-lip′ă-ră). A woman who has never borne children. [L. *nullus,* none, + *pario,* to bear]

nul·li·par·i·ty (nŭl-i-par′i-tē). Condition of having borne no children.

nul·lip·a·rous (nŭl-ip′ă-rŭs). Never having borne children.

num·ber (nŭm′ber). **1.** A symbol expressive of a certain value or of a specific quantity determined by count. **2.** The place of any unit in a series.

    atomic n. (Z), the number of protons in the nucleus of an atom; it indicates the position of the element in the periodic system.

    atomic mass n., the mass of the atom of a particular isotope relative to hydrogen-1 (or to one twelfth the mass of carbon-12), generally very close to the whole number represented by the sum of the protons and neutrons in the atomic nucleus of the isotope; it is not to be confused with the atomic weight of an element, which may include a number of isotopes in natural proportion.

    Avogadro's n. (N_A, lambda), the n. of molecules in one gram-molecular weight (1 mol) of any compound; defined as the number of atoms in 0.0120 kg of pure carbon-12; equivalent to 6.0221367×10^{23}. SYN Avogadro's constant.

    Hogben n., unique personal identifying number constructed by using a sequence of digits for birth date, sex, birthplace, and other identifiers; invented by and named for Lancelot Hogben, British mathematician; Hogben n.'s are the basis for identification n.'s in many primary care facilities and are used in many record linkage systems.

    linking n., a property of a long biopolymer (such as duplex DNA) equal to the number of twists (related to the frequency of turns around the central axis of the helix) plus the writhing n.

    MIM n., the catalog assignment for a mendelian trait in the MIM system. If the initial digit is 1, the trait is deemed autosomal dominant; if 2, autosomal recessive; if 3, then X-linked. Wherever a trait defined in this dictionary has a MIM n. the n. from the tenth edition of MIM is given in square brackets with or without an asterisk as appropriate *e.g.,* Pelizaeus-Merzbacher disease [MIM*169500] is a well-established, autosomal, dominant, mendelian disorder.

    stoichiometric n. (ν), the n. associated with a reactant or product participating in a defined chemical reaction; usually an integer.

    turnover n., the number of substrate molecules converted into product in an enzyme-catalyzed reaction under saturating conditions per unit time per unit quantity of enzyme; *e.g.,* $k_{cat} = V_{max}/[E_{total}]$.

numb·ness (nŭm′nes). Indefinite term for abnormal sensation, including absent or reduced sensory perception as well as paresthesias.

num·mu·lar (nŭm′yū-ler). **1.** Discoid or coin-shaped; denoting thick mucopurulent sputum, so

called because of the disc shape assumed when it is flattened on the bottom of a sputum mug containing water or transparent disinfectant. **2.** Arranged like stacks of coins, denoting the lining up of the red blood cells into rouleaux formation. [L. *nummulus,* small coin, dim. of *nummus,* coin]

nurse (ners). **1.** To breast feed. **2.** To provide care of the sick. **3.** One who is educated in the scientific basis of nursing under defined standards of education and is concerned with the diagnosis and treatment of human responses to actual or potential health problems. [O. Fr. *nourice,* fr. L. *nutrix,* wet-nurse, nurse, fr. *nutrio,* to suckle, to tend]

    clinical n. specialist, a registered n. with at least a master's degree who has advanced education in a particular area of clinical practice such as oncology or psychiatry.

    general duty n., n. who accepts assignment to any unit of a hospital other than an intensive care unit.

    licensed practical n., a n. who has graduated from an accredited school of practical (vocational) nursing, passed the state examination for licensure and been licensed to practice by a state authority. Program is generally one year in length.

    private duty n., (1) a n. who is not a member of a hospital staff, but is hired on a fee-for-service basis to care a patient; **(2)** a n. who specializes in the care of patients with diseases of a particular class, *e.g.,* surgical cases, tuberculosis, children's diseases.

    registered n., a n. who has graduated from an accredited nursing program, has passed the state exam for licensure, and been registered and licensed to practice by a state authority.

    scrub n., a n. who has scrubbed arms and hands, donned sterile gloves and, usually, a sterile gown, and assists an operating surgeon, primarily by passing instruments.

    wet n., a woman who breast-feeds a child not her own.

nurse prac·ti·tion·er (ners prak-tish′ŭ-ner). A registered nurse with at least a master's degree in nursing and advanced education in the primary care of particular groups of clients. Capable of independent practice in a variety of settings.

nurs·ing (ner′sing). **1.** Feeding an infant at the breast; tending and caring for a child. **2.** The scientific application of principles of care related to prevention of illness and care during illness.

nursing facility. health care facility for patients who require long-term nursing or rehabilitation services; formerly known as a nursing home. SYN long-term care facility.

nursing home. Former term for nursing facility. SEE nursing facility.

nu·ta·tion (nū-tā′shŭn). The act of nodding, especially involuntary nodding. [L. *annuo,* to nod]

nu·tri·ent (nū′trē-ent). A constituent of food necessary for normal physiologic function. [L. *nutriens,* fr. *nutrio,* to nourish]

nu·tri·tion (nū-trish′ŭn). **1.** A function of living plants and animals, consisting in the taking in and metabolism of food material whereby tissue is built up and energy liberated. **2.** The study of the

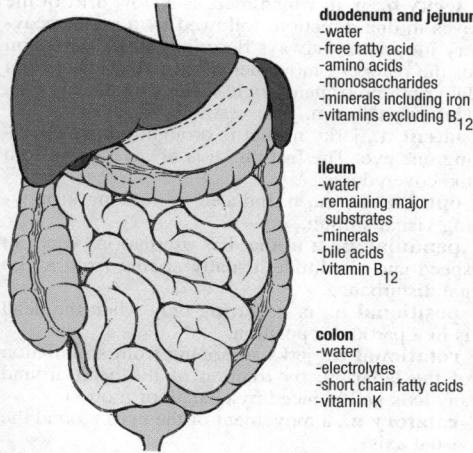

duodenum and jejunum
-water
-free fatty acid
-amino acids
-monosaccharides
-minerals including iron
-vitamins excluding B$_{12}$

ileum
-water
-remaining major
  substrates
-minerals
-bile acids
-vitamin B$_{12}$

colon
-water
-electrolytes
-short chain fatty acids
-vitamin K

nutrient absorption: gastrointestinal tract sites

food and liquid requirements of human beings or animals for normal physiologic function, including energy, need, maintenance, growth, activity, reproduction, and lactation. [L. *nutritio*, fr. *nutrio*, to nourish]

total parenteral n. (TPN), n. maintained entirely by intravenous injection or other nongastrointestinal route.

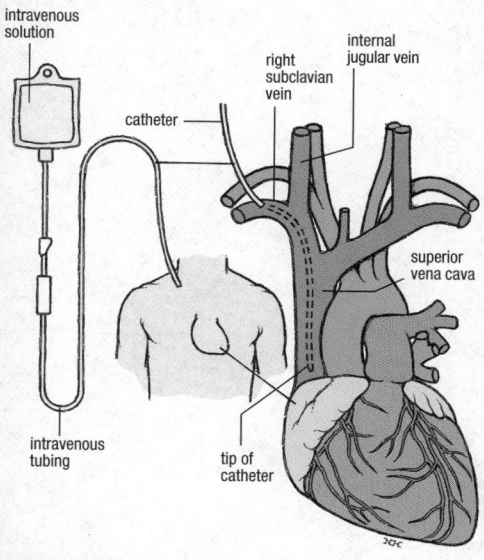

intravenous
solution

catheter

right
subclavian
vein

internal
jugular vein

superior
vena cava

intravenous
tubing

tip of
catheter

total parenteral nutrition: with catheter entering the circulation at the right subclavian vein

nu·tri·tive (nū′tri-tiv). **1.** Pertaining to nutrition. **2.** Capable of nourishing.

nu·tri·ture (nū′tri-chūr). State or condition of the nutrition of the body; state of the body with regard to nourishment. [L. *nutritura*, a nursing, fr. *nutrio*, to nourish]

nyct-. SEE nycto-.

nyc·tal·gia (nik-tal′jē-ă). Denoting especially the osteocopic pains of syphilis occurring at night. [nyct- + G. *algos*, pain]

nyc·ta·lo·pia (nik-tă-lō′pē-ă). Decreased ability to see in reduced illumination. Seen in patients with impaired rod function; often associated with a deficiency of vitamin A. SYN night blindness. [nyct- + G. *alaos*, obscure, + *ōps*, eye]

nyc·ter·ine (nik′ter-īn, -in). **1.** By night. **2.** Dark or obscure. [G. *nykterinos*]

nycto-, nyct-. Night, nocturnal. SEE ALSO noct-. [G. *nyx*]

nyc·to·hem·e·ral (nik-tō-hē′mer-ăl). Both daily and nightly. [nycto- + G. *hēmera*, day]

nyc·to·phil·ia (nik-tō-fil′ē-ă). Preference for the night or darkness. SYN scotophilia. [nycto- + G. *philos*, fond]

nyc·to·pho·bia (nik-tō-fō′bē-ă). Morbid fear of night or or the dark. SYN scotophobia. [nycto- + G. *phobos*, fear]

nym·pha, pl. **nym·phae** (nim′fă, nim′fē). One of the labia minora. [Mod. L., fr. G. *nymphē*, a bride]

nym·phec·to·my (nim-fek′tō-mē). Surgical removal of hypertrophied labia minora. [nympha + G. *ektomē*, excision]

nym·phi·tis (nim-fī′tis). Inflammation of the labia minora. [nympha + G. *-itis*, inflammation]

nympho-, nymph-. The nymphae (labia minora). [L. *nympha*]

nym·pho·ma·nia (nim-fō-mā′nē-ă). An insatiable impulse to engage in sexual behavior in a female; the counterpart of satyriasis in a male. [nympho- + G. *mania*, frenzy]

nym·pho·ma·ni·a·cal (nim′fō-mă-nī′ă-kăl). Pertaining to, or exhibiting, nymphomania.

nym·phon·cus (nim-fong′kŭs). Swelling or hypertrophy of one or both labia minora. [nympho- + G. *onkos*, tumor]

nym·phot·o·my (nim-fot′ō-mē). Incision into the labia minora or the clitoris. [nympho- + G. *tomē*, incision]

nys·tag·mic (nis-tag′mik). Relating to or suffering from nystagmus.

nys·tag·mi·form (nis-tag′mi-fōrm). SYN nystagmoid.

nys·tag·mo·graph (nis-tag′mō-graf). An apparatus for measuring the amplitude, periodicity, and velocity of ocular movements in nystagmus, by measuring the change in the resting potential of the eye as the eye moves. [nystagmus + G. *graphō*, to write]

nys·tag·mog·ra·phy (nis-tag-mog′ră-fē). The technique of recording nystagmus.

nys·tag·moid (nis-tag′moyd). Resembling nystagmus. SYN nystagmiform. [nystagmus + G. *eidos*, resemblance]

nys·tag·mus (nis-tag′mŭs). Rhythmical oscillation of the eyeballs, either pendular or jerky. [G. *nystagmos*, a nodding, fr. *nystazō*, to be sleepy, nod]

    caloric n., jerky n. induced by labyrinthine stimulation with hot or cold water in the ear.

    congenital n., (1) n. present at birth or caused

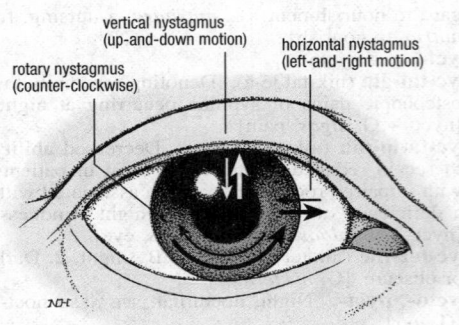

vertical nystagmus
(up-and-down motion)

horizontal nystagmus
(left-and-right motion)

rotary nystagmus
(counter-clockwise)

nystagmus: the thick arrows indicate the slower, first phase

by lesions sustained *in utero* or at the time of birth; **(2)** inherited n., usually X-linked, without associated neurologic lesions and nonprogressive. **(3)** the n. associated with albinism, achromatopsia, and hypoplasia of the macula.

conjugate n., a n. in which the two eyes move simultaneously in the same direction.

dissociated n., a n. in which the movements of the two eyes are dissimilar in direction, amplitude, and periodicity.

fixation n., n. aggravated or induced by ocular fixation, arising as optokinetic n., or resulting from midbrain lesions.

jerky n., n. in which there is a slow drift of the eyes in one direction, followed by a rapid recovery movement, always described in the direction of the recovery movement; it usually arises from labyrinthine or neurologic lesions or stimuli.

labyrinthine n., SYN vestibular n.

latent n., jerky n. that is brought out by covering one eye. The fast phase is always away from the covered eye.

optokinetic n., n. induced by looking at moving visual stimuli.

pendular n., a n. that has oscillations equal in speed and amplitude, usually arising from a visual disturbance.

positional n., n. occurring only when the head is in a particular position.

rotational n., jerky n. arising from stimulation of the labyrinth by rotation of the head around any axis and induced by change of motion.

rotatory n., a movement of the eyes around the visual axis.

vertical n., an up-and-down oscillation of the eyes.

vestibular n., n. resulting from physiological stimuli to the labyrinth that may be rotatory, caloric, compressive, or galvanic, or due to labyrinthal lesions. SYN labyrinthine n.

nyx•is (nik′sis). A pricking; paracentesis. [G.]

O

Ω omega. SEE omega.

O 1. oxygen; orotidine. **2.** opening (in formulas for electrical reactions). **3.** a blood group in the ABO system. See ABO blood group, Blood Groups appendix. **4.** An abbreviation derived from *ohne Hauch* (without a film), used as a designation for: 1) antigens that occur in the bacterial cell, in contrast to those in the flagella; 2) specific antibodies for such somatic antigens; 3) the agglutinative reaction between somatic antigen and its antibody.

OAE otoacoustic *emissions*, under *emission*.

OB obstetrics.

ob·dor·mi·tion (ob-dōr-mish′ŭn). Numbness of an extremity, due to pressure on the sensory nerve. [L. *ob-dormio*, pp. *-itus*, to sleep]

obe·li·ac (ō-bē′lē-ak). Relating to the obelion.

obe·li·on (ō-bē′lē-on). A craniometric point on the sagittal suture between the parietal foramina near the lambdoid suture. [G. *obelos*, a spit]

obese (ō-bēs′). Excessively fat. SYN corpulent. [L. *obesus*, fat, partic. adj., fr. *ob-edo*, pp. *-esus*, to eat away, devour]

obe·si·ty (ō-bē′si-tē). An abnormal increase of fat in the subcutaneous connective tissues. SYN adiposity (1), corpulence, corpulency.

  morbid o., o. sufficient to prevent normal activity or physiologic function, or to cause the onset of a pathologic condition.

obex (ō′beks) [NA]. The point on the midline of the dorsal surface of the medulla oblongata that marks the caudal angle of the rhomboid fossa or fourth ventricle. It corresponds to a small, transverse medullary fold overhanging the calamus scriptorius. [L. barrier]

OB/GYN obstetrics and gynecology.

ob·ject choice. PSYCHOANALYSIS The object (usually a person) upon which psychic energy is centered.

ob·jec·tive (ob-jek′tiv). **1.** The lens or lenses in the lower end of the body tube of a microscope. **2.** Viewing events or phenomena as they exist in the external world, impersonally, or in an unprejudiced way; open to observation by oneself and by others. Cf. subjective. [L. *ob- jicio*, pp. *-jectus*, to throw before]

  achromatic o., an o. that is corrected for two colors chromatically, and one color spherically.

  apochromatic o., an o. in which chromatic aberration is corrected for three colors and spherical aberration is corrected for two.

  immersion o., a high power o. used with a drop of oil between the lens and the specimen on the slide, allowing a greater numerical aperture; similar lenses are available for use with water as the immersing liquid.

ob·li·gate (ob′li-gāt). Without an alternative system or pathway. [L. *ob-ligo*, pp. *-atus*, to bind to]

ob·lique (ob-lēk′). **1.** Slanting; deviating from the perpendicular, horizontal, sagittal, or coronal plane of the body. **2.** RADIOGRAPHY A projection that is neither frontal nor lateral. [L. *obliquus*]

ob·liq·ui·ty (ob-lik′wi-tē). SYN asynclitism.

  Litzmann o., inclination of the fetal head so

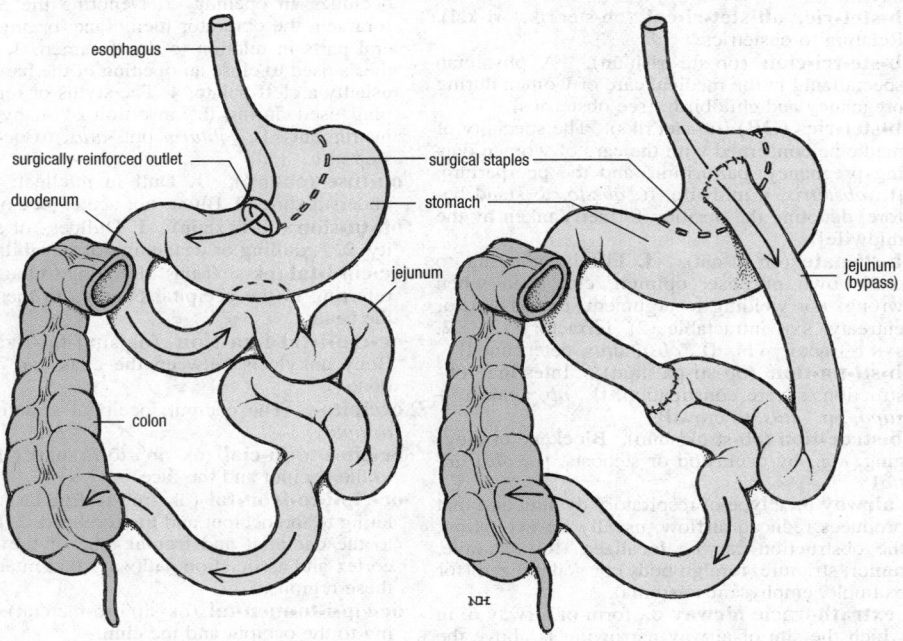

esophagus
surgically reinforced outlet
duodenum
surgical staples
stomach
jejunum
colon
jejunum (bypass)

NH

surgical procedures to control obesity: (A) vertical banded gastroplasty, (B) gastric bypass

that the biparietal diameter is oblique in relation to the plane of the pelvic brim, the posterior parietal bone presenting to the parturient canal. SYN posterior asynclitism.

Nägele o., inclination of the fetal head in cases of flat pelvis, so that the biparietal diameter is oblique in relation to the plane of the pelvic brim, the anterior parietal bone presenting to the parturient canal.

ob·lit·er·a·tion (ob-lit-er-ā'shŭn). **1.** Blotting out, especially by filling of a natural space or lumen by fibrosis or inflammation. **2.** RADIOLOGY Disappearance of the contour of an organ when the adjacent tissue has the same x-ray absorption. [L. *oblittero,* to blot out]

ob·lon·ga·ta (ob-long-gā'tă). SYN *medulla* oblongata. [L. fem. of *oblongatus,* from *oblongus,* rather long]

OBS. SYN organic brain *syndrome.*

ob·ses·sion (ob-sesh'ŭn). A recurrent and persistent idea, thought, or impulse to carry out an act that is ego-dystonic, that is experienced as senseless or repugnant, and that the individual cannot voluntarily suppress. [L. *obsideo,* pp. -*sessus,* to besiege, fr. *sedeo,* to sit]

impulsive o., an o. accompanied by action, sometimes becoming a mania.

inhibitory o., an o. involving an impediment to action, usually representing a phobia.

ob·ses·sive-com·pul·sive. Having a tendency to perform certain repetitive acts or ritualistic behavior to relieve anxiety, as in obsessive-compulsive neurosis (*e.g.,* a compulsive, ritualistic need to wash one's hands many dozens of times per day).

ob·stet·ric, ob·stet·ri·cal (ob-stet'rik, -ri-kăl). Relating to obstetrics.

ob·ste·tri·cian (ob-stě-trish'ŭn). A physician specializing in the medical care of women during pregnancy and childbirth. [see obstetrics]

ob·stet·rics (OB) (ob-stet'riks). The specialty of medicine concerned with the care of women during pregnancy, parturition, and the puerperium. [L. *obstetrix,* a midwife, fr. *ob-sto,* to stand before, denoting the position formerly taken by the midwife]

ob·sti·nate (ob'sti-năt). **1.** Firmly adhering to one's own purpose, opinion, etc. even when wrong; not yielding to argument, persuasion, or entreaty. SYN intractable (2), refractory (2). **2.** SYN refractory (1). [L. *obstinatus,* determined]

ob·sti·pa·tion (ob-sti-pā'shŭn). Intestinal obstruction; severe constipation. [L. *ob,* against, + *stipo,* pp. -*atus,* to crowd]

ob·struc·tion (ob-strŭk'shŭn). Blockage or clogging, *e.g.,* by occlusion or stenosis. [L. *obstructio*]

airway o., a type of respiratory dysfunction that produces reduced airflow, usually on expiration; the obstruction can be localized (for example, tumor, stricture, foreign body) or generalized (for example, emphysema, asthma).

extrathoracic airway o., form of airway o. in which the site of airway narrowing is above the thoracic inlet. It can be variable (*e.g.,* reduction in inspiratory but not expirator flows) or fixed (reduction in both inspiratory and expiratory flows).

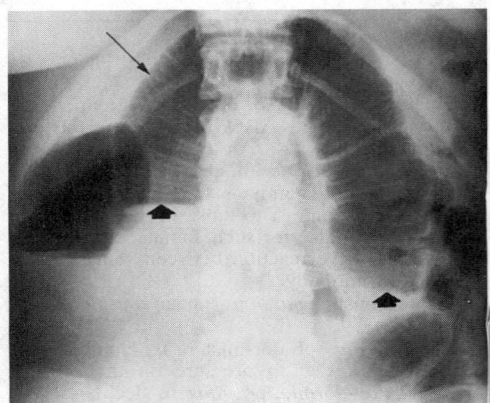

small bowel obstruction: plain, erect radiograph of the abdomen reveals dilated, air-filled loops of small bowel; the obstruction is due to adhesions

intrathoracic airway o., form of airway o. in which the site of airway narrowing is below the thoracic inlet. It can be variable (*e.g.,* reduction in expiratory but not inspiratory flows) or fixed (reduction in both inspiratory and expiratory flows).

ob·tund (ob-tŭnd'). To dull or blunt, especially to blunt sensation or deaden pain. [L. *ob-tundo,* pp. -*tusus,* to beat against, blunt]

ob·tu·ra·tion (ob-tū-rā'shŭn). Obstruction or occlusion. [see obturator]

ob·tu·ra·tor (ob'tū-rā-tŏr). **1.** Any structure that occludes an opening. **2.** Denoting the obturator foramen, the obturator membrane, or any of several parts in relation to this foramen. **3.** A prosthesis used to close an opening of the hard palate, usually a cleft palate. **4.** The stylus or removable plug used during the insertion of many tubular instruments. [L. *obturo,* pp. -*atus,* to occlude or stop up]

ob·tuse (ob-tūs'). **1.** Dull in intellect; of slow understanding. **2.** Blunt; not acute. [see obtund]

ob·tu·sion (ob-tū'zhŭn). **1.** Dullness of sensibility. **2.** A dulling or deadening of sensibility.

oc·cip·i·tal (ok-sip'i-tăl). Relating to the occiput. referring to the occipital bone or to the back of the head.

oc·cip·i·tal·i·za·tion (ok'sip'i-tăl-i-zā'shŭn). Bony ankylosis between the atlas and occipital bone.

△**occipito-.** The occiput, occipital structures. [L. *occiput*]

oc·cip·i·to·fa·cial (ok-sip'i-tō-fā'shăl). Relating to the occiput and the face.

oc·cip·i·to·fron·tal (ok-sip'i-tō-frŭn'tăl). **1.** Relating to the occiput and the forehead. **2.** Relating to the occipital and frontal lobe of the cerebral cortex and association pathways that interconnect these regions.

oc·cip·i·to·men·tal (ok-sip'i-tō-men'tăl). Relating to the occiput and the chin.

oc·ci·put, gen. **oc·cip·i·tis** (ok'si-put, ok-sip'i-tis) [NA]. The back of the head. [L.]

oc·clude (ŏ-klūd'). **1.** To close or bring together.

2. To enclose, as in an occluded virus. [see occlusion]

oc•clu•sal (ŏ-klū′zăl). **1.** Pertaining to occlusion or closure. **2.** DENTISTRY Pertaining to the contacting surfaces of opposing occlusal units (teeth or occlusion rims), or the masticating surfaces of the posterior teeth.

oc•clu•sion (ŏ-klū′zhŭn). **1.** The act of closing or the state of being closed. **2.** In chemistry, the absorption of a gas by a metal or the inclusion of one substance within another (as in a gelatinous precipitate). **3.** Any contact between the incising or masticating surfaces of the upper and lower teeth. **4.** The relationship between the occlusal surfaces of the maxillary and mandibular teeth when they are in contact. [L. *oc- cludo*, pp. *-clusus*, to shut up, fr. *ob., against,* + *claudo,* to close]

abnormal o., an arrangement of the teeth which is not considered to be within the normal range of variation.

afunctional o., a malocclusion which does not permit normal function of the dentition.

balanced o., the simultaneous contacting of the upper and lower teeth on the right and left and in the anterior and posterior occlusal areas in centric and eccentric positions within the functional range.

centric o., (1) the relation of opposing occlusal surfaces which provides the maximum contact and/or intercuspation; (2) the o. of the teeth when the mandible is in centric relation to the maxillae.

coronary o., blockage of a coronary vessel, usually by thrombosis or atheroma, often leading to myocardial infarction.

distal o., (1) a tooth occluding in a position distal to normal; SYN retrusive o. (2). (2) SYN distoclusion.

eccentric o., any o. other than centric.

functional o., (1) any tooth contacts made within the functional range of the opposing teeth surfaces; (2) o. which occurs during function.

hyperfunctional o., occlusal stress of tooth or teeth exceeding normal physiologic demands.

mesial o., (1) o. in which the mandibular teeth articulate with the maxillary teeth in a position anterior to normal; SYN mesio-occlusion. (2) SYN mesioclusion.

neutral o., (1) an arrangement of teeth such that the maxillary and mandibular first permanent molars are in normal anteroposterior relation; SYN normal o. (2). (2) SYN neutroclusion.

normal o., (1) that arrangement of teeth and their supporting structure which is usually found in health and which approaches an ideal or standard arrangement; (2) SYN neutral o. (1).

pathogenic o., an occlusal relationship capable of producing pathologic changes in the supporting tissues.

physiologic o., o. in harmony with functions of the masticatory system.

protrusive o., o. which results when the mandible is protruded forward from centric position.

retrusive o., (1) a biting relationship in which the mandible is forcefully or habitually placed more distally than the patient's centric o.; (2) SYN distal o. (1).

traumatogenic o., a malocclusion capable of producing injury to the teeth and/or associated structures.

oc•clu•sive (ŏ-klū′siv). Serving to close; denoting a bandage or dressing that closes a wound and excludes it from the air.

oc•cult (ŏ-kŭlt′, ok′ŭlt). **1.** Hidden; concealed; not manifest. **2.** Denoting a disease or condition (bleeding, infection) that is clinically inapparent, though it may be inferred from indirect evidence or identified by special tests. SEE occult *blood.* **3.** ONCOLOGY A clinically unidentified primary tumor with recognized metastases. [L. *oc-culo,* pp. *-cultus,* to cover, hide]

ochrom•e•ter (ō-krom′ĕ-ter). An instrument for determining the capillary blood pressure; one of two adjacent fingers is compressed by a rubber balloon until blanching of the skin occurs, after which the force necessary to accomplish this color change is read in millimeters of mercury. [G. *ōchros,* pale yellow, + *metron,* measure]

ochro•no•sis (o-kron-ō′sis). A condition observed in persons with alkaptonuria, characterized by pigmentation of the cartilages; may also affect the sclera, mucous membrane of the lips, and skin of the ears, face, and hands, and cause standing urine to be dark-colored and contain pigmented casts; pigmentation from oxidized homogentisic acid; cartilage degeneration results in osteoarthritis. [G. *ōchros,* pale yellow, + *nosos,* disease]

ochro•not•ic (ō-kron-ot′ik). Relating to or characterized by ochronosis.

△**oct-, octi-, octo-, octa-.** Eight. [G. *oktō,* L. *octo*]

oc•tan (ok′tan). Applied to fever, the paroxysms of which recur every eighth day, the day of a paroxysm being counted as the first in the computation. [L. *octo,* eight]

△**octi-.** SEE oct-.

△**octo-.** SEE oct-.

oc•u•lar (ok′yū-lăr). **1.** SYN ophthalmic. **2.** The eyepiece of a microscope, the lens or lenses at the observer end of a microscope, by means of which the image focused by the objective is viewed. [L. *oculus,* eye]

oc•u•lar•ist (ok′yū-lăr-ist). One skilled in the design, fabrication, and fitting of artificial eyes and the making of prostheses associated with the appearance or function of the eyes. [L. *oculus,* eye]

oc•u•li (ok′yū-lī). Plural of oculus. [L.]

oc•u•list (ok′yū-list). SYN ophthalmologist. [L. *oculus,* eye]

△**oculo-.** The eye, ocular. SEE ALSO ophthalmo-. [L. *oculus*]

oc•u•lo•cu•ta•ne•ous (ok′yū-lō-kyū-tā′nē-ŭs). Relating to the eyes and the skin.

oc•u•lo•dyn•ia (ok′yū-lō-din′ē-ă). Pain in the eyeball. [ophthalmo- + G. *algos,* pain]

oc•u•lo•fa•cial (ok-yū-lō-fā′shăl). Relating to the eyes and the face.

oc•u•log•ra•phy (ok-yū-log′ră-fē). A method of recording eye position and movements. [oculo- + G. *graphē,* a writing]

oc•u•lo•gy•ria (ok′yū-lō-jī′rē-ă). The limits of rotation of the eyeballs. [oculo- + G. *gyros,* circle]

oc·u·lo·gy·ric (ok′yū-lō-jī′rik). Referring to rotation of the eyeballs; characterized by oculogyria.

oc·u·lo·mo·tor (ok′yū-lō-mō′tŏr). Pertaining to the o. cranial nerve. [L. *oculomotorius*, fr. oculo- + L. *motorius*, moving]

oc·u·lo·na·sal (ok′yū-lō-nā′săl). Relating to the eyes and the nose. [oculo- + L. *nasus*, nose]

oc·u·lo·pleth·ys·mog·ra·phy (ok′yū-lō-pleth-iz-mog′ră-fē). Indirect measurement of the hemodynamic significance of internal carotid artery stenosis or occlusion by demonstration of an ipsilateral delay in the arrival of ocular pressure transmitted from branches of the ophthalmic artery. [oculo- + G. *plēthymos*, increase, + *graphē*, to write]

oc·u·lo·pneu·mo·pleth·ys·mog·ra·phy (ok′yū-lō-nū′mō-pleth-iz-mog′ră-fē). A method of bilateral measurement of ophthalmic artery pressure that reflects pressure and flow in the internal carotid artery. SEE oculoplethysmography.

oc·u·lo·pu·pil·lary (ok′yū-lō-pū′pi-lār-ē). Pertaining to the pupil of the eye.

oc·u·lo·sym·pa·thet·ic (ok′ū-lō-sim-pa-the′tik). Pertaining to the sympathetic pathway to the eye, damage to which produces Horner's *syndrome*.

oc·u·lo·zy·go·mat·ic (ok′yū-lō-zī-gō-mat′ik). Relating to the orbit or its margin and the zygomatic bone.

oc·u·lus, gen. and pl. **oc·u·li** (ok′yū-lŭs, -lī) [NA]. SYN eye (1). [L.]

△**ocy-**. SEE oxy-.

OD overdose; optical *density* (see absorbance).

od. A force assumed to be exerted upon the nervous system by magnets. [G. *hodos*, way]

△**-odes.** Having the form of, resembling. [G. *eidos*, form, resemblance]

△**odont-, odonto-**. A tooth, teeth. [G. *odous* (*odont-*)]

odon·tal·gia (ō-don-tal′jē-ă). SYN toothache. [odont- + G. *algos*, pain]

odon·tal·gic (ō-don-tal′jik). Relating to or marked by toothache.

odon·tec·to·my (ō-don-tek′tō-mē). Removal of teeth by the reflection of a mucoperiosteal flap and excision of bone from around the root or roots before the application of force to effect the tooth removal. [odont- + G. *ektomē*, excision]

△**odonto-**. SEE odont-.

odon·to·blast (ō-don′tō-blast). One of the dentin-forming cells, derived from mesenchyme of neural crest origin, lining the pulp cavity of a tooth. [odonto- + G. *blastos*, sprout, germ]

odon·to·blas·to·ma (ō-don′tō-blas-tō′mă). 1. A tumor composed of neoplastic epithelial and mesenchymal cells that may differentiate into cells able to produce calcified tooth substances. 2. An odontoma in its early formative stage. [odontoblast + G. *-oma*, tumor]

odon·to·clast (ō-don′tō-klast). One of the cells believed to produce resorption of the roots of the deciduous teeth. [odonto- + G. *klastos*, broken]

odon·to·dys·pla·sia (ō-don′tō-dis-plā′zē-ă). A developmental disturbance of one or of several adjacent teeth, of unknown etiology, characterized by deficient formation of enamel and dentin which results in an abnormally large pulp chamber and imparts a ghostlike radiographic image to the teeth; such teeth exhibit delayed eruption into the oral cavity.

odon·to·gen·e·sis (ō-don-tō-jen′ĕ-sis). The process of development of the teeth. SYN odontogeny, odontosis. [odonto- + G. *genesis*, production]

odon·tog·e·ny (ō-don-toj′ĕ-nē). SYN odontogenesis.

odon·toid (ō-don′toyd). 1. Shaped like a tooth. 2. Relating to the toothlike o. process of the second cervical vertebra. [odont- + G. *eidos*, resemblance]

odon·tol·o·gy (ō-don-tol′ŏ-jē). SYN dentistry. [odonto- + G. *logos*, study]

odon·tol·y·sis (ō-don-tol′i-sis). SYN erosion (3). [odonto- + G. *lysis*, dissolution]

odon·to·ma (ō-don-tō′mă). 1. A tumor of odontogenic origin. 2. A hamartomatous odontogenic tumor composed of enamel, dentin, cementum, and pulp tissue that may or may not be arranged in the form of a tooth. [odonto- + G. *-oma*, tumor]

   ameloblastic o., a benign mixed odontogenic tumor composed of an undifferentiated component histologically identical to an ameloblastoma and a well differentiated component identical to an odontoma.

   complex o., an o. in which the various odontogenic tissues are organized in a haphazard arrangement with no resemblance to teeth.

   compound o., an o. in which the odontogenic tissues are organized and resemble anomalous teeth.

odon·to·neu·ral·gia (ō-don′tō-nū-ral′jē-ă). Facial neuralgia caused by a carious tooth.

odon·ton·o·my (ō-don-ton′ō-mē). Dental nomenclature. [odonto- + G. *onoma*, name]

odon·top·a·thy (ō-don-top′ă-thē). Any disease of the teeth or of their sockets. [odonto- + G. *pathos*, suffering]

odontoplasty (ō-dŏn′tō-plăs-tē). Reshaping of a portion of a tooth; may be performed for therapeutic or cosmetic purposes. [odonto- + -plasty]

odon·to·sis (ō-don-tō′sis). SYN odontogenesis.

odon·tot·o·my (ō-don-tot′ō-mē). Cutting into the crown of a tooth. [odonto- + G. *tomē*, incision]

odor (ō′dŏr). Emanation from any substance that stimulates the olfactory cells in the organ of smell. SYN smell (3). [L.]

△**odyn-, odyno-**. Pain. [G. *odynē*]

odyn·a·cu·sis (ō-din′ă-kū′sis). Hypersensitiveness of the organ of hearing, so that noises cause actual pain. [odyn- + G. *akouō*, to hear]

ody·nom·e·ter (ō-di-nom′ĕ-ter). SYN algesiometer. [odyno- + G. *metron*, measure]

odyn·o·pha·gia (ō-din-ō-fā′jē-ă). Pain on swallowing. [odyno- + G. *phagō* to eat]

△**oe-**. For words so beginning and not found here, see e-.

oe·di·pism (ed′i-pizm). 1. Self-infliction of injury to the eyes, usually an attempt at evulsion. 2. Manifestation of the Oedipus complex. [*Oedipus*, G. myth. char.]

oer·sted (er′sted). A unit of magnetic field intensity; the magnetic field intensity that exerts a force of 1 dyne on unit magnetic pole; equal to

BLOOD CELLS

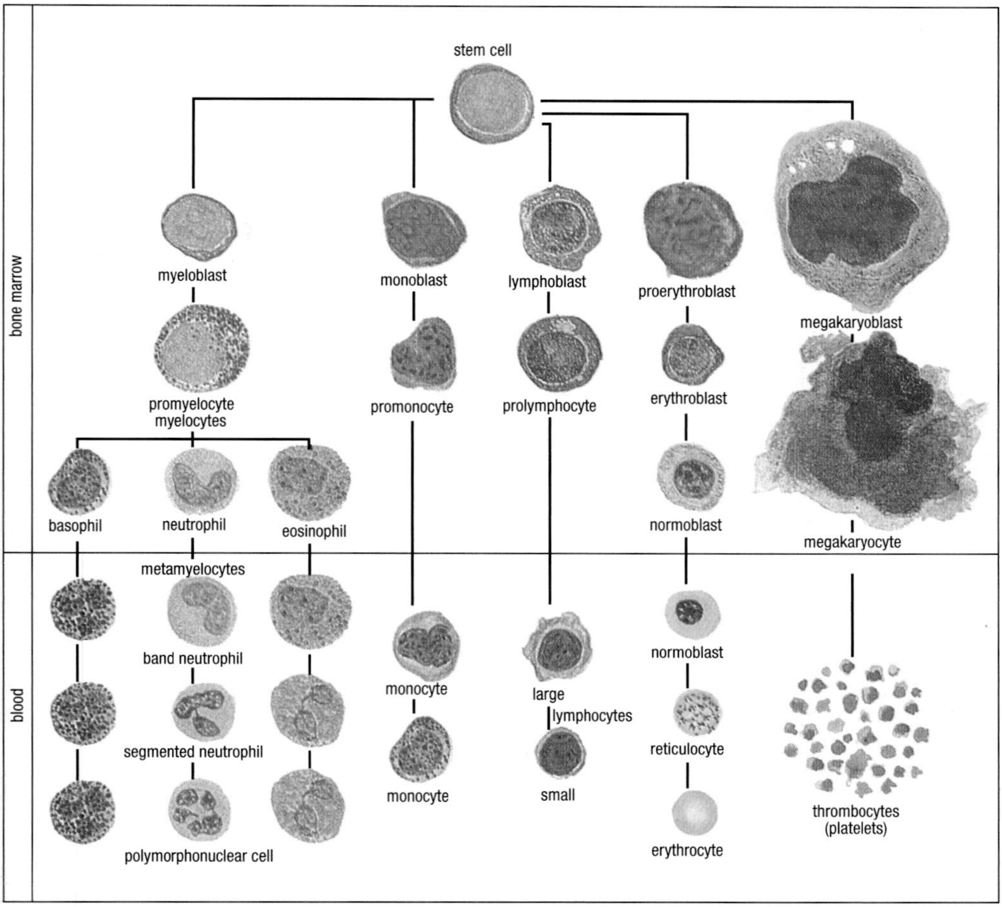

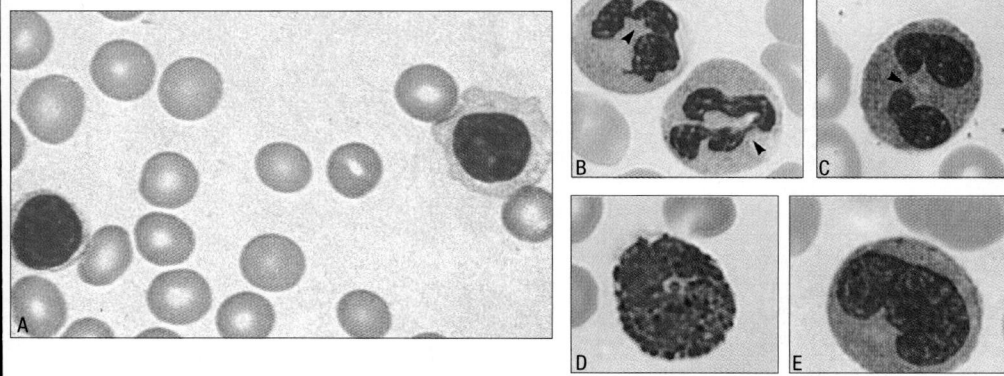

stem cell

bone marrow

myeloblast monoblast lymphoblast proerythroblast

megakaryoblast

promyelocyte monomyelocytes promonocyte prolymphocyte erythroblast

basophil neutrophil eosinophil

normoblast

megakaryocyte

blood

metamyelocytes

band neutrophil

monocyte

large lymphocytes

normoblast

segmented neutrophil

monocyte small

reticulocyte

polymorphonuclear cell

erythrocyte

thrombocytes (platelets)

blood cells: developmental series (simplified scheme)

blood cells: (A) stained smear of normal blood showing a small **lymphocyte** (left) and a large lymphocyte (right); (B) **neutrophils** showing a somewhat granular cytoplasm and lobulated nuclei (arrows); (C) **eosinophils** with large pink granules and sausage-shaped nuclei (arrow); (D) **basophil** with dense, dark, large granules; (E) **monocyte** characterized by large size, acentric, kidney-shaped nucleus, and lack of specific granules

ABNORMALITIES OF ERYTHROCYTES

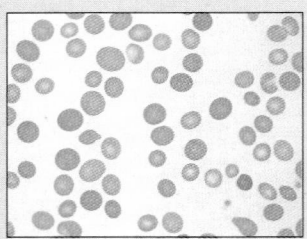

anisocytosis

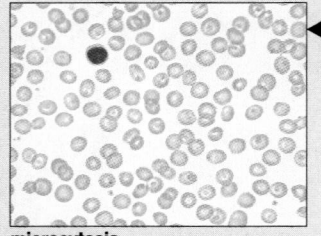

microcytosis

◄ shown in heterozygous thalassemia (thalassemia minor)

poikilocytosis

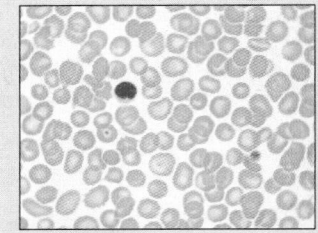

macrocytosis

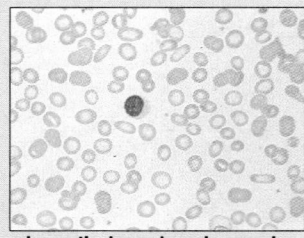

microcytic, hypochromic anemia

showing poikilocytosis ►

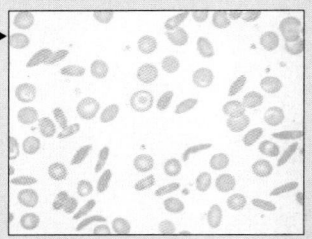

sickle cell anemia

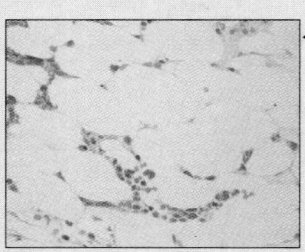

aplastic anemia

◄ marrow smear showing absence of red cell, white cell, and platelet precursors; cells present are lymphocytes

slide showing poikilocytosis and absence of platelets, but no signs of hemolysis (reduced number of RBCs, presence of reticulocytes = immature RBCs pushed into circulation to replace hemolyzed RBCs) ►

peripheral blood smear showing oval macrocytes and a hypersegmented neutrophil ◄

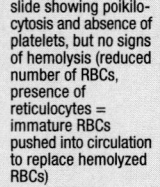

hemolytic anemia

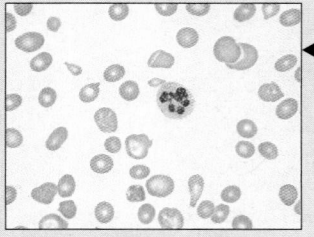

pernicious anemia

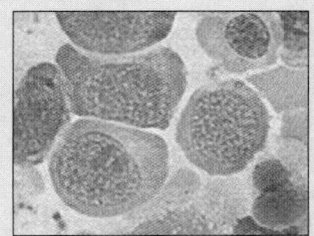

pernicious anemia: in bone marrow

organisms

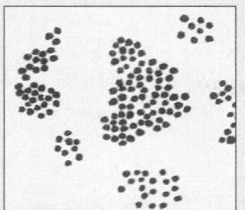

staphylococci

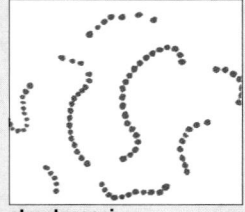

streptococci

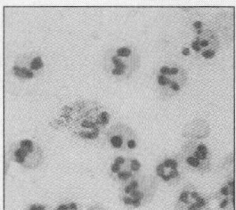

gonococci

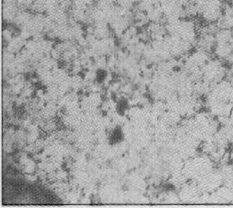

Mycobacterium tuberculosis

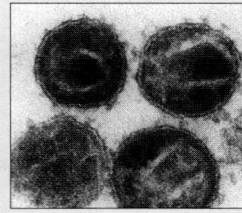

AIDS virus

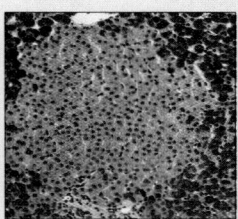

hepatitis B

skin infections

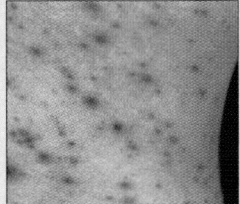

varicella (chicken pox)

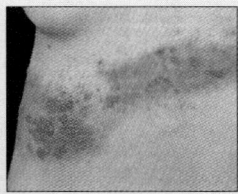

zoster

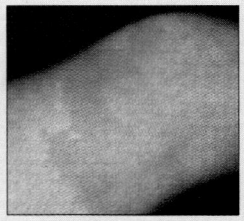

Lyme disease (erythema chronicum migrans)

cutaneous parasitic infestations

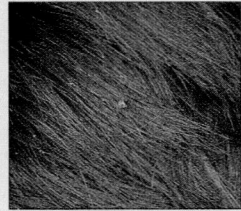

pediculosis capitis

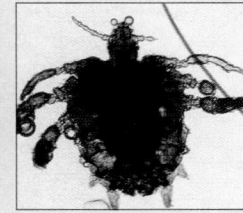

pediculosis pubis

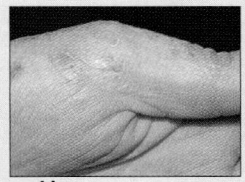

scabies

sexually transmitted diseases (STDs)

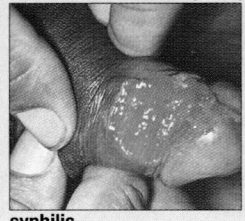

syphilis

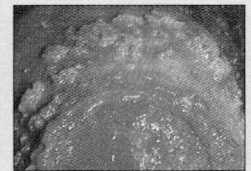

condyloma acuminatum (genital wart)

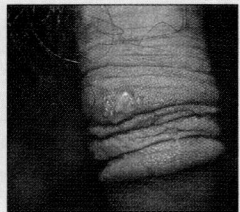

HSV-2 (genital herpes)

PLATES

primary lesions

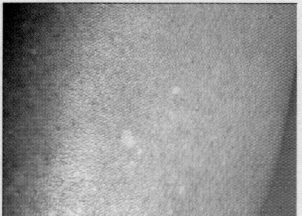

macule

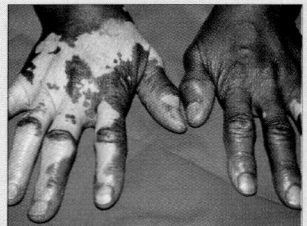

patch

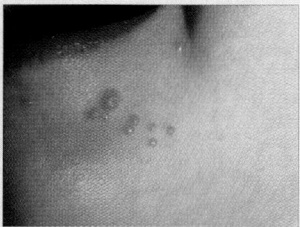

papule

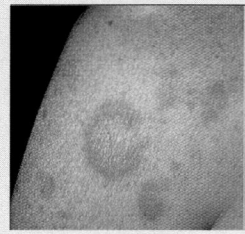

plaque

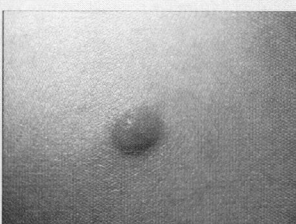

nodule

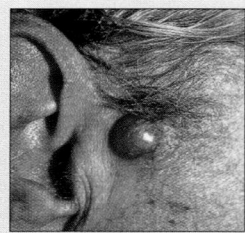

tumor

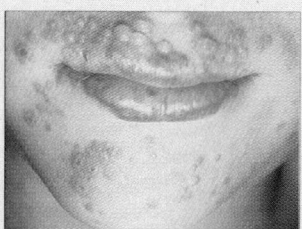

vesicle

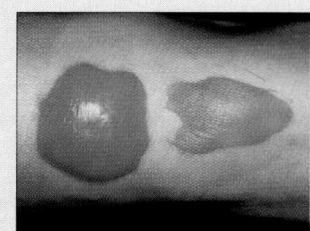

bulla

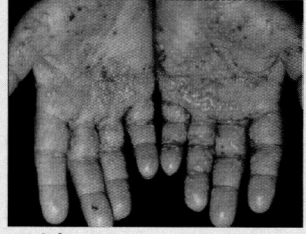

pustule

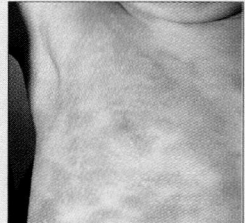

wheal

SECONDARY AND VASCULAR LESIONS

secondary lesions

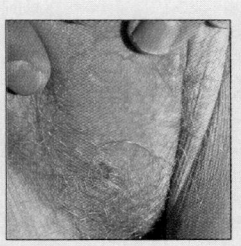

erosion

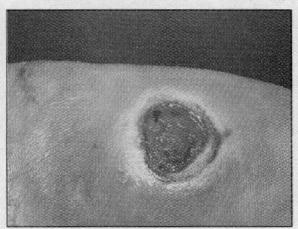

ulcer

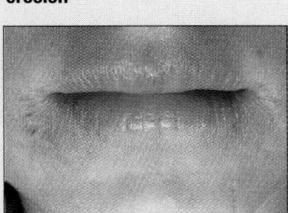

fissure

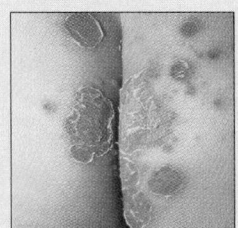

scale

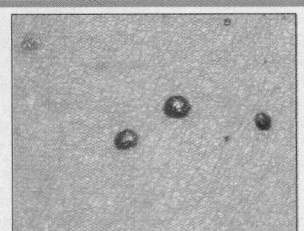

crust

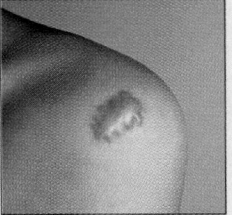

keloid

vascular lesions

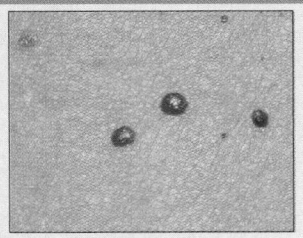

cherry angioma

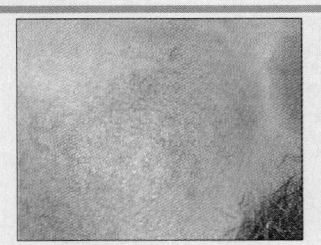

telangiectasia

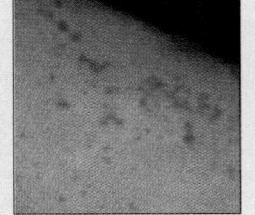

petechia

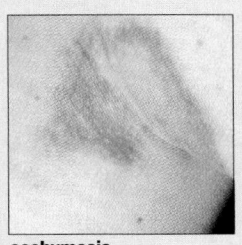

ecchymosis

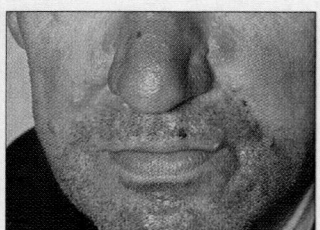

rosacea

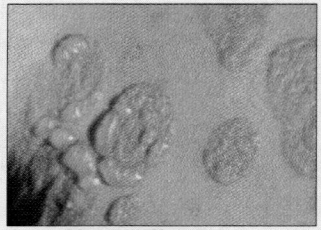

dermatitis herpetiformis

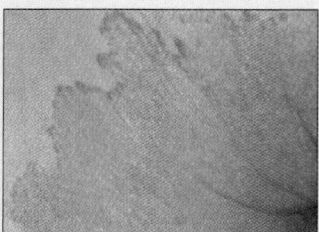

tinea corporis

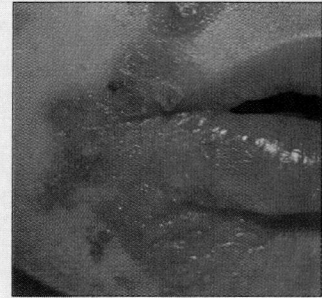

impetigo

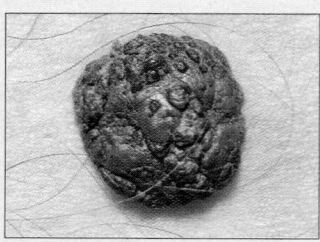

seborrheic keratoses

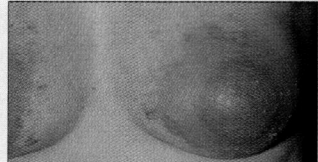

contact dermatitis

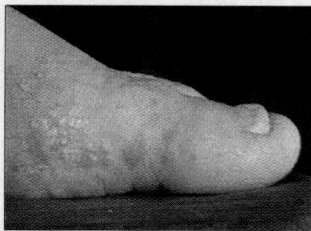

tinea pedis

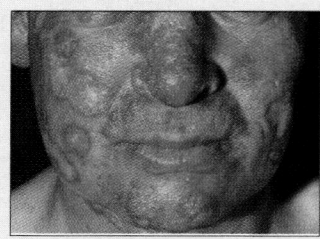

lupus erythematosus

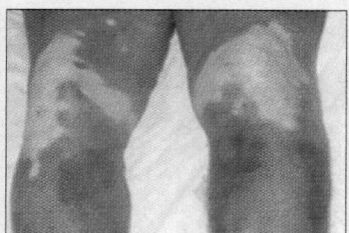

purpura fulminans

actinic keratoses

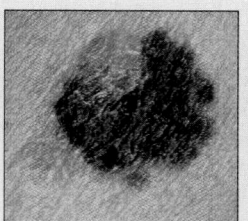

malignant melanoma: showing uneven pigmentation

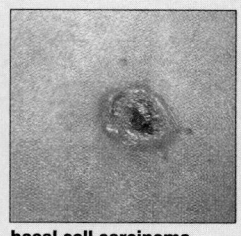

basal cell carcinoma

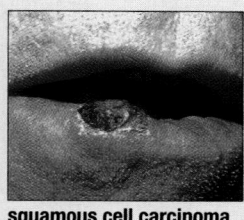

squamous cell carcinoma

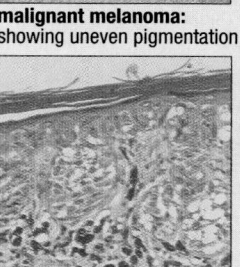

nodular melanoma: tumor cells invade the dermis

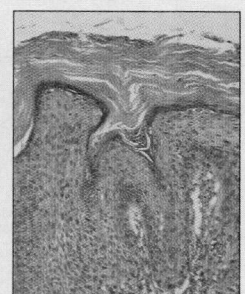

Bowen's disease

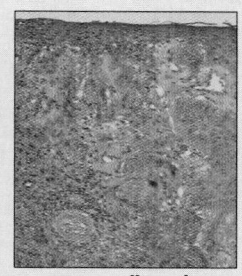

squamous cell carcinoma: invasive tumor

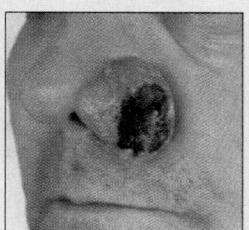

keratoacanthoma: of the nose

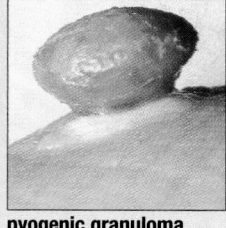

pyogenic granuloma

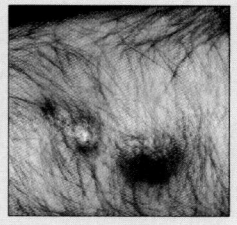

Kaposi's sarcoma

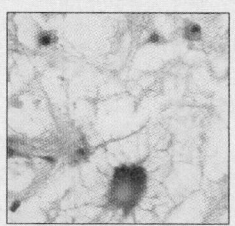

liposarcoma

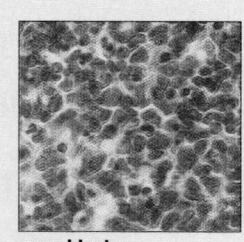

neuroblastoma

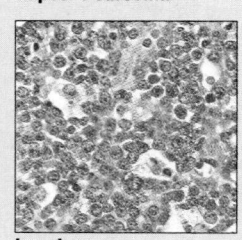

lymphoma

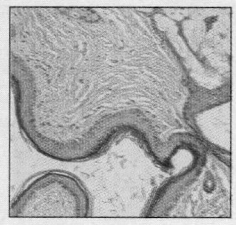

teratoma

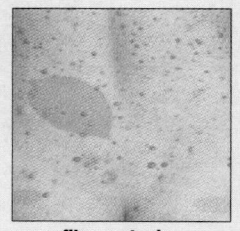

neurofibromatosis

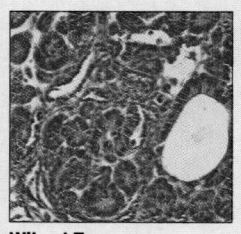

Wilms' Tumor

PLATES

endoscopy is the examination of a body cavity with a flexible endoscope to examine within for diagnostic or treatment purpose; fiberoptics in the endoscope conduct bright, cool light along a curved path, allowing illumination of tissues and structures within the body; the endoscope often contains small instruments such as biopsy snares; the photographs on these two pages were taken with a camera that attaches to the examiner's end of the instrument

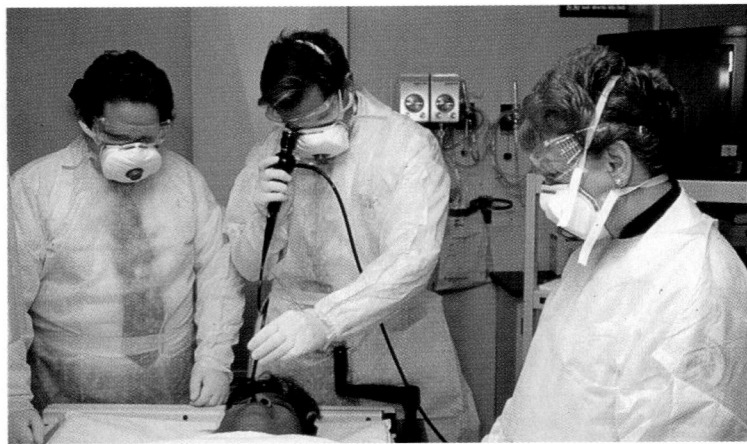

bronchoscopy team performing procedure

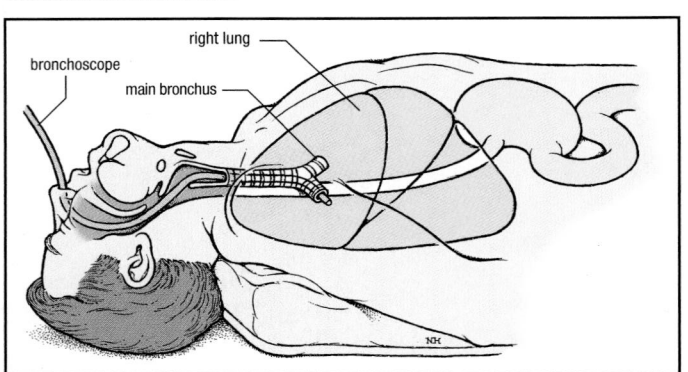

the **bronchoscope** is introduced nasally and slowly led down the trachea until the desired level is reached

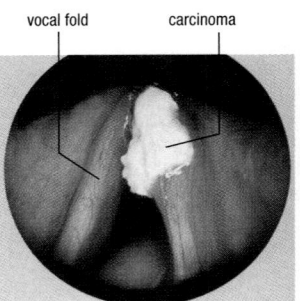

laryngeal carcinoma: the bronchoscope is an effective tool in the diagnosis of pathological conditions

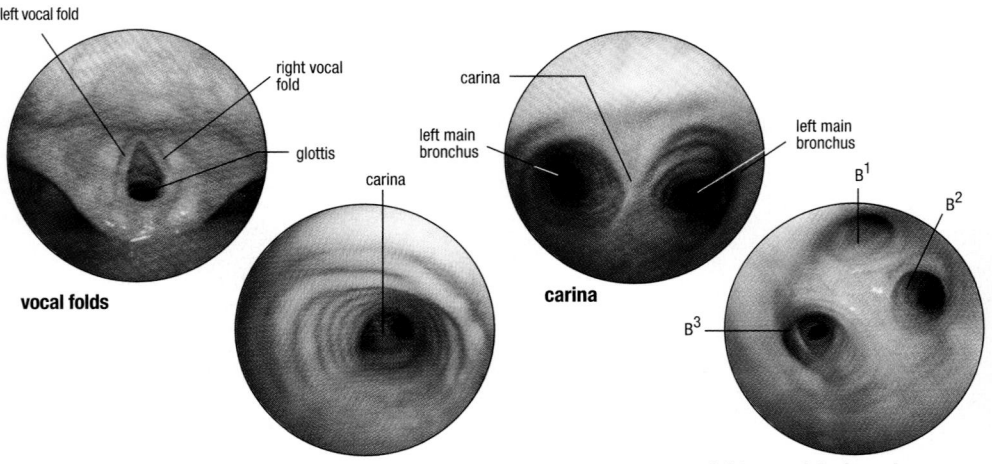

vocal folds

entire trachea and the carina

carina

right upper lobe bronchus

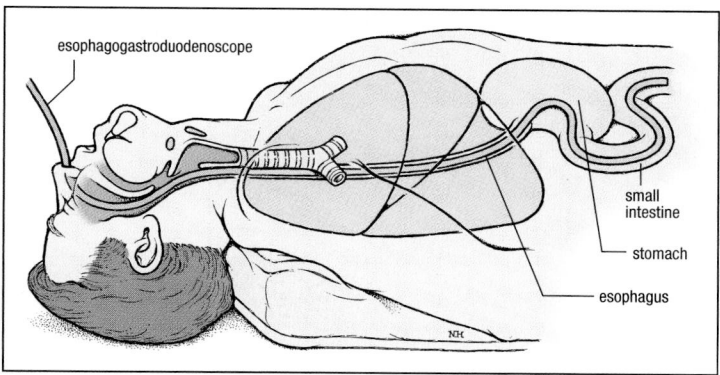

esophagogastroduodenoscope

small intestine

stomach

esophagus

the **esophagogastroduodenoscope** is introduced nasally or orally and slowly led down the gastrointestinal tract until the desired level is reached; it is used for evaluating pathological conditions and performing minimally invasive corrective procedures

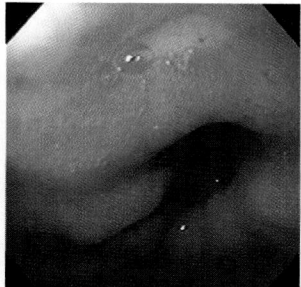

A

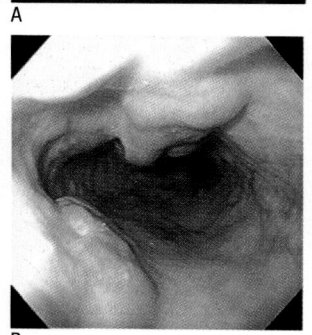

B

various pathologies as viewed through the esophagogastrodoudenoscope: (A) **gastritis**, (B) **esophageal varices**

various pathologies as viewed through the colonoscope: (C) **diverticulosis**, (D) **ulcerative colitis**, (E) **colon polypectomy**

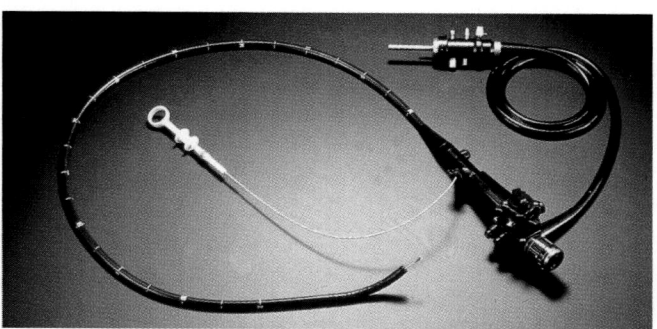

the **colonoscope**, an instrument for viewing and photographing the lower gastrointestinal track, is introduced anally and, like other endoscopes, is used for evaluating pathological conditions and performing minimally invasive corrective procedures

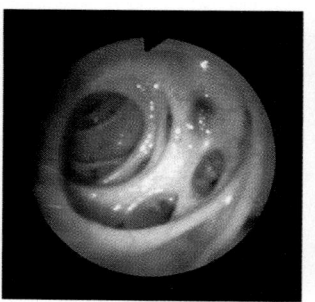

C

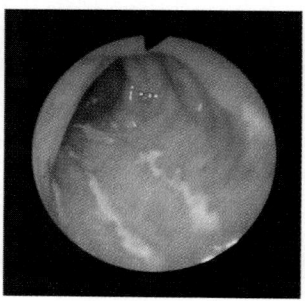

D

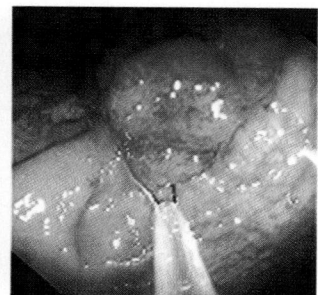

E

PLATES

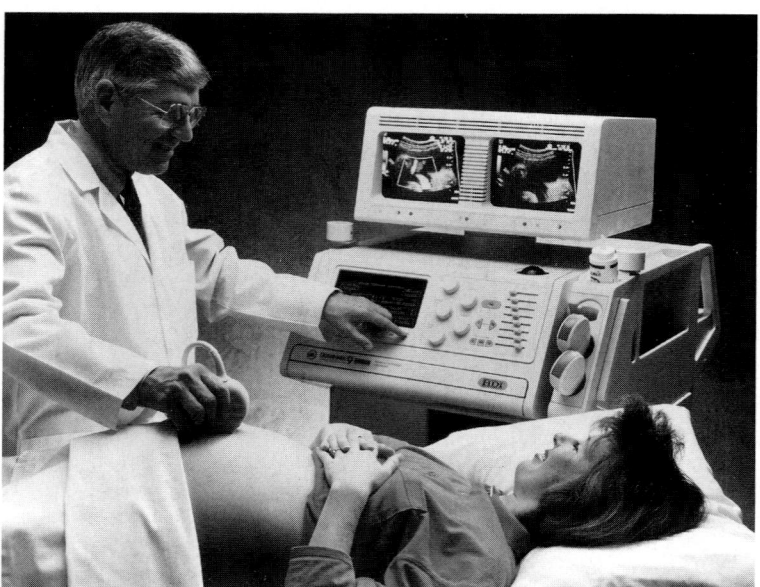

during **obstetrical sonography** an ultrasound image of the pregnant uterus is created in order to determine fetal development

energy in the form of sound waves is reflected off internal organs or, during pregnancy, the fetus, and transformed into an image on a TV-type monitor ▶

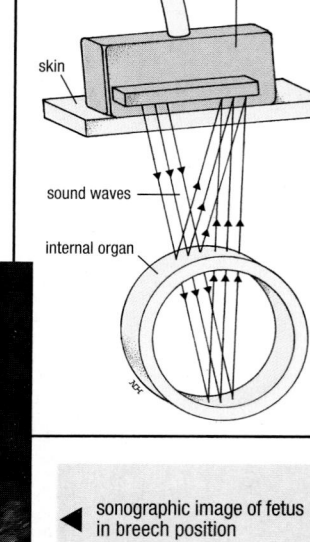

transducer

skin

sound waves

internal organ

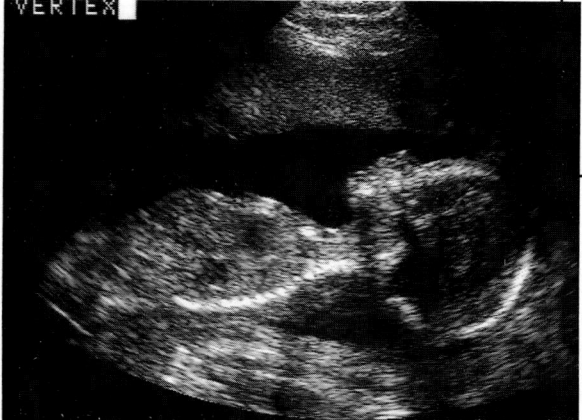

◀ sonographic image of fetus in breech position

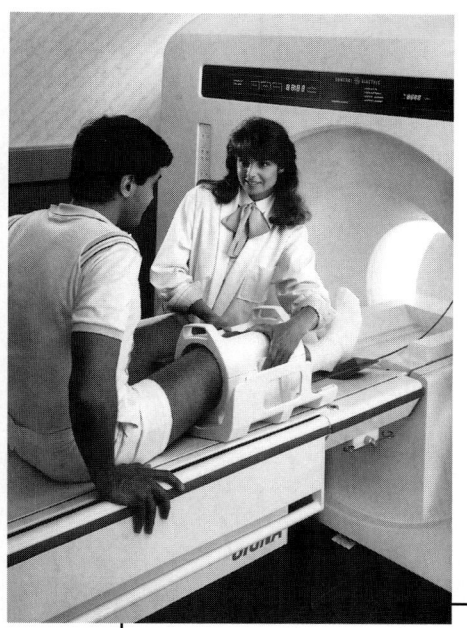

magnetic resonance imaging (MRI) is a nonionizing (non-x-ray) imaging technique using magnetic fields and radio frequency waves to visualize anatomical structures-- useful in detecting joint, tendon, and vertebral disc disorders

◀ **MRI unit**

the patient is positioned within a magnetic field as radiowave signals are conducted through the selected body part; energy is absorbed by tissues and then released

▼

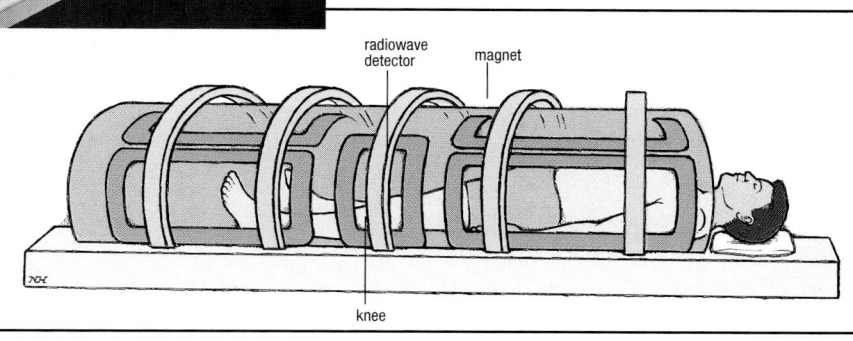

radiowave detector

magnet

knee

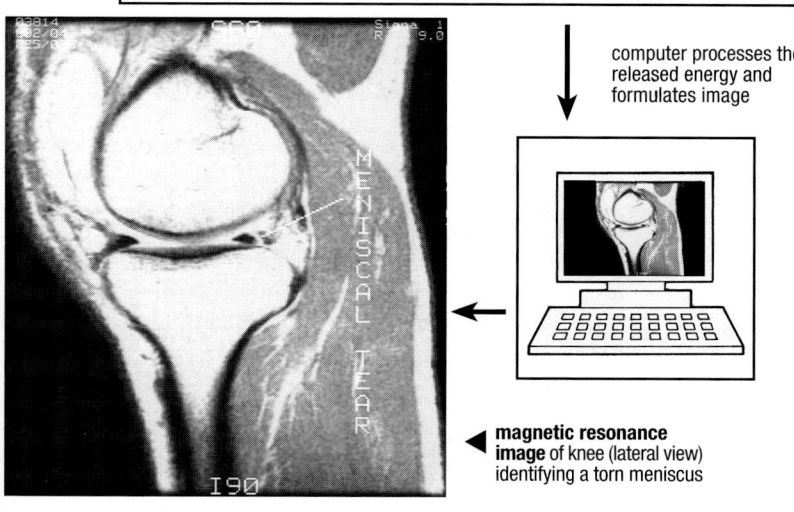

computer processes the released energy and formulates image

magnetic resonance image of knee (lateral view) identifying a torn meniscus

PLATES

nuclear medicine imaging is a diagnostic imaging technique using injected or ingested radioactive isotopes and a gamma-camera for determining size, shape, location, and function of various body parts

thyroid uptake and image is a nuclear image involving scanning of the thyroid ▶ to visualize the radioactive accumulation of previously injected isotopes to detect thyroid nodules or tumors

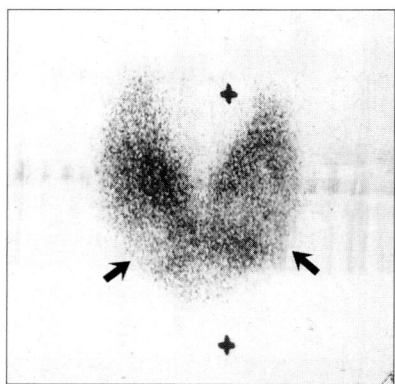

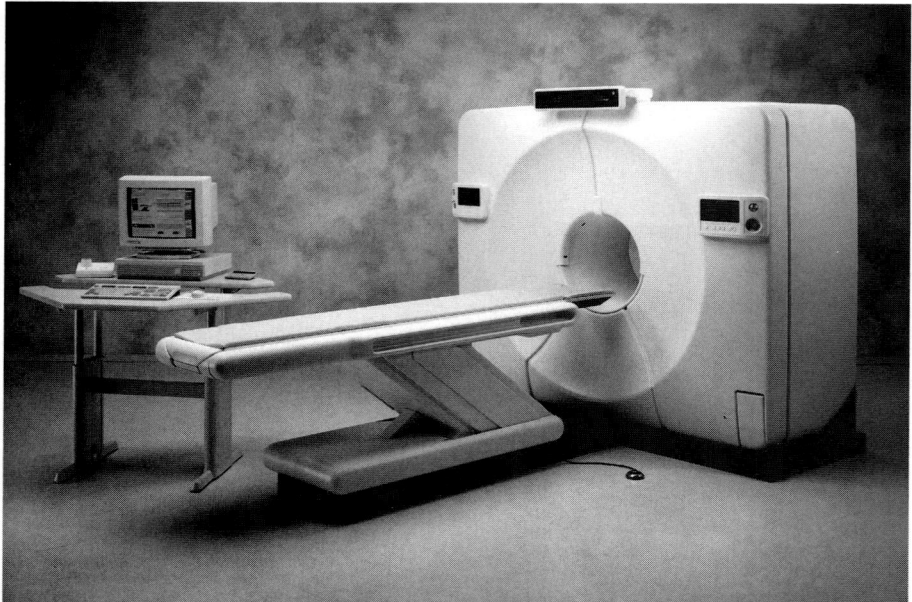

positron emission tomography combines nuclear medicine and computed tomography to produce images of brain anatomy and corresponding physiology--used to study conditions such as stroke, Alzheimer's disease, epilepsy, metabolic brain disorders, and chemistry of nerve transmissions in the brain

warm colors (red and yellow) indicate a higher rate of metabolism and brain activity in the normal ▶ brain (A) when compared with the brain of the patient with Alzheimer's (B)

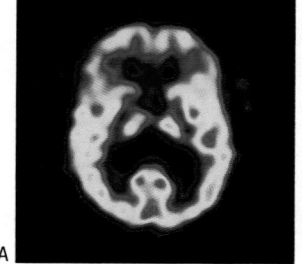

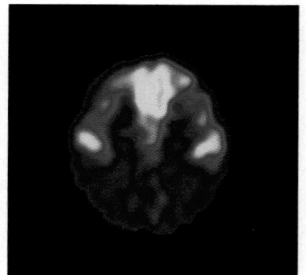

A   B

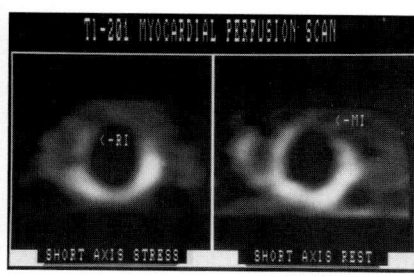

▶ **myocardial perfusion stress scan** is a nuclear scan of the heart taken before and after the induction of controlled physical exercise (treadmill or bicycle) or a pharmaceutical agent that produces the effect of exercise stress in patients unable to ambulate

lung scan is a nuclear scan of the lung used to detect abnormalities of perfusion (blood flow) or ventilation (respiration); commonly called a V / Q (ventilation / perfusion) scan ▼

(A) gamma-camera used to produce nuclear lung scan; (B) and (C) show a posterior lung scan in a patient with an embolus in the right lung; ventilation image (B) shows a normal pattern; absence of blood flow to the right lung is apparent on perfusion scan (C) ▶

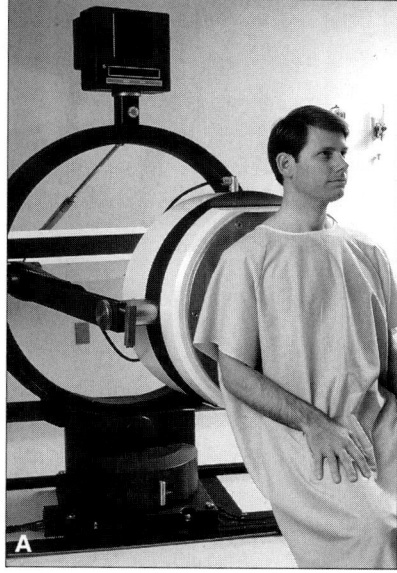

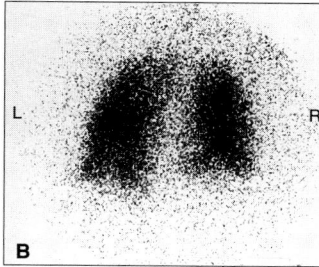

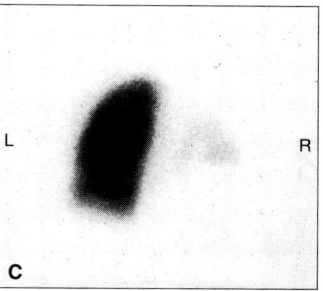

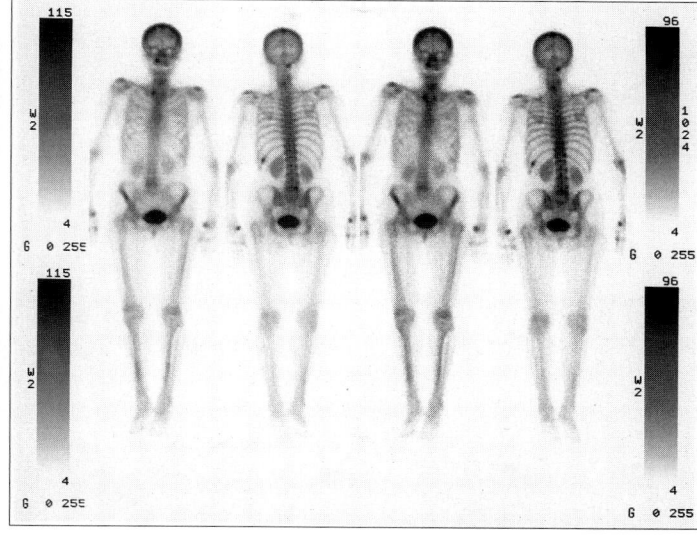

◀ a **bone scan** is a nuclear scan of bone tissue to detect abnomalies such as tumors and malignancies; below is an example of a full-body bone scan

PLATES

computed tomography (CT) is a radiologic procedure using a machine called a scanner to examine a body site by taking a series of cross-sectional images one slice at a time in a full-circle rotation; a computer then calcutes and converts the rates of absorption and density of the x-rays into a picture on a screen

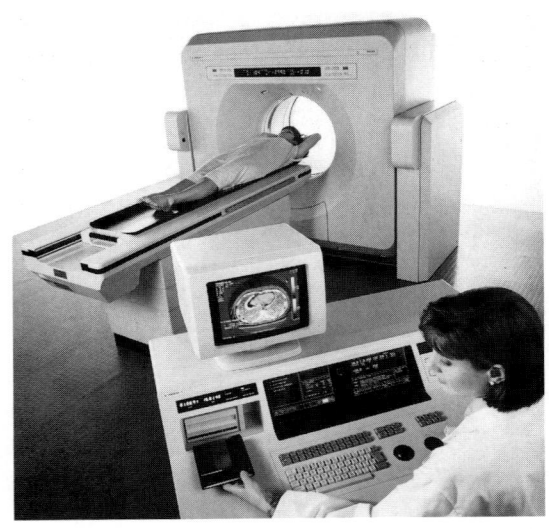

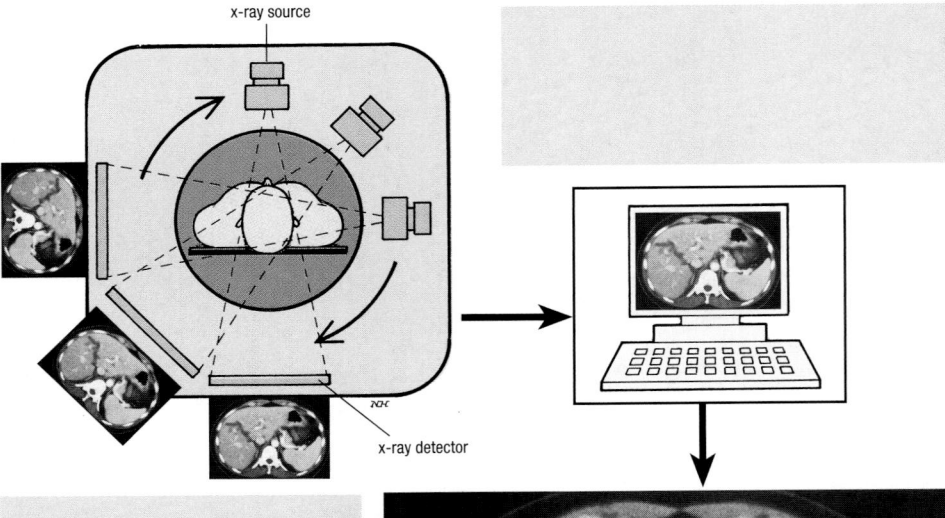

x-ray source

x-ray detector

CT scan of a patient involved in a motor vehicle accident demonstrates a jagged laceration (arrows) extending from posterior to inferior vena cava (V) through right lobe of the liver (L); (S), spleen

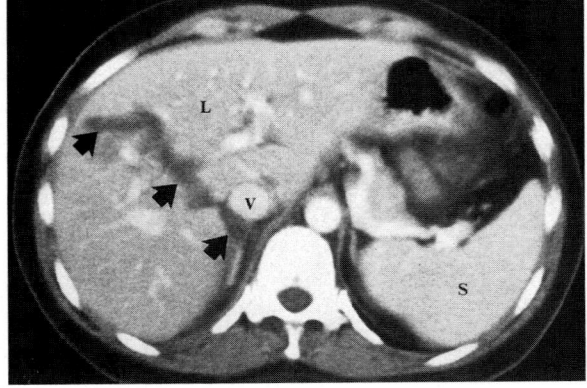

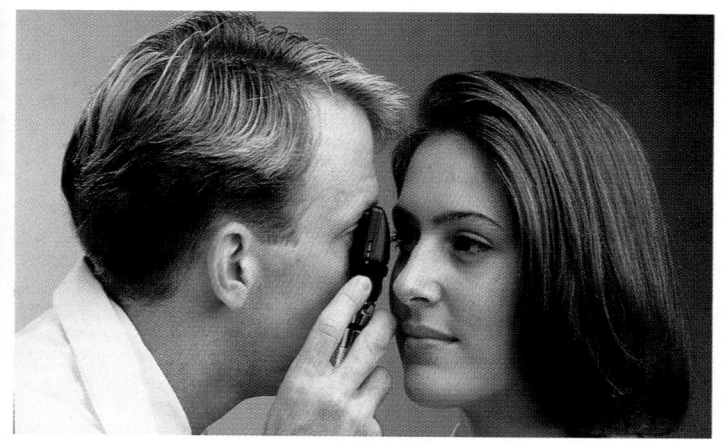

doctor examining patient using ophthalmoscope

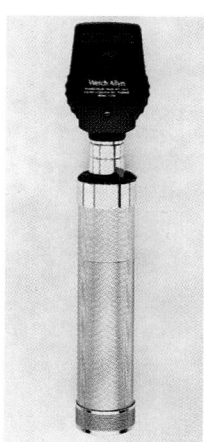

ophthalmoscope

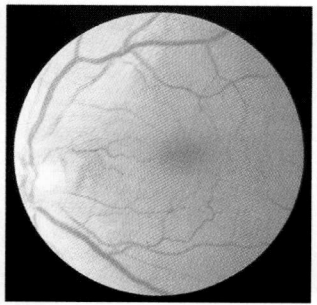

normal retina

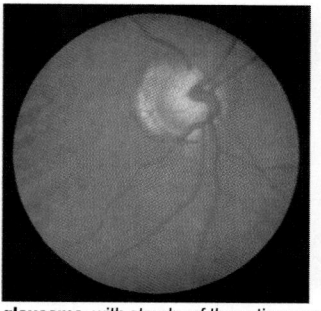

glaucoma: with atrophy of the optic nerve

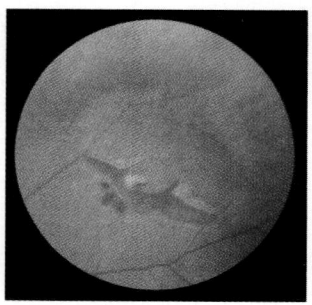

retinal tear

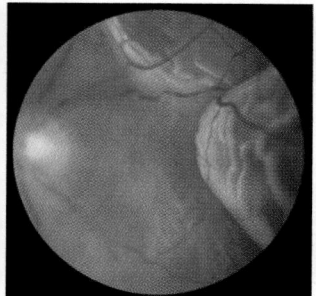

retinal detachment

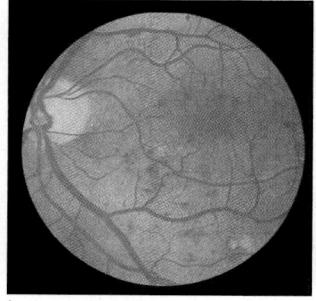

diabetic retinopathy: showing neovascularization

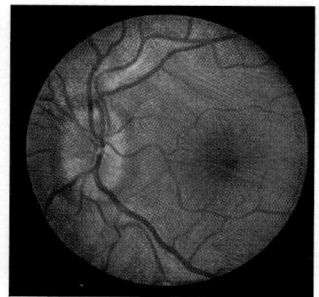

papilledema: with conspicuous retinal folding

PLATES

OTOSCOPY

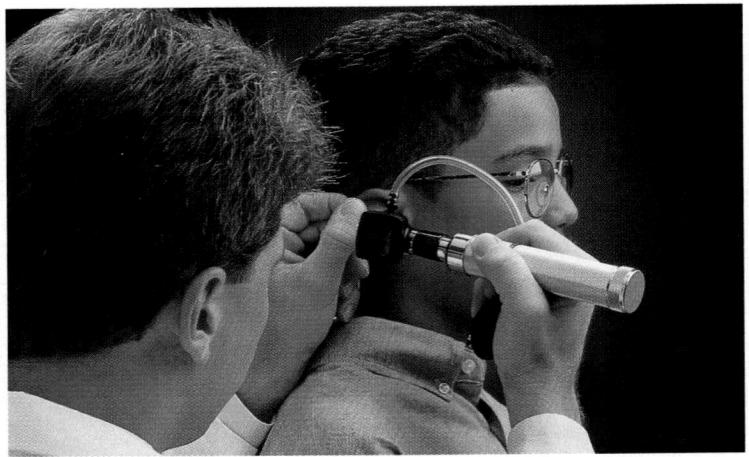

doctor examining patient using otoscope

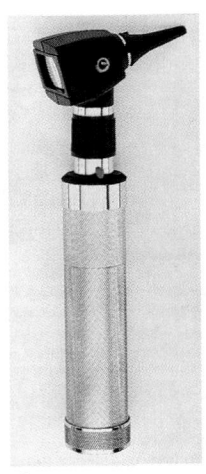

otoscope

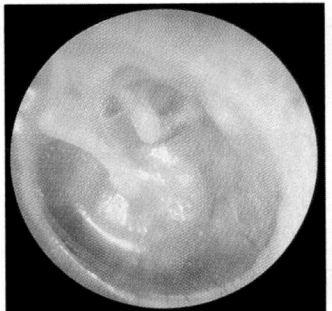

normal tympanic membrane

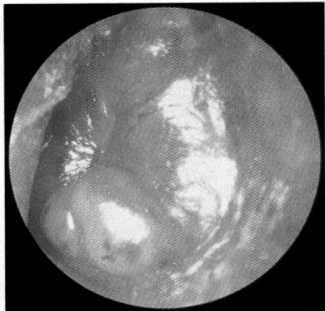

otitis media

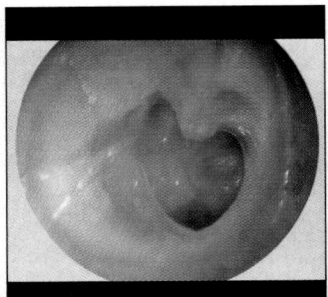

perforation

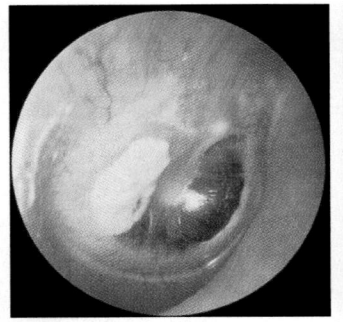

tympanosclerosis

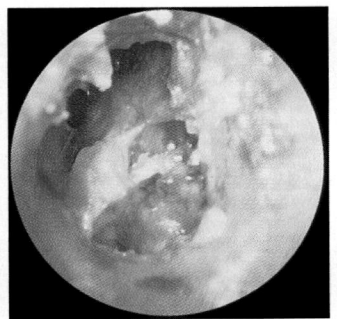

cholesteatoma

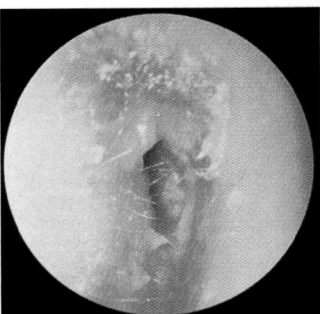

otitis externa

(1000/4π) A·m⁻¹. [Hans-Christian *Oersted*, Danish physicist, 1777–1851]

of·fi·cial (ŏ-fish'ăl). Authoritative; denoting a drug or a chemical or pharmaceutical preparation recognized as standard in the pharmacopeia. Cf. officinal. [L. *officialis*, fr. *officium*, a favor, service, fr. *opus*, work, + *facio*, to do]

of·fic·i·nal (ŏ-fis'i-năl). Denoting a chemical or pharmaceutical preparation kept in stock, in contrast to magistral (prepared extemporaneously according to a physician's prescription). [L. *officina*, shop]

Ohm (Ω), Georgi S., German physicist, 1787–1854. SEE ohm.

ohm (ōm). The practical unit of electrical resistance; the resistance of any conductor allowing 1 ampere of current to pass under the electromotive force of 1 volt. [G.S. *Ohm*]

oh·ne Hauch (ō'nă howch). Term used to designate the nonspreading growth of nonflagellated bacteria on agar media; also applied to somatic agglutination. SEE ALSO O *antigen*. [Ger. without breath]

˃oi-. For words so beginning and not found here, see e-.

˃-oid. Resemblance to, joined properly to words formed from G. roots; equivalent to Eng. -form. [G. *eidos*, form, resemblance]

oid·i·o·my·cin (ō-id'ē-ō-mī'sin). An antigen used to demonstrate cutaneous hypersensitivity in patients infected with Candida; one of a series of antigens used to demonstrate an immunocompromised patient's capacity to react to any cutaneous antigen. [oidium + G. *mykēs*, fungus, + -in]

oil. An inflammable fluid, of fatty consistence and unctuous feel, that is insoluble in water, soluble or insoluble in alcohol, and freely soluble in ether. o.'s are variously classified as animal, vegetable, and mineral o.'s according to their source (the mineral o.'s probably being of remote animal and vegetable origin); into fatty (fixed) and volatile o.'s; and into drying and nondrying (fatty) o.'s, the former becoming gradually thicker when exposed to the air and finally drying to a varnish, the latter not drying but liable to become rancid on exposure. Many of the o.'s, both fixed and volatile, are used in medicine. For individual o.'s, see the specific names.

essential o.'s, plant products, usually somewhat volatile, giving the odors and tastes characteristic of the particular plant; usually, the steam distillates of plants or oils of plants obtained by pressing out the rinds of a particular plant. SEE ALSO volatile o.

ethereal o., SYN volatile o.

fatty o., an o. derived from both animals and plants; chemically, a glyceride of a fatty acid which, by substitution of the glycerine with an alkaline base, is converted into a soap; a fatty o., in contrast to a volatile o., is permanent and not capable of distillation.

volatile o., a substance of oily consistency and feel, derived from a plant and containing the principles to which the odor and taste of the plant are due (essential o.); in contrast to a fatty o., a volatile o. evaporates when exposed to the air and thus is capable of distillation. SYN ethereal o.

oint·ment (oynt'ment). A semisolid preparation usually containing medicinal substances and intended for external application. SYN salve, unguent. [O. Fr. *oignement*; L. *unguo*, pp. *unctus*, to smear]

△-ol. Suffix denoting that a substance is an alcohol or a phenol.

o·le·ag·i·nous (ō-lē-aj'i-nŭs). Oily or greasy. [L. *oleagineus*, pertaining to *olea*, the olive tree]

ole·ate (ō'lē-āt). **1.** A salt of oleic acid. **2.** A pharmacopeial preparation consisting of a combination or solution of an alkaloid or metallic base in oleic acid, used as an inunction.

olec·ra·non (ō-lek'ră-non, ō'lē-krā'non) [NA]. The prominent curved proximal extremity of the ulna, the upper and posterior surface of which gives attachment to the tendon of the triceps muscle, the anterior surface entering into the formation of the trochlear notch. SYN elbow bone, point of elbow. [G. the head or point of the elbow, fr. *ōlenē*, ulna, + *kranion*, skull, head]

ole·fin (ō'lē-fin). SYN alkene.

△oleo-. Oil. SEE ALSO eleo-. [L. *oleum*]

▯ol·fac·tion (ol-fak'shŭn). **1.** The sense of smell. SYN smell (2). **2.** The act of smelling. SYN osphresis. [L. *ol- facio*, pp. *-factus*, to smell]

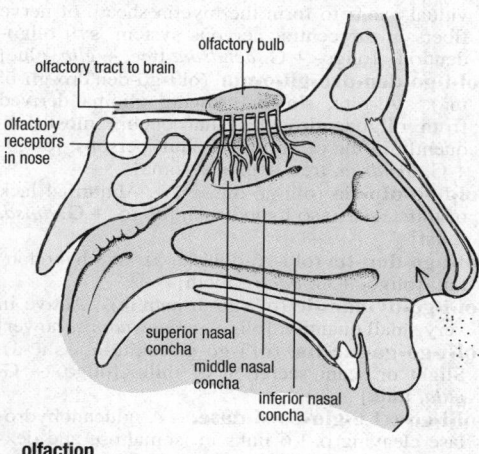

olfactory bulb
olfactory tract to brain
olfactory receptors in nose
superior nasal concha
middle nasal concha
inferior nasal concha

olfaction

ol·fac·to·ry (ol-fak'tŏ-rē). Relating to the sense of smell. SYN osphretic. [see olfaction]

△olig-. SEE oligo-.

ol·i·ge·mia (ol-i-gē'mē-ă). A deficiency of blood in the body or any organ or tissue. [oligo- + G. *haima*, blood]

ol·i·ge·mic (ol-i-gē'mik). Pertaining to or characterized by oligemia.

△oligo-, olig-. **1.** A few, a little; too little, too few. **2.** CHEMISTRY Used in contrast to "poly-" in describing polymers; *e.g.*, oligosaccharide. [G. *oligos*, few]

ol·i·go·am·ni·os (ol'i-gō-am'nē-os). SYN oligohydramnios. [oligo- + amnion]

ol·i·go·cys·tic (ol'i-gō-sis'tik). Consisting of only a few cysts. [oligo- + G. *kystis*, bladder, cyst]

ol·i·go·dac·ty·ly, ol·i·go·dac·tyl·ia (ol'i-gō-dak'ti-lē, -dak-til'ē-ă). Presence of fewer than five digits on one or more limbs. [oligo- + G. *daktylos,* finger or toe]

ol·i·go·den·dria (ol'i-gō-den'drē-ă). SYN oligodendroglia.

🔲 **ol·i·go·den·dro·cyte** (ol'i-gō-den'drō-sīt). A cell of the oligodendroglia.

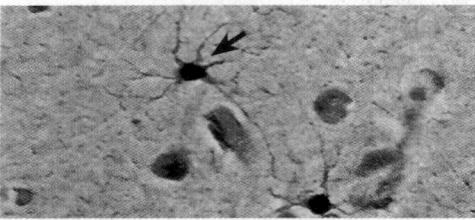

oligodendrocyte (arrow)

ol·i·go·den·drog·lia (ol'ĭ-gō-den-drog'lē-ă). One of the three types of glia cells (the other two being macroglia or astrocytes, and microglia) that, together with nerve cells, compose the tissue of the central nervous system. O. cells are characterized by variable numbers of veillike or sheetlike processes that are wrapped each around individual axons to form the myelin sheath of nerve fibers in the central nervous system. SYN oligodendria. [oligo- + G. *dendron,* tree, + *glia,* glue]

ol·i·go·den·dro·gli·o·ma (ol'i-gō-den'drō-glī-ō'mă). A rare, slowly growing glioma derived from oligodendrocytes that occurs most frequently in the cerebrum of adult persons. [oligo- + G. *dendron,* tree, + glia, + -oma]

ol·i·go·dip·sia (ol'i-gō-dip'sē-ă). Abnormal lack of thirst. SEE ALSO hypodipsia. [oligo- + G. *dipsa,* thirst]

ol·i·go·don·tia (ol'i-gō-don'shē-ă). SYN hypodontia. [oligo- + G. *odous,* tooth]

ol·i·go·dy·nam·ic (ol'i-gō-dī-nam'ik). Active in very small quantity. [oligo- + G. *dynamis,* power]

ol·i·go·ga·lac·tia (ol'i-gō-gă-lak'tē-ă, -shē-ă). Slight or scant secretion of milk. [oligo- + G. *gala,* milk]

ol·i·go-α1,6-glu·co·si·dase. A glucanohydrolase cleaving α-1,6 links in isomaltose and dextrins produced from starch and glycogen by α-amylase; secreted into the duodenum; a deficiency of this enzyme leads to defects in intestinal digestion of limit dextrins. SEE ALSO sucrose α-D-glucohydrolase.

ol·i·go·hy·dram·ni·os (ol'i-gō-hī-dram'nē-os). The presence of an insufficient amount of amniotic fluid (less than 300 ml at term). SYN oligoamnios. [oligo- + G. *hydōr,* water, + amnion]

ol·i·go·men·or·rhea (ol'i-gō-men-ō-rē'ă). Scanty menstruation. [oligo- + menorrhea]

ol·i·go·mor·phic (ol'-i-gō-mōr'fik). Presenting few changes of form; not polymorphic. [oligo- + G. *morphē,* form]

ol·i·go·nu·cle·o·tide (ol'i-gō-nū'klē-ō-tīd). A compound made up of the condensation of a small number (typically fewer than twenty) of nucleotides. Cf. polynucleotide.

ol·i·gop·nea (ol'i-gop-nē'ă, -gop'nē-ă). SYN hypopnea. [oligo- + G. *pnoē,* breath]

ol·i·go·pty·a·lism (ol'i-gō-tī'ă-lizm, ol'i-gop-tī'). A scanty secretion of saliva. [oligo- + G. *ptyalon,* saliva]

ol·i·go·gor·ia (ol-i-gō'rē-ă). An abnormal indifference toward or dislike of persons or things. [G. *oligōria,* negligence, slight esteem, fr. *oligos,* little, + *ōra,* care, regard]

ol·i·go·sac·cha·ride (ol'i-gō-sak'ă-rīd). A compound made up of the condensation of a small number of monosaccharide units. Cf. polysaccharide.

ol·i·go·sper·mia, ol·i·go·sper·ma·tism (ol-i-gō-sper'mē-ă, -mă-tizm). A subnormal concentration of spermatozoa in the penile ejaculate. [oligo- + G. *sperma,* seed]

ol·i·go·sy·nap·tic (ol'i-gō-si-nap'tik). Referring to neural conduction pathways that are interrupted by only a few synaptic junctions, *i.e.,* made up of a sequence of only few nerve cells, in contrast to polysynaptic pathways. SYN paucisynaptic.

ol·i·go·tro·phia, ol·i·got·ro·phy (ol'i-gō-trō'fē-ă, -got'rō-fē). Deficient nutrition. [oligo- + G. *trophē,* nourishment]

ol·i·gu·ria (ol-i-gū'rē-ă). Scanty urine production. [oligo- + G. *ouron,* urine]

oli·va, pl. **oli·'vae** (ō-lī'vă, -vē) [NA]. A smooth oval prominence of the ventrolateral surface of the medulla oblongata lateral to the pyramidal tract, corresponding to the inferior olivary nucleus. SYN corpus olivare, olive (1). [L.]

ol·i·vary (ol'i-vār-ē). 1. Relating to the oliva. 2. Relating to or shaped like an olive.

ol·ive (ol'iv). 1. SYN oliva. 2. Common name for a tree of the genus *Olea* (family Oleaceae) or its fruit. [L. *oliva*]

ol·i·vif·u·gal (ol'i-vif'yū-găl). In a direction away from the olive. [oliva + L. *fugio,* to flee]

ol·i·vip·e·tal (ol'i-vip'ĕ-tăl). In a direction toward the olive. [oliva + L. *peto,* to seek]

ol·i·vo·pon·to·cer·e·bel·lar (ol'i-vō-pon'tō-sār-ĕ-bel'ar). Relating to the olivary nucleus, basis pontis, and cerebellum.

△**-ology.** SEE -logia.

△**-oma.** A tumor or neoplasm. [G. *-ōma*]

△**-omata.** Plural of -oma.

omega (ō-mā'gă). 1. Twenty-fourth and last letter of the Greek alphabet (ω). 2. Ohm.

omen·tal (ō-men'tăl). Relating to the omentum. SYN epiploic.

omen·tec·to·my (ō-men-tek'tō-mē). Resection or excision of the omentum. [omentum + G. *ektomē,* excision]

omen·ti·tis (ō-men-tī'tis). Peritonitis involving the omentum. [L. *omentum* + G. *-itis,* inflammation]

△**omento-, oment-.** The omentum. SEE ALSO epiplo-. [L. *omentum*]

omen·to·fix·a·tion (ō-men'tō-fik-sā'shŭn). SYN omentopexy.

omen·to·pexy (ō-men'tō-pek-sē). 1. Suture of the greater omentum to the abdominal wall to induce collateral portal circulation. 2. Suture of the omentum to another organ to increase arterial circulation. SEE ALSO omentoplasty. SYN omentofixation. [omento- + G. *pēxis,* fixation]

omen·to·plas·ty (ō-men'tō-plas-tē). Use of the

greater omentum to cover or fill a defect, augment arterial or portal venous circulation, absorb effusions, or increase lymphatic drainage. SEE ALSO omentopexy. [omento- + G. *plastos*, formed]

omen·tor·rha·phy (ō-men-tōr'ă-fē). Suture of an opening in the omentum. [omento- + G. *rhaphē*, suture]

omen·tum, pl. **omen·ta** (ō-men'tŭm, -tă) [NA]. A fold of peritoneum passing from the stomach to another abdominal organ. [L. the membrane that encloses the bowels]

  greater o., a peritoneal fold passing from the greater curvature of the stomach to the transverse colon, hanging like an apron in front of the intestines. SYN caul (2), cowl, velum (3).

  lesser o., a peritoneal fold passing from the margins of the porta hepatis and the bottom of the fissure of the ductus venosus to the lesser curvature of the stomach and to the the upper border of the duodenum for a distance of about 2 cm beyond the gastroduodenal pylorus.

OML orbitomeatal *line*.

om·niv·o·rous (om-niv'ŏ-rŭs). Living on food of all kinds, upon both animal and vegetable food. [L. *omnis*, all, + *voro*, to eat]

omo-. The shoulder (sometimes including the upper arm). [G. *ōmos*, shoulder]

omphal-, omphalo-. The umbilicus, the navel. [G. *omphalos*, navel (umbilicus)]

om·pha·lec·to·my (om-fă-lek'tō-mē). Excision of the umbilicus or of a neoplasm connected with it. [omphal- + G. *ektomē*, excision]

om·phal·el·co·sis (om'fal-el-kō'sis). Ulceration at the umbilicus. [omphal- + G. *helkōsis*, ulceration]

om·phal·ic (om-fal'ik). SYN umbilical. [G. *omphalos*, umbilicus]

om·pha·li·tis (om-fă-lī'tis). Inflammation of the umbilicus and surrounding parts.

omphalo-. SEE omphal-.

om·phal·o·cele (om'fal-ō-sēl, om'fă-lō-). Congenital herniation of viscera into the base of the umbilical cord, with a covering membranous sac of peritoneum-amnion. SEE ALSO umbilical *hernia*. SYN exomphalos (3), exumbilication (3). [omphalo- + G. *kēlē*, hernia]

om·pha·lo·en·ter·ic (om'fă-lō-en-tār-ik). Relating to the umbilicus and the intestine.

om·pha·lo·mes·en·ter·ic (om'fă-lō-mez-en-tār'ik). 1. Term denoting relationship of the midgut to the yolk sac. As the head and tail folds of the embryo continue to form, this relationship is diminished and is represented by a narrow yolk stalk or vitelline duct. 2. Relating to the vitelline duct.

om·pha·lo·phle·bi·tis (om'fă-lō-fle-bī'tis). Inflammation of the umbilical veins. [omphalo- + G. *phleps*, vein, + *-itis*, inflammation]

om·pha·lor·rha·gia (om'fă-lō-rā'jē-ă). Bleeding from the umbilicus. [omphalo- + G. *rhēgnymi*, to burst forth]

om·pha·lor·rhea (om'fă-lō-rē'ă). A serous discharge from the umbilicus. [omphalo- + G. *rhoia*, flow]

om·pha·lor·rhex·is (om'fă-lō-rek'sis). Rupture

of the umbilical cord during childbirth. [omphalo- + G. *rhēxis*, rupture]

om·pha·lo·site (om'fă-lō-sīt). Underdeveloped twin of allantoangiopagous twin; joined by umbilical vessels. [omphalo- + G. *sitos*, food]

om·pha·lo·spi·nous (om'fă-lō-spī'nŭs). Denoting a line connecting the umbilicus and the anterior superior spine of the ilium, on which lies McBurney's point.

om·pha·lot·o·my (om-fă-lot'ō-mē). Cutting of the umbilical cord at birth. [omphalo- + G. *tomē*, incision]

onan·ism (ō'nan-izm). **1.** Withdrawal of the penis before ejaculation, in order to prevent conception. **2.** Incorrectly, masturbation. [*Onan*, son of Judah, who practiced it. Genesis 38:9]

△**oncho-.** SEE onco-.

△**onco-, oncho-.** A tumor. [G. *onkos*, bulk, mass]

on·co·cyte (ong'kō-sīt). A large, granular, acidophilic tumor cell containing numerous mitochondria; a neoplastic oxyphil cell. [onco- + G. *kytos*, cell]

on·co·fe·tal (ong-kō-fē'tăl). Relating to tumor-associated substances present in fetal tissue, as o. antigens.

on·co·gene (ong'kō-jēn). **1.** Any of a family of genes which under normal circumstances code for proteins involved in cell growth or regulation (*e.g.*, protein kinases, GTPases, nuclear proteins, growth factors) but may foster malignant processes if mutated or activated by contact with retroviruses. Oncogenes often work in concert to produce cancer, and their action may be exacerbated by retroviruses, jumping genes, or inherited genetic mutations. SEE antioncogene. **2.** Found in certain DNA tumor viruses. It is required for viral replication. [onco- + gene]

on·co·gen·e·sis (ong-kō-jen'ĕ-sis). Origin and growth of a neoplasm. [onco- + G. *genesis*, production]

on·co·gen·ic (ong-kō-jen'ik). SYN oncogenous.

on·cog·en·ous (ong-koj'ĕ-nŭs). Causing, inducing, or being suitable for the formation and development of a neoplasm. SYN oncogenic.

on·col·o·gist (ong-kol'ō-jist). A specialist in oncology.

on·col·o·gy (ong-kol'ō-jē). The study or science dealing with the physical, chemical, and biologic properties and features of neoplasms, including causation, pathogenesis, and treatment. [onco- + G. *logos*, study]

on·col·y·sis (ong-kol'i-sis). Destruction of a neoplasm; sometimes used with reference to the reduction of any swelling or mass. [onco- + G. *lysis*, dissolution]

on·co·lyt·ic (ong-kō-lit'ik). Pertaining to, characterized by, or causing oncolysis.

on·cor·na·vi·rus·es (ong-kōr'nă-vī'rŭs-ez). SYN Oncovirinae.

on·co·sis (ong-kō'sis). The formation of one or more neoplasms or tumors. [G. *onkōsis*, swelling, fr. *onkos*, bulk, mass]

on·cot·ic (ong-kot'ik). Relating to or caused by edema or any swelling (oncosis).

on·cot·o·my (ong-kot'ō-mē). Rarely used term for incision of an abscess, cyst, or other tumor. [onco- + G. *tomē*, incision]

on

on·co·tro·pic (ong′kō-trop′ik). Manifesting a special affinity for neoplasms or neoplastic cells. [onco- + G. *tropē*, a turning]

On·co·vir·i·nae (ong-kō-vir′i-nē). A subfamily of viruses (family Retroviridae) composed of the RNA tumor viruses that contain two identical plus stranded RNA molecules. SYN oncornaviruses.

on·co·vi·rus (ong′kō-vī′rŭs). Any virus of the subfamily Oncovirinae. SEE ALSO oncogenic *virus*.

△**-one.** Suffix indicating a ketone (–CO–) group.

onei·ric (ō-nī′rik). **1.** Pertaining to dreams. **2.** Pertaining to the clinical state of oneirophrenia. [G. *oneiros*, dream]

onei·rism (ō-nī′rizm). A waking dream state. [G. *oneiros*, dream]

onei·ro·dyn·ia (ō-nī-rō-din′ē-ă). Rarely used term for an unpleasant or painful dream. [G. *oneiros*, dream, + *odynē*, pain]

onei·ro·phre·nia (ō-nī-rō-frē′nē-ă). A state in which hallucinations occur, caused by such conditions as prolonged deprivation of sleep, sensory isolation, and a variety of drugs. [G. *oneiros*, dream, + *phrēn*, mind]

onei·ros·co·py (ō-nī-ros′kŏ-pē). The diagnosis of a patient's mental state by an analysis of the person's dreams. [G. *oneiros*, dream, + *skopeō*, to examine]

△**-onium.** Suffix indicating a positively charged radical; *e.g.,* ammonium, NH_4^+.

△**onko-.** SEE onco-.

on·lay (on′lā). **1.** A metal (usually gold) cast restoration of the occlusal surface of a posterior tooth or the lingual surface of an anterior tooth, the entire surface of which is in dentin without side walls; retention in the anterior tooth is by pins and in the posterior by pins and/or boxes in retentive grooves in the buccal and lingual walls. **2.** A graft applied on the exterior of a bone.

on·o·mat·o·ma·nia (on′ō-mat-ō-mā′nē-ă). An abnormal impulse to dwell upon certain words and their supposed significance, or to frantically try to recall a particular word. [G. *onoma*, name, + *mania*, frenzy]

on·o·mat·o·pho·bia (on′ō-mat-ō-fō′bē-ă). Abnormal dread of certain words or names because of their supposed significance. [G. *onoma*, name, + *phobos*, fear]

on·to·gen·e·sis (on-tō-jen′ĕ-sis). SYN ontogeny.

on·to·ge·net·ic, on·to·gen·ic (on′tō-jĕ-net′ik, -jen′ik). Relating to ontogeny.

on·tog·e·ny (on-toj′ĕ-nē). Development of the individual, as distinguished from phylogeny, which is evolutionary development of the species. SYN ontogenesis. [G. *ōn*, being, + *genesis*, origin]

△**onych-.** SEE onycho-.

on·y·chal·gia (on-i-kal′jē-ă). Pain in the nails. [onycho- + G. *algos*, pain]

on·y·cha·tro·phia, on·ych·at·ro·phy (on′i-kă-trō′fē-ă, on-ik-at′rō-fē). Atrophy of the nails. [onycho- + G. *atrophia*, atrophy]

on·y·chaux·is (on-i-kawk′sis). Marked overgrowth of the fingernails or toenails. [onycho- + G. *auxē*, increase]

on·y·chec·to·my (on-i-kek′tō-mē). Ablation of a toenail or fingernail. [onycho- + G. *ektomē*, excision]

onych·ia (ō-nik′ē-ă). Inflammation of the matrix of the nail. SYN onychitis. [onycho- + G. *-ia*, condition]

on·y·chi·tis (on-i-kī′tis). SYN onychia.

△**onycho-, onych-.** A finger nail, a toenail. [G. *onyx*, nail]

on·y·choc·la·sis (on-i-kok′lă-sis). Breaking of the nails. [onycho- + G. *klasis*, breaking]

on·y·cho·dys·tro·phy (on′i-kō-dis′trō-fē). Dystrophic changes in the nails occurring as a congenital defect or due to any illness or injury that may cause a malformed nail. [onycho- + G. *dys-*, bad, + *trophē*, nourishment]

on·y·cho·graph (on′i-kō-graf). An instrument for recording the capillary blood pressure as shown by the circulation under the nail. [onycho- + G. *graphō*, to write]

on·y·cho·gry·po·sis (on′i-kō-gri-pō′sis). Enlargement with increased thickening and curvature of the fingernails or toenails. [onycho- + G. *grypōsis*, a curvature]

on·y·cho·het·er·o·to·pia (on′i-kō-het-er-ō-tō′pē-ă). Abnormal placement of nails.

on·y·choid (on′i-koyd). Resembling a fingernail in structure or form. [onycho- + G. *eidos*, resemblance]

on·y·chol·y·sis (on-i-kol′i-sis). Loosening of the nails, beginning at the free border, and usually incomplete. [onycho- + G. *lysis*, loosening]

on·y·cho·ma (on-i-kō′mă). A tumor arising from the nail bed. [onycho- + G. *-ōma*, tumor]

on·y·cho·ma·de·sis (on′i-kō-mă-dē′sis). Complete shedding of the nails, usually associated with systemic disease. [onycho- + G. *madēsis*, a growing bald, fr. *madaō*, to be moist, (of hair) fall off]

on·y·cho·ma·la·cia (on′i-kō-mă-lā′shē-ă). Abnormal softness of the nails. [onycho- + G. *malakia*, softness]

on·y·cho·my·co·sis (on′i-kō-mī-kō′sis). Very common fungus infections of the nails, causing thickening, roughness, and splitting, often caused by *Trichophyton rubrum* or *T. mentagrophytes*, *Candida* in the immunodeficient, and molds in the elderly. [onycho- + G. *mykēs*, fungus, + *-ōsis*, condition]

on·y·cho·path·ic (on′i-kō-path′ik). Relating to or suffering from any disease of the nails.

on·y·chop·a·thy (on-i-kop′ă-thē). Any disease of the nails. SYN onychosis. [onycho- + G. *pathos*, suffering]

on·y·choph·a·gy, on·y·cho·pha·gia (on-i-kof′ă-jē, on′i-kō-fā′jē-ă). Habitual nailbiting. [onycho- + G. *phagō*, to eat]

on·y·cho·plas·ty (on′i-kō-plas-tē). A corrective or plastic operation on the nail matrix. [onycho- + G. *plastos*, formed, shaped]

on·y·chor·rhex·is (on′i-kō-rek′sis). Abnormal brittleness of the nails with splitting of the free edge. [onycho- + G. *rhēxis*, a breaking]

on·y·cho·schiz·ia (on′i-kō-skiz′ē-ă). Splitting of the nails in layers. [onycho- + G. *schizō*, to divide, + *-ia*, condition]

on·y·cho·sis (on-i-kō′sis). SYN onychopathy.

on·y·chot·il·lo·ma·nia (on′i-kot′i-lō-mā′nē-ă).

A tendency to pick at the nails. [onycho- + G. *tillō*, to pluck, + *mania*, insanity]

on·y·chot·o·my (on-i-kot'ō-mē). Incision into a toenail or fingernail. [onycho- + G. *tomē*, cutting]

on·yx (on'iks). SYN nail. [G. nail]

oo-. Egg, ovary. SEE ALSO oophor-, ovario-, ovi-, ovo-. [G. *ōon*, egg. OO-]

oo·cyst (ō'ō-sist). The encysted form of the fertilized macrogamete, or zygote, in coccidian Sporozoea in which sporogonic multiplication occurs; results in the formation of sporozoites, infectious agents for the next stage of the sporozoan life cycle. [G. *ōon*, egg, + *kystis*, bladder]

oo·cyte (ō'ō-sīt). The immature ovum. [G. *ōon*, egg, + *kytos*, a hollow (cell)]

primary o., an o. during its growth phase and before it completes the first maturation division.

secondary o., an o. in which the first meiotic division is completed; the second meiotic division usually stops short of completion unless fertilization occurs.

oo·gen·e·sis (ō-ō-jen'ĕ-sis). Process of formation and development of the ovum. SYN ovigenesis. [G. *ōon*, egg, + *genesis*, origin]

oo·ge·net·ic (ō-ō-jĕ-net'ik). Producing ova. SYN ovigenetic, ovigenic.

oo·go·ni·um, pl. **oo·go·nia** (ō-ō-gō'nē-ŭm, -ă). **1.** Primitive germ cells; proliferate by mitotic division. **2.** In fungi, the female gametangium bearing one or more oospores. [G. *ōon*, egg, + *gonē*, generation]

oo·ki·ne·sis, oo·ki·ne·sia (ō'ō-ki-nē'sis, -zē-ă). Chromosomal movements of the egg during maturation and fertilization. [G. *ōon*, egg, + *kinēsis*, movement]

oo·ki·nete (ō'ō-ki-net', -kī'ne't). The motile zygote of the malarial organism that penetrates the mosquito stomach to form an oocyst under the outer gut lining; the contents of the oocyst subsequently divide to produce numerous sporozoites. [G. *ōon*, egg, + *kinētos*, motile]

oo·lem·ma (ō-ō-lem'ă). Plasma membrane of the oocyte. [G. *ōon*, egg, + *lemma*, sheath]

oophor-, oophoro-. The ovary. SEE ALSO oo-, ovario-. [Mod. L. *oophoron*, ovary, fr. G. *ōophoros*, egg-bearing]

ooph·o·rec·to·my (ō-of-ōr-ek'tō-mē). SYN ovariectomy. [G. *ōon*, egg, + *phoros*, bearing, + *ektomē*, excision]

ooph·or·i·tis (ō-of-ōr-ī'tis). Inflammation of an ovary. SYN ovaritis. [G. *ōon*, egg, + *phoros*, a bearing, + *-itis*, inflammation]

oophoro-. SEE oophor-.

ooph·o·ro·cys·tec·to·my (ō-of'ōr-ō-sis-tek'tō-mē). Excision of an ovarian cyst.

ooph·o·ro·cys·to·sis (ō-of'ōr-ō-sis-tō'sis). Ovarian cyst formation.

ooph·o·ro·hys·ter·ec·to·my (ō-of'ōr-ō-his-ter-ek'tō-mē). SYN ovariohysterectomy.

ooph·or·on (ō-of'ōr-on). SYN ovary. [G. *ōon*, egg, + *phoros*, bearing]

ooph·o·ro·pexy (ō-of'ōr-ō-pek-sē). Surgical fixation or suspension of an ovary. [oophoro- + G. *pēxis*, fixation]

ooph·o·ro·plas·ty (ō-of'ōr-ō-plas-tē). Plastic operation upon an ovary. [oophoro- + G. *plastos*, formed, shaped]

ooph·or·os·to·my (ō-of-ōr-os'tō-mē). SYN ovariostomy. [oophoro- + G. *stoma*, mouth]

ooph·or·ot·o·my (ō-of-ōr-ot'ō-mē). SYN ovariotomy. [oophoro- + G. *tomē*, incision]

oo·plasm (ō'ō-plazm). Protoplasmic portion of the ovum. [G. *ōon*, egg, + *plasma*, a thing formed]

oo·tid (ō'ō-tid). The nearly mature ovum after the first meiotic division has been completed and the second initiated; in most higher mammals, the second meiotic division is not completed unless fertilization occurs. [G. *ōotidion*, a diminutive egg. See -id (2)]

opac·i·fi·ca·tion (ō-pas'i-fi-kā'shŭn). **1.** The process of making opaque. **2.** The formation of opacities. [L. *opacus*, shady]

opac·i·ty (ō-pas'i-tē). **1.** A lack of transparency; an opaque or nontransparent area. **2.** On a radiograph, a more transparent area is interpreted as an o. to x-rays in the body. **3.** Mental dullness. [L. *opacitas*, shadiness]

opaque (ō-pāk'). Impervious to light; not translucent or only slightly so. Cf. radiopaque. [Fr. fr. L. *opacus*, shady]

open·ing (ō'pen-ing). SYN aperture. SEE ALSO aperture, fossa, ostium, orifice.

o. of external acoustic meatus, the orifice of the external acoustic meatus in the tympanic portion of the temporal bone.

o. of internal acoustic meatus, the inner opening of the internal acoustic meatus on the posterior surface of the petrous part of the temporal bone.

pharyngeal o. of auditory tube, an opening in the upper part of the nasopharynx about 1.2 cm behind the posterior extremity of the inferior concha on each side.

o. of pulmonary trunk, the o. of the pulmonary trunk from the right ventricle, guarded by the pulmonary valve.

saphenous o., the opening in the fascia lata inferior to the medial part of the inguinal ligament through which the saphenous vein passes to enter the femoral vein. SYN fossa ovalis (2).

tympanic o. of auditory tube, an opening in the anterior part of the tympanic cavity below the canal for the tensor tympani muscle.

op·er·a·ble (op'er-ă-bl). Denoting a patient or condition on which a surgical procedure can be performed with a reasonable expectation of cure or relief.

op·er·ant (op'er-ănt). In conditioning, any behavior or specific response chosen by the experimenter; its frequency is intended to increase or decrease by the judicious pairing with it of a reinforcer when it occurs. SYN target response.

op·er·ate (op'er-āt). **1.** To work upon the body by the hands or by means of cutting or other instruments to correct a surgical problem. **2.** To cause a movement of the bowels; said of a laxative or cathartic remedy. [L. *operor*, pp. -atus, to work, fr. *opus*, work]

op·er·a·tion (op-er-ā'shŭn). **1.** Any surgical procedure. **2.** The act, manner, or process of functioning. SEE ALSO method, procedure, technique.

Bassini's o., an o. for an inguinal hernia repair; after reduction of the hernia, the sac is twisted,

op

ligated, and cut off, then a new inguinal canal is made by uniting the edge of the internal oblique muscle to the inguinal ligament, placing on this the cord, and covering the latter by the external oblique muscle.

Baudelocque's o., an incision through the posterior cul-de-sac of the vagina for the removal of the ovum, in extrauterine pregnancy.

Blalock-Taussig o., an o. for congenital malformations of the heart, in which an abnormally small volume of blood passes through the pulmonary circuit; blood from the systemic circulation is directed to the lungs by anastomosing the right or left subclavian artery to the right or left pulmonary artery.

bloodless o., an o. performed with negligible loss of blood.

Bricker o., an o. utilizing an isolated segment of ileum to collect urine from the ureters and conduct it to the skin surface.

Caldwell-Luc o., an intraoral procedure for opening into the maxillary antrum through the supradental (canine) fossa above the maxillary premolar teeth.

Cotte's o., SYN presacral *neurectomy*.

Dandy o., SEE third *ventriculostomy*, trigeminal *rhizotomy*.

Daviel's o., extracapsular cataract extraction.

debulking o., excision of a major part of a malignant tumor which cannot be completely removed, so as to enhance the effectiveness of subsequent radio- or chemotherapy.

Dupuy-Dutemps o., a modified dacryocystorhinostomy for stenosis of the lacrimal duct.

Elliot's o., trephining of the eyeball at the corneoscleral margin to relieve tension in glaucoma.

Estlander o., use of an Estlander flap in plastic surgery of the lips.

filtering o., a surgical procedure for creation of a fistula between the anterior chamber of the eye and the subconjunctival space in treatment of glaucoma.

flap o., (1) SYN flap *amputation*. (2) DENTAL SURGERY An o. in which a portion of the mucoperiosteal tissues is surgically detached from the underlying bone or impacted tooth for better access and visibility in exploring the area covered by the tissue. SEE ALSO flap.

Fothergill's o., SYN Manchester o.

Frazier-Spiller o., SEE trigeminal *rhizotomy*.

Fredet-Ramstedt o., SYN *pyloromyotomy*.

Glenn's o., anastomosis between the superior vena cava and the right main pulmonary artery to increase pulmonary blood flow as a palliative correction for tricuspid atresia.

Graefe's o., (1) removal of cataract by a limbal incision with capsulotomy and iridectomy. (2) iridectomy for glaucoma.

Halsted's o., (1) an o. for the radical correction of inguinal hernia; (2) SYN radical *mastectomy*.

Hartmann's o., resection of the rectosigmoid colon beginning at or just above the peritoneal reflection and extending proximally, with closure of the rectal stump and end-colostomy.

Hill o., repair of hiatus hernia; narrowing the esophagogastric junction and attaching it to the right medial arcuate ligament.

Hoffa's o., in congenital dislocation of the hip, hollowing out the acetabulum and reduction of the head of the femur after severing the muscles inserted into the upper portion of the bone.

Hofmeister's o., partial gastrectomy with closure of a portion of the lesser curvature and retrocolic anastomosis of the remainder to jejunum.

Kasai o., SYN portoenterostomy.

Kelly's o., (1) correction of retroversion of the uterus by plication of uterosacral ligaments; (2) correction of urinary stress incontinence by vaginally placing sutures beneath the bladder neck.

Kondoleon o., excision of strips of subcutaneous connective tissue for the relief of elephantiasis.

Kraske's o., removal of the coccyx and excision of the left wing of the sacrum in order to afford approach for resection of the rectum for cancer or stenosis.

Lambrinudi o., a form of triple arthrodesis done in such a manner as to prevent foot-drop such as occurs in poliomyelitis.

Manchester o., a vaginal o. for prolapse of the uterus, consisting of cervical amputation and parametrial fixation (cardinal ligaments) anterior to the uterus. SYN Fothergill's o. [*Manchester,* England]

Mayo's o., an o. for the radical cure of umbilical hernia; the neck of the sac is exposed by two elliptical incisions, the gut is returned to the abdomen, the sac and adherent omentum are cut away, and the fascial edges of the opening are overlapped with mattress sutures.

McVay's o., repair of inguinal and femoral hernias by suture of the transversus abdominis muscle and its associated fasciae (transversus layer) to the pectineal ligament.

Miles' o., combined abdominoperineal resection for carcinoma of the rectum.

morcellation o., vaginal hysterectomy in which the uterus is removed in multiple pieces after being split or partitioned.

Mustard o., correction, at the atrial level, of hemodynamic abnormality due to transposition of the great arteries by an intraatrial baffle to direct pulmonary venous blood through the tricuspid orifice into the right ventricle and the systemic venous blood through the mitral valve into the left ventricle.

Naffziger o., orbital decompression for severe malignant exophthalmos by removal of the lateral and superior orbital walls.

Ogura o., orbital decompression by removal of the floor of the orbit through an opening made in the supradental (canine) fossa.

Payne o., a jejunoileal bypass for morbid obesity utilizing end-to-side anastomosis of the upper jejunum to the terminal ileum, with closure of the proximal end of the bypassed intestine.

Pomeroy's o., excision of a ligated portion of the fallopian tubes.

Potts' o., direct side-to-side anastomosis between aorta and pulmonary artery as a palliative procedure in congenital malformation of the heart.

Putti-Platt o., a procedure for recurrent dislocation of shoulder joint.

Ramstedt o., SYN pyloromyotomy.

Scott o., a jejunoileal bypass for morbid obesity utilizing end-to-end anastomosis of the upper jejunum to the terminal ileum, with the bypassed intestine closed proximally and anastomosed distally to the colon.

second-look o., exploratory celiotomy within a year after apparently curative resection of intra-abdominal cancer, in patients with no sign or symptom of recurrence, to resect an occult tumor if present.

Smith-Indian o., a surgical technique for removal of cataract within the capsule.

Soave o., endorectal pull-through for treatment of congenital megacolon.

Stookey-Scarff o., SEE third *ventriculostomy*.

subcutaneous o., an o., as for the division of a tendon, performed without incising the skin other than by a minute opening made by the entering knife.

talc o., an obsolete o. in which magnesium silicate (talc) powder is applied to the epicardium to create a sterile granulomatous pericarditis and thus promote pericardial anastomoses with the coronary circulation. SYN poudrage (2).

Wertheim's o., a radical o. for carcinoma of the uterus in which as much as possible of the vagina is excised and there is wide lymph node excision.

Whipple's o., SYN pancreatoduodenectomy.

Whitehead's o., excision of hemorrhoids by two circular incisions above and below involved veins, allowing normal mucosa to be pulled down and sutured to anal skin.

op•er•a•tive (op′er-ă-tiv). **1.** Relating to, or effected by means of an operation. **2.** Active or effective.

op•er•a•tor (op′er-ā-tor). **1.** One who performs an operation or operates equipment. **2.** GENETICS A sequence of DNA that interacts with a repressor of operon to control the expression of adjacent structural genes. SEE operator *gene*. **3.** A symbol representing a mathematical operation. [L. worker, fr. *operor*, to work]

oper•cu•lar (ō-per′kyū-lăr). Relating to an operculum.

oper•cu•li•tis (ō-perk-yū-lī′tis). Originating under an operculum. [operculum + G. -*itis*, inflammation]

oper•cu•lum, gen. **oper•cu•li,** pl. **oper•cu•la** (ō-per′kyū-lŭm, -lī, -lă). **1.** Anything resembling a lid or cover. **2** [NA]. ANATOMY The portions of the frontal, parietal, and temporal lobes bordering the lateral sulcus and covering the insula. **3.** Mucus sealing the endocervical canal of the uterus after conception has taken place. **4.** PARASITOLOGY The lid or caplike cover of the shell opening of operculated freshwater snails in the subclass Prosobranchiata, and of the eggs of certain trematode and cestode parasites. **5.** The attached flap in the tear of retinal detachment. **6.** The mucosal flap partially or completely covering an unerupted tooth. [L. cover or lid, fr. *operio*, pp. *opertus*, to cover]

ophi•a•sis (ō-fī′ă-sis). A form of alopecia areata in which the loss of hair occurs in bands along the scalp margin partially or completely encircling the head. [G., fr. *ophis*, snake]

oph•ri•tis (of-rī′tis). Dermatitis in the region of the eyebrows. [G. *ophrys*, eyebrow, + -*itis*, inflammation]

oph•ry•on (of′rē-on). The point on the midline of the forehead just above the glabella (1). [G. *ophrys*, eyebrow]

oph•ry•o•sis (of-rē-ō′sis). Spasmodic twitching of the upper portion of the orbicularis palpebrarum muscle causing a wrinkling of the eyebrow. [G. *ophrys*, eyebrow, + -*osis*, condition]

△**ophthalm-.** SEE ophthalmo-.

oph•thal•mia (of-thal′mē-ă). **1.** Severe, often purulent, conjunctivitis. **2.** Inflammation of the deeper structures of the eye. [G.]

  Egyptian o., SYN trachoma.

  gonorrheal o., acute purulent conjunctivitis due to *Neisseria gonorrhoeae*.

  granular o., SYN trachoma.

  o. neonato′rum, a conjunctival inflammation occurring within the first 10 days of life; causes include *Neisseria gonorrhoeae, Staphylococcus, Streptococcus pneumoniae,* and *Chlamydia trachomatis.* SYN infantile purulent conjunctivitis.

  purulent o., purulent conjunctivitis, usually of gonorrheal origin.

  sympathetic o., a serous or plastic uveitis caused by a perforating wound of the uvea followed by a similar severe reaction in the other eye that may lead to bilateral blindness.

oph•thal•mic (of-thal′mik). Relating to the eye. SYN ocular (1). [G. *ophthalmikos*]

△**ophthalmo-, ophthalm-.** Relationship to the eye. SEE ALSO oculo-. [G. *ophthalmos*]

oph•thal•mo•dy•na•mom•e•ter (of-thal′mō-dī-nă-mom′ĕ-ter). An instrument to measure the blood pressure in the retinal vessels. [ophthalmo- + G. *dynamis*, power, + *metron*, measure]

oph•thal•mo•dy•na•mom•e•try (of-thal′mō-dī-nă-mom′ĕ-trē). The measurement of blood pressure in the retinal vessels by means of an ophthalmodynamometer. [ophthalmo- + G. *dynamis*, power, + *metron*, measure]

oph•thal•mo•lith (of-thal′mō-lith). SYN dacryolith. [ophthalmo- + G. *lithos*, stone]

oph•thal•mol•o•gist (of-thal-mol′ō-jist). A specialist in ophthalmology. SYN oculist.

oph•thal•mol•o•gy (of-thal-mol′ō-jē). The medical specialty concerned with the eye, its diseases, and refractive errors. [ophthalmo- + G. *logos*, study]

oph•thal•mo•ma•la•cia (of-thal′mō-mă-lā′shē-ă). Abnormal softening of the eyeball. [ophthalmo- + G. *malakia*, softness]

oph•thal•mom•e•ter (of-thal-mom′ĕ-ter). SYN keratometer. [ophthalmo- + G. *metron*, measure]

oph•thal•mo•my•co•sis (of-thal′mō-mī-kō′sis). Any disease of the eye or its appendages caused by a fungus. [ophthalmo- + G. *mykēs*, fungus, + -*osis*, condition]

oph•thal•mop•a•thy (of-thal-mop′ă-thē). Any disease of the eyes. [ophthalmo- + G. *pathos*, suffering]

  external o., any disease of the conjunctiva, cornea, or adnexa of the eye.

internal o., any disease of the internal structures of the eyeball.

oph·thal·mo·ple·gia (of-thal-mō-plē′jē-ă). Paralysis of one or more of the ocular muscles. [ophthalmo- + G. *plēgē*, stroke]

    chronic progressive external o., a specific type of slowly worsening weakness of the ocular muscles, usually associated with a pigmentary retinopathy. SEE Kearns-Sayre *syndrome*, oculopharyngeal *dystrophy*.

    exophthalmic o., o. with protrusion of the eyeballs due to increased water content of orbital tissues incidental to thyroid disorders, usually hyperthyroidism.

    o. exter′na, paralysis affecting one or more of the extrinsic eye muscles. SYN external o.

    external o., SYN o. externa.

    o. inter′na, paralysis affecting only the sphincter muscle of the pupil and the ciliary muscle. SYN internal o.

    internal o., SYN o. interna.

    nuclear o., o. due to a lesion of the nuclei of origin of the motor nerves of the eye.

oph·thal·mo·ple·gic (of-thal-mō-plē′jik). Relating to or marked by ophthalmoplegia.

oph·thal·mo·scope (of-thal′mō-skōp). A device for studying the interior of the eyeball through the pupil. [ophthalmo- + G. *skopeō*, to examine]

    direct o., an instrument designed to visualize the interior of the eye, with the instrument relatively close to the subject's eye and the observer viewing an upright magnified image.

    indirect o., an instrument designed to visualize the interior of the eye, with the instrument at arm's length from the subject's eye and the observer viewing an inverted image through a convex lens located between the instrument and the subject's eye.

oph·thal·mo·scop·ic (of′thal-mō-skop′ik). Relating to examination of the interior of the eye.

oph·thal·mos·co·py (of-thal-mos′kŏ-pē). Examination of the fundus of the eye by means of the ophthalmoscope.

oph·thal·mo·vas·cu·lar (of-thal′mō-vas′kyū-lăr). Relating to the blood vessels of the eye.

-opia. Vision. [G. *ōps*, eye]

opi·ate (ō′pē-āt). Any preparation or derivative of opium.

opi·oid (ō′pē-oyd). A narcotic substance, either natural or synthetic.

opis·the·nar (ō-pis′thē-nar). Dorsum of the hand. [G. back of the hand, from *opisthen*, behind, + *thenar*, palm of the hand]

opis·thi·on (ō-pis′thē-on) [NA]. The middle point on the posterior margin of the foramen magnum, opposite the basion. [G. *opisthios*, posterior]

opistho-. Backward, behind, dorsal. [G. *opisthen*, at the rear, behind]

op·is·thot·on·ic (op-is-thot′ō-nik, ō-pis′thō-ton′ik). Relating to or characterized by opisthotonos.

op·is·thot·o·nos, op·is·thot·o·nus (op-is-thot′ō-nŭs). A tetanic spasm in which the spine and extremities are bent with convexity forward, the body resting on the head and the heels. [opistho- + G. *tonos*, tension, stretching]

op·por·tun·is·tic (op′ŏr-tū-nis′tik). **1.** Denoting an organism capable of causing disease only in a host whose resistance is lowered, *e.g.,* by other diseases or by drugs. **2.** Denoting a disease caused by such an organism.

op·sin. The protein portion of the rhodopsin molecule; at least three separate o.'s are located in cone cells.

op·sin·o·gen (op-sin′ō-jen). A substance that stimulates the formation of opsonin, such as the antigen contained in a suspension of bacteria used for immunization. SYN opsogen. [opsonin + -gen]

op·si·u·ria (op-sē-ū′rē-ă). A more rapid excretion of urine during fasting than after a full meal. [G. *opsi*, late, + *ouron*, urine]

op·so·clo·nus (op′sō-klō′nŭs). Rapid, irregular, nonrhythmic movements of the eye in horizontal and vertical directions. [G. *ōps, ōpos*, eye, + *klonos*, confused motion]

op·so·gen (op′sō-jen). SYN opsinogen.

op·so·ma·nia (op′sō-mā′nē-ă). A longing for a particular article of diet, or for highly seasoned food. [G. *opson*, seasoning, + *mania*, frenzy]

op·son·ic (op-son′ik). Relating to opsonins or to their utilization.

op·so·nin (op′sŏ-nin). A substance that binds to antigens, enhancing phagocytosis. [G. *opson*, boiled meat, provisions, fr. *hepsō*, to boil, + -in]

    normal o., that normally present in the blood without stimulation by a specific antigen; it is relatively thermolabile and reacts with various organisms.

    specific o., antibodies formed in response to stimulation by a specific antigen, either as a result of an attack of a disease, or injections with a suitably prepared suspension of the specific microorganism.

op·so·ni·za·tion (op′sŏ-nī-zā′shŭn). The process by which bacteria are altered in such a manner that they are more readily and more efficiently engulfed by phagocytes.

op·so·no·cy·to·pha·gic (op′sŏ-nō-sī′tō-fā′jik). Pertaining to the increased efficiency of phagocytic activity of the leukocytes in blood that contains specific opsonin. [opsonin + G. *kytos*, hollow (cell), + *phagō*, to eat]

op·so·nom·e·try (op-sŏ-nom′ě-trē). Determination of the opsonic index or the opsonocytophagic activity.

op·tic, op·ti·cal (op′tik, op′ti-kăl). Relating to the eye, vision, or optics. [G. *optikos*]

op·ti·cian (op-tish′an). One who practices opticianry.

op·ti·cian·ry (op-tish′an-rē). The professional practice of filling prescriptions for ophthalmic lenses, dispensing spectacles, and making and fitting contact lenses.

optico-. SEE opto-.

op·ti·co·cil·i·a·ry (op′ti-kō-sil′ē-ār-ē). Relating to the optic and ciliary nerves.

op·ti·co·pu·pil·lary (op′ti-kō-pyū′pi-lār-ē). Relating to the optic nerve and the pupil.

op·tics (op′tiks). The science concerned with the properties of light, its refraction and absorption, and the refracting media of the eye in that relation. [G. *optikos*, fr. *ōps*, eye]

opto-, optico-. Optical; optic; ocular. [G. *optikos,* optical, from *ōps,* eye]

op•tom•e•ter (op-tom′ĕ-ter). An instrument for determining the refraction of the eye. [opto- + G. *metron,* measure]

op•tom•e•trist (op-tom′ĕ-trist). One who practices optometry.

op•tom•e•try (op-tom′ĕ-trē). **1.** The profession concerned with the examination of the eyes and related structures to determine the presence of vision problems and eye disorders, and with the prescription and adaptation of lenses and other optical aids or the use of visual training for maximum visual efficiency. **2.** The use of an optometer.

op•to•my•om•e•ter (op′tō-mī-om′ĕ-ter). An instrument for determining the relative power of the extrinsic muscles of the eye. [opto- + G. *mys,* muscle, + *metron,* measure]

ora (ō′ră). Plural of L. *os,* the mouth. [L.]

ora, pl. **orae** (ō′ră, ō′rē) [NA]. An edge or a margin. [L.]

or•ad (ad-ō′răl). **1.** In a direction toward the mouth. **2.** Situated nearer the mouth in relation to a specific reference point; opposite of aborad. [L. *os,* mouth, + *ad,* to]

oral (ōr′ăl). Relating to the mouth. [L. *os (or-),* mouth]

oral•i•ty (ōr-al′i-tē). FREUDIAN PSYCHOLOGY the psychic organization derived from, and characteristic of, the oral period of psychosexual development.

or•ange wood. A soft wood used in dentistry for placement of bridges, crowns, etc. by biting pressure, also used as a burnishing point in the polishing of root surfaces.

or•bic•u•lar (or-bik′yū-lăr). Similar in form to an orb; circular in form. [L. *orbiculus,* a small disk, dim. of *orbis,* circle]

or•bic•u•la•re (ōr-bik-yū-lā′rē). SYN lenticular *process* of incus. [L., fr. *orbiculus,* a small disk]

or•bi•cu•lus cil•i•ar•is (ōr-bik′yū-lŭs sil-ē-ār′is) [NA]. The darkly pigmented posterior zone of the ciliary body continuous with the retina at the ora serrata. SYN ciliary disk, ciliary ring, pars plana. [Mod. L.]

or•bit (ōr′bit). The bony cavity containing the eyeball and its adnexa; it is formed of parts of the frontal, maxillary, sphenoid, lacrimal, zygomatic, ethmoid, and palatine bones. SYN orbita [NA], orbital cavity.

or•bi•ta, gen. **or•bi•tae** (ōr′bi-tă, -tē) [NA]. SYN orbit. [L. a wheel-track, fr. *orbis,* circle]

or•bi•tal (ōr′bi-tăl). Relating to the orbits.

or•bi•ta•le (or-bi-tā′lē). CEPHALOMETRICS The lowermost point in the lower margin of the bony orbit that may be felt under the skin. [L. of an orbit]

or•bi•tog•ra•phy (ōr-bi-tog′ră-fē). Radiographic evaluation of the orbit. [L. *orbita,* orbit, + G. *graphō,* to write]

or•bi•to•na•sal (ōr′bi-tō-nā′săl). Relating to the orbit and the nose or nasal cavity.

or•bi•to•nom•e•ter (ōr′bi-tō-nom′ĕ-ter). An instrument that measures the resistance offered to pressing the eyeball backwards into its socket. [L. *orbita,* orbit, + G. *metron,* measure]

or•bi•to•nom•e•try (ōr′bi-tō-nom′ĕ-trē). Measurement by means of the orbitonometer.

or•bi•tot•o•my (ōr-bi-tot′ō-mē). Surgical incision into the orbit. [L. *orbita,* orbit, + *tomē,* a cutting]

Or•bi•vi•rus (ōr′bi-vī-rŭs). A genus of viruses of vertebrates that multiply in insects, including Colorado tick fever virus of man. [L. *orbis,* ring, + virus]

or•ce•in (ōr′sē-in). A natural dye derived from ᴏʀcinol which is used in various histologic staining methods.

△**orchi-, orchido-, orchio-.** The testes. [G. *orchis,* testis]

or•chi•al•gia (ōr-kē-al′jē-ă). Pain in the testis. SYN testalgia. [orchi- + G. *algos,* pain]

or•chi•dec•to•my (ōr-ki-dek′tō-mē). SYN orchiectomy.

or•chid•ic (ōr-kid′ik). Relating to the testis.

△**orchido-.** SEE orchi-.

or•chi•dom•e•ter (ōr-ki-dom′ĕ-ter). **1.** A caliper device used to measure the size of testes. **2.** A set of sized models of testes for comparison of testicular development. [orchido- + G. *metron,* measure]

or•chi•ec•to•my (ōr-kē-ek′tō-mē). Removal of one or both testes. SYN orchidectomy, testectomy. [orchi- + G. *ektomē,* excision]

or•chi•ep•i•did•y•mi•tis (ōr′kē-ep′i-did′i-mī′tis). Inflammation of the testis and epididymis. [orchi- + epididymis, + G. *-itis,* inflammation]

△**orchio-.** SEE orchi-.

or•chi•o•cele (ōr′kē-ō-sēl). A testis retained in the inguinal canal. [orchio- + G. *kēlē,* hernia, tumor]

or•chi•op•a•thy (ōr-kē-op′ă-thē). Disease of a testis. [orchio- + G. *pathos,* suffering]

or•chi•o•pexy (ōr′kē-ō-pek′sē). Surgical treatment of an undescended testicle by freeing it and implanting it into the scrotum. SYN cryptorchidopexy. [orchio- + G. *pēxis,* fixation]

or•chi•o•plas•ty (ōr′kē-ō-plas-tē). Surgical reconstruction of the testis. [orchio- + G. *plastos,* formed]

or•chi•ot•o•my (ōr-kē-ot′ō-mē). Incision into a testis. [orchio- + G. *tomē,* incision]

or•chis, pl. **or•chis•es** (ōr′kis, ōr′ki-sēz). SYN testis. [G. testis, an orchid]

or•chit•ic (ōr-kit′ik). Denoting orchitis.

or•chi•tis (ōr-kī′tis). Inflammation of the testis. SYN testitis. [orchi- + G. *-itis,* inflammation]

Ord orotidine.

or•der (ōr′der). **1.** In biological classification, the division just below the class (or subclass) and above the family. **2.** In a reaction, the sum of the exponents of all the concentration terms in that reaction's rate expression. [L. *ordo,* regular arrangement]

or•der•ly (ōr′der-lē). An attendant in a hospital unit who assists in the care of patients.

or•di•nate (ōr′di-nāt). In a plane cartesian coordinate system, the vertical axis (y).

orex•i•gen•ic (ŏ-rek-si-jen′ik). Appetite-stimulating.

or•gan (ōr′găn). Any part of the body exercising a specific function, as of respiration, secretion, digestion. SYN organum [NA], organon. [L. *orga-num,* fr. G. *organon,* a tool, instrument]

accessory o.'s of the eye, the eyelids, with lashes and eyebrows, lacrimal apparatus, conjunctival sac, and extrinsic muscles of the eyeball.

circumventricular o.'s, four small areas at the base of the brain that are outside the blood-brain barrier. They are neurohypophysis, area postrema, organum vasculosum of the lamina terminalis, and subfornical organ (SFO).

Corti's o., SYN spiral o.

critical o., the o. or physiologic system that for a given source of radiation would first reach its legally defined maximum permissible radiation exposure as the dose of radiopharmaceutical is increased.

enamel o., a circumscribed mass of ectodermal cells budded off from the dental lamina; it develops ameloblast layer of cells that produce the enamel cap of a developing tooth.

end o., the special structure containing the terminal of a nerve fiber in peripheral tissue such as muscle, tissue, skin, mucous membrane, or glands.

genital o.'s, the organs of reproduction or generation, external and internal. SYN genitalia, genitals.

Golgi tendon o., a proprioceptive sensory nerve ending embedded among the fibers of a tendon, often near the musculotendinous junction; it is activated by any increase of tension in the tendon, caused either by active contraction or passive stretch of the corresponding muscle. SYN neurotendinous spindle.

sense o.'s, the organs of special sense, including the eye, ear, olfactory organ, taste organs, and the accessory structures associated with these organs.

spiral o., a prominent ridge of highly specialized epithelium in the floor of the cochlear duct overlying the basilar membrane of cochlea, containing one inner row and three outer rows of hair cells, or cells of Corti (the auditory receptor cells innervated by the cochlear nerve) supported by various columnar cells: the pillars of Corti, cells of Hensen, and cells of Claudius; the spiral o. is partly overhung by an awning-like shelf, the tectorial membrane, the free marginal zone of which is covered by a gelatinous substance in which the stereocilia of the outer hair cells are embedded. SYN Corti's o.

target o., a tissue or o. upon which a hormone exerts its action; generally, a tissue or organ with appropriate receptors for a hormone. SYN target (3).

vestibular o., collective term for the utricle, saccule, and semicircular ducts of the membranous labyrinth, each having a patch of ciliated receptor epithelium innervated by the vestibular nerve.

vestigial o., a rudimentary structure in humans corresponding to a functional structure or o. in the lower animals.

or•ga•na (ōr′gă-nă). Plural of organum.

or•gan•elle (or′gă-nel). One of the specialized parts of a protozoan or tissue cell; mitochondria,

the Golgi apparatus, nucleus and centrioles, granular and agranular endoplasmic reticulum, vacuoles, microsomes, lysosomes, plasma membrane, and certain fibrils, as well as plastids of plant cells. SYN organoid (3). [G. *organon,* organ, + Fr. *-elle,* dim. suffix, fr. L. *-ella*]

or•gan•ic (ōr-gan′ik). 1. Relating to an organ. 2. Relating to or formed by an organism. 3. Organized; structural. 4. SEE organic *compound.* [G. *organikos*]

or•ga•nism (ōr′gă-nizm). Any living individual, whether plant or animal, considered as a whole.

hypothetical mean o. (HMO), a hypothetical o. whose characters are the means of the positive characters of the organisms which belong to the same taxon as the HMO, as opposed to the calculated mean o.

pleuropneumonia-like o.'s (PPLO), the original name given to a group of bacteria which did not possess cell walls; these o.'s, isolated from man and other animals, soil, and sewage, are now assigned to the order Mycoplasmatales.

or•ga•ni•za•tion (ōr′gan-i-zā′shŭn). 1. An arrangement of distinct but mutually dependent parts. 2. The conversion of coagulated blood, exudate, or dead tissue into fibrous tissue.

Joint Commission on Accreditation of Healthcare O.'s (JCAHO), a private, nonprofit o. that awards accreditation to any health care facility that voluntarily meets its standards.

peer-review o. (PRO), an o. that contracts with the Health Care Financing Administration (which pays for health care to Medicare patients) to review the need for and quality of care given to Medicare patients, and to monitor the accuracy of assigned DRGs submitted by the health care facility as the basis for reimbursement for services provided.

preferred provider o. (PPO), a health care o. that negotiates set rates of reimbursement with participating health care providers for services to insured clients. This is a type of prospective payment system. SEE health maintenance organization.

or•ga•nize (ōr′gan-īz). To provide with, or to assume, a structure.

or•ga•niz•er (ōr′gan-ī-zer). 1. A group of cells on the dorsal lip of the blastopore, which induce differentiation of cells in the embryo and control growth and development of adjacent parts. 2. Any group of cells having such a controlling influence, the effects being brought about through the action of an evocator.

△**organo-.** Organ; organic. [G. *organon*]

or•gan•o•gel (ōr-gan′ō-jel). A hydrogel with an organic liquid instead of water as the dispersion means.

or•ga•no•gen•e•sis (ōr′gă-nō-jen′ĕ-sis). Formation of organs during development. SYN organogeny. [organo- + G. *genesis,* origin]

or•ga•no•ge•net•ic, or•ga•no•gen•ic (ōr′gă-nō-jĕ-net′ik, -jen′ik). Relating to organogenesis.

or•ga•nog•e•ny (ōr-gan-oj′ĕ-nē). SYN organogenesis.

or•gan•oid (ōr′gă-noyd). 1. Resembling in superficial appearance or in structure any of the organs or glands of the body. 2. Composed of glandular or organic elements, and not of a single tissue; pertaining to certain neoplasms that contain cytologic and histologic elements arranged in a pattern that closely resembles that of a normal organ. SEE ALSO histoid. **3.** SYN organelle. [organo- + G. *eidos,* resemblance]

or•ga•no•meg•a•ly (ōr′gă-nō-meg′ă-lē). SYN visceromegaly.

or•gan•o•mer•cur•i•al (ōr-gan′ō-mer-kyū′rē-ăl). Any organic mercurial compound; *e.g.,* merbromin, thimerosal.

or•ga•no•me•tal•lic (ōr′gă-nō-me-tal′ik). Denoting an organic compound containing one or more metallic atoms in its structure.

or•ga•non, pl. **or•ga•na** (ōr′gă-non, ōr′gă-nă). SYN organ. [G. organ]

or•ga•no•phos•phates (ōr-gă-nō-fos′fāts). Phosphorus-containing organic compounds which phosphorylate cholinesterase and thus irreversibly inhibit it. Used as insecticides; have also been used as war gases.

or•ga•no•tro•phic (ōr′gă-nō-trof′ik). **1.** Pertaining to the nourishment of an organ. **2.** Pertaining to a microorganism that uses organic sources as a reducing power. [organo- + G. *trophē,* nourishment]

or•ga•no•tro•pic (ōr′gă-nō-trop′ik). Pertaining to or characterized by organotropism.

or•ga•not•ro•pism (ōr-gă-not′rō-pizm). The special affinity of particular drugs, pathogens, or metastatic tumors for particular organs or their component parts. Cf. parasitotropism. [organo- + G. *tropē,* a turning]

or•gan-spe•cif•ic. Denoting or pertaining to a serum produced by the injection of the cells of a certain organ or tissue that, when injected into another animal, destroys the cells of the corresponding organ.

or•ga•num, pl. **or•ga•na** (ōr′gă-nŭm, ōr′gă-nă) [NA]. SYN organ, organ. [L. tool, instrument]

or•gasm (ōr′gazm). The peak state of excitement in the sexual act. SYN climax (2). [G. *orgaō,* to swell, be excited]

or•gas•mic, or•gas•tic (ōr-gaz′mik, -gas′tik). Relating to, characteristic of, or tending to produce an orgasm.

or•i•en•ta•tion (ōr-ē-en-tā′shŭn). **1.** The recognition of one's temporal, spatial, and personal relationships and environment. **2.** The relative position of an atom with respect to one to which it is connected. [Fr. *orienter,* to set toward the East, fr. L. *sol oriens,* the rising sun]

  topographical o., determination of the position of objects and settings and the route to a desired location.

  visual o., awareness of the location of objects in the environment and their relationship to one another and to the person viewing them.

or•i•fice (or′i-fis). Any aperture or opening. SYN orificium [NA]. [L. *orificium*]

  aortic o., the opening from the left ventricle into the ascending aorta; it is guarded by the aortic valve.

  cardiac o., the trumpet-shaped opening of the esophagus into the stomach.

  external urethral o., (1) the slitlike opening of the urethra in the glans penis; **(2)** the external orifice of the urethra (in the female) in the vestibule, usually upon a slight elevation, the papilla urethrae.

  ileocecal o., the opening of the terminal ileum into the large intestine at the transition between the cecum and the ascending colon.

  internal urethral o., the internal opening or orifice of the urethra, at the anterior and inferior angle of the trigone.

  mitral o., an atrioventricular opening which leads from the left atrium into the left ventricle of the heart.

  pyloric o., the opening between the stomach and the superior part of the duodenum.

  tricuspid o., an atrioventricular opening which leads from the right atrium into the right ventricle of the heart.

  ureteric o., the opening of the ureter in the bladder, situated one at each lateral angle of the trigone; wide gaping of the o. usually indicates vesicoureteral reflux.

  vaginal o., the narrowest portion of the canal, in the floor of the vestibule posterior to the urethral orifice.

or•i•fi•cial (ōr-i-fish′ăl). Relating to an orifice of any kind.

or•i•fi•ci•um, pl. **or•i•fi•cia** (ōr-i-fish′ē-ŭm, -ă) [NA]. SYN orifice, orifice. [L.]

or•i•gin (ōr′i-jin). **1.** The less movable of the two points of attachment of a muscle, that which is attached to the more fixed part of the skeleton. **2.** The starting point of a cranial or spinal nerve. The former have two o.'s: the **ental o., deep o.,** or **real o.,** the cell group in the brain or medulla whence the fibers of the nerve begin, and the **ectal o., superficial o.,** or **apparent o.,** the point where the nerve emerges from the brain. [L. *origo,* source, beginning, fr. *orior,* to rise]

Orn ornithine or its radical.

or•ni•thine (Orn) (ōr′ni-thēn, -thin). The amino acid formed when L-arginine is hydrolyzed by arginase; an important intermediate in the urea cycle; elevated levels seen in certain defects of the urea cycle.

or•ni•thi•nu•ria (ōr′ni-thi-nū′rē-ă). Excretion of excessive amounts of ornithine in the urine.

Or•ni•thod•o•ros (ōr-ni-thod′ŏ-rŭs). A genus of soft ticks, several species of which are vectors of pathogens of various relapsing fevers. [G. *ornis* (*ornith-*), bird, + *doros,* a leather bag]

or•ni•tho•sis (ōr-ni-thō′sis). SYN psittacosis. [G. *ornis* (*ornith-*), bird, + *-osis,* condition]

Oro orotic acid or orotate.

△**oro-. 1.** The mouth. [L. *os, oris,* mouth] **2.** Obsolete alternative spelling is orrho-. SEE sero-. [G. *orrhos,* whey; serum]

or•o•dig•i•to•fa•cial (ōr′ō-dij′i-tō-fā′shăl). Relating to the mouth, fingers, and face.

or•o•fa•cial (ōr-ō-fā′shăl). Relating to the mouth and face.

or•o•lin•gual (ōr-ō-ling′gwăl). Relating to the mouth and tongue.

or•o•na•sal (ōr-ō-nā′săl). Relating to the mouth and nose.

or•o•pha•ryn•ge•al (ōr-ō-fă-rin′jē-ăl). Relating to the oropharynx.

or•o•phar•ynx (ōr′ō-far′ingks). The portion of

the pharynx that lies posterior to the mouth; it is continuous above with the nasopharynx via the pharyngeal isthmus and below with the laryngopharynx. [L. *os* (*or*-), mouth]

or·o·so·mu·coid (ōr′ō-sō-myū′koyd). α_1-acid glycoprotein; increased plasma levels are associated with inflammation.

or·o·tate (Oro) (ōr′ō-tāt). A salt or ester of orotic acid.

orot·ic ac·id (Oro) (ōr-ot′ik). An important intermediate in the formation of the pyrimidine nucleotides; elevated in certain inherited defects of pyrimidine biosynthesis.

orot·i·dine (O, Ord) (ō-rot′i-dēn). Orotic acid-3-β-D-ribonucleoside; uridine-6-carboxylic acid; elevated in cases of orotidinuria.

◇**orth-.** SEE ortho-.

or·the·sis (ōr-thē′sis). SYN orthosis. [ortho- + -*esis*, process]

or·thet·ics (ōr-thet′iks). SYN orthotics.

◇**ortho-, orth-.** **1.** Straight, normal, in proper order. **2.** CHEMISTRY Italicized prefix denoting that a compound has two substitutions on adjacent carbon atoms in a benzene ring. For terms beginning *ortho-* or *o-*, see the specific name. [Gr. *orthos* correct]

or·tho·cho·rea (ōr′thō-kōr-ē′ă). A form of chorea in which the spasms occur only or chiefly when the patient is in the erect posture.

or·tho·chro·mat·ic (ōr′thō-krō-mat′ik). Denoting any tissue or cell that stains the color of the dye used, *i.e.,* the same color as the dye solution with which it is stained. [ortho- + G. *chrōma*, color]

or·tho·cy·to·sis (ōr′thō-sī-tō′sis). A condition in which all of the cellular elements in the circulating blood are mature forms, irrespective of the proportions of various types and total numbers. [ortho- + G. *kytos*, cell, + -*osis*, condition]

or·tho·de·ox·ia (ōr′thō-dē-ok′sē-ă). Fall in arterial blood oxygen upon assuming the upright posture.

or·tho·don·tics (ōr-thō-don′tiks). That branch of dentistry concerned with the correction and prevention of irregularities and malocclusion of the teeth. [ortho- + G. *odous*, tooth]

or·tho·dont·ist. A dental specialist who practices orthodontics.

or·tho·dro·mic (ōr-thō-drō′mik). Denoting the propagation of an impulse along an axon in the normal direction. Cf. antidromic. [ortho- + G. *dromos*, course]

or·thog·nath·ia (ōr-thō-nath′ē-ă). The study of the causes and treatment of conditions related to malposition of the bones of the jaws. [ortho- + G. *gnathos*, jaw]

or·thog·nath·ic, or·thog·na·thous (ōr-thō-nath′ik, ōr-thog′năthŭs). **1.** Relating to orthognathia. **2.** Having a face without projecting jaw, one with a gnathic index below 98. [ortho- + G. *gnathos*, jaw]

or·tho·grade (ōr′thō-grād). Walking or standing erect; denoting the posture of human beings; opposed to pronograde. [ortho- + L. *gradior*, pp. *gressus*, to walk]

or·tho·ker·a·tol·o·gy (ōr′thō-ker-ă-tol′ŏ-jē). A method of molding the cornea with contact lenses

to improve unaided vision. [ortho- + G. *keras*, horn (cornea), + *logos*, science]

or·tho·ker·a·to·sis (ōr′thō-ker-ă-tō′sis). Formation of an anuclear keratin layer, as in the normal epidermis. [ortho- + G. *keras*, horn, + -*osis*, condition]

or·tho·me·chan·i·cal (ōr-thō-mě-kan′i-kăl). Pertaining to braces, prostheses, orthotic devices, and appliances. [ortho- + mechanical]

or·tho·mo·lec·u·lar (ōr′thō-mō-lek′yū-lăr). A therapeutic approach designed to provide an optimum molecular environment for body functions, with particular reference to the optimum concentrations of substances normally present in the body.

Or·tho·myx·o·vir·i·dae (ōr′thō-mik-sō-vir′i-dē). The family of viruses that comprises the three groups of influenza viruses, types A, B, and C. The only recognized genus is *Influenzavirus*, which comprises the strains of virus types A and B, both of which are subject to mutation resulting in epidemics. Influenza virus type C differs from types A and B somewhat and probably belongs to a separate genus. SEE ALSO *Influenzavirus*.

or·tho·pae·dics, or·tho·pe·dics (ōr-thō-pē′diks). The medical specialty concerned with the preservation, restoration, and development of form and function of the musculoskeletal system, extremities, spine, and associated structures by medical, surgical, and physical methods. [ortho- + G. *pais* (*paid*-), child]

or·tho·pe·dics. SEE orthopaedics.

or·tho·per·cus·sion (ōr′thō-per-kŭsh′ŭn). Very light percussion of the chest, used to determine the size of the heart.

or·tho·pho·ria (ōr-thō-fōr′ē-ă). Absence of heterophoria; the condition of binocular fixation in which the lines of sight meet at a distant or near point of reference in the absence of a fusion stimulus. [ortho- + G. *phora*, motion]

or·tho·phor·ic (ōr-thō-fōr′ik). Pertaining to orthophoria.

or·tho·phos·phate (ōr-thō-fos′fāt). A salt or ester of orthophosphoric acid.

inorganic o. (P_i, P_1), any ion or salt form of phosphoric acid.

or·tho·phos·phor·ic ac·id (ōr′thō-fos-fōr′ik). Phosphoric acid, $O=P(OH)_3$, distinguished by ortho- from meta- and pyrophosphoric acids.

or·thop·nea (ōr-thop-nē′ă, ōr-thop′nē-ă). Discomfort in breathing that is brought on or aggravated by lying flat. Cf. platypnea. [ortho- + G. *pnoē*, a breathing]

or·thop·ne·ic (or′thop-ne′ik). Relating to or characterized by orthopnea.

Or·tho·pox·vi·rus (ōr-thō-poks′vī-rŭs). The genus of the family Poxviridae which comprises the viruses of alastrim, vaccinia, variola, cowpox, ectromelia, monkeypox, and rabbitpox.

or·tho·psy·chi·a·try (ōr′thō-sī-kī′ă-trē). A cross-disciplinary science combining child psychiatry, developmental psychology, pediatrics, and family care devoted to the discovery, prevention, and treatment of mental and psychological disorders in children and adolescents.

or·thop·tic (ōr-thop′tik). Relating to orthoptics.

or·thop·tics (ōr-thop′tiks). The study and treatment of defective binocular vision, of defects in the action of the ocular muscles, or of faulty visual habits. [*ortho-* straightened + G. *optikos*, sight]

or·tho·scope (ōr′thō-skōp). **1.** An instrument by means of which one is able to draw the outlines of the various normas of the skull. [ortho- + G. *skopeō*, to view]

or·tho·sis, pl. **or·tho·ses** (ōr-thō′sis, -sēz). An external orthopaedic appliance, as a brace or splint, that prevents or assists movement of the spine or the limbs. SYN orthesis. [G. *orthōsis*, a making straight]

or·tho·stat·ic (ōr-thō-stat′ik). Relating to an erect posture or position.

or·thot·ics (ōr-thot′iks). The science concerned with the making and fitting of orthopaedic appliances. SYN orthetics.

or·tho·tist (or′thō-tist). A maker and fitter of orthopaedic appliances.

or·thot·o·nos, or·thot·o·nus (ōr-thot′ŏ-nos, -ŏnŭs). A form of tetanic spasm in which the neck, limbs, and body are held fixed in a straight line. [ortho- + G. *tonos*, tension]

or·tho·top·ic (ōr-thō-top′ik). In the normal or usual position. [ortho- + G. *topos*, place]

or·tho·tro·pic (ōr-thō-trop′ik). Extending or growing in a straight, especially a vertical, direction. [ortho- + G. *tropē*, a turn]

Os osmium.

  external os of uterus, the vaginal opening of the uterus.

  os multan′gulum ma′jus, SYN trapezium.

os, gen. **os·sis,** pl. **os·sa** (os, os′is, os′ă) [NA]. SYN bone. For histological description, see bone. [L. bone]

  o. incisi′vum [NA], the anterior and inner portion of the maxilla, which in the fetus and sometimes in the adult is a separate bone; the incisive suture runs from the incisive canal between the lateral incisor and the canine tooth. SYN incisive bone, intermaxillary bone, premaxillary bone.

  o. intermetatar′seum, a supernumerary bone at the base of the first metatarsal, or between the first and second metatarsal bones, usually fused with one or the other or with the medial cuneiform bone.

  o. trigo′num [NA], an independent ossicle sometimes present in the tarsus; usually it forms part of the talus, constituting the lateral tubercle of the posterior process. SYN triangular bone.

os, gen. **o′ris,** pl. **ora.** 1 [NA]. The mouth. **2.** Term applied sometimes to an opening into a hollow organ or canal, especially one with thick or fleshy edges. [L. mouth]

  incompetent cervical o., a defect in the strength of the internal o. allowing premature dilation of the cervix.

osche-, oscheo-. The scrotum. [G. *oschē*]

os·che·al (os′kē-ăl). SYN scrotal.

os·che·i·tis (os-kē-ī′tis). Inflammation of the scrotum. [osche- + G. *-itis*, inflammation]

os·che·o·hy·dro·cele (os-kē-ō-hī′drō-sēl). Scrotal hydrocele. [oscheo- + G. *hydōr*, water, + *kēlē*, tumor]

os·che·o·plas·ty (os′kē-ō-plas-tē). SYN scrotoplasty. [oscheo- + *plastos*, formed]

os·cil·la·tion (os-i-lā′shŭn). **1.** A to-and-fro movement. **2.** A stage in inflammation in which the accumulation of leukocytes in small vessels arrests the passage of blood and there is simply a to-and-fro movement at each cardiac contraction. [L. *oscillatio*, fr. *oscillo*, to swing]

os·cil·lom·e·ter (os-i-lom′ĕ-ter). An apparatus for measuring oscillations of any kind, especially those of the bloodstream in sphygmometry. [L. *oscillo*, to swing, + G. *metron*, measure]

os·cil·lo·met·ric (os′i-lō-met′rik). Relating to the oscillometer or the records made by its use.

os·cil·lom·e·try (os-i-lom′ĕ-trē). The measurement of oscillations of any kind with an oscillometer.

os·cil·lop·sia (os-i-lop′sē-ă). The subjective sensation of oscillation of objects viewed. SYN oscillating vision. [L. *oscillo*, to swing, + G. *opsis*, vision]

os·cu·lum, pl. **os·cu·la** (os′kyū-lŭm, -lă). A pore or minute opening. [L. dim. of *os*, mouth]

△**-ose. 1.** CHEMISTRY A terminator usually indicating a carbohydrate. **2.** Suffix appended to some Latin stems, with significance of the more common -ous (2). [L. *-osus*, full of, abounding] **3.** Full of, having much of.

△**-oses.** Plural of -osis.

OSHA Occupational Safety and Health Administration of the U.S. Department of Labor, responsible for establishing and enforcing safety and health standards in the workplace.

△**-osis,** pl. **-oses.** A process, condition, or state, usually abnormal or diseased colon; production of an abnormal substance, increase of a normal substance, or parasitic infestation. [G.]

os·mic ac·id (oz′mik). A volatile caustic and strong oxidizing agent; colorless crystals, poorly soluble in water, but soluble in organic solvents; the aqueous solution is a fat and myelin stain and a general fixative for electron microscopy.

os·mics (oz′miks). The science of olfaction. [G. *osmē*, smell]

os·mi·dro·sis (oz-mi-drō′sis). SYN bromidrosis. [G. *osmē*, smell, + *hidrōs*, sweat]

os·mi·um (Os) (oz′mē-ŭm). A metallic element of the platinum group, atomic no. 76, atomic wt. 190.2. [G. *osmē*, smell, because of the strong odor of the tetroxide]

△**osmo-. 1.** Osmosis. [G. *ōsmos*, impulsion] **2.** Smell, odor. [G. *osmē*]

os·mo·lal·i·ty (os-mō-lal′i-tē). The concentration of a solution expressed in osmoles of solute particles per kilogram of solvent.

os·mo·lar (os-mō′lăr). SYN osmotic.

os·mo·lar·i·ty (os-mō-lār′i-tē). The osmotic concentration of a solution expressed as osmoles of solute per liter of solution.

os·mole (os′mōl). The molecular weight of a solute, in grams, divided by the number of ions or particles into which it dissociates in solution.

osmometry (ŏz-mŏm′ĕ-trē). Technique used to determine the number of solute particles in solution by measuring changes in colligative property. [osmo- + -metry]

os·mo·re·cep·tor (os′mō-rē-sep′ter, -tōr). **1.** A receptor in the central nervous system (probably the hypothalamus) that responds to changes in the osmotic pressure of the blood. [G. *osmos,* impulsion] **2.** A receptor that receives olfactory stimuli. [G. *osmē,* smell]

os•mo•reg•u•la•to•ry (os-mō-reg′yū-lă-tōr-ē). Influencing the degree and rapidity of osmosis.

os•mose (os′mōs). To move through a membrane by osmosis.

os•mo•sis (os-mō′sis). The process by which solvent tends to move through a semipermeable membrane from a solution of lower to a solution of higher osmolal concentration of the solutes to which the membrane is relatively impermeable. [G. *ōsmos,* a thrusting, an impulsion]

    reverse o., movement of solvent in the opposite direction from o.

os•mot•ic (os-mot′ik). Relating to osmosis. SYN osmolar.

△**osphresio-.** Odor; sense of smell. [G. *osphrēsis,* smell]

os•phre•sis (os-frē′sis). SYN olfaction. [G. *osphrēsis,* smell]

os•phret•ic (os-fret′ik). SYN olfactory.

os•sa (os′ă). Plural of L. *os,* bone. [L.]

os•se•in, os•se•ine (os′ē-in). SYN collagen. [L. *os,* bone]

△**osseo-.** Bony. SEE ALSO ossi-, osteo-. [L. *osseus*]

os•se•o•car•ti•lag•i•nous (os′ē-ō-kar-ti-laj′i-nŭs). Relating to, or composed of, both bone and cartilage. SYN osteocartilaginous.

os•se•o•mu•cin (os′ē-ō-myū′sin). The ground substance of bony tissue.

os•se•ous (os′ē-ŭs). Bony, of bone-like consistency or structure. SYN osteal. [L. *osseus*]

△**ossi-.** Bone. SEE ALSO osseo-, osteo-. [L. *os*]

os•si•cle (os′i-kl). A small bone; specifically, one of the bones of the tympanic cavity or middle ear. SYN ossiculum [NA], bonelet. [L. *ossiculum,* dim. of *os,* bone]

🔲**auditory o.'s,** the small bones of the middle ear; they are articulated to form a chain for the transmission of sound from the tympanic membrane to the oval window. SYN ear bones, ossicula auditus.

os•sic•u•la (ŏ-sik′yū-lă). Plural of ossiculum. [L.]

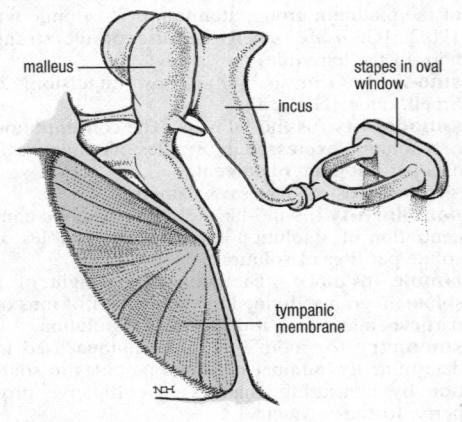

malleus

stapes in oval window

incus

tympanic membrane

auditory ossicles

ossicula auditus, SYN auditory *ossicles,* under *ossicle.*

os•sic•u•lar (ŏ-sik′yū-lăr). Pertaining to an ossicle.

os•sic•u•lec•to•my (os′i-kyū-lek′tō-mē). Removal of one or more of the ossicles of the middle ear. [L. *ossiculum,* ossicle, + G. *ektomē,* excision]

os•sic•u•lot•o•my (os′i-kyū-lot′ō-mē). Division of one of the processes of the ossicles of the middle ear, or of a fibrous band causing ankylosis between any two ossicles. [L. *ossiculum,* ossicle, + G. *tomē,* incision]

os•sic•u•lum, pl. **os•sic•u•la** (ŏ-sik′yū-lŭm, -lă) [NA]. SYN ossicle. [L. dim. of *os,* bone]

os•sif•er•ous (ŏ-sif′er-ŭs). Containing or producing bone. [ossi- + L. *fero,* to bear]

os•sif•ic (o-sif′ik). Relating to a change into, or formation of, bone.

os•si•fi•ca•tion (os′i-fi-kā′shŭn). **1.** The formation of bone. **2.** A change into bone. [L. *ossificatio,* fr. *os,* bone, + *facio,* to make]

    endochondral o., formation of osseous tissue by the replacement of calcified cartilage; long bones grow in length by endochondral o. at the epiphysial cartilage plate where osteoblasts form bone trabeculae on a framework of calcified cartilage.

    membranous o., intramembranous o., development of osseous tissue within mesenchymal tissue without prior cartilage formation, such as occurs in the frontal and parietal bones.

    metaplastic o., the formation of irregular foci of bone (sometimes including bone marrow) in various soft structures, such as the muscles, lungs, brain, and other sites where osseous tissue is abnormal.

os•si•fy (os′i-fī). To form bone or convert into bone. [ossi- + L. *facio,* to make]

△**ost-.** SEE osteo-.

os•te•al (os′tē-ăl). SYN osseous. [G. *osteon,* bone]

os•te•al•gia (os-tē-al′jē-ă). Pain in a bone. SYN osteodynia. [osteo- + G. *algos,* pain]

os•te•al•gic (os-tē-al′jik). Relating to or marked by bone pain.

os•tec•to•my (os-tek′tō-mē). **1.** Surgical removal of bone. **2.** DENTISTRY Resection of supporting osseous structure to eliminate periodontal pockets. [osteo- + G. *ektomē,* excision]

os•te•in, os•te•ine (os′tē-in). SYN collagen. [G. *osteon,* bone]

os•te•it•ic (os-tē-it′ik). Relating to or affected by osteitis. SYN ostitic.

os•te•i•tis (os-tē-ī′tis). Inflammation of bone. SYN ostitis. [osteo- + G. *-itis,* inflammation]

    caseous o., tuberculous caries in bone.

    central o., (1) SYN osteomyelitis. **(2)** SYN endosteitis.

    o. defor′mans, SYN Paget's *disease* (1).

    o. fibro′sa cys′tica, increased osteoclastic resorption of calcified bone with replacement by fibrous tissue, due to primary hyperparathyroidism or other causes of the rapid mobilization of mineral salts. SYN Recklinghausen's disease of bone.

    o. pubis (ŏs-tē-ī′tĭs pyū′bĭs), painful inflammation of the pubic bones near the midline, sometimes due to repeated overload of the adductor muscles or repetitive stress activities.

sclerosing o., fusiform thickening or increased density of bones, of unknown cause.

os·tem·py·e·sis (os'tem-pī-ē'sis). Suppuration in bone. [osteo- + G. *empyēsis,* suppuration]

osteo-, ost-, oste-. Bone. SEE ALSO osseo-, ossi-. [G. *osteon*]

os·te·o·an·a·gen·e·sis (os'tē-ō-an-ă-jen'ě-sis). Regeneration of bone. [osteo- + G. *ana,* again, + *genesis,* generation]

os·te·o·ar·thri·tis (os'tē-ō-ar-thrī'tis). Arthritis characterized by erosion of articular cartilage, which becomes soft, frayed, and thinned with eburnation of subchondral bone and outgrowths of marginal osteophytes; pain and loss of function result; mainly affects weight-bearing joints, is more common in overweight and older persons. SYN degenerative joint disease, hypertrophic arthritis, osteoarthrosis.

os·te·o·ar·throp·a·thy (os'tē-ō-ar-throp'ă-thē). A disorder affecting bones and joints. [osteo- + G. *arthron,* joint, + *pathos,* suffering]

hypertrophic pulmonary o., expansion of the distal ends, or the entire shafts, of the long bones, sometimes with erosions of the articular cartilages and thickening and villous proliferation of the synovial membranes, and frequently clubbing of fingers; the disorder occurs in chronic pulmonary disease, in heart disease, and occasionally in other acute and chronic disorders. SYN Bamberger-Marie disease.

os·te·o·ar·thro·sis (os'tē-ō-ar-thrō'sis). SYN osteoarthritis. [osteo- + G. *arthron,* joint, + -*osis,* condition]

os·te·o·blast (os'tē-ō-blast). A bone-forming cell that is derived from mesenchyme (fibroblast) and forms an osseous matrix in which it becomes enclosed as an osteocyte. [osteo- + G. *blastos,* germ]

os·te·o·blas·tic (os'tē-ō-blas'tik). Relating to the osteoblasts; describes any region of increased radiographic bone density, in particular, metastases that stimulate o. activity.

os·te·o·blas·to·ma (os'tē-ō-blas-tō'mă). An uncommon benign tumor of osteoblasts with areas of osteoid and calcified tissue, occurring most frequently in the spine of a young person.

os·te·o·car·ti·lag·i·nous (os'tē-ō-kar-ti-laj'i-nŭs). SYN osseocartilaginous.

os·te·o·chon·dri·tis (os'tē-ō-kon-drī'tis). Inflammation of a bone and its cartilage. [osteo- + G. *chondros,* cartilage, + -*itis,* inflammation]

o. dis'secans, complete or incomplete separation of a portion of joint cartilage and underlying bone, usually involving the knee, associated with epiphyseal aseptic necrosis.

os·te·o·chon·dro·dys·tro·phy (os'tē-ō-kon'drō-dis'trō-fē). SYN chondro-osteodystrophy.

os·te·o·chon·dro·ma (os'tē-ō-kon-drō'mă). A

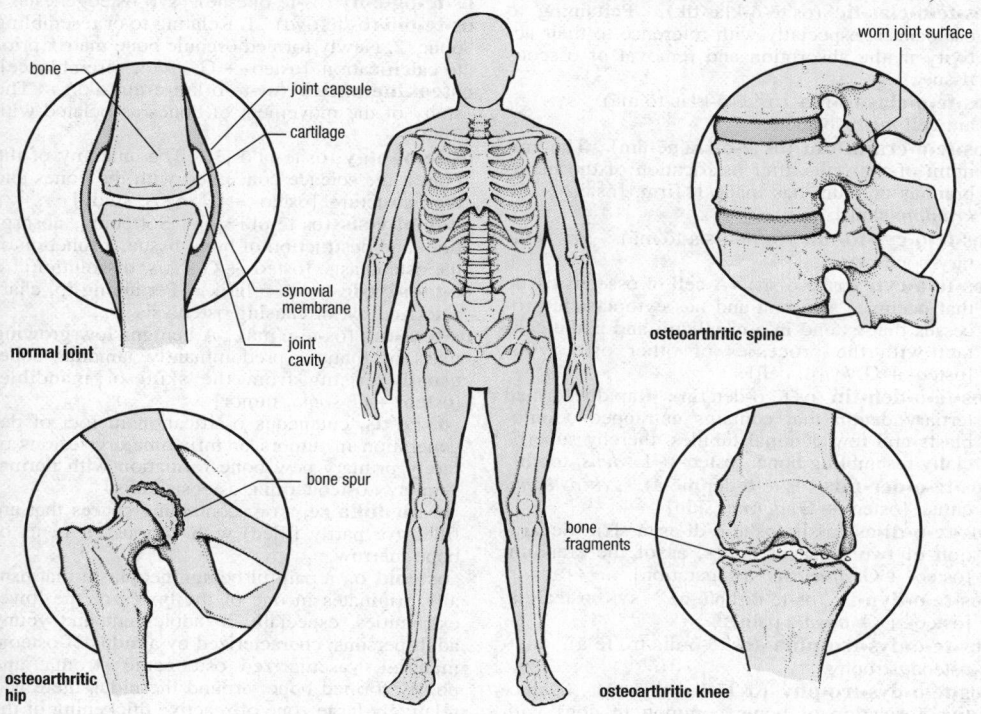

bone — joint capsule — cartilage — synovial membrane — joint cavity — **normal joint** — worn joint surface — **osteoarthritic spine** — bone spur — **osteoarthritic hip** — bone fragments — **osteoarthritic knee**

osteoarthritis: problems associated with osteoarthritis and some sites where they commonly occur; a healthy joint is shown in top left corner

benign cartilaginous neoplasm that consists of a pedicle of normal bone covered with a rim of proliferating cartilage cells; multiple o.'s are inherited and referred to as hereditary multiple exostoses. [osteo- + G. *chondros,* cartilage, + *-oma,* tumor]

os•te•o•chon•dro•sar•co•ma (os′tē-ō-kon′drō-sar-kō′mă). Chondrosarcoma arising in bone. Sarcomas in bone containing foci of neoplastic cartilage as well as bone are classified as osteogenic sarcomas. [osteo- + G. *chondros,* cartilage, + *sarx,* flesh, + *-oma,* tumor]

os•te•o•chon•dro•sis (os′tē-ō-kon-drō′sis). Any of a group of disorders of one or more ossification centers in children, characterized by degeneration or aseptic necrosis followed by reossification; includes the various forms of epiphysial aseptic necrosis. [osteo- + G. *chondros,* cartilage, + *-osis,* condition]

os•te•oc•la•sis, os•te•o•cla•sia (os′tē-ok′lă-sis, os′tē-ō-klā′zē-ă). Intentional fracture of a bone in order to correct deformity. [osteo- + G. *klasis,* fracture]

os•te•o•clast (os′tē-ō-klast). **1.** A large multinucleated cell, possibly of monocytic origin, with abundant acidophilic cytoplasm, functioning in the absorption and removal of osseous tissue. SYN osteophage. **2.** An instrument used to fracture a bone to correct a deformity. [osteo- + G. *klastos,* broken]

os•te•o•clas•tic (os′tē-ō-klas′tik). Pertaining to osteoclasts, especially with reference to their activity in the absorption and removal of osseous tissue.

os•te•o•clas•to•ma (os′tē-ō-klas-tō′mă). SYN giant cell *tumor* of bone.

os•te•o•cra•ni•um (os′tē-ō-krā′nē-ŭm). The cranium of the fetus after ossification of the membranous cranium has made it firm. [osteo- + G. *kranion,* skull]

os•te•o•cys•to•ma (os′tē-ō-sis-tō′mă). SYN solitary bone *cyst.*

os•te•o•cyte (os′tē-ō-sīt). A cell of osseous tissue that occupies a lacuna and has cytoplasmic processes that extend into canaliculi and make contact with the processes of other osteocytes. [osteo- + G. *kytos,* cell]

os•te•o•den•tin (os′tē-ō-den′tin). Rapidly formed tertiary dentin that contains entrapped odontoblasts and few dentinal tubules, thereby superficially resembling bone. [osteo- + L. *dens,* tooth]

os•te•o•der•mia (os′tē-ō-der′mē-ă). SYN *osteoma cutis.* [osteo- + G. *derma,* skin]

os•te•o•di•as•ta•sis (os′tē-ō-dī-as′tă-sis). Separation of two adjacent bones, as of the cranium. [osteo- + G. *diastasis,* a separation]

os•te•o•dyn•ia (os-tē-ō-din′ē-ă). SYN ostealgia. [osteo- + G. *odynē,* pain]

os•te•o•dys•tro•phia (os′tē-ō-dis-trō′fē-ă). SYN osteodystrophy.

os•te•o•dys•tro•phy (os′tē-ō-dis′trō-fē). Defective formation of bone; common in dogs with chronic nephritis. SYN osteodystrophia. [osteo- + G. *dys,* difficult, imperfect, + *trophē,* nourishment]

renal o., generalized bone changes resembling

osteomalacia and rickets or osteitis fibrosa, occurring in chronic renal failure.

os•te•o•ec•ta•sia (os′tē-ō-ek-tā′zē-ă). Bowing of bones, particularly of the legs. [osteo- + G. *ektasis,* a stretching]

os•te•o•fi•bro•ma (os′tē-ō-fī-brō′mă). A benign lesion of bone, probably not a true neoplasm, consisting of connective tissue in which there are small foci of osteogenesis.

os•te•o•fi•bro•sis (os′tē-ō-fī-brō′sis). Fibrosis of bone, mainly involving red bone marrow.

os•te•o•gen (os′tē-ō-jen). A bone matrix-producing tissue or layer. [osteo- + G. *-gen,* producing]

os•te•o•gen•e•sis (os′tē-ō-jen′ĕ-sis). The formation of bone. SYN osteogeny, osteosis (2). [osteo- + G. *genesis,* production]

   o. imperfec′ta, abnormal fragility and plasticity of bone, with recurring fractures on trivial trauma; variable associated features include deformity of long bones, blueness of sclerae [MIM 166200], laxity of ligaments, and otosclerosis. In **o. imperfecta congenita**, a more severe form [MIM 166230], the fractures occur before or at birth; in **o. imperfecta tarda**, a less severe form, the fractures occur later in childhood. SYN brittle bones.

os•te•o•gen•ic, os•te•o•ge•net•ic (os′tē-ō-jen′ik, -jĕ-net′ik). Relating to osteogenesis. SYN osteogenous.

os•te•og•e•nous (os-tē-oj′ĕ-nŭs). SYN osteogenic.

os•te•og•e•ny (os-tē-oj′ĕ-nē). SYN osteogenesis.

os•te•oid (os′tē-oyd). **1.** Relating to or resembling bone. **2.** Newly formed organic bone matrix prior to calcification. [osteo- + G. *eidos,* resemblance]

osteokinematics (os-te-o-kin-e-mat-iks). The study of the movement of bones associated with joints.

os•te•ol•o•gy (os′tē-ol′ŏ-jē). The anatomy of the bones; the science concerned with the bones and their structure. [osteo- + G. *logos,* study]

os•te•ol•y•sis (os-tē-ol′i-sis). Softening, absorption, and destruction of bony tissue, a function of the osteoclasts. [osteo- + G. *lysis,* dissolution]

os•te•o•lyt•ic (os-tē-ō-lit′ik). Pertaining to, characterized by, or causing osteolysis.

os•te•o•ma (os-tē-ō′mă). A benign slow-growing mass of mature, predominantly lamellar bone, usually arising from the skull or mandible. [osteo- + G. *-oma,* tumor]

   o. cu′tis, cutaneous ossification in foci of degeneration in tumors or inflammatory lesions or rarely primary new bone formation with normal skin. SYN osteodermia, osteosis cutis.

   o. medulla′re, an o. containing spaces that are filled (or partly filled) with various elements of bone marrow.

   osteoid o., a painful benign neoplasm that usually originates in one of the bones of the lower extremities, especially in adolescent and young adult persons; characterized by a nidus of osteoid material, vascularized osteogenic stroma, and poorly formed bone; around the nidus there is a relatively large zone of reactive thickening of the cortex.

   o. spongio′sum, an o. that consists chiefly of cancellous bone tissue.

os•te•o•ma•la•cia (os′tē-ō-mă-lā′shē-ă). A

disease characterized by a gradual softening and bending of the bones with varying severity of pain; softening occurs because the bones contain osteoid tissue which has failed to calcify due to lack of vitamin D or renal tubular dysfunction. SYN adult rickets, late rickets. [osteo- + G. *malakia*, softness]

infantile o., juvenile o., SYN rickets.

os·te·o·ma·lac·ic (os′tē-ō-mă-lā′sik). Relating to, or suffering from, osteomalacia.

os·te·o·ma·toid (os-tē-ō′mă-toyd). An abnormal nodule or small mass of overgrowth of bone; lesions are not neoplasms but anomalous outpouchings of the cortex, and are more properly termed exostoses. [osteoma + G. *eidos*, appearance, form]

os·te·o·mere (os′tē-ō-mēr). One of the series of bone segments, such as the vertebrae. [osteo- + G. *meros*, a part]

os·te·o·my·e·li·tis (os′tē-ō-mī-ĕ-lī′tis). Inflammation of the bone marrow and adjacent bone. SYN central osteitis (1). [osteo- + G. *myelos*, marrow, + -*itis*, inflammation]

os·te·o·my·e·lo·dys·pla·sia (os′tē-ō-mī′ĕ-lō-displā′-zē-ă). A disease characterized by enlargement of the marrow cavities of the bones, thinning of the osseous tissue, leukopenia, and irregular fever. [osteo- + G. *myelos*, marrow, + dysplasia]

os·te·on, os·te·one (os′tē-on, -ōn). A central canal containing blood capillaries and the concentric osseous lamellae around it occurring in compact bone. SYN haversian system. [G. *osteon*, bone]

os·te·o·ne·cro·sis (os′tē-ō-ne-krō′sis). The death of bone in mass, as distinguished from caries ("molecular death") or relatively small foci of necrosis in bone. [osteo- + G. *nekrōsis*, death]

os·te·o·path (os′tē-ō-path). SYN osteopathic *physician*.

os·te·o·path·ia (os′tē-ō-path′ē-ă). SYN osteopathy (1).

os·te·o·path·ic (os-tē-ō-path′ik). Relating to osteopathy.

os·te·op·a·thy (os-tē-op′ă-thē). 1. Any disease of bone. SYN osteopathia. 2. A school of medicine based upon a concept of the normal body as a vital machine capable, when in correct adjustment, of making its own remedies against infections and other toxic conditions; practitioners use the diagnostic and therapeutic measures of conventional medicine in addition to manipulative measures. SYN osteopathic medicine. [osteo- + G. *pathos*, suffering]

os·te·o·pe·nia (os′tē-ō-pē′nē-ă). 1. Decreased calcification or density of bone; a descriptive term applicable to all skeletal systems in which such a condition is noted; carries no implication about causality. 2. Reduced bone mass due to inadequate osteoid synthesis. [osteo- + G. *penia*, poverty]

os·te·o·per·i·os·ti·tis (os′tē-ō-per′ē-os-tī′tis). Inflammation of the periosteum and of the underlying bone.

os·te·o·pe·tro·sis (os′tē-ō-pe-trō′sis) [MIM* 166600]. Excessive formation of dense trabecular bone and calcified cartilage, especially in long bones, leading to obliteration of marrow spaces and to anemia, with myeloid metaplasia and hepatosplenomegaly, beginning in infancy and with progressive deafness and blindness. [osteo- + G. *petra*, stone, + -*osis*, condition]

os·te·o·phage (os′tē-ō-fāj). SYN osteoclast (1). [osteo- + G. *phagō*, to eat]

os·te·o·phle·bi·tis (os′tē-ō-fle-bī′tis). Inflammation of the veins of a bone. [osteo- + G. *phleps*, vein, + -*itis*, inflammation]

os·te·o·phy·ma (os-tē-ō-fī′mă). SYN osteophyte. [osteo- + G. *phyma*, tumor]

os·te·o·phyte (os′tē-ō-fīt). A bony outgrowth or protuberance. SYN osteophyma. [osteo- + G. *phyton*, plant]

os·te·o·plas·ty (os′tē-ō-plas-tē). 1. Bone grafting; reparative or plastic surgery of the bones. 2. DENTISTRY Resection of osseous structure to achieve acceptable gingival contour. [osteo- + G. *plastos*, formed]

os·te·o·poi·ki·lo·sis (os′tē-ō-poy-ki-lō′sis). Mottled or spotted bones caused by widespread foci of compact bone in the substantia spongiosa. [osteo- + G. *poikilos*, dappled, + -*osis*, condition]

os·te·o·po·ro·sis (os′tē-ō-pō-rō′sis). Reduction in the quantity of bone or atrophy of skeletal tissue; occurs in postmenopausal women and elderly men, resulting in bone trabeculae that are scanty, thin, and without osteoclastic resorption. [osteo- + G. *poros*, pore, + -*osis*, condition]

os·te·o·po·rot·ic (os′tē-ō-pŏ-rot′ik). Pertaining to, characterized by, or causing a porous condition of the bones.

os·te·o·ra·di·o·ne·cro·sis (os′tē-ō-rā′dē-ō-ne-krō′sis). Necrosis of bone produced by ionizing radiation; may be planned or unplanned. [osteo- + radionecrosis]

os·te·or·rha·phy (os-tē-ōr′ă-fē). Wiring together the fragments of a broken bone. SYN osteosuture. [osteo- + G. *rhaphē*, suture]

os·te·o·sar·co·ma (os′tē-ō-sar-kō′mă). SYN osteogenic *sarcoma*.

os·te·o·scle·ro·sis (os′tē-ō-skle-rō′sis). Abnormal hardening or eburnation of bone. [osteo- + G. *sklērōsis*, hardness]

os·te·o·scle·rot·ic (os′tē-ō-skle-rot′ik). Relating to, due to, or marked by hardening of bone substance.

os·te·o·sis (os-tē-ō′sis). 1. A morbid process in bone. 2. SYN osteogenesis. [osteo- + G. -*osis*, condition]

o. cu′tis, SYN osteoma cutis.

os·te·o·su·ture (os-tē-ō-sū′chūr). SYN osteorrhaphy.

os·te·o·syn·the·sis (os-tē-ō-sin′thē-sis). Internal fixation of a fracture by means of a mechanical device, such as a pin, screw, or plate.

os·te·o·throm·bo·sis (os′tē-ō-throm-bō′sis). Thrombosis in one or more of the veins of a bone.

os·te·o·tome (os′tē-ō-tōm). An instrument for use in cutting bone. [osteo- + G. *tomē*, incision]

os·te·ot·o·my (os-tē-ot′ō-mē). Cutting a bone, usually by means of a saw or chisel. [osteo- + G. *tomē*, incision]

os·te·o·tribe (os′tē-ō-trīb). An instrument for

OS

crushing off bits of necrosed or carious bone. [osteo- + G. *tribō*, to bruise, to grind down]

os•te•o•trite (os′tē-ō-trīt). An instrument with conical or olive-shaped tip having a cutting surface, resembling a dental bur, used for the removal of carious bone. [osteo- + L. *tritus*, a grinding, a wearing off]

os•tia (os′tē-ă). Plural of ostium. [L.]

os•ti•al (os′tē-ăl). Relating to any orifice, or ostium.

os•ti•tic (os-tī′tik). SYN osteitic.

os•ti•tis (os-tī′tis). SYN osteitis.

os•ti•um, pl. **os•tia** (os′tē-ŭm, -ă) [NA]. A small opening, especially one of entrance into a hollow organ or canal. [L. door, entrance, mouth]

   abdominal o. of uterine tube, the fimbriated or ovarian extremity of an oviduct.

   uterine o. of uterine tubes, the uterine opening of the oviduct.

os•to•mate (os′tō-māt). Term for one who has an ostomy. [L. *ostium,* mouth]

os•to•my (os′tō-mē). **1.** An artificial stoma or opening into the urinary or gastrointestinal canal, or the trachea. **2.** Any operation by which a permanent opening is created between two hollow organs or between a hollow viscus and the skin externally, as in tracheostomy. [L. *ostium,* mouth]

△**ot-.** The ear. SEE ALSO auri-. [G. *ous*]

otal•gia (ō-tal′jē-ă). SYN earache. [ot- + G. *algos,* pain]

otal•gic (ō-tal′jik). **1.** Relating to otalgia, or earache. **2.** A remedy for earache.

oth•er-di•rect•ed (odh′er-di-rek′ted). Pertaining to a person readily influenced by the attitudes of others.

otic (ō′tik). Relating to the ear. [G. *otikos,* fr. *ous,* ear]

otit•ic (ō-tit′ik). Relating to otitis.

oti•tis (ō-tī′tis). Inflammation of the ear. [ot- + G. *-itis,* inflammation]

   adhesive o., inflammation of the middle ear caused by prolonged auditory tube dysfunction resulting in permanent retraction of the eardrum and obliteration of the middle ear space.

   o. externa, SYN swimmer's *ear.*

   o. inter′na, SYN labyrinthitis.

▮**o. me′dia,** inflammation of the middle ear, or tympanum.

   reflux o. me′dia, o. media caused by passage of nasopharyngeal secretions through the auditory tube.

   secretory o. me′dia, SYN serous o.

   serous o., inflammation of middle ear mucosa, often accompanied by accumulation of fluid, secondary to auditory tube obstruction. SYN secretory o. media.

△**oto-.** The ear. SEE ALSO auri-. [G. *ous*]

oto•ceph•a•ly (ō-tō-sef′ă-lē). Malformation characterized by markedly defective development of the lower jaw (micrognathia or agnathia) and the union or close approach of the ears (synotia) on the front of the neck. [oto- + G. *kephalē,* head]

oto•co•nia, sing. **oto•co•ni•um** (ō-to-kō′nē-ă, -ŭm). SYN statoliths.

oto•cra•ni•al (ō-tō-krā′nē-ăl). Relating to the otocranium.

oto•cra•ni•um (ō′tō-krā′nē-um). The bony case

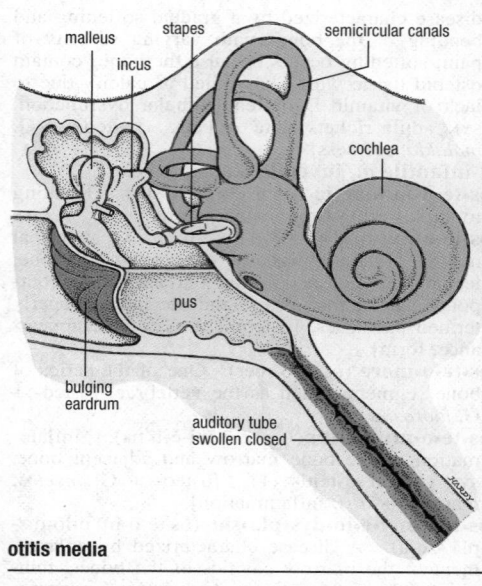

otitis media

of the internal and middle ear, consisting of the petrous portion of the temporal bone. [oto- + G. *kranion,* cranium]

oto•cyst (ō′tō-sist). **1.** Embryonic auditory vesicle. **2.** A balancing organ, analogous to the utricle of mammals, possessed by certain invertebrates and containing grains of calcareous material or of sand. [oto- + G. *kystis,* a bladder]

oto•dyn•ia (ō-tō-din′ē-ă). SYN earache. [oto- + G. *odynē,* pain]

oto•en•ceph•a•li•tis (ō′tō-en-sef-ă-lī′tis). Inflammation of the brain by extension of the process from the middle ear and mastoid cells. [oto- + G. *enkephalos,* brain, + *-itis,* inflammation]

oto•gen•ic, otog•e•nous (ō′tō-jen′ik, ō-toj′ĕ-nŭs). Of otic origin; originating within the ear, especially from inflammation of the ear. [oto- + G. *-gen,* producing]

oto•lar•yn•gol•o•gist (ō′tō-lar-ing-gol′ŏ-jist). A physician who specializes in otolaryngology.

oto•lar•yn•gol•o•gy (ō′tō-lar-ing-gol′ŏ-jē). The combined specialties of diseases of the ear and larynx, often including upper respiratory tract and many diseases of the head and neck, tracheobronchial tree, and esophagus. [oto- + G. *larynx,* + *logos,* study]

oto•log•ic (ō′tō-loj′ik). Relating to otology.

otol•o•gist (ō-tol′ŏ-jist). A specialist in otology.

otol•o•gy (ō-tol′ŏ-jē). The branch of medical science concerned with the study, diagnosis, and treatment of diseases of the ear and related structures. [oto- + G. *logos,* study]

oto•mu•cor•my•co•sis (ō-tō-myū′kōr-mī-kō′sis). Mucormycosis of the ear.

△**-otomy.** SEE -tomy.

oto•my•co•sis (ō′tō-mī-kō′sis). An infection due to a fungus in the external auditory canal, usually unilateral, with scaling, itching, and pain as the primary symptoms.

otop·a·thy (ō-top′ă-thē). Any disease of the ear. [oto- + G. *pathos,* suffering]

oto·pha·ryn·ge·al (ō′tō-fa-rin′jē-ăl). Relating to the middle ear and the pharynx.

oto·plas·ty (ō′tō-plas-tē). Reparative or plastic surgery of the auricle of the ear. [oto- + G. *plastos,* formed]

oto·rhi·no·lar·yn·gol·o·gy (ō′tō-rī′nō-lar-ing-gol′ō-jē). The combined specialties of diseases of the ear, nose, and larynx; including diseases of related structures of the head and neck. SEE ALSO otolaryngology. [oto- + G. *rhis,* nose, + *larynx,* larynx, + *logos,* study]

otor·rhea (ō-tō-rē′ă). A discharge from the ear. [oto- + G. *rhoia,* flow]

oto·scle·ro·sis (ō′tō-sklē-rō′sis). A new formation of spongy bone about the stapes and fenestra vestibuli (ovalis), resulting in progressively increasing deafness, without signs of disease in the auditory tube or tympanic membrane. [oto- + G. *sklērōsis,* hardening]

oto·scope (ō′tō-skōp). An instrument for examining the drum membrane or auscultating the ear. [oto- + G. *skopeō,* to view]

otos·co·py (ō-tos′kŏ-pē). Inspection of the ear, especially of the drum membrane. [oto- + G. *skopeō,* to view]

   pneumatic o., inspection of the ear with a device capable of varying air pressure against the eardrum. Imparting movement to the tympanic membrane suggests normal middle ear compliance; the lack of movement indicates either increased impedance or eardrum perforation.

otos·te·al (ō-tos′tē-ăl). Relating to the ossicles of the ear. [oto- + G. *osteon,* bone]

oto·tox·ic (ō′tō-tok′sik). Having a toxic action upon the ear. [oto- + G. *toxikon,* poison]

oto·tox·ic·i·ty (ō-tō-tok-sis′i-te). The property of being ototoxic.

ounce (owns). A weight containing 480 gr., or $\frac{1}{12}$ pound troy and apothecaries' weight, or $437\frac{1}{2}$ gr., $\frac{1}{16}$ pound avoirdupois. The apothecary oz. (used in the USP) contains 8 dr. and is equivalent to 31.10349 g; the avoirdupois oz. is equivalent to 28.35 g. [L. *uncia,* the twelfth part (of a pound or foot) hence also inch]

-ous. 1. Chemical suffix attached to the name of an element in one of its lower valencies. Cf. -ic (1). **2.** Having much of. [L. *-osus,* full of, abounding]

out·pa·tient (owt′pā′shent). A patient treated in a hospital dispensary or clinic instead of in a room or ward.

out·put (owt′put). The quantity produced, ejected, or excreted of a specific entity in a specified period of time or per unit time, *e.g.,* urinary sodium o.; the opposite of intake or input.

ova (ō′vă). Plural of ovum. [L.]

ov·al·bu·min (ō-văl-byū′min). The chief protein occurring in the white of egg and resembling serum albumin; also found in phosphorylated form. SYN albumen, egg albumin.

oval·o·cyte (ō′văl-ō-sīt). SYN elliptocyte. [L. *ovalis,* oval, + G. *kytos,* cell]

oval·o·cy·to·sis (ō′vă-lō-sī-tō′sis). SYN elliptocytosis.

ovar·i·al·gia (ō-var-ē-al′jē-ă). Pain in an ovary. [ovario- + G. *algos,* pain]

ovar·i·an (ō-var′ē-an). Relating to the ovary.

ovar·i·ec·to·my (ō-var-ē-ek′tō-mē). Excision of one or both ovaries. SYN oophorectomy. [ovario- + G. *ektomē,* excision]

△**ovario-, ovari-.** Ovary. SEE ALSO oo-, oophor-. [L. *ovarium*]

ovar·i·o·cele (ō-var′ē-ō-sēl). Hernia of an ovary. [ovario- + G. *kēlē,* hernia]

ovar·i·o·cen·te·sis (ō-var′ē-ō-sen-tē′sis). Puncture of an ovary or an ovarian cyst. [ovario- + G. *kentēsis,* puncture]

ovar·i·o·cy·e·sis (ō-var′ē-ō-sī-ē′sis). SYN ovarian *pregnancy.* [ovario- + G. *kyēsis,* pregnancy]

ovar·i·o·hys·ter·ec·to·my (ō-var′ē-ō-his-ter-ek′tō-mē). Removal of ovaries and uterus. SYN oophorohysterectomy. [ovario- + G. *hystera,* uterus, + *ektomē,* excision]

ovar·i·or·rhex·is (ō-var′ē-ō-rek′sis). Rupture of an ovary. [ovario- + G. *rhēxis,* rupture]

ovar·i·o·sal·pin·gec·to·my (ō-var′ē-ō-sal-pin-jek′tō-mē). Operative removal of an ovary and the corresponding oviduct. [ovario- + salpingectomy]

ovar·i·o·sal·pin·gi·tis (ō-var′ē-ō-sal-pin-jī′tis). Inflammation of ovary and oviduct. [ovario- + salpingitis]

ovar·i·os·to·my (ō-var-ē-os′tō-mē). Establishment of a temporary fistula for drainage of a cyst of the ovary. SYN oophorostomy. [ovario- + G. *stoma,* mouth]

ovar·i·ot·o·my (ō-var-ē-ot′ō-mē). An incision into an ovary, *e.g.,* a biopsy or a wedge excision. SYN oophorotomy. [ovario- + G. *tomē,* incision]

ova·ri·tis (ō-vă-rī′tis). SYN oophoritis.

ovar·i·um, pl. **ova·ria** (ō-vār′ē-ŭm, -ă) [NA]. SYN ovary. [Mod. L. fr. *ovum,* egg]

ova·ry (ō′vă-rē). One of the paired female reproductive glands containing the ova or germ cells; the o. stroma is a vascular connective tissue containing numbers of ovarian follicles enclosing the ova; surrounding this stroma is a more condensed layer called the tunica albuginea. SYN ovarium [NA], oophoron. [Mod. L. *ovarium,* fr. *ovum,* egg]

   polycystic o., enlarged cystic o.'s, pearl white in color, with thickened tunica albuginea, characteristic of the Stein-Leventhal syndrome; clinical features are abnormal menses, obesity, and evidence of masculinization, such as hirsutism.

over·bite (ō′ver-bīt). SYN vertical *overlap.*

over·com·pen·sa·tion (ō′ver-kom-pen-sā′shŭn). **1.** An exaggeration of personal capacity by which one overcomes a real or imagined inferiority. **2.** The process in which a psychologic deficiency inspires exaggerated correction. SEE compensation.

over·cor·rec·tion (ō′ver-kŏ-rek′shŭn). In behavior modification treatment programs, especially those involving mentally retarded individuals, overlearning the desired target behavior beyond the set criterion to assure that the behavior will continue to meet the established criterion when the post-learning decrements and forgetting occur.

OV

over·den·ture (ō-ver-den'chŭr). SYN overlay *denture*.

over·de·ter·mi·na·tion (o'ver-dē-ter'min-ā'shŭn). PSYCHOANALYSIS Ascribing the cause of a single behavioral or emotional reaction, mental symptom, or dream to the operation of two or more forces (*e.g.*, ascribing an emotional outburst not only to the immediate precipitant but also to a lingering inferiority complex).

over·dom·i·nance (ō-ver-dom'i-năns). That state in which the heterozygote has greater phenotype value and perhaps is more fit than the homozygous state for either of the alleles that it comprises. Cf. balanced *polymorphism*.

over·dom·i·nant (ō-ver-dom'i-nănt). Denoting heterozygous states that exhibit overdominance.

over·drive (ō-ver-drīv). An electrophysiologic pacing technique to exceed the rate of an abnormal pacemaker and so capture the territory controlled by that pacemaker (usually atrial).

over·jet, over·jut (ō'ver-jet, ō'ver-jŭt). SYN horizontal *overlap*.

over·lap (ō'ver-lap). **1.** Suturing of one layer of tissue above or under another to gain strength. **2.** An extension or projection of one tissue over another.

    horizontal o., the projection of the upper anterior and/or posterior teeth beyond their antagonists in a horizontal direction. SYN overjet, overjut.

    vertical o., (1) the extension of the upper teeth over the lower teeth in a vertical direction when the opposing posterior teeth are in contact in centric occlusion; **(2)** the distance that teeth lap over their antagonists vertically; **(3)** the relationship of the maxillary incisors to the mandibular incisors when the incisal edges pass each other in centric occlusion. SYN overbite.

over·rid·ing (ō'ver-rī'ding). **1.** Slippage of the lower fragment of a broken long bone upward and alongside the proximal portion. **2.** Denoting a fetal head which is palpable above the symphysis because of cephalopelvic disproportion.

over·shoot (ō'ver-shūt). **1.** Any response to a step change in some factor, that is greater than the steady-state response to the new level of that factor; common in systems in which inertia or a time lag in negative feedback outweighs any damping that may be present. **2.** Momentary reversal of the membrane potential of a cell (inside becoming positive rather than negative relative to the outside) during an action potential.

over·win·ter·ing (ō'ver-win'ter-ing). Persistence of an infectious agent in its vector for extended periods, such as the cooler winter months, during which the vector has no opportunity to be reinfected or to infect another host.

△**ovi-.** Egg. SEE ALSO oo-, ovo-. [L. *ovum*]

ovi·ci·dal (ō-vi-sī'dăl). Causing death of the ovum. [ovi- + L. *caedo,* to kill]

ovi·du·cal (ō-vi-dū'kăl). SYN oviductal.

ovi·duct (ō'vi-dŭkt). SYN uterine *tube*. [ovi- + L. *ductus,* a leading, fr. *duco,* pp. *ductus,* to lead]

ovi·duc·tal (ō-vi-dŭk'tăl). Relating to a uterine tube. SYN oviducal.

ovif·er·ous (ō-vif'er-ŭs). Carrying, containing, or producing ova. [ovi- + L. *fero,* to carry]

ovi·form (ō'vi-fōrm). SYN ovoid (2).

ovi·gen·e·sis (ō-vi-jen'ĕ-sis). SYN oogenesis.

ovi·ge·net·ic, ovi·gen·ic (ō-vi-jĕ-net'ik, -jen'ik). SYN oogenetic.

△**ovo-.** Egg. SEE ALSO oo-, ovi-. [L. *ovum*]

ovoid (ō'voyd). **1.** An oval or egg-shaped form. **2.** Resembling an egg. SYN oviform. [ovo- + G. *eidos,* resemblance]

ovo·plasm (ō'vō-plazm). Protoplasm of an unfertilized egg.

ovo·sis·ton (ō-vō-sis'ton). An oral contraceptive that consists of a mixture of a progestin and an estrogen.

ovo·tes·tis (ō'vō-tes'tis). Gonad in which both testicular and ovarian components are present; a form of hermaphroditism.

o·vu·lar (ov'yū-lăr, ō'vyū-). Relating to an ovule.

o·vu·la·tion (ov'yū-lā'shŭn, ō'vyū-). Release of an ovum from the ovarian follicle.

o·vu·la·to·ry (ov'yū-lă-tō-rē, ō'vyū-). Relating to ovulation.

o·vule (ov'yūl, ō'vyū-). **1.** The ovum of a mammal, especially while still in the ovarian follicle. **2.** A small beadlike structure bearing a fancied resemblance to an o. SYN ovulum. [Mod. L. *ovulum,* dim. of L. *ovum,* egg]

o·vu·lo·cy·clic (ov'yū-lō-sī'klik, ō'vyū-). Denoting any recurrent phenomenon associated with and occurring at a certain time within the ovulatory cycle, as, for example, ovulocyclic porphyria.

o·vu·lum, pl. **ovu·la** (ov'yū-lŭm, ō'vyū-; -lă). SYN ovule.

ovum, gen. **ovi**, pl. **ova** (ō'vŭm, -vī, -vă). The female sex cell. When fertilized by a spermatozoon, an o. is capable of developing into a new individual of the same species; during maturation, the o., like the spermatozoon, undergoes a halving of its chromosomal complement so that, at its union with the male gamete, the species number of chromosomes (46 in humans) is maintained. [L. egg]

    Peters' o., an o. with a presumptive fertilization age of about 13 days; for many years, it was one of very few young human embryos recovered in good condition and its study furnished many facts regarding early embryonic changes.

△**oxa-.** Combining form inserted in names of organic compounds to signify the presence or addition of oxygen atom(s) in a chain or ring (as in ethers), not appended to either (as in ketones and aldehydes). SEE ALSO hydroxy-, oxo-, oxy-. [English *oxygen*]

ox·a·late (ok'să-lāt). A salt of oxalic acid.

ox·a·le·mia (ok-să-lē'mē-ă). The presence of an abnormally large amount of oxalate in the blood. [oxalate + G. *haima,* blood]

ox·al·ic ac·id (ok-sal'ik). An acid found in many plants and vegetables; used as a hemostatic in veterinary medicine, but toxic when ingested by man; also used in the removal of ink and other stains, and as a general reducing agent; salts of o. a. are found in renal calculi; accumulates in cases of primary hyperoxaluria.

ox·a·lo·a·ce·tic ac·id (ok'să-lō-ă-sē'tik). A ketodicarboxylic acid and important intermediate in the tricarboxylic acid cycle.

ox·a·lo·suc·cin·ic ac·id (ok'să-lō-sŭk-sin'ik). An enzyme-bound intermediate of the tricarboxylic acid cycle.

ox·a·lu·ria (ok-să-lū'rē-ă). SYN hyperoxaluria. [oxalate + G. *ouron,* urine]

ox·a·lyl·u·rea (ok'să-lil-yū-rē'ă). The cyclic (end-to-end) amide anhydride of oxaluric acid; an oxidation product of uric acid.

ox·i·dant (ok'si-dant). The substance that is reduced and that, therefore, oxidizes the other component of an oxidation-reduction system.

ox·i·dase (ok'si-dās). One of a group of enzymes that bring about organic reactions in which O_2 acts as an acceptor (of H or of electrons).

ox·i·da·tion (ok-si-dā'shŭn). **1.** Combination with oxygen; increasing the valence of an atom or ion by the loss from it of hydrogen or of one or more electrons. **2.** BACTERIOLOGY The aerobic dissimilation of substrates with the production of energy and water; the transfer of electrons is accomplished via the respiratory chain, which utilizes oxygen as the final electron acceptor.

ox·i·da·tion-re·duc·tion. Any chemical oxidation or reduction reaction, which must, *in toto,* comprise both oxidation and reduction; the basis for calling all oxidative enzymes (formerly oxidases) oxidoreductases. Often shortened to "redox."

ox·i·da·tive (ok-si-dā'tiv). Having the power to oxidize; denoting a process involving oxidation.

ox·ide (ok'sīd). A compound of oxygen with another element or a radical.

ox·i·dize (ok'si-dīz). To combine or cause an element or radical to combine with oxygen or to lose electrons.

ox·i·do·re·duc·tase (ok'si-dō-rē-dŭk'tās). An enzyme (EC class 1) catalyzing an oxidation-reduction reaction. Trivial names for o.'s include dehydrogenase, reductase, oxidase, oxygenase, peroxidase, and hydroxylase. SEE ALSO oxidase.

ox·ime (ok'sēm). A compound resulting from the action of hydroxylamine, NH_2OH, on a ketone or an aldehyde to yield the group =N–OH attached to the former carbonyl carbon atom.

ox·im·e·ter (ok-sim'ě-ter). An instrument for determining photoelectrically the oxygen saturation of a sample of blood.

   pulse o., a spectrophotometric device that noninvasively estimates saturation of arterial oxyhemoglobin (SaO₂) by use of selected wavelengths of light.

ox·im·e·try (ok-sim'ě-trē). Measurement with an oximeter of the oxygen saturation of hemoglobin in a sample of blood.

oxo-. Prefix denoting addition of oxygen; used in place of keto- in systematic nomenclature. SEE ALSO hydroxy-, oxa-, oxy-.

3-ox·o·ac·yl-ACP re·duc·tase (ok'sō-as'il). An enzyme of the fatty acid synthase complex.

3-ox·o·ac·yl-ACP syn·thase. An enzyme participating in fatty acid synthesis.

17-ox·o·ste·roids (ok-sō-stēr'oydz). SYN 17-ketosteroids.

oxy-. 1. Shrill; sharp, pointed; quick (incorrectly used for ocy-, from G. *ōkys,* swift). **2.** CHEMISTRY Combining form denoting the presence of oxy-

gen, either added or substituted, in a substance. SEE ALSO hydroxy-, oxa-, oxo-. [G. *oxys,* keen]

ox·y·ce·phal·ic, ox·y·ceph·a·lous (ok-sē-se-fal'ik, -sef'ă-lŭs). Relating to or characterized by oxycephaly. SYN acrocephalic, acrocephalous.

ox·y·ceph·a·ly (ok-sē-sef'ă-lē). A type of craniosynostosis in which there is premature closure of the lambdoid and coronal sutures, resulting in an abnormally high, peaked, or conically shaped skull. SYN acrocephalia, acrocephaly. [G. *oxys,* pointed, + *kephalē,* head]

ox·y·chro·mat·ic (ok'sē-krō-mat'ik). SYN acidophilic. [G. *oxys,* sour, acid, + *chrōma,* color]

11-ox·y·cor·ti·coids (ok-sē-kōr'ti-koydz). Corticosteroids bearing an alcohol or ketonic group on carbon-11; *e.g.,* cortisone, cortisol.

ox·y·es·the·sia (ok'sē-es-thē'zē-ă). SYN hyperesthesia. [G. *oxys,* acute, + *aisthēsis,* sensation]

ox·y·gen (O) (ok'sē-jen). **1.** A gaseous element, atomic no. 8, atomic wt. 15.9994 on basis of ^{12}C = 12.0000; an abundant and widely distributed chemical element, which combines with most of the other elements to form oxides and is essential to animal and plant life. **2.** The molecular form of o., O_2. **3.** A medicinal gas that contains not less than 99.0%, by volume, of O_2. [G. *oxys,* sharp, acid and *genes,* forming]

   hyperbaric o., high pressure o., o. at a pressure greater than 1 atmosphere.

ox·y·gen·ase (ok-sē-jĕ-nās). One of a group of enzymes (EC subclass 1.13) catalyzing direct incorporation of O_2 into substrates. Cf. dioxygenase, monooxygenases.

ox·y·gen·ate (ok'sē-jĕ-nāt). To accomplish oxygenation.

ox·y·gen·a·tion (ok'sē-jĕ-nā'shŭn). Addition of oxygen to any chemical or physical system.

   extracorporeal-membrane o. (ECMO), a system to augment alveolar ventilation by gaseous diffusion across membranes outside the patient's body.

ox·y·geu·sia (ok-sē-gū'sē-ă). SYN hypergeusia. [G. *oxys,* acute, + *geusis,* taste]

ox·y·heme (ok'sē-hēm). SYN hematin.

ox·y·he·mo·chro·mo·gen (ok'sē-hēm'ō-krō'mō-jen). SYN hematin.

ox·y·he·mo·glo·bin (ok'sē-hē-mō-glō'bin). Hemoglobin in combination with oxygen, the form of hemoglobin present in arterial blood, scarlet or bright red when dissolved in water.

ox·y·my·o·glo·bin (MbO₂) (ok'sē-mī-ō-glō'bin). Myoglobin in its oxygenated form, analogous in structure to oxyhemoglobin. SEE ALSO myoglobin.

ox·yn·tic (ok-sin'tik). Acid-forming, *e.g.,* the parietal cells of the gastric glands. [G. *oxynō,* to sharpen, make sour, acid]

ox·y·phil, ox·y·phile (ok'sē-fil, -fīl). **1.** Oxyphil *cell.* **2.** SYN eosinophilic *leukocyte.* **3.** SYN oxyphilic. [G. *oxys,* sour, acid, + *philos,* fond]

ox·y·phil·ic (ok-sē-fil'ik). Having an affinity for acid dyes; denoting certain cell or tissue elements. SYN oxyphil (3), oxyphile.

ox·y·pho·nia (ok-sē-fō'nē-ă). Shrillness or high pitch of the voice. [G. *oxys,* sharp, + *phōnē,* voice]

ox·y·ta·lan (ok-sit'ă-lan). A type of connective tissue fiber histochemically distinct from colla-

OX

gen or elastic fibers described in the periodontal ligament and gingivae. [G. *oxys,* acid, + *talas,* suffering, resisting; coined term probably intended to mean "resistant to acid hydrolysis"]

ox•y•to•cia (ok-sē-tō′sē-ă). Rapid parturition. [G. *okytokos,* swift birth]

ox•y•to•cic (ok-sē-tō′sik). **1.** Hastening childbirth. **2.** SYN parturifacient (2).

ox•y•to•cin (ok-sē-tō′sin). A nonapeptide neurohypophysial hormone that causes myometrial contractions at term and promotes milk release during lactation; used for the induction or stimulation of labor, in the management of postpartum hemorrhage and atony, and to relieve painful breast engorgement. [G. *okytokos,* swift birth]

ox•y•u•ri•a•sis (ok-sē-yū-rī′ă-sis). Infection with nematode parasites of the genus *Oxyuris.*

ox•y•u•ri•cide (ok′sē-yū′ri-sīd). An agent that destroys pinworms. [oxyurid + L. *caedo,* to kill]

ox•y•u•rid (ok-sē-yū′rid). Common name for members of the family Oxyuridae. [see *Oxyuris*]

Ox•y•u•ri•dae (ok-sē-yū′ri-dē). A family of parasitic nematodes found in the large intestine or cecum of vertebrates and the intestine of invertebrates, especially insects and millipedes.

Ox•y•u•ris (ok′sē-yū′ris). A genus of nematodes commonly called seatworms or pinworms (although the pinworm of humans is the closely related form, *Enterobius vermicularis*). [G. *oxys,* sharp, + *oura,* tail]

△**-oyl.** Suffix denoting an acyl radical; -yl replaces -ic in acid names.

oze•na (ō-zē′nă). A disease characterized by intranasal crusting, atrophy, and fetid odor. [G. *ozaina,* a fetid polypus, fr. *ozō,* to smell]

ozone (ō′zōn). O_3; a powerful oxidizing agent; air containing a perceptible amount of O_3 formed by an electric discharge or by the slow combustion of phosphorus; also formed by the action of solar UV radiation on atmospheric O_2. [G. *ozō,* to smell]

P

π, Π. pi. SEE pi.

φ, Φ. phi. SEE phi.

Ψ. psi. SEE psi.

P_CO2, pCO2 partial pressure (tension) of carbon dioxide. SEE partial *pressure*.

P_i inorganic *orthophosphate*.

P_1 parental *generation*.

P_B barometric *pressure*.

P In nucleic acid terminology, symbol for phosphoric residue.

p 1. pupil; optic *papilla*. **2.** In polynucleotide symbolism, phosphoric ester or phosphate. **3.** pico- (2); momentum (in italics). **4.** CYTOGENETICS The short arm of a chromosome. [fr. Fr. *petit*, small]

Pa (periapical film) pascal; protactinium.

PABA. *p*-aminobenzoic acid.

pac·chi·o·ni·an (pak-ē-ō′nē-an). Attributed to or described by Antonio Pacchioni (1665–1726).

pace·fol·low·er (pās′fawl-ō-er). Any cell in excitable tissue that responds to stimuli from a pacemaker.

pace·mak·er (pās′mā-ker). **1.** Biologically, any rhythmic center that establishes a pace of activity. **2.** An artificial regulator of rate activity. **3.** CHEMISTRY The substance whose rate of reaction sets the pace for a series of chain reactions. [L. *passus*, step, pace]

artificial p., any device that substitutes for the normal p. and controls the rhythm of the organ; especially an electronic cardiac p., which may be implanted in the chest, with electrodes attached to the external cardiac surface, or passed through the venous circulation into the right side of the heart (pervenous p.).

demand p., a form of artificial p. usually implanted into cardiac tissue because its output of electrical stimuli can be inhibited by endogenous cardiac electrical activity.

fixed-rate p., an artificial p. that emits electrical stimuli at a constant frequency.

runaway p., rapid heart rates over 140/min caused by electronic circuit instability in an implanted pulse generator.

subsidiary atrial p., secondary source for rhythmic control of the heart, available for controlling cardiac activity if the sinoatrial pacemaker fails; located within the crista terminalis and atrial free wall near the inferior vena cava.

wandering p., a disturbance of the normal cardiac rhythm in which the site of the controlling p. shifts from beat to beat, usually between the sinus and A-V nodes, often with gradual sequential changes in P waves between upright and inverted in a given ECG lead.

pachy-. Thick. [G. *pachys*, thick]

pach·y·bleph·a·ron (pak′ē-blef′ă-ron). Thickening of the tarsal border of the eyelid. [pachy- + G. *blepharon*, eyelid]

pach·y·ce·phal·ic, pach·y·ceph·a·lous (pak′ē-se-fal′ik, -sef′ă-lŭs). Relating to or marked by pachycephaly.

pach·y·ceph·a·ly (pak-i-sef′ă-lē). Abnormal thickness of the skull. [pachy- + G. *kephalē*, head]

pach·y·chei·lia, pach·y·chi·lia (pak-i-kī′lē-ă). Swelling or abnormal thickness of the lips. [pachy- + G. *cheilos*, lip]

pach·y·chro·mat·ic (pak′ē-krō-mat′ik). Having a coarse chromatin reticulum.

pach·y·dac·ty·ly (pak-i-dak′ti-lē). Enlargement of the fingers or toes, especially extremities; often seen in neurofibromatosis. [pachy- + G. *daktylos*, finger or toe]

pach·y·der·ma (pak-i-der′mă). Abnormally thick skin. SEE ALSO elephantiasis. [pachy- + G. *derma*, skin]

p. laryn′gis, a circumscribed connective tissue hyperplasia at the posterior commissure of the larynx.

pach·y·der·mat·o·cele (pak′ē-der-mat′ō-sēl). SYN *cutis* laxa. [pachy- + G. *derma*, skin, + *kēlē*, tumor]

pach·y·glos·sia (pak-i-glos′ē-ă). An enlarged thick tongue. [pachy- + G. *glōssa*, tongue]

pach·y·gy·ria (pak-i-jī′rē-ă). Condition in which the convolutions of the cerebral cortex are abnormally large; there are fewer sulci than normal and in some cases the amount of brain substance is somewhat increased. [pachy- + G. *gyros*, circle]

pach·y·lep·to·men·in·gi·tis (pak′i-lep′tō-men-in-jī′tis). Inflammation of all the membranes of the brain or spinal cord. [G. *pachys*, thick, + *leptos*, thin, + *mēninx* (*mēning-*), membrane, + *-itis*, inflammation]

pach·y·men·in·gi·tis (pak′i-men′in-jī′tis). Inflammation of the dura mater. SYN perimeningitis. [pachy- + G. *mēninx*, membrane, + *-itis*, inflammation]

pach·y·me·nin·gop·a·thy (pak′ē-mě-ning-gop′ă-thē). Disease of the dura mater. [pachy- + G. *mēninx* (*mēning-*), membrane, + *pathos*, disease]

pach·y·me·ninx (pak′i-mē′ningks). The dura mater. [pachy- + G. *mēninx*, membrane]

pa·chyn·sis (pă-kin′sis). Any pathologic thickening. [G. a thickening]

pa·chyn·tic (pă-kin′tic). Relating to pachynsis.

pach·y·o·nych·ia (pak′ē-ō-nik′ē-ă). Abnormal thickness of the fingernails or toenails. [pachy- + G. *onyx*, nail]

pach·y·per·i·os·ti·tis (pak′i-per′ē-ōs-tī′tis). Proliferative thickening of the periosteum caused by inflammation. [pachy- + periostitis]

pach·y·per·i·to·ni·tis (pak′i-per′i-tō-nī′tis). Inflammation of the peritoneum with thickening of the membrane. [pachy- + peritonitis]

pach·y·pleu·ri·tis (pak′ē-plū-rī′tis). Inflammation of the pleura with thickening of the membrane. [pachy- + pleura + G. *-itis*, inflammation]

pach·y·sal·pin·gi·tis (pak′ē-sal-pin-jī′tis). SYN chronic interstitial *salpingitis*.

pach·y·sal·pin·go·o·va·ri·tis (pak-i-sal′pin-gō-ō-va-rī′tis). Chronic parenchymatous inflammation of the ovary and ovarian (fallopian) tube. [pachy- + salpinx + Mod. L. *ovarium*, ovary, + G. *-itis*, inflammation]

pach·y·so·mia (pak-i-sō′mē-ă). Pathologic thickening of the soft parts of the body, notably in acromegaly. [pachy- + G. *sōma*, body]

pach·y·tene (pak′i-tēn). The stage of prophase in meiosis in which pairing of homologous chromosomes is complete; longitudinal cleavage occurs in each chromosome to form two sister chromatids so that each homologous chromosome pair becomes a set of four intertwined chromatids. [pachy- + G. *tainia,* band, tape]

pach·y·vag·i·nal·i·tis (pak′i-vaj′i-năl-ī′tis). Chronic inflammation with thickening of the tunica vaginalis testis. [pachy- + Mod. L. (tunica) *vaginalis,* + G. *-itis,* inflammation]

pach·y·vag·i·ni·tis (pak′i-vaj′i-nī′tis). Chronic vaginitis with thickening and induration of the vaginal walls. [pachy- + vagina + G. *-itis,* inflammation]

pa·ci·ni·an (pa-sin′ē-an, pa-chin′). Attributed to or described by Filippo Pacini (1812–1883).

pack (pak). **1.** To fill, stuff, or tampon. **2.** To enwrap or envelop the body in a sheet, blanket, or other covering. **3.** To apply a dressing or covering to a surgical site. **4.** The items used above. [M.E. *pak,* fr. Germanic]

pack·er (pak′er). **1.** An instrument for tamponing. **2.** SYN plugger.

pack·ing (pak′ing). **1.** Filling a natural cavity, a wound, or a mold with some material. **2.** The material so used. **3.** The application of a pack.

PACS *p*icture *a*rchive and *c*ommunication *s*ystem, a computer network for digitized radiologic images and reports.

pad. **1.** Soft material forming a cushion, used in applying or relieving pressure on a part, or in filling a depression so that dressings can fit snugly. **2.** A more or less encapsulated body of fat or some other tissue serving to fill a space or act as a cushion in the body.

  abdominal p., SYN laparotomy p.

  dinner p., a p. of moderate thickness placed over the pit of the stomach before the application of a plaster jacket; after the plaster has set the p. is removed, leaving space for varying degrees of abdominal distention.

  fat p., SEE fat-pad.

  knuckle p.'s, (1) an autosomal dominant trait, in which thick p.'s of skin appear over the proximal phalangeal joints; occasionally associated with leukonychia and deafness or Dupuytren's contracture; (2) a callus reaction in persons predisposed to producing callus and as the result of occupational or self-inflicted trauma.

  laparotomy p., a p. made from several layers of gauze folded into a rectangular shape; used as a sponge or packing material in surgery. SYN abdominal p.

  retromolar p., a cushioned mass of tissue, frequently pear-shaped, located on the alveolar process of the mandible behind the area of the last natural molar tooth.

△**paed-.** SEE ped-.

PAGE *p*oly*a*crylamide *g*el *e*lectrophoresis.

△**-pagus.** Conjoined twins, the first element of the word denoting the parts fused. SEE ALSO -didymus, -dymus. [G. *pagos,* something fixed, fr. *pēgnymi,* to fasten together]

pain (pān). **1.** An unpleasant sensation associated with actual or potential tissue damage, and mediated by specific nerve fibers to the brain where its conscious appreciation may be modified by various factors. **2.** Term used to denote a painful uterine contraction occurring in childbirth. [L. *poena,* a fine, a penalty]

  after-p.'s, SEE afterpains.

  bearing-down p., a uterine contraction accompanied by straining and tenesmus; usually appearing in the second stage of labor.

  expulsive p.'s, effective labor p.'s, associated with contraction of the uterine muscle.

  growing p.'s, aching p.'s, frequently felt at night, in the limbs of growing children; attributed variously to growth, rheumatic state, faulty posture, fatigue, or ill-defined psychic causes.

  hunger p., cramp in the epigastrium associated with hunger.

  intermenstrual p., (1) pelvic discomfort occurring approximately at the time of ovulation, usually at the midpoint of the menstrual cycle; (2) SYN mittelschmerz.

  labor p.'s, rhythmical uterine contractions which under normal conditions increase in intensity, frequency, and duration, culminating in vaginal delivery of the infant.

  phantom limb p., SEE phantom *limb.*

  psychogenic p., somatoform p.; p. which is associated or correlated with a psychological, emotional, or behavioral stimulus. SYN psychalgia (2).

  referred p., p. at a site other than the actual location of trauma or disease.

  somatic p., p. originating in the skin, ligaments, muscles, bones, or joints.

  visceral p., p. resulting from injury or disease in an organ in the thoracic or abdominal cavity.

pair (pār). Two objects considered together because of similarity, for a common purpose, or because of some attracting force between them.

  base p., the complex of two heterocyclic nucleic acid bases, one a pyrimidine and the other a purine, brought about by hydrogen bonding between the purine and the pyrimidine; base pairing is the essential element in the structure of DNA. Usually guanine is paired with cytosine (G·C), and adenine with thymine (A·T) or uracil (A·U). The sequence of the complementary bases in either strand of a two-stranded DNA molecule codes for amino acids used in the manufacture of proteins. Trios of bases (codons) specify each of 20 amino acids. During protein synthesis (translation), messenger RNA and ribosomes read the order of amino acids from strings of DNA to create protein chains, which are then released into the cell.

  conjugate acid-base p., in prototonic solvents, acetic acid), two molecular species differing only in the presence or absence of a hydrogen ion; the basis of buffer action.

pal·a·tal (pal′ă-tăl). Relating to the palate or the palate bone. SYN palatine.

pal·ate (pal′ăt). The bony and muscular partition between the oral and nasal cavities. SYN palatum [NA]. [L. *palatum,* palate]

  bony p., a concave elliptical bony plate, constituting the roof of the oral cavity, formed of the palatine process of the maxilla and the horizontal plate of the palatine bone on either side.

cleft p., a congenital fissure in the median line of the p., often associated with cleft lip. Often occurs as a feature of a syndrome or generalized condition, *e.g.,* diastrophic dwarfism or spondyloepiphyseal dysplasia congenita; its general genetic behavior resembles that of cleft *lip.* SYN palatoschisis.

hard p., (1) the anterior part of the palate, consisting of the bony p. covered above by the mucous membrane of the floor of the nasal cavity and below by the mucoperiosteum of the roof of the mouth which contains the palatine vessels, nerves, and mucous glands; **(2)** CEPHALOMETRICS A line connecting the anterior and posterior nasal spines to represent the position of the bony p.

occult cleft p., lack of closure in the bone of the hard p. or muscle of the soft p., but with full closure of the overlying surface tissues. SYN submucous cleft p.

soft p., the posterior muscular portion of the palate, forming an incomplete septum between the mouth and the oropharynx, and between the oropharynx and the nasopharynx. SYN velum palatinum ✶ [NA].

submucous cleft p., SYN occult cleft p.

pal·a·tine (pal′ă-tīn). SYN palatal.

pal·a·ti·tis (pal-ă-tī′tis). Inflammation of the palate.

palato-. Palate. [L. *palatum,* palate]

pal·a·to·glos·sal (pal′ă-tō-glos′ăl). Relating to the palate and the tongue, or to the palatoglossus muscle.

pal·a·tog·na·thous (pal′ă-tog′nă-thŭs). Having a cleft palate. [palato- + G. *gnathos,* jaw]

pal·a·to·max·il·lary (pal′ă-tō-mak′si-lār-ē). Relating to the palate and the maxilla.

pal·a·to·na·sal (pal-ă-tō-nā′sal). Relating to the palate and the nasal cavity.

pal·a·to·pha·ryn·ge·al (pal′ă-tō-fa-rin′jē-ăl). Relating to palate and pharynx.

pal·a·to·pha·ryn·gor·rha·phy (pal′ă-tō-far′in-gōr′ă-fē). SYN staphylopharyngorrhaphy. [palato- + pharynx + G. *rhaphē,* suture]

pal·a·to·plas·ty (pal′ă-tō-plas-tē). Surgery of the palate to restore form and function. SYN staphyloplasty, uranoplasty. [palato- + G. *plassō,* to form]

pal·a·to·ple·gia (pal′ă-tō-plē′jē-ă). Paralysis of the muscles of the soft palate. [palato- + G. *plēgē,* stroke]

pal·a·tor·rha·phy (pal-ă-tōr′ă-fē). Suture of a cleft palate. SYN staphylorrhaphy, uranorrhaphy. [palato- + G. *rhaphē,* suture]

pal·a·tos·chi·sis (pal-ă-tos′ki-sis). SYN cleft *palate.* [palato- + G. *schisis,* fissure]

pa·la·tum, pl. **pa·la·′ti** (pă-lā′tŭm, -tī) [NA]. SYN palate. [L.]

paleo-, pale-. Old, primitive, primary, early. [G. *palaios,* old, ancient]

pa·le·o·cer·e·bel·lum (pā′lē-ō-ser′ĕ-bel′ŭm) [NA]. Phylogenetic term referring to the portion of the cerebellum including most of the vermis and the adjacent zones of the cerebellar hemispheres rostral to the primary fissure; p. is equated with the anterior lobe and corresponds to the zone of distribution of the spinocerebellar tracts and is sometimes called spinocerebellum;

in phylogenetic age, it is thought to be intermediate between the archicerebellum and the neocerebellum. SYN spinocerebellum. [paleo- + L. *cerebellum*]

pa·le·o·cor·tex (pā′lē-ō-kōr′teks). The phylogenetically oldest part of the cortical mantle of the cerebral hemisphere, represented by the olfactory cortex.

pa·le·o·ki·net·ic (pā′lē-ō-ki-net′ik). Denoting the primitive motor mechanisms underlying muscular reflexes and automatic, stereotyped movements. [paleo- + G. *kinetikos,* relating to movement]

pa·le·o·pa·thol·o·gy (pā′lē-ō-pa-thol′ō-jē). The science of disease in prehistoric times as revealed in bones, mummies, and archaeologic artifacts. [paleo- + pathology]

pa·le·o·stri·a·tal (pā′lē-ō-strī-ā′tăl). Relating to the paleostriatum.

pa·le·o·stri·a·tum (pā′lē-ō-strī-ā′tŭm). Term denoting the globus pallidus and expressing the hypothesis that this component of the striate body developed earlier in evolution than the "neostriatum" or striatum (caudate nucleus and putamen) and that it is a diencephalic derivative. [paleo- + L. *striatum*]

pa·le·o·thal·a·mus (pā′lē-ō-thal′ă-mŭs). The intralaminar nuclei, believed to have been the earliest components of the thalamus to evolve; they lack reciprocal connections with the isocortex.

pal·i·ki·ne·sia, pal·i·ci·ne·sia (pal-i-ki-nē′zē-ă, -si-nē′zē-ă). Involuntary repetition of movements. [G. *palin,* again, + *kinēsis,* movement]

pal·i·la·lia (pal-i-lā′lē-ă). SYN paliphrasia. [G. *palin,* again, + *lalia,* a form of speech]

pal·in·drome (pal′in-drōm). MOLECULAR BIOLOGY A self-complementary nucleic acid sequence; a sequence identical to its complementary strand, if both are "read" in the same 5′- to 3′ direction, or inverted repeating sequences running in opposite directions (but same 5′- to 3′- direction) on either side of an axis of symmetry; p.'s occur at sites of important reactions. [G. *palindromos,* a running back]

pal·in·dro·mia (pal-in-drō′mē-ă). A relapse or recurrence of a disease. [G. *palindromos,* a running back, + *-ia,* condition]

pal·in·drom·ic (pal-in-drom′ik). Recurring.

pal·i·nop·sia (pal-i-nop′sē-ă). Abnormal recurring visual hallucinations. [G. *palin,* again, + *opsis,* vision]

pal·i·phra·sia (pal-i-frā′zē-ă). In speech, involuntary repetition of words or sentences. SEE ALSO echolalia. SYN palilalia. [G. *palin,* again, + *phrasis,* speech]

pal·la·di·um (Pd) (pă-lā′dē-ŭm). A metallic element resembling platinum, atomic no. 46, atomic wt. 106.42. [fr. the asteroid, Pallas; G. *Pallas,* goddess of wisdom]

pall·an·es·the·sia (pal′an-es-thē′zē-ă). Absence of pallesthesia. SYN apallesthesia. [G. *pallō,* to quiver, + *anaisthēsia,* insensibility]

pall·es·the·sia (pal′es-thē′zē-ă). The appreciation of vibration, a form of pressure sense; most acute when a vibrating tuning fork is applied over a bony prominence. [G. *pallō,* to quiver, + *aisthēsis,* sensation]

pa

pall·es·thet·ic (pal-es-thet′ik). Pertaining to pallesthesia.

pal·li·al (pal′ē-ăl). Relating to the pallium.

pal·li·ate (pal′ē-āt). To reduce the severity of; to relieve slightly. SYN mitigate. [L. *palliatus* (adj.), dressed in a *pallium,* cloaked]

pal·li·a·tive (pal-ē-ă-tiv). Reducing the severity of; denoting the alleviation of symptoms without curing the underlying disease.

pal·li·dal (pal′i-dăl). Relating to the pallidum.

pal·li·dec·to·my (pal′i-dek′tō-mē). Excision or destruction of the globus pallidus, usually by stereotaxy. [pallidum + G. *ektomē,* excision]

pal·li·do·an·sot·o·my (pal′i-dō-an-sot′ō-mē). Production of lesions in the globus pallidus and ansa lenticularis.

pal·li·dot·o·my (pal-i-dot′ō-mē). A destructive operation on the globus pallidus, done to relieve involuntary movements or muscular rigidity. [pallidum + G. *tomē,* incision]

pal·li·dum (pal′i-dŭm). SYN *globus* pallidus. [L. *pallidus,* pale]

pal·li·um (pal′ē-ŭm) [NA]. The cerebral cortex with the subjacent white substance. SYN mantle (2). [L. cloak]

pal·lor (pal′ŏr). Paleness, as of the skin. [L.]

palm (pahm, pawlm). The flat of the hand; the flexor or anterior surface of the hand, exclusive of the thumb and fingers; the opposite of the dorsum. SYN palma [NA]. [L. *palma*]

pal·ma, pl. **pal·mae** (pawl′mă, pawl′mē) [NA]. SYN palm, palm. [L.]

pal·mar (pawl′măr). Referring to the palm of the hand; volar. [L. *palmaris,* fr. *palma*]

palm·ic (pal′mik). Beating; throbbing; relating to a palmus.

pal·mit·o·le·ic ac·id (pal′mi-tō-lē′ik). A monounsaturated 16-carbon acid; one of the common constituents of the triacylglycerols of human adipose tissue.

pal·mus, pl. **pal·mi** (pal′mŭs, -mī). **1.** SYN facial *tic.* **2.** Rhythmical fibrillary contractions in a muscle. SEE ALSO jumping *disease.* **3.** The heart beat. [G. *palmos,* pulsation, quivering]

pal·pa·ble (pal′pă-bl). **1.** Perceptible to touch; capable of being palpated. **2.** Evident; plain. [see palpation]

pal·pate (pal′pāt). To examine by feeling and pressing with the palms of the hands and the fingers.

pal·pa·tion (pal-pā′shŭn). **1.** Examination with the hands, feeling for organs, masses, or infiltration of a part of the body, feeling the heart or pulse beat, vibrations in the chest, etc. SYN touch (2). **2.** Touching, feeling, or perceiving by the sense of touch. [L. *palpatio,* fr. *palpo,* pp. *-atus,* to touch, stroke]

pal·pe·bra, pl. **pal·pe·brae** (pal-pē′bră, pē′brē) [NA]. SYN eyelid. [L.]

pal·pe·bral (pal′pē-brăl). Relating to an eyelid or the eyelids.

pal·pi·ta·tion (pal-pi-tā′shŭn). Forcible or irregular pulsation of the heart, perceptible to the patient, usually with an increase in frequency or force, with or without irregularity in rhythm. SYN trepidatio cordis. [L. *palpito,* to throb]

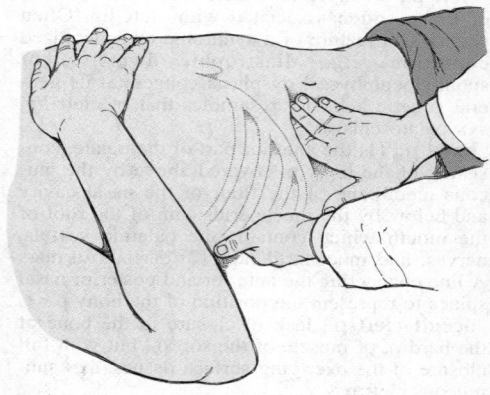

palpation of liver

pal·sy (pawl′zē). Paralysis or paresis. [a corruption of O. Fr. fr. L. and G. *paralysis*]

Bell's p., unilateral weakness or paralysis of facial muscles, due to trauma or disease of the facial nerve. SEE ALSO paralysis.

birth p., any motor abnormality in the infant caused by or attributed to the birthing process; includes obstetrical paralysis, infantile hemiplegia, etc.

bulbar p., flaccid paralysis of the motor units of any or all cranial nerves. Bulbar p.'s may also be identifed by the specific nerve affected, such as facial p. or hypoglossal p. SEE ALSO cranial *nerves,* under *nerve.*

cerebral p., defect of motor power and coordination related to damage of the brain.

cyclist's p., paresthesia of the ulnar nerve in cyclists resulting from leaning on the handlebars for an extended period. SYN ulnar nerve compression syndrome.

Erb p., a type of brachial birth p. in which there is paralysis of the muscles of the upper arm and shoulder girdle (deltoid, biceps, brachialis, and brachioradialis muscles) due to a lesion of the upper trunk of the brachial plexus or of the roots of the fifth and sixth cervical roots. SYN Duchenne-Erb paralysis, Erb paralysis.

facial p., SYN facial *paralysis.*

Klumpke p., a type of brachial birth p. in which there is paralysis of the muscles of the distal forearm and hand (all ulnar innervated muscles, plus more distal radial and median-innervated muscles), due to a lesion of the lower trunk of the brachial plexus, or of the C8 and T1 cervical roots.

obstetrical p., a brachial plexus lesion sustained by the infant during the birthing process; three types are recognized: 1) upper plexus type, affects the shoulder and upper arm (Erb p.); 2) total plexus type, involves the whole arm; 3) lower plexus type, involves the forearm and hand (Klumpke p.). SYN obstetrical paralysis.

pseudobulbar p., spastic paralysis of the bulbar musculature due to bilateral impairment of corticobulbar upper motor neuron fibers.

pam·pin·i·form (pam-pin′i-fōrm). Having the shape of a tendril; denoting a vinelike structure. [L. *pampinus,* a tendril, + *forma,* form]

pan-. All, entire (properly affixed to words derived from G. roots). SEE ALSO pant-. [G. *pas,* all]

pan·a·cea (pan-ă-sē′ă). A cure-all; a remedy claimed to be curative of all diseases. [G. *panakeia,* universal remedy, fr. Panacea, Aesculapius' daughter]

pan·ag·glu·ti·nins (pan-ă-glū′ti-ninz). Agglutinins that react with all human erythrocytes. [pan + L. *agglutino,* to glue]

pan·an·gi·i·tis (pan′an-jē-ī′tis). Inflammation involving all the coats of a blood vessel. [pan- + angiitis]

pan·ar·thri·tis (pan-ar-thrī′tis). **1.** Inflammation involving all the tissues of a joint. **2.** Inflammation of all the joints of the body.

pan·at·ro·phy (pan-at′rō-fē). **1.** Atrophy of all the parts of a structure. **2.** General atrophy of the body.

pan·car·di·tis (pan-kar-dī′tis). Inflammation of all the structures of the heart.

pan·co·lec·to·my (pan′kō-lek′tō-mē). Extirpation of the entire colon.

pan·cre·as, pl. **pan·cre·a·ta** (pan′krē-as, pan-krē-ā′tă) [NA]. An elongated lobulated retroperitoneal gland extending from the duodenum to the spleen; it consists of a flattened head (caput) within the duodenal concavity, an elongated three-sided body extending transversely across the abdomen, and a tail in contact with the spleen. The gland secretes from its exocrine part pancreatic juice that is discharged into the intestine, and from its endocrine part the internal secretions, insulin and glucagon. [G. *pankreas,* the sweetbread, fr. *pas* (*pan*), all, + *kreas,* flesh]

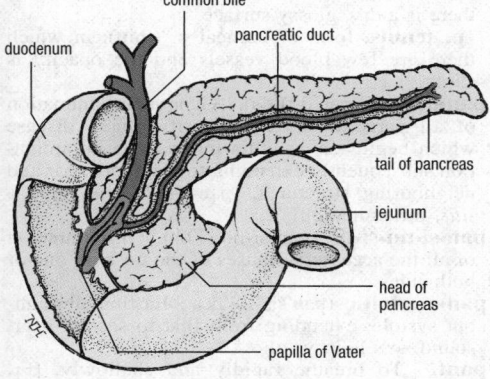

pancreas (and part of duodenum)

pancreat-, pancreatico-, pancreato-, pancreo-. The pancreas. [G. *pankreas,* pancreas]

pan·cre·a·tal·gia (pan′krē-ă-tal′jē-ă). Pain arising from the pancreas or felt in or near the region of the pancreas. [pancreat- + G. *algos,* pain]

pan·cre·a·tec·to·my (pan′krē-ă-tek′tō-mē). Excision of the pancreas. [pancreat- + G. *ektomē,* excision]

pan·cre·at·ic (pan-krē-at′ik). Relating to the pancreas.

pancreatico-. SEE pancreat-.

pan·cre·at·i·co·du·o·de·nal (pan-krē-at′i-kō-dū′ō-dē′năl, -dū-ŏd′ĕ-năl). Relating to the pancreas and the duodenum.

pan·cre·a·ti·tis (pan′krē-ă-tī′tis). Inflammation of the pancreas.

  acute hemorrhagic p., an acute inflammation of the pancreas accompanied by the formation of necrotic areas and hemorrhages into the substance of the gland; clinically marked by sudden severe abdominal pain, nausea, fever, and leukocytosis; areas of fat necrosis are present on the surface of the pancreas and in the omentum due to the action of the escaped pancreatic enzyme (trypsin and lipase).

  chronic fibrosing p., inflammation of the pancreas consisting of fibrosis, acinar atrophy, and calcification. Clinically, it follows a protracted course with relapses and remissions, and is usually due to alcohol abuse or malnutrition.

  chronic relapsing p., repeated exacerbations of p. in patient with chronic inflammation of that organ.

pancreato-. SEE pancreat-.

pan·cre·at·o·du·o·de·nec·to·my (pan-krē-at′ō-dū-ō-dē-nek′tō-mē, pan′krē-ă-tō-). Excision of all or part of the pancreas together with the duodenum. SYN Whipple's operation.

pan·cre·at·o·du·o·de·nos·to·my (pan-krē-at′ō-dū-ō-dē-nos′tō-mē, pan′krē-ă-tō-). Surgical anastomosis of a pancreatic duct, cyst, or fistula to the duodenum.

pan·cre·at·o·gas·tros·to·my (pan-krē-at′ō-gas-tros′tō-mē, pan′krē-ă-tō-). Surgical anastomosis of a pancreatic cyst or fistula to the stomach.

pan·cre·a·to·gen·ic, pan·cre·a·tog·en·ous (pan′krē-ă-tō-jen′ik, -toj′ĕ-nŭs). Of pancreatic origin; formed in the pancreas. [pancreato- + G. *genesis,* origin]

pan·cre·a·tog·ra·phy (pan′krē-ă-tog′ră-fē). Radiographic demonstration of the pancreatic ducts, after retrograde injection of radiopaque material into the distal duct. [pancreato- + G. *graphō,* to write]

pan·cre·at·o·li·thec·to·my (pan-krē-at′ō-li-thek′tō-mē, pan′krē-ă-tō-). SYN pancreatolithotomy. [pancreato- + G. *lithos,* stone, + *ektomē,* excision]

pan·cre·at·o·li·thi·a·sis (pan-krē-at′ō-li-thī′ă-sis, pan′krē-ă-tō-). Stones in the pancreas, usually found in the pancreatic duct system.

pan·cre·at·o·li·thot·o·my (pan-krē-at′ō-li-thot′ō-mē, pan′krē-ă-tō-). Removal of a pancreatic concretion. SYN pancreatolithotomy. [pancreato- + G. *lithos,* stone, + *tomē,* incision]

pan·cre·a·tol·y·sis (pan′krē-ă-tol′i-sis). Destruction of the pancreas. [pancreato- + G. *lysis,* dissolution]

pan·cre·a·to·lyt·ic (pan′krē-ă-tō-lit′ik). Denoting pancreatolysis.

pan·cre·a·top·a·thy (pan′krē-ă-top′ă-thē). Any disease of the pancreas. [pancreato- + G. *pathos,* suffering]

pan·cre·a·tot·o·my (pan′krē-ă-tot′ō-mē). Incision of the pancreas. [pancreato- + G. *tomē,* incision]

pan·cre·a·tro·pic (pan′krē-ă-trop′ik). Exerting an action on the pancreas. [pancreat- + G. *tropikos*, relating to a turning]

pan·cre·li·pase (pan-krē-lip′ās, -lī′pās). A concentrate of pancreatic enzymes standardized for lipase content; a lipolytic used for substitution therapy.

△**pancreo-.** SEE pancreat-.

pan·cy·to·pe·nia (pan′sī-tō-pē′nē-ă). Pronounced reduction in the number of erythrocytes, all types of white blood cells, and the blood platelets in the circulating blood. [pan- + G. *kytos*, cell, + *penia*, poverty]

pan·dem·ic (pan-dem′ik). Denoting a disease affecting or attacking the population of an extensive region, country, continent; extensively epidemic. [pan- + G. *dēmos*, the people]

pan·en·ceph·a·li·tis (pan′en-sef-ă-lī′tis). A diffuse inflammation of the brain.

   subacute sclerosing p. (SSPE), a rare chronic, progressive encephalitis that affects primarily children and young adults, caused by the measles virus. Characterized by a history of primary measles infection before the age of two years, followed by several asymptomatic years, and then gradual, progressive psychoneurological deterioration, consisting of personality change, seizures, myoclonus, ataxia, photosensitivity, ocular abnormalities, spasticity, and coma. Characteristic periodic activity is seen on EEG; pathologically, the white matter of both the hemispheres and brainstem are affected, as well as the cerebral cortex, and eosinophilic inclusion bodies are present in the cytoplasm nuclei of neurons and glial cells. Death usually occurs within three years.

pan·en·do·scope (pan-en′dō-skōp). An illuminated instrument for inspection of the interior of the urethra as well as the bladder by means of a Foroblique lens system. [pan- + G. *endon*, within, + *skopeō*, to view]

pan·es·the·sia (pan-es-thē′zē-ă). The sum of all the sensations experienced by a person at one time. SEE ALSO cenesthesia. [pan- + G. *aisthēsis*, sensation]

pang. A sudden sharp, brief pain.

pan·hy·po·pi·tu·i·tar·ism (pan-hī′pō-pi-tū′i-tă-rizm). A state in which the secretion of all anterior pituitary hormones is inadequate or absent. SYN hypophysial cachexia.

pan·ic (pan′ik). Extreme and unreasoning anxiety and fear, often accompanied by disturbed breathing, increased heart activity, vasomotor changes, sweating, and a feeling of dread. SEE anxiety. [fr. G. myth. char., *Pan*]

   homosexual p., an acute, severe attack of anxiety based on unconscious conflicts regarding homosexuality.

pan·im·mu·ni·ty (pan-i-myū′ni-tē). A general immunity to all infectious diseases.

pan·my·e·loph·thi·sis (pan′mī-ĕ-lof′thi-sis). SYN myelophthisis (2).

pan·my·e·lo·sis (pan′mī-ĕ-lō′sis). Myeloid metaplasia with abnormal immature blood cells in the spleen and liver, associated with myelofibrosis. [pan- + G. *myelos*, marrow, + -*osis*, condition]

pan·nic·u·lec·to·my (pa-nik-yū-lek′tō-mē). Sur-

gical excision of redundant panniculus adiposus, usually of the abdomen. [panniculus + G. *ektomē*, a cutting out]

pan·nic·u·li·tis (pă-nik′yū-lī′tis). Inflammation of subcutaneous adipose tissue. [panniculus + G. -*itis*, inflammation]

   α-1 antitrypsin deficiency p., painful subcutaneous nodules in severe antitrypsin deficiency.

   relapsing febrile nodular nonsuppurative p., nodular fat necrosis of a variety of possible causes.

   subacute migratory p., non-scarring plaques of changing configuration on the lateral aspect of one or both legs, of many months duration.

pan·nic·u·lus, pl. **pan·nic·u·li** (pă-nik′yū-lŭs, -lī) [NA]. A sheet or layer of tissue. [L. dim. of *pannus*, cloth]

   p. adipo′sus [NA], the superficial fascia which contains an abundance of fat deposit in its areolar substance.

   p. carno′sus, the skeletal muscle layer in the superficial fascia represented in humans by the platysma muscle; it is much more extensive in lower mammals.

pan·nus, pl. **pan·ni** (pan′ŭs, pan′ī). A membrane of granulation tissue covering a normal surface: **1.** The articular cartilages in rheumatoid arthritis and in chronic granulomatous diseases such as tuberculosis; **2.** The cornea in trachoma. SEE ALSO corneal p. [L. cloth]

   corneal p., fibrovascular connective tissue that proliferates in the anterior layers of the peripheral cornea in inflammatory corneal disease, particularly trachoma in which the p. involves the superior cornea.

   p. crassus, form of corneal p. (thick) in which there are many blood vessels and the opacity is very dense.

   p. siccus, form of corneal p. (dry) in which there is a dry, glossy surface.

   p. tenuis, form of corneal p. (thin) in which there are few blood vessels and the opacity is slight.

pan·o·ti·tis (pan′ō-tī′tis). General inflammation of all parts of the ear; specifically, a disease which begins as an otitis interna, the inflammation subsequently extending to the middle ear and neighboring structures. [pan- + G. *ous*, ear, + -*itis*, inflammation]

pan·si·nu·si·tis (pan-sī-nŭ-sī′tis). Inflammation of all the accessory sinuses of the nose on one or both sides.

pan·sys·tol·ic (pan′sis-tol′ik). Lasting throughout systole, extending from first to second heart sound. SYN holosystolic.

pant. To breathe rapidly and shallowly. [Fr. *panteler,* to gasp]

△**pant-, panto-.** Entire. SEE ALSO pan-. [G. *pas*, all]

pan·tal·gia (pan-tal′jē-ă). Pain involving the entire body. [pant- + G. *algos*, pain]

△**panto-.** SEE pant-.

pan·to·mo·gram (pan′tō-mō-gram). A panoramic radiographic record of the maxillary and mandibular dental arches and their associated structures, obtained by a pantomograph. [pan- + tomogram]

pan·to·mo·graph (pan′tō-mō-graf). A panoramic radiographic instrument that permits visualization of the entire dentition, alveolar bone, and contiguous structures on a single extraoral film.

pan·to·mog·ra·phy (pan-tō-mog'ră-fē). A method of radiography by which a radiograph (pantomogram) of the maxillary and mandibular dental arches and their contiguous structures may be obtained on a single film.

pan·to·the·nate (pan-tō-then'āt). A salt or ester of pantothenic acid.

pan·to·then·ic ac·id (pan-tō-then'ik). The β-alanine amide of pantoic acid. A growth substance widely distributed in plant and animal tissues, and essential for growth of a number of organisms; deficiency in diet causes a dermatitis in chicks and rats and achromotrichia in the latter; a precursor to coenzyme A.

PAP peroxidase *antiperoxidase* complex, 3'-phosphoadenosine 5'-phosphate. SEE PAP *technique*.

pa·pil·la, pl. **pa·pil·lae** (pă-pil'ă, -pil'ē) [NA]. Any small, nipplelike process. SYN teat (3). [L. a nipple, dim. of *papula,* a pimple]

  conical papillae, numerous projections on the dorsum of the tongue, scattered among the filiform papillae and similar to them, but shorter.

  dental p., a projection of the mesenchymal tissue of the developing jaw into the cup of the enamel organ; its outer layer becomes a layer of specialized columnar cells, the odontoblasts, that form the dentin of the tooth.

  dermal papillae, the superficial projections of the dermis (corium) that interdigitate with recesses in the overlying epidermis; they contain vascular loops and specialized nerve endings, and are arranged in ridgelike lines best developed in the hand and foot.

  filiform papillae, numerous elongated conical keratinized projections on the dorsum of the tongue.

  foliate papillae, numerous projections arranged in several transverse folds upon the lateral margins of the tongue just in front of the palatoglossus muscle.

  fungiform papillae, numerous minute elevations on the dorsum of the tongue, of a fancied mushroom shape, the tip being broader than the base; the epithelium of many of these papillae has taste buds.

  hair p., SYN p. pili.

  incisive p., a slight elevation of the mucosa at the anterior extremity of the raphe of the palate.

  interdental p., the gingiva that fills the interproximal space between two adjacent teeth.

  lacrimal p., a slight projection from the margin of each eyelid near the medial commissure, in the center of which is the lacrimal punctum (opening of the lacrimal duct).

  lingual p., (1) one of numerous variously shaped projections of the mucous membrane of the dorsum of the tongue; **(2)** the lingual portion of the gingiva filling the interproximal space between adjacent teeth; in molar and premolar areas, there may be separate lingual and buccal interdental papillae. SEE ALSO interdental p.

  optic p. (p), SYN optic *disk.*

  p. pi'li, a knoblike indentation of the bottom of the hair follicle, upon which the hair bulb fits like a cap; it is derived from the corium and contains vascular loops for the nourishment of the hair root. SYN hair p.

  parotid p., the projection at the opening of the parotid duct into the vestibule of the mouth opposite the neck of the upper second molar tooth.

  renal p., the apex of a renal pyramid that projects into a minor calyx; some 10 to 25 openings of papillary ducts occur on its tip, forming the area cribrosa.

  retrocuspid p., a small tissue tag located on the mandibular gingiva lingual to the cuspid teeth; considered a normal anatomic structure.

  tactile p., one of the papillae of the dermis containing a tactile cell or corpuscle.

  urethral p., p. urethra'lis, the slight projection often present in the vestibule of the vagina marking the urethral orifice.

  p. valla'ta [NA], SYN vallate p.

  vallate p., one of eight or ten projections from the dorsum of the tongue forming a row anterior to and parallel with the sulcus terminalis; each p. is surrounded by a circular trench (fossa) having a slightly raised outer wall (vallum); on the sides of the vallate p. and the opposed margin of the vallum are numerous taste buds. SYN p. vallata [NA].

pap·il·lary, pap·il·late (pap'i-lār-ē, -i-lāt). Relating to, resembling, or provided with papillae.

pap·il·lec·to·my (pap-i-lek'tō-mē). Surgical removal of any papilla. [papilla + G. *ektomē,* excision]

pa·pil·le·de·ma (pă-pil-e-dē'mă). Edema of the optic disk, often due to increased intracranial pressure. SYN choked disk. [papilla + edema]

pa·pil·li·form (pă-pil'i-fōrm). Resembling or shaped like a papilla.

pap·il·li·tis (pap-i-lī'tis). **1.** Optic neuritis with swelling of the optic disk. **2.** Inflammation of the renal papilla. [papilla + G. *-itis,* inflammation]

△**papillo-.** A papilla, papillary. [L. *papilla*]

pap·il·lo·ad·e·no·cys·to·ma (pap'i-lō-ad'ĕ-nō-sis-tō'mă). A benign epithelial neoplasm characterized by glands or glandlike structures, formation of cysts, and finger-like projections of neoplastic cells covering a core of fibrous connective tissue.

pap·il·lo·car·ci·no·ma (pap'i-lō-kar-si-nō'mă). **1.** A papilloma that has become malignant. **2.** A carcinoma that is characterized by papillary, finger-like projections of neoplastic cells in association with cores of fibrous stroma as a supporting structure. [papilla + G. *karkinōma,* cancer]

pap·il·lo·ma (pap-i-lō'mă). A circumscribed benign epithelial tumor projecting from the surrounding surface and consisting of villous or arborescent outgrowths of fibrovascular stroma covered by neoplastic cells. SYN papillary tumor, villoma. [papilla + G. *-oma,* tumor]

pap·il·lo·ma·to·sis (pap'i-lō-mă-tō'sis). **1.** The development of numerous papillomas. **2.** Papillary projections of the epidermis forming a microscopically undulating surface.

  laryngeal p., multiple squamous papillomas of the larynx in young children, usually due to infection by the human papilloma virus, which may

pa

be transmitted at birth from maternal condylomata.

pap·il·lo·ma·tous (pap-i-lō′mă-tŭs). Relating to a papilloma.

Pa·pil·lo·ma·vi·rus (pap-i-lō′mă-vī-rŭs). A genus of viruses containing DNA and including the papilloma and wart viruses of humans and other animals, some of which are associated with induction of carcinoma. Over 70 types are known to infect humans and are differentiated by DNA homology.

pap·il·lo·ret·i·ni·tis (pap′i-lō-ret-i-nī′tis). SYN neuroretinitis.

pap·il·lot·o·my (pă-pi-lot′ō-mē). An incision into the major duodenal papilla. [papilla + G. *tomē*, incision]

Pa·po·va·vir·i·dae (pă-po′vă-vir′i-dē). A family of small, antigenically distinct viruses that replicate in nuclei of infected cells; most have oncogenic properties. The family includes the genera *Papillomavirus* and *Polyomavirus*. [*papilloma* + *polyoma* + *vacuolating*]

pa·po·va·vi·rus (pă-pō′vă-vī′rŭs). Any virus of the family Papovaviridae.

Pappenheimer bod·ies. See under body.

pap·u·lar (pap′yū-lăr). Relating to papules.

pap·u·la·tion (pap-yū-lā′shŭn). The formation of papules.

ⓘ **pap·ule** (pap′yūl). A small, circumscribed, solid elevation on the skin. [L. *papula*, pimple]

   piezogenic pedal p., pressure-induced papules of the heel, occurring probably as a result of herniation of fat tissue.

   pruritic urticarial p.'s and plaques of pregnancy (PUPPP), intensely pruritic papulovesicles that begin on the abdomen in the third trimester and spread peripherally, resolves rapidly after delivery and does not affect the fetus.

△**papulo-.** Papule. [L. *papula*, papule]

pap·u·lo·er·y·them·a·tous (pap′yū-lō-er-i-them′ă-tŭs, -thē′mă-tŭs). Denoting an eruption of papules on an erythematous surface.

pap·u·lo·pus·tu·lar (pap′yū-lō-pŭs′tū-lăr). Denoting an eruption composed of papules and pustules.

pa·pu·lo·sis (pap-yū-lō′sis). The occurrence of numerous widespread papules.

pap·u·lo·squa·mous (pap′yū-lō-skwā′mŭs). Denoting an eruption composed of both papules and scales. [papulo- + L. *squamosus*, scaly (squamous)]

pap·u·lo·ve·sic·u·lar (pap′yū-lō-ve-sik′yū-lăr). Denoting an eruption composed of papules and vesicles.

pap·y·ra·ceous (pap-i-rā′shŭs). Like parchment or paper. [L. *papyraceus*, made of *papyrus*]

par. A pair; specifically a pair of cranial nerves, *e.g.,* p. nonum, ninth pair, glossopharyngeal; p. vagum, the vagus or tenth pair. [L. equal]

para (par′ă). A woman who has given birth to one or more infants. Para followed by a roman numeral or preceded by a Latin prefix (primi-, secundi-, terti-, quadri-, etc.) designates the number of times a pregnancy has culminated in a single or multiple birth; *e.g.,* **para I**, primipara; a woman who has given birth for the first time; **para II**, secundipara; a woman who has given

birth for the second time to one or more infants. Cf. gravida. [L. *pario*, to bring forth]

△**para-.** **1.** Prefix denoting a departure from the normal. **2.** Prefix denoting involvement of two like parts or a pair. **3.** Adjacent, alongside, near, etc. **4.** CHEMISTRY an italicized prefix denoting two substitutions in the benzene ring arranged symmetrically, *i.e.,* linked to opposite carbon atoms in the ring. For words beginning with *para-* or *p-*, see the specific name. [G. alongside of, near]

par·a·bal·lism (par-ă-bal′izm). Severe jerking movements of both legs. [para- + G. *ballismos*, jumping about]

par·a·bi·o·sis (par-ă-bī-ō′sis). **1.** Fusion of whole eggs or embryos, as occurs in conjoined twins. **2.** Surgical joining of the vascular systems of two organisms. [para- + G. *biōsis*, life]

par·a·bi·ot·ic (par-ă-bī-ot′ik). Relating to, or characterized by, parabiosis.

par·a·bu·lia (par-ă-bū′lē-ă). Perversion of volition or will in which one impulse is checked and replaced by another. [para- + G. *boulē*, will]

par·a·ca·se·in (par-ă-kā′sē-in). The compound produced by the action of rennin upon κ-casein, which precipitates with calcium ion as the insoluble curd.

par·a·ce·nes·the·sia (par′ă-sē-nes-thē′zē-ă). Deterioration in one's sense of bodily well-being, *i.e.,* of the normal functioning of one's organs. [para- + G. *koinos*, common, + *aisthēsis*, feeling]

par·a·cen·te·sis (par′ă-sen-tē′sis). The passage into a cavity of a trocar and cannula, needle, or other hollow instrument for the purpose of removing fluid; variously designated according to the cavity punctured. SYN tapping (2). [G. *parakentēsis*, a tapping for dropsy, fr. *para*, beside, + *kentēsis*, puncture]

par·a·cen·tet·ic (par-ă-sen-tet′ik). Relating to paracentesis.

par·a·cer·vi·cal (par-ă-ser′vi-kăl). Connective tissue adjacent to the uterine cervix.

par·a·cer·vix (par-ă-ser′viks) [NA]. The connective tissue of the pelvic floor extending from the fibrous subserous coat of the cervix of the uterus laterally between the layers of the broad ligament.

par·a·chol·er·a (par-ă-kol′er-ă). A disease resembling Asiatic cholera but due to a vibrio specifically different from *Vibrio cholerae*.

par·a·chor·dal (par-ă-kōr′dăl). Alongside the anterior portion of the notochord in the embryo; designating the bilateral cartilaginous bars that enter into the formation of the base of the skull. [para- + G. *chordē*, cord]

par·a·chro·ma (par-ă-krō′mă). Abnormal coloration of the skin. SYN parachromatosis. [para- + G. *chrōma*, color]

par·a·chro·ma·to·sis (par-ă-krō-mă-tō′sis). SYN parachroma.

Par·a·coc·cid·i·oi·des bra·sil·i·en·sis (par′ă-kok-sid-ē-oy′dēz bră-sil-ē-en′sis). A dimorphic fungus that causes paracoccidioidomycosis.

par·a·coc·cid·i·oi·din (par′ă-kok-sid-ē-oy′din). Antigen prepared from the fungus, *Paracoccidioides brasiliensis;* used for demonstrating present or past infection and identifying endemic areas.

par·a·coc·cid·i·oi·do·my·co·sis (par'ă-kok-sid-ē-oy'dō-mī-kō'sis). A chronic mycosis characterized by primary pulmonary lesions with dissemination to many visceral organs, conspicuous ulcerative granulomas of the buccal and nasal mucosa with extensions to the skin, and generalized lymphangitis; caused by *Paracoccidioides brasiliensis*. SYN Almeida's disease, Lutz-Splendore-Almeida disease, paracoccidioidal granuloma, South American blastomycosis.

par·a·co·li·tis (par'ă-kō-lī'tis). Inflammation of the peritoneal coat of the colon.

par·a·crine (par'ă-krin). Relating to a kind of hormone function in which the effects of the hormone are restricted to the local environment. Cf. endocrine. [para- + G. *krinō*, to separate]

par·a·cu·sis, par·a·cu·sia (par'ă-kū'sis, -kū'sē-ă). **1.** Impaired hearing. **2.** Auditory illusions or hallucinations. [para- + G. *akousis*, hearing]

par·a·cys·tic (par-ă-sis'tik). Alongside or near a bladder, specifically the urinary bladder. [para- + G. *kystis*, bladder]

par·a·cys·ti·tis (par'ă-sis-tī'tis). Inflammation of the connective tissue and other structures about the urinary bladder. [para- + G. *kystis*, bladder, + -*itis*, inflammation]

par·a·did·y·mis, pl. **par·a·did·y·mi·des** (par'ă-did'i-mis, -di-dim'i-dēz) [NA]. A small body sometimes attached to the front of the lower part of the spermatic cord above the head of the epididymis; the remnants of tubules of the mesonephros. SYN parepididymis. [para- + G. *didymos*, twin, in pl. *didymoi*, testes]

par·a·dip·sia (par-ă-dip'sē-ă). An abnormal desire to consume fluids, without regard to bodily need. [para- + G. *dipsa*, thirst]

par·a·dox (par'ă-doks). That which is apparently, though not actually, inconsistent with or opposed to the known facts in any case. [G. *paradoxos*, incredible, beyond belief, fr. *doxa*, belief]

 Weber's p., if a muscle is loaded beyond its power to contract, it may elongate.

par·af·fi·no·ma (par'ă-fi-nō'mă). A tumefaction, usually a granuloma, caused by the prosthetic or therapeutic injection of paraffin into the tissues. SEE ALSO lipogranuloma.

par·a·gan·glia (par-ă-gang'glē-ă). Plural of paraganglion.

par·a·gan·gli·o·ma (par'ă-gang-glē-ō'mă). A neoplasm usually derived from the chromoreceptor tissue of a paraganglion, such as the carotid body, or the medulla of the adrenal gland; the latter is usually termed a chromaffinoma or pheochromocytoma.

par·a·gan·gli·on, pl. **par·a·gan·glia** (par-ă-gang'glē-on, -ă). A small, roundish body containing chromaffin cells; a number of such bodies may be found retroperitoneally near the aorta and in organs such as the kidney, liver, heart, and gonads. SYN chromaffin body.

par·a·geu·sia (par-ă-gyū'sē-ă, -jū'sē-ă). Disordered or abnormal sense of taste. [para- + G. *geusis*, taste]

par·a·geu·sic (par-ă-gyū'sik). Relating to parageusia.

par·a·gram·ma·tism (par-ă-gram'ă-tizm). SYN paraphasia.

par·a·graph·ia (par-ă-graf'ē-ă). **1.** Loss of the power of writing from dictation, although the words are heard and comprehended. **2.** Writing one word when another is intended. [para- + G. *graphō*, to write]

par·a·hor·mone (par-ă-hōr'mōn). A substance, product of ordinary metabolism, not produced for a specific purpose, that acts like a hormone in modifying the activity of some distant organ; *e.g.*, the action of carbon dioxide on the control of breathing.

par·a·ker·a·to·sis (par'ă-ker-ă-tō'sis). Retention of nuclei in the cells of the stratum corneum of the epidermis, observed in many scaling dermatoses such as psoriasis and subacute or chronic dermatitis.

par·a·ki·ne·sia, par·a·ki·ne·sis (par'ă-ki-nē'zē-ă, -ki-nē'sis). Any motor abnormality. [para- + G. *kinēsis*, movement]

par·a·la·lia (par-ă-lā'lē-ă). Any speech defect; especially one in which one letter is habitually substituted for another. [para- + G. *lalia*, talking]

par·a·lex·ia (par-ă-lek'sē-ă). Misapprehension of written or printed words, other meaningless words being substituted for them in reading. [para- + G. *lexis*, speech]

par·al·ge·sia (par-al-jē'zē-ă). Painful paresthesia; any disorder or abnormality of the sense of pain. [para- + G. *algēsis*, the sense of pain]

par·al·lac·tic (par-ă-lak'tik). Relating to a parallax.

par·al·lax (par'ă-laks). The apparent displacement of an object that follows a change in the position from which it is viewed. [G. alternately, fr. *par-allassō*, to make alternate, fr. *allos*, other]

par·al·ler·gic (par-ă-ler'jik). Denoting an allergic state in which the body becomes predisposed to nonspecific stimuli following original sensitization with a specific allergen.

par·a·lo·gia, pa·ral·o·gism, pa·ral·o·gy (par-ă-lō'jē-ă, pă-ral'ō-jizm, -ral'ō-jē). False reasoning, involving self-deception. [G. *paralogia*, a fallacy, fr. *para*, beside, + *logos*, reason]

pa·ral·y·sis, pl. **pa·ral·y·ses** (pă-ral'i-sis, -sēz). **1.** Loss of power of voluntary movement in a muscle through injury to or disease of its nerve supply. **2.** Loss of any function, as sensation, secretion, or mental ability. [G. fr. para- + *lysis*, a loosening]

 acute ascending p., a p. of rapid course beginning in the legs and involving progressively the trunk, arms, and neck, ending sometimes in death in from one to three weeks.

 bulbar p., SYN progressive bulbar p.

 central p., p. due to a lesion in the brain or spinal cord.

 compression p., p. due to external pressure on a nerve.

 Duchenne-Erb p., SYN Erb *palsy*.

 Erb p., SYN Erb *palsy*.

 facial p., paresis or p. of the facial muscles, usually unilateral, due to lesion of the facial nerve involving the nucleus or the facial nerve or a supranuclear lesion in the cerebrum or upper brainstem. SYN facial palsy, facioplegia, prosopoplegia.

familial periodic p., inherited muscle disorder manifested as recurrent episodes of marked generalized weakness. SEE hyperkalemic periodic p., hypokalemic periodic p., normokalemic periodic p.

hyperkalemic periodic p., a form of periodic p. in which the serum potassium level is elevated during attacks; onset occurs in infancy, attacks are frequent but relatively mild, and myotonia is often present.

hypokalemic periodic p. [type I MIM 17066, *170600, *311700], periodic p. in which the serum potassium level is low during attacks; attacks may be precipitated by cold, high carbohydrate meal, or alcohol, may last hours to days, and may cause respiratory p.

immunological p., lack of specific antibody production after exposure to large doses of the antigen; immunological p. disappears when the antigen is eliminated.

Landry's p., SYN acute idiopathic *polyneuritis.*

mixed p., combined motor and sensory p.

motor p., loss of the power of muscular contraction.

musculospiral p., p. of the muscles of the forearm due to injury of the radial (musculospiral) nerve.

normokalemic periodic p. [type III MIM 170600], periodic p. in which the serum potassium level is within normal limits during attacks; there is often severe quadriplegia, usually improved by the administration of sodium salts;

obstetrical p., SYN obstetrical *palsy.*

periodic p., term for a group of diseases characterized by recurring episodes of muscular weakness or flaccid p. without loss of consciousness, speech, or sensation; attacks begin when the patient is at rest, and there is apparent good health between attacks. SEE hyperkalemic periodic p., hypokalemic periodic p., normokalemic periodic p.

pressure p., p. due to compression of a nerve, nerve trunk, or spinal cord.

progressive bulbar p., progressive weakness and atrophy of the muscles of the tongue, lips, palate, pharynx, and larynx; most often caused by motor neuron disease. SYN bulbar p.

pseudobulbar p., p. of the lips and tongue, simulating progressive bulbar p., but due to supranuclear lesions with bilateral involvement of the upper motor neurons; characterized by speech and swallowing difficulties, emotional instability, and spasmodic, mirthless laughter.

sensory p., loss of sensation; anesthesia.

sleep p., brief episodic loss of voluntary movement that occurs when falling asleep (hypnagogic sleep p.) or when awakening (hypnopompic sleep p.). One of the narcoleptic tetrad.

spinal p., loss of motor power due to a lesion of the spinal cord.

supranuclear p., p. due to lesions above the primary motor neurons.

tick p., an ascending p. caused by the continuing presence of *Dermacentor* and *Ixodes* ticks attached in the occipital region or on the upper neck of humans, often hidden under long hair.

Todd's p., p. of temporary duration (normally not more than a few days) that occurs in the limb or limbs involved in jacksonian epilepsy after the seizure.

vasomotor p., SYN vasoparesis.

par·a·lyt·ic (par-ă-lit'ik). Relating to paralysis or suffering from paralysis.

par·a·ly·zant (pă-ral'i-zant). **1.** Causing paralysis. **2.** Any agent, such as curare, that causes paralysis.

par·a·lyze (par'ă-līz). To render incapable of movement.

Par·a·me·ci·um (par-ă-mē'shē-ŭm, -sē-ŭm). An abundant genus of freshwater holotrichous ciliates, characteristically slipper-shaped and often large enough to be visible to the naked eye; commonly used for genetic and other studies. [G. *paramēkēs,* rather long, fr. *mēkos,* length]

par·a·med·ic (par-ă-med'ik). A person trained and certified to provide emergency medical care.

par·a·med·i·cal (par-ă-med'i-kăl). **1.** Related to the medical profession in an adjunctive capacity, *e.g.,* denoting allied health fields such as physical therapy, speech pathology, etc. **2.** Relating to a paramedic.

par·a·me·nia (par-ă-mē'nē-ă). Any disorder or irregularity of menstruation. [para- + G. *mēn,* month]

pa·ram·e·ter (pă-ram'ĕ-ter). One of many dimensions or ways of measuring or describing an object or evaluating a subject: **1.** MATHEMATICS An arbitrary constant that can possess different values, each value defining other expressions. **2.** STATISTICS A term used to define a characteristic of a population, in contrast to a sample from that population. **3.** PSYCHOANALYSIS Any tactic, other than interpretation, used by the analyst to further the patient's progress. [para- + G. *metron,* measure]

par·a·me·tri·al (par-ă-mē'trē-ăl). Pertaining to the parametrium.

par·a·met·ric (par-ă-met'rik). Relating to the parametrium, or structures immediately adjacent to the uterus.

par·a·me·trit·ic (par'ă-me-trit'ik). Relating to parametritis.

par·a·me·tri·tis (par'ă-me-trī'tis). Inflammation of the tissue adjacent to the uterus, particularly in the broad ligament. SYN pelvic cellulitis. [parametrium + G. *-itis,* inflammation]

par·a·me·tri·um, pl. **par·a·me·tria** (par-ă-mē'trē-ŭm, -ă) [NA]. The connective tissue of the pelvic floor extending from the fibrous subserous coat of the supracervical portion of the uterus laterally between the layers of the broad ligament. [para- + G. *mētra,* uterus]

par·a·mim·ia (par-ă-mim'ē-ă). The use of gestures unsuited to the words which they accompany. [para- + G. *mimia,* imitation]

par·am·ne·sia (par-am-nē'zē-ă). False recollection, as of events that have never occurred. [para- + G. *amnēsia,* forgetfulness]

par·am·y·loi·do·sis (par-am'ĭ-loy-dō'sis). **1.** Deposition in tissues of an amyloidlike protein in primary amyloidosis or in atypical amyloidosis of multiple myeloma. **2.** Various hereditary amyloidoses (Portuguese amyloidosis, Indiana amyloidosis) characterized by progressive hypertrophic polyneuritis with sensory changes, ataxia, paresis, and muscle atrophy due to amyloid deposits in peripheral and visceral nerves.

par•a•my•o•to•nia (par'ă-mī-ō-tō'nē-ă). An atypical form of myotonia.

congenital p., p. congen'ita [MIM*168300], a nonprogressive myotonia induced by exposure of muscles to cold; there are episodes of intermittent flaccid paralysis, but no atrophy or hypertrophy of muscles; autosomal dominant inheritance. There is a variant autosomal dominant form [MIM*168350] in which cold is not a provoking factor.

Par•a•myx•o•vir•i•dae (par-ă-mik'sō-vir'i-dē). A family of RNA-containing viruses. Three genera are recognized: *Paramyxovirus, Morbillivirus,* and *Pneumovirus,* all of which cause cell fusion and produce cytoplasmic eosinophilic inclusions.

Par•a•myx•o•vi•rus (par-ă-mik'sō-vī-rŭs). A genus of viruses that includes Newcastle disease, mumps, and parainfluenza viruses (types 1 to 4).

par•a•ne•o•pla•sia (par'ă-nē-ō-plā'zē-ă). Hormonal, neurological, hematological, and other clinical and biochemical disturbances associated with malignant neoplasms but not directly related to invasion by the primary tumor or its metastases.

par•a•ne•o•plas•tic (par'ă-nē-ō-plas'tik). Relating to or characteristic of paraneoplasia.

par•a•neph•ric (par-ă-nef'rik). **1.** Relating to the paranephros. **2.** SYN pararenal.

par•a•neph•ros, pl. **par•a•neph•roi** (par-ă-nef'ros, -nef'roy). SYN suprarenal *gland.* [para- + G. *nephros,* kidney]

par•a•noia (par-ă-noy'ă). A disorder characterized by the presence of systematized delusions, often of a persecutory character involving being followed, poisoned, or harmed by other means, in an otherwise intact personality. SEE ALSO paranoid *personality.* [G. derangement, madness, fr. para- + *noeō,* to think]

par•a•noid (par'ă-noyd). **1.** Relating to or characterized by paranoia. **2.** Having delusions of persecution.

par•a•no•mia (par-ă-nō'mē-ă). A form of aphasia in which objects are called by the wrong names. [para- + G. *onoma,* name]

par•a•nu•cle•ar (par-ă-nū'klē-ăr). **1.** SYN paranucleate. **2.** Outside, but near the nucleus.

par•a•nu•cle•ate (par'ă-nū'klē-āt). Relating to or having a paranucleus. SYN paranuclear (1).

par•a•nu•cle•us (par-ă-nū'klē-ŭs). An accessory nucleus or small mass of chromatin lying outside, though near, the nucleus.

par•a•op•er•a•tive (par-ă-op'er-ă-tiv). SYN perioperative.

par•a•pa•re•sis (par-ă-pă-rē'sis). Weakness affecting the lower extremities. [para- + paresis]

par•a•pa•ret•ic (par-ă-pă-ret'ik). **1.** Relating to paraparesis. **2.** A person with paraparesis.

par•a•pha•sia (par-ă-fā'zē-ă). A form of aphasia in which a person has lost the ability to speak correctly, substituting one word for another, and jumbling words and sentences unintelligibly. SYN jargon (2), paragrammatism, paraphrasia. [para- + G. *phasis,* speech]

par•a•pha•sic (par-ă-fā'sik). Relating to paraphasia.

pa•ra•phia (pa-rā'fē-ă). Any disorder of the sense of touch. SYN parapsia, pseudesthesia (1). [para- + G. *haphē,* touch]

par•a•phil•ia (par-ă-fil'ē-ă). A mental disorder characterized by socially proscribed sexual practices. [para- + G. *philos,* fond]

par•a•phi•mo•sis (par'ă-fī-mō'sis). Painful constriction of the glans penis by a phimotic foreskin, which has been retracted behind the corona. [para- + G. phimosis]

par•a•phra•sia (par-ă-frā'zē-ă). SYN paraphasia. [para- + G. *phrasis,* speech]

par•a•plec•tic (par-ă-plek'tik). SYN paraplegic. [G. *paraplēktikos,* paralyzed]

par•a•ple•gia (par-ă-plē'jē-ă). Paralysis of both lower extremities and, generally, the lower trunk. [para- + G. *plēgē,* a stroke]

par•a•ple•gic (par-ă-plē'jik). Relating to or suffering from paraplegia. SYN paraplectic.

par•a•prax•ia (par-ă-prak'sē-ă). A condition analogous to paraphasia and paragraphia in which there is a defective performance of purposive acts; *e.g.,* slips of the tongue, or mislaying of objects. [para- + G. *praxis,* a doing]

par•a•pro•tein ((par-ă-prō'tēn). **1.** A monoclonal immunoglobulin of the blood plasma, produced by a clone of plasma cells arising from the abnormal rapid multiplication of a single cell. Paraprotein in serum may be seen in a variety of malignant, benign, or nonneoplastic diseases. **2.** SYN monoclonal *immunoglobulin.* [para + protein, fr. G. *protos,* first]

par•a•pro•tein•e•mia (par'ă-prō-tēn-ē'mē-ă). The presence of abnormal proteins in the blood.

pa•rap•sia (pă-rap'sē-ă). SYN paraphia. [para- + G. *hapsis,* touch]

par•a•pso•ri•a•sis (par'ă-sō-rī'ă-sis). A heterogenous group of skin disorders including pityriasis lichenoides and small and large plaque variants.

par•a•psy•chol•o•gy (par'ă-sī-kol'ō-jē). The study of extrasensory perception, such as thought transference (telepathy) and clairvoyance.

par•a•re•flex•ia (par'ă-rē-flek'sē-ă). A condition characterized by abnormal reflexes.

par•a•re•nal (par-ă-rē'năl). Near or adjacent to the kidneys. SYN paranephric (2).

par•a•ro•san•i•lin (par'ă-rō-san'i-lin) [C.I. 42500]. A biologic stain used in Schiff's reagent to detect cellular DNA (Feulgen stain), mucopolysaccharides (PAS stain), and proteins (ninhydrin-Schiff stain).

par•a•rhyth•mia (par-ă-ridh'mē-ă). A cardiac dysrhythmia in which two independent rhythms coexist, but not as a result of A-V block; p. thus includes parasystole and A-V dissociation (2), but not complete A-V block. [para- + G. *rhythmos,* rhythm]

par•a•si•noi•dal (par'ă-sī-noy'dăl). Near a sinus, particularly a cerebral sinus.

par•a•site (par'ă-sīt). **1.** An organism that lives on or in another and draws its nourishment therefrom. **2.** In the case of a fetal inclusion or conjoined twins, the usually incomplete twin that derives its support from the more nearly normal autosite. [G. *parasitos,* a guest, fr. *para,* beside, + *sitos,* food]

facultative p., an organism that may either lead an independent existence or live as a p., in contrast to obligate p.

heterogenetic p., a p. whose life cycle involves an alternation of generations.

heteroxenous p., a p. that has more than one obligatory host in its life cycle.

incidental p., a p. that normally lives on a host other than its present host.

obligate p., a p. that cannot lead an independent nonparasitic existence, in contrast to facultative p.

specific p., a p. that habitually lives in its present host and is particularly adapted for the host species.

temporary p., an organism accidentally ingested that survives briefly in the intestine.

par·a·si·te·mia (păr′ă-sī-tē′mē-ă). The presence of parasites in the circulating blood; used especially with reference to malarial and other protozoan forms, and microfilariae.

par·a·sit·ic (par-ă-sit′ik). 1. Relating to or of the nature of a parasite. 2. Denoting organisms that normally grow only in or on the living body of a host.

par·a·sit·i·ci·dal (par′ă-sit-i-sī′dăl). Destructive to parasites.

par·a·sit·i·cide (par-ă-sit′i-sīd). An agent that destroys parasites. [parasite + L. *caedo,* to kill]

par·a·sit·ism (par′ă-si-tizm). A symbiotic relationship in which one species (the parasite) benefits at the expense of the other (the host). Cf. mutualism, commensalism, symbiosis, metabiosis.

par·a·si·tize (par′ă-si-tīz). To invade as a parasite.

par·a·si·to·gen·ic (par′-ă-sī-tō-jen′ik). 1. Caused by certain parasites. 2. Favoring parasitism. [parasite + G. *-gen,* producing]

par·a·si·tol·o·gist (par′ă-sī-tol′ŏ-jist). One who specializes in the science of parasitology.

par·a·si·tol·o·gy (par′ă-sī-tol′ō-jē). The branch of biology and of medicine concerned with all aspects of parasitism. [parasite + G. *logos,* study]

par·a·sit·o·sis (par′ă-sī-tō′sis). Infestation or infection with parasites.

par·a·si·to·tro·pic (par′ă-sī-tō-trop′ik). Pertaining to or characterized by parasitotropism.

par·a·si·tot·ro·pism (par′ă-sī-tot′rō-pizm). The special affinity of particular drugs or other agents for parasites rather than for their hosts, including microparasites that infect a larger parasite. Cf. organotropism. [parasite + G. *trope,* a turning]

par·a·som·nia (par-ă-som′nē-ă). Any dysfunction associated with sleep, *e.g.,* somnambulism, pavor nocturnus, enuresis, or nocturnal seizures.

par·a·sta·sis (par-ă-stā′sis). 1. A reciprocal relationship among causal mechanisms that can compensate for, or mask defects in, each other. 2. GENETICS A relationship between non-alleles (classified by some as a form of epistasis). [G. standing shoulder to shoulder]

par·a·sym·pa·thet·ic (par-ă-sim-pa-thet′ik). Pertaining to a division of the autonomic nervous system. SEE autonomic nervous *system.*

par·a·sym·pa·tho·lyt·ic (par-ă-sim′pă-thō-lit′ik). Relating to an agent that annuls or antagonizes the effects of the parasympathetic nervous system; *e.g.,* atropine.

par·a·sym·pa·tho·mi·met·ic (par-ă-sim′pă-thō-mi-met′ik). Relating to drugs or chemicals having an action resembling that caused by stimulation of the parasympathetic nervous system. SEE ALSO cholinomimetic. [para- + G. *sympatheia,* sympathy, + *mimētikos,* imitative]

par·a·sy·nap·sis (par′ă-si-nap′sis). Union of chromosomes side to side in the process of reduction. [para- + G. *synapsis,* a connection, junction]

par·a·sy·no·vi·tis (par′ă-si-nō-vī′tis). Inflammation of the tissues immediately adjacent to a joint. [para- + synovitis]

par·a·sys·to·le (par-ă-sis′tō-lē). A second automatic rhythm existing simultaneously with normal sinus or other dominant rhythm, the parasystolic center being protected from the dominant rhythm's impulses so that its basic rhythm is undisturbed, although it may be manifest in the ECG only at various multiples of its basic periodicity. [para- + G. *systolē,* a contracting]

par·a·ten·on (par-ă-ten′on). The tissue, fatty or synovial, between a tendon and its sheath. [para- + G. *tenōn,* tendon]

par·a·thy·roid (par-ă-thī′royd). 1. Adjacent to the thyroid gland. 2. SYN parathyroid *gland.*

par·a·thy·roid·ec·to·my (pa′ră-thī-roy-dek′to-mē). Excision of the parathyroid glands. [parathyroid + G. *ektomē,* excision]

par·a·thy·ro·tro·pic, par·a·thy·ro·tro·phic (par′ă-thī-rō-trop′ik, -trof′ik). Influencing the growth or activity of the parathyroid glands. [parathyroid + G. *trope,* a turning; *trophē,* nourishment]

par·a·tope (par′ă-tōp). That part of an antibody molecule composed of the variable regions of both the light and heavy chains that combine with the antigen. [para- + -tope]

par·a·ty·phoid (par-ă-tī′foyd). SYN paratyphoid *fever.*

par·a·vag·i·ni·tis (par′ă-vaj-i-nī′tis). Inflammation of the connective tissue alongside the vagina.

par·ax·i·al (par-ak′sē-ăl). By the side of the axis of any body or part.

par·ax·on (par-ak′son). A collateral branch of an axon. [para- + G. *axōn,* axis]

pa·ren·chy·ma (pă-reng′ki-mă). 1. The distinguishing or specific cells of a gland or organ, contained in and supported by the connective tissue framework, or stroma. 2. The endoplasm of a protozoan cell. [G. anything poured in beside, fr. *parencheō,* to pour in beside]

pa·ren·chy·ma·ti·tis (pă-reng′ki-mă-tī′tis). Inflammation of the parenchyma or differentiated substance of a gland or organ.

par·en·chym·a·tous (par′eng-kim′ă-tŭs). Relating to the parenchyma.

par·en·ter·al (pă-ren′ter-ăl). By some other means than through the gastrointestinal tract; referring particularly to the introduction of substances into an organism by intravenous, subcutaneous, intramuscular, or intramedullary injection. [para- + G. *enteron,* intestine]

par·ep·i·did·y·mis (par'ep'i-did'i-mis). SYN par-adidymis.

pa·re·sis (pă-rē'sis, par'ĕ-sis). **1.** Partial or incomplete paralysis. **2.** A disease of the brain, syphilitic in origin, marked by progressive dementia, tremor, speech disturbances, and increasing muscular weakness; in a large proportion of cases there is a preliminary stage of irritability often followed by exaltation and delusions of grandeur. SYN Bayle's disease. [G. a letting go, slackening, paralysis, fr. *paritēmi*, to let go]

par·es·the·sia (par-es-thē'zē-ă). An abnormal sensation, such as of burning, pricking, tickling, or tingling. [para- + G. *aisthēsis*, sensation]

par·es·thet·ic (par-es-thet'ik). Relating to or marked by paresthesia; denoting numbness and tingling in an extremity which usually occurs on the resumption of the blood flow to a nerve following temporary pressure or mild injury.

pa·ret·ic (pa-ret'ik). Relating to or suffering from paresis.

pa·reu·nia (par-yū'nē-ă). SYN coitus. [G. *pareunos*, lying beside, fr. *para*, beside, + *eunē*, a bed]

par·i·es, gen. **pa·ri·e'etis**, pl. **pa·ri·e·tes** (par'i-ēz, pā'rī-ēz; pă-rī'ĕ-tēz) [NA]. SYN wall. [L. wall]

pa·ri·e·tal (pă-rī'ĕ-tăl). **1.** Relating to the wall of any cavity. **2.** SYN somatic (1). **3.** SYN somatic (2). **4.** Relating to the parietal bone.

△**parieto-**. A wall (of the body, *e.g.*, the abdominal wall); a parietal bone. [L. *paries*, wall]

pa·ri·e·tog·ra·phy (pa-rī'ē-tog'ră-fē). Rarely used term for a radiographic examination of the wall of the stomach using a combination of pneumoperitoneum and intraluminal air and barium. [parieto- + G. *graphē*, a writing]

par·i·ty (par'i-tē). The condition of having given birth to an infant or infants, alive or dead; a multiple birth is considered as a single parous experience. [L. *pario*, to bear]

par·kin·so·ni·an (par-kin-sō'nē-an). Relating to or the suffering from parkinsonism (1).

par·kin·son·ism (par'kin-son-izm). **1.** A neurological syndrome usually resulting from deficiency of the neurotransmitter dopamine as the consequence of degenerative, vascular, or inflammatory changes in the basal ganglia; characterized by rhythmical muscular tremors, rigidity of movement, festination, droopy posture, and masklike facies. SYN Parkinson's disease. **2.** A syndrome similar to p. appearing as a side effect of certain antipsychotic drugs. [J. *Parkinson*]

par·om·pha·lo·cele (par-om'fă-lō-sēl). **1.** A tumor near the umbilicus. **2.** A hernia through a defect in the abdominal wall near the umbilicus. [para- + G. *omphalos*, umbilicus, + *kēlē*, tumor, hernia]

▯**par·o·nych·ia** (par-ō-nik'ē-ă). Suppurative inflammation of the nail fold surrounding the nail plate; may be due to bacteria or fungi, most commonly staphylococci and streptococci. [para- + G. *onyx*, nail]

par·o·nych·i·al (par-ō-nik'ē-ăl). Relating to paronychia.

par·o·öph·o·ron (par-ō-of'ōr-on) [NA]. Remnants of the tubules and glomeruli of the lower part of the mesonephros appearing as a few scat-

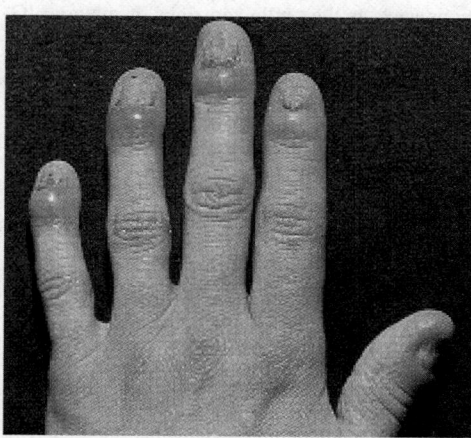

paronychia: chronic form

tered tubules in the broad ligament between the epoöphoron and the uterus. Its equivalent in the male is the paradidymis. [para- + oophoron, ovary]

par·or·chid·i·um (par-ōr-kid'ē-ŭm). SYN testis ectopia. [para- + G. *orchis*, testis]

par·o·rex·ia (par-ō-rek'sē-ă). An abnormal or disordered appetite. [para- + G. *orexis*, appetite]

par·os·mia (par-oz'mē-ă). Any disorder of the sense of smell, especially subjective perception of nonexistent odors. [para + G. *osmē*, sense of smell]

par·os·te·o·sis, par·os·to·sis (par'os-tē-ō'sis, -os-tō'sis). **1.** Development of bone in an unusual location, as in the skin. **2.** Abnormal or defective ossification. [para- + G. *osteon*, bone, + *-osis*, condition]

pa·rot·ic (pă-rot'ik). Near or beside the ear. [para- + G. *ous*, ear]

pa·rot·id (pă-rot'id). Situated near the ear; denoting several structures in this neighborhood. Usually refers to the p. salivary gland. [G. *parōtis* (*parōtid-*), the gland beside the ear, fr. *para*, beside, + *ous* (*ōt-*), ear]

pa·rot·i·dec·to·my (pă-rot'i-dek'tō-mē). Surgical removal of the parotid gland. [parotid + G. *ektomē*, excision]

pa·rot·i·di·tis (pă-rot-i-dī'tis). Inflammation of the parotid gland. SYN parotitis.

 epidemic p., an acute infectious and contagious disease caused by a *Paramyxovirus* and characterized by fever, inflammation and swelling of the parotid gland, sometimes of other salivary glands, and occasionally by inflammation of the testis, ovary, pancreas, or meninges. SYN mumps.

par·o·ti·tis (par-o-tī'tis). SYN parotiditis.

par·ous (par'ŭs). Pertaining to parity. [L. *pario*, to bear]

par·o·var·i·an (par-ō-var'ē-an). **1.** Relating to the paroöphoron. **2.** Beside or in the neighborhood of the ovary.

par·ox·ysm (par'ok-sizm). **1.** A sharp spasm or convulsion. **2.** A sudden onset of a symptom or disease, especially one with recurrent manifestations such as the chills and rigor of malaria. [G. *paroxysmos*, fr. *paroxynō*, to sharpen, irritate, fr. *oxys*, sharp]

par·ox·ys·mal (par-ok-siz′măl). Relating to or occurring in paroxysms.

pars, pl. **par·tes** (pars, par′tēz) [NA]. A part; a portion. [L. *pars* (*part-*) a part]

   p. amor′pha, the part of the nucleolus that occupies irregular spaces in the nucleolonema and contains finely filamentous substance. SEE ALSO p. granulosa.

   p. granulo′sa, the granular and filamentous part of the nucleolonema of the nucleolus.

   p. pla′na, SYN orbiculus ciliaris.

   p. tympanica [NA], tympanic portion of the temporal bone, forming the greater part of the wall of the external acoustic meatus.

   p. uteri′na placen′tae [NA], the part of the placenta derived from the uterine tissue. SEE ALSO placenta. SYN maternal placenta.

pars-pla·ni·tis (parz′plă-nī′tis). A clinical syndrome consisting of inflammation of the peripheral retina and/or pars plana, exudation into the overlying vitreous base, and edema of the optic disk and adjacent retina.

part. A portion.

   cardiac p. of stomach, the area of the stomach close to the esophageal opening (cardiac orifice or cardia) which contains the cardiac glands.

   convoluted p. of kidney lobule, proximal and distal convoluted tubules and the associated renal corpuscles supplied by branches of the interlobular arteries. SYN labyrinth (3).

   petrous p. of internal carotid artery, the part of the internal carotid artery in the carotid canal; its branches are carotidotympanic arteries and the artery of the pterygoid canal.

   petrous p. of temporal bone, the part of the temporal bone that contains the structures of the inner ear and the second part of the internal carotid artery; in antenatal life it appears as a separate ossification center.

part. aeq. Abbreviation for L. *partes aequales*, in equal parts (amounts).

par·the·no·gen·e·sis (par′the-nō-jen′ĕ-sis). A form of nonsexual reproduction, or agamogenesis, in which the female reproduces its kind without fecundation by the male. [G. *parthenos*, virgin, + *genesis*, product]

par·ti·cle (par′ti-kl). A very small piece or portion of anything. [L. *particula*, dim. of *pars*, part]

   alpha p. (alpha), a p. consisting of two neutrons and two protons, with a positive charge (2e$^+$); emitted energetically from the nuclei of unstable isotopes of high atomic number (elements of mass number from 82 up); identical to the helium nucleus.

   beta p., an electron, either positively (positron, β$^+$) or negatively (negatron, β$^-$) charged, emitted during beta decay of a radionuclide. SYN beta ray.

   Dane p.'s, the larger spherical forms of hepatitis-associated antigens; they comprise the virion of hepatitis B virus.

   elementary p., (1) SYN platelet. **(2)** one of the units occurring on the matrical surface of mitochondrial cristae; the p.'s may be concerned with the electron transport system.

par·tic·u·late (par-tik′yū-lāt). Relating to or occurring in the form of fine particles.

par·tic·u·lates (par-tik′yū-lats). Formed elements, discrete bodies, as contrasted with the surrounding liquid or semiliquid material; *e.g.,* granules or mitochondria in cells.

par·tu·ri·ent (par-tū′rē-ent). Relating to or in the process of childbirth. [L. *parturio*, to be in labor]

par·tu·ri·fa·cient (par-tūr-ē-fā′shent). **1.** Inducing or accelerating labor. **2.** An agent that induces or accelerates labor. SYN oxytocic (2). [L. *parturio*, to be in labor, + *facio*, to make]

par·tu·ri·om·e·ter (par-tūr-ē-om′ĕ-ter). Device for determining the force of the uterine contractions in childbirth. [L. *parturitio*, parturition, + G. *metron*, measure]

par·tu·ri·tion (par-tūr-ish′ŭn). SYN childbirth. [L. *parturitio*, fr. *parturio*, to be in labor]

part. vic. Abbreviation for L. *partibus vicibus*, in divided doses.

par·vo·cel·lu·lar (par-vi-sel′yū-lăr). Relating to or composed of cells of small size. [L. *parvus*, small, + Mod. L. *cellularis*, cellular]

Par·vo·vir·i·dae (par-vō-vir′i-dē). A family of small viruses containing single-stranded DNA. Three genera are recognized: *Parvovirus*, *Densovirus*, and *Dependovirus*, which includes the adeno-associated satellite virus.

Par·vo·vi·rus (par′vō-vī-rŭs). A genus of viruses that replicate autonomously in suitable cells. [L. *parvus*, small, + virus]

Par·vo·vi·rus B 19. A small DNA virus belonging to the family Parvoviridae that is associated with erythema infectiosum (fifth disease) and aplastic crisis in patients with hemolytic anemia.

Pascal, Blaise, French scientist, 1623–1662. SEE pascal; P.'s *law*.

pas·cal (Pa) (pas′kăl). A derived unit of pressure or stress in the SI system, expressed in newtons per square meter; equal to 10^{-5} bar or 7.50062×10^{-3} torr. [B. *Pascal*]

pas·sive (pas′iv). Not active; submissive. [L. *passivus*, fr. *patior*, to endure]

pas·siv·ism (pas′iv-izm). An attitude of submission, particularly in sexual relations. [see passive]

paste (pāst). A soft semisolid of firmer consistency than pap but soft enough to flow slowly and not to retain its shape. [L. *pasta*]

Pas·teu·rel·la (pas-ter-el′ă). A genus of aerobic to facultatively anaerobic, nonmotile bacteria containing small, Gram-negative, ellipsoidal to elongated rods which, with special methods, show bipolar staining. These organisms are parasites of humans and other animals. [L. *Pasteur*]

   P. multoci′da, a species that causes fowl cholera and hemorrhagic septicemia in warm-blooded animals and may infect dog or cat bites or scratches and cause cellulitis and septicemia in humans with chronic disease. Most common pathogen associated with cat and dog bites. It is the type species of the genus *P.*

   P. pes′tis, SYN *Yersinia pestis.*

   P. pseudotuberculo′sis, SYN *Yersinia pseudotuberculosis.*

pas·teu·rel·la, pl. **pas·teu·rel·lae** (pas-ter-el′ă, pas-ter-el′ē). A vernacular term used to refer to any member of the genus *Pasteurella.*

pas·teur·el·lo·sis (pas'ter-ĕ-lō'sis). Infection with bacteria of the genus *Pasteurella*.

pas·teur·i·za·tion (pas'ter-i-zā'shŭn). The heating of milk, wines, fruit juices, etc., for about 30 minutes at 68°C (154.4°F) whereby living bacteria are destroyed but the flavor or bouquet is preserved; the spores are unaffected, but are kept from developing by immediately cooling the liquid to 10°C (50°F) or lower. SEE ALSO sterilization. [L. *Pasteur*]

patch. A small circumscribed area differing in color or structure from the surrounding surface.

   cotton-wool p.'s, white, fuzzy areas on the surface of the retina (accumulations of cellular organelles) caused by damage (usually infarction) of the retinal fiber layer.

   Peyer's p.'s, collections of many lymphoid follicles closely packed together, forming oblong elevations on the mucous membrane of the small intestine.

pa·tel·la, gen. and pl. **pa·tel·lae** (pa-tel'ă, -ē) [NA]. The large sesamoid bone, in the combined tendon of the extensors of the leg, covering the anterior surface of the knee. SYN kneecap. [L. a small plate, the kneecap, dim. of *patina,* a shallow disk, fr. *pateo,* to lie open]

   p. alta, a p. with an abnormally high position relative to the joint line of the knee.

   ballotable p. (ba-lŏt'abl), a condition in which the patella can be balloted because of an effusion of blood or fluid in the capsule of the knee joint. SYN floating p.

   floating p., SYN ballotable p.

   squinting p., a p. that is medially rotated.

pa·tel·lar (pa-tel'ăr). Relating to the patella.

pat·el·lec·to·my (pat'ĕ-lek'tō-mē). Excision of the patella. [patella + G. *ektomē,* excision]

pa·tel·li·form (pa-tel'i-fōrm). Of the shape of the patella.

pa·ten·cy (pā'ten-sē). The state of being freely open or exposed.

pa·tent (pā'tent, pā'tent). Open or exposed. SYN patulous. [L. *patens,* pres. p. of *pateo,* to lie open]

path-, -pathy, patho-, path·ic. Disease. [G. *pathos,* feeling, suffering, disease]

path·er·gy (path'er-jē). Those reactions resulting from a state of altered activity, both allergic (immune) and nonallergic. [G. *pathos,* disease, + *ergon,* work]

path·find·er (path'fīn-der). A filiform bougie for introduction through a narrow stricture and to serve as a guide for the passage of a larger sound or catheter.

patho-. SEE path-.

path·o·bi·ol·o·gy (path'ō-bī-ol'ō-jē). Pathology with emphasis more on the biological than on the medical aspects.

path·o·clis·is (path-ō-klis'is). A specific tendency to sensitivity to special toxins; a tendency for toxins to attack certain organs. [patho- + G. *klisis,* bending, proneness]

path·o·gen (path'ō-jen). Any virus, microorganism, or other substance causing disease. [patho- + G. *-gen,* to produce]

   behavioral p., the personal habits and lifestyle behaviors of an individual that are associated with an increased risk of physical illness and dysfunction. Cf. behavioral *immunogen.*

path·o·gen·e·sis (path-ō-jen'ĕ-sis). The pathologic, physiologic, or biochemical mechanism resulting in the development of a disease or morbid process. Cf. etiology. [patho- + G. *genesis,* production]

path·o·gen·ic, path·o·ge·net·ic (path-ō-jen'ik, -jĕ-net'ik). Causing disease or abnormality. SYN morbific, nosogenic, nosopoietic.

path·o·ge·nic·i·ty (path'ō-jĕ-nis'i-tē). The condition or quality of being pathogenic, or the ability to cause disease.

path·og·no·mon·ic (path'og-nō-mon'ik). Characteristic or indicative of a disease; denoting especially one or more typical symptoms, findings, or pattern of abnormalities specific for a given disease and not found in any other condition. [see pathognomony]

path·o·log·ic, path·o·log·i·cal (path-ō-loj'ik, -i-kăl). **1.** Pertaining to pathology. **2.** Morbid or diseased; resulting from disease.

pa·thol·o·gist (pa-thol'ō-jist). A specialist in pathology; a physician who practices, evaluates, or supervises diagnostic tests, using materials removed from living or dead patients, and functions as a laboratory consultant to clinicians, or who conducts experiments or other investigations to determine the causes or nature of disease changes.

pa·thol·o·gy (pa-thol'ō-jē). The medical science, and specialty practice, concerned with all aspects of disease, but with special reference to the essential nature, causes, and development of abnormal conditions, as well as the structural and functional changes that result from the disease processes. [patho- + G. *logos,* study, treatise]

   anatomical p., the subspecialty of p. that pertains to the gross and microscopic study of organs and tissues removed for biopsy or during postmortem examination, and also the interpretation of the results of such study. SYN pathological anatomy.

   cellular p., (1) the interpretation of diseases in terms of cellular alterations; **(2)** sometimes used as a synonym for cytopathology (1).

   clinical p., (1) any part of the medical practice of p. as it pertains to the care of patients; **(2)** the subspecialty in p. concerned with the theoretical and technical aspects of chemistry, immunohematology, microbiology, parasitology, immunology, hematology, and other fields as they pertain to the diagnosis of disease.

   comparative p., the p. of diseases of animals, especially in relation to human p.

   oral p., the branch of dentistry concerned with the etiology, pathogenesis, and clinical, gross, and microscopic aspects of oral and paraoral disease, including oral soft tissues, the teeth, jaws, and salivary glands.

   speech p., the science concerned with functional and organic speech defects and disorders.

   surgical p., a field in anatomical p. concerned with examination of tissues removed from living patients for the purpose of diagnosis of disease and guidance in the care of patients.

path·o·mi·me·sis (path'ō-mi-mē'sis). Mimicry

of a disease or dysfunction, whether intentional or unconscious. [patho- + G. *mimēsis,* imitation]

path·o·phys·i·ol·o·gy (path'ō-fiz-ē-ol'ō-jē). Derangement of function seen in disease; alteration in function as distinguished from structural defects.

pa·tho·sis (pă-thō'sis). Rarely used term for a state of disease, diseased condition, or disease entity. [patho- + G. *-osis,* condition]

path·way (path'wā). **1.** A collection of axons establishing a conduction route for nerve impulses from one group of nerve cells to another group or to an effector organ composed of muscle or gland cells. **2.** Any sequence of chemical reactions leading from one compound to another; if taking place in living tissue, usually referred to as a biochemical pathway.

common p. of coagulation, a part of the coagulation system where the intrinsic and extrinsic p.'s converge to activate factor X. Coagulation factors X, V, II, and fibrinogen are part of this p. Both the APTT and PT test the integrity of this system.

Embden-Meyerhof p., the anaerobic glycolytic p. by which D-glucose (most notably in muscle) is converted to lactic acid. Cf. glycolysis.

extrinsic coagulation p., a part of the coagulation p. that is activated by contact of factor VII in the blood with tissue factor (TF), an integral membrane protein of extravascular plasma membranes. The integrity of this p. can be tested by the prothrombin time (PT).

intrinsic coagulation p., a part of the coagulation p. that is activated by contact of coagulation proteins with negatively charged surfaces. All components are within the blood stream and include factors XII, XI, IX, VII, HMWK, and prekallikrein. The activated partial thromboplastin time tests for abnormalities in this pathway.

pentose phosphate p., a secondary p. for the oxidation of D-glucose (not occurring in skeletal muscle), generating reducing power (NADPH) in the cytoplasm outside the mitochondria and synthesizing pentoses and a few other sugars. This p. is defective in certain inherited diseases, *e.g.,* glucose-6-phosphate dehydrogenase deficiency. SYN Dickens shunt.

△**-pathy.** SEE path-.

pa·tient (pā'shent). One who is suffering from disease, injury, abnormal state, or mental disorder. Cf. case (1). [L. *patiens,* pres. p. of *patior,* to suffer]

pat·ri·lin·e·al (pat-ri-lin'ē-ăl). Related to descent through the male line; inheritance of the Y chromosome is exclusively patrilineal. [L. *pater,* father, + *linea,* line]

pat·tern (pat'ern). **1.** A design. **2.** DENTISTRY A form used in making a mold, as for an inlay or partial denture framework.

butterfly p., bilateral, symmetric, pulmonary alveolar opacities sparing the periphery, on chest radiographs; usually caused by pulmonary edema.

ground-glass p., radiographic or CT appearance of hazy opacity which does not obscure underlying anatomic detail.

honeycomb p., dense, slightly irregular circular shadows, most common next to the pleura at the lung base, on chest radiographs or CT; caused by chronic interstitial fibrosis of diverse causes.

miliary p., a chest radiographic pattern of fine, rounded opacities, typical of hematogenous dissemination of tuberculosis.

mosaic p., on high-resolution CT scans of the lungs, a p. of brighter and darker regions corresponding to differences in perfusion or aeration; found in some cases of chronic thromboembolism or of bronchiolitis obliterans. Cf. oligemia.

pat·u·lous (pat'yū-lŭs). SYN patent. [L. *patulus,* fr. *pateo,* to lie open]

pau·ci·bac·il·lary (paw-sē-bas'i-lār-ē). Made up of, or denoting the presence of, few bacilli.

pau·ci·sy·nap·tic (paw'sē-si-nap'tik). SYN oligosynaptic. [L. *paucus,* few, + synapse]

pause (pawz). Temporary stop. [G. *pausis,* cessation]

apneic p., cessation of air flow for more than 10 seconds. SEE sleep *apnea.*

compensatory p., the p. following an extrasystole, when the p. is long enough to compensate for the prematurity of the extrasystole; the short cycle ending with the extrasystole plus the p. following the extrasystole together equal two of the regular cycles.

postextrasystolic p., the somewhat prolonged cycle immediately following an extrasystole.

preautomatic p., a temporary p. in cardiac activity before an automatic pacemaker escapes. SEE ALSO escape.

respiratory p., cessation of air flow for less than 10 seconds. SEE sleep *apnea.*

sinus p., a spontaneous interruption in the regular sinus rhythm, the p. lasting for a period that is not an exact multiple of the sinus cycle. SEE ALSO sinus *arrest.*

pav·or noc·tur·nus (pā'vōr nok-ter'nŭs). SYN night-terrors. [L.]

Pb lead (plumbum).

PBG. porphobilinogen.

PCA patient-controlled *analgesia.*

pCa. A way of reporting calcium ion levels; equal to $-\log[Ca^{2+}]$.

PCH paroxysmal cold *hemoglobinuria.*

PCIS patient *c*are *i*nformation *s*ystem, the interactive computer system used to store medical records in a hospital.

PCR polymerase chain *reaction.*

PCWP Abbreviation for pulmonary capillary wedge *pressure.*

PD phenyldichloroarsine.

Pd palladium.

PDLL poorly differentiated lymphocytic *lymphoma.*

peak (pēk). The top or upper limit of a graphic tracing or of any variable. [M.E. *peke, pike,* fr. Sp. *pico,* beak, fr. L. *picus,* magpie]

kilovolt p., the highest voltage applied across an X-ray tube; it influences the penetrating power of the X-ray beam.

pearl (perl). **1.** A concretion formed around a grain of sand or other foreign body within the shell of certain mollusks. **2.** One of a number of small, tough masses, such as mucus occurring in the sputum in asthma.

epithelial p., SYN keratin p.

keratin p., a focus of central keratinization within concentric layers of abnormal squamous cells; seen in squamous cell carcinoma. SYN epithelial p.

peau d'orange (pō-dŏ-rahnj'). A swollen pitted skin surface overlying carcinoma of the breast in which there is both stromal infiltration and lymphatic obstruction with edema. [Fr. orange peel]

pec·cant (pek'ant). Unhealthy; producing disease. [L. *peccans* (*-ant-*), pres. p. of *pecco*, to sin]

pec·ten (pek'ten). **1** [NA]. A structure with comblike processes or projections. **2.** SYN anal p. [L. comb]

  anal p., the middle third of the anal canal. SYN p. analis [NA], pecten (2).

  p. ana'lis [NA], SYN anal p.

  p. pu'bis, the continuation on the superior ramus pubis of the linea terminalis, forming a sharp ridge.

pec·ten·i·tis (pek-ten-ī'tis). Inflammation of the sphincter ani. [L. *pecten*, a comb, + G. *-itis*, inflammation]

pec·ten·o·sis (pek-ten-ō'sis). Exaggerated enlargement of the pecten band.

pec·ti·nate (pek'ti-nāt). **1.** Combed; comb-shaped. SYN pectiniform. **2.** In fungi, used to describe a particular type of branching hyphae in cultures of dermatophytes.

pec·tin·e·al (pek-tin'ē-ăl). Ridged; relating to the os pubis or to any comblike structure.

pec·tin·i·form (pek-tin'i-fōrm). SYN pectinate (1).

pec·to·ral (pek'tŏ-răl). Relating to the chest. [L. *pectoralis; fr. pectus,* breast bone]

pec·to·ril·o·quy (pek-tō-ril'ō-kwē). Increased transmission of the voice sound through the pulmonary structures, so that it is clearly audible on auscultation of the chest; usually indicates consolidation of the underlying lung parenchyma. [L. *pectus,* chest, + *loquor,* to speak]

pec·tus, gen. **pec·to·ris,** pl. **pec·to·ra** (pek'tŭs, pek'tō-ris, pek'tō-ră) [NA]. SYN chest. [L.]

  p. carina'tum, flattening of the chest on either side with forward projection of the sternum resembling the keel of a boat. SYN chicken breast, pigeon breast.

  p. excava'tum, a hollow at the lower part of the chest caused by a backward displacement of the xiphoid cartilage. SYN funnel breast, funnel chest.

△**ped-, pedi-, pedo-. 1.** Child. [G. *pais,* child] **2.** Foot, feet. [L. *pes,* foot]

ped·al (ped'ăl). Relating to the feet, or to any structure called pes. [L. *pedalis,* fr. *pes* (*ped-*), a foot]

ped·er·as·ty (ped'er-as-tē). Sexual relations between a man and a boy. [G. *paiderastia; fr. pais* (*paid-*), boy, + *eraō*, to long for]

pe·de·sis (pē-dē'sis). SYN brownian *movement.* [G. *pēdēsis*, a leaping]

△**pedi-.** SEE ped-.

pe·di·at·ric (pē-dē-at'rik). Relating to pediatrics. [G. *pais* (*paid-*), child, + *iatrikos,* relating to medicine]

pe·di·a·tric·ian (pē'dē-ă-trish'ăn). A specialist in pediatrics.

pe·di·at·rics (pē-dē-at'riks). The medical specialty concerned with the study and treatment of children in health and disease during development from birth through adolescence. [G. *pais* (*paid-*), child, + *iatreia,* medical treatment]

ped·i·cel (ped'i-sel). The secondary process of a podocyte, which helps form the visceral capsule of a renal corpuscle. SYN foot process, footplate (2), foot-plate. [Mod. L. *pedicellus,* dim. of L. *pes,* foot]

ped·i·cel·late (ped'i-sel-lāt). SYN pediculate.

ped·i·cel·la·tion (ped'i-sĕ-lā'shŭn). Formation of a pedicle or peduncle.

ped·i·cle (ped'ĭ-kl). **1.** A constricted portion or stalk. SYN pediculus (1) [NA]. **2.** A stalk by which a nonsessile tumor is attached to normal tissue. SYN pedunculus [NA], peduncle (2). **3.** A stalk through which a flap receives nourishment until its transfer to another site results in the nourishment coming from that site. [L. *pediculus,* dim. of *pes,* foot]

pe·dic·u·lar (pĕ-dik'yū-lăr). Relating to pediculi, or lice. [L. *pedicularis*]

pe·dic·u·late (pĕ-dik'yū-lāt). Not sessile, having a pedicle or peduncle. SYN pedicellate, pedunculate. [L. *pediculatus*]

pe·dic·u·la·tion (pĕ-dik'yū-lā'shŭn). Infestation with lice. [L. *pediculus,* louse]

pe·dic·u·li (pĕ-dik'yū-lī). Plural of pediculus. [L.]

pe·dic·u·li·cide (pĕ-dik'yū-li-sīd). An agent used to destroy lice. [L. *pediculus,* louse, + *caedo,* to kill]

pe·dic·u·lo·sis (pĕ-dik'yū-lō'sis). The state of being infested with lice. [L. *pediculus,* louse, + G. *-osis,* condition]

⬛**p. pu'bis,** infestation with the pubic or crab louse, *Pthirus pubis,* especially in pubic hair, causing pruritus and maculae ceruleae.

pe·dic·u·lous (pĕ-dik'yū-lŭs). Infested with lice.

Pe·dic·u·lus (pĕ-dik'yū-lŭs). A genus of parasitic lice that live in the hair and feed periodically on blood. Important species include *P. humanus* var. *capitis,* the head louse of man; *P. humanus* var. *corporis* (also called *P. corporis*), the body louse or clothes louse, which lives and lays eggs (nits) in clothing and feeds on the human body; and *P. pubis.* [L.]

pe·dic·u·lus, pl. **pe·dic·u·li** (pĕ-dik'yū-lŭs, -lī) [NA]. **1.** SYN pedicle (1). [L. pedicle] **2.** A louse. SEE *Pediculus.* [L.]

ped·i·gree (ped'i-grē). Ancestral line of descent, especially as diagrammed on a chart to show ancestral history; used in genetics to analyze inheritance. [M.E. *pedegra* fr. O.Fr. *pie de grue,* foot of crane]

△**pedo-.** SEE ped-.

pe·do·don·tics (pē-dō-don'tiks). The branch of dentistry concerned with the dental care and treatment of children. [G. *pais,* child, + *odous,* tooth]

pe·do·don·tist (pē-dō-don'tist). A dentist who practices pedodontics.

ped·o·dy·na·mom·e·ter (ped'ō-dī-nă-mom'ĕ-ter). An instrument for measuring the strength of the leg muscles. [L. *pes* (*ped-*), foot, + G. *dynamis*, force, + G. *metron*, measure]

pe•do•mor•phism (pē-dō-mōr′fizm). Description of adult behavior in terms appropriate to child behavior. [G. *pais* (*paid*), child, + *morphē*, form]

pe•do•phil•ia (pē-dō-fil′ē-ă). An abnormal sexual attraction to children in an adult. [G. *pais*, child, + *philos*, fond]

pe•do•phil•ic (pē-dō-fil′ik). Relating to or exhibiting pedophilia.

pe•dun•cle (pe-dŭng′kl, pē′dŭng-kl). **1.** In neuroanatomy, term loosely applied to a variety of stalklike connecting structures in the brain, composed either exclusively of white matter (*e.g.*, cerebellar p.) or of white and gray matter (*e.g.*, cerebral p. **2.** SYN pedicle (2). [Mod. L. *pedunculus*, dim. of *pes*, foot]

cerebellar p., pedunculus cerebellaris inferior, medius, and superior.

cerebral p., Large bundles of corticofugal fibers forming the *crus* cerebri, plus the midbrain tegmentum; the substantia nigra, while a part of the base of the p. (basis pedunculi), is considered a structure separating the midbrain tegmentum from the crus cerebri. SEE ALSO *crus* cerebri.

inferior cerebellar p., large paired bundles of nerve fibers which develop on the dorsolateral surfaces of the upper medulla, extend under the lateral recesses of the rhomboid fossa and curve dorsally into the cerebellum medial to the middle cerebellar peduncle; composed of a larger (lateral) bundle, the restiform body, and a small (medial) bundle, the juxtarestiform body. Fibers forming this composite bundle originate from spinal neurons and medullary relay nuclei. The largest constituent (restiform body) is crossed fibers from the inferior olive; it also contains the dorsal spinocerebellar tract and cerebellar projections from the lateral reticular nucleus, the accessory cuneate nucleus, the paramedian reticular nuclei and the perihypoglossal nuclei. Vestibulocerebellar fibers are placed medially in the inferior cerebellar p. and are usually separately identified as the juxtarestiform body.

inferior thalamic p., a large fiber bundle emerging from the anterior part of the thalamus in the ventral direction, in part joining the medial fibers of the internal capsule, in other part curving laterally around the medial margin of the capsule into the innominate substance. Many of its fibers establish a reciprocal connection of the mediodorsal nucleus of the thalamus with the orbital gyri of the frontal lobe, but numerous other fibers constitute a conduction system from the amygdala and olfactory cortex to the mediodorsal nucleus. SEE ALSO *ansa* peduncularis.

lateral thalamic p., the massive group of fibers that emerges from the laterodorsal side of the thalamus to join the corona radiata; it reciprocally connects the lateral nucleus and the geniculate bodies of the thalamus with the corresponding regions of the cerebral cortex.

middle cerebellar p., the largest of three paired cerebellar p.'s, composed mainly of fibers that originate in the pontine nuclei, cross the midline in the ventral part of pons, and emerge on the

opposite side as a massive bundle arching dorsally along the lateral side of the pontine tegmentum into the cerebellum; its fibers are distributed chiefly to the cortex of the cerebellar hemisphere.

superior cerebellar p., a large bundle of nerve fibers that originate from the dentate and interpositus nuclei and emerges from the cerebellum in the rostral direction, along the lateral wall of the fourth ventricle. The bundle submerges from the dorsal surface of the brainstem into the mesencephalic tegmentum, where all of its fibers cross in the massive decussation of the superior cerebellar p.'s. Part of the bundle terminates in the contralateral red nucleus; the bulk of the fibers continue rostrally to parts of the ventral intermediate nucleus of thalamus, ventral posterolateral nucleus of thalamus, and central lateral nucleus of thalamus.

thalamic p., pedunculus thalami inferior, lateralis, and ventralis.

ventral thalamic p., the massive system of fiber bundles emerging through the ventral, lateral, and anterior borders of the thalamus to join the internal capsule and parts of the corona radiata; it contains the fibers reciprocally connecting the ventral thalamic nuclei with the precentral and postcentral gyri of the cerebral cortex.

pe•dun•cu•lar (pĕ-dŭng′kyū-lăr). Relating to a pedicle or peduncle.

pe•dun•cu•late (pĕ-dŭng′kyū-lāt). SYN pediculate.

pe•dun•cu•lot•o•my (pe-dŭng′kyū-lot′ō-mē). **1.** A total or partial section of a cerebral peduncle. **2.** A mesencephalic pyramidal tractotomy. [peduncle + G. *tomē*, incision]

pe•dun•cu•lus, pl. **pe•dun•cu•li** (pe-dŭng′kyū-lŭs, -kyū-lī) [NA]. SYN pedicle (2). [Mod. L. dim. of *pes*, foot]

PEEP positive end-expiratory *pressure*.

intrinsic PEEP, SYN auto-positive end-expiratory *pressure*.

occult PEEP, SYN auto-positive end-expiratory *pressure*.

peer re•view. Assessment of research proposals, manuscripts submitted for publication, or a physician's clinical practice by other physicians or scientists in the same field.

PEFR peak *flowmeter*.

pe•li•o•sis (pē-lē-ō′sis, pel-). SYN purpura. [G. *peliōsis*, a livid spot, livor]

p. hep′atis, the presence throughout the liver of blood-filled cavities which may become lined by endothelium or become organized; a feature of bacillary angiomatosis, caused by *Rochalimaea henselae* in immunocompromised persons.

pel•lag•ra (pĕ-lag′ră, pĕ-lā′gră). An affection characterized by diarrhea, dermatitis, and dementia due to dietary deficiency of niacin. [It. *pelle*, skin, + *agra*, rough]

pel•lag•rous (pĕ-lag′rŭs). Relating to or suffering from pellagra.

pel•let (pel′et). **1.** A pilule, or very small pill. **2.** A small rod-shaped dosage form composed essentially of pure steroid hormones in compressed form, intended for subcutaneous implantation in body tissues; serves as a depot providing for the slow release of the hormone over an extended period of time. [Fr. *pelote;* L. *pila,* a ball]

pel·li·cle (pel'i-kl). **1.** Literally and nonspecifically, a thin skin. **2.** A film or scum on the surface of a liquid. **3.** Cell boundary of sporozoites and merozoites among members of the protozoan subphylum Apicomplexa (Sporozoa), consisting of an outer unit membrane and an inner layer of two unit membranes. [L. *pellicula,* dim of *pellis,* skin]

pel·lu·cid (pe-lū'sid). Allowing the passage of light. [L. *pellucidus*]

pel·ta·tion (pel-tā'shŭn). Protection provided by inoculation with an antiserum or with a vaccine. [L. *pelta,* a light shield, fr. G. *peltē*]

△**pelvi-, pelvio-, pelvo-.** The pelvis. Cf. pyelo-. [L. *pelvis,* basin (pelvis)]

pel·vic (pel'vik). Relating to a pelvis.

pel·vic di·rec·tion (pel'vik dī-rek'shŭn). The direction of the axis of the pelvis.

pel·vi·ceph·a·lom·e·try (pel'vi-sef-ă-lom'ĕ-trē). Measurement of the female pelvic diameters in relation to those of the fetal head. [pelvi- + G. *kephalē,* head, + *metron,* measure]

pel·vi·fix·a·tion (pel-vi-fik-sā'shŭn). Surgical attachment of a floating pelvic organ to the wall of the pelvic cavity.

pel·vi·li·thot·o·my (pel'vi-li-thot'ō-mē). SYN pyelolithotomy. [pelvi- + G. *lithos,* stone, + *tomē,* incision]

pel·vim·e·ter (pel-vim'ĕ-ter). Calipers for measuring the diameters of the pelvis.

pel·vim·e·try (pel-vim'ĕ-trē). Measurement of the diameters of the pelvis. [pelvi- + G. *metron,* measure]

△**pelvio-.** SEE pelvi-.

pel·vi·o·plas·ty (pel'vē-ō-plas-tē). **1.** Symphysiotomy or pubiotomy for enlargement of the female pelvic outlet. **2.** SYN pyeloplasty. [pelvio- + G. *plastos,* formed]

pel·vi·ot·o·my, pel·vit·o·my (pel'vē-ot'ō-mē). **1.** SYN symphysiotomy. **2.** SYN pubiotomy. **3.** SYN pyelotomy. [pelvio- + G. *tomē,* incision]

pel·vi·per·i·to·ni·tis (pel-vē-per-i-tō-nī'tis). SYN pelvic *peritonitis.*

pel·vis, pl. **pel·ves** (pel'vis, pel'vēz). **1** [NA]. The massive cup-shaped ring of bone, with its ligaments, at the lower end of the trunk, formed of the hip bone (the pubic bone, ilium, and ischium) on either side and in front, and of the sacrum and the coccyx posteriorly. **2.** Any basinlike or cup-shaped cavity, as the p. of the kidney. [L. basin]

android p., a masculine or funnel-shaped p.

anthropoid p., an apelike p., with a long anteroposterior diameter and a narrow transverse diameter.

assimilation p., a deformity in which the transverse processes of the last lumbar vertebra are fused with the sacrum, or the last sacral with the first coccygeal body.

beaked p., SYN osteomalacic p.

brachypellic p., a p. in which the transverse diameter is more than 1 cm longer but less than 3 cm longer than the anteroposterior diameter.

contracted p., a p. with less than normal measurements in any diameter.

cordate p., cordiform p., a p. with sacrum

projecting forward between the ilia, giving to the brim a heart shape.

dolichopellic p., a p. in which the anteroposterior diameter is longer than the transverse.

false p., SYN greater p.

flat p., a p. in which the anteroposterior diameter is uniformly contracted, the sacrum being dislocated forward between the iliac bones.

frozen p., a condition in which the true p. is indurated throughout, especially by carcinoma.

funnel-shaped p., a p. in which the pelvic inlet dimensions are normal, but the outlet is contracted in the transverse or in both transverse and anteroposterior diameters.

greater p., the expanded portion of the p. above the brim. SYN false p.

gynecoid p., the normal female p.

p. jus'to ma'jor, a symmetrical p. with greater than normal measurements in all diameters.

p. jus'to mi'nor, a p. of the female type, but with all its diameters smaller than normal.

juvenile p., a p. justo minor in which the bones are slender.

kyphotic p., backward curvature of the lumbar spine causing contraction of pelvic measurements.

lesser p., the cavity of the p. below the brim or superior aperture.

masculine p., (1) a p. justo minor in which the bones are large and heavy; (2) a slight degree of funnel-shaped p. in the woman, in which the shape approximates that of the male p.

osteomalacic p., a pelvic deformity in osteomalacia; the pressure of the trunk on the sacrum and lateral pressure of the femoral heads produce a pelvic aperture that is three-cornered or has the shape of a heart or a cloverleaf, while the pubic bone becomes beak shaped. SYN beaked p.

platypellic p., flat oval p., in which the transverse diameter is more than 3 cm longer than the anteroposterior diameter.

platypelloid p., simple flat p.

Prague p., SYN spondylolisthetic p.

rachitic p., a contracted and deformed p., most commonly a flat p., occurring from rachitic softening of the bones in early life.

renal p., a flattened funnel-shaped expansion of the upper end of the ureter receiving the calices, the apex being continuous with the ureter.

Rokitansky's p., SYN spondylolisthetic p.

scoliotic p., a deformed p. associated with lateral curvature of the spine.

split p., a p. in which the symphysis pubis is absent, the pelvic bones being separated; usually associated with exstrophy of the bladder.

spondylolisthetic p., a p. whose brim is more or less occluded by a forward dislocation of the body of the lower lumbar vertebra. SYN Prague p., Rokitansky's p.

△**pelvo-.** SEE pelvi-.

pem·phi·goid (pem'fi-goyd). **1.** Resembling pemphigus. **2.** A disease resembling pemphigus but significantly distinguishable histologically (nonacantholytic) and clinically (generally benign course). [G. *pemphix,* blister, + *eidos,* resemblance]

bullous p., a chronic, generally benign disease,

most commonly of old age, characterized by tense nonacantholytic bullae in which serum antibodies are localized to the epidermal basement membrane, causing detachment of the entire thickness of the epidermis.

cicatricial p., a chronic disease that produces adhesions and progressive cicatrization and shrinkage of the conjunctival, oral, and vaginal mucous membranes.

pem•phi•gus (pem'fi-gŭs). **1.** Auto-immune bullous diseases with acantholysis: p. vulgaris, p. foliaceus, p. erythematosus, or p. vegetans. **2.** A nonspecific term for blistering skin diseases. [G. *pemphix*, a blister]

p. erythemato'sus, an eruption involving sun-exposed skin, especially the face; the lesions are scaling erythematous macules and blebs.

p. folia'ceus, a generally chronic form of p. in which extensive exfoliative dermatitis may be present in addition to the bullae.

p. gangreno'sus, (1) SYN *dermatitis* gangrenosa infantum. **(2)** SYN bullous *impetigo* of newborn.

p. vulga'ris, a serious form of p., occurring in middle age, in which cutaneous bullae and oral erosions may be localized a few months before becoming generalized; blisters break easily and are slow to heal; results from the action of autoimmune antibodies that localize to intercellular sites of stratified squamous epithelium.

pe•nes. Plural of penis.

pen•e•trance (pen'ĕ-trans). The frequency, expressed as a fraction or percentage, of individuals who are phenotypically affected, among persons of an appropriate genotype; factors affecting expression may be environmental, or due to purely random variation; contrasted with hypostasis where the condition has a genetic origin and therefore tends to cause correlation in relatives. [see penetration]

△**-penia.** Deficiency. [G. *penia,* poverty]

Pen•i•cil•li•um (pen-i-sil'ē-ŭm). A genus of fungi species of which yield various antibiotic substances and biologicals. [see penicillus]

pen•i•cil•lus, pl. **pe•ni•cil•li** (pen-i-sil'ŭs, -sil'ī). **1** [NA]. One of the tufts formed by the repeated subdivision of the minute arterial twigs in the spleen. **2.** In fungi, one of the branched conidiophores bearing chains of conidia in *Penicillium* species. [L. paint brush]

pe•nile (pē'nīl). Relating to the penis.

pe•nis, pl. **pe•nes** (pē'nis) [NA]. The organ of copulation in the male; it is formed of three columns of erectile tissue, two arranged laterally on the dorsum (corpora cavernosa p.) and one median below (corpus spongiosum); the urethra traverses the latter; the extremity (glans p.) is formed by an expansion of the corpus spongiosum, and is more or less completely covered by a free fold of skin (preputium). SYN phallus. [L. tail]

pe•nis•chi•sis (pē-nis'ki-sis). A fissure of the penis resulting in an abnormal opening into the urethra, either above (epispadias), below (hypospadias), or to one side (paraspadias). [L. *penis* + G. *schisis,* fissure]

pen•nate (pen'āt). Feathered; resembling a feather. SYN penniform. [L. *pennatus,* fr. *penna,* feather]

pen•ni•form (pen'i-fŏrm). SYN pennate. [L. *penna,* feather, + *forma,* form]

△**penta-.** five. [G. *pente,* five]

pen•tose (pen'tōs). A monosaccharide containing five carbon atoms in the molecule.

pen•to•su•ria (pen-tō-sū'rē-ă). The excretion of one or more pentoses in the urine.

alimentary p., the urinary excretion of L-arabinose and L-xylose, as the result of the excessive ingestion of fruits containing these pentoses.

pen•tyl (pen'til). **1.** SYN amyl. **2.** The $CH_3(CH_2)_3CH_2$– moiety.

penumbra. RADIOLOGY The blurred margin of an image. SYN geometric unsharpness.

pep•lo•mer (pep'lō-mer). A part or subunit of the peplos of a virion, the assemblage of which produces the complete peplos, produced from the peplos by detergent treatment. [see peplos]

pep•los (pep'lōs). The coat or envelope of lipoprotein material that surrounds certain virions. [G. an outer garment worn by women]

pep•sin•o•gen (pep-sin'ō-jen). A proenzyme formed and secreted by the chief cells of the gastric mucosa; the acidity of the gastric juice and pepsin itself remove 42 amino acid residues from p. to form active pepsin. SYN propepsin. [pepsin + G. *-gen,* producing]

pep•tic (pep'tik). Relating to the stomach, to gastric digestion, or to pepsin A. [G. *peptikos,* fr. *peptō,* to digest]

pep•ti•dase (pep'ti-dās). Any enzyme capable of hydrolyzing one of the peptide links of a peptide; *e.g.,* carboxypeptidases, aminopeptidases.

pep•tide (pep'tīd). A compound of two or more amino acids in which a carboxyl group of one is united with an amino group of another, with the elimination of a molecule of water, thus forming a peptide bond, –CO–NH–; *i.e.,* a substituted amide.

corticotropin-like intermediate-lobe p. (CLIP), product of propiomelanocortin with unknown function.

gastric inhibitory p. (GIP), SYN gastric inhibitory *polypeptide.*

pep•ti•der•gic (pep-ti-der'jik). Referring to nerve cells or fibers that are believed to employ small peptide molecules as their neurotransmitter. [peptide + G. *ergon,* work]

pep•ti•do•gly•can (pep'ti-dō-glī'kan). A compound containing amino acids (or peptides) linked to sugars, with the latter preponderant. Cf. glycopeptide.

pep•ti•doid (pep'ti-doyd). A condensation product of two amino acids involving at least one condensing group other than the α-carboxyl or α-amino group; *e.g.,* glutathione.

pep•ti•do•lyt•ic (pep'ti-dō-lit'ik). Causing the cleavage or digestion of peptides. [peptide + G. *lytikos,* solvent]

pep•ti•dyl di•pep•ti•dase A (pep'ti-dil). A hydrolase cleaving C-terminal dipeptides from a variety of substrates, including angiotensin I, which is converted to angiotensin II and histidylleucine. An important step in the metabolism of certain vasopressor agents.

Pep·to·coc·cus (pep'tō-kok'ŭs). A genus of nonmotile, anaerobic, chemoorganotrophic bacteria containing Gram-positive, spherical cells that occur singly, in pairs, tetrads, or irregular masses, rarely in short chains. They are frequently found in association with pathologic conditions. The type species is *P. niger.* [G. *peptō,* to digest, + *kokkos,* berry]

pep·to·gen·ic, pep·tog·e·nous (pep-tō-jen'ik, pep-toj'ĕ-nŭs). **1.** Producing peptones. **2.** Promoting digestion.

pep·tol·y·sis (pep-tol'i-sis). The hydrolysis of peptones.

pep·to·lyt·ic (pep-tō-lit'ik). **1.** Pertaining to peptolysis. **2.** Denoting an enzyme or other agent that hydrolyses peptones.

pep·tone (pep'tōn). Descriptive term applied to intermediate polypeptide products, formed in partial hydrolysis of proteins, that are soluble in water, diffusible, and not coagulable by heat; used in bacterial culture media.

pep·ton·ic (pep-ton'ik). Relating to or containing peptone.

pep·to·ni·za·tion (pep'ton-i-zā'shŭn). Conversion by enzymic action of native protein into soluble peptone.

Pep·to·strep·to·coc·cus (pep'tō-strep-tō-kok'ŭs). A genus of nonmotile, anaerobic, chemoorganotrophic bacteria containing spherical to ovoid, Gram-positive cells which occur in pairs and short or long chains. These organisms are found in normal and pathologic female genital tracts and blood in puerperal fever, in respiratory and intestinal tracts of normal humans and other animals, in the oral cavity, and in pyogenic infections, putrefactive war wounds, and appendicitis; they may be pathogenic. The type species is *P. anaerobius.* [G. *peptō,* to digest, + *streptos,* curved, + *kokkos,* berry]

per-. **1.** Through; denoting intensity. **2.** CHEMISTRY More or most, with respect to the amount of a given element or radical contained in a compound; the degree of substitution for hydrogen, as in peroxides, peroxy acids (*e.g.,* hydrogen peroxide, peroxyformic acid). SEE ALSO peroxy-. [L. through, throughout, extremely]

per·ac·id (per-as'id). An acid containing a peroxide group (–O–OH); *e.g.,* peracetic acid.

per·a·cute (per-ă-kyut'). Very acute; said of a disease. [L. *peracutus,* very sharply]

per an·um (per ā'nŭm). By or through the anus. [L.]

per·cept (per'sept). **1.** That which is perceived; the complete mental image, formed by the process of perception, of an object or idea. **2.** CLINICAL PSYCHOLOGY A single unit of perceptual report, such as one of the responses to an inkblot in the Rorschach test. [L. *perceptum,* a thing perceived]

per·cep·tion (per-sep'shun). The mental process of becoming aware of or recognizing an object or idea; primarily cognitive rather than affective or conative, although all three aspects are manifested.

    depth p., the visual ability to judge depth or distance.

    extrasensory p. (ESP), p. by means other than

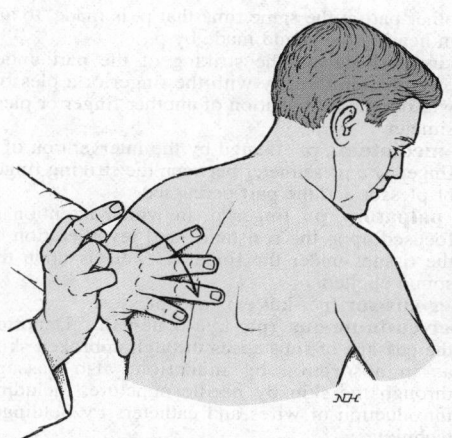

percussion: distal phalanx of left middle finger is pressed firmly against chest wall parallel with ribs; a short, quick blow is struck at the base of the distal phalanx of the middle finger with the tip of the middle finger of the right hand

through the ordinary senses; *e.g.,* telepathy, clairvoyance, precognition.

    figure-ground p., differentiation between foreground and background forms and objects.

    speech p., identification of speech sounds, mainly from acoustic cues.

per·cep·tive (per-sep'tiv). Relating to or having a higher than normal power of perception.

per·cep·tiv·i·ty (per-sep-tiv'i-tē). The power of perception.

per·co·la·tion (per-kō-lā'shŭn). **1.** SYN filtration. **2.** Extraction of the soluble portion of a solid mixture by passing a solvent liquid through it. **3.** Passage of saliva or other fluids into the interface between tooth structure and restoration; sometimes induced by thermal changes. [L. *percolatio,* fr. per- + *colare,* to strain]

per con·tig·u·um (per kon-tig'yū-ŭm). In contiguity; denoting the mode by which an inflammation or other morbid process spreads into an adjacent contiguous structure. [per- + L. *contiguus,* touching, fr. *tango,* to touch]

per con·tin·u·um (per kon-tin'yū-ŭm). In continuity; continuous; denoting the mode by which an inflammation or other morbid process spreads from one part to another through continuous tissue. [per- + L. *continuus,* holding together, continuous, fr. *teneo,* to hold]

per·cuss (per-kŭs'). To perform percussion.

per·cus·sion (per-kŭsh'ŭn). **1.** A diagnostic procedure designed to determine the density of a part by the sound produced by tapping the surface with the finger or a plessor; performed primarily over the chest to determine presence of normal air content in the lungs and over the abdomen to evaluate air in the loops of intestine. **2.** A form of massage, consisting of repeated blows or taps of varying force. [L. *percussio,* fr. *per-cutio,* pp. *-cussus,* to beat, fr. *quatio,* to shake, beat]

    auscultatory p., auscultation of the chest or

other part at the same time that p. is made, to aid in hearing the sound made by p.

immediate p., the striking of the part under examination directly with the finger or a plessor, without the intervention of another finger or plessimeter.

mediate p., p. effected by the intervention of a finger or a plessimeter between the striking finger or plessor and the part percussed.

palpatory p., finger p. in which attention is focused upon the resistance and reverberation of the tissues under the finger as well as upon the sound elicited.

per·cus·sor (per-kŭs'er). SYN plessor.

per·cu·ta·ne·ous (per-kyū-tā'nē-ŭs). Denoting the passage of substances through unbroken skin, as in absorption by inunction; also passage through the skin by needle puncture, including introduction of wires and catheters by Seldinger technique.

per·en·ceph·a·ly (per-en-sef'ă-lē). A condition marked by one or more cerebral cysts. [G. *pēra,* a purse, a wallet, + *enkephalos,* brain]

per·fec·tion·ism (per-fek'shŭn-izm). A tendency to set rigid high standards of performance for oneself.

per·fo·rat·ed (per'fō-rāt-ed). Pierced with one or more holes. [L. *perforatus,* fr. *per-foro,* pp. *-atus,* to bore through]

▣ **per·fo·ra·tion** (per-fō-rā'shŭn). Abnormal opening in a hollow organ or viscus. SYN tresis. [see perforated]

per·fo·rin (per'fōr-in). A protein found in the cytoplasmic granules of both T cytotoxic lymphocytes and natural killer cells, implicated in target cell lysis. [L. *per-foro,* to bore, pierce, + -in]

performance (per-for-mans). Organized patterns of behavior that are characteristic or expected of a person in a given situation.

p. areas, activities of daily living, work or other productive activity, play, and leisure that determine a person's functional abilities and define human activity.

p. components, sensorimotor, cognitive, psychosocial, and psychological elements of functional p. that are required for successful engagement in p. areas and that are evaluated and addressed during intervention for the purpose of improving p.

p. context, the physical, social, and cultural features of the environment that influence p. of meaningful and purposeful life tasks of daily life.

per·fuse (per-fyŭs'). To force blood or other fluid to flow from the artery through the vascular bed of a tissue or to flow through the lumen of a hollow structure (*e.g.,* an isolated renal tubule). [L. *perfusio,* fr. per- + *fusio,* a pouring]

per·fu·sion (per-fyū'zhŭn). **1.** The act of perfusing. **2.** The flow of blood or other perfusate per unit volume of tissue, as in ventilation/perfusion ratio.

△**peri-.** Around, about, near. Cf. circum-. [G. around]

per·i·ad·e·ni·tis (per'ē-ad-ĕ-nī'tis). Inflammation of the tissues surrounding a gland. [peri- + G. *adēn,* gland, + *-itis,* inflammation]

p. muco'sa necrot'ica recur'rens, SYN *aphthae* major, under *aphtha.*

per·i·an·gi·tis (per'ē-an-jī'tis). Inflammation of the adventitia of a blood vessel or of the tissues surrounding it or a lymphatic vessel. SEE ALSO periarteritis, periphlebitis, perilymphangitis. SYN perivasculitis. [peri- + G. *angeion,* a vessel, + *-itis,* inflammation]

per·i·a·or·ti·tis (per'ē-ā-ōr-tī'tis). Inflammation of the adventitia of the aorta and of the tissues surrounding it.

per·i·ap·i·cal (per-ē-ap'i-kăl). **1.** At or around the apex of a root of a tooth. **2.** Denoting the periapex.

per·i·ap·pen·di·ci·tis (per'ē-ă-pen-di-sī'tis). Inflammation of the tissue surrounding the vermiform appendix.

per·i·ar·te·ri·tis (per'ē-ar-ter-ī'tis). Inflammation of the adventitia of an artery.

p. nodo'sa, SYN *polyarteritis* nodosa.

per·i·ar·thri·tis (per'ē-ar-thrī'tis). Inflammation of the parts surrounding a joint. [peri- + arthritis]

per·i·bron·chi·o·li·tis (per'i-brong'kē-ō-lī'tis). Inflammation of the tissues surrounding the bronchioles.

per·i·bron·chi·tis (per'i-brong-kī'tis). Inflammation of the tissues surrounding the bronchi or bronchial tubes.

per·i·car·dia (per-i-kar'dē-ă). Plural of pericardium.

per·i·car·di·ac, per·i·car·di·al (per-i-kar'dē-ak, -dē-ăl). **1.** Surrounding the heart. **2.** Relating to the pericardium.

per·i·car·di·cen·te·sis (per-i-kar'dē-sen-tē'sis). Needle drainage of the pericardium, usually accompanied by placement of an indwelling catheter for continuing drainage.

per·i·car·di·ec·to·my (per'i-kar-dē-ek'tō-mē). Excision of a portion of the pericardium. [pericardium + G. *ektomē,* excision]

per·i·car·di·o·per·i·to·ne·al (per-i-kar'dē-ō-per-i-tō-nē'ăl). Relating to the pericardial and peritoneal cavities.

per·i·car·di·o·phren·ic (per-i-kar'dē-ō-fren'ik). Relating to the pericardium and the diaphragm. [pericardium + G. *phrēn,* diaphragm]

per·i·car·di·o·pleur·al (per-i-kar'dē-ō-plūr'ăl). Relating to the pericardial and pleural cavities.

per·i·car·di·or·rha·phy (per'i-kar-dē-ōr'ă-fē). Suture of the pericardium. [pericardium + G. *rhaphē,* suture]

per·i·car·di·os·to·my (per'i-kar-dē-os'tō-mē). Establishment of an opening into the pericardium. [pericardium + G. *stoma,* mouth]

per·i·car·di·ot·o·my (per'i-kar-dē-ot'ō-mē). Incision into the pericardium. [pericardium + G. *tomē,* incision]

per·i·car·dit·ic (per'i-kar-dit'ik). Relating to pericarditis.

per·i·car·di·tis (per'i-kar-dī'tis). Inflammation of the pericardium.

adhesive p., p. with adhesions between the two pericardial layers, between the pericardium and heart, or between the pericardium and neighboring structures.

constrictive p., postinflammatory thickening and scarring of the membrane producing constric-

tion of the cardiac chambers; may be acute, subacute, or chronic. Formerly called chronic constrictive p.

p. with effusion, pericardial inflammation producing excess pericardial fluid.

fibrinous p., acute p. with fibrinous exudate.

internal adhesive p., SYN concretio cordis.

p. oblit´erans, inflammation of the pericardium
leading to adhesion of the two layers, obliterating
the sac. SEE ALSO adhesive p.

postpericardiotomy p., a syndrome characterized by fever, substernal chest pain, and pericardial rub following cardiac surgery.

per·i·car·di·um, pl. **per·i·car·dia** (per-i-kar´dē-
ŭm, -ă) [NA]. The fibroserous membrane, consisting of mesothelium and submesothelial connective tissue, covering the heart and beginnings
of the great vessels. It is a closed sac having two
layers: the visceral layer (epicardium), immediately surrounding the heart, and the outer parietal
layer, forming the sac, composed of strong fibrous tissue, the fibrous p. fibrosum, lined with
serous membrane, serous pericardium. SYN heart
sac, theca cordis. [L. fr. G. *pericardion,* the
membrane around the heart]

per·i·cho·lan·gi·tis (per´i-kō-lan-jī´tis). Inflammation of the tissues around the bile ducts. [peri-
+ G. *cholē,* bile, + *angeion,* vessel, + *-itis,* inflam-
mation]

per·i·chon·dral, per·i·chon·dri·al (per-i-kon´
drăl, -kon´drē-ăl). Relating to the perichondrium.

per·i·chon·dri·tis (per´i-kon-drī´tis). Inflammation of the perichondrium.

per·i·chon·dri·um (per-i-kon´drē-ŭm) [NA].
The dense, irregular connective tissue membrane
around cartilage. [peri- + G. *chondros,* cartilage]

per·i·chrome (per´i-krōm). Denoting a nerve cell
in which the chromophil substance, or stainable
material, is scattered throughout the cytoplasm.
[peri- + G. *chrōma,* a color]

per·i·co·li·tis (per´i-kō-lī´tis). Inflammation of
the connective tissue or peritoneum surrounding
the colon. SYN serocolitis.

per·i·col·pi·tis (per´i-kol-pī´tis). SYN perivagini-
tis. [peri- + G. *kolpos,* bosom (vagina), + *-itis,*
inflammation]

per·i·cor·o·ni·tis (per-i-kōr-o-nī´tis). Inflammation around the crown of a tooth, usually one that
is incompletely erupted into the oral cavity. [peri-
+ L. *corona,* crown, + G. *-itis,* inflammation]

per·i·cra·ni·tis (per´i-krā-nī´tis). Inflammation
of the pericranium.

per·i·cra·ni·um (per´i-krā´nē-ŭm) [NA]. The
periosteum of the skull. [peri- + G. *kranion,*
skull]

per·i·cys·tic (per´i-sis´tik). **1.** Surrounding the
urinary bladder. **2.** Surrounding the gallbladder.
3. Surrounding a cyst. SYN perivesical. [peri- +
G. *kystis,* bladder]

per·i·cys·ti·tis (per´i-sis-tī´tis). Inflammation of
the tissues surrounding a bladder, especially the
urinary bladder.

per·i·cyte (per´i-sīt). One of the slender mesen-
chymal-like cells found in close association with
the outside wall of postcapillary venules; it is
relatively undifferentiated and may become a fi-

broblast, macrophage, or smooth muscle cell. SYN
adventitial cell. [peri- + G. *kytos,* cell]

per·i·derm, per·i·der·ma (per´i-derm, -i-der´
mă). The outermost layer of the epidermis of the
embryo and fetus to the sixth month of intrauterine life; desquamated epitrichial cells are a considerable component of the vernix caseosa. SYN
epitrichium. [peri- + G. *derma,* skin]

per·i·des·mi·tis (per´i-dez-mī´tis). Inflammation
of the connective tissue surrounding a ligament.
[peri- + G. *desmos,* band, + *-itis,* inflammation]

per·i·des·mi·um (per-i-dez´mē-ŭm). The connective tissue membrane surrounding a ligament.
[peri- + G. *desmion (desmos),* band]

per·i·did·y·mi·tis (per´i-did-i-mī´tis). Inflammation of the perididymis.

per·i·di·ver·tic·u·li·tis (per´i-dī´ver-tik´yū-lī´tis).
Inflammation of the tissues around an intestinal
diverticulum.

per·i·du·o·de·ni·tis (per´i-dū´ō-dē-nī´tis). Inflammation around the duodenum.

per·i·en·ceph·a·li·tis (per´ē-en-sef-ă-lī´tis). Inflammation of the cerebral membranes, particularly leptomeningitis or inflammation of the pia
mater with involvement of the underlying cortex.
[peri- + G. *enkephalos,* brain]

per·i·en·ter·i·tis (per´ē-en-ter-ī´tis). Inflammation of the peritoneal coat of the intestine. SYN
seroenteritis.

per·i·e·soph·a·gi·tis (per´ē-e-sof´ă-jī´tis). Inflammation of the tissues surrounding the esophagus.

per·i·fol·lic·u·li·tis (per´i-fŏ-lik´yū-lī´tis). The
presence of an inflammatory infiltrate surrounding hair follicles; frequently occurs in conjunction with folliculitis.

per·i·gas·tri·tis (per´i-gas-trī´tis). Inflammation
of the peritoneal coat of the stomach.

per·i·glot·tis (per-i-glot´is). The mucous membrane of the tongue. [G. *periglōttis,* covering of
the tongue]

per·i·hep·a·ti·tis (pĕr´i-hep-ă-tī´tis). Inflammation of the serous, or peritoneal, covering of the
liver. [peri- + G. *hēpar,* liver, + *-itis,* inflamma-
tion]

per·i·je·ju·ni·tis (per´i-jĕ-jū-nī´tis). Inflammation around the jejunum.

per·i·kar·y·on, pl. **per·i·kar·ya** (per-i-kar´ē-on,
-ă). **1.** The cytoplasm around the nucleus, such as
that of the cell body of nerve cells. **2.** The body
of the odontoblast, excluding the dentinal fiber. **3.**
The cell body of the nerve cell, as distinguished
from its axon and dendrites. [peri- + G. *karyon,*
kernel]

per·i·lab·y·rin·thi·tis (per´i-lab´ĭ-rin-thī´tis). Inflammation of the parts about the labyrinth.

per·i·lymph (per´i-limf). The fluid contained
within the osseus labyrinth, surrounding and protecting the membranous labyrinth; perilymph resembles extracellular fluid in composition (sodium salts are the predominant positive electrolyte) and, via the perilymphatic duct, is in continuity with cerebrospinal fluid. SYN perilympha
[NA].

per·i·lym·pha (per´i-lim´fă) [NA]. SYN perilymph. [peri- + L. *lympha,* a clear fluid (lymph)]

per·i·lym·phan·gi·tis (per´i-lim-fan-jī´tis). Inflammation of the tissues surrounding a lymphatic vessel.

per·i·lym·phat·ic (per'i-lim-fat'ik). 1. Surrounding a lymphatic structure (node or vessel). 2. The spaces and tissues surrounding the membranous labyrinth of the inner ear.

per·i·men·in·gi·tis (per'i-men-in-jī'tis). SYN pachymeningitis.

pe·rim·e·ter (pe-rim'ĕ-ter). 1. A circumference, edge, or border. 2. An instrument, usually half a circle or sphere, used to measure the field of vision. [G. *perimetros*, circumference, fr. *peri*, around, + *metron*, measure]

per·i·met·ric (per-i-met'rik). 1. Surrounding the uterus; relating to the perimetrium. SYN periuterine. [G. *peri*, around, + *mētra*, uterus] 2. Relating to the circumference of any part or area. [G. *perimetros*, circumference] 3. Relating to perimetry.

per·i·me·trit·ic (per-i-me-trit'ik). Relating to or marked by perimetritis.

per·i·me·tri·tis (per'i-me-trī'tis). SYN metroperitonitis. [perimetrium + G. *-itis*, inflammation]

per·i·me·tri·um, pl. **per·i·me·tria** (per-i-mē'trē-ŭm, -ă) [NA]. The serous (peritoneal) coat of the uterus. [peri- + G. *mētra*, uterus]

pe·rim·e·try (pe-rim'ĕ-trē). 1. The determination of the limits of the visual field. 2. The mapping of the sensitivity contours of the visual field. [G. *perimetros*, circumference]

per·i·mol·y·sis (per-ē-mol'i-sis). Decalcification of the teeth from exposure to gastric acid in individuals with chronic vomiting. [=perimylolysis, fr. peri- + G. *mylos*, molar + *lysis*, loosening, dissolving, fr. *luō*, to loosen]

per·i·my·e·li·tis (per'i-mī-ĕ-lī'tis). SYN endosteitis.

per·i·my·o·si·tis (per'i-mī-ō-sī'tis). Inflammation of the loose cellular tissue surrounding a muscle. SYN perimysiitis (2), perimysitis.

per·i·my·si·al (per-i-mis'ē-ăl, -miz'ē-ăl). Relating to the perimysium; surrounding a muscle.

per·i·my·si·i·tis, per·i·my·si·tis (per'i-mis-ē-ī'tis, -mī-sī'tis). 1. Inflammation of the perimysium. 2. SYN perimyositis.

per·i·my·si·um, pl. **per·i·my·sia** (per-i-mis'ē-ŭm, -miz'ē-ŭm; -ē-ă) [NA]. The fibrous sheath enveloping each of the primary bundles of skeletal muscle fibers. [peri- + G. *mys*, muscle]

per·i·na·tal (per-i-nā'tăl). Occurring during, or pertaining to, the periods before, during, or after the time of birth; *i.e.*, before delivery from the 28th week of gestation through the first 7 days after delivery. [peri- + L. *natus*, pp. of *nascor*, to be born]

per·i·na·tol·o·gist (per-i-nā-tol'ō-jist). An obstetrician who subspecializes in perinatology.

per·i·na·tol·o·gy (per-i-nā-tol'ō-jē). A subspecialty of obstetrics concerned with care of the mother and fetus during pregnancy, labor, and delivery, particularly when the mother and/or fetus are at a high risk for complications. SYN perinatal medicine.

per·i·ne·al (per'i-nē'ăl). Relating to the perineum.

⌂**perineo-.** The perineum. [L. fr. G. *perineos, perinaion*]

per·i·ne·o·cele (per-i-nē'ō-sēl). A hernia in the perineal region, either between the rectum and the vagina or the rectum and the bladder, or alongside the rectum. [perineo- + G. *kēlē*, hernia]

per·i·ne·o·plas·ty (per-i-nē'ō-plas-tē). Plastic surgery of the perineum. [perineum + G. *plastos*, formed]

per·i·ne·or·rha·phy (per-i-nē-ōr'ă-fē). Suture of the perineum, performed in perineoplasty. [perineum + G. *rhaphē*, a sewing]

per·i·ne·o·scro·tal (per-i-nē'ō-skrō'tăl). Relating to the perineum and the scrotum.

per·i·ne·os·to·my (per-i-nē-os'tō-mē). Urethrostomy through the perineum. [perineo- + G. *stoma*, mouth]

per·i·ne·ot·o·my (per-i-nē-ot'ō-mē). Incision into the perineum to facilitate childbirth. SEE ALSO episiotomy.

per·i·ne·o·vag·i·nal (per-i-nē'ō-vaj'i-năl). Relating to the perineum and the vagina.

per·i·neph·ri·al (per'i-nef'rē-ăl). Relating to the perinephrium.

per·i·neph·ri·tis (per'i-ne-frī'tis). Inflammation of perinephric tissue.

per·i·neph·ri·um, pl. **per·i·neph·ria** (per'i-nef'rē-ŭm, -nef'rē-ă). The connective tissue and fat surrounding the kidney. [peri- + G. *nephros*, kidney]

per·i·ne·um, pl. **per·i·nea** (per'i-nē'ŭm, -nē'ă). 1 [NA]. The area between the thighs extending from the coccyx to the pubis and lying below the pelvic diaphragm. 2. The external surface of the central tendon of the perineum, lying between the vulva and the anus in the female and the scrotum and the anus in the male. [L. fr. G. *perineon, perinaion*]

per·i·neu·ri·al (per'i-nū'rē-ăl). Relating to the perineurium.

per·i·neu·ri·tis (per'i-nū-rī'tis). Inflammation of the perineurium. SEE ALSO adventitial *neuritis*.

per·i·neu·ri·um, pl. **per·i·neu·ria** (per-i-nū'rē-ŭm, -rē-ă). One of the supporting structures of peripheral nerve trunks, consisting of layers of flattened cells and collagenous connective tissue, which surround the nerve fasciculi and form the major diffusion barrier within the nerve; with the endoneurium and epineurium, composes the peripheral nerve stroma. [L. fr. peri- + G. *neuron*, nerve]

pe·ri·od (pēr'ē-ŏd). 1. A certain duration or division of time. 2. One of the stages of a disease, *e.g.*, p. of incubation, p. of convalescence. SEE ALSO stage, phase. 3. Colloquialism for menses. [G. *periodos*, a way round, a cycle, fr. *peri*, around, + *hodos*, way]

eclipse p., the time between infection by (or induction of) a bacteriophage, or other virus, and the appearance of mature virus within the cell; an interval of time during which infective viral material cannot be recovered.

ejection p., SYN sphygmic *interval*.

extrinsic incubation p. (eks-trin'sik), time required for the development of a disease agent in a vector, from the time of uptake of the agent to the time when the vector is infective.

fertile p., the p. in a regularly menstruating

woman's cycle, during which conception is most likely.

incubation p., (1) time interval between invasion of the body by an infecting organism and the appearance of the first sign or symptom it causes; SYN incubative stage, latent p. (2), latent stage, prodromal stage. (2) in a disease vector, the p. between entry of the disease organism and the time at which the vector is capable of transmitting the disease to another human host.

induction p., the p. required for a specific agent to produce a disease; the interval from the causal action of a factor to initiation of disease; the interval between an initial injection of antigen and the appearance of demonstrable antibodies in the blood.

isoelectric p., the p. occurring in the electrocardiogram between the end of the S wave and the beginning of the T wave during which electrical forces neutralize each other so that there is no difference in potential under the two electrodes.

isometric p. of cardiac cycle, that p. in which the muscle fibers do not shorten although the cardiac muscle is excited and the pressure in the ventricles rises, extending from the closure of the atrioventricular valves to the opening of the semilunar valves (isovolumic constriction) or the reverse (isovolumic relaxation).

latency p., SYN latency *phase*.

latent p., (1) the p. elapsing between the application of a stimulus and the response, *e.g.,* contraction of a muscle; (2) SYN incubation p. (1).

menstrual p., SYN menses.

prepatent p., PARASITOLOGY The p. equivalent to the incubation period of microbial infections; it is biologically different, however, because the parasite is undergoing developmental stages in the host.

refractory p., (1) the p. following effective stimulation, during which excitable tissue such as heart muscle and nerve fails to respond to a stimulus of threshold intensity (*i.e.,* excitability is depressed); (2) a period of temporary psychophysiologic resistance to further sexual stimulation which occurs immediately following orgasm.

synthesis p., the p. of the cell cycle when there is synthesis of DNA and histone; it occurs between Gap_1 and Gap_2.

Wenckebach p., a sequence of cardiac cycles in the electrocardiogram ending in a dropped beat due to A-V block, the preceding cycles showing progressively lengthening P-R intervals; the P-R interval following the dropped beat is again shortened.

pe·ri·od·ic (pēr-ē-od′ik). **1.** Recurring at regular intervals. **2.** Denoting a disease with regularly recurring exacerbations or paroxysms.

per·i·o·dic·i·ty (pēr′ē-ō-dis′i-tē). Tendency to recurrence at regular intervals.

per·i·o·don·tal (per′ē-ō-don′tăl). Around a tooth. [peri- + G. *odous,* tooth]

per·i·o·don·tia (per′ē-ō-don′shē-ă). **1.** Plural of periodontium. **2.** SYN periodontics.

per·i·o·don·tics (per′ē-ō-don′tiks). The branch of dentistry concerned with the study of the normal tissues and the treatment of abnormal conditions of the tissues immediately about the teeth. SYN periodontia (2). [peri- + G. *odous,* tooth]

per·i·o·don·tist (per′ē-ō-don′tist). A dentist who specializes in periodontics.

per·i·o·don·ti·tis (per′ē-ō-don-tī′tis). **1.** Inflammation of the periodontium. **2.** A chronic inflammatory disease of the periodontium occurring in response to bacterial plaque on the adjacent teeth; characterized by gingivitis, destruction of the alveolar bone and periodontal ligament, apical migration of the epithelial attachment resulting in the formation of periodontal pockets, and ultimately loosening and exfoliation of the teeth. [periodontium + G. *-itis,* inflammation]

juvenile p., a degenerative periodontal disease of adolescents in which the periodontal destruction is out of proportion to the local irritating factors present on the adjacent teeth; inflammatory changes become superimposed, and bone loss, migration, and extrusion are observed. Two forms are recognized: 1) localized, in which the destruction is limited to the incisors and first molars; 2) generalized, involving all of the teeth. SYN periodontosis.

per·i·o·don·ti·um, pl. **per·i·o·don·tia** (per′ē-ō-don′shē-ŭm, -shē-ă) [NA]. SYN periodontal *ligament.* [L. fr. peri- + G. *odous,* tooth]

per·i·o·don·to·cla·sia (per′ē-ō-don-tō-klā′zē-ă). Destruction of periodontal tissues, gingiva, pericementum, alveolar bone, and cementum. [periodontium + *klasis,* breaking]

per·i·o·don·to·sis (per′ē-ō-don-tō′sis). SYN juvenile *periodontitis.* [periodontium + G. *-osis,* condition]

per·i·o·nych·ia (per-ē-ō-nik′ē-ă). **1.** Inflammation of the perionychium. **2.** Plural of perionychium.

per·i·o·nych·i·um, pl. **per·i·o·nych·ia** (per-ē-ō-nik′ē-ŭm, -nik′ē-ă). SYN eponychium (2). [peri- + G. *onyx,* nail]

per·i·o·o·pho·ri·tis (per′ē-ō-of′ō-rī′tis). Inflammation of the peritoneal covering of the ovary. SYN periovaritis. [peri- + Mod. L. *oophoron,* ovary, + *-itis,* inflammation]

per·i·o·o·pho·ro·sal·pin·gi·tis (per′ē-ō-of′ō-rō-sal-pin-jī′tis). Inflammation of the peritoneum and other tissues around the ovary and oviduct. [peri- + Mod. L. *oophoron,* ovary, + *salpinx,* trumpet, + *-itis,* inflammation]

per·i·op·er·a·tive (per-ē-op′er-ă-tiv). Around the time of operation. SYN paraoperative.

per·i·or·bit (per-ē-ōr′bit). SYN periorbita.

pe·ri·or·bi·ta (per′ē-ōr′bi-tă) [NA]. The periosteum of the orbit. SYN periorbit. [peri- + L. *orbita,* orbit]

per·i·or·bi·tal (per-ē-ōr′bi-tăl). **1.** Relating to the periorbita. **2.** SYN circumorbital.

per·i·or·chi·tis (per′ē-ōr-kī′tis). Inflammation of the tunica vaginalis testis. [peri- + G. *orchis,* testis, + *-itis,* inflammation]

pe·ri·os·tea (per-ē-os′tē-ă). Plural of periosteum.

per·i·os·te·al (per-ē-os′tē-ăl). Relating to the periosteum.

per·i·os·te·i·tis (per′ē-os-tē-ī′tis). SYN periostitis.

△**periosteo-.** The periosteum. [Mod. L. *periosteum*]

per·i·os·te·o·ma (per′ē-os′tē-ō′mă). A neoplasm derived from the periosteum. SYN periosteophyte.

per·i·os·te·o·my·e·li·tis (per-ē-os′tē-ō-mī-ĕ-lī′tis). Inflammation of the entire bone, with the periosteum and marrow. [periosteo- + G. *myelos,* marrow, + *-itis,* inflammation]

per·i·os·te·o·phyte (per-ē-os′te-ō-fīt). SYN periosteoma. [periosteo- + G. *phyton,* growth]

per·i·os·te·o·sis (per′ē-os-tē-ō′sis). The formation of a periosteoma. SYN periostosis.

per·i·os·te·ot·o·my (per′ē-os-tē-ot′ō-mē). The operation of cutting through the periosteum to the bone. [periosteo- + G. *tomē,* incision]

per·i·os·te·um, pl. **pe·ri·os·tea** (per-ē-os′tē-ŭm, -ă) [NA]. The thick fibrous membrane covering the entire surface of a bone except its articular cartilage. In young bones, it consists of two layers: an inner cellular layer that is osteogenic, forming new bone tissue, and an outer fibrous connective tissue layer conveying the blood vessels and nerves supplying the bone; in older bones, the osteogenic layer is reduced. SEE ALSO perichondral *bone.* [Mod. L. fr. G. *periosteon,* ntr. of adj. *periosteos,* around the bones, fr. *peri,* around, + *osteon,* bone]

per·i·os·ti·tis (per′ē-os-tī′tis). Inflammation of the periosteum. SYN periosteitis.

per·i·os·to·sis, pl. **per·i·os·to·ses** (per′ē-os-tō′sis, -sēz). SYN periosteosis.

per·i·o·va·ri·tis (per′ē-ō-vă-rī′tis). SYN perioophoritis.

per·i·pach·y·men·in·gi·tis (per′i-pak′ē-men-in-jī′tis). Inflammation of the area between the dura and bony covering of the central nervous system. [peri- + pachymeninx (dura mater) + G. *-itis,* inflammation]

per·i·pan·cre·a·ti·tis (per′i-pan′krē-ă-tī′tis). Inflammation of the peritoneal coat of the pancreas.

pe·riph·er·ad (pĕ-rif′ĕ-rad). In a direction toward the periphery. [G. *periphereia,* periphery, + L. *ad,* to]

pe·riph·e·ral (pĕ-rif′ĕ-răl). **1.** Relating to or situated at the periphery. **2.** Situated nearer the periphery of an organ or part of the body in relation to a specific reference point; opposite of central (centralis). SYN eccentric (3).

pe·riph·e·ry (pĕ-rif′ĕ-rē). **1.** The part of a body away from the center; the outer part or surface. **2.** SYN denture *border.* [G. *periphereia,* fr. *peri,* around, + *pherō,* to carry]

per·i·phle·bi·tis (per′i-fle-bī′tis). Inflammation of the outer coat of a vein or of the tissues surrounding it. [peri- + G. *phleps,* vein, + *-itis,* inflammation]

per·i·po·ri·tis (per′i-pŏ-rī′tis). Miliary papules and papulovesicles with staphylococcic infection; most frequently on the face and in infants. [peri- + G. *poros,* pore, + *-itis,* inflammation]

per·i·proc·ti·tis (per′i-prok-tī′tis). Inflammation of the areolar tissue about the rectum. SYN perirectitis.

per·i·pros·ta·ti·tis (per′i-pros-tă-tī′tis). Inflammation of the tissues surrounding the prostate.

per·i·py·le·phle·bi·tis (per-i-pī′lĕ-fle-bī′tis). Inflammation of the tissues around the portal vein. [peri- + G. *pylē,* gate, + *phleps,* vein, + *-itis,* inflammation]

per·i·rec·ti·tis (per′i-rek-tī′tis). SYN periproctitis.

per·i·rhi·zo·cla·sia (per′ē-rī-zō-klā′zē-ă). Inflammatory destruction of tissues immediately around the root of a tooth. [peri- + G. *rhiza,* root, -o- + *klasis,* destruction]

per·i·sal·pin·gi·tis (per-i-sal-pin-jī′tis). Inflammation of the peritoneum covering the uterine tube. [peri- + G. *salpinx,* trumpet, + *-itis,* inflammation]

per·i·sal·pinx (per′i-sal′pingks). The peritoneal covering of the uterine tube. [peri- + G. *salpinx* (*salping-*), trumpet]

per·i·scop·ic (per′i-skop′ik). Denoting that which gives the ability to see objects to one side as well as in the direct axis of vision. [peri- + G. *skopeō,* to view]

per·i·sig·moi·di·tis (per′i-sig-moy-dī′tis). Inflammation of the connective tissues surrounding the sigmoid flexure, giving rise to symptoms, referable to the left iliac fossa, similar to those of perityphlitis in the right iliac fossa.

per·i·sper·ma·ti·tis (per′i-sper-mă-tī′tis). Inflammation of the tissues around the spermatic cord.

per·i·splanch·ni·tis (per′i-splangk-nī′tis). Inflammation surrounding any viscus or viscera. [peri- + G. *splanchna,* viscera, + *-itis,* inflammation]

per·i·sple·ni·tis (per′i-sple-nī′tis). Inflammation of the peritoneum covering the spleen.

per·i·spon·dy·li·tis (per-i-spon-di-lī′tis). Inflammation of the tissues about a vertebra. [peri- + G. *spondylos,* vertebra, + *-itis,* inflammation]

per·i·stal·sis (per-i-stal′sis). The movement of the intestine or other tubular structure, characterized by waves of alternate circular contraction and relaxation of the tube by which the contents are propelled onward. SYN vermicular movement. [peri- + G. *stalsis,* constriction]

  mass p., forcible peristaltic movements of short duration, occurring only three or four times a day, which move the contents of the large intestine from one division to the next, as from the ascending to the transverse colon.

  reversed p., a wave of intestinal contraction in a direction the reverse of normal, by which the contents of the intestine are forced backward. SYN antiperistalsis.

per·i·stal·tic (per-i-stal′tik). Relating to peristalsis.

pe·ris·to·le (pĕ-ris′tō-lē). The tonic activity of the walls of the stomach whereby the organ contracts about its contents; contrasting with the peristaltic waves passing from the cardia toward the pylorus (peristalsis). [peri- + G. *stellō,* to contract]

per·i·stol·ic (per-i-stol′ik). Relating to peristole.

per·i·tec·to·my (per′i-tek′tō-mē). **1.** The removal of a paracorneal strip of the conjunctiva for the relief of corneal disease. **2.** SYN circumcision (2). [peri- + G. *ektomē,* excision]

pe·ri·ten·di·ne·um, pl. **pe·ri·ten·di·nea** (per-i-ten-din′ē-ŭm, -ē-ŭ) [NA]. One of the fibrous sheaths surrounding the primary bundles of fibers in a tendon. [L. fr. peri- + G. *tenōn,* tendon]

per·i·ten·di·ni·tis (per′i-ten-di-nī′tis). Inflammation of the sheath of a tendon. SYN peritenontitis.

per·i·ten·on·ti·tis (per′i-ten-on-tī′tis). SYN peritendinitis.

per·i·the·li·um, pl. **per·i·the·li·a** (per-i-thē′lē-ŭm, -ă). The connective tissue that surrounds smaller vessels and capillaries. [peri- + G. *thēlē,* nipple]

per·i·thy·roi·di·tis (per′i-thī-roy-dī′tis). Inflammation of the capsule or tissues surrounding the thyroid gland.

pe·rit·o·my (pe-rit′ō-mē). **1.** A circumcorneal incision through the conjunctiva. **2.** SYN circumcision (1). [G. *peritomē,* fr. *peri,* around, + *tomē,* incision]

per·i·to·ne·al (per′i-tō-nē′ăl). Relating to the peritoneum.

△**peritoneo-.** The peritoneum. [L. *peritoneum*]

per·i·to·ne·o·cen·te·sis (per′i-tō-nē′ō-sen-tē′sis). Paracentesis of the abdomen. [peritoneum + G. *kentēsis,* puncture]

per·i·to·ne·oc·ly·sis (per′i-tō-nē-ok′li-sis). Irrigation of the abdominal cavity. [peritoneum, + G. *klysis,* a washing out]

per·i·to·ne·o·per·i·car·di·al (per′i-tō-nē′ō-per′i-kar′dē-ăl). Relating to the peritoneum and the pericardium.

per·i·to·ne·o·pexy (per′i-tō-nē′ō-pek-sē). A suspension or fixation of the peritoneum. [peritoneum + G. *pēxis,* fixation]

per·i·to·ne·o·plas·ty (per′i-tō-nē′ō-plas-tē). Loosening adhesions and covering the raw surfaces with peritoneum to prevent reformation. [peritoneum + G. *plastos,* formed]

per·i·to·ne·o·scope (per′i-tō-nē′ō-skōp). SYN laparoscope. [peritoneum + G. *skopeō,* to view]

per·i·to·ne·os·co·py (per′i-tō-nē-os′kŏ-pē). Examination of the contents of the peritoneum with a peritoneoscope passed through the abdominal wall. SEE ALSO laparoscopy. SYN abdominoscopy, celioscopy, ventroscopy.

per·i·to·ne·ot·o·my (per′i-tō-nē-ot′ō-mē). Incision of the peritoneum. [peritoneum + G. *tomē,* incision]

per·i·to·ne·um, pl. **pe·ri·to·nea** (per′i-tō-nē′ŭm, -ă) [NA]. The serous membrane, consisting of mesothelium and connective tissue, that lines the abdominal cavity and covers most of the viscera contained therein; it forms two sacs: the peritoneal (or greater) sac and the omental bursa (lesser sac) connected by the epiploic foramen. [Mod. L. fr. G. *peritonaion,* fr. *periteinō,* to stretch over]

per·i·to·ni·tis (per′i-tō-nī′tis). Inflammation of the peritoneum.

  adhesive p., a form of p. in which a fibrinous exudate occurs, matting together the intestines and various other organs.

  chemical p., p. due to the escape of bile, contents of the gastrointestinal tract, or pancreatic juice into the peritoneal cavity; the contents of the fluid causes chemical injury, shock, and peritoneal exudation.

  gas p., inflammation of the peritoneum accompanied by an intraperitoneal accumulation of gas.

  meconium p., p. caused by intestinal perforation in the fetus or newborn; associated with congenital obstruction or fibrocystic disease of the pancreas.

  pelvic p., generalized inflammation of the peri-

toneum surrounding the uterus and fallopian tubes. SYN pelviperitonitis.

per·i·ton·sil·li·tis (per′i-ton′si-lī′tis). Inflammation of the connective tissue above and behind the tonsil.

pe·rit·ri·chal, pe·rit·ri·chate, per·i·trich·ic (pe-rit′ri-kăl, -rit′ri-kāt, per-i-trik′ik). SYN peritrichous (2).

pe·rit·ri·chous (pe-rit′ri-kŭs). **1.** Relating to cilia or other appendicular organs projecting from the periphery of a cell. **2.** Having flagella uniformly distributed over a cell; used especially with reference to bacteria. SYN peritrichal, peritrichate, peritrichic. [peri- + G. *thrix,* hair]

per·i·u·re·ter·i·tis (per′i-yū-rē′ter-ī′tis). Inflammation of the tissues about a ureter. [peri- + ureter + G. -*itis,* inflammation]

per·i·u·re·thri·tis (per′i-yū-rē-thrī′tis). Inflammation of the tissues about the urethra. [peri- + urethra + G. -*itis,* inflammation]

per·i·u·ter·ine (per′i-yū′ter-in). SYN perimetric (1).

per·i·vag·i·ni·tis (per′i-vaj-i-nī′tis). Inflammation of the connective tissue around the vagina. SYN pericolpitis.

per·i·vas·cu·li·tis (per′i-vas-kū-lī′tis). SYN periangitis.

per·i·ves·i·cal (per-i-ves′i-kăl). SYN pericystic. [peri- + L. *vesica,* bladder]

per·i·vis·cer·i·tis (per′i-vis-er-ī′tis). Inflammation surrounding any viscus or viscera. [peri- + L. *viscera,* internal organs, + G. -*itis,* inflammation]

per·me·a·bil·i·ty (per′mē-ă-bil′i-tē). The property of being permeable.

per·me·a·ble (per′mē-ă-bl). Permitting the passage of substances (*e.g.,* liquids, gases, heat), as through a membrane or other structure. SYN pervious. [L. *permeabilis* (see permeate)]

per·me·ase (per′mē-ās). Any of a group of membrane-bound carriers (enzymes) that effect the transport of solute through a semipermeable membrane.

per·me·ate (per′mē-āt). **1.** To pass through a membrane or other structure. **2.** That which can so pass. [L. *permeo,* to pass through]

per·me·a·tion (per-mē-ā′shŭn). The process of spreading through or penetrating, as the extension of a malignant neoplasm by proliferation of the cells continuously along the blood vessels or lymphatics. [L. *per-meo,* pp. -*meatus,* to pass through]

per·ni·cious (per-nish′ŭs). Destructive; harmful; denoting a disease of severe character and usually fatal without appropriate treatment. [L. *perniciosus,* destructive, fr. *pernicies,* destruction]

△**pero-.** Maimed, malformed. [G. *pēros*]

pe·ro·dac·ty·ly, pe·ro·dac·tyl·ia (pē-rō-dak′ti-lē, -dak-til′ē-ă). Congenital deformity of fingers and toes. [pero- + G. *daktylos,* finger or toe]

pe·ro·me·lia, pe·rom·e·ly (pē-rō-mē′lē-ă, pĕ-rom′ĕ-lē). Severe congenital malformations of extremities, including absence of hand or foot. [pero- + G. *melos,* limb]

per·o·ne·al (per-ō-nē′ăl). Relating to the fibula, to the lateral side of the leg, or to the muscles there present. [L. *peroneus,* fr. G. *peronē,* fibula]

per·o·ral (per-ō′răl). Through the mouth, denoting a method of medication or an approach. [L. *per,* through, + *os* (*or-*), mouth]

per os. By or through the mouth, denoting a method of medication. [L.]

⌂**peroxi-.** SEE peroxy-.

per·ox·i·das·es (per-ok'si-dās-ez) [EC subclass 1.11]. Enzymes in animal and plant tissues that catalyze the dehydrogenation (oxidation) of various substances in the presence of hydrogen peroxide, which acts as hydrogen acceptor, being converted to water in the process.

horseradish p., an enzyme used in immunohistochemistry to label the antigen-antibody complex.

per·ox·ide (per-ok'sīd). That oxide of any series that contains the greatest number of oxygen atoms.

per·ox·i·some (per-ok'si-sōm). A membrane-bound organelle occurring in nearly all eukaryotic cells that often contains oxidative enzymes relating to the formation and degradation of H_2O_2. SYN microbody. [peroxide + G. *sōma,* body]

⌂**peroxy-.** Prefix denoting the presence of an extra O atom, as in peroxides, peroxy acids.

per·ox·yl (per-ok'sil). H–O–O; one of the free radicals presumed formed as a result of the bombardment of tissue by high-energy radiation.

per rec·tum (per rek'tŭm). By or through the rectum, denoting a method of examination or treatment. [L.]

per·salt (per'sawlt). CHEMISTRY Any salt that contains the greatest possible amount of the acid radical.

per·sev·er·a·tion (per-sev-er-ā'shŭn). **1.** The constant repetition of a meaningless word or phrase. **2.** The duration of a mental impression, measured by the rapidity with which one impression follows another as determined by the revolving of a two-colored disk. **3.** CLINICAL PSYCHOLOGY The uncontrollable repetition of a previously appropriate or correct response, even though the repeated response has since become inappropriate or incorrect. [L. *persevero,* to persist]

per·sis·tence (per-sis'tens). **1.** Obstinate continuation of characteristic behavior. **2.** Survival in spite of opposition or adverse environmental conditions. [L. *persisto,* to abide, stand firm]

per·so·na (per-sō'nă). A term that embodies the total constellation of physical, psychological, and behavioral attributes of each unique individual; in jungian psychology, the outer aspect of character, as opposed to anima (2); the assumed personality used to mask the true one. [L. *persona,* actor's mask; character, role, prob. fr. Etruscan]

per·son·al·i·ty (per-sŏn-al'i-tē). **1.** The unique self; the organized system of attitudes and behavioral predispositions by which one feels, thinks, acts, and impresses and establishes relationships with others. **2.** An individual with a particular p. pattern.

antisocial p., a p. disorder characterized by a continuous and persistent pattern of aggressive behavior in which the rights of others are violated. SEE psychopath, sociopath.

authoritarian p., a cluster of p. traits reflecting a desire for security and order, *e.g.,* rigidity, un-

questioning obedience, scapegoating, desire for structured lines of authority.

avoidant p., a p. characterized by a hypersensitivity to potential rejection, humiliation, or shame, an unwillingness to enter into relationships without unusually strong guarantees of uncritical acceptance, social withdrawal in spite of a desire for affection and acceptance, and low self-esteem.

compulsive p., a p. characterized by rigidity, extreme inhibition, perfectionism, and excessive concern with conformity and adherence to standards of conscience either for the individual or for others.

cyclothymic p., a p. disorder in which a person experiences regularly alternating periods of elation and depression, usually not related to external circumstances.

dependent p., a p. disorder in which a person passively allows others to assume responsibility for making decisions.

inadequate p., a p. disorder, characterized by personal and social ineptness plus emotional and physical instability, which renders the individual unable to cope with the normal vicissitudes of life.

masochistic p., a p. disorder in which the individual accepts exploitation and sacrifices self-interest while at the same time feeling morally superior or feigning moral superiority, attempting to elicit sympathy, and inducing guilt in others.

multiple p., a dissociative disorder in which two or more distinct conscious p.'s alternately prevail in the same person, without any p. being aware of the others.

paranoid p., a p. disorder characterized by hypersensitivity, rigidity, unwarranted suspicion, jealousy, and a tendency to blame others and ascribe evil motives to them; though neither a neurosis nor psychosis, it interferes with the individual's ability to maintain interpersonal relationships.

passive-aggressive p., a p. disorder in which aggressive feelings are manifested in passive ways, especially through mild obstructionism and stubbornness.

schizoid p., a disorder characterized by social withdrawal, emotional coldness or aloofness, and indifference to praise or criticism from others.

schizotypical p., a personality disorder characterized by eccentricities in thinking, appearance, and behavior; although not psychotic, individuals with such a disorder hold ideas that are considered unusual and have difficulty relating to others.

type A p., type B p., SEE type A *behavior,* type B *behavior.*

pers·pi·ra·tion (pers-pi-rā'shŭn). **1.** The excretion of fluid by the sweat glands of the skin. SYN diaphoresis, sudation, sweating. SEE ALSO sweat. **2.** All fluid loss through normal skin, whether by sweat gland secretion or by diffusion through other skin structures. **3.** The fluid excreted by the sweat glands; it consists of water containing sodium chloride and phosphate, urea, ammonia, ethereal sulfates, creatinine, fats, and other waste products; the average daily quantity is estimated at about 1500 g. SYN sudor. SEE ALSO sweat (1). [L. *per-spiro,* pp. *-atus,* to breathe everywhere]

insensible p., p. that evaporates before it is perceived as moisture on the skin; the term sometimes includes evaporation from the lungs.

sensible p., p. excreted in large quantity, or when there is much humidity in the atmosphere, so that it appears as moisture on the skin.

per•tech•ne•tate (per-tek-ne-tāt). Anionic form of technetium used widely in nuclear scanning; ^{99m}Tc04.

per tu•bam (per tū′băm). Through a tube. [L.]

per•tus•sis (per-tŭs′is). An acute infectious inflammation of the larynx, trachea, and bronchi caused by *Bordetella pertussis;* characterized by recurrent bouts of spasmodic coughing that continues until the breath is exhausted, then ending in a noisy inspiratory stridor (the "whoop") caused by laryngeal spasm. SYN whooping cough. [L. *per,* very (intensive), + *tussis,* cough]

per vi•as na•tu•ra•les (per vī′as nach′er-ā′lēz). Through the natural passages; *e.g.,* denoting a normal delivery, as opposed to cesarean section, or the passage in stool of a foreign body instead of its surgical removal. [L.]

per•vi•ous (per′vē-ŭs). SYN permeable. [L. *pervius,* fr. *per,* through, + *via,* a way]

pes, gen. **pe•dis,** pl. **pe•des** (pes, pē′dis, -dēz). 1 [NA]. SYN foot (1). **2.** Any footlike or basal structure or part. **3.** Talipes. In this sense, p. is always qualified by a word expressing the specific type. [L.]

  p. anseri′nus, (1) SYN intraparotid *plexus* of facial nerve. **(2)** the combined tendinous expansions of the sartorius, gracilis, and semitendinosus muscles at the medial border of the tuberosity of the tibia.

  p. cavus, condition characterized by increased height of the foot's medial longitudinal arch.

  p. pla′nus, SYN *talipes* planus.

pes•sa•ry (pes′ă-rē). **1.** An appliance of varied form, introduced into the vagina to support the uterus or to correct any displacement. **2.** A medicated vaginal suppository. [L. *pessarium,* fr. G. *pessos,* an oval stone used in certain games]

pest. SYN plague (2). [L. *pestis*]

pes•ti•cide (pes′ti-sīd). General term for an agent that destroys fungi, insects, rodents, or any other pest.

pes•ti•lence (pes′ti-lens). **1.** SYN plague (2). **2.** A virulent outbreak of any disease. [L. *pestilentia*]

pes•ti•len•tial (pes-ti-len′shăl). Relating to or tending to produce a pestilence.

pes•tle (pes′l). An instrument in the shape of a rod with one rounded and weighted extremity, used for bruising, breaking, grinding, and mixing substances in a mortar. [L. *pistillum,* fr. *pinso,* or *piso,* to pound]

PET positron emission *tomography.*

△**peta-.** Prefix used in the SI and metric systems to signify one quadrillion (10^{15}).

△**-petal.** Seeking; movement toward the part indicated by the main portion of the word. [L. *peto,* to seek, strive for]

pe•te•chi•ae, sing. **pe•te•chia** (pe-tē′kē-ē, pē-tek′-; pe-tē′kē-ă). Minute hemorrhagic spots, of pinpoint to pinhead size, in the skin, which are not

blanched by diascopy. [Mod. L. form of It. *petecchie*]

  calcaneal p., traumatic hemorrhage into the stratum corneum of the heel which may persist for several weeks as centrally confluent black dots.

pe•te•chi•al (pē-tē′kē-ăl, pē-tek′-). Relating to, accompanied by, or characterized by petechiae.

pet•i•o•late, pet•i•o•lat•ed (pet′ē-ō-lāt, -lāt-ed). Having a stem or pedicle. [L. *petiolus*]

pe•ti•o•lus (pe-tī′ō-lŭs). A stem or pedicle. [L. dim. of *pes* (foot), the stalk of a fruit]

pet•ri•fac•tion (pet-ri-fak′shŭn). Fossilization, as in conversion into stone. [L. *petra,* rock + *facio,* to make]

△**petro-.** Stone; stonelike hardness. [L. *petra,* rock; G. *petros,* stone]

pet•ro•mas•toid (pet′rō-mas′toyd). Relating to the petrous and the squamous portions of the temporal bone, which are usually united at birth by the petrosquamosal suture.

pet•ro•oc•cip•i•tal (pet′rō-ok-sip′i-tăl). Denoting the cranial suture between the occipital bone and the petrous portion of the temporal.

pe•tro•sa, pl. **pe•tro•sae** (pe-trō′să, -sē). The petrous portion of the temporal bone. [L. fr. *petra,* rock]

pe•tro•sal (pe-trō′săl). Relating to the petrosa. SYN petrous (2).

pet•ro•si•tis (pet-rō-sī′tis). An inflammation involving the petrous portion of the temporal bone and its air cells.

pet•ro•sphe•noid (pet′rō-sfē′noyd). Relating to the petrous portion of the temporal bone and to the sphenoid bone.

pet•ro•squa•mo•sal, pet•ro•squa•mous (pet′rō-skwā-mō′săl, -skwā′mŭs). Relating to the petrous and the squamous portions of the temporal bone.

pet•rous (pet′rŭs, pē′trŭs). **1.** Of stony hardness. **2.** SYN petrosal. [L. *petrosus,* fr. *petra,* a rock]

pex•is (pek′sis). Fixation of substances in the tissues. [G. *pēxis,* fixation]

△**-pexy.** Fixation, usually surgical. [G. *pēxis,* fixation]

PF platelet *factor* 4.

PFT pulmonary function *test.*

pg picogram.

Ph phenyl.

pH Symbol for the negative logarithm of the H$^+$ ion concentration (measured in moles per liter); a solution with pH 7.00 is neutral at 22°C, one with a pH of more than 7.0 is alkaline, and one with a pH lower than 7.00 is acid. At a temperature of 37°C, neutrality is at a pH value of 6.8. [p (power or potency) of H$^+$]

PHA phytohemagglutinin.

△**phaco-.** **1.** Lens-shaped, relating to a lens; **2.** Birthmark; as in phacomatosis. [G. *phakos,* lentil (lens), anything shaped like a lentil]

phac•o•an•a•phy•lax•is (fak′ō-an-ă-fī-lak′sis). Hypersensitivity to protein of the lens of the eye.

phac•o•cele (fak′ō-sēl). Hernia of the lens of the eye through the sclera. [phaco- + G. *kēlē,* hernia]

phac•o•e•mul•si•fi•ca•tion (fak′ō-ē-mŭl-si-fi-kā′shŭn). A method of emulsifying and aspirating a cataract with a low frequency ultrasonic needle.

phac•o•er•y•sis (fak-ō-er′i-sis). Extraction of the

lens of the eye by means of a suction cup called the erysophake. [phaco- + G. *erysis,* pulling, drawing off]

pha·coid (fak'oyd). Of lentil shape. [phaco- + G. *eidos,* resemblance]

pha·col·y·sis (fă-kol'i-sis). Operative breaking down and removal of the lens. [phaco- + G. *lysis,* dissolution]

pha·co·lyt·ic (fak-ō-lit'ik). Characterized by or referring to phacolysis.

pha·co·ma (fa-kō'mă). A hamartoma found in phacomatosis; often refers to a retinal hamartoma in tuberous sclerosis. SYN phakoma. [phaco- + G. *-oma,* tumor]

pha·co·ma·la·cia (fak'ō-mă-lā'shē-ă). Softening of the lens, as may occur in hypermature cataract. [phaco- + G. *malakia,* softness]

phac·o·ma·to·sis (fak'ō-mă-tō'sis). A generic term for a group of hereditary diseases characterized by hamartomas involving multiple tissues; *e.g.,* von Hippel-Lindau's disease, neurofibromatosis, Sturge-Weber syndrome, tuberous sclerosis. SYN phakomatosis. [Van der Hoeve's coinage fr. G. *phakos,* mother-spot]

phac·o·scope (fak'ō-skōp). An instrument in the form of a dark chamber for observing the changes in the lens during accommodation. [phaco- + G. *skopeō,* to view]

△**phaeo-.** SEE pheo-.

phae·o·hy·pho·my·co·sis (fē'ō-hī'fō-mī-kō'sis). A group of superficial and deep infections caused by fungi that form pigmented hyphae and yeastlike cells in tissue. [G. *phaios,* dusky, + *hyphē,* web, + mycosis]

phage (fāj). SYN bacteriophage.

△**-phage, -phagia, -phagy.** Eating, devouring. [G. *phagō,* to eat]

phag·e·de·na (faj-ĕ-dē'nă). An ulcer that rapidly spreads peripherally, destroying the tissues as it increases in size. [G. *phagedaina,* a canker]

phag·e·den·ic (faj-ĕ-den'ik). Relating to or having the characteristics of phagedena.

△**phago-.** Eating, devouring. [G. *phagō,* to eat]

phag·o·cyte (fag'ō-sīt). A cell possessing the property of ingesting bacteria, foreign particles, and other cells. P.'s are divided into two general classes: 1) microphages, polymorphonuclear leukocytes that ingest chiefly bacteria; 2) macrophages, mononucleated cells (histiocytes and monocytes) that are largely scavengers, ingesting dead tissue and degenerated cells. [phago- + G. *kytos,* cell]

phag·o·cyt·ic (fag-ō-sit'ik). Relating to phagocytes or phagocytosis.

phag·o·cy·tin (fag-ō-sī'tin). A very labile bactericidal substance that may be isolated from polymorphonuclear leukocytes.

phag·o·cy·tize (fag'ō-si-tīz). SYN phagocytose.

phag·o·cy·tol·y·sis (fag'ō-sī-tol'i-sis). 1. Destruction of phagocytes, or leukocytes, occurring in the process of blood coagulation or as the result of the introduction of certain antagonistic foreign substances into the body. 2. A spontaneous breaking down of the phagocytes, preliminary to the liberation of complement. [phagocyte + G. *lysis,* dissolution]

phag·o·cy·to·lyt·ic (fag'ō-sī-tō-lit'ik). Relating to phagocytolysis.

phag·o·cy·tose (fag'ō-si-tōz). To perform phagocytosis, denoting the action of phagocytic cells. SYN phagocytize.

phag·o·cy·to·sis (fag'ō-sī-tō'sis). The process of ingestion and digestion by cells of solid substances, *e.g.,* other cells, bacteria, bits of necrosed tissue, foreign particles. SEE ALSO endocytosis. [phagocyte + G. *-osis,* condition]

phag·o·ly·so·some (fag-ō-lī'sō-sōm). A body formed by union of a phagosome or ingested particle with a lysosome having hydrolytic enzymes.

phag·o·some (fag'ō-sōm). A vesicle that forms around a particle (bacterial or other) within the phagocyte that engulfed it, separates from the cell membrane, and then fuses with and receives the contents of cytoplasmic granules (lysosomes), thus forming a phagolysosome in which digestion of the engulfed particle occurs. [phago- + G. *sōma,* body]

phag·o·type (fag'ō-tīp). MICROBIOLOGY A subdivision of a species distinguished from other strains therein by sensitivity to a certain bacteriophage or set of bacteriophages. [phago- + G. *typos,* type]

△**-phagy.** SEE -phage.

△**phako-.** For words so beginning and not listed here, see phaco-.

pha·ko·ma (fa-kō'mă). SYN phacoma.

phak·o·ma·to·sis (fak'ō-mă-tō'sis). SYN phacomatosis.

pha·lan·ge·al (fă-lan'jē-ăl). Relating to a phalanx.

phal·an·gec·to·my (fal-an-jek'tō-mē). Excision of one or more of the phalanges of hand or foot. [phalang- + G. *ektomē,* excision]

pha·lanx, gen. **pha·lan·gis,** pl. **pha·lan·ges** (fā'langks, fă-langks'; fă-lan'jis; -jēz). 1 [NA]. One of the long bones of the digits, 14 in number for each hand or foot, two for the thumb or great toe, and three each for the other four digits; designated as proximal, middle, and distal, beginning from the metacarpus. 2. One of a number of cuticular plates, arranged in several rows, on the surface of the spiral organ (of Corti), which are the heads of the outer row of pillar cells and of phalangeal cells. [L. fr. G. *phalanx* (*-ang-*), line of soldiers, bone between two joints of the fingers and toes]

△**phall-, phalli-, phallo-.** The penis. [G. *phallos*]

phal·lec·to·my (fal-ek'tō-mē). Surgical removal of the penis. [phall- + G. *ektomē,* excision]

phal·lic (fal'ik). 1. Relating to the penis. 2. PSYCHOANALYSIS Relating to the penis, especially during the phases of infantile psychosexuality. SEE ALSO phallic *phase.* [G. *phallos,* penis]

△**phallo-.** SEE phall-.

phal·lo·camp·sis (fal-ō-kamp'sis). Curvature of the erect penis. SEE ALSO chordee. [phallo- + G. *kampsis,* a bending]

phal·lo·dyn·ia (fal-ō-din'ē-ă). Pain in the penis. [phallo- + G. *odynē,* pain]

phal·loi·din (fă-loy'din). Best known of the toxic cyclic peptides produced by the poisonous mushroom, *Amanita phalloides;* closely related to amanitin.

phal·lo·plas·ty (fal′ō-plas-tē). Surgical reconstruction of the penis. [phallo- + G. *plastos,* formed]

phal·lot·o·my (fal-ot′ō-mē). Surgical incision into the penis. [phallo- + G. *tomē,* a cutting]

phal·lus, pl. **phalli** (fal′ŭs, fal′ī). SYN penis. [L.; G. *phallos*]

phan·ta·sia (fan-tā′zē-ă). SYN fantasy. [G. appearance]

phan·tasm (fan′tazm). The mental imagery produced by fantasy. SYN phantom (1). [G. *phantasma,* an appearance]

phan·tas·ma·go·ria (fan-taz-mă-gōr′ē-ă). A fantastic sequence of haphazardly associative imagery.

phan·tom (fan′tŏm). **1.** SYN phantasm. **2.** A model, especially a transparent one, of the human body or any of its parts. **3.** RADIOLOGY A mechanical or computer-originated model for predicting irradiation dosage deep in the body. [G. *phantasma,* an appearance]

phar·ma·ceu·tic, phar·ma·ceu·ti·cal (far-mă-sū′tik, sū′ti-kăl). Relating to pharmacy or to pharmaceutics. [G. *pharmakeutikos,* relating to drugs]

phar·ma·ceu·tics (far-mă-sū′tiks). **1.** SYN pharmacy (1). **2.** The science of pharmaceutical systems, *i.e.,* preparations, dosage forms, etc.

phar·ma·cist (far′mă-sist). One who is licensed to prepare and dispense drugs and compounds and is knowledgeable concerning their properties. [G. *pharmakon,* a drug]

pharmaco-. Drugs. [G. *pharmakon,* medicine]

phar·ma·co·di·ag·no·sis (far′mă-kō-dī-ag-nō′sis). Use of drugs in diagnosis.

phar·ma·co·dy·nam·ic (far′mă-kō-dī-nam′ik). Relating to drug action, particularly at the receptor level.

phar·ma·co·dy·nam·ics (far′mă-kō-dī-nam′iks). The study of uptake, movement, binding, and interactions of pharmacologically active molecules at their tissue site(s) of action. [pharmaco- + G. *dynamis,* force]

pharmacoeconomics. Science dealing with the description and analysis of the costs of drug therapy to health care systems and society.

pharmacoepidemiology. The application of epidemiologic knowledge, methods, and reasoning to the study of the effects and uses of pharmacologic treatments in a defined time, space, and population. SEE epidemiology, pharmacology.

phar·ma·co·ge·net·ics (far′mă-kō-jĕ-net′iks). The study of genetically determined variations in responses to drugs in humans or in laboratory organisms.

phar·ma·cog·no·sy (far-mă-kog′nō-sē). A branch of pharmacology concerned with the physical characteristics and botanical and animal sources of crude drugs. [pharmaco- + G. *gnosis,* knowledge]

phar·ma·co·ki·net·ic (far′mă-kō-ki-net′ik). Relating to the disposition of drugs in the body (*i.e.,* their absorption, distribution, metabolism, and elimination).

phar·ma·co·ki·net·ics (far′mă-kō-ki-net′iks).

Study of the movement of drugs within biological systems, as affected by absorption, distribution, metabolism, and secretion; particularly the rates of such movements. [pharmaco- + G. *kinēsis,* movement]

phar·ma·co·log·ic, phar·ma·co·log·i·cal (far′mă-kō-loj′ik, -loj′i-kăl). **1.** Relating to pharmacology or to the composition, properties, and actions of drugs. **2.** PHYSIOLOGY A dose of a chemical agent that is so much larger or more potent than would occur naturally that it might have qualitatively different effects. Cf. homeopathic (2), physiologic (4).

phar·ma·col·o·gist (far-mă-kol′ō-jist). A specialist in pharmacology.

phar·ma·col·o·gy (far-mă-kol′ō-jē). The science concerned with drugs, their sources, appearance, chemistry, actions, and uses. [pharmaco- + G. *logos,* study]

Phar·ma·co·pe·ia, Phar·ma·co·poe·ia (far′mă-kō-pē′ă). A work containing monographs of therapeutic agents, standards for their strength and purity, and their formulations. The various national pharmacopeias are referred to by abbreviations, of which the most frequently encountered are *USP,* the Pharmacopeia of the United States of America (United States Pharmacopeia); and *BP,* British Pharmacopoeia. [G. *pharmakopoiia,* fr. *pharmakon,* a medicine, + *poieo,* to make]

phar·ma·co·pe·ial (far′mă-kō-pē′ăl). Relating to the Pharmacopeia; denoting a drug in the list of the Pharmacopeia. SEE ALSO official.

phar·ma·co·ther·a·py (far′mă-kō-thār′ă-pē). Treatment of disease by means of drugs. SEE ALSO chemotherapy. [pharmaco- + G. *therapeia,* therapy]

phar·ma·cy (far′mă-sē). **1.** The practice of preparing and dispensing drugs and the delivery of pharmaceutical care. SYN pharmaceutics (1). **2.** A drugstore. [G. *pharmakon,* drug]

pharmakinetics. The mathematical characterization of the disposition of a drug in the body over time. Used to help understand and interpret blood levels and to adjust dosage and interval for maximum therapeutic results and minimum toxic effects.

△**pharyng-.** SEE pharyngo-.

pha·ryn·ge·al (fă-rin′jē-ăl). Relating to the pharynx. [Mod. L. *pharyngeus*]

phar·yn·gec·to·my (far′in-jek′tō-mē). Resection of the pharynx. [pharyng- + G. *ektomē,* excision]

pha·ryn·ges (fă-rin′jēz). Plural of pharynx.

phar·gis·mus (far-in-jiz′mŭs). Spasm of the muscles of the pharynx. SYN pharyngospasm.

phar·yn·git·ic (far-in-jit′ik). Relating to pharyngitis.

phar·yn·gi·tis (far-in-jī′tis). Inflammation of the mucous membrane and underlying parts of the pharynx. [pharyng- + G. *-itis,* inflammation]

△**pharyngo-, pharyng-.** The pharynx. [Mod. L. fr. G. *pharynx*]

pha·ryn·go·cele (fă-ring′gō-sēl). A diverticulum from the pharynx. [pharyngo- + G. *kēlē,* hernia]

pha·ryn·go·ep·i·glot·tic, pha·ryn·go·ep·i·glot·tid·e·an (fă-ring′gō-ep′i-glot′ik, -glo-tid′ē-an). Relating to the pharynx and the epiglottis.

pha·ryn·go·e·soph·a·ge·al (fă-ring′gō-ē-sof′ă-jē'ăl). Relating to the pharynx and the esophagus.

pha·ryn·go·glos·sal (fă-ring'gō-glos'ăl). Relating to the pharynx and the tongue.

pha·ryn·go·la·ryn·ge·al (fă-ring'gō-lă-rin'jē-ăl). Relating to both the pharynx and the larynx.

pha·ryn·go·lar·yn·gi·tis (fă-ring'gō-lar-in-jī'tis). Inflammation of both the pharynx and the larynx.

pha·ryn·go·lith (fă-ring'gō-lith). A concretion in the pharynx. [pharyngo- + G. *lithos,* stone]

pha·ryn·go·my·co·sis (fă-ring'gō-mī-kō'sis). Invasion of the mucous membrane of the pharynx by fungi. [pharyngo- + G. *mykēs,* a fungus]

pha·ryn·go·na·sal (fă-ring'gō-nā'săl). Relating to the pharynx and the nasal cavity.

pha·ryn·go·plas·ty (fă-ring'gō-plas-tē). Plastic surgery of the pharynx. [pharyngo- + G. *plastos,* formed]

pha·ryn·go·ple·gia (fă-ring'gō-plē'jē-ă). Paralysis of the muscles of the pharynx. [pharyngo- + G. *plēgē,* stroke]

pha·ryn·go·scope (fă-ring'gō-skōp). An instrument like a laryngoscope, used for inspection of the mucous membrane of the pharynx. [pharyngo- + G. *skopeō,* to view]

phar·yn·gos·co·py (far'ing-gos'kŏ-pē). Inspection and examination of the pharynx. [pharyngo- + G. *skopeō,* to view]

pha·ryn·go·spasm (fă-ring'gō-spazm). SYN pharyngismus.

pha·ryn·go·ste·no·sis (fă-ring'gō-ste-nō'sis). Stricture of the pharynx. [pharyngo- + G. *stenōsis,* a narrowing]

phar·yn·got·o·my (far'ing-got'ō-mē). Any cutting operation upon the pharynx either from without or from within. [pharyngo- + G. *tomē,* incision]

phar·ynx, gen. **pha·ryn·gis,** pl. **pha·ryn·ges** (far'ingks, fă-rin'jis, fă-rin'jēz) [NA]. The upper expanded portion of the digestive tube, between the esophagus below and the mouth and nasal cavities above and in front. [Mod. L. fr. G. *pharynx (pharyng-),* the throat, the joint opening of the gullet and windpipe]

phase (fāz). **1.** A stage in the course of change or development. **2.** A homogeneous, physically distinct, and separable portion of a heterogeneous system; *e.g.,* oil, gum, and water are three p.'s of an emulsion. **3.** The time relationship between two or more events. **4.** A particular part of a recurring time pattern or wave form. SEE ALSO stage, period. [G. *phasis,* an appearance]

anal p., in psychoanalytic personality theory, the stage of psychosexual development, occurring when a child is between 1 and 3 years, during which activities, interests, and concerns center on the anal zone.

aqueous p., the water portion of a system consisting of two liquid p.'s, one mainly water, the other a liquid immiscible with water (*e.g.,* benzene, ether).

external p., the medium or fluid in which a disperse is suspended. SYN dispersion medium.

genital p., in psychoanalytic personality theory, the final stage of psychosexual development, occurring during puberty, in which the individual's psychosexual development is so organized that

sexual gratification can be achieved from genital-to-genital contact and the capacity exists for a mature affectionate relationship with another individual. SEE ALSO phallic p.

internal p., the particles contained in a colloid solution.

latency p., in psychoanalytic personality theory, the period of psychosexual development in children, extending from about age 5 to the beginning of adolescence around age 12, during which the apparent cessation of sexual preoccupation stems from a strong, aggressive blockade of libidinal and sexual impulses in an effort to avoid oedipal relationships; during this p., boys and girls are inclined to choose friends and join groups of their own sex. SYN latency period.

luteal p., that portion of the menstrual cycle extending from the time of formation of the corpus luteum to the onset of menses, usually 14 days in length; **short luteal p.,** a period of 10 days or less between ovulation and the onset of menses, frequently associated with infertility.

oedipal p., in psychoanalysis, a stage in the psychosexual development of the child, characterized by erotic attachment to the parent of the opposite sex, repressed because of fear of the parent of the same sex; usually occurring between the ages of 3 and 6 years.

oral p., in psychoanalytic personality theory, the earliest stage in psychosexual development, lasting through the first 18 months of life, during which the oral zone is the center of the infant's needs, expression, gratification, and pleasurable erotic experiences; has a strong influence on the organization and development of the child's psyche.

phallic p., in psychoanalytic personality theory, the stage in psychosexual development, occurring when a child is between 2 and 6 years of age, during which interest, curiosity, and pleasurable experiences are centered around the penis in boys and the clitoris in girls. SEE ALSO genital p.

radial growth p., the early pattern of growth of cutaneous malignant melanoma, in which tumor cells spread laterally in the epidermis.

vertical growth p., spread of melanoma cells from the epidermis into the dermis and later the subcutis, from which site metastasis may take place.

vulnerable p., a period in the cardiac cycle during which an ectopic impulse may lead to repetitive activity such as flutter or fibrillation of the affected chamber.

△**phen-, pheno-. 1.** Appearance. **2.** CHEMISTRY Combining form denoting derivation from benzene (phenyl-). [fr. G. *phainō,* to appear, show forth]

phen·ac·e·tur·ic ac·id (fĕ-nas-ĕ-tūr'ik). An end product of the metabolism of phenylated fatty acids with even numbers of carbon atoms. SYN phenylaceturic acid.

△**pheno-.** SEE phen-.

phe·no·copy (fē'nō-kop'ē). **1.** A set of clinical and laboratory characteristics that would ordinarily warrant the diagnosis of a specific genetic abnormality, but are of environmental rather than genetic etiology. **2.** A condition of environmental etiology that mimics one usually of genetic etiology. [G. *phainō*, to display, + copy]

phe·nol·u·ria (fē-nol-yū′rē-ă). The excretion of phenols in the urine.

phe·nom·e·non, pl. **phe·nom·e·na** (fĕ-nom′ĕ-non, -nă). **1.** A symptom; an occurrence of any sort, whether ordinary or extraordinary, in relation to a disease. **2.** Any unusual fact or occurrence. [G. *phainomenon*, fr. *phainō*, to cause to appear]

AFORMED p., as induced pulsus alternans progresses, a state in which alternating heart depolarizations fail to eject any blood, thus allowing longer diastolic filling; the subsequent beat is then able to produce a significant ejection; at high rates the cardiac minute volume and blood pressure may appear normal. [*A*lternating *f*ailure *o*f *r*esponse, *m*echanical, to *e*lectrical *d*epolarization]

Anrep p., homeometric autoregulation of the heart whereby cardiac performance improves as the afterload (aortic pressure) is increased.

Austin Flint p., the murmur of relative mitral stenosis during significant aortic regurgitation owing to narrowing of the mitral orifice by pressure of the aortic regurgitant flow on the anterior mitral leaflet. SYN Austin Flint murmur.

dawn p., abrupt increases in fasting levels of plasma glucose concentrations between 5 and 9 AM in the absence of antecedent hypoglycemia; occurs in diabetic patients receiving insulin therapy.

declamping p., shock or hypotension following abrupt release of clamps from a large portion of the vascular bed, as from the aorta; apparently caused by transient pooling of blood in a previously ischemic area. SYN declamping shock.

Donath-Landsteiner p., the hemolysis which results in a sample of blood of a subject with paroxysmal hemoglobinuria when the sample is cooled to around 5°C and then warmed again.

gap p., a short period in the cycle of the atrioventricular or intraventricular conduction allowing passage of an impulse which at other times would be blocked in transit.

generalized Shwartzman p., when both the primary injection of endotoxin-containing filtrate and the secondary injection are given intravenously 24 hours apart, the animal usually dies within 24 hours after the second inoculation. This reaction has no immunological basis.

gestalt p., SEE gestalt.

Jod-Basedow p., induction of thyrotoxicosis in a previously euthyroid individual as a result of exposure to large quantities of iodine; occurs most often in areas of endemic iodine-deficient goiter and in patients with multinodular goiter; also can develop following use of iodine-containing agents for diagnostic studies.

Marcus Gunn p., SYN jaw-winking *syndrome.*

on-off p., a phase in the treatment of Parkinson's disease with *l*-dopa, in which there is a rapid fluctuation of akinetic (off) and choreoathetotic (on) states.

paradoxical diaphragm p., in pyopneumothorax, hydropneumothorax, and some cases of injury, the diaphragm on the affected side rises during inspiration and falls during expiration.

psi p., a p. that includes both psychokinesis and extrasensory perception; the extrasensory mental processes involved in the alleged ability to send or receive telepathic messages.

quellung p., SYN Neufeld capsular *swelling.*

Raynaud's p., a reaction to cold chracterized by intermittent bilateral attacks of ischemia of the fingers or toes marked by severe pallor, numbness, and pain.

rebound p., (1) SYN Stewart-Holmes *sign.* **(2)** generally, any p. in which a variable that has been displaced from its normal state by a disturbing influence temporarily deviates from normal in the opposite direction when the disturbing influence is suddenly removed, before finally stabilizing at its normal state.

Shwartzman p., a rabbit injected intradermally with a small quantity of lipopolysaccharide (endotoxin) followed by a second intravenous injection 24 hours later develops a hemorrhagic and necrotic lesion at the site of the first injection. SEE ALSO generalized Shwartzman p.

Somogyi p., a rebound p. of reactive hyperglycemia following a period of relative hypoglycemia, which may be subclinical and difficult to detect; the hyperglycemia induces use of more insulin, thus aggravating the problem.

staircase p., SYN treppe.

Tyndall p., the visibility of floating particles in gases or liquids when illuminated by a ray of sunlight and viewed at right angles to the illuminating ray.

phe·no·type (fē′nō-tīp). Manifestation of a genotype or the combined manifestation of several different genotypes. The discriminating power of the p. in identifying the genotype depends on its level of subtlety; thus special methods of detecting carriers distinguish them from normal subjects from whom they are inseparable on simple physical examination. P. is the immediate cause of genetic disease and object of genetic selection. [G. *phainō*, to display, + *typos*, model]

phe·no·typ·ic (fē′nō-tip′ik, fen-ō-). Relating to phenotype.

phe·no·zy·gous (fē′nō-zī′gŭs, fe-noz′i-gŭs). Having a narrow cranium as compared with the width of the face, so that when the skull is viewed from above, the zygomatic arches are visible. [G. *phainō*, to show, + *zygon*, yoke]

phen·yl (Ph, Φ) (fen′il). The univalent radical, C_6H_5-, of benzene.

phen·yl·a·ce·tic ac·id (fen′il-ă-sē′tik). An abnormal product of phenylalanine catabolism, appearing in the urine of individuals with phenylketonuria.

phen·yl·a·ce·tur·ic ac·id (fen′il-as-ĕ-tūr′ik). SYN phenaceturic acid.

phen·yl·al·a·nin·ase (fen-il-al′ă-nin-ās). Phenylalanine 4- monooxygenase.

phen·yl·al·a·nine (F) (fen-il-al′ă-nēn). One of the common amino acids in proteins; a nutritionally essential amino acid.

p. 4-monooxygenase, an enzyme that catalyzes the oxidation of L-phenylalanine to L-tyrosine; a deficiency results in phenylketonuria.

phen·yl·di·chlo·ro·ar·sine (PD) (fen′il-dī-klōr-ō-ar′sēn). $C_6H_5As_5Cl_2$; a toxic liquid that has been used as a blister and vomiting agent by certain military and police organizations; it was first used in a limited manner in World War I.

phen·yl·ke·to·nu·ria (PKU) (fen′il-kē′tō-nū′rē-ă). Congenital deficiency of phenylalanine 4-monooxygenase [MIM*261600] or occasionally of dihydropherine reductase [MIM*261630] or of dihydrobiopterin synthetase [MIM*261640]; it causes inadequate formation of L-tyrosine, elevation of serum L-phenylalanine, urinary excretion of phenylpyruvic acid and other derivatives, and accumulation of phenylalanine and its metabolites, which can produce brain damage resulting in severe mental retardation, often with seizures, other neurologic abnormalities such as retarded myelination, and deficient melanin formation leading to hypopigmentation of the skin and eczema. Cf. hyperphenylalaninemia. [phenyl + ketone + G. *ouron*, urine]

phen·yl·lac·tic ac·id (fen-il-lak′tik). A product of phenylalanine catabolism, appearing prominently in the urine in individuals with phenylketonuria.

phe·nyl·py·ru·vic ac·id (fen′il-pī-rū″vik). The transaminated product of the action of phenylalanine aminotransferase; elevated in the urine in individuals with phenylketonuria.

phen·yl·thi·o·hy·dan·to·in (fen′il-thī′ō-hī-dan′tō-in). The compound formed from an amino acid in the Edman method of protein degradation, in which phenylisothiocyanate reacts with the amino moiety of the N-terminal amino acid to form a phenylthiocarbamoyl peptide or protein, on which weak acids act to release the p. containing the N-terminal amino acid.

⬦**pheo-.** **1.** Prefix denoting the same substituents on a phorbin or phorbide (porphyrin) residue as are present in chlorophyll, excluding any ester residues and Mg. **2.** Combining form meaning gray, dark-colored. [G. *phaios*, dusky]

phe·o·chrome (fē′ō-krōm). **1.** SYN chromaffin. **2.** Staining darkly with chromic salts. [G. *phaios*, dusky, + *chrōma*, color]

phe·o·chro·mo·cyte (fē-ō-krō′mō-sīt). A chromaffin cell of a sympathetic paraganglion, medulla of an adrenal gland, or of a pheochromocytoma. [pheochrome + G. *kytos*, cell]

phe·o·chro·mo·cy·to·ma (fē′ō-krō′mō-sī-tō′mă). A functional chromaffinoma, usually benign, derived from adrenal medullary tissue cells and characterized by the secretion of catecholamines, resulting in hypertension, which may be paroxysmal and associated with attacks of palpitation, headache, nausea, dyspnea, anxiety, pallor, and profuse sweating. SEE ALSO paraganglioma.

phe·re·sis (fe-rē′sis). A procedure in which blood is removed from a donor, separated, and a portion retained, with the remainder returned to the donor. SEE ALSO leukapheresis, plateletpheresis, plasmapheresis. [G. *aphairesis*, a taking away, a withdrawal]

pher·o·mones (fer′ō-mōnz). A type of ectohormone secreted by an individual and perceived by a second individual of the same species, thereby producing a change in the sexual or social behav-

ior of that individual. [G. *pherō*, to carry, + *hormaō*, to excite, stimulate]

phi (Φ) (fī). **1.** The 21st letter of the Greek alphabet (φ). **2.** (Φ) Phenyl; potential energy; magnetic flux. **3.** (φ) Plane angle; volume fraction; quantum yield; the dihedral angle of rotation about the $N–C_α$ bond associated with a peptide bond.

Phi·a·loph·o·ra (fī-ă-lof′ŏ-ră). A genus of fungi of which at least two species, *P. verrucosa* and *P. dermatitidis*, cause chromoblastomycosis. [G. *phialē*, a broad, flat vessel, + *phoreō*, to carry]

⬦**-phil, -phile, -philic, -philia.** Affinity for, craving for. [G. *philos*, fond, loving; *phileō*, to love]

phil·trum, pl. **phil·tra** (fil′trŭm, -tră). **1.** A philter or love potion. **2** [NA]. The infranasal depression; the groove in the midline of the upper lip. [L., fr. G. *philtron*, a love-charm, depression on upper lip, fr. *phileō*, to love]

phi·mo·sis, pl. **phi·mo·ses** (fī-mō′sis, -sēz). Narrowness of the opening of the prepuce, preventing its being drawn back over the glans. [G. a muzzling, fr. *phimos*, a muzzle]

phi·mot·ic (fī-mot′ik). Pertaining to phimosis.

⬦**phleb-.** SEE phlebo-.

phleb·ec·ta·sia (fleb-ek-tā′zē-ă). Vasodilation of the veins. SYN venectasia. [phlebo- + G. *ektasis*, a stretching]

phle·bec·to·my (fle-bek′tō-mē). Excision of a segment of a vein, performed sometimes for the cure of varicose veins. SEE ALSO strip (2). SYN venectomy. [phlebo- + G. *ektomē*, excision]

phle·bit·ic (fle-bit′ik). Relating to phlebitis.

phle·bi·tis (fle-bī′tis). Inflammation of a vein. [phlebo- + G. *-itis*, inflammation]

   septic p., inflammation of a vein due to bacterial infection.

⬦**phlebo-, phleb-.** Vein [G. *phleps*]

phleb·o·cly·sis (flĕ-bok′li-sis). Intravenous injection of an isotonic solution of dextrose or other substances in quantity. [phlebo- + G. *klysis*, a washing out]

phleb·o·gram (fleb′ō-gram). A tracing of the jugular or other venous pulse. SYN venogram (2). [phlebo- + G. *gramma*, something written]

phleb·o·graph (fleb′ō-graf). A venous sphygmograph; an instrument for making a tracing of the venous pulse. [phlebo- + G. *graphō*, to write]

phle·bog·ra·phy (fle-bog′ră-fē). **1.** The recording of the venous pulse. **2.** SYN venography. [phlebo- + G. *graphē*, a writing]

phleb·o·lith (fleb′ō-lith). A calcific deposit in a venous wall or thrombus; commonly seen on abdominal radiographs in the lower pelvic region. [phlebo- + G. *lithos*, stone]

phleb·o·li·thi·a·sis (fleb′ō-li-thī′ă-sis). The formation of phleboliths.

phle·bo·ma·nom·e·ter (fleb′ō-mă-nom′ĕ-ter). A manometer for measuring venous blood pressure.

phleb·o·phle·bos·to·my (fleb′ō-fle-bos′tō-mē). SYN venovenostomy.

phleb·o·plas·ty (fleb′ō-plas-tē). Repair of a vein. [phlebo- + G. *plastos*, formed]

phle·bor·rha·phy (fle-bōr′ă-fē). Suture of a vein. [phlebo- + G. *rhaphē*, seam]

phleb·o·scle·ro·sis (fleb′ō-skle-rō′sis). Fibrous

hardening of the walls of the veins. SYN venosclerosis. [phlebo- + G. *sklērōsis,* hardening]

phle·bos·ta·sis (fle-bos′tă-sis). **1.** Abnormally slow motion of blood in veins, usually with venous distention. **2.** Treatment of congestive heart failure by compressing proximal veins of the extremities with tourniquets. SYN venostasis. [phlebo- + G. *stasis,* a standing still]

phleb·o·ste·no·sis (fleb′ō-stĕ-nō′sis). Narrowing of the lumen of a vein from any cause. [phlebo- + G. *stenōsis,* a narrowing]

phleb·o·throm·bo·sis (fleb′ō-throm-bō′sis). Thrombosis, or clotting, in a vein without primary inflammation. [phlebo- + thrombosis]

phle·bot·o·mist (fle-bot′ō-mist). An individual trained and skilled in phlebotomy.

Phle·bot·o·mus (fle-bot′ō-mŭs). A genus of very small bloodsucking sandflies of the subfamily Phlebotominae, family Psychodidae. [phlebo- + G. *tomos,* cutting]

phle·bot·o·my (fle-bot′ō-mē). Incision into a vein for the purpose of drawing blood. SYN venesection, venotomy. [phlebo- + G. *tomē,* incision]

phlegm (flem). **1.** Abnormal amounts of mucus, especially as expectorated from the mouth. **2.** One of the four humors of the body, according to the ancient Greek humoral doctrine. [G. *phlegma,* inflammation]

phleg·ma·sia (fleg-mā′zē-ă). Obsolete term for inflammation, especially when acute and severe. [G. fr. *phlegma,* inflammation]

phleg·mat·ic (fleg-mat′ik). Relating to the heavy one of the four ancient Greek humors (see phlegm), and therefore calm, apathetic, unexcitable. [G. *phlegmatikos,* relating to phlegm]

phleg·mon·ous (fleg′mon-ŭs). Denoting phlegmon.

phlyc·te·na, pl. **phlyc·te·nae** (flik-tē′nă, -nē). A small vesicle, especially one of a number of small blisters following a first degree burn. [G. *phlyktaina,* a blister made by a burn]

phlyc·te·nar (flik′tē-năr). Relating to or marked by the presence of phlyctenae.

phlyc·te·noid (flik′tē-noyd). Resembling a phlyctena. [G. *phlyktaina,* blister, + *eidos,* resemblance]

phlyc·ten·u·la, pl. **phlyc·ten·u·lae** (flik-ten′yū-lă). A small red nodule of lymphoid cells, with ulcerated apex, occurring in the conjunctiva. SYN phlyctenule. [Mod. L. dim. of G. *phlyktaina,* blister]

phlyc·ten·u·lar (flik-ten′yū-lăr). Relating to a phlyctenula.

phlyc·ten·ule (flik′ten-yūl). SYN phlyctenula.

phlyc·ten·u·lo·sis (flik-ten′yū-lō′sis). A nodular hypersensitive affection of corneal and conjunctival epithelium due to endogenous toxin.

pho·bia (fō′bē-ă). Any objectively unfounded morbid dread or fear that arouses a state of panic. The word is used as a combining form in many terms expressing the object that inspires the fear. [G. *phobos,* fear]

   alcoholism, alcoholophobia.

   blood, hemophobia.

   cancer, cancerophobia, carcinophobia.

   childbirth, tocophobia.

   cold, psychrophobia.

   confinement, claustrophobia.

   death, thanatophobia.

   disease, nosophobia, pathophobia.

   disorder, ataxiophobia.

   error, hamartophobia.

   excrement, coprophobia.

   fatigue, ponophobia, kopophobia.

   fever, pyrexiophobia.

   food, cibophobia.

   glass, crystallophobia, hyalophobia.

   hair, trichophobia, trichopathophobia.

   heat, thermophobia.

   infection, molysmophobia.

   itching, acarophobia.

   lice, pediculophobia, phthiriophobia.

   light, photophobia.

   malignancy, cancerophobia, carcinophobia.

   pain, algophobia.

   poisoning, toxicophobia, iophobia.

   pregnancy, maieusiophobia.

   radiation, radiophobia.

   school p., a young child's sudden aversion to or fear of attending school, usually considered a manifestation of separation anxiety.

   self, autophobia.

   sexual intercourse, coitophobia, cypridophobia.

   sexually transmitted disease, cypridophobia, venereophobia.

   sleep, hypnophobia.

   stuttering, laliophobia.

   teeth, odontophobia.

   time, chronophobia.

   vaccination, vaccinophobia.

   water, aquaphobia.

pho·bic (fō′bik). Pertaining to or characterized by phobia.

pho·bo·pho·bia (fō-bō-fō′bē-ă). Morbid dread of developing some phobia. [G. *phobos,* fear]

pho·co·me·lia, pho·com·e·ly (fō-kō-mē′lē-ă, fō-kom′ĕ-lē). Defective development of arms or legs, or both, so that the hands and feet are attached close to the body, resembling the flippers of a seal. [G. *phōkē,* a seal, + *melos,* extremity]

△**phon-.** SEE phono-.

pho·nal (fō′năl). Relating to sound or to the voice. [G. *phōnē,* voice]

phon·as·the·nia (fō-nas-thē′nē-ă). Difficult or abnormal voice production, the enunciation being too high, too loud, or too hard. [phon- + G. *astheneia,* weakness]

pho·na·tion (fō-nā′shŭn). The utterance of sounds by means of vocal folds. [G. *phōnē,* voice]

pho·na·tory (fō′nă-tōr-ē). Relating to phonation.

pho·neme (fō′nēm). The smallest sound unit which, in terms of the phonetic sequences of sound, controls meaning. [G. *phōnēma,* a voice]

pho·nen·do·scope (fō-nen′dō-skōp). A stethoscope that intensifies the auscultatory sounds by means of two parallel resonating plates, one resting on the patient's chest or attached to a stethoscope tube, the other vibrating in unison with it. [phon- + G. *endon,* within, + *skopeō,* to view]

pho·net·ic (fō-net′ik). Relating to speech or to the voice. SEE ALSO phonic. [G. *phōnētikos*]

pho•net•ics (fō-net′iks). The science of speech and of pronunciation.

pho•ni•at•rics (fō-nē-at′riks). A branch of medicine concerned with the diagnosis and treatment of voice and speech disorders. [phon- + G. *iatrikos,* of the healing art]

phon•ic (fon′ik, fō′nik). Relating to sound or to the voice. SEE ALSO phonetic.

△**phono-, phon-.** Sound, speech, or voice sounds. [G. *phōnē*]

pho•no•an•gi•og•ra•phy (fō′nō-an-jē-og′ră-fē). Recording and analysis of the audible frequency-intensity components of the bruit of turbulent arterial blood flow through a stenotic lesion. [phono- + G. *angeion,* vessel, + *graphō,* to write]

pho•no•car•di•o•gram (fō-nō-kar′dē-ō-gram). A record of the heart sounds made by means of a phonocardiograph.

pho•no•car•di•o•graph (fō-nō-kar′dē-ō-graf). An instrument, utilizing microphones, amplifiers, and filters, for graphically recording the heart sounds, which are displayed on an oscilloscope or analog tracing.

pho•no•car•di•og•ra•phy (fō′nō-kar-dē-og′ră-fē). **1.** Recording of the heart sounds with a phonocardiograph. **2.** The science of interpreting phonocardiograms. [phono- + G. *kardia,* heart, + *graphō,* to record]

pho•no•cath•e•ter (fō-nō-kath′ĕ-ter). A cardiac catheter with diminutive microphone housed in its tip, for recording sounds and murmurs from within the heart and great vessels.

pho•no•gram (fō′nō-gram). A graphic curve depicting the duration and intensity of a sound. [phono- + G. *gramma,* diagram]

pho•nom•e•ter (fō-nom′ĕ-ter). An instrument for measuring the pitch and intensity of sounds. [phono- + G. *metron,* measure]

pho•no•my•oc•lo•nus (fō′nō-mī-ok′lō-nŭs). Clonic spasms of muscles in response to aural stimuli. [phono- + G. *mys,* muscle, + *klonos,* tumult]

pho•nop•a•thy (fō-nop′ă-thē). Any disease of the vocal organs affecting speech. [phono- + G. *pathos,* suffering]

phonophoresis (fō-nō-fōr-e′sĭs). Introduction of anti-inflammatory drugs through the skin by the use of ultrasound. SEE ALSO iontophoresis. [phono- + G. *phorēsis,* a carrying]

pho•no•pho•tog•ra•phy (fō′nō-fō-tog′ră-fē). The recording on a moving photographic plate of the movements imparted to a diaphragm by sound waves. [phono- + photography]

pho•nop•sia (fō-nop′sē-ă). A condition in which the hearing of certain sounds gives rise to a subjective sensation of color. [phono- + G. *opsis,* vision]

pho•no•re•cep•tor (fō′nō-rē-sep′ter). A receptor for sound stimuli.

△**phor-.** SEE phoro-.

pho•re•sis (fōr′ē-sis, fō-rē′sis). **1.** SYN electrophoresis. **2.** A biological association in which one organism is transported by another. [G. *phorēsis,* a being borne]

phor•ia (fōr′ē-ă). The relative directions assumed by the eyes during binocular fixation of a given object in the absence of an adequate fusion stimulus. SEE cyclophoria, esophoria, exophoria, heterophoria, hyperphoria, hypophoria, orthophoria. [G. *phora,* a carrying, motion]

△**phoro-, phor-.** Carrying, bearing; a carrier, a bearer; phobia. [G. *phoros,* carrying, bearing]

△**phos-.** Light. [G. *phōs*]

phos•gene (fos′jēn). Carbonic dichloride, $COCl_2$; a colorless liquid below 8.2°C, but an extremely poisonous gas at ordinary temperatures; more than 80% of World War I chemical agent fatalities were caused by p.

△**phosph-, phospho-, phosphor-, phosphoro-.** Prefixes indicating the presence of phosphorus in a compound. See phospho- for specific usage of that prefix. [G. *phōs,* light; *phoros,* carrying]

phos•pha•tase (fos′fă-tās). Any of a group of enzymes (EC sub-subclass 3.1.3) that liberate inorganic phosphate from phosphoric esters.

 acid p., a p. with an optimum pH of less than 7.0, notably present in the prostate gland.

 alkaline p., a p. with an optimum pH of above 7.0 present ubiquitously; low levels of this enzyme are seen in cases of hypophosphatasia.

phos•phate (fos′fāt). A salt or ester of phosphoric acid. For individual p.'s not listed here, see under the name of the base.

 high energy p.'s, those p.'s that, on hydrolysis, yield an unusually large amount of energy; *e.g.,* nucleotide polyphosphates such as ATP, enol p.'s such as phospho*enol*pyruvate.

phos•pha•te•mia (fos-fă-tē′mē-ă). An abnormally high concentration of inorganic phosphates in the blood. [phosphate + G. *haima,* blood]

phos•phat•ic (fos-fat′ik). Relating to or containing phosphates.

phos•phat•i•dyl•glyc•er•ol (fos-fă-tī′dĭl-glis′er-ol). A constituent in human amniotic fluid that denotes fetal lung maturity when present in the last trimester.

phos•pha•tu•ria (fos-fă-tū′rē-ă). Excessive excretion of phosphates in the urine. [phosphate + G. *ouron,* urine]

phos•phene (fos′fēn). Sensation of light produced by mechanical or electrical stimulation of the peripheral or central optic pathway of the nervous system. [G. *phōs,* light, + *phainō,* to show]

phos•phide (fos′fīd). A compound of phosphorus with valence −3; *e.g.,* sodium phosphide, Na_3P.

△**phospho-.** Prefix for *O*-phosphono-, which may replace the suffix phosphate; *e.g.,* glucose phosphate is *O*-phosphonoglucose or phosphoglucose. SEE ALSO phosph-.

3′-phos•pho•aden•o•sine 5′-phos•phate (PAP) (fos′fō-a-den′ō-sēn). A product in sulfuryl transfer reactions.

phos•pho•am•i•dase (fos-fō-am′i-dās). An enzyme catalyzing the hydrolysis of phosphorus-nitrogen bonds.

phos•pho•am•ides (fos-fō-am′īdz). Amides of phosphoric acid (phosphoramidic acids) and their salts or esters.

phos•pho•cre•a•tine (fos-fō-krē′ă-tēn). A phosphagen; a compound of creatine with phosphoric acid; a source of energy in the contraction of vertebrate muscle, its breakdown furnishing phosphate for the resynthesis of ATP from ADP by creatine kinase. SYN creatine phosphate.

phos·pho·di·es·ter·as·es (fos'fō-dī-es'ter-ās-ez). Enzymes (EC sub-subclass 3.1.4) cleaving phosphodiester bonds, such as those in cAMP or between nucleotides in nucleic acids, liberating smaller poly- or oligonucleotide units or mononucleotides but not inorganic phosphate.

phos·pho·e·nol·pyr·u·vic ac·id (fos'fō-ē'nol-pī-rū'vik). The phosphoric ester of pyruvic acid in the latter's enol form; an intermediate in the conversion of glucose to pyruvic acid and an example of a high energy phosphate ester.

phos·pho·glyc·er·ides (fos-fō-glis'er-īdz). Acylglycerol and diacylglycerol phosphates; constituents of nerve tissue, and involved in fat transport and storage.

phos·pho·li·pase (fos-fō-lip'ās). An enzyme that catalyzes the hydrolysis of a phospholipid. SYN lecithinase.

phos·pho·lip·id (fos-fō-lip'id). A lipid containing phosphorus, thus including the lecithins and other phosphatidyl derivatives, sphingomyelin, and plasmalogens; the basic constituents of biomembranes.

phos·pho·mu·tase (fos-fō-myū'tās). One of a number of enzymes that catalyze intramolecular transfer.

phos·pho·ne·cro·sis (fos-fō-ne-krō'sis). Necrosis of the osseous tissue of the jaw, as a result of poisoning by inhalation of phosphorus fumes, occurring especially in persons with prolonged occupational exposure. [phosphorus + G. *nekrōsis*, death (necrosis)]

phos·pho·pro·tein (fos-fō-prō'tēn). A protein containing phosphoryl groups attached directly to the side chains of some of its constituent amino acids.

phos·phor (fos'fōr). A chemical substance that transforms incident electromagnetic or radioactive energy into light, as in scintillation radioactivity determinations or radiographic intensifying screens or image amplifiers. [G. *phōs*, light, + *phoros*, bearing]

phosphor-, phosphoro-. SEE phosph-.

phos·pho·res·cence (fos-fŏ-res'ens). The quality or property of emitting light without active combustion or the production of heat, generally as the result of prior exposure to radiation, which persists after the inciting cause is removed. [G. *phōs*, light, + *phoros*, bearing]

phos·pho·res·cent (fos'fŏ-res'ent). Having the property of phosphorescence.

5-phos·pho-α-D-ri·bo·syl 1-py·ro·phos·phate (PRPP). 5-Phosphoribosyl 1-diphosphate; D-Ribose carrying a phosphate group on ribose carbon-5 and a pyrophosphate group on ribose carbon-1; an intermediate in the formation of the pyrimidine and purine nucleotides as well as NAD^+.

phos·phor·ic ac·id (fos-fōr'ik). A strong acid of industrial importance; dilute solutions have been used as urinary acidifiers and as dressings to remove necrotic debris. In dentistry, it comprises about 60% of the liquid used in zinc phosphate and silicate cements; solutions are used for conditioning enamel surfaces prior to applications of various types of resins.

phos·phor·ism (fos'fōr-izm). Chronic poisoning with phosphorus.

phos·pho·rol·y·sis (fos-fŏ-rol'i-sis). A reaction analogous to hydrolysis except that the elements of phosphoric acid, rather than of water, are added in the course of splitting a bond.

phos·pho·rous (fos'fōr-ŭs, fos-fōr'ŭs). **1.** Relating to, containing, or resembling phosphorus. **2.** Referring to phosphorus in its lower (+3) valence state.

phos·pho·rus (fos'fōr-ŭs). A nonmetallic chemical element, atomic no. 15, atomic wt. 30.973762, occurring extensively in nature, always in chemical combination; the elemental form is extremely poisonous, causing intense inflammation and fatty degeneration; repeated inhalation of p. fumes may cause necrosis of the jaw (phosphonecrosis). [G. *phosphoros*, fr. *phōs*, light, + *phoros*, bearing]

phos·pho·rus-32. Radioactive phosphorus isotope; beta emitter with half-life of 14.28 days; used as tracer in metabolic studies and in the treatment of certain diseases of the osseous and hematopoietic systems.

phos·pho·ryl·ase (fos-fōr'i-lās). A phosphorylated enzyme cleaving poly(1,4-α-D-glucosyl)$_n$ with inorganic phosphate to form poly(1,4-α-D-glucosyl)$_{n-1}$ and α-D-glucose 1-phosphate.

 p. phosphatase, an enzyme catalyzing the conversion of one p. *a* into two p. *b*, with the release of four phosphates.

phos·pho·ryl·a·tion (fos'fōr-i-lā'shŭn). Addition of phosphate to an organic compound, such as glucose to produce glucose monophosphate, through the action of a phosphotransferase (phosphorylase) or kinase.

 oxidative p., formation of high energy phosphoric bonds from the energy released by the dehydrogenation (*i.e.*, oxidation) of various substrates.

phos·pho·sug·ar (fos-fō-shug'er). A phosphorylated saccharide; any sugar containing an alcoholic group esterified with phosphoric acid.

phos·pho·tung·stic ac·id (PTA) (fos-fō-tŭng' stik). A mixture of phosphoric and tungstic acids, approximately 24 WO_3, 2 H_3PO_4, 48 H_2O; a protein precipitant and reagent for arginine, lysine, histidine, and cystine; used with hematoxylin for nuclear and muscle staining; also used in electron microscopy as a stain for collagen and as a negative stain.

phot-. SEE photo-.

pho·tal·gia (fō-tal'jē-ă). Light-induced pain, especially of the eyes. SYN photodynia. [phot- + G. *algos*, pain]

pho·tic (fō'tik). Relating to light.

pho·tism (fō'tizm). Production of a sensation of light or color by a stimulus to another sense organ, such as of hearing, taste, or touch.

photo-, phot-. Light. [G. *phōs* (*phōt*-)]

pho·to·ab·la·tion (fō'tō-ab-lā'shun). The process of photoablative decomposition of tissue by laser light, *e.g.*, in photorefractive keratectomy.

pho·to·bi·ot·ic (fō'tō-bī-ot'ik). Living or flourishing only in the light. [photo- + G. *bios*, life]

pho·to·cat·a·lyst (fō-tō-kat'ă-list). A substance that helps bring about a light-catalyzed reaction;

e.g., chlorophyll. [photo- + G. *katalysis,* dissolution (catalysis)]

pho·to·chem·i·cal (fō-tō-kem'i-kăl). Denoting chemical changes caused by or involving light.

pho·to·che·mo·ther·a·py (fō'tō-kem-ō-thār'ă-pē, -kē-mō-). SYN photoradiation.

pho·to·co·ag·u·la·tion (fō'tō-kō-ag'yū-lā'shŭn). A method by which a beam of electromagnetic energy is directed to a desired tissue under visual control; localized coagulation results from absorption of light energy and its conversion to heat or conversion of tissue to plasma (atoms stripped of electrons). [photo- + L. *coagulo,* pp. *-atus,* to curdle]

pho·to·co·ag·u·la·tor (fō'tō-kō-ag'yū-lā'ter, tōr). The apparatus used in photocoagulation.

pho·to·der·ma·ti·tis (fō'tō-der-mă-tī'tis). Dermatitis caused or elicited by exposure to sunlight; may be phototoxic or photoallergic, and can result from topical application, ingestion, inhalation, or injection of mediating phototoxic or photoallergic material. SEE ALSO photosensitization. SYN actinic dermatitis, actinodermatitis. [photo- + G. *derma,* skin, + *-itis,* inflammation]

photodetector (fo-to-di-tek-ter). A device in a spectrophotometer that responds to photons in a manner usually proportional to the number of photons striking its light-sensitive surface.

pho·to·dis·tri·bu·tion (fō'tō-dis-tri-byū'shŭn). Areas on the skin that receive the greatest amount of exposure to sunlight, and which are involved in eruptions due to photosensitivity.

pho·to·dyn·ia (fō-tō-din'ē-ă). SYN photalgia. [photo- + G. *odynē,* pain]

pho·to·e·lec·tric (fō'tō-ē-lek'trik). Denoting electronic or electric effects produced by the action of light.

pho·to·flu·o·rog·ra·phy (fō'tō-flūr-og'ră-fē). Miniature radiographs made by contact photography of a fluoroscopic screen, formerly used in mass radiographic examination of the lungs. SYN fluorography. [photo- + L. *fluor,* a flow, + G. *graphē,* a writing]

pho·to·gas·tro·scope (fō'tō-gas'trō-skōp). An instrument for taking photographs of the interior of the stomach. [photo- + G. *gastēr,* stomach, + *skopeō,* to view]

pho·to·gen·ic, pho·tog·e·nous (fō-tō-jen'ik, fō-toj'ĕ-nŭs). Denoting or capable of photogenesis.

pho·to·in·ac·ti·va·tion (fō'tō-in-ak-ti-vā'shŭn). Inactivation by light; *e.g.,* as in the treatment of herpes simplex by local application of a photoactive dye followed by exposure to a fluorescent lamp.

pho·to·lu·mi·nes·cent (fō'tō-lū-mi-nes'ent). Having the ability to become luminescent upon exposure to visible light. [photo- + L. *lumen,* light]

pho·tol·y·sis (fō-tol'i-sis). Decomposition of a chemical compound by the action of light. [photo- + G. *lysis,* dissolution]

pho·to·lyt·ic (fō-tō-lit'ik). Pertaining to photolysis.

pho·to·mi·cro·graph (fō'tō-mī'krō-graf). An enlarged photograph of an object viewed with a microscope, as distinguished from microphoto-

graph. SYN micrograph. [photo- + G. *mikros,* small, + *graphē,* a record]

pho·to·mi·crog·ra·phy (fō'tō-mī-krog'ră-fē). The production of a photomicrograph.

pho·to·my·oc·lo·nus (fō'tō-mī-ok'lō-nŭs). Clonic spasms of muscles in response to visual stimuli. [photo- + G. *mys,* muscle, + *klonos,* confused motion]

pho·ton (gamma) (fō'ton). PHYSICS A corpuscle of energy or particle of light; a quantum of light or other electromagnetic radiation.

pho·to·per·cep·tive (fō'tō-per-sep'tiv). Capable of both receiving and perceiving light.

pho·to·pho·bia (fō-tō-fō'bē-ă). Morbid dread and avoidance of light. Although often an expression of undue anxiety about the eyes, photosensitivity and photalgia, past or present, should be considered. [photo- + G. *phobos,* fear]

pho·to·pho·bic (fō-tō-fō'bik). Relating to or suffering from photophobia.

pho·toph·thal·mia (fō'tof-thal'mē-ă). Keratoconjunctivitis caused by ultraviolet energy, as in snow blindness, exposure to an ultraviolet lamp, arc welding, or the short circuit of a high-tension electric current. SEE ALSO photoretinopathy. [photo- + G. *ophthalmos,* eye]

pho·to·pia (fō-tō'pē-ă). SYN photopic *vision.* [photo- + G. *opsis,* vision]

pho·top·ic (fō-top'ik). Pertaining to photopic vision.

pho·top·sia (fō-top'sē-ă). A subjective sensation of lights, sparks, or colors due to electrical or mechanical stimulation of the ocular system. SYN photopsy. [photo- + G. *opsis,* vision]

pho·top·sin (fō-top'sin). The protein moiety (opsin) of the pigment (iodopsin) in the cones of the retina.

pho·top·sy (fō-top'sē). SYN photopsia.

pho·to·ptar·mo·sis (fō'tō-tar-mō'sis). Reflex sneezing that occurs when bright light stimulates the retina. [photo- + G. *ptarmos,* a sneezing, + *-osis,* condition]

pho·to·ra·di·a·tion (fō'tō-rā-dē-ā'shŭn). Treatment of cancer by intravenous injection of a photosensitizing agent, such as hematoporphyrin, followed by exposure to visible light of superficial tumors or of deep tumors by a fiberoptic probe. SYN photochemotherapy, photoradiation therapy.

pho·to·re·ac·tion (fō'tō-rē-ak'shŭn). A reaction caused or affected by light; *e.g.,* a photochemical reaction, photolysis, photosynthesis, phototropism, thymine dimer formation.

pho·to·re·ac·ti·va·tion (fō'tō-rē-ak-ti-vā'shŭn). Activation by light of something or of some process previously inactive or inactivated.

pho·to·re·cep·tive (fō'tō-rē-sep'tiv). Functioning as a photoreceptor.

pho·to·re·cep·tor (fō'tō-rē-sep'ter, tōr). A receptor that is sensitive to light, *e.g.,* a retinal rod or cone. [photo- + L. *re-cipio,* pp. *-ceptus,* to receive, fr. *capio,* to take]

pho·to·ret·i·ni·tis (fō'tō-ret'i-nī'tis). SEE photoretinopathy.

pho·to·ret·i·nop·a·thy (fō'tō-ret'i-nop'ă-thē). A macular burn from excessive exposure to sunlight or other intense light (*e.g.,* the flash of a short circuit); characterized subjectively by reduced visual acuity. [photo- + retina, + G. *pathos,* suffering]

pho•to•scan (fō′tō-skan). SYN scintiscan.

pho•to•sen•si•ti•za•tion (fō′tō-sen-si-ti-zā′shŭn). **1.** Sensitization of the skin to light, usually due to the action of certain drugs, plants, or other substances; may occur shortly after administration of the drug (phototoxic sensitivity), or may occur only after a latent period of days to months (photoallergic sensitivity, or photoallergy). **2.** SYN photodynamic *sensitization.*

pho•to•sta•ble (fō′tō-stā-bl). Not subject to change upon exposure to light.

pho•to•steth•o•scope (fō-tō-steth′ō-skōp). Device that converts sound into flashes of light; used for continuous observation of the fetal heart.

pho•to•syn•the•sis (fō-tō-sin′thĕ-sis). **1.** The compounding or building up of chemical substances under the influence of light. **2.** The process by which green plants, using chlorophyll and the energy of sunlight, produce carbohydrates from water and carbon dioxide, liberating molecular oxygen in the process. [photo- + G. *synthesis,* a putting together]

pho•to•tax•is (fō-tō-tak′sis). Reaction of living protoplasm to the stimulus of light, involving bodily motion of the whole organism toward (**positive p.**) or away from (**negative p.**) the stimulus. Cf. phototropism. [photo- + G. *taxis,* orderly arrangement]

pho•to•ther•a•py (fō-tō-thār′ă-pē). Treatment of disease by means of light rays. SYN light treatment.

pho•to•tim•er (fō-tō-tīm′ĕr). An electronic device in radiography that measures the radiation that has passed through the patient and terminates the x-ray exposure when it is sufficient to form an image.

pho•tot•ro•pism (fō-to′trō-pizm). Movement of a part of an organism toward (**positive p.**) or away from (**negative p.**) the stimulus of light. Cf. phototaxis. [photo- + G. *trope,* a turning]

pho•tu•ria (fō-tū′rē-ă). The passage of phosphorescent urine. [photo- + G. *ouron,* urine]

⊃phren-. SEE phreno-.

phre•nal•gia (fre-nal′jē-ă). **1.** SYN psychalgia (1). **2.** Pain in the diaphragm. [phren- + G. *algos,* pain]

phre•net•ic (frĕ-net′ik). **1.** Frenzied; maniacal. **2.** An individual exhibiting such behavior. [G. *phrenitikos,* frenzied]

⊃phreni-. SEE phreno-.

⊃-phrenia. 1. The diaphragm. **2.** The mind. SEE phreno-. [G. *phrēn,* the diaphragm, mind, heart (as seat of emotions]

phren•ic (fren′ik). **1.** SYN diaphragmatic. **2.** Relating to the mind.

phren•i•cec•to•my (fren-i-sek′tō-mē). Exsection of a portion of the phrenic nerve, to prevent reunion such as may follow phrenicotomy. SYN phrenicoexeresis. [phreni- + G. *ektomē,* excision]

phren•i•cla•sia (fren-i-klā′zē-ă). Crushing of a section of the phrenic nerve to produce a temporary paralysis of the diaphragm. SYN phrenicotripsy. [phreni- + G. *klasis,* a breaking away]

phren•i•co•col•ic (fren′i-kō-kol′ik). Relating to the diaphragm and the colon.

phren•i•co•ex•er•e•sis (fren′i-kō-ek-ser′ĕ-sis). SYN phrenicectomy. [phrenico- + G. *exairesis,* a taking out, fr. *haireō,* to take, grasp]

phren•i•co•gas•tric (fren′i-kō-gas′trik). Relating to the diaphragm and the stomach.

phren•i•co•he•pa•tic (fren′i-kō-he-pa′tik). Relating to the diaphragm and the liver.

phren•i•cot•o•my (fren-i-kot′ō-mē). Section of the phrenic nerve in order to induce unilateral paralysis of the diaphragm, which is then pushed up by the abdominal viscera and exerts compression upon a diseased lung. [phrenico- + G. *tomē,* incision]

phren•i•co•trip•sy (fren′i-kō-trip′sē). SYN phreniclasia. [phrenico- + G. *tripsis,* a rubbing]

⊃phreno-, phren-, phreni-, phrenico-. The diaphragm; the mind; the phrenic nerve. [G. *phrēn,* diaphragm, mind, heart (as seat of emotions)]

phren•o•car•dia (fren-ō-kar′dē-ă). Precordial pain and dyspnea of psychogenic origin, often a symptom of anxiety neurosis. SEE cardiac *neurosis.* [phreno- + G. *kardia,* heart]

phren•o•ple•gia (fren-ō-plē′jē-ă). Paralysis of the diaphragm. [phreno- + G. *plēgē,* stroke]

phren•op•to•sia (fren-op-tō′sē-ă). An abnormal sinking down of the diaphragm. [phreno- + G. *ptōsis,* a falling]

phryn•o•der•ma (frin-ō-der′mă). A follicular hyperkeratotic eruption thought to be due to deficiency of vitamin A. [G. *phrynos,* toad, + *derma,* skin]

Phthi•rus (thī′rŭs). SEE *Pthirus.* [L. *phthir;* G. *phtheir,* a louse]

phy•co•my•co•sis (fī′kō-mī′kō-sis). SYN zygomycosis.

phy•lax•is (fī-lak′sis). Protection against infection. [G. a guarding, protection]

phyl•lo•qui•none (K) (fil-ō-kwin′ōn). Vitamin K_1 or $K_1(20)$; 2-methyl-3-phytyl-1,4-naphthoquinone; 3-phytylmenaquinone; isolated from alfalfa; also prepared synthetically; major form of vitamin K found in plants. SYN phylloquinone K, vitamin K_1, vitamin $K_1(20)$.

phyl•lo•qui•none K (-kwi′nōn). SYN phylloquinone.

⊃phylo-. Tribe, race; a taxonomic phylum. [G. *phylon,* tribe]

phy•lo•gen•e•sis (fī-lō-jen′ĕ-sis). SYN phylogeny. [phylo- + G. *genesis,* origin]

phy•lo•ge•net•ic, phy•lo•gen•ic (fī′lō-jĕ-net′ik, -jen′ik). Relating to phylogenesis.

phy•log•e•ny (fī-loj′ĕ-nē). The evolutionary development of species, as distinguished from ontogeny, development of the individual. SYN phylogenesis.

phy•lum, pl. **phy•la** (fī′lŭm, fī′lă). A taxonomic division below the kingdom and above the class. [Mod. L. fr. G. *phylon,* tribe]

phy•ma (fī′mă). A nodule or small rounded tumor of the skin. [G. a tumor]

phy•ma•to•sis (fī-mă-tō′sis). The growth or presence of phymas or small nodules in the skin.

phy•sal•i•form (fi-sal′i-fōrm). Like a bubble or small bleb. [G. *physallis,* bladder, bubble, + L. *forma,* form]

ph

phys·a·lis (fis'ă-lis). A vacuole in a giant cell found in certain malignant neoplasms, such as chordoma. [G. *physallis,* a bladder]

phys·e·al (fiz'ē-ăl). Pertaining to the physis, or growth cartilage area, separating the metaphysis and the epiphysis.

△**physi-.** SEE physio-.

phys·i·at·rics (fiz-ē-at'riks). **1.** Old term for physical *therapy.* **2.** Rehabilitation management. [G. *physis,* nature, + *iatrikos,* healing]

phys·i·a·trist (fiz-ī'ă-trist). A physician who specializes in physical medicine.

phys·i·a·try (fi-zī'ă-trē). SYN physical *medicine.*

phys·i·cal (fiz'i-kăl). Relating to the body, as distinguished from the mind. [Mod. L. *physicalis,* fr. G. *physikos*]

phy·si·cian (fi-zish'ŭn). **1.** A doctor; a person who has been educated, trained, and licensed to practice the art and science of medicine. **2.** A practitioner of medicine, as contrasted with a surgeon. [Fr. *physicien,* a natural philosopher]

admitting p., p. who formally and legally accepts a patient for admission to a health care facility.

attending p., p. who is formally and legally responsible for a patient's care throughout the stay in a health care facility.

osteopathic p., a practitioner of osteopathy. SYN osteopath.

primary care p., p. in family practice, internal medicine, obstetrics/gynecology, or pediatrics who is a patient's first contact for health care in an ambulatory setting. SEE ALSO health care provider.

phys·i·co·chem·i·cal (fiz'i-kō-kem'i-kăl). Relating to the field of physical chemistry.

phys·ics (fiz'iks). The branch of science concerned with the phenomena of matter and energy and their interactions.

△**physio-, physi-.** **1.** Physical, physiological. **2.** Natural, relating to physics. [G. *physis,* nature]

phys·i·o·gen·ic (fiz'ē-ō-jen'ik). Related to or caused by physiologic activity. [physio- + G. *genesis,* origin]

phys·i·og·no·my (fiz-ē-og'nō-mē). **1.** The physical appearance of one's face, countenance, or habitus, especially regarded as an indication of character. **2.** Estimation of one's character and mental qualities by a study of the face and other external bodily features. [physio- + G. *gnōmōn,* a judge]

phys·i·o·log·ic, phys·i·o·log·i·cal (fiz-ē-ō-loj'ik, -loj'i-kăl). **1.** Relating to physiology. **2.** Normal, as opposed to pathologic; denoting the various vital processes. **3.** Denoting something that is apparent from its functional effects rather than from its anatomical structure; *e.g.,* a p. sphincter. **4.** Denoting a dose or the effects of such a dose (of a chemical agent that either is or mimics a hormone, neurotransmitter, or other naturally occurring agent) that is within the range of concentrations or potencies that would occur naturally. Cf. homeopathic (2), pharmacologic (2).

phys·i·ol·o·gist (fiz-ē-ol'ō-jist). A specialist in physiology.

phys·i·ol·o·gy (fiz-ē-ol'ō-jē). The science concerned with the normal vital processes of animal and vegetable organisms, especially as to how things normally function in the living organism rather than to their anatomical structure, their biochemical composition, or how they are affected by drugs or disease. [L. or G. *physiologia,* fr. G. *physis,* nature, + *logos,* study]

exercise p., subfield of p. related to responses and adaptations in body function and structure with acute and chronic exposure to exercise. SEE ALSO physiology.

phys·i·o·ther·a·peu·tic (fiz'ē-ō-thār-ă-pyū'tik). Pertaining to physical *therapy.*

phys·i·o·ther·a·pist (fiz'ē-ō-thār'ă-pist). A physical therapist. SEE physical *therapy* (2).

phys·i·o·ther·a·py (fiz'ē-ō-thār'ă-pē). SYN physical *therapy* (1). [physio- + G. *therapeia,* treatment]

phy·sique (fi-zēk'). constitutional type; the physical or bodily structure; the "build." [Fr.]

△**physo-.** **1.** Tendency to swell or inflate. **2.** Relation to air or gas. [G. *physaō,* to inflate, distend]

phy·so·cele (fī'sō-sēl). **1.** A circumscribed swelling due to the presence of gas. **2.** A hernial sac distended with gas. [physo- + G. *kēlē,* tumor, hernia]

phy·so·me·tra (fī-sō-mē'tră). Distention of the uterine cavity with air or gas. [physo- + G. *mētra,* uterus]

phy·so·py·o·sal·pinx (fī'sō-pī-ō-sal'pingks). Pyosalpinx accompanied by a formation of gas in an ovarian (fallopian) tube. [physo- + G. *pyon,* pus, + *salpinx,* trumpet]

△**phyt-.** SEE phyto-.

△**phyto-, phyt-.** Plants. [G. *phyton,* a plant]

phy·to·ag·glu·ti·nin (fī'tō-ă-glū'ti-nin). A lectin that causes agglutination of erythrocytes or of leukocytes.

phy·to·be·zoar (fī-tō-bē'zōr). A gastric concretion formed of vegetable fibers, with the seeds and skins of fruits, and sometimes starch granules and fat globules. SYN food ball. [phyto- + bezoar]

phy·to·der·ma·ti·tis (fī'tō-der-mă-tī'tis). Dermatitis caused by various mechanisms including mechanical and chemical injury, allergy, or photosensitization (phytophotodermatitis) at skin sites previously exposed to plants.

phy·to·hem·ag·glu·ti·nin (PHA) (fī'tō-hēm-ă-glū'ti-nin). A phytomitogen from plants that agglutinates red blood cells. The term is commonly used specifically for the lectin obtained from the red kidney bean (*Phaseolus vulgaris*) which is also a mitogen. SYN phytolectin.

phy·toid (fī'toyd). Resembling a plant; denoting an animal having many of the biologic characteristics of a vegetable. [G. *phytōdēs,* fr. *phyton,* plant, + *eidos,* resemblance]

phy·tol (fī'tol). An unsaturated primary alcohol derived from the hydrolysis of chlorophyll; a constituent of vitamins E and K_1.

phy·to·lec·tin (fī-tō-lek'tin). SYN phytohemagglutinin.

phy·to·mi·to·gen (fī-tō-mī'tō-jen). A mitogenic lectin causing lymphocyte transformation accompanied by mitotic proliferation of the resulting blast cells identical to that produced by antigenic stimulation; *e.g.,* phytohemagglutinin, concanavalin A.

phy·to·phlyc·to·der·ma·ti·tis (fī′tō-flik′tō-der-mă-ti′tis). SYN meadow *dermatitis*. [phyto- + G. *phlyktaina*, blister, + dermatitis]

phy·to·pho·to·der·ma·ti·tis (fī′tō-fō′tō-der-mă-ti′tis). Phytodermatitis resulting from photosensitization.

phy·to·tox·ic (fī-tō-tok′sik). **1.** Poisonous to plant life. **2.** Pertaining to a phytotoxin.

phy·to·tox·in (fī-tō-tok′sin). A substance similar in its properties to an extracellular bacterial toxin. [phyto- + G. *toxikon*, poison]

PI Periodontal *Index*.

pI The pH value for the isoelectric *point* of a given substance.

pi (π) (pī). **1.** The 16th letter of the Greek alphabet (π, Π). **2.** Symbol for osmotic pressure. **3.** MATHEMATICS symbol for the product of a series. **4.** Symbol for the ratio of the circumference of a circle to its diameter (approximately 3.14159265).

pia (pī′ă, pē′ă). SYN pia mater. [L. fem. of *pius*, tender]

pia-a·rach·ni·tis (pī′ă-ă-rak-nī′tis). SYN leptomeningitis.

pia-a·rach·noid (pī′ă-ă-rak′noyd, pē′ă-). SYN leptomeninges.

pi·al (pī′al, pē′al). Relating to the pia mater.

pia mat·er (pī′ă mā′ter, pē′ă mah′ter). A delicate vasculated fibrous membrane firmly adherent to the glial capsule of the brain (**p. m. cranialis [encephali]** [NA]) and spinal cord (**p. m. spinalis** [NA] or membrana limitans gliae); following exactly the outer markings of the cerebrum and also the ependymal lining circumference of the choroid membranes and plexus, it invests the cerebellum but not so intimately as it does the cerebrum, not dipping down into all the smaller sulci. The p. m. and the arachnoid are collectively called leptomeninges, as distinguished from dura mater or pachymeninx. SYN pia. [L. tender, affectionate mother, mistransl. of Arabic *umm raqīqah*, delicate covering or protection]

pi·an (pē-an′, pī′an). SYN yaws.

pi·a·rach·noid (pī′ă-rak′noyd). SYN leptomeninges.

pi·ca (pī′kă, pē′kă). An appetite for substances not fit as food or of no nutritional value; clay, dried paint, starch. [L. *pica*, magpie]

pico-. **1.** Small. **2 (p).** Prefix used in the SI and metric systems to signify one-trillionth (10^{-12}). SYN bicro-. [It. *piccolo*]

pi·co·gram (pg) (pī′kō-gram, pē′kō-gram). One-trillionth of a gram.

pi·co·ka·tal (pkat) (pī′kō-kat′ăl; pē′ko-kat′ăl). One trillionth of a katal (10^{-12} katal).

pi·com·e·ter (pm) (pī′kō-mē-ter). One-trillionth of a meter. SYN bicron.

pi·co·mole (pmol) (pē′kō-mōl; pī′kō-mōl). One-trillionth of a mole (10^{-12} mole).

Pi·cor·na·vir·i·dae (pi-kōr-nă-vir′i-dē). A family of very small viruses having a core of single-stranded RNA. Numerous species (including the polioviruses, coxsackieviruses, and echoviruses) are included in the family. There are four accepted genera: *Enterovirus, Rhinovirus, Cardiovirus*, and *Aphthovirus*. [It. *piccolo*, very small, + RNA + -viridae]

pi·cor·na·vi·rus (pi-kōr-nă-vī′rŭs). A virus of the family Picornaviridae.

pic·ro·car·mine (pik-rō-kar′min, -mēn). SEE picrocarmine *stain*.

PID Abbreviation for pelvic inflammatory *disease*.

pie·bald·ism (pī′bawld-izm). SYN piebaldness.

pie·bald·ness (pī′bawld-ness) [MIM*172800]. Patchy absence of the pigment of scalp hair, giving a streaked appearance; patches of vitiligo may be present in other areas due to absence of melanocytes. May be associated with neurological defects [MIM*172850] or eye cahnges [MIM 172870]. SYN piebald skin, piebaldism.

pie·dra (pē-ā′dră). A fungus disease of the hair characterized by the formation of numerous waxy, small, firm, nodular masses on the hair shaft. [Sp. a stone]

  white p., p. of the beard, moustache, and genital areas, as well as the scalp, caused by *Trichosporon beigelii* and found in South America, Europe, and Japan; characterized by soft, mucilaginous, white to light brown nodules, within as well as on the hairs.

pi·e·ses·the·sia (pī-ē-ses-thē′zē-ă). SYN pressure *sense*. [G. *piesis*, pressure, + *aisthēsis*, sensation]

PIF prolactin-inhibiting *factor*.

pig·ment. **1.** Any coloring matter, as that of the red blood cells, hair, iris, etc., or the stains used in histologic or bacteriologic work, or that in paints. **2.** A medicinal preparation for external use, applied to the skin like paint or coloring agents used in paints. [L. *pigmentum*, paint]

  bile p.'s, coloring matter in the bile derived from porphyrins by rupture of a methane bridge; *e.g.,* bilirubin, biliverdin.

  formalin p., a p. formed when acid aqueous solutions of formaldehyde act on blood-rich tissues.

  respiratory p.'s, the oxygen-carrying (colored) substances in blood and tissues (hemoglobin, myoglobin, hemocyanin, etc.).

  visual p.'s, the photopigments in the retinal cones and rods that absorb light and initiate the visual process.

  wear-and-tear p., lipofuscin that accumulates in aging or atrophic cells as a residue of lysosomal digestion.

pig·men·tary (pig′men-tār-ē). Relating to a pigment.

pig·men·ta·tion (pig-men-tā′shŭn). Coloration, either normal or pathologic, of the skin or tissues resulting from a deposit of pigment.

pig·ment·ed (pig′men-ted). Colored as the result of a deposit of pigment.

pig·men·to·ly·sin (pig-men-tol′i-sin). An antibody causing destruction of pigment. [L. *pigmentum*, pigment, + G. *lysis*, a loosening]

pig·men·tum ni·grum (pig-men′tŭm nī′grŭm). Melanin of the choroid coat of the eye.

PIH prolactin-inhibiting *hormone*.

pi·lar, pi·la·ry (pī′lăr, pil′ă-rē). SYN hairy. [L. *pilus*, hair]

pile (pīl). **1.** A series of plates of two different metals imposed alternately one on the other, separated by a sheet of material moistened with a dilute acid solution, used to produce a current of electricity. [L. *pila,* pillar] **2.** An individual hemorrhoidal tumor. SEE hemorrhoids. [L. *pila,* ball]

    sentinel p., a circumscribed thickening of the mucous membrane at the lower end of a fissure of the anus.

pi·le·ous (pī′lē-ŭs). SYN hairy. [L. *pilus,* hair]

piles (pīlz). SYN hemorrhoids. [L. *pila,* a ball]

pi·li (pī′lī) [NA]. Plural of pilus. [L.]

pill. A small globular mass of some coherent but soluble substance, containing a medicinal substance to be swallowed. [L. *pilula;* dim. of *pila,* ball]

    pep p.'s, colloquialism for tablets containing a central nervous system stimulant, especially amphetamine.

pil·lar (pil′ăr). A structure or part having a resemblance to a column or pillar. [L. *pila*]

    p.'s of fauces, SEE palatoglossal *arch,* palatopharyngeal *arch.*

    p.'s of fornix, the columna fornicis and crus fornicis.

pill-roll·ing (pil′rōl′ing). A circular movement of the opposed tips of the thumb and the index finger appearing as a form of tremor in paralysis agitans.

△**pilo-.** Hair. [L. *pilus*]

pi·lo·be·zoar (pī-lō-bē′zōr). SYN trichobezoar. [pilo- + bezoar]

pi·lo·cys·tic (pī′lō-sis′tik). Denoting a dermoid cyst containing hair. [pilo- + G. *kystis,* bladder]

pi·lo·e·rec·tion (pī′lō-ē-rek′shŭn). Erection of hair due to action of arrectores pilorum muscles.

pi·loid (pī′loyd). Hairlike; resembling hair. [pilo- + G. *eidos,* resemblance]

pi·lo·jec·tion (pī-lō-jek′shŭn). Process of shooting shafts of stiff mammalian hair into a saccular aneurysm in the brain in order to produce thrombosis. [pilo- + injection]

pi·lo·ma·trix·o·ma (pī′lō-mā-trik-sō′mă). A benign solitary hair follicle tumor containing cells resembling basal cell carcinoma and areas of epithelial necrosis. [pilo- + matrix + G. *-oma,* tumor]

pi·lo·mo·tor (pī′lō-mō′ter). Moving the hair; denoting the arrectores pilorum muscles of the skin and the postganglionic sympathetic nerve fibers innervating these small smooth muscles. [pilo- + L. *motor,* mover]

pi·lo·ni·dal (pī-lō-nī′dăl). Denoting the presence of hair in a dermoid cyst or in a sinus opening on the skin. [pilo- + L. *nidus,* nest]

pi·lose (pī′lōs). SYN hairy. [L. *pilosus*]

pi·lo·se·ba·ceous (pī′lō-sē-bā′shŭs). Relating to the hair follicles and sebaceous glands. [pilo- + L. *sebum,* suet]

pi·lus, pl. **pi·li** (pī′lŭs, pī′lī). **1** [NA]. One of the fine, keratinized filamentous epidermal growths arising from the skin of the body of mammals except the palms, soles, and flexor surfaces of the joints; the full length and texture of the hair varies markedly in different body sites. h SYN hair (1). **2.** A fine filamentous appendage, somewhat analogous to the flagellum, that occurs on some bacteria. SYN fimbria (2). SEE ALSO conjugative *plasmid.* [L.]

    pi′li tor′ti, a condition in which many hair shafts are twisted on the long axis, congenital or acquired as a result of distortion of the follicles

from a scarring inflammatory process, mechanical stress, or cicatrizing alopecia; the hair shafts resemble spangles in reflected light, are brittle, and break at varying lengths with many areas appearing bald with a dark stubble; as a developmental defect it can be manifested in such syndromes as Bjornstad's, Crandall's, and Menkes'. SYN twisted hairs.

pi·mel·ic ac·id (pī-mel′ik). An intermediate in the oxidation of oleic acid in some microorganisms; a precursor of biotin.

△**pimelo-.** Fat, fatty. [G. *pimelē,* soft fat, lard, fr. *piar,* fat]

pim·ple (pim′pl). A papule or small pustule; usually meant to denote an inflammatory lesion of acne.

PIN Abbreviation for prostatic intraepithelial *neoplasia.*

pin. Rod used in surgical treatment of bone fractures. SEE ALSO nail. [O.E. *pinn,* fr. L. *pinna,* feather]

pince·ment (pans-mon′). A pinching manipulation in massage. [Fr. pinching]

▌**pinch.** OCCUPATIONAL THERAPY Grip between fingers at the most distal joints.

    lateral pinch, OCCUPATIONAL THERAPY pinch between the tip pad of the thumb and the lateral surface of the index finger at the proximal interphalangeal (PIP) joints.

    palmar pinch, OCCUPATIONAL THERAPY pinch between the pad of the thumb and the pads of the index and middle fingers.

    tip pinch, OCCUPATIONAL THERAPY pinch between the tips of the index finger and the thumb.

pin·e·al (pin′ē-ăl). **1.** Shaped like a pine cone. SYN piniform. **2.** Pertaining to the pineal body. [L. *pineus,* relating to the pine, *pinus*]

pin·e·al·ec·to·my (pin′ē-ă-lek′tō-mē). Removal of the pineal body. [pineal + G. *ektomē,* excision]

pin·e·a·lo·cyte (pin-ē′al-ō-sīt). A cell of the pineal body with long processes ending in bulbous expansions. P.'s receive a direct innervation from sympathetic neurons that form recognizable synapses. [pineal + G. *kytos,* cell]

pin·e·a·lo·ma (pin′ē-ă-lō′mă). A term that has been variably used to designate germ cell tumors, pineocytomas and pineoblastomas of the pineal gland. [pineal + G. *-oma,* tumor]

pin·e·o·blas·to·ma (pin′ē-ō-blas-tō′mă). A poorly differentiated tumor of the pineal gland consisting of small cells with a scant amount of cytoplasms and often forming pseudorosettes. [pineal + G. *blastos,* germ, + *-oma,* tumor]

pin·guec·u·la, pin·guic·u·la (ping-gwek′yū-lă -gwik′-). A yellowish accumulation of connective tissue that thickens the conjunctiva; occurs in the aged. [L. *pinguiculus,* fattish, fr. *pinguis,* fat]

pin·i·form (pin′i-fōrm, pī′ni-). SYN pineal (1). [L. *pinus,* pine, + *forma,* form]

pink·eye (pink′ī). **1.** SYN acute contagious *conjunctivitis.* **2.** SYN infectious bovine *keratoconjunctivitis.* **3.** In horses, a form of equine viral arteritis.

pin·na, pl. **pin·nae** (pin′ă, pin′ē). **1.** SYN auricle (1). **2.** A feather, wing, or fin. [L. *pinna* or *penna,* a feather, in pl. a wing]

pin·nal (pin′ăl). Relating to the pinna.

pin•o•cyte (pin′ō-sīt, pī′nō-). A cell that exhibits pinocytosis. [G. *pineō,* to drink, + *kytos,* cell]

pin•o•cy•to•sis (pin′ō-sī-tō′sis, pī′nō-). The cellular process of actively engulfing liquid, a phenomenon in which minute incuppings or invaginations are formed in the surface of the cell membrane and close to form fluid-filled vesicles; it resembles phagocytosis. [pinocyte + G. *-osis,* condition]

pin•o•some (pin′ō-sōm, pī′nō-). A fluid-filled vacuole formed by pinocytosis. [G. *pineō,* to drink, + *sōma,* body]

pint (pīnt). A measure of quantity (U.S. liquid), containing 16 fluid ounces, 28.875 cubic inches; 473.1765 cc. An imperial p. contains 20 British fluid ounces, 34.67743 cubic inches; 568.2615 cc.

pin•ta (pin′tă, pēn′tă). A disease caused by a spirochete, *Treponema carateum,* and characterized by a small primary papule followed by an enlarging plaque and disseminated secondary macules of varying color called pintids that finally become white. [Sp. painted]

pin•worm (pin′werm). A member of the genus *Enterobius* or related nematodes causing intestinal parasitism in a large variety of vertebrates, including man (*Enterobius vermicularis* (the human p.). SYN seatworm.

pi•pette, pi•pet (pĭ-pet′, pī-pet′). A graduated tube (marked in ml) used to transport a definite volume of a gas or liquid in laboratory work. [Fr. dim. of *pipe,* pipe]

pir•i•form (pir′i-fōrm, pī′rē-). Pear-shaped. [L. *pirum,* pear, + *forma,* form]

pis•i•form (pis′i-fōrm). Pea-shaped or pea-sized. [L. *pisum,* pea, + *forma,* appearance]

pit. **1.** Any natural depression on the surface of the body, such as the axilla. Cf. dimple. **2.** One of the pinhead-sized depressed scars following the pustule of acne, chickenpox, or smallpox (pockmark). **3.** A sharp-pointed depression in the enamel surface of a tooth, due to faulty or incomplete calcification or formed at the confluent point of two or more lobes of enamel. **4.** To indent, as by pressure of the finger on the edematous skin; to become indented, said of the edematous tissues when pressure is made with the fingertip. [L. *puteus*]

   anal p., SYN proctodeum (1).

   auditory p.'s, paired depressions, one on either side of the head of the embryo, marking the location of the future auditory vesicles.

   granular p.'s, pits on the inner surface of the skull, along the course of the superior sagittal sinus, in which are lodged the arachnoidal granulations.

   iris p.'s, colobomas affecting the stroma of the iris with pigment epithelium intact.

   lens p.'s, the paired depressions formed in the superficial ectoderm of the embryonic head as the lens placodes sink in toward the optic cup; the external openings of the p.'s are closed as the lens vesicles are formed.

   nail p.'s, small punctate depressions on the surface of the nail plate due to defective nail formation; seen in psoriasis and other disorders.

   nasal p.'s, the paired depressions formed when

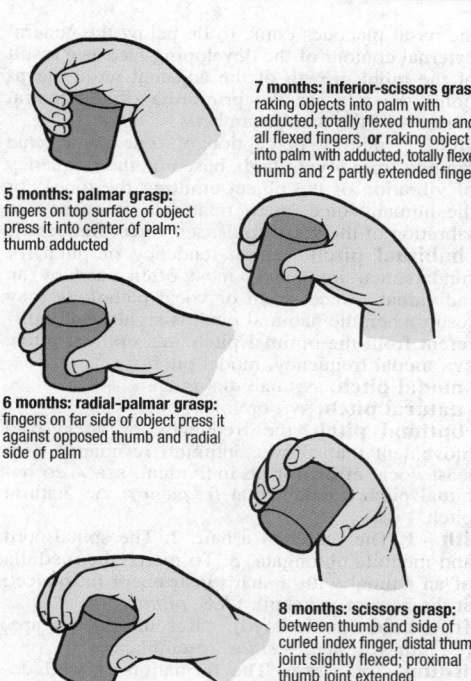

7 months: inferior-scissors grasp: raking objects into palm with adducted, totally flexed thumb and all flexed fingers, **or** raking object into palm with adducted, totally flexed thumb and 2 partly extended fingers

5 months: palmar grasp: fingers on top surface of object press it into center of palm; thumb adducted

6 months: radial-palmar grasp: fingers on far side of object press it against opposed thumb and radial side of palm

7 months: radial-palmar grasp: wrist straight

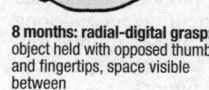

8 months: scissors grasp: between thumb and side of curled index finger, distal thumb joint slightly flexed; proximal thumb joint extended

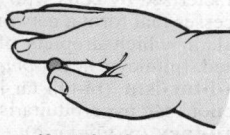

9 months: inferior-pincer grasp: between ventral surfaces of thumb and index finger, distal thumb joint extended; beginning thumb opposition

8 months: radial-digital grasp: object held with opposed thumb and fingertips, space visible between

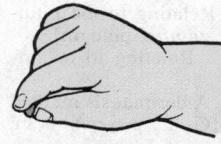

10 months: pincer grasp: between distal pads of thumb and index finger, distal thumb joint slightly flexed; thumb opposed

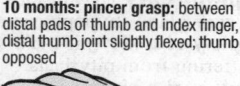

9 months: radial-digital grasp: wrist extended

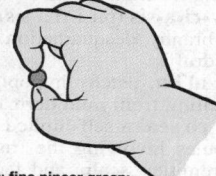

12 months: fine pincer grasp: between fingertips or fingernails; distal thumb joint flexed

pinch and grasp patterns

the nasal placodes come to lie below the general external contour of the developing face as a result of the rapid growth of the adjacent nasal elevations; the p.'s are the primordia of the rostral portions of the nasal chambers.

pitch. Auditory perception of tone on a scale ranging from low to high, based on the frequency of vibration of the object emitting the tone. For the human voice, pitch relates to frequency of vibration of the vocal folds. SEE voice, frequency.

habitual pitch, central tendency of pitch, or fundamental frequency, most often used by an individual. Voice strain or vocal pathology may result when the habitual pitch is significantly different from the optimal pitch. SEE optimal pitch. SYN modal frequency, modal pitch.

modal pitch, SYN habitual pitch.

natural pitch, SYN optimal pitch.

optimal pitch, the frequency of vocal fold movement that allows optimum resonance with least vocal effort for an individual. SEE ALSO habitual pitch, fundamental *frequency.* SYN natural pitch.

pith. 1. The center of a hair. 2. The spinal cord and medulla oblongata. 3. To pierce the medulla of an animal with a sharp instrument introduced at the base of the skull. [A.S. *pitha*]

pith·e·coid (pith'ĕ-koyd). Resembling an ape. [G. *pithēkos,* ape, + *eidos,* resemblance]

pit·ting. DENTISTRY The formation of well defined, relatively deep depressions in a surface, usually used in describing defects in surfaces (often golds, solder joints, or amalgam). It may arise from a variety of causes, although the clinical occurrence is often associated with corrosion. SEE ALSO pitting *edema,* nail *pits,* under *pit.*

pi·tu·i·cyte (pi-tū'i-sīt). The primary cell of the posterior lobe of the pituitary gland, a fusiform cell closely related to neuroglia. [pituitary + G. *kytos,* cell]

pi·tu·i·cy·to·ma (pi-tū'i-sī-tō'mă). A rare gliogenous neoplasm derived from pituicytes, occurring in the posterior lobe of the pituitary gland and characterized by cells with small nuclei and long processes that form a network of cytoplasmic material, in which droplets of fat may be demonstrated. [pituicyte + G. *-oma,* tumor]

pi·tu·i·tar·ism (pi-tū'i-tār-izm). Pituitary dysfunction. SEE hyperpituitarism, hypopituitarism.

pi·tu·i·tary (pi-tū'i-tār-ē). Relating to the pituitary gland (hypophysis). [L. *pituita,* phlegm]

pit·y·ri·a·sic (pit-i-rī'ă-sik). Relating to or suffering from pityriasis.

pit·y·ri·a·sis (pit-i-rī'ă-sis). A dermatosis marked by branny desquamation. [G. fr. *pityron,* bran, dandruff]

p. al'ba, patchy hypopigmentation of the skin resulting from mild dermatitis.

p. ro'sea, a self-limited eruption of macules or papules involving the trunk and less frequently extremities, scalp, and face; the lesions are usually oval and follow the crease lines of the skin; the onset is frequently preceded by a single larger scaling lesion known as the herald patch.

p. ru'bra, SYN exfoliative *dermatitis.*

p. ru'bra pila'ris, an uncommon chronic pruritic eruption of the hair follicles, which become

firm, red, surmounted with a horny plug, and often confluent to form scaly plaques.

p. versic'olor, SYN *tinea* versicolor.

pit·y·roid (pit'i-royd). SYN furfuraceous. [G. *pityrōdēs,* branlike, fr. *pityron,* bran, + *eidos,* resemblance]

Pit·y·ro·spo·rum (pit-i-ros'pō-rŭm, pit'i-rō-spō'rŭm). A genus of fungi found in dandruff and seborrheic dermatitis. [G. *pityron,* bran, + *sporos,* seed]

PIVKA *protein* induced by vitamin K absence.

pix·el (pik'sel). A contraction for picture element, a two-dimensional representation of a volume element (voxel) in the display of the CT or MR image, usually 512 by 512 or 256 by 256 pixels respectively.

PK *pyruvate* kinase.

pkat picokatal.

PKU phenylketonuria.

pkV, pkv Abbreviation for peak kilovoltage, the nominal voltage setting of an x-ray machine.

pkv SEE pkV.

pla·ce·bo (plă-sē'bō). **1.** A medicinally inactive substance given as a medicine for its suggestive effect. **2.** An inert compound identical in appearance to material being tested in experimental research, which may or may not be known to the physician and/or patient, administered to distinguish between drug action and suggestive effect of the material under study. [L. I will please, future of *placeo*]

pla·cen·ta (plă-sen'tă) [NA]. Organ of metabolic interchange between fetus and mother. It has a portion of embryonic origin, derived from the outermost embryonic membrane (chorion frondosum), and a maternal portion formed by a modification of the part of the uterine mucosa (decidua basalis) in which the chorionic vesicle is implanted. Within the p., the chorionic villi, with their contained capillaries carrying blood of the embryonic circulation, are exposed to maternal blood in the intervillous spaces in which the villi lie; no direct mixing of fetal and maternal blood occurs, but the intervening tissue (the placental membrane) is sufficiently thin to permit the absorption of nutritive materials, oxygen, and some harmful substances, like viruses, into the fetal blood and the release of carbon dioxide and nitrogenous waste from it. At term, the human p. is disk shaped, about 4 cm in thickness and 18 cm in diameter, and averages about ⅙ to ⅐ the weight of the fetus; its fetal surface is smooth, being formed by the adherent amnion, with the umbilical cord normally attached near its center; the maternal surface of a detached p. is rough because of the torn decidual tissue adhering to the chorion and shows lobular elevations called cotyledons or lobes. [L. a cake]

p. accre'ta, the abnormal adherence of the chorionic villi to the myometrium, associated with partial or complete absence of the decidua basalis and, in particular, the stratum spongiosum.

battledore p., a p. in which the umbilical cord is attached at the border; so-called because of the fancied resemblance to the racquet (racket) used in battledore, a precursor to badminton.

bidiscoidal p., a p. with two separate disc-

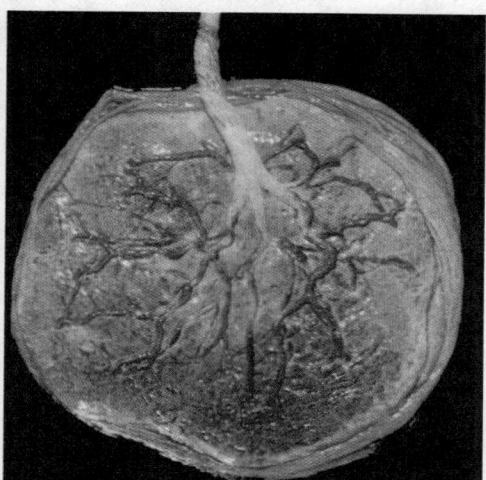

placenta: with umbilical cord

shaped portions attached to opposite walls of the uterus, normal for certain monkeys and shrews, and occasionally found in humans.

p. circumvalla′ta, a cup-shaped p. with raised edges, having a thick, round, white, opaque ring around its periphery; a portion of the decidua separates the margin of the p. from its chorionic plate; the remainder of the chorionic surface is normal in appearance, but the fetal vessels are limited in their course across the p. by the ring. SEE ALSO p. marginata, p. reflexa.

p. fenestra′ta, a p. in which there are areas of thinning, sometimes extending to entire absence of placental tissue.

fetal p., p. feta′lis, the chorionic portion of the placenta, containing the fetal blood vessels, from which the funis develops; specifically, in humans, it develops from the chorion frondosum.

hemochorial p., the type of p., as in humans and some rodents, in which maternal blood is in direct contact with the chorion.

hemoendothelial p., the type of p., as in rabbits, in which the trophoblast becomes so attenuated that, by light microscopy, maternal blood appears to be separated from fetal blood only by the endothelium of the chorionic capillaries.

p. incre′ta, a form of p. accreta in which the chorionic villi invade the myometrium.

p. margina′ta, a p. with raised edges, less pronounced than the p. circumvallata. SEE ALSO p. reflexa.

maternal p., SYN *pars uterina placentae.*

p. membrana′cea, an abnormally thin p. covering an unusually large area of the uterine lining.

p. pre′via, the condition in which the p. is implanted in the lower segment of the uterus, extending to the margin of the internal os of the cervix or partially or completely obstructing the os. SYN placental presentation.

p. reflex′a, an anomaly of the p. in which the margin is thickened so as to appear turned back

upon itself. SEE ALSO p. circumvallata, p. marginata.

p. spu′ria, a mass of placental tissue which has no vascular connection with the main p.

pla·cen·tal (pla-sen′tăl). Relating to the placenta.

plac·en·ta·tion (plas-en-tā′shŭn). The structural organization and mode of attachment of fetal to maternal tissues in the formation of the placenta. Types of p. are defined under placenta.

plac·en·ti·tis (plas-en-tī′tis). Inflammation of the placenta.

plac·en·to·ma (plas-en-tō′mă). SYN deciduoma.

plac·ode (plak′ōd). Local thickening in the embryonic ectoderm layer; the cells of the p. ordinarily constitute a primordial group from which a sense organ or ganglion develops. [G. *plakōdēs,* fr. *plax,* anything flat or broad, + *eidos,* like]

pla·fond (plă-fon′). A ceiling, especially the ceiling of the ankle joint, *i.e.,* the articular surface of the distal end of the tibia. [Fr. ceiling]

△**plagio-.** Oblique, slanting. [G. *plagios*]

pla·gi·o·ce·phal·ic (plă′jē-ō-se-fal′ik). Relating to or marked by plagiocephaly.

pla·gi·o·ceph·a·ly (plă′jē-ō-sef′ă-lē). An asymmetric craniostenosis due to premature closure of the lambdoid and coronal sutures on one side; characterized by an oblique deformity of the skull. [G. *plagios,* oblique, + *kephalē,* head]

plague (plāg). **1.** Any disease of wide prevalence or of excessive mortality. **2.** An acute infectious disease caused by *Yersinia pestis* and marked by high fever, toxemia, prostration, a petechial eruption, lymph node enlargement, and pneumonia, or hemorrhage from the mucous membranes; primarily a disease of rodents, transmitted to humans by fleas that have bitten infected animals. In humans the disease takes one of four clinical forms: bubonic *p.,* septicemic *p.,* pneumonic *p.,* or ambulant *p..* SYN pest, pestilence (1). [L. *plaga,* a stroke, injury]

bubonic p., the usual form of p. marked by inflammatory enlargement of the lymphatic glands in the groins, axillae, or other parts.

hemorrhagic p., the hemorrhagic form of bubonic p.

pneumonic p., a rapidly progressive and frequently fatal form of p. in which there are areas of pulmonary consolidation, with chill, pain in the side, bloody expectoration, and high fever.

△**plan-.** SEE plano-.

pla·na (plā′nă). Plural of planum. [L.]

plane (plān). **1.** A flat surface. SEE planum. **2.** An imaginary surface formed by extension through any axis or two definite points in reference especially to craniometry and to pelvimetry. [L. *planus,* flat]

canthomeatal p., p. passing through the two lateral angles of the eye and the center of the external acoustic meatus; this p. lies approximately midway between the Frankfort and the supraorbitomeatal p.'s.

coronal p., a vertical p. at right angles to a sagittal p., dividing the body into anterior and posterior portions. SYN frontal p.

datum p., an arbitrary p. used as a base from which to make craniometric measurements.

equatorial p., in metaphase of mitosis, the p.

pl

that touches all of the centromeres and their spindle attachments.

frontal p., SYN coronal p.

horizontal p., SYN transverse p.

interspinal p., a horizontal plane passing through the anterior superior iliac spines; it marks the boundary between the lateral and umbilical regions superiorly and the inguinal and pubic regions inferiorly.

median p., a vertical p. through the midline of the body that divides the body into right and left halves. SYN midsagittal p.

midsagittal p., SYN median p.

nuchal p., the external surface of the squamous part of the occipital bone below the superior nuchal line, giving attachment to the muscles of the back of the neck.

orbital p., the orbital surface of the maxilla, lying perpendicular to the orbitomeatal p. at the orbitale.

orbitomeatal p., a standard craniometric reference p. passing through the right and left porion and the left orbitale; drawn on the profile radiograph or photograph from the superior margin of the acoustic meatus to the orbitale.

p. of pelvic canal, SYN pelvic *axis.*

pelvic p. of greatest dimensions, the p. extending from the middle of the posterior surface of the pubic symphysis to the junction of the second and third sacral vertebrae, and laterally passing through the ischial bones over the middle of the acetabulum.

pelvic p. of least dimensions, the p. that extends from the end of the sacrum to the inferior border of the pubic symphysis; it is bounded posteriorly by the end of the sacrum, laterally by the ischial spines, and anteriorly by the inferior border of the pubic symphysis.

sagittal p., originally (and strictly speaking) the sagittal plane is the median plane, and any other plane parallel to it is a parasagittal plane; in contemporary usage and in a broad sense, s. p. is used for any p. parallel to the median, *i.e.,* as a synonym for parasagittal.

sternal p., a p. indicated by the front surface of the sternum.

subcostal p., a horizontal plane passing through the inferior limits of the costal margin, *i.e.,* the tenth costal cartilages; it marks the boundary between the hypochondriac and epigastric regions superiorly and the lateral and umbilical regions inferiorly.

supraorbitomeatal p., a p. passing the superior orbital margins and the superior margin of the external acoustic meatuses; it makes an angle of approximately 25 to 30 degrees with the Frankfort p. and is the p. in which routine CT (computed tomography) scans of the brain are made.

temporal p., a slightly depressed area on the side of the cranium, below the inferior temporal line, formed by the temporal and parietal bones, the greater wing of the sphenoid, and a part of the frontal bone.

transverse p., a p. across the body at right angles to the coronal and sagittal p.'s. SYN horizontal p.

⚠ **plani-.** SEE plano-.

pla·nig·ra·phy (pla-nig′ră-fē). SYN tomography. [L. *planum,* plane, + G. *graphē,* a writing]

plan·ing (plān′ing). SYN dermabrasion.

⚠ **plano-, plan-, plani-.** **1.** A plane; flat, level. [L. *planum,* plane; *planus,* flat] **2.** Wandering. [G. *planos,* roaming]

pla·no·cel·lu·lar (plā-nō-sel′yū-lăr). Relating to or composed of flat cells. [L. *planus,* flat, + cellular]

pla·no·con·cave (plā′nō-kon′kāv). Flat on one side and concave on the other; denoting a lens of that shape.

pla·no·con·vex (plā′nō-kon′veks). Flat on one side and convex on the other; denoting a lens of that shape.

pla·nog·ra·phy (pla-nog′ră-fē). SYN tomography.

pla·no·val·gus (plā-nō-val′gŭs). A condition in which the longitudinal arch of the foot is flattened and everted. [plano- + L. *valgus,* turned outward]

plan·ta, gen. and pl. **plan·tae** (plan′tă, plan′tē) [NA]. SYN sole. [L.]

plan·tal·gia (plan-tal′jē-ă). Pain on the plantar surface of the foot over the plantar fascia. [L. *planta,* sole of foot, + G. *algos,* pain]

plan·tar (plan′tăr). Relating to the sole of the foot. [L. *plantaris*]

plantarflexion (plăn-tăr-flěk′shŭn). Extension of the ankle, pointing of the foot and toes.

plan·ti·grade (plan′ti-grād). Walking with the entire sole and heel of the foot on the ground, as do man and bears. [L. *planta,* sole, + *gradior,* to walk]

pla·num, pl. **pla·na** (plā′nŭm, plā′nă). A plane or flat surface. SEE ALSO plane. [L. plane]

ℹ **plaque** (plak). **1.** A patch or small differentiated area on a body surface (*e.g.,* skin, mucosa, or arterial endothelium) or on the cut surface of an organ such as the brain. **2.** An area of clearing in a flat confluent growth of bacteria or tissue cells. **3.** A sharply defined zone of demyelination characteristic of multiple sclerosis. **4.** SEE dental p. [Fr. a plate]

bacterial p., DENTISTRY A mass of filamentous microorganisms and large variety of smaller forms attached to the surface of a tooth which, depending on bacterial activity and environmental factors, may give rise to caries, calculus, or inflammatory changes in adjacent tissue. SYN dental p. (2).

dental p., (1) the noncalcified accumulation mainly of oral microorganisms and their products, that adheres tenaciously to the teeth and is not readily dislodged; (2) SYN bacterial p.

Hollenhorst p.'s, glittering, orange-yellow, atheromatous emboli in the retinal arterioles that contain cholesterin crystals and originate in the carotid artery or great vessels.

neuritic p., SYN senile p.

senile p., a spherical mass composed primarily of amyloid fibrils and interwoven neuronal processes, frequently, although not exclusively, observed in Alzheimer's disease. SYN neuritic p.

⚠ **-plasia.** Formation (especially of cells). SEE plasma-. [G. *plassō,* to form]

plasm (plazm). SYN plasma.

plas•ma (plaz′mă). **1.** The fluid (noncellular) portion of the circulating blood, as distinguished from the serum obtained after coagulation. SYN blood p. **2.** The fluid portion of the lymph. **3.** A "fourth state of matter" in which, owing to elevated temperature (*ca.* 10^6 degrees), atoms have broken down to form free electrons and more or less stripped nuclei; produced in the laboratory in connection with hydrogen fusion (thermonuclear) research. SYN plasm. [G. something formed]

  blood p., SYN plasma (1).

  normal human p., sterile p. obtained by pooling approximately equal amounts of the liquid portion of citrated whole blood from eight or more adult humans who have been certified as free from any disease which is transmissible by transfusion, and treating it with ultraviolet irradiation to destroy possible bacterial and viral contaminants.

plasma-, plasmat-, plasmato-, plasmo-. Formative, organized; plasma. [G. *plasma*, something formed]

plas•ma•blast (plaz′mă-blast). Precursor of the plasma cell. [plasma + G. *blastos*, germ]

plas•ma•crit (plaz′mă-krit). A measure of the percentage of the volume of blood occupied by plasma, in contrast to a hematocrit. [plasma + G. *krino*, to separate]

plas•ma•cyte (plaz′mă-sīt). SYN plasma *cell.*

plas•ma•cy•to•ma (plaz′mă-sī-tō′mă). A discrete, presumably solitary mass of neoplastic plasma cells in bone or in one of various extramedullary sites; in humans, such lesions are probably the initial phase of developing plasma cell myeloma. [plasmacyte + G. *-oma,* tumor]

plas•ma•cy•to•sis (plaz′mă-sī-tō′sis). **1.** Presence of plasma cells in the circulating blood. **2.** Presence of unusually large proportions of plasma cells in the tissues or exudates. [plasmacyte + G. *-osis,* condition]

plas•ma•ki•nins (plaz′mă-kīn′inz). A group of highly active oligopeptides found in sera that act upon smooth muscle of blood vessels, uterus, bronchi, etc.; *e.g.,* bradykinin, kallidin.

plas•ma•lem•ma (plaz-mă-lem′ă). SYN cell *membrane.* [plasma + G. *lemma,* husk]

plas•mal•o•gens (plaz-mal′ō-jenz). Generic term for glycerophospholipids in which the glycerol moiety bears a 1-alkenyl or 1-alkyl ether group.

plas•ma•phe•re•sis (plaz′mă-fĕ-rē′sis). Removal of whole blood from the body, separation of its cellular elements by centrifugation, and reinfusion of them suspended in saline or some other plasma substitute, thus depleting the body's own plasma without depleting its cells. [plasma + G. *aphairesis,* a withdrawal]

plas•ma•phe•ret•ic (plaz′mă-fĕ-ret′ik). Relating to plasmapheresis.

plasmat-. SEE plasma-.

plas•mat•ic (plaz-mat′ik). Relating to plasma. SYN plasmic.

plas•mic (plaz′mik). SYN plasmatic.

plas•mid (plaz′mid). A genetic particle physically separate from the chromosome of the host cell (chiefly bacterial) that can stably function and replicate; not essential to the cell's basic functioning. SYN extrachromosomal element, extrachromosomal genetic element. [cyto*plasm* + -id]

  bacteriocinogenic p.'s, bacterial p.'s responsible for the elaboration of bacteriocins. SYN bacteriocinogens.

  conjugative p., a p. that can effect its own intercellular transfer by means of conjugation; this transfer is accomplished by a bacterium being rendered a donor, usually with specialized pili.

  F p., the prototype conjugative p. associated with conjugation in the K-12 strain of *Escherichia coli.* SYN F factor.

  nonconjugative p., a p. that cannot effect conjugation and self-transfer to another bacterium (bacterial strain); transfer depends upon mediation of another (and conjugative) p.

  resistance p.'s, p.'s carrying genes responsible for antibiotic (or antibacterial drug) resistance among bacteria (notably Enterobacteriaceae); they may be conjugative or nonconjugative p.'s, the former possessing transfer genes (resistance transfer factor) lacking in the latter.

plas•min (plaz′min). An enzyme hydrolyzing peptides and esters of L-arginine and L-lysine, and converting fibrin to soluble products; p. is responsible for the dissolution of blood clots. SYN fibrinase (2), fibrinolysin.

plas•min•o•gen (plaz-min′ō-jen). **1.** A precursor of plasmin. There is an autosomal dominant deficiency of p. [MIM*173350] that may promote thrombosis. SEE plasmin.

plasmo-. SEE plasma-.

plas•mo•dia (plaz-mō′dē-ă). Plural of plasmodium. [L.]

plas•mo•di•al (plaz-mō′dē-ăl). **1.** Relating to a plasmodium. **2.** Relating to any species of the genus *Plasmodium.*

Plas•mo•di•um (plaz-mō′dē-ŭm). A genus of the protozoan family Plasmodiidae, blood parasites of vertebrates; includes the causal agents of malaria, with an asexual cycle occurring in liver and red blood cells of vertebrates and a sexual cycle in mosquitoes, the latter cycle resulting in the production of large numbers of infective sporozoites in the salivary glands of the vector, which are transmitted when the mosquito bites and draws blood. [Mod. L. from G. *plasma,* something formed, + *eidos,* appearance]

  P. falcip′arum, *Laverania falciparum,* a species that is the causal agent of falciparum (malignant tertian) malaria; infected erythrocytes are normal or contracted in size and are likely to contain basophilic granules and red dots (Maurer's clefts or dots); multiple infection is extremely frequent and causes bouts of fever somewhat irregularly since the parasites' cycles of multiplication are usually asynchronous.

  P. mala′riae, a species that is the causal agent of quartan malaria; infected erythrocytes are normal or slightly contracted in size, usually with no stippling (the two most important characteristics that distinguish it from *P. vivax*), although extremely fine Ziemann's dots may be observed; multiple infection is extremely rare, thus bouts of fever occur fairly regularly at 72-hour intervals.

  P. ova′le, a species that is the agent of the least

common form of human malaria; SchHufner's dots are abundant and appear early, host cells are normal or only slightly enlarged, and only about 8 to 10 grapelike merozoites are produced; fever is tertian (every 48 hours), and relapses are infrequent.

P. vi'vax, a species that is the most common malarial parasite of human beings except in west Africa; affected red blood cells are pale, enlarged, and contain SchHufner's dots in the later stages of growth; causes bouts of fever fairly regularly at 48-hour intervals; but multiple infection is common.

plas•mo•di•um, pl. **plas•mo•dia** (plaz-mō'dē-ŭm, -dē-ă). A protoplasmic mass containing several nuclei, resulting from multiplication of the nucleus with cell division. [Mod. L. fr. G. *plasma,* something formed, + *eidos,* appearance]

plas•mog•a•my (plaz-mog'ă-mē). Union of two or more cells with preservation of the individual nuclei; formation of a plasmodium. [plasmo- + G. *gamos,* marriage]

plas•mol•y•sis (plaz-mol'i-sis). **1.** Dissolution of cellular components. **2.** Shrinking of plant cells by osmotic loss of cytoplasmic water. [plasmo- + G. *lysis,* dissolution]

plas•mo•lyt•ic (plaz-mō-lit'ik). Relating to plasmolysis.

plas•mon (plaz'mon). The total of the extrachromosomal genetic properties of the eukaryotic cell cytoplasm. [cyto*plasm* + -on]

plas•mor•rhex•is (plaz-mō-rek'sis). The splitting open of a cell from the pressure of the protoplasm.

plas•mos•chi•sis (plaz-mos'ki-sis). The splitting of protoplasm into fragments. [plasmo- + G. *schisis,* a cleaving]

plas•mo•tro•pic (plaz-mō-trop'ik). Pertaining to or manifesting plasmotropism.

plas•mot•ro•pism (plaz-mot'rō-pizm). A condition in which the bone marrow, spleen, and liver are sites for the destruction of the erythrocytes, as opposed to destruction in the circulating blood. [plasmo- + G. *tropē,* a turning]

plas•ter. 1. A solid preparation which can be spread when heated, and which becomes adhesive at the temperature of the body; used to keep the edges of a wound in apposition, to protect raw surfaces, and, when medicated, to redden or blister the skin or to apply drugs to the surface to obtain their systemic effects. **2.** DENTISTRY Colloquialism for p. of Paris. [L. *emplastrum;* G. *emplastron,* plaster or mold]

plas•tic (plas'tik). **1.** Capable of being formed or molded. **2.** A material that can be shaped by pressure or heat to the form of a cavity or mold. [G. *plastikos,* relating to molding]

plas•tic•i•ty (plas-tis'i-tē). The capability of being formed or molded; the quality of being plastic.

plas•tid (plas'tid). **1.** One of the differentiated structures in cytoplasm of plant cells where photosynthesis or other cellular processes are carried on; p.'s contain DNA and are self-replicating. SYN trophoplast. **2.** One of the granules of foreign or differentiated matter in cells: food particles, fat, waste material, chromatophores, and

trichocysts. **3.** A self-duplicating virus-like particle that multiplies within a host cell, such as kappa particles in certain paramecia. [G. *plastos,* formed, + -id]

plas•ty (plas'tē). Surgical procedure for repair of a defect or restoration of form and/or function of a part. [G. *plastos,* formed]

△**-plasty.** Molding, shaping or the result thereof, of a surgical procedure. [G. *plastos,* formed, shaped]

plate (plāt). **1.** ANATOMY A thin, flat, structure, such as a lamina or lamella. **2.** A metal bar applied to a fractured bone in order to maintain the ends in apposition. **3.** The agar layer within a Petri dish or similar vessel. **4.** To form a very thin layer of a bacterial culture by streaking it on the surface of an agar p. (usually within a Petri dish) in order to isolate individual organisms from which a colonial clone will develop. [O.Fr. *plat,* a flat object, fr. G. *platys,* flat, broad]

anal p., the anal portion of the cloacal p.

axial p., the primitive streak of an embryo.

buttress p., a metal p. used to support the internal fixation of a fracture.

cribriform p. of ethmoid bone, a horizontal p. from which are suspended the labyrinth, one on either side, and the p. perpendicularis in the center; it fits into the ethmoidal notch of the frontal bone and supports the olfactory lobes of the cerebrum, being pierced with numerous openings for the passage of the olfactory nerves. SYN lamina cribrosa ossis ethmoidalis [NA], cribrum.

cutis p., SYN dermatome (2).

epiphysial p., the disc of cartilage between the metaphysis and the epiphysis of an immature long bone permitting growth in length. SYN cartilago epiphysialis [NA], epiphysial cartilage.

equatorial p., the assembly of chromosomes in mitosis.

flat p., JARGON an abdominal radiograph made with the subject supine and without contrast medium.

floor p., ventral midline thinning of the developing neural tube, a continuity between the basal laminae of either side; opposite of roof plate. SYN ventral p.

lateral p., a nonsegmented mass of mesoderm on the lateral periphery of the embryonic disk.

medullary p., SYN neural p.

motor p., a motor endplate.

muscle p., SYN myotome (2).

neural p., the unpaired neuroectodermal region of the early embryo's dorsal surface which in later development is transformed into the neural tube and neural crest. SYN medullary p.

neutralization p., a metal p. used for the internal fixation of a long bone fracture to neutralize the forces producing displacement.

roof p., the thin layer of the embryonic neural tube connecting the alar p.'s dorsally.

ventral p., SYN floor p.

plate•let (plāt'let). An irregularly shaped disklike cytoplasmic fragment of a megakaryocyte that is shed in the marrow sinus and subsequently found in the peripheral blood where it functions in clotting. A p. contains granules in the central part (granulomere) and, peripherally, clear protoplasm (hyalomere), but no definite nucleus; is about one-third to one-half the size of an erythrocyte. SYN blood disk, elementary particle (1), thrombocyte, thromboplastid (1). [see plate]

plate·let·phe·re·sis (plāt′let-fĕ-rē′sis). Removal of blood from a donor with replacement of all blood components except platelets. [platelet + G. *aphairesis*, a withdrawal]

plat·i·num (Pt) (plat′i-nŭm). A metallic element, atomic no. 78, atomic wt. 195.08, used for making small parts for chemical apparatus because of its resistance to acids; in powdered form (**p. black**) it is an important catalyst in hydrogenation. A derivative, cisplatin, is used as an antineoplastic agent. [Mod. L., originally *platina*, fr. Sp. *plata*, silver]

platy-. Width; flatness. [G. *platys*, flat, broad]

plat·y·ba·sia (plat-i-bā′sē-ă). A developmental anomaly of the skull or an acquired softening of the skull bones so that the floor of the posterior cranial fossa bulges upward in the region about the foramen magnum. [*platy-* + G. *basis*, ground]

plat·y·ceph·a·ly (plat′i-sef′ă-lē). Flatness of the skull, a condition in which the vertical cranial index is below 70. [*platy-* + G. *kephalē*, head]

plat·y·hel·minth (plat-i-hel′minth). Common name for any flatworm of the phylum Platyhelminthes; any cestode (tapeworm) or trematode (fluke). [*platy-* + G. *helmins*, worm]

Plat·y·hel·min·thes (plat′i-hel-min′thēz). A phylum of flatworms that are bilaterally symmetric, flattened, and acelomate. Parasitic species of medical importance are in the subclass Cestoda (the true tapeworms) of the class Cestoidea, and in the subclass Digenea (the digenetic flukes) of the class Trematoda.

pla·typ·nea (plă-tip′nē-ă). Difficulty in breathing when erect, relieved by recumbency. Cf. orthopnea. [*platy-* + G. *pnoē*, a breathing]

plat·y·spon·dyl·ia, plat·y·spon·dyl·i·sis (plat-i-spon-dil′ē-ă, plat′i-spon-dil′i-sis). Flatness of the bodies of the vertebrae. [*platy-* + G. *spondylos*, vertebra]

pled·get (plej′et). A tuft of wool, cotton, or lint.

-plegia. Paralysis. [G. *plēgē*, stroke]

pleio-. Rarely used alternative spelling for pleo-.

plei·o·tro·pic (plī-ō-trop′ik). Denoting, or characterized by, pleiotropy.

plei·ot·ro·py, plei·o·tro·pia (plī-ot′rō-pē, plī′ō-trō′pē-ă). Production by a single mutant gene of apparently unrelated multiple effects at the clinical or phenotypic level. [*pleio-* + G. *tropos*, turning]

pleo-. More. [G. *pleiōn*]

ple·o·cy·to·sis (ple′ō-sī-tō′sis). Presence of more cells than normal, often denoting leukocytosis and especially lymphocytosis or round cell infiltration. [*pleo-* + G. *kytos*, cell, + *-ōsis*, condition]

ple·o·mas·tia, ple·o·ma·zia (plē-ō-mas′tē-ă, -mā′zē-ă). SYN polymastia. [*pleo-* + G. *mastos*, breast]

ple·o·mor·phic (plē-ō-mōr′fik). **1.** SYN polymorphic. **2.** Among fungi, having two or more spore forms; also used to describe a sterile mutant dermatophyte resulting from degenerative changes in culture.

ple·o·mor·phism (plē-ō-mōr′fizm). SYN polymorphism. [*pleo-* + G. *morphē*, form]

ple·o·mor·phous (plē-ō-mōr′fŭs). SYN polymorphic.

ple·o·nasm (plē′ō-nazm). Excess in number or size of parts. [G. *pleonasmos*, exaggeration, excessive, fr. *pleiōn*, more]

ple·on·os·te·o·sis (plē′on-os-tē-ō′sis). Superabundance of bone formation. [*pleo-* + G. *osteon*, bone, + *-osis*, condition]

pless-, plessi-. A striking, especially percussion. [G. *plēssō*, to strike]

ples·sim·e·ter (ple-sim′ĕ-ter). An oblong flexible plate used in mediate percussion by being placed against the surface and struck with the plessor. SYN pleximeter, plexometer. [G. *plēssō*, to strike, + *metron*, measure]

ples·sor (ples′er). A small hammer, usually with soft rubber head, used to tap the part directly, or with a plessimeter, in percussion of the chest or other part. SYN percussor, plexor. [G. *plēssō*, to strike]

pleth·o·ra (pleth′ō-ră). **1.** SYN hypervolemia. **2.** An excess of any of the body fluids. SYN repletion (2). [G. *plēthōrē*, fullness, fr. *plēthō*, to become full]

pleth·o·ric (ple-thōr′ik, pleth′ō-rik). Relating to plethora. SYN sanguine (1), sanguineous (2).

ple·thys·mo·graph (plĕ-thiz′mō-graf). A device for measuring and recording changes in volume of a part, organ, or whole body. [G. *plēthysmos*, increase, + *graphō*, to write]

pleth·ys·mog·ra·phy (pleth-iz-mog′ră-fē). Measuring and recording changes in volume of an organ or other part of the body by a plethysmograph. [G. *plēthysmos*, increase, + *graphē*, a writing]

pleth·ys·mom·e·try (pleth-iz-mom′ĕ-trē). Measuring the fullness of a hollow organ or vessel, as of the pulse. [G. *plēthysmos*, increase, + *metron*, measure]

pleur-, pleuro-, pleura-. Rib, side, pleura. [G. *pleura*; a rib, the side]

pleu·ra, gen. and pl. **pleu·rae** (plūr′ă, plūr′ē) [NA]. The serous membrane enveloping the lungs and lining the walls of the pleural cavity. [G. *pleura*, a rib, pl. the side]

pleu·ral (plūr′ăl). Relating to the pleura.

pleur·a·poph·y·sis (plūr′ă-pof′i-sis). A rib, or the process on a cervical or lumbar vertebra corresponding thereto. [*pleur-* + G. *apophysis*, process, offshoot]

pleur·ec·to·my (plū-rek′tō-mē). Excision of pleura, usually parietal. [*pleur-* + G. *ektomē*, excision]

pleu·ri·sy (plūr′i-sē). Inflammation of the pleura. SYN pleuritis. [L. *pleurisis*, fr. G. *pleuritis*]

  adhesive p., SYN dry p.

  diaphragmatic p., SYN epidemic *pleurodynia.*

  dry p., p. with a fibrinous exudation, without an effusion of serum, resulting in adhesion between the opposing surfaces of the pleura. SYN adhesive p., fibrinous p., plastic p.

  fibrinous p., SYN dry p.

  interlobular p., inflammation limited to the pleura in the sulci between the pulmonary lobes.

  plastic p., SYN dry p.

purulent p., p. with empyema.

serofibrinous p., the more common form of p., characterized by a fibrinous exudate on the surface of the pleura and an extensive effusion of serous fluid into the pleural cavity.

serous p., SYN p. with effusion.

p. with effusion, p. accompanied by serous exudation. SYN serous p.

pleu·rit·ic (plū-rit′ik). Pertaining to pleurisy.

pleu·ri·tis (plū-rī′tis). SYN pleurisy. [G. fr. *pleura,* side, + *-itis,* inflammation]

⌂**pleuro-.** SEE pleur-.

pleu·ro·cele (plūr′ō-sēl). SYN pneumonocele. [pleuro- + G. *kēlē,* hernia]

pleu·ro·cen·te·sis (plūr′ō-sen-tē′sis). SYN thoracentesis. [pleuro- + G. *kentēsis,* puncture]

pleu·ro·cen·trum (plūr′ō-sen′trŭm). One of the lateral halves of the body of a vertebra. [pleuro- + G. *kentron,* center]

pleu·roc·ly·sis (plūr-ok′li-sis). Washing out of the pleural cavity. [pleuro- + G. *klysis,* a washing out]

pleu·rod·e·sis (plūr-od′e-sis). The creation of a fibrous adhesion between the visceral and parietal layers of the pleura, obliterating the pleural cavity; it is performed surgically by abrading the pleura or by inserting a sterile irritant into the pleural canal in cases of recurrent spontaneous pneumothorax, malignant pleural effusion, and chylothorax. [pleuro- + G. *desis,* a binding together]

pleu·ro·dyn·ia (plūr-ō-din′ē-ă). **1.** Pleuritic pain in the chest. **2.** A painful affection of the tendinous attachments of the thoracic muscles, usually of one side only. SYN costalgia. [pleuro- + G. *odynē,* pain]

epidemic p., an acute infectious disease usually occurring in epidemic form, characterized by paroxysms of pain, usually in the chest, and associated with strains of coxsackievirus type B. SYN Bornholm disease, devil's grip, diaphragmatic pleurisy, epidemic myalgia, epidemic myositis, myositis epidemica acuta.

pleu·ro·gen·ic (plūr-ō-jen′ik). Of pleural origin; beginning in the pleura. SYN pleurogenous (1). [pleuro- + G. *-gen,* producing]

pleu·rog·e·nous (plūr-oj′ĕ-nŭs). **1.** SYN pleurogenic. **2.** In fungi, denoting spores or conidia developed on the sides of a conidiophore or hypha.

pleu·rog·ra·phy (plūr-og′ră-fē). Radiography of the pleural cavity after injecting contrast medium. [pleuro- + G. *graphō,* to write]

pleu·ro·hep·a·ti·tis (plūr′ō-hep-ă-tī′tis). Hepatitis with extension of the inflammation to the neighboring portion of the pleura. [pleuro- + G. *hēpar,* liver, + *-itis,* inflammation]

pleu·ro·lith (plūr′ō-lith). A concretion in the pleural cavity. [pleuro- + G. *lithos,* stone]

pleu·rol·y·sis (plūr-ol′i-sis). Locating pleural adhesions by the aid of an endoscope and then dividing them with the electric cautery. [pleuro- + G. *lysis,* dissolution]

pleu·ro·per·i·car·di·al (plūr′ō-per-i-kar′dē-ăl). Relating to both pleura and pericardium.

pleu·ro·per·i·car·di·tis (plūr′ō-per-i-kar-dī′tis). Combined inflammation of the pericardium and of the pleura. [pleuro- + pericardium + G. *-itis,* inflammation]

pleu·ro·per·i·to·ne·al (plūr′ō-per-i-tō-nē′ăl). Relating to both pleura and peritoneum.

pleu·ro·pul·mo·nary (plūr-ō-pul′mō-ner-ē). Relating to the pleura and the lungs.

pleu·rot·o·my (plū-rot′ō-mē). SYN thoracotomy. [pleuro- + G. *tomē,* incision]

pleu·ro·vis·cer·al (plūr′ō-vis′er-ăl). SYN visceropleural.

plex·al (plek′săl). Relating to a plexus.

plex·ect·o·my (plek-sek′tō-mē). Surgical excision of a plexus. [plexus + G. *ektomē,* excision]

plex·i·form (plek′si-fōrm). Weblike, or resembling or forming a plexus. [plexus + L. *forma,* form]

plex·im·e·ter (plek-sim′i-ter). SYN plessimeter. [G. *plēxis,* stroke]

plex·i·tis (plek-sī′tis). Inflammation of a plexus.

plex·o·gen·ic (plek′sō-jen-ik). Giving rise to weblike or plexiform structures. [plexus + G. *-gen,* producing]

plex·om·e·ter (plek-som′ĕ-ter). SYN plessimeter.

plex·or (plek′ser). SYN plessor. [G. *plēxis,* stroke]

plex·us, pl. **plex·us, plex·us·es** (plek′sŭs, -sŭs-ez) [NA]. A network or interjoining of nerves and blood vessels or of lymphatic vessels. [L. a braid]

areolar venous p., a venous p. in the areola surrounding the nipple, formed by the mammary veins, and sending its blood to the lateral thoracic vein. SYN Haller's circle (2).

autonomic plexuses, p.'s of nerves in relation to blood vessels and viscera, the component fibers of which are sympathetic, parasympathetic, and sensory.

brachial p., a complex web of spinal nerves arising from the cervical spine which innervate the upper extremities.

cardiac p., a wide-meshed network of anastomosing cardiopulmonary and splanchnic nerves arising from the afferent and autonomic nerve fibers (sympathetic) and vagus (parasympathetic) nerves, surrounding the arch of the aorta, the pulmonary artery, and continuing to the atria, ventricles, and coronary vessels.

celiac (nervous) p., the most substantial, superior portion of the abdominal aortic plexus lying anterior to the aorta at the level of origin of the celiac trunk (vertebral level T-12); the celiac ganglia lie within the plexus; it is formed by contributions from the greater splanchnic and vagus (especially the posterior or right vagus) nerves and communicating branches to and from the superior mesenteric and renal plexuses and ganglia; most sympathetic, parasympathetic and visceral afferent fibers serving the abdominal viscera pass through this plexus.

cervical p., formed by loops joining the adjacent ventral primary rami of the first four cervical nerves and receiving gray communicating rami from the superior cervical ganglion; it lies deep to the sternocleidomastoid muscle, and sends out numerous cutaneous, muscular, and communicating rami.

choroid p., a vascular proliferation or fringe of

the tela choroidea in the third, fourth and lateral cerebral ventricles; it secretes cerebrospinal fluid thereby regulating to some degree the intraventricular pressure.

coccygeal p., a small p. formed by the fifth sacral and the coccygeal nerves; it gives origin to the anococcygeal nerves.

intraparotid p. of facial nerve, the diverging branches of the facial nerve passing through the substance of the parotid gland, connected by numerous looped anastomoses. SYN pes anserinus (1).

lymphatic p., a p. of lymphatic capillaries, usually without valves, that opens into one or more larger lymphatic vessels.

lumbar p., (1) a nervous p., formed by the ventral rami of the first four lumbar nerves; it lies in the substance of the psoas muscle; (2) a lymphatic p. formed of about twenty lymph nodes and connecting vessels situated along the lower portion of the aorta and the common iliac vessels.

myenteric p., a p. of unmyelinated fibers and postganglionic autonomic cell bodies lying in the muscular coat of the esophagus, stomach, and intestines; it communicates with the subserous and submucous p.'s, all subdivisions of the enteric p.

nerve p., a p. formed by the interlacing of nerves by means of numerous communicating branches.

pampiniform p., a p. formed, in the male, by veins from the testicle and epididymis, consisting of eight or ten veins lying in front of the ductus deferens and forming part of the spermatic cord; in the female the ovarian veins form this p. between the layers of the broad ligament; in the male it is part of the thermoregulatory system of the testis, helping to keep the testis at a constant temperature slightly lower than the other body temperature.

periarterial p., an autonomic p. that accompanies an artery, surrounding it in a network of autonomic nerve fibers.

pulmonary p., one of two autonomic p.'s, anterior and posterior, at the hilus of each lung, formed by cardiopulmonary splanchnic nerves of the sympathetic trunk and bronchial branches of the vagus nerve; from them various branches accompany the bronchi and arteries into the lung.

sacral p., interconnected roots of the L4-S4 spinal nerves that innervate the lower extremities. SEE ALSO brachial p.

submucosal p., a ganglicated p. of unmyelinated nerve fibers, derived chiefly from the superior mesenteric p., ramifying in the intestinal submucosa.

tympanic p., a p. on the promontory of the labyrinthine wall of the tympanic cavity, formed by the tympanic nerve, an anastomotic branch of the facial, and sympathetic branches from the internal carotid p.; it supplies the mucosa of the middle ear, mastoid cells, and auditory (eustachian) tube, and gives off the lesser superficial petrosal nerve to the otic ganglion.

pli•ca, gen. and pl. **pli•cae** (plī′kă, plī′sē). **1** [NA]. One of several anatomical structures in which there is a folding over of the parts. **2.** SYN

false *membrane.* SEE ALSO fold. [Mod. L. a plait or fold]

p. aryepiglot′tica [NA], SYN aryepiglottic *fold.*

pli′cae circula′res [NA], the numerous folds of the mucous membrane of the small intestine, running transversely for about two-thirds of the circumference of the gut. SYN circular folds.

p. interureter′ica [NA], SYN interureteric *fold.*

p. lacrima′lis [NA], SYN lacrimal *fold.*

pli′cae palma′tae [NA], SYN palmate *folds,* under *fold.*

p. semiluna′ris conjuncti′vae, (1) [NA], the semilunar fold formed by the palpebral conjunctiva at the medial angle of the eye; (2) a fold of the conjunctival mucous membrane found in many animals; normally partially hidden in the medial canthus of the eye when at rest, it may be extended to cover part or all of the cornea in a winking-like action to clean the cornea, as in birds. SYN semilunar conjunctival fold.

p. spira′lis duc′tus cys′tici [NA], SYN spiral *fold* of cystic duct.

p. vestibula′ris [NA], SYN vestibular *fold.*

p. voca′lis [NA], SYN vocal *fold.*

pli•cate (plī′kāt). Folded; pleated; tucked.

pli•ca•tion (plī-kā′shŭn, pli-). A folding or putting together in pleats; specifically, an operation for reducing the size of a hollow viscus by taking folds or tucks in its walls. [L. *plico,* pp. *-atus,* to fold]

pli•cot•o•my (plī-kot′ō-mē). Division of the plica mallearis. [plica + G. *tomē,* incision]

△**-ploid.** Multiple in form; its combinations are used both adjectivally: and substantively of a (specified) multiple of chromosomes. [G. *-plo-,* -fold, + *-ides,* in form; L. *-ploïdeus*]

ploi•dy (ploy′dē). The number of haploid sets in a cell. Gametes normally contain one; autosomal cells two. SEE ALSO polyploidy. [-ploid + -y, condition]

plug (plŭg). Any mass filling a hole or closing an orifice.

epithelial p., a mass of epithelial cells temporarily occluding an embryonic opening; the term is most commonly used with reference to the external nares.

mucous p., a mass of mucus and cells filling the cervical canal between periods or during pregnancy; a mass of mucous occluding a main or lobar bronchus.

plug•ger. A dental instrument used for condensing gold (foil), amalgam, or any plastic material in a cavity, operated by hand or by mechanical means. SYN packer (2).

plum•bism (plŭm′bizm). SYN lead *poisoning.* [L. *plumbum,* lead]

plum•bum (plŭm′bŭm). SYN lead. [L.]

△**pluri-.** Several, more. SEE ALSO multi-, poly-. [L. *plus, pluris*]

plu•ri•glan•du•lar (plū-ri-glan′dū-lăr). Denoting several glands or their secretions. SYN polyglandular.

plu•rip•o•tent, plu•ri•po•ten′tial (plū-rip′ō-tent, plū′rē-pō-ten′shăl). **1.** Having the capacity to affect more than one organ or tissue. **2.** Not fixed as to potential development.

plu•to•ni•um (Pu) (plū-tō′nē-ŭm). A transuranium artificial radioactive element, atomic no. 94, atomic wt. 244.064. The best-known α-emitting isotope is ^{239}Pu (half-life 24,110 years) which, like ^{235}U, is fissionable and can be used in atomic bombs and nuclear power plants; ^{238}Pu (half-life 87.74 years) is used as an energy source in pacemakers. Pu ions are bone seekers; ingestion is a radiation hazard as with radium and radiostrontium. [planet, *Pluto*]

Pm promethium.

pM picomolar (10^{-12} M).

pm picometer.

P mit·ra·le (mī-trā′lē). Broad, notched P waves in several or many leads of the electrocardiogram with a prominent late negative component to the P wave in lead V$_1$; it is characteristic of overload of the left atrium such as occurs in disease of the mitral valve. SYN P sinistrocardiale.

PML progressive multifocal *leukoencephalopathy*.

pmol picomole.

PMS premenstrual *syndrome*.

△**-pnea.** Breath, respiration. [G. *pneō*, to breathe]

△**pneo-.** Combining form denoting breath or respiration. SEE ALSO pneum-, pneumo-. [G. *pneō*, to breathe]

△**pneum-, pneuma-, pneumat-, pneumato-.** Presence of air or gas, the lungs, or breathing. SEE ALSO pneo-, pneumo-. [G. *pneuma, pneumatos,* air, breath]

pneu·marth·ro·gram (nū-marth′rō-gram). Film records of pneumarthrography.

pneu·marth·rog·ra·phy (nū-marth-rog′ră-fē). Radiographic examination of a joint following the introduction of air, with or without another contrast medium.

pneu·mar·thro·sis (nū-mar-thrō′sis). Presence of air in a joint. [G. *pneuma,* air, + *arthron,* joint, + *-osis,* condition]

pneu·mat·ic (nū-mat′ik). **1.** Relating to air or gas, or to a structure filled with air. **2.** Relating to respiration. [G. *pneumatikos*]

pneu·mat·ic an·ti·shock gar·ment. An inflatable suit used to apply pressure to the peripheral circulation, thus reducing blood flow and fluid exudation into tissues, to maintain central blood flow in the presence of shock. SYN military anti-shock trousers.

pneu·ma·ti·za·tion (nū′mă-ti-zā′shŭn). The development of air cells such as those of the mastoid and ethmoidal bones. [G. *pneuma,* air]

△**pneumato-.** SEE pneum-.

pneu·ma·to·car·dia (nū′mă-tō-kar′dē-ă). Presence of air bubbles or gas in the blood of the heart; produced by air embolism.

pneu·ma·to·cele (nū′mă-tō-sēl). **1.** An emphysematous or gaseous swelling. **2.** SYN pneumonocele. **3.** A thin-walled cavity within the lung, one of the characteristic sequelae of staphylococcus pneumonia. [G. *pneuma,* air, + *kēlē,* tumor, hernia]

pneu·ma·tor·rha·chis (nū-mă-tōr′ă-kis). SYN pneumorrhachis. [G. *pneuma,* air, + *rhachis,* spine]

pneu·ma·to·sis (nū-mă-tō′sis). Abnormal accumulation of gas in any tissue or part of the body. [G. a blowing out]

p. cystoi′des intestina′lis, a condition of unknown cause characterized by the occurrence of gas cysts in the intestinal mucous membrane; may produce intestinal obstruction. SYN intestinal emphysema.

pneu·ma·tu·ria (nū-mă-tū′rē-ă). The passage of gas or air from the urethra during or after urination, resulting from decomposition of bladder urine or, more commonly, from an intestinal fistula. [G. *pneuma,* air, + *ouron,* urine]

△**pneumo-, pneumon-, pneumono-.** The lungs, air or gas, respiration, or pneumonia. SEE ALSO aer-, pneo-, pneum-. [G. *pneumōn, pneumonos,* lung]

pneu·mo·ar·throg·ra·phy (nū′mō-ar-throg′ră-fē). Radiography of a joint after injection of air and usually a water-soluble contrast medium. [G. *pneuma,* air, + *arthron,* joint, + *graphō,* to write]

pneu·mo·car·di·al (nū′mō-kar′dē-ăl). SYN cardiopulmonary.

pneu·mo·cele (nū′mō-sēl). SYN pneumonocele.

pneu·mo·cen·te·sis (nū′mō-sen-tē′sis). SYN pneumonocentesis.

pneu·mo·ceph·a·lus (nū-mō-sef′ă-lŭs). Presence of air or gas within the cranial cavity. [G. *pneuma,* air, + *kephalē,* head]

pneu·mo·coc·cal (nū-mō-kok′ăl). Pertaining to or containing the pneumococcus.

pneu·mo·coc·ce·mia (nū′mō-kok-sē′mē-ă). The presence of pneumococci in the blood. [pneumococcus + G. *haima,* blood]

pneu·mo·coc·ci·dal (nū′mō-kok-sī′dăl). Destructive to pneumococci. [pneumococcus + L. *caedo,* to kill]

pneu·mo·coc·co·sis (nū′mō-kok-ō′sis). Rarely used term for infection with pneumococci.

pneu·mo·coc·co·su·ria (nū′mō-kok-o-sū′rē-ă). The presence of pneumococci or their specific capsular substance in the urine. [pneumococcus + G. *ouron,* urine]

pneu·mo·coc·cus, pl. **pneu·mo·coc·ci** (nū-mō-kok′ŭs, -kok′sī). SYN *Streptococcus pneumoniae.* [G. *pneumōn,* lung, + *kokkos,* berry (coccus)]

pneu·mo·co·ni·o·sis, pneu·mo·ko·ni·o·sis, pl. **pneu·mo·co·ni·o·ses** (nū′mō-kō-nē-ō′sis, -sēz). Inflammation commonly leading to fibrosis of the lungs caused by the inhalation of dust in various occupations; characterized by pain in the chest, cough with little or no expectoration, dyspnea, reduced thoracic excursion, sometimes cyanosis, and fatigue after slight exertion; degree of disability depends on the types of particles inhaled, as well as the level of exposure to them. [G. *pneumōn,* lung, + *konis,* dust, + *-osis,* condition]

pneu·mo·cra·ni·um (nū-mō-krā′nē-ŭm). Air present between the cranium and the dura mater; the term is commonly used to indicate extradural or subdural air. [G. *pneuma,* air, + -o- + *kranion,* skull]

Pneu·mo·cys·tis ca·ri·nii (nū-mō-sis′tis kă-rī′nē-ī). The microorganism that causes interstitial plasma cell pneumonia in immunodeficient persons, particularly those with AIDS. [G. *pneuma,* air, breathing, + *kystis,* bladder, pouch]

pneu·mo·cys·tog·ra·phy (nū′mō-sis-tog′ră-fē). Radiography of the bladder following injection of air. [G. *pneuma*, air, + *kystis*, bladder, + *graphō*, to write]

pneu·mo·cys·to·sis (nū′mō-sis-tō′sis). SYN *Pneumocystis carinii pneumonia.*

pneu·mo·der·ma (nū-mō-der′mă). SYN subcutaneous *emphysema*. [G. *pneuma*, air, + -o- + derma, skin]

pneu·mo·dy·nam·ics (nū′mō-dī-nam′iks). The mechanics of respiration. [G. *pneuma*, breath, + *dynamis*, force]

pneu·mo·en·ceph·a·lo·gram (nū′mō-en-sef′ă-lō-gram). Radiographs obtained by pneumoencephalography.

pneu·mo·gas·tric (nū-mō-gas′trik). Relating to the lungs and the stomach. SYN gastropulmonary. [G. *pneumōn*, lung, + *gastēr*, stomach]

pneu·mo·gram (nū′mō-gram). **1.** The record or tracing made by a pneumograph. **2.** Radiographic record of pneumography. [G. *pneumōn*, lung, + *gramma*, a drawing]

pneu·mo·graph (nū′mō-graf). Generic term for any device that records respiratory excursions from movements on the body surface. [G. *pneumōn*, lung, + *graphō*, to write]

pneu·mog·ra·phy (nū-mog′ră-fē). **1.** Examination with a pneumograph. **2.** A general term indicating radiography after injection of air. SYN pneumoradiography. [G. *pneumōn*, lung, + *graphō*, to write]

pneu·mo·he·mo·per·i·car·di·um (nū′mō-hē-mō-per-i-kar′dē-ŭm). SYN hemopneumopericardium.

pneu·mo·he·mo·thor·ax (nū′mō-hē-mō-thōr′aks). SYN hemopneumothorax.

pneu·mo·hy·dro·me·tra (nū′mō-hī-drō-mē′tră). The presence of gas and serum in the uterine cavity. [G. *pneuma*, air, + *hydōr* (*hydr-*), water, + *mētra*, uterus]

pneu·mo·hy·dro·per·i·car·di·um (nū′mō-hī′drō-păr-i-kar′dē-ŭm). SYN hydropneumopericardium.

pneu·mo·hy·dro·per·i·to·ne·um (nū′mō-hī-drō-per-i-tō-nē′ŭm). SYN hydropneumoperitoneum.

pneu·mo·hy·dro·thor·ax (nū-mō-hī-drō-thōr′aks). SYN hydropneumothorax.

pneu·mo·ko·ni·o·sis. SEE pneumoconiosis.

pneu·mo·lith (nū′mō-lith). A calculus in the lung. [G. *pneumōn*, lung, + *lithos*, stone]

pneu·mo·li·thi·a·sis (nū-mō-li-thī′ă-sis). Formation of calculi in the lungs.

pneu·mo·me·di·as·ti·num (nū′mō-mē′dē-ă-stī′nŭm). Escape of air into mediastinal tissues, usually from interstitial emphysema or from a ruptured pulmonary bleb. [G. *pneuma*, air, + mediastinum]

pneu·mo·my·e·log·ra·phy (nū′mō-mī′ĕ-log′ră-fē). Rarely used radiographic examination of spinal canal after injection of air or gas into the subarachnoid space. [G. *pneuma*, air, + *myelos*, marrow, + *graphō*, to write]

pneumon-. SEE pneumo-.

pneu·mo·nec·to·my (nū′mō-nek′tō-mē). Removal of all pulmonary lobes from a lung in one operation. [G. *pneumōn*, lung, + *ektomē*, excision]

pneu·mo·nia (nū-mō′nē-ă). Inflammation of the lung parenchyma characterized by consolidation of the affected part, the alveolar air spaces being filled with exudate, inflammatory cells, and fibrin. Most cases are due to infection by bacteria or viruses, a few to inhalation of chemicals or trauma to the chest wall, and a small minority to rickettsias, fungi, and yeasts. Distribution may be lobar, segmental, or lobular; when lobular, in association with bronchitis, it is termed bronchopneumonia. SEE ALSO pneumonitis. [G. fr. *pneumōn*, lung, + -ia, condition]

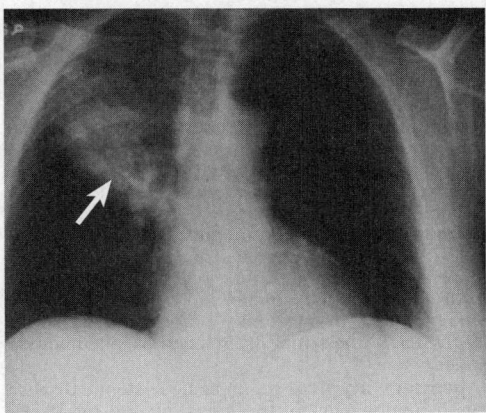

lobar pneumonia: chest x-ray showing pulmonary infiltrates (arrow) in upper lobe of right lung

apex p., apical p., p. of the apex or apices.

aspiration p., bronchopneumonia resulting from the inhalation of foreign material, usually food particles or vomit, into the bronchi; p. developing secondary to the presence in the airways of fluid, blood, saliva, or gastric contents.

atypical p., SYN primary atypical p.

bronchial p., SYN bronchopneumonia.

double p., lobar p. involving both lungs.

eosinophilic p., an immunologic disorder characterized by radiologic evidence of infiltrates accompanied by either peripheral blood eosinophilia or histopathologic evidence of eosinophilic infiltrates in lung tissue.

hypostatic p., p. resulting from infection developing in the dependent portions of the lungs due to decreased ventilation of those areas, with resulting failure to drain bronchial secretions; occurs primarily in the aged or those debilitated by disease who lie in the same position for long periods.

influenzal p., (1) p. complicating influenza; **(2)** p. due to *Haemophilus influenzae.*

interstitial plasma cell p., SYN *Pneumocystis carinii* p.

lipid p., lipoid p., pulmonary condition marked by inflammatory and fibrotic changes in the lungs due to the inhalation of various oily or fatty substances, particularly liquid petrolatum, or resulting from accumulation in the lungs of endogenous lipid material, either cholesterol from obstructive pneumonitis or following fracture of a bone; phagocytes containing lipid are usually present.

lobar p., p. affecting one or more lobes, or part of a lobe, of the lung in which the consolidation is virtually homogeneous; commonly due to infection by *Streptococcus pneumoniae;* sputum is scanty and usually of a rusty tint from altered blood.

mycoplasmal p., SYN primary atypical p.

Pittsburgh p., a variant of Legionnaires' disease caused by *Legionella micdadei.*

***Pneumocystis carinii* p.,** pneumonia resulting from infection with *Pneumocystis carinii,* frequently seen in the immunologically compromised, such as persons with AIDS, or steroid-treated individuals, the elderly, or premature or debilitated babies. Throughout the alveolar walls and pulmonary septa there is a diffuse infiltration of mononuclear inflammatory cells, chiefly plasma cells and macrophages, as well as a few lymphocytes. Helmet-shaped organisms can be demonstrated in sputum and tissue specimens with silver stains. Patients may be only slightly febrile (or even afebrile) but are likely to be extremely weak, dyspneic, and cyanotic. This is a major cause of morbidity among patients with AIDS. SYN interstitial plasma cell p., pneumocystosis.

primary atypical p., an acute systemic disease with involvement of the lungs, caused by *Mycoplasma pneumoniae* and marked by high fever, cough, relatively few physical signs, and scattered densities on x-rays; usually associated with development of cold agglutinins and antibodies to the bacteria. SYN atypical p., mycoplasmal p.

rheumatic p., p. rarely occurring in severe acute rheumatic fever; consolidation occurs, the lungs being of a rubbery consistency, with fibrin exudate and small hemorrhages, as well as edema from left ventricle failure.

usual interstitial p. of Liebow, a progressive inflammatory condition starting with diffuse alveolar damage and resulting in fibrosis and honeycombing over a variable time period; also a common feature of collagen-vascular diseases.

pneu•mon•ic (nū-mon'ik). **1.** SYN pulmonary. **2.** Relating to pneumonia.

pneu•mo•ni•tis (nū-mō-nī'tis). Inflammation of the lungs. SEE ALSO pneumonia. SYN pulmonitis. [G. *pneumōn,* lung, + -*itis,* inflammation]

hypersensitivity p., chronic progressive form of pneumonia with wheezing, dyspnea, diffuse infiltrates seen on radiographs; occurs following exposure to any of a variety of antigens, sometimes occupational and many names are given to cases with known types of exposure (such as farmer's lung, maple bark stripper's lung, chicken plucker's lung, bagassosis, byssinosis, humidifier lung, etc.); can progress to irreversible interstitial fibrotic disease with restrictive pattern on pulmonary function, but in early disease most manifestations are reversible if offending antigen is identified and removed from environment.

△**pneumono-.** SEE pneumo-.

pneu•mo•no•cele (nū-mōn'ō-sēl). Protrusion of a portion of the lung through a defect in the chest wall. SYN pleurocele, pneumatocele (2), pneumocele.

pneu•mo•no•cen•te•sis (nū'mō-nō-sen-tē'sis). Rarely used term for paracentesis of the lung. SYN pneumocentesis. [G. *pneumōn,* lung, + *kentēsis,* puncture]

pneu•mo•no•coc•cal (nū'mō-nō-kok'ăl). Relating to or associated with *Streptococcus pneumoniae.*

pneu•mo•no•cyte (nū'mō-nō-sīt). Nonspecific term referring to cells lining alveoli in the respiratory part of the lung. [G. *pneumōn,* lung, + *kytos,* cell]

phagocytic p., an alveolar phagocyte containing hemosiderin, carbon, or other foreign particles.

pneu•mo•no•pexy (nū'mō-nō-pek-sē). Fixation of the lung by suturing the costal and pulmonary pleurae or otherwise causing adhesion of the two layers. [G. *pneumōn,* lung, + *pēxis,* fixation]

pneu•mo•nor•rha•phy (nū-mō-nōr'ă-fē). Suture of the lung. [G. *pneumōn,* lung, + *rhaphē,* suture]

pneu•mo•not•o•my (nū-mō-not'ō-mē). Incision of the lung. SYN pneumotomy. [G. *pneumōn,* lung, + *tomē,* incision]

pneu•mo•or•bi•tog•ra•phy (nū'mō-ōr'bi-tog'ră-fē). Radiographic visualization of the orbital contents following injection of a gas, usually air.

pneu•mo•per•i•car•di•um (nū'mō-per-i-kar'dē-ŭm). Presence of gas in the pericardial sac. [G. *pneuma,* air, + pericardium]

pneu•mo•per•i•to•ne•um (nū'mō-per-i-tō-nē'ŭm). Presence of air or gas in the peritoneal cavity as a result of disease, or produced artificially in the abdomen to achieve exposure during laparoscopy and laporoscopic surgery for treatment of pulmonary or intestinal tuberculosis, bronchiectasis, tuberculous empyema, and certain other conditions. [G. *pneuma,* air, + peritoneum]

pneu•mo•per•i•to•ni•tis (nū'mō-per-i-tō-nī'tis). Inflammation of the peritoneum with an accumulation of gas in the peritoneal cavity. [G. *pneuma,* air, + peritonitis]

pneu•mo•pleu•ri•tis (nū'mō-plū-rī'tis). Pleurisy with air or gas in the pleural cavity. [G. *pneuma,* air, + pleur- + -*itis,* inflammation]

pneu•mo•py•e•log•ra•phy (nū'mō-pī-ĕ-log'ră-fē). Radiography of the kidney after air or gas has been injected into the renal pelvis. [G. *pneuma,* air, + *pyelos,* pelvis, + *graphō,* to write]

pneu•mo•py•o•thor•ax (nū'mō-pī-ō-thōr'aks). SYN pyopneumothorax.

pneu•mo•ra•di•og•ra•phy (nu'mo-ra-dĭ-og'ră-fē). SYN pneumography (2).

pneu•mo•ret•ro•per•i•to•ne•um (nū'mō-ret'rō-per-i-tō-nē'ŭm). Escape of air into the retroperitoneal tissues.

pneu•mor•rha•chis (nū-mō-rā'kis, nū-mōr'ă-kis). The presence of gas in the spinal canal. SYN pneumatorrhachis. [G. *pneuma,* air, + *rhachis,* spinal column]

pneu•mo•tach•o•gram (nū-mō-tak'ō-gram). A recording of respired gas flow as a function of time, produced by a pneumotachograph. [G. *pneuma,* air, + *tachys,* swift, + *gramma,* something written]

pneu•mo•tach•o•graph (nū-mō-tak'ō-graf). An

instrument for measuring the instantaneous flow of respiratory gases. SYN pneumotachometer.

pneu•mo•ta•chom•e•ter (nū′mō-tă-kom′ĕ-ter). SYN pneumotachograph. [G. *pneuma,* air, + -o- + *tachys,* swift, + *metron,* measure]

pneu•mo•thor•ax (nū-mō-thōr′aks). The presence of air or gas in the pleural cavity. [G. *pneuma,* air, + thorax]

  artificial p., p. produced by the injection of air, or a more slowly absorbed gas such as nitrogen, into the pleural space to collapse the lung.

  open p., a free communication between the atmosphere and the pleural space either via the lung or through the chest wall. SYN sucking wound.

  spontaneous p., p. occurring secondary to parenchymal lung disease, usually from an emphysematous bulla which ruptures or occasionally from a lung abscess.

pneu•mot•o•my (nū-mot′ō-mē). SYN pneumonotomy.

PNF proprioceptive neuromuscular *facilitation.*

PNH paroxysmal nocturnal *hemoglobinuria.*

PNP platelet neutralization *procedure.*

PNPB positive-negative pressure *breathing.*

Po polonium.

pock (pok). The specific pustular cutaneous lesion of smallpox. [A.S. *poc,* a pustule]

pock•et (pok′et). **1.** A cul-de-sac or pouchlike cavity. **2.** A diseased gingival attachment; a space between the inflamed gum and the surface of a tooth, limited apically by an epithelial attachment. **3.** To enclose within a confined space, as the stump of the pedicle of an ovarian or other abdominal tumor between the lips of the external wound. **4.** A collection of pus in a nearly closed sac. **5.** To approach the surface at a localized spot, as with the thinned out wall of an abscess which is about to rupture. [Fr. *pochette*]

pock•mark (pok′mark). The small depressed scar left after the healing of the smallpox pustule.

pod-, podo-. Foot, foot-shaped. Cf. ped-. [G. *pous, podos*]

po•dag•ra (pō-dag′ră). Severe pain in the foot, especially that of typical gout in the great toe. [G. fr. *pous,* foot, + *agra,* a seizure]

po•dal•gia (pō-dal′jē-ă). Pain in the foot. SYN pododynia, tarsalgia. [pod- + G. *algos,* pain]

po•dal•ic (pō-dal′ik). Relating to the foot. [G. *pous (pod-),* foot]

pod•ar•thri•tis (pod-ar-thrī′tis). Inflammation of any of the tarsal or metatarsal joints. [pod- + arthritis]

pod•e•de•ma (pod-e-dē′mă). Edema of the feet and ankles.

po•di•a•tric (pō-dī′ă-trik). Relating to podiatry.

po•di•a•trist (pō-dī′ă-trist). A practitioner of podiatry. SYN chiropodist. [pod- + G. *iatros,* physician]

po•di•a•try (pō-dī′ă-trē). The specialty concerned with the diagnosis and/or medical, surgical, mechanical, physical, and adjunctive treatment of the diseases, injuries, and defects of the human foot. SYN chiropody, podiatric medicine. [pod- + G. *iatreia,* medical treatment]

podo-. SEE pod-.

po•do•cyte (pod′ō-sīt). An epithelial cell of the visceral layer of Bowman's capsule in the renal corpuscle, attached to the outer surface of the glomerular capillary basement membrane by cytoplasmic foot processes (pedicels); believed to play a role in the ultrafiltration of blood. [podo- + G. *kytos,* a hollow (cell)]

pod•o•dy•na•mom•e•ter (pod′ō-dī′nă-mom′ĕ-ter). An instrument for measuring the strength of the muscles of the foot or leg. [podo- + G. *dynamis,* force, + *metron,* measure]

pod•o•dyn•ia (pod-ō-din′ē-ă). SYN podalgia. [podo- + G. *odynē,* pain]

pod•o•gram (pod′ō-gram). An imprint of the sole of the foot, showing the contour and the condition of the arch, or an outline tracing. [podo- + G. *gramma,* written]

pod•o•mech•a•no•ther•a•py (pod-ō-mek′ă-nō-thār′ă-pē). Treatment of foot conditions with mechanical devices; *e.g.,* arch supports, orthoses.

po•go•ni•on (pō-gō′ni-on). In craniometry, the most anterior point on the mandible in the midline; the most anterior, prominent point on the chin. SYN mental point. [G. dim. of *pōgōn,* beard]

pOH. The negative logarithm of the OH⁻ concentration (in moles per liter).

-poiesis. Production; producing. [G. *poiēsis,* a making]

poikilo-. Irregular, varied. [G. *poikilos,* many colored, varied]

poi•ki•lo•blast (poy′ki-lō-blast). A nucleated red blood cell of irregular shape. [poikilo- + G. *blastos,* germ]

poi•ki•lo•cyte (poy′ki-lō-sīt). A red blood cell of irregular shape. [poikilo- + G. *kytos,* cell]

poi•ki•lo•cy•the•mia (poy′ki-lō-sī-thē′mē-ă). SYN poikilocytosis. [poikilocyte + G. *haima,* blood]

poi•ki•lo•cy•to•sis (poy′ki-lō-sī-tō′sis). The presence of poikilocytes in the peripheral blood. SYN poikilocythemia. [poikilocyte + G. -*osis,* condition]

poi•ki•lo•der•ma (poy′ki-lō-der′mă). A variegated hyperpigmentation and telangiectasia of the skin, followed by atrophy. [poikilo- + G. *derma,* skin]

poi•ki•lo•ther•mic, poi•ki•lo•ther•mal, poi•ki•lo•ther•mous (poy′ki-lō-ther′mic, -măl, -mŭs). **1.** Varying in temperature according to the temperature of the surrounding medium; denoting the so-called cold-blooded animals, such as the reptiles and amphibians, and the plants. **2.** Capable of existence and growth in mediums of varying temperatures. [poikilo- + G. *thermē,* heat]

point (poynt). **1.** SYN punctum. **2.** A sharp end or apex. **3.** A slight projection. **4.** A stage or condition reached, as the boiling p. **5.** To become ready to open, said of an abscess or to boil the wall of which is becoming thin and is about to break. [Fr.; L. *punctum,* fr. *pungo,* pp. *punctus,* to pierce]

  p. A, SYN subspinale.

  alveolar p., SYN prosthion.

  anterior focal p., the p. where parallel rays from the retina are focused.

  auricular p., SYN auriculare.

  axial p., SYN nodal p.

  p. B, SYN supramentale.

break-even p., the p. in sales volume at which total revenues equal total costs. Sales volume below the break-even p. will cause a negative cash flow (loss); sales volume above the break-even p. will result in a profit. This point is calculated to help determine whether a new test or procedure should be offered by a health care provider based on projected sales volume.

Cannon's p., the location in the mid-transverse colon at which innervation by superior and inferior mesenteric plexuses overlap at the junction of the primitive midgut and hindgut, frequently resulting in narrowing evident on barium enema.

cardinal p.'s, (1) the four p.'s in the pelvic inlet toward one of which the occiput of the baby is usually directed in case of head presentation: two sacroiliac articulations and the two iliopectineal eminences corresponding to the acetabula; **(2)** six p.'s of a compound optical system: the anterior focal p., the posterior focal p., the two principal p.'s, and the two nodal p.'s.

conjugate p., a p. so related to another that an object at one is imaged at the other.

craniometric p.'s, fixed p.'s on the skull used as landmarks in craniometry.

p. of elbow, SYN olecranon.

far p., that p. in conjugate focus with the retina when the eye is not accommodating.

p. of fixation, the p. on the retina at which the rays coming from an object regarded directly are focused.

focal p., SEE anterior focal p., posterior focal p.

gutta-percha p.'s, cones of a gutta percha compound used for filling root canals in conjunction with a cement, paste, or plastic.

incident p., the p. at which a light ray enters an optical system.

isoelectric p. (pI), the pH at which an amphoteric substance, such as protein or an amino acid, is electrically neutral.

isosbestic p., in applied spectroscopy, a wavelength at which absorbance of two substances, one of which can be converted into the other, is the same.

J p., the p. marking the end of the QRS complex and the beginning of the ST segment in the electrocardiogram.

jugal p., SYN jugale.

McBurney's p., a site one-third the distance from the anterior superior iliac spine (ASIS) to the umbilicus that with deep palpation produces rebound tenderness indicating appendicitis. SEE ALSO appendicitis.

melting p. (T_m), (1) the temperature at which a solid becomes a liquid; **(2)** the temperature at which 50% of a macromolecule becomes denatured.

mental p., SYN pogonion.

motor p., a p. on the skin where the application of an electrical stimulus, via an electrode, will cause the contraction of an underlying muscle.

nasal p., SYN nasion.

near p., that p. in conjugate focus with the retina when the eye exerts maximal accommodation.

nodal p., one of two p.'s in a compound optical system so related that a ray directed toward the first p. will appear to have passed through the second p. parallel to its original direction. SYN axial p.

p. of ossification, SYN center of ossification.

posterior focal p., the p. of a compound optical system where parallel rays entering the system are focused.

pressure p., a cutaneous locus having pressure-sensitive elements that, when compressed, produce a sensation of pressure.

principal p., one of two p.'s on an optic axis so related that an object at one is exactly imaged at the other without magnification, minification, or inversion.

trigger p., pathological condition characterized by a small, hypersensitive area located within muscles or fasciae. SYN trigger area, trigger zone.

zygomaxillary p., SYN zygomaxillare.

poin•til•lage (pwan-tē-yazh′). A massage manipulation with the tips of the fingers. [Fr. dotting, stippling]

poise (poyz, pwahz). In the CGS system, the unit of viscosity equal to 1 dyne-second per square centimeter and to 0.1 pascal-second. [J. *Poiseuille*]

poi•son (poy′zŭn). Any substance, either taken internally or applied externally, that is injurious to health or dangerous to life. [Fr., fr. L. *potio*, potion, draught]

poi•son•ing (poy′zŏn-ing). **1.** The administering of poison. **2.** The state of being poisoned. SYN intoxication (1).

bacterial food p., a term commonly used to refer to conditions limited to enteritis or gastroenteritis (excluding the enteric fevers and the dysenteries) caused by bacterial multiplication per se or by a soluble bacterial exotoxin.

blood p., SEE septicemia, pyemia.

carbon monoxide p., a potentially fatal acute or chronic intoxication caused by inhalation of carbon monoxide gas which competes favorably with oxygen for binding with hemoglobin (carboxyhemoglobinemia) and thus interferes with the transportation of oxygen and carbon dioxide by the blood.

djenkol p., p. believed to result from eating excessive amounts of a bean, *Pitecolobium lobatum;* symptoms are pain in the renal region, dysuria, and later anuria; the djenkol bean has a high vitamin B content and is used for food despite its toxic qualities.

food p., poisoning in which the active agent is contained in ingested food.

lead p., acute or chronic intoxication by lead or any of its salts; symptoms of **acute lead p.** usually are those of acute gastroenteritis in adults or encephalopathy in children; **chronic lead p.** is manifested chiefly by anemia, constipation, colicky abdominal pain, neuropathy with paralysis, especially wrist-drop involving the extensor muscles of the forearm, bluish lead line of the gums, and interstitial nephritis; saturnine gout, convulsions, and coma may occur. SYN plumbism.

mercury p., a disease usually caused by the ingestion of mercury or mercury compounds, which are toxic in relation to their ability to produce mercuric ions; usually **acute mercury p.** is associated with ulcerations of the stomach and intestine and toxic changes in the renal tubules; anuria and anemia may occur; usually **chronic mercury p.** is a result of industrial p. and causes gastrointestinal or central nervous system manifestations including stomatitis, diarrhea, ataxia, tremor, hyperreflexia, sensorineural impairment, and emotional instability (Mad Hatter syndrome). SYN hydrargyria, hydrargyrism, mercurialism.

mushroom p., SEE mycetism.

scombroid p., p. from ingestion of heat-stable toxins produced by bacterial action on inadequately preserved dark-meat fish of the order Scombroidea (tuna, bonito, mackerel, albacore, skipjack); characterized by epigastric pain, nausea and vomiting, headache, thirst, difficulty in swallowing, and urticaria.

poi·son·ous (poy′zŭn-ŭs). Characterized by, having the characteristics of, or containing a poison. SYN toxic (1), venenous.

POL physician office *laboratory*.

po·lar (pō′lăr). 1. Relating to a pole. 2. Having poles, said of certain nerve cells having one or more processes. [Mod. L. *polaris,* fr. *polus,* pole]

po·lar·i·ty (pō-lar′i-tē). 1. The property of having two opposite poles, as that possessed by a magnet. 2. The possession of opposite properties or characteristics. 3. The direction or orientation of positivity relative to negativity. 4. The direction along a polynucleotide chain; or any biopolymer, or macro-structure (*e.g.,* microtubules). [Mod. L. *polaris,* polar]

po·lar·i·za·tion (pō′lăr-i-zā′shŭn). 1. ELECTRICITY Coating of an electrode with a thick layer of hydrogen bubbles, with the result that the flow of current is weakened or arrested. 2. A change effected in a ray of light passing through certain media, whereby the transverse vibrations occur in one plane only, instead of in all planes as in an ordinary light ray. 3. Development of differences in potential between two points in living tissues, as between the inside and outside of a cell wall.

pole (pōl). 1. One of the two points at the extremities of the axis of any organ or body. 2. Either of the two points on a sphere at the greatest distance from the equator. 3. One of the two points in a magnet or an electric battery or cell having extremes of opposite properties; the negative p. a cathode, the positive p. an anode. SYN polus [NA]. [L. *polus,* the end of an axis, pole, fr. G. *polos*]

animal p., the point in a telolecithal egg opposite the yolk, where most of the protoplasm is concentrated and where the nucleus is located; from this region, the polar bodies are extruded during maturation. SYN germinal p.

cephalic p., the head end of the fetus.

frontal p. of cerebrum, the most anterior promontory of each cerebral hemisphere.

germinal p., SYN animal p.

occipital p. of cerebrum, the most posterior promontory of each cerebral hemisphere; the apex of the occipital lobe.

pelvic p., the breech end of the fetus.

temporal p. of cerebrum, the most prominent part of the anterior extremity of the temporal lobe

of each cerebral hemisphere, a short distance below the fissure of Sylvius.

vegetal p., vegetative p., the part of a telolecithal egg where the bulk of the yolk is situated.

vitelline p., the vegetative p. of an ovum.

po·lice·man (pō-lēs′man). An instrument, usually a rubber-tipped rod, for removing solid particles from a glass container.

po·lio (pō′lē-ō). Abbreviated term for poliomyelitis.

△ **polio-.** Gray; gray matter (substantia grisea). [G. *polios*]

po·li·o·clas·tic (pō′lē-ō-klas′tik). Destructive to gray matter of the nervous system. [polio- + G. *klastos,* broken]

po·li·o·dys·tro·phia (pō′lē-ō-dis-trō′fē-ă). SYN poliodystrophy.

p. cer′ebri progressi′va infan′tilis [MIM* 203700], familial progressive spastic paresis of extremities with progressive mental deterioration, with development of seizures, blindness and deafness, beginning during the first year of life, and with destruction and disorganization of nerve cells of the cerebral cortex.

po·li·o·dys·tro·phy (pō′lē-ō-dis′trō-fē). Wasting of the gray matter of the nervous system. SYN poliodystrophia. [polio- + G. *dys-,* bad, + *trophē,* nourishment]

po·li·o·en·ceph·a·li·tis (pō′lē-ō-en-sef′ă-lī′tis). Inflammation of the gray matter of the brain, either of the cortex or of the central nuclei; as contrasted to inflammation of the white matter. [polio- + G. *enkephalos,* brain, + *-tis,* inflammation]

po·li·o·en·ceph·a·lo·me·nin·go·my·e·li·tis (pō′lē-ō-en-sef′ă-lō-mĕ-ning′gō-mī-ĕ-lī′tis). Inflammation of the gray matter of the brain and spinal cord and of the meningeal covering of the parts. [polio- + G. *enkephalos,* brain, + *mēninx,* membrane, + *myelon,* marrow, + *-itis,* inflammation]

po·li·o·en·ceph·a·lo·my·e·li·tis (pō′lē-ō-en-sef′ă-lō-mī′ĕ-lī′tis). SYN poliomyeloencephalitis.

po·li·o·en·ceph·a·lop·a·thy (pō′lē-ō-en-sef′ă-lop′ă-thē). Any disease of the gray matter of the brain. [polio- + G. *enkephalos,* brain, + *pathos,* suffering]

po·li·o·my·e·li·tis (pō′lē-ō-mī′ĕ-lī′tis). An inflammatory process involving the gray matter of the cord. [polio- + G. *myelos,* marrow, + *-itis,* inflammation]

acute anterior p., inflammation of the anterior cornua of the spinal cord; an acute infectious disease caused by the poliomyelitis virus and marked by fever, pains, and gastroenteric disturbances, followed by a flaccid paralysis of one or more muscular groups, and later by atrophy.

acute bulbar p., poliomyelitis virus infection affecting nerve cells in the medulla oblongata and producing paralysis of the lower motor cranial nerves.

po·li·o·my·e·lo·en·ceph·a·li·tis (pō′lē-ō-mī′ĕ-lō-en-sef′ă-lī′tis). Acute anterior poliomyelitis with pronounced cerebral signs. SYN polioencephalomyelitis. [polio- + G. *myelon,* marrow, + *enkephalos,* brain, + *-itis,* inflammation]

po·li·o·my·e·lop·a·thy (pō′lē-ō-mī′ĕ-lop′ă-thē)

Any disease of the gray matter of the spinal cord. [polio- + G. *myelon,* marrow, + *pathos,* suffering]

po•li•o•sis (po-lē-ō′sis). A patchy absence or lessening of melanin in hair of the scalp, brows, or lashes, due to lack of pigment in the epidermis; it occurs in several hereditary syndromes but may be caused by inflammation, irradiation, or infection such as herpes zoster. [G., fr. *polios,* gray]

po•li•o•vi•rus hom•i•nis (pō′lē-ō-vī′rŭs hom′i-nis). SYN poliomyelitis *virus.*

pol•itz•er•i•za•tion (pol′it-zer-i-zā′shŭn). Inflation of the auditory tube and middle ear by the Politzer method.

pol•len (pol′en). Microspores of seed plants carried by wind or insects prior to fertilization; important in the etiology of hay fever and other allergies. [L. fine dust, fine flour]

pol•le•no•sis (pol-ĕ-nō′sis). SYN pollinosis.

pol•lex, gen. **pol•li•cis,** pl. **pol•li•ces** (pol′eks, pol′i-sis, -sēz) [NA]. SYN thumb. [L.]

pol•li•ci•za•tion (pol′i-si-zā′shŭn). Construction of a substitute thumb. [L. *pollex,* thumb, + *-ize,* to make like, + *-ation,* state]

pol•li•no•sis (pol-i-nō′sis). Hay fever excited by the pollen of various plants. SYN pollenosis. [L. *pollen,* pollen, + G. *-osis,* condition]

pol•lu•tant (pŏ-lū′tănt). An undesired contaminant that results in pollution.

pol•lu•tion (pŏ-lū′shŭn). Rendering unclean or unsuitable by contact or mixture with an undesired contaminant. [L. *pollutio,* fr. *pol-luo,* pp. *-lutus,* to defile]

air p., contamination of air by smoke, particulate matter, and harmful gases, mainly oxides of carbon, sulfur, and nitrogen, as from automobile exhausts, industrial emissions, and burning rubbish. SEE ALSO smog.

noise p., annoying or physiologically damaging environmental sound levels, as from automobile engines, industrial machinery, and amplified music.

po•lo•ni•um (Po) (pō-lō′nē-ŭm). A radioactive element, atomic no. 84, isolated from pitchblende; the longest-lived isotope is ^{209}Po (half-life 102 years); ^{210}Po is radium F (half-life 138.38 days), the only readily accessible isotope. [L. fr. *Polonia,* Poland, native country of Marie Curie, who, with her husband Pierre, discovered the substance]

po•lus, pl. **po•li** (pō′lŭs, -lī) [NA]. SYN pole. [L. pole]

△**poly-.** **1.** Many; multiplicity. Cf. multi-, pluri-. **2.** CHEMISTRY Prefix meaning "polymer of," as in polypeptide, polysaccharide, polynucleotide; often used with symbols, as in poly(A) for poly(adenylic acid), poly(Lys) for poly(L-lysine). [G. *polys,* much, many]

pol•y•ad•e•ni•tis (pol′ē-ad-ĕ-nī′tis). Inflammation of many lymph nodes, especially with reference to the cervical group.

pol•y•ad•e•nop•a•thy (pol′ē-ad-ĕ-nop′ă-thē). Adenopathy affecting many lymph nodes.

pol•y•a•mine (pol-ē-am′ēn). Class name for substances of the general formula $H_2N(CH_2)_nNH_2$, $H_2N(CH_2)_nNH(CH_2)_nNH_2$, $H_2N(CH_2)_nNH-(CH_2)_nNH(CH_2)_nNH_2$, where n = 3, 4, or 5. Many p.'s arise by bacterial action on protein; many are

normally occurring body constituents of wide distribution, or are essential growth factors for microorganisms. [G. *polys,* much, many + amine]

pol•y(amine) (pol-ē-ă-mēn, am′ēn). A polymer of an amine. SEE poly- (2).

pol•y•an•gi•i•tis (pol′ē-an-jē-ī′tis). Inflammation of multiple blood vessels involving more than one type of vessel, *e.g.,* arteries and veins, arterioles and capillaries.

pol•y•an•i•on (pol-ē-an′ī-on). Anionic sites on proteoglycans in the renal glomeruli that restrict filtration of anionic molecules and facilitate filtration of cationic proteins; loss of p. may cause albuminuria in lipoid nephrosis.

pol•y•ar•ter•i•tis (pol′ē-ar-ter-ī′tis). Simultaneous inflammation of a number of arteries.

p. nodo′sa, segmental inflammation, with infiltration by eosinophils, and necrosis of medium-sized or small arteries, most common in males, with varied symptoms related to involvement of arteries in the kidneys, muscles, gastrointestinal tract, and heart. SYN Kussmaul's disease, periarteritis nodosa.

pol•y•ar•thric (pol-ē-ar′thrik). SYN multiarticular.

pol•y•ar•thri•tis (pol′ē-ar-thrī′tis). Simultaneous inflammation of several joints. [poly- + G. *arthron,* joint, + *-itis,* inflammation]

epidemic p., a mild febrile illness of humans in Australia characterized by polyarthralgia and rash, caused by the Ross River virus and transmitted by mosquitoes.

pol•y•ar•tic•u•lar (pol-ē-ar-tik′yū-lăr). SYN multiarticular. [poly- + L. *articulus,* joint]

pol•y•ba•sic (pol-ē-bās′ik). Having more than one replaceable hydrogen atom, denoting an acid with a basicity greater than 1.

pol•y•blast (pol′ē-blast). One of a group of ameboid, mononucleated, wandering phagocytic cells found in inflammatory exudates. [poly- + G. *blastos,* germ]

pol•y•chon•dri•tis (pol′ē-kon-drī′tis). A widespread disease of cartilage. [poly- + G. *chondros,* cartilage, + *-itis,* inflammation]

relapsing p., a hereditary degenerative disease of cartilage producing a bizarre form of arthritis, with collapse of the ears, the cartilaginous portion of the nose, and the tracheobronchial tree; death may occur from chronic infection or suffocation because of loss of stability in the tracheobronchial tree.

pol•y•chro•ma•sia (pol′ē-krō-mā′zē-ă). SYN polychromatophilia.

pol•y•chro•mat•ic (pol-ē-krō-mat′ik). Multicolored.

pol•y•chro•mat•o•cyte (pol′ē-krō-mat′ō-sīt). SYN polychromatophil (2).

pol•y•chro•ma•to•phil, pol•y•chro•ma•to•phile (pol-ē-krō′mă-tō-fil, -fīl). **1.** Staining readily with acid, neutral, and basic dyes; denoting certain cells, especially certain red blood cells. SYN polychromatophilic. **2.** A young or degenerating erythrocyte that manifests acid and basic staining affinities. SYN polychromatocyte. [poly- + G. *chrōma,* color, + *phileō,* to love]

pol•y•chro•ma•to•phil•ia (pol-ē-krō′mă-tō-fil′ē-ă). **1.** A tendency of certain cells, such as the red blood cells in pernicious anemia, to stain with basic and also acid dyes. **2.** Condition characterized by the presence of many red blood cells that have an affinity for acid, basic, or neutral stains. SYN polychromasia.

pol•y•chro•ma•to•phil•ic (pol-ē-krō′mă-tō-fil′ik). SYN polychromatophil (1).

pol•y•chro•me•mia (pol-ē-krō-mē′mē-ă). An increase in the total amount of hemoglobin in the blood.

pol•y•clin•ic (pol-ē-klin′ik). A dispensary for the treatment and study of diseases of all kinds. [poly- + G. *klinē*, bed]

pol•y•clo•nal (pol-ē-klō′năl). IMMUNOCHEMISTRY Pertaining to proteins from more than a single clone of cells, in contradistinction to monoclonal.

pol•y•clo•nia (pol′ē-klō′nē-ă). SYN *myoclonus* multiplex. [poly- + G. *klonos*, tumult]

pol•y•co•ria (pol-ē-kŏ′rē-ă). The presence of two or more pupils in one iris. [poly- + G. *korē*, pupil]

pol•y•crot•ic (pol-ē-krot′ik). Relating to or marked by polycrotism.

po•lyc•ro•tism (pol-ik′rō-tizm). A condition in which the sphygmographic tracing shows several upward breaks in the descending wave. [poly- + G. *krotos*, a beat]

pol•y•cy•e•sis (pol′ē-sī-ē′sis). SYN multiple *pregnancy*. [poly- + G. *kyēsis*, pregnancy]

pol•y•cys•tic (pol-ē-sis′tik). Composed of many cysts.

pol•y•cy•the•mia (pol′ē-sī-thē′mē-ă). An increase above the normal in the number of red cells in the blood. SYN erythrocythemia. [poly- + G. *kytos*, cell, + *haima*, blood]

  compensatory p., a secondary p. resulting from anoxia, *e.g.,* in congenital heart disease, pulmonary emphysema, or prolonged residence at a high altitude.

  p. hyperton′ica, p. associated with hypertension, but without splenomegaly.

  relative p., a relative increase in the number of red blood cells as a result of loss of the fluid portion of the blood.

  p. ru′bra, SYN p. vera.

  p. ve′ra, a chronic form of polycythemia of unknown cause; characterized by bone marrow hyperplasia, an increase in blood volume as well as in the number of red cells, redness or cyanosis of the skin, and splenomegaly. SYN erythremia, Osler's disease (1), Osler-Vaquez disease, p. rubra.

pol•y•dac•ty•ly (pol-ē-dak′ti-lē). Presence of more than five digits on hand or foot. [poly- + G. *daktylos,* finger]

pol•y•dip•sia (pol-ē-dip′sē-ă). Excessive thirst that is relatively prolonged. [poly- + G. *dipsa,* thirst]

pol•y•dys•pla•sia (pol′ē-dis-plā′zē-ă). Tissue development abnormal in several respects. [poly- + G. *dys-,* bad, + *plasis,* a molding]

poly•en•do•crin•op•athy (pol′ē-en′dō-krĭn-op′ă-thē). A disease usually caused by insufficiency of multiple endocrine glands. SEE multiple endocrine deficiency *syndrome.*

pol•y•e•no•ic ac•ids (pol-ē-en′ik). Fatty acids with more than one double bond in the carbon chain; *e.g.,* linoleic, linolenic, and arachidonic acids.

pol•y•er•gic (pol-ē-er′jik). Capable of acting in several different ways. [poly- + G. *ergon,* work]

pol•y•es•the•sia (pol-ē-es-thē′zē-ă). A disorder of sensation in which a single touch or other stimulus is felt as several. [poly- + G. *aisthēsis,* sensation]

pol•y•ga•lac•tia (pol′ē-gă-lak′tē-ă, -shē-ă). Excessive secretion of breast milk, especially at the weaning period. [poly- + G. *gala,* milk]

pol•y•ga•lac•tu•ro•nase (pol′ē-gă-lak′tū-ron-ās). Pectin depolymerase; an enzyme catalyzing the random hydrolysis of 1,4-α-D-galactosiduronic linkages in pectate and other galacturonans.

pol•y•gene (pol′ē-jēn). One of many genes that contribute to the phenotypic value of a measurable phenotype.

pol•y•gen•ic (pol-ē-jen′ik). Relating to a hereditary disease or normal characteristic controlled by the added effects of genes at multiple loci.

pol•y•glan•du•lar (pol-ē-glan′dū-lăr). SYN pluriglandular.

pol•y•graph (pol′ē-graf). **1.** An instrument to obtain simultaneous tracings from several different sources; *e.g.,* radial and jugular pulse, apex beat of the heart, phonocardiogram, electrocardiogram. The ECG is nearly always included for timing. **2.** An instrument for recording changes in respiration, blood pressure, galvanic skin response, and other physiological changes while the person is questioned about some matter or asked to give associations to relevant and irrelevant words; the physiological changes are presumed to be indicators of emotional reactions, and thus whether the person is telling the truth. SYN lie detector. [poly- + G. *graphō,* to write]

pol•y•gy•ria (pol-ē-jī′rē-ă). Condition in which the brain has an excessive number of convolutions. [poly- + G. *gyros,* circle, gyre]

pol•y•hi•dro•sis (pol′ē-hī-drō′sis). SYN hyperhidrosis.

pol•y•hy•dram•ni•os (pol′ē-hī-dram′nē-os). Excess amount of amniotic fluid. [poly- + G. *hydōr,* water, + amnion]

pol•y•hy•dric (pol-ē-hī′drik). Containing more than one hydroxyl group, as in polyhydric alcohols and polyhydric acids.

pol•y•i•dro•sis (pol′ē-i-drō′sis). SYN hyperhidrosis.

pol•y•lep•tic (pol-ē-lep′tik). Denoting a disease occurring in many paroxysms, *e.g.,* malaria, epilepsy. [poly- + G. *lēpsis,* a seizing]

pol•y•mas•tia (pol-ē-mas′tē-ă). In humans, a condition in which more than two breasts are present. SYN hypermastia (1), pleomastia, pleomazia. [poly- + G. *mastos,* breast]

pol•y•me•lia (pol-ē-mē′lē-ă). A developmental defect in which there are supernumerary limbs or parts of limbs. [poly- + G. *melos,* limb]

pol•y•men•or•rhea (pol-ē-men-ō-rē′ă). Occurrence of menstrual cycles of greater than usual frequency. [poly- + G. *mēn,* month, + *rhoia,* flow]

pol•y•mer (pol′i-mer). A substance of high molecular weight, made up of a chain of repeated units sometimes called "mers." [see -mer (1)]

po

pol•y•mer•ase (po-lim'er-ās). General term for any enzyme catalyzing a polymerization, as of nucleotides to polynucleotides, thus belonging to EC class 2, the transferases.

pol•y•me•ria (pol-ē-mēr'ē-ă). Condition characterized by an excessive number of parts, limbs, or organs of the body. [poly- + G. *meros,* part]

pol•y•mer•ic (pol-i-mer'ik). **1.** Having the properties of a polymer. **2.** Relating to or characterized by polymeria. **3.** Rarely used synonym for polygenic.

po•lym•er•i•za•tion (po-lim'er-i-za'shŭn). A reaction in which a high-molecular-weight product is produced by successive additions to or condensations of a simpler compound.

po•lym•er•ize (pol'i-mer-īz, po-lim'er-īz). To bring about polymerization.

pol•y•mor•phic (pol-ē-mōr'fik). Occurring in more than one morphologic form. SYN multiform, pleomorphic (1), pleomorphous, polymorphous. [G. *polymorphos,* multiform]

pol•y•mor•phism (pol-ē-mōr'fizm). Occurrence in more than one form; existence in the same species or other natural group of more than one morphologic type. SYN pleomorphism.

balanced p., a unilocal trait in which two alleles are maintained at stable frequencies because the heterozygote is more fit than either of the homozygotes. SEE ALSO overdominance.

DNA p., a condition in which one of two different but normal nucleotide sequences can exist at a particular site in DNA.

restriction fragment length p. (RFLP), used in genetic analysis of populations or individual relationships. In regions of the human genome not coding for proteins there is often wide sequence variety between individuals that can be measured.

restriction-site p., DNA p. in which the sequence of one form of the p. contains a recognition site for a particular endonuclease, but the sequence of the other form lacks such a site.

pol•y•mor•pho•cel•lu•lar (pol-ē-mōr'fō-sel'yū-lăr). Relating to or formed of cells of several different kinds. [G. *polymorphos,* multiform, + L. *cellula,* cell]

pol•y•mor•pho•nu•cle•ar (pol'ē-mōr-fō-nū'klē-ăr). Having nuclei of varied forms; denoting a variety of leukocyte. [G. *polymorphos,* multiform, + L. *nucleus,* kernel]

pol•y•mor•phous (pol-ē-mōr'fŭs). SYN polymorphic.

pol•y•my•al•gia (pol'ē-mī-al'jē-ă). Pain in several muscle groups. [poly- + G. *mys,* muscle, + *algos,* pain]

pol•y•my•oc•lo•nus (pol'ē-mī-ok'lō-nŭs). SYN *myoclonus* multiplex.

pol•y•my•o•si•tis (pol'ē-mī-ō-sī'tis). Inflammation of a number of voluntary muscles simultaneously. [poly- + G. *mys,* muscle, + *-itis,* inflammation]

pol•y•ne•sic (pol-i-nē'sik). Occurring in many separate foci; denoting certain forms of inflammation or infection. [poly- + G. *nēsos,* island]

pol•y•neu•ral (pol-ē-nū'răl). Relating to, supplied by, or affecting several nerves. [poly- + G. *neuron,* nerve]

pol•y•neu•ral•gia (pol'ē-nū-ral'jē-ă). Neuralgia of several nerves simultaneously.

pol•y•neu•ri•tis (pol'ē-nū-rī'tis). SYN polyneuropathy (2).

acute idiopathic p., a neurological syndrome, probably an immune-mediated disorder, often a sequela of certain virus infections, marked by paresthesia of the limbs and muscular weakness or a flaccid paralysis; the characteristic laboratory finding is increased protein in the cerebrospinal fluid without increase in cell count. SYN Landry syndrome, Landry's paralysis.

pol•y•neu•rop•a•thy (pol'ē-nū-rop'ă-thē). **1.** A disease process involving a number of peripheral nerves (literal sense). **2.** A nontraumatic generalized disorder of peripheral nerves, affecting the distal fibers most severely, with proximal shading (*e.g.,* the feet are affected sooner or more severely than the hands), and typically symmetrically; most often affects motor and sensory fibers almost equally, but can involve either one solely or very disproportionately; classified as axon degenerating (axonal), or demyelinating; many causes, particularly metabolic and toxic; familial or sporadic in nature. SYN polyneuritis. SYN multiple neuritis. [poly- + G. *neuron,* nerve, + *pathos,* disease]

progressive hypertrophic p., SYN Dejerine-Sottas *disease.*

pol•y•nu•cle•ar, pol•y•nu•cle•ate (pol-ē-nū'klē-ăr, -klē-āt). SYN multinuclear.

pol•y•nu•cle•o•ti•das•es (pol'ē-nū'klē-ō-ti'dās-ez). Enzymes catalyzing the hydrolysis of polynucleotides to oligonucleotides or to mononucleotides.

pol•y•nu•cle•o•tide (pol-ē-nū'klē-ō-tīd). A linear polymer containing an indefinite (usually large) number of nucleotides, linked from one ribose (or deoxyribose) to another via phosphoric residues. Cf. oligonucleotide.

pol•y•o•don•tia (pol-ē-ō-don'shē-ă). Presence of supernumerary teeth. [poly- + G. *odous,* tooth]

pol•y•on•co•sis, pol•y•on•cho•sis (pol'ē-ong-kō'sis). Formation of multiple tumors. [poly- + G. *onkos,* tumor, + *-osis,* condition]

pol•y•o•nych•ia (pol-ē-ō-nik'ē-ă). Presence of supernumerary nails on fingers or toes. [poly- + G. *onyx,* nail]

pol•y•o•pia, pol•y•op•sia (pol'ē-ō'pē-ă, -op'sē-ă). The perception of several images of the same object. SYN multiple vision. [poly- + G. *ōps,* eye]

pol•y•or•chism, pol•y•or•chid•ism (pol-ē-ōr'kizm, -ōr'kid-izm). Presence of one or more supernumerary testes. [poly- + G. *orchis,* testis]

pol•y•os•tot•ic (pol'ē-os-tot'ik). Involving more than one bone. [poly- + G. *osteon,* bone]

pol•y•o•tia (pol-ē-ō'shē-ă). Presence of a supernumerary auricle on one or both sides of the head. [poly- + G. *ous,* ear]

pol•y•ov•u•lar (pol-ē-ō'vyū-lăr). Containing more than one ovum.

pol•y•ov•u•la•tory (pol-ē-ō'vyū-lă-tōr-ē). Discharging several ova in one ovulatory cycle.

pol•yp (pol'ip). A general descriptive term applied to any mass of tissue that bulges or projects outward or upward from the normal surface level, thereby being macroscopically visible as a hemispheroidal, spheroidal, or irregular moundlike structure growing from a relatively broad base or a slender stalk; p.'s may be neoplasms, foci of inflammation, degenerative lesions, or malformations. SYN polypus. [L. *polypus*; G. *polypous*, contr. fr. G. *polys*, many, + *pous*, foot]

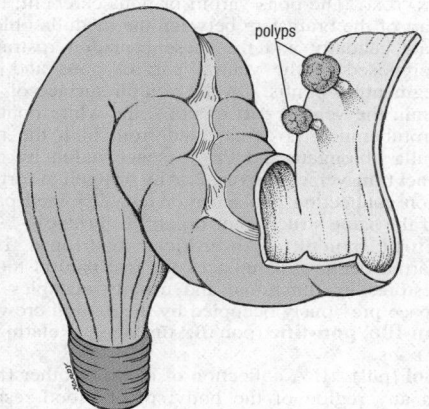

polyps

polyps: in sigmoid region of large intestine

adenomatous p., a p. that consists of benign neoplastic tissue derived from glandular epithelium.

fibrinous p., a misnomer for a mass of fibrin retained within the uterine cavity after childbirth.

hyperplastic p., a benign small sessile p. of the large bowel showing lengthening and cystic dilation of mucosal glands; also applied to non-neoplastic gastric mucosal p.'s. SYN metaplastic p.

metaplastic p., SYN hyperplastic p.

regenerative p., a hyperplastic p. of the gastric mucosa.

vascular p., a bulging or protruding angioma of the nasal mucous membrane.

pol•y•pec•to•my (pol-i-pek′tō-mē). Excision of a polyp. [polyp + G. *ektomē*, excision]

pol•y•pep•tide (pol-ē-pep′tīd). A peptide formed by the union of an indefinite (usually large) number of amino acids by peptide links (–NH–CO–).

gastric inhibitory p. (GIP), a peptide hormone, secreted by the stomach, that stimulates insulin release as part of the digestive process; GIP inhibits the secretion of acids and of pepsin. SYN gastric inhibitory peptide.

vasoactive intestinal p. (VIP), a p. hormone secreted most commonly by non-beta islet cell tumors of the pancreas, producing copious watery diarrhea and fecal electrolyte loss, particularly hypokalemia; VIP increases the rates of glycogenolysis; stimulates pancreatic bicarbonate secretion.

pol•y•pha•gia (pol-ē-fā′jē-ă). Excessive eating; gluttony. [poly- + G. *phagō*, to eat]

pol•y•phar•ma•cy (pol-ē-far′mă-sē). The administration of many drugs at the same time.

pol•y•pho•bia (pol-ē-fō′bē-ă). Morbid fear of many things; a condition marked by the presence of many phobias. [poly- + G. *phobos*, fear]

pol•y•phra•sia (pol-ē-frā′zē-ă). Extreme talkativeness. SEE logorrhea. [poly- + G. *phrasis*, speech]

pol•y•phy•let•ic (pol′ē-fī-let′ik). **1.** Derived from more than one source, or having several lines of descent, in contrast to monophyletic. **2.** HEMATOLOGY Relating to polyphyletism.

po•ly•pi (pol′i-pī). Plural of polypus.

pol•y•plas•tic (pol-ē-plas′tik). **1.** Formed of several different structures. **2.** Capable of assuming several forms. [poly- + G. *plastikos*, plastic]

pol•yp•loid (pol′ē-ployd). Characterized by or pertaining to polyploidy.

pol•y•ploi•dy (pol′ē-ploy′dē). The state of a cell nucleus containing three or more haploid sets. Cells containing three, four, five, or six multiples are referred to, respectively, as triploid, tetraploid, pentaploid, hexaploid, etc. [poly- + G. *ploidēs*, in form]

pol•yp•nea (pol-ip-nē′ă). SYN tachypnea. [poly- + G. *pnoia*, breath]

pol•yp•oid (pol′i-poyd). Resembling a polyp in gross features. [polyp + G. *eidos*, resemblance]

po•lyp•or•ous (pol-ip′ōr-ŭs). SYN cribriform. [poly- + G. *poros*, pore]

pol•yp•o•sis (pol′i-pō′sis). Presence of several polyps. [polyp + G. *-osis*, condition]

multiple intestinal p., **(1)** begins usually in late childhood; polyps increase in numbers, causing symptoms of chronic colitis, and carcinoma of the colon almost invariably develops in untreated cases; autosomal dominant inheritance. In the Gardner syndrome there are extracolonic changes (desmoid tumors, etc.); **(2)** hamartomatous p. of the small or large intestine, Peutz-Jeghers syndrome [MIM*175200] with melanin spots on the lips, less common; **(3)** [MIM 175400–], miscellaneous, rare, and doubtful occurrences.

pol•y•pous (pol′i-pŭs). Pertaining to, manifesting the gross features of, or characterized by the presence of a polyp or polyps.

pol•yp•tych•i•al (pol-ē-tik′ē-ăl). Folded or arranged so as to form more than one layer. [G. *polyptychos*, having many folds or layers, fr. poly- + *ptychē*, fold or layer]

pol•y•pus, pl. **po•ly•pi** (pol′i-pŭs, -pī). SYN polyp. [L.]

pol•y•ra•dic•u•li•tis (pol′ē-ra-dik′yū-lī′tis). SYN polyradiculopathy.

pol•y•ra•dic•u•lo•my•op•a•thy (pol′ē-ra-dik′yū-lō-mī-op′ă-thē). Coexisting polyradiculopathy and myopathy.

pol•y•ra•dic•u•lo•neu•rop•a•thy (pol-ē-ra-dik′yū-lō-nū-rop′ă-thē). Coexisting polyradiculopathy and polyneuropathy.

pol•y•ra•dic•u•lop•a•thy (pol-ē-ra-dik′yū-lop′ă-thē). Diffuse root involvement; seen with, among other disorders, diabetic neuropathy (diabetic polyradiculopathy). SYN polyradiculitis.

pol•y•ri•bo•somes (pol-ē-rī′bō-sōmz). Two or more ribosomes connected by a molecule of messenger RNA. SYN polysomes.

pol•y•sac•char•ide (pol-ē-sak′ă-rīd). A carbohydrate containing a large number of saccharide groups; *e.g.,* starch. Cf. oligosaccharide. SYN glycan.

po

pol•y•ser•o•si•tis (pol′ē-sēr-ō-sī′tis). Chronic inflammation with effusions in several serous cavities resulting in fibrous thickening of the serosa and constrictive pericarditis. [poly- + L. *serum,* serum, + G. *-itis,* inflammation]

   familial paroxysmal p. [MIM*249100], transient recurring attacks of abdominal pain, fever, pleurisy, arthritis, and rash; the condition is asymptomatic between attacks.

pol•y•si•nu•si•tis (pol′ē-sī-nŭ-sī′tis). Simultaneous inflammation of two or more sinuses.

pol•y•somes (pol′ē-sōmz). SYN polyribosomes.

pol•y•so•mia (pol-ē-sō′mē-ă). Fetal malformation involving two or more imperfect and partially fused bodies. [poly- + G. *sōma,* body]

pol•y•so•mic (pol-ē-sō′mik). Pertaining to or characterized by polysomy.

pol•y•som•no•gram (pol-ē-som′nō-gram). The recorded physiologic function(s) obtained in polysomnography. [poly- + L. *somnus,* sleep, + G. *gramma,* diagram]

pol•y•som•nog•ra•phy (pol′ē-som-nog′ră-fē). Simultaneous and continuous monitoring of relevant normal and abnormal physiological activity during sleep. [poly- + L. *somnus,* sleep, + G. *graphō,* to write]

pol•y•so•my (pol-ē-sō′mē). State of a cell nucleus in which a specific chromosome is represented more than twice. Cells containing three, four, or five homologous chromosomes are referred to, respectively, as trisomic, tetrasomic, or pentasomic. Cf. polyploidy. [poly- + G. *sōma,* body (chromosome)]

pol•y•sper•mia, pol•y•sper•mism (pol-ē-sper′mē-ă, -sper′mizm). **1.** SYN polyspermy. **2.** An abnormally profuse spermatic secretion.

pol•y•sper•my (pol′ē-sper-mē). The entrance of more than one spermatozoon into the ovum. SYN polyspermia (1), polyspermism.

pol•y•stich•ia (pol-ē-stik′ē-ă). Arrangement of the eyelashes in two or more rows. [poly- + G. *stichos,* row]

pol•y•sym•brach•y•dac•ty•ly (pol′ē-sim-brak-ē-dak′ti-lē). Malformation of the hand or foot in which the shortened digits are syndactylous and polydactylous. [poly- + symbrachydactyly]

pol•y•syn•ap•tic (pol′ē-si-nap′tik). Referring to neural pathways formed by a chain of a large number of synaptically connected nerve cells, as distinguished from oligosynaptic conduction systems. SYN multisynaptic.

pol•y•syn•dac•ty•ly (pol′ē-sin-dak′ti-lē). Syndactyly of several fingers or toes.

pol•y•ten•di•ni•tis (pol′ē-ten-di-nī′tis). Inflammation of several tendons.

pol•y•the•lia (pol-ē-thē′lē-ă). Presence of supernumerary nipples, either on the breast or elsewhere on the body. SYN hyperthelia. [poly- + G. *thēlē,* nipple]

pol•y•to•mog•ra•phy (pol-i-tō-mog′ră-fē). Body section radiography using a machine designed to effect complex motion; images a thinner tissue plane compared to simple linear or circular tomography.

pol•y•trich•ia (pol-ē-trik′ē-ă). Excessive hairiness. [poly- + G. *thrix* (*trich-*), hair]

pol•y•u•ria (pol-ē-yū′rē-ă). Excessive excretion of urine resulting in profuse micturition. [poly- + G. *ouron,* urine]

pol•y•va•lent (pol-ē-vā′lent). **1.** SYN multivalent. **2.** Pertaining to a polyvalent antiserum.

POMC pro-opiomelanocortin.

pons, pl. **pon•tes** (ponz, pon′tēz). **1** [NA]. NEUROANATOMY The pons varolii or pons cerebelli; that part of the brainstem between the medulla oblongata caudally and the mesencephalon rostrally, composed of the ventral part of pons and the tegmentum pontis. On the ventral surface of the brain the ventral part of pons, the white pontine protuberance, is demarcated from both the medulla oblongata and the mesencephalon by distinct transverse grooves. **2.** Any bridgelike formation connecting two more or less disjoined parts of the same structure or organ. [L. bridge]

pon•tic (pon′tik). An artificial tooth on a fixed partial denture; it replaces the lost natural tooth, restores its functions, and usually occupies the space previously occupied by the natural crown.

pon•tile, pon•tine (pon′tīl, -tīn; -tēn). Relating to a pons.

pool (pūl). **1.** A collection of blood or other fluid in any region of the body; p. of blood results from dilation and retardation of the circulation in the capillaries and veins of the part. **2.** A combination of resources. [A.S. *pōl*]

pop•lit•e•al (pop-lit′ē-ăl, pop-li-tē′ăl). Relating to the popliteal fossa.

pop•u•la•tion (pop-yū-lā′shŭn). Statistical term denoting all the objects, events, or subjects in a particular class. Cf. sample (1). [L. *populus,* a people, nation]

POR problem-oriented *record.*

pore (pōr). **1.** An opening, hole, perforation, or foramen. A pore, meatus, or foramen. **2.** SYN sweat p. [G. *poros,* passageway]

   dilated p., an enlarged follicular opening of the skin, with a keratinous plug and occasional lanugo or mature hair.

   sweat p., the surface opening of the duct of a sweat gland. SYN pore (2).

por•en•ce•pha•lia (pōr′en-se-fā′lē-ă). SYN porencephaly.

por•en•ce•phal•ic (pōr′en-se-fal′ik). Relating to or characterized by porencephaly. SYN porencephalous.

por•en•ceph•a•li•tis (pōr′en-sef-ă-lī′tis). Chronic inflammation of the brain with the formation of cavities in the organ's substance. [G. *poros,* pore, + *enkephalos,* brain, + *-itis,* inflammation]

por•en•ceph•a•lous (pōr-en-sef′ă-lŭs). SYN porencephalic.

por•en•ceph•a•ly (pōr-en-sef′ă-lē). The occurrence of cavities in the brain substance, communicating usually with the lateral ventricles. SYN porencephalia. [G. *poros,* pore, + *enkephalos,* brain]

po•ri (pō′rī). Plural of porus.

po•ro•ker•a•to•sis (pō′rō-ker-ă-tō′sis). A rare dermatosis in which there is a thickening of the stratum corneum with an annular keratotic rim or cornoid lamella surrounding progressive centrifugal atrophy; cutaneous carcinoma has been reported to arise in the lesions. [G. *poros,* pore, + keratosis]

po•ro•ma (pō-rō′mă). **1.** SYN callosity. **2.** SYN exostosis. **3.** Induration following a phlegmon. **4.** A tumor of cells lining the skin openings of sweat glands. [G. *pōrōma*, callus, fr. *pōros*, stone]

eccrine p., a p. or acrospiroma of the eccrine sweat glands, usually occurring on the sole of the foot.

po•ro•sis, pl. **po•ro•ses** (pō-rō′sis, -sēz). A porous condition. SYN porosity (1). [L. *porosus*, porous]

po•ros•i•ty (pō-ros′i-tē). **1.** SYN porosis. **2.** A perforation. [G. *poros*, pore]

po•rous (pō′rŭs). Having openings that pass directly or indirectly through the substance.

por•pho•bi•lin (pōr′fō-bī′lin). General term denoting intermediates between the monopyrrole, porphobilinogen, and the cyclic tetrapyrrole of heme (a porphin derivative).

por•pho•bi•lin•o•gen (PBG) (pōr′fō-bī-lin′ō-jen). A porphyrin precursor of porphyrinogens, porphyrins, and heme; found in the urine in large quantities in cases of acute or congenital porphyria.

por•phyr•ia (pōr-fir′ē-ă). A group of disorders involving heme biosynthesis, characterized by excessive excretion of porphyrins or their precursors; may be inherited or may be acquired, as from the effects of certain chemical agents (*e.g.,* hexachlorobenzene).

acute intermittent p., acute p., SYN intermittent acute p.

congenital erythropoietic p. [MIM*263700], enhanced porphyrin formation by erythroid cells in bone marrow, leading to severe porphyrinuria, often with hemolytic anemia and persistent cutaneous photosensitivity; caused by a deficiency of uroporphyrinogen III cosynthetase.

p. cuta′nea tar′da [MIM*176090, MIM*176100], familial or sporadic p. characterized by liver dysfunction and photosensitive cutaneous lesions, with hyperpigmentation and scleroderma-like changes in the skin, and increased excretion of uroporphyrin; caused by a deficiency of uroporphyrinogen decarboxylase induced in sporadic cases by chronic alcoholism. SYN symptomatic p.

erythropoietic p., a classification of p. that includes congenital erythropoietic p. and erythropoietic protoporphyria.

hepatic p. [MIM*176100.0002], a category of p. that includes p. cutanea tarda, variegate p., and coproporphyria.

intermittent acute p. (IAP) [MIM*176000], p. caused by hepatic overproduction of δ-aminolevulinic acid, with greatly increased urinary excretion of it and of porphobilinogen, due to a deficiency of porphobilinogen deaminase; characterized by intermittent acute attacks of hypertension, abdominal colic, psychosis, and polyneuropathy, but with no photosensitivity; exacerbation caused by ingestion of certain drugs (*e.g.,* barbiturates). SYN acute intermittent p., acute p.

symptomatic p., SYN p. cutanea tarda.

variegate p. [MIM*176200], p. characterized by abdominal pain and neuropsychiatric abnormalities, by dermal sensitivity to light and mechanical trauma, by increased fecal excretion of

proto- and coproporphyrin, and by increased urinary excretion of δ-aminolevulinic acid, porphobilinogen, and porphyrins; due to a deficiency of protoporphyrinogen oxidase.

por•phy•rin•o•gens (pōr-fi-rin′ō-jenz). Intermediates in the biosynthesis of heme; certain p. are elevated in certain porphyrias.

por•phy•rins (pōr′fi-rinz). Pigments widely distributed throughout nature (*e.g.,* heme, bile pigments, cytochromes) consisting of four pyrroles joined in a ring (porphin) structure.

por•phy•ri•nu•ria (pōr′fir-i-nū′rē-ă). Excretion of porphyrins and related compounds in the urine. SYN purpurinuria.

por•ta, pl. **por•tae** (pōr′tă, -tē). **1.** SYN hilum (1). **2.** SYN interventricular *foramen.* [L. gate]

p. hep′atis [NA], a transverse fissure on the visceral surface of the liver between the caudate and quadrate lobes, lodging the portal vein, hepatic artery, hepatic nerve plexus, hepatic ducts, and lymphatic vessels. SYN caudal transverse fissure, portal fissure.

por•ta•ca•val (pōr′tă-kā′văl). Concerning the portal vein and the inferior vena cava.

por•tal (pōr′tăl). **1.** Relating to any porta or hilus, specifically to the porta hepatis and the p. vein. **2.** The point of entry into the body of a pathogenic microorganism. [L. *portalis*, pertaining to a porta (gate)]

por•tio, pl. **por•ti•o•nes** (pōr′shē-ō, -ō′nēz) [NA]. A part. [L. portion]

por•tion (pōr′shun). Part or division.

supravaginal p. of cervix, the part of the cervix of the uterus lying above the attachment of the vagina.

vaginal p. of cervix, the part of the cervix uteri contained within the vagina.

△**porto-.** Portal. [L. *porta,* gate]

por•to•bil•i•o•ar•te•ri•al (pōr′tō-bil′ē-ō-ar-tēr′ē-ăl). Relating to the portal vein, biliary ducts, and hepatic artery, which have similar distributions.

por•to•en•ter•os•to•my (pōr′tō-en-ter-os′tō-mē). An operation for biliary atresia in which a Roux-en-Y loop of jejunum is anastomosed to the hepatic end of the divided extravascular portal structures, including rudimentary bile ducts. SYN Kasai operation.

por•to•gram (pōr′tō-gram). Radiographic record of portography. [porto- + G. *gramma,* a writing]

por•tog•ra•phy (pōr-tog′ră-fē). Delineation of the portal circulation by roentgenograms, using radiopaque material, usually introduced into the spleen or into the portal vein at operation. [porto- + G. *graphō,* to write]

por•to•sys•tem•ic (pōr′tō-sis-tem′ik). Relating to connections between the portal and systemic venous systems.

po•si•tion (pŏ-zish′ŭn). **1.** An attitude, posture, or place occupied. **2.** Posture or attitude assumed by a patient for comfort and to facilitate the performance of diagnostic, surgical, or therapeutic procedures. **3.** In obstetrics, the relation of an arbitrarily chosen portion of the fetus to the right or left side of the mother; with each presentation there may be a right or left p.; the fetal occiput, chin, and sacrum are the determining points of p. in vertex, face, and breech presentations, respectively. Cf. presentation. [L. *positio,* a placing, position, fr. *pono,* to place]

anatomical p., the erect p. of the body with the face directed forward (skull aligned in orbitomeatal or Frankfort plane); the arms at the side and the palms of the hands directed forward; the terms posterior, anterior, lateral, medial, etc., are applied to the parts as they stand related to each other and to the axis of the body when in this p.

Bozeman's p., knee-elbow p., the patient being strapped to supports.

close pack p., joint position in which contact between the articulation structures is maximal. SYN joint extension.

flank p., a lateral recumbent p., but with the lower leg flexed, the upper leg extended, and convex extension of the upper side of the body; used for nephrectomy.

Fowler's p., an inclined p. obtained by raising the head of the bed about 60 to 90 cm to promote better dependent drainage after an abdominal operation.

frontoanterior p., a cephalic presentation of the fetus with its forehead directed toward the right (**right frontoanterior**, RFA) or to the left (**left frontoanterior**, LFA) of the acetabulum of the mother.

frontoposterior p., a cephalic presentation of the fetus with its forehead directed toward the right (**right frontoposterior**, RFP) or to the left (**left frontoposterior**, LFP) sacroiliac articulation of the mother.

frontotransverse p., a cephalic presentation of the fetus with its forehead directed toward the right (**right frontotransverse**, RFT) or to the left (**left frontotransverse**, LFT) iliac fossa of the mother.

genucubital p., SYN knee-elbow p.

genupectoral p., SYN knee-chest p.

knee-chest p., a prone posture resting on the knees and upper part of the chest, assumed for gynecologic or rectal examination. SYN genupectoral p.

knee-elbow p., a prone p. resting on the knees and elbows, assumed for gynecologic or rectal examination or operation. SYN genucubital p.

lateral recumbent p., SYN Sims' p.

lithotomy p., a supine p. with buttocks at the end of the operating table, the hips and knees being fully flexed with feet strapped in p.

Mayo-Robson's p., a supine p. with a thick pad under the loins, causing a marked lordosis in this region; used in operations on the gallbladder.

mentoanterior p., a cephalic presentation of the fetus with its chin pointing to the right (**right mentoanterior**, RMA) or to the left (**left mentoanterior**, LMA) acetabulum of the mother.

mentoposterior p., a cephalic presentation of the fetus with its chin pointing to the right (**right mentoposterior**, RMP) or to the left (**left mentoposterior**, LMP) sacroiliac articulation of the mother.

mentotransverse p., a cephalic presentation of the fetus with its chin pointing to the right (**right mentotransverse**, RMT) or to the left (**left mentotransverse**, LMT) iliac fossa of the mother.

occipitoanterior p., a cephalic presentation of

the fetus with its occiput turned toward the right (**right occipitoanterior**, ROA) or to the left (**left occipitoanterior**, LOA) acetabulum of the mother.

occipitoposterior p., a cephalic presentation of the fetus with its occiput turned toward the right (**right occipitoposterior**, ROP) or to the left (**left occipitoposterior**, LOP) sacroiliac joint of the mother.

occipitotransverse p., a cephalic presentation of the fetus with its occiput turned toward the right (**right occipitotransverse**, ROT) or to the left (**left occipitotransverse**, LOT) iliac fossa of the mother.

occlusal p., the relationship of the mandible and maxillae when the jaws are closed and the teeth are in contact; it may or may not coincide with centric occlusion.

open-packed p., (1) position of the joint at which its bones are maximally congruent. (2) SYN flexion.

physiologic rest p., the usual p. of the mandible when the patient is resting comfortably in the upright p. and the condyles are in a neutral unstrained p. in the glenoid fossae. SYN postural p., postural resting p.

postural p., postural resting p., SYN physiologic rest p.

Rose's p., the patient lies supine with the head falling down over the end of the table; used in operations within the mouth or pharynx.

sacroanterior p., a breech presentation of the fetus with the sacrum pointing to the right (**right sacroanterior**, RSA) or to the left (**left sacroanterior**, LSA) acetabulum of the mother.

sacroposterior p., a breech presentation of the fetus with the sacrum pointing to the right (**right sacroposterior**, RSP) or to the left (**left sacroposterior**, LSP) sacroiliac articulation of the mother.

sacrotransverse p., a breech presentation of the fetus with its sacrum pointing to the right (**right sacrotransverse**, RST) or to the left (**left sacrotransverse**, LST) sacroiliac articulation of the mother.

Sims' p., a p. to facilitate a vaginal examination, the patient lying on the side with the under arm behind the back, the thighs flexed, the upper one more than the lower. SYN lateral recumbent p.

Valentine's p., a supine p. on a table with double inclined plane so as to cause flexion at the hips; used to facilitate urethral irrigation.

pos•i•tive (poz′i-tiv). **1.** Affirmative; definite; not negative. **2.** MATHEMATICS Having a value more than zero. **3.** PHYSICS, CHEMISTRY Having an electric charge resulting from a loss or deficit of electrons, hence able to attract or gain electrons. **4.** MEDICINE Denoting a response to a diagnostic maneuver or laboratory study that indicates the presence of the disease or condition tested for. [L. *positivus,* settled by arbitrary agreement, fr. *pono,* pp. *positus,* to set, place]

pos•i•tron (β^+) (poz′i-tron). A subatomic particle of mass and charge equal to the electron but of opposite (*i.e.,* positive) charge.

po•so•log•ic (pō-sō-loj′ik). Relating to posology.

po•sol•o•gy (pō-sol′ō-jē). The branch of pharmacology and therapeutics concerned with a determination of the doses of remedies; the science of dosage. [G. *posos*, how much, + *logos*, study]

post-. After, behind, posterior; opposite of anti-. Cf. meta-. [L. *post*]

post·ax·i·al (pōst-ak′sē-ăl). **1.** Posterior to the axis of the body or any limb, the latter being in the anatomical position. **2.** Denoting the portion of a limb bud that lies caudal to the axis of the limb: the ulnar aspect of the upper limb and the fibular aspect of the lower limb.

post·bra·chi·al (pōst′brā′kē-ăl). On or in the posterior part of the upper arm.

post·ca·va (pōst′kā′vă). SYN inferior *vena cava*.

post·ca·val (pōst′kā′văl). Relating to the inferior vena cava.

post·ci·bal (pōst-sī′băl). After a meal or the taking of food. [L. *cibum*, food]

post·co·i·tal (pōst-kō′i-tăl). After coitus.

post·co·i·tus (pōst-kō′i-tŭs). The time immediately after coitus.

post·cor·dial (pōst′kŏr′jăl). Posterior to the heart. [L. *cor* (*cord*-), heart]

post·cu·bi·tal (pōst′kyū′bi-tăl). On or in the posterior or dorsal part of the forearm.

post·duc·tal (pōst-dŭk′tăl). Relating to that part of the aorta distal to the aortic opening of the ductus arteriosus.

pos·te·ri·or (pos-tēr′ē-ŏr). **1.** After, in relation to time or space. **2** [NA]. HUMAN ANATOMY Denoting the back surface of the body. Often used to indicate the position of one structure relative to another, *i.e.*, nearer the back of the body. SYN dorsal (2). **3.** Near the tail or caudal end of certain embryos. **4.** An undesirable and confusing substitute for caudal in quadrupeds; in veterinary anatomy, p. is used only to denote some structures of the head. [L. comparative of *posterus*, following]

postero-. Posterior; at the back of. [L. *posterior*]

pos·ter·o·an·te·ri·or (pos′ter-ō-an-tēr′ē-ŏr). A term denoting the direction of view or progression, from posterior to anterior, through a part.

pos·ter·o·ex·ter·nal (pos′ter-ō-ek-ster′năl). SYN posterolateral.

pos·ter·o·in·ter·nal (pos′ter-ō-in-ter′năl). SYN posteromedial.

pos·ter·o·lat·er·al (pos′ter-ō-lat′ĕ-răl). Behind and to one side, specifically to the outer side. SYN posteroexternal.

pos·ter·o·me·di·al (pos′ter-ō-mē′dē-ăl). Behind and to the inner side. SYN posterointernal.

pos·ter·o·me·di·an (pos′ter-ō-mē′dē-an). Occupying a central position posteriorly.

pos·ter·o·su·pe·ri·or (pos′ter-ō-sū-pē′rē-ŏr). Situated behind and at the upper part.

post·es·trus, post·es·trum (pōst-es′trŭs, -trŭm). The period in the estrus cycle following estrus; characterized by the growth of the corpus luteum and physiologic changes related to the production of progesterone.

post·gan·gli·on·ic (pōst′gang-glē-on′ik). Distal to or beyond a ganglion; referring to the unmyelinated nerve fibers originating from cells in an autonomic ganglion.

pos·thi·o·plas·ty (pos′thē-ō-plas-tē). Surgical reconstruction of the prepuce. [G. *posthion*, dim. form of *posthē*, prepuce, + *plastos*, formed]

pos·thi·tis (pos-thī′tis). Inflammation of the prepuce. [G. *posthē*, prepuce, + *-itis*, inflammation]

post·hyp·not·ic (pōst-hip-not′ik). Following hypnotism; denoting an act suggested during hypnosis that is to be carried out at some time after the hypnotized subject is awakened.

post·ic·tal (pōst-ik′tăl). Following a seizure, *e.g.*, epileptic.

post·ma·ture (pōst-mă-tūr′, mă-tyūr′). Referring to a fetus that remains in the uterus longer than the normal gestational period; *i.e.*, longer than 42 weeks (288 days) in humans.

post·men·o·pau·sal (pōst-men-ō-paw′săl). Relating to the period following the menopause.

post·mor·tem (pōst-mŏr′tem). **1.** Pertaining to or occurring during the period after death. **2.** Colloquialism for autopsy (1). [post- + L. acc. case of *mors* (*mort*-), death]

post·na·sal (pōst′nā′săl). **1.** Posterior to the nasal cavity. **2.** Relating to the posterior portion of the nasal cavity.

post·na·tal (pōst-nā′tăl). Occurring after birth. [L. *natus*, birth]

post·op·er·a·tive (pōst-op′er-ă-tiv). Following an operation.

post·o·ral (pos-tō′răl). In the posterior part of, or posterior to, the mouth. [L. *os* (*or*-), mouth]

post·par·tum (pōst-par′tŭm). After childbirth. Cf. antepartum, intrapartum. [L. *partus*, birth (noun), fr. *pario*, pp. *partus*, to bring forth]

post·pran·di·al (pōst-pran′dē-ăl). Following a meal. [L. *prandium*, breakfast]

post·pu·ber·al, post·pu·ber·tal (pōst-pū′ber-ăl, -ber-tăl). SYN postpubescent.

post·pu·bes·cent (pōst-pū-bes′ent). Subsequent to the period of puberty. SYN postpuberal, postpubertal.

post·sphyg·mic (pōst-sfig′mik). Occurring after the pulse wave. [G. *sphygmos*, pulse]

post·tib·i·al (pōst′tib′ē-ăl). Posterior to the tibia; situated in the posterior portion of the leg.

post·trau·mat·ic (pōst-traw-mat′ik). Occurring after trauma, and, by implication, caused by it.

pos·tu·late (pos′tyū-lăt). A proposition that is taken as self-evident or assumed without proof as a basis for further analysis. SEE ALSO hypothesis, theory. [L. *postulo*, pp. *-atus*, to demand]

pos·tur·al (pos′tyū-răl, pos′cher-ăl). Relating to or affected by posture.

pos·ture (pos′chŭr, pos′cher). The position of the limbs or the carriage of the body as a whole. [L. *positura*, fr. *pono*, pp. *positus*, to place]

post·val·var, post·val·vu·lar (pōst-val′văr, -val′vyū-lăr). Relating to a position distal to the pulmonary or aortic valves.

po·ta·ble (pō′tă-bl). Drinkable; fit to drink. [L. *potabilis*, fr. *poto*, to drink]

po·tas·si·um (K) (pō-tas′ē-ŭm). An alkaline metallic element, atomic no. 19, atomic wt. 39.0983, occurring abundantly in nature but always in combination; its salts are used medicinally. For organic p. salts not listed below, see the name of the anion. SYN kalium. [Mod. L., fr. Eng. potash (fr. pot + ashes) + *-ium*]

    p. sodium tartrate, KNaC$_4$H$_4$O$_6$; a mild saline cathartic, used as an ingredient in compound effervescent powders.

po•ten•cy (pō'ten-sē). **1.** Power, force, or strength; the condition or quality of being potent. **2.** Specifically, sexual p. **3.** In therapeutics, the relative pharmacological activity of a compound. [L. *potentia,* power]

po•tent (pō'tent). **1.** Possessing force, power, strength. **2.** Indicating the ability of a primitive cell to differentiate. SEE ALSO totipotent, pluripotent. **3.** PSYCHIATRY Possessing sexual potency.

po•ten•tial (pō-ten'shăl). **1.** Capable of doing or being, although not yet doing or being; possible, but not actual. **2.** A state of tension in an electric source enabling it to do work under suitable conditions; in relation to electricity, p. is analogous to the temperature in relation to heat. [L. *potentia,* power, potency]

action p., the change in membrane p. occurring in nerve, muscle, or other excitable tissue when excitation occurs.

chemical p. (μ), a measure of how the Gibbs free energy of a phase depends on any change in the composition of that phase.

excitatory postsynaptic p., the change in p. which is produced in the membrane of the next neuron when an impulse which has an excitatory influence arrives at the synapse; it is a local change in the direction of depolarization; summation of these p.'s can lead to discharge of an impulse by the neuron.

inhibitory postsynaptic p., the change in p. produced in the membrane of the next neuron when an impulse which has an inhibitory influence arrives at the synapse; it is a local change in the direction of hyperpolarization; the frequency of discharge of a given neuron is determined by the extent to which impulses that lead to excitatory postsynaptic p.'s predominate over those that cause inhibitory postsynaptic p.'s.

membrane p., the p. inside a cell membrane, measured relative to the fluid just outside; it is negative under resting conditions and becomes positive during an action p.

oscillatory p., the variable voltage in the positive deflection of the electroretinogram (B-wave) of the dark-adapted eye arising from amacrine cells.

spike p., the main wave in the action p. of a nerve; it is followed by negative and positive afterpotentials.

visual evoked p., voltage fluctuations that may be recorded from the occipital area of the scalp as the result of retinal stimulation by a light flashing at ¼-second intervals; commonly summated and averaged by computer.

zoonotic p., the p. for infections of subhuman animals to be transmissible to humans.

po•ten•ti•a•tion (pō-ten'shē-ā'shŭn). Interaction between two or more drugs or agents resulting in a pharmacologic response greater than the sum of individual responses to each drug or agent.

po•tion (pō'shŭn). A draft or large dose of liquid medicine. [L. *potio, potus,* fr. *poto,* to drink]

pouch (powch). A pocket or cul-de-sac.

Hartmann's p., a spheroid or conical p. at the junction of the neck of the gallbladder and the cystic duct.

Kock p., a continent ileostomy with a reservoir and valved opening fashioned from doubled loops of ileum.

Rathke's p., SYN pituitary *diverticulum.*

rectouterine p., a pocket formed by the deflection of the peritoneum from the rectum to the uterus. SYN excavatio rectouterina [NA], cul-de-sac (2).

rectovesical p., a pocket formed by the deflection of the peritoneum from the rectum to the bladder in the male. SYN excavatio rectovesicalis [NA].

uterovesical p., a pocket formed by the deflection of the peritoneum from the bladder to the uterus in the female.

pou•drage (pū-drahzh'). **1.** Powdering. **2.** SYN talc *operation.* [F.]

poul•tice (pōl'tis). A soft magma or mush prepared by wetting various powders or other absorbent substances with oily or watery fluids, sometimes medicated, and usually applied hot to the surface; it exerts an emollient, relaxing, or stimulant, counterirritant effect upon the skin and underlying tissues. [L. *puls (pult-),* a thick pap; G. *poltos*]

pound (pownd). A unit of weight, containing 12 ounces, apothecaries' weight, or 16 ounces, avoirdupois; equivalent to 2.2046 kg. [A.S. *pund;* L. *pondus,* weight]

pow•der. 1. A dry mass of minute separate particles of any substance. **2.** PHARMACEUTICS A homogenous dispersion of finely divided, relatively dry, particulate matter consisting of one or more substances. **3.** A single dose of a powdered drug, enclosed in an envelope of folded paper. **4.** To reduce a solid substance to a state of very fine division. [Fr. *poudre;* L. *pulvis*]

pow•er. 1. OPTICS The refractive vergence of a lens. **2.** PHYSICS, ENGINEERING The rate at which work is done.

carbon dioxide combining p., a measurement of the total CO_2 that can be bound as HCO_2 at a P_{CO_2} of 40 mmHg at 25 C by serum, plasma, or whole blood.

muscular p., ability of muscles to produce force at a given time.

resolving p., (1) definition of a lens; in a microscope objective lens it is calculated by dividing the wavelength of the light used by twice the numerical aperture of the objective. (2) analogies to other modalities, *e.g.,* two-point discrimination in neurological examination. (3) SYN resolution (2).

pox (poks). **1.** An eruptive disease, usually qualified by a descriptive prefix; *e.g.,* smallpox, cowpox, chickenpox. See the specific term. **2.** An eruption, first papular then pustular, occurring in chronic antimony poisoning. **3.** Archaic or colloquial term for syphilis. [var. of pl. *pocks*]

Pox•vir•i•dae (poks-vir'i-dē). A family of large complex viruses, with a marked affinity for skin tissue, that are pathogenic for man and other animals. a number of genera are recognized including: *Orthopoxvirus, Avipoxvirus, Capripoxvirus, Leporipoxvirus,* and *Parapoxvirus.*

pox•vi•rus (poks'vī-rŭs). Any virus of the family Poxviridae.

PP pyrophosphate.

PPCA proserum prothrombin conversion *accelerator*.

PPLO pleuropneumonia-like *organisms*, under *organism*.

ppm parts per million.

PPO 2,5-diphenyloxazole, a liquid scintillator; preferred provider *organization*.

PPPPPP A mnemonic of 6 P's designating the symptom complex of acute arterial occlusion. [*p*ain, *p*allor, *p*araesthesia, *p*ulselessness, *p*aralysis, *p*rostration]

PPS prospective payment *system*.

P pul·mo·na·le (pul-mō-nā'lē). Tall, narrow, peaked P waves in electrocardiographic leads II, III, and aVF, and often a prominent initial positive P wave component in V₁; it is characteristic of right atrial enlargement, such as occurs in pulmonary disease and tricuspid stenosis.

PPV. positive pressure *ventilation*.

Pr 1. presbyopia. **2.** praseodymium; propyl.

PRA plasma renin *activity*; phosphoribosylamine.

prac·tice (prak'tis). The exercise of the profession of medicine or one of the allied health professions. [Mediev. L. *practica*, business, G. *praktikos*, pertaining to action]

  family p., a specialty of medicine in which the physician takes responsibility for the health and medical care of all members of a family group, regardless of age or gender, but usually does limited amounts of obstetrics and surgery.

  group p., the cooperative p. of medicine by a group of physicians, each of whom as a rule specializes in some particular field; such a group often shares a common suite of consulting rooms, laboratories, staff, equipment, etc.

prac·ti·tion·er (prak-tish'ŭn-er). A person who practices medicine or one of the allied health care professions.

  respiratory care p. (RCP), an allied health professional who works under the direction of a physician, educating patients, treating, assessing patient response to therapy and the need for continued therapy, managing and monitoring patients with deficiencies and abnormalities of cardiopulmonary function; term is applied by states to individuals licensed to practice.

△**prae-.** SEE pre-.

prag·ma·tism (prag'mă-tizm). A philosophy emphasizing practical applications and consequences of beliefs and theories, that the meaning of ideas or things is determined by the testability of the idea in real life. [G. *pragma* (*pragmat-*), thing done]

pran·di·al (pran'dē-ăl). Relating to a meal. [L. *prandium*, breakfast]

pra·se·o·dym·i·um (Pr) (prā-sē-ō-dim'ē-ŭm). An element of the lanthanide or "rare earth" group; atomic no. 59, atomic wt. 140.90765. [G. *prasios*, leekgreen, fr. *prason*, a leek, + *didymos*, twin]

praxis (prăk'sĭs). OCCUPATIONAL THERAPY Conception and planning of a motor act in response to an environmental demand. [G., practice, activity]

PRE progressive-resistance *exercise*.

△**pre-.** Anterior; before (in time or space). SEE ALSO ante-, pro- (1). [L. *prae*]

pre·ag·o·nal (prē-ag'ō-năl). Immediately preceding death. [pre- + G. *agōn*, struggle (agony)]

pre·an·es·thet·ic (prē-an-es-thet'ik). Before anesthesia.

pre·ax·i·al (prē-ak'sē-ăl). **1.** Anterior to the axis of the body or a limb, the latter being in the anatomical position. **2.** Denoting the portion of a limb bud which lies cranial to the axis of the limb: the radial aspect of the upper limb and the tibial aspect of the lower limb.

pre·can·cer (prē-kan'ser). A lesion from which a malignant neoplasm is believed to develop in a significant number of instances, and which may or may not be recognizable clinically or by microscopic changes in the affected tissue.

pre·can·cer·ous (prē-kan'ser-ŭs). Pertaining to any lesion that is interpreted as precancer. SYN premalignant.

pre·cap·il·lary (prē-kap'i-lār-ē). Preceding a capillary; an arteriole or venule.

pre·car·ti·lage (prē-kar'ti-lij). A closely packed aggregation of mesenchymal cells just prior to their differentiation into embryonic cartilage.

pre·ca·va (prē-kā'vă). SYN superior *vena* cava.

pre·cip·i·ta·ble (prē-sip'i-tă-bl). Capable of being precipitated.

pre·cip·i·tant (prē-sip'i-tant). Anything causing a precipitation from a solution.

pre·cip·i·tate (prē-sip'i-tāt). **1.** To cause a substance in solution to separate as a solid. **2.** A solid separated out from a solution or suspension; a floc or clump, such as that resulting from the mixture of a specific antigen and its antibody. **3.** Accumulation of inflammatory cells on the corneal endothelium in uveitis (keratic precipitates). [L. *praecipito*, pp. *-atus*, to cast headlong]

  keratic p.'s, inflammatory cells on the corneal endothelium.

pre·cip·i·ta·tion (prē-sip-i-tā'shŭn). **1.** The process of formation of a solid previously held in solution or suspension in a liquid. **2.** The phenomenon of clumping of proteins in serum produced by the addition of a specific precipitin. [see precipitate]

pre·cip·i·tin (prē-sip'i-tin). An antibody that under suitable conditions combines with and causes its specific and soluble antigen to precipitate from solution.

pre·cip·i·tin·o·gen (prē-sip-i-tin'ō-jen). **1.** An antigen that stimulates the formation of specific precipitin when injected into an animal body. **2.** A precipitable soluble antigen. [precipitin + G. *-gen*, producing]

pre·ci·sion (prē-sĭ'zhun). **1.** The quality of being sharply defined or stated; one measure of precision is the number of distinguishable alternatives to a measurement. **2.** STATISTICS The inverse of the variance of a measurement or estimate. **3.** Reproducibility of a quantifiable result; an indication of the random error.

pre·clin·i·cal (prē-klin'i-kăl). **1.** Before the onset of disease. **2.** A period in medical education before the student becomes involved with patients and clinical work.

pre·co·cious (prē-kō'shŭs). Developing unusually early or rapidly. [L. *praecox*, premature]

pre·coc·i·ty (prē-kos'i-tē). Unusually early or

pr

rapid development of mental or physical traits. [see precocious]

pre•cog•ni•tion (prē-kog-nish'ŭn). Advance knowledge, by means other than the normal senses, of a future event; a form of extrasensory perception. [L. *praecogito,* to ponder before]

pre•con•scious (prē-kon'shŭs). PSYCHOANALYSIS One of the three divisions of the psyche, the other two being the conscious and unconscious; includes all ideas, thoughts, past experiences, and other memory impressions that with effort can be consciously recalled. Cf. foreconscious.

pre•con•vul•sive (prē-kon-vŭl'siv). Denoting the stage in an epileptic paroxysm preceding convulsions (*e.g.,* aura).

pre•cor•dia (prē-kōr'dē-ă). The epigastrium and anterior surface of the lower part of the thorax. [L. *praecordia* (ntr. pl. only), the diaphragm, the entrails, fr. *prae,* before, + *cor* (*cord-*), heart]

pre•cor•di•al (prē-kōr'dē-ăl). Relating to the precordia.

pre•cor•di•um (prē-kōr'dē-ŭm). Singular of precordia.

pre•cu•ne•ate (prē-kū'nē-āt). Relating to the precuneus.

pre•cu•ne•us (prē-kū'nē-ŭs) [NA]. A division of the medial surface of each cerebral hemisphere between the cuneus and the paracentral lobule; it lies above the subparietal sulcus and is bounded anteriorly by the marginal part of the cingulate sulcus and posteriorly by the parietooccipital sulcus. SYN quadrate lobe (3). [pre- + L. *cuneus,* a wedge]

pre•cur•sor (prē-ker'ser). That which precedes another or from which another is derived, applied especially to a physiologically inactive substance that is converted to an active enzyme, vitamin, hormone, etc., or to a chemical substance that is built into a larger structure in the course of synthesizing the latter. [L. *praecursor,* fr. *prae-,* pre- + *curro,* to run]

pre•de•cid•u•al (prē-dē-sid'yū-ăl). Relating to the premenstrual or secretory phase of the menstrual cycle.

pre•den•tin (prē-den'tin). The organic fibrillar matrix of the dentin before its calcification.

pre•di•a•be•tes (prē'dī-ă-bē'tēz). A state of potential diabetes mellitus, with normal glucose tolerance but with an increased risk of developing diabetes, (*e.g.,* family history).

pre•di•as•to•le (prē-dī-as'tō-lē). The interval in the cardiac rhythm immediately preceding diastole. SYN late systole.

pre•di•a•stol•ic (prē-dī-ă-stol'ik). Late systolic, relating to the interval preceding cardiac diastole.

pre•di•ges•tion (prē-dī-jes'chŭn). The artificial initiation of digestion of proteins (proteolysis) and starches (amylolysis) before they are eaten.

pre•dis•pose (prē'dis-pōz). To render susceptible.

pre•dis•po•si•tion (prē'dis-pō-zish'ŭn). A condition of special susceptibility to a disease.

pre•duc•tal (prē-dŭk'tăl). Relating to that part of the aorta proximal to the aortic opening of the ductus arteriosus.

pre•e•clamp•sia (prē-ē-klamp'sē-ă). Development of hypertension with proteinuria or edema, or both, due to pregnancy or the influence of a recent pregnancy; it usually occurs after the 20th week of gestation, but may develop before this time in the presence of trophoblastic disease. [pre- + G. *eklampsis,* a shining forth (eclampsia)]

pre•ex•ci•ta•tion (prē'ek-sī-tā'shŭn). Premature activation of part of the ventricular myocardium by an impulse that travels by an anomalous path and so avoids physiological delay in the atrioventricular junction; an intrinsic part of the Wolff-Parkinson-White syndrome.

pre•gan•gli•on•ic (prē'gang-glē-on'ik). Situated proximal to or preceding a ganglion; referring specifically to the preganglionic motor neurons of the autonomic nervous system (located in the spinal cord and brainstem) and the preganglionic, myelinated nerve fibers by which they are connected to the autonomic ganglia.

preg•nan•cy (preg'nan-sē). The condition of a female after conception until the birth of the baby. SYN gestation. [L. *praegnans* (*praegnant-*), pregnant, fr. *prae,* before, + *gnascor,* pp. *natus,* to be born]

    abdominal p., the implantation and development of a fertilized ovum in the peritoneal cavity, usually following early rupture of a tubal p.; very rarely, primary implantation may occur in the peritoneal cavity. SYN abdominocyesis (1).

    ampullar p., tubal p. situated near the midportion of the oviduct.

    cervical p., the implantation and development of the impregnated ovum in the cervical canal.

    combined p., coexisting uterine and ectopic p.

    cornual p., the implantation and development of the impregnated ovum in one of the cornua of the uterus.

    ectopic p., the development of an impregnated ovum outside the cavity of the uterus. SYN eccyesis.

    false p., a condition in which some signs and symptoms suggest pregnancy, although the woman is not pregnant. SYN pseudocyesis, pseudopregnancy (1).

    interstitial p., SYN intramural p.

    intraligamentary p., p. within the broad ligament.

    intramural p., development of the fertilized ovum in the uterine portion of the uterine tube. SYN interstitial p.

    multiple p., condition of bearing two or more fetuses simultaneously. SYN polycyesis.

    ovarian p., development of an impregnated ovum in an ovarian follicle. SYN ovariocyesis.

    secondary abdominal p., a condition in which the embryo or fetus continues to grow in the abdominal cavity after its expulsion from the uterine tube or other seat of its primary development. SYN abdominocyesis (2).

    tubal p., development of an impregnated ovum in the uterine tube.

    tuboabdominal p., development of an ectopic p. partly in the uterine tube and partly in the abdominal cavity.

    tubo-ovarian p., development of the ovum at the fimbriated extremity of the uterine tube and involving the ovary.

preg•nane (preg'nān). Parent hydrocarbon of the

progesterones, pregnane alcohols, ketones, and several adrenocortical hormones.

preg•nane•di•ol (preg-nān-dī′ol). The chief steroid metabolite of progesterone; it is biologically inactive and occurs as p. glucuronate in the urine.

preg•nane•di•one (preg-nān-dī′ŏn). A metabolite of progesterone, formed in relatively small quantities, that occurs in 5α and 5β isomeric forms.

preg•nane•tri•ol (preg-nān-trī′ol). A urinary metabolite of 17-hydroxyprogesterone and a precursor in the biosynthesis of cortisol; its excretion is enhanced in certain diseases of the adrenal cortex and following administration of corticotropin.

preg•nant. Denoting a gestating female. SYN gravid. [see pregnancy]

pre•hen•sile (prē-hen′sil). Adapted for taking hold of or grasping. [L. *prehendo*, pp. -*hensus*, to lay hold of, seize]

pre•hen•sion (prē-hen′shŭn). The act of grasping, or taking hold of.

pre•hor•mone (prē-hōr′mōn). A glandular secretory product, having little or no inherent biological potency, that is converted peripherally to an active hormone. Cf. prohormone.

pre•ic•tal (prē-ik′tăl). Occurring before a seizure or stroke. [pre- + L. *ictus*, a stroke]

pre•in•duc•tion (prē-in-dŭk′shŭn). A modification in the third generation resulting from the action of environment on the germ cells of one or both individuals of the grandparental generation. An effect from the action of environment on the germ cells of progenitors upon their grandchildren. [L. *prae*, before, + *inductio*, a bringing in, fr. *induco*, to lead in]

pre•kal•li•kre•in (prē-kal-ĭ-krē′in). A plasma glycoprotein which in complex with kininogen serves as a cofactor in the activation of factor XII. P. also serves as the proenzyme for plasma kallikrein. SYN Fletcher factor.

preleukemia. SYN myelodysplastic *syndrome.*

pre•load (prē′lōd). **1.** The load to which a muscle is subjected before shortening. **2.** SYN ventricular p.

    ventricular p., the pressure stretching the ventricular walls at the onset of ventricular contraction, expressed in terms of the wall stress at this moment, related to the tension per unit cross-sectional area in the ventricular muscle fibers that balances this transmural pressure at the moment before contraction begins. SYN preload (2).

pre•ma•lig•nant (prē-mă-lig′nănt). SYN precancerous.

pre•ma•ture (prē-mă-tūr′, -chūr). **1.** Occurring before the usual or expected time. **2.** Denoting an infant born less than 37 weeks (8-1/2 months) after conception. [L. *praematurus*, too early, fr. *prae*-, pre- + *maturus*, ripe (mature)]

pre•ma•tu•ri•ty (prē-mă-tūr′i-tē, -chūr′i-tē). **1.** The state of being premature. **2.** DENTISTRY Deflective occlusal contact.

pre•med•i•ca•tion (prē′med-i-kā′shŭn). **1.** Administration of drugs before induction of general anesthesia to allay apprehension, produce sedation, and facilitate the administration of anesthetic. **2.** Drugs used for such purposes.

pre•men•stru•al (prē-men′strū-ăl). Relating to the period of time preceding menstruation.

pre•men•stru•um (prē-men′strū-ŭm). The few days preceding menstruation. [pre- + L. *menstruum*, ntr. of *menstruus*, monthly, pertaining to menstruation]

pre•mo•lar (prē-mō′lăr). **1.** Anterior to a molar tooth. **2.** A bicuspid tooth.

pre•mon•o•cyte (prē-mon′ō-sīt). An immature monocyte not normally seen in the circulating blood. SYN promonocyte.

pre•mor•bid (prē-mōr′bid). Preceding the occurrence of disease. [pre- + L. *morbidus*, ill, fr. *morbus*, disease]

pre•mu•ni•tion (pre-mū-nish′ŭn). A state of existing resistance of a host to infection or reinfection with a parasite; used especially in malaria epidemiology. [L. *praemunitio*, fortification in advance, fr. *prae*-, + *munio*, to fortify]

pre•mu•ni•tive (pre-mū′ni-tiv). Relating to premunition.

pre•my•e•lo•blast (prē-mī′ĕ-lō-blast). The earliest recognizable precursor of the myeloblast.

pre•my•e•lo•cyte (prē-mī′ĕ-lō-sīt). SYN promyelocyte.

pre•na•tal (prē-nā′tăl). Preceding birth. SYN antenatal. [pre- + L. *natus*, born]

pre•ne•o•plas•tic (prē′nē-ō-plas′tik). Preceding the formation of any neoplasm, benign or malignant. [pre- + G. *neos*, new, + *plastikos*, formative]

pre•op•er•a•tive (prē-op′er-ă-tiv). Preceding an operation.

pre•os•te•o•blast (prē-os′tē-ō-blast). SYN osteoprogenitor *cell.*

pre•ox•y•gen•a•tion (prē′ok-sĕ-jĕ-nā′shŭn). Denitrogenation with 100% oxygen prior to induction of general anesthesia.

pre•po•ten•tial (prē-pō-ten′shăl). A gradual rise in potential between action potentials as a phasic swing in electric activity of the cell membrane, which establishes its rate of automatic activity, as in the ureter or cardiac pacemaker.

pre•psy•chot•ic (prē-sī-kot′ik). **1.** Relating to the period before the onset of psychosis. **2.** Denoting a potential for a psychotic episode, one that appears imminent under continued stress.

pre•pu•ber•al, pre•pu•ber•tal (prē-pyū′ber-ăl, -ber-tăl). Before puberty.

pre•pu•bes•cent (prē-pyū-bes′ent). Immediately prior to the commencement of puberty.

pre•puce (prē′pūs). The free fold of skin that covers more or less completely the glans penis. SYN preputium [NA], foreskin. [L. *praeputium*, foreskin]

    p. of clitoris, the external fold of the labia minora, forming a cap over the clitoris.

pre•pu•ti•al (pre-pyū′shē-ăl). Relating to the prepuce.

pre•pu•ti•ot•o•my (prē-pyū′shē-ot′ō-mē). Incision of prepuce. [preputium + G. *tomē*, incision]

pre•pu•ti•um, pl. **pre•pu•tia** (prē-pyū′shē-ŭm, shē-ă) [NA]. SYN prepuce. [L. *praeputium*]

♻**presby-, presbyo-.** Old age. SEE ALSO gero-. [G. *presbys*, old man]

pres•by•a•cu•sia. SEE presbyacusis.

pres•by•a•cu•sis, pres•by•a•cu•sia (prez′bē-ă-kū'sis). Loss of ability to perceive or discriminate sounds as a part of the aging process; the pattern and age of onset may vary. [presby- + G. *akousis,* hearing]

pres·by·o·pia (Pr) (prez-bē-ō'pē-ă). The physiologic loss of accommodation in the eyes in advancing age, said to begin when the near point has receded beyond 22 cm (9 inches). [presby- + G. *ōps,* eye]

pres·by·op·ic (prez'bē-op'ik, -ō'pik). Relating to or suffering from presbyopia.

pre·scribe (prē-skrīb'). To give directions, either orally or in writing, for the preparation and administration of a remedy to be used in the treatment of any disease. [L. *prae-scribo,* pp. *-scriptus,* to write before]

pre·scrip·tion (prē-skrip'shŭn). **1.** A written formula for the preparation and administration of any remedy. **2.** A medicinal preparation compounded according to formulated directions, consisting of four parts: 1) *superscription,* consisting of the word *recipe,* take, or its sign, ℞; 2) *inscription,* the main part of the p., containing the names and amounts of the drugs ordered; 3) *subscription,* directions for mixing the ingredients and designation of the form (pill, powder, solution, etc.) in which the drug is to be made; 4) *signature,* directions to the patient regarding the dose and times of taking the remedy. [L. *praescriptio;* see prescribe]

  exercise p., formulation of individualized exercise program based on exercise frequency, intensity, and duration with consideration for the specificity of the training response. SEE ALSO prescription, specificity of training *principle.*

pre·se·nile (prē-sē'nīl). Prior to the usual onset of senility.

pre·se·nil·i·ty (prē-sĕ-nil'i-tē). Premature old age; the condition of an individual, not old in years, who displays the physical and mental characteristics of old age but not to the extent of senility. [pre- + L. *senilis,* old]

pre·sent (prē-zent'). **1.** To precede or appear first at the os uteri, said of the part of the fetus first felt during examination. **2.** To appear for examination, treatment, etc., said of a patient. [L. *praesens (-sent-),* pres. p. of *prae-sum,* to be before, be at hand]

pre·sen·ta·tion (prē'zen-tā'shŭn, prez'). That part of the fetus presenting at the superior strait of the maternal pelvis; occiput, chin, and sacrum are, respectively, the determining points in vertex, face, and breech p. SEE ALSO position (3). See also entries under position. [see present]

  breech p., p. of any part of the pelvic extremity of the fetus, the nates, knees, or feet; more properly only of the nates; frank breech p. occurs when the fetus presents by the pelvic extremity; the thighs may be flexed and the legs extended over the anterior surfaces of the body; in **full breech p.,** the thighs may be flexed on the abdomen and the legs upon the thighs, in **footling p., foot p.** the feet may be the lowest part; in **incomplete foot p., incomplete knee p.,** one leg may retain the position which is typical of one of the above-mentioned presentations, while the other foot or knee may present.

  brow p., SEE cephalic p.

  cephalic p., p. of any part of the fetal head, usually the upper and back part as a result of flexion such that the chin is in contact with the thorax in vertex p.; there may be degrees of flexion so that the presenting part is the large fontanel in sincipital p., the brow in brow p., or the face in face p.

  face p., SEE cephalic p.

  footling p., foot p., SEE breech p.

  frank breech p., SEE breech p.

  incomplete foot p., SEE breech p.

  knee p., SEE breech p.

  placental p., SYN *placenta* previa.

  shoulder p., transverse p. with the shoulder as the presenting part.

  sincipital p., SEE cephalic p.

  transverse p., an abnormal p., neither head nor breech, in which the fetus lies transversely in the uterus across the axis of the parturient canal.

  vertex p., SEE cephalic p.

pre·ser·va·tive (prē-zer'vă-tiv). A substance added to food products or to an organic solution to prevent chemical change or bacterial action.

pre·so·mite (prē-sō'mīt). Relating to the embryonic stage before the appearance of somites (before day 19 in the human).

pre·sphyg·mic (prē-sfig'mik). Preceding the pulse beat; denoting a brief interval following the filling of the ventricles with blood before their contraction forces open the semilunar valves, corresponding to the isovolumic contraction period. [pre- + G. *sphygmos,* pulse]

pres·sor (pres'er, -ōr). Exciting to vasomotor activity; producing increased blood pressure; denoting afferent nerve fibers which, when stimulated, excite vasoconstrictors which increase peripheral resistance. SYN hypertensor. [L. *premo,* pp. *pressus,* to press]

pres·so·re·cep·tive (pres'ō-rē-sep'tiv). Capable of receiving as stimuli changes in pressure, especially changes of blood pressure. SYN pressosensitive.

pres·so·re·cep·tor (pres'ō-rē-sep'ter, -tōr). SYN baroreceptor.

pres·so·sen·si·tive (pres-ō-sen'si-tiv). SYN pressoreceptive.

pres·sure (presh'ŭr). **1.** A stress or force acting in any direction against resistance. **2** (P, frequently followed by a subscript indicating location). In physics and physiology, the force per unit area exerted by a gas or liquid against the walls of its container or that would be exerted on a wall immersed at that spot in the middle of a body of fluid. The p. can be considered either relative to some reference p., such as that of the ambient atmosphere (imagined to be on the other side of the wall), or in absolute terms (relative to a perfect vacuum). [L. *pressura,* fr. *premo,* pp. *pressus,* to press]

  abdominal p., p. surrounding the bladder; estimated from rectal, gastric, or intraperitoneal p.

  auto-positive end-expiratory p. (auto-PEEP), developing in the periphery of the lung as a consequence of incomplete emptying of lung units due to inadequate expiratory time. SYN intrinsic PEEP, occult PEEP.

back p., p. exerted upstream in the circulation as a result of obstruction to forward flow, as when congestion in the pulmonary circulation results from stenosis of the mitral valve or failure of the left ventricle.

barometric p. (P_B), the absolute p. of the ambient atmosphere, varying with weather, altitude, etc.; expressed in millibars (meteorology) or mm Hg or torr (respiratory physiology); at sea level, one atmosphere (atm, 760 mm Hg or torr) is equivalent to: 14.69595 lb/sq in, 1013.25 millibars, 1013.25×10^6 dynes/cm^2, and, in SI units, 101,325 pascals (Pa).

bilevel positive airway p. (BiPAP), a mode of mechanical ventilatory support in which two levels of continuous positive airway p. (CPAP) are delivered to the patient: (1) inspiratory positive airway p. (IPAP); (2) expiratory positive airway p. (EPAP) . h

blood p., the p. or tension of the blood within the systemic arteries, maintained by the contraction of the left ventricle, the resistance of the arterioles and capillaries, the elasticity of the arterial walls, as well as the viscosity and volume of the blood; expressed as relative to the ambient atmospheric p.

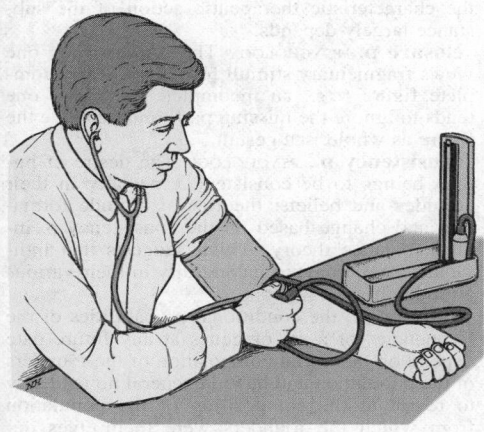

gauging **blood pressure**

central venous p. (CVP), the p. of the blood within the venous system in the superior and inferior vena cava, normally between 4 and 10 cm of water; it is depressed in circulatory shock and deficiencies of circulating blood volume, and increased with cardiac failure and congestion of the venous circulation.

cerebrospinal p., the p. of the cerebrospinal fluid, normally 100 to 150 mm of water, relative to the ambient atmospheric p.

continuous positive airway p. (CPAP), a technique of respiratory therapy, in either spontaneously breathing or mechanically ventilated patients, in which airway p. is maintained above atmospheric p. throughout the respiratory cycle by pressurization of the ventilatory circuit.

diastolic p., the intracardiac p. during or resulting from diastolic relaxation of a cardiac cham-

ber; the lowest arterial blood p. reached during any given ventricular cycle.

effective osmotic p., that part of the total osmotic p. of a solution that governs the tendency of its solvent to pass across a boundary, usually a semipermeable membrane.

intracranial p. (ICP), p. within the cranial cavity.

intraocular p., the p. of the intraocular fluid (usually measured in millimeters of mercury) with a manometer.

maximum expiratory p. (MEP), the maximum p. within the alveoli that occurs during a forceful expiration; the measurement is made when the lungs are full.

maximum inspiratory p. (MIP), the maximum p. within the alveoli that occurs during inspiration; the measurement of MIP provides a global assessment of inspiratory muscle function.

negative end-expiratory p. (NEEP), a subatmospheric p. at the airway at the end of expiration.

oncotic p., the osmotic p. attributed to proteins and other macromolecules.

osmotic p. (Π), the p. that must be applied to a solution to prevent the passage into it of solvent when solution and pure solvent are separated by a membrane permeable only to the solvent.

partial p., the p. exerted by a single component of a mixture of gases, commonly expressed in mm Hg or torr; for a gas dissolved in a liquid, the partial p. is that of a gas that would be in equilibrium with the dissolved In respiratory physiology, symbolized by P, followed by subscripts denoting location and/or chemical species (*e.g.,* P_{CO_2}, P_{O_2}, $P_{A_{CO_2}}$).

plateau p., the equilibrium p. between airways and alveoli in a patient-ventilator system; it is considered to be at least a close approximation of alveolar p.

positive end-expiratory p. (PEEP), a technique used in respiratory therapy in which airway p. greater than atmospheric p. is achieved at the end of exhalation by introduction of a mechanical impedance to exhalation.

pulmonary capillary wedge p. (PCWP), the p. obtained when a catheter is passed from the right side of the heart into pulmonary artery as far as it will go and "wedged" into an end artery. The p. distal to the wedged catheter is an approximation of cardiac left atrial p. The p. recorded with the balloon deflated is pulmonary artery p.

pulse p., the variation in blood p. occurring in an artery during the cardiac cycle; it is the difference between the systolic or maximum and diastolic or minimum p.'s.

standard p., the absolute p. to which gases are referred under standard conditions (STPD), *i.e.,* 760 mm Hg, 760 torr, or 101,325 newtons/m^2 (*i.e.,* 101,325 Pa).

systolic p., the intracardiac p. during or resulting from systolic contraction of a cardiac chamber; the highest arterial blood pressure reached during any given ventricular cycle.

trans-airway p., the p. gradient between the inside of the lung (the alveolus) and the outside of the lung (the pleural space).

wedge p., the intravascular pressure reading obtained when a fine catheter is advanced until it completely occludes a small blood vessel or is sealed in place by inflation of a small cuff; commonly measured in the lung to estimate left atrial pressure.

zero end-expiratory p. (ZEEP), airway p. which, at the end of expiration, equals atmospheric p.

pre•sup•pu•ra•tive (prē-sŭp′yū-rā-tiv). Denoting an early stage in an inflammation prior to the formation of pus.

pre•syn•ap•tic (prē′si-nap′tik). Pertaining to the area on the proximal side of a synaptic cleft.

pre•sys•to•le (prē-sis′tō-lē). That part of diastole immediately preceding systole.

pre•sys•tol•ic (prē-sis-tol′ik). Late diastolic, relating to the interval immediately preceding systole.

pre•tar•sal (prē-tar′săl). Denoting the anterior, or inferior, portion of the tarsus.

prev•a•lence (prev′ă-lens). The number of cases of a disease existing in a given population at a specific period of time (*period p.*) or at a particular moment in time (*point p.*).

pre•ven•tive (prē-ven′tiv). SYN prophylactic (1). [L. *prae-venio,* pp. -*ventus,* to come before, prevent]

pre•vi•us (prē′vē-ŭs). Obstructing; denoting anything blocking the passages in childbirth. [L. *prae,* before, + *via,* way]

Pre•vo•tel•la (prev′ō-tel′ah). A genus of Gramnegative, nonmotile, nonsporeforming, obligately anaerobic, chemoorganotrophic, and pleomorphic rods.

P. melani′noge′nica, a species found in the mouth, feces, infections of the mouth, soft tissue, respiratory tract, urogenital tract, and the intestinal tract. Implicated in periodontal disease; seen in aspiration pneumonitis. The type species of *Prevotella.* SYN *Bacteroides melaninogenicus.*

PRF prolactin-releasing *factor.*

PRH prolactin-releasing *hormone.*

pri•a•pism (prī′ă-pizm). Persistent erection of the penis, accompanied by pain and tenderness, resulting from a pathologic condition rather than sexual desire. [see priapus]

pri•mal (prī′măl). **1.** First or primary. **2.** SYN primordial (2).

pri•mal scene. PSYCHOANALYSIS The actual or fantasized observation by a child of sexual intercourse, particularly between its parents.

pri•mary (prī′mār-ē). **1.** The first or foremost, as a disease or symptoms to which others may be secondary or occur as complications. **2.** Relating to the first stage of growth or development. SEE primordial. [L. *primarius,* fr. *primus,* first]

pri•mate (prī′māt). An individual of the order Primates. [L. *primus,* first]

pri•mi•grav•i•da (prī-mi-grav′i-dă). SEE gravida. [L. fr. *primus,* first, + *gravida,* a pregnant woman]

pri•mip•a•ra (prī-mip′ă-ră). SEE para. [L. fr. *primus,* first, + *pario,* to bring forth]

pri•mi•par•i•ty (prī-mi-par′i-tē). Condition of being a primipara.

pri•mip•a•rous (prī-mip′ă-rŭs). Denoting a primipara.

prim•i•tive (prim′i-tiv). SYN primordial (2). [L. *primitivus,* fr. *primus,* first]

pri•mor•dia (prī-mōr′dē-ă). Plural of primordium.

pri•mor•di•al (prī-mōr′dē-ăl). **1.** Relating to a primordium. **2.** Relating to a structure in its first or earliest stage of development. SYN primal (2), primitive.

pri•mor•di•um (prī-mōr′-dē-ŭm). An aggregation of cells in the embryo indicating the first trace of an organ or structure. SYN anlage (1). [L. origin, fr. *primus,* first, + *ordior,* to begin]

prin•ceps, pl. **prin•ci•pes** (prin′seps, -si-pēz). Principal. ANATOMY Term used to distinguish the largest or most important of several arteries. [L. chief, fr. *primus,* first, + *capio,* to take, choose]

prin•ci•ple (prin′si-pl). **1.** A general or fundamental doctrine or tenet. SEE ALSO law, rule, theorem. **2.** The essential ingredient in a substance, especially one that gives it its distinctive quality or effect. [L. *principium,* a beginning, fr. *princeps,* chief]

active p., a constituent of a drug, usually an alkaloid or glycoside, upon the presence of which the characteristic therapeutic action of the substance largely depends.

closure p., PSYCHOLOGY The p. that when one views fragmentary stimuli forming a nearly complete figure (*e.g.,* an incomplete rectangle) one tends to ignore the missing parts and perceive the figure as whole. SEE gestalt.

consistency p., PSYCHOLOGY The desire of human beings to be consistent, especially in their attitudes and beliefs; theories of attitude formation and change based on the consistency p. include balance theory, which suggests that individuals seek to avoid incongruity in their various attitudes.

founder p., the conditional probabilities of the frequencies of a set of genes at any future date depend on the initial composition of the founders of the population and have in general no tendency to revert to the composition of the population from which the founders were themselves derived.

overload p., EXERCISE SCIENCE fundamental p. of training stating that exercise at an intensity above that normally attained will induce highly specific adaptations enabling the body to function more efficiently. Overload is applied by manipulating combinations of training frequency, intensity, and duration.

pain-pleasure p., PSYCHOANALYSIS The concept that one tends to seek pleasure and avoid pain; a term borrowed by experimental psychology to denote the same tendency of an animal in a learning situation. SYN pleasure p.

pleasure p., SYN pain-pleasure p.

reality p., the concept that the pleasure p. in personality development is modified by the demands of external reality; the p. or force that compels the growing child to adapt to the demands of external reality.

reversibility p., EXERCISE SCIENCE p. stating that training adaptations are lost at a relatively rapid rate when a person terminates participation in an exercise program. SYN detraining.

specificity of training p., EXERCISE SCIENCE concept that specific exercise elicits specific adaptations, creating specific training effects. The effects are most effectively induced by training the specific muscles involved in the desired performance.

pri•on (prī'on). SYN prion *protein.* [proteinaceous infectious particle]

prism (prizm). A transparent solid, with sides that converge at an angle, that deflects a ray of light toward the thickest portion (the base) and splits white light into its component colors; in spectacles, a p. corrects ocular muscle imbalance. [G. *prisma*]

pris•ma, pl. **pris•ma•ta** (priz'mă, priz'mah-tă). A structure resembling a prism. [G. something sawed, a prism]

pris'mata adamanti'na, the calcified, microscopic rods radiating from the surface of the dentin, forming the substance of the enamel of a tooth.

prism bar. A graduated series of p. b.'s mounted on a frame and used in ocular diagnosis.

pri•va•cy (prī'vă-sē). **1.** Being apart from others; seclusion; secrecy. **2.** Especially in psychiatry and clinical psychology, respect for the confidential nature of the therapist-patient relationship.

PRO. peer-review *organization.*

Pro proline or its radicals.

pro-. 1. Before, forward. SEE ALSO ante-, pre-. **2.** CHEMISTRY Prefix indicating precursor of. SEE ALSO -gen. [L. and G. *pro*]

pro•ac•cel•er•in (prō-ak-sel'er-in). SYN *factor* V.

pro•ac•ti•va•tor (prō-ak'ti-vā-ter). A substance that, when chemically split, yields a fragment (activator) capable of rendering another substance enzymatically active.

prob•a•bil•i•ty. 1. A measure, ranging from zero to 1, of the degree of belief in a hypothesis or statement. **2.** The limit of the relative frequency of an event in a sequence of N random trials as N approaches infinity.

pro•bac•te•ri•o•phage (prō-bak-tēr'ē-ō-fāj). The stage of a temperate bacteriophage in which the genome is incorporated in the genetic apparatus of the bacterial host. SYN prophage.

pro•band (prō'band). HUMAN GENETICS The patient or member of the family that brings a family under study. SYN index case. [L. *probo,* to test, prove]

probe (prōb). **1.** A slender rod of flexible material, with blunt bulbous tip, used for exploring sinuses, fistulas, other cavities, or wounds. **2.** A device or agent used to detect or explore a substance; *e.g.,* a molecule used to detect the presence of a specific fragment of DNA or RNA or of a specific bacterial colony. **3.** To enter and explore, as with a p. [L. *probo,* to test]

pro•bi•o•sis (prō-bī-ō'sis). An association of two organisms that enhances the life processes of both. Cf. antibiosis (1), symbiosis, mutualism. [pro- + G. *biōsis,* life]

pro•bi•ot•ic (prō-bī-ot'ik). Relating to probiosis.

pro•cap•sid (prō-kap'sid). A protein shell lacking a virus genome.

pro•car•box•y•pep•ti•dase (prō'kar-bok-sē-pep'ti-dās). Inactive precursor of a carboxypeptidase.

pro•car•y•ote (pro-kar'ē-ōt). SYN prokaryote. [pro- + G. *karyon,* kernel, nut]

pro•car•y•ot•ic (prō'kar-ē-ot'ik). SYN prokaryotic.

pro•ce•dure (prō-sē'jŭr). Act or conduct of diagnosis, treatment, or operation. SEE ALSO method, operation, technique.

commando p., an operation for malignant tumors of the floor of the oral cavity, involving resection of portions of the mandible in continuity with the oral lesion and radical neck dissection.

endorectal pull-through p., removal of diseased rectal mucosa along with resection of the lower bowel, followed by anastomosis of the proximal stump to the anus, in order to spare rectal muscle function.

loop electrocautery excision p. (LEEP), electrocautery excisional biopsy of abnormal cervical tissue.

platelet neutralization p. (PNP), a p. based on the ability of platelets to bypass the effect of a lupus anticoagulant by correcting prolonged coagulation times in various phospholipid-dependent test systems; the disrupted platelet membranes in the freeze-thawed platelet suspension neutralize phospholipid antibodies in the plasma of patients with lupus anticoagulant; after mixing the patient plasma with the freeze-thawed platelet suspension, the activated partial thromboplastin time will be corrected when compared with the original baseline activated partial thromboplastin time.

Puestow p., longitudinal pancreaticojejunostomy for treatment of chronic pancreatitis.

pro•cen•tri•ole (prō-sen'trē-ōl). The early phase in development *de novo* of centrioles or basal bodies from the centrosphere; p.'s form in relation to deuterosomes (p. organizers).

pro•ce•phal•ic (prō-se-fal'ik). Relating to the anterior part of the head. [pro- + G. *kephalē,* head]

pro•cess (pros'es, prō'ses). **1.** In anatomy, a projection or outgrowth. SYN processus [NA]. **2.** A method or mode of action used in the attainment of a certain result. **3.** An advance, progress, or method as of a disease. SEE processus. **4.** A pathologic condition or disease. **5.** In dentistry, a series of operations that convert a wax pattern, such as that of a denture base, into a solid denture base of another material. [L. *processus,* an advance, progress, process, fr. *pro-cedo,* pp. -*cessus,* to go forward]

acromial p., SYN acromion.

alveolar p., the projecting ridge on the inferior surface of the body of the maxilla containing the tooth sockets; the term is also applied to the superior aspect of the body of the mandible, containing the tooth sockets of the lower jaw.

caudate p., a narrow band of hepatic tissue connecting the caudate and right lobes of the liver posterior to the porta hepatis.

ciliary p., one of the radiating pigmented ridges, usually seventy in number, on the inner surface of the ciliary body, increasing in thickness as they advance from the orbiculus ciliaris to the external border of the iris; these, together with the folds (plicae) in the furrows between them, constitute the corona ciliaris.

clinoid p., one of three pairs of bony projections from the sphenoid bone: anterior clinoid p., the recurved posterior angle of the lesser wing; middle clinoid p., a little spur of bone on the body of the sphenoid, posterolateral to the tuberculum sellae; posterior clinoid p., a spur of bone at each superior angle of the dorsum sellae.

complex learning p.'s, those p.'s that require the use of symbolic manipulations, as in reasoning.

condylar p., the articular process of the ramus of the mandible; it includes the head of the mandible, the neck of the mandible and pterygoid fovea. SYN condyloid p.

condyloid p., SYN condylar p.

coracoid p., a long curved projection from the neck of the scapula overhanging the glenoid cavity; it gives attachment to the short head of the biceps, the coracobrachialis, and the pectoralis minor muscles, and the conoid and coracoacromial ligaments.

coronoid p., a sharp triangular projection from a bone; coronoid p. of the mandible, the triangular anterior process of the mandibular ramus, giving attachment to the temporal muscle; coronoid p. of the ulna, a bracketlike projection from the anterior portion of the proximal extremity of the ulna; its anterior surface gives attachment to the brachialis, its proximal surface enters into the formation of the trochlear notch.

dendritic p., SYN dendrite (1).

ensiform p., SYN xiphoid p.

falciform p., a continuation of the inner border of the sacrotuberous ligament upward and forward on the inner aspect of the ramus of the ischium. SYN falciform ligament.

foot p., SYN pedicel.

funicular p., the tunica vaginalis surrounding the spermatic cord.

lenticular p. of incus, a knob at the tip of the long limb of the incus which articulates with the stapes. SYN orbiculare.

mandibular p., SYN mandibular arch.

mastoid p., the nipplelike projection of the petrous part of the temporal bone. SYN mastoid bone.

maxillary p., a thin plate of irregular form projecting from the middle of the upper border of the inferior concha, articulating with the maxilla bone and partly closing the orifice of the maxillary sinus.

odontoid p. of epistropheus, SYN dens (2).

orbital p., the anterior and larger of the two processes at the upper extremity of the vertical plate of the palatine bone, articulating with the maxilla, ethmoid, and sphenoid bones.

palatine p., in the embryo, medially directed shelves from the oral surface of the maxillae; they develop into the secondary palate after midline fusion.

primary p., PSYCHOANALYSIS The mental p. directly related to the functions of the primitive life forces associated with the id and characteristic of unconscious mental activity; marked by unorganized, illogical thinking and by the tendency to

seek immediate discharge and gratification of instinctual demands. Cf. secondary p.

pterygoid p., a long process extending downward from the junction of the body and greater wing of the sphenoid bone on either side; it is formed of two plates (lateral and medial), united anteriorly but separated below to form the pterygoid notch; the pterygoid fossa is formed by the divergence of these two plates posteriorly.

secondary p., PSYCHOANALYSIS The mental p. directly related to the learned and acquired functions of the ego and characteristic of conscious and preconscious mental activities; marked by logical thinking and by the tendency to delay gratification by regulation of the discharge of instinctual demands. Cf. primary p.

spinous p., (1) the dorsal projection from the center of a vertebral arch; (2) SYN sphenoidal spine.

styloid p., SEE styloid p. of radius, styloid p. of ulna, styloid p. of temporal bone.

styloid p. of radius, a thick, pointed, palpable projection on the lateral side of the distal extremity of the radius.

styloid p. of temporal bone, a slender pointed projection running downward and slightly forward from the base of the inferior surface of the petrous portion of the temporal bone where it joins the tympanic portion; it gives attachment to the styloglossus, stylohyoid, and stylopharyngeus muscles and the stylohyoid and stylomandibular ligaments.

styloid p. of ulna, a cylindrical, pointed palpable projection from the medial and posterior aspect of the head of the ulna, to the tip of which is attached the ulnar collateral ligament of the wrist.

supracondylar p., an occasional spine projecting from the anteromedial surface of the humerus about 5 cm above the medial epicondyle to which it is joined by a fibrous band. The supracondylar foramen thus formed transmits the brachial artery and median nerve.

temporal p., the posterior projection of the zygomatic bone articulating with the zygomatic process of the temporal bone to form the zygomatic arch.

transverse p., a bony protrusion on either side of the arch of a vertebra, from the junction of the lamina and pedicle, which functions as a lever for attached muscles.

vocal p. of arytenoid cartilage, the lower end of the anterior margin of the arytenoid cartilage to which the vocal cord is attached.

xiphoid p., the cartilage at the lower end of the sternum. SYN ensiform p., xiphisternum, xiphoid cartilage.

zygomatic p. of maxilla, the rough projection from the maxilla that articulates with the zygomatic bone.

processing. The activity of effecting a series of changes in something so as to achieve a particular result.

perceptual processing, the organization of sensory input into meaningful patterns.

sensory processing, interpreting and organizing varied stimuli, including those acquired by the tactile, proprioceptive, visual, vestibular, auditory, gustatory, and olfactory senses. SEE ALSO sensory *integration*, sensory awareness.

pro•ces•sus, pl. **pro•ces•sus** (prō-ses'ŭs) [NA]. SYN process (1). [L. see process]

  p. vaginalis of peritoneum, a peritoneal diverticulum in the embryonic lower anterior abdominal wall that traverses the inguinal canal; in the male it forms the tunica vaginalis testis and normally loses its connection with the peritoneal cavity; a persistent p. vaginalis in the female is known as the canal of Nuck.

pro•chon•dral (prō-kon'drăl). Denoting a developmental stage prior to the formation of cartilage. [pro- + G. *chondros*, cartilage]

pro•chy•mo•sin (prō-kī'mō-sin). The precursor of chymosin. SYN prorennin, renninogen, rennogen.

pro•ci•den•tia (pros-i-den'shē-ă, prō'si-). A sinking down or prolapse of any organ or part. [L. a falling forward, fr. *procido*, to fall forward]

pro•col•la•gen (prō-kol'ă-jen). Soluble precursor of collagen formed by fibroblasts and other cells in the process of collagen synthesis.

pro•con•ver•tin (prō-kon-ver'tin). SYN *factor VII*.

pro•cre•ate (prō'krē-āt). To beget; to produce by the sexual act. [L. *pro-creo*, pp. *-creatus*, to beget]

pro•cre•a•tion (prō-krē-ā'shŭn). SYN reproduction (2).

pro•cre•a•tive (prō'krē-ā-tiv). Having the power to beget or procreate.

⌂**proct-.** SEE procto-.

proc•tal•gia (prok-tal'jē-ă). Pain at the anus, or in the rectum. SYN proctodynia, rectalgia. [proct- + G. *algos*, pain]

proc•ta•tre•sia (prok-tă-trē'zē-ă). SYN anal *atresia*. [proct- + G. *a-* priv. + *trēsis*, a boring]

proc•tec•to•my (prok-tek'tō-mē). Surgical resection of the rectum. SYN rectectomy. [proct- + G. *ektomē*, excision]

proc•ti•tis (prok-tī'tis). Inflammation of the mucous membrane of the rectum. SYN rectitis. [proct- + G. *-itis*, inflammation]

⌂**procto-, proct-.** Anus; (more frequently) rectum; Cf. recto-. [G. *prōktos*]

proc•to•cele (prok'tō-sēl). Prolapse or herniation of the rectum. SYN rectocele. [procto- + G. *kēlē*, tumor]

proc•to•cly•sis (prok-tok'li-sis). Slow, continuous administration of saline solution by instillation into the rectum and sigmoid colon. SYN Murphy drip. [procto- + G. *klysis*, a washing out]

proc•to•coc•cy•pexy (prok-tō-kok'si-pek-sē). Suture of a prolapsing rectum to the tissues anterior to the coccyx. SYN rectococcypexy. [procto- + G. *kokkyx*, coccyx, + *pēxis*, fixation]

proc•to•co•lec•to•my (prok'tō-kō-lek'tō-mē). Surgical removal of the rectum together with part or all of the colon. [procto- + G. *kolon*, colon, + *ektomē*, excision]

proc•to•co•lo•nos•co•py (prok'tō-kō'lō-nos'kŏ-pē). Inspection of the interior of the rectum and colon. [procto- + G. *kolon*, colon, + *skopeō*, to view]

proc•to•col•po•plas•ty (prok'tō-kol'pō-plas-tē).

Surgical closure of a rectovaginal fistula. [procto- + G. *kolpos*, bosom (vagina), + *plastos*, formed]

proc•to•cys•to•plas•ty (prok'tō-sis'tō-plas-tē). Surgical closure of a rectovesical fistula. [procto- + G. *kystis*, bladder, + *plastos*, formed]

proc•to•cys•tot•o•my (prok'tō-sis-tot'ō-mē). Incision into the bladder from the rectum. [procto- + G. *kystis*, bladder, + *tomē*, incision]

proc•to•de•al (prok'tō-dē-ăl). Relating to the proctodeum.

proc•to•de•um, pl. **proc•to•dea** (prok-tō-dē'ŭm, -dē'ă). **1.** An ectodermally lined depression under the root of the tail, adjacent to the terminal part of the embryonic hindgut; at its bottom, proctodeal ectoderm and cloacal endoderm form the cloacal plate. When this epithelial plate ruptures, the anal and urogenital external orifices are established. SYN anal pit. **2.** Terminal portion of the insect alimentary canal. [L. fr. G. *prōktos*, anus + *hodaios*, on the way, fr. *hodos*, a way]

proc•to•dyn•ia (prok'tō-din'ē-ă). SYN proctalgia. [procto- + G. *odynē*, pain]

proc•to•log•ic (prok-tō-loj'ik). Relating to proctology.

proc•tol•o•gist (prok-tol'ō-jist). A specialist in proctology.

proc•tol•o•gy (prok-tol'ō-jē). Surgical specialty concerned with the anus and rectum and their diseases. [procto- + G. *logos*, study]

proc•to•pa•ral•y•sis (prok'tō-pa-ral'i-sis). Paralysis of the anus, leading to incontinence of feces.

proc•to•pexy (prok'tō-pek-sē). Surgical fixation of a prolapsing rectum. SYN rectopexy. [procto- + G. *pēxis*, fixation]

proc•to•plas•ty (prok'tō-plas-tē). Plastic surgery of the anus or rectum. SYN rectoplasty. [procto- + G. *plastos*, formed]

proc•to•ple•gia (prok'tō-plē'jē-ă). Paralysis of the anus and rectum occurring with paraplegia. [procto- + G. *plēgē*, stroke]

proc•top•to•sia, proc•top•to•sis (prok-top-tō'sē-ă, -tō'sis). Prolapse of the rectum and anus. [procto- + G. *ptōsis*, a falling]

proc•tor•rha•phy (prok-tōr'ă-fē). Repair by suture of a lacerated rectum or anus. [procto- + G. *rhaphē*, suture]

proc•tor•rhea (prok-tō-rē'ă). A mucoserous discharge from the rectum. [procto- + G. *rhoia*, a flow]

proc•to•scope (prok'tō-skōp). A rectal speculum. SYN rectoscope. [procto- + G. *skopeō*, to view]

proc•tos•co•py (prok-tos'kŏ-pē). Visual examination of the rectum and anus, as with a proctoscope.

proc•to•sig•moi•dec•to•my (prok'tō-sig-moy-dek'tō-mē). Excision of the rectum and sigmoid colon. [procto- + sigmoid, + G. *ektomē*, excision]

proc•to•sig•moi•di•tis (prok'tō-sig-moy-dī'tis). Inflammation of the sigmoid colon and rectum. [procto- + sigmoid + G. *-itis*, inflammation]

proc•to•sig•moi•dos•co•py (prok'tō-sig-moy-dos'kŏ-pē). Direct inspection through a sigmoidoscope of the rectum and sigmoid colon. [procto- + sigmoid + G. *skopeō*, to view]

proc•to•spasm (prok'tō-spazm). **1.** Spasmodic stricture of the anus. **2.** Spasmodic contraction of the rectum. [procto- + G. *spasmos*, spasm]

proc·to·ste·no·sis (prok'tō-stĕ-nō'sis). Stricture of the rectum or anus. SYN rectostenosis. [procto- + G. *stenōsis,* a narrowing]

proc·tos·to·my (prok-tos'tō-mē). The formation of an artificial opening into the rectum. SYN rectostomy. [procto- + G. *stoma,* mouth]

proc·tot·o·my (prok-tot'ō-mē). An incision into the rectum. SYN rectotomy. [procto- + G. *tomē,* incision]

proc·to·tre·sia (prok-tō-trē'zē-ă). Operation for correction of an imperforate anus. [procto- + G. *trēsis,* a boring]

proc·to·val·vot·o·my (prok'tō-val-vot'ō-mē). Incision of rectal valves.

pro·dro·mal (prō-drō'măl, prod'rō'măl). Relating to a prodrome. SYN prodromic, prodromous.

pro·drome (prō'drōm). An early or premonitory symptom of a disease. [G. *prodromos,* a running before, fr. pro- + *dromos,* a running, a course]

pro·dro·mic, pro·dro·mous (prō-drō'-mik, prod'rō-; -mŭs). SYN prodromal.

pro·drug (prō'drŭg). A class of drugs, the pharmacologic action of which results from conversion by metabolic processes within the body (biotransformation).

pro·duct (prod'ŭkt). **1.** Anything produced or made, either naturally or artificially. **2.** MATHEMATICS The result of multiplication. [L. *productus,* fr. *pro-duco,* pp. *-ductus,* to lead forth]

cleavage p., a substance resulting from the splitting of a molecule into two or more simpler molecules.

double p., the p. of systolic blood pressure multiplied by the heart frequency; a measure of heart work load. SEE ALSO Robinson *index.*

fibrin/fibrinogen degradation p.'s, several poorly characterized small peptides that result from the action of plasmin on fibrinogen and fibrin in the fibrinolytic process.

fission p., an atomic species produced in the course of the fission of a larger atom such as ^{235}U.

orphan p.'s, drugs, biologicals, and medical devices (including diagnostic *in vitro* tests) that may be useful in uncommon or rare diseases but which are not considered commercially viable. SYN orphan drugs.

spallation p., an atomic species produced in the course of the spallation of any atom.

substitution p., a p. obtained by replacing one atom or group in a molecule with another atom or group.

pro·duc·tive (prō-dŭk'tiv). Producing or capable of producing; denoting especially an inflammation leading to the production of new tissue with or without an exudate. [see product]

pro·en·zyme (prō-en'zīm). The precursor of an enzyme, requiring some change (usually the hydrolysis of an inhibiting fragment that masks an active grouping) to render it active; *e.g.,* pepsinogen, trypsinogen, profibrinolysin. SYN zymogen.

pro·e·ryth·ro·blast (prō-ĕ-rith'rō-blast). SYN pronormoblast.

pro·e·ryth·ro·cyte (prō-ĕ-rith'rō-sīt). The precursor of an erythrocyte; an immature red blood cell with a nucleus.

pro·es·tro·gen (prō-es'trō-jen). A substance that acts as an estrogen only after it has been metabolized in the body to an active compound.

pro·fi·bri·nol·y·sin (prō'fī-bri-nol'i-sin). SEE plasmin.

pro·file (prō'fīl). **1.** An outline or contour, especially one representing a side view of the human head. SYN norma [NA]. **2.** A summary, brief account, or record. [It. *profilo,* fr. L. *pro,* forward, + *filum,* thread, line (contour)]

biochemical p., a combination of biochemical tests usually performed with automated instrumentation upon admission of a patient to a hospital or clinic.

personality p., (1) a method by which the results of psychological testing are presented in graphic form; (2) a vignette or brief personality description.

test p., a combination of laboratory tests usually performed by automated methods and designed to evaluate organ systems of patients upon admission to a hospital or clinic.

pro·gas·trin (prō-gas'trin). Precursor of gastric secretion in the mucous membrane of the stomach.

pro·ge·nia (prō-jē'nē-ă). SYN prognathism. [pro- + L. *gena,* cheek]

pro·gen·i·tor (prō-jen'i-ter, -tōr). A precursor, ancestor; one who begets. [L.]

prog·e·ny (proj'ĕ-nē). Offspring; descendants. [L. *progenies,* fr. *progigno,* to beget]

pro·ge·ria (prō-jēr'ē-ă) [MIM*176670]. A condition in which normal development in the first year is followed by gross retardation of growth, with a senile appearance characterized by dry wrinkled skin, total alopecia, and birdlike facies; genetics unclear. SYN Hutchinson-Gilford disease. [pro- + G. *gēras,* old age]

pro·ges·ta·tion·al (prō'jes-tā'shŭn-ăl). **1.** Favoring pregnancy; conducive to gestation; capable of stimulating the uterine changes essential for implantation and growth of a fertilized ovum. **2.** Referring to progesterone, or to a drug with progesterone-like properties.

pro·ges·ter·one (prō-jes'ter-ōn). 4-Pregnene-3,20-dione; an antiestrogenic steroid, believed to be the active principle of the corpus luteum, isolated from the corpus luteum and placenta or synthetically prepared; used to correct abnormalities of the menstrual cycle, as a contraceptive, and to control habitual abortion. SYN corpus luteum hormone, luteohormone, progestational hormone.

pro·ges·tin (prō-jes'tin). **1.** A hormone of the corpus luteum. **2.** Generic term for any substance, natural or synthetic, that effects some or all of the biological changes produced by progesterone. [pro- + gestation + -in]

pro·ges·to·gen (prō-jes'tō-jen). **1.** Any agent capable of producing biological effects similar to those of progesterone; most p.'s are steroids like the natural hormones. **2.** A synthetic derivative from testosterone or progesterone that has some of the physiologic activity and pharmacologic effects of progesterone; progesterone is antiestrogenic, whereas some p.'s have estrogenic or androgenic properties in addition to progestational activity. [pro- + gestation + G. *-gen,* producing]

pro·glos·sis (prō-glos'is). The anterior portion, or tip, of the tongue. [pro- + G. *glōssa,* tongue]

pro·glot·tid (prō-glot'id). One of the segments of a tapeworm, containing the reproductive organs. SYN proglottis. [pro- + G. *glōssa,* tongue]

pro·glot·tis, pl. **pro·glot·ti·des** (prō-glot'is, -i-dēz). SYN proglottid.

prog·nath·ic (prog-nath'ik, -nā'thik). **1.** Having a projecting jaw; having a gnathic index above 103. **2.** Denoting a forward projection of either or both of the jaws relative to the craniofacial skeleton. SYN prognathous. [pro- + G. *gnathos,* jaw]

prog·na·thism (prog'nă-thizm). The condition of being prognathic; abnormal forward projection of one or of both jaws beyond the established normal relationship with the cranial base; the mandibular condyles are in their normal rest relationship to the temporomandibular joints. SYN progenia.

prog·na·thous (prog'nă-thŭs). SYN prognathic.

prog·no·sis (prog-nō'sis). A forecast of the probable course and/or outcome of a disease. [G. *prognōsis,* fr. *pro,* before, + *gignōskō,* to know]

prog·nos·tic (prog-nos'tik). **1.** Relating to prognosis. **2.** A symptom upon which a prognosis is based, or one indicative of the likely outcome. [G. *prognōstikos*]

prog·nos·ti·cate (prog-nos'ti-kāt). To give a prognosis.

prog·nos·ti·cian (prog-nos-tish'ŭn). One skilled in prognosis.

pro·gram. **1.** A formal set of procedures for conducting an activity. **2.** An ordered list of instructions directing a computer to carry out a desired sequence of operations required to solve a problem.

individualized education program (IEP), an education program tailored to a particular individual with a disability, whose provision is mandated by law. SEE ALSO Individuals with Disabilities Education Act.

pro·gran·u·lo·cyte (prō-gran'yū-lō-sīt). SYN promyelocyte.

pro·gress·ive (prō-gres'iv). Going forward; advancing; denoting the course of a disease, especially, when unqualified, an unfavorable course.

pro·hor·mone (prō-hōr'mōn). An intraglandular precursor of a hormone; *e.g.,* proinsulin. Cf. prehormone.

pro·in·su·lin (prō-in'sŭ-lin). A single-chain precursor of insulin.

pro·jec·tion (prō-jek'shŭn). **1.** A pushing out; an outgrowth or protuberance. **2.** The referring of a sensation to the object producing it. **3.** A defense mechanism by which a repressed complex in the individual is denied and conceived as belonging to another person, as when faults which the person tends to commit are perceived in or attributed to others. **4.** The conception by the consciousness of a mental occurrence belonging to the self as of external origin. **5.** Localization of visual impressions in space. **6.** NEUROANATOMY The system or systems of nerve fibers by which a group of nerve cells discharges its nerve impulses ("projects") to one or more other cell groups. **7.**

The image of a three-dimensional object on a plane, as in a radiograph. **8.** RADIOGRAPHY Standardized views of parts of the body, described by body part position, the direction of the x-ray beam through the body part, or by eponym. [L. *projectio;* fr. *pro- jicio,* pp. *-jectus,* to throw before]

anteroposterior p., SYN AP p.

AP p., the alternative frontal radiographic p., used mainly in bedside or portable radiography. SYN anteroposterior p.

cross-table lateral p., lateral p. radiography of a supine subject using a horizontal x-ray beam.

decubitus p., RADIOLOGY Procedure in which a patient to be x-rayed is placed in a decubitus position, with the x-ray beam directed horizontally.

occipitomental p., SYN Waters' p.

PA p., the standard frontal chest film p.; radiographic skull p. with the petrous ridge superimposed on the orbits.

Rhese p., oblique radiographic view of the skull to show the optic foramen.

Waters' p., a PA radiographic view of the skull made with the orbitomeatal line at an angle of 37° from the plane of the film, to show the orbits and maxillary sinuses. SYN occipitomental p.

pro·kar·y·ote (prō-kar'ē-ōt). A member of the superkingdom Prokaryotae; an organism consisting of a single cell, or a precellular organism, which lacks a nuclear membrane, paired organized chromosomes, a mitotic mechanism for cell division, microtubules, and mitochondria. SEE ALSO eukaryote. SYN procaryote.

pro·kar·y·ot·ic (prō'kar-ē-ot'ik). Pertaining to or characteristic of a prokaryote. SYN procaryotic.

pro·la·bi·um (prō-lā'bē-ŭm). **1.** The exposed carmine margin of the lip. **2.** The isolated central soft-tissue segment of the upper lip in the embryonic state and in an unrepaired complete cleft palate. [pro- + L. *labium,* lip]

pro·lac·tin (prō-lak'tin). A protein hormone of the anterior lobe of the hypophysis that stimulates the secretion of milk and possibly, during pregnancy, breast growth. SYN lactogenic hormone. [pro- + L. *lac, lact-,* milk, + -in]

pro·lac·ti·no·ma (prō-lak-ti-nō'mă). SYN prolactin-producing adenoma.

pro·lac·to·lib·er·in (prō-lak-tō-lib'er-in). A substance of hypothalamic origin that stimulates the release of prolactin. SYN prolactin-releasing factor, prolactin-releasing hormone. [prolactin + L. *libero,* to free, + -in]

pro·lac·to·stat·in (prō-lak-tō-stat'in). A substance of hypothalamic origin capable of inhibiting the synthesis and release of prolactin. SYN prolactin-inhibiting factor, prolactin-inhibiting hormone. [prolactin + G. *stasis,* standing still, + -in]

pro·lapse (prō-laps'). **1** (prō-laps'). To sink down, said of an organ or other part. **2** (prō'laps). A sinking of an organ or other part, especially its appearance at a natural or artificial orifice. SEE ALSO procidentia, ptosis. [L. *prolapsus,* a falling]

first degree p., form of cervical p. where the cervix of the prolapsed uterus is well within the vaginal orifice.

mitral valve p., excessive retrograde movement of one or both mitral valve leaflets into the left atrium during left ventricular systole, often allowing mitral regurgitation; responsible for the click-murmur of Barlow syndrome, and rarely may be due to rheumatic carditis, a connective tissue disorder such as Marfan's syndrome or ruptured chorda tendinea ("flail mitral leaflet").

second degree p., form of cervical p. where the cervix is at or near the introitus.

third degree p., form of cervical p. (procidentia uteri) where the cervix protrudes well beyond the vaginal orifice.

p. of umbilical cord, presentation of part of the umbilical cord ahead of the fetus; it may cause fetal death due to compression of the cord between the presenting part of the fetus and the maternal pelvis.

p. of the uterus, downward movement of the uterus due to laxity and atony of the muscular and fascial structures of the pelvic floor, usually resulting from injuries of childbirth or advanced age.; p. occurs in three forms. SEE **first degree p.**, **second degree p.**, **third degree p.**.

pro·lec·tive (prō′lek-tiv). Pertaining to data collected by planning in advance proportional mortality ratio. Number of deaths from a given cause in a specified period, per 100 or per 1000 total deaths. [pro- + L. *lego*, pp. *lectum*, to gather]

pro·lep·sis (prō-lep′sis). Recurrence of the paroxysm of a periodical disease at regularly shortening intervals. [G. *prolēpsis*, anticipation]

pro·lep·tic (prō-lep′tik). Relating to prolepsis.

pro·li·dase (prō′li-dās). SYN *proline* dipeptidase.

pro·lif·er·ate (prō-lif′ĕ-rāt). To grow and increase in number by means of reproduction of similar forms. [L. *proles*, offspring, + *fero*, to bear]

pro·lif·er·a·tion (prō-lif-ĕ-rā′shŭn). Growth and reproduction of similar cells.

pro·lif·er·a·tive, pro·lif·er·ous (prō-lif′er-ă-tiv, -er-ŭs). Increasing the numbers of similar forms.

pro·lig·er·ous (prō-lij′er-ŭs). Germinating; producing offspring. [L. *proles*, offspring, + *gero*, to bear]

pro·li·nase (prō′li-nās). SYN *prolyl* dipeptidase.

pro·line (Pro) (prō′lēn). An amino acid found in proteins, especially the collagens.

p. dipeptidase, an enzyme cleaving aminoacyl-L-proline bonds in dipeptides containing a C-terminal prolyl residue; a deficiency of this enzyme results in hyperimidodipeptiduria. SYN prolidase.

p. iminopeptidase [EC 3.4.11.5], a hydrolase cleaving L-proline residues from the N-terminal position in peptides.

pro·lyl (prō′lil). The acyl radical of proline.

p. dipeptidase, an enzyme cleaving L-prolyl-amino acid bonds in dipeptides containing N-terminal prolyl residues. SYN prolinase.

pro·mas·ti·gote (prō-mas′ti-gōt). The flagellate stage of a trypanosomatid protozoan in which the flagellum arises from a kinetoplast in front of the nucleus and emerges from the anterior end of the organism; usually an extracellular phase, as in the insect intermediate host (or in culture) of *Leishmania* parasites. [pro- + G. *mastix*, whip]

pro·meg·a·lo·blast (prō-meg′ă-lō-blast). The

earliest of four maturation stages of the megaloblast. SEE erythroblast.

pro·met·a·phase (prō-met′ă-fāz). The stage of mitosis or meiosis in which the nuclear membrane disintegrates and the centrioles reach the poles of the cell, while the chromosomes continue to contract.

pro·me·thi·um (Pm) (prō-mē′thē-ŭm). A radioactive element of the rare earth series, atomic no. 61; [145]Pm has the longest known half-life (17.7 years). [*Prometheus*, a Titan of G. myth who stole fire to give to mortals]

prom·i·nence (prom′i-nens). ANATOMY Tissues or parts that project beyond a surface. [L. *prominentia*]

laryngeal p., the projection on the anterior portion of the neck formed by the thyroid cartilage of the larynx; serves as an external indication of the level of the fifth cervical vertebra. SYN Adam's apple.

pro·mon·o·cyte (prō-mon′ō-sīt). SYN premonocyte.

prom·on·to·ry (prom′on-tō-rē). An eminence or projection. A projection of a part. [L. *promontorium*]

pro·mot·er (prō-mō′ter). **1.** CHEMISTRY A substance that increases the activity of a catalyst. **2.** MOLECULAR BIOLOGY A DNA sequence at which RNA polymerase binds and initiates transcription.

pro·mo·tion (prō-mō′shŭn). Stimulation of tumor induction, following initiation, by a promoting agent which may of itself be noncarcinogenic.

pro·my·e·lo·cyte (prō-mī′ĕ-lō-sīt). **1.** The developmental stage of a granular leukocyte between the myeloblast and myelocyte, when a few specific granules appear in addition to azurophilic ones. **2.** A large uninuclear cell occurring in the circulating blood of persons with myelocytic leukemia. SYN premyelocyte, progranulocyte. [pro- + G. *myelos*, marrow, + *kytos*, cell]

pro·na·si·on (prō-nā′zē-on). The point of the angle between the septum of the nose and the surface of the upper lip, found at the point where a tangent applied to the nasal septum meets the upper lip. [pro- + L. *nasus*, nose]

pro·nate (prō′nāt). **1.** To assume, or to be placed in, a prone position. **2.** To perform pronation of the forearm or foot. [L. *pronatus*, fr. *prono*, pp. *-atus*, to bend forward, fr. *pronus*, bent forward]

pro·na·tion (prō-nā′shŭn). The condition of being prone; the act of assuming or of being placed in a prone position.

rearfoot p., SYN hindfoot *valgus*.

pro·na·tor (prō-nā′ter, tōr). A muscle which turns a part into the prone position. SEE muscle. [L.]

prone (prōn). Denoting: **1.** Denoting the position of the body when lying face downward. **2.** The position of hand or foot with volar surface downward. [L. *pronus*, bending down or forward]

pro·neph·ros, pl. **pro·neph·roi** (prō-nef′ros, -roy). **1.** The definitive excretory organ of primitive fishes. **2.** In the embryos of higher vertebrates, a vestigial structure consisting of a series of tortuous tubules emptying into the cloaca by way of the primary nephric duct; in the human embryo, the p. is a very rudimentary and temporary structure, followed by the mesonephros and still later by the metanephros. [pro- + G. *nephros,* kidney]

pro•nor•mo•blast (prō-nōr′mō-blast). The earliest of four stages in development of the normoblast. SEE ALSO erythroblast. SYN proerythroblast, rubriblast.

pro•nu•cle•us, pl. **pro•nu•clei** (prō-nū′klē-ŭs, -klē-ī). **1.** One of a pair of nuclei undergoing fusion in karyogamy. **2.** EMBRYOLOGY The nuclear material of the head of the spermatozoon (**male p.**) or of the ovum (**female p.**), after the ovum has been penetrated by the spermatozoon; each p. normally carries a haploid set of chromosomes, so that the merging of the pronuclei in fertilization reestablishes the diploidy.

pro•opi•o•mel•a•no•cor•tin (POMC) (prō-ō′pē-ō-mel′ă-nō-kōr′tin). A large molecule found in the anterior and intermediate lobes of the pituitary gland, the hypothalamus, and other parts of the brain as well as in the lungs, gastrointestinal tract, and placenta; the precursor of ACTH, CLIP, β-LPH, γ-MSH, β-endorphin, and met-enkephalin.

pro•o•tic (prō-ō′tik). In front of the ear. [pro- + G. *ous,* ear]

prop•a•gate (prop′ă-gāt). **1.** To reproduce; to generate. **2.** To move along a fiber, *e.g.,* propagation of the nerve impulse. [L. *propago,* pp. -*atus,* to generate, reproduce]

prop•a•ga•tion (prop-ă-gā′shŭn). The act of propagating.

prop•a•ga•tive (prop-ă-gā′tiv). Relating to or concerned in propagation; denoting the sexual part of an animal or plant as distinguished from the soma.

pro•pane (prō′pān). $CH_3CH_2CH_3$; one of the alkane series of hydrocarbons.

pro•pep•sin (prō-pep′sin). SYN pepsinogen.

pro•per•din (prō-per′din). A group of proteins involved in resistance to infection that participate, in conjunction with other factors, in an alternate pathway to the activation of the terminal components of complement. SEE ALSO properdin *system, component* of complement. [pro- + L. *perdo,* to destroy]

pro•phage (prō′fāj). SYN probacteriophage.

pro•phase (prō′fāz). The first stage of mitosis or meiosis, consisting of linear contraction and increase in thickness of the chromosomes (each composed of two chromatids) accompanied by migration of the two daughter centrioles and their asters toward the poles of the cell. [G. *prophasis,* from *prophainō,* to foreshadow]

pro•phy•lac•tic (prō-fi-lak′tik). **1.** Preventing disease; relating to prophylaxis. SYN preventive. **2.** An agent that acts to prevent a disease. [G. *prophylaktikos;* see prophylaxis]

pro•phy•lax•is, pl. **pro•phy•lax•es** (prō-fi-lak′sis, -sēz). Prevention of disease or of a process that can lead to disease. [Mod. L. fr. G. *prophylassō,* to guard before, take precaution]

pro•pi•o•nate (prō′pē-ō-nāt). A salt or ester of propionic acid.

Pro•pi•on•i•bac•te•ri•um (prō-pē-on-i-bak-tēr′ē-ŭm). A genus of nonmotile, nonsporeforming,

anaerobic to aerotolerant bacteria containing Gram-positive rods which are usually pleomorphic, diphtheroid, or club-shaped with one end rounded, the other tapered or pointed. The cells usually occur singly, in pairs, in V and Y configurations, short chains, or clumps. These organisms occur in dairy products, on human skin, and in the intestinal tracts of humans and other animals. They may be pathogenic. The type species is *P. freudenreichii.*

pro•pi•on•ic ac•id (prō-pē-on′ik). methylacetic acid; ethylformic acid; found in sweat.

pro•pos•i•tus, pl. **pro•po•si•ti** (prō′poz′i-tŭs, -tī). **1.** Proband distinguished by sex. **2.** A premise; an argument. [L. fr. *propono,* pp. -*positus,* to lay out, propound]

pro•pri•e•tary name (prō-prī′ĕ-tār-ē). The protected brand name or trademark, registered with the U.S. Patent Office, under which a manufacturer markets a product. It is written with a capital initial letter and is often further distinguished by a superscript R in a circle (®). Cf. generic name, nonproprietary name. [L. *proprietarius*]

pro•pri•o•cep•tion (prō-prē-ō-sep′shun). A sense or perception, usually at a subconscious level, of the movements and position of the body and especially its limbs, independent of vision; this sense is gained primarily from input from sensory nerve terminals in muscles and tendons (muscle spindles) and the fibrous capsule of joints combined with input from the vestibular apparatus. SEE ALSO exteroceptor.

pro•pri•o•cep•tive (prō′prē-ō-sep′tiv). Capable of receiving stimuli originating in muscles, tendons, and other internal tissues. [L. *proprius,* one's own, + *capio,* to take]

pro•pri•o•cep•tor (prō′prē-ō-sep′ter). One of a variety of sensory end organs (such as the muscle spindle and Golgi's tendon organ) in muscles, tendons, and joint capsules.

prop•to•sis (prop-tō′sis). SYN exophthalmos. [G. *proptōsis,* a falling forward]

prop•tot•ic (prop-tot′ik). Referring to proptosis.

pro•pul•sion (prō-pŭl′shŭn). The tendency to fall forward; responsible for the festination in paralysis agitans. [G. *pro-pello,* pp. -*pulsus,* to drive forth]

pro•pyl (Pr) (prō′pil). The alkyl radical of propane, $CH_3CH_2CH_2-$.

  p. alcohol, ethylcarbinol; a solvent for resins and cellulose esters.

pro•py•lene (prō′pi-lēn). Methylethylene; a gaseous olefinic hydrocarbon.

pro rat. aet. Abbreviation for L. *pro ratione aetatis,* according to (patient's) age.

pro re na•ta (prō rē nā′tä). As the occasion arises; as necessary. [L.]

pro•ren•nin (prō-ren′in). SYN prochymosin.

pro•ru•bri•cyte (prō-rū′bri-sīt). Basophilic normoblast. SEE erythroblast. [pro- + rubricyte]

pro•se•cre•tin (prō-sē-krē′tin). Unactivated secretin.

pro•sect (prō-sekt′). To dissect a cadaver or any part, that it may serve for a demonstration of anatomy before a class. [L. *pro-seco,* pp. -*sectus,* to cut]

pro•sec•tor (prō′sek′ter). One who prosects, or

prepares the material for a demonstration of anatomy before a class.

pros·en·ceph·a·lon (pros-en-sef′ă-lon) [NA]. The anterior primitive cerebral vesicle and the most rostral of the three primary brain vesicles of the embryonic neural tube; it subdivides to form the diencephalon and telencephalon. SYN forebrain. [G. *prosō*, forward, + *enkephalos*, brain]

pros·o·dem·ic (pros-ō-dem′ik). Denoting a disease that is transmitted directly from person to person. [G. *prosō*, forward, + *dēmos*, people]

△**prosop-.** SEE prosopo-.

pros·o·pag·no·sia (pros′ō-pag-nō′sē-ă). Difficulty in recognizing familiar faces. [prosop- + G. *a-* priv. + *gnōsis*, recognition]

pros·o·pal·gia (pros-ō-pal′jē-ă). SYN trigeminal *neuralgia*. [prosop- + G. *algos*, pain]

pros·o·pal·gic (pros-ō-pal′jik). Relating to or suffering from trigeminal neuralgia.

pros·o·pla·sia (pros-ō-plā′zē-ă). Progressive transformation, such as the change of cells of the salivary ducts into secreting cells. SEE cytomorphosis. [G. *prosō*, forward, + *plasis*, a molding]

△**prosopo-, prosop-.** The face. SEE ALSO facio-. [G. *prosōpon*]

pros·o·po·di·ple·gia (pros′ō-pō-dī-plē′jē-ă). Paralysis affecting both sides of the face. [prosopo- + diplegia]

pros·o·po·neu·ral·gia (pros′ō-pō-nū-ral′jē-ă). SYN trigeminal *neuralgia*.

pros·o·po·ple·gia (pros′ō-pō-plē′jē-ă). SYN facial *paralysis*. [prosopo- + G. *plēgē*, stroke]

pros·o·po·ple·gic (pros′ō-pō-plē′jik). Relating to, or suffering from, facial paralysis.

pros·o·pos·chi·sis (pros-ō-pos′ki-sis). Congenital facial cleft from mouth to the inner canthus of the eye. [prosopo- + G. *schisis*, fissure]

pros·o·po·spasm (pros-ō-pō-spazm). SYN facial *tic*. [prosopo- + G. *spasmos*, spasm]

pros·ta·no·ic ac·id (pros′tă-nō-ik). The 20-carbon acid that is the skeleton of the prostaglandins.

△**prostat-.** SEE prostato-.

pros·ta·ta (pros′tah-tă) [NA]. SYN prostate. [Mod. L. from G. *prostatēs*, one standing before]

pros·ta·tal·gia (pros-tă-tal′jē-ă). A rarely used term for pain in the area of the prostate gland. [prostat- + G. *algos*, pain]

pros·tate (pros′tāt). A chestnut-shaped body, surrounding the beginning of the urethra in the male, that consists of two lateral lobes connected anteriorly by an isthmus and posteriorly by a middle lobe lying above and between the ejaculatory ducts. In structure, the prostate consists of 30 to 50 compound tubuloalveolar glands between which is abundant stroma consisting of collagen and elastic fibers and many smooth muscle bundles. The secretion of the glands is a milky fluid that is discharged by excretory ducts into the prostatic urethra at the time of the emission of semen. SYN prostata [NA], prostate gland.

pros·ta·tec·to·my (pros-tă-tek′tō-mē). Removal of a part or all of the prostate. [prostat- + G. *ektomē*, excision]

pros·tat·ic (pros-tat′ik). Relating to the prostate.

pros·ta·tism (pros′tă-tizm). A syndrome, occurring mostly in older men, usually caused by en-largement of the prostate gland and manifested by irritative (nocturia, frequency, decreased voided volume, sensory urgency, and urgency incontinence) and obstructive (hesitancy, decreased stream, terminal dribbling, double voiding, and urinary retention) symptoms.

pros·ta·ti·tis (pros-tă-tī′tis). Inflammation of the prostate. [prostat- + G. *-itis*, inflammation]

△**prostato-, prostat-.** The prostate gland. [Med. L. *prostata* fr. G. *prostatēs*, one who stands before, protects]

pros·ta·to·cys·ti·tis (pros′tă-tō-sis-tī′tis). Inflammation of the prostate and the bladder; cystitis by extension of inflammation from the prostatic urethra. [prostato- + G. *kystis*, bladder, + *-itis*, inflammation]

pros·ta·to·li·thot·o·my (pros′tă-tō-li-thot′ō-mē, pros-tat′ō-). Incision of the prostate for removal of a calculus. [prostato- + G. *lithos*, stone, + *tomē*, incision]

pros·ta·to·meg·a·ly (pros′tă-tō-meg′ă-lē). Enlargement of the prostate gland. [prostato- + G. *megas*, large]

pros·ta·tor·rhea (pros′tă-tō-rē′ă). An abnormal discharge of prostatic fluid. [prostato- + G. *rhoia*, a flow]

pros·ta·tot·o·my (pros′tă-tot′ō-mē). An incision into the prostate. [prostato- + G. *tomē*, incision]

pros·ta·to·ve·sic·u·lec·to·my (pros′tă-tō-ve-sik′yū-lek′tō-mē). Surgical removal of the prostate gland and seminal vesicles.

pros·ta·to·ve·sic·u·li·tis (pros′tă-tō-ve-sik′yū-lī′tis). Inflammation of the prostate gland and seminal vesicles.

pros·the·sis, pl. **pros·the·ses** (pros′thē-sis, -sēz; pros-thē′sis). Fabricated substitute for a diseased or missing part of the body. [G. an addition]

  surgical p., an appliance prepared as an aid or as a part of a surgical proceeding, such as a heart valve or cranial plate.

pros·thet·ic (pros-thet′ik). **1.** Relating to a prosthesis or to an artificial part. **2.** SEE prosthetic *group*.

pros·thet·ics (pros-thet′iks). The art and science of making and adjusting artificial parts of the human body.

pros·the·tist (pros′the-tist). One skilled in constructing and fitting prostheses.

pros·thi·on (pros′thē-on). The most anterior point on the maxillary alveolar process in the midline. SYN alveolar point. [G. ntr. of *prosthios*, foremost]

pros·tho·don·tics (pros-thō-don′tiks). The science of and art of providing suitable substitutes for the coronal portions of teeth, or for one or more lost or missing teeth and their associated parts, in order that impaired function, appearance, comfort, and health of the patient may be restored. [L. *prosthodontia*, fr. G. *prosthesis* + *odous* (*odont-*), tooth]

pros·tho·don·tist (pros-thō-don′tist). A dentist engaged in the practice of prosthodontics.

pros·tra·tion (pros-trā′shŭn). A marked loss of strength, as in exhaustion. [L. *pro-sterno*, pp. *-stratus*, to strew before, overthrow]

△**prot-.** SEE proteo-, proto-.

prot·ac·tin·i·um (Pa) (prō-tak-tin′ē-ŭm). A radioactive element, atomic no. 91, atomic wt. 231.03588, formed in the decay of uranium and thorium; its longest-lived isotope, ^{231}Pa, has a half-life of 32,500 years. [G. *prōtos*, first]

prot•a•mine (prō′tă-mēn, -min). Any of a class of proteins found in fish spermatozoa in combination with nucleic acid; neutralizes anticoagulant action of heparin.

pro•ta•no•pia (prō′tă-nō′pē-ă). A form of dichromatism characterized by absence of the red-sensitive pigment in cones, decreased luminosity for long wavelengths of light, and confusion in recognition of red and green. [G. *prōtos,* first, + *a-*priv. + *ōps* (*ōp-*) eye]

pro•te•an (prō′tē-an). Changeable in form; having the power to change body form, like the ameba. [G. *Prōteus,* a god having the power to change his form]

pro•te•ase (prō′tē-ās). Descriptive term for proteolytic enzymes, both endopeptidases and exopeptidases.

pro•tein (prō′tēn, prō′tē-in). Macromolecules consisting of long sequences of α-amino acids [$H_2N–CHR–COOH$] in peptide (amide) linkage (elimination of H_2O between the α-NH_2 and α-COOH of successive residues). P. is three-fourths of the dry weight of most cell matter and is involved in structures, hormones, enzymes, muscle contraction, immunological response, and essential life functions. The amino acids involved are generally the 20 α-amino acids (glycine, L-alanine, etc.) recognized by the genetic code. Crosslinks yielding globular forms of p. are often effected through the –SH groups of two sulfur-containing L-cysteinyl residues, as well as by noncovalent forces (hydrogen bonds, lipophilic attractions, etc.). [G. *prōtos,* first, + -in]

acyl carrier p. (ACP), one of the p.'s of the complex in cytoplasm that contains all of the enzymes required to convert acetyl-CoA (and, in certain cases, butyryl-CoA or propionyl-CoA) and malonyl-CoA to palmitic acid. This complex is tightly bound together in mammalian tissues and in yeast, but that from *Escherichia coli* is readily dissociated. The ACP thus isolated is a heat-stable p. with a molecular weight of about 10,000. It contains a free –SH that binds the acyl intermediates in the synthesis of fatty acids as thioesters. This –SH group is part of a 4′-phosphopantetheine, added to the apoprotein by ACP phosphodiesterase, which thus plays the same role that it does in coenzyme A. ACP is involved in every step of the fatty acid synthetic process.

androgen binding p. (ABP), a p. secreted by testicular Sertoli cells along with inhibin and müllerian inhibiting substance. Androgen binding p. probably maintains a high concentration of androgen in the seminiferous tubules.

antiviral p. (AVP), a human or animal factor, induced by interferon in virus-infected cells, which mediates interferon inhibition of virus replication.

cAMP receptor p. (CRP), SYN catabolite (gene) activator p.

catabolite (gene) activator p. (CAP), a p. that can be activated by cAMP, whereupon it affects the action of RNA polymerase by binding it with it or near it on the DNA to be transcribed. SYN cAMP receptor p.

conjugated p., p. attached to some other molecule or molecules (not amino acid in nature) otherwise than as a salt. SEE ALSO prosthetic *group.* Cf. simple p.

C-reactive p. (CRP), a β-globulin found in the serum of various persons with certain inflammatory, degenerative, and neoplastic diseases; although the p. is not a specific antibody, it precipitates *in vitro* the C polysaccharide present in all types of pneumococci.

p. induced by vitamin K absence (PIVKA), nonfunctional p. precursors of the prothrombin group of coagulation factors (Factors II, VII, IX, X). They are synthesized in the liver in the absence of vitamin K and lack the carboxyl (COOH⁻) group needed to bind the factor to a phospholipid surface.

nonspecific p., a p. substance that elicits a response not mediated by specific antigen-antibody reaction.

plasma p.'s, dissolved p.'s (more than 100) of blood plasma, mainly albumins and globulins (normally 6 to 8 g/100 ml); they hold fluid in blood vessels by osmosis and include antibodies and blood-clotting p.'s.

prion p., small, infectious proteinaceous particle, of non-nucleic acid composition; the causative agent of four spongiform encephalopathies in humans: kuru, Creutzfeldt-Jakob disease, Gerstmann-Straussler-Scheinker syndrome, and fatal familial insomnia. The gene encoding for the PrP is found on chromosome 20. SYN prion.

receptor p., an intracellular p. (or p. fraction) that has an affinity for a known stimulus to cellular activity, such as a steroid hormone or adenosine 3′,5′-cyclic phosphate.

p. S, a vitamin K-dependent antithrombotic p. that functions as a cofactor with activated p. C.

simple p., p. that yields only α-amino acids or their derivatives by hydrolysis; *e.g.,* albumins, globulins, glutelins, prolamines, albuminoids, histones, protamines. Cf. conjugated p.

pro•tein•a•ceous (prō′tē-nā′shŭs, prō′tē-i-nā′shŭs). Resembling a protein; possessing, to some degree, the physicochemical properties characteristic of proteins.

pro•tein•o•sis (pro-tē-nō′sis, prō′tē-i-nō′sis). A state characterized by disordered protein formation and distribution, particularly as manifested by the deposition of abnormal proteins in tissues. [protein + G. *-osis,* condition]

pulmonary alveolar p., a chronic progressive lung disease of adults, characterized by alveolar accumulation of granular proteinaceous material that is PAS-positive and lipid rich, with little inflammatory cellular exudate; the cause is unknown.

pro•tein•u•ria (prō-tē-nū′rē-ă, prō′tē-i-nū′rē-ă). **1.** Presence of urinary protein in concentrations greater than 0.3 g in a 24-hour urine collection or in concentrations greater than 1 g/l in a random urine collection on two or more occasions at least 6 hours apart; specimens must be clean-voided midstream or obtained by catheterization. **2.** SYN albuminuria. [protein + G. *ouron,* urine]

Bence Jones p., presence of Bence Jones protein in the urine, indicative of multiple myeloma, amyloidosis, or Waldenström's macroglobulinemia.

gestational p., the presence of p. during or under the influence of pregnancy in the absence of hypertension, edema, renal infection, or known intrinsic renovascular disease.

isolated p., p. in a patient who is asymptomatic, has normal renal function and urinary sediment, and has no manifestation of systemic disease upon initial examination.

nonisolated p., p. associated with other abnormalities.

△**proteo-, prot-.** Protein.

pro·te·o·gly·cans (prō′tē-ō-glī′kanz). Glycoaminoglycans (mucopolysaccharides) bound to protein chains in covalent complexes; occur in the extracellular matrix of connective tissue.

pro·te·o·lip·ids (prō′tē-ō-lip′idz). A class of lipid-soluble proteins found in brain tissue, insoluble in water but soluble in chloroform-methanol-water mixtures.

pro·te·ol·y·sis (prō-tē-ol′i-sis). The decomposition of protein; primarily via the hydrolysis of peptide bonds, both enzymatically and nonenzymatically. [proteo- + G. *lysis,* dissolution]

pro·te·o·lyt·ic (prō′tē-ō-lit′ik). Relating to or effecting proteolysis.

pro·te·o·met·a·bol·ic (prō′tē-ō-met′ă-bol′ik). Relating to the metabolism of proteins.

pro·te·ose (prō′tē-ōs). A nondescript mixture of intermediate products of proteolysis between protein and peptone.

Pro·teus (prō′tē-ŭs). A genus of motile, peritrichous, nonsporeforming, aerobic to facultatively anaerobic bacteria containing Gram-negative rods. Coccoid forms, filaments, and spheroplasts occur under certain conditions. The metabolism is fermentative, producing acid. *P.* occurs primarily in fecal matter and in putrefying materials. [G. *Prōteus,* a sea god, who had the power to change his form]

P. morgan′ii, a species found in the intestinal canal and in normal and diarrheal stools.

P. vulgar′is, the type species of the genus *P.,* found in putrefying materials and in abscesses; certain strains are agglutinated by the serum of persons with typhus and other rickettsial diseases (Weil-Felix reaction). SEE ALSO Weil-Felix *reaction.*

pro·throm·bin (prō-throm′bin). A glycoprotein formed and stored in the parenchymal cells of the liver and present in blood in a concentration of approximately 20 mg/100 ml. In the presence of thromboplastin and calcium ion, p. is converted to thrombin, which in turn converts fibrinogen to fibrin, this process resulting in coagulation of blood; a deficiency of p. leads to impaired blood coagulation.

pro·throm·bin·ase (prō-throm′bi-nās). SYN *factor* X.

pro·tist (prō′tist). A member of the kingdom Protista.

Pro·tis·ta (prō-tis′ta). A kingdom of both plant-like and animal-like eucaryotic unicellular organisms, either in the form of solitary organisms,

e.g., protozoa, or colonies of cells lacking true tissues. [G. ntr. pl. of *prōtistos,* the first of all]

△**proto-, prot-.** The first in a series; the highest in rank (properly prefixed to words derived from G. roots). [G. *prōtos,* first]

pro·to·col (prō′tō-kol). **1.** A precise and detailed plan for the study of a biomedical problem or for a regimen of therapy, especially cancer chemotherapy. **2.** A record of findings in an experiment or investigation, especially an autopsy.

Pro·toc·tis·ta (prō-tok-tis′tă). A kingdom of eukaryotes incorporating the algae and the protozoans that comprise the presumed ancestral stocks of the fungi, plant, and animal kingdoms; they lack the developmental pattern stemming from a blastula, typical of animals, the pattern of embryo development typical of plants, and development from spores as in the fungi. Included are the nucleated algae and seaweeds, the flagellated water molds, slime molds and slime nets, and the protozoa; unicellular, colonial, and multicellular organisms are included, but the complex development of tissues and organs of plants and animals is absent. [G. *prōtos,* the first, + *ktizō,* to create]

pro·to·di·a·stol·ic (prō′tō-dī-ă-stol′ik). Early diastolic, relating to the beginning of cardiac diastole.

pro·to·du·o·de·num (prō′tō-dū-ō-dē′nŭm, -dū-od′ĕ-nŭm). The first part of the duodenum which extends from the gastroduodenal pylorus as far as the major duodenal papilla and develops from the caudal foregut of the embryo; it has no plicae circulares and is the seat of the duodenal glands.

pro·ton (prō′ton). The positively charged unit of the nuclear mass; p.'s form part (or in hydrogen-1 the whole) of the nucleus of the atom around which the negative electrons revolve. [G. ntr. of *prōtos,* first]

pro·to-on·co·gene (prō-tō-on′kō-jēn). A gene present in the normal human genome, that appears to have a role in normal cellular physiology and is often involved in regulation of normal cell growth or proliferation; as a result of somatic mutations these genes may become oncogenic. SEE ALSO oncogene.

pro·to·path·ic (prō-tō-path′ik). Denoting a supposedly primitive set or system of peripheral sensory nerve fibers conducting a low order of pain and temperature sensibility which is poorly localized. Cf. epicritic. [proto- + G. *pathos,* suffering]

pro·to·plasm (prō′tō-plazm). **1.** Living matter, the substance of which animal and vegetable cells are formed. SEE ALSO cytoplasm, nucleoplasm. **2.** The total cell material, including cell organelles. Cf. cytoplasm, cytosol, hyaloplasm. [proto- + G. *plasma,* thing formed]

pro·to·plast (prō′tō-plast). A bacterial cell from which the rigid cell wall has been completely removed; the bacterium loses its characteristic form. [proto- + G. *plastos,* formed]

pro·to·por·phyr·ia (prō′tō-pōr-fir′ē-ă). Enhanced fecal excretion of protoporphyrin.

erythropoietic p. [MIM*177000], a benign disorder of porphyrin metabolism due to a deficiency of ferrochelatase and characterized by enhanced fecal excretion of protoporphyrin and increased protoporphyrin IX in red blood cells, plasma, and feces; solar urticaria or eczema develops on exposure to sunlight.

pro·to·troph (prō′tō-trof, -trōf). A bacterial strain that has the same nutritional requirements as the wild-type strain from which it was derived. [proto- + G. *trophē,* nourishment]

pro·to·type (prō′tō-tīp). The primitive form; the first form to which subsequent individuals of the class or species conform. [proto- + G. *typos,* type]

pro·to·ver·te·bra (prō′tō-ver′tĕ-bră). The caudal half of each sclerotomal concentration, which is the primordium of the centrum of a vertebra. SYN provertebra.

Pro·to·zoa (prō-tō-zō′ă). Formerly considered a phylum, now regarded as a subkingdom of the animal kingdom, including all of the so-called acellular or unicellular forms. They consist of a single functional cell unit or aggregation of nondifferentiated cells, loosely held together and not forming tissues. [proto- + G. *zōon,* animal]

pro·to·zo·al (prō-tō-zō′ăl). SYN protozoan (2).

pro·to·zo·an (prō-tō-zō′an). **1.** A member of the phylum Protozoa. SYN protozoon. **2.** Relating to protozoa. SYN protozoal.

pro·to·zo·i·a·sis (prō′tō-zō-ī′ă-sis). Infection with protozoans.

pro·to·zo·ol·o·gy (prō′tō-zō-ol′ō-jē). The science concerned with all aspects of the biology and human interest in protozoa. [protozoa + G. *logos,* study]

pro·to·zo·on, pl. **pro·to·zoa** (prō-tō-zō′on, -zō′ă). SYN protozoan (1).

pro·to·zo·o·phage (prō-tō-zō′ō-fāj). A phagocyte that ingests protozoa. [protozoa + G. *phagō,* to eat]

pro·trac·tion (prō-trak′shŭn). DENTISTRY The extension of teeth or other maxillary or mandibular structures into a position anterior to normal. [see protractor]

pro·trac·tor (prō-trak′ter, -tōr). A muscle drawing a part forward, as antagonistic to a retractor. [L. *pro-traho,* pp. *-tractus,* to draw forth]

pro·tru·sion (prō-trū′zhŭn). **1.** The state of being thrust forward or projected. **2.** DENTISTRY A position of the mandible forward from centric relation. [L. *protrusio*]

pro·tu·ber·ance (prō-tū′ber-ans). A swelling or knoblike outgrowth. A bulging, swelling, or protruding part. SYN protuberantia [NA]. [Mod. L. *protuberantia*]

pro·tu·be·ran·tia (prō-tū-ber-an′shē-ă) [NA]. SYN protuberance. SEE ALSO protuberance, prominence, eminence. [Mod. L. fr. *protubero,* to swell out, fr. *tuber,* a swelling]

pro·ver·te·bra (prō-ver′tĕ-bră). SYN protovertebra.

Pro·vi·den·cia (prov′i-den′sē-ă). A genus of motile, peritrichous, nonsporeforming, aerobic or facultatively anaerobic bacteria containing Gram-negative rods. These organisms occur particularly in urinary tract infections and in small outbreaks and sporadic cases of diarrheal disease.

P. alcalifa′ciens, a species found in extraintestinal sources, particularly in urinary tract infections; it has also been isolated from small out-

breaks and sporadic cases of diarrheal disease; it is the type species of the genus *P.*

P. rettger′i, species that is found in chicken cholera and human gastroenteritis.

P. stuar′tii, a species isolated from urinary tract infections and from small outbreaks and sporadic cases of diarrheal disease.

pro·vi·rus (prō-vī′rŭs). The precursor of an animal virus; theoretically analogous to the prophage in bacteria, the p. being integrated in the nucleus of infected cells.

△**prox-.** SEE proximo-.

△**proxi-.** SEE proximo-.

prox·i·mad (prok′si-mad). In a direction toward a proximal part, or toward the center; not distad. [L. *proximus,* nearest, next, + *ad,* to]

prox·i·mal (prok′si-măl). **1.** Nearest the trunk or the point of origin, said of part of a limb, of an artery or a nerve, etc., so situated. **2.** SYN mesial. **3.** DENTAL ANATOMY Denoting the surface of a tooth in relation with its neighbor, whether mesial or distal, *i.e.,* nearer to or farther from the antero-posterior median plane. [Mod. L. *proximalis,* fr. L. *proximus,* nearest, next]

prox·i·mate (prok′si-māt). Immediate; next; proximal.

△**proximo-, proxi-, prox-.** Proximal. [L. *proximus,* nearest, next (to)]

prox·i·mo·a·tax·ia (prok′si-mō-ă-tak′sē-ă). Ataxia or lack of muscular coordination in the proximal portions of the extremities, *i.e.,* arms and thighs. Cf. acroataxia. [proximo- + ataxia]

pro·zone (prō′zōn). A phenomenon in which visible agglutination and precipitation do not occur in mixtures of specific antigen and antibody because of antibody excess.

PRPP 5-phospho-α-D-ribosyl 1-pyrophosphate.

pru·rig·i·nous (prū-rij′i-nŭs). Relating to or suffering from prurigo. [L. *pruriginosus,* having the itch]

pru·ri·go (prū-rī′gō). A chronic disease of the skin marked by a persistent eruption of papules that itch intensely. [L. itch, fr. *prurio,* to itch]

p. mi′tis, a mild form of a chronic dermatitis characterized by recurring, intensely itching papules and nodules, probably atopic.

p. nodula′ris, an eruption of hard nodules (Picker's nodules) in the skin caused by rubbing and accompanied by intense itching.

p. sim′plex, a mild form of p. having a pronounced tendency to relapse.

pru·rit·ic (prū-rit′ik). Relating to pruritus.

pru·ri·tus (prū-rī′tŭs). **1.** SYN itching. **2.** SYN itch (1). [L. an itching, fr. *prurio,* to itch]

p. a′ni, itching at the anus; may be associated with seborrheic dermatitis, candidosis, or external hemorrhoids, or occur in systemic disease.

aquagenic p., intense itching produced by brief contact with water at any temperature without visible changes in the skin.

bath p., itching produced by inadequate rinsing off of soap or by overdrying of skin from excessive bathing. SYN bath itch.

essential p., itching that occurs independently of skin lesions.

p. seni′lis, senile p., itching associated with dryness of the skin in the aged.

symptomatic p., itching occurring as a symptom of some systemic disease.

p. vul′vae, itching of the external female genitalia, caused by seborrheic dermatitis, allergy to local contactants, senile atrophy of the vulva, or systemic disease.

Prus·sian blue [C.I. 77510]. SYN Berlin blue.

PSA prostate-specific *antigen.*

△**psammo-.** Sand. [G. *psammos*]

psam·mous (sam′ŭs). Sandy. [G. *psammos,* sand]

△**pseud-.** SEE pseudo-.

pseud·a·graph·ia (su-dă-graf′e-ă). Partial agraphia in which one can do no original writing, but can copy correctly. SYN pseudoagraphia. [pseud- + G. *a-* priv. + *graphō,* to write]

Pseud·al·les·che·ria boy·dii (sūd′al-es-kē′re-ă boy′dē-ī). A species of fungus that causes eumycotic mycetoma and pseudallescheriasis; its conidial (asexual) state is *Scedosporium apiospermum.*

pseud·al·les·che·ri·a·sis (sūd′al-es-kē′ri-ă-sis). A variety of clinical diseases resulting from infection with *Pseudallescheria boydii; e.g.,* pulmonary colonization, fungoma, and invasive pneumonitis, as well as mycotic keratitis, endophthalmitis, endocarditis, meningitis, sinusitis, brain abscesses, cutaneous and subcutaneous infections, and disseminated systemic infections.

pseud·an·ky·lo·sis (sū-dang′ki-lō′sis). SYN fibrous *ankylosis.*

pseud·ar·thro·sis (sū-dar-thrō′sis). A new, false joint arising at the site of an ununited fracture. SYN false joint, pseudoarthrosis. [pseud- + G. *arthrōsis,* a joint]

pseud·es·the·sia (sū-des-thē′zē-ă). 1. SYN paraphia. 2. A subjective sensation not arising from an external stimulus. 3. SYN phantom *limb.* [pseud- + G. *aisthēsis,* sensation]

△**pseudo- (psi), pseud-.** False (often used about a deceptive resemblance). [G. *pseudēs*]

pseu·do·a·graph·ia (sū′dō-ă-graf′e-ă). SYN pseudagraphia.

pseu·do·al·lel·ic (sū′dō-ă-le′lik). Relating to pseudoallelism.

pseu·do·al·lel·ism (sū-dō-ă-lē′lizm). Relationship of two or more loci that are difficult to distinguish from a single locus by classical genetic analysis.

pseu·do·a·ne·mia (sū′dō-ă-nē′mē-ă). Pallor of the skin and mucous membranes without the blood changes of anemia. SYN false anemia.

pseu·do·ar·thro·sis (sū′dō-ar-thrō′sis). SYN pseudarthrosis.

pseu·do·bul·bar (sū-dō-bŭl′bar). Denoting a supranuclear paralysis of the bulbar nerves.

pseu·do·car·ti·lage (sū-dō-kar′ti-lij). SYN chondroid *tissue* (1).

pseu·do·cast (sū′dō-kast). SYN false *cast.*

pseu·do·chan·cre (sū-dō-shang′ker). A nonspecific indurated sore, usually located on the penis, resembling a chancre.

pseu·do·cho·rea (sū-dō-kōr-e′ă). A spasmodic disorder or extensive tic resembling chorea.

pseu·do·chro·mes·the·sia (sū′dō-krō-mes-thē′zē-ă). 1. An anomaly in which each vowel in the printed word is seen as colored. SEE ALSO photism. 2. SYN color *hearing.* [pseudo- + G. *chrōma,* color, + *aisthēsis,* sensation]

pseu·do·co·arc·ta·tion (sū′dō-kō-ark-tā′shŭn). Distortion, often with slight narrowing, of the aortic arch at the level of insertion of the ligamentum arteriosum.

pseu·do·croup (sū-dō-krūp′). SYN *laryngismus stridulus.*

pseu·do·cryp·tor·chism (sū-dō-krip′tōr-kizm). A condition in which the testes descend to the scrotum but intermittently retreat into the inguinal canal. [pseudo- + G. *kryptos,* hidden, + *orchis,* testis]

pseu·do·cy·e·sis (sū′dō-sī-ē′sis). SYN false *pregnancy.* [pseudo- + G. *kyēsis,* pregnancy]

pseu·do·cyl·in·droid (sū-dō-sil′in-droyd). A shred of mucus or other substance in the urine resembling a renal cast.

pseu·do·cyst (sū′dō-sist). 1. An accumulation of fluid in a cystlike loculus, but without an epithelial or other membranous lining. SYN adventitious cyst. 2. A cyst whose wall is formed by a host cell and not by a parasite. 3. A mass of 50 or more *Toxoplasma* bradyzoites, found within a host cell, frequently in the brain; a true cyst enclosed in its own membrane within the host cell that may rupture to release particles that form new cysts. [pseudo- + G. *kystis,* bladder]

pseu·do·de·men·tia (sū′dō-dē-men′shē-ă). A condition resembling dementia but usually due to a depressive disorder rather than brain dysfunction.

pseu·do·diph·the·ria (sū′dō-dif-thēr′ē-ă). SYN diphtheroid (1).

pseu·do·e·de·ma (sū′dō-e-dē′mă). A puffiness of the skin not due to a fluid accumulation. [pseudo- + G. *oidēma,* a swelling (edema)]

pseu·do·fol·lic·u·li·tis (sū′dō-fo-lik-yū-lī′tis). Erythematous follicular papules or, less commonly, pustules resulting from close shaving of curly hair; tips of growing hairs reenter the skin producing ingrown hairs; p. of the beard area is very common in blacks.

pseu·do·frac·ture (sū-dō-frak′chūr). A condition in which a radiograph shows formation of new bone with thickening of periosteum at site of an injury to bone.

pseu·do·gan·gli·on (sū-dō-gang′glē-on). A localized thickening of a nerve trunk having the appearance of a ganglion.

pseu·do·geu·ses·the·sia (sū′dō-gyū-ses-thē′zē-ă). SYN color *taste.* [pseudo- + G. *geusis,* taste, + *aisthēsis,* sensation]

pseu·do·geu·sia (sū-dō-gyū′sē-ă). A subjective taste sensation not produced by an external stimulus. [pseudo- + G. *geusis,* taste]

pseu·do·gout (sū′dō-gowt). [MIM*118600]. Acute episodes of synovitis caused by deposits of calcium pyrophosphate crystals rather than urate crystals as in true gout; associated with articular chondrocalcinosis.

pseu·do·he·ma·tu·ria (sū′dō-hem-ă-tū′rē-ă -he-mă-). A red pigmentation of urine caused by certain foods or drugs, and thus not actually hematuria. SYN false hematuria.

pseu·do·her·maph·ro·dite (sū′dō-her-maf′rō-dīt). An individual exhibiting pseudohermaphroditism.

pseu·do·her·maph·ro·dit·ism (sū′dō-her-maf′rō-dī-tizm). A state in which the individual is of an unambiguous gonadal sex (*i.e.,* possesses either testes or ovaries) but has ambiguous external genitalia. SYN false hermaphroditism.

female p. [MIM*264270], p. with skeletal and genital anomalies but with female gonads and an XX karyotype. SYN androgyny (1).

pseu·do·hy·per·kal·e·mia (sū′dō-hī′per-kal-ē′ē-ă). A spurious elevation of the serum concentration of potassium occurring when potassium is released in vitro from cells in a blood sample collected for a potassium measurement. This may be a consequence of disease (*i.e.,* myeloproliferative disorders with marked leukocytosis or thrombocytosis) or as a result of improper collection technique with in vitro hemolysis. [pseudo- + G. *hyper*, above + L. *kalium*, potassium, G. *haima*, blood]

pseu·do·hy·per·par·a·thy·roid·ism (sū′dō-hī′per-par-ă-thī′roy-dizm). Hypercalcemia in a patient with a malignant neoplasm in the absence of skeletal metastases or primary hyperparathyroidism; believed to be due to formation of parathyroid-like hormone by nonparathyroid tumor tissue.

pseu·do·hy·per·tro·phic (sū′dō-hī-per-trof′ik). Relating to or marked by pseudohypertrophy.

pseu·do·hy·per·tro·phy (sū′dō-hī-per′trō-fē). Increase in size of an organ or a part, due not to increase in size or number of the specific functional elements but to that of some other tissue, fatty or fibrous.

pseu·do·hy·po·a·cu·sis (sū′dō-hī′pō-ă-kū′sis). Apparent loss of hearing without an organic disorder or with insufficient pathological evidence to explain the extent of the loss; usually due to conversion disorder or malingering.

pseu·do·hy·po·na·tre·mia (sū′dō-hī-pō-nă-trē′mē-ă). A low serum sodium concentration due to volume displacement by massive hyperlipidemia or hyperproteinemia; also used to describe the low serum sodium concentration which may occur with high blood glucose.

pseu·do·hy·po·par·a·thy·roid·ism (sū′dō-hī′pō-par-ă-thī′roid-izm) [MIM*103500]. A disorder resembling hypoparathyroidism, with high serum phosphate and low calcium levels, but with normal or elevated serum parathyroid hormone levels; due to lack of end-organ responsiveness to parathyroid hormone.

pseu·do·ic·ter·us (sū-dō-ik′ter-ŭs). Yellowish discoloration of the skin not due to bile pigments, as in Addison's disease. SYN pseudojaundice.

pseu·do·i·so·chro·mat·ic (sū′dō-ī-sō-krō-mat′ik). Apparently of the same color; denoting certain charts containing colored spots mixed with figures printed in confusion colors; used in testing for color vision deficiency.

pseu·do·jaun·dice (sū-dō-jawn′dis). SYN pseudoicterus.

pseu·do·lo·gia (sū-dō-lō′jē-ă). Pathological lying in speech or writing. [pseudo- + G. *logos*, word]

p. phantas′tica, a fantastic account of a patient's exploits, which the patient appears to believe.

pseu·do·ma·lig·nan·cy (sū′dō-mă-lig′nan-sē). A benign tumor that appears, clinically or histologically, to be a malignant neoplasm. SEE ALSO pseudotumor.

pseu·do·ma·nia (sū-dō-mā′nē-ă). **1.** A factitious mental disorder. **2.** A mental disorder in which the patient falsely claims to have committed a crime. **3.** Generally, the morbid impulse to falsify or lie, as in pseudologia.

pseu·do·mem·brane (sū-dō-mem′brān). SYN false *membrane.*

pseu·do·mem·bra·nous (sū-dō-mem′bră-nŭs). Relating to or marked by the presence of a false membrane.

pseu·do·mo·nad (sū-dō-mō′nad). A vernacular term used to refer to any member of the genus *Pseudomonas.*

Pseu·do·mo·nas (sū-dō-mō′nas). A genus of motile, polar-flagellate, non-spore-forming, strictly aerobic bacteria containing straight or curved Gram-negative rods. They occur commonly in soil and in fresh water and marine environments. Some species are involved in human infections. [pseudo- + G. *monas,* unit, mónad]

pseu·do·myx·o·ma (sū′dō-mik-sō′mă). A gelatinous mass resembling a myxoma but composed of epithelial mucus.

p. peritone′i, the accumulation of large quantities of mucoid or mucinous material in the peritoneal cavity, either as a result of rupture of a mucocele of the appendix, or rupture of benign or malignant cystic neoplasms of the ovary.

pseu·do·ne·o·plasm (sū-dō-nē′ō-plazm). SYN pseudotumor.

pseu·do·pap·il·le·de·ma (sū′dō-pap-il-e-dē′mă). Anomalous elevation of the optic disk; seen in severe hyperopia and optic nerve drusen.

pseu·do·pa·ral·y·sis (sū′dō-pă-ral′i-sis). Apparent paralysis due to voluntary inhibition of motion because of pain, to incoordination, or other cause, but without actual paralysis. SYN pseudoparesis (1).

arthritic general p., a disease, occurring in arthritic subjects, having symptoms resembling those of general paresis, the lesions of which consist of diffuse changes of a degenerative and noninflammatory character due to intracranial atheroma.

pseu·do·par·a·ple·gia (sū′dō-par-ă-plē′jē-ă). Apparent paralysis in the lower extremities, in which the tendon and skin reflexes and the electrical reactions are normal; the condition is sometimes observed in rickets.

pseu·do·pa·re·sis (sū′dō-pa-rē′sis, -par′ĕ-sis). **1.** SYN pseudoparalysis. **2.** A condition marked by the pupillary changes, tremors, and speech disturbances suggestive of early paresis, in which, however, the serologic tests are negative.

pseu·do·pe·lade (sū′dō-pĕ-lahd′). A scarring type of alopecia; usually occurs in scattered irregular patches; of uncertain cause. [pseudo- + Fr. *pelade*, disease that causes sporadic falling of hair]

pseu·do·plate·let (sū-dō-plāt′let). Any of the fragments of neutrophils which may be mistaken for platelets, especially in peripheral blood smears of leukemic patients.

pseu·do·pod (sū'dō-pod). SYN pseudopodium.

pseu·do·po·di·um, pl. **pseu·do·po·dia** (sū-dō-pō'dē-ŭm, -pō'-dē-ă). A temporary protoplasmic process, put forth by an ameboid stage or amebic protozoan for locomotion or for prehension of food. SYN pseudopod. [pseudo- + G. *pous,* foot]

pseu·do·pol·yp (sū-dō-pol'ip). A projecting mass of granulation tissue, large numbers of which may develop in ulcerative colitis; may become covered by regenerating epithelium.

pseu·do·preg·nan·cy (sū-dō-preg'nan-sē). **1.** SYN false *pregnancy.* **2.** A condition in which symptoms resembling those of pregnancy are present, but which is not pregnancy.

pseu·do·pte·ryg·i·um (sū'dō-tĕ-rij'ē-ŭm). Adhesion of the conjunctiva to the cornea, occurring after injury.

pseu·dop·to·sis (sū-dō-tō'sis, sū-dop'tō-sis). A condition resembling an inability to elevate the eyelid, due to blepharophimosis, blepharochalasis, or some other affection. SYN false blepharoptosis. [pseudo- + G. *ptōsis,* a falling]

pseu·do·re·ac·tion (sū'dō-rē-ak'shŭn). A false reaction; one not due to specific causes in a given test.

pseu·do·rick·ets (sū-dō-rik'ets). SYN renal *rickets.*

pseu·do·ro·sette (sū'dō-rō-zet'). Perivascular radial arrangement of neoplastic cells around a small blood vessel. SEE rosette (2).

pseu·do·scar·la·ti·na (sū'dō-skar-lă-tē'nă). Erythema with fever, due to causes other than *Streptococcus pyogenes.*

pseu·dos·mia (sū-doz'mē-ă). Subjective sensation of an odor that is not present. [pseudo- + G. *osmē,* smell]

pseu·do·stra·bis·mus (sū'dō-stra-biz'mŭs). The appearance of strabismus caused by epicanthus, abnormality in interorbital distance, or corneal light reflex not corresponding to the center of the pupil. [pseudo- + G. *strabismos,* a squinting]

pupillotonic p., SYN Adie *syndrome.*

pseu·do·tu·mor (sū'dō-tū-mer). **1.** An enlargement of nonneoplastic character which clinically resembles a true neoplasm so closely as to often be mistaken for such. **2.** A condition, commonly associated with obesity in young females, of cerebral edema with narrowed small ventricles but with increased intracranial pressure and frequently papilledema. SYN pseudoneoplasm.

inflammatory p., a tumorlike mass in the lungs or other sites, composed of fibrous or granulation tissue infiltrated by inflammatory cells.

pseu·do·u·ri·dine (Ψ, Q) (sū-dō-yū'ri-dēn, -din). 5-β-D-ribosyluracil; a naturally occurring isomer of uridine found in transfer ribonucleic acids; unique in that the ribosyl is attached to carbon (C-5) rather than to nitrogen; excreted in urine.

pseu·do·xan·tho·ma elas·ti·cum (sū'dō-zan-thō'mă e-las'ti-kŭm) [MIM*177850, MIM*264800, MIM*264810]. An inherited disorder of connective tissue characterized by yellowish plaques on the neck, axillae, abdomen, and thighs, associated with angioid streaks of the retina and similar elastic tissue degeneration and calcification in arteries.

psi (Ψ) (sī) **1.** The 23rd letter of the Greek alphabet. **2.** Symbol for pseudouridine; pseudo-; psychology; wave function; the dihedral angle of rotation about the C_1–C_α bond associated with a peptide bond.

P sin·is·tro·car·di·a·le (sin-is-trō-kar-dē-ā'lē). SYN P mitrale.

psit·ta·co·sis (sit-ă-kō'sis). An infectious disease in psittacine birds and humans caused by the bacterium *Chlamydia psittaci.* Avian infections are mainly inapparent or latent, although acute disease does occur; human infections may result in mild disease with a flulike syndrome or in severe disease, with symptoms of bronchopneumonia. SYN ornithosis, parrot fever. [G. *psittakos,* a parrot, + *-osis,* condition]

pso·rel·co·sis (sō-rel-kō'sis). Cutaneous ulceration resulting from scabies. [G. *psōra,* itch, + *helkōsis,* ulceration]

pso·ri·a·sic (sō-rī'ă-sik). SYN psoriatic.

pso·ri·a·si·form (sō-rī'ă-si-fōrm). Resembling psoriasis.

pso·ri·a·sis (sō-rī'ă-sis). A common inherited condition characterized by the eruption of reddish, silvery-scaled maculopapules, predominantly on the elbows, knees, scalp, and trunk. [G. *psōriasis,* fr. *psōra,* the itch]

pso·ri·at·ic (sō-rē-at'ik). Relating to psoriasis. SYN psoriasic.

PSV pressure support *ventilation.*

△**psych-.** SEE psycho-.

psy·chal·gia (sī-kal'jē-ă). **1.** Distress attending a mental effort, noted especially in melancholia. SYN phrenalgia (1). **2.** SYN psychogenic *pain.* [psych- + G. *algos,* pain]

psy·cha·tax·ia (sī-kă-tak'sē-ă). Mental confusion; inability to fix one's attention or to make any continued mental effort. [psych- + G. *ataxia,* confusion]

psy·che (sī'kē). Term for the subjective aspects of the mind, self, soul; the psychological or spiritual as distinct from the bodily nature of persons. [G. mind, soul]

△**psyche-.** SEE psycho-.

psy·che·del·ic (sī-kĕ-del'ik). **1.** Pertaining to a category of drugs with mainly central nervous system action, said to be the expansion or heightening of consciousness, *e.g.,* LSD, hashish, mescaline. **2.** A hallucinogenic substance, visual display, music, or other sensory stimulus having such action. [psyche- + G. *dēloō,* to manifest]

psy·chi·at·ric (sī-kē-at'rik). Relating to psychiatry.

psy·chi·a·trist (sī-kī'ă-trist). A physician who specializes in psychiatry.

psy·chi·a·try (sī-kī'ă-trē). **1.** The medical specialty concerned with the diagnosis and treatment of mental disorders. **2.** The diagnosis and treatment of mental disorders. For some types of p. not listed below, see also subentries under therapy, psychotherapy, psychoanalysis. [psych- + G. *iatreia,* medical treatment]

community p., p. focusing on the detection, prevention, early treatment, and rehabilitation of individuals with emotional disorders and social deviance as they develop in the community.

contractual p., psychiatric intervention voluntarily assumed by the patient, who is prompted by his personal difficulties or suffering and who retains control over his participation with the psychiatrist.

dynamic p., SYN psychoanalytic p.

forensic p., legal p., the application of p. in courts of law, *e.g.,* in determinations for commitment, competency, fitness to stand trial, responsibility for crime.

psychoanalytic p., psychiatric theory and practice emphasizing the principles of psychoanalysis. SYN dynamic p.

social p., an approach to psychiatric theory and practice emphasizing the cultural and sociological aspects of mental disorder and treatment; the application of p. to social problems. SEE ALSO community p.

psy•chic (sī′kik). **1.** Relating to the phenomena of consciousness, mind, or soul. **2.** A person supposedly endowed with the power of communicating with spirits. [G. *psychikos*]

△**psycho-, psych-, psyche-.** The mind; mental; psychological. [G. *psychē,* soul, mind]

psy•cho•ac•tive (sī-kō-ak′tiv). Possessing the ability to alter mood, anxiety, behavior, cognitive processes, or mental tension; usually applied to pharmacologic agents.

psy•cho•a•nal•y•sis (sī′kō-ă-nal′i-sis). **1.** A method of psychotherapy, originated by Freud, designed to bring preconscious and unconscious material to consciousness primarily through the analysis of transference and resistance. SYN psychoanalytic therapy. SEE ALSO freudian p. **2.** A method of investigating total mental life, conscious and unconscious, of a person with a mental disorder, employing interpretation of resistance and transference, free association, and dream analysis. **3.** An integrated body of observations and theories on personality development, motivation, and behavior. **4.** A school of psychotherapy, as in jungian or freudian p. [psycho- + analysis]

freudian p., the theory and practice of p. and psychotherapy as developed by Sigmund Freud, based on: 1) his theory of personality, which postulates that psychic life is made up of instinctual and socially acquired forces, or the id, the ego, and a superego; 2) his discovery that the free-associated technique of verbalizing for the analyst all thoughts reveals the areas of conflict within a patient's personality; 3) that the vehicle for gaining this insight and readjusting one's personality is the learning a patient does, first developing a stormy emotional bond with the analyst (transference relationship) and next successfully learning to break this bond.

jungian p., the theory of psychopathology and the practice of psychotherapy, according to the principles of C. G. Jung, which emphasized human beings' symbolic nature, and differs from freudian p. especially in placing less significance upon instinctual (sexual) urges. SYN analytical psychology.

psy•cho•an•a•lyst (sī-kō-an′ă-list). A psycho-

therapist, usually a psychiatrist or clinical psychologist, trained in psychoanalysis and employing its methods in the treatment of emotional disorders.

psy•cho•an•a•lyt•ic (sī′kō-an-ă-lit′ik). Pertaining to psychoanalysis.

psy•cho•bi•ol•o•gy (sī′kō-bī-ol′ō-jē). The study of the interrelationships of the biology and psychology in cognitive functioning, including intellectual, memory, and related neurocognitive processes.

psy•cho•del•ic (sī-kō-del′-ik). A property of a drug or chemical which produces hallucinations or other bizarre aberrations in mental functioning. SYN hallucinogenic.

psy•cho•di•ag•no•sis (sī′kō-dī-ag-nō′sis). **1.** Any method used to discover the factors which underlie behavior, especially maladjusted or abnormal behavior. **2.** A subspecialty within clinical psychology that emphasizes the use of psychological tests and techniques for assessing psychopathology.

psy•cho•dra•ma (sī′kō-drah-mā). A method of psychotherapy in which patients act out their personal problems by spontaneously enacting without rehearsal diagnostically specific roles in dramatic performances put on before their patient peers.

psy•cho•dy•nam•ics (sī′kō-dī-nam′iks). The systematized study and theory of the psychological forces that underlie human behavior, emphasizing the interplay between unconscious and conscious motivation and the functional significance of emotion. SEE ALSO role-playing. [psycho- + G. *dynamis,* force]

psy•cho•gen•e•sis (sī-kō-jen′ĕ-sis). The origin and development of the psychic processes including mental, behavioral, emotional, personality, and related psychological processes. [psycho- + G. *genesis,* origin]

psy•cho•gen•ic, psy•cho•ge•net•ic (sī-kō-jen′ik, -jĕ-net′ik). **1.** Of mental origin or causation. **2.** Relating to emotional and related psychological development or to psychogenesis.

psy•cho•ki•ne•sis, psy•cho•ki•ne•sia (sī′kō-ki-nē′sis, -nē′zē-ă). **1.** The influence of mind upon matter, as the use of mental "power" to move or distort an object. **2.** Impulsive behavior. [psycho- + G. *kinēsis,* movement]

psy•cho•lin•guis•tics (sī′kō-ling-gwi′stiks). Study of a host of psychological factors associated with speech, including voice, attitudes, emotions, and grammatical rules, that affect communication and understanding of language. [psycho- + L. *lingua,* tongue]

psy•cho•log•ic, psy•cho•log•i•cal (sī-kō-loj′ik, -loj′i-kăl). **1.** Relating to psychology. **2.** Relating to the mind and its processes. SEE psychology.

psy•chol•o•gist (sī-kol′ō-jist). A specialist in psychology licensed to practice professional psychology (*e.g.,* clinical p.), or qualified to teach psychology as a scholarly discipline (academic p.), or whose scientific specialty is a subfield of psychology (research p.).

psy•chol•o•gy (Ψ) (sī-kol′ō-jē). The profession (*e.g.,* clinical p.), scholarly discipline (academic p.), and science (research p.) concerned with the behavior of humans and animals, and related mental and physiological processes. [psycho- + G. *logos,* study]

analytical p., SYN jungian *psychoanalysis.*

behavioral p., SYN behaviorism.

clinical p., a branch of p. that specializes in both discovering new knowledge and in applying the art and science of p. to persons with emotional or behavioral disorders; subspecialities include clinical child p. and pediatric p.

community p., the application of p. to community programs, *e.g.,* in the schools, correctional and welfare systems, and community mental health centers.

criminal p., the study of the mind and its workings in relation to crime. SEE forensic p.

developmental p., the study of the psychological, physiological, and behavioral changes in an organism that occur from birth to old age.

dynamic p., a psychologic approach that concerns itself with the causes of behavior.

environmental p., the study and application by behavioral scientists and architects of how changes in physical space and related physical stimuli impact upon the behavior of individuals. SEE ALSO personal *space.*

experimental p., (1) a subdiscipline within the science of p. that is concerned with the study of conditioning, learning, perception, motivation, emotion, language, and thinking; (2) also used in relation to subject-matter areas in which experimental, in contrast to correlational or socioexperiential, methods are emphasized.

forensic p., the application of p. to legal matters in a court of law.

genetic p., a science dealing with the evolution of behavior and the relation to each other of the different types of mental activity.

gestalt p., SEE gestaltism.

individual p., a theory of human behavior emphasizing humans' social nature, strivings for mastery, and drive to overcome, by compensation, feelings of inferiority.

medical p., the branch of p. concerned with the application of psychologic principles to the practice of medicine; the application of clinical p. or clinical health p., usually in a hospital setting.

psy•cho•met•rics (sī-kō-met′riks). SYN psychometry.

psy•chom•e•try (sī-kom′ĕ-trē). The discipline pertaining to psychological and mental testing, and to any quantitative analysis of an individual's psychological traits or attitudes or mental processes. SYN psychometrics. [psycho- + G. *metron,* measure]

psy•cho•mo•tor (sī-kō-mō′ter). **1.** Relating to the psychological processes associated with muscular movement, and to the production of voluntary movements. **2.** Relating to the combination of psychic and motor events, including disturbances. [psycho- + L. *motor,* mover]

psy•cho•neu•ro•sis (sī′kō-nū-rō′sis). SYN neurosis.

psy•cho•neu•rot•ic (sī′kō-nū-rot′ik). Pertaining to or suffering from psychoneurosis.

psy•cho•path (sī′kō-path). Former designation for an individual with an antisocial type of personality disorder. SEE ALSO antisocial *personality,* sociopath. [psycho- + G. *pathos,* disease]

psy•cho•path•ic (sī-kō-path′ik). Relating to or characteristic of psychopathy.

psy•cho•pa•thol•o•gy (sī′kō-pă-thol′ō-jē). **1.** The science concerned with the pathology of the mind and behavior. **2.** The science of mental and behavioral disorders, including psychiatry and abnormal psychology. [psycho- + G. *pathos,* disease, + *logos,* study]

psy•cho•phar•ma•ceu•ti•cals (sī′kō-far-mă-sū′ti-kălz). Drugs used in the treatment of emotional disorders.

psy•cho•phar•ma•col•o•gy (sī′kō-far′mă-kol′ō-jē). **1.** The use of drugs to treat mental and psychological disorders. **2.** The science of drug-behavior relationships. [psycho- + G. *pharmakon,* drug, + *logos,* study]

psy•cho•phys•i•cal (sī-kō-fiz′i-kăl). **1.** Relating to the mental perception of physical stimuli. SEE psychophysics. **2.** SYN psychosomatic.

psy•cho•phys•ics (sī-kō-fīz′iks). The science of the relation between the physical attributes of a stimulus and the measured, quantitative attributes of the mental perception of that stimulus.

psy•cho•phys•i•o•log•ic (sī′kō-fiz-ē-ō-loj′ik). **1.** Pertaining to psychophysiology. **2.** Denoting a psychosomatic illness. **3.** Denoting a somatic disorder with significant emotional or psychological etiology.

psy•cho•phys•i•ol•o•gy (sī′kō-fiz-ē-ol′ō-jē). The science of the relation between psychological and physiological processes.

psy•cho•sen•so•ry, psy•cho•sen•so•ri•al (sī′kō-sen′sōr-ē, -sen-sōr′ē-ăl). **1.** Denoting the mental perception and interpretation of sensory stimuli. **2.** Denoting a hallucination which by effort of mind is able to distinguish from reality.

psy•cho•sex•u•al (sī-kō-sek′shū-ăl). Pertaining to the relationships among the emotional, mental physiologic, and behavioral components of sex or sexual development.

psy•cho•sis, pl. **psy•cho•ses** (sī-kō′sis, -sēz). **1.** A mental and behavioral disorder causing gross distortion or disorganization of a person's mental capacity, affective response, and capacity to recognize reality, communicate, and relate to others to the degree of interfering with the person's capacity to cope with the ordinary demands of everyday life. **2.** Generic term for any of the so-called insanities, the most common forms being the schizophrenias. **3.** A severe emotional and behavioral disorder. [G. an animating]

affective p., p. with predominant affective features.

drug p., p. following or precipitated by ingestion of a drug.

hysterical p., (1) a psychotic disturbance with predominantly hysterical symptoms; (2) a mental disorder resembling conversion hysteria but of psychotic severity; (3) a brief reactive p., often culture bound.

ICU p., psychotic episode(s) occurring within 24 hours after entering the ICU in individuals with no previous history of p.; related to sleep deprivation, overstimulation and time spent on life support systems.

infection-exhaustion p., a p. following an acute infection, shock, or chronic intoxication; begins as delirium followed by pronounced mental confusion with hallucinations and unsystematized delusions, and sometimes stupor.

Korsakoff's p., SYN Korsakoff's *syndrome.*

manic-depressive p., SYN bipolar *disorder.*

polyneuritic p., SYN Korsakoff's *syndrome.*

postpartum p., an acute mental disorder with depression in the mother following childbirth.

schizo-affective p., psychotic disturbance in which there is a mixture of schizophrenic and manic-depressive symptoms.

senile p., mental disturbance occurring in old age and related to degenerative cerebral processes.

situational p., a transitory but severe emotional disorder caused in a predisposed person by a seemingly unbearable situation.

psy·cho·so·cial (sī-kō-sō'shăl). Involving both psychological and social aspects; *e.g.,* age, education, marital history.

psy·cho·so·mat·ic (sī'kō-sō-mat'ik). Pertaining to the influence of the mind or higher functions of the brain (emotions, fears, desires, etc.) upon the functions of the body, especially in relation to bodily disorders or disease. SEE psychophysiologic. SYN psychophysical (2). [psycho- + G. *sōma,* body]

psy·cho·so·mi·met·ic (sī-kō'sō-mi-met'ik). SYN psychotomimetic.

psy·cho·stim·u·lant (sī-kō-stim'yū-lant). An agent with antidepressant or mood-elevating properties.

psy·cho·sur·gery (sī-kō-ser'jer-ē). The treatment of mental disorders by operation upon the brain, *e.g.,* lobotomy.

psy·cho·ther·a·peu·tics (sī'kō-thār-ă-pyū'tiks). SYN psychotherapy.

psy·cho·ther·a·pist (sī-kō-thār'ă-pist). A person, usually a psychiatrist or clinical psychologist, professionally trained and engaged in psychotherapy. Currently, the term is also applied to social workers, nurses, and others whose state licensing practice acts include psychotherapy.

psy·cho·ther·a·py (sī-kō-thār'ă-pē). Treatment of emotional, behavioral, personality, and psychiatric disorders based primarily upon verbal or nonverbal communication and interventions with the patient, in contrast to treatments utilizing chemical and physical measures. SEE psychoanalysis, psychiatry, psychology, therapy. SYN psychotherapeutics. [psycho- + G. *therapeia,* treatment]

psy·chot·ic (sī-kot'ik). Relating to or affected by psychosis.

psy·chot·o·gen·ic (sī-kot-ō-jen'ik). Capable of inducing psychosis; particularly referring to drugs of the LSD series and similar substances.

psy·chot·o·mi·met·ic (sī-kot'ō-mi-met'ik). **1.** A drug or substance that produces psychological and behavioral changes resembling those of psychosis; *e.g.,* LSD. **2.** Denoting such a drug or substance. SYN psychosomimetic. [psychosis + G. *mimetikos,* imitative]

psy·cho·tro·pic (sī-kō-trop'ik). Capable of affecting the mind, emotions, and behavior; denot-

ing drugs used in the treatment of mental illnesses. [psycho- + G. *tropē,* a turning]

△**psychro-.** Cold. SEE ALSO cryo-, crymo-. [G. *psychros*]

psy·chro·al·gia (sī-krō-al'jē-ă). A painful sensation of cold. [psychro- + G. *algos,* pain]

psy·chrom·e·try (sī-krom'ĕ-trē). The calculation of relative humidity and water vapor pressures from wet and dry bulb temperatures and barometric pressure; whereas relative humidity is the value ordinarily employed, the vapor pressure is the measurement of physiological significance. SYN hygrometry. [psychro- + G. *metron,* measure]

psy·chro·phile, psy·chro·phil (sī'krō-fīl). An organism which grows best at a low temperature (0 to 32°C; 32 to 86°F), with optimum growth occurring at 15 to 20°C (59 to 68°F). [psychro- + G. *phileō,* to love]

psy·chro·phil·ic (sī-krō-fil'ik). Pertaining to a psychrophile. [psychro- + G. *phileō,* to love]

psy·chro·phore (sī'krō-fōr). A double catheter through which cold water is circulated to apply cold to the urethra or another canal or cavity. [psychro- + G. *phoros,* bearing]

PT physical *therapy* or physical therapist; prothrombin *time.*

Pt platinum.

PTA plasma thromboplastin *antecedent*; phosphotungstic acid; percutaneous transluminal *angioplasty.*

PTAH phosphotungstic acid *hematoxylin.*

△**pter-, ptero-.** wing; feather. [G. *pteron,* wing, feather]

pter·i·on (tē'rē-on). A craniometric point in the region of the sphenoid fontanelle, at the junction of the greater wing of the sphenoid, the squamous portion of the temporal, the frontal, and the parietal bones; it intersects the course of the anterior division of the middle meningeal artery. [G. *pteron,* wing]

pte·ryg·i·um (tĕ-rij'ē-ŭm). **1.** A triangular patch of hypertrophied bulbar subconjunctival tissue, extending from the medial canthus to the border of the cornea or beyond, with apex pointing toward the pupil. **2.** Forward growth of the cuticle over the nail plate, seen most commonly in lichen planus. **3.** An abnormal skin web. [G. *pterygion,* anything like a wing, a disease of the eye, dim. of *pteryx,* wing]

△**pterygo-.** Wing-shaped, usually relating to the pterygoid process. [G. *pteryx, pterygos,* wing]

pter·y·goid (ter'i-goyd). Wing-shaped; resembling a wing; a term applied to various anatomical parts relating to the sphenoid bone. [G. *pteryx* (*pteryg-*), wing, + *eidos,* resemblance]

pter·y·go·man·dib·u·lar (ter'i-gō-man-dib'yū-lăr). Relating to the pterygoid process and the mandible.

pter·y·go·max·il·lary (ter'i-gō-mak'si-lār-ē). Relating to the pterygoid process and the maxilla.

pter·y·go·pal·a·tine (ter'i-gō-pal'ă-tīn). Relating to the pterygoid process and the palatine bone.

PTHC percutaneous transhepatic *cholangiography.*

Pthir·us (thī'rŭs). A genus of lice formerly grouped in the genus *Pediculus.* The main species is *P. pubis*, the crab or pubic louse, a parasite that infests the pubes and adjacent hairy parts of the body. Often incorrectly spelled *Phthirus* or *Phthirius*. [irreg. fr. G. *phtheir*, louse]

pto·maine (tō'mān). An indefinite term applied to poisonous substances, *e.g.*, toxic amines, formed in the decomposition of protein by the decarboxylation of amino acids by bacterial action. [G. *ptōma*, a corpse]

ptosed (tōst). SYN ptotic.

pto·sis, pl. **pto·ses** (tō'sis, tō'sēz). **1.** A sinking down or prolapse of an organ. **2.** SYN blepharoptosis. [G. *ptōsis*, a falling]

△**-ptosis.** A sinking down or prolapse of an organ. [G. *ptōsis*, a falling]

pto·tic (tot'ik). Relating to or marked by ptosis. SYN ptosed.

PTT partial thromboplastin *time*.

pty·a·lec·ta·sis (tī'ă-lek'tă-sis). SYN sialectasis. [ptyal- + G. *ektasis*, a stretching out]

pty·a·lism (tī'al-izm). SYN sialism. [G. *ptyalismos*, spitting]

pty·a·lo·cele (tī'ă-lō-sēl). SYN ranula (2).

Pu plutonium.

pu·bar·che (pyū-bar'kē). Onset of puberty, particularly as manifested by the appearance of pubic hair. [puberty + G. *archē*, beginning]

pu·ber·al, pu·ber·tal (pyū'ber-ăl, -ber-tăl). Relating to puberty.

pu·ber·ty (pyū'ber-tē). Sequence of events by which a child becomes a young adult, characterized by the beginning of gametogenesis, secretion of gonadal hormones, development of secondary sexual characteristics and reproductive functions; sexual dimorphism is accentuated. [L. *pubertas*, fr. *puber*, grown up]

 precocious p., condition in which pubertal changes begin at an unexpectedly early age.

pu·bes (pyū'bēz). **1.** The area above the external genitals where hair growth signals puberty. **2** [NA]. One of the pubic hairs; the hair of the pubic region. [L. *pubes*, the hair on the genitals; the genitals]

pu·bes·cence (pyū-bes'ens). **1.** The approach of the age of puberty or sexual maturity. [L. *pubesco*, to attain puberty] **2.** Presence of downy or fine, short hair. [L. *pubes*, pubic hair]

pu·bes·cent (pyū-bes'ent). Pertaining to pubescence.

pu·bic (pyū'bik). Relating to the pubes or to the pubic bone.

pu·bi·ot·o·my (pyū-bē-ot'ō-mē). Severance of the pubic bone a few centimeters lateral to the symphysis, in order to increase the capacity of a contracted pelvis sufficiently to permit the passage of a living child. SYN pelviotomy (2), pelvitomy. [L. *pubis*, pubic bone, + G. *tomē*, incision]

pubis (pyū'bis). [NA] Official alternate term for os pubis, the pubic bone.

△**pubo-.** Pubic, pubes. [L. *pubes*]

pu·bo·pros·tat·ic (pyū'bō-pros-tat'ik). Relating to the pubic bone and the prostate.

pu·bo·rec·tal (pyū'bō-rek'tăl). Relating to the pubic bone and the rectum.

pu·bo·ves·i·cal (pyū'bō-ves'i-kăl). Relating to the pubic bone and the bladder.

pu·den·dal (pyū-den'dăl). Relating to the external genitals. SYN pudic.

pu·den·dum, pl. **pu·den·da** (pyū-den'dŭm, -dă). The external genitals, especially the female genitals (vulva). Used also in the plural. [L. ntr. of *pudendus*, particip. adj. of *pudeo*, to feel ashamed]

pu·dic (pyū'dik). SYN pudendal. [L. *pudicus*, modest]

pu·er·pera, pl. **pu·er·per·ae** (pyū-er'per-ă, -per-ē). A woman who has just given birth. [L., fr. *puer*, child, + *pario*, to bring forth]

pu·er·per·al (pyū-er'per-ăl). Relating to the puerperium, or period after childbirth. SYN puerperant (1).

pu·er·per·ant (pyū-er'per-ant). **1.** SYN puerperal. **2.** A puerpera.

pu·er·pe·ri·um, pl. **pu·er·pe·ria** (pyū-er-pēr'ē-ŭm, -ē-ă). Period from the termination of labor to complete involution of the uterus, usually defined as 42 days. [L. childbirth, fr. *puer*, child, + *pario*, to bring forth]

Pu·lex (pyū'leks). A genus of fleas (family Pulicidae, order Siphonaptera). [L. flea]

pu·lic·i·cide, pu·li·cide (pyū-lis'i-sīd, pyū'li-sīd). A chemical agent destructive to fleas. [L. *pulex* (*pulic-*), flea, + *caedo*, to kill]

pul·mo, gen. **pul·mo·nis**, pl. **pul·mo·nes** (pŭl' mō, pŭl-mō'nis, -mō'nēz) [NA]. SYN lung. [L.]

△**pulmo-, pulmon-, pulmono-.** The lungs. SEE ALSO pneum-, pneumo-. [L. *pulmo*, lung]

pul·mo·a·or·tic (pŭl'mō-ā-ōr'tik). Relating to the pulmonary artery and the aorta.

pul·mo·nary (pŭl'mō-nār-ē). Relating to the lungs, to the pulmonary artery, or to the aperture leading from the right ventricle into the pulmonary artery. SYN pneumonic (1), pulmonic. [L. *pulmonarius*, fr. *pulmo*, lung]

pul·mon·ic (pŭl-mon'ik). SYN pulmonary.

pul·mo·ni·tis (pŭl-mō-nī'tis). SYN pneumonitis.

pulp (pŭlp). **1.** A soft, moist, coherent solid. SYN pulpa [NA]. **2.** SYN dental p. **3.** SYN chyme. [L. *pulpa*, flesh]

 dead p., SYN necrotic p.

 dental p., dentinal p., the soft tissue within the pulp cavity, consisting of connective tissue containing blood vessels, nerves and lymphatics, and at the periphery a layer of odontoblasts capable of internal repair of the dentin. SYN pulp (2), tooth p.

 necrotic p., necrosis of the dental p. which clinically does not respond to thermal stimulation; the tooth may be asymptomatic or sensitive to percussion and palpation. SYN dead p., nonvital p.

 nonvital p., SYN necrotic p.

 red p., splenic p. seen grossly as a reddish brown substance, due to its abundance of red blood cells, consisting of splenic sinuses and the tissue intervening between them (splenic cords).

 splenic p., the soft cellular substance of the spleen.

 tooth p., SYN dental p.

 vital p., a p. composed of viable tissue, either normal or diseased, that responds to electric stimuli and to heat and cold.

white p., that part of the spleen that consists of nodules and other lymphatic concentrations.

pul·pa (pŭl′pă) [NA]. SYN pulp (1). [L. pulp]

pul·pal (pŭl′păl). Relating to the pulp.

pulp·ec·to·my (pŭl-pek′tō-mē). Removal of the entire pulp structure of a tooth, including the pulp tissue in the roots. [L. *pulpa,* pulp, + G. *ektomē,* excision]

pul·pi·fac·tion (pŭl-pi-fak′shŭn). Reduction to a pulpy condition. [L. *pulpa,* pulp, + *facio,* pp. *factus,* to make]

pulp·i·tis (pŭl-pī′tis). Inflammation of the pulp of a tooth. [L. *pulpa,* pulp, + G. *-itis,* inflammation]

   hyperplastic p., hyperplastic granulation tissue growing out of the exposed pulp chamber of a grossly decayed tooth.

   irreversible p., inflammation of the dental pulp from which the pulp is unable to recover; clinically, may be asymptomatic or characterized by pain which persists after thermal stimulation.

pulp·ot·o·my (pŭl-pot′ō-mē). Removal of a portion of the pulp structure of a tooth, usually the coronal portion. SYN pulp amputation. [L. *pulpa,* pulp, + G. *tomē,* incision]

pulpy (pŭl′pē). In the condition of a soft, moist solid.

pul·sate (pŭl′sāt). To throb or beat rhythmically; said of the heart or an artery. [L. *pulso,* pp. *-atus,* to beat]

pul·sa·tile (pŭl′să-til). Throbbing or beating.

pul·sa·tion (pŭl-sā′shŭn). A throbbing or rhythmical beating, as of the pulse or the heart. [L. *pulsatio,* a beating]

pulse (pŭls). Palpable rhythmic expansion of an artery, produced by the increased volume of blood thrown into the vessel by the contraction of the heart. A p. may also at times occur in a vein or a vascular organ, such as the liver. SYN pulsus. [L. *pulsus*]

   alternating p., mechanical alternation, a pulse regular in time but with alternate beats stronger and weaker, often detectable only with the sphygmomanometer and usually indicating serious myocardial disease. SYN pulsus alternans.

   anacrotic p., anadicrotic p., a p. wave showing one or more notches or indentations on its rising limb that are sometimes detectable by palpation.

   apical p., a p. heard directly over the apex of the heart by use of a stethoscope.

   bigeminal p., a p. in which the beats occur in pairs. SYN coupled p., pulsus bigeminus.

   bisferious p. (bis-fer′ē-ŭs), an arterial p. with peaks that may be palpable. SYN pulsus bisferiens.

   cannonball p., SYN water-hammer p.

   coupled p., SYN bigeminal p.

   dicrotic p., a p. which is marked by a double beat, the second, due to a palpable dicrotic wave, being weaker than the first.

   hard p., a p. that strikes forcibly against the tip of the finger and is with difficulty compressed, suggesting hypertension.

   jugular p., the venous p. as observed in the jugular veins of the neck, usually the deep jugular veins.

   oxygen p. (V̇O₂ HR), volume of oxygen consumed by the body per heartbeat.

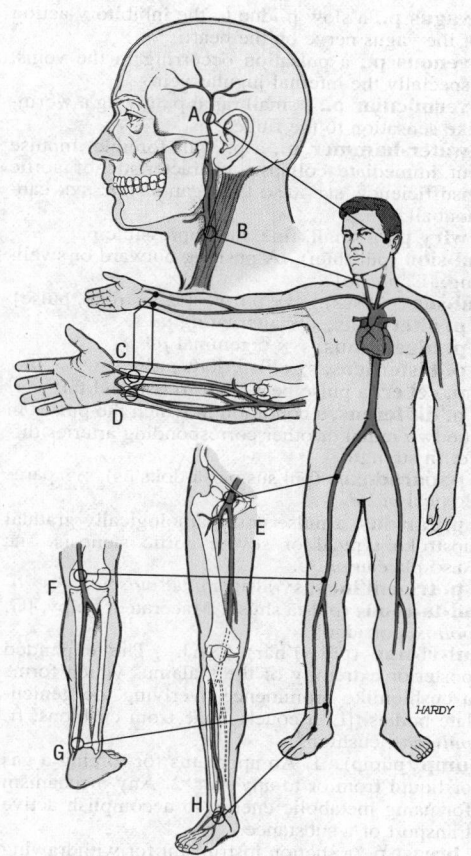

peripheral pulses: (A) temporal, (B) carotid, (C) radial, (D) ulnar, (E) femoral, (F) popliteal, (G) posterior tibial, (H) dorsalis pedis

   paradoxical p., a reversal of the normal variation in the p. volume with respiration, the p. becoming weaker with inspiration and stronger with expiration; characteristic of cardiac tamponade and rare in constrictive pericarditis. So called because these changes are independent of changes in the cardiac rate as measured directly or by electrocardiogram. SYN pulsus paradoxus.

   plateau p., a slow, sustained p.

   Quincke's p., the capillary p. as appreciated in the finger and toenails during aortic regurgitation; ebb and flow is seen. SYN Quincke's sign.

   Riegel's p., a p. that diminishes in volume during expiration.

   thready p., a small fine p., feeling like a small cord or thread under the finger.

   trigeminal p., a p. in which the beats occur in trios, a pause following every third beat. SYN pulsus trigeminus.

   undulating p., a p. in which there is a succession of waves rather than discrete pulsations.

pu

vagus p., a slow p. due to the inhibitory action of the vagus nerve on the heart.

venous p., a pulsation occurring in the veins, especially the internal jugular vein.

vermicular p., a small rapid p., giving a worm-like sensation to the finger.

water-hammer p., a p. with forcible impulse but immediate collapse, characteristic of aortic insufficiency. SEE ALSO Corrigan's *sign.* SYN cannonball p.

wiry p., a small, fine, incompressible p.

pul·sion (pŭl'shŭn). A pushing outward or swelling. [L. *pulsio*]

pul·sus (pŭl'sŭs). SYN pulse. [L. a stroke, pulse]

p. alter′nans, SYN alternating *pulse.*

p. bigem′inus, SYN bigeminal *pulse.*

p. bisfer′iens, SYN bisferious *pulse.*

p. cel′er, a pulse beat swift to rise and fall.

p. dif′ferens, a condition in which the pulses in the two radial or other corresponding arteries differ in strength.

p. paradoxus (pŭl'sŭs pār-ă-doks'ŭs), SYN paradoxical *pulse.*

p. tar′dus, a pulse with pathologically gradual upstroke typical of severe aortic stenosis. SEE ALSO plateau *pulse.*

p. trigem′inus, SYN trigeminal *pulse.*

pul·ta·ceous (pŭl-tā'shŭs). Macerated; pulpy. [G. *poltos,* porridge]

pul·vi·nar (pŭl-vī'năr) [NA]. The expanded posterior extremity of the thalamus which forms a cushionlike prominence overlying the geniculate bodies. [L. a couch made from cushions, fr. *pulvinus,* cushion]

pump (pŭmp). **1.** An apparatus for forcing a gas or liquid from or to any part. **2.** Any mechanism for using metabolic energy to accomplish active transport of a substance.

breast p., a suction instrument for withdrawing milk from the breast.

calcium p., a membranal protein that can transport calcium ions across the membrane using energy from ATP.

hydrogen p., molecular mechanism for acid secretion from gastric parietal cells based on the activity of a H^+-K^+-ATPase.

intra-aortic balloon p., a pump connected to a balloon inserted into the descending aorta as a counterpulsation device to provide temporary cardiac assistance in left ventricular failure.

proton p., molecular mechanism for the net transport of protons across a membrane; usually involves the activity of an ATPase.

sodium p., a biologic mechanism that uses metabolic energy from ATP to achieve active transport of sodium across a membrane; sodium p.'s expel sodium from most cells of the body, sometimes coupled with the transport of other substances, and also serve to move sodium across multicellular membranes such as renal tubule walls.

sodium-potassium p., a membrane-bound transporter that maintains the high potassium and low sodium intracellular concentrations relative to the extracellular medium. This exchange is accomplished at the expense of cellular energy in the form of ATP.

stomach p., an apparatus for removing the contents of the stomach by means of suction.

pump-ox·y·gen·a·tor (pŭmp-ok'si-je-nā'ter). A mechanical device that can substitute for both the heart (pump) and the lungs (oxygenator) during open heart surgery.

punch·drunk (pŭnch'drŭnk). SEE punchdrunk *syndrome.*

punc·ta (pŭngk'tă). Plural of punctum. [L.]

punc·tate (pŭngk'tāt). Marked with points or dots differentiated from the surrounding surface by color, elevation, or texture. [L. *punctum,* a point]

punc·ti·form (pŭngk'ti-fōrm). Very small but not microscopic, having a diameter of less than 1 mm. [L. *punctum,* a point, + *forma,* shape]

punc·tum, gen. **punc·ti,** pl. **punc·ta** (pŭngk'tŭm, -tī, -tă) [NA]. **1.** The tip of a sharp process. **2.** A minute round spot differing in color or otherwise in appearance from the surrounding tissues. **3.** A point on the optic axis of an optical system. SEE ALSO point. SYN point (1). [L. a prick, point, pp. ntr. of *pungo,* to prick, used as noun]

p. ce′cum, the blind spot in the visual field corresponding to the location of the optic disk.

lacrimal p., the minute circular opening of the lacrimal canaliculus, on the margin of each eyelid near the medial commissure.

p. vasculo′sum, one of the minute dots seen on section of the brain, due to small drops of blood at the cut extremities of the arteries.

punc·ture (pŭnk'chŭr). **1.** To make a hole with a small pointed object, such as a needle. **2.** A prick or small hole made with a pointed instrument. [L. *punctura,* fr. *pungo,* pp. *punctus,* to prick]

cisternal p., passage of a hollow needle through the posterior atlantooccipital membrane into the cisterna cerebellomedullaris.

lumbar p., a p. into the subarachnoid space of the lumbar region to obtain spinal fluid for diagnostic or therapeutic purposes. SYN rachicentesis, rachiocentesis, spinal tap.

sternal p., removal of bone marrow from the manubrium by needle.

tracheoesophageal p. (TEP, TEP TEP), surgical p. connecting the trachea and esophagus. In laryngectomies, the p., in combination with a prosthetic valve, allows exhaled air from the lungs to enter the esophagus for production of speech.

PUO Pyrexia of unknown (or undetermined) origin.

pu·pa, pl. **pu·pae** (pyū'pă, -pē). The stage of insect metamorphosis following the larva and preceding the imago. [L. *pupa,* doll]

pu·pil (p) (pyū'pĭl). The circular orifice in the center of the iris, through which light rays enter the eye. SYN pupilla [NA]. [L. *pupilla*]

Adie's p., SYN Adie *syndrome.*

amaurotic p., p. in an eye that is blind because of ocular or optic nerve disease; this p. will not contract to light except when the normal fellow eye is stimulated with light.

Argyll Robertson p., a form of reflex iridoplegia characterized by miosis, irregular shape, and a loss of the direct and consensual pupillary reflex to light, with normal pupillary constriction to a near vision effort (light-near dissociation); often present in tabetic neurosyphilis.

fixed p., a stationary pupil unresponsive to all stimuli.

Holmes-Adie p., SYN Adie *syndrome.*

Horner's p., constricted p. due to impairment of sympathetic nerve innervation of the dilator muscle of the pupil. SEE ALSO Horner's *syndrome.*

Hutchinson's p., dilation of the p. on the side of the lesion as part of a third nerve palsy; often due to herniation of the uncus of the temporal lobe through the tentorial notch.

pinhole p., an extremely constricted p.

tonic p., a general term for a p. with delayed, slow, long-lasting contractions to light and to a near vision effort, often with light-near dissociation; due to denervation and aberrant reinnervation of the iris sphincter; seen in various autonomic neuropathies and in Adie *syndrome.*

pu·pil·la, pl. **pu·pil·lae** (pyū-pil′ă, pyū-pil′ē) [NA]. SYN pupil. [L. dim. of *pupa,* a girl or doll]

pu·pil·lary (pyū′pi-lār-ē). Relating to the pupil.

△**pupillo-.** The pupils. [L. *pupilla,* pupil]

pu·pil·lom·e·ter (pyū′pi-lom′ĕ-ter). An instrument for measuring and recording the diameter of the pupil. [pupillo- + G. *metron,* measure]

pu·pil·lom·e·try (pyū′pi-lom′ĕ-trē). Measurement of the pupil.

pu·pil·lo·mo·tor (pyū′pĭ-lō-mō′ter). Relating to the autonomic nerve fibers that supply the smooth muscle of the iris. [pupillo- + L. *motor,* mover]

pu·pil·lo·sta·tom·e·ter (pyū′pi-lō-stă-tom′ĕ-ter). An instrument for measuring the distance between the centers of the pupils. [pupillo- + G. *statos,* placed, + *metron,* measure]

PUPPP *p*ruritic *u*rticarial *p*apules and *p*laques of *p*regnancy, an intensely pruritic, occasionally vesicular, eruption of the trunk and arms appearing in the third trimester of pregnancy; spontaneous involution occurs within 10 days of term.

pur·ga·tion (per-gā′shŭn). Evacuation of the bowels with the aid of a purgative or cathartic. SYN catharsis (1). [L. *purgatio*]

pur·ga·tive (per′gă-tiv). An agent used for purging the bowels. SEE ALSO cathartic (2). [L. *purgativus,* purging]

purge (perj). **1.** To cause a copious evacuation of the bowels. **2.** A cathartic remedy. [L. *purgo,* to cleanse, fr. *purus,* pure, + *ago,* to do]

pu·rine (pyūr′ēn, -rin). The parent substance of adenine, guanine, and other naturally occurring in "bases"; not known to exist as such in mammals.

pur·ple (per′pl). A color formed by a mixture of blue and red. For individual purple dyes see specific name. [L. *purpura*]

visual p., SYN rhodopsin.

pur·pu·ra (pŭr′pū-ră). A condition characterized by hemorrhage into the skin. Appearance of the lesions varies with the type of p., the duration of the lesions, and the acuteness of the onset. The color is first red, gradually darkens to purple, fades to a brownish yellow, and usually disappears in 2 or 3 weeks; color of residual permanent pigmentation depends largely on the type of unabsorbed pigment of the extravasated blood; extravasations may occur also into the mucous

membranes and internal organs. SYN peliosis. [L. fr. G. *porphyra,* purple]

allergic p., nonthrombocytopenic p. due to sensitization to foods, drugs, and insect bites. SYN anaphylactoid p. (1).

anaphylactoid p., (1) SYN allergic p. **(2)** SYN Henoch-Schönlein p.

fibrinolytic p., p. in which the bleeding is associated with rapid fibrinolysis of the clot.

🔲 **p. ful′minans,** a severe and rapidly fatal form of p. hemorrhagica, occurring especially in children, with hypotension, fever, and disseminated intravascular coagulation, usually following an infectious illness.

p. hemorrhag′ica, SYN idiopathic thrombocytopenic p.

Henoch-Schönlein p., an eruption of nonthrombocytopenic purpuric lesions due to dermal leukocytoclastic vasculitis with IgA in vessel walls associated with joint pain and swelling, colic, and passage of bloody stools, and occurring characteristically in young children; glomerulonephritis may occur during an initial episode or develop later. SYN anaphylactoid p. (2).

idiopathic thrombocytopenic p. (ITP), a systemic illness characterized by extensive ecchymoses and hemorrhages from mucous membranes and very low platelet counts; resulting from destruction in the spleen of platelets to which an autoimmune globulin is bound; childhood cases, which often follow viral infection, are mild and transitory; in adults, bleeding may be recurrent and severe. SYN immune thrombocytopenic p., p. hemorrhagica, thrombopenic p.

immune thrombocytopenic p., SYN idiopathic thrombocytopenic p.

nonthrombocytopenic p., SYN p. simplex.

p. seni′lis, the occurrence of petechiae and ecchymoses on the atrophic skin of the legs in aged and debilitated subjects.

p. sim′plex, the eruption of petechiae or larger ecchymoses, usually unaccompanied by constitutional symptoms and not associated with systemic illness. SYN nonthrombocytopenic p.

thrombocytopenic p., SEE idiopathic thrombocytopenic p.

thrombopenic p., SYN idiopathic thrombocytopenic p.

thrombotic thrombocytopenic p., a rapidly fatal or occasionally protracted disease with varied symptoms in addition to p., including signs of central nervous system involvement, due to formation of fibrin or platelet thrombi in arterioles and capillaries in many organs.

pur·pu·ric (pŭr-pū′rik). Relating to or affected with purpura.

pur·pu·ri·nu·ria (per′pyū-ri-nū′rē-ă). SYN porphyrinuria.

pu·ru·lence, pu·ru·len·cy (pyūr′ŭ-lens, -len-sē; pyūr′yū-lens). The condition of containing or forming pus. [L. *purulentia,* a festering, fr. *pus* (*pur-*), pus]

pu·ru·lent (pyūr′ŭ-lent, pyūr′yū-). Containing, consisting of, or forming pus.

pu·ru·loid (pyūr′ŭ-loyd). Resembling pus.

pus (pŭs). A fluid product of inflammation containing leukocytes and the debris of dead cells and tissue elements. [L.]

blue p., p. tinged with pyocyanin, a product of *Pseudomonas aeruginosa*.

pus·tu·lar (pŭs′chū-lăr). Relating to or marked by pustules.

pus·tu·la·tion (pŭs′chū-lā′shŭn). The formation or the presence of pustules.

pus·tule (pŭs′chūl). A small, circumscribed elevation of the skin, containing purulent material. [L. *pustula*]

pus·tu·lo·sis (pŭs-chū-lō′sis). **1.** An eruption of pustules. **2.** Term occasionally used to designate acropustulosis. [L. *pustula*, pustule, + G. *-osis*, condition]

p. palmar′is et plantar′is, a sterile pustular eruption of the fingers and toes, variously attributed to dyshidrosis, pustular psoriasis, and unidentified bacterial infection. SYN acrodermatitis continua, acrodermatitis perstans, dermatitis repens.

pu·ta·men (pyū-tā′men) [NA]. The outer, larger, and darker gray of the three portions into which the lenticular nucleus is divided by laminae of white fibers; it is connected with the caudate nucleus by bridging bands of gray substance that penetrate the internal capsule. Its histological structure is similar to that of the caudate nucleus together with which it composes the striatum. SEE ALSO striate *body*. [L. that which falls off in pruning, fr. *puto*, to prune]

pu·tre·fac·tion (pyū-tri-fak′shŭn). Decomposition or rotting, the breakdown of organic matter usually by bacterial action, resulting in the formation of other substances of less complex constitution with the evolution of ammonia or its derivatives and hydrogen sulfide; characterized usually by the presence of toxic or malodorous products. SYN decay (2), decomposition. [L. *putre-facio*, pp. *-factus*, to make rotten]

pu·tre·fac·tive (pyū-tri-fak′tiv). Relating to or causing putrefaction.

pu·tre·fy (pyū′tri-fī). To cause to become, or to become, putrid.

pu·tres·cence (pyū-tres′ens). The state of putrefaction.

pu·tres·cent (pyū-tres′ent). Denoting, or in the process of, putrefaction. [L. *putresco*, to grow rotten, fr. *puter*, rotten]

pu·tres·cine (pyū-tres′ēn). A poisonous polyamine formed from the amino acid arginine during putrefaction; found in urine and feces.

pu·trid (pyū′trid). **1.** In a state of putrefaction. **2.** Denoting putrefaction. [L. *putridus*]

PUVA oral administration of *p*soralen and subsequent exposure to long wavelength *u*ltra*v*iolet light (*uv-a*); used to treat psoriasis.

py·ar·thro·sis (pī-ar-thrō′sis). SYN suppurative *arthritis*. [G. *pyon*, pus, + *arthrōsis*, a jointing]

△**pycno-.** SEE pykno-.

△**pyel-.** SEE pyelo-.

py·e·lec·ta·sis, py·e·lec·ta·sia (pī-ĕ-lek′tă-sis, pī-ĕ-lek-tā′zē-ă). Dilation of the pelvis of the kidney. [pyel- + G. *ektasis*, extension]

py·e·lit·ic (pī-ĕ-lit′ik). Relating to pyelitis.

py·e·li·tis (pī-ĕ-lī′tis). Inflammation of the renal pelvis. [pyel- + G. *-itis*, inflammation]

△**pyelo-, pyel-.** Pelvis, usually the renal pelvis. [G. *pyelos*, trough, tub, vat]

py·e·lo·cal·i·ce·al (pī′ĕ-lō-kal′i-sē′ăl). Relating to the renal pelvis and calices.

py·e·lo·cys·ti·tis (pī-ĕ-lō-sis-tī′tis). Inflammation of the renal pelvis and the bladder. [pyelo- + G. *kystis*, bladder, + *-itis*, inflammation]

py·e·lo·flu·o·ros·co·py (pī′ĕ-lō-flūr-os′kŏ-pē). Fluoroscopic examination of the renal pelves and ureters, following administration of contrast medium. [pyelo- + L. *fluo*, to flow, + G. *skopeō*, to view]

py·el·o·gram (pī′el-ō-gram). A radiograph or series of radiographs of the renal pelvis and ureter, following injection of contrast medium.

py·e·log·ra·phy (pī′ĕ-log′ră-fē). Radiologic study of the kidney, ureters, and usually the bladder, performed with the aid of a contrast agent either injected intravenously, or directly through a ureteral or nephrostomy catheter or percutaneously. SYN pyeloureterography, ureteropyelography. [pyelo- + G. *graphō*, to write]

py·e·lo·li·thot·o·my (pī′ĕ-lō-li-thot′ō-mē). Operative removal of a calculus from the kidney through an incision in the renal pelvis. SYN pelvilithotomy. [pyelo- + G. *lithos*, stone, + *tomē*, incision]

py·e·lo·ne·phri·tis (pī′ĕ-lō-ne-frī′tis). Inflammation of the renal parenchyma, calices, and pelvis, particularly due to local bacterial infection. [pyelo- + G. *nephros*, kidney, + *-itis*, inflammation]

py·e·lo·plas·ty (pī′e-lō-plas-tē). Surgical reconstruction of the kidney pelvis to correct an obstruction. SYN pelvioplasty (2). [pyelo- + G. *plastos*, formed]

py·e·los·co·py (pī-ĕ-los′kŏ-pē). Fluoroscopic observation of the pelvis and calices of the kidney, and the ureter, after the injection through the ureter of a radiopaque solution. [pyelo- + G. *skopeō*, to view]

py·e·los·to·my (pī-ĕ-los′tō-mē). Formation of an opening into the kidney pelvis to establish urinary drainage. [pyelo- + G. *stoma*, mouth]

py·e·lot·o·my (pī-ĕ-lot′ō-mē). Incision into the pelvis of the kidney. SYN pelviotomy (3), pelvitomy. [pyelo- + G. *tomē*, incision]

py·e·lo·u·re·ter·ec·ta·sis (pī′ĕ-lō-yū-rē′ter-ek′tă-sis). Dilation of kidney pelvis and ureter, seen in hydronephrosis due to obstruction in the lower urinary tract. [pyelo- + ureter + G. *ektasis*, stretching]

py·e·lo·u·re·ter·og·ra·phy (pī′ĕ-lō-yū-rē′ter-og′ră-fē). SYN pyelography.

py·e·lo·ve·nous (pī′ĕ-lō-vē′nŭs). Relating to the renal pelvis and renal veins. Denoting the passage of urine from the renal pelvis into the renal veins, because of increased intrapelvic pressure. [pyelo- + venous]

py·em·e·sis (pī-em′ĕ-sis). The vomiting of pus. [G. *pyon*, pus, + *emesis*, vomiting]

py·e·mia (pī-ē′mē-ă). Septicemia due to pyogenic organisms causing multiple abscesses. [G. *pyon*, pus, + *haima*, blood]

py·e·mic (pī-ē′mik). Relating to or suffering from pyemia.

py·en·ceph·a·lus (pī-en-sef′ă-lŭs). SYN pyocephalus. [G. *pyon*, pus, + *enkephalos*, brain]

py·e·sis (pī-ē′sis). SYN suppuration. [G. *pyon*, pus, + *-esis*, condition or process]

pyg·my (pig′mē) [MIM*177850, MIM*177860, MIM*265850]. A physiologic dwarf; especially one of a race of similar people, such as the p.'s of central Africa. [G. *pygmaios*, dwarfish, fr. *pygmē*, fist, also a measure of length from elbow to knuckles]

△**pyk-.** SEE pykno-.

pyk·nic (pik′nik). Denoting a constitutional body type characterized by well-rounded external contours and ample body cavities; virtually synonymous with endomorphic. [G. *pyknos*, thick]

△**pykno-, pyk-.** Thick, dense, compact. [G. *pyknos*]

pyk·no·mor·phous (pik′nō-mōr′fŭs). Denoting a cell or tissue that stains deeply because the stainable material is closely packed. [pykno- + G. *morphē*, form, shape]

pyk·no·sis (pik-nō′sis). A thickening or condensation; specifically, a condensation and reduction in size of the cell or its nucleus, usually associated with hyperchromatosis; nuclear p. is a stage of necrosis. [pykno- + G. *-osis*, condition]

pyk·not·ic (pik-not′ik). Relating to or characterized by pyknosis.

py·le·phle·bi·tis (pī′lē-fle-bī′tis). Inflammation of the portal vein or any of its branches. [G. *pylē*, a gate, + *phleps*, vein, + *-itis*, inflammation]

py·le·throm·bo·phle·bi·tis (pī-lē-throm′bō-phle-bī′tis). Inflammation of the portal vein with the formation of a thrombus. [G. *pylē*, gate, + *thrombos*, a clot, + *phleps*, vein, + *-itis*, inflammation]

py·le·throm·bo·sis (pī′lē-throm-bō′sis). Thrombosis of the portal vein or its branches. [G. *pylē*, gate, + *thrombos*, a clot, + *-osis*, condition]

△**pylor-.** SEE pyloro-.

py·lo·rec·to·my (pī′lōr-ek′tō-mē). Excision of the pylorus. SYN gastropylorectomy, pylorogastrectomy. [pylor- + G. *ektomē*, excision]

py·lo·ri (pī-lōr′ī). Plural of pylorus. [L.]

py·lor·ic (pī-lōr′ik). Relating to the pylorus.

py·lo·ri·ste·no·sis (pī-lōr′i-ste-nō′sis). Stricture or narrowing of the orifice of the pylorus. SYN pylorostenosis. [pylor- + G. *stenōsis*, a narrowing]

△**pyloro-, pylor-.** The pylorus. [G. *pyloros*, gatekeeper]

py·lo·ro·du·o·de·ni·tis (pī-lōr′ō-dū′od-ĕ-nī′tis). Inflammation involving the pyloric outlet of the stomach and the duodenum. [pyloro- + duodenitis]

py·lo·ro·gas·trec·to·my (pī-lōr′ō-gas-trek′tō-mē). SYN pylorectomy.

py·lo·ro·my·ot·o·my (pī-lōr′ō-mī-ot′ō-mē). Longitudinal incision through the anterior wall of the pyloric canal to the level of the submucosa, to treat hypertrophic pyloric stenosis. SYN Fredet-Ramstedt operation, Ramstedt operation. [pyloro- + G. *mys*, muscle, + *tomē*, incision]

py·lo·ro·plas·ty (pī-lōr′ō-plas-tē). Widening of the pyloric canal and any adjacent duodenal stricture by means of a longitudinal incision closed transversely. [pyloro- + G. *plastos*, formed]

py·lo·ro·spasm (pī-lōr′ō-spazm). Spasmodic contraction of the pylorus.

py·lo·ro·ste·no·sis (pī-lōr′ō-stĕ-nō′sis). SYN pyloristenosis.

py·lo·ros·to·my (pī-lō-ros′tō-mē). Establishment of a fistula from the abdominal surface into the stomach near the pylorus. [pyloro- + G. *stoma*, mouth]

py·lo·rot·o·my (pī-lō-rot′ō-mē). Incision of the pylorus. [pyloro- + G. *tomē*, incision]

py·lo·rus, pl. **py·lo·ri** (pī-lōr′ŭs, pī-lōr′ī) [NA]. **1.** A muscular or myovascular device to open (musculus dilator) and to close (musculus sphincter) an orifice or the lumen of an organ. **2.** The muscular tissue surrounding and controlling the aboral outlet of the stomach. [L. fr. G. *pylōros*, a gatekeeper, the pylorus, fr. *pylē*, gate, + *ouros*, a warder]

△**pyo-.** Suppuration, accumulation of pus. [G. *pyon*, pus]

py·o·cele (pī′ō-sēl). An accumulation of pus in the scrotum. [pyo- + G. *kēlē*, tumor, hernia]

py·o·ceph·a·lus (pī′ō-sef′ă-lŭs). A purulent effusion within the cranium. SYN pyencephalus. [pyo- + G. *kephalē*, head]

py·o·che·zia (pī-ō-kē′zē-ă). A discharge of pus from the bowel. [pyo- + G. *chezō*, to defecate]

py·o·coc·cus (pī′ō-kok′ŭs). One of the cocci causing suppuration, especially *Streptococcus pyogenes*. [pyo- + G. *kokkos*, berry (coccus)]

py·o·col·po·cele (pī-ō-kol′pō-sēl). A vaginal tumor or cyst containing pus. [pyo- + G. *kolpos*, bosom (vagina), + *kēlē*, tumor, hernia]

py·o·col·pos (pī-ō-kol′pos). Accumulation of pus in the vagina. [pyo- + G. *kolpos*, bosom (vagina)]

py·o·cy·an·ic (pī′ō-sī-an′ik). Relating to blue pus or the organism that causes blue pus, *Pseudomonas aeruginosa*. [pyo- + G. *kyanos*, blue]

py·o·cy·a·no·gen·ic (pī′ō-sī′ă-nō-jen′ik). Causing blue pus. [pyo- + G. *kyanos*, blue, + *-gen*, producing]

py·o·cyst (pī′ō-sist). A cyst with purulent contents. [pyo- + G. *kystis*, bladder]

py·o·der·ma (pī-ō-der′mă). Any pyogenic infection of the skin; may be primary, as impetigo, or secondary to a previously existing condition. [pyo- + G. *derma*, skin]

  p. gangreno′sum, a chronic, noninfective eruption of spreading, undermined ulcers showing central healing, with diffuse dermal neutrophil infiltration; often associated with ulcerative colitis.

py·o·gen·e·sis (pī′ō-jen′ĕ-sis). SYN suppuration. [pyo- + G. *genesis*, production]

py·o·gen·ic, py·o·ge·net·ic (pī-ō-jen′ik, -jĕ-net′ik). Pus-forming; relating to pus formation.

py·o·he·mo·tho·rax (pī′ō-hē-mō-thōr′aks). Presence of pus and blood in the pleural cavity. [pyo- + G. *haima*, blood, + thorax]

py·oid (pī′oyd). Resembling pus. [G. *pyōdēs*, fr. *pyon*, pus, + *eidos*, resemblance]

py·o·me·tra (pī-ō-mē′tră). Accumulation of pus in the uterine cavity. [pyo- + G. *mētra*, uterus]

py·o·me·tri·tis (pī′ō-mē-trī′tis). Inflammation of uterine musculature associated with pus in the uterine cavity. [pyo- + G. *mētra*, womb, + *-itis*, inflammation]

py

py·o·my·o·si·tis (pī′ō-mī-ō-sī′tis). Abscesses, carbuncles, or infected sinuses lying deep in muscles. [pyo- + G. *mys,* muscle, + *-itis,* inflammation]

py·o·ne·phri·tis (pī-ō-ne-frī′tis). Suppurative inflammation of the kidney. [pyo- + G. *nephros,* kidney, + *-itis,* inflammation]

py·o·neph·ro·li·thi·a·sis (pī′ō-nef′rō-li-thī′ă-sis). Presence in the kidney of pus and calculi. [pyo- + G. *nephros,* kidney, + *lithos,* stone, + *-iasis,* condition]

py·o·ne·phro·sis (pī′ō-ne-frō′sis). Distention of the pelvis and calices of the kidney with pus, usually associated with obstruction. SYN nephropyosis. [pyo- + G. *nephros,* kidney, + *-osis,* condition]

pyo·ova·ri·um (pī′ō-ō-var′ē-ŭm). Presence of pus in the ovary; an ovarian abscess.

py·o·per·i·car·di·tis (pī′ō-per-i-kar-dī′tis). Suppurative inflammation of the pericardium.

py·o·per·i·car·di·um (pī′ō-per-i-kar′dē-ŭm). An accumulation of pus in the pericardial sac.

py·o·per·i·to·ne·um (pī′ō-per-i-tō-nē′ŭm). An accumulation of pus in the peritoneal cavity. [G. *pyon,* pus]

py·o·per·i·to·ni·tis (pī′ō-per-i-tō-nī′tis). Suppurative inflammation of the peritoneum. [pyo- + peritonitis]

py·o·phy·so·me·tra (pī′ō-fī-sō-mē′tră). Presence of pus and gas in the uterine cavity. [pyo- + G. *physa,* air, + *mētra,* uterus]

py·o·pneu·mo·cho·le·cys·ti·tis (pī′ō-nū′mō-kō′lē-sis-ī′tis). Combination of pus and gas in an inflamed gallbladder caused by gas-producing organisms or by the entry of gas from the duodenum through the biliary tree. [pyo- + G. *pneuma,* air, + cholecystitis]

py·o·pneu·mo·hep·a·ti·tis (pī′ō-nū′mō-hep-ă-tī′tis). Combination of pus and gas in the liver, usually in association with an abscess. [pyo- + G. *pneuma,* air, + hepatitis]

py·o·pneu·mo·per·i·car·di·um (pī′ō-nū′mō-per-i-kar′dē-ŭm). Presence of pus and gas in the pericardial sac. [pyo- + G. *pneuma,* air, + pericardium]

py·o·pneu·mo·per·i·to·ne·um (pī′ō-nū′mō-per-i-tō-nē′ŭm). Presence of pus and gas in the peritoneal cavity. [pyo- + G. *pneuma,* air, + peritoneum]

py·o·pneu·mo·per·i·to·ni·tis (pī′ō-nū′mō-per-i-tō-nī′tis). Peritonitis with gas-forming organisms or with gas introduced from a ruptured bowel. [pyo- + G. *pneuma,* air, + peritonitis]

py·o·pneu·mo·tho·rax (pī′ō-nū-mō-thōr′aks). The presence of gas together with a purulent effusion in the pleural cavity. SYN pneumopyothorax. [pyo- + G. *pneuma,* air, + thorax]

py·o·poi·e·sis (pī′ō-poy-ē′sis). SYN suppuration. [pyo- + G. *poiēsis,* a making]

py·o·poi·et·ic (pī′ō-poy-et′ik). Pus-producing.

py·o·py·e·lec·ta·sis (pī′ō-pī-ĕ-lek′tă-sis). Dilation of the renal pelvis with pus-producing inflammation. [pyo- + G. *pyelos,* pelvis, + *ektasis,* a stretching]

py·or·rhea (pī-ō-rē′ă). A purulent discharge. [pyo- + G. *rhoia,* a flow]

py·o·sal·pin·gi·tis (pi′o-sal-pin-ji′tis). Suppura-

tive inflammation of the fallopian tube. [pyo- + salpingitis]

py·o·sal·pin·go-ooph·o·ri·tis (pī-ō-sal′ping-gō-ō-of′ō-rī′tis). Suppurative inflammation of the fallopian tube and the ovary. [pyo- + G. *salpinx,* trumpet (tube), + oophoritis]

py·o·sal·pinx (pī-ō-sal′pingks). Distention of a fallopian tube with pus. [pyo- + G. *salpinx,* trumpet (tube)]

py·o·sis (pī-ō′sis). SYN suppuration. [G.]

py·o·tho·rax (pī-ō-thōr′aks). Empyema in a pleural cavity.

py·o·u·ra·chus (pī-ō-yū′ră-kŭs). A purulent accumulation in the urachus.

py·o·u·re·ter (pī-ō-yū-rē′ter). Distention of a ureter with pus.

pyr·a·mid (pir′ă-mid). **1.** A term applied to a number of anatomical structures having a more or less pyramidal shape. SYN pyramis [NA]. **2.** An obsolete term denoting the petrous portion of the temporal bone. [G. *pyramis (pyramid-),* a pyramid]

   anterior p., SYN p. of medulla oblongata.

🔲 **eating-right p.,** USDA guidelines for sound nutrition that categorize foods that make similar nutrient contributions with emphasis on grains, vegetables, and fruits; food sources high in animal protein, lipids, and dairy products are downplayed.

   Ferrein's p., SYN medullary *ray.*

   p. of light, a triangular area at the anterior inferior part of the tympanic membrane, running from the umbo to the periphery, where there is seen a bright reflection of light. SYN cone of light, light reflex (3), red reflex.

   malpighian p., SYN renal p.

   p. of medulla oblongata, an elongated, white prominence on the ventral surface of the medulla oblongata on either side along the anterior median fissure, corresponding to the pyramidal tract. SYN pyramis medullae oblongatae [NA], anterior p.

   medullary p., SYN renal p.

   renal p., one of a number of pyramidal masses seen on longitudinal section of the kidney; collectively, they constitute the renal medulla, and contain part of the secreting tubules and the collecting tubules. SYN pyramis renalis [NA], malpighian p., medullary p.

   p. of vermis, a subdivision of the inferior vermis of the cerebellum between the tuber and the uvula.

py·ram·i·dal (pi-ram′i-dal). **1.** Of the shape of a pyramid. **2.** Relating to any anatomical structure called pyramid.

pyr·a·mis, pl. **py·ra·mi·des** (pir′ă-mis, pi-ram′i-dēz) [NA]. SYN pyramid (1). [Mod. L. fr. G. pyramid]

   p. medul′lae oblonga′tae [NA], SYN *pyramid of medulla oblongata.*

   p. rena′lis, pl. **pyram′ides rena′les** [NA], SYN renal *pyramid.*

pyr·a·nose (pir′ă-nōs, pī′-). A cyclic form of a sugar in which the oxygen bridge forms a pyran.

py·ret·ic (pī-ret′ik). SYN febrile. [G. *pyretikos*]

△ **pyreto-.** Fever. SEE ALSO pyro- (1). [G. *pyretos,* fever, fr. *pyr,* fire]

py·rex·ia (pī-rek′sē-ă). SYN fever. [G. *pyrexis,* feverishness]

   p. of unknown origin, SYN *fever* of unknown origin.

py·rex·i·al (pī-rek′sē-ăl). Relating to fever.

pyr·i·dox·al 5′-phos·phate. a coenzyme essential to many reactions in tissue, notably transaminations and amino acid decarboxylations.

pyr·i·dox·a·mine (pir-i-dok′să-mēn). The amine of pyridoxine which has a similar physiologic action. SEE pyridoxine.

4-pyr·i·dox·ic ac·id (pir-i-dok′sik). The principal product of the metabolism of pyridoxal, appearing in the urine.

pyr·i·dox·ine (pir-i-dok′sēn, -sin). The original vitamin B₆, which term now includes pyridoxal and pyridoxamine, associated with the utilization of unsaturated fatty acids. Deficiency may result in increased irritability, convulsions, and peripheral neuritis. The hydrochloride is used in pharmaceutical preparations; the chief form in vegetables.

py·rim·i·dine (pī-rim′i-dēn). A heterocyclic substance, the formal parent of several "bases" present in nucleic acids (uracil, thymine, cytosine) as well as of the barbiturates.

pyro-. 1. fire, heat, or fever. SEE ALSO pyreto-. **2.** CHEMISTRY Combining form denoting derivatives formed by removal of water (usually by heat) to form anhydrides. SEE ALSO anhydro-. [G. *pyr,* fire]

py·ro·gen (pī′rō-jen). A fever-inducing agent that causes a rise in temperature; p.'s are produced by bacteria, molds, viruses, and yeasts, and commonly occur in distilled water. [pyro- + G. -*gen,* producing]

   endogenous p. (EP), proteins that induce fever. Several have been identified, including cytokines formed by components of the immune system, especially macrophages.

   exogenous p.'s, drugs or substances that are formed by microorganisms and induce fever. Among the latter are lipopolysaccharides and lipoteichoic acid.

py·ro·gen·ic (pī-rō-jen′ik). Causing fever.

py·ro·glob·u·lins (pī-rō-glob′yū-linz). Serum proteins (immunoglobulins), usually associated with multiple myeloma or macroglobulinemia, which precipitate irreversibly when heated to 56°C.

py·rol·y·sis (pī-rol′i-sis). Decomposition of a substance by heat. [pyro- + G. *lysis,* dissolution]

py·ro·ma·nia (pī-rō-mā′nē-ă). A morbid impulse to set fires. [pyro- + G. *mania,* frenzy]

py·ro·nin (pī′rō-nin). A fluorescent red basic xanthene dye, used in combination with methyl green for differential staining of RNA (red) and DNA (green); also used as a tracking dye for RNA in electrophoresis.

py·ro·pho·bia (pī-rō-fō′bē-ă). Morbid dread of fire. [pyro- + G. *phobos,* fear]

py·ro·phos·pha·tase (pī-rō-fos′fă-tās). Any enzyme cleaving a pyrophosphate bond between two phosphoric groups, leaving one on each of the two fragments.

py·ro·phos·phate (PP) (pī-rō-fos′fāt). A salt of pyrophosphoric acid; accumulates in cases of hypophosphatasia; sometimes referred to as inorganic p. (PP_i).

py·ro·sis (pī-rō′sis). Substernal pain or burning sensation, usually associated with regurgitation of acid-peptic gastric juice into the esophagus. SYN heartburn. [G. a burning]

pyr·role (pir′ōl). A heterocyclic compound found in many biologically important substances. SYN azole, imidole.

pyr·rol·i·dine (pi-rol′i-dēn). **1.** Pyrrole to which four H atoms have been added; the structural basis of proline and hydroxyproline. **2.** A class of alkaloids containing a p. (1) moiety or a p. derivative.

py·ru·vate (pī′rū-vāt). A salt or ester of pyruvic acid.

   p. kinase (PK), phospho*enol*pyruvate kinase; a phosphotransferase catalyzing transfer of phosphate from phospho*enol*pyruvate to ADP, forming ATP and p.; other nucleoside phosphates can participate in the reaction; a key step in glycolysis; a deficiency in p. kinase will lead to hemolytic anemia.

py·ru·vic ac·id (pī-rū′vik). An intermediate compound in the metabolism of carbohydrate; in thiamin deficiency, its oxidation is retarded and it accumulates in the tissues. SEE phosphoenolpyruvic acid.

py·u·ria (pī-yū′rē-ă). Presence of pus in the urine when voided. [G. *pyon,* pus, + *ouron,* urine]

Q

Q coulomb; quantity; quaternary; glutamine; glutaminyl; pseudouridine; coenzyme Q; electric charge; the second product formed in an enzyme-catalyzed reaction.

Q̇ blood flow. SEE flow (3). [quantity + an overdot denoting the time derivative]

Q_{CO_2} Symbol for the microliters STPD of CO_2 given off per milligram of tissue per hour.

q 1. CYTOGENETICS Long arm of a chromosome (in contrast to p for the short arm). **2.** Abbreviation for [L.] *quodque*, each, every. **3.** Symbol for heat.

QA quality assurance.

QNS quantity not sufficient (amount of specimen submitted to laboratory is inadequate to perform test requested).

quack (kwak). SYN charlatan. [Abbreviation of quacksalver, Dutch *quack*, to boast + *salf*, cream]

quad·rant (kwah′drant). One quarter of a circle. ANATOMY Roughly circular areas are divided for descriptive purposes into q.'s. The abdomen is divided into right upper and lower, and left upper and lower q.'s by a horizontal and a vertical line intersecting at the umbilicus. Q.'s of the ocular fundus (superior and inferior nasal, superior and inferior temporal) are demarcated by a horizontal and a vertical line intersecting at the optic disk. The tympanic membrane is divided into anterosuperior, anteroinferior, posterosuperior, and posteroinferior q.'s by a line drawn across the diameter of the drum in the axis of the handle of the malleus and another intersecting the first at right angles at the umbo. [L. *quadrans*, a quarter]

quad·rate (kwah′drāt). Having four equal sides; square. [L. *quadratus*, square]

quadri-. Four. [L. *quattuor*]

quad·ri·ba·sic (kwah-dri-bā′sik). Denoting an acid having four hydrogen atoms that are replaceable by atoms or radicals of a basic character.

quad·ri·ceps (kwah′dri-seps). Having four heads; denoting a muscle of the thigh, q. femoris muscle, and one of the calf, q. surae muscle, or the combined gastrocnemius (with two heads), soleus, and plantaris, more commonly called triceps surae muscle, the plantaris being counted as a separate muscle. [L. fr. quadri- + *caput*, head]

quad·ri·gem·i·nal (kwah′dri-jem′i-năl). Fourfold. [quadri- + L. *geminus*, twin]

quad·ri·ge·mi·num (kwah′dri-jem′i-nŭm). One of the quadrigeminal bodies.

quad·ri·pa·re·sis (kwah′dri-pă-rē′sis). SYN tetraparesis.

quad·ri·ple·gia (kwah′dri-plē′jē-ă). Paralysis of all four limbs. SYN tetraplegia. [quadri- + G. *plēgē*, stroke]

quad·ri·ple·gic (kwah′dri-plē′jik). Pertaining to or afflicted with quadriplegia.

quad·ri·va·lent (kwah-dri-vā′lent). Having the combining power (valency) of four. SYN tetravalent.

quad·rup·let (kwah′drŭp-let, kwă-drū′plet). One of four children born at one birth. [L. *quadruplus*, fourfold]

quality assurance (QA). An institutional program designed to assess the success of the total

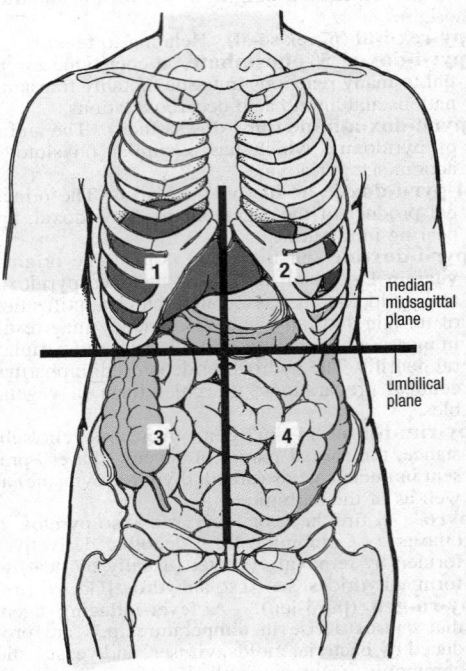

quadrants: (1) right superior, (2) left superior, (3) right inferior, (4) left inferior

organization in achieving its goals. SEE ALSO quality *control*.

quan·tile (kwon′til). Division or distribution into equal, ordered subgroups; deciles are tenths, quartiles are quarters, quintiles are fifths, terciles are thirds, centiles are hundredths. [L. *quantum*, how much, + *-ilis*, adj. suffix]

quan·tum, pl. **quan·ta** (kwahn′tŭm, -tă). **1.** A unit of radiant energy (ε) varying according to the frequency (ν) of the radiation. **2.** A certain definite amount. [L. how much]

quar·an·tine (kwar′an-tēn). The isolation of a person with a known or possible contagious disease. [It. *quarantina* fr. L. *quadraginta*, forty]

quark (qwark). A fundamental particle believed to be the primary constituent of all mesons and baryons; q.'s have a charge that is a fraction of 1 electron charge and interact through electromagnetic and nuclear forces. Six varieties are thought to exist with the unusual names of up, down, strange, charmed, bottom, and top. [a word of indeterminate sense used by James Joyce in his novel *Finnegans Wake*]

quart (kwōrt). **1.** A measure of fluid capacity; the fourth part of a gallon; the equivalent of 0.9468 liter. **2.** A dry measure holding a little more than the fluid measure. [L. *quartus*, fourth]

quar·tan (kwōr′tan). Recurring every fourth day, including the first day of an episode in the computation, *i.e.*, after a free interval of two days. SEE malariae *malaria*. [L. *quartanus*, relating to a fourth (thing)]

quartz (kwôrts). A crystalline form of silicon dioxide used in chemical apparatus and in optical and electric instruments.

qua·si·dom·i·nance (kwā-si-dom'i-nans). Simulation by a recessive trait of the pedigree of dominant inheritance (*i.e.*, recurrence in several generations) by repeated, and often occult, consanguineous matings.

qua·si·dom·i·nant (kwā-si-dom'i-nănt). Denoting a trait in an inbred pedigree that exhibits quasidominance.

qua·ter·na·ry (Q) (kwah'ter-nār-ē, kwah-ter'nĕ-rē). **1.** Denoting a chemical compound containing four elements. **2.** Fourth in a series. **3.** Relating to organic compounds in which some central atom is attached to four functional groups. **4.** Referring to a level of structure of macromolecules in which more than one biopolymer is present. [L. *quaternarius*,, fr. *quaterni*, four each, fr. *quattuor*, four, + -*arius*, adj. suffix]

quench·ing (kwench'ing). **1.** The process of extinguishing, removing, or diminishing a physical property such as heat or light. **2.** In beta liquid scintillation counting, the shifting of the energy spectrum from a true to a lower energy; it is caused by a variety of interfering materials in the counting solution. **3.** The process of stopping a chemical or enzymatic reaction. [M. E. *quenchen*, fr. O.E. *ācwencan*]

ques·tion·naire (kwes-chŭn-âr'). A list of questions submitted orally or in writing to obtain personal information or statistically useful data.

Holmes-Rahe q., a survey to measure, in life change units, the stressfulness of various life events such as an acute illness, bankruptcy, death of a loved one, etc.

Quick, Armand J., U.S. physician, 1894–1978. SEE Q.'s *method, test.*

quick (kwik). **1.** Pregnant with a child whose fetal movements are recognizable. **2.** A sensitive part, painful to touch. [A.S. *cwic*, living]

quick·en·ing (kwik'ĕn-ing). Signs of life felt by the mother as a result of the fetal movements, usually noted from 16 to 20 weeks of pregnancy. [A.S. *cwic*, living]

qui·es·cent (kwi-es'ent). At rest or inactive.

quin·sy (kwin'zē). SYN peritonsillar *abscess*. [M.E. *quinsie* (*quinesie*), a corruption of L. *cynanche*, sore throat]

quin·tan (kwin'tan). Recurring every fifth day, including the first day of an episode in the computation, *i.e.*, after a free interval of three days. [L. *quintus*, fifth]

quin·tu·plet (kwin-tŭp'let). One of five children born at one birth. [L. *quintuplex*, fivefold]

quod·que (q.) Each, every. [L.]

quo·tid·i·an (kwō-tid'ē-ăn). Daily; occurring every day. SEE quotidian *malaria*. [L. *quotidianus*, daily, fr. *quot*, as many as, + *dies*, day]

quo·tient (kwo'shĕnt). The number of times one amount is contained in another. SEE ALSO index (2), ratio. [L. *quoties*, how often]

achievement q., a ratio, percentile rating, or related q. denoting the amount a child has learned in relation to peers of his or her age or level of education.

cognitive laterality q., test for difference in cognitive performance of left and right sides of the brain.

intelligence q. (IQ), the psychologist's index of intelligence as one part of a two-part determination, the other part being an index of adaptive behavior. IQ is ordinarily expressed as a ratio between the person's score on a given test and the score which the average individual of comparable age attained on the same test.

respiratory q., the steady state ratio of carbon dioxide produced by tissue metabolism to oxygen consumed in the same metabolism; for the whole body, normally about 0.82 under basal conditions; in the steady state, the respiratory q. is equal to the respiratory exchange ratio.

qu

R

ρ rho. SEE rho.

℞ Symbol for *recipe* in a prescription. SEE prescription (2).

R$_f$, R$_F$. Symbol denoting movement of a substance in paper chromatography *r*elative to the solvent *f*ront; equal to the migration distance of a substance divided by the migration distance of the solvent front.

r racemic, occasionally used in naming compounds in place of the more common DL- or (±)-, as "r-alanine" (more often as the prefix rac-); roentgen; radius.

Ra radium.

rab•bet•ing (rab'et-ing). Making congruous stepwise cuts on apposing bone surfaces for stability after impaction. [Fr. *raboter,* to plane]

rab•id. Relating to or suffering from rabies. [L. *rabidus,* raving, mad]

ra•bies (rā'bēz). Highly fatal infectious disease transmitted by the bite of infected animals including dogs, cats, skunks, wolves, foxes, raccoons, and bats, and caused by a neurotropic lyssavirus that replicates in the central nervous system and the salivary glands. The symptoms are excitement, aggressiveness, and madness, followed by paralysis and death. Characteristic cytoplasmic inclusion bodies (Negri bodies) found in many of the neurons are an aid to rapid laboratory diagnosis. SYN hydrophobia. [L. rage, fury, fr. *rabio,* to rave, to be mad]

△**rac-.** Prefix for racemic.

rac•e•mase (rā'sē-mās). An enzyme capable of catalyzing racemization, *i.e.,* inversions of asymmetric groups; when more than one center of asymmetry is present, "epimerase" is used.

rac•e•mate (rā'sē-māt). A racemic compound, or the salt or ester of such a compound. SEE ALSO racemic.

ra•ceme (rā-sēm'). An optically inactive chemical compound. SEE ALSO racemic.

ra•ce•mic (r) (rā-sē'mik, -sem'ik). Denoting a mixture of optically active compounds that is itself optically inactive, being composed of an equal number of dextro- and levorotatory substances, which are separable.

rac•e•mi•za•tion (rā'sē-mi-zā'shŭn, ras-mi-). Partial conversion of one enantiomorph into another (as an L-amino acid to the corresponding D-amino acid) so that the specific optical rotation is decreased, or even reduced to zero, in the resulting mixture.

rac•e•mose (ras'ĕ-mōs). Branching, with nodular terminations; resembling a bunch of grapes. [L. *racemosus,* full of clusters]

△**rachi-, rachio-.** The spine. [G. *rhachis,* spine, backbone]

ra•chi•al (rā'kē-ăl). SYN spinal.

ra•chi•cen•te•sis (rā-kē-sen-tē'sis). SYN lumbar puncture. [rachi- + G. *kentēsis,* puncture]

ra•chid•i•al (rā-kid'ē-ăl). SYN spinal.

ra•chi•graph (rā'kē-graf). A graph for recording the curves of the vertebrae. [rachi- + G. *graphō,* to write]

ra•chil•y•sis (ră-kil'i-sis). Forcible correction of lateral curvature of the spine by lateral pressure against the convexity of the curve. [rachi- + G. *lysis,* a loosening]

△**rachio-.** SEE rachi-.

ra•chi•o•cen•te•sis (rā-kē-ō-sen-tē'sis). SYN lumbar *puncture.* [rachio- + G. *kentēsis,* puncture]

ra•chi•om•e•ter (rā-kē-om'ĕ-ter). An instrument for measuring the curvature of the spine, natural or pathologic, of the spinal column. [rachio- + G. *metron,* measure]

ra•chi•ot•o•my (rā-kē-ot'ō-mē). SYN laminotomy. [rachio- + G. *tomē,* incision]

ra•chis, pl. **rach•i•des, ra•chis•es** (rā'kis, rā'ki-dēz, rak-). SYN vertebral *column.* [G. spine, backbone]

ra•chis•chi•sis (ră-kis'ki-sis). **1.** Embryologic failure of fusion of vertebral arches and neural tube with consequent exposure of neural tissue at surface; spina bifida cystica with myelocele or myeloschisis. **2.** Spinal dysraphism. [G. *rhachis,* spine, + *schisis,* division]

ra•chit•ic (ră-kit'ic). Relating to or suffering from rickets (rachitis).

ra•chi•tis (ră-kī'tis). SYN rickets. [G. *rhachitis*]

rach•i•to•gen•ic (ră-kit-ō-jen'ik). Producing or causing rickets. [rachitis + G. *genesis,* production]

rad 1. The unit for the dose absorbed from ionizing radiation, equivalent to 100 ergs per gram of tissue; 100 rad = 1 Gy. **2.** Radian. **3.** Racemic.

ra•dar•ky•mog•ra•phy (rā'dar-kī-mog'ră-fē). An obsolete procedure involving the video tracking of heart motion by means of image intensification and closed circuit television during fluoroscopy; enabled cardiac motion to be measured by reproducible linear graphic tracing.

ra•dec•to•my (rā-dek'tō-mē). SYN root *amputation.* [L. *radix,* root, + G. *ektomē,* excision]

ra•di•a•bil•i•ty (rā'dē-ă-bil'i-tē). The property of being radiable.

ra•di•a•ble (rā'dē-ă-bl). Capable of being penetrated or examined by rays, especially by x-rays.

ra•di•ad (rā'dē-ad). In a direction toward the radial side.

ra•di•al (rā'dē-ăl). **1.** Relating to the radius (bone of the forearm), to any structures named from it, or to the radial or lateral aspect of the upper limb as compared to the ulnar or medial aspect. **2.** Relating to any radius. **3.** Radiating; diverging in all directions from any given center. SYN brachio- (2). [L. *radialis,* fr. *radius,* ray, lateral bone of the forearm]

ra•di•an (rad) (rā'dē-ăn). A supplementary SI unit of plane angle. [L. *radius,* ray]

ra•di•ant (rā'dē-ant). **1.** Giving out rays. **2.** A point from which light radiates to the eye.

ra•di•ate (rā'dē-āt). **1.** To spread out in all directions from a center. **2.** To emit radiation. [L. *radio,* pp. *-atus,* to shine]

ra•di•a•tio, pl. **ra•di•a•ti•o•nes** (rā-dē-ā'shē-ō, -shē-ō'nēz). NEUROANATOMY A term applied to any one of the thalamocortical fiber systems that together compose the corona radiata of the cerebral hemisphere's white matter (*e.g.,* optic radiation, acoustic radiation, etc.). SYN radiation (3). [L.]

r. acus′tica [NA], SYN acoustic *radiation*.

r. cor′poris callo′si [NA], SYN *radiation* of corpus callosum.

r. op′tica [NA], SYN optic *radiation*.

r. pyramida′lis, SYN pyramidal *radiation*.

ra·di·a·tion (rā′dē-ā′shŭn). **1.** The act or condition of diverging in all directions from a center. **2.** The sending forth of light, short radio waves, ultraviolet or x-rays, or any other rays for treatment or diagnosis or for other purpose. Cf. irradiation (2). **3.** SYN radiatio. **4.** A ray. **5.** Radiant energy or a radiant beam. [L. *radiatio,* fr. *radius,* ray, beam]

acoustic r., the fibers that pass from the medial geniculate body to the transverse temporal gyri of the cerebral cortex by way of the sublentiform part of the internal capsule. SYN radiatio acustica [NA].

background r., irradiation from environmental sources, including the earth's crust, the atmosphere, cosmic rays, and ingested radionuclides in the body.

braking r., SYN Bremsstrahlung r.

Bremsstrahlung r. (brĕmz′strah-lŭng), a high-speed electron from the cathode stream is slowed down and pulled off course by the positive pull of the target, this represents a loss of energy which is given up as heat and an x-ray photon. Most x-rays in medicine and dentistry are of Bremsstrahlung origin. SYN braking r. [Ger. *Bremse,* brake, + *Strahlung,* radiation]

characteristic r., when an incoming electron from the cathode stream that has enough energy to overcome the binding energy of electrons in the inner shells of the target material knocks the electron out of its shell, the outer electrons fall into the inner shell, giving up energy in the form of x-radiation. Produced at levels of greater than 69.5 kilovolts.

r. of corpus callosum, the spreading out of the fibers of the corpus callosum in the centrum semiovale of each cerebral hemisphere. SYN radiatio corporis callosi [NA].

corpuscular r., r. consisting of streams of subatomic particles such as protons, electrons, neutrons, etc.

electromagnetic r., wavelike energy propagated through matter or space. Varies widely in wavelength, frequency, photon energy, and properties. Is natural or artificial and includes radiowaves, microwaves, visible light, ultraviolet light, x-rays, gamma rays, and cosmic r. SYN electromagnetic spectrum.

heterogeneous r., r. consisting of different frequencies, various energies, or a variety of particles.

homogeneous r., r. consisting of a narrow band of frequencies, the same energy, or a single type of particle.

ionizing r., corpuscular (*e.g.,* neutrons, electrons) or electromagnetic (*e.g.,* gamma) r. of sufficient energy to ionize the irradiated material.

optic r., the massive, fanlike fiber system passing from the lateral geniculate body of the thalamus to the visual cortex; the fibers follow the retrolenticular and sublenticular limbs of the internal capsule into the corona radiata but they curve back along the lateral wall of the temporal and occipital horns of the lateral ventricle to the striate cortex on the medial surface and pole of the occipital lobe. SYN radiatio optica [NA].

pyramidal r., corticospinal fibers passing from the cortex into the pyramid. SYN radiatio pyramidalis.

rad·i·cal (rad′i-kăl). **1.** CHEMISTRY A group of elements or atoms usually passing intact from one compound to another, but usually incapable of prolonged existence in a free state (*e.g.,* methyl, CH_3); in chemical formulas, a r. is often distinguished by being enclosed in parentheses or brackets. **2.** Thorough or extensive; relating or directed to the extirpation of the root or cause of a morbid process; *e.g.,* a r. operation. **3.** Denoting treatment by extreme, drastic, or innovative, as opposed to conservative, measures. **4.** SYN free r. [L. *radix* (*radic-*), root]

free r., a radical in its (usually transient) uncombined state; an atom or atom group carrying an unpaired electron and no charge. Free r.'s may be involved as short-lived, highly active intermediates in various reactions in living tissue, notably in photosynthesis. The free radical nitric oxide, NO·, plays an important role in vasodilation. SYN radical (4).

ra·di·ces (rā-dī′sēz). Plural of radix.

rad·i·cle (rad′i-kl). A rootlet or structure resembling one, as the r. of a *vein,* a minute veinlet joining with others to form a vein, or the r. of a *nerve,* a nerve fiber which joins others to form a nerve. [L. *radicula,* dim. of *radix,* root]

rad·i·cot·o·my (rad-i-kot′ō-mē). SYN rhizotomy. [L. *radix* (*radic-*), root, + G. *tomē,* incision]

⌂**radicul-.** SEE radiculo-.

ra·dic·u·la (ră-dik′yū-lă). A spinal nerve root. [L. dim of *radix,* root]

ra·dic·u·lal·gia (ra-dik′yū-lal′jē-ă). Neuralgia due to irritation of the sensory root of a spinal nerve. [radicul- + G. *algos,* pain]

ra·dic·u·lar (ra-dik′yū-lăr). **1.** Relating to a radicle. **2.** Pertaining to the root of a tooth.

ra·dic·u·lec·to·my (ra-dik′yū-lek′tō-mē). SYN rhizotomy. [radicul- + G. *ektomē,* excision]

ra·dic·u·li·tis (ra-dik-yū-lī′tis). SYN radiculopathy. [radicul- + G. *-itis,* inflammation]

⌂**radiculo-, radicul-.** Radicle; radicular. [L. *radicula,* radicle, dim. of *radix,* root]

ra·dic·u·lo·gang·li·o·ni·tis (ra-dik′yū-lō-gang′glē-ō-nī′tis). Involvement of roots and ganglia.

ra·dic·u·lo·me·nin·go·my·e·li·tis (ra-dik′yū-lō-mē-ning′gō-mī-ĕ-lī′tis). SYN rhizomeningomyelitis.

ra·dic·u·lo·my·e·lop·a·thy (ra-dik′yū-lō-mī′ĕ-lop′ă-thē). SYN myeloradiculopathy.

ra·dic·u·lo·neu·rop·a·thy (ra-dik′yū-lō-nū-rop′ă-thē). Disease of the spinal nerve roots and nerves.

ra·dic·u·lop·a·thy (ra-dik′yū-lop′ă-thē). Disorder of the spinal nerve roots. SYN radiculitis. [radiculo- + G. *pathos,* suffering]

ra·di·ec·to·my (rā-dē-ek′tō-mē). SYN root *amputation.* [L. *radix,* root, + G. *ektomē,* excision]

ra·dii (rā′dē-ī). Plural of radius. [L.]

radio-. **1.** Radiation, chiefly (in medicine) gamma or x-ray. **2.** SYN radioactive. **3.** SYN radius. [L. *radius,* ray]

ra·di·o·ac·tive (rā′dē-ō-ak′tiv). Possessing radioactivity. SYN radio- (2).

ra·di·o·ac·tiv·i·ty (rā′dē-ō-ak-tiv′i-tē). The property of some atomic nuclei of spontaneously emitting gamma rays or subatomic particles (alpha and beta rays).

artificial r., the r. of isotopes created by the bombardment of naturally occurring isotopes by subatomic particles, or high levels of x- or gamma radiation.

ra·di·o·au·tog·ra·phy (rā′dē-ō-aw-tog′ră-fē). SYN autoradiography.

ra·di·o·bi·cip·i·tal (rā′dē-ō-bī-sip′i-tăl). Relating to the radius and the biceps muscle.

ra·di·o·bi·ol·o·gy (rā′dē-ō-bī-ol′ō-jē). The study of the biological effects of ionizing radiation upon living tissue. Cf. radiopathology.

ra·di·o·car·di·o·gram (rā′dē-ō-kar′dē-ō-gram). A graphic record of the concentration of injected radioisotope within the cardiac chambers.

ra·di·o·car·di·og·ra·phy (rā′dē-ō-kar-dē-og′ră-fē). The technique of recording or interpreting radiocardiograms.

ra·di·o·car·pal (rā′dē-ō-kar′păl). **1.** Relating to the radius and the bones of the carpus. **2.** On the radial or lateral side of the carpus.

ra·di·o·chem·is·try (rā′dē-ō-kem′is-trē). **1.** The science of using radionuclides to synthesize labeled compounds for biochemical or biological research, or radiopharmaceuticals for clinical diagnostic studies. **2.** The study of methods of labeling compounds with radionuclides.

ra·di·o·cin·e·ma·tog·ra·phy (rā′dē-ō-sĭ-nē-mă-tog′ră-fē). Taking a motion picture of the movements of organs or other structures as revealed by x-ray fluoroscopic examination. [radio- + G. *kinēma,* motion, + *graphō,* to write]

ra·di·o·cur·a·ble (rā′dē-ō-kyūr′ă-bl). Curable by irradiation therapy.

ra·di·o·dense (rā′dē-ō-dens). SYN radiopaque.

ra·di·o·den·si·ty (rā′dē-ō-den′si-tē). SYN radiopacity.

ra·di·o·der·ma·ti·tis (rā′dē-ō-der-mă-tī′tis). Dermatitis due to exposure to x-rays or gamma rays causing ionization of tissue water with changes resembling thermal injury.

ra·di·o·di·ag·no·sis (rā′dē-ō-dī-ag-nō′sis). Diagnosis using x-rays; or, more broadly, diagnostic imaging, including radiology, ultrasound, and magnetic resonance.

ra·di·o·fre·quen·cy (rā′dē-o-frē′kwen-sē). **1.** Radiant energy of a certain frequency range; *e.g.,* radio and television employ radiant energy having a frequency between 10^5–10^{11} Hz, while diagnostic x-rays have a frequency in the range of 3×10^{18} Hz. **2.** MAGNETIC RESONANCE IMAGING The energy applied to switch or create a gradient in the magnetic field.

ra·di·o·graph (rā′dē-ō-graf). A negative image on photographic film made by exposure to x-rays or gamma rays that have passed through matter or tissue. SYN roentgenogram, roentgenograph. [radio- + G. *graphō,* to write]

bitewing r., intraoral dental film adapted to show the coronal portion and cervical third of the root of the teeth in near occlusion; especially useful in detecting interproximal caries and determining alveolar septal height.

panoramic r., a radiographic view of the maxillae and mandible extending from the left to the right glenoid fossae.

periapical r., a r. demonstrating tooth apices and surrounding structures in a particular intraoral area.

ra·di·og·raph·er (rā-dē-og′ră-fĕr). A technician trained to position patients and take radiographs or perform other radiodiagnostic procedures.

ra·di·og·ra·phy (rā′dē-og′ră-fē). Examination of any part of the body for diagnostic purposes by means of x-rays with the record of the findings usually impressed upon a photographic film. SYN roentgenography.

advanced multiple-beam equalization r. (AMBER), a variant of scanning equalization r. using several x-ray beams.

digital r., computed radiography or computer processing of a digitized image from a conventional image-intensifier and video camera. SEE DSA.

electron r., radiographic imaging in which x-radiation is converted to a latent image and subsequently recovered by a printing process. SEE xeroradiography.

magnification r., r. using a microfocal x-ray tube and increased subject-film distance to provide magnification of the subject without loss of sharpness or increase in radiation exposure.

scanning equalization r., an electronically enhanced method of radiography in which a small x-ray beam is scanned over the patient while its attenuation is measured, providing feedback to modulate beam intensity in order to equalize average x-ray film exposure.

serial r., making several x-ray exposures of a single region over a period of time, as in angiography.

ra·di·o·im·mu·ni·ty (rā′dē-ō-i-myū′ni-tē). Lessened sensitivity to radiation.

ra·di·o·im·mu·no·as·say (rā′dē-ō-im′u-nō-as′sā). An immunological (immunochemical) procedure that uses the competition between radioisotope-labeled antigen (hormone) or other substance and unlabeled antigen for antiserums, resulting in quantitation of the unlabeled antigen; any method for detecting or quantitating antigens or antibodies using radiolabeled reactants.

ra·di·o·im·mu·no·dif·fu·sion (rā′dē-ō-im′yū-nō-di-fyū′zhŭn). A method for the study of antigen-antibody reactions by gel diffusion using radioisotope-labeled antigen or antibody.

ra·di·o·im·mu·no·elec·tro·pho·re·sis (rā′dē-ō-im′yū-nō-ē-lek′trō-fō-rē′sis). Immunoelectrophoresis in which the antigen or antibody is labeled with a radioisotope.

ra·di·o·im·mu·no·pre·cip·i·ta·tion (rā′dē-ō-im′yū-nō-prē-sip-i-tā′shŭn). Immunoprecipitation utilizing a radioisotope-labeled antibody or antigen.

ra·di·o·i·so·tope (rā′dē-ō-ī′sō-tōp). An isotope that changes to a more stable state by emitting radiation.

ra·di·o·le·sion (rā′dē-ō-lē′zhŭn). A lesion produced by ionizing radiation.

ra·di·o·li·gand (rā′dē-ō-lig′and). A molecule with a radionuclide tracer attached; usually used for radioimmunoassay procedures. [radio- + L. *ligandus,* that which is to be bound, fr. *ligo,* to bind]

ra·di·o·log·ic, ra·di·o·log·i·cal (rā-dē-ō-log′ik, -loj′i-kăl). Pertaining to radiology.

ra·di·ol·o·gist (rā-dē-ol′ō-jist). A physician trained in the diagnostic and/or therapeutic use of x-rays and radionuclides, radiation physics, and biology; a diagnostic r. is also trained in diagnostic ultrasound and magnetic resonance imaging and applicable physics.

ra·di·ol·o·gy (rā-dē-ol′ō-jē). **1.** The science of high energy radiation and of the sources and the chemical, physical, and biologic effects of such radiation; the term usually refers to the diagnosis and treatment of disease. **2.** The scientific discipline of medical imaging using ionizing radiation, radionuclides, nuclear magnetic resonance, and ultrasound. [radio- + G. *logos,* study]

ra·di·o·lu·cen·cy (rā-dē-ō-lū′sen-sē). The state of being radiolucent.

ra·di·o·lu·cent (rā-dē-ō-lū′sent). Relatively penetrable by x-rays or other forms of radiation. Cf. radiopaque. [radio- + L. *lucens,* shining]

ra·di·om·e·ter (rā-dē-om′ĕ-ter). A device for determining the penetrative power of x-rays. [radio- + G. *metron,* measure]

ra·di·o·mi·met·ic (rā′dē-ō-mi-met′ik). Imitating the biologic effects of radiation, as in the case of chemicals such as nitrogen mustards. [radio- + G. *mimētikos,* imitative]

ra·di·o·ne·cro·sis (rā′dē-ō-ne-krō′sis). Necrosis due to radiation; *e.g.,* after excessive exposure to x- or gamma rays.

ra·di·o·neu·ri·tis (rā′dē-ō-nū-rī′tis). Neuritis caused by prolonged or repeated exposure to x-rays or radium.

ra·di·o·nu·clide (rā′dē-ō-nū′klīd). An isotope of artificial or natural origin that exhibits radioactivity. R.'s are used in diagnostic imaging and cancer therapy.

ra·di·o·pac·i·ty (rā′dē-ō-pas′i-tē). State of being radiopaque. SYN radiodensity.

ra·di·o·paque (rā-dē-ō-pāk′). Exhibiting relative opacity to, or impenetrability by, x-rays or any other form of radiation. Cf. radiolucent. SYN radiodense. [radio- + Fr. opaque fr. L. *opacus,* shady]

ra·di·o·pa·thol·o·gy (rā′dē-ō-path-ol′ō-jē). A branch of radiology or pathology concerned with the effects of radiation on cells and tissues. Cf. radiobiology.

ra·di·o·pel·vim·e·try (rā′dē-ō-pel-vim′ĕ-trē). Radiographic measurement of the pelvis. SEE pelvimetry.

ra·di·o·re·cep·tor (rā′dē-ō-rē-sep′ter). **1.** A receptor that normally responds to radiant energy such as light or heat. **2.** A receptor used as a binding agent for unlabeled and radiolabeled analyte in a type of competitive binding assay called radioreceptor assay.

ra·di·o·re·sis·tant (rā′dē-ō-rē-zis′tant). Indicates cells or tissues that are less affected than average mammalian cells on exposure to radiation; when applied to neoplasms, indicates less susceptibility to damage from therapeutic radiation than the surrounding host tissues.

ra·di·o·sen·si·tive (rā′dē-ō-sen′si-tiv). Readily affected by radiation. Cf. radioresistant.

ra·di·o·sen·si·tiv·i·ty (rā′dē-ō-sen-si-tiv′i-tē). The condition of being readily affected by radiant energy.

ra·di·o·te·lem·e·try (rā′dē-ō-tĕ-lem′ĕ-trē). SEE telemetry, biotelemetry.

ra·di·o·ther·a·peu·tic (rā′dē-ō-thăr-ă-pyū′tik). Relating to radiotherapy or to radiotherapeutics.

ra·di·o·ther·a·peu·tics (rā′dē-ō-thăr-ă-pyū′tiks). The study and use of radiotherapeutic agents.

ra·di·o·ther·a·pist (rā′dē-ō-thăr′ă-pist). One who practices radiotherapy or is versed in radiotherapeutics.

ra·di·o·ther·a·py (rā′dē-ō-thăr′ă-pē). The medical specialty concerned with the use of electromagnetic or particulate radiation in the treatment of disease.

    mantle r., r. with protection of uninvolved radiosensitive structures or organs.

ra·di·o·ther·my (rā′dē-ō-ther′mē). Diathermy effected by heat from radiant sources. [radio- + G. *thermē,* heat]

ra·di·o·tox·e·mia (rā′dē-ō-tok-sē′mē-ă). Radiation sickness caused by the products of disintegration produced by the action of x-rays or other forms of radioactivity and by the depletion of certain cells and enzyme systems from the organism. [radio- + G. *toxikon,* poison, + *haima,* blood]

ra·di·o·trans·par·ent (rā′dē-ō-trans-par′ent). Allowing relatively free transmission of radiant energy.

ra·di·o·trop·ic (rā′dē-ō-trop′ik). Affected by radiation. [radio- + G. *tropē,* a turning]

ra·di·sec·to·my (rā-dē-sek′tō-mē). SYN root *amputation.* [L. *radix,* root, + G. *ektomē,* excision]

ra·di·um (Ra) (rā′dē-ŭm). A metallic element, atomic no. 88, extracted in very minute quantities from pitchblende; an alkaline earth metal with properties similar to those of barium. Its therapeutic action is similar to that of x-rays. [L. *radius,* ray]

ra·di·us, gen. and pl. **ra·dii** (rā′dē-ŭs, rā′dē-ī). **1.** [NA]. The lateral and shorter of the two bones of the forearm. **2.** A straight line passing from the center to the periphery of a circle. SYN radio- (3). [L. spoke of a wheel, rod, ray]

    ra′dii len′tis [NA], 9 to 12 faint lines on the anterior and posterior surfaces of the lens that radiate from the poles toward the equator; they mark the lines along which the ends of lens fibers abut. SYN lens stars (1).

ra·dix, gen. **ra·di·cis,** pl. **ra·di·ces** (rā′diks, rā-di′sis, rā′di-sēz or rā-dī′sēz) [NA]. **1.** SYN *root* of tooth. **2.** The hypothetical size of the birth cohort in a life table, commonly 1000 or 100,000. [L.]

ra·don (Rn) (rā′don). A gaseous radioactive element, atomic no. 86, resulting from the breakdown of radium; ^{222}Rn is medically significant as an alpha-emitter with a half-life of 3.8235 days; it is used in the treatment of certain malignancies. Poorly ventilated homes in some parts of the country accumulate a dangerous amount of naturally occurring radon gas. [from radium]

rale (rahl). An extraneous sound heard on auscultation of breath sounds; used by some to denote rhonchus and by others for crepitation. [Fr. rattle]

amphoric r., sound heard through the stethoscope associated with the movement of fluid in a lung cavity communicating with a bronchus.

cavernous r., a resonating, bubbling sound caused by air entering a cavity partly filled with fluid.

crepitant r., a fine bubbling or crackling sound produced by air mixing with very thin secretions in the smaller bronchial tubes.

dry r., a harsh or musical breath sound produced by a constriction in a bronchial tube or the presence of a viscid secretion narrowing the lumen.

gurgling r., coarse sound heard over large cavities or over trachea nearly filled with secretions.

moist r., a bubbling r. caused by air mixing with a fluid exudate in the bronchial tubes or a cavity.

sibilant r., a whistling sound caused by air moving through a viscid secretion narrowing the lumen of a bronchus.

sonorous r., a cooing or snoring sound often produced by the vibration of a projecting mass of viscid secretion in a large bronchus.

ra•mal (rā′măl). Relating to a ramus.

ra•mi (rā′mī). Plural of ramus. [L.]

ram•i•fi•ca•tion (ram′i-fi-kā′shŭn). The process of dividing into a branchlike pattern.

ram•i•fy (ram′i-fī). To split into a branchlike pattern. [L. *ramus,* branch, + *facio,* to make]

ram•i•sec•tion (ram-i-sek′shŭn). Section of the rami communicantes of the sympathetic nervous system. [L. *ramus,* branch, + L. *sectio,* section]

ram•i•tis (ram-ī′tis). Inflammation of a ramus. [L. *ramus,* branch, + G. *-itis,* inflammation]

ram•u•lus, pl. **ram•u•li** (ram′yū-lŭs, -lī). A small branch or twig; one of the terminal divisions of a ramus. [L. dim. of *ramus,* a branch]

ra•mus, pl. **ra•mi** (rā′mŭs, rā′mī) [NA]. **1.** SYN branch. **2.** One of the primary divisions of a nerve or blood vessel. SEE ALSO artery, nerve. **3.** A part of an irregularly shaped bone (less slender than a "process") that forms an angle with the main body (*e.g.,* ramus of mandible). **4.** One of the primary divisions of a cerebral sulcus. [L.]

ran•cid (ran′sid). Having a disagreeable odor and taste, usually characterizing fat undergoing oxidation or bacterial decomposition to more volatile odoriferous substances. [L. *rancidus,* stinking, rank]

range (rānj). A statistical measure of the dispersion or variation of values determined by the endpoint values themselves or the difference between them; *e.g.,* in a group of children aged 6, 8, 9, 10, 13, and 16, the r. would be from 6 to 16 or, alternately, 10 (16 minus 6). [O.Fr. *rang,* line fr. Germanic]

normal r., SYN reference r.

reference r., the usual r. of test values for a healthy population. SYN normal r.

target heart rate r., SYN training-sensitive *zone.*

therapeutic r., refers to either the dosage r. or blood plasma or serum concentration expected to achieve therapeutic effects.

range of motion (ROM). 1. the measured beginning and terminal angles, as well as the total degrees of r.o.m., traversed by a joint moved by active muscle contraction or by passive movement. **2.** joint movement (active, passive, or a combination of both) carried out to assess, preserve, or increase the arc of joint r.o.m.

ra•nine (rā′nīn). **1.** Relating to the frog. **2.** Relating to the undersurface of the tongue. [L. *rana,* frog]

ran•u•la (ran′yū-lă). **1.** Hypoglottis. **2.** Any cystic tumor of the undersurface of the tongue or floor of the mouth, especially one of the floor of the mouth due to obstruction of the duct of the sublingual glands. SYN ptyalocele, sialocele, sublingual cyst. [L. tadpole, dim. of *rana,* frog]

ran•u•lar (ran′yū-lăr). Relating to a ranula.

RAO right anterior oblique, a radiographic projection.

rape (rāp). **1.** Sexual intercourse by force, duress, intimidation, or without legal consent (as with a minor). **2.** The performance of such an act. [L. *rapio,* to seize, to drag away]

ra•phe (rā′fē) [NA]. The line of union of two contiguous, bilaterally symmetrical structures. [G. *rhaphē,* suture, seam]

anogenital r., in the male embryo the line of closure of the genital folds and swellings extending from the anus to the tip of the penis; it is differentiated in the adult into three regions: perineal r., scrotal r., and penile r.

palatine r., a rather narrow, low elevation in the center of the hard palate that extends from the incisive papilla posteriorly over the entire length of the mucosa of the hard palate.

penile r., the continuation of the r. of the scrotum onto the underside of the penis.

perineal r., the central anteroposterior line of the perineum, most marked in the male, being continuous with the r. of the scrotum.

scrotal r., a central line, like a cord, running over the scrotum from the anus to the root of the penis; it marks the position of the septum scroti.

rap•port (rap-ōr′). **1.** A feeling of relationship, especially when characterized by emotional affinity. **2.** A conscious feeling of accord, trust, empathy, and mutual responsiveness between two or more persons (*e.g.,* physician and patient) that fosters the therapeutic process. [Fr.]

rar•e•fac•tion (rār-ĕ-fak′shŭn). The process of becoming light or less dense; the condition of being light; opposed to condensation. [L. *rarus,* rare, + *facio,* to make]

RAS reticular activating *system.*

rash. Lay term for a cutaneous eruption. [O. Fr. *rasche,* skin eruption, fr. L. *rado,* pp. *rasus,* to scratch, scrape]

diaper r., SYN diaper *dermatitis.*

drug r., SYN drug *eruption.*

heat r., SYN *miliaria* rubra.

ras•pa•to•ry (ras′pă-tōr-ē). A surgical instrument used to smooth the edges of a divided bone. [L. *raspatorium*]

RAST radioallergosorbent *test.*

rat. A rodent of the genus *Rattus*, involved in the spread of some diseases, including bubonic plague.

  albino r.'s, r.'s with white fur and pink eyes; used extensively in laboratory experiments.

rate (rāt). **1.** A measurement of an event or process in terms of its relation to some fixed standard; measurement is expressed as the ratio of one quantity to another (*e.g.*, velocity, distance per unit time). **2.** A measure of the frequency of an event in a defined population; the components of a r. are: the numerator (number of events); the denominator (population at risk of experiencing the event); the specified time in which the events occur; and usually a multiplier, a power of 10, which makes it possible to express the rate as a whole number. [L. *ratum,* a reckoning (see ratio)]

  attack r., a cumulative incidence rate used for particular groups observed for limited periods under special circumstances, such as during an epidemic.

  birth r., a summary r. based on the number of live births in a population over a given period, usually one year; the numerator is the number of live births, the denominator is the midyear population.

  case fatality r., the proportion of individuals contracting a disease that die of that disease.

  concordance r., the rate of occurrence of a trait, behavior, or action in members of a specified group that are concordant for a trait of interest. Broadly, it is taken as evidence of causal connection.

  death r., an estimate of the proportion of the population that dies during a specified period, usually a year; the numerator is the number of people dying, the denominator is the number in the population, usually an estimate of the number at the midperiod. SYN mortality r., mortality (2).

  erythrocyte sedimentation r. (ESR), the rate of settling of red blood cells in anticoagulated blood; increased r.'s are often associated with anemia or inflammatory states.

  fatality r., the death r. observed in a designated series of persons affected by a simultaneous event such as a disaster.

  five-year survival r., the proportion of patients still alive five years after a diagnosis or form of treatment is completed. Usually applied to statistics of survival of cancer patients, since, after five years, recurrences are less likely.

  glomerular filtration r. (GFR), the volume of water filtered out of the plasma through glomerular capillary walls into Bowman's capsules per unit time; it is considered to be equivalent to inulin clearance.

  growth r., absolute or relative growth increase, expressed per unit of time.

  heart r., r. of the heart's beat, recorded as the number of beats per minute.

  infant mortality r., a measure of the r. of deaths of liveborn infants before their first birthday; the numerator is the number of infants under one year of age born alive in a defined region during a calendar year who die before they are one year old; the denominator is the total number of live births.

  mitotic r., the proportion of cells in a tissue that are undergoing mitosis, expressed as a mitotic index or, roughly, as the number of cells in mitosis in each microscopic high-power field in tissue sections.

  morbidity r., the proportion of patients with a particular disease during a given year per given unit of population.

  mortality r., SYN death r.

  mutation r., the probability (or proportion) of progeny genes with a particular component of the genome not present in either biological parent; usually expressed as the number of mutants per generation occurring at one gene or locus.

  neonatal mortality r., the number of deaths in the first 28 days of life divided by the number of live births occurring in the same population during the same period of time.

  pulse r., r. of the pulse as observed in an artery; recorded as beats per minute.

  respiration r., frequency of breathing, recorded as the number of breaths per minute.

  sedimentation r., the sinking velocity of blood cells, *i.e.*, the degree of rapidity with which the red cells sink in a mass of drawn blood.

  slew r., in electronic pacemaker function, the maximum rate of change of an amplifier output voltage; important variable affecting heart function as controlled by an electronic pacemaker.

rating of perceived exertion (RPE). subjective numerical rating (range 6–19) of exercise intensity based on how an individual feels in relation to level of physiologic stress. An RPE of 13 or 14 (exercise that feels "somewhat hard") coincides with an exercise heart rate of about 70% maximum. SYN Borg scale.

RPE scale	
6	
7	very, very light
8	
9	very light
10	
11	fairly light
12	
13	somewhat hard
14	
15	hard
16	
17	very hard
18	
19	very, very hard

scale of perceived exertion

ra·tio (ra′shē-ō). An expression of the relation of one quantity to another (*e.g.*, of a proportion or rate). SEE ALSO index (2), quotient. [L. *ratio (ra-*

tion-) a reckoning, reason, fr. *reor,* pp. *ratus,* to reckon, compute]

accommodative convergence-accommodation r. (AC/A), the amount of convergence (measured in prism diopters of convergence) divided by the amount of accommodation (measured in diopters) required to direct both eyes upon an object.

albumin-globulin r., the r. of albumin to globulin in the serum or in the urine in kidney disease; the normal r. in the serum is approximately 1.55.

ALT:AST r., the r. of serum alanine aminotransferase to serum aspartate aminotransferase; elevated serum levels of both enzymes characterize hepatic disease; when both levels are abnormally elevated and the ALT:AST r. is greater than 1.0, severe hepatic necrosis or alcoholic hepatic disease is likely; when the r. is less than 1.0, an acute nonalcoholic hepatic condition is favored.

amylase-creatinine clearance r., a test for the diagnosis of acute pancreatitis; it is determined by measuring amylase and creatinine in serum and urine.

cardiothoracic r., the r. of the horizontal diameter of the heart to the inner diameter of the rib cage at its widest point as determined on a chest roentgenogram.

cup:disc r., the r. between the diameter of the cupped or depressed central zone of the optic disc and the diameter of the entire disc; normally less than 1:3, it is increased in glaucoma.

extraction r. (E), the fraction of a substance removed from the blood flowing through the kidney.

IRI/G r., the r. of immunoreactive insulin to serum or plasma glucose.

lecithin/sphingomyelin r., a r. used to determine fetal pulmonary maturity, found by testing the amniotic fluid; when the lungs are mature, lecithin exceeds sphingomyelin by 2 to 1.

M:E r., the r. of myeloid to erythroid precursors in bone marrow; normally it varies from 2:1 to 4:1; an increased r. is found in infections, chronic myelogenous leukemia, or erythroid hypoplasia; a decreased r. may mean a depression of leukopoiesis or normoblastic hyperplasia depending on the overall cellularity of the bone marrow.

molecular weight r. (M_r), SYN molecular *weight.*

nuclear:cytoplasmic r., the r. of the volume of the cell's nucleus to the volume of the cytoplasm. In general, as blood cells mature, the N:C r. decreases.

respiratory exchange r., the r. of the net output of carbon dioxide to the simultaneous net uptake of oxygen at a given site, both expressed as moles or STPD volumes per unit time.

segregation r., GENETICS the proportion of progeny of a particular genotype or phenotype from actual matings of specified genotypes. The test of a mendelian hypothesis is the comparison of the segregation r. with the mendelian r.

sex r., (1) the r. of male to female progeny at some specified stage of the life cycle, notably at

conception (primary), at birth (secondary), or at any stage between birth and death (tertiary); **(2)** the r. of the numbers of males to females affected by a particular disease or trait.

signal-to-noise r., the relative intensity of a signal to the random variation in signal intensity, or noise; used to evaluate many imaging techniques and electronic systems.

therapeutic r., the r. of the maximally tolerated dose of a drug to the minimal curative or effective dose; LD_{50} divided by ED_{50}.

ventilation/perfusion r. ($\dot{V}a/\dot{Q}$), the r. of alveolar ventilation to simultaneous alveolar capillary blood flow in any part of the lung; because both ventilation and perfusion are expressed per unit volume of tissue and per unit time, which cancel, the units become liters of gas per liter of blood.

zeta sedimentation r., the r. of the zetacrit to the hematocrit, normally 0.41 to 0.54 (41 to 54%); it is a sensitive indicator of the erythrocyte sedimentation rate (ESR) and is unaffected by anemia.

ra·tion·al (rash'ŭn-ăl). **1.** Pertaining to reasoning or to the higher thought processes; based on objective or scientific knowledge, in contrast to empirical (1). **2.** Influenced by reasoning rather than by emotion. **3.** Having the reasoning faculties; not delirious or comatose. [L. *rationalis,* fr. *ratio,* reason]

ra·tion·al·i·za·tion (ra-shŭn-ăl-i-zā'shŭn). A psychoanalytic defense mechanism through which irrational behavior, motives, or feelings are made to appear reasonable. [L. *ratio,* reason]

RAV Rous-associated *virus.*

ray (rā). **1.** A beam of light, heat, or other form of radiation. The r.'s from radium and other radioactive substances are produced by a spontaneous disintegration of the atom; they are electrically charged particles or electromagnetic waves of extremely short wavelength. **2.** A part or branch that extends radially from a structure. [L. *radius*]

beta r., SYN beta *particle.*

grenz r. (grents), very soft x-r.'s, closely allied to the ultraviolet r.'s in their wavelength (*i.e.,* long) and in their biologic action upon tissues; they are produced by a specially built vacuum tube with a hot cathode operating from a transformer delivering not more than 8 kw. [Ger. *Grenze,* borderline, boundary]

medullary r., the center of the renal lobule, which has the shape of a small, steep pyramid, consisting of straight tubular parts; these may be either ascending or descending limbs of the nephronic loop or collecting tubules. SYN Ferrein's pyramid.

roentgen r., SYN x-ray.

x-r., SEE x-ray.

rbc, RBC red blood *cell*; red blood count.

RBF renal blood flow. SEE effective renal blood *flow.*

RBRVS Resource Based Relative Value Scale.

RCP respiratory care *practitioner.*

RDA recommended daily *allowance.*

Re rhenium.

△**re-.** Prefix meaning again or backward. [L.]

re•act (rē-akt′). To take part in or to undergo a chemical reaction. [Mod. L. *reactus*]

re•ac•tance (X) (rē-ak′tans). The weakening of an alternating electric current by passage through a coil of wire or a condenser.

re•ac•tant (rē-ak′tant). A substance taking part in a chemical reaction.

re•ac•tion (rē-ak′shŭn). **1.** The response of a muscle or other living tissue or organism to a stimulus. **2.** The color change effected in litmus and certain other organic pigments by contact with substances such as acids or alkalies; also the property that such substances possess of producing this change. **3.** In chemistry, the intermolecular action of two or more substances upon each other, whereby these substances are caused to disappear, new ones being formed in their place (chemical r.). **4.** In immunology, *in vivo* or *in vitro* action of antibody on specific antigen, with or without involvement of complement or other components of the immunological system. [L. *re-*, again, backward, + *actio,* action]

acute situational r., SYN stress r.

adverse r., any undesirable or unwanted consequence of a preventive, diagnostic, or therapeutic procedure or regimen.

adverse drug r. (ADR), any noxious, unintended, and undesired effect of a drug after its administration for prophylaxis, diagnosis, or therapy. SYN adverse drug event.

alarm r., the various phenomena, *e.g.,* stimulated endocrine activity, which the body exhibits as an adaptive response to injury or stress; first phase of the general adaptation syndrome.

allergic r., a local or general r. of an organism following contact with a specific allergen to which it has been previously exposed and sensitized.

anamnestic r., augmented production of an antibody due to previous response of the subject to stimulus by the same antigen.

antigen-antibody r., the phenomenon, occurring *in vitro* or *in vivo*, of antibody combining with antigen of the type that stimulated the formation of the antibody, thereby resulting in agglutination, precipitation, complement fixation, greater susceptibility to ingestion and destruction by phagocytes, or neutralization of exotoxin. SEE ALSO skin *test*.

anxiety r., a psychological r. or experience involving the apprehension of danger accompanied by a feeling of dread and such physical symptoms as an increase in the rate of breathing, sweating, and tachycardia, in the absence of a clearly identifiable fear stimulus; when chronic, it is called generalized anxiety *disorder*. SEE ALSO panic *attack.*

Bence Jones r., the classic means of identifying Bence Jones protein, which precipitates when urine containing it is gradually warmed to 45° to 70°C, and redissolves as the urine is heated to near boiling.

bi-bi r., a r. catalyzed by a single enzyme in which two substrates and two products are involved; the ping-pong mechanism may be involved in such a r. Cf. mechanism.

biuret r., the formation of biuret, which gives a violet color due to the r. of a polypeptide of more than three amino acids with $CuSO_4$ in strongly alkaline solution; used for the detection and quantitation of polypeptides or protein in biological fluids.

catastrophic r., the disorganized behavior that is the response to a severe shock or threatening situation with which the person cannot cope.

cell-mediated r., immunological r. of the delayed type, involving chiefly T lymphocytes, important in host defense against infection, in autoimmune diseases, and in transplant rejection. SEE ALSO skin *test*.

chain r., a self-perpetuating r. in which a product of one step in the r. itself serves to bring about the next step in the r., and so on. Cf. autocatalysis.

constitutional r., a generalized r. in contrast to a focal or local r.; in allergy the immediate or delayed response, following the introduction of an allergen, occurring at sites remote from that of injection.

conversion r., SYN conversion *hysteria.*

cross r., a specific r. between an antiserum and an antigen complex other than the antigen complex that evoked the various specific antibodies of the antiserum. It is due to the fact that each complex includes among its antigenic determinants at least one that is also included in the other complex.

cytotoxic r., an immunologic (allergic) r. in which noncytotropic IgG or IgM antibody combines with specific antigen on cell surfaces; the resulting complex initiates the activation of complement which causes cell lysis or other damage, or, in the absence of complement, may lead to phagocytosis or may enhance T lymphocyte involvement.

r. of degeneration (DR), the electrical r. in a degenerated nerve and the muscles supplied by it; characterized by absence of response to both galvanic and faradic stimulus in the nerve and to faradic stimulus in the muscles.

delayed r., a local or generalized immune response that begins 24 to 48 hours after exposure to an antigen. SEE cell-mediated r.

dissociative r., r. characterized by such dissociative behavior as amnesia, fugues, sleepwalking, and dream states.

dystonic r., a state of abnormal tension or muscle tone, similar to dystonia, produced as a side effect of certain antipsychotic medication; a severe form, where the eyes appear to roll up into the head, is called oculogyric crisis.

eye-closure pupil r., a constriction of both pupils when an effort is made to close eyelids forcibly held apart. A variant of the pupil response to near vision.

false-negative r., an erroneous or mistakenly negative response.

false-positive r., an erroneous or mistakenly positive response.

focal r., a r. which occurs at the point of entrance of an infecting organism or of an injection, as in the Arthus phenomenon. SYN local r.

general adaptation r., SEE general adaptation *syndrome.*

re

graft versus host r. (GVHR), clinical and histologic changes of graft versus host disease occurring in a specific organ.

Herxheimer's r., an inflammatory r. induced in certain cases of treponemal infection (syphilis, Lyme disease) by treatment with Salvarsan, mercury, or antibiotics; believed to be due to a rapid release of treponemal antigen with an associated allergic reaction in the patient. SYN Jarisch-Herxheimer r.

immediate r., local or generalized immune response that begins within a few minutes to about an hour after exposure to an antigen to which the individual has been sensitized. SEE ALSO skin *test*, wheal-and-erythema r.

immune r., antigen-antibody r. indicating a certain degree of resistance.

intracutaneous r., intradermal r., a r. following the injection of antigen into the skin of a sensitive subject, such as in the case of the tuberculin test.

Jarisch-Herxheimer r., SYN Herxheimer's r.

leukemoid r., SEE leukemoid reaction.

local r., SYN focal r.

mixed agglutination r., immune agglutination in which the aggregates contain cells of two different kinds but with common antigenic determinants; when used to identify isoantigens, the test cells are exposed to appropriate isoantibody, washed, and then mixed with indicator erythrocytes that combine with free sites on the test cell-attached isoantibody.

Neufeld r., SYN Neufeld capsular *swelling*.

ninhydrin r., a test for proteins, peptones, peptides, and amino acids possessing free carboxyl and α-amino groups that is based upon the r. with triketohydrinene hydrate; a blue color r. is used to quantitate free amino acids.

polymerase chain r. (PCR) (po-lim′er-ās), an enzymatic method for the repeated copying and amplification of the two strands of DNA of a particular gene sequence. It is widely used in the detection of HIV.

In vivo, DNA polymerase facilitates the replication of DNA. During replication, a helical DNA molecule "unzips" and the polymerase moves along one strand mediating the addition of free nucleotides to form complementary base pairs with the nucleotides on the strand. The laboratory technique known as polymerase chain reaction exploits the capacity of DNA polymerase to assemble new DNA. The polymerase is added to a mixture of free nucleotides and primers. Primers are specially prepared units containing both RNA and DNA with a free terminus where the polymerase will react. The short sequence of DNA to be amplified is flanked by two primers. Once the reaction begins, the polymerase churns out multiple copies of the target sequence, which can then be recovered for analysis. PCR is used as a forensic tool, one which is more accurate by one or two magnitudes than DNA fingerprinting.

quellung r., (1) SYN Neufeld capsular *swelling*. **(2)** if pneumococcal organisms, India ink, and specific antisera are mixed, the antibodies present in the sera will bind to the polysaccharide antigens of the pneumococcal capsule and the capsule will appear more opaque and swollen. [Ger. *Quellung,* swelling]

Schultz-Charlton r., the specific blanching of a scarlatinal rash at the site of intracutaneous injection of scarlatina antiserum.

serum r., SYN serum *sickness*.

specific r., the phenomena produced by an agent that is identical with or immunologically related to the one that has stimulated an immune response.

stress r., an acute emotional r. related to extreme environmental stress. SYN acute situational r.

symptomatic r., an allergic response similar to the original one, but occurring after the use of a test or therapeutic dose of an allergen or atopen.

Weil-Felix r., SYN Weil-Felix *test*.

Wernicke's r., in hemianopia, a r. due to damage of the optic tract, consisting in loss of pupillary constriction when the light is directed to the blind side of the retina; pupillary constriction is maintained when light stimulates the normal side. SYN Wernicke's sign.

wheal-and-erythema r., the characteristic immediate r. observed in the skin test; within 10 to 15 minutes after injection of antigen (allergen), an irregular, blanched, elevated wheal appears, surrounded by an area of erythema (flare). SYN wheal-and-flare r.

wheal-and-flare r., SYN wheal-and-erythema r.

re•ac•ti•vate (rē-ak′ti-vāt). **1.** To render active again. **2.** In particular, of an inactivated immune serum to which normal serum (complement) is added.

re•ac•tiv•i•ty (rē-ak-tiv′i-tē). **1.** The property of reacting, chemically or in any other sense. **2.** The process of reacting.

read•through (rēd′thrū). MOLECULAR BIOLOGY Transcription of a nucleic acid sequence beyond its normal termination sequence.

re•a•gent (rē-ā′jent). Any substance added to a solution of another substance to participate in a chemical reaction. [Mod. L. *reagens*]

re•al•i•ty aware•ness. The ability to distinguish external objects as being different from oneself.

re•al•i•ty test•ing. See under testing.

ream•er (rē′mer). A rotating finishing or drilling tool used to shape or enlarge a hole. [A.S. *ryman,* to widen]

re•breath•ing (rē-brēdh′ing). Inhalation of part or all of gases previously exhaled.

re•cal•ci•fi•ca•tion (rē-kal′si-fi-kā′shŭn). Restoration to the tissues of lost calcium salts.

re•call (rē′kawl). The process of remembering thoughts, words, and actions of a past event in an attempt to recapture actual happenings.

re•ca•nal•i•za•tion (rē-kan′ăl-i-zā′shŭn). **1.** Restoration of a lumen in a blood vessel following thrombotic occlusion, by organization of the thrombus with formation of new channels. **2.** Spontaneous restoration of the continuity of the lumen of any occluded duct or tube, as with postvasectomy r.

re•cep•tac•u•lum, pl. **re•cep•tac•u•la** (rē′septak′yū-lŭm, -lă). A receptacle. SYN reservoir. [L.

fr. *re-cipio,* pp. *-ceptus,* to receive, fr. *capio,* to take]

re•cep•tor (rē-sep'tŏr, tōr). **1.** A structural protein molecule on the cell surface or within the cytoplasm that binds to a specific factor, such as a hormone, antigen, or neurotransmitter. **2.** Any of the sensory nerve endings in the skin, deep tissues, viscera, and special sense organs. [L. receiver, fr. *recipio,* to receive]

  adrenergic r.'s, reactive components of effector tissues, most of which are innervated by the sympathetic nervous system. Such r.'s can be activated by norepinephrine, epinephrine, and adrenergic drugs; r. activation results in a change in effector tissue function, such as contraction of arteriolar muscles or relaxation of bronchial muscles. SYN adrenoreceptors.

  α-**adrenergic r.'s,** adrenergic r.'s in effector tissues capable of selective activation by methoxamine and blockade by phenoxybenzamine. Their activation results in physiological responses such as increased peripheral vascular resistance, mydriasis, and contraction of pilomotor muscles.

  β-**adrenergic r.'s,** adrenergic r.'s in effector tissues capable of selective activation by isoproterenol and blockade by propranolol. Their activation results in physiological responses such as increases in cardiac rate and force of contraction (β_1), and relaxation of bronchial and vascular smooth muscle (β_2).

  cholinergic r.'s, chemical sites in effector cells or at synapses through which acetylcholine exerts its action.

  opiate r.'s, regions of the brain which have the capacity to bind morphine; some, along the aqueduct of Sylvius and in the centromedian nucleus, are in areas related to pain, but others, as in the striatum, are not related.

  stretch r.'s, r.'s that are sensitive to elongation, especially those in Golgi tendon organs and muscle spindles, but also those found in visceral organs such as the stomach, small intestine, and urinary bladder.

  T-cell r. (TCR), an adhesion molecule on the membrane of T-lymphocytes that serves as the receptor for antigen bound to antigen-presenting cells (APC) via MHC molecules. It is expressed in a complex with CD3. It is in close proximity to the MHC-restricted r. (CD4 or CD8). SYN T-lymphocyte antigen r.

  T-lymphocyte antigen r., SYN T-cell r.

re•cess (rē'ses). A small hollow or indentation. SYN recessus [NA]. [L. *recessus*]

  epitympanic r., the upper portion of the tympanic cavity above the tympanic membrane; it contains the head of the malleus and the body of the incus.

re•ces•sion (rē-sesh'ŭn). A withdrawal or retreating. SEE ALSO retraction. [L. *recessio* (see recessus)]

  tendon r., surgical displacement of the tendon of an eye muscle posterior to its anatomic insertion.

re•ces•sive (rē-ses'iv). **1.** Drawing away; receding. **2.** GENETICS Denoting a trait due to a particular allele that does not manifest itself in the presence of other alleles that generate traits dominant to it.

re•ces•sus, pl. **re•ces•sus** (rē-ses'ŭs) [NA]. SYN recess. [L. a withdrawing, a receding]

re•cid•i•va•tion (rē-sid-i-vā'shŭn). Relapse of a disease, a symptom, or a behavioral pattern such as an illegal activity for which one was previously imprisoned. [L. *recidivus,* falling back, recurring; fr. *re-* cido, to fall back]

re•cid•i•vism (rē-sid'i-vizm). The tendency of an individual toward recidivation. [L. *recidivus,* recurring]

re•cid•i•vist (rē-sid'i-vist). A person who tends toward recidivation.

rec•i•pe (res'i-pē). **1.** The superscription of a prescription, usually indicated by the sign ℞. **2.** A prescription or formula. [L. imperative of *recipio,* to receive]

rec•li•na•tion (rek-li-nā'shŭn). Turning the cataractous lens over into the vitreous to displace it from the line of vision. [L. *reclino,* pp. *-atus,* to bend back]

re•com•bi•nant (rē-kom'bi-nant). **1.** A progeny that has received chromosomal parts from different parental strains as a result of uncorrected crossing over. **2.** Pertaining to or denoting such organisms. **3.** In linkage analysis, the change of coupling phase at two loci during meiosis. If two syntenic, nonallelic genes are inherited from the same parent, they must be in coupling.

re•com•bi•nant DNA. Altered DNA resulting from the insertion into the chain, by chemical, enzymatic, or biological means, of a sequence (a whole or partial chain of DNA) not originally (biologically) present in that chain.

re•com•bi•na•tion (rē-kom-bi-nā'shŭn). **1.** The process of reuniting of parts that had become separated. **2.** The reversal of coupling phase in meiosis as gauged by the resulting phenotype. SEE ALSO recombinant.

rec•ord (rek'erd). **1.** MEDICINE A chronologic written account that includes a patient's initial complaint(s) and medical history, the physician's physical findings, the results of diagnostic tests and procedures, and any therapeutic medications and/or procedures. **2.** DENTISTRY A registration or desired jaw relations in a plastic material or on a device to permit these relationships to be transferred to an articulator. [M.E. *recorden,* fr. O.Fr. *recorder,* fr. L. *re-cordor,* to remember, fr. *re-,* back, again, + *cor,* heart]

  anesthesia r., a written account of drugs administered, procedures undertaken, and physiologic responses during the course of surgical or obstetrical anesthesia.

  computer-based patient r., electronic health r. that integrates all of a patient's health care information into a database for accessibility; the CPR supports patient care decision making and research. SEE ALSO Computer-Based Patient Record Institute.

  health r., formerly known as the medical r.; a comprehensive r. containing all the information in the medical r. but also covering all aspects of the patient's physical, mental, and social health.

  hospital r., the medical r. generated during hospitalization, containing a history and physical ex-

re

amination report, physicians' progress notes and treatment orders, notes of nurses' observations and treatments administered, reports of laboratory tests, x-ray and other diagnostic studies, surgical procedures, consultants' opinions, and a discharge summary or autopsy record.

   medical r., SEE record (1).

   problem-oriented r. (POR), a system of record keeping in which a list of the patient's problems is made and all history, physical findings, and laboratory data pertinent to each problem are placed under that heading; especially useful for outpatient records of patients with many problems who are followed for long periods.

   unit r., single, comprehensive collection of all health care data for all episodes of care for a patient.

recorded detail. The visible sharpness of features on a radiograph (for example, bone trabeculae or pulmonary markings).

re•cru•des•cence (rē-krū-des′ens). Resumption of a morbid process or its symptoms after a period of remission. [L. *re-crudesco,* to become raw again, break out afresh, fr. *crudus,* raw, harsh]

re•cru•des•cent (rē-krū-des′ent). Becoming active again, relating to a recrudescence.

re•cruit•ment (rē-krūt′ment). **1.** AUDIOLOGY The unequal reaction of the ear to equal steps of increasing intensity, measured in decibels, with greater than normal increment in perceived loudness. **2.** The bringing into activity of additional motor neurons, causing greater activity in response to increased duration of the stimulus applied to a given receptor or afferent nerve. SEE ALSO irradiation. **3.** The adding of parallel channels of flow in any system. [Fr. *recrutement,* fr. L. *re-cresco,* pp. *-cretus,* to grow again]

⌂**rect-.** SEE recto-.

rec•tal (rek′tăl). Relating to the rectum.

rec•tal•gia (rek-tal′jē-ă). SYN proctalgia.

rec•tec•to•my (rek-tek′tō-mē). SYN proctectomy.

rec•ti•fy (rek′ti-fī). **1.** To correct. **2.** To purify or refine by distillation; usually implies repeated distillations. [L. *rectus,* right, straight]

rec•ti•tis (rek-tī′tis). SYN proctitis.

⌂**recto-, rect-.** The rectum. SEE ALSO procto-. [L. *rectum,* fr. *rectus,* straight]

rec•to•cele (rek′tō-sēl). SYN proctocele. [recto- + G. *kēlē,* tumor, hernia]

rec•to•coc•cy•pexy (rek-tō-kok′si-pek-sē). SYN proctococcypexy.

rec•to•pexy (rek′tō-pek-sē). SYN proctopexy.

rec•to•plas•ty (rek′tō-plas-tē). SYN proctoplasty.

rec•to•scope (rek′tō-skōp). SYN proctoscope.

rec•to•sig•moid (rek′tō-sig′moyd). The rectum and sigmoid colon considered as a unit; the term is also applied to the junction of the sigmoid colon and rectum.

rec•to•ste•no•sis (rek′tō-stĕ-nō′sis). SYN proctostenosis.

rec•tos•to•my (rek-tos′tō-mē). SYN proctostomy.

rec•tot•o•my (rek-tot′ō-mē). SYN proctotomy.

rec•tum, pl. **rec•tums, rec•ta** (rek′tŭm, rek′tă) [NA]. The terminal portion of the digestive tube, extending from the rectosigmoid junction to the anal canal. [L. *rectus,* straight, pp. of *rego,* to make straight]

re•cum•bent (rē-kŭm′bent). Leaning; reclining; lying down. [L. *recumbo,* to lie back, recline, fr. *re-,* back, + *cubo,* to lie]

re•cu•per•ate (rē-kū′per-āt). To undergo recuperation. [L. *recupero* (or *recip-*), pp. *-atus,* to take again, recover]

re•cur•rence (rē-kŭr′ens). **1.** A return of the symptoms in the course of a disease, following improvement or remission. **2.** SYN relapse. **3.** Appearance of a genetic trait in a relative of a proband. [L. *re-curro,* to run back, recur]

re•cur•rent (rē-kŭr′ent). **1.** ANATOMY Turning back on itself. **2.** Denoting symptoms or lesions reappearing after an intermission or remission.

re•cur•va•tion (rē-ker-vā′shŭn). A backward bending or flexure. [L. *re-curvus,* bent back]

re•din•te•gra•tion (rē′din-tĕ-grā′shŭn). **1.** The restoration of lost or injured parts. **2.** Restoration to health. **3.** The recalling of a whole experience on the basis only of some item or portion of the original stimulus or circumstances of the experience. [L. *red-integro,* pp. *-atus,* to make whole again, renew, fr. *integer,* untouched, entire]

re•dox (rēd′oks). Contraction of reduction-oxidation.

re•duce (rē-dūs′). **1.** To perform reduction (1). **2.** CHEMISTRY To initiate reduction (2). [L. *re-duco,* to lead back, restore, reduce]

re•duc•i•ble (rē-dūs′i-bl). Capable of being reduced.

re•duc•tant (rē-dŭk′tant). The substance that is oxidized in the course of reduction.

re•duc•tase (rē-dŭk′tās). An enzyme that catalyzes a reduction; since all enzymes catalyze reactions in either direction, any r. can, under the proper conditions, behave as an oxidase and vice versa, hence the term oxidoreductase. For individual r.'s, see the specific names.

re•duc•tion (rē-dŭk′shŭn). **1.** The restoration, by surgical or manipulative procedures, of a part to its normal anatomical relation. SYN repositioning. **2.** CHEMISTRY A reaction involving a gain of one or more electrons by a substance. [L. *reductio,* fr. *re-duco,* pp. *ductus,* to lead back]

   r. of chromosomes, the process during meiosis whereby one member of each homologous pair of chromosomes is distributed to a sperm or ovum; the diploid set of chromosomes (46 in humans) is thus reduced to the haploid set in each gamete; union of the sperm and ovum restores the diploid or somatic number in the one-cell zygote.

   closed r. of fractures, r. by manipulation of bone, without incision in the skin.

   open r. of fractures, r. by manipulation of bone, after incision in skin and muscle over the site of the fracture.

re•du•pli•ca•tion (rē′dū′pli-kā′shŭn). **1.** A redoubling. **2.** A duplication or doubling, as of the sounds of the heart in certain morbid states or the presence of two instead of a normally single part. **3.** A fold or duplicature. [L. *reduplicatio,* fr. *re-* again, + *duplico,* to double, fr. *duplex,* two-fold]

Red•u•vi•i•dae (rē-dū-vī′i-dē). A family of predatory insects, the assassin bugs; it includes the subfamily Triatominae, the kissing or conenosed bugs, whose type genus *Triatoma* includes species that are vectors of *Trypanosoma cruzi.*

reef•ing (rēf′ing). Surgically reducing the extent of a tissue by folding it and securing with sutures, as in plication.

re•en•try (rē-en′trē). Return of the same impulse into a zone of heart muscle that it has recently activated, sufficiently delayed that the zone is no longer refractory, as seen in most ectopic beats, reciprocal rhythms, and most tachycardias.

re•fine (rē-fīn′). To free from impurities.

re•flec•tion (rē-flek′shŭn). 1. The act of reflecting. 2. That which is reflected. 3. PSYCHOTHERAPY A technique in which a patient's statements are repeated, restated, or rephrased in order that the patient will continue to explore and expound on emotionally significant content. [L. *reflexio,* a bending back]

re•flec•tor (rē-flek′ter). Any surface that reflects light, heat, or sound.

re•flex (rē′fleks). 1. An involuntary reaction in response to a stimulus applied to the periphery and transmitted to the nervous centers in the brain or spinal cord. Most of the deep r.'s listed as subentries are stretch or myotatic r.'s, elicited by striking a tendon or bone, causing stretching, even slight, of the muscle which then contracts as a result of the stimulus applied to its proprioceptors. SEE ALSO phenomenon. 2. A reflection. 3. SYN consensual. [L. *reflexus,* pp. of *re-flecto,* to bend back]

accommodation r., increased convexity of the lens, due to contraction of the ciliary muscle and relaxation of the suspensory ligament, to maintain a distinct retinal image.

Achilles r., Achilles tendon r., a contraction of the calf muscles when the tendo calcaneus is sharply struck. SYN ankle r., triceps surae r.

anal r., contraction of the internal sphincter gripping the finger passed into the rectum.

ankle r., SYN Achilles r.

auditory r., any r. occurring in response to a sound, *e.g.,* cochleopalpebral r.

auropalpebral r., brisk closure of the eyes in reaction to sudden presentation of a loud noise. SYN Moro's r.

basal joint r., opposition and adduction of the thumb with flexion at its metacarpophalangeal joint and extension at its interphalangeal joint, when firm passive flexion of the third, fourth, or fifth finger is made; the r. is present normally but is absent in pyramidal lesions. SYN finger-thumb r., Mayer's r.

Bechterew-Mendel r., percussion of the dorsum of the foot causes flexion of the toes; present in a pyramidal lesion. SYN Mendel-Bechterew r.

biceps r., contraction of the biceps brachii muscle when its tendon of insertion is struck.

Brain's r., SYN quadripedal extensor r.

carotid sinus r., a normal r. relating to the carotid sinus syndrome, which results from hypersensitivity or hyperactivation of the carotid sinus.

celiac plexus r., arterial hypotension coincident with surgical manipulations in the upper abdomen during general anesthesia.

Chaddock r., SYN Chaddock sign.

chain r., a series of r.s, each serving as a stimulus for the next.

ciliospinal r., SYN pupillary-skin r.

cochleopalpebral r., a form of the wink r. in which there is a contraction, sometimes very slight, of the orbicularis palpebrarum muscle when a sudden noise is made close to the ear; it is absent in labyrinthine disease with total deafness. SYN startle r. (2).

conditioned r. (CR), a r. that is gradually developed by training and association through the frequent repetition of a definite stimulus. SEE conditioning.

conjunctival r., closure of the eyes in response to irritation of the conjunctiva.

corneal r., (1) a contraction of the eyelids when the cornea is lightly touched with a camel-hair pencil; **(2)** reflection of light from the surface of the cornea.

cough r., the r. which mediates coughing in response to irritation of the larynx or tracheobronchial tree.

cremasteric r., a drawing up of the scrotum and testicle of the same side when the skin over Scarpa's triangle or on the inner side of the thigh is scratched.

crossed r., a r. movement on one side of the body in response to a stimulus applied to the opposite side.

crossed extension r., r. extension of the joints of an extremity accompanying a flexion r. in the contralateral extremity, induced by application to the contralateral extremity of a painful stimulus distally.

darwinian r., the tendency of young infants to grasp a bar and hang suspended. Cf. grasping r.

deep r., an involuntary muscular contraction following percussion of a tendon or bone. SYN jerk (2).

digital r., SYN Hoffmann's *sign* (2).

diving r., a r. by which immersing the face or body in water, especially cold water, tends to cause bradycardia and peripheral vasoconstriction; relatively minor in most humans.

enterogastric r., peristaltic contraction of the small intestine induced by the entrance of food into the stomach. SEE ALSO gastrocolic r.

finger-thumb r., SYN basal joint r.

flexor r., flexion of ankle, knee, and hip when the foot is painfully stimulated; the crossed extension r. occurs in association with it.

gag r., contact of a foreign body with the mucous membrane of the fauces causes retching or gagging.

gastrocolic r., a mass movement of the contents of the colon, frequently preceded by a similar movement in the small intestine, that sometimes occurs immediately following the entrance of food into the stomach.

gastroileac r., opening of the ileocolic valve induced by entrance of food into the stomach.

grasp r., SYN grasping r.

grasping r., an involuntary flexion of the fingers to tactile or tendon stimulation on the palm of the hand, producing an uncontrollable grasp; physiologic in the newborn, otherwise usually associated with frontal lobe lesions. Cf. darwinian r. SYN grasp r.

Hering-Breuer r., the effects of afferent impulses from the pulmonary vagi in the control of respiration, *e.g.,* inflation of the lungs arrests inspiration, with expiration then ensuing, while deflation of the lungs brings on inspiration.

Hoffmann's r., SYN Hoffmann's *sign* (2).

intrinsic r., a r. muscular contraction elicited by the application of a stimulus, usually stretching, to the muscle itself as opposed to a muscular contraction caused by an extrinsic stimulus, *e.g.,* skin, as in the abdominal skin r.'s.

jaw r., a spasmodic contraction of the temporal muscles following a downward tap on the loosely hanging mandible.

knee r., SYN patellar r.

knee-jerk r., SYN patellar r.

latent r., a r. which must be considered normal but which usually appears only under some pathologic circumstance that lowers its threshold.

light r., (1) SYN pupillary r. (2) a red glow reflected from the fundus of the eye when a light is cast upon the retina, as in retinoscopy; (3) SYN *pyramid* of light.

lip r., a pouting movement of the lips provoked in young infants by tapping near the angle of the mouth.

Mayer's r., SYN basal joint r.

Mendel-Bechterew r., SYN Bechterew-Mendel r.

myotatic r., tonic contraction of the muscles in response to a stretching force, due to stimulation of muscle proprioceptors. SYN stretch r.

Moro's r., SYN auropalpebral r.

nasal r., sneezing caused by irritation of the nasal mucous membrane.

orienting r., an aspect of attending in which an organism's initial response to a change or to a novel stimulus is such that the organism becomes more sensitive to the stimulation; *e.g.,* dilation of the pupil of the eye in response to dim light. SYN orienting response.

palatal r., palatine r., swallowing r. induced by stimulation of the palate.

parachute r., SYN startle r. (1).

paradoxical r., any r. in which the usual response is reversed or does not conform to the pattern characteristic of the particular r.

patellar r., a sudden contraction of the anterior muscles of the thigh, caused by a smart tap on the patellar tendon while the leg hangs loosely at a right angle with the thigh. SYN knee r., knee-jerk r., quadriceps r.

pharyngeal r., (1) SYN swallowing r. (2) SYN vomiting r.

pilomotor r., contraction of the smooth muscle of the skin resulting in "gooseflesh" caused by mild application of a tactile stimulus or by local cooling.

plantar r., the response to tactile stimulation of the ball of the foot, normally plantar flexion of the toes; the pathologic response is Babinski's *sign* (1).

protective laryngeal r., closure of the glottis to prevent entry of foreign substances into the respiratory tract.

pupillary r., change in diameter of the pupil as a reflex response to any type of stimulus; *e.g.,* constriction caused by light. SYN light r. (1).

pupillary-skin r., dilation of the pupil following scratching of the skin of the neck. SYN ciliospinal r.

quadriceps r., SYN patellar r.

quadripedal extensor r., extension of the arm of a hemiplegic patient when turned prone as if on all fours. SYN Brain's r.

red r., SYN *pyramid* of light.

rooting r., in infants, rubbing or scratching about the mouth causes a puckering of the lips.

Rossolimo's r., flicking the tops of the toes from the plantar surface causes flexion of the toes in lesions of the pyramidal tracts. SYN Rossolimo's sign.

snout r., pouting or pursing of the lips induced by light tapping of closed lips near the midline; seen in defective pyramidal innervation of facial musculature.

spinal r., a r. arc involving the spinal cord. SEE reflex *arc*.

startle r., (1) the r. response of an infant (contraction of the limb and neck muscles) when allowed to drop a short distance through the air or startled by a sudden noise or jolt; SYN parachute r. (2) SYN cochleopalpebral r.

statokinetic r., a r. which, through stimulation of the receptors in the neck muscles and semicircular canals, brings about movements of the limbs and eyes appropriate to a given movement of the head in space.

stretch r., SYN myotatic r.

superficial r., any r., *e.g.,* the abdominal or cremasteric r., which is elicited by stimulation of the skin.

swallowing r., the act of swallowing (second stage) induced by stimulation of the palate, fauces, or posterior pharyngeal wall. SYN pharyngeal r. (1).

tendon r., a myotatic or deep r. in which the muscle stretch receptors are stimulated by percussing the tendon of a muscle.

tonic neck r., a brainstem-level r. that may produce positional changes of all limbs in response to active or passive head turning or to flexion/extension of the head.

triceps r., a sudden contraction of the triceps muscle caused by a smart tap on its tendon when the forearm hangs loosely at a right angle with the arm.

triceps surae r., SYN Achilles r.

unconditioned r., an instinctive r. not dependent on previous learning or experience.

vestibulospinal r., the influence of vestibular stimulation on body posture.

vomiting r., vomiting (contraction of the abdominal muscles with relaxation of the cardiac sphincter of the stomach and of the muscles of the throat) elicited by a variety of stimuli, especially one applied to the region of the fauces. SYN pharyngeal r. (2).

wink r., general term for r. closure of eyelids caused by any stimulus.

re·flex·o·gen·ic (rē-flek-sō-jen′ik). Causing a reflex.

re·flex·o·graph (rē-flek′sō-graf). An instrument for graphically recording a reflex. [reflex + G. *graphō,* to write]

re·flex·om·e·ter (rē-flek-som′ĕ-ter). An instrument for measuring the force necessary to excite a reflex. [reflex + G. *metron*, measure]

re·flux (rē′flŭks). 1. A backward flow. SEE ALSO regurgitation. 2. CHEMISTRY To boil without loss of vapor because of the presence of a condenser that returns vapor as liquid. [L. *re-*, back, + *fluxus*, a flow]

   esophageal r., gastroesophageal r., SEE gastroesophageal reflux *disease*.

   hepatojugular r., an elevation of venous pressure visible in the jugular veins and measurable in the veins of the arm, produced in active or impending congestive heart failure by firm pressure with the flat hand over the liver.

   ureterorenal r., backward flow of urine from ureter into renal pelvis.

   vesicoureteral r., backward flow of urine from bladder into ureter.

re·fract (rē-frakt′). 1. To change the direction of a ray of light. 2. To detect an error of refraction and to correct it by means of lenses. [L. *refringo*, pp. *-fractus*, to break up]

re·frac·tion (rē-frak′shŭn). 1. The deflection of a ray of light when it passes from one medium into another of different optical density; in passing from a denser into a rarer medium it is deflected away from a line perpendicular to the surface of the refracting medium; in passing from a rarer to a denser medium it is bent toward this perpendicular line. 2. The act of determining the nature and degree of the refractive errors in the eye and correction of them by lenses. SYN refringence. [L. *refractio* (see refract)]

   double r., the property of having more than one refractive index according to the direction of the transmitted light. SYN birefringence.

   dynamic r., r. of the eye during accommodation.

re·frac·tion·ist (rē-frak′shŭn-ist). A person trained to measure the refraction of the eye and to determine the proper corrective lenses.

re·frac·tive (rē-frak′tiv). 1. Pertaining to refraction. 2. Having the power to refract. SYN refringent.

re·frac·tiv·i·ty (rē-frak-tiv′i-tē). Refractive power.

re·frac·tom·e·ter (rē-frak-tom′ĕ-ter). An instrument for measuring the degree of refraction in translucent substances, especially the ocular media. SEE refractive *index*. [refraction + G. *metron*, measure]

re·frac·tom·e·try (rē-frak-tom′ĕ-trē). 1. Measurement of the refractive index. 2. Use of a refractometer to determine the refractive error of the eye.

re·frac·to·ry (rē-frak′tōr-ē). 1. Resistant to treatment, as of a disease. SYN intractable (1), obstinate (2). 2. SYN obstinate (1). [L. *refractarius*, fr. *refringo*, pp. *-fractus*, to break in pieces]

re·frac·ture (rē-frak′chūr). Breaking a bone that has united after a previous fracture. [re- + fracture]

re·fresh (rē-fresh′). 1. To renew; to cause to recuperate. 2. To perform revivification (2). [O. Fr. *re-frescher*]

re·frig·er·ant (rē-frij′er-ănt). 1. Cooling; reducing slight fever. 2. An agent that gives a sensation of coolness or relieves feverishness. [L. *re-frigero*, pp. *-atus*, pr. p. *-ans*, to make cold, fr. *frigus* (*frigor-*), cold]

re·frig·er·a·tion (rē-frij-er-ă′shŭn). The act of cooling or reducing fever. [L. *refrigeratio* (see refrigerant)]

re·frin·gence (rē-frin′jens). SYN refraction.

re·frin·gent (rē-frin′jent). SYN refractive.

re·fu·sion (rē-fū′zhŭn). Return of the circulation of blood which has been temporarily cut off by ligature of a limb. [L. *re-fundo*, pp. *-fusus*, to pour back]

re·gen·er·a·tion (rē′jen-er-ă′shŭn). 1. Reproduction or reconstitution of a lost or injured part. SYN neogenesis. 2. A form of asexual reproduction; *e.g.,* when a worm is divided into two or more parts, each segment is regenerated into a new individual. [L. *regeneratio* (see regenerate)]

reg·i·men (rej′i-men). A program, including drugs, which regulates aspects of one's life-style for a hygienic or therapeutic purpose; a program of treatment; sometimes mistakenly called regime. [L. direction, rule]

re·gio, gen. **re·gi·o·nis,** pl. **re·gi·o·nes** (rē′jē-ō, -ō′nis, -ō′nēz) [NA]. SYN region. [L.]

re·gion (rē′jŭn). 1. An often arbitrarily limited portion of the surface of the body. SEE ALSO space, zone. 2. A portion of the body having a special nervous or vascular supply, or a part of an organ having a special function. SEE ALSO area, space, spatium, zone. SYN regio [NA]. [L. *regio*]

⊞ **abdominal r.'s,** the topographical subdivisions of the abdomen; based on subdividing the abdomen by the transpyloric, interspinous and midclavicular planes; including the right and left hypochondriac, right and left lateral, right and left inguinal, and the unpaired epigastric, umbilical and pubic regions.

   r.'s of back, the topographical regions of the back of the trunk, including the vertebral r., sacral r., scapular r., infrascapular r., and lumbar r.

   r.'s of chest, the topographical divisions of the chest: presternal, mammary, inframammary, and axillary. SEE pectoral r.

   chromosomal r., that part of a chromosome defined either by anatomical details, notably banding, or by its linkages (linkage group).

   epigastric r., the region of the abdomen located between the costal margins and the subcostal plane.

   r.'s of face, the topographical subdivisions of the face, including nasal, oral, mental, orbital, infraorbital, buccal, and zygomatic.

   r.'s of head, the topographical division of the cranium in relation to the bones of the cranial vault; the regions include frontal, parietal, occipital, and temporal.

   hinge r., (1) that part of a tRNA structure that is deformed, bending a "cloverleaf" (two-dimensional) model to form an "L" model (crystal form, as seen by electron microscopy); (2) in an immunoglobulin, a short sequence of amino acids that lies between two longer sequences and allows the latter to bend about the former.

   hypochondriac r., the region on each side of

re

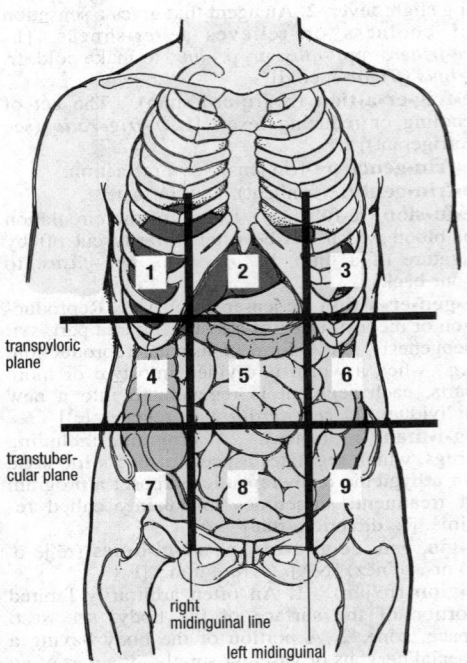

transpyloric plane

transtubercular plane

right midinguinal line

left midinguinal line

abdominal regions: (1) right hypochondriac, (2) epigastric, (3) left hypochondriac, (4) right lateral (lumbar), (5) umbilical, (6) left lateral (lumbar), (7) right iliac, (8) hypogastric (suprapubic), (9) left iliac

the abdomen covered by the costal cartilages; it is lateral to the epigastric region.

inguinal r., the topographical area of the inferior abdomen related to the inguinal canal, lateral to the pubic region. SYN groin (1).

r. of interest, in computed tomography or other computerized imaging, an interactively selected portion of the image, whose individual or average pixel values can be displayed numerically.

r.'s of lower limb, the topographical divisions of the lower limb: gluteal, thigh (or femoral), knee, leg (or crural), ankle, and foot.

r.'s of neck, the topographical subdivisions of the neck. SYN neck (1).

pectoral r., the region of the chest demarcated by the outline of the pectoralis major muscle. SEE ALSO r.'s of chest.

pubic r., the lower central region of the abdomen below the umbilical region.

sural r., the muscular swelling of the back of the leg below the knee, formed chiefly by the bellies of the gastrocnemius and soleus muscles. SYN calf.

r.'s of upper limb, the topographic divisions of the upper limb: deltoid, arm, elbow, forearm, carpal region, and hand.

re·gion·al (rē′jŭn-ăl). Relating to a region.

re·gi·o·nes (rē′jē-ō′nēz). Plural of regio. [L.]

registration. The reception of external stimuli; the capacity to perform this activity.

sensory registration, the ability to receive input and select that which will receive attention and that which will be inhibited from consciousness.

registry. Database on patients who share a particular characteristic; common registries include cancer, trauma, and implants; data are used to assess the quality of care, monitor trends, and do research.

re·gres·sion (rē-gresh′ŭn). **1.** A subsidence of symptoms. **2.** A relapse; a return of symptoms. **3.** Any retrograde movement or action. **4.** A return to a more primitive mode of behavior due to an inability to function adequately at a more adult level. **5.** The tendency for offspring of exceptional parents to possess characteristics closer to those of the general population. **6.** An unconscious defense mechanism by which there occurs a return to earlier patterns of adaptation. **7.** The distribution of one random variable given particular values of other variables relevant to it, *e.g.,* a formula for the distribution of weight as a function of height and chest circumference. [L. *regredior,* pp. *-gressus,* to go back]

re·gres·sive (rē-gres′iv). Relating to or characterized by regression.

reg·u·la·tion (reg′yū-lā′shŭn). **1.** Control of the rate or manner in which a process progresses or a product is formed. **2.** EXPERIMENTAL EMBRYOLOGY The power of a pregastrula embryo to continue approximately normal development after a part or parts have been manipulated or destroyed. [L. *regula,* a rule]

reg·u·lon (reg′yū-lon). A set of structural genes all with the same gene regulation, whose gene products are involved in the same reaction pathway.

re·gur·gi·tant (rē-ger′ji-tant). Regurgitating flowing backward.

re·gur·gi·tate (rē-ger′ji-tāt). **1.** To flow backward. **2.** To expel the contents of the stomach in small amounts, short of vomiting. [L. *re-,* back, + *gurgito,* pp. *-atus,* to flood, fr. *gurges* (*gurgit-*), a whirlpool]

re·gur·gi·ta·tion (rē-ger′ji-tā′shŭn). **1.** A backward flow, as of blood through an incompetent valve of the heart. **2.** The return of gas or small amounts of food from the stomach. [L. *regurgitatio* (see regurgitate)]

valvular r., a leaky state of one or more of the cardiac valves, the valve not closing tightly and blood therefore regurgitating through it. SYN valvular insufficiency.

re·ha·bil·i·ta·tion (rē′hă-bil-i-tā′shŭn). Spontaneous or therapeutic restoration, after disease, illness, or injury, of the ability to function in a normal or near normal manner. [L. *rehabilitare,* pp. *-tatus,* to make fit, fr. *re-* + *habilitas,* ability]

aural r., procedures to enhance the communication capacity of persons with hearing impairments, such as auditory training, lip reading, and hearing aid orientation.

psychiatric r., service and support provided with limited professional intervention, to assist persons with long-term psychiatric disabilities in self-directed, self-satisfying functional life tasks.

re·hears·al (rē-her′săl). A process associated

with enhancing short-term and long-term memory wherein newly presented information, such as a name or a list of words, is repeated to oneself one or more times in order not to forget it.

re·hy·dra·tion (rē-hī-drā′shŭn). The return of water to a system after its loss.

re·im·plan·ta·tion (rē′im-plan-tā′shŭn). SYN replantation.

re·in·fec·tion (rē-in-fek′shŭn). A second infection by the same microorganism, after recovery from or during the course of a primary infection.

re·in·force·ment (rē-in-fōrs′ment). 1. An increase of force or strength; denoting specifically the increased sharpness of the patellar reflex when the patient at the same time closes the fist tightly or pulls against the flexed fingers or contracts some other set of muscles. 2. DENTISTRY A structural addition or inclusion used to give additional strength in function; *e.g.,* bars in plastic denture base. 3. CONDITIONING The totality of the process in which the conditioned stimulus is followed by presentation of the unconditioned stimulus which itself elicits the response to be conditioned. SEE ALSO reinforcer.

re·in·forc·er (rē-in-fōrs′er). In conditioning, a pleasant or satisfaction-yielding (**positive r.**) or painful or unsatisfying (**negative r.**), stimulus, object, or stimulus event that is obtained upon the performance of a desired or predetermined operant. SEE ALSO reinforcement (3). SYN reward.

re·in·ner·va·tion (rē-in-ner-vā′shŭn). Restoration of nerve control of a paralyzed muscle or other effector organ by means of regrowth of nerve fibers, either spontaneously or after anastomosis.

re·in·te·gra·tion (rē′in-tĕ-grā′shŭn). In the mental health professions, the return to well-adjusted functioning following disturbances due to mental illness.

re·jec·tion (rē-jek′shŭn). 1. The immunological response to incompatibility in a transplanted organ. 2. A refusal to accept, recognize, or grant; a denial. 3. Elimination of small ultrasonic echoes from display. [L. *rejectio,* a throwing back]

  allograft r. (al′lō-graft), the r. of tissue transplanted between two genetically different individuals of the same species. R. is caused by T lymphocytes responding to the foreign major histocompatibility complex of the graft. SYN homograft.

re·lapse (rē′laps). Return of the manifestations of a disease after an interval of improvement. SYN recurrence (2). [L. *re-labor,* pp. *-lapsus,* to slide back]

re·la·tion (rē-lā′shŭn). 1. An association or connection between or among people or objects. SEE ALSO relationship. 2. DENTISTRY The mode of contact of teeth or the positional relationship of oral structures. [L. *relatio,* a bringing back]

  spatial r., position of an object in r. to another.

re·la·tion·ship (rē-lā′shŭn-ship). The state of being related, associated, or connected.

  blood r., SYN consanguinity.

  object r., BEHAVIORAL SCIENCES the emotional bond between an individual and another person (or between two groups), as opposed to the individual's or group's interest in self.

re·lax·ant (rē-lak′sănt). 1. Relaxing; causing relaxation; reducing tension, especially muscular tension. 2. An agent that reduces muscular tension or produces skeletal muscle paralysis, usually referred to as a muscle r.

  muscular r., an agent that relaxes striated muscle; includes drugs acting at the brain and/or spinal cord level or directly on muscle to decrease tone, as well as the neuromuscular r.'s.

re·lax·a·tion (rē-lak-sā′shŭn). 1. Loosening, lengthening, or lessening of tension in a muscle. 2. MAGNETIC RESONANCE IMAGING The decay in magnetization of tissue after the direction of the surrounding magnetic field is changed; the different rates of r. for individual nuclei and tissues are used to provide contrast in imaging. [L. *relaxatio* (see relax)]

  longitudinal r., MAGNETIC RESONANCE IMAGING the return of the magnetic dipoles of the hydrogen nuclei (magnetization vector) to equilibrium parallel to the magnetic field, after they have been flipped 90°; varies in rate in different tissues, taking up to 15 seconds for water. SEE TI.

  transverse r., MAGNETIC RESONANCE IMAGING the rapid decay of the nuclear magnetization vector at right angles to the magnetic field after the 90° pulse is turned off; the signal is called free induction decay. SEE T2. Cf. longitudinal r.

re·learn·ing (rē-lern′ing). The process of regaining a skill or ability that has been partially or entirely lost; savings involved in r., as compared with original learning, give an index of the degree of retention.

re·lieve (rē-lēv′). To free wholly or partly from pain or discomfort, either physical or mental. [through O. Fr. fr. L. *re-levo,* to lift up, lighten]

REM rapid eye *movements,* under *movement.*

rem *roentgen*-equivalent-*man.* See entries under roentgen.

rem·e·dy (rem′ĕ-dē). An agent that cures disease or alleviates its symptoms. [L. *remedium,* fr. *re-,* again, + *medeor,* cure]

re·min·er·al·i·za·tion (rē′min′er-ăl-i-zā′shŭn). 1. The return to the body or a local area of necessary mineral constituents lost through disease or dietary deficiencies; commonly used in referring to the content of calcium salts in bone. 2. DENTISTRY A process enhanced by the presence of fluoride whereby partially decalcified enamel, dentin, and cementum become recalcified by mineral replacement.

re·mis·sion (rē-mish′ŭn). 1. Abatement or lessening in severity of the symptoms of a disease. 2. The period during which such abatement occurs. [L. *remissio,* fr. *re-mitto,* pp. *-missus,* to send back, slacken, relax]

re·mit·tence (rē-mit′ens). A temporary amelioration, without actual cessation, of symptoms.

re·mit·tent (rē-mit′ent). Characterized by temporary periods of abatement of the symptoms of a disease.

re·mod·el·ing (rē-mod′el-ing). A cyclical process by which bone maintains a dynamic steady state through sequential resorption and formation of a small amount of bone at the same site; unlike the process of modeling, the size and shape of remodeled bone remain unchanged.

ren, gen. **re·nis**, pl. **re·nes** (ren, rē′nis, rē′nēz) [NA]. SYN kidney. [L.]

re·nal (rē′năl). SYN nephric.

△**reni-**. SEE reno-.

ren·i·form (ren′i-fōrm). SYN nephroid.

re·nin (rē′nin). An enzyme that converts angiotensinogen to angiotensin I. SYN angiotensinogenase.

ren·i·por·tal (ren′i-pōr′tăl). **1.** Relating to the hilum of the kidney. **2.** Relating to the portal, or venous capillary circulation in the kidney. [reni- + L. *porta,* gate]

ren·nin (ren′in). SYN chymosin.

ren·nin·o·gen, ren·no·gen (rĕ-nin′ō-jen, ren′ō-jen). SYN prochymosin. [rennin + G. -*gen,* producing]

△**reno-, reni-**. The kidney. SEE ALSO nephro-. [L. *ren*]

re·no·gen·ic (rē-nō-jen′ik). Originating in or from the kidney.

re·no·gram (rē′nō-gram). The assessment of renal function by external radiation detectors after the administration of a radiopharmaceutical that is filtered and excreted by the kidney. [reno- + G. *gramma,* something written]

re·nog·ra·phy (rē-nog′ră-fē). Radiography of the kidney.

re·no·meg·a·ly (rē′nō-meg′ă-lē). Enlargement of the kidney.

re·no·pri·val (rē-nō-prī′văl). Relating to, characterized by, or resulting from total loss of kidney function or from removal of all functioning renal tissue. [reno- + L. *privus,* deprived of]

re·no·tro·phic (rē-nō-trof′ik). Relating to any agent influencing the growth or nutrition of the kidney or to the action of such an agent. SYN nephrotrophic, nephrotropic. [reno- + G. *trophē,* nourishment]

re·no·vas·cu·lar (rē-nō-vas′kyū-ler). Pertaining to the blood vessels of the kidney, denoting especially disease of these vessels.

Re·o·vir·i·dae (rē-ō-vir′i-dē). A family of double-stranded RNA viruses, comprising six genera: *Reovirus, Orbivirus, Rotavirus,* cytoplasmic polyhidrosis virus group (*Cypovirus*), and two plant reovirus groups (*Phytoreovirus, Fijivirus*). [*Res*piratory *E*nteric *O*rphan + viridae]

Re·o·vi·rus (rē′ō-vī′rŭs). A genus of viruses recovered from children with mild fever and sometimes diarrhea, and from children with no apparent infection; a causative relationship to illness has not been proven.

re·pair (rē-pār′). Restoration of diseased or damaged tissues naturally by healing processes or artificially, as by surgical means. [M.E.,fr. O.Fr.,fr. L. *re-paro,* fr. *re-,* back, again, + *paro,* prepare, put in order]

chemical r., conversion of a free radical to a stable molecule.

re·pel·lent (rē-pel′ent). **1.** Capable of driving off or repelling; repulsive. **2.** An agent that drives away or prevents annoyance or irritation by insect pests. **3.** An astringent or other agent that reduces swelling. [L. *re-pello,* pp. -*pulsus,* to drive back]

rep·e·ti·tion-com·pul·sion (rep-e-tish′ŭn-kŏm-pŭl′shŭn). PSYCHOANALYSIS The tendency to repeat earlier experiences or actions, in an unconscious effort to achieve belated mastery over them; a morbid need to repeat a particular behavior such as handwashing or repeated checking to see if the door is locked.

re·plant (rē′plant). **1.** To perform replantation. **2.** A part or organ so replaced or about to be so replaced.

re·plan·ta·tion (rē-plan-tā′shŭn). Replacement of an organ or part back in its original site and reestablishing its circulation. SYN reimplantation. [L. *re-,* again, + *planto,* pp. -*atus,* to plant, fr. *planta,* a sprout, slip]

re·ple·tion (rē-plē′shŭn). **1.** SYN hypervolemia. **2.** SYN plethora (2). [L. *repletio,* fr. *re-pleo,* pp. -*pletus,* to fill up]

rep·li·case (rep′li-kās). Descriptive term for RNA-directed RNA polymerase (EC 2.7.7.48) associated with replication of RNA viruses.

rep·li·cate (rep′li-kāt). **1.** One of several identical processes or observations. **2.** To repeat; to produce an exact copy.

rep·li·ca·tion (rep-li-kā′shŭn). **1.** The execution of an experiment or study more than once so as to confirm the original findings, increase precision, and obtain a closer estimate of sampling error. **2.** Autoreproduction, as in mitosis or cellular biology. SEE autoreproduction. **3.** DNA-directed DNA synthesis. [L. *replicatio,* a reply, fr. *replico,* pp. -*atus,* to fold back]

rep·li·ca·tor (rep′li-kā-ter). The specific site of a bacterial genome (chromosome) at which replication begins.

rep·li·con (rep′li-kon). **1.** A segment of a chromosome (or of the DNA of a chromosome or similar entity) that can replicate, with its own initiation and termination codons, independently of the chromosome in which it may be located. **2.** The replication unit; several are found per DNA in eukaryotic systems. [*replic*ation + -on]

re·po·lar·i·za·tion (rē′pō-lăr-i-zā′shŭn). The process whereby the membrane, cell, or fiber, after depolarization, is polarized again, with positive charges on the outer and negative charges on the inner surface.

re·po·si·tion·ing (rē′pō-zish′ŭn-ing). SYN reduction (1).

re·pos·i·tor (rē-poz′i-ter, -tōr). An instrument used to reposition a displaced organ.

re·pressed (rē-prest′). Subjected to repression.

re·pres·sion (rē-presh′ŭn). **1.** PSYCHOTHERAPY The active process or defense mechanism of keeping out and ejecting, banishing from consciousness, ideas or impulses that are unacceptable to it. **2.** Decreased expression of some gene product. [L. *re-primo,* pp. -*pressus,* to press back, repress]

re·pres·sor (rē-pres′er). The product of a regulator or r. gene.

active r., a r. that combines directly with an operator gene to repress the operator and its structural genes, thus repressing protein synthesis; an active r. may be repressed by an inducer, with resulting protein synthesis; a homeostatic mechanism for regulation of inducible enzyme systems.

inactive r., a r. that cannot combine with an

operator gene until it has combined with a core-pressor (usually a product of a protein pathway); after activation, the r. arrests production of the proteins controlled by the operator gene; a home-ostatic mechanism for regulation of repressible enzyme systems. SYN aporepressor.

re·pro·duc·i·bil·i·ty (rē-prō-dus'i-bil'i-tē). **1.** Ability to cause to exist again or to present again. **2.** Ability to duplicate measurements over long periods of time by different laboratories.

re·pro·duc·tion (rē-prō-dŭk'shŭn). **1.** The recall and presentation in the mind of the elements of a former impression. **2.** The total process by which organisms produce offspring. SYN generation (1), procreation. [L. *re-*, again, + *pro-duco*, pp. *-duc-tus*, to lead forth, produce]

asexual r., r. other than by union of male and female sex cells.

cytogenic r., r. by means of unicellular germ cells; includes both sexual r. and asexual r. by means of spores.

sexual r., r. by union of male and female ga-metes to form a zygote. SYN gamogenesis, syn-genesis.

somatic r., asexual r. by fission or budding of somatic cells.

re·pro·duc·tive (rē'prō-dŭk'tiv). Relating to re-production.

rep·ti·lase (rep'til-as). An enzyme found in the venom of *Bothrops atrox* that clots fibrinogen by splitting off its fibrinopeptide. [reptile + -ase]

re·pul·sion (rē-pŭl'shŭn). **1.** The act of repelling or driving apart, in contrast to attraction. **2.** Strong dislike; aversion; repugnance. **3.** Coupling phase of genes at linked loci that are borne on opposite chromosomes. [L. *re-pello*, pp. *-pulsus*, to drive back]

RES reticuloendothelial *system.*

re·sect (rē-sekt'). **1.** To cut off, especially to cut off the articular ends of one or both bones form-ing a joint. **2.** To excise a segment of a part. [L. *re-seco*, pp. *sectus*, to cut off]

re·sect·a·ble (rē-sek'tă-bl). Amenable to resec-tion.

re·sec·tion (rē-sek'shŭn). **1.** Removal of articular ends of one or both bones forming a joint. **2.** SYN excision (1).

gum r., SYN gingivectomy.

root r., SYN apicoectomy.

transurethral r., endoscopic removal of the prostate gland or bladder lesions, usually for re-lief of prostatic obstruction or treatment of blad-der malignancies.

wedge r., removal of a wedge-shaped portion of the ovary; used in the treatment of virilizing disorders of ovarian origin, such as the polycystic ovarian syndrome.

re·sec·to·scope (rē-sek'tō-skōp). A special endo-scopic instrument for the transurethral electrosur-gical removal of lesions involving the bladder, prostate gland, or urethra.

re·serve (rē-zerv'). Something available but held back for later use. [L. *re-servo*, to keep back, reserve]

alkali r., the sum total of the basic ions (mainly bicarbonates) of the blood and other body fluids which, acting as buffers, maintain the normal pH of the blood.

breathing r., the difference between the pul-monary ventilation (*i.e.*, the volume of air breathed under ordinary resting conditions) and the maximum breathing capacity.

cardiac r., the work which the heart is able to perform beyond that required under the ordinary circumstances of daily life, depending upon the state of the myocardium and the degree to which, within physiologic limits, the cardiac muscle fi-bers can be stretched by the volume of blood reaching the heart during diastole.

res·er·voir (rez'ĕv-wor). SYN receptaculum. [Fr.]

r. of infection, living or nonliving material in or on which an infectious agent multiplies and/or develops and is dependent for its survival in na-ture.

r. of spermatozoa, the site where spermatozoa are stored; the distal portion of the tail of the epididymis and the beginning of the ductus defer-ens.

res·i·dent (rez'i-dent). **1.** A house officer at-tached to a hospital for clinical training. **2.** Patient residing in a nursing facility. [L. *resideo*, to re-side]

re·sid·ua (rē-zid'yū-ă). Plural of residuum.

re·sid·u·al (rē-zid'yū-ăl). Relating to or of the nature of a residue.

res·i·due (rez'i-dū). That which remains after removal of one or more substances. SYN resid-uum. [L. *residuum*]

re·sid·u·um, pl. **re·sid·ua** (rē-zid'yū-ŭm, -yū-ă). SYN residue. [L. ntr. of *residuus*, left behind, remaining, fr. *re- sideo*, to sit back, remain be-hind]

res·in (rez'in). **1.** An amorphous brittle substance consisting of the hardened secretion of a number of plants, probably derived from a volatile oil and similar to a stearoptene. **2.** SYN rosin. **3.** A pre-cipitate formed by the addition of water to certain tinctures. **4.** A broad term used to indicate or-ganic substances insoluble in water. [L. *resina*]

anion-exchange r., SEE *anion* exchange.

autopolymer r., autopolymerizing r., any r. that can be polymerized by chemical catalysis rather than by the application of heat; used in dentistry for dental restoration, denture repair, and impression trays. SYN cold cure r., cold-cur-ing r.

cation-exchange r., SEE cation exchange.

cold cure r., cold-curing r., SYN autopolymer r.

ion-exchange r., SEE *anion* exchange, cation exchange, ion exchange *chromatography.*

res·in·ous (rez'i-nŭs). Relating to or derived from a resin.

re·sis·tance (rē-zis'tans). **1.** A passive force ex-erted in opposition to another active force. **2.** The opposition in a conductor to the passage of a current of electricity, whereby there is a loss of energy and a production of heat; specifically, the potential difference in volts across the conductor per ampere of current flow; unit: ohm. Cf. imped-ance (1). **3.** The opposition to flow of a fluid through one or more passageways; units are usu-ally those of pressure difference per unit flow. Cf.

impedance (2). **4.** PSYCHOANALYSIS An individual's unconscious defense against bringing repressed thoughts to consciousness. **5.** The ability of red blood cells to resist hemolysis and to preserve their shape under varying degrees of osmotic pressure in the blood plasma. **6.** The natural or acquired ability of an organism to maintain its immunity to or to resist the effects of an antagonistic agent, *e.g.,* pathogenic microorganism, toxin, drug. [L. *re-sisto,* to stand back, withstand]

airway r., PHYSIOLOGY the r. to flow of gases during ventilation due to obstruction or turbulent flow in the upper and lower airways; to be differentiated during inhalation from r. to inflation due to decreases in pulmonary or thoracic compliance.

drug r., the capacity of disease-causing pathogens to withstand drugs previously toxic to them; achieved by spontaneous mutation or through selective pressure after exposure to the drug in question.

insulin r., diminished effectiveness of insulin in lowering blood sugar levels; arbitrarily defined as requiring 200 units or more of insulin per day to prevent hyperglycemia or ketosis; usually due to insulin binding by antibodies, but abnormalities in insulin receptors on cell surfaces also occur; associated with obesity, ketoacidosis, infection, and certain rare conditions.

mutual r., SYN antagonism.

systemic vascular r., an index of arteriolar compliance or constriction throughout the body; equal to the blood pressure divided by the cardiac output.

res•o•lu•tion (rez-ō-lū'shŭn). **1.** The arrest of an inflammatory process without suppuration; the absorption or breaking down and removal of the products of inflammation or of a new growth. **2.** The optical ability to distinguish detail such as the separation of closely adjacent objects. SYN resolving power (3). [L. *resolutio,* a slackening, fr. *re-solvo,* pp. *-solutus,* to loosen, relax]

re•solve (rē-zolv'). To return or cause to return to the normal, particularly without suppuration, said of a phlegmon or other form of inflammation. [L. *resolvo,* to loosen]

res•o•nance (rez'ō-nans). **1.** Sympathetic or forced vibration of air in the cavities above, below, in front of, or behind a source of sound; in speech, modification of the quality (*e.g.,* tone) of a sound by the passage of air through the chambers of the nose, pharynx, and head, without increasing the intensity of the sound. **2.** The sound obtained on percussing a part that can vibrate freely. **3.** The intensification and hollow character of the voice sound obtained on auscultating over a cavity. **4.** CHEMISTRY The manner in which electrons or electric charges are distributed among the atoms in compounds that are planar and symmetrical, particularly those with conjugated (alternating) double bonds; the existence of r. in the latter case lowers the energy content and increases the stability of a compound. **5.** The natural or inherent frequency of any oscillating system. **6.** SYN resonant *frequency.* [L. *resonantia,* echo, fr. *re-sono,* to resound, to echo]

amphoric r., a hollow sound produced by percussing over a pulmonary cavity or pneumothorax.

electron spin r. (ESR), a spectrometric method, based on measurement of electron spins and magnetic moments, for detecting and estimating free radicals in reactions and in biological systems.

nuclear magnetic r. (NMR), the phenomenon in which certain atomic nuclei possessing a magnetic moment will precess around the axis of a strong external magnetic field, the frequency of precession being specific for each nucleus and the strength of the magnetic field; spinning nuclei induce their own oscillating magnetic fields and therefore emit electromagnetic radiation that can produce a detectable signal. NMR is used as a method of identifying covalent bonds and is applied clinically in magnetic resonance *imaging.*

skodaic r., a peculiar, high-pitched sound, less musical than that obtained over a cavity, elicited by percussion just above the level of a pleuritic effusion.

tympanitic r., SYN tympany.

vesicular r., the sound obtained on percussing over the normal lungs.

vesiculotympanitic r., a peculiar, partly tympanitic, partly vesicular sound, obtained on percussion in cases of pulmonary emphysema.

vocal r. (VR), the voice sounds as heard on auscultation of the chest.

re•sorb (rē-sōrb'). To reabsorb; to absorb what has been excreted, as an exudate or pus. [L. *re-sorbeo,* to suck back]

re•sorp•tion (rē-sōrp'shŭn). **1.** The act of resorbing. **2.** A loss of substance by lysis, or by physiologic or pathologic means.

res•pi•ra•ble (re-spīr'ă-bl, res'pĭ-ră-bl). Capable of being breathed.

🛈**res•pi•ra•tion** (res-pi-rā'shŭn). **1.** A fundamental process of life, characteristic of both plants and animals, in which oxygen is used to oxidize organic fuel molecules, providing a source of energy as well as carbon dioxide and water. In green plants, photosynthesis is not considered r. **2.** SYN ventilation (2). [L. *respiratio,* fr. *re-spiro,* pp. *-atus,* to exhale, breathe]

abdominal r., breathing effected mainly by the action of the diaphragm.

aerobic r., a form of r. in which molecular oxygen is consumed and carbon dioxide and water are produced.

anaerobic r., a form of r. in which molecular oxygen is not consumed; *e.g.,* nitrate r., sulfate r.

artificial r., SYN artificial *ventilation.*

assisted r., SYN assisted *ventilation.*

Biot's r., abrupt, irregular alternating periods of apnea with constant rate and depth of breathing, as that resulting from lesions due to increased intracranial pressure. SYN Biot's breathing.

Biot's r., completely irregular breathing pattern, with continually variable rate and depth of breathing; results from lesions in the respiratory centers in the brainstem, extending from the dorsomedial medulla caudally to the obex.

Cheyne-Stokes r., the pattern of breathing with gradual increase in depth and sometimes in rate to a maximum, followed by a decrease re-

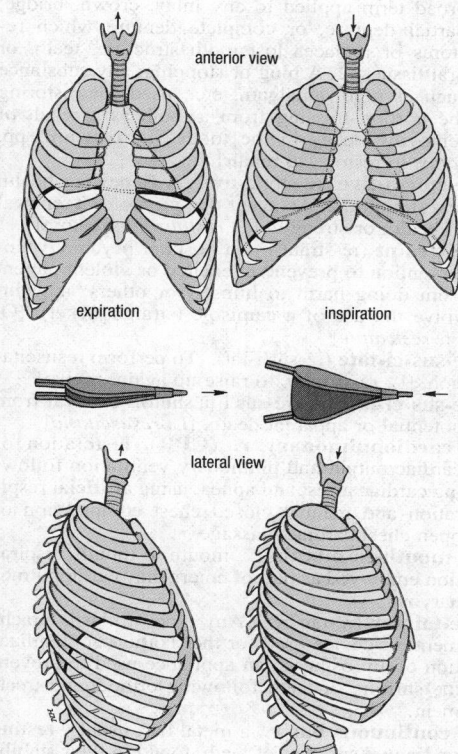

anterior view

expiration

inspiration

lateral view

expiration

inspiration

respiration

sulting in apnea; the cycles ordinarily are 30 seconds to 2 minutes in duration, with 5 to 30 seconds of apnea; seen with bilateral deep febrile hemisphere lesions, with metabolic encephalopathy and, characteristically, in coma from affection of the nervous centers of respiration.

cogwheel r., the inspiratory sound being broken into two or three by silent intervals.

controlled r., SYN controlled *ventilation.*

diffusion r., maintenance of oxygenation during apnea by intratracheal insufflation of oxygen at high flow rates.

electrophrenic r., the rhythmical electrical stimulation of the phrenic nerve by an electrode applied to the skin at the motor points of the phrenic nerve; it is used in paralysis of the respiratory center resulting from acute bulbar poliomyelitis.

external r., the exchange of respiratory gases in the lungs as distinguished from internal or tissue r.

internal r., SYN tissue r.

Kussmaul r., deep, rapid r. characteristic of diabetic or other causes of acidosis.

mouth-to-mouth r., a method of artificial ventilation involving an overlap of the patient's mouth (and nose in small children) with the operator's mouth to inflate the patient's lungs by blowing, followed by an unassisted expiratory phase brought about by elastic recoil of the patient's chest and lungs; repeated 12 to 16 times a minute; where the nose is not covered by the operator's mouth, the nostrils must be closed by pinching.

paradoxical r., deflation of the lung during inspiration and inflation of the lung during the phase of expiration; seen in the lung on the side of an open pneumothorax.

tissue r., the interchange of gases between the blood and the tissues. SYN internal r.

vesicular r., the respiratory murmur heard on auscultating over the normal lung. SYN vesicular murmur.

res•pi•ra•tor (res'pi-rā-ter, -tōr). **1.** An appliance fitting over the mouth and nose, used for the purpose of excluding dust, smoke, or other irritants, or of otherwise altering the air before it enters the respiratory passages. SYN inhaler (1). **2.** An apparatus for administering artificial respiration, especially for a prolonged period, in cases of paralysis or inadequate spontaneous ventilation.

Drinker r., a mechanical r. in which the body except the head is encased within a metal tank, which is sealed at the neck with an airtight gasket; artificial respiration is induced by making the air pressure inside alternately negative and positive. SYN iron lung.

res•pi•ra•to•ry (res'pi-ră-tōr-ē, rĕ-spīr'ă-tōr-ē). Relating to respiration.

res•pi•rom•e•ter (res-pǐ-rom'ĕ-ter). **1.** An instrument for measuring the extent of the respiratory movements. **2.** An instrument for measuring oxygen consumption or carbon dioxide production, usually of an isolated tissue. [L. *respiro,* to breathe, + G. *metron,* measure]

re•sponse (rē-spons'). **1.** The reaction of a muscle, nerve, gland, or other excitable tissue to a stimulus. **2.** Any act or behavior, or its constituents, that a living organism is capable of emitting. Reflexes are usually excluded because they are typically elicited by a specifiable (unconditioned or natural) stimulus rather than emitted under circumstances in which the stimulus was not specifiable. [L. *responsus,* an answer]

conditioned r., a r. already in an individual's repertoire but which, through repeated pairings with its natural stimulus, has been acquired or conditioned anew to a previously neutral or conditioned stimulus. SEE conditioning. Cf. unconditioned r.

evoked r., an alteration in the electrical activity of a region of the nervous system through which an incoming sensory stimulus is passing.

flight or fight r., SEE emergency *theory.*

galvanic skin r. (GSR), a measure of changes in emotional arousal recorded by attaching electrodes to any part of the skin and recording changes in moment-to-moment perspiration and related autonomic nervous system activity.

hunting r., alternating vasodilatation and vaso-

re

constriction in one or more extremities during application of ice or generalized hypothermia.

immune r., (1) any r. of the immune system to an antigen including antibody production and/or cell-mediated immunity; (2) the r. of the immune system to an antigen (immunogen) that leads to the condition of induced sensitivity; the immune r. to the initial antigenic exposure (primary immune response) is detectable, as a rule, only after a lag period of from several days to two weeks; the immune r. to a subsequent stimulus (secondary immune response) by the same antigen is more rapid than in the case of the primary immune r.

orienting r., SYN orienting *reflex*.

primary immune r., SEE immune r.

secondary immune r., SEE immune r.

target r., SYN operant.

triple r., the triphasic r. to the firm stroking of the skin: Phase 1 is the sharply demarcated erythema that follows a momentary blanching of the skin, and is the result of release of histamine from the mast cells. Phase 2 is the intense red flare extending beyond the margins of the line of pressure but in the same configuration, and is the result of arteriolar dilation. Phase 3 is the appearance of a line wheal in the configuration of the original stroking.

unconditioned r., a r., such as salivation, which is a part of the animal or human repertoire. Cf. conditioned r.

rest. 1. Quiet; repose. [A.S. *raest*] **2.** To repose; to cease from work. [A.S. *raestan*] **3.** A group of cells or a portion of fetal tissue that has become displaced and lies embedded in tissue of another character. [L. *restare*, to remain] **4.** DENTISTRY An extension from a prosthesis that affords vertical support for a restoration.

adrenal r., SYN accessory *adrenal*.

bed r., maintenance of the recumbent position, in bed, to minimize activity and help recovery from disease; formerly used extensively in treatment of tuberculosis, myocardial infarction, and other diseases.

wolffian r., remnants of the wolffian duct in the female genital tract that give rise to cysts; *e.g.,* Gartner's cyst.

re•ste•no•sis (rē′sten-ō-sis). Recurrence of stenosis after corrective surgery on the heart valve; narrowing of a structure (usually a coronary artery) following the removal or reduction of a previous narrowing. [re-, + G. *stenōsis,* a narrowing]

res•ti•form (res′ti-fōrm). Ropelike; rope-shaped; referring to the restiform body, the larger (lateral) part of the inferior cerebellar peduncle; contains fibers from the spinal cord (spinocerebellar) and medulla (cuneo-, olivo-, reticulocerebellar, etc.) to cerebellum. [L. *restis,* rope, + *forma,* form]

rest•i•tope (res′ti-tōp). The part of the T cell receptor that associates with the class II major histocompatibility molecule. [*rest*riction + -tope]

res•ti•tu•tion (res-ti-tū′shŭn). OBSTETRICS The return of the rotated head of the fetus to its natural relation with the shoulders after its emergence from the vulva. [L. *restitutio,* act of restoring]

res•to•ra•tion (res-tō-rā′shŭn). DENTISTRY **1.** A broad term applied to any inlay, crown, bridge, partial denture, or complete denture which restores or replaces lost tooth structure, teeth, or oral tissues. **2.** A plug or stopping; any substance such as gold, amalgam, etc., used for restoring the portion missing from a tooth as a result of removing decay in the tooth. [L. *restauro,* pp. *-atus,* to restore, to repair]

re•stor•a•tive (re-stōr′ă-tiv). **1.** Renewing health and strength. **2.** An agent that promotes a renewal of health or strength. [L. *restauro,* to restore]

re•straint (rē-strānt′). In hospital psychiatry, intervention to prevent an excited or violent patient from doing harm to himself or others; may involve the use of a camisole (straightjacket). [O. Fr. *restrainte*]

re•sus•ci•tate (rē-sŭs′i-tāt). To perform resuscitation. [L. *re-suscito,* to raise up again, revive]

re•sus•ci•ta•tion (rē-sŭs′i-tā′shŭn). Revival from potential or apparent death. [L. *resuscitatio*]

cardiopulmonary r. (CPR), restoration of cardiac output and pulmonary ventilation following cardiac arrest and apnea, using artificial respiration and manual closed chest compression or open chest cardiac massage.

mouth-to-mouth r., mouth-to-mouth respiration employed as part of emergency cardiopulmonary r.

re•tain•er (rē-tān′er). Any type of clasp, attachment, or device used for the fixation or stabilization of a prosthesis; an appliance used to prevent the shifting of teeth following orthodontic treatment.

continuous bar r., a metal bar, usually resting on lingual surfaces of teeth, to aid in their stabilization and to act as indirect r.'s.

re•tar•da•tion (rē-tahr-dā′shŭn). Slowness or limitation of development.

mental r., subaverage general intellectual functioning that originates during the developmental period and is associated with impairment in adaptive behavior. Mental r. classification requires assignment of an index for performance relative to a person's peers on two interrelated criteria: measured intelligence (IQ) and overall socioadaptive behavior. In general an IQ of 70 or below indicates mental retardation. SYN amentia (1).

retch. To make an involuntary effort to vomit. [A.S. *hraecan,* to hawk]

retch•ing. Gastric and esophageal movements of vomiting without expulsion of vomitus. SYN dry vomiting, vomiturition.

re•te, pl. **re•tia** (rē′tē; rē′shē-ă, -tē-ă) [NA]. **1.** SYN network (1). **2.** A structure composed of a fibrous network or mesh. [L. a net]

r. cuta′neum co′rii, the network of vessels parallel to the surface between the corium and the tela subcutanea.

r. mirab′ile [NA], a vascular network interrupting the continuity of an artery or vein, such as occurs in the glomeruli of the kidney (arterial) or in the liver (venous).

r. ova′rii, a transient network of cells in the developing ovary; homologous to the r. testis.

r. subpapilla′re, the network of vessels between the papillary and reticular strata of the corium.

r. tes′tis [NA], the network of canals at the termination of the straight tubules in the mediastinum testis.

re•ten•tion (rē-ten′shŭn). **1.** The keeping in the body of what normally belongs there, especially the retaining of food and drink in the stomach. **2.** The keeping in the body of what normally should be discharged, as urine or feces. **3.** Retaining that which has been learned so that it can be utilized later as in recall, recognition, or, if r. is partial, relearning. SEE ALSO memory. **4.** Resistance to dislodgement. **5.** DENTISTRY A passive period following treatment when a patient is wearing an appliance or appliances to maintain or stabilize the teeth in the new position into which they have been moved. [L. *retentio,* a holding back]

re•tia (rē′shē-ă, -tē-ă). Plural of rete. [L.]

re•ti•al (rē′shē-ăl). Relating to a rete.

reticul-. SEE reticulo-.

re•tic•u•la (re-tik′yū-lă). Plural of reticulum. [L.]

re•tic•u•lar, re•tic•u•lated (re-tik′yū-lăr, -lāt-ed). Relating to a reticulum.

re•tic•u•la•tion (re-tik-yū-lā′shŭn). The presence or formation of a reticulum or network, such as that observed in red blood cells during active regeneration of blood. Also used to describe a chest radiographic pattern.

re•tic•u•lin (re-tik′yū-lin). The chemical substance of reticular fibers, regarded as type III collagen (with its associated proteoglygans and structural glycoproteins).

reticulo-, reticul-. Reticulum; reticular. [L. *reticulum,* a small net, dim. of *rete,* a net]

reticulocyte (rĕ-tik′kyu-lō-sīt). A young red cell (erythrocyte) that contains no nucleus but has residual RNA. The RNA can be visualized as granules or filaments when the cell is stained supravitally with new methylene blue. Normally, new red cells are released from the bone marrow to the peripheral blood as reticulocytes. They mature, loosing the filamentous RNA in about 2 days. Reticulocytes compose about 1% of circulating red cells. Increased concentrations are associated with hemolytic anemias and blood loss. Decreased concentrations are associated with ineffective erythropoiesis, aplastic anemia and hypocellularity of erythroid precursors in the bone marrow. SEE ALSO reticulocyte production *index,* erythroblast. [reticulo- + G. kytos, cell]

re•tic•u•lo•cy•to•pe•nia (re-tik′yū-lō-sī-tō-pē′nē-ă). Paucity of reticulocytes in the blood. SYN reticulopenia. [reticulocyte + G. *penia,* poverty]

re•tic•u•lo•cy•to•sis (re-tik′yū-lō-sī-tō′sis). An increase in the number of circulating reticulocytes above the normal, which is less than 1% of the total number of red blood cells; it occurs during active blood regeneration (stimulation of red bone marrow) and in certain anemias, especially congenital hemolytic anemia. [reticulocyte + G. *-osis,* condition]

re•tic•u•lo•en•do•the•li•al (re-tik′yū-lō-en-dō-thē′lē-ăl). Denoting or referring to reticuloendothelium.

re•tic•u•lo•en•do•the•li•um (re-tik′yū-lō-en-dō-thē′lē-ŭm). The cells making up the reticuloendothelial system. [reticulo- + endothelium]

re•tic•u•lo•his•ti•o•cy•to•ma (re-tik′yū-lō-his′tē-ō-sī-tō′mă). A solitary skin nodule composed of glycolipid-containing multinucleated large histiocytes; multiple lesions sometimes occur in association with arthritis. [reticulo- + histiocytoma]

re•tic•u•lo•pe•nia (re-tik′yū-lō-pē′nē-ă). SYN reticulocytopenia.

re•tic•u•lo•sis (re-tik-yū-lō′sis). An increase in histiocytes, monocytes, or other reticuloendothelial elements. [reticulo- + G. *-osis,* condition]

   benign inoculation r., SYN cat-scratch *disease.*

re•tic•u•lum, pl. **re•tic•u•la** (re-tik′yū-lŭm, -lă). **1.** A fine network formed by cells, or formed of certain structures within cells or of connective tissue fibers between cells. **2.** SYN neuroglia. **3.** The second compartment of the stomach of a ruminant, a comparatively small chamber communicating with the rumen; sometimes called the honeycomb because of the characteristic structure of its wall. [L. dim of *rete,* a net]

   agranular endoplasmic r., endoplasmic r. that is lacking in ribosomal granules; involved in synthesis of complex lipids and fatty acids, detoxification of drugs, carbohydrate synthesis, and sequestering of Ca^{++}.

   endoplasmic r. (ER), the network of cytoplasmic tubules or flattened sacs (cisternae) with (rough ER) or without (smooth ER) ribosomes on the surface of their membranes in eukaryotes.

   granular endoplasmic r., endoplasmic r. in which ribosomal granules are applied to the cytoplasmic surface of the cisternae; involved in the synthesis and secretion of protein via membrane-bound vesicles to the extracellular space. SYN ergastoplasm.

   sarcoplasmic r., the endoplasmic r. of skeletal and cardiac muscle; the complex of vesicles, tubules, and cisternae forming a continuous structure around striated myofibrils, with a repetition of structure within each sarcomere.

   stellate r., a network of epithelial cells disposed in a fluid-filled compartment in the center of the enamel organ between the outer and inner enamel epithelium.

   trabecular r., the network of fibers (pectinate ligaments) at the iridocorneal angle between the anterior chamber of the eye and the venous sinus of the sclera; it contains spaces between the fibers that are involved in drainage of the aqueous humor, and is composed of two portions: the corneoscleral part, the part attached to the sclera, and the uveal part, the part attached to the iris.

ret•i•form (ret′i-fōrm). Resembling a net or network. [L. *rete,* network]

retin-. SEE retino-.

ret•i•na (ret′i-nă) [NA]. The light-sensitive membrane forming the innermost layer of the eyeball. Grossly, the r. consists of three parts: optic part of retina, ciliary part of retina, and iridial part of retina. The optic part, the physiologic portion that receives the visual light rays, is further divided into two parts, pigmented part (pigment epithelium) and nervous part, which are arranged in the following layers: 1) pigment epithelium; 2) layer of rods and cones; 3) external limiting lamina, actually a row of junctional complexes; 4) external nuclear lamina; 5) external plexiform lamina; 6) internal nuclear lamina; 7) internal plexiform lamina; 8) ganglionic cell lamina; 9) lamina of nerve fibers; 10) internal limiting lamina. Layers 2 through 10 comprise the nervous part. At the posterior pole of the visual axis is the macula, in the center of which is the fovea, the area of acute vision. Here layers 6, 7, 8, and 9 and blood vessels are absent, and only elongated cones are present. About 3 mm medial to the fovea is the optic disk, where axons of the ganglionic cells converge to form the optic nerve. The ciliary and iridial parts of the r. are forward prolongations of the pigmented layer and a layer of supporting columnar or epithelial cells over the ciliary body and the posterior surface of the iris, respectively. [Mediev. L. prob. fr. L. *rete,* a net]

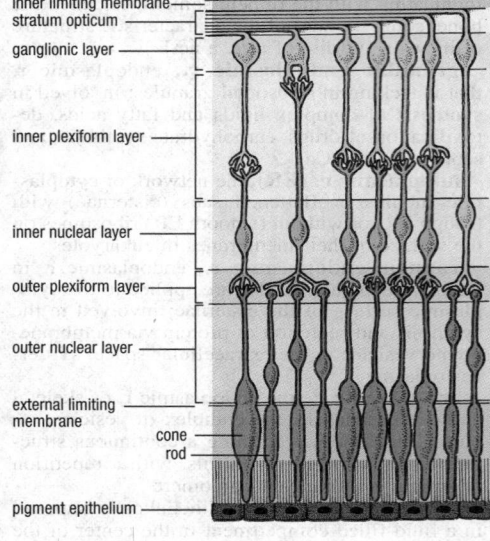

inner limiting membrane
stratum opticum
ganglionic layer
inner plexiform layer
inner nuclear layer
outer plexiform layer
outer nuclear layer
external limiting membrane
cone
rod
pigment epithelium

layers of the retina

detached r., syn retinal *detachment.*

shot-silk r., the appearance of numerous wavelike, glistening reflexes, like the shimmer of silk, observed sometimes in the r. of a young person.

ret•i•nac•u•lum, gen. **ret•i•nac•u•li,** pl. **ret•i•nac•u•la** (ret-i-nak′yū-lŭm, -lī, -lă) [NA]. A frenum, or a retaining band or ligament. [L. a band, a halter, fr. *retineo,* to hold back]

r. cu′tis [NA], one of the numerous small fibrous strands that extend through the superficial fascia attaching the deep surface of the dermis to the underlying deep fascia determining the mobility of the skin over the deep structures. syn r. of skin.

retinacula of extensor muscles, see inferior extensor r., superior extensor r.

extensor r., a strong fibrous band formed as a thickening of the antebrachial deep fascia, stretching obliquely across the back of the wrist, attaching deeply to ridges on the dorsal aspect of the radius, triquetral and pisiform bones, binding

down the extensor tendons of the fingers and thumb.

flexor r. of lower limb, a wide band passing from the medial malleolus to the medial and upper border of the calcaneus and to the plantar surface as far as the navicular bone; it holds in place the tendons of the tibialis posterior, flexor digitorum longus, and flexor hallucis longus.

inferior extensor r., a Y-shaped ligament restraining the extensor tendons of the foot distal to the ankle joint.

peroneal r., superior and inferior fibrous bands retaining the tendons of the peroneus longus and brevis in position as they cross the lateral side of the ankle. syn retinacula of peroneal muscles.

retinacula of peroneal muscles, syn peroneal r.

r. of skin, syn r. cutis.

superior extensor r., the ligament that binds down the extensor tendons proximal to the ankle joint; it is continuous with (a thickening of) the deep fascia of the leg.

r. ten′dinum, a ligamentous structure to restrain tendons, such as the flexor or extensor retinacula, or the annular parts of the digital fibrous sheaths.

ret•i•nal (ret′i-năl). **1.** Relating to the retina. **2.** Retinaldehyde; most commonly referring to the all-*trans* form.

r. isomerase, an isomerase that catalyzes the *cis-trans*-interconversion of all-*trans*-retinal-(aldehyde) to 11-*cis*-retinal(aldehyde); a part of the vision cycle.

11-*cis*-ret•i•nal. The isomer of retinaldehyde that can combine with opsin to form rhodopsin; it is formed from 11-*trans*-retinal by retinal isomerase.

ret•i•nal•de•hyde (ret-i-nal′dĕ-hīd). Retinol oxidized to a terminal aldehyde; a carotene released (as all-*trans*-retinal(aldehyde)) in the bleaching of rhodopsin by light and the dissociation of opsin in the vision cycle. syn retinene.

ret•i•nene (ret′i-nēn). syn retinaldehyde.

ret•i•ni•tis (ret-i-nī′tis). Inflammation of the retina. [retina + G. -*itis,* inflammation]

exudative r., r. exudati′va, a chronic abnormality characterized by deposition of cholesterol and cholesterol esters in outer retinal layers and subretinal space. In adults, often preceded by uveitis; in children, often preceded by retinal vascular abnormalities.

r. pigmento′sa, a hereditary progressive abiotrophy of the neuroepithelium, with atrophy and pigmentary infiltration of the inner layers of the retina. syn pigmentary retinopathy.

r. prolif′erans, syn proliferative *retinopathy.*

⌂**retino-, retin-.** The retina. [Med. L. *retina*]

ret•i•no•blas•to•ma (ret′i-nō-blas-tō′mă) [MIM* 180200, MIM*180201, MIM*180202]. Malignant ocular neoplasm of childhood, usually occurring before the third year of life, composed of primitive retinal small round cells with deeply staining nuclei and of elongate cells forming rosettes. In familial forms, the disease is commonly bilateral and multiple within an eye; in sporadic cases, rarely so. [retino- + G. *blastos,* germ, + -*oma,* tumor]

ret•i•no•cho•roid (ret′i-nō-kō′royd). SYN chorioretinal.

ret•i•no•cho•roid•i•tis (ret′i-nō-kō-roy-dī′tis). Inflammation of the retina extending to the choroid. SYN chorioretinitis, choroidoretinitis. [retinochoroid + G. -itis, inflammation]

bird shot r., bilateral diffuse retinal vasculitis with depigmentation of multiple areas of the choroid and retinal pigment epithelium posterior to the ocular equator, often with an associated papillitis or optic atrophy; vitiligo occurs occasionally.

r. juxtapapilla′ris, r. close to the optic disk. SYN Jensen's disease.

ret•i•no•ic ac•id (ret-i-nō′ik). Vitamin A_1 acid; retinaldehyde in which the terminal –CHO has been oxidized to a –COOH; used topically in the treatment of acne; plays an important role in growth and differentiation. SYN vitamin A_1 acid.

ret•i•noids (ret′i-noydz). A class of keratolytic drugs derived from retinoic acid and used for treatment of severe acne and psoriasis.

ret•i•nol (ret′i-nol). vitamin A_1 alcohol; an intermediate in the vision cycle, it also plays a role in growth and differentiation.

r. dehydrogenase, an oxidoreductase catalyzing interconversion of retinal and NADH to retinol and NAD⁺.

ret•i•no•pap•il•li•tis (ret′i-nō-pap-i-lī′tis). Inflammation of the retina extending to the optic disk.

ret•i•nop•a•thy (ret-i-nop′ă-thē). Noninflammatory degenerative disease of the retina. [retino- + G. pathos, suffering]

⚅ **diabetic r.,** retinal changes occurring in diabetes of long duration, marked by hemorrhages, microaneurysms, and sharply defined waxy deposits, or by proliferative retinopathy.

hypertensive r., a retinal condition occurring in accelerated vascular hypertension, marked by arteriolar constriction, flame-shaped hemorrhages, cotton-wool patches, star-figure edema at the macula, and papilledema.

leukemic r., appearance of the retina in all types of leukemia, characterized by engorgement and tortuosity of veins, scattered hemorrhages, and edema of the retina and disk.

pigmentary r., SYN retinitis pigmentosa.

r. of prematurity, abnormal replacement of the sensory retina by fibrous tissue and blood vessels, occurring mainly in premature infants having a birth weight of less than 1500 g who are placed in a high-oxygen environment.

proliferative r., neovascularization of the retina extending into the vitreous humor. SYN retinitis proliferans.

sickle cell r., a condition marked by dilation and tortuosity of retinal veins, and by microaneurysms and retinal hemorrhages; advanced stages may show neovascularization, vitreous hemorrhage, or retinal detachment.

ret•i•no•pexy (ret′i-nō-pek′sē). A procedure to repair a detached retina by holding it in place; e.g., by producing chorioretinal adhesions by freezing ("retinal cryopexy"). [retino- + G. pēxis, fixation]

ret•i•nos•chi•sis (ret-i-nos′ki-sis). Degenerative splitting of the retina, with cyst formation between the two layers. [retino- + G. schisis, division]

senile r., r. occurring most often in the elderly and affecting the outer plexiform layer.

ret•i•no•scope (ret′i-nō-skōp). An optical device used to illuminate a subject's retina during retinoscopy. [retino- + G. skopeō, to view]

ret•i•nos•co•py (ret′i-nos′kŏ-pē). A method of determining errors of refraction by illuminating the retina and observing the rays of light emerging from the eye. SYN shadow test, skiascopy. [retino- + G. skopeō, to view]

re•trac•tile (rē-trak′til). Retractable; capable of being drawn back.

re•trac•tion (rē-trak′shŭn). 1. A shrinking, drawing back, or pulling apart. 2. Posterior movement of teeth, usually with the aid of an orthodontic appliance. [L. retractio, a drawing back]

re•trac•tor (rē-trak′ter, -tōr). 1. An instrument for drawing aside the edges of a wound or for holding back structures adjacent to the operative field. 2. A muscle that draws a part backward.

re•treat from re•al•i•ty. Substitution of imaginary satisfactions or fantasy for relations with the real world.

re•trench•ment (rē-trench′-ment). The cutting away of superfluous tissue. [F. re-, back, + trancher, to cut]

re•triev•al (rē-trē′văl). The third stage in the memory process, after encoding and storage, involving mental processes associated with bringing stored information back into consciousness. SEE ALSO memory.

△ **retro-.** Prefix, to words formed from L. roots, denoting backward or behind. [L. back, backward]

ret•ro•cal•ca•ne•o•bur•si•tis (re′trō-kal-kā′nē-ō-ber-sī′tis). SYN achillobursitis. [retro- + L. calcaneum heel, + bursitis]

ret•ro•ces•sion (re-trō-sesh′ŭn). 1. A going back; a relapse. 2. Cessation of the external symptoms of a disease followed by signs of involvement of some internal organ or part. 3. Denoting a position of the uterus or other organ farther back than is normal. [L. retro-cedo, pp. -cessus, to go back, retire]

ret•ro•clu•sion (re-trō-klū′zhŭn). A form of acupressure for the arrest of bleeding; the needle is passed through the tissues above the cut end of the artery, is turned around, and then is passed backward beneath the vessel to come out near the point of entrance. [retro- + L. claudo (cludo) to close]

ret•ro•col•lis (re-trō-kol′is). SYN retrocollic spasm.

ret•ro•cur•sive (re′trō-ker′siv). Running backward. [retro- + L. cursus, a running]

ret•ro•de•vi•a•tion (re′trō-dē-vē-ā′shŭn). A backward bending or inclining.

ret•ro•dis•place•ment (re′trō-dis-plās′ment). Any backward displacement, such as retroversion or retroflexion of the uterus.

ret•ro•flex•ion (re-trō-flek′shŭn). Backward bending, as of the uterus when the corpus is bent back, forming an angle with the cervix.

ret•ro•gnath•ic (re-trō-nath′ik). Denoting a state

re

in which the mandible is located posterior to its normal position in relation to the maxillae.

ret·ro·gnath·ism (re-trō-nath′izm). A condition of facial disharmony in which one or both jaws are posterior to normal in their craniofacial relationships; usually used in reference to the mandible. [retro- + G. *gnathos,* jaw]

ret·ro·grade (ret′rō-grād). **1.** Moving backward. **2.** Degenerating; reversing the normal order of growth and development. [L. *retrogradus,* fr. retro- + *gradior,* to go]

ret·ro·gres·sion (re-trō-gresh′ŭn). SYN cataplasia. [L. *retrogressus,* fr. *retrogradior,* to go backwards]

ret·ro·jec·tion (re-trō-jek′shŭn). The washing out of a cavity by the backward flow of an injected fluid. [L. *retro,* backward, + *jacio,* to throw]

ret·ro·per·i·to·ni·tis (ret′rō-per-i-tō-nī′tis). Inflammation of the cellular tissue behind the peritoneum.

ret·ro·phar·ynx (re′trō-făr′ingks). The posterior part of the pharynx.

ret·ro·pla·sa (ret-rō-plā′zē-ă). That state of cell or tissue in which activity is decreased below that considered normal; associated with retrogressive changes (*e.g.,* injury, degeneration, death, necrosis). [retro- + G. *plasis,* a molding]

ret·ro·posed (re′trō-pōzd). Denoting retroposition. [retro- + L. *pono,* pp. *positus,* to place]

ret·ro·po·si·tion (re′trō-pō-zish′ŭn). Simple backward displacement of a structure or organ, as the uterus, without inclination, bending, retroversion, or retroflexion. [retro- + L. *positio,* a placing]

ret·ro·pos·on (re-trō-pōs′on). A transposition of sequences in a DNA that does not originate in the DNA but in an mRNA that is transcribed back into the genomic DNA by reverse transcription. [retro- + L. *pono,* pp. *positum,* to place, + -on]

ret·ro·pul·sion (re-trō-pŭl′shŭn). **1.** An involuntary backward walking or running, occurring in patients with the parkinsonian syndrome. **2.** A pushing back of any part. [retro- + L. *pulsio,* a pushing, fr. *pello,* pp. *pulsus,* beat, drive]

ret·ro·spon·dy·lo·lis·the·sis (re′trō-spon′di-lō-lis-thē′sis). Slipping posteriorly of the body of a vertebra, bringing it out of line with the adjacent vertebrae. [retro- + G. *spondylos,* vertebra, + *olisthēsis,* a slipping]

ret·ro·ver·si·o·flex·ion (re-trō-ver′sē-ō-flek′shŭn, -ver′zhō-). Combined retroversion and retroflexion of the uterus.

ret·ro·ver·sion (re-trō-ver′zhŭn). **1.** A turning backward, as of the uterus. **2.** Condition in which the teeth are located in a more posterior position than is normal. [retro- + L. *verto,* pp. *versus,* to turn]

ret·ro·vert·ed (re′trō-ver-ted). Denoting retroversion.

Ret·ro·vir·i·dae (re-trō-vir′i-dē). A family of viruses grouped in three subfamilies: Oncovirinae (HTLV-I, HTLV-II RNA tumor viruses), Spumavirinae (foamy viruses), and Lentivirinae (HIV-like viruses, visna and related agents).

ret·ro·vi·rus (re′trō-vī′rŭs). Any virus of the family Retroviridae. A virus with RNA core genetic material; requires the enzyme reverse transcriptase in order to convert its RNA into proviral DNA.

re·tru·sion (rē-trū′zhŭn). **1.** Retraction of the mandible from any given point. **2.** The backward movement of the mandible. [L. *retrudo,* pp. *-trusus,* to push back]

re·vas·cu·lar·i·za·tion (rē-vas′kyū-lăr-i-zā′shŭn). Reestablishment of blood supply to a part.

re·ver·sal (rē-ver′săl). **1.** A turning or changing to the opposite direction, as of a process, disease, symptom, or state. **2.** The changing of a dark line or a bright one of the spectrum into its opposite. **3.** Denoting the difficulty of some persons in distinguishing the lowercase printed or written letter *p* from *q* or *g, b* from *d,* or *s* from *z.* **4.** PSYCHOANALYSIS The change of an instinct or affect into its opposite, as from love into hate. [L. *reverto,* pp. *-versus,* to turn back or about]

   narcotic r., the use of narcotic antagonists, such as naloxone, to terminate the action of narcotics.

   pressure r., cessation of anesthesia by hyperbaric pressure; of major importance in understanding the mode of action of anesthetics.

   relaxant r., use of acetylcholinesterase inhibitors to terminate the action of nondepolarizing neuromuscular relaxants.

   sex r., a process whereby the sexual identity of an individual is changed from one sex to the other (*e.g.,* by a combination of surgical, pharmacologic, and psychiatric procedures); it may also occur in the life history of pseudohermaphroditic individuals whose sex at birth was uncertain; initially reared as members of one gender or sex role, such individuals may, upon subsequent medical examination and advice, be reared thereafter as members of the opposite gender or sex role.

re·ver·sion (rē-ver′zhŭn). **1.** The manifestation in an individual of certain characteristics, peculiar to a remote ancestor, which have been suppressed during one or more of the intermediate generations. **2.** The return to the original phenotype, either by reinstatement of the original genotype (true r.) or by a mutation at a site different from that of the first mutation which cancels the effect of the first mutation (suppressor mutation). [L. *reversio* (see reversal)]

re·ver·tant (rē-ver′tant). In microbial genetics, a mutant that has reverted to its former genotype (true reversion) or to the original phenotype by means of a suppressor mutation. [L. *revertans,* pros. p. of *reverto,* to turn back]

re·viv·i·fi·ca·tion (rē-viv′i-fi-kā′shŭn). **1.** Renewal of life and strength. **2.** Refreshening the edges of a wound by paring or scraping to promote healing. SYN vivification. [L. *re-,* again, + *vivo,* to live, + *facio,* to make]

re·vul·sion (rē-vŭl′shŭn). **1.** SYN counterirritation. **2.** SYN derivation (1). [L. *revulsio,* act of pulling away, fr. *revello,* pp. *-vulsus,* to pluck or pull away]

re·ward (rē-ward′). SYN reinforcer.

RFLP restriction fragment length *polymorphism.*

RFP right frontoposterior position.

RFT right frontotransverse position.

Rh 1. rhodium. **2.** See Rh blood group, Blood Groups appendix.

⌂**rhabd-.** SEE rhabdo-.

⌂**rhabdo-, rhabd-.** Rod; rod-shaped (rhabdoid). [G. *rhabdos*]

rhab·doid (rab′doyd). Rod-shaped. [rhabdo- + G. *eidos*, resemblance]

rhab·do·my·o·blast (rab-dō-mī′ō-blast). Large round, spindle-shaped, or strap-shaped cells with deeply eosinophilic fibrillar cytoplasm which may show cross striations; found in some rhabdomyosarcomas. [rhabdo- + G. *mys*, muscle, + *blastos*, germ]

rhab·do·my·ol·y·sis (rab′dō-mī-ol′i-sis). An acute, fulminating, potentially fatal disease of skeletal muscle that entails destruction of muscle as evidenced by myoglobinemia and myoglobinuria. [rhabdo- + G. *mys*, muscle, + *lysis*, loosening]

rhab·do·my·o·ma (rab′dō-mī-ō′mă). A benign neoplasm derived from striated muscle, occurring in the heart in children, probably as a hamartomatous process. [rhabdo- + G. *mys*, muscle, + *-oma*, tumor]

rhab·do·my·o·sar·co·ma (rab′dō-mī-ō-sar-kō′mă). A malignant neoplasm derived from skeletal (striated) muscle, classified as embryonal alveolar (composed of loose aggregates of small round cells) or pleomorphic (containing rhabdomyoblasts). SYN rhabdosarcoma. [rhabdo- + G. *mys*, muscle, + *sarkōma*, sarcoma]

  embryonal r.'s, malignant neoplasms occurring in children, consisting of loose, spindle-celled tissue with rare cross-striations, and arising in many parts of the body in addition to skeletal muscles.

rhab·do·sar·co·ma (rab′dō-sar-kō′mă). SYN rhabdomyosarcoma.

Rhab·do·vir·i·dae (rab′dō-vir′i-dē). A family of rod- or bullet-shaped viruses of vertebrates, insects, and plants, including rabies virus.

rhab·do·vi·rus (rab′dō-vī′rŭs). Any virus of the family Rhabdoviridae.

rhag·a·des (rag′ă-dēz). Chaps, cracks, or fissures occurring at mucocutaneous junctions; seen in vitamin deficiency diseases and in congenital syphilis. [G. *rhagas*, pl. *rhagades*, a crack]

rheg·ma (reg′mă). A rent or fissure. [G. breakage]

rheg·ma·tog·e·nous (reg-mă-toj′ĕ-nŭs). Arising from a bursting or fractionating of an organ. [G. *rhēgma*, breakage, + *-gen*, producing]

rhe·ni·um (Re) (rē′nē-ŭm). A metallic element of the platinum group; atomic wt. 186.207, atomic no. 75. [Mod. L., fr. L. *Rhenus*, Rhine river]

⌂**rheo-.** Blood flow; electrical current. [G. *rheos*, stream, current, flow]

rhe·o·base (rē′ō-bās). The minimal strength of an electrical stimulus of indefinite duration that is able to cause excitation of a tissue, *e.g.*, muscle or nerve. SEE ALSO chronaxie. [rheo- + G. *basis*, a base]

rhe·o·ba·sic (rē-ō-bā′sik). Pertaining to or having the characteristics of a rheobase.

rhe·ol·o·gy (rē-ol′ō-jē). The study of the deformation and flow of materials. [rheo- + G. *logos*, study]

rhe·om·e·try (rē-om′ĕ-trē). Measurement of electrical current or blood flow.

rhe·os·to·sis (rē-os-tō′sis). A hypertrophying and condensing osteitis which tends to run in longitudinal streaks or columns, like wax drippings on a candle, and which involves a number of the long bones. [rheo- + G. *osteon*, bone, + *-osis*, condition]

rhe·o·tax·is (rē-ō-tak′sis). A form of positive barotaxis, in which a microorganism in a fluid is impelled to move against the current flow of its medium. [rheo- + G. *taxis*, orderly arrangement]

rhe·ot·ro·pism (rē-ot′rō-pizm). A movement contrary to the motion of a current, involving part of an organism, rather than the organism as a whole, as in rheotaxis. [rheo- + G. *tropos*, a turning]

rhes·to·cy·the·mia (res′tō-sī-thē′mē-ă). The presence of broken down red blood cells in the peripheral circulation. [G. *rhaiō*, to destroy, + *kytos*, a hollow (a cell), + *haima*, blood]

rheum (rūm). A mucous or watery discharge. [G. *rheuma*, a flux]

rheu·mat·ic (rū-mat′ik). Relating to or characterized by rheumatism. [G. *rheumatikos*, subject to flux, fr. *rheuma*, flux]

rheu·ma·tid (rū′mă-tid). Rheumatic nodules or other eruptions which may accompany rheumatism. [G. *rheum*, flux, + *-id (1)*]

rheu·ma·tism (rū′mă-tizm). Indefinite term applied to various conditions with pain or other symptoms of articular origin or related to other elements of the musculoskeletal system. [G. *rheumatismos*, rheuma, a flux]

  articular r., SYN arthritis.

  inflammatory r., rheumatoid arthritis or other cause of joint inflammation.

  lumbar r., SYN lumbago.

  nodose r., (1) SYN rheumatoid *arthritis*. **(2)** an acute or subacute articular r., accompanied by the formation of nodules on the tendons, ligaments, and periosteum in the neighborhood of the affected joints.

rheu·ma·toid (rū′mă-toyd). Resembling r. arthritis in one or more features. [G. *rheuma*, flux, + *eidos*, resemblance]

rheu·ma·tol·o·gist (rū-mă-tol′ō-jist). A specialist in rheumatology.

rheu·ma·tol·o·gy (rū-mă-tol′ō-jē). The medical specialty concerned with the study, diagnosis, and treatment of rheumatic conditions. [G. *rheuma*, flux, + *logos*, study]

RhIG Rh-immune *globulin*.

⌂**rhin-, rhino-.** The nose. [G. *rhis*]

rhi·nal (rī′năl). SYN nasal.

rhi·nal·gia (rī-nal′jē-ă). Pain in the nose. SYN rhinodynia. [rhin- + G. *algos*, pain]

rhin·e·de·ma (rī′ne-dē′mă). Swelling of the nasal mucous membrane. [rhin- + G. *oidēma*, swelling]

rhin·en·ce·phal·ic (rī′nen-se-fal′ik). Relating to the rhinencephalon.

rhin·en·ceph·a·lon (rī′nen-sef′ă-lon). Collective term denoting the parts of the cerebral hemisphere directly related to the sense of smell: the olfactory bulb, olfactory peduncle, olfactory tubercle, and olfactory or piriform cortex including the cortical nucleus of the amygdala. SEE ALSO limbic *system*. [rhin- + G. *enkephalos*, brain]

rhi·ni·tis (rī-nī′tis). Inflammation of the nasal mucous membrane. [rhin- + G. *-itis*, inflammation]

   acute r., an acute catarrhal inflammation of the mucous membrane of the nose, marked by sneezing, lacrimation, and a profuse secretion of watery mucus; usually associated with infection by one of the common cold viruses. SYN coryza.

   allergic r., r. associated with hay fever.

   atrophic r., chronic r. with thinning of the mucous membrane; often associated with crusts and foul-smelling discharge.

   hypertrophic r., chronic r. with permanent thickening of the mucous membrane.

   vasomotor r., congestion of nasal mucosa without infection or allergy.

△**rhino-.** SEE rhin-.

rhi·no·cele (rī′nō-sēl). Cavity (ventricle) of the rhinencephalon, the primitive olfactory part of the telencephalon. [rhino- + G. *koilia*, a hollow]

rhi·no·ceph·a·ly, rhi·no·ce·pha·lia (rī′nō-sef′ă-lē, -se-fā′lē-ă). Rhinencephaly; a form of cyclopia in which the nose is represented by a fleshy protuberance arising above the slitlike orbits, and the rhinencephalic lobes of the telencephalon are poorly developed. [rhino- + G. *kephalē*, head]

Rhi·no·clad·i·el·la (rī′nō-klad-ē-el′ă). A genus of dematiaceous fungi that cause chromoblastomycosis. SEE ALSO *Phialophora*.

rhi·no·clei·sis (rī-nō-klī′sis). SYN rhinostenosis. [rhino- + G. *kleisis*, a closure]

rhi·no·dyn·ia (rī-nō-din′ē-ă). SYN rhinalgia. [rhino- + G. *odynē*, pain]

rhi·nog·e·nous (rī-noj′ĕ-nŭs). Originating in the nose. [rhino- + G. *-gen*, producing]

rhi·no·ky·pho·sis (rī′nō-kī-fō′sis). A humpback deformity of the nose. [rhino- + G. *kyphōsis*, humped condition]

rhi·no·la·lia (rī′nō-lā′lē-ă). Nasalized speech. SYN rhinophonia. [rhino- + G. *lalia*, talking]

rhi·no·lith (rī′nō-lith). A calcareous concretion in the nasal cavity often around foreign body. [rhino- + G. *lithos*, stone]

rhi·no·li·thi·a·sis (rī′nō-li-thī′ă-sis). The presence of a nasal calculus. [rhinolith + G. *-iasis*, condition]

rhi·nol·o·gist (rī-nol′ō-jist). A specialist in diseases of the nose.

rhi·nol·o·gy (rī-nol′ō-jē). The branch of medical science concerned with the nose and its diseases. [rhino- + G. *logos*, study]

rhi·no·ma·nom·e·ter (rī′nō-mă-nom′ĕ-ter). A manometer used to determine the presence and amount of nasal obstruction, and the nasal air pressure and flow relationships. [rhino- + manometer]

rhi·no·ma·nom·e·try (rī′nō-mă-nom′ĕ-trē). **1.** The use of a rhinomanometer. **2.** The study and measurement of nasal air flow and pressures.

rhi·no·my·co·sis (rī′nō-mī-kō′sis). Fungus infection of the nasal mucous membranes. [rhino- + mycosis]

rhi·no·ne·cro·sis (rī′nō-ne-krō′sis). Necrosis of the bones of the nose. [rhino- + necrosis]

rhi·nop·a·thy (rī-nop′ă-thē). Disease of the nose. [rhino- + G. *pathos*, suffering]

rhi·no·pho·nia (rī′nō-fō′nē-ă). SYN rhinolalia. [rhino- + G. *phōnē*, voice]

rhi·no·phy·ma (rī′nō-fī′mă). Hypertrophy of the nose with follicular dilation, resulting from hyperplasia of sebaceous glands with fibrosis and increased vascularity. [rhino- + G. *phyma*, tumor, growth]

rhi·no·plas·ty (rī′nō-plas-tē). **1.** Repair of a defect of the nose with tissue taken from elsewhere. **2.** Plastic surgery to change the shape or size of the nose. [rhino- + G. *plastos*, formed]

rhi·nor·rhea (rī-nō-rē′ă). A discharge from the nasal mucous membrane. [rhino- + G. *rhoia*, flow]

   cerebrospinal fluid r., a discharge of cerebrospinal fluid from the nose.

   gustatory r., watery nasal discharge associated with stimulation of the sense of taste.

rhi·no·sal·pin·gi·tis (rī′nō-sal-pin-jī′tis). Inflammation of the mucous membrane of the nose and auditory tube. [rhino- + G. *salpinx*, tube, + *-itis*, inflammation]

rhi·no·scle·ro·ma (rī′nō-sklē-rō′mă). A chronic granulomatous process involving the nose, upper lip, mouth, and upper air passages; it may involve the external auditory meatus and is believed to be due to a specific bacterium, possibly a strain of *Klebsiella*. [rhino- + G. *sklērōma*, an induration]

rhi·no·scope (rī′nō-skōp). A small mirror attached at a suitable angle to a rodlike handle, used in posterior rhinoscopy.

rhi·no·scop·ic (rī′nō-skop′ik). Relating to the rhinoscope or to rhinoscopy.

rhi·nos·co·py (rī-nos′kŏ-pē). Inspection of the nasal cavity. [rhino- + G. *skopeō*, to view]

   anterior r., inspection of the anterior portion of the nasal cavity with or without the aid of a nasal speculum.

   median r., inspection of the roof of the nasal cavity and openings of the posterior ethmoid cells and sphenoidal sinus by means of a long-bladed nasal speculum or nasopharyngoscope.

   posterior r., inspection of the nasopharynx and posterior portion of the nasal cavity by means of the rhinoscope, or with a nasopharyngoscope. SEE ALSO nasopharyngoscopy.

rhi·no·ste·no·sis (rī′nō-ste-nō′sis). Nasal obstruction. SYN rhinocleisis. [rhino- + G. *stenōsis*, a narrowing]

rhi·not·o·my (rī-not′ō-mē). **1.** Any cutting operation on the nose. **2.** Operative procedure in which the nose is incised along one side so that it may be turned away to provide full vision of the nasal passages for radical sinus operations. [rhino- + G. *tomē*, incision, cutting]

Rhi·no·vi·rus (rī′nō-vī′rŭs). A genus of acid-labile viruses associated with the common cold. There are more than 110 antigenic types.

rhi·no·vi·rus. Any virus of the genus *Rhinovirus*.

rhizo-. Combining form denoting root. [G. *rhiza*]

rhi·zoid (rī′zoyd). **1.** Rootlike. **2.** Irregularly branching, like a root; denoting a form of bacterial growth. **3.** In fungi, the rootlike hyphae which arise at the nodes of the hyphae of *Rhizopus* species. [rhizo- + G. *eidos,* resemblance]

rhi·zo·me·lia (rī-zō-mē′lē-ă). **1.** Disproportion in the length of the most proximal segment of the limbs (upper arms and thighs). **2.** A disorder involving the shoulder and hip joint. [rhizo- + G. *melos,* limb]

rhi·zo·me·nin·go·my·e·li·tis (rī′zō-mĕ-ning′gō-mī-ĕ-lī′tis). Inflammation of the nerve roots, the meninges, and the spinal cord. SYN radiculomeningomyelitis. [rhizo- + G. *mēninx,* membrane, + *myelon,* marrow, + *-itis,* inflammation]

Rhi·zop·o·da (rī-zō-pō′dă). A superclass in the subphylum Sarcodina that includes the amebae of humans, having pseudopodia of various forms but without axial filaments. [rhizo + G. *pous* (*pod*-), foot]

Rhi·zo·pus (rī-zō′pŭs). A genus of fungi of which some species cause zygomycosis in humans.

rhi·zot·o·my (rī-zot′ō-mē). Section of the spinal nerve roots for the relief of pain or spastic paralysis. SYN radicotomy, radiculectomy. [G. *rhiza,* root, + *tomē,* section]

    trigeminal r., division or section of a sensory root of the fifth cranial nerve, accomplished through a subtemporal (Frazier-Spiller operation), suboccipital (Dandy operation), or transtentorial approach.

rho (ρ) (rō). **1.** 17th letter of the Greek alphabet. **2.** Population correlation coefficient; symbol for density.

rhod-. SEE rhodo-.

rho·di·um (Rh) (rō′dē-ŭm). A metallic element, atomic no. 45, atomic wt. 102.90550. [Mod. L. fr. G. *rhodon,* a rose]

rhodo-, rhod-. Rosy, red color. [G. *rhodon,* rose]

rho·do·gen·e·sis (rō′dō-jen′ĕ-sis). The production of rhodopsin by the combination of 11-*cis*-retinal and opsin in the dark. [rhodopsin + G. *genesis,* production]

rho·do·phy·lac·tic (rō′dō-fī-lak′tik). Relating to rhodophylaxis.

rho·do·phy·lax·is (rō′dō-fī-lak′sis). The action of the pigment cells of the choroid in preserving or facilitating the reproduction of rhodopsin. [rhodopsin + G. *phylaxis,* a guarding]

rho·dop·sin (rō-dop′sin). A red thermolabile protein found in the rods of the retina; it is bleached by the action of light, which converts it to opsin and all-*trans*-retinal, and is restored in the dark by rhodogenesis; the dominant protein in the plasma membrane of rod cells. SYN visual purple.

rhomb·en·ceph·a·lon (rom-ben-sef′ă-lon) [NA]. That part of the developing brain that is the most caudal of the three primary vesicles of the embryonic neural tube; secondarily divided into metencephalon and myelencephalon; the r. includes the pons, cerebellum, and medulla oblongata. SYN hindbrain. [rhombo- + G. *enkephalos,* brain]

rhom·bic (rom′bik). **1.** SYN rhomboid. **2.** Relating to the rhombencephalon.

rhom·bo·cele (rom′bō-sēl). SYN rhomboidal *sinus.* [rhombo- + G. *koilia,* a hollow]

rhom·boid, rhom·boi·dal (rom′boyd, rom-boy′dăl). Resembling a rhomb; *i.e.,* an oblique parallelogram, but having unequal sides. SYN rhombic (1). [rhombo- + G. *eidos,* appearance]

rhon·chal, rhon·chi·al (rong′kăl, rong′kē-ăl). Relating to or characteristic of a rhonchus.

rhon·chus, pl. **rhon·chi** (rong′kŭs, -kī). An added sound with a musical pitch occurring during inspiration or expiration, heard on auscultation of the chest, and caused by air passing through bronchi that are narrowed by inflammation, spasm of smooth muscle, or presence of mucus in the lumen; if low-pitched, it is called **sonorous r.**; if high-pitched, with a whistling or squeaky quality, **sibilant r..** [L. fr. G. *rhenchos,* a snoring]

rhythm (rith′ŭm). **1.** Measured time or motion; the regular alternation of two or more different or opposite states. **2.** SYN rhythm *method.* **3.** Regular occurrence of an electrical event in the electroencephalogram. SEE ALSO wave. **4.** Sequential beating of the heart generated by a single beat or sequence of beats. [G. *rhythmos*]

    alpha r., (1) a wave pattern in the encephalogram in the frequency band of 8 to 13 Hz; **(2)** the posterior dominant 8–13 Hz r. in the awake, relaxed person with closed eyes. SYN alpha wave.

    atrioventricular junctional r., the cardiac r. when the heart is controlled by the A-V junction (including node); arising in the A-V junction, the impulse ascends to the atria and descends to the ventricles, each at varying speeds depending on site of the pacemaker.

    beta r., a wave pattern in the electroencephalogram in the frequency band of 18 to 30 Hz. SYN beta wave.

    bigeminal r., cardiac r. in which each beat of the dominant rhythm (sinus or other) is followed by a premature beat, with the result that the heartbeats occur in pairs (bigeminy). SYN coupled r.

    cantering r., SYN gallop.

    coupled r., SYN bigeminal r.

    delta r., a wave pattern in the electroencephalogram in the frequency band of 1.5 to 4.0 Hz. SYN delta wave (2).

    escape r., three or more consecutive impulses at a rate not exceeding the upper limit of the inherent pacemaker.

    gallop r., SYN gallop.

    idioventricular r., a slow independent ventricular r. under control of an ectopic ventricular center. SYN ventricular r.

    junctional r., r.'s originating anywhere within the A-V junction. Formerly, "A-V nodal" or simply "nodal" r.'s.

    quadrigeminal r., a cardiac arrhythmia in which the heartbeats are grouped in fours, each usually composed of one sinus beat followed by three extrasystoles, but a repetitive group of four of any composition is quadrigeminal.

    scapulohumeral r., coordinated rotational movement of the scapula that accompanies abduction and adduction of the humerus.

    sinus r., normal cardiac r. proceeding from the sinoatrial node.

    theta r., a wave pattern in the electroencephalo-

normal sinus rhythm (NSR)

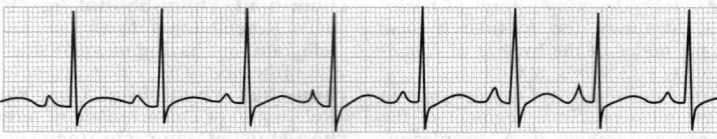

bradycardia

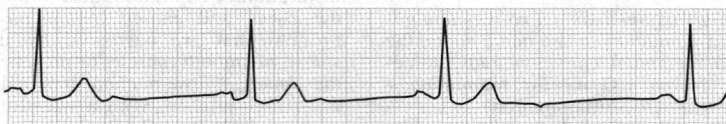

fibrillation (ventricular)

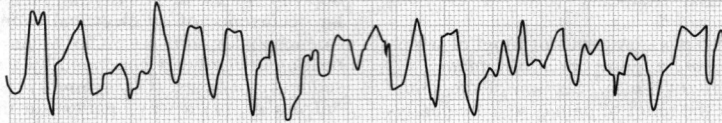

flutter (atrial)

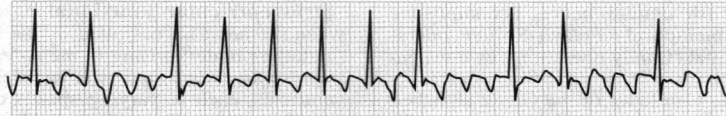

heart block

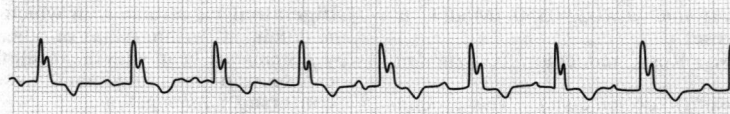

premature ventricular contraction (PVC)

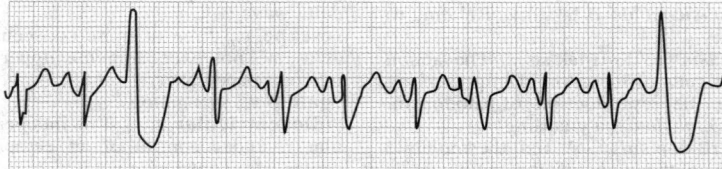

tachycardia (sinus)

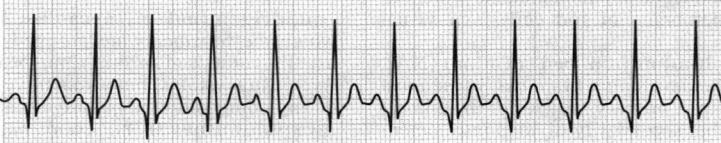

rhythm: electrocardiogram tracings showing common types of arrhythmia

gram in the frequency band of 4 to 7 Hz. SYN theta wave.

trigeminal r., a cardiac arrhythmia in which the beats are grouped in trios, usually composed of a sinus beat followed by two extrasystoles. SYN trigeminy.

ventricular r., SYN idioventricular r.

rhyt·i·dec·tomy (rit-i-dek′tō-mē). Elimination of wrinkles from, or reshaping of, the face by excising any excess skin and tightening the remainder; the so-called face-lift. SYN rhytidoplasty. [G. *rhytis* (*rhytid-*), a wrinkle, + ectomy]

rhyt·i·do·plas·ty (rit′i-dō-plas-tē). SYN rhytidectomy. [G. *rhytis,* a wrinkle, + *plastos,* formed]

rhyt·i·do·sis (rit-i-dō′sis). **1.** Wrinkling of the face to a degree disproportionate to age. **2.** Laxity and wrinkling of the cornea, an indication of approaching death. SYN rutidosis. [G. a wrinkling, fr. *rhytis,* a wrinkle, + *-osis,* condition]

Rib ribose. SYN costa (1).

rib. One of the twenty-four elongated curved bones forming the main portion of the bony wall of the chest. [A.S. *ribb*]

bicipital r., fusion of first thoracic r. with cervical vertebra.

cervical r., a supernumerary rib articulating with a cervical vertebra, usually the seventh, but not reaching the sternum anteriorly. SEE ALSO cervical rib *syndrome.* SYN costa cervicalis [NA].

false r.'s, five lower ribs on either side that do not articulate with the sternum directly. SYN costae spuriae [NA].

floating r.'s, the two lower ribs on either side that are not attached anteriorly. SYN costae fluitantes [NA], vertebral r.'s.

lumbar r., an occasional r. articulating with the transverse process of the first lumbar vertebra.

slipping r., subluxation of a r. cartilage, with costochondral separation.

true r.'s, seven upper ribs on either side whose cartilages articulate directly with the sternum. SYN costae verae [NA].

vertebral r.'s, SYN floating r.'s.

ribo-. 1. Ribose. **2.** As an italicized prefix to the systematic name of a monosaccharide, *ribo-* indicates that the configuration of a set of three consecutive CHOH groups is that of ribose. [German *Ribose,* alt. from arabinose, fr. *gum arabic* + *-ose*]

ri·bo·nu·cle·ase (RNase) (rī-bō-nū′klē-ās). A transferase or phosphodiesterase that catalyzes the hydrolysis of ribonucleic acid.

ri·bo·nu·cle·ic ac·id (RNA) (rī′bō-nū-klē′ik). A macromolecule consisting of ribonucleoside residues connected by phosphate bonds, concerned in the control of cellular chemical process, especially protein synthesis. RNA is found in all cells, in both nuclei and cytoplasm, and also in many viruses.

messenger RNA (mRNA), the RNA reflecting the exact nucleoside sequence of the genetically active DNA and carrying the "message" of the latter, coded in its sequence, to the cytoplasmic areas where protein is made in amino acid sequences specified by the mRNA, and hence primarily by the DNA; viral RNA's are considered to be natural messenger RNA's.

nuclear RNA (nRNA), rNA found in nuclei, or associated with DNA, or with nuclear structures (nucleoli).

ribosomal RNA, the RNA of ribosomes and polyribosomes.

soluble RNA (sRNA), SYN transfer RNA. [soluble in molar salt]

transfer RNA (tRNA), short-chain RNA molecules present in cells in at least 20 varieties, each variety capable of combining with a specific amino acid (see aminoacyl-tRNA). By joining (through their anticodons) with particular spots (codons) along the messenger RNA molecule and carrying their amino acyl residues along, they lead to the formation of protein molecules with a specific amino acid arrangement. SYN soluble RNA.

ri·bo·nu·cle·o·pro·tein (RNP) (rī′bō-nū′klē-ō-prō′tēn). A combination of ribonucleic acid and protein.

ri·bo·nu·cle·o·side (rī-bō-nū′klē-ō-sīd). A nucleoside in which the sugar component is ribose; the common r.'s of RNA are adenosine, cytidine, guanosine, and uridine.

ri·bo·nu·cle·o·tide (rī-bō-nū′klē-ō-tīd). A nucleotide (nucleoside phosphate) in which the sugar component is ribose; the major r.'s of RNA are adenylic acid, cytidylic acid, guanylic acid, and uridylic acid.

ri·bose (Rib) (rī′bōs). The pentose present in ribonucleic acid; epimers of D-r. are D-arabinose, D-xylose, and L-lyxose.

ri·bose-5-phos·phate. Ribose phosphorylated on carbon-5; an intermediate in the pentose phosphate pathway.

r.-5-p. isomerase, an enzyme catalyzing interconversion of D-ribose 5-phosphate and D-ribulose 5-phosphate; of importance in ribose metabolism and in the pentose phosphate pathway.

ri·bo·some (rī′bō-sōm). A granule of ribonucleoprotein, 120 to 150 Å in diameter, that is the site of protein synthesis from aminoacyl-tRNAs as directed by mRNAs.

ri·bo·su·ria (rī-bō-sū′rē-ă). The enhanced urinary excretion of D-ribose; commonly one manifestation of muscular dystrophy. [ribose + G. *ouron,* urine]

ri·bo·syl (rī′bō-sil). The radical formed by loss of the hemiacetal OH group from either of the two cyclic forms of ribose.

ri·bo·thy·mi·dine (T) (rī-bō-thī′mi-dēn). 5-methyluridine; the ribosyl analog of thymidine (deoxyribosylthymine); a nucleoside found in small amounts in ribonucleic acids.

ri·bo·thy·mi·dyl·ic ac·id (rTMP, TMP) (rī′bō-thī-mi-dil′ik). Ribothymidine 5′-phosphate; the ribose analog of thymidylic acid; a rare component of transfer RNAs.

rick·ets (rik′ets). A disease due to vitamin-D deficiency and characterized by overproduction and deficient calcification of osteoid tissue, with associated skeletal deformities, disturbances in growth, and hypocalcemia. SYN infantile osteomalacia, juvenile osteomalacia, rachitis. [E. *wrick,* to twist]

adult r., SYN osteomalacia.

late r., SYN osteomalacia.

renal r., a form of r. occurring in children in association with and apparently caused by renal disease with hyperphosphatemia. SYN pseudorickets.

vitamin D-resistant r., a group of disorders characterized by hypophosphatemic osteomalacia; heritable renal tubular disorders and abnormalities in vitamin-D metabolism occur in some patients.

Rick•ett•sia (ri-ket'sē-ă). A genus of bacteria containing small (nonfilterable), often pleomorphic, coccoid to rod-shaped, Gram-negative organisms that usually occur intracytoplasmically in lice, fleas, ticks, and mites; pathogenic species are parasitic in man and other animals, causing epidemic typhus, murine or endemic typhus, Rocky Mountain spotted fever, tsutsugamushi disease, rickettsialpox, and other diseases; type species is *R. prowazekii*. [Howard T. *Ricketts*]

R. ak'ari, a species causing human rickettsialpox, a mild, acute febrile disease; transmitted by the house mouse mite, *Liponyssoides sanguineus*.

R. conorii, a widespread African species probably causing boutonneuse fever in humans, transmitted by various ticks.

R. prowazek'ii, a species causing epidemic and recrudescent typhus, transmitted by body lice; type species of the genus *R*.

R. ricketts'ii, the agent of Rocky Mountain spotted fever and geographic variants of its; transmitted by infected ixodid ticks, especially *Dermacentor andersoni* and *D. variabilis*.

R. tsutsugamu'shi, a species causing tsutsugamushi disease and scrub typhus; transmitted by trombiculid mites.

rick•ett•si•al (ri-ket'sē-ăl). Pertaining to or caused by rickettsiae.

rick•ett•si•al•pox (ri-ket'sē-ăl-poks'). Infection with *Rickettsia akari*, which is spread by mites from reservoir in mice; a benign, self-limited febrile illness.

rick•ett•si•o•sis (ri-ket-sē-ō'sis). Infection with rickettsiae.

ridge (rij). **1.** A (usually rough) linear elevation. SEE ALSO crest. **2.** DENTISTRY Any linear elevation on the surface of a tooth. **3.** The remainder of the alveolar process and its soft tissue covering after the teeth are removed. [A. S. *hyrcg*, back, spine]

dental r., the prominent border of a cusp or margin of a tooth.

epidermal r.'s, ridges of the epidermis of the palms and soles, where the sweat pores open. SYN skin r.'s.

genital r., SYN gonadal r.

gonadal r., an elevation of thickened mesothelium and underlying mesenchyme on the ventromedial border of the embryonic mesonephros; the primordial germ cells become embedded in it, establishing it as the primordium of the testis or ovary. SYN genital r.

mammary r., bandlike thickening of ectoderm in the embryo extending on either side from just below the axilla to the inguinal region; in human embryos, the mammary glands arise from primordia in the thoracic part of the r. SYN mammary fold, milk line.

mesonephric r., a r. which, in early human embryos, comprises the entire urogenital r.; however, later in development a more medial genital r., the potential gonad, is demarcated from it. SEE ALSO urogenital r. SYN mesonephric fold.

rete r.'s, downward thickening of the epidermis between the dermal papillae; peg is a misnomer because the dermal papillae are cylindrical but the epidermal thickening between papillae is not.

skin r.'s, SYN epidermal r.'s.

urogenital r., one of the paired longitudinal r.'s developing in the dorsal body wall of the embryo on either side of the dorsal mesentery; the r. is formed at first by the growing mesonephros and later by the mesonephros and the gonad.

right-foot•ed (rīt'fŭt-ed). SYN dextropedal.

right-hand•ed (rīt'hand-ed). Denoting the habitual or more skillful use of the right hand for writing and most manual operations. SYN dextral.

ri•gid•i•ty (ri-jid'i-tē). **1.** Stiffness or inflexibility. SYN rigor (1). **2.** PSYCHIATRY, CLINICAL PSYCHOLOGY An aspect of personality characterized by an individual's resistance to change. [L. *rigidus*, rigid, inflexible]

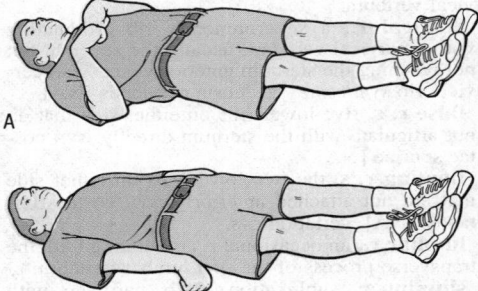

rigidity: (A) decorticate, (B) decerebrate

catatonic r., r. associated with catatonic psychotic states in which all muscles exhibit flexibilitas cerea.

clasp-knife r., SYN clasp-knife *spasticity*.

cogwheel r., a type of r. seen in parkinsonism in which the muscles respond with cogwheel-like jerks to the use of constant force in bending the limb.

decerebrate r., a postural change that occurs in some comatose patients, consisting of episodes of opisthotonos, rigid extension of the limbs, internal rotation of the upper extremities, and marked plantar flexion of the feet; produced by a variety of metabolic and structural brain disorders. SEE ALSO decorticate r.

decorticate r., a unilateral or bilateral postural change, consisting of the upper extremities flexed and adducted and the lower extremities in rigid extension; due to structural lesions of the thalamus, internal capsule, or cerebral white matter.

postmortem r., SYN rigor mortis.

rig•or (rig'er). **1.** SYN rigidity (1). **2.** SYN chill (2). [L. stiffness]

r. mor'tis, stiffening of the body, from 1 to 7 hours after death, from hardening of the muscular tissues in consequence of the coagulation of the myosinogen and paramyosinogen; it disappears after 1 to 6 days, or when decomposition begins. SYN postmortem rigidity.

rim. A margin, border, or edge, usually circular in form.

ri•ma, gen. and pl. **ri•mae** (rī′mă, rī′mē) [NA]. A slit or fissure, or narrow elongated opening between two symmetrical parts. [L. a slit]

r. glot′tidis [NA], the interval between the true vocal cords.

r. o′ris [NA], the mouth slit; the aperture of the mouth.

r. palpebra′rum [NA], the lid slit, or fissure between the eye lids. SYN palpebral fissure.

r. vestib′uli [NA], the interval between the false vocal cords or vestibular folds.

ri•mose (rī′mōs). Fissured; marked by cracks in all directions, like the crackle of porcelain. [L. *rimosus,* fr. *rima,* a fissure]

rim•u•la (rim′yū-lă). A minute slit or fissure. [L. dim. of *rima*]

ring. 1. A circular band surrounding a wide central opening; a ring-shaped or circular structure surrounding an opening or level area. 2. ANATOMY Annulus; sometimes anulus when used as an official alternate Nomina Anatomica term. 3. The closed chain of atoms in a cyclic compound; commonly used for "cyclic" or "cycle." 4. A marginal growth on the upper surface of a broth culture of bacteria, adhering to the sides of the test tube in the form of a circle. SYN annulus [NA], anulus★ [NA]. [A.S. *hring*]

anterior limiting r., the periphery of the cornea marking the termination of Descemet's membrane and the anterior border of the trabecular meshwork; an important landmark in gonioscopy. SYN Schwalbe's r.

Bandl's r., SYN pathologic retraction r.

benzene r., the closed-chain arrangement of the carbon and hydrogen atoms in the benzene molecule. SEE ALSO cyclic *compound.*

ciliary r., SYN orbiculus ciliaris.

conjunctival r., a narrow ring at the junction of the periphery of the cornea with the conjunctiva. SYN annulus conjunctivae [NA].

constriction r., (1) spastic stricture of the uterine cavity resulting when a zone of muscle goes into local tetanic contraction and forms a tight constriction about some part of the fetus; (2) SYN amniotic *bands,* under *band.*

deep inguinal r., the opening in the transversalis fascia through which the ductus deferens (or round ligament in the female) and gonadal vessels enter the inguinal canal. Located midway between anterior superior iliac spine and pubic tubercle, it is bounded medially by the lateral umbilical ligament (inferior epigastric vessels) and inferiorly by the inguinal ligament. Indirect inguinal hernias exit the abdominal cavity via the deep inguinal r. SYN annulus inguinalis profundus [NA], annulus abdominalis.

Kayser-Fleischer r., a greenish yellow pigmented r. encircling the cornea just within the corneoscleral margin, seen in hepatolenticular degeneration, due to copper deposited in Descemet's membrane.

pathologic retraction r., a constriction located at the junction of the thinned lower uterine segment with the thick retracted upper uterine segment, resulting from obstructed labor; this is one of the classic signs of threatened rupture of the uterus. SYN Bandl's r.

physiologic retraction r., a ridge on the inner uterine surface at the boundary line between the upper and lower uterine segment that occurs in the course of normal labor.

Schwalbe's r., SYN anterior limiting r.

superficial inguinal r., the slit-like opening in the aponeurosis of the external oblique muscle of the abdominal wall through which the spermatic cord (round ligament in the female) and inguinal hernias emerge from the inguinal canal. SYN annulus inguinalis superficialis [NA].

tympanic r., in the fetus, a more or less complete bony ring at the medial end of the cartilaginous external acoustic meatus, to which is attached the tympanic membrane. SYN annulus tympanicus [NA], tympanic bone.

umbilical r., an opening in the linea alba through which pass the umbilical vessels in the fetus; in young embryos it is relatively nearer to the pubes, but gradually ascends to the center of the abdomen; it is closed in the adult, its site being indicated by the umbilicus or navel. SYN annulus umbilicalis [NA].

vascular r., anomalous arteries (aortic arches) congenitally encircling the trachea and esophagus, at times producing pressure symptoms.

ring-knife (ring-nīf). A circular or oval ring with internal cutting edge, for shaving off tumors in the nasal and other cavities.

ring•worm (ring′werm). SYN tinea.

risk. The probability that an event will occur.

empiric r., r. that is based on empirical evidence alone, without any appeal to formal theory or surmise.

recurrence r., r. that a disease will occur elsewhere in a pedigree, given that at least one member of the pedigree (the proband) exhibits the disease.

RIST radioimmunosorbent *test.*

ri•sus ca•ni•nus (rī′sŭs kā-nī′nŭs). The semblance of a grin caused by facial spasm, especially in tetanus. SYN cynic spasm, sardonic grin. [L. *risus,* laugh + *caninus,* dog like]

rit•u•al (rich′ū-ăl). PSYCHIATRY, PSYCHOLOGY Any psychomotor activity (*e.g.,* morbid handwashing) performed by an individual to relieve anxiety or forestall its development; typically seen in obsessive-compulsive disorder. [L. *ritualis,* fr. *ritus,* rite]

ri•val•ry (rī′văl-rē). Competition between two or more individuals for the same object or goal. [L. *rivalis,* competitor, rival]

sibling r., jealous competition among children, especially for the attention, affection, and esteem of their parents; by extension, a factor in both normal and abnormal competitiveness throughout life.

riz•i•form (riz′i-fōrm). Resembling rice grains. [Fr. *riz,* rice]

RLL right lower lobe (of lung).

RLQ right lower quadrant (of abdomen).

RL

RMA right mentoanterior position.

RML right middle lobe (of lung).

RMP right mentoposterior position.

RMT right mentotransverse position.

Rn radon.

RNA ribonucleic acid. For terms bearing this abbreviation, see subentries under ribonucleic acid.

RNase ribonuclease. For terms bearing this abbreviation, see subentries under ribonuclease.

RNA splic•ing. SYN splicing (2).

RNP ribonucleoprotein.

ROA right occipitoanterior position.

ro•bot•ic (rō-bot′ik). Pertaining to or characteristic of a robot, an automatic mechanical device designed to duplicate a human function without direct human operation. [Czech *robot*, robot, fr. *robota*, drudgery, + -ic]

rod. 1. A straight slender cylindrical structure or device. For surgical rods, see also under nail; pin. **2.** The photosensitive, outward-directed process of a rhodopsin-containing r. cell in the external granular layer of the retina; many millions of such r.'s, together with the cones, form the photoreceptive layer of r.'s and cones. SYN rod cell. [A.S. *rōd*]

    Auer r.'s, SYN Auer *bodies*, under *body*.

    basal r., SYN costa (2).

ro•den•ti•cide (rō-den′ti-sīd). An agent lethal to rodents. [rodent + L. *caedo*, to kill]

Roentgen, Wilhelm K., German physicist and Nobel laureate, 1845–1923; discovered x-rays. SEE roentgen; roentgen *ray*.

roent•gen (r) (rent′gen, rent′chen). The international unit of exposure dose for x-rays or gamma rays; that quantity of radiation that will produce in 1 cm of air at STP, or 0.001293 g of air, 2.08×10^9 ions of both signs, each totaling 1 electrostatic unit (e.s.u.) of charge; in the MKS system this is 2.58×10^{-4} coulombs per kg of air. [W. K. *Roentgen*]

    r.-equivalent-man (rem), a unit of dose equivalent quantity of ionizing radiation of any type that produces in human subjects the same biologic effect as one rad of x-rays or gamma rays; the number of rems is equal to the absorbed dose, measured in rads, multiplied by the quality factor of the radiation in question.100 rem = 1 Sv.

roent•gen•o•gram (rent′gen-ō-gram). SYN radiograph.

roent•gen•o•graph (rent′gen-ō-graf). SYN radiograph.

roent•gen•og•ra•phy (rent′ge-nog′ră-fē). SYN radiography.

roent•gen•ol•o•gist (rent′gen-ol′ō-jist). A person skilled in the diagnostic or therapeutic application of roentgen rays; a radiologist.

roent•gen•ol•o•gy (rent′gen-ol′ō-jē). The study of roentgen rays in all their applications. Radiology is the preferred term in the context of medical imaging.

ro•lan•dic (rō-lan′dik). Relating to or described by Luigi Rolando.

role (rōl). The pattern of behavior that one exhibits in relationship to significant persons with whom one has or had primary relationships. [Fr.]

    gender r., the sex of a child assigned by a

parent; when opposite to the child's anatomical sex (*e.g.*, due to genital ambiguity at birth or to the parents' strong wish for a child of the opposite sex), the basis is set for postpubertal dysfunctions. SEE sex r., sex *reversal*.

    occupational r., a function undertaken to provide the context for organizing one's time for work, play, and rest.

    sex r., the degree to which an individual acts out a stereotypical masculine or feminine r. in everyday behavior. Cf. gender r.

    sick r., in medical sociology, the familially or culturally accepted behavior pattern or r. which one is permitted to exhibit during illness or disability, including sanctioned absence from school or work and a submissive, dependent relationship to family, health care personnel, and significant others.

role-play•ing. A psychotherapeutic method used in psychodrama to understand and treat emotional conflicts through the enactment or reenactment of stressful interpersonal events. SEE ALSO psychodrama.

ROM range of motion.

rom•berg•ism (rom′berg-izm). SYN Romberg's *sign*.

ron•geur (rawn-zhĕr′). A strong biting forceps for nipping away bone. [Fr. *ronger*, to gnaw]

roof (rūf). A covering or rooflike structure; *e.g.*, a tectorium, tectum, tegmen, tegmentum, integument. [A.S. *hrōf*]

roof•plate (rūf′plāt). SEE roof *plate*.

root (rūt). **1.** The primary or beginning portion of any part, as of a nerve at its origin from the brainstem or spinal cord. **2.** SYN r. of tooth. **3.** The descending underground portion of a plant; it absorbs water and nutrients, provides support, and stores nutrients. For r.'s of pharmacological significance not listed below, see specific names. [A.S. rot]

    cranial r. of accessory nerve, the r.'s of the accessory nerve which arise from the medulla; the nerve fibers of the cranial r. join the intracranial portion of the vagus nerve and are distributed to the pharyngeal plexus, providing the motor innervation of the soft palate (except the tensor veli palati) and the pharynx.

    dorsal r., the sensory root of a spinal nerve, having a dorsal r. ganglion containing the nerve cell bodies of the fibers conveyed by the root in its distal end.

    hair r., the part of a hair that is embedded in the hair follicle, its lower succulent extremity capping the dermal papilla pili in the deep bulbous portion of the follicle.

    r. of lung, all the structures entering or leaving the lung at the hilum, forming a pedicle invested with the pleura; includes the bronchi, pulmonary artery and veins, bronchial arteries and veins, lymphatics, and nerves.

    r. of nail, the proximal end of the nail, concealed under a fold of skin.

    r. of penis, the proximal attached part of the penis, including the two crura and the bulb.

    r. of tongue, the posterior attached portion of the tongue.

    r. of tooth, that part of a tooth below the neck,

covered by cementum rather than enamel, and attached by the periodontal ligament to the alveolar bone. SYN radix (1) [NA], root (2).

ventral r., the motor root of a spinal nerve.

ROP right occipitoposterior position.

ro•sa•cea (rō-zā′shē-ă). Chronic vascular and follicular dilation involving the nose and contiguous portions of the cheeks with erythema, hyperplasia of sebaceous glands, deep-seated papules and pustules, and telangiectasia. SYN acne erythematosa, acne rosacea. [L. *rosaceus,* rosy]

ro•sa•ry (rō′zer-ē). A beadlike arrangement or structure.

rachitic r., a row of beading at the junction of the ribs with their cartilages, often seen in rachitic children.

rose ben•gal (rōz′ ben′gal) [C.I. 45440]. A fluorescein derivative used as a biologic stain.

ro•se•o•la (rō-zē′ō-lă). A symmetrical eruption of small, closely aggregated patches of rose-red color. It is believed to be caused by human herpesvirus type 6. SEE ALSO *exanthema* subitum. [Mod. L. dim. of L. *roseus,* rosy]

epidemic r., SYN rubella.

r. infan′tilis, r. infan′tum, SYN *exanthema* subitum.

syphilitic r., usually the first eruption of syphilis, occurring 6 to 12 weeks after the initial lesion.

ro•sette (rō-zet′). **1.** The quartan malarial parasite *Plasmodium malariae* in its segmented or mature phase. **2.** A grouping of cells characteristic of neoplasms of neuroblastic or neuroectodermal origin; a number of nuclei form a ring from which neurofibrils, which can be demonstrated by silver impregnation, extend to interlace in the center. **3.** Roselike coiling of the uterus among certain pseudophyllidean tapeworms, such as *Diphyllobothrium latum.* [Fr. a little rose]

ros•in (roz′in). The solid resin obtained after steam distillation of crude balsam from species of *Pinus;* used in plasters to render them adhesive and also in ointments to render them locally stimulating. SYN resin (2).

ros•tel•lum (ros-tel′ŭm). The anterior fixed or invertible portion of the scolex of a tapeworm, frequently provided with a row (or several rows) of hooks. [L. dim. of *rostrum,* a beak]

ros•trad (ros′trad). **1.** In a direction toward any rostrum. **2.** Situated nearer a rostrum or the snout end of an organism in relation to a specific reference point; opposite of caudad (2). [L. *rostrum,* beak, + *-ad,* toward]

ros•tral (ros′trăl). Relating to any rostrum or anatomical structure resembling a beak. [L. *rostralis,* fr. *rostrum,* beak]

ros•trate (ros′trāt). Having a beak or hook. [L. *rostratus*]

ros•trum, pl. **ros•tra, ros•trums** (ros′trŭm, -tră) [NA]. Any beak-shaped structure. [L. a beak]

ROT right occipitotransverse position.

rot. To decay or putrify. [A.S. *rotian*]

ro•ta•tion (rō-tā′shŭn). **1.** Turning or movement of a body round its axis. **2.** A recurrence in regular order of certain events, such as the symptoms of a periodic disease. [L. *rotatio,* fr. *roto,* pp. *rotatus,* to revolve, rotate]

molecular r., one-hundredth of the product of the specific r. of an optically active compound and its molecular weight.

optical r., the change in the plane of polarization of polarized light of a given wavelength upon passing through optically active substances; measured in terms of specific rotation by polarimetry, an important tool in chemical structural work, especially on carbohydrates.

ro•ta•tor (rō-tā′ter, -tōr). A muscle by which a part can be turned circularly. [L. See rotation]

Ro•ta•vi•rus (rō′tă-vī′rŭs). A genus of RNA viruses that includes the human gastroenteritis viruses (a major cause of infant diarrhea throughout the world). SYN gastroenteritis virus type B. [L. *rota,* wheel, + virus]

ro•to•sco•li•o•sis (rō′tō-skō-lē-ō′sis). Combined lateral and rotational deviation of the vertebral column. [L. *roto,* to rotate, + G. *skoliōsis,* crookedness]

ro•to•tome (rō′tō-tōm). A rotating cutting instrument used in arthroscopic surgery.

rough•age (rŭf′ij). Anything in the diet, *e.g.,* bran, serving as a bulk stimulant of intestinal peristalsis.

round•worm (rownd′werm). A nematode member of the phylum Nematoda, commonly confined to the parasitic forms.

RPE rating of perceived exertion.

RPF renal plasma flow. SEE effective renal plasma *flow.*

RPI reticulocyte production *index.*

rpm revolutions per minute.

RPO right posterior oblique, a radiographic projection.

-rrhagia. Excessive or unusual discharge. [G. *rhēgnymi,* to burst forth]

-rrhaphy. Surgical suturing. [G. *rhaphē,* suture]

-rrhea. A flowing; a flux. [G. *rhoia,* a flow]

rRNA ribosomal ribonucleic acid.

RSA right sacroanterior position.

RSD reflex sympathetic *dystrophy.*

RSP right sacroposterior position.

RST right sacrotransverse position.

RSV Rous sarcoma *virus.*

rTMP ribothymidylic acid.

Ru ruthenium.

rub (rŭb). Friction encountered in moving one body over another.

friction r., SYN friction *sound.*

pleuritic r., a friction sound produced by the rubbing together of inflamed surfaces of the parietal and visceral pleurae.

ru•be•do (rū-bē′dō). A temporary redness of the skin. [L. redness, fr. *ruber,* red]

ru•be•fa•cient (rū-bē-fā′shent). **1.** Causing a reddening of the skin. **2.** A counterirritant that produces erythema when applied to the skin surface. [L. *rubi-facio,* fr. *ruber,* red, + *facio,* to make]

ru•be•fac•tion (rū-bē-fak′shŭn). Erythema of the skin caused by local application of a counterirritant. [see rubefacient]

ru•bel•la (rū-bel′ă). An acute exanthematous disease caused by rubella virus (*Rubivirus*), with enlargement of lymph nodes, but usually with little fever or constitutional reaction; a high incidence of birth defects in children results from maternal infection during the first several months of fetal life (congenital rubella syndrome). SYN epidemic roseola, German measles, third disease. [L. *rubellus,* fem. *-a,* reddish, dim. of *ruber,* red]

ru•be•o•la (rū-bē′ō-lă, -bē-ō′lă). SYN measles (1). [Mod. L. dim. of *ruber,* red, reddish]

ru•be•o•sis (rū-bē-ō′sis). Reddish discoloration, as of the skin. [L. *ruber,* red, + G. *-osis,* condition]

  r. i′ridis diabet′ica, neovascularization of the anterior surface of the iris in diabetes mellitus.

ru•bes•cent (rū-bes′ent). Reddening. [L. *rubesco,* pr. p. *rubescens,* to become red]

ru•bid•i•um (rū-bid′ē-ŭm). An alkali element, atomic no. 37, atomic wt. 85.4678; its salts have been used in medicine for the same purposes as the corresponding sodium or potassium salts. [L. *rubidus,* reddish, dark red, fr. *rubeo,* to be red]

ru•bid•o•my•cin (rū-bid′ō-mī-sin). An antibiotic used as an antineoplastic; similar to doxorubicin in antitumor activity and in exhibiting cumulative cardiotoxicity. SYN daunorubicin.

Ru•bi•vi•rus (rū′bi-vī′rŭs). A genus of viruses that includes the rubella virus. [*rubella* + virus]

ru•bor (rū′bōr). Redness of skin or mucous membrane, as one of the four signs of hyperemia or inflammation (r., calor, dolor, tumor) enunciated by Celsus. [L.]

ru•bre•dox•ins (rū-brĕ-dok′sinz). Ferredoxins without acid-labile sulfur and with the iron in a typical mercaptide coordination.

ru•bri•blast (rū′bri-blast). SYN pronormoblast. [L. *ruber,* red, + G. *blastos,* germ]

ru•bri•cyte (rū′bri-sīt). Polychromatic normoblast. SEE erythroblast. [L. *ruber,* red, + *kytos,* cell]

ru•di•ment (rū′di-ment). 1. An organ or structure that is incompletely developed. 2. The first indication of a structure in the course of ontogeny. SYN rudimentum [NA]. [L. *rudimentum,* a beginning, fr. *rudis,* unformed]

ru•di•men•ta•ry (rū-di-men′tār-ē). Relating to a rudiment. SYN abortive (2).

ru•di•men•tum, pl. **ru•di•men•ta** (rū′di-men′ tŭm, -tă) [NA]. SYN rudiment, rudiment. [L.]

ru•fous (rū′fŭs). SYN erythristic. [L. *rufus,* reddish]

ru•ga, pl. **ru•gae** (rū′gă, rū′gē) [NA]. A fold, ridge, or crease; a wrinkle. [L. a wrinkle]

  rugae of stomach, characteristic folds of the gastric mucosa, especially evident when the stomach is contracted.

ru•gine (rū-zhēn′). 1. SYN periosteal *elevator.* 2. A raspatory. [Fr.]

ru•gose (rū′gōs). Marked by rugae; wrinkled. SYN rugous. [L. *rugosus*]

ru•gos•i•ty (rū-gos′i-tē). 1. The state of being thrown into folds or wrinkles. 2. A ruga.

ru•gous (rū′gŭs). SYN rugose.

RUL right upper lobe (of lung).

rule (rūl). A criterion, standard, or guide governing a procedure, arrangement, action, etc. SEE ALSO law, principle, theorem. [O. Fr. *reule,* fr. L. *regula,* a guide, pattern]

  American Law Institute r., a test of criminal responsibility (1962): "a person is not responsible for criminal conduct if at the time of such conduct as a result of mental disease or defect he lacks substantial capacity either to appreciate the wrongfulness of his conduct or to conform his conduct to the requirements of law."

  r. of bigeminy, r. that a ventricular premature beat will follow the beat terminating a long cycle. Sudden prolongation of the ventricular cycle, by changing the refractoriness in the conduction system, causes a peripheral region of bidirectional block to become transiently unidirectional and thus opens potential pathways for reentry to occur.

  Durham r., an American test of criminal responsibility (1954): "an accused is not criminally responsible if his unlawful act was the product of mental disease or mental defect."

  M'Naghten r., the classic English test of criminal responsibility (1843): "to establish a defense on the ground of insanity, it must be clearly proved that, at the time of committing the act, the party accused was laboring under such a defect of reasoning, from disease of the mind, as not to know the nature and quality of the act he was doing, or if he did know it, that he did not know he was doing what was wrong."

  New Hampshire r., pioneering American test of criminal responsibility (1871): "if the [criminal] act was the offspring of insanity, a criminal intent did not produce it."

  r. of nines, method used in calculating body surface area involved in burns whereby values of 9 or 18% of surface area are assigned to specific regions as follows: Head and neck, 9%; anterior thorax, 18%; posterior thorax, 18%; arms, 9% each; legs, 18% each; perineum 1%.

  Ogino-Knaus r., the time in the menstrual period when conception is most likely to occur is at about midway between two menstrual periods; fertilization of the ovum is least likely just before or just after menstruation; the basis for the rhythm method of contraception.

  r. of outlet, an obstetric r. for determining whether the pelvic outlet will permit the passage of a fetus; the sum of the posterior sagittal diameter and the transverse diameter of the outlet must equal at least 15 cm if a normal-sized baby is to pass.

  Westgard r.'s, a quality control protocol that allows detection of random and systematic error. The protocol includes the 12s, 13s, 22s, R4s, 41s, and 10x r.'s.

ru•pia (rū′pē-ă). 1. Ulcers of late secondary syphilis, covered with yellowish or brown crusts. 2. SYN yaws. 3. Term occasionally used to designate a very scaly, heaped-up, and secondarily infected psoriatic lesion. [G. *rhypos,* filth]

ru•pi•al (rū′pē-ăl). Relating to rupia.

rup•ture (rŭp′chūr). 1. SYN hernia. 2. A solution of continuity or a tear; a break of any organ or other of the soft parts. [L. *ruptura,* a fracture (of limb or vein), fr. *rumpo,* pp. *ruptus,* to break]

RUQ right upper quadrant (of abdomen).

rusts (rŭsts). Species of *Puccinia* and other microbes comprising important pathogens of plants, especially cereal grains; they are important allergens for humans when inhaled in large numbers, as in harvesting processes.

ru·the·ni·um (Ru) (rū-thē′nē-ŭm).　A metallic element of the platinum group; atomic no. 44, atomic wt. 101.07; ^{106}Ru, with a half-life of 1.020 years, has been used in the treatment of certain eye problems. [Mediev. L. *Ruthenia,* Russia, where first obtained]

ru·ti·do·sis (rū-ti-dō′sis). SYN rhytidosis.

RV residual *volume*.

S

σ, Σ sigma. SEE sigma.

S 1. sacral vertebra (S1 to S5); spherical or spherical *lens*; Svedberg *unit*. **2.** siemens; sulfur; entropy in thermodynamics; substrate in the Michaelis-Menton mechanism; percentage saturation of hemoglobin (when followed by subscript O_2 or CO); serine; one of the two stereochemical designations (in italics) in the Cahn-Ingold-Prelog system. **3.** Designation of a rare human antigen (hemagglutinogen) related genetically to the MNSs blood group. See Blood Groups appendix.

S_1 first heart *sound*.
S_2 second heart *sound*.
S_3 third heart *sound*.
S_4 fourth heart *sound*.
S_f flotation *constant*.

s L. *sinister*, left; L. *semis*, half; second; as a subscript, denotes steady *state*.

s selection *coefficient*; sedimentation *coefficient*.

S-A sinuatrial.

sab·u·lous (sab'yū-lŭs). Sandy; gritty. [L. *sabulosus*, fr. *sabulum*, coarse sand]

sac (sak). **1.** A pouch or bursa. SEE sacculus. **2.** An encysted abscess at the root of a tooth. **3.** The capsule of a tumor, or envelope of a cyst. SYN saccus [NA]. [L. *saccus*, a bag]

allantoic s., the dilated distal portion of the allantois; it forms part of the placenta in many mammals.

alveolar s., terminal dilation of the alveolar ducts that give rise to alveoli in the lung; a small air chamber in the pulmonary tissue from which the pulmonary alveoli project like bays and into which an alveolar duct opens; SYN sacculus alveolaris [NA].

amniotic s., SYN amnion.

conjunctival s., the space bound by the conjunctival membrane between the palpebral and bulbar conjunctiva, into which the lacrimal fluid is secreted; it opens anteriorly between the eyelids. SYN saccus conjunctivae [NA].

dental s., the outer connective tissue envelope surrounding a developing tooth; also applied to the mesenchymal concentration that is the primordium of the s. SEE ALSO dental *follicle*.

endolymphatic s., the dilated blind extremity of the endolymphatic duct. SYN saccus endolymphaticus [NA].

heart s., SYN pericardium.

hernial s., the peritoneal envelope of a hernia.

lacrimal s., the upper portion of the nasolacrimal duct into which empty the two lacrimal canaliculi; empty. SYN saccus lacrimalis [NA], dacryocyst, tear s.

tear s., SYN lacrimal s.

yolk s., in humans and other mammals, the s. of extraembryonic membrane that is located ventral to the embryonic disk and, after formation of the gut tube, is connected to the midgut; by the second month of development, this connection has become the narrow yolk stalk; the yolk s. is the first hematopoietic organ of the embryo, and its vitelline circulation plays an important role in the early embryonic circulation. SYN umbilical vesicle.

sac·cad·ic (să-kad'ik). Jerky.

sac·cate (sak'āt). Relating to a sac. [L. *saccus*, sac]

△**sacchar-.** SEE saccharo-.

△**sacchari-.** SEE saccharo-.

sac·cha·rides (sak'ă-rīdz). A group of carbohydrates that includes the sugars. S. are classified as mono-, di-, tri-, and polysaccharides according to the number of saccharide units ($C_6H_{10}O_5$) composing them. SEE ALSO carbohydrates.

sac·cha·rif·er·ous (sak'ă-rif'er-ŭs). Producing sugar.

△**saccharo-, sacchar-, sacchari-.** Combining forms denoting sugar (saccharide). [G. *sak-char-on*, sugar]

sac·cha·ro·lyt·ic (sak'ă-rō-lit'ik). Capable of hydrolyzing or otherwise breaking down a sugar molecule. [saccharo- + G. *lysis*, loosening]

sac·cha·ro·met·a·bol·ic (sak'ă-rō-met'ă-bol'ik). Relating to saccharometabolism.

sac·cha·ro·me·tab·o·lism (sak-ă-rō-mě-tab'ō-lizm). Metabolism of sugar; the process of utilization of sugar in cells.

sac·cha·rose (sak'ă-rōs). SYN sucrose.

sac·ci·form (sak'si-fōrm). Pouched; sac-shaped. SYN saccular. [L. *saccus*, sack, + *forma*, form]

sac·cu·lar (sak'yū-lăr). SYN sacciform.

sac·cu·la·tion (sak'yū-lā'shŭn). **1.** A structure formed by a group of sacs. **2.** The formation of a sac or pouch.

sac·cule (sak'yūl). SYN sacculus. [L. *sacculus*]

s. of larynx, a small diverticulum provided with mucous glands extending upward from the ventricle of the larynx between the vestibular fold and the lamina of the thyroid cartilage. SYN sacculus laryngis [NA].

sac·cu·lo·co·chle·ar (sak'yū-lō-kok'lē-ăr). Relating to the sacculus and the membranous cochlea.

sac·cu·lus, pl. **sac·cu·li** (sak'yū-lŭs, -lī). **1** [NA]. The smaller of the two membranous sacs in the vestibule of the labyrinth, lying in the spherical recess; it is connected with the cochlear duct by a very short tube, the ductus reuniens, and with the utriculus by the beginning of the ductus endolymphaticus and the ductus utriculosaccularis that joins it. **2.** The immense bag-shaped structure formed by peptidoglycans as part of the cell wall of certain microorganisms. SYN saccule. [L. dim. of *saccus*, sac]

s. alveola'ris, pl. **sacculi alveola'res** [NA], SYN alveolar *sac*.

s. laryn'gis [NA], SYN *saccule* of larynx.

sac·cus, pl. **sac·ci** (sak'ŭs, sak'sī) [NA]. SYN sac. [L. a bag, sack]

s. conjuncti'vae [NA], SYN conjunctival *sac*.

s. endolymphat'icus [NA], SYN endolymphatic *sac*.

s. lacrima'lis [NA], SYN lacrimal *sac*.

△**sacr-.** SEE sacro-.

sa·crad (sā'krad). In the direction of the sacrum. [sacr- + L. *ad*, to]

sa·cral (sā'krăl). Relating to or in the neighborhood of the sacrum.

sa·cral·gia (sā-kral'jē-ă). Pain in the sacral region. SYN sacrodynia. [sacr- + G. *algos*, pain]

sa·crec·to·my (sā-krek'tō-mē). Resection of a portion of the sacrum to facilitate an operation. [sacr- + G. *ektomē*, excision]

⌂**sacro-, sacr-.** Muscular substance; resemblance to flesh. [L. *os sacrum*, sacred bone]

sa·cro·coc·cyg·e·al (sā-krō-kok-sij'ē-ăl). Relating to both sacrum and coccyx.

sa·cro·dyn·ia (sā'krō-din'ē-ă). SYN sacralgia. [sacro- + G. *odynē*, pain]

sa·cro·il·i·ac (sā-krō-il'ē-ak). Relating to the sacrum and the ilium.

sa·cro·lum·bar (sā'krō-lŭm'băr). SYN lumbosacral.

sa·cro·sci·at·ic (sā'krō-sī-at'ik). Relating to both sacrum and ischium.

sa·cro·spi·nal (sā'krō-spī'năl). Relating to the sacrum and the vertebral column above.

sa·cro·ver·te·bral (sā'krō-ver'tē-brăl). Relating to the sacrum and the vertebrae above.

sa·crum, pl. **sa·cra** (sā'krŭm, sā'kră) [NA]. The segment of the vertebral column forming part of the pelvis; a broad, slightly curved, spade-shaped bone, thick above, thinner below, closing in the pelvic girdle posteriorly; it is formed by the fusion of five originally separate sacral vertebrae; it articulates with the last lumbar vertebra, the coccyx, and the hip bone on either side. [L. (lit. sacred bone), neuter of *sacer* (sacr-), sacred]

SAD seasonal affective *disorder*.

sad·dle (sad'l). **1.** A structure shaped like, or suggestive of, a seat or s. used in horseback riding. SYN sella. **2.** SYN denture *base*.

sa·dism (sā'dizm, sad'izm). A form of perversion, often sexual in nature, in which a person finds pleasure in inflicting abuse and maltreatment. Cf. masochism. [Marquis de *Sade*, 1740–1814, confessedly addicted to the practice]

sa·dist (sā'dist, sad'ist). One who practices sadism.

sa·dis·tic (să-dis'tik). Pertaining to or characterized by sadism.

sa·do·mas·och·ism (sā-dō-mas'ō-kizm, sad-o-). A form of perversion marked by enjoyment of cruelty and/or humiliation, both received and dispensed. [sadism + masochism]

sag·it·tal (saj'i-tăl). **1.** Resembling an arrow. **2.** In an anteroposterior direction, referring to a sagittal plane or direction. [L. *sagitta*, an arrow]

sa·lic·y·late (să-lis'i-lāt). **1.** A salt or ester of salicylic acid. **2.** To treat foodstuffs with salicylic acid as a preservative.

sal·i·cyl·ic ac·id (sal-i-sil'ik). A component of aspirin, derived from salicin and made synthetically; used externally as a keratolytic agent, antiseptic, and fungicide.

sal·i·cyl·ism (sal'i-sil-izm). Poisoning by salicylic acid or any of its compounds.

sa·line (sā'lēn, -līn). **1.** Relating to, of the nature of, or containing salt; salty. **2.** A salt solution, usually sodium chloride. [L. *salinus*, salty, fr. *sal*, salt]

　physiological s., an isotonic aqueous solution of salts, containing 0.9% sodium chloride.

sa·li·va (să-lī'vă). A clear, tasteless, odorless, slightly acid (pH 6.8) viscid fluid, consisting of the secretion from the parotid, sublingual, and submandibular salivary glands and the mucous glands of the oral cavity; its function is to keep the mucous membrane of the mouth moist, to lubricate the food during mastication, and to convert starch into maltose. SYN spittle. [L. akin to G. *sialon*]

sal·i·vant (sal'i-vant). **1.** Causing a flow of saliva. **2.** An agent that increases the flow of saliva. SYN salivator.

sal·i·vary (sal'i-vār-ē). Relating to saliva. SYN sialic, sialine. [L. *salivarius*]

sal·i·vate (sal'i-vāt). To cause an excessive flow of saliva.

sal·i·va·tion (sal'i-vā'shŭn). SYN sialism.

sal·i·va·tor (sal'i-vā-ter). SYN salivant (2).

Sal·mo·nel·la (sal'mō-nel'ă). A genus of aerobic to facultatively anaerobic bacteria containing Gram-negative rods that are either motile or nonmotile. They are pathogenic for humans and other animals. The type species is *S. choleraesuis*. [Daniel E. *Salmon*, U.S. pathologist, 1850–1914]

　S. enterit'idis, a widely distributed species that occurs in humans and in domestic and wild animals, especially rodents.

　S. ty'phi, a species that causes typhoid fever in humans and is transmitted in contaminated water and food. SYN typhoid bacillus.

　S. typhimu'rium, a species causing food poisoning in humans; it is a natural pathogen of all warm-blooded animals and is also found in snakes.

　S. typho'sa, former name for *S. typhi*.

sal·mo·nel·lo·sis (sal'mō-nel-ō'sis). Infection with bacteria of the genus *Salmonella*. Patients with sickle cell anemia and compromised immune systems are particularly susceptible. [*Salmonella* + G. -*osis*, condition]

⌂**salping-.** SEE salpingo-.

sal·pin·gec·to·my (sal-pin-jek'tō-mē). Removal of the uterine tube. SYN tubectomy. [salping- + G. *ektomē*, excision]

sal·pin·ges (sal-pin'jēz). Plural of salpinx.

sal·pin·gi·an (sal-pin'jē-ăn). Relating to the uterine tube or to the auditory tube.

sal·pin·git·ic (sal-pin-jit'ik). Relating to salpingitis.

sal·pin·gi·tis (sal-pin-jī'tis). Inflammation of the uterine or the auditory tube. [salping- + G. -*itis*, inflammation]

　chronic interstitial s., s. in which fibrosis or mononuclear cell infiltration involves all layers of the uterine or auditory tube. SYN pachysalpingitis.

　s. isth'mica nodo'sa, a condition of the uterine tube characterized by nodular thickening of the tunica muscularis of the isthmic portion of the tube enclosing gland-like or cystic duplications of the lumen. SYN adenosalpingitis.

⌂**salpingo-, salping-.** A tube (usually the uterine or auditory tubes). SEE ALSO tubo-. Cf. tubo-. [G. *salpinx*, trumpet (tube)]

sal·pin·go·cele (sal-ping'gō-sēl). Hernia of a uterine tube. [salpingo- + G. *kēlē*, hernia]

sal·pin·gog·ra·phy (sal-ping-gog'ră-fē). Radiography of the uterine tubes after the injection of radiopaque contrast medium. [salpingo- + G. *graphō*, to write]

sal·pin·gol·y·sis (sal-ping-gol'i-sis). Freeing the uterine tube from adhesions. [salpingo- + G. *lysis*, loosening]

sal·pin·go·o·o·pho·rec·to·my (sal-ping'gō-ō-of-ō-rek'tō-mē). Removal of the ovary and its uterine tube.

sal·pin·go·o·o·pho·ri·tis (sal-ping'gō-ō-of-ō-rī'tis). Inflammation of both uterine tube and ovary.

sal·pin·go·o·oph·o·ro·cele (sal-ping'gō-ō-of'ō-rō-sēl). Hernia of both ovary and uterine tube.

sal·pin·go·per·i·to·ni·tis (sal-ping'gō-per-i-tō-nī'tis). Inflammation of the uterine tube, perisalpinx, and peritoneum. [salpingo- + peritonitis]

sal·pin·go·pexy (sal-ping'gō-pek-sē). Operative fixation of an oviduct. [salpingo- + G. *pēxis*, fixation]

sal·pin·go·plas·ty (sal-ping'gō-plas-tē). Plastic surgery of the uterine tubes. SYN tuboplasty. [salpingo- + G. *plastos*, formed]

sal·pin·gor·rha·phy (sal-ping-gōr'ă-fē). Suture of the uterine tube. [salpingo- + G. *rhaphē*, stitching]

sal·pin·gos·to·my (sal-ping-gos'tō-mē). Establishment of an artificial opening in a uterine tube primarily as surgical treatment for an ectopic pregnancy. [salpingo- + G. *stoma*, mouth]

sal·pin·got·o·my (sal-ping-got'ō-mē). Incision into a uterine tube. [salpingo- + G. *tomē*, incision]

sal·pinx, pl. **sal·pin·ges** (sal'pingks, sal-pin'jēz). **1** [NA]. ✗official alternate term for uterine *tube*. **2.** ✗official alternate term for auditory *tube*. [G. a trumpet (tube)]

salt. 1. A compound formed by the interaction of an acid and a base, the ionizable hydrogen atoms of the acid being replaced by the positive ion of the base. **2.** Sodium chloride, the prototypical s. **3.** A saline cathartic, especially magnesium sulfate, sodium sulfate, or Rochelle s.; often denoted by the plural, salts. [L. *sal*]

bile s.'s, the s. forms of bile acids; *e.g.,* taurocholate, glycocholate.

effervescent s.'s, preparations made by adding sodium bicarbonate and tartaric and citric acids to the active s.; when thrown into water the acids break up the sodium bicarbonate, setting free the carbonic acid gas.

sal·ta·tion (sal-tā'shŭn). A dancing or leaping, as in a disease (*e.g.,* chorea) or physiologic function (*e.g.,* saltatory conduction). [L. *saltatio*, fr. *salto*, pp. *-atus*, to dance, fr. *salio*, to leap]

sal·ta·to·ry (sal'tă-tōr-ē). Pertaining to, or characterized by, saltation.

salt·ing out. The precipitation of a protein from its solution by saturation or partial saturation with such neutral salts as sodium chloride, magnesium sulfate, or ammonium sulfate.

sa·lu·bri·ous (să-lū'brē-ŭs). Healthful, usually in reference to climate. [L. *salubris*, healthy, fr. *salus*, health]

sal·u·re·sis (sal-yū-rē'sis). Excretion of sodium in the urine. [L. *sal*, salt, + G. *ourēsis*, uresis (urination)]

sal·u·ret·ic (sal-yū-ret'ik). Facilitating the renal excretion of sodium.

sal·u·tary (sal'yū-tār-ē). Healthful; wholesome. [L. *salutaris*]

salve (sav). SYN ointment. [A.S. *sealf*]

sa·mar·i·um (Sm) (să-mār'ē-ŭm). A metallic element of the lanthanide group, atomic no. 62, atomic wt. 150.36. [bands indicating its presence first found in the spectrum of *samarskite,* a mineral named after Col. von Samarski, 19th century Russian mine official]

sam·ple. 1. A selected subset of a population; a sample may be random or nonrandom (haphazard); representative or nonrepresentative. **2.** A specimen of a whole entity small enough to involve no threat or damage to the whole; an aliquot. [M.E. *ensample,* fr. L. *exemplum,* example]

sam·pling. The policy of inferring the behavior of a whole batch by studying a fraction of it. [MF *essample,* fr. L. *exemplum,* taking out]

biological sampling, denotes sampling that can be taken without jeopardy to the whole organism (*e.g.,* for hematological or biochemical study).

random sampling, a selection of elements by a formal randomizing device for purposes of inference about a population in such a way that the probability of each possible outcome may be precisely specified in advance; the inferences are necessarily stochastic.

san·a·to·ri·um (san'ă-tōr'ē-ŭm). An institution for the treatment of chronic disorders and a place for recuperation under medical supervision. Cf. sanitarium. [Mod. L. neuter of *sanatorius,* curative, fr. *sano,* to cure, heal]

san·a·to·ry (san'ă-tōr-ē). Health-giving; conducive to health. [Mod. L. *sanatorius*]

sand. The fine granular particles of quartz and other crystalline rocks, or a gritty material resembling s. [A.S.]

urinary s., multiple small calculous particles passed in the urine of patients with nephrolithiasis; each particle is usually too small to cause significant symptoms or to be identified as a true calculus.

sane (sān). Of sound mind; mentally healthy. [L. *sanus*]

△**sangui-, sanguin-, sanguino-.** Blood, bloody. [G. *sanguis*]

san·gui·fa·ci·ent (sang-gwi-fā'shent). SYN hemopoietic. [sangui- + L. *facio,* to make]

san·guif·er·ous (sang-gwif'er-ŭs). Conveying blood. SYN circulatory (2). [sangui- + L. *fero,* to carry]

san·gui·fi·ca·tion (sang'gwi-fi-kā'shŭn). SYN hemopoiesis. [sangui- + L. *facio,* to make]

san·guine (sang'gwin). **1.** SYN plethoric. **2.** Formerly, denoting a temperament characterized by a light, fair complexion, full pulse, good digestion, optimistic outlook, and a quick but not lasting temper. SYN sanguineous (3). [L. *sanguineus*]

san·guin·e·ous (sang-gwin'ē-ŭs). **1.** Relating to blood; bloody. **2.** SYN plethoric. **3.** SYN sanguine (2). [L. *sanguineus*]

san·guin·o·lent (sang-gwin'ō-lent). Bloody; tinged with blood. [L. *sanguinolentus*]

san·gui·no·pu·ru·lent (sang'gwi-nō-pū'rū-lent).

Denoting exudate or matter containing blood and pus. [sanguino- + L. *purulentus,* festering (suppurative), fr. *pus,* pus]

san·guiv·or·ous (sang-gwiv′er-ŭs). Bloodsucking, as applied to certain bats, leeches, insects, etc. [sangui- + L. *voro,* to devour]

sa·ni·es (sā′nē-ēz). A thin, blood-stained, purulent discharge. [L.]

sa·ni·o·pu·ru·lent (sā′nē-ō-pū′rū-lent). Characterized by bloody pus. [L. *sanies,* thin, bloody matter, + *purulentus,* festering (suppurative), fr. *pus,* pus]

sa·ni·o·se·rous (sā′nē-ō-sēr′ŭs). Characterized by blood-tinged serum.

sa·ni·ous (sā′nē-ŭs). Relating to sanies; ichorous and blood-stained.

san·i·tar·i·an (san-i-tār′ē-ăn). One who is skilled in sanitation and public health. [L. *sanitas,* health, fr. *sanus,* sound]

san·i·tar·i·um (san-i-tār′ē-ŭm). A health resort. Cf. *sanatorium.* [L. *sanitas,* health]

san·i·tary (san′i-tār-ē). Healthful; conducive to health; usually in reference to a clean environment. [L. *sanitas,* health]

san·i·ta·tion (san-i-tā′shŭn). Use of measures designed to promote health and prevent disease; development and establishment of conditions in the environment favorable to health. [L. *sanitas,* health]

san·i·ti·za·tion (san′i-ti-zā′shŭn). The process of making something sanitary.

san·i·ty (san′i-tē). Soundness of mind, emotions, and behavior; of a sound degree of mental health. [L. *sanitas,* health]

sa·phe·nous (să-fē′nŭs). Relating to or associated with a saphenous vein; denoting a number of structures in the thigh and leg. [see saphena]

△**sapo-, sapon-.** Soap. [L. *sapo*]

sap·o·na·ceous (sap-ō-nā′shŭs). Soapy; relating to or resembling soap.

sa·pon·i·fi·ca·tion (să-pon′i-fi-kā′shŭn). Conversion into soap, denoting the hydrolytic action of an alkali upon fat, especially on triacylglycerols. [sapo- (sapon-) + L. *facio,* to make]

sap·o·nins (sap′ō-ninz). Glycosides of plant origin characterized by properties of foaming in water and of lysing cells; powerful surfactants; many have antibiotic activities.

sap·phism (saf′izm). SYN lesbianism. [*Sapphō,* homosexual Greek poet, queen of the island of Lesbos]

△**sapr-.** SEE sapro-.

△**sapro-, sapr-.** Rotten, putrid, decayed. [G. *sapros*]

sap·robe (sap′rōb). An organism that lives upon dead organic material. This term is preferable to saprophyte, since bacteria and fungi are no longer regarded as plants. [sapro- + G. *bios,* life]

sa·pro·bic (sap-rō′bik). Pertaining to a saprobe.

sap·ro·gen (sap′rō-jen). An organism living on dead organic matter and causing the decay thereof. [sapro- + G. *-gen,* producing]

sap·ro·gen·ic, sa·prog·e·nous (sap-rō-jen′ik, să-proj′ĕ-nŭs). Causing or resulting from decay.

sap·ro·phyte (sap′rō-fīt). An organism that grows on dead organic matter, plant or animal. SEE saprobe. [sapro- + G. *phyton,* plant]

sap·ro·phyt·ic (sap-rō-fit′ik). Relating to a saprophyte.

sap·ro·zo·ic (sap-rō-zō′ik). Living in decaying organic matter; especially denoting certain protozoa. [sapro- + G. *zōikos,* relating to animals]

sap·ro·zo·o·no·sis (sap′rō-zō-ō-nō′sis). A zoonosis the agent of which requires both a vertebrate host and a nonanimal (food, soil, plant) reservoir or developmental site for completion of its cycle. [sapro- + G. *zōon,* animal, + *nosos,* disease]

Sar·ci·na (sar′si-nă). A genus of nonmotile, strictly anaerobic bacteria containing Gram-positive cocci, which divide in three perpendicular planes, producing regular packets of eight or more cells. Saprophytic and facultatively parasitic species occur. The type species is *S. ventriculi.* [L. *sarcina,* a pack, bundle, fr. *sarcio,* to mend, patch]

△**sarco-.** denoting muscular substance or a resemblance to flesh. [G. *sarx* (sark-), flesh]

sar·co·blast (sar′kō-blast). SYN myoblast. [sarco- + G. *blastos,* germ]

Sar·co·di·na (sar′kō-dī′nă, -dē′nă). The amebae; a subphylum of protozoa possessing pseudopodia or locomotive protoplasmic flow for movement. Most species are free-living. [Mod. L. fr. G. *sarx,* flesh]

sar·coid (sar′koyd). SYN sarcoidosis. [sarco- + G. *eidos,* resemblance]

sar·coid·o·sis (sar-koy-dō′sis). A systemic granulomatous disease of unknown cause, especially involving the lungs with resulting fibrosis, but also involving lymph nodes, skin, liver, spleen, eyes, phalangeal bones, and parotid glands; granulomas are composed of epithelioid and multinucleated giant cells with little or no necrosis. SYN Besnier-Boeck-Schaumann disease, Besnier-Boeck-Schaumann syndrome, sarcoid. [sarcoid + G. *-osis,* condition]

sar·co·lem·ma (sar′kō-lem′ă). The plasma membrane of a muscle fiber; formerly, the delicate connective tissue of the endomysium was included under this term by some. [sarco- + G. *lemma,* husk]

sar·co·lem·mal, sar·co·lem·mic, sar·co·lem·mous (sar′kō-lem′ăl, -lem′ik, -lem′ŭs). Relating to the sarcolemma.

sar·co·ma (sar-kō′mă). A connective tissue neoplasm, usually highly malignant, formed by proliferation of mesodermal cells. [G. *sarkōma,* a fleshy excrescence, fr. *sarx,* flesh, + *-oma,* tumor]

  alveolar soft part s., a malignant tumor formed of a reticular stroma of connective tissue enclosing aggregates of large round or polygonal cells; occurs in subcutaneous and fibromuscular tissues.

  ameloblastic s., SYN ameloblastic *fibrosarcoma.*

  botryoid s., a polypoid form of embryonal rhabdomyosarcoma which occurs in children, most frequently in the urogenital tract, characterized by the formation of grossly apparent grapelike clusters of neoplastic tissue; neoplasms of this type grow relatively rapidly and are highly malignant.

  endometrial stromal s., a term sometimes

sa

used for a relatively rare s. believed to be a form of endometriosis in which the lesions form multiple foci in the myometrium and in vascular spaces in other sites, and which consist of histologic and cytologic elements that resemble those of the endometrial stroma.

   granulocytic s., a malignant tumor of immature myeloid cells, frequently subperiosteal, associated with or preceding granulocytic leukemia. SEE ALSO chloroma. SYN myeloid s.

   ❚Kaposi's s., malignant neoplasm of primitive vasoformative tissue, occurring in the skin and sometimes in lymph nodes or viscera; manifested by cutaneous lesions consisting of reddish-purple to dark-blue macules, plaques, or nodules; seen most commonly in men over 60 years of age and as an opportunistic disease in AIDS patients.

   myeloid s., SYN granulocytic s.

   osteogenic s., the most common and malignant of bone s.'s, which arises from bone-forming cells and affects chiefly the ends of long bones; its greatest incidence is in the age group between 10 and 25 years. SYN osteosarcoma.

   telangiectatic osteogenic s., a lytic cystic variant of osteogenic s. composed of aneurysmal blood-filled spaces lined by sarcoma cells producing osteoid.

sar•co•ma•toid (sar-kō′mă-toyd). Resembling a sarcoma. [sarcoma + G. *eidos,* resemblance]

sar•co•ma•to•sis (sar′kō-mă-tō′sis). Occurrence of several sarcomatous growths on different parts of the body. [sarcoma + G. *-osis,* condition]

sar•com•a•tous (sar-kō′mă-tŭs). Relating to or of the nature of sarcoma.

sar•co•mere (sar′kō-mēr). The segment of a myofibril between two adjacent Z lines, representing the functional unit of striated muscle. [sarco- + G. *meros,* part]

sar•co•plasm (sar′kō-plazm). The nonfibrillar cytoplasm of a muscle fiber. [sarco- + G. *plasma,* a thing formed]

sar•co•plas•mic (sar-kō-plaz′mik). Relating to sarcoplasm.

sar•co•poi•et•ic (sar′kō-poy-et′ik). Forming muscle. [sarco- + G. *poiēsis,* a making]

Sar•cop•tes sca•biei (sar-kop′tēz skā-bē-ē′ī). The itch mite, varieties of which are distributed worldwide and affect humans and many animals. The mite burrows into the skin and lays eggs within the burrow; intense itching and rash develop near the burrow in about a month. SEE scabies, mange. [sarco- + G. *koptō,* to cut; L. *scabies,* scurf]

sar•cop•tic (sar-kop′tik). Of, relating to, or caused by mites of the genus *Sarcoptes* or other members of the family Sarcoptidae.

sar•cop•tid (sar-kop′tid). Common name for members of the Sarcoptidae, a family of mites that includes the genera *Sarcoptes, Knemidokoptes,* and *Notoedres.*

sar•co•sis (sar-kō′sis). **1.** An abnormal increase of flesh. **2.** A multiple growth of fleshy tumors. **3.** A diffuse sarcoma involving the whole of an organ. [G. *sarkōsis,* the growth of flesh, fr. *sarx,* flesh]

sar•cos•to•sis (sar-kos-tō′sis). Ossification of

muscular tissue. [sarco- + G. *osteon,* bone, + *-osis,* condition]

sar•cot•ic (sar-kot′ik). **1.** Relating to sarcosis. **2.** Causing an increase of flesh.

sar•co•tu•bules (sar-kō-tū′būlz). The continuous system of membranous tubules in striated muscle that corresponds to the smooth endoplasmic reticulum of other cells.

sar•cous (sar′kŭs). Relating to muscular tissue; fleshy. [G. *sarx,* flesh]

sar•don•ic grin (sar-don′ik). SYN risus caninus.

sat saturated.

sat•el•lite (sat′ĕ-līt). **1.** A minor structure accompanying a more important or larger one; *e.g.,* a vein accompanying an artery, or a small or secondary lesion adjacent to a larger one. **2.** The posterior member of a pair of gregarine gamonts in syzygy, several of which may be found in some species. [L. *satelles* (*sattelit-*), attendant]

   chromosome s., a small chromosomal segment separated from the main body of the chromosome by a secondary constriction; in humans it is usually associated with the short arm of an acrocentric chromosome.

sat•el•lit•o•sis (sat′ĕ-lī-tō′sis). **1.** A condition marked by an accumulation of neuroglia cells around the neurons of the central nervous system; often as a prelude to neuronophagia. **2.** The presence of satellite, smaller structures or lesions. [L. *satelles* (*satellit-*), an attendant, + G. *-ōsis,* condition]

sa•ti•a•tion (sā-shē-ā′shŭn). The state produced by fulfillment of a specific need, such as hunger or thirst. [L. *satio,* pp. *-atus,* to fill, satisfy]

sat. sol., sat. soln. Abbreviation for saturated *solution.*

sat•u•rate (satch′ŭ-rāt). **1.** To impregnate to the greatest possible extent. **2.** To neutralize; to satisfy all the chemical affinities of a substance (as by converting all double bonds to single bonds). **3.** To dissolve a substance up to that concentration beyond which the addition of more results in two phases. [L. *saturo,* pp. *-atus,* to fill, fr. *satur,* sated]

sat•u•ra•tion (satch-ŭ-rā′shŭn). **1.** Impregnation of one substance by another to the greatest possible extent. **2.** Neutralization, as of an acid by an alkali. **3.** That concentration of a dissolved substance that cannot be exceeded. **4.** OPTICS SEE saturated *color.* **5.** Filling of all the available sites on an enzyme molecule by its substrate, or on a hemoglobin molecule by oxygen (symbol S_{O_2}) or carbon monoxide (symbol S_{CO}). [L. *saturatio,* fr. *saturo,* to fill, fr. *satis,* enough]

   secondary s., a technique of nitrous oxide anesthesia consisting of an abrupt curtailment of the oxygen in the inhaled mixture to produce a deep plane of anesthesia, following which oxygen is administered to correct hypoxia.

   transferrin s., a calculation, expressed in percent, of the amount of transferrin that is bound to iron. It is determined by measuring serum iron and total iron binding capacity: serum iron X 100 = percent s. TIBC. It is helpful in differentiating anemias. A low transferrin s. is associated with iron deficiency states; a high s. is associated with excess iron.

sat•ur•nine (sat′er-nīn). **1.** Relating to lead. **2.** Due to or symptomatic of lead poisoning. [Mediev. L. *saturninus,* fr. *saturnus,* lead, fr. L. *saturnus,* the god and planet Saturn]

sat•y•ri•a•sis (sat-i-rī′ă-sis). Satyromania; excessive sexual excitement and behavior in the male; the counterpart of nymphomania in the female. [G. *satyros,* a satyr]

sau•cer•i•za•tion (saw′ser-i-zā′shŭn). Excavation of tissue to form a shallow depression, performed in wound treatment to facilitate drainage from infected areas.

sax•i•tox•in (sak-si-tok′sin). A potent neurotoxin found in shellfish, such as the mussel or the clam, produced by the dinoflagellate *Gonyaulax catenella,* which is ingested by the shellfish; the cause of poisoning from eating California sea mussel, scallops, and Alaskan butterclams.

Sb antimony.

SBE subacute bacterial *endocarditis.*

Sc scandium.

scab (skab). A crust formed by coagulation of blood, pus, serum, or a combination of these, on the surface of an ulcer, erosion, or other type of wound. [A.S. *scaeb*]

scab•i•ci•dal (skā-bi-sī′dăl). Destructive to scabies mites.

scab•i•cide (skā′bi-sīd). An agent lethal to scabies mites.

█ **sca•bies** (skā′bē-ēz). An eruption due to the mite *Sarcoptes scabiei* var. *hominis;* the female of the species burrows into the skin, producing a vesicular eruption with intense pruritus between the fingers, on the male genitalia, buttocks, and elsewhere on the trunk and extremities. [L. *scabo,* to scratch]

sca•la, pl. **sca•lae** (skā′lă, -lē) [NA]. One of the cavities of the cochlea winding spirally around the modiolus. [L. a stairway]

  s. me′dia, SYN cochlear *duct.*

  s. tym′pani [NA], the division of the spiral canal of the cochlea lying on the basal side of the spiral lamina.

  s. vestib′uli [NA], the division of the spiral canal of the cochlea lying on the apical side of the spiral lamina and vestibular membrane. SYN vestibular canal.

scald (skawld). **1.** To burn by contact with a hot liquid or steam. **2.** The lesion resulting from such contact. [L. *excaldo,* to wash in hot water]

scale (skāl). **1.** A standardized test for measuring psychological, personality, or behavioral characteristics. SEE ALSO test. **2.** SYN squama. **3.** A small thin plate of horny epithelium cast off from the skin. **4.** To desquamate. **5.** To remove tartar from the teeth. [L. *scala,* a stairway]

  absolute s., SYN Kelvin s.

  activities of daily living s., a s. to score physical activity and its limitations, based on answers to simple questions about mobility, self-care, grooming, etc; widely used in geriatrics, rheumatology, etc.

  adaptive behavior s.'s, a behavioral assessment device to quantify the levels of skills of mentally retarded and developmentally delayed individuals in interacting with the environment; consists of three developmentally related factors: 1) personal self-sufficiency, *e.g.,* eating, dressing; 2) community self-sufficiency, *e.g.,* shopping, communicating; 3) personal and social responsibility, *e.g.,* use of leisure time, job performance. SEE intelligence.

  Binet s., a measure of intelligence designed for both children and adults.

  Borg s., SYN rating of perceived exertion.

  Celsius s., a temperature s. that is based upon the triple point of water (defined to be 273.16 K) and assigned the value of 0.01°C; this has replaced the centigrade scale because the triple point of water can be more accurately measured than the ice point; for most practical purposes, the two s.'s are equivalent.

  coma s., a clinical s. to assess impaired consciousness; assessment may include motor responsiveness, verbal performance, and eye opening, as in the Glasgow (Scotland) c.s., or the same three items and dysfunction of cranial nerves, as in the Maryland (U.S.) c.s.

  Fahrenheit s., a thermometer s. in which the freezing point of water is 32°F and the boiling point of water 212°F; 0°F indicates the lowest temperature Fahrenheit could obtain by a mixture of ice and salt in 1724; °C = (5/9)(°F − 32).

  French s. (Fr), a s. for grading sizes of sounds, tubules, and catheters as based on a measurement of $\frac{1}{3}$ mm and equaling 1 fr on the scale (*e.g.,* 3 fr = 1 mm).

  Karnofsky s., a performance s. for rating a person's usual activities; used to evaluate a patient's progress after a therapeutic procedure.

  Kelvin s., temperature scale in which the triple point of water is assigned the value of 273.16 K; °C = K − 273.15. SYN absolute s.

  Likert s., a method of measuring attitudes that asks respondents to indicate their degree of agreement or disagreement with statements, according to a three- or five-point scoring system, *e.g.,* "strongly agree," "no opinion" or "strongly disagree."

  Stanford-Binet intelligence s., a standardized test for the measurement of intelligence consisting of a series of questions, graded according to the intelligence of normal children at different ages, the answers to which indicate the mental age of the person tested; primarily used with children, but also contains norms for adults standardized against adult age levels. SYN Binet test.

  Wechsler intelligence s.'s, continuously revised and updated standardized s.'s for the measurement of general intelligence in preschool children (Wechsler preschool and primary s. of intelligence), in children (Wechsler intelligence s. for children), and in adults (Wechsler adult intelligence s.).

sca•le•nec•to•my (skā′lĕ-nek′tō-mē). Resection of the scalene muscles. [scalene + G. *ektomē,* excision]

sca•le•not•o•my (skā′lĕ-not′ō-mē). Division or section of the anterior scalene muscle. [scalene + G. *tomē,* incision]

scal•ing (skā′ling). DENTISTRY Removal of accretions from the crowns and roots of teeth by use of special instruments.

scal•lop•ing (skal′ō-ping). A series of indenta-

SC

tions or erosions on a normally smooth margin of a structure.

scalp (skalp). The skin and subcutaneous tissue, normally hair bearing, covering the neurocranium. [M. E. fr. Scand. *skalpr,* sheath]

scal·pel (skal'pl). A knife used in surgical dissection. [L. *scalpellum;* dim. of *scalprum,* a knife]

scal·prum (skal'prŭm). **1.** A large strong scalpel. **2.** A raspatory. [L. chisel, penknife, fr. *scalpo,* pp. *scalptus,* to carve]

scaly (skā'lē). SYN squamous.

scan (skan). **1.** To survey by traversing with an active or passive sensing device. **2.** The image, record, or data obtained by scanning, usually identified by the technology or device employed; *e.g.,* CT s., radionuclide s., ultrasound s., etc. **3.** Abbreviated form of scintiscan, usually identified by the organ or structure examined; *e.g.,* brain s., bone s., etc.

⚕bone s., x-ray examination of bone after injection of radioactive material, to identify areas of injury, disease, or regeneration.

Meckel s., use of technetium-99m pertechnetate in a s. of the gastric mucosa to detect ectopic gastric mucosa in Meckel's diverticulum; the pertechnetate anion is secreted by epithelial cells in the gastric mucosa.

sector s., ULTRASONOGRAPHY a system in which the transducer or transmitted ultrasound beam is rotated through an angle, resulting in a pie-shaped image.

⚕ventilation-perfusion s., a lung function test, especially useful in the diagnosis of pulmonary embolism, employing an inhaled radionuclide for ventilation and an intravenous radionuclide for perfusion; their respective distributions in the lung are recorded scintigraphically.

scan·di·um (Sc) (skan'dē-ŭm). A metallic element, atomic no. 21, atomic wt. 44.955910. [L. *Scandia,* Scandinavia, where discovered]

scan·ner (skan'er). A device or instrument that scans.

scan·ning (skan'ing). The act of imaging by traversing with an active or passive sensing device, often identified by the technology or device employed.

scan·o·gram (skan'ō-gram). A radiographic technique for showing true dimensions by moving a narrow orthogonal beam of x-rays along the length of the structure being measured, *e.g.,* the lower extremities. [scan- + G. *gramma,* something written]

sca·pha (skaf'ă, skā'fă) [NA]. The longitudinal furrow between the helix and the antihelix of the auricle. [L. fr. G. *skaphē,* skiff]

△scapho-. A scapha, scaphoid. [G. *skaphē,* skiff, boat]

scaph·o·ce·phal·ic (skaf-ō-se-fal'ik). Denoting or relating to scaphocephaly.

scaph·o·ceph·a·lism (skaf-ō-sef'ă-lizm). SYN scaphocephaly.

scaph·o·ceph·a·ly (skaf-ō-sef'ă-lŭs). Craniosynostosis involving the sagittal suture, resulting in a long, narrow cranial vault; sometimes accompanied by mental retardation. SYN cymbocephaly, sagittal synostosis, scaphocephalism, tectocephaly. [scapho- + G. *kephalē,* head]

scaph·oid (skaf'oyd). Boat-shaped; hollowed. SEE scaphoid *bone.* SYN navicular. [scapho- + G. *eidos,* resemblance]

scap·u·la, gen. and pl. **scap·u·lae** (skap'yū-lă, -lē) [NA]. A large triangular flattened bone lying over the ribs, posteriorly on either side, articulating laterally with the clavicle at the acromioclavicular joint and the humerus at the glenohumeral joint. It forms a functional joint with the chest wall, the scapulothoracic joint. SYN shoulder blade. [L. *scapulae,* the shoulder blades]

    s. ala'ta, SYN winged s.

scaphoid s., a s. in which the vertebral border below the level of the spine presents concavity instead of the normal convexity; the **scaphoid type of s.** (Graves) is a s. in which the vertebral border between the spine and the teres major process is either straight or tends toward concavity.

    winged s., condition wherein the medial border of the scapula protrudes away from the thorax; the protrusion is posterior and lateral, as the scapula rotates out; caused by paralysis of the serratus anterior muscle. SYN s. alata.

scap·u·lar (skap'yū-lăr). Relating to the scapula.

scap·u·lec·to·my (skap'yū-lek'tō-mē). Excision of the scapula. [scapula + G. *ektomē,* excision]

△scapulo-. Scapula, scapular. [L. *scapulae,* shoulder blades]

scap·u·lo·cla·vic·u·lar (skap'yū-lō-klă-vik'yū-lăr). **1.** SYN acromioclavicular. **2.** SYN coracoclavicular.

scap·u·lo·hu·mer·al (skap'yū-lō-hyū'mer-ăl). Relating to both scapula and humerus. SEE ALSO glenohumeral.

scap·u·lo·pexy (skap'yū-lō-pek-sē). Operative fixation of the scapula to the chest wall or to the spinous process of the vertebrae. [scapulo- + G. *pēxis,* fixation]

scapulothoracic (ST) (skap-yu-lo-tho-ras-ik). Relating to the scapula and the dorsal thorax. SEE shoulder *complex.*

sca·pus, pl. **sca·pi** (skā'pŭs, -pī). A shaft or stem. [L. shaft, stalk]

scar (skar). The fibrous tissue replacing normal tissues destroyed by injury or disease. [G. *eschara,* scab]

scar·i·fi·ca·tion (skar-i-fi-kā'shŭn). The making of a number of superficial incisions in the skin. [L. *scarifico,* to scratch, fr. G. *skariphos,* a style for sketching]

scar·i·fi·ca·tor (skar'i-fi-kā-tŏr). An instrument for scarification, consisting of a number of concealed spring-projected cutting blades, set near together, that make superficial incisions in the skin.

scar·la·ti·na (skar'lă-tē'nă). An acute exanthematous disease, caused by infection with streptococcal organisms producing erythrogenic toxin, marked by fever and other constitutional disturbances, and a generalized eruption of closely aggregated points or small macules of a bright red color followed by desquamation; mucous membrane of the mouth and fauces is usually also involved. SYN scarlet fever. [through It. fr. Mediev. L. *scarlatum,* scarlet, a scarlet cloth]

    anginose s., s. angino'sa, a form of s. in which

the throat affection is unusually severe. SYN Fothergill's disease (2).

   s. hemorrhag′ica, a form of s. in which blood extravasates into the skin and mucous membranes, giving to the eruption a dusky hue; frequent bleeding from the nose and into the intestine also occurs.

scar·la·ti·nal (skar-lă-tē′năl). Relating to scarlatina.

scar·la·ti·ni·form (skar-lă-tē′ni-fōrm, -tin′i-fōrm). Resembling scarlatina, denoting a rash. SYN scarlatinoid (1).

scar·la·ti·noid (skar-lă-tē′noyd, skar-lat′i-noyd). **1.** SYN scarlatiniform. **2.** SYN Filatov-Dukes' disease. [scarlatina + G. eidos, resemblance]

sca·te·mia (skă-tē′mē-ă). Intestinal autointoxication. [scato- + G. haima, blood]

⚠**scato-.** Feces. SEE ALSO copro-, sterco-. [G. skōr (skat-), excrement]

scat·o·log·ic (skat-ō-loj′ik). Pertaining to scatology.

sca·tol·o·gy (skă-tol′o-jē). **1.** The scientific study and analysis of feces, for physiologic and diagnostic purposes. SYN coprology. **2.** The study relating to the psychiatric aspects of excrement or excremental (anal) function. [scato- + G. logos, study]

sca·tos·co·py (skă-tos′kŏ-pē). Examination of the feces for purposes of diagnosis. [scato- + G. skopeō, to view]

scat·ter (skat′er). **1.** A change in direction of a photon or subatomic particle, as the result of a collision or interaction. **2.** The secondary radiation resulting from the interaction of primary radiation with matter.

Sce·do·spor·i·um ap·i·o·sper·mum (sē-dō-spōr′ē-ŭm ā-pē-os′per-mŭm). The imperfect state of the fungus *Pseudallescheria boydii,* one of the fungi that cause mycetoma in humans.

sche·ma, pl. **sche·ma·ta** (skē′mă, skē-mah′tă). **1.** A plan, outline, or arrangement. SYN scheme. **2.** In sensorimotor theory, the organized unit of cognitive experience. [G. schēma, shape, form]

scheme (skēm). SYN schema (1).

   body scheme, a kinesthetic awareness of body parts and the relationship of those parts to one another and to objects in the environment. SYN kinesthetic awareness.

schin·dy·le·sis (skin-dī-lē′sis) [NA]. SYN wedge-and-groove *joint.* [G. schindylēsis, splintering]

⚠**schisto-.** Cleft, division. SEE ALSO schizo-. [G. schistos, split]

schis·to·ce·lia (skis-tō-sē′lē-ă). Congenital fissure of the abdominal wall. [schisto- + G. koilia, a hollow]

schis·to·cor·mia (skis-tō-kōr′mē-ă). Congenital clefting of the trunk, the lower extremities of the fetus usually being imperfectly developed. SYN schistosomia. [schisto- + G. kormos, trunk of a tree]

schis·to·cyte (skis′tō-sīt). A variety of poikilocyte that owes its abnormal shape to fragmentation occurring as the cell flows through damaged small vessels. [schisto- + G. kytos, cell]

schis·to·cy·to·sis (skis′tō-sī-tō′sis). The occurrence of many schistocytes in the blood.

schis·to·glos·sia (skis-tō-glos′ē-ă). Congenital fissure or cleft of the tongue. [schisto- + G. glōssa, tongue]

Schis·to·so·ma (skis-tō-sō′mă). A genus of trematodes, including the blood flukes that cause schistosomiasis; characterized by elongate shape, marked sexual dimorphism, location in the smaller blood vessels of their host, and utilization of water snails as intermediate hosts. [schisto- + G. sōma, body]

   S. haemato′bium, the vesical blood fluke, a species that occurs as a parasite in the portal system and mesenteric veins of the bladder (causing human schistosomiasis haematobium) and rectum; found throughout Africa and the Middle East; intermediate hosts are *Bulinus truncatus* and other snails.

   S. japon′icum, the Oriental or Japanese blood fluke, a species that causes schistosomiasis japonica, with extensive pathology from encapsulation of the eggs, particularly in the liver. The intermediate hosts are amphibious snails; other animals, such as pigs, oxen, cattle, and dogs, serve as reservoir hosts.

   S. manso′ni, a common species characterized by large eggs with a strong lateral spine and transmitted by planorbid snails of the genus *Biomphalaria;* causes schistosomiasis mansoni.

schis·to·some (skis′tō-sōm). Common name for a member of the genus *Schistosoma.*

schis·to·so·mia (skis-tō-sō′mē-ă). SYN schistocormia. [schisto- + G. sōma, body]

schis·to·so·mi·a·sis (skis′tō-sō-mī′ă-sis). Infection with a species of *Schistosoma;* manifestations of this often chronic and debilitating disease vary with the infecting species but depend in large measure upon tissue reaction (granulation and fibrosis) to the eggs deposited in venules and in the hepatic portals, the latter resulting in portal hypertension and esophageal varices, as well as liver damage leading to cirrhosis. SEE tropical *diseases,* under *disease.*

   ectopic s., a clinical form of s. that occurs outside of the normal site of parasitism (mesenteric vein or hepatic portals).

   s. haemato′bium, infection with *Schistosoma haematobium,* the eggs of which invade the urinary tract, causing cystitis and hematuria, and possibly an increased likelihood of bladder cancer. SYN endemic hematuria.

   s. japon′ica, Japanese s., infection with *Schistosoma japonicum,* characterized by dysenteric symptoms, painful enlargement of the liver and spleen, dropsy, urticaria, and progressive anemia.

   s. manso′ni, infection with *Schistosoma mansoni,* the eggs of which invade the wall of the large intestine and the liver, causing irritation, inflammation, and ultimately fibrosis. SYN Manson's disease.

schis·to·tho·rax (skis-tō-thōr′aks). Congenital cleft of the chest wall. [schisto- + G. thōrax, thorax]

⚠**schiz-.** SEE schizo-.

schiz·am·ni·on (skiz-am′nē-on). An amnion developing, as in the human embryo, by the formation of a cavity within the inner cell mass. [schiz- + amnion]

SC

schiz·ax·on (skiz-ak′son). An axon divided into two branches. [schiz- + G. *axōn*, axis]

⚠**schizo-, schiz-**. Split, cleft, division; schizophrenia. SEE ALSO schisto-. [G. *schizō*, to split or cleave]

schiz·o·af·fec·tive (skiz′ō-ă-fek′tiv). Having an admixture of symptoms suggestive of both schizophrenia and affective (mood) disorder.

schiz·o·gen·e·sis (skiz-ō-jen′ĕ-sis). Reproduction by fission. SYN fissiparity. [schizo- + G. *genesis*, origin]

schi·zog·o·ny (ski-zog′ō-nē). Multiple fission in which the nucleus first divides and then the cell divides into as many parts as there are nuclei; called merogony if daughter cells are merozoites, sporogony if daughter cells are sporozoites, or gametogony if daughter cells are gametes. [schizo- + G. *gonē*, generation]

schiz·o·gy·ria (skiz-ō-jī′rē-ă, -jir′ē-ă). Deformity of the cerebral convolutions marked by occasional interruptions of their continuity. [schizo- + G. *gyros*, circle (convolution)]

schiz·oid (skiz′oyd). Socially isolated, withdrawn, having few (if any) friends or social relationships; resembling the personality features characteristic of schizophrenia, but in a milder form. SEE ALSO schizoid *personality*. [schizo-(phrenia), + G. *eidos*, resemblance]

schiz·ont (skiz′ont). A sporozoan trophozoite (vegetative form) that reproduces by schizogony, producing a varied number of daughter trophozoites or merozoites. [schizo- + G. *ōn (ont-)*, a being]

schiz·o·nych·ia (skiz-ō-nik′ē-ă). Splitting of the nails. [schizo- + G. *onyx*, nail]

schiz·o·pha·sia (skiz-ō-fā′zē-ă). The disordered speech (word salad) of the schizophrenic individual. [schizo- + G. *phasis*, speech]

schiz·o·phre·nia (skiz-ō-frē′nē-ă, skits′ō-). A term, coined by Bleuler synonymous with and replacing dementia praecox; a common type of psychosis, characterized by a disorder in perception, content of thought, and thought processes (hallucinations and delusions), and extensive withdrawal of one's interest from other people and the outside world, and the investment of it in one's own; now considered a group or spectrum of schizophrenic disorders rather than as a single entity. [schizo- + G. *phrēn*, mind]

  catatonic s., s. characterized by marked disturbance, which may involve stupor, negativism, rigidity, excitement, or posturing; sometimes there is rapid alteration between the extremes of excitement and stupor. Associated features include stereotypic behavior, mannerisms, and waxy flexibility; mutism is particularly common.

  disorganized s., a severe form of s. characterized by the predominance of incoherence, blunted, inappropriate or silly affect, and the absence of systematized delusions. SYN hebephrenic s.

  hebephrenic s., SYN disorganized s.

  latent s., a preexisting susceptibility for developing overt s. under strong emotional stress.

  paranoid s., s. characterized predominantly by delusions of persecution and megalomania.

  residual s., blunted or inappropriate affect, social withdrawal, eccentric behavior, or loose associations, but without prominent psychotic symptoms, as the remains of former psychotic symptoms of s.

schiz·o·phren·ic (skiz-ō-fren′ik, -frē′nik, skits-ō-). Relating to, characteristic of, or suffering from one of the schizophrenias.

schiz·o·trich·ia (skiz-ō-trik′ē-ă). A splitting of the hairs at their ends. [schizo- + G. *thrix*, hair]

schwan·no·ma (shwah-nō′mă). A benign, encapsulated neoplasm in which the fundamental component is structurally identical to a syncytium of Schwann cells; the neoplastic cells proliferate within the endoneurium, and the perineurium forms the capsule. The neoplasm may originate from a peripheral or sympathetic nerve or from various cranial nerves. SEE ALSO neurofibroma. SYN neurilemoma. [Theodor *Schwann* + -oma]

schwan·no·sis (shwah-nō′sis). A nonneoplastic proliferation of Schwann cells in the perivascular spaces of the spinal cord; seen particularly in older patients, especially those with diabetes mellitus.

sci·age (sē-ahzh′). A to-and-fro, sawlike movement of the hand in massage. [Fr. *scie*, saw]

sci·at·ic (sī-at′ik). **1.** Relating to or situated in the neighborhood of the ischium or hip. Ischial or sciatic. SYN ischiadic, ischial, ischiatic. **2.** Relating to sciatica. [Mediev. L. *sciaticus*, a corruption of G. *ischiadikos*, fr. *ischion*, the hip joint]

sci·at·i·ca (sī-at′i-kă). Pain in the lower back and hip radiating down the back of the thigh into the leg, initially attributed to sciatic nerve dysfunction (hence the term), but now known to usually be due to herniated lumbar disk compromising the L5 or S1 root. [see sciatic]

sci·ence (sī′ens). **1.** The branch of knowledge that produces theoretical explanations of natural phenomena based on experiments and observations. **2.** An area of such knowledge that is restricted to explaining a limited class of phenomena. [L. *scientia*, knowledge, fr. *scio*, to know]

  occupational s., the study of the effects of occupation upon human behavior.

scin·ti·cis·tern·og·ra·phy (sin′ti-sis-tern-og′ră-fē). Cisternography performed with a radiopharmaceutical and recorded with a stationary imaging device.

scin·ti·gram (sin′ti-gram). SYN scintiscan. [L. *scintilla*, spark, + G. *gramma*, something written]

scin·ti·graph·ic (sin′ti-graf′ik). Relating to or obtained by scintigraphy.

scin·tig·ra·phy (sin-tig′ră-fē). A diagnostic procedure consisting of the administration of a radionuclide with an affinity for the organ or tissue of interest, followed by recording the distribution of the radioactivity with a stationary or scanning external scintillation camera.

scin·til·la·tion (sin-ti-lā′shŭn). **1.** Flashing or sparkling; a subjective sensation as of sparks or flashes of light. **2.** In radiation measurement, the light produced by an ionizing event in a phosphor, as in a crystal or liquid scintillator. SEE ALSO scintillation *counter*. [L. *scintilla*, a spark]

scin·til·la·tor (sin′ti-lā-ter, -tōr). A substance that emits visible light when hit by a subatomic particle or x- or gamma ray. SEE ALSO scintillation *counter.*

scin·ti·pho·tog·ra·phy (sin′ti-fō-tog′ră-fē). The process of obtaining a photographic recording of the distribution of an internally administered radiopharmaceutical with the use of a gamma camera.

scin·ti·scan (sin′ti-skan). The record obtained by scintigraphy. SEE ALSO scan. SYN photoscan, scintigram.

scin·ti·scan·ner (sin′ti-skan′er). The apparatus used to make a scintiscan.

scir·rhous (skir′us, sir′). Hard; relating to a scirrhus.

scis·sion (sizh′ŭn). **1.** A separation, division, or splitting, as in fission. **2.** SYN cleavage (2). [L. *scissio,* fr. *scindo,* pp. *scissus,* to cleave]

scis·su·ra, pl. **scis·su·rae** (si-sū′ră, -rē). **1.** Cleft or fissure. **2.** A splitting. SYN scissure. [L.]

scis·sure (sish′ūr). SYN scissura.

△**scler-.** SEE sclero-.

scle·ra, pl. **scle·ras, scler·ae** (sklēr′ă, -ăz, -ē) [NA]. A portion of the fibrous tunic forming the outer envelope of the eye, except for its anterior sixth, which is the cornea. SYN sclerotica. [Mod. L. fr. G. *sklēros,* hard]

scler·ad·e·ni·tis (sklēr′ad-ĕ-nī′tis). Inflammatory induration of a gland. [scler- + G. *adēn,* gland, + *-itis,* inflammation]

scle·ral (sklēr′ăl). Relating to the sclera. SYN sclerotic (2).

scle·rec·ta·sia (sklēr-ek-tā′zē-ă). Localized bulging of the sclera. [scler- + G. *ektasis,* an extension]

scle·rec·to·my (sklĕ-rek′tō-mē). **1.** Excision of a portion of the sclera. **2.** Removal of the fibrous adhesions formed in chronic otitis media. [scler- + G. *ektomē,* excision]

scle·re·de·ma (sklēr-e-dē′mă). Hard nonpitting edema of the skin of the dorsal aspect of the upper body and extremities, giving a waxy appearance and no sharp demarcation. [scler- + G. *oidēma,* a swelling (edema)]

   s. adulto′rum, a benign spreading induration of the skin and subcutaneous tissue, possibly streptococcal in origin, that may follow a febrile illness, with thickening of the skin by collagen and mucin deposit.

scle·re·ma (sklĕ-rē′mă). Induration of subcutaneous fat. [scler- + edema]

   s. neonato′rum, s. appearing at birth or in early infancy, usually in premature and hypothermic infants, as sharply demarcated and yellowish white indurated plaques that usually involve the cheeks, buttocks, shoulders, and calves; subcutaneous fat has a high proportion of saturated fatty acids; microscopically, there is thickening of interlobular fibrous tissue and formation of triglyceride crystals and foreign body giant cells; prognosis is poor for widespread lesions, but localized lesions may resolve slowly over a period of many months.

scle·ri·tis (sklĕ-rī′tis). Inflammation of the sclera.

   anterior s., inflammation of the sclera adjacent to the cornea.

   posterior s., inflammation, often monocular, of

the sclera adjacent to the optic nerve, with frequent extension to the retina and choroid.

△**sclero-, scler-.** Hardness (induration), sclerosis, relationship to sclera. [G. *sklēros,* hard]

scle·ro·blas·te·ma (sklēr-ō-blas-tē′mă). The embryonic tissue entering into the formation of bone. [sclero- + G. *blastēma,* sprout]

scle·ro·cho·roid·i·tis (sklēr′ō-kō-roy-dī′tis). Inflammation of the sclera and choroid.

scle·ro·con·junc·ti·val (sklēr′ō-kon-jŭngk-tī′văl). Relating to the sclera and the conjunctiva.

scle·ro·cor·nea (sklēr-ō-kōr′nē-ă). **1.** The cornea and sclera regarded as forming together the hard outer coat of the eye, the fibrous tunic of the eye. **2.** A congenital anomaly in which the whole or part of the cornea is opaque and resembles the sclera; other ocular abnormalities are frequently present.

scle·ro·dac·ty·ly, scle·ro·dac·tyl·ia (sklēr-ō-dak′ti-lē, -dak-til′ē-ă). SYN acrosclerosis. [sclero- + G. *daktylos,* finger or toe]

■**scle·ro·der·ma** (sklēr-ō-der′mă). Thickening and induration of the skin caused by new collagen formation, with atrophy of pilosebaceous follicles; either a manifestation of progressive systemic sclerosis or localized (morphea). SYN dermatosclerosis. [sclero- + G. *derma,* skin]

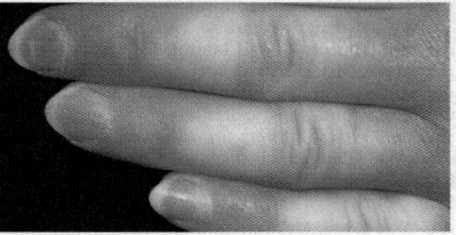

scleroderma: early stage

   localized s., SYN morphea.

scle·rog·e·nous, scle·ro·gen·ic (skle-roj′ĕ-nŭs, sklēr-ō-jen′ik). Producing hard or sclerotic tissue; causing sclerosis. [sclero- + G. *-gen,* producing]

scle·roid (sklēr′oyd). Indurated or sclerotic, of unusually firm texture, leathery, or of scar-like texture. SYN sclerosal, sclerous. [sclero- + G. *eidos,* resemblance]

scle·ro·i·ri·tis (sklēr′ō-ī-rī′tis). Inflammation of both sclera and iris.

scle·ro·ker·a·ti·tis (sklēr′ō-ker-ă-tī′tis). Inflammation of the sclera and cornea. [sclero- + G. *keras,* horn]

scle·ro·ker·a·to·i·ri·tis (sklēr-ō-ker′ă-tō-ī-rī′tis). Inflammation of sclera, cornea, and iris.

scle·ro·ma (skle-rō′mă). A circumscribed indurated focus of granulation tissue in the skin or mucous membrane. [G. *sklērōma,* an induration]

   respiratory s., rhinoscleroma in which the lesion involves the mucous membrane of the greater part or all of the upper respiratory tract.

scle·ro·ma·la·cia (sklēr′ō-mă-lā′shē-ă). Degenerative thinning of the sclera, occurring in persons with rheumatoid arthritis and other collagen disorders. [sclero- + G. *malakia,* a softening]

SC

scle·ro·mere (sklēr′ō-mēr). **1.** Any metamere of the skeleton, such as a vertebral segment. **2.** Caudal half of a sclerotome. [sclero- + G. *meros*, part]

scle·ro·nych·ia (sklēr-ō-nik′ē-ă). Induration and thickening of the nails. [sclero- + G. *onyx*, nail, + *-ia*, condition]

scle·ro·o·o·pho·ri·tis (sklēr′ō-ō-of′ō-rī′tis). Inflammatory induration of the ovary. [sclero- + Mod. L. *oophoron*, ovary + G. *-itis*, inflammation]

scle·roph·thal·mia (sklēr-of-thal′mē-ă). An abnormality in which most of the normally transparent cornea resembles the opaque sclera. [sclero- + G. *ophthalmos*, eye]

scle·ro·pro·tein (sklēr-ō-prō′tēn). SYN albuminoid (3).

scle·ro·sal (sklĕ-rō′săl). SYN scleroid.

scle·ro·sant (sklĕ-rō′sant). An injectable irritant used to treat varices by producing thrombi in them.

scle·rose (sklĕ-rōz′). To harden; to undergo sclerosis.

scle·ro·sis, pl. **scle·ro·ses** (sklĕ-rō′sis, -sēz). **1.** SYN induration (2). **2.** In neuropathy, induration of nervous and other structures by a hyperplasia of the interstitial fibrous or glial connective tissue. [G. *sklērōsis*, hardness]

   amyotrophic lateral s. (ALS), a disease of the motor tracts of the lateral columns and anterior horns of the spinal cord, causing progressive muscular atrophy, increased reflexes, fibrillary twitching, and spastic irritability of muscles; associated with a defect in superoxide dismutase. SYN Aran-Duchenne disease, Charcot's disease, Cruveilhier's disease, Duchenne-Aran disease, Lou Gehrig's disease, progressive muscular atrophy.

   arterial s., SYN arteriosclerosis.

   multiple s. (MS), common demyelinating disorder of the central nervous system, causing patches of sclerosis (plaques) in the brain and spinal cord; occurs primarily in young adults; clinical manifestations depend upon the location and size of the plaques; typical symptoms include visual loss, diplopia, nystagmus, dysarthria, weakness, paresthesias, bladder abnormalities, and mood alterations; characteristically, the symptoms show exacerbations and remissions.

   primary lateral s., considered by many to be a subgroup of motor neuron disease; a slowly progressive degenerative disorder of the motor neurons of the cerebral cortex, resulting in widespread weakness on an upper motor neuron basis; spasticity, hyperreflexia, and Babinski signs are present, but not fasciculation potentials, nor any electrodiagnostic evidence of a lower motor neuron lesion.

scle·ro·ste·no·sis (sklēr-ō-ste-nō′sis). Induration and contraction of the tissues. [sclero- + G. *stenōsis*, a narrowing]

scle·ros·to·my (sklĕ-ros′tō-mē). Surgical perforation of the sclera, as for the relief of glaucoma. [sclero- + G. *stoma*, mouth]

scle·ro·ther·a·py (sklēr-ō-thār′ă-pē). Treatment involving the injection of a sclerosing solution into vessels or tissues.

scle·rot·ic (sklĕ-rot′ik). **1.** Relating to or characterized by sclerosis. **2.** SYN scleral.

scle·rot·i·ca (sklĕ-rot′i-kă). SYN sclera. [Mod. L. *scleroticus*, hard]

scle·ro·tome (sklēr′ō-tōm). **1.** A knife used in sclerotomy. **2.** The group of mesenchymal cells emerging from the ventromedial part of a mesodermic somite and migrating toward the notochord. Sclerotomal cells from adjacent somites become merged in intersomitically located masses that are the primordia of the centra of the vertebrae. [sclero- + G. *tomē*, a cutting]

scle·rot·o·my (sklĕ-rot′ō-mē). An incision through the sclera. [sclero- + G. *tomē*, incision]

scle·rous (sklēr′ŭs). SYN scleroid. [G. *sklēros*, hard]

sco·lex, pl. **scol·e·ces, scol·i·ces** (skō′leks, skō′le-sēz, skō′li-sēz). The head or anterior end of a tapeworm attached by suckers, and frequently by rostellar hooks, to the wall of the intestine. [G. *skōlēx*, a worm]

sco·li·o·ky·pho·sis (skō′lē-ō-kī-fō′sis). Lateral and posterior curvature of the spine. [G. *scolios*, curved, + *kyphōsis*, kyphosis]

◨ **sco·li·o·sis** (skō-lē-ō′sis). Abnormal lateral curvature of the vertebral column. Depending on the etiology, there may be one curve, or primary and secondary compensatory curves; s. may be "fixed" as a result of muscle and/or bone deformity or "mobile" as a result of unequal muscle contraction. [G. *skoliōsis*, a crookedness]

sco·li·ot·ic (skō′lē-ot′ik). Relating to or suffering from scoliosis.

△**-scope.** Viewing, staring; an instrument for viewing but extended to include other methods of examination (*e.g.*, stethoscope). [G. *skopeō*, to view]

sco·po·phil·ia (skō-pō-fil′ē-ă). SYN voyeurism. [G. *skopeō*, to view, + *philos*, fond]

sco·po·pho·bia (skō-pō-fō′bē-ă). Morbid dread of being stared at. [G. *skopeō*, to view, + *phobos*, fear]

△**-scopy.** An action or activity involving the use of in instrument for viewing. [G. *skopeō*, to view]

scor·bu·tic (skōr-byū′tik). Relating to, suffering from, or resembling scurvy (scorbutus).

scor·bu·ti·gen·ic (skōr-byū-ti-jen′ik). Scurvy-producing.

scor·di·ne·ma (skōr′di-nē′mă). Heaviness of the head with yawning and stretching, occurring as a prodrome of an infectious disease. [G. *skordinēma*, yawning]

score (skōr). An evaluation, usually expressed numerically, of status, achievement, or condition in a given set of circumstances. [M. E. *scor*, notch, tally]

   Apgar s., evaluation of a newborn infant's physical status by assigning numerical values (0 to 2) to each of 5 criteria: 1) heart rate, 2) respiratory effort, 3) muscle tone, 4) response stimulation, and 5) skin color; a score of 8 to 10 indicates the best possible condition.

   Dubowitz s., a method of clinical assessment of gestational age in the newborn that includes neurological criteria for the infant's maturity and other physical criteria to determine the gestational age of the infant; useful from birth to 5 days of life.

△**scoto-.** Darkness. [G. *skotos*]

sco•to•ma, pl. **sco•to•ma•ta** (skō-tō′mă, skō-tō′mă-tă). **1.** An isolated area of varying size and shape, within the visual field, in which vision is absent or depressed. **2.** A blind spot in psychological awareness. [G. *skotōma*, vertigo, fr. *skotos*, darkness]

annular s., a circular s. surrounding the center of the field of vision. SEE ring s.

cecocentral s., a s. involving the optic disk area (blind spot) and the papillomacular fibers; there are three forms: 1) the cecocentral defect which extends from the blind spot toward or into the fixation area; 2) angioscotoma; 3) glaucomatous nerve-fiber bundle s., due to involvement of nerve-fiber bundles at the edge of the optic disk.

central s., a s. involving the fixation point.

color s., an area of depressed color vision in the visual field.

mental s., absence of insight into, or inability to comprehend, items relative to a subject whose content is highly emotional to the individual. SYN blind spot (2).

negative s., a s. that appears as a blank or black patch in the visual field.

peripheral s., a s. outside of the central 30 degrees of the visual field.

physiologic s., the negative s. in the visual field, corresponding to the optic disk. SYN blind spot (1).

positive s., a s. that is perceived as a black spot within the field of vision.

relative s., a s. in which there is visual depression but not complete loss of light perception.

ring s., an annular area of blindness in the visual field surrounding the fixation point in pigmentary degeneration of the retina and in glaucoma.

scintillating s., a localized area of blindness edged by brilliantly colored shimmering lights (teichopsia); usually a prodromal symptom of migraine. SEE ALSO fortification *spectrum*.

sco•tom•a•tous (skō-tō′mă-tŭs). Relating to scotoma.

sco•tom•e•ter (skō-tom′ĕ-ter). An instrument for determining the size, shape, and intensity of a scotoma.

sco•tom•e•try (skō-tom′ĕ-trē). The plotting and measuring of a scotoma. [scoto- + G. *metron*, measure]

scot•o•phil•ia (skō-tō-fil′ē-ă). SYN nyctophilia. [scoto- + G. *philos*, fond]

scot•o•pho•bia (skō-tō-fō′bē-ă). SYN nyctophobia. [scoto- + G. *phobos*, fear]

sco•to•pia (skō-tō′pē-ă). SYN scotopic *vision*. [scoto- + G. *opsis*, vision]

sco•top•ic (skō-tō′pik, -top′ik). Referring to low illumination to which the eye is dark-adapted. SEE scotopic *vision*.

sco•top•sin (skō-top′sin). The protein moiety of the pigment in the rods of the retina.

scot•ty dog (scot′tē dawg). The fancied appearance of the articular facets on oblique radiographs of the lumbar spine; the neck of the s. d. is the pars interarticularis, site of the most common defect in spondylolysis.

screen (skrēn). **1.** A sheet of any substance used to shield an object from any influence, such as heat, light, x-rays, etc. **2.** A sheet upon which an image is projected. **3.** PSYCHOANALYSIS Concealment, as one image or memory concealing another. SEE ALSO screen *memory*. **4.** To examine, evaluate; to process a group to select or separate certain individuals from it. **5.** A thin layer of crystals that converts x-rays to light photons to expose film; used in a cassette to produce radiographic images on film. [Fr. *écran*]

fluorescent s., a s. coated with fluorescent crystals such as the calcium tungstate used in the fluoroscope.

screen•ing (skrēn′ing). **1.** To screen (5). **2.** Examination of a group of usually asymptomatic individuals to detect those with a high probability of having a given disease, typically by means of an inexpensive diagnostic test. **3.** In the mental health professions, initial patient evaluation that includes medical and psychiatric history, mental status evaluation, and diagnostic formulation to determine the patient's suitability for a particular treatment modality.

carrier s., indiscriminate examination of members of a population to detect heterozygotes for serious disorders and counsel about the risks of marriages with other carriers, and by antenatal diagnosis where a married couple are both carriers.

familial s., s. directed at close relatives of probands with diseases that may lie latent, as in age-dependent dominant traits, or that may involve risk to progeny, as X-linked traits.

scro•bic•u•late (skrō-bik′yū-lāt). Pitted; marked with minute depressions. [L. *scrobiculus;* dim. of *scrobis,* a trench]

scrof•u•lo•der•ma (skrof′yū-lō-der′mă). Tuberculosis resulting from extension into the skin from underlying atypical mycobacterial infection, most commonly of cervical lymph nodes. [scrofula + G. *derma*, skin]

scro•tal (skrō′tăl). Relating to the scrotum. SYN oscheal.

scro•tec•to•my (skrō-tek′tō-mē). Removal of all or part of scrotum. [scrotum, + G. *ektomē*, excision]

scro•ti•tis (skrō-tī′tis). Inflammation of the scrotum.

scro•to•plas•ty (skrō′tō-plas-tē). Surgical reconstruction of the scrotum. SYN oscheoplasty. [scrotum + G. *plastos*, formed]

scro•tum, pl. **scro•ta, scro•tums** (skrō′tŭm, -tă, -tŭmz) [NA]. A musculocutaneous sac containing the testes; it is formed of skin, containing a network of nonstriated muscular fibers (the dartus or dartus fascia), which also forms the scrotal septum internally. [L.]

scru•ple (skrū′pl). An apothecaries' weight of 20 grains or one-third of a dram. [L. *scrupulus,* a small sharp stone, a weight, the 24th part of an ounce, a scruple, dim. of *scrupus,* a sharp stone]

scurf (skerf). SYN dandruff. [A.S.]

scur•vy (sker′vē). A disease marked by inanition, debility, anemia, edema of the dependent parts, a

SC

spongy condition (sometimes with ulceration) of the gums, and hemorrhages into the skin and from the mucous membranes; due to a diet lacking vitamin C. [fr. A.S. *scurf*]

infantile s., osteopathia hemorrhagica infantum; a cachectic condition in infants, resulting from malnutrition and marked by pallor, fetid breath, coated tongue, diarrhea, and subperiosteal hemorrhages; probably a combination of s. and rickets due to combined deficiency of vitamins C and D. SYN Barlow's disease.

scute (skūt). A thin lamina or plate. SYN scutum (1). [L. *scutum,* shield]

scu•ti•form (skū'ti-fōrm). Shield-shaped. [L. *scutum,* shield, + *forma,* form]

scu•tu•lar (skū'tyū-lăr). Relating to a scutulum.

scu•tu•lum, pl. **scu•tu•la** (skū'tyū-lŭm, -lă; skū' chū-lŭm). A yellow, saucer-shaped crust, the characteristic lesion of favus, consisting of a mass of hyphae and spores. [L. dim. of *scutum,* shield]

scu•tum, pl. **scu•ta** (skū'tŭm, -tă). **1.** SYN scute. **2.** In ixodid (hard) ticks, a plate that largely or entirely covers the dorsum of the male and forms an anterior shield behind the capitulum of the female or immature ticks. [L. shield]

scyb•a•la (sib'ă-lă). Plural of scybalum.

scyb•a•lous (sib'ă-lŭs). Relating to scybala.

scyb•a•lum, pl. **scyb•a•la** (sib'ă-lŭm, -lă). A hard, round mass of inspissated feces. [G. *skybalon,* excrement]

scy•phoid (sī'foyd). Cup-shaped. [G. *skyphos,* cup, + *eidos,* resemblance]

SDA specific dynamic *action.*

Se selenium.

search•er (ser'cher). A form of sound used to determine the presence of a calculus in the bladder.

sea•sick•ness (sē'sik-nes). A form of motion sickness caused by the motion of a floating platform, such as a ship, boat, or raft. SYN mal de mer.

seat•worm (sēt'werm). SYN pinworm.

△**seb-.** SEE sebo-.

se•ba•ceous (sē-bā'shŭs). Relating to sebum; oily; fatty. [L. *sebaceus*]

se•bif•er•ous (sē-bif'er-ŭs). Producing sebaceous matter. [sebi- + L. *fero,* to bear]

△**sebo-, seb-, sebi-.** Sebum, sebaceous. [L. *sebum,* suet, tallow]

seb•o•lith (seb'ō-lith). A concretion in a sebaceous follicle. [sebo- + G. *lithos,* stone]

seb•or•rhea (seb-ō-rē'ă). Overactivity of the sebaceous glands, resulting in an excessive amount of sebum. [sebo- + G. *rhoia,* a flow]

s. facie′i, s. of face, s. oleosa affecting especially the nose and forehead.

s. furfura′cea, SYN s. sicca (1).

s. sic′ca, (1) an accumulation on the skin, especially the scalp, of dry scales; SYN s. furfuracea. **(2)** SYN dandruff.

seb•or•rhe•ic (seb-ō-rē'ik). Relating to seborrhea.

se•bum (sē'bŭm). The secretion of the sebaceous glands. [L. tallow]

sec second.

se•cre•ta (se-krē'tă). Secretions. [L. neuter pl. of *secretus,* pp. of *se-cerno,* to separate]

se•cre•ta•gogue (se-krē'tă-gog). An agent that promotes secretion; *e.g.,* acetylcholine, gastrin, secretin. [secreta + G. *agōgos,* drawing forth]

se•cre•tase (sē-krē'tās). A term used to describe a proteinase that acts on amyloid precursor protein to produce peptides that are soluble and do not precipitate to produce amyloid.

se•crete (se-krēt'). To elaborate or release products of cellular metabolism (enzymes, mucus, waste products). [L. *se-cerno,* pp. *-cretus,* to separate]

se•cre•tin (se-krē'tin). A hormone, formed by the epithelial cells of the duodenum under the stimulus of acid contents from the stomach, that incites secretion of pancreatic juice; used as an aid in the diagnosis of pancreatic exocrine disease and as an adjunct in obtaining desquamated pancreatic cells for cytological examination. [secrete + -in]

se•cre•tion (se-krē'shŭn). **1.** Production by a cell or aggregation of cells (a gland) of a physiologically active substance and its movement out of the cell or organ in which it is formed. **2.** The solid, liquid, or gaseous product of cellular or glandular activity that is stored up in or utilized by the organism in which it is produced. Cf. excretion. [L. *se-cerno,* pp. *-cretus,* to separate]

secretoinhibitory (se-kre-to-in-hib-itor-e). Restraining or curbing secretion.

se•cre•to•mo•tor, se•cre•to•mo•tory (se-krē'tō-mō'ter, -mō'ter-ē). Stimulating secretion. [secrete = *motor,* mover]

se•cre•tor (se-krē'ter, tōr). An individual whose bodily fluids (saliva, semen, vaginal secretions) contain a water-soluble form of the antigens of the ABO blood group.

se•cre•to•ry (se-krēt'ě-rē, sē'krě-tōr-ē). Relating to secretion or the secretions.

sec•tio, pl. **sec•ti•o•nes** (sek'shē-ō, sek-shē-ō'nēz) [NA]. ANATOMY, A subdivision or segment. [L.]

sec•tion (sek'shŭn). **1.** The act of cutting. **2.** A cut or division. **3.** A segment or part of any organ or structure delimited from the remainder. **4.** A cut surface. **5.** A thin slice of tissue, cells, microorganisms, or any material for examination under the microscope. [L. *sectio,* a cutting, fr. *seco,* to cut]

abdominal s., SYN celiotomy.

cesarean s., incision through the abdominal wall and the uterus (abdominal hysterotomy) for extraction of the fetus.

cross s., (1) a planar or two-dimensional view, diagram, or image of the internal structure of the body, part of the body, or any anatomic structure afforded by slicing, actually or through imaging (radiographic, magnetic, or microscopic) techniques, the body or structure along a particular plane; **(2)** the slice or section of a given thickness created by actual serial parallel cuts through a structure or by the application of imaging technique.

frozen s., a thin slice of tissue cut from a frozen specimen, often used for rapid microscopic diagnosis.

longitudinal s., a cross s. attained by slicing in any plane parallel to the long or vertical axis, actually or through imaging techniques, the body or any part of the body or anatomic structure. Longitudinal sections include, but are not limited to, median, sagittal, and coronal sections.

median s., a cross s. obtained by slicing in the median plane, actually or through imaging techniques, the body or any part of the body which occupies or crosses the median plane or by slicing any generally symmetrical anatomic structure, such as a finger or a cell, in its midline. Since actual sectioning the median plane results in a right and a left half, an anatomical median s. may be a two-dimensional view of the cut surface on the medial aspect of either half.

oblique s., a diagonal cross s. attained by slicing, actually or through imaging techniques, the body or any part of the body or anatomic structure, in any plane which does not parallel the longitudinal axis or intersect it at a right angle, *i.e.,* which is neither longitudinal (vertical) nor transverse (horizontal).

perineal s., any cutting through the perineum, either lateral or median lithotomy or external urethrotomy.

Saemisch's s., procedure of transfixing the cornea beneath an ulcer and then cutting from within outward through the base.

serial s., one of a number of consecutive microscopic s.'s.

thin s., ultrathin s., a s. of tissue for electron microscopic examination; the specimen is fixed, typically in glutaraldehyde and/or in osmium tetroxide, embedded in a plastic resin, and sectioned at less than 0.1 μm in thickness with a glass or diamond knife in an ultramicrotome.

transverse s., a cross s. obtained by slicing, actually or through imaging techniques, the body or any part of the body structure, in a horizontal plane, *i.e.,* a plane which intersects the longitudinal axis at a right angle. Since actual sectioning in the transverse plane results in an inferior and a superior portion, an anatomical transverse section may be a two-dimensional view of the cut surface on the inferior aspect of the superior portion, or of the superior aspect of the inferior portion. By convention, in medical imaging transverse sections demonstrate the former unless otherwise stated.

sec•ti•o•nes (sek-shē-ō′nēz). Plural of sectio.

sec•tor•an•o•pia (sek′tŏr-an-ō′pē-ă). Loss of vision in a sector of the visual field. [sector + G. *an-* priv. + *opsis,* vision]

se•cun•di•grav•i•da (sek′ŭn-di-grav′i-dă). SEE gravida.

se•cun•dines (sek′ŭn-dēnz). SYN afterbirth. [L. *secundinae,* the afterbirth]

se•cun•dip•a•ra (sek′ŭn-dip′ă-ră). SEE para.

se•date (sĕ-dāt′). To bring under the influence of a sedative. [L. *sedatus;* see sedation]

se•da•tion (sĕ-dā′shŭn). **1.** The act of calming, especially by the administration of a sedative. **2.** The state of being calm. [L. *sedatio,* to calm, allay]

sed•a•tive (sed′ă-tiv). **1.** Calming; quieting. **2.** A drug that quiets nervous excitement; designated according to the organ or system upon which specific action is exerted; *e.g.,* cardiac, cerebral,

nervous, respiratory, spinal. [L. *sedativus;* see sedation]

sed•i•ment (sed′i-ment). **1.** Insoluble material that tends to sink to the bottom of a liquid, as in hypostasis. **2.** To cause the formation of a sediment or deposit, as in the case of centrifugation or ultracentrifugation. SYN sedimentate. [L. *sedimentum,* a settling, fr. *sedeo,* to sit, settle down]

sed•i•men•tate (sed′i-men-tāt). SYN sediment (2).

sed•i•men•ta•tion (sed′i-men-tā′shŭn). Formation of a sediment.

sed•i•men•ta•tor (sed′i-men-tā′ter, tōr). A centrifuge.

sed•i•men•tom•e•ter (sed′ĭ-men-tom′ĕ-ter). A photographic apparatus for the automatic recording of the blood sedimentation rate. [sediment + G. *metron,* measure]

seed (sēd). **1.** The reproductive body of a flowering plant; the mature ovule. SYN semen (2). **2.** BACTERIOLOGY To inoculate a culture medium with microorganisms. [A.S. *soed*]

seg•ment. 1. A section; a part of an organ or other structure delimited naturally, artificially, or by invagination from the remainder. SEE ALSO metamere. **2.** A territory of an organ having independent function, supply, or drainage. **3.** To divide and redivide into minute equal parts. SYN segmentum [NA]. [L. *segmentum,* fr. *seco,* to cut]

anterior ocular s., that portion of the eye comprising the cornea, iris, lens, and their associated chambers and adnexa.

bronchopulmonary s., the largest subdivision of a lobe of the lung; it is supplied by a direct tertiary (lobular) bronchus and a tertiary branch of the pulmonary artery; it is separated from adjacent segments by connective tissue septa.

internodal s., the portion of a myelinated nerve fiber between two successive nodes. SYN internode.

posterior s. of eyeball, the large space between the lens and the retina; it is filled with the vitreous body.

uterine s.'s, (1) lower: the isthmus of the uterus, the lower extremity of which joins with the cervical canal and, during pregnancy, expands to become the lower part of the uterine cavity; **(2)** upper: the main portion of the body of the gravid uterus, the contraction of which furnishes the chief expulsory force in labor.

seg•men•tec•to•my (seg-men-tek′tō-mē). Excision of a segment of any organ or gland.

seg•men•tum, pl. **seg•men•ta** (seg-men′tŭm, -tă) [NA]. SYN segment. [L. segment]

seg•re•ga•tion (seg-rĕ-gā′shŭn). **1.** Removal of certain parts from a mass, *e.g.,* those with infectious diseases. **2.** Separation of contrasting characters in the offspring of heterozygotes. **3.** Separation of the paired state of genes, which occurs at the reduction division of meiosis; only one member of each somatic gene pair is normally included in each sperm or ovum. **4.** Progressive restriction of potencies in the zygote to the following embryo. [L. *segrego,* pp. *-atus,* to set apart from the flock, separate]

sei•zure (sē′zher). **1.** An attack; the sudden onset of a disease or of certain symptoms. **2.** An epileptic attack. SYN convulsion (2). [O. Fr. *seisir,* to grasp, fr. Germanic]

absence s., a brief s. characterized by arrest of activity and occasionally clonic movements. There is loss of consciousness or slowing of thought. The EEG typically shows generalized spike wave discharges greater than 2.5 Hz. More prolonged absence seizures may have automatisms.

complex partial s., a partial s. with impairment of consciousness without features of a generalized s. Complex partial s.'s are commonly associated with automatisms.

generalized tonic-clonic s., a generalized s. characterized by the sudden onset of tonic contraction of the muscles often associated with a cry or moan, and frequently resulting in a fall to the ground. The tonic phase of the s. gradually gives way to clonic convulsive movements occurring bilaterally and synchronously before slowing and eventually stopping, followed by a variable period of unconsciousness and gradual recovery. SYN generalized tonic-clonic epilepsy, grand mal.

jacksonian s., a s. originating in or near the rolandic neocortex, which clinically involves one part of the body; s. spread is accompanied by progressive spread to other parts of the body on the same side; may become generalized. SYN jacksonian epilepsy.

partial s., s. characterized by localized cerebral ictal onset. The symptoms experienced are dependent on the cortical area of ictal onset or seizure spread.

psychomotor s., SYN psychomotor *epilepsy.*

se·lec·tion (sĕ-lek'shŭn). The combined effect of the causes and consequences of genetic factors that determine the average number of progeny of a species that attain sexual maturity. [L. *se-ligo,* to separate, select, fr. *se,* apart, + *lego,* to pick out]

artificial s., interference with natural s. by purposeful breeding of animals or plants of specific genotype or phenotype to produce a strain with desired characteristics.

natural s., "survival of the fittest," the principle that in nature those individuals best able to adapt to their environment will survive and reproduce, while those less able will die without progeny; and the genes carried by the survivors will increase in frequency. This principle is heuristic rather than rigorous since it cannot be tested, the outcome being tautologous with the empirical definition of fitness.

sexual s., a form of natural s. in which, according to Darwin's theory, the male or female is attracted by certain characteristics, form, color, behavior, etc., in the opposite sex; thus modifications of a special nature are brought about in the species.

se·le·ni·um (Se) (sĕ-lē'nē-ŭm). A metallic element chemically similar to sulfur, atomic no. 34, atomic wt. 78.96; an essential trace element toxic in large quantities; required for glutathione peroxidase and a few other enzymes; [75]Se (half-life equal to 119.78 days) is used in scintography of the pancreas and parathyroid glands. [G. *selēnē,* moon]

self. 1. A sum of the attitudes, feelings, memories, traits, and behavioral predispositions that make up the personality. 2. The individual as represented in his or her own awareness and in his or her environment. 3. IMMUNOLOGY An individual's autologous cell components as contrasted with non-s., or foreign, constituents; discrimination by the immune system between s. and non-s. protects against an attack on the host's own antigenic constituents. The mechanism of recognition of s. from non-s. is unknown, but serves to protect from an immunologic attack on the host's own antigenic constituents, as opposed to immune system destruction or elimination of foreign antigens.

self-a·ware·ness. Realization of one's ongoing feeling and emotional experience; a major goal of all psychotherapy.

self-con·trol. 1. Self-regulation of one's behavior in accordance with personal beliefs, goals, attitudes and societal expectations. 2. Use by an individual of active coping strategies to deal with problem situations, in contrast to passive conditioning strategies which do things to the individual and require no action by the person.

self-lim·it·ed. Denoting a disease that tends to cease after a definite period; *e.g.,* pneumonia.

self-love. SYN narcissism.

sel·la (sel'ă). SYN saddle (1). [L. saddle]

s. tur'cica [NA], a saddle-like bony prominence on the upper surface of the body of the sphenoid bone, constituting the middle part of the butterfly-shaped middle cranial fossa; it includes the tuberculum sellae anteriorly and the dorsum sellae posteriorly; with its covering of dura mater it constitutes the hypophysial fossa which accommodates the hypophysis or pituitary gland.

sel·lar (sel'ăr). Relating to the sella turcica.

se·man·tics (se-man'tiks). A branch of semiotics: 1. The study of the significance and development of the meaning of words. 2. The study concerned with the relations between signs and their referents; the relations between the signs of a system; and human behavioral reaction to signs, including unconscious attitudes, influences of social institutions, and epistemological and linguistic assumptions. [G. *sēmainō,* to show]

se·men, pl. **sem·i·na, se·mens** (sē'men, sē-mi'nă, sē'menz). 1 [NA]. The penile ejaculate; a thick, yellowish-white, viscid fluid containing spermatozoa; a mixture produced by secretions of the testes, seminal vesicles, prostate, and bulbourethral glands. SYN sperm (2) [NA], seminal fluid. 2. SYN seed (1). [L. *semen (semin-),* seed (of plants, men, animals)]

se·me·nu·ria (sē-mĕ-nū'rē-ă). The excretion of urine containing semen. SYN seminuria, spermaturia.

△**semi-.** One-half. Cf. hemi-. [L. *semis,* half]

sem·i·ca·nal (sem'ē-kă-nal'). A half canal; a deep groove on the edge of a bone which, uniting with a similar groove or part of an adjoining bone, forms a complete canal.

sem·i·co·ma. SEE semicomatose.

sem·i·com·a·tose. An imprecise term for a state of drowsiness and inaction, in which more than ordinary stimulation may be required to evoke a response, and the response may be delayed or incomplete. SYN semiconscious.

sem·i·con·scious. SYN semicomatose.

sem·i·lu·nar (sem-ē-lū′năr). SYN lunar (2). [semi- + L. *luna,* moon]

sem·i·nal (sem′i-năl). **1.** Relating to the semen. **2.** Original or influential of future developments.

sem·i·na·tion (sem-i-nā′shŭn). SYN insemination.

sem·i·nif·er·ous (sem′i-nif′er-ŭs). Carrying or conducting the semen; denoting the tubules of the testis. [L. *semen,* seed (semen) + *fero,* to carry]

sem·i·no·ma (sem-i-nō′mă). A radiosensitive malignant neoplasm usually arising from germ cells in the testis of young male adults which metastasizes to the paraortic lymph nodes; a counterpart of dysgerminoma of the ovary. [L. *semen,* seed (semen) + G. *-oma,* tumor]

    spermacytic s., a relatively slow-growing, locally invasive type of testicular s. that does not metastasize and has no ovarian counterpart.

sem·i·nu·ria (sē-mi-nū′rē-ă). SYN semenuria.

sem·i·per·me·a·ble (sem-ē-per′mē-ă-bl). Freely permeable to water (or other solvent) but relatively impermeable to solutes.

sem·i·sul·cus (sem′ē-sŭl′kŭs). A slight groove on the edge of a bone or other structure, which, uniting with a similar groove on the corresponding adjoining structure, forms a complete sulcus.

sem·i·syn·thet·ic (sem′ē-sin-thet′ik). Describing the process of synthesizing a particular chemical utilizing a naturally occurring chemical as a starting material, thus obviating part of a total synthesis.

se·nes·cence (se-nes′ens). The state of being old. [L. *senesco,* to grow old, fr. *senex,* old]

se·nes·cent (sē-nes′ent). Growing old.

se·nile (sē′nīl, sen′īl). Relating to or characteristic of old age. [L. *senilis*]

se·nil·i·ty (se-nil′i-tē). Old age; a general term for a variety of mental disorders occurring in old age which consist of two broad categories, organic and psychological disorders. [see senile]

sen·sate (sen′sāt). Able to perceive touch and other sensations; used in reference to patients who have had partial nerve or spinal cord injuries.

sen·sa·tion (sen-sā′shŭn). A feeling; the translation into consciousness of the effects of a stimulus exciting any of the organs of sense. [L. *sensatio,* perception, feeling, fr. *sentio,* to perceive, feel]

    girdle s., SYN zonesthesia.

    objective s., a s. caused by a verifiable stimulus.

    referred s., a s. felt in one place in response to a stimulus applied in another.

    subjective s., a s. not readily referable to a denotably verifiable stimulus.

sense (sens). The faculty of perceiving any stimulus. [L. *sentio,* pp. *sensus,* to feel, to perceive]

    s. of equilibrium, the s. that makes possible a normal physiologic posture.

    kinesthetic s., SYN myesthesia.

    muscular s., SYN myesthesia.

    position s., SYN posture s.

    posture s., the ability to recognize the position

in which a limb is passively placed, with the eyes closed. SYN position s.

    pressure s., the faculty of discriminating various degrees of pressure on the surface. SYN baresthesia, piesesthesia.

    special s., one of the five senses related respectively to the organs of sight, hearing, smell, taste, and touch.

    visceral s., the perception of the existence of the internal organs. SYN splanchnesthesia, splanchnesthetic sensibility.

sen·si·bil·i·ty (sen-si-bil′i-tē). The consciousness of sensation; the capability of perceiving sensible stimuli. [L. *sensibilitas*]

    dissociation s., the loss of the pain and the thermal senses with preservation of tactile sensibility or vice versa.

    epicritic s., SEE epicritic.

    proprioceptive s., SEE proprioceptive.

    protopathic s., SEE protopathic.

    splanchnesthetic s., SYN visceral *sense.*

sen·si·ble (sen′si-bl). **1.** Perceptible to the senses. **2.** Capable of sensation. **3.** SYN sensitive. **4.** Having reason or judgment; intelligent. [L. *sensibilis,* fr. *sentio,* to feel, perceive]

sen·si·tive (sen′si-tiv). **1.** Capable of perceiving sensations. **2.** Responding to a stimulus. **3.** Acutely perceptive of interpersonal situations. **4.** One who is readily hypnotizable. **5.** Readily undergoing a chemical change, with but slight change in environmental conditions, as a s. reagent. **6.** IMMUNOLOGY Denoting: 1) a sensitized *antigen;* 2) a person (or animal) rendered susceptible to immunological reactions by previous exposure to the antigen concerned. **7.** MICROBIOLOGY Denoting a microorganism that is susceptible to inhibition or destruction by a given antimicrobial agent. SYN sensible (3).

sen·si·tiv·i·ty (sen-si-tiv′i-tē). SYN susceptibility (2). **1.** The ability to appreciate by one or more of the senses. **2.** State of being sensitive. **3.** CLINICAL PATHOLOGY The proportion of individuals with a given disease or condition in which a test intended to identify that disease or condition yields positive results. S. (%) = number of diseased individuals with a positive test × 100 total number of diseased individuals tested. Cf. specificity (2). [L. *sentio,* pp. *sensus,* to feel]

sen·si·ti·za·tion (sen′si-ti-zā′shŭn). Immunization, especially with reference to antigens (immunogens) not associated with infection; the induction of acquired sensitivity or of allergy.

    autoerythrocyte s., SEE autoerythrocyte sensitization *syndrome.*

    covert s., aversive conditioning or training to abolish an unwanted behavior, during which the patient is taught to imagine unpleasant and related aversive consequences while engaging in the unwanted habit.

    photodynamic s., the action by which certain substances, notably fluorescing dyes (acridine, eosin, methylene blue, rose bengal) absorb visible light and emit the energy at wavelengths that are deleterious to microbes or other organisms in the dye-containing suspension, or selectively destroy cancer cells sensitized by intravenous porphyrin

se

and exposed to red laser light. SYN photosensitization (2).

sen·si·tize (sen'si-tīz). To render sensitive; to induce acquired sensitivity, to immunize. SEE ALSO sensitized *antigen*.

sen·sor (sen'sŏr). A device designed to respond to physical stimuli such as temperature, light, magnetism, or movement, and transmit resulting impulses for interpretation, recording, movement, or operating control. [see sense]

△**sensori-.** Sensory. [L. *sensorius*]

sen·so·ri·al (sen-sōr'ē-ăl). Relating to the sensorium.

sen·so·ri·mo·tor (sen'sōr-i-mō'ter). Both sensory and motor; denoting a mixed nerve with afferent and efferent fibers.

sen·so·ri·um, pl. **sen·so·ria**, **sen·so·ri·ums** (sen-sōr'ē-ŭm, -ă, -ŭmz). **1.** An organ of sensation. **2.** The hypothetical "seat of sensation." **3.** PSYCHOLOGY Consciousness; sometimes used as a generic term for the intellectual and cognitive functions. [Late L.]

sen·so·ry (sen'sŏ-rē). Relating to sensation. [L. *sensorius*, fr. *sensus*, sense]

sensory awareness. The ability to receive and differentiate sensory stimuli.

sen·su·al (sen'shū-ăl). **1.** Relating to the body and the senses, as distinguished from the intellect or spirit. **2.** Denoting bodily or sensory pleasure, not necessarily sexual. [L. *sensualis,* endowed with feeling]

sen·tient (sen'shent, sen'shē-ent). Capable of, or characterized by, sensation. [L. *sentiens,* pres. p. of *sentio,* to feel, perceive]

sep·sis, pl. **sep·ses** (sep'sis, -sēz). The presence of various pus-forming and other pathogenic organisms, or their toxins, in the blood or tissues; septicemia is a common type of s. [G. *sēpsis,* putrefaction]

△**sept-.** SEE septi-, septico-, septo-.

sep·ta (sep'tă). Plural of septum. [L.]

sep·tal (sep'tăl). Relating to a septum.

sep·tate (sep'tāt). Having a septum; divided into compartments. [L. *saeptum,* septum]

sep·tec·to·my (sep-tek'tō-mē). Operative removal of the whole or a part of a septum, specifically of the nasal septum. [L. *saeptum,* septum, + G. *ektomē,* excision]

△**septi-, sept-.** Seven. [L. *septem*]

sep·tic (sep'tik). Relating to or caused by sepsis.

sep·ti·ce·mia (sep-ti-sē'mē-ă). Systemic disease caused by the multiplication of microorganisms in the circulating blood; formerly called "blood poisoning". SEE ALSO pyemia. SYN septic fever. [G. *sēpsis,* putrefaction, + *haima,* blood]

  cryptogenic s., a form of s. in which no primary focus of infection can be found.

  puerperal s., a severe bloodstream infection resulting from an obstetric delivery or procedure.

sep·ti·ce·mic (sep-ti-sē'mik). Relating to, suffering from, or resulting from septicemia.

△**septico-, septic-.** Sepsis, septic. [G. *sēptikos,* putrifying, fr. *sēpsis,* putrefaction]

sep·ti·co·py·e·mia (sep'ti-kō-pī-ē'mē-ă). Pyemia and septicemia occurring together.

sep·ti·co·py·e·mic (sep'ti-kō-pī-ē'mik). Relating to septicopyemia.

△**septo-, sept-.** Septum. [L. *saeptum*]

sep·to·mar·gi·nal (sep'tō-mar'ji-năl). Relating to the margin of a septum, or to both a septum and a margin.

sep·to·na·sal (sep'tō-nā'săl). Relating to the nasal septum.

sep·to·plas·ty (sep'tō-plas-tē). Operation to correct defects or deformities of the nasal septum, often by alteration or partial removal of supporting structures. [septo- + G. *plastos,* formed]

sep·to·rhi·no·plas·ty (sep-tō-rī'nō-plas-tē). Combined operation to repair defects or deformities of the nasal septum and of the external nasal pyramid. [septo- + G. *rhis,* nose, + *plastos,* formed]

sep·tos·to·my (sep-tos'tō-mē). Surgical creation of a septal defect. [septo- + G. *stoma,* mouth]

sep·tu·lum, pl. **sep·tu·la** (sep'tyū-lŭm, -lă). A minute septum. [Mod. L. dim. of *septum*]

sep·tum, gen. **sep·ti**, pl. **sep·ta** (sep'tŭm, -tī, -tă). **1** [NA]. A thin wall dividing two cavities or masses of softer tissue. SEE transparent s. **2.** In fungi, a wall; usually a cross-wall in a hypha. [L. *saeptum,* a partition]

  atrioventricular s., the small part of the membranous s. of the heart just above the septal cusp of the tricuspid valve that separates the right atrium from the left ventricle.

  interalveolar s., (**1**) the tissue intervening between two adjacent pulmonary alveoli; it consists of a close-meshed capillary network covered on both surfaces by very thin alveolar epithelial cells; (**2**) one of the bony partitions between the tooth sockets.

  interatrial s., the wall between the atria of the heart.

  interdental s., the bony portion separating two adjacent teeth in a dental arch.

  intermuscular s., a term applied to aponeurotic sheets separating various muscles of the limbs; these are anterior and posterior crural, lateral and medial femoral, lateral and medial humeral.

  interventricular s., the wall between the ventricles of the heart.

  nasal s., the wall dividing the nasal cavity into halves; it is composed of a central supporting skeleton covered on each side by a mucous membrane.

  rectovaginal s., the fascial layer between the vagina and the lower part of the rectum.

  rectovesical s., a fascial layer that extends superiorly from the central tendon of the perineum to the peritoneum between the prostate and rectum.

  s. pe·nis [NA], the portion of the tunica albuginea incompletely separating the two corpora cavernosa of the penis.

  scrotal s., an incomplete wall of connective tissue and nonstriated muscle (dartos fascia) dividing the scrotum into two sacs, each containing a testis.

  transparent s., a thin plate of brain tissue, containing nerve cells and numerous nerve fibers, that is stretched like a flat, vertical sheet between the column and body of fornix below, the corpus callosum above and anteriorly; it is usually fused in the median plane with its partner on the opposite side so as to form a thin, median partition between the left and right frontal horn of the lateral ventricles; in less than 10% of humans there is a blind, slitlike, fluid-filled space between the two transparent septa, the cavity of s. pellucidum. The transparent s. is continuous ventralward through the interval between the corpus callosum and the anterior commissure with the precommissural septum and subcallosal gyrus.

se·que·la, pl. **se·que·lae** (sē-kwel′ă, sē-kwel′ē). A condition following as a consequence of a disease. [L. *sequela*, a sequel, fr. *sequor*, to follow]

se·quence (sē′kwens). The succession, or following, of one thing or event after another. [L. *sequor*, to follow]

    coding s., the portion of DNA that codes for transcription of messenger RNA. SEE exon.

    insertion s.'s, discrete DNA s.'s which are repeated at various sites on a bacterial chromosome, certain plasmids, and bacteriophages; insertion s.'s can move from one site to another on the chromosome, to another plasmid in the same bacterium, or to a bacteriophage.

    regulatory s., any DNA s. that is responsible for the regulation of gene expression, such as promoters and operators.

se·quence lad·der. The array of bands, made conspicuous by labeling, formed when DNA fragmented by endonucleases is subject to gel electrophoresis; corresponds to the nucleotide sequence.

se·ques·tra (sē-kwes′tră). Plural of sequestrum.

se·ques·tral (sē-kwes′trăl). Relating to a sequestrum.

se·ques·tra·tion (sē-kwes-trā′shŭn). **1.** Formation of a sequestrum. **2.** Loss of blood or of its fluid content into spaces within the body so that it is withdrawn from the circulating volume, resulting in hemodynamic impairment, hypovolemia, hypotension, and reduced venous return to the heart. [L. *sequestratio*, fr. *sequestro*, pp. *-atus*, to lay aside]

    bronchopulmonary s., a congenital anomaly in which a mass of lung tissue becomes isolated, during development, from the rest of the lung; the bronchi in the mass are usually dilated or cystic and are not connected with the bronchial tree; it is supplied by a branch of the aorta.

se·ques·trec·to·my (sē-kwes-trek′tō-mē). Operative removal of a sequestrum. [sequestrum + G. *ektomē*, excision]

se·ques·trum, pl. **se·ques·tra** (sē-kwes′trŭm, -tră). A piece of necrotic tissue, usually bone, that has become separated from the surrounding healthy tissue. [Mod. L. use of Mediev. L. *sequestrum*, something laid aside, fr. L. *sequestro*, to lay aside, separate]

se·quoi·o·sis (sē-kwoy-ō′sis). Extrinsic allergic alveolitis caused by inhalation of redwood sawdust containing spores of *Graphium*, *Pullularia*, *Aureobasidium*, and other fungi. [*Sequoia* (genus name) for *Sequoah* (George Guess), Cherokee scholar, + G. *-osis*, condition]

SER somatosensory evoked response. SEE ALSO evoked *response*.

Ser serine and its radical.

ser·al·bu·min (sēr-al-byū′min). SYN serum *albumin*.

se·ries, pl. **se·ries** (sēr′ēz). **1.** A succession of similar objects following one another in space or time. **2.** CHEMISTRY A group of substances, either elements or compounds, having similar properties or differing from each other in composition by a constant ratio. [L. fr. *sero*, to join together]

    aromatic s., all the compounds derived from benzene, or similar cyclic compounds that obey Hückel's rule.

    erythrocytic s., the cells in the various stages of development in the red bone marrow leading to the formation of the erythrocyte, *e.g.*, erythroblasts, normoblasts, erythrocytes.

    granulocytic s., the cells in the several stages of development in the bone marrow leading to the mature granulocyte of the circulation, *e.g.*, myeloblasts, different stages of the myelocyte, granulocytes.

    lymphocytic s., lymphoid s., the cells at various states in the development in lymphoid tissue of the mature lymphocytes, *e.g.*, lymphoblasts, young lymphocytes, mature lymphocytes.

    myeloid s., the granulocytic and the erythrocytic s.

    thrombocytic s., the cells of successive stages in thrombocytic (platelet) development in the bone marrow, *e.g.*, thromboblasts, thrombocytes.

    upper gastrointestinal s. (UGIS), a fluoroscopic-radiographic examination of the esophagus, stomach, and duodenum; a contrast medium, usually barium sulfate, is introduced.

ser·ine (S, Ser) (ser′ēn). One of the amino acids occurring in proteins.

sero-. Serum, serous. [L. *serum*, whey]

se·ro·co·li·tis (sēr′ō-kō-lī′tis). SYN pericolitis. [Mod. L. *serosa*, serous membrane, + colitis]

seroconversion (sēr-ō-kŭn-vŭr′zhun). Process by which, after exposure to etiologic agent of a disease, the blood changes from a negative to a positive serum marker for that specific disease.

se·ro·di·ag·no·sis (sēr′ō-dī-ag-nō′sis). Diagnosis by means of a reaction using blood serum or other serous fluids in the body (serologic tests).

se·ro·en·ter·i·tis (sēr′ō-en-ter-ī′tis). SYN perienteritis. [Mod. L. *serosa*, serous membrane, + enteritis]

se·ro·ep·i·de·mi·ol·o·gy (sēr′ō-ep-i-dē-mē-ol′ō-jē). Epidemiological study based on the detection of infection by serological testing.

se·ro·fi·brin·ous (sēr-ō-fī′bri-nŭs). Denoting an exudate composed of serum and fibrin.

se·ro·fi·brous (sēr-ō-fī′brŭs). Relating to a serous membrane and a fibrous tissue.

se·ro·log·ic (sēr-ō-loj′ik). Relating to serology.

se·rol·o·gy (sē-rol′ō-jē). The branch of science concerned with serum, especially with specific immune or lytic serums; to measure either antigens or antibodies in sera. [sero- + G. *logos*, study]

se·ro·ma (sē-rō′mă). A mass or tumefaction caused by the localized accumulation of serum within a tissue or organ. [sero- + G. *-oma*, tumor]

se·ro·mem·bra·nous (sēr′ō-mem′bră-nŭs). Relating to a serous membrane.

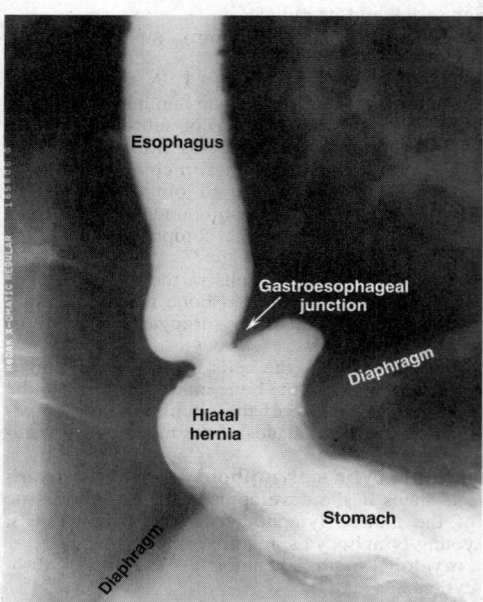

upper gastrointestinal series: radiograph showing hiatal hernia

---

se•ro•mu•coid (sēr-ō-myū′koyd). General term for a mucoprotein (glycoprotein) from serum.

se•ro•mu•cous (sēr-ō-myū′kŭs). Pertaining to a mixture of watery and mucinous material, such as that of certain glands.

se•ro•neg•a•tive (sēr-ō-neg′ă-tiv). Lacking an antibody of a specific type in serum; denoting absence of prior infection with a specific agent, disappearance of antibodies after treatment of a disease, or absence of antibody usually found in a given syndrome.

se•ro•pos•i•tive (sēr-ō-poz′i-tiv). Containing antibody of a specific type in serum; denoting presence of immunological evidence of a specific infection or presence of a diagnostically useful antibody.

se•ro•pu•ru•lent (sēr-ō-pū′rū-lent). Composed of or containing both serum and pus; denoting a discharge of thin watery pus (seropus).

se•ro•pus (sēr′ō-pŭs). Purulent serum, *i.e.,* pus largely diluted with serum.

se•ro•sa (se-rō′să). **1.** The outermost coat or serous layer of a visceral structure that lies in the body cavities of abdomen or thorax; it consists of a surface layer of mesothelium reinforced by irregular fibroelastic connective tissue. **2.** The outermost of the extraembryonic membranes, which encloses the embryo and all its other membranes; it consists of ectoderm reinforced by somatic mesoderm; the serosa of mammalian embryos is frequently called the trophoderm. SYN membrana serosa (2). SEE ALSO chorion. SYN membrana serosa (1), serous membrane. [fem. of Mod. L. *serosus,* serous]

se•ro•san•guin•e•ous (sēr′ō-sang-gwin′ē-ŭs).

Denoting an exudate or a discharge composed of or containing serum and also blood.

se•ro•se•rous (sēr-ō-sēr′ŭs). **1.** Relating to two serous surfaces. **2.** Denoting a suture, as of the intestine, in which the edges of the wound are infolded so as to bring the two serous surfaces in apposition.

se•ro•si•tis (sēr-ō-sī′tis). Inflammation of a serous membrane.

se•ros•i•ty (se-ros′i-tē). **1.** A serous fluid or a serum. **2.** The condition of being serous. **3.** The serous quality of a liquid.

se•ro•syn•o•vi•tis (sēr′ō-sin-ō-vī′tis). Synovitis attended with a copious serous effusion.

se•ro•ther•a•py (sēr-ō-thār′ă-pē). Treatment of an infectious disease by injection of an antitoxin or serum containing specific antibody.

se•ro•to•ner•gic (sēr-ō-tō-ner′jik, sĕr-). Related to the action of serotonin or its precursor L-tryptophan. [serotonin + G. *ergon,* work]

se•ro•to•nin (sēr-ō-tō′nin). A vasoconstrictor, liberated by platelets, that inhibits gastric secretion and stimulates smooth muscle; also acts as a neurotransmitter, present in the central nervous system, many peripheral tissues and cells, and carcinoid tumors. SYN 5-hydroxytryptamine. [sero- + G. *tonos,* tone, tension, + -in]

se•ro•type (sēr′ō-tīp). SYN serovar.

se•rous (sēr′ŭs). Relating to, containing, or producing serum or a substance having a watery consistency.

se•ro•vac•ci•na•tion (sēr′ō-vak-si-nā′shŭn). A process for producing mixed immunity by the injection of a serum, to secure passive immunity, and by vaccination with a modified or killed culture to acquire active immunity later.

se•ro•var (sēr′ō-var). A subdivision of a species or subspecies distinguishable from other strains therein on the basis of antigenic character. SYN serotype. [sero- + *variant*]

ser•pig•i•nous (ser-pij′i-nŭs). Creeping; denoting an ulcer or other cutaneous lesion that extends with a wavy or serpent-like border. [Mediev. L. *serpigo- (-gin-),* ringworm, fr. L. *serpo,* to creep]

ser•pi•go (ser-pī′gō). **1.** SYN tinea. **2.** SYN herpes. **3.** Any creeping or serpiginous eruption. [Mediev. L. *serpigo (-gin-),* ringworm, fr. L. *serpo,* to creep]

ser•rate, ser•rat•ed (ser′āt, -ā′ted). Toothed. [L. *serratus,* fr. *serra,* a saw]

ser•ra•tion (se-rā′shŭn). **1.** The state of being serrated or notched. **2.** Any one of the processes in a serrate or dentate formation. [L. *serra,* saw]

serre•fine (ser-e-fēn′). A small spring forceps used for approximating the edges of a wound or for temporarily closing an artery during an operation. [Fr.]

se•rum, pl. **se•rums, se•ra** (sēr′ŭm, -ŭmz, -ă). **1.** A clear, watery fluid, especially that moistening the surface of serous membranes, or exuded in inflammation of any of those membranes. **2.** The fluid portion of the blood obtained after removal of the fibrin clot and blood cells, distinguished from the plasma in circulating blood. Sometimes used as a synonym for antiserum or antitoxin. [L. whey]

    antilymphocyte s. (ALS), antiserum against

lymphocytes, used to suppress rejection of grafts or organ transplants.

Coombs' s., syn antihuman *globulin*.

immune s., syn antiserum.

muscle s., the fluid remaining after the coagulation of muscle plasma and the separation of myosin.

nonimmune s., a s. from a subject that is not immune; a s. that is free of antibodies to a given antigen.

normal s., a nonimmune s., usually with reference to a s. obtained prior to immunization.

polyvalent s., an antiserum obtained by inoculating an animal with several antigens or species or strains of bacteria.

se•rum•al (sēr'ŭm-ăl). Relating to or derived from serum.

se•rum-fast (sēr'ŭm-fast). **1.** Pertaining to a serum in which there is little or no change in the titer of antibody, even under conditions of treatment or immunologic stimulation. **2.** Resistant to the destructive effect of sera.

se•rum glu•tam•ic-py•ru•vic trans•am•i•nase (SGPT). syn alanine aminotransferase.

ses•a•moid (ses'ă-moyd). **1.** Resembling in size or shape a grain of sesame. **2.** Denoting a sesamoid bone. [G. *sēsamoeidēs,* like sesame]

ses•qui•hy•drates (ses-kwi-hī'drāts). Compounds crystallizing with (nominally) 1.5 molecules of water.

ses•sile (ses'il). Having a broad base of attachment; not pedunculated. [L. *sessilis,* low-growing, fr. *sedeo,* pp. *sessus,* to sit]

set. **1.** A readiness to perceive or to respond in some way; an attitude which facilitates or predetermines an outcome; *e.g.,* prejudice or bigotry. **2.** To reduce a fracture; *i.e.,* to bring the bones back into a normal position or alignment.

minimum data s. (MDS), smallest number of data that can be collected and still positively identify the patient.

se•ta, pl. **set•ae** (sē'tă, -tē). A bristle or a slender, stiff, bristle-like structure. [L. *saeta* or *seta,* a stiff hair or bristle]

se•ta•ceous (sē-tā'shŭs). **1.** Having bristles. **2.** Resembling a bristle. [L. *seta,* a bristle]

se•ton (sē'tŏn). A wisp of threads, a strip of gauze, a length of wire, or other foreign material passed through the subcutaneous tissues or a cyst to form a sinus or fistula. [L. *seta,* bristle]

sex (seks). **1.** The biological character or quality that distinguishes male and female from one another as expressed by analysis of the individual's gonadal, morphological (internal and external), chromosomal, and hormonal characteristics. Cf. gender. **2.** The physiological and psychological processes within an individual which prompt behavior related to procreation or erotic pleasure. [L. *sexus*]

sex-in•flu•enced. Denoting a class of genetic disorders in which the same genotype has differing manifestations in the two sexes. SEE ALSO sex-influenced *inheritance.*

sex-lim•it•ed. Occurring in one sex only. SEE sex-limited *inheritance.*

sex-linked. SEE sex *linkage.*

sex•ol•o•gy (sek-sol'ō-jē). The study of all aspects of sex and, in particular, sexual behavior. [L. *sexus,* sex, + G. *logos,* study]

sex•u•al (sek'shū-ăl). **1.** Relating to sex; genital. **2.** A person as perceived by his or her s. attractiveness, tendencies, and overall sexuality. [L. *sexualis,* fr. *sexus,* sex]

sex•u•al•i•ty (sek-shū-al'i-tē). **1.** The sum of a person's sexual behaviors and tendencies, and the strength of such tendencies. **2.** One's degree of sexual attractiveness. **3.** The quality of having sexual functions or implications.

infantile s., PSYCHOANALYSIS the body of theories concerning psychosexual development in infants and children; encompasses the overlapping oral, anal, and phallic phases during the first five years of life.

sex•u•al pref•er•ence. The biologic sex preferred in one's sexual partners.

SGOT serum glutamic-oxaloacetic *transaminase.*

SGPT serum glutamic-pyruvic transaminase.

SH sulfhydryl.

shaft. An elongated rodlike structure, as the part of a long bone between the epiphysial extremities. syn diaphysis [NA]. [A.S. *sceaft*]

shank. **1.** The tibia; the shin; the leg. **2.** The portion of an instrument that connects the cutting or functional portion to a handle; with rotary tools, such as burs and drills, the end that fits into the chuck. [A.S. *sceanca*]

shap•ing (shāp'ing). In operant conditioning, when the operant response is not in the organism's repertoire, a procedure in which the experimenter breaks down the response into those parts which appear most frequently, begins reinforcing them, and then slowly and successively withholds the reinforcer until more and more of the operant is emitted.

sheath (shēth). **1.** Any enveloping structure, such as the membranous covering of a muscle, nerve, or blood vessel; any sheathlike structure. syn vagina (1). **2.** The prepuce of male animals, especially of the horse. **3.** A specially designed tubular instrument through which special obturators or cutting instruments can be passed, or through which blood clots, tissue fragments, calculi, etc. can be evacuated. **4.** A tube used as an orthodontic appliance, usually on molars. [A.S. *scaeth*]

carotid s., the dense fibrous investment of the carotid artery, internal jugular vein, and vagus nerve on each side of the neck, deep to the sternocleidomastoid muscle; the layers of cervical fascia blend with it. syn vagina carotica [NA].

common flexor s., the synovial sheath that surrounds the eight tendons of the superficial and deep flexors of the digits of the hand as they pass through the carpal canal; it is commonly continuous with the digital sheath of the little finger.

crural s., syn femoral s.

dentinal s., a layer of tissue relatively resistant to the action of acids, which forms the walls of the dentinal tubules.

dural s., an extension of the dura mater that ensheathes the roots of spinal nerves or, more particularly, the vagina nervi optici.

fascial s. of eyeball, a condensation of connective tissue on the outer aspect of the sclera from which it is separated by a narrow cleftlike epi-

sh

scleral space; the sheath is attached to the sclera near the sclerocorneal junction and blends with the fascia of the extraocular muscles.

femoral s., the fascia enclosing the femoral vessels, formed by the transversalis fascia anteriorly and the iliac fascia posteriorly; two septa divide the s. into three compartments, the lateral of which contains the femoral artery and the femoral branch of the genitofemoral nerve, the middle the femoral vein, and the medial is the femoral canal. SYN crural s.

Henle's s., SYN endoneurium.

intertubercular s., the extension of the synovial membrane of the shoulder joint downward in the intertubercular groove to surround the tendon of the long head of the biceps.

Mauthner's s., SYN axolemma.

myelin s., the lipoproteinaceous envelope in vertebrates surrounding most axons of more than 0.5-μm diameter; it consists of a double plasma membrane wound tightly around the axon in a variable number of turns, and supplied by oligodendroglia cells (in the brain and spinal cord) or Schwann cells (in peripheral nerves).

root s., one of the epidermic layers of the hair follicle: external root s. is continuous with the stratum basale and stratum spinosum of the epidermis; internal root s. comprises the cuticle of the internal roots, Huxley's layer, and Henle's layer.

s. of Schwann, SYN neurilemma.

synovial s., SEE synovial s.'s of digits of hand, synovial s.'s of digits of foot.

synovial s.'s of digits of foot, similar in structure to the corresponding sheaths of the hand.

synovial s.'s of digits of hand, the synovial sheaths that enclose the flexor tendons of the fingers and line the inside of the fibrous tendon sheaths.

shield (shēld). A protecting screen; lead sheet for protecting the operator and patient from x-rays. [A.S. *scild*]

embryonic s., a thickened area of the embryonic blastoderm from which the embryo develops.

nipple s., a cap or dome placed over the nipple to protect it during nursing.

shift. SYN change. SEE ALSO deviation.

antigenic s., mutation, *i.e.,* sudden change in molecular structure of RNA/DNA in microorganisms, especially viruses, which produces new strains of the microorganism; hosts previously exposed to other strains have little or no acquired immunity to the new strain.

axis s., SYN axis *deviation.*

chloride s., when CO_2 enters the blood from the tissues, it passes into the red blood cell and is converted by carbonate dehydratase to bicarbonate (HCO_3^-); HCO_3^- ion passes out into the plasma while Cl^- migrates into the red blood cell. Reverse changes occur in the lungs when CO_2 is eliminated from the blood.

Doppler s., the magnitude of the frequency change in hertz when sound and observer are in relative motion away from or toward each other. SEE ALSO Doppler *effect.*

s. to the left, (1) a marked increase in the

percentage of immature neutrophils in the circulating blood; **(2)** SEE maturation *index.*

luteoplacental s., the change in site of production of the estrogen and progesterone essential for human pregnancy from the corpus luteum to the placenta; after the sixth week of pregnancy, a human placenta can produce enough of these hormones to prevent abortion despite ovariectomy.

s. to the right, (1) in a differential count of white blood cells in the peripheral blood, the absence of young and immature forms; **(2)** SEE maturation *index.*

Shi•gel•la (shē-gel′lă). A genus of nonmotile, aerobic to facultatively anaerobic bacteria containing Gram-negative nonencapsulated rods. The normal habitat is the intestinal tract of humans and of higher apes; all species cause dysentery. [Kiyoshi *Shiga*]

S. boy′dii, a species found only in feces of symptomatic individuals; occurs in a low proportion of cases of bacillary dysentery.

S. dysenter′iae, a species causing dysentery in humans and in monkeys, found only in feces of symptomatic individuals; the type species of the genus *S.* SYN Shiga-Kruse bacillus.

S. flexne′ri, a species found in the feces of symptomatic individuals and of convalescents or carriers; the most common cause of dysentery epidemics and sometimes of infantile gastroenteritis. Sometimes sexually transmitted through anal intercourse. SYN Flexner's bacillus.

S. son′nei, a species causing mild dysentery and also summer diarrhea in children. SYN Sonne bacillus.

shig•el•lo•sis (shig-ĕ-lō′sis). Bacillary dysentery caused by bacteria of the genus *Shigella,* often occurring in epidemic patterns; an opportunistic infection of people with AIDS.

shin. 1. The anterior aspect of the leg, from knee to ankle. **2.** SYN anterior *border* of tibia. [A.S. *scina*]

saber s., the sharp-edged, anteriorly convex tibia in congenital syphilis.

shin•gles (shing′glz). SYN *herpes* zoster. [L. *cingulum,* girdle]

shin-splints. Tenderness and pain with induration and swelling in the anterior tibial compartment, particularly following athletic overexertion by the untrained.

shock (shok). **1.** A sudden physical or mental disturbance. **2.** A state of profound mental and physical depression consequent upon severe physical injury or an emotional disturbance. **3.** A severe disturbance of hemodynamics in which the circulatory system fails to maintain adequate perfusion of vital organs; may be due to reduction of blood volume (hemorrhage, dehydration), cardiac failure, or dilation of the vascular system in toxemia or septicemia. **4.** The abnormally palpable impact, appreciated by a hand on the chest wall, of an accentuated heart sound. [Fr. *choc,* fr. Germanic]

anaphylactic s., a severe, often fatal form of s. characterized by smooth muscle contraction and capillary dilation initiated by cytotropic (IgE class) antibodies. SEE ALSO anaphylaxis, serum *sickness.*

anaphylactoid s., a reaction that is similar to anaphylactic s., but which does not require the incubation period characteristic of induced sensitivity (anaphylaxis); it is unrelated to antigen-antibody reactions.

cardiogenic s., s. resulting from decline in cardiac output secondary to serious heart disease, usually myocardial infarction.

chronic s., the state of peripheral circulatory insufficiency developing in elderly patients with a debilitating disease, *e.g.,* carcinoma; a subnormal blood volume makes the patient susceptible to hemorrhagic s. as a result of even a moderate blood loss such as may occur during an operation.

cultural s., a form of stress associated with the beginning of an individual's assimilation into a new and vastly different culture.

declamping s., SYN declamping *phenomenon.*

hemorrhagic s., hypovolemic s. resulting from acute hemorrhage, characterized by hypotension, tachycardia, pale, cold, and clammy skin, and oliguria.

hypovolemic s., s. caused by a reduction in volume of blood, as from hemorrhage or dehydration.

insulin s., severe hypoglycemia produced by administration of insulin, manifested by sweating, tremor, anxiety, vertigo, and diplopia, followed by delirium, convulsions, and collapse.

septic s., (1) s. associated with sepsis, usually associated with abdominal and pelvic infection complicating trauma or operations; **(2)** s. associated with septicemia caused by Gram-negative bacteria.

serum s., anaphylactic or anaphylactoid s. caused by the injection of antitoxic or other foreign serum.

shell s., SYN battle *fatigue.*

toxic s., SEE toxic shock *syndrome.*

short·sight·ed·ness (shŏrt′sīt-ed-nes). SYN myopia.

shot·ty. Having a consistency like pieces of shot; consisting of small firm discrete nodules; said of lymph nodes palpated through the skin.

shoul·der (shōl). **1.** The lateral portion of the scapular region, where the scapula joins with the clavicle and humerus and is covered by the rounded mass of the deltoid muscle. **2.** Shoulder joint. **3.** DENTISTRY The ledge formed by the junction of the gingival and axial walls in extracoronal restorative preparations. [A.S. *sculder*]

Little League shoulder, fracture of the growth plate of the humeral head in the adolescent, resulting from repetitive rotational stresses during the act of pitching a baseball.

shoul·der blade (shōl′der blād). SYN scapula.

show (shō). An appearance. **1.** First appearance of blood in beginning menstruation. **2.** Sign of impending labor, characterized by the discharge from the vagina of a small amount of blood-tinged mucus representing the extrusion of the mucous plug which has filled the cervical canal during pregnancy. [A.S. *sceáwe*]

shunt (shŭnt). **1.** To bypass or divert. **2.** A bypass or diversion of accumulations of fluid to an absorbing or excreting system by fistulation or a mechanical device. SEE ALSO bypass. [M.E. *shunten,* to flinch]

arteriovenous s., the passage of blood directly from arteries to veins, without going through the capillary network.

Blalock-Taussig s., a palliative subclavian artery to pulmonary artery anastomosis.

Dickens s., SYN pentose phosphate *pathway.*

jejunoileal s., SYN jejunoileal *bypass.*

left-to-right s., a diversion of blood from the left side of the heart to right (as through a septal defect), or from the systemic circulation to the pulmonary (as through a patent ductus arteriosus).

mesocaval s., (1) anastomosis of the side of the superior mesenteric vein to the proximal end of the divided inferior vena cava, for control of portal hypertension; **(2)** h-shunt anastomosis of the inferior vena cava to the superior mesenteric vein, using a synthetic conduit or autologous vein.

peritoneovenous s., a s., usually by a catheter, between the peritoneal cavity and the venous system.

portacaval s., (1) surgical anastomosis between portal and systemic veins; **(2)** surgical anastomosis between the portal vein and the vena cava, as in an Eck fistula.

Rapoport-Leubering s., a shunt of the glycolytic pathway in which 1,3 diphosphoglycerate (1,3-DPG) is converted to 2,3-DPG. 2,3-DPG enhances the release of oxygen from hemoglobin to the tissues.

right-to-left s., the passage of blood from the right side of the heart into the left (as through a septal defect), or from the pulmonary artery into the aorta (as through a patent ductus arteriosus); such a shunt can occur only when the pressure on the right side exceeds that in the left.

splenorenal s., anastomosis of the splenic vein to the left renal vein, usually end-to-side, for control of portal hypertension.

transjugular intrahepatic portosystemic s. (TIPS), an interventional radiology procedure to relieve portal hypertension.

SI International System of Units (Système International d'Unités).

Si silicon.

sI. 6-mercaptopurine ribonucleoside (or 6-thioinosine).

△**sial-.** SEE sialo-.

si·al·ad·e·ni·tis (sī′al-ad-ĕ-nī′tis). Inflammation of a salivary gland. SYN sialoadenitis. [sial- + G. *adēn,* gland, + -*itis,* inflammation]

si·al·a·gogue (sī-al′ă-gog). **1.** Promoting the flow of saliva. **2.** An agent having this action (*e.g.,* anticholinesterase agents). SYN sialogogue. [sial- + G. *agōgos,* drawing forth]

si·al·ec·ta·sis (sī′ă-lek′tă-sis). Dilation of a salivary duct. SYN ptyalectasis. [sial- + G. *ektasis,* a stretching]

si·al·em·e·sis, si·al·e·me·sia (sī′al-em′ē-sis, -ĕ-mē′zē-ă). Vomiting of saliva, or vomiting caused by or accompanying an excessive secretion of saliva. [sial- + G. *emesis,* vomiting]

si·al·ic (sī-al′ik). SYN salivary.

si·al·ic ac·ids (sī-al'ik). Esters and other *N*- and *O*-acyl derivatives of neuraminic acid.

si·al·i·dase (sī-al'i-dās). An enzyme that cleaves terminal acylneuraminic residues from 2,3-, 2,6-, and 2,8 linkages in oligosaccharides, glycoproteins, or glycolipids; present as a surface antigen in myxoviruses; used in histochemistry to selectively remove sialomucins, as from bronchial mucous glands and the small intestine; a deficiency of this enzyme will result in sialidosis.

si·al·i·do·sis (sī-al-i-dō'sis). SYN cherry-red spot myoclonus *syndrome.*

si·a·line (sī'ă-lēn). SYN salivary.

si·a·lism, si·a·lis·mus (sī'ă-lizm, sī'ă-liz'mŭs). An excess secretion of saliva. SYN ptyalism, salivation, sialorrhea, sialosis. [G. *sialismos*]

⌂**sialo-, sial-.** Saliva, salivary glands. [G. *sialon*]

si·a·lo·ad·e·nec·to·my (sī'ă-lō-ad-ĕ-nek'tō-mē). Excision of a salivary gland. [sialo- + G. *adēn*, gland, + *ektomē*, excision]

si·a·lo·ad·e·ni·tis (sī'ă-lō-ad-ĕ-nī'tis). SYN sialadenitis.

si·a·lo·ad·e·not·o·my (sī'ă-lō-ad-ĕ-not'ŏ-mē). Incision of a salivary gland. [sialo- + G. *adēn*, gland, + *tomē*, incision]

si·a·lo·an·gi·ec·ta·sis (sī'ă-lō-an-jē-ek'tă-sis). Dilation of salivary ducts. [sialo- + G. *angeion*, vessel, + *ektasis*, a stretching]

si·a·lo·an·gi·i·tis (sī'ă-lō-an-jē-ī'tis). Inflammation of a salivary duct. [sialo- + G. *angeion*, vessel, + *-itis*, inflammation]

si·a·lo·cele (sī'ă-lō-sēl). SYN ranula (2). [sialo- + G. *kēlē*, tumor]

si·a·lo·do·chi·tis (sī'ă-lō-dō-kī'tis). Inflammation of the duct of a salivary gland. [sialo- + G. *dochē*, receptacle, + *-itis*, inflammation]

si·a·lo·do·cho·plas·ty (sī'ă-lō-dō'kŏ-plas'tē). Repair of a salivary duct. [sialo- + G. *dochē*, receptacle, + *plassō*, to fashion]

si·a·log·e·nous (sī'ă-loj'ĕ-nŭs). Producing saliva. SEE ALSO sialagogue. [sialo- + G. *-gen*, producing]

si·a·lo·gogue (sī-al'ă-gog). SYN sialagogue.

si·a·lo·gram (sī-al'ō-gram). The recorded display following sialography. [sialo- + G. *gramma*, a writing]

si·a·log·ra·phy (sī-ă-log'ră-fē). Radiography of the salivary glands and ducts after the introduction of contrast medium into the ducts. [sialo- + G. *graphō*, to write]

si·a·lo·lith (sī'ă-lō-lith). A salivary calculus. [sialo- + G. *lithos*, stone]

si·a·lo·li·thi·a·sis (sī'ă-lō-li-thī'ă-sis). The formation or presence of a salivary calculus. [sialolith + G. *-iasis*, condition]

si·a·lo·li·thot·o·my (sī'ă-lō-li-thot'ō-mē). Incision of a salivary duct or gland to remove a calculus. [sialolith + G. *tomē*, incision]

si·a·lor·rhea (sī'ă-lō-rē'ă). SYN sialism. [sialo- + G. *rhoia*, a flow]

si·a·los·che·sis (sī'ă-los'kĕ-sis). Suppression of the secretion of saliva. [sialo- + G. *schesis*, retention]

si·a·lo·sis (sī'ă-lō'sis). SYN sialism.

si·a·lo·ste·no·sis (sī'ă-lō-ste-nō'sis). Stricture of a salivary duct. [sialo- + G. *stenōsis*, a narrowing]

sib. A member of a sibship. SYN sibling.

sib·i·lant (sib'i-lănt). Hissing or whistling in character; denoting a form of rhonchus. [L. *sibilans* (*-ant*-), pres. p. of *sibilo*, to hiss]

sib·ling. SYN sib. [A. S. *sib*, relation, + *-ling*, diminutive]

sib·ship. **1.** The reciprocal state between individuals who have the same pair of parents. **2.** All progeny of one pair of parents. [A.S. *sib*, relationship]

sic·cant (sik'ant). **1.** Drying; removing moisture from surrounding substances. **2.** A substance with such properties. SYN siccative. [L. *siccans* (*-ant*-), pres. p. of *sicco*, pp. *-atus*, to dry]

sic·ca·tive (sik'ă-tiv). SYN siccant.

sick (sik). **1.** Unwell; suffering from disease. **2.** SYN nauseated. [A.S. *seóc*]

sick·le·mia (sik-lē'mē-ă). Presence of sickle- or crescent-shaped erythrocytes in peripheral blood; seen in sickle cell anemia and sickle cell trait.

sick·ling (sik'ling). Production of sickle-shaped erythrocytes in the circulation, as in sickle cell anemia.

sick·ness (sik'nes). SYN disease (1).

acute African sleeping s., SYN Rhodesian *trypanosomiasis.*

African sleeping s., SEE Gambian *trypanosomiasis*, Rhodesian *trypanosomiasis.*

air s., a form of motion s. caused by flying in an airplane.

altitude s., a syndrome caused by low inspired oxygen pressure (as at high altitude) and characterized by nausea, headache, dyspnea, malaise, and insomnia; in severe instances, pulmonary edema and adult respiratory distress syndrome can occur; SYN Acosta's disease, mountain s.

car s., a form of motion s. caused by riding on a train or in an automobile or bus.

chronic mountain s., loss of high altitude tolerance after prolonged exposure (*e.g.*, by residence), characterized by extreme polycythemia, exaggerated hypoxemia, and reduced mental and physical capacity; relieved by descent. SYN Monge's disease.

decompression s., a symptom complex caused by the escape from solution in the body fluids of nitrogen bubbles absorbed originally at high atmospheric pressure, as a result of abrupt reduction in atmospheric pressure (either rapid ascent to high altitude or return from a compressed-air environment); it is characterized by headache, pain in the arms, legs, joints, and epigastrium, itching of the skin, vertigo, dyspnea, coughing, choking, vomiting, weakness and sometimes paralysis, and severe peripheral circulatory collapse. SYN caisson disease.

morning s., the nausea and vomiting of early pregnancy. SYN nausea gravidarum.

motion s., the syndrome of pallor, nausea, weakness, and malaise, which may progress to vomiting and incapacitation, caused by stimulation of the semicircular canals during travel or motion as on a boat, plane, train, car, swing, or rotating amusement ride. SYN kinesia.

mountain s., SYN altitude s.

radiation s., a systemic condition caused by substantial whole-body irradiation, seen after nuclear explosions or accidents, rarely after radiotherapy. Manifestations depend on dose, ranging from anorexia, nausea, vomiting, and mild leukopenia, to thrombocytopenia with hemorrhage, severe leukopenia with infection, anemia, central nervous system damage, and death.

serum s., an immune complex disease appearing 1-2 weeks after injection of a foreign serum or serum protein, with local and systemic reactions such as urticaria, fever, general lymphadenopathy, edema, arthritis, and occasionally albuminuria or severe nephritis. SYN serum disease, serum reaction.

sleeping s., SEE Gambian *trypanosomiasis,* Rhodesian *trypanosomiasis.*

side ef•fect. A result of drug or other therapy in addition to or in extension of the desired therapeutic effect; usually, but not necessarily, connoting an undesirable effect.

⌂**sidero-.** Iron. [G. *siDēros*]

sid•er•o•blast (sid′er-ō-blast). An erythroblast containing granules of ferritin stained by the Prussian blue reaction. [sidero- + G. *blastos,* germ]

sid•er•o•cyte (sid′er-ō-sīt). An erythrocyte containing granules of free iron, as detected by the Prussian blue reaction, in the blood of normal fetuses, where they constitute from 0.10 to 4.5% of the erythrocytes. [sidero- + G. *kytos,* cell]

sid•er•o•fi•bro•sis (sid′er-ō-fī-brō′sis). Fibrosis associated with small foci in which iron is deposited.

sid•er•o•pe•nia (sid′er-ō-pē′nē-ă). An abnormally low level of serum iron. [sidero- + G. *penia,* poverty]

sid•er•o•pe•nic (sid′er-ō-pē′nik). Characterized by sideropenia.

sid•er•o•phage (sid′er-ō-fāj). SYN siderophore. [sidero- + G. *phagō,* to eat]

sid•er•o•phil, sid•er•o•phile (sid′er-ō-fil, -fīl). 1. Absorbing iron. SYN siderophilous. 2. A cell or tissue that contains iron. [sidero- + G. *philos,* fond]

sid•er•oph•i•lous (sid-er-of′i-lŭs). SYN siderophil (1).

sid•er•o•phore (sid′er-ō-fōr). A large extravasated mononuclear phagocyte containing granules of hemosiderin, found in the sputum or in the lungs of individuals with longstanding pulmonary congestion from left ventricular failure. SYN siderophage. [sidero- + G. *phoros,* bearing]

sid•er•o•sil•i•co•sis (sid′er-ō-sil′i-kō′sis). Silicosis due to inhalation of dust containing iron and silica. SYN silicosiderosis. [sidero- + silicosis]

sid•er•o•sis (sid-er-ō′sis). 1. A form of pneumoconiosis due to the presence of iron dust. 2. Discoloration of any part by disposition of an iron pigment; usually called hemosiderosis. 3. An excess of iron in the circulating blood. 4. Degeneration of the retina, lens, and uvea as a result of the deposition of iron. [sidero- + G. *-osis,* condition]

sid•er•ot•ic (sid-er-ot′ik). Related to siderosis; pigmented by iron or containing an excess of iron.

SIDS sudden infant death *syndrome.*

sie•mens (S) (sē′menz). The SI unit of electrical conductance; the conductance of a body with an electrical resistance of 1 ohm, allowing 1 ampere of current to flow per volt applied; equal to 1 mho. SYN mho. [Sir William *Siemens,* Ger. born British engineer, 1823–1883]

sie•vert (Sv) (sē′vert). The SI unit of ionizing radiation effective dose, equal to the absorbed dose in gray, weighted for both the quality of radiation in question and the tissue response to that radiation. The unit is the joule per kilogram and 1 Sv = 100 rem. SEE effective *dose.*

sight (sīt). The ability or faculty of seeing. SEE ALSO vision. [A.S. *gesihth*]

sigma (sig′mă). 1. The 18th letter of the Greek alphabet (σ, Σ). 2. (σ) reflection *coefficient*; standard *deviation*; a factor in prokaryotic RNA initiation; surface *tension*. 3. (Σ) Summation of a series.

sig•moid (sig′moyd). Resembling in outline the letter S or one of the forms of the Greek sigma. [G. *sigma,* the letter S, + *eidos,* resemblance]

⌂**sigmoid-.** SEE sigmoido-.

⌂**sig•moi•dec•to•my** (sig-moy-dek′tō-mē). Excision of the sigmoid colon. [sigmoid- + G. *ektomē,* excision]

sig•moid•i•tis (sig-moy-dī′tis). Inflammation of the sigmoid colon. [sigmoid- + G. *-itis,* inflammation]

⌂**sigmoido-, sigmoid-.** Sigmoid, usually the sigmoid colon. [G. *sigma,* the letter S, + *eidos,* resemblance]

sig•moi•do•pexy (sig-moy′dō-pek-sē). Operative attachment of the sigmoid colon to a firm structure to correct rectal prolapse. [sigmoido- + G. *pēxis,* fixation]

sig•moi•do•proc•tos•to•my (sig-moy′dō-proktos′tō-mē). Anastomosis between the sigmoid colon and the rectum. SYN sigmoidorectostomy. [sigmoido- + G. *prōktos,* anus, + *stoma,* mouth]

sig•moi•do•rec•tos•to•my (sig-moy′dō-rek-tos′ tō-mē). SYN sigmoidoproctostomy.

sig•moi•do•scope (sig-moy′dō-skōp). An endoscope for viewing the cavity of the sigmoid colon. [sigmoido- + G. *skopeō,* to view]

sig•moi•dos•co•py (sig′moy-dos′kŏ-pē). Inspection, through an endoscope, of the interior of the sigmoid colon.

sig•moi•dos•to•my (sig′moy-dos′tō-mē). Establishment of an artificial anus by opening into the sigmoid colon. [sigmoido- + G. *stoma,* mouth]

sig•moi•dot•o•my (sig′moy-dot′ō-mē). Surgical opening of the sigmoid. [sigmoido- + G. *tomē,* incision]

sign (sīn). 1. Any abnormality indicative of disease, discoverable on examination of the patient; an objective symptom of disease, in contrast to a symptom which is a subjective s. of disease. 2. An abbreviation or symbol. 3. In psychology, any object or artifact (stimulus) that represents a specific thing or conveys a specific idea to the person who perceives it. [L. *signum,* mark]

Babinski's s., (1) extension of the great toe and abduction of the other toes instead of the normal flexion reflex to plantar stimulation, considered indicative of pyramidal tract involvement ("positive" Babinski); (2) in hemiplegia, weakness of the platysma muscle on the affected side, as is evident in such actions as blowing or opening the mouth; (3) when the patient is lying supine with arms crossed on the front of the chest, and attempts to assume the sitting posture, the thigh on the side of an *organic* paralysis is flexed and the heel raised, whereas the limb on the sound side remains flat; (**4**) in hemiplegia, the forearm on the affected side turns to a pronated position when placed in a position of supination.

Bamberger's s., (**1**) jugular pulse in tricuspid insufficiency; (**2**) SYN allochiria. (**3**) dullness on percussion at the angle of the scapula, clearing up as the patient leans forward, indicating pericarditis with effusion.

Battle's s., ecchymosis over the mastoid process, suggestive of basal skull fracture.

Beevor's s., with paralysis of the lower portions of the recti abdominis muscles the umbilicus moves upward.

Biernacki's s., analgesia to percussion of the ulnar nerve in tabes dorsalis and dementia paralytica.

Blumberg's s., pain felt upon sudden release of steadily applied pressure on a suspected area of the abdomen, indicative of peritonitis.

Braxton Hicks s., irregular uterine contractions occurring after the third month of pregnancy.

Broadbent's s., a retraction of the thoracic wall, synchronous with cardiac systole, visible anywhere, but particularly in the left posterior axillary line; a s. of adherent pericardium.

Brudzinski's s., (**1**) in meningitis, on passive flexion of the leg on one side, a similar movement occurs in the opposite leg; (**2**) in meningitis, if the neck is passively flexed, flexion of the legs occurs.

Chaddock s., when the external malleolar skin area is irritated, extension of the great toe occurs in cases of organic disease of the corticospinal reflex paths. SYN Chaddock reflex.

Chvostek's s., facial irritability in tetany, unilateral spasm of the orbicularis oculi or oris muscle being excited by a slight tap over the facial nerve just anterior to the external auditory meatus.

clenched fist s., in angina pectoris, pressing of the clenched fist against the chest to indicate the constricting, pressing quality of the pain.

Comby's s., an early s. of measles, consisting of thin, whitish patches on the gums and buccal mucous membrane, formed of desquamating epithelial cells.

Comolli's s., in cases of fracture of the scapula, a typical triangular cushion-like swelling appears, corresponding to the outline of the scapula.

conventional s.'s, s.'s that acquire their function through social (linguistic) custom; *e.g.,* words, mathematical symbols.

Corrigan's s., a full, hard pulse followed by a sudden collapse easily palpated and occurring in aortic regurgitation.

Cruveilhier-Baumgarten s., a murmur over the umbilicus often in the presence of caput medusae, resulting from portal hypertension, usually with hepatic cirrhosis; recanalization of the umbilical vein with reverse blood flow from the liver into the abdominal wall veins creates the murmur.

Cullen's s., periumbilical darkening of the skin

from blood, a s. of intraperitoneal hemorrhage, especially in ruptured ectopic pregnancy.

Dalrymple's s., retraction of the upper eyelid in Graves' disease, causing abnormal wideness of the palpebral fissure.

Delbet's s., in a case of aneurysm of a main artery, maintenance of healthy tissue distally indicates efficient collateral circulation despite the fact that the pulse has disappeared.

doll's eye s., reflex movement of the eyes in the opposite direction to that in which the head is moved, *e.g.,* the eyes being lowered as the head is raised, and the reverse (Cantelli's sign); an indication of functional integrity of the brainstem tegmental pathways and cranial nerves involved in eye movement.

drawer s., in a knee examination, abnormal forward or backward sliding of the tibia with respect to the femur indicating laxity or tear of the anterior (forward slide) or posterior (backward slide) cruciate ligaments of the knee. SYN drawer test.

Ebstein's s., in pericardial effusion, obtuseness of the cardiohepatic angle on percussion.

Erb-Westphal s., abolition of the patellar tendon reflex, in tabes and certain other diseases of the spinal cord, and occasionally also in brain disease. SYN Westphal's s.

Ewart's s., in large pericardial effusions, an area of dullness with bronchial breathing and bronchophony below the angle of the left scapula.

eyelash s., in a case of apparent unconsciousness due to functional disease, such as conversion hysteria, stroking the eyelashes will occasion movement of the lids, but no such reflex will occur in case of severe organic brain lesion such as apoplexy, fracture of the skull, or other traumatism.

Friedreich's s., in adherent pericardium, sudden collapse of the previously distended veins of the neck at each diastole of the heart.

Goldstein's toe s., increased space between the great toe and its neighbor, seen in Down syndrome and occasionally in cretinism.

Goodell's s., softening of the cervix as an indication of pregnancy.

Graefe's s., in Grave's disease, lag of the upper eyelid as it follows the rotation of the eyeball downward. SYN von Graefe's s.

Gunn's s., (**1**) compression of the underlying vein at arteriovenous crossings seen ophthalmoscopically in arteriolar sclerosis; (**2**) on alternate stimulation with light, the pupil of an eye with optic nerve transmission defect constricts poorly or even dilates when stimulated (a relative afferent pupillary defect). SYN Marcus Gunn's s.

halo s., elevation of the subcutaneous fat layer over the fetal skull in a dead or dying fetus; said to be the most common radiologic sign of fetal death.

Hill's s., in aortic insufficiency, greater systolic blood pressure in the legs than in the arms; normal arterial systolic pressure in the leg is 10 to 20 mm of Hg above that in the arm, whereas in aortic insufficiency the difference may be 60 to 100 mm of Hg.

Hoffmann's s., (**1**) in latent tetany mild mechanical stimulation of the trigeminal nerve causes severe pain; (2) flexion of the terminal phalanx of the thumb and of the second and third phalanges of one or more of the fingers when the volar surface of the terminal phalanx of the fingers is flicked. SYN digital reflex, Hoffmann's reflex.

Homans' s., slight pain at the back of the knee or calf when the ankle is slowly and gently dorsiflexed (with the knee bent), indicative of incipient or established thrombosis in the veins of the leg. SEE ALSO thrombosis.

Joffroy's s., disorder of the arithmetical faculty (the person being unable to do simple sums in addition or multiplication) in the early stages of organic brain disease.

Kehr's s., pain referred to the left shoulder, due to splenic rupture.

Kernig's s., when the subject lies upon the back and the thigh is flexed to a right angle with the axis of the trunk, complete extension of the leg on the thigh is impossible; present in various forms of meningitis.

Kussmaul's s., in constrictive pericarditis, a paradoxical increase in venous distention and pressure during inspiration.

Leri's s., voluntary flexion of the elbow is impossible in a case of hemiplegia when the wrist on that side is passively flexed.

Lhermitte's s., sudden electric-like shocks extending down the spine on flexing the head.

Macewen's s., percussion of the skull gives a cracked-pot sound in cases of hydrocephalus.

Marcus Gunn's s., SYN Gunn's s.

McBurney's s., tenderness at site two-thirds of the distance between the umbilicus and the anterior-superior iliac spine; seen in appendicitis.

Murphy's s., pain on palpation of the right subcostal area during inspiration frequently associated with acute cholecystitis.

Musset's s., in incompetence of the aortic valve, rhythmical nodding of the head, synchronous with the heart beat.

Nikolsky's s., a peculiar vulnerability of the skin in pemphigus vulgaris; the apparently normal epidermis may be separated at the basal layer and rubbed off when pressed with a sliding motion.

Osler's s., SYN Osler *node*.

Payr's s., pain on pressure over the sole of the foot; a s. of thrombophlebitis.

physical s., a s. that is evident on inspection or elicited by auscultation, percussion, or palpation.

pyramid s., any of the symptoms indicating a morbid condition of the pyramidal tracts, such as the Babinski or Gordon s., spastic spinal paralysis, foot clonus, etc.

Quincke's s., SYN Quincke's *pulse*.

Remak's s., dissociation of the sensations of touch and of pain in tabes dorsalis and polyneuritis.

Romberg's s., with feet approximated, the patient stands with eyes open and then closed; if closing the eyes increases the unsteadiness, a loss of proprioceptive control is indicated, and the sign is positive. SYN rombergism.

Rossolimo's s., SYN Rossolimo's *reflex*.

Russell's s., abrasions and scars on the backs of the hands of individuals with bulimia, usually due to manual attempts to induce vomiting.

Saenger's s., a lost light reflex of the pupil returns after a short time in the dark, noted in cerebral syphilis but absent in tabes dorsalis.

Schwartze s., vascularization of the promontory of the middle ear resulting in a rosy glow that can be seen through the eardrum; a sign of otosclerosis. SEE ALSO otosclerosis. SYN promontory flush.

scimitar s., a curvilinear structure seen roentgenographically in the lung and associated with anomalous pulmonary venous drainage, suggesting the sickle shape of a Turkish saber; also used to refer to the scalloped shape of the sacrum in spinal dysraphism with anterior meningocele.

setting sun s., retraction of the upper lid without upgaze so that the iris seems to "set" below the lower lid; suggestive of neurologic damage in the newborn, but usually clears up without sequelae.

silhouette s. of Felson, in pulmonary radiology, the obliteration of a normal air-soft tissue interface, such as the cardiac silhouette, when fluid fills the adjacent part of the lung.

Steinberg thumb s., in Marfan's syndrome, when the thumb is held across the palm of the same hand, it projects well beyond the ulnar surface of the hand.

Stellwag's s., infrequent and incomplete blinking in Graves' disease.

Stewart-Holmes s., in cerebellar disease, the inability to check a movement when passive resistance is suddenly released. SYN rebound phenomenon (1).

string s., in pediatric gastrointestinal radiology, the narrowed pyloric canal seen with congenital pyloric stenosis; also used to describe a narrowed segment in Crohn's disease on small bowel series.

Tinel's s., distally radiating pain or paresthesia caused by tapping over the site of a superficial nerve, indicating inflammation or irritation of the nerve.

Trendelenburg's s., in congenital dislocation of the hip or in hip abductor weakness, the pelvis of a standing subject will sag on the side opposite to the dislocation when the foot on the normal side is raised from the floor; without dislocation or weakness, the pelvis will rise on the side of the flexed hip and knee.

Trousseau's s., in latent tetany, the occurrence of carpopedal spasm accompanied by paresthesia elicited when the upper arm is compressed, as by a tourniquet or a blood pressure cuff.

vital s.'s, objective measurements of temperature, pulse, respirations, and blood pressure as a means of assessing general health and cardiorespiratory function.

von Graefe's s., SYN Graefe's s.

Wernicke's s., SYN Wernicke's *reaction*.

Westphal's s., SYN Erb-Westphal s.

wrist s., in Marfan's syndrome, when the wrist is gripped with the opposite hand, the thumb and fifth finger overlap appreciably.

sig·na·ture (sig′nă-chūr, -tūr). The part of a prescription containing the directions to the patient. [Mediev. L. *signatura,* fr. L. *signum,* a sign, mark]

sign language. A system of manual communication used by the deaf. True sign languages such as American Sign Language (ASL) have a complete representation of morphology, semantics, and syntax.

SIH somatotropin release-inhibiting *hormone.*

si·lent (sī'lent). Producing no detectable signs or symptoms, said of certain diseases or morbid processes.

sil·i·ca (sil'ĭ-kă). SiO_2; the chief constituent of sand, hence of glass. SYN silicon dioxide. [Mod. L. fr. L. *silex* (*silic-*), flint]

sil·i·ca·to·sis (sil'i-kă-tō'sis). SYN silicosis.

sil·i·con (Si) (sil'i-kon). A very abundant nonmetallic element, atomic no. 14, atomic wt. 28.0855, occurring in nature as silica and silicates; in pure form, used as a semiconductor and in solar batteries; also found in certain polysaccharide structures in mammary tissue. [L. *silex,* flint]

sil·i·con di·ox·ide. SYN silica.

sil·i·cone (sil'i-kōn). A polymer of organic silicon oxides, which may be a liquid, gel, or solid, depending on the extent of polymerization; used in surgical implants, in intracorporeal tubes to conduct fluids, as dental impression material, as a grease or sealing substance, as a coating on the inside of glass vessels for blood collection, and in various ophthalmological procedures.

sil·i·co·pro·te·i·no·sis (sil'i-kō-prō'tē-i-nō'sis). An acute pulmonary disorder, radiographically and histologically similar to pulmonary alveolar proteinosis, resulting from relatively short exposure to high concentrations of silica dust; pulmonary symptoms are of rapid onset and the condition is invariably fatal.

sil·i·co·sid·er·o·sis (sil'i-kō-sid'er-ō'sis). SYN siderosilicosis.

sil·i·co·sis (sil-i-kō'sis). A form of pneumoconiosis resulting from occupational exposure to and inhalation of silica dust over a period of years; characterized by a slowly progressive fibrosis of the lungs, which may result in impairment of lung function; s. predisposes to pulmonary tuberculosis. SYN silicatosis. [L. *silex,* flint, + *-osis,* condition]

sil·i·co·tu·ber·cu·lo·sis (sil'i-kō-tū-ber-kyū-lō'sis). Silicosis associated with tuberculous pulmonary lesions.

sil·ver (Ag). L. argentum; a metallic element, atomic no. 47, atomic wt. 107.8682. Many salts have clinical applications. [A.S. *seolfor*]

sil·ver im·preg·na·tion. Silver complexes employed to demonstrate reticulin in normal and diseased tissues, as well as neuroglia, neurofibrillae, argentaffin cells, and Golgi apparatus.

si·mi·lia si·mi·li·bus cur·an·tur (si-mil'ē-ă si-mil'i-bŭs kūr-an'tūr). The homeopathic formula expressing the law of similars, the doctrine that any drug capable of producing morbid symptoms in the healthy will remove similar symptoms occurring as an expression of disease. Another reading of the formula, employed by Hahnemann, the founder of homeopathy, is *similia similibus*

curentur, let likes be cured by likes. [L. likes are cured by likes]

sim·u·la·tion (sim-yū-lā'shŭn). **1.** Imitation; said of a disease or symptom that resembles another, or of the feigning of illness as in factitious illness or malingering. **2.** RADIATION THERAPY Using a geometrically similar radiographic system or computer to plan the location of therapy ports. [L. *simulatio,* fr. *simulo,* pp. *-atus,* to imitate, fr. *similis,* like]

si·mul·tan·ag·no·sia (sī-mŭl-tan-ag-nō'sē-ă). Inability to recognize multiple elements in a visual presentation, *i.e.,* one object or some elements of a scene can be appreciated but not the display as a whole. [simultaneous + agnosia]

SIMV spontaneous intermittent mandatory *ventilation,* synchronized intermittent mandatory *ventilation.*

sin·cip·i·tal (sin-sip'i-tăl). Relating to the sinciput.

sin·ci·put, pl. **sin·cip·i·ta, sin·ci·puts** (sin'siput, sin-sip'i-tă). The anterior part of the head just above and including the forehead. [L. half of the head]

sin·ew (sin'ū). SYN tendon. [A.S. *sinu*]

sin·is·ter (si-nis'ter) [NA]. Left. [L.]

sin·is·trad (sin'is-trad, si-nis'trad). Toward the left side. [L. *sinister,* left, + *ad,* to]

sin·is·tral (sin'is-trăl, sī-nis'trăl). **1.** Relating to the left side. **2.** Denoting a left-handed person.

sin·is·tral·i·ty (sin-is-tral'i-tē). The condition of being left-handed.

⌂**sinistro-.** Left, toward the left. [L. *sinister*]

sin·is·tro·car·dia (sin'is-trō-kar'dē-ă). Leftward displacement of the heart beyond its normal position. [sinistro- + G. *kardia,* heart]

sin·is·tro·ce·re·bral (sin'is-trō-ser'ĕ-brăl). Relating to the left cerebral hemisphere. [sinistro- + L. *cerebrum,* brain]

sin·is·tro·gy·ra·tion (sin'is-trō-jī-rā'shŭn). SYN sinistrotorsion. [sinistro- + L. *gyratio,* a turning around (gyration)]

sin·is·tro·man·u·al (sin'is-trō-man'yū-ăl). SYN left-handed. [sinistro- + L. *manus,* hand]

sin·is·trop·e·dal (sin-is-trop'ĕ-dăl). Denoting one who uses the left leg by preference. SYN left-footed. [sinistro- + L. *pes* (*ped-*), foot]

sin·is·tro·tor·sion (sin'is-trō-tōr'shŭn). A turning or twisting to the left. SYN levorotation (2), levotorsion (1), sinistrogyration. [sinistro- + L. *torsio,* a twisting (torsion)]

si·no·pul·mo·nary (sī'nō-pŭl'mŏ-nār-ē). Relating to the paranasal sinuses and the pulmonary airway.

si·nu·a·tri·al (S-A) (sin'yū-ā'trē-ăl, sī'nū-). Relating to the sinus venosus and the right atrium of the heart.

si·nus, pl. **si·nus, si·nus·es** (sī'nŭs, -ĕz). **1** [NA]. A channel for the passage of blood or lymph, without the coats of an ordinary vessel; *e.g.,* blood passages in the gravid uterus or those in the cerebral meninges. **2** [NA]. A cavity or hollow space in bone or other tissue. **3** [NA]. A dilation in a blood vessel. **4.** A fistula or tract leading to a suppurating cavity. [L. *sinus,* cavity, channel, hollow]

  anal sinuses, (1) the grooves between the anal

columns; (2) pockets or crypts in the columnar zone of the anal canal between the anocutaneous line and the anorectal line; the sinuses give the mucosa a scalloped appearance.

aortic s., the space between the superior aspect of each cusp of the aortic valve and the dilated portion of the wall of the ascending aorta, immediately above each cusp.

carotid s., a slight dilation of the common carotid artery at its bifurcation into external and internal carotids; it contains baroreceptors which, when stimulated, cause slowing of the heart, vasodilation, and a fall in blood pressure and is innervated primarily by the glossopharyngeal nerve.

cavernous s., a paired dural venous s. on either side of the sella turcica, the two being connected by anastomoses, the anterior and posterior intercavernous s., in front of and behind the hypophysis, respectively, making thus the circular s.; the cavernous s. is unique among dural venous sinuses in being trabeculated; coursing within the sinus are the internal carotid artery and the abducent nerve.

circular s., (1) dural venous formation which surrounds the hypophysis, composed of right and left cavernous sinuses and the intercavernous sinuses; (2) a venous s. at the periphery of the placenta; (3) SYN s. venosus sclerae.

coccygeal s., a fistula opening in the region of the coccyx, being the result of incomplete closure of the caudal end of the neurenteric canal. SEE ALSO pilonidal s.

coronary s., a short trunk receiving most of the cardiac veins, beginning at the junction of the great cardiac vein and the oblique vein of the left atrium, running in the posterior part of the coronary sulcus and emptying into the right atrium between the inferior vena cava and the atrioventricular orifice.

dermal s., a s. lined with epidermis and skin appendages extending from the skin to some deeper-lying structure, most frequently the spinal cord.

dural venous sinuses, endothelium-lined venous channels in the dura mater. SYN venous sinuses.

frontal s., a hollow paranasal sinus formed on either side in the lower part of the squama of the frontal bone; it communicates by the ethmoidal infundibulum with the middle meatus of the nasal cavity of the same side.

intercavernous sinuses, the anterior and posterior anastomoses between the cavernous s.'s, passing anterior and posterior to the hypophysis and forming, with the cavernous sinuses, the circular s. (1).

lactiferous s., a circumscribed spindle-shaped dilation of the lactiferous duct just before it enters the nipple. In nursing mothers this dilatation stores a droplet of milk which is expressed by compression as the infant begins to suckle; this is thought to encourage continual suckling while the let-down reflex ensues.

lymphatic s., the channels in a lymph node crossed by a reticulum of cells and fibers and bounded by littoral cells; there are subcapsular, trabecular, and medullary s.'s.

maxillary s., the largest of the paranasal sinuses occupying the body of the maxilla, communicating with the middle meatus of the nose.

occipital s., an unpaired dural venous s. commencing at the confluence of the sinuses and passing downward in the base of the falx cerebelli to the foramen magnum.

paranasal sinuses, the paired air-filled cavities in the bones of the face lined by mucous membrane continuous with that of the nasal cavity; these s.'s are the frontal, sphenoidal, maxillary, and ethmoidal.

parasinoidal sinuses, SYN lateral venous lacunae, under lacuna.

pilonidal s., a fistula or pit in the sacral region, communicating with the exterior, containing loose, broken-off body hairs which may act as a foreign body producing chronic inflammation.

prostatic s., the groove on either side of the urethral crest in the prostatic part of the urethra into which the prostatic ducts open.

renal s., the cavity of the kidney, containing the calices and pelvis of the ureter and the segmental vessels embedded within a fatty matrix. The renal sinuses cause the kidneys to appear hollow or C-shaped on cross section or medical imaging.

rhomboidal s., a dilation of the central canal of the spinal cord in the lumbar region. SYN rhombocele.

sigmoid s., the S-shaped dural venous s. lying deep to the mastoid process of the temporal bone and immediately posterior to the petrous temporal bone; it is continuous with the transverse s. and empties into the internal jugular vein as it passes through the jugular foramen.

sphenoidal s., one of a pair of paranasal sinuses in the body of the sphenoid bone communicating with the upper posterior nasal cavity or sphenoethmoidal recess.

sphenoparietal s., a paired dural venous s. beginning on the parietal bone, running along the sphenoidal ridges and emptying into the cavernous s.

splenic s., an elongated venous channel, 12 to 40 μm wide, lined by rod-shaped cells.

straight s., an unpaired dural venous s. in the posterior part of the falx cerebri where it is attached to the tentorium cerebelli; it is formed anteriorly by the merging of the great cerebral vein with the inferior sagittal sinus, and passes horizontally and posteriorly to the confluence of sinuses. SYN tentorial s.

tarsal s., a hollow or canal formed by the groove of the talus and the interosseous groove of the calcaneus which is occupied by the interosseous talocalcaneal ligament.

tentorial s., SYN straight s.

terminal s., the vein bounding the area vasculosa in the blastoderm.

transverse s., a paired dural venous s. that drains the confluence of sinuses, running along the occipital attachment of the tentorium cerebelli and terminating in the sigmoid s.

transverse pericardial s., a passage in the pericardial sac between the origins of the great

si

vessels, *i.e.,* posterior to the intrapericardial portions of the pulmonary trunk and ascending aorta and anterior to the superior vena cava and superior to the atria; it is formed as a result of the flexure of the heart tube, partially approximating the great venous and arterial vessels.

tympanic s., a depression in the tympanic cavity posterior to the tympanic promontory.

uterine s., a small, irregular vascular channel in the endometrium, of a type that forms during pregnancy.

uteroplacental sinuses, irregular vascular spaces in the zone of the chorionic attachment to the decidua basalis.

s. of the vena cava, the portion of the cavity of the right atrium of the heart that receives the blood from the venae cavae; it is separated from the rest of the atrium by the crista terminalis.

s. veno′sus [NA], a cavity at the caudal end of the embryonic cardiac tube in which the veins from the intra- and extraembryonic circulatory arcs unite; in the course of development it forms the portion of the right atrium known in adult anatomy as the sinus of the vena cava.

s. veno′sus scle′rae [NA], the vascular structure encircling the anterior chamber of the eye and through which the aqueous is returned to the blood circulation. SYN circular s. (3), Schlemm's canal.

venous sinuses, SYN dural venous sinuses.

si•nus•i•tis (sī-nŭ-sī′tis). Inflammation of the lining membrane of any sinus, especially of one of the paranasal sinuses. [sinus + G. *-itis,* inflammation]

si•nus•oid (sī′nŭ-soyd). **1.** Resembling a sinus. **2.** Sinusoidal capillary; a thin-walled terminal blood vessel having a more variable and larger caliber than an ordinary capillary; its endothelial cells have large gaps and the basal lamina is either discontinuous or absent. [sinus + G. *eidos,* resemblance]

si•nus•oi•dal (sī-nŭ-soy′dăl). Relating to a sinusoid.

si•nus•ot•o•my (sin-ŭ-sot′ŏ-mē). Incision into a sinus. [sinus + G. *tomē,* incision]

si•phon (sī′fŏn). A tube bent into two unequal lengths, used to remove fluid from a cavity or vessel by atmospheric pressure and gravity. [G. *siphōn,* tube]

si•phon•age (sī′fŏn-ij). Emptying of the stomach or other cavity by means of a siphon.

SIRD source-to-image-receptor *distance.*

si•re•no•me•lia (sī′rĕ-nō-mē′lē-ă). Union of the legs with partial or complete fusion of the feet. [L. *siren,* G. *seirēn,* a siren]

sis•ter. In Great Britain: **1.** The title of a head nurse in a public hospital or in a ward or the operating room of a hospital; **2.** Any registered nurse in private practice.

site (sīt). A place or location. SYN situs. [L. *situs*]

active s., that portion of an enzyme molecule at which the actual reaction proceeds; one or more residues or atoms in a spatial arrangement that permits interaction with the substrate.

allosteric s., postulated as the place on an enzyme, other than the active s., where a compound, which may be the ultimate product of the

biosynthetic pathway involving the enzyme, may bind and influence the activity of the enzyme by changing the enzyme's conformation.

cleavage s., SYN restriction s.

fragile s. [MIM*136540-136670], a nonstaining gap at a specific point on a chromosome, usually involving both chromatids, always at the same point on chromosomes of different cells from an individual or kindred.

privileged s., an anatomic area lacking lymphatic drainage, such as the brain, cornea, and hamster cheek pouch, in which heterologous tumors may grow because the host does not become sensitized.

restriction s., a s. in nucleic acid in which the bordering bases are of such a type as to leave them vulnerable to the cleaving action of an endonuclease. SYN cleavage s.

switching s., the break point in a DNA sequence at which a gene segment unites with another gene segment, as in the production of the immunoglobulins.

△**sito-.** Food, grain. [G. *sitos, sition*]

si•to•tax•is (sī-tō-tak′sis). SYN sitotropism. [sito- + G. *taxis,* orderly arrangement]

si•tot•ro•pism (sī-tot′rō-pizm). Turning of living cells to or away from food. SYN sitotaxis. [sito- + G. *tropē,* a turning]

si•tus (sī′tŭs). SYN site. [L.]

s. inver′sus, reversal of position or location, referring particularly to left-right reversal of thoracic viscera.

siz•er (sī′zer). A cylinder of variable diameter, with rounded ends, used to measure the internal diameter of the bowel in preparation for stapling.

SK streptokinase.

skat•ole (skat′ōl). An indole derivative formed in the intestine by bacterial decomposition and found in fecal matter, to which it imparts its characteristic odor.

skat•ox•yl (skă-tok′sil). An indole derivative formed in the intestine by the oxidation of skatole; some undergoes conjugation in the body with sulfuric or gluronic acids and is excreted in the urine in conjugated form.

skel•e•tal (skel′ĕ-tăl). Relating to the skeleton.

skel•e•ton (skel′ĕ-tŏn). **1.** The bony framework of the body in vertebrates (endoskeleton) or the hard outer envelope of insects (exoskeleton or dermoskeleton). **2.** All the dry parts remaining after the destruction and removal of the soft parts; this includes ligaments and cartilages as well as bones. **3.** All the bones of the body taken collectively. **4.** A rigid or semirigid nonosseous structure which functions as the supporting framework of a particular structure. [G. *skeletos,* dried, ntr. *skeleton,* a mummy, a skeleton]

appendicular s., the bones of the limbs including the shoulder and pelvic girdles.

axial s., articulated bones of head and vertebral column, *i.e.,* head and trunk, as opposed to the appendicular skeleton, the articulated bones of the upper and lower limbs.

△**skia-.** Shadow; superseded by radio-. [G. *skia*]

ski•as•co•py (skī-as′kŏ-pē). SYN retinoscopy.

skilled-nursing facility (SNF). nursing facility providing 24-hour nonacute nursing care.

skin. The membranous protective covering of the body, consisting of the epidermis and corium (dermis). SYN cutis [NA]. [A.S. *scinn*]

piebald s., SYN piebaldness.

shagreen s., an oval-shaped nevoid plaque, skin-colored or occasionally pigmented, smooth or crinkled, appearing on the trunk or lower back in early childhood; sometimes seen with other signs of tuberous sclerosis.

■**skull** (skŭl). The bones of the head collectively. In a more limited sense, the neurocranium, the bony braincase containing the brain, excluding the bones of the face (viscero-cranium). SYN cranium [NA]. [Early Eng. *skulle,* a bowl]

skull•cap (skŭl'kap). SYN calvaria.

SLE systemic *lupus* erythematosus.

sleep (slēp). A physiologic state of relative unconsciousness and inaction of the voluntary muscles, the need for which recurs periodically. The stages of sleep have been variously defined in terms of depth (light, deep), EEG characteristics (delta waves, synchronization), physiological characteristics (REM, NREM), and presumed anatomical level (pontine, mesencephalic, rhombencephalic, rolandic, etc.). [A.S. *slaep*]

paradoxical s., a deep s., with a brain wave pattern more like that of waking states than of other states of s., which occurs during rapid eye movement s.

slide (slīd). A rectangular glass plate on which is placed an object to be examined under the microscope.

sling. A supporting bandage or suspensory device; especially a loop suspended from the neck and supporting the flexed forearm.

slit•lamp. In ophthalmology, an instrument consisting of a microscope combined with a rectangular light source that can be narrowed into a slit. SYN biomicroscope.

slough (slŭf). **1.** Necrosed tissue separated from the living structure. **2.** To separate from the living tissue, said of a dead or necrosed part. [M.E. *slughe*]

Sm samarium.

small•pox (smawl'poks). An acute eruptive contagious disease caused by a poxvirus (*Orthopoxvirus*) and marked by chills, fever, and an eruption papules which become umbilicated vesicles, develop into pustules, dry, and form scabs that on falling off, leave a permanent marking of the skin (pock marks). The virus was declared extinct in 1979, having been eradicated by vaccination, and is now of mainly historical interest. SYN variola. [E. *small pocks,* or pustules]

smear (smēr). A thin specimen for microscopic examination; it is usually prepared by spreading liquid or semisolid material uniformly onto a glass slide, fixing it, and staining it before examination.

cytologic s., a type of cytologic specimen made by smearing a sample (obtained by a variety of methods from a number of sites), then fixing it and staining it, usually with 95% ethyl alcohol and Papanicolaou stain.

fast s., a cytologic smear containing material from the vaginal pool and pancervical scrapings, mixed and prepared on one microscopic slide,

smeared, and fixed immediately; used principally for routine screening of ovaries, endometrium, cervix, vagina, and hormonal states.

Pap s., a s. of vaginal or cervical cells obtained for cytological study.

smeg•ma (smeg'mă). A foul-smelling pasty accumulation of desquamated epidermal cells and sebum that has collected in moist areas of the genitalia. [G. unguent]

smeg•ma•lith (smeg'mă-lith). A calcareous concretion in the smegma. [smegma + G. *lithos,* stone]

smell. **1.** To scent; to perceive by means of the olfactory apparatus. **2.** SYN olfaction (1). **3.** SYN odor.

smog. A hazy and often highly irritating atmosphere resulting from a mixture of fog with smoke and other air pollutants. [smoke + fog]

Sn tin.

△**sn-.** Prefix meaning stereospecifically numbered; a system of numbering the glycerol carbon atoms in lipids, so that the locant numbers remain constant regardless of chemical substitutions, as opposed to systematic numbering.

snap. A click; a short sharp sound; said especially of cardiac sounds.

closing s., the accentuated first heart sound of mitral stenosis, related to closure of the abnormal valve.

opening s., a sharp, high-pitched click in early diastole, usually best heard between the cardiac apex and the lower left sternal border, related to opening of the abnormal valve in cases of mitral stenosis.

snare (snār). An instrument for removing polyps and other projections from a surface, especially within a cavity; it consists of a wire loop passed around the base of the tumor and gradually tightened. [A.S. *snear,* a cord]

sneeze (snēz). **1.** To expel air from the nose and mouth by an involuntary spasmodic contraction of the muscles of expiration. **2.** An act of sneezing; a reflex excited by an irritation of the mucous membrane of the nose or, sometimes, by a bright light striking the eye. [A.S. *fneōsan*]

SNF skilled-nursing facility.

snore (snōr). **1.** A rough, rattling inspiratory noise produced by vibration of the pendulous palate, or sometimes of the vocal cords, during sleep or coma. SEE ALSO stertor, rhonchus. **2.** To breathe noisily, or with a s. [A.S. *snora*]

snorting. SYN nasal *emission.*

snuff (snŭf). **1.** To inhale forcibly through the nose. **2.** Finely powdered tobacco used by inhalation through the nose or applied to the gums. **3.** Any medicated powder applied by insufflation to the nasal mucous membrane. [echoic]

snuf•fles (snŭf'lz). Obstructed nasal respiration, especially in the newborn infant, sometimes due to congenital syphilis.

SOAP *s*ubjective, *o*bjective, *a*ssessment, and *p*lan; used in problem-oriented records for organizing follow-up data, evaluation, and planning.

soap (sōp). The sodium or potassium salts of long chain fatty acids (*e.g.,* sodium stearate); used for cleansing purposes and as an excipient in the making of pills and suppositories. [A.S. *sape,* L. *sapo,* G. *sapōn*]

so•cial•i•za•tion (sō'shăl-i-zā'shŭn). **1.** The process of learning attitudes and interpersonal and interactional skills which are in conformity with the values of one's society. **2.** In a group therapy setting, a way of learning to participate effectively in the group. [L. *socius,* partner, companion]

△**socio-.** Social, society. [L. *socius,* companion]

so•ci•o•cen•tric (sō'sē-ō-sen'trik). Outgoing; reactive to the social or cultural milieu. [socio- + L. *centrum,* center]

so•ci•o•gen•e•sis (sō'sē-ō-jen'ĕ-sis). The origin of social behavior from past interpersonal experiences. [socio- + G. *genesis,* origin]

so•ci•o•path (sō'sē-ō-path). Former designation for a person with an antisocial personality type of disorder. SEE ALSO antisocial *personality,* psychopath.

sock•et (sok'et). **1.** The hollow part of a joint; the excavation in one bone of a joint which receives the articular end of the other bone. **2.** Any hollow or concavity into which another part fits, as the eye s. [thr. O. Fr. fr. L. *soccus,* a shoe, a sock]

tooth s., a socket in the alveolar process of the maxilla or mandible, into which each tooth fits and is attached by means of the periodontal ligament. SYN alveolus (4) [NA].

so•di•um (sō'dē-ŭm). A metallic element, atomic no. 11, atomic weight 22.989768; an alkali metal oxidizing readily in air or water; its salts are extensively used in medicine and industry. For organic s. salts not listed below, see under the name of the organic acid portion. SYN natrium. [Mod. L. fr. *soda*]

s. borate, $Na_2B_4O_7 \cdot 10H_2O$; used in lotions, gargles, mouthwashes, and as a detergent.

sod•om•ist, sod•om•ite (sod'ŏ-mist, -mīt). One who practices sodomy. [G. *sodomitēs,* an inhabitant of the biblical city of Sodom, which was destroyed by fire because of the wickedness of its people]

sod•o•my (sod'ŏm-ē). A term denoting a number of sexual practices variously proscribed by law, especially bestiality, oral-genital contact, and anal intercourse. [see sodomist]

sol. 1. A collodial dispersion of a solid in a liquid. Cf. gel. **2.** Abbreviation for solution.

sol•a•tion (sol-ā'shŭn). COLLOIDAL CHEMISTRY The transformation of a gel into a sol, as by melting gelatin.

sole (sōl). The plantar surface or under part of the foot. SYN planta [NA]. [A.S.]

sol•id. 1. Firm; compact; not fluid; without interstices or cavities; not cancellous. **2.** A body that retains its form when not confined; one that is not fluid, neither liquid nor gaseous. [L. *solidus*]

sol•u•bil•i•ty (sol-yū-bil'i-tē). The property of being soluble.

sol•u•ble (sol'yū-bl). Capable of being dissolved. [L. *solubilis,* fr. *solvo,* to dissolve]

sol•ute (sol'yūt, sō'lūt). The dissolved substance in a solution. [L. *solutus,* dissolved, pp. of *solvo,* to dissolve]

so•lu•tion (sō-lū'shŭn). **1.** The incorporation of a solid, a liquid, or a gas in a liquid or noncrystal-

line solid resulting in a homogeneous single phase. SEE dispersion, suspension. **2.** Generally, an aqueous s. of a nonvolatile substance. **3.** An aqueous s. of a nonvolatile substance is called a solution or liquor; an aqueous s. of a volatile substance is a water (aqua); an alcoholic s. of a nonvolatile substance is a tincture (tinctura); an alcoholic s. of a volatile substance is a spirit (spiritus); a s. in vinegar is a vinegar (acetum); a s. in glycerin is a glycerol (glyceritum); a s. in wine is a wine (vinum); a s. of sugar in water is a syrup (syrupus); a s. of a mucilaginous substance is a mucilage (mucilago); a s. of an alkaloid or metallic oxide in oleic acid is an oleate (oleatum). **4.** The termination of a disease by crisis. **5.** A break, cut, or laceration of the solid tissues. SEE s. of contiguity, s. of continuity. [L. *solutio*]

colloidal s., a dispersoid, emulsoid, or suspensoid.

s. of contiguity, the breaking of contiguity; a dislocation or displacement of two normally contiguous parts.

s. of continuity, division of bones or soft parts that are normally continuous, as by a fracture, a laceration, or an incision. SYN dieresis.

disclosing s., a s. that selectively stains all soft debris, pellicle, and bacterial plaque on teeth; used as an aid in identifying bacterial plaque after rinsing with water.

normal s., SEE normal (3).

ophthalmic s.'s, sterile s.'s, free from foreign particles and suitably compounded and dispensed for instillation into the eye.

saline s., (1) a s. of any salt; **(2)** specifically, isotonic or physiologic sodium chloride s.; 0.85 to 0.9 g/100 ml water.

saturated s. (sat. sol., sat. soln.), a s. that contains all of a solute capable of being dissolved in the solvent; a substance in equilibrium with excess undissolved substance.

standard s., standardized s., a s. of known concentration, used as a standard of comparison or analysis.

supersaturated s., a s. containing more of the solid than the liquid would ordinarily dissolve; it is made by heating the solvent when the substance is added, and on cooling the latter is retained without precipitation; addition of a crystal or solid of any kind usually results in precipitation of the excess solute, leaving a saturated s.

test s., a s. of some reagent, in definite strength, used in chemical analysis or testing.

volumetric s. (VS), a s. made by mixing measured volumes of the components.

sol•vent. A liquid that holds another substance in solution, *i.e.,* dissolves it. [L. *solvens,* pres. p. of *solvo,* to dissolve]

so•ma (sō'mă). **1.** The axial part of the body, *i.e.,* head, neck, trunk, and tail, excluding the limbs. **2.** All of an organism with the exception of the germ cells. SEE ALSO body. **3.** The body of a nerve cell, from which axons, dendrites, etc. project. [G. *sōma,* body]

so•mas•the•nia (sō-mas-thē'nē-ă). SYN somatasthenia.

△**somat-.** SEE somato-.

so•ma•tag•no•sia (sō'mă-tag-nō'sē-ă). SYN somatotopagnosis. [somat- + G. *a*- priv. + *gnōsis*, recognition]

so•ma•tal•gia (sō-mă-tal′jē-ă). **1.** Pain in the body. **2.** Pain due to organic causes, as opposed to psychogenic pain. [somat- + G. *algos*, pain]

so•ma•tas•the•nia (sō′mă-tas-thē′nē-ă). A condition of chronic physical weakness and fatigability. SYN somasthenia. [somat- + G. *astheneia*, weakness]

so•ma•tes•the•sia (sō′mă-tes-thē′zē-ă). Bodily sensation, the conscious awareness of the body. SYN somesthesia. [somat- + G. *aisthēsis*, sensation]

so•mat•es•the•tic (sō′mat-es-thet′ik). Relating to somatesthesia.

so•mat•ic (sō-mat′ik). **1.** Relating to the soma or trunk, the wall of the body cavity, or the body in general. SYN parietal (2). **2.** Relating to or involving the skeleton or skeletal (voluntary) muscle and the innervation of the latter, as distinct from the viscera or visceral (involuntary) muscle and its (autonomic) innervation. SYN parietal (3). **3.** Relating to the vegetative, as distinguished from the generative, functions. [G. *sōmatikos*, bodily]

so•ma•ti•za•tion (sō′mat-i-zā′shŭn). The process by which psychological needs are expressed in physical symptoms. SEE ALSO somatization *disorder.*

△**somato-, somat-, somatico-.** The body, bodily. [G. *sōma*, body]

so•ma•to•chrome (sō′mă-tō-krōm). Denoting the group of neurons or nerve cells in which there is an abundance of cytoplasm completely surrounding the nucleus. [somato- + G. *chrōma*, color]

so•ma•to•crin•in (sō′mă-tō-crin′in). Hypothalamic growth hormone-releasing hormone, GHRH. [somato- + G. *krinō*, to secrete, + -in]

so•ma•to•gen•ic (sō′mă-tō-jen′ik). **1.** Originating in the soma or body under the influence of external forces. **2.** Having origin in body cells. [somato- + G. *genesis*, origin]

so•ma•to•lib•er•in (sō′mă-tō-lib′er-in). A decapeptide released by the hypothalamus, which induces the release of human growth hormone (somatotropin). SYN growth hormone-releasing factor, growth hormone-releasing hormone, somatotropin-releasing factor, somatotropin-releasing hormone. [somatotropin + L. *libero*, to free, + -in]

so•ma•to•mam•mo•tro•pin (sō′mă-tō-mam′ō-trō-pin). A peptide hormone, closely related to somatotropin in its biological properties, produced by the normal placenta and by certain neoplasms. [somato- + L. *mamma*, breast, + G. *tropē*, a turning, + -in]

  human chorionic s. (HCS), SYN human placental *lactogen.*

so•ma•to•me•din (sō′mă-tō-mē′din). A peptide synthesized in the liver, and probably in the kidney, that is capable of stimulating certain anabolic processes in bone and cartilage, such as synthesis of DNA, RNA, and protein and the sulfation of mucopolysaccharides; secretion and/or biological activity of s. is known to be dependent on somatotropin. [*somato*tropin + *me*-*d*iator + -in]

so•ma•to•path•ic (sō′mă-tō-path′ik). Relating to

bodily or organic illness, as distinguished from mental (psychologic) disorder. [somato- + G. *pathos*, suffering]

so•ma•to•plasm (sō′mă-tō-plazm, sō-mat′ō-). Aggregate of all the forms of specialized protoplasm entering into the composition of the body, other than germ plasm. [somato- + G. *plasma*, something formed]

so•ma•to•pleure (sō′mă-tō-plūr). Embryonic layer formed by association of the parietal layer of the lateral plate mesoderm with the ectoderm. [somato- + G. *pleura*, side]

so•ma•to•psy•chic (sō′mă-tō-sī′kik). Relating to the body-mind relationship; the study of the effects of the body upon the mind, as opposed to psychosomatic, which refers to the effects of mind on body. [somato- + G. *psychē*, soul]

so•ma•to•psy•cho•sis (sō′mă-tō-sī-kō′sis). An emotional disorder associated with an organic disease. [somato- + G. *psychōsis*, an animating]

so•ma•to•sen•so•ry (sō-mă-tō-sen′sō-rē). Sensation relating to the body's superficial and deep parts as contrasted to specialized senses such as sight.

so•ma•to•sex•u•al (sō′mă-tō-sek′shū-ăl). Denoting the somatic aspects of sexuality as distinguished from its psychosexual aspects.

so•ma•to•stat•in (sō′mă-tō-stat′in). A tetradecapeptide capable of inhibiting the release of somatotropin, insulin, and gastrin. SYN growth hormone-inhibiting hormone, somatotropin release-inhibiting factor, somatotropin release-inhibiting hormone. [somatotropin + G. *stasis*, a standing still, + -in]

so•ma•to•stat•i•no•ma (sō′mă-tō-stat-i-nō′mă). A somatostatin-secreting tumor of the pancreatic islets.

so•ma•to•ther•a•py (sō′mă-tō-thār′ă-pē). **1.** Therapy directed at physical disorders. **2.** PSYCHIATRY A variety of therapeutic interventions employing chemical or physical, as opposed to psychological, methods.

so•ma•to•top•ag•no•sis (sō′mă-tō-top′ag-nō′sis). The inability to identify any part of one's own or another's body. Cf. autotopagnosia. SYN somatagnosia. [somato- + top- + G. *a*- priv. + G. *gnōsis*, knowledge]

so•ma•to•top•ic (sō-mă-tō-top′ik). Relating to somatotopy.

so•ma•tot•o•py (sō-mă-tot′ō-pē). The topographic association of positional relationships of receptors in the body via respective nerve fibers to their terminal distribution in specific functional areas of the cerebral cortex; the continuation of these positional relationships in all stages of the ascent of nerve fibers through the central nervous system enables the brain and spinal cord to function on a basis of spatially designated units. [somato- + G. *topos*, place]

so•ma•to•tropes (sō-mă-tō-trōps). A subclass of pituitary acidophilic cells; site of synthesis of growth hormone.

so•ma•to•troph (sō′mă-tō-trof). A cell of the adenohypophysis that produces somatotropin.

so•ma•to•tro•phic (sō′mă-tō-trof′ik). SYN somatotropic. [somato- + G. *trophē*, nourishment]

so•ma•to•tro•pic (sō′mă-tō-trop′ik). Having a

stimulating effect on body growth. SYN somato-trophic. [somato- + G. *trope*, a turning]

so•ma•to•tro•pin (sō'mă-tō-trō'pin). A protein hormone of the anterior lobe of the pituitary, produced by the acidophil cells, that promotes body growth, fat mobilization, and inhibition of glucose utilization; diabetogenic when present in excess; a deficiency of s. is associated with a number of types of dwarfism. SYN growth hormone, pituitary growth hormone, somatotropic hormone. [for *somatotrophin*, fr. somato- + G. *trophe* nourishment; corrupted to -*tropin* and reanalyzed as fr. G. *trope*, a turning]

so•ma•to•type (sō'mă-tō-tīp). **1.** The constitutional or body type of an individual. **2.** The constitutional or body type associated with a particular personality type.

som•es•the•sia (sō-mes-thē'zē-ă). SYN somatesthesia.

so•mite (sō'mīt). One of the paired, metamerically arranged cell masses formed in the early embryonic paraxial mesoderm; commencing in the third or early fourth week in the region of the hindbrain, they develop in a caudal direction until 42 pairs are formed; their presence is considered evidence that metameric segmentation is a vertebrate characteristic. [G. *sōma*, body, + -*ite*]

som•nam•bu•lism (som-nam'byū-lizm). **1.** A disorder of sleep involving complex motor acts which occurs primarily during the first third of the night but not during rapid eye movement sleep. **2.** A form of hysteria in which purposeful behavior is forgotten. [L. *somnus*, sleep, + *ambulo*, to walk]

som•ni•fa•cient (som-ni-fā'shent). SYN soporific (1). [L. *somnus*, sleep, + *facio*, to make]

som•nif•er•ous (som-nif'er-ŭs). SYN soporific (1). [L. *somnus*, sleep, + *fero*, to bring]

som•nil•o•quence, som•nil•o•quism (som-nil'ō-kwens, -kwizm). **1.** Talking or muttering in one's sleep. **2.** SYN somniloquy. [L. *somnus*, sleep, + *loquor*, to talk]

som•nil•o•quy (som-nil'ō-kwē). Talking under the influence of hypnotic suggestion. SYN somniloquence (2), somniloquism. [L. *somnus*, sleep, + *loquor*, to speak]

som•nip•a•thy (som-nip'ă-thē). **1.** Any sleep disorder. **2.** SYN hypnotism (1). [L. *somnus*, sleep, + G. *pathos*, suffering]

som•no•cin•e•ma•tog•ra•phy (som'nō-sin-ĕ-mă-tog'ră-fē). The process or technique of recording movements during sleep.

som•no•lence, som•no•len•cy (som'nō-lens, -len-sē). **1.** An inclination to sleep. **2.** A condition of obtusion. [L. *somnolentia*]

som•no•lent (som'nō-lent). **1.** Drowsy; sleepy; inclined to sleep. **2.** In a condition of incomplete sleep; semicomatose. SYN somnolescent. [L. *somnus*, sleep]

som•no•les•cent (som-nō-les'ent). SYN somnolent.

son•ic (son'ik). Of, pertaining to, or determined by sound; *e.g.*, s. vibration. [L. *sonus*, sound]

son•i•ca•tion (son-i-kā'shŭn). The process of disrupting biologic materials by use of sound wave energy.

son•i•fi•ca•tion (son'i-fi-kā'shŭn). The production of sound, or of sound waves.

son•o•gram (son'ō-gram). SYN ultrasonogram. [L. *sonus*, sound, + G. *gramma*, a drawing]

son•o•graph (son'ō-graf). SYN ultrasonograph. [L. *sonus*, sound, + G. *graphō*, to write]

so•nog•ra•pher (sŏ-nog'ră-fer). SYN ultrasonographer.

so•nog•ra•phy (sŏ-nog'ră-fī). SYN ultrasonography. [L. *sonus*, sound. + G. *graphō*, to write]

so•por (sō'pōr). An unnaturally deep sleep. [L.]

so•po•rif•ic (sō-pōr-if'ik, sop'ōr-). **1.** Causing sleep. SYN somnifacient, somniferous. **2.** An agent that produces sleep. [L. *sopor*, deep sleep, + *facio*, to make]

sor•be•fa•cient (sōr-bĕ-fā'shent). **1.** Causing absorption. **2.** An agent that causes or facilitates absorption. [L. *sorbeo*, to suck up, + *facio*, to make]

sor•des (sōr'dēz). A dark brown or blackish crustlike collection on the lips, teeth, and gums of a person with dehydration associated with a chronic debilitating disease. [L. filth, fr. *sordeo*, to be foul]

sore (sōr). **1.** A wound, ulcer, or any open skin lesion. **2.** Painful; aching; tender. [A.S. *sār*]
  bed s., SEE bedsore.
  canker s.'s, SYN aphtha (2).
  cold s., colloquialism for *herpes* simplex.
  pressure s., SYN decubitus *ulcer*.
  tropical s., SYN cutaneous *leishmaniasis*.

sorp•tion (sōrp'shŭn). Adsorption or absorption.

souf•fle (sū'fl). A soft, blowing sound heard on auscultation. [Fr. *souffler*, to blow]
  cardiac s., a soft, puffing heart murmur.
  fetal s., a blowing murmur, synchronous with the fetal heart beat, sometimes only systolic and sometimes continuous, heard on auscultation over the pregnant uterus.
  uterine s., a blowing sound, synchronous with the cardiac systole of the mother, heard on auscultation of the pregnant uterus.

sound (sownd). **1.** The vibrations produced by a sounding body, transmitted by the air or other medium, and perceived by the internal ear. **2.** An elongated cylindrical, usually curved, instrument of metal, used for exploring the bladder or other cavities of the body, for dilating strictures of the urethra, esophagus, or other canal, for calibrating the lumen of a body cavity, or for detecting the presence of a foreign body in a body cavity. **3.** To explore or calibrate a cavity with a s. **4.** Whole; healthy; not diseased or injured.
  adventitious lung s.'s, breath s.'s that are not normally heard, and that fall into one of two categories: (1) continuous: musical-type s.'s with a persistent pitch (for example, wheezes, rhonchi); (2) discontinuous: intermittent, crackling, or bubbling s.'s (rales).
  bowel s.'s, relatively high-pitched abdominal s.'s caused by propulsion of intestinal contents through the lower alimentary tract.
  first heart s. (S$_1$), occurs with ventricular systole and is mainly produced by closure of the atrioventricular valves.
  fourth heart s. (S$_4$), the s. produced in late diastole in association with ventricular filling due

to atrial systole and related to reduced ventricular compliance. It may be normal at older ages but is nearly always abnormal at younger ages. It is common in ventricular hypertrophy, particularly with hypertension, and is almost invariable during acute myocardial infarction. Fourth heart s.'s may arise from the right or left ventricle or both.

friction s., the s., heard on auscultation, made by the rubbing of two opposed serous surfaces roughened by an inflammatory exudate, or, if chronic, by nonadhesive fibrosis. SYN friction rub.

hippocratic succussion s., a splashing s. elicited by shaking a patient with hydro- or pyopneumothorax, the physician's ear being applied to the chest.

Korotkoff s.'s, s.'s heard during blood pressure determination. S.'s originating within the blood passing through the vessel or produced by a vibrating motion of the arterial wall.

second heart s. (S₂), the second s. heard on auscultation of the heart; signifies the beginning of diastole and is due to closure of the semilunar valves.

splitting of heart s.'s, the production of major components of the first and second heart s.'s (rarely the third and fourth) due to contribution by the left-sided and right-sided valves; thus, the first heart s. would have a mitral and a tricuspid component and the second heart s. has an aortic and pulmonic component. The latter are best appreciated during respiration, with inspiration delaying the pulmonic component and producing an earlier aortic component.

succussion s., the noise made by fluid with overlying air when shaken, such as occurs with gastric dilation or with fluid and air in a pleural cavity (hydropneumothorax).

third heart s. (S₃), occurs in early diastole and corresponds with the end of the first phase of rapid ventricular filling; normal in children and younger people but abnormal in others.

space (spās). Any demarcated portion of the body, either an area of the surface, a segment of the tissues, or a cavity. SEE ALSO area, region, zone. SYN spatium [NA]. [L. *spatium,* room, space]

alveolar dead s., the difference between physiologic dead s. and anatomical dead s.; it represents that part of the physiologic dead s. resulting from ventilation of relatively underperfused or nonperfused alveoli; it differs specifically in being placed so as to fill and empty in parallel with functional alveoli, rather than being interposed in the conducting tubes between functional alveoli and the external environment.

anatomical dead s., the volume of the conducting airways from the nose and mouth to the level at which inspired gas exchanges oxygen and carbon dioxide with pulmonary capillary blood; formerly presumed to extend down to the beginning of alveolar epithelium in the respiratory bronchioles, but more recent evidence indicates that effective gas exchange extends some distance up the thicker-walled conducting airways because of rapid longitudinal mixing. Cf. alveolar dead s., physiologic dead s.

apical s., the s. between the alveolar wall and

the apex of the root of a tooth where an alveolar abscess usually has its origin.

capsular s., the slitlike s. between the visceral and parietal layers of the capsule of the renal corpuscle; it opens into the proximal tubule of the nephron at the neck of the tubule.

cartilage s., SYN cartilage *lacuna.*

central palmar s., the more medial of the central palmar spaces, bounded medially by the hypothenar compartment; related distally to the synovial tendon sheaths of digits 3 and 4 and proximally to the common flexor sheath.

corneal s., one of the stellate s.'s between the lamellae of the cornea, each of which contains a cell or corneal corpuscle. SYN lacuna (4).

dead s., (1) a cavity, potential or real, remaining after the closure of a wound which is not obliterated by the operative technique; (2) SEE anatomical dead s., physiologic dead s.

episcleral s., the space between the fascial sheath of the eyeball and the sclera.

freeway s., the s. between the occluding surfaces of the maxillary and mandibular teeth when the mandible is in physiologic resting position. SYN interocclusal distance (2).

haversian s.'s, s.'s in bone formed by the enlargement of haversian canals.

intercostal s., an interval between the ribs, occupied by intercostal muscles, veins, arteries and nerves.

interpleural s., SYN mediastinum (2).

interproximal s., the s. between adjacent teeth in a dental arch; it is divided into the embrasure occlusal to the contact area, and the septal s. gingival to the contact area.

interradicular s., the s. between the roots of multirooted teeth.

intervillous s.'s, the s.'s containing maternal blood, located between placental villi; they are lined with syncytiotrophoblast.

Kiernan's s., interlobular s. in the liver.

mediastinal s., SYN mediastinum (2).

medullary s., the central cavity and the cellular intervals between the trabeculae of bone, filled with marrow.

perilymphatic s., space between the bony and membranous portions of the labyrinth.

personal s., a term used in the behavioral sciences to denote the physical area immediately surrounding an individual who is in proximity to one or more others, whether known or unknown, and which serves as a body buffer zone in such interpersonal transactions.

physiologic dead s., the sum of anatomic and alveolar dead s.; the dead s. calculated when the carbon dioxide pressure in systemic arterial blood is used instead of that of alveolar gas in Bohr's equation; it is a virtual or apparent volume that takes into account the impairment of gas exchange because of uneven distributions of lung ventilation and perfusion.

plantar s., one of four areas between fascial layers in the foot, where pus may be confined when the foot is infected.

pleural s., SYN pleural *cavity.*

Poiseuille's s., SYN still *layer.*

retroperitoneal s., the space between the parietal peritoneum and the muscles and bones of the posterior abdominal wall.

retropubic s., the area of loose connective tissue between the bladder with its related fascia and the pubis and anterior abdominal wall.

subarachnoid s., the s. between the arachnoidea and pia mater, traversed by delicate fibrous trabeculae and filled with cerebrospinal fluid. Since the pia mater immediately adheres to the surface of the brain and spinal cord, the s. is greatly widened wherever the brain surface exhibits a deep depression (for example, between the cerebellum and medulla); such widenings are called cisternae. The large blood vessels supplying the brain and spinal cord lie in the subarachnoid s.

subchorial s., the part of the placenta adjacently beneath the chorionic plate; it joins with irregular channels to form the marginal lakes. SYN subchorial lake.

subdural s., an artificial s. created by the separation of the arachnoid from the dura as the result of trauma or some pathologic process; in the healthy state, the arachnoid is attached to the dura and a subdural s. does not naturally occur.

zonular s.'s, the spaces between the fibers of the ciliary zonule at the equator of the lens of the eye.

spacer. An extension device for a metered-dose inhaler; it is designed to eliminate the need for hand-breath coordination and to reduce the deposition of large aerosol particles in the upper airway.

spasm (spazm). A sudden involuntary contraction of one or more muscle groups; includes cramps, contractures. SYN muscle s., spasmus. [G. *spasmos*]

carpopedal s., s. of the feet and hands observed in hyperventilation, calcium deprivation, and tetany: flexion of the hands at the wrists and of the fingers at the metacarpophalangeal joints and extension of the fingers at the phalangeal joints; the feet are dorsiflexed at the ankles and the toes plantar flexed. SYN carpopedal contraction.

clonic s., alternate involuntary contraction and relaxation of a muscle.

cynic s., SYN risus caninus.

facial s., SYN facial *tic.*

habit s., SYN tic.

intention s., a spasmodic contraction of the muscles occurring when a voluntary movement is attempted.

muscle s., SYN spasm.

nodding s., (1) in infants, a drop of the head on the chest due to loss of tone in the neck muscles as in epilepsia nutans, or to tonic spasm of anterior neck muscles as in West's syndrome; (2) in adults, a nodding of the head from clonic s.'s of the sternomastoid muscles. SYN spasmus nutans (1).

retrocollic s., torticollis in which the s. affects the posterior neck muscles. SYN retrocollis.

saltatory s., a spasmodic affection of the muscles of the lower extremities.

tonic s., a continuous involuntary muscular contraction.

tonoclonic s., convulsive contraction of muscles.

torsion s., SYN dystonia.

△**spasmo-.** Spasm. [G. *spasmos*]

spas·mod·ic (spaz-mod′ik). Relating to or marked by spasm. [G. *spasmōdes,* convulsive, fr. *spasmos,* + *eidos,* form]

spas·mol·y·sis (spaz-mol′i-sis). The arrest of a spasm or convulsion. [spasmo- + G. *lysis,* dissolution]

spas·mo·lyt·ic (spaz′mō-lit′ik). **1.** Relating to spasmolysis. **2.** Denoting a chemical agent that relieves smooth muscle spasms.

spas·mus (spaz′mŭs). SYN spasm. [L. fr. G. *spasmos,* spasm]

s. nu′tans, (1) SYN nodding *spasm.* (2) a fine nystagmus, sometimes rotary, sometimes monocular, associated with head-nodding movements.

spas·tic (spas′tik). **1.** SYN hypertonic (1). **2.** Relating to spasm or to spasticity. [L. *spasticus,* fr. G. *spastikos,* drawing in]

spas·tic·i·ty (spas-tis′i-tē). A state of increased muscular tone with exaggeration of the tendon reflexes.

clasp-knife s., initial increased resistance to stretch of the extensor muscles of a joint that give way rather suddenly allowing the joint then to be easily flexed; the rigidity is due to an exaggeration of the stretch reflex. SYN clasp-knife rigidity.

spa·tial (spā′shăl). Relating to space or a space.

spa·ti·um, pl. **spa·tia** (spā′shē-ŭm, -shē-ă) [NA]. SYN space. [L.]

spat·u·late (spach′ū-lāt). **1.** Shaped like a spatula. **2.** To manipulate or mix with a spatula. **3.** To incise the cut end of a tubular structure longitudinally and splay it open, to allow creation of an elliptical anastomosis of greater circumference than would be possible with conventional transverse or oblique (bevelled) end-to-end anastomoses.

spay (spā). To remove the ovaries of an animal. [Gael. *spoth,* castrate, or G. *spadōn,* eunuch]

SPCA serum prothrombin conversion *accelerator.*

spe·cial·ist (spesh′ă-list). One who devotes professional attention to a particular specialty or subject area.

spe·cial·i·za·tion (spesh′ă-li-zā′shŭn). **1.** Professional attention limited to a particular specialty or subject area for study, research, and/or treatment. **2.** SYN differentiation (1).

spe·cial·ty (spesh′al-tē). The particular subject area or branch of medical science to which one devotes professional attention. [L. *specialitas* fr. *specialis,* special]

spe·ci·a·tion (spē-shē-ā′shŭn). The evolutionary process by which diverse species of animals or plants are formed from a common ancestral stock.

spe·cies, pl. **spe·cies** (spē′shēz). **1.** A biological division between the genus and a variety or the individual; a group of organisms that generally bear a close resemblance to one another in the more essential features of their organization, and breed effectively producing fertile progeny. **2.** A class of pharmaceutical preparations consisting of a mixture of dried plants, not pulverized, but in sufficiently fine division to be conveniently used in the making of extemporaneous decoctions or infusions, as a tea. [L. appearance, form, kind, fr. *specio*, to look at]

spe·cies-spe·cif·ic. Characteristic of a given species; serum that is produced by the injection of immunogens into an animal, and that acts only upon the cells, protein, etc., of a member of the same species as that from which the original antigen was obtained.

spe·cif·ic (spĕ-sif'ik). **1.** Relating to a species. **2.** Relating to an individual infectious disease, one caused by a special microorganism. **3.** A remedy having a definite therapeutic action in relation to a particular disease or symptom, as quinine in relation to malaria. [L. *specificus* fr. *species* + *facio*, to make]

spec·i·fic·i·ty (spes-i-fis'i-tē). **1.** The condition or state of being specific, of having a fixed relation to a single cause or to a definite result; manifested in the relation of a disease to its pathogenic microorganism, of a reaction to a certain chemical union, or of an antibody to its antigen or the reverse. **2.** CLINICAL PATHOLOGY The proportion of individuals who do not have a disease or condition and in whom a test intended to identify that disease or condition yields negative results. Cf. sensitivity (2).

diagnostic s., (1) the probability (P) that, given the absence of disease (D), a normal test result (T) excludes disease; *i.e.,* P(T/D). (2) s. (%) = number of individuals without the disease who test negative × 100 ÷ total number of individuals tested without the disease.

relative s., the s. of a medical screening test as determined by comparison with the same type of test (*e.g.,* s. of a new serological test relative to s. of an established serological test).

spec·i·men (spes'ĭ-men). A small part, or sample, of any substance or material obtained for testing. [L. fr. *specio*, to look at]

SPECT single photon emission computed *tomography.*

spec·ta·cles (spek'tĭ-klz). Lenses set in a frame that holds them in front of the eyes, used to correct errors of refraction or to protect the eyes. The parts of the s. are the *lenses;* the *bridge* between the lenses, resting on the nose; the *rims* or *frames,* encircling the lenses; the *sides* or *temples* that pass on either side of the head to the ears; the *bows,* the curved extremities of the temples; the *shoulders,* short bars attached to the rims or the lenses and jointed with the sides. SYN eyeglasses, glasses (1). [L. *specto,* pp. *-atus,* to watch, observe]

spec·tra (spek'tră). Plural of spectrum. [L.]

spec·tral (spek'trăl). Relating to a spectrum.

spec·trin (spek'trin). A filamentous contractile protein that together with actin and other cytoskeleton proteins forms a network that gives the red blood cell membrane its shape and flexibility; a defect or deficiency of s. is associated with hereditary spherocytosis and hereditary elliptocytosis; the principal component of the membrane skeleton of red cells.

spectro-. A spectrum. [L. *spectrum,* an image]

spec·trom·e·ter (spek-trom'ĕ-ter). An instrument for determining the wavelength or energy of light or other electromagnetic emission. [spectro- + G. *metron,* measure]

spec·trom·e·try (spek-trom'ĕ-trē). The procedure of observing and measuring the wavelengths of light or other electromagnetic emissions.

spec·tro·pho·tom·e·ter (spek'trō-fō-tom'ĕ-ter). An instrument for measuring the intensity of light of a definite wavelength transmitted by a substance or a solution, giving a quantitative measure of the amount of material in the solution absorbing the light; a colorimeter with a choice of wavelength and photometric measurement. [spectro- + photometer]

spec·tro·pho·tom·e·try (spek'trō-fō-tom'ĕ-trē). Analysis by means of a spectrophotometer.

atomic absorption s., determination of concentration by the ability of atoms to absorb radiant energy of specific wavelengths.

reflectance s., a quantitative spectrophotometric technique in which light is reflected from the surface of a colorimetric reaction and is then used to measure the amount of the reaction product.

spec·tro·scope (spek'trō-skōp). An instrument for resolving light from any luminous body into its spectrum, and for the analysis of the spectrum so formed. It consists of a prism that refracts the light or a grating for diffraction of the light, an arrangement for rendering the rays parallel, and a telescope that magnifies the spectrum. [spectro- + G. *skopeō,* to view]

spec·tro·scop·ic (spek-trō-skop'ik). Relating to or performed by means of a spectroscope.

spec·tros·co·py (spek-tros'kŏ-pē). Observation and study of spectra of absorbed or emitted light by means of a spectroscope.

spec·trum, pl. **spec·tra, spec·trums** (spek'trŭm, -ă, -ŭmz). **1.** The range of colors presented when white light is resolved into its constituent colors by being passed through a prism or through a diffraction grating: red, orange, yellow, green, blue, indigo, and violet, arranged in increasing frequency of vibration or decreasing wavelength. **2.** The range of pathogenic microorganisms against which an antibiotic or other antibacterial agent is active. **3.** The plot of intensity vs. wavelength of light emitted or absorbed by a substance, usually characteristic of the substance and used in qualitative and quantitative analysis. **4.** The range of wavelengths presented when a beam of radiant energy is subjected to dispersion and focused. [L. an image, fr. *specio,* to look at]

absorption s., the s. observed after light has passed through, and been partially absorbed by, a solution or translucent substance; many molecular groupings have characteristic light absorption patterns, which can be used for detection and quantitative assay.

broad s., a term indicating activity of an antibiotic against a wide variety of microorganisms.

electromagnetic s., SYN electromagnetic *radiation.*

fortification s., the zigzag banding of light, resembling the walls of fortified medieval towns, that marks the margin of the scintillating scotoma of migraine.

line s., an emission spectrum of elements in

sp

which the emitted light bands cover a very narrow range of energies.

visible s., that part of electromagnetic radiation that is visible to the human eye; it extends from extreme red, 7606 Å (760.6 nm), to extreme violet, 3934 Å (393.4 nm).

spec•u•lum, pl. **spec•u•la** (spek′yū-lŭm, -lă). An instrument for enlarging the opening of any canal or cavity in order to facilitate inspection of its interior. [L. a mirror, fr. *specio,* to look at]

eye s., an instrument for keeping the eyelids apart during inspection of or operation on the eye. SYN blepharostat.

speech. Talk; the use of the voice in conveying ideas. [A.S. *spaec*]

alaryngeal s., production of s. using a sound source other than the larynx, as in esophageal s. or use of an artificial larynx. SEE esophageal s. SEE ALSO artificial *larynx.*

automatic s., overlearned or low-content language that can be produced with little awareness of meaning, such as consecutive numbers, days of the week, verses, prayers, expletives, or other common expressions. SYN nonpropositional s.

esophageal s., a technique for speaking after total laryngectomy; consists of swallowing air and regurgitating it, producing a vibration in the hypopharynx.

mirror s., a reversal of the order of syllables in a word, analogous to mirror writing.

nonpropositional s., SYN automatic s.

propositional s., intellectual, rational use of language for specific communication goals. SEE automatic s.

scanning s., measured or metered, often slow s.

spontaneous s., spoken language that occurs without prompting or during an unstructured interview.

staccato s., an abrupt utterance, each syllable being enunciated separately; noted especially in multiple sclerosis.

subvocal s., slight movements of the muscles of s. related to thinking but producing no sound.

speed (spēd). The magnitude of velocity without regard to direction. Cf. velocity.

sperm [NA]. **1.** SYN spermatozoon. **2.** SYN semen (1). [G. *sperma,* seed]

⚠**sperma-, spermato-, spermo-.** Semen, spermatozoa. [G. *sperma,* seed]

sperm-as•ter (sperm′as-ter). Cytocentrum with astral rays in the cytoplasm of an inseminated ovum; it is brought in by the penetrating spermatozoon and evolves into the mitotic spindle of the first cleavage division. [sperm + G. *astēr,* a star (aster)]

sper•mat•ic (sper-mat′ik). Relating to the sperm or semen.

sper•ma•tid (sper′mă-tid). A cell in a late stage of the development of the spermatozoon; it is a haploid cell derived from the secondary spermatocyte and evolves by spermiogenesis into a spermatozoon. [spermat- + -*id* (2)]

⚠**spermato-.** SEE sperma-.

sper•ma•to•blast (sper′mă-tō-blast). SYN spermatogonium. [spermato- + G. *blastos,* germ]

sper•ma•to•cele (sper′mă-tō-sēl). Cyst of the ep-

ididymis containing spermatozoa. [spermato- + G. *kēlē,* tumor]

sper•ma•to•ci•dal (sper′mă-tō-sī′dăl). Destructive to spermatozoa. SYN spermicidal.

sper•ma•to•cide (sper′mă-tō-sīd). An agent destructive to spermatozoa. SYN spermicide. [spermato- + L. *caedo,* to kill]

sper•ma•to•cy•tal (sper-mă-tō-sī′tăl). Relating to spermatocytes.

sper•ma•to•cyte (sper′mă-tō-sīt). Parent cell of a spermatid, derived by mitotic division from a spermatogonium. [spermato- + G. *kytos,* cell]

primary s., the s. derived by a growth phase from a spermatogonium, and that undergoes the first division of meiosis.

secondary s., the s. derived from a primary s. by the first meiotic division; each secondary s. produces two spermatids by the second meiotic division.

sper•ma•to•cy•to•gen•e•sis (sper′mă-tō-sī′tō-jen′ĕ-sis). SYN spermatogenesis.

sper•ma•to•gen•e•sis (sper′mă-tō-jen′ĕ-sis). The entire process by which spermatogonial stem cells divide and differentiate into spermatozoa. SEE ALSO spermiogenesis. SYN spermatocytogenesis. [spermato- + G. *genesis,* origin]

sper•ma•to•gen•ic (sper′mă-tō-jen′ik). Relating to spermatogenesis; sperm-producing. SYN spermatopoietic (1).

sper•ma•to•go•ni•um (sper′mă-tō-gō′nē-ŭm). The primitive sperm cell derived by mitotic division from the germ cell; increasing several times in size, it becomes a primary spermatocyte. SEE ALSO spermatid. SYN spermatoblast. [spermato- + G. *gonē,* generation]

sper•ma•toid (sper′mă-tōid). **1.** Resembling a sperm, a sperm tail, or semen. **2.** A male or flagellated form of the malarial microparasite. [spermato + G. *eidos,* form]

sper•ma•tol•y•sis (sper-mă-tol′i-sis). Destruction, with dissolution, of spermatozoa. [spermato + G. *lysis,* dissolution]

sper•ma•to•lyt•ic (sper′mă-tō-lit′ik). Relating to spermatolysis.

sper•ma•to•poi•et•ic (sper′mă-tō-poy-et′ik). **1.** SYN spermatogenic. **2.** Secreting semen. [spermato- + G. *poieō,* to make]

sper•ma•tor•rhea (sper′mă-tō-rē′ă). An involuntary discharge of semen, without orgasm. [spermato- + G. *rhoia,* a flow]

sper•ma•to•zo•al, sper•ma•to•zo•an (sper′mă-tō-zō′ăl, -zō′ăn). Relating to spermatozoa.

sper•ma•to•zo•on, pl. **sper•ma•to•zoa** (sper′mă-tō-zō′on, -zō′ă). The male gamete or sex cell that contains the genetic information to be transmitted by the male, exhibits autokinesia, and is able to effect zygosis with an ovum. The human s. is composed of a head and a tail, the tail being divisible into a neck, a middle piece, a principal piece, and an end piece; the head, 4 to 6 μm in length, is a broadly oval, flattened body containing the nucleus; the tail is about 55 μm in length. SYN sperm (1) [NA]. [G. *sperma,* seed, + *zōon* animal]

sper•ma•tu•ria (sper-mă-tū′rē-ă). SYN semenuria.

sper•mia (sper′mē-ă). Plural of spermium.

sper·mi·ci·dal (sper-mi-sī′dăl). SYN spermatocidal.

sper·mi·cide (sper′mi-sīd). SYN spermatocide.

sper·mi·duct (sper′mi-dŭkt). **1.** SYN *ductus* deferens. **2.** SYN ejaculatory *duct.*

sper·mi·o·gen·e·sis (sper′mē-ō-jen′ĕ-sis). That segment of spermatogenesis during which immature spermatids become spermatozoa. [sperm- + G. *genesis*, origin]

sper·mi·um, pl. **sper·mia** (sper′mē-ŭm, -ă). The mature male germ cell or spermatozoon.

ˀspermo-. SEE sperma-.

sper·mo·lith (sper′mō-lith). A concretion in the ductus deferens. [spermo- + G. *lithos*, stone]

SPF sun protection *factor.*

sphac·e·late (sfas′ĕ-lāt). To become gangrenous or necrotic. [G. *sphakelos*, gangrene]

sphac·e·la·tion (sfas-ĕ-lā′shŭn). **1.** The process of becoming gangrenous or necrotic. **2.** Gangrene or necrosis. [G. *sphakelos*, gangrene]

sphac·el·ism (sfas′ĕ-lizm). The condition manifested by a sphacelus.

sphac·e·lo·der·ma (sfas′ĕ-lō-der′mă). Gangrene of the skin. [G. *sphakelos*, gangrene, + *derma*, skin]

sphac·e·lous (sfas′ĕ-lŭs). Sloughing, gangrenous, or necrotic.

sphac·e·lus (sfas′ĕ-lŭs). A mass of sloughing, gangrenous, or necrotic matter. [G. *sphakelos*, gangrene]

sphe·ni·on (sfē′nē-on). The tip of the sphenoidal angle of the parietal bone; a craniometric point. [Mod. L. fr. G. *sphēn*, wedge, + dim. *-iōn*]

ˀspheno-. Wedge, wedge-shaped; the sphenoid bone. [G. *sphēn*, wedge]

sphe·no·ceph·a·ly (sfē′nō-sef′ă-lē). Condition characterized by a deformation of the skull giving it a wedge-shaped appearance. [spheno- + G. *kephalē*, head]

sphe·noid (sfē′noyd). **1.** SYN sphenoidal. **2.** SYN sphenoid *bone.* [G. *sphēnoeidēs*, fr. *sphēn*, wedge, + *eidos*, resemblance]

sphe·noi·dal (sfē-noy′dăl). **1.** Relating to the sphenoid bone. **2.** Wedge-shaped. SYN sphenoid (1).

sphe·noid·i·tis (sfē-noy-dī′tis). **1.** Inflammation of the sphenoid sinus. **2.** Necrosis of the sphenoid bone. [sphenoid + G. *-itis*, inflammation]

sphe·noi·dot·o·my (sfē′noy-dot′ō-mē). Any operation on the sphenoid bone or sinus. [sphenoid + G. *tomē*, a cutting]

sphe·nor·bit·al (sfē-nōr′bi-tăl). Denoting the portions of the sphenoid bone contributing to the orbits.

sphe·not·ic (sfē-nō′tik). Relating to the sphenoid bone and the bony case of the ear. [spheno- + G. *ous*, ear]

sphere (sfēr). A ball or globular body. [G. *sphaira*]

  attraction s., SYN astrosphere.

ˀsphero-. Spherical, a sphere. [G. *sphaira*, globe]

sphe·ro·cyte (sfēr′ō-sīt). A small, spherical red blood cell. [sphero- + G. *kytos*, cell]

sphe·ro·cy·to·sis (sfēr′ō-sī-tō′sis). Presence of sphere-shaped red blood cells in the blood. [spherocyte + G. *-osis*, condition]

  hereditary s. [MIM*182900], a congenital defect of spectrin [MIM*182860], the main component of the erythrocyte cell membrane, which becomes abnormally permeable to sodium, resulting in thickened and almost spherical erythrocytes that are fragile and susceptible to spontaneous hemolysis, with decreased survival in the circulation; results in chronic anemia with reticulocytosis, episodes of mild jaundice due to hemolysis, and acute crises with gallstones, fever, and abdominal pain. SYN familial jaundice, spherocytic anemia.

sphe·roid, sphe·roi·dal (sfēr′oyd, sfir-; sfē-royd′ăl). Shaped like a sphere. [L. *spheroideus*]

sphe·ro·pha·ki·a (sfēr-ō-fā′kē-ă). A congenital bilateral aberration in which the lenses are small, spherical, and subject to subluxation; may occur as an independent anomaly or may be associated with the Weill-Marchesani syndrome. [sphero- + G. *phakos*, lens]

sphinc·ter (sfingk′ter). A muscle that encircles a duct, tube or orifice in such a way that its contraction constricts the lumen or orifice; it is the closing component of a pylorus (the outer component is the s. dilator). SYN sphincter muscle. [G. *sphinktēr*, a band or lace]

  anatomical s., an accumulation of muscular circular fibers or specially arranged oblique fibers the function of which is to reduce partially or totally the lumen of a tube, the orifice of an organ, or the cavity of a viscus; the closing component of a pylorus.

  cardiac s., a physiologic sphincter at the esophagogastric junction.

  extrinsic s., a s. provided by circular muscular fibers extraneous to the organ.

  s. of hepatopancreatic ampulla, the smooth muscle sphincter of the hepatopancreatic ampulla within the duodenal papilla.

  intrinsic s., a thickening of the circular fibers of the muscular coat of an organ.

  lower esophageal s. (LES), musculature of the gastroesophageal junction that is tonically active except during swallowing.

  s. of Oddi, a valvelike muscular sheath surrounding the distal pancreatic and common bile ducts as they enter the duodenum together.

  s. of Oddi dysfunction, structural or functional abnormality of the sphincter of Oddi that interferes with bile drainage.

  physiological s., a section of a tubular structure that acts as if it has a band of circular muscle to constrict it, although no such specialized structure can be found on morphological examination.

  s. pupil′lae, a ring of smooth muscle fibers surrounding the pupillary border of the iris. SYN musculus sphincter pupillae [NA], sphincter muscle of pupil.

  pyloric s., a thickening of the circular layer of the gastric musculature encircling the gastroduodenal junction. SYN musculus sphincter pylori [NA].

  s. ure′thrae, *origin,* ramus of pubis; *insertion,* with fellow in median raphe behind and in front of urethra; *action,* constricts membranous urethra; *nerve supply,* pudendal. SYN musculus sphincter urethrae [NA].

  s. vesi′cae, the complete collar of smooth muscle cells of the neck of the urinary bladder which extends distally to surround the preprostatic portion of the male urethra. There is not a comparable structure in the neck of the female bladder; the internal urethral s. may exist to prevent reflux of semen into bladder. SYN musculus sphincter vesicae.

sphinc·ter·al (sfingk'ter-ăl). Relating to a sphincter.

sphinc·ter·al·gia (sfingk-ter-al'jē-ă). Pain in the sphincter ani muscles. [sphincter + G. *algos*, pain]

sphinc·ter·ec·to·my (sfingk-ter-ek'tō-mē). **1.** Excision of a portion of the pupillary border of the iris. **2.** Dissecting away any sphincter muscle. [sphincter + G. *ektomē*, excision]

sphinc·ter·is·mus (sfingk-ter-iz'mŭs). Spasmodic contraction of the sphincter ani muscles.

sphinc·ter·i·tis (sfingk'ter-ī'tis). Inflammation of any sphincter.

sphinc·ter·ol·y·sis (sfingk-ter-ol'i-sis). An operation for freeing the iris from the cornea in anterior synechia involving only the pupillary border. [sphincter, + G. *lysis*, loosening]

sphinc·ter·o·plas·ty (sfingk'ter-ō-plas-tē). Plastic surgery of any sphincter muscle. [sphincter + G. *plastos*, formed]

sphinc·ter·ot·o·my (sfingk-tĕ-rot'ō-mē). Incision or division of a sphincter muscle. [sphincter + G. *tomē*, incision]

sphin·go·lip·id (sfing'gō-lip-id). Any lipid containing a long-chain base like that of sphingosine (*e.g.*, ceramides, cerebrosides, gangliosides, sphingomyelins); a constituent of nerve tissue.

sphin·go·lip·i·do·sis (sfing'gō-lip-i-dō'sis). Collective designation for a variety of diseases characterized by abnormal sphingolipid metabolism, *e.g.*, gangliosidosis, Gaucher's disease, Niemann-Pick disease. SYN sphingolipodystrophy.

sphin·go·lip·o·dys·tro·phy (sfing'gō-lip-ō-dis'trō-fē). SYN sphingolipidosis.

sphin·go·my·e·lin phos·pho·di·es·ter·ase (sfing'gō-mī'ĕ-lin). An enzyme catalyzing hydrolysis of sphingomyelin to *N*-acylsphingosine (a ceramide) and phosphocholine; a deficiency of this enzyme is associated with type I Niemann-Pick disease.

sphin·go·my·e·lins (sfing'gō-mī'ĕ-linz). A group of phospholipids, found in brain, spinal cord, kidney, and egg yolk, containing 1-phosphocholine (choline *O*-phosphate) combined with a ceramide.

sphin·go·sine (sfing'gō-sēn). The principal long-chain base found in sphingolipids.

△**sphygm-.** SEE sphygmo-.

sphyg·mic (sfig'mik). Relating to the pulse.

△**sphyg·mo-, sphygm-.** Pulse. [G. *sphygmos*]

sphyg·mo·chron·o·graph (sfig'mō-kron'ō-graf). A modified sphygmograph that represents graphically the time relations between the beat of the heart and the pulse; one recording the character of the pulse as well as its rapidity. [sphygmo- + G. *chronos*, time, + *graphō*, to write]

sphyg·mo·gram (sfig'mō-gram). The graphic curve made by a sphygmograph. [sphygmo- + G. *gramma*, something written]

sphyg·mo·graph (sfig'mō-graf). An instrument consisting of a lever, the short end of which rests on the radial artery at the wrist, its long end being provided with a stylet which records on a moving ribbon of paper the excursions of the pulse. [sphygmo- + G. *graphō*, to write]

sphyg·mo·graph·ic (sfig-mō-graf'ik). Relating to or made by a sphygmograph; denoting the s. tracing, or sphygmogram.

sphyg·moid (sfig'moyd). Pulselike; resembling the pulse. [sphygmo- + G. *eidos*, resemblance]

sphyg·mo·ma·nom·e·ter (sfig'mō-mă-nom'ĕ-ter). An instrument for measuring arterial blood pressure consisting of an inflatable cuff, inflating bulb, and a gauge showing the blood pressure. SYN sphygmometer. [sphygmo- + G. *manos*, thin, scanty, + *metron*, measure]

sphyg·mo·ma·nom·e·try (sfig'mō-mă-nom'ĕ-trē). Determination of the blood pressure by means of a sphygmomanometer.

sphyg·mom·e·ter (sfig-mom'ĕ-ter). SYN sphygmomanometer.

sphyg·mos·co·py (sfig-mos'kŏ-pē). Examination of the pulse. [sphygmo- + G. *skopeō*, to view]

spic·u·lar (spik'yū-lăr). Relating to or having spicules.

spic·ule (spik'yūl). A small needle-shaped body. [L. *spiculum*, dim. of *spica*, or *spicum*, a point]

spi·der (spī'der). **1.** An arthropod of the order Araneida characterized by four pairs of legs; a cephalothorax; a globose, smooth abdomen; and a complex of web-spinning spinnerets. Among the venomous s.'s are the black widow s., *Latrodectus mactans*, and the brown recluse s., *Loxosceles reclusus*. **2.** SYN spider *angioma*. [O. E. *spinnan*, to spin]

  arterial s., SYN spider *angioma*.

  vascular s., SYN spider *angioma*.

spi·der-burst (spī'der-berst). Radiating dull red capillary lines on the skin of the leg, usually without any visible or palpable varicose veins, but nevertheless due to deep-seated venous dilation; sometimes referred to as skyrocket capillary ectasis. [*spider*web + sun*burst*]

spi·ge·li·an (spī-jē'lē-an). Relating to or described by Spigelius (Adrian van der Spieghel, 1578–1625).

spike. **1.** A brief electrical event of 3 to 25 msec that gives the appearance in the electroencephalogram of a rising and falling vertical line. **2.** ELECTROPHORESIS A sharply angled upward deflection on a densitometric tracing.

△**spin-.** SEE spino-.

spi·na, gen. and pl. **spi·nae** (spī'nă, -nē). **1** [NA]. SYN vertebral *column*. **2.** SYN vertebral *column*. [L. a thorn, the backbone, spine]

▪ **s. bif'ida,** embryologic failure of fusion of one or more vertebral arches; subtypes of spina bifida are based upon degree and pattern of deformity associated with neuroectoderm involvement.

  s. bif'ida cys'tica, s. bifida associated with a meningeal cyst (meningocele) or a cyst containing both meninges and spinal cord (meningomyelocele) or only spinal cord (myelocele).

  s. bif'ida occul'ta, s. bifida in which there is a spinal defect, but no protrusion of the cord or its membrane, although there is often some abnormality in their development.

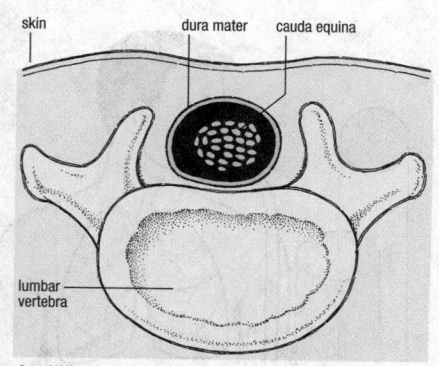

spina bifida occulta

spi·nal (spī'năl). **1.** Relating to any spine or spinous process. **2.** Relating to the vertebral column. SYN rachial, rachidial. [L. *spinalis*]

spi·nate (spī'nāt). Spined; having spines.

spin·dle (spin'dl). Any fusiform cell or structure. [A.S.]

central s., a central group of microtubules (continuous fibers) that course uninterrupted, between the asters, in contrast to the microtubules attached to the individual chromosomes (s. fibers).

cleavage s., the s. formed during the cleavage of a zygote or its blastomeres.

Krukenberg's s., a vertical fusiform area of melanin pigmentation on the posterior surface of the central cornea.

mitotic s., the fusiform figure characteristic of a dividing cell; it consists of microtubules (s. fibers), some of which become attached to each chromosome at its centromere and appear to be involved in chromosomal movement; other microtubules (continuous fibers) pass from pole to pole. SYN nuclear s.

neuromuscular s., a fusiform end organ in skeletal muscle in which afferent and a few efferent nerve fibers terminate; this sensory end organ is particularly sensitive to passive stretch of the muscle in which it is enclosed.

neurotendinous s., SYN Golgi tendon *organ.*

nuclear s., SYN mitotic s.

spine (spīn). **1.** A short, sharp, thornlike process of bone; a spinous process. **2.** SYN vertebral *column.* **3.** The bar or stay in a horse's hoof. [L. *spina*]

alar s., SYN sphenoidal s.

angular s., SYN sphenoidal s.

anterior nasal s., a pointed projection at the anterior extremity of the intermaxillary suture; the tip, as seen on a lateral cephalometric radiograph, is used as a cephalometric landmark.

bamboo s., RADIOLOGY The appearance of the thoracic or lumbar spine with ankylosing spondylitis.

cleft s., SEE *spina bifida.*

dendritic s.'s, variably long excrescences of nerve cell dendrites, varying in shape from small knobs to thornlike or filamentous processes, usually more numerous on distal dendrite arborizations than on the proximal part of dendritic

trunks; they are a preferential site of synaptic axodendritic contact; sparse or absent in some types of nerve cells (motor neurons, the large cells of the globus pallidus, stellate cells of the cerebral cortex), exceedingly numerous in others such as the pyramidal cells of the cerebral cortex and the Purkinje cells of the cerebellar cortex. SYN gemmule (2).

ischial s., a pointed process from the posterior border of the ischium on a level with the lower border of the acetabulum; gives attachment to the sacrospinous ligament; the pudendal nerve passes dorsal to the ischial s., which is palpable per vagina or rectum, and thus is used as a target for the needle-tip in administering a pudendal nerve block.

mental s., a slight projection, sometimes two, in the middle line of the posterior surface of the body of the mandible, giving attachment to the geniohyoid muscle (below) and the genioglossus (above). SYN genial tubercle.

nasal s.'s, spina nasalis anterior, posterior, and ossis frontalis.

nasal s. of frontal bone, a projection from the center of the nasal part of the frontal bone, which lies between and articulates with the nasal bones and the perpendicular plate of the ethmoid.

neural s., the middle point of the neural arch of the typical vertebra, represented by the spinous process.

palatine s.'s, the longitudinal ridges along the palatine grooves on the inferior surface of the palatine process of the maxilla.

poker s., stiff s. resulting from widespread joint immobility or overwhelming muscle spasm as might occur in osteomyelitis of a vertebra or a rheumatoid spondylitis.

posterior nasal s., the sharp posterior extremity of the nasal crest of the hard palate.

s. of scapula, the prominent triangular ridge on the dorsal aspect of the scapula, providing attachment for the trapezius and deltoid muscles and separating the supra- and infraspinous fossae.

sphenoidal s., a posterior and downward projection from the greater wing of the sphenoid bone on either side, located posterolateral to the foramen spinosum, so named for its proximity to the sphenoidal s.; gives attachment to the sphenomandibular ligament. SYN alar s., angular s., spinous process (2).

trochlear s., a spicule of bone arising from the edge of the trochlear fovea, giving attachment to the pulley of the superior oblique muscle of the eyeball.

spinn·bar·keit (spin'bahr-kīt). The property of cervical mucus that permits it to be drawn out in strings; indicative of estrogenic effect, and most pronounced during the ovulatory period. [Ger. *Spinnbarkeit,* viscosity, ability to form a thread]

⚠**spino-, spin-. 1.** The spine. **2.** Spinous. [L. *spina*]

spi·no·bul·bar (spī'nō-bŭl'bar). SYN bulbospinal.

spi·no·cer·e·bel·lum (spī'nō-sār-ĕ-bel'ŭm). SYN paleocerebellum.

spi·nous (spī'nŭs). Relating to, shaped like, or having a spine or spines.

⚠**spir-.** SEE spiro-.

spi•rad•e•no•ma (spī-rad-ĕ-nō′mă). A benign tumor of sweat glands. [G. *speira*, coil, + adenoma]

spi•ral (spī′răl). **1.** Coiled; winding around a center like a watch spring; winding and ascending like a wire spring. **2.** A structure in the shape of a coil. [Mediev. L. *spiralis*, fr. G. *speira*, a coil]

spi•ril•lar (spī-ril′ăr). S-shaped; referring to a bacterial cell with an S shape.

Spi•ril•lum (spī-ril′ŭm). A genus of large, rigid, helical, Gram-negative bacteria which are motile by means of bipolar fascicles of flagella. [Mod. L. dim. of L. *spira*, coil, fr. G. *speira*]
   S. mi′nus, a species of uncertain taxonomic classification that causes a form of rat-bite fever (sodoku). This species has never been cultured.

spi•ril•lum, pl. **spi•ril•la** (spī-ril′ŭm, -ă). A member of the genus *Spirillum*.

spir•it (spir′it). **1.** An alcoholic liquor stronger than wine, obtained by distillation. **2.** Any distilled liquid. **3.** An alcoholic or hydroalcoholic solution of volatile substances; some s.'s are used as flavoring agents, others have medicinal value. [L. *spiritus*, a breathing, life soul, fr. *spiro*, to breathe]
   aromatic ammonia s., a hydroalcoholic solution containing approximately 2% ammonia and 4% ammonium carbonate and the aromatics: lemon oil, lavender oil, and myristica oil. Used mainly by inhalation to produce reflex stimulation in persons who have fainted or are at risk of syncope.

△**spiro-, spir-.** **1.** Coil, coil-shaped. [G. *speira*] **2.** Breathing. [L. *spiro*, to breathe]

Spi•ro•chae•ta (spī′rō-kē′tă). A genus of motile bacteria containing Gram-negative, flexible, undulating, spiral-shaped rods which may or may not possess flagelliform, tapering ends. These organisms are motile by means of a creeping motion over the surfaces of supporting objects. They are not parasitic but are found free-living in fresh- or seawater slime; they are commonly found in sewage and foul waters. [Mod. L. fr. G. *speira*, a coil, + *chaitē*, hair]

spi•ro•chet•e•mia (spī′rō-kē-tē′mē-ă). Presence of spirochetes in the blood. [spirochete + G. *haima*, blood]

spi•ro•gram (spī′rō-gram). The tracing made by the spirograph.

spi•ro•graph (spī′rō-graf). A device for representing graphically the depth and rapidity of respiratory movements. [L. *spiro*, to breathe, + G. *graphō*, to write]

spi•rom•e•ter (spī-rom′ĕ-ter). A gasometer used for measuring respiratory gases; usually understood to consist of a counterbalanced cylindrical bell sealed by dipping into a circular trough of water. [L. *spiro*, to breathe, + G. *metron*, measure]

▯**spi•rom•e•try** (spī-rom′ĕ-trē). Making pulmonary measurements with a spirometer.
   closed circuit s., measurement of CO_2 and O_2 in inspired and expired air by means of a device that, along with the subject's respiratory tract, forms a closed circuit.
   open circuit s., measurement of the volume and rate of respiratory air flow by a device into which the subject expels inspired room air.

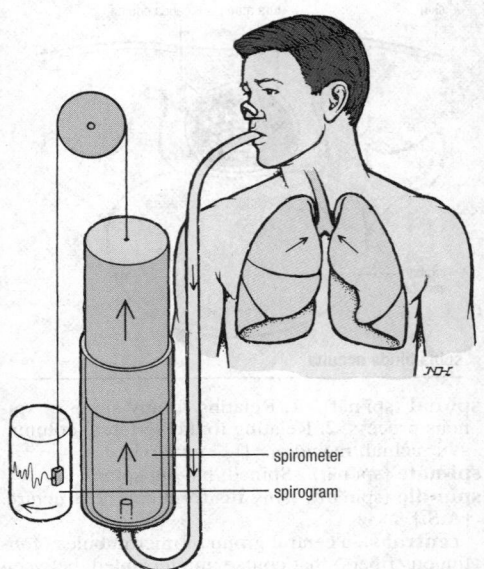

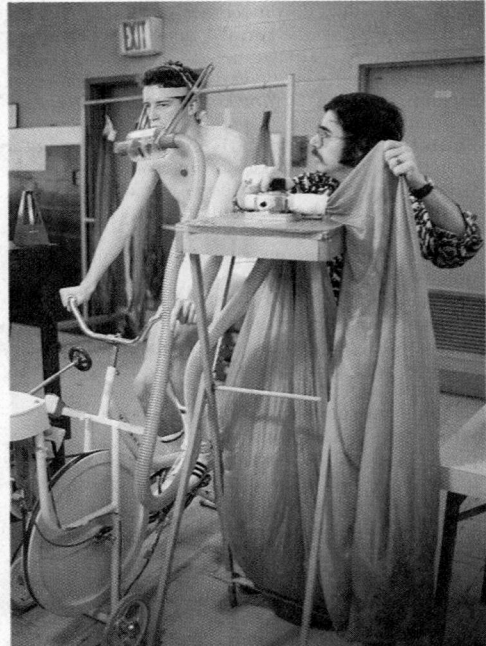

spirometry: (top) principle of closed-circuit spirometry; (bottom) measurement of oxygen uptake using open-circuit spirometry (bag technique) during stationary cycle ergometer exercise

spis•si•tude (spis′i-tūd). The state of being inspissated; the condition of a fluid thickened almost to a solid by evaporation or inspissation. [L. *spissitudo*, fr. *spissus*, thick]

spit·tle (spit'l). SYN saliva. [A.S. *spātl*]

splanchn-. SEE splanchno-.

splanch·nap·o·phys·i·al, splanch·nap·o·phys·e·al (splangk'nă-pō-fiz'ē-ăl). Relating to a splanchnapophysis.

splanch·na·poph·y·sis (splangk'nă-pof'i-sis). An apophysis of the typical vertebra, on the side opposite to the neural apophysis, or any bony process, giving attachment to a viscus or part of the alimentary tract. [splanchn- + G. *apophysis*, offshoot]

splanch·nec·to·pia (splangk-nek-tō'pē-ă). Displacement of any of the viscera. [splanchn- + G. *ektopos*, out of place]

splanch·nes·the·sia (splangk-nes-thē'zē-ă). SYN visceral *sense*. [splanch- + G. *aisthēsis*, sensation]

splanch·nic (splangk'nik). SYN visceral.

splanch·ni·cec·to·my (splangk-ni-sek'tō-mē). Resection of the splanchnic nerves and usually of the celiac ganglion as well. [splanchni- + G. *ektomē*, excision]

splanch·ni·cot·o·my (splangk-ni-kot'ō-mē). Section of a splanchnic nerve or nerves, a surgical procedure formerly used in the treatment of hypertension. [splanchni- + G. *tomē*, incision]

splanchno-, splanchn-, splanchni-. The viscera. SEE ALSO viscero-. [G. *splanchnon*, viscus]

splanch·no·cele (splangk'nō-sēl). **1.** The primitive body cavity or celom in the embryo. [G. *koilos*, hollow] **2.** Hernia of any of the abdominal viscera. [G. *kēlē*, hernia]

splanch·nog·ra·phy (splangk-nog'ră-fē). A treatise on or description of the viscera. [splanchno- + G. *graphō*, to write]

splanch·no·lith (splangk'nō-lith). An intestinal calculus. [splanchno- + G. *lithos*, stone]

splanch·no·meg·a·ly (splangk-nō-meg'ă-lē). SYN visceromegaly. [splanchno- + G. *megas*, large]

splanch·nop·a·thy (splangk-nop'ă-thē). Any disease of the abdominal viscera. [splanchno- + G. *pathos*, disease]

splanch·no·pleure (splangk'nō-plūr). The embryonic layer formed by association of the visceral layer of the lateral plate mesoderm with the endoderm. [splanchno- + G. *pleura*, side]

splanch·nop·to·sis, splanch·nop·to·sia (splangk'nō-tō'sis, -tō'sē-ă). SYN visceroptosis. [splanchno- + G. *ptōsis* a falling]

splanch·no·scle·ro·sis (splangk'nō-skle-rō'sis). Hardening, through connective tissue overgrowth, of any of the viscera. [splanchno- + G. *sklērōsis*, hardening]

splanch·no·skel·e·tal (splangk-nō-skel'ĕ-tăl). SYN visceroskeletal.

splanch·no·skel·e·ton (splangk-nō-skel'ĕ-tŏn). SYN visceroskeleton (2).

splanch·no·tribe (splangk'nō-trīb). An instrument resembling a large angiotribe used for occluding the intestine temporarily, prior to resection. [splanchno- + G. *tribō*, to rub, bruise]

spleen (splēn). A large vascular lymphatic organ lying in the upper part of the abdominal cavity on the left side, between the stomach and diaphragm, composed of white and red pulp; the white consists of lymphatic nodules and diffuse lymphatic tissue; the red consists of venous sinusoids between which are splenic cords; the stroma of both red and white pulp is reticular fibers and cells. A framework of fibroelastic trabeculae extending from the capsule subdivides the structure into poorly defined lobules. It is a blood-forming organ in early life and later a storage organ for red corpuscles and platelets; because of the large number of macrophages, it also acts as a blood filter, both identifying and destroying effete erythrocytes. SYN lien ★ [NA]. [G. *splēn*]

accessory s., one of the small globular masses of splenic tissue occasionally found in the region of the spleen, in one of the peritoneal folds or elsewhere. SYN lien accessorius.

diffuse waxy s., a condition of amyloid degeneration of the s., affecting chiefly the extrasinusoidal tissue spaces of the pulp.

floating s., a s. that is palpable because of excessive mobility from a relaxed or lengthened pedicle rather than because of enlargement. SYN lien mobilis, movable s.

movable s., SYN floating s.

sago s., amyloidosis in the s. affecting chiefly the malpighian bodies.

waxy s., amyloidosis of the s.

splen-. SEE spleno-.

sple·nec·to·my (splē-nek'tō-mē). Removal of the spleen. [splen- + G. *ektomē*, excision]

sple·nec·to·pia, sple·nec·to·py (splen'ek-tō'pē-ă, splē-nek'tō-pē). **1.** Displacement of the spleen, as in a floating spleen. **2.** The presence of rests of splenic tissue, usually in the region of the spleen. [splen- + G. *ektopos*, out of place]

splen·ic (splen'ik). Relating to the spleen. SYN lienal.

sple·ni·tis (splē-nī'tis). Inflammation of the spleen. [splen- + G. *-itis*, inflammation]

sple·ni·um, pl. **sple·nia** (splē'nē-ŭm, -ă). **1.** A compress or bandage. **2** [NA]. A structure resembling a bandaged part. [Mod. L. fr. G. *splēnion*, bandage]

s. cor'poris callo'si [NA], SYN s. of corpus callosum.

s. of corpus callosum, the thickened posterior extremity of the corpus callosum. SYN corporis s. callosi [NA].

spleno-, splen-. The spleen. [G. *splēn*]

sple·no·cele (splē'nō-sēl). **1.** SYN splenoma. **2.** A splenic hernia. [spleno- + G. *kēlē*, tumor, hernia]

sple·no·he·pa·to·meg·a·ly, sple·no·he·pa·to·me·ga·lia (splē'nō-hep'ă-tō-meg'ă-lē, -mĕ-gā'ē-ă). Enlargement of both spleen and liver. [spleno- + G. *hēpar*, liver, + *megas*, large]

sple·noid (splē'noyd). Resembling the spleen. [spleno- + G. *eidos*, resemblance]

sple·no·ma (splē-nō'mă). General nonspecific term for an enlarged spleen. SYN splenocele (1). [spleno- + G. *-oma*, tumor]

sple·no·ma·la·cia (splē'nō-mă-lā'shē-ă). Softening of the spleen. [spleno- + G. *malakia*, softness]

sple·no·med·ul·lary (splē-nō-med'ŭ-lār-ē). SYN splenomyelogenous. [spleno- + L. *medulla*, marrow]

sple·no·meg·a·ly, sple·no·me·ga·lia (splē-nō-meg'ă-lē, -mĕ-gā'lē-ă). Enlargement of the spleen. SYN megalosplenia. [spleno- + G. *megas* (*megal*-), large]

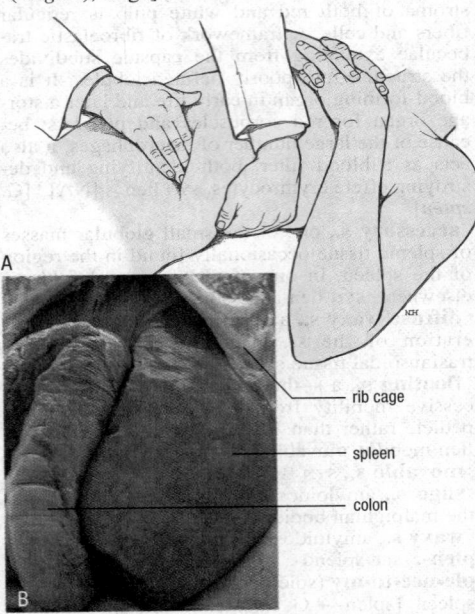

A

B

splenomegaly: (A) showing palpation technique used in diagnosis; (B) splenomegaly due to granulocytic leukemia (weight of spleen: 9 lbs. 2 oz.)

rib cage

spleen

colon

congestive s., enlargement of the spleen due to passive congestion; sometimes used as a synonym for Banti's syndrome.

hemolytic s., s. associated with congenital hemolytic jaundice.

hyperreactive malarious s., a syndrome characterized by persistent splenomegaly, exceptionally high serum IgM and malaria antibody levels, and hepatic sinusoidal lymphocytosis. SYN tropical splenomegaly syndrome.

sple·no·my·e·log·e·nous (splē′nō-mī-ĕ-loj′ĕ-nŭs). Originating in the spleen and bone marrow, denoting a form of leukemia. SYN splenomedullary. [spleno- + G. *myelos*, marrow, + -*gen*, producing]

sple·no·my·e·lo·ma·la·cia (splē′nō-mī′ĕ-lō-mă-lā′shē-ă). Pathologic softening of the spleen and bone marrow. [spleno- + G. *myelos*, marrow, + *malakia*, softness]

sple·nop·a·thy (splē-nop′ă-thē). Any disease of the spleen. [spleno- + G. *pathos*, suffering]

sple·no·pexy, sple·no·pex·ia (splē′nō-pek-sē, splē-nō-pek′sē-ă). Suturing in place an ectopic or floating spleen. SYN splenorrhaphy (2). [spleno- + G. *pēxis*, fixation]

sple·no·por·tog·ra·phy (splē′nō-pōr-tog′ră-fē). Introduction of radiopaque material into the spleen to obtain an x-ray visualization of the portal vessel of the portal circulation. [spleno- + portography]

sple·nop·to·sis, sple·nop·to·sia (splē-nop-tō′sis, -tō′sē-ă). Downward displacement of the spleen,

as in a floating spleen. [spleno- + G. *ptōsis*, falling]

sple·nor·rha·gia (splē′nō-rā′jē-ă). Hemorrhage from a ruptured spleen. [spleno- + G. *rhēgnymi*, to burst forth]

sple·nor·rha·phy (splē-nōr′ă-fē). **1.** Suturing a ruptured spleen. **2.** SYN splenopexy. [spleno- + G. *rhaphē*, suture]

sple·not·o·my (splē-not′ō-mē). **1.** Anatomy or dissection of the spleen. **2.** Surgical incision of the spleen. [spleno- + G. *tomē*, incision]

sple·no·tox·in (splē-nō-tok′sin). A cytotoxin specific for cells of the spleen. [spleno- + G. *toxikon*, poison]

splic·ing (splīs′ing). **1.** Attachment of one DNA molecule to another. SYN gene splicing. **2.** Removal of introns from mRNA precursors and the reattachment or annealing of exons. SYN RNA splicing.

splint. 1. An appliance for preventing movement of a joint or for the fixation of displaced or movable parts. **2.** The s. bone, or fibula. [Middle Dutch *splinte*]

active s., SYN dynamic s.

air s., a plastic s. inflated by air used to immobilize part or all of an extremity.

airplane s., a complicated s. that holds the arm in abduction at about shoulder level with the forearm midway in flexion, generally with an axillary strut for support.

anchor s., a s. used for fracture of the jaw, with wires around teeth and a rod to hold it in place.

Anderson s., a skeletal traction s. with pins inserted into proximal and distal ends of a fracture; reduction is obtained by an external plate attached to the pins.

backboard s., a board s. with slots for fixation by straps; shorter ones are used for neck injuries, longer ones for back injuries.

Balkan s., SYN Balkan *frame*.

coaptation s., a short s. designed to prevent overriding of the ends of a fractured bone, usually supplemented by a longer s. to fix the entire limb.

contact s., a slotted plate, held by screws, used in the treatment of fracture of long bones.

Denis Browne s., a light aluminum s. applied to the lateral aspect of the leg and foot; used for clubfoot.

dynamic s., a s. utilizing springs or elastic bands that aids in movements initiated by the patient by controlling the plane and range of motion. SYN active s., functional s. (1).

Frejka pillow s., a pillow s. used for abduction and flexion of the femurs in treatment of congenital hip dysplasia or dislocation in infants.

functional s., (1) SYN dynamic s. **(2)** the joining of two or more teeth into a rigid unit by means of fixed restorations that cover all or part of the abutment teeth.

interdental s., a s. for a fractured jaw, consisting of two metal or acrylic resin bands wired to the teeth of the upper and lower jaws, respectively, and then fastened together to keep the jaws immovable.

labial s., an appliance of plastic, metal, or in combination, made to conform to the outer aspect of the dental arch and used in the management of jaw and facial injuries.

ladder s., a flexible s. consisting of two stout parallel wires with finer cross wires.

pillow s., a s. that is inflatable or that is made from unusually bulky fabric.

surgical s., general term for a device used to maintain tissues in a new position following surgery.

Thomas s., a long leg s. extending from a ring at the hip to beyond the foot, allowing traction to a fractured leg, for emergencies and transportation.

split·ting. CHEMISTRY The cleavage of a covalent bond, fragmenting the molecule involved.

spm A gene that leads to *sup*pression and *mut*ation of mutants that are unstable.

spo·dog·e·nous (spŏ-doj'ĕ-nŭs). Caused by waste material. [G. *spodos*, ashes, + *-gen*, producing]

spon·dee (spon'dē). A bisyllabic word with generally equivalent stress on each of the two syllables; used in the testing of speech hearing. [Fr.]

spondyl-. SEE spondylo-.

spon·dy·lal·gia (spon-di-lal'jē-ă). Pain in the spine. [spondyl- + G. *algos*, pain]

spon·dy·lar·thri·tis (spon'dil-ar-thrī'tis). Inflammation of the intervertebral articulations. [spondyl- + G. *arthron*, joint, + *-itis*, inflammation]

spon·dy·lit·ic (spon-di-lit'ik). Relating to spondylitis.

spon·dy·li·tis (spon-di-lī'tis). Inflammation of one or more of the vertebrae. [spondyl- + G. *-itis*, inflammation]

ankylosing s., arthritis of the spine, resembling rheumatoid arthritis, that may progress to bony ankylosis with lipping of vertebral margins; the disease is more common in the male, often with the rheumatoid factor absent and the HLA antigen present. There is a striking association with the B27 tissue type and the strong familial aggregation suggests an important genetic factor. SYN rheumatoid s.

s. defor'mans, arthritis and osteitis deformans involving the spinal column; marked by nodular deposits at the edges of the intervertebral disks with ossification of the ligaments and bony ankylosis of the intervertebral articulations, it results in a rounded kyphosis with rigidity. SYN Bechterew's disease.

rheumatoid s., SYN ankylosing s.

tuberculous s., tuberculous infection of the spine associated with a sharp angulation of the spine at the point of disease. SYN Pott's disease.

△**spondylo-, spondyl-.** The vertebrae. [G. *spondylos*, vertebra]

⚑ **spon·dy·lo·lis·the·sis** (spon'di-lō-lis-thē'sis). Forward movement of the body of one of the lower lumbar vertebrae on the vertebra below it, or upon the sacrum. [spondylo- + G. *olisthēsis*, a slipping and falling]

spon·dy·lo·lis·thet·ic (spon'di-lō-lis-thet'ik). Relating to or marked by spondylolisthesis.

spon·dy·lol·y·sis (spon-di-lol'i-sis). Degeneration or deficient development of the articulating part of a vertebra. [spondylo- + G. *lysis*, loosening]

spon·dy·lop·a·thy (spon-di-lop'ă-thē). Any disease of the vertebrae or spinal column. [spondylo- + G. *pathos*, suffering]

spon·dy·lo·py·o·sis (spon'di-lō-pī-ō'sis). Suppurative inflammation of one or more of the vertebral bodies. [spondylo- + G. *pyōsis*, suppuration]

spon·dy·los·chi·sis (spon-di-los'ki-sis). Embryologic failure of fusion of vertebral arch. SEE *spina bifida*. [spondylo- + G. *schisis*, fissure]

spon·dy·lo·sis (spon-di-lō'sis). Ankylosis of the vertebra; often applied nonspecifically to any lesion of the spine of a degenerative nature. [G. *spondylos*, vertebra]

spon·dy·lo·syn·de·sis (spon'di-lō-sin-dē'sis). SYN spinal *fusion*. [spondylo- + G. *syndesis*, binding together]

sponge (spŭnj). **1.** Absorbent material, such as gauze or prepared cotton, used to absorb fluids. **2.** A member of the phylum Porifera, the cellular endoskeleton of which is a source of commercial s.'s. [G. *spongia*]

contraceptive s., a resilient, hydrophilic s. of polyurethane foam impregnated with a spermicide; contraception is achieved by action of the spermicide.

spon·gi·form (spŭn'ji-fōrm). SYN spongy.

△**spongio-.** Sponge, sponglike, spongy. [G. *spongia*]

spon·gi·o·blast (spŭn'jē-ō-blast). A neuroepithelial, filiform ependyma cell extending across the entire thickness of the wall of the brain or spinal

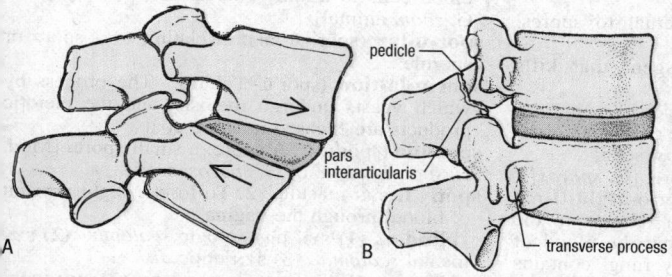

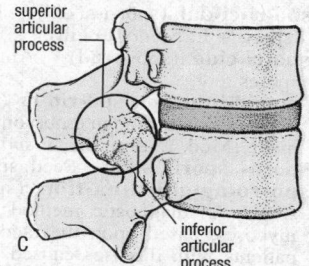

spondylolisthesis: (A) showing forward slippage of lumbar vertebrae; **spondylolysis:** (B) showing fracture of pars interarticularis; **spondylosis:** (C) showing fixation of the articular processes

cord, *i.e.,* from the internal to the external limiting membrane; s.'s become neuroglial and ependymal cells. SEE ALSO glioblast. [spongio- + G. *blastos,* germ]

spon•gi•o•blas•to•ma (spŭn'jē-ō-blas-tō'mă). **1.** A glioma consisting of cells (elongated, spindle-shaped, and sometimes pleomorphic, with one or two fibrillary processes) that resemble the embryonic spongioblasts, occurring normally around the neural canal of the human embryo; it grows relatively slowly, usually originating in the brainstem, optic chiasm, or infundibulum, and infiltrates adjacent structures or causes compression of the third and fourth ventricle. [spongioblast + G. *-oma* tumor]

spon•gi•o•cyte (spŭn'jē-ō-sīt). **1.** A neuroglial cell. **2.** A cell in the zona fasciculata of the adrenal containing many droplets of lipid material which, after staining with hematoxylin and eosin, show pronounced vacuolization. [spongio- + G. *kytos,* cell]

spon•gi•oid (spŭn'jē-oyd). SYN spongy. [spongio- + G. *eidos,* resemblance]

spon•gi•ose (spŭn'jē-ōs). Resembling or characteristic of a sponge. [L. *spongiosus*]

spon•gi•o•sis (spŭn-jē-ō'sis). Inflammatory intercellular edema of the epidermis.

spon•gi•o•si•tis (spŭn-jē-ō-sī'tis). Inflammation of the corpus spongiosum, or corpus cavernosum urethrae.

spongy (spŭn'jē). Of spongelike texture or appearance. SYN spongiform, spongioid.

△**spor-.** SEE sporo-.

spo•rad•ic (spō-rad'ik). **1.** Denoting a temporal pattern of disease occurrence in an animal or human population in which the disease occurs only rarely and without regularity. SEE ALSO endemic, epidemic, epizootic. **2.** Occurring irregularly, haphazardly. [G. *sporadikos,* scattered]

spo•ran•gi•um (spō-ran'jē-ŭm). A saclike structure (a cell) within a fungus, in which asexual spores are borne by progressive cleavage. [L. fr. G. *sporos,* seed, + *angeion,* vessel]

spore (spōr). **1.** The asexual or sexual reproductive body of fungi or sporozoan protozoa. **2.** A cell of a plant lower in organization than the seed-bearing spermatophytic plants. **3.** A resistant form of certain species of bacteria. **4.** The highly modified reproductive body of certain protozoa, as in the phyla Microspora and Myxozoa. [G. *sporos,* seed]

spo•ri•ci•dal (spōr-i-sī'dăl). Lethal to spores. [spori- + L. *caedo,* to kill]

spo•ri•cide (spōr'i-sīd). An agent that kills spores.

spo•rid•i•um, pl. **spo•rid•ia** (spō-rid'ē-ŭm, -ă). A protozoan spore; an embryonic protozoan organism. [Mod. L. dim., fr. G. *sporos,* seed]

△**sporo-, spori-, spor-.** Seed, spore. [G. *sporos*]

spo•ro•ag•glu•ti•na•tion (spōr'ō-ă-glū-ti-nā'shŭn). A diagnostic method in relation to the mycoses, based upon the fact that the blood of patients with diseases caused by fungi contains specific agglutinins that cause clumping of the spores of these organisms.

spo•ro•blast (spōr'ō-blast). An early stage in the development of a sporocyst prior to differentia-

tion of the sporozoites. SEE ALSO oocyst, sporocyst (2). [sporo- + G. *blastos,* germ]

spo•ro•cyst (spōr'ō-sist). **1.** A larval form of digenetic trematode (fluke) that develops in the body of its molluscan intermediate host, usually a snail. SEE ALSO cercaria. **2.** A secondary cyst that develops within the oocyst of Coccidia, a group of sporozoans that includes many of the most important disease agents of domestic animals and fowl. [sporo- + G. *kystis,* bladder]

spo•ro•gen•e•sis (spōr-ō-jen'ĕ-sis). SYN sporogony. [sporo- + G. *genesis,* production]

spo•rog•e•nous (spŏ-roj'ĕ-nŭs). Relating to or involved in sporogony.

spo•rog•e•ny (spŏ-roj'ĕ-nē). SYN sporogony.

spo•rog•o•ny (spŏ-rog'ŏ-nē). The formation of sporozoites in sporozoan protozoa, a process of asexual division within the sporoblast, which becomes the sporocyst within an oocyst; follows fusion of gametes (gametogony) and zygote (sporont) formation. SYN sporogenesis, sporogeny. [sporo- + G. *goneia,* generation]

spo•ront (spōr'ont). The zygote stage within the oocyst wall in the life cycle of coccidia; gives rise to sporoblasts, which form sporocysts, within which the infective sporozoites are produced. [sporo- + G. *ōn (ont-),* being]

Spo•ro•thrix (spōr'ō-thriks). A genus of dimorphic imperfect fungi, including *S. schenckii,* an organism of worldwide distribution and the causative agent of sporotrichosis in humans and animals. [Mod. L., fr. G. *sporos,* seed, + *thrix,* hair]

spo•ro•tri•cho•sis (spōr'ō-tri-kō'sis). A chronic cutaneous mycosis spread by way of the lymphatics and caused by inoculation of *Sporothrix schenckii,* typically rare in tissue sections but rapidly growing in cultures. The disease may remain localized or may become generalized, involving bones, joints, lungs, and the central nervous system; lesions may be granulomatous or suppurative, ulcerative, or draining.

spo•ro•zo•ite (spōr-ō-zō'īt). One of the minute elongated bodies resulting from the repeated division of the oocyst during sporogony. In the case of the malarial parasite, it is the form that is concentrated in the salivary glands and introduced into the blood by the bite of a mosquito; it enters the liver cells (exoerythrocytic cycle), whose progeny, the merozoites, infect the red blood cells to initiate clinical malaria. [sporo- + G. *zōon,* animal]

spor•u•lar (spōr'yū-lăr). Relating to a spore or sporule.

spor•u•la•tion (spōr'ū-lā'shŭn). The process by which yeasts undergo meiosis, and the meiotic products are encased in spore coats.

spor•ule (spōr'ūl). A spore; a small spore. [Mod. L. *sporula;* dim. of G. *sporos,* seed]

spot. 1. SYN macula. **2.** To lose a slight amount of blood through the vagina.

   blind s., (1) SYN physiologic *scotoma.* **(2)** SYN mental *scotoma.* **(3)** SYN optic *disk.*

   blue s., (1) SYN *macula* cerulea. **(2)** SYN mongolian s.

   cherry-red s., the ophthalmoscopic appearance of the normal choroid beneath the fovea centralis, appearing as a red s. surrounded by white retinal edema in central artery closure or lipid infiltration in sphingolipidosis.

Fordyce's s.'s, a condition marked by the presence of numerous small, yellowish-white bodies or granules on the inner surface and vermilion border of the lips; histologically the lesions are ectopic sebaceous glands.

hot s., a region in a gene in which there is a putatively high rate of mutation.

hypnogenic s., a pressure-sensitive point on the body of certain susceptible persons, which, when pressed, causes the induction of sleep.

liver s., SYN senile *lentigo.*

mongolian s., any of a number of dark-bluish or mulberry-colored rounded or oval s.'s on the sacral region due to the ectopic presence of scattered melanocytes in the dermis. These congenital lesions are frequent in black, Native American, and Asian children from 2 to 12 years, after which time they gradually recede; they do not disappear on pressure and are sometimes mistaken for bruises from child abuse. SYN blue s. (2).

rose s.'s, characteristic exanthema of typhoid fever; 10–20 small pink papules on the lower trunk lasting a few days and leaving hyperpigmentation.

sprain (sprān). **1.** An injury to a ligament when the joint is carried through a range of motion greater than normal, but without dislocation or fracture. **2.** To cause a s. of a joint.

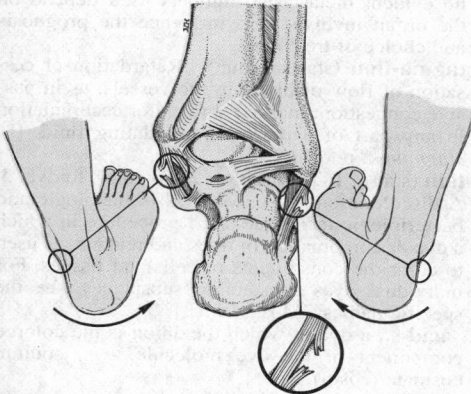

sprain: involving ankle ligaments

spray (sprā). A jet of liquid in fine drops, coarser than a vapor; it is produced by forcing the liquid from the minute opening of an atomizer, mixed with air.

sprue (sprū). **1.** Primary intestinal malabsorption with steatorrhea. **2.** DENTISTRY Wax or metal used to form the aperture(s) for molten metal to flow into a mold to make a casting; also, the metal that later fills the s. hole(s). [D. *spruw*]

nontropical s., s. occurring in persons away from the tropics; usually called celiac disease; due to gluten-induced enteropathy.

tropical s., s. occurring in the tropics, often associated with enteric infection and nutritional

deficiency, and frequently complicated by folate deficiency with macrocytic anemia. SYN tropical diarrhea.

spud (spŭd). A triangular knife used for removing foreign bodies from the cornea.

spur (sper). SYN calcar. [A.S. *spora*]

  bone s., SYN heel s.

  calcaneal s., SYN heel s.

  heel s., an abnormal bony growth on the calcaneus. SYN bone s., calcaneal s.

spu·ri·ous (spū'rē-ŭs). False; not genuine. [L. *spurius*]

spu·tum, pl. **spu·ta** (spū'tŭm, -tă). **1.** Expectorated matter, especially mucus or mucopurulent matter expectorated in diseases of the air passages. SEE ALSO expectoration (1). **2.** An individual mass of such matter. [L. *sputum,* fr. *spuo,* pp. *sputus,* to spit]

  nummular s., a thick, coherent mass expectorated in globular shape which does not run at the bottom of the cup but forms a discoid mass resembling a coin.

  rusty s., a reddish brown, blood-stained expectoration characteristic of pneumonococcal lobar pneumonia.

SQ subcutaneous.

squa·ma, pl. **squa·mae** (skwā'mă, skwā'mē). **1.** A thin plate of bone. **2.** An epidermal scale. SYN scale (2), squame. [L. a scale]

squa·mate (skwā'māt). SYN squamous.

squame (skwām). SYN squama.

squamo-. Squama, squamous. [L. *squama,* a scale]

squa·mo·sa, pl. **squa·mo·sae** (skwā-mō'să, -sē). The squamous parts of the frontal, occipital, or temporal bone, especially the latter. [L. *squamosus,* scaly, fr. *squama,* scale]

squa·mo·sal (skwā-mō'săl). Relating especially to the squamous part of the temporal bone.

squa·mous (skwā'mŭs). Relating to or covered with scales. SYN scaly, squamate. [L. *squamosus*]

squa·mo·zy·go·mat·ic (skwā'mō-zī-gō-mat'ik). Relating to the squamous part of the temporal bone and the zygomatic process of the temporal bone.

squint (skwint). SYN strabismus.

Sr strontium.

SRH somatotropin-releasing *hormone.*

sRNA soluble RNA. See entries under ribonucleic acid.

SRS slow-reacting *substance.*

SSPE subacute sclerosing *panencephalitis.*

SSRI selective serotonin reuptake *inhibitor.*

ST scapulothoracic.

sta·bi·late (stā'bi-lāt). A sample of organisms preserved alive on a single occasion.

sta·bile (stā'bīl, -bil). Steady; fixed; denoting: 1) certain constituents of serum unaffected by moderate heating or prolonged storage; 2) an electrode held steadily on a part during the passage of an electric current. Cf. labile. [L. *stabilis*]

sta·bil·i·ty (stă-bil'i-tē). The condition of being stable or resistant to change.

  denture s., the quality of a denture to be firm, steady, constant, and resist change of position when functional forces are applied. SYN stabilization (2).

endemic s., a situation in which all factors influencing disease occurrence are relatively stable, resulting in little fluctuation in disease incidence over time; changes in one or more of these factors (*e.g.,* reduction in proportion of individuals with immunity from exposure to infectious agent) can lead to an unstable situation in which major disease outbreaks occur. SYN enzootic s.

   enzootic s., SYN endemic s.

sta·bi·li·za·tion (stā′bĭ-li-zā′shŭn). **1.** The accomplishment of a stable state. **2.** SYN denture *stability.*

sta·ble (stā′bl). Steady; not varying; resistant to change. SEE ALSO stabile.

staff. 1. A specific group of workers. **2.** SYN director (1). [A.S. *staef*]

   attending s., physicians and surgeons who are members of a hospital s. and regularly attend their patients at the hospital; may also supervise and teach house s., fellows, and medical students.

   consulting s., specialists affiliated with a hospital who serve in an advisory capacity to the attending s.

   house s., physicians and surgeons in specialty training at a hospital who care for the patients under the direction and responsibility of the attending s.

staff of Aes·cu·la·pi·us. A rod with only one serpent encircling it and without wings; symbol of medicine and emblem of the American Medical Association, Royal Army Medical Corps (Britain), and Royal Canadian Medical Corps. SEE ALSO caduceus. [L. *Aesculapius,* G. *Asklēpios,* god of medicine]

stage (stāj). **1.** A period in the course of a disease; a description of the extent of involvement of a disease process or the status of a patient with a specific disease, as of the distribution and extent of dissemination of a malignant neoplastic disease; also, the act of determining the s. of a disease, especially cancer. SEE ALSO period. **2.** The part of a microscope on which the microscope slide bears the object to be examined. **3.** A particular step, phase, or position in a developmental process. For psychosexual stages, see entries under phase. [M.E. thr. O. Fr. *estage,* standing-place, fr. L. *sto,* pp. *status,* to stand]

   algid s., the s. of collapse in cholera.

   cold s., the s. of chill in a malarial paroxysm.

   end s., the late, fully developed phase of a disease.

   exoerythrocytic s., developmental s. of the malaria parasite (*Plasmodium*) in liver parenchyma cells of the vertebrate host before erythrocytes are invaded. The initial generation produces cryptozoites, the next generation metacryptozoites; reinfection of liver cells from blood cells apparently does not occur.

   imperfect s., a mycological term used to describe the asexual life cycle phase of a fungus.

   incubative s., SYN incubation *period* (1).

   intuitive s., PSYCHOLOGY a s. of development, usually occurring between 4 and 7 years of age, in which the most prominent aspects of the stimuli to which a child is exposed, rather than any form of logical thought, determine the child's thought processes.

s.'s of labor, SEE labor.

latent s., SYN incubation *period* (1).

perfect s., a mycological term used to describe the sexual life cycle phase of a fungus in which spores are formed after nuclear fusion.

preconceptual s., PSYCHOLOGY the s. of development in an infant's life, prior to actual conceptual thinking, in which sensorimotor activity predominates.

prodromal s., SYN incubation *period* (1).

Tanner s., a s. of puberty in the Tanner growth chart, based on pubic hair growth, development of genitalia in boys, and breast development in girls.

tumor s., the extent of the spread of a malignant neoplasm from its site of origin. SEE ALSO TNM *staging.*

stag·ing (stāj′ing). **1.** The determination or classification of distinct phases or periods in the course of a disease or pathological process. **2.** The determination of the specific extent of a disease process in an individual patient.

   Jewett and Strong s., s. of bladder carcinoma: O, noninvasive; A, with submucosal invasion; B, with muscle invasion; C, with invasion of perivascular fat; D, with lymph node metastasis.

   TNM s., a system of clinicopathologic evaluation of tumors based on the extent of tumor involvement at the primary site (T, followed by a number indicating size and depth of invasion), and lymph node involvement (N) and metastasis (M), each followed by a number starting at 0 for no evident metastasis; numbers used depend on the organ involved and influence the prognosis and choice of treatment.

stag·na·tion (stag-nā′shŭn). Retardation or cessation of flow of blood in the vessels, as in passive congestion; marked slowing or accumulation in any part of a normally circulating fluid. [L. *stagnum,* a pool]

stain (stān). **1.** To discolor. **2.** To color; to dye. **3.** A discoloration. **4.** A dye used in histologic and bacteriologic technique. **5.** A procedure in which a dye or combination of dyes and reagents is used to color the constituents of cells and tissues. For individual dyes or staining substances, see the specific names. [M.E. *steinen*]

   acid s., a dye in which the anion is the colored component of the dye molecule, *e.g.,* sodium eosinate (eosin).

   basic s., a dye in which the cation is the colored component of the dye molecule that binds to anionic groups of nucleic acids ($PO_4\equiv$) or acidic mucopolysaccharides.

   basic fuchsin-methylene blue s., a s. for intact epoxy sections; semithick sections of plastic-embedded tissues have nuclei stained purple; collagen, elastic lamina, and connective tissue are stained blue; mitochondria, myelin, and lipid droplets are stained red; cytoplasm, smooth muscle cells, axoplasm, and chondroblast are stained pink.

   C-banding s., a selective chromosome banding s. used in human cytogenetics, employing Giemsa s. after most of the DNA is denatured or extracted by treatment with alkali, acid, salt, or heat; only heterochromatic regions close to the centromeres and rich in satellite DNA stain, with the exception of the Y chromosome, whose long arm usually stains throughout.

contrast s., a dye used to color one portion of a tissue or cell which remained unaffected when the other part was stained by a dye of different color.

double s., a mixture of two dyes, each of which stains different portions of a tissue or cell.

fluorescent s., a s. or staining procedure using a fluorescent dye or substance that will combine selectively with certain tissue components and that will then fluoresce upon irradiation with ultraviolet or violet-blue light.

G-banding s., a chromosome-staining technique used in human cytogenetics to identify individual chromosomes, which produces characteristic bands; it utilizes acetic acid, proteolytic enzymes, salts, heat, detergents, or urea, and finally Giemsa s.; chromosome bands appear similar to those fluorochromed by Q-banding s.

Giemsa s., compound of methylene blue-eosin and methylene blue used for demonstrating Negri bodies, *Tunga* species, spirochetes and protozoans, and differential staining of blood smears; also used for chromosomes, sometimes after hydrolyzing the cytologic preparation in hot hydrochloric acid, and for showing chromosome G bands.

Golgi's s., any of several methods for staining nerve cells, nerve fibers, and neuroglia using fixation and hardening in formalin-osmic-dichromate combinations for various times, followed by impregnation with silver nitrate.

Gram's s., a method for differential staining of bacteria; smears are fixed by flaming, stained in a solution of crystal violet, treated with iodine solution, rinsed, decolorized, and then counterstained with safranin O; Gram-positive organisms stain purple-black and Gram-negative organisms stain pink; useful in bacterial taxonomy and identification, and also in indicating fundamental differences in cell wall structure.

hematoxylin and eosin s., the most generally useful staining method for tissues; nuclei are stained a deep blue-black with hematoxylin, and cytoplasm is stained pink after counterstaining with eosin, usually in water.

immunofluorescent s., s. resulting from combination of fluorescent antibody with antigen specific for the antibody portion of the fluorochrome conjugate.

intravital s., a s. which is taken up by living cells after parenteral administration, *e.g.,* intravenously or subcutaneously.

iodine s., a s. to detect amyloid, cellulose, chitin, starch, carotenes, and glycogen, and to stain amebas by virtue of their glycogen; feces and other wet preparations are stained directly with Lugol's iodine solution; smears are treated with Schaudinn's fixative and then stained with alcoholic iodine, followed by Heidenhain's iron hematoxylin.

metachromatic s., a s., such as methylene blue, thionine, or azure A, that interacts chemically with certain histologic or cytologic structures, yielding a color different from that of the stain.

multiple s., a mixture of several dyes each having an independent selective action on one or more portions of the tissue.

negative s., s. forming an opaque or colored background against which the object to be demonstrated appears as a translucent or colorless area; in electron microscopy, an electron opaque material, such as phosphotungstic acid or sodium phosphotungstate, is used to give detail as to surface structure.

neutral s., a compound of an acid s. and a basic s., such as the eosinate of methylene blue, in which the anion and cation each contains a chromophore group.

nuclear s., a s. for cell nuclei, usually based on the binding of a basic dye to DNA or nucleohistone.

Papanicolaou s., a multichromatic s. used principally on exfoliated cytologic specimens and based on aqueous hematoxylin with multiple counterstaining dyes in 95% ethyl alcohol, giving great transparency and delicacy of detail; important in cancer screening, especially of gynecologic smears.

picrocarmine s., a red crystalline powder derived from a solution of carmine, ammonia, and picric acid which is evaporated, leaving the powder (soluble in water); it produces excellent staining of keratohyaline granules.

port-wine s., SYN *nevus* flammeus.

positive s., direct binding of a dye with a tissue component to produce contrast; in electron microscopy, heavy metals like uranyl and lead salts are used to bind to selective cell constituents to produce increased density to the electron beam, *i.e.,* contrast.

Puchtler-Sweat s.'s, SEE Puchtler-Sweat s. for basement membranes, Puchtler-Sweat s. for hemoglobin and hemosiderin.

Puchtler-Sweat s. for basement membranes, a staining method using resorcin-fuchsin and nuclear fast red solutions after Carnoy's fixative; basement membranes are gray to black and nuclei pink to red.

Puchtler-Sweat s. for hemoglobin and hemosiderin, a complex staining method in which, on a yellow background, hemoglobin is stained red, hemosiderin blue to green and elastic fibers are pink.

Q-banding s., a fluorescent s. for chromosomes which produces specific banding patterns for each pair of homologous chromosomes; the acridine dye derivative, quinacrine hydrochloride, or other derivatives like quinacrine mustard dihydrochloride produces a green-yellow fluorescence at pH 4.5 in chromosome segments rich in constitutive heterochromatin with deoxyadenylate-deoxythymidilate (A-T) bases of DNA; centromeric regions of human chromosomes 3, 4, and 13 are specifically stained, as are satellites of some acrocentric chromosomes and the end of the long arm of the Y chromosome.

R-banding s., a reverse Giemsa chromosome banding method that produces bands complementary to G-bands; induced by treatment with high temperature, low pH, or acridine orange staining; often used together with G-banding on human karyotype to determine whether there are deletions.

selective s., a s. that colors one portion of a tissue or cell exclusively or more deeply than the remaining portions.

silver protein s., a silver proteinate complex used in staining nerve fibers, nerve endings, and flagellate protozoa; also used to demonstrate phagocytosis in living animals by the cells of the reticuloendothelial system.

supravital s., a procedure in which living tissue is removed from the body and cells are placed in a nontoxic dye solution so that their vital processes may be studied.

trichrome s., staining combinations which usually contain three dyes of contrasting colors selected to stain connective tissue, muscle, cytoplasm, and nuclei in bright colors; generally, tissue sections are first dyed in iron hematoxylin before being treated with the other dyes.

vital s., a s. applied to cells or parts of cells while they are still living.

Wright's s., a staining mixture of eosinates of polychromed methylene blue used in staining of blood smears.

stain•ing (stān′ing). **1.** The act of applying a stain. SEE ALSO stain. **2.** DENTISTRY Modification of the color of the tooth or denture base.

progressive s., a procedure in which s. is continued until the desired intensity of coloring of tissue elements is attained.

regressive s., a type of s. in which tissues are overstained and the excess dye is then removed selectively until the desired intensity is obtained.

stair•case (stār′kās). A series of reactions that follow one another in progressively increasing or decreasing intensity, so that a chart shows a continuous rise or fall. SEE treppe.

stal•ag•mom•e•ter (stal-ăg-mom′ē-ter). An instrument for determining exactly the number of drops in a given quantity of liquid; used as a measure of the surface tension of a fluid (the lower the tension, the smaller the drops and, consequently, the more numerous in a given quantity of the fluid). [G. *stalagma*, a drop, + *metron*, measure]

stalk (stawk). A narrowed connection with a structure or organ.

allantoic s., the narrow connection between the intraembryonic portion of the allantois and the extraembryonic allantoic vesicle.

infundibular s., SYN infundibular *stem.*

pineal s., the attachment of the pineal body to the roof of the third ventricle; it contains the pineal recess of the third ventricle.

pituitary s., a process comprising the tuberal part investing the infundibular stem that attaches the hypophysis to the tuber cinereum at the base of the brain.

yolk s., the narrowed connection between the intraembryonic gut and the yolk sac; its walls are splanchnopleure. SYN omphalomesenteric duct.

stam•mer•ing (stam′er-ing). **1.** A speech disorder characterized by hesitation and repetition of words, or by mispronunciation or transposition of

certain consonants, especially *l*, *r*, and *s*. **2.** Sounds other than speech, that are similar to stammering.

stan•dard•i•za•tion (stan′dard-i-zā′shŭn). **1.** The making of a solution of definite strength so that it may be used for comparison and in tests. **2.** Making any drug or other preparation conform to the type or standard. **3.** A set of techniques used to remove as far as possible the effects of differences in the age or other confounding variables when comparing two or more populations.

stand•still. Cessation of activity.

stan•nous (stan′ŭs). Relating to tin, especially when in combination in its lower valency. [L. *stannum*, tin]

stan•num (stan′ŭm). SYN tin. [L.]

sta•pe•dec•to•my (stā-pĕ-dek′tō-mē). Operation to remove the stapes footplate in whole or part with replacement of the stapes superstructure (crura) by metal or plastic prosthesis; used for otosclerosis with stapes fixation to overcome a conductive hearing loss. [stapes + G. *ektomē*, excision]

sta•pe•di•al (stā-pē′dē-ăl). Relating to the stapes.

sta•pe•di•o•te•not•o•my (stā-pē′dē-ō-tĕ-not′ŏ-mē). Division of the tendon of the stapedius muscle. [stapedius + G. *tenōn*, tendon, + *tomē*, incision]

sta•pes, pl. **sta•pes, sta•pe•des** (stā′pēz, stā′pē-dēz) [NA]. The smallest of the three auditory ossicles; its base, or footpiece, fits into the vestibular (oval) window, while its head is articulated with the lenticular process of the long limb of the incus. SYN stirrup. [Mod. L. stirrup]

△**staphyl-.** SEE staphylo-.

staph•y•lec•to•my (staf-i-lek′tō-mē). SYN uvulectomy. [staphyl- + G. *ektomē*, excision]

staph•yl•e•de•ma (staf′il-e-dē′mă). Edema of the uvula. [staphyl- + G. *oidēma*, swelling (edema)]

staph•y•line (staf′i-līn, -lēn). SYN botryoid.

sta•phyl•i•on (stă-fil′ē-on). The midpoint of the posterior edge of the hard palate; a craniometric point. [G. dim. of *staphylē*, a bunch of grapes]

△**staphylo-, staphyl-.** Resemblance to a grape or a bunch of grapes, hence relating usually to staphylococci or to the uvula palatina. [G. *staphylē*, bunch of grapes]

staph•y•lo•coc•cal (staf′i-lō-kok′ăl). Relating to or caused by any organism of the genus *Staphylococcus.*

staph•y•lo•coc•ce•mia (staf′i-lō-kok-sē′mē-ă). The presence of staphylococci in the circulating blood. [staphylo- + G. *haima*, blood]

◪**staph•y•lo•coc•ci** (staf′i-lō-kok′sī). Plural of staphylococcus.

staph•y•lo•coc•co•sis, pl. **staph•y•lo•coc•co•ses** (staf′i-lō-kok-ō′sis, -sēz). Infection by species of the bacterium *Staphylococcus.*

Sta•phy•lo•coc•cus (staf′i-lō-kok′ŭs). A genus of nonmotile, non-spore-forming, aerobic to facultatively anaerobic bacteria containing Gram-positive, spherical cells which divide in more than one plane to form irregular clusters. Coagulase-positive strains produce a variety of toxins and are therefore potentially pathogenic and may cause food poisoning. These organisms are usually susceptible to antibiotics such as the β-lactam and macrolide antibiotics, tetracyclines, novobiocin, and chloramphenicol but are resistant to polymyxin and polyenes. They are found on the skin, in skin glands, on the nasal and other mucous membranes of warm-blooded animals, and in a variety of food products. The type species is *S. aureus.* [staphylo- + G. *kokkos,* a berry]

S. au'reus, a common species found especially on nasal mucous membrane and skin (hair follicles); it causes furunculosis, cellulitis, pyemia, pneumonia, osteomyelitis, endocarditis, suppuration of wounds, other infections, and food poisoning; also a cause of infection in burn patients. Humans are the chief reservoir. The type species of the genus *S.*

S. pyog'enes al'bus, a name formerly applied to the organisms which are now regarded as the mutants of *S. aureus* that form white colonies.

staph•y•lo•coc•cus, pl. **staph•y•lo•coc•ci** (staf'i-lō-kok'ŭs, kok'sī). A vernacular term used to refer to any member of the genus *Staphylococcus.*

staph•y•lo•der•ma (staf'i-lō-der'mă). Pyoderma due to staphylococci. [staphylo- + G. *derma,* skin]

staph•y•lo•der•ma•ti•tis (staf'i-lō-der-mă-tī'tis). Inflammation of the skin due to the action of staphylococci.

staph•y•lo•di•al•y•sis (staf'i-lō-dī-al'i-sis). SYN uvuloptosis. [staphylo- + G. *dialysis,* a separation]

staph•y•lo•ki•nase (staf'i-lō-kī'nās). A microbial metalloenzyme from *Staphylococcus aureus,* with action similar to that of urokinase and streptokinase, that can convert plasminogen to plasmin but requires Ca²⁺; separated in forms A, B, and C.

staph•y•lol•y•sin (staf-i-lol'i-sin). **1.** A hemolysin elaborated by a staphylococcus. **2.** An antibody causing lysis of staphylococci.

staph•y•lo•ma (staf-i-lō'mă). A bulging of the cornea or sclera containing uveal tissue. [staphylo- + G. *-ōma,* tumor]

anterior s., a bulging near the anterior pole of the eyeball. SYN corneal s.

corneal s., SYN anterior s.

equatorial s., a s. occurring in the area of exit of the vortex veins. SYN scleral s.

posterior s., a bulging near the posterior pole of the eyeball due to degenerative changes in severe myopia.

scleral s., SYN equatorial s.

staph•y•lom•a•tous (staf-i-lō'mă-tŭs). Relating to or marked by staphyloma.

staph•y•lo•phar•yn•gor•rha•phy (staf'i-lō-far-in-gōr'ă-fē). Surgical repair of defects in the uvula or soft palate and the pharynx. SYN palatopharyngorrhaphy. [staphylo- + pharynx + G. *rhaphē,* suture]

staph•y•lo•plas•ty (staf'i-lō-plas-tē). SYN palatoplasty. [staphylo- + G. *plassō,* to form]

staph•y•lop•to•sis (staf'i-lop-tō'sis). SYN uvuloptosis. [staphylo- + G. *ptōsis,* a falling]

staph•y•lor•rha•phy (staf-i-lōr'ă-fē). SYN palatorrhaphy. [staphylo- + G. *rhaphē,* suture]

staph•y•lo•tox•in (staf'i-lō-tok'sin). The toxin elaborated by any species of *Staphylococcus.* [staphylo- + G. *toxikon,* poison]

sta•pling (stāp'ling). Use of a stapling device that unites two tissues, such as the two ends of bowel, by applying a row or circle of staples.

gastric s., partitioning of the stomach by rows of staples; used to treat morbid obesity.

star. Any star-shaped structure. SEE ALSO aster, astrosphere, stella, stellula. [A.S. *steorra*]

daughter s., one of the figures forming the diaster. SYN polar s.

lens s.'s, (1) SYN *radii* lentis, under *radius.* **(2)** congenital cataracts with opacities along the suture lines of the lens; may be anterior or posterior, or both.

polar s., SYN daughter s.

venous s., a small, red nodule formed by a dilated vein in the skin; caused by increased venous pressure.

starch. A high molecular-weight polysaccharide built up of D-glucose residues in α-1,4 linkage, differing from cellulose in the presence of α- rather than β-glucoside linkages, that exists in most plant tissues; converted into dextrin when subjected to the action of dry heat, and into dextrin and D-glucose by amylases and glucoamylases in saliva and pancreatic juice; used as a dusting powder, an emollient, and an ingredient in medicinal tablets; chief storage carbohydrate in most higher plants. [A.S. *stearc,* strong]

starve. 1. To suffer from lack of food. **2.** To deprive of food so as to cause suffering or death. **3.** Formerly, to die of cold. [A.S. *steorfan,* to die]

sta•sis, pl. **sta•ses** (stā'sis, stas'is; -ēz). Stagnation of the blood or other fluids. [G. a standing still]

papillary s., obsolete term for papilledema.

pressure s., SYN traumatic *asphyxia.*

stat. Referring to a diagnostic or therapeutic procedure that is to be performed immediately. [L. *statim,* immediately]

⌂-stat. An agent intended to keep something from changing or moving. [G. *statēs,* stationary]

state (stāt). A condition, situation, or status. [L. *status,* condition, state]

clonic s., movement marked by repetitive muscle contractions and relaxations in rapid succession.

dreamy s., the semiconscious s. associated with an epileptic attack.

excited s., the condition of an atom or molecule after absorbing energy, which may be the result of exposure to light, electricity, elevated temperature, or a chemical reaction; such activation may be a necessary prelude to a chemical reaction or to the emission of light.

ground s., the normal, inactivated s. of an atom from which, on activation, the singlet, triplet, and other excited s.'s are derived.

multiple ego s.'s, various psychological organizational s.'s reflecting different personas or life experiences.

refractory s., subnormal excitability immediately following a response to previous excitation; the s. is divided into absolute and relative phases.

steady s. (s), (1) a s. obtained in moderate muscular exercise, when the removal of lactic acid by oxidation keeps pace with its production, the oxygen supply being adequate, and the muscles do not go into debt for oxygen; **(2)** any condition in which the formation or introduction of substances just keeps pace with their destruction or removal so that all volumes, concentrations, pressures, and flows remain constant; **(3)** in enzyme kinetics, conditions such that the rate of change in the concentration of any enzyme species (*e.g.*, free enzyme or the enzyme-substrate binary complex) is zero or much less than the rate of formation of product. [often subscript s or ss]

twilight s., a condition of disordered consciousness during which actions may be performed without the conscious volition of the individual and with no memory of such actions.

sta•tim (stă′tim). At once; immediately. [L.]

sta•tis•tics (stă-tis′tiks). **1.** A collection of numerical values, items of information, or other facts which are numerically grouped into definite classes and subject to analysis, particularly analysis of the probability that the resulting empirical findings are due to chance. **2.** The science and art of collecting, summarizing and analyzing data that are subject to random variation.

vital s., systematically tabulated information concerning births, marriages, divorces, separations, and deaths, based on the numbers of official registrations of these vital events; the branch of s. concerned with such data.

stat•o•a•cou•stic (stat′ō-ă-kū′stik). Relating to equilibrium and hearing. SYN vestibulocochlear (2). [G. *statos*, standing, + *akoustikos*, acoustic]

stat•o•co•nia, sing. **stat•o•co•ni•um** (stat′ō-kō′nē-ă, -nē-ŭm) [NA]. SYN statoliths. [L. fr. G. *statos*, standing, *konis*, dust]

stat•o•liths (stat′ŏ-liths). Crystalline particles of calcium carbonate and a protein adhering to the gelatinous membrane of the maculae of the utricle and saccule. SYN statoconia [NA], otoconia. [G. *statos*, standing, + *lithos*, stone]

stat•ure (statch′er). The height of a person. [L. *statura*, fr. *statuo*, pp. *statutus*, to cause to stand]

sta•tus (stā′tŭs, stat′ŭs). A state or condition. [L. a way of standing]

s. asthmat′icus, a condition of severe, prolonged asthma.

s. epilep′ticus, repeated seizure or a seizure prolonged for at least 30 minutes; may be convulsive (tonic-clonic), nonconvulsive (absence or complex partial) or partial (epilepsia partialis continuans) or subclinical (electrographic status epilepticus).

stau•ri•on (staw′rē-on). A craniometric point at the intersection of the median and transverse palatine sutures. [G. dim. of *stauros*, cross]

STD sexually transmitted *disease*.

steal (stēl). Diversion of blood via alternate routes or reversed flow, from a vascularized tissue to one deprived by proximal arterial obstruction. [M.E. *stelen*, fr. A.S. *stelan*]

subclavian s., obstruction of the subclavian artery proximal to the origin of the vertebral artery; blood flow through the vertebral artery is reversed and the subclavian artery thus "steals" cerebral blood, causing symptoms of vertebrobasilar insufficiency (subclavian steal syndrome); manifest during vigorous use of an upper extremity.

ste•ap•sin (stē-ap′sin). SYN *triacylglycerol* lipase.

△**stear-.** SEE stearo-.

ste•a•rate (stē′ă-rāt). A salt of stearic acid.

△**stearo-, stear-.** Combining form denoting fat. SEE ALSO steato-. [G. *stear*, tallow]

ste•a•ti•tis (stē-ă-tī′tis). Inflammation of adipose tissue. [G. *stear* (*steat-*), tallow, + *-itis,* inflammation]

△**steato-.** fat. SEE stearo-. [G. *stear* (*steat-*), tallow]

ste•a•to•cys•to•ma (stē′ă-tō-sis-tō′mă). A cyst with sebaceous gland cells in its wall.

ste•a•tol•y•sis (stē-ă-tol′i-sis). The hydrolysis or emulsion of fat in the process of digestion. [steato- + G. *lysis*, dissolution]

ste•a•to•ly•tic (stē-ă-tō-lit′ik). Relating to steatolysis.

ste•a•to•ne•cro•sis (stē′ă-tō-ne-krō′sis). SYN fat *necrosis*. [steato- + G. *nekrōsis*, death]

ste•a•to•py•ga, ste•a•to•py•gia (stē′ă-tō-pī′gă, -pij′ē-ă). Excessive accumulation of fat on the buttocks. [steato- + G. *pygē*, buttocks]

ste•a•to•py•gous (stē-ă-top′ă-gŭs). Having excessively fat buttocks.

ste•a•tor•rhea (stē′ă-tō-rē′ă). Passage of fat in large amounts in the feces due to failure to digest and absorb it; occurs in pancreatic disease and the malabsorption syndromes; an absence of bile acids will increase s. [steato- + G. *rhoia,* a flow]

ste•a•to•sis (stē-ă-tō′sis). **1.** SYN adiposis. **2.** SYN fatty *degeneration*. [steato- + G. *-osis,* condition]

steg•no•sis (steg-nō′sis). **1.** A stoppage of any of the secretions or excretions. **2.** A constriction or stenosis. [G. stoppage]

stel•la, pl. **stel•lae** (stel′ă, -ē). A star or star-shaped figure. [L.]

stel•late (stel′āt). Star-shaped. [L. *stella,* a star]

stel•lu•la, pl. **stel•lu•lae** (stel′yū-lă, -lē). A small star or star-shaped figure. [L. dim. of *stella,* star]

stem. A supporting structure similar to the stalk of a plant.

brain s., SEE brainstem.

infundibular s., the neural component of the pituitary stalk that contains nerve tracts passing from the hypothalamus to the pars nervosa. SYN infundibular stalk.

ste•ni•on (sten′ē-on). The termination in either temporal fossa of the shortest transverse diameter of the skull; a craniometric point. [G. *stenos,* narrow, + dim. *-iōn*]

△**steno-.** Narrowness, constriction; opposite of eury-. [G. *stenos,* narrow]

sten•o•car•dia (sten-ō-kar′dē-ă). SYN *angina* pectoris. [steno- + G. *kardia,* heart]

sten•o•ceph•a•lous, sten•o•ce•phal•ic (sten-ō-sef′ă-lŭs, -se-fal′ik). Pertaining to, or characterized by, stenocephaly.

sten•o•ceph•a•ly (sten-ō-sef′ă-lē). Marked narrowness of the head. [steno- + G. *kephalē,* head]

sten•o•cho•ria (sten-ō-kō′rē-ă). Abnormal contraction of any canal or orifice, especially of the lacrimal ducts. [G. *stenochōria,* narrowness, fr. steno- + *chōra,* place, room]

sten•o•pe•ic, sten•o•pa•ic (stĕn-ō-pē′ik, sten-ō-pā′ik). Provided with a narrow opening or slit, as in s. spectacles. [steno- + G. *opē,* opening]

ste•nosed (sten′ōzd). Narrowed; contracted: strictured.

ste•no•sis, pl. **ste•no•ses** (ste-nō'sis, -sēz). A stricture of any canal; especially, a narrowing of one of the cardiac valves. [G. *stenōsis*, a narrowing]

  aortic s., pathologic narrowing of the aortic valve orifice.

  congenital pyloric s., SYN hypertrophic pyloric s.

  hypertrophic pyloric s., muscular hypertrophy of the pyloric sphincter, associated with projectile vomiting appearing in the second or third week of life, usually in males. SYN congenital pyloric s.

  idiopathic hypertrophic subaortic s., left ventricular outflow obstruction due to hypertrophy, usually congenital, of the ventricular septum.

  laryngeal s., narrowing or stricture of any or all areas of the larynx; may be congenital or acquired.

  mitral s. (MS), pathologic narrowing of the orifice of the mitral valve.

  pulmonary s., narrowing of the opening into the pulmonary artery from the right ventricle.

  pyloric s., narrowing of the gastric pylorus, especially by congenital muscular hypertrophy or scarring resulting from a peptic ulcer. SEE ALSO hypertrophic pyloric s.

  spinal s., abnormal narrowing of the spinal canal, often with compression of the spinal cord.

  subaortic s., congenital narrowing of the outflow tract of the left ventricle by a ring of fibrous tissue or by hypertrophy of the muscular septum below the aortic valve.

  supravalvar s., narrowing of the aorta above the aortic valve by a constricting ring or shelf, or by coarctation or hypoplasia of the ascending aorta.

  tricuspid s., pathologic narrowing of the orifice of the tricuspid valve.

sten•o•sto•mia (sten-ō-stō'mē-ă). Narrowness of the oral cavity. [steno- + G. *stoma,* mouth]

sten•o•ther•mal (sten-ō-ther'măl). Thermostable through a narrow temperature range; able to withstand only slight changes in temperature. [steno- + G. *thermē,* heat]

sten•o•tho•rax (sten'ō-thōr'aks). A narrow, contracted chest. [steno- + thorax]

ste•not•ic (ste-not'ik). Narrowed; affected with stenosis.

Stent, C., English dentist, †1901. SEE stent.

stent. 1. Device used to maintain a bodily orifice or cavity during skin grafting, or to immobilize a skin graft after placement. **2.** Slender thread, rod, or catheter, lying within the lumen of tubular structures, used to provide support during or after their anastomosis, or to assure patency of an intact but contracted lumen. [C. *Stent*]

step. 1. DENTISTRY A dovetailed or similarly shaped projection of a cavity prepared in a tooth into a surface perpendicular to the main part of the cavity for the purpose of preventing displacement of the restoration (filling) by the force of mastication. **2.** A change in direction resembling a stairstep in a line, a surface, or the construction of a solid body.

step-down transformer. device used in radiol-

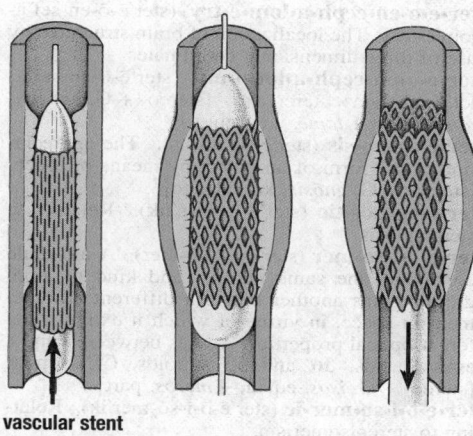

vascular stent

ogy to decrease the voltage coming into the x-ray tube.

ste•pha•ni•al (ste-fā'nē-ăl). Pertaining to the stephanion.

ste•pha•ni•on (ste-fā'nē-on). A craniometric point where the coronal suture intersects the inferior temporal line. [G. dim. of *stephanos,* crown]

step-up transformer. device used in radiology to increase the voltage coming into an x-ray tube.

△**sterco-.** Feces. SEE ALSO copro-, scato-. [L. *stercus,* excrement]

ster•co•bi•lin (ster'kō-bī'lin, -bil'in). A brown degradation product of hemoglobin, present in the feces. SEE ALSO bilirubinoids.

ster•co•lith (ster'kō-lith). SYN coprolith. [sterco- + G. *lithos,* stone]

ster•co•ra•ceous (ster-kō-rā'shŭs). Relating to or containing feces. SYN stercoral, stercorous.

ster•co•ral (ster'kō-răl). SYN stercoraceous.

ster•co•ro•ma (ster-kō-rō'mă). SYN coproma. [sterco- + G. *-oma,* tumor]

ster•co•rous (ster'kō-rŭs). SYN stercoraceous.

ster•cus (ster'kŭs). SYN feces. [L. feces, excrement]

△**stereo-. 1.** A solid; a solid condition or state. **2.** Spatial qualities, three-dimensionality. [G. *stereos,* solid]

ster•e•o•ar•throl•y•sis (ster'ē-ō-ar-throl'i-sis). Production of a new joint with mobility in cases of bony ankylosis. [stereo- + G. *arthron,* joint, + *lysis,* loosening]

ster•e•o•cam•pim•e•ter (ster'ē-ō-kam-pim'ĕ-ter). An apparatus for studying the central visual fields while the fellow eye holds fixation. [stereo- + L. *campus,* field, + G. *metron,* measure]

ster•e•o•chem•i•cal (ster'ē-ō-kem'i-kăl). Relating to stereochemistry.

ster•e•o•chem•is•try (ster-ē-ō-kem'is-trē). The branch of chemistry concerned with the spatial three-dimensional relations of atoms in molecules, *i.e.,* the positions the atoms in a compound bear in relation to one another in space.

ster•e•o•e•lec•tro•en•ceph•a•log•ra•phy (ster-ē-ō-ē-lek'trō-en-sef-ă-log'ră-fē). Recording of electrical activity in three planes of the brain, *i.e.,* with surface and depth electrodes.

st

ster·e·o·en·ceph·a·lom·e·try (ster′ē-ō-en-sef′ă-lom′ĕ-trē). The localization of brain structures by use of three-dimensional coordinates.

ster·e·o·en·ceph·a·lot·o·my (ster′ē-ō-en-sef′ă-lot′ō-mē). SYN stereotaxy. [stereo- + G. *encephalos,* brain, + *tomē,* a cutting]

ster·e·og·no·sis (ster′ē-og′nō′sis). The appreciation of the form of an object by means of touch. [stereo- + G. *gnōsis,* knowledge]

ster·e·og·nos·tic (ster′ē-og-nos′tik). Relating to stereognosis.

ster·e·o·i·so·mer (ster′ē-ō-ī′sō-mer). A molecule containing the same number and kind of atom groupings as another but in a different arrangement in space, in virtue of which it exhibits different optical properties; *e.g.,* as between D and L amino acids, 5α and 5β steroids. Cf. isomer. [stereo- + G. *isos,* equal, + *meros,* part]

ster·e·o·i·so·mer·ic (ster′ē-ō-ī-sō-mer′ik). Relating to stereoisomerism.

ster·e·o·i·som·er·ism (ster′ē-ō-ī-som′er-izm). Molecular asymmetry, isomerism involving different spatial arrangements of the same groups. SEE ALSO stereoisomer.

ster·e·om·e·try (ster-ē-om′ĕ-trē). **1.** Measurement of a solid object or the cubic capacity of a vessel. **2.** Determination of the specific gravity of a liquid.

ster·e·op·a·thy (ster-ē-op′ă-thē). Persistent stereotyped thinking.

ster·e·o·ra·di·og·ra·phy (ster′ē-ō-rā-dē-og′ră-fē). Preparation of a pair of radiographs with appropriate shift of the x-ray tube or film so that the images can be viewed stereoscopically to give a three-dimensional appearance.

ster·e·o·scop·ic (ster′ē-ō-skop′ik). Relating to a stereoscope, or giving the appearance of three dimensions.

ster·e·os·co·py (ster-ē-os′kŏ-pē). An optical technique by which two images of the same object are blended into one, giving a three-dimensional appearance to the single image.

ster·e·o·tac·tic, ster·e·o·tax·ic (ster′ē-ō-tak′tik, -tak′sik). Relating to stereotaxis or stereotaxy.

ster·e·o·tax·is (ster′ē-ō-tak′sis). **1.** Three-dimensional arrangement. **2.** Stereotropism, but applied more exactly when the organism as a whole, rather than a part only, reacts. **3.** SYN stereotaxy. [stereo- + G. *taxis,* orderly arrangement]

ster·e·o·taxy (ster′ē-ō-tak′sē). A precise method of destroying deep-seated brain structures located by use of three-dimensional coordinates. SYN stereoencephalotomy, stereotactic surgery, stereotaxic surgery, stereotaxis (3).

ster·e·o·tro·pic (ster′ē-ō-trop′ik). Relating to or exhibiting stereotropism.

ster·e·ot·ro·pism (ster′ē-ot′rō-pizm). Growth or movement of a plant or animal toward (**positive s.**) or away from (**negative s.**) a solid body, usually applied when a part of the organism rather than the whole reacts. [stereo- + G. *tropos,* a turning]

ster·e·o·typy (ster′ē-ō-tī-pē). **1.** Maintenance of one attitude for a long period. **2.** Constant repetition of certain meaningless gestures or movements, as in certain forms of schizophrenia. [stereo- + G. *typos,* impression, type]

ste·ric (ster′ik, stēr-). Pertaining to stereochemistry.

ster·ile (ster′il). Relating to or characterized by sterility. [L. *sterilis,* barren]

ste·ril·i·ty (stĕ-ril′i-tē). **1.** In general, the incapability of fertilization or reproduction. **2.** Condition of being aseptic, or free from all living microorganisms and their spores. [L. *sterilitas*]

ster·il·i·za·tion (ster′ĭ-li-zā′shŭn). **1.** The act or process by which an individual is rendered incapable of fertilization or reproduction, as by vasectomy, partial salpingectomy, or castration. **2.** The destruction of all microorganisms in or about an object, as by steam (flowing or pressurized), chemical agents (alcohol, phenol, heavy metals, ethylene oxide gas), high-velocity electron bombardment, ultraviolet light radiation.

ster·il·ize (ster′ĭ-līz). To produce sterility.

ster·il·iz·er (ster′i-lī-zer). An apparatus for rendering objects sterile.

△**stern-.** SEE sterno-.

ster·na (ster′nă). Plural of sternum.

ster·nal (ster′năl). Relating to the sternum.

ster·nal·gia (ster-nal′jē-ă). Pain in the sternum or the sternal region. SYN sternodynia. [stern- + G. *algos,* pain]

ster·ne·bra, pl. **ster·ne·brae** (ster′nē-bră, -brē). One of the four segments of the primordial sternum of the embryo by the fusion of which the body of the adult sternum is formed. [Mod. L. fr. stern(um) + (vert)ebra]

△**ster·no-, stern-.** The sternum, sternal. [G. *sternon,* chest]

ster·no·cla·vic·u·lar (ster′nō-kla-vik′yū-lăr). Relating to the sternum and the clavicle.

ster·no·clei·do·mas·toid (ster′nō-klī′dō-mas′toyd). Relating to sternum, clavicle, and mastoid process.

ster·no·cos·tal (ster′nō-kos′tăl). Relating to the sternum and the ribs. [L. *costa,* rib]

ster·no·dyn·ia (ster-nō-din′ē-ă). SYN sternalgia. [sterno- + G. *odynē,* pain]

ster·no·glos·sal (ster-nō-glos′ăl). Denoting muscular fibers that occasionally pass from the sternohyoid muscle to join the hyoglossal muscle.

ster·noid (ster′noyd). Resembling the sternum. [sterno- + G. *eidos,* resemblance]

ster·no·pa·gia (ster-nō-pā′jē-ă). Condition shown by conjoined twins united at the sterna or more extensively at the ventral walls of the chest. SEE conjoined *twins,* under *twin.* [sterno- + G. *pagos,* something fixed]

ster·no·per·i·car·di·al (ster′nō-per′i-kar′dē-ăl). Relating to the sternum and the pericardium.

ster·nos·chi·sis (ster-nos′ki-sis). Congenital cleft of the sternum. [sterno- + G. *schisis,* a cleaving]

ster·not·o·my (ster-not′ō-mē). Incision into or through the sternum. [sterno- + G. *tomē,* incision]

ster·no·ver·te·bral (ster′nō-ver′tĕ-brăl). Relating to the sternum and the vertebrae; denoting the true ribs, or the seven upper ribs on either side, which articulate with the vertebrae and with the sternum. SYN vertebrosternal.

ster·num, gen. **ster·ni**, pl. **ster·na** (ster′nŭm, -nī, -nă) [NA]. A long, flat bone, articulating with the cartilages of the first seven ribs and with the clavicle, that forms the middle part of the anterior wall of the thorax; it consists of three portions: the corpus or body, the manubrium, and the xiphoid process. SYN breast bone. [Mod. L. fr. G. *sternon,* the chest]

ster·nu·ta·tion (ster′nū-tā′shŭn). The act of sneezing. [L. *sternutatio,* fr. *sternuo (sternuto),* pp. *sternutatus,* to sneeze]

ste·roid (stēr′oyd, ster′oyd). **1.** Pertaining to the steroids. SYN steroidal. Cf. steroids. **2.** One of the steroids. **3.** Generic designation for compounds closely related in structure to the steroids, such as sterols, bile acids, cardiac glycosides, and precursors of the D vitamins.

   anabolic s., prescription drug abused by some athletes to increase muscle mass; functions in a manner similar to that of the chief male hormone, testosterone. Masculinizing effects are minimized by synthetically manipulating chemical structure to emphasize tissue-building, nitrogen-retaining processes. SEE ALSO ergogenic *aid.* SYN androgenic s.

   androgenic s., SYN anabolic s.

ste·roi·dal (stēr′oy-dăl, ster′). SYN steroid (1).

ste·roi·do·gen·e·sis (stēr′oy-dō-jen′ĕ-sis, ster′). The formation of steroids; commonly referring to the biological synthesis of steroid hormones, but not to the production of such compounds in a chemical laboratory. [steroid + G. *genesis,* production]

ste·roids (stēr′oydz, ster-). A large family of chemical substances, comprising many hormones, body constituents, and drugs, each containing the tetracyclic cyclopenta[*a*]phenanthrene skeleton.

ste·rol (stēr′ol). A steroid with one OH (alcohol) group; the systematic names contain either the prefix hydroxy- or the suffix -ol, *e.g.,* cholesterol, ergosterol.

ster·tor (ster′tōr). A noisy inspiration occurring in coma or deep sleep, sometimes due to obstruction of the larynx or upper airways. [L. *sterto,* to snore]

ster·to·rous (ster′tōr-ŭs). Relating to or characterized by stertor or snoring.

⟩steth-. SEE stetho-.

⟩stetho-, steth-. The chest. [G. *stēthos*]

steth·o·go·ni·om·e·ter (steth′ō-gō-nē-om′ĕ-ter). An apparatus for measuring the curvatures of the thorax. [stetho- + G. *gōnia,* angle, + *metron,* measure]

steth·o·scope (steth′ō-skōp). An instrument originally devised by Laënnec for aid in hearing the respiratory and cardiac sounds in the chest, but now modified in various ways and used in auscultation of any of vascular or other sounds anywhere in the body. [stetho- + G. *skopeō,* to view]

steth·o·scop·ic (steth-ō-skop′ik). **1.** Relating to or effected by means of a stethoscope. **2.** Relating to an examination of the chest.

ste·thos·co·py (stĕ-thos′kŏ-pē). **1.** Examination of the chest by means of auscultation, either mediate or immediate, and percussion. **2.** Mediate auscultation with the stethoscope.

steth·o·spasm (steth′ō-spazm). Spasm of the chest.

sthe·nia (sthē′nē-ă). A condition of activity and apparent force, as in an acute sthenic fever. [G. *sthenos,* strength, + *-ia,* condition]

sthen·ic (sthen′ik). Active; marked by sthenia; said of a fever with strong bounding pulse, high temperature, and active delirium.

△stheno-. Strength, force, power. [G. *sthenos*]

stib·i·al·ism (stib′ē-ă-lizm). Chronic antimonial poisoning. [L. *stibium,* antimony]

stig·ma, pl. **stig·mas, stig·ma·ta** (stig′mă, -mă-tă). **1.** Visible evidence of a disease. **2.** SYN follicular s. **3.** Any spot or blemish on the skin. **4.** A bleeding spot on the skin, which is considered a manifestation of conversion hysteria. **5.** The orange pigmented eyespot of certain chlorophyll-bearing protozoa, such as *Euglena viridis,* which serves as a light filter by absorbing certain wavelengths. **6.** A mark of shame or discredit. [G. a mark. fr. *stizō,* to prick]

   follicular s., the point where the graafian follicle is about to rupture on the surface of the ovary. SYN stigma (2).

   malpighian stigmas, the points of entrance of the smaller veins into the larger veins of the spleen.

stig·mat·ic (stig-mat′ik). Relating to or marked by a stigma.

stig·ma·tism (stig′mă-tizm). The condition of having a stigma. SYN stigmatization (1).

stig·ma·ti·za·tion (stig′mă-ti-zā′shŭn). **1.** SYN stigmatism. **2.** Production of stigmas, especially of a hysterical nature. **3.** Debasement of a person by the attribution of a negatively toned characteristic or other stigma.

stil·bene (stil′bēn). **1.** An unsaturated hydrocarbon, the nucleus of stilbestrol and other synthetic estrogenic compounds. **2.** A class of compounds based on s. (1).

still·birth (stil′berth). The birth of an infant that has died prior to delivery.

still·born (stil′bōrn). Born dead; denoting an infant dead at birth.

sti·lus (stī′lŭs). SEE stylus.

stim·u·lant (stim′yū-lănt). **1.** Stimulating; exciting to action. **2.** An agent that arouses organic activity, strengthens the action of the heart, increases vitality, and promotes a sense of well-being; classified according to the parts upon which they chiefly act: cardiac, respiratory, gastric, hepatic, cerebral, spinal, vascular, genital, etc. SYN stimulator. SEE ALSO stimulus. [L. *stimulans,* pres. p. of *stimulo,* pp. *-atus,* to goad, incite, fr. *stimulus,* a goad]

   diffusible s., a s. that produces a rapid but temporary effect.

   general s., a s. that affects the entire body.

   local s., a s. whose action is confined to the part to which it is applied.

stim·u·la·tion (stim-yū-lā′shŭn). **1.** Arousal of the body or any of its parts or organs to increased functional activity. **2.** The condition of being stimulated. **3.** NEUROPHYSIOLOGY The application of a stimulus to a responsive structure, such as a nerve or muscle, regardless of whether the strength of the stimulus is sufficient to produce excitation. [see stimulant]

stim·u·la·tor (stim′yū-lā-ter, -tōr). SYN stimulant (2).

long-acting thyroid s. (LATS), a substance, found in the blood of some hyperthyroid patients, that exerts a prolonged stimulatory effect on the thyroid gland; associated in plasma with the IgG (7S γ-globulin) fraction and seems to be an antibody or, perhaps, an immune complex.

stim•u•lus, pl. **stim•u•li** (stim'yū-lŭs, -lī). **1.** A stimulant. **2.** That which can elicit or evoke action (response) in a muscle, nerve, gland or other excitable tissue, or cause an augmenting action upon any function or metabolic process. [L. a goad]

adequate s., a s. to which a particular receptor responds effectively and that gives rise to a characteristic sensation; *e.g.,* light and sound waves that stimulate, respectively, visual and auditory receptors.

conditioned s., (1) a s. applied to one of the sense organs which are an essential and integral part of the neural mechanism underlying a conditioned reflex; **(2)** a neutral s., when paired with the unconditioned s. in simultaneous presentation to an organism, capable of eliciting a given response.

discriminant s., a s. which can be differentiated from all other s. in the environment because it has been, and continues to serve as, an indicator of a potential reinforcer.

heterologous s., a s. that acts upon any part of the sensory apparatus or nerve tract.

homologous s., a s. that acts only on the nerve terminations in a special sense organ.

inadequate s., a s. too weak to evoke a response.

threshold s., a s. of threshold strength, *i.e.,* one just strong enough to excite. SEE ALSO adequate s.

unconditioned s., a s. that elicits an unconditioned response; *e.g.,* food is an unconditioned s. for salivation, which in turn is an unconditioned response in a hungry animal.

sting. 1. Sharp momentary pain, most commonly produced by the puncture of the skin by many species of arthropods, including hexapods, myriapods, and arachnids; can also be produced by jellyfish, sea urchins, sponges, mollusks, and several species of venomous fish, such as the stingray, toadfish, rabbitfish, and catfish. SEE ALSO bites. **2.** The venom apparatus of a stinging animal, consisting of a chitinous spicule or bony spine and a venom gland or sac. **3.** To introduce (or the process of introducing) a venom by stinging. [O.E. *stingan*]

stip•pling (stip'ling). **1.** A speckling of a blood cell or other structure with fine dots when exposed to the action of a basic stain, due to the presence of free basophil granules in the cell protoplasm. **2.** An orange peel appearance of the attached gingiva. **3.** A roughening of the surfaces of a denture base to stimulate natural gingival s.

stir•rup (ster'ŭp, stir'ŭp). SYN stapes. [A.S. *stirāp*]

stitch. 1. A sharp sticking pain of momentary duration. **2.** A single suture. **3.** SYN suture (2). [A.S. *stice,* a pricking]

STM short-term *memory.*

stoi•chi•o•met•ric (stoy'kē-ō-met'rik). Pertaining to stoichiometry.

stoi•chi•om•e•try (stoy-kē-om'ĕ-trē). Determination of the relative quantities of the substances concerned in any chemical reaction; *e.g.,* with the laws of definite proportions in chemistry, as in the molar proportions in a reaction. [G. *stoicheion,* element, + *metron,* measure]

stoke (stōk). A unit of kinematic viscosity, that of a fluid with a viscosity of 1 poise and a density of 1 g/ml; equal to 10^{-4} square meter per second. [Sir George Gabriel *Stokes*]

△**stom-.** SEE stomato-.

sto•ma, pl. **sto•mas, sto•ma•ta** (stō'mă, stō'maz, stō'mă-tă). **1.** A minute opening or pore. **2.** An artificial opening between two cavities or canals, or between such and the surface of the body. [G. a mouth]

stoma blast. sound produced by forceful expiration of air through a tracheal stoma.

stom•ach (stŭm'ŭk). A large, irregularly piriform sac between the esophagus and the small intestine, lying just beneath the diaphragm. Its wall has four coats or tunics: mucous, submucous, muscular, and peritoneal; the muscular coat is composed of three layers, the fibers running longitudinally in the outer, circularly in the middle, and obliquely in the inner layer. SYN gaster [NA], ventriculus (1)★. [G. *stomachos,* L. *stomachus*]

cascade s., a radiographic description: when contrast material is swallowed while the patient is in the upright position, the gastric fundus acts as a reservoir until contrast overflows (cascades) into the antrum; a normal variant in a horizontal s.

hourglass s., a condition in which there is a central constriction of the wall of the s. dividing it into two cavities, cardiac and pyloric.

leather-bottle s., marked thickening and rigidity of the s. wall, with reduced capacity of the lumen although often without obstruction; nearly always due to scirrhous carcinoma, as in linitis plastica.

water-trap s., a ptotic and dilated s., having a relatively high (though normally placed) pyloric outlet which is held up by the gastrohepatic ligament.

stom•ach•al (stŭm'ă-kăl). Relating to the stomach.

sto•mal (stō'măl). Relating to a stoma.

△**stomat-.** SEE stomato-.

sto•ma•ta (stō'mă-tă). Alternate plural of stoma.

sto•ma•tal•gia (stō-mă-tal'jē-ă). Pain in the mouth. SYN stomatodynia. [stomat- + G. *algos,* pain]

sto•ma•ti•tis (stō-mă-tī'tis). Inflammation of the mucous membrane of the mouth. [stomat- + G. -*itis,* inflammation]

angular s., SYN angular *cheilitis.*

aphthous s., SYN aphtha (2).

gangrenous s., s. characterized by necrosis of oral tissue. SEE noma.

s. medicamento′sa, inflammatory alterations of the oral mucosa associated with a systemic drug allergy; lesions may consist of erythema, vesicles, bullae, ulcerations, or angioneurotic edema.

primary herpetic s., first infection of oral tissues with herpes simplex virus; characterized by gingival inflammation, vesicles, and ulcers.

recurrent herpetic s., reactivation of herpes simplex virus infection, characterized by vesicles and ulceration limited to the hard palate and attached gingiva.

recurrent ulcerative s., SYN aphtha (2).

ulcerative s., SYN aphtha (2).

◁**stomato-, stomat-, stom-.** Mouth. [G. *stoma*]

sto·ma·to·cy·to·sis (stō′mă-tō-sī-tō′sis). A hereditary deformation of red blood cells, which are swollen and cup-shaped, causing congenital hemolytic anemia. SEE ALSO Rh null *syndrome*.

sto·ma·to·dyn·ia (stō′mă-tō-din′ē-ă). SYN stomatalgia. [stomato- + G. *odynē*, pain]

sto·ma·to·ma·la·cia (stō′mă-tō-mă-lā′shē-ă). Pathologic softening of any of the structures of the mouth. [stomato- + G. *malakia*, softness]

sto·ma·to·my·co·sis (stō′mă-tō-mī-kō′sis). Disease of the mouth due to the presence of a fungus. [stomato- + G. *mykēs*, fungus, + *-osis*, condition]

sto·ma·to·ne·cro·sis (stō′mă-tō-nĕ-krō′sis). SYN noma. [stomato- + G. *nekrōsis*, death]

sto·ma·top·a·thy (stō-mă-top′ă-thē). Any disease of the oral cavity. [stomato- + G. *pathos*, suffering]

sto·ma·to·plas·tic (stō′mă-tō-plas′tik). Relating to stomatoplasty.

sto·ma·to·plas·ty (stō′mă-tō-plas-tē). Plastic surgery of the mouth. [stomato- + G. *plastos*, formed]

sto·ma·tor·rha·gia (stō′mă-tō-rā′jē-ă). Bleeding from the gums or other part of the oral cavity. [stomato- + G. *rhēgnymi*, to burst forth]

sto·mo·de·al (stō′mō-dē′ăl). Relating to a stomodeum.

sto·mo·de·um (stō-mō-dē′ŭm). **1.** A midline ectodermal depression ventral to the embryonic brain and surrounded by the mandibular arch; when the buccopharyngeal membrane disappears, it becomes continuous with the foregut and forms the mouth. **2.** The anterior portion of the insect alimentary canal. [Mod. L. fr. G. *stoma*, mouth, + *hodaios*, on the way, fr. *hodos*, a way]

◁**-stomy.** Artificial or surgical opening. SEE stomato-. [G. *stoma*, mouth]

stone (stōn). **1.** SYN calculus. **2.** An English unit of weight of the human body, equal to 14 pounds. [A.S. *stān*]

tear s., SYN dacryolith.

stool (stūl). **1.** A discharging of the bowels. **2.** The matter discharged at one movement of the bowels. SYN evacuation (2). SYN movement (2). [A.S. *stōl*, seat]

stor·age (stōr′ij). The second stage in the memory process, following encoding and preceding retrieval, involving mental processes associated with retention of stimuli that have been registered and modified by encoding. SEE memory.

STORCH. Acronym for *s*yphilis, *t*oxoplasmosis, *o*ther infections, *r*ubella, *c*ytomegalovirus infection, and *h*erpes simplex; fetal infections that can cause congenital malformations. SEE ALSO TORCH.

sto·ri·form (stōr′i-fōrm). Having a cartwheel pattern, as of spindle cells with elongated nuclei

radiating from a center. [L. *storea*, woven mat, + *-formis*, form]

storm (stōrm). An exacerbation of symptoms or a crisis in the course of a disease.

thyroid s., SYN thyrotoxic *crisis*.

STPD Symbol indicating that a gas volume has been expressed as if it were at standard temperature (0°C), standard pressure (760 mm Hg absolute), dry; under these conditions a mole of gas occupies 22.4 liters.

stra·bis·mal (stra-biz′măl). Relating to or affected with strabismus.

stra·bis·mus (stra-biz′mŭs). A manifest lack of parallelism of the visual axes of the eyes. SYN crossed eyes, heterotropia, heterotropy, squint. [Mod. L., fr. G. *strabismos*, a squinting]

comitant s., a condition in which the degree of s. is the same in all directions of gaze.

convergent s., SYN esotropia.

divergent s., SYN exotropia.

vertical s., a form of s. in which the visual axis of one eye deviates upward (s. sursum vergens) or downward (s. deorsum vergens).

strain (strān). **1.** A population of homogeneous organisms possessing a set of defined characters; in bacteriology, the set of descendants that retains the characteristics of the ancestor; members of a s. that subsequently differ from the original isolate are regarded as belonging either to a sub-strain of the original s., or to a new s. **2.** Specific host cell(s) designed or selected to optimize production of recombinant products. [A.S. *stryand; strēon*, gain, begetting] **3.** To make an effort to the limit of one's strength. **4.** To injure by over-use or improper use. **5.** An act of straining. **6.** Injury resulting from s. or overuse. **7.** The change in shape that a body undergoes when acted upon by an external stress. **8.** To filter; to percolate. [L. *stringere*, to bind]

strait (strāt). A narrow passageway. **inferior s.,** *apertura pelvis inferior;* **superior s.,** *apertura pelvis superior.* [M.E. *streit* thr. O. Fr. fr. L. *strictus*, drawn together, tight]

strait·jack·et (strāt′jak-et). A garment-like device with long sleeves that can be secured to restrain a violently disturbed person.

stran·gle (strang′gl). To suffocate; to choke; to compress the trachea so as to prevent sufficient passage of air. [G. *strangaloō*, to choke, fr. *strangalē*, a halter]

stran·gu·lat·ed (strang′gyū-lā-ted). Constricted so as to prevent sufficient passage of air, as through the trachea, or to cut off venous return and/or arterial air flow, as in the case of a hernia. [L. *strangulo*, pp. *-atus*, to choke, fr. G. *strangaloō*, to choke (strangle)]

stran·gu·la·tion (strang′gyū-lā′shŭn). The act of strangulating or the condition of being strangulated, in any sense.

stran·gu·ry (strang′gyū-rē). Difficulty in micturition, the urine being passed drop by drop with pain and tenesmus. [G. *stranx* (strang-), something squeezed out, a drop, + *ouron*, urine]

strap. **1.** A strip of adhesive plaster. **2.** To apply overlapping strips of adhesive plaster. [A.S. *stropp*]

stra·ta (strā′tă, strat′ă). Plural of stratum.

strat·i·fi·ca·tion (strat'i-fi-kā'shŭn). The process or result of separating a sample into subsamples according to specified criteria such as age or occupational groups. [L. *stratum,* layer, + *facio,* to make]

strat·i·fied (strat'i-fīd). Arranged in the form of layers or strata.

stra·tig·ra·phy (stra-tig'ră-fē). SYN tomography. [L. *stratum,* layer, + G. *graphē,* a writing]

stra·tum, gen. **stra·ti,** pl. **stra·ta** (strat'ŭm, tă; strā'tŭm; tī). One of the layers of differentiated tissue, the aggregate of which forms any given structure, such as the retina or the skin. SEE ALSO lamina, layer. [L. *sterno,* pp. *stratus,* to spread out, strew, ntr. of pp. as noun, *stratum,* a bed cover, layer]

s. **basa′le, (1)** the outermost layer of the endometrium which undergoes only minimal changes during the menstrual cycle; SYN basal layer. **(2)** SYN s. basale epidermidis.

s. **basa′le epider′midis,** the deepest layer of the epidermis, composed of dividing stem cells and anchoring cells. SYN s. basale (2).

s. **compac′tum,** the superficial layer of decidual tissue in the pregnant uterus, in which the interglandular tissue preponderates.

s. **corneum epidermidis,** [NA] the outermost layer of the epidermis, consisting of nonliving, nonnucleated, fully keratinized epithelial cells about to be lost by desquamation. SYN corneal layer, horny layer.

s. **functiona′le,** the endometrium except for the s. basale; formerly believed to be lost during menstruation but now considered to be only partially disrupted.

s. **lu′cidum,** a layer of lightly staining corneocytes in the deepest level of the s. corneum; found primarily in the thick epidermis of the palmar and plantar skin. SYN clear layer of epidermis.

malpighian s., the living layer of the epidermis comprising the s. basale, s. spinosum, and s. granulosum.

s. **spino′sum epider′midis,** the layer of polyhedral cells in the epidermis; shrinkage artifacts and adhesion of these cells at their desmosomal junctions give a spiny or prickly appearance. SYN prickle cell layer, spinous layer.

s. **spongio′sum,** the middle layer of the endometrium formed chiefly of dilated glandular structures; it is flanked by the compacta on the luminal side and the basalis on the myometrial side.

streak (strēk). A line, stria, or stripe, especially one that is indistinct or evanescent. [A.S. *strica*]

meningitic s., a line of redness resulting from drawing a point across the skin, especially notable in cases of meningitis.

primitive s., an ectodermal ridge in the midline at the caudal end of the embryonic disk from which arises the intraembryonic mesoderm; achieved by inward and then lateral migration of cells; in human embryos, it appears on day 15 and gives a cephalocaudal axis to the developing embryo.

stream·ing (strēm'ing). SEE streaming *movement.*

strength. 1. The quality of being strong or powerful. **2.** The degree of intensity. **3.** The property of materials by which they endure the application of force without yielding or breaking. **4.** OCCUPATIONAL THERAPY Demonstration of degree of muscle power when movement is resisted, as with objects or gravity.

ionic s. (I), symbolized as $\Gamma/2$ or I and set equal to $0.5\Sigma m_i z_i^2$, where m_i equals the molar concentration and z_i the charge of each ion present in solution; if molar concentrations (c_i) are used instead of molality (and the solution is dilute), then $I = 0.5(1/\rho_o)\Sigma c_i z_i^2$ where ρ_o is the density of the solvent; a number of biochemically important events (*e.g.,* protein solubility and rates of enzyme action) vary with the ionic s. of a solution.

streph·o·sym·bo·lia (stref'ō-sim-bō'lē-ă). **1.** Generally, the perception of objects reversed as if in a mirror. **2.** Specifically, difficulty in distinguishing written or printed letters that extend in opposite directions but are otherwise similar, such as *p* and *d,* or related kinds of mirror reversal. [G. *strephō,* to turn, + *symbolon,* a mark or sign]

strep·ti·ce·mia (strep-ti-sē'mē-ă). SYN streptococcemia.

⚠**strepto-.** Curved or twisted (usually relating to organisms thus described). [G. *streptos,* twisted, fr. *strephō,* to twist]

Strep·to·ba·cil·lus (strep-tō-ba-sil'ŭs). A genus of nonmotile, non-spore-forming, aerobic to facultatively anaerobic bacteria containing Gram-negative, pleomorphic cells which vary from short rods to long, interwoven filaments which have a tendency to fragment into chains of bacillary and coccobacillary elements. The type species, *S. moniliformis.,* causes Haverhill fever and rat-bite fever. [strepto- + bacillus]

strep·to·coc·cal (strep'tō-kok'ăl). Relating to or caused by any organism of the genus *Streptococcus.*

strep·to·coc·ce·mia (strep'tō-kok-sē'-mē-ă). The presence of streptococci in the blood. SYN strepticemia, streptosepticemia. [streptococcus + G. *haima,* blood]

🔲**strep·to·coc·ci** (strep'tō-kok'sī). Plural of streptococcus.

strep·to·coc·cic (strep'tō-kok'sik). Relating to or caused by any organism of the genus *Streptococcus.*

Strep·to·coc·cus (strep-tō-kok'ŭs). A genus of nonmotile, non-spore-forming, aerobic to facultatively anaerobic bacteria containing Gram-positive, spherical, or ovoid cells which occur in pairs or short or long chains. These organisms occur regularly in the mouth and intestines of humans and other animals, in dairy and other food products, and in fermenting plant juices. Some species are pathogenic. [strepto- + G. *kokkos,* berry (coccus)]

S. mu′tans, a species associated with the production of dental caries in humans and in some other animals and with subacute endocarditis.

S. pneumo′niae, a species of Gram-positive, lancet-shaped diplococci frequently occurring in pairs or chains. Virulent forms are enclosed in type-specific polysaccharide capsules. Normal inhabitants of the respiratory tract, and the cause of lobar pneumonia, otitis media, meningitis, sinusitis, and other infections. SYN pneumococcus.

S. pyog′enes, a species found in the human mouth, throat, and respiratory tract and in inflammatory exudates, bloodstream, and lesions in human diseases; it is sometimes found in the udders of cows and in dust from sickrooms, hospital wards, schools, theaters, and other public places; it causes the formation of pus or even fatal septicemias.

S. vir′idans, a name applied not to a distinct species but rather to the group of α-hemolytic streptococci as a whole; viridans streptococci have been isolated from the mouth and intestines of humans, the intestines of horses, the milk and feces of cows, milk products, and the sputum and lungs.

strep•to•coc•cus, pl. **strep•to•coc•ci** (strep′tō-kok′ŭs, -kok′sī). A term used to refer to any member of the genus *Streptococcus*.

α-streptococci, streptococci that form a green variety of reduced hemoglobin in the area of the colony on a blood agar medium.

β-hemolytic streptococci, those that produce active hemolysins (O and S) which cause a zone in the blood agar medium in the area of the colony; β-hemolytic streptococci are divided into groups (A to O) on the basis of cell wall C carbohydrate (see Lancefield *classification*); Group A includes strains that cause human infections such as streptococcal pharyngitis, impetigo, erysipelas, otitis media, and wound infections, and that can stimulate production of autoimmune globulins that cause acute rheumatic fever and acute glomerulonephritis. The more than 20 extracellular substances elaborated by strains of β-hemolytic streptococci include erythrogenic toxin (elaborated only by lysogenic strains), deoxyribonuclease (streptodornase), hemolysins (streptolysins O and S), hyaluronidase, and streptokinase.

strep•to•ki•nase (SK) (strep-tō-kī′nās). An extracellular metalloenzyme from hemolytic streptococci that cleaves plasminogen, producing plasmin, which causes the liquefaction of fibrin; usually used in conjunction with streptodornase in the removal of clots.

strep•to•ly•sin (strep-tol′i-sin). A hemolysin produced by streptococci.

Strep•to•my•ces (strep-tō-mī′sēz). A genus of nonmotile, aerobic, Gram-positive bacteria that grow in the form of a much-branched mycelium; conidia are produced in chains on aerial hyphae. These organisms (several hundred species in the genus) are predominantly saprophytic soil forms; some are parasitic on plants or animals; many produce antibiotics. The type species is *S. albus*. [strepto- + G. *mykēs,* fungus]

strep•to•sep•ti•ce•mia (strep′tō-sep-ti-sē′mē-ă). SYN streptococcemia.

stress (stres). **1.** Reactions of the body to forces of a deleterious nature, infections, and various abnormal states that tend to disturb its normal physiologic equilibrium (homeostasis). **2.** DENTISTRY The forces set up in teeth, their supporting structures, and structures restoring or replacing teeth as a result of the force of mastication. **3.** The force or pressure applied or exerted between portions of a body or bodies, generally expressed in pounds per square inch. **4.** In rheology, the force in a material transmitted per unit area to adjacent layers. **5.** PSYCHOLOGY A physical or psychological stimulus such as very high heat, public criticism, or another noxious agent or experience which, when impinging upon an individual, produces psychological strain or disequilibrium. [L. *strictus,* tight, fr. *stringo,* to draw together]

life s., events or experiences that produce severe strain, *e.g.,* failure on the job, marital separation, loss of a love object.

stres•sor. PSYCHIATRY Any event or situation that induces emotional distress in a given patient.

stress shield•ing. Osteopenia occurring in bone as the result of removal of normal stress from the bone by an implant.

stretch•er. A litter, usually a sheet of canvas stretched to a frame with four handles, used for transporting the sick or injured. [A.S. *streccan,* to stretch]

stri•a, gen. and pl. **stri•ae** (strī′ă, strī′ē). **1.** A stripe, band, streak, or line, distinguished by color, texture, depression, or elevation from the tissue in which it is found. SYN striation (1). **2.** SYN striae cutis distensae. [L. channel, furrow]

stri′ae atroph′icae, SYN striae cutis distensae.

stri′ae cu′tis disten′sae, bands of thin wrinkled skin, initially red but becoming purple and white, which occur commonly on the abdomen, buttocks, and thighs at puberty and/or during and following pregnancy, and result from atrophy of the dermis and overextension of the skin; also associated with ascites and Cushing's syndrome. SYN lineae atrophicae, linear atrophy, stria (2), striae atrophicae.

stri′ae gravida′rum, striae cutis distensae related to pregnancy.

lateral longitudinal s., a thin longitudinal band of nerve fibers accompanied by gray matter, near each outer edge of the upper surface of the corpus callosum under cover of the cingulate gyrus.

medial longitudinal s., a thin longitudinal band of nerve fibers accompanied by gray matter, running along the surface of the corpus callosum on either side of the median line. Together with the lateral longitudinal s. it forms part of a thin layer of gray matter on the dorsal surface of the corpus callosum, the indusium griseum, a rudimentary component of the hippocampus.

medullary s. of thalamus, a narrow, compact fiber bundle that extends along the line of attachment of the roof of the third ventricle to the thalamus on each side and terminates posteriorly in the habenular nucleus. It is composed of fibers originating in the septal area, the anterior perforated substance, the lateral preoptic nucleus, and the medial segment of the globus pallidus.

medullary striae of fourth ventricle, slender fascicles of fibers extending transversely below the ependymal floor of the ventricle from the median sulcus to enter the inferior cerebellar peduncle. They arise from the arcuate nuclei on the ventral surface of the medullary pyramid.

terminal s., a slender, compact fiber bundle that connects the amygdala (amygdaloid body) with the hypothalamus and other basal forebrain regions. Originating from the amygdala, the bundle passes first caudalward in the roof of the temporal horn of the lateral ventricle; it follows the medial side of the caudate nucleus forward in the floor of the ventricle's central part (or body) until it reaches the interventricular foramen, in the posterior wall of which it curves steeply down to enter the hypothalamus, with fibers passing both rostral and caudal to the anterior commissure. Coursing caudalward in the medial part of the hypothalamus, the bundle terminates in the anterior and ventromedial hypothalamic nuclei.

stri·ate (strī'āt). Striped; marked by striae. [L. *striatus,* furrowed]

stri·a·tion (strī-ā'shŭn). 1. SYN stria (1). 2. A striate appearance. 3. The act of streaking or making striae.

stri·a·to·ni·gral (strī-ā-tō-nī'grăl). Referring to the efferent connection of the striatum with the *substantia* nigra.

stri·a·tum (strī-ā'tŭm). Collective name for the caudate nucleus and putamen which together with the globus pallidus or pallidum form the striate body. [L. neut. of *striatus,* furrowed]

stric·ture (strik'chŭr). A circumscribed narrowing or stenosis of a tube, duct, or hollow structure, such as the esophagus or urethra, usually consisting of cicatricial contracture or deposition of abnormal tissue. May be congenital or acquired. If acquired, may result from infection, trauma, muscular spasm, or mechanical or chemical irritation. [L. *strictura,* fr. *stringo,* pp. *strictus,* to draw tight, bind]

stric·tur·ot·o·my (strik-chūr-ot'ō-mē). Surgical opening or division of a stricture. [stricture + G. *tomē,* incision]

stri·dor (strī'dōr). A high-pitched, noisy respiration, like the blowing of the wind; a sign of respiratory obstruction, especially in the trachea or larynx. [L. a harsh, creaking sound]

 congenital s., crowing inspiration occurring at birth or within the first few months of life; sometimes without apparent cause and sometimes due to abnormal flaccidity of epiglottis or arytenoids.

 expiratory s., a singing sound due to the semiapproximated vocal folds offering resistance to the escape of air.

 inspiratory s., a crowing sound during the inspiratory phase of respiration due to pathology involving the epiglottis or larynx.

strid·u·lous (strid'yū-lŭs). Having a shrill or creaking sound. [L. *stridulus,* fr. *strideo,* to creak, to hiss]

strip. 1. To express the contents from a collapsible tube or canal, such as the urethra, by running the finger along it. SYN milk (4). 2. Subcutaneous excision of a vein in its longitudinal axis, performed with a stripper. 3. Any narrow piece, relatively long and of uniform width. [A.S. *strypan,* to rob]

stro·bi·la (strō'bi-lă, -lē), pl. **stro·bi·lae** (strō'bi-lă, -lē). A chain of segments, less the scolex and unsegmented neck portion, of a tapeworm. [G. *stobilē,* a twist of lint]

stroke (strōk). 1. Term denoting the sudden development of focal neurological deficits usually related to impaired cerebral blood flow; more appropriate terms indicate the nature of the disturbance; *e.g.,* thrombosis, hemorrhage, or embolism. 2. A pulsation. 3. To pass the hand or any instrument gently over a surface. 4. A gliding movement over a surface. [A.S. *strāc*]

 heat s., SEE heatstroke.

 sun s., SEE sunstroke.

stro·ma, pl. **stro·ma·ta** (strō'mă, strō'mă-tă) [NA]. 1. The framework, usually of connective tissue, of an organ, gland, or other structure, as distinguished from the parenchyma or specific substance of the part. 2. Aqueous phase of chloroplasts; *i.e.,* chloroplast matrix. [G. *strōma,* bed]

stro·mal (strō'măl). Stromatic; relating to the stroma of an organ or other structure.

stro·muhr (strōm'ūr). An instrument for measuring the quantity of blood that flows per unit of time through a blood vessel. [Ger. *Strom,* stream, + *Uhr,* clock]

Stron·gy·loi·des (stron-ji-loy'dēz). The threadworm, a genus of small nematode parasites commonly found in the small intestine of mammals (particularly ruminants). Human infection is chiefly by *S. stercoralis* or *S. fuelleborn.* Fatal infection in infants produces the condition known as swollen belly disease or syndrome, which causes grossly distended abdomens. [G. *strongylos,* round, + *eidos,* resemblance]

stron·gy·loi·di·a·sis (stron'ji-loy-dī'ă-sis). Infection with soil-borne nematodes of the genus *Strongyloides,* considered to be a parthenogenetic parasitic female. Larvae passed to the soil develop through 4 larval instars to form free-living adults or develop from first and second free-living stages into infective third-stage strongyliform or filariform larvae, which penetrate the skin or enter the buccal mucosa via drinking water. Most serious human infections and nearly all fatalities commonly follow immunosuppression by steroids, ACTH, or other agents, or in AIDS.

stron·ti·um (Sr) (stron'shē-ŭm). A metallic element, atomic no. 38, atomic wt. 87.62; one of the alkaline earth series and similar to calcium in chemical and biological properties. Various salts of s. are used therapeutically for their anions; *e.g.,* s. bromide, iodide, lactate. [*Strontian,* a town in Scotland]

stroph·u·lus (strof'yū-lŭs). SYN *miliaria* rubra. [Mod. L. dim. of G. *strophus,* colic]

struc·tur·al (strŭk'chūr-ăl). Relating to the structure of a part; having a structure. SYN anatomical (2).

struc·ture (strŭk'chūr). 1. The arrangement of the details of a part; the manner of formation of a part. 2. A tissue or formation made up of different but related parts. 3. CHEMISTRY The configuration and interconnections of the atoms in a given molecule. [L. *structura,* fr. *struo,* pp. *structus,* to build]

 tuboreticular s., tubules 20–30 nm in length that lie within cisterns of smooth endoplasmic reticulum; observed in connective tissue diseases such as SLE, and in various cancers and virus infections.

stru·ma, pl. **stru·mae** (strū'mă, -mē). SYN goiter. [L. a scrofulous tumor, fr. *struo,* to pile up, build]

Hashimoto's s., SYN Hashimoto's *thyroiditis.*

s. lymphomato′sa, SYN Hashimoto's *thyroiditis.*

s. ova′rii, a rare ovarian tumor, regarded as teratomatous, in which thyroid tissue has surpassed the other elements; occasionally associated with hyperthyroidism.

stru•mec•to•my (strū-mek′tō-mē). Surgical removal of all or a portion of a goitrous tumor. [struma + G. *ektomē,* excision]

stru•mi•form (strū′mi-fōrm). Resembling a goiter. [struma + L. *forma,* form]

stru•mi•tis (strū-mī′tis). Inflammation, with swelling, of the thyroid gland. SEE ALSO thyroiditis. [struma + G. *-itis,* inflammation]

stru•mous (strū′mŭs). Denoting or characteristic of a struma.

strych•nine (strik′nin, -nēn, -nīn). An alkaloid from *Strychnos nux-vomica;* colorless crystals of intensely bitter taste, nearly insoluble in water. It stimulates all parts of the central nervous system, and was formerly used as a stomachic, an antidote for depressant poisons, and in the treatment of myocarditis. S. blocks the inhibitory neurotransmitter, glycine, and thus can cause convulsions. It is a potent chemical capable of producing acute or chronic poisoning.

strych•nin•ism (strik′nin-izm). Chronic strychnine poisoning, the symptoms being those that arise from central nervous system stimulation; the first signs are tremors and twitching, progressing to severe convulsions and respiratory arrest.

study (stŭd′ē). Research, detailed examination, and/or analysis of an organism, object, or phenomena. [L. *studium,* study, inquiry]

   cross-over s., a s. in which the subject is switched from the experimental to the control procedure (or vice versa).

   cross-sectional s., a s. in which groups of individuals of different types are composed into one large sample and studied at only a single point in time (*e.g.,* a survey in which all voters, regardless of age, religion, gender, or geographic location, are sampled in one day). SYN synchronic s.

   diachronic s., a s. of the natural course of a life or disorder in which a cohort of subjects is serially observed over a period of time and no assumptions need be made about the stability of the system.

   synchronic s., SYN cross-sectional s.

stump (stŭmp). **1.** The extremity of a limb left after amputation. **2.** The pedicle remaining after removal of the tumor attached to it. [M.e. *stumpe*]

stu•por (stū′per). A state of impaired consciousness in which the individual shows a marked diminution in reactivity to environmental stimuli; only continual stimulation arouses the individual. [L. fr. *stupeo,* to be stunned]

stu•por•ous (stū′per-ŭs). Relating to or marked by stupor.

stut•ter•ing (stŭt′er-ing). A phonatory or articulatory disorder, characteristically beginning in childhood, with intense anxiety about the efficiency of oral communications, and characterized by hesitations, repetitions, and prolongations of sounds and syllables, interjections, broken words,

circumlocutions, and words produced with excess tension.

   urinary s., frequent involuntary interruption occurring during the act of urination.

sty, stye, pl. **sties, styes** (stī, stīz). SYN *hordeolum* externum.

sty•let, sty•lette (stī′let, stī-let′). **1.** A flexible metallic rod inserted in the lumen of a flexible catheter to stiffen it and give it form during its passage. **2.** A slender probe. SYN stylus (3), stilus. [It. *stilletto,* a dagger; dim. of L. *stilus* or *stylus,* a stake, a pen]

△**stylo-.** Styloid (specifically the styloid process of the temporal bone). [G. *stylos,* pillar, post]

sty•lo•hy•al (stī-lō-hī′ăl). Relating to the styloid process of the temporal bone and to the hyoid bone.

sty•loid (stī′loyd). Peg-shaped; denoting one of several slender bony processes. [stylo- + G. *eidos,* resemblance]

sty•loi•di•tis (stī-loy-dī′tis). Inflammation of a styloid process.

sty•lus, sti•lus (stī′lŭs, stī′lŭs). **1.** Any pencil-shaped structure. **2.** A pencil-shaped medicinal preparation for external application. **3.** SYN stylet. [L. *stilus* or *stylus,* a stake or pen]

stype (stīp). A tampon. [G. *stypē,* tow]

styp•tic (stip′tik). **1.** Having an astringent or hemostatic effect. **2.** An astringent agent used topically to stop bleeding. [G. *styptikos,* astringent]

△**sub-.** Prefix to words formed from L. roots, denoting beneath, less than the normal or typical, inferior. Cf. hypo-. [L. *sub,* under]

sub•a•cute (sŭb-ă-kyūt′). Between acute and chronic; denoting the course of a disease of moderate duration or severity.

sub•ap•i•cal (sŭb-ap′i-kăl). Below the apex of any part.

sub•a•tom•ic (sŭb-ă-tom′ik). Pertaining to particles making up the intraatomic structure; *e.g.,* protons, electrons, neutrons.

sub•ax•i•al (sŭb-ak′sē-ăl). Below the axis of the body or any part.

sub•car•ti•lag•i•nous (sŭb′kar-ti-laj′i-nŭs). **1.** Partly cartilaginous. **2.** Beneath a cartilage.

sub•class (sŭb′klas). In biologic classification, a division between class and order.

sub•clin•i•cal (sŭb-klin′i-kăl). Denoting the presence of a disease without manifest symptoms; may be an early stage in the evolution of a disease.

sub•con•scious (sŭb-kon′shŭs). **1.** Not wholly conscious. **2.** Denoting an idea or impression which is present in the mind, but of which there is at the time no conscious knowledge or realization.

sub•con•scious•ness (sŭb-kon′shŭs-nes). **1.** Partial unconsciousness. **2.** The state in which mental processes take place without the conscious perception of the individual.

sub•cor•tex (sŭb-kōr′teks). Any part of the brain lying below the cerebral cortex, and not itself organized as cortex.

sub•cor•ti•cal (sŭb-kōr′ti-kăl). Relating to the subcortex; beneath the cerebral cortex.

sub•crep•i•tant (sub-krep′i-tănt). Nearly, but not frankly, crepitant; denoting a rale.

SU

sub·cul·ture (sŭb-kŭl′chūr). **1.** A culture made by transferring to a fresh medium microorganisms from a previous culture; a method used to prolong the life of a particular strain where there is a tendency to degeneration in older cultures or to transfer organisms to a medium containing nutrients, reagents, dyes, or other substances to favor growth or facilitate identification. **2.** To make a fresh culture with material obtained from a previous one.

sub·cu·ta·ne·ous (SQ) (sŭb-kyū-tā′nē-ŭs). Beneath the skin. SYN hypodermic. [sub- + L. *cutis*, skin]

sub·duce, sub·duct (sŭb-dūs′, sŭb-dŭkt′). To pull or draw downward. [L. *sub-duco*, pp. *-ductus*, to lead away]

sub·en·do·the·li·um (sŭb′en-dō-thē′lē-ŭm). The connective tissue between the endothelium and inner elastic membrane in the intima of arteries.

sub·ep·en·dy·mo·ma (sŭb-ep-en-di-mō′mă). Discrete lobulated ependymal nodules in the walls of the anterior third or posterior fourth ventricles commonly found at autopsy.

sub·fam·i·ly (sŭb-fam′i-lē). In biologic classification, a division between family and tribe or between family and genus.

sub·fer·til·i·ty (sŭb-fer-til′i-tē). Less than normal capacity for reproduction.

sub·ge·nus (sŭb-jē′nŭs). In biologic classification, a division between genus and species.

sub·glos·sal (sŭb-glos′ăl). Below or beneath the tongue. SYN sublingual.

sub·grun·da·tion (sŭb-grŭn-dā′shŭn). The depression of one fragment of a broken cranial bone below the other. [sub- + A.S. *grund*, bottom, foundation]

su·bic·u·lum, pl. **su·bic·u·la** (sū-bik′yū-lŭm, sŭ-bik′; -lă). **1.** A support or prop. **2.** The zone of transition between the parahippocampal gyrus and Ammon's horn of the hippocampus. [L. dim. of *subex*, support]

sub·il·i·ac (sŭb-il′ē-ak). **1.** Below the ilium. **2.** Relating to the subilium.

sub·il·i·um (sŭb-il′ē-ŭm). The portion of the ilium contributing to the acetabulum.

sub·in·fec·tion (sŭb-in-fek′shŭn). A secondary infection occurring in one exposed to and successfully resisting an epidemic of another infectious disease.

sub·in·vo·lu·tion (sŭb-in-vō-lū′shŭn). Arrest of the normal involution of the uterus following childbirth with the organ remaining abnormally large.

sub·ja·cent (sŭb-jā′sent). Below or beneath another part. [L. *sub-jaceo*, to lie under]

sub·jec·tive (sŭb-jek′tiv). **1.** Perceived by the individual only and not evident to the examiner; said of certain symptoms, such as pain. **2.** Colored by one's personal beliefs and attitudes. Cf. objective (2). [L. *subjectivus*, fr. *subjicio*, to throw under]

sub·king·dom (sŭb-king′dom). In biologic classification, a division between kingdom and phylum.

sub·la·tion (sŭb-lā′shŭn). Detachment, elevation, or removal of a part. [L. *sublatio*, a lifting up]

sub·le·thal (sŭb-lē′thăl). Not quite lethal.

sub·li·mate (sŭb′lim-āt). **1.** To perform or accomplish sublimation. **2.** Any substance that has been submitted to sublimation. [L. *sublimo*, pp. *-atus*, to raise on high, fr. *sublimis*, high]

sub·li·ma·tion (sŭb-lim-ā′shŭn). **1.** The process of converting a solid into a gas without passing through a liquid state; analogous to distillation. **2.** PSYCHOANALYSIS An unconscious defense mechanism in which unacceptable instinctual drives and wishes are modified into more personally and socially acceptable channels.

sub·lim·i·nal (sŭb-lim′i-năl). Below the threshold of perception or excitation; below the limit or threshold of consciousness. [sub- + L. *limen* (*limin-*), threshold]

sub·lin·gual (sŭb-ling′gwăl). SYN subglossal.

sub·lux·a·tion (sŭb-lŭk-sā′shŭn). An incomplete luxation or dislocation; though a relationship is altered, contact between joint surfaces remains. [sub- + L. *locatio*, luxation (dislocation)]

sub·man·dib·u·lar (sŭb-man-dib′yū-lăr). Beneath the mandible or lower jaw. SYN submaxillary (2).

sub·max·il·la (sŭb-mak-sil′ă). SYN mandible.

sub·max·il·lary (sŭb-mak′si-lār-ē). **1.** SYN mandibular. **2.** SYN submandibular.

sub·mi·cro·scop·ic (sŭb′mī-krō-skop′ik). Too minute to be visible with a light microscope. SYN ultramicroscopic.

sub·mu·co·sa (sŭb-mū-kō′să). A layer of tissue beneath a mucous membrane; the layer of connective tissue beneath the tunica mucosa. SYN tela submucosa [NA].

sub·na·si·on (sŭb-nā′zē-on). The point of the angle between the septum of the nose and the surface of the upper lip.

sub·nu·cle·us (sŭb-nū′klē-ŭs). A secondary nucleus.

sub·or·der (sŭb-ōr′der). In biologic classification, a division between order and family.

sub·pap·u·lar (sŭb-pap′yū-lăr). Denoting the eruption of few and scattered papules, in which the lesions are very slightly elevated, being scarcely more than macules.

sub·phy·lum (sŭb-fī′lŭm). In biologic classification, a division between phylum and class.

sub·scrip·tion (sŭb-skrip′shŭn). The part of a prescription preceding the signature, in which are the directions for compounding. [L. *subscriptio*, fr. *subscribo*, pp. *-scriptus*, to write under, subscribe]

sub·si·dence (sŭb-sī′dens). Sinking or settling in bone, as of a prosthetic component of a total joint implant.

sub·spi·na·le (sŭb-spi-nā′lē). CEPHALOMETRICS The most posterior midline point on the premaxilla between the anterior nasal spine and the prosthion. SYN point A.

sub·stance (sŭb′stans). Stuff; material. SYN substantia [NA], matter. [L. *substantia*, essence, material, fr. *sub- sto*, to stand under, be present]

blood group-specific s.'s A and B, solution of complexes of polysaccharides and amino acids that reduces the titer of anti-A and anti-B isoagglutinins in serum from group O persons; used to render group O blood reasonably safe for transfusion into persons of group A, B, or AB, but does not affect any incompatibility that results from various other factors, such as Rh.

compact s., SYN compact *bone*.

controlled s., a s. subject to the Controlled Substances Act (1970), which regulates the prescribing and dispensing, as well as the manufacturing, storage, sale, or distribution of s.'s assigned to five schedules according to their 1) potential for or evidence of abuse, 2) potential for psychic or physiologic dependence, 3) contributing a public health risk, 4) harmful pharmacologic effect, or 5) role as a precursor of other controlled s.'s.

cortical s., SYN cortical *bone*.

gelatinous s., the apical part of the posterior horn (dorsal horn; posterior gray column) of the spinal cord's gray matter, composed largely of very small nerve cells; its gelatinous appearance is due to its very low content of myelinated nerve fibers.

gray s., SYN gray *matter*.

ground s., the amorphous material in which structural elements occur; in connective tissue, it is composed of proteoglycans, plasma constituents, metabolites, water, and ions present between cells and fibers.

medullary s., (1) the lipid material present in the myelin sheath of nerve fibers; **(2)** medulla of bones and other organs. SYN substantia medullaris (2).

Nissl s., the material consisting of granular endoplasmic reticulum and ribosomes that occurs in nerve cell bodies and dendrites. SYN Nissl bodies, Nissl granules.

s. P, a peptide neurotransmitter composed of eleven amino acid residues normally present in minute quantities in the nervous system and intestines of humans and various animals and found in inflamed tissue, that is primarily involved in pain transmission and is one of the most potent compounds affecting smooth muscle (dilation of blood vessels and contraction of intestine) and thus presumed to play a role in inflammation.

reticular s., (1) a filamentous plasmatic material, beaded with granules, demonstrable by means of vital staining in the immature red blood cells; **(2)** SYN reticular *formation*.

slow-reacting s. (SRS), slow-reacting s. of anaphylaxis, a leukotriene of low molecular weight which is released in anaphylactic shock and produces slower and more prolonged contraction of muscle than does histamine; it is active in the presence of antihistamines (but not epinephrine) and seems not to occur preformed in mast cells, but as a result of an antigen-antibody reaction on the granules.

spongy s., SYN substantia spongiosa.

threshold s., any material (*e.g.,* glucose) that is excreted in the urine only when its plasma concentration exceeds a certain value, termed its threshold.

white s., SYN white *matter*.

sub·stan·tia, pl. **sub·stan·ti·ae** (sŭb-stan'shē-ă, -shē-ē) [NA]. SYN substance. [L.]

s. al′ba [NA], SYN white *matter*.

s. compac′ta [NA], SYN compact *bone*.

s. cortica′lis [NA], SYN cortical *bone*.

s. gris′ea [NA], SYN gray *matter*.

s. medulla′ris, (1) SYN medulla. **(2)** SYN medullary *substance*.

s. ni′gra [NA], a large cell mass, crescentic on transverse section, extending forward over the dorsal surface of the crus cerebri from the rostral border of the pons into the subthalamic region; it is composed of a dorsal stratum of closely spaced pigmented (*i.e.,* melanin-containing) cells, the pars compacta, and a larger ventral region of widely scattered cells, the pars reticulata; the pars compacta in particular includes numerous cells that project forward to the striatum (caudate nucleus and putamen) and contain dopamine, which acts as the transmitter substance at their synaptic endings; other, apparently nondopaminergic cells of the s. nigra project to a rostral part of the ventral nucleus of thalamus, to the middle layers of the superior colliculus, and to restricted parts of the reticular formation of the midbrain; the nigrostriatal projection is reciprocated by a massive striatonigral fiber system with multiple neurotransmitters, chief among which is γ-aminobutyric acid (GABA); s. n. receives smaller afferent projections from the subthalamic nucleus, the lateral segment of the globus pallidus, the dorsal nucleus of the raphe and the pedunculopontine nucleus of the midbrain. The pars reticulata forms part of the output system for the striate body. The s. n. is involved in the metabolic disturbances associated with Parkinson's disease and Huntington's disease.

s. spongio′sa [NA], bone in which the spicules or trabeculae form a three-dimensional latticework (cancellus) with the interstices filled with embryonal connective tissue or bone marrow. SYN cancellous bone, spongy bone (1), spongy substance, trabecular bone.

sub·sti·tu·tion (sŭb-sti-tū'shŭn). **1.** CHEMISTRY The replacement of an atom or group in a compound by another atom or group. **2.** PSYCHOANALYSIS An unconscious defense mechanism by which an unacceptable or unattainable goal, object, or emotion is replaced by one that is more acceptable or attainable; the process is more acute and direct, and less subtle, than sublimation. [L. *substitutio,* to put in place of another]

sub·strate (S) (sŭb'strāt). **1.** The substance acted upon and changed by an enzyme; the reactant considered to be attacked in a chemical reaction. **2.** The base on which an organism lives or grows; *e.g.,* the s. on which microorganisms and cells grow in cell culture. [L. *sub-sterno,* pp. *-stratus,* to spread under]

sub·struc·ture (sŭb-strŭk'chūr). A tissue or structure wholly or partly beneath the surface.

sub·tha·lam·ic (sŭb-thă-lam'ik). Related to the subthalamus region or to the subthalamic nucleus.

sub·thal·a·mus (sŭb-thal'ă-mŭs). That part of the diencephalon that lies wedged between the thalamus on the dorsal side and the cerebral peduncle ventrally, lateral to the dorsal half of the hypothalamus from which it cannot be sharply delineated. It is composed of the subthalamic nucleus (corpus luysi), the zona incerta, and the fields of Forel; laterally it expands in a winglike

SU

fashion into the reticular nucleus of the thalamus; caudally it is continuous with the midbrain tegmentum.

sub·tribe (sŭb-trīb). In biologic classification, a division between tribe and genus.

sub·un·gual, sub·un·gui·al (sŭb-ŭng'gwăl, sŭb-ŭng'gwi-ăl). Beneath the finger or toe nail. SYN hyponychial (1). [L. *unguis,* nail]

sub·vag·i·nal (sŭb-vaj'i-năl). 1. Below the vagina. 2. On the inner side of any tubular membrane serving as a sheath.

suc·ci·nyl-CoA (sŭk'sin-il). SYN succinyl-coenzyme A.

suc·ci·nyl-co·en·zyme A (sŭk'si-nil-kō-en'zīm ā). The condensation product of succinic acid and CoA; one of the intermediates of the tricarboxylic acid cycle and a precursor in the synthesis of heme. SYN succinyl-CoA.

suc·cor·rhea (sŭk-ō-rē'ă). An abnormal increase in the secretion of a digestive fluid. [L. *succus,* juice, + G. *rhoia,* a flow]

suc·cu·bus (sŭk'yū-bŭs). A demon, in female form, believed to have sexual intercourse with a man during sleep. Cf. incubus. [L. *succubo,* to lie under]

su·crase (sū'krās). SYN sucrose α-D-glucohydrolase.

su·crose (sū'krōs). A nonreducing disaccharide made up of D-glucose and D-fructose obtained from sugar cane, *Saccharum officinarum* (family Gramineae), from several species of sorghum, and from the sugar beet, *Beta vulgaris* (family Chenopodiaceae); the common sweetener, used in pharmacy in the manufacture of syrup, confections, etc. SYN saccharose.

su·crose α-D-glu·co·hy·dro·lase. An enzyme hydrolyzing sucrose and maltose in a complex with isomaltase; hence, hydrolyzes both sucrose and isomaltose; found in the intestinal mucosa; a deficiency of this enzyme results in defective digestion of sucrose and linear α1,4-glucans. SYN sucrase.

su·cro·se·mia (sū-krō-sē'mē-ă). The presence of sucrose in the blood. [sucrose + G. *haima,* blood]

su·cro·su·ria (sū-krō-sū'rē-ă). The excretion of sucrose in the urine. [sucrose + G. *ouron,* urine]

suc·to·ri·al (sŭk-tō'rē-ăl). Relating to suction, or the act of sucking; adapted for sucking.

su·da·men, pl. **su·dam·i·na** (sū-dā'men, -dam'i-nă). A minute vesicle due to retention of fluid in a sweat follicle, or in the epidermis. [Mod. L., fr. L. *sudo,* to sweat]

su·dam·i·nal (sū-dam'i-năl). Relating to sudamina.

su·dan·o·phil·ic (sū-dan-ō-fil'ik). Staining easily with Sudan dyes, usually referring to lipids in tissues.

su·dan·o·pho·bic (sū-dan-ō-fō'bik). Denoting tissue that fails to stain with a Sudan or fat-soluble dye.

Su·dan yel·low. Metadioxyazobenzene; a yellow stain for fats.

su·da·tion (sū-dā'shŭn). SYN perspiration (1). [L. *sudatio,* fr. *sudo,* pp. *-atus,* to sweat]

su·do·mo·tor (sū-dō-mō'ter). Denoting the autonomic (sympathetic) nerves that stimulate the

sweat glands to activity. [L. *sudor,* sweat, + *motor,* mover]

su·dor (sū'dōr). SYN perspiration (3). [L.]

△**sudor-.** Sweat, perspiration. [L. *sudor*]

su·dor·al (sū'dōr'ăl). Relating to perspiration.

su·do·re·sis (sū-dō-rē'sis). Profuse sweating. [sudor- + G. *-ēsis,* condition]

su·do·rif·er·ous (sū-dō-rif'er-ŭs). Carrying or producing sweat. [sudor- + L. *fero,* to bear]

su·do·rif·ic (sū-dō-rif'ik). Causing sweat. [sudor- + L. *facio,* to make]

su·do·rip·a·rous (sū-dō-rip'ă-rŭs). Secreting sweat. [sudor- + L. *pario,* to produce]

suf·fo·cate (sŭf'ō-kāt). 1. To impede respiration; to asphyxiate. 2. To be unable to breathe; to suffer from asphyxiation. [L. *suffoco* (*subf-*), pp. *-atus,* to choke, strangle]

suf·fo·ca·tion (sŭf-ō-kā'shŭn). The act or condition of suffocating or of asphyxiation.

suf·fu·sion (sŭ-fyū'zhŭn). 1. The act of pouring a fluid over the body. 2. A reddening of the surface. 3. The condition of being wet with a fluid. 4. SYN extravasate (2). [L. *suffusio,* fr. *suffundo* (*subf-*), to pour out]

sug·ar (shu-ger). One of the sugars; *q.v.,* pharmaceutical forms are compressible s. and confectioner's s. SEE ALSO sugars. [G. *sakcharon;* L. *saccharum*]

  blood s., SEE glucose.

  brain s., D-galactose. SEE galactose.

  deoxy s., a s. containing fewer oxygen atoms than carbon atoms and in which, consequently, one or more carbons in the molecule lack an attached hydroxyl group.

  fruit s., D-fructose. SEE fructose.

  invert s., a mixture of equal parts of D-glucose and D-fructose produced by hydrolysis of sucrose (inversion).

  milk s., SYN lactose.

sug·ars (shug'erz). Those carbohydrates (saccharides) having the general composition $(CH_2O)_n$ and simple derivatives thereof. S. are generally identifiable by the ending -ose or, if in combination with a nonsugar (aglycon), -oside or -osyl. S., especially D-glucose, are the chief source of energy by oxidation in nature, and they and their derivatives in polymeric form are major constituents of mucoproteins, bacterial cell walls, and plant structural material (*e.g.,* cellulose). S. are often found in combination with steroids (steroid glycosides) and other aglycons.

sug·gest·i·bil·i·ty (sŭg-jes'tĭ-bil'i-tē). Responsiveness or susceptibility to a psychological process such as a hypnotic command whereby an idea is induced into, or adopted by, an individual without argument, command, or coercion.

sug·gest·i·ble (sŭg-jes'tĭ-bl). Susceptible to suggestion.

sug·ges·tion (sŭg-jes'chŭn). The implanting of an idea in the mind of another by some word or act on one's part, the subject's conduct or physical condition being influenced to some degree by the implanted idea. SEE ALSO autosuggestion. [L. *sug-gero* (*subg-*), pp. *-gestus,* to bring under, supply]

  posthypnotic s., s. given to a subject who is under hypnosis for certain actions to be performed after he or she is "awakened" from the hypnotic trance.

sug·gil·la·tion (sŭg-ji-lā'shŭn, sŭj-i-). A bruise or livedo. SEE ALSO contusion. [L. *sugillo*, pp. *-atus*, to beat black and blue]

SUI. stress urinary *incontinence*.

su·i·cide (sū'i-sīd). **1.** The act of taking one's own life. **2.** A person who commits such an act. [L. *sui*, self, + *caedo*, to kill]

sul·cal (sŭl'kăl). Relating to a sulcus.

sul·cate (sŭl'kāt). Grooved; furrowed; marked by a sulcus or sulci.

sul·cus, gen. and pl. **sul·ci** (sŭl'kŭs, sŭl'sī). **1** [NA]. One of the grooves or furrows on the surface of the brain, bounding the several convolutions or gyri; a fissure. SEE ALSO fissure. **2** [NA]. Any long narrow groove, furrow, or slight depression. SEE ALSO groove. **3.** A groove or depression in the oral cavity or on the surface of a tooth. [L. a furrow or ditch]

    calcarine s., a deep fissure on the medial aspect of the cerebral cortex, extending on an arched line from the isthmus of the fornicate gyrus back to the occipital pole, marking the border between the lingual gyrus below and the cuneus above it. The cortex in the depth of the sulcus corresponds to the horizontal meridian of the contralateral half of the visual field.

    central s., a double-S-shaped fissure extending obliquely upward and backward on the lateral surface of each cerebral hemisphere at the boundary between frontal and parietal lobes.

    cingulate s., a fissure on the mesial surface of the cerebral hemisphere, bounding the upper surface of the cingulate gyrus (callosal convolution); the anterior portion is called the pars subfrontalis; the posterior portion which curves up to the superomedial margin of the hemisphere and borders the paracentral lobule posteriorly, the pars marginalis.

    collateral s., a long, deep sagittal fissure on the undersurface of the temporal lobe, marking the border between the fusiform gyrus laterally and the hippocampal and lingual gyri medially; the great depth of the collateral s. results in a bulging of the floor of the occipital and temporal horn of the lateral ventricle, the collateral eminence.

    gingival s., the space between the surface of the tooth and the free gingiva.

    hippocampal s., a shallow groove between the dentate gyrus and the parahippocampal gyrus; the remains of a fissure extending deep into the hippocampus between Ammon's horn and the dentate gyrus which becomes obliterated during fetal development.

    inferior temporal s., the s. on the basal aspect of the temporal lobe that separates the fusiform gyrus from the inferior temporal gyrus on its lateral side.

    intraparietal s., a horizontal s. extending back from the postcentral s. over some distance, then dividing perpendicularly into two branches so as to form, with the postcentral s., a figure H. It divides the parietal lobe into superior and inferior parietal lobules.

    lateral cerebral s., the deepest and most prominent of the cortical fissures, extending from the anterior perforated substance first laterally at the deep incisure between the frontal and temporal lobes, then back and slightly upward over the lateral aspect of the cerebral hemisphere, with the superior temporal gyrus as its lower bank, the insula forming its greatly expanded floor. Two short side branches, the ramus anterior and ramus ascendens, divide the inferior frontal gyrus into an orbital part, triangular part, and opercular part.

    s. ma'tricis un'guis, the cutaneous furrow in which the lateral border of the nail is situated. SYN groove of nail matrix.

    olfactory s., the sagittal s. on the inferior or orbital surface of each frontal lobe of the cerebrum, demarcating the straight gyrus from the orbital gyri, and covered on the orbital surface by the olfactory bulb and tract.

    parieto-occipital s., a very deep, almost vertically oriented fissure on the medial surface of the cerebral cortex, marking the border between the parietal lobe and the cuneus of the occipital lobe; its lower part curves forward and fuses with the anterior extent of the calcarine fissure (sulcus calcarinus); the great depth of this combined fissure causes a bulge in the medial wall of the occipital horn of the lateral ventricle, the calcar avis.

    postcentral s., the s. that demarcates the postcentral gyrus from the superior and inferior parietal lobules.

    posterolateral s., a longitudinal furrow on either side of the posterior median s. of the spinal cord marking the line of entrance of the posterior nerve roots.

    precentral s., an interrupted fissure anterior to and in general parallel with the central s., marking the anterior border of the precentral gyrus.

    rhinal s., the shallow rostral continuation of the collateral s. that delimits the rostral part of the parahippocampal gyrus from the fusiform or lateral occipitotemporal gyrus. One of the oldest sulci of the pallium, it marks the border between the neocortex and the allocortical (olfactory).

    scleral s., a slight groove on the external surface of the eyeball indicating the line of union of the sclera and cornea or limbus of cornea.

    superior temporal s., the longitudinal s. that separates the superior and middle temporal gyri.

    s. termina'lis [NA], **(1)** s. terminalis linguae [NA]; a V-shaped groove, with apex pointing backward, on the surface of the tongue, marking the separation between the oral, or horizontal, and the pharyngeal, or vertical, parts; **(2)** s. terminalis atrii dextri [NA]; a groove on the surface of the right atrium of the heart, marking the junction of the primitive sinus venosus with the atrium.

△**sulf-, sulfo-. 1.** Prefix denoting that the compound to the name of which it is attached contains a sulfur atom. This spelling (rather than sulph-, sulpho-) is preferred by the American Chemical Society and has been adopted by the USP and NF, but not by the BP. **2.** Prefix form of sulfonic acid or sulfonate.

sul·fa·tase (sŭl'fă-tās). **1.** Trivial name for enzymes in EC group 3.1.6, the sulfuric ester hydrolases, which catalyze the hydrolysis of sulfuric esters (sulfates) to the corresponding alcohols plus inorganic sulfate. **2.** SYN arylsulfatase.

sul·fa·tides (sŭl′fă-tīdz). Cerebroside sulfuric esters containing one or more sulfate groups in the sugar portion of the molecule.

sul·fa·tion (sŭl-fā′shŭn). Addition of sulfate groups as esters to preexisting molecules.

sulf·he·mo·glo·bin (sŭlf-hē′mō-glō-bin). SYN sulfmethemoglobin.

sulf·he·mo·glo·bi·ne·mia (sulf-hē′mō-glō-bi-nē′mē-ă). A morbid condition due to the presence of sulfhemoglobin in the blood; it is marked by a persistent cyanosis, but the blood count does not reveal any abnormality in blood cells; it is thought to be caused by the action of hydrogen sulfide absorbed from the intestine.

sulf·hy·dryl (SH) (sŭlf-hī′dril). The radical –SH; contained in glutathione, cysteine, coenzyme A, lipoamide (all in the reduced state), and in mercaptans (R–SH).

sul·fide (sŭl′fīd). A compound of sulfur in which the sulfur has a valence of −2.

sul·fite ox·i·dase. A liver oxidoreductase (hemoprotein) catalyzing the reaction of inorganic sulfite ion with O_2 and water to produce sulfate ion and H_2O_2; a lower activity of this enzyme is observed in cases of molybdenum cofactor deficiency.

sulf·met·he·mo·glo·bin (sŭlf-met-hē′mō-glō-bin). The complex formed by H_2S (or sulfides) and ferric ion in methemoglobin. SYN sulfhemoglobin.

△**sulfo-.** SEE sulf-.

sul·fo·nate (sŭl′fō-nāt). A salt or ester of sulfonic acid.

sul·fone (sŭl-fōn). A compound of the general structure R′–SO₂–R″.

sul·fon·ic ac·id (sŭl-fon′ik). Any of the compounds in which a hydrogen atom of a CH group is replaced by the s. a. group, –SO₃H; general formula: R–SO₃H.

sul·fo·trans·fer·ase (sŭl-fō-trans′fer-ās). Generic term for enzymes in EC sub-subclass 2.8.2 catalyzing the transfer of a sulfate group from 3′-phosphoadenylyl sulfate (active sulfate) to the hydroxyl group of an acceptor.

sulf·ox·ide (sŭl-fok′sīd). The sulfur analog of a ketone, R′–SO–R″.

sul·fur (S) (sŭl′fer). An element, atomic no. 16, atomic wt. 32.066, that combines with oxygen to form s. dioxide (SO_2) and s. trioxide (SO_3), and these with water to make strong acids, and with many metals and nonmetallic elements to form sulfides; mildly laxative; used externally in the treatment of skin diseases. [L. *sulfur*, brimstone, sulfur]

sul·fur-35. A radioactive sulfur isotope; a beta emitter with a half-life of 87.2 days; used as a tracer in the study of metabolism of cysteine, cystine, methionine, etc.; also used to estimate, with labeled sulfate, extracellular fluid volumes.

sul·fur·yl (sŭl′fŭr-il). Bivalent radical, –SO₂–.

△**sulph-, sulpho-.** SEE sulf-.

sum·ma·tion (sŭm-ā′shŭn). The aggregation of a number of similar neural impulses or stimuli. [Mediev. L. *summatio,* fr. *summo,* pp. *-atus,* to sum up, fr. L. *summa,* sum]

sun·burn (sŭn′bern). Erythema with or without blistering caused by exposure to critical amounts of ultraviolet light, usually within the range of 260 to 320 nm in sunlight (UVB).

sun·down·ing (sŭn′down-ing). The onset or exacerbation of delirium during the evening or night with improvement or disappearance during the day; most often seen in mid and later stages of dementing disorders, such as Alzheimer's disease.

sun·screen (sŭn′skrēn). A topical product that protects the skin from ultraviolet-induced erythema and resists washing off; its use also reduces formation of solar keratoses and may prevent ultraviolet-B-induced skin cancer and wrinkling.

sun·stroke (sŭn′strōk). A form of heatstroke resulting from undue exposure to the sun's rays, probably caused by the action of actinic rays combined with high temperature; symptoms are those of heatstroke, but often without fever.

△**super-.** (Properly prefixed to words of L. derivation) denoting in excess, above, superior, or in the upper part of; often the same usage as L. *supra-.* Cf. hyper-. [L. *super,* above, beyond]

su·per·ac·tiv·i·ty (sū-per-ak-tiv′i-tē). Abnormally great activity. SYN hyperactivity (1).

su·per·a·cute (sū′per-ă-kyūt′). Extremely acute; marked by extreme severity of symptoms and rapid progress, as of the course of a disease.

su·per·cil·i·ary (sū-per-sil′ē-ār-ē). Relating to or in the region of the eyebrow.

su·per·cil·i·um, pl. **su·per·cil·ia** (sū′per-sil′ē-ŭm, -ă) [NA]. **1.** SYN eyebrow. **2.** An individual hair of the eyebrow. [L. fr. *super,* above, + *cilium,* eyelid]

su·per·duct (sūper-dŭkt). To elevate or draw upward. [L. *super-duco,* pp. *-ductus,* to lead over]

su·per·e·go (sū-per-ē′gō). PSYCHOANALYSIS One of the three components of the psychic apparatus in the freudian structural framework, the other two being the ego and the id. It is an outgrowth of the ego that has identified itself unconsciously with important persons, such as parents, from early life, and which results from incorporating the values and wishes of these persons and subsequently societal norms as part of one's own standards to form the "conscience."

su·per·ex·ci·ta·tion (sū′per-ek-sī-tā′shŭn). **1.** The act of exciting or stimulating unduly. **2.** A condition of extreme excitement or stimulation.

su·per·fi·cial (sū-per-fish′ăl). **1.** Cursory; not thorough. **2.** Pertaining to or situated near the surface. **3.** SYN superficialis. [L. *superficialis,* fr. *superficies,* surface]

su·per·fi·ci·a·lis (sū′per-fish-ē-ā′lis) [NA]. Situated nearer the surface of the body in relation to a specific reference point. SYN superficial (3). [L.]

su·per·fi·cies (su-per-fish′ĭ-ēz). Outer surface; facies. [L. the top surface, fr. *super,* above, + *facies,* figure, form]

su·per·in·duce (sū′per-in-dūs). To induce or bring on in addition to something already existing.

su·per·in·fec·tion (sū′per-in-fek′shŭn). A new infection in addition to one already present.

su·per·in·vo·lu·tion (sū′per-in-vō-lū′shŭn). An

extreme reduction in size of the uterus, after childbirth, below the normal size of the nongravid organ. SYN hyperinvolution.

su•pe•ri•or (sū-pēr'ē-ōr). **1.** Situated above or directed upward. **2** [NA]. HUMAN ANATOMY Situated nearer the vertex of the head in relation to a specific reference point; opposite of inferior. SYN cranial (2). [L. comparative of *superus,* above]

su•per•mo•til•i•ty (sū'per-mō-til'ī-tē). SYN hyperkinesis.

su•per•nu•mer•ary (sū-per-nū'mer-ār-ē). Exceeding the normal number. [super- + L. *numerus,* number]

su•per•o•lat•er•al (sū-per-ō-lat'er-ăl). At the side and above.

su•per•ox•ide (sū-per-oks'īd). An oxygen free radical, O_2^-, which is toxic to cells.

s. dismutase, an enzyme that catalyzes the dismutation reaction, $2O_2^- + 2H^+ \rightarrow H_2O_2 + O_2$; a deficiency is associated with amyotrophic lateral sclerosis.

su•per•sat•u•rate (sū-per-sach'ŭ-rāt). To make a solution hold more of a salt or other substance in solution than it will dissolve when in equilibrium with that salt in the solid phase; such solutions are usually unstable with respect to precipitating the excess salt or substance and becoming saturated.

su•per•scrip•tion (sū'per-skrip'shŭn). The beginning of a prescription, consisting of the injunction, *recipe,* take, usually denoted by the sign ℞. [L. *super-scribo,* pp. *-scriptus,* to write upon or over]

su•per•son•ic (sū'per-son'ik). **1.** Pertaining to or characterized by a speed greater than the speed of sound. **2.** Pertaining to sound vibrations of high frequency, above the level of human audibility. SEE ALSO ultrasonic. [super- + L. *sonus,* sound]

su•per•struc•ture (sū-per-strŭk'chūr). A structure above the surface.

su•pi•nate (sū'pi-nāt). **1.** To assume, or to be placed in, a supine (face upward) position. **2.** To perform supination of the forearm or of the foot. [L. *supino,* pp. *-atus,* to bend backwards, place on back, fr. *supinus,* supine]

su•pi•na•tion (sū'pi-nā'shŭn). The condition of being supine; the act of assuming or of being placed in a supine position.

rearfoot s., SYN hindfoot *varus.*

su•pine (sū-pīn'). **1.** Denoting the body when lying face upward; opposite of prone. **2.** Supination of the forearm or of the foot. [L. *supinus*]

sup•pos•i•to•ry (sŭ-poz'i-tōr-ē). A small, solid body shaped for ready introduction into one of the orifices of the body other than the oral cavity (*e.g.,* rectum, urethra, vagina), made of a substance, usually medicated, which is solid at ordinary temperatures but melts at body temperature. [L. *suppositorium,* fr. *suppositorius,* placed underneath]

sup•pres•sion (sŭ-presh'ŭn). **1.** Deliberately excluding from conscious thought. Cf. repression. **2.** Arrest of the secretion of a fluid, such as urine or bile. Cf. retention (2). **3.** Checking of an abnormal flow or discharge, as in s. of a hemorrhage. **4.** The effect of a second mutation, which overwrites a phenotypic change caused by a pre-

vious mutation at a different point on the chromosome. SEE epistasis. **5.** Inhibition of vision in one eye when dissimilar images fall on corresponding retinal points. [L. *subprimo* (*subp*-), pp. *-pressus,* to press down]

sup•pu•rate (sŭp'yŭr-āt). To form pus. [L. *suppuro* (*subp*-), pp. *-atus,* to form *pus* (*pur*), pus]

sup•pu•ra•tion (sŭp'yŭ-rā'shŭn). The formation of pus. SYN pyesis, pyogenesis, pyopoiesis, pyosis. [L. *suppuratio* (see suppurate)]

sup•pu•ra•tive (sŭp'yŭr-ă-tiv). Forming pus.

△**supra-.** A position above the part indicated by the word to which it is joined; in this sense, the same as super-; opposite of infra-. [L. *supra,* on the upper side]

su•pra•bulge (sū'pră-bŭlj). The portion of the crown of a tooth that converges toward the occlusal surface of the tooth.

su•pra•cho•roid (sū-pră-kō'royd). On the outer side of the choroid of the eye.

su•pra•cos•tal (sū-pră-kos'tăl). Above the ribs.

su•pra•cris•tal (sū-pră-kris'tăl). Above a crest or ridge; specifically used to denote a line or plane across the summits of the iliac crests.

su•pra•duc•tion (sū-pră-dŭk'shŭn). The upward rotation of one eye. SYN sursumduction.

su•pra•lim•i•nal (sū-pră-lim'i-năl). More than just perceptible; above the threshhold for conscious awareness. Cf. subliminal. [supra- + L. *limen,* threshold]

su•pra•max•il•lary (sū-pră-mak'si-lār-ē). Above the maxilla.

su•pra•men•ta•le (sū'pră-men-tā'lē). CEPHALOMETRICS The most posterior midline point, above the chin, on the mandibula between the infradentale and the pogonion. SYN point B. [supra- + L. *mentum,* chin]

su•pra•nu•cle•ar (sū-pră-nū'klē-er). Above (cranial to) the level of the motor neurons of the spinal or cranial nerves; the pathways the suprasegmental nerve fibers follow to reach the motor cell bodies in the brainstem; as used in clinical neurology, s. indicates disorders of movement caused by destruction or functional impairment of brain structures other than the motor neurons, such as the motor cortex, pyramidal tract, or striate body; *e.g.,* supranuclear palsy, as distinguished from the nuclear (or flaccid, or "lower motor neuron") paralysis that results from destruction or functional impairment of the motor neurons or their axons in a peripheral nerve.

su•pra•oc•clu•sion (sū'pră-ō-klū'zhŭn). An occlusal relationship in which a tooth extends beyond the occlusal plane.

su•pra•scle•ral (sū-pră-sklēr'ăl). On the outer side of the sclera, denoting the s. or perisclerotic space between the sclera and the fascia bulbi.

su•pra•ven•tric•u•lar (sū-pră-ven-trik'yū-lăr). Above the ventricles; especially applied to rhythms originating from centers proximal to the ventricles, namely in the atrium, A-V node, or A-V junction, in contrast to rhythms arising in the ventricles themselves.

su•pra•ver•sion (sū-pră-ver'zhŭn). **1.** A turning (version) upward. **2.** DENTISTRY The position of a tooth when it is out of the line of occlusion in an occlusal direction; a deep overbite. **3.** OPHTHAL-

SU

MOLOGY Binocular conjugate rotation upward. [supra- + L. *verto*, pp. *versus*, to turn]

su•ral (sū'răl). Relating to the calf of the leg.

sur•face (ser'făs). The outer part of any solid. SYN face (2), facies (2). [F. fr. L. *superficius*, see superficial]

sur•face-ac•tive (ser'făs-ak'tiv). Indicating the property of certain agents of altering the physicochemical nature of surfaces and interfaces, bringing about lowering of interfacial tension; they usually possess both lipophilic and hydrophilic groups. SEE ALSO surfactant.

sur•fac•tant (ser-fak'tănt). **1.** A surface-active agent, including substances commonly referred to as wetting agents, surface tension depressants, detergents, dispersing agents, and emulsifiers. **2.** Those surface-active agents forming a monomolecular layer over pulmonary alveolar surfaces; lipoproteins that include lecithins and sphingomyelins that stabilize alveolar volume by reducing surface tension and altering the relationship between surface tension and surface area. [*surface active agent*]

sur•geon (ser'jŭn). A physician who treats disease, injury, and deformity by operation or manipulation. [G. *cheirougos*; L. *chirurgus*]

   dental s., a general practitioner of dentistry; a dentist with the D.D.S. or D.M.D. degree.

sur•gery (ser'jer-ē). **1.** The branch of medicine concerned with the treatment of disease, injury, and deformity by operation or manipulation. **2.** The performance or procedures of an operation. [L. *chirurgia*; G. *cheir*, hand, + *ergon*, work]

   ambulatory s., operative procedures performed on patients who are admitted to and discharged from a hospital on the same day.

   aseptic s., the performance of an operation with sterilized hands, instruments, etc., and utilizing precautions against the introduction of infectious microorganisms from without.

   closed s., s. without incision into skin, *e.g.*, reduction of a fracture or dislocation.

   cosmetic s., s. in which the principal purpose is to improve the appearance, usually with the connotation that the improvement sought is beyond the normal appearance, and its acceptable variations, for the age and the ethnic origin of the patient.

   open heart s., operative procedure(s) performed on or within the exposed heart, usually with cardiopulmonary bypass.

   oral s., the branch of dentistry concerned with the diagnosis and surgical and adjunctive treatment of diseases, injuries, and deformities of the oral and maxillofacial region.

   orthopaedic s., the branch of s. that embraces the treatment of acute and chronic disorders of the musculoskeletal system, including injuries, diseases, dysfunction and deformities in the extremities and spine.

   plastic s., the surgical specialty or procedure concerned with the restoration, construction, reconstruction, or improvement in the shape and appearance of body structures that are missing, defective, damaged, or misshapen.

   reconstructive s., SEE plastic s.

   same-day s., ambulatory surgery.

stereotactic s., SYN stereotaxy.

stereotaxic s., SYN stereotaxy.

sur•gi•cal (ser'ji-kăl). Relating to surgery.

sur•ro•gate (ser'ŏ-gāt). **1.** A person who functions in another's life as a substitute for some third person such as a relative who assumes the nurturing and other responsibilities of the absent parent. **2.** A person who reminds one of another person so that one uses the first as an emotional substitute for the second. [L. *surrogo*, to put in another's place]

sur•sum•duc•tion (ser-sŭm-dŭk'shŭn). SYN supraduction. [L. *sursum*, upward, + *duco*, pp. -*ductus*, to draw]

sur•sum•ver•sion (ser-sŭm-ver'zhŭn). The act of rotating the eyes upward. [L. *sursum*, upward, + *verto*, pp. *versus*, to turn]

sur•veil•lance (ser-vā'lans). **1.** The collection, collation, analysis, and dissemination of data; a type of observational study that involves continuous monitoring of disease occurrence within a population. **2.** Ongoing scrutiny, generally using methods distinguished by practicability, uniformity, rapidity, rather than complete accuracy. [Fr. *surveiller*, to watch over, fr. L. *super-* + *vigilo*, to watch]

   immune s., A theory that the immune system destroys tumor cells which are constantly arising during the life of the individual. SYN immunological s.

   immunological s., SYN immune s.

sus•cep•ti•bil•i•ty (su-sep-ti-bil'i-tē). **1.** Likelihood of an individual to develop ill effects from an external agent, such as *Mycobacterium tuberculosis*, high altitude, or ambient temperature. **2.** Likelihood that a given pathogenic microorganism will be inhibited or killed by a given microbial agent. SYN sensitivity. **3.** MAGNETIC RESONANCE IMAGING The loss of magnetization signal caused by rapid phase dispersion because of marked local inhomogeneity of the magnetic field, as with the multiple air–soft tissue interfaces in the lung; s. measurement can estimate calcium content in trabecular bone.

sus•pen•sion (sŭs-pen'shŭn). **1.** A temporary interruption of any function. **2.** A hanging from a support, as used in the treatment of spinal curvatures or during the application of a plaster jacket. **3.** Fixation of an organ, such as the uterus, to other tissue for support. **4.** The dispersion through a liquid of a solid in finely divided particles of a size large enough to be detected by purely optical means; if the particles are too small to be seen by microscope but still large enough to scatter light (Tyndall phenomenon), they will remain dispersed indefinitely and are then called a colloidal s. **5.** A class of pharmacopeial preparations of finely divided, undissolved drugs (*e.g.*, powders for s.) dispersed in liquid vehicles for oral or parenteral use. [L. *suspensio*, fr. *suspendo*, pp. -*pensus*, to hang up, suspend]

sus•pen•soid (sŭs-pen'soyd). A colloidal solution in which the disperse particles are solid and lyophobe or hydrophobe, and are therefore sharply demarcated from the fluid in which they are suspended. [suspension + G. *eidos*, resemblance]

sus•pen•so•ry (sŭs-pen'sŏ-rē). **1.** Suspending;

supporting; denoting a ligament, a muscle, or other structure that keeps an organ or other part in place. **2.** A supporter applied to uplift a dependent part, such as the scrotum or a pendulous breast.

sus·ten·tac·u·lar (sŭs-ten-tak′yū-lăr). Relating to a sustentaculum; supporting.

sus·ten·tac·u·lum, pl. **sus·ten·tac·u·la** (sŭs′ten-tak′yū-lŭm, -lă) [NA]. A structure that serves as a stay or support to another. [L. a prop, fr. *sustento*, to hold upright]

su·tu·ra, pl. **su·tu·rae** (sū-tū′ră, -rē) [NA]. SYN suture. [L. a sewing, a suture, fr. *suo*, pp. *sutus*, to sew]

su·tur·al (sū′chūr-ăl). Relating to a suture in any sense.

su·ture (sū′chūr). **1.** A form of fibrous joint in which two bones formed in membrane are united by a fibrous membrane continuous with the periosteum. **2.** To unite two surfaces by sewing. SYN stitch (3). **3.** The material (silk thread, wire, catgut, etc.) with which two surfaces are kept in apposition. **4.** The seam so formed, a surgical s. SYN sutura [NA]. [L. *sutura*, a seam]

apposition s., a s. of the skin only. SYN coaptation s.

approximation s., a s. that pulls together the deep tissues.

atraumatic s., a s. swaged onto the end of an eyeless needle.

blanket s., a continuous lock-stitch used to approximate the skin of a wound.

bridle s., a s. passed through the superior rectus muscle to rotate the globe downward in eye surgery.

buried s., any s. placed entirely below the surface of the skin.

button s., a s. in which the threads are passed through the holes of a button and then tied; used to reduce the danger of the threads cutting through the flesh.

coaptation s., SYN apposition s.

cobbler's s., SYN doubly armed s.

continuous s., an uninterrupted series of stitches using one s.; the stitching is fastened at each end by a knot. SYN uninterrupted s.

coronal s., the line of junction of the frontal with the two parietal bones of the skull.

cranial s.'s, the sutures between the bones of the skull.

Czerny-Lembert s., an intestinal s. in two rows combining the Czerny s. (first) and the Lembert s. (second).

Czerny's s., the first row of the Czerny-Lembert intestinal s.; the needle enters the serosa and passes out through the submucosa or muscularis, and then enters the submucosa or muscularis of the opposite side and emerges from the serosa.

dentate s., SYN serrate s.

doubly armed s., a s. with a needle attached at both ends. SYN cobbler's s.

Faden s., a s. placed between an ocular rectus muscle and the posterior sclera to limit excessive action of the eyeball. [Ger. *Faden,* thread, twine]

false s., one whose opposing margins are smooth or present only a few ill-defined projections.

far-and-near s., a s. consisting of alternate near and far stitches, used to approximate fascial edges.

frontal s., the suture between the two halves of the frontal bone, usually obliterated by about the sixth year; if persistent it is called a metopic s.

Frost s., intermarginal s. between the eyelids to protect the cornea.

glover's s., a continuous s. in which each stitch is passed through the loop of the preceding one.

Halsted's s., a s. placed through the subcuticular fascia; used for exact skin approximation.

harmonic s., SYN plane s.

implanted s., passage of a pin through each lip of the wound parallel to the line of incision, the pins then being looped together with s.'s.

intermaxillary s., the line of union of the two maxillae.

internasal s., line of union between the two nasal bones.

interparietal s., SYN sagittal s.

interrupted s., a single stitch fixed by tying ends together.

lambdoid s., line of union between the occipital and the parietal bones.

Lembert s., the second row of the Czerny-Lembert intestinal s.; an inverting s. for intestinal surgery, used either as a continuous s. or interrupted s., producing serosal apposition and including the collagenous submucosal layer but not entering the lumen of the intestine.

mattress s., a s. utilizing a double stitch that forms a loop about the tissue on both sides of a wound, producing eversion of the edges when tied.

metopic s., a persistent frontal suture, sometimes discernible a short distance above s. frontonasalis.

plane s., a simple firm apposition of two smooth surfaces of bones, without overlap, as seen in the lacrimomaxillary suture. SYN harmonic s.

purse-string s., a continuous s. placed in a circular manner either for inversion (as for an appendiceal stump) or closure (as for a hernia).

relaxation s., a s. so arranged that it may be loosened if the tension of the wound becomes excessive.

retention s., a heavy reinforcing s. placed deep within the muscles and fasciae of the abdominal wall to relieve tension on the primary s. line and thus obviate postoperative wound disruption. SYN tension s.

sagittal s., line of union between the two parietal bones. SYN interparietal s.

serrate s., one whose opposing margins present deep sawlike indentations, as most of the sagittal suture. SYN dentate s.

squamoparietal s., the articulation of the parietal with the squamous portion of the temporal bone.

squamous s., a scalelike suture, one whose opposing margins are scalelike and overlapping;

tension s., SYN retention s.

transfixion s., (1) a criss-cross stitch so placed

SU

as to control bleeding from a tissue surface or small vessel when tied; (2) a s. used to fix the columella to the nasal septum.

uninterrupted s., SYN continuous s.

wedge-and-groove s., SYN wedge-and-groove *joint.*

su•tur•ec•to•my (sū-chūr-ek′tō-mē). Removal of cranial suture.

SV simian *virus*, numbered serially; *e.g.,* SV1.

Sv sievert.

Svedberg of flo•ta•tion. SYN flotation *constant.*

swab (swob). A wad of cotton, gauze, or other absorbent material attached to the end of a stick or clamp, used to apply or remove a substance from a surface.

swal•low (swawl′ō). To pass anything through the fauces, pharynx, and esophagus into the stomach; to perform deglutition. [A.S. *swelgan*]

somatic s., a swallowing pattern with muscular contractions which appear to be under control of the person at a subconscious level; distinguished from visceral s.

supraglottic s., therapeutic technique to prevent aspiration during swallowing, involving voluntary closure of the vocal folds before and after a swallow. The patient holds the breath, swallows with breath held, then coughs when the s. is finished, before inhaling again.

visceral s., the immature swallowing pattern of an infant or a person with tongue thrust, resembling peristaltic wavelike muscular contractions observed in the gut; adult or mature swallowing is more volitional and therefore somatic.

sweat (swet). **1.** Especially sensible perspiration. **2.** To perspire. [*A.S. swāt*]

sweat•ing (swet′ing). SYN perspiration (1).

swell•ing (swel′ing). **1.** An enlargement, *e.g.,* a protuberance or tumor. **2.** EMBRYOLOGY A primordial elevation that develops into a fold, ridge, or process.

brain s., a pathologic entity, localized or generalized, characterized by an increase in bulk of brain tissue, due to expansion of the intravascular (congestion) or extravascular (edema) compartments that may coexist or may occur separately and be clinically indistinguishable; clinical manifestations depend on disturbed neuronal function

due to local s., shifting of intracranial structures, and the effects of intracranial hypertension or circulatory disturbance.

cloudy s., s. of cells due to injury to the membranes affecting ionic transfer; causes an accumulation of intracellular water. SYN hydropic degeneration, parenchymatous degeneration.

Neufeld capsular s., increase in opacity and visibility of the capsule of capsulated organisms exposed to specific agglutinating anticapsular antibodies. SYN Neufeld reaction, quellung phenomenon, quellung reaction (1), quellung test.

sy•co•ma (sī-kō′mă). **1.** A pendulous figlike growth. **2.** A large soft wart. [G. *sykōma,* fr. *sykon,* fig, + *-oma,* tumor]

sy•co•si•form (sī-kō′si-fōrm). Resembling sycosis.

sy•co•sis (sī-kō′sis). A pustular folliculitis, particularly of the bearded area. [G. *sykōsis,* fr. *sykōn,* fig, + *-osis,* condition]

lupoid s., a papular or pustular inflammation of the hair follicles of the beard, followed by punctuate scarring and loss of the hair.

syl•vi•an (sil′vē-an). Relating to Franciscus or Jacobaeus Sylvius or to any of the structures described by either of them.

sym-. SEE syn-.

sym•bal•lo•phone (sim-bal′ō-fōn). A stethoscope having two chest pieces, designed to lateralize sound and produce a stereophonic effect. [G. *symballō,* to throw together, + *phōnē,* sound]

sym•bi•on, sym•bi•ont (sim′bē-on, -ont). An organism associated with another in symbiosis. SYN mutualist, symbiote. [G. *symbion,* neut. of *symbiōs,* living together]

sym•bi•o•sis (sim-bī-ō′sis). **1.** The biological association of two or more species to their mutual benefit. Cf. commensalism, parasitism. **2.** The mutual cooperation or interdependence of two persons, as mother and infant, or husband and wife; sometimes used to denote excessive or pathological interdependence of two persons. [G. *symbiōsis,* state of living together, fr. sym- + *bios,* life, + *-osis,* condition]

sym•bi•ote (sim′bī-ōt). SYN symbion.

sym•bi•ot•ic (sim-bī-ot′ik). Relating to symbiosis.

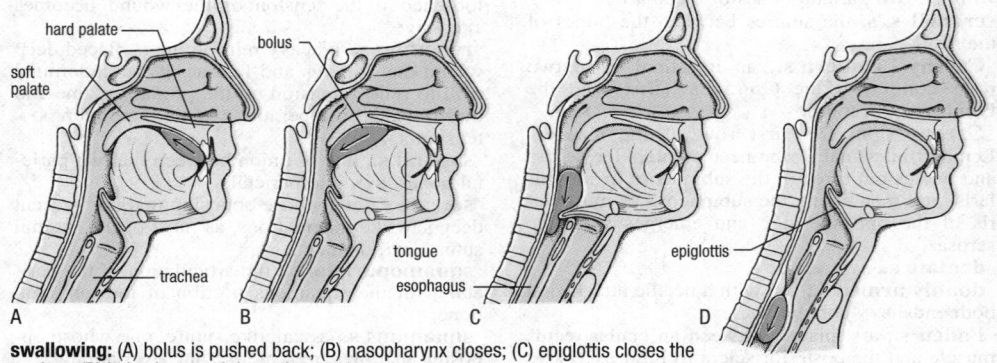

hard palate
bolus
soft palate
tongue
esophagus
trachea
epiglottis

A   B   C   D

swallowing: (A) bolus is pushed back; (B) nasopharynx closes; (C) epiglottis closes the trachea; (D) bolus is moved down the esophagus

sym•bleph•a•ron (sim-blef′ă-ron). Adhesion of one or both eyelids to the eyeball, partial or complete, resulting from burns or other trauma but rarely congenital. [sym- + G. *blepharon,* eyelid]

sym•bol•ism (sim′bō-lizm). **1.** PSYCHOANALYSIS The process involved in the disguised representation in consciousness of unconscious or repressed contents or events. **2.** A mental state in which one regards everything that happens as symbolic of one's own thoughts. **3.** The description of the emotional life and experiences in abstract terms.

sym•bol•i•za•tion (sim′bō-li-zā′shŭn). An unconscious mental mechanism whereby one object or idea is represented by another.

sym•brach•y•dac•ty•ly (sim-brak′i-dak′ti-lē). Condition in which abnormally short fingers are joined or webbed in their proximal portions. [sym- + G. *brachys,* short, + *daktylos,* finger]

sym•me•try (sim′ĕ-trē). Equality or correspondence in form of parts distributed around a center or an axis, at the extremities or poles, or on the opposite sides of any body. [G. *symmetria,* fr. sym- + *metron,* measure]

△**sympath-, sympatheto-, sympathico-, sympatho-.** The sympathetic part of the autonomic nervous system. [see sympathetic]

sym•pa•thec•to•my (sim-pă-thek′tō-mē). Excision of a segment of a sympathetic nerve or of one or more sympathetic ganglia. [sympath- + G. *ektomē,* excision]

    periarterial s., sympathetic denervation by arterial decortication.

    presacral s., SYN presacral *neurectomy.*

sym•pa•thet•ic (sim-pă-thet′ik). **1.** Relating to or exhibiting sympathy. **2.** Denoting the sympathetic part of the autonomic nervous system. [G. *sympathētikos,* fr. *sympatheō,* to feel with, sympathize, fr. *syn,* with, + *pathos,* suffering]

sym•pa•thet•o•blast (sim-pă-thet′ō-blast). SYN sympathoblast.

△**sympathico-.** SEE sympath-.

sym•path•i•co•blast (sim-path′i-kō-blast). SYN sympathoblast.

sym•path•i•co•lyt•ic (sim-path′i-kō-lit′ik). SYN sympatholytic.

sym•path•i•co•mi•met•ic (sim-path′i-kō-mi-met′ik). SYN sympathomimetic.

sym•path•i•co•to•nia (sim-path′i-kō-tō′nē-ă). A condition in which there is increased tonus of the sympathetic system and a marked tendency to vascular spasm and high blood pressure; opposed to vagotonia. [sympathico- + G. *tonos,* tone, tension]

sym•path•i•co•ton•ic (sim-path′i-kō-ton′ik). Relating to or characterized by sympathicotonia.

sym•path•i•co•trip•sy (sim-path′i-kō-trip′sē). Operation of crushing a sympathetic ganglion. [sympathico- + G. *tripsis,* a rubbing]

△**sympatho-.** SEE sympath-.

sym•pa•tho•ad•re•nal (sim′pă-thō-ă-drē′năl). Relating to the sympathetic part of the autonomic nervous system and the medulla of the adrenal gland, as the postganglionic neurons.

sym•pa•tho•blast (sim′pă-thō-blast). A primitive cell derived from the neural crest glia; with the pheochromoblasts, s.'s enter into the formation of the adrenal medulla and sympathetic ganglia. SYN

sympathetoblast, sympathicoblast. [sympatho- + G. *blastos,* germ]

sym•pa•tho•go•nia (sim′pă-thō-gō′nē-ă). The completely undifferentiated cells of the sympathetic nervous system. [sympatho- + G. *gonē,* seed]

sym•pa•tho•lyt•ic (sim′pă-thō-lit′ik). Denoting antagonism to or inhibition of adrenergic nerve activity. SEE ALSO adrenergic blocking *agent,* antiadrenergic. SYN sympathicolytic. [sympatho- + G. *lysis,* a loosening]

sym•pa•tho•mi•met•ic (sim′pă-thō-mi-met′ik). Denoting mimicking of action of the sympathetic system. SEE ALSO adrenomimetic. SYN sympathicomimetic. [sympatho- + G. *mimikos,* imitating]

sym•pa•thy (sim′pă-thē). **1.** The mutual relation, physiologic or pathologic, between two organs, systems, or parts of the body. **2.** Mental contagion, as seen in mass hysteria or in the yawning induced by seeing another person yawn. **3.** An expressed sensitive appreciation or emotional concern for and sharing of the mental and emotional state of another person. Cf. empathy (1). [G. *sympatheia,* fr. sym- + *pathos,* suffering]

sym•pha•lan•gism, sym•pha•lan•gy (sim-fal′ an-jizm, sim-fal′an-jē). **1.** SYN syndactyly. **2.** Ankylosis of the finger or toe joints. [sym- + phalanx]

sym•phys•i•al, sym•phys•e•al (sim-fiz′ē-ăl). Grown together; relating to a symphysis; fused.

sym•phys•i•on (sim-fiz′ē-on). A craniometric point, the most anterior point of the alveolar process of the mandible.

sym•phys•i•ot•o•my, sym•phys•e•ot•o•my (sim-fiz-ē-ot′ō-mē). Division of the pubic joint to increase the capacity of a contracted pelvis sufficiently to permit passage of a living child. SYN pelviotomy (1), pelvitomy, synchondrotomy. [symphysis + G. *tomē,* incision]

sym•phy•sis, gen. **sym•phy•ses** (sim′fi-sis, -sēz). **1** [NA]. Form of cartilaginous joint in which union between two bones is effected by means of fibrocartilage. **2.** A union, meeting point, or commissure of any two structures. **3.** A pathologic adhesion or growing together. [G. a growing together]

    mental s., the fibrocartilaginous union of the two halves of the mandible in the fetus; it becomes an osseous union during the first year.

    pubic s., the firm fibrocartilaginous joint between the two pubic bones.

sym•po•dia (sim-pō′dē-ă). Condition characterized by union of the feet. SEE ALSO sirenomelia. [sym- + G. *pous,* foot]

sym•port (sim′pōrt). Coupled transport of two different molecules or ions through a membrane in the same direction by a common carrier mechanism (symporter). Cf. antiport, uniport. [sym- + L. *porto,* to carry]

symp•tom (simp′tŏm). Any morbid phenomenon or departure from the normal in structure, function, or sensation, experienced by the patient and indicative of disease. SEE ALSO phenomenon (1), reflex (1), sign (1), syndrome. [G. *symptōma*]

    accessory s., a s. that usually but not always accompanies a certain disease, as distinguished from a pathognomonic s. SYN concomitant s.

sy

cardinal s., the primary or major s. of diagnostic importance.

concomitant s., SYN accessory s.

constitutional s., a s. indicating a systemic effect of a disease; *e.g.,* weight loss.

deficiency s., manifestation of a lack, in varying degrees, of some substance (*e.g.,* hormone, enzyme, vitamin) necessary for normal structure and/or function of an organism.

localizing s., a s. indicating clearly the seat of the morbid process.

objective s., a s. that is evident to the observer.

pathognomonic s., a s. that, when present, points unmistakably to the presence of a certain definite disease.

reflex s., a disturbance of sensation or function in an organ or part more or less remote from the morbid condition giving rise to it; *e.g.,* muscle spasm due to joint inflammation.

subjective s., a s. apparent only to the patient.

withdrawal s.'s, a group of morbid s.'s, predominantly erethistic, occurring in an addict who is deprived of the accustomed dose of the addicting agent.

symp•to•mat•ic (simp-tō-mat'ik). Indicative; relating to or constituting the aggregate of symptoms of a disease.

symp•tom•a•tol•o•gy (simp'tō-mă-tol'ō-jē). **1.** The science of the symptoms of disease, their production, and the indications they furnish. **2.** The aggregate of symptoms of a disease. [symptom + G. *logos,* study]

symp•to•mat•o•lyt•ic (simp'tō-mat-ō-lit'ik). Removing symptoms. [symptom + G. *lytikos,* dissolving]

symp•to•sis (sim-tō'sis). A localized or general wasting of the body. [G. a falling together, collapse, fr. *syn,* together, + *ptōsis,* a falling]

△**syn-.** Together, with, joined; appears as sym- before b, p, ph, or m; corresponds to L. *con-.* [G. *syn,* with, together]

syn•apse, pl. **syn•aps•es** (sin'aps, sĭ-naps'; sĭ-nap' sēz). The functional membrane-to-membrane contact of the nerve cell with another nerve cell, an effector (muscle, gland) cell, or a sensory receptor cell. The s. subserves the transmission of nerve impulses, commonly from a club-shaped axon terminal (the presynaptic element) to the circumscripta patch of the receiving cell's plasma membrane (the postsynaptic element) on which the s. occurs. In most cases the impulse is transmitted by means of a chemical transmitter substance (such as acetylcholine, γ-aminobutyric acid, dopamine, norepinephrine) released into a synaptic cleft that separates the presynaptic from the postsynaptic membrane; the transmitter is stored in synaptic vesicles in the presynaptic element. In other s.'s transmission takes place by direct propagation of the bioelectrical potential from the presynaptic to the postsynaptic membrane. [syn- + G. *hapto,* to clasp]

syn•ap•sis (si-nap'sis). The point-for-point pairing of homologous chromosomes during the prophase of meiosis. [G. a connection, junction]

syn•ap•tic (si-nap'tik). **1.** Relating to a synapse. **2.** Relating to synapsis.

syn•ap•to•some (si-nap'tō-sōm). Membrane-bound sac containing synaptic vesicles that breaks away from axon terminals when brain tissue is homogenized under controlled conditions; such particles can be separated from other subcellular particles by differential and density gradient centrifugation. [synapse + G. *sōma,* body]

syn•ar•thro•dia (sin'ar-thrō'dē-ă). SYN fibrous *joint.*

syn•ar•thro•di•al (sin-ar-thrō'dē-ăl). Relating to synarthrosis; denoting an articulation without a joint cavity.

syn•ar•thro•phy•sis (sin-ar-thrō-fī'sis). The process of ankylosis. [syn- + G. *arthron,* joint, + *physis,* growth]

syn•ar•thro•sis, pl. **syn•ar•thro•ses** (sin'ar-thrō' sis, -sēz). In the BNA, this class of joints has included those that in the NA are classified as articulatio fibrosa (fibrous joint) and articulatio cartilaginis (cartilaginous joint). SEE joint. [G. fr. *syn,* together, + *arthrōsis,* articulation]

syn•can•thus (sin-kan'thŭs). Adhesion of the eyeball to orbital structures. [syn- + L. *canthus,* wheel]

syncephalus (sin-sef'ă-lŭs). Conjoined twins having a single head with two bodies. [syn- + G. *kephalē,* head]

syn•ceph•a•ly (sin-sef'ă-lē). The condition exhibited by a syncephalus.

syn•chei•ria (sin-kī'rē-ă). A form of dyscheiria in which the subject refers a stimulus applied to one side of the body to both sides. [syn- + G. *cheir,* hand]

syn•chon•dro•se•ot•o•my (sin-kon'drō-sē-ot'ō-mē). Operation of cutting through a synchondrosis; specifically, cutting through the sacroiliac ligaments and forcibly closing the pubic arch; used in the treatment of exstrophy of the bladder. [synchondrosis + G. *tomē,* cutting]

syn•chon•dro•sis, pl. **syn•chon•dro•ses** (sin' kon-drō'sis, -sēz) [NA]. A union between two bones formed either by hyaline cartilage or fibrocartilage. SYN synchondrodial joint. [Mod. L. fr. G. *syn,* together, + *chondros,* cartilage, + *-osis,* condition]

syn•chon•dro•to•my (sin-kon-drot'ō-mē). SYN symphysiotomy.

syn•chro•nia (sin-krō'nē-ă). **1.** SYN synchronism. **2.** Origin, development, involution, or functioning of tissues or organs at the usual time for such an event. Cf. heterochronia. [syn- + G. *chronos,* time]

syn•chron•ic (sin'krōn-ik). Referring to the study of the natural history of a disease by its state and distribution in a population at one time.

syn•chro•nism (sin'krō-nizm). Occurrence of two or more events at the same time; the condition of being simultaneous. SYN synchronia (1). [syn- + G. *chronos,* time]

syn•chro•nous (sin'krō-nŭs). Occurring simultaneously. [G. *synchronos*]

syn•chy•sis (sin'kĭ-sis). Collapse of the collagenous framework of the vitreous humor, with liquefaction of the vitreous body. [G. a mixing together, fr. syn- + *chysis,* a pouring]

s. scintil'lans, an appearance of glistening spots in the eye, due to cholesterol crystals floating in a fluid vitreous.

syn·clit·ic (sin-klit′ik). Relating to or marked by synclitism.

syn·cli·tism (sin′kli-tizm). Condition of parallelism between the planes of the fetal head and of the pelvis, respectively. [G. *syn-klinō,* to incline together]

syn·clo·nus (sin′klō-nŭs). Clonic spasm or tremor of several muscles. [syn- + G. *klonos,* tumult]

syn·co·pal (sin′kō-păl). Relating to syncope. SYN syncopic.

syn·co·pe (sin′kŏ-pē). Loss of consciousness and postural tone caused by diminished cerebral blood flow. [G. *synkopē,* a cutting short, a swoon]

    carotid sinus s., s. resulting from overactivity of the carotid sinus; attacks may be spontaneous or produced by pressure on a sensitive carotid sinus.

    laryngeal s., a paroxysmal neurosis characterized by attacks of coughing, with unusual sensations, as of tickling, in the throat, followed by a brief period of unconsciousness.

    postural s., s. upon assuming an upright position; caused by failure of normal vasoconstrictive mechanisms.

    vasodepressor s., faintness or loss of consciousness due to reflex reduction in blood pressure.

syn·cop·ic (sin-kop′ik). SYN syncopal.

syn·cy·tial (sin-sish′ăl, -sish′ē-ăl, -sit′ē-ăl). Relating to a syncytium.

syn·cy·ti·o·tro·pho·blast (sin-sish′ē-ō-trō′fō-blast). The syncytial outer layer of the trophoblast; site of synthesis of human chorionic gonadotropin. SEE ALSO trophoblast. SYN syntrophoblast. [syncytium + trophoblast]

syn·cy·ti·um, pl. **syn·cy·tia** (sin-sish′ē-ŭm, -ă; -sit′ē-ŭm). A multinucleated protoplasmic mass formed by the secondary union of originally separate cells. [Mod. L. fr. syn- + G. *kytos,* cell]

syn·dac·tyl·ia, syn·dac·ty·lism (sin-dak-til′ē-ă, -dak′ti-lizm). SYN syndactyly.

syn·dac·ty·lous (sin-dak′ti-lŭs). Having fused or webbed fingers or toes.

syn·dac·ty·ly (sin-dak′ti-lē). Any degree of webbing or fusion of fingers or toes, involving soft parts only or including bone structure. SYN symphalangism (1), symphalangy, syndactylia, syndactylism. [syn- + G. *daktylos,* finger or toe]

syn·de·sis (sin-dē′sis). SYN arthrodesis. [syn- + G. *desis,* a binding]

△**syndesm-.** SEE syndesmo-.

syn·des·mec·to·my (sin-dez-mek′tō-mē). Cutting away a section of a ligament. [syndesm- + G. *ektomē,* excision]

syn·des·mec·to·pia (sin-dez-mek-tō′pē-ă). Displacement of a ligament. [syndesm- + G. *ektopos,* out of place]

syn·des·mi·tis (sin-dez-mī′tis). Inflammation of a ligament. [syndesm- + G. *-itis,* inflammation]

△**syndesmo-, syndesm-.** Ligament, ligamentous. [G. *syndesmos,* a fastening, fr. *syndeō,* to bind]

syn·des·mo·di·al (sin-des-mō′dē-ăl). SYN syndesmotic.

syn·des·mo·pexy (sin-dez′mō-pek-sē). The joining of two ligaments, or attachment of a ligament in a new place. [syndesmo- + G. *pēxis,* fixation]

syn·des·mo·phyte (sin-dez′mō-fīt). An osseous excrescence attached to a ligament. [syndesmo- + G. *phyton,* plant]

syn·des·mo·plas·ty (sin-dez′mō-plas-tē). Rarely used term for plastic surgery of a ligament. [syndesmo- + G. *plastos,* formed]

syn·des·mor·rha·phy (sin-dez-mōr′ă-fē). Suture of ligaments. [syndesmo- + G. *rhaphē,* suture]

syn·des·mo·sis, pl. **syn·des·mo·ses** (sin′dez-mō′sis, -sēz) [NA]. A form of fibrous joint in which opposing surfaces that are relatively far apart are united by ligaments. SYN syndesmodial joint, syndesmotic joint. [syndesmo- + G. *-osis,* condition]

syn·des·mot·ic (sin-des-mot′ik). Relating to syndesmosis. SYN syndesmodial.

syn·des·mot·o·my (sin-dez-mot′ō-mē). Surgical division of a ligament. [syndesmo- + G. *tomē,* incision]

syn·drome (sin′drōm). The aggregate of signs and symptoms associated with any morbid process, and constituting together the picture of the disease. SEE ALSO disease. [G. *syndromē,* a running together, tumultuous concourse; (in med.) a concurrence of symptoms, fr. *syn,* together, + *dromos,* a running]

    acquired immunodeficiency s., SYN AIDS.

    Adams-Stokes s., a s. characterized by slow or absent pulse, vertigo, syncope, convulsions, and sometimes Cheyne-Stokes respiration; usually as a result of advanced A-V block or sick sinus syndrome. SYN Adams-Stokes disease, Morgagni's disease, Spens' s., Stokes-Adams s.

    Adie s. [MIM*100300], an idiopathic postganglionic denervation of the parasympathetically innervated intraocular muscles, usually complicated by signs of aberrant regeneration of these nerves: a weak light reaction with segmental palsy of iris sphincter, a strong, slow near response. Deep tendon reflexes are often asymmetrically reduced. SEE ALSO tonic *pupil.* SYN Adie's pupil, Holmes-Adie pupil, Holmes-Adie s., pupil-lotonic pseudostrabismus.

    adrenogenital s., generic designation for a group of disorders caused by adrenocortical hyperplasia or malignant tumors and characterized by masculinization of women, feminization of men, or precocious sexual development of children; representative of excessive or abnormal secretory patterns of adrenocortical steroids, especially those with androgenic or estrogenic effects.

    adult respiratory distress s. (ARDS), acute lung injury from a variety of causes, characterized by interstitial and/or alveolar edema and hemorrhage as well as perivascular pulmonary edema associated with hyaline membrane, proliferation of collagen fibers, and swollen epithelium with increased pinocytosis. SYN wet lung (2), white lung.

    Ahumada-Del Castillo s., unphysiological lactation and amenorrhea not following pregnancy characterized by hyperprolactinemia and a pituitary adenoma.

    alcohol amnestic s., an amnestic s. resulting from alcoholism; alcoholic "blackouts." Cf. Korsakoff's s.

    amenorrhea-galactorrhea s., unphysiologic

sy

lactation from endocrinological causes or from a pituitary tumor.

amnestic s., (1) SYN Korsakoff's s. **(2)** an organic brain s. with short term (but not immediate) memory disturbance, regardless of the etiology.

anterior tibial compartment s., ischemic necrosis of the muscles of the anterior tibial compartment of the leg, presumed due to compression of arteries by swollen muscles following unaccustomed exertion.

antiphospholipid antibody s., a tendency for recurrent thrombosis together with recurrent abortion, thrombocytopenia, and neurologic disease, with antibodies against certain negatively charged phospholipids such as cardiolipin, phosphatidylserine, and phosphatidylethanolamine.

autoerythrocyte sensitization s., a condition, usually occurring in women, in which the individual bruises easily (purpura simplex) and the ecchymoses tend to enlarge and involve adjacent tissues, resulting in pain in the affected parts; thought to be a form of localized autosensitization. SYN Gardner-Diamond s.

Ayerza's s., sclerosis of the pulmonary arteries in chronic cor pulmonale; associated with severe cyanosis, it is a condition resembling polycythemia vera but resulting from primary pulmonary arteriosclerosis or primary pulmonary hypertension and characterized by plexiform lesions of arterioles. SYN Ayerza's disease.

bare lymphocyte s., absence of HLA antigens on peripheral mononuclear cells, which may result in immunodeficiency.

**basal cell nevus ⸢s. [MIM*109400], a s. of myriad basal cell nevi with development of basal cell carcinomas in adult life, odontogenic keratocysts, erythematous pitting of the palms and soles, calcification of the cerebral falx, and frequently skeletal anomalies, particularly ribs that are bifid or broadened anteriorly; autosomal dominant inheritance.

Bauer's s., aortitis and aortic endocarditis as a little-recognized manifestation of rheumatoid arthritis.

Beckwith-Wiedemann s. [MIM*130650], exomphalos, macroglossia, and gigantism, often with neonatal hypoglycemia; autosomal recessive inheritance.

Besnier-Boeck-Schaumann s., SYN sarcoidosis.

Beuren s., supravalvular aortic stenosis with multiple areas of peripheral pulmonary arterial stenosis, mental retardation, and dental anomalies.

blind loop s., cluster of symptoms that results from the overgrowth of bacteria in a surgically bypassed segment of the intestine. Primary symptoms are fat malabsorption and vitamin B_{12} and folate deficiencies.

Boerhaave's s., spontaneous rupture of the lower esophagus, a variant of Mallory-Weiss s.

carcinoid s., a combination of symptoms and lesions usually produced by the release of serotonin from carcinoid tumors of the gastrointestinal tract that have metastasized to the liver; consists of irregular mottled blushing, flat angiomas of the skin, acquired tricuspid and pulmonary stenosis

often with regurgitation, diarrhea, bronchial spasm, mental aberration, and excretion of large quantities of 5-hydroxyindoleacetic acid.

carotid sinus s., stimulation of a hyperactive carotid sinus, causing a marked fall in blood pressure due to vasodilation, cardiac slowing, or both; syncope with or without convulsions or A-V block may occur.

⬛carpal tunnel s., the most common nerve entrapment s., characterized by nocturnal hand paresthesia and pain, and sometimes sensory loss and wasting in the median hand distribution; caused by entrapment of the median nerve at the wrist, within the carpal tunnel.

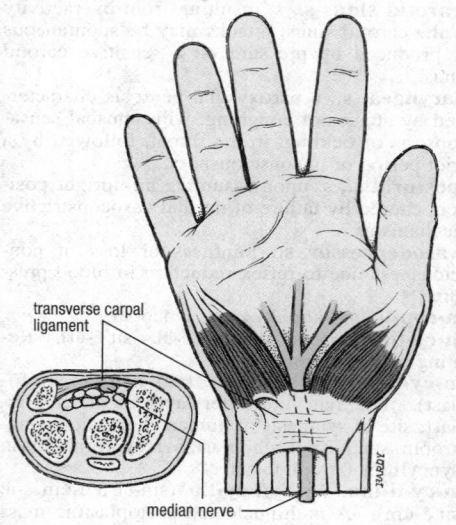

transverse carpal ligament

median nerve

carpal tunnel syndrome

central cord s., quadriparesis most severely involving the distal upper extremities, with or without sensory loss and bladder dysfunction, usually due to ischemia from osteophytic or traumatic compression of the central part of the cervical spinal cord and/or artery.

cervical rib s., 1) arterial thoracic outlet s. in which the subclavian artery is compromised by a fully formed cervical rib, and 2) true neurogenic thoracic outlet s. in which the proximal lower trunk of the brachial plexus is compromised by a radiolucent band extending from a rudimentary cervical rib to the first rib.

Cestan-Chenais s., contralateral hemiplegia, hemianesthesia, and loss of pain and temperature sensibility, with ipsilateral hemiasynergia and lateropulsion, paralysis of the larynx and soft palate, enophthalmia, miosis, and ptosis, due to lesions of the brainstem.

Chandler s., iris atrophy with corneal edema.

Charcot's s., SYN intermittent *claudication*.

cherry-red spot myoclonus s., a neuronal storage disorder in children characterized by a cherry red spot at the macula, progressive myoclonus, and easily controlled seizures; the result of sialidase deficiency. SYN sialidosis.

Chinese restaurant s., development of chest pain, feelings of facial pressure, and sensation of burning over variable portions of the body surface after ingestion of food containing monosodium L-glutamate (MSG) by persons sensitive to this food additive.

chromosomal s., general designation for s.'s due to chromosomal aberrations; typically associated with mental retardation and multiple congenital anomalies.

chromosomal instability s.'s, chromosomal breakage s.'s, a group of mendelian conditions associated with chromosomal instability and breakage *in vitro;* they often manifest an increased tendency to certain types of malignancies. SEE fragile X *chromosome, xeroderma* pigmentosum.

Cobb s., cutaneous angiomas, usually in a dermatomal distribution on the trunk, associated with vascular abnormality of the spinal cord and resulting neurologic symptoms.

Cogan-Reese s., SYN iridocorneal endothelial s.

compartment s., condition in which increased intramuscular pressure in a confined anatomical space brought on by overactivity or trauma impedes blood flow and function of tissues within that space. SYN compression s. (2).

compression s., (1) SYN crush s. **(2)** SYN compartment s.

Conn's s., SYN primary *aldosteronism.*

CREST s., a variant of scleroderma characterized by *c*alcinosis, *R*aynaud's phenomenon, *e*sophageal motility disorders, *s*clerodactyly, and *t*elangiectasia.

cri-du-chat s., cat-cry s., a disorder due to deletion of the short arm of chromosome 5, characterized by microcephaly, hypertelorism, antimongoloid palpebral fissures, epicanthal folds, micrognathia, strabismus, mental and physical retardation, and a characteristic high-pitched catlike whine.

Crigler-Najjar s. [MIM*218800], a defect in ability to form bilirubin glucuronide due to deficiency of bilirubin-glucuronide glucuronosyltransferase; characterized by familial nonhemolytic jaundice and, in its severe form, by irreversible brain damage in infancy that resembles kernicterus and may be fatal. SYN Crigler-Najjar disease.

crocodile tears s., a flow of tears, usually unilateral, upon eating or the anticipation of eating; this happens when nerve fibers originally destined for a salivary gland are damaged and regrow, aberrantly, into the lacrimal gland.

crush s., the shocklike state that follows release of a limb or limbs or the trunk and pelvis after a prolonged period of compression, as by a heavy weight; characterized by suppression of urine, probably the result of damage to the renal tubules by myoglobin from the damaged muscles. SYN compression s. (1).

Cushing's s., a disorder resulting from increased level of adrenocortical hormones, due to any of several causes: ACTH-dependent adrenocortical hyperplasia or tumor, ectopic ACTH-secreting tumor, or excessive administrations of steroids; characterized by truncal obesity, moon face, acne, abdominal striae, hypertension, decreased carbohydrate tolerance, protein catabolism, psychiatric disturbances, and osteoporosis, amenorrhea, and hirsutism in females; when associated with an ACTH producing adenoma, called Cushing's disease. SYN Cushing's basophilism.

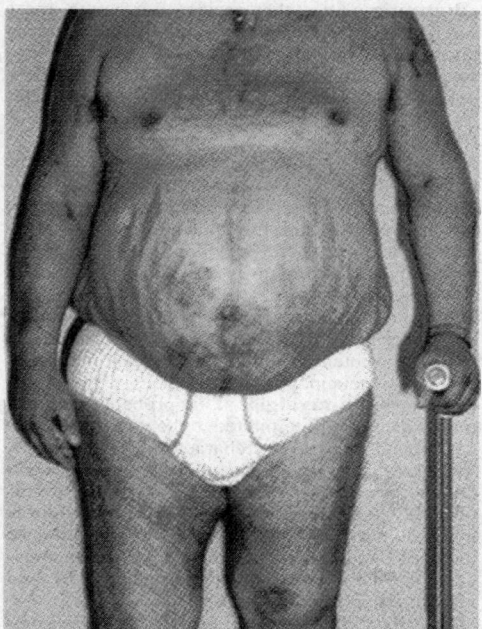

Cushing's syndrome: note abdominal obesity and striae

Cushing's s. medicamentosa, a variable number of the signs and symptoms of Cushing's s.; produced by the chronic administration of large doses of any steroid that is a potent glucocorticoid.

Dandy-Walker s. [MIM*304340], developmental anomaly of the fourth ventricle associated with atresia of the foramina of Luschka and Magendie that results in cerebellar hypoplasia, hydrocephalus, and posterior fossa cyst formation.

dialysis encephalopathy s., a progressive, often fatal, diffuse encephalopathy occurring in patients on chronic hemodialysis. SYN dialysis dementia.

disk s., a constellation of symptoms and signs, including pain, paresthesias, sensory loss, weakness, and impaired reflexes, due to a compressive radiculopathy caused by intervertebral disk pressure.

Down s., a chromosomal dysgenesis syndrome consisting of a variable constellation of abnormalities caused by triplication or translocation of chromosome 21. The abnormalities include mental retardation, retarded growth, flat hypoplastic face with short nose, prominent epicanthic skin folds, small, low-set ears with prominent antihe-

sy

lix, fissured and thickened tongue, laxness of joint ligaments, pelvic dysplasia, broad hands and feet, stubby fingers, and transverse palmar crease. Lenticular opacities and heart disease are common. The incidence of leukemia is increased and Alzheimer's disease is almost inevitable by age 40. SYN trisomy 21 s.

dumping s., a s. that occurs after eating, most often seen in patients with shunts of the upper alimentary canal; characterized by flushing, sweating, dizziness, weakness, and vasomotor collapse, occasionally with pain and headache; results from rapid passage of large amounts of food into the small intestine, with an osmotic effect removing fluid from plasma and causing hypovolemia. SYN postgastrectomy s.

dyskinesia s. (dis-ki-nē′zē-ă), clearance of mucus is sluggish and bronchiectasis is prevalent and intractable. There is evidence that the defect lies in dynein, a protein in the cilia.

dysplastic nevus s. [MIM*155600], clinically atypical nevi having variable pigmentation and ill defined borders, with an increased risk for development of cutaneous malignant melanoma; biopsies show melanocytic dysplasia.

eosinophilia-myalgia s., a probable autoimmune disorder precipitated by contaminated L-tryptophan tablets, and characterized by fatigue, low-grade fever, myalgias, muscle tenderness and cramps, weakness, paresthesias of the extremities, and skin indurations; marked eosinophilia is noted on peripheral blood studies, serum aldolase increased and biopsies of peripheral nerve, muscle, skin, and fascia show microangiopathy and inflammation in connective tissue.

fetal alcohol s., a specific pattern of fetal malformation with growth deficiency, craniofacial anomalies, and limb defects, found among offspring of mothers who are chronic alcoholics; mental retardation is often demonstrated later.

folded-lung s., collapse of part of the lung caught between shrinking fibrous pleural scars, sometimes resulting from pleural asbestosis. SYN round atelectasis.

fragile X s., SEE fragile X *chromosome.*

Ganser's s., a psychotic-like condition, without the symptoms and signs of a traditional psychosis, occurring typically in prisoners who feign insanity; *e.g.,* such a person, when asked to multiply 6 by 4, will give 23 as the answer, or will call a key a lock.

Gardner-Diamond s., SYN autoerythrocyte sensitization s.

gay bowel s., gastrointestinal discomfort experienced by homosexual males; includes abdominal pain, cramps, bloating, flatulence, nausea, vomiting, or diarrhea caused by enteric bacteria, viruses, fungi, zooparasites, or trauma.

general adaptation s., a term introduced by Hans Selye to describe marked physiological changes in various organ systems of the body, especially the pituitary-endocrine system, as a result of exposure to prolonged physical or psychological stress.

Gilles de la Tourette's s. [MIM*137580], SYN Tourette s.

Gowers' s., s. consisting of palpitation, chest pain, respiratory difficulties, and disturbances in gastric motility; once attributed to vagal stimulation, now considered psychogenic (anxiety neurosis).

gray s., gray baby s., gray appearance of an infant at birth and during the neonatal period which can be caused by transplacental toxic effects of the drug chloramphenicol taken by the mother during late pregnancy; the s. may be fatal.

Hallervorden-Spatz s., a disorder characterized by dystonia with other extrapyramidal dysfunctions appearing in the first two decades of life; associated with large amounts of iron in the globus pallidus and substantia nigra.

Hamman's s., spontaneous mediastinal emphysema, resulting from rupture of alveoli. SYN Hamman's disease.

Harada's s., bilateral retinal edema, uveitis, choroiditis, and retinal detachment, with temporary or permanent deafness, graying of the hair (poliosis), and alopecia; related to the Vogt-Koyanagi s. and sympathetic ophthalmia.

Hartnup s., SYN Hartnup *disease.*

hemolytic uremic s., hemolytic anemia and thrombocytopenia occurring with acute renal failure. In children, characterized by sudden onset of gastrointestinal bleeding, hematuria, oliguria, and microangiopathic hemolytic anemia in association with intestinal infection by *Shigella, Salmonella,* or *E. coli* srain O157:H7; in adults, associated with complications of pregnancy following normal delivery, or associated with oral contraceptive use or with infection.

hepatorenal s., hepatonephoric s., the occurrence of acute renal failure in patients with disease of the liver or biliary tract.

Holmes-Adie s., SYN Adie s.

Horner's s., ptosis, miosis, and anhidrosis on the side of a sympathetic palsy. Enophthalmos is more apparent than real. The affected pupil is visibly slow to dilate in dim light; due to a lesion of the cervical sympathetic chain or its central pathways.

Hunt's s. [MIM*159700], **(1)** an intention tremor beginning in one extremity, gradually increasing in intensity, and subsequently involving other parts of the body; **(2)** facial paralysis, otalgia, and herpes zoster resulting from viral infection of the seventh cranial nerve and geniculate ganglion; **(3)** a form of juvenile paralysis agitans associated with primary atrophy of the pallidal system. SYN Ramsay Hunt's s. (1).

Hurler's s. [MIM*252800], mucopolysaccharidosis in which there is a deficiency of α-L-iduronidase, an accumulation of an abnormal intracellular material, and excretion of dermatan sulfate and heparan sulfate in the urine; with severe abnormality in development of skeletal cartilage and bone, with dwarfism, kyphosis, deformed limbs, limitation of joint motion, spadelike hand, corneal clouding, hepatosplenomegaly, mental retardation, and gargoyle-like facies.

hypereosinophilic s., persistent peripheral eosinophilia with later infiltration into bone marrow, heart, and other organ systems; accompanied by nocturnal sweating, coughing, anorexia and weight loss, itching and various skin lesions, and symptoms of Löffler's endocarditis.

hyperimmunoglobulin E s., an immunodeficiency disorder characterized by high levels of plasma IgE concentrations, a leukocyte chemotactic defect, and recurrent staphylococcal infections of the skin, upper respiratory tract, and other sites.

hyperkinetic s., a condition marked by pathologically excessive energy seen sometimes in young children with brain injury, mental illness, and attention deficit disorder, and in epileptics; hypermotility and emotional instability are the chief characteristics; distractibility, inattention, and lack of shyness and of fear are common accompaniments.

hypophysial s., SYN *dystrophia* adiposogenitalis.

impingement s., chronic shoulder pain and disability due to trauma to the rotator cuff (particularly the supraspinatus tendon) by surrounding bony processes and ligaments, such as occurs during performance of overhead work.

iridocorneal endothelial s., s. of glaucoma, iris atrophy, decreased corneal endothelium, anterior peripheral synechia, and multiple iris nodules. SYN Cogan-Reese s., iris-nevus s.

iris-nevus s., SYN iridocorneal endothelial s.

Irvine-Gass s., macular edema, aphakia, and vitreous humor adherent to incision for cataract extraction.

jaw-winking s. [MIM*154600], an increase in the width of the palpebral fissures during chewing, sometimes with a rhythmic elevation of the upper lid when the mouth is open and ptosis when the mouth is closed. SYN Marcus Gunn phenomenon, Marcus Gunn s.

Joubert's s. [MIM*213300], agenesis of the cerebellar vermis, characterized clinically by attacks of tachypnea or prolonged apnea, abnormal eye movements, ataxia, and mental retardation.

Kanner's s., SYN infantile *autism*.

Kartagener's s. [MIM*244400], complete situs inversus associated with bronchiectasis and chronic sinusitis associated with ciliary dysmotility and impaired ciliary mucus transport in the respiratory epithelium. SYN Kartagener's triad.

Kawasaki's s., a polymorphous erythematous febrile, sometimes epidemic, disease of unknown etiology occurring in children, especially under two years of age; accompanied by conjunctivitis, pharyngitis, strawberry tongue, cervical lymphadenopathy, occasionally fatal arteritis with coronary artery aneurysm formation, and characteristic desquamation of perineum, fingers, and toes. SYN mucocutaneous lymph node s.

Kearns-Sayre s. [MIM*165100], a form of chronic progressive external ophthalmoplegia with associated cardiac conduction defects, short stature, and hearing loss; a sporadically ocurring mitochondrial myopathy presenting in childhood.

Kimmelstiel-Wilson s., nephrotic syndrome and hypertension in diabetics, associated with diabetic glomerulosclerosis. SYN Kimmelstiel-Wilson disease.

Klinefelter's s., a chromosomal anomaly with chromosome count 47, XXY sex chromosome constitution; patients are male in development but have seminiferous tubule dysgenesis, elevated urinary gonadotropins, gynecomastia, and eunuchoid habitus. SYN XXY s.

Korsakoff's s., an alcohol amnestic s. characterized by confusion and severe impairment of memory, especially for recent events, for which the patient compensates by confabulation; typically encountered in chronic alcoholics; delirium tremens may precede the s., and Wernicke's s. often coexists; the precise pathogenesis is uncertain, but direct toxic effects of alcohol are probably less important than severe nutritional deficiencies often associated with chronic alcoholism. SYN amnestic s. (1), Korsakoff's psychosis, polyneuritic psychosis.

Landau-Kleffner s., childhood disorder characterized by generalized and psychomotor seizures associated with acquired aphasia; multifocal spikes and spike and wave discharges in the electroencephalogram. SYN acquired epileptic aphasia.

Landry s., SYN acute idiopathic *polyneuritis*.

Lennox s., SYN Lennox-Gastaut s.

Lennox-Gastaut s., a generalized myoclonic astatic epilepsy in children, with mental retardation, resulting from various cerebral afflictions such as perinatal hypoxia, cerebral hemorrhage, encephalitides, maldevelopment or metabolic disorders of the brain; characterized by multiple seizure types (generalized tonic, atonic, myoclonic, tonic-clonic, and atypical absence) and background slowing and slow spike and wave pattern on EEG; patients are usually mentally retarded or developmentally delayed. SYN Lennox s.

LEOPARD s., a hereditary s. consisting of *l*entigines (multiple), *e*lectrocardiographic abnormalities, *o*cular hypertelorism, *p*ulmonary stenosis, *a*bnormalities of genitalia, *r*etardation of growth, and *d*eafness (sensorineural).

Leriche's s., aortoiliac occlusive *disease* producing distal ischemic symptoms and signs.

Lev's s., bundle branch block in a patient with normal myocardium and normal coronary arteries resulting from fibrosis or calcification including the conducting system; affects the membranous septum, the apex of the muscular septum, and often the mitral and aortic valve rings.

Libman-Sacks s., SYN Libman-Sacks *endocarditis*.

locked-in s., basis pontis infarct resulting in tetraplegia, horizontal ophthalmoplegia, dysphagia, and facial diplegia with preserved consciousness; caused by basilar artery occlusion.

Lutembacher's s., a congenital cardiac abnormality consisting of a defect of the interatrial septum, mitral stenosis, and enlarged right atrium.

Mad Hatter s., gastrointestinal and central nervous system manifestations of chronic mercury poisoning, including stomatitis, diarrhea, ataxia, tremor, hyperreflexia, sensorineural impairment, and emotional instability; previously seen in workers in lead manufacturing who put mercury-containing materials in their mouths to make them more pliable. [fr. char. in *Alice in Wonderland*]

sy

malabsorption s., a state characterized by diverse features such as diarrhea, weakness, edema, lassitude, weight loss, poor appetite, protuberant abdomen, pallor, bleeding tendencies, paresthesias, and muscle cramps, caused by any of several conditions in which there is ineffective absorption of nutrients, *e.g.,* sprue, gluten-induced enteropathy, gastroileostomy, tuberculosis, and certain fistulas.

Mallory-Weiss s., laceration of the lower end of the esophagus associated with bleeding, or penetration into the mediastinum, with subsequent mediastinitis; caused usually by severe retching and vomiting.

Marcus Gunn s., SYN jaw-winking s.

Marfan's s. [MIM*154700], a s. of congenital changes in the mesodermal and ectodermal tissues, skeletal changes (arachnodactyly, long limbs, laxness of joints), ectopia lentis, and vascular defects (particularly aneurysm of the aorta, dissecting or diffuse); marked iris transillumination is due to a deficiency of posterior epithelium pigment.

Mauriac's s., dwarfism with obesity and hepatosplenomegaly in children with poorly controlled diabetes mellitus.

May-White s., progressive myoclonus epilepsy with lipomas, deafness, and ataxia; probably a familial form of mitochondrial encephalomyopathy.

McCune-Albright s., polyostotic fibrous dysplasia with irregular brown patches of cutaneous pigmentation and endocrine dysfunction, especially precocious puberty in girls. SEE ALSO pseudohypoparathyroidism.

megacystic s., a combination of a large smooth thin-walled bladder, vesicoureteral regurgitation, and dilated ureters.

milk-alkali s., a chronic disorder of the kidneys, reversible in its early stages, induced by ingestion of large amounts of calcium and alkali in the therapy of peptic ulcer; can progress to renal failure.

Morgagni's s. [MIM*144800], hyperostosis frontalis interna in elderly women, with obesity and neuropsychiatric disorders of uncertain cause; at least sometimes familial. SYN metabolic craniopathy.

Morton's s., congenital shortening of the first metatarsal causing metatarsalgia.

mucocutaneous lymph node s., SYN Kawasaki's s.

multiple endocrine deficiency s., acquired deficiency of the function of several endocrine glands, usually on an autoimmune basis.

multiple mucosal neuroma s., multiple submucosal neuromas or neurofibromas of the tongue, lips, and eyelids in young persons; sometimes associated with tumors of the thyroid or adrenal medulla, or with subcutaneous neurofibromatosis.

myasthenic s. (MS), a disorder of neuromuscular transmission marked primarily by limb and girdle weakness, absent deep tendon reflexes, dry mouth, and impotence; due to an immunological disorder; often, especially in males, a paraneoplastic syndrome linked to small cell carcinoma of the lung.

myelodysplastic s., a primary, neoplastic, pluripotential stem-cell disorder characterized by peripheral blood cytopenias and prominent maturation abnormalities in the bone marrow. The disease evolves progressively and may transform into leukemia. Classified by the French-American-British (FAB) system into five groups. SEE ALSO French-American-British *classification* system. SYN chronic erythremic myelosis, preleukemia, smoldering leukemia.

myeloproliferative s.'s [MIM*159595], a group of conditions that result from a disorder in the rate of formation of cells of the bone marrow, including chronic granulocytic leukemia, erythremia, myelosclerosis, panmyelosis, and erythremic myelosis and erythroleukemia.

myofacial pain-dysfunction s., dysfunction of the masticatory apparatus related to spasm of the muscles of mastication precipitated by occlusal disharmony or alteration in vertical dimension of the jaws, and exacerbated by emotional stress; characterized by pain in the preauricular region, muscle tenderness, popping noise in the temporomandibular joint, and limitation of jaw motion. SYN temporomandibular joint pain-dysfunction s., TMJ s.

Naegeli s. [MIM*161000], reticular skin pigmentation, diminished sweating, hypodontia, and hyperkeratosis of the palms and soles.

Nelson s., a s. of hyperpigmentation, third nerve damage, and enlarging sella turcica caused by pituitary adenomas presumably present before adrenalectomy for Cushing's s. but enlarging and symptomatic afterward. SYN postadrenalectomy s.

nephritic s., the clinical symptoms of acute glomerulonephritis, particularly hematuria, hypertension, and renal failure.

nephrotic s., a clinical state characterized by edema, albuminuria, decreased plasma albumin, doubly refractile bodies in the urine, and usually increased blood cholesterol; lipid droplets may be present in the cells of the renal tubules, but the basic lesion is increased permeability of the glomerular capillary basement membranes, of unknown cause or resulting from glomerulonephritis, diabetic glomerulosclerosis, systemic lupus erythematosus, amyloidosis, renal vein thrombosis, or hypersensitivity to various toxic agents. SYN nephrosis (3).

neural crest s., s. consisting of loss of pain sensibility, autonomic dysfunction, pupillary abnormalities, neurogenic anhidrosis, vasomotor instability, aplasia of dental enamel, meningeal thickening, hyperflexion, and a degree of albinism; may reflect developmental abnormalities of the neural crest.

neuroleptic malignant s., hyperthermia with extrapyramidal and autonomic disturbances which may result in death, following the use of neuroleptic agents.

Oppenheim's s., SYN *amyotonia* congenita (1).

organic brain s., a constellation of behavioral or psychological signs and symptoms including problems with attention, concentration, memory, confusion, anxiety, and depression caused by transient or permanent dysfunction of the brain. SYN OBS.

overuse s., injury caused by accumulated microtraumatic stress placed on a structure or body area.

Pancoast s., lower trunk brachial plexopathy and Horner s. due to malignant tumor in the region of the superior pulmonary sulcus.

paraneoplastic s., a s. directly resulting from a malignant neoplasm, but not resulting from the presence of tumor cells in the affected parts.

Parinaud's s., paralysis of conjugate upward gaze with a lesion at the level of the superior colliculi; Bell's phenomenon is present.

Parinaud's oculoglandular s., unilateral conjunctival granuloma with preauricular adenopathy in tularemia, chancre, and tuberculosis.

patellofemoral s., chronic knee pain due to failure of the patella to glide smoothly in its groove on the femur, as a result of structural misalignment or deviant traction by the quadriceps tendon. SEE ALSO *chondromalacia* patellae.

pickwickian s., a combination of severe, grotesque obesity, somnolence, and general debility, theoretically resulting from hypoventilation induced by the obesity; hypercapnia, pulmonary hypertension and cor pulmonale can result. [after the "fat boy" in Dickens's *Pickwick Papers*]

Pierre Robin s. [MIM*261800], micrognathia and abnormal smallness of the tongue, often with cleft palate, severe myopia, congenital glaucoma, and retinal detachment.

Pins' s., dullness, diminution of vocal fremitus and of the vesicular murmur, and a slight distant blowing sound, heard in the posteroinferior region of the chest on the left side, in cases of pericardial effusion; there is sometimes also a fine rale in this region, but all the adventitious auscultatory signs disappear when the patient assumes the genupectoral position.

Plummer-Vinson s., iron deficiency anemia, dysphagia, esophageal web, and atrophic glossitis.

polycystic ovary s. [MIM*184700], a condition commonly characterized by hirsutism, obesity, menstrual abnormalities, infertility, and enlarged ovaries; thought to reflect excessive androgen secretion of ovarian origin.

postadrenalectomy s., SYN Nelson s.

postcommissurotomy s., SYN postpericardiotomy s.

postconcussion s., progressive deterioration of cognitive function following repeated brain trauma.

postgastrectomy s., SYN dumping s.

postpericardiotomy s., pericarditis, with or without fever and often in repeated episodes, weeks to months after cardiac surgery. SYN postcommissurotomy s.

posttraumatic s., a clinical disorder that often follows head injury, characterized by headache, dizziness, neurasthenia, hypersensitivity to stimuli, and diminished concentration.

preexcitation s., SYN Wolff-Parkinson-White s.

premenstrual s. (PMS), in some women of reproductive age, the regular monthly experience of physiological and emotional distress, usually during the several days preceding menses; characterized by nervousness, depression, fluid retention, and weight gain. SYN premenstrual tension.

pulmonary dysmaturity s., a respiratory disorder occurring in premature infants who are incapable of normal pulmonary ventilation and who often die of hypoxia after an illness of 6 to 8 weeks; the lungs contain widespread focal emphysematous blebs and the parenchyma has thickened alveolar walls.

punchdrunk s., a condition seen in boxers, often years after retirement, and presumably caused by repeated cerebral injury, characterized by weakness in the lower limbs, unsteadiness of gait, slowness of muscular movements, tremors of hands, dysarthria, and slow cerebration.

Putnam-Dana s., SYN subacute combined *degeneration* of the spinal cord.

Ramsay Hunt's s., (1) SYN Hunt's s. **(2)** SYN *herpes* zoster oticus.

Raynaud's s., idiopathic paroxysmal bilateral cyanosis of the digits due to arterial and arteriolar contraction; caused by cold or emotion. SEE ALSO Raynaud's *phenomenon*. SYN Raynaud's disease.

Reiter's s., the association of urethritis, iridocyclitis, mucocutaneous lesions, and arthritis, sometimes with diarrhea; one or more of these conditions may recur at intervals of months or years, but the arthritis may be persistent. SYN Reiter's disease.

Rett's s. [MIM*312750], a progressive s. of autism, dementia, ataxia, and purposeless hand movements; associated with hyperammonemia, principally in girls.

Reye's s., an acquired encephalopathy of young children that follows an acute febrile illness, usually influenza or varicella infection; characterized by recurrent vomiting, agitation, and lethargy, which may lead to coma with intracranial hypertension; ammonia and serum transaminases are elevated; death may result from edema of the brain and resulting cerebral herniation. Strongly associated with aspirin use. SYN hepatic encephalopathy (2).

Rh null s. [MIM*269150], a lack of all Rh antigens, compensated hemolytic anemia, and stomatocytosis.

Russell's s., failure of infants and young children to thrive due to suprasellar lesions, commonly astrocytomas of the anterior third ventricle; although the growth hormone may be elevated, the child is emaciated and has loss of body fat.

scapulocostal s., pain of insidious development in the upper or posterior part of the shoulder radiating into the neck and occiput, down the arm, or around the chest; there may be numbness or tingling in the fingers; attributed to an alteration from the normal relationship between the scapula and posterior wall of the thorax.

Sertoli-cell-only s. [MIM*305700], the absence from the seminiferous tubules of the testes of germinal epithelium, Sertoli cells alone being present; there is sterility due to azoospermia but Leydig cells are normal; the output of gonadotrophins in the urine is increased.

Sheehan's s., hypopituitarism arising from a

severe circulatory collapse postpartum, with resultant pituitary necrosis.

short bowel s., complex of symptoms that can result whenever the absorptive surface of the small bowel is reduced, such as in multiple small bowel resections. Symptoms include diarrhea, weight loss, malabsorption, hypocalcemia, hypomagnesemia and other electrolyte abnormalities, and anemia. SYN short gut s.

short gut s., SYN short bowel s.

shoulder-girdle s., SYN neuralgic *amyotrophy.*

Shy-Drager s. [MIM*146500], a progressive disorder involving the autonomic system, characterized by hypotension, external ophthalmoplegia, iris atrophy, incontinence, anhidrosis, impotence, tremor, and muscle wasting.

sick building s., a s. of nonspecific symptoms including fatigue, headache, dry eyes and throat, and nasal problems, occurring mostly in office workers; attributed to low-level exposures to substances used in building and interior construction; most symptoms lessen during off-work periods.

Sjögren's s., keratoconjunctivitis sicca, dryness of mucous membranes, telangiectasias or purpuric spots on the face, and bilateral parotid enlargement seen in menopausal women and often associated with rheumatoid arthritis, Raynaud's phenomenon, and dental caries; there are changes in the lacrimal and salivary glands resembling those of Mikulicz' disease. [H. S. C. Sjögren]

snapping hip s., a snapping sensation either heard or felt during hip motion.

Spens' s., SYN Adams-Stokes s.

Stevens-Johnson s., a bullous form of erythema multiforme which may be extensive, involving the mucous membranes and large areas of the body; it may produce serious subjective symptoms and may have a fatal termination.

Stewart-Treves s., angiosarcoma arising in an arm affected by postmastectomy lymphedema.

stiff-man s., a chronic, progressive central nervous system disorder of unknown cause, associated with fluctuating painful muscle spasm and rigidity involving muscles of the limbs, trunk, and neck.

Stockholm s., a form of bonding between a captive and captor in which the captive begins to identify with, and may even sympathize with, the captor. [*Stockholm,* Sweden, where early cases reported]

Stokes-Adams s., SYN Adams-Stokes s.

sudden infant death s. (SIDS), abrupt and inexplicable death of an apparently healthy infant; various theories have been advanced to explain such deaths (*e.g.,* sleep-induced apnea, laryngospasm, overwhelming infectious disease) but none has been generally accepted or demonstrated at autopsy. SYN crib death.

sump s., a complication of side-to-side choledochoduodenostomy in which the lower end of the common bile duct at times acts as a diverticulum, resulting in stasis, trapping of food particles, and infection.

superior vena cava s., obstruction of the superior vena cava or its main tributaries by benign or malignant lesions, causing edema and engorgement of the vessels of the face, neck, and arms,

nonproductive cough, and dyspnea; bluish looking venous stars may be found in the early phases, overlying the large veins to which they are tributary, but they tend to diminish in size and disappear after collateral circulation has been reestablished.

Swyer-James s., (1) SYN unilateral lobar *emphysema.* **(2)** hyperlucency of one lung from obliterating bronchiolitis, usually caused by adenovirus infection in childhood, with decreased size and vascularity of the lung; distinguished from other causes of unilateral hyperlucency by demonstration of air trapping without central obstruction.

tachycardia-bradycardia s., alternating periods of slow and rapid heart beat; often associated with disturbances of both sinoatrial and atrioventricular conduction.

Takayasu's s., SYN Takayasu's *arteritis.*

Taussig-Bing s., complete transposition of the aorta, which arises from the right ventricle, with a left-sided pulmonary artery overriding the left ventricle, and with high ventricular septal defect, right ventricular hypertrophy, anteriorly situated aorta, and posteriorly situated pulmonary artery.

tegmental s., a s. usually caused by a vascular lesion in the tegmentum; marked by contralateral hemiplegia and ipsilateral ocular paresis.

temporomandibular joint pain-dysfunction s., SYN myofacial pain-dysfunction s.

testicular feminization s. [MIM*313700], a type of male pseudohermaphroditism characterized by female external genitalia, incompletely developed vagina often with rudimentary uterus and fallopian tubes, female habitus at puberty but with scanty or absent axillary and pubic hair and amenorrhea, and testes present within the abdomen or in the inguinal canals or labia majora; epididymis and vas deferens are usually present; androgens and estrogens are formed, but target tissues are largely unresponsive to androgens; individuals are sex chromatin-negative and have a normal male karyotype; there is a defect in the androgen receptor protein.

thoracic outlet s. (TOS), collective title for a number of conditions attributed to compromise of blood vessels or nerve fibers (brachial plexus) at any point between the base of the neck and the axilla; classified on the basis of the structure known or presumed to be compromised, and divided into two main groups: vascular and neurologic.

thrombocytopenia-absent radius s. [MIM* 270400], congenital absence of the radius associated with thrombocytopenia that is symptomatic in infancy but later improves; congenital heart disease and renal anomalies occur in some cases; autosomal recessive inheritance.

TMJ s., SYN myofacial pain-dysfunction s.

Tolosa-Hunt s., cavernous sinus s. produced by an idiopathic granuloma.

TORCH s., a group of infections with similar clinical manifestations, although symptoms may vary in degree and time of appearance: *t*oxoplasmosis, *o*ther infections, *r*ubella, *c*ytomegalovirus infection, and *h*erpes simplex. These infections might be associated with underlying HIV infection.

Tourette s., a tic disorder appearing in childhood, characterized by multiple motor tics and vocal tics present for more than one year. Obsessive-compulsive behavior, attention-deficit disorder, and other psychiatric disorders may be associated; coprolalia and echolalia rarely occur; autosomal dominant inheritance. SYN Gilles de la Tourette's s.

toxic shock s. (TSS), infection with toxin-producing staphylococci, occurring most often in the vagina of menstruating women using superabsorbent tampons and characterized by high fever, vomiting, diarrhea, a scarlatiniform rash followed by desquamation, and decreasing blood pressure and shock, which can result in death; hyperemia of the conjunctival, oropharyngeal, and vaginal mucous membranes also occurs.

trisomy 21 s., SYN Down s.

tropical splenomegaly s., SYN hyperreactive malarious *splenomegaly.*

Turner's s., a s. with chromosome count 45 and only one X chromosome; buccal and other cells are usually sex chromatin-negative; anomalies include dwarfism, webbed neck, valgus of elbows, pigeon chest, infantile sexual development, and amenorrhea; the ovary has no primordial follicles and may be represented only by a fibrous streak. SYN XO s.

ulnar nerve compression s., SYN cyclist's *palsy.*

VACTERL s., abnormalities of *v*ertebrae, *a*nus, *c*cardiovascular tree, *t*rachea, *e*sophagus, *r*enal system, and *l*imb buds associated with administration of sex steroids during early pregnancy.

van Buchem's s. [MIM*239100], an inherited skeletal dysplasia, with mandibular enlargement and thickening of the diaphyses and calvaria, and increased serum alkaline phosphatase; autosomal recessive inheritance.

vanishing lung s., progressive decrease of radiographic opacity of the lung caused by accelerated development of emphysema or rapid cystic destruction of the lung from infection.

Vernet's s., a s. characterized by paralysis of the motor components of the glossopharyngeal, vagus, and accessory cranial nerves as they lie in the posterior fossa; it is most commonly the result of head injury.

Waterhouse-Friderichsen s., a condition due to meningococcemia, occurring mainly in children under 10 years of age, characterized by vomiting, diarrhea, extensive purpura, cyanosis, tonoclonic convulsions, and circulatory collapse, usually with meningitis and hemorrhage into the adrenal glands.

Weber's s., midbrain tegmentum lesion characterized by ipsilateral oculomotor nerve paresis and contralateral paralysis of the extremities, face, and tongue.

Weill-Marchesani s. [MIM*277600], ectopia lentis (lens abnormally round and small), short stature, and brachydactyly; recessive autosomal inheritance.

Wernicke-Korsakoff s., the coexistence of Wernicke's and Korsakoff's s.'s.

Wernicke's s., a condition frequently encountered in chronic alcoholics, largely due to thiamin deficiency and characterized by disturbances in ocular motility, pupillary alterations, nystagmus, and ataxia with tremors; an organic-toxic psychosis is often an associated finding, and Korsakoff's s. often coexists; characteristic cellular pathology found in several areas of the brain. SYN Wernicke's disease, Wernicke's encephalopathy.

Wissler's s., high intermittent fever, irregularly recurring macular and maculo-papular eruption of the face, chest and limbs, leukocytosis, arthralgia, occasionally eosinophilia, and raised erythrocyte sedimentation rate; occurs in children and adolescents, with varying duration.

withdrawal s., a substance-specific s. that follows the cessation of, or reduction in, intake of a psychoactive substance previously used regularly. The s. that develops varies according to the psychoactive substance used. Common symptoms include anxiety, restlessness, irritability, insomnia, and impaired attention.

Wolff-Parkinson-White s. [MIM*194200], an electrocardiographic pattern sometimes associated with paroxysmal tachycardia; it consists of short P-R interval (usually 0.1 second or less; occasionally normal) together with a prolonged QRS complex with a slurred initial component (delta wave). SYN preexcitation s.

Wyburn-Mason s., arteriovenous malformation on the cerebral cortex, retinal arteriovenous angioma and facial nevus, usually occurring in mentally retarded individuals.

XO s., SYN Turner's s.

XXY s., SYN Klinefelter's s.

XYY s., a chromosomal anomaly with chromosome count 47, with a supernumerary Y chromosome; controversial evidence associates tallness, aggressiveness, and acne with this condition.

Zollinger-Ellison s. [MIM*131100], peptic ulceration with gastric hypersecretion and non-beta cell tumor of the pancreatic islets, sometimes associated with familial polyendocrine adenomatosis.

syn•drom•ic (sin-drom′ik, -drō′mik). Relating to a syndrome.

syn•ech•ia, pl. **syn•ech•i•ae** (si-nek′ē-ă, -kē-ē; si-nĕ′kē-ă). Any adhesion; specifically, adhesion of an inflamed iris to the cornea (anterior s.) or lens (posterior s.). [G. *synecheia,* continuity, fr. *syn,* together, + *echō,* to have, hold]

syn•ech•i•ot•o•my (si-nek′ē-ot′ō-mē). Division of synechiae. [synechia + G. *tomē,* incision]

syn•en•ceph•a•lo•cele (sin-en-sef′ă-lō-sēl). Protrusion of brain substance through a defect in the skull, with adhesions preventing reduction. [syn- + G. *enkephalos,* brain, + *kēlē,* hernia]

syn•er•e•sis (si-ner′ĕ-sis). 1. The contraction of a gel, *e.g.,* a blood clot, by which part of the dispersion medium is squeezed out. 2. Degeneration of the vitreous humor with loss of gel consistency to become partially or completely fluid. [G. *synairesis,* a taking or drawing together]

syn•er•gism (sin′er-jizm). Coordinated or correlated action of two or more structures, agents, or physiologic processes so that the combined action is greater than the sum of each acting separately. Cf. antagonism. SYN synergy. [G. *synergia*, fr. *syn*, together, + *ergon*, work]

syn•er•gist (sin'er-jist). A structure, agent, or physiologic process that aids the action of another. Cf. antagonist.

syn•er•gy (sin'er-jē). SYN synergism.

syn•es•the•sia (sin-es-thē'zē-ă). A condition in which a stimulus, in addition to exciting the usual and normally located sensation, gives rise to a subjective sensation of different character or localization; *e.g.*, color hearing, color taste. [syn- + G. *aisthēsis*, sensation]

syn•es•the•si•al•gia (sin'es-thē-zē-al'jē-ă). Painful synesthesia.

syn•ga•my (sin'gă-mē). Conjugation of the gametes in fertilization. [syn- + G. *gamos*, marriage]

syn•ge•ne•ic (sin'jĕ-nē'ik). Relating to genetically identical individuals. SYN isogeneic, isogenic, isologous, isoplastic. [G. *syngenēs*, congenital]

syn•gen•e•sis (sin-jen'ĕ-sis). SYN sexual *reproduction*. [syn- + G. *genesis*, origin]

syn•ge•net•ic (sin-jĕ-net'ik). Relating to syngenesis.

syn•graft (sin'graft). A tissue or organ transplanted between genetically identical individuals. SYN isogeneic graft, isograft, isologous graft, isoplastic graft.

syn•i•ze•sis (sin-i-zē'sis). **1.** Closure or obliteration of the pupil. **2.** The massing of chromatin at one side of the nucleus that occurs usually at the beginning of synapsis. [G. collapse]

syn•kar•y•on (sin-kar'ē-on). The nucleus formed by the fusion of the two pronuclei in karyogamy. [syn- + G. *karyon*, kernel (nucleus)]

syn•ki•ne•sis (sin-ki-nē'sis). Involuntary movement accompanying a voluntary one, as the movement of a closed eye following that of the uncovered one, or the movement occurring in a paralyzed muscle accompanying motion in another part. [syn- + G. *kinēsis*, movement]

syn•ki•net•ic (sin-ki-net'ik). Relating to or marked by synkinesis.

syn•o•nych•ia (sin-ō-nik'ē-ă). Fusion of two or more nails of the digits, as in syndactyly. [sin- + G. *onyx* (onych-), nail]

syn•oph•thal•mia (sin-of-thal'mē-ă). SYN cyclopia. [syn- + G. *ophthalmos*, eye]

syn•or•chi•dism, syn•or•chism (sin-ōr'ki-dizm, sin-ōr'kizm). Congenital fusion of the testes in the abdomen or scrotum. [syn- + G. *orchis*, testis]

syn•os•che•os (sin-os'kē-os). Partial or complete adhesion of the penis and scrotum, a malformation in hermaphroditism. [syn- + G. *oschē*, scrotum]

syn•os•to•sis (sin-os-tō'sis). Osseous union between the bones forming a joint. SYN bony ankylosis, true ankylosis. [syn- + G. *osteon*, bone, + *-osis*, condition]

 sagittal s., SYN scaphocephaly.

syn•os•tot•ic (sin-os-tot'ik). Relating to synostosis.

sy•no•tia (si-nō'shē-ă). Fusion or abnormal approximation of the lobes of the ears in otocephaly. [syn- + G. *ous*, ear]

syn•o•vec•to•my (sin-ō-vek'tō-mē). Excision of a portion or all of the synovial membrane of a joint. SYN villusectomy. [synovia + G. *ektomē*, excision]

syn•o•via (si-nō'vē-ă) [NA]. SYN synovial *fluid*. [Mod. L., a word coined by Paracelsus, fr. G. *syn*, together, + *ōon* (L. *ovum*), egg]

syn•o•vi•al (si-nō'vē-ăl). **1.** Relating to, containing, or consisting of synovia. **2.** Relating to the membrana synovialis.

syn•o•vi•o•ma (si-nō-vē-ō'mă). A tumor of synovial origin involving joint or tendon sheath. [synovium + G. *-oma*, tumor]

syn•o•vi•tis (sin-ō-vī'tis). Inflammation of a synovial membrane, especially that of a joint; in general, when unqualified, the same as arthritis. [synovia + G. *-itis*, inflammation]

 bursal s., SYN bursitis.

 dry s., s. with little serous or purulent effusion. SYN s. sicca.

 pigmented villonodular s., diffuse outgrowths of synovial membrane of a joint, usually the knee, composed of synovial villi and fibrous nodules infiltrated by hemosiderin- and lipid-containing macrophages and multinucleated giant cells; the condition may be inflammatory, although recurrence is likely to follow incomplete removal.

 purulent s., SYN suppurative *arthritis*.

 serous s., s. with a large effusion of nonpurulent fluid.

 s. sic'ca, SYN dry s.

 tendinous s., SYN tenosynovitis.

syn•o•vi•um (si-nō'vē-ŭm). SYN synovial *membrane*.

syn•ten•ic (sin-ten'ik). Pertaining to synteny.

syn•te•ny (sin'ten-ē). The relationship between two genetic loci (not genes) represented on the same chromosomal pair or (for haploid chromosomes) on the same chromosome; an anatomic rather than a segregational relationship. [syn- + G. *tainia*, ribbon]

syn•thase (sin'thās). Trivial name used in Enzyme Commission Report for a lyase reaction going in the reverse direction (NTP-independent). For individual s.'s, see the specific names. SEE ALSO synthetase.

syn•the•sis, pl. **syn•the•ses** (sin'thĕ-sis, -sēz). **1.** A building up, putting together, composition. **2.** CHEMISTRY The formation of compounds by the union of simpler compounds or elements. **3.** Stage in the cell *cycle* in which DNA is synthesized as a preliminary to cell division. [G. fr. *syn*, together, + *thesis*, a placing, arranging]

 activity s., the process of combining component parts of the human and nonhuman environment so as to design an activity suitable for evaluation or intervention.

syn•the•size (sin'thĕ-sīz). To make something by synthesis, *i.e.*, synthetically.

syn•the•tase (sin'thĕ-tās). An enzyme catalyzing the synthesis of a specific substance. For individual s.'s, see the specific names.

syn•thet•ic (sin-thet'ik). Relating to or made by synthesis.

syn•ton•ic (sin-ton'ik). Having even tone or temperament; a personality trait characterized by a high degree of emotional responsiveness to the environment. [G. *syntonos,* in harmony, fr. *syn,* together, + *tonos,* tone]

syn·tro·pho·blast (sin-trō′fō-blast, -trof′ō-). SYN syncytiotrophoblast.

syn·tro·pic (sin-trop′ik). Relating to syntropy.

syn·tro·py (sin′trō-pē). **1.** The tendency sometimes seen in two diseases to coalesce into one. **2.** The state of harmonious association with others. **3.** ANATOMY A number of similar structures inclined in one general direction; *e.g.,* the spinous processes of a series of vertebrae, the ribs. [syn- + G. *tropē,* a turning]

⌂**syphil-.** SEE syphilo-.

syph·i·lid (sif′i-lid). Any of the several kinds of cutaneous and mucous membrane lesions of secondary and tertiary syphilis, but most commonly denoting the former. [syphilis + *-id* (1)]

▪**syph·i·lis** (sif′i-lis). An acute and chronic infectious disease caused by *Treponema pallidum* and transmitted by direct contact, usually through sexual intercourse. After an incubation period of 12 to 30 days, the first symptom is a chancre (a painless, indurated ulcer), followed by slight fever and other constitutional symptoms (*primary s.*), followed by a skin eruption of various appearances with mucous patches and generalized lymphadenopathy (*secondary s.*), and subsequently by the formation of gummas, cellular infiltration, and functional abnormalities usually resulting from cardiovascular and central nervous system lesions (*tertiary s.*). [Mod. L. *syphilis* (*syphilid-*), (?) fr. a poem, *Syphilis sive Morbus Gallicus,* by Fracastorius, *Syphilus* being a shepherd and principal char.]

congenital s., s. acquired by the fetus *in utero,* thus present at birth.

primary s., the first stage of s. SEE syphilis.

secondary s., the second stage of s. SEE syphilis.

syph·i·lit·ic (sif-i-lit′ik). Relating to, caused by, or suffering from syphilis. SYN luetic.

⌂**syphilo-, syphil-, syphili-.** Syphilis. [see syphilis]

syph·i·lo·ma (sif-i-lō′mă). SYN gumma. [syphilo- + G. *-oma,* tumor]

⌂**syring-.** SEE syringo-.

syr·ing·ad·e·no·ma (sir′ing-ad-ĕ-nō′mă). A benign sweat gland tumor showing glandular differentiation typical of secretory cells. SYN syringoadenoma. [syring- + G. *adēn,* gland, + *-oma,* tumor]

sy·ringe (sĭ-rinj′, sir′inj). An instrument used for injecting or withdrawing fluids. [G. *syrinx,* pipe or tube]

chip s., a tapered metal tube through which air is forced from a rubber bulb or pressure tank to blow debris from, or to dry, a cavity in preparing teeth for restoration.

control s., a type of Luer-Lok s. with thumb and finger rings attached to the proximal end of the barrel and to the tip of the plunger, allowing operation of the s. with one hand. SYN ring s.

dental s., a breech-loading metal cartridge s. into which fits a hermetically sealed glass cartridge containing anesthetic solution.

fountain s., an apparatus consisting of a reservoir for holding fluid, to the bottom of which is attached a tube with a suitable nozzle; used for vaginal or rectal injections, irrigating wounds, etc., the force of the flow being regulated by the height of the reservoir above the point of discharge.

hypodermic s., a small s. with a barrel (which may be calibrated), perfectly matched plunger, and tip; used with a hollow needle for subcutaneous injections and for aspiration. SYN hypodermic (3).

Luer s., a glass s. with a metal tip and locking device to secure the needle; used for hypodermic and intravenous injections and phlebotomy.

probe s., a s. with an olive-shaped tip, used in treatment of diseases of the lacrimal passages.

ring s., SYN control s.

rubber-bulb s., a s. with a hollow rubber bulb and cannula provided with a check valve, used to obtain a jet of air or water.

sy·rin·gec·to·my (si-rin-jek′tō-mē). SYN fistulectomy. [syring- + G. *ektomē,* excision]

sy·rin·gi·tis (si-rin-jī′tis). Inflammation of the auditory tube. [syring- + G. *-itis,* inflammation]

⌂**syringo-, syring-.** A syrinx; syringeal. [G. *syrinx,* pipe or tube]

sy·rin·go·ad·e·no·ma (sĭ-ring′gō-ad-ĕ-nō′mă). SYN syringadenoma.

sy·rin·go·bul·bia (sĭ-ring′gō-bŭl′bē-ă). A fluid-filled cavity of the brainstem, analogous to syringomyelia. [syringo- + L. *bulbus,* bulb (medulla oblongata)]

sy·rin·go·car·ci·no·ma (sĭ-ring′gō-kar-si-nō′mă). A malignant epithelial neoplasm which has undergone cystic change (cystic carcinoma). [syringo- + carcinoma]

sy·rin·go·cele (sĭ-ring′gō-sēl). **1.** SYN central canal. **2.** A meningomyelocele in which there is a cavity in the ectopic spinal cord. [syringo- + G. *koilia,* a hollow]

sy·rin·go·cys·tad·e·no·ma (sĭ-ring′gō-sis-tad-ĕ-nō′mă). A cystic benign sweat gland tumor. [syringo- + cystadenoma]

sy·rin·go·cys·to·ma (sĭ-ring′gō-sis-tō′mă). SYN hidrocystoma. [syringo- + cystoma]

sy·rin·go·ma (si-ring-gō′mă). A benign, often multiple, sometimes eruptive neoplasm of the sweat gland ducts composed of very small round cysts. [syringo- + G. *-ōma,* tumor]

sy·rin·go·me·nin·go·cele (sĭ-ring′gō-mĕ-ning′gō-sēl). A form of spina bifida in which the dorsal sac consists chiefly of membranes, with very little cord substance, enclosing a cavity that communicates with a syringomyelic cavity. [syringo- + meningocele]

sy·rin·go·my·e·lia (sĭ-ring′gō-mī-ē′lē-ă). The presence in the spinal cord of longitudinal cavities lined by dense, gliogenous tissue, which are not caused by vascular insufficiency. S. is marked clinically by pain and paresthesia, followed by muscular atrophy of the hands and analgesia with thermoanesthesia of the hands and arms, but with the tactile sense preserved; later marked by painless whitlows, spastic paralysis in the lower extremities, and scoliosis of the lumbar spine. Some cases are associated with low-grade astrocytomas or vascular malformations of the spinal cord. SYN hydrosyringomyelia, Morvan's disease. [syringo- + G. *myelos,* marrow]

sy•rin•go•my•e•lo•cele (sĭ-ring′gō-mī′ĕ-lō-sēl). A form of spina bifida, consisting in a protrusion of the membranes and spinal cord through a dorsal defect in the vertebral column, the fluid of the syrinx of the cord being increased and expanding the cord tissue into a thin-walled sac which then expands through the vertebral defect. [syringo- + myelocele]

sy•rin•got•o•my (si-rin-got′ō-mē). SYN fistulotomy.

syr•inx, pl. **sy•ring•es** (sir′ingks, sĭ-rin′jēz). **1.** A rarely used synonym for fistula. **2.** A pathologic tube-shaped cavity in the brain or spinal cord. **3.** The lower part of the bird trachea, which produces vocal sounds. [G. a tube, pipe]

syr•up (ser′ŭp, sir′ŭp). **1.** Refined molasses; the uncrystallizable saccharine solution left after the refining of sugar. **2.** Any sweet fluid; a solution of sugar in water in any proportion. **3.** A liquid preparation of medicinal or flavoring substances in a concentrated aqueous solution of a sugar, usually sucrose; when the s. contains a medicinal substance, it is termed a medicated s. [Mod. L. *syrupus,* fr. Ar. *sharāb*]

sys•tem (sis′tĕm). **1.** A consistent and complex whole made up of correlated and semi-independent parts. A complex of anatomical structures functionally related. **2.** The entire organism seen as a complex organization of parts. **3.** Any complex of structures anatomically related (*e.g.*, vascular s.) or functionally related (*e.g.*, digestive s.). **4.** A scheme of medical theory. SEE ALSO apparatus, classification, system. **5.** S. followed by one or more letters denotes specific amino acid transporters; s. N is a sodium-dependent transporter specific for amino acids such as L-glutamine, L-asparagine, and L-histidine; s. y⁺ is a sodium-independent transporter of cationic amino acids. SYN systema [NA]. [G. *systēma,* an organized whole]

  alimentary s., SYN digestive s.

  autonomic nervous s., that part of the nervous system which represents the motor innervation of smooth muscle, cardiac muscle, and gland cells. It consists of two physiologically and anatomically distinct, mutually antagonistic components: the sympathetic and parasympathetic divisions. In both of these the pathway of innervation consists of a synaptic sequence of two motor neurons, one of which lies in the spinal cord or brainstem as the preganglionic neuron, the thin but myelinated axon of which emerges with an outgoing spinal or cranial nerve and synapses with one or more of the postganglionic neurons composing the autonomic ganglia; the unmyelinated postganglionic fibers in turn innervate the smooth muscle, cardiac muscle, or gland cells. The preganglionic neurons of the sympathetic part lie in the intermediolateral cell column of the thoracic and upper two lumbar segments of the spinal gray matter; those of the parasympathetic part compose the visceral motor (visceral efferent) nuclei of the brainstem as well as the lateral column of the second to fourth sacral segments of the spinal

cord. The ganglia of the sympathetic division are the paravertebral ganglia of the sympathetic trunk and the prevertebral or collateral ganglia; those of the parasympathetic division lie either near the organ to be innervated or as intramural ganglia within the organ itself except in the head, where there are four discrete parasympathetic ganglia (ciliary, otic, pterygopalatine, and submandibular). Impulse transmission from preganglionic to postganglionic neuron is mediated by acetylcholine in both the sympathetic and parasympathetic parts; transmission from the postganglionic fiber to the visceral effector tissues is classically said to be by acetylcholine in the parasympathetic part and by noradrenalin in the sympathetic part; recent evidence suggests the existence of further noncholinergic, nonadrenergic classes of postganglionic fibers.

  Bethesda s., a comprehensive s. for reporting findings on cervical Papanicolaou smears; includes observations on the adequacy of the specimen, benign cellular changes (inflammation, infection), changes in squamous or glandular epithelial cells reflecting atypia or malignancy, and hormonal status. [*Bethesda,* Maryland, site of NIH]

  cardiovascular s., the heart and blood vessels considered as a whole.

  centimeter-gram-second s. (CGS, cgs), the scientific s. of expressing the fundamental physical units of length, mass, and time, and those units derived from them, in centimeters, grams, and seconds; currently being replaced by the International System of Units based on the meter, kilogram, and second.

  central auditory nervous s. (CANS), auditory neural pathway from the cochleas to the auditory cortex. SEE vestibulocochlear *nerve.* SYN eighth cranial nerve.

  central nervous s. (CNS), the brain and the spinal cord.

  circulatory s., SYN vascular s.

  conducting s. of heart, the s. of atypical cardiac muscle fibers comprising the sinoatrial node, internodal tracts, atrioventricular node and bundle, the bundle branches, and their terminal ramifications into the Purkinje network; sometimes also called cardionector.

  ▣ **digestive s.,** the digestive tract from the mouth to the anus with all its associated glands and organs. SYN alimentary s.

  endocrine s., collective designation for those tissues capable of secreting hormones.

  extrapyramidal motor s., literally: all of the brain structures affecting bodily (somatic) movement, excluding the motor neurons, the motor cortex, and the pyramidal (corticobulbar and corticospinal) tract. Despite its very wide literal connotation, the term is commonly used to denote in particular the striate body (basal ganglia), its associated structures (substantia nigra; subthalamic nucleus), and its descending connections with the midbrain.

  foot-pound-second s. (FPS, fps), a s. of absolute units based on the foot, pound, and second.

  genital s., the complex s. consisting of the male or female gonads, associated ducts, and external genitalia dedicated to the function of reproducing the species. SYN reproductive s.

genitourinary s., SYN urogenital s.

haversian s., SYN osteon.

hematopoietic s., the blood-making organs; in the embryo at different ages these are the yolk sac, liver, thymus, spleen, lymph nodes, and bone marrow; after birth they are principally the bone marrow, spleen, thymus, and lymph nodes.

heterogeneous s., CHEMISTRY a s. that contains various distinct and mechanically separable parts or phases; *e.g.,* a suspension or an emulsion.

homogeneous s., CHEMISTRY a s. whose parts cannot be mechanically separated, and is therefore uniform throughout and possesses in every part identically physical properties; *e.g.,* a solution of sodium chloride in water.

hypothalamohypophysial portal s., SYN portal hypophysial *circulation.*

immune s., an intricate complex of interrelated cellular, molecular, and genetic components which provides a defense (immune response) against foreign organisms or substances and aberrant native cells.

International S. of Units, SEE International System of Units.

limbic s., collective term denoting a heterogeneous array of brain structures at or near the edge (limbus) of the medial wall of the cerebral hemisphere, in particular the hippocampus, amygdala, and fornicate gyrus; the term is often used so as to include also the interconnections of these structures, as well as their connections with the septal area, the hypothalamus, and a medial zone of mesencephalic tegmentum. By way of the latter connections, the limbic s. exerts an important influence upon the endocrine and autonomic motor s.'s; its functions also appear to affect motivational and mood states.

lymphatic s., the bodily system concerned with the circulation of lymph and the production of lymphocytes; it consists of lymphatic vessels, nodes, and lymphoid tissue (spleen, tonsils, thymus, and other lymphoid structures); it empties into the veins at the level of the superior aperture of the thorax.

masticatory s., the organs and structures primarily functioning in mastication: the jaws, teeth with their supporting structures, temporomandibular joint, muscles of mastication, tongue, lips, cheeks, and oral mucosa.

metameric nervous s., that part of the nervous s. which innervates body structures developed in ontogeny from the segmentally arranged somites or, in the head region, branchial arches. The term implies reference to the neural mechanisms intrinsic to the spinal cord and brainstem (represented by the sensory nuclei, motoneuronal cell groups, and their associated interneurons in the reticular formation); by strict definition it should exclude the autonomic nervous system.

metric s., a s. of weights and measures, universal for scientific use, based upon the meter, the gram, and the liter.

mononuclear phagocyte s., a widely distributed collection of both free and fixed macrophages derived from bone marrow precursor cells

by way of monocytes; their substantial phagocytic activity is mediated by immunoglobulin and the serum complement system. In both connective and lymphoid tissue, they may occur as free and fixed macrophages; in the sinusoids of the liver, as Kupffer cells; in the lung, as alveolar macrophages; and in the nervous system, as microglia.

movement s., (1) a physiological system that functions to produce motion of the whole body or of its component parts. (2) the functional interction of structures that contribute to the act of moving.

muscular s., all the muscles of the body collectively.

nervous s., the entire nerve apparatus, composed of a central part, the brain and spinal cord, and a peripheral part, the cranial and spinal nerves, autonomic ganglia, and plexuses.

neuromuscular s., the muscles of the body collectively and the nerves supplying them.

parasympathetic nervous s., SEE autonomic nervous s.

peripheral nervous s., the peripheral part of the nervous system external to the brain and spinal cord from their roots to their peripheral terminations. This includes the ganglia, both sensory and autonomic and any plexuses through which the nerve fibers run. SEE ALSO autonomic nervous s.

portal s., a s. of vessels in which blood, after passing through one capillary bed, is conveyed through a second capillary network, as in the hepatic portal system in which blood from the intestines passes through the liver sinusoids.

properdin s., an immunological s. that is the alternative pathway for complement, composed of several distinct proteins that react in a serial manner and activate C3 (third component of complement); the s. can be activated, in the absence of specific antibody, by bacterial endotoxins, and a variety of polysaccharides and lipopolysaccharides.

prospective payment s. (PPS), arrangement mandated by the Tax Equity and Fiscal Responsibility Act of 1982 (TERFA) to control Medicare costs; payment for services provided to a Medicare patient is fixed and adjusted annually by the Health Care Financing Administration (HCFA); payment is based on assigned diagnosis-related groups (DRGs).

renin-angiotensin-aldosterone s., the hormones, renin, angiotensin, and aldosterone work together to regulate blood pressure. A sustained fall in blood pressure causes the kidney to release renin. This is converted to angiotensin in the circulation. Angiotensin then raises blood pressure directly by arteriolar constriction and stimulates the adrenal glands to produce aldosterone which promotes sodium and water retention by kidney, such that blood volume and blood pressure increase.

reproductive s., SYN genital s.

respiratory s., all the air passages from the nose to the pulmonary alveoli.

reticular activating s. (RAS), a physiological term denoting that part of the brainstem reticular formation that plays a central role in the organism's bodily and behavioral alertness; it extends as a diffusely organized neural apparatus through the central region of the brainstem into the subthalamus and the intralaminar nuclei of the thalamus; by its ascending connections it affects the function of the cerebral cortex in the sense of behavioral responsiveness; its descending (reticulospinal) connections transmit its activating influence upon bodily posture and reflex mechanisms (*e.g.*, muscle tonus), in part by way of the gamma motor neurons. SEE ALSO reticular *formation*.

reticuloendothelial s. (RES), an obsolescent term sometimes applied to the lymphatic s., the mononuclear phagocytic s., or both.

stomatognathic s., all of the structures involved in speech and in the reception, mastication, and deglutition of food. SEE ALSO masticatory s.

sympathetic nervous s., (1) originally, the entire autonomic nervous s.; **(2)** the sympathetic part of the nervous system. SEE ALSO autonomic nervous s.

urinary s., SYN urogenital s.

i urogenital s., includes all the organs concerned in reproduction and in the formation and discharge of urine. SYN genitourinary s., urinary s.

vascular s., the cardiovascular and lymphatic s.'s collectively. SYN circulatory s.

sys•te•ma (sis'tē'mă) [NA]. SYN system. SEE ALSO system, apparatus. [L. fr. G. *systēma*]

sys•tem•at•ic name. As applied to chemical substances, a s. n. is composed of specially coined or selected words or syllables, each of which has a precisely defined chemical structural meaning, so that the structure may be derived from the name.

sys•tem•ic (sis-tem'ik). Relating to a system; specifically somatic, relating to the entire organism as distinguished from any of its individual parts.

sys•to•le (sis'tō-lē). Contraction of the heart, especially of the ventricles, by which the blood is driven through the aorta and pulmonary artery to traverse the systemic and pulmonary circulations, respectively; its occurrence is indicated physically by the first sound of the heart heard on auscultation, by the palpable apex beat, and by the arterial pulse. [G. *systolē*, a contracting]

aborted s., a loss of the systolic beat in the radial pulse through weakness of the ventricular contraction.

electrical s., the duration of the QRS-T complex (*i.e.,* from the earliest Q wave to the end of the latest T wave on the ECG).

late s., SYN prediastole.

premature s., SYN extrasystole.

sys•tol•ic (sis-tol'ik). Relating to, or occurring during cardiac systole.

sys•trem•ma (sis-trem'ă). A muscular cramp in the calf of the leg, the contracted muscles forming a hard ball. [G. anything twisted]

T

τ tau. SEE tau.

θ, Θ theta. SEE theta.

T 1. ribothymidine; tension (T+, increased tension; T−, diminished tension); tera-; tritium; threonine; torque; transmittance. **2.** As a subscript, refers to tidal *volume*. **3.** Thoracic vertebra (T1 to T12); tocopherol. **4.** Tesla, the unit of magnetic field strength.

T1. MAGNETIC RESONANCE The time for 63% of longitudinal relaxation to occur; the value is a function of magnetic field strength and the chemical environment of the hydrogen nucleus.

T2. MAGNETIC RESONANCE The time for 63% of transverse relaxation to occur; the value is a function of magnetic field strength and the chemical environment of the hydrogen nucleus.

T absolute *temperature* (kelvin).

T_m *temperature* midpoint (kelvin); melting *point*.

t metric ton; time.

t temperature (Celsius); tritium.

t_m *temperature* midpoint (Celsius).

Ta tantalum.

tab·a·nid (tab′ă-nid). Common name for flies of the family Tabanidae. [L. *tabanus*, gadfly]

ta·bes (tā′bēz). Progressive wasting or emaciation. [L. a wasting away]

  t. dorsalis, SYN tabetic *neurosyphilis*.

  t. mesenter′ica, tuberculosis of the mesentery and retroperitoneal lymph nodes.

ta·bes·cent (ta-bes′ent). Characteristic of tabes. [L. *tabesco*, to waste away, fr. *tabes*, a wasting away]

ta·bet·ic (ta-bet′ik). Relating to or suffering from tabes, especially tabes dorsalis.

ta·bet·i·form (ta-bet′i-fōrm). Resembling tabes, especially tabes dorsalis. [irreg. formed fr. L. *tabes*, a wasting, + *forma*, form]

tab·la·ture (tab-lă-chūr). The state of division of the cranial bones into two plates separated by the diploë. [L. *tabula*, tablet]

ta·ble (tā′bl). **1.** One of the two plates or laminae, separated by the diploë, into which the cranial bones are divided. **2.** An arrangement of data in parallel columns, showing the essential facts in a readily appreciable form. [L. *tabula*]

  life t., a representation of the probable years of survivorship of a defined population of subjects.

ta·ble·spoon (tā′bl-spūn). A large spoon, used as a measure of the dose of a medicine, equivalent to about 4 fluidrams or ½ fluidounce or 15 ml.

tablet. A solid dosage form containing medicinal substances with or without suitable diluents; it may vary in shape, size, and weight, and may be classed according to the method of manufacture, as molded tablet and compressed tablet. [Fr. *tablette*, L. *tabula*]

  enteric coated tablet, a tablet coated with a substance that delays release of the medication until the tablet has passed through the stomach and into the intestine (enteron).

  hypodermic tablet, a compressed or molded tablet that dissolves completely in water to form an injectable solution.

  sustained-action tablet, a drug in tablet form

that provides the required dosage initially and then maintains or repeats it at desired intervals. SYN sustained-release tablet.

  sustained-release tablet, SYN sustained-action tablet.

ta·boo, ta·bu (tă-bū′). Restricted, prohibited, or forbidden; set apart for religious or ceremonial purposes. [Tongan, set apart]

ta·bo·pa·re·sis (tā′bō-pă-rē′sis, -par′ē-sis). A condition in which the symptoms of tabes dorsalis and general paresis are associated.

tab·u·lar (tab′yū-lăr). **1.** Tablelike. **2.** Arranged in the form of a table (2). [L. *tabularis*, fr. *tabula*, table]

tache (tash). A circumscribed discoloration of the skin or mucous membrane, such as a macule or freckle. [Fr. spot]

ta·chet·ic (tă-ket′ik). Marked by bluish or brownish spots. [Fr. *tache*, spot]

ta·chom·e·ter (tă-kom′ĕ-ter). An instrument for measuring speed or rate; *e.g.*, revolutions of a shaft, heart rate (cardiotachometer), arterial blood flow (hemotachometer), respiratory gas flow (pneumotachometer). [G. *tachos*, speed, + *metron*, measure]

△**tachy-.** Rapid. [G. *tachys*, quick,]

tach·y·ar·rhyth·mia (tak′ē-ă-ridh′mē-ă). Any disturbance of the heart's rhythm, regular or irregular, resulting by convention in a rate over 100 beats per minute during physical examination. [tachy- + G. *a-* priv. + *rhythmos*, rhythm]

tach·y·car·dia (tak′i-kar′dē-ă). Rapid beating of the heart, conventionally applied to rates over 100 per minute. SYN tachyrhythmia. [tachy- + G. *kardia*, heart]

  atrial chaotic t., multifocal origin of tachycardia within the atrium; often confused with atrial fibrillation during physical examination.

  bidirectional ventricular t., ventricular t. in which the QRS complexes in the electrocardiogram are alternately mainly positive and mainly negative; many such cases may represent ventricular t. with alternating forms of aberrant ventricular conduction.

  ectopic t., a t. originating in a focus other than the sinus node, *e.g.*, atrial, A-V junctional, or ventricular t.

  paroxysmal t., recurrent attacks of t., with abrupt onset and often also abrupt termination, originating from an ectopic focus which may be atrial, A-V junctional, or ventricular.

tach·y·car·di·ac (tak-i-kar′dē-ak). Relating to or suffering from excessively rapid action of the heart.

tach·y·crot·ic (tak′i-krot′ik). Relating to, causing, or characterized by a rapid pulse. [tachy- + G. *krotos*, a striking]

tach·yp·nea (tak-ip-nē′ă). Rapid breathing. SYN polypnea. [tachy- + G. *pnoē* (*pnoiē*), breathing]

tach·y·rhyth·mia (tak-i-ridh′mē-ă). SYN tachycardia. [tachy- + G. *rhythmos*, rhythm]

ta·chys·ter·ol (tă-kis′ter-ōl). Sterol(s) formed by ultraviolet irradiation of any 5,7-diene-3β-sterol.

ta

When reduced to the 5,7-diene (or 5,7,22-triene) form, antirachitic action appears.

tac•tile (tak′til). Relating to touch or to the sense of touch. [L. *tactilis,* fr. *tango,* pp. *tactus,* to touch]

tac•tom•e•ter (tak-tom′ĕ-ter). SYN esthesiometer. [L. *tactus,* touch, + G. *metron,* measure]

tac•tu•al (tak′chūl). Relating to or caused by touch.

TAD transient acantholytic *dermatosis.*

Tae•nia (tē′nē-ă). A genus of cestodes that formerly included most of the tapeworms, but is now restricted to those species infecting carnivores with cysticerci found in tissues of various herbivores, rodents, and other animals of prey. SEE ALSO tapeworm. [see taenia]

   T. sagina′ta, the beef, hookless, or unarmed tapeworm of humans, acquired by eating insufficiently cooked flesh of cattle infected with *Cysticercus bovis.*

   T. so′lium, the pork, armed, or solitary tapeworm of humans, acquired by eating insufficiently cooked pork infected with *Cysticercus cellulosae;* hatching of ova within the human intestine may result in establishment of cysticerci in human tissues, resulting in cysticercosis.

tae•nia (tē′nē-ă). **1.** A coiled bandlike anatomical structure. SEE tenia (1). **2.** Common name for a tapeworm, especially of the genus *Taenia.* SYN tenia (2). [L., fr. G. *tainia,* band, tape, a tapeworm]

tae•ni•a•sis (tē-nī′i-sĭs). Infection with cestodes of the genus *Taenia.*

tae•ni•id (tē-nē′id). Common name for a member of the family Taeniidae.

tae•ni•oid (tē′nē-oyd). Denoting members of the genus *Taenia.*

TAF tumor angiogenic *factor.*

tag. 1. SEE label, tracer. **2.** A small outgrowth or polyp.

   sentinel t., projecting edematous skin at the lower end of an anal fissure.

   skin t., (1) a polypoid outgrowth of both epidermis and dermal fibrovascular tissue; **(2)** common terminology for any small benign cutaneous lesion. SYN acrochordon, soft wart.

tail (tāl). **1.** Any tail, or tail-like structure, or tapering or elongated extremity of an organ or other part. **2.** VETERINARY ANATOMY A free appendage representing the caudal end of the vertebral column; covered by skin and hair, feathers, or scales. SYN cauda [NA]. [A.S. *taegl*]

   t. of pancreas, the left extremity of the pancreas within the lienorenal ligament.

ta•lar (tā′lăr). Relating to the talus.

tal•co•sis (tal-kō′sis). A pulmonary disorder related to silicosis, occurring in workers exposed to talc mixed with silicates; characterized by restrictive or obstructive disorders of breathing or the two in combination. [talc + G. -osis, condition]

tal•i•ped•ic (tal-i-ped′ik). Clubfooted.

tal•i•pes (tal′i-pēz). Any deformity of the foot involving the talus. [L. *talus,* ankle, + *pes,* foot]

   t. calcaneoval′gus, t. calcaneus and t. valgus combined; the foot is dorsiflexed, everted, and abducted. SEE clubfoot.

   t. calcaneova′rus, t. calcaneus and t. varus

combined; the foot is dorsiflexed, inverted, and adducted. SEE clubfoot.

   t. calca′neus, a deformity due to weakness or absence of the calf muscles, in which the axis of the calcaneus becomes vertically oriented; commonly seen in poliomyelitis. SYN calcaneus (2).

   t. ca′vus, an exaggeration of the normal arch of the foot.

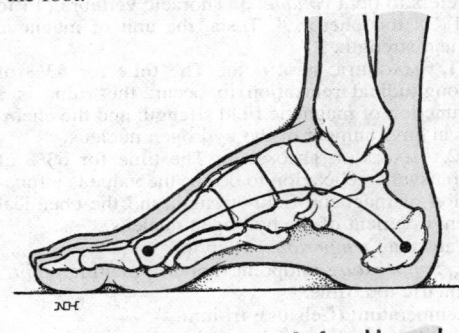

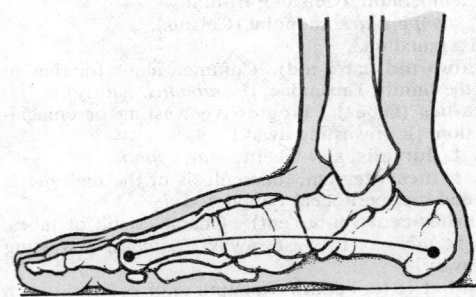

talipes cavus (top) and **talipes planus** (bottom)

   t. equinoval′gus, t. equinus and t. valgus combined; the foot is plantiflexed, everted, and abducted. SEE clubfoot. SYN equinovalgus.

   t. equinova′rus, t. equinus and t. varus combined; the foot is plantiflexed, inverted, and adducted. SYN clubfoot, equinovarus.

   t. equi′nus, permanent extension of the foot so that only the ball rests on the ground; it is commonly combined with t. varus.

   t. planus, a condition in which the longitudinal arch is broken down, the entire sole touching the ground. SYN flatfoot, pes planus.

   t. val′gus, permanent eversion of the foot, the inner side alone of the sole resting on the ground; it is usually combined with a breaking down of the plantar arch.

   t. va′rus, inversion of the foot, the outer side of the sole only touching the ground; usually some degree of t. equinus is associated with it, and often t. cavus.

talo-. The talus. [L. *talus,* ankle, ankle bone]

ta•lo•cru•ral (tā′lō-krū′răl). Relating to the talus and the bones of the leg; denoting the ankle joint.

ta•lus, gen. **ta•li** (tā′lŭs, -lī) [NA]. The bone of the foot that articulates with the tibia and fibula to form the ankle joint. SYN ankle bone, ankle (3). [L. ankle bone, heel]

tam•pon. 1. A cylinder or ball of cotton-wool,

gauze, or other loose substance; used as a plug or pack in a canal or cavity to restrain hemorrhage, absorb secretions, or maintain a displaced organ in position. **2.** To insert such a plug or pack. [O. Fr.]

tam·pon·ade, tam·pon·age (tam-pŏ-nād′, tam′pŏ-nij). The insertion of a tampon.

  cardiac t., compression of the heart due to critically increased volume of fluid in the pericardium.

tan·gen·ti·al·i·ty (tan-jen′shē-al′i-tē). A disturbance in the associative thought process in which one tends to digress readily from one topic under discussion to other topics which arise in the course of associations; observed in bipolar disorder and schizophrenia and certain types of organic brain disorders. Cf. circumstantiality. [off on a tangent, fr. L. *tango,* to touch]

Tanner growth chart. See under chart.

Tanner stage. See under stage.

tan·ta·lum (Ta) (tan′tă-lŭm). A heavy metal of the vanadium group, atomic no. 73, atomic wt. 180.9479; used in surgical prostheses because of its noncorrosive properties. [G. mythical king of Lydia *Tantalus*]

tan·trum (tan′trŭm). A fit of bad temper, especially in children.

tap. 1. To withdraw fluid from a cavity by means of a trocar and cannula, hollow needle, or catheter. **2.** To strike lightly with the finger or a hammerlike instrument in percussion or to elicit a tendon reflex. **3.** A light blow. **4.** An East Indian fever of undetermined nature. **5.** An instrument to cut threads in a hole in bone prior to inserting a screw. [M.E. *tappe,* fr. A.S. *taeppa*]

  spinal t., SYN lumbar *puncture*.

ta·pe·tum, pl. **ta·pe·ta** (tă-pē′tŭm, -tă). **1.** In general, any membranous layer or covering. **2.** NEUROANATOMY A thin sheet of fibers in the lateral wall of the temporal and occipital horns of the lateral ventricle, continuous with the corpus callosum. [L. *tapeta,* a carpet]

tape·worm (tāp′werm). An intestinal parasitic worm, adults of which are found in the intestine of vertebrates. T.'s consist of a scolex, variously equipped with spined or sucking structures by which the worm is attached to the intestinal wall of the host, and strobila having several to many proglottids that lack a digestive tract at any stage of development. The ovum, entering the intestine of an appropriate intermediate host, hatches and the hexacanth penetrates the gut wall and develops into a specific larval form (*e.g.,* cysticercoid, cysticercus, hydatid, strobilocercus), which develops into an adult when the intermediate host is ingested by the proper final host.

ta·pote·ment (tă-pot-mawn′). A massage movement consisting in striking with the side of the hand, usually with partly flexed fingers. SYN tapping (1). [Fr. fr. *tapoter,* to tap]

tap·ping (tap′ing). **1.** SYN tapotement. **2.** SYN paracentesis.

  pressure t., SYN intermittent *compression* (1).

TAR thrombocytopenia and absent radius. SEE thrombocytopenia-absent radius *syndrome*.

ta·ran·tu·la (tă-ran′chū-lă). A very large, hairy spider, considered highly venomous and often

greatly feared; the bite, however, is usually no more harmful than a bee sting. [see tarantism]

tar·dive (tar′div). Late; tardy.

tar·get (tar′get). **1.** An object fixed as goal or point of examination. **2.** In the ophthalmometer, the mire. **3.** SYN target *organ.* **4.** Anode of an x-ray tube. SEE ALSO x-ray. [It. *targhetta,* a small shield]

△**tars-.** SEE tarso-.

tar·sal (tar′săl). Relating to a tarsus in any sense.

tar·sa·le, pl. **tar·sa·lia** (tar-sā′lē, tar-sā′lē-ă). Any tarsal bone. [Mod. L. fr. G. *tarsos,* sole of the foot]

tars·al·gia (tar-sal′jē-ă). SYN podalgia. [tarsus + G. *algos,* pain]

tars·ec·to·my (tar-sek′tō-mē). Excision of the tarsus of the foot or a segment of the tarsus of an eyelid. [tarsus + G. *ektomē,* excision]

tar·si·tis (tar-sī′tis). **1.** Inflammation of the tarsus of the foot. **2.** Inflammation of the tarsal border of an eyelid.

△**tarso-, tars-.** A tarsus. [See tarsus]

tar·so·cla·sia, tar·soc·la·sis (tar-sō-klā′zē-ă, tar-sok′lă-sis). Instrumental fracture of the tarsus, for the correction of talipes equinovarus. [tarso- + G. *klasis,* a breaking]

tar·so·ma·la·cia (tar′sō-mă-lā′shē-ă). Softening of the tarsal cartilages of the eyelids. [tarso- + G. *malakia,* softness]

tar·so·meg·a·ly (tar-sō-meg′ă-lē). A congenital maldevelopment and overgrowth of a tarsal or carpal bone. [tarso- + G. *megas,* large]

tar·so·met·a·tar·sal (TMT) (tar-sō-met′ă-tar′săl). Relating to the tarsal and metatarsal bones; denoting the articulations between the two sets of bones, and the ligaments in relation thereto.

tar·so·pha·lan·ge·al (tar-sō-fă-lan′jē-ăl). Relating to the tarsus and the phalanges.

tar·sor·rha·phy (tar-sōr′ă-fē). The suturing together of the eyelid margins, partially or completely, to shorten the palpebral fissure or to protect the cornea in keratitis or in paralysis of the orbicularis oculi muscle. [tarso- + G. *rhaphē,* suture]

tar·sot·o·my (tar-sot′ō-mē). **1.** Incision of the tarsal cartilage of an eyelid. **2.** Any operation on the tarsus of the foot. [tarso- + G. *tomē,* incision]

tar·sus, gen. and pl. **tar·si** (tar′sŭs, -sī) [NA]. **1.** As a division of the skeleton, the seven tarsal bones of the instep. SEE tarsal *bones,* under *bone.* **2.** The fibrous plates giving solidity and form to the edges of the eyelids; often erroneously called tarsal or ciliary cartilages. [G. *tarsos,* a flat surface, sole of the foot, edge of eyelid]

tar·tar (tar′tăr). **1.** A crust on the interior of wine casks, consisting essentially of potassium bitartrate. **2.** A white, brown, or yellow-brown deposit at or below the gingival margin of teeth, chiefly hydroxyapatite in an organic matrix. SYN dental calculus (2). [Mediev. L. *tartarum,* ult. etym. unknown]

taste (tāst). **1.** To perceive through the medium of the gustatory nerves. **2.** The sensation produced by a suitable stimulus applied to the gustatory nerve endings in the tongue. [It. *tastare;* L. *tango,* to touch]

  color t., a form of synesthesia in which the

color sense and t. are associated, with stimulation of either sense inducing a subjective sensation in the associated sense. SYN pseudogeusesthesia.

TAT thematic apperception *test*.

tat·too (tă-tū′). **1.** A deliberate decorative implanting or injecting of indelible pigments into the skin or the tinctorial effect of accidental implantation. **2.** To produce such an effect. [Tahiti, *tatu*]

   amalgam t., a bluish-black or gray macular lesion of the oral mucous membrane caused by accidental implantation of silver amalgam into the tissue during tooth restoration or extraction.

tau (τ) (tow). **1.** The 19th letter of the Greek alphabet (τ). **2.** Tele; relaxation *time*. **3.** A protein that associates with microtubules and other elements of the cytoskeleton; t. accelerates tubulin polymerization and stabilizes microtubules; t. is also found in the plaque observed in individuals with Alzheimer's disease.

tau·ro·cho·lic ac·id (taw-rō-kō′lik). A compound of cholic acid and taurine, involving the carboxyl group of the former and the amino of the latter; a common bile salt in carnivores.

tau·to·mer·ic (taw-tō-mer′ik). **1.** Relating to the same part. **2.** Relating to or marked by tautomerism. [G. *tautos,* the same, + *meros,* part]

tau·tom·er·ism (taw-tom′er-izm). A phenomenon in which a chemical compound exists in two forms of different structure (isomers) in equilibrium, the two forms differing, usually, in the position of a hydrogen atom. [G. *tautos,* the same, + *meros,* part]

taxa (tak′să). Plural of taxon.

tax·is (tak′sis). **1.** Reduction of a hernia or of a dislocation of any part by means of manipulation. **2.** Systematic classification or orderly arrangement. **3.** The reaction of protoplasm to a stimulus, by virtue of which animals and plants are led to move or act in certain definite ways in relation to their environment; the various kinds of t. are designated by a prefix denoting the stimulus governing them; *e.g.,* chemotaxis, electrotaxis, thermotaxis. [G. orderly arrangement]

tax·on, pl. **taxa** (tak′son, tak′să). The name given to a particular level or grouping in a systematic classification of living things or organisms (taxonomy). [G. *taxis,* order, arrangement, + -on]

tax·o·nom·ic (tak-sō-nom′ik). Relating to taxonomy.

tax·on·o·my (tak-sawn′ŏ-mē). The systematic classification of living things or organisms. Kingdoms of living organisms are divided into groups (taxa) to show degrees of similarity or presumed evolutionary relationships, with the higher categories being larger, more inclusive, and more broadly defined, the lower categories being more restricted, with fewer species more closely related. The divisions below kingdom are, in descending order: phylum, class, order, family, genus, species, and subspecies (variety). Infra- and supra- or sub- and super- categories can be used when needed; additional categories, such as tribe, section, level, group, etc., are also used. [G. *taxis,* orderly arrangement, + *nomos,* law]

TB tuberculosis.

Tb terbium.

TBV total blood volume.

Tc. T cytotoxic *cells,* under *cell.*

Tc technetium.

TCR T-cell *receptor.*

TDD Telephone Device for the Deaf.

TDP ribothymidine 5′-diphosphate. The thymidine analog is dTDP.

TE In magnetic resonance spin echo pulse sequences, the time to echo, when the magnetization signal is sampled.

Te 1. ELECTRODIAGNOSIS Abbreviation denoting tetanic contraction. **2.** Symbol for tellurium.

tear (tār). A discontinuity in substance of a structure. Cf. laceration.

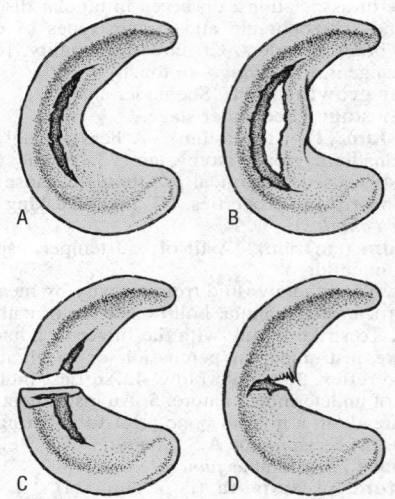

meniscal tears: (A) longitudinal, (B) bucket-handle, (C) horizontal, (D) parrot beak

   bucket-handle t., (1) a t. in the central part of a semilunar cartilage. **(2)** a t. in one of the menisci of a knee joint, near the rim and following its curvature, which can allow a flap of cartilage to impede movement of the joint.

   horizontal t., a t. of articular cartilage roughly perpendicular to the long axis of the bone.

   longitudinal t., a t. of articular cartilage roughly parallel to the long axis of the bone.

   Mallory-Weiss t., SYN Mallory-Weiss *lesion.*

   parrot's beak t., an injury to articular cartilage resulting in the separation of a narrow, curved wedge resembling a parrot's beak.

tear (tēr). The fluid secreted by the lacrimal glands by means of which the conjunctiva and cornea are kept moist. [A.S. *teár*]

teardrop (ter). **1.** A drop of the fluid secreted by the lacrimal glands. **2.** A red cell with a pear shape, where the constricted end narrows to a point. [Anglo-Saxon tear, teahor, taeher, Old Norse tar]

tear·ing (tēr′ing). SYN epiphora.

tease (tēz). To separate the structural parts of a tissue by means of a needle, in order to prepare it for microscopic examination. [A. S. *taesan*]

tea·spoon (tē′spūn). A small spoon, holding

about 1 dram (or about 5 ml) liquid; used as a measure in the dosage of fluid medicines.

teat (tēt). **1.** SYN nipple. **2.** SYN breast. **3.** SYN papilla. [A.S. *tit*]

tech·ne·ti·um (Tc) (tek-nē'shē-um). An artificial radioactive element, atomic no. 43, atomic wt. 99, produced by bombardment of molybdenum by deuterons; also a product of the fission of ^{235}U; used extensively as a radiographic tracer in imaging studies of internal organs. [G. *technetos*, artificial]

tech·ne·ti·um-99m. A radioisotope of technetium which decays by isomeric transition, emitting an essentially monoenergetic gamma ray of 142 keV with a half-life of 6.01 hr. It is used to prepare radiopharmaceuticals for scanning the brain, parotid, thyroid, lungs, blood pool, liver, heart, spleen, kidney, lacrimal drainage apparatus, bone, and bone marrow.

tech·nic (tek-nik'). SYN technique.

tech·ni·cian (tek-nish'ŭn). SYN technologist. [G. *technē*, an art]

  pulmonary function t., SYN pulmonary function *technologist.*

tech·nique (tek-nēk'). The manner of performance, or the details, of any surgical operation, experiment, or mechanical act. SEE ALSO method, operation, procedure. SYN technic. [Fr., fr. G. *technikos*, relating to *technē*, art, skill]

  Ficoll-Hypaque t., a density-gradient centrifugation t. for separating lymphocytes from other formed elements in the blood; the sample is layered onto a Ficoll-sodium metrizoate gradient of specific density; following centrifugation, lymphocytes are collected from the plasma-Ficoll interface.

  fluorescent antibody t., a procedure to test for antigen with a fluorescent antibody by one of two methods: *direct*, in which immunoglobulin (antibody) conjugated with a fluorescent dye is added to tissue and combines with specific antigen (microbe, or other), the resulting antigen-antibody complex being located by fluorescence microscopy; or *indirect*, in which unlabeled immunoglobulin (antibody) is added to tissue and combines with specific antigen, after which the antigen-antibody complex may be labeled with fluorescein-conjugated anti-immunoglobulin antibody, the resulting triple complex then being located by fluorescence microscopy.

  immunoperoxidase t., an immunologic test that utilizes antibodies chemically conjugated to the enzyme peroxidase.

  Kleihauer-Betke t., procedure used to determine the concentration of fetal cells in maternal circulation.

  Ouchterlony t., a t. in which both reaction partners (antigen and antibody) are allowed to diffuse to each other in a gel in a precipitation reaction.

  PAP t., an unlabeled antibody peroxidase method which reacts both with the rabbit antihorseradish peroxidase antibody and free horseradish peroxidase to form a soluble complex of peroxidase antiperoxidase or PAP; a uniquely sensitive immunohistochemical method that is applicable to paraffin-embedded tissues.

  rebreathing t., use of a breathing or anesthesia circuit in which exhaled air is subsequently inhaled either with or without absorption of CO_2 from the exhaled air.

  Seldinger t., a method of percutaneous insertion of a catheter into a blood vessel or space, such as an abscess cavity: a needle is used to puncture the structure and a guide wire is threaded through the needle; when the needle is withdrawn, a catheter is threaded over the wire; the wire is then withdrawn, leaving the catheter in place.

tech·nol·o·gist (tek-nol'ŏ-jist). One trained in and using the techniques of a profession, art, or science. SYN technician.

  nuclear medicine t., an individual skilled in injecting and following the course of radioisotopes in the diagnosing of disease.

  pulmonary function t., individual trained to perform pulmonary function tests for the diagnostic assessment and monitoring of cardiopulmonary disorders. SYN pulmonary function technician.

  radiologic t., an individual skilled in the use of ionizing radiation to produce diagnostic images.

tec·tal (tek'tăl). Relating to a tectum.

tec·to·ceph·a·ly (tek'tō-sĕ-fal'ik). SYN scaphocephaly.

tec·to·ri·al (tek-tōr'ē-ăl). Relating to or characteristic of a tectorium.

tec·to·ri·um (tek-tōr'ē-ŭm). **1.** An overlying structure. **2.** SYN tectorial *membrane* of cochlear duct. [L. an overlying surface (plaster, stucco), fr. *tego*, pp. *tectus*, to cover]

tec·to·spi·nal (tek-tō-spī'năl). Denoting nerve fibers passing from the mesencephalic tectum to the spinal cord.

tec·tum, pl. **tec·ta** (tek'tŭm, tek'tă) [NA]. Any rooflike covering or structure. [L. roof, roofed structure, fr. *tego*, pp. *tectus*, to cover]

teeth (tēth). Plural of tooth.

teeth·ing (tē'thing). Eruption or "cutting" of the teeth, especially of the deciduous teeth.

teg·men, gen. **teg·mi·nis**, pl. **teg·mi·na** (teg' men, -mi-nis, -mi-nă) [NA]. A structure that covers or roofs over a part. [L. a covering, fr. *tego*, to cover]

  t. mastoi'deum, the lamina of bone roofing over the mastoid cells.

  t. tym'pani [NA], the roof of the middle ear, formed by the thinned anterior surface of the petrous portion of the temporal bone. Its anterior edge is inserted into the petrosquamous fissure so that it can be seen as a wedge of bone subdividing that fissure into a squamotympanic and a petrotympanic fissure.

  t. ventric'uli quar'ti [NA], roof of fourth ventricle, formed in its upper part by the superior medullary velum stretching between the two brachia conjunctiva (superior cerebellar peduncles), in its lower part by the inferior medullary velum composed of the choroid membrane and choroid plexus of the fourth ventricle.

teg·men·tal (teg-men'tăl). Relating to, characteristic of, or placed or oriented toward a tegmentum or tegmen.

teg·men·tum, pl. **teg·men·ta** (teg-men'tŭm, -tă)

[NA]. **1.** A covering structure. **2.** SYN mesencephalic t. [L. covering structure, fr. *tego,* to cover]

mesencephalic t., that major part of the substance of the mesencephalon or midbrain that extends from the substantia nigra to the level of the cerebral aqueduct. SYN tegmentum (2) [NA].

rhombencephalic t., the portion of the pons continuous with the mesencephalic t.; it consists of reticular formation, tracts, and cranial nerve nuclei, and forms the dorsal part of the pons (pars dorsalis pontis).

teg•u•ment (teg'yū-ment). **1.** SYN integument. **2.** SYN integument (2). [L. *tegumentum,* a collat. form of *tegmentum*]

teg•u•men•tal, teg•u•men•ta•ry (teg-yū-men'tăl, teg-yū-men'tă-rē). Relating to the integument.

tei•cho•ic ac•ids (tī-kō'ik). One of two classes (the other being the muramic acids or mucopeptides) of polymers constituting the cell walls of Gram-positive bacteria, but also found intracellularly.

tei•chop•sia (tī-kop'sē-ă). The jagged, shimmering visual sensation resembling the fortifications of a walled medieval town; the scintillating scotoma of migraine. [G. *teichos,* wall, + *opsis,* vision]

△**tel-, tele-, telo-.** Distance, end, other end. [G. *tēle,* distant, *telos,* end]

te•la, gen. and pl. **te•lae** (tē'lă, tē'lē). **1.** Any thin weblike structure. **2.** A tissue; especially one of delicate formation. [L. a web]

choroid t. of fourth ventricle, the sheet of pia mater covering the lower part of the ependymal roof of the fourth ventricle.

choroid t. of third ventricle, a double fold of pia mater, enclosing subarachnoid trabeculae, between the fornix above and the epithelial roof of the third ventricle and the thalami below; at each lateral margin is a vascular fringe projecting into the choroidal fissure of the lateral ventricle; on its undersurface are several small vascular projections filling the folds of the ependymal roof of the third ventricle.

t. subcuta'nea [NA], SYN superficial *fascia.*

t. submuco'sa [NA], SYN submucosa.

🔢**tel•an•gi•ec•ta•sia** (tel-an'jē-ek-tā'zē-ă). Dilation of the previously existing small or terminal vessels of a part. [G. *telos,* end, + *angeion,* vessel, + *ektasis,* a stretching out]

essential t., (1) localized capillary dilation of undetermined origin; (2) SYN *angioma* serpiginosum.

spider t., SYN spider *angioma.*

tel•an•gi•ec•ta•sis, pl. **tel•an•gi•ec•ta•ses** (tel-an'jē-ek'tă-sis, -sēz). A lesion formed by a dilated capillary or terminal artery, most commonly on the skin. SEE telangiectasia.

tel•an•gi•ec•tat•ic (tel-an'jē-ek-tat'ik). Relating to or marked by telangiectasia.

tel•an•gi•o•sis (tel'an-jē-ō'sis). Any disease of the capillaries and terminal arterioles.

△**tele-.** SEE tel-.

tel•e•can•thus (tel-ĕ-kan'thŭs). Increased distance between the medial canthi of the eyelids. [G. *tēle,* distant, + *kanthos,* canthus]

tel•e•di•ag•no•sis (tel'ĕ-dī-ag-nō'sis). Detection of a disease by evaluation of data transmitted to a

receiving station, a process normally involving patient-monitoring instruments and a transfer link to a diagnostic center at some distance from the patient.

te•lem•e•try (tĕ-lem'ĕ-trē). The science of measuring a quantity, transmitting the results by radio signals to a distant station, and there interpreting, indicating, and/or recording the results. SEE ALSO biotelemetry.

tel•en•ce•phal•ic (tel'en-se-fal'ik). Relating to the telencephalon or endbrain.

tel•en•ceph•a•lon (tel-en-sef'ă-lon) [NA]. The anterior division of the prosencephalon, which develops into the olfactory lobes, the cortex of the cerebral hemispheres, and the subcortical telencephalic nuclei, and the basal ganglia (nuclei), particularly the striatum and the amygdala. SYN endbrain. [G. *telos,* end, + *enkephalos,* brain]

tel•e•o•mi•to•sis (tel'ē-ō-mī-tō'sis). A completed mitosis. [G. *teleos,* complete, + mitosis]

tel•e•op•sia (tel-ē-op'sē-ă). An error in judging the distance of objects arising from lesions in the parietal temporal region. [G. *tēle,* distant, + *opsis,* vision]

tel•e•or•gan•ic (tel'ē-ōr-gan'ik). Manifesting life. [G. *teleos,* complete, + *organikos,* organic]

te•lep•a•thy (tĕ-lep'ă-thē). Transmittal and reception of thoughts by means other than through the normal senses, as a form of extrasensory perception. [G. *tēle,* distant, + *pathos,* feeling]

Telephone Device for the Deaf (TDD, TT, TTY). Telephone accessory that transmits and receives text over standard telephone lines. Also referred to as teletypewriter (TTY) and text telephone (TT). SEE assistive listening *device.*

tel•e•ra•di•og•ra•phy (tel-ĕ-rā-dē-og'ră-fē). Radiography with the x-ray tube positioned about 2 m from the film thereby securing practical parallelism of the x-rays to minimize geometric distortion; the standard configuration for chest radiography. SYN teleroentgenography. [G. *tēle,* distant, + radiography]

tel•e•ra•di•ol•o•gy (tel-ĕ-rā-dē-ol'ō-jē). The interpretation of digitized diagnostic images transmitted over telephone lines. [tele- + radiology]

tel•er•gy (tel'er-jē). SYN automatism. [G. *tēle,* far off, + *ergon,* work]

tel•e•roent•gen•og•ra•phy (tel'ĕ-rent-gen-og'ră-fē). SYN teleradiography.

tel•e•ther•a•py (tel-ĕ-thār'ă-pē). Radiation therapy administered with the source at a distance from the body. [G. *tēle,* distant, + *therapeia,* treatment]

tel•lu•ric (tĕ-lūr'ik). **1.** Relating to or originating in the earth. **2.** Relating to the element tellurium, especially in its 6+ valence state. [L. *tellus* (*tellur-*), the earth]

tel•lu•ri•um (Te) (tel-ū'rē-ŭm). A rare semimetallic element, atomic no. 52, atomic wt. 127.60, belonging to the sulfur group. [L. *tellus* (*tellur-*), the earth]

△**telo-.** SEE tel-.

tel•o•den•dron (tel-ō-den'dron). The terminal arborization of an axon. [G. *telos,* end, + *dendron,* tree]

tel•o•gen (tel'ō-jen). Resting phase of hair cycle. [G. *telos,* end, + *-gen,* producing]

tel·o·lec·i·thal (tel-ō-les′i-thăl). Denoting an ovum in which a large amount of deuteroplasm accumulates at the vegetative pole, as in the eggs of birds and reptiles. [G. *telos,* end, + G. *lekithos,* yolk]

tel·o·mere (tel′ō-mēr). The distal end of a chromosome arm; telomeres undergo dramatic changes during the progression of cancer. [G. *telos,* end, + *meros,* part]

tel·o·phase (tel′ō-fāz). The final stage of mitosis or meiosis that begins when migration of chromosomes to the poles of the cell has been completed; the chromosomes progressively lengthen while the nuclear membranes of the two daughter nuclei are reconstructed and a cell membrane at the equator completes the separation of the two daughter cells. [G. *telos,* end, + *phasis,* appearance]

tem·per. **1.** Disposition; in general, any characteristic or particular state of mind. SYN temperament (2). **2.** A display of irritation or anger. SEE tantrum. **3.** To treat metal by application of heat, as in annealing or quenching.

tem·per·a·ment (tem′per-ă-ment). **1.** The psychological and biological organization peculiar to the individual, including one's character or personality predispositions, which influence the manner of thought and action and general views of life. **2.** SYN temper (1). [L. *temperamentum,* proper measure, moderation, disposition]

tem·per·ance (tem′per-ans). Moderation in all things; especially, abstinence from the use of alcoholic beverages. [L. *temperantia,* moderation]

tem·per·ate (tem′per-ăt). Moderate; restrained in the indulgence of any appetite or activity.

tem·per·a·ture (tem′per-ă-chŭr). The sensible intensity of heat of any substance; the manifestation of the average kinetic energy of the molecules making up a substance due to heat agitation. SEE ALSO scale. [L. *temperatura,* due measure, temperature, fr. *tempero,* to proportion duly]

  absolute t. (*T*), t. reckoned in Kelvins from absolute zero.

  core t., the t. of the interior of the body.

  critical t., the t. of a gas above which it is no longer possible by use of any pressure, however great, to convert it into a liquid.

  effective t., a comfort index or scale which takes into account the t. of air, its moisture content, and movement.

  t. midpoint (T_m, t_m), the midpoint in the change in optical properties (absorbance, rotation) of a structured polymer (*e.g.,* DNA) with increasing t.

  standard t., a t. of 0°C or 273.15° absolute (Kelvin).

tem·plate (tem′plăt). **1.** A pattern or guide that determines the shape of a substance. **2.** Metaphorically, the specifying nature of a macromolecule, usually a nucleic acid or polynucleotide, with respect to the primary structure of the nucleic acid or polynucleotide or protein made from it *in vivo* or *in vitro.* **3.** DENTISTRY A curved or flat plate utilized as an aid in setting teeth. **4.** An outline used to trace teeth, bones, or soft tissue in order to standardize their form. **5.** A pattern or guide that determines the specificity of antibody

globulins. [Fr. *templet,* temple of a loom, fr. L. *templum,* small timber]

tem·ple (tem′pl). **1.** The area of the temporal fossa on the side of the head above the zygomatic arch. **2.** The part of a spectacle frame passing from the rim backward over the ear. [L. *tempus* (*tempor*-), time, the temple]

tem·po·la·bile (tem-pō-lā′bil, -bīl). Undergoing spontaneous change or destruction during the passage of time. [L. *tempus,* time, + *labilis,* perishable]

tem·po·ral (tem′pŏ-răl). **1.** Relating to time; limited in time; temporary. **2.** Relating to the temple. [L. *temporalis,* fr. *tempus* (*tempor*-), time, temple]

△**temporo-.** Temporal (2). [L. *temporalis,* temporal]

tem·po·ro·man·dib·u·lar (tem′pŏ-rō-man-dib′yū-lăr). Relating to the temporal bone and the mandible; denoting the joint of the lower jaw. SYN temporomaxillary (2).

tem·po·ro·max·il·lary (tem′pŏ-rō-mak′si-lār′ē). **1.** Relating to the regions of the temporal and maxillary bones. **2.** SYN temporomandibular.

tem·po·sta·bile, tem·po·sta·ble (tem-pō-stā′bil, -stā′bl). Not subject to spontaneous alteration or destruction. [L. *tempus,* time + *stabilis,* stable]

tem·pus, gen. **tem·po·ris,** pl. **tem·po·ra** (tem′pŭs, -pŏ-ris, -pŏ-ră). **1.** The temple. **2.** SYN time. [L. time]

TEN toxic epidermal *necrolysis.*

te·na·cious (tĕ-nā′shŭs). Having the capacity to stick or adhere. [L. *tenax* (*tenac*-), fr. *teneo,* to hold]

te·nac·u·lum, pl. **te·nac·u·la** (tĕ-nak′yū-lŭm, -lă). A surgical clamp designed to hold or grasp tissue during dissection. [L. a holder, fr. *teneo,* to hold]

te·nal·gia (te-nal′jē-ă). Pain referred to a tendon. SYN tenodynia, tenontodynia. [G. *tenōn,* tendon, + *algos,* pain]

ten·der. Sensitive or painful as a result of pressure or contact that is not sufficient to cause discomfort in normal tissues. [L. *tener,* soft, delicate]

ten·der·ness (ten′der-nes). The condition of being tender.

  rebound t., t. felt when pressure, particularly pressure on the abdomen, is suddenly released.

ten·di·ni·tis (ten-di-ni′tis). SYN tendonitis.

ten·di·no·plas·ty (ten′din-ō-plas-tē). SYN tenontoplasty. [Mediev. L. *tendo* (*tendin*-), tendon, + G. *plastos,* formed]

ten·di·no·su·ture (ten′di-nō-sū′chūr). SYN tenorrhaphy.

ten·di·nous (ten′di-nŭs). Relating to, composed of, or resembling a tendon.

ten·do, gen. **ten·di·nis,** pl. **ten·di·nes** (ten′dō, -di-nis, -di-nēz) [NA]. SYN tendon. For gross and histological description, see tendon. [Mediev. L., fr. L. *tendo,* to stretch out, extend]

  t. calca′neus [NA], the tendon of insertion of the triceps surae (gastrocnemius and soleus) into the tuberosity of the calcaneus. SYN Achilles tendon, heel tendon.

△**tendo-.** A tendon. SEE ALSO teno-. [L. *tendo*]

ten·dol·y·sis (ten-dol′i-sis). Release of a tendon

from adhesions. SYN tenolysis. [tendo- + G. *lysis,* dissolution]

ten·don (ten'dŏn). A fibrous cord or band of variable length that connects a muscle with its bony attachment or other structure; it may unite with the muscle at its extremity or may run along the side or in the center of the muscle for a longer or shorter distance, receiving the muscular fibers along its lateral border. It consists of fascicles of very densely arranged, almost parallel collagenous fibers, rows of elongated fibrocytes, and a minimum of ground substance. SYN tendo [NA], sinew. [L. *tendo*]

  Achilles t., SYN *tendo* calcaneus.

  hamstring t., SEE hamstring.

  heel t., SYN *tendo* calcaneus.

ten·don·i·tis (ten-dō-nī'tis). Inflammation of a tendon. SYN tendinitis, tenonitis (2), tenontitis, tenositis.

ten·do·plas·ty (ten'dō-plas-tē). SYN tenontoplasty.

ten·do·syn·o·vi·tis (ten'dō-si-nō-vī'tis). SYN tenosynovitis.

ten·dot·o·my (ten-dot'ō-mē). SYN tenotomy.

ten·do·vag·i·nal (ten-dō-vaj'i-năl). Relating to a tendon and its sheath. [tendo- + L. *vagina,* sheath]

ten·do·vag·i·ni·tis (ten'dō-vaj-i-nī'tis). SYN tenosynovitis. [tendo- + L. *vagina,* sheath, + G. *-itis,* inflammation]

te·nec·to·my (tĕ-nek'tō-mē). Resection of part of a tendon. SYN tenonectomy. [G. *tenōn,* tendon, + *ektomē,* excision]

te·nes·mic (tĕ-nez'mik). Relating to or marked by tenesmus.

te·nes·mus (te-nez'mŭs). A painful spasm of the anal sphincter with an urgent desire to evacuate the bowel or bladder, involuntary straining, and the passage of little fecal matter or urine. [G. *teinesmos,* ineffectual effort to defecate, fr. *teinō,* to stretch]

te·nia, pl. **te·ni·ae** (tē'nē-ă, tē'nē-ē). 1. Any anatomical bandlike structure. 2. SYN taenia (2). [L. fr. G. *tainia,* band, tape, a tapeworm]

  t. choroi'dea [NA], the somewhat thickened line along which a choroid membrane or plexus is attached to the rim of a brain ventricle.

  te'niae co'li [NA], the three bands in which the longitudinal muscular fibers of the large intestine, except the rectum, are collected; these are the mesocolic t., situated at the place corresponding to the mesenteric attachment; the free t., opposite the mesocolic t.; and the omental t., at the place corresponding to the site of adhesion of the greater omentum to the transverse colon.

te·ni·a·cide (tē'nē-ă-sīd). An agent destructive to tapeworms. [L. *taenia,* tapeworm, + *caedo,* to kill]

ten·i·al (ten'ē-ăl). 1. Relating to a tapeworm. 2. Relating to one of the structures called tenia.

te·ni·a·sis (tē-nī'ă-sis). Presence of a tapeworm in the intestine.

△**teno-, tenon-, tenont-, tenonto-.** Tendon. SEE ALSO tendo-. [G. *tenōn*]

te·no·de·sis (tĕ-nod'ē-sis, ten'ō-dē'sis). Stabilizing a joint by anchoring the tendons which move that joint. [teno- + G. *desis,* a binding]

ten·o·dyn·ia (ten-ō-din'ēă). SYN tenalgia. [teno- + G. *odynē,* pain]

ten·ol·y·sis (ten-ol'i-sis). SYN tendolysis.

ten·o·my·o·plas·ty (ten-ō-mī'ō-plas-tē). SYN tenontomyoplasty.

ten·o·my·ot·o·my (ten-ō-mī-ot'ō-mē). SYN myotenotomy.

△**tenon-.** SEE teno-.

ten·o·nec·to·my (ten-ō-nek'tō-mē). SYN tenectomy. [tenon- + G. *ektomē,* excision]

ten·o·ni·tis (ten-ō-nī'tis). 1. Inflammation of Tenon's capsule or the connective tissue within Tenon's space. 2. SYN tendonitis. [tenont- + G. *-itis,* inflammation]

ten·on·ti·tis (ten'on-tī'tis). SYN tendonitis. [tenont- + G. *-itis,* inflammation]

△**tenonto-.** SEE teno-.

te·non·to·dyn·ia (te-non'tō-din'ē-ă). SYN tenalgia.

te·non·to·my·o·plas·ty (te-non'tō-mī'ō-plas-tē). A combined tenontoplasty and myoplasty, used in the radical correction of a hernia. SYN tenomyoplasty. [tenonto- + G. *mys,* muscle, + *plastos,* formed]

te·non·to·plas·ty (te-non'tō-plas-tē). Reparative or plastic surgery of the tendons. SYN tendinoplasty, tendoplasty, tenoplasty. [tenonto- + G. *plastos,* formed]

ten·o·phyte (ten'ō-fīt). Bony or cartilaginous growth in or on a tendon. [teno- + G. *phyton,* plant]

ten·o·plas·ty (ten'ō-plas-tē). SYN tenontoplasty.

ten·o·re·cep·tor (ten'ō-rē-sep'ter, -tōr). A receptor in a tendon, activated by increased tension.

te·nor·rha·phy (te-nōr'ă-fē). Suture of the divided ends of a tendon. SYN tendinosuture, tenosuture. [teno- + G. *rhaphē,* suture]

ten·o·si·tis (ten-ō-sī'tis). SYN tendonitis.

ten·os·to·sis (ten-os-tō'sis). Ossification of a tendon. [teno- + G. *osteon,* bone, + *-osis,* condition]

ten·o·sus·pen·sion (ten'ō-sŭs-pen'shŭn). Using a tendon as a suspensory ligament, sometimes as a free graft or in continuity.

ten·o·su·ture (ten-ō-sū'chūr). SYN tenorrhaphy.

ten·o·syn·o·vec·to·my (ten'ō-sin-ō-vek'tō-mē). Excision of a tendon sheath. [teno- + synovia + G. *ektomē,* excision]

ten·o·syn·o·vi·tis (ten'ō-sin-ō-vī'tis). Inflammation of a tendon and its enveloping sheath. SYN tendinous synovitis, tendosynovitis, tendovaginitis, tenovaginitis. [teno- + synovia + G. *-itis,* inflammation]

  de Quervain's t., inflammatory stenosing t. of the abductor pollicis longus and extensor pollicis brevis tendons.

  localized nodular t., SYN giant cell *tumor* of tendon sheath.

  villous t., a condition resembling pigmented villonodular synovitis but arising in periarticular soft tissue rather than in joint synovia; occurs most commonly in the hands.

te·not·o·my (te-not'ō-mē). The surgical division of a tendon for relief of a deformity caused by congenital or acquired shortening of a muscle, as in clubfoot or strabismus. SYN tendotomy. [teno- + G. *tomē,* incision]

graduated t., partial incisions of the tendon of an eye muscle for correction of strabismus.

subcutaneous t., division of a tendon by means of a small pointed knife introduced through skin and subcutaneous tissue without an open operation.

ten•o•vag•i•ni•tis (ten′ō-vaj-i-nī′tis). SYN tenosynovitis. [teno- + L. *vagina,* sheath, + G. *-itis,* inflammation]

ten•sion (ten′shŭn). **1.** The act of stretching. **2.** The condition of being stretched or tense, or a stretching or pulling force. **3.** The partial pressure of a gas, especially that of a gas dissolved in a liquid such as blood. **4.** Mental, emotional, or nervous strain; strained relations or barely controlled hostility between persons or groups. [L. *tensio,* fr. *tendo,* pp. *tensus,* to stretch]

arterial t., the blood pressure within an artery.

ocular t. (Tn), resistance of the tunics of the eye to deformation; it can be estimated digitally or measured by means of a tonometer.

premenstrual t., SYN premenstrual *syndrome.*

surface t. (σ, gamma), the expression of intermolecular attraction at the surface of a liquid, in contact with air or another gas, a solid, or another immiscible liquid, tending to pull the molecules of the liquid inward from the surface; dimensional formula: mt^{-2}.

tissue t., a theoretical condition of equilibrium or balance between the tissues and cells whereby overaction of any part is restrained by the pull of the mass.

ten•sor, pl. **ten•so•res** (ten′sōr, ten-sō′rēz). A muscle the function of which is to render a part firm and tense. [Mod. L. fr. L. *tendo,* pp. *tensus,* to stretch]

tent. 1. Canopy used in various types of inhalation therapy to control humidity and concentration of oxygen in inspired air. **2.** Cylinder of some material, usually absorbent, introduced into a canal or sinus to maintain its patency or to dilate it. **3.** To elevate or pick up a segment of skin, fascia, or tissue at a given point, giving it the appearance of a t. [L. *tendo,* pp. *tensus,* to stretch]

ten•ta•cle (ten′tă-kl). A slender process for feeling, prehension, or locomotion in invertebrates. [Mod. L. *tentaculum,* a feeler, fr. *tento,* to feel]

ten•to•ri•al (ten-tō′rē-ăl). Relating to a tentorium.

ten•to•ri•um, pl. **ten•to•ria** (ten-tō′rē-ŭm, -rē-ă) [NA]. A membranous cover or horizontal partition. [L. tent, fr. *tendo,* to stretch]

t. cerebel′li [NA], a strong fold of dura mater roofing over the posterior cranial fossa with an anterior median opening, the tentorial notch, through which the midbrain passes; the t. cerebelli is attached along the midline to the falx cerebri and separates the cerebellum from the basal surface of the occipital and temporal lobes of the cerebral hemisphere.

TEP tracheoesophageal *puncture.*

tera- (T). 1. Prefix used in the SI and metric systems to signify one trillion. **2.** Denoting a teras. SEE ALSO terato-. [G. *teras,* monster]

ter•as, pl. **ter•a•ta** (ter′as, ter′ă-tă). Fetus with deficient, redundant, misplaced, or grossly misshapen parts. [G.]

ter•at•ic (ter-at′ik). Relating to a teras.

ter•a•tism (ter′ă-tizm). SYN teratosis. [G. *teratisma,* fr. *teras*]

△**terato-.** A teras. SEE ALSO tera- (2). [G. *teras,* monster]

ter•a•to•blas•to•ma. A tumor containing embryonic tissue differing from a teratoma in that not all germ layers are present.

ter•a•to•car•ci•no•ma (ter′ă-tō-kar-si-nō′mă). **1.** A malignant teratoma, occurring most commonly in the testis. **2.** A malignant epithelial tumor arising in a teratoma.

te•rat•o•gen (ter′ă-tō-jen). A drug or other agent that causes abnormal fetal development. [terato- + G. *-gen,* producing]

ter•a•to•gen•e•sis (ter′ă-tō-jen′ĕ-sis). The origin or mode of production of a malformed fetus; the disturbed growth processes involved in the production of a malformed neonate. [terato- + G. *genesis,* origin]

ter•a•to•gen•ic, ter•a•to•ge•net•ic (ter′ă-tō-jen′ik, -jĕ-net′ik). **1.** Relating to teratogenesis. **2.** Causing abnormal embryonic development.

ter•a•to•ge•nic•i•ty (ter′ă-tō-jĕ-nis′i-tē). The property or capability of producing fetal malformation. [terato- + G. *genesis,* generation]

ter•a•toid (ter′ă-toyd). Resembling a teras. [G. *teratōdēs,* fr. *teras* (*terat-*), monster, + *eidos,* resemblance]

ter•a•to•log•ic (ter′ă-tō-loj′ik). Relating to teratology.

ter•a•tol•o•gy (ter-ă-tol′ō-jē). The branch of science concerned with the production, development, anatomy, and classification of malformed fetuses. SEE ALSO dysmorphology. [terato- + G. *logos,* study]

ter•a•to•ma (ter-ă-tō′mă). A neoplasm composed of multiple tissues, including tissues not normally found in the organ in which it arises. T.'s occur most frequently in the ovary, where they are usually benign and form dermoid cysts; in the testis, where they are usually malignant; and, uncommonly, in other sites, especially the midline of the body. SYN teratoid tumor. [terato- + G. *-oma,* tumor]

ter•a•tom•a•tous (ter′ă-tō′mă-tŭs). Relating to or of the nature of a teratoma.

ter•a•to•sis (ter′ă-tō′sis). An anomaly producing a teras. SYN teratism. [terato- + G. *-osis,* condition]

ter•bi•um (Tb) (ter′bē-ŭm). A metallic element of the lanthanide or rare earth series, atomic no. 65, atomic wt. 158.92534. [fr. *Ytterby,* a village in Sweden]

te•res, gen. **ter•e•tis,** pl. **ter•e•tes** (ter′ēz, -tēr-; ter′ĕ-tis; ter′ĕ-tēz). Round and long; denoting certain muscles and ligaments. [L. round, smooth, fr. *tero,* to rub]

term. 1. A definite or limited period. **2.** A name or descriptive word or phrase. [L. *terminus,* a limit, an end]

ter•mi•nal (ter′mi-năl). **1.** Relating to the end; final. **2.** Relating to the extremity or end of any body; *e.g.,* the end of a biopolymer. **3.** A termination, extremity, end, or ending. [L. *terminus,* a boundary, limit]

axon t.'s, the somewhat enlarged, often club-shaped endings by which axons make synaptic contacts with other nerve cells or with effector cells (muscle or gland cells). Axon t.'s contain neurotransmitters of various kinds, sometimes more than one. SEE ALSO synapse. SYN end-feet, neuropodia, terminal boutons, boutons terminaux.

ter·mi·na·tion (ter'mi-nā′shŭn). An end or ending. A termination or ending, particularly a nerve ending. [L. *terminatio*]

ter·na·ry (ter'nār-ē). Denoting or composed of three compounds, elements, molecules, etc. [L. *ternarius,* of three]

ter·pene (ter'pēn). One of a class of hydrocarbons with an empirical formula of $C_{10}H_{16}$, occurring in essential oils and resins.

ter·race (ter'as). To suture in several rows, in closing a wound through a considerable thickness of tissue. [thr. O. Fr. fr. L. *terra,* earth]

ter·ri·to·ri·al·i·ty (ter'i-tōr-ē-al′i-tē). **1.** The tendency of individuals or groups to defend a particular domain or sphere of interest or influence. **2.** The tendency of an individual animal to define a finite space as its own habitat from which it will fight off trespassing animals of its own species.

ter·tian (ter'shăn). Recurring every third day, counting the day of an episode as the first; actually, occurring every 48 hours or every other day. [L. *tertianus,* fr. *tertius,* third]

Tesla, Nikola, Serbian-American electrical engineer, 1856–1943. SEE tesla.

tesla (T) (tes′lă). In the SI system, the unit of magnetic flux density expressed as $kg\ sec^{-2}\ A^{-1}$; equal to one weber per square meter. [N. *Tesla*]

tes·sel·lat·ed (tes′ĕ-lāt-ed). Made up of small squares; checkered. [L. *tessella,* a small square stone]

test. 1. To prove; to try a substance; to determine the chemical nature of a substance by means of reagents. **2.** A method of examination, as to determine the presence or absence of a definite disease or of some substance in any of the fluids, tissues, or excretions of the body, or to determine the presence or degree of a psychological or behavioral trait. **3.** A reagent used in making a t. SEE ALSO assay, reaction, reagent, scale, stain. [L. *testum,* an earthen vessel]

achievement t., a standardized t. used to measure acquired learning, in contrast to an intelligence t., which is an index of potential learning ability.

acid perfusion t., SYN Bernstein t.

acidified serum t., lysis of the patient's red cells in acidified fresh serum, specific for paroxysmal nocturnal hemoglobinuria.

Adson's t., a t. for thoracic outlet syndrome; the patient is seated, with head extended and turned to the side of the lesion; with deep inspiration there is a diminution or total loss of radial pulse on the affected side. Not all patients with a positive Adson's test have thoracic outlet syndrome.

alternate cover t., a t. to detect phoria or strabismus; attention is directed to a small fixation object, and one eye is covered for several sec-

onds; then the cover is moved quickly to the other eye; if the eye moves when it is uncovered, a strabismus or phoria is present.

Ames t., a screening t. for possible carcinogens using strains of *Salmonella typhimurium* that are unable to synthesize histidine; if the test substance produces mutations that regain the ability to synthesize histidine, the substance is carcinogenic.

aptitude t., an occupation-oriented intelligence t. used to evaluate a person's abilities, talents, and skills; particularly valuable in vocational counseling.

association t., a word (stimulus word) is spoken to the subject, who is to reply immediately with another word (reaction word) suggested by the first; used as a diagnostic aid in psychiatry and psychology.

Bárány's caloric t., a t. for vestibular function, made by irrigating the external auditory meatus with either hot or cold water; this normally causes stimulation of the vestibular apparatus, resulting in nystagmus and past-pointing; in vestibular disease, the response may be reduced or absent. SYN caloric t.

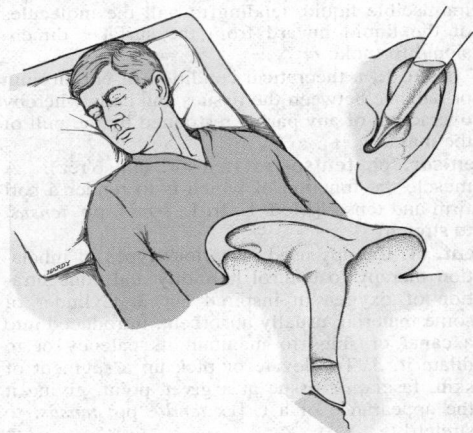

Bárány's caloric test: for vestibular function

Bender gestalt t., a psychological t. used by neurologists and clinical psychologists to measure a person's ability to visually copy a set of geometric designs; useful for measuring visuospatial and visuomotor coordination to detect brain damage.

Benedict's t., a copper-reduction t. for glucose in urine.

bentiromide t., a t. of pancreatic exocrine function that does not require duodenal intubation: orally administered bentiromide is cleaved by chymotrypsin within the lumen of the small intestine, releasing *p*-aminobenzoic acid which is absorbed and excreted in the urine; diminished urinary excretion of *p*-aminobenzoic acid suggests pancreatic insufficiency.

bentonite flocculation t., a flocculation t. for rheumatoid arthritis in which sensitized bentonite particles are added to inactivated serum; the t. is positive if half of the particles are clumped while the other half remain in suspension.

Bernstein t., a t. to establish that substernal pain is due to reflux esophagitis, performed by instillation of a weak hydrochloric acid solution directly into the lower esophagus. SYN acid perfusion t.

Betke-Kleihauer t., a slide t. for the presence of fetal red blood cells among those of the mother.

Binet t., SYN Stanford-Binet intelligence *scale.*

biuret t., a t. for the determination of serum proteins, based on the reaction of an alkaline copper reagent with substances containing two or more peptide bonds to produce a violet-blue color.

breath-holding t., a rough index of cardiopulmonary reserve measured by the length of time that a subject can voluntarily stop breathing; normal duration is 30 seconds or more; diminished cardiac or pulmonary reserve is indicated by a duration of 20 seconds or less.

bromphenol t., a colorimetric t. for measurement of protein, albumin, and globulin in the urine by use of reagent strips.

caloric t., SYN Bárány's caloric t.

cancer antigen 125 t., t. for cell-surface antigen found on derivatives of coelomic epithelium. Elevated levels of this antigen are associated with ovarian malignancy and benign pelvic disease such as endometriosis.

chi-square t. (kī), a statistical method of assessing the significance of a difference, as when the data from two or more samples are represented by a discrete number such as the numbers of females and males attending each of two colleges.

complement-fixation t., an immunological t. for determining the presence of a particular antigen or antibody when one of the two is known to be present, based on the fact that complement is "fixed" in the presence of antigen and its specific antibody.

Coombs' t., a t. for antibodies, the so-called anti-human globulin t. using either the direct or indirect Coombs' t.'s.

cover-uncover t., a t. to detect strabismus; the patient's attention is directed to a small fixation object, one eye is covered and after a few seconds, uncovered; if the uncovered eye moves to see the picture, strabismus is present.

Crampton t., a test for physical condition and resistance; a record is made of the pulse and the blood pressure in the recumbent and in the standing position, and the difference is graded from the theoretical perfection of 100 (seldom attained) downward (a reading of 75 is considered excellent, 65 poor).

Denver Developmental Screening T., a scale used by psychologists and pediatricians to assess the developmental, intellectual, motor, and social maturity of children at any age level from birth to adolescence.

Dick t., an intracutaneous t. of susceptibility to the erythrogenic toxin of *Streptococcus pyogenes* responsible for the rash and other manifestations of scarlet fever.

differential ureteral catheterization t., a study performed to determine various functional parameters of one kidney compared to the other; ureteral catheters are inserted at cystoscopy into the ureter or renal pelvis bilaterally, and simultaneous measurements are made of urine flow rate, insulin, or PAH (if infused), endogenous creatinine, or various urinary solutes.

dilute Russell's viper venom t. (DRVVT), a t. used to confirm the presence of a lupus anticoagulant.

dinitrophenylhydrazine t., a screening t. for maple syrup urine disease; the addition of 2,4-dinitrophenylhydrazine in HCl to urine gives a chalky white precipitate in the presence of ketoacids.

discontinuation t., a t. to determine whether a certain drug is responsible for a reaction by observation of a remission of symptoms following cessation of its use.

drawer t., SYN drawer *sign.*

Dugas' t., in the case of an injured shoulder, if the elbow cannot be made to touch the chest while the hand rests on the opposite shoulder, the injury is a dislocation and not a fracture of the humerus.

E-rosette t., a t. to identify T lymphocytes by mixing purified blood lymphocytes with serum and sheep erythrocytes; rosettes of erythrocytes form around human T lymphocytes on incubation.

exercise stress t., SYN stress t.

fern t., (1) a t. for estrogenic activity; cervical mucus smears form a fern pattern at those times when estrogen secretion is elevated, as at the time of ovulation; (2) a t. to detect ruptured amniotic membranes.

finger-nose t., a t. of voluntary eye-motor coordination of the upper limb(s); the subject is asked to slowly touch the tip of the nose with the extended index finger; assesses cerebellar function.

finger-to-finger t., a t. for coordination and position sense of the upper limbs; the subject is asked to approximate the ends of the index fingers; assesses cerebellar function.

Fishberg concentration t., a t. of renal water conservation; after overnight fluid deprivation, morning urine samples are collected and specific gravity is measured.

fluorescent treponemal antibody-absorption t., a sensitive and specific serologic t. for syphilis using a suspension of the Nichols strain of *Treponema pallidum* as antigen; the presence or absence of antibody in the patient's serum is indicated by an indirect fluorescent antibody technique.

Folin's t., (1) a quantitative t. for uric acid by means of the color produced with phosphotungstic acid and a base; (2) a quantitative t. for urea; the urea is decomposed by boiling with magnesium chloride, and the freed ammonia is measured.

fragility t., a t. that measures the resistance of erythrocytes to hemolysis in hypotonic saline solutions; erythrocytes to be tested are added to varying concentrations of saline and beginning

te

and complete hemolysis are measured; in hereditary spherocytosis, the fragility of the erythrocytes is markedly increased, whereas in thalassemia and sickle cell anemia, the fragility of the erythrocytes is usually reduced.

functional t., assessment of an individual's ability to move a body part actively, against resistance, and in a specific movement pattern.

gel diffusion precipitin t.'s, precipitin t.'s in which the immune precipitate forms in a gel medium (usually agar) into which one or both reactants have diffused; generally classified in two types, in one dimension, and in two dimensions.

Goodenough draw-a-man t., a brief t. for assessing an individual's level of intelligence based on how accurately drawn and how many elements are included when a child or adult is given a pencil and sheet of white paper and asked to draw a man. Also called the Goodenough draw-a-person t. and, in its current form, the Goodenough-Harris drawing t.

graded exercise t. (GXT), multistage exercise testing (usually on treadmill or bicycle ergometer) in which exercise intensity is progressively increased (graded) through levels that bring the test subject to a self-imposed fatigue level.

Guthrie t., bacterial inhibition assay for direct measurement of serum phenylalanine; in widespread use for detection of phenylketonuria in the newborn.

Hardy-Rand-Ritter t., a t. for color vision deficiency using pseudoisochromatic cards. These excellent cards have not been reprinted by the American Optical Co. since the plates were accidentally destroyed in 1965.

head-dropping t., a t. used in the diagnosis of disease of the extrapyramidal or striatal system (*e.g.,* parkinsonism, Wilson's disease); with the patient supine and relaxed, the examiner briskly lifts the head with the right hand and then allows it to drop upon the palm of the left hand; the head of a normal person drops suddenly like a dead weight, whereas, in striatal disease the head falls slowly, gently, and almost hesitantly.

Hemoccult t., a qualitative t. for occult blood in stool based upon detecting the peroxidase activity of hemoglobin; a t. kit can be used at home and the specimen mailed to a laboratory for evaluation.

Histalog t., a t. for measurement of maximal production of gastric acidity or anacidity; it is similar to the histamine t., but uses Histalog (betazole hydrochloride), an analogue of histamine.

histamine t., a t. for maximal production of gastric acidity or anacidity; after preliminary administration of an antihistamine, histamine acid phosphate is injected subcutaneously, followed by analysis of gastric contents. SEE ALSO Histalog t.

17-hydroxycorticosteroid t., a t., dependent on the Porter-Silber reaction, that is used as a measure of adrenocortical function and is performed on urine. Low values are seen in Addison's disease and hypopituitarism; high values are seen in Cushing's syndrome and extreme stress.

immunologic pregnancy t., a general term for t.'s for detection of increased human chorionic gonadotropin in plasma or urine by immunologic techniques including latex particle agglutination, hemagglutination inhibition, radioimmunoassay, and radioreceptor assays.

indirect hemagglutination t., SYN passive *hemagglutination.*

Ishihara t., a t. for color vision deficiency that utilizes a series of pseudoisochromatic plates on which numbers or letters are printed in dots of primary colors surrounded by dots of other colors; the figures are discernible by individuals with normal color vision.

^{131}I uptake t., a t. of thyroid function in which ^{131}I-iodide is given orally; after 24 hours, the amount present in the thyroid gland is measured and compared with normal values.

Korotkoff's t., a t. of collateral circulation; while the artery above an aneurysm is compressed, the blood pressure in the distal circulation is estimated; if it is fairly high, the collateral circulation is good.

Kveim t., an intradermal t. for the detection of sarcoidosis, done by injecting Kveim antigen (obtained from spleens of persons with sarcoidosis) and examining skin biopsies after three and six weeks; a positive t. is indicated by typical nodules showing evidence of sarcoid tissue.

Lachman t., a maneuver to detect deficiency of the anterior cruciate ligament; with the knee flexed 20 to 30°, the tibia is displaced anteriorly relative to the femur; a soft endpoint or greater than 4 millimeters of displacement is positive (abnormal).

LE cell t., *in vitro* incubation of blood or bone marrow of patients with systemic lupus erythematosus, or action of their serum on normal leukocytes, causes formation of characteristic LE cells. SYN lupus erythematosus cell t.

lepromin t., a t. utilizing an intradermal injection of a lepromin, to classify the stage of leprosy. It differentiates tuberculoid leprosy, in which there is a positive delayed reaction at the injection site, from lepromatous leprosy, in which there is no reaction.

leukocyte esterase t. (LET), a chemical t. for the presence of lysed or intact white blood cells in urine, performed with a dipstick as part of routine urinalysis; serves as an adjunct to microscopic examination of urinary sediment, and used to screen asymptomatic persons for urinary tract infection, especially chlamydial urethritis.

lupus band t., a direct immunofluorescent technique for demonstrating a band of immunoglobulins at the dermal-epidermal junction of the skin of patients with lupus erythematosus.

lupus erythematosus cell t., SYN LE cell t.

Mantoux t., SEE tuberculin t.

Master t., an early and long-used exercise challenge to identify ischemic heart disease using a pair of nine inch steps with a platform on top, the number of trips by the patient arbitrarily chosen and related to age and body weight. SEE ALSO two-step exercise t. SYN Master's two-step exercise t.

Master's two-step exercise t., SYN Master t.

McMurray t., rotation of the tibia on the femur to determine injury to meniscal structures.

metabisulfite t., a t. for sickle cell hemoglobin (Hb S); deoxygenation of cells containing Hb S is enhanced by addition of sodium metabisulfite to the blood, causing sickling visible on a slide; certain other abnormal hemoglobins (Hb C_{Harlem} and Hb I) also sickle in this t.

Minnesota multiphasic personality inventory t., a questionnaire type of psychological test for ages 16 and over, with 550 true-false statements coded in 4 validity and 10 personality scales which may be administered in both an individual or group format. SYN Minnesota Multiphasic Personality Inventory.

mixed agglutination t., SEE mixed agglutination *reaction.*

mixed lymphocyte culture t., a t. for histocompatibility of HL-A antigens in which donor and recipient lymphocytes are mixed in culture; the degree of incompatibility is indicated by the number of cells that have undergone transformation and mitosis, or by the uptake of radioactive isotope-labeled thymidine.

Moloney t., a t. to detect a high degree of sensitivity to diphtheria toxoid; more than a minimal local reaction to toxoid given intradermally indicates that prophylactic toxoid should be administered in fractional doses at suitable intervals.

multiple puncture tuberculin t., a kind of tine t. SEE tuberculin t.

neutralization t., SYN protection t.

nitroprusside t., a qualitative t. for cystinuria; following the addition of sodium cyanide to the urine, the further addition of nitroprusside produces a red-purple color if the cyanide has reduced any cystine present to cysteine.

Pap t., microscopic examination of cells exfoliated or scraped from a mucosal surface after staining with Papanicolaou's stain; used especially for detection of cancer of the uterine cervix.

parallax t., measurement of the deviation in strabismus by the alternate cover t. combined with neutralization of the deviation using prisms.

patch t., a t. of skin sensitiveness: a small piece of paper, tape, or a cup, wet with a dilute solution or suspension of t. material, is applied to skin of the upper back or upper outer arm and after 48 hours the area previously covered is compared with the uncovered surface; an erythematous reaction with vesicles occurs if the substance causes contact allergy. SEE ALSO photo-patch t.

Patrick's t., a t. to determine the presence or absence of disease in the hip (acetabulofemoral) joint; with the patient supine, the hip and knee are flexed and the external malleolus is placed above the patella of the opposite leg; when the knee is depressed, pain is elicited in disease of the hip joint.

photo-patch t., a t. of contact photosensitization: after application of a patch with the suspected sensitizer for 48 hours to two sites, if there is no reaction, one area is exposed to a weak erythema dose of sunlight or ultraviolet light; if positive, a more severe reaction with vesiculation develops at the exposed patch area than the nonexposed skin patch site.

plasmacrit t., a serologic screening method for syphilis; heparinized blood is centrifuged in a capillary tube and the plasma thus separated with cardiolipin antigen. The presence of flocculation should not be regarded as conclusively diagnostic, but a negative result excludes the likelihood of syphilis.

precipitin t., an *in vitro* t. in which antigen is in soluble form and precipitates when it combines with added specific antibody in the presence of an electrolyte. SEE ALSO gel diffusion precipitin t.'s.

protection t., a t. to determine the antimicrobial activity of a serum by inoculating a susceptible animal with a mixture of the serum and the virus or other microbe being tested. SYN neutralization t.

prothrombin t., a quantitative t. for prothrombin in the blood based on the clotting time of oxalated blood plasma in the presence of thromboplastin and calcium chloride; measures the integrity of the extrinsic and common pathways of coagulation. SEE ALSO prothrombin *time.* SYN Quick's method, Quick's t.

pulmonary function t. (PFT), the assessment (from various breathing maneuvers) that provides information about airflow, lung volumes, and the diffusion of gas; the assessment of airflow is made from spirometry, peak flow meters, and the body plethysmograph; the assessment of lung volumes requires the measurement of functional residual capacity and of slow vital capacity; the assessment of diffusing capacity is usually made by the single-breath carbon monoxide technique. Other PFTs include exercise, bronchial provocation, and pressure-volume assessment.

pulp t., SYN vitality t.

Queckenstedt-Stookey t., compression of the jugular vein in a healthy person causes an increase in the pressure of the spinal fluid in the lumbar region within 10 to 12 seconds; when there is a block of subarachnoid channels, compression of the vein causes little or no increase of pressure in the cerebrospinal fluid.

quellung t., SYN Neufeld capsular *swelling.*

Quick's t., SYN prothrombin t.

radioallergosorbent t. (RAST), a radioimmunoassay t. to detect IgE-bound allergens responsible for tissue hypersensitivity: the allergen is bound to insoluble material and the patient's serum is reacted with this conjugate; if the serum contains antibody to the allergen, it will be complexed to the allergen.

radioimmunosorbent t. (RIST), a competition t., performed *in vitro*, used to measure IgE specific for a particular antigen. Known amounts of radiolabeled IgE compete with the patient's unlabeled IgE to bind to a surface coated with anti-IgE. The reduction in radiolabeled IgE due to the presence of IgE in the patient's serum can be determined by comparison to known IgE standards; thus, the amount of the patient's total serum IgE can be determined.

Rapoport t., a differential ureteral catheterization t. used to evaluate suspected renovascular hypertension; urine specimens from each kidney are obtained by bilateral ureteral catheterization, and the tubular rejection fraction ratio is determined by measuring concentrations of sodium and creatinine in the urine from each kidney.

Rinne's t., a vibrating tuning fork is held alternately with the base touching the mastoid process and with the prongs near the external ear. Normally the sound can be heard by air conduction longer than by bone conduction; the reverse phenomenon indicates conductive hearing loss in the ear tested.

rubella HI t., a hemagglutination inhibition (HI) t. for rubella, often performed routinely as part of a prenatal workup of the pregnant woman; the presence of any detectable HI titer in the absence of disease indicates previous infection and immunity to reinfection.

Saundby's t., a t. for blood in the stool with hydrogen peroxide and benzidine; a dark blue color denotes the presence of blood.

Schick t., a t. for susceptibility to *Corynebacterium diphtheriae* toxin. Schick test toxin is injected into the skin; individuals lacking toxin-neutralizing antibodies may have a positive reaction, which consists of an area of redness.

Schiller's t., a t. for nonglycogen-containing areas of the portio vaginalis of the cervix, which may be the site of early carcinoma; such areas fail to stain dark brown with iodine solution.

Schilling t., a procedure for determining the amount of vitamin B_{12} excreted in the urine using cyanocobalamin tagged with a radioisotope of cobalt.

scratch t., a form of skin t. in which antigen is applied through a scratch in the skin.

screening t., any testing procedure designed to separate people or objects according to a fixed characteristic or property.

shadow t., SYN retinoscopy.

SISI t., the sounding of a tone 20 dB above threshold, followed by a series of 200-msec tones 1 dB louder; perception of these is indicative of cochlear damage.

skin t., a method for determining induced sensitivity (allergy) by applying an antigen (allergen) to, or inoculating it into, the skin; induced sensitivity (allergy) to the specific antigen is indicated by an inflammatory reaction of one of two general kinds: 1) immediate, appears in minutes to an hour or so and in general is dependent upon circulating immunoglobulins (antibodies); 2) delayed, appears in 12 to 48 hours and is not dependent upon these soluble substances but upon cellular response and infiltration.

sniff t., FLUOROSCOPY a t. for diaphragmatic function; paradoxical motion of a hemidiaphragm when a patient sniffs vigorously shows phrenic nerve paralysis or paresis of the hemidiaphragm. If rapid upward movement of the diaphragm occurs on brisk sniffing in the supine position, it is highly suggestive of paralysis of the diaphragm.

solubility t., a screening t. for sickle cell hemoglobin (Hb S), which is reduced by dithionite and is insoluble in concentrated inorganic buffer; addition of blood showing Hb S to buffer and dithionite causes opacity of the solution.

spot t. for infectious mononucleosis, a slide t. widely used for the diagnosis of infectious

mononucleosis; when horse red cells are agglutinated by patient serum (previously treated with guinea pig kidney, which adsorbs confounding antibodies), the presumptive diagnosis is infectious mononucleosis.

stress t., systematic use of exercise for (1) ECG and other cardiac function evaluations, and (2) to evaluate the physiological adjustments to metabolic demands that exceed the resting requirement. SEE graded exercise t. SYN exercise stress t.

thematic apperception t. (TAT), a projective psychological t. in which the subject is asked to tell a story about standard ambiguous pictures depicting life-situations to reveal personal attitudes and feelings.

Thompson's t., the urine, in a case of gonorrhea, is passed into two glasses in succession; if gonococci and mucous threads are found only in the first glass the probability is that the process is limited to the anterior urethra. SYN two-glass t.

three-glass t., the male patient empties his bladder into a series of 3-ounce test tubes, and the contents of the first and the last are examined; the first tube contains the washings from the anterior urethra, the second, material from the bladder, and the last, material from the posterior urethra, prostate, and seminal vesicles.

thyrotropin-releasing hormone stimulation t., TRH stimulation t., a t. of pituitary response to injection of thyrotropin-releasing hormone, which normally stimulates pituitary secretion of thyroid-stimulating hormone (TSH, thyrotropin), used primarily to distinguish pituitary from hypothalamic causes of thyroid disorders; TSH does not rise in cases of pituitary dysfunction, but does rise in cases of hypothalamic disorders.

tilt t., any measurement of response during tilting of the body usually head up but also head down. The t. may be monitored by catheterization, echocardiography, electrophysiologic measurements, electrocardiography, or mechanocardiography.

tine t., SEE tuberculin t.

tolbutamide t., a t. to detect insulin-producing tumors; after a 1-g intravenous dose of tolbutamide, plasma insulin and glucose are measured at intervals up to 3 hr; higher insulin responses and lower glucose values characterize patients with such tumors.

Trendelenburg's t., a t. of the valves of the leg veins; the leg is raised above the level of the heart until the veins are empty and is then rapidly lowered; in varicosity and incompetence of the valves the veins will at once become distended, but placement of a tourniquet around the leg will prevent distention of veins below the incompetent perforators or valves below the tourniquet.

tuberculin t., a skin t. in which tuberculin or its purified protein derivative (PPD) is injected into the skin; the t. is read on the basis of local induration occurring in 48–72 hours.

two-glass t., SYN Thompson's t.

two-step exercise t., a t. used mainly for coronary insufficiency; significant depression of RS-T in the electrocardiogram is considered abnormal and suggests coronary insufficiency.

VDRL t., a flocculation t. for syphilis, using

cardiolipin-lecithin-cholesterol antigen as developed by the Venereal Disease Research Laboratory of the United States Public Health Service.

vitality t., a group of thermal and electrical t.'s used to aid in assessment of dental pulp health. SYN pulp t.

Weil-Felix t., a t. for the presence and type of rickettsial disease based on the agglutination of X-strains of *Proteus vulgaris* with suspected rickettsia in a patient's blood serum. SYN Weil-Felix reaction.

Western blot t., a serum electrophoretic analysis used to identify proteins.

tes•tal•gia (tes-tal′jē-ă). SYN orchialgia. [testis + G. *algos*, pain]

tes•tec•to•my (tes-tek′tō-mē). SYN orchiectomy. [testis + G. G. *ektomē*, excision]

tes•tes (tes′tēz). Plural of testis. [L.]

tes•ti•cle (tes′tĭ-kl). SYN testis. [L. *testiculus*, dim. of *testis*]

tes•tic•u•lar (tes-tik′yū-lăr). Relating to the testes.

test•ing. SEE test.

histocompatibility t., a t. system for HLA antigens, of major importance in transplantation.

limit t., OCCUPATIONAL THERAPY attempts to approach or exceed established boundaries or guidelines for purposes of challenge or control.

reality t., in psychiatry and psychology, the ego function by which the objective or real world and one's subjectively sensed relationship to it are evaluated and appreciated; the ability to distinguish internal from external events.

tes•tis, pl. **tes•tes** (tes′tis, -tēz) [NA]. One of the two male reproductive glands, located in the cavity of the scrotum. SYN didymus, orchis, testicle. [L.]

ectopic t., a variant of undescended t. wherein testicular position is outside the usual pathway of descent. SEE ALSO testis *ectopia*.

undescended t., a t. that has failed to descend into the scrotum; there are palpable and nonpalpable variants.

tes•ti•tis (tes-tī′tis). SYN orchitis.

tes•tos•ter•one (tes-tos′tĕ-rōn). The most potent naturally occurring androgen, formed in greatest quantities by the interstitial cells of the testes, and possibly secreted also by the ovary and adrenal cortex; used in the treatment of hypogonadism, cryptorchism, certain carcinomas, and menorrhagia.

test types. Letters of various sizes used to test visual acuity.

tetan-. SEE tetano-.

te•tan•ic (te-tan′ik). 1. Relating to or marked by a sustained muscular contraction, as in tetanus. 2. An agent, such as strychnine, that in poisonous doses produces tonic muscular spasm. [G. *tetanikos*]

te•tan•i•form (te-tan′i-fōrm). SYN tetanoid (1).

tet•a•nig•e•nous (tet-ă-nij′ĕ-nŭs). Causing tetanus or tetaniform spasms. [tetanus + G. *-gen*, producing]

tet•a•nism (tet′ă-nizm). SYN neonatal *tetany*.

tet•a•ni•za•tion (tet′ă-ni-zā′shŭn). 1. The act of tetanizing the muscles. 2. A condition of tetaniform spasm.

tet•a•nize (tet′ă-nīz). To stimulate a muscle by a rapid series of stimuli so that the individual muscular responses (contractions) are fused into a sustained contraction; to cause tetanus (2) in a muscle.

⚠**tetano-, tetan-.** Combining forms denoting tetanus, tetany. [G. *tetanos*, convulsive tension]

tet•a•node (tet′ă-nōd). Denoting the quiet interval between the recurrent tonic spasms in tetanus. [G. *tetanōdēs*]

tet•a•noid (tet′ă-noyd). 1. Resembling or of the nature of tetanus. SYN tetaniform. 2. Resembling tetany. [tetano- + G. *eidos*, resemblance]

tet•a•no•spas•min (tet′ă-nō-spaz′min). The neurotoxin of *Clostridium tetani*, which causes the characteristic signs and symptoms of tetanus; chief action is on the anterior horn cells, and the spasms seem to be due to action at inhibitory synapses.

tet•a•nus (tet′ă-nŭs). 1. A disease marked by painful tonic muscular contractions, caused by the neurotropic toxin (tetanospasmin) of *Clostridium tetani* acting upon the central nervous system. 2. A sustained muscular contraction caused by a series of nerve stimuli repeated so rapidly that the individual muscular responses are fused; producing a sustained tetanic contraction. SEE emprosthotonos, opisthotonos. [L. fr. G. *tetanos*, convulsive tension]

benign t., a disorder marked by intermittent tonic muscular contractions of the extremities, especially the hands and feet (carpopedal spasm), accompanied by paresthesias and, when severe, by crowing respirations due to laryngospasm and seizures; results from hypocalcemia, caused by various disorders, including gastrointestinal abnormalities. SYN intermittent cramp (2).

cephalic t., a type of local tetanus that follows wounds to the face and head; after a brief incubation (1–2 days) the facial and ocular muscles become paretic yet undergo repeated tetanic spasms. The throat and tongue muscles may also be affected.

drug t., tonic spasms caused by strychnine or other tetanic. SYN toxic t.

intermittent t., SYN tetany.

t. neonatorum (nē-ō-nā′tōr-ŭm), t. occurring in newborn infants, usually due to infection of umbilical area with *Clostridium tetani*, often a result of ritualistic practices; has high fatality rate (about 60%).

puerperal t., t. occurring during the puerperium from infection of the obstetric wound.

toxic t., SYN drug t.

traumatic t., t. following infection of a wound.

tet•a•ny (tet′ă-nē). A clinical neurological syndrome characterized by muscle twitches, cramps, and carpopedal spasm, and when severe, laryngospasm and seizures; these findings reflect irritability of the central and peripheral nervous systems, usually resulting from low serum levels of ionized calcium or, rarely, magnesium. Causes include hyperventilation, hypoparathyroidism, rickets, and uremia. SYN intermittent cramp (1), intermittent tetanus. [G. *tetanos*, tetanus]

duration t. (DT), a tonic spasm occurring in

degenerated muscles upon application of a strong galvanic current.

gastric t., t. associated with a gastric disorder, especially with loss of HCl by vomiting.

hyperventilation t., t. caused by forced overbreathing, due to a reduction in CO_2 in the blood.

neonatal t., hypocalcemic t. occurring in neonates or young infants, due to transient functional hypoparathyroidism in consumption of cow's milk (high phosphorus content). SYN tetanism.

parathyroid t., t. due to lack of parathyroid function, spontaneous or following excision of the parathyroid glands.

△**tetra-.** Four. [G. *tetra-,* four]

tet·ra·crot·ic (tet'ră-krot'ik). Denoting a pulse curve with four upstrokes in the cycle. [tetra- + G. *krotos,* a striking]

tet·rad. 1. A group of four things having something in common such as a deformity with four features *e.g.,* Fallot's tetralogy. SYN tetralogy. **2.** CHEMISTRY A quadrivalent element. **3.** In heredity, a bivalent chromosome that divides into four during meiosis. [G. *tetras* (*tetrad-*), the number four]

tet·ra·dac·tyl (tet-ră-dak'til). Having only four fingers or toes on a hand or foot. [tetra- + G. *daktylos,* finger or toe]

△**tetrahydro-.** Prefix denoting attachment of four hydrogen atoms; *e.g.,* tetrahydrofolate, H_4folate.

te·tral·o·gy (tet-ral'ō-jē). SYN tetrad (1). [G. *tetralogia*]

t. of Fallot, a set of congenital cardiac defects including ventricular septal defect, pulmonic valve stenosis or infundibular stenosis, and dextroposition of the aorta so that it overrides the ventricular septum and receives venous as well as arterial blood. Right ventricular hypertrophy is considered part of the tetralogy although it is reactive to the other defects.

tet·ra·mer·ic, te·tram·er·ous (tet'ră-mer'ik, tĕ-tram'ĕ-rŭs). Having four parts, or parts arranged in groups of four, or capable of existing in four forms. [tetra- + G. *meros,* part]

tet·ra·pa·re·sis (tet'ră-pă-rē'sis). Weakness of all four extremities. SYN quadriparesis.

tet·ra·pep·tide (tet'ră-pep'tīd). A compound of four amino acids in peptide linkage.

tet·ra·ple·gia (tet'ră-plē'jē-ă). SYN quadriplegia. [tetra- + G. *plēgē,* stroke]

tet·ra·ploid (tet'ră-ployd). SEE polyploidy. [G. *tetraploos,* fourfold, + *eidos,* form]

tet·ra·sac·cha·ride (tet'ră-sak'ă-rīd). A sugar containing four molecules of a monosaccharide.

tet·ra·so·mic (tet'ră-sō'mik). Relating to a cell nucleus in which one chromosome is represented four times while all others are present in the normal number. [tetra- + chromosome]

tet·ra·va·lent (tet'ră-vā'lent). SYN quadrivalent. [tetra- + L. *valentia,* strength]

tet·rose (tet'rōs). A monosaccharide containing only four carbon atoms in the main chain.

tex·ti·form (teks'tĭ-fōrm). Weblike. [L. *textum,* something woven]

tex·tur·al (teks'chŭr-ăl). Relating to the texture of the tissues.

tex·ture (teks'chūr). The composition or structure of a tissue or organ. [L. *textura,* fr. *texo,* pp. *textus,* to weave]

TF tuning *fork.*

Th thorium; T helper *cells,* under *cell.*

△**thalam-.** SEE thalamo-.

thal·a·men·ceph·a·lon (thal'ă-men-sef'ă-lon). That part of the diencephalon comprising the thalamus and its associated structures. [thalamus + G. *enkephalos,* brain]

tha·lam·ic (tha-lam'ik). Relating to the thalamus.

△**thalamo-, thalam-.** The thalamus. [G. *thalamos,* bedroom (thalamus)]

thal·a·mo·cor·ti·cal (thal'ă-mō-kōr'ti-kăl). Relating to the efferent connections of the thalamus with the cerebral cortex.

thal·a·mot·o·my (thal-ă-mot'ō-mē). Destruction of a selected portion of the thalamus by stereotaxy for the relief of pain, involuntary movements, epilepsy, and, rarely, emotional disturbances. [thalamus + G. *tomē,* incision]

thal·a·mus, pl. **thal·a·mi** (thal'ă-mŭs, -mī) [NA]. The large, ovoid mass of gray matter that forms the larger dorsal subdivision of the diencephalon; it is placed medial to the internal capsule and the body and tail of the caudate nucleus. Its medial aspect forms the dorsal half of the lateral wall of the third ventricle; its dorsal surface can be subdivided into a lateral triangle forming the floor of the body (central part) of the lateral ventricle, and a medial triangle covered by the velum interpositum; its taillike caudal part curves ventralward around the posterolateral aspect of the cerebral peduncle and ends in the lateral geniculate body. The t. is composed of a large number of anatomically and functionally distinct cell groups or nuclei, usually classified as 1) sensory relay nuclei (ventral posterior nucleus, lateral and medial geniculate body) each receiving a modally specific sensory conduction system and in turn projecting each to the corresponding primary sensory area of the cortex; 2) "secondary" relay nuclei (ventral intermediate nucleus and ventral anterior nucleus) receiving fibers from the medial segment of the globus pallidus, the contralateral deep cerebellar nuclei (*i.e.,* cerebellothalamic fibers) and the pars reticulata of the substantia nigra which project to various regions of the motor cortex; 3) a nucleus associated with the limbic system: the composite anterior nucleus receiving the mamillothalamic tract and projecting to the fornicate gyrus; 4) association nuclei (medial dorsal nucleus, lateral nucleus including the large pulvinar) each projecting to a particular large expanse of association cortex; 5) the midline and intralaminar nuclei or "nonspecific" nuclei (centromedian nucleus, central lateral nucleus, paracentral nucleus, nucleus reuniens). [G. *thalamos,* a bed, bedroom]

⬛**thal·as·se·mia, thal·as·sa·ne·mia** (thal-ă-sē'mē-ă, thă-las-ă-nē'mē-ă). Any of a group of inherited disorders of hemoglobin metabolism in which there is impaired synthesis of one or more of the polypeptide chains of globin; several genetic types exist, and the corresponding clinical picture may vary from barely detectable hematologic abnormality to severe and fatal anemia. [G. *thalassa,* the sea, + *haima,* blood]

α t., t. due to one of two or more genes that depress synthesis of α-globin chains.

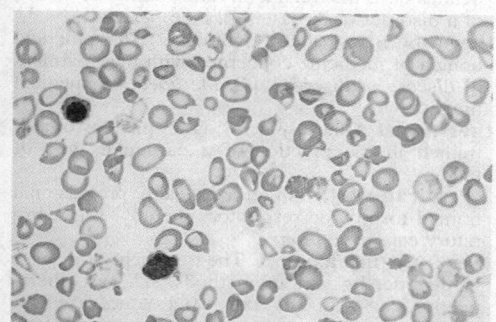

thalassemia: a blood film from a patient with homozygous β-thalassemia (250 x original magnification; Wright-Giemsa stain)

β t., t. due to one of two or more genes that depress (partially or completely) synthesis of β-globin chains.

β-δ t., t. due to a gene that depresses synthesis of both β- and δ-globin chains.

t. ma′jor [MIM*141800-142310 passim], the syndrome of severe anemia resulting from the homozygous state of one of the t. genes or one of the hemoglobin Lepore genes with onset, in infancy or childhood, of pallor, icterus, weakness, splenomegaly, cardiac enlargement, thinning of inner and outer tables of skull, microcytic hypochromic anemia with poikilocytosis, anisocytosis, stippled cells, target cells, and nucleated erythrocytes; types of hemoglobin are variable and depend on the gene involved. SYN Cooley's anemia.

t. mi′nor [MIM*141800-142310 passim], the heterozygous state of a t. gene or a hemoglobin Lepore gene; usually asymptomatic and quite variable hematologically, with target cells, mild hypochromic microcytosis, and often slightly reduced hemoglobin level with slightly increased erythrocyte count; types of hemoglobin are variable and depend on the gene involved.

thal•lic (thal′lik). Denoting conidia produced with no enlargement or growth after delimitation by septa in the hypha (thallus); the entire parent cell becomes an arthroconidium.

thal•li•um (Tl) (thal′ē-ŭm). A white metallic element, atomic no. 81, atomic wt. 204.3833; ^{201}Tl (half-life equal to 3.038 days) is used to scan the myocardium. [G. *thallos,* a green shoot (it gives a green line in the spectrum)]

thal•lus (thal′ŭs). A simple plant or fungus body which is devoid of roots, stems, and leaves. The vegetative growth of a fungus. [G. *thallos,* a young shoot]

thanato-. Death. SEE ALSO necro-. [G. *thanatos,* death]

than•a•to•bi•o•log•ic (than′ă-tō-bī-ō-loj′ik). Relating to the processes involved in life and death. [thanato- + G. *bios,* life, + *logos,* study]

than•a•to•gno•mon•ic (than′ă-tō-nō-mon′ik). Of fatal prognosis, indicating the approach of death. [thanato- + G. *gnōmē,* a sign]

than•a•toid (than′ă-toyd). 1. Resembling death. 2. Deadly. [thanato- + G. *eidos,* resemblance]

than•a•tol•o•gy (than-ă-tol′ō-jē). The branch of science concerned with the study of death and dying. [thanato- + G. *logos,* study]

the•ca, pl. **the•cae** (thē′kă, thē′sē). A sheath or capsule. [G. *thēkē,* a box]

    t. cor′dis, SYN pericardium.

    t. follic′uli, the wall of a vesicular ovarian follicle. SEE ALSO *tunica* externa.

the•cal (thē′kăl). Relating to a sheath, especially a tendon sheath. [see theca]

the•ci•tis (thē-sī′tis). Inflammation of the sheath of a tendon. [G. *thēkē,* box (sheath), + -*itis,* inflammation]

the•co•ma (thē-kō′mă). A neoplasm derived from ovarian mesenchyme, consisting chiefly of spindle-shaped cells that frequently contain small droplets of fat; it may form considerable quantities of estrogens, thereby resulting in precocious development of secondary sexual features in prepubertal girls, or hyperplasia of the endometrium in older patients. [G. *thēkē,* box (theca), + -*oma,* tumor]

△**thel-.** SEE thelo-.

the•lar•che (thē-lar′kē). The beginning of development of the breasts in the female. [thel- + G. *archē,* beginning]

the•le•plas•ty (thē′lē-plas-tē). SYN mammillaplasty. [thel- + G. *plastos,* formed]

the•li•um, pl. **the•lia** (thē′lē-ŭm, -lē-ă). 1. A nipple-like structure. 2. A cellular layer. 3. SYN nipple. [Mod. L., fr. G. *thēlē,* nipple]

△**thelo-, thel-.** The nipples. Cf. mamil-. [G. *thēlē*]

the•lor•rha•gia (thē-lō-rā′jē-ă). Bleeding from the nipple. [thelo- + G. *rhēgnymi,* to burst forth]

the•nar (thē′nar). 1 [NA]. SYN thenar *eminence.* 2. Applied to any structure in relation with the thenar eminence or its underlying collective components. [G. the palm of the hand]

the•o•rem (thē′ō-rem). A proposition that can be proved, and so is established as a law or principle. SEE ALSO law, principle, rule.

the•o•ry (thē′ōr-ē). A reasoned explanation of known facts or phenomena that serves as a basis of investigation by which to reach the truth. SEE ALSO hypothesis, postulate. [G. *theōria,* a beholding, speculation, theory, fr. *theōros,* a beholder]

    adsorption t. of narcosis, that a drug becomes concentrated at the surface of the cell as a result of adsorption, and thus alters permeability and metabolism.

    Arrhenius-Madsen t., that the reaction of an antigen with its antibody is a reversible reaction, the equilibrium being determined according to the law of mass action by the concentrations of the reacting substances.

    Brønsted t., that an acid is a substance, charged or uncharged, liberating hydrogen ions in solution, and that a base is a substance that removes them from solution; useful in the concept of weak electrolytes and buffers. Cf. Brønsted *acid,* Brønsted *base.*

    clonal selection t., a t. which states that each lymphocyte has membrane-bound immunoglobulin receptors specific for a particular antigen and once the receptor is engaged, proliferation of the

th

cell occurs such that a clone of antibody producing cells (plasma cell) is produced.

decay t., a t. of forgetting based on the premise that an engram or memory trace dissipates progressively with time during the interval when it is not activated.

emergency t., a t. of the emotions, advanced by W.B. Cannon, that animal and human organisms respond to emergency situations by increased sympathetic nervous system activity including an increased catecholamine production with associated increases in blood pressure, heart and respiratory rates, and skeletal muscle blood flow.

gate-control t., a theory to explain the mechanism of pain; small-fiber afferent stimuli, particularly pain, entering the substantia gelatinosa can be modulated by large-fiber afferent stimuli and descending spinal pathways so that their transmission to ascending spinal pathways is blocked (gated).

information t., BEHAVIORAL SCIENCES a system for studying the communication process through the detailed analysis, often mathematical, of all aspects of the process including the encoding, transmission, and decoding of signals; not concerned in any direct sense with the meaning of a message.

lipoid t. of narcosis, that narcotic efficiency parallels the coefficient of partition between oil and water, and that lipoids in the cell and on the cell membrane absorb the drug because of this affinity.

membrane expansion t., that adsorption of anesthetics into membranes so alters membrane volume and/or configuration that membrane function is affected in such a way as to produce anesthesia.

omega-oxidation t., that the oxidation of fatty acids commences at the CH_3 group, *i.e.,* the terminal or omega-group; beta-oxidation then proceeds at both ends of the fatty acid chain.

quantum t., that energy can be emitted, transmitted, and absorbed only in discrete quantities (quanta), so that atoms and subatomic particles can exist only in certain energy states.

recapitulation t., that individuals in their embryonic development pass through stages similar in general structural plan to the stages their species passed through in its evolution; more technically phrased, the t. that ontogeny is an abbreviated recapitulation of phylogeny. SYN law of recapitulation.

somatic mutation t. of cancer, that cancer is caused by a mutation or mutations in the body cells (as opposed to germ cells), especially nonlethal mutations associated with increased proliferation of the mutant cells.

Young-Helmholtz t. of color vision, a t. that there are three color-perceiving elements in the retina: red, green, and blue. Perception of other colors arises from the combined stimulation of these elements; deficiency or absence of any one of these elements results in inability to perceive that color and a misperception of any other color of which it forms a part.

ther•a•peu•tic (thār-ă-pyū′tik). Relating to therapeutics or to the treatment, remediating, or curing of a disorder or disease. [G. *therapeutikos*]

ther•a•peu•tics (thār-ă-pyū′tiks). The practical branch of medicine concerned with the treatment of disease or disorder. [G. *therapeutikē,* medical practice]

ther•a•pist (thār′ă-pist). One professionally trained in the practice of a particular type of therapy.

respiratory t., An allied health professional trained to provide respiratory therapy. SEE respiratory care *practitioner.*

ther•a•py (thār′ă-pē). **1.** The treatment of disease or disorder by various methods. SEE ALSO therapeutics. **2.** PSYCHIATRY, CLINICAL PSYCHOLOGY Psychotherapy. SEE ALSO psychotherapy, psychiatry, psychology, psychoanalysis. [G. *therapeia,* medical treatment]

aversion t., a form of behavior t. that pairs an unpleasant stimulus with undesirable behavior(s) so that the patient learns to avoid the latter.

behavior t., an offshoot of psychotherapy involving the use of procedures and techniques associated with conditioning and learning for the treatment of a variety of psychological conditions.

client-centered t., a system of nondirective psychotherapy based on the assumption that the client (patient) both has the internal resources to improve and is in the best position to resolve personality dysfunction.

cognitive t., any of a variety of techniques in psychotherapy that utilizes guided self-discovery, imaging, self-instruction, symbolic modeling, and related forms of explicitly elicited cognitions as the principal mode of treatment.

cold t., SYN cryokinetics.

compression t., use of circumferential elastic tubing, bandages, or a custom garment to apply pressure in such conditions as burns, lymphedema, edema, and venous stasis.

cytoreductive t., t. with the intention of reducing the number of cells in a lesion, usually a malignancy.

electroconvulsive t. (ECT), SYN electroshock t.

electroshock t. (EST), a form of treatment of mental disorders in which convulsions are produced by the passage of an electric current through the brain. SYN electroconvulsive t.

family t., a type of group psychotherapy in which a family in conflict meets as a group with the therapist and explores its relationships and processes; focus is on the resolution of current issues between members rather than on individual members.

gene t., the process of inserting a gene into an organism to replace or repair gene function to treat a disease or genetic defect.

gestalt t., a type of psychotherapy, used with individuals or groups, that emphasizes treatment of the person as a whole: the individual's biological component parts and their organic functioning, perceptual configuration, and interrelationships with the external world.

helium t., the use of a helium-gas mixture (usually helium and oxygen) in the management of obstruction of the airways; the density of helium is much lower than that of either air or oxygen; as a result, the gaseous mixture will move past an airway obstruction more easily.

hyperbaric oxygen t., treatment in which oxygen is provided in a sealed chamber at an ambient pressure greater than 1 atmosphere.

milieu t., psychiatric treatment employing manipulation of the social environment for the benefit of the patient.

myofunctional t., SPEECH PATHOLOGY any technique used to promote normal patterns of tongue movement and swallowing; primarily used to ameliorate tongue thrust. SEE tongue thrust. SYN tongue thrust t.

occupational t., therapeutic use of self-care, work, and recreational activities to increase independent function, enhance development, prevent disability and achieve optimum quality of life.

photoradiation t., SYN photoradiation.

physical t. (PT), (1) treatment of pain, disease, or injury by physical means; SYN physiotherapy. **(2)** the health profession concerned with promotion of health, with prevention of physical disabilities, with evaluation and rehabilitation of persons disabled by pain, disease, or injury, and with treatment by physical therapeutic measures as opposed to medical, surgical, or radiologic measures.

play t., a type of t. used with children in which they can express or reveal their problems and fantasies by playing with dolls or other toys, drawing, etc.

psychoanalytic t., SYN psychoanalysis (1).

radiation t., treatment with x-rays or radionuclides.

rational t., therapeutic procedures based on the premise that lack of information or illogical thought patterns are basic causes of a patient's difficulties.

replacement t., t. designed to compensate for a lack or deficiency arising from inadequate nutrition, from certain dysfunctions (*e.g.,* glandular hyposecretion), or from losses (*e.g.,* hemorrhage); replacement may be physiological or may entail administration of a substitute (*e.g.,* a synthetic estrogen in place of estradiol).

respiratory t., care and treatment intended to support respiration or to reverse abnormalities of the respiratory system. SEE respiratory *care.*

shock t., SEE electroshock t.

substitution t., replacement t., particularly when replacement is not physiological but entails administration of a substitute.

tongue thrust t., SYN myofunctional t.

transtracheal oxygen t., a method of oxygen delivery via a catheter inserted into the second tracheal interspace.

therm-. SEE thermo-.

ther•mal (ther′măl). Pertaining to heat.

ther•mal•ge•sia (ther-mal-jē′zē-ă). High sensibility to heat; pain caused by a slight degree of heat. [therm- + G. *algēsis,* sense of pain]

ther•mal•gia (ther-mal′jē-ă). Burning pain. SEE ALSO causalgia. [therm- + G. *algos,* pain]

therm•an•al•ge•sia (therm′an-al-jē′zē-ă). SYN thermoanesthesia. [therm- + analgesia]

therm•an•es•the•sia (therm′an-es-thē′zē-ă). SYN thermoanesthesia.

therm•es•the•sia (therm-es-thē′zē-ă). SYN thermoesthesia.

therm•es•the•si•om•e•ter (therm′es-thē-zē-om′ĕ-ter). SYN thermoesthesiometer.

△**thermo-, therm-.** Heat. [G. *thermē,* heat; *thermos,* warm or hot]

ther•mo•an•al•ge•sia (ther′mō-an′al-jē′zē-ă). SYN thermoanesthesia.

ther•mo•an•es•the•sia (ther′mō-an-es-thē′zē-ă). Loss of the temperature sense or of the ability to distinguish between heat and cold; insensibility to heat or to temperature changes. SYN thermanalgesia, thermanesthesia, thermoanalgesia. [thermo- + G. *an-* priv. + *aisthēsis,* sensation]

ther•mo•chem•is•try (ther-mō-kem′is-trē). The interrelation of chemical action and heat.

ther•mo•co•ag•u•la•tion (ther′mō-kō-ag-yū-lā′shŭn). The process of converting tissue into a gel by heat.

ther•mo•cou•ple (ther-mō-kŭp′l). A device for measuring slight changes in temperature, consisting of two wires of different metals, one wire being kept at a certain low temperature, the other in the tissue or other material whose temperature is to be measured; a thermoelectric current set up is measured by a potentiometer.

ther•mo•dif•fu•sion (ther′mō-di-fyū′zhŭn). Diffusion of fluids, either gaseous or liquid, as influenced by the temperature of the fluid.

ther•mo•du•ric (ther-mō-dū′rik). Resistant to the effects of exposure to high temperature; used especially with reference to microorganisms. [thermo- + L. *durus,* hard, enduring]

ther•mo•dy•nam•ics (ther′mō-dī-nam′iks). **1.** The branch of physicochemical science concerned with heat and energy and their conversions one into the other involving mechanical work. **2.** The study of the flow of heat. [thermo- + G. *dynamis,* force]

ther•mo•es•the•sia (ther′mō-es-thē′zē-ă). The ability to distinguish differences of temperature. SYN thermesthesia. [thermo- + G. *aisthēsis,* sensation]

ther•mo•es•the•si•om•e•ter (ther′mō-es-thē′zē-om′ĕ-ter). An instrument for testing the temperature sense, consisting of a metal disk with thermometer attached, by which the exact temperature of the disk at the time of application may be known. SYN thermesthesiometer. [thermo- + G. *aisthēsis,* sensation, + *metron,* measure]

ther•mo•ex•ci•to•ry (ther′mō-ek-sī′tŏ-rē). Stimulating the production of heat.

ther•mo•gen•e•sis (ther′mō-jen′ĕ-sis). The production of heat; specifically the physiologic process of heat production in the body. [thermo- + G. *genesis,* production]

ther•mo•ge•net•ic, ther•mo•gen•ic (ther′mō-je-net′ik, -jen′ik). **1.** Relating to thermogenesis. **2.** SYN calorigenic (2).

ther•mo•gram (ther′mō-gram). **1.** A regional temperature map of the surface of a part of the body, obtained by infrared sensing device; it measures radiant heat, and thus subcutaneous blood flow, if the environment is constant. **2.** The record made by a thermograph. [thermo- + G. *gramma*, a writing]

ther·mo·graph (ther'mō-graf). An instrument or device used in producing a thermogram. [thermo- + G. *graphō*, to write]

ther·mog·ra·phy (ther-mog'ră-fē). The technique for making a thermogram.

ther·mo·in·hib·i·to·ry (ther'mō-in-hib'i-tōr-ē). Inhibiting or arresting thermogenesis.

ther·mo·la·bile (ther-mō-lā'bīl, -bil). Subject to alteration or destruction by heat. [thermo- + L. *labilis*, perishable]

ther·mol·y·sis (ther-mol'i-sis). 1. Loss of body heat by evaporation, radiation, etc. 2. Chemical decomposition by heat. [thermo- + G. *lysis*, dissolution]

ther·mo·lyt·ic (ther-mō-lit'ik). 1. Relating to thermolysis. 2. An agent promoting heat dissipation.

ther·mo·mas·sage (ther'mō-mă-sahzh'). Combination of heat and massage in physical therapy.

ther·mom·e·ter (ther-mom'ĕ-ter). An instrument for indicating the temperature of any substance; usually a sealed vacuum tube containing mercury, which expands with heat and contracts with cold, its level accordingly rising or falling in the tube, with the exact degree of variation of level being indicated by a scale. SEE ALSO scale. [thermo- + G. *metron*, measure]

    clinical t., a small, self-registering t., consisting of a simple scaled glass tube containing mercury, used for taking the temperature of the body.

    resistance t., a device measuring temperature by the change of the electrical resistance of a metal wire.

    self-registering t., a t. in which the maximum or minimum temperature, during the period of observation, is registered.

ther·mo·met·ric (ther-mō-met'rik). Relating to thermometry or to a thermometer reading.

ther·mom·e·try (ther-mom'ĕ-trē). The measurement of temperature. [thermo- + G. *metron*, measure]

ther·mo·phile, ther·mo·phil (ther'mō-fīl, -fil). An organism that thrives at a temperature of 50°C or higher. [thermo- + G. *phileō*, to love]

ther·mo·phil·ic (ther-mō-fil'ik). Pertaining to a thermophile.

ther·mo·phore (ther'mō-fōr). 1. An arrangement for applying heat to a part; consists of a water heater, a tube conveying hot water to a coil, and another tube conducting the water back to the heater. 2. A flat bag containing certain salts that produce heat when moistened; used as a substitute for the hot-water bag. [thermo- + G. *phoros*, bearing]

ther·mo·re·cep·tor (ther'mō-rē-sep'ter, -tōr). A receptor that is sensitive to heat.

ther·mo·reg·u·la·tion (ther'mō-reg-yū-lā'shŭn). Temperature control, as by a thermostat.

ther·mo·sta·bile, ther·mo·sta·ble (ther-mō-stā'bil, -stā'bl). Not readily subject to alteration or destruction by heat. [thermo- + L. *stabilis*, stable]

ther·mo·ste·re·sis (ther'mō-stĕ-rē'sis). The abstraction or deprivation of heat. [thermo- + G. *steresis*, deprivation, loss]

ther·mo·tac·tic, ther·mo·tax·ic (ther-mō-tak'tik, tak'sik). Relating to thermotaxis.

ther·mo·tax·is (ther-mō-tak'sis). 1. Reaction of living protoplasm to the stimulus of heat. Cf. thermotropism. 2. Regulation of the temperature of the body. [thermo- + G. *taxis*, orderly arrangement]

ther·mo·ther·a·py (ther'mō-thār'ă-pē). Treatment of disease by therapeutic application of heat. [thermo- + G. *therapeia*, treatment]

ther·mo·to·nom·e·ter (ther'mō-tō-nom'ĕ-ter). An instrument for measuring the degree of thermosystaltism, or muscular contraction under the influence of heat. [thermo- + G. *tonos*, tone, tension, + *metron*, measure]

ther·mot·ro·pism (ther-mot'rō-pizm). The motion by a part of an organism (*e.g.*, leaves or stems) toward or away from a source of heat. Cf. thermotaxis. [thermo- + G. *tropē*, a turning]

the·ta (θ, Θ) (thā'ta). 1. The 8th letter in the Greek alphabet (θ, Θ). 2. Symbol for angle. 3. The eighth in a series; denotes the position of a substituent located on the eighth atom from the carboxyl or other functional group.

△**thia-.** The replacement of carbon by sulfur in a ring or chain. Cf. thio-. [G. *theion*]

thi·a·min (thī'ă-min). A heat-labile and water-soluble vitamin contained in milk, yeast, and in the germ and husk of grains; also artificially synthesized; essential for growth; a deficiency of t. is associated with beriberi and Wernicke-Korsakoff's syndrome. SYN vitamin B₁. [*thia-* + vitamin]

thi·a·zides (thī'ă-zīdz). Abbreviated form of benzothiadiazides.

thi·a·zin (thī'ă-zin). Parent substance of a family of biological blue dyes; *e.g.*, methylene blue, thionine, toluidine blue.

thick·ness (thik'nes). 1. The measure of the depth of something, as opposed to its length or width. 2. A layer or stratum.

    Breslow's t., maximal t. of a primary cutaneous melanoma measured in tissue sections from the top of the epidermal granular layer, or from the ulcer base (if the tumor is ulcerated), to the bottom of the tumor; metastatic rates correlate closely with tumor t.

thi·e·mia (thī-ē'mē-ă). The presence of sulfur in the circulating blood. [G. *theion*, sulfur, + *haima*, blood]

thi·e·nyl·al·a·nine (thī'ē-nil-al'ă-nēn). A compound structurally similar to phenylalanine that inhibits the growth of *Escherichia coli*, presumably by competitive inhibition of enzymes for which L-phenylalanine is the substrate.

thigh (thī). The part of the inferior limb between the hip and the knee.

thig·mes·the·sia (thig-mes-thē'zē-ă). Sensibility to touch. [G. *thigma*, touch, + *aisthēsis*, sensation]

thig·mo·tax·is (thig-mō-tak'sis). A form of barotaxis; denoting the reaction of plant or animal protoplasm to contact with a solid body. Cf. thigmotropism. [G. *thigma*, touch, + *taxis*, orderly arrangement]

thig·mot·ro·pism (thig-mot'rō-pizm). A movement toward or away from a touch stimulus on the part of a portion of an organism, such as leaves or tendrils. Cf. thigmotaxis. [G. *thigma*, touch, + *trope*, a turning]

think•ing. The act of reasoning.

    abstract t., t. in terms of concepts and general principles (*e.g.,* perceiving a table and a chair as furniture), as contrasted with concrete t.

    concrete t., t. of objects or ideas as specific items rather than as an abstract representation of a more general concept, as contrasted with abstract t. (*e.g.,* perceiving a chair and a table as individual useful items and not as members of the general class, furniture).

    prelogical t., a concrete type of t., characteristic of children and primitives, to which schizophrenic persons sometimes regress.

think•ing through. The psychological process of understanding, with insight, one's own behavior.

thio-. Prefix denoting the replacement of oxygen by sulfur in a compound. Cf. thia-. [G. *theion*, sugar]

thi•o•ac•id (thī-ō-as'id). An organic acid in which one or more of the oxygen atoms have been replaced by sulfur atoms; *e.g.,* thiosulfuric acid.

-thioic ac•id. Suffix denoting the radical, —C(S)OH or —C(O)SH, the sulfur analog of a carboxylic acid.

thi•ol•trans•a•cet•y•lase A (thī'ol-trans-ă-set'ĭ-lās). SYN dihydrolipoamide acetyltransferase.

thi•ol•y•sis (thī-ol'ĭ-sis). The cleavage of a chemical bond with the addition of coenzyme A to one part; analogous to hydrolysis and phosphorolysis.

-thione. Suffix denoting the radical =C=S, the sulfur analog of a ketone.

thi•on•ic (thī-on'ik). Relating to sulfur.

thi•o•nine (thī'ō-nin) [C.I. 52000]. Dark-green powder, giving a purple solution in water; useful as a basic stain in histology for chromatin and mucin because of its metachromatic properties.

thi•o•sul•fate (thī-ō-sŭl'fāt). $S_2O_3^=$; the anion of thiosulfuric acid; elevated in individuals with a molybdenum cofactor deficiency.

thi•o•sul•fur•ic ac•id (thī'ō-sŭl-fyūr'ik). $H_2S_2O_3$; sulfuric acid in which an atom of oxygen has been replaced by one of sulfur.

thioxo-. Prefix indicating =S in a thioketone.

third-party payer. Institution or company that provides reimbursement to health care providers for services rendered to a third party (the patient).

thirst. A desire to drink associated with uncomfortable sensations in the mouth and pharynx. [A.S. *thurst*]

thix•o•la•bile (thik-sō-lā'bil, -bīl). Susceptible to thixotropy.

thix•o•tro•pic (thik-sō-trop'ik). Pertaining to, or characterized by, thixotropy.

thix•ot•ro•py (thik-sot'rō-pē). The property of certain gels of becoming less viscous when shaken or subjected to shearing forces and returning to the original viscosity upon standing. [G. *thixis*, a touching, + *trope*, turning]

thorac-. SEE thoraco-.

tho•ra•cal•gia (thōr-ă-kal'jē-ă). Pain in the chest. SYN thoracodynia. [thoraco- + G. *algos*, pain]

tho•ra•cen•te•sis (thōr-ă-sen-tē'sis). Paracentesis

of the pleural cavity. SYN pleurocentesis, thoracocentesis. [thoraco- + G. *kentēsis*, puncture]

tho•rac•ic (thō-ras'ik). Relating to the thorax.

thoracico-. SEE thoraco-.

thoraco-, thorac-, thoracico-. The chest (thorax). [G. *thōrax*]

tho•ra•co•a•cro•mi•al (thōr'ă-kō-ă-krō'mē-ăl). Relating to the acromion and the thorax; denoting especially the thoracoacromial *artery.* SYN acromiothoracic.

tho•ra•co•ce•los•chi•sis (thōr'ă-kō-sē-los'ki-sis). A congenital fissure of the trunk embracing both the thoracic and abdominal cavities. SYN thoracogastroschisis. [thoraco- + G. *koilia*, belly, + *schisis*, fissure]

tho•ra•co•cen•te•sis (thōr'ă-kō-sen-tē'sis). SYN thoracentesis.

tho•ra•co•cyl•lo•sis (thōr'ă-kō-si-lō'sis). A deformity of the chest. [thoraco- + G. *kyllōsis*, a crippling]

tho•ra•co•cyr•to•sis (thōr'ă-kō-ser-tō'sis). Abnormally wide curvature of the chest wall. [thoraco- + G. *kyrtōsis*, a being crooked]

tho•ra•co•dyn•ia (thōr'ă-kō-din'ē-ă). SYN thoracalgia. [thoraco- + G. *odynē*, pain]

tho•ra•co•gas•tros•chi•sis (thōr'ă-kō-gas-tros'ki-sis). SYN thoracoceloschisis. [thoraco- + G. *gastēr*, belly, + *schisis*, fissure]

tho•ra•co•lum•bar (thōr'ă-kō-lŭm'bar). **1.** Relating to the thoracic and lumbar portions of the vertebral column. **2.** Relating to the origins of the sympathetic division of the autonomic nervous system. SEE autonomic nervous *system.*

tho•ra•col•y•sis (thōr-ă-kol'i-sis). Breaking up of pleural adhesions. [thoraco- + G. *lysis*, dissolution]

tho•ra•com•e•ter (thōr-ă-kom'ĕ-ter). An instrument for measuring the circumference of the chest or its variations in respiration. [thoraco- + G. *metron*, measure]

tho•ra•co•my•o•dyn•ia (thōr'ă-kō-mī-ō-din'ē-ă). Pain in the muscles of the chest wall. [thoraco- + G. *mys*, muscle, + *odynē*, pain]

tho•ra•co•plas•ty (thōr'ă-kō-plas-tē). An operation that reduces intrathoracic space. [thoraco- + G. *plastos*, formed]

    conventional t., resection of ribs to allow inward retraction of the chest wall to reduce size of the pleural space; may be used in the treatment of empyema.

tho•ra•cos•chi•sis (thōr-ă-kos'ki-sis). Congenital fissure of the chest wall. [thoraco- + G. *schisis*, fissure]

tho•ra•co•scope (thō-rak'ō-skōp). A scope for viewing intrathoracic structures; may be video assisted. [thoraco- + G. *skopeō*, to view]

tho•ra•cos•co•py (thōr-ă-kos'kŏ-pē). Examination of the pleural cavity with an endoscope. [thoraco- + G. *skopeō*, to view]

tho•ra•co•ste•no•sis (thōr'ă-kō-stĕ-nō'sis). Narrowness of the chest. [thoraco- + G. *stenōsis*, narrowing]

tho•ra•cos•to•my (thōr-ă-kos'tō-mē). Establishment of an opening into the chest cavity, as for the drainage of an empyema. [thoraco- + G. *stoma*, mouth]

tho•ra•cot•o•my (thōr-ă-kot'ō-mē). Incision into

the chest wall. SYN pleurotomy. [thoraco- + G. *tomē*, incision]

🔲 **tho•rax**, gen. **tho•ra•cis**, pl. **tho•ra•ces** (thō'raks, thō'rā-sis, -rā'sēz) [NA]. The upper part of the trunk between the neck and the abdomen; it is formed by the 12 thoracic vertebrae, the 12 pairs of ribs, the sternum, and the muscles and fasciae attached to these; below, it is separated from the abdomen by the diaphragm; it contains the chief organs of the circulatory and respiratory systems. [L. fr. G. *thōrax*, breastplate, the chest, fr. *thōrēssō*, to arm]

tho•ri•um (Th) (thōr'ē-ŭm). A radioactive metallic element; atomic no. 90, atomic wt. 232.0381. ^{232}Th, the only naturally occurring nuclide, with a half-life of 14×10^9 years, is used in colloidal form in electron microscopy as a stain for acid mucopolysaccharides. [*Thor*, Norse god of thunder]

Thr Symbol for threonine or its radical forms.

thread•worm (thred'werm). Common name for species of the genus *Strongyloides;* sometimes applied to any of the smaller parasitic nematodes.

three•o•nine (T, Thr) (thrē'ō-nēn). One of the naturally occurring amino acids, included in the structure of most proteins, and nutritionally essential in the diet of humans and other mammals.

thresh•old (thresh'ōld). **1.** The point at which a stimulus first produces a sensation. **2.** The lower limit of perception of a stimulus. **3.** The minimal stimulus that produces excitation of any structure. **4.** SYN limen. [A.S. *therxold*]

  acoustic reflex t. (ART), lowest sound intensity required to elicit contraction of the stapedius muscle in the middle ear.

  anaerobic t., a point, during exercise of increasing intensity, when a measurable increase in venous lactic acid levels occurs in conjunction with an exponential increase in respiratory frequency.

  lactate t., highest level of exercise intensity or oxygen uptake that is not associated with an increase in measurable levels of blood lactates.

  ventilatory t., point at which the relation between minute ventilation and oxygen consumption varies from linearity during progressive increases in oxygen demand required by exercise. SEE lactate t.

thrill. A vibration accompanying a cardiac or vascular murmur that can be palpated. SEE ALSO fremitus.

  diastolic t., a t. felt over the precordium or over a blood vessel during ventricular diastole.

  hydatid t., the peculiar trembling or vibratory sensation felt on palpation of a hydatid cyst. SYN hydatid fremitus.

  presystolic t., a t. immediately preceding the ventricular contraction, that is sometimes felt on palpation over the apex of the heart.

  systolic t., a t. felt over the precordium or over a blood vessel during ventricular systole.

thrix (thriks). SYN hair (2). [G.]

throat (thrōt). **1.** The fauces and pharynx. SYN gullet. **2.** The anterior aspect of the neck. **3.** Any narrowed entrance into a hollow part. [A.S. *throtu*]

  sore t., a condition characterized by pain or

discomfort on swallowing; it may be due to any of a variety of inflammations of the tonsils, pharynx, or larynx.

throb. **1.** To pulsate. **2.** A beating or pulsation.

△**thromb-.** SEE thrombo-.

throm•bas•the•nia (throm-bas-thē'nē-ă). An abnormality of platelets characteristic of Glanzmann's t. SYN thromboasthenia. [thromb- + G. *astheneia*, weakness]

  Glanzmann's t. [MIM*273800], a hemorrhagic diathesis characterized by normal or prolonged bleeding time, normal coagulation time, defective clot retraction, normal platelet count but morphologic or functional abnormality of platelets; defect in platelet membrane glycoprotein IIb-IIIa complex. SYN Glanzmann's disease.

throm•bec•to•my (throm-bek'tō-mē). The excision of a thrombus. [thromb- + G. *ektomē*, excision]

throm•bi (throm'bī). Plural of thrombus.

throm•bin. **1.** An enzyme (proteinase), formed in shed blood, that converts fibrinogen into fibrin by hydrolyzing peptides (and amides and esters) of L-arginine; formed from prothrombin by the action of prothrombinase (factor Xa, another proteinase). **2.** A sterile protein substance prepared from prothrombin of bovine origin through interaction with thromboplastin in the presence of calcium; causes clotting of whole blood, plasma, or a fibrinogen solution; used as a topical hemostatic for capillary bleeding with or without fibrin foam in general and plastic surgical procedures.

△**thrombo-, thromb-.** Blood clot; coagulation; thrombin. [G. *thrombos*, clot (thrombus)]

throm•bo•an•gi•i•tis (throm'bō-an-ji-ī'tis). Inflammation of the intima of a blood vessel, with thrombosis. [thrombo- + G. *angeion*, vessel, + -*itis*, inflammation]

  t. oblit'erans, inflammation of the entire wall and connective tissue surrounding medium-sized arteries and veins, especially of the legs of young and middle-aged men; associated with thrombotic occlusion and commonly resulting in gangrene. SYN Buerger's disease.

throm•bo•ar•te•ri•tis (throm'bō-ar-ter-ī'tis). Arterial inflammation with thrombus formation.

throm•bo•as•the•nia (throm'bō-as-thē'nē-ă). SYN thrombasthenia.

throm•bo•clas•tic (throm-bō-klas'tik). SYN thrombolytic.

throm•bo•cyst, throm•bo•cys•tis (throm'bō-sist, -sis'tis). A membranous sac enclosing a thrombus. [thrombo- + G. *kystis*, a bladder]

throm•bo•cyte (throm'bō-sīt). SYN platelet. [thrombo- + G. *kytos*, cell]

throm•bo•cy•the•mia (throm'bō-sī-thē'mē-ă). SYN thrombocytosis. [thrombocyte + G. *haima*, blood]

throm•bo•cy•top•a•thy (throm'bō-sī-top'ă-thē). General term for any disorder of the coagulating mechanism that results from dysfunction of the blood platelets. [thrombocyte + G. *pathos*, suffering]

throm•bo•cy•to•pe•nia (throm'bō-sī-tō-pē'nē-ă). A condition in which there is an abnormally small number of platelets in the circulating blood.

SYN thrombopenia. [thrombocyte + G. *penia*, poverty]

essential t., a primary form of t., in contrast to secondary forms that are associated with metastatic neoplasms, tuberculosis, and leukemia involving the bone marrow, or with direct suppression of bone marrow by the use of chemical agents, or with other conditions.

throm·bo·cy·to·poi·e·sis (throm′bō-sī-tō-poy-ē′sis). The process of formation of thrombocytes or platelets. [thrombocyte + G. *poiēsis*, a making]

throm·bo·cy·to·sis (throm′bō-sī-tō′sis). An increase in the number of platelets in the circulating blood. SYN thrombocythemia. [thrombocyte + G. -*osis*, condition]

throm·bo·e·las·to·gram (throm′bō-ē-las′tō-gram). Registration of coagulation process by a thromboelastograph.

throm·bo·e·las·to·graph (throm′bō-ē-las′tō-graf). Apparatus for registering elastic variations of a thrombus during the process of coagulation. [thromb- + G. *elastreō*, to push, + *graphō*, to write]

throm·bo·em·bo·lism (throm′bō-em′bō-lizm). Embolism from a thrombus. [thrombo- + G. *embolismos*, embolism]

throm·bo·end·ar·ter·ec·to·my (throm′bō-end-ar-ter-ek′tō-mē). An operation that involves opening an artery, removing an occluding thrombus along with the intima and atheromatous material, and leaving a clean, fresh plane internal to the adventitia. [thrombo- + endarterectomy]

throm·bo·gen·ic (throm-bō-jen′ik). **1.** Relating to thrombogen. **2.** Causing thrombosis or coagulation of the blood.

throm·boid (throm′boyd). Resembling a thrombus. [thrombo- + G. *eidos*, resemblance]

throm·bo·ki·nase (throm-bō-kī′nās). SYN thromboplastin.

throm·bo·lym·phan·gi·tis (throm′bō-lim-fan-jī′tis). Inflammation of a lymphatic vessel with the formation of a lymph clot.

throm·bol·y·sis (throm-bol′i-sis). Liquefaction or dissolving of a thrombus. [thrombo- + G. *lysis*, a dissolving]

throm·bo·lyt·ic (throm-bō-lit′ik). Breaking up or dissolving a thrombus. SYN thromboclastic.

throm·bon. An all-inclusive term for circulating thrombocytes (blood platelets) and the cellular forms from which they arise (thromboblasts or megakaryocytes).

throm·bop·a·thy (throm-bop′ă-thē). A nonspecific term applied to disorders of blood platelets resulting in defective thromboplastin, without obvious change in the appearance or number of platelets. [thrombo- + G. *pathos*, disease]

throm·bo·pe·nia (throm-bō-pē′nē-ă). SYN thrombocytopenia.

throm·bo·phil·ia (throm-bō-fil′ē-ă). A disorder of the hemopoietic system in which there is a tendency to the occurrence of thrombosis. [thrombo- + G. *philos*, fond]

throm·bo·phle·bi·tis (throm′bō-flē-bī′tis). Venous inflammation with thrombus formation. [thrombo- + G. *phleps*, vein, + -*itis*, inflammation]

throm·bo·plas·tid (throm-bō-plas′tid). **1.** SYN

platelet. **2.** A nucleated spindle cell in submammalian blood. [thrombo- + G. plastos, formed]

throm·bo·plas·tin (throm-bō-plas′tin). A substance present in tissues, platelets, and leukocytes necessary for the coagulation of blood; in the presence of calcium ions t. is necessary for the conversion of prothrombin to thrombin, an important step in coagulation of blood. SYN platelet tissue factor, thrombokinase.

throm·bo·poi·e·sis (throm′bō-poy-ē′sis). Precisely, the process of a clot forming in blood, but generally used with reference to the formation of blood platelets (thrombocytes). [thrombo- + G. *poiēsis*, a making]

throm·bosed (throm′bōsd). **1.** Clotted. **2.** Denoting a blood vessel that is the seat of thrombosis.

throm·bo·sis, pl. **throm·bo·ses** (throm-bō′sis, -sēz). Formation or presence of a thrombus; clotting within a blood vessel which may cause infarction of tissues supplied by the vessel. [G. *thrombōsis*, a clotting, fr. *thrombos*, clot]

coronary t., coronary occlusion by thrombus formation, usually the result of atheromatous changes in the arterial wall and usually leading to myocardial infarction.

mural t., the formation of a thrombus in contact with the endocardial lining of a cardiac chamber, or a large blood vessel, if not occlusive.

throm·bo·sta·sis (throm-bos′tă-sis). Local arrest of the circulation by thrombosis. [thrombo- + G. *stasis*, a standing]

throm·bot·ic (throm-bot′ik). Relating to, caused by, or characterized by thrombosis.

throm·box·ane (throm′bok-sān). The formal parent of the thromboxanes; prostanoic acid in which the –COOH has been reduced to –CH$_3$ and an oxygen atom has been inserted between carbons 11 and 12.

throm·box·anes (throm′bok-sānz). A group of compounds, included in the eicosanoids, formally based on thromboxane, but with the terminal COOH group present; biochemically related to the prostaglandins and formed from them. T. are so named from their influence on platelet aggregation and the formation of the oxygen-containing six-membered ring (pyran or oxane). Like the prostaglandins, individual t. (abbreviated TX) are designated by letters (A, B, C, etc.) and subscripts indicating structural features.

throm·bus, pl. **throm·bi** (throm′bŭs, -bī). A clot in the cardiovascular system formed during life from constituents of blood; it may be occlusive or attached to the vessel or heart wall without obstructing the lumen (mural t.). [L. fr. G. *thrombos*, a clot]

mural t., a t. formed on and attached to a diseased patch of endocardium, not on a valve or on one side of a large blood vessel. SEE ALSO parietal t.

obstructive t., a t. due to obstruction in the vessel from compression or other cause.

parietal t., an arterial t. adhering to one side of the wall of the vessel. SEE ALSO mural t.

thrush (thrŭsh). Infection of the oral tissues with *Candida albicans;* often an opportunistic infection in persons with AIDS or other conditions that depress the immune system.

thu·li·um (Tm) (thū'lē-ŭm). A metallic element of the lanthanide series, atomic no. 69, atomic wt. 168.93421. [L. *Thule*, the earliest name for Scandinavia]

thumb (thŭmb). The first digit on the radial side of the hand. SYN pollex [NA]. [A.S. *thuma*]

  bowler's t., compression of the digital nerve on the medial aspect of the t. resulting in paresthesia of the t.

  gamekeeper's t., rupture of the volar ligament at the first metacarpophalangeal joint due to forceful abduction of the thumb while extended.

  tennis t., tendinitis with calcification in the tendon of the long flexor of the t. (flexor pollicis longus) caused by friction and strain as in tennis playing, but also occurring in other exercises in which the t. is subject to repeated pressure or strain.

△**thym-.** SEE thymo-.

thy·mec·to·my (thī-mek'tō-mē). Removal of the thymus gland. [thymus + G. *ektomē*, excision]

△**thymi-.** SEE thymo-.

△**-thymia.** Mind, soul, emotions. SEE ALSO thymo- (2). [G. *thymos*, the mind or heart as the seat of strong feelings or passion]

thy·mic (thī'mik). Relating to the thymus gland.

thy·mi·co·lym·phat·ic (thī'mi-kō-lim-fat'ik). Relating to the thymus and the lymphatic system.

thy·mi·dine (dThd) (thī'mi-dēn). 1-(2-deoxyribosyl)thymine; one of the four major nucleosides in DNA (the others being deoxyadenosine, deoxycytidine, and deoxyguanosine). SYN deoxythymidine.

thy·mi·dine 5'-di·phos·phate (dTDP). Thymidine esterified at its 5' position with diphosphoric acid.

thy·mine (thī'mēn, -min). A constituent of thymidylic acid and DNA; elevated in hyperuracilthyminuria.

thy·mi·tis (thī-mī'tis). Inflammation of the thymus gland.

△**thymo-, thym-, thymi-.** 1. The thymus. [G. *thymos*] 2. Mind, soul, emotions. [G. *thymos*, the mind or heart as the seat of strong feelings or passions] 3. Wart, warty. [G. *thymos, thymion*]

thy·mo·cyte (thī'mō-sīt). A cell that develops in the thymus, seemingly from a stem cell of bone marrow and of fetal liver, and is the precursor of the thymus-derived lymphocyte (T lymphocyte) that effects cell-mediated (delayed type) sensitivity. [thymus + G. *kytos*, cell]

thy·mo·gen·ic (thī-mō-jen'ik). Of affective origin. [G. *thymos*, mind, + *genesis*, origin]

thy·mo·ki·net·ic (thī'mō-ki-net'ik). Activating the thymus gland. [thymus + G. *kinēsis*, movement]

thy·mo·ma (thī-mō'mă). A neoplasm in the anterior mediastinum, originating from thymic tissue, usually benign, and frequently encapsulated; occasionally invasive, but metastases are extremely rare. [thymus + G. *-oma*, tumor]

thy·mo·pri·val, thy·mo·priv·ic, thy·mo·pri··vous (thī-mō-prī'văl, -priv'ik, -prī'vŭs). Relating to or marked by premature atrophy or removal of the thymus. [thymus + L. *privus*, deprived of]

thy·mus, pl. **thy·mi, thy·mus·es** (thī'mŭs, thī'mī). [NA] A primary lymphoid organ, located in the superior mediastinum and lower part of the neck, that is necessary in early life for the normal development of immunological function. It reaches its greatest relative weight shortly after birth and its greatest absolute weight at puberty; it then begins to involute, and much of the lymphoid tissue is replaced by fat. The t. consists of two irregularly shaped parts united by a connective tissue capsule. Each part is partially subdivided by connective tissue septa into lobules, which consist of an inner medullary portion, continuous with the medullae of adjacent lobules, and an outer cortical portion. SYN thymus gland. [G. *thymos*, excrescence, sweetbread]

△**thyr-.** SEE thyro-.

△**thyro-, thyr-.** The thyroid gland. [see thyroid]

thy·ro·a·pla·sia (thī'rō-ă-plā'zē-ă). Anomalies observed in individuals with congenital defects of the thyroid gland and deficiency of its secretion. [thyro- + G. *a-* priv. + *plasis*, a molding]

thy·ro·ar·y·te·noid (thī'rō-ar'i-tē'noyd). Relating to the thyroid and arytenoid cartilages. SEE thyroarytenoid *muscle*.

thy·ro·cele (thī'rō-sēl). A tumor of the thyroid gland, such as a goiter. [thyro- + G. *kēlē*, tumor]

thy·ro·ep·i·glot·tic (thī'rō-ep-i-glot'ik). Relating to the thyroid cartilage and the epiglottis.

thy·ro·gen·ic, thy·rog·e·nous (thī-rō-jen'ik, -roj'ĕ-nŭs). Of thyroid gland origin. [thyroid + G. *-gen*, producing]

thy·ro·glob·u·lin (thī-rō-glob'yū-lin). 1. A thyroid hormone-containing protein, usually stored in the colloid within the thyroid follicles; biosynthesis of thyroid hormone entails iodination of the L-tyrosyl moieties of this protein. A defect in t. will lead to hypothyroidism. 2. A substance obtained by the fractionation of thyroid glands from the hog, *Sus scrofula*, containing not less than 0.7% of total iodine; used as a thyroid hormone in the treatment of hypothyroidism.

thy·ro·glos·sal (thī-rō-glos'ăl). Relating to the thyroid gland and the tongue, denoting especially an embryological duct.

thy·ro·hy·al (thī-rō-hī'ăl). The greater cornu of the hyoid bone.

thy·ro·hy·oid (thī-rō-hī'oyd). Relating to the thyroid cartilage and the hyoid bone. SEE thyrohyoid *muscle*.

thy·roid (thī'royd). 1. Resembling a shield; denoting a gland (thyroid gland) and a cartilage of the larynx (thyroid cartilage) having such a shape. 2. The cleaned, dried, and powdered t. gland obtained from one of the domesticated animals used for food and containing 0.17 to 0.23% of iodine; used in the treatment of hypothyroidism, cretinism and myxedema, in certain cases of obesity, and in skin disorders. [G. *thyreoeidēs*, fr. *thyreos*, an oblong shield, + *eidos*, form]

thy·roid·ec·to·my (thī-roy-dek'tō-mē). Removal of the thyroid gland. [thyroid + G. *ektomē*, excision]

thy·roid·i·tis (thī-roy-dī'tis). Inflammation of the thyroid gland. [thyroid + G. *-itis*, inflammation]

  chronic atrophic t., replacement of the thyroid gland by fibrous tissue, the commonest cause of myxedema in older persons.

  Hashimoto's t., diffuse infiltration of the thyroid gland with lymphocytes, resulting in diffuse goiter, progressive destruction of the parenchyma and hypothyroidism. SYN Hashimoto's disease, Hashimoto's struma, struma lymphomatosa.

Riedel's t., a rare fibrous induration of the thyroid gland, with adhesion to adjacent structures, which may cause tracheal compression.

subacute granulomatous t., t. with round cell (usually lymphocytes) infiltration, destruction of thyroid cells, epithelial giant cell proliferation, and evidence of regeneration; thought by some to be a reflection of a systemic infection and not an example of true chronic t.

thy·ro·lib·er·in (thī-rō-lib′er-in). A tripeptide hormone from the hypothalamus, which stimulates the anterior lobe of the hypophysis to release thyrotropin. SYN thyrotropin-releasing hormone. [thyrotropin + L. *libero,* to free, + -in]

thy·ro·meg·a·ly (thī-rō-meg′ă-lē). Enlargement of the thyroid gland. [thyro- + G. *megas,* large]

thy·ro·nine (thī′rō-nēn, -nin). An amino acid with a diphenyl ether group in the side chain; occurs in proteins only in the form of iodinated derivatives (iodothyronines), such as thyroxine.

thy·ro·par·a·thy·roid·ec·to·my (thī′rō-par-ă-thī′roy-dek′tō-mē). Excision of thyroid and parathyroid glands.

thy·ro·pri·val (thī-rō-prī′văl). Relating to thyroprivia, denoting hypothyroidism produced by disease or thyroidectomy. [thyro- + L. *privus,* deprived of]

thy·rop·to·sis (thī-rop-tō′sis). Downward dislocation of the thyroid gland. [thyro- + G. *ptōsis,* a falling]

thy·rot·o·my (thī′rot′ō-mē). **1.** Any cutting operation on the thyroid gland. **2.** SYN laryngofissure. [thyro- + G. *tomē,* a cutting]

thy·ro·tox·ic (thī-rō-tok′sik). Denoting thyrotoxicosis.

thy·ro·tox·i·co·sis (thī′rō-tok-si-kō′sis). The state produced by excessive quantities of endogenous or exogenous thyroid hormone. [thyro- + G. *toxikon,* poison, + -osis, condition]

thy·ro·troph (thī′rō-trof). A cell in the anterior lobe of the pituitary that produces thyrotropin.

thy·ro·tro·phic (thī-rō-trof′ik). SYN thyrotropic. [thyro- + G. *trophē,* nourishment]

thy·rot·ro·phin (thī-rot′rō-fin, thī-rō-trō′fin). SYN thyrotropin.

thy·ro·tro·pic (thī-rō-trop′ik). Stimulating or nurturing the thyroid gland. SYN thyrotrophic. [thyro- + G. *tropē,* a turning]

thy·rot·ro·pin (thī-rot′rō-pin, thī-rō-trō′pin). A glycoprotein hormone produced by the anterior lobe of the hypophysis which stimulates the growth and function of the thyroid gland; it also is used as a diagnostic test to differentiate primary and secondary hypothyroidism. SYN thyroid-stimulating hormone, thyrotrophin. [for thyrotrophin, fr. thyro- + G. *trophē,* nourishment; corrupted to -tropin, and reanalyzed as fr. G. *tropē,* a turning]

thy·rox·ine, thy·rox·in (thī-rok′sēn, -sin). The active iodine compound existing normally in the thyroid gland and extracted therefrom in crystalline form for therapeutic use; also prepared syn-

thetically; used for the relief of hypothyroidism, cretinism, and myxedema.

TI. The delay time between the inverting pulse and the "read" pulse in the inversion recovery experiment, in magnetic resonance imaging.

Ti titanium.

TIA transient ischemic *attack.*

TIBC total iron binding *capacity.*

tib·ia, gen. and pl. **tib·i·ae** (tib′ē-ă, tib′ē-ē) [NA]. The medial and larger of the two bones of the leg, articulating with the femur, fibula, and talus. SYN shin bone. [L. the large shinbone]

saber t., deformity of the t. occurring in tertiary syphilis or yaws, the bone having a marked forward convexity as a result of the formation of gummas and periostitis.

t. val′ga, SYN *genu* valgum.

t. va′ra, SYN *genu* varum.

tib·i·al (tib′ē-ăl). Relating to the tibia or to any structure named from it; also denoting the medial or tibial aspect of the lower limb. [L. *tibialis*]

△**tibio-.** The tibia. [L. *tibia,* the large shinbone]

tic (tik). Habitual, repeated contraction of certain muscles, resulting in stereotyped individualized actions that can be voluntarily suppressed for only brief periods, *e.g.,* clearing the throat, sniffing, pursing the lips, excessive blinking; especially prominent when the person is under stress; there is no known pathologic substrate. SEE ALSO spasm. SYN habit spasm. [Fr.]

t. douloureux (dū-lū-rě′), SYN trigeminal *neuralgia.* [Fr. painful]

facial t., involuntary twitching of the facial muscles, sometimes unilateral. SYN facial spasm, palmus (1), prosopospasm.

tick (tik). An acarine of the families Ixodidae (hard t.'s) or Argasidae (soft t.'s), which contain many bloodsucking species that are important pests of humans and domestic birds and mammals, and that probably exceed all other arthropods in the number and variety of disease agents that they transmit. Some important t.'s are *Amblyomma americanum* (Lone Star t.), *Boophilus* (cattle t.'s), *Dermacentor andersoni* (Rocky Mountain spotted fever or wood t.), *D. variabilis* (American dog t.), and *Ixodes pacificus* (California black-legged t.).

tid·al (tī′dăl). Relating to or resembling the tides, alternately rising and falling.

tide (tīd). An alternate rise and fall, ebb and flow, or an increase or a decrease. [A.S. *tīd,* time]

acid t., a temporary increase in the acidity of the urine occurring during fasting.

alkaline t., a period of urinary neutrality or even alkalinity after meals due to withdrawal of hydrogen ion for the purpose of secretion of the highly acid gastric juice.

fat t., an increase in the fat content of blood and lymph following a meal.

tim·bre (tam′br, tim′br). The distinguishing quality of a sound, by which one may determine its source. [Fr.]

time (t) (tīm). **1.** That relation of events which is expressed by the terms past, present, and future, and measured by units such as minutes, hours, days, months, or years. **2.** A certain period during

ti

which something definite or determined is done. SYN tempus (2). [A.S. *tima*]

activated clotting t. (ACT), the most common test used for coagulation t. in cardiovascular surgery.

activated partial thromboplastin t. (aPTT), the t. needed for plasma to form a fibrin clot following the addition of calcium and a phospholipid reagent; used to evaluate the intrinsic clotting system.

bleeding t., the t. interval between the appearance of the first drop of blood and the removal of the last drop following puncture of the ear lobe or the finger, usually 1 to 3 minutes; it is prolonged in cases of thrombocytopenia, diminished prothrombin, phosphorus poisoning, or chloroform poisoning, and in some liver diseases; it is normal in hemophilia.

coagulation t., the t. required for blood to coagulate; prolonged in hemophilia and in the presence of obstructive jaundice, some anemias and leukemias, and some of the infectious diseases.

forced expiratory t. (FET), the t. taken to expire a given volume or a given fraction of vital capacity during measurement of forced vital capacity; subscripts specify the exact parameters measured.

half-t., SEE half-time.

inertia t., the interval elapsing between the reception of the stimulus from a nerve and the contraction of the muscle.

kaolin clotting t. (KCT), a sensitive test of platelet-poor plasma for detecting lupus anticoagulants in mixtures of plasmas taken from patients and from control groups; kaolin initiates clotting via the contact factors and subsequently involves the other factors in the intrinsic pathway of coagulation.

left ventricular ejection t. (LVET), the t. measured clinically from onset to incisural notch of the carotid or other pulse; properly the time of ejection of blood from the left ventricle beginning with aortic valve opening and ending with aortic valve closure.

partial thromboplastin t. (PTT), SEE activated partial thromboplastin t.

prothrombin t. (PT), the t. required for clotting after thromboplastin and calcium are added in optimal amounts to blood of normal fibrinogen content; if prothrombin is diminished, the clotting t. increases; used to evaluate the extrinsic clotting system. SEE ALSO prothrombin *test.*

reaction t., the interval between the presentation of a stimulus and the responsive reaction to it.

relaxation t. (τ), the time required for the substrate in an enzymatic or chemical reaction to fall to 1/e of its initial value.

repetition t. (TR), MAGNETIC RESONANCE IMAGING the t. between repetitions of the pulse sequence.

tissue thromboplastin inhibition t., a test used to identify lupus anticoagulant; the thromboplastin source used in the prothrombin test is diluted to increase sensitivity to inhibitors.

turnaround t., the interval between the order-

ing of a clinical laboratory test or other diagnostic procedure and the reporting of results.

tin (Sn) (tin). A metallic element, atomic no. 50, atomic wt. 118.710. SYN stannum. [AS, tin]

tinct. L. *tinctura,* tincture.

tinc·to·ri·al (tingk-tōr′ē-ăl). Relating to coloring or staining. [L. *tinctorius,* fr. *tingo,* to dye]

tinc·ture (tingk′chŭr). An alcoholic or hydroalcoholic solution prepared from vegetable materials or from chemical substances. [see *tinctura*]

tin·ea (tin′ē-ă). A fungus infection (dermatophytosis) of the keratin component of hair, skin, or nails. Genera of fungi causing such infection are *Microsporum, Trichophyton,* and *Epidermophyton.* SYN ringworm, serpigo (1). [L. worm, moth]

t. bar′bae, t. of the beard, occurring as a follicular infection or as a granulomatous lesion; the primary lesions are papules and pustules. SYN folliculitis barbae, t. sycosis.

t. cap′itis, a common form of fungus infection of the scalp caused by various species of *Microsporum* and *Trichophyton* on or within hair shafts, occurring almost exclusively in children and characterized by irregularly placed and variously sized patches of apparent baldness because of hairs breaking off at the surface of the scalp, scaling, black dots, and occasionally erythema and pyoderma.

t. circina′ta, SYN t. corporis.

■**t. cor′poris,** a well-defined, scaling, macular eruption of dermatophytosis that frequently forms annular lesions and may appear on any part of the body. SYN t. circinata.

t. cru′ris, a form of t. imbricata occurring in the genitocrural region, including the inner side of the thighs, the perineal region, and the groin. SYN eczema marginatum, jock itch.

t. imbrica′ta, an eruption consisting of a number of concentric rings of overlapping scales forming papulosquamous patches scattered over the body; it occurs in tropical climates and is caused by the fungus *Trichophyton concentricum.*

t. ke′rion, an inflammatory fungus infection of the scalp and beard, marked by pustules and a boggy infiltration of the surrounding parts; most commonly caused by *Microsporum audouinii.*

■**t. pe′dis,** dermatophytosis of the feet, especially of the skin between the toes, caused by one of the dermatophytes, usually a species of *Trichophyton* or *Epidermophyton;* the disease consists of small vesicles, fissures, scaling, maceration, and eroded areas between the toes and on the plantar surface of the foot; other skin areas may be involved. SYN athlete's foot.

t. syco′sis, SYN t. barbae.

t. un′guium, ringworm of the nails due to a dermatophyte.

t. versic′olor, an eruption of tan or brown branny patches on the skin of the trunk, often appearing white, in contrast with hyperpigmented skin after exposure to the summer sun; caused by growth of *Malassezia furfur* in the stratum corneum with minimal inflammatory reaction. SYN pityriasis versicolor.

tin·ni·tus (ti-nī′tŭs). A sensation of noises (ringing, whistling, booming, etc.) in the ears. [L. a jingling, fr. *tinnio,* pp. *tinnitus,* to jingle, clink]

TIPS transjugular intrahepatic portosystemic *shunt*.

tir•ing (tīr′ing). SYN cerclage. [Eng. tire]

tis•sue (tish′ū). A collection of similar cells and the intercellular substances surrounding them. There are four basic tissues in the body: 1) epithelium; 2) the connective tissues, including blood, bone, and cartilage; 3) muscle tissue; and 4) nerve tissue. [Fr. *tissu*, woven, fr. L. *texo*, to weave]

　adenoid t., SYN lymphatic t.

　adipose t., a connective t. consisting chiefly of fat cells surrounded by reticular fibers and arranged in lobular groups or along the course of one of the smaller blood vessels. SYN fat (1).

　areolar t., loose, irregularly arranged connective t. that consists of collagenous and elastic fibers, a protein polysaccharide ground substance, and connective t. cells (fibroblasts, macrophages, mast cells, and sometimes fat cells, plasma cells, leukocytes, and pigment cells).

　bone t., SYN osseous t.

　cancellous t., latticelike or spongy osseous t.

　chondroid t., (1) in an adult, t. resembling cartilage; SYN pseudocartilage. **(2)** in an embryo, an early stage in cartilage formation.

　chromaffin t., a cellular t., vascular and well supplied with nerves, made up chiefly of chromaffin cells; it is found in the medulla of the suprarenal glands and, in smaller collections, in the paraganglia.

　connective t., the supporting or framework t. of the animal body, formed of fibrous and ground substance with more or less numerous cells of various kinds; it is derived from the mesenchyme, and this in turn from the mesoderm; the varieties of connective t. are: areolar or loose; adipose; dense, regular or irregular, white fibrous; elastic; mucous; and lymphoid t.; cartilage; and bone; the blood and lymph may be regarded as connective t.'s the ground substance of which is a liquid. SYN interstitial t.

　elastic t., a form of connective t. in which the elastic fibers predominate; it constitutes the ligamenta flava of the vertebrae and the ligamentum nuchae, especially of quadrupeds; it occurs also in the walls of the arteries and of the bronchial tree, and connects the cartilages of the larynx.

　erectile t., a t. with numerous vascular spaces that may become engorged with blood.

　fibrous t., a t. composed of bundles of collagenous white fibers between which are rows of connective t. cells; the tendons, ligaments, aponeuroses, and some of the membranes, such as the dura mater.

　granulation t., vascular connective t. forming granular projections on the surface of a healing wound, ulcer, or inflamed surface. SEE ALSO granulation.

　indifferent t., undifferentiated, nonspecialized, embryonic t.

　interstitial t., SYN connective t.

　lymphatic t., lymphoid t., a three-dimensional network of reticular fibers and cells the meshes of which are occupied in varying degrees of density with lymphocytes; there is nodular, diffuse, and loose lymphatic t. SYN adenoid t.

　mucous connective t., a type of connective t. little differentiated beyond the mesenchymal stage; its ground substance of glycoproteins is abundant and contains fine collagenous fibers and fibroblasts; in its most characteristic form, it appears in the umbilical cord as Wharton's jelly.

　muscular t., a t. characterized by the ability to contract upon stimulation; its three varieties are skeletal, cardiac, and smooth. SEE muscle. SYN flesh (2).

　myeloid t., bone marrow consisting of the developmental and adult stages of erythrocytes, granulocytes, and megakaryocytes in a stroma of reticular cells and fibers, with sinusoidal vascular channels.

　osseous t., a connective t., the matrix of which consists of collagen fibers and ground substance and in which are deposited calcium salts (phosphate, carbonate, and some fluoride) in the form of an apatite. SYN bone t.

　reticular t., retiform t., a t. in which the argyrophilic collagenous fibers form a network and that usually has a network of reticular cells associated with the fibers.

　subcutaneous t., a layer of loose, irregular, connective t. immediately beneath the skin and closely attached to the corium by coarse fibrous bands, the retinacula cutis; it contains fat cells except in the auricles, eyelids, penis, and scrotum.

ti•ta•ni•um (Ti) (tī-tā′nē-ŭm). A metallic element, atomic no. 22, atomic wt. 47.88, used as an implant in dental work because of its uniquely high level of biocompatibility. [*Titans,* in G. myth., sons of Earth]

ti•ter (tī′ter). The standard of strength of a volumetric test solution; the assay value of an unknown measure by volumetric means. [Fr. *titre,* standard]

ti•trate (tī′trāt). To analyze volumetrically by a solution (the titrant) of known strength to an end point.

ti•tra•tion (tī-trā′shŭn). Volumetric analysis by addition of definite amounts of a test solution to a solution of the substance being assayed. [Fr. *titre,* standard]

tit•u•ba•tion (tit-yū-bā′shŭn). **1.** A staggering or stumbling in trying to walk. **2.** A tremor or shaking of the head, of cerebellar origin. [L. *titubo,* pp. *-atus,* to stagger]

Tl thallium.

TLC thin-layer *chromatography*; total lung *capacity.*

TLD thermoluminescent *dosimeter.*

Tm thulium; transport *maximum.*

TMJ Colloquial for temporomandibular joint *dysfunction.*

TMP ribothymidylic acid; trimethoprim; sometimes for deoxyribothymidylic acid.

TMT tarsometatarsal.

T-my•co•plas•ma. SYN *Ureaplasma.*

Tn 1. ocular *tension.* **2.** troponin.

TNM Abbreviation for tumor-node-metastasis. SEE TNM *staging.*

TNTC too numerous to count (indicating the finding of a large number of discrete objects, usually cells in a urine specimen, of which precise enumeration is not practicable).

tocainide hydrochloride (to-ka-nid). An oral antiarrhythmic agent, similar in action to lidocaine, used in the treatment of ventricular arrhythmias.

⚠**toco-.** Childbirth. [G. *tokos,* birth]

toc•o•dy•na•graph (tō-kō-dī′nă-graf, tok-ō-). A recording of the force of uterine contractions. [toco- + G. *dynamis,* force, + *graphē,* a writing]

toc•o•dy•na•mom•e•ter (tō′kō-dī-nă-mom′ĕ-ter, tok′ō-). An instrument for measuring the force of uterine contractions. [toco- + G. *dynamis,* force, + *metron,* measure]

to•cog•ra•phy (tō-kog′ră-fē). The process of recording uterine contractions. [toco- + G. *graphō,* to write]

to•co•lyt•ic (tō-kō-lit′ik). Denoting any pharmacological agent used to arrest uterine contractions; often used in an attempt to arrest premature labor contractions. [G. *tokos,* childbirth, labor, + *lysis,* loosening]

to•coph•er•ol (**T**) (tō-kof′er-ōl). **1.** A generic term for vitamin E and compounds chemically related to it, with or without biological activity. **2.** A methylated tocol or methylated tocotrienol.

toe (tō). One of the digits of the feet. [A.S. *ta*]

hammer t., permanent flexion at the midphalangeal joint of one or more of the t.'s.

Morton's t., metatarsal pain caused by compression of sensory nerves by the metatarsal heads, sometimes with neuroma formation.

turf t., sprain and subsequent inflammation of the first metatarsophalangeal joint.

toe-drop (tō′drop). Inability to dorsiflex the toes, usually due to paralysis of the toe extensor muscles.

toe•nail (tō′nāl). SEE nail.

To•ga•vir•i•dae (tō-gă-vir′i-dē). A family of viruses that includes the following genera: *Alphavirus,* which includes eastern equine encephalitis, western equine encephalitis, Venezuelan equine encephalitis, and the rubella virus (*Rubivirus*).

to•ga•vi•rus (tō′gă-vī′rŭs). Any virus of the family Togaviridae. [L. *toga,* garment covering, + virus]

toi•let (toy-let′). **1.** Cleansing of the obstetrical patient after childbirth or of a wound after an operation preparatory to the application of the dressing. **2.** DENTISTRY Cavity debridement, the final step before placing a restoration in a tooth whereby the cavity is cleaned and all debris is removed. [Fr. *toilette*]

pulmonary t., cleansing of the trachea and bronchial tree.

⚠**toko-.** SEE toco-.

tol•er•ance (tol′er-ăns). **1.** The ability to endure or be less responsive to a stimulus, especially over a period of continued exposure. **2.** The power of resisting the action of a poison or of taking a drug continuously or in large doses without injurious effects. [L. *tolero,* pp. *-atus,* to endure]

cross t., the resistance to one or several effects of a compound as a result of t. developed to a pharmacologically similar compound.

immunologic t., lack of immune response to

antigen. Theories of t. induction include clonal deletion and clonal anergy. In clonal deletion, the actual clone of cells is eliminated whereas in clonal anergy the cells are present but nonfunctional.

tol•er•ant (tol′er-ănt). Having the property of tolerance.

tol•er•o•gen•ic (tol′er-ō-jen′ik). Producing immunologic tolerance.

⚠**-tome.** **1.** A cutting instrument, the first element in the compound usually indicating the part that the instrument is designed to cut. **2.** Segment, part, section. **3.** Tomography. **4.** Surgery. [G. *tomos,* cutting, sharp; a cutting (section or segment)]

to•men•tum, to•men•tum ce•re•bri (tō-men′tŭm, tō-men′tŭm ser′ĕ-brī). The numerous small blood vessels passing between the cerebral surface of the pia mater and the cortex of the brain. [L. a stuffing for cushions]

to•mo•gram (tō′mō-gram). A radiograph obtained by tomography. [G. *tomos,* a cutting (section) + *gramma,* a writing]

to•mo•graph (tō′mō-graf). The radiographic equipment used in tomography. [G. *tomos,* a cutting (section), + *graphō,* to write]

to•mog•ra•phy (tō-mog′ră-fē). Making a radiographic image of a selected plane by means of reciprocal linear or curved motion of the x-ray tube and film cassette; images of all other planes are blurred ("out of focus") by being relatively displaced on the film. SYN planigraphy, planography, stratigraphy.

⏹**computed t.** (**CT**), imaging anatomical information from a cross-sectional plane of the body, each image generated by a computer synthesis of x-ray transmission data obtained in many different directions in a given plane. SYN computerized axial t.

computerized axial t. (**CAT**), SYN computed t.

high-resolution computed t. (**HRCT**), computed t. with narrow collimation to reduce volume-averaging and an edge-enhancing reconstruction algorithm to sharpen the image, sometimes with a restricted field of view to minimize the size of pixels in the region imaged; used particularly for lung imaging.

⏹**positron emission t.** (**PET**), tomographic images formed by computer analysis of photons detected from annihilation of positrons emitted by radionuclides incorporated into biochemical substances; the images, often quantitated with a color scale, show the uptake and distribution of the substances in the tissue, permitting analysis and localization of metabolic and physiological function.

single photon emission computed t. (**SPECT**), tomographic imaging of metabolic and physiological functions in tissues, the image being formed by computer synthesis of photons of a single energy emitted by radionuclides administered in suitable form to the patient.

⚠**-tomy.** A cutting operation. SEE ALSO -ectomy. [G. *tomē,* incision]

tone (tōn). **1.** A musical sound. **2.** The character of the voice expressing an emotion. **3.** The tension present in resting muscles. **4.** Firmness of the tissues; normal functioning of all the organs. **5.** To perform toning. [G. *tonos,* tone, or a tone]

muscle t., (1) the internal state of muscle-fiber tension within individual muscles and muscle groups. **(2)** degree of muscle tension or resistance during rest or in response to stretching.

pure t., an audible t. that can be represented by a sine wave; an oscillation showing only one frequency of vibration, with no overtones or harmonics. SEE ALSO conduction, sine *wave.*

tongue (tŭng). **1.** A mobile mass of muscular tissue covered with mucous membrane, occupying the cavity of the mouth and forming part of its floor, constituting also by its posterior portion the anterior wall of the pharynx. It bears the organ of taste and assists in mastication, deglutition, and articulation. SYN lingua (1) [NA], glossa. **2.** A tonguelike structure. SYN lingua (2) [NA]. [A.S. *tunge*]

bifid t., a structural defect of the t. in which the extremity is divided longitudinally for a greater or lesser distance. SEE ALSO diglossia. SYN cleft t.

black t., black to yellowish-brown discoloration of the dorsum of the t. due to staining by exogenous material such as the components of tobacco; usually superimposed on hairy t. SYN lingua nigra, melanoglossia.

cleft t., SYN bifid t.

coated t., a t. with a whitish layer on its upper surface, composed of epithelial debris, food particles, and bacteria; often an indication of indigestion or of fever.

fissured t., a painless condition of the t. characterized by numerous grooves or furrows on the dorsal surface.

geographic t., idiopathic, asymptomatic erythematous circinate macules, often bounded peripherally by a white band, as a result of atrophy of the filiform papillae; with time the lesions resolve, coalesce, and change in distribution; frequently associated with fissured t.'s. SYN erythema migrans, erythema migrans linguae, glossitis areata exfoliativa, lingua geographica.

hairy t., a t. with abnormal elongation of the filiform papillae, resulting in a thickened furry appearance. SYN glossotrichia, trichoglossia.

strawberry t., a t. with a whitish coat through which the enlarged fungiform papillae project as red points, characteristic of scarlet fever and mucocutaneous lymph node syndrome.

tongue crib. An appliance used to control visceral (infantile) swallowing and tongue thrusting and to encourage the mature or somatic tongue posture and function.

tongue-swal·low·ing. A slipping back of the tongue against the pharynx, causing choking.

tongue thrust. The infantile pattern of the suckle-swallow movement in which the tongue is placed between the incisor teeth or the alveolar ridges during the initial stage of swallowing, resulting sometimes in an anterior open bite.

tongue-tie. SYN ankyloglossia.

ton·ic (ton′ik). **1.** In a state of continuous unremitting action; denoting especially a muscular contraction. **2.** Invigorating; increasing physical or mental tone or strength. **3.** A remedy purported to restore enfeebled function and promote vigor and a sense of well-being qualified, according to the organ or system on which they are presumed to act, as cardiac, digestive, hematic, vascular, nervine, uterine, general, etc. [G. *tonikos,* fr. *tonos,* tone]

to·nic·i·ty (tō-nis′i-tē). **1.** A state of normal tension of the tissues by virtue of which the parts are kept in shape, alert, and ready to function in response to a suitable stimulus. In the case of muscle, it refers to a state of continuous activity or tension beyond that related to the physical properties; *i.e.,* it is active resistance to stretch; in skeletal muscle it is dependent upon the efferent innervation. SYN tonus. **2.** The osmotic pressure or tension of a solution, usually relative to that of blood. SEE ALSO isotonicity. [G. *tonos,* tone]

ton·i·co·clon·ic (ton-i-kō-klon′ik). Both tonic and clonic, referring to muscular spasms. SYN tonoclonic.

△**tono-.** Tone, tension, pressure. [G. *tonos*]

ton·o·clon·ic (ton-ō-klon′ik). SYN tonicoclonic.

ton·o·fi·bril (ton-ō-fī′bril). One of a system of fibers found in the cytoplasm of epithelial cells. SEE cytoskeleton.

ton·o·fil·a·ment (ton-ō-fil′ă-ment). A structural cytoplasmic protein, bundles of which together form a tonofibril; t.'s are made up of a variable number of related proteins, keratins, and are found in all epithelial cells.

ton·o·graph (ton′ō-graf, tō′nō-). A recording tonometer. [tono- + G. *graphō,* to write]

to·nog·ra·phy (tō-nog′ră-fē). Continuous measurement of intraocular pressure by means of a recording tonometer, in order to determine the facility of aqueous outflow.

to·nom·e·ter (tō-nom′ĕ-ter). **1.** An instrument for determining pressure or tension, especially determining ocular tension. **2.** A vessel for equilibrating a liquid (*e.g.,* blood) with a gas, usually at a controlled temperature. [tono- + G. *metron,* measure]

applanation t., an instrument for determining ocular tension by application of a small, flat disk to the cornea.

Mueller electronic t., a Schiötz type t. that electronically indicates the extent of corneal indentation; may also have an attached recorder for continuous pressure readings (tonography).

pneumatic t., a recording applanation t. operated by compressed gas.

to·nom·e·try (tō-nom′ĕ-trē). **1.** Measurement of the tension of a part, *e.g.,* intravascular tension or blood pressure. **2.** Measurement of ocular tension.

ton·o·plast (tō′nō-plast, ton′ō-). An intracellular structure or vacuole. [tono- + G. *plastos,* formed]

to·no·top·ic (tō-nō-top′ik). Denoting a spatial arrangement of structures such that certain tone frequencies are transmitted, as in the auditory pathway. [tono- + G. *topos,* place]

to·no·tro·pic (tō-nō-trop′ik). Denoting the shortening of the resting length of a muscle. [G. *tonikos, tonos,* tone, + *tropos,* a turning]

ton·sil (ton′sil). **1.** Any collection of lymphoid tissue. **2.** SYN palatine t. [L. *tonsilla,* a stake, in pl. the tonsils]

cerebellar t., a rounded lobule on the undersurface of each cerebellar hemisphere, continuous medially with the uvula of the cerebellar vermis. SYN tonsilla cerebelli [NA].

faucial t., SYN palatine t.

lingual t., a collection of lymphoid follicles on the posterior or pharyngeal portion of the dorsum of the tongue. SYN tonsilla lingualis [NA].

palatine t., a large, oval mass of lymphoid tissue embedded in the lateral wall of the oral pharynx on either side between the pillars of the fauces. SYN tonsilla palatina [NA], tonsilla [NA], faucial t., tonsil (2).

pharyngeal t., a collection of more or less closely aggregated lymphoid nodules on the posterior wall and roof of the nasopharynx, the hypertrophy of which constitutes the morbid condition called adenoids.

ton·sil·la, pl. **ton·sil·lae** (ton-sil′ă, -ē) [NA]. SYN palatine *tonsil*. [L. (see tonsil)]

  t. cerebel′li [NA], SYN cerebellar *tonsil*.

  t. lingua′lis [NA], SYN lingual *tonsil*.

  t. palati′na [NA], SYN palatine *tonsil*.

ton·sil·lar, ton·sil·lary (ton′si-lăr, ton′si-lă-rē). Relating to a tonsil, especially the palatine tonsil.

ton·sil·lec·to·my (ton′si-lek′tō-mē). Removal of the entire tonsil. [tonsil + G. *ektomē,* excision]

ton·sil·li·tis (ton′si-lī′tis). Inflammation of a tonsil, especially of the palatine tonsil. [tonsil + G. *-itis,* inflammation]

△**tonsillo-.** Tonsil. [L. *tonsilla*]

ton·sil·lo·lith (ton-sil′ō-lith). A calcareous concretion in a distended tonsillar crypt. [tonsillo- + G. *lithos,* stone]

ton·sil·lot·o·my (ton′si-lot′ō-mē). The cutting away of a portion or all of a hypertrophied faucial tonsil. [tonsillo- + G. *tomē,* incision]

to·nus (tō′nŭs). SYN tonicity (1). [L., fr. G. *tonos*]

Tooth, Howard H., English physician, 1856–1925. SEE Charcot-Marie-T. *disease.*

■**tooth,** pl. **teeth** (tūth, tēth). One of the hard conical structures set in the alveoli of the upper and lower jaws, used in mastication and assisting in articulation. A t. is a dermal structure composed of dentin and encased in cementum on the anatomic root and enamel on its anatomic crown. It consists of a root buried in the alveolus, a neck covered by the gum, and a crown, the exposed portion. In the center is the pulp cavity filled with a connective tissue reticulum containing a jelly-like substance (dental pulp) and blood vessels and nerves that enter through a canal at the apex of the root. The 20 deciduous teeth, or primary teeth, appear between the 6th and 9th and the 24th month of life; these exfoliate and are replaced by the 32 permanent teeth appearing between the 5th and 7th year and the 17th to 23rd year. There are four kinds of teeth: incisor, canine, premolar, and molar. SYN dens (1) [NA]. [A.S. *tōth*]

  baby t., SYN deciduous t.

  bicuspid t., SYN premolar t.

  buck t., an anterior t. in labioversion.

  canine t., a t. having a crown of thick conical shape and a long, slightly flattened conical root; there are two canine teeth in each jaw, one on either side adjacent to the distal surface of the

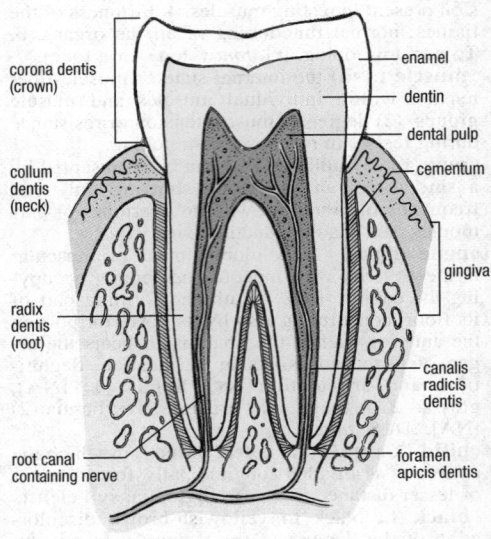

lateral incisors, in both the deciduous and the permanent dentition. SYN dens caninus [NA], canine (3), cuspid (2), eye t.

  deciduous t., one of the first set of teeth, comprising 20 in all, that erupts between the mean ages of 6 and 28 months of life. SYN dens deciduus [NA], baby t., deciduous dentition, milk t., primary dentition, primary t., temporary t.

  eye t., SYN canine t.

  Horner's teeth, incisor teeth having a horizontal, hypoplastic groove.

  Hutchinson's teeth, the teeth of congenital syphilis in which the incisal edge is notched and narrower than the cervical area. SEE ALSO Hutchinson's crescentic *notch.*

  impacted t., (1) a t. whose normal eruption is prevented by adjacent teeth or bone; (2) a t. that has been driven into the alveolar process or surrounding tissue as a result of trauma.

  incisor t., a t. with a chisel-shaped crown and a single conical tapering root; there are four of these teeth in the anterior part of each jaw, in both the deciduous and the permanent dentitions. SYN dens incisivus [NA].

  milk t., SYN deciduous t.

  molar t., a t. having a somewhat quadrangular crown with four or five cusps on the grinding surface; the root is bifid in the lower jaw, but there are three conical roots in the upper jaw; there are six molars in each jaw, three on either side behind the premolars in the permanent dentition; in the deciduous dentition there are but four molars in each jaw, two on either side behind the canines. SYN dens molaris [NA], molar (2).

  pegged t., a conical t. whose sides converge from the cervical to the incisal region.

  permanent t., one of the 32 teeth belonging to the second, or permanent, dentition; eruption of the permanent teeth begins from the 5th to the 7th

tooth: and supporting tissues

Figure labels: corona dentis (crown), collum dentis (neck), radix dentis (root), root canal containing nerve, enamel, dentin, dental pulp, cementum, gingiva, canalis radicis dentis, foramen apicis dentis

year, and is not completed until the 17th to the 23rd year, when the last of the wisdom teeth appears. SYN dens permanens [NA], second t., secondary dentition.

premolar t., a t. usually having two tubercles or cusps on the grinding surface and a flattened root, single in the lower jaw and upper second premolar, and furrowed in the upper first premolar. There are four premolars in each jaw, two on either side between the canine and the molars; there are no premolars in the deciduous dentition. SYN dens premolaris [NA], bicuspid t.

primary t., SYN deciduous t.

second t., SYN permanent t.

temporary t., SYN deciduous t.

Turner's t., enamel hypoplasia involving a solitary permanent t.; related to infection in the primary t. that preceded it or to trauma during odontogenesis.

wisdom t., SYN third *molar*.

tooth·ache (tūth′āk). Pain in a tooth due to the condition of the pulp or periodontal ligament resulting from caries, infection, or trauma. SYN dentalgia, odontalgia.

▷**top-.** SEE topo-.

top·ag·no·sis (top-ag-nō′sis). Inability to localize tactile sensations. SYN topoanesthesia. [top- + G. *a*- priv. + *gnōsis*, recognition]

to·pal·gia (tō-pal′jē-ă). Pain localized in one spot; a symptom occurring in neuroses whereby localized pain, without evident organic basis, is experienced. [top- + G. *algos*, pain]

top·es·the·sia (top′es-thē′zē-ă). The ability to localize a light touch applied to any part of the skin. [top- + G. *aisthēsis*, sensation]

to·pha·ceous (tō-fā′shŭs). Sandy; gritty; pertaining to or manifesting the features of a tophus. [L. *tophaceus*]

to·phus, pl. **to·phi** (tō′fŭs, tō′fī). **1.** SEE gouty t. **2.** A salivary calculus, or tartar. [L. a calcareous deposit from springs, tufa]

gouty t., a deposit of uric acid and urates in periarticular fibrous tissue, cartilage of the external ear, or kidney, in gout.

top·i·cal (top′i-kăl). Relating to a definite place or locality; local. [G. *topikos*, fr. *topos*, place]

▷**topo-, top-.** Place, topical. [G. *topos*]

top·o·an·es·the·sia (top′ō-an-es-thē′zē-ă, tō′pō-). SYN topagnosis. [topo- + anesthesia]

to·pog·ra·phy (tō-pog′ră-fē). ANATOMY The description of any part of the body, especially in relation to a definite and limited area of the surface. [topo- + G. *graphē*, a writing]

top·o·nar·co·sis (top′ō-nar-kō′sis). A localized cutaneous anesthesia. [topo- + narcosis]

TORCH toxoplasmosis, *o*ther infections, *r*ubella, *c*ytomegalorvirus infection, and *h*erpes simplex. SEE TORCH *syndrome*.

tor·pid (tŏr′pid). Inactive; sluggish. [L. *torpidus*, fr. *torpeo*, to be sluggish]

tor·por (tŏr′per, pōr). Inactivity, sluggishness. [L. sluggishness, numbness]

torque (T) (tŏrk). **1.** A rotatory force. **2.** DENTISTRY A torsion force applied to a tooth to produce or maintain crown or root movement. [L. *torqueo*, to twist]

torsade de pointes (tŏr-săd dĕ pwant′). "Twist-ing of the points," a form of ventricular tachycardia nearly always due to medications and characterized by a long QT interval and a "short-long-short" sequence in the beat preceding its onset. The QRS complexes during this rhythm tend to show a series of complexes points up followed by complexes points down, often with a narrow waist between. [Fr. *torsade*, fringe, twist, or coil, + *pointe*, point or tip (euphonious for "wave burst")]

tor·sion (tŏr′shŭn). **1.** A twisting or rotation of a part upon its long axis. **2.** Twisting of the cut end of an artery to arrest hemorrhage. **3.** Rotation of the eye around its anteroposterior axis. SEE ALSO intorsion, extorsion, dextrotorsion, levotorsion. [L. *torsio*, fr. *torqueo*, to twist]

tor·si·ver·sion (tŏr-si-ver′shŭn). A malposition of a tooth in which it is rotated on its long axis. SYN torsoclusion (2).

tor·so (tŏr′sō). The trunk; the body without relation to head or extremities. [It.]

tor·so·clu·sion (tŏr′sō-klū-zhŭn). **1.** Acupressure performed by entering the needle in the tissues parallel with the artery, then turning it so that it crosses the artery transversely, and passing it into the tissues on the opposite side of the vessel. **2.** SYN torsiversion. [L. *torqueo*, to twist, + *claudo* or *cludo*, to close]

tor·ti·col·lar (tŏr-ti-kol′ăr). Relating to or marked by torticollis.

tor·ti·col·lis (tŏr-ti-kol′is). A contraction, often spasmodic, of the muscles of the neck, chiefly those supplied by the spinal accessory nerve; the head is drawn to one side and usually rotated so that the chin points to the other side. SYN wry neck, wryneck. [L. *tortus*, twisted, + *collum*, neck]

tor·tu·ous (tŏr′chū-ŭs). Having many curves; full of turns and twists. [L. *tortuosus*, fr. *torqueo*, to twist]

Tor·u·lop·sis. A genus of yeasts with smaller blastoconidia (2 to 4 mm) with a wide attachment to the parent cell; the species *T. glabrata* is the causative agent of torulopsosis, usually in immunocompromised hosts.

tor·u·lop·so·sis (tŏr-ū-lop′sō-sis). A usually opportunistic infection caused by *Torulopsis glabrata* and seen in patients with severe underlying disease or in immunocompromised patients; the disease may be bronchopulmonary, genitourinary, or septicemic. SEE *Torulopsis*.

tor·u·lus, pl. **tor·u·li** (tŏr′yū-lŭs, -lī). A minute elevation or papilla. [L. dim. of *torus*, a protuberance, swelling]

to·rus, pl. **to·ri** (tō′rŭs, tō′rī). **1.** A geometrical figure formed by the revolution of a circle round the base of any of its arcs, such as the convex molding at the base of a pillar. **2** [NA]. A rounded swelling, such as that caused by a contracting muscle. [L. swelling, knot, bulge]

TOS thoracic outlet *syndrome*.

to·ti·po·ten·cy, to·ti·po·tence (tō-ti-pō′ten-sē, tō-tip′ō-tens). The ability of a cell to differentiate into any type of cell and thus form a new organism or regenerate any part of an organism. [L. *totus*, entire, + *potentia*, power]

to•ti•po•tent, to•ti•po•ten•tial (tō-tip′ŏ-tent, tō′ti-pō-ten′shăl). Relating to totipotency.

touch (tŭch). **1.** The sense by which slight contact with the skin or mucous membrane is perceived. **2.** SYN palpation (1). [Fr. *toucher*]

tour•ni•quet (tūr′ni-ket). An instrument for temporarily arresting the flow of blood to or from a distal part by pressure applied with an encircling device. [Fr. fr. *tourner*, to turn]

△ **tox-.** SEE toxico-.

tox•e•mia (tok-sē′mē-ă). **1.** Clinical manifestations observed during certain infectious diseases, assumed to be caused by toxins and other noxious substances elaborated by the infectious agent. **2.** The clinical syndrome caused by toxic substances in the blood. **3.** A lay term referring to the hypertensive disorders of pregnancy. [G. *toxikon*, poison, + *haima*, blood]

tox•e•mic (tok-sē′mik). Pertaining to, affected by, or manifesting the features of toxemia.

△ **toxi-.** SEE toxico-.

tox•ic (tok′sik). **1.** SYN poisonous. **2.** Pertaining to a toxin. [G. *toxikon*, an arrow-poison]

tox•ic•i•ty (tok-sis′i-tē). The state of being poisonous.

  oxygen t., a body disturbance resulting from breathing high partial pressures of oxygen; characterized by visual and hearing abnormalities, unusual fatigue while breathing, muscular twitching, anxiety, confusion, incoordination, and convulsions.

△ **toxico-, tox-, toxi-, toxo-.** Poison, toxin. [G. *toxikon*, bow, hence (arrow) poison]

Tox•i•co•den•dron (tok′si-kō-den′dron). A genus of poisonous plants (also known as *Rhus*) with fruits and foliage that contain urushiol, which produces a contact dermatitis (rhus dermatitis); species include poison ivy (*T. radicans*), poison oak (*T. diversilobum*), and poison sumac (*T. vernix*) [toxico- + G. *dendron*, tree]

tox•i•co•gen•ic (tok′si-kō-jen′ik). **1.** Producing a poison. **2.** Caused by a poison. [toxico- + G. *-gen*, producing]

tox•i•co•log•ic (tok′si-kō-loj′ik). Relating to toxicology.

tox•i•col•o•gist (tok-si-kol′ŏ-jist). A specialist or expert in toxicology.

tox•i•col•o•gy (tok-si-kol′ŏ-jē). The science of poisons, including their source, chemical composition, action, tests, and antidotes. [toxico- + G. *logos*, study]

tox•i•co•sis (tok-si-kō′sis). Any disease of toxic origin. [toxico- + G. *-osis*, condition]

  endogenic t., SYN autointoxication.

tox•i•gen•ic (tok-si-jen′ik). SYN toxinogenic.

tox•in (tok′sin). A noxious or poisonous substance that is formed or elaborated during the metabolism and growth of certain microorganisms and some higher plant and animal species. [G. *toxikon*, poison]

  botulinus t., a potent neurotoxin from *Clostridium botulinum*.

  erythrogenic t., SYN streptococcus erythrogenic t.

  extracellular t., SYN exotoxin.

  intracellular t., SYN endotoxin.

  streptococcus erythrogenic t., a culture filtrate of lysogenized group A strains of β-hemolytic streptococci, erythrogenic when inoculated into the skin of persons susceptible to scarlet fever, and neutralized by antibodies that appear during scarlet fever convalescence. SYN erythrogenic t.

  tetanus t., the neurotropic, heat-labile exotoxin of *Clostridium tetani* and the cause of tetanus; it is one of the most poisonous substances known, and seems to function by blocking inhibitory synaptic impulses.

tox•in•ic (tok-sin′ik). Relating to a toxin.

tox•i•no•gen•ic (tok′si-nō-jen′ik). Producing a toxin, said of an organism. SYN toxigenic. [toxin + G. *-gen*, producing]

△ **toxo-.** SEE toxico-.

tox•o•ca•ri•a•sis (tok′sō-kă-rī′ă-sis). Infection with nematodes of the genus *Toxocara;* parenterally migrating larvae, chiefly of *Toxocara canis*, may cause visceral larva migrans; ocular involvement results in a solitary granuloma in the retina, peripheral inflammatory masses, or chronic endophthalmitis.

tox•oid (tok′soyd). A toxin that has been treated (commonly with formaldehyde) so as to destroy its toxic property but retain its antigenicity, *i.e.*, its capability of stimulating the production of antitoxin antibodies and thus of producing an active immunity. For specific toxoids, see entries under vaccine. [toxin + G. *eidos*, resemblance]

tox•o•phore (tok′sō-fōr). Denoting the atomic group of the toxin molecule which carries the poisonous principle. [toxo- + G. *phoros*, bearing]

tox•oph•o•rous (tok-sof′ăr-ŭs). Relating to the toxophore group of the toxin molecule.

Tox•o•plas•ma gon•dii (tok-sō-plaz′mă gon′dē-ī). An abundant, widespread sporozoan species that is an intracellular, non-host-specific parasite in a great variety of vertebrates. It develops its sexual cycle, leading to oocyst production, exclusively in cats and other felids; proliferative stages (tachyzoites) and tissue cysts (containing bradyzoites) develop in a wide variety of animal species. [G. *toxon*, bow or arc, + *plasma*, anything formed]

tox•o•plas•mo•sis (tok′sō-plaz-mō′sis). Disease caused by the protozoan parasite *Toxoplasma gondii*, which can produce a variety of syndromes in humans. Prenatally acquired infection can result in abnormalities such as microcephalus or hydrocephalus at birth, jaundice with hepatosplenomegaly or meningoencephalitis in early childhood, or delayed ocular lesions such as chorioretinitis in later childhood. Postnatally acquired human infections typically remain subclinical; if clinical disease does occur, symptoms include fever, lymphadenopathy, headache, myalgia, and fatigue, with eventual recovery, except in the immunocompromised patient where fatal encephalitis often develops.

  acquired t. in adults, a form of t. that may result in fever, encephalomyelitis, chorioretinopathy, maculopapular rash, arthralgia, myalgia, myocarditis, and pneumonitis; a lymphadenopathic form seems to be more prevalent in adults, and such persons may manifest fever, lymphadenopathy, malaise, and headache, a form frequently found in patients with AIDS.

congenital t., transmitted *in utero* to the fetus, observed as three syndromes: 1) acute: most of the organs contain foci of necrosis in association with fever, jaundice, hydrocephaly, encephalomyelitis, pneumonitis, cutaneous rash, ophthalmic lesions, hepatomegaly, and splenomegaly; 2) subacute: most of the lesions are partly healed or calcified, but those in the brain and eye seem to remain active, inasmuch as chorioretinitis is observed in more than 80% of diseased infants; 3) chronic: usually not recognized during the newborn period, but chorioretinitis and cerebral lesions may be detected weeks to years later.

tox•o•py•rim•i•dine (toks′ō-pi-rim′i-dēn). One of the products resulting from the hydrolysis of thiamin by thiaminase and appearing in the urine; a competitive inhibitor of pyridoxal.

TPN, TPNH triphosphopyridine *nucleotide* and its reduced form (the oxidized form is TPN⁺).

TPN total parenteral *nutrition*.

TR repetition *time*.

tra•bec•u•la, gen. and pl. **tra•bec•u•lae** (tră-bek′ yū-lă, -lē). **1.** One of the supporting bundles of fibers traversing the substance of a structure, usually derived from the capsule or one of the fibrous septa. **2.** A small piece of the spongy substance of bone usually interconnected with other similar pieces. **3.** HISTOPATHOLOGY A band of neoplastic tissue two or more cells wide. [L. dim. of *trabs,* a beam]

tra•bec•u•lar (tră-bek′yū-lăr). Relating to or containing trabeculae.

tra•bec•u•lo•plas•ty (tră-bek′yū-lō-plas-tē). Photocoagulation of the trabecular meshwork of the eye using the laser in the treatment of glaucoma.

tra•bec•u•lot•o•my (tră-bek-yū-lot′ō-mē). Surgical opening of the sinus venosus sclerae (canal of Schlemm) to treat glaucoma. [trabekula + G. *tomē,* incision]

trac•er (trā′ser). **1.** An element or compound containing atoms that can be distinguished from their normal counterparts by physical means (*e.g.,* radioactivity assay or mass spectrography) and can thus be used to follow (trace) the metabolism of the normal substances. **2.** A colored substance (*e.g.,* a dye) used as a t. to follow the flow of water. **3.** An instrument used in dissecting out nerves and blood vessels. **4.** A mechanical device with a marking point attached to one jaw and a graph plate or tracing plate attached to the other jaw; used to record the direction and extent of movements of the mandible. SEE ALSO tracing (2). [M.E. track, fr. O. Fr. *tracier,* to make one's way, fr. L. *traho,* pp. *tractum,* to draw, + *-er,* agent suffix]

△ **trache-.** SEE tracheo-.

◨ **tra•chea,** pl. **tra•che•ae** (trā′kē-ă, -kē-ē) [NA]. The air tube extending from the larynx into the thorax (level of the fifth or sixth thoracic vertebra) where it bifurcates into the right and left main bronchi. The t. is composed of from 16 to 20 rings of hyaline cartilage connected by a membrane (annular ligament); posteriorly, the rings are deficient for one-fifth to one-third of their circumference, the interval forming the membranous wall being closed by a fibrous membrane containing smooth muscular fibers. In-

ternally, the mucosa is composed of a pseudostratified ciliated columnar epithelium with mucous goblet cells; numerous small mixed mucous and serous glands occur, the ducts of which open to the surface of the epithelium. SYN windpipe. [G. *tracheia artēria,* rough artery]

tra•che•al (trā′kē-ăl). Relating to the trachea.

tra•che•i•tis (trā-kē-ī′tis). Inflammation of the lining membrane of the trachea. SYN trachitis. [trachea + G. *-itis,* inflammation]

△ **trachel-.** SEE trachelo-.

trach•e•lec•to•my (trak-ĕ-lek′tō-mē). SYN cervicectomy. [trachel- + G. *ektomē,* excision]

trach•e•lism, trach•e•lis•mus (trak′ĕ-lizm, -liz′ mŭs). A bending backward of the neck, such as sometimes ushers in an epileptic attack. [G. *trachēlismos,* a seizing by the throat]

trach•e•li•tis (trak-ĕ-lī′tis). SYN cervicitis.

△ **trachelo-, trachel-.** Neck. [G. *trachēlos*]

trach•e•lo•dyn•ia (trak′ĕ-lō-din′ē-ă). SYN cervicodynia. [trachelo- + G. *odynē,* pain]

trach•e•lor•rha•phy (trak-ĕ-lōr′ă-fē). Repair by suture of a laceration of the cervix uteri. [trachelo- + G. *rhaphē,* suture]

trach•e•lot•o•my (trak-ĕ-lot′ō-mē). SYN cervicotomy. [trachelo- + G. *tomē,* incision]

△ **tracheo-, trache-.** The trachea. [see trachea]

tra•che•o•aer•o•cele (trā′kē-ō-ār′ō-sēl). An air cyst in the neck caused by distention of a tracheocele. [tracheo- + G. *aēr,* air, + *kēlē,* hernia]

tra•che•o•bron•chi•al (trā′kē-ō-brong′kē-ăl). Relating to both trachea and bronchi, denoting especially a set of lymph nodes.

tra•che•o•bron•chi•tis (trā′kē-ō-brong-kī′tis). Inflammation of the mucous membrane of the trachea and bronchi.

tra•che•o•bron•chos•co•py (trā′kē-ō-brong-kos′ kŏ-pē). Inspection of the interior of the trachea and bronchi. [tracheo- + bronchus, + G. *skopeō,* to view]

tra•che•o•cele (trā′kē-ō-sēl). A protrusion of the mucous membrane through a defect in the wall of the trachea. [tracheo- + G. *kēlē,* hernia]

tra•che•o•e•soph•a•ge•al (trā′kē-ō-ē-sof′ă-jē′ăl). Relating to the trachea and the esophagus.

tra•che•o•la•ryn•ge•al (trā′kē-ō-lă-rin′jē-ăl). Relating to the trachea and the larynx.

tra•che•o•ma•la•cia (trā′kē-ō-mă-lā′shē-ă). Degeneration of elastic and connective tissue of the trachea. [tracheo- + G. *malakia,* softness]

tra•che•o•meg•a•ly (trā′kē-ō-meg′ă-lē). An abnormally dilated trachea which may, like bronchiectasis, result from infection or prolonged positive pressure ventilation. [tracheo- + G. *megas* (*megal-*), large]

tra•che•o•path•ia, tra•che•op•a•thy (trā′kē-ō-path′ē-ă, -op′ă-thē). Any disease of the trachea. [tracheo- + G. *pathos,* disease]

tra•che•o•pha•ryn•ge•al (trā′kē-ō-fă-rin′jē-ăl). Relating to both trachea and pharynx; denoting an occasional band of muscular fibers passing from the inferior constrictor of the pharynx to the trachea.

tra•che•oph•o•ny (trā-kē-of′ō-nē). The hollow voice sound heard in auscultating over the trachea. SEE ALSO bronchophony. [tracheo- + G. *phōnē,* voice]

tra·che·o·plas·ty (trā′kē-ō-plas-tē). Plastic surgery of the trachea. [tracheo- + G. *plastos*, formed]

tra·che·or·rha·gia (trā-kē-ō-rā′jē-ă). Hemorrhage from the mucous membrane of the trachea. [tracheo- + G. *rhēgnymi*, to burst forth]

tra·che·os·chi·sis (trā-kē-os′ki-sis). A fissure into the trachea. [tracheo- + G. *schisis*, fissure]

tra·che·o·scop·ic (trā-kē-ō-skop′ik). Relating to tracheoscopy.

tra·che·os·co·py (trā-kē-os′kŏ-pē). Inspection of the interior of the trachea. [tracheo- + G. *skopeō*, to examine]

tra·che·o·ste·no·sis (trā′kē-ō-stĕ-nō′sis). Narrowing of the lumen of the trachea. [tracheo- + G. *stenōsis*, constriction]

tra·che·os·to·my (trā′kē-os′tō-mē). SYN tracheotomy. [tracheo- + G. *stoma*, mouth]

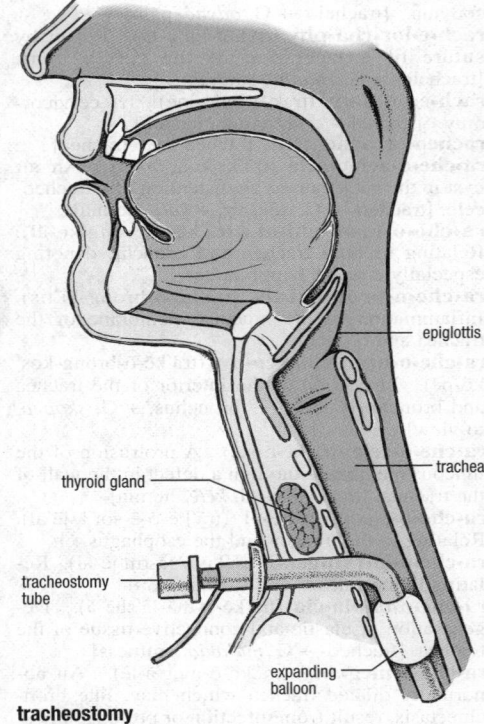

thyroid gland
tracheostomy tube
epiglottis
trachea
expanding balloon

tracheostomy

tra·che·ot·o·my (trā-kē-ot′ō-mē). The operation of opening into the trachea, usually intended to be temporary. SYN tracheostomy. [tracheo- + G. *tomē*, incision]

tra·chi·tis (trā-kī′tis). SYN tracheitis.

tra·cho·ma (tră-kō′mă). Chronic inflammation and hypertrophy of the conjunctiva, marked by the formation of minute grayish or yellowish translucent granules, caused by *Chlamydia trachomatis*. SYN Egyptian ophthalmia, granular ophthalmia. [G. *trachōma*, fr. *trachys*, rough, harsh]

tra·chom·a·tous (tră-kō′mă-tŭs). Relating to or suffering from trachoma.

trac·ing (trās′ing). **1.** A graphic reproduction of the outline or salient features of a physical object or structure. SEE ALSO curve. **2.** Any graphic display of electrical or mechanical events in normal or diseased tissues or organs, as detected or measured by diagnostic instruments. SEE ALSO curve. **3.** DENTISTRY A line or lines, scribed on a table or plate by a pointed instrument, representing a record of movements of the mandible; may be extraoral (made outside the oral cavity) or intraoral (made within the oral cavity).

tract (trakt). An elongated area, *e.g.,* path, track, way. SEE ALSO fascicle. SYN tractus. [L. *tractus*, a drawing out]

   alimentary t., SYN digestive t.

   anterior spinocerebellar t., a bundle of fibers originating in the base of the posterior horn and zona intermedia throughout lumbosacral segments of the spinal cord, crossing to the opposite side and ascending in a peripheral position in the ventral half of the lateral funiculus. In its ascent through the rhombencephalon, the tract curves sharply dorsalward along the rostral border of the trigeminal motor nucleus, entering the cerebellum in a caudal direction over the dorsal surface of the superior cerebellar peduncle, and terminating as mossy fibers in the granular layer of the cortex of the cerebellar vermis. The bundle conveys proprioceptive and exteroceptive information largely from the opposite lower extremity.

   digestive t., the passage leading from the mouth to the anus through the pharynx, esophagus, stomach, and intestine. SYN alimentary canal, alimentary t.

   gastrointestinal t., (G.I. t.) the stomach, small intestine, and large intestine; often used as a synonym of digestive t.

   genital t., the genital passages of the urogenital apparatus.

   iliotibial t., a fibrous reinforcement of the fascia lata on the lateral surface of the thigh, extending from the crest of the ilium to the lateral condyle of the tibia.

   optic t., the continuation of the optic nerve fibers beyond their hemidecussation in the optic chiasm; each of the two symmetrical optic t.'s is composed of fibers originating from the temporal half of the retina of the ipsilateral eye and a nearly equal number of fibers from the nasal half of the contralateral retina; it forms a compact, somewhat flattened fiber band passing caudolaterally alongside the base of the hypothalamus and over the basal surface of the crus cerebri; most of its fibers terminate in the lateral geniculate body; a smaller number of fibers enter the brachium of the superior colliculus, to terminate in the superior colliculus and the pretectal region.

   posterior spinocerebellar t., a compact bundle of heavily myelinated, thick fibers at the periphery of the dorsal half of the lateral funiculus of the spinal cord, originating in the ipsilateral thoracic nucleus (column of Clarke) and ascending by way of the inferior cerebellar peduncle. Terminals end as mossy fibers in the granular layer of the cortex of the cerebellar vermis. The bundle conveys largely proprioceptive information originating from the annulospiral nerve endings surrounding muscle spindles and from Golgi tendon organs.

pyramidal t., a massive bundle of fibers originating from pyramidal cells in the precentral motor and premotor area, and the postcentral gyrus. Fibers from these cortical regions descend through the internal capsule, the middle third of the crus cerebri, and the ventral part of the pons to emerge on the ventral surface of the medulla oblongata as the pyramis. Continuing caudally, most of the fibers cross to the opposite side in the pyramidal decussation and descend in the spinal cord as the lateral pyramidal t., which distributes its fibers to interneurons of the spinal gray matter. Interruption of the pyramidal tract at or below its cortical origin causes impairment of movement in the opposite body-half, especially severe in the arm and leg and characterized by muscular weakness, spasticity and hyperreflexia, and a loss of discrete finger and hand movements. Babinski's sign is associated with this condition of hemiplegia.

respiratory t., the air passages from the nose to the pulmonary alveoli, through the pharynx, larynx, trachea, and bronchi.

reticulospinal t., collective term denoting a variety of fiber tracts descending to the spinal cord from the reticular formation of the pons and medulla oblongata. Part of these fibers conduct impulses from the neural mechanisms regulating autonomic functions to the corresponding somatic and visceral motor neurons of the spinal cord; others form links in nonpyramidal motor mechanisms affecting muscle tonus, reflex activity, and somatic movement.

solitary t., a slender, compact fiber bundle extending longitudinally through the dorsolateral region of the medullary tegmentum, surrounded by the nucleus of the solitary t., below the obex decussating over the central canal, and descending into the upper cervical segments of the spinal cord. It is composed of primary sensory fibers that enter with the vagus, glossopharyngeal, and facial nerves, and in part convey information from stretch receptors and chemoreceptors in the walls of the cardiovascular, respiratory, and intestinal tracts; in rostral parts of the tract impulses are generated by the receptor cells of the taste buds in the mucosa of the tongue. Its fibers are distributed to the nucleus of the solitary tract.

spinothalamic t., a large ascending fiber bundle in the ventral half of the lateral funiculus of the spinal cord, arising from cells in the posterior horn at all levels of the cord, which cross within their segments of origin in the white commissure. The spinothalamic t. continues from the spinal cord into the brainstem, occupying a ventrolateral position and issuing numerous fibers to the rhombencephalic and mesencephalic reticular formation, to the lateral part of the central gray substance of the mesencephalon, and to the deep and intermediate layers of the superior colliculus; the fibers that remain form the true spinothalamic t., which enters the diencephalon and ends in the nucleus ventralis posterior (caudal part) and intra-laminar nuclei of the thalamus. In its ascent in the spinal cord the t. is composed of a dorsal part, the lateral spinothalamic t., which conveys impulses associated with pain and temperature sensation, and a more ventral part, the anterior spinothalamic t., involved in tactile sensation.

urinary t., the passage from the pelvis of the kidney to the urinary meatus through the ureters, bladder, and urethra.

vestibulospinal t., a fiber bundle originating from the lateral vestibular nucleus which descends uncrossed into the anterior funiculus of the spinal cord; the t. extends throughout the length of the cord, distributing fibers at all levels to the medial part of the anterior horn. Excitatory impulses conveyed by the vestibulospinal t. increase extensor muscle tone.

trac•tion (trak′shŭn). **1.** The act of drawing or pulling, as by an elastic or spring force. **2.** A pulling or dragging force exerted on a limb in a distal direction. [L. *tractio,* fr. *traho,* pp. *tractus,* to draw]

external t., a pulling force created by using fixed anchorage (*e.g.,* a headcap or bed frame) outside the oral cavity; principally used in the management of midfacial fractures.

internal t., a pulling force created by using one of the cranial bones, above the point of fracture, for anchorage.

skeletal t., t. pull on a bone structure mediated through pin or wire inserted into the bone to reduce a fracture of long bones. SYN skeletal extension.

skin t., t. on an extremity by means of adhesive tape or other types of strapping applied to the limb.

trac•tot•o•my (trak-tot′ō-mē). Interruption of a nerve tract in the brainstem or spinal cord. [L. *tractus,* tract, + G. *tomē,* incision]

trac•tus, gen. and pl. **trac•tus** (trak′tŭs). SYN tract. [L. a drawing, drawing out, extent, tract, fr. *traho,* pp. *tractus,* to draw]

tra•gal (trā′găl). Relating to the tragus.

tra•gi (trā′jī). **1.** Plural of tragus. **2** [NA]. The hairs growing at the entrance to the external acoustic meatus.

tra•gus (trā′gŭs). **1** [NA]. A tonguelike projection of the cartilage of the auricle in front of the opening of the external acoustic meatus and continuous with the cartilage of this canal. SYN hircus (3). **2.** SEE tragi (2). [G. *tragos,* goat, in allusion to the hairs growing on the part, like a goatee]

training. An organized system of education, instruction, or discipline.

athletic training, provision of comprehensive health care services to athletes, including pre-event preparation, evaluation of illnesses and injuries, first aid and emergency care, rehabilitation, and other, related services.

circuit training, SYN circuit resistance training.

circuit resistance training (CRT), modification of standard strength training emphasizing relatively light load (40–60% of maximum strength) and continuous exercise to provide a more general conditioning to improve body composition, muscular strength and endurance, and cardiovascular fitness. SYN circuit training, circuit weight training.

circuit weight training, SYN circuit resistance △ training.

trait (trāt). A qualitative characteristic; a discrete attribute as contrasted with metrical character. A t. is amenable to segregation rather than quantitative analysis; it is an attribute of phenotype, not of genotype. [Fr. from L. *tractus,* a drawing out, extension]

categorical t., GENETICS A feature that can conveniently and effectively be analyzed by sorting into classes either because there is no satisfactory way of measuring it or because it falls into natural classes so that the variation among classes far exceeds that within classes; existence of categories suggests but does not prove the operation of a major, simple, underlying cause.

chromosomal t., a t. dependent on a recurrent chromosomal aberration.

codominant t., SEE codominant.

dominance of t.'s, an expression of the apparent physiologic relationship existing between two or more genes that may occupy the same chromosomal locus (alleles). At a specific locus there are three possible combinations of two allelic genes, *A* and *a*: two homozygous (*AA* and *aa*) and one heterozygous (*Aa*). If a heterozygous individual presents only the hereditary characteristic determined by gene *A*, but not *a*, *A* is said to be dominant and *a* recessive; in this case, *AA* and *Aa*, although genotypically distinct, should be phenotypically indistinguishable. If *AA*, *Aa*, and *aa* are distinguishable, each from the others, *A* and *a* are codominant.

dominant t., an outstanding mental or physical characteristic; SEE dominance of t.'s.

intermediate t., a measurable t. in which there is some evidence of the operation of a simple major cause, but in which the variation within the putative categories is such as to cause overlap and hence ambiguity in classification of any particular reading.

marker t., a t. that may be of little importance in itself but which by association, linkage, or other means facilitates the detection, anticipation, or understanding of a disease or (for genetic diseases) the localization of the causative gene on the karyotype.

nonpenetrant t., a genetic t. that is not phenotypically manifest because of nongenetic factors; it therefore does not include recessivity, epistasis, hypostasis, or parastasis but does include environmental factors and pure random effects such as lyonization.

recessive t., SEE dominance of t.'s.

threshold t., a t. that falls into natural groups that originate not in categorically distinct causes but in whether or not the outcome attains critical values; *e.g.,* gallstones may result from a categorical cause or from unusual levels of causal factors that themselves show no evidence of grouping.

trance (trans). An altered state of consciousness as in hypnosis, catalepsy, or ecstasy. [L. *transeo,* to go across]

tran·quil·iz·er (trang′kwi-lī-zer). A drug that promotes tranquility without sedating or depressant effects.

△**trans-.** **1.** Prefix denoting across, through, beyond; opposite of *cis-.* **2.** GENETICS Denoting the location of two genes on opposite chromosomes of a homologous pair. **3.** ORGANIC CHEMISTRY A form of geometric isomerism in which the atoms attached to two carbon atoms, joined by double bonds, are located on opposite sides of the molecule. **4.** BIOCHEMISTRY A prefix to a group name in an enzyme name or a reaction denoting transfer of that group from one compound to another. [L. *trans,* through, across]

trans·a·cet·y·lase (trans-ă-set′i-lās). SYN acetyltransferase.

trans·a·cet·y·la·tion (trans′ă-set-i-lā′shŭn). Transfer of an acetyl group ($CH_3CO–$), from one compound to another; such reactions, usually involving formation of acetyl-CoA, occur notably in the initiation of the tricarboxylic acid cycle by the transfer of an acetyl group to oxaloacetate to form citrate.

trans·ac·yl·as·es (trans-as′i-lā-sez). SYN acyltransferases.

trans·al·do·la·tion (trans′al-dō-lā′shŭn). A reaction involving the transfer of an aldol group from one compound to another; such reactions generally involve the sugar phosphates and occur in the phosphogluconate oxidation pathway of carbohydrate catabolism.

trans·am·i·di·na·tion (trans-am′i-di-nā′shŭn). A reaction involving the transfer of an amidine group from one compound to another; the amidine donor is generally L-arginine and the reaction is of significance in the biosynthesis of creatine.

trans·am·i·nas·es (trans-am′i-nās-ez). SYN aminotransferases.

serum glutamic-oxaloacetic t. (SGOT), SYN *aspartate* aminotransferase.

trans·am·i·na·tion (trans-am′i-nā′shŭn). The reaction between an amino acid and an α-keto acid through which the amino group is transferred from the former to the latter.

trans·ca·lent (trans-kā′lent). SYN diathermanous. [trans- + L. *caleo,* to be warm]

trans·car·bam·o·y·las·es (trans-kar-bam′ō-i-lā-sez). SYN carbamoyltransferases.

trans·car·box·yl·as·es (trans-kar-boks′i-lās-ez). SYN carboxyltransferases.

trans·co·bal·a·mins (trans-kō-bal′ă-minz). Substances included in "R binder," the name given a family of cobalamin-binding proteins; deficiencies have been associated with low serum cobalamin levels, and can lead to megaloblastic anemia.

trans·cor·ti·cal (tranz-kōr′ti-kăl). **1.** Across or through the cortex of the brain, ovary, kidney, or other organ. **2.** From one part of the cerebral cortex to another; denoting the various association tracts.

trans·cor·tin (trans-kōr′tin). An α₂-globulin in blood that binds cortisol and corticosterone; the principal corticosteroid-binding protein in the plasma. SYN corticosteroid-binding globulin.

tran·scrip·tase (tran-skrip′tās). A polymerase associated with the process of transcription; especially the DNA-dependent RNA polymerase. [L. *transcribo*, pp. *transcriptum*, to copy, + -ase]

reverse t., RNA-dependent DNA polymerase, present in virions of RNA tumor viruses.

tran•scrip•tion (tran-skrip′shŭn). Transfer of genetic code information from one kind of nucleic acid to another, especially with reference to the process by which a base sequence of messenger RNA is synthesized (by an RNA polymerase) on a template of complementary DNA.

trans•cy•to•sis (trans-sī-tō′sis). A mechanism for transcellular transport in which a cell encloses extracellular material in an invagination of the cell membrane to form a vesicle (endocytosis), then moves the vesicle across the cell to eject the material through the opposite cell membrane by the reverse process (exocytosis). SYN vesicular transport.

trans•duc•tion (trans-dŭk′shŭn). **1.** Transfer of genetic material (and its phenotypic expression) from one cell to another by viral infection. **2.** A form of genetic recombination in bacteria. **3.** Conversion of energy from one form to another. [trans- + L. *duco*, pp. *ductus*, to lead across]

abortive t., t. in which the genetic fragment from the donor bacterium is not integrated in the genome of the recipient bacterium, and, when the latter divides, is transmitted to only one of the daughter cells.

complete t., t. in which the transferred genetic fragment is fully integrated in the genome of the recipient bacterium.

tran•sec•tion (tran-sek′shŭn). **1.** A cross-section. **2.** Cutting across. SYN transsection. [trans- + L. *seco*, pp. *sectus*, to cut]

trans•fec•tion (trans-fek′shŭn). A method of gene transfer utilizing infection of a cell with nucleic acid (as from a retrovirus) resulting in subsequent viral replication in the transfected cell. [trans- + in*fection*]

trans•fer. **1.** Process of removal or transferral. **2.** A condition in which learning in one situation influences learning in another situation. SYN transmission (1). [L. *trans-fero*, to bear across]

embryo t., after artificial insemination *in vitro*, the fertilized ovum is transferred at the blastocyst stage to the recipient's uterus or oviduct.

trans•fer•as•es (trans′fer-ās-ez). Enzymes transferring one-carbon groups, acyl and glucosyl residues, alkyl or aryl groups, nitrogenous groups, phosphorus-containing groups, and sulfur-containing groups.

trans•fer•ence (trans-fer′ens). **1.** Conveyance of an object from one place to another. **2.** Shifting of symptoms from one side of the body to the other, as seen in certain cases of conversion hysteria. **3.** Displacement of affect from one person or one idea to another. **4.** PSYCHOANALYSIS generally applied to the projection of feelings, thoughts, and wishes onto the analyst, who has come to represent some person from the patient's past.

trans•fer•rin (trans-fer′in). **1.** A nonheme β_1-globulin of the plasma, capable of associating reversibly with up to 1.25 µg of iron per g, and acting therefore as an iron-transporting protein. **2.** A glycoprotein, found in mammalian milk (lactoferrin) and egg white (conalbumin, ovotransfer-

rin), that binds and transports iron (Fe^{3+}). [trans- + L. *ferrum*, iron, + -ia]

trans•fer-RNA. See entries under ribonucleic acid.

trans•fix•ion (trans-fik′shŭn). A maneuver in amputation in which the knife is passed from side to side through the soft parts, close to the bone, and the muscles are then divided from within outward. [L. *transfixio* (see transfix)]

trans•for•ma•tion (trans-fōr-mā′shŭn). **1.** SYN metamorphosis. **2.** A change of one tissue into another, as cartilage into bone. **3.** In metals, a change in phase and physical properties in the solid state caused by heat treatment. **4.** MICROBIAL GENETICS Transfer of genetic information between bacteria by means of "naked" intracellular DNA fragments derived from bacterial donor cells and incorporated into a competent recipient cell. [L. *trans-formo*, pp. *-atus*, to transform]

trans•fuse (trans-fyūz′). To perform transfusion.

trans•fu•sion (trans-fyū′zhŭn). **1.** Transfer of blood or a blood component from one individual (donor) to another (recipient). **2.** Intravascular injection of physiologic saline solution. [L. *trans-fundo*, pp. *-fusus*, to pour from one vessel to another]

direct t., t. of blood from the donor to the recipient, either through a tube connecting their blood or by suturing the vessels together. SYN immediate t.

exchange t., removal of most of a patient's blood followed by introduction of an equal amount from donors. SYN substitution t., total t.

immediate t., SYN direct t.

indirect t., t. into a patient of blood previously obtained from a donor and stored in a suitable container.

reciprocal t., an attempt to confer immunity by transfusing blood taken from a donor into a receiver suffering from the same affection, the balance being maintained by transfusing an equal amount from the receiver to the donor.

substitution t., SYN exchange t.

total t., SYN exchange t.

twin-twin t., direct vascular anastomosis, arterial or venous, between the placental circulations of twins.

trans•hi•a•tal (trans-hī-ā′tăl). By way of a hiatus; said of a surgical procedure.

tran•sil•i•ent (tran-sil′yent, -zil-). Jumping across; passing over; pertaining to those cortical association fibers in the brain that pass from one convolution to another nonadjacent one. [L. *transilio*, to leap across, fr. *salio*, to leap]

trans•ke•to•la•tion (trans′kē-tō-lā′shŭn). A reaction involving the transfer of a ketole group from one compound to another.

trans•la•tion (trans-lā′shŭn). **1.** A change or conversion into another form. **2.** The process by which messenger RNA, transfer RNA, and ribosomes effect the production of protein from amino acids. **3.** DENTISTRY The movement of a tooth through alveolar bone without change in axial inclination. [L. *translatio*, a transferring, fr. *trans- fero*, pp. *-latus*, to carry across]

trans•lo•ca•tion (trans-lō-kā′shŭn). **1.** Transposition of two segments between nonhomologous chromosomes as a result of abnormal breakage and refusion of reciprocal segments. **2.** Transport of a metabolite across a biomembrane. [trans- + L. *locatio,* placement, fr. *loco,* to place]

balanced t., t. of the long arm of an acrocentric chromosome to another chromosome; an individual with a balanced t. has a normal diploid genome and is clinically normal but has a chromosome count of 45 and as a result of asymmetrical meiosis may have children lacking the genes on the translocated segment or have them in trisomy.

reciprocal t., t. without demonstrable loss of genetic material.

robertsonian t., t. in which the centromeres of two acrocentric chromosomes appear to have fused, forming an abnormal chromosome consisting of the long arms of two different chromosomes; if the t. is balanced, the individual is clinically normal but a carrier of the t.; if the t. is unbalanced, the individual is trisomic for the long arm of a chromosome. SYN centric fusion. [W.R.B. *Robertson,* U.S. geneticist, *1881]

unbalanced t., condition resulting from fertilization of a gamete containing a t. chromosome by a normal gamete; if this abnormality is compatible with life, the individual has 46 chromosomes but a segment of the t. chromosome is represented three times in each cell and a partial or complete trisomic state exists.

trans·meth·yl·ase (trans-meth'i-lās). SYN methyltransferase.

trans·meth·yl·a·tion (trans'meth-i-lā'shŭn). Transfer of a methyl group from one compound to another.

trans·mi·gra·tion (trans-mī-grā'shŭn). Movement from one site to another; may entail the crossing of some usually limiting barrier, as in the passage of blood cells through the walls of the vessels (diapedesis). [L. *transmigro,* pp. *-atus,* to remove from one place to another]

trans·mis·si·ble (trans-mis'i-bl). Capable of being transmitted (carried across) from one person to another, as a t. disease, an infectious or contagious disease.

trans·mis·sion (trans-mish'ŭn). **1.** SYN transfer. **2.** The conveyance of disease from one person to another. **3.** The passage of a nerve impulse across an anatomic cleft, as in autonomic or central nervous system synapses and at neuromuscular junctions, by activation of a specific chemical mediator that stimulates or inhibits the structure across the synapse. **4.** In general, passage of energy through a material. [L. *transmissio,* a sending across]

horizontal t., t. of infectious agents from an infected individual to a susceptible contemporary, in contradistinction to vertical t.

iatrogenic t., t. of infectious agents due to medical interference (*e.g.,* t. by contaminated needles).

vertical t., (**1**) t. of a virus (*e.g.,* RNA tumor virus) by means of the genetic apparatus of a cell in which the viral genome is integrated; (**2**) for infectious agents in general, t. of an agent from an individual to its offspring. *i.e.,* from one generation to the next. Cf. horizontal t.

trans·mu·ral (trans-myū'răl). Through any wall,

as of the body or of a cyst or any hollow structure. [trans- + L. *murus,* wall]

trans·mu·ta·tion (trans-myū-tā'shŭn). A change; transformation. SYN conversion (1). [L. *transmuto,* pp. *-atus,* to change, transmute]

trans·pep·ti·dase (trans-pep'ti-dās). An enzyme catalyzing a transpeptidation reaction.

trans·pep·ti·da·tion (trans'pep-ti-dā'shŭn). A reaction involving the transfer of one or more amino acids from one peptide chain to another, as by transpeptidase action, or of a peptide chain itself, as in bacterial cell wall synthesis.

trans·phos·pho·ryl·a·tion (trans'fos-fōr-i-lā'shŭn). A reaction involving the transfer of a phosphoric group from one compound to another, often with the involvement of ATP.

tran·spi·ra·tion (trans-pi-rā'shŭn). Passage of water vapor through the skin or any membrane. SEE ALSO insensible *perspiration.* [trans- + L. *spiro,* pp. *-atus,* to breathe]

trans·plant (tranz'plant). **1.** To transfer from one part to another, as in grafting and transplantation. **2.** The tissue or organ in grafting and transplantation. SEE ALSO graft. [trans- + L. *planto,* to plant]

trans·plan·ta·tion (tranz-plan-tā'shŭn). Implanting in one part a tissue or organ taken from another part or from another individual. SEE ALSO graft. [L. *trans-planto,* pp. *-atus,* to transplant]

bone marrow t., grafting of bone marrow tissue; of value in aplastic anemia, primary immunodeficiency, and acute leukemia (following total body irradiation).

trans·port (trans'pōrt). The movement or transference of biochemical substances in biologic systems. [L. *transporto,* to carry over, fr. trans- + *porto,* to carry]

active t., the passage of ions or molecules across a cell membrane, not by passive diffusion but by an energy-consuming process against an electrochemical gradient.

axoplasmic t., transport by way of flow of axoplasm toward cell soma (retrograde) or toward axon terminal (anterograde).

hydrogen t., the transfer of hydrogen from one metabolite (hydrogen donor) to another (hydrogen acceptor) through the action of an enzyme system; the donor is thus oxidized and the acceptor reduced.

mucociliary t., movement of mucus and mucoid fluid through the bronchial tree by the action of cilia.

vesicular t., SYN transcytosis.

trans·pos·ase (tranz-pōz'ās). An enzyme that is required for transposition of DNA segments. [L. *trans-pono,* pp. *trans-positum,* to set across, transfer, + -ase]

trans·pose (tranz-pōz). To transfer one tissue or organ to the place of another and *vice versa.* [L. *trans-pono,* pp. *-positus,* to place across, transfer]

trans·po·si·tion (tranz-pō-zish'ŭn). **1.** Removal from one place to another; metathesis. **2.** The condition of being transposed to the wrong side of the body, as in t. of the viscera, in which the viscera are located opposite their normal position. **3.** Positioning of teeth out of their normal sequence in an arch.

t. of the great vessels, congenital malformation in which the aorta arises from the morphologic right ventricle and the pulmonary artery from the morphologic left ventricle resulting in two separate and parallel circulations. The condition is lethal unless some communication exists between the systemic and pulmonic circulation after birth; the life-sustaining communication may be an intra-atrial passage or a patent ductus arteriosus.

trans•po•son (trans-pō'son). A segment of DNA which has a repeat of an insertion sequence element at each end that can migrate from one plasmid to another within the same bacterium, to a bacterial chromosome, or to a bacteriophage. [L. *transpono,* pp. *transpositum,* to transfer, + -on]

trans•sec•tion (trans-sek'shŭn). SYN transection.

trans•sex•u•al (trans-sek'shū-ăl). **1.** A person with the external genitalia and secondary sexual characteristics of one sex, but whose personal identification and psychosocial configuration is that of the opposite sex; a study of morphologic, genetic, and gonadal structure may be genitally congruent or incongruent. **2.** Denoting or relating to such a person. **3.** Relating to medical and surgical procedures designed to alter a patient's external sexual characteristics so that they resemble those of the opposite sex.

trans•sex•u•al•ism (tranz-sek'shū-ă-lizm). **1.** The state of being a transsexual. **2.** The desire to change one's anatomic sexual characteristics to conform physically with one's perception of self as a member of the opposite sex.

tran•su•date (tran'sū-dāt). Any fluid (solvent and solute) that has passed through a presumably normal membrane, such as the capillary wall, as a result of imbalanced hydrostatic and osmotic forces; characteristically low in protein unless there has been secondary concentration. Cf. exudate. SYN transudation (2). [trans- + L. *sudo,* pp. -*atus,* to sweat]

tran•su•da•tion (tran-sū-dā'shŭn). **1.** Passage of a fluid or solute through a membrane by a hydrostatic or osmotic pressure gradient. **2.** SYN transudate. [see transudate]

trans•u•re•ter•o•u•re•ter•os•to•my (tranz-yū-rē'ter-ō-yū-rē-ter-os'tō-mē). Anastomosis of the transected end of one ureter into the intact contralateral ureter, by direct or elliptical end-to-side technique. SEE ALSO ureteroureterostomy.

trans•vec•tor (trans-vek'tŏr, tōr). An animal that transmits a toxic substance that it does not produce, but that may be accumulated from animal (dinoflagellate) or plant (algae) sources.

trans•verse (trans-vers'). Crosswise; lying across the long axis of the body or of a part. [L. *transversus*]

trans•ver•sec•to•my (trans-ver-sek'tō-mē). Resection of the transverse process of a vertebra. [transverse + G. *ektomē,* excision]

trans•ver•sion (trans-ver'zhŭn). **1.** Substitution in DNA and RNA of a pyrimidine for a purine, or vice versa, by mutation. **2.** DENTISTRY The eruption of a tooth in a position normally occupied by another; transposition of a tooth.

trans•ves•tism (trans-ves'tizm). The practice of dressing or masquerading in the clothes of the opposite sex; especially the adoption of feminine mannerisms and costume by a male. SYN transvestitism. [trans- + L. *vestio,* to dress]

trans•ves•tite (trans-ves'tīt). A person who practices transvestism.

trans•ves•ti•tism (trans-ves'ti-tizm). SYN transvestism.

tra•pe•zi•al (tra-pē'zē-ăl). Relating to any trapezium.

tra•pe•zi•form (tra-pē'zi-form). SYN trapezoid (1).

tra•pe•zi•um, pl. **tra•pe•zia, tra•pe•zi•ums** (tra-pē'zē-ŭm, -ă). **1.** A four-sided geometrical figure having no two sides parallel. **2.** The lateral (radial) bone in the distal row of the carpus; it articulates with the first and second metacarpals, scaphoid, and trapezoid bones. SYN greater multangular bone, os multangulum majus, trapezium bone. [G. *trapezion,* a table or counter, a trapezium, dim. of *trapeza,* a table, fr. *tra-* (= *tetra-*), four, + *pous* (*pod-*), foot]

tra•pe•zi•us (tra-pē'zē-ŭs). SYN trapezius *muscle.*

trap•e•zoid (trap'ĕ-zoyd). **1.** Resembling a trapezium. SYN trapeziform. **2.** A geometrical figure resembling a trapezium except that two of its opposite sides are parallel. **3.** SYN trapezoid *bone.* [G. *trapeza,* table, + *eidos,* resemblance]

△**traum-.** SEE traumato-.

trau•ma, pl. **trau•ma•ta, trau•mas** (traw'mă, -mă-tă). An injury, physical or mental. SYN traumatism. [G. wound]

  birth t., **(1)** physical injury to an infant during its delivery; **(2)** the supposed emotional injury, inflicted by events incident to birth, upon an infant which allegedly appears in symbolic form in patients with mental illness.

  psychic t., an upsetting experience precipitating or aggravating an emotional or mental disorder.

trau•mas•the•nia (traw-mas-thē'nē-ă). Nervous exhaustion following an injury. [traum- + G. *astheneia,* weakness]

trau•ma•ta (traw'mă-tă). Plural of trauma.

trau•mat•ic (traw-mat'ik). Relating to or caused by trauma. [G. *traumatikos*]

trau•ma•tism (traw'mă-tizm). SYN trauma.

△**traumato-, traumat-, traum-.** Wound, injury. [G. *trauma*]

trau•ma•top•nea (traw'mă-top-nē'ă). Passage of air in and out through a wound of the chest wall. [traumato- + G. *pnoē,* breath]

tra•verse (trav'ers). COMPUTED TOMOGRAPHY One complete linear movement of the gantry across the object being scanned. [M.E., fr. O.Fr., fr. L.L. *transverso,* fr. L. *trans-verto,* to turn across]

treat (trēt). To manage a disease by medicinal, surgical, or other measures; to care for a patient medically or surgically. [Fr. *traiter,* fr. L. *tracto,* to drag, handle, perform]

treat•ment (trēt'ment). Medical or surgical management of a patient. SEE ALSO therapy, therapeutics. [Fr. *traitement* (see treat)]

  light t., SYN phototherapy.

  neurodevelopmental t., a therapeutic method involving hands-on intervention to facilitate normal movement patterns necessary for the acquisition of functional skills.

  palliative t., t. to alleviate symptoms without curing the disease.

tr

prophylactic t., the institution of measures designed to protect a person from an attack of a disease to which he or she has been, or is liable to be, exposed.

shock t., SEE electroshock *therapy.*

Trem·a·to·da (trem′ă-tō′dă). A class in the phylum Platyhelminthes (the flatworms), consisting of flukes with a leaf-shaped body and two muscular suckers, and an acelomate parenchyma-filled body cavity. Flukes of interest to human or veterinary medicine are members of the order Digenea, with complete life cycles involving embryonic multiplication in a mollusk as their first intermediate host. [G. *trēmatōdēs,* full of holes, fr. *trēma,* a hole, + *eidos,* appearance]

trem·a·tode, trem·a·toid (trem′ă-tōd, trem′ă-toyd). **1.** Common name for a fluke of the class Trematoda. **2.** Relating to a fluke of the class Trematoda.

trem·or (trem′er, -ōr). **1.** Repetitive, often regular, oscillatory movements caused by alternate, or synchronous, but irregular contraction of opposing muscle groups; usually involuntary. **2.** Minute ocular movement occurring during fixation on an object. SYN trepidation (1). [L. a shaking]

  alternating t., a form of hyperkinesia characterized by regular, symmetrical, to-and-fro movements (at about 4 per second) that are produced by patterned, alternating contraction of muscles and their antagonists.

  essential t., an action t. of 4–8 Hz frequency that usually begins in early adult life and is limited to the upper limbs and head; called familial when it appears in several family members.

  flapping t., SYN asterixis.

  intention t., a t. that occurs during the performance of precise voluntary movements, caused by disorders of the cerebellum or its connections. SYN volitional t. (2).

  pill-rolling t., resting t. of the thumb and fingers seen in Parkinson disease.

  resting t., a coarse, rhythmic t. 3–5 Hz frequency, usually confined to hands and forearms, that appears when the limbs are relaxed, and disappears with active limb movements; characteristic of Parkinson disease.

  senile t., an essential t. that becomes symptomatic in the elderly.

  volitional t., (1) a t. that can be arrested by a strong effort of the will; **(2)** SYN intention t.

trem·u·lous (trem′yū-lŭs). Characterized by tremor.

trend of thought. Thinking with a tendency toward or centering on a particular idea with a particular affect.

tre·pan (trē-pan′). SYN trephine. [G. *trypanon,* a borer]

trep·a·na·tion (trep-ă-nā′shŭn). SYN trephination.

treph·i·na·tion (tref-i-nā′shŭn). Removal of a circular piece ("button") of cranium by a trephine. SYN trepanation.

tre·phine (trē-fīn′, -fēn′). **1.** A cylindrical or crown saw used for the removal of a disc of bone, especially from the skull, or of other firm tissue as that of the cornea. **2.** To remove a disc of bone or other tissue by means of a t. SYN trepan. [contrived fr. L. *tres fines,* three ends]

trep·i·dant (trep′i-dant). Marked by tremor. [L. *trepidans,* pres. p. of *trepido,* to tremble, to be agitated]

trep·i·da·tio cor·dis (trep-i-dā′shē-ō kōr′dis). SYN palpitation.

trep·i·da·tion (trep-i-dā′shŭn). **1.** SYN tremor. **2.** Anxious fear. [L. *trepidatio,* fr. *trepido,* to tremble, to be agitated]

Trep·o·ne·ma (trep-ō-nē′mă). A genus of anaerobic bacteria (order Spirochaetales) consisting of cells, 3 to 8 μm in length, with acute, regular, or irregular spirals and no obvious protoplasmic structure. A terminal filament may be present. They stain with difficulty except with Giemsa's stain or silver impregnation. Some species are pathogenic and parasitic for humans and other animals, generally producing local lesions in tissues. [G. *trepō,* to turn, + *nēma,* thread]

  T. pal′lidum, a species that causes syphilis in humans.

  T. perten′ue, a species that causes yaws; patients with this disease give positive results in serologic screening tests for syphilis.

trep·o·ne·ma·to·sis (trep′ō-nē-mă-tō′sis). SYN treponemiasis.

trep·o·neme (trep′ō-nēm). A vernacular term used to refer to any member of the genus *Treponema.*

trep·o·ne·mi·a·sis (trep′ō-nē-mī′ă-sis). Infection caused by *Treponema.* SYN treponematosis.

trep·o·ne·mi·ci·dal (trep′ō-nē′mi-sī′dăl). Destructive to any species of *Treponema,* but usually with reference to *T. pallidum.* SYN antitreponemal. [*Treponema* + L. *caedo,* to kill]

trep·pe (trep′eh). A phenomenon in cardiac muscle: if a number of stimuli of the same intensity are sent into the muscle after a quiescent period, the first few contractions of the series show a successive increase in amplitude (strength). SYN staircase phenomenon. [Ger. *Treppe,* staircase]

tre·sis (trē′sis). SYN perforation. [G. *trēsis,* a boring]

△**tri-.** Three. Cf. tris-. [L. and G.]

tri·a·ce·tic ac·id (trī-ă-sē′tik). A compound formed by condensation of acetyl and malonyl CoA's in the course of fatty acid synthesis.

tri·ac·yl·glyc·er·ol (trī-as′il-glis′er-ol). Glycerol esterified at each of its three hydroxyl groups by a fatty (aliphatic) acid. SYN fat (4), triglyceride.

  t. lipase, the fat-splitting enzyme in pancreatic juice; it hydrolyzes t. to produce a diacylglycerol and a fatty acid anion; a deficiency of the hepatic enzyme results in hypercholesterolemia and hypertriglyceridemia. SYN steapsin.

tri·ad (trī′ad). **1.** A collection of three things having something in common. **2.** The transverse tubule and the terminal cisternae on each side of it in skeletal muscle fibers. **3.** SYN portal t. **4.** The father, mother, and child relationship projectively experienced in group psychotherapy. [G. *trias* (*triad*-), the number 3, fr. *treis,* three]

  acute compression t., the rising venous pressure, falling arterial pressure, and decreased heart sounds of pericardial tamponade.

  Charcot's t., (1) in multiple (disseminated)

sclerosis, the three symptoms: nystagmus, tremor, and scanning speech; **(2)** combination of jaundice, fever, and upper abdominal pain that occurs as a result of cholangitis.

Fallot's t., SYN *trilogy* of Fallot.

Hutchinson's t., parenchymatous keratitis, labyrinthine disease, and Hutchinson's teeth, significant of congenital syphilis.

Kartagener's t., SYN Kartagener's *syndrome*.

portal t., branches of the portal vein, hepatic artery, and the biliary ducts bound together in the perivascular fibrous capsule or portal tract as they ramify within the substance of the liver. SYN triad (3).

Saint's t., the concurrence of hiatal hernia, diverticulosis, and cholelithiasis.

tri·age (trē'ahzh). Medical screening of patients to determine their relative priority for treatment; the separation of a large number of casualties, in military or civilian disaster medical care, into three groups: 1) those who cannot be expected to survive even with treatment; 2) those who will recover without treatment; 3) the highest priority group, those who will not survive without treatment. [Fr. sorting]

tri·an·gle (trī'ang-gl). ANATOMY, SURGERY a three-sided area with arbitrary or natural boundaries. SEE ALSO trigonum. [L. *triangulum,* fr. *tri-*, three, + *angulus,* angle]

t. of auscultation, space bounded by the lower border of the trapezius, the latissimus dorsi, and the medial margin of the scapula, where the absence of musculature allows respiratory sounds to be heard clearly with a stethoscope.

Bryant's t., in fracture of the neck of the femur, to determine upward displacement of the trochanter, lines are drawn on the body to form a t.: line *a* is drawn around the body at the level of the anterior superior iliac spines; line *b*, perpendicular to line *a*, is drawn to the greater trochanter of the femur; line *c* is drawn from the trochanter to the iliac spine; upward displacement is measured along line *b*. SYN iliofemoral t.

Calot's t., t. bounded by the cystic artery, cystic duct, and hepatic duct; its dissection early in cholecystectomy safeguards essential structures, should there be anatomic variations from the norm.

carotid t., a space bounded by the superior belly of the omohyoid muscle, anterior border of the sternocleidomastoid, and posterior belly of the digastric; it contains the bifurcation of the common carotid artery.

Codman's t., RADIOLOGY the interface between growing bone tumor and normal bone, presenting as an incomplete triangle formed by periosteum.

digastric t., SYN submandibular t.

Einthoven's t., an imaginary equilateral t. with the heart at its center, its equal sides representing the three standard limb leads of the electrocardiogram.

Farabeuf's t., the t. formed by the internal jugular and facial veins and the hypoglossal nerve.

femoral t., a triangular space at the upper part of the thigh, bounded by the sartorius and adductor longus muscles and the inguinal ligament,

with a floor formed laterally by the iliopsoas muscle and medially by the pectineus muscle; the branches of the femoral nerve are distributed within the femoral t.; it is bisected by the femoral vessels, which enter the adductor canal at its apex. SYN trigonum femorale [NA], Scarpa's t.

Hesselbach's t., SYN inguinal t.

iliofemoral t., SYN Bryant's t.

inguinal t., the triangular area in the lower abdominal wall bounded by the inguinal ligament below, the border of the rectus abdominis medially and the inferior epigastric vessels (lateral umbilical fold) laterally. It is the site of direct inguinal hernia. SYN trigonum inguinale [NA], Hesselbach's t., inguinal trigone.

Langenbeck's t., a t. formed by lines drawn from the anterior superior iliac spine to the surface of the greater trochanter and to the surgical neck of the femur; a penetrating wound in this area probably involves the joint.

Lesser's t., the space between the bellies of the digastric muscle and the hypoglossal nerve.

lumbar t., an area in the posterior abdominal wall bounded by the edges of the latissimus dorsi and external oblique muscles and the iliac crest; herniations occasionally occur here. SYN trigonum lumbale [NA], Petit's lumbar t.

lumbocostoabdominal t., an irregular area bounded by the serratus posterior inferior, obliquus externus, obliquus internus, and erector spinae muscles.

Macewen's t., SYN suprameatal t.

muscular t., the t. bounded by the sternocleidomastoid muscle, the superior belly of the omohyoid muscle, and the anterior midline of the neck; the infrahyoid muscles occupy most of it. SYN trigonum musculare [NA].

Petit's lumbar t., SYN lumbar t.

t. of safety, the area at the lower left sternal border where the pericardium is not covered by lung (pericardial notch); preferred site for aspiration of pericardial fluid.

Scarpa's t., SYN femoral t.

submandibular t., the t. of the neck bounded by the mandible and the two bellies of the digastric muscle; it contains the submandibular gland. SYN trigonum submandibulare [NA], digastric t.

supraclavicular t., the t. bounded by the clavicle, the omohyoid muscle, and the sternocleidomastoid muscle; it contains the subclavian artery and vein.

suprameatal t., a t. formed by the root of the zygomatic arch, the posterior wall of the bony external acoustic meatus, and an imaginary line connecting the extremities of the first two lines; used as a guide in mastoid operations. SYN Macewen's t.

vesical t., SYN *trigone* of bladder.

Tri·at·o·ma (trī-ă-tō'mă). A genus of insects that includes important vectors of *Trypanosoma cruzi,* such as *T. dimidiata, T. infestans,* and *T. maculata.*

tri·ba·sic (trī-bā'sik). Having three titratable hydrogen atoms; denoting an acid with a basicity of 3.

tribe (trīb). In biological classification, an occasionally used division between the family and the genus; often the same as the subfamily. [L. *tribus*]

tri·bra·chia (trī-brā′kē-ă). Condition seen in conjoined twins when the fusion has merged the adjacent arms to form a single one, so that there are only three arms for the two bodies. SEE conjoined *twins*, under *twin*. [tri- + G. *brachiōn,* arm]

TRIC *trachoma* and *inclusion conjunctivitis.*

tri·ceps (trī′seps). Three-headed; denoting especially two muscles: t. brachii and t. surae. SEE muscle. [L. fr. *tri-,* three, + *caput,* head]

△**trich-.** SEE tricho-.

△**trichi-.** SEE tricho-.

△**-trichia.** Condition or type of hair. [G. *thrix* (*trich-*), hair, + *-ia,* condition]

tri·chi·a·sis (trī-kī′ă-sis). A condition in which the hair adjacent to a natural orifice turns inward and causes irritation; *e.g.,* in inversion of an eyelid (entropion), eyelashes irritate the eye. [trich- + G. *-iasis,* condition]

trich·i·lem·mo·ma (trik′i-le-mō′mă). A benign tumor derived from outer root sheath epithelium of a hair follicle, consisting of cells with pale-staining cytoplasm containing glycogen; multiple t.'s are present on the face in Cowden's disease. [trichi- + G. *lemma,* husk, + *-ōma,* tumor]

tri·chi·na, pl. **tri·chi·nae** (tri-kī′nă, -nē). A larval worm of the genus *Trichinella;* the infective form in pork. [Mod. L., fr. G. *thrix* (*trich-*), a hair]

Trich·i·nel·la (trik′i-nel′ă). A nematode genus in the aphasmid group that causes trichinosis in humans and carnivores. [Mod. L. fr. trichina + dim. suffix *-ella*]

trich·i·no·sis (trik-i-nō′sis). The disease resulting from ingestion of raw or inadequately cooked pork or other meat that contains encysted larvae of the nematode parasite *Trichinella spiralis.* The initial symptoms are abdominal pain, cramping, and diarrhea, associated with the development of the parasites in the small intestine. Once the larval parasites invade muscular tissue, a second set of symptoms is manifest, including facial and periorbital edema, myalgia, fever, pruritus, urticaria, conjunctivitis, and signs of myocarditis. [*Trichinella* (trichina) + G. *-osis,* condition]

tri·chi·nous (trik′i-nŭs). Infected with trichina worms.

tri·chi·tis (tri-kī′tis). Inflammation of the hair bulbs. [trich- + G. *-itis,* inflammation]

tri·chlo·ride (trī-klōr′īd). A chloride having three chlorine atoms in the molecule; *e.g.,* PCl_3.

(2,4,5-tri·chlo·ro·phen·oxy) ace·tic ac·id (trī-klōr-ō-fe-nok′sē). A herbicide and defoliant synthesized by condensation of chloracetic acid and 2,4,5-trichlorophenol, used as the principal constituent of Agent Orange.

△**tricho-, trich-, trichi-.** The hair; a hairlike structure. [G. *thrix* (*trich-*)]

trich·o·be·zoar (trik-ō-bē′zōr). A hair cast in the stomach or intestinal tract. SYN hair ball, pilobezoar. [tricho- + bezoar]

trich·o·cla·sia, trich·choc·la·sis (trik-ō-klā′zē-ă, tri-kok′lă-sis). SYN *trichorrhexis* nodosa. [tricho- + G. *klasis,* breaking off]

trich·o·dis·co·ma (trik′ō-dis-kō′mă). Elliptical parafollicular mesenchymal hamartomas. SYN haarscheibe tumor.

trich·o·ep·i·the·li·o·ma (trik′ō-ep-i-thē-lē-ō′mă) [MIM*132700]. Multiple small benign nodules, occurring mostly on the skin of the face, derived from basal cells of hair follicles enclosing small keratin cysts. [tricho- + epithelioma]

desmoplastic t., a solitary, hard, annular, centrally depressed papule, occurring usually in women on the face, consisting of dermal strands of basaloid cells and small keratinous cysts within sclerotic desmoplastic stroma.

trich·o·glos·sia (trik-ō-glos′ē-ă). SYN hairy *tongue.* [tricho- + G. *glōssa,* tongue]

trich·oid (trik′oyd). Hairlike. [tricho- + G. *eidos,* resemblance]

trich·o·lith (trik′ō-lith). A concretion on the hair; the lesion of piedra. [tricho- + G. *lithos,* stone]

trich·o·lo·gia (trik-ō-lō′jē-ă). A nervous habit of plucking at the hair. [G. *trichologeō,* to pluck hairs, fr. tricho- + *legō,* to pick out, gather]

trich·o·meg·a·ly (trik′ō-meg′ă-lē). Congenital condition characterized by abnormally long eyelashes; associated with dwarfism. [tricho- + G. *megas,* large]

trich·o·mo·na·cide (trik-ō-mō′nă-sīd). An agent that is destructive to *Trichomonas* organisms.

trich·o·mon·ad (trik-ō-mō′nad). Common name for members of the family Trichomonadidae.

Trich·o·mon·as (trik-ō-mō′nas). A genus of parasitic protozoan flagellates causing trichomoniasis. [tricho- + G. *monas,* single (unit)]

T. te′nax, a species that lives as a commensal in the mouth of humans and other primates, especially in the tartar around the teeth or in the defects of carious teeth.

T. vagina′lis, a species frequently found in the vagina and urethra of women, in whom it causes trichomonal vaginitis, and in the urethra and prostate gland of men.

trich·o·mo·ni·a·sis (trik′ō-mō-nī′ă-sis). Disease caused by infection with a protozoan of the genus *Trichomonas;* often used to designate t. vaginitis.

trich·o·my·co·sis (trik′ō-mī-kō′sis). A disease of the hair caused by *Nocardia* or *Corynebacterium.* [tricho- + G. *mykēs,* fungus, + G. *-osis,* condition]

t. axilla′ris, *Corynebacterium* infection of axillary and pubic hairs with development of yellow (flava), black (nigra), or red (rubra) concretions around the hair shafts; frequently asymptomatic. SYN lepothrix, trichonodosis.

trich·o·no·car·di·o·sis (trik′ō-nō-kar′dē-ō′sis). An infection of hair shafts, especially of the axillary and pubic regions, with nocardiae. Yellow, red, or black concretions develop around the infected hair shafts and contain the causative agent and, frequently, micrococci. SEE ALSO trichomycosis, trichomycosis axillaris. [tricho- + *Nocardia* + G. *-osis,* condition]

trich·o·no·do·sis (trik′ō-nō-dō′sis). SYN *trichomycosis* axillaris. [tricho- + L. *nodus,* node (swelling), + G. *-osis,* condition]

trich·o·no·sis (trik′ō-nō′sis). SYN trichopathy.

trich·o·path·ic (trik-ō-path′ik). Relating to any disease of the hair.

tri·chop·a·thy (tri-kop′ă-thē). Any disease of the

hair. SYN trichonosis, trichosis. [tricho- + G. *pathos,* suffering]

tri•choph•a•gy (tri-kof'ă-jē). Habitual biting of the hair. [tricho- + G. *phagō,* to eat]

trich•o•phyt•ic (trik-ō-fit'ik). Relating to trichophytosis.

trich•o•phy•tid (tri-kof'i-tid, trik-ō-fī'tid). An eruption remote from the site of infection, which is the expression of allergic response to *Trichophyton* infection. [tricho- + G. *phyton,* plant, + -*id* (1)]

trich•o•phy•to•be•zoar (trik'ō-fī'tō-bē'zōr). A mixed hair and food ball, consisting of vegetable fibers, seeds and skins of fruits, and animal hair matted together to form a ball in the stomach of humans or animals. [tricho- + G. *phyton,* plant, + bezoar]

Trich•o•phy•ton (tri-kof'i-tŏn). A genus of pathogenic fungi causing dermatophytosis in humans and animals; species attack the hair, skin, and nails. [tricho- + G. *phyton,* plant]

  T. concen'tricum, an anthropophilic species which is the causative agent of tinea imbricata; it closely resembles the branching mycelium of *T. schoenleinii.*

  T. mentagrophy'tes, a zoophilic small-spored ectothrix species that causes infection of the hair, skin, and nails; it is a cause of ringworm in dogs, horses, rabbits, mice, rats, chinchillas, foxes, and humans (especially tinea pedis with severe inflammation, and tinea cruris).

  T. ru'brum, a widely distributed anthropophilic species that causes persistent infections of the skin, especially tinea pedis and tinea cruris, and in the nails that are unusually resistant to therapy.

  T. schoenlei'nii, species of dermatophyte causing favus in humans; it produces tunnels within the hair shaft which are filled with air bubbles after the hyphae disintegrate.

  T. ton'surans, species that causes epidemic dermatophytosis; the most common cause of tinea capitis in the U.S., forming black dots where hair breaks off at the skin surface.

  T. viola'ceum, an anthropophilic species that causes black-dot ringworm or favus infection of the scalp.

trich•o•phyt•o•sis (trik'ō-fī-tō'sis). Superficial fungus infection caused by species of *Trichophyton.* [tricho- + G. *phyton,* plant, + -*osis,* condition]

trich•o•pti•lo•sis (trik'ō-ti-lō'sis, tri-kop-ti-lō'sis). A condition of splitting of the shaft of the hair, giving it a feathery appearance. [tricho- + G. *ptilōsis,* plumage, + -*osis,* condition]

trich•or•rhex•is (trik-ō-rek'sis). A condition in which the hairs tend to break or split. [tricho- + G. *rhēxis,* a breaking]

  t. invagina'ta, SYN bamboo *hair.*

  t. nodo'sa, a congenital or acquired condition in which minute nodes are formed in the hair shafts; splitting and breaking, complete or incomplete, may occur at these nodes. SYN clastothrix, trichoclasia, trichoclasis.

tri•chos•chi•sis (tri-kos'ki-sis). The presence of broken or split hairs. SEE ALSO trichorrhexis. [tricho- + G. *schisis,* a cleaving]

tri•cho•sis (tri-kō'sis). SYN trichopathy. [tricho- + G. -*osis,* condition]

Tri•cho•spo•ron (tri-kos'pō-ron, trik-ō-spōr'on). A genus of imperfect fungi that possess branching septate hyphae with arthroconidia and blastoconidia; these organisms are part of the normal flora of the intestinal tract of humans. *T. beigelii* is the causative agent of white piedra or trichosporosis and fatal fungemia in immunocompromised patients. [tricho- + G. *sporos,* seed (spore)]

trich•o•sta•sis spi•nu•lo•sa (tri-kos'tă-sis spī'nū-lō'să). A condition in which hair follicles are blocked with a keratin plug containing lanugo hairs. [tricho- + G. *stasis,* a standing; L. *spinulosus,* thorny]

trich•o•til•lo•ma•nia (trik'ō-til-ō-mā'nē-ă). A compulsion to pull out one's own hair. [tricho- + G. *tillo,* pull out, + *mania,* insanity]

tri•chro•mat•ic (trī-krō-mat'ik). **1.** Having, or relating to, the three primary colors, red, green, and blue. **2.** Capable of perceiving the three primary colors; having normal color vision. SYN trichromic.

tri•chro•ma•top•sia (trī-krō'mă-top'sē-ă). Normal color vision; the ability to perceive the three primary colors. [tri- + G. *chrōma,* color, + *opsis,* vision]

tri•chro•mic (trī-krō'mik). SYN trichromatic.

trich•u•ri•a•sis (trik-ū-rī'ă-sis). Infection with nematodes of the genus *Trichuris.* In humans, intestinal parasitization by *T. trichiura* is usually asymptomatic; in massive infections it frequently induces diarrhea or rectal prolapse.

Trich•u•ris (tri-kū'ris). A genus of aphasmid nematodes related to the trichina worm, *Trichinella spiralis,* and having a body with a slender, elongated, anterior portion threaded into the mucosa of the colon or large intestine of the host and a thick posterior portion bearing reproductive organs and their products. [tricho- + G. *oura,* tail]

  T. trichiu'ra, the whipworm of humans, a species that causes trichuriasis; the body is filiform and slender in the anterior three-fifths, and more robust posteriorly; females are 4 or 5 cm long, males are shorter (with coiled caudal extremity and a single eversible spicule); eggs are barrel-shaped, 50 to 56 by 20 to 22 μm, with double shell and translucent knobs at each of the two poles; humans are the only susceptible hosts and usually acquire infection by direct finger-to-mouth contact or by ingestion of soil, water, or food that contains larvated eggs (development in the soil takes 3 to 6 weeks under proper conditions of warmth and moisture, hence distribution is chiefly tropical); larvae escape from eggs in the ileum, mature in approximately a month, and then pass directly into the cecum without undergoing a parenteral migration as occurs with *Ascaris lumbricoides;* adults may persist for 2 to 7 years.

tri•cip•i•tal (trī-sip'i-tăl). Having three heads; denoting a triceps muscle.

tri•cor•nute (tri-kōr'nūt). Having three cornua or horns. [tri- + L. *cornutus,* horned, fr. *cornu,* a horn]

tri•crot•ic (trī-krot'ik). Thrice-beating; marked

tr

by three waves in the arterial pulse tracing. [tri- + G. *krotos,* a beat]

tri·cus·pid, tri·cus·pi·dal, tri·cus·pi·date (trī-kŭs′pid, -kŭs′pi-dăl, -kŭs′pi-dāt). **1.** Having three points, prongs, or cusps, as the tricuspid valve of the heart. **2.** Having three tubercles or cusps, as the second upper molar tooth (occasionally) and the upper third molar (usually).

tri·den·tate (trī-den′tāt). Three-toothed; three-pronged. [tri- + L. *dentatus,* toothed]

tri·der·mic (trī-der′mik). Relating to or derived from the three primary germ layers of the embryo: ectoderm, endoderm, and mesoderm. [tri- + G. *derma,* skin]

tri·fid (trī′fid). Split into three. [L. *trifidus,* three-cleft]

tri·fur·ca·tion (trī-fŭr-kā′shŭn). **1.** A division into three branches. **2.** The area where the tooth roots divide into three distinct portions. [tri- + L. *furca,* fork]

tri·gas·tric (trī-gas′trik). Having three bellies; denoting a muscle with two tendinous interruptions. [tri- + G. *gastēr,* belly]

tri·gem·i·ny (trī-jem′i-nē). SYN trigeminal *rhythm.* [L. *trigeminus,* threefold]

tri·glyc·er·ide (trī-glis′er-īd). SYN triacylglycerol.

tri·go·na (trī-gō′nă). Plural of trigonum. [L.]

trig·o·nal (trig′ō-năl). Triangular; relating to a trigonum.

tri·gone (trī′gōn). **1.** SYN trigonum. **2.** The first three dominant cusps (protocone, paracone, and metacone), taken collectively, of an upper molar tooth. [L. *trigonum,* fr. G. *trigōnon,* triangle]

   t. of bladder, a triangular smooth area at the base of the bladder between the openings of the two ureters and that of the urethra. SYN trigonum vesicae [NA], vesical triangle.

   inguinal t., SYN inguinal *triangle.*

   vertebrocostal t., a triangular area in the diaphragm near the lateral arcuate ligament that is devoid of muscle fibers; it is covered by pleura superiorly and by peritoneum inferiorly.

tri·go·nid (trī-gon′id, -gō′nid). The first three dominant cusps, taken collectively, of a lower molar tooth. SEE ALSO trigone. [see *trigonum*]

tri·go·ni·tis (trī′gō-nī′tis). Inflammation of the urinary bladder, localized in the trigone. [trigone + G. *-itis,* inflammation]

trig·o·no·ce·phal·ic (trig′ō-nō-se-fal′ik). Pertaining to trigonocephaly.

trig·o·no·ceph·a·ly (trig′ō-nō-sef′ă-lē, trī′gō-nō-). Malformation characterized by a triangular configuration of the skull, due in part to premature synostosis of the cranial bones with compression of the cerebral hemispheres. [trigone + G. *kephalē,* head]

tri·go·num, pl. **tri·go·na** (trī-gō′nŭm, -nă). Any triangular area. SEE triangle. SYN trigone (1). [L., fr. G. *trigōnon,* a triangle]

   t. femora′le [NA], SYN femoral *triangle.*

   t. inguina′le [NA], SYN inguinal *triangle.*

   t. lumba′re [NA], SYN lumbar *triangle.*

   t. muscula′re [NA], SYN muscular *triangle.*

   t. submandibula′re [NA], SYN submandibular *triangle.*

   t. vesi′cae [NA], SYN *trigone* of bladder.

tri·labe (trī′lāb). A three-pronged forceps for removal of foreign bodies from the bladder. [tri- + G. *labē,* a handle, hold]

tri·lam·i·nar (trī-lam′i-nar). Having three laminae.

tri·lo·bate, tri·lobed (trī-lō′bāt, trī′lobd). Having three lobes.

tri·loc·u·lar (trī-lok′yū-lăr). Having three cavities or cells.

tril·o·gy (tril′ō-jē). A triad of related entities. [G. *trilogia,* fr. tri- + *logos,* study, discourse]

   t. of Fallot, a set of congenital defects including pulmonic stenosis, atrial septal defect, and right ventricular hypertrophy. SYN Fallot's triad.

tri·mes·ter (trī′mes-ter, trī-mes′ter). A period of 3 months; one-third of the length of a pregnancy. [L. *trimestris,* of three-month duration]

tri·meth·yl·a·mine (trī-meth′il-am′ēn). A degradation product, often by putrefaction, of nitrogenous plant and animal substances such as beet sugar residue or herring brine; in the body, it probably results from decomposition of choline.

tri·meth·yl·am·i·nur·ia (trī-meth′il-am-i-nūr′ē-ă). Increased excretion of trimethylamine in urine and sweat, with characteristic offensive, fishy body odor.

tri·nu·cle·o·tide (trī-nū′klē-ō-tīd). A combination of three adjacent nucleotides, free or in a polynucleotide or nucleic acid molecule; often used with specific reference to the unit (codon or anticodon) specifying a particular amino acid in expression of the genetic code.

tri·ose (trī′ōs). A three-carbon monosaccharide; *e.g.,* glyceraldehyde and dihydroxyacetone.

tri·ose·phos·phate isom·er·ase (trī′ōs-fos′fāt). An isomerizing enzyme that catalyzes the reversible interconversion of D-glyceraldehyde 3-phosphate and dihydroxyacetone phosphate, a reaction of importance in glycolysis and gluconeogenesis; a deficiency of this enzyme will result in hemolytic anemia and severe neurological deficits.

tri·ox·ide (trī-oks′īd). A molecule containing three atoms of oxygen.

tri·ple·gia (trī-plē′jē-ă). Paralysis of an upper and a lower extremity and of the face, or of both extremities on one side and of one on the other. [tri- + G. *plēgē,* stroke]

trip·let. 1. One of three children delivered at the same birth. **2.** A set of three similar objects, as a compound lens in a microscope, formed of three planoconvex lenses. **3.** SYN codon.

   nonsense t., **(1)** a trinucleotide (codon) in which a base change to a termination codon results in premature termination of the growing polypeptide chain and, consequently, incomplete protein molecules; **(2)** a termination codon.

trip·loid (trip′loyd). Pertaining to or characteristic of triploidy. [tri- + -ploid]

trip·loi·dy (trip′loy-dē). The presence of three haploid sets of chromosomes, instead of two, in all cells; results in fetal or neonatal death.

trip·lo·pia (trip-lō′pē-ă). Visual defect in which three images of the same object are seen. SYN triple vision. [G. *triploos,* triple, + *opsis,* sight]

△**tris-.** Chemical prefix indicating three of the substituents that follow, independently linked. Cf. tri-.

tris•mus (triz′mŭs). Persistent contraction of the masseter muscles due to failure of central inhibition; often the initial manifestation of generalized tetanus. SYN lockjaw. [L. fr. G. *trismos,* a creaking, rasping]

tri•so•mic (trī-sō′mik). Relating to trisomy.

tri•so•my (trī′sō-mē). The state of an individual or cell with an extra chromosome instead of the normal pair of homologous chromosomes; in humans, the state of a cell containing 47 normal chromosomes. For various types of trisomy syndrome, see under *syndrome.* [tri- + (chromo)-some]

tri•splanch•nic (trī-splangk′nik). Relating to the three visceral cavities: skull, thorax, and abdomen. [tri- + G. *splanchnon,* viscus]

tri•stich•ia (trī-stik′i-ă). Presence of three rows of eyelashes. [G. *tristichos,* in three rows, fr. *tri-,* three, + *stichos,* row]

tri•sul•cate (trī-sŭl′kāt). Marked by three grooves.

tri•ta•nom•a•ly (trī′tă-nom′ă-lē). A type of partial color deficiency due to a deficiency or abnormality of blue-sensitive retinal cones. [G. *tritos,* third, + *anōmalia,* irregularity]

trit•an•o•pia (trī′tă-nō′pē-ă). Deficient color perception in which there is an absence of blue-sensitive pigment in the retinal cones. [G. *tritos,* third, + *an-* priv. + *ōps,* eye]

trit•i•um (T, *t*) (trit′ē-ŭm, trish′-). SYN hydrogen-3.

trit•u•ra•ble (trit′yū-ră-bl). Capable of being triturated.

trit•u•rate (trit′yū-rāt). **1.** To accomplish trituration. **2.** A triturated substance.

trit•u•ra•tion (trit-yū-rā′shŭn). **1.** The act of reducing a drug to a fine powder and incorporating it thoroughly with sugar of milk by rubbing the two together in a mortar. **2.** Mixing of dental amalgam in a mortar and pestle or with a mechanical device. [L. *trituratio,* fr. *trituro,* to thresh, fr. *tero,* pp. *tritus,* to rub]

tri•va•lence, tri•va•len•cy (trī-vā′lens, -len-sē). The property of being trivalent.

tri•va•lent (trī-vā′lent). Having the combining power (valence) of 3.

triv•i•al name. A name of a chemical, no part of which is necessarily used in a systematic sense; *i.e.,* it gives little or no indication as to chemical structure. Such names are common for drugs, hormones, proteins, and other biologicals, and are used by the general public. Examples are water, aspirin, chlorophyll, heme, methotrexate, folic acid, caffeine, thyroxine, epinephrine, barbital, etc.; also common abbreviations for chemically defined substances, such as ACTH, MSH, BAL, DDT, which are spoken as such and not in terms of the words they represent. Trivial names are often assigned arbitrarily to chemical compounds, especially from natural sources, before the chemical structures are known.

tRNA Abbreviation for transfer RNA.

tro•car (trō′kar). An instrument for withdrawing fluid from a cavity, or for use in paracentesis; it consists of a metal tube (cannula) into which fits an obturator with a sharp three-cornered tip, which is withdrawn after the instrument has been pushed into the cavity; the name t. is usually applied to the obturator alone, the entire instrument being designated t. and cannula. [Fr. *trocart,* fr. *trois,* three, + *carre,* side (of a sword blade)]

tro•chan•ter (trō-kan′ter). One of two bony prominences developed from independent osseous centers near the upper extremity of the femur. [G. *trochantēr,* a runner, fr. *trechō,* to run]

   greater t., a strong process at the proximal and lateral part of the shaft of the femur, overhanging the root of the neck; it gives attachment to the gluteus medius and minimus, piriformis, obturator internus and externus, and gemelli muscles.

   lesser t., a pyramidal process projecting from the medial and proximal part of the shaft of the femur at the line of junction of the shaft and the neck; it receives the insertion of the psoas major and iliacus (iliopsoas) muscles.

tro•chan•ter•i•an, tro•chan•ter•ic (trō-kan-ter′ē-an, -ter′ik). Relating to a trochanter; especially the greater trochanter.

tro•che (trōk, trō′kē). A small, disk-shaped or rhombic body composed of solidifying paste containing an astringent, antiseptic, or demulcent drug, used for local treatment of the mouth or throat, the t. being held in the mouth until dissolved. SYN lozenge. [L. *trochiscus,* fr. G. *trochiskos,* a little wheel, fr. *trochos,* a wheel]

troch•lea, pl. **troch•le•ae** (trok′lē-ă, -lē-ē) [NA]. **1.** A structure serving as a pulley. **2.** A smooth articular surface of bone upon which another glides. **3.** A fibrous loop in the orbit, near the nasal process of the frontal bone, through which passes the tendon of the superior oblique muscle of the eye. [L. pulley, fr. G. *trochileia,* a pulley, fr. *trechō,* to run]

troch•le•ar (trok′lē-ar). **1.** Relating to a trochlea, especially the trochlea of the superior oblique muscle of the eye. **2.** SYN trochleiform.

troch•le•i•form (trok′lē-i-fōrm). Pulley-shaped. SYN trochlear (2).

tro•choid (trō′koyd). Revolving; rotating; denoting a revolving or wheel-like articulation. [G. *trochōdēs,* fr. *trochos,* wheel, + *eidos,* resemblance]

Trom•bic•u•la (trom-bik′yū-lă). The chigger mite, a genus of mites whose larvae (chiggers, red bugs) include pests of humans and other animals, and vectors of rickettsial and probably viral diseases.

trom•bic•u•li•a•sis (trom-bik-yū-lī′ă-sis). Infestation by mites of the genus *Trombicula.*

trom•bic•u•lid (trom-bik′yū-lid). Common name for members of the family Trombiculidae.

Trom•bic•u•li•dae (trom-bik-ū-lī′dē). A family of mites whose larvae (redbugs, rougets, harvest mites, scrub mites, or chiggers) are parasitic on vertebrates and whose nymphs and adults are bright red and free-living, living on insect eggs or minute organisms in the soil. The six-legged larvae are barely visible red or orange parasites that attach to the skin for a few days to a month, producing an exceedingly irritating reaction. Chiggers of the genus *Leptotrombidium* transmit tsutsugamushi disease, caused by *Rickettsia tsutsugamushi.*

Tr

△**troph-.** SEE tropho-.

troph•ec•to•derm (trof-ek′tō-derm). Outermost layer of cells in the mammalian blastodermic vesicle, which will make contact with the endometrium and take part in establishing the embryo's means of receiving nutrition; the cell layer from which the trophoblast differentiates. [troph- + ectoderm]

tro•phe•sic (trō-fē′sik). Pertaining to trophesy.

troph•e•sy (trof′ĭě-sē). The results of any disorder of the trophic nerves.

tro•phic (trof′ik, trō′fik). **1.** Relating to or dependent upon nutrition. **2.** Resulting from interruption of nerve supply. [G. *trophē,* nourishment]

△**-trophic.** Nutrition. Cf. -tropic. [G. *trophē,* nourishment]

△**tropho-, troph-.** Food, nutrition. [G. *trophē,* nourishment]

troph•o•blast (trof′ō-blast, trō′fō-blast). The mesectodermal cell layer covering the blastocyst that erodes the uterine mucosa and through which the embryo receives nourishment from the mother; the cells do not enter into the formation of the embryo itself, but contribute to the formation of the placenta. The t. develops processes that later receive a core of vascular mesoderm and are then known as the chorionic villi; the t. soon becomes two-layered, differentiating into the syncytiotrophoblast, an outer layer consisting of a multinucleated protoplasmic mass (syncytium), and the cytotrophoblast, the inner layer next to the mesoderm in which the cells retain their membranes. [tropho- + G. *blastos,* germ]

troph•o•blas•tic (trō-fō-blas′tik). Relating to the trophoblast.

troph•o•der•ma•to•neu•ro•sis (trof′ō-der′mă-tō-nū-rō′sis). Cutaneous trophic changes due to neural involvement.

troph•o•neu•ro•sis (trof′ō-nū-rō′sis). A trophic disorder, such as atrophy, hypertrophy, or a skin eruption, occurring as a consequence of disease or injury of the nerves of the part. [tropho- + G. *neuron,* nerve, + *-osis,* condition]

troph•o•neu•rot•ic (trof-ō-nū-rot′ik). Relating to a trophoneurosis.

troph•o•plast (trof′ō-plast). SYN plastid (1). [tropho- + G. *plastos,* formed]

troph•o•tax•is (trof-ō-tak′sis). SYN trophotropism. [tropho- + G. *taxis,* arrangement]

troph•o•tro•pic (trof-ō-trop′ik). Relating to trophotropism.

tro•phot•ro•pism (trō-fot′rō-pizm). Chemotaxis of living cells in relation to nutritive material; it may be positive (toward nutritive material) or negative (away from nutritive material). SYN trophotaxis. [tropho- + G. *trope,* a turning]

troph•o•zo•ite (trof-ō-zō′īt). The ameboid, vegetative, asexual form of certain Sporozoea, such as the schizont of the plasmodia of malaria and related parasites. [tropho- + G. *zōon,* animal]

△**-trophy.** Food, nutrition. [G. *trophē,* nourishment]

tro•pia (trō′pē-ă). Abnormal deviation of the eye. SEE strabismus. [G. *trope,* a turning]

△**-tropic.** A turning toward, having an affinity for. Cf. -trophic. [G. *trope,* a turning]

tro•pism (trō′pizm). The phenomenon, observed in living organisms, of moving toward (**positive t.**) or away from (**negative t.**) a focus of light, heat, or other stimulus; usually applied to the movement of a portion of the organism as opposed to taxis, the movement of an entire organism. [G. *trope,* a turning]

viral t., the specificity of a virus for a particular host tissue, determined in part by the interaction of viral surface structures with host cell-surface receptors.

tro•po•col•la•gen (trō-pō-kol′ă-jen, trop′ō-). The fundamental units of collagen fibrils, consisting of three helically arranged polypeptide chains.

tro•po•my•o•sin (trō-pō-mī′ō-sin). A fibrous protein extractable from muscle; sometimes specified as t. B to distinguish it from t. A (paramyosin) prominent in mollusks.

troponin (Tn) (trō′pō-nĭn). A complex of three proteins, troponin-C (TnC), troponin-I (TnI), troponin-T (TnT), present in striated muscle. Together, these proteins function as regulators of muscle contraction. There are a number of isoforms. The cardiac isoform of TnT is specific for cardiac muscle; the blood level of TnT rises within 4 hours after myocardial damage and remains elevated for 10–14 days after an acute myocardial infarction. Measurement of this protein is valuable in the early diagnosis of MI and in monitoring the effectiveness of thrombolytic therapy after an MI.

Trp tryptophan and its radicals.

trun•cal (trŭng′kăl). Relating to the trunk of the body or to any arterial or nerve trunk, etc.

trun•cate (trŭng′kāt). Truncated; cut across at right angles to the long axis, or appearing to be so cut. [L. *trunco,* pp. *-atus,* to maim, cut off]

trun•cus, gen. and pl. **trun•ci** (trŭng′kŭs, -kī). SYN trunk. [L. stem, trunk]

  t. brachiocepha′licus [NA], SYN brachiocephalic *trunk.*

  t. celi′acus [NA], SYN celiac *trunk.*

  t. costocervica′lis [NA], SYN costocervical *trunk.*

  persistent t. arterio′sus, a congenital cardiovascular deformity resulting from failure of development of the spiral septum and consisting of a common arterial trunk opening out of both ventricles, the pulmonary arteries being given off from the ascending common trunk.

  t. pulmona′lis [NA], SYN pulmonary *trunk.*

  t. sympath′icus [NA], SYN sympathetic *trunk.*

  t. thyrocervica′lis [NA], SYN thyrocervical *trunk.*

  t. vaga′lis [NA], SYN vagal *trunk.*

trunk (trŭnk). **1.** The body (trunk or torso), excluding the head and extremities. **2.** A primary nerve, vessel, or collection of tissue before its division. **3.** A large collecting lymphatic vessel. SYN truncus. [L. *truncus*]

  brachiocephalic t., *origin,* arch of aorta; *branches,* right subclavian and right common carotid; occasionally it gives off the thyroidea ima. SYN truncus brachiocephalicus [NA].

  celiac t., *origin,* abdominal aorta just below diaphragm; *branches,* left gastric, common hepatic, splenic. SYN truncus celiacus [NA], arteria celiaca, celiac artery.

costocervical t., a short artery that arises from the subclavian artery on each side and divides into deep cervical and superior intercostal branches, the latter dividing usually to form the first and second posterior intercostal arteries. SYN truncus costocervicalis [NA], costocervical artery.

pulmonary t., *origin,* right ventricle of heart; *distribution,* it divides into the right pulmonary artery and the left pulmonary artery, which enter the corresponding lungs and branch along with the segmental bronchi. SYN truncus pulmonalis [NA], arteria pulmonalis, pulmonary artery.

◼**sympathetic t.,** one of the two long ganglionated nerve strands alongside the vertebral column that extend from the base of the skull to the coccyx; they are connected to each spinal nerve by gray rami and receive fibers from the spinal cord through white rami connecting with the thoracic and upper lumbar spinal nerves. SYN truncus sympathicus [NA].

thyrocervical t., a short arterial t. arising from the subclavian artery, giving rise to the suprascapular (which may instead arise directly from the subclavian artery) and terminating by dividing into the ascending cervical and inferior thyroid arteries. SYN truncus thyrocervicalis [NA].

vagal t., one of the two nerve bundles, anterior and posterior, into which the esophageal plexus continues as it passes through the diaphragm. SYN truncus vagalis [NA].

truss (trŭs). An appliance designed to prevent the return of a reduced hernia or the increase in size of an irreducible hernia; it consists of a pad attached to a belt and kept in place by a spring or straps. [Fr. *trousser,* to tie up, to pack]

try·pan·o·ci·dal (tri-pan′ō-sī′dăl, trip′ă-nō-). Destructive to trypanosomes.

try·pan·o·cide (tri-pan′ō-sīd, trip′ă-nō-). An agent that kills trypanosomes. [trypanosome + L. *caedo,* to kill]

Try·pan·o·so·ma (tri-pan′ō-sō′mă, trip′ă-nō-). A genus of asexual digenetic protozoan flagellates that are parasitic in the blood plasma of many vertebrates and as a rule have an intermediate host, a bloodsucking invertebrate, such as a leech, tick, or insect; pathogenic species cause trypanosomiasis in humans. [G. *trypanon,* an auger, + *sōma,* body]

T. bru′cei gambien′se, a subspecies causing Gambian trypanosomiasis; transmitted by tsetse flies, especially *Glossina palpalis.* SYN *T. gambiense.*

T. bru′cei rhodesien′se, a subspecies causing Rhodesian trypanosomiasis; it is transmitted by tsetse flies, especially *Glossina morsitans;* various game animals can act as reservoir hosts. SYN *T. rhodesiense.*

T. cru′zi, a species that causes South American trypanosomiasis; transmission and infection are common only where the triatomine bug vector defecates while taking blood, as the bug feces contains the infective agents that are scratched into the skin or brought in contact with mucosal surfaces. Trypomastigotes are found in the blood; heart muscle and other organs are attacked.

T. gambien′se, SYN *T. brucei gambiense.*

T. rhodesien′se, SYN *T. brucei rhodesiense.*

try·pan·o·some (tri-pan′ō-sōm, trip′ă-nō-). Common name for any member of the genus *Trypanosoma* or of the family Trypanosomatidae. [G. *trypanon,* an auger, + *sōma,* body]

try·pan·o·so·mi·a·sis (tri-pan′ō-sō-mī′ă-sis, trip′ă-nō-). Any disease caused by a trypanosome.

acute t., SYN Rhodesian t.

African t., a serious endemic disease in tropical Africa, of two types: Gambian or West African t. and Rhodesian or East African t.

chronic t., SYN Gambian t.

Cruz t., SYN South American t.

Gambian t., a chronic disease of humans caused by *Trypanosoma brucei gambiense* in Africa; characterized by splenomegaly, drowsiness, an uncontrollable urge to sleep, and the development of psychotic changes; basal ganglia and cerebellar involvement commonly lead to chorea and athetosis; the terminal phase of the disease is characterized by wasting, anorexia, and emaciation that gradually leads to coma and death, usually from intercurrent infection. SYN chronic t.

Rhodesian t., a disease of humans caused by *Trypanosoma brucei rhodesiense* in eastern Africa; it is clinically similar to Gambian t. but of shorter duration and more acute in form; patients suffer repeated episodes of pyrexia, become anemic, and die commonly from cardiac failure. SYN acute African sleeping sickness, acute t.

South American t., t. caused by *Trypanosoma* (or *Schizotrypanum) cruzi* and transmitted by certain species of reduviid (triatomine) bugs. In its acute form, it is seen most frequently in young children, with swelling of the skin at the site of entry, most often the face, and regional lymph node enlargement; in its chronic form it can assume several aspects, commonly cardiomyopathy, but megacolon and megaesophagus also occur; natural reservoirs include domestic, domiciliated, and wild mammals. SYN Chagas-Cruz disease, Cruz t.

try·pan·o·so·mic (tri-pan-ō-sō′mik, trip′ă-nō-). Relating to trypanosomes, especially denoting infection by such organisms.

try·pan·o·so·mid (tri-pan′ō-sō-mid). A skin lesion resulting from immunologic changes from trypanosome disease. [trypanosome + G. *-id* (1)]

tryp·sin (trip′sin). A proteolytic enzyme formed in the small intestine from trypsinogen by the action of enteropeptidase; a serine proteinase that hydrolyzes peptides, amides, and esters.

tryp·sin·o·gen, tryp·so·gen (trip-sin′ō-jen, trip′sō-jen). An inactive protein secreted by the pancreas that is converted into trypsin by the action of enteropeptidase.

tryp·tic (trip′tik). Relating to trypsin, as t. digestion.

tryp·to·phan (Trp, W) (trip′tō-fan). The L-isomer is a component of proteins; a nutritionally essential amino acid.

t. 2,3-dioxygenase, an oxidoreductase catalyzing the reaction of L-t. and O_2 to produce L-*N*-formylkynurenine; an adaptive enzyme, the level (in the liver) being controlled by adrenal hormones; a step in t. catabolism; also, a step in the synthesis of NAD^+ from t. SYN tryptophanase (1).

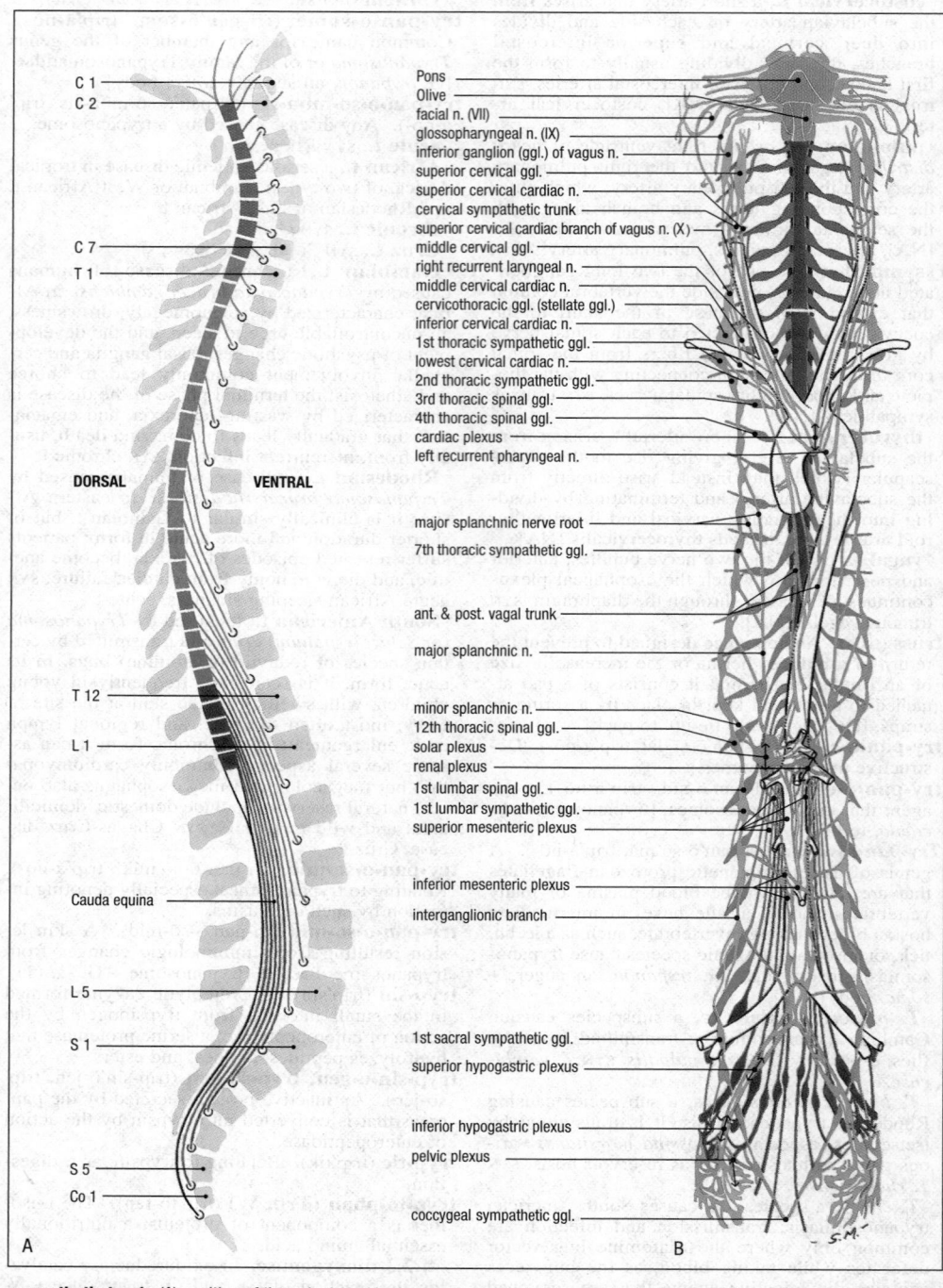

C 1
C 2

C 7
T 1

DORSAL   VENTRAL

T 12
L 1

Cauda equina

L 5

S 1

S 5
Co 1

A

Pons
Olive
facial n. (VII)
glossopharyngeal n. (IX)
inferior ganglion (ggl.) of vagus n.
superior cervical ggl.
superior cervical cardiac n.
cervical sympathetic trunk
superior cervical cardiac branch of vagus n. (X)
middle cervical ggl.
right recurrent laryngeal n.
middle cervical cardiac n.
cervicothoracic ggl. (stellate ggl.)
inferior cervical ggl.
1st thoracic sympathetic ggl.
lowest cervical cardiac n.
2nd thoracic sympathetic ggl.
3rd thoracic spinal ggl.
4th thoracic spinal ggl.
cardiac plexus
left recurrent pharyngeal n.

major splanchnic nerve root
7th thoracic sympathetic ggl.

ant. & post. vagal trunk

major splanchnic n.

minor splanchnic n.
12th thoracic spinal ggl.
solar plexus
renal plexus
1st lumbar spinal ggl.
1st lumbar sympathetic ggl.
superior mesenteric plexus

inferior mesenteric plexus

interganglionic branch

1st sacral sympathetic ggl.
superior hypogastric plexus

inferior hypogastric plexus
pelvic plexus

coccygeal sympathetic ggl.

B

sympathetic trunk: (A) position of the spinal cord in the vertebral canal; (B) sympathetic trunk and its relationship to the spinal nerves and their branches; (different colors indicate spinal cord segments and nerve roots in relation to segments of the vertebral column); cervical: brown, thoracic: red, sacral: green, coccygeal: purple

tryp·to·pha·nase (trip′to-fă-nās). **1.** SYN *trypto-phan* 2,3-dioxygenase. **2.** An enzyme found in bacteria that catalyzes the cleavage of L-trypto-phan to indole, pyruvic acid, and ammonia; pyri-doxal phosphate is a coenzyme.

tryp·to·pha·nu·ria (trip′tō-fă-nū′rē-ă). En-hanced urinary excretion of tryptophan.

tset·se (tset′sē, tsē′tsē). SEE *Glossina*. [S. African native name]

TSI thyroid-stimulating *immunoglobulins*, under *immunoglobulin*.

TSS toxic shock *syndrome*.

TSTA tumor-specific transplantation *antigens*, under *antigen*.

TT, TTY Telephone Device for the Deaf.

t$_i$/t$_{tot}$ duty *cycle*.

tu·ba, gen. and pl. **tu·bae** (tū′bă, tū′bē). SYN tube. [L. a straight trumpet]

tub·al (tū′băl). Relating to a tube, especially the uterine tube.

tube (tūb). **1.** A hollow cylindrical structure or canal. **2.** A hollow cylinder or pipe. SYN tuba. [L. *tubus*]

   auditory t., a tube leading from the tympanic cavity to the nasopharynx; it consists of an osse-ous (posterolateral) portion at the tympanic end, and a fibrocartilaginous (anteromedial) portion at the pharyngeal end; where the two portions join, in the region of the sphenopetrosal fissure, is the narrowest portion of the tube (isthmus); the audi-tory t. permits equalization of pressure within the tympanic cavity and ambient air pressure. SYN eustachian t., salpinx (2).

   Carlen's t., a double-lumen, flexible endobron-chial t. used for bronchospirometry, for isolation of one lung to prevent contamination or secre-tions from the contralateral lung, or for ventila-tion of one lung.

   chest t., a t. introduced into the intrapleural space to evacuate air or pleural fluid.

   drainage t., a t. introduced into a wound or cavity to facilitate removal of a fluid.

   endobronchial t., a single- or double-lumen t. with an inflatable cuff at the distal end that, after being passed through the larynx and trachea, is positioned so that ventilation is restricted to one lung; a single-lumen t. is placed in the mainstem bronchus of the lung; a double-lumen t. is posi-tioned at the tracheal carina to permit ventilation of either or both lungs.

   endotracheal t., SYN tracheal t.

   eustachian t., SYN auditory t.

   fallopian t., SYN uterine t.

   feeding t., a flexible t. passed through the oral pharynx and into the esophagus and stomach, through which liquid food is fed.

   Levin t., a t. introduced through the nose into the upper alimentary canal, to facilitate intestinal decompression.

   Miller-Abbott t., a t. with two lumens, one ending in a small collapsible balloon and the other in a metallic tip with numerous perfora-tions; used for intestinal decompression.

   molybdenum target t., an x-ray t. with an anode surface made of molybdenum instead of tungsten, used in mammography.

   Moss t., (1) a triple-lumen, nasogastric, feed-ing-decompression t. that utilizes a gastric bal-loon to occlude the cardioesophageal junction, with simultaneous esophageal aspiration and in-tragastric feeding; **(2)** a double-lumen, gastric la-vage t. that provides continuous delivery of saline via a small bore, with simultaneous aspiration of fluid and some particles via a large bore.

   nasogastric t., a stomach t. passed through the nose.

   nasotracheal t., a tracheal t. inserted through the nasal passages.

   nephrostomy t., a t. placed in the renal collect-ing system for drainage, diagnostic tests, or re-moval of calculi. May be placed through a percu-taneous route or during an open surgical proce-dure.

   orotracheal t., a tracheal t. inserted through the mouth.

   Sengstaken-Blakemore t., a t. with three lu-mens, one for drainage of the stomach and two for inflation of attached gastric and esophageal balloons; used for emergency treatment of bleed-ing esophageal varices.

   stomach t., a flexible t. passed into the stomach for lavage or feeding.

   test t., a round-bottomed, cylindrical vessel, usually of transparent glass, in which laboratory tests involving liquids are performed.

   Tovell t., an armored tracheal t. with a wire spiral embedded in the wall to prevent obstruc-tion of the lumen when the t. is compressed and kinking when the t. is bent at a sharp angle.

   tracheal t., a flexible t. inserted nasally, orally, or through a tracheotomy into the trachea to pro-vide an airway, as in tracheal intubation. SYN endotracheal t.

   tracheotomy t., a curved t. used to keep the opening free after tracheotomy. May be metal or plastic.

   tympanostomy t., a small t. inserted through the tympanic membrane after myringotomy to aerate the middle ear; often used for serous otitis media.

   uterine t., one of the t.'s leading on either side from the upper or outer extremity of the ovary, which is largely enveloped by its expanded infun-dibulum, to the fundus of the uterus; it consists of infundibulum, ampulla, isthmus, and uterine parts. SYN salpinx (1)☆, fallopian t., gonaduct (2), oviduct.

tu·bec·to·my (tū-bek′tō-mē). SYN salpingectomy. [L. *tuba*, tube, + G. *ektomē*, excision]

tu·ber, pl. **tu·bera** (tū′ber, tū′ber-ă). **1** [NA]. A localized swelling; a knob. **2.** A short, fleshy, thick, underground stem of plants, such as the potato. [L. protuberance, swelling]

   t. cine′reum [NA], a prominence of the base of the hypothalamus, bordered caudally by the mamillary bodies, rostrally by the optic chiasm, and laterally by the optic tract, extending ven-trally into the infundibulum and hypophysial stalk.

tu·ber·cle (tū′ber-kl). **1.** A nodule, especially in an anatomical, not pathologic, sense. SYN tuber-culum (1) [NA]. **2.** A circumscribed, rounded, solid elevation on the skin, mucous membrane, or surface of an organ. SYN tuberculum (1) [NA]. **3.**

tu

A slight elevation from the suface of a bone giving attachment to a muscle or ligament. SYN tuberculum (1) [NA]. **4.** DENTISTRY A small elevation arising on the surface of a tooth. **5.** A granulomatous lesion due to infection by *Mycobacterium tuberculosis*. T.'s tend to be fairly well circumscribed, spheroidal, firm lesions that consist of three irregularly outlined but moderately distinct zones: 1) an inner focus of necrosis, coagulative at first, and then becoming caseous; 2) a middle zone that consists of a dense accumulation of large mononuclear phagocytes (macrophages), frequently arranged radially, resembling an epithelium and hence termed epithelioid cells; multinucleated giant cells of Langhans type may also be present; 3) an outer zone of numerous lymphocytes, and a few monocytes and plasma cells. Indistinguishable lesions may occur in diseases caused by other agents. [L. *tuberculum*, dim. of *tuber*, a swelling]

auricular t., a small projection from the upper end of the posterior portion of the incurved free margin of the helix. SYN darwinian t.

darwinian t., SYN auricular t.

dissection t., SYN postmortem *wart*.

fibrous t., a t. in which fibroblasts proliferate about the periphery (and into the cellular zones), eventually resulting in a rim or wall of cellular fibrous tissue or collagenous material around the t.

genial t., SYN mental *spine*.

Ghon's t., calcification seen in pulmonary parenchyma (usually mid-lung area) and hilar nodes resulting from earlier, usually childhood, infection with tuberculosis. SYN Ghon's focus, Ghon's primary lesion.

hard t., a t. lacking necrosis.

hyaline t., a form of fibrous t. in which the cellular fibrous tissue and collagenous fibers become altered and merged into a fairly homogeneous, acellular, deeply acidophilic, firm mass.

intervenous t., the slight projection on the wall of the right atrium between the orifices of the venae cavae.

t. of rib, the knob on the posterior surface of a rib, at the junction of its neck and shaft, which articulates with the transverse process of the vertebra, which corresponds in number to the rib, forming a costotransverse joint.

soft t., a t. showing caseous necrosis.

t. of trapezium, a prominent ridge on the trapezium forming the lateral border of the groove in which runs the tendon of the flexor carpi radialis.

△**tubercul-.** SEE tuberculo-.

tu·ber·cu·la (tū-ber′kyū-lă). Plural of tuberculum.

tu·ber·cu·lar, tu·ber·cu·late, tu·ber·cu·lat·ed (tū-ber′kyū-lăr, -lāt, -lāt-ed). Pertaining to or characterized by tubercles or small nodules. Cf. tuberculous.

tu·ber·cu·lid (tū-ber′kyū-lid). A lesion of the skin or mucous membrane resulting from hypersensitivity to mycobacterial antigens disseminated from a distant site of active tuberculosis. [tubercul- + G. -*id* (1)]

papular t., SYN *lichen* scrofulosorum.

papulonecrotic t., dusky-red papules followed by crusting and ulceration primarily on the extremities and predominantly in young adults with a deep focus of tuberculosis or with a history of preceding infection.

tu·ber·cu·lin (tū-ber′kyū-lin). A glycerin-broth culture of *Mycobacterium tuberculosis* evaporated to $^1/_{10}$ volume at 100°C and filtered; used chiefly for diagnostic tests.

Koch's old t., Koch's original t., SEE tuberculin.

Koch's original t.,

tu·ber·cu·li·tis (tū-ber-kyū-lī′tis). Inflammation of any tubercle. [tubercul- + G. -*itis,* inflammation]

△**tuberculo-, tubercul-.** A tubercle, tuberculosis. [L. *tuberculum,* tubercle]

tu·ber·cu·lo·cele (tū-ber′kyū-lō-sēl). Tuberculosis of the testes. [tuberculo- + G. *kēlē,* tumor, hernia]

tu·ber·cu·lo·fi·broid (tū-ber′kyū-lō-fī′broyd). A discrete, well-circumscribed, usually spheroidal, moderately to extremely firm, encapsulated nodule that is formed during the process of healing in a focus of tuberculous granulomatous inflammation.

tu·ber·cu·loid (tū-ber′kyū-loyd). Resembling tuberculosis or a tubercle. [tuberculo- + G. *eidos,* resemblance]

tu·ber·cu·lo·ma (tū-ber-kyū-lō′mă). A rounded tumorlike but nonneoplastic mass, usually in the lungs or brain, due to localized tuberculous infection. [tuberculo- + G. -*oma,* tumor]

tu·ber·cu·lo·sis (TB) (tū-ber-kyū-lō′sis). A specific disease caused by the presence of *Mycobacterium tuberculosis*, which may affect almost any tissue or organ of the body, the most common seat of the disease being the lungs; the anatomical lesion is the tubercle, which can undergo caseation necrosis; general symptoms are those of sepsis: hectic fever, sweats, and emaciation; often progressive with high mortality if not treated. An opportunistic infection of persons with compromised immune systems, including those with AIDS. There is also a high incidence among IV drug abusers. [tuberculo- + G. -*osis,* condition]

acute t., a rapidly fatal disease due to the general dissemination of tubercle bacilli in the blood, resulting in the formation of miliary tubercles in various organs and tissues, and producing symptoms of profound toxemia. SYN disseminated t.

cutaneous t., pathologic lesions of the skin caused by *Mycobacterium tuberculosis*.

t. cu′tis verruco′sa, a tuberculous skin lesion having a warty surface with a chronic inflammatory base. SEE ALSO postmortem *wart*. SYN tuberculous wart.

disseminated t., SYN acute t.

enteric t., a complication of cavitary pulmonary t. usually resulting from expectoration and swallowing of bacilli that then infect areas of the digestive tract. SEE ALSO tuberculous *enteritis*.

open t., pulmonary t., tuberculous ulceration, or other form in which the tubercle bacilli are present in the excretions or secretions; in the lung, usually the result of cavity formation.

primary t., first infection by *Mycobacterium*

tuberculosis, typically seen in children but also occurs in adults, characterized in the lungs by the formation of a primary complex consisting of small peripheral pulmonary focus with spread to hilar or paratracheal lymph nodes; may cavitate or heal with scarring or may progress.

secondary t., t. found in adults and characterized by lesions near the apex of an upper lobe, which may cavitate or heal with scarring without spreading to lymph nodes; theoretically, secondary t. may be due to exogenous reinfection or to reactivation of a dormant endogenous infection.

tu·ber·cu·lo·stat·ic (tū-ber′kyū-lō-stat′ik). Relating to an agent that inhibits the growth of tubercle bacilli. [tuberculo- + G. *statikos,* causing to stand]

tu·ber·cu·lous (tū-ber′kyū-lŭs). Relating to or affected by tuberculosis. Cf. tubercular.

tu·ber·cu·lum, pl. **tu·ber·cu·la** (tū-ber′kyū-lŭm, -lă) [NA]. **1.** SYN tubercle (1), tubercle (2), tubercle (3). **2.** A circumscribed, rounded, solid elevation on the skin, mucous membrane, or surface of an organ. **3.** A slight elevation from the surface of a bone giving attachment to a muscle or ligament. [L. dim. of *tuber,* a knob, swelling, tumor]
t. arthrit′icum, (1) SYN Heberden's *nodes,* under *node.* **(2)** any gouty concretion in or around a joint.

tu·ber·os·i·tas (tū′ber-os′i-tas). SYN tuberosity. [LL., fr. L., *tuberosus,* full of lumps, fr. *tuber,* a knob]

tu·ber·os·i·ty (tū′ber-os′i-tē). A large tubercle or rounded elevation, especially from the surface of a bone. SYN tuberositas.

tu·ber·ous (tū′ber-ŭs). Knobby, lumpy, or nodular; presenting many tubers or tuberosities. [L. *tuberosus*]

△**tubo-.** Tubular, a tube. SEE ALSO salpingo-. [L. *tubus, tuba,* tube]

tu·bo·o·var·i·an (tū′bō-ō-vā′rē-an). Relating to the uterine (fallopian) tube and the ovary.

tu·bo·plas·ty (tū′bō-plas-tē). SYN salpingoplasty.

tu·bo·tor·sion (tū′bō-tōr-shŭn). Twisting of a tubular structure, such as an oviduct. [tubo- + L. *torsio,* torsion]

tu·bo·tym·pan·ic, tu·bo·tym·pa·nal (tū′bō-tim-pan′ik, -tim′pă-năl). Relating to the auditory tube and the tympanic cavity of the ear.

tu·bo·u·ter·ine (tū′bō-ū′ter-in). Relating to a uterine tube and the uterus.

tu·bule (tū′byūl). A small tube. SYN tubulus. [L. *tubulus,* dim. of *tubus,* tube]
convoluted t., either of two coiled segments of the renal t.; the proximal convoluted tubule leads from the capsule of the kidney to the straight portion of the proximal t.; the distal convoluted t. is formed from the ascending limb of Henle's loop and ends in a collecting t.
dentinal t.'s, SYN *canaliculi* dentales, under *canaliculus.*
renal t.'s, SEE convoluted t.
seminiferous t., the tubulus seminifer contortus or the tubulus seminifer rectus.
straight seminiferous t., the continuation of the t. seminifer contortus which becomes straight just before entering the mediastinum to form the rete testis. SYN vasa recta (2).

T t., the transverse t. that passes from the sarcolemma across a myofibril of striated muscle; it is the intermediate t. of the triad.

tu·bu·li (tū′byū-lī). Plural of tubulus.

tu·bu·lin (tū′byū-lin). A protein subunit of microtubules; it is a dimer composed of two globular polypeptides, α-tubulin and β-tubulin. SEE ALSO dynein.

tu·bu·lo·cyst (tū′byū-lō-sist). A cyst formed by the dilation of any occluded canal or tube. SYN tubular cyst.

tu·bu·lor·rhex·is (tū′byū-lō-rek′sis). A pathologic process characterized by necrosis of the epithelial lining in localized segments of renal tubules, with focal rupture or loss of the basement membrane. [tubule + G. *rhēxis,* a breaking]

tu·bu·lus, pl. **tu·bu·li** (tū′byū-lŭs, -lī). SYN tubule. [L. dim. of *tubus,* a pipe]

tu·bus, pl. **tu·bi** (tū′bŭs, -bī). A tube or canal. [L.]

tu·la·re·mia (tū-lă-rē′mē-ă). A disease caused by *Francisella tularensis* and transmitted to humans from rodents through the bite of a deer fly, *Chrysops discalis,* and other bloodsucking insects; can also be acquired directly through the bite of an infected animal or through handling of an infected animal carcass; symptoms consist of fever and swelling and suppuration of the lymph nodes draining the site of infection; rabbits are an important reservoir host. [*Tulare,* Lake and County, CA, + G. *haima,* blood]

tu·me·fac·tion (tū-mĕ-fak′shŭn). **1.** A swelling. **2.** SYN tumescence. [see tumefacient]

tu·me·fy (tū′mĕ-fī). To swell or to cause to swell.

tu·mes·cence (tū-mes′ens). The condition of being or becoming tumid. SYN tumefaction (2), turgescence. [L. *tumesco,* to begin to swell]

tu·mes·cent (tū-mes′ent). Denoting tumescence. SYN turgescent.

tu·mid (tū′mid). Swollen, as by congestion, edema, hyperemia. SYN turgid. [L. *tumidus*]

tu·mor (tū′mŏr). **1.** Any swelling or tumefaction. **2.** SYN neoplasm. **3.** One of the four signs of inflammation (t., calor, dolor, rubor) enunciated by Celsus. [L. *tumor,* a swelling]
adenomatoid t., a small benign t. of the male epididymis and female genital tract, consisting of fibrous tissue enclosing glandlike spaces lined by mesothelial cells. SYN adenofibromyoma, Recklinghausen's t.
adenomatoid odontogenic t., a benign epithelial odontogenic t. appearing radiographically as a well-circumscribed, radiolucent-radiopaque lesion usually surrounding the crown of an impacted tooth in an adolescent or young adult; characterized histologically by columnar cells organized in a ductlike configuration interspersed with spindle-shaped cells and amyloidlike deposition that gradually undergoes dystrophic calcification. SYN ameloblastic adenomatoid t.
ameloblastic adenomatoid t., SYN adenomatoid odontogenic t.
amyloid t., SYN nodular *amyloidosis.*
benign t., a t. that does not form metastases and does not invade and destroy adjacent normal tissue.
Brenner t., a benign neoplasm of the ovary,

consisting chiefly of fibrous tissue that contains nests of cells resembling transitional type epithelium, as well as glandlike structures that contain mucin; origin is controversial, but it may arise from Walthard's cell rest; ordinarily found incidentally in ovaries removed for other reasons, especially in postmenopausal women.

t. burden, The total mass of tumor tissue carried by a patient with cancer.

carcinoid t., a neoplasm composed of cells of medium size, with moderately small vesicular nuclei; neoplastic cells are frequently palisaded at the periphery of small groups. Such neoplasms occur in the gastrointestinal tract, the lungs, and other sites, with approximately 90% in the appendix. SEE ALSO carcinoid *syndrome*. SYN argentaffinoma.

chromaffin t., SYN chromaffinoma.

connective t., any t. of the connective tissue group, such as osteoma, fibroma, sarcoma.

dermoid t., SYN dermoid *cyst*.

desmoid t., SYN desmoid (2).

embryonal t., embryonic t., a neoplasm, usually malignant, which arises during intrauterine or early postnatal development from an organ rudiment or immature tissue; it forms immature structures characteristic of the part from which it arises, and may form other tissues as well. The term includes neuroblastoma and Wilms' t., and is also used to include certain neoplasms presenting in later life, this usage being based on the belief that such t.'s arise from embryonic rests. SEE ALSO teratoma. SYN embryoma.

endometrioid t., a t. of the ovary containing epithelial or stromal elements resembling t.'s of the endometrium.

Ewing's t., a malignant neoplasm which occurs usually before the age of 20 years and involves bones of the extremities, with a predilection for the metaphysis. SYN endothelial myeloma.

giant cell t. of bone, a soft, reddish-brown, sometimes malignant, osteolytic t. composed of multinucleated giant cells and ovoid or spindle-shaped cells, occurring most frequently in an end of a long tubular bone of young adults. SYN giant cell myeloma, osteoclastoma.

giant cell t. of tendon sheath, a nodule arising commonly from the flexor sheath of the fingers and thumb; composed of fibrous tissue, lipid- and hemosiderin-containing macrophages, and multinucleated giant cells. SYN localized nodular tenosynovitis.

glomus t. [MIM*138000], an unusual vascular neoplasm composed of specialized pericytes, usually in nodular masses, which occurs almost exclusively in the skin; it is exquisitely tender and may be so painful that patients voluntarily immobilize an extremity. SEE ALSO glomangioma.

glomus jugulare t., SYN chemodectoma.

granular cell t., a microscopically specific, generally benign t., often involving peripheral nerves in skin, mucosa, or connective tissue, derived from Schwann cells; the abundant cytoplasm contains lysosomal granules, the cells infiltrate between adjacent tissues although growth is slow, and adjacent surface epithelium may show hyperplasia.

granulosa cell t., a benign or malignant t. of the ovary arising from the membrana granulosa of the ovarian (graafian) follicle and frequently secreting estrogen. SYN folliculoma (1).

haarscheibe t., SYN trichodiscoma. [Ger. *Haar,* hair, + *Scheibe,* disk]

heterologous t., a t. composed of a tissue unlike that from which it springs.

homologous t., a t. composed of tissue of the same sort as that from which it springs.

Hürthle cell t., a neoplasm of the thyroid gland composed of polyhedral acidophilic cells, thought by some to be oncocytes; it may be benign or malignant, the behavior of the latter depending on the general microscopic pattern, whether follicular, papillary, or undifferentiated. SEE ALSO Hürthle cell *adenoma*. SYN Hürthle cell carcinoma.

Krukenberg's t., a metastatic carcinoma of the ovary, usually bilateral and secondary to a mucous carcinoma of the stomach, which contains signet-ring cells filled with mucus.

malignant t., a t. that invades surrounding tissues, is usually capable of producing metastases, may recur after attempted removal, and is likely to cause death of the host unless adequately treated. SEE ALSO cancer.

melanotic neuroectodermal t. of infancy, a benign neoplasm of neuroectodermal origin that most often involves the anterior maxilla of infants in the first year of life. It presents clinically as a rapidly growing blue-black lesion producing a destructive radiolucency; histologically, it is characterized by small, round, undifferentiated t. cells interspersed with larger polyhedral melanin-producing cells arranged in an alveolar configuration.

mixed t., a t. composed of two or more varieties of tissue.

oncocytic hepatocellular t., SYN fibrolamellar liver cell *carcinoma*.

organoid t., a t. of complex structure, glandular in origin, containing epithelium and connective tissue.

papillary t., SYN papilloma.

phantom t., accumulation of fluid in the interlobar spaces of the lung, secondary to congestive heart failure, radiologically simulating a neoplasm.

pilar t. of scalp, a benign solitary t. of the scalp in elderly women that may ulcerate.

Recklinghausen's t., SYN adenomatoid t.

squamous odontogenic t., a benign epithelial odontogenic t. thought to arise from the epithelial cell rests of Malassez; appears clinically as a radiolucent lesion closely associated with the tooth root and histologically as islands of squamous epithelium enclosed by a peripheral layer of flattened cells.

teratoid t., SYN teratoma.

triton t., a peripheral nerve t. with striated muscle differentiation, seen most often in neurofibromatosis.

Wilms' t., a malignant renal t. of young children, composed of small spindle cells and various other types of tissue, including tubules and, in some cases, structures resembling fetal glomeruli, and striated muscle and cartilage. Often inherited as an autosomal dominant trait [MIM*194070, *194080, *194090].

tu·mor·i·ci·dal (tū′mŏr-i-sī′dăl). Denoting an agent destructive to tumors. [tumor + L. *caedo,* to kill]

tu·mor·i·gen·e·sis (tū′mŏr-i-jen′ĕ-sis). Production of a new growth or growths. [tumor + G. *genesis,* origin]

tu·mor·i·gen·ic (tū′mŏr-i-jen′ik). Causing or producing tumors.

Tun·ga pen·e·trans (tŭng′ă pen′ĕ-tranz). A member of the flea family, Tungidae, commonly known as chigger flea, sand flea, chigoe, or jigger; the minute female penetrates the skin, frequently under the toenails; as she becomes distended with eggs to about pea size, a painful ulcer with inflammation develops at the site.

tung·sten (W) (tŭng′sten). A metallic element, atomic no. 74, atomic wt. 183.85. SYN wolfram, wolframium. [Swed. *tung,* heavy, + *sten,* stone]

tu·nic (tū′nik). Coat or covering; one of the enveloping layers of a part, especially one of the coats of a blood vessel or other tubular structure. SYN tunica [NA]. [L. *tunica*]

   vascular t. of eye, the vascular, pigmentary, or middle coat of the eye, comprising the choroid, ciliary body, and iris.

tu·ni·ca, pl. **tu·ni·cae** (tū′ni-kă, -sē) [NA]. SYN tunic. [L. a coat]

   t. albugin′ea [NA], a dense white collagenous tunic surrounding a structure.

   t. albuginea of testis, a thick white fibrous membrane forming the outer coat of the testis.

   t. exter′na [NA], **(1)** the outer of two or more enveloping layers of any structure; **(2)** specifically, the outer fibroelastic coat of a blood or lymph vessel.

   t. in′tima [NA], the innermost coat of a blood or lymphatic vessel; it consists of endothelium, usually a thin fibroelastic subendothelial layer, and an inner elastic membrane or longitudinal fibers.

   t. me′dia [NA], the middle, usually muscular, coat of an artery or other tubular structure. SYN media (1).

   t. pro′pria, the special envelope of a part as distinguished from the peritoneal or other investment common to several parts.

   t. reflex′a, the reflected layer of the t. vasculosa testis that lines the scrotum.

   t. vagina′lis tes′tis [NA], the serous sheath of the testis and epididymis, derived from the peritoneum; it consists of outer parietal and inner visceral serous layers.

   t. vasculo′sa, any vascular layer.

tun·nel (tŭn′ĕl). An elongated passageway, usually open at both ends.

   carpal t., the passageway deep to the transverse carpal ligament between tubercles of the scaphoid and trapezoid bones on the radial side and the pisiform and hook of the hamate on the ulnar side, through which the median nerve and the flexor tendons of the fingers and thumb pass. SYN canalis carpi [NA].

   Corti's t., the spiral canal in the organ of Corti, formed by the outer and inner pillar cells or rods

of Corti; it is filled with fluid and occasionally crossed by nonmedullated nerve fibers. SYN Corti's canal.

tur·bid (ter′bid). Cloudy, as by sediment or insoluble matter in a solution. [L. *turbidus,* confused, disordered]

tur·bi·dim·e·try (ter-bi-dim′ĕ-trē). A method for determining the concentration of a substance in a solution by the degree of cloudiness or turbidity it causes or by the degree of clarification it induces in a turbid solution. [turbidity + G. *metron,* measure]

tur·bid·i·ty (ter-bid′i-tē). The quality of being turbid, of losing transparency because of sediment or insoluble matter. [L. *turbiditas,* fr. *turbidus,* turbid]

tur·bi·nate (ter′bi-nāt). **1.** Shaped like a top. **2.** Any of the turbinated bones. SEE inferior nasal *concha,* middle nasal *concha,* superior nasal *concha,* supreme nasal *concha.*

tur·bi·nat·ed (ter′bi-nāt-ed). Scroll-shaped. [L. *turbinatus,* shaped like a top]

tur·bi·nec·to·my (ter′bi-nek′tō-mē). Surgical removal of a turbinated bone. [turbinate + G. *ektomē,* excision]

tur·bi·not·o·my (ter′bi-not′ō-mē). Incision into or excision of a turbinated body. [turbinate + G. *tomē,* incision]

tur·ges·cence (ter-jes′ens). SYN tumescence. [L. *turgesco,* to begin to swell, fr. *turgeo,* to swell]

tur·ges·cent (ter-jes′ent). SYN tumescent.

tur·gid (ter′jid). SYN tumid. [L. *turgidus,* swollen, fr. *turgeo,* to swell]

tur·gor (ter′gōr). Fullness. [L., fr. *turgeo,* to swell]

tu·ris·ta (tū-rēs′tă). SYN traveler's *diarrhea.* [Sp. tourist]

tus·sal (tŭs′ăl). SYN tussive.

tus·sis (tŭs′is). A cough. [L.]

tus·sive (tŭs′siv). Relating to a cough. SYN tussal. [L. *tussis,* a cough]

twin. 1. One of two children born at one birth. **2.** Double; growing in pairs. [A.S. *getwin,* double]

   allantoidoangiopagous t.'s, unequal monochorial t.'s with fusion of their allantoic vessels within the placenta; the lesser t. is essentially a parasite on the placental circulation of the larger t.

   conjoined t.'s, monozygotic t.'s with varying extent of union and different degrees of residual duplication. The various types of union are named by the use of a prefix designating the region that is united and adding the suffix *-pagus,* meaning fused (*e.g.,* craniopagus, thoracopagus); the various types of residual duplication are named by designating the parts duplicated and adding the suffix *-didymus,* or *-dymus,* meaning twin (*e.g.,* cephalodidymus, cephalodymus).

   dizygotic t.'s, t.'s derived from two separate zygotes. SYN fraternal t.'s, heterologous t.'s.

   enzygotic t.'s, SYN monozygotic t.'s.

   fraternal t.'s, SYN dizygotic t.'s.

   heterologous t.'s, SYN dizygotic t.'s.

   identical t.'s, SYN monozygotic t.'s.

   monoamniotic t.'s, t.'s within a common amnion; such t.'s are monovular in origin and may be conjoined.

monozygotic t.'s, t.'s resulting from a single fertilized ovum that at an early stage of development becomes separated into independently growing cell aggregations giving rise to two individuals of the same sex and identical genetic constitution. SYN enzygotic t.'s, identical t.'s.

Siamese t.'s, a much publicized pair of conjoined t.'s born in Siam in the 19th century; this term has since come into general lay usage for any type of conjoined t.'s.

twinge (twinj). A sudden momentary sharp pain.

twin·ning. Production of equivalent structures by division; the tendency of divided parts to assume symmetrical relations.

twitch. 1. To jerk spasmodically. 2. A momentary spasmodic contraction of a muscle fiber. [A.S. *twiccian*]

ty·lec·to·my (tī-lek′tō-mē). Surgical removal of a localized swelling or tumor. SEE ALSO lumpectomy. [G. *tylē,* lump, + *ektomē,* excision]

ty·lo·ma (tī-lō′mă). SYN callosity. [G. a callus]

ty·lo·sis, pl. **ty·lo·ses** (tī-lō′sis, -sēz). Formation of a callosity (tyloma). [G. a becoming callous]

ty·lot·ic (tī-lot′ik). Relating to or marked by tylosis.

△**tympan-.** SEE tympano-.

tym·pa·nal (tim′pă-năl). **1.** SYN tympanic (1). **2.** Resonant. **3.** SYN tympanitic (2).

tym·pa·nec·to·my (tim′pă-nek′tō-mē). Excision of the tympanic membrane. [tympan- + G. *ektomē,* excision]

tym·pan·ic (tim-pan′ik). **1.** Relating to the tympanic cavity or membrane. SYN tympanal (1). **2.** Resonant. **3.** SYN tympanitic (2).

tym·pa·nism (tim′pă-nizm). SYN tympanites.

tym·pa·ni·tes (tim-pă-nī′tēz). Swelling of the abdomen from gas in the intestinal or peritoneal cavity. SYN meteorism, tympanism. [L. fr. G. *tympanitēs,* an edema in which the belly is stretched like a drum, *tympanon*]

tym·pa·nit·ic (tim-pă-nit′ik). **1.** Referring to tympanites. SYN tympanous. **2.** Denoting the quality of sound elicited by percussing over the inflated intestine or a large pulmonary cavity. SYN tympanal (3), tympanic (3).

tym·pa·ni·tis (tim-pă-nī′tis). SYN myringitis.

△**tympano-, tympan-, tympani-.** Tympanum, tympanites. [G. *tympanon,* drum]

tym·pa·no·cen·te·sis (tim′pă-nō-sen-tē′sis). Puncture of the tympanic membrane with a needle to aspirate middle ear fluid. [tympano- + G. *kentēsis,* puncture]

▊**tympanogram** (tim′pah-nō-gram). A visual depiction (*e.g.,* a printout) of the relative compliance and impedance of the structures of the middle ear in response to pressure changes in the external ear canal.

tympanometry. Measurement of the pressure-compliance function of the eardrum using an immitance instrument (audiometer).

tym·pa·no·plas·ty (tim′pă-nō-plas-tē). Operative correction of a damaged middle ear. [tympano- + G. *plassō,* to form]

tym·pan·os·to·my (tim-pan-os′tō-mē). SYN myringotomy. [tympano- + G. *ostium,* mouth]

tym·pa·not·o·my (tim′pă-not′ō-mē). SYN myringotomy. [tympano- + G. *tomē,* incision]

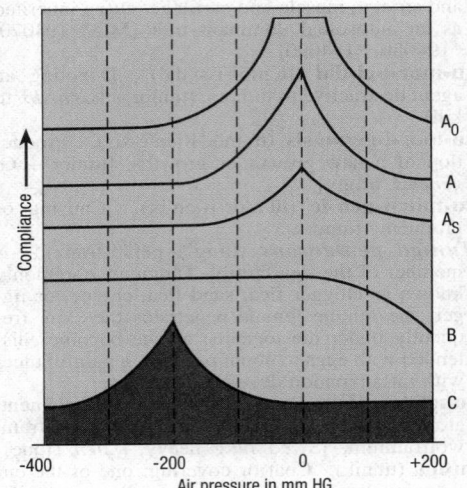

tympanogram: five typical tympanograms illustrating various conditions of the middle ear: type A is typical of normal middle ear; type A$_S$ is associated with stiffness of stapes; type A$_O$ is associated with interruptions in the chain of bones or flaccidity of the eardrum membrane; type B suggests fluid in the middle ear space; type C suggests that the pressure within the middle ear space is below atmospheric pressure

tym·pa·nous (tim′pă-nŭs). SYN tympanitic (1).

tym·pa·ny (tim′pă-nē). A low-pitched, resonant, drumlike note obtained by percussing the surface of a large air-containing space, such as the distended abdomen or the thorax with or without pneumothorax. SYN tympanitic resonance.

type (tīp). **1.** The usual form, or a composite form, that all others of the class resemble more or less closely; a model, denoting especially a disease or a symptom complex giving the stamp or characteristic to a class. SEE ALSO constitution, habitus, personality. **2.** CHEMISTRY A substance in which the arrangement of the atoms in a molecule may be taken as representative of other substances in that class. [G. *typos,* a mark, a model]

basic personality t., (1) an individual's unique, covert, or underlying personality propensities, whether or not they are behaviorally manifest or overt; (2) personality characteristics of an individual which are also shared by a majority of the members of a social group.

blood t., SEE blood type.

wild t., a gene, phenotype, or genotype that is overwhelmingly common among those possible at a locus of interest, and therefore presumably not harmful.

△**typhl-.** SEE typhlo-.

typh·lec·ta·sis (tif-lek′tă-sis). Dilation of the cecum. [G. *typhlon,* cecum, + *ektasis,* a stretching out]

typh·lec·to·my (tif-lek′tō-mē). SYN cecectomy.

typh·len·ter·i·tis (tif′len-ter-ī′tis). SYN cecitis.

typh·li·tis (tif′lī′tis). SYN cecitis.

△**typhlo-, typhl-.** **1.** The cecum. SEE ALSO ceco-. [G. cecum] **2.** Blindness. [G. *typhlos,* blind]

typh·lo·dic·li·di·tis (tif-lō-dik-li-dī′tis). Inflammation of the ileocecal valve. [G. *typhlon*, cecum, + *diklis* (*diklid-*), double-folding (of doors), + *-itis*, inflammation]

typh·lo·en·ter·i·tis (tif′lō-en-ter-ī′tis). SYN cecitis.

typh·lo·li·thi·a·sis (tif′lō-li-thī′ă-sis). Presence of fecal concretions in the cecum. [G. *typhlon*, cecum, + *lithos*, stone]

typh·lo·pexy, typh·lo·pex·ia (tif′lō-pek-sē, tif-lō-pek′sē-ă). SYN cecopexy.

typh·lor·rha·phy (tif-lōr′ă-fē). SYN cecorrhaphy.

typh·lo·sis (tif-lō′sis). SYN blindness. [G. *typhlos*, blind]

typh·los·to·my (tif-los′tō-mē). SYN cecostomy.

typh·lot·o·my (tif-lot′ō-mē). SYN cecotomy.

ty·phoid (tī′foyd). **1.** Typhus-like; stuporous from fever. **2.** SYN typhoid *fever*. [typhus + G. *eidos*, resemblance]

ty·phoi·dal (tī-foyd′ăl). Relating to or resembling typhoid fever.

ty·phous (tī′fŭs). Relating to typhus.

ty·phus (tī′fŭs). A group of acute infectious and contagious diseases, caused by rickettsiae that are transmitted by arthropods, and occurring in two principal forms: epidemic t. and endemic (murine) t. Also called jail, camp, or ship fever. SYN camp fever (1). [G. *typhos*, smoke, stupor]

  endemic t., SYN murine t.

  epidemic t., t. caused by *Rickettsia prowazekii* and spread by body lice; marked by high fever, mental and physical depression, and a macular and papular eruption; lasts for about two weeks and occurs when large crowds are brought to-

gether and personal hygiene is at a low ebb; recrudescences can occur.

  mite t., SYN tsutsugamushi *disease*.

  murine t., a milder form of epidemic t. caused by *Rickettsia typhi* and transmitted to humans by rat or mouse fleas. SYN endemic t.

  recrudescent t., SYN Brill-Zinsser *disease*.

  scrub t., SYN tsutsugamushi *disease*.

  tick t., SYN boutonneuse *fever*.

  tropical t., SYN tsutsugamushi *disease*.

typ·ing (tīp′ing). Classification according to type. [see type]

  HLA t., tests done in order to determine if a patient has antibodies against a potential donor's HLA antigens. The presence of antibodies means that a graft will be rejected. Also used to establish paternity and in forensic medicine.

Tyr tyrosine and its radicals.

ty·ro·ke·to·nu·ria (tī′rō-kē-tō-nū′rē-ă). The urinary excretion of ketonic metabolites of tyrosine, such as *p*-hydroxyphenylpyruvic acid.

ty·ro·ma (tī-rō′mă). A caseous tumor. [G. *tyros*, cheese, + *-ōma*, tumor]

ty·ro·sine (Tyr, Y) (tī′rō-sēn, -sin). An α-amino acid present in most proteins.

ty·ro·si·nu·ria (tī′rō-si-nū′rē-ă). The excretion of tyrosine in the urine. [tyrosine + G. *ouron*, urine]

ty·ro·sy·lu·ria (tī′rō-si-lū′rē-ă). Enhanced urinary excretion of certain metabolites of tyrosine, such as *p*-hydroxyphenylpyruvic acid; present in tyrosinosis, scurvy, pernicious anemia, and other diseases.

ty

U

ʊ. SEE upsilon.

U 1. unit. 2. kilurane; uranium; uridine in polymers; uracil; internal *energy*; urinary concentration, followed by subscripts indicating location and chemical species.

ubi·qui·nol (yū'bi-kwī'nol, yū-bik'wi-nol). The reduction product of a ubiquinone.

ubi·qui·none (yū'bi-kwī'nōn, yū-bik'wi-nōn). A 2,3-dimethoxy-5-methyl-1,4-benzoquinone with a multiprenyl side chain; a mobile component of electron transport. SEE ALSO coenzyme Q.

ubiq·ui·tin (yū-bik'kwi-tin). A small protein found in all cells of higher organisms and one whose structure has changed minimally during evolutionary history; involved in histone modification and intracellular protein breakdown.

UDP *uridine* 5'-diphosphate.

UDPglu·cose-hex·ose-1-phos·phate uri·dyl·yl·trans·fer·ase. An enzyme that catalyzes the reversible reaction of α-D-glucose 1-phosphate UDPgalactose to produce UDPglucose and α-D-galactose 1-phosphate.

UGIS upper gastrointestinal *series*.

ul·cer (ŭl'ser). A lesion on the surface of the skin or on a mucous surface, caused by superficial loss of tissue, usually with inflammation. SYN ulcus. [L. *ulcus* (*ulcer-*), a sore, ulcer]

   anastomotic u., an u. of jejunum, after gastroenterostomy.

   chronic u., a longstanding u. with fibrous scar tissue in the floor of the u.

   cold u., a small, gangrenous u. on the extremities; due to defective circulation.

   Curling's u., an u. of the duodenum in a patient with extensive superficial burns, intracranial lesions, or severe bodily injury. SYN stress u.

   ▣ **decubitus u.,** breakdown of skin and underlying tissues caused by constant pressure and inadequate oxygenation. SEE decubitus. SYN bedsore, pressure sore.

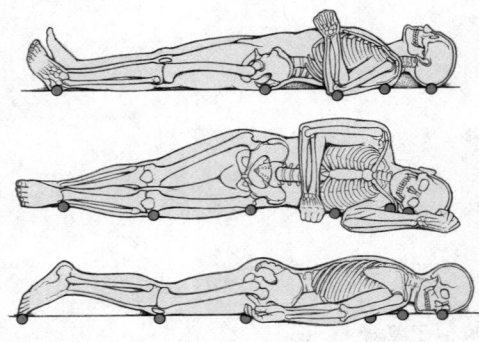

decubitus ulcer: most common sites due to proximity of bone to skin

   dendritic corneal u., keratitis caused by herpes simplex virus.

   gravitational u., a chronic u. of the leg with impaired healing because of the incompetence of the valves of varicose veins; the venous return

stagnates and creates hypoxemia. SEE ALSO varicose u.

   hard u., SYN chancre.

   Hunner's u., a focal and often multiple lesion involving all layers of the bladder wall in chronic interstitial cystitis; the surface epithelium is destroyed by inflammation and the initially pale lesion cracks and bleeds with distention of the bladder.

   Meleney's u., undermining u. of the skin and subcutaneous tissues, usually following an operation, caused by a synergistic interaction between microaerophilic nonhemolytic streptococci and aerobic hemolytic staphylococci.

   peptic u., an u. of the alimentary mucosa, usually in the stomach or duodenum, exposed to acid gastric secretion.

   perforated u., an u. extending through the wall of an organ.

   phagedenic u., a rapidly spreading u. attended by the formation of extensive sloughing.

   recurrent aphthous u.'s, SYN aphtha (2).

   rodent u., a slowly enlarging ulcerated basal cell carcinoma, usually on the face.

   soft u., SYN chancroid.

   stercoral u., an u. of the colon due to pressure and irritation of retained fecal masses.

   steroid u., an u., usually on the leg or foot, developing from a wound in patients undergoing long-term steroid therapy; results from the wound-healing inhibitory effects characteristic of steroids.

   stomal u., an intestinal u. occurring after gastrojejunostomy in the jejunal mucosa near the opening (stoma) between the stomach and the jejunum.

   stress u., SYN Curling's u.

   trophic u., u. resulting from cutaneous sensory denervation.

   tropical u., (1) the lesion occurring in cutaneous leishmaniasis; **(2)** tropical phagedenic ulceration caused by a variety of microorganisms, including mycobacteria; common in northern Nigeria.

   varicose u., the loss of skin surface in the drainage area of a varicose vein, usually in the leg, resulting from stasis and infection.

   venereal u., SYN chancroid.

ul·ce·ra (ŭl'ser-ă). Plural of ulcus.

ul·cer·ate (ŭl'ser-āt). To form an ulcer.

ul·cer·a·tion (ŭl-ser-ā'shŭn). 1. The formation of an ulcer. 2. An ulcer or aggregation of ulcers.

ul·cer·a·tive (ŭl'ser-ă-tiv). Relating to, causing, or marked by an ulcer or ulcers.

ul·cer·ous (ŭl'ser-ŭs). Relating to, affected with, or containing an ulcer. [L. *ulcerosus*]

ul·cus, pl. **ul·ce·ra** (ŭl'kŭs, ŭl'ser-ă). SYN ulcer. [L.]

△**ule-.** SEE ulo-.

uler·y·the·ma (ū'ler-i-thē'mă). Scarring with erythema. [G. *oulē,* scar, + *erythēma,* redness of the skin]

ul·na, gen. and pl. **ul·nae** (ŭl'nă, ŭl'nē) [NA]. The medial and larger of the two bones of the forearm. SYN cubitus (2) [NA]. [L. elbow, arm, fr. G. *ōlenē*]

ul•nad (ŭl′nad). In a direction toward the ulna. [ulna + L. *ad,* to]

ul•nar (ŭl′năr). Relating to the ulna, or to any of the structures (artery, nerve, etc.) named from it; relating to the ulnar or medial aspect of the upper limb.

♻**ulo-, ule-.** **1.** Scar, scarring. [G. *oulē*] **2.** The gums. SEE ALSO gingivo-. [G. *oulon*] **3.** Curly. [G. *oulo-, ouli-,* woolly.]

ulo•der•ma•ti•tis (ū′lō-der-mă-tī′tis). Inflammation of the skin resulting in destruction of tissue and the formation of scars. [G. *oulē,* scar, + *derma,* skin, + *-itis,* inflammation]

uloid (yū′loyd). **1.** Resembling a scar. **2.** A scarlike lesion due to a degenerative process in deeper layers of skin. [G. *oulē,* scar + *eidos,* resemblance]

♻**ultra-.** Excess, exaggeration, beyond. [L. beyond]

ul•tra•cen•tri•fuge (ŭl′tră-sen′tri-fyūj). A highspeed centrifuge by means of which large molecules, *e.g.,* of protein or nucleic acids, are caused to sediment at practicable rates.

ul•tra•di•an (ŭl-trā′dē-ăn). Relating to biologic variations or rhythms occurring in cycles more frequent than every 24 hours. Cf. circadian, infradian. [ultra- + L. *dies,* day]

ul•tra•fil•tra•tion (ŭl′tră-fil-trā′shŭn). Filtration through a semipermeable membrane or any filter that separates colloid solutions from crystalloids or separates particles of different size in a colloid mixture.

ul•tra•li•ga•tion (ŭl-tră-lī-gā′shŭn). Ligation of a blood vessel beyond the point where a branch is given off.

ul•tra•mi•cro•scop•ic (ŭl′tră-mī-krō-skop′ik). SYN submicroscopic.

ul•tra•mi•cro•tome (ŭl-tră-mī′krō-tōm). A microtome used in cutting sections 0.1 μm thick, or less, for electron microscopy.

ul•tra•son•ic (ŭl-tră-son′ik). Relating to energy waves similar to those of sound but of higher frequencies (above 30,000 Hz). [ultra- + L. *sonus,* sound]

ul•tra•son•ics (ŭl-tră-son′iks). The science and technology of ultrasound, its characteristics and phenomena.

ul•tra•son•o•gram (ŭl-tră-son′ō-gram). The image obtained by ultrasonography. SEE ALSO echogram. SYN sonogram.

ul•tra•son•o•graph (ŭl-tră-son′ō-graf). Computerized instrument used to create an image using ultrasound. SYN sonograph. [ultra- + L. *sonus,* sound, + G. *graphō,* to write]

ul•tra•so•nog•ra•pher (ŭl′tră-sŏ-nog′ră-fer). A person who performs and interprets ultrasonographic examinations. SYN sonographer.

ul•tra•so•nog•ra•phy (ŭl′tră-sŏ-nog′ră-fē). The location, measurement, or delineation of deep structures by measuring the reflection or transmission of high frequency or ultrasonic waves. Computer calculation of the distance to the sound-reflecting or absorbing surface plus the known orientation of the sound beam gives a two-dimensional image. SEE ALSO ultrasound. SYN

echography, sonography. [ultra- + L. *sonus,* sound, + G. *graphō,* to write]

▯**Doppler u.,** application of the Doppler effect in ultrasound to detect movement of scatterers (usually red blood cells) by the analysis of the change in frequency of the returning echoes.

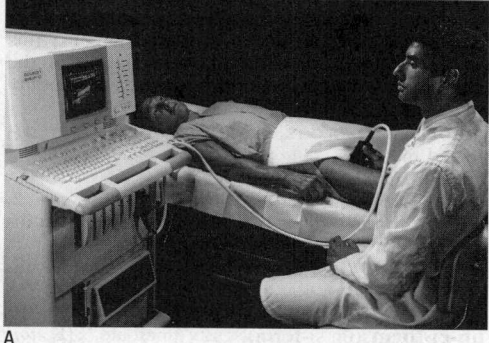

A

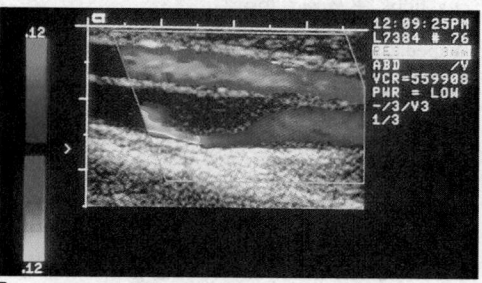

B

Doppler ultrasonography: (A) vascular imaging (B) color flow Doppler showing femoral vein thrombus

duplex u., the combination of real-time and Doppler u.

gray-scale u., the display of the ultrasound echo amplitude or signal intensity as different shades of gray, improving image quality compared to the obsolete black-and-white presentation.

ul•tra•sound (ŭl′tră-sownd). Sound having a frequency greater than 30,000 Hz.

diagnostic u., the use of u. to obtain images for medical diagnostic purposes.

ul•tra•vi•o•let (ŭl-tră-vī′ō-let). Denoting electromagnetic rays at higher frequency than the violet end of the visible spectrum.

ul•tra•vi•rus (ŭl′tră-vī′rŭs). SYN virus (2).

um•bil•i•cal (ŭm-bil′i-kăl). Relating to the umbilicus. SYN omphalic.

um•bil•i•cate, um•bil•i•cat•ed (ŭm-bil′i-kāt, -kāt-ed). Of navel shape; pitlike; dimpled. [L. *umbilicatus*]

um•bil•i•ca•tion (ŭm-bil-i-kā′shŭn). **1.** A pit or navel-like depression. **2.** Formation of a depression at the apex of a papule, vesicle, or pustule.

um•bil•i•cus, pl. **um•bil•i•ci** (ŭm-bil′i-kŭs, ŭm-bi-lī-kŭs; -i-sī, -lī′kī) [NA]. The pit in the center of the abdominal wall marking the point where the umbilical cord entered in the fetus. SYN navel. [L. navel]

um·bo, gen. **um·bo·nis,** pl. **um·bo·nes** (ŭm′bō, um-bō′nis, um-bō′nēz). **1** [NA]. A projecting point of a surface. **2.** SYN u. of tympanic membrane. [L. boss of a shield, a knob]

u. of tympanic membrane, the projection on the inner surface of the tympanic membrane at the end of the manubrium of the malleus; this corresponds to the most depressed point of the membrane, viewed laterally, that is commonly called the umbo. SYN umbo (2).

umbra. RADIOLOGY An image with sharply defined margins.

UMP *uridine* 5′-monophosphate.

△**un-. 1.** Not, akin to L. *in-* and G. *a-, an-.* **2.** Reversal, removal, release, deprivation. **3.** An intensive action. [M.E.]

un·cal (ŭng′kăl). Denoting or relating to the uncus.

un·ci (ŭn′sī). Plural of uncus.

un·ci·form (ŭn′si-fōrm). SYN uncinate. [L. *uncus,* hook, + *forma,* form]

un·ci·nate (ŭn′si-nāt). **1.** Hooklike or hook-shaped. **2.** Relating to an uncus or, specifically, to the u. gyrus (2) or a process of the pancreas or of a vertebra. SYN unciform. [L. *uncinatus*]

un·con·scious (ŭn-kon′shŭs). **1.** Not conscious. **2.** PSYCHOANALYSIS The psychic structure comprising the drives and feelings of which one is unaware. SYN insensible (1).

collective u., JUNGIAN PSYCHOLOGY the combined engrams or memory potentials inherited from an individual's phylogenetic past.

un·con·scious·ness (ŭn-kon′shŭs-ness). An imprecise term for severely impaired awareness of self and the surrounding environment; most often used as a synonym for coma or unresponsiveness.

un·co·ver·te·bral (ŭn-kō-ver′tĕ-brăl). Pertaining to or affecting the uncinate process of a vertebra.

unc·tion (ŭngk′shŭn). The action of anointing or rubbing with an ointment or oil. [L. *unctio,* fr. *ungo,* pp. *unctus,* to anoint]

unc·tu·ous (ŭngk′shū-ŭs, -chū-ŭs). Greasy or oily. [L. *unctuosus,* fr. *unctio,* unction]

un·cus, pl. **un·ci** (ŭn′kŭs, ŭn′sī) [NA]. **1.** Any hook-shaped process or structure. **2.** The anterior, hooked extremity of the parahippocampal gyrus on the basomedial surface of the temporal lobe; the anterior face of the u. corresponds to the olfactory cortex, its ventral surface to the entorhinal area; deep to the uncus lies the amygdala (amygdaloid body). SYN uncinate gyrus. [L. a hook, fr. G. *onkos*]

un·der·bite (ŭn′der-bīt). A nontechnical term applied to mandibular underdevelopment or to excessive maxillary development.

un·der·drive pac·ing (ŭn′der-drīv pās′ing). Electrical stimulation of the heart at a rate lower than that of an existing tachycardia; designed to capture the heart between beats, *i.e.,* to interrupt a reentry pathway in order to terminate the tachycardia.

un·der·shoot (ŭn′der-shūt). A temporary decrease below the final steady-state value that may occur immediately following the removal of an influence that had been raising that value, *i.e.,* overshoot in a negative direction.

underwater weighing. assessment of body volume by measuring an individual's weight in air and weight under water; loss in scale weight (corrected for water density) equals body volume. Body density (ratio of body mass to volume) is then used to compute percent body fat. SYN hydrostatic weighing.

un·dif·fer·en·ti·at·ed (ŭn′dif-er-en′shē-ā-ted). Not differentiated; *e.g.,* primitive, embryonic, immature, or having no special structure or function.

un·du·late (ŭn′dū-lāt). Having an irregular, wavy border; denoting the shape of a bacterial colony. [Mod. L. *undula,* dim. of *unda,* wave]

un·du·li·po·di·um, pl. **un·du·li·po·dia** (ŭn′dū-li-pō′dē-um, -ă). A flexible whiplike intracellular extension of many eukaryotic cells, with a characteristic arrangement of nine paired peripheral microtubules and one central pair; it appears to grow out from a basal body (kinetosome) in the cell. Both the cilium and the eukaryotic flagellum (not the bacterial flagellum, which lacks the 9 + 2 pattern) are considered u. [LL. *undulo,* to move in waves, fr. L. *unda,* wave, + Mod.L. *podium,* fr. G. *podion,* dim. of *pous,* foot]

un·gual (ŭng′gwăl). Relating to a nail or the nails. SYN unguinal. [L. *unguis,* nail]

un·guent (ŭng′gwent). SYN ointment. [L. *unguentum*]

un·gues (ŭng′gwēz). Plural of unguis.

un·gui·nal (ŭng′gwi-năl). SYN ungual.

un·guis, pl. **un·gues** (ŭng′gwis, -gwēz) [NA]. SYN nail. [L.]

△**uni-.** One, single, not paired; corresponds to G. *mono-.* [L. *unus*]

uni·cam·er·al, uni·cam·er·ate (yū-nē-kam′ĕ-răl, -kam′ĕ-rāt). SYN monolocular.

uni·cel·lu·lar (yū-ni-sel′yū-lăr). Composed of but one cell, as in the protozoa (or protozoans); for such u. organisms capable of undertaking life processes independently of other cells, the term acellular is also used.

uni·cor·nous (yū′ni-kōr′nŭs). Having but one horn, or cornu. [L. *unicornis,* fr. uni- + *cornu,* horn]

uni·ger·mi·nal (yū-ni-jer′mi-năl). Relating to a single germ or ovum, *e.g.,* monozygotic. SYN monozygotic, monozygous.

uni·glan·du·lar (yū-ni-glan′dū-lăr). Involving, relating to, or containing but one gland.

uni·lat·e·ral (yū-ni-lat′ĕ-răl). Confined to one side only.

uni·lo·bar (yū-ni-lō′băr). Having but one lobe.

uni·lo·cal (yū-ni-lō′kăl). Strictly, denoting a trait in which the genetic component is contributed exclusively by one locus; in practice, any trait in which the contribution from one locus is so large that the data are readily interpreted as mendelian.

uni·loc·u·lar (yū-ni-lok′yū-lăr). Having but one compartment or cavity, as in a fat cell. [uni- + L. *loculus,* compartment]

uni·mo·lec·u·lar (yū′ni-mō-lek′yū-lăr). Denoting a single molecule.

un·ion (yūn′yŭn). **1.** The joining or amalgamation of two or more bodies. **2.** The structural adhesion or growing together of the edges of a wound. [L. *unus,* one]

faulty u., SYN fibrous u. SEE vicious u.

fibrous u., u. of fracture by fibrous tissue. SEE nonunion, vicious u. SYN faulty u.

primary u., SYN *healing* by first intention.

secondary u., SYN *healing* by second intention.

vicious u., u. of the ends of a broken bone resulting in a deformity or a crooked limb; frequently used interchangeably with faulty u.

uni•pen•nate (yū-ni-pen′āt). **1.** Having a feather arrangement on one side; resembling one-half of a feather. **2.** Denoting certain muscles with fibers running at an acute angle from one side of a tendon. [uni- + L. *penna,* feather]

uni•po•lar (yū-ni-pō′lăr). **1.** Having but one pole; denoting a nerve cell from which the branches project from one side only. **2.** Situated at one extremity only of a cell.

uni•port (yū′ni-pōrt). Transport of a molecule or ion through a membrane by a carrier mechanism (uniporter), without known coupling to any other molecule or ion transport. Cf. antiport, symport. [uni- + L. *porto,* to carry]

unit (U) (yū′nit). **1.** One; a single person or thing. **2.** A standard of measure, weight, or any other quality, by multiplications or fractions of which a scale or system is formed. **3.** A group of persons or things considered as a whole because of mutual activities or functions. **4.** SYN international u. [L. *unus,* one]

absolute u., a u. whose value is constant regardless of place or time and not dependent on gravitation.

Ångström u. (Å), SEE angstrom.

antigen u., the smallest amount of antigen that, in the presence of specific antiserum, will fix 1 complement u.

antitoxin u., a u. expressing the strength or activity of an antitoxin; in general, determined with reference to a preserved standard preparation of antitoxin. SEE ALSO L *doses,* under *dose.*

atomic mass u. (amu), a u. of mass by definition equal to $\frac{1}{12}$ of the mass of an atom of carbon-12, which equals $1.6605402 \times 10^{-27}$ kg; in terms of energy, 1 amu equals 931.49432 MeV. Cf. dalton.

base u.'s, the fundamental u.'s of length, mass, time, electric current, thermodynamic temperature, amount of substance, and luminous intensity in the International System of Units (SI); the names and symbols of the u.'s for these quantities are meter (m), kilogram (kg), second (s), ampere (A), kelvin (K), mole (mol), and candela (cd). SEE ALSO International System of Units.

Bethesda u., a measure of inhibitor activity: the amount of inhibitor that will inactivate 50% or 0.5 unit of a coagulation factor during the incubation period. [*Bethesda,* MD]

Bodansky u., that amount of phosphatase that liberates 1 mg of phosphorus as inorganic phosphate during the first hour of incubation with a buffered substrate containing sodium β-glycerophosphate.

British thermal u. (BTU), the quantity of heat required to raise one pound of water from 3.9°C to 4.4°C; equal to 251.996 calories or to 1055.056 joules.

centimeter-gram-second u. (CGS, cgs), CGS u., an absolute u. of the centimeter-gram-second system.

colony-forming u. (CFU), a stem cell in culture capable of proliferating and differentiating into more mature cells. If the CFU is committed to a specific cell line it is designated by an additional letter to indicate its commitment; *e.g.,* CFU-E is committed to erythroid maturation; CFU-GM is committed to granulocyte/monocyte maturation.

complement u., the smallest amount (highest dilution) of complement that will cause hemolysis of a u. of red blood cells in the presence of a hemolysin u.

coronary care u. (CCU), a group of beds within a hospital set aside for the care of patients having or suspected of having myocardial infarction.

critical care u. (CCU), SYN intensive care u.

foot-pound-second u. (FPS, fps), FPS u., an absolute u. of the foot-pound-second system.

hemolysin u., hemolytic u., the smallest quantity (highest dilution) of inactivated immune serum (hemolysin) that will sensitize the standard suspension of erythrocytes so that the standard complement will cause complete hemolysis.

Holzknecht u. (H), an obsolete u. of x-ray dosage equal to one-fifth of the erythema dose.

intensive care u. (ICU), a hospital facility for provision of intensive nursing and medical care of critically ill patients, characterized by high quality and quantity of continuous nursing and medical supervision and by use of sophisticated monitoring and resuscitative equipment; may be organized for the care of specific patient groups, *e.g.,* neonatal or newborn ICU, neurological ICU, pulmonary ICU. SYN critical care u.

international u., the amount of a substance, such as a drug, hormone, vitamin, enzyme, etc., that produces a specific effect as defined by an international body and accepted internationally. SYN unit (4).

International System of U.'s, SEE International System of Units.

Kienböck's u. (X), an obsolete u. of x-ray dosage equivalent to $\frac{1}{10}$ the erythema dose.

motor u., a single somatic motor neuron and the group of muscle fibers innervated by it.

u. of penicillin (international), the penicillin activity of 0.6 μg of penicillin G.

physiologic u., (1) the ultimate (hypothetical) vital u. of protoplasm, as conceived by Spencer; (2) the smallest division of an organ that will perform its function; *e.g.,* the uriniferous tubule.

Somogyi u., a measure of the level of activity of amylase in blood serum, as analyzed by means of the Somogyi method (the most frequently used procedure).

Svedberg u. (S), a sedimentation constant of 1 $\times 10^{-13}$ seconds.

toxic u., a u. formerly synonymous with minimal lethal dose but which, because of the instability of toxins, is now measured in terms of the quantity of standard antitoxin with which the toxin combines. SEE ALSO L *doses*, under *dose*, minimal lethal *dose*. SYN toxin u.

toxin u., SYN toxic u.

USP u., a u. as defined and adopted by the *United States Pharmacopeia*.

workload u. (WLU), a u. of work used to calculate productivity. Health care organizations may use billable procedures or patient visits.

Uni•ted States Adopt•ed Names (USAN). Designation for nonproprietary names (for drugs) adopted by the USAN Council in cooperation with the manufacturers concerned; the designation USAN is applicable only to nonproprietary names coined since June 1961.

Uni•ted States Phar•ma•co•pe•ia (USP). SEE Pharmacopeia.

Uni•ted States Pub•lic Health Ser•vice (USPHS). A bureau of the Department of Health and Human Services, served by a corps of medical officers presided over by the Surgeon General, concerned with scientific research, domestic and insular quarantine, administration of government hospitals, publication of sanitary reports, and statistics; associated with it are the National Institutes of Health, Centers for Disease Control and Prevention, and other units.

uni•va•lence, uni•va•len•cy (yū-ni-vā′lens, -vā′len-sē). SYN monovalence.

uni•va•lent (yū-ni-vā′lent). SYN monovalent (1).

universal precautions. An approach to infection control in which all human blood, tissue, and certain fluids are treated as if known to be infectious for HIV, HBV, and other blood-borne pathogens.

un•my•e•li•nat•ed (ŭn-mī′ĕ-li-nā-ted). Denoting nerve fibers (axons) lacking a myelin sheath. SYN amyelinated, amyelinic.

un•of•fi•cial (ŭn-ŏ-fish′ăl). Denoting a drug that is not listed in the United States Pharmacopeia or the National Formulary.

un•phys•i•o•log•ic (ŭn-fis′ē-ō-loj′ik). Pertaining to conditions in the organism which are abnormal; can be used to refer to subjecting the body to abnormal amounts of substances normally present.

un•san•i•tary (ŭn-san′i-tār-ē). SYN insanitary.

un•sat•u•rat•ed (ŭn-sach′ŭr-āt-ed). **1.** Not saturated; denoting a solution in which the solvent is capable of dissolving more of the solute. **2.** Denoting a chemical compound in which all the affinities are not satisfied, so that still other atoms or radicals may be added to it. **3.** ORGANIC CHEMISTRY Denoting compounds containing double and/or triple bonds.

un•stri•at•ed (ŭn-strī′āt-ed). Without striations; not striped; denoting the structure of the smooth or involuntary muscles.

UPJ ureteropelvic *junction*.

up•reg•u•la•tion. Opposite of down-regulation.

up•si•lon (υ) (up′si-lon). **1.** The 20th letter in the Greek alphabet. **2.** kinematic *viscosity*.

up•take (ŭp′tāk). The absorption by a tissue of some substance (food material, mineral) its permanent or temporary retention.

ura•chal (yūr′ă-kăl). Relating to the urachus.

ura•chus (yūr′ă-kŭs). That portion of the reduced allantoic stalk between the apex of the bladder and the umbilicus median umbilical ligament. [G. *ourachos*, the urinary canal of a fetus]

ura•cil (U) (yūr′ă-sil). A pyrimidine (base) present in ribonucleic acid.

△**uranisco-.** SEE urano-.

ura•ni•um (U) (yū-rā′nē-ŭm). A radioactive metallic element, atomic no. 92, atomic wt. 238.0289, occurring mainly in pitchblende and notable for its two isotopes: ^{238}U and ^{235}U (99.2745% and 0.720%, respectively, the rest being made up by ^{234}U), ^{235}U being the first substance ever shown capable of supporting a self-sustaining chain reaction. [G. myth. character, *Uranus*]

△**urano-, uranisco-.** The hard palate. [G. *ouranos*, sky vault, *ouraniskos*, roof of mouth (palate)]

ura•no•plas•ty (yū′ră-nō-plas-tē). SYN palatoplasty.

ura•nor•rha•phy (yū′ră-nōr′ă-fē). SYN palatorrhaphy. [urano- + G. *rhaphē*, suture]

ura•nos•chi•sis (yū′ră-nos′ki-sis). Cleft of the hard palate. [urano- + G. *schisis*, fissure]

ura•no•staph•y•los•chi•sis (yū′ră-nō-staf′i-los′ki-sis). Cleft of the soft and hard palates. [urano- + G. *staphylē*, uvula, + *schisis*, fissure]

ura•nyl (yūr′ă-nil). The ion, UO_2^{2+}; uranyl acetate is used in electron microscopy.

urar•thri•tis (yū-rar-thrī′tis). Gouty inflammation of a joint. [urate + arthritis]

urate (yūr′āt). A salt of uric acid.

u. oxidase, a copper-containing, oxygen-requiring oxidoreductase that oxidizes uric acid; used in the clinical diagnosis of increased uric acid levels. SYN uricase.

ura•te•mia (yū-rā-tē′mē-ă). The presence of urates, especially sodium urate, in the blood. [urate + G. *haima*, blood]

ura•to•sis (yū-rā-tō′sis). Any morbid condition due to the presence of urates in the blood or tissues.

ura•tu•ria (yū-rā-tū′rē-ă). The passage of an increased amount of urates in the urine. [urate + G. *ouron*, urine]

Urd uridine.

ur•de•fens•es (ūr′dē-fens-ez). Fundamental beliefs essential for human psychological integrity; *e.g.*, religion, science.

△**ure-, urea-, ureo-.** Urea; urine. SEE ALSO urin-, uro-. [G. *ouron*, urine]

urea (yū-rē′ă). The chief end product of nitrogen metabolism in mammals, formed in the liver, by means of the Krebs-Henseleit cycle, and excreted in normal adult human urine in the amount of about 32 g a day (about 6/7 of the nitrogen excreted from the body). It has been used as a diuretic in kidney function tests, and topically for various dermatitides. [G. *ouron*, urine]

ure•a•gen•e•sis (yū-rē-ă-jen′ĕ-sis). Formation of urea, usually referring to the metabolism of amino acids to urea. SYN ureapoiesis. [urea + G. *genesis*, production]

Ure•a•plas•ma (yū-rē′ă-plaz′mă). A genus of microaerophilic to anaerobic, nonmotile bacteria containing Gram-negative, predominantly coccoidal to coccobacillary elements, approximately 0.3 μm in diameter, which frequently grow in short filaments. These organisms hydrolyze urea with production of ammonia, and are found in the human genitourinary tract, occasionally in the pharynx and rectum. In males, they are associated with nongonococcal urethritis and prostatitis; in females, with genitourinary tract infections and reproductive failure. The type species is *U. urealyticum.* SYN T-mycoplasma.

ure•a•poi•e•sis (yū-rē′ă-poy-ē′sis). SYN ureagenesis. [urea + G. *poiēsis,* a making]

ure•ase (yūr′ē-ās). An enzyme that catalyzes the hydrolysis of urea to carbon dioxide and ammonia; used as an antitumor enzyme; it is present in intestinal bacteria and accounts for most of the ammonia generated from urea in mammals.

ure•de•ma (yū-re-dē′mă). Edema due to infiltration of urine into the subcutaneous tissues. [G. *ouron,* urine, + *oidēma,* swelling]

urel•co•sis (yū-rel-kō′sis). Ulceration of any part of the urinary tract. [G. *ouron,* urine, + *helkōsis,* ulceration]

ure•mia (yū-rē′mē-ă). **1.** An excess of urea and other nitrogenous waste in the blood. **2.** The complex of symptoms due to severe persisting renal failure that can be relieved by dialysis. SYN azotemia. [G. *ouron,* urine, + *haima,* blood]

ure•mic (yū-rē′mik). Relating to uremia.

ure•mi•gen•ic (yū-rē-mi-jen′ik). **1.** Of uremic origin or causation. **2.** Causing or resulting in uremia.

△**ureo-.** SEE ure-.

ure•si•es•the•sia (yū-rē′si-es-thē′zē-ă). The desire to urinate. SYN uriesthesia. [G. *ourēsis,* a urinating, + *aisthēsis,* sensation]

ure•sis (yū-rē′sis). SYN urination. [G. *ourēsis*]

ure•ter (yū-rē′ter, yū′rē-ter) [NA]. The thick-walled tube that conducts the urine from the renal pelvis to the bladder; it consists of an abdominal part and a pelvic part, is lined with transitional epithelium surrounded by smooth muscle, both circular and longitudinal, and is covered externally by a tunica adventitia. [G. *ourētēr,* urinary canal]

ure•ter•al (yū-rē′tĕ-răl). Relating to the ureter. SYN ureteric.

ure•ter•al•gia (yū-rē-ter-al′jē-ă). Pain in the ureter. [ureter + G. *algos,* pain]

ure•ter•cys•to•scope (yū-rē′ter-sis′tō-skōp). SYN ureterocystoscope.

ure•ter•ec•ta•sia (yū-rē′ter-ek-tā′zē-ă). Dilation of a ureter. [ureter + G. *ektasis,* a stretching out]

ure•ter•ec•to•my (yū-rē-ter-ek′tō-mē). Excision of a segment or all of a ureter. [ureter + G. *ektomē,* excision]

ure•ter•ic (yū-rē-ter′ik). SYN ureteral.

ure•ter•i•tis (yū-rē-ter-ī′tis). Inflammation of a ureter.

△**uretero-.** The ureter. [G. *ourētēr,* urinary canal]

ure•ter•o•cele (yū-rē′ter-ō-sēl). Saccular dilation of the terminal portion of the ureter which protrudes into the lumen of the urinary bladder, probably due to a congenital stenosis of the ureteral meatus. [uretero- + G. *kēlē,* hernia]

ure•ter•o•ce•lor•ra•phy (yū-rē′ter-ō-se-lōr′ă-fē). Excision and suturing of a ureterocele performed through an open cystotomy incision. [ureterocele + G. *raphē,* suture]

ure•ter•o•co•los•to•my (yū-rē′ter-ō-kō-los′tō-mē). Implantation of the ureter into the colon. [uretero- + G. *kolon,* colon, + *stoma,* mouth]

ure•ter•o•cys•to•scope (yū-rē′ter-ō-sis′tō-skōp). A cystoscope with an attachment for catheterization of the ureters; the catheter is passed into the ureter when its orifice is brought into view with the cystoscope. SYN uretercystoscope. [uretero- + G. *kystis,* bladder, + *skopeō,* to view]

ure•ter•o•cys•tos•to•my (yū-rē′ter-ō-sis-tos′tō-mē). SYN ureteroneocystostomy. [uretero- + G. *kystis,* bladder, + *stoma,* mouth]

ure•ter•o•en•ter•os•to•my (yū-rē′ter-ō-en-ter-os′tō-mē). Formation of an opening between a ureter and the intestine. [uretero- + G. *enteron,* intestine, + *stoma,* mouth]

ure•ter•og•ra•phy (yū-rē′ter-og′ră-fē). Radiography of the ureter after the direct injection of contrast medium. [uretero- + G. *graphē,* a writing]

ure•ter•o•il•e•o•ne•o•cys•tos•to•my (yū-rē′ter-ō-il′ē-ō-nē′ō-sis-tos′tō-mē). Restoration of the continuity of the urinary tract by anastomosis of the upper segment of a partially destroyed ureter to a segment of ileum, the lower end of which is then implanted into the bladder. [uretero- + ileum + G. *neos,* new, + *hystis,* bladder, + *stoma,* mouth]

ure•ter•o•il•e•os•to•my (yū-rē′ter-ō-il-ē-os′tō-mē). Implantation of a ureter into an isolated segment of ileum which drains through an abdominal stoma. [uretero- + ileum + G. *stoma,* mouth]

ure•ter•o•li•thi•a•sis (yū-rē′ter-ō-li-thī′ă-sis). The formation or presence of a calculus or calculi in one or both ureters. [ureterolith + G. *-iasis,* condition]

ure•ter•o•li•thot•o•my (yū-rē′ter-ō-li-thot′ō-mē). Removal of a stone lodged in a ureter. [ureterolith + G. *tomē,* incision]

ure•ter•ol•y•sis (yū′rē-ter-ol′i-sis). Surgical freeing of the ureter from surrounding disease or adhesions. [uretero- + G. *lysis,* a loosening]

ure•ter•o•ne•o•cys•tos•to•my (yū-rē′ter-ō-nē′ō-sis-tos′tō-mē). An operation whereby a ureter is implanted into the bladder. SYN ureterocystostomy. [uretero- + G. *neos,* new, + *kystis,* bladder, + *stoma,* mouth]

ure•ter•o•ne•phrec•to•my (yū-rē′ter-ō-nĕ-frek′tō-mē). SYN nephroureterectomy. [uretero- + G. *nephros,* kidney, + *ektomē,* excision]

ure•ter•o•plas•ty (yū-rē′ter-ō-plas-tē). Surgical reconstruction of the ureters. [uretero- + G. *plastos,* formed]

ure•ter•o•py•e•li•tis (yū-rē′ter-ō-pī-ĕ-lī′tis). Inflammation of the pelvis of a kidney and its ureter. [uretero- + G. *pyelos,* pelvis, + *-itis,* inflammation]

ure•ter•o•py•e•log•ra•phy (yū-rē′ter-ō-pī′ĕ-log′ră-fē). SYN pyelography.

ure•ter•o•py•e•lo•plasty (yū-rē′ter-ō-pī′ĕ-lō-plas-tē). Surgical reconstruction of the ureter and of the pelvis of the kidney, usually for congenital ureteropelvic junction obstruction. [uretero- + G. *pyelos,* pelvis, + *plastos,* formed]

ure•ter•o•py•e•los•to•my (yū-rē′ter-ō-pī-ĕ-los′tō-mē). Formation of a junction of the ureter and

ur

the renal pelvis. [uretero- + pelvis, + *stoma*, mouth]

ure•ter•o•py•o•sis (yū-rē'ter-ō-pī-ō'sis). An accumulation of pus in the ureter. [uretero- + G. *pyōsis*, suppuration]

ure•ter•or•rha•gia (yū-rē'ter-ō-rā'jē-ă). Hemorrhage from a ureter. [uretero- + G. *rhēgnymi*, to burst forth]

ure•ter•or•rha•phy (yū-rē-ter-ōr'ă-fē). Suture of a ureter. [uretero- + G. *rhaphē*, suture]

ure•ter•o•sig•moi•dos•to•my (yū-rē'ter-ō-sig-moy-dos'tō-mē). Implantation of the ureter into the sigmoid colon.

ure•ter•os•to•my (yū-rē-ter-os'tō-mē). Establishment of an external opening into the ureter. [uretero- + G. *stoma*, mouth]

ure•ter•ot•o•my (yū-rē-ter-ot'ō-mē). Incision and stenting of a narrow ureter. [uretero- + G. *tomē*, incision]

ure•ter•o•u•re•ter•os•to•my (yū-rē'ter-ō-yū-rē'ter-os'tō-mē). Establishment of an anastomosis between the two ureters or between two segments of the same ureter. SEE ALSO transureteroureterostomy.

ure•ter•o•ves•i•cos•to•my (yū-rē'ter-ō-ves-i-kos'tō-mē). Surgical joining of a ureter to the bladder. [uretero- + L. *vesica*, bladder, + *stoma*, mouth]

△**urethr-**. SEE urethro-.

ure•thra (yū-rē'thră). A canal leading from the bladder, discharging the urine externally. SYN urogenital canal. [G. *ourēthra*]

ure•thral (yū-rē'thrăl). Relating to the urethra.

ure•thral•gia (yū-rē-thral'jē-ă). Pain in the urethra. SYN urethrodynia. [urethr- + G. *algos*, pain]

ure•threc•to•my (yūr-ĕ-threk'tō-mē). Excision of a segment or of the entire urethra. [urethr- + G. *ektomē*, excision]

ure•threm•or•rha•gia (yū-rē'threm-ō-rā'jē-ă). Bleeding from the urethra. SYN urethrorrhagia. [urethr- + G. *haima*, blood, + *rhēgnymi*, to burst forth]

ure•thrism, ure•thris•mus (yū'rē-thrizm, -thriz'mŭs). Irritability or spasmodic stricture of the urethra. SYN urethrospasm.

ure•thri•tis (yū-rē-thrī'tis). Inflammation of the urethra. [ureth- + G. *-itis*, inflammation]

  u. petrif'icans, u., sometimes of gouty origin, in which there is a deposit of calcareous matter in the wall of the urethra.

△**urethro-, urethr-**. The urethra. [G. *ourēthra*]

ure•thro•bul•bar (yū-rē'thrō-bŭl'băr). SYN bulbourethral.

ure•thro•cele (yū-rē'thrō-sēl). Prolapse of the female urethra. [urethro- + G. *kēlē*, tumor, hernia]

ure•thro•cys•tom•e•try (yū-rē'thrō-sis-tom'ĕ-trē). A procedure that simultaneously measures pressures in urinary bladder and urethra. [urethro- + G. *kystis*, bladder, + *metron*, measure]

ure•thro•dyn•ia (yū-rē-thrō-din'ē-ă). SYN urethralgia. [urethro- + G. *odynē*, pain]

ureth•ro•per•i•ne•o•scro•tal (yū-rē'thrō-pe-rī-nē-ō-skrō'tăl). Relating to the urethra, perineum, and scrotum.

ure•thro•plasty (yu-re-thro-plas-te). Surgical repair of hypospadias or epispadias. [urethro- + G. *plastos*, formed]

ure•thror•rha•gia (yū-rē-thrō-rā'jē-ă). SYN urethremorrhagia.

ure•thror•rha•phy (yū-rē-thrōr'ă-fē). Suture of the urethra. [urethro- + G. *rhaphē*, suture]

ure•thror•rhea (yū-rē-thrō-rē'ă). An abnormal discharge from the urethra. [urethro- + G. *rhoia*, a flow]

ure•thro•scope (yū-rē'thrō-skōp). An instrument for viewing the interior of the urethra. [urethro- + G. *skopeō*, to view]

ure•thro•scop•ic (yū-rē-thrō-skop'ik). Relating to the urethroscope or to urethroscopy.

ure•thros•co•py (yū-rē-thros'kŏ-pē). Inspection of the urethra with a urethroscope.

ure•thro•spasm (yū-rē'thrō-spazm). SYN urethrism.

ure•thro•stax•is (yū-rē'thrō-stak'sis). Oozing of blood from the urethra. [urethro- + G. *staxis*, trickling]

ure•thro•ste•no•sis (yū-rē'thrō-ste-nō'sis). Stricture of the urethra. [urethro- + G. *stenōsis*, a narrowing]

ure•thros•to•my (yū-rē-thros'tō-mē). Surgical formation of a permanent opening between the urethra and the skin. [urethro- + G. *stoma*, mouth]

ure•throt•o•my (yū-rē-throt'ō-mē). Surgical incision of a stricture of the urethra. [urethro- + G. *tomē*, incision]

ure•thro•ves•i•co•pexy (yū-rē'thrō-ves'i-kŏ-pek-sē). Surgical suspension of the urethra and the base of the bladder from the posterior surface of the pubic symphysis (or anterior abdominal wall or Cooper's ligament) for correction of urinary stress incontinence. [urethro- + L. *vesica*, bladder, + G. *pexis*, fixation]

△**-uretic**. Urine. [G. *ourētikos*, relating to the urine]

ur•gen•cy (er'jen-sē). A strong desire to void.

  motor u., u. from overactive detrusor function.

  sensory u., u. due to vesicourethral hypersensitivity.

ur•hi•dro•sis (yūr-hi-drō'sis). SYN uridrosis.

△**uri-, uric-, urico-**. Uric acid. [G. *ouron*, urine]

uric (yūr'ik). Relating to urine.

uric ac•id. 2,6,8-Trioxypurine; white crystals, poorly soluble, contained in solution in the urine of mammals; sometimes solidified in small masses as stones or crystals or in larger concretions as calculi; with sodium and other bases it forms urates; elevated levels associated with gout.

uri•case (yūr'i-kās). SYN *urate* oxidase.

△**urico-**. SEE uri-.

uri•col•y•sis (yūr-i-kol'i-sis). Decomposition of uric acid. [urico- + G. *lysis*, a loosening]

uri•co•lyt•ic (yūr'i-kō-lit'ik). Relating to or effecting the hydrolysis of uric acid.

uri•co•su•ria (yū'ri-kō-sū'rē-ă). Excessive amounts of uric acid in the urine. [urico- + G. *ouron*, urine]

uri•dine (Urd) (yūr'i-dēn). Uracil ribonucleoside; one of the major nucleosides in RNAs; as the pyrophosphate (UDP, UDPG, etc.), u. is active in sugar metabolism.

  u. 5'-diphosphate (UDP), uridine 5'-pyrophosphate; a condensation product of uridine and pyrophosphoric acid.

u. 5′-monophosphate (UMP), SYN uridylic acid.

u. 5′-triphosphate (UTP), u. esterified with triphosphoric acid at its 5′-position; the immediate precursor of uridylic acid residues in RNA.

uri·dro·sis (yū-ri-drō′sis). The excretion of urea or uric acid in the sweat. SYN urhidrosis. [uri- + G. *hidrōs,* sweat]

uri·dyl·ic ac·id (yūr-i-dil′ik). Uridine esterified by phosphoric acid, precursor for the biosynthesis of other pyrimidine nucleotides. SYN uridine 5′-monophosphate.

uri·es·the·sia (yūri-es-thē′zē-ă). SYN uresiesthesia.

△**urin-, urino-.** Urine. SEE ALSO ure-, uro-. [G. *ouron*]

uri·nal (yū′rin-ăl). A vessel into which urine is passed.

uri·nal·y·sis (yū-ri-nal′i-sis). Analysis of the urine.

uri·nary (yūr′i-nār-ē). Relating to urine.

uri·nate (yūr′i-nāt). To pass urine. SYN micturate.

uri·na·tion (yūr′i-nā′shŭn). The passing of urine. SYN miction, micturition (1), uresis.

urine (yūr′in). The fluid and dissolved substances excreted by the kidney. [L. *urina;* G. *ouron*]

   residual u., u. remaining in the bladder at the end of micturition in cases of prostatic obstruction, bladder atony, etc.

△**urino-.** SEE urin-.

uri·nog·e·nous (yūr-i-noj′ĕ-nŭs). **1.** Producing or excreting urine. **2.** Of urinary origin. SYN urogenous.

uri·no·ma (yūr′i-nō′mă). A cystic collection of extravasated urine.

uri·nom·e·try (yūr-i-nom′ĕ-trē). The determination of the specific gravity of the urine.

uri·nos·co·py (yūr-i-nos′kŏ-pē). SYN uroscopy.

△**uro-.** Urine. SEE ALSO ure-, urin-. [G. *ouron*]

uro·bi·lin (yūr-ō-bī′lin, -bil′in). A uroporphyrin; an acyclic tetrapyrrole that is one of the natural breakdown products of heme; a urinary pigment that gives a varying orange-red coloration to urine.

uro·bi·li·ne·mia (yū′rō-bil-i-nē′mē-ă). The presence of urobilins in the blood.

uro·bi·lin·o·gen (yūr-ō-bī-lin′ō-jen). Precursor of urobilin.

uro·bi·lin·u·ria (yū′rō-bil-i-nū′rē-ă). The presence in the urine of urobilins in excessive amount, formed mainly from hemoglobin.

ur·o·can·ate (yūr′ō-kă-nāt). A salt or ester of urocanic acid.

u. hydratase, an enzyme catalyzing the reaction of water with urocanic acid, a step in L-histidine catabolism; this enzyme is absent in cases of urocanic aciduria.

uro·can·ic ac·id (yūr-ō-kan′ik). An acid derived from the oxidative deamination of L-histidine; present in sweat; elevated levels are observed in cases of urocanate hydratase deficiency.

uro·cele (yū′rō-sēl). Extravasation of urine into the scrotal sac. [uro- + G. *kēlē,* hernia]

uro·che·sia (yū-rō-kē′zē-ă). Passage of urine from the anus. [uro- + G. *chezō,* to defecate]

uro·chrome (yūr′ō-krōm). The principal pigment of urine, a compound of urobilin and a peptide of unknown structure.

uro·dyn·ia (yūr-ō-din′ē-ă). Pain on urination. [uro- + G. *odynē,* pain]

uro·fla·vin (yūr-ō-flā′vin). A fluorescent product of riboflavin catabolism, or perhaps riboflavin itself, found in mammalian urine and feces.

ur·o·fol·li·tro·pin (yūr-ō-fol′i-trō-pin). A preparation of gonadotropin extracted from the urine of postmenopausal women, used in conjunction with human chorionic gonadotropin to induce ovulation. SEE ALSO menotropins.

uro·gas·trone (yūr-ō-gas′trōn). A fluorescent pigment extracted from urine; an inhibitor of gastric secretion and motility. Cf. enterogastrone.

uro·gen·i·tal (yū′rō-jen′i-tăl). SYN genitourinary.

urog·e·nous (yū-roj′ĕ-nŭs). SYN urinogenous.

uro·gram (yūr′ō-gram). The radiographic record obtained by urography.

urog·ra·phy (yū-rog′ră-fē). Radiography of any part (kidneys, ureters, or bladder) of the urinary tract. SEE ALSO pyelography. [uro- + G. *graphō,* to write]

   antegrade u., radiography following percutaneous injection of contrast agent with a needle or catheter into the renal calices or pelvis (antegrade pyelography), or into the urinary bladder (antegrade cystography).

   cystoscopic u., SYN retrograde u.

🛈**intravenous u., excretory u.,** radiography of kidneys, ureters, and bladder following injection of contrast medium into a peripheral vein.

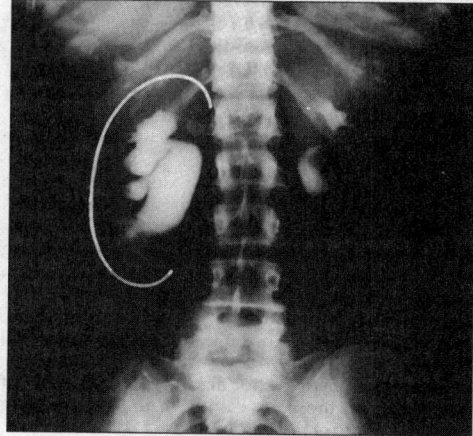

urography: intravenous urogram showing collection of contrast media in the kidney displays an extraordinary amount of material, indicating right-sided hydronephrosis caused by obstruction in the ureter

   retrograde u., radiography of the urinary tract following injection of contrast medium directly into the bladder, ureter, or renal pelvis. SYN cystoscopic u.

uro·ki·nase (yūr-ō-kī′nās). SYN plasminogen *activator.*

uro·li·thi·a·sis (yū-rō-li-thī′ă-sis). Presence of calculi in the urinary system.

uro·lith·ic (yū-rō-lith'ik). Relating to urinary calculi.

uro·log·ic, uro·log·i·cal (yū-rō-loj'ik, i-kăl). Relating to urology.

urol·o·gist (yū-rol'ō-jist). A specialist in urology.

urol·o·gy (yū-rol'ō-jē). The medical specialty concerned with the study, diagnosis, and treatment of diseases of the genitourinary tract. [uro- + G. *logos,* study]

uron·cus (yū-rong'kŭs). A urinary cyst; a circumscribed area of extravasation of urine. [uro- + G. *onkos,* mass (tumor)]

uro·ne·phro·sis (yū'rō-ne-frō'sis). SYN hydronephrosis.

urop·a·thy (yū-rop'ă-thē). Any disorder involving the urinary tract. [uro- + G. *pathos,* suffering]

obstructive u., any pathologic condition, anatomic or functional, of the urinary tract caused by obstruction.

uro·phan·ic (yūr-ō-fan'ik). Appearing in the urine; denoting any constituent, normal or pathologic, of the urine. [uro- + G. *phainō,* to appear]

uro·poi·e·sis (yū'rō-poy-ē'sis). The production or secretion and excretion of urine. [uro- + G. *poiēsis,* a making]

uro·poi·et·ic (yū'rō-poy-et'ik). Relating or pertaining to uropoiesis.

uro·por·phy·rin (yūr-ō-pōr'fi-rin). **1.** Porphyrin excreted in the urine in porphyrinuria. **2.** Class name for all porphyrins containing 4 acetic acid groups and 4 propionic acid groups in positions 1 through 8. SEE ALSO porphyrinogens.

ur·o·por·phy·rin·o·gen (yūr'ō-pōr-fi-rin'ō-jen). SEE porphyrinogens.

ur·o·ra·di·ol·o·gy (yū'rō-rā-dē-ol'ŏ-jē). The study of the radiology of the urinary tract.

uros·che·sis (yū-ros'kē-sis). **1.** Retention of urine. **2.** Suppression of urine. [uro- + G. *schesis,* a checking]

uro·scop·ic (yūr-ō-skop'ik). Relating to uroscopy.

uros·co·py (yū-ros'kŏ-pē). Examination of the urine, usually by means of a microscope. SYN urinoscopy. [uro- + G. *skopeō,* to view]

uro·sep·sis (yūr-ō-sep'sis). **1.** Sepsis resulting from the decomposition of extravasated urine. **2.** Sepsis from obstruction of infected urine. [uro- + G. *sēpsis,* decomposition]

u·ro·the·li·um (yū-rō-thē'lē-ŭm). The epithelial lining of the urinary tract. [uro- + epithelium]

ur·o·thor·ax (yūr-ō-thōr'aks). The presence of urine in the thoracic cavity, usually following complex multiple organ injuries.

ur·ti·cant (er'ti-kant). Producing a wheal or other similar itching agent. [L. *urtica,* nettle; see urtica]

ur·ti·car·ia (er'ti-kar'i-ă). An eruption of itching wheals, usually of systemic origin; it may be due to a state of hypersensitivity to foods or drugs, foci of infection, physical agents (heat, cold, light, friction), or psychic stimuli. SYN hives (1), urtication (3). [L. *urtica*]

cholinergic u., a form of physical or nonallergic u. initiated by heat (*e.g.,* hot baths, physical exercise, pyrexia, exposure to sun or to a warm room) or by excitement; the rather distinctive lesions consist of pruritic areas 1 to 2 mm in diam-

eter surrounded by bright red macules. SYN heat u.

cold u., hypersensitivity to cold leading to superficial vascular reaction manifested by transient itching, erythema, and hives. SEE ALSO hyphothermia.

u. endem'ica, u. epidem'ica, u. caused by the nettling hairs of certain caterpillars.

giant u., SYN angioedema.

heat u., SYN cholinergic u.

u. medicamento'sa, an urticarial form of drug eruption.

papular u., a sensitivity reaction to insect bites, especially human and pet fleas, seen mostly in young children as wheals followed by papules on exposed areas. SYN lichen urticatus.

u. pigmento'sa, cutaneous mastocytosis resulting from an excess of mast cells in the superficial dermis, producing a chronic eruption characterized by flat or slightly elevated brownish papules which urticate when stroked.

solar u., a form of u. resulting from exposure to specific light spectra; *e.g.,* sunlight; some patients have passive-transfer antibodies and others do not.

ur·ti·car·i·al, ur·ti·car·i·ous (er-ti-kar'ē-ăl, -kar'ē-ŭs). Relating to or marked by urticaria.

ur·ti·cate (er'ti-kāt). **1.** To perform urtication. **2.** Marked by the presence of wheals. [L. *urticatus*]

ur·ti·ca·tion (er-ti-kā'shŭn). **1.** Whipping with nettles to induce counterirritation, formerly used in the treatment of peripheral paralysis. **2.** A burning sensation resembling that produced by urticaria or resulting from nettle poisoning. **3.** SYN urticaria. [L. *urticatio*]

USAN United States Adopted Names.

USP United States Pharmacopeia. SEE Pharmacopeia.

USPHS United States Public Health Service.

uter-. SEE utero-.

uter·ine (yū'ter-in, yū'ter-īn). Relating to the uterus.

in utero (in yū'ter-ō). Within the womb; not yet born. [L.]

utero-, uter-. The uterus. SEE ALSO hystero- (1), metr-. [L. *uterus*]

uter·o·cys·tos·to·my (yū'ter-ō-sis-tos'tō-mē). Formation of a communication between the uterus (cervix) and the bladder. [utero- + G. *kystis,* bladder, + *stoma,* mouth]

uter·o·fix·a·tion (yū'ter-ō-fik-sā'shŭn). SYN hysteropexy.

uter·om·e·ter (yū-ter-om'ĕ-ter). SYN hysterometer.

uter·o·pexy (yū'ter-ō-pek-sē). SYN hysteropexy.

uter·o·plas·ty (yū'ter-ō-plas-tē). Plastic surgery of the uterus. SYN hysteroplasty, metroplasty. [utero- + G. *plastos,* formed]

uter·o·sal·pin·gog·ra·phy (yū'ter-ō-sal-pin-gog'ră-fē). SYN hysterosalpingography.

uter·o·scope (yū'ter-ō-skōp). SYN hysteroscope.

uter·os·co·py (yū-ter-os'kŏ-pē). SYN hysteroscopy.

uter·ot·o·my (yū-ter-ot'ō-mē). SYN hysterotomy.

uter·o·ton·ic (yū'ter-ō-ton'ik). **1.** Giving tone to the uterine muscle. **2.** An agent that overcomes relaxation of the muscular wall of the uterus. [utero- + G. *tonos,* tone, tension]

uter·o·tu·bog·ra·phy (yū′ter-ō-tū-bog′ră-fē). SYN hysterosalpingography.

uter·us, pl. **uteri** (yū′ter-ŭs, yū′ter-ī) [NA]. The hollow muscular organ in which the impregnated ovum is developed into the child; it consists of a main portion (body) with an elongated lower part (neck), at the extremity of which is the opening (os). The upper rounded portion of the u., opposite the os, is the fundus, at each extremity of which is the horn marking the part where the uterine tube joins the u. and through which the ovum reaches the uterine cavity after leaving the ovary. The organ is supported in the pelvic cavity by the broad ligaments, round ligaments, cardinal ligaments, and rectouterine and vesicouterine folds or ligaments. SYN metra, womb. [L.]

bicornate u., a u. that is more or less completely divided into two lateral horns as a result of imperfect fusion of the paramesonephric ducts; it differs from septate u., in which there is no external mark of separation; in u. bicornis, the cervix may be single (uterus bicornis unicollis) or double (uterus bicornis bicollis).

cordiform u., an incomplete u. bicornis with a wedge-shaped depression at the fundus.

Couvelaire u., extravasation of blood into the uterine musculature and beneath the uterine peritoneum in association with severe forms of abruptio placentae.

u. didel′phys, double u. with double cervix and double vagina; due to failure of the paramesonephric ducts to unite. [G. *di-,* two, + *delphys,* womb]

duplex u., any u. with double lumen (u. didelphys, u. bicornis bicollis, or septate u.).

gravid u., the condition of the u. in pregnancy.

masculine u., SYN prostatic *utricle.*

septate u., a u. divided into two cavities by an anteroposterior septum.

unicorn u., a u. in which only one lateral half exists, the other half being undeveloped or absent.

UTI urinary tract *infection.*

UTP *uridine 5′-triphosphate.*

utri·cle (yū′tri-kl). The larger of the two membranous sacs in the vestibule of the labyrinth, lying in the elliptical recess; from it arise the semicircular ducts. SYN utriculus [NA].

prostatic u., a minute pouch in the prostate opening on the summit of the seminal colliculus, the analogue of the uterus and vagina in the female. SYN utriculus prostaticus [NA], masculine uterus, vesica prostatica.

utric·u·lar (yū-trik′yū-lăr). Relating to or resembling a utricle.

utric·u·li (yū-trik′yū-lī). Plural of utriculus.

utric·u·li·tis (yū-trik-yū-lī′tis). **1.** Inflammation of the internal ear. **2.** Inflammation of the prostatic utricle. [utriculus + G. *-itis,* inflammation]

utric·u·lo·sac·cu·lar (yū-trik′yū-lō-sak′yū-lăr). Relating to the utricle and the saccule of the labyrinth, denoting especially a duct connecting the two structures.

utric·u·lus, pl. **utric·u·li** (yū′trik′yū-lŭs, -lī) [NA]. SYN utricle. SEE ALSO vestibular *organ.* [L. dim. of *uter,* leather bag]

u. prostat′icus [NA], SYN prostatic *utricle.*

UV, uv. ultraviolet.

uve·al (yū′vē-ăl). Relating to the uvea.

uve·it·ic (yū-vē-it′ik). Relating to the uvea.

uve·i·tis, pl. **uve·i·ti·des** (yū-vē-ī′tis, -it′ī-dēz). Inflammation of the uveal tract: iris, ciliary body, and choroid. [uvea + G. *-itis,* inflammation]

heterochromic u., anterior uveitis and depigmentation of the iris.

sympathetic u., a bilateral inflammation of the uveal tract caused by a perforating wound of one eye that injures the uvea.

uve·o·scle·ri·tis (yū′vē-ō-sklē-rī′tis). Inflammation of the sclera involved by extension from the uvea.

uvi·form (yū′vi-fōrm). SYN botryoid. [L. uva, grape, + *forma,* form]

uvu·la, pl. **uvu·lae** (yū′vyū-lă, -lē) [NA]. An appendant fleshy mass; a structure bearing a fancied resemblance to the palatine u. [Mod. L. dim. of L. *uva,* a grape, the uvula]

u. of bladder, a slight projection into the cavity of the bladder, usually more prominent in old men, just behind the urethral opening, marking the location of the middle lobe of the prostate.

u. cerebel′li, SYN u. vermis.

palatine u., a conical projection from the posterior edge of the middle of the soft palate, composed of connective tissue containing a number of racemose glands, and some muscular fibers (uvulae muscle).

u. ver′mis [NA], elevation on the vermis of the cerebellum, lying between the two tonsils anterior to the pyramis. SYN u. cerebelli.

uvu·lar (yū′vyū-lăr). Relating to the uvula.

uvu·lec·to·my (yū-vyū-lek′tō-mē). Excision of the uvula. SYN staphylectomy. [uvula + G. *ektomē,* excision]

uvu·li·tis (yū-vyū-lī′tis). Inflammation of the uvula.

uvu·lop·to·sis (yū′vyū-lop-tō′sis). Relaxation or elongation of the uvula. SYN staphylodialysis, staphyloptosis. [uvulo- + G. *ptōsis,* a falling]

uvu·lot·o·my (yū-vyū-lot′ō-mē). Any cutting operation on the uvula. [uvulo- + G. *tomē,* a cutting]

UV

V

V **1.** vision; volt; with subscript 1, 2, 3, etc., the abbreviation for unipolar electrocardiogram leads. **2.** vanadium; valine; volume, frequently with subscripts denoting location, chemical species, and/or conditions.

V̇ **1.** gas flow, frequently with subscripts indicating location and chemical species. SEE flow (3). **2.** ventilation (3), frequently with a subscript. See entries under ventilation (3). [volume + overdot denoting time derivative]

V̇$_A$. alveolar *ventilation.*

V$_{max}$ maximum *velocity.*

v **1.** volt; initial rate velocity; velocity; *vel* [L, or]. **2.** As a subscript, refers to venous *blood.*

v̄. As a subscript, refers to mixed venous (pulmonary arterial) blood.

V-A ventriculoatrial.

vac•ci•nal (vak′si-năl). Relating to vaccine or vaccination.

vac•ci•nate (vak′si-nāt). To administer a vaccine.

vac•ci•na•tion (vak′si-nā′shŭn). The act of administering a vaccine.

vac•cine (vak′sēn, vak-sēn′). Any preparation intended for active immunological prophylaxis; *e.g.,* preparations of killed microbes of virulent strains or living microbes of attenuated (variant or mutant) strains, or microbial, fungal, plant, protozoal, or metazoan derivatives or products. [L. *vaccinus,* relating to a cow]

autogenous v., a v. made from a culture of the patient's own bacteria.

diphtheria toxoid, tetanus toxoid, and pertussis v., a v. available in three forms: 1) diphtheria and tetanus toxoids plus pertussis v. (DTP); 2) tetanus and diphtheria toxoids, adult type (Td); and 3) tetanus toxoid (T); used for active immunization against diphtheria, tetanus, and whooping cough.

Haemophilus influenzae **type B v.,** a conjugate of oligosaccharides of the capsular antigen of *H. influenzae* type B and diphtheria CRM protein.

human diploid cell v., an iodinated virus vaccine used for protection against rabies vaccine usually prepared in the human diploid cell WI-38.

inactivated poliovirus v., SEE poliovirus v.'s (1).

live v., v. prepared from living, attenuated organisms.

multivalent v., SYN polyvalent v.

oral poliovirus v., SEE poliovirus v.'s (2).

poliovirus v.'s, (1) inactivated poliovirus v. (IPV), an aqueous suspension of inactivated strains of poliomyelitis virus (types 1, 2, and 3) used by injection; has largely been replaced by the oral v.; **(2)** oral poliovirus v. (OPV), an aqueous suspension of live, attenuated strains of poliomyelitis virus (types 1, 2, and 3) given orally for active immunization against poliomyelitis.

polyvalent v., a v. prepared from cultures of two or more strains of the same species or microorganism. SYN multivalent v.

stock v., a v. made from a stock microbial strain, in contradistinction to an autogenous v.

subunit v., a v. which, through chemical extraction, is free of viral nucleic acid and contains only specific protein subunits of a given virus; such v.'s are relatively free of the adverse reactions (*e.g.,* influenza virus) associated with v.'s containing the whole virion.

vac•u•o•lar (vak-yū-ō′lăr). Relating to or resembling a vacuole.

vac•u•o•late, vac•u•o•lat•ed (vak′yū-ō-lāt, -lāt′ ed). Having vacuoles.

vac•u•o•la•tion (vak′yū-ō-lā′shŭn). **1.** Formation of vacuoles. **2.** The condition of having vacuoles. SYN vacuolization.

vac•u•ole (vak′yū-ōl). **1.** A minute space in any tissue. **2.** A clear space in the substance of a cell, sometimes degenerative in character, sometimes surrounding an englobed foreign body and serving as a temporary cell stomach for the digestion of the body. [Mod. L. *vacuolum,* dim. of L. *vacuum,* an empty space]

vac•u•o•li•za•tion (vak′yū-ō-li-zā′shŭn). SYN vacuolation.

vac•u•tome (vak′yū-tōm). Electrodermatome that applies suction to the skin to raise it before an advancing blade, usually for taking a split-thickness skin graft. [vacuum + G. *tomē,* a cutting]

vac•u•um (vak′ūm). An empty space, one practically exhausted of air or gas. [L. ntr. of *vacuus,* empty]

va•gal (vā′găl). Relating to the vagus nerve.

va•gi (vā′gī, -jī). Plural of vagus.

△**vagin-.** SEE vagino-.

va•gi•na, gen. and pl. **va•gi•nae** (vă-jī′nă, -nē). **1.** SYN sheath (1). **2** [NA]. The genital canal in the female, extending from the uterus to the vulva. [L. sheath, the vagina]

v. carot′ica [NA], SYN carotid *sheath.*

vag•i•nal (vaj′i-năl). Relating to the vagina or to any sheath. [Mod. L. *vaginalis*]

vag•i•nate (vaj′i-nāt). **1.** To ensheathe; to enclose in a sheath. **2.** Ensheathed; provided with a sheath.

vag•i•nec•to•my (vaj-i-nek′tō-mē). Excision of the vagina or a segment thereof. SYN colpectomy. [vagina + G. *ektomē,* excision]

vag•i•nis•mus (vaj-i-niz′mŭs). Painful spasm of the vagina preventing intercourse. [vagina + L. *-ismus,* action, condition]

vag•i•ni•tis, pl. **vag•i•ni•ti•des** (vaj-i-nī′tis, -nī′ti-dēz). Inflammation of the vagina. [vagina + G. *-itis,* inflammation]

adhesive v., inflammation of vaginal mucosa with adhesions of the vaginal walls to each other.

atrophic v., thinning and atrophy of the vaginal epithelium usually resulting from diminished estrogen stimulation; a common occurrence in postmenopausal women.

senile v., atrophic v. resulting from withdrawal of estrogen stimulation of mucosa, often assuming the form of adhesive v.

trichomonal v., acute v. caused by infection with *Trichomonas vaginalis,* which does not invade tissues but provokes an intense local inflammatory reaction in the vagina, cervix, and sometimes the urethra; infection is sexually transmitted; symptoms include frothy green or brown discharge, vulvar itching and irritation, and dysuria.

△**vagino-, vagin-.** The vagina. SEE ALSO colpo-. [L. *vagina*, sheath]

vag•i•no•cele (vaj′i-nō-sēl). SYN colpocele (1).

vag•i•no•dyn•ia (vaj′i-nō-din′ē-ă). Vaginal pain. SYN colpodynia.

vag•i•no•fix•a•tion (vaj′i-nō-fik-sā′shŭn). Suture of a relaxed and prolapsed vagina to the abdominal wall. SYN colpopexy, vaginopexy.

vag•i•no•my•co•sis (vaj′i-nō-mī-kō′sis). Vaginal infection due to a fungus.

vag•i•nop•a•thy (vaj-i-nop′ă-thē). Any diseased condition of the vagina. [vagino- + G. *pathos*, suffering]

vag•i•no•per•i•ne•o•plas•ty (vaj′i-nō-per-i-nē′ō-plas-tē). Plastic surgery of the perineum involving the vagina. SYN colpoperineoplasty. [vagino- + perineum, + G. *plastos*, formed]

vag•i•no•per•i•ne•or•rha•phy (vaj′i-nō-per-i-nē-ōr′ă-fē). Repair of a lacerated vagina and perineum. SYN colpoperineorrhaphy. [vagino- + perineum, + G. *rhaphē*, suture]

vag•i•no•per•i•ne•ot•o•my (vaj′i-nō-per-i-nē-ot′ō-mē). Division of the posterior aspect of the vagina and adjacent portion of the perineum to facilitate childbirth. [vagino- + perineum, + G. *tomē*, incision]

vag•i•no•pexy (vaj′i-nō-pek-sē). SYN vaginofixation.

vag•i•no•plas•ty (vaj′i-nō-plas-tē). Plastic surgery of the vagina. SYN colpoplasty. [vagino- + G. *plastos*, formed]

vag•i•nos•co•py (vaj-i-nos′kŏ-pē). Inspection of the vagina, usually with an instrument.

vag•in•o•sis. Disease of the vagina.

bacterial v., infection of the vagina apparently caused by *Gardnerella vaginalis* and other anaerobes. Characterized by excessive, sometimes malodorous, discharge.

vag•i•not•o•my (vaj-i-not′ō-mē). A cutting operation in the vagina. SYN colpotomy.

va•gi•tus uter•i•nus (va-jī′tŭs yū-ter-ī′nŭs). Crying of the fetus while still within the uterus, possible when the membranes have been ruptured and air has entered the uterine cavity. [L. fr. *vagio*, to squall; L. fr. *uterus*, womb]

△**vago-.** The vagus nerve. [L. *vagus*]

va•gol•y•sis (vā-gol′i-sis). Surgical destruction of the vagus nerve. [vago- + G. *lysis*, a loosening]

va•go•lyt•ic (vā-gō-lit′ik). **1.** Pertaining to or causing vagolysis. **2.** A therapeutic or chemical agent that has inhibitory effects on the vagus nerve. **3.** Denoting an agent having such effects.

va•go•mi•met•ic (vā′gō-mi-met′ik). Mimicking the action of the efferent fibers of the vagus nerve.

va•got•o•my (vā-got′ō-mē). Division of the vagus nerve. [vago- + G. *tomē*, incision]

va•go•tro•pic (vā-gō-trop′ik). Attracted by, hence acting upon, the vagus nerve. [vago- + G. *tropos*, turning]

va•go•va•gal (vā′gō-vā′găl). Pertaining to a process that utilizes both afferent and efferent vagal fibers.

va•gus, gen. and pl. **va•gi** (vā′gŭs; vā′gī, -jī). SYN vagus *nerve*. [L. wandering, so-called because of the wide distribution of the nerve]

Val valine and its radicals.

va•lence, va•len•cy (vā′lens, -len-sē). The combining power of one atom of an element (or a radical), that of the hydrogen atom being the unit of comparison, determined by the number of electrons in the outer shell of the atom (v. electrons); *e.g.*, in HCl, chlorine is monovalent; in H_2O, oxygen is bivalent; in NH_3, nitrogen is trivalent. [L. *valentia*, strength]

val•gus (val′gŭs). Descriptive of any of the paired joints of the extremities with a static angular deformity in which the bone distal to the joint deviates laterally from the longitudinal axis of the proximal bone, and from the midline of the body, when the subject is in anatomical position. The adjective v. is attached sometimes to the name of the joint (cubitus v.) and sometimes to the name of the part just distal to the joint (hallux v.). The gender of the adjective matches that of the Latin noun to which it is joined; thus, cubitus, hallux, metatarsus, pes, talipes *valgus*; coxa, manus, talipomanus *valga*; genu *valgum*. [Mod. L. turned outward, fr. L. bowlegged]

hindfoot v., eversion of the calcaneus relative to the tibia. SYN rearfoot pronation.

va•line (Val, V) (val′in). 2-Amino-3-methylbutanoic acid; the L-isomer is a constituent of most proteins; a nutritionally essential amino acid.

val•late (val′āt). Bordered with an elevation, as a cupped structure; denoting especially certain lingual papillae. SEE ALSO circumvallate. [L. *vallo*, pp. *-atus*, to surround with, fr. *vallum*, a rampart]

val•lec•u•la, pl. **val•lec•u•lae** (vă-lek′yū-lă, -lē) [NA]. A crevice or depression on any surface. [L. dim. of *vallis*, valley]

val•ue (val′yū). A particular quantitative determination. For v.'s not given below, see the specific name. SEE ALSO index, number. [M.E., fr. O.Fr., fr. L. *valeo*, to be of value]

buffer v., the power of a substance in solution to absorb acid or alkali without change in pH; this is highest at a pH value equal to the pK_a value of the acid of the buffer pair.

normal v.'s, a set of laboratory test v.'s used to characterize apparently healthy individuals; now replaced by reference v.'s.

phenotypic v., QUANTITATIVE GENETICS The metrical quantity of some trait associated with a particular phenotype.

predictive v., an expression of the likelihood that a given test result correlates with the presence or absence of disease. A positive predictive v. is the ratio of patients with the disease who test positive to the entire population of individuals with a positive test result; a negative predictive v. is the ratio of patients without the disease who test negative to the entire population of individuals with a negative test.

reference v.'s, a set of laboratory test v.'s obtained from an individual or group in a defined state of health; this term replaces normal v.'s, since it is based on a defined state of health rather than on apparent health.

threshold limit v., the maximum concentration of a chemical recommended by the American

va

Conference of Government Industrial Hygienists for repeated exposure without adverse health effects on workers.

val•va, pl. **val•vae** (val′vă, -vē) [NA]. SYN valve. [L. one leaf of a double door]

val•val, val•var (val′văl, val′văr). Relating to a valve.

val•vate (val′vāt). Relating to or provided with a valve. SYN valvular.

valve (valv). **1.** A fold of the lining membrane of a canal or other hollow organ serving to retard or prevent a reflux of fluid. **2.** Any reduplication of tissue or flaplike structure resembling a v. SEE ALSO valvule, plica. SYN valva [NA]. [L. *valva*]

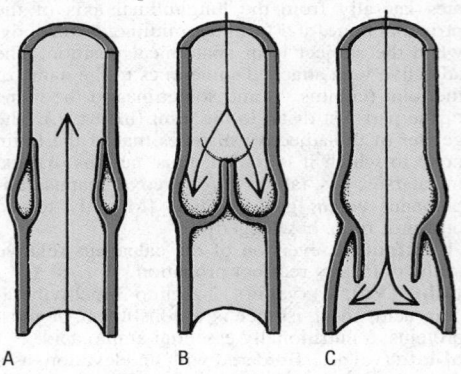

A   B   C

valve: in a healthy vein the valves allow blood to travel toward heart (A) while keeping blood from flowing back away from heart (B); valves in varicose veins (C) no longer function properly, thus allowing blood to travel back toward extremities

aortic v., the v. between the left ventricle and the ascending aorta, consisting of three fibrous semilunar cusps (valvules). They are named in accordance with their embryonic derivation: the anteriorly located cusp is the right cusp (above which the right coronary artery arises), the left posteriorly positioned cusp is the left cusp (above which the left coronary artery arises), and the right posteriorly positioned cusp is the posterior or noncoronary cusp.

atrioventricular v.'s, SEE tricuspid v., mitral v.

ball v., any of a variety of prosthetic cardiac v.'s consisting of a ball within a retaining cage affixed to the orifice; when appropriately sized, used in aortic, mitral, or tricuspid position.

bicuspid v., SYN mitral v.

congenital v., an abnormal lining fold obstructing a passage.

v. of coronary sinus, a delicate fold of endocardium at the opening of the coronary sinus into the right atrium.

Heyer-Pudenz v., a v. used in the shunting procedure for hydrocephaly; consisting of a catheter-v. system in which the ventricular catheter leads the cerebrospinal fluid into a one-way pump through which the cerebrospinal fluid passes down the distal catheter into the right atrium of the heart.

ileocecal v., the bilabial prominence of the terminal ileum into the large intestine at the cecocolic junction as seen in cadavers; in the living individual it appears as a truncated cone with a star-shaped orifice. SYN ileocolic v.

ileocolic v., SYN ileocecal v.

mitral v., the v. closing the orifice between the left atrium and left ventricle of the heart; its two cusps are called anterior and posterior. SYN bicuspid v.

parachute mitral v., congenital deformity of the mitral v. characterized by the presence of a single papillary muscle from which the chordae of both v. leaflets divide; the condition often produces a stenosis as the combined result of the tugging action of the chordae on, and the subsequent narrowing between, the leaflets.

pulmonary v., the v. at the entrance to the pulmonary trunk from the right ventricle; it consists of semilunar cusps (valvules) which are usually arranged in the adult in right anterior, left anterior, and posterior positions; however, they are named in accordance with their embryonic derivation; thus the posteriorly located cusp is designated as the left cusp, the right anteriorly located cusp is designated the right cusp and the left anteriorly positioned cusp is called the anterior cusp.

semilunar v., a heart v. composed of a set of three semilunar cusps (valvules); hence both the aortic and pulmonary valves are semilunar v.'s.

tricuspid v., the v. closing the orifice between the right atrium and right ventricle of the heart; its three cusps are called anterior, posterior, and septal.

urethral v.'s, folds in the urethral mucous membrane.

vesicoureteral v., a lock mechanism in the wall of the intravesical portion of the ureter that normally prevents urinary reflux.

val•vo•plas•ty (val′vō-plas-tē). Surgical reconstruction of a deformed cardiac valve, for the relief of stenosis or incompetence. SYN valvuloplasty. [valve + G. *plastos,* formed]

val•vot•o•my (val-vot′ō-mē). **1.** Cutting through a stenosed cardiac valve to relieve the obstruction. SYN valvulotomy. **2.** Incision of a valvular structure. [valve + G. *tomē,* incision]

val•vu•la, pl. **val•vu•lae** (val′vyū-lă, -lē) [NA]. SYN valvule. [Mod. L. dim. of *valva*]

val•vu•lar (val′vyū-lăr). SYN valvate.

val•vule (val′vūl). A valve, especially one of small size. SYN valvula [NA]. [L. *valvula*]

val•vu•li•tis (val-vyū-lī′tis). Inflammation of a valve, especially a heart valve. [Mod. L. *valvula,* valve, + G. *-itis,* inflammation]

val•vu•lo•plas•ty (val′vyū-lō-plas′tē). SYN valvoplasty.

val•vu•lot•o•my (val-vyū-lot′ō-mē). SYN valvotomy (1).

va•na•di•um (V) (vă-nā′dē-ŭm). A metallic element, atomic no. 23, atomic wt. 50.9415; a bioelement, its deficiency can result in abnormal bone growth and a rise in cholesterol and triglyceride levels. [*Vanadis,* Scand. goddess]

v. group, Those elements resembling vanadium in chemical and metallurgical properties; included with vanadium are niobium and tantalum.

va•na•di•um group. See under vanadium.

va·nil·lism (vă-nil′izm). **1.** Symptoms of irritation of the skin, nasal mucous membrane, and conjunctiva from which workers with vanilla sometimes suffer. **2.** Infestation of the skin by sarcoptiform mites found in vanilla pods.

va·nil·lyl·man·del·ic ac·id (VMA) (van′i-lil-man-del′ik, vă-nil′il-). The major urinary metabolite of adrenal and sympathetic catecholamines; elevated in most patients with pheochromocytoma.

va·por (vā′per). **1.** Molecules in the gaseous phase of a solid or liquid substance exposed to a gas. **2.** A visible emanation of fine particles of a liquid. **3.** A medicinal preparation to be administered by inhalation. [L. steam]

va·por·i·za·tion (vā-pōr-i-zā′shŭn). **1.** The change of a solid or liquid to a state of vapor. **2.** The therapeutic application of a vapor.

va·por·ize (vā′-per-īz). **1.** To convert a solid or liquid into a vapor. **2.** To apply a vapor therapeutically.

va·por·iz·er (vā′per-īz-er). **1.** An apparatus for reducing medicated liquids to a state of vapor suitable for inhalation or application to accessible mucous membranes. SEE ALSO nebulizer, atomizer. **2.** A device for volatilizing liquid anesthetics.

V̇a/Q̇ ventilation/perfusion *ratio.*

var·i·a·ble (var′ē-ă-bl). **1.** That which is inconstant, which can or does change, as contrasted with a constant. **2.** Deviating from the type in structure, form, physiology, or behavior. [L. *vario,* to vary, change, differ]

var·i·ance (var′ē-ans). **1.** The state of being variable, different, divergent, or deviate; a degree of deviation. **2.** A measure of the variation shown by a set of observations, defined as the sum of squares of deviations from the mean, divided by the number of degrees of freedom in the set of observations.

var·i·ant (var′ē-ant). **1.** That which, or one who, is variable. **2.** Having the tendency to alter or change, exhibit variety or diversity, not conform, or differ from the type.

var·i·a·tion (var-ē-ā′shŭn). Deviation from the type, especially the parent type, in structure, form, physiology, or behavior. [L. *variatio,* fr. *vario,* to change, vary]

var·i·ca·tion (var-i-kā′shŭn). Formation or presence of varices.

var·i·ce·al (var-ĭ-sē′ăl, vă-ris′ē-ăl). Of or pertaining to a varix.

⌐**var·i·cel·la** (var-i-sel′ă). An acute contagious disease, usually occurring in children, caused by the varicella-zoster virus and marked by a sparse eruption of papules, which become vesicles and then pustules, usually with mild constitutional symptoms; incubation period is about 14 to 17 days. SYN chickenpox. [Mod. L. dim. of *variola*]

var·i·cel·li·form (var-ĭ-sel′ĭ-fōrm). Resembling varicella.

va·ri·ces (var′i-sēz). Plural of varix.

var·i·ci·form (var′ĭ-si-fōrm, vă-ris′ĭ-fōrm). Resembling a varix.

⌐**varico-.** A varix, varicose, varicosity. [L. *varix,* a dilated vein]

var·i·co·bleph·a·ron (var′i-kō-blef′ă-ron). A varicosity of the eyelid. [varico- + G. *blepharon,* eyelid]

var·i·co·cele (var′i-kō-sēl). A condition manifested by abnormal dilation of the veins of the spermatic cord, caused by incompetent valves in the internal spermatic vein and resulting in impaired drainage of blood into the spermatic cord veins when the patient assumes the upright position. [varico- + G. *kēlē,* tumor, hernia]

var·i·co·ce·lec·to·my (var′i-kō-sē-lek′tō-mē). Operation for the correction of a varicocele by ligature and excision and by ligation of the dilated veins. [varicocele + G. *ektomē,* excision]

var·i·cog·ra·phy (var′ĭ-kog′ră-fē). Radiography of the veins after injection of contrast medium into varicose veins. [varico- + G. *graphō,* to write]

var·i·com·pha·lus (var-i-kom′fă-lŭs). A swelling formed by varicose veins at the umbilicus. [varico- + G. *omphalos,* navel]

var·i·co·phle·bi·tis (var′i-kō-flĕ-bī′tis). Inflammation of varicose veins. [varico- + G. *phleps,* vein, + *-itis,* inflammation]

var·i·cose (var′i-kōs). Relating to, affected with, or characterized by varices or varicosis.

var·i·co·sis, pl. **var·i·cos·es** (var-i-kō′sis, -sēz). A dilated or varicose state of a vein or veins. [varico- + G. *-osis,* condition]

var·i·cos·i·ty (var-i-kos′i-tē). A varix or varicose condition.

var·i·cot·o·my (var-i-kot′ō-mē). An operation for varicose veins by subcutaneous incision. [varico- + G. *tomē,* a cutting]

va·ric·u·la (vă-rik′yū-lă). A varicose condition of the veins of the conjunctiva. SYN conjunctival varix. [L. dim. of *varix*]

var·i·cule (var′i-kyūl). A small varicose vein ordinarily seen in the skin; may be associated with venous stars, venous lakes, or larger varicose veins. [L. *varicula,* dim. of *varix*]

va·ri·o·la (vă-rī′ō-lă). SYN smallpox. [Med. L. dim of L. *varius,* spotted]

va·ri·o·lar (vă-rī′ō-lăr). Relating to smallpox. SYN variolous.

var·i·o·late (var′ē-ō-lāt). **1.** To inoculate with smallpox. **2.** Pitted or scarred, as if by smallpox.

var·i·ol·i·form (vă-rī′ō-li-fōrm, var-ē-ō′li-fōrm). SYN varioloid. [variola + L. *forma,* form]

va·ri·o·loid (var′ē-ō-loyd). Resembling smallpox. SYN varioliform. [variola + G. *eidos,* resemblance]

va·ri·o·lous (vă-rī′ō-lŭs). SYN variolar.

var·ix, pl. **va·ri·ces** (var′iks, var′i-sēz). **1.** A dilated vein. **2.** An enlarged and tortuous vein, artery, or lymphatic vessel. [L. *varix* (*varic-*), a dilated vein]

> **aneurysmal v.,** dilation and tortuosity of a vein resulting from an acquired communication with an adjacent artery.

> **conjunctival v.,** SYN varicula.

⌐**esophageal varices,** longitudinal venous varices at the lower end of the esophagus as a result of portal hypertension; they are superficial and liable to ulceration and massive bleeding.

var·nish (dental). Solutions of natural resins and gums in a suitable solvent, of which a thin coating is applied over the surfaces of the cavity

va

preparations before placement of restorations, used as a protective agent for the tooth against constituents of restorative materials. SYN vernix.

var·us (va′rŭs). Descriptive of any of the paired joints of the extremities with a static angular deformity in which the bone distal to the joint deviates medially from the longitudinal axis of the proximal bone, and toward the midline of the body, when the subject is in anatomical position. The adjective v. is attached sometimes to the name of the joint (cubitus v.) and sometimes to the name of the body part just distal to the joint (hallux v.). The gender of the adjective matches that of the Latin noun to which it is joined; thus, cubitus, hallux, metatarsus, pes, talipes *varus;* coxa, manus, talipomanus *vara;* genu *varum.* Cf. valgus. [Mod. L. bent inward, fr. L. knock-kneed]

  hindfoot v., inversion of the calcaneus relative to the tibia. SYN rearfoot supination.

vas, gen. **va′sis,** pl. **va·sa,** gen. and pl. **va·so·rum** (vas, vā′sis, vā′să, vā-sō′rŭm) [NA]. A duct or canal conveying any liquid, such as blood, lymph, chyle, or semen. SEE ALSO vessel. [L. a vessel, dish]

  v. af′ferens, pl. **va′sa afferen′tia** [NA], SYN afferent glomerular *arteriole.*

  v. def′erens, pl. **va′sa deferen′tia,** SYN *ductus* deferens.

  v. ef′ferens, pl. **va′sa efferen′tia** [NA], **(1)** a vein carrying blood away from a part; **(2)** SYN efferent glomerular *arteriole.* **(3)** SYN efferent *ductules* of testis, under *ductule.*

  va′sa lymphat′ica [NA], SYN lymph *vessels,* under *vessel.*

  va′sa pre′via, umbilical vessels presenting in advance of the fetal head, usually traversing the membranes and crossing the internal cervical os.

  va′sa rec′ta, (1) straight vessels into which the efferent arteriole of the juxtamedullary glomeruli breaks up; they form a leash of vessels which, arising at the bases of the pyramids, run through the renal medulla toward the apex of each pyramid, then reverse direction in a hairpin turn, and run straight back again toward the base of the pyramid as venae rectae; **(2)** SYN straight seminiferous *tubule.*

  va′sa vaso′rum [NA], small arteries distributed to the outer and middle coats of the larger blood vessels, and their corresponding veins.

△**vas-.** A vas, blood vessel. SEE ALSO vasculo-, vaso-. [L. *vas*]

va·sa (vā′să). Plural of vas.

va·sal (vā′săl). Relating to a vas or to vasa.

vas·cu·lar (vas′kyū-lăr). Relating to or containing blood vessels. [L. *vasculum,* a small vessel, dim. of *vas*]

vas·cu·lar·i·ty (vas-kyū-lar′i-tē). The condition of being vascular.

vas·cu·lar·i·za·tion (vas′kyū-lăr-i-zā′shŭn). The formation of new blood vessels in a part.

vas·cu·lar·ized (vas′kyū-lăr-īzd). Rendered vascular by the formation of new vessels.

vas·cu·la·ture (vas′kyū-lă-chūr). The vascular network of an organ.

vas·cu·li·tis (vas-kyū-lī′tis). SYN angiitis.

  cutaneous v., an acute form of v. which may affect the skin only, but also may involve other

organs, with a polymorphonuclear infiltrate in the walls of and surrounding small (dermal) vessels. Nuclear fragments are formed by karyorrhexis of the neutrophils. SEE ALSO leukocytoclastic v.

  leukocytoclastic v., cutaneous acute v. characterized clinically by palpable purpura, especially of the legs, and histologically by exudation of the neutrophils and sometimes fibrin around dermal venules, with nuclear dust and extravasation of red cells; may be limited to the skin or involve other tissues as in Henoch-Schönlein purpura. SEE ALSO cutaneous v. [G. *leukos,* white, + *kytos,* cell, + *klastos,* broken, fr. *klao,* to break]

△**vasculo-.** A blood vessel. SEE ALSO vas-, vaso-. [L. *vasculum,* a small vessel, dim. of *vas*]

vas·cu·lo·my·e·li·nop·a·thy (vas′kyū-lō-mī-ĕ-li-nop′ă-thē). Small cerebral vessel vasculopathy with subsequent perivascular demyelination, presumably due to circulating immune complexes.

vas·cu·lop·a·thy (vas-kyū-lop′ă-thē). Any disease of the blood vessels. [vasculo- + G. *pathos,* disease]

va·sec·to·my (va-sek′tō-mē). Excision of a segment of the vas deferens, performed in association with prostatectomy, or to produce sterility. SYN deferentectomy, gonangiectomy. [vas- + G. *ektomē,* excision]

vas·i·fac·tion (vas-i-fak′shŭn). SYN angiopoiesis.

vas·i·fac·tive (vas-i-fak′tiv). SYN angiopoietic.

vas·i·form (vas′i-fōrm). Having the shape of a vas or tubular structure.

vas·i·tis (va-sī′tis). SYN deferentitis.

△**vaso-.** Vas, blood vessel. SEE ALSO vas-, vasculo-. [L. *vas,* a vessel]

va·so·ac·tive (vā-sō-ak′tiv, vas-ō-). Influencing the tone and caliber of blood vessels.

va·so·con·stric·tion (vā′sō-kon-strik′shŭn, vas′ō-). Narrowing of the blood vessels.

va·so·con·stric·tive (vā′sō-kon-strik′tiv, vas′ō-). **1.** Causing narrowing of the blood vessels. **2.** SYN vasoconstrictor (1).

va·so·con·stric·tor (vā′sō-kon-strik′ter, vas′ō-). **1.** An agent that causes narrowing of the blood vessels. SYN vasoconstrictive (2). **2.** A nerve, stimulation of which causes vascular constriction.

va·so·de·pres·sion (vā′sō-dē-presh′ŭn, vas′ō). Reduction of tone in blood vessels with vasodilation and resulting lowered blood pressure.

va·so·de·pres·sor (vā′sō-dē-pres′er, vas′ō). **1.** Producing vasodepression. **2.** An agent that produces vasodepression.

va·so·di·la·ta·tion (vā′sō-dil-ă-tā′shŭn, vas′ō-). SYN vasodilation.

va·so·di·la·tion (vā′sō-dī-lā′shŭn, vas-ō-). widening of the lumen of blood vessels. SYN vasodilatation.

va·so·di·la·tive (vā′sō-dī-lā′tiv, vas′ō-). **1.** Causing dilation of the blood vessels. **2.** SYN vasodilator (1).

va·so·di·la·tor (vā′sō-dī-lā′ter, vas′ō-). **1.** An agent that causes dilation of the blood vessels. SYN vasodilative (2). **2.** A nerve, stimulation of which results in dilation of the blood vessels.

va·so·ep·i·did·y·mos·to·my (vā′sō-ep-i-did-i-mos′tō-mē, vas′ō-). Surgical anastomosis of the vasa deferentia to the epididymis, to bypass an obstruction at the level of the mid to distal epididymis or proximal vas. [vaso- + epididymis + G. *stoma*, mouth]

va·so·for·ma·tion (vā-sō-fōr-mā′shŭn, vas-ō-). SYN angiopoiesis.

va·so·for·ma·tive (vā-sō-fōr′mă-tiv, vas-ō-). SYN angiopoietic.

va·so·gan·gli·on (vā-sō-gang′glē-on, vas-ō-). A mass of blood vessels.

va·sog·ra·phy (vā-sog′ră-fē). Radiography of the vas deferens to determine patency, by injecting contrast medium into its lumen either transurethrally or by open vasotomy. [vas + G. *graphō*, to write]

va·so·hy·per·ton·ic (vā′sō-hī-per-ton′ik, vas′ō-). Relating to increased arteriolar tension or vasoconstriction. [vaso- + G. *hyper*, over, + *tonos*, tone]

va·so·hy·po·ton·ic (vā′sō-hī-po-ton′ik, vas′ō-). Relating to reduced arteriolar tension or vasodilation. [vaso- + G. *hypo*, under, + *tonos*, tone]

va·so·in·hib·i·tor (vā′sō-in-hib′i-ter, vas′ō-). An agent that restricts or prevents the functioning of the vasomotor nerves.

va·so·in·hib·i·to·ry (vā′sō-in-hib′i-tōr-ē, vas′ō-). Restraining vasomotor action.

va·so·li·ga·tion (vā′sō-li-gā′shŭn, vas′ō-). Ligation of the vas deferens, usually after its division.

va·so·mo·tion (vā-sō-mō′shŭn, vas-ō-). Change in caliber of a blood vessel. SYN angiokinesis.

va·so·mo·tor (vā-sō-mō′ter, vas-ō-). 1. Causing dilation or constriction of the blood vessels. 2. Denoting the nerves which have this action. SYN angiokinetic.

va·so·neu·rop·a·thy (vā′sō-nū-rop′ă-thē, vas′ō-). Any disease involving both the nerves and blood vessels. [vaso- + G. *neuron*, nerve, + *pathos*, suffering]

va·so·or·chi·dos·to·my (vā′sō-ōr-ki-dos′tō-mē, vas′ō-). Reestablishment of the interrupted seminiferous channels by uniting the tubules of the epididymis or of the rete testis to the divided end of the vas deferens. [vaso- + G. *orchis*, testis, + *stoma*, mouth]

va·so·pa·ral·y·sis (vā′sō-pă-ral′i-sis, vas′ō-). Paralysis, atonia, or hypotonia of blood vessels.

va·so·pa·re·sis (vā′sō-pă-rē′sis, -par′ē-sis, vas′ō-). A mild degree of vasoparalysis. SYN vasomotor paralysis. [vaso- + G. *paresis*, weakness]

va·so·pres·sin (vā-sō-pres′in, vas-ō-). A nonapeptide neurohypophysial hormone related to oxytocin and vasotocin; synthetically prepared or obtained from the posterior lobe of the pituitary of healthy domestic animals. In pharmacological doses v. causes contraction of smooth muscle, notably that of all blood vessels; large doses may produce cerebral or coronary arterial spasm. SYN antidiuretic hormone. [vaso- + L. *premo*, pp. *pressum*, to press down, + -in]

 arginine v. (AVP) [8-arginine]vasopressin; [Arg⁸]vasopressin; v. containing an arginyl residue in position 8 (as in chickens and most mammals, including humans); porcine v. has a lysyl residue at position 8. All are vasopressors.

va·so·pres·sor (vā-sō-pres′er, vas-ō-). 1. Producing vasoconstriction and a rise in systemic arterial pressure. 2. An agent that has this effect.

va·so·punc·ture (vā-sō-pŭnk′chūr, vas-ō-). The act of puncturing a vessel with a needle.

va·so·re·flex (vā-sō-rē′fleks, vas′ō-). A reflex that influences the caliber of blood vessels.

va·so·re·lax·a·tion (vā′sō-rē-lak-sā′shŭn, vas-ō). Reduction in tension of the walls of the blood vessels.

va·so·sec·tion (vā-sō-sek′shŭn, vas-ō-). SYN vasotomy.

va·so·sen·so·ry (vā-sō-sen′ser-ē, vas-ō-). 1. Relating to sensation in the blood vessels. 2. Denoting sensory nerve fibers innervating blood vessels.

va·so·spasm (vā′sō-spazm, vas′ō-). Contraction or hypertonia of the muscular coats of the blood vessels. SYN angiospasm.

va·so·spas·tic (vā-sō-spas′tik, vas-ō-). Relating to or characterized by vasospasm. SYN angiospastic.

va·so·stim·u·lant (va-sō-stim′yū-lant). 1. Exciting vasomotor action. 2. An agent that excites the vasomotor nerves to action. 3. SYN vasotonic (2).

va·sos·to·my (vă-sos′tō-mē). Establishment of an artificial opening into the deferent duct. [vaso- + G. *stoma*, mouth]

va·sot·o·my (vā-sot′ō-mē). Incision into or division of the vas deferens. SYN vasosection. [vaso- + G. *tomē*, incision]

va·so·to·nia (vā-sō-tō′nē-ă, vas-ō-). The tone of blood vessels, particularly the arterioles. SYN angiotonia. [vaso- + G. *tonos*, tone]

va·so·ton·ic (vā-sō-ton′ik, vas-ō-). 1. Relating to vascular tone. 2. An agent that increases vascular tension. SYN vasostimulant (3).

va·so·tro·phic (vā-sō-trof′ik, vas-ō-). Relating to the nutrition of the blood vessels or the lymphatics. [vaso- + G. *trophē*, nourishment]

va·so·tro·pic (vā-sō-trō′pik, vas-ō-). Tending to act on the blood vessels. [vaso- + G. *tropē*, a turning]

va·so·va·gal (vā-sō-vā′găl, vas-ō-). Relating to the action of the vagus nerve upon the blood vessels.

va·so·va·sos·to·my (vā′sō-vă-sos′tō-mē, vas′ō-). Surgical anastomosis of vasa deferentia, to restore fertility in a previously vasectomized male. [vaso- + vaso- + G. *stoma*, mouth]

va·so·ve·sic·u·lec·to·my (vā′sō-vĕ-sik-yū-lek′tō-mē, vas′ō-). Excision of the vas deferens and seminal vesicles. [vaso- + L. *vesicula*, vesicle, + G. *ektomē*, excision]

VC colored *vision*; vital *capacity*.

V̇CO₂ carbon dioxide production.

VCUG voiding cystourethrogram.

VDRL Abbreviation for Venereal Disease Research Laboratories. SEE VDRL *test*.

vec·tion (vek′shŭn). Transference of the agents of disease from an infected to an uninfected individual by a vector. [L. *vectio*, conveyance]

vec·tor (vek′ter, tōr). 1. An invertebrate animal capable of transmitting an infectious agent among vertebrates. 2. Anything having magnitude, direction, and sense; it can be represented by a straight line of appropriate length and direction. 3. The net electrical axis of the heart (represented by an arrow) whose length is proportional to the magnitude of the electrical force, whose direction gives the direction of the force, and whose tip represents the positive pole of the force. **4.** DNA such as a chromosome or plasmid that autonomously replicates in a cell to which another DNA segment may be inserted and be itself replicated, as in cloning. **5.** SYN recombinant v. [L. *vector,* a carrier]

biological v., a v., such as the *Anopheles* mosquito for malarial agents or the tsetse fly for agents of African sleeping sickness, in which the agent multiplies prior to being transmitted to another host.

cloning v., an autonomously replicating plasmid or phage with regions that are not essential for its propagation in bacteria and into which foreign DNA can be inserted; this foreign DNA is replicated and propagated as if it were a normal component of the v.

expression v., a v. (plasmid, yeast, or animal virus genome) used experimentally to introduce foreign genetic material into a propagatable host cell in order to replicate and amplify the foreign DNA sequences as a recombinant molecule (recombinant DNA cloning of sequences).

mechanical v., a v. that conveys pathogens to a susceptible individual without essential biological development of the pathogens in the v., as in the transfer of septic organisms on the feet or mouth parts of the housefly.

recombinant v., a v. into which a foreign DNA has been inserted. SYN vector (5).

vec•tor•car•di•o•gram (vek′tōr-kar′dē-ō-gram). A graphic representation of the magnitude and direction of the heart's action currents in the form of vector loops.

vec•tor•car•di•og•ra•phy (vek′tōr-kar-dē-og′ră-fē). **1.** A variant of electrocardiography in which the heart's activation currents are represented by vector loops. **2.** The study and interpretation of vectorcardiograms.

vec•to•ri•al (vek-tōr′ē-ăl). Relating in any way to a vector.

veg•an (veg′an). A strict vegetarian; *i.e.,* one who consumes no animal or dairy products of any type. Cf. vegetarian.

veg•e•ta•ble (vej′tă-bl, vej′ě-tă-bl). **1.** A plant, specifically one used for food. **2.** Relating to plants, as distinguished from animals or minerals. SYN vegetal (1). [M.E., fr. L. *vegetabilis* (see vegetation)]

veg•e•tal (vej′ě-tăl). **1.** SYN vegetable (2). **2.** Denoting the vital functions common to plants and animals, such as respiration, metabolism, growth, and generation, distinguished from those peculiar to animals, such as conscious sensation and the mental faculties.

veg•e•tar•i•an (vej-ě-tār′ē-ăn). One whose diet is restricted to foods of vegetable origin, excluding primarily animal meats. Cf. vegan.

veg•e•ta•tion (vej-ě-tā′shŭn). **1.** The process of growth in plants. **2.** A condition of sluggishness, comparable to the inactivity of plant life. **3.** A growth or excrescence of any sort. **4.** Specifically, a clot, composed largely of fused blood platelets, fibrin, and sometimes microorganisms, adherent to a diseased heart orifice or valve, and

often initiated by infection of the structures involved. [Mod. L. *vegetatio,* growth]

veg•e•ta•tive (vej′ě-tā-tiv). **1.** Growing or functioning involuntarily or unconsciously, after the assumed manner of vegetable life; denoting especially a state of grossly impaired consciousness, as after severe head trauma or brain disease, in which an individual is incapable of voluntary or purposeful acts and only responds reflexively to painful stimuli. **2.** Resting; not active; denoting the stage of a cell or its nucleus in which the process of karyokinesis is quiescent. [see vegetation]

ve•hi•cle (vē′hi-kl). **1.** An excipient or a menstruum; a substance, usually without therapeutic action, used as a medium to give bulk for the administration of medicines. **2.** An inanimate substance (*e.g.,* food, milk, dust, clothing, instrument) by which or upon which an infectious agent passes from an infected to a susceptible host. [L. *vehiculum,* a conveyance, fr. *veho,* to carry]

veil (vāl). **1.** SYN velum (1). **2.** SYN caul (1). [L. *velum*]

Veil•lo•nel•la (vā′yō-nel′ă). A genus of nonmotile, non-spore-forming, anaerobic bacteria containing small Gram-negative cocci which occur as diplococci and in masses. These organisms are parasitic in the mouth and the intestinal and respiratory tracts of humans and other animals. [Adrien *Veillon,* French bacteriologist, 1864–1931]

vein (vān). A blood vessel carrying blood toward the heart; all the veins except the pulmonary carry dark or oxygenated blood. SYN vena [NA]. [L. *vena*]

accessory cephalic v., a variable v. that passes along the radial border of the forearm to join the cephalic v. near the elbow.

accessory hemiazygos v., formed by the union of the fourth to seventh left posterior intercostal v.'s, passes along the side of the bodies of the fifth, sixth, and seventh thoracic vertebrae, then crosses the midline behind the aorta, esophagus, and thoracic duct, and empties into the azygos v., sometimes in common with the hemiazygos v.

accessory vertebral v., a v. that accompanies the vertebral v. but passes through the foramen of the transverse process of the seventh cervical vertebra and opens independently into the brachiocephalic v.

angular v., a short v. at the medial angle of the eye, formed by the supraorbital and supratrochlear v.'s and continuing as the facial v.

anterior cardinal v.'s, SEE cardinal v.'s.

anterior cerebral v., a small v. that parallels the anterior cerebral artery and drains into the basal v.

anterior intercostal v.'s, tributaries to the musculophrenic or internal thoracic v.'s from the anterior portions of intercostal spaces.

anterior labial v.'s, tributaries of the femoral or external pudendal v.'s draining the mons pubis and anterior labia majora.

anterior vertebral v., the small v. that accompanies the ascending cervical artery; it opens below into the vertebral v.

appendicular v., the tributary of the ileocolic v. that accompanies the appendicular artery.

arcuate v.'s of kidney, v.'s that parallel the arcuate arteries, receive blood from interlobular v.'s and straight venules, and terminate in interlobar v.'s.

ascending lumbar v., paired, vertical v. of the posterior abdominal wall, adjacent and parallel to the vertebral column, posterior to the origin of the psoas major muscle; it connects the common iliac, iliolumbar, and lumbar v.'s in the paravertebral line, the right v. joining the right subcostal v. to form the azygos v., the left v. uniting with the left subcostal v. to form the hemiazygos v.

axillary v., a continuation of the basilic and brachial v.'s running from the lower border of the teres major muscle to the outer border of the first rib where it becomes the subclavian v.

azygos v., arises from the merger of the right ascending lumbar v. with the right subcostal v. and often a communication with the inferior vena cava; ascends through the aortic hiatus of the diaphragm or its right crus; it runs along the right side of the thoracic vertebral bodies in the posterior mediastinum, and terminates by arching anteriorly over the root of the right lung to enter the posterior aspect of the superior vena cava. SYN azygos (2).

basal v. of Rosenthal, a large v. passing caudally and dorsally along the medial surface of the temporal lobe from which it receives tributaries; it empties into the great cerebral v. (of Galen) from the lateral side.

basilic v., arises from the ulnar side of the dorsal venous network of the hand; it curves around the medial side of the forearm, communicates with the cephalic v. via the median cubital v., and passes up the medial side of the arm to join the axillary v.

basivertebral v., one of a number of v.'s in the spongy substance of the bodies of the vertebrae, emptying into the anterior internal vertebral venous plexus.

brachial v.'s, venae comitantes of the brachial artery which empty into the axillary v.

brachiocephalic v.'s, formed by the union of the internal jugular and subclavian v.'s; other tributaries of the right brachiocephalic v. are the right vertebral and internal thoracic v.'s, and the right lymphatic duct; other tributaries of the left brachiocephalic v. are the left vertebral, internal thoracic, superior intercostal, thyroidea ima, and various anterior pericardial, bronchial, mediastinal v.'s, and the thoracic duct. SYN innominate v.'s.

bronchial v.'s, many v.'s running in front of and behind the bronchi and uniting into two main trunks which empty on the right side into the azygos v., on the left into the accessory hemiazygos or the left superior intercostal v.

v. of bulb of penis, a tributary of the internal pudendal v. that drains the bulb of the penis.

capillary v., SYN venule.

cardinal v.'s, the major systemic venous channels in adult primitive vertebrates and in the embryos of higher vertebrates; the **anterior cardinal v.'s** are the major drainage channels from the cephalic part of the body, and the **posterior cardinal v.'s,** from the caudal part; the **common cardinal v.'s,** formed by the anastomosis of the anterior and posterior cardinal v.'s, are the main systemic return channels to the heart.

cavernous v.'s of penis, the cavernous venous spaces in the erectile tissue of the penis.

central v.'s of liver, the terminal branches of the hepatic v.'s that lie centrally in the hepatic lobules and receive blood from the liver sinusoids.

central v. of retina, formed by union of the retinal v.'s and accompanies the artery of the same name in the optic nerve.

central v. of suprarenal gland, the single draining v. of the gland; it receives a number of medullary v.'s; on the right side it empties directly into the inferior vena cava and on the left into the left renal v.

cephalic v., arises at the radial border of the dorsal venous rete of the hand, passes upward in front of the elbow and along the lateral side of the arm; it empties into the upper part of the axillary v.

ciliary v.'s, several small v.'s, anterior and posterior, coming from the ciliary body and emptying into the superior and inferior ophthalmic veins.

v. of cochlear canaliculus, it drains the cochlea, sacculus, and part of the utricules, and empties into the superior bulb of the jugular v. by accompanying the perilymphatic duct through the cochlear canaliculus.

common basal v., the tributary to the inferior pulmonary v. (right and left) that receives blood from the superior and inferior basal v.'s.

common facial v., a short vessel formed by the union of the facial v. and the retromandibular v., emptying into the jugular v.; considered to be a continuation of the facial v. in the NA.

conjunctival v.'s, the v.'s of the conjunctiva which drain primarily to the ophthalmic v.'s.

costoaxillary v., one of a number of anastomotic v.'s connecting the intercostal v.'s of the first to seventh intercostal spaces with the lateral thoracic or the thoracoepigastric v.

cystic v.'s, v.'s, usually anterior and posterior, which drain the neck of the gallbladder and cystic duct, along which they pass to enter the right branch of the portal v.; they communicate extensively with surrounding v.'s of the stomach, duodenum and pancreas.

deep cerebral v.'s, the numerous v.'s draining the deep structures of the cerebral hemispheres; they empty into the tributaries of the great cerebral v.

deep cervical v., large v. running with the artery of the same name between the semispinalis capitis and semispinalis cervicis, draining the deep muscles at the back of the neck and emptying into the brachiocephalic or the vertebral v.

deep dorsal v. of clitoris, a tributary of the vesical venous plexus; it runs a course deep to the fascia on the dorsum of the clitoris.

deep dorsal v. of penis, a vein on the dorsum of the penis deep to the fascia of the penis; it is a tributary to the prostatic venous plexus.

ve

deep facial v., the communicating v. that passes from the pterygoid venous plexus of the infratemporal fossa to the facial v.; it is devoid of valves.

deep femoral v., the v. that accompanies the deep femoral artery, receiving perforating v.'s from the lateral and posterior aspects of the thigh. It joins the femoral v. in the femoral triangle, usually in common with the medial and lateral circumflex femoral v.'s.

deep lingual v., the principal v. of the tongue that accompanies the deep lingual artery and joins the lingual v. It drains the body and apex of the tongue, running posteriorly near the median plane; often visible through the mucosa on the underside of the tongue, to each side of the frenulum.

deep v. of penis, the v. deep to the deep fascia on the dorsum of the penis. It enters the prostatic plexus by passing through a gap between the arcuate pubic ligament and the transverse perineal ligament.

deep v.'s of clitoris, the v.'s that pass from the dorsum of the clitoris to join the vesical plexus.

diploic v., one of the v.'s in the diploë of the cranial bones, connected with the cerebral sinuses by emissary v.'s; the main diploic v.'s are the frontal, anterior temporal, posterior temporal, and occipital.

dorsal scapular v., the vena comitans of the descending scapular artery; it is a tributary to the subclavian or the external jugular v.

emissary v., one of the channels of communication between the venous sinuses of the dura mater and the v.'s of the diploë and the scalp. SYN emissary (2).

episcleral v.'s, a series of small venules in the sclera close to the corneal margin that empty into the anterior ciliary v.'s.

esophageal v.'s, series of v.'s draining the submucous venous plexus of the esophagus; proceding inferiorly from the cervical portion of the esophagus, they drain to the inferior thyroid v., the superior intercostal v.'s, the azygos, accessory hemiazygos and hemiazygos v.'s, all of which are ultimately tributaries of the superior vena cava; the most inferior esophageal v.'s, from the cardiac portion of the esophagus, drain via the esophageal branches of the left gastric v., a tributary of the portal v. Thus, the submucosal v.'s of the inferior esophagus form a portocaval anastomoses, and are subject to the formation of varicosities in portal hypertension.

ethmoidal v.'s, v.'s that accompany the anterior and posterior ethmoidal arteries and pass into the superior ophthalmic v.; they drain the ethmoidal sinuses.

external nasal v.'s, several vessels that drain the external nose, emptying into the angular or facial v.

external pudendal v.'s, these correspond to the arteries of the same name; they empty into the great saphenous v. or directly into the femoral v., and receive the superficial dorsal v. of the penis (or clitoris) and the anterior scrotal (or labial) v.'s.

facial v., a continuation of the angular v. at the medial angle of the eye; it passes diagonally downward and outward, uniting with the retromandibular v. below the border of the lower jaw before emptying into the internal jugular v.

femoral v., a continuation of the popliteal v.; it accompanies the femoral artery through the adductor canal and into the femoral triangle where it lies within the femoral sheath; it becomes the external iliac v. as it passes deep to inguinal ligament.

fibular v.'s, SYN peroneal v.'s.

great cardiac v., begins at the apex of the heart (where it anastomoses with the middle cardiac v.), runs first with the anterior interventricular artery as it ascends the anterior interventricular groove, then turns to the left as it approaches or reaches the coronary groove to run with the circumflex branch of the left coronary artery; it merges with the oblique v. of the left atrium to form the coronary sinus.

great cerebral v. of Galen, a large, unpaired v. formed by the junction of the two internal cerebral v.'s in the caudal part of the tela choroidea of the third ventricle; it passes caudally between the splenium of the corpus callosum and the pineal gland, curving dorsally to merge with the inferior sagittal sinus to form the straight sinus.

hemiazygos v., formed by the merger of the left ascending lumbar v. with the left subcostal v. or a communication from the inferior vena cava, it pierces the left crus of the diaphragm, ascends along the left side of the bodies of the lower thoracic vertebrae, opposite the eighth vertebra, crosses the midline behind the aorta, thoracic duct, and esophagus, and empties into the azygos v., sometimes in common with the accessory hemiazygos v.

hepatic v.'s, the v.'s that drain the liver; they collect blood from the central v.'s and terminate in three large v.'s opening into the inferior vena cava below the diaphragm and several small inconstant v.'s entering the vena cava at more inferior levels.

hepatic portal v., SYN portal v.

highest intercostal v., the v. draining the first intercostal space into either the vertebral or the brachiocephalic v.

ileal v.'s, SEE jejunal and ileal v.'s.

ileocolic v., a large tributary of the superior mesenteric v. that runs parallel to the ileocolic artery and drains the terminal ileum, appendix, cecum, and the lower part of the ascending colon.

iliolumbar v., accompanying the artery of the same name, anastomosing with the lumbar and deep circumflex iliac v.'s, and emptying into the internal iliac v.

inferior basal v., tributary to the common basal v. draining the medial and posterior part of the inferior lobe in each lung.

inferior cerebral v.'s, numerous cerebral v.'s that drain the undersurface of the cerebral hemispheres and empty into the cavernous and transverse sinuses.

inferior epigastric v., corresponds to the artery of the same name and empties into the external iliac v. just proximal to the inguinal ligament.

inferior labial v., a tributary of the facial v. draining the lower lip.

inferior thalamostriate v.'s, v.'s draining the thalamus and striate body exiting the anterior perforated substance; tributary to the basal v. SYN striate v.'s.

innominate v.'s, SYN brachiocephalic v.'s.

intercapitular v.'s, the v.'s connecting the dorsal and palmar v.'s in the hand, or the dorsal and plantar v.'s in the foot.

interlobar v.'s of kidney, the v.'s in the kidney that parallel the interlobar arteries, receiving blood from arcuate v.'s, and terminate in the renal v.

interlobular v.'s of kidney, they parallel the interlobular arteries and drain the peritubular capillary plexus, emptying into the arcuate v.'s.

interlobular v.'s of liver, the terminal branches of the portal v. that course in the portal canals between the conceptual liver lobules and empty into the liver sinusoids.

intermediate basilic v., the medial branch of the median antebrachial v. which joins the basilic v.

intermediate cephalic v., the lateral branch of the median antebrachial v. that joins the cephalic v. near the elbow.

internal auditory v.'s, SYN labyrinthine v.'s.

internal cerebral v.'s, paired v.'s passing caudally near the midline in the tela choroidea of the third ventricle, formed by the union of the choroid v., thalamostriate (terminal) v., and v. of septum pellucidum, and uniting caudally so as to form the great cerebral v.

internal iliac v., runs from the upper border of the greater sciatic notch to the brim of the pelvis where it joins the external iliac v. to form the common iliac v.; it drains most of the territory supplied by the internal iliac artery.

internal pudendal v., a tributary of the internal iliac v. that accompanies the internal pudendal artery as a single or double vessel. It drains the perineum.

intervertebral v., one of numerous v.'s accompanying the spinal nerves through the intervertebral foramina, draining spinal cord and vertebral venous plexuses, and emptying in the neck into the vertebral v., in the thorax into the intercostal v.'s, in the lumbar and sacral regions into the lumbar and sacral v.'s.

jejunal and ileal v.'s, the v.'s that drain the jejunum and ileum; they terminate in the superior mesenteric v.

v.'s of kidney, the tributaries of the renal v. that drain the kidney; they parallel the arteries in the kidney and consist of interlobular, arcuate, and interlobar v.'s.

v.'s of knee, the v.'s that accompany the genicular arteries; they drain blood from the structures around the knee, terminating in the popliteal v.

labyrinthine v.'s, one or more v.'s accompanying the labyrinthine artery; they drain the internal ear, pass out through the internal acoustic meatus, and empty into the transverse sinus or the inferior petrosal sinus. SYN internal auditory v.'s.

lacrimal v., small v. which drains the lacrimal gland, passing posteriorly through the orbit with the lacrimal artery to empty into the superior ophthalmic v.

lateral sacral v.'s, several v.'s that receive the drainage of the sacral venous plexus and sacral intervertebral v.'s, then accompany the corresponding artery and empty into the internal iliac v. on each side.

left gastric v., arises from a union of v.'s from both surfaces of the cardia of the stomach and an esophageal tributary from the cardiac portion of the esophagus; it runs in the lesser omentum and empties into the portal v. SEE ALSO esophageal v.'s.

left umbilical v., the v. that returns the blood from the placenta to the fetus; traversing the umbilical cord, it enters the fetal body at the umbilicus and passes thence into the liver, where it is joined by the portal v.; its blood then flows by way of the ductus venosus and the inferior vena cava to the right atrium.

lingual v., receives blood from the tongue, sublingual and submandibular glands, and muscles of the floor of the mouth; empties into the internal jugular or the facial v.

lumbar v.'s, v.'s accompanying the lumbar arteries, which drain the posterior body wall and the lumbar vertebral venous plexuses, and terminate anteriorly as follows: the first and second in the ascending lumbar v., the third and fourth in the inferior vena cava, and the fifth in the iliolumbar v.; all communicate via the ascending lumbar v.'s.

maxillary v., the posterior continuation of the pterygoid plexus; it joins the superficial temporal vein to form the retromandibular vein.

median antebrachial v., it begins at the base of the dorsum of the thumb, curves around the radial side, ascends the middle of the forearm, and just below the bend of the elbow divides into the intermediate basilic and intermediate cephalic v.'s; sometimes it divides lower down, one branch going to the basilic v., the other to the intermediate v. of the elbow.

median cubital v., a v. which passes across the anterior aspect of the elbow from the cephalic v. to the basilic v.; commonly this v. is replaced by intermediate basilic and intermediate cephalic v.'s. The median cubital v. is often used for venipuncture.

median sacral v., an unpaired v. accompanying the middle sacral artery receiving blood from the sacral venous plexus and emptying into the left common iliac v.

mediastinal v.'s, several small v.'s from the mediastinum emptying into the brachiocephalic v.'s or the superior vena cava.

meningeal v.'s, v.'s that accompany the meningeal arteries; they communicate with venous sinuses and diploic v.'s and drain into regional v.'s outside the cranial vault.

middle cardiac v., begins at the apex of the heart (where it anastomoses with the great cardiac v.), and ascends within the posterior interventricular sulcus to the coronary sinus.

middle meningeal v.'s, the venae comitantes of the middle meningeal artery that empty into the pterygoid plexus.

middle temporal v., it arises near the lateral angle of the eye and joins the superficial temporal v.'s to form the retromandibular v.

musculophrenic v.'s, the v.'s that accompany the musculophrenic artery and drain blood from the upper abdominal wall and anterior portions of the lower intercostal spaces and the diaphragm.

nasofrontal v., the v. located in the anterior medial part of the orbit that connects the superior ophthalmic v. with the angular v.

oblique v. of left atrium, a small v. on the posterior wall of the left atrium which merges with the great cardiac v. to form the coronary sinus; it is developed from the left common cardinal v., and occasionally persists as a left superior vena cava.

obturator v., formed by the union of tributaries draining the hip joint and the obturator and adductor muscles of the thigh; it enters the pelvis by the obturator canal as venae comitantes of the obturator artery and empties into the internal iliac v.

occipital v., drains the occipital region and empties into the internal jugular v. or the suboccipital plexus.

occipital cerebral v.'s, the superior cerebral v.'s draining the occipital cortex and emptying into the superior sagittal sinus and the transverse sinus.

palatine v., drains the palatine regions and empties into the facial v.

palpebral v.'s, v.'s draining the superior eyelid posteriorly as tributaries of the superior ophthalmic v.

pancreatic v.'s, v.'s draining the pancreas, emptying into the splenic v. and the superior mesenteric v.

pancreaticoduodenal v.'s, v.'s that accompany the superior and inferior pancreaticoduodenal arteries, emptying into the superior mesenteric or portal v.

paraumbilical v.'s, several small v.'s arising from cutaneous v.'s about the umbilicus running along the round ligament of the liver, and terminating as accessory portal v.'s in the substance of this organ; they constitute a portocaval anastomosis and are subject to varicosity during portal hypertension; varicose paraumbilical v.'s form the "caput medusae."

parotid v.'s, branches draining part of the parotid gland and emptying into the retromandibular v.

pectoral v.'s, v.'s draining the pectoral muscles and emptying directly into the subclavian v.

perforating v.'s, the v.'s that accompany the perforating arteries from the profunda femoris artery; they drain blood from the vastus lateralis and hamstring muscles and terminate in the profunda femoris v.

pericardiacophrenic v.'s, the v.'s accompanying the pericardiacophrenic artery and emptying into the brachiocephalic v.'s or superior vena cava.

pericardial v.'s, several small v.'s from the pericardium emptying into the brachiocephalic v.'s or superior vena cava.

peroneal v.'s, venae comitantes of the peroneal artery; they join the posterior tibial v.'s to enter the popliteal v. syn fibular v.'s.

pharyngeal v.'s, several v.'s from the pharyngeal venous plexus emptying into the internal jugular v.

popliteal v., formed at the lower border of the popliteus muscle by the union of the anterior and posterior tibial v.'s, ascends through the popliteal space where it receives the lesser saphenous v. and passes through the adductor hiatus, entering the adductor canal as the femoral v.

portal v., a wide short v. formed by the superior mesenteric and splenic v. posterior to the neck of the pancreas, ascending in front of the inferior vena cava, and dividing at the right end of the porta hepatis into right and left branches, which ramify within the liver. syn hepatic portal v.

posterior v. of left ventricle, arises on the diaphragmatic surface of the heart near the apex, runs to the left and parallel to the posterior interventricular sulcus, and empties in the coronary sinus.

posterior intercostal v.'s, v.'s draining the intercostal spaces posteriorly; those of the first 1-C space drain into the brachiocephalic v.'s; from spaces 2–3 they drain into right and left superior intercostal v.'s; from the 4th to the 11th spaces on the right they are tributaries of the azygos v.; on the left they empty into either the hemiazygos or accessory hemiazygos v.'s.

posterior labial v.'s, they pass posteriorly from the labia majora and minora to the internal pudendal v.'s.

prepyloric v., a tributary of the right gastric v. that passes anterior to the pylorus at its junction with the duodenum.

v. of pterygoid canal, a v. accompanying the nerve and artery through the pterygoid canal and emptying into the pharyngeal venous plexus.

pulmonary v.'s, four v.'s, two on each side, conveying oxygenated blood from the lungs to the left atrium of the heart. Those from the left lung and the inferior v. from the right lung are lobar v.'s, each draining a single lobe with the corresponding name; the right superior pulmonary v. drains both the superior and middle lobes of the right lung.

pyloric v., syn right gastric v.

radial v.'s, venae comitantes of the radial artery continuing from those of the radial aspect of the deep palmar arch, draining into the venae comitantes of the brachial artery in the cubital fossa.

renal v.'s, large v.'s formed at the renal hilus by the merger of the segmental v.'s anterior to the corresponding arteries; they open at right angles into the inferior vena cava at the level of the second lumbar vertebra. The left renal v. receives the left suprarenal v. and the left gonadal v., and passes through the angle between the abdominal aorta and superior mesenteric artery where it may be compressed.

retromandibular v., formed by the union of the superficial temporal and maxillary v.'s in front of the ear; runs posterior to the ramus of the mandible through the parotid gland, and unites with the posterior auricular v. to form the external jugular v.; it usually has a large communicating branch with the facial v.

right gastric v., it receives v.'s from both surfaces of the upper portion of the stomach, runs to the right along the lesser curvature of the stomach, and empties into the portal v. SYN pyloric v.

scleral v.'s, small v.'s draining the sclera; they are tributaries to the anterior ciliary v.'s.

short gastric v.'s, small vessels that drain the fundus and left portion of the stomach wall and empty into the splenic v.

sigmoid v.'s, the several tributaries of the inferior mesenteric v. that drain the sigmoid colon.

small cardiac v., an inconstant vessel, accompanying the right coronary artery in the coronary sulcus, from the right margin of the right ventricle, and emptying into the coronary sinus or the middle cardiac v.

spinal v.'s, the v.'s that drain the spinal cord; they form a plexus on the surface of the cord from which v.'s pass along the spinal roots to the internal vertebral venous plexus.

spiral v. of modiolus, the v. running a spiral course in the modiolus of the cochlea; it is tributary to both the labyrinthine v. and the v. of the cochlear canaliculus.

splenic v., arises by the union of several small v.'s at the hilum on the anterior surface of the spleen with the short gastric and left gastroepiploic v.'s; passes backward through the splenorenal ligament to the left kidney, then runs behind the upper border of the pancreas to the neck of the pancreas where it joins the superior mesenteric v. to form the portal v.

stellate v.'s, SYN *venulae* stellatae, under *venula.*

sternocleidomastoid v., it arises in the sternocleidomastoid muscle and accompanies the sternocleidomastoid branch of the occipital artery; it drains into the internal jugular or superior thyroid v.

striate v.'s, SYN inferior thalamostriate v.'s.

stylomastoid v., it drains the tympanic cavity, traverses the facial canal exiting via the stylomastoid foramen, and empties into the retromandibular v.

subclavian v., the direct continuation of the axillary v. at the lateral border of the first rib; it passes medially to join the internal jugular v. and form the brachiocephalic v. on each side.

subcutaneous v.'s of abdomen, the network of superficial v.'s of the abdominal wall that empty into the thoracoepigastric, superficial epigastric, or superior epigastric v.'s and form portocaval anastomoses through their communications with the paraumbilical v.'s.

sublingual v., v. which accompanies the sublingual artery in the floor of the mouth, lateral to the hypoglossal nerve; it may join the deep lingual v. to form the lingual v., or join the vena comitans nervi hypoglossi.

submental v., a v. situated below the chin, anastomosing with the sublingual v., connecting with the anterior jugular v., and emptying into the facial v.

superficial dorsal v.'s of penis, a pair of v.'s

on the dorsum of the penis superficial to the fascia penis; they are tributaries of the external pudendal v.'s on each side.

superficial epigastric v., drains the lower and medial part of the anterior abdominal wall and empties into the great saphenous v.

superficial v., one of a number of v.'s that course in the subcutaneous tissue and empty into deep v.'s; they form prominent systems of vessels in the limbs and are usually not accompanied by arteries.

superior basal v., tributary to the common basal v. draining the lateral and anterior part of the inferior lobe of each lung.

superior cerebral v.'s, numerous (8 to 10) v.'s that drain the dorsal convexity of the cortical hemisphere and empty into the superior sagittal sinus, curving rostrally in passing through the subdural space so as to enter the sinus at an acute forward angle.

superior epigastric v.'s, the venae comitantes of the artery of the same name, tributaries of the internal thoracic v.

superior labial v., v.'s taking blood from the upper lip and discharging into the facial v.

superior thalamostriate v., a long v. passing forward in the groove between the thalamus and caudate nucleus, covered by the lamina affixa, receiving the transverse caudate v.'s along its lateral side, and joining at the caudal wall of Monro's foramen with the choroidal v. and v. of septum pellucidum to form the internal cerebral v.

superior v. of vermis, a v. draining part of the superior part of the cerebellum; it runs on the superior surface of the vermis to terminate in the internal cerebral v.

supraorbital v., drains the front of the scalp and unites with the supratrochlear v.'s to form the angular v.

suprascapular v., v. that accompanies the suprascapular artery and empties into the external jugular v.

supratrochlear v.'s, several v.'s that drain the front part of the scalp and unite with the supraorbital v. to form the angular v.

surface thalamic v.'s, SYN *venae* directae laterales, under *vena.*

v.'s of temporomandibular joint, several small tributaries to the retromandibular v. from the temporomandibular joint.

thalamostriate v.'s, SEE inferior thalamostriate v.'s, superior thalamostriate v.

thoracoacromial v., corresponding to the artery of the same name, empties into the axillary v., sometimes by a common trunk with the cephalic v.

thoracoepigastric v., one of two v.'s, sometimes a single v., arising from the region of the superficial epigastric v. and opening into the axillary or the lateral thoracic v., thus forming an anastomotic or collateral pathway between tributaries of the inferior and superior venae cavae.

thymic v.'s, a number of small v.'s from the thymus emptying into the left brachiocephalic v.

tracheal v.'s, several small venous trunks from

ve

the trachea, emptying into the brachiocephalic v.'s or the superior vena cava.

transverse cervical v.'s, venae comitantes of the corresponding arteries, emptying into the external jugular v. or sometimes into the subclavian v. SYN transverse v.'s of neck.

transverse facial v., a tributary of the superficial temporal or retromandibular v.'s, anastomosing with the facial v. SYN transverse v. of face.

transverse v. of face, SYN transverse facial v.

transverse v.'s of neck, SYN transverse cervical v.'s.

tympanic v.'s, v.'s exiting from the tympanic cavity through the petrotympanic fissure with the chorda tympani and emptying into the retromandibular v.

ulnar v.'s, venae comitantes of the ulnar artery, continuing from those of the superficial palmar arch and joining with those of the radial artery to form the brachial veins in the cubital fossa.

umbilical v., SEE left umbilical v.

uterine v.'s, two v.'s on each side which arise from the uterine venous plexus, pass through a part of the broad ligament and then through a peritoneal fold, and empty into the internal iliac v.

varicose v.'s, permanent dilation and tortuosity of v.'s, most commonly seen in the legs, probably as a result of congenitally incomplete valves; there is a predisposition to varicose v.'s among persons in occupations requiring long periods of standing, and in pregnant women.

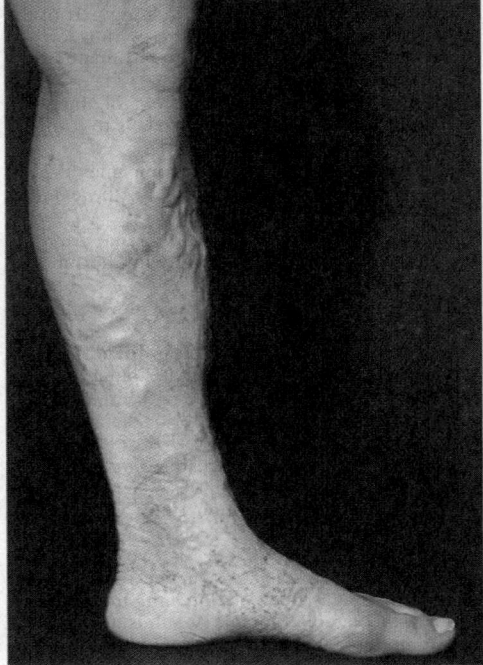

varicose veins

vertebral v., a v. derived from tributaries (ve-

nae comitantes) which run through the foramina in the transverse processes of the first six cervical vertebrae and form a plexus around the vertebral artery; it empties as a single trunk into the brachiocephalic v.'s.

v.'s of vertebral column, includes the internal and external vertebral venous plexuses, the basivertebral v.'s, and the anterior and posterior spinal v.'s.

vesical v.'s, v.'s that drain the vesical venous plexus; they join the internal iliac v.'s.

vestibular v.'s, v.'s draining the saccule and utricle; they are tributaries of both the labyrinthine v.'s and the v. of the vestibular aqueduct.

v. of vestibular aqueduct, a small v. accompanying the endolymphatic duct; it drains much of the vestibular portion of the labyrinth and terminates in the inferior petrosal sinus.

v. of vestibular bulb, the v. draining the bulb of the vestibule; a tributary of the internal pudendal v.

vortex v.'s, several v.'s (usually four) from the vascular tunic formed of v.'s accompanying the posterior ciliary arteries and the ciliary body; then drain into the superior or inferior ophthalmic v. SYN vorticose v.'s.

vorticose v.'s, SYN vortex v.'s.

ve·la (vē′lă). Plural of velum.

ve·la·men, pl. **ve·lam·i·na** (vě-lā′men, vě-lam′i-nă). SYN velum (1). [L. a veil]

vel·a·men·tous (vel-ă-men′tŭs). Expanded in the form of a sheet or veil.

ve·lar (vē′lăr). Relating to any velum, especially the velum palatinum.

vel·lus (vel′ŭs). **1.** Fine nonpigmented hair covering most of the body. **2.** A structure that is fleecy or soft and woolly in appearance. [L. fleece]

ve·loc·i·ty (v) (vě-los′i-tē). Rate and direction of movement; specifically, distance traveled or quantity converted per unit time in a given direction. [L. velocitas, fr. velox (veloc-), quick, swift]

maximum v. (V_{max}), (1) the maximum rate of an enzyme-catalyzed reaction that can be achieved by progressively increasing the substrate concentration at a given enzyme concentration; in cases of substrate inhibition, V_{max} is an extrapolated value in the absence of such inhibition; **(2)** the maximum initial rate of shortening of a myocardial fiber that can be obtained under zero load; used to evaluate the contractility of the fiber.

vel·o·pha·ryn·ge·al (vē′lō-fă-rin′jē-ăl). Pertaining to the soft palate (velum palatinum) and the posterior nasopharyngeal wall.

ve·lum, pl. **ve·la** (vē′lŭm, -lă). **1.** Any structure resembling a veil or curtain. SYN veil (1), velamen. **2.** SYN caul (1). **3.** SYN greater omentum. **4.** Any serous membrane or membranous envelope or covering. [L. veil, sail]

inferior medullary v., a thin sheet of white matter, hidden by the cerebellar tonsil, attached along the peduncle of the flocculus and, at or near the midline, to the nodulus of the vermis; it is continuous caudally with the epithelial lamina and choroid plexus of the fourth ventricle.

superior medullary v., the thin layer of white matter stretching between the two superior cerebellar peduncles, forming the roof of the superior recess of the fourth ventricle.

v. palati′num [NA], ✴official alternate term for soft *palate*.

ve•na, gen. and pl. **ve•nae** (vē′nă, -nē) [NA]. SYN vein. [L.]

venae comitan′tes, [NA] a pair of veins, occasionally more, that closely accompany an artery in such a manner that the pulsations of the artery aid venous return.

ve′nae direc′tae latera′les [NA], one or more veins running a subependymal course in a coronal plane over the thalamus, terminating in the internal cerebral vein. SYN surface thalamic veins.

inferior v. cava (IVC), receives the blood from the lower limbs and the greater part of the pelvic and abdominal organs; it begins at the level of the fifth lumbar vertebra on the right side by the merger of the right and left common iliac veins, pierces the diaphragm at the level of the eighth thoracic vertebra, and empties into the posteroinferior aspect of the right atrium of the heart. SYN postcava.

superior v. cava, returns blood from the head and neck, upper limbs, and thorax to the posterosuperior aspect of the right atrium; formed in the superior mediastinum by union of the two brachiocephalic veins. SYN precava.

ve•na•ca•vog•ra•phy (vē′nă-kā-vog′ră-fē). Angiography of a vena cava. SYN cavography.

⟩vene-. **1.** The veins, venous. SEE ALSO veno-. [L. *vena,* vein] **2.** venom. [L. *venenum,* poison]

ve•nec•ta•sia (ve-nek-tā′sē-ă). SYN phlebectasia.

ve•nec•to•my (ve-nek′tō-mē). SYN phlebectomy.

ve•neer (vĕ-nēr′). **1.** A thin surface layer laid over a base of common material. **2.** DENTISTRY A layer of tooth-colored material, usually porcelain or acrylic resin, attached to and covering the surface of a metal crown or natural tooth structure. [Fr. *fournir,* to furnish]

ven•e•na•tion (ven-ĕ-nā′shŭn, vē-nĕ-). Poisoning, as from a sting or bite. [L. *veneno,* pp. -*atus,* to poison, fr. *venenum,* poison]

ven•e•nous (ven′ĕ-nŭs). SYN poisonous. [L. *venenosus*]

ve•ne•re•al (ve-nēr′ē-ăl). Relating to or resulting from sexual intercourse. [L. *Venus* (*vener-*), goddess of love]

ven•e•sec•tion (ven-ē-sek′shŭn). SYN phlebotomy. [L. *vena,* vein, + *sectio,* a cutting]

⟩veni-. SEE veno-.

ven•i•punc•ture (ven′i-pŭnk-chūr, vē′ni-). The puncture of a vein, usually to withdraw blood or inject a solution.

⟩veno-, veni-. The veins. SEE ALSO vene- (1). [L. *vena*]

ve•no•gram (vē′nō-gram). **1.** Radiograph of opacified veins. **2.** SYN phlebogram. [veno- + G. *gramma,* a writing]

ve•nog•ra•phy (vē-nog′ră-fē). Radiographic demonstration of a vein, after the injection of contrast medium. SYN phlebography (2). [veno- + G. *graphō,* to write]

ven•om (ven′ŏm). A poisonous fluid secreted by snakes, spiders, scorpions, and other cold-blooded animals. [M. Eng. and O. Fr. *venim,* fr. L. *venenum,* poison]

ve•no•mo•tor (vē′nō-mō′ter). Causing change in the caliber of a vein. [veno- + L. *motor,* a move]

ve•no•scle•ro•sis (vē′nō-skle-rō′sis). SYN phlebosclerosis.

ve•nos•i•ty (vē-nos′i-tē). **1.** A venous state; a condition in which the bulk of the blood is in the veins at the expense of the arteries. **2.** The unaerated condition of venous blood.

ve•nos•ta•sis (vē-nō-stā′sis, vē-nos′tă-sis). SYN phlebostasis. [veno- + G. *stasis,* a standing]

ve•nos•to•my (vē-nos′tō-mē). SYN cutdown.

ve•not•o•my (vē-not′ō-mē). SYN phlebotomy.

ve•nous (vē′nŭs). Relating to a vein or to the veins. [L. *venosus*]

ve•nous re•turn. The blood returning to the heart via the great veins and coronary sinus.

ve•no•ve•nos•to•my (vē′nō-vē-nos′tō-mē). The formation of an anastomosis between two veins. SYN phlebophlebostomy. [veno- + veno- + G. *stoma,* mouth]

vent. An opening into a cavity or canal, especially one through which the contents of such a cavity are discharged, as the anus. [O. Fr. *fente,* a chink, cleft]

ven•ter (ven′ter). **1.** SYN abdomen. **2** [NA]. SYN belly (2). **3.** One of the great cavities of the body. **4.** The uterus. [L. *venter* (*ventr-*), belly]

ven•ti•late (ven′ti-lāt). To aerate, or oxygenate, the blood in the pulmonary capillaries. SYN air (2). [L. *ventilo,* pp. -*atus,* to fan, fr. *ventus,* the wind]

ven•ti•la•tion (ven-ti-lā′shŭn). **1.** Replacement of air or other gas in a space by fresh air or gas. **2.** Movement of gas(es) into and out of the lungs. SYN respiration (2). **3** (V̇). In physiology, the tidal exchange of air between the lungs and the atmosphere that occurs in breathing. SEE ALSO respiration. [see ventilate]

alveolar v. (V̇$_A$), the volume of gas expired from the alveoli to the outside of the body per minute; calculated as the respiratory frequency (f) multiplied by the difference between tidal volume and the dead space ($V_T - V_D$); units: ml/min BTPS.

ℹ️artificial v., application of mechanically or manually generated pressures, usually positive, to gas(es) in or about the airway as a means of producing gas exchange between the lungs and surrounding atmosphere. SYN artificial respiration.

assist-control v., artificial respiration in which inspiration is produced automatically after a set interval if the person has not already begun to inspire. Cf. assisted v., controlled v.

assisted v., application of mechanically or manually generated positive pressure to gas(es) in or about the airway during inhalation as a means of augmenting movement of gases into the lungs. SYN assisted respiration.

continuous positive pressure v., SYN controlled mechanical v.

controlled v., intermittent application of mechanically or manually generated positive pressure to gas(es) in or about the airway as a means of forcing gases into the lungs in the absence of spontaneous ventilatory efforts. SYN controlled respiration.

ve

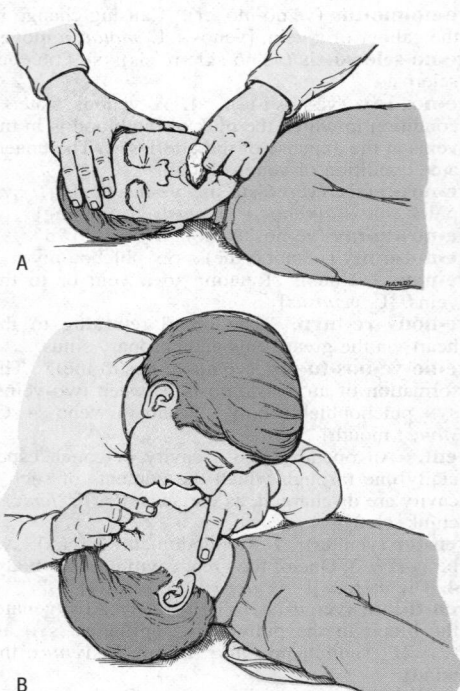

artificial ventilation: (A) attempt to remove any foreign matter in mouth with index finger wrapped in cloth or a handkerchief; (B) tilting head back and pinching nose, give two slow breaths into the victim's mouth with lips making a tight seal; breathe into victim until chest gently rises

controlled mechanical v. (CMV), artificial v. in which all inspirations are provided by positive pressure applied to the airway. SYN continuous positive pressure breathing, continuous positive pressure v., intermittent positive pressure breathing, intermittent positive pressure v.

high-frequency v. (HFV), a technique of positive pressure ventilation in which ventilating rates are above normal with ventilating volumes that are below normal; there are three basic modes: (1) high-frequency positive pressure v. (HFPPV), which uses respiratory rates between 60 and 100 breaths per minute; (2) high-frequency jet v. (HFJV), which uses rates about 100 and 400 to 600 breaths per minute; and (3) high-frequency oscillatory v. (HFOV), which uses rates in the thousands.

intermittent mandatory v. (IMV), mechanical application of positive pressure at a predetermined frequency to the airway to increase tidal volume.

intermittent positive pressure v. (IPPV), SYN controlled mechanical v.

manual v., intermittent manual compression of a gas-filled reservoir bag to force gases into a patient's lungs and thus maintain oxygenation

and carbon dioxide elimination during apnea or hypoventilation.

maximum voluntary v. (MVV), the volume of air breathed when an individual breathes as deeply and as quickly as possible for a given time. SYN maximum breathing capacity.

mechanical v., use of automatically cycling devices to generate airway pressures; employed in assisted or controlled v.

negative pressure v., a method of ventilatory support which creates a negative extrathoracic pressure and thus creates a more negative pleural pressure, as a result of which transpulmonary pressure is increased.

positive pressure v. (PPV), a mode of ventilatory support in which compressed gas is delivered under positive pressure (usually by a mechanical ventilator) into the patient's lungs.

pressure support v. (PSV), a mode of mechanical v. that provides a set amount of positive airway pressure; the patient's ventilatory demands determine the inspiratory time, peak inspiratory flow, volume, and rate.

pulmonary v., respiratory minute volume, *i.e.,* the total volume of gas per minute inspired (V_I) or expired (V_E) expressed in liters per minute; differs from alveolar v. by including the exchange of dead space gas.

spontaneous intermittent mandatory v. (SIMV), intermittent mandatory v. spontaneously initiated by the patient, to increase tidal volume, and subsequently synchronized with patient's respiratory cycle. SYN synchronized intermittent mandatory v.

synchronized intermittent mandatory v. (SIMV), SYN spontaneous intermittent mandatory v.

ventilator (ven-til-a-tor). An apparatus for producing mechanical ventilation, especially for a prolonged period, in cases of paralysis or of inadequate spontaneous ventilation.

pressure ventilator, a device designed to deliver inspired gas into the lungs until a preset level of pressure is reached.

volume ventilator, a device for delivering a preset volume of inspired gas into the lungs; within specified limits, the volume is independent of the pressure required to deliver that volume.

ven•trad (ven'trad). Toward the ventral aspect; opposed to dorsad. [L. *venter,* belly, + *ad,* to]

ven•tral (ven'trăl). **1.** Pertaining to the belly or to any venter. **2.** SYN anterior (1). **3.** VETERINARY ANATOMY The undersurface of an animal; often used to indicate the position of one structure relative to another, *i.e.,* situated nearer the undersurface of the body. [L. *ventralis*]

ven•tri•cle (ven'tri-kl). A normal cavity, as of the brain or heart. SYN ventriculus (2). [L. *ventriculus,* dim. of *venter,* belly]

fourth v., a cavity of irregular shape extending from the obex rostralward to its communication with the sylvian aqueduct, enclosed between the cerebellum dorsally and the rhombencephalic tegmentum ventrally, having a rhomboid-shaped floor (rhomboid fossa) and a tentlike roof which in its caudal part is formed by the tela choroidea and the posterior medullary velum, in its middle

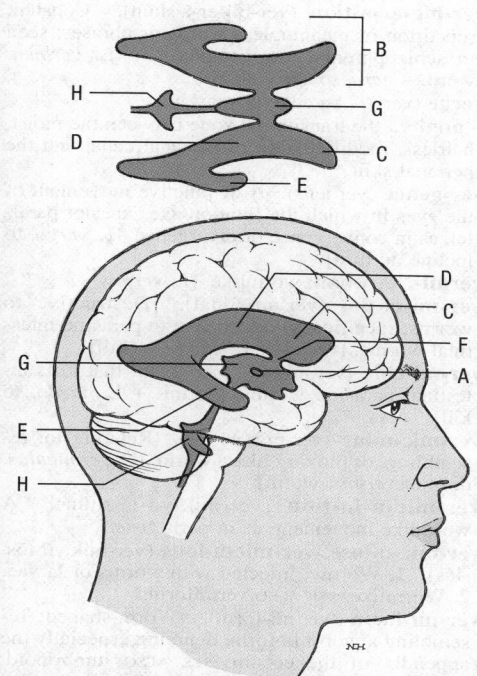

ventricles of the brain (superior and lateral views): (A) massa intermedia, (B) left lateral ventricle, (C) anterior horn of right lateral ventricle, (D) central part of right lateral ventricle, (E) inferior horn of right lateral ventricle, (F) interventricular foramen, (G) third ventricle, (H) fourth ventricle

part by the white matter of the cerebellum, and in its narrowing rostral part (recessus superior) by the anterior medullary velum. The fourth v. reaches its greatest width at the pontomedullary transition, where it expands laterally behind the cerebellar peduncles into the spoutlike lateral recess, and its greatest height at the fastigial recess, which reaches up into the cerebellar white matter. Direct communication of the brain's v. system and the subarachnoid space is established at the level of the fourth v. by a median opening in the tela choroidea, the medial aperture of Magendie's foramen, which opens into the cerebellomedullary cistern, and on both sides by the lateral aperture or foramen of Luschka, which connects the lateral recess with the interpeduncular cistern.

lateral v., a cavity shaped somewhat like a horseshoe in conformity with the general shape of the hemisphere; each lateral v. communicates with the third v. through the interventricular foramen of Monro, and expands from there forward into the frontal lobe as the anterior horn as well as caudally over the thalamus as the central part or cella media which, behind the thalamus, curves ventrally and laterally, then forward into the temporal lobe as the inferior horn; from the apex of the curve a variably sized posterior horn extends back into the white matter of the occipital lobe. The large choroid plexus of the lateral v.

invades the cella media and the inferior horn (but not the anterior and posterior horn) from the medial side.

left v., the lower chamber on the left side of the heart that receives the arterial blood from the left atrium and drives it by the contraction of its walls into the aorta.

right v., the lower chamber on the right side of the heart which receives the venous blood from the right atrium and drives it by the contraction of its walls into the pulmonary artery.

third v., a narrow, vertically oriented, irregularly quadrilateral cavity in the midplane, extending from the lamina terminalis to the rostral opening of the mesencephalic aqueduct. This v. communicates at its rostrodorsal corner with each of the two lateral v.'s through the left and right interventricular foramen of Monro. Its narrow roof is formed by the tela choroidea which is attached on either side to the tenia thalami; its lateral wall by the medial surface of the thalamus and, below the hypothalamic sulcus, by the hypothalamus, which also forms its floor. In lateral profile, the third v. exhibits a number of recesses: in its floor, from before backward, 1) the preoptic recess in the acute angle between the base of the lamina terminalis and the dorsum of the optic chiasm, 2) the infundibular recess extending ventrally into the infundibulum but not into the hypophysial stalk, and 3) the mamillary or inframamillary recess caused by the protrusion of the mamillary bodies into the v. From its dorsocaudal corner, the pineal recess extends caudally into the pineal stalk.

ven•tric•u•lar (ven-trik′yū-lăr). Relating to a ventricle, in any sense.

ven•tric•u•li•tis (ven-trik-yū-lī′tis). Inflammation of the ventricles of the brain. [ventricle + G. *-itis,* inflammation]

△**ventriculo-.** A ventricle. [L. *ventriculus*]

ven•tric•u•lo•a•tri•al (V-A) (ven-trik′yū-lō-ā′trē-ăl). Relating to both ventricles and atria, especially to the sequential passage of conduction in the retrograde direction from ventricle to atrium.

ven•tric•u•lo•cis•ter•nos•to•my (ven-trik′yū-lō-sis′ter-nos′tō-mē). An artificial opening between the ventricles of the brain and the cisterna magna. SEE ALSO shunt (2). [ventriculo- + L. *cisterna,* cistern, + G. *stoma,* mouth]

ven•tric•u•log•ra•phy (ven-trik-yū-log′ră-fē). **1.** Radiographic demonstration of the cerebral ventricles by direct injection of air or contrast medium. **2.** Demonstration of the contractility of the cardiac ventricles by recording serially the distribution of intravenously injected radionuclide or that of radiographic contrast medium injected through an intracardiac catheter. **3.** Visualization by roentgenography of a cardiac ventricle by injection of radiopaque contrast material. [ventriculo- + G. *graphē,* a writing]

ven•tric•u•lo•mas•toi•dos•to•my (ven-trik′yū-lō-mas′toy-dos′tō-mē). Establishment of a communication between the lateral cerebral ventricle and the mastoid antrum by means of a polythene tube for the relief of hydrocephalus. SEE ALSO shunt (2). [ventriculo- + mastoid, + G. *stoma,* mouth]

ve

ven·tric·u·lo·nec·tor (ven-trik′yū-lō-nek′ter, -tōr). SYN atrioventricular *bundle.* [ventriculo- + L. *necto,* to join]

ven·tric·u·lo·plas·ty (ven-trik′yū-lō-plas-tē). Any surgical procedure to repair a defect of one of the ventricles of the heart. [ventriculo- + G. *plastos,* formed]

ven·tric·u·lo·punc·ture (ven-trik′yū-lō-pŭnk′chūr). Insertion of a needle into a ventricle.

ven·tric·u·los·co·py (ven-trik-yū-los′kŏ-pē). Direct inspection of a ventricle with an endoscope. [ventriculo- + G. *skopeō,* to view]

ven·tric·u·los·to·my (ven-trik-yū-los′tō-mē). Establishment of an opening in a ventricle, usually from the third ventricle to the subarachnoid space to relieve hydrocephalus. SEE ALSO shunt (2). [ventriculo- + G. *stoma,* mouth]

    third v., an operation to establish an opening from the third ventricle to the prechiasmal and interpeduncular cisterns (Stookey-Scarff operation) or from the third ventricle to the interpeduncular cistern (Dandy operation).

ven·tric·u·lo·sub·a·rach·noid (ven-trik′yū-lō-sŭb-ă-rak′noyd). Relating to the space occupied by the cerebrospinal fluid. [ventriculo- + subarachnoid]

ven·tric·u·lot·o·my (ven-trik-yū-lot′ō-mē). Incision into a ventricle; *e.g.,* into the cerebral third ventricle for the relief of hydrocephalus or into a cardiac ventricle to surgically correct an abnormality. [ventriculo- + G. *tomē,* incision]

ven·tric·u·lus, pl. **ven·tric·u·li** (ven-trik′yū-lŭs, -lī). **1** [NA]. ✴official alternate term for stomach. **2** [NA]. ✴official alternate term for ventricle. [L. dim. of *venter,* belly]

ven·tri·duc·tion (ven-tri-dŭk′shŭn). Drawing toward the abdomen or abdominal wall.

△**ventro-.** Ventral. [L. *venter,* belly]

ven·tros·co·py (ven-tros′kŏ-pē). SYN peritoneoscopy. [ventro- + G. *skopeō,* to view]

ven·trot·o·my (ven-trot′ō-mē). SYN celiotomy. [ventro- + G. *tomē,* incision]

ven·u·la, pl. **ven·u·lae** (ven′yū-lă, -lē) [NA]. SYN venule. [L. dim. of *vena,* vein]

    ven′ulae stella′tae [NA], the star-shaped groups of venules in the renal cortex. SYN stellate veins, stellate venules.

ven·u·lar (ven′yū-lăr). Pertaining to venules.

ven·ule (ven′yūl, vē′nūl). A venous radicle continuous with a capillary. SYN venula [NA], capillary vein.

    high endothelial postcapillary v.'s, v.'s in the lymph nodes, tonsils, and Peyer's patches that have a high-walled endothelium through which blood lymphocytes migrate into the lymphatic parenchyma.

    pericytic v.'s, SYN postcapillary v.'s.

    postcapillary v.'s, the microvasculature immediately following the capillaries, ranging in size from 10 to 50 μm, and characterized by investment of pericytes; they are the site of extravasation of blood cells, are particularly sensitive to histamine, and are believed to be important in blood-interstitial fluid exchanges. SYN pericytic v.'s.

    stellate v.'s, SYN *venulae* stellatae, under *venula.*

ver·big·er·a·tion (ver-bij-er-ā′shŭn). Constant repetition of meaningless words or phrases; seen in schizophrenia. SYN cataphasia. [L. *verbum,* word, + *gero,* to carry about]

verge (verj). An edge or margin.

    anal v., the transitional zone between the moist, hairless, modified skin of the anal canal and the perianal skin.

ver·gence (ver′jens). A disjunctive movement of the eyes in which the fixation axes are not parallel, as in convergence or divergence. [L. *vergo,* to incline, to turn]

△**vermi-.** A worm; wormlike. [L. *vermis*]

ver·mi·ci·dal (ver′mi-sī′dăl). Destructive to worms; specifically, destructive to parasitic intestinal worms. [vermi- + L. *caedo,* to kill]

ver·mi·cide (ver′mi-sīd). An agent that kills intestinal parasitic worms. [vermi- + L. *caedo,* to kill]

ver·mic·u·lar (ver-mik′yū-lăr). Relating to, resembling, or moving like a worm. [L. *vermiculus,* dim. of *vermis,* worm]

ver·mic·u·la·tion (ver-mik-yū-lā′shŭn). A wormlike movement, as in peristalsis.

ver·mic·u·lose, ver·mic·u·lous (ver-mik′yū-lōs, -lŭs). **1.** Wormy; infected with worms or larvae. **2.** Wormlike. SEE ALSO vermiform.

ver·mi·form (ver′mi-fōrm). Worm-shaped; resembling a worm in form, denoting especially the appendix of the cecum. SEE ALSO lumbricoid. [vermi- + L. *forma,* form]

ver·mil·ion·ec·to·my (ver-mil-yon-ek′tō-mē). Excision of the vermilion border. [vermilion border + G. *ektomē,* cutting out]

ver·min (ver′min). Parasitic insects, such as lice and bedbugs. [L. *vermis,* a worm]

ver·mi·na·tion (ver-mi-nā′shŭn). **1.** The production or breeding of worms or larvae. **2.** Infestation with vermin.

ver·min·ous (ver′mi-nŭs). Relating to, caused by, or infested with worms, larvae, or vermin. [L. *verminosus,* wormy]

ver·mis, pl. **ver·mes** (ver′mis, -mēz). **1.** A worm; any structure or part resembling a worm in shape. **2** [NA]. The narrow middle zone between the two hemispheres of the cerebellum; the portion projecting above the level of the hemispheres on the upper surface is called the superior v.; the lower portion, sunken between the two hemispheres and forming the floor of the vallecula, is the inferior v. [L. worm]

ver·nix (ver′niks). SYN varnish (dental). [Mod. L.]

    v. caseo′sa, the fatty substance, consisting of desquamated epithelial cells, lanugo hairs, and sebaceous matter, which covers the skin of the fetus.

ver·ru·ca, pl. **ver·ru·cae** (vĕ-rū′kă, -sē). A flesh-colored growth characterized by circumscribed hypertrophy of the papillae of the corium, with thickening of the malpighian, granular, and keratin layers of the epidermis, caused by human papilloma virus; also applied to epidermal verrucous tumors of nonviral etiology. SYN verruga, wart. [L.]

    v. necrogen′ica, SYN postmortem *wart.*

v. perua′na, v. peruvia′na, SYN *verruga* peruana.

v. pla′na, a smooth, flat, flesh-colored wart of small size, occurring in groups, seen especially on the face of the young; often associated with common warts of the hands, due to human papilloma virus, commonly, types 3 and 10. SYN flat wart.

v. planta′ris, SYN plantar *wart*.

ver·ru·ci·form (vĕ-rū′si-fōrm). Wart-shaped. [L. *verruca,* wart, + *forma,* form]

ver·ru·cose (vĕ-rū′kōs). Resembling a wart; denoting wartlike elevations. [L. *verrucosus*]

ver·ru·ga (vĕ-rū′gă). SYN verruca. [Sp.]

v. perua′na, a late, eruptive stage of bartonellosis; characterized by soft conical or pedunculated vascular papules on the skin or mucous membranes, resolving without scars after a few months. SYN Peruvian wart, verruca peruana, verruca peruviana.

ver·sion (ver′zhŭn, -shŭn). **1.** Displacement of the uterus, with tilting of the entire organ without bending upon itself; such displacement may be anteversion, retroversion, or lateroversion. **2.** Change of position of the fetus in the uterus, occurring spontaneously or effected by manipulation. **3.** SYN inclination. **4.** Conjugate rotation of the eyes in the same direction; such rotation may be dextroversion, levoversion, supraversion, or infraversion. [L. *verto,* pp. *versus,* to turn]

bimanual v., turning of the baby *in utero,* performed by the hands acting upon both extremities of the fetus; it may be external v. or combined v.

cephalic v., v. in which the fetus is turned so that the head presents; can be external cephalic v. or internal cephalic v. SEE ALSO external cephalic v., internal cephalic v.

combined v., bipolar v. by means of one hand in the vagina, the other on the abdominal wall.

external cephalic v., v. performed entirely by external manipulation. SEE ALSO cephalic v.

internal cephalic v., v. performed by means of one hand within the vagina. SEE ALSO cephalic v.

pelvic v., v. by means of which a transverse or oblique presentation is converted into a pelvic presentation by manipulating the buttocks of the fetus.

podalic v., a manual procedure that results in a podalic extraction.

spontaneous v., turning of the fetus effected by the unaided contraction of the uterine muscle.

ver·te·bra, gen. and pl. **ver·te·brae** (ver′tĕ-bră, -brē) [NA]. One of the segments of the spinal column; in human beings there are usually 33 vertebrae, 7 cervical, 12 thoracic, 5 lumbar, 5 sacral (fused into one bone, the sacrum), and 4 coccygeal (fused into one bone, the coccyx). [L. joint, fr. *verto,* to turn]

basilar v., the lowest lumbar v.

cranial v., a segment of the skull regarded as homologous with a segment of the vertebral column.

v. denta′ta, SYN axis (5).

v. pla′na, spondylitis with reduction of vertebral body to a thin disk.

ver·te·bral (ver′tĕ-brăl). Relating to a vertebra or the vertebrae.

Ver·te·bra·ta (ver-tĕ-brah′tă, -brā′tă). The vertebrates, a major division of the phylum Chordata, consisting of those animals with a dorsal hollow nerve cord enclosed in a cartilaginous or bony spinal column; includes several classes of fishes, and the amphibians, reptiles, birds, and mammals. [L. *vertebratus,* jointed]

ver·te·brate (ver′tĕ-brāt). **1.** Having a vertebral column. **2.** An animal having vertebrae.

ver·te·brec·to·my (ver′tĕ-brek′tō-mē). Resection of a vertebral body. [vertebra + G. *ektomē,* excision]

⌂ vertebro-. A vertebra, vertebral. [L. *vertebra*]

ver·te·bro·chon·dral (ver′tĕ-brō-kon′drăl). Denoting the three false ribs (eighth, ninth, and tenth), which are connected with the vertebrae at one extremity and the costal cartilages at the other, these cartilages not articulating directly with the sternum. SYN vertebrocostal (2). [vertebro- + G. *chondros,* cartilage]

ver·te·bro·cos·tal (ver′tĕ-brō-kos′tăl). **1.** SYN costovertebral. **2.** SYN vertebrochondral. [vertebro- + L. *costa,* rib]

ver·te·bro·ster·nal (ver′tĕ-brō-ster′năl). SYN sternovertebral.

ver·tex, pl. **ver·ti·ces** (ver′teks, ver′ti-sēz). **1** [NA]. The topmost point of the vault of the skull, a landmark in craniometry. **2.** OBSTETRICS The portion of the fetal head bounded by the planes of the trachelobregmatic and biparietal diameters, with the posterior fontanel at the apex. [L. whirl, whorl]

ver·ti·cal (ver′ti-kăl). **1.** Relating to the vertex, or crown of the head. **2.** Perpendicular. **3.** Denoting any plane or line that passes longitudinally through the body in the anatomical position.

ver·ti·cil. A collection of similar parts radiating from a common axis. SYN vortex (1), whorl (4). [L. *verticillus,* the whirl of a spindle, dim. of *vertex,* a whirl]

ver·ti·cil·late (ver′ti-sil′āt). Disposed in the form of a verticil.

ver·tig·i·nous (ver-tij′i-nŭs). Relating to or suffering from vertigo.

ver·ti·go (ver′ti-gō, ver-tī′gō). **1.** A sensation of spinning or whirling motion. V. implies a definite sensation of rotation of the subject or of objects about the subject in any plane. **2.** Imprecisely used as a general term to describe dizziness. [L. *vertigo* (*vertigin*-), dizziness, fr. *verto,* to turn]

auditory v., SYN Ménière's *disease.*

benign paroxysmal postural v., a recurrent, brief form of postural v. occurring in clusters; believed to result from displaced remnants of utricular otoconia.

benign positional v., brief attacks of paroxysmal v. and nystagmus that occur solely with certain head movements or positions, *e.g.,* with neck extension; due to labyrinthine dysfunction. SYN postural v. (1).

gastric v., v. symptomatic of disease of the stomach.

labyrinthine v., SYN Ménière's *disease.*

ocular v., dizziness attributed to refractive errors or imbalance of the extrinsic muscles.

organic v., v. due to brain damage.

postural v., (1) SYN benign positional v. **(2)**

ve

light-headedness that appears particularly in elderly people with change of position, usually from lying or sitting to standing; due to orthostatic hypotension.

△**vesic-.** SEE vesico-.

ve·si·ca, gen. and pl. **ve·si·cae** (věs-ī'kă, věs-ī'sē, -kē). **1** [NA]. SYN bladder. **2.** Any hollow structure or sac, normal or pathologic, containing a serous fluid. [L.]

   v. bilia'ris [NA], SYN gallbladder.

   v. prostat'ica, SYN prostatic *utricle.*

   v. urina'ria [NA], SYN urinary *bladder.*

ves·i·cal (ves'i-kăl). Relating to any bladder, but usually the urinary bladder.

ves·i·cant (ves'i-kănt). An agent that produces a vesicle.

ves·i·ca·tion (ves-i-kā'shŭn). SYN vesiculation (1).

🔳 **ves·i·cle** (ves'i-kl). **1.** SYN vesicula. **2.** A small, circumscribed elevation of the skin containing fluid. SEE ALSO bleb, blister, bulla. **3.** A small sac containing liquid or gas. [L. *vesicula,* a blister, dim. of *vesica,* bladder]

   acrosomal v., a v. derived from the Golgi apparatus during spermiogenesis; together with the acrosomal granule within, it spreads in a thin layer over the pole of the nucleus to form the acrosomal cap.

   air v.'s, SYN pulmonary *alveolus.*

   allantoic v., the hollow portion of the allantois.

   auditory v., one of the paired sacs of invaginated ectoderm that develop into the membranous labyrinth of the internal ear. SYN otic v.

   blastodermic v., SYN blastocyst.

   cerebral v., each of the three divisions of the early embryonic brain (prosencephalon, mesencephalon, and rhombencephalon). SYN primary brain v.

   lens v., in the embryo, the ectodermal invagination that forms opposite the optic cup; it is the primordium of the lens of the eye.

   ophthalmic v., in the embryo, one of the paired evaginations from the ventrolateral walls of the forebrain from which the sensory and pigment layers of the retina develop.

   otic v., SYN auditory v.

   primary brain v., SYN cerebral v.

   seminal v., one of two folded, sacculated, glandular diverticula of the ductus deferens; its secretion is one of the components of the semen. SYN gonecyst, gonecystis, seminal gland.

   synaptic v.'s, the small (average diameter 30 nm), intracellular, membrane-bound v.'s near the presynaptic membrane of a synaptic junction, containing the transmitter substance which, in chemical synapses, mediates the passage of nerve impulses across the junction. SEE ALSO synapse.

   umbilical v., SYN yolk *sac.*

△**vesico-, vesic-.** A vesica, vesicle. SEE ALSO vesiculo-. [L. *vesica,* bladder]

ves·i·co·cele (ves'i-kō-sēl). SYN cystocele.

ves·i·coc·ly·sis (ves'i-kok'li-sis). Washing out, or lavage, of the urinary bladder. [vesico- + G. *klysis,* a washing out]

ves·i·co·pus·tu·lar (ves'i-kō-pŭs'tyū-lăr). Pertaining to a vesicopustule. SYN vesiculopustular (1).

ves·i·co·rec·tos·to·my (ves'i-kō-rek-tos'tō-mē). Surgical urinary tract diversion by anastomosis of the posterior bladder wall to the rectum. SYN cystorectostomy. [vesico- + rectum + G. *stoma,* mouth]

ves·i·co·sig·moi·dos·to·my (ves'ĭ-kō-sig-moy-dos'tō-mē). Operative formation of a communication between the bladder and the sigmoid colon. [vesico- + sigmoid + G. *stoma,* mouth]

ves·i·co·spi·nal (ves'i-kō-spī'năl). Relating to the urinary bladder and the spinal cord; denoting the neural mechanisms that control retention and evacuation of urine by the bladder, located in the second lumbar and second sacral segment, respectively, of the spinal cord.

ves·i·cos·to·my (ves'i-kos'tō-mē). SYN cystostomy. [vesico- + G. *stoma,* mouth]

ves·i·cot·o·my (ves'i-kot'ō-mē). SYN cystotomy.

ve·sic·u·la, gen. and pl. **ve·sic·u·lae** (vě-sik'yū-lă, -lē). A small bladder or bladder-like structure. SYN vesicle (1). [L. blister, vesicle, dim. of *vesica,* bladder]

ve·sic·u·lar (vě-sik'yū-lăr). **1.** Relating to a vesicle. **2.** Characterized by or containing vesicles. SYN vesiculate (2), vesiculous.

ve·sic·u·late (vě-sik'yū-lāt). **1.** To become vesicular. **2.** SYN vesicular (2).

ve·sic·u·la·tion (vě-sik'yū-lā'shŭn). **1.** The formation of vesicles. SYN blistering, vesication. **2.** SYN inflation. **3.** Presence of a number of vesicles.

ve·sic·u·lec·to·my (vě-sik'yū-lek'tō-mē). Resection of a portion or all of each of the seminal vesicles. [L. *vesicula,* vesicle, + G. *ektomē,* excision]

ve·sic·u·li·form (vě-sik'yū-li-fōrm). Resembling a vesicle.

ve·sic·u·li·tis (vě-sik-yū-lī'tis). Inflammation of any vesicle; especially of a seminal vesicle. [L. *vesicula,* vesicle, + G. *-itis,* inflammation]

△**vesiculo-.** A vesicle. [L. *vesicula,* vesicle, dim. of *vesica,* bladder]

ve·sic·u·lo·cav·ern·ous (vě-sik'yū-lō-kav'er-nŭs). Both vesicular and cavernous; denoting: **1.** An auscultatory sound having both a vesicular and a cavernous quality; **2.** The structure of certain neoplasms.

ve·sic·u·log·ra·phy (vě-sik-yū-log'ră-fē). Radiographic contrast study of the seminal vesicles. [vesiculo- + G. *graphō,* to write]

ve·sic·u·lo·pap·u·lar (vě-sik'yū-lō-pap'yū-lăr). Pertaining to or consisting of a combination of vesicles and papules, or of papules becoming increasingly edematous with sufficient collection of fluid to form vesicles.

ve·sic·u·lo·pros·ta·ti·tis (vě-sik'yū-lō-pros'tă-tī'tis). Inflammation of the bladder and prostate. [vesiculo- + prostate + G. *-itis,* inflammation]

ve·sic·u·lo·pus·tu·lar (vě-sik'yū-lō-pŭs'tyū-lăr). **1.** SYN vesicopustular. **2.** Pertaining to a mixed eruption of vesicles and pustules.

ve·sic·u·lot·o·my (vě-sik-yū-lot'ō-mē). Surgical incision of the seminal vesicles. [vesiculo- + G. *tomē,* incision]

ve·sic·u·lo·tu·bu·lar (vě-sik'yū-lō-tū'byū-ler). Denoting an auscultatory sound having both a vesicular and a tubular quality.

ve·sic·u·lo·tym·pan·ic (vĕ-sik′yū-lō-tim-pan′ik). Denoting a percussion sound having both a vesicular and a tympanic quality.

ve·sic·u·lous (vĕ-sik′yū-lŭs). SYN vesicular (2).

ves·sel (ves′ĕl). A structure conveying or containing a fluid, especially a liquid. SEE ALSO vas. [O. Fr. fr. L. *vascellum*, dim. of *vas*]

   afferent v., any artery conveying blood to a part.

   blood v., SEE blood vessel.

   chyle v., SYN lacteal (2).

   collateral v., (1) a branch of an artery running parallel with the parent trunk; (2) a v. that runs in parallel with another v., nerve, or other long structure.

   efferent v., SYN efferent glomerular *arteriole*.

   lacteal v., SYN lacteal (2).

   lymph v.'s, the v.'s that convey the lymph; they anastomose freely with each other. SYN vasa lymphatica [NA].

   nutrient v., SYN nutrient *artery*.

ves·tib·u·la (ves-tib′yū-lă). Plural of vestibulum.

ves·tib·u·lar (ves-tib′yū-lăr). **1.** Relating to a vestibule, especially the vestibule of the ear. **2.** Interpreting stimuli from the inner ear receptors regarding head position and movement.

ves·ti·bule (ves′ti-būl). **1.** A small cavity or a space at the entrance of a canal. **2.** Specifically, the central, somewhat ovoid, cavity of the osseous labyrinth communicating with the semicircular canals posteriorly and the cochlea anteriorly. SYN vestibulum [NA]. [L. *vestibulum*]

   aortic v., the anterosuperior portion of the left ventricle of the heart immediately below the aortic orifice, having fibrous walls and affording room for the segments of the closed aortic valve.

   v. of nose, the anterior part of the nasal cavity, especially that enclosed by cartilage.

   oral v., that part of the mouth bounded anteriorly and laterally by the lips and the cheeks, posteriorly and medially by the teeth and/or gums, and above and below by the reflections of the mucosa from the lips and cheeks to the gums.

   v. of vagina, the space behind the glans clitoridis and between the labia minora, containing the openings of the vagina, urethra, and ducts of the greater vestibular glands.

vestibulo-. Vestibule, vestibulum. [L. *vestibulum*]

ves·tib·u·lo·co·chle·ar (ves-tib′yū-lō-kok′lē-ăr). **1.** Relating to the vestibulum and cochlea of the ear. **2.** SYN statoacoustic.

ves·tib·u·lo·plas·ty (ves-tib′yū-lō-plas-tē). Any of a series of surgical procedures designed to restore alveolar ridge height by lowering muscles attaching to the buccal, labial, and lingual aspects of the jaws. [vestibulo- + G. *plassō*, to form]

ves·tib·u·lot·o·my (ves-tib′yū-lot′ō-mē). Operation for an opening into the vestibule of the labyrinth. [vestibulo- + G. *tomē*, incision]

ves·tib·u·lum, pl. **ves·tib·u·la** (ves-tib′yū-lŭm, -lă) [NA]. SYN vestibule. [L. antechamber, entrance court]

ves·tige (ves′tij). A trace or a rudimentary structure; the degenerated remains of any structure which occurs as an entity in the embryo or fetus. [L. *vestigium*]

ves·tig·i·al (ves-tij′ē-ăl). Relating to a vestige.

vet·er·i·nar·i·an (vet′ĕ-rin-ār′ē-ăn). A person who holds an academic degree in veterinary medicine; a licensed practitioner of veterinary medicine. [see veterinary]

vet·er·i·nary (vet′ĕ-rin-ār-ē). Relating to the diseases of animals. [L. *veterinarius,* fr. *veterina,* beast of burden]

VHDL very high density lipoprotein. SEE lipoprotein.

vi·a·bil·i·ty (vī-ă-bil′i-tē). Capability of living; the state of being viable; usually connotes a fetus that has reached 500 g in weight and 20 gestational weeks. [Fr. *viabilité* fr. L. *vita*, life]

vi·a·ble (vī′ă-bl). Capable of living; denoting a fetus sufficiently developed to live outside the uterus. [Fr. fr. *vie*, life, fr. L. *vita*]

Vib·rio (vib′rē-ō). A genus of motile (occasionally nonmotile), non-spore-forming, aerobic to facultatively anaerobic, Gram-negative bacteria containing short curved or straight rods which occur singly or which are occasionally united into S-shapes or spirals. Some of these organisms are saprophytes in water and soil; others are parasites or pathogens. The type species is *V. cholerae*. [L. *vibro,* to vibrate]

   V. alginolyt′icus, a species associated with wound and ear infections, and with bacteremia in immunocompromised and burn patients.

   V. chol′erae, a species that produces a soluble exotoxin and is the cause of cholera in humans; it is the type species of the genus *V.* SYN comma bacillus, Koch's bacillus (2).

   V. fe′tus, former name for *Campylobacter fetus*.

   V. fluvia′lis, a species similar to strains of *Aeromonas,* associated with diarrheal disease in humans.

   V. furnis′sii, an aerogenic strain, similar to *V. fluvialis,* associated with diarrheal disease and outbreaks of gastroenteritis.

   V. mim′icus, a species similar to *V. cholerae,* isolated from human stool in diarrheal disease and from human ear infections.

   V. parahaemolyt′icus, a marine species that causes gastroenteritis and bloody diarrhea, usually from eating contaminated shellfish.

   V. vulnif′icus, a species capable of causing cutaneous lesions in an immunocompromised patient; usually contracted from contaminated oysters; also a cause of wound infections.

vib·rio (vib′rē-ō). A member of the genus *Vibrio*.

vib·ri·o·sis, pl. **vib·ri·o·ses** (vib-rē-ō′sis). Infection caused by bacteria of the genus *Vibrio*.

vi·bris·sa, gen. and pl. **vi·bris·sae** (vī-bris′ă, vī-bris′ē) [NA]. One of the hairs growing at the nares, or vestibule of the nose. [L. found only in pl. *vibrissae,* fr. *vibro,* to quiver]

vi·bro·car·di·o·gram (vī′brō-kar′dē-ō-gram). A graphic record of chest vibrations produced by hemodynamic events of the cardiac cycle; the record provides an indirect, externally recorded measurement of isovolumic contraction and ejection times. [L. *vibro,* to shake, + G. *kardia,* heart, + *gramma,* a drawing]

vi·car·i·ous (vī-ker′ē-ŭs). Acting as a substitute; occurring in an abnormal situation. [L. *vicarius,* from *vicis,* supplying place of]

VI

vid·i·an (vid′ē-an). Named after or described by Vidius (Guido Guidi, 1500–1569).

vig·il·am·bu·lism (vij-i-lam′byū-lizm). A condition of unconsciousness regarding one's surroundings, with automatism, resembling somnambulism but occurring in the waking state. [L. *vigil,* awake, alert, + *ambulo,* to walk about]

vil·li (vil′ī). Plural of villus.

vil·lo·ma (vi-lō′mă). SYN papilloma.

vil·lose (vil′ōs). SYN villous (2).

vil·lo·si·tis (vil-ō-sī′tis). Inflammation of the villous surface of the placenta. [villous + G. -*itis* inflammation]

vil·los·i·ty (vi-los′i-tē). Shagginess; an aggregation of villi.

vil·lous (vil′ŭs). **1.** Relating to villi. **2.** Shaggy; covered with villi. SYN villose.

vil·lus, pl. **vil·li** (vil′ŭs, vil′ī). **1.** A projection from the surface, especially of a mucous membrane. If the projection is minute, as from a cell surface, it is termed a microvillus. **2.** An elongated dermal papilla projecting into an intraepidermal vesicle or cleft. SEE festooning. [L. shaggy hair (of beasts)]

   arachnoid villi, tufted prolongations of pia-arachnoid that protrude through the meningeal layer of the dura mater and have a thin limiting membrane; collections of arachnoid v. form arachnoid granulations that lie in venous lacunae at the margin of the superior sagittal sinus; the spongy tissue of the a. v. contains tubules that serve as one-way valves for transfer of cerebrospinal fluid from the subarachnoid space to the venous system. Both a. v. and the granulations formed from them are major sites of fluid transfer. SEE ALSO arachnoid *granulations,* under *granulation.*

   chorionic villi, vascular processes of the chorion of the embryo entering into the formation of the placenta.

   intestinal villi, projections (0.5 to 1.5 mm in length) of the mucous membrane of the intestine; they are leaf-shaped in the duodenum and become shorter, more finger-shaped, and sparser in the ileum.

vil·lus·ec·to·my (vil-ŭs-ek′tō-mē). SYN synovectomy. [villus + G. *ektomē,* excision]

vi·men·tin (vī-men′tin). The major polypeptide that copolymerizes with other subunits to form the intermediate filament cytoskeleton of mesenchymal cells; they may have a role in maintaining the internal organization of certain cells.

vin·cu·lum, pl. **vin·cu·la** (ving′kū-lŭm, -lă) [NA]. A frenum, frenulum, or ligament. [L. a fetter, fr. *vincio,* to bind]

   vincula of tendons, fibrous bands that extend from the flexor tendons of the fingers and toes to the capsules of the interphalangeal joints and to the phalanges; they convey small vessels to the tendons.

vin·e·gar (vin′ĕ-găr). Impure dilute acetic acid, made from wine, cider, malt, etc. [Fr. *vinaigre,* fr. *vin,* wine, + *aigre,* sour]

vi·nyl (vī′nil). The hydrocarbon radical, $CH_2=CH-$. SYN ethenyl.

vi·o·let (vī′ō-let). The color evoked by wavelengths of the visible spectrum shorter than 450

nm. For individual violet dyes, see the specific name. [L. *viola*]

   visual v., SYN iodopsin.

VIP vasoactive intestinal *polypeptide.*

vi·po·ma (vi-pō′mă). An endocrine tumor, usually originating in the pancreas, which produces a vasoactive intestinal polypeptide believed to cause profound cardiovascular and electrolyte changes with vasodilatory hypotension, watery diarrhea, hypokalemia, and dehydration. [*v*asoactive *i*ntestinal *p*olypeptide + G. -*ōma,* tumor]

vi·ral (vī′răl). Of, pertaining to, or caused by a virus.

vi·re·mia (vī-rē′mē-ă). The presence of a virus in the bloodstream. [virus + G. *haima,* blood]

vir·gin (ver′jin). **1.** A person who has never had sexual intercourse. **2.** Unused; uncontaminated. SYN virginal (2). [L. *virgo (virgin-),* maiden]

vir·gin·al (ver′ji-năl). **1.** Relating to a virgin. **2.** SYN virgin (2). [L. *virginalis*]

vir·gin·i·ty (ver-jin′i-tē). The virgin state. [L. *virginitas*]

△-**viridae.** A virus family. [L. *vir,* fr. *virus,* venom]

vir·ile (vir′il). **1.** Relating to the male sex. **2.** Manly, strong, masculine. **3.** Possessing masculine traits. [L. *virilis,* masculine, fr. *vir,* a man]

vir·i·les·cence (vir-i-les′ens). Assumption of male characteristics by a female.

vir·i·lism (vir′i-lizm). Possession of mature masculine somatic characteristics by a girl, woman, or prepubescent male; may be present at birth or may appear later; commonly the result of gonadal or adrenocortical dysfunction, or of androgenic therapy. [L. *virilis,* masculine]

vi·ril·i·ty (vi-ril′i-tē). The condition or quality of being virile. [L. *virilitas,* manhood, fr. *vir,* man]

vir·i·li·za·tion (vir′i-li-zā′shŭn). Production or acquisition of virilism.

vir·i·liz·ing (vir′i-līz-ing). Causing virilism.

△-**virinae.** Suffix used in naming a subfamily of viruses.

vi·ri·on (vī′rē-on, vir′ē-on). The complete virus particle that is structurally intact and infectious.

vi·rol·o·gist (vī-rol′ō-jist). A specialist in virology.

vi·rol·o·gy (vī-rol′ō-jē, vi-). The study of viruses and of viral disease. [virus + G. *logos,* study]

vi·ru·ci·dal (vī-rŭ-sī′dăl). Destructive to a virus.

vi·ru·cide (vī-rŭ-sīd). An agent active against virus infections. [virus + L. *caedo,* to kill]

vir·u·lence (vēr′yū-lĕns). The disease-evoking power of a pathogen; numerically expressed as the ratio of the number of cases of overt infection to the total number infected, as determined by immunoassay. [L. *virulentia,* fr. *virulentus,* poisonous]

vir·u·lent (vir′ū-lent). Extremely toxic, denoting a markedly pathogenic microorganism. [L. *virulentus,* poisonous]

vir·u·lif·er·ous (vī-rŭ-lif′er-ŭs). Conveying virus.

vir·u·ria (vī-rŭ′rē-ă). Presence of viruses in the urine. [virus + G. *ouron,* urine]

vi·rus, pl. **vi·rus·es** (vī′rŭs). **1.** Formerly, the specific agent of an infectious disease. **2.** Specifically, a term for a group of infectious agents which with few exceptions are capable of passing through fine filters that retain most bacteria, are usually not visible through the light microscope, lack independent metabolism, and are incapable of growth or reproduction apart from living cells. They have a prokaryotic genetic apparatus but differ sharply from bacteria in other respects. The complete particle usually contains only DNA or RNA, not both, and is usually covered by a protein shell or capsid that protects the nucleic acid. They range in size from 15 mm up to several hundred mm. Classification of v.'s depends upon characteristics of virions as well as upon mode of transmission, host range, symptomatology, and other factors. For v.'s not listed below, see the specific name. SYN ultravirus. **3.** Relating to or caused by a v., as a virus disease. [L. poison]

adenoidal-pharyngeal-conjunctival v., SYN adenovirus.

amphotropic v., an oncornavirus that does not produce disease in its natural host but does replicate in tissue culture cells of the host species and also in cells from other species.

attenuated v., a variant strain of a pathogenic v., so modified as to excite the production of protective antibodies, yet not producing the specific disease.

avian leukosis-sarcoma v., SYN avian leukosis-sarcoma *complex* (2).

B19 v., a human parvovirus associated with arthritis and arthralgia and a number of specific clinical entities, including erythema infectiosum and aplastic crisis in the presence of hemolytic anemia.

bacterial v., a v. which "infects" bacteria; a bacteriophage.

Bornholm disease v., SYN epidemic pleurodynia v.

California v., a serologic group of the genus *Bunyavirus,* comprising over 14 strains including La Crosse and Tahyna v., and the type strain, California v., which causes encephalitis, chiefly in the age group 4 to 14 years.

CELO v., a v. with characteristics of adenovirus, and similar to quail bronchitis v.

chickenpox v., SYN varicella-zoster v.

Coe v., a v. serologically identical with the A-21 strain of coxsackievirus; the cause of a common-cold-like disease in military recruits.

Colorado tick fever v., a v. of the genus *Orbivirus,* found in the Rocky Mountain region of the United States and transmitted by the tick, *Dermacentor andersoni;* it causes Colorado tick fever.

Coxsackie v., SEE Coxsackievirus.

croup-associated v., parainfluenza v. type 2. SEE parainfluenza viruses.

cytopathogenic v., a v. whose multiplication leads to degenerative changes in the host cell.

defective v., a v. particle that contains insufficient nucleic acid to provide for production of all essential viral components.

dengue v., a v. of the genus *Flavivirus;* the etiologic agent of dengue in humans and also occurring in monkeys and chimpanzees, usually as inapparent infection; four serotypes are recognized; transmission is effected by mosquitoes of the genus *Aedes.*

DNA v., a major group of animal v.'s in which the core consists of deoxyribonucleic acid (DNA); it includes parvoviruses, papovaviruses, adenoviruses, herpesviruses, poxviruses, and other unclassified DNA v.'s.

EB v., SYN Epstein-Barr v.

Ebola v., a v. morphologically similar to but antigenically distinct from Marburg v., in the family Filoviridae, which causes viral hemorrhagic fever.

ECHO v., an enterovirus isolated from humans; while there are many inapparent infections, certain of the several serotypes are associated with fever and aseptic meningitis, and some appear to cause mild respiratory disease. SYN echovirus.

ecotropic v., an oncornavirus that does not produce disease in its natural host but does replicate in tissue culture cells derived from the host species.

encephalomyocarditis v., a picornavirus, probably of rodents; occasionally causes febrile illness with central nervous system involvement in humans.

enteric viruses, v.'s of the genus Enterovirus.

enteric orphan viruses, enteroviruses isolated from humans and other animals, "orphan" implying lack of known association with disease when isolated; many v.'s of the group are now known to be pathogenic; they include ECBO viruses, ECHO viruses, and ECSO viruses.

epidemic gastroenteritis v., a RNA v., about 27 nm in diameter, which has not been cultured *in vitro;* it is the cause of epidemic nonbacterial gastroenteritis; at least five antigenically distinct serotypes have been recognized, including the Norwalk agent. These viruses are classified with the Caliciviruses in the family Caliciviridae. SYN gastroenteritis v. type A.

epidemic keratoconjunctivitis v., an adenovirus (type 8) causing epidemic keratoconjunctivitis, especially among shipyard workers, and also associated with outbreaks of swimming pool conjunctivitis.

epidemic parotitis v., SYN mumps v.

epidemic pleurodynia v., a coxsackievirus, type B, that causes epidemic pleurodynia. SYN Bornholm disease v.

Epstein-Barr v. (EBV), a herpesvirus that causes infectious mononucleosis and is also found in cell cultures of Burkitt's lymphoma; associated with nasopharyngeal carcinoma. SYN EB v., human herpesvirus 4.

fixed v., rabies v. whose virulence for rabbits has been stabilized by numerous passages through this experimental host. SEE ALSO street v.

foamy viruses, retroviruses found in primates and other mammals; so named because of lacelike changes produced in monkey kidney cells; syncytia are also produced.

gastroenteritis v. type A, SYN epidemic gastroenteritis v.

gastroenteritis v. type B, SYN *Rotavirus.*

German measles v., SYN rubella v.

HA1 v., SYN hemadsorption v. type 1. SEE parainfluenza viruses.

HA2 v., SYN hemadsorption v. type 2. SEE parainfluenza viruses.

vi

helper v., a v. whose replication renders it possible for a defective v. or a virusoid (also present in the host cell) to develop into a fully infectious agent.

hemadsorption v. type 1, parainfluenza v. type 3. SEE parainfluenza viruses. SYN HA1 v.

hemadsorption v. type 2, parainfluenza v. type 1. SEE parainfluenza viruses. SYN HA2 v.

hepatitis A v. (HAV), an RNA virus, the causative agent of viral hepatitis type A. SYN infectious hepatitis v.

hepatitis B v. (HBV), a DNA virus, the causative agent of viral hepatitis type B. SYN serum hepatitis v.

hepatitis C v. (HCV), a non-A, non-B RNA v. causing posttransfusion hepatitis.

hepatitis D v., a small "defective" RNA v. that requires the presence of hepatitis B v. for replication. The clinical course is variable but is usually more severe than other hepatitides. SYN delta agent, delta antigen, hepatitis delta v.

hepatitis delta v. (HDV), SYN hepatitis D v.

hepatitis E v. (HEV), an RNA v. that is the principal cause of enterically transmitted, waterborne, or epidemic non-A, non-B hepatitis occurring primarily in Asia and Africa.

herpes v., SEE herpesvirus.

herpes simplex v. (HSV), SEE *herpes* simplex.

herpes zoster v., SYN varicella-zoster v.

▣**human immunodeficiency v. (HIV),** human T-cell lymphotropic v. type III; a cytopathic retrovirus that is the etiologic agent of acquired immunodeficiency syndrome (AIDS). SYN lymphadenopathy-associated v.

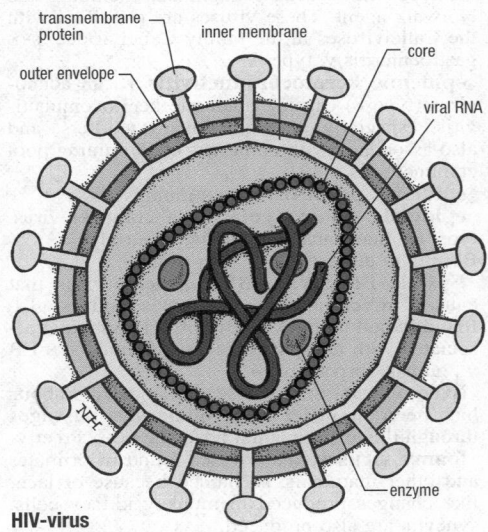

HIV-virus

human papilloma v. (HPV), DNA v. of the genus *Papillomavirus;* certain types cause cutaneous and genital warts in humans, including verruca vulgaris and condyloma acuminatum; other types are associated with severe cervical intraepithelial neoplasia and anogenital and laryngeal carcinomas. Over 70 types have been character-

ized on the basis of DNA relatedness. SYN infectious papilloma v.

human T-cell lymphoma/leukemia v. (HTLV), a group of viruses (subfamily Oncovirinae, family Retroviridae) that are lymphotropic with a selective affinity for the helper/inducer cell subset of T lymphocytes and that are associated with adult T-cell leukemia and lymphoma.

infectious hepatitis v., SYN hepatitis A v.

infectious papilloma v., SYN human papilloma v.

influenza viruses, v.'s which cause influenza and influenzalike infections of humans and other animals; v.'s included are influenza v. types A and B of the genus *Influenzavirus,* causing, respectively, influenza A and B and influenza v. type C, which probably belongs to a separate genus and causes influenza C.

Japanese B encephalitis v., a v. of the genus *Flavivirus* (group B arbovirus) normally present in humans, especially in children, as an inapparent infection, but may cause febrile response and sometimes encephalitis.

Korean hemorrhagic fever v., SEE *Hantavirus.*

Lassa v., an arenavirus that causes Lassa fever, an acute febrile disease with a high mortality.

lymphadenopathy-associated v. (LAV), SYN human immunodeficiency v.

lymphocytic choriomeningitis v., an RNA v. that causes lymphocytic choriomeningitis; infection may be inapparent, but sometimes the v. causes influenzalike disease, meningitis, or, rarely, meningoencephalomyelitis.

Marburg v., an RNA-containing v., genus *Filovirus,* first recognized at Marburg University (Germany), where it was the cause of a highly fatal hemorrhagic fever among laboratory workers and handlers of green monkeys.

masked v., a v. ordinarily occurring in the host in a noninfective state, but which may be activated and demonstrated by special procedures such as blind passage in experimental animals.

measles v., an RNA v. of the genus *Morbillivirus* that causes measles and is transmitted via the respiratory tract; possesses hemagglutinating, hemadsorbing, and hemolyzing properties. SYN rubeola v.

Mokola v., a rabies-related v. of the genus *Lyssavirus,* which has caused fatal neurological disease.

mumps v., a v. of the genus *Paramyxovirus* causing parotitis, sometimes with complications of orchitis, oophoritis, pancreatitis, meningoencephalitis and others, and transmitted by infectious salivary secretions. SYN epidemic parotitis v.

naked v., a v. consisting only of a nucleocapsid; *i.e.,* one that does not possess an enclosing envelope.

Norwalk v., a v. associated with acute viral gastroenteritis and probably belonging to the calicivirus group.

oncogenic v., a v. of one of the two groups of tumor-inducing v.'s: the RNA tumor v.'s, which are well defined and rather homogeneous, or the DNA v.'s, which are more diverse. SYN tumor v.

orphan viruses, v.'s, such as the enteric orphan v.'s, which when originally found were not specifically associated with disease; a number of these have since been shown to be pathogenic.

parainfluenza viruses, v.'s of the genus *Paramyxovirus*, of four types: type 1 (hemadsorption v. type 2), which includes sendai v., causes acute laryngotracheitis in children and occasionally adults; type 2 (croup-associated v.) is associated especially with acute laryngotracheitis or croup in young children and minor upper respiratory infections in adults; type 3 (hemadsorption v. type 1; shipping fever v.) has been isolated from small children with pharyngitis, bronchiolitis, and pneumonia, and causes occasional respiratory infection in adults; type 4 has been isolated from a very few children with minor respiratory illness.

poliomyelitis v., the picornavirus (genus *Enterovirus*) causing poliomyelitis in humans; the route of infection is the alimentary tract, but the v. may enter the bloodstream and nervous system, sometimes causing paralysis of the limbs and, rarely, encephalitis; many infections are inapparent; serologic types 1, 2, and 3 are recognized, type 1 being responsible for most paralytic poliomyelitis and most epidemics. SYN poliovirus hominis.

rabies v., a large bullet-shaped v. of the genus *Lyssavirus*, in the family Rhabdoviridae, that is the causative agent of rabies.

respiratory enteric orphan v., a nonenveloped icosahedral virus whose genome consists of double stranded RNA, belonging to the family Reoviridae, frequently found in both the respiratory and enteric tract.

RNA v., a group of v.'s in which the core consists of RNA; a major group of animal v.'s that includes the families Picornaviridae, Reoviridae, Togaviridae, Flaviviridae, Bunyaviridae, Arenaviridae, Paramyxoviridae, Retroviridae, Coronaviridae, Orthomyxoviridae, and Rhabdoviridae.

RNA tumor viruses, v.'s of the subfamily Oncovirinae.

Ross River v., a mosquito-borne alphavirus, family Togaviridae, that causes epidemic polyarthritis.

Rous-associated v. (RAV), a leukemia v. of the leukosis-sarcoma complex which by phenotypic mixing with a defective (noninfectious) strain of Rous sarcoma v. effects production of infectious sarcoma v. with envelope antigenicity of the RAV.

Rous sarcoma v. (RSV), a sarcoma-producing v. of the avian leukosis-sarcoma complex identified by Rous in 1911.

rubella v., an RNA v. of the genus *Rubivirus;* the agent causing rubella (German measles) in humans. SYN German measles v.

rubeola v., SYN measles v.

serum hepatitis v., SYN hepatitis B v.

simian v. (SV), any of a number of v.'s, belonging to various families, isolated from monkeys or from cultures of monkey cells.

Sindbis v., the type species of the genus *Alphavirus*, usually transmitted by mosquitoes of the genus *Culex;* and causative agent of Sindbis fever. [village in Egypt where first isolated]

slow v., a v., or a viruslike agent, etiologically associated with a disease having a long incubation period of months to years with a gradual onset frequently terminating in severe illness and/or death.

smallpox v., SYN variola v.

St. Louis encephalitis v., a group B arbovirus often causing inapparent infection but sometimes encephalitis; the v. has been isolated from birds in Panama and from several mosquito species, especially *Psorophora*.

street v., an isolate of rabies v. from a naturally infected domestic animal.

tick-borne encephalitis v., an arbovirus of the genus *Flavivirus* that occurs in Central Europe and the republics of the former Soviet Union in two subtypes, causing two forms of encephalitis in humans: tick-borne encephalitis (Central European subtype) and tick-borne encephalitis (Eastern subtype); the vectors are ticks of the genus *Ixodes*.

tumor v., SYN oncogenic v.

varicella-zoster v., a herpesvirus, morphologically identical to herpes simplex v., that causes varicella (chickenpox) and herpes zoster; varicella results from a primary infection, herpes zoster from secondary invasion or by reactivation of infection which has been latent for years. SYN chickenpox v., herpes zoster v., human herpesvirus 3.

variola v., a poxvirus of the genus *Orthopoxvirus*, the pathogen of smallpox in humans. SYN smallpox v.

xenotropic v., a retrovirus that does not produce disease in its natural host and replicates only in tissue culture cells derived from a different species.

△**-virus.** A genus of viruses.

vi•rus•oid (vī′rŭs-oyd). A plant pathogen resembling a viroid but having a much larger circular or linear RNA segment and a capsid. [virus + G. *eidos*, resembling]

vi•rus shed•ding. Excretion of virus by any route from the infected host; route and duration of excretion vary according to the pathogenesis of the infection or disease.

vis•cera (vis′er-ă). Plural of viscus. SYN vitals.

vis•cer•ad (vis′er-ad). In a direction toward the viscera. [viscera + L. *ad*, to]

vis•cer•al (vis′er-ăl). Relating to the viscera. SYN splanchnic.

vis•cer•al•gia (vis-er-al′jē-ă). Pain in any viscus. [viscero- + G. *algos*, pain]

△**viscero-.** The viscera. SEE ALSO splanchno-. [L. *viscus*, pl. *viscera*, the internal organs]

vis•cer•o•gen•ic (vis′er-ō-jen′ik). Of visceral origin; denoting a number of sensory and other reflexes. [viscero- + G. *-gen*, producing]

vis•cer•o•in•hib•i•to•ry (vis′er-ō-in-hib′i-tōr-ē). Restricting or arresting the functional activity of the viscera.

vis•cer•o•meg•a•ly (vis′er-ō-meg′ă-lē). Abnormal enlargement of the viscera, such as may be seen in acromegaly and other disorders. SYN orga-

vi

nomegaly, splanchnomegaly. [viscero- + G. *megas,* large]

vis•cer•o•mo•tor (vis'er-ō-mō'ter). **1.** Relating to or controlling movement in the viscera; denoting the autonomic nerves innervating the viscera, especially the intestines. **2.** Denoting a movement having a relation to the viscera; referring to reflex muscular contractions of the abdominal wall in cases of visceral disease.

vis•cer•o•pleu•ral (vis'er-ō-plū'răl). Relating to the pleural and the thoracic viscera. SYN pleurovisceral.

vis•cer•op•to•sis, vis•cer•op•to•sia (vis'er-op-tō' sis, -tō'sē-ă). Descent of the viscera from their normal positions. SYN splanchnoptosis, splanchnoptosia. [viscero- + G. *ptōsis,* a falling]

vis•cer•o•sen•sory (vis'er-ō-sen'sōr-ē). Relating to the sensory innervation of internal organs.

vis•cer•o•skel•e•tal (vis-er-ō-skel'ĕ-tăl). Relating to the visceroskeleton. SYN splanchnoskeletal.

vis•cer•o•skel•e•ton (vis-er-ō-skel'ĕ-tŏn). **1.** Any bony or cartilaginous formation in an organ, as in the cartilaginous rings of the trachea and bronchi. **2.** The bony framework protecting the viscera, such as the ribs and sternum, the pelvic bones, and the anterior portion of the skull. SYN splanchnoskeleton.

vis•cer•o•so•mat•ic (vis'er-ō-sō-mat'ik). Relating to the viscera and the body. [viscero- + G. *sōma,* body]

vis•cer•o•tro•phic (vis'er-ō-trof'ik). Relating to any trophic change determined by visceral conditions. [viscero- + G. *trophē,* nourishment]

vis•cer•o•tro•pic (vis'er-ō-trop'ik). Affecting the viscera. [L. *viscera* internal organs, + G. *tropē,* a turning]

vis•cid (vis'id). Sticky; glutinous. [L. *viscidus,* stick, fr. *viscum,* birdlime]

vis•cid•i•ty (vi-sid'i-tē). Stickiness; adhesiveness.

vis•cos•i•ty (vis-kos'i-tē). In general, the resistance to flow or alteration of shape by any substance as a result of molecular cohesion; most frequently applied to liquids as the resistance of a fluid to flow because of a shearing force. [L. *viscositas,* fr. *viscosus,* viscous]

    kinematic v. (ν, υ), a measure used in studies of fluid flow; the dynamic viscosity, μ, in poises divided by the density of the material; units: stokes.

vis•cous (vis'kŭs). Sticky; marked by high viscosity. [see viscid, viscosity]

vis•cus, pl. **vis•cera** (vis'kŭs, vis'er-ă). An organ of the digestive, respiratory, urogenital, and endocrine systems as well as the spleen, the heart, and great vessels; hollow and multilayered walled organs studied in splanchnology. [L. the soft parts, internal organs]

vi•sion (vizh'ŭn). The act of seeing. SEE ALSO sight. [L. *visio,* fr. *video,* pp. *visus,* to see]

    achromatic v., SYN achromatopsia.

    binocular v., v. with a single image, by both eyes simultaneously.

    central v., v. stimulated by an object imaged on the fovea centralis. SYN direct v.

    chromatic v., SYN chromatopsia.

    colored v. (VC), SYN chromatopsia.

    direct v., SYN central v.

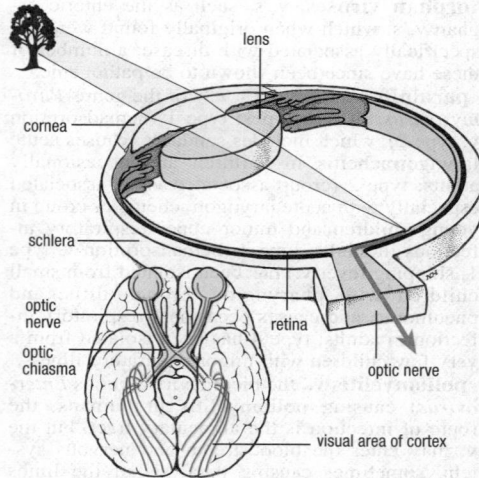

vision: light passes through the cornea and is focused onto the retina by the lens; cells in the retina then transmit this information though the optic nerve to the visual area of the cortex.

    double v., SYN diplopia.

    indirect v., SYN peripheral v.

    multiple v., SYN polyopia.

    night v., SYN scotopic v.

    oscillating v., SYN oscillopsia.

    peripheral v., v. resulting from retinal stimulation beyond the macula. SYN indirect v.

    photopic v., v. when the eye is light-adapted. SEE light *adaptation,* light-adapted *eye.* SYN photopia.

    scotopic v., v. when the eye is dark-adapted. SEE ALSO dark *adaptation,* dark-adapted *eye.* SYN night v., scotopia.

    stereoscopic v., the single perception of a slightly different image from each eye.

    triple v., SYN triplopia.

    tubular v., a constriction of the visual field, as though one were looking through a hollow cylinder or tube. SYN tunnel v.

    tunnel v., SYN tubular v.

vi•su•al (vizh'ū-ăl). **1.** Relating to vision. **2.** Denoting a person who learns and remembers more readily through sight than through hearing. [Late L. *visualis,* fr. *visus,* vision]

visual neglect. inattention to visual stimuli occurring in the space on the involved side of the body.

vi•su•og•no•sis (vizh'yū-og-nō'sis). Recognition and understanding of visual impressions. [L. *visus,* vision, + G. *gnōsis,* knowledge]

vis•u•o•mo•tor (vizh'yū-ō-mō'ter). Denoting the ability to synchronize visual information with physical movement, *e.g.,* driving a car.

vi•su•o•sen•so•ry (vizh'yū-ō-sen'sōr-ē). Pertaining to the perception of visual stimuli.

vis•u•o•spa•tial (viz'yū-ō-spā'shăl). Denoting the ability to comprehend and conceptualize visual representations and spatial relationships in learning and performing a task.

vi•tal (vīt-ăl). Relating to life. [L. *vitalis,* fr. *vita,* life]

vi•tal•i•ty (vīt-al′i-tē). Vital force or energy.

vi•ta•lom•e•ter (vī-tă-lom′ĕ-ter). An electrical device for determining the vitality of the tooth pulp.

vi•tal red [C.I. 23570]. Trisodium salt of a sulfonated diazo dye, used as a vital stain.

vi•tals (vīt′ălz). SYN viscera.

vi•ta•mer (vī′tă-mer). One of two or more similar compounds capable of fulfilling a specific vitamin function in the body; *e.g.,* niacin, niacinamide.

vi•ta•min (vīt′ă-min). One of a group of organic substances, present in minute amounts in natural foodstuffs, that are essential to normal metabolism; insufficient amounts in the diet may cause deficiency diseases. [L. *vita,* life, + amine]

v. A, (1) any β-ionone derivative, except provitamin A carotenoids, possessing qualitatively the biological activity of retinol; deficiency interferes with the production and resynthesis of rhodopsin, thereby causing night blindness, and produces a keratinizing metaplasia of epithelial cells that may result in xerophthalmia, keratosis, susceptibility to infections, and retarded growth; **(2)** the original v. A, now known as retinol.

v. A$_1$ acid, SYN retinoic acid.

v. B, a group of water-soluble substances originally considered as one v.

v. B$_1$, SYN thiamin.

v. B$_6$, pyridoxine and related compounds (pyridoxal; pyridoxamine).

v. B$_{12}$, generic descriptor for compounds exhibiting the biological activity of cyanocobalamin (cyanocob(III)alamin). The physiologically active v. B$_{12}$ coenzymes are methylcobalamin and deoxyadenosinecobalamine. A deficiency of v. B$_{12}$ causes megaloblastic anemia with or without peripheral neuropathy, and is often associated with certain methylmalonic acidurias. SEE pernicious *anemia.*

v. B complex, a pharmaceutical term applied to drug products containing a mixture of the B v.'s, usually B$_1$ (thiamine), B$_2$ (riboflavin), B$_3$ (nicotinamide), and B$_6$ (pyridoxine).

v. C, SYN ascorbic acid.

v. D, generic descriptor for all steroids exhibiting the biological activity of ergocalciferol or cholecalciferol, the antirachitic v.'s. They promote the proper utilization of calcium and phosphorus, thereby producing growth, together with proper bone and tooth formation, in young children.

v. D$_2$, SYN ergocalciferol.

v. D$_3$, SYN cholecalciferol.

v. E, generic descriptor of tocol and tocotrienol derivatives possessing the biological activity of α-tocopherol; contained in various oils (wheat germ, cotton-seed, palm, rice) and whole grain cereals where it constitutes the nonsaponifiable fraction, also in animal tissue (liver, pancreas, heart) and lettuce; deficiency produces resorption or abortion in female rats and sterility in males.

fat-soluble v.'s, those v.'s, soluble in fat solvents (nonpolar solvents) and relatively insoluble in water, marked in chemical structure by the presence of large hydrocarbon moieties in the molecule; *e.g.,* v.'s A, D, E, K.

v. K, generic descriptor for compounds with the biological activity of phylloquinone; fat-soluble, thermostable compounds found in alfalfa, hog liver, fish meal, and vegetable oils, essential for the formation of normal amounts of prothrombin.

v. K$_1$, v. K$_1$(20), SYN phylloquinone.

v. K$_2$, v. K$_2$(30), SYN menaquinone-6.

v. P, a mixture of bioflavonoids extracted from plants (especially citrus fruits). It reduces the permeability and fragility of capillaries and is useful in the treatment of certain cases of purpura that are resistant to v. C therapy.

vi•tel•line (vī-tel′in, -ēn). Relating to the vitellus. SEE yolk *sac.*

vi•tel•lus (vī-tel′ŭs). SYN yolk (1). [L.]

vi•ti•a•tion (vish-ē-ā′shŭn). A change that impairs utility or reduces efficiency. [L. *vitiatio* fr. *vitio,* pp. *vitiatus,* to corrupt, fr. *vitium,* vice]

vit•i•lig•i•nes (vit-i-lij′i-nēz). Plural of vitiligo.

vit•i•lig•i•nous (vit-i-lij′i-nŭs). Relating to or characterized by vitiligo.

vit•i•li•go, pl. **vit•i•lig•i•nes** (vit-i-lī′gō, vit-i-lij′i-nēz). The appearance on otherwise normal skin of nonpigmented white patches of varied sizes; hair in the affected areas is usually white. Epidermal melanocytes are completely lost in depigmented areas by an autoimmune process. [L. a skin eruption, fr. *vitium,* blemish, vice]

vit•rec•to•my (vi-trek′tō-mē). Removal of the vitreous by means of an instrument that simultaneously removes vitreous by suction and cutting and replaces it with saline or some other fluid. [vitreous + G. *ektomē,* excision]

vit•re•i•tis (vit-rē-ī′tis). Inflammation of the corpus vitreum. SYN hyalitis. [L. *vitreus,* glassy, + G. *-itis,* inflammation]

△ **vitreo-.** Vitreous. [L. *vitreus,* glassy]

vit•re•o•den•tin (vit′rē-ō-den′tin). Dentin of a particularly brittle character.

vit•re•o•ret•i•nal (vit′rē-ō-ret′i-năl). Pertaining to the retina and the vitreous body.

vit•re•ous (vit′rē-ŭs). **1.** Glassy; resembling glass. **2.** SYN vitreous *body.* [L. *vitreus,* glassy, fr. *vitrum,* glass]

persistent anterior hyperplastic primary v., a unilateral congenital abnormality occurring in full-term infants; characterized by a retrolental fibrovascular membrane formed by persistent primary v. with remnants of the hyaloid artery and tunica vasculosa lentis; associated with leukokoria, microphthalmos, shallow anterior chamber, and elongated ciliary processes.

persistent posterior hyperplastic primary v., a unilateral congenital anomaly in full-term infants; associated with a congenital retinal fold and a v. membranous stalk containing remnants of the hyaloid artery.

vit•re•um (vit′rē-ŭm). SYN vitreous *body.* [L. ntr. of *vitreus,* glassy]

vit•ri•fi•ca•tion (vit′ri-fi-kā′shŭn). Conversion of dental porcelain (frit) to a glassy substance by heat and fusion. [L. *vitrium,* glassy, + *facio,* to make]

△ **vivi-.** Living. [L. *vivus,* alive]

viv•i•fi•ca•tion (viv′i-fi-kā′shŭn). SYN revivification (2). [L. *vivifico,* pp. *-atus,* fr. *vivus,* alive, + *facio,* to make]

vi•vip•a•rous (vī-vip′ă-rŭs). Giving birth to living young, in distinction to oviparous, or egg-laying. [vivi- + L. *pario,* to bear]

viv•i•sec•tion (viv-i-sek′shŭn). Any cutting operation on a living animal for purposes of experimentation; often extended to denote any form of animal experimentation. [vivi- + section]

viv•i•sec•tion•ist, viv•i•sec•tor (vi-vi-sek′shŭn-ist, -tōr; vi-vi-sek′tŏr). One who practices vivisection.

VLDL very low density lipoprotein. SEE lipoprotein.

VMA vanillylmandelic acid.

$\mathring{V}O_2$ oxygen *consumption.*

vo•cal (vō′kăl). Pertaining to the voice or the organs of speech. [L. *vocalis*]

vocal fry. SYN glottal fry.

$\mathring{V}O_2$ **/HR (oxygen pulse)** oxygen pulse.

voice (voys). The sound made by air passing out through the larynx and upper respiratory tract, the vocal folds being approximated. [L. *vox*]

  gravel v., SYN glottal fry.

void (voyd). To evacuate urine or feces.

vo•la (vō′lă). Palm of the hand or sole of the foot. [L.]

vo•lar (vō′lăr). Referring to the vola; denoting either the palm of the hand or sole of the foot.

vol•a•tile (vol′ă-til). **1.** Tending to evaporate rapidly. **2.** Tending toward violence, explosiveness, or rapid change. [L. *volatilis,* fr. *volo,* to fly]

vol•a•til•i•za•tion (vol′ă-til-i-zā′shŭn). SYN evaporation. [fr. L. *volatilis,* volatile, fr. *volo,* pp. *volatus,* to fly]

vo•li•tion (vō-lish′ŭn). The conscious impulse to perform any act or to abstain from its performance; voluntary action. [L. *volo,,* to wish]

vo•li•tion•al (vo-lish′ŭn-ăl). Done by an act of will; relating to volition.

vol•ley (vol′ē). A synchronous group of impulses induced simultaneously by artificial stimulation of either nerve fibers or muscle fibers. [Fr. *volée,* fr. L. *volo,* to fly]

volt (v, V) (vōlt). The unit of electromotive force; the electromotive force that will produce a current of 1 ampere in a circuit that has a resistance of 1 ohm; *i.e.,* joule per coulomb. [Alessandro *Volta,* It. physicist, 1745–1827]

volt•age (vōl′tej). Electromotive force, pressure, or potential expressed in volts.

volt•am•pere (vōlt′am-pēr). A unit of electrical power; the product of 1 volt by 1 ampere; equivalent to 1 watt or $^1/_{1000}$ kilowatt.

vol•ume (V) (vol′yŭm). Space occupied by matter, expressed usually in cubic millimeters, cubic centimeters, liters, etc. SEE ALSO capacity, water. [L. *volumen,* something rolled up, scroll, fr. *volvo,* to roll]

  v. at ATPS, a v. of gas at ambient (A) temperature (T) (room temperature) and barometric pressure (P) saturated (S) with water vapor.

  v. at BTPS, a v. of gas saturated (S) with water vapor at 37°C (body (B) temperature (T)) and the ambient environmental barometric pressure (P).

  v. at STPD, a v. of gas, at the standard (S)

temperature (T) of 0°C, a barometric pressure (P) of 760 mm Hg, and dry (D).

  closing v., the lung v. at which the flow from the lower parts of the lungs becomes severely reduced or stops during expiration, presumably because of airway closure; measured by the sharp rise in expiratory concentration of a tracer gas that had been inspired at the beginning of a breath that started from residual volume.

  compressible v., the volume of gas compressed (and therefore lost) in the mechanical ventilator circuit per delivered pressure; most systems have compressible volume loss factors of 3 to 5 ml/cm H_2O; some newer mechanical ventilators calculate the loss factor and monitor gas delivery so that the set volume is the volume that actually enters the patient's airway.

  end-diastolic v., the amount of blood in the ventricle immediately before a cardiac contraction begins; a measurement of cardiac filling between beats, related to diastolic function.

  end-systolic v., the amount of blood in the ventricle at the end of the cardiac ejection period and immediately preceding the beginning of ventricular relaxation; a measurement of the adequacy of cardiac emptying, related to systolic function.

  expiratory reserve v. (ERV), the maximal v. of air (about 1000 ml) that can be expelled from the lungs after a normal expiration. SYN reserve air, supplemental air.

  forced expiratory v. (FEV), the maximal v. that can be expired in a specific time interval when starting from maximal inspiration.

  inspiratory reserve v. (IRV), the maximal v. of air that can be inspired after a normal inspiration; the inspiratory capacity less the tidal v. SYN complementary air.

  mean corpuscular v. (MCV), the average v. of red cells, calculated from the hematocrit and the red cell count, in erythrocyte indices.

  minute v., the v. of any gas or fluid moved per minute; *e.g.,* cardiac output or the respiratory minute v.

  partial v., the actual v. occupied by one species of molecule or particle in a solution; the reciprocal of the density of the molecule.

  rebreathing v., the v. of exhaled gas reinhaled on inspiration as a result of the presence of a breathing apparatus; this v. is also referred to as instrument dead space.

  residual v. (RV), the v. of air remaining in the lungs after a maximal expiratory effort. SYN residual air, residual capacity.

  respiratory minute v., the minute v. of breathing; the product of tidal v. times the respiratory frequency. SEE pulmonary *ventilation.*

  resting tidal v., the tidal v. under normal conditions, *i.e.,* in the absence of exercise or other conditions that stimulate breathing.

  standard v., the v. of an ideal gas at standard temperature and pressure, approximately 22.414 liters.

  stroke v., the v. pumped out of one ventricle of the heart in a single beat.

  tidal v., the v. of air that is inspired or expired

in a single breath during regular breathing. SYN tidal air.

vol•u•met•ric (vol-yū-met′rik). Relating to measurement by volume.

vol•un•tary (vol′ŭn-tār-ē). Relating or acting in obedience to the will; not obligatory. [L. *voluntarius*, fr. *voluntas*, will, fr. *volo*, to wish]

vo•lute (vō-lūt). Rolled up; convoluted. [L. *voluta*, a scroll, fr. *volvo*, pp. *volutus*, to roll]

vol•vu•lus (vol′vyū-lŭs). A twisting of the intestine causing obstruction. [L. *volvo*, to roll]

vo•mer, gen. **vo•me•ris** (vō′mer, vō′mer-is) [NA]. A flat bone of trapezoidal shape forming the inferior and posterior portion of the nasal septum; it articulates with the sphenoid, ethmoid, two maxillae, and two palatine bones. [L. ploughshare]

vo•mer•ine (vō′mer-ēn). Relating to the vomer.

vom•it. 1. To eject matter from the stomach through the mouth. **2.** Vomitus; the matter so ejected. SYN vomitus (2). [L. *vomo*, pp. *vomitus*, to vomit]

vom•it•ing (vom′i-ting). The ejection of matter from the stomach through the esophagus and mouth. SYN emesis (1), vomitus (1).

 dry v., SYN retching.

 fecal v., vomitus with appearance and/or odor of feces suggestive of long-standing distal small bowel or colonic obstruction. SYN copremesis, stercoraceous v.

 pernicious v., uncontrollable v.

 v. of pregnancy, v. occurring in the early months of pregnancy.

 projectile v., expulsion of the contents of the stomach with great force.

 psychogenic v., v. associated with emotional distress and anxiety.

 retention v., v. due to mechanical obstruction, usually hours after ingestion of a meal.

 stercoraceous v., SYN fecal v.

vom•i•tu•ri•tion (vom′i-tū-rish′ŭn). SYN retching.

vom•i•tus (vom′i-tŭs). **1.** SYN vomiting. **2.** SYN vomit (2). [L. a vomiting, vomit]

vor•tex, pl. **vor•ti•ces** (vōr′teks, vōr′ti-sēz). **1.** SYN verticil. **2.** SYN whorl (5). **3.** SYN v. lentis. [L. whirlpool, whorl, fr. *verto* or *vorto*, to turn around]

 v. len′tis, one of the stellar figures on the surface of the lens of the eye. SYN vortex (3).

 v. of heart, a spiral arrangement of muscular fibers at the apex of the heart. SYN whorl (2).

vox•el (vok′sel). A contraction for volume element, which is the basic unit of CT or MR reconstruction; represented as a pixel in the display of the CT or MR image.

voy•eur (vwah-yer′). One who practices voyeurism.

voy•eur•ism (vwah-yer′izm). The practice of obtaining sexual pleasure by looking at the naked body or genitals of another or at erotic acts between others. SYN scopophilia. [Fr. *voir*, to see]

VR vocal *resonance.*

VS volumetric *solution.*

vul•ga•ris (vŭl-gā′ris). Ordinary; of the usual type. [L. fr. *vulgus*, a crowd]

vul•sel•la, vul•sel•lum (vŭl-sel′ă, -lŭm). SYN vulsella *forceps.* [L. pincers, fr. *vello*, pp. *vulsus*, to pluck]

vul•va, pl. **vul′vae** (vŭ′vă). [NA] The external genitalia of the female, composed of the mons pubis, the labia majora and minora, the clitoris, the vestibule of the vagina and its glands, and the opening of the urethra and of the vagina. [L. a wrapper or covering, seed covering, womb, fr. *volvo*, to roll]

vul•var, vul•val (vŭl′văr, vŭl′văl). Relating to the vulva.

vul•vec•to•my (vŭl-vek′tō-mē). Excision (either partial, complete, or radical) of the vulva. [vulva + G. *ektomē*, excision]

vul•vi•tis (vŭl-vī′tis). Inflammation of the vulva. [vulva + G. *-itis*, inflammation]

vulvo-. The vulva. [L. *vulva*]

vul•vo•vag•i•ni•tis (vŭl′vō-vaj-i-nī′tis). Inflammation of both vulva and vagina.

W

W tungsten; watt; tryptophan.

waist (wāst). The portion of the trunk between the ribs and the pelvis. [A.S. *waext*]

walk. **1.** To move on foot. **2.** The characteristic manner in which one moves on foot. SEE ALSO gait. [M.E. *walken*, fr. O.E. *wealcen*, to roll]

walk·ing (wo'king). Characteristic of sequential movement or progression in steps.

   chromosome w., sequential isolation of overlapping sequences of DNA; with this procedure large regions of the chromosome can be spanned.

wall (wawl). An investing part enclosing a cavity such as the chest or abdomen, or covering a cell or any anatomical unit. A wall, as of the chest, abdomen, or any hollow organ. SYN paries [NA]. [L. *vallum*]

   cell w., the outer layer or membrane of some animal and plant cells; in the latter, it is mainly cellulose.

   chest w., in respiratory physiology, the total system of structures outside the lungs that move as a part of breathing; it includes the rib cage, diaphragm, abdominal w., and abdominal contents. SYN thoracic w.

   parietal w., the body w. or the somatopleure from which it is formed.

   splanchnic w., the w. of one of the viscera or the splanchnopleure from which it is formed.

   thoracic w., SYN chest w.

wal·le·ri·an (waw-ler'ē-an). Relating to or described by A.V. Waller.

wall-eye (wawl'ī). **1.** SYN exotropia. **2.** Absence of color in the iris, or leukoma of the cornea.

wan·der·ing (wahn'der-ing). Moving about; not fixed; abnormally motile. [A.S. *wandrian*, to wander]

Wang·i·el·la (wang-gē-el'ă). A dematiaceous genus of fungi; *W. dermatitidis* is an etiological agent of phaeohyphomycosis.

ward (wōrd). A large room or hall in a hospital containing a number of beds. SEE ALSO unit. [A.S. *weard*]

wart (wōrt). SYN verruca.

   anatomical w., SYN postmortem w.

   flat w., SYN *verruca* plana.

   genital w., SYN *condyloma* acuminatum.

   mosaic w., plantar growth of numerous closely aggregated w.'s forming a mosaic appearance, frequently caused by human papilloma virus type 2.

   necrogenic w., SYN postmortem w.

   Peruvian w., SYN *verruga* peruana.

   pitch w., a precancerous keratotic epidermal tumor, common among workers in pitch and coal tar derivatives.

   plantar w., an often painful w. on the sole; usually caused by human papilloma virus type 1. SYN verruca plantaris.

   postmortem w., a tuberculous warty growth (tuberculosis cutis verrucosa) on the hand of one who performs postmortem examinations. SYN anatomical w., dissection tubercle, necrogenic w., verruca necrogenica.

   soft w., SYN skin *tag*.

   telangiectatic w., SYN angiokeratoma.

   tuberculous w., SYN *tuberculosis* cutis verrucosa.

   venereal w., SYN *condyloma* acuminatum.

wash (wosh). A solution used to clean or bathe a part.

wash-out (wosh-out). A technique for eliminating (washing out) a specific substance.

   open-circuit nitrogen wash-out, a gas-dilution technique for measuring the functional residual capacity (FRC); the subject breathes 100% oxygen to wash out the resident nitrogen.

was·tage (hōz). Decay, loss, or dimunition of something.

   fetal w., loss of an embryo or fetus through spontaneous abortion or stillbirth; usually expressed as a rate per 1000 pregnancies with respect to a particular cause, such as maternal infection or drug addiction.

wast·ing (wāst'ing). **1.** SYN emaciation. **2.** Denoting a disease characterized by emaciation.

   salt w., inappropriately large renal excretion of salt despite the apparent need of the body to retain it.

wa·ter (wah'ter). **1.** H_2O; a clear, odorless, tasteless liquid, solidifying at 32°F (0°C and R), and boiling at 212°F (100°C, 80°R), that is present in all animal and vegetable tissues and dissolves more substances than any other liquid. SEE ALSO volume. **2.** Euphemism for urine. **3.** A pharmacopeial preparation of a clear, saturated aqueous solution (unless otherwise specified) of volatile oils, or other aromatic or volatile substances, prepared by processes involving distillation or solution (agitation followed by filtration). [A.S. *waeter*]

   w. of crystallization, w. of constitution that unites with certain salts and is essential to their arrangement in crystalline form; *e.g.*, $CuSO_4 \cdot 5H_2O$.

   w. of metabolism, the w. formed in the body by oxidation of the hydrogen of the food, the greatest amount being produced in the metabolism of fat (about 117 g/100 g of fat).

   mineral w., w. that contains appreciable amounts of certain salts, which give it therapeutic properties.

wa·ter·fall (wah'ter-fawl). A term used to describe flow in vascular beds where lateral pressure tending to collapse vessels greatly exceeds venous pressure. Flow is independent of venous pressure and occurs only when arterial pressure exceeds lateral pressure.

wa·ters (wah'ters). Colloquialism for amniotic *fluid*.

   bag of w., See entries under bag.

   false w., a leakage of fluid prior to or in beginning labor, before the rupture of the amnion.

wa·ter·shed. **1.** The area of marginal blood flow at the extreme periphery of a vascular bed. **2.** Slopes in the abdominal cavity, formed by projections of the lumbar vertebrae and the pelvic brim that determine the direction in which a free effusion will gravitate when the body is in a supine position.

watt (W) (waht). The SI unit of electrical power; the power available when the current is 1 ampere and the electromotive force is 1 volt; equal to 1 joule (10^7 ergs) per second or 1 voltampere. [James *Watt,* Scot. engineer, 1736–1819]

wave (wāv). **1.** A movement of particles in an elastic body, whether solid or fluid, whereby an advancing series of alternate elevations and depressions, or expansions and condensations, is produced. **2.** The elevation of the pulse, felt by the finger, or represented graphically in the curved line of the sphygmograph. **3.** The complete cycle of changes in the level of a source of energy that is repetitively varying with respect to time; in the electrocardiogram and the electroencephalogram the w. is essentially a voltage-time graph. SEE ALSO rhythm. [A.S. *wafian,* to fluctuate]

alpha w., SYN alpha *rhythm.*

beta w., SYN beta *rhythm.*

brain w., colloquialism for electroencephalogram.

delta w., (1) a premature upstroke of the QRS complex due to an atrioventricular bypass tract as in WPW syndrome; (2) SYN delta *rhythm.*

excitation w., a w. of altered electrical conditions that is propagated along a muscle fiber preparatory to its contraction.

P w., the first complex of the electrocardiogram, representing depolarization of the atria; if the P w. is retrograde or ectopic in axis or form, it is labeled P′.

postextrasystolic T w., the modified T w. of the beat immediately following an extrasystole.

pulse w., the progressive expansion of the arteries occurring with each contraction of the left ventricle of the heart.

Q w., the initial deflection of the QRS complex when such deflection is negative (downward).

R w., the first positive (upward) deflection of the QRS complex in the electrocardiogram; successive upward deflections within the same QRS complex are labeled R′, R″, etc.

S w., a negative (downward) deflection of the QRS complex following an R w.; successive downward deflections within the same QRS complex are labeled S′, S″, etc.

sine w., a symmetric wave representing one complete cycle of a single-frequency oscillation; the displacement of mass over time described by using a function from trigonometry, the sine. SEE ALSO pure *tone.*

T w., the next deflection in the electrocardiogram following the QRS complex; represents ventricular repolarization.

theta w., SYN theta *rhythm.*

Traube-Hering w.'s, SYN Traube-Hering *curves,* under *curve.*

U w., a positive w. following the T w. of the electrocardiogram.

V w., a large pressure w. visible in recordings from either atrium or its incoming veins, normally produced by venous return but becoming very large when blood regurgitates through the A-V valve beyond the chamber from which the recording is made.

wave•length (lambda) (wāv′length). The distance from one point on a wave (frequently shaped like a sine curve) to the next point in the same phase; *i.e.,* from peak to peak or from trough to trough.

wax•ing, wax•ing-up (wak′sing). The contouring of a pattern in wax, generally applied to the shaping in wax of the contours of a trial denture or a crown prior to casting in metal.

Wb weber.

WBC white blood *cell.*

WDLL well-differentiated lymphocytic *lymphoma.*

wean (wēn). To implement weaning. [A.S. *wenian*]

wean•ing (sēn′ing). **1.** Permanent deprivation of breast milk and commencement of nourishment with other food. **2.** Gradual withdrawal of a patient from dependence on a life support system or other form of therapy.

web (wĕb). A tissue or membrane bridging a space. SEE ALSO tela. [A.S.]

web•bing (web′ing). Congenital condition apparent when adjacent structures are joined by a broad band of tissue not normally present to such a degree.

Weber, Ernst H., German physiologist and anatomist, 1795–1878. SEE W.'s *paradox;* Fechner-Weber *law;* W.-Fechner *law.*

Weber, Sir Hermann, English physician, 1823–1918. SEE Weber's *syndrome.*

we•ber (Wb) (web′er). SI unit of magnetic flux, equal to volt-seconds (V·s). [Wilhelm E. *Weber*]

weight (wāt). The product of the force of gravity, defined internationally as 9.80665 m/s^2, times the mass of the body. [A.S. *gewiht*]

apothecaries' w., a system of w.'s based upon the w. of a grain of wheat; now superseded by the metric system (based on grams). One grain is the equivalent of 64.8 milligrams. One scruple contains 20 grains; one dram contains 60 grains; one apothecary ounce contains 8 drams (480 grains); one apothecary pound contains 12 ounces (5760 grains).

atomic w. (at wt, AW), the mass in grams of 1 mol (6.02×10^{23}, atoms) of an atomic species; the mass of an atom of a chemical element in relation to the mass of an atom of carbon-12 (^{12}C), which is set equal to 12.000, thus a ratio and therefore dimensionless (although the actual mass, numerically the same, is sometimes expressed in daltons); not necessarily the w. of any individual atom of an element, since most elements are made up of several isotopes of different masses. SEE ALSO molecular w.

avoirdupois w., a system of w.'s based on the grain; 7000 grains equal 256 drams, or 16 ounces, or 1 pound.

birth w., in humans, the first w. of an infant obtained within less than the first 60 completed minutes after birth; a full-size infant is one weighing 2500 g or more; a low birth w. is less than 2500 g.

molecular w. (mol wt, MW), the sum of the atomic w.'s of all the atoms constituting a mole-

we

cule; the mass of a molecule relative to the mass of a standard atom, now ^{12}C (taken as 12.000). Relative molecular mass (M_r) is the mass relative to the dalton and has no units. SEE ALSO atomic w. SYN molecular weight ratio, relative molecular mass.

welt (wĕlt). SYN wheal. [O.E. *waelt*]

wen (wĕn). Old term for pilar *cyst.* [A.S.]

West·ern blot, West·ern blot·ting. SYN Western blot *analysis.* SEE immunoblot.

ℹ️**wheal** (hwēl). A circumscribed, evanescent papule or irregular plaque of edema of the skin, appearing as an urticarial lesion, slightly reddened, often changing in size and shape and extending to adjacent areas, and usually accompanied by intense itching; produced by intradermal injection or test, or by exposure to allergenic substances in susceptible persons. SYN hives (2), welt. [A.S. *hwēle*]

wheeze (hwēz). **1.** To breathe with difficulty and noisily. **2.** A whistling, squeaking, musical, or puffing sound made by air passing through the fauces, glottis, or narrowed tracheobronchial airways in difficult breathing. [A.S. *hwēsan*]

whip·lash (hwip′lash). SEE whiplash *injury.*

white (hwīt). The color resulting from commingling of all the rays of the spectrum; the color of chalk or of snow. SYN albicans (1). [A.S. *hwīt*]

Whitehead, Walter, English surgeon, 1840–1913. SEE W.'s *operation.*

white·head (hwīt′hed). **1.** SYN milium. **2.** SYN closed *comedo.*

whit·low (hwit′lō). SYN felon. [M.E. *whitflawe*]

   herpetic w., painful herpes simplex virus infection of a finger from direct inoculation of the unprotected perionychial fold, often accompanied by lymphangitis and regional adenopathy, lasting up to several weeks; most common in physicians, dentists, and nurses as a result of exposure to the virus in a patient's mouth.

WHO World Health Organization.

whoop (hoop). The loud sonorous inspiration in pertussis with which the paroxysm of coughing terminates, due to spasm of the larynx (glottis).

whorl (hwerl). **1.** A turn of the spiral cochlea of the ear. **2.** SYN *vortex* of heart. **3.** A turn of a concha nasalis. **4.** SYN verticil. **5.** An area of hair growing in a radial manner suggesting whirling or twisting. SYN vortex (2). SEE hair w.'s. **6.** One of the distinguishing patterns in Galton's system of classification of fingerprints.

   hair w.'s, a spiral arrangement of the hairs, as at the crown of the head.

whorled (hwerld). Marked by or arranged in whorls. SEE ALSO turbinate, verticillate.

wind·burn (wind′bern). Erythema of the face due to exposure to wind.

win·dow (win′dō). SYN fenestra.

   oval w., SYN *fenestra* vestibuli.

   round w., SYN *fenestra* cochleae.

   tachycardia w., in paroxysmal tachycardia of the reentry type, the interval of time (the window) between the earliest and latest premature activation that can excite the paroxysm.

wind·pipe (wind′pīp). SYN trachea.

wind-suck·ing. A more severe form of crib-

biting where air is ingested abnormally and forcefully by swallowing. SEE aerophagia.

wing. 1. The anterior appendage of a bird. **2.** ANATOMY Ala. SYN ala.

   greater w. of sphenoid bone, strong squamous processes extending in a broad superolateral curve from the body of the sphenoid bone. The greater w. presents these surfaces (facies): 1) cerebral surface: forms anterior third of the floor of the lateral portion of the middle cranial fossa; 2) temporal surface: forms the deepest portion of the temporal fossa; 3) infratemporal surface, forms the "roof" of the infratemporal fossa; 4) orbital surface: forms posterolateral wall of orbit. The greater w. forms the inferior border of the supraorbital fissure, and is perforated at its root by the foramina rotundum ovale and spinosum and the pterygoid canal.

   lesser w. of sphenoid bone, one of a bilateral pair of triangular, pointed plates extending laterally from the anterolateral body of the sphenoid bone. Forming the posteriormost portion of the floor of the anterior cranial fossa, their sharp posterior edge forms the sphenoidal ridge separating anterior and middle cranial fossae. The medial end of the lesser w. attaches to the body by means of two pedicles, thus forming the optic canal. The w. itself forms the superior margin of the supraorbital fissure.

   w. of nose, the outer, more or less flaring, wall of each nostril.

wink (wink). To close and open the eyes rapidly; an involuntary act by which the tears are spread over the conjunctiva, keeping it moist. [A.S. *wincian*]

wir·ing (wīr′ing). Fastening together the ends of a broken bone by wire sutures.

wiry (wīr′ē). Resembling or having the feel of a wire; filiform and hard; denoting a variety of pulse.

with·draw·al (with-draw′ăl). **1.** The act of removal or retreat. **2.** A psychological and/or physical syndrome caused by the abrupt cessation of the use of a drug in a habituated individual. **3.** The therapeutic process of discontinuing a drug so as to avoid w. (2). **4.** A pattern of behavior observed in schizophrenia and depression, characterized by a pathological retreat from interpersonal contact and social involvement and leading to self-preoccupation.

WLU workload *unit.*

wob·ble (wah′bl). MOLECULAR BIOLOGY Unorthodox pairing between the base at the 5′ end of an anticodon and the base that pairs with it (in the 3′-position of the codon).

wolff·i·an (wulf′ē-an). Relating to or described by Kaspar Wolff.

wolf·ram, wolf·ram·i·um (wulf′ram, wulf-ram′ē-ŭm). SYN tungsten. [from *wolframite*]

womb (woom). SYN uterus. [A.S. the belly]

word sal·ad (werd sal′ăd). A jumble of meaningless and unrelated words emitted by persons with certain kinds of schizophrenia.

work·ing out (werk′ing). PSYCHOANALYSIS The stage in the treatment process in which the patient's personal history and psychodynamics are uncovered.

work·ing through. PSYCHOANALYSIS The process of obtaining additional insight and personality changes in a patient through repeated and varied examination of a conflict or problem; the interactions between free association, resistance, interpretation, and working out are the chief parts of this process.

World Health Or·ga·ni·za·tion (WHO). A unit of the United Nations devoted to international health problems.

Worm, Ole, Danish anatomist, 1588–1654. SEE wormian *bones,* under *bone.*

worm (werm). **1.** ANATOMY Any structure resembling a w., *e.g.,* the midline part of the cerebellum. **2.** SYN lyssa (1). **3.** Any member of the separate phyla Annelida (the segmented or true w.'s), the Nematoda (roundworms), and the Platyhelminthes (flatworms). Important species include *Dracunculus medinensis* (dragon, guinea, Medina, or serpent w.), *Enterobius vermicularis* (seat w. or pinworm), *Loa loa* (African eye w.), *Oxyspirura mansoni* (Manson's eye w.), and *Trichinella spiralis* (pork or trichina w.). For some types of w.'s not listed as subentries here (because they are usually written as one word), see the full name. [A.S. *wyrm*]

wor·mi·an (werm'ē-an). Relating to or described by Ole Worm.

wound (wūnd). **1.** Trauma to any of the tissues of the body, especially that caused by physical means and with interruption of continuity. **2.** A surgical incision. [O.E. *wund*]

 abraded w., SYN abrasion (1).

 avulsed w., a w. caused by or resulting from avulsion.

 gutter w., a tangential w. that makes a furrow without perforating the skin.

 incised w., a clean cut, as by a sharp instrument.

 nonpenetrating w., injury, especially within the thorax or abdomen, produced without disruption of the surface of the body.

 open w., a w. in which the tissues are exposed to the air.

 penetrating w., a w. with disruption of the body surface that extends into underlying tissue or into a body cavity.

 perforating w., a w. with an entrance and exit opening.

 puncture w., a w. in which the opening is relatively small as compared to the depth, as produced by a narrow pointed object.

 sucking w., SYN open *pneumothorax.*

W-plas·ty. Surgery to prevent the contracture of a straight-line scar; the edges of the wound are trimmed in the shape of a W, or a series of W's, and closed in a zig-zag manner.

wrist (rist). The proximal segment of the hand consisting of the carpal bones and the associated soft parts. SYN carpus (1) [NA]. [A.S. wrist joint, ankle joint]

w.-drop, Paralysis of the extensors of the wrist and fingers; most often caused by lesion of the radial nerve. SYN drop hand.

wry·neck (rī'nek). SYN torticollis.

Wuch·er·e·ria (vū-ker-e'rē-ă). A genus of filarial nematodes characterized by adult forms that live

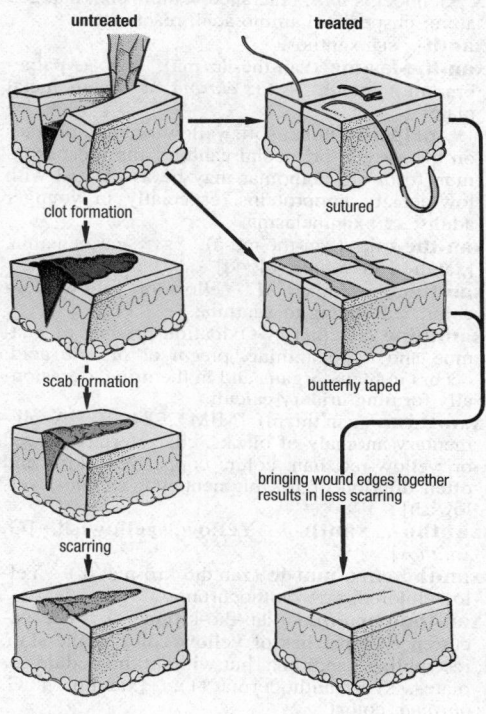

untreated — treated

clot formation — sutured

scab formation — butterfly taped

bringing wound edges together results in less scarring

scarring

wound healing

chiefly in lymphatic vessels and produce large numbers of embryos or microfilariae that circulate in the bloodstream (microfilaremia), often appearing in the peripheral blood at regular intervals. The extreme form of this infection (wuchereriasis or filariasis) is elephantiasis or pachydermia.

 W. bancrof'ti, the bancroftian filaria, transmitted to humans (apparently the only definitive host) by mosquitoes, especially *Culex quinquefasciatus* and *Aedes pseudoscutellaris,* but also by several other species of *Culex, Aedes, Anopheles,* and *Mansonia,* depending on the specific geographic area; adults are white, threadlike worms, and the microfilariae are ensheathed, with rounded anterior end and tapered, nonnucleated tail; the adult worms inhabit the larger lymphatic vessels (*e.g.,* in the extremities, breasts, spermatic cord, and retroperitoneal tissues) and the sinuses of lymph nodes, where they sometimes cause temporary obstruction to the flow of lymph and slight or moderate degrees of inflammation.

wu·cher·e·ri·a·sis (vū'ker-ē-rī'ă-sis). Infection with worms of the genus *Wuchereria.* SEE ALSO filariasis.

WU

X Kienböck's *unit*; reactance; xanthosine; halogen atom; unspecified amino acid; reactance.

⌂**xanth-.** SEE xantho-.

xan·the·las·ma (zan-thĕ-laz′mă). SYN x. palpebrarum. [xanth- + G. *elasma*, a beaten metal plate]

x. **palpebra′rum,** soft, yellow-orange, plaques on the eyelids or medial canthus, the most common form of xanthoma; may be associated with low-density lipoproteins, especially in younger adults. SYN xanthelasma.

xan·the·mia (zan-thē′mē-ă). SYN carotenemia. [xanth- + G. *haima*, blood]

xan·thic (zan′thik). **1.** Yellow or yellowish in color. **2.** Relating to xanthine.

xan·thine (zan′thēn). Oxidation product of guanine and hypoxanthine, precursor of uric acid; occurs in many organs and in the urine, occasionally forming urinary calculi.

xan·thism (zan′thizm) [MIM*278400]. A pigmentary anomaly of blacks, characterized by red or yellow-red hair color, copper-red skin, and often dilution of iris pigment. [G. *xanthos,* yellowish]

⌂**xantho-, xanth-.** Yellow, yellowish. [G. *xanthos*]

xan·tho·chro·mat·ic (zan′thō-krō-mat′ik). Yellow-colored. SYN xanthochromic.

xan·tho·chro·mia (zan-thō-krō′mē-ă). The occurrence of patches of yellow color in the skin, resembling xanthoma, but without the nodules or plates. SYN xanthoderma (1). [xantho- + G. *chrōma,* color]

xan·tho·chro·mic (zan-thō-krō′mik). SYN xanthochromatic.

xan·tho·der·ma (zan-thō-der′mă). **1.** SYN xanthochromia. **2.** Any yellow coloration of the skin. [xantho- + G. *derma,* skin]

xan·tho·gran·u·lo·ma (zan′thō-gran′yū-lō′mă). A peculiar infiltration of retroperitoneal tissue by lipid macrophages, occurring most commonly in women.

xan·tho·ma (zan-thō′mă). A yellow nodule or plaque, especially of the skin, composed of lipid-laden histiocytes. [xantho- + G. *-oma,* tumor]

x. **dissemina′tum,** a rare benign normolipemic disorder of adults with coalescent cutaneous x.'s composed of non-X histiocytes on flexural surfaces, often with mild diabetes insipidus.

eruptive x., the sudden appearance of groups of waxy, yellow or yellowish-brown papules with an erythematous halo, especially over extensors of the elbows and knees, and on the back and buttocks of patients with severe hyperlipemia, often familial or, more rarely, in severe diabetes.

x. **mul′tiplex,** SYN xanthomatosis.

x. **pla′num,** a form marked by the occurrence of yellow, flat bands or minimally palpable rectangular plates in the corium, either normolipemic or associated with type IIa or III hyperlipoproteinemia.

x. **tubero′sum,** xanthomatosis associated with familial type II, and occasionally type III, hyperlipoproteinemia.

verrucous x., histocytosis Y; a papilloma of the oral mucosa and skin in which squamous epithelium covers connective tissue papillae filled with large foamy histiocytes.

xan·tho·ma·to·sis (zan-thō-mă-tō′sis). Widespread xanthomas, especially on the elbows and knees, that sometimes affect mucous membranes and are sometimes associated with metabolic disturbances. SYN lipid granulomatosis, lipoid granulomatosis, xanthoma multiplex.

x. **bul′bi,** ulcerative fatty degeneration of the cornea after injury.

xan·thom·a·tous (zan-thō′mă-tŭs). Relating to xanthoma.

Xan·tho·mo·nas (zan-thō-mō′nas). Genus of the family Pseudomonadaceae; aerobic, Gram-negative, chemoorganotrophic, straight bacilli which exhibit motility by flagella. Type species is *Xanthomonas campestris.*

X. maltophil′ia, a species found primarily in clinical specimens but also in water, milk, and frozen food. Frequent cause of infections in hospitalized and immunocompromised humans.

xan·tho·phyll (zan′thō-fil). (3*R*,3′*R*, 6′*R*)-β-ε-Carotene-3′,3′-diol; oxygenated derivative of carotene; a yellow plant pigment, occurring also in egg yolk and corpus luteum. SYN lutein (2).

xan·thop·sia (zan-thop′sē-ă). A condition in which objects appear yellow; may occur in picric acid and santonin poisoning, in jaundice, and in digitalis intoxication. [xantho- + G. *opsis,* vision]

xan·tho·sine (X, Xao) (zan′thō-sēn, -sin). The deamination product of guanosine (O replacing $-NH_2$).

xan·tho·sis (zan-thō′sis). A yellowish discoloration of degenerating tissues, especially seen in malignant neoplasms. [xantho- + G. *-osis,* condition]

Xao xanthosine.

Xe xenon.

⌂**xeno-.** Strange; foreign material; parasite. SEE hetero-, allo-. [G. *xenos,* guest, host, stranger, foreign]

xen·o·bi·ot·ic (zen′ō-bī-ot′ik). A pharmacologically, endocrinologically, or toxicologically active substance not endogenously produced and therefore foreign to an organism.

xen·o·di·ag·no·sis (zen′ō-dī-ag-nō′sis). **1.** A method of diagnosing acute or early *Trypanosoma cruzi* infection (Chagas' disease) in humans. Infection-free triatomine bugs are fed on the suspected person and the trypanosome is identified by microscopic examination of the intestinal contents of the bug after a suitable incubation period. **2.** A similar method of biological diagnosis based upon experimental exposure of a parasite-free normal host capable of allowing the organism in question to multiply, enabling it to be more easily and reliably detected.

xen·o·gen·e·ic (zen′ō-jĕ-nē′ik). Heterologous, with respect to tissue grafts, especially when donor and recipient belong to widely separated species. SYN xenogenic (2), xenogenous (2). [xeno- + G. *-gen,* producing]

xen•o•gen•ic (zen-ō-jen′ik). **1.** Originating outside of the organism, or from a foreign substance that has been introduced into the organism. SYN xenogenous (1). **2.** SYN xenogeneic. [xeno- + G. -gen, producing]

xe•nog•e•nous (zĕ-noj′ĕ-nŭs). **1.** SYN xenogenic (1). **2.** SYN xenogeneic.

xen•o•graft (zen′ō-graft). A graft transferred from an animal of one species to one of another species. SYN heterograft, heterologous graft.

xe•non (Xe) (zē′non). A gaseous element, atomic no. 54, atomic wt. 131.29; present in minute proportion in the atmosphere; produces general anesthesia in concentrations of 70 vol.%. [G. xenos, a stranger]

xe•non-133. A radioisotope of xenon with a gamma emission at 81 keV and a physical half-life of 5.243 days; used in the study of pulmonary function and organ blood flow.

xen•o•par•a•site (zen-ō-par′ă-sīt). An ecoparasite that becomes pathogenic in consequence of weakened resistance on the part of its host.

xen•o•pho•bia (zen-ō-fō′bē-ă). Morbid fear of strangers. [xeno- + G. phobos, fear]

Xen•o•psyl•la (zen-op-sil′ă). A genus of fleas parasitic on the rat and involved in the transmission of bubonic plague. *X. cheopis* serves as a potent vector of *Yersinia pestis*; *X. astia* and *X. braziliensis* are also efficient vectors of plague. [xeno- + G. psylla, flea]

△**xero-.** Dry. [G. xeros]

xer•o•chi•lia (zēr-ō-kī′lē-ă). Dryness of lips. [xero- + G. cheilos, lip]

xe•ro•der•ma (zēr′ō-der′mă). A mild form of ichthyosis characterized by excessive dryness of the skin due to slight increase of the horny layer and diminished water content of the stratum corneum from decreased perspiration, wind, or low humidity; seen with aging, atopic dermatitis, vitamin A deficiency, etc. [xero- + G. derma, skin]

  x. pigmento′sum [MIM*278700], an eruption of exposed skin occurring in childhood and characterized by photosensitivity with severe sunburn in infancy and the development of numerous pigmented spots resembling freckles, larger atrophic lesions eventually resulting in glossy white thinning of the skin surrounded by telangiectases, and multiple solar keratoses which undergo malignant change at an early age. Severe ophthalmic and neurologic abnormalities are also found.

xe•ro•gram (zē′rō-gram). SYN xeroradiograph.

xe•rog•ra•phy (zēr-og′ră-fē). SYN xeroradiography.

xe•ro•ma (zē-rō′mă). SYN xerophthalmia.

xe•roph•thal•mia (zēr-of-thal′mē-ă). Excessive dryness of the conjunctiva and cornea, which lose their luster and become keratinized; may be due to local disease or to a systemic deficiency of vitamin A. SYN xeroma. [xero- + G. ophthalmos, eye]

xe•ro•ra•di•o•graph (zē-rō-rā′dē-ō-graf). The permanent record made by xeroradiography. SYN xerogram.

xe•ro•ra•di•og•ra•phy (zē′rō-rā′dē-og′ră-fē). Radiography using a specially coated charged plate instead of x-ray film, developing with a dry powder rather than liquid chemicals, and transferring the powder image onto paper for a permanent record; edge enhancement is inherent. SYN xerography.

xe•ro•sis (zē-rō′sis). Pathologic dryness of the skin (xeroderma), the conjunctiva (xerophthalmia), or mucous membranes. [xero- + G. -osis, condition]

xe•ro•sto•mia (zēr′ō-stō′mē-ă). A dryness of the mouth, having a varied etiology, resulting from diminished or arrested salivary secretion, or asialism. [xero- + G. stoma, mouth]

xe•rot•ic (zē-rot′ik). Dry; affected with xerosis.

X-in•ac•ti•va•tion. SYN lyionization.

△**xiph-.** SEE xipho-.

xiph•i•ster•nal (zif-i-ster′năl). Relating to the xiphoid process.

xiph•i•ster•num (zif′i-ster′nŭm). SYN xiphoid process. [xiphoid + G. sternon, chest]

△**xipho-, xiph-, xiphi-.** Xiphoid, usually the processus xiphoideus. [G. xiphos, sword]

xi•phoid (zif′oyd). Sword-shaped; applied especially to the xiphoid process. SYN ensiform. [xipho- + G. eidos, appearance]

xi•phoi•di•tis (zif′oy-dī′tis). Inflammation of the xiphoid process of the sternum. [xiphoid + G. -itis, inflammation]

X-linked. Pertaining to genes borne on the X chromosome. Commonly but erroneously used synonymously with sex-linked, which would also comprise Y-linked traits.

x-ray. 1. The ionizing electromagnetic radiation emitted from a highly evacuated tube, resulting from the excitation of the inner orbital electrons by the bombardment of the target anode with a stream of electrons from a heated cathode. **2.** Ionizing electromagnetic radiation produced by the excitation of the inner orbital electrons of an atom by other processes, such as nuclear delay and its sequelae. **3.** A radiograph. SYN roentgen ray.

xy•lose (zī′lōs). An aldopentose, isomeric with ribose, obtained by fermentation or hydrolysis of carbohydrate.

xy•lu•lose (zī′lū-lōs). *threo*-pentulose; A ketopentose that appears in the urine in cases of essential pentosuria; it is also an intermediate in the glucuronate pathway.

xys•ma (ziz′mă). Membranous shreds in the feces. [G. filings, shavings, fr. *xyō*, to scrape]

Y

Y yttrium; tyrosine; pyrimidine nucleoside.

y⁺. SEE system (5).

yaw (yau). An individual lesion of the eruption of yaws.

 mother y., a large granulomatous lesion, considered to be the initial lesion in yaws, most commonly present on the hand, leg, or foot. SYN buba madre, frambesioma.

yawn (yaun). **1.** To gape. **2.** An involuntary opening of the mouth, usually accompanied by a movement of respiration; it may be a sign of drowsiness or of vital depression, as after hemorrhage, but is often caused by suggestion. [A.S. *gānian*]

yaws (yawz). An infectious tropical disease caused by *Treponema pertenue* and characterized by the development of crusted granulomatous ulcers on the extremities; may involve bone, but, unlike syphilis, does not produce central nervous system or cardiovascular pathology. SYN boubas, bubas, granuloma tropicum, pian, rupia (2). [of Caribbean origin; similar to Calinago *yaya*, the disease]

Yb ytterbium.

years of po•ten•tial life lost. Measure of the relative impact of various diseases and lethal forces on society, computed by estimating the years that people would have lived if they had not died prematurely from injury, cancer, heart disease, etc.

yeast (yēst). A general term denoting true fungi of the family Saccharomycetaceae that are widely distributed in substrates that contain sugars (such as fruits), and in soil, animal excreta, the vegetative parts of plants, etc. Because of their ability to ferment carbohydrates, some y.'s are important to the brewing and baking industries. [A.S. *gyst*]

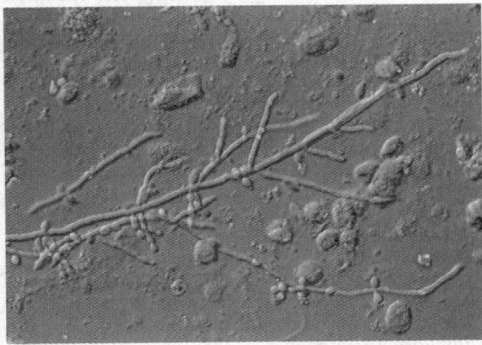

yeast

Yer•sin•ia (yer-sin′ē-ă). A genus of motile and nonmotile, non-spore-forming bacteria containing Gram-negative, unencapsulated, ovoid to rod-shaped cells. These organisms are parasitic on humans and other animals. The type species is *Y.*

pestis. [A. J. E. *Yersin,* Swiss bacteriologist, 1862–1943]

 Y. enterocolit′ica, a species that causes yersiniosis in humans; it is found in the feces and lymph nodes of sick and healthy animals, including humans, and in material contaminated with feces.

 Y. pes′tis, a species causing plague in humans, rodents, and many other mammalian species, and transmitted from rat to rat and from rat to human host by the rat flea, *Xenopsylla;* it is the type species of the genus *Y.* SYN *Pasteurella pestis.*

 Y. pseudotuberculo′sis, a species causing pseudotuberculosis in birds, rodents, and rarely in humans. SYN *Pasteurella pseudotuberculosis.*

yer•sin•i•o•sis (yer-sin-ē-ō′sis). A common human infectious disease caused by *Yersinia enterocolitica* and marked by diarrhea, enteritis, pseudoappendicitis, ileitis, erythema nodosum, and sometimes septicemia or acute arthritis.

yield (yēld). The amount or quantity produced or returned, often measured as a percent of the starting material; *e.g.,* a y. in an enzyme preparation is equal to the units of enzyme activity recovered at the end of the preparation divided by the total units observed in the starting material.

 quantum y. (φ), the number of molecules transformed (*e.g.,* via a reaction) per quantum of light absorbed; the inverse of the quantum requirement.

-yl. Chemical suffix signifying that the substance is a radical by loss of an H atom (*e.g.,* alkyl, methyl, phenyl) or OH group (*e.g.,* acyl, acetyl, carbamoyl).

-ylene. Chemical suffix denoting a bivalent hydrocarbon radical (*e.g.,* methylene, –CH_2–) or possessing a double bond (*e.g.,* ethylene, $CH_2=CH_2$).

Y-link•age. The state of a genetic factor (gene) being borne on the Y chromosome. This idea is analogous with X-linkage but since the Y chromosome does not fully take part in chiasma formation and recombination, it not amenable to analysis by conventional linkage methods.

yoke (yōk). SYN jugum (1). [A.S. *geoc*]

yolk (yōk, yōlk). **1.** One of the types of nutritive material stored in the ovum for the nutrition of the embryo; y. is particularly abundant and conspicuous in the eggs of birds. SYN vitellus. **2.** Fatty material found in the wool of sheep; when extracted and purified, it becomes lanolin. [A.S. *geolca; geolu,* yellow]

yt•ter•bi•um (Yb) (i-ter′bē-ŭm). A metallic element of the lanthanide group; atomic no. 70, atomic wt. 173.04. ¹⁶⁹Yb, with a half-life of 32.03 days, has been used in cisternography and in brain scans. [*Ytterby,* village in Sweden]

yt•tri•um (Y) (it′rē-ŭm). A metallic element, atomic no. 39, atomic wt. 88.90585. [*Ytterby,* village in Sweden]

Z benzyloxycarbonyl; atomic *number*; symbol for an amino acid that is either glutamic acid, glutamine, or a substance that yields glutamic acid on acid hydrolysis of peptides; carbobenzoxy.

ZEEP zero end-expiratory *pressure*.

Zeit•geist (zīt′gīst). PSYCHOLOGY The climate of opinion, conventions of thought, covert influences, and unquestioned assumptions that are implicit in a given culture, the arts, or science at any time, and in which the individual operates and thus is influenced. [Ger. *Zeit,* time, + *Geist,* spirit]

zep•to-. Prefix used in the SI and metric systems to signify 10^{-21}.

ze•ro (zē′rō). **1.** The figure 0, indicating the absence of magnitude, or nothing. **2.** THERMOMETRY The point from which the figures on the scale start in one or the other direction; in the Celsius and Réeaumur scales, z. indicates the freezing point for distilled water; in the Fahrenheit scale, it is 32° below the freezing point of water. [Sp. fr. Ar. *sifr,* cipher]

  absolute z., the lowest possible temperature, that at which the form of translational motion constituting heat is assumed no longer to exist, determined as −273.15°C or 0 Kelvin.

ze•ta (zāt′a). **1.** Sixth letter of the Greek alphabet, ζ **2.** CHEMISTRY The sixth in a series, *e.g.,* the sixth carbon from a functional group. **3.** Electrokinetic potential.

ze•ta•crit (zā′tă-krit). The packed cell volume produced by vertical centrifugation of blood in capillary tubes, allowing controlled compaction and dispersion of red blood cells; read with a hematocrit to produce the zeta sedimentation ratio.

zinc (zingk). A metallic element, atomic no. 30, atomic wt. 65.39; an essential bioelement; a number of salts of z. are used in medicine; a cofactor in many proteins. [Ger. *Zink*]

zinc-65. A radioactive zinc isotope that decays mainly by K-capture with a half-life of 243.8 days; used as a tracer in studies of zinc metabolism.

zir•co•ni•um (Zr) (zir-kō′nē-ŭm). A metallic element, atomic no. 40, atomic wt. 91.224; widely distributed in nature, but never found in quantity in any one place. [*zircon,* a mineral, fr. Ar. *zarkūn,* cinnabar, Pers, *zargun,* goldlike]

zo-. SEE zoo-.

zo•ac•an•tho•sis (zō′ă-kan-thō′sis). A cutaneous eruption due to introduction into the human skin of hair, bristles, stingers, etc., of lower animals. [G. *zōon,* animal, + acanthosis]

zo•an•throp•ic (zō-an-throp′ik). Relating to or marked by zoanthropy.

zo•an•thro•py (zō-an′thrō-pē). A delusion that one is an animal, such as a dog. [G. *zōon,* animal, + *anthrōpos,* man]

zo•na, pl. **zo•nae** (zō′nă, zō′nē). **1.** SYN zone. **2.** SYN *herpes* zoster. [L. fr. G. *zōnē,* a girdle, one of the zones of the sphere]

  z. arcua′ta, SYN arcuate *zone.*

  z. fascicula′ta, the layer of radially arranged cell cords in the cortex of the suprarenal gland, between the z. glomerulosa and z. reticularis; secretes cortisol and dehydroepiandrosterone.

  z. glomerulo′sa, the outer layer of the cortex of the suprarenal gland just beneath the capsule; secretes aldosterone.

  z. ophthal′mica, herpes zoster in the distribution of the ophthalmic nerve.

  z. orbicula′ris [NA], fibers of the articular capsule of the hip joint encircling the neck of the femur. SYN orbicular zone.

  z. pectina′ta, SYN pectinate *zone.*

  z. pellu′cida, a layer consisting of microvilli of the oocyte, cellular processes of follicular cells, and an intervening substance rich in glycoprotein; it appears homogeneous and translucent under the light microscope. SYN pellucid zone.

  z. reticula′ris, the inner layer of the cortex of the adrenal gland, where the cell cords anastomose in a netlike fashion.

  z. tec′ta, SYN arcuate *zone.*

  z. vasculo′sa, SYN vascular *zone.*

zone (zōn). A segment; any encircling or beltlike structure, either external or internal, longitudinal or transverse. SEE ALSO area, band, region, space, spot. SYN zona (1). [L. *zona*]

  arcuate z., the inner third of the basilar membrane of the cochlear duct extending from the tympanic lip of the osseous spiral lamina to the outer pillar cell of the spiral organ (of Corti). SYN zona arcuata, zona tecta.

  ciliary z., the outer, wider z. of the anterior surface of the iris, separated from the pupillary z. by the collarette.

  comfort z., the temperature range between 28°C and 30°C at which the naked body is able to maintain the heat balance without either shivering or sweating; in the clothed body the range is from 13°C to 21°C.

  epileptogenic z., a cortical region which on stimulation reproduces the patient's spontaneous seizure or aura.

  erogenous z.'s, erotogenic z.'s, areas of the body, such as genitals and nipples, which elicit sexual arousal when stimulated.

  hemorrhoidal z., the part of the anal canal that contains the rectal venous plexus.

  orbicular z., SYN *zona* orbicularis.

  pectinate z., the outer two-thirds of the basilar membrane of the cochlear duct. SYN zona pectinata.

  pellucid z., SYN *zona* pellucida.

  pupillary z., the central region of the anterior surface of the iris located between the collarette and the pupillary margin.

  training-sensitive z., level of exercise heart rate, usually 70–85% of maximum, required to induce training improvements in aerobic fitness. Exercise heart rates below the 70% threshold are generally offset by extending exercise duration. SYN target heart rate range.

  transitional z., (1) the equatorial region of the lens of the eye where the anterior epithelial cells become transformed into lens fibers; (2) that portion of a scleral contact lens between the corneal and scleral sections.

trigger z., SYN trigger *point.*

vascular z., an area in the external acoustic meatus where a number of minute blood vessels enter from the mastoid bone. SYN zona vasculosa.

zo•nes•the•sia (zōn-es-thē′zē-ă). A sensation as if a cord were drawn around the body, constricting it. SYN girdle sensation. [G. *zōnē,* girdle, + *aisthēsis,* sensation]

zo•nif•u•gal (zō-nif′yū-găl). Passing from within any region outward; as in mapping out an area of disturbed sensation, when the stimulus is first applied to the affected region and is carried into the area where sensation is normal. [L. *zona,* zone, + *fugio,* to flee]

zon•ing (zōn′ing). The occurrence of a stronger reaction in a lesser amount of suspected serum, observed sometimes in serologic tests used in the diagnosis of syphilis, and probably the result of high antibody titer.

zo•nip•e•tal (zō-nip′ĕ-tăl). Passing from without toward and into any region, as in mapping out an area of disturbed sensation, when the stimulus begins in a normal area and is carried into the affected region. [L. *zona,* zone, + *peto,* to seek]

zon•og•ra•phy (zō-nog′ră-fē). A form of tomography with a relatively thick plane of focus; especially used in renal radiography. [zone + G. *graphō,* to write]

zo•nu•la, pl. **zo•nu•lae** (zō′nyū-lă, zon′yū-; -lē) [NA]. SYN zonule. [L. dim. of *zona,* zone]

zo•nu•lar (zō′nyū-lăr, zon′yū-). Relating to a zonula.

zon•ule (zō′nyūl, zon′yūl). A small zone. SYN zonula [NA].

ciliary z., a series of delicate meridional fibers arising from the inner surface of the orbiculus ciliaris that run in bundles between, and in a very thin layer over, the ciliary processes; at the inner border of the corona, the fibers diverge into two groups that are attached to the capsule on the anterior and posterior surfaces of the lens close to the equator; the spaces between these two layers of fibers are filled with aqueous humor. SYN suspensory ligament of lens.

zo•nu•li•tis (zō-nyū-lī′tis). Inflammation of the zonule of Zinn, or suspensory ligament of the lens of the eye. [zonule + G. *-itis,* inflammation]

zo•nu•lol•y•sis, zo•nu•ly•sis (zō′nyū-lol′i-sis, -lī′sis). Dissolution of the zonula ciliaris by enzymes (α-chymotrypsin) to facilitate surgical removal of a cataract. [zonule + G. *lysis,* dissolution]

△zoo-, zo-. Animal, animal life. [G. *zōon*]

zo•o•e•ras•tia (zō′ō-ĕ-ras′tē-ă). SYN bestiality. [zoo- + G. *erastēs,* lover]

zo•o•graft (zō′ō-graft). A graft of tissue from an animal to a human.

zo•o•graft•ing (zō-ō-graft′ing). SYN zooplasty.

zo•oid (zō′oyd). **1.** Resembling an animal; an organism or object with an animal-like appearance. **2.** An animal cell capable of independent existence or movement, as the ovum or a spermatozoon, or the segment of a tapeworm. **3.** An individual of a colonial invertebrate, such as a

coral. [G. *zoōdēs,* fr. *zōon,* animal, + *eidos,* resemblance]

zo•o•lag•nia (zō-ō-lag′nē-ă). Sexual attraction toward animals. [zoo- + G. *lagneia,* lust]

zo•o•no•sis (zō-ō-nō′sis). An infection or infestation shared in nature by humans and other animals that are the normal or usual host; a disease of humans acquired from an animal source. SEE ALSO anthropozoonosis, metazoonosis, saprozoonosis. [zoo- + G. *nosos,* disease]

zo•o•par•a•site (zō-ō-par′ă-sīt). An animal parasite; an animal existing as a parasite.

zo•oph•i•lism (zō-of′i-lizm). Fondness for animals, especially an extravagant fondness for them.

zo•o•pho•bia (zō-ō-fō′bē-ă). Morbid fear of animals. [zoo- + G. *phobos,* fear]

zo•o•plas•ty (zō′ō-plas-tē). Grafting of tissue from an animal to a human. SYN zoografting.

zo•o•tox•in (zō-ōtok′sin). A substance, resembling the bacterial toxins in its antigenic properties, found in the fluids of certain animals; *e.g.,* in snake venom, the secretions of poisonous insects, eel blood.

zos•ter (zos′ter). SYN herpes zoster. [G. *zōstēr,* a girdle]

zos•ter•oid (zos′ter-oyd). Resembling herpes zoster. [zoster + G. *eidos,* resemblance]

Z-plas•ty. Surgery to elongate a contracted scar or to rotate tension 90°; the middle line of a Z-shaped incision is made along the line of greatest tension or contraction, and triangular flaps are raised on opposite sides of the two ends and transposed.

Zr zirconium.

zwit•ter•i•ons (tsvit′er-ī-onz). SYN dipolar *ions,* under *ion.* SEE ALSO zwitter *hypothesis.* [Ger. *Zwitter,* hermaphrodite, mongrel + ion]

△zyg-. SEE zygo-.

zy•gal (zī′găl). Relating to or shaped like a zygon or yoke; H-shaped.

△zygo-, zyg-. A yoke, a joining. [G. *zygon,* yoke, *zygōsis,* a joining]

zy•go•ma (zī-gō′mă). **1.** SYN zygomatic *bone.* **2.** SYN zygomatic *arch.* [G. a bar, bolt, the os jugale, fr. *zygon,* yoke]

zy•go•mat•ic (zī′gō-mat′ik). Relating to the zygomatic bone.

zy•go•max•il•la•re (zī′gō-mak-si-lā′rē). A craniometric point located externally at the lowest extent of the zygomaticomaxillary suture. SYN zygomaxillary point.

Zy•go•my•ce•tes (zī′gō-mī-sē′tēz). A class of fungi characterized by sexual reproduction resulting in the formation of a zygospore, and asexual reproduction by means of nonmotile spores called sporangiospores or conidia. [zygo- + G. *mykēs* (*mykēt-*), fungus]

zy•go•my•co•sis (zī′gō-mī-kō′sis). A fungous infection associated with genera of the class Zygomycetes, *e.g., Absidia, Mortierella, Mucor, Rhizopus.* The genera *Conidiobolus* and *Basidiobolus* have species that are also causative agents. SYN mucormycosis, phycomycosis.

zy•gon (zī′gon). The short crossbar connecting the branches of a zygal fissure. [G. crossbar, yoke]

zy•go•ne•ma (zī-g-ō-nē′mă).   SYN zygotene. [zygo- + G. *nēma,* thread]

zy•go•sis (zī-gō′sis).   True conjugation or sexual union of two unicellular organisms, consisting essentially in the fusion of the nuclei of the two cells. [G. a joining]

zy•gos•i•ty (zī-gos′i-tē).   The nature of the zygotes from which individuals are derived; *e.g.,* whether by division of one zygote (monozygotic), in which case they will be genetically identical, or from two separate fertilized ova (dizygotic).

zy•gote (zī′gōt).   **1.** The diploid cell resulting from union of a sperm and an ovum. Cf. conceptus. **2.** The individual that develops from a fertilized ovum. [G. *zygōtos,* yoked]

zy•go•tene (zī′gō-tēn).   The stage of prophase in meiosis in which precise point-for-point pairing of homologous chromosomes begins. SYN zygonema. [zygo- + G. *tainia* (L. *taenia*), band]

zy•got•ic (zī-got′ik).   Pertaining to a zygote, or to zygosis.

△ **zym-.**   SEE zymo-.

△ **zymo-, zym-.**   Fermentation, enzymes. [G. *zymē,* leaven]

zy•mo•deme (zī′mō-dēm).   An isoenzyme pattern, as identified by isoenzyme electrophoresis. [zymo- + G. *dēmos,* populace]

zy•mo•gen (zī′mō-jen).   SYN proenzyme.

zy•mo•gen•e•sis (zī-mō-jen′ĕ-sis).   Transformation of a proenzyme (zymogen) into an active enzyme. [zymo- + G. *genesis,* production]

zy•mo•gen•ic (zī-mō-jen′ik).   **1.** Relating to a zymogen or to zymogenesis. **2.** Causing fermentation.

zy

CONTENTS: THE APPENDICES

APPENDICES

TABLE OF ELEMENTS AND THEIR ATOMIC WEIGHTS

Element	Symbol	Atomic Number	Atomic Weight	Element	Symbol	Atomic Number	Atomic Weight
Actinium	Ac	89	227.0278*	Magnesium	Mg	12	24.3050
Aluminum	Al	13	26.981539	Manganese	Mn	25	54.93805
Americium	Am	95	243.0614*	Mendelevium	Md	101	258.10*
Antimony	Sb	51	121.75	Mercury	Hg	80	200.59
Argon	Ar	18	39.948	Molybdenum	Mo	42	95.94
Arsenic	As	33	74.92159	Neodymium	Nd	60	144.24
Astatine	At	85	209.9871*	Neon	Ne	10	20.1797
Barium	Ba	56	137.327	Neptunium	Np	93	237.0482*
Berkelium	Bk	97	247.0703*	Nickel	Ni	28	58.69
Beryllium	Be	4	9.012182	Niobium	Nb	41	92.90638
Bismuth	Bi	83	208.98037	Nitrogen	N	7	14.00674
Boron	B	5	10.811	Nobelium	No	102	259.1009*
Bromine	Br	35	79.904	Osmium	Os	76	190.2
Cadmium	Cd	48	112.411	Oxygen	O	8	15.9994
Calcium	Ca	20	40.078	Palladium	Pd	46	106.42
Californium	Cf	98	251.0796*	Phosphorus	P	15	30.973762
Carbon	C	6	12.011	Platinum	Pt	78	195.08
Cerium	Ce	58	140.115	Plutonium	Pu	94	244.0642*
Cesium	Cs	55	132.90543	Polonium	Po	84	208.9824*
Chlorine	Cl	17	35.4527	Potassium	K	19	39.0983
Chromium	Cr	24	51.9961	Praseodymium	Pr	59	140.90765
Cobalt	Co	27	58.93320	Promethium	Pm	61	144.9127*
Copper	Cu	29	63.546	Protactinium	Pa	91	231.0359*
Curium	Cm	96	247.0703*	Radium	Ra	88	226.0254*
Dysprosium	Dy	66	162.50	Radon	Rn	86	222.0176*
Einsteinium	Es	99	252.083*	Rhenium	Re	75	186.207
Erbium	Er	68	167.26	Rhodium	Rh	45	102.90550
Europium	Eu	63	151.965	Rubidium	Rb	37	85.4678
Fermium	Fm	100	257.0951*	Ruthenium	Ru	44	101.07
Fluorine	F	9	18.9984032	Samarium	Sm	62	150.36
Francium	Fr	87	223.0197*	Scandium	Sc	21	44.955910
Gadolinium	Gd	64	157.25	Selenium	Se	34	78.96
Gallium	Ga	31	69.723	Silicon	Si	14	28.0855
Germanium	Ge	32	72.61	Silver	Ag	47	107.8682
Gold	Au	79	196.96654	Sodium	Na	11	22.989768
Hafnium	Hf	72	178.49	Strontium	Sr	38	87.62
Helium	He	2	4.002602	Sulfur	S	16	32.066
Holmium	Ho	67	164.93032	Tantalum	Ta	73	180.9479
Hydrogen	H	1	1.00794	Technetium	Tc	43	97.9072*
Indium	In	49	114.82	Tellurim	Te	52	127.60
Iodine	I	53	126.90447	Terbium	Tb	65	158.92534
Iridium	Ir	77	192.22	Thallium	Tl	81	204.3833
Iron	Fe	26	55.947	Thorium	Th	90	232.0381
Krypton	Kr	36	83.80	Thulium	Tm	69	168.93421
Lanthanum	La	57	138.9055	Tin	Sn	50	118.710
Lawrencium	Lr	103	262.11*	Titanium	Ti	22	47.88
Lead	Pb	82	207.2	Tungsten	W	74	183.85
Lithium	Li	3	6.941	Unnilquadium	Unq	104	216.11*
Lutetium	Lu	71	174.967	Unnilpentium	Unp	105	262.114*

Element	Symbol	Atomic Number	Atomic Weight	Element	Symbol	Atomic Number	Atomic Weight
Unnihexium	Unh	106	263.118*	Ytterbium	Yb	70	173.04
Unnilseptium	Uns	107	262.12*	Yttrium	Y	39	88.90585
Uranium	U	92	238.0289	Zinc	Zn	30	65.39
Vanadium	V	23	50.9415	Zirconium	Zr	40	91.224
Xenon	Xe	54	131.29				

*Relative atomic mass of the isotope of that element with the longest known half-life.

From Budavari S, O'Neil MJ, Smith A, Heckelman PE, & Kinnear JF, eds. The Merck index: an encyclopedia of chemicals, drugs, and biologicals, 12th ed. Whitehouse Station, NJ: Merck & Co., Inc., 1996.

COMPARATIVE TEMPERATURE SCALES

Celsius °C	Fahrenheit °F	Kelvin °K

To convert Celsius or Fahrenheit to Kelvin:

C to K: add 273.16
10°C to K: $10 + 273.16 = 283.16$ K

F to K: convert to C, add 273.16
63°F = 17.2°C + $273.16 = 290.36$ K

To convert Fahrenheit to Celsius, Celsius to Fahrenheit:

Above 0°C or 32°F

F to C: subtract 32, multiply by 5, divide by 9
63°F to C: $63 - 32 = 31 \times 5 = 155 \div 9 = 17.2$°C

C to F: multiply by 9, divide by 5, add 32
37°C to F: $37 \times 9 = 333 \div 5 = 66.6 + 32 = 98.6$°F

WEIGHTS AND MEASURES

Scale of the Metric System and SI

Prefix	Symbol	Power	Multiple or Submultiple
exa-	E	10^{18}	1,000,000,000,000,000,000
peta-	P	10^{15}	1,000,000,000,000,000
tera-	T	10^{12}	1,000,000,000,000
giga	G	10^{9}	1,000,000,000
mega-	M	10^{6}	1,000,000
kilo-	k	10^{3}	1,000
hecto-	h	10^{2}	100
deca-	da	10^{1}	10
UNIT			**1**
deci-	d	10^{-1}	0.1
centi-	c	10^{-2}	0.01
milli-	m	10^{-3}	0.001
micro-	μ	10^{-6}	0.000001
nano-	n	10^{-9}	0.000000001
pico-	p	10^{-12}	0.000000000001
femto-	f	10^{-15}	0.000000000000001
atto-	a	10^{-18}	0.000000000000000001

SI Base Units

Quantity	Name	Symbol
length	meter	m
mass*	kilogram†	kg
time	second	s
electric current	ampere	A
thermodynamic temperature	kelvin‡	K
luminous intensity	candela	cd
amount of substance	mole	mol

* In commercial and everyday use, "weight" usually means mass; when speaking of a person's weight, the quantity referred to is mass.

† For historic reasons, kilogram is the only base unit with a prefix. Multiples and submultiples of the kilogram are formed by attaching the appropriate prefix to the stem word "gram" (for example, milligram) and the appropriate prefix symbol to the symbol "g" (for example, mg.).

‡ The degree Celsius (°C) is still widely accepted usage for expressing temperature and temperature intervals. Celsius (formerly centigrade) temperatture is converted to kelvin (K) thermodynamic temperature by adding 273.16 to the Celsius scale. For temperature interval, 1°C equals K.

Some SI Derived Units
Expressed in Terms of Base Units

Quantity	Name	Symbol
area	square meter	m^2
volume*	cubic meter	m^3
specific volume	cubic meter per kilogram	m^3/kg
speed, velocity	meter per second	m/s
acceleration	meter per second squared	m/s^2
mass density	kilogram per cubic meter	kg/m^3
concentration	mole per cubic meter	mol/m^3
luminance	candela per square meter	cd/m^2

*Liter (L, 1). 10^{-3} m^3, is regarded as a special name for the cubic decimeter, which is preferred for high-accuracy measurement.

Some SI Derived Units with Special Names

Quantity	Name	Symbol	Expression
frequency	hertz	Hz	s^{-1}
force	newton	N	$m\ kg\ s^{-2}$
pressure, stress	pascal	Pa	$m^{-1}\ kg\ s^{-2}$
energy	joule	J	$m^2\ kg\ s^{-2}$
power	watt	W	$m^2\ kg\ s^{-3}$
quantity of electricity, electric charge	coulomb	C	$s\ A$
electric potential, electromotive force	volt	V	$m^2\ kg\ s^{-3}\ A^{-1}$
capacitance	farad	F	$m^{-2}\ kg^{-1}s^4\ A^2$
electrical resistance	ohm	Ω	$m^2\ kg^{-2}\ A^{-2}$
electrical conductance	siemens	S	$m^{-2}\ kg\ s^{-2}\ A^{-1}$
magnetic flux	weber	Wb	$m^2\ kg\ s^{-2}\ A^{-1}$
magnetic flux density	tesla	T	$kg\ s^{-2}\ A^{-1}$
activity of radionuclide	becquerel*	Bq	s^{-1}
absorbed dose of radiation	gray†	Gy	$m^2\ s^{-2}$
exposure (x and γ radiation)	coulomb per kilogram‡	C kg	$kg^{-1}\ s\ A$

*Replacing the curie (Ci), 3.7×10^{10} s^{-1}.

†Replacing the rad (rad), 10^{-2} J kg^{-1}.

‡Replacing the roentgen (R), 2.58×10^{-4} C kg^{-1}.

Measures of Length

Micrometers	Millimeters	Centimeters	Meters	Kilometers	Miles	Yards	Feet	Inches
1	0.001	10^{-4}						0.000039
10^3	1	10^{-1}					0.00328	0.03937
10^4	10	1	0.01			0.0109	0.03281	0.3937
254,000	25.4	2.54	0.0254			0.0278	0.0833	1
	304.8	30.48	0.3048			0.333	1	12
10^6	10^3	10^2	1	0.001	0.0006213	1.0936	3.2808	39.37
914,400	914.40	91.44	0.9144	0.009	0.0005681	1	3	36
10^9	10^6	10^5	10^3	1	0.6215	1093.6121	3280.8	
			1609.0	1.609	1	1760.0	5280.0	

To convert (approximately):

Millimeters to inches: multiply by 10, divide by 254
Inches to millimeters: multiply by 254, divide by 10

Centimeters to feet: multiply by 10, divide by 305
Feet to centimeters: multiply by 305, divide by 10

Meters to yards: multiply by 70, divide by 64
Yards to meters: multiply by 64, divide by 70

Kilometers to miles: multiply by 5, divide by 8
Miles to kilometers: multiply by 8, divide by 5

Measures of Mass (Weight)

Avoirdupois Weights

Grains	Drams	Ounces	Pounds	Metric Equivalents		
				Milligrams	Grams	Kilograms
1	0.0366	0.0023	0.00014	64.8	0.0648	0.000065
27.34	1	0.0625	0.0039		1.772	0.001772
437.5	16	1	0.0625		28.350	0.028350
7,000	256	16	1		453.5924	0.453592
0.0154				1	0.001	
15.4324	0.5648	0.0353	0.002205	1000	1	0.001
15,432.358	564.32	35.27	2.2046		1000	1

To convert (approximately):

Kilograms to pounds: multiply by 1000, divide by 454
Pounds to kilograms: multiply by 454, divide by 1000

Grams to ounces: multiply by 20, divide by 567
Ounces to grams: multiply by 567, divide by 20

Apothecaries' Weights

Grains	Scruples	Drams	Ounces	Pounds	Metric Equivalents Milligrams	Grams	Kilograms
1	0.05	0.0167	0.0021	0.00017	64.8	0.0648	0.000065
20	1	0.333	0.042	0.0035		1.296	0.001296
60	3	1	0.125	0.0104		3.888	0.000389
480	24	8	1	0.0833		31.103	0.031103
5,760	288	96	12	1		373.2418	0.373242
0.0154					1	0.001	
15.4324		0.2576	0.0322	0.0027	1000	1	0.001
15,432.358		257.2	32.15	2.6792		1000	1

Measures of Capacity

Apothecaries' Measures

Minims	Fluid Drams	Fluid Ounces	Pints	Quarts	Gallons	Metric Equivalents Liters	Milliliters
1	0.0166	0.002	0.00013			0.0006	0.06161
60	1	0.125	0.0078	0.0039		0.0037	3.6967
480	8	1	0.0625	0.0312	0.0078	0.0296	29.5737
7,680	128	16	1	0.5	0.125	0.4732	473.166
15,360	256	32	2	1	0.25	0.9464	946.358
61,440	1024	128	8	4	1	3.7854	3785.434
16,230	270.52	33.8418	2.1134	1.0567	0.2642	1	1000
16.23	0.2705	0.0338	0.00212	0.00106	0.000265	0.001	1

To convert (approximately):

Liters to gallons: multiply by 264, divide by 1000
Gallons to liters: divide by 264, multiply by 1000

Liters to pints: multiply by 21, divide by 10
Pints to liters: multiply by 10, divide by 21

Approximate Household Measures and Weights*

Teaspoons	Tablespoons	Cups or Glasses	Drams	Fluid Ounces	Milliliters	Grams
1			1	0.167	5	5
3	1		4	0.50	15	15
48	16	1	64	8	237	240

*A drop is a measure of uncertain quantity, depending on the nature of the liquid as well as the shape of the container and of the opening from which the liquid falls. One drop of water is roughly equivalent to 1 minim.

RECOMMENDED DIETARY ALLOWANCES

Food and Nutrition Board, National Academy of Sciences—National Research Council Recommended Dietary Allowances,[a] Revised 1989

Designed for the maintenance of good nutrition of practically all healthy people in the United States

Category	Age (years) or Condition	Weight[b] (kg)	Weight[b] (lb)	Height[b] (cm)	Height[b] (in)	Protein (g)	Vitamin A (µg RE)[c]	Vitamin D (µg)[d]	Vitamin E (mg α-TE)[e]	Vitamin K (µg)	Vitamin C (mg)	Thiamin (mg)	Riboflavin (mg)	Niacin (mg NE)[f]	Vitamin B$_6$ (mg)	Folate (µg)	Vitamin B$_{12}$ (µg)	Calcium (mg)	Phosphorus (mg)	Magnesium (mg)	Iron (mg)	Zinc (mg)	Iodine (µg)	Selenium (µg)
Infants	0.0–0.5	6	13	60	24	13	375	7.5	3	5	30	0.3	0.4	5	0.3	25	0.3	400	300	40	6	5	40	10
	0.5–1.0	9	20	71	28	14	375	10	4	10	35	0.4	0.5	6	0.6	35	0.5	600	500	60	10	5	50	15
Children	1–3	13	29	90	35	16	400	10	6	15	40	0.7	0.8	9	1.0	50	0.7	800	800	80	10	10	70	20
	4–6	20	44	112	44	24	500	10	7	20	45	0.9	1.1	12	1.1	75	1.0	800	800	120	10	10	90	20
	7–10	28	62	132	52	28	700	10	7	30	45	1.0	1.2	13	1.4	100	1.4	800	800	170	10	10	120	30
Males	11–14	45	99	157	62	45	1,000	10	10	45	50	1.3	1.5	17	1.7	150	2.0	1,200	1,200	270	12	15	150	40
	15–18	66	145	176	69	59	1,000	10	10	65	60	1.5	1.8	20	2.0	200	2.0	1,200	1,200	400	12	15	150	50
	19–24	72	160	177	70	58	1,000	10	10	70	60	1.5	1.7	19	2.0	200	2.0	1,200	1,200	350	10	15	150	70
	25–50	79	174	176	70	63	1,000	5	10	80	60	1.5	1.7	19	2.0	200	2.0	800	800	350	10	15	150	70
	51+	77	170	173	68	63	1,000	5	10	80	60	1.2	1.4	15	2.0	200	2.0	800	800	350	10	15	150	70
Females	11–14	46	101	157	62	46	800	10	8	45	50	1.1	1.3	15	1.4	150	2.0	1,200	1,200	280	15	12	150	45
	15–18	55	120	163	64	44	800	10	8	55	60	1.1	1.3	15	1.5	180	2.0	1,200	1,200	300	15	12	150	50
	19–24	58	128	164	65	46	800	10	8	60	60	1.1	1.3	15	1.6	180	2.0	1,200	1,200	280	15	12	150	55
	25–50	63	138	163	64	50	800	5	8	65	60	1.1	1.3	15	1.6	180	2.0	800	800	280	15	12	150	55
	51+	65	143	160	63	50	800	5	8	65	60	1.0	1.2	13	1.6	180	2.0	800	800	280	10	12	150	55
Pregnant						60	800	10	10	65	70	1.5	1.6	17	2.2	400	2.2	1,200	1,200	300	30	15	175	65
Lactating	1st 6 months					65	1,300	10	12	65	95	1.6	1.8	20	2.1	280	2.6	1,200	1,200	355	15	19	200	75
	2nd 6 months					62	1,200	10	11	65	90	1.6	1.7	20	2.1	260	2.6	1,200	1,200	340	15	16	200	75

[a] The allowances, expressed as average daily intakes over time, are intended to provide for individual variations among most normal persons as they live in the United States under usual environmental stresses. Diets should be based on a variety of common foods in order to provide other nutrients for which human requirements have been less well defined. See text for detailed discussion of allowances and of nutrients not tabulated.

[b] Weights and heights of Reference Adults are actual medians for the U.S. population of the designated age, as reported by NHANES II. The median weights and heights of those under 19 years of age were taken from Hamill et al. (1979). The use of these figures does not imply that the height-to-weight ratios are ideal.

[c] Retinol equivalents. 1 retinol equivalent = 1 µg retinol or 6 µg β-carotene. See text for calculation of vitamin A activity of diets as retinol equivalents.

[d] As cholecalciferol. 10 µg cholecalciferol = 400 IU of vitamin D.

[e] α-Tocopherol equivalents. 1 mg d-α tocopherol = 1 α-TE. See text for variation in allowances as calculation of vitamin E activity of the diet as α-tocopherol equivalents.

[f] 1 NE (niacin equivalent) is equal to 1 mg of niacin or 60 mg of dietary tryptophan.

From National Academy of Sciences. Recommended dietary allowances, 10th ed. Washington DC: National Academy Press, 1989.

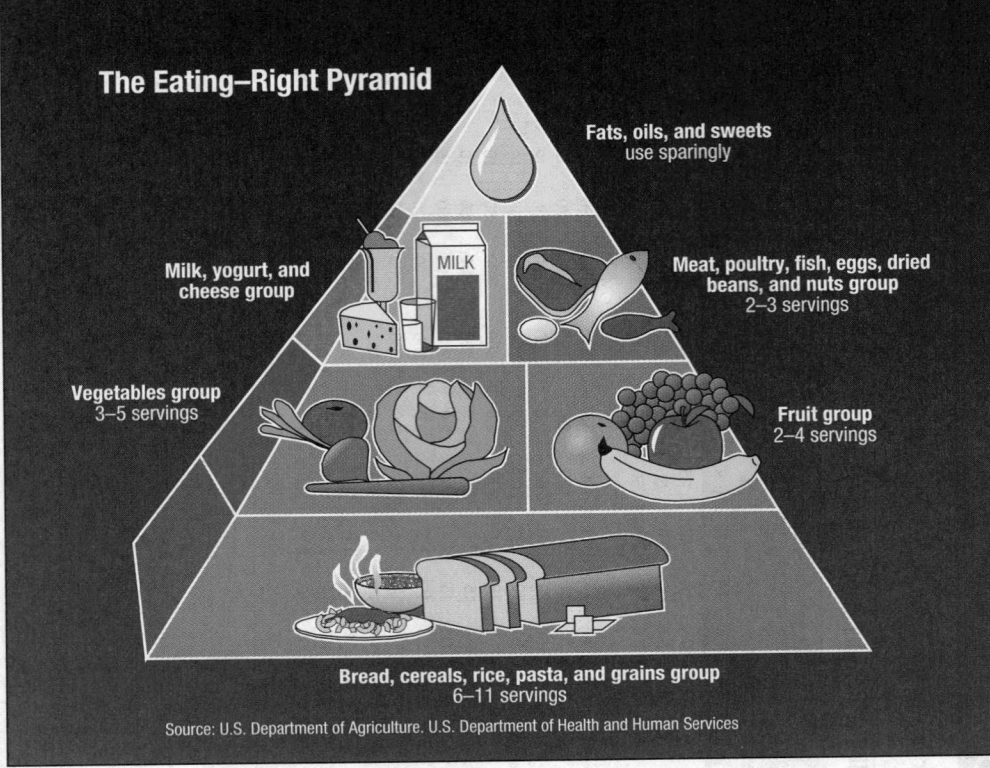

The Eating–Right Pyramid

Fats, oils, and sweets
use sparingly

MILK

Milk, yogurt, and
cheese group

Meat, poultry, fish, eggs, dried
beans, and nuts group
2–3 servings

Vegetables group
3–5 servings

Fruit group
2–4 servings

Bread, cereals, rice, pasta, and grains group
6–11 servings

Source: U.S. Department of Agriculture. U.S. Department of Health and Human Services

Milk, yogurt, and cheese	1 cup milk or yogurt	or	1-1/2 oz natural cheese	or	2 oz processed cheese
Meat, poultry, fish, eggs, dried beans, and nuts	2-3 oz cooked lean meat, poultry, or fish	or	1/2 cup cooked dried beans, or 1 egg, or 2 tbsp. peanut butter equals 1 oz lean meat		
Vegetables	1 cup raw leafy vegetables	or	1/2 cup nonleafy vegetables cooked or chopped raw	or	3/4 cup vegetable juice
Fruit	1 medium apple, banana, or orange	or	1/2 cup chopped, cooked, or canned fruit	or	3/4 cup fruit juice
Bread, cereals, rice, pasta, and grains	1 slice bread	or	1 oz ready-to-eat cereal	or	1/2 cup cooked cereal, rice, or pasta

The six food groups are depicted in the dietary pyramid. The serving-portions chart provides examples of what constitutes a serving in each group. Developed by the U.S. Department of Agriculture, these guidelines facilitate planning of a healthful daily diet.

CLINICAL DECISION ALGORITHM: ROUTE OF NUTRITION SUPPORT

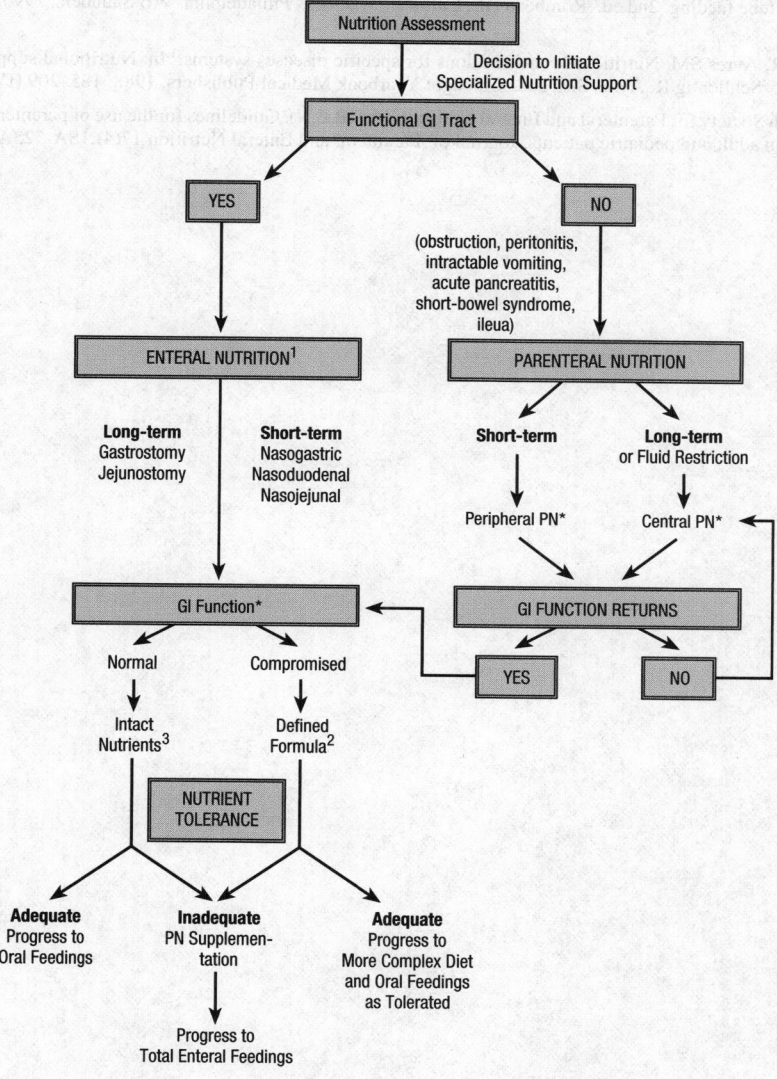

In outline form, this figure depicts the selection process for choosing the route of nutrition support in adult patients.

The major considerations for selecting the feeding route and nutrition support formula include gastrointestinal function (1,2), expected duration of nutrition therapy, aspiration risk, and the potential for—or actual development of—organ dysfunction.

GI: gastrointestinal; PN: parenteral nutrition.

*Formulation of enteral and parenteral solutions should be made considering organ function (e.g., cardiac, renal, respiratory, hepatic).

[1]Feedings may be more appropriate distal to the pylorus if the patient is at increased aspiration risk.

[2]Elemental low/high fat content, lactose-free, fiber-rich, and modular formulas should be provided according to patient's GI tolerance. See specific conditions for formula guidelines.

[3]Polymeric, complete formulas or pureed diets are appropriate.

1. Gander P, Jones S, Jacobs DO, et al. Administration and delivery of enteral nutrition. In: Clinical nutrition: Enteral and tube feeding. 2nd ed. Rombeau HL, Caldwell MD, eds. Philadelphia: WB Saunders, 1990; 192–203 (IV).

2. Schlichtig R, Ayres SM. Nutritional considerations for specific diseases systems. In: Nutritional support of the critically ill. Schlichtig R, Ayres SM, eds. Chicago: Yearbook Medical Publishers, 1988; 185–209 (IV).

From American Society for Parenteral and Enteral Nutrition (A.S.P.E.N). Guidelines for the use of parenteral and enteral nutrition in adult and pediatric patients. Journal of Parenteral and Enteral Nutrition 17(4):1SA-52SA.

HEIGHT-WEIGHT TABLES (ENGLISH-METRIC)

Men					Women				
Height		**Small Frame (lb)**	**Medium Frame (lb)**	**Large Frame (lb)**	**Height**		**Small Frame (lb)**	**Medium Frame (lb)**	**Large Frame (lb)**
Feet	Inches				Feet	Inches			
5	2	128–134	131–141	138–150	4	10	102–111	109–121	118–131
5	3	130–136	133–143	140–153	4	11	103–113	111–123	120–134
5	4	132–138	135–145	142–156	5	0	104–115	113–126	122–137
5	5	134–140	137–148	144–160	5	1	106–118	115–129	125–140
5	6	136–142	139–151	146–164	5	2	108–121	118–132	128–143
5	7	138–145	142–154	149–168	5	3	111–124	121–135	131–147
5	8	140–148	145–157	152–172	5	4	114–127	124–138	134–151
5	9	142–151	148–160	155–176	5	5	117–130	127–141	137–155
5	10	144–154	151–163	158–180	5	6	120–133	130–144	140–159
5	11	146–157	154–166	161–184	5	7	123–136	133–147	143–163
6	0	149–160	157–170	164–188	5	8	126–139	136–150	146–167
6	1	152–164	160–174	168–192	5	9	129–142	139–153	149–170
6	2	155–168	164–178	172–197	5	10	132–145	142–156	152–173
6	3	158–172	167–182	176–202	5	11	135–148	145–159	155–176
6	4	162–176	171–187	181–207	6	0	138–151	148–162	158–179

Weight according to frame (ages 25 to 59) for men wearing indoor clothing weighing 5 lb, shoes with one-inch heels; for women, indoor clothing weighing 3 lb, shoes with one-inch heels.

Men				Women			
Height (cm)	**Small Frame (kg)**	**Medium Frame (kg)**	**Large Frame (kg)**	**Height (cm)**	**Small Frame (kg)**	**Medium Frame (kg)**	**Large Frame (kg)**
157.5	58.2–60.9	59.4–64.1	62.7–68.2	147.5	46.4–50.5	49.5–55.0	53.6–59.5
160	59.1–61.8	60.5–65.0	63.6–69.5	150	46.8–51.4	50.5–55.9	54.5–60.9
162.5	60.0–62.7	61.4–65.9	64.5–70.9	152.5	47.3–52.3	51.4–57.3	55.5–62.3
165	60.9–63.7	62.3–67.3	65.5–72.7	155	48.2–53.6	52.3–58.6	56.8–63.6
167.5	61.8–64.5	63.2–68.6	66.4–74.5	157.5	49.1–55.0	53.6–60.0	58.2–65.0
170	62.7–65.9	64.5–70.0	67.7–76.4	160	50.5–56.4	55.0–61.4	59.5–66.8
173	63.6–67.3	65.9–71.4	69.1–78.2	162.5	51.8–57.7	56.4–62.7	60.9–68.6
175	64.5–68.6	67.3–72.7	70.5–80.0	165	53.2–59.1	57.7–64.1	62.3–70.5
178	65.4–70.0	68.6–74.1	71.8–81.8	167.5	54.5–60.5	59.1–65.5	63.6–72.3
180	66.4–71.4	70.0–75.5	73.2–83.6	170	55.9–61.8	60.5–66.8	65.0–74.1
183	67.7–72.7	71.4–77.3	74.5–85.6	173	57.3–63.2	61.8–68.2	66.4–75.9
185.5	69.1–74.5	72.7–79.1	76.4–87.3	175	58.6–64.5	63.2–69.5	67.7–77.3
188	70.5–76.4	74.5–80.9	78.2–89.5	178	60.0–65.9	64.5–70.9	69.1–78.6
190.5	71.8–78.2	75.9–82.7	80.0–91.8	180	61.4–67.3	65.9–72.3	70.5–80.0
193	73.6–80.0	77.7–85.0	82.3–94.1	183	62.3–68.6	67.3–73.6	71.8–81.4

*The 1983 Metropolitan Height-Weight Tables are based on the 1979 Build Study.

The values are statistical computations from individuals ranging from 25 to 59 years of weights by height and body frame at which mortality has been found to be lowest or longevity the highest. Metropolitan Life does not advocate the use of the term "ideal," which has different meanings to various individuals, because the term was used originally in their 1942 to 1943 tables. If one wishes to use these tables in the sense that they are "ideal" in terms of lowest mortality, they are "appropriate" in that context. These tables do not provide weights related to minimizing illness, optimizing job performance, or creating the best appearance.

From Statistical bulletin, New York: Metropolitan Life Insurance Company, 1983.

Factors for converting nutrients expressed in metric or milliequivalent units into International System (SI) units.

1. Definitions

a. Equivalent weight (EW) = atomic weight of element/valence of ionic form. Example with magnesium: atomic wt = 24, valence = 2+; therefore EW = 12

b. Quantity of an electrolyte in milliequivalents per liter (mEq/1) = mg of electrolyte/L/EW. Example: 48 mg of magnesium/L/12 = 4 mEq/L

c. Quantity of an electrolyte in md/dl = (mEq/L × EW)/10

d. To convert mg/dl (= mg%) of an electrolyte to mEq/L mg/dl × 10/EW = mEq/L

e. 1 mol = 1 molecular or atomic weight of element or compound in grams (GMWt). In solutions this is usually expressed as moles per liter; i.e., 1 mol/L = 1 M; 1 mM (mmol) = 1 mol × 10^{-3}; 1 μM (μmol) = 1 mol × 10^{-6}; 1 nM (nmol) = 1 mol × 10^{-9}

f. (1) To convert mEq/L of an electrolyte or other ions in solution to mmol/L: mEq/L divided by valence = mmol/L; e.g., (a) 2 mEq/L of magnesium (Mg^{2+}) = 2/2 = 1 mmol/L; e.g., (b) 140 mEq Na^+/L = 140/L = 140 mmol/L

(2) To convert mg/dl to mmol/L: (mg/dl × 10/EW) divided by valence = mmol/L; e.g., 2 mg/dl of magnesium = (2 × 10/12) divided by 2 = 0.83 mmol/L

(3) For organic substances: mmol/L = wt in mg/L/MW (in mg)

2. SI units for expressing clinical laboratory data

These units are now widely used and are increasingly required for publication of scientific data in physical, biologic, and biomedical publications. Extensive SI conversion tables have been published together with an explanation of the rationale for their use and technical aspects of usage.

Table 1. The base units of interest in physical quantities used in clinical chemistry

Quantity	Base Unit
mass	kiolgram
time	second
amount	mole
length	meter

A derived unit for energy is the kjoule (kJ) 4.18 kJ = 1 kcal
1 MJ = 239 kcal

Table 2. Prefixes and symbols for decimal multiples and submultiples

Factor	Prefix	Symbol	Factor	Prefix	Symbol
10^9	giga	G	10^{-3}	milli	m
10^6	mega	M	10^{-6}	micro	μ
10^3	kilo	k	10^{-9}	nano	n
10^2	hecto	h	10^{-12}	pico	p
10^1	deka	da	10^{-15}	femto	f
10^{-1}	deci	d	10^{-18}	atto	a
10^{-2}	centi	c			

Table 3. Conversion factors for selected compounds of nutrition interest*

Component	(1) Present Unit	(2) Conversion Factor	(3) SI Unit Symbol	(4) Mass Conversion Factor
Albumin (s)	g/dl	10	g/L	—
Aluminum (s)	μg/L	37.04	nmol/L	μg/27 = mol
Amino acid nitrogen (p)	md/dl	0.714	mmol/L	mg/14 = mmol
Ascorbic acid (p)	mg/dl	56.78	μmol/L	mg/176 = mmol
Calcium (s)	mg/dl	0.250	mmol/L	mg/40 = mmol
Calcium (s)	mEq/dl	0.500	mmol/L	mEq/2 = mmol
β-Carotene (s)	μ/dl	0.0186	μmol/L	ug/536.85 umol
Chloride (s)	mEq/L	1.00	mmol/L	mEq = mmol
Cholesterol (p)	mg/dl	0.0259	mmol/L	mg/386.6 = mmol
Copper (s)	μd/dl	0.157	μmol/L	μg/63.5 = umol
Cyanocobalamin (B_{12})	pg/ml	0.738	pmol/L	pg/1355 = pmol
Ethanol (p)	mg/dl	0.217	mmol/L	mg/46 = mmol
Folic acid	ng/ml	2.265	nmol/L	ng/441.4 = nmol
Glucose (p)	mg/dl	0.0555	mmol/L	mg/180.2 = mmol
Iron (s)	μg/dl	0.179	μmol/L	μg/55.9 = umol
Phosphate (p) (as phosphorus)	mg/dl	0.323	mmol/L	mg/31 = mmol
Potassium (s)	mEq/L	1.000	mmol/L	mEq = mmol
Potassium	mg/dl	0.256	mmol/L	mg/39.1 = mmol
Magnesium (s)	mg/dl	0.411	mmol/L	mg/24.3 = mmol
Pyridoxal (B)	ng/ml	5.981	nmol/L	ng/167 = nmol
Retinol (p,s)	μg/dl	0.0349	μmol/L	μg/286 = umol
Riboflavin (s)	μg/dl	26.57	nmol/L	μ/376 = nmol
Sodium (s)	mEq/L	1.00	mmol/L	mEq = nmol
Thiamin HCl (U)	μg/24 hr	0.00298	μmol/d	μg/337 = umol
α-Tocopherol (p)	mg/dl	23.22	μmol/L	μg/431 = umol
Vitamin D_3	μg/dl	26.01	nmol/L	μg/384 = umol
Calcidiol	ng/ml	2.498	nmol/L	ng/400 = nmol
Zinc (s)	μg/dl	0.153	μmol/L	μg/65.4 = umol

*To convert metric or equivalent unit per unit volume (column 1) to SI units per liter (column 3), multiply by the conversion factor in column 2. Column 1 abbreviations: p = plasma; s = serum; B = blood; U = urine.

From Shils ME, Olson JA, Shike M. Modern nutrition in health and disease, 8th ed. Malvern, PA: Lea & Febiger, 1994.

GLASGOW COMA SCALE

Monitored Performance	Reaction	Score
Eye Opening	Spontaneous	4
	Open when spoken to	3
	Open at pain stimulus	2
	No reaction	1
Verbal Performance	Coherent	5
	Confused, disoriented	4
	Disconnected words	3
	Unintelligible sounds	2
	No verbal reaction	1
Motor Responsiveness	Follows instructions	6
	Intentional pain-avoidance	5
	Large motor movement	4
	Flexor synergism	3
	Extensor synergism	2
	No reaction	1

APPENDICES

John Moulds, MT(ASCP) SBP

In this appendix, and in the related terms defined in the dictionary proper, *blood group* is used to refer to an entire blood group system consisting of heritable antigens whose specificity is controlled by a series of allelic genes. Most blood components, i.e., erythrocytes, leukocytes, platelets, or plasma protein, possess heritable antigens that have been identified as belonging to systems. Traditionally, blood group is used predominantly in reference to erythrocyte antigens. The terms *blood type* and *phenotype* are used to refer to a specific reaction pattern to testing antisera within a system. The term *blood group factor* is used to refer to a specific antigen within a system. This usage is not universal. It should be noted that in current literature, a single system may be referred to in the plural (i.e., ABO blood groups), and the term *blood group* may be assigned to a single phenotype (i.e., blood group A).

Each blood group is defined in terms of reaction to the original antisera with which the system was discovered, with modification or extension as required by the discovery of additional antisera proven to be related to the same system. A new blood group antigen or factor can be defined by showing that it is detected by an antiserum with reactions different from those of previously known antisera. If it is shown that the new antigen is genetically independent of known blood group systems, it may qualify as a prototype antigen for a new blood group. Alternatively, if it can be shown that the new antigen is controlled by a gene allelic to one of the known blood group genes, it is assigned to the blood group system of its alleles.

In the blood group definitions, emphasis has been placed on identification of symbols for genes, antigens, antisera, and phenotypes. These often appear in the literature without specification that they refer to a blood group. Attention is called to the general convention, followed here, that symbols for genes and genotypes are set in italics, whereas symbols for gene products or antigens, antisera, and phenotypes are set in roman type. In the Rh-Hr terminology for the Rh blood group, roman type is used to designate antigen substances, and boldface type is used to designate serological factors and their corresponding antibodies. These are in wide use but are not consistently followed by all authors.

Nomenclature

The designation of blood group systems and antigens has been based upon alphabetical assignment of names or initials of first antibody producer, reactive or nonreactive red cell source or derivation of name, location, or discovering institution. The International Society of Blood Transfusion (ISBT) developed a Working Party on Terminology of Red Cell Surface Antigens to establish a uniform nomenclature, while not modifying historical designations and guidelines. Part of the Working Party's charge is to review periodically the available data and report additions, alterations, or deletions to those blood group antigens considered extinct. In addition, the Working Party developed a nomenclature coding system, based on order of discovery of the blood group systems, to aid in the computerization of data. Reports of the Working Party are published in *Vox Sanguinis* (1990; 58:152–169, 1993; 65:77–80).

Currently, there are 22 blood group systems. Each system is serologically, immunochemically, and genetically proven to be the product of distinct independent genes. The Rh system has 47 separate antigens, while others (i.e., P, Xg, Hh, and Kx systems) have only one antigen associated with them. Table 1 lists the approved system names, abbreviated symbol, and numerical designation developed by the ISBT. For clinical considerations, the ABO and Rh are of most importance; others are useful for genetic linkage or red cell membrane protein studies.

In addition to the defined blood group systems, there are other blood group antigens that fail, as of yet, to fit the system criteria. Some are loosely associated by serological and immunochemical reactivity, but insufficient data exist to classify them as a system. Hence they are referred to as *collections* (Table 2).

A second set of antigens occurring with a high incidence in the random population are collectively referred to as *high incidence* or *public* antigens. These occur in almost all individuals but are absent in a few. The antibodies usually have been found in the serum of patients lacking the antigen who have become immunized by transfusion or pregnancy. There are 11 distinct high incidence antigens, and some of the symbols applied to public antigens include: Vel, Lan, At[a], Jr[a] and JMH.

The third set of erythrocyte antigens, each defined by a specific antiserum, are uncommon, and each is found only in members of a very few families. Because of their rarity, they are often referred to as *low incidence* or *private* antigens. The antibodies usually have been found in the serum of patients who have received transfusions or in mothers of infants with hemolytic disease of the newborn (HDN). They are often named for the family in which they were first discovered. There are 36 distinct low incidence antigens, and some symbols assigned to the private antigens are: By, Sw[a], Bi[a], Hey, NFLD, RAS, HJK and ELO.

Table 1. Designation of Blood Group Systems

System Name	Symbol	System No.	No. Antigens	System Name	Symbol	System No.	No. Antigens
ABO	ABO	001	4	Xg	XG	012	1
MNS	MNS	002	37	Scianna	SC	013	3
P	P1	003	1	Dombrock	DO	014	5
Rh	RH	004	47	Colton	CO	015	3
Lutheran	LU	005	18	Landsteiner-Weiner	LW	016	3
Kell	KEL	006	21	Chido/Rogers	CH/RG	017	9
Lewis	LE	007	3	Hh	H	018	1
Duffy	FY	008	6	Kx	XK	019	1
Kidd	JK	009	3	Gerbich	GE	020	7
Diego	DI	010	2	Cromer	CR	021	10
Yt	YT	011	2	Knops	KN	022	5

Table 2. Designations of Collections

Collection Name	Symbol	No.	No. of Associated Antigens
Indian	IN	203	2
Cost	COST	205	2
Ii	I	207	2
Er	ER	208	2
		209	3
		210	2
Wright	WR	211	2

Show-Hong Duh, Ph.D., D.A.B.C.C. / Gladys Alonsozana, M.D.

Reference range values are for apparently healthy individuals and often overlap significantly with values for persons who are sick. Actual values may vary significantly due to differences in assay methodologies and standardization. Institutions may also set up their own reference ranges based on the particular populations that they serve; thus there can be regional differences. Consequently, values reported by individual laboratories may differ from those listed in this appendix.

All values are given in conventional and SI units. However, where the SI units have not been widely accepted, conventional units are used. In case of the heterogenous nature of the materials measured or uncertainty of the exact molecular weight of the compounds, the SI system cannot be followed, and mass per volume is used as the unit of concentration.

ABBREVIATIONS

ACD, acid-citrate-dextrose; **CHF**, congestive heart failure; **Cit**, citrate; **CNS**, central nervous system; **CSF**, cerebrospinal fluid; **cyclic AMP**, adenosine 3': 5'- cyclic phosphate; **EDTA**, ethylenediaminetetraacetic acid; **HDL**, high-density lipoprotein; **Hep**, heparin; **LDL-C**, low-density lipoprotein-cholesterol; **Ox**, oxalate; **RBC**, red blood cell(s); **RIA**, radioimmunoassay; **SD**, standard deviation

REFERENCES

Reference Intervals. In: Tietz Textbook of Clinical Chemistry. 2nd ed. Burtis CA, Ashwood ER, eds. Philadelphia: WB Saunders, 1994.

Hematologic Values. In: Clinical Hematology and Fundamentals of Hemostasis. 2nd ed. Harmening DM, ed. Philadelphia: FA Davis, 1992.

National Cholesterol Education Program. Report of the expert panel on detection, evaluation, and treatment of high blood cholesterol in adults. Arch Intern Med 1988;148:36-69.

Department of Pathology. Clinical Chemistry Laboratory: Reference Range Values in Clinical Chemistry. Professional services manual. Baltimore: University of Maryland Medical System, 1993.

Triglyceride, High Density Lipoprotein, and Coronary Heart Disease. National Institutes of Health Consensus Statement, NIH Consensus Development Conference, 1992;10 (2).

Tests	Conventional Units	SI Units
Acetaminophen, serum or plasma (Hep or EDTA)		
Therapeutic	10–30 μg/mL 66–199 μmol/L	
Toxic	>200 μg/mL	>1324 μmol/L
Acetone		
Serum		
Qualitative	Negative	Negative
Quantitative	0.3–2.0 mg/dL	3–20 mg/L
Urine		
Qualitative	Negative	Negative
N-Acetylprocainamide, serum or plasma (Hep or EDTA); trough		
Therapeutic	5–30 μg/mL	18–108 μmol/L
Toxic	>40 μg/mL	>144 μmol/L
Acid hemolysis test (Ham)	No hemolysis	No hemolysis
Adrenocorticotropin (ACTH), plasma		
6 AM	10–80 pg/mL	10–80 ng/L
6 PM	<50 pg/mL	<50 ng/L
Alanine aminotransferase (see Transaminase)		
Albumin		
Serum		
Adult	3.5–5.0 g/dL	35–50 g/L
>60 y	3.4–4.8 g/dL	34–48 g/L
	Avg. of 0.3 g/dL higher in upright individuals	Avg. of 3 g/L higher in upright individuals
Urine		
Qualitative	Negative	Negative
Quantitative	10–100 mg/24 h	10–100 mg/24 h
CSF	10–30 mg/dL	100–300 mg/L
*Aldolase, serum	0–11 U/L (30°C)	Same
Aldosterone		
Serum		
Supine	3–10 ng/dL	0.08–0.3 nmol/L
Standing		
Male	6–22 ng/dL	0.17–0.61 nmol/L
Female	5–30 ng/dL	0.14–0.8 nmol/L
Urine	3–20 μg/24 h	8.3–55 nmol/24 h
Alpha amino nitrogen		
Serum	3.0–5.5 mg/dL	2.1–3.9 mmol/L
Urine	50–200 mg/24 h	3.6–14.3 nmol/24 h
Amikacin, serum or plasma (EDTA)		
Therapeutic		
Peak	25–35 μg/mL	43–60 μmol/L
Trough		
Less severe infection	1–4 μg/mL	1.7–6.8 μmol/L
Life-threatening infection	4–8 μg/mL	6.8–13.7 μmol/L
Toxic		
Peak	>35–40 μg/mL	>60–68 μmol/L
Trough	>10–15 μg/mL	>17–26 μmol/L
δ-Aminolevulinic acid, urine	1.3–7.0 mg/24 h	10–53 μmol/24 h
Amitriptyline, serum or plasma (Hep or EDTA); trough (≥12 h after dose)		

*Test values are method dependent.

APPENDICES

Tests	Conventional Units		SI Units	
Therapeutic	120–250 ng/mL		433–903 nmol/L	
Toxic	>500 ng/mL		>1805 nmol/L	
Ammonia nitrogen				
Plasma	15–45 µg/dL		11–32 µmol/L	
Urine	140–1500 mg/d		10–107 mmol/d	
*Amylase				
Serum	25–125 mIU/mL		25–125 U/L	
Urine	1–17 U/h		Same	
Amylase/creatinine clearance ratio	1–4%		0.01–0.04	
Anion gap	8–16 mEq/L		8–16 mmol/L	
Arsenic				
Whole blood (Hep)	0.2–6.2 µg/dL		0.03–0.83 µmol/L	
Chronic poisoning	10–50 µg/dL		1.33–6.65 µmol/L	
Acute poisoning	60–930 µg/dL		7.98–124 µmol/L	
Urine, 24 h	5–50 µg/d		0.07–0.67 µmol/d	
Ascorbic acid, blood	0.4–1.5 mg/dL		23–85 µmol/L	
Aspartate aminotransferase (see Transaminase)				
Base excess, blood	0 ± 2 mEq/L		0 ± 2 mmol/L	
Bicarbonate, serum	23–29 mEq/L		23–29 mmol/L	
Bile acids, serum	0.3–3.0 mg/dL		3.0–30.0 mg/L	
*Bilirubin				
Serum				
Adults				
Conjugated	0.0–0.3 mg/dL		0–5 µmol/L	
Unconjugated	0.01–1.1mg/dL		0–19 µmol/L	
Delta	0–0.2 mg/dL		0–3 µmol/L	
Total	0.2–1.3 mg/L		3–22 µmol/L	
Neonates				
Conjugated	0–0.6 mg/dL		0–10 µmol/L	
Unconjugated	0.6–10.5 mg/dL		10–180 µmol/L	
Total	1.0–10.5 mg/dL		1.7–180 µmol/L	
Urine, qualitative	Negative		Negative	
Bone marrow, differential cell count	Range (%)	Average (%)	Range	Average
Myeloblasts	0.3–5.0	2.0	0.003–0.05	0.02
Promyelocytes	1.0–8.0	5.0	0.01–0.08	0.05
Myelocytes				
Neutrophilic	5.0–19.0	12.0	0.05–0.19	0.12
Eosinophilic	0.5–3.0	1.5	0.005–0.03	0.015
Basophilic	0.0–0.5	0.3	0.00–0.005	0.003
Metamyelocytes	13.0–32.0	22.0	0.13–0.32	0.22
Polymorphonuclear neutrophils	7.0–30.0	20.0	0.07–0.30	0.20
Polymorphonuclear eosinophils	0.5–4.0	2.0	0.005–0.04	0.02
Polymorphonuclear basophils	0.0–0.7	0.2	0.00–0.007	0.002
Lymphocytes	3.0–17.0	10.0	0.03–0.17	0.10
Plasma cells	0.0–2.0	0.4	0.00–0.02	0.004
Monocytes	0.5–5.0	2.0	0.005–0.05	0.02
Reticulum cells	0.1–2.0	0.2	0.001–0.02	0.002
Megakaryocytes	0.3–3.0	0.4	0.003–0.03	0.004
Pronormoblasts	1.0–8.0	4.0	0.01–0.08	0.04
Normoblasts	7.0–32.0	18.0	0.07–0.32	0.18

*Test values are method dependent.

Tests	Conventional Units	SI Units
Cadmium, whole blood (Hep)	0.1–0.5 µg/dL	0.89–4.45 nmol/L
Toxic	10–300 µg/dL	0.89–26.70 µmol/L
Cadmium, urine, 24 h	<15 µg/d	<0.13 µmol/d
Calcium, serum	8.4–10.2 mg/dL	2.1–2.6 mmol/L
	(Slightly higher in children)	(Slightly higher in children)
Calcium, ionized, serum	4.65–5.28 mg/dL	1.16–1.32 mmol/L
Calcium, urine		
Low-calcium diet	<150 mg/24 h	<3.8 nmol/24 h
Usual diet; trough	<250 mg/24 h	<6.3 nmol/24 h
Carbamazepine, serum or plasma (Hep or EDTA)		
Therapeutic	8–12 µg/mL	34–51 µmol/L
Toxic	>15 µg/mL	>63 µmol/L
Carbon dioxide, total, serum/ plasma (Hep)	22–29 mmol/L (lower in children)	Same
Carbon dioxide tension (Pco₂), blood	35–45mm Hg	35–45 mm Hg
Carbon monoxide as carboxyhemoglobin (HbCO), whole blood (EDTA)		
Nonsmokers	0.5–1.5% total Hb	0.005–0.015 HbCO fraction
Smokers		
1–2 packs/d	4–5% total Hb	0.04–0.05 HbCO fraction
>2 packs/d	8–9% total Hb	0.08–0.09 HbCO fraction
Toxic	>20% total Hb	>0.20 HbCO fraction
Lethal	>50% total Hb	>0.5 HbCO fraction
Carotene, serum	40–200 µg/dL	0.74–3.72 µmol/L
*Catecholamines, urine		
Epinephrine	<10 µg/24 h	<55 nmol/24 h
Norepinephrine	<100 µg/24 h	<590 nmol/24 h
Total free catecholamines	4–126 µg/24 h	24–745 nmol/24 h (as norepinephrine)
Total metanephrines	0.1–1.6 mg/24 h	0.5–8.1 µmol/24 h (as metanephrine)

Cell counts (Coulter)	Percentage	Absolute	
Erythrocytes			
Males	4.7–6.1 × 10⁶/µL		4.7–6.1 × 10¹²/L
Females	4.2–5.4 × 10⁶/µL		4.2–5.4 × 10¹²/L
Children (varies with age)	3.8–5.5 × 10⁶/µL		3.8–5.5 × 10¹²/L
Leukocytes			
Total	4.8–10.8 × 10³/µL		4.8–10.8 × 10⁹/L
Differential	*Percentage*	*Absolute*	
Myelocytes	0	0/µL	0/L
Band neutrophils	3–5	150–400/µL	150–400 × 10⁶/L
Segmented neutrophils	54–62	3000–5800/µL	3000–5800 × 10⁶/L
Lymphocytes	25–33	1500–3000/µL	1500–3000 × 10⁶/L
Monocytes	3–7	300–500/µL	300–500 × 10⁶/L
Eosinophils	1–3	50–250/µL	50–250 × 10⁶/L
Basophils	0–0.75	15–50/µL	15–50 × 10⁶/L
Platelets	150–450 × 10³/µL	150–450 × 10⁹/L	
Reticulocytes	25,000–75,000/µL	25–75 × 10⁹/L	
	0.5–1.5% of erythrocytes		
Cells, CSF	<5/µL (all mononucleocytes)		Same

*Test values are method dependent.

Tests	Conventional Units	SI Units
*Ceruloplasmin, serum	23–44 mg/dL	230–440 mg/L
Chloramphenicol, serum or plasma (Hep or EDTA); trough		
Therapeutic	10–25 µg/mL	31–77 µmol/L
Toxic	>25 µg/mL	>77 µmol/L
Chloride		
Serum	96–106 mmol/L	Same
Sweat		
Normal	0–30 mmol/L	Same
Cystic fibrosis	60–200 mmol/L	Same
Urine, 24 h (vary greatly with Cl intake)		
Infant	2–10 mmol/d	Same
Child	14–50 mmol/d	Same
Adults	110–250 mmol/d	Same
CSF	120–130 mmol/L (20 mmol/L higher than serum)	Same
Cholesterol, serum	Recommended desirable range: <200 mg/dL	Recommended desirable range: <5.2 mmol/L
	Borderline range: 200–239 mg/dL	Borderline range: 5.2–6.2 mmol/L
Cholinesterase		
Serum	0.5–1.3 pH units	0.5–1.3 pH units
Erythrocytes	0.5–1.0 pH unit	0.5–1.0 pH unit
*Chorionic gonadotropin, β-subunit (β-hCG)		
Serum or plasma (EDTA)		
Male and nonpregnant female	<3.0 IU/L	Same
Female, postconception		
7-10 d	>3.0 IU/L	Same
30 d	100–5000 IU/L	Same
40 d	>2000 IU/L	Same
10 wk	50,000–140,000 IU/L	Same
14 wk	10,000–50,000 IU/L	Same
Trophoblastic disease	>100,000 IU/L	Same
Urine, 24 h		
Male and nonpregnant female	0 IU/d	Same
Pregnancy (wk)		
6th	13,000 U/d (mean)	Same
8th	30,000 U/d (mean)	Same
12–14th	105,000 U/d (mean)	Same
16th	46,000 U/d (mean)	Same
Thereafter	5,000–20,000 U/d (mean)	Same
Clonazepam, serum or plasma (Hep or EDTA); trough		
Therapeutic	15–60 ng/mL	48–190 nmol/L
Toxic	>80 ng/mL	>254 nmol/L
Coagulation tests		
Antithrombin III (synthetic substrate)	80–120% of normal	0.8–1.2 of normal
Bleeding time (Duke)	0–6 min	0–6 min
Bleeding time (Ivy)	1–6 min	1–6 min
Bleeding time (template)	2.3–9.5 min	2.3–9.5 min
Clot retraction, qualitative	Begins in 30–60 min Complete in 24 h	Begins in 30–60 min Complete in 24 h

*Test values are method dependent.

Tests	Conventional Units	SI Units
Coagulation time (Lee-White)	5–15 min (glass tubes) 19–60 min (siliconized tubes)	5–15 min (glass tubes) 19–60 min (siliconized tubes)
Cold hemolysin test (Donath-Landsteiner)	No hemolysis	No hemolysis
Complement components		
Total hemolytic complement activity, plasma (EDTA)	75–160 U/mL or >33% of plasma CH50	75–160 kU/L Fraction of CH50 : >0.33
Total complement decay rate (functional), plasma (EDTA)	10–20% Deficiency: >50%	Fraction decay rate: 0.10–0.20 >0.50
$C1_q$, serum	5.1–7.9 mg/dL	51–79 mg/L
$C1_r$, serum	2.2–4.6 mg/dL	22–46 mg/L
$C1_s$(C1 esterase), serum	2.1–4.1 mg/dL	21–41 mg/L
C2, serum	1.9–2.5 mg/dL	19–25 mg/L
C3, serum	83–177 mg/dL	830–1770 mg/L
C4, serum	12–36 mg/dL	120–360 mg/L
C5, serum	3.8–9.0 mg/dL	38–90 mg/L
C6, serum	4.0–7.2 mg/dL	40–72 mg/L
C7, serum	4.9–7.0 mg/dL	49–70 mg/L
C8, serum	4.3–6.3 mg/dL	43–63 mg/L
C9, serum	4.7–6.9 mg/dL	47–69 mg/L
Coombs' test		
Direct	Negative	Negative
Indirect	Negative	Negative
Copper		
Serum		
Males	70–140 µg/dL	11–22 µmol/L
Females	85–155 µg/dL	13–24 µmol/L
Urine	0–50 µg/24 h	0–0.80 µmol/24 h
Corpuscular values of erythrocytes (values are for adults; in children, values vary with age)		
Mean corpuscular hemoglobin (MCH)	27–31 pg	0.42–0.48 fmol
Mean corpuscular hemoglobin concentration (MCHC)	33–37 g/dL	330–370 g/L
Mean corpuscular volume (MCV)	80-96 µ³ 80-96 fL	
Cortisol		
Plasma		
8 AM	5–23 µg/dL	138–635 nmol/L
4 PM	3–16 µg/dL	82–441 nmol/L
10 PM	<50% of 8 AM value	<0.5 of 8 AM value
Free, urine	10–100 µg/24 h	27.6–276 mmol/24 h
Creatine		
Serum	0.2–0.8 mg/dL	15–61 µmol/L
Urine		
Males	0–40 mg/24 h	0–0.30 mmol/24 h
Females	0–100 mg/24 h (Higher in children and pregnant women)	0– 0.76 mmol/24 h (Higher in children and pregnant women)
*†Creatine kinase, serum (CK, CPK)		
White		
Male	60–320 U/L (37°C)	Same

*Test values are method dependent.
†Test values are race dependent.

Tests	Conventional Units	SI Units
Female	50–200 U/L (37°C)	Same
Black		
Male	130–450 U/L (37°C)	Same
Female	60–270 U/L (37°C)	Same
*Creatine kinase MB isoenzyme, serum	0–5 ng/mL	Same
*Creatinine enzymatic		
Serum or plasma, adult		
Male	0.7–1.3 mg/dL	62–115 µmol/L
Female	0.6–1.1 mg/dL	53–97 µmol/L
Urine		
Male	14–26 mg/kg body weight/24 h	0.12–0.23 mmol/kg body weight/24h
Female	11–20 mg/kg body weight/24 h	0.10–0.18 mmol/kg body weight/24 h
*Creatinine clearance, enzymatic		
Males	90–139 mL/min/1.73 m²	0.87–1.34 mL/s/m²
Females	80–125 mL/min/1.73 m²	0.77–1.2 mL/s/m²
Cryoglobulins, serum	0	0
Cyanide		
Serum		
Nonsmokers	0.004 mg/L	0.15 µmol/L
Smokers	0.006 mg/L	0.23 µmol/L
Nitroprusside therapy	0.01–0.06 mg/L	0.38–2.30 µmol/L
Toxic	>0.1 mg/L	>3.84 µmol/L
Whole blood (Ox)		
Nonsmokers	0.016 mg/L	0.61 µmol/L
Smokers	0.041 mg/L	1.57 µmol/L
Nitroprusside therapy	0.05–0.5 mg/L	1.92–19.20 µmol/L
Toxic	>1 mg/L	>38.40 µmol/L
Cyclic AMP		
Plasma (EDTA)		
Males	4.6–8.6 ng/mL	14–26 nmol/L
Females	4.3–7.6 ng/mL	13–23 nmol/L
Urine, 24 h	0.3–3.6 mg/d or 0.29–2.1 mg/g creatinine	1.0–10.9 µmol/d or 100–723 µmol/mol creatinine
Cystine or cysteine, urine, qualitative	Negative	Negative
*C-Peptide, serum	0.78–1.89 ng/mL	0.26–0.62 nmol/L
*C-Reactive protein, serum		
Cord blood	1–35 µg/dL 10–350 µg/L	
Adult	6.8–820 µg/dL	68–8200 µg/L
*≠Cyclosporine, whole blood		
Therapeutic, trough	100–200 ng/mL	83–166 nmol/L
Dehydroepiandrosterone, urine	<15% of total 17–ketosteroids	<15% of total 17–ketosteroids
Males	0.2–2.0 mg/24 h	0.7–6.9 µmol/24 h
Females	0.2–1.8 mg/24 h	0.7–6.2 µmol/24 h
Desipramine, serum or plasma (Hep or EDTA); trough (12 h after dose)		
Therapeutic	75–300 ng/mL	281–1125 nmol/L
Toxic	>400 ng/mL	>1500 nmol/L
Diazepam, serum or plasma (Hep or EDTA); trough		
Therapeutic	100–1000 ng/mL	0.35–3.51 µmol/L

*Test values are method dependent.
≠Actual therapeutic range should be adjusted for individual patient.

Tests	Conventional Units	SI Units
Toxic	>5000 ng/mL	>17.55 µmol/L
Digitoxin, serum or plasma (Hep or EDTA); 6 h after dose		
Therapeutic	20–35 ng/mL	26–46 nmol/L
Toxic	>45 ng/mL	>59 nmol/L
Digoxin, serum or plasma (Hep or EDTA); 12 h after dose		
Therapeutic		
CHF	0.8–1.5 ng/mL	1.0–1.9 nmol/L
Arrhythmias	1.5–2.0 ng/mL	1.9–2.6 nmol/L
Toxic		
Adult	>2.5 ng/mL	>3.2 nmol/L
Child	>3.0 ng/mL	>3.8 nmol/L
Disopyramide, serum or plasma (Hep or EDTA); trough		
Therapeutic arrhythmias		
Atrial	2.8–3.2 µg/mL	8.3–9.4 µmol/L
Ventricular	3.3–7.5 µg/mL	9.7–22 µmol/L
Toxic	>7 µg/mL >20.7 µmol/L	
Doxepin, serum or plasma (Hep or EDTA); trough (≥ 12 h after dose)		
Therapeutic	30–150 ng/mL	107–537 nmol/L
Toxic	>500 ng/mL	>1790 nmol/L
Electrophoresis, CSF	Predominantly albumin	Predominantly albumin
Estrogens, urine		
Males		
Estrone	3–8 µg/24 h	11–30 nmol/24 h
Estradiol	0–6 µg/24 h	0–22 nmol/24 h
Estriol	1–11 µg/24 h	3–38 nmol/24 h
‡Total	4–25 µg/24 h	14–90 nmol/24 h
Females		
Estrone	4–31 µg/24 h	15–115 nmol/24 h
Estradiol	0–14 µg/24 h	0–51 nmol/24 h
Estriol	0–72 µg/24 h	0–250 nmol/24 h
‡Total	5–100 µg/24 h	18–360 nmol/24 h
	(Markedly increased during pregnancy)	(Markedly increased during pregnancy)
Ethanol, whole blood (Ox) or serum		
Depression of CNS	>100 mg/dL	>21.7 mmol/L
Fatalities reported	>400 mg/dL	>86.8 mmol/L
Ethosuximide, serum or plasma (Hep or EDTA); trough		
Therapeutic	40–100 µg/mL	283–708 µmol/L
Toxic	>150 µg/mL	>1062 µmol/L
Euglobulin lysis time	2–6 h at 37°C	2–6 h at 37°C
Factor VIII and other coagulation factors	70–150% of normal	0.70–1.5 of normal
Fibrin split products (Thrombo–Wellco test)	<10 µg/mL	<10mg/L
Fibrinogen	200–400 mg/dL	5.9–11.7 µmol/L

‡Assuming a mixture of estrone, estradioles, and estriol in a molecular proportion of 2:1:2.

APPENDICES

Tests	Conventional Units	SI Units
Fibrinolysins	0	Same
Partial thromboplastin time, activated (APTT)	20–35 sec	Same
Prothrombin consumption	Over 80% consumed in 1 h	Over 0.80 consumed in 1 h
Prothrombin content	100% (calculated from prothrombin time)	1.0 (calculated from prothrombin time)
Prothrombin time (one stage)	12.0–14.0 sec	Same
Tourniquet test	Ten or fewer petechiae in a 2.5 cm circle after 5 min	Same
Fat, fecal, F, 72 h		
Infant, breast–fed	<1 g/d	Same
0–6 y	<2 g/d	Same
Adult	<7 g/d	Same
Adult (fat–free diet)	<4 g/d	Same
§Fatty acids, total, serum	190–420 mg/dL	7–15 mmol/L
Nonesterified, serum	8–25 mg/dL	0.30–0.90 mmol/L
Ferritin, serum		
Males	20–250 ng/mL	20–250 µg/L
Females	10–120 ng/mL (higher if postmenopausal)	10–120 µg/L (higher if postmenopausal)
Ferritin values of <20 ng/mL (20 µg/L) have been reported to be generally associated with depleted iron stores		
Fibrinogen, plasma	200–400 mg/dL	5.9–11.7 µmol/L
Fluoride		
Plasma (Hep)	0.01–0.2 µg/mL	0.5–10.5 µmol/L
Urine	0.2–1.1 µg/mL	10.5–57.9 µmol/L
Urine, occupational exposure	<8 µg/mL	<421 µmol/L
Folate, serum	2.2–17.3 ng/mL	5.0–39.2 nmol/L
Erythrocytes	169–707 ng/mL	451–1602 nmol/L
*Follicle-stimulating hormone (FSH), serum		
Males	2.0–17.7 mIU/mL	2.0–17.7 IU/L
Females		
Follicular phase	3.6–16.0 mIU/mL	Same
Midcycle peak	8.1–28.9 mIU/mL	Same
Luteal phase	1.8–11.7 mIU/mL	Same
Postmenopause	22.9–167 mIU/mL	Same
Gastrin, serum		
Males	<100 pg/mL	<100 ng/L
Females	<75 pg/mL	<75 ng/L
Gentamicin, serum or plasma (EDTA)		
Therapeutic		
Peak		
Less severe infection	5–8 µg/mL	10.4–16.7 µmol/L
Severe infection	8–10 µg/mL	16.7–20.9 µmol/L
Trough		
Less severe infection	<1 µg/mL	<2.1 µmol/L
Moderate infection	<2 µg/mL	<4.2 µmol/L
Severe infection	<2–4 µg/mL	<4.2–8.4 µmol/L
Toxic		
Peak	>10–12 µg/mL	>21–25 µmol/L
Trough	>2–4 µg/mL	>4.2–8.4 µmol/L

*Test values are method dependent.

§"Fatty acids" include a mixture of different aliphatic acids of varying molecular weight; a mean molecular weight of 284 daltons has been assumed.

Tests	Conventional Units	SI Units
Glucose (fasting)		
Blood	60–100 mg/dL	3.33–5.55 mmol/L
Plasma or serum	70–115 mg/dL	3.89–6.38 mmol/L
Glucose, 2 h postprandial, serum	<120 mg/dL	<6.7 mmol/L
Glucose, urine		
Quantitative	<500 mg/24 h	<2.8 mmol/24 h
Qualitative	Negative	Negative
Glucose, CSF	50–75 mg/dL (20 mg/dL less than serum)	2.8–4.2 mmol/L (1.1 mmol/L less than serum)
*Glucose-6-phosphate dehydrogenase (G-6-PD) in erythrocytes, whole blood (ACD, EDTA, or Hep)	12.1 ± 2.1 U/g Hb (SD) 351 ± 60.6 U/10^{12} RBC	0.78 ± 0.13 mU/mol Hb 0.35 ± 0.06 nU/RBC
	4.11 ± 0.71 U/mL RBC	4.11 ± 0.71 kU/L RBC
*γ-Glutamyltransferase		
Males	≤50 U/L (37°C)	Same
Females	≤30 U/L (37°C)	Same
Glutethimide, serum		
Therapeutic	2–6 µg/mL	9–28 µmol/L
Toxic	>5 µg/mL	>23 µmol/L
Growth hormone, serum	0–10 ng/mL	0–10 µg/L
Haptoglobin, serum	26–185 mg/dL	260–1850 mg/L
Haptoglobin (as hemoglobin binding capacity)	40–336 mg/dL	0.4–36 g/L
HDL-cholesterol (HDL-C), serum or plasma (EDTA)	Recommended desirable range: >40 mg/dL	Recommended desirable range: >1.04 mmol/L
Borderline: 35–40 mg/dL		
Hematocrit		
Males	42–52%	0.42–0.52
Females	37–47%	0.37–0.47
Newborns	53–65%	0.53–0.65
Children (varies with age)	30–43%	0.30–0.43
Hemoglobin (Hb)		
Males	14.0–18.0 g/dL	2.17–2.79 mmol/L
Females	12.0–16.0 g/dL	1.86–2.48 mmol/L
Newborns	17.0–23.0 g/dL	2.64–3.57 mmol/L
Children (varies with age)	11.2–16.5 g/dL	1.74–2.56 mmol/L
Hemoglobin, fetal	≥1 y old: < 2% of total Hb	≥1 y old: < 2% of total Hb
Hemoglobin, plasma	0–5.0 mg/dL	0–0.8 µmol/L
Hemoglobin and myoglobin, urine, qualitative	Negative	Negative
Hemoglobin electrophoresis, whole blood (EDTA, Cit or Hep)		
HbA	96–98.6%	0.96–0.986 Hb fraction
HbA$_{1c}$	5.3–7.5%	0.053–0.075 Hb fraction
HbA$_2$	1.5–3.5%	0.015–0.035 Hb fraction
HbF	<2%	<0.02 Hb fraction
Homogentisic acid, urine, qualitative	Negative	Negative
*Hydroxybutyric dehydrogenase serum (HBD)	0–180 mU/mL (30°C)	0–180 U/L (30°C)
17-Hydroxycorticosteroids		
Plasma	8–18 µg/dL	0.22–0.50 µmol/L

*Test values are method dependent.

Tests	Conventional Units	SI Units
Urine		
Males	3–9 mg/24 h	8.3–25 μmol/24 h (as cortisol)
Females	2–8 mg/24 h	5.5–22 μmol/24 h (as cortisol)
5-Hydroxyindoleacetic acid, urine		
Qualitative	Negative	Negative
Quantitative	2–6 mg/24 h	10.4–31.2 μmol/24 h
Imipramine, serum or plasma (Hep or EDTA); trough (≥12 h after dose)		
Therapeutic	125–250 ng/mL	446–893 nmol/L
Toxic	>500 ng/mL	>1785 nmol/L
*Immunoglobulins, serum		
IgG	723–1685 mg/dL	7.2–16.9 g/L
IgA	69–382 mg/dL	0.69–3.8 g/L
IgM	63–277 mg/dL	0.63–2.8 g/L
IgD	0–8 mg/dL	0–80 mg/L
IgE	0–380 IU/mL 0–380 kIU/L	
Immunoglobulin G (IgG), CSF	0.5–6.1 mg/dL	0.5–6.1 g/L
Insulin, plasma (fasting)	5–25 μU/mL 36–179 pmol/L	
*Iron, serum		
Males	65–170 μg/dL	11.6–30.4 μmol/L
Females	50–170 μg/dL	9.0–30.4 μmol/L
Iron binding capacity, serum		
Total 250–450 mg/24 h	45–81 μmol/L 43–73	43–73
Saturation	20–55%	0.20–0.55
*Isoenzymes, serum by agarose gel electrophoresis		
Fraction 1	14–26% of total	0.14–0.26 fraction of total
Fraction 2	29–39% of total	0.29–0.39 fraction of total
Fraction 3	20–26% of total	0.20–0.26 fraction of total
Ketosteroids, urine		
Males	8–20 mg/24 h	28–70 μmol/24 h
Females	6–15 mg/24 h (decrease with age)	21–52 μmol/24 h (decrease with age)
L-Lactate		
Plasma (NaF)		
Venous	4.5–19.8 mg/dL	0.5–2.2 mmol/L
Arterial	4.5–14.4 mg/dL	0.5–1.6 mmol/L
Whole blood (Hep), at bed rest		
Venous	8.1–15.3 mg/dL	0.9–1.7 mmol/L
Arterial	3–7 mg/dL	0.36–0.75 mmol/L
Urine, 24 h	496–1982 mg/d	5.5–22 mmol/d
CSF	<25.5 mg/dL <2.8 mmol/L	
*Lactate dehydrogenase (LDH)		
Total (L→P), 37°C, serum		
Newborn	290–775 U/L Same	
Neonate	545–2000 U/L	Same
Infant	180–430 U/L Same	
Child	110–295 U/L Same	
Adult	100–190 U/L Same	
>60 y	110–210 U/L Same	

*Test values are method dependent.

Tests	Conventional Units	SI Units
Fraction 4	8–16% of total	0.08–0.16 fraction of total
Fraction 5	6–16% of total	0.06–0.16 fraction of total
*Lactate dehydrogenase, CSF	10% of serum value	0.10 fraction of serum value
LDL-cholesterol (LDL–C), calculated, serum or plasma (EDTA)	Recommended desirable range for adults: <130 mg/dL	<3.37 mmol/L
Lead,		
Whole blood (Hep)	<10 µg/dL	<0.48 µmol/L
Urine, 24 h	<80 µg/d	<0.39 µmol/d
Lecithin–sphingomyelin (L/S) ratio, amniotic fluid	2.0–5.0 indicates probable fetal lung maturity; > 3.5 in diabetics	Same
*Leucine aminopeptidase, serum	14–40 mU/mL (30°C)	14–40 U/L (30°C)
Lidocaine, serum or plasma (Hep or EDTA); 45 min after bolus dose		
Therapeutic	1.5–6.0 µg/mL	6.4–26 µmol/L
Toxic		
CNS, cardiovascular depression	6–8 µg/mL	26–34.2 µmol/L
Seizures, obtundation, decreased cardiac output	>8 µg/mL	>34.2 µmol/L
*Lipase, serum	23–208 U/L (37°C)	23–208 U/L (37°C)
Lithium, serum or plasma (Hep or EDTA); 12 h after last dose		
Therapeutic	0.6–1.2 mEq/L	0.6–1.2 mmol/L
Toxic	>2 mEq/L	>2 mmol/L
Lorazepam, serum or plasma (Hep or EDTA), therapeutic	50–240 ng/mL	156–746 nmol/L
*Luteinizing hormone (LH), serum		
Males	0.9–10.6 mIU/mL	0.9–10.6 IU/L
Females		
Follicular phase	1.1–11.1 mIU/mL	1.1–11.1 IU/L
Midcycle peak	17.5–72.9 mIU/mL	17.5–72.9 IU/L
Luteal phase	0.4–15.1 mIU/mL	0.4–15.1 IU/L
Postmenopausal	6.8–46.6 mIU/mL	6.8–46.6 IU/L
Magnesium		
Serum	1.3–2.1 mEq/L	0.65–1.05 mmol/L
	1.6–2.5 mg/dL	16–25 mg/L
Urine	6.0–10.0 mEq/24 h	3.0–5.0 mmol/24 h
Mercury		
Whole blood (EDTA)	0.6–59 µg/L	<0.29 µmol/L
Urine, 24 h	<20 µg/d	<0.1 µmol/d
Toxic	>150 µg/d	>0.75 µmol/d
Metanephrines (see Catecholamines)		
Methemoglobin (MetHb, hemoglobin), whole blood (EDTA, Hep or ACD)	0.06–0.24 g/dL or 0.78 ± 0.37% of total Hb (SD)	9.3–37.2 µmol/L or Mass fraction of total Hb: 0.008 ± 0.0037 (SD)
Methotrexate, serum or plasma (Hep or EDTA)		
Therapeutic	Variable	Variable

*Test values are method dependent.

Tests	Conventional Units	SI Units
Toxic		
post IV infusion	24 h <5 µmol/L	Same
48 h	<0.5 µmol/L	Same
72 h	<0.05 µmol/L	Same
Myelin basic protein, CSF	<2.5 mg/mL	<2.5 µg/L
Nortriptyline, serum or plasma		
(Hep or EDTA);		
trough (≥12 h after dose)		
Therapeutic	50–150 ng/mL	190–570 nmol/L
Toxic	>500 ng/mL	>1900 nmol/L
*5′-Nucleotidase, serum	2–17 U/L	Same
Occult blood, feces, random	Negative (<2 mL blood/ 150 g stool/d)	Negative (<13.3 mL blood/ kg stool/d)
Qualitative, urine, random	Negative	Negative
Osmolality		
Serum	275–295 mOsm/kg serum water	285–295 mmol/kg serum water
Urine	50–1200 mOsm/kg water	38–1400 mmol/kg water
Ratio, urine/serum	1.0–3.0, 3.0–4.7 after 12 h fluid restriction	Same
Osmotic fragility of erythrocytes	Begins in 0.45–0.39% NaCl	Begins in 77–67 mmol/L NaCl
	Complete in 0.33– 0.30% NaCl	Complete in 56–51 mmol/L NaCl
Oxazepam, serum or plasma		
(Hep or EDTA),		
therapeutic	0.2–1.4 µg/mL	0.70–4.9 µmol/L
Oxygen, blood		
Capacity	16–24 vol% (varies with hemoglobin)	7.14–10.7 mmol/L (varies with hemoglobin)
Content		
Arterial	15–23 vol%	6.69–10.3 mmol/L
Venous	10–16 vol%	4.46–7.14 mmol/L
Saturation		
Arterial and capillary	95–98% of capacity	0.95–0.98 of capacity
Venous	60–85% of capacity	0.60–0.85 of capacity
Tension		
pO_2 arterial and capillary	83–108 mm Hg	Same
Venous	35–45 mm Hg	Same
P50, blood	25–29 mm Hg (adjusted to pH 7.4)	3.33–3.86 kPa
Pentobarbital, serum or plasma		
(Hep or EDTA);		
trough		
Therapeutic		
Hypnotic	1–5 µg/mL	4–22 µmol/L
Therapeutic coma	20–50 µg/mL	88–221 µmol/L
Toxic	>10 µg/mL	>44 µmol/L
pH		
Blood, arterial	7.35–7.45	Same
Urine	4.6–8.0 (depends on diet)	Same
Phenacetin, plasma (EDTA)		
Therapeutic	1–30 µg/mL	6–167 µmol/L
Toxic	50–250 µg/mL	279–1395 µmol/L

*Test values are method dependent.

Tests	Conventional Units	SI Units
Phenobarbital, serum or plasma (Hep or EDTA); trough		
Therapeutic	15–40 µg/mL	65–170 µmol/L
Toxic		
Slowness, ataxia, nystagmus	35–80 µg/mL	151–345 µmol/L
Coma with reflexes	65–117 µg/mL	280–504 µmol/L
Coma without reflexes	>100 µg/mL	>430 µmol/L
Phenolsulfonphthalein excretion (PSP), urine	28–51% in 15 min	0.28–0.51 in 15 min
	13–24% in 30 min	0.13–0.24 in 30 min
	9–17% in 60 min	0.09–0.17 in 60 min
	3–10% in 2 h	0.03–0.10 in 2 hr
	(After injection of 1 mL PSP intravenously)	(After injection of 1 mL PSP intravenously)
Phenylalanine, serum	0.8–1.8 mg/dL	48–109 µmol/L
Phenylpyruvic acid, urine, qualitative	Negative	Negative
Phenytoin, serum or plasma (Hep or EDTA); trough		
Therapeutic	10–20 µg/mL	40–79 µmol/L
Toxic	>20 µg/mL	>79 µmol/L
*Phosphatase, acid, prostatic, serum RIA	<3.0 ng/mL	<3.0 µg/L
*Phosphatase, alkaline		
Leukocyte	Total score: 14–100	Total score: 14–100
Serum (ALP)	20–90 mU/mL (30°C)	20–90 U/L (30°C)
	(Values are higher in children)	(Values are higher in children)
Phosphate, inorganic, serum		
Adults	2.7–4.5 mg/dL	0.87–1.45 mmol/L
Children	4.5–5.5 mg/dL	1.45–1.78 mmol/L
Phosphatidylglycerol (PG), amniotic fluid		
Fetal lung immaturity	Absent	Same
Fetal lung maturity	Present	Same
Phospholipids, serum	125–275 mg/dL	1.25–2.75 g/L
Phosphorus, urine	0.4–1.3 g/24 h	12.9–42 mmol/24 h
Porphobilinogen, urine		
Qualitative	Negative	Negative
Quantitative	<2.0 mg/24 h	<9 µmol/24 h
Porphyrins, urine		
Coproporphyrin	34–230 µg/24 h	52–351 nmol/24 h
Uroporphyrin	<50 µg/24 h	<60 nmol/24 h
Potassium, plasma (Hep)		
Males	3.5–4.5 mEq/L	3.5–4.5 mmol/L
Females	3.4–4.4 mEq/L	3.4–4.4 mmol/L
Potassium		
Serum		
Premature		
Cord	5.0–10.2 mEq/L	5.0–10.2 mmol/L
48 h	3.0–6.0 mEq/L	3.0–6.0 mmol/L
Newborn, cord	5.6–12.0 mEq/L	5.6–12.0 mmol/L
Newborn	3.7–5.9 mEq/L	3.7–5.9 mmol/L
Infant	4.1–5.3 mEq/L	4.1–5.3 mmol/L
Child	3.4–4.7 mEq/L	3.4–4.7 mmol/L

*Test values are method dependent.

APPENDICES

Tests	Conventional Units	SI Units
Adult	3.5–5.1 mEq/L	3.5–5.1 mmol/L
Urine, 24 h	25–125 mEq/d, varies with diet	25–125 mmol/d; varies with diet
CSF	70% of plasma level or 2.5–3.2 mEq/L; rises with plasma hyperosmolality	0.70 of plasma level or 2.5–3.2 mmol/L; rises with plasma hyperosmolality
Pregnanediol, urine		
Males	0–1.9 mg/24 h	0–5.9 µmol/24 h
Females		
Follicular phase	<2.6 mg/24 h	<8 µmol/24 h
Luteal phase	2.6–10.6 mg/24 h	8–33 µmol/24 h
Postmenopausal phase	0.2–1.0 mg/24 h	6.2–3.1 µmol/24 h
Pregnanetriol, urine	0.4–2.5 mg/24 h in adults	1.2–7.5 µmol/24 h in adults
Pressure, CSF	70–180 mm H_2O	Same
Primidone, serum or plasma (Hep or EDTA); trough		
Therapeutic	5–12 µg/mL	23–55 µmol/L
Toxic	>15 µg/mL	>69 µmol/L
Procainamide, serum or plasma (Hep or EDTA); trough		
Therapeutic	4–10 µg/mL	17–42 µmol/L
Toxic (also consider effect of metabolite (NAPA)	>10–12 µg/mL	>42–51 µmol/L
*Prolactin, serum		
Males	1.58–23.12 ng/mL	1.58–23.12 µg/L
Females	<0.6–27.33 ng/mL	<0.6–27.33 µg/L
Propoxyphene, plasma (EDTA)		
Therapeutic	0.1–0.4 µg/mL	0.3–1.2 µmol/L
Toxic	>0.5 µg/mL	>1.5 µmol/L
Propranolol, serum or plasma (Hep or EDTA); trough		
Therapeutic	50–100 ng/mL	193–386 nmol/L
*Protein, serum		
Total	6.4–8.3 g/dL	64–83 g/L
Albumin	3.9–5.1 g/dL	39–51 g/L
Globulin		
α_1	0.2–0.4 g/dL	2–4 g/L
α_2	0.5–0.9 g/dL	5–9 g/L
β	0.6–1.1 g/dL	6–11 g/L
γ	0.7–1.7 g/dL	7–17 g/L
Protein		
Urine		
Qualitative	Negative	Negative
Quantitative	50–80 mg/24 h (at rest)	Same
CSF, total	15–40 mg/dL	150–400 mg/dL
Protoporphyrin, free, erythrocyte	17–77 µg/dL packed RBC	0.3–1.37 µmol/L packed RBC
Pyruvate, blood	0.3–0.9 mg/dL	34–103 µmol/L
Quinidine, serum or plasma (Hep or EDTA); trough		
Therapeutic	2–5 µg/mL	6–15 µmol/L
Toxic	>6 µg/mL	>18 µmol/L

*Test values are method dependent.

Tests	Conventional Units	SI Units
Salicylates, serum or plasma (Hep or EDTA); trough		
Therapeutic	150–300 µg/mL	1.09–2.17 mmol/L
Toxic	>500 µg/mL	>3.62 mmol/L
Sedimentation rate		
Wintrobe		
Males	0–10 mm in 1 h	0–5 mm/h
Females	0–20 mm in 1 h	0–15 mm/H
Westergren		
Males	0–15 mm in 1 h	0–15 mm/h
Females	0–20 mm in 1 h	0–20 mm/h
Sodium		
Serum or plasma (Hep)		
Premature		
Cord	116–140 mEq/L	116–140 mmol/L
48 h	128–148 mEq/L	128–148 mmol/L
Newborn, cord	126–166 mEq/L	126–166 mmol/L
Newborn	134–144 mEq/L	134–144 mmol/L
Infant	139–146 mEq/L	139–146 mmol/L
Child	138–145 mEq/L	138–145 mmol/L
Adult	136–146 mEq/L	136–146 mmol/L
Urine, 24 h	40–220 mEq/d (diet dependent)	40–220 mmol/d (diet dependent)
Sweat		
Normal	10–40 mEq/L	10–40 mmol/L
Cystic fibrosis	70–190 mEq/L	70–190 mmol/L
Specific gravity	1.002–1.030	Same
Sulfates, inorganic, serum	0.8–1.2 mg/dL	83–125 µmol/L
*Testosterone, plasma		
Males	300–1000 ng/dL	10.4–34.7 nmol/L
Females	20–75 ng/dL	0.69–2.6 nmol/L
Pregnant females	3–4 times the adult level	Same
Theophylline, serum or plasma (Hep or EDTA)		
Therapeutic		
Bronchodilator	8–20 µg/mL	44–111 µmol/L
Prem. apnea	6–13 µg/mL	33–72 µmol/L
Toxic	>20 µg/mL	>110 µmol/L
Thiocyanate		
Serum or plasma (EDTA)		
Nonsmoker	1–4 µg/mL	17–69 µmol/L
Smoker	3–12 µg/mL	52–206 µmol/L
Therapeutic after nitroprusside infusion	6–29 µg/mL	103–499 µmol/L
Urine		
Nonsmoker	1–4 mg/d	17–69 µmol/d
Smoker	7–17 mg/d	120–292 µmol/d
Thiopental, serum or plasma (Hep or EDTA); trough		
Hypnotic	1.0–5.0 µg/mL	4.1–20.7 µmol/L
Coma	30–100 µg/mL	124–413 µmol/L
Anesthesia	7–130 µg/mL	29–536 µmol/L
Toxic concentration	>10 µg/mL	>41 µmol/L
*Thyroid-stimulating hormone (TSH), serum	0.32–5 µIU/L	0.32–5 mIU/L

*Test values are method dependent.

Tests	Conventional Units	SI Units
Thyroxine (T₄) serum	5–12 µg/dL (varies with age, higher in children and pregnant women)	65–155 nmol/L (varies with age, higher in children and pregnant women)
Thyroxine, free, serum	0.8–2.3 ng/dL	10.3–31 pmol/L
Thyroxine binding globulin (TBG), serum (as thyroxine)	1.5–3.4 mg/dL	15–34 mg/L
Tobramycin, serum or plasma (Hep or EDTA)		
Therapeutic		
Peak		
Less severe infection	5–8 µg/mL	11–17 µmol/L
Severe infection	8–10 µg/mL	17–21 µmol/L
Trough		
Less severe infection	<1 µg/mL	<2 µmol/L
Moderate infection	<2 µg/mL	<4 µmol/L
Severe infection	<2–4 µg/mL	<4–9 µmol/L
Toxic		
Peak	>10–12 µg/mL	>21–26 µmol/L
Trough	>2–4 µg/mL	>4–9 µmol/L
*Transaminase, serum		
AST (asparate aminotransferase, SGOT)	5–40 U/L (37°C)	Same
ALT (alanine aminotransferase, SGPT)	7–56 U/L (37°C)	Same
Transferrin, serum		
Newborn	130–275 mg/dL	1.30–2.75 g/L
Adult	220–400 mg/dL	2.20–4.00 g/L
>60 y	180–380 mg/dL	1.80–3.80 g/L
Triglycerides, serum, fasting		
Males	40–160 mg/dL	0.45–1.81 mmol/L
Females	35–135 mg/dL	0.4–1.53 mmol/L
Triiodothyronine, total (T₃) serum	150–250 ng/dL	1.54–3.08 nmol/L
*Triiodothyronine (T₃) uptake, resin (T₃RU)	24–34% uptake	0.24–0.34 uptake
Urea nitrogen, serum	7–18 mg/dL	2.5–6.4 mmol Urea/L
Urea nitrogen/creatinine ratio, serum	12:1 to 20:1	48–80 urea/creatinine mole ratio
Uric acid		
Serum, enzymatic		
Male	4.5–8.0 mg/dL	0.27–0.47 mmol/L
Female	2.5–6.2 mg/dL	0.15–0.37 mmol/L
Child	2.0–5.5 mg/dL	0.12–0.32 mmol/L
*Urine	250–750 mg/24 h (with normal diet)	1.48–4.43 mmol/24 h (with normal diet)
Urobilinogen, urine	0.1–0.8 Ehrlich unit/2 h	Same
	0.5–4.0 mg/24 h	Same
Valproic acid, serum or plasma (Hep or EDTA); trough		
Therapeutic	50–100 µg/mL	347–693 µmol/L
Toxic	>100 µg/mL	>693 µmol/L

*Test values are method dependent.

Tests	Conventional Units	SI Units
Vancomycin, serum or plasma (Hep or EDTA)		
Therapeutic		
Peak	20–40 µg/mL	14–28 µmol/L
Trough	5–10 µg/mL	3–7 µmol/L
Toxic	>80–100 µg/mL	>55–69 µmol/L
Vanillylmandelic acid (VMA), urine (4-hydroxy-3-methoxymandelic acid)	1.4–6.5 mg/24 h	7–33 µmol/d
Viscosity, serum	1.4–1.8 times water	Same
Vitamin A, serum	30–80 µg/dL	1.05–2.8 µmol/L
Vitamin B_{12}, serum	100–700 pg/mL	74–516 pmol/L
Vitamin E, serum		
Normal	5–18 µg/mL	11.6–46.4 µmol/L
Therapeutic	30–50 µg/mL	69.6–116 µmol/L
Zinc, serum	70–150 µg/mL	10.7–22.9 µmol/L

COMMONLY PRESCRIBED DRUGS AND THEIR APPLICATIONS

Compiled by Marjorie Canfield Willis

This alphabetical index of commonly prescribed drugs (trade and generic) is based on listings of new and refill prescriptions dispensed in the United States in 1995. The names of trade drugs are capitalized; their generic names accompany them in parentheses. Names of generic drugs are set in lower case. Common classifications for each drug are identified.

NAME	CLASSIFICATION
Accupril (quinapril hydrochloride)	antihypertensive; angiotensin-converting enzyme (ACE) inhibitor
acetaminophen and codeine	analgesic, antipyretic
Adalat CC (nifedipine)	antianginal; antihypertensive; calcium channel blocker
Advil (ibuprofen)	analgesic; nonsteroidal anti-inflammatory (NSAID)
albuterol	bronchodilator; β-2-adrengenic agonist
allopurinol	antigout; xanthine oxidase inhibitor
alprazolam	antianxiety
Altace (ramipril)	antihypertensive; angiotensin-converting enzyme (ACE) inhibitor
Ambien (zolpidem tartrate)	hypnotic; sedative
amitriptyline hydrochloride	antidepressanta; tricyclic
amoxicillin trihydrate	antibiotic
ampicillin	antibiotic
Amoxil (amoxicillin trihydrate)	antibiotic
atenolol	antihypertensive; antianginal; β-adrenergic blocker
Ativan (lorazepam)	antianxiety; hypnotic; sedative
Atrovent (ipratropium bromide)	anticholinergic; bronchodilator
Augmentin (amoxicillin/clavulanic acid)	antibiotic
Axid (nizatidine)	antiulcer; histamine-2 antagonist
Azmacort (triamcinolone)	inhaled anti-inflammatory; corticosteroid
Bactrim (co-trimoxazole)	antibiotic
Bactroban (mupirocin)	antibiotic
Beconase AQ (beclomethasone dipropionate)	anti-inflammatory; corticosteroid (nasal)
benazepril hydrochloride	angiotensin-converting enzyme (ACE) inhibitor; antihypertensive
Biaxin (clarithromycin)	antibiotic
BuSpar (buspirone hydrochloride)	antianxiety
Calan SR (verapamil hydrochloride)	antianginal; antiarrhythmic; calcium channel blocker
Capoten (captopril)	antihypertensive; angiotensin-converting enzyme (ACE) inhibitor
Carafate (sucralfate)	antiulcer
Cardizem CD (diltiazem hydrochloride)	antianginal; calcium channel blocker
Cardura (doxazosin mesylate)	antihypertensive; α-adrenergic blocker
carisoprodol	skeletal muscle relaxant
Ceclor (cefaclor)	antibiotic
cefpodoxime proxetil	antibiotic
cefaclor	antibiotic
Ceftin (cefuroxime)	antibiotic
Cefzil (cefprozil)	antibiotic
cephalexin	antibiotic
cimetidine	antiulcer; histamine-2 antagonist
Cipro (ciprofloxacin hydrochloride)	antibiotic
Claritin (loratadine)	antihistamine
Claritin-D (loratadine and pseudoephedrine)	antihistamine/decongestant combination
clonidine	antihypertensive
co-trimoxazole	antibiotic
Coumadin Sodium (warfarin sodium)	anticoagulant
cyclobenzaprine hydrochloride	skeletal muscle relaxant
Cycrin (medroxyprogesterone acetate)	progestin; contraceptive
Darvocet-N 100 (propoxyphene and acetaminophen)	analgesic; antipyretic

NAME	CLASSIFICATION
Daypro (oxaprozin)	nonsteroidal anti-inflammatory (NSAID)
Deltasone (prednisone)	anti-inflammatory;corticosteroid
Demulen 1/35–28 (ethinyl estradiol and ethynodiol diacetate)	oral contraceptive
Depakote (valproic acid)	anticonvulsant
Desogen (ethinyl estradiol and desogestrel)	oral contraceptive
DiaBeta (glyburide)	antidiabetic; oral hypoglycemic
diazepam	antianxiety; anticonvulsant; sedative
dicyclomine hydrochloride	antispasmodic
Diflucan (fluconazole)	antifungal
Dilacor (diltiazem hydrochloride)	antianginal; calcium channel blocker
Dilantin (phenytoin)	anticonvulsant; antiarrhythmic
dicloxacillin sodium	antibiotic
doxycycline hyclate	antibiotic
Duricef (cefadroxil monohydrate)	antibiotic
Dyazide (hydrochlorothiazide and triamterene)	diuretic
E.E.S. (erythromycin)	antibiotic
Effexor (venlafaxine)	antidepressant
Elocon (mometasone furoate)	topical anti-inflammatory; corticosteroid
Ery-Tab (erythromycin)	antibiotic
Erythrocin Stearate (erythromycin)	antibiotic
erythromycin	antibiotic
Estrace Oral (estradiol)	estrogen derivative
Estraderm (estradiol)	topical estrogen derivative
ferrous sulfate	iron salt
Fiorinal with Codeine (butalbital compound and codeine)	analgesic, narcotic; barbiturate
Flonase (fluticasone propionate)	corticosteroid; nasal anti-inflammatory
Floxin (ofloxacin)	antibiotic
folic acid	vitamin
furosemide	diuretic
gemfibrozil	antilipemic
glipizide	antidiabetic; oral hypoglycemic
Glucotrol (glipizide)	antidiabetic; oral hypoglycemic
glyburide	antidiabetic; oral hypoglycemic
Glynase Prestab (glyburide)	antidiabetic; oral hypoglycemic
guaifenesin and phenylpropanolamine	decongestant; expectorant
Hismanal (astemizole)	antihistamine
Humulin (insulin preparation)	antidiabetic
hydrochlorothiazide	diuretic
hydrocodone and acetaminophen	analgesic, narcotic; antipyretic
hydrocortisone	anti-inflammatory; corticosteroid
Hytrin (terazosin)	antihypertensive; α-adrenergic blocking agent
ibuprofen	analgesic; nonsteroidal anti-inflammatory (NSAID)
imipramine hydrochloride	antidepressant; tricyclic
Imitrex (sumatriptan succinate)	antimigraine agent
K-Dur (potassium chloride)	potassium salt; electrolyte supplement
Klonopin (clonazepam)	anticonvulsant; antianxiety
Klor-Con 10 (potassium chloride)	potassium salt; electrolyte supplement
Lanoxin (digoxin)	cardiotonic; antiarrhythmic
Lasix Oral (furosemide)	diuretic
Lescol (fluvastatin)	antilipemic agent
Levoxyl (levothyroxine sodium)	thyroid product
lithium carbonate	antimanic agent
Lo/Ovral-28 (ethinyl estradiol and norgestrel)	oral contraceptive
Lodine (etodolac)	analgesic, nonsteroidal anti-inflammatory (NSAID)
Loestrin-FE 1.5/30 (ethinyl estradiol and norethindrone)	oral contraceptive
Lopressor (metoprolol)	antihypertensive; antianginal; β-adrenergic blocker
Lorabid (loracarbef)	antibiotic

NAME	CLASSIFICATION
lorazepam	antianxiety; hypnotic; sedative
Lorcet 10/650 (hydrocodone and acetaminophen)	analgesic, narcotic; antipyretic
Lotensin (benazepril hydrochloride)	angiotensin-converting enzyme (ACE) inhibitor; antihypertensive
Lotrisone (betamethasone dipropionate and clotrimazole)	antifungal; anti-inflammatory
Lozol (indapamide)	diuretic
Macrobid (nitrofurantoin)	antibiotic
meclizine hydrochloride	antiemetic; antihistamine
medroxyprogesterone	progestin; contraceptive
methylphenidate hydrochloride	central nervous system stimulant
methylprednisolone	anti-inflammatory; corticosteroid
metoprolol	antihypertensive; antianginal; β-adrenergic blocker
Mevacor (lovastatin)	antilipemic
metronidazole	antibiotic
Micronase (glyburide)	antidiabetic; oral hypoglycemic
Monopril (fosinopril)	angiotensin-converting enzyme (ACE) inhibitor; antihypertensive
Motrin (ibuprofen)	analgesic; nonsteroidal anti-inflammatory (NSAID)
Naprosyn (naproxen)	analgesic, nonsteroidal anti-inflammatory (NSAID); antipycetic
naproxen	analgesic, nonsteroidal anti-inflammatory (NSAID); antipyretic
Nasacort (triamcinolone)	nasal anti-inflammatory; corticosteroid
neomycin, polymyxin b and hydrocortisone	antibiotic; corticosteroid
Nitro-Dur (nitroglycerin)	antianginal; coronary vasodilator
nitroglycerin	antianginal coronary vasodilator
Nitrostat (nitroglycerin)	antianginal; coronary vasodilator
Nizoral (ketoconazole)	antifungal
nortriptyline hydrochloride	antidepressant; tricyclic
Norvasc (amlodipine)	antihypertensive; antianginal; calcium channel blocker
nystatin	antifungal
Ortho-Cept 28 (ethinyl estradiol and desogestrel)	oral contraceptive
Ortho-Novum 1/35–28 (ethinyl estradiol and norethindrone)	oral contraceptive
Ortho-Novum 7/7/7–28 (ethinyl estradiol and norethindrone)	oral contraceptive
Oruvail (ketoprofen)	analgesic; nonsteroidal anti-inflammatory (NSAID)
Paxil (paroxetine)	antidepressant
Penicillin VK (penicillin v potassium)	antibiotic
Pepcid (famotidine)	antiulcer; histamine-2 antagonist
Phenergan (promethazine hydrochloride)	antiemetic; antihistamine; sedative
phenobarbital	anticonvulsant; hypnotic; sedative
potassium chloride	potassium salt; electrolyte supplement
Pravachol (pravastatin sodium)	antilipemic
prednisone	anti-inflammatory; corticosteroid
Premarin (conjugated estrogens)	estrogen derivative
Prilosec (omeprazole)	gastric acid secretion inhibitor
Prinivil (lisinopril)	antihypertensive; angiotensin-converting enzyme (ACE) inhibitor
Procardia XL (nifedipine)	antianginal; antihypertensive; calcium channel blocker
promethazine and codeine	antihistamine; antitussive
Propacet (propoxyphene and acetaminophen)	analgesic; narcotic
propoxyphene napsylate and acetaminophen	analgesic
propranolol hydrochloride	antianginal; antiarrhythmic; amtihypertensive; antimigraine
Propulsid (cisapride)	antiemetic; gastrointestinal stimulant

NAME	CLASSIFICATION
Proventil (albuterol)	bronchodilator; β-2-adrengenic agonist
Provera (medroxyprogesterone acetate)	contraceptive; progestin
Prozac (fluoxetine hydrochloride)	antidepressant
Relafen (nabumetone)	nonsteroidal anti-inflammatory (NSAID)
Retin-A (tretinoin)	acne product
Ritalin (methylphenidate hydrochloride)	central nervous system stimulant
Roxicet (oxycodone and acetaminophen)	analgesic, narcotic; antipyretic
Seldane (terfenadine)	antihistamine
Seldane-D (terfenadine and pseudoephedrine)	antihistamine/decongestant
Serevent (salmeterol xinafoate)	inhaled bronchodilator; β-2-adrengenic agonist
Sumycin (tetracycline)	antibiotic; acne product
Suprax (cefixime)	antibiotic
Synthroid (levothyroxine sodium)	thyroid product
Tegretol (carbamazepine)	anticonvulsant; miscellaneous
temazepam	hypnotic; sedative
Tenormin (atenolol)	antianginal; β-adrenergic blocker
Terazol (terconazole)	vaginal antifungal
tetracycline	antibiotic
Theo-Dur (theophylline)	antiasthmatic; bronchodilator
Timoptic (timolol maleate)	ophthalmic β-adrenergic blocker; antiglaucoma
Toprol-XL (metoprolol)	antianginal; antihypertensive; β-adrenergic blocker
Toradol (ketorolac tromethamine)	analgesic; nonsteroidal anti-inflammatory (NSAID)
trazodone hydrochloride	antidepressant
Trental (pentoxifylline)	blood-viscosity–reducing agent
Tri-Levlen 28 (ethinyl estradiol and levonorgestrel)	oral contraceptive
triamcinolone	anti-inflammatory; corticosteroid
triamtereme and hydrochlorothiazide (HCTZ)	diuretic
trimethoprim-sulfamethoxazole	antibiotic
Trimox (amoxicillin trihydrate)	antibiotic
Triphasil-28 (ethinyl estradiol and levonorgestrel)	oral contraceptive
Tylenol with Codeine (acetaminophen and codeine)	analgesic, narcotic, antipyretic
Ultram (tramadol hydrochloride)	analgesic, non-narcotic
Valium (diazepam)	antianxiety; anticonvulsant; sedative
Vancenase AQ (beclomethasone dipropionate)	nasal anti-inflammatory; corticosteroid
Vanceril (beclomethasone dipropionate)	inhaled anti-inflammatory; corticosteroid
Vantin (cefpodoxime proxetil)	antibiotic
Vasotec (enalapril)	antihypertensive; angiotensin-converting enzyme (ACE) inhibitor
Veetids (penicillin v potassium)	antibiotic
Ventolin aerosol (albuterol)	inhaled bronchodilator; β-2-adrengic agonist
verapamil hydrochloride	antianginal; antiarrhythmic; calcium channel blocker
Verelan (verapamil hydrochloride)	antianginal; antiarrhythmic; calcium channel blocker
Vicodin (hydrocodone and acetaminophen)	analgesic, narcotic; antipyretic
Voltaren (diclofenac sodium)	analgesic; nonsteroidal anti-inflammatory (NSAID)
Xanax (alprazolam)	antianxiety agent
Zantac (ranitidine hydrochloride)	antiulcer; histamine-2 antagonist
Zestril (lisinopril)	antihypertensive; angiotensin-converting enzyme (ACE) inhibitor
Zithromax (azithromycin dihydrate)	antibiotic
Zocor (simvastatin)	antilipemic
Zoloft (sertraline hydrochloride)	antidepressant
Zovirax (acyclovir)	antiviral

REFERENCES

Lance LL, Lacy C, Goldman MP, eds. Quick look drug book. Baltimore: Williams & Wilkins, 1996.

Top 200 drugs of 1995. Pharmacy Times 1996; April: 27–36.

COMMON ABBREVIATIONS USED IN MEDICAL ORDERS

Word	Abbreviation	Meaning
ana	āā, aa	of each
ante cibum	a.c.	before meals or food
ad	ad	to, up to
ad libitum	ad lib.	at pleasure
ante meridiem	A.M.	morning
ampulla	amp	ampul
aqua	aq.	water
aqua destillata	aq. dest.	distilled water
aurio dextra	a.d.	right ear
aurio laeva	a.l.	left ear
aurio sinister	a.s.	left ear
aures utrae	a.u.	each ear
bis in die	b.i.d.	twice daily
bowel movement	b.m.	bowel movement
blood pressure	b.p.	blood pressure
cong	c.	gallon
cum	c̄	with
capsula	caps.	capsule
–	cc.	cubic centimeter
compositus	comp.	compound
dies	d.	day
dilue	dil.	dilute
dispensa	disp.	dispense
divide	div.	divide
dentur tales doses	d.t.d.	give of such a dose
elixir	el.	elixir
–	e.m.p.	as directed
et	et	and
–	ex aq.	in water
fac, fiat, fiant	f., ft.	make, let be made
Food and Drug Administration	FDA	Food and Drug Administration
gramma	Gm., g.	gram
granum	gr.	grain
gutta	gtt.	a drop
hora	h.	hour
hora somni	h.s., hor. som.	at bedtime
–	i.m., I.M.	intramuscular
–	i.v.	intravenous
liquor	liq.	a liquor, solution
–	mcg.	microgram
–	mg.	milligram
–	ml.	milliliter
misce	M.	mix
more dictor	m.dict.	as directed
mixtura	mixt.	a mixture
National Formulary	N.F.	National Formulary
numerus	no.	number
nocturnal	noc.	in the night
non repetatur	non. rep.	do not repeat, no refills
octarius	O, Oct.	a pint
oculus dexter	o.d.	right eye
oculus laevus	o.l.	left eye
oculus sinister	o.s.	left eye
oculos uterque	o.u.	each eye
post cibos	p.c., post. cib.	after meals
post meridiem	P.M.	afternoon or evening
per os	p.o.	by mouth

Word	Abbreviation	Meaning
pro re nata	p.r.n.	as needed
pulvis	pulv.	a powder
quoque alternis die	q.a.d.	every other day
–	q.d.	every day
quiaque hora	q.h.	every hour
quater in die	q.i.d.	four times a day
–	q.o.d.	every other day
quantam sufficiat	q.s.	a sufficient quantity
–	q.s. ad	a sufficient quantity to make
quam volueris	q.v.	as much as you wish
recipe	℞	take, a recipe
repetatur	rep.	let it be repeated
sine	s̄, s	without
secundum artem	s.a.	according to art
saturatus	sat.	saturated
signa	Sig.	label, or let it be printed
solutio	sol.	solution
–	solv.	dissolve
semis	s̄s̄, sss	one-half
si opus sit	s.o.s.	if there is need
statim	stat.	at once, immediately
suppositorium	supp.	suppository
syrupus	syr.	syrup
tabella	tab.	tablet
–	tal.	such
–	tal. dos.	such doses
ter in die	t.i.d.	three times a day
tincture	tr., tinct.	tincture
tritura	trit.	triturate
–	tsp.	teaspoonful
unguentum	ung.	ointment
United States Adopted Names	USAN	official adopted names
United States Pharmacopeia	U.S.P.	United States Pharmacopeia
ut dictum	ut. dict.	as directed
while awake	w.a.	while awake

[NOTE: The listing of commonly used abbreviations is included as an aid in interpreting medical orders.]

From The American drug index. St. Louis: Facts and Comparisons, 1993.

α alpha; Bunsen's solubility coefficient; first in a series; specific rotation term

A adenosine (or adenylic acid) (in polynucleotides); alveolar gas (subscript); anterior; assessment ampere

A absorbance

Å angstrom; Ångström unit

a (specific) absorption (coefficient) (usually italic); (total) acidity; area; (systemic) arterial (blood) (subscript); asymmetric; atto-

AA amino acid; aminoacyl

AB abortion

Ab antibody

ABG arterial blood gas

abl Abelson murine (mouse) leukemia virus

ABLB alternate binaural loudness balance (test)

ABMS American Board of Medical Specialists

ABR abortus-Bang-ring (test); auditory brainstem response (audiometry)

abs feb [L.] absente febre; when fever is absent

λ-Abu λ-aminobutyric acid

ABVD Adriamycin (doxorubicin), bleomycin, vinblastine, (and) dacarbazine

AC acetate; acromioclavicular; atriocarotid

aC arabinosylcytosine

Ac acetyl; actinium

ac acetyl; [L.] ante cibum; before a meal

AC/A accommodation convergence-accommodation (ratio)

ACE angiotensin-converting enzyme

ACEI angiotensin-converting enzyme inhibitor

AcG accelerator globulin

ac-g accelerator globulin

Ach acetylcholine

aCL anticardiolipin (antibody)

ACP acyl carrier protein; American College of Physicians

ACS American College of Surgeons

ACTH adrenocorticotropic hormone (corticotropin)

add. [L.] adde; (please) add

Ade adenine

ADH antidiuretic hormone

adhib [L.] adhibendus; to be administered

ADL activities (of) daily living

admov [L.] admove; apply

Ado adenosine

ADP adenosine 5'-diphosphate

ad sat [L.] ad saturatum, ad saturandum; to saturation

adst feb [L.] adstante febre; when fever is present

ad us. ext [L.] ad usum externum; for external use

adv [L.] adversum; against

A-E above-the-elbow (amputation)

AFORMED alternating failure of response, mechanical, (to) electrical depolarization

AFP α-fetoprotein

Ag antigen; [L.] argentum; silver

agit. ante us. [L.] agita ante usum; shake before using

agit. bene [L.] agita bene; shake well

A/G R albumin-globulin ratio

AHF antihemophilic factor

AHG antihemophilic globulin

AID artificial insemination donor

AIDS acquired immunodeficiency syndrome

AIH artificial insemination by husband; artificial insemination, homologous

A-K above-the-knee (amputation)

Al aluminum

Ala alanine (or its mono- or diradical)

alb albumin

ALA σ-aminolevulinic acid

ALD adrenoleukodystrophy

ALL acute lymphocytic leukemia

ALS antilymphocyte serum

ALT alanine aminotransferase

alt hor [L.] alternis horis; every other hour

Am americium

AMP adenosine monophosphate (adenylic acid)

amu atomic mass unit

ANF antinuclear factor

ANS autonomic nervous system

ANUG acute necrotizing ulcerative gingivitis

AP anterior posterior

A & P auscultation and percussion

APA antipernicious anemia (factor)

APC acetylsalicylic (acid), phenacetin, (and) caffeine (combined as an antipyretic and analgesic); antigen-presenting cell

A-P-C adenoidal-pharyngeal-conjunctival (virus)

aPS antiphospholipid antibody syndrome

APTT activated partial thromboplastin time

Ar argon

araC arabinosylcytosine (cytarabine)

ARC AIDS-related complex

ARDS adult respiratory distress syndrome

Arg arginine (or its mono- or diradical)

ARV AIDS-related virus

As arsenic

ASD atrial septal defect

ASHD arteriosclerotic heart disease

Asn asparagine (or its mono- or diradical)

Asp aspartic (acid) (or its radical forms)

AST aspartate aminotransferase

At astatine

ATL adult T-cell leukemia; adult T-cell lymphoma

atm (standard) atmosphere

ATP adenosine 5′-triphosphate

ATPase adenosine triphosphatase

ATPD ambient temperature (and) pressure, dry

ATPS ambient temperature (and) pressure, saturated (with water vapor)

at. wt. atomic weight

Au [L.] aurum; gold

Au Ag Australia antigen

AV arteriovenous

A-V arteriovenous; atrioventricular (block, bundle, conduction, dissociation, extrasystole)

AVN atrioventricular nodal (extrasystole)

AVP antiviral protein

AW atomic weight
A&W alive and well
ax. axis
AZT azidothymidine (zidovudine)
b blood (subscript)
B barometric (pressure) (subscript); boron
Ba barium
BADL basic activities (of) daily life
BAER brainstem auditory evoked response
BAL British anti-Lewisite (dimercaprol); bronchoalveolar lavage
BALB binaural alternate loudness balance (test)
BBB blood-brain barrier
BCG bacille bilié de Calmette-Guérin (vaccine); ballistocardiograph
BCP biochemistry panel
Be beryllium
B-E below-the-elbow (amputation)
Bi bismuth
bib. [L.] bibe; (please) drink
BIB. [L.] bibe; (please) drink
BID [L.] bis in die; twice (in) a day
BIDS brittle (hair), impaired (intelligence), decreased (fertility), (and) short (stature)
BIPAP bilevel positive airway pressure
Bk berkelium
BMR basal metabolic rate
BP blood pressure; boiling point; British Pharmacopoeia
BPF bronchopleural fistula
BPH benign prostatic hypertrophy/hyperplasia
Bq becquerel (SI unit of radionuclide activity)
Br bromine
BRP bathroom privileges
BS blood sugar
BSA body surface area
BSER brainstem evoked response (audiometry)
BSP brom(o)sulfophthalein (liver function)
BT bleeding time
BTPS body temperature, (ambient) pressure, saturated (with water vapor)
BTU British thermal unit
BUN blood urea nitrogen
Bx biopsy
C calorie (large); carbon; Celsius; centigrade; clearance (rate, renal) (followed by a subscript); compliance; concentration; cylindrical (lens); cytidine
c calorie (small); capillary (blood) (subscript); centi-
C&S culture and sensitivity
ca [L.] circa; (about, approximately)
c-a cardioarterial
Ca calcium; cathodal; cathode
CA cancer; carcinoma; cardiac arrest; chronologic age; croup-associated (virus); cytosine arabinoside
CABG coronary artery bypass graft
CAD coronary artery disease
cal calorie (small)
Cal calorie (large)
cAMP cyclic AMP (adenosine monophosphate)

cap capsule
CAP catabolite (gene) activator protein
CAT computerized axial tomography
CBC complete blood (cell) count
CBG corticosteroid-binding globulin
Cbz carbobenzoxy (chloride)
C.C. cardiac catheterization
C.C. chief complaint
CCNU chloroethylcyclohexylnitrosourea (lomustine)
CCU coronary care unit; critical care unit
cd candela
Cd cadmium
CDC Centers (for) Disease Control
cDNA complementary DNA
CDP cytidine 5'-diphosphate
Ce cerium
CEA carcinoembryonic antigen
CELO chicken embryo lethal orphan (virus)
CEP congenital erythropoietic porphyria
Cf californium
CF coupling factor
CG chorionic gonadotropin
CGA catabolite gene activator
cgs centimeter-gram-second (system, unit)
CGS centimeter-gram-second (system, unit)
Ch1 Christchurch (chromosome)
CHF congestive heart failure
μCi microcurie
Ci curie
CI color index; Colour Index
CIB [L.] cibus; food
CIN cervical intraepithelial neoplasia
CIQ cognitive laterality quotient
CIS carcinoma in situ
Cl chlorine
CL cardiolipin
CLL chronic lymphocytic leukemia
cM centimorgan
Cm curium
CMC carpometacarpal
CMI cell-mediated immunity
CML chronic myelogenous leukemia
CMP cytidine 5'-phosphate (or any cytidine monophosphate)
CMV controlled mechanical ventilation; cytomegalovirus
CNS central nervous system
Co cobalt
CO cardiac output
c/o complains of
CoA coenzyme A
COG center of gravity
conA concanavalin A
cont. rem. [L.] continuetur remedium; let the medicine be continued
COPD chronic obstructive pulmonary disease

CP cerebral palsy; chest pain
CPAP continuous (or constant) positive airway pressure
CPD cephalopelvic disproportion
CPM continuous passive motility
CPPB continuous (or constant) positive-pressure breathing
CPPV continuous positive-pressure ventilation
CPR cardiopulmonary resuscitation
cps cycles per second
Cr chromium; creatinine
CR conditioned reflex; crown-rump (length)
CRD chronic respiratory disease
CRH corticotropin-releasing hormone
CRL crown-rump length
CRP cross-reacting protein
CRST calcinosis (cutis), Raynaud's (phenomenon), sclerodactyly, (and) telangiectasia (syndrome)
Cs cesium
CSF cerebrospinal fluid
CT computed tomography
CTP cytidine 5'-triphosphate
Cu [L.] cuprum; copper
cu mm cubic millimeter
CV cardiovascular
CVA cerebral vascular accident (older classical term for stroke)
CVP central venous pressure
CVS chorionic villus sampling
CXR chest x-ray
Cyd cytidine
cyl cylinder; cylindrical (lens)
Cys cysteine
Cyt cytosine
δ delta
Δ delta
d day
d deci-
d deuterium
d- dextrorotatory
D dead (space gas) (subscript); deciduous; deuterium; diffusing (capacity); dihydrouridine (in nucleic acids); diopter; [L.] dexter; right (opposite of left); vitamin D potency of cod liver oil
da deca-
dA deoxyadenosine
DA developmental age
dAdo deoxyadenosine
dAMP deoxyadenylic acid
DANS 1-dimethylaminonaphthalene-5-sulfonic acid
dB decibel
db decibel
DC, D/C discharge; discontinue
DC Dental Corps
D & C dilation and curettage
DCG dacryocystography
DCI dichloroisoproterenol
dCMP deoxycytidylic acid

DDT dichlorodiphenyltrichloroethane (chlorophenothane)
D & E dilation and evacuation
def decayed, extracted, (or) filled (deciduous "baby" teeth)
DEF decayed, extracted, (or) filled (permanent "adult" teeth)
deglut [L.] degluttiatur; (please) swallow
DES diethylstilbestrol
det [L.] detur; (please) give
DET diethyltryptamine
DEV duck embryo vaccine; duck embryo virus
df decayed (and) filled (deciduous "baby" teeth)
DF decayed (and) filled (permanent "adult" teeth)
dGMP deoxyguanosine monophosphate (deoxyguanylic acid)
DIC disseminated intravascular coagulation
dieb alt [L.] diebus alternis; every other day
dim. [L.] dimidius; one-half
DIP desquamative interstitial pneumonia
dir. prop. [L.] directione propria; with proper direction
div in par aeq [L.] divide in partes aequales; (please) divide into equal parts
DJD degenerative joint disease
dk deca-, deka-
dM decimorgan
dmf decayed, missing, (or) filled (deciduous "baby" teeth)
DMF decayed, missing, (or) filled (permanent "adult" teeth)
DMSO dimethyl sulfoxide
DMT N,N-dimethyltryptamine
DN dibucaine number
DNA deoxyribonucleic acid
DNAase deoxyribonucleic acid nuclease
DNase deoxyribonuclease
DNAse deoxyribonuclease
DNP deoxyribonucleoprotein; 2,4-dinitrophenol
DNR do not resuscitate
DNS Director (of) Nursing Service(s)
DO Doctor (of) Osteopathy
DOA dead on arrival
DOC deoxycholic acid
DOC deoxycorticosterone
DOM 2,5-dimethoxy-4-methylamphetamine
2,3-DPG 2,3-diphosphoglycerate
DPI dry powder inhaler
DPN diphosphopyridine nucleotide
DPT dipropyltryptamine
dr dram
DR degeneration reaction; reaction (of) degeneration (muscle fibers)
DRE digital rectal exam
DRG diagnosis-related group
DRVVT dilute Russell's viper venom test
D-S Doerfler-Stewart (test)
DSA digital subtraction angiography
dT deoxythymidine
DT delirium tremens; duration (of) tetany
dTDP deoxythymidine 5'-diphosphate
dThd thymidine

DTIC (dimethyltrizeno)imidazole carboxamide (dacarbazine)

dTMP deoxythymidylic acid

DTP diphtheria-tetanus (toxoids)-pertussis (vaccine); distal tingling (on) percussion (Tinel's sign)

DTPA diethylenetriamine pentaacetic acid

DTR deep tendon reflex

dTTP deoxythymidine 5′-triphosphate

dur dol [L.] durante dolore; while pain lasts

DVT deep vein thrombosis

Dy dysprosium

Dx diagnosis

ε epsilon; molar absorption coefficient

E exa-; extraction (ratio)

EB Epstein-Barr (virus)

EBV Epstein-Barr virus

ECF extracellular fluid

ECF-A eosinophilic chemotactic factor (of) anaphylaxis

ECG electrocardiogram

ECHO echocardiagram

ECHO enterocytopathogenic human orphan (virus)

ECMO extracorporeal-membrane oxygenation (pronounced ek mo)

ECS electrocerebral silence

ECT electroconvulsive therapy

ECU emergency care unit

ED effective dose

EDC estimated date of confinement

EDTA ethylenediaminetetraacetic acid (edathamil, edetic acid)

EEG electroencephalogram

EENT eye, ear, nose, (and) throat

EGD esophagogastroduodenoscopy

EIA enzyme immunoassay

EKG [German] Elektrokardiogramme electrocardiogram

EKY electrokymogram

ELISA enzyme-linked immunoadsorbent assay

EMC encephalomyocarditis (virus)

EMF electromotive force

EMG electromyogram; exomphalos, macroglossia, (and) gigantism (syndrome)

emp [L.] emplastrum; plaster; [L.] ex modo praescripto; in the manner prescribed

ENG electronystagmography

ENT ear, nose, (and) throat

EOG electro-oculography

EPAP expiratory positive airway pressure

Er erbium

ER emergency room; endoplasmic reticulum

ERBF effective renal blood flow

ERCP endoscopic retrograde cholangiopancreatography

ERG electroretinogram

ERPF effective renal plasma flow

ERV expiratory reserve volume

Es einsteinium

ESEP extreme somatosensory evoked potential

ESP extrasensory perception

ESR electron spin resonance; erythrocyte sedimentation rate

ESWL extracorporeal shock wave lithotripsy
ETOH ethyl alcohol
Eu europium
ev electron-volt
eV electron-volt
f femto- (one-quadrillionth [10–15]); (respiratory) frequency
F Fahrenheit; faraday (constant); fertility (factor); field (of vision); filial (generation); fluorine; force; fractional (concentration); free (energy)
F1.2 (prothrombin) fragment 1.2
Fab fragment (of immunoglobulin G involved in) antigen binding
FAD flavin(e) adenine dinucleotide
FANA fluorescent antinuclear antibody (test)
FBS fasting blood sugar
Fe [L.] ferrum; iron
FEF forced expiratory flow
FET forced expiratory time
FEV forced expiratory volume
FF filtration fraction
FFD focus-film distance
FH family history
FIA fluorescent immunoassay
FIGLU formiminoglutamic (acid)
fl oz fluid ounce
Fm fermium
FMN flavin(e) mononucleotide
fps foot-pound-second (system, unit)
FPS foot-pound-second (system, unit)
Fr francium; French (gauge, scale)
FRC functional residual capacity (of lungs)
FRF follicle-stimulating hormone-releasing factor
FRS first-rank symptom
Fru fructose
FS frozen section
FSH follicle-stimulating hormone
FSH-RF follicle-stimulating hormone-releasing factor
FSH-RH follicle-stimulating hormone-releasing hormone
FTA-ABS fluorescent treponemal antibody-absorption (test)
FUO fever (of) unknown origin
FVC forced vital capacity
Fw F wave (fibrillary wave; flutter wave) gamma; Ostwald's solubility coefficient; the third in a series
Fx fracture
μg microgram
g gram
G giga-; glucose (as in UDPG, uridinediphosphoglucose); gravitation (newtonian constant of); guanosine (or guanylic acid) residues in polynucleotides, as in poly(G)
G 1 gap 1
G 2 gap 2
Ga gallium
GABA γ-aminobutyric acid
Gal galactose
Gd gadolinium
GDP mannose-1-phosphate guanylyltransferase

Ge germanium
GERD gastroesophageal reflux disease
GFR glomerular filtration rate
GH glenohumeral; growth hormone
GHRF growth hormone-releasing factor
GH-RF growth hormone-releasing factor
GHRH growth hormone-releasing hormone
GH-RH growth hormone-releasing hormone
GI Gingival Index; gastrointestinal
GIP gastric inhibitory polypeptide
GLC gas-liquid chromatography
Gln glutamine; glutaminyl
Glu glutamic acid; glutamyl
Gly glycine; glycyl
gm gram
GMP guanosine monophosphate (guanylic acid)
GnRH gonadotropin-releasing hormone
GOT glutamic-oxaloacetic transaminase (aspartate aminotransferase)
GPI Gingival-Periodontal Index
GPT glutamic-pyruvic transaminase
grad. [L.] gradatim; gradually
GSH reduced glutathione
GSR galvanic skin response
GSSG oxidized glutathione
GTP guanosine 5′-triphosphate
gtt [L.] guttae; drops, (plural of the abbreviation gt)
GTT glucose tolerance test
GU genitourinary
Guo guanosine
guttat [L.] guttatim; drop by drop
Gy gray (unit of absorbed dose of ionizing radiation)
GYN gynecology
h hecto-
h hour
h Planck's constant
α-h the right-handed helical form assumed by many proteins
H henry; hydrogen; hyperopia; hyperopic
1H hydrogen-1 (protium, light hydrogen)
2H hydrogen-2 (deuterium, heavy hydrogen)
3H hydrogen-3 (tritium, radioactive hydrogen)
H+ hydrogen ion
Ha hahnium
HA hyaluronic acid
HAA hepatitis-associated antigen
HAV hepatitis A virus
Hb hemoglobin
HbA adult hemoglobin
HbA1 major (component of) adult hemoglobin
HbA2 minor (fraction of) adult hemoglobin
HbAS heterozygosity for hemoglobin A and hemoglobin S (sickle cell trait)
HBcAg hepatitis B core antigen
HbCO carboxyhemoglobin
HBe hepatitis B early (antigen)

HBeAb hepatitis B early antibody
HBeAg hepatitis B early antigen
HbF fetal hemoglobin
HbO₂ oxyhemoglobin; oxygenated hemoglobin
HbS sickle-cell hemoglobin
HBsAb hepatitis B surface antibody
HBsAg hepatitis B surface antigen
HBV hepatitis B virus
HCG human chorionic gonadotropin
HCS human chorionic somatomammotropin (hormone) (human placental lactogen)
Hct hematocrit
hd [L.] hora decubitus; at bedtime
HDL high-density lipoprotein
HDRV human diploid (cell strain) rabies vaccine
HDV human delta virus
He helium
HEENT head, eyes, ears, nose, throat
HEMPAS hereditary erythroblastic multinuclearity (associated with) positive acidified serum
Hf hafnium
HFJV high-frequency jet ventilation
HFOV high-frequency oscillatory ventilation
HFPPV high-frequency positive pressure ventilation
HFV high-frequency ventilation
Hg [L.] hydrargyrum; water-silver; mercury
HGB hemoglobin
HGH human (pituitary) growth hormone
HHA hepatitis-associated antigen
HI hemagglutination inhibition (test, titer)
His histidine
His- histidyl
-His histidino
HIV human immunodeficiency virus
Hl hyperopia, latent
HLA human lymphocyte antigen
Hm hyperopia, manifest (hypermetropia)
HMG human menopausal gonadotropin
HMO health maintenance organization
HMWK high molecular weight kininogen (Fletcher factor)
Ho holmium
hor decub [L.] hora decubitus; at bedtime
H & P history and physical
HPI history of present illness
HPL human placental lactogen
HPV human papilloma virus
HRT hromone replacement therapy
HSV herpes simplex virus
Ht hyperopia, total; height
5-HT 5-hydroxytryptamine (serotonin)
HTLV human T-cell lymphocytotrophic virus; human T-cell lymphoma/leukemia virus
HTLV-III human T-cell lymphotropic virus (type) III
HTN hypertension
HVL half-value layer
Hx history

APPENDICES

Hz hertz
I inspired (gas) (subscript); iodine
123I iodine-123 (radioisotope)
125I iodine-125
131I iodine-131
IADL instrumental activities (of) daily living
IAP intermittent acute porphyria
ICD implantable cardioverter defibrillator
ICD International Classification of Diseases of the World Health Organization
ICDA International Classification of Diseases, Adapted for Use in the United States
ICF intracellular fluid
ICP intracranial pressure
ICSH interstitial cell-stimulating hormone
ICU intensive care unit
ID infective dose; intradermal
I & D incision and drainage
IDDM insulin-dependent diabetes mellitus
IDU idoxuridine
IF initiation factor; intrinsic factor
IFN interferon
Ig immunoglobulin
IGF insulin-like growth factor
IH infectious hepatitis
IL interleukin
ILA insulin-like activity
Ile isoleucine (or its radical, isoleucyl)
IM internal medicine; intramuscular (injection site, or) intramuscularly
IMP impression
IMP inosine monophosphate (inosinic acid)
IMV intermittent mandatory ventilation
in d [L.] in dies; daily
In indium
Ino inosine
INR international normalized ratio
int cib [L.] inter cibos; between meals
IOL intraocular lens implant
IOML infraorbitomeatal line
IP inpatient
IP interphalangeal (joint, keratosis); intraperitoneal, intraperitoneally
IPAP inspiratory positive airway pressure
IPPB intermittent positive-pressure breathing
IPPV intermittent positive-pressure ventilation
IPV inactivated poliovirus vaccine
IQ intelligence quotient
Ir iridium
IRV inspiratory reserve volume
ISI International Sensitivity Index
ITP idiopathic thrombocytopenic purpura; inosine 5′-triphosphate
IU International Unit
IUCD intrauterine contraceptive device
IUD intrauterine device
IV intravenous, intravenously; intraventricular
IVP intravenous pyelogram

J joule
J flux (density)
k kilo-
K [Modern L.] kalium potassium; kelvin (SI fundamental unit of temperature)
kat katal (enzyme unit of measurement)
kc kilocycle
kcal kilocalorie
KCT kaolin clotting time
kg kilogram
Kr krypton
17-KS 17-ketosteroid
KUB kidney, ureter, bladder
kv kilovolt
kVp kilovolt peak
μl microliter
l liter
L inductance; left; [L.] limes; a boundary, a limit; liter
L left
La lanthanum
LA lupus anticoagulant
LATS long-acting thyroid stimulator
LAV lymphadenopathy-associated virus
lb pound
LBT lupus band test
LCAT lecithin-cholesterol acyltransferase (deficiency)
LCM lymphocytic choriomeningitis (virus)
LD lethal dose
LDH lactate dehydrogenase
LDL low-density lipoprotein
LE left eye; lupus erythematosus
LEEP loop electrosurgical excision procedure
LETS large external transformation-sensitive (fibronectin)
LFA left frontoanterior (fetal position)
LFP left frontoposterior (fetal position)
LFT left frontotransverse (fetal position)
LH luteinizing hormone
LH/FSH-RF luteinizing hormone/follicle-stimulating hormone-releasing factor
LH-RF luteinizing hormone-releasing factor
LH-RH luteinizing hormone-releasing hormone
Li lithium
LLETZ loop electrosurgical excision procedure
LLQ lower left quadrant
LM Licentiate (in) Midwifery
LMA left mentoanterior (fetal position)
LMP left mentoposterior (fetal position)
LMT left mentotransverse (fetal position)
LNPF lymph node permeability factor
LOA left occipitoanterior (fetal position)
LOP left occipitoposterior (fetal position)
LOT left occipitotransverse (fetal position)
LP lumbar puncture
LPH lipotropic pituitary hormone (lipotropin)
Lr lawrencium

LRH luteinizing (hormone)-releasing hormone
LSA left sacroanterior (fetal position)
LSD lysergic acid diethylamide
LSP left sacroposterior (fetal position)
L/S R lecithin/sphingomyelin ratio
LST left sacrotransverse (fetal position)
LTB laryngotracheobronchitis
LTH luteotropic hormone
LTM long-term memory
Lu lutetium
LUQ left upper quadrant (of abdomen)
LVET left ventricular ejection time
Lw (former symbol for) lawrencium (now Lr)
L & W living and well
Lys lysine (or its radicals in peptides)
μ mu; micro-
m mass; meter; milli-; minim; molar; moles (per liter)
m- meta-
M mega-, meg-; molar; moles (per liter); morgan; myopic; myopia; molar; moles (per liter)
μμ micromicro-
μm micrometer
mμ millimicron
mA milliampere
MA mental age
MAA macroaggregated albumin
M + Am compound myopic astigmatism
man. pr. [L.] mane primo; early morning, first thing in the morning
MAO monoamine oxidase
MAOI monoamine oxidase inhibitor
mA-s milliampere-second
Mb myoglobin
MBC maximum breathing capacity
MbCO carbon monoxided myoglobin
MbO$_2$ oxymyoglobin (myoglobin in its combination with O$_2$)
MC Medical Corps
MCH mean cell hemoglobin
MCHC mean cell hemoglobin concentration
mCi millicurie
MCP metacarpophalangeal
MCV mean cell volume
Md mendelevium
MD muscular dystrophy
MDF myocardial depressant factor
MDI metered-dose inhaler
Me methyl
MEDLARS Medical Literature Analysis and Retrieval System
MEP maximal expiratory pressure
mEq; meq milliequivalent
Met methionine (or its radicals in peptides)
MET metabolic equivalent (of) task
met-Hb methemoglobin
met-Mb metmyoglobin
MEV million electron-volts (106 ev)

Mg magnesium
MHC major histocompatibility complex
mho siemens unit
mHz megahertz
MI myocardial infarction
MID minimal infecting dose
MIP maximum inspiratory pressure
MK menaquinone (vitamin K2)
MKS, mks meter-kilogram-second (system, unit)
MLC mixed lymphocyte culture (test)
MLD minimal lethal dose
mm millimeter
mmol millimole
MMPI Minnesota Multiphasic Personality Inventory (test)
MMR measles-mumps-rubella (vaccine)
Mn manganese
Mo molybdenum
MO medical officer; mineral oil
mol mole
mol wt molecular weight
MOPP Mustargen (mechlorethamine hydrochloride), Oncovin (vincristine sulfate), procarbazine hydrochloride, and prednisone
mor dict [L.] more dicto; in the manner stated
mor sol [L.] more solito; as usual, as customary
MPD maximal permissible dose
MPS mononuclear phagocyte system
MR milk-ring (test)
Mr molecular (weight) ratio
MRA magnetic resonance angiography
MRD, mrd minimal reacting dose
MRI magnetic resonance imaging
mRNA messenger RNA
ms millisecond
MS multiple sclerosis; musculoskeletal
msec millisecond
MSG monosodium glutamate
MSH melanocyte-stimulating hormone
MTP metatarsophalangeal (joint)
Mu Mache unit
mV millivolt
Mv mendelevium
MVE Murray Valley encephalitis (virus)
MVP mitral valve prolapse
MVV maximal voluntary ventilation
MW molecular weight
My myopia
ν nu; kinematic viscosity
n index of refraction; nano-
N newton; nitrogen; normal (concentration)
N normal
Na [Modern L.] natrium; sodium
NAD nicotinamide adenine dinucleotide
NAD+ nicotinamide adenine dinucleotide (oxidized form)
NADH nicotinamide adenine dinucleotide (reduced form)

NADP nicotinamide adenine dinucleotide phosphate
NADP+ nicotinamide adenine dinucleotide phosphate (oxidized form)
NADPH nicotinamide adenine dinucleotide phosphate (reduced form)
NAME nevi, atrial (myxoma), myxoid (neurofibromas, and) ephelides (syndrome)
NANB non-A, non-B (hepatitis)
Nb niobium
NBT nitroblue tetrazolium (test)
NCV nerve conduction velocity
Nd neodymium
Ne neon
NEEP negative end-expiratory pressure
NF National Formulary
ng nanogram
NG nasogastric
NGF nerve growth factor (antigen)
Ni nickel
NIDDM non–insulin-dependent diabetes mellitus
NIH National Institutes (of) Health
NK natural killer (cell)
NKA no known allergy
NKDA no known drug allergy
NLM National Library (of) Medicine
nm nanometer
NMN nicotinamide mononucleotide
NMR nuclear magnetic resonance (imaging)
No nobelium
noc maneq [L.] nocte maneque; at night and in the morning
Np neptunium
NPN nonprotein nitrogen
NPO nothing by mouth
NREM non–rapid eye movement (sleep)
nRNA nuclear RNA
NSAID nonsteroidal anti-inflammatory drug
NSR normal sinus rhythm
NUG necrotizing ulcerative gingivitis
Ω omega; ohm
O [L.] oculus; an eye; opening (in formulas for electrical reactions); oxygen; objective
OAV oculoauriculovertebral (dysplasia, syndrome)
OB obstetrics
OB/GYN obstetrics (and) gynecology
OBS organic brain syndrome
OD Doctor (of) Optometry; [L.] oculus dexter; the right eye; overdose, overdosage
ODD oculodentodigital (dysplasia, syndrome)
Oe oersted (centimeter-gram-second unit of magnetic field strength)
OFD orofaciodigital (dysostosis, syndrome)
OH occupational history
OKT Ortho-Kung T (cell)
OML orbitomeatal line
OMM ophthalmomandibulomelic (dysplasia, syndrome)
omn hor [L.] omni hor ; at every hour
OMS organic mental syndrome
OP outpatient
OPV oral (attenuated) poliovirus vaccine

OR operating room
ORD optical rotatory dispersion
ORIF open reduction, internal fixation
Orn ornithine (or its radical)
Oro orotate; orotic acid
Os osmium
OSHA Occupational Safety (and) Health Administration
OT occupational therapy; (Koch's) old tuberculin
OTC over the counter (nonprescription drug)
OXT oxytocin
oz ounce
p pico-; pupil
P partial (pressure); peta- one quadrillion (1015); phosphorus; phosphoric (residue); plasma (concentration); pressure; plan; posterior; pulse
32P phosphorus-32
P1 first parental (generation)
Pa pascal; protactinium
PA posterior anterior
PABA p-aminobenzoic acid; para-aminobenzoic acid
PaCO₂ arterial partial pressure of carbon dioxide
PAF platelet-aggregating (or -activating) factor
PAH p-aminohippuric (acid); para-aminohippuric (acid)
PaO₂ partial (pressure of) arterial oxygen
PAP Papanicolaou test (smear)
PAR postanesthetic recovery
part. aeq. [L.] partes aequales; equal parts (amounts)
part. vic. [L.] partitis vicibus; in divided doses
PAS p-aminosalicylic (acid), para-aminosalicylic (acid)
PASA p-aminosalicylic acid, para-aminosalicylic acid
Pb [L.] plumbum; lead
PBG porphobilinogen
PBI protein-bound iodine (test)
PCB polychlorinated biphenyl
Pco₂ partial pressure (tension) of carbon dioxide
PCP phencyclidine
Pd palladium
PD prism diopter
PDA patent ductus arteriosus
PDLL poorly differentiated lymphocytic lymphoma
PE physical examination
PEEP positive end-expiratory pressure
PEFR peak expiratory flow rate
per by
PERRLA pupils equal, round, and reactive to light and accomodation
PET positron emission tomography
PF peak flow
PF4 platelet factor 4
PFT pulmonary function test
pg picogram
PGA prostaglandin A
PGB prostaglandin B
PGE prostaglandin E
PGF prostaglandin F

APPENDICES

pH hydrogen ion concentration: p (power) of [H+]10
Ph phenyl
PH past history
Ph1 Philadelphia (chromosome)
PHA phytohemagglutinin (antigen)
Phe phenylalanine (or its radical)
PhG [L.] Pharmacopoeia Germanica; German Pharmacopeia
PI present illness
PID pelvic inflammatory disease
PIF prolactin-inhibiting factor
PIH pregnancy-induced hypertension
pK negative logarithm of the ionization constant (Ka) of an acid
PK pyruvate kinase
PKU phenylketonuria
pm picometer
Pm promethium
PMH past medical history
PMS premenstrual syndrome
PNP platelet neutralization procedure
PNPB positive-negative pressure breathing
PNS peripheral nervous system
Po polonium
PO_2, pO_2 partial pressure (tension) of oxygen
POEMS polyneuropathy, organomegaly, endocrinopathy, monoclonal (protein, and) skin (changes) (syndrome)
polio poliomyelitis (pl—)
POMP prednisone, Oncovin (vincristine sulfate), methotrexate, and Purinethol (6-mercaptop-urine)
POR problem-oriented (medical) record
post op postoperation
PP pyrophosphate
PPBS postprandial blood sugar
PPCA proserum prothrombin conversion accelerator
PPD (Siebert) purified protein derivative (of tuberculin)
PPLO pleuropneumonia-like organism
ppm parts per million
PPO 2,5-diphenyloxazole
PPPPP pain, pallor, pulse (loss), paresthesia, paralysis
PPPPPP pain, pallor, paraesthesia, pulselessness, paralysis, prostration
PPV positive pressure ventilation
Pr praseodymium; presbyopia
PR [L.] per rectum; rectally
PRA plasma renin activity
pre op preoperation
PRF prolactin-releasing factor
PRL prolactin
PRN [L.] pro re nata; as needed, as required
pro rat. aet. [L.] pro ratione aetatis; according to (patient's) age
Pro proline (or its radicals)
PSA prostate-specific antigen
PSG polysomnography
PSP phenolsulfonphthalein (phenol red)

PSV pressure supported ventilation
pt patient
Pt platinum
PT physical therapy; prothrombin time
PTA plasma thromboplastin antecedent
PTAH phosphotungstic acid hematoxylin
PTCA percutaneous transluminal coronary angioplasty
PTH parathyroid hormone
PTT partial thromboplastin time
PTU propylthiouracil
Pu plutonium
PUO pyrexia (of) unknown (or uncertain or undetermined) origin
PUPPP pruritic urticarial papules (and) plaques (of) pregnancy
PUVA (oral administration of) psoralen (and subsequent exposure to) ultraviolet light of A wavelength (uv-a)
PV per vagina
PVC polyvinyl chloride; premature ventricular contraction
PVP polyvinylpyrrolidone (povidone)
Px physical examination
Q volume of blood flow; coulomb
QCO$_2$ microliters of CO_2 given off per milligram of dry weight of tissue per hour
q2h [L.] quaque dua horas; every two hours
ql [L.] quantum libet; as much as desired
qns [L.] quantum non sufficiat; quantity not sufficient
Qo oxygen consumption
QO$_2$ oxygen consumption
qt quart
r racemic; roentgen
R gas constant (8.315 joules); (organic) radical; Réaumur (scale); [L.] recipe; (please) take; resistance determinant (plasmid); resistance (electrical); resistance (unit) (in the cardiovascular system); resolution;respiration; respiratory (exchange ratio); roentgen; right
Ra radium
rad radian
RAS reticular activating system
RAST radioallergosorbent test
RAV Rous-associated virus
RAW resistance, airway
Rb rubidium
RBC, rbc red blood cell; red blood (cell) count
RBF renal blood flow
RD reaction (of) degeneration; reaction (of) denervation
Re rhenium
RE right ear; right eye
rem roentgen-equivalent-man
REM rapid eye movement (sleep); reticular erythematous mucinosis
rep roentgen-equivalent-physical
RES reticuloendothelial system
RF release factor; rheumatoid factor
RFA right frontoanterior (fetal position)
RFLP restriction fragment length polymorphism
RFP right frontoposterior (fetal position)
RFT right frontotransverse (fetal position)
Rh Rhesus (Rh blood group); rhodium

RH releasing hormone
RIA radioimmunoassay
Rib ribose
RLL right lower lobe (of lung)
RLQ right lower quadrant (of abdomen)
RMA right mentoanterior (fetal position)
RML right middle lobe (of lung)
RMP right mentoposterior (fetal position)
RMT right mentotransverse (fetal position)
Rn radon
RNA ribonucleic acid
RNase ribonuclease
RNP ribonucleoprotein
R/O rule out
ROA right occipitoanterior (fetal position)
ROM range of motion
ROP right occipitoposterior (fetal position)
ROS review of symptoms
ROT right occipitotransverse (fetal position)
RP retrograde pyelogram
RPF renal plasma flow
rpm revolutions per minute
RPR rapid plasma reagent (test)
RQ respiratory quotient
rRNA ribosomal RNA
RRR regular rate and rhythm
Rs resolution
RS respiratory syncytial (virus)
RSA right sacroanterior (fetal position)
RSP right sacroposterior (fetal position)
RST right sacrotransverse (fetal position)
RSV Rous-sarcoma virus; respiratory syncytial virus
RTC return to clinic
rTMP ribothymidylic acid
RTO return to office
Ru ruthenium
RUL right upper lobe (of lung)
RUQ right upper quadrant (of the abdomen)
RV residual volume
σ sigma; reflection coefficient; standard deviation
s [L.] semis; half; steady state (subscript); [L.] sinister; left (opposite of "right"; does not mean "remaining")
S [L.] sinister; left (opposite of "right"; does not mean "remaining"); saturation of hemoglobin (percentage of) (followed by subscript O_2 or CO_2); siemens; spherical; spherical (lens); sulfur; Svedberg (unit); subjective
S-A sinoatrial (block)
SaO₂ oxygen saturation (of) arterial (oxyhemoglobin)
sat. saturated
sat. sol. saturated solution
Sb [L.] stibium; antimony
SBE subacute bacterial endocarditis
sc subcutaneous, subcutaneously
Sc scandium

SC sternoclavicular; subcutaneous, subcutaneously
SD standard deviation; streptodornase
SDA specific dynamic action
Se selenium
Sf Svedberg flotation (constant, unit)
SGOT serum glutamic-oxaloacetic transaminase (aspartate aminotransferase)
SGPT serum glutamic-pyruvic transaminase (alanine aminotransferase)
SH serum hepatitis
SH social history
Si silicon
SI [French] Système International d'Unités International System of Units
SID source-to-image(-receptor) distance
SIDS sudden infant death syndrome
SIMV spontaneous intermittent mandatory ventilation; synchronized intermittent mandatory
ventilation
SIRD source-to-image-receptor distance
SISI small-increment (or short-increment) sensitivity index (test)
SK streptokinase
SLE systemic lupus erythematosus
Sm samarium
SMA sequential multiple analyzer
Sn [L.] stannum; tin
SOAP subjective (data), objective (data), assessment, (and) plan (problem-oriented record)
SOB shortness of breath
SPCA serum prothrombin conversion accelerator (factor VII)
SPECT single photon emission computed tomography
SPF sun protection (or protective) factor
sp gr specific gravity
sph spherical (lens)
spm suppression (and) mutation
spp species (when plural); (plural of the abbreviation sp)
SQ subcutaneous
Sr strontium
SR systems review
SRF somatotropin-releasing factor
SRF-A slow-reacting factor (of) anaphylaxis
SRIF somatotropin-release inhibiting factor
sRNA soluble RNA
SRS slow-reacting substance (of anaphylaxis)
SRS-A slow-reacting substance (of) anaphylaxis
ss one-half
ST scapulothoracic
STD sexually transmitted disease
STEL short-term exposure limit
STH somatotropic hormone
STM short-term memory
STPD standard temperature (0C) (and) pressure (760 mm Hg absolute), dry
suppos suppository
Sv sievert (unit)
SV sievert (unit); stroke volume
Sx symptom
t metric ton; temperature (Celsius); tritium
α-T α-tocopherol

APPENDICES

T temperature, absolute (Kelvin); tension (intraocular); tera-; tesla; tetanus (toxoid vaccine); tidal (volume) (subscript); tocopherol; transverse (tubule); tritium; tumor (antigen)

T$_3$ 3,5,3′-triiodothyronine

T$_4$ tetraiodothyronine (thyroxine)

T− decreased tension (pressure)

T+ increased tension (pressure)

Ta tantalum

T & A tonsillectomy and adenoidectomy

TAB therapeutic abortion; typhoid, (paratyphoid) A, (and paratyphoid) B (vaccine)

TAD transient acantholytic dermatosis

TAF tumor angiogenesis factor

TAR thrombocytopenia (with) absent radii (syndrome)

TAT thematic apperception test

Tb terbium

TB tuberculosis

TBP thyroxine-binding protein

TBV total blood volume

Tc technetium

99mTc technetium-99m

TCN talocalcaneonavicular (joint)

Td tetanus-diphtheria (toxoid adult type vaccine)

TDP ribothymidine 5′-diphosphate

Te tellurium

TEDD total end-diastolic diameter

TEDS thrombo-embolic disease stockings

TEE transesophageal echocardiogram

TEN toxic epidermal necrolysis

TESD total end-systolic diameter

Th thorium

Thr threonine (or its radicals)

ti/ttot duty cycle

Ti titanium

TIA transient ischemic attack

TITh 3,5,3′-triiodothyronine

Tl thallium

TLC thin-layer chromatography; total lung capacity

TLV threshold-limit value

tm temperature midpoint (Celsius)

Tm thulium; tubular maximal (excretory capacity of kidneys)

Tm temperature midpoint (Kelvin)

TM transport maximum

TM tympanic membrane

TMJ temporomandibular joint (dysfunction)

TMP ribothymidine 5′-monophosphate

TMT tarsometatarsal

Tn (ocular) tension; (intraocular) tension, normal

TNM tumor, node, metastasis (tumor staging)

TORCH toxoplasmosis, other (infections), rubella, cytomegalorvirus (infection, and) herpes (simplex) (titer)

TPA tissue plasminogen activator

TPHA Treponema pallidum hemagglutination (test)

TPI Treponema pallidum immobilization (test)

TPN total parenteral nutrition

TPR temperature, pulse, respiration
tr tincture
Tr treatment
TRH thyrotropin-releasing hormone (stimulation test)
TRIC trachoma inclusion conjunctivitis (organism)
tRNA transfer RNA
Trp tryptophan (and its radicals)
TSH thyroid-stimulating hormone (stimulation test)
TSS toxic shock syndrome
TSTA tumor-specific transplantation antigen
TU toxic unit, toxin unit
TURP transurethral resection of the prostate
TV tidal volume
Tx treatment; traction
Tyr tyrosine (and its radicals)
U unit; uranium; uridine (in polymers); urinary (concentration)
UA urinalysis
UCHD usual childhood diseases
UDP uridine diphosphate
UGIS upper gastrointestinal series
UMP uridine monophosphate (uridylic acid)
Urd uridine
URI upper respiratory infection
USPHS United States Public Health Service
UTI urinary tract infection
UTP uridine triphosphate
v venous (blood); volt
V vanadium; vision; visual (acuity); volt; volume (frequently with subscripts denoting location, chemical species, and conditions) ventilation; gas flow (frequently with subscripts indicating location and chemical species); ventilation;
V1 V6 the unipolar precordial electrocardiogram chest leads
VA viral antigen
A alveolar ventilation
V-A ventriculoatrial
Val valine (and its radicals)
a/ ventilation/perfusion ratio
VATER vertebral (defects), (imperforate) anus, tracheoesophageal (fistula with) esophageal (atresia, and) radial and renal (dysplasia) (complex)
VC vision, color; vital capacity
VCE vagina, ectocervix, endocervix
VCU voiding cystourethrogram
VD (physiologic) dead (space)
VDRL Venereal Disease Research Laboratory (test)
VHDL very-high-density lipoprotein
VIP vasoactive intestinal polypeptide
vipoma vasoactive intestinal polypeptide (+G.—ma, a tumor); (vi-pm)
VLDL very-low-density lipoprotein
VMA vanillylmandelic acid (test)
Vmax maximal velocity
VP vasopressin
VR vocal resonance
VS vital signs; volumetric solution
VSD ventricular septal defect

VT tidal volume
W watt; [German] Wolfram tungsten
Wb weber
WBC white blood cell; white blood (cell) count
WDLL well differentiated lymphocytic (or lymphatic) lymphoma
WDWN well developed, well nourished
WHO World Health Organization
wk week
WNL within normal limits
WR Wassermann reaction
wt weight
X xanthosine
Xao xanthosine
Xe xenon
133Xe xenon-133
Y yttrium
Yb ytterbium
y.o. year old
yr year
Z carbobenzoxy (chloride)
ZEEP zero end-expiratory pressure
Zn zinc
65Zn zinc-65
Zr zirconium
ZSR zeta sedimentation ratio
− negative
+ positive

SYMBOLS

Angles, Triangles, and Circles

$\wedge$	above • diastolic blood pressure (anesthesa records) • elevated • enlarged • improved • increased • superior (position) • upper		$\Delta+$	time interval
			ΔA	change in absorbance
			ΔdB	difference in decibels
$\vee$	below • decreased • deficiency • deficit • depressed • deteriorated • diminished • down • inferior (position) • lower • systolic blood pressure (anesthesia records)		ΔP	change in (intraocular) pressure
			ΔpH	change in pH
			Δt	time interval
			$\Delta H,\ H's\Delta$	Hesselbach's triangle
$>$	causes • demonstrates • distal • followed by • derived from • greater than • indicates • larger than • leads to • more severe than • produces • radiates to • radiating to • results in • reveals • shows • to • toward • worse than • yields		◯	respiration (anesthesia records)
			♀	female • female sex
			♂	male • male sex
			(A), (ax)	axilla (temperature)
$<$	caused by • derived from • less severe than • less than • produced by • proximal • smaller than		(H), (h)	hypodermic • hypodermically
			(IM)	intramuscular • intramuscularly
$\angle$	angle • flexion • flexor		(IV)	intravenous • intravenously
$\angle\!\!\!\!\diagup$	angle of entry		(L)	left
$\angle\!\!\!\!\diagdown$	angle of exit		(M)	murmur
$\llcorner$	factorial product • right lower quadrant		(m)	by mouth • mouth (temperature) • murmur
$\ulcorner$	right upper quadrant		$\sqrt{}$ (m)	factitial murmur
$\urcorner$	left upper quadrant		(o)	by mouth • oral • orally
$\lrcorner$	left lower quadrant		(R)	rectal • rectally • rectum (temperature) • right
Δ	anion gap • centrad prism • change • delta gap • heat • increment • occipital triangle • prism diopter • temperature (anesthesia records)		(X)	end of anesthesia (anesthesia records) • end of operation

Arrows

↑ above • elevated • elevation • enlarged • gas • greater than • improved • increase • increased • increases • more than • rising • superior (position) • up • upper

↑g increasing • rising

↑V increase due to in vivo effect (lab)

↓ below • decrease • decreased • deficiency • deficit • depressed • depression • deteriorated • deteriorating • diminished •

diminution • down • falling • inferior (position) • less than • low • lower • normal plantar reflex • precipitate • precipitates

↓g decreasing • diminishing • falling • lowering

↓V decrease due to in vivo effect (lab)

↗ deviated • displaced • increasing

↘ decreasing

→ approaches limit of • causes • demonstrates • direction of flow or reaction •
distal • due to • followed by • indicates •
leads to • produces • radiating to • results in • reveals • shows • to • to right •
toward • yields

← caused by • derived from • direction of flow
or reaction • due to • produced by • resulting from • secondary to • to left

↑↑ extensor response (Babinski sign) • positive Babinski • testes undescended

↓↓ down bilaterally • plantar response
(Babinski sign) • testes descended

↑↓ reversible reaction • up and down

⇆, ⇌ reversible (chemical) reaction

Genetic Symbols

□ male

○ female

◊ sex unspecified

□─○ mating

□─○ consanguinity

□┬○ illegitimacy

I □┬○ parents and offspring, in
II □ ○ generations

□┬○ dizygotic twins

□┬○ monozygotic twins

④ ③ number of children of sex indicated

□□○ adopted individuals

☉ abortion or stillbirth, sex unspecified

□ ○ normal individuals

□ ♀ individual died without leaving offspring

□┬○ no issue

■ ● affected individuals

■ ●
↗ ↗ proband or propositus

□□ examined professionally • normal for
trait

□ not examined • dubiously reported to
have trait

□▌ not examined • reliably reported to
have trait

■ ◑ heterozygotes for autosomal recessive

⊙ carrier of sex-linked recessive

☒ ∅ death

Numbers

0 completely absent (pulse) • no response (reflexes)

+1, 1+ markedly impaired (pulse)

1+ low normal or somewhat diminished
(reflexes) • slight reaction or trace
(lab tests)

+2, 2+ moderately impaired (pulse)

2+ average or normal (reflexes) • notica-
ble reaction or trace (lab tests)

+3, 3+ slightly impaired (pulse)

3+ moderate reaction (lab tests) • more
brisk than average (reflexes)

+4, 4+ normal (pulse)

4+ hyperactive (reflexes) • large amount
(lab tests) • pronounced reaction (lab
tests) • very brisk (reflexes)

Ī bowel movement (numeral indicates
number of stools in a given period)

1x once • one time

2x, x2 twice • two times

3x etc. three times, etc.

Arabic	Roman		Arabic	Roman
0			17	XVII
1	I, i		18	XVIII
2	II, ii		19	XIX
3	III, iii		20	XX
4	IV, iv		30	XXX
5	V, v		40	XL
6	VI, vi		50	L
7	VII, vii		60	LX
8	VIII, viii		70	LXX
9	IX, ix		80	LXXX
10	X, x		90	XC
11	XI, xi		100	C
12	XII, xii		1,000	M
13	XIII, xiii		5,000	$\overline{V}$
14	XIV, xiv		10,000	$\overline{X}$
15	XV		100,000	$\overline{C}$
16	XVI		1,000,000	$\overline{M}$

Plus, Minus, and Equivalencies

+   acid (reaction) • added to • convex lens • decreased or diminished (reflexes) • excess • less than 50% inhibition of hemolysis (Wassermann) • low normal (reflexes) • markedly impaired (pulse) • mild (severity) • plus • plus (slightly more than stated amount) • positive (lab tests) • present • slight reaction or trace (lab) • sluggish (reflexes) • somewhat diminished (reflexes)

(+)   significant • uncommon or uncertain mode of inheritance

(+)ive   positive

+ to ++   slight pain

++   average (reflexes) • 50% inhibition of hemolysis (Wassermann) • moderate (pain, severity) • moderately impaired (pulse) • normally active (reflexes) *also* ‡ • noticeable reaction or trace (lab tests)

+++   increased reflexes • 75% inhibition of hemolysis (Wassermann) • moderate amount • moderate reaction (lab tests) • moderately hyperactive (reflexes) • moderately severe (pain, severity) • more brisk than average (reflexes) • slightly impaired (pulse)

++++   complete inhibition of hemolysis (Wassermann) • large amount (lab tests) • markedly hyperactive reflexes • markedly severe (pain, severity) • normal (pulse) • pronounced reaction (lab test) • very brisk (reflexes)

−   absent • alkaline (reaction) • concave lens • deficiency • deficient • minus • negative (lab test) • none • subtract • without

(−)   insignificant

±   doubtful • either positive or negative • equivocal (reflexes, qualitative tests) • flicker (reflexes) • indefinite • more or less • plus or minus • possibly significant • questionable • suggestive • variable • very slight (reaction, severity, trace) • with or without

(±)   possibly significant

± to +   minimal pain

APPENDICES

∓	minus or plus	≢	not identical • not identical with
‡	moderate (severity) • normally active (reflexes) *also* ++	≒	nearly equal to
#	fracture • gauge • number • pound(s) • weight	≐	approximately equal
~	about • approximate • approximately • proportionate to	≅	approximately • approximately equals • congruent to
≈	approximately equal • nearly equal to	≑	approaches
=	equal • equals • equal to	⟂	equilateral
≠	does not equal • not equal • not equal to • unequal	≜	equiangular
⌣	combined with	>	greater than
⬭	equivalent	<	less than
⬭̸	not equivalent to	≯	not greater than
≡	identical • identical with	≮	not less than
		≥, ⩾	greater than or equal to
		≤, ⩽	less than or equal to

Primes, Checks, and Dots

?	doubtful • equivocal (reflexes) • flicker (reflexes) *also* ± • not tested (severity) • possible • questionable • question of • suggested • suggestive (severity) • unknown	√d	checked • observed
!	factorial product	√g, √ing	checking
†	death • deceased	√qs	voided sufficient quanity
/	divided by • either meaning • extension • extensor • fraction • of • per • to	√	radical root
′	foot • hour • univalent	²√	square root
″	bivalent • ditto • inch • minute • second (¹/₆₀ degree)	³√	cube root
‴	line (¹/₁₂ inch) • trivalent	*	birth • multiplication sign (genetics) • not verified • presumed • supposed
√	check • observe for • urine • voided (urine)	°	degree • measurement (¹/₃₆₀ of circle) • severity (burns, wounds) • temperature • time (hour)
√·	urine and defecation • voided and bowels moved	:	is to • ratio
√c̄	check with	⋯	no data (in given category)
		∴	therefore
		∵	because • since
		::	as • equality between ratios • proportion • porportionate to

Statistical Symbols

α	probability of Type I error • significance level		ρ	population correlation coefficient
β	probability of Type II error		s	sample standard deviation
$1-\beta$	power of statistical test		s^2	sample variance
$nCk; \binom{n}{k}$	binomial coefficient • number of combination of n things taken k at a time		SE	standard error of estimate
			σ	population standard deviation
			σ^2	population variance
χ^2	chi-squared statistic		$\sigma_{diff.}$	standard error of difference between scores
E	expected frequency in cell of contingency table		$\sigma_{est.}$	standard error of estimate
$E(X)$	expected value of random variable X		$\sigma_{meas.}$	standard error of measurement
F	F statistic (variance ratio)		$\sum_{i=1}^{n} x_i, \Sigma_i \overset{n}{=} x_i$	$x_1 + x_2 + ... + x_n$
f	frequency		t	Student's t statistic • Student's test variable
H_0	null hypothesis			
H_1	alternative hypothesis		θ	latent trait
μ	population mean		U	Mann-Whitney rank sum statistic
N	population size		W	Wilcoxson rank sum statistic
n	sample size		$\overline{X}$	sample mean
$n!$	n factorial		$|x|$	absolute value of x
O	observed frequency in a contingency table		$\sqrt{x}$	square root of x
ϕ	ability continuum • phi coefficient		z	standard score
P	probability		$=$	equal
p	probability of success in independent trials		$\neq$	not equal
			$\approx$	approximately equal
$P(A)$	probability that event A ocurrs		$>$	greater than
$P(A\backslash B)$	conditional probability that A occurs given that B has occurred		$\ngtr$	not greater than
			$<$	less than
r	sample correlation coefficient, usually the Pearson product-moment correlation		$\nless$	not less than
			$\geq, \geqslant$	greater than or equal to
r^2	coefficient of determination		$\leq, \leqslant$	less than or equal to
r_s	Spearman rank correlation coefficient		∞	infinity

From Stedman's abbreviations, acronyms, and symbols. Baltimore: Williams & Wilkins, 1992.

APPENDICES

DIAGNOSIS-RELATED GROUPS (DRGS)

DRG	Description
1	Craniotomy, Age Greater than 17 Except for Trauma
2	Craniotomy for Trauma, Age Greater than 17
3	Craniotomy, Age 0–17
4	Spinal Procedures
5	Extracranial Vascular Procedures
6	Carpal Tunnel Release
7	Peripheral and Cranial Nerve and Other Nervous System Procedures with CC
8	Peripheral and Cranial Nerve and Other Nervous System Procedures without CC
9	Spinal Disorders and Injuries
10	Nervous System Neoplasms with CC
11	Nervous System Neoplasms without CC
12	Degenerative Nervous System Disorders
13	Multiple Sclerosis and Cerebellar Ataxia
14	Specific Cerebrovascular Disorders Except Transient Ischemic Attack
15	Transient Ischemic Attack and Precerebral Occlusions
16	Nonspecific Cerebrovascular Disorders with CC
17	Nonspecific Cerebrovascular Disorders without CC
18	Cranial and Peripheral Nerve Disorders with CC
19	Cranial and Peripheral Nerve Disorders without CC
20	Nervous System Infection Except Viral Meningitis
21	Viral Meningitis
22	Hypertensive Encephalopathy
23	Nontraumatic Stupor and Coma
24	Seizure and Headache, Age Greater than 17 with CC
25	Seizure and Headache, Age Greater than 17 without CC
26	Seizure and Headache, Age 0–17
27	Traumatic Stupor and Coma, Coma Greater than One Hour
28	Traumatic Stupor and Coma, Coma Less than One Hour, Age Greater than 17 with CC
29	Traumatic Stupor and Coma, Coma Less than One Hour, Age Greater than 17 without CC
30	Traumatic Stupor and Coma, Coma Less than One Hour, Age 0–17
31	Concussion, Age Greater than 17 with CC
32	Concussion, Age Greater than 17 without CC
33	Concussion, Age 0–17
34	Other Disorders of Nervous System with CC
35	Other Disorders of Nervous System without CC

DRG	Description
36	Retinal Procedures
37	Orbital Procedures
38	Primary Iris Procedures
39	Lens Procedures with or without Vitrectomy
40	Extraocular Procedures except Orbit, Age Greater than 17
41	Extraocular Procedures Except Orbit, Age 0–17
42	Intraocular Procedures Except Retina, Iris and Lens
43	Hyphema
44	Acute Major Eye Infections
45	Neurological Eye Disorders
46	Other Disorders of the Eye, Age Greater than 17 with CC
47	Other Disorders of the Eye, Age Greater than 17 without CC
48	Other Disorders of the Eye, Age 0–17
49	Major Head and Neck Procedures
50	Sialoadenectomy
51	Salivary Gland Procedures except Sialoadenectomy
52	Cleft Lip and Palate Repair
53	Sinus and Mastoid Procedures, Age Greater than 17
54	Sinus and Mastoid Procedures, Age 0–17
55	Miscellaneous Ear, Nose, Mouth, and Throat Procedures
56	Rhinoplasty
57	T and A Procedures except Tonsillectomy and/or Adenoidectomy Only, Age Greater than 17
58	T and A Procedures except Tonsillectomy and/or Adenoidectomy Only, Age 0–17
59	Tonsillectomy and/or Adenoidectomy Only, Age Greater than 17
60	Tonsillectomy and/or Adenoidectomy Only, Age 0–17
61	Myringotomy with Tube Insertion, Age Greater than 17
62	Myringotomy with Tube Insertion, Age 0–17
63	Other Ear, Nose, Mouth, and Throat OR Procedures
64	Ear, Nose, Mouth, and Throat Malignancy
65	Disequilibrium
66	Epistaxis
67	Epiglottitis
68	Otitis Media and URI, Age Greater than 17 with CC
69	Otitis Media and URI, Age Greater than 17 without CC
70	Otitis Media and URI, Age 0–17
71	Laryngotracheitis
72	Nasal Trauma and Deformity
73	Other Ear, Nose, Mouth, and Throat Diagnoses, Age Greater than 17

DRG	Description
74	Other Ear, Nose, Mouth, and Throat Diagnoses, Age 0–17
75	Major Chest Procedures
76	Other Respiratory System OR Procedures with CC
77	Other Respiratory System OR Procedures without CC
78	Pulmonary Embolism
79	Respiratory Infections and Inflammations, Age Greater than 17 with CC
80	Respiratory Infections and Inflammations, Age Greater than 17 without CC
81	Respiratory Infections and Inflammations, Age 0–17
82	Respiratory Neoplasms
83	Major Chest Trauma with CC
84	Major Chest Trauma without CC
85	Pleural Effusion with CC
86	Pleural Effusion without CC
87	Pulmonary Edema and Respiratory Failure
88	Chronic Obstructive Pulmonary Disease
89	Simple Pneumonia and Pleurisy, Age Greater than 17 with CC
90	Simple Pneumonia and Pleurisy, Age Greater than 17 without CC
91	Simple Pneumonia and Pleurisy, Age 0–17
92	Interstitial Lung Disease with CC
93	Interstitial Lung Disease without CC
94	Pneumothorax with CC
95	Pneumothorax without CC
96	Bronchitis and Asthma, Age Greater than 17 with CC
97	Bronchitis and Asthma, Age Greater than 17 without CC
98	Bronchitis and Asthma, Age 0–17
99	Respiratory Signs and Symptoms with CC
100	Respiratory Signs and Symptoms without CC
101	Other Respiratory System Diagnoses with CC
102	Other Respiratory System Diagnoses without CC
103	Heart Transplant
104	Cardiac Valve Procedures with Cardiac Catheterization
105	Cardiac Valve Procedures without Cardiac Catheterization
106	Coronary Bypass with Cardiac Catheterization
107	Coronary Bypass without Cardiac Catheterization
108	Other Cardiothoracic Procedures
109	No Longer Valid
110	Major Cardiovascular Procedures with CC
111	Major Cardiovascular Procedures without CC
112	Percutaneous Cardiovascular Procedures
113	Amputation for Circulatory System Disorders except Upper Limb and Toe

DRG	Description
114	Upper Limb and Toe Amputation for Circulatory System Disorders
115	Permanent Cardiac Pacemaker Implant with Acute Myocardial Infarction, Heart Failure, or Shock
116	Other Permanent Cardiac Pacemaker Implant or AICD Lead or Generator Procedure
117	Cardiac Pacemaker Revision except Device Replacement
118	Cardiac Pacemaker Device Replacement
119	Vein Ligation and Stripping
120	Other Circulatory System OR Procedures
121	Circulatory Disorders with Acute Myocardial Infarction and Cardiovascular Complication, Discharged Alive
122	Circulatory Disorders with Acute Myocardial Infarction without Cardiovascular Complication, Discharged Alive
123	Circulatory Disorders with Acute Myocardial Infarction, Expired
124	Circulatory Disorders except Acute Myocardial Infarction with Cardiac Catheterization and Complex Diagnosis
125	Circulatory Disorders except Acute Myocardial Infarction with Cardiac Catheterization without Complex Diagnosis
126	Acute and Subacute Endocarditis
127	Heart Failure and Shock
128	Deep Vein Thrombophlebitis
129	Cardiac Arrest, Unexplained
130	Peripheral Vascular Disorders with CC
131	Peripheral Vascular Disorders without CC
132	Atherosclerosis with CC
133	Atherosclerosis without CC
134	Hypertension
135	Cardiac Congenital and Valvular Disorders, Age Greater than 17 with CC
136	Cardiac Congenital and Valvular Disorders, Age Greater than 17 without CC
137	Cardiac Congenital and Valvular Disorders, Age 0–17
138	Cardiac Arrhythmia and Conduction Disorders with CC
139	Cardiac Arrhythmia and Conduction Disorders without CC
140	Angina Pectoris
141	Syncope and Collapse with CC
142	Syncope and Collapse without CC
143	Chest Pain
144	Other Circulatory System Diagnoses with CC
145	Other Circulatory System Diagnoses without CC
146	Rectal Resection with CC
147	Rectal Resection without CC
148	Major Small and Large Bowel Procedures with CC

APPENDICES

DRG	Description
149	Major Small and Large Bowel Procedures without CC
150	Peritoneal Adhesiolysis with CC
151	Peritoneal Adhesiolysis without CC
152	Minor Small and Large Bowel Procedures with CC
153	Minor Small and Large Bowel Procedures without CC
154	Stomach, Esophageal, and Duodenal Procedures, Age Greater than 17 with CC
155	Stomach, Esophageal, and Duodenal Procedures, Age Greater than 17 without CC
156	Stomach, Esophageal, and Duodenal Procedures, Age 0–17
157	Anal and Stomal Procedures with CC
158	Anal and Stomal Procedures without CC
159	Hernia Procedures except Inguinal and Femoral, Age Greater than 17 with CC
160	Hernia Procedures except Inguinal and Femoral, Age Greater than 17 without CC
161	Inguinal and Femoral Hernia Procedures, Age Greater than 17 with CC
162	Inguinal and Femoral Hernia Procedures, Age Greater than 17 without CC
163	Hernia Procedures, Age 0–17
164	Appendectomy with Complicated Principal Diagnosis with CC
165	Appendectomy with Complicated Principal Diagnosis without CC
166	Appendectomy without Complicated Principal Diagnosis with CC
167	Appendectomy without Complicated Principal Diagnosis without CC
168	Mouth Procedures with CC
169	Mouth Procedures without CC
170	Other Digestive System OR Procedures with CC
171	Other Digestive System OR Procedures without CC
172	Digestive Malignancy with CC
173	Digestive Malignancy without CC
174	GI Hemorrhage with CC
175	GI Hemorrhage without CC
176	Complicated Peptic Ulcer
177	Uncomplicated Peptic Ulcer with CC
178	Uncomplicated Peptic Ulcer without CC
179	Inflammatory Bowel Disease
180	GI Obstruction with CC
181	GI Obstruction without CC
182	Esophagitis, Gastroenteritis, and Miscellaneous Digestive Disorders, Age Greater than 17 with CC
183	Esophagitis, Gastroenteritis, and Miscellaneous Digestive Disorders, Age Greater than 17 without CC
184	Esophagitis, Gastroenteritis, and Miscellaneous Digestive Disorders, Age 0–17
185	Dental and Oral Diseases except Extractions and Restorations, Age Greater than 17
186	Dental and Oral Diseases except Extractions and Restorations, Age 0–17
187	Dental Extractions and Restorations
188	Other Digestive System Diagnoses, Age Greater than 17 with CC
189	Other Digestive System Diagnoses, Age Greater than 17 without CC
190	Other Digestive System Diagnoses, Age 0–17
191	Pancreas, Liver, and Shunt Procedures with CC
192	Pancreas, Liver, and Shunt Procedures without CC
193	Biliary Tract Procedures except Only Cholecystectomy with or without Common Duct Exploration with CC
194	Biliary Tract Procedures except Only Cholecystectomy with or without Common Duct Exploration without CC
195	Cholecystectomy with Common Duct Exploration with CC
196	Cholecystectomy with Common Duct Exploration without CC
197	Cholecystectomy except by Laparoscope without Common Duct Exploration with CC
198	Cholecystectomy except by Laparoscope without Common Duct Exploration without CC
199	Hepatobiliary Diagnostic Procedure for Malignancy
200	Hepatobiliary Diagnostic Procedure for Nonmalignancy
201	Other Hepatobiliary or Pancreas OR Procedures
202	Cirrhosis and Alcoholic Hepatitis
203	Malignancy of Hepatobiliary System or Pancreas
204	Disorders of Pancreas except Malignancy
205	Disorders of Liver except Malignancy, Cirrhosis and Alcoholic Hepatitis with CC
206	Disorders of Liver except Malignancy, Cirrhosis, and Alcoholic Hepatitis without CC
207	Disorders of the Biliary Tract with CC
208	Disorders of the Biliary Tract without CC
209	Major Joint and Limb Reattachment Procedures of Lower Extremity
210	Hip and Femur Procedures except Major Joint Procedures, Age Greater than 17 with CC
211	Hip and Femur Procedures except Major Joint Procedures, Age Greater than 17 without CC
212	Hip and Femur Procedures except Major Joint Procedures, Age 0–17

DRG	Description
213	Amputation for Musculoskeletal System and Connective Tissue Disorders
214	Back and Neck Procedures with CC
215	Back and Neck Procedures without CC
216	Biopsies of Musculoskeletal System and Connective Tissue
217	Wound Debridement and Skin Graft except Hand for Musculoskeletal and Connective Tissue Disorders
218	Lower Extremity and Humerus Procedures except Hip, Foot, and Femur, Age Greater than 17 with CC
219	Lower Extremity and Humerus Procedures except Hip, Foot, and Femur, Age Greater than 17 without CC
220	Lower Extremity and Humerus Procedures except Hip, Foot, and Femur, Age 0–17
221	Knee Procedures with CC
222	Knee Procedures without CC
223	Major Shoulder/Elbow Procedures or Other Upper Extremity Procedures with CC
224	Major Shoulder/Elbow Procedures or Other Upper Extremity Procedures without CC
225	Foot Procedures
226	Soft Tissue Procedures with CC
227	Soft Tissue Procedures without CC
228	Major Thumb or Joint Procedures or Other Hand or Wrist Procedures with CC
229	Major Thumb or Joint Procedures or Other Hand or Wrist Procedures without CC
230	Local Excision and Removal of Internal Fixation Devices of Hip and Femur
231	Local Excision and Removal of Internal Fixation Devices except Hip and Femur
232	Arthroscopy
233	Other Musculoskeletal System and Connective Tissue OR Procedures with CC
234	Other Musculoskeletal System and Connective Tissue OR Procedures without CC
235	Fractures of Femur
236	Fractures of Hip and Pelvis
237	Sprains, Strains, and Dislocations of Hip, Pelvis, and Thigh
238	Osteomyelitis
239	Pathological Fractures and Musculoskeletal and Connective Tissue Malignancy
240	Connective Tissue Disorders with CC
241	Connective Tissue Disorders without CC
242	Septic Arthritis
243	Medical Back Problems
244	Bone Diseases and Specific Arthropathies with CC
245	Bone Diseases and Specific Arthropathies without CC

DRG	Description
246	Nonspecific Arthropathies
247	Signs and Symptoms of Musculoskeletal System and Connective Tissue
248	Tendinitis, Myositis, and Bursitis
249	Aftercare, Musculoskeletal System and Connective Tissue
250	Fractures, Sprains, Strains, and Dislocations of Forearm, Hand, and Foot, Age Greater than 17 with CC
251	Fractures, Sprains, Strains, and Dislocations of Forearm, Hand and Foot, Age Greater than 17 without CC
252	Fractures, Sprains, Strains, and Dislocations of Forearm, Hand, and Foot, Age 0–17
253	Fractures, Sprains, Strains, and Dislocations of Upper Arm and Lower Leg except Foot, Age Greater than 17 with CC
254	Fractures, Sprains, Strains, and Dislocations of Upper Arm and Lower Leg except Foot, Age Greater than 17 without CC
255	Fractures, Sprains, Strains, and Dislocations of Upper Arm and Lower Leg except Foot, Age 0–17
256	Other Musculoskeletal System and Connective Tissue Diagnoses
257	Total Mastectomy for Malignancy with CC
258	Total Mastectomy for Malignancy without CC
259	Subtotal Mastectomy for Malignancy with CC
260	Subtotal Mastectomy for Malignancy without CC
261	Breast Procedure for Nonmalignancy except Biopsy and Local Excision
262	Breast Biopsy and Local Excision for Nonmalignancy
263	Skin Grafts and/or Debridement for Skin Ulcer or Cellulitis with CC
264	Skin Grafts and/or Debridement for Skin Ulcer or Cellulitis without CC
265	Skin Grafts and/or Debridement except for Skin Ulcer or Cellulitis with CC
266	Skin Grafts and/or Debridement except for Skin Ulcer or Cellulitis without CC
267	Perianal and Pilonidal Procedures
268	Skin, Subcutaneous Tissue, and Breast Plastic Procedures
269	Other Skin, Subcutaneous Tissue, and Breast Procedures with CC
270	Other Skin, Subcutaneous Tissue, and Breast Procedures without CC
271	Skin Ulcers
272	Major Skin Disorders with CC
273	Major Skin Disorders without CC
274	Malignant Breast Disorders with CC
275	Malignant Breast Disorders without CC

APPENDICES

DRG	Description
276	Nonmalignant Breast Disorders
277	Cellulitis, Age Greater than 17 with CC
278	Cellulitis, Age Greater than 17 without CC
279	Cellulitis, Age 0–17
280	Trauma to Skin, Subcutaneous Tissue, and Breast, Age Greater than 17 with CC
281	Trauma to Skin, Subcutaneous Tissue, and Breast, Age Greater than 17 without CC
282	Trauma to Skin, Subcutaneous Tissue, and Breast, Age 0–17
283	Minor Skin Disorders with CC
284	Minor Skin Disorders without CC
285	Amputation of Lower Limb for Endocrine, Nutritional, and Metabolic Disorders
286	Adrenal and Pituitary Procedures
287	Skin Grafts and Wound Debridement for Endocrine, Nutritional, and Metabolic Disorders
288	OR Procedures for Obesity
289	Parathyroid Procedures
290	Thyroid Procedures
291	Thyroglossal Procedures
292	Other Endocrine, Nutritional, and Metabolic OR Procedures with CC
293	Other Endocrine, Nutritional, and Metabolic OR Procedures without CC
294	Diabetes, Age Greater than 35
295	Diabetes, Age 0–35
296	Nutritional and Miscellaneous Metabolic Disorders, Age Greater than 17 with CC
297	Nutritional and Miscellaneous Metabolic Disorders, Age Greater than 17 without CC
298	Nutritional and Miscellaneous Metabolic Disorders, Age 0–17
299	Inborn Errors of Metabolism
300	Endocrine Disorders with CC
301	Endocrine Disorders without CC
302	Kidney Transplant
303	Kidney, Ureter, and Major Bladder Procedures for Neoplasm
304	Kidney, Ureter, and Major Bladder Procedures for Neoplasms with CC
305	Kidney, Ureter, and Major Bladder Procedures for Neoplasms without CC
306	Prostatectomy with CC
307	Prostatectomy without CC
308	Minor Bladder Procedures with CC
309	Minor Bladder Procedures without CC
310	Transurethral Procedures with CC
311	Transurethral Procedures without CC
312	Urethral Procedures, Age Greater than 17 with CC
313	Urethral Procedures, Age Greater than 17 without CC
314	Urethral Procedures, Age 0–17
315	Other Kidney and Urinary Tract OR Procedures
316	Renal Failure

DRG	Description
317	Admission for Renal Dialysis
318	Kidney and Urinary Tract Neoplasms with CC
319	Kidney and Urinary Tract Neoplasms without CC
320	Kidney and Urinary Tract Infections, Age Greater than 17 with CC
321	Kidney and Urinary Tract Infections, Age Greater than 17 without CC
322	Kidney and Urinary Tract Infections, Age 0–17
323	Urinary Stones with CC and/or ESW Lithotripsy
324	Urinary Stones without CC
325	Kidney and Urinary Tract Signs and Symptoms, Age Greater than 17 with CC
326	Kidney and Urinary Tract Signs and Symptoms, Age Greater than 17 without CC
327	Kidney and Urinary Tract Signs and Symptoms, Age 0–17
328	Urethral Stricture, Age Greater than 17 with CC
329	Urethral Stricture, Age Greater than 17 without CC
330	Urethral Stricture, Age 0–17
331	Other Kidney and Urinary Tract Diagnoses, Age Greater than 17 with CC
332	Other Kidney and Urinary Tract Diagnoses, Age Greater than 17 without CC
333	Other Kidney and Urinary Tract Diagnoses, Age 0–17
334	Major Male Pelvic Procedures with CC
335	Major Male Pelvic Procedures without CC
336	Transurethral Prostatectomy with CC
337	Transurethral Prostatectomy without CC
338	Testes Procedures for Malignancy
339	Testes Procedures for Nonmalignancy, Age Greater than 17
340	Testes Procedures for Nonmalignancy, Age 0–17
341	Penis Procedures
342	Circumcision, Age Greater than 17
343	Circumcision, Age 0–17
344	Other Male Reproductive System OR Procedures for Malignancy
345	Other Male Reproductive System OR Procedures Except for Malignancy
346	Malignancy of Male Reproductive System with CC
347	Malignancy of Male Reproductive System without CC
348	Benign Prostatic Hypertrophy with CC
349	Benign Prostatic Hypertrophy without CC
350	Inflammation of the Male Reproductive System
351	Sterilization, Male

DRG	Description
352	Other Male Reproductive System Diagnoses
353	Pelvic Evisceration, Radical Hysterectomy, and Radical Vulvectomy
354	Uterine and Adnexal Procedures for Nonovarian/Adnexal Malignancy with CC
355	Uterine and Adnexal Procedures for Nonovarian/Adnexal Malignancy without CC
356	Female Reproductive System Reconstructive Procedures
357	Uterine and Adnexal Procedures for Ovarian or Adnexal Malignancy
358	Uterine and Adnexal Procedures for Nonmalignancy with CC
359	Uterine and Adnexal Procedures for Nonmalignancy without CC
360	Vagina, Cervix, and Vulva Procedures
361	Laparoscopy and Incisional Tubal Interruption
362	Endoscopic Tubal Interruption
363	D and C, Conization and Radioimplant for Malignancy
364	D and C, Conization except for Malignancy
365	Other Female Reproductive System OR Procedures
366	Malignancy of Female Reproductive System with CC
367	Malignancy of Female Reproductive System without CC
368	Infections of Female Reproductive System
369	Menstrual and Other Female Reproductive System Disorders
370	Cesarean Section with CC
371	Cesarean Section without CC
372	Vaginal Delivery with Complicating Diagnoses
373	Vaginal Delivery without Complicating Diagnoses
374	Vaginal Delivery with Sterilization and/or D and C
375	Vaginal Delivery with OR Procedure except Sterilization and/or D and C
376	Postpartum and Postabortion Diagnoses without OR Procedure
377	Postpartum and Postabortion Diagnoses with OR Procedure
378	Ectopic Pregnancy
379	Threatened Abortion
380	Abortion without D and C
381	Abortion with D and C, Aspiration Curettage, or Hysterotomy
382	False Labor
383	Other Antepartum Diagnoses with Medical Complications
384	Other Antepartum Diagnoses without Medical Complications
385	Neonates, Died or Transferred to Another Acute Care Facility

DRG	Description
386	Extreme Immaturity or Respiratory Distress Syndrome of Neonate
387	Prematurity with Major Problems
388	Prematurity without Major Problems
389	Full-Term Neonate with Major Problems
390	Neonate with Other Significant Problems
391	Normal Newborn
392	Splenectomy, Age Greater than 17
393	Splenectomy, Age 0–17
394	Other OR Procedures of the Blood and Blood-Forming Organs
395	Red Blood Cell Disorders, Age Greater than 17
396	Red Blood Cell Disorders, Age 0–17
397	Coagulation Disorders
398	Reticuloendothelial and Immunity Disorders with CC
399	Reticuloendothelial and Immunity Disorders without CC
400	Lymphoma and Leukemia with Major OR Procedures
401	Lymphoma and Nonacute Leukemia with Other OR Procedure with CC
402	Lymphoma and Nonacute Leukemia with Other OR Procedure without CC
403	Lymphoma and Nonacute Leukemia with CC
404	Lymphoma and Nonacute Leukemia without CC
405	Acute Leukemia without Major OR Procedure, Age 0–17
406	Myeloproliferative Disorders or Poorly Differentiated Neoplasms with Major OR Procedures with CC
407	Myeloproliferative Disorders or Poorly Differentiated Neoplasms with Major OR Procedures without CC
408	Myeloproliferative Disorders or Poorly Differentiated Neoplasms with Other OR Procedures
409	Radiotherapy
410	Chemotherapy without Acute Leukemia as Secondary Diagnosis
411	History of Malignancy without Endoscopy
412	History of Malignancy with Endoscopy
413	Other Myeloproliferative Disorders or Poorly Differentiated Neoplasm Diagnoses with CC
414	Other Myeloproliferative Disorders or Poorly Differentiated Neoplasm Diagnoses without CC
415	OR Procedure for Infectious and Parasitic Diseases
416	Septicemia, Age Greater than 17
417	Septicemia, Age 0–17
418	Postoperative and Posttraumatic Infections
419	Fever of Unknown Origin, Age Greater than 17 with CC

APPENDICES

DRG	Description
420	Fever of Unknown Origin, Age Greater than 17 without CC
421	Viral Illness, Age Greater than 17
422	Viral Illness and Fever of Unknown Origin, Age 0–17
423	Other Infectious and Parasitic Diseases Diagnoses
424	OR Procedures with Principal Diagnosis of Mental Illness
425	Acute Adjustment Reactions and Disturbances of Psychosocial Dysfunction
426	Depressive Neuroses
427	Neuroses Except Depressive
428	Disorders of Personality and Impulse Control
429	Organic Disturbances and Mental Retardation
430	Psychoses
431	Childhood Mental Disorders
432	Other Mental Disorder Diagnoses
433	Alcohol/Drug Abuse or Dependence, Left against Medical Advice
434	Alcohol/Drug Abuse or Dependence, Detoxification or Other Symptomatic Treatment with CC
435	Alcohol/Drug Abuse or Dependence, Detoxification or Other Symptomatic Treatment without CC
436	Alcohol/Drug Dependence with Rehabilitation Therapy
437	Alcohol/Drug Dependence with Combined Rehabilitation and Detoxification Therapy
438	No Longer Valid
439	Skin Grafts for Injuries
440	Wound Debridements for Injuries
441	Hand Procedures for Injuries
442	Other OR Procedures for Injuries with CC
443	Other OR Procedures for Injuries without CC
444	Traumatic Injury, Age Greater than 17 with CC
445	Traumatic Injury, Age Greater than 17 without CC
446	Traumatic Injury, Age 0–17
447	Allergic Reactions, Age Greater than 17
448	Allergic Reactions, Age 0–17
449	Poisoning and Toxic Effects of Drugs, Age Greater than 17 with CC
450	Poisoning and Toxic Effects of Drugs, Age Greater than 17 without CC
451	Poisoning and Toxic Effects of Drugs, Age 0–17
452	Complications of Treatment with CC
453	Complications of Treatment without CC
454	Other Injury, Poisoning and Toxic Effect Diagnoses with CC
455	Other Injury, Poisoning and Toxic Effect Diagnoses without CC
456	Burns, Transferred to Another Acute Care Facility

DRG	Description
457	Extensive Burns without OR Procedure
458	Nonextensive Burns with Skin Graft
459	Nonextensive Burns with Wound Debridement or Other OR Procedure
460	Nonextensive Burns without OR Procedure
461	OR Procedures with Diagnoses of Other Contact with Health Services
462	Rehabilitation
463	Signs and Symptoms with CC
464	Signs and Symptoms without CC
465	Aftercare with History of Malignancy as Secondary Diagnosis
466	Aftercare without History of Malignancy as Secondary Diagnosis
467	Other Factors Influencing Health Status
468	Extensive OR Procedure Unrelated to Principal Diagnosis
469	Principal Diagnosis Invalid as Discharge Diagnosis
470	Ungroupable
471	Bilateral or Multiple Major Joint Procedures of Lower Extremity
472	Extensive Burns with OR Procedure
473	Acute Leukemia without Major OR Procedure, Age Greater than 17
474	No Longer Valid
475	Respiratory System Diagnosis with Ventilator Support
476	Prostatic OR Procedure Unrelated to Principal Diagnosis
477	Nonextensive OR Procedure Unrelated to Principal Diagnosis
478	Other Vascular Procedures with CC
479	Other Vascular Procedures without CC
480	Liver Transplant
481	Bone Marrow Transplant
482	Tracheostomy for Face, Mouth, and Neck Diagnosis
483	Tracheostomy Except for Face, Mouth, and Neck Diagnoses
484	Craniotomy for Multiple Significant Trauma
485	Limb Reattachment, Hip and Femur Procedures for Multiple Significant Trauma
486	Other OR Procedures for Multiple Significant Trauma
487	Other Multiple Significant Trauma
488	HIV with Extensive OR Procedure
489	HIV with Major Related Condition
490	HIV with or without Other Related Condition
491	Major Joint and Limb Reattachment Procedures of Upper Extremity
492	Chemotherapy with Acute Leukemia as Secondary Diagnosis
493	Laparoscopic Cholecystectomy without Common Duct Exploration with CC
494	Laparoscopic Cholecystectomy without Common Duct Exploration without CC
495	Lung Transplant

1. Muscles of the Shoulder

Muscle	Origin	Insertion	Nerve	Action
Deltoid	Lateral third of clavicle, acromion, and spine of scapula	Deltoid tuberosity of humerus	Axillary n.	Abducts, adducts, flexes, extends, and rotates arm medially
Supraspinatus	Supraspinous fossa of scapula	Superior facet of greater tubercle of humerus	Suprascapular n.	Abducts arm
Infraspinatus	Infraspinous fossa	Middle facet of greater tubercle of humerus	Suprascapular n.	Rotates arm laterally
Subscapularis	Subscapular fossa	Lesser tubercle of humerus	Upper and lower subscapular n.	Rotates arm medially
Teres major	Dorsal surface of inferior angle of scapula	Medial lip of intertubercular groove of humerus	Lower subscapular n.	Adducts and rotates arm medially
Teres minor	Upper portion of lateral border of scapula	Lower facet of greater tubercle of humerus	Axillary n.	Rotates arm laterally
Latissimus dorsi	Spines of T7–T12 thoracolumbar fascia, iliac crest, ribs 9–12	Floor of bicipital groove of humerus	Thoracodorsal n.	Adducts, extends, and rotates arm medially

2. Muscles of the Arm

Muscle	Origin	Insertion	Nerve	Action
Coracobra-chialis	Coracoid process	Middle third of medial surface of humerus	Musculocuta-neous n.	Flexes and adducts arm
Biceps brachii	Long head, supraglenoid tubercle; short head, coracoid process	Radial tuberosity of radius	Musculocuta-neous n.	Flexes arm and forearm, supinates forearm
Brachialis	Lower anterior surface of humerus	Coronoid process of ulna and ulnar tuberosity	Musculocuta-neous n.	Flexes forearm
Triceps	Long head, infraglenoid tubercle; lateral head, superior to radial groove of humerus; medial head, inferior to radial groove	Posterior surface of olecranon process of ulna	Radial n.	Extends forearm
Anconeus	Lateral epicondyle of humerus	Olecranon and upper posterior surface of ulna	Radial n.	Extends forearm

APPENDICES

3. Muscles of the Anterior Forearm

Muscle	Origin	Insertion	Nerve	Action
Pronator teres	Medial epicondyle and coronoid process of ulna	Middle of lateral side of radius	Median n.	Pronates forearm
Flexor carpi radialis	Medial epicondyle of humerus	Bases of second and third metacarpals	Median n.	Flexes forearm, flexes and abducts hand
Palmaris longus	Medial epicondyle of humerus	Flexor retinaculum, palmar aponeurosis	Median n.	Flexes hand and forearm
Flexor carpi ulnaris	Medial epicondyle, medial olecranon, and posterior border of ulna	Pisiform, hook of hamate, and base of fifth metacarpal	Ulnar n.	Flexes and adducts hand, flexes forearm
Flexor digitorum superficialis	Medial epicondyle, coronoid process, oblique line of radius	Middle phalanges of finger	Median n.	Flexes proximal interphalangeal joints, flexes hand and forearm
Flexor digitorum profundus	Anteromedial surface of ulna, interosseous membrane	Bases of distal phalanges of fingers	Ulnar and median nn.	Flexes distal interphalangeal joints and hand
Flexor pollicis longus	Anterior surface of radius, interosseous membrane, and coronoid process	Base of distal phalanx of thumb	Median n.	Flexes thumb
Pronator quadratus	Anterior surface of distal ulna	Anterior surface of distal radius	Median n.	Pronates forearm

4. Muscles of the Posterior Forearm

Muscle	Origin	Insertion	Nerve	Action
Brachioradialis	Lateral supracondylar ridge of humerus	Base of radial styloid process	Radial n.	Flexes forearm
Extensor carpi radialis longus	Lateral supracondylar ridge of humerus	Dorsum of base of second metacarpal	Radial n.	Extends and abducts hand
Extensor carpi radialis brevis	Lateral epicondyle of humerus	Posterior base of third metacarpal	Radial n.	Extends fingers and abducts hands
Extensor digitorum	Lateral epicondyle of humerus	Extensor expansion, base of middle and digital phalanges	Radial n.	Extends fingers and hand

(continued)

Muscle	Origin	Insertion	Nerve	Action
Extensor digiti minimi	Common extensor tendon and interosseous membrane	Extensor expansion, base of middle and distal phalanges	Radial n.	Extends little finger
Extensor carpi ulnaris	Lateral epicondyle and posterior surface of ulna	Base of fifth metacarpal	Radial n.	Extends and adducts hand
Supinator	Lateral epicondyle, radial collateral and annular ligaments	Lateral side of upper part of radius	Radial n.	Supinates forearm
Abductor pollicis longus	Interosseous membrane, middle third of posterior surfaces of radius and ulna	Lateral surface of base of first metacarpal	Radial n.	Abducts thumb and hand
Extensor pollicis longus	Interosseous membrane and middle third of posterior surface of ulna	Base of distal phalanx of thumb	Radial n.	Extends distal phalanx of thumb and abducts hand
Extensor pollicis brevis	Interosseous membrane and posterior surface of middle third of radius	Base of proximal phalanx of thumb	Radial n.	Extends proximal phalanx of thumb and abducts hand
Extensor indicis	Posterior surface of ulna and interosseous membrane	Extensor expansion of index finger	Radial n.	Extends index finger

5. Muscles of the Hand

Muscle	Origin	Insertion	Nerve	Action
Abductor pollicis brevis	Flexor retinaculum, scaphoid, and trapezium	Lateral side of base of proximal phalanx of thumb	Median n.	Abducts thumb
Flexor pollicis brevis	Flexor retinaculum and trapezium	Base of proximal phalanx of thumb	Median n.	Flexes thumb
Opponens pollicis	Flexor retinaculum and trapezium	Lateral side of first metacarpal	Median n.	Opposes thumb to other digits
Adductor pollicis	Capitate and bases of second and third metacarpals (oblique head); palmar surface of third metacarpal (transverse head)	Medial side of base of proximal phalanx of the thumb	Ulnar n.	Adducts thumb

(continued)

Muscle	Origin	Insertion	Nerve	Action
Palmaris brevis	Medial side of flexor retinaculum, palmar aponeurosis	Skin of medial side of palm	Ulnar n.	Wrinkles skin on medial side of palm
Abductor digiti minimi	Pisiform and tendon of flexor carpi ulnaris	Medial side of base of proximal phalanx of little finger	Ulnar n.	Abducts little finger
Flexor digiti minimi brevis	Flexor retinaculum and hook of hamate	Medial side of base of proximal phalanx of little finger	Ulnar n.	Flexes proximal phalanx of little finger
Opponens digiti minimi	Flexor retinaculum and hook of hamate	Medial side of fifth metacarpal	Ulnar n.	Opposes little finger
Lumbricals (4)	Lateral side of tendons of flexor digitorum profundus	Lateral side of extensor expansion	Median (two lateral) and ulnar (two medial) nn.	Flex metacar-pophalangeal joints and extend interphalangeal joints
Dorsal interossei (4)	Adjacent sides of metacarpal bones	Lateral sides of bases of proximal phalanges; extensor expansion	Ulnar n.	Abduct fingers; flex metacar-pophalangeal joints; extend interphalangeal joints
Palmar interossei (3)	Medial side of second metacarpal; lateral sides of fourth and fifth metacarpals	Base of proximal phalanges in same sides as their origins; extensor expansion	Ulnar n.	Adduct fingers; flex metacarpo-phalangeal joints; extend interphalangeal joints

6. Muscles of the Gluteal Region

Muscle	Origin	Insertion	Nerve	Action
Gluteus maximus	Ilium; sacrum; coccyx; sacrotuberous ligament	Gluteal tuberosity; iliotibial tract	Inferior gluteal n.	Extends and rotates thigh laterally
Gluteus medius	Ilium between iliac crest, and anterior and posterior gluteal lines	Greater trochanter	Superior gluteal n.	Abducts and rotates thigh medially
Gluteus minimus	Ilium between anterior and inferior gluteal lines	Greater trochanter	Superior gluteal n.	Abducts and rotates thigh medially
Tensor fasciae latae	Iliac crest; anterior-superior iliacs pine	Iliotibial tract	Superior gluteal n.	Flexes, abducts, and rotates thigh medially

(continued)

Muscle	Origin	Insertion	Nerve	Action
Piriformis	Pelvic surface of sacrum; sacrotuberous ligament	Upper end of greater trochanter	Sacral n. (S1–S2)	Rotates thigh laterally
Obturator internus	Ischiopubic rami; obturator membrane	Greater trochanter	N. to obturator internus	Abducts and rotates thigh laterally
Superior gemellus	Ischial spine	Obturator internus tendon	N. to obturator internus	Rotates thigh laterally
Inferior gemellus	Ischial tuberosity	Obturator internus tendon	N. to quadratus femoris	Rotates thigh laterally
Quadratus femoris	Ischial tuberosity	Intertro-chanteric crest	N. to quadratus femoris	Rotates thigh laterally

7. Posterior Muscles of the Thigh*

Muscle	Origin	Insertion	Nerve	Action
Semitendinosus	Ischial tuberosity	Medial surface of upper part of tibia	Tibial portion of sciatic n.	Extends thigh; flexes and rotates leg medially
Semimembra-nosus	Ischial tuberosity	Medial condyle of tibia	Tibial portion of sciatic n.	Extends thigh; flexes and rotates leg medially
Biceps femoris	Long head from ischial tuberosity; short head from linea aspera and upper supracondylar line	Head of fibula	Tibial (long head) and common peroneal (short head) divisions of sciatic n.	Extends thigh; flexes and rotates leg laterally

*These three muscles collectively are called hamstrings.

8. Anterior Muscles of the Thigh

Muscle	Origin	Insertion	Nerve	Action
Iliacus	Iliac fossa; ala of sacrum	Lesser trochanter	Femoral n.	Flexes and rotates thigh medially (with psoas major)
Sartorius	Anterior-superior iliac spine	Upper medial side of tibia	Femoral n.	Flexes and rotates thigh laterally; flexes and rotates leg medially
Rectus femoris	Anterior-inferior iliac spine; posterior-superior rim of acetabulum	Base of patella; tibial tuberosity	Femoral n.	Flexes thigh; extends leg
Vastus medialis	Intertro-chanteric line; linea aspera; medial inter-muscular septum	Medial side of patella; tibial tuberosity	Femoral n.	Extends leg

(continued)

Muscle	Origin	Insertion	Nerve	Action
Vastus lateralis	Intertrochanteric line; greater trochanter; linea aspera; gluteal tuberosity; lateral intermuscular septum	Lateral side of patella; tibial tuberosity	Femoral n.	Extends leg
Vastus intermedius	Upper shaft of femur; lower lateral intermuscular septum	Upper border of patella; tibial tuberosity	Femoral n.	Extends leg

9. Medial Muscles of the Thigh

Muscle	Origin	Insertion	Nerve	Action
Adductor longus	Body of pubis below its crest	Middle third of linea aspera	Obturator n.	Adducts and flexes thigh
Adductor brevis	Body and inferior pubic ramus	Pectineal line; upper part of linea aspera	Obturator n.	Adducts and flexes thigh
Adductor magnus	Ischiopubic ramus; ischial tuberosity	Linea aspera; medial supracondylar line; adductor tubercle	Obturator and sciatic n.n.	Adducts, flexes, and extends thigh
Pectineus	Pectineal line of pubis	Pectineal line of femur	Obturator and femoral nn.	Adducts and flexes thigh
Gracilis	Body and inferior pubic ramus	Medial surface of upper quarter of tibia	Obturator n.	Adducts and flexes thigh; flexes and rotates leg medially
Obturator externus	Margin of obturator foramen and obturator membrane	Intertrochanteric fossa of femur	Obturator n.	Rotates thigh laterally

10. Anterior and Lateral Muscles of the Leg

Muscle	Origin	Insertion	Nerve	Action
Anterior:				
Tibialis anterior	Lateral tibial condyle; interosseous membrane	First cuneiform; first metatarsal	Deep peroneal n.	Dorsiflexes and inverts foot
Extensor hallucis longus	Middle half of anterior surface of fibula; interosseous membrane	Base of distal phalanx of big toe	Deep peroneal n.	Extends big toe; dorsiflexes and inverts foot

(continued)

Muscle	Origin	Insertion	Nerve	Action
Extensor digitorum longus	Lateral tibial condyle; upper two-thirds of fibula; interosseous membrane	Bases of middle and distal phalanges	Deep peroneal n.	Extends toes; dorsiflexes foot
Peroneus tertius	Distal one-third of fibula; interosseous membrane	Base of fifth metatarsal	Deep peroneal n.	Dorsiflexes and everts foot
Lateral:				
Peroneus longus	Lateral tibial condyle; head and upper lateral side of fibula	Base of first metatarsal; medial cuneiform	Superficial peroneal n.	Everts and plantar flexes foot
Peroneus brevis	Lower lateral side of fibula; intermuscular septa	Base of fifth metatarsal	Superficial peroneal n.	Everts and plantar flexes foot

11. Posterior Muscles of the Leg

Muscle	Origin	Insertion	Nerve	Action
Superficial group:				
Gastrocnemius	Lateral (lateral head) and medial (medial head) femoral condyles	Posterior aspect of calcaneus via tendo calcaneus	Tibial n.	Flexes knee; plantar flexes foot
Soleus	Upper fibula head; soleal line on tibia	Posterior aspect of calcaneus via tendo calcaneus	Tibial n.	Plantar flexes foot
Plantaris	Lower lateral supracondylar line	Posterior surface of calcaneus	Tibial n.	Flexes and rotates leg medially
Deep group:				
Popliteus	Lateral condyle of femur; popliteal ligament	Upper posterior side of tibia	Tibial n.	Flexes and rotates leg medially
Flexor hallucis longus	Lower two-thirds of fibula; interosseous membrane; intermuscular septa	Base of distal phalanx of big toe	Tibial n.	Flexes distal phalanx of big toe
Flexor digitorum longus	Middle posterior aspect of tibia	Distal phalanges of lateral four toes	Tibial n.	Flexes lateral four toes; plantar flexes foot

(continued)

APPENDICES

Muscle	Origin	Insertion	Nerve	Action
Tibialis posterior	Interosseous membrane; upper parts of tibia and fibula	Tuberosity of navicular; sustentacula tali; three cuneiforms; cuboid; bases of metatarsals 2–4	Tibial n.	Plantar flexes and inverts foot

12. Muscles of the Foot

Muscle	Origin	Insertion	Nerve	Action
Dorsum of foot:				
Extensor digitorum brevis	Dorsal surface of calcaneus	Tendons of extensor digitorum longus	Deep peroneal n.	Extends toes
Extensor hallucis brevis	Dorsal surface of calcaneus	Base of proximal phalanx of big toe	Deep peroneal n.	Extends big toe
Sole of foot:				
Abductor hallucis	Medial tubercle of calcaneus	Base of proximal phalanx of big toe	Medial plantar n.	Abducts big toe
Flexor digitorum brevis	Medial tubercle of calcaneus	Middle phalanges of lateral four toes	Medial plantar n.	Flexes middle phalanges of lateral four toes
Abductor digiti minimi	Medial and lateral tubercles of calcaneus	Proximal phalanx of little toe	Lateral plantar n.	Abducts little toe
Quadratus plantae	Medial and lateral side of calcaneus	Tendons of flexor digitorum longus	Lateral plantar n.	Aids in flexing toes
Lumbricals (4)	Tendons of flexor digitorum longus	Proximal phalanges; extensor expansion	First by medial plantar n.; lateral three by lateral plantar n.	Flex metatarso-phalangeal joints and extend interphalangeal joints
Flexor hallucis brevis	Cuboid; third cuneiform	Proximal phalanx of big toe	Medial plantar n.	Flexes big toe
Adductor hallucis:				
Oblique head	Bases of metatarsals 2–4	Proximal phalanx of big toe	Lateral plantar n.	Adducts big toe
Transverse head	Capsule of lateral four metatarso-phalangeal joints			

(continued)

Muscle	Origin	Insertion	Nerve	Action
Flexor digiti minimi brevis	Base of metatarsal 5	Proximal phalanx of little toe	Lateral plantar n.	Flexes little toe
Plantar interossei (3)	Medial sides of metatarsals 3–5	Medial sides of base of proximal phalanges 3–5	Lateral plantar n.	Adduct toes; flex proximal and extend distal phalanges
Dorsal interossei (4)	Adjacent shafts of metatarsals	Proximal phalanges of second toes (medial and lateral sides), and third and fourth toes (lateral sides)	Lateral plantar n.	Abduct toes; flex proximal, and extend distal phalanges

13. Muscles of the Throacic Wall

Muscle	Origin	Insertion	Nerve	Action
External intercostals	Lower border of ribs	Upper border of rib below	Intercostal n.	Elevate ribs in inspiration
Internal intercostals	Lower border of ribs	Upper border of rib below	Intercostal n.	Depress ribs; interchondral part elevates ribs
Innermost intercostals	Lower border of ribs	Upper border of rib below	Intercostal n.	Elevate ribs
Transverse thoracic	Posterior surface of lower sternum and xiphoid	Inner surface of costal cartilages 2–6	Intercostal n.	Depresses ribs
Subcostalis	Inner surface of lower ribs near their angles	Upper borders of ribs 2 or 3 below	Intercostal n.	Elevates ribs
Levator costarum	Transverse processes of T7–T11	Subjacent ribs between tubercle and angle	Dorsal primary rami of C8–T11	Elevates ribs

14. Muscles of the Anterior Abdominal Wall

Muscle	Origin	Insertion	Nerve	Action
External oblique	External surface of lower eight ribs (5–12)	Anterior half of iliac crest; anterior superior iliac spine; pubic tubercle; linea alba	Intercostal n. (T7–T11); subcostal n. (T12)	Compresses abdomen; flexes trunk; active in forced expiration
Internal oblique	Lateral two-thirds of inguinal ligament; iliac crest; thoracolumbar fascia	Lower four costal cartilages; linea alba; pubic crest; pectineal line	Intercostal n. (T7–T11); subcostal n. (T12); iliohypogastric and ilioinguinal nn. (L1)	Compresses abdomen; flexes trunk; active in forced expiration

APPENDICES

(continued)

Muscle	Origin	Insertion	Nerve	Action
Transverse	Lateral one-third of inguinal ligament; iliac crest; thoracolumbar fascia; lower six costal cartilages	Linea alba; pubic crest; pectineal line	Intercostal n. (T7–T12); subcostal n. (T12); iliohypogastric and ilioinguinal nn. (L1)	Compresses abdomen; depresses ribs
Rectus abdominis	Pubic crest and pubic symphysis	Xiphoid process and costal cartilages 5–7	Intercostal n. (T7–T11); subcostal n. (T12)	Depresses ribs; flexes trunk
Pyramidalis	Pubic body	Linea alba	Subcostal n. (T12)	Tenses linea alba
Cremaster	Middle of inguinal ligament; lower margin of internal oblique muscle	Pubic tubercle and crest	Genitofemoral n.	Retracts testis

15. Muscles of the Posterior Abdominal Wall

Muscle	Origin	Insertion	Nerve	Action
Quadratus lumborum	Transverse processes of L3–L5; iliolumbar ligament; iliac crest	Lower border of last rib; transverse processes of L1–L3	Subcostal n.; L1–L3	Depresses rib 12; flexes trunk laterally
Psoas major	Transverse processes, intervertebral disks and bodies of T12–L5	Lesser trochanter	L2–L3	Flexes thigh and trunk
Psoas minor	Bodies and intervertebral disks of T12–L1	Pectineal line; iliopectineal eminence	L1	Aids in flexing of trunk

16. Superficial Muscles of the Back

Muscle	Origin	Insertion	Nerve	Action
Trapezius	External occipital protuberance, superior nuchal line, ligamentum nuchae, spines of C7–T12	Spine of scapula, acromion, and lateral third of clavicle	Spinal accessory n., C3–C4	Adducts, rotates, elevates, and depresses scapula
Levator scapulae	Transverse processes of C1–C4	Medial border of scapula	Nerves to levator scapulae, C3–C4, dorsal scapular n.	Elevates scapula

(continued)

Muscle	Origin	Insertion	Nerve	Action
Rhomboid minor	Spines of C7–T1	Root of spine of scapula	Dorsal scapular n., C5	Adducts scapula
Rhomboid major	Spines of T2–T5	Medial border of scapula	Dorsal scapular n.	Adducts scapula
Latissimus dorsi	Spines of T5–T12, thoracodorsal fascia, iliac crest, ribs 9–12	Floor of bicipital groove of humerus	Thoracodorsal n.	Adducts, extends, and rotates arm medially
Serratus posterior-superior	Ligamentum nuchae, supraspinal ligament, and spines of C7–T3	Upper border of ribs 2–5	Intercostal n., T1–T4	Elevates ribs
Serratus posterior-inferior	Supraspinous ligament and spines of T11–L3	Lower border of ribs 9–12	Intercostal n., T9–T12	Depresses ribs

17. Suboccipital Muscles

Muscle	Origin	Insertion	Nerve	Action
Rectus capitis posterior major	Spine of axis	Lateral portion of inferior nuchal line	Suboccipital n.	Extends, rotates, and flexes head laterally
Rectus capitis posterior minor	Posterior tubercle of atlas	Occipital bone below inferior nuchal line	Suboccipital n.	Extends and flexes head laterally
Obliquus capitis superior	Transverse process of atlas	Occipital bone above inferior nuchal line	Suboccipital n.	Extends, rotates, and flexes head laterally
Obliquus capitis inferior	Spine of axis	Transverse process of atlas	Suboccipital n.	Extends head and rotates it laterally

18. Muscles of the Neck

Muscle	Origin	Insertion	Nerve	Action
Cervical muscles:				
Platysma	Superficial fascia over upper part of deltoid and pectoralis major	Mandible; skin and muscles over mandible and angle of mouth	Facial n.	Depresses lower jaw and lip and angle of mouth; wrinkles skin of neck
Sterno-cleidomastoid	Manubrium sterni and medial one-third of clavicle	Mastoid process and lateral one-half of superior nuchal line	Spinal accessory n.; C2–C3 (sensory)	Singly turns face toward opposite side; together flex head, raise thorax

APPENDICES

(continued)

Muscle	Origin	Insertion	Nerve	Action
Suprahyoid muscles:				
Digastric	Anterior belly from digastric fossa of mandible; posterior belly from mastoid notch	Intermediate tendon attached to body of hyoid	Posterior belly by facial n.; anterior belly by mylohyoid n. of trigeminal n.	Elevates hyoid and tongue; depresses mandible
Mylohyoid	Mylohyoid line of mandible	Median raphe and body of hyoid bone	Mylohyoid n. of trigeminal n.	Elevates hyoid and tongue; depresses mandible
Stylohyoid	Styloid process	Body of hyoid	Facial n.	Elevates hyoid
Geniohyoid	Genial tubercle of mandible	Body of hyoid	C1 via hypoglossal n.	Elevates hyoid and tongue
Infrahyoid muscles:				
Sternohyoid	Manubrium sterni and medial end of clavicle	Body of hyoid	Ansa cervicalis	Depresses hyoid and larynx
Sternothyroid	Manubrium sterni; first costal cartilage	Oblique line of thyroid cartilage	Ansa cervicalis	Depresses thyroid cartilage and larynx
Thyrohyoid	Oblique line of thyroid cartilage	Body and greater horn of hyoid	C1 via hypoglossal n.	Depresses and retracts hyoid and larynx
Omohyoid	Inferior belly from medial lip of suprascapular notch and suprascapular ligament; superior belly from intermediate tendon	Inferior belly to intermediate tendon; superior belly to body of hyoid	Ansa cervicalis	Depresses and retracts hyoid and larynx

19. Prevertebral Muscles

Muscle	Origin	Insertion	Nerve	Action
Lateral vertebral:				
Anterior scalene	Transverse processes of CV3–CV6	Scalene tubercle on first rib	Lower cervical (C5–C8)	Elevates first rib; bends neck
Middle scalene	Transverse processes of CV2–CV7	Upper surface of first rib	Lower cervical (C5–C8)	Elevates first rib; bends neck
Posterior scalene	Transverse processes of CV4–CV6	Outer surface of second rib	Lower cervical (C6–C8)	Elevates second rib; bends neck

(continued)

Muscle	Origin	Insertion	Nerve	Action
Anterior vertebral:				
Longus capitus	Transverse processes of CV3–CV6	Basilar part of occipital bone	C1–C4	Flexes and rotates head
Longus colli (L. cervicis)	Transverse processes and bodies of CV3–TV3	Anterior tubercle of atlas; bodies of CV2–CV4; transverse process of CV5–CV6	C2–C6	Flexes and rotates head
Rectus capitis anterior	Lateral mass of atlas	Basilar part of occipital bone	C1–C2	Flexes and rotates head
Rectus capitis lateralis	Transverse process of atlas	Jugular process of occipital bone	C1–C2	Flexes head laterally

20. Muscles of Facial Expression

Muscle	Origin	Insertion	Nerve	Action
Occipito-frontalis	Superior nuchal line; upper orbital margin	Epicranial aponeurosis	Facial n.	Elevates eyebrows; wrinkles forehead (surprise)
Corrugator supercilii	Medial supraorbital margin	Skin of medial eyebrow	Facial n.	Draws eyebrows downward medially (anger, frowning)
Orbicularis oculi	Medial orbital margin; medial palpebral ligament; lacrimal bone	Skin and rim of orbit; tarsal plate; lateral palpebral raphe	Facial n.	Closes eyelids (squinting)
Procerus	Nasal bone and cartilage	Skin between eyebrows	Facial n.	Wrinkles skin over bones (sadness)
Nasalis	Maxilla lateral to incisive fossa	Ala of nose	Facial n.	Draws ala of nose toward septum
Depressor septi*	Incisive fossa of maxilla	Ala and nasal septum	Facial n.	Constricts nares
Orbicularis oris	Maxilla above incisor teeth	Skin of lip	Facial n.	Closes lips
Levator anguli oris	Canine fossa of maxilla	Angle of mouth	Facial n.	Elevates angle of mouth medially (disgust)
Levator labii superioris	Maxilla above infraorbital foramen	Skin of upper lip	Facial n.	Elevates upper lip; dilates nares (disgust)
Levator labii superioris alaeque nasi*	Frontal process of maxilla	Skin of upper lip	Facial n.	Elevates ala of nose and upper lip

APPENDICES

(continued)

Muscle	Origin	Insertion	Nerve	Action
Zygomaticus major	Zygomatic arch	Angle of mouth	Facial n.	Draws angle of mouth backward and upward (smile)
Zygomaticus minor	Zygomatic arch	Angle of mouth	Facial n.	Elevates upper lip
Depressor labii inferioris	Mandible below mental foramen	Orbicularis oris and skin of lower lip	Facial n.	Depresses lower lip
Depressor anguli oris	Oblique line of mandible	Angle of mouth	Facial n.	Depresses angle of mouth
Risorius	Fascia over masseter	Angle of mouth	Facial n.	Retracts angle of mouth (false smile)
Buccinator	Mandible; pterygomandibular raphe; alveolar processes	Angle of mouth	Facial n.	Presses cheek to keep it taut
Mentalis	Incisive fossa of mandible	Skin of chin	Facial n.	Elevates and protrudes lower lip
Auricularis anterior, superior, and posterior*	Temporal fascia; epicranial aponeurosis; mastoid process	Anterior, superior, and posterior sides of auricle	Facial n.	Retract and elevate ear

*Indicates less important muscles.

21. Muscles of Mastication

Muscle	Origin	Insertion	Nerve	Action
Temporalis	Temporal fossa	Coronoid process and ramus of mandible	Trigeminal n.	Elevates and retracts mandible
Masseter	Lower border and medial surface of zygomatic arch	Lateral surface of coronoid process, ramus and angle of mandible	Trigeminal n.	Elevates mandible
Lateral pterygoid	Superior head from infratemporal surface of sphenoid; inferior head from lateral surface of lateral pterygoid plate of sphenoid	Neck of mandible; articular disk and capsule of temporo-mandibular joint	Trigeminal n.	Protracts (protrudes) and depresses mandible

(continued)

Muscle	Origin	Insertion	Nerve	Action
Medial pterygoid	Tuber of maxilla; medial surface of lateral pterygoid plate; pyramidal process of palatine bone	Medial surface of angle and ramus of mandible	Trigeminal n.	Protracts (protrudes) and elevates mandible

The jaws are opened by the lateral pterygoid muscle and are closed by the temporalis, masseter, and medial pterygoid muscles.

22. Muscles of Eye Movement

Muscle	Origin	Insertion	Nerve	Action
Superior rectus	Common tendinous ring	Sclera just behind cornea	Oculomotor n.	Elevates eyeball
Inferior rectus	Common tendinous ring	Sclera just behind cornea	Oculomotor n.	Depresses eyeball
Medial rectus	Common tendinous ring	Sclera just behind cornea	Oculomotor n.	Adducts eyeball
Lateral rectus	Common tendinous ring	Sclera just behind cornea	Abducens n.	Abducts eyeball
Levator palpebrae superioris	Lesser wing of sphenoid above and anterior to optic canal	Tarsal plate and skin of upper eyelid	Oculomotor n.	Elevates upper eyelid
Superior oblique	Body of sphenoid bone above optic canal	Sclera beneath superior rectus	Trochlear n.	Rotates downward and medially; depresses adducted eye
Inferior oblique	Floor of orbit lateral to lacrimal groove	Sclera beneath lateral rectus	Oculomotor n.	Rotates upward and laterally; elevates adducted eye

23. Muscles of the Palate

Muscle	Origin	Insertion	Nerve	Action
Tensor veli palatini	Scaphoid fossa; spine of sphenoid; cartilage of auditory tube	Tendon hooks around hamulus of medial pterygoid plate to insert into aponeurosis of soft palate	Mandibular branch of trigeminal n.	Tenses soft palate
Levator veli palatini	Petrous part of temporal bone; cartilage of auditory tube	Aponeurosis of soft palate	Vagus n. via pharyngeal plexus	Elevates soft palate
Palatoglossus	Aponeurosis of soft palate	Dorsolateral side of tongue	Vagus n. via pharyngeal plexus	Elevates tongue
Palato-pharyngeus	Aponeurosis of soft palate	Thyroid cartilage and side of pharynx	Vagus n. via pharyngeal plexus	Elevates pharynx; closes nasopharynx

(continued)

Muscle	Origin	Insertion	Nerve	Action
Musculus uvulae	Posterior nasal spine of palatine bone; palatine aponeurosis	Mucous membrane of uvula	Vagus n. via pharyngeal plexus	Elevates uvula

24. Muscles of the Tongue

Muscle	Origin	Insertion	Nerve	Action
Styloglossus	Styloid process	Side and inferior aspect of tongue	Hypoglossal n.	Retracts and elevates tongue
Hyoglossus	Body and greater horn of hyoid bone	Side and inferior aspect of tongue	Hypoglossal n.	Depresses and retracts tongue
Genioglossus	Genial tubercle of mandible	Inferior aspect of tongue; body of hyoid bone	Hypoglossal n.	Protrudes and depresses tongue
Palatoglossus	Aponeurosis of soft palate	Dorsolateral side of tongue	Vagus n. via pharyngeal plexus	Elevates tongue

25. Muscles of the Pharynx

Muscle	Origin	Insertion	Nerve	Action
Circular muscles:				
Superior constrictor	Medial pterygoid plate; pterygoid hamulus; pterygo-mandibular raphe; mylohyoid line of mandible; side of tongue	Median raphe and phryngeal tubercle of skull	Vagus n. via pharyngeal plexus	Constricts upper pharynx
Middle constrictor	Greater and lesser horns of hyoid; stylohyoid ligament	Median raphe	Vagus n. via pharyngeal plexus	Constricts lower pharynx
Inferior constrictor	Arch of cricoid and oblique line of thyroid cartilages	Median raphe of pharynx	Vagus n. via pharyngeal plexus, recurrent and external laryngeal n.	Constricts lower pharynx
Longitudinal muscles:				
Stylo-pharyngeus	Styloid process	Thyroid cartilage and muscles of pharynx	Glossopharyn-geal n.	Elevates pharynx and larynx

(continued)

Muscle	Origin	Insertion	Nerve	Action
Palato-pharyngeus	Hard palate; aponeurosis of soft palate	Thyroid cartilage and muscles of pharynx	Vagus n. via pharyngeal plexus	Elevates pharynx and closes nasopharynx
Salpingo-pharyngeus	Cartilage of auditory tube	Muscles of pharynx	Vagus n. via pharyngeal plexus	Elevates nasopharynx; opens auditory tube

26. Muscles of the Larynx

Muscle	Origin	Insertion	Nerve	Action on Vocal Cord
Cricothyroid	Arch of cricoid cartilage	Inferior horn and lower lamina of thyroid cartilage	External laryngeal n.	Tenses
Posterior cricoarytenoid	Posterior surface of lamina of cricoid cartilage	Muscular process of arytenoid cartilage	Recurrent laryngeal n.	Abducts
Lateral cricoarytenoid	Arch of cricoid cartilage	Muscular process of arytenoid cartilage	Recurrent laryngeal n.	Adducts
Transverse arytenoid	Posterior surface of arytenoid cartilage	Opposite arytenoid cartilage	Recurrent laryngeal n.	Adducts
Oblique arytenoid	Muscular process of arytenoid cartilage	Apex of opposite arytenoid	Recurrent laryngeal n.	Adducts
Aryepiglottic	Apex of arytenoid cartilage	Side of epiglottic cartilage	Recurrent laryngeal n.	Adducts
Thyroarytenoid	Inner surface of thyroid lamina	Anterolateral surface of arytenoid cartilage	Recurrent laryngeal n.	Adducts, relaxes
Thyroepiglottic	Anteromedial surface of lamina of thryoid cartilate	Lateral margin of epiglottic cartilage	Recurrent laryngeal n.	Adducts
Vocalis	Anteromedial surface of lamina of thyroid cartilage	Vocal process	Recurrent laryngeal n.	Adducts and tenses

From Chung KW. Gross anatomy, 3rd ed. Baltimore: Williams & Wilkins, 1995.

APPENDICES

NORMAL RANGE OF MOTION (IN DEGREES) ACCORDING TO VARIOUS AUTHORS*

Joint	AAOS	Boone and Azen	Clark	CMA	Daniels and Worthing-ham	Dorinson and Wagner	Esch and Lepley	Gerhardt and Russe	Hoppen-feld	JAMA	Kapandji	Kendall and McCreary	Wiechec and Krusen
Shoulder													
Flexion	180	167	130	170	–	180	170	170	–	150	180	180	180
Extension	60	62	80	30	50	45	60	50	45	40	50	45	45
Abduction	180	184	180	170	–	180	170	170	180	150	180	180	180
Internal rotation	70	69	90†	60†	90	90	80	80	55	40†	95	70	90
External rotation	90	104	40†	80†	90	90	90	90	45	90†	80	–	90
Horizontal abduction	–	45	–	–	–	–	–	30	–	–	–	–	–
Horizontal adduction	135	140	–	–	–	–	–	135	–	–	–	–	–
Elbow													
Flexion	150	143	150	135	160	145	150	150	150	150	145	145	135
Radioulnar													
Pronation	80	76	50	75	90	80	90	80	90	80	85	90	90
Supination	80	82	90	85	90	70	90	90	90	80	90	90	90
Wrist													
Flexion	80	76	80	70	90	80	90	60	80	70	85	80	60
Extension	70	75	70	65	90	55	70	50	70	60	85	70	55
Radial deviation	20	22	15	20	25	20	20	20	20	20	15	20	35
Ulnar deviation	30	36	30	40	65	40	30	30	30	30	–	35	75

Hip													
Flexion	120	125	120	100	135	125	130	125	125	110	120	122	120
Extension	45	10	30	30	30	15	45	50	15	30	20	10	30
Abduction	45	45	40	40	50	45	45	45	45	50	55	46	45
Adduction	–	10	20	20	30	15	15	20	0	30	45	27	30
Internal rotation	–	45	30	40	35	45	33	30	45	35	20	47	45
External rotation	–	45	60	50	45	45	36	50	45	50	45	47	45
Knee													
Flexion	135	140	160	120	135	130	135	140	130	135	145	143	135
Ankle													
Plantar Flexion	55	45	50	40	50	45	65	45	45	50	50	56	50
Dorsiflexion	30	20	30	20	20	20	10	20	–	15	15	13	20
Subtalar Joint													
Inversion	–	35	30	30	–	40	30	50	–	35	–	37	35
Eversion	–	20	30	20	–	20	15	20	–	20	–	26	15

*References for the normal values: American Academy of Orthopaedic Surgeons. Joint motion: Method of measuring and recording. Chicago: AAOS, 1965; Boone DC, Azen SP. Normal range of motion in male subjects. J Bone Joint Surg 1979; 61A: 756; Clark WA. A system of joint measurement. J Orthop Surg 1920; 2:687; Commission of California Medical Association (CMA) and The Industrial Accident Commission of the State of California: Evaluation of industrial disability. New York: Oxford University Press, 1960; Daniels L, Worthingham C. Muscle testing: Techniques of manual examination. 3rd ed. Philadelphia: WB Saunders, 1972; Dorinson SM, Wagner ML. An exact technique for clinically measuring and recording joint motion. 1948; Arch Phys Med 29:468; Esch D, Lepley M. Evaluation of joint motion: Methods of measurement and recording. Minneapolis: University of Minnesota Press, 1974; Gerhardt JJ, Russe OA. International SFTR method of measuring and recording joint motion. Bern: Huber, 1975; Hoppenfeld S. Physical examination of the spine and extremities. New York: Appleton-Century-Crofts, 1976; Journal of the American Medical Association: A guide to the evaluation of permanent impairment of the extremities and back. JAMA 1958: (special edition) 1; Kapandji LA. Physiology of the joints. Vols. 1 and 2, 2nd ed. London: Churchill Livingstone, 1970; Kendall FP, McCreary EK. Muscles, testing and function, 3rd ed. Baltimore: Williams & Wilkins, 1983; Wiechec FJ, Krusen FH. A new method of joint measurement and a review of the literature. Am J Surg 1939; 43:659.

†Measurements obtained with the shoulder in 0 degrees of abduction.

From Rothstein JM, Roy SH, Wolf SL. The rehabilitation specialist's handbook. Philadelphia: F. A. Davis Company, 1991.

APPENDICES

Anatomic Planes

A plane is a flat surface formed by making a cut (imaginary or real) through the body or a part of it. In radiography, various planes are used as points of reference that assist in localizing areas of the body to permit specific centering guidelines. The major anatomic planes used in radiographic positioning are as follows:

Longitudinal plane
Made by cutting along the long (longitudinal) axis of the body or body part. In the erect position, this plane is termed *vertical* and is perpendicular to the horizontal.

Transverse plane
Made by cutting across the body or body part crosswise (at a right angle to the long axis). If the patient is erect, this plane is termed *horizontal* (parallel to the horizon).

Midsagittal or median plane
Longitudinal plane made by cutting from front (anterior) to back (posterior) along the median line of the body and along the sagittal suture of the skull.

Sagittal plane
Longitudinal plane made by cutting from front (anterior) to back (posterior) on either side of the sagittal suture and parallel to the midsagittal or median plane.

Coronal plane
Longitudinal plane made by cutting lengthwise from side to side through the head and body (or body part) along the coronal suture of the skull or parallel to it. The coronal suture lies behind the frontal bone and extends toward the sides of the skull.

Transpyloric plane
Transverse plane made by cutting across the body from one side to the other at the level of the 9th costal cartilages. The plane is situated about halfway between the superior border of the sternum (manubrial, or sternal, notch) and the symphysis pubis (junction of the two anterior or superior portions of the pubic bones). The name of this plane reflects the fact that it should cut across the pylorus of the stomach.

Midcoronal (midaxillary) plane
Longitudinal plane made by cutting through the head and body along the coronal suture of the head and extending the cut down the body.

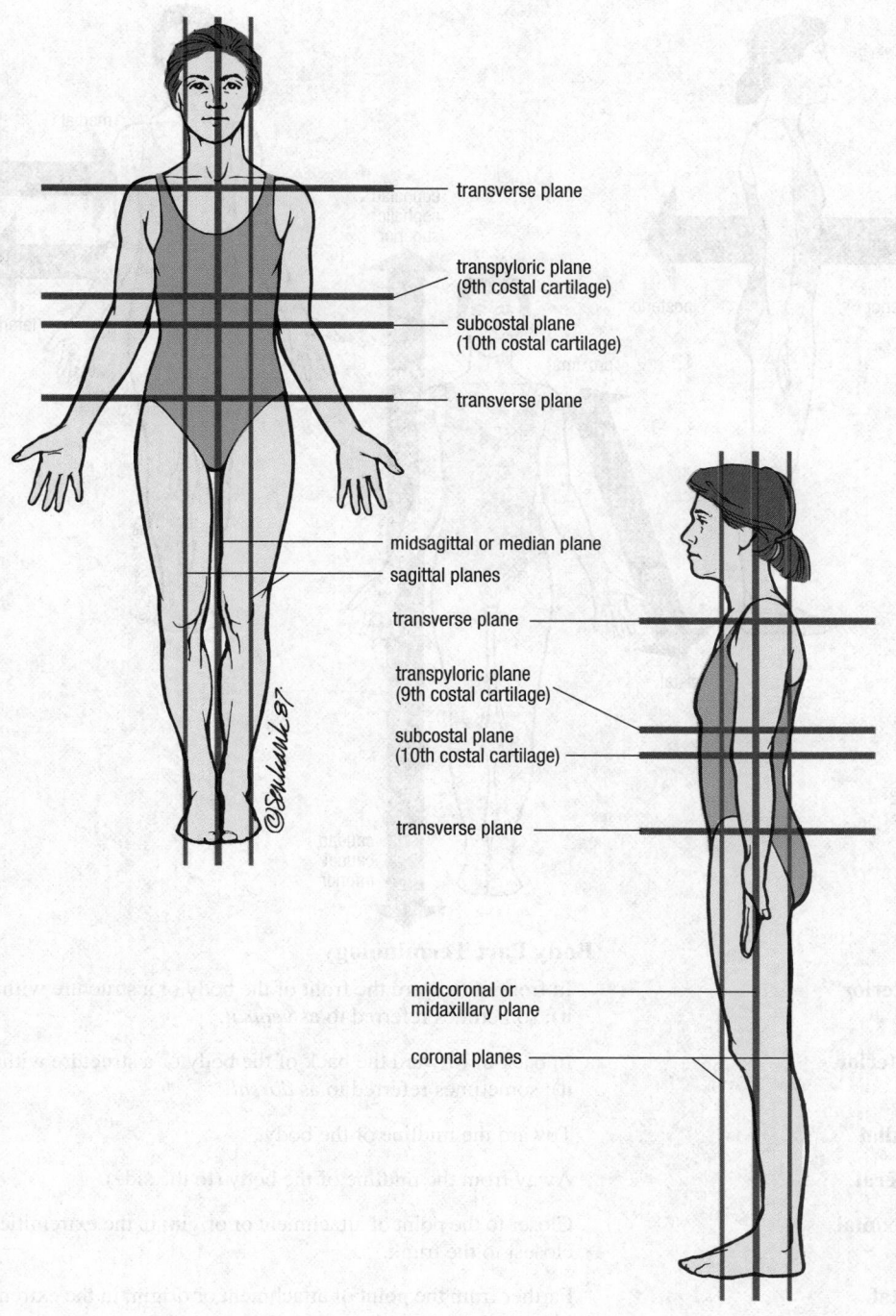

transverse plane

transpyloric plane
(9th costal cartilage)

subcostal plane
(10th costal cartilage)

transverse plane

midsagittal or median plane

sagittal planes

transverse plane

transpyloric plane
(9th costal cartilage)

subcostal plane
(10th costal cartilage)

transverse plane

midcoronal or
midaxillary plane

coronal planes

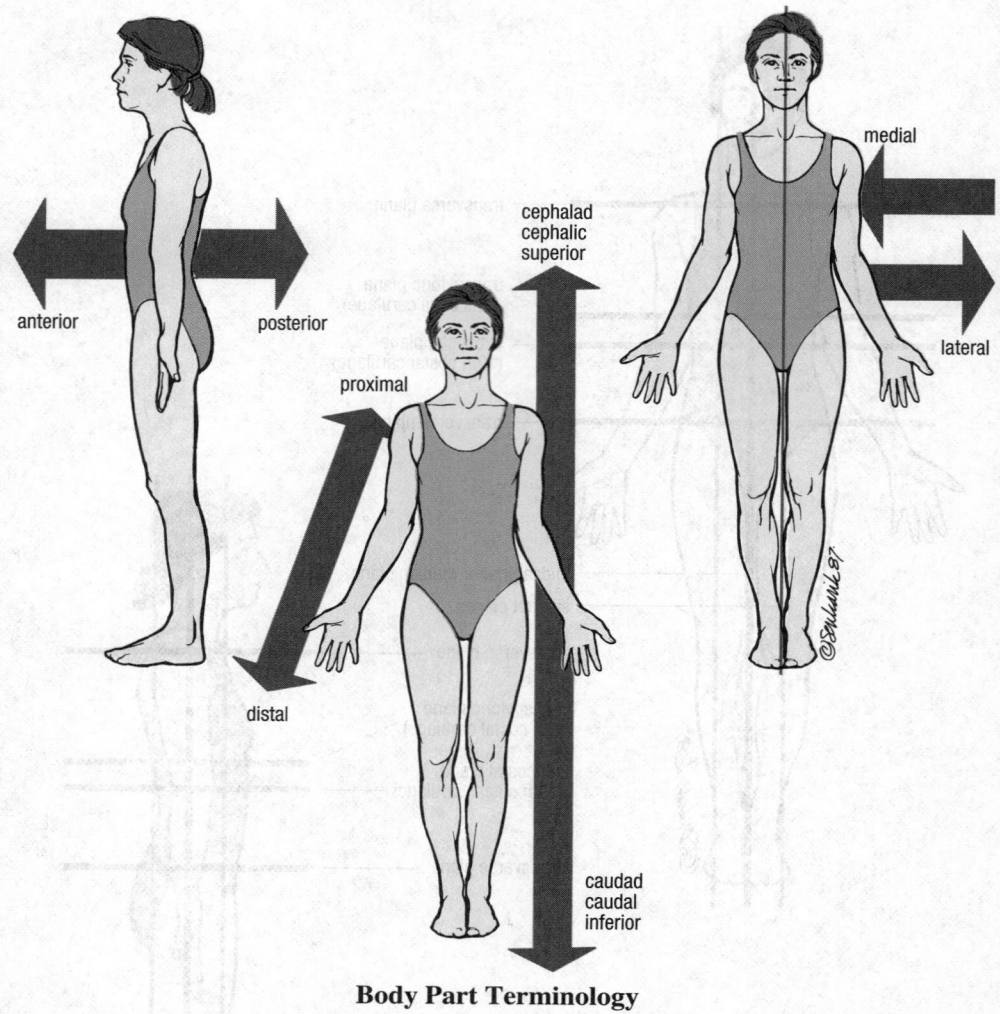

Body Part Terminology

Anterior	In front of (toward the front of the body or a structure within it); sometimes referred to as *ventral*.
Posterior	In back of (toward the back of the body or a structure within it); sometimes referred to as *dorsal*.
Medial	Toward the midline of the body.
Lateral	Away from the midline of the body (to the side).
Proximal	Closer to the point of attachment or origin; in the extremities, closest to the trunk.
Distal	Farther from the point of attachment or origin; in the extremities, farthest from the trunk.
Cephalad, cephalic, superior	Toward the head or the upper part of a structure.
Caudad, caudal, inferior	Away from the head or the lower part of a structure (literally means "toward the tail").

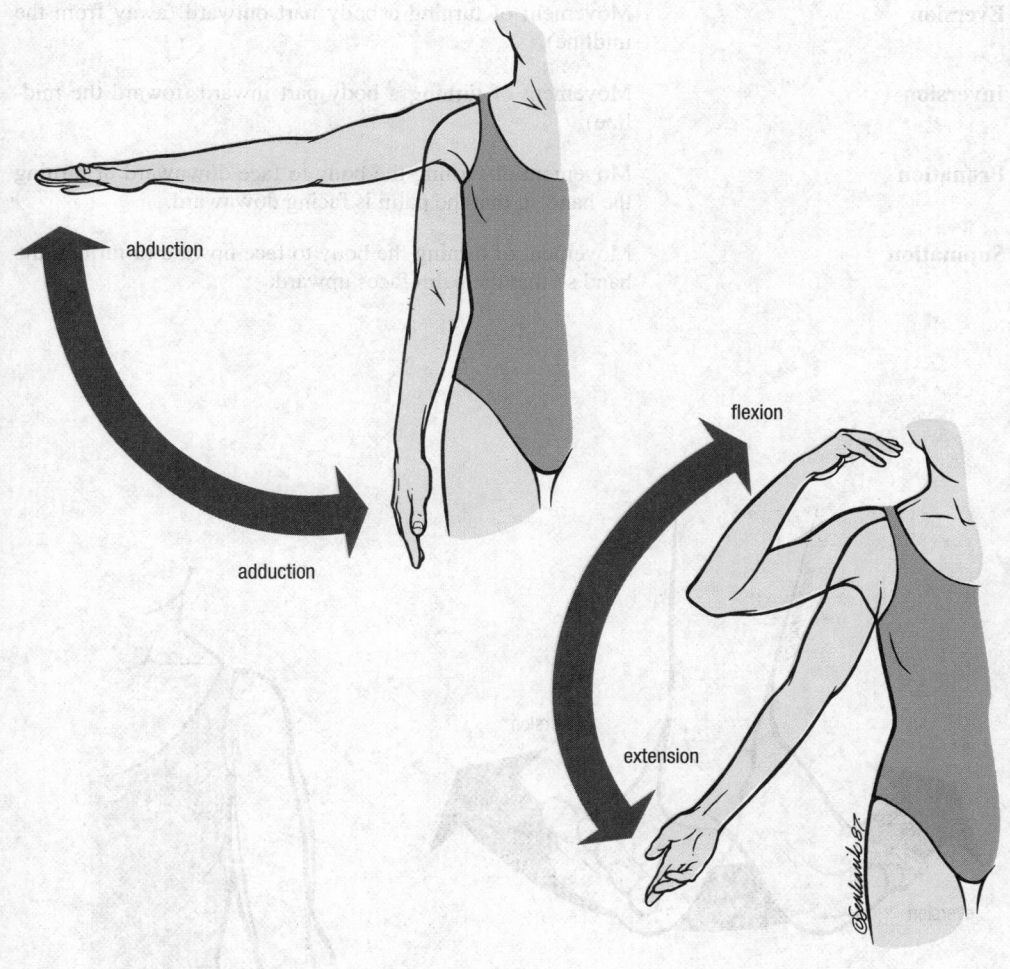

Body Movement

Abduction   Movement of a limb or body part further from or away from the midline of the body.

Adduction   Movement of a limb or body part closer to or toward the midline of the body.

Extension   Straightening of a joint or extremity so that the angle between contiguous (adjoining) bones is increased.

Flexion   Bending of a joint or extremity so that the angle between contiguous (adjoining) bones is decreased.

Eversion   Movement of turning a body part outward (away from the midline).

Inversion   Movement of turning a body part inward (toward the midline).

Pronation   Movement of turning the body to face downward or turning the hand so that the palm is facing downward.

Supination   Movement of turning the body to face upward or turning the hand so that the palm faces upward.

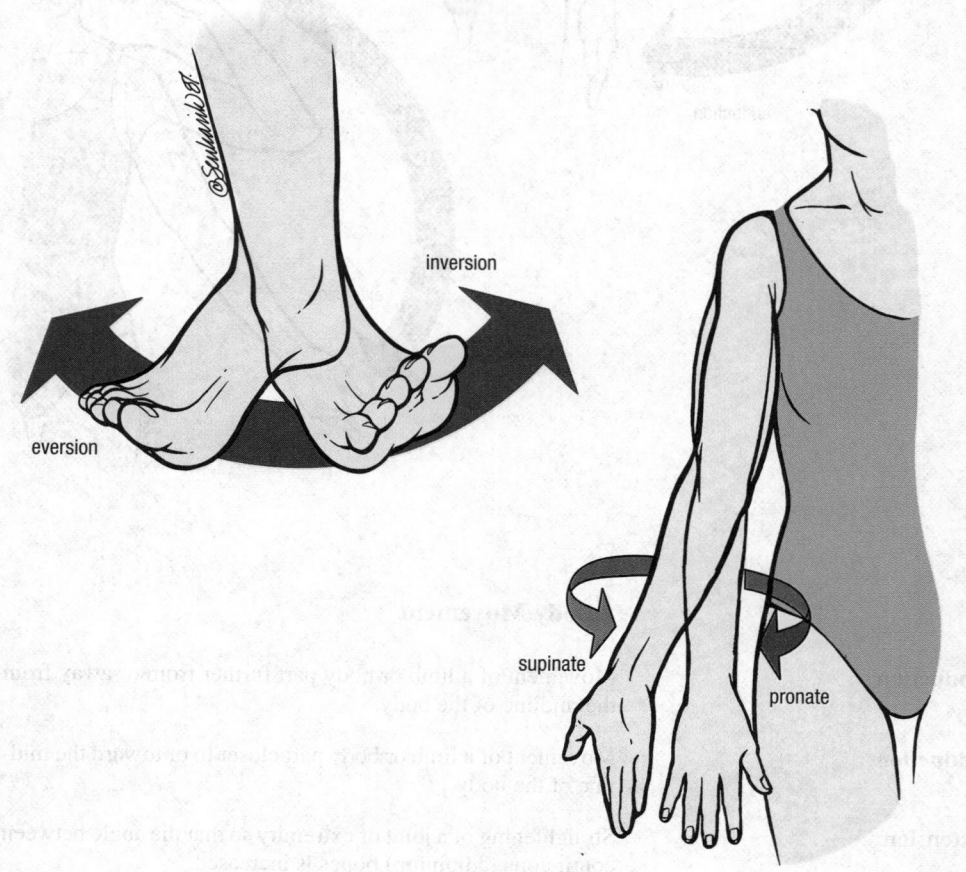

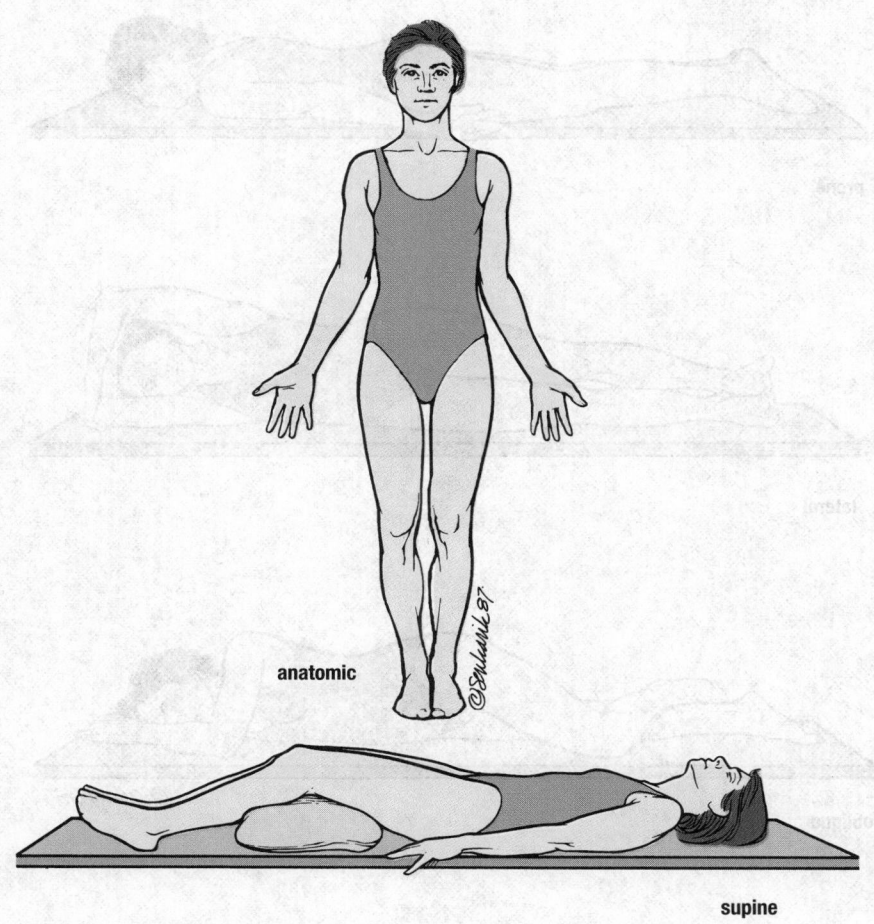

anatomic

supine

Positioning Terminology

Anatomic position

Position of the body when the subject is facing the front in the erect position with the arms and legs fully extended. The palms of the hands are facing forward and the feet are together. In radiography, this term is used as the reference position of the body to describe the various different positions.

Supine position

Position in which the subject is lying on the back with the face up. Sometimes referred to as the *dorsal recumbent* (lying down) or *dorsal decubitus* position, since the back (dorsal surface) of the body is dependent (nearer the table).

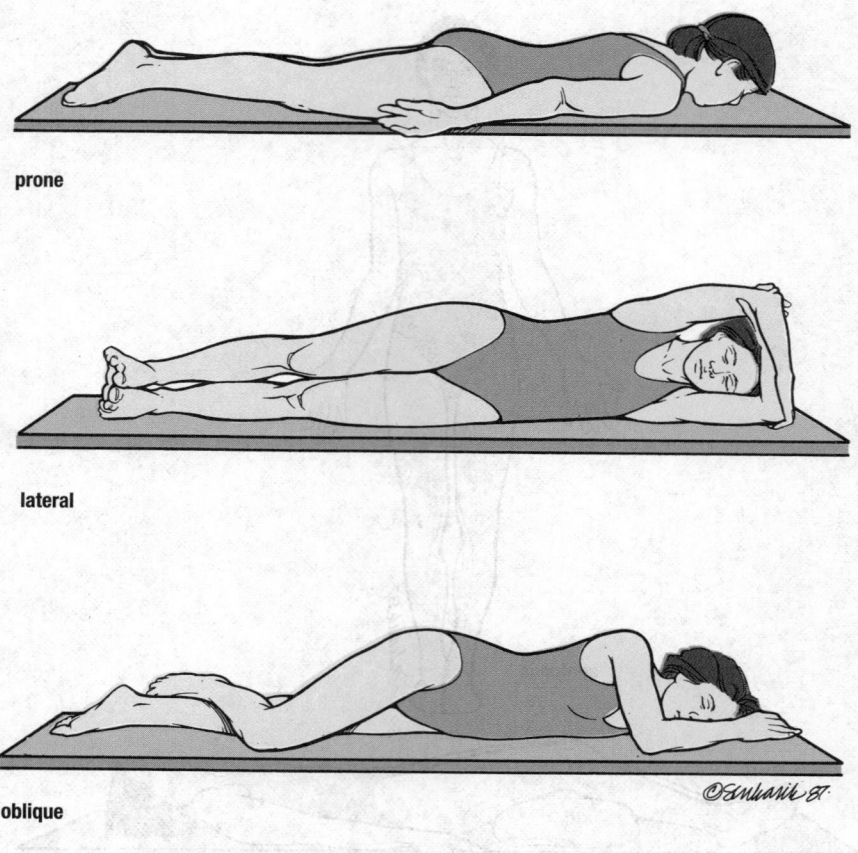

prone

lateral

oblique

Prone position

Position in which the subject is lying face down on the front of the body. Sometimes referred to as the *ventral recumbent* or *ventral decubitus* position, since the front (ventral surface) of the body is dependent (nearer the table).

Lateral position

Position in which the side of the subject is next to the film. A lateral position is named by the side of the subject that is situated adjacent to the film. Sometimes referred to as an *erect lateral* if the subject is sitting or standing and a *lateral recumbent* or *lateral decubitus* if the subject is lying down.

Oblique position

Position in which the subject is neither prone nor supine, but rotated somewhere in between. In radiographic terminology, the subject is in a posterior oblique position if some part of the posterior surface of the body is closer to the film, and in an anterior oblique position if some part of the anterior surface of the body is closer to the film.

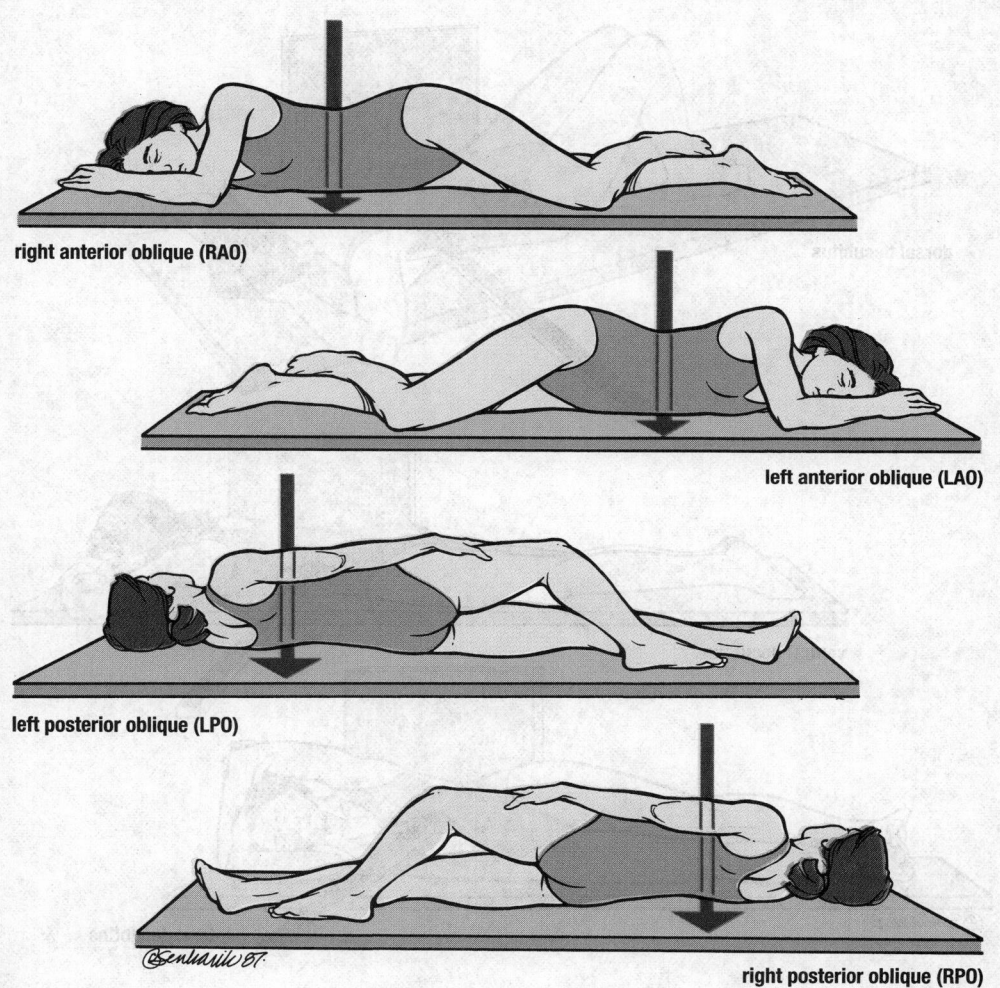

right anterior oblique (RAO)

left anterior oblique (LAO)

left posterior oblique (LPO)

right posterior oblique (RPO)

Right anterior oblique (RAO)   Patient is lying semiprone (face down) on the radiographic table or standing facing a vertical grid device with the *right* side closer to the film.

Left anterior oblique (LAO)   Patient is lying semiprone (face down) on the radiographic table or standing facing a vertical grid device with the *left* side closer to the film.

Right posterior oblique (RPO)   Patient is lying semisupine (face up) on the radiographic table or standing facing away from a vertical grid device with the *right* side closest to the film.

Left posterior oblique (LPO)   Patient is lying semisupine (face up) on the radiographic table or standing with the back against a vertical grid device with the *left* side closer to the film.

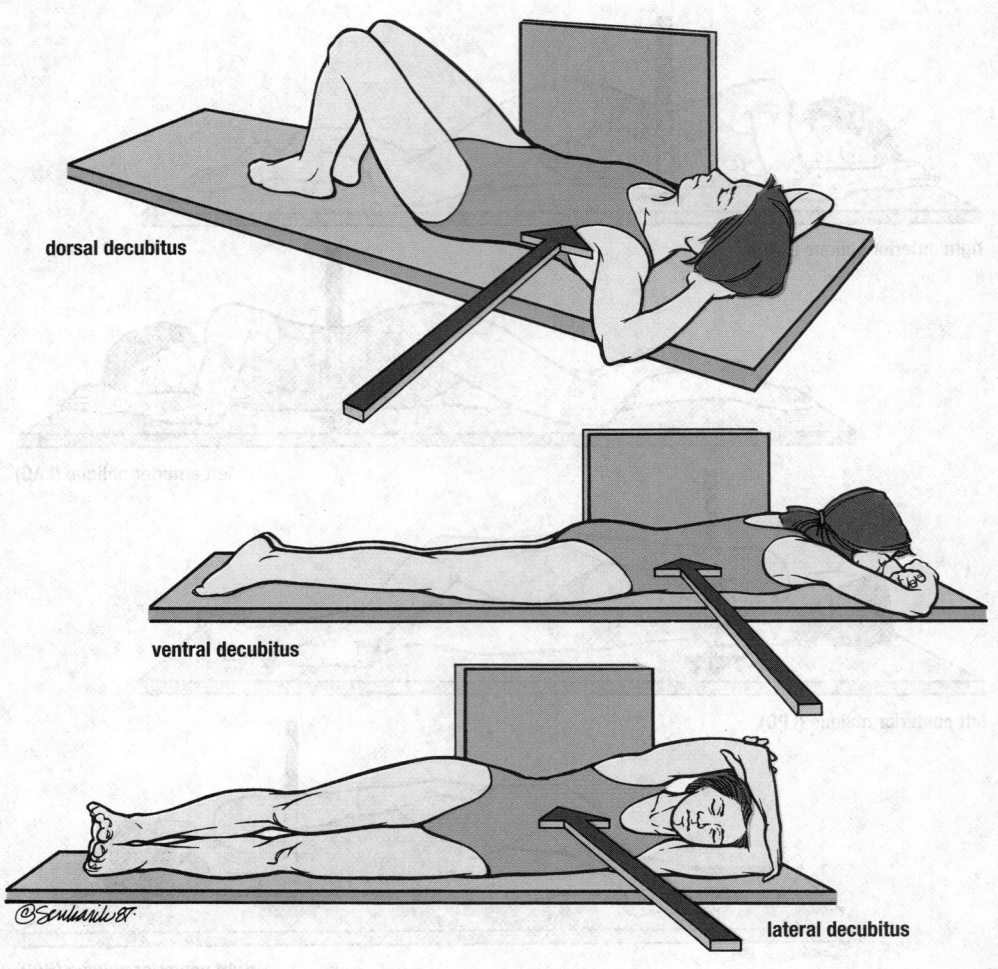

dorsal decubitus

ventral decubitus

lateral decubitus

Decubitus position	Patient is lying down, and the central ray is horizontal (parallel to the floor).
Dorsal decubitus	Patient is lying supine (face up) on the radiographic table or on a stretcher placed next to a vertical grid device. The x-ray beam enters from one side of the patient and exits the other.
Ventral decubitus	Patient is lying prone (face down) on the radiographic table or on a stretcher placed next to a vertical grid device. The x-ray beam enters from one side of the patient and exits the other.
Lateral decubitus	Patient is lying on either side on the radiographic table or on a stretcher placed next to a vertical grid device. For a *left* lateral decubitus, the patient is lying on the *left* side with the *right* side up, while for a *right* lateral decubitus, the patient is lying on the *right* side with the *left* side up. The x-ray beam passes through the patient from front to back or back to front, depending on whether the patient is facing toward or away from the radiographic tube.

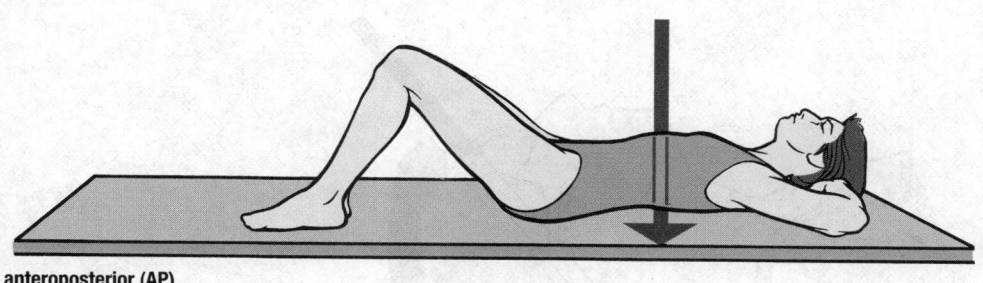

anteroposterior (AP)

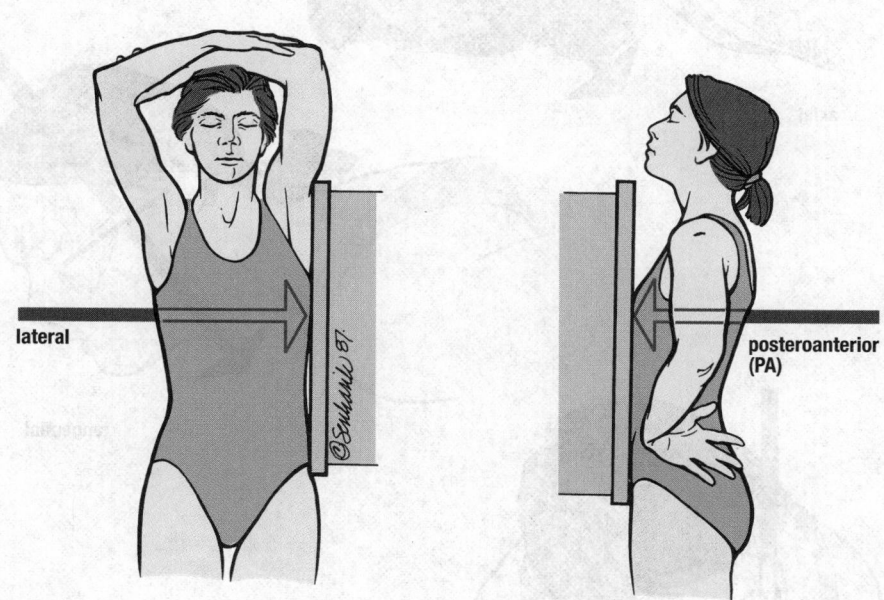

lateral

posteroanterior (PA)

Radiographic Projections

In radiography, the term *projection* is described by the path along which the x-rays travel from the radiographic tube through the subject to the image receptor.

Anteroposterior (AP) projection Patient is either supine (face up) on the radiographic table (dorsal decubitus) or erect with the back against a vertical grid device. The x-ray beam enters the front (anterior) surface of the body and exists the back (posterior) surface.

Posteroanterior (PA) projection Patient is either prone (face down) on the radiographic table (ventral decubitus) or erect facing a vertical grid device. The x-ray beam enters the back (posterior) surface of the body and exits the front (anterior) surface.

Lateral projection Patient is lying on either side on the radiographic table (lateral decubitus) or standing with either side against a vertical grid device. The lateral projection is always named by the side of the patient that is placed next to the film.

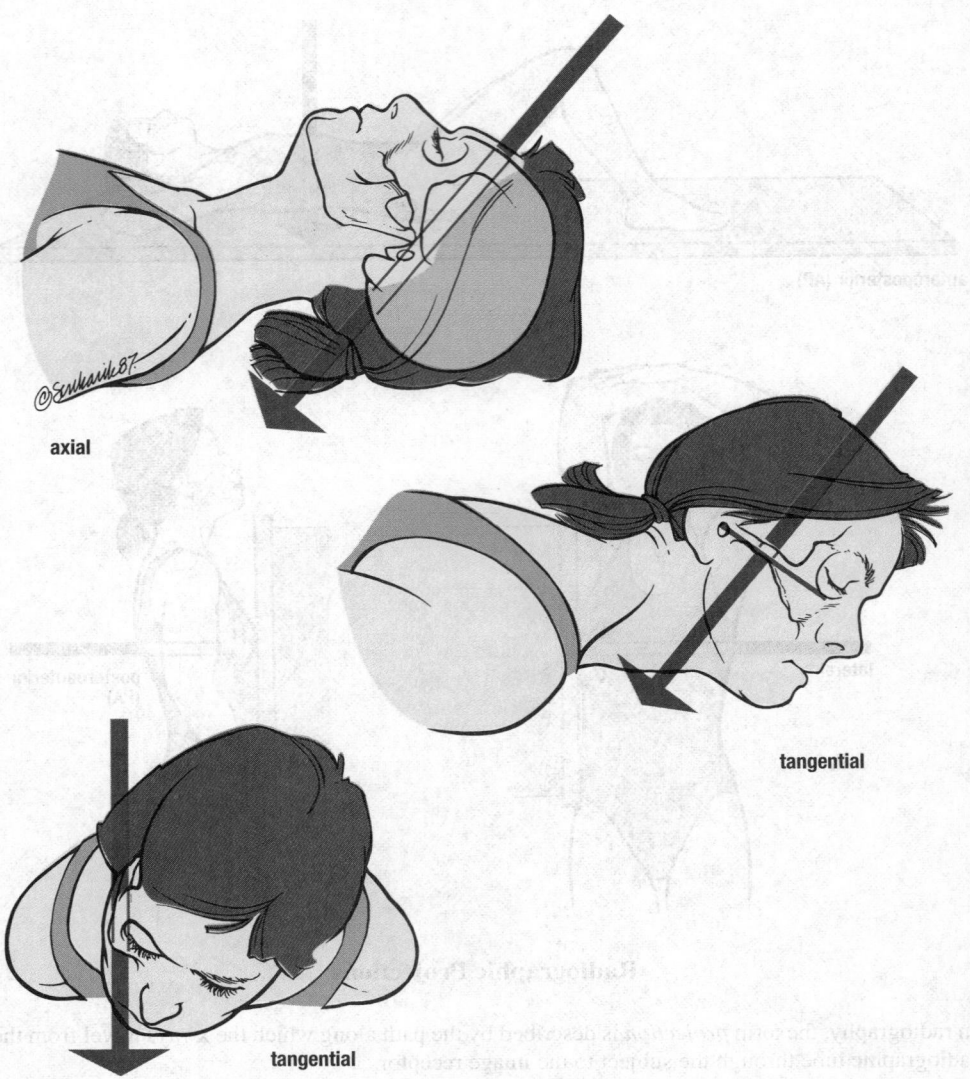

axial

tangential

tangential

Oblique projection	Patient is rotated into a position that does not produce either a frontal (AP or PA) or lateral projection.
Axial projection	Any projection in which there is longitudinal angulation of the central ray with respect to the long axis of the body part.
Tangential projection	Any projection in which the central ray passes between or passes by (skims) body parts to project an anatomic structure in profile and free of superimposition.

From Eisenberg RL, Dennis CA, & May CR. Radiographic positioning, 2nd ed. Boston: Little, Brown, 1995.

0 to 180 system: This system, first described by Silver, is probably the most widely used system of notating and recording range of motion measurements. The starting position (the anatomical position) for all movements except pronation and supination is considered to be 0. Movements then proceed toward 180 degrees.

180 to 0 system: According to Clark, who first described this system, the anatomical position is designated as the 180-degree position for all joints. Movements toward flexion approach 180 degrees, and movements toward extension or past the 180-degree or neutral position approach 0 degrees. Movements in the frontal plane also approach 0 degrees. External rotation movements approach 180 degrees, and internal rotation movements approach zero.

360-degree system: This system, first described by West, is similar to the 180- to 0-degree system in that the neutral starting position for most joints is designated as 180 degrees. Movements of flexion are toward 0 degrees, and movements beyond the neutral position are toward 360 degrees.

SFTR system of recording range of motion values: The SFTR (abbreviation for sagittal, frontal, transverse, and rotation) system combines the 0 to 180 method for notating range-of-motion (ROM) measurements with a systematic set of rules for recording these measurements. The following rules guide the use of the SFTR system. All joint motions are measured from the anatomical position. All joint motions and positions are recorded in the three basic planes (sagittal, frontal, and transverse). Motions of internal and external rotation are recorded as rotations.

All motions are recorded with three numbers. Motions leading away from the body are recorded first, and motions leading toward the body are recorded last. The starting position is recorded in the middle and is usually 0. For example, an elbow that can be hyperextended 10 degrees and flexed 140 degrees would be recorded as S 10-0-140. The *S* indicates motion in the sagittal plane. All fixed positions, such as ankyloses, are recorded with two numbers. For example, an elbow that is ankylosed at a position of 30 degrees of flexion would be recorded as S 0-30. Lateral bending and rotation of the spine to the left is recorded first and motions to the right are recorded last.

REFERENCES

1. Silver D: Measurement of the range of motion in joints. J Bone Joint Surg 21:569, 1923.

2. Clark WA: A system of joint measurement. J Orthop Surg 2:687, 1920.

3. West CC: Measurement of joint motion. Arch Phys Med 26:414, 1945.

4. Gerhardt JJ, Russe OA. International SFTR method of measuring and recording joint motion. Bern: Huber, 1975.

5. Gerhardt JJ. Clinical measurements of joint motion and position in the neutral-zero method and SFTR: Basic principles. Int Rehab Med 1983; 5:161–164.

From Rothstein JM, Roy SH, Wolf SL. The rehabilitation specialist's handbook. Philadelphia: F. A. Davis Company, 1991.

DUBOIS' BODY SURFACE AREA CHART

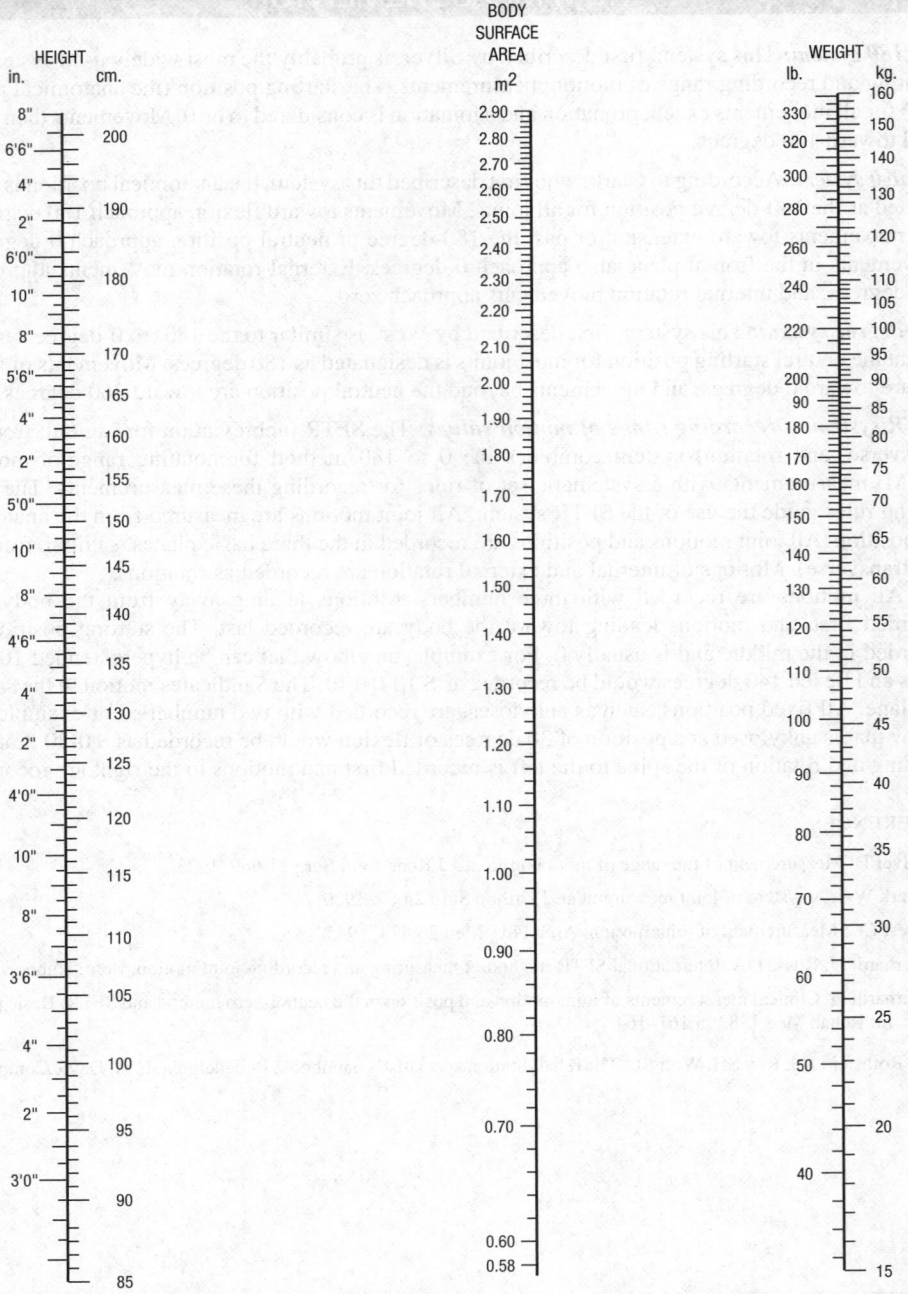

To determine body surface area, draw a straight line from the point on the height scale indicating the subject's height to the point on the weight scale indicating the subject's weight. The point where the line crosses the body surface scale will indicate the subject's body surface area. For example, for a subject 170 cm tall and weighing 75 kg, body surface area will total 1.90 m².

LUNG VOLUME COMPARTMENTS AND SUBDIVISIONS (BASED ON A VOLUME-TIME SPIROGRAM)

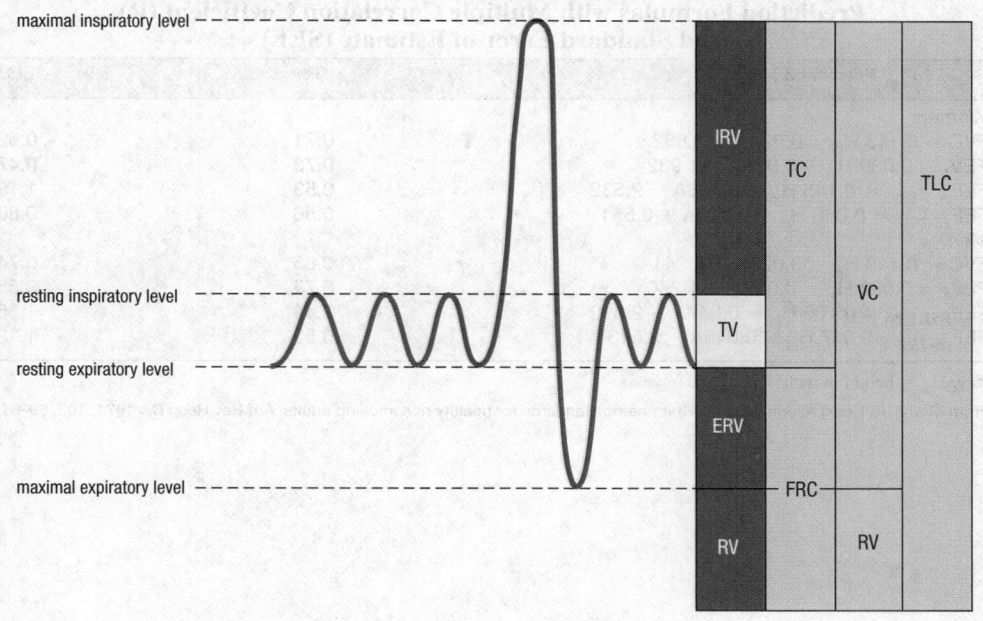

ERV: Expiratory reserve volume; the maximal amount of air that can be exhaled from the resting end-tidal (end-expiratory) position.

FRC: Functional residual capacity; the volume of air in the lungs at tidal volume end-expiratory position, or the sum of RV and ERV.

IC: Inspiratory capacity; the maximum volume of air that can be inhaled from the tidal volume end-expiratory position, or the sum of IRV and TV. This capacity usually makes up 60–70% of the vital capacity in health individuals.

IRV: Inspiratory reserve volume; the maximal amount of air inhaled from the end-inspiratory position.

RV: Residual volume; that volume of air remaining in the lungs after maximal exhalation, or TLC − VC.

TLC: Total lung capacity; the sum of all volume compartments or the volume of air in the lungs after maximal inspiration.

TV: Tidal volume; that volume of air inhaled or exhaled with each breath during quiet breathing.

VC: Vital capacity; the maximum volume of air exhaled from the point of maximum inspiration. VC can also be described as the sum of the TV, IRV, and ERV. In healthy individuals, VC makes up about 70% of total lung volume.

From Wanger J. Pulmonary function testing. Baltimore: Williams & Wilkins, 1992: 64. Modified from Forster RE, DuBois AB, Briscoe WA, Fisher AB. The lung: Physiologic basis of pulmonary function tests, 3rd ed. Chicago: Year Book Medical Publishers, 1986.

APPENDICES

Prediction Formulas with Multiple Correlation Coefficient (R) and Standard Error of Estimate (SEE)

Prediction Formula	R	SEE
Women		
$FVC = 0.115\ H_{in} - 0.024A - 2.852$	0.71	0.52
$FEV_1 = 0.089\ H_{in} - 0.025A - 1.932$	0.73	0.47
$FEF_{200-1200} = 0.145\ H_{in} - 0.036A - 2.532$	0.53	1.19
$FEF_{25-75\%} = 0.060\ H_{in} - 0.030A + 0.551$	0.56	0.80
Men		
$FVC = 0.148\ H_{in} - 0.025A - 4.241$	0.65	0.74
$FEV_1 = 0.092\ H_{in} - 0.032A - 1.260$	0.73	0.55
$FEF_{200-1200} = 0.109\ H_{in} - 0.047A + 2.010$	0.44	1.66
$FEF_{25-75\%} = 0.047\ H_{in} - 0.045A + 2.513$	0.53	1.12

Key: H_{in} = height in inches; A = age in years

From Morris JF, Koski A, Johnson LC. Spirometric standards for healthy nonsmoking adults. Am Rev Resp Dis 1971; 103, 59–61.

PREDICTION NOMOGRAMS FOR NORMAL ADULTS

Male

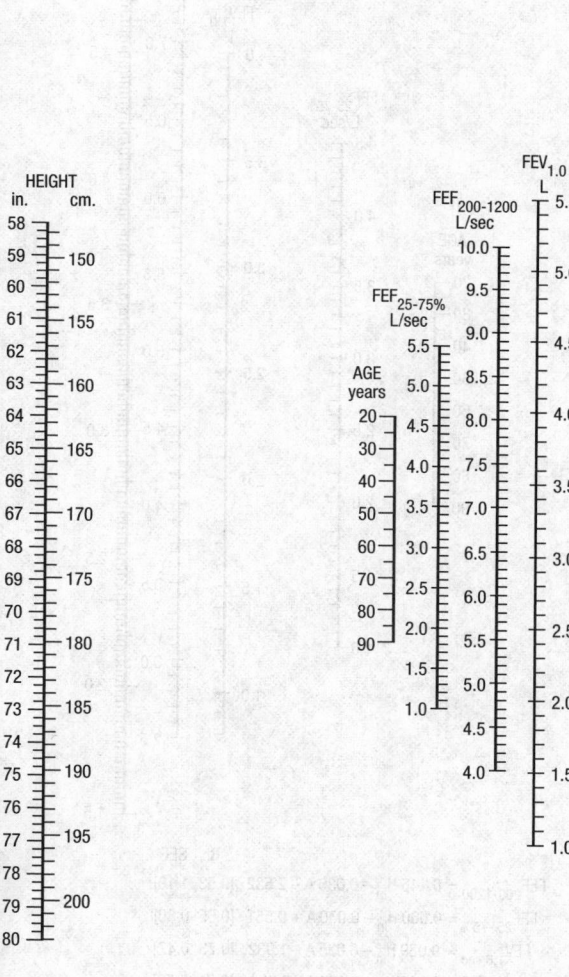

$$FEF_{200\text{-}1200} = 0.109\ H_{in} - 0.047\ A + 2.010 \quad [0.44\ 1.66]$$
$$FEF_{25\text{-}75\%} = 0.047\ H_{in} - 0.045\ A + 2.513 \quad [0.53\ 1.12]$$
$$FEV_{1.0\ sec} = 0.092\ H_{in} - 0.032\ A - 1.260 \quad [0.73\ 0.55]$$
$$FVC = 0.148\ H_{in} - 0.025\ A - 4.241 \quad [0.65\ 0.74]$$

From Morris JF, Koski A, Johnson LC. Spirometric standards for healthy nonsmoking adults. Am Rev Resp Dis 1971;103, 59–61.

APPENDICES

Female

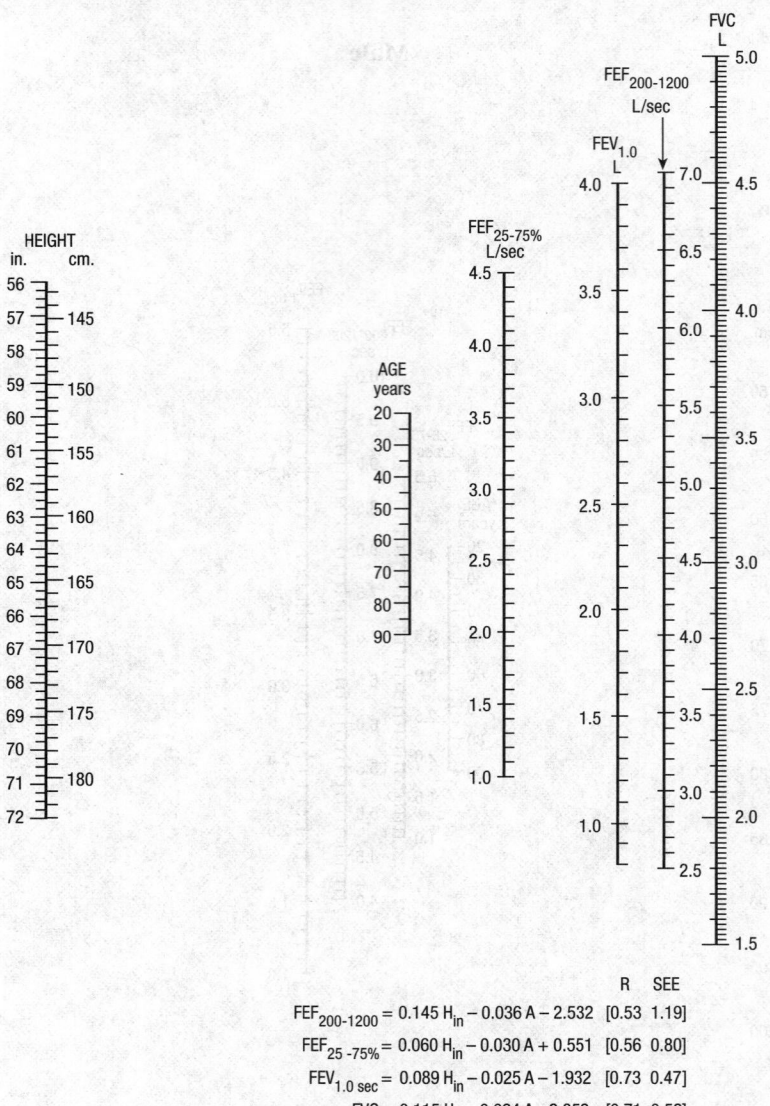

$$FEF_{200-1200} = 0.145\,H_{in} - 0.036\,A - 2.532 \quad [0.53 \; 1.19]$$

$$FEF_{25-75\%} = 0.060\,H_{in} - 0.030\,A + 0.551 \quad [0.56 \; 0.80]$$

$$FEV_{1.0\,sec} = 0.089\,H_{in} - 0.025\,A - 1.932 \quad [0.73 \; 0.47]$$

$$FVC = 0.115\,H_{in} - 0.024\,A - 2.852 \quad [0.71 \; 0.52]$$

From Morris JF, Koski A, Johnson LC. Spirometric standards for healthy nonsmoking adults. Am Rev Resp Dis 1971;103, 59–61.

CLASSIC TEXTBOOK METHOD OF BLOOD GAS INTERPRETATION

Status	pH	Pco₂	HCO₃⁻	BE
RESPIRATORY ACIDOSIS				
Uncompensated	↓ 7.35	↑ 45	Normal	Normal
Partially compensated	↓ 7.35	↑ 45	↑ 27	↑ +2
Compensated	7.35–7.45	↑ 45	↑ 27	↑ +2
RESPIRATORY ALKALOSIS				
Uncompensated	↑ 7.45	↓ 35	Normal	Normal
Partially compensated	↑ 7.45	↓ 35	↓ 22	↓ −2
Compensated	7.40–7.45	↓ 35	↓ 22	↓ −2
METABOLIC ACIDOSIS				
Uncompensated	↓ 7.35	Normal	↓ 22	↓ −2
Partially compensated	↓ 7.35	↓ 35	↓ 22	↓ −2
Compensated	7.35–7.40	↓ 35	↓ 22	↓ −2
METABOLIC ALKALOSIS				
Uncompensated	↑ 7.45	Normal	↑ 27	↑ +2
Partially compensated*	↑ 7.45	↑ 45	↑ 27	↑ +2
Compensated*	7.40–7.45	↑ 45	↑ 27	↑ +2
COMBINED RESPIRATORY AND METABOLIC ACIDOSIS	↓ 7.35	↑ 45	↓ 22	↓ −2
COMBINED RESPIRATORY AND METABOLIC ALKALOSIS	↑ 7.45	↓ 35	↑ 27	↑ +2

*In general, partially compensated or compensated metabolic alkalosis is rarely seen clinically because of the body's mechanism to prevent hypoventilation.

From Kacmarek RM, Mack CW, Dimas S. The essentials of respiratory care, 3rd ed. St. Louis, MO: Mosby-Year Book, 1990.

Since medical history and examination cannot reliably identify all patients infected with HIV or other blood-borne pathogens, blood and body-fluid precautions should be consistently used for *all* patients. This approach, previously recommended by CDC and referred to as "universal blood and body-fluid precautions" or "universal precautions," should be used in the care of *all* patients, especially including those in emergency-care settings in which the risk of blood exposure is increased and the infection status of the patient is usually unknown.

1. All health-care workers should routinely use appropriate barrier precautions to prevent skin and mucous-membrane exposure when contact with blood or other body fluids of any patient is anticipated. Gloves should be worn for touching blood and body fluids, mucous membranes, or non-intact skin of all patients, for handling items or surfaces soiled with blood or body fluids, and for performing venipuncture and other vascular access procedures. Gloves should be changed after contact with each patient. Masks and protective eyewear or face shields should be worn during procedures that are likely to generate droplets of blood or other body fluids to prevent exposure of mucous membranes of the mouth, nose and eyes. Gowns or aprons should be worn during procedures that are likely to generate splashes of blood or other body fluids.

2. Hands and other skin surfaces should be washed immediately and thoroughly if contaminated with blood or other body fluids. Hands should be washed immediately after gloves are removed.

3. All health-care workers should take precautions to prevent injuries caused by needles, scalpels, and other sharp instruments or devices during procedures; when cleaning used instruments; during disposal of used needles; and when handling sharp instruments after procedures. To prevent needlestick injuries, needles should not be recapped, purposely bent or broken by hand, removed from disposable syringes, or otherwise manipulated by hand. After they are used, disposable syringes and needles, scalpel blades, and other sharp items should be placed in puncture-resistant containers for disposal; the puncture-resistant containers should be located as close as practical to the use area. Large-bore reusable needles should be placed in a puncture-resistant container for transport to the reprocessing area.

4. Although saliva has not been implicated in HIV transmission, to minimize the need for emergency mouth-to-mouth resuscitation, mouthpieces, resuscitation bags, or other ventilation devices should be available for use in areas in which the need for resuscitation is predictable.

5. Health-care workers who have exudative lesions or weeping dermatitis should refrain from all direct patient care and from handling patient-care equipment until the condition resolves.

6. Pregnant health-care workers are not known to be at greater risk of contracting HIV infection than health-care workers who are not pregnant; however, if a health-care worker develops HIV infection during pregnancy, the infant is at risk of infection resulting from perinatal transmission. Because of this risk, pregnant health-care workers should be especially familiar with and strictly adhere to precautions to minimize the risk of HIV transmission.

Precautions for Invasive Procedures

In this document, an invasive procedure is defined as surgical entry into tissues, cavities, or organs or repair of major traumatic injuries 1) in an operating or delivery room, emergency department, or outpatient setting, including both physicians' and dentists' offices; 2) cardiac catheterization and angiographic procedures; 3) a vaginal or cesarean delivery or other invasive obstetric procedure during which bleeding may occur; or 4) the manipulation, cutting, or removal of any oral or perioral tissues, including tooth structure, during which bleeding occurs or the potential for bleeding exists. The universal blood and body-fluid precautions listed above, combined with the precautions listed below, should be the minimum precautions for *all* such invasive procedures.

1. All health-care workers who participate in invasive procedures must routinely use appropriate barrier precautions to prevent skin and mucous-membrane contact with blood and other body fluids of all patients. Gloves and surgical masks must be worn for all invasive procedures. Protective eyewear or face shields should be worn for procedures that commonly result in the generation of droplets, splashing of blood or other body fluids, or the generation of bone chips. Gowns or aprons made of materials that provide an effective barrier should be worn during invasive procedures that are likely to result in the splashing of blood or other body fluids. All health-care workers who perform or assist in vaginal or cesarean deliveries should wear gloves and gowns when handling the placenta or the infant until blood and amniotic fluid have been removed from the infant's skin and should wear gloves during post-delivery care of the umbilical cord.

2. If a glove is torn or a needlestick or other injury occurs, the glove should be removed and a new glove used as promptly as patient safety permits; the needle or instrument involved in the incident should also be removed from the sterile field.

Precautions for Dentistry

Blood, saliva, and gingival fluid from *all* dental patients should be considered infective. Special emphasis should be placed on the following precautions for preventing transmission of bloodborne pathogens in dental practice in both institutional and non-institutional settings.

1. In addition to wearing gloves for contact with oral mucous membranes of all patients, all dental workers should wear surgical masks and protective eyewear or chin-length plastic face shields during dental procedures in which splashing or spattering of blood, saliva, or gingival fluids is likely. Rubber dams, high-speed evacuation, and proper patient positioning, when appropriate, should be utilized to minimize generation of droplets and spatter.

2. Handpieces should be sterilized after use with each patient, since blood, saliva, or gingival fluid of patients may be aspirated into the handpiece or waterline. Handpieces that cannot be sterilized should at least be flushed, the outside surface cleaned and wiped with a suitable chemical germicide, and then rinsed. Handpieces should be flushed at the beginning of the day and after use with each patient. Manufacturers' recommendations should be followed for use and maintenance of waterlines and check valves and for flushing of handpieces. The same precautions should be used for ultrasonic scalers and air/water syringes.

3. Blood and saliva should be thoroughly and carefully cleaned from material that has been used in the mouth (e.g., impression materials, bite registration), especially before polishing and grinding intra-oral devices. Contaminated materials, impressions, and intra-oral devices should also be cleaned and disinfected before being handled in the dental laboratory and before they are placed in the patient's mouth. Because of the increasing variety of dental materials used intra-orally, dental workers should consult with manufacturers as to the stability of specific materials when using disinfection procedures.

4. Dental equipment and surfaces that are difficult to disinfect (e.g., light handles or x-ray-unit heads) and that may become contaminated should be wrapped with impervious-backed paper, aluminum foil, or clear plastic wrap. The coverings should be removed and discarded, and clean coverings should be put in place after use with each patient.

Precautions for Autopsies or Morticians' Services

In addition to the universal blood and body-fluid precautions listed above, the following precautions should be used by persons performing postmortem procedures:

1. All persons performing or assisting in postmortem procedures should wear gloves, masks, protective eyewear, gowns, and waterproof aprons.

2. Instruments and surfaces contaminated during postmortem procedures should be decontaminated with an appropriate chemical germicide.

Precautions for Dialysis

Patients with end-stage renal disease who are undergoing maintenance dialysis and who have HIV infection can be dialyzed in hospital-based or free-standing dialysis units using conventional infection-control precautions. Universal blood and body-fluid precautions should be used when dialyzing *all* patients.

Strategies for disinfecting the dialysis fluid pathways of the hemodialysis machine are targeted to control bacterial contamination and generally consist of using 500–750 parts per million (ppm) of sodium hypochlorite (household bleach) for 30–40 minutes or 1.5%–2.0% formaldehyde overnight. In addition, several chemical germicides formulated to disinfect dialysis machines are commercially available. None of these protocols or procedures need to be changed for dialyzing patients infected with HIV.

Patients infected with HIV can be dialyzed by either hemodialysis or peritoneal dialysis and do not need to be isolated from other patients. The type of dialysis treatment (i.e., hemodialysis or peritoneal dialysis) should be based on the needs of the patient. The dialyzer may be discarded after each use. Alternatively, centers that reuse dialyzers (i.e., a specific single-use dialyzer is issued to a specific patient, removed, cleaned, disinfected, and reused several times on the same patient only) may include HIV-infected patients in the dialyzer-reuse program. An individual dialyzer must never be used on more than one patient.

Precautions for Laboratories

Blood and other body fluids from *all* patients should be considered infective. To supplement the universal blood and body-fluid precautions listed above, the following precautions are recommended for health-care workers in clinical laboratories:

1. All specimens of blood and body fluids should be put in a well-constructed container with a secure lid to prevent leaking during transport. Care should be taken when collecting each specimen to avoid contaminating the outside of the container and of the laboratory form accompanying the specimen.

2. All persons processing blood and body-fluid specimens (e.g., removing tops from vacuum tubes) should wear gloves. Masks and protective eyewear should be worn if mucous-membrane contact with blood or body fluids is anticipated. Gloves should be changed and hands washed after completion of specimen processing.

3. For routine procedures, such as histologic and pathologic studies or microbiologic culturing, a biological safety cabinet is not necessary. However, biological safety cabinets (Class I or II) should be used whenever procedures are conducted that have a high potential for generating droplets. These include activities such as blending, sonicating, and vigorous mixing.

4. Mechanical pipetting devices should be used for manipulating all liquids in the laboratory. Mouth pipetting must not be done.

5. Use of needles and syringes should be limited to situations in which there is no alternative, and the recommendations for preventing injuries with needles outlined under universal precautions should be followed.

6. Laboratory work surfaces should be decontaminated with an appropriate chemical germicide after a spill of blood or other body fluids and when work activities are completed.

7. Contaminated materials used in laboratory tests should be decontaminated before reprocessing or be placed in bags and disposed of in accordance with institutional policies for disposal of infective waste.

8. Scientific equipment that has been contaminated with blood or other body fluids should be decontaminated and cleaned before being repaired in the laboratory or transported to the manufacturer.

9. All persons should wash their hands after completing laboratory activities and should remove protective clothing before leaving the laboratory.

Implementation of universal blood and body-fluid precautions for all patients eliminates the need for warning labels on specimens since blood and other body fluids from all patients should be considered infective.

Courtesy of the Centers for Disease Control and Prevention, Atlanta, GA.

INFECTION CONTROL FOR THE DENTAL OFFICE: A CHECKLIST

Immunization
- Health care workers should have appropriate immunizations such as that for hepatitis B virus.

Before Patient Treatment
- Obtain a thorough medical history
- Disinfect prostheses and appliances received from the laboratory
- Place disposable coverings to prevent contamination of surfaces, or disinfect surfaces after treatment
- Set out supplies and instruments needed for procedure
- Flush waterlines before connecting handpiece, syringe, or scalers

During Patient Treatment
- Treat all patients as potentially infectious
- Use protective attire and barrier techniques when contact with body fluids or mucous membranes is anticipated
  —Wear gloves
  —Wear mask
  —Wear protective eyewear
  —Wear uniforms, laboratory coats, or gowns
- Open intraorally contaminated x-ray film packets in the darkroom with disposable gloves without touching the films
- Use aseptic technique to retrieve additional items
- Minimize formation of droplets, spatters, and aerosols
- Use a rubber dam to isolate the tooth and field when appropriate
- Use high-volume vacuum evacuation
- Protect hands
  —Wash hands before gloving and after gloves are removed
  —Change gloves between each patient
  —Discard gloves that are torn, cut, or punctured
  —Avoid hand injuries
- Avoid injury with sharp instruments and needles
  —Handle sharp items carefully
  —Do not bend or break disposable needles
  —If needles are not recapped, place in separate field. If recapping is necessary, use a method that protects hands from injury, such as a holder for the cap.
  —Place sharp items in appropriate containers

After Patient Treatment
- Wear heavy-duty rubber gloves
- Clean instruments thoroughly
- Heat-sterilize instruments
  —Sterilize instruments that penetrate soft tissue or bone
  —Sterilize, whenever possible, all instruments that come in contact with oral mucous membranes, body fluids, or those that have been contaminated with secretions of patients. Otherwise, use appropriate chemical sterilization.
  —Wrap instruments for sterilization whenever possible to maintain sterility until use. Do not reuse single-use wraps.
  —Monitor the sterilizer with biological monitors
- Clean handpieces, dental units, and ultrasonic scalers
  —Flush handpieces, dental units, ultrasonic scalers, and air/water syringes between patients

—Clean and sterilize air/water syringes or use disposable tips
—Clean and sterilize ultrasonic scalers if possible; otherwise, disinfect them appropriately
—Clean and sterilize handpieces
—Process single-use water delivery systems according to manufacturers directions
• Handle sharp instruments with caution
—Place disposable needles, scalpels, and other sharp items intact into puncture-resistant containers before disposal
• Replace any disposable surface covers on environmental surfaces
• Decontaminate environmental surfaces
—Wipe work surfaces with absorbent toweling to remove debris, and dispose of this toweling appropriately
—Disinfect with suitable chemical disinfectant
—Change protective coverings on light handles, x-ray unit head, and other items
• Decontaminate supplies and materials
—Rinse and disinfect impressions, bite registrations, and appliances to be sent to the laboratory
• Communicate infection control program to dental laboratory
• Dispense a small amount of pumice in a disposable container for individual use on each case and discard any excess
• Remove contaminated wastes appropriately
—Pour blood, suctioned fluids, and other liquid waste into drain connected to a sanitary sewer system
—Place solid waste contaminated with blood or saliva in sealed, sturdy impervious bags; dispose according to local government regulations
• Remove gloves and wash hands

Daily
• Flush cleansing solution through evacuation lines, and clean or replace the unit's solid waste filter trap
• Flush waterlines for 2–3 minutes after periods of nonuse if waterlines were not drained
• If in-line water filters are used, change daily
• For in-line check valves, change daily or as directed by manufacturer

Overnight
• If possible, drain waterlines for dry storage for periods of nonuse (overnight, weekends)

Weekly
• Clean and disinfect main evacuation trap
• Clean and disinfect inside and outside of drawers and cabinets
• Perform weekly disinfection procedures on waterlines as directed by manufacturer

Adapted from Cottone JA, Terezhalmy GT, Molinari JA. Practical infection control in dentistry, 2nd. ed. Baltimore: Williams & Wilkins, 1996.

AIDS-INDICATOR CONDITIONS

REPORTED IN 1995, BY AGE GROUP, UNITED STATES

AIDS-indicator Conditions	Adults/ adolescents No.	(%)[1]	Children <13 years old No.	(%)[1]
Bacterial infections, multiple or recurrent	NA[2]		123	(15)
Candidiasis of bronchi, trachea, or lungs	736	(1)	18	(2)
Candidiasis of esophagus				
Definitive diagnosis	3,136	(4)	56	(7)
Presumptive diagnosis	2,286	(3)	69	(9)
Carcinoma, invasive cervical	166	(0)	NA[3]	
Coccidioidomycosis, disseminated or extrapulmonary	140	(0)	—	—
Cryptococcosis, extrapulmonary	1,626	(2)	7	(1)
Cryptosporidiosis, chronic intestinal	760	(1)	27	(3)
Cytomegalovirus disease other than retinitis	1,611	(2)	48	(6)
Cytomegalovirus retinitis				
Definitive diagnosis	1,003	(1)	7	(1)
Presumptive diagnosis	491	(1)	1	(0)
Herpes simplex, with esophagitis, pneumonitis, or chronic mucocutaneous ulcers	1,927	(3)	46	(6)
Histoplasmosis, disseminated or extrapulmonary	309	(0)	—	—
HIV encephalopathy (dementia)	1,872	(3)	132	(17)
HIV wasting syndrome	6,618	(9)	146	(18)
Immunosuppression, severe HIV-related[4]	62,292	(85)	NA[3]	
Isosporiasis, chronic intestinal	39	(0)	—	—
Kaposi's sarcoma				
Definitive diagnosis	2,067	(3)	1	(0)
Presumptive diagnosis	662	(1)	—	—
Lymphoid interstitial pneumonia and/or pulmonary lymphoid hyperplasia				
Definitive diagnosis	NA[2]		45	(6)
Presumptive diagnosis	NA[2]		102	(13)
Lymphoma, Burkitt's (or equivalent term)	197	(0)	2	(0)
Lymphoma, immunoblastic (or equivalent term)	742	(1)	7	(1)
Lymphoma, primary in brain	277	(0)	3	(0)
Mycobacterium avium or M. Kensasii, disseminated or extrapulmonary				
Definitive diagnosis	1,745	(2)	41	(5)
Presumptive diagnosis	297	(0)	9	(1)
M. tuberculosis, disseminated or extrapulmonary				
Definitive diagnosis	435	(1)	2	(0)
Presumptive diagnosis	90	(0)	—	—
M. tuberculosis, pulmonary				
Definitive diagnosis	1,383	(2)	NA[3]	
Presumptive diagnosis	306	(0)	NA[3]	
Mycobacterial disease, other, disseminated or extrapulmonary				
Definitive diagnosis	315	(0)	7	(1)
Presumptive diagnosis	90	(0)	4	(1)
Pneumocystis cerinii pneumonia				
Definitive diagnosis	8,654	(12)	143	(18)
Presumptive diagnosis	4,442	(6)	69	(9)
Pneumonia, recurrent				
Definitive diagnosis	1,417	(2)	NA[3]	
Presumptive diagnosis	412	(1)	NA[3]	
Progressive multifocal leukoencephalopathy	327	(0)	4	(1)
Salmonella septicemia, recurrent	78	(0)	NA[5]	

AIDS-indicator Conditions	Adults/ adolescents		Children <13 years old	
	No.	(%)[1]	No.	(%)[1]
Toxoplasmosis of brain				
Definitive diagnosis	806	(1)	5	(1)
Presumptive diagnosis	744	(1)	4	(1)

[1]Percentages are based upon 73,380 adult/adolescent and 800 pediatric cases reported to CDC in 1995. The sum of percentages is greater than 100 because some patients have more than one condition.

[2]Not applicable as indicator of AIDS in adults/adolescents.

[3]Not applicable as indicator of AIDS in children.

[4]Defined as $CD4^+$ T-lymphocyte count of less than 200 cells/μL or a $CD4^+$ percentage less than 14 in adults/adolescents who meet the AIDS surveillance case definition.

[5]Tabulated above in "bacterial infections, multiple or recurrent."

Courtesy of the Centers for Disease Control and Prevention, Atlanta, GA.

American Academy of Audiology
8201 Greensboro Dr., Ste. 300
McLean, VA 22102
(800) AAA-2336
(703) 610–9022
(703) 610–9005 [fax]
http://www.audiology.com

**American Academy of Anesthesiologists'
Assistants**
PO Box 33876
Decatur, GA 30032
(no permanent telephone number)

American Academy of Physician Assistants
950 N. Washington St.
Alexandria, VA 22314–1552
(703) 836–2272

**American Alliance for Health, Physical
Education, Recreation, and Dance**
1900 Association Dr.
Reston, VA 20191
(703) 476–3400

American Association of Blood Banks
8101 Glenbrook Rd.
Bethesda, MD 20814
(301) 907–6977

American Association of Dental Schools
1625 Massachusetts Ave. NW
Washington, DC 20036
(202) 667–9433

**American Association of Diabetes
Educators**
444 N. Michigan Ave., Ste. 1240
Chicago, IL 60611
(800) 338–3633

American Association of Medical Assistants
20 N. Wacker Dr., Ste. 1575
Chicago, IL 60606
(312) 899–1500

**American Association for Medical
Transcription**
PO Box 576187
Modesto, CA 95357–6187
(800) 982–2182

American Association for Respiratory Care
11030 Ables La.
Dallas, TX 75229
(214) 243–2772

**American Board of Cardiovascular
Perfusion**
207 N. 25th Ave.
Hattiesburg, MS 39401
(601) 582–3309

American College of Clinical Pharmacy
3101 Broadway, Ste. 380
Kansas City, MO 64111
(816) 531–2177

American College of Sports Medicine
401 W. Michigan St.
Indianapolis, IN 46202
(317) 637–9200

American Dental Assistants Association
203 N. LaSalle St., Ste. 1320
Chicago, IL 60601–1225
(312) 541–1550

American Dental Association
211 E. Chicago Ave.
Chicago, IL 60611
(312) 440–2500
http://www.ada.org

American Dental Hygienists Association
444 N. Michigan Ave., Ste. 3400
Chicago, IL 60611
(312) 440–8900
http://www.adha.org

American Dietetic Association
216 W. Jackson Blvd., Ste. 800
Chicago, IL 60606–6995
(312) 899–0040

American Electroencephalographic Society
PO Box 30
Bloomfield, CT 06002
(203) 243–3977

**American Health Information Management
Association**
919 N. Michigan Ave., Ste. 1400
Chicago, IL 60611–1683
(312) 787–2672
info@ahima.mhs.compuserve.com

American Hospital Association
1 N. Franklin
Chicago, IL 60606
(312) 422–3000

American Medical Electroencephalographic Association
850 Elm Grove Rd.
Elm Grove, WI 53122
(414) 784–3646

American Occupational Therapy Association
PO Box 31220
Bethesda, MD 20824–1220
(301) 652–2682
(301) 652–7111 [fax]
(800) 377–8555 [TDD]

American Pharmaceutical Association
2215 Constitution Ave. NW
Washington, DC 20037
(202) 628–4410

American Physical Therapy Association
1111 N. Fairfax St.
Alexandria, VA 22314–1488
(703) 684–2782
(800) 999–2782
SVCCTR@apta.org

American Registry of Radiologic Technologists
1255 Northland Dr.
Mendota Heights, MN 55120
(612) 687-0048

American Society for Clinical Laboratory Science
7910 Woodmont Ave., Ste. 530
Bethesda, MD 20814
(301) 657–2768
(301) 657–2909 [fax]

American Society for Clinical Nutrition
9650 Rockville Pike
Bethesda, MD 20814–3998
(301) 530–7110

American Society of Clinical Pathologists
2100 W. Harrison St.
Chicago, IL 60612
(312) 738–1336

American Society of Echocardiography
4101 Lake Boone Trail, Ste. 201
Raleigh, NC 27607
(919) 787–5181

American Society of Electroneurodiagnostic Technologists
204 W. Seventh St.
Carroll, IA 51401
(712) 792–2978

American Society of Extra-Corporeal Technology
11480 Sunset Hills Rd., Ste. 210E
Reston, VA 22090
(703) 435–8556

American Society for Parenteral and Enteral Nutrition
8630 Fenton St., Ste. 412
Silver Spring, MD 20910
(301) 587–6315

American Society of Radiologic Technologists
15000 Central Ave. SE
Albuquerque, NM 87123–3917
(505) 298–4500
(505) 298–5063 [fax]

American Speech-Language-Hearing Association
10801 Rockville Pike
Rockville, MD 20852
(301) 897–5700
(301) 571–0457 [fax]

American Thoracic Society
1740 Broadway
New York, NY 10019–4374
(212) 315–8700
Mhansen@lungUSA.org

Association for Anesthesiologists' Assistants Education
PO Box 49713
Atlanta, GA 30359
(404) 727–5910

Association of Medical Illustrators
1819 Peachtree St. NE, Ste. 560
Atlanta, GA 30309
(404) 350–7900

Association of Surgical Technologists
7108-C S. Alton Way
Englewood, CO 80112
(303) 694–9130

Board of Pharmaceutical Specialties
2215 Constitution Ave. NW
Washington, DC 20037
(202) 429-7542

Commission on Dietetic Registration
216 W. Jackson Blvd., Ste. 800
Chicago, IL 60606
(313) 899–0040
ext. 5500

**Joint Commission on Allied Health
Personnel in Ophthalmology**
2025 Woodlane Dr.
St. Paul, MN 55125–2995
(612) 731–2944

**National Association of Emergency Medical
Technicians**
102 W. Leake
Clinton, MS 39056
(800) 346–2368

National Athletic Trainers Association
2952 Stemmons Fwy.
Dallas, TX 75247
(214) 637–6282
http://www.nata.org

**National Board of Nutrition Support
Certification**
8630 Fenton St., Ste. 412
Silver Spring, MD 20910
(301) 587-6315
(301) 587-2365 [fax]

National Board for Respiratory Care
8310 Nieman Rd.
Lenexa, KS 66214
(913) 599–4200
nbrc-info@nbrc.org

**National Certification Agency for Medical
Laboratory Personnel**
PO Box 15945-289
Lenexa, KS 66285
(913) 438-5110
(913) 541-0156 [fax]

**National Registry of Emergency Medical
Technicians**
6610 Busch Blvd.
PO Box 2933
Columbus, OH 43229
(614) 888–4484

Society of Diagnostic Medical Sonographers
12770 Coit Rd., Ste. 508
Dallas, TX 75251
(214) 239–7367

Society of Vascular Technology
4601 Presidents Dr., Ste. 260
Lanham, MD 20706
(301) 459–7550

ART Accredited Record Technician

ATC Athletic Trainer Certified

BB(ASCP) Technologist in Blood Banking (certified by American Society of Clinical Pathologists)

BCNP Board Certified Nuclear Pharmacist

BCNSP Board Certified Nutrition Support Pharmacist (certified by Board of Pharmaceutical Specialties)

BCPS Board Certified Pharmacotherapy Specialist

C(ASCP) Technologist in Chemistry (certified by American Society of Clinical Pathologists)

CCC-A Certificate of Clinical Competence in Audiology

CCC-SLP Certificate of Clinical Competence in Speech-Language Pathology

CCS Cardiopulmonary Certified Specialist (certified by American Physical Therapy Association), Certified Coding Specialist

CDA Certified Dental Assistant

CDE Certified Diabetes Educator (certified by American Association of Diabetes Educators)

CDT Certified Dental Laboratory Technician

CLA Certified Laboratory Assistant

CLDir(NCA) Clinical Laboratory Director (certified by National Certification Agency for Medical Laboratory Personnel)

CLPlb(NCA) Clinical Laboratory Phlebotomist (certified by National Certification Agency for Medical Laboratory Personnel)

CLS Clinical Laboratory Scientist

CLS(NCA) Clinical Laboratory Scientist (certified by National Certification Agency for Medical Laboratory Personnel)

CLSp(CG)(NCA) Clinical Laboratory Specialist in Cytogenetics (certified by National Certification Agency for Medical Laboratory Personnel)

CLSp(H)(NCA) Clinical Laboratory Specialist in Hematology (certified by National Certification Agency for Medical Laboratory Personnel)

CLSup(NCA) Clinical Laboratory Supervisor (certified by National Certification Agency for Medical Laboratory Personnel)

CLT Certified Laboratory Technician or Clinical Laboratory Technician

CLT(NCA) Certified Laboratory Technician (certified by National Certification Agency for Medical Laboratory Personnel)

CMA Certified Medical Assistant

CMT Certified Medical Transcriptionist

CNM Certified Nurse Midwife

CNMT Certified Nuclear Medicine Technologist

CNSD Certified Nutrition Support Dietician (certified by National Board of Nutrition Support Certification)

CNSN Certified Nutrition Support Nurse

CNSP Certified Nutrition Support Physician

COMT Certified Ophthalmic Medical Technologist

COTA Certified Occupational Therapy Assistant

CPFT Certified Pulmonary Function Technologist (certified by National Board for Respiratory Care)

CRNA Certified Registered Nurse Anesthetist

CRTT Certified Respiratory Therapy Technician (certified by National Board for Respiratory Care)

CT(ASCP) Cytotechnologist (certified by American Society of Clinical Pathologists)

CTR Certified Tumor Registrar

DC Doctor of Chiropractic

DDS Doctor of Dental Surgery

DLM(ASCP) Diplomate in Laboratory Management (certified by American Society of Clinical Pathologists)

DMD Doctor of Dental Medicine

DNS Doctor of Nursing Services

DO Doctor of Optometry (also seen as OD)

DO Doctor of Osteopathy

DP Doctor of Podiatry

DPH Doctor of Public Health, Doctor of Public Hygiene

DPM Doctor of Physical Medicine, Doctor of Podiatric Medicine

ECS Electrophysiologic Certified Specialist (certified by American Physical Therapy Association)

EFDA Expanded Function Dental Auxiliary

FACP Fellow, American College of Physicians

FACS Fellow, American College of Surgeons

FACSM Fellow, American College of Sports Medicine

FADA Fellow, American Dietetic Association

FNP Family Nurse Practitioner

GCS Geriatric Certified Specialist (certified by American Physical Therapy Association)

GNP Gerontological Nurse Practitioner

H(ASCP) Technologist in Hematology (certified by American Society of Clinical Pathologists)

HP(ASCP) Hemapheresis practitioner (certified by American Society of Clinical Pathologists)

HT Histologic Technologist

HT(ASCP) Histologic Technician (certified by American Society of Clinical Pathologists)

HTL(ASCP) Histotechnologist (certified by American Society of Clinical Pathologists)

I(ASCP) Technologist in Immunology (certified by American Society of Clinical Pathologists)

LPN Licensed Practical Nurse

LVN Licensed Vocational Nurse

M(ASCP) Technologist in Microbiology (certified by American Society of Clinical Pathologists)

MD Doctor of Medicine

MLT Medical Laboratory Technician

MLT(ASCP) Medical Laboratory Technician (certified by American Society of Clinical Pathologists)

MT Medical Technologist

MT(ASCP) Medical Technologist (certified by American Society of Clinical Pathologists)

NCS Neurologic Certified Specialist (certified by American Physical Therapy Association)

NM(ASCP) Technologist in Nuclear Medicine (certified by American Society of Clinical Pathologists)

NP Nurse Practitioner

OCS Orthopaedic Certified Specialist (certified by American Physical Therapy Association)

OD Doctor of Optometry (also seen as DO)

OTR Occupational Therapist Registered

PA Physician's Assistant

PBT(ASCP) Phlebotomy Technician (certified by American Society of Clinical Pathologists)

PCS Pediatric Certified Specialist (certified by American Physical Therapy Association)

PharmD Doctor of Pharmacy

PhD Doctor of Philosophy

PhG Graduate in Pharmacy

PNP Pediatric Nurse Practitioner

PT Physical Therapist

PTA Physical Therapy Assistant

RD Registered Dietician (certified by Commission on Dietetic Registration)

RD, CS Registered Dietician, Clinical

RDCS Registered Diagnostic Cardiac Sonographer

RDMS Registered Diagnostic Medical Sonographer

RDH Registered Dental Hygienist

RDMS Registered Diagnostic Medical Sonographer

R. EEGT. Registered Electroencephalographic Technologist

R. EPT. Registered Evoked Potential Technologist

RMA Registered Medical Assistant

RN Registered Nurse

RPFT Registered Pulmonary Function Technologist (registered by National Board for Respiratory Care)

RPh Registered Pharmacist

RPSGT Registered Polysomnographic Technologist

RRA Registered Record Administrator

RRT Registered Respiratory Therapist (registered by National Board for Respiratory Care)

RT Radiologic Technologist, Respiratory Therapist

RT(ARRT) Registered Technologist (certified by American Registry of Radiologic Technologists)

RT(CT) Registered Technologist in Computed Tomography

RT(CV) Registered Technologist in Cardiovascular Interventional Technology

RT(M) Registered Technologist in Mammography

RT(MR) Registered Technologist in Magnetic Resonance Imaging

RT(N) Registered Technologist in Nuclear Medicine

RT(R) Registered Technologist in Radiography

RT(T) Registered Technologist in Radiation Therapy

RTT Respiratory Therapy Technician

RVT Registered Vascular Technologist

SBB(ASCP) Specialist in Blood Banking (certified by American Society of Clinical Pathologists)

SC(ASCP) Specialist in Chemistry (certified by American Society of Clinical Pathologists)

SCS Sports Certified Specialist (certified by American Physical Therapy Association)

SCT(ASCP) Specialist in Cytotechnology (certified by American Society of Clinical Pathologists)

SH(ASCP) Specialist in Hematology (certified by American Society of Clinical Pathologists)

SI(ASCP) Specialist in Immunology (certified by American Society of Clinical Pathologists)

SM(ASCP) Specialist in Microbiology (certified by American Society of Clinical Pathologists)

APPENDICES

ARGENTINA

Buenos Aires
Educational Adviser
Fulbright Commission
American Embassy-USIS
Unit 4330
APO AA 34034-0001

AUSTRALIA

Canberra
Educational Information Officer
Australian-American
Educational Foundation
USIS/American Embassy
APO AP 96549

Melbourne
Co-ordinator, Volunteer
Educational Advisors/Melbourne
USIS/US Consulate-General,
Melbourne
APO AP 96551

Perth
US Consulate - Perth
USIS-Educational Adviser
Unit 11021
APO AP 96530

Sydney
Educational Advising
USIS: AMCONGEN
PSC 280
Unit #11026
APO AP 96554

AUSTRIA

Vienna
Educational Adviser
ZAS
Wu Wien
Augasse 2-6
A-1190 Vienna AUSTRIA

Vienna
Student Counselor
Austrian-American Educational
Commission
(Fulbright Commission)
Schmidgasse 14
A-1082 Vienna, AUSTRIA

BAHRAIN

Manama
AMIDEAST
P.O. Box 10410
Manama, BAHRAIN

BELGIUM

Brussels
Educational Adviser
USIS/CEE/ABL
APO AE 09724

BRITISH VIRGIN ISLANDS

Road Town
Educational Adviser
H. Lavity Stoutt Community
*College
Paraquita Bay
P.O. Box 3097
Road Town, Tortola
BRITISH VIRGIN ISLANDS

CHINA

Beijing
Chinese Service Center for
Scholarly Exchange,
Information Division
No. 15 Xue Yuan Road
Beijing 100083, CHINA

Chengdu
Educational Adviser
Center for International Education
Information
Chengdu Univ. of Science & Technology
Xingnanmenwai Moziqiao
Chengdu, Sichuan Province

Chongqing
Educational Adviser
Study Abroad Training Department
Sichuan Foreign Languages Institute
Shapingba
Chongqing, Sichuan Province
CHINA 630031

Dalian
Educational Adviser
TOEFL Office and Educational
Advising Center
Dalian Foreign Language Institute
No. 110 Nanshan Road,
Zhongshan District
Dalian, Liaoning 116001 CHINA

Guangzhou
Educational Adviser
Guangdong Education Service of
International Exchanges
Room 1101, 11th Floor
Gaojiao (Higher Education) Building
No. 723 East Dongfeng Road
Guangzhou, Guangdong 510080 CHINA

Guangzhou
Guangzhou Service Center for
Scholarly Exchange
Room 208, 2nd Floor
Gaojiao (Higher Education) Building
No. 723 East Dongfeng Road
Guangzhou, Guangdong 510080 CHINA

Ningbo
Chinese Service Center for
Scholarly Exchange
Ningbo Branch
No. 100 Xiaowen Street
Ningbo, Zhejiang 315000 CHINA

Shanghai
Educational Adviser
Shanghai Educational Information
Center for International Exchanges
Shanghai Intl. Studies University
No. 410 East Ti Yu Hui Road
Shanghai 200083 CHINA

Xi'an
Educational Adviser
Study Abroad Training Department
Xi'an Foreign Languages Institute
Wujiafen
Xi'an, Shaanxi 710061 CHINA

CZECH REPUBLIC

Prague
Educational Adviser
AIA-Academic Information Agency
House of International Relations
Senovazne nam. 24
110 00 Praha 1
CZECH REPUBLIC

Prague
Educational Adviser
USIS
c/o AMCONGEN (PRG)
P.O. Box 5630
APO AE 09213

Prague
Educational Adviser
IREX
Narodni trida 3
11142 Praha 1
CZECH REPUBLIC

DENMARK

Copenhagen
American Embassy in
Copenhagen
Att: Fulbright Commission
APO AE 09716

DOMINICA

Roseau
Educational Adviser
National Documentation Centre
c/o Ministry of Education and
Sports
Gov't Headquarters
Roseau, DOMINICA

DOMINICAN REPUBLIC

Santiago de los Caballeros
American Embassy
USIS
Unit 5543
APO AA 34041-5543
c/o BNC Santiago, D.R.

Santo Domingo
American Embassy
Unit 5543
APO AA 34041-5543
c/o Educational Advising (ECO)

EGYPT, ARAB REPUBLIC OF

Alexandria
USIS (for AMIDEAST/Alexandria)
Unit 64900
Box 24
APO AE 09839-4900

Cairo
USIS (for AMIDEAST/Cairo)
Unit 64900
Box 24
APO AE 09839-4900

FINLAND

Helsinki
FUSEEC Educational Adviser
USIS - FUSEEC
American Embassy - Helsinki
PSC 78, Box H
APO AE 09723

Joensuu
Dir. of International Relations
University of Joensuu
Box 111
FIN-80101 Joensuu
FINLAND

Jyvaskyla
International Study Coord.
University of Jyvaskyla
P.O. Box 35
FIN-40351 Jyvaskyla
FINLAND

APPENDICES

Tampere
Educational Adviser
University of Tampere
P.O. Box 607
33101 Tampere
FINLAND

FRANCE

Paris
Educational Adviser
AMEMBASSY PARIS (USIS)
PSC 116 (E-301 FACEE)
APO AE 09777

GERMANY, FEDERAL REPUBLIC OF

Berlin
Exchanges Specialist
USIS/USBER
APO AE 09235

Berlin
US Embassy Office Berlin
Unit # 26738
USIS/AH/Exchanges
APO AE 09235-5500

Bonn
Educational Adviser
Unit 21701
USIS/Box 380
APO AE 09080

Cologne
Educational Adviser
USIS/Cologne
c/o American Embassy Bonn
APO AE 09080

Frankfurt
Exchanges Specialist
USIS Frankfurt
PSC 115
APO AE 09213-0115

Hamburg
Exchanges Specialist
USIS/Hamburg
c/o American Consulate General
APO AE 09215

Leipzig
America House Leipzig
Attn.: Educational Spec.
PSC 120, Box 1000
APO AE 09265

Munich
Exchanges Specialist
AM CON GEN/USIS Munich
Unit 24 718
APO AE 09178

GREECE

Athens
Educational Adviser
U.S. Educational Foundation in Greece
USIS/American Embassy
APO AE 09842

Thessaloniki
Fulbright Adviser
American Center
34 Mitropoleos Street
546 23 Thessaloniki, GREECE

HONG KONG

Shatin
IIE/Hong Kong
US Consulate, Hong Kong
PSC 464, Box 30
FPO AP 96522-0002

HUNGARY

Budapest
Educational Adviser
Szabo Ervin Library
Szabo Ervin ter 1
1371 Budapest
HUNGARY

Budapest
USIS BUDAPEST AE
UNIT 1320
APO AE 09213-1320

Debrecen
Educational Adviser
P.O. Box 39
Debrecen
H-4010
HUNGARY

Miskolc
Educational Adviser
Central Library
University of Miskolc
Egyetemvaros
3515 Miskolc
HUNGARY

Pecs
Educational Adviser
International English Center
Maria u. 9
7621 Pecs, HUNGARY

Szeged
Educational Adviser
Central Library
Jozsef Attila University
SZEGED Pf. 393
H-6701 HUNGARY

Veszprem
Educational Adviser
Central Library
University of Veszprem
10 Egyetem St.
8200 Veszprem
HUNGARY

ICELAND

Reykjavik
Educational Adviser
Amembassy Reykjavik
Fulbright Office
FPO AE 09728

INDONESIA

Jakarta
EAS/USIS/Box 5
Unit 8136
American Embassy - Jakarta
APO AP 96520-8136

Medan
USIS, American Embassy
Box 5
APO AP 96520

Surabaya
Educational Advising Serv.-Surbaya
USIS
American Embassy
Box 5
APO AP 96520

IRELAND

Dublin
Educational Adviser
USIS/Dublin
Department of State
Washington, DC 20521-5290

ISRAEL

Tel Aviv
Educational Adviser
USIEF (USIS)
Unit 7228
APO AE 09830

East Jerusalem
PAO for Student Counsel
American Consulate General
(for AMIDEAST/Jerusalem)
APO AE 09830

ITALY

Bologna
Educational Adviser
Associazione di Cultura e
di Studio Italo-Americana
Via del Belmeloro, 11
40126 Bologna, ITALY

Florence
Educational Adviser
USIS/Florence
APO AE 09624

Genoa
Educational Adviser
USIS/Genoa Box G
APO AE 09624

Milan
Educational Adviser
USIS/Milan Box M
APO AE 09624

Naples
Educational Adviser
USIS/Naples
APO AE 09624

Palermo
Educational Adviser
USIS/Palermo
c/o AMEMBASSY Rome - P
APO AE 09624

Rome
Educational Adviser
Comm. for Educational and Cultural
Exchange between Italy and USA
USIS/American Embassy
APO AE 09624

Trieste
Educational Adviser/Trieste
Comm. for Educational and Cultural
Exchange between Italy and U.S.A.
USIS/American Embassy
APO AE 09624

Turin
Educational Adviser/Turin
Comm. for Educational and Cultural
Exchange between Italy and U.S.A.
USIS/American Embassy
APO AE 09624

JAMAICA

Kingston
Student Counselor
USIS/Kingston
Department of State
Washington DC 20521-3210

APPENDICES

JAPAN

Tokyo
Educational Information Service
The Japan-US Educational Comm.
US Embassy
Unit 45005, Box 215
APO AP 96337-0001

JORDAN

Amman
CAO
American Embassy
(For AMIDEAST)
APO AE 09892

Irbid
AMIDEAST
Branch Counseling Services
Yarmouk University
Irbid, JORDAN

KOREA

Pusan
Pusan American Center Library
American Consulate, Pusan
Unit 15485
APO AP 96259-0002

Seoul
Cultural Affairs Officer
The Korean-American
Educational Commission
USIS/American Embassy-Seoul
UNIT 15550 - APO AP 96205-0001

LAOS

Vientiane
USIS VIENTIANE
AMEMB BOX V
APO AP 96546

LUXEMBOURG

Luxembourg
American Studies Center
Centre Universitaire de Luxembourg
162A avenue de la Faiencerie
L-1511 Luxembourg
Grand-Duche de LUXEMBOURG

MALAYSIA

Kuala Lumpur
Educational Adviser
US Embassy Kuala Lumpur
APO AP 96535-9998

Pulau Pinang
Educational Adviser
US Embassy,Kuala Lumpur
APO AP 96536-9998

NETHERLANDS

Amsterdam
Educational Adviser
USIA American Embassy
PSC 71 Box 1000
APO AE 09715
Attn. Educational Adviser

NEW ZEALAND

Auckland
Educational Adviser
USIS/AUCKLAND LIB
PSC 467, Box 99
FPO AP 96531-1099

Wellington
Educational Adviser
NZ-US Educational Foundation
c/o American Embassy
FPO AP 96531

NORWAY

Oslo
AMembassy Oslo
Fulbright Norway
PSC 69, Box 10000
APO New York 09707

PHILIPPINES

Manila
The Cultural Attache (PAEF)
American Embassy, Manila
APO AP 96440

POLAND

Warsaw
Educational Adviser
Polish-US Fulbright Comm.
APO AE 09213-5010

PORTUGAL

Lisbon
Educational Adviser
Luso-American Educational
Commission (Fulbright)
USIS/American Embassy
APO AE 09726

ROMANIA

Bucharest
Educational Adviser
US Embassy Bucharest
APO AE 09213

...poca
...tional Adviser
...OS Foundation
...Iarului, No. 5
...Box 1084
...Cluj-Napoca
...MANIA

Educational Adviser
Soros Foundation
P.O. Box 6-1356
Iasi, IS 6600 ROMANIA

Timisoara
Educational Adviser
Fundatia Soros
Timisoara
Str. Semenic 10
Timisoara 1900 ROMANIA

SAUDI ARABIA

Dhahran
American Consulate General
Attn. Educational Adviser
USIS/Dhahran
Unit 66803
APO AE 09858-6803

Jeddah
American Consulate General-USIS
Attn. Educational Adviser
Unit 62112
APO AE 09811 - 2112

Riyadh
U.S. Embassy/USIS
Attn: Educational Adviser
Unit 61307
APO AE 09803 - 1307

SINGAPORE

Singapore
Student Adviser
USIS/Student Advising Service
American Embassy,Singapore
PSC 470, Box USIS
FPO AP 96534-0001

SLOVAK REPUBLIC

Bratislava
Educational Adviser
SAIA-Slovak Academic Information
Agency
Hviezdoslavovo nam. 14
813 29 Bratislava
SLOVAK REPUBLIC

SLOVENIA

Ljubljana
Educational Adviser
USIS
American Embassy
Cankarjeva 11
61000 Ljubljana, SLOVENIA

SOUTH AFRICA

Cape Town
Educational Adviser
USIS/Cape Town
Department of State
Washington, DC 20521-2480

Durban
Educational Adviser
USIS/Durban
Department of State
Washington, DC 20521-2490

Johannesburg
Educational Adviser
USIS/Johannesburg
Department of State
Washington, DC 20521-2500

Pretoria
Educational Adviser
U.S.I.S.
P.O. Box 9536
Embassy of the United States of
America
Pretoria 0001
SOUTH AFRICA

SPAIN

Barcelona
Academic Advising Office
US Consulate Barcelona
PSC 61, Box 0005
APO AE 09642

Madrid
Educational Adviser
Fulbright Commission
USIS/American Embassy
APO AE 09642

SWEDEN

Stockholm
Educational Adviser/CAO-CEEUS
American Embassy (Stockholm)
Department of State
Washington, D.C. 20521-5750

Stockholm
Educational Adviser
Sweden-America Foundation
Box 5280
S-102 46 Stockholm, SWEDEN

SWITZERLAND

Bern
Educational Adviser
USIS/Bern
Department of State
Washington,DC 20521-5110

Bern
Schweizerische Zentralstelle
fur Hochschulwesen
Seidenweg 68
CH-3012 Bern, SWITZERLAND

Geneva
Educational Adviser
Geneva America Center
P.O. Box
CH-1202 Geneva, SWITZERLAND

SYRIA

Damascus
AMIDEAST
P.O. Box 2313
Damascus, SYRIA

TAIWAN

Taipei
AIT/CIS Taipei (FSE)
c/o Department of State
Washington DC 20521-4170

THAILAND

Bangkok
Cultural Affairs Office
American Embassy/USIS Box 48
APO AP 96546

Bangkok
Institute of International
Education
G.P.O. Box 2050
Bangkok 10501, THAILAND

Bangkok
Educational Advisory Division
Bangkok Bank Public Co., Ltd.
333 Silom Road
and/or
P.O. Box 95 B.M.C.
Bangkok 10000
THAILAND

Bangkok
Education Abroad Division
Office of the Civil Service Comm.
Pitsanuloke Road
Bangkok 10300, THAILAND

Chiang Mai
BPAO - Chiang Mai
American Embassy - USIS
Box 48
APO AP 96546

Khon Kaen
Educational Adviser
Khon Kaen University
PO Box 31
Khon Kaen THAILAND 40002

TURKEY

Ankara
CAO
American Embassy/Ankara
PSC 93 Box 5000
APO AE 09823

Istanbul
Educational Adviser
USIS/AMCONGEN/IST.
PSC 97, Box 0002
APO AE 09827-0002

Izmir
Educational Adviser
USIS Izmir
Am Con Gen
PSC 88 Box 5000
APO AE 09821

UNITED ARAB EMIRATES

Abu Dhabi
Educational Adviser
USIS/Abu Dhabi
Department of State
Washington DC 20521-6010

Dubai
Educational Adviser
USIS/Dubai
Department of State
Washington, DC 20521-6020

UNITED KINGDOM

London
Educational Adviser/Fulbright
PSC 801 Box 62
FPO AE 09498-4062